THE

Biomedical

Engineering

HANDBOOK

Editor-in-Chief
JOSEPH D. BRONZINO
Trinity College
Hartford, Connecticut

 CRC PRESS   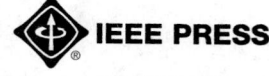 **IEEE PRESS**

A CRC Handbook Published in Cooperation with IEEE Press

Library of Congress Cataloging-in-Publication Data

The biomedical engineering handbook / editor-in-chief, Joseph D. Bronzino.
    p.   cm. — (The electrical engineering handbook series)
    Includes bibliographical references and index.
    ISBN 0-8493-8346-3
    1. Biomedical engineering—Handbooks, manuals, etc.   I. Bronzino,
Joseph D., 1937– . II. Series.
    [DNLM: 1. Biomedical Engineering—handbooks. QT 29 B615 1995]
  R856.15.B86 1995
  610′.28—dc20
  DNLM/DLC
  For Library of Congress   95-6294
                                                  CIP

No claim to original U.S. Government works
International Standard Book Number 0-8493-8346-3
Library of Congress Card Number 95-6294
Printed in the United States of America 2 3 4 5 6 7 8 9 0
Printed on acid-free paper

Introduction

In the 20th century, technological innovation has progressed at such an accelerated pace that it has permeated almost every facet of our lives. This is especially true in the field of medicine and the delivery of health care services. Today, in most developed countries, the modern hospital has emerged as the center of a technologically sophisticated health care system serviced by an equally technologically sophisticated staff.

With almost continual technological innovation driving medical care, engineering professionals have become intimately involved in many medical ventures. As a result, the discipline of biomedical engineering has emerged as an integrating medium for two dynamic professions, medicine and engineering. In the process, biomedical engineers have become actively involved in the design, development, and utilization of materials, devices (such as ultrasonic lithotripsy, pacemakers, etc.), and techniques (such as signal and image processing, artificial intelligence, etc.) for clinical research, as well as the diagnosis and treatment of patients. Thus many biomedical engineers now serve as members of health care delivery teams seeking new solutions for the difficult health care problems confronting our society. The purpose of this handbook is to *provide a central core of knowledge from those fields encompassed by the discipline of biomedical engineering.* Before presenting this detailed information, it is important to provide a sense of the evolution of the modern health care system and identify the diverse activities biomedical engineers perform to assist in the diagnosis and treatment of patients.

Evolution of the Modern Health Care System

Before 1900, medicine had little to offer the average citizen, since its resources consisted mainly of the physician, his education, and his "little black bag." In general, physicians seemed to be in short supply, but the shortage had rather different causes than the current crisis in the availability of health care professionals. Although the costs of obtaining medical training were relatively low, the demand for doctors' services also was very small, since many of the services provided by the physician also could be obtained from experienced amateurs in the community. The home was typically the site for treatment and recuperation, and relatives and neighbors constituted an able and willing nursing staff. Babies were delivered by midwives, and those illnesses not cured by home remedies were left to run their natural, albeit frequently fatal, course. The contrast with contemporary health care practices, in which specialized physicians and nurses located within the hospital provide critical diagnostic and treatment services, is dramatic.

The changes that have occurred within medical science originated in the rapid developments that took place in the applied sciences (chemistry, physics, engineering, microbiology, physiology, pharmacology, etc.) at the turn of the century. This process of development was characterized by intense interdisciplinary cross-fertilization, which provided an environment in which medical research was able to take giant strides in developing techniques for the diagnosis and treatment of disease. For example, in 1903, Willem Einthoven, the Dutch physiologist, devised the first electrocardiograph to measure the electrical activity of the heart. In applying discoveries in the physical sciences to the analysis of a biologic process, he initiated a new age in both cardiovascular medicine and electrical measurement techniques.

New discoveries in medical sciences followed one another like intermediates in a chain reaction. However, the most significant innovation for clinical medicine was the development of x-rays. These "new kinds of rays," as their discoverer W. K. Roentgen described them in 1895, opened the "inner man" to medical inspection. Initially, x-rays were used to diagnose bone fractures and dislocations, and in the process, x-ray machines became commonplace in most urban hospitals. Separate departments of radiology were established, and their influence spread to other departments throughout the hospital. By the 1930s, x-ray visualization of practically all organ systems of the body had been made possible through the use of barium salts and a wide variety of radiopaque materials.

X-ray technology gave physicians a powerful tool that, for the first time, permitted accurate diagnosis of a wide variety of diseases and injuries. Moreover, since x-ray machines were too cumbersome and expensive for local doctors and clinics, they had to be placed in health care centers or hospitals. Once there, x-ray technology essentially triggered the transformation of the hospital from a passive receptacle for the sick to an active curative institution for all members of society.

For economic reasons, the centralization of health care services became essential because of many other important technological innovations appearing on the medical scene. However, hospitals remained institutions to dread, and it was not until the introduction of sulfanilamide in the mid-1930s and penicillin in the early 1940s that the main danger of hospitalization, i.e., cross-infection among patients, was significantly reduced. With these new drugs in their arsenals, surgeons were permitted to perform their operations without prohibitive morbidity and mortality due to infection. Furthermore, even though the different blood groups and their incompatibility were discovered in 1900 and sodium citrate was used in 1913 to prevent clotting, full development of blood banks was not practical until the 1930s, when technology provided adequate refrigeration. Until that time, "fresh" donors were bled and the blood transfused while it was still warm.

Once these surgical suites were established, the employment of specifically designed pieces of medical technology assisted in further advancing the development of complex surgical procedures. For example, the Drinker respirator was introduced in 1927 and the first heart-lung bypass in 1939. By the 1940s, medical procedures heavily dependent on medical technology, such as cardiac catheterization and angiography (the use of a cannula threaded through an arm vein and into the heart with the injection of radiopaque dye for the x-ray visualization of lung and heart vessels and valves), were developed. As a result, accurate diagnosis of congenital and acquired heart disease (mainly valve disorders due to rheumatic fever) became possible, and a new era of cardiac and vascular surgery was established.

Following World War II, technological advances were spurred on by efforts to develop superior weapon systems and establish habitats in space and on the ocean floor. As a by-product of these efforts, the development of medical devices accelerated and the medical profession benefited greatly from this rapid surge of "technological finds." Consider the following examples:

1. Advances in solid-state electronics made it possible to map the subtle behavior of the fundamental unit of the central nervous system—the neuron—as well as to monitor various physiologic parameters, such as the electrocardiogram, of patients in intensive care units.
2. New prosthetic devices became a goal of engineers involved in providing the disabled with tools to improve their quality of life.
3. Nuclear medicine—an outgrowth of the atomic age—emerged as a powerful and effective approach in detecting and treating specific physiologic abnormalities.

4. Diagnostic ultrasound based on sonar technology became so widely accepted that ultrasonic studies are now part of the routine diagnostic workup in many medical specialties.
5. "Spare parts" surgery also became commonplace. Technologists were encouraged to provide cardiac assist devices, such as artificial heart valves and artificial blood vessels, and the artificial heart program was launched to develop a replacement for a defective or diseased human heart.
6. Advances in materials have made the development of disposable medical devices, such as needles and thermometers, as well as implantable drug delivery systems, a reality.
7. Computers similar to those developed to control the flight plans of the *Apollo* capsule were used to store, process, and cross-check medical records, to monitor patient status in intensive care units, and to provide sophisticated statistical diagnoses of potential diseases correlated with specific sets of patient symptoms.
8. Development of the first computer-based medical instrument, the computerized axial tomography scanner, revolutionized clinical approaches to noninvasive diagnostic imaging procedures, which now include magnetic resonance imaging and positron emission tomography as well.

The impact of these discoveries and many others has been profound. The health care system consisting primarily of the "horse and buggy" physician is gone forever, replaced by a technologically sophisticated clinical staff operating primarily in "modern" hospitals designed to accommodate the new medical technology. This evolutionary process continues, with advances in biotechnology and tissue engineering altering the very nature of the health care delivery system itself.

The Field of Biomedical Engineering

Today, many of the problems confronting health professionals are of extreme interest to engineers because they involve the design and practical application of medical devices and systems—processes that are fundamental to engineering practice. These medically related design problems can range from very complex large-scale constructs, such as the design and implementation of automated clinical laboratories, multiphasic screening facilities (i.e., centers that permit many clinical tests to be conducted), and hospital information systems, to the creation of relatively small and "simple" devices, such as recording electrodes and biosensors, that may be used to monitor the activity of specific physiologic processes in either a research or clinical setting. They encompass the many complexities of remote monitoring and telemetry, including the requirements of emergency vehicles, operating rooms, and intensive care units. The American health care system, therefore, encompasses many problems that represent challenges to certain members of the engineering profession called *biomedical engineers*.

Biomedical Engineering: A Definition

Although what is included in the field of biomedical engineering is considered by many to be quite clear, there are some disagreements about its definition. For example, consider the terms *biomedical engineering, bioengineering*, and *clinical* (or *medical*) *engineering* which have been defined in Pacela's *Bioengineering Education Directory* [Quest Publishing Co., 1990]. While Pacela defines *bioengineering* as the broad umbrella term used to describe this entire field, *bioengineering* is usually defined as a basic research–oriented activity closely related to biotechnology and genetic engineering, i.e., the modification of animal or plant cells, or parts of cells, to improve plants or animals or to develop new microorganisms for beneficial ends. In the food industry, for example, this has meant the improvement of strains of yeast for fermentation. In agriculture, bioengineers may be concerned with the improvement of crop yields by treatment of plants with organisms to reduce frost damage. It is clear that bioengineers of the future will have a tremendous impact on the quality of human life, the potential of this specialty is difficult to imagine. Consider the following activities of bioengineers:

- Development of improved species of plants and animals for food production
- Invention of new medical diagnostic tests for diseases
- Production of synthetic vaccines from clone cells
- Bioenvironmental engineering to protect human, animal, and plant life from toxicants and pollutants
- Study of protein-surface interactions
- Modeling of the growth kinetics of yeast and hybridoma cells
- Research in immobilized enzyme technology
- Development of therapeutic proteins and monoclonal antibodies

In reviewing the above-mentioned terms, however, *biomedical engineering* appears to have the most comprehensive meaning. Biomedical engineers apply electrical, mechanical, chemical, optical, and other engineering principles to understand, modify, or control biologic (i.e., human and animal) systems, as well as design and manufacture products that can monitor physiologic functions and assist in the diagnosis and treatment of patients. When biomedical engineers work within a hospital or clinic, they are more properly called *clinical engineers*.

Activities of Biomedical Engineers

The breadth of activity of biomedical engineers is significant. The field has moved significantly from being concerned primarily with the development of medical devices in the 1950s and 1960s and to include a more wide-ranging set of activities. As illustrated below, the field of biomedical engineering now includes many new career areas, each of which is presented in this *Handbook*. These areas include

- Application of engineering system analysis (physiologic modeling, simulation, and control) to biologic problems
- Detection, measurement, and monitoring of physiologic signals (i.e., *biosensors* and *biomedical instrumentation*)
- Diagnostic interpretation via signal-processing techniques of bioelectric data
- Therapeutic and rehabilitation procedures and devices (rehabilitation engineering)
- Devices for replacement or augmentation of bodily functions (*artificial organs*)
- Computer analysis of patient-related data and clinical decision making (i.e., medical informatics and artificial intelligence)
- Medical imaging, i.e., the graphic display of anatomic detail or physiologic function
- The creation of new biologic products (i.e., *biotechnology* and *tissue engineering*)

Typical pursuits of biomedical engineers, therefore, include

- Research in new materials for implanted artificial organs
- Development of new diagnostic instruments for blood analysis
- Computer modeling of the function of the human heart
- Writing software for analysis of medical research data
- Analysis of medical device hazards for safety and efficacy
- Development of new diagnostic imaging systems
- Design of telemetry systems for patient monitoring
- Design of biomedical sensors for measurement of human physiologic systems variables
- Development of expert systems for diagnosis of diseases
- Design of closed-loop control systems for drug administration

- Modeling of the physiologic systems of the human body
- Design of instrumentation for sports medicine
- Development of new dental materials
- Design of communication aids for the handicapped
- Study of pulmonary fluid dynamics
- Study of the biomechanics of the human body
- Development of material to be used as replacement for human skin

Biomedical engineering, then, is an interdisciplinary branch of engineering that ranges from theoretical, nonexperimental undertakings to state-of-the-art applications. It can encompass research, development, implementation, and operation. Accordingly, like medical practice itself, it is unlikely that any single person can acquire expertise that encompasses the entire field. Yet, because of the interdisciplinary nature of this activity, there is considerable interplay and overlapping of interest and effort between them. For example, biomedical engineers engaged in the development of biosensors may interact with those interested in prosthetic devices to develop a means to detect and use the same bioelectric signal to power a prosthetic device. Those engaged in automating the clinical chemistry laboratory may collaborate with those developing expert systems to assist clinicians in making decisions based on specific laboratory data. The possibilities are endless.

Perhaps a greater potential benefit occurring from the use of biomedical engineering is identification of the problems and needs of our present health care system that can be solved using existing engineering technology and systems methodology. Consequently, the field of biomedical engineering offers hope in the continuing battle to provide high-quality health care at a reasonable cost; and if properly directed toward solving problems related to preventive medical approaches, ambulatory care services, and the like, biomedical engineers can provide the tools and techniques to make our health care system more effective and efficient.

Joseph D. Bronzino
Editor-in-Chief

The Discipline of Biomedical Engineering

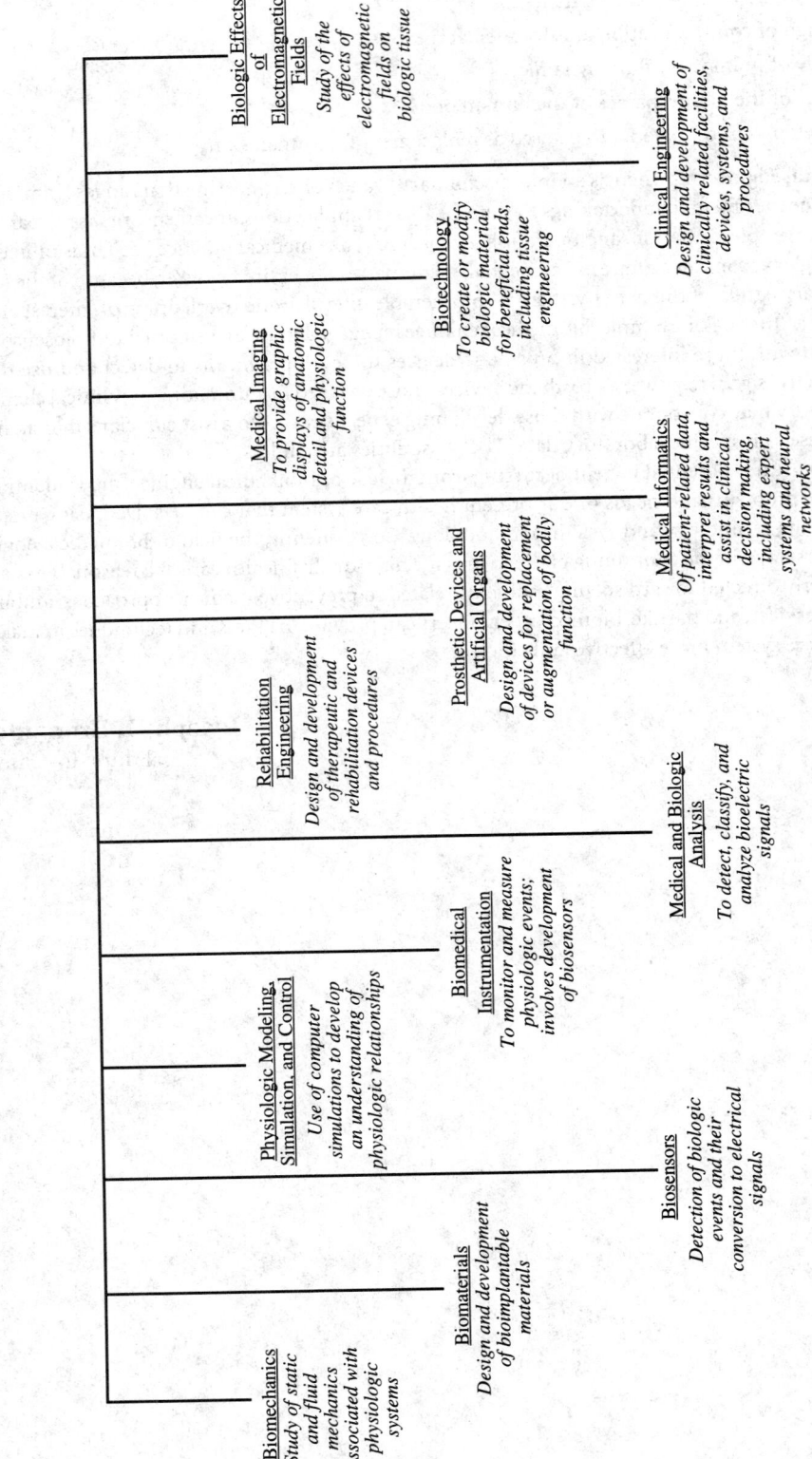

Biomechanics
Study of static and fluid mechanics associated with physiologic systems

Biomaterials
Design and development of bioimplantable materials

Physiologic Modeling, Simulation, and Control
Use of computer simulations to develop an understanding of physiologic relationships

Biosensors
Detection of biologic events and their conversion to electrical signals

Biomedical Instrumentation
To monitor and measure physiologic events; involves development of biosensors

Rehabilitation Engineering
Design and development of therapeutic and rehabilitation devices and procedures

Medical and Biologic Analysis
To detect, classify, and analyze bioelectric signals

Prosthetic Devices and Artificial Organs
Design and development of devices for replacement or augmentation of bodily function

Medical Imaging
To provide graphic displays of anatomic detail and physiologic function

Medical Informatics
Of patient-related data, interpret results and assist in clinical decision making, including expert systems and neural networks

Biotechnology
To create or modify biologic material for beneficial ends, including tissue engineering

Biologic Effects of Electromagnetic Fields
Study of the effects of electromagnetic fields on biologic tissue

Clinical Engineering
Design and development of clinically related facilities, devices, systems, and procedures

Editor-in-Chief

Joseph D. Bronzino, Ph.D., P.E., Vernon Roosa Professor of Applied Science at Trinity College, Hartford, Connecticut, and director of the Biomedical Engineering Program at the Hartford Graduate Center, teaches graduate and undergraduate courses in biomedical engineering in the fields of clinical engineering, electrophysiology, signal analysis, and computer applications in medicine. He earned his B.S. in electrical engineering from Worcester Polytechnic Institute, M.S. in electrical engineering from the Naval Postgraduate School, and Ph.D. in electrical engineering also from Worcester Polytechnic Institute. Deeply concerned with the discipline of biomedical engineering, as well as with ethical and economic issues related to the application of technology to the delivery of health care, Dr. Bronzino has written and lectured internationally. He is the author of over 180 articles and six books: *Technology for Patient Care* (C.V. Mosby, 1977), *Computer Applications for Patient Care* (Addison-Wesley, 1982), *Biomedical Engineering: Basic Concepts and Instrumentation* (PWS Publishing Co., 1986), *Expert Systems: Basic Concepts and Applications* (Research Foundation of the State University of New York, 1989), *Medical Technology and Society: An Interdisciplinary Perspective* (MIT Press, 1990), and *Management of Medical Technology* (Butterworth/Heinemann, 1992). Dr. Bronzino is a fellow of both the Institute of Electrical and Electronic Engineers (IEEE) and the American Institute of Medical and Biological Engineering (AIMBE), a past president of the IEEE Engineering in Medicine and Biology Society (EMBS), a past chairman of the Biomedical Engineering Division of the American Society for Engineering Education, and a charter member of the Connecticut Academy of Science and Engineering (CASE). Dr. Bronzino has extensive experience in the formulation of public policy regarding the utilization and regulation of medical technology. He has served as a past chairman of both the IEEE Health Care Engineering Policy Committee (HCEPC) and the IEEE Technical Policy Council in Washington, D.C.

Advisory Board

Contributors

James J. Abbas
Catholic University of America
Washington, D.C.

Patrick Aebischer
Lausanne University Medical School
Lausanne, Switzerland

Hashem Odeh Al-Fadel
King Faisal Specialist Hospital and
    Research Center
Riyadh, Saudi Arabia

Robert C. Allen
Emory University
Atlanta, Georgia

Kai-Nan An
Mayo Clinic
Rochester, Minnesota

John G. Aunins
Merck Research Laboratories
Rahway, New Jersey

Dennis D. Autio
Oregon Health Sciences University
Portland, Oregon

Praphulla K. Bajpai
University of Dayton
Dayton, Ohio

Gary J. Baker
Stanford University
Stanford, California

D. C. Barber
University of Sheffield
Sheffield, United Kingdom

Berj L. Bardakjian
University of Toronto
Toronto, Canada

Roger C. Barr
Duke University
Durham, North Carolina

Pamela J. Hoyes Beehler
University of Texas at Arlington
Arlington, Texas

Khosrow Behbehani
University of Texas at Arlington and
    University of Texas Southwestern
    Medical Center at Dallas
Arlington, Texas

Ravi Bellamkonda
Lausanne University Medical School
Lausanne, Switzerland

Jan E. W. Beneken
Eindhoven University of Technology
Eindhoven, the Netherlands

Edward J. Berbari
Indiana University/Purdue University
Indianapolis, Indiana

François Berthiaume
Shriners Burns Institute
Cambridge, Massachusetts

Anna M. Bianchi
St. Raffaele Hospital
Milan, Italy

William G. Billotte
Wright State University
Dayton, Ohio

Jeffrey S. Blair
IBM Health Care Solutions
Atlanta, Georgia

G. Faye Boudreaux-Bartels
University of Rhode Island
Kingston, Rhode Island

Bruce R. Bowman
Edentec Corporation
Eden Prairie, Minnesota

Joseph D. Bronzino
Trinity College/The Hartford
    Graduate Center
Hartford, Connecticut

Susan V. Brooks
University of Michigan
Ann Arbor, Michigan

Mark E. Bruley
ECRI
Plymouth Meeting, Pennsylvania

Richard P. Buck
University of North Carolina
Chapel Hill, North Carolina

Thomas F. Budinger
University of California at Berkeley
Berkeley, California

Thomas J. Burkholder
University of California and Veterans
    Administration Medical Centers
San Diego, California

Robert D. Butterfield
IVAC Corporation
San Diego, California

Joseph P. Cammarota
Naval Air Warfare Center
Warminster, Pennsylvania

Thomas R. Canfield
Argonne National Laboratory
Argonne, Illinois

Ewart R. Carson
City University
London, United Kingdom

Sergio Cerutti
Polytechnic University
Milan, Italy

A. Enis Çetin
Bilkent University and Koç University
Ankara, Turkey

K. B. Chandran
University of Iowa
Iowa City, Iowa

Wei Chen
Center for Magnetic Resonance
    Research and the University of
    Minnesota Medical School
Minneapolis, Minnesota

David A. Chesler
Massachusetts General Hospital and
    Harvard University Medical
    School
Boston, Massachusetts

Joseph A. Chinn
Carbomedics, Inc.
Austin, Texas

Howard Jay Chizeck
Case Western Reserve University
Cleveland, Ohio

C. K. Chou
City of Hope National Medical
    Center
Durante, California

Chih-Chang Chu
Cornell University
Ithaca, New York

Arthur Ciarkowski
U.S. Food and Drug Administration
Rockville, Maryland

Ben M. Clopton
University of Washington
Seattle, Washington

Vivian H. Coates
ECRI
Plymouth Meeting, Pennsylvania

Claudio Cobelli
University of Padua
Padua, Italy

Robin Coger
Massachusetts General Hospital,
    Harvard University Medical
    School, and the Shriners Burns
    Institute
Boston, Massachusetts

Arnon Cohen
Ben-Gurion University
Beer Sheva, Israel

Neil M. Cole
University of Michigan
Ann Arbor, Michigan

Clark K. Colton
Massachusetts Institute of
    Technology
Cambridge, Massachusetts

Steven Conolly
Stanford University
Stanford, California

Rory A. Cooper
University of Pittsburgh and
    Highland Drive Veterans Affairs
    Medical Center
Pittsburgh, Pennsylvania

Derek G. Cramp
City University
London, United Kingdom

Barbara Y. Croft
University of Virginia
Charlottesville, Virginia

Ian A. Cunningham
Victona Hospital, the John Robarts
    Research Institute, and the
    University of Western Ontario
London, Canada

Yadin David
Texas Children's Hospital
Houston, Texas

Roy B. Davis
Newington Children's Hospital
Newington, Connecticut

Benoit M. Dawant
Vanderbilt University
Nashville, Tennessee

Peter A. DeLuca
Newington Children's Hospital
Newington, Connecticut

Kennerly H. Digges
George Washington University
Charlottesville, Virginia

Philip B. Dobrin
Hines VA Hospital and Loyola
    University Medical Center
Hines, Illinois

Cathryn R. Dooly
University of Maryland
College Park, Maryland

Paul D. Drumheller
Gore Hybrid Technologies, Inc.
Flagstaff, Arizona

Gary Drzewiecki
Rutgers University
Piscataway, New Jersey

Edwin G. Duffin
Medtronic, Inc.
Minneapolis, Minnesota

Graham A. Dunn
Kings College London
London, United Kingdom

Dominique M. Durand
Case Western Reserve University
Cleveland, Ohio

Jeffrey L. Eggleston
Valleylab, Inc..
Boulder, Colorado

Edward Elson
Walter Reed Army Institute of
    Research
Washington, D.C.

John Denis Enderle
University of Connecticut
Storrs, Connecticut

John A. Faulkner
University of Michigan
Ann Arbor, Michigan

K. Whittaker Ferrara
Riverside Research Institute
New York, New York

Stanley M. Finkelstein
University of Minnesota
Minneapolis, Minnesota

J. Michael Fitzmaurice
U.S. Department of Health and
    Human Services
Rockville, Maryland

Ross Flewelling
Nellcor Incorporated
Pleasant, California

Michael Forde
Medtronic, Inc.
Minneapolis, Minnesota

Kenneth R. Foster
University of Pennsylvania
Philadelphia, Pennsylvania

Lisa E. Freed
Massachusetts Institute of
Technology and Harvard
University
Cambridge, Massachusetts

Michael J. Furey
Virginian Polytechnic and State
University
Blacksburg, Virginia

Pierre M. Galletti
Brown University
Providence, Rhode Island

Catherine Garbay
Laboratoire TIMC/IMAG
Grenoble, France

Leslie A. Geddes
Purdue University
West Lafayette, Indiana

V. K. Goel
University of Iowa
Iowa City, Iowa

John W. Goethe
The Institute of Living
Hartford, Connecticut

Richard L. Goldberg
University of North Carolina
Chapel Hill, North Carolina

Wallace Grant
Virginia Polytechnic Institute and
State University
Blacksburg, Virginia

Walter J. Greenleaf
Greenleaf Medical Systems
Palo Alto, California

Michael L. Gullikson
Texas Children's Hospital
Houston, Texas

Jon Gunderson
University of Illinois at Urbana/
Champaign
Champaign, Illinois

Alan R. Hargens
University of California at San Diego
San Diego, California

Russell S. Heinrich
Georgia Institute of Technology
Atlanta, Georgia

Scott L. Hendricks
Virginia Polytechnic Institute and
State University
Blacksburg, Virginia

Kaj-Åge Henneberg
University of Montreal
Montreal, Canada

Craig S. Henriquez
Duke University
Durham, North Carolina

Douglas Hobson
University of Pittsburgh
Pittsburgh, Pennsylvania

Robert M. Hochmuth
Duke University
Durham, North Carolina

Thomas V. Holohan
Agency for Health Care Policy
and Research
U.S. Public Health Service
Bethesda, Maryland

Joanne Hopmeyer
Georgia Institute of Technology
Atlanta, Georgia

Xiaoping Hu
Center for Magnetic Resonance
Research and the University of
Minnesota Medical School
Minneapolis, Minnesota

Jeffrey A. Hubbell
California Institute of Technology
Pasadena, California

H. David Humes
University of Michigan
Ann Arbor, Michigan

Bernard F. Hurley
University of Maryland
College Park, Maryland

Sheik N. Imrhan
University of Texas at Arlington
Arlington, Texas

Marcos Intaglietta
University of California at San Diego
La Jolla, California

Michel Jaffrin
Université de Technologie de
Compiègne
Compiègne, France

Hugo O. Jauregui
Rhode Island Hospital
Providence, Rhode Island

Arthur T. Johnson
University of Maryland
College Park, Maryland

Christopher R. Johnson
University of Utah
Salt Lake City, Utah

G. Allan Johnson
Duke University Medical Center
Durham, North Carolina

Stephen B. Johnson
Columbia-Presbyterian Medical
Center
New York, New York

Richard D. Jones
Christchurch Hospital
Christchurch, New Zealand

Craig T. Jordan
Somatix Therapy Corp.
Alameda, California

Thomas M. Judd
Texas Children's Hospital
Houston, Texas

Millard M. Judy
Baylor Research Institute
Dallas, Texas

Philip F. Judy
Brigham and Women's Hospital and
Harvard University Medical School
Boston, Massachusetts

Kurt Kaczmarek
University of Wisconsin
Madison, Wisconsin

Robert Kaiser
University of Washington
Seattle, Washington

J. Lawrence Katz
Case Western Reserve University
Cleveland, Ohio

Kenton R. Kaufman
Children's Hospital
San Diego, California

J. C. Keller
University of Iowa
Iowa City, Iowa

Peter L. M. Kerkhof
University of Utrecht
Utrecht, the Netherlands

Gilson Khang
Korea Research Institute of Chemical
Technology
Chungnam, Korea

Sung S. Kim
Korea Research Institute of Chemical
Technology
Chungnam, Korea

Tae Ho Kim
Harvard University and
Children's Hospital
Boston, Massachusetts

Albert I. King
Wayne State University
Detroit, Michigan

Manfred R. Koller
Aastrom Biosciences, Inc.
Ann Arbor, Michigan

George V. Kondraske
University of Texas at Arlington
Arlington, Texas

Hayrettin Köymen
Bilkent University and Koç University
Ankara, Turkey

David N. Ku
Georgia Institute of Technology
Atlanta, Georgia

Casimir A. Kulikowski
Rutgers University
New Brunswick, New Jersey

Luis G. Kun
Cedars-Sinai Medical Center
Los Angeles, California

Kenneth K. Kwong
Massachusetts General Hospital and
Harvard University Medical
School
Boston, Massachusetts

Roderic Lakes
University of Iowa
Iowa City, Iowa

Robert S. Langer
Massachusetts Institute of
Technology
Cambridge, Massachusetts

Douglas A. Lauffenburger
Massachusetts Institute of
Technology
Cambridge, Massachusetts

Swamy Laxminarayan
New Jersey Institute of Technology
Newark, New Jersey

Joseph M. Le Doux
Rutgers University
Piscataway, New Jersey

Ann L. Lee
Merck Research Laboratories
Rahway, New Jersey

Hae B. Lee
Korea Research Institute of Chemical
Technology
Chungnam, Korea

Shu-Tung Li
ReGen Biologics, Inc.
Franklin Lakes, New Jersey

Richard L. Lieber
University of California and Veterans
Administration Medical Centers
San Diego, California

Edwin N. Lightfoot
University of Wisconsin
Madison, Wisconsin

Chung-Chiun Liu
Case Western Reserve University
Cleveland, Ohio

A. Llinás
Javeriana University
Bogotá, Colombia

Murray H. Loew
George Washington University
Washington, D.C.

Michael W. Long
University of Michigan
Ann Arbor, Michigan

Marilyn Lord
Kings College London
London, United Kingdom

Michael J. Lysaght
CytoTherapeutics, Inc.
Providence, Rhode Island

Albert Macovski
Stanford University
Stanford, California

Lucia T. Mainardi
Polytechnic University of Milan
Milan, Italy

Jaakko Malmivuo
Tampere University of Technology
Tampere, Finland

Wolf von Maltzahn
University of Texas at Arlington
Arlington, Texas

Vasilis Z. Marmarelis
University of Southern California
Los Angeles, California

Robert E. Mates
SUNY University at Buffalo
Buffalo, New York

Kenneth J. Maxwell
Departure Technology
Forth Worth, Texas

Joseph P. McClain
Walter Reed Army Medical Center
Washington, D.C.

Andrew D. McCulloch
University of California at San Diego
La Jolla, California

Ken McDermott
U.S. Food and Drug Administration
Rockville, Maryland

Larry V. McIntire
Rice University
Houston, Texas

Yitzhak Mendelson
Worcester Polytechnic Institute
Worcester, Massachusetts

Evangelia Micheli-Tzanakou
Rutgers University
Piscataway, New Jersey

David J. Mooney
Massachusetts Institute of
Technology
Cambridge, Massachusetts

John Moran
Baxter Healthcare Corporation
McGaw Park, Illinois

Jeffrey R. Morgan
Massachusetts General Hospital,
Harvard University Medical
School, and the Shriners Burns
Institute
Cambridge, Massachusetts

Robert L. Morris
Oregon Health Sciences University
Portland, Oregon

Wayne A. Morse
Spacelabs Medical, Inc.
Redmond, Washington

Jack G. Mottley
University of Rochester
Rochester, New York

Karen M. Mudry
The Whitaker Foundation
Washington, D.C.

Edward P. Mueller
U.S. Food and Drug Administration
Rockville, Maryland

Robin Murray
University of Rhode Island
Kingston, Rhode Island

Joachim H. Nagel
University of Miami
Coral Gables, Florida

Tatsuo Nakamura
Kyoto University
Kyoto, Japan

Brian A. Naughton
Advanced Tissue Sciences, Inc.
La Jolla, California

Michael R. Neuman
Case Western Reserve University
Cleveland, Ohio

Abraham Noordergraaf
University of Pennsylvania
Philadelphia, Pennsylvania

Pirkko Nykänen
VTT Information Technology
Tampere, Finland

P. Äke Öberg
Linköping University Hospital
Linköping, Sweden

Banu Onaral
Drexel University
Philadelphia, Pennsylvania

Sylvia Õunpuu
Newington Children's Hospital
Newington, Connecticut

Joseph L. Palladino
Trinity College
Hartford, Connecticut

Bernhard Ø. Palsson
University of Michigan
Ann Arbor, Michigan

Joon B. Park
University of Iowa
Iowa City, Iowa

S-H. Park
University of Southern California
Los Angles, California

Mohamad Parnianpour
Ohio State University
Columbus, Ohio

Maqbool Patel
Center for Magnetic Resonance
Research and the University of
Minnesota Medical School
Minneapolis, Minnesota

Charles W. Patrick, Jr.
Rice University
Houston, Texas

Robert Patterson
University of Minnesota
Minneapolis, Minnesota

A. William Paulsen
West Virginia University
Morgantown, West Virginia

John Pauly
Stanford University
Stanford, California

P. Hunter Peckham
Case Western Reserve University and
Veterans Affairs Medical Center
Cleveland, Ohio

Athina P. Petropulu
Drexel University
Philadelphia, Pennsylvania

Roland N. Pittman
Virginia Commonwealth University
Richmond, Virginia

Robert Plonsey
Duke University
Durham, North Carolina

Charles Polk
University of Rhode Island
Kingston, Rhode Island

Chi-Sang Poon
Harvard University/Massachusetts
Institute of Technology
Cambridge, Massachusetts

Aleksander S. Popel
Johns Hopkins University
Baltimore, Maryland

Dejan B. Popović
University of Miami and University
of Belgrade
Miami, Florida

T. Allan Pryor
University of Utah
Salt Lake City, Utah

Gerard Reach
Hôpital Hotel-Dieu Paris
Paris, France

Pat Ridgely
Medtronic, Inc.
Minneapolis, Minnesota

Richard L. Roa
Baylor University Medical Center
Dallas, Texas

Charles J. Robinson
University of Pittsburgh and
Highland Drive Veterans Affairs
Medical Center
Pittsburgh, Pennsylvania

Barry Romich
Prentke Romich Company
Wooster, Ohio

Gerson Rosenberg
Pennsylvania State University
Hershey, Pennsylvania

Bradley J. Roth
National Institute of Health
Bethesda, Maryland

Carl F. Rothe
Indiana University
Indianapolis, Indiana

J. O. Rowan
Glasgow Royal Infirmary
Glasgow, United Kingdom

Alan J. Russell
University of Pittsburgh
Pittsburgh, Pennsylvania

Maria Pia Saccomani
University of Padua
Padua, Italy

Rangarajan Sampath
Rice University
Houston, Texas

Niilo Saranummi
VTT Information Technology
Tampere, Finland

John Schenck
General Electric Corporate Research
    and Development Center
Schenectady, New York

Daniel J. Schneck
Virginia Polytechnic and State
    University
Blacksburg, Virginia

Edward Schuck
EdenTec Corporation
Eden Prairie, Minnesota

Soumitra Sengupta
Columbia University
New York, New York

S. W. Shalaby
Clemson University
Clemson, South Carolina

David Sherman
Johns Hopkins University
Baltimore, Maryland

Yasuhiko Shimizu
Kyoto University
Kyoto, Japan

Artin A. Shoukas
Johns Hopkins University
Baltimore, Maryland

Robert E. Shroy, Jr.
Picker International
Highland Heights, Ohio

Brian Smith
Case Western Reserve University
Cleveland, Ohio

Stephen W. Smith
Duke University
Durham, North Carolina

Susan S. Smith
Southwestern PT
Dallas, Texas

Francis A. Spelman
University of Washington
Seattle, Washington

Charles R. Steele
Stanford University
Stanford, California

George Stetten
Duke University
Durham, North Carolina

Mark Strauss
University of Illinois at Urbana/
    Champaign
Champaign, Illinois

Maria A. Stuchly
University of Victoria
Victoria, Canada

Ron Summers
City University
London, United Kingdom

Srikanth Sundaram
Rutgers University
Piscataway, New Jersey

Karl Syndulko
UCLA School of Medicine
Los Angeles, California

Willis A. Tacker
Purdue University
West Lafayette, Indiana

Nitish V. Thakor
Johns Hopkins University
Baltimore, Maryland

William D. Timmons
University of Akron
Akron, Ohio

Jason A. Tolomeo
Stanford University
Stanford, California

Mehmet Toner
Massachusetts General Hospital,
    Harvard University Medical
    School, and the Shriners Burns
    Institute
Boston, Massachusetts

Elaine Trefler
University of Pittsburgh
Pittsburgh, Pennsylvania

Benjamin M. W. Tsui
University of North Carolina
Chapel Hill, North Carolina

Alan Turner-Smith
King's College London
London, United Kingdom

Kamil Ugurbil
Center for Magnetic Resonance
    Research and the University of
    Minnesota Medical School
Minneapolis, Minnesota

Shiro Usai
Toyohashi University of Technology
Toyohashi, Japan

Joseph P. Vacanti
Harvard University and
    Children's Hospital
Boston, Massachusetts

Robert F. Valentini
Brown University
Providence, Rhode Island

Henry F. VanBrocklin
University of California at Berkeley
Berkeley, California

Michael S. Van Lysel
University of Wisconsin Medical
    School
Madison, Wisconsin

Gary Van Zant
University of Kentucky Medical
    Center
Lexington, Kentucky

Gregg Vanderheiden
University of Wisconsin at Madison
Madison, Wisconsin

Anthony Varghese
Johns Hopkins Medical Institute
Baltimore, Maryland

Paul J. Vasta
University of Texas at Arlington
Arlington, Texas

David C. Viano
Wayne State University
Detroit, Michigan

Chenzhao Vierheller
University of Pittsburgh
Pittsburgh, Pennsylvania

J. Leonel Villavicencio
Walter Reed Army and Bethesda
    Naval Centers
Bethesda, Maryland

David B. Volkin
Merck Research Laboratories
Rahway, New Jersey

Gregory I. Voss
IVAC Corporation
San Diego, California

Jafar Vossoughi
University of the District
    of Columbia
Washington, D.C.

Gordana Vunjak-Novakovic
Massachusetts Institute
    of Technology
Cambridge, Massachusetts

Alvin Wald
Columbia-Presbyterian Medical Center
New York, New York

Richard E. Waugh
University of Rochester
Rochester, New York

James C. Weaver
Massachusetts Institute
    of Technology
Cambridge, Massachusetts

Robert M. Winslow
University of California at
    San Diego
La Jolla, California

Eileen A. Woodruff
PA Consulting Group
Hightstown, New Jersey

Martin J. Yaffe
University of Toronto
Toronto, Canada

Ioannis V. Yannas
Massachusetts Institute of
    Technology
Cambridge, Massachusetts

David M. Yarmush
Rutgers University
Piscataway, New Jersey

Martin L. Yarmush
Rutgers University, Massachusetts
    General Hospital, Harvard
    University Medical School, and the
    Shriners Burns Institute
Piscataway, New Jersey

Ajit P. Yoganathan
Georgia Institute of Technology
Atlanta, Georgia

Daniel A. Zahner
Rutgers University
Piscataway, New Jersey

Deborah E. Zetes
Stanford University
Stanford, California

Xiaohong Zhou
Duke University Medical Center
Durham, North Carolina

Craig Zupke
Massachusetts General Hospital and
    the Shriners Burns Institute
Cambridge, Massachusetts

Andrew L. Zydney
University of Colorado at Boulder
Boulder, Colorado

Contents

SECTION III   Biomechanics

SECTION IV Biomaterials

SECTION V Biomedical Sensors

SECTION VI   Biomedical Signal Analysis

SECTION VII   Imaging

SECTION VIII Medical Instruments and Devices

SECTION IX　Biologic Effects of Nonionizing Electromagnetic Fields

SECTION X　Biotechnology

SECTION XI   Tissue Engineering

SECTION XII   Prostheses and Artificial Organs

SECTION XIII   Rehabilitation Engineering

SECTION XIV   Human Performance Engineering

SECTION XV Physiologic Modeling, Simulation, and Control

SECTION XVI Clinical Engineering

SECTION XVII Medical Informatics

SECTION XVIII Artificial Intelligence

SECTION XIX   Regulations and Organizations

THE

Biomedical

Engineering

HANDBOOK

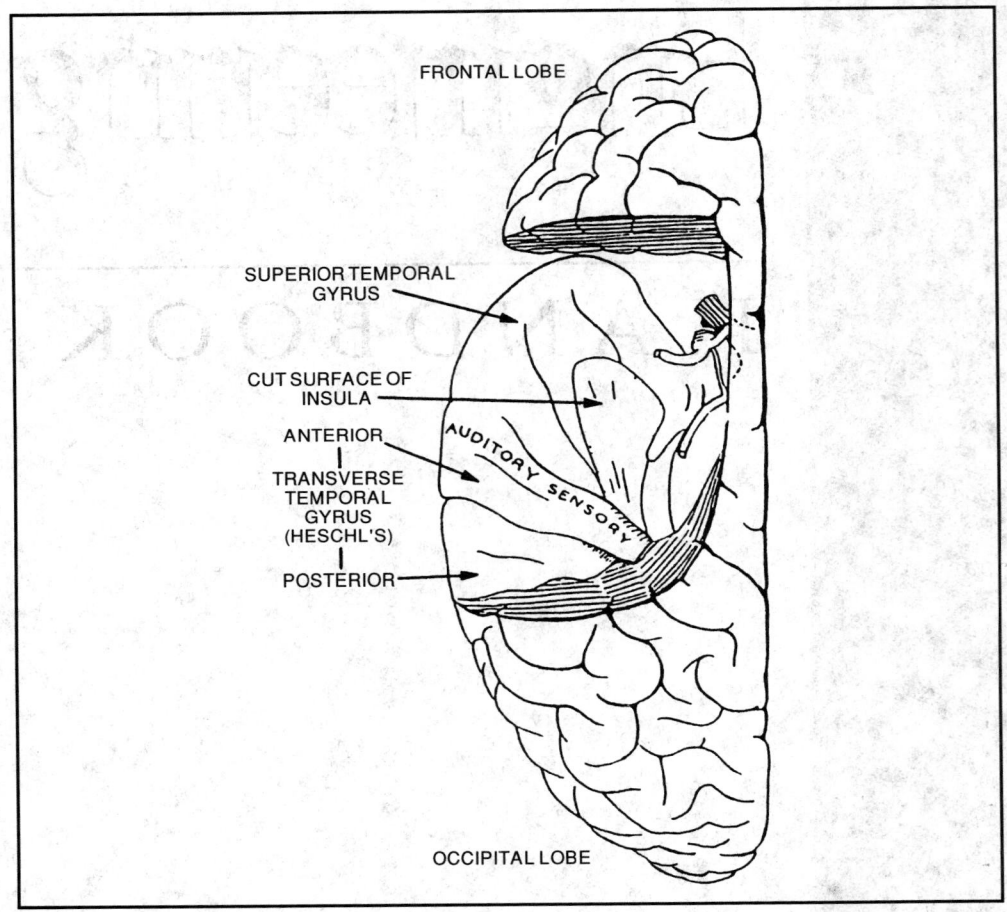

A view of the human cerebral cortex showing the underlying auditory cortex.

Physiologic Systems

Robert Plonsey
Duke University

THE CONTENT OF THIS *HANDBOOK* is devoted to the subject of *biomedical engineering*. We understand biomedical engineering to involve the application of engineering science and technology to problems arising in medicine and biology. In principle, the intersection of each engineering discipline (i.e., electrical, mechanical, chemical, etc.) with each discipline in medicine (i.e., cardiology, pathology, neurology, etc.) or biology (i.e., biochemistry, pharmacology, molecular biology, cell biology, etc.) is a potential area of biomedical engineering application. As such, the discipline of biomedical engineering is potentially very extensive. However, at least to date, only a few of the afore-mentioned "intersections" contain active areas of research and/or development. The most significant of these are described in this *Handbook*.

While the application of engineering expertise to the life sciences requires an obvious knowledge of contemporary technical theory and its applications, it also demands an adequate knowledge and understanding of relevant medicine and biology. It has been argued that the most challenging part of finding engineering solutions to problems lies in the formulation of the solution in engineering terms. In biomedical engineering, this usually demands a full understanding of the life science substrate as well as the quantitative methodologies.

This section is devoted to an overview of the major physiologic systems of current interest to biomedical engineers, on which their work is based. The overview may contain useful definitions, tables of basic physiologic data, and an introduction to the literature. Obviously these chapters must be extremely brief. However, our goal is an introduction that may enable the reader to clarify some item of interest or to indicate a way to pursue further information. Possibly the reader will find the greatest value in the references to more extensive literature.

This section contains seven chapters, and these describe each of the major organ systems of the human body. Thus we have chapters describing the cardiovascular, endocrine, nervous, visual, gastrointestinal, and respiratory systems. While each author is writing at an introductory and tutorial level, the audience is assumed to have some technical expertise, and consequently, mathematical descriptions are not avoided. All authors are recognized as experts on the system which they describe, but all are also biomedical engineers.

The authors in this section noted that they would have liked more space but recognized that the main focus of this *Handbook* is on "engineering." Hopefully, readers will find this introductory section helpful to their understanding of later chapters of this *Handbook* and, as noted above, to at least provide a starting point for further investigation into the life sciences.

1

An Outline of Cardiovascular Structure and Function

Daniel J. Schneck
Virginia Polytechnic Institute and State University

Because not every cell in the human body is near enough to the environment to easily exchange with it mass (including nutrients, oxygen, carbon dioxide, and the waste products of metabolism), energy (including heat), and momentum, the physiologic system is endowed with a major highway network—organized to make available thousands of miles of access tubing for the transport to and from a differential neighborhood (on the order of 10 μm or less) of any given cell whatever it needs to sustain life. This highway network, called the *cardiovascular system*, includes a pumping station, the heart; a working fluid, blood; a complex branching configuration of distributing and collecting pipes and channels, blood vessels; and a sophisticated means for both intrinsic (inherent) and extrinsic (autonomic and endocrine) control.

1.1 The Working Fluid: Blood

Accounting for about $8\pm1\%$ of total body weight, averaging 5200 ml, blood is a complex, heterogeneous suspension of formed elements—the *blood cells*, or *hematocytes*—suspended in a continuous, straw-colored fluid called *plasma*. Nominally, the composite fluid has a mass density of 1.057 ± 0.007 g/cm^3, and it is three to six times as viscous as water. The hematocytes (Table 1.1) include three basic types of cells: red blood cells (erythrocytes, totaling nearly 95% of the formed elements), white blood cells (leukocytes, averaging $<0.15\%$ of all hematocytes), and platelets (thrombocytes, on the order of 5% of all blood cells). Hematocytes are all derived in the active ("red") bone marrow (about 1500 g) of adults from undifferentiated stem cells called *hemocytoblasts*, and all reach ultimate maturity via a process called *hematocytopoiesis*.

The primary function of erythrocytes is to aid in the transport of blood gases—about 30 to 34% (by weight) of each cell consisting of the oxygen- and carbon dioxide–carrying protein hemoglobin $(64,000 \le \text{MW} \le 68,000)$ and a small portion of the cell containing the enzyme carbonic anhydrase, which catalyzes the reversible formation of carbonic acid from carbon dioxide and water. The primary function of leukocytes is to endow the human body with the ability to identify and dispose of foreign substances such as infectious organisms) that do not belong there—agranulocytes (lympho-

TABLE 1.1   Hematocytes

Cell Type	Number of Cells per mm³ Blood*	Corpuscular Diameter (μm)*	Corpuscular Surface Area (μm²)*	Corpuscular Volume (μm³)*	Mass Density (g/cm³)*	Percent Water*	Percent Protein*	Percent Extractives*†
Erythrocytes (red blood cells)	4.2–5.4 ×10⁶ ♀ 4.6–6.2 ×10⁶ ♂ (5 ×10⁶)	6–9 (7.5) Thickness 1.84–2.84 "Neck" 0.81–1.44	120–163 (140)	80–100 (90)	1.089–1.100 (1.098)	64–68 (66)	29–35 (32)	1.6–2.8 (2)
Leukocytes (white blood cells)	4000–11000 (7500)	6–10	300–625	160–450	1.055–1.085	52–60 (56)	30–36 (33)	4–18 (11)
Granulocytes								
Neutrophils: 55–70% WBC (65%)	2–6 × 10³ (4875)	8–8.6 (8.3)	422–511 (467)	268–333 (300)	1.075–1.085 (1.080)	—	—	—
Eosinophils: 1–4% WBC (3%)	45–480 (225)	8–9 (8.5)	422–560 (491)	268–382 (321)	1.075–1.085 (1.080)	—	—	—
Basophils: 0–1.5% WBC (1%)	0–113 (75)	7.7–8.5 (8.1)	391–500 (445)	239–321 (278)	1.075–1.085 (1.080)	—	—	—
Agranulocytes								
Lymphocytes: 20–35% WBC (25%)	1000–4800 (1875)	6.75–7.34 (7.06)	300–372 (336)	161–207 (184)	1.055–1.070 (1.063)	—	—	—
Monocytes: 3–8% WBC (6%)	100–800 (450)	9–9.5 (9.25)	534–624 (579)	382–449 (414)	1.055–1.070 (1.063)	—	—	—
Thrombocytes (platelets)	1.4 (♂)–5 2.14 (♀)–5 ×10⁵ (2.675 × 10⁵)	2–4 (3) Thickness 0.9–1.3	16–35 (25)	5–10 (7.5)	1.04–1.06 (1.05)	60–68 (64)	32–40 (36)	Neg.

*Normal physiologic range, with "typical" value in parentheses.
†Extractives include mostly minerals (ash), carbohydrates, and fats (lipids).

cytes and monocytes) essentially doing the "identifying" and granulocytes (neutrophils, basophils, and eosinophils) essentially doing the "disposing." The primary function of platelets is to participate in the blood clotting process.

Removal of all hematocytes from blood by centrifugation or other separating techniques leaves behind the aqueous (91% water by weight, 94.8% water by volume), saline (0.15 N) suspending medium called *plasma*—which has an average mass density of 1.035 ± 0.005 g/cm^3 and a viscosity $1\frac{1}{2}$ to 2 times that of water. Some 6.5 to 8% by weight of plasma consists of the plasma proteins, of which there are three major types—albumin, the globulins, and fibrinogen—and several of lesser prominence (Table 1.2).

TABLE 1.2 Plasma

Constituent	Concentration Range (mg/dl plasma)	Typical Plasma Value (mg/dl)	Molecular Weight Range	Typical Value	Typical size (nm)
Total protein, 7% by weight	6400–8300	7245	21,000–1,200,000	—	—
Albumin (56% TP)	2800–5600	4057	66,500–69,000	69,000	15 × 4
α_1-*Globulin* (5.5% TP)	300–600	400	21,000–435,000	60,000	5–12
α_2-*Globulin* (7.5% TP)	400–900	542	100,000–725,000	200,000	50–500
β-*Globulin* (13% TP)	500–1230	942	90,000–1,200,000	100,000	18–50
γ-*Globulin* (12% TP)	500–1800	869	150,000–196,000	150,000	23 × 4
Fibrinogen (4% TP)	150–470	290	330,000–450,000	390,000	(50–60) × (3–8)
Other (2% TP)	70–210	145	70,000–1,000,000	200,000	(15–25) × (2–6)
Inorganic ash, 0.95% by weight	930–1140	983	20–100	—	— (Radius)
Sodium	300–340	325	—	22.98977	0.102 (Na$^+$)
Potassium	13–21	17	—	39.09800	0.138 (K$^+$)
Calcium	8.4–11.0	10	—	40.08000	0.099 (Ca^{2+})
Magnesium	1.5–3.0	2	—	24.30500	0.072 (Mg^{2+})
Chloride	336–390	369	—	35.45300	0.181 (Cl$^-$)
Bicarbonate	110–240	175	—	61.01710	0.163 (HCO$_3^-$)
Phosphate	2.7–4.5	3.6	—	95.97926	0.210 (HPO$_4^{2-}$)
Sulfate	0.5–1.5	1.0	—	96.05760	0.230 (SO$_4^{2-}$)
Other	0–100	80.4	20–100	—	0.1–0.3
Lipids (fats), 0.80% by weight	541–1000	828	44,000–3,200,000	= Lipoproteins	Up to 200 or more
Cholesterol (34% TL)	12–105 "free" 72–259 esterified, 84–364 "total"	59 224 283	386.67	Contained mostly in intermediate to LDL β-lipoproteins; higher in women	
Phospholipid (35% TL)	150–331	292	690–1010	Contained mainly in HDL to VHDL α_1-lipoproteins	
Triglyceride (26% TL)	65–240	215	400–1370	Contained mainly in VLDL α_2-lipoproteins and chylomicrons	
Other (5% TL)	0–80	38	280–1500	Fat-soluble vitamins, prostaglandins, fatty acids	
Extractives, 0.25% by weight	200–500	259	—	—	—
Glucose	60–120, fasting	90	—	180.1572	0.86 D
Urea	20–30	25	—	60.0554	0.36 D
Carbohydrate	60–105	83	180.16–342.3	—	0.74–0.108 D
Other	11–111	61	—	—	—

The primary functions of albumin are to help maintain the osmotic (oncotic) transmural pressure differential that ensures proper mass exchange between blood and interstitial fluid at the capillary level and to serve as a transport carrier molecule for several hormones and other small biochemical constituents (such as some metal ions). The primary functions of the globulin class of proteins are to act as transport carrier molecules (mostly of the α and β class) for large biochemical substances, such as fats (lipoproteins) and certain carbohydrates (muco- and glycoproteins) and heavy metals (mineraloproteins), and to work together with leukocytes in the body's immune system. The latter function is primarily the responsibility of the γ class of immunoglobulins, which have antibody activity. The primary function of fibrinogen is to work with thrombocytes in the formation of a blood clot—a process also aided by one of the most abundant of the lesser proteins, prothrombin (MW ≃ 62,000).

Of the remaining 2% or so (by weight) of plasma, just under half (0.95%, or 983 mg/dl plasma) consists of minerals (inorganic ash), trace elements, and electrolytes, mostly the cations sodium, potassium, calcium, and magnesium and the anions chlorine, bicarbonate, phosphate, and sulfate—the latter three helping as buffers to maintain the fluid at a slightly alkaline pH between 7.35 and 7.45 (average 7.4). What is left, about 1087 mg of material per deciliter of plasma, includes: (1) mainly (0.8% by weight) three major types of fat, i.e., cholesterol (in a free and esterified form), phospholipid (a major ingredient of cell membranes), and triglyceride, with lesser amounts of the fat-soluble vitamins (A, D, E, and K), free fatty acids, and other lipids, and (2) "extractives" (0.25% by weight), of which about two-thirds includes glucose and other forms of carbohydrate, the remainder consisting of the water-soluble vitamins (B-complex and C), certain enzymes, nonnitrogenous and nitrogenous waste products of metabolism (including urea, creatine, and creatinine), and many smaller amounts of other biochemical constituents—the list seeming virtually endless.

Removal from blood of all hematocytes and the protein fibrinogen (by allowing the fluid to completely clot before centrifuging) leaves behind a clear fluid called *serum*, which has a density of about 1.018 ± 0.003 g/cm^3 and a viscosity up to $1\frac{1}{2}$ times that of water. A glimpse of Tables 1.1 and 1.2, together with the very brief summary presented above, nevertheless gives the reader an immediate appreciation for why blood is often referred to as the "river of life." This river is made to flow through the vascular piping network by two central pumping stations arranged in series: the left and right sides of the human heart.

1.2 The Pumping Station: The Heart

Barely the size of the clenched fist of the individual in whom it resides—an inverted, conically shaped, hollow muscular organ measuring 12 to 13 cm from base (top) to apex (bottom) and 7 to 8 cm at its widest point and weighing just under 0.75 lb (about 0.474% of the individual's body weight, or some 325 g)—the human heart occupies a small region between the third and sixth ribs in the central portion of the thoracic cavity of the body. It rests on the diaphragm, between the lower part of the two lungs, its base-to-apex axis leaning mostly toward the left side of the body and slightly forward. The heart is divided by a tough muscular wall—the interatrial-interventricular septum—into a somewhat crescent-shaped right side and cylindrically shaped left side (Fig. 1.1), each being one self-contained pumping station, but the two being connected in series. The left side of the heart drives oxygen-rich blood through the aortic semilunar outlet valve into the *systemic circulation*, which carries the fluid to within a differential neighborhood of each cell in the body—from which it returns to the right side of the heart low in oxygen and rich in carbon dioxide. The right side of the heart then drives this oxygen-poor blood through the pulmonary semilunar (pulmonic) outlet valve into the *pulmonary circulation*, which carries the fluid to the lungs—where its oxygen supply is replenished and its carbon dioxide content is purged before it returns to the left side of the heart to begin the cycle all over again. Because of the anatomic proximity of the heart to the lungs, the right side of the heart does not have to work very hard to drive blood through the pulmonary circulation, so it functions as a low-pressure ($P \leq 40$ mmHg gauge) pump compared with the left side

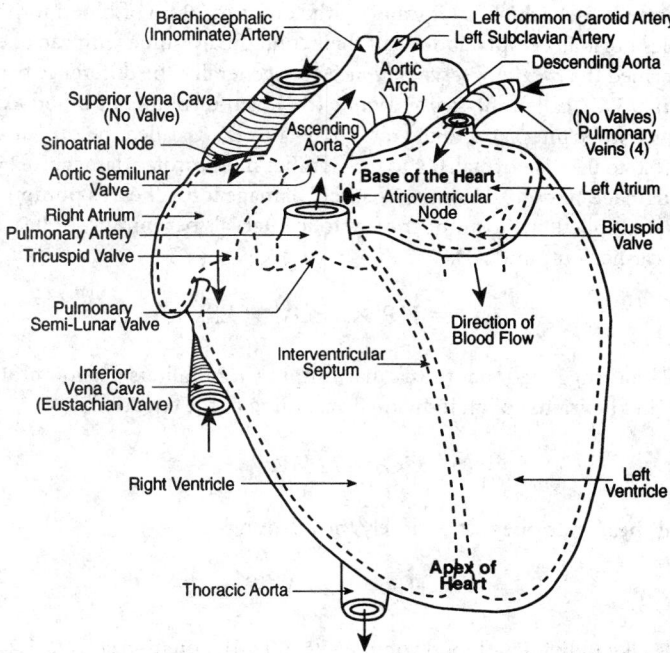

FIGURE 1.1.   Anterior view of the human heart showing the four chambers, the inlet and outlet valves, the inlet and outlet major blood vessels, the wall separating the right side from the left side, and the two cardiac pacing centers—the sinoatrial node and the atrioventricular node. Boldface arrows show the direction of flow through the heart chambers, the valves, and the major vessels.

of the heart, which does most of its work at a high pressure (up to 140 mmHg gauge or more) to drive blood through the entire systemic circulation to the furthest extremes of the organism.

Each cardiac (heart) pump is further divided into two chambers: a smaller upper receiving chamber, or atrium (auricle), separated by a one-way valve from a lower discharging chamber, or ventricle, which is about twice the size of its corresponding atrium. In order of size, the somewhat spherically shaped left atrium is the smallest chamber—holding about 45 ml of blood (at rest), operating at pressures on the order of 0 to 25 mmHg gauge, and having a wall thickness of about 3 mm. The pouch-shaped right atrium is next (63 ml of blood, 0 to 10 mmHg gauge of pressure, 2-mm wall thickness), followed by the conical/cylindrically shaped left ventricle (100 ml of blood, up to 140 mmHg gauge of pressure, variable wall thickness up to 12 mm) and the crescent-shaped right ventricle (about 130 ml of blood, up to 40 mmHg gauge of pressure, and a wall thickness on the order of one-third that of the left ventricle, up to about 4 mm). All together, then, the heart chambers collectively have a capacity of some 325 to 350 ml, or about 6.5% of the total blood volume in a "typical" individual—but these values are nominal, since the organ alternately fills and expands, contracts, and then empties as it generates a *cardiac output*.

During the 480-ms or so filling phase—diastole—of the average 750-ms cardiac cycle, the inlet valves of the two ventricles (3.8-cm-diameter tricuspid valve from right atrium to right ventricle; 3.1-cm-diameter bicuspid or mitral valve from left atrium to left ventricle) are open, and the outlet valves (2.4-cm-diameter pulmonary valve and 2.25-cm-diameter aortic semilunar valve, respectively) are closed—the heart ultimately expanding to its end-diastolic-volume (EDV), which is on the order of 140 ml of blood for the left ventricle. During the 270-ms emptying phase—systole—electrically induced vigorous contraction of cardiac muscle drives the intraventricular pressure up, forcing the one-way inlet valves closed and the unidirectional outlet valves open as the heart contracts to its end-systolic-volume (ESV), which is typically on the order of 70 ml of blood for the left ventricle. Thus the ventricles normally empty about half their contained volume with each heart beat, the remainder being termed the *cardiac reserve volume*. More generally, the difference between the *actual* EDV and the *actual* ESV, called the *stroke volume* (SV), is the volume of blood expelled from the heart during each systolic interval, and the ratio of SV to EDV is called the *cardiac ejection fraction*, or *ejection ratio* (0.5 to 0.75 is normal, 0.4 to 0.5 signifies mild cardiac damage, 0.25 to 0.40 implies moderate heart damage, and <0.25 warns of severe damage to the heart's pumping ability). If the stroke volume is multiplied by the number of systolic intervals per minute, or heart rate (HR), one obtains the total cardiac output (CO):

$$CO = HR \times (EDV - ESV) \tag{1.1}$$

Dawson [1991] has suggested that the cardiac output (in milliliters per minute) is proportional to the weight W (in kilograms) of an individual according to the equation

$$CO = 224W^{3/4} \tag{1.2}$$

and that "normal" heart rate obeys very closely the relation

$$HR = 229W^{-1/4} \tag{1.3}$$

For a "typical" 68.7-kg individual (blood volume = 5200 ml), Equations (1.1), (1.2), and (1.3) yield CO = 5345 ml/min, HR = 80 beats/min (cardiac cycle period = 754 ms) and SV = CO/HR = $224W^{3/4}/229W^{-1/4} = 0.978W = 67.2$ ml/beat, which are very reasonable values. Furthermore, assuming this individual lives about 75 years, his or her heart will have cycled over 3.1536 billion times, pumping a total of 0.2107 billion liters of blood (55.665 million gallons, or 8134 quarts per day)—all of it emptying into the circulatory pathways that constitute the vascular system.

1.3 The Piping Network: Blood Vessels

The vascular system is divided by a microscopic capillary network into an upstream, high-pressure, efferent arterial side (Table 1.3)—consisting of relatively thick-walled, viscoelastic tubes that carry blood away from the heart—and a downstream, low-pressure, afferent venous side (Table 1.4)—consisting of correspondingly thinner (but having a larger caliber) elastic conduits that return blood back to the heart. Except for their difference in thickness, the walls of the largest arteries and veins consist of the same three distinct, well-defined, and well-developed layers. From innermost to outermost, these layers are (1) the thinnest *tunica intima*, a continuous lining (the vascular endothelium) consisting of a single layer of simple squamous (thin, sheetlike) endothelial cells "glued" together by a polysaccharide (sugar) intercellular matrix, surrounded by a thin layer of subendothelial connective tissue interlaced with a number of circularly arranged elastic fibers to form the subendothelium, and separated from the next adjacent wall layer by a thick elastic band called the *internal elastic lamina*, (2) the thickest *tunica media*, composed of numerous circularly arranged elastic fibers, especially prevalent in the largest blood vessels on the arterial side (allowing them to expand during systole and to recoil passively during diastole), a significant amount of smooth muscle cells arranged in spiraling layers around the vessel wall, especially prevalent in medium-sized arteries and arterioles (allowing them to function as control points for blood distribution), and some interlacing collagenous connective tissue, elastic fibers, and intercellular mucopolysaccharide substance (extractives), all separated from the next adjacent wall layer by another thick elastic band called the *external elastic lamina*, and (3) the medium-sized *tunica adventitia*, an outer vascular sheath consisting entirely of connective tissue.

The largest blood vessels, such as the aorta, the pulmonary artery, the pulmonary veins, and others, have such thick walls that they require a separate network of tiny blood vessels—the vasa

TABLE 1.3 Arterial System*

Blood Vessel Type	(Systemic) Typical Number	Internal Diameter Range	Length Range†	Wall Thickness	Systemic Volume	(Pulmonary) Typical Number	Pulmonary Volume
Aorta	1	1.0–3.0 cm	30–65 cm	2–3 mm	156 ml	—	—
Pulmonary artery	—	2.5–3.1 cm	6–9 cm	2–3 mm	—	1	52 ml
Wall morphology: Complete tunica adventitia, external elastic lamina, tunica media, internal elastic lamina, tunica intima, subendothelium, endothelium, and vasa vasorum vascular supply							
Main branches	32	5 mm–2.25 cm	3.3–6 cm	≃2 mm	83.2 ml	6	41.6 ml
(Along with the aorta and pulmonary artery, the largest, most well-developed of all blood vessels)							
Large arteries	288	4.0–5.0 mm	1.4–2.8 cm	≃1 mm	104 ml	64	23.5 ml
(A well-developed tunica adventitia and vasa vasorum, although wall layers are gradually thinning)							
Medium arteries	1152	2.5–4.0 mm	1.0–2.2 cm	≃0.75 mm	117 ml	144	7.3 ml
Small arteries	3456	1.0–2.5 mm	0.6–1.7 cm	≃0.50 mm	104 ml	432	5.7 ml
Tributaries	20,736	0.5–1.0 mm	0.3–1.3 cm	≃0.25 mm	91 ml	5184	7.3 ml
(Well-developed tunica media and external elastic lamina, but tunica adventitia virtually nonexistent)							
Small rami	82,944	250–500 μm	0.2–0.8 cm	≃125 μm	57.2 ml	11,664	2.3 ml
Terminal branches	497,664	100–250 μm	1.0–6.0 mm	≃60 μm	52 ml	139,968	3.0 ml
(A well-developed endothelium, subendothelium, and internal elastic lamina, plus about two to three 15-μm-thick concentric layers forming just a very thin tunica media; no external elastic lamina)							
Arterioles	18,579,456	25–100 μm	0.2–3.8 mm	≃20–30 μm	52 ml	4,094,064	2.3 ml
Wall morphology: More than one smooth muscle layer (with nerve association in the outermost muscle layer), a well-developed internal elastic lamina; gradually thinning in 25- to 50-μm vessels to a single layer of smooth muscle tissue, connective tissue, and scant supporting tissue.							
Metarterioles	238,878,720	10–25 μm	0.1–1.8 mm	≃5–15 μm	41.6 ml	157,306,536	4.0 ml
(Well-developed subendothelium; discontinuous contractile muscle elements; one layer of connective tissue)							
Capillaries	16,124,431,360	3.5–10 μm	0.5–1.1 mm	≃0.5–1 μm	260 ml	3,218,406,696	104 ml
(Simple endothelial tubes devoid of smooth muscle tissue; one-cell-layer-thick walls)							

*Values are approximate for a 68.7-kg individual having a total blood volume of 5200 ml.

†Average uninterrupted distance between branch origins (except aorta and pulmonary artery, which are total length).

TABLE 1.4 Venous System

Blood Vessel Type	(Systemic) Typical Number	Internal Diameter Range	Length Range	Wall Thickness	Systemic Volume	(Pulmonary) Typical Number	Pulmonary Volume
Postcapillary venules	4,408,161,734	8–30 µm	0.1–0.6 mm	1.0–5.0 µm	166.7 ml	306,110,016	10.4 ml
(Wall consists of thin endothelium exhibiting occasional pericytes (pericapillary connective tissue cells) which increase in number as the vessel lumen gradually increases)							
Collecting venules	160,444,500	30–50 µm	0.1–0.8 mm	5.0–10 µm	161.3 ml	8,503,056	1.2 ml
(One complete layer of pericytes, one complete layer of veil cells (veil-like cells forming a thin membrane), occasional primitive smooth muscle tissue fibers that increase in number with vessel size)							
Muscular venules	32,088,900	50–100 µm	0.2–1.0 mm	10–25 µm	141.8 ml	3,779,136	3.7 ml
(Relatively thick wall of smooth muscle tissue)							
Small collecting veins	10,241,508	100–200 µm	0.5–3.2 mm	$\approx$30 µm	329.6 ml	419,904	6.7 ml
(Prominent tunica media of continuous layers of smooth muscle cells)							
Terminal branches	496,900	200–600 µm	1.0–6.0 mm	30–150 µm	206.6 ml	34,992	5.2 ml
(A well-developed endothelium, subendothelium, and internal elastic lamina; well-developed tunica media but fewer elastic fibers than corresponding arteries and much thinner walls)							
Small veins	19,968	600 µm–1.1 mm	2.0–9.0 mm	$\approx$0.25 mm	63.5 ml	17,280	44.9 ml
Medium veins	512	1–5 mm	1–2 cm	$\approx$0.50 mm	67.0 ml	144	22.0 ml
Large veins	256	5–9 mm	1.4–3.7 cm	$\approx$0.75 mm	476.1 ml	48	29.5 ml
(Well-developed wall layers comparable to large arteries but about 25% thinner)							
Main branches	224	9.0 mm–2.0 cm	2.0–10 cm	$\approx$1.00 mm	1538.1 ml	16	39.4 ml
(Along with the vena cava and pulmonary veins, the largest, most well-developed of all blood vessels)							
Vena cava	1	2.0–3.5 cm	20–50 cm	$\approx$1.50 mm	125.3 ml	—	—
Pulmonary veins	—	1.7–2.5 cm	5–8 cm	$\approx$1.50 mm	—	4	52 ml

Wall morphology: Essentially the same as comparable major arteries but a much thinner tunica intima, a much thinner tunica media, and a somewhat thicker tunica adventitia; contains vasa vasorum

Total systemic blood volume: 4394 ml—84.5% of total blood volume; 19.5% in arteries (~3:2 large:small), 5.9% in capillaries, 74.6% in veins (~3:1 large:small); 63% of volume is in vessels greater than 1 mm internal diameter

Total pulmonary blood volume: 468 ml—9.0% of total blood volume; 31.8% in arteries, 22.2% in capillaries, 46% in veins; 58.3% of volume is in vessels greater than 1 mm internal diameter; remainder of blood in heart, about 338 ml (6.5% of total blood volume)

vasorum—just to service the vascular tissue itself. As one moves toward the capillaries from the arterial side (see Table 1.3), the vascular wall keeps thinning, as if it were shedding 15-μm-thick, onion-peel-like concentric layers, and while the percentage of water in the vessel wall stays relatively constant at 70% (by weight), the ratio of elastin to collagen decreases (actually reverses)—from 3:2 in large arteries (9% elastin, 6% collagen, by weight) to 1:2 in small tributaries (5% elastin, 10% collagen)—and the amount of smooth muscle tissue increases from 7.5% by weight of large arteries (the remaining 7.5% consisting of various extractives) to 15% in small tributaries. By the time one reaches the capillaries, one encounters single-cell-thick endothelial tubes—devoid of any smooth muscle tissue, elastin, or collagen—downstream of which the vascular wall gradually "reassembles itself," layer-by-layer, as it directs blood back to the heart through the venous system (see Table 1.4).

Blood vessel structure is directly related to function. The thick-walled large arteries and main *distributing branches* are designed to withstand the pulsating 80 to 130 mmHg blood pressures that they must endure. The smaller elastic *conducting vessels* need only operate under steadier blood pressures in the range 70 to 90 mmHg, but they must be thin enough to penetrate and course through organs and tissues without unduly disturbing the anatomic integrity of the mass involved. Controlling arterioles operate at blood pressures between 45 and 70 mmHg but are heavily endowed with smooth muscle tissue (hence their being referred to as *muscular vessels*) so that they may be actively shut down when flow to the capillary bed they service is to be restricted (for whatever reason), and the smallest capillary *resistance vessels* (which operate at blood pressures on the order of 10 to 45 mmHg) are designed to optimize conditions for transport to occur between blood and the surrounding interstitial fluid. Traveling back up the venous side, one encounters relatively steady blood pressures continuously decreasing from around 30 mmHg all the way down to near zero, so these vessels can be thin-walled without significant consequence. However, the low blood pressure, slower, steady (time-independent) flow, thin walls, and larger caliber that characterize the venous system cause blood to tend to "pool" in veins, allowing them to act somewhat like reservoirs. It is not surprising, then, that at any given instant, one normally finds about two-thirds of the total human blood volume residing in the venous system, the remaining one-third being divided among the heart (6.5%), the microcirculation (7% in systemic and pulmonary capillaries), and the arterial system (19.5 to 20%).

In a global sense, then, one can think of the human cardiovascular system—using an electrical analogy—as a voltage source (the heart), two capacitors (a large venous system and a smaller arterial system), and a resistor (the microcirculation taken as a whole). Blood flow and the dynamics of the system represent electrical inductance (inertia), and useful engineering approximations can be derived from such a simple model. The cardiovascular system is designed to bring blood to within a capillary size of each and every one of the more than 10^{14} cells of the body—but *which* cells receive blood at any given time, *how much* blood they get, the *composition* of the fluid coursing by them, and related physiologic considerations are all matters that are not left up to chance.

1.4 Cardiovascular Control

Blood flows through organs and tissues either to nourish and sanitize them or to be itself processed in some sense—e.g., to be oxygenated (pulmonary circulation), stocked with nutrients (splanchnic circulation), dialyzed (renal circulation), cooled (cutaneous circulation), filtered of dilapidated red blood cells (splenic circulation), and so on. Thus any given vascular network normally receives blood according to the metabolic needs of the region it perfuses and/or the function of that region as a blood treatment plant and/or thermoregulatory pathway. However, it is not feasible to expect that our physiologic transport system can be "all things to all cells all of the time"—especially when resources are scarce and/or time is a factor. Thus the distribution of blood is further prioritized according to three basic criteria: (1) how essential the perfused region is to the maintenance of life itself (e.g., we can survive without an arm, a leg, a stomach, or even a large portion of our small intestine but not without a brain, a heart, and at least one functioning kidney and lung, (2) how essential the perfused region is in allowing the organism to respond to a life-threatening situation (e.g., digesting a meal is among the least of the body's concerns in a "fight or flight" circumstance), and (3) how well the perfused region can function and survive on a decreased supply of blood (e.g., some tissues—like striated skeletal and smooth muscle—have significant anaerobic capability; others—like several forms of connective tissue—can function quite effectively at a significantly decreased metabolic rate when necessary; some organs—like the liver—are larger than they really need to be; and some anatomic structures—like the eyes, ears, and limbs—have duplicates, giving them a built-in redundancy).

Within this generalized prioritization scheme, control of cardiovascular function is accomplished by mechanisms that are based either on the inherent physicochemical attributes of the tissues and organs themselves—so-called intrinsic control—or on responses that can be attributed to the effects on cardiovascular tissues of other organ systems in the body (most notably the autonomic nervous system and the endocrine system)—so-called extrinsic control. For example, the accumulation of wastes and depletion of oxygen and nutrients that accompany the increased rate of metabolism in an active tissue both lead to an *intrinsic* relaxation of local precapillary sphincters (rings of muscle)—with a consequent widening of corresponding capillary entrances—which reduces the local resistance to flow and thereby allows more blood to perfuse the active region. On the other hand, the *extrinsic* innervation by the autonomic nervous system of smooth muscle tissue in the walls of arterioles allows the central nervous system to completely shut down the flow to entire vascular beds (such as the cutaneous circulation) when this becomes necessary (such as during exposure to extremely cold environments).

In addition to prioritizing and controlling the *distribution* of blood, physiologic regulation of cardiovascular function is directed mainly at four other variables: cardiac output, blood pressure, blood volume, and blood composition. From Equation (1.1) we see that cardiac output can be increased by increasing the heart rate (a chronotropic effect), increasing the end-diastolic volume (allowing the heart to fill longer by delaying the onset of systole), decreasing the end-systolic volume (an inotropic effect), or doing all three things at once. Indeed, under the extrinsic influence of the sympathetic nervous system and the adrenal glands, HR can triple—to some 240 beats/min if necessary—EDV can increase by as much as 50%—to around 200 ml or more of blood—and ESV can decrease a comparable amount (the cardiac reserve)—to about 30 to 35 ml or less. The combined result of all three effects can lead to over a sevenfold increase in cardiac output—from the normal 5 to 5.5 liters/min to as much as 40 to 41 liters/min or more for very brief periods of strenuous exertion.

The control of blood pressure is accomplished mainly by adjusting at the arteriolar level the downstream resistance to flow—an increased resistance leading to a rise in arterial backpressure, and vice versa. This effect is conveniently quantified by a fluid-dynamic analogue to Ohm's famous $E = IR$ law in electromagnetic theory, voltage drop E being equated to fluid pressure drop ΔP, electric current I corresponding to flow—cardiac output (CO)—and electric resistance R being associated with an analogous vascular "peripheral resistance" (PR). Thus one may write

$$\Delta P = (\text{CO})(\text{PR}) \tag{1.4}$$

Normally, the total systemic peripheral resistance is 15 to 20 mmHg/liter/min of flow but can increase significantly under the influence of the vasomotor center located in the medulla of the brain, which controls arteriolar muscle tone.

The control of blood volume is accomplished mainly through the excretory function of the kidney. For example, antidiuretic hormone (ADH) secreted by the pituitary gland acts to prevent renal fluid loss (excretion via urination) and thus increases plasma volume, whereas perceived extracellular fluid overloads such as those which result from the peripheral vasoconstriction response to cold stress lead to a sympathetic/adrenergic receptor–induced renal diuresis (urination) that tends to decrease plasma volume—if not checked, to sometimes dangerously low dehydration levels. Blood composition, too, is maintained primarily through the activity of endocrine hormones and enzymes that enhance or repress specific biochemical pathways. Since these pathways are too numerous to itemize here, suffice it to say that in the body's quest for homeostasis and stability, virtually nothing is left to chance, and every biochemical end can be arrived at through a number of alternative means. In a broader sense, as the organism strives to maintain life, it coordinates a wide variety of different functions, and central to its ability to do just that is the role played by the cardiovascular system in transporting mass, energy, and momentum.

Defining Terms

Atrioventricular (AV) node: A highly specialized cluster of neuromuscular cells at the lower portion of the right atrium leading to the interventricular septum; the AV node delays sinoatrial, (SA) node–generated electrical impulses momentarily (allowing the atria to contract first) and then conducts the depolarization wave to the bundle of His and its bundle branches.

Autonomic nervous system: The functional division of the nervous system that innervates most glands, the heart, and smooth muscle tissue in order to maintain the internal environment of the body.

Cardiac muscle: Involuntary muscle possessing much of the anatomic attributes of skeletal voluntary muscle and some of the physiologic attributes of involuntary smooth muscle tissue; SA node–induced contraction of its interconnected network of fibers allows the heart to expel blood during systole.

Chronotropic: Affecting the periodicity of a recurring action, such as the slowing (bradycardia) or speeding up (tachycardia) of the heartbeat that results from extrinsic control of the SA node.

Endocrine system: The system of ductless glands and organs secreting substances directly into the blood to produce a specific response from another "target" organ or body part.

Endothelium: Flat cells that line the innermost surfaces of blood and lymphatic vessels and the heart.

Homeostasis: A tendency to uniformity or stability in an organism by maintaining within narrow limits certain variables that are critical to life.

Inotropic: Affecting the contractility of muscular tissue, such as the increase in cardiac *power* that results from extrinsic control of the myocardial musculature.

Precapillary sphincters: Rings of smooth muscle surrounding the entrance to capillaries where they branch off from upstream metarterioles. Contraction and relaxation of these sphincters close and open the access to downstream blood vessels, thus controlling the irrigation of different capillary networks.

Sinoatrial (SA) node: Neuromuscular tissue in the right atrium near where the superior vena cava joins the posterior right atrium (the sinus venarum); the SA node generates electrical impulses that initiate the heartbeat, hence its nickname the cardiac "pacemaker."

Stem cells: A generalized parent cell spawning descendants that become individually specialized.

Acknowledgments

The author gratefully acknowledges the assistance of Professor Robert Hochmuth in the preparation of Table 1.1 and the Radford Community Hospital for their support of the Biomedical Engineering Program at Virginia Tech.

References

Bhagavan NV. 1992. Medical Biochemistry. Boston, Jones and Bartlett.

Beall HPT, Needham D, Hochmuth RM. 1993. Volume and osmotic properties of human neutrophils. Blood 81(10):2774–2780.

Caro CG, Pedley TJ, Schroter RC, Seed WA. 1978. The Mechanics of the Circulation. New York, Oxford University Press.

Chandran KB. 1992. Cardiovascular Biomechanics. New York, New York University Press.

Frausto da Silva JJR, Williams RJP. 1993. The Biological Chemistry of the Elements. New York, Oxford University Press/Clarendon.

Dawson TH. 1991. Engineering Design of the Cardiovascular System of Mammals. Englewood Cliffs, NJ, Prentice-Hall.

Duck FA. 1990. Physical Properties of Tissue. San Diego, Academic Press.

Kaley G, Altura BM (eds). Microcirculation, vol I (1977), vol II (1978), vol III (1980). Baltimore, University Park Press.

Kessel RG, Kardon RH. 1979. Tissues and Organs—A Text-Atlas of Scanning Electron Microscopy. San Francisco, WH Freeman.

Lentner C (ed). Geigy Scientific Tables, vol 3: Physical Chemistry, Composition of Blood, Hematology and Somatometric Data, 8th ed. 1984. New Jersey, Ciba-Geigy.

———Vol 5: Heart and Circulation, 8th ed. 1990. New Jersey, Ciba-Geigy.

Schneck DJ. 1990. Engineering Principles of Physiologic Function. New York, New York University Press.

Tortora GJ, Grabowski SR. 1993. Principles of Anatomy and Physiology, 7th ed. New York, HarperCollins.

2

Endocrine System

Derek G. Cramp
City University, London

Ewart R. Carson
City University, London

The body, if it is to achieve optimal performance, must possess mechanisms for sensing and responding appropriately to numerous biologic cues and signals in order to control and maintain its internal environment. This role is effected by the interaction of the endocrine and neural systems. The endocrine contribution is achieved through a highly sophisticated set of communication and control systems involving signal generation, propagation, recognition, transduction, and response. The signal entities are chemical messengers or hormones that are distributed through the body by the blood circulation to their respective target organs to modify their activity in some fashion.

Endocrinology has a comparatively long history, but real advances in understanding of endocrine mechanisms and control have been highly dependent on methods that permit measurement of the minute amounts of the various circulating hormones reliably, relatively simply, and at low cost. The breakthrough came in the late 1960s when Berson and Yalow developed and promoted sensitive methods of competitive protein binding and radioimmunoassay that superseded existing cumbersome bioassay methods.

Since then, much knowledge has accrued not only of the physiology of individual endocrine glands but also of the neural control of the pituitary gland and the overall feedback control of the endocrine system. This has been facilitated at a practical level by developments in cellular and molecular biology and recombinant DNA technology. However, theoretical and quantitative approaches using mathematical modeling also have been of value in gaining a greater understanding of endocrinology. This brief exposition can only describe the salient features of this fascinating domain, but it is hoped that it may nevertheless stimulate a further interest.

2.1 Endocrine System: Hormones, Signals, and Communication

Endocrine cells secrete hormones that act locally or at a distance, having been carried in the bloodstream (classic endocrine activity) or secreted into the gut lumen (lumocrine activity) to act on target cells that are distributed elsewhere in the body. Hormones can be classified broadly into three

0-8493-8346-3/95/$0.00+$.50

groups according to their physicochemical characteristics: steroid hormones derived from choles- terol, peptide and protein hormones, and those derived from the aromatic amino acid tyrosine. The peptide and protein hormones are essentially hydrophilic and are therefore able to circulate in the blood in the free state; however, the more hydrophobic lipid-derived molecules have to be carried in the circulation bound to specific transport proteins.

Figure 2.1 and Table 2.1 show, in schematic and descriptive form, respectively, details of the major endocrine glands of the body and the endocrine pathways. The endocrine and nervous system are physically and functionally linked by a specific region of the brain called the *hypothalamus*, which

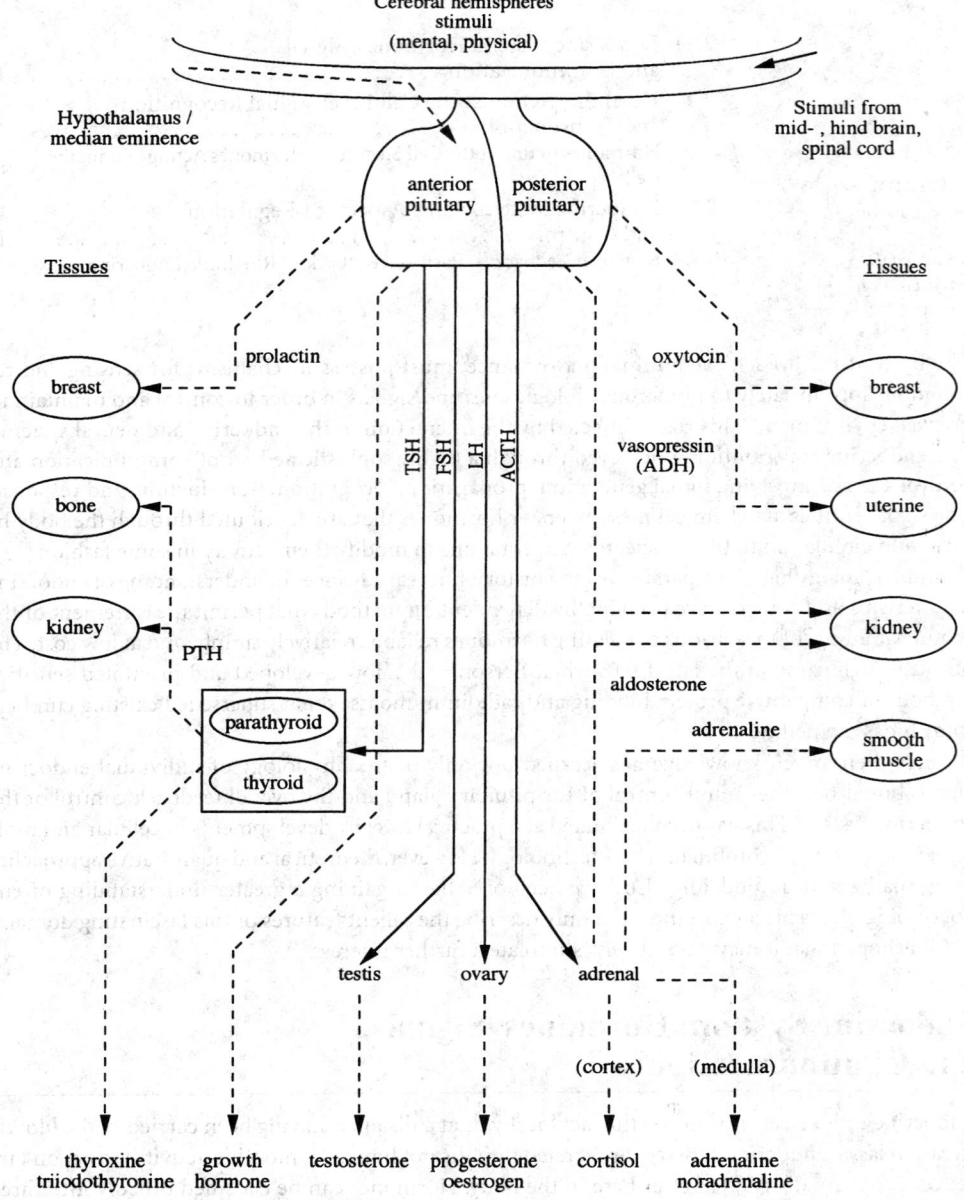

FIGURE 2.1   Representation of the forward pathways of pituitary and target gland hormone release and ac- tion: ——— trophic hormones; – – – – tissue-affecting hormones.

TABLE 2.1   Main Endocrine Glands and the Hormones They Produce and Release

Gland	Hormone	Chemical Characteristics
Hypothalamus/median eminence	Thyrotropin-releasing hormone (TRH)	⎫
	Somatostatin	⎪
	Gonadotropin-releasing hormone	├ Peptides
	Growth hormone–releasing hormone	⎪
	Corticotropin-releasing hormone	⎭
	Prolactin inhibitor factor	Amine
Anterior pituitary	Thyrotropin (TSH)	⎫
	Luteinizing hormone	├ Glycoproteins
	Follicle-stimulating hormone (FSH)	⎭
	Growth hormone	⎫
	Prolactin	├ Proteins
	Adrenocorticotropin (ACTH)	⎭
Posterior pituitary	Vasopressin (antidiuretic hormone, ADH)	⎫ Peptides
	Oxytocin	⎭
Thyroid	Triidothyronine (T_3)	⎫ Tyrosine derivatives
	Thyroxine (T_4)	⎭
Parathyroid	Parathyroid hormone (PTH)	Peptide
Adrenal cortex	Cortisol	⎫ Steroids
	Aldosterone	⎭
Adrenal medulla	Epinephrine	⎫ Catecholamines
	Norepinephrine	⎭
Pancreas	Insulin	⎫
	Glucagon	├ Proteins
	Somatostatin	⎭
Gonads: Testes	Testosterone	⎫
Ovaries	Oestrogen	├ Steroids
	Progesterone	⎭

lies immediately above the pituitary gland, to which it is connected by an extension called the *pituitary stalk*. The integrating function of the hypothalamus is mediated by cells that possess the properties of both nerve and processes that carry electrical impulses and on stimulation can release their signal molecules into the blood. Each of the hypothalamic neurosecretory cells can be stimulated by other nerve cells in higher regions of the brain to secrete specific peptide hormones or releasing factors into the adenohypophyseal portal vasculature. These hormones can then specifically stimulate or suppress the secretion of a second hormone from the anterior pituitary.

These pituitary hormones in the circulation interact with their target tissues, which, if endocrine glands, are stimulated to secrete further (third) hormones that feed back to inhibit the release of the pituitary hormones. It will be seen from Fig. 2.1 and Table 2.1 that the main targets of the pituitary are the adrenal cortex, the thyroid, and the gonads. These axes provide good examples of the control of pituitary hormone release by negative-feedback inhibition; e.g., adrenocorticotropin (ACTH), luteinizing hormone (LH), and follicle-stimulating hormone (FSH) are selectively inhibited by different steroid hormones, as is thyrotropin (TSH) release by the thyroid hormones.

In the case of growth hormone (GH) and prolactin, the target tissue is not an endocrine gland and thus does not produce a hormone; then the feedback control is mediated by inhibitors. Prolactin is under dopamine inhibitory control, whereas hypothalamic releasing and inhibitory factors control GH release. The two posterior pituitary (neurohypophyseal) hormones oxytocin and vasopressin are synthesized in the supraoptic and paraventricular nuclei and are stored in granules at the end of the nerve fibers in the posterior pituitary. Oxytocin is subsequently secreted in response to peripheral stimuli from the cervical stretch receptors or the suckling receptors of the breast. In a like manner, antidiuretic hormone (ADH, vasopressin) release is stimulated by the altered activity of hypothalamic osmoreceptors responding to changes in plasma solute concentrations.

It will be noted how the hypothalamus, pituitary, and other endocrine glands together form a complex hierarchical regulatory system composed of several endocrine axes. There is no doubt that the anterior pituitary occupies a central position in the control of hormone secretion, and because of its important role, it was often called the "conductor of the endocrine orchestra." However, the release of pituitary hormones is mediated by complex feedback control, and thus the pituitary should be regarded as having essentially a permissive role rather than having the overall control of the endocrine system.

2.2 Hormone Action at the Cell Level: Signal Recognition and Transduction

The ability of target glands or tissues to respond to hormonal signals depends on the ability of the cells to recognize the signal. This role is played by specific receptor proteins unique for a particular hormone that bind with high affinity, thus enabling the cell not only to recognize the hormonal signal but also to respond in a preprogrammed fashion. It is useful to classify the site of such action into two groups: those hormones which act at the cell surface without, generally, traversing the cell membrane and those which actually enter the cell before effecting a response.

Hormones Acting at the Cell Surface

Most peptide and protein hormones are hydrophilic and thus unable to traverse the lipid-containing cell membrane and must act through activation of receptor proteins on the cell surface. When these receptors are activated by the binding of an extracellular signal ligand, the ligand-receptor complex initiates a series of protein interactions within or adjacent to the inner surface of the plasma membrane, which in turn bring about changes in intracellular activity. This can be brought about in one of two ways. The first involves altering the activity of a plasma membrane–bound enzyme, which in turn increases (or sometimes decreases) the concentration of an intracellular mediator, the so-called second messenger. The activation of other types of cell surface receptors can lead to changes in the plasma membrane electrical potential and thus the membrane permeability, resulting in altered transmembrane transport of ions or metabolites, the second method.

Adaptation to a high concentration of a signal ligand in a time-dependent reversible manner enables cells to respond to changes in the concentration of a ligand instead of to its absolute concentration. Adaptation can occur in several ways. Ligand binding can inactivate a cell surface receptor either by inducing its internalization and degradation or by causing the receptor to adopt an inactive conformation. Alternatively, it may result from the changes in one of the nonreceptor proteins involved in signal transduction following receptor activation.

The peptide and protein hormones circulate at very low concentrations relative to other proteins in the blood plasma. These low concentrations are reflected in the very high affinity and specificity of the receptor sites, which permit recognition of the relevant hormones amid the profusion of protein molecules in the circulation.

The cell surface receptors for peptide hormones are linked functionally to a cell membrane–bound enzyme that acts as the catalytic unit. As the hormone binds at the receptor site, it is coupled through a regulatory protein, a transducer, to the enzyme adenyl cyclase, which catalyzes the formation of cyclic adenosine monophosphate (cAMP) from adenosine triphosphate (ATP). If the hormone is thought of as the "first messenger," cAMP can be regarded as the "second messenger," capable of triggering a cascade of intracellular biochemical events that can lead either to a rapid secondary response such as altered ion transport, enhanced metabolic pathway flux, or steroidogenesis or to a slower response such as DNA, RNA, and protein synthesis resulting in cell growth or cell division.

The adenylate cyclase reaction is rapid, and the increased concentration of intracellular cAMP is short, since it is rapidly hydrolyzed by phosphodiesterase group enzymes. The continual and rapid removal from the cytosol of cAMP and free calcium ions makes for both the rapid increase and decrease of these intracellular mediators when the cells respond to signals. Rising cAMP concentrations affect cells by stimulating cAMP-dependent protein kinases to phosphorylate specific target proteins. These effects are reversible because phosphorylated proteins are rapidly dephosphorylated when the concentration of cAMP falls.

The action of thyrotropin-releasing hormone (TRH), parathyroid hormone (PTH), and epinephrine is catalyzed by adenyl cyclase, and this can be regarded as the "classic" reaction. However, there are variants. Thyrotropin and vasopressin modulate an activity of phospholipase C that catalyzes the conversion of phosphatidylinositol to diacylglycerol and inositol-1,4,5-triphosphate, which act as the second messengers. They mobilize bound intracellular calcium and activate a protein kinase, which in turn alters the activity of other calcium-dependent enzymes within the cell.

Increased concentrations of free calcium ions affect cellular events by binding to and altering the molecular conformation of calmodulin; the resulting calcium ion–calmodulin complex can activate many different target proteins, including calcium ion–dependent protein kinases. Each cell type has a characteristic set of target proteins that are so regulated by cAMP-dependent kinases and/or calmodulin that it will respond in a specific way to an alteration in cAMP or calcium ion concentrations. In this way, cAMP or calcium ions act as second messengers in such a way as to allow the original extracellular signal not only to be greatly amplified but, as important, also to be made specific for each cell type.

The action of the important glucoregulatory hormone insulin depends on the activation of the membrane enzyme tyrosine kinase catalyzing the phosphorylation of tyrosyl residues of proteins. This effects changes in the activity of calcium-sensitive enzymes, leading to enhanced movement of glucose and fatty acids across the cell membrane and modulating their intracellular metabolism. The binding of insulin to its receptor site has been studied extensively; the receptor complex has been isolated and characterized. Such work highlighted an interesting aspect of feedback control at the cell level: the ability of peptide hormones to regulate the concentration of cell surface receptors. After activation, the receptor population becomes desensitized, or "down-regulated," leading to a decreased availability of receptors and thus a modulation of transmembrane events.

The hormonal activities of GH and prolactin influence cellular gene transcription and translation of messenger RNA by complex mechanisms.

Hormones Acting Within the Cell

Steroid hormones are small hydrophobic molecules derived from cholesterol that are solubilized by binding reversibly to specify carrier proteins in the blood plasma. Once released from their carrier proteins, they have to pass through the plasma membrane of the target cell and bind, again reversibly, to steroid hormone receptor proteins in the cytosol. The protein component of the steroid hormone–receptor complex acquires an affinity for DNA in the cell nucleus, where it binds to nuclear chromatin and regulates the transcription of a small number of genes. These gene products may, in turn, activate other genes and produce a secondary response, thereby amplifying the initial effect of the hormone. Each steroid hormone is recognized by a separate receptor protein, but this same receptor protein has the capacity to regulate several different genes in different target cells. This, of course, suggests that the nuclear chromatin of each cell type is organized so that only the appropriate genes are made available for regulation by the hormone-receptor complex. The thyroid hormone triiodothyronine (T_3) also acts, though by a different mechanism than the steroids, at the cell nucleus level.

2.3 Endocrine System: Some Aspects of Regulation and Control

From the foregoing sections it is clear that the endocrine system exhibits complex dynamics and involves many levels of control and regulation. Hormones are chemical signals released from a hierarchy of endocrine glands and propagated through the circulation to a hierarchy of cell types. The integration of this system depends on a series of what systems engineers call "feedback loops"; feedback is a reflection of mutual dependence of the system variables: variable x affects variable y, and y affects x. Further, it is essentially a closed-loop system in which the feedback of information from the system output to the input has the capacity to maintain homeostasis. A diagrammatic representation of the ways in which hormone action is controlled is shown in Fig. 2.2. One example of this control structure arises in the context of the thyroid hormones. In this case, TRH, secreted by the hypothalamus, triggers the anterior pituitary into the production of TSH. The target gland is the thyroid, which produces T_3 and thyroxine (T). The complexity of control includes both direct and indirect feedback of T_3 and T_4, as outlined in Fig. 2.2, together with TSH feedback on to the hypothalamus.

Negative Feedback

If an increase in y causes a change in x which tends to decrease y, feedback is said to be *negative*; in other words, the signal output induces a response that feeds back to the signal generator to decrease its output. This is the most common form of control in physiologic systems, and examples are many. For instance, as mentioned earlier, the anterior pituitary releases trophic or stimulating hormones that act on peripheral endocrine glands such as the adrenals or thyroid or to gonads to produce hormones that act back on the pituitary to decrease the secretion of the trophic hormones. These are examples of what is called *long-loop feedback* (see Fig. 2.2.). The trophic hormones of the pituitary are also regulated by feedback action at the level of their releasing factors. *Ultrashort-loop feedback* is also described. There are numerous examples also of *short-loop feedback*, the best being the reciprocal relation between insulin and blood glucose concentrations, as depicted in Fig. 2.3. In this case, elevated glucose concentration (and positive rate of change, implying not only proportional but also

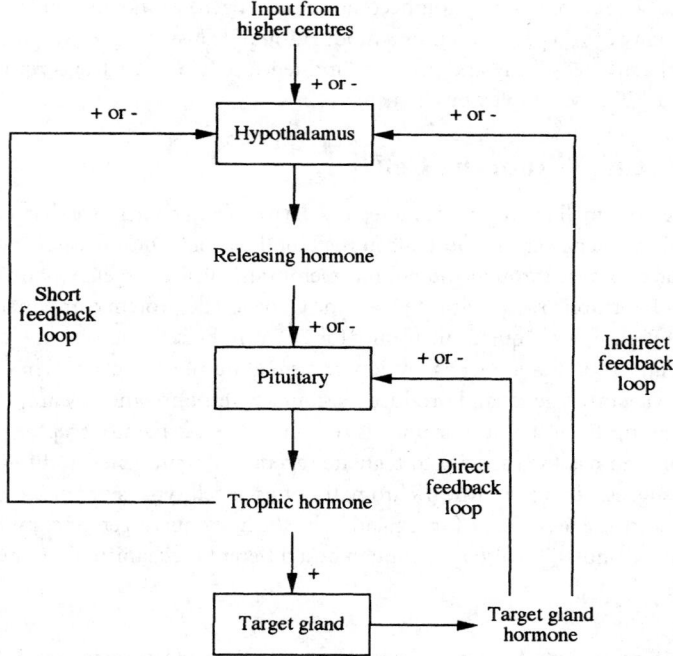

FIGURE 2.2   Illustration of the complexity of hormonal feedback control (+ indicates a positive or augmenting effect; − indicates a negative or inhibiting effect).

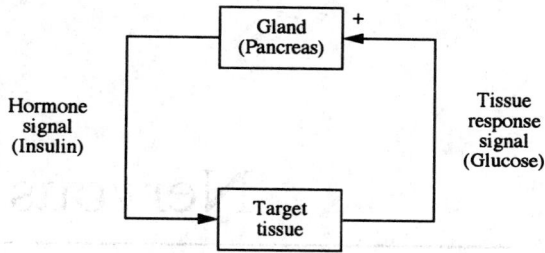

FIGURE 2.3 The interaction of insulin as an illustration of negative feedback within a hormonal control system.

derivative control) has a positive effect on the pancreas, which secretes insulin in response. This has an inhibiting effect on glucose metabolism, resulting in a reduction of blood glucose toward a normal concentration, in other words, classic negative-feedback control.

Positive Feedback

If an increase in y causes a change in x which tends to increase y, feedback is said to be *positive*; in other words, a further signal output is evoked by the response it induces or provokes. This is intrinsically an unstable system, but there are physiologic situations where such control is valuable. In the positive-feedback situation, the signal output will continue until no further response is required. Suckling provides an example; stimulation of nipple receptors by the suckling child provokes an increased oxytocin release from the posterior pituitary with a corresponding increase in milk flow. Removal of the stimulus causes cessation of oxytocin release.

Rhythmic Endocrine Control

Many hormone functions exhibit rhythmicity in the form of pulsatile release of hormones. The most common is the approximately 24-hour cycle (circadian or diurnal rhythm). For instance, blood sampling at frequent intervals has shown that ACTH is secreted episodically, each secretory burst being followed 5 to 10 minutes later by cortisol secretion. These episodes are most frequent in the early morning, with plasma cortisol concentrations highest around 7 to 8 A.M. and lowest around midnight. ACTH and cortisol secretion vary inversely, and the parallel circadian rhythm is probably due to a cyclic change in the sensitivity of the hypothalamic feedback center to circulating cortisol. Longer cycles are also known, e.g., the infradian menstrual cycle.

It is clear that such inherent rhythms are important in endocrine communication and control, suggesting that its physiologic organization is based not only on the structural components of the system but also on the dynamics of their interactions. The rhythmic, pulsatile nature of release of many hormones is a means whereby time-varying signals can be encoded, thus allowing large quantities of information to be transmitted and exchanged rapidly in a way that small, continuous changes in threshold levels would not allow.

References

De Groot LJ (ed). 1989. Endocrinology. 2nd ed. Philadelphia, WB Saunders.
Norman AW, Litwak G. 1987. Hormones. San Diego, Academic Press.
McIntosh JEA, McIntosh RP. 1980. Mathematical Modelling and Computers in Endocrinology. Berlin, Springer Verlag.

3

Nervous System

Evangelia
Micheli-Tzanakou
Rutgers University

The nervous system, unlike other organ systems, is concerned primarily with signals, information encoding and processing, and control rather than manipulation of energy. It acts like a communication device whose components use substances and energy in processing signals and in reorganizing them, choosing, and commanding, as well as in developing and learning. A central question that is often asked is how nervous systems work and what are the principles of their operation. In an attempt to answer this question, we will, at the same time, ignore other fundamental questions, such as those relating to anatomic or neurochemical and molecular aspects. We will concentrate rather on relations and transactions between neurons and their assemblages in the nervous system. We will deal with neural signals (encoding and decoding), the evaluation and weighting of incoming signals, and the formulation of outputs. A major part of this chapter is devoted to higher aspects of the nervous system, such as memory and learning, rather than individual systems, such as vision and audition, which are treated extensively elsewhere in this *Handbook*.

3.1 Definitions

Nervous systems can be defined as organized assemblies of nerve cells as well as nonnervous cells. Nerve cells, or *neurons*, are specialized in the generation, integration, and conduction of incoming signals from the outside world or from other neurons and deliver them to other excitable cells or to *effectors* such as muscle cells. Nervous systems are easily recognized in higher animals but not in the lower species, since the defining criteria are difficult to apply.

A central nervous system (CNS) can be distinguished easily from a peripheral nervous system (PNS), since it contains most of the motor and nucleated parts of neurons that innervate muscles and other effectors. The PNS contains all the sensory nerve cell bodies, with some exceptions, plus local *plexuses*, local *ganglia*, and peripheral axons that make up the *nerves*. Most sensory axons go all the way into the CNS, while the remaining sensory axons relay in peripheral plexuses. Motor axons originating in the CNS innervate effector cells.

The nervous system has two major roles: (1) to regulate, acting homeostatically in restoring some conditions of the organism after some external stimulus, and (2) to act to alter a preexisting condition by replacing it or modifying it. In both cases—regulation or initiation of a process—learning can be superimposed. In most species, learning is a more or less adaptive mechanism, combining and timing species-characteristic acts with a large degree of evolution toward perfection.

The nervous system is a complex structure for which realistic assumptions have led to irrelevant oversimplifications. One can break the nervous system down into four components: sensory transducers, neurons, axons, and muscle fibers. Each of these components gathers, processes, and transmits information impinging on it from the outside world, usually in the form of complex stimuli. The processing is carried out by exitable tissues—neurons, axons, sensory receptors, and muscle fibers. Neurons are the basic elements of the nervous system. If put in small assemblies or clusters, they form neuronal assemblies or neuronal networks communicating with each other either chemically via *synaptic junctions* or electrically via *tight* junctions. The main characteristics of a cell are the *cell body*, or *soma*, which contains the *nucleus*, and a number of processes originating from the cell body, called the *dendrites*, which reach out to surroundings to make contacts with other cells. These contacts serve as the incoming information to the cell, while the outgoing information follows a conduction path, the axon. The incoming information is integrated in the cell body and generates its action potential at the *axon hillock*. There are two types of outputs that can be generated and therefore two types of neurons: those which generate *graded* potentials that attenuate with distance and those which generate *action* potentials. The latter travel through the axon, a thin, long process that passively passes the action potential or rather a train of action potentials without any attenuation (*all-or-none effect*). A number of action potentials is often called a *spike train*. A threshold built into the hillock, depending on its level, allows or stops the generation of the spike train. Axons usually terminate on other neurons by means of *synaptic terminals* or *boutons* and have properties similar to those of an electric cable with varying diameters and speeds of signal transmission. Axons can be of two types: *myelinated* or *unmyelinated*. In the former case, the axon is surrounded by a thick fatty material, the myelin sheath, which is interrupted at regular intervals by gaps called the *nodes of Ranvier*. These nodes provide for the *saltatory* conduction of the signal along the axon. The axon makes functional connections with other neurons at synapses on either the cell body, the dendrites, or the axons. There exist two kinds of synapses: *excitatory* and *inhibitory*, and as the names imply, they either increase the *firing* frequency of the postsynaptic neurons or decrease it, respectively.

Sensory receptors are specialized cells that, in response to an incoming stimulus, generate a corresponding electrical signal, a graded receptor potential. Although the mechanisms by which the sensory receptors generate receptor potentials are not known exactly, the most plausible scenario is that an external stimulus alters the membrane permeabilities. The receptor potential, then, is the change in intracellular potential relative to the *resting* potential.

It is important to notice here that the term *receptor* is used in physiology to refer not only to sensory receptors but also, in a different sense, to proteins that bind neurotransmitters, hormones, and other substances with great affinity and specificity as a first step in starting up physiologic responses. This receptor is often associated with nonneural cells that surround it and form a *sense organ*. The forms of energy converted by the receptors include mechanical, thermal, electromagnetic, and chemical energy. The particular form of energy to which a receptor is most sensitive is called its *adequate stimulus*. The problem of how receptors convert energy into action potentials in the sensory nerves has been the subject of intensive study. In the complex sense organs such as those concerned with hearing and vision, there exist separate receptor cells and synaptic junctions between receptors and afferent nerves. In other cases, such as the cutaneous sense organs, the receptors are specialized. Where a stimulus of constant strength is applied to a receptor repeatedly, the frequency of the action potentials in its sensory nerve declines over a period of time. This phenomenon is known as *adaptation*; if the adaptation is very rapid, then the receptors are called *phasic*; otherwise, they are called *tonic*.

Another important issue is the *coding* of sensory information. Action potentials are similar in all nerves, although there are variations in their speed of conduction and other characteristics. However, if the action potentials were the same in most cells, then what makes the visual cells sensitive to light and not to sound and the touch receptors sensitive to touch and not to smell? And how can we tell if these sensations are strong or not? These sensations depend on what is called the *doctrine of specific nerve energies*, which has been questioned over time by several researchers. No matter where a particular sensory pathway is stimulated along its course to the brain, the sensation produced is referred to the location of the receptor. This is the *law of projections*. An example of this law is the "phantom limb," in which an amputee complains about an itching sensation in the amputated limb.

3.2 Functions of the Nervous System

The basic unit of integrated activity is the *reflex arc*. This arc consists of a sense organ, an afferent neuron, one or more synapses in a central integrating station (or sympathetic ganglion), an efferent neuron, and an effector. The simplest reflex arc is the *monosynaptic* one, which has only one synapse between the afferent and efferent neurons. With more than one synapse, the reflex arc is called *polysynaptic*. In each of these cases, activity is modified by both spatial and temporal facilitation, occlusion, and other effects.

In mammals, the connection between afferent and efferent somatic neurons is found either in the brain or in the spinal cord. The Bell-Magendie law dictates that in the spinal cord the dorsal roots are sensory, while the ventral roots are motor. The action potential message that is carried by an axon is eventually fed to a muscle, to a secretory cell, or to the dendrite of another neuron. If an axon is carrying a graded potential, its output is too weak to stimulate a muscle, but it can terminate on a secretory cell or dendrite. The latter can have as many as 10,000 inputs. If the endpoint is a motor neuron, which has been found experimentally in the case of fibers from the primary endings, then there is a lag between the time when the stimulus was applied and when the response is obtained from the muscle. This time interval is called the *reaction time* and in humans is approximately 20 ms for a stretch reflex. The distance from the spinal cord can be measured, and since the conduction velocities of both the efferent and afferent fibers are known, another important quality can be calculated: the *central delay*. This delay is the portion of the reaction time that was spent for conduction to and from the spinal cord. It has been found that muscle spindles also make connections that cause muscle contraction via polysynaptic pathways, while the afferents from secondary endings make connections that excite extensor muscles. When a motor neuron sends a burst of action potentials to its skeletal muscle, the amount of contraction depends largely on the discharge frequency but also on many other factors, such as the history of the load on the muscle and the load itself. The *stretch error* can be calculated from the desired motion minus the actual stretch. If this error is then fed back to the motor neuron, its discharge frequency is modified appropriately. This corresponds to one of the three feedback loops that are available locally. Another loop corrects for overstretching beyond the point that the muscle or tendon may tear. Since a muscle can only contract, it must be paired with another muscle (*antagonist*) in order to effect the return motion. Generally speaking, a flexor muscle is paired with an extensor muscle that cannot be activated simultaneously. This means that the motor neurons that affect each one of these are not activated at the same time. Instead, when one set of motor neurons is activated, the other is inhibited, and vice versa. When movement involves two or more muscles that normally cooperate by contracting simultaneously, the excitation of one causes facilitation of the other *synergistic* members via cross-connections. All these networks form feedback loops. An engineer's interpretation of how these loops work would be to assume dynamic conditions, as is the case in all parts of the nervous system. This has little value in dealing with stationary conditions, but it provides for an ability to adjust to changing conditions.

The nervous system, as mentioned earlier, is a control system of processes that adjust both internal and external operations. As humans, we have experiences that change our perceptions of events in our environment. The same is true for higher animals, which, besides having an internal environment the status of which is of major importance, also share an external environment of utmost richness and variety. Objects and conditions that have direct contact with the surface of an animal directly affect the future of the animal. Information about changes at some point provides a prediction of possible future status. The amount of information required to represent changing conditions increases as the required temporal resolution of detail increases. This creates a vast amount of data to be processed by any finite system. Considering the fact that the information reaching sensory receptors is too extensive and redundant, as well as modified by external interference (noise), the nervous system has a tremendously difficult task to accomplish. Enhanced responsiveness to a particular stimulus can be produced by structures that either increase the energy converging on a receptor or increase the effectiveness of coupling of a specific type of stimulus with its receptor. Different species have sensory systems that respond to stimuli that are important to them for survival. Often one nervous system responds to conditions that are not sensed by another nervous system. The transduction, processing, and transmission of signals in any nervous system produce a survival mechanism for an organism but only after these signals have been further modified by effector organs. Although the nerve impulses that drive a muscle, as explained earlier, are discrete events, a muscle twitch takes much longer to happen, a fact that allows for their responses to overlap and produce a much smoother output. Neural control of motor activity of skeletal muscle is accomplished entirely by the modification of muscle excitation, which involves changes in velocity, length, stiffness, and heat production. The importance of accurate timing of inputs and the maintenance of this timing across several synapses is obvious in sensory pathways of the nervous system. Cells are located next to other cells that have overlapping or adjacent receptive or motor fields. The dendrites provide important and complicated sites of interactions as well as channels of variable effectiveness for excitatory inputs, depending on their position relative to the cell body. Among the best examples are the cells of the medial superior olive in the auditory pathway. These cells have two major dendritic trees extending from opposite poles of the cell body. One receives synaptic inhibitory input from the ipsilateral cochlear nucleus, the other from the contralateral nucleus that normally is an excitatory input. These cells deal with the determination of the azimuth of a sound. When a sound is present on the contralateral side, most cells are excited, while ipsilateral sounds cause inhibition. It has been shown that the cells can go from complete excitation to full inhibition with a difference of only a few hundred milliseconds in arrival time of the two inputs.

The question then arises: How does the nervous system put together the signals available to it so that a determination of output can take place? To arrive at an understanding of how the nervous system intergrades incoming information at a given moment of time, we must understand that the processes that take place depend both on cellular forms and a topologic architecture and on the physiologic properties that relate input to output. That is, we have to know the *transfer* functions or *coupling* functions. Integration depends on the weighting of inputs. One of the important factors determining weighting is the area of synaptic contact. The extensive dendrites are the primary integrating structures. Electronic spread is the means of mixing, smoothing, attenuating, delaying, and summing postsynaptic potentials. The spatial distribution of input is often not random but systematically restricted. Also, the wide variety of characteristic geometries of synapses is no doubt important not only for the weighting of different combinations of inputs. When repeated stimuli are presented at various intervals at different junctions, increasing synaptic potentials are generated if the intervals between them are not too short or too long. This increase is due to a phenomenon called *facilitation*. If the response lasts longer than the interval between impulses, such that the second response rises from the residue of the first, then it is temporal summation. If, in addition, the response increment due to the second stimulus is larger than the preceding one, then it is facilitation. Facilitation is an important function of the nervous system and is found in quite different forms and durations ranging from a few milliseconds to tenths of seconds. Facilitation may grade from forms of sensitization to learning, especially at long intervals. A special case is the so-called *posttetanic potentiation* that is the result of high-frequency stimulation for long periods of time (about 10 seconds). This is an interesting case, since no effects can be seen during stimulation, but afterwards, any test stimulus at various intervals creates a marked increase in response up to many times more than the "tetanic" stimulus. *Antifacilitation* is the phenomenon where a decrease of response from the neuron is observed at certain junctions due to successive impulses. Its mechanism is less understood than facilitation. Both facilitation and antifacilitation may be observed on the same neuron but in different functions of it.

3.3 Representation of Information in the Nervous System

Whenever information is transferred between different parts of the nervous system, some communication paths have to be established, and some parameters of impulse firing relevant to communication must be set up. Since what is communicated is nothing more than impulses—spike trains—the only basic variables in a train of events are the number and intervals between spikes. With respect to this, the nervous system acts like a pulse-coded analog device, since the intervals are continuously graded. There exists a distribution of interval lengths between individual spikes, which in any sample can be expressed by the shape of the interval histogram. If one examines different examples, their distributions differ markedly. Some histograms look like Poisson distributions; some others exhibit gaussian or bimodal shapes. The coefficient of variation—expressed as the standard deviation over the mean—in some cases is constant, while in others it varies. Some other properties depend on the sequence of longer and shorter intervals than the mean. Some neurons show no linear dependence; some others show positive or negative correlations of successive intervals. If a stimulus is delivered and a discharge from the neuron is observed, a *poststimulus time histogram* can be used, employing the onset of the stimulus as a reference point and averaging many responses in order to reveal certain consistent features of temporal patterns. Coding of information can then be based on the average frequency, which can represent relevant gradations of the input. Mean frequency is the code in most cases, although no definition of it has been given with respect to measured quantities, such as averaging time, weighting functions, and forgetting functions. Characteristic transfer functions have been found, which suggests that there are several distinct coding principles in addition to the mean frequency. Each theoretically possible code becomes a candidate code as long as there exists some evidence that is readable by the system under investigation. Therefore, one has to first test for the availability of the code by imposing a stimulus that is considered "normal." After a response has been observed, the code is considered to be available. If the input is then changed to different levels of one parameter and changes are observed at the postsynaptic level, the code is called *readable*. However, only if both are formed in the same preparation and no other parameter is available and readable can the code be said to be the *actual* code employed. Some such parameters are

1. Time of firing
2. Temporal pattern
3. Number of spikes in the train
4. Variance of interspike intervals
5. Spike delays or latencies
6. Constellation code

The latter is a very important parameter, especially when used in conjunction with the concept of *receptive fields* of units in the different sensory pathways. The unit receptors do not need to have highly specialized abilities to permit encoding of a large number of distinct stimuli. Receptive fields are topographic and overlap extensively. Any given stimulus will excite a certain constellation of receptors and is therefore encoded in the particular set that is activated. A large degree of uncertainty prevails and requires the brain to operate probabilistically. In the nervous system there exists a large amount of *redundancy*, although neurons might have different thresholds. It is questionable, however, if these units are entirely equivalent, although they share parts of their receptive fields. The nonoverlapping parts might be of importance and critical to sensory function. On the other hand, redundancy does not necessarily mean unspecified or random connectivity. Rather, it allows for greater sensitivity and resolution, improvement of signal-to-noise ratio, while at the same time it provides stability of performance.

Integration of large numbers of converging inputs to give a single output can be considered as an averaging or probabilistic operation. The "decisions" made by a unit depend on its inputs, or some intrinsic states, and reaching a certain threshold. This way every unit in the nervous system can make a decision when it changes from one state to a different one. A theoretical possibility also exists that a mass of randomly connected neurons may constitute a trigger unit and that activity with a sharp threshold can spread through such a mass redundancy. Each part of the nervous system, and in particular the receiving side, can be thought of as a filter. Higher-order neurons do not merely pass their information on, but instead they use convergence from different channels, as well as divergence of the same channels and other processes, in order to modify incoming signals. Depending on the structure and coupling functions of the network, what gets through is determined. Similar networks exist at the output side. They also act as filters, but since they formulate decisions and commands with precise *spatiotemporal* properties, they can be thought of as *pattern generators*.

3.4 Lateral Inhibition

This discussion would be incomplete without a description of a very important phenomenon in the nervous system. This phenomenon, called *lateral inhibition*, is used by the nervous system to improve spatial resolution and contrast. The effectiveness of this type of inhibition decreases with distance. In the retina, for example, lateral inhibition is used extensively in order to improve contrast. As the stimulus approaches a certain unit, it first excites neighbors of the recorded cell. Since these neighbors inhibit that unit, it responds by a decrease in firing frequency. If the stimulus is exactly over the recorded unit, this unit is excited and fires above its normal rate, and as the stimulus moves out again, the neighbors are excited, while the unit under consideration fires less. If we now examine the output of all the units as a whole and at once while half the considered array is stimulated and the other half is not, we will notice that at the point of discontinuity of the stimulus going from stimulation to nonstimulation, the firing frequencies of the two halves have been differentiated to the extreme at the stimulus edge, which has been enhanced. The neuronal circuits responsible for lateral shifts are relatively simple. Lateral inhibition can be considered to give the negative of the second spatial derivative of the input stimulus. A second layer of neurons could be constructed to perform this spacial differentiation on the input signal to detect the edge only. It is probably lateral inhibition that explains the psychophysical illusion known as *Mach bands*. It is probably the same principle that operates widely in the nervous system to enhance the sensitivity to contrast in the visual system in particular and in all other modalities in general. Through the years, different models have been developed to describe lateral inhibition mathematically, and various methods of analysis have been employed. Such methods include

  Functional notations
  Graphic solutions
  Tabular solution
  Taylor's series expansions
  Artificial neural network modeling

These models include both one-dimensional examination of the phenomenon and two-dimensional treatment, where a two-dimensional array is used as a stimulus. This two-dimensional treatment is justified because most of the sensory receptors of the body form two-dimensional maps (receptive fields). In principle, if a one-dimensional lateral inhibition system is linear, one can extend the analysis to two dimensions by means of superposition. The two-dimensional array can be thought of as a function $f(x, y)$, and the lateral inhibition network itself is embodied in a separate $N \times N$ array, the central square of which has a positive value and can be thought of as a direct input from an incoming axon. The surrounding squares have negative values that are higher than the corner values, which are also negative. The method consists of multiplying the input signal values $f(x, y)$ and their contiguous values by the lateral inhibitory network's weighting factors to get a corresponding $g(x, y)$. Figure 3.1 presents an example of such a process. The technique illustrated here is used in the contrast enhancement of photographs. The objective is the same as that of the nervous system: to improve image sharpness without introducing too much distortion. This technique requires storage of each picture element and lateral "inhibitory" interactions between adjacent ele-

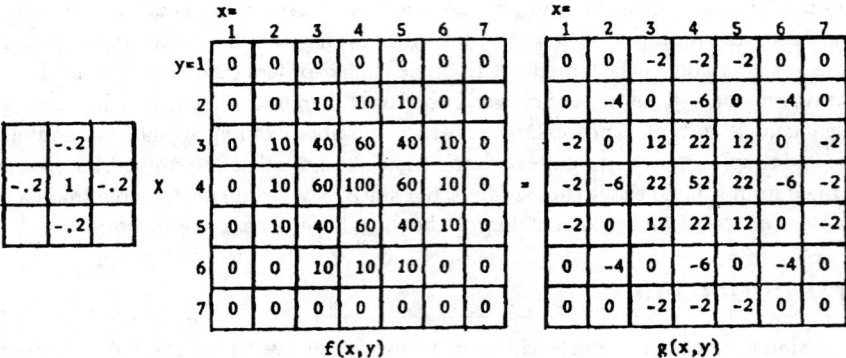

FIGURE 3.1   An example of two-dimensional lateral inhibition. On the left, the 3 × 3 array corresponds to the values of the synaptic junctions weighting coefficients. For simplicity, the corner weights are assumed to be zero. $g(x, y)$ represents the output matrix after lateral inhibition has been applied to the input matrix.

ments. Since a picture may contain millions of elements, high-speed computers with large-scale memories are required.

At a higher level, similar algorithms can be used to evaluate decision-making mechanisms. In this case, many inputs from different sensory systems are competing for attention. The brain evaluates each one of the inputs as a function of the remaining ones. One can picture a decision-making mechanism resembling a "locator" of stimulus peaks. The final output depends on what weights are used at the inputs of a push-pull mechanism. Thus a decision can be made depending on the weights an individual's brain is applying to the incoming information about a situation under consideration. The most important information is heavily weighted, while the rest is either totally masked or weighted very lightly.

3.5 Higher Functions of the Nervous System

Pattern Recognition

One way of understanding human perception is to study the mechanisms of information processing in the brain. The recognition of patterns of sensory input is one of the functions of the brain, a task accomplished by neuronal circuits, the *feature extractors*. Although such neuronal information is more likely to be processed globally by a large number of neurons, in animals, single-unit recording is one of the most powerful tools in the hands of a physiologist. Most often, the concept of the *receptive field* is used as a method of understanding sensory information processing. In the case of the visual system, one could call the receptive field a well-defined region of the visual field which, when stimulated, will change the firing rate of a neuron in the visual pathway. The response of that neuron will usually depend on the distribution of light in the receptive field. Therefore, the information collected by the brain from the outside world is transformed into spatial as well as temporal patterns of neuronal activity.

The question often asked is how do we perceive and recognize faces, objects, and scenes. Even in those cases where only noisy representations exist, we are still able to make some inference as to what the pattern represents. Unfortunately, in humans, single-unit recording, as mentioned above, is impossible. As a result, one has to use other kinds of measurements, such as *evoked potentials (EPs)*. Although physiologic in nature, EPs are still far away from giving us information at the neuronal level. Yet EPs have been used extensively as a way of probing the human (and animal) brains because of their noninvasive character. EPs can be considered to be the result of integrations of the neuronal activity of many neurons some place in the brain. This gross potential can then be used as a measure of the response of the brain to sensory input.

The question then becomes: Can we somehow use this response to influence the brain in producing patterns of activity that we want? None of the efforts of the past closed this loop. How do we explain then the phenomenon of selective attention by which we selectively direct our attention to something of interest and discard the rest? And what happens with the evolution of certain species that change appearance according to their everyday needs? All these questions tend to lead to the fact that somewhere in the brain there is a loop where previous knowledge or experience is used as a feedback to the brain itself. This feedback then modifies the ability of the brain to respond is a different way to the same stimulus the next time it is presented. In a way, then, the brain creates mental "images" independent of the stimulus which tend to modify the representation of the stimulus in the brain.

This section describes some efforts in which different methods have been used in trying to address the difficult task of feedback loops in the brain. However, no attempt will be made to explain or even postulate where these feedback loops might be located. If one considers the brain as a huge set of neural nets, then one question has been debated for many years: What is the role of the individual neuron in the net, and what is the role of each network in the holistic process of the brain? More specifically, does the neuron act as an analyzer or a detector of specific features, or does it merely reflect the characteristic response of a population of cells of which it happens to be a member? What invariant relationships exist between sensory input and the response of a single neuron, and how much can be "read" about the stimulus parameters from the record of a single EP? In turn, then, how much feedback can one use from a single EP in order to influence the stimulus, and how successful can that influence be? Many physiologists express doubts that simultaneous observations of large numbers of individual neuronal activities can be readily interpreted. The main question we are asking is: Can a feedback process influence and modulate the stimuli patterns so that they appear optimal? If this is proven to be true, it would mean that we can reverse the pattern-recognition process, and instead of recognizing a pattern, we would be able to create a pattern from a vast variety of possible patterns. It would be like creating a link between our brain and a computer; equivalent to a brain-computer system network. Figure 3.2 is a schematic representation of such a process

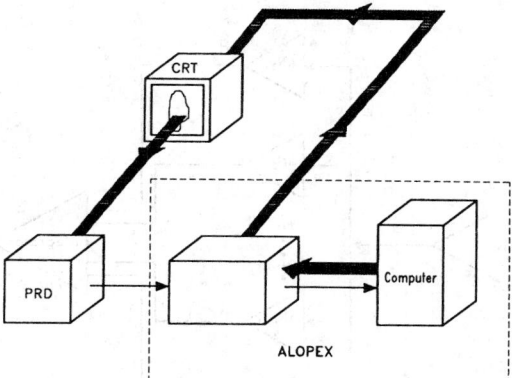

FIGURE 3.2 An ALOPEX system. The stimulus is presented on the CRT. The observer or any pattern-recognition device (PRD) faces the CRT; the subject's response is sent to the ALOPEX interface unit, where it is recorded and integrated, and the final response is sent to the computer. The computer calculates the values of the new pattern to be presented on the CRT according to the ALOPEX algorithm, and the process continues until the desired pattern appears on the CRT. At this point, the response is considered to be optimal and the process stops.

involved in what we call the *feedback loop* of the system. The pattern-recognition device (PRD) is connected to an ALOPEX system (a computer algorithm and an image processor in this case) and faces a display monitor where different-intensity patterns can be shown. Thin arrows representing response information and heavy arrows representing detailed pattern information are generated by the computer and relayed by the ALOPEX system to the monitor. ALOPEX is a set of algorithms described in detail elsewhere in this handbook. If this kind of arrangement is used for the determination of visual receptive fields of neurons, then the PRD is nothing more than the brain of an experimental animal. This way the neuron under investigation does its own selection of the best stimulus or trigger feature and reverses the role of the neuron from being a feature extractor to becoming a feature generator, as mentioned earlier. The idea is to find the response of the neuron to a stimulus and use this response as a positive feedback in the directed evaluation of the initially random pattern. Thus the cell involved filters out the key trigger features from the stimulus and reinforces them with the feedback.

As a generalization of this process, one might consider that a neuron N receives a visual input from a pattern P which is transmitted in a modified form P' to an analyzer neuron AN (or even a complex of neurons), as shown in Fig. 3.3. The analyzer responds with a scalar variable R that is then fed back to the system, and the pattern is modified accordingly. The process continues in small steps until there is an almost perfect correlation between the original pattern (template) and the one that neuron N indirectly created. This integrator sends the response back to the original modifier. The integrator need not be a linear summator. It could take any nonlinear form, a fact that is a more realistic representation of the visual cortex. One can envision the input patterns as templates preexisting in the memory of the system, a situation that might come about with visual experience. For a "naive" system, any initial pattern will do. As experience is gained, the patterns become less random. If one starts with a pattern that has some resemblance to one of the preexisting patterns, evolution will take its course. In nature, there might exist a mechanism similar to that of ALOPEX. By filtering the characteristics most important for the survival of the species, changes would be triggered. Perception, therefore, could be considered to be an interaction between sensory inputs and

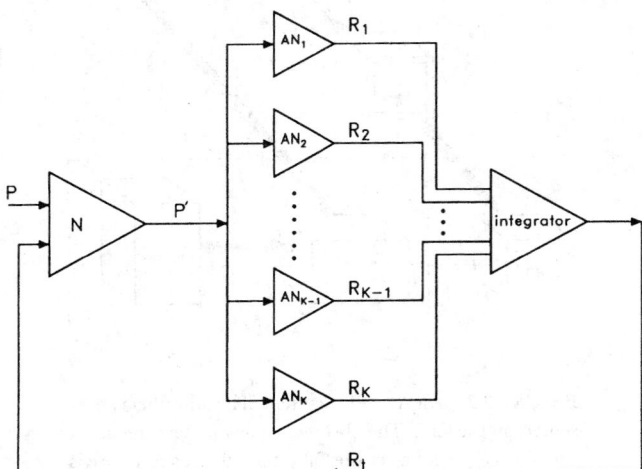

FIGURE 3.3 Diagrammatic representation of the ALOPEX "inverse" pattern-recognition scheme. Each neuron represents a feature analyzer that responds to the stimulus with a scalar quantity R called the *response*. R is then fed back to the system, and the pattern is modified accordingly. This process continues until there is a close correlation between the desired output and the original pattern.

past experience in the form of templates stored in the memory of the perceiver and specific to the perceiver's needs. These templates are modifiable with time and adjusted accordingly to the input stimuli. With this approach, the neural nets and ensembles of nets under observation generate patterns that describe their thinking and memory properties. The normal flow of information is reversed and controls the afferent systems.

The perception processes as well as feature extraction or suppression of images or objects can be ascribed to specific neural mechanisms due to some sensory input or even due to some "wishful thinking" of the PRD. If it is true that the association cortex is affecting the sensitivity of the sensory cortex, then an ALOPEX mechanism is what one needs to close the loop for memory and learning.

Memory and Learning

If we try to define what memory is, we will face the fact that memory is not a single mental faculty but is rather composed of multiple abilities mediated by separate and distinct brain systems. Memory for a recent event can be expressed *explicitly* as a conscious recollection or *implicitly* as a facilitation of test performance without conscious recollection. The major distinction between these two memories is that explicit or *declarative* memory depends on limbic and diencephalic structures and provides the basis for recollection of events, while implicit or *nondeclarative* memory supports skills and habit learning, single conditioning, and the well-researched phenomenon of *priming*.

Declarative memory refers to memory of recent events and is usually assessed by tests of recall or recognition for specific single items. When the list of items becomes longer, a subject not only learns about each item on the list but also makes associations about what all these items have in common; i.e., the subject learns about the category that the items belong to. Learning lead to changes that increase or decrease the effectiveness of impulses arriving at the junctions between neurons, and the cumulative effect of these changes constitutes memory. Very often a particular pattern of neural activity leads to a result that occurs some time after that activity has ended. Learning then requires some means of relating the activity that is to be changed to the evaluation that can be made only by the delayed consequence. This phenomenon in physics is called *hysteresis* and refers to any modifications of future actions due to past actions. *Learning* then could be defined as change in any neuronal response resulting from previous experiences due to an external stimulus. Memory, in turn, would be the maintenance of these changes over time. The collection of neural changes representing memory is commonly known as the *engram*, and a major part of recent work has been to identify and locate engrams in the brain, since specific parts of the nervous system are capable of specific types of learning. The view of memory that has recently emerged is that information storage is tied to specific processing areas that are engaged during learning. The brain is organized so that separate regions of neocortex simultaneously carry out computations on specific features or characteristics of the external stimulus, no matter how complex that stimulus might be. If the brain learns specific properties or features of the stimulus, then we talk about the *nonassociative memory*. Associated with this type of learning is the phenomenon of *habituation*, in which if the same stimulus is presented repeatedly, the neurons respond less and less, while the introduction of a new stimulus increases the sensitization of the neuron. If the learning includes two related stimuli, then we talk about associative learning. This type of learning can be of two types: *classic conditioning* and *operant conditioning*. The first deals with relationships among stimuli, while the latter deals with the relationship of the stimulus to the animal's own behavior. In humans, there exist two types of memory: *short-term* and *long-term memories*. The best way to study any physiologic process in humans, and especially memory, is to study its pathology. The study of amnesia has provided strong evidence distinguishing between these types of memory. Amnesic patients can keep a short list of numbers in mind for several minutes if they pay attention to the task. The difficulty comes when the list becomes longer, especially if the amount to be learned exceeds the brain capacity of what can be held in immediate memory. It could be that this happens because more systems have to be involved and that temporary information storage may occur within each brain area where stable changes in synaptic efficacy can eventually develop.

Plasticity within existing pathways can account for most of the observations, and short-term memory occurs too quickly for it to require any major modifications of neuronal pathways. The capacity of long-term memory requires the integrity of the medial temporal and diencephalic regions in conjunction with neurons for storage of information. Within the domain of long-term memory, amnesic patients demonstrate intact learning and retention of certain motor, perceptual, and cognitive skills and intact priming effects. These patients do not exhibit any learning deficits but have no conscious awareness of prior study sessions or recognition of previously presented stimuli.

Priming effects can be tested by presenting words and then providing either the first few letters of the word or the last part of the word for recognition by the patient. Normal subjects, as expected, perform better than amnesic subjects. However, if these patients are instructed to "read" the incomplete word instead of memorizing it, then they perform as well as the normal individuals. Also, these amnesic patients perform well if words are cued by category names. Thus priming effects seem to be independent of the processes of recall and recognition memory, which is also observed in normal subjects. All this evidence supports the notion that the brain has organized its memory functions around fundamentally different information storage systems. In perceiving a word, a preexisting array of neurons is activated that have concurrent activities that produce perception, and priming is one of these functions.

Memory is not fixed immediately after learning but continues to grow toward stabilization over a period of time. This stabilization is called *consolidation of memory*. Memory consolidation is a *dynamic* feature of long-term memory, especially the declarative memory, but it is neither an automatic process with fixed lifetime nor is it determined at the time of learning. It is rather a process of reorganization of stored information. As time passes, some not yet consolidated memories fade out by remodeling the neural circuitry that is responsible for the original representation or by establishing new representations, since the original one can be forgotten.

The problems of learning and memory are studied continuously and with increased interest these days, especially because artificial systems such as neural networks can be used to mimic functions of the nervous system.

References

Cowan WM, Cuenod M (eds). 1975. Use of Axonal Transport for Studies of Neuronal Connectivity. New York, Elsevier.

Deutsch S, Micheli-Tzanakou E. 1987. Neuroelectric Systems. New York, NYU Press.

Ganong WF. 1989. Review of Medical Physiology, 14th ed. Norwalk, CT, Appleton and Lange.

Hartzell HC. 1981. Mechanisms of slow postsynaptic potentials. Nature 291:593.

McMahon TA. 1984. Muscles, Reflexes and Locomotion. Princeton, NJ, Princeton University Press.

Partridge LD, Partridge DL. 1993. The Nervous System: Its Function and Interaction with the World. Cambridge, MA, MIT Press.

Shepherd GM. 1978. Microcircuits in the nervous system. Sci Am 238(2):92–103.

4

Vision System

George Stetten
Duke University

David Marr, an early pioneer in computer vision, defined *vision* as extracting ". . . from images of the external world a description that is useful for the viewer and not cluttered with irrelevant information" [Marr, 1982]. Advances in computers and video technology in the past decades have created the expectation that artificial vision should be realizable. The nontriviality of the task is evidenced by the continuing proliferation of new and different approaches to computer vision without any observable application in our everyday lives. Actually, computer vision is already offering practical solutions in industrial assembly and inspection, as well as for military and medical applications, so it seems we are beginning to master some of the fundamentals. However, we have a long way to go to match the vision capabilities of a 4-year-old child. In this chapter we will explore what is known about how nature has succeeded at this formidable task—that of interpreting the visual world.

4.1 Fundamentals of Vision Research

Research into biologic visual systems has followed several distinct approaches. The oldest is psychophysics, in which human and animal subjects are presented with visual stimuli and their responses recorded. Important early insights also were garnered by correlating clinical observations of visual defects with known neuroanatomic injury. In the past 50 years, a more detailed approach to understanding the mechanisms of vision has been undertaken by inserting small electrodes deep within the living brain to monitor the electrical activity of individual neurons and by using dyes and biochemical markers to track the anatomic course of nerve tracts. This research has led to a detailed and coherent, if not complete, theory of a visual system capable of explaining the discrimination of form, color, motion, and depth. This theory has been confirmed by noninvasive radiologic techniques that have been used recently to study the physiologic responses of the visual system, including positron emission tomography [Zeki et al., 1991] and functional magnetic resonance imaging [Belliveau et al., 1992; Cohen and Bookheimer, 1994], although these noninvasive techniques provide far less spatial resolution and thus can only show general regions of activity in the brain.

4.2 A Modular View of the Vision System

The Eyes

Movement of the eyes is essential to vision, not only allowing rapid location and tracking of objects but also preventing stationary images on the retina, which are essentially invisible. Continual movement of the image on the retina is essential to the visual system.

The eyeball is spherical and therefore free to turn in both the horizontal and vertical directions. Each eye is rotated by three pairs of mutually opposing muscles, innervated by the oculomotor nuclei in the brainstem. The eyes are coordinated as a pair in two useful ways: turning together to find and follow objects and turning inward to allow adjustment for parallax as objects become closer. The latter is called *convergence.*

The optical portion of the eye, which puts an image on the retina, is closely analogous to a photographic or television camera. Light enters the eye, passing through a series of transparent layers— the cornea, the aqueous humor, the lens, and the vitreous body—to eventually project on the retina.

The *cornea,* the protective outer layer of the eye, is heavily innervated with sensory neurons, triggering the blink reflex and tear duck secretion in response to irritation. The cornea is also an essential optical element, supplying two-thirds of the total refraction in the eye. Behind the cornea is a clear fluid, the *aqueous humor,* in which the central aperture of the iris, the pupil, is free to constrict or dilate. The two actions are accomplished by opposing sets of muscles.

The *lens,* a flexible transparent object behind the iris, provides the remainder of refraction necessary to focus an image on the retina. The ciliary muscles surrounding the lens can increase the lens' curvature, thereby decreasing its focal length and bringing nearer objects into focus. This is called *accommodation.* When the ciliary muscles are at rest, distant objects are in focus. There are no contradictory muscles to flatten the lens. This depends simply on the elasticity of the lens, which decreases with age. Behind the lens is the *vitreous humor,* consisting of a semigelatinous material filling the volume between the lens and the retina.

The Retina

The retina coats the back of the eye and is therefore spherical, not flat, making optical magnification constant at 3.5 degrees of scan angle per millimeter. The retina is the neuronal front end of the visual system, the image sensor. In addition, it accomplishes the first steps in edge detection and color analysis before sending the processed information along the optic nerve to the brain. The retina contains five major classes of cells, roughly organized into layers. The dendrites of these cells each occupy no more than 1 to 2 mm^2 in the retina, limiting the extent of spatial integration from one layer of the retina to the next.

First come the *receptors,* which number approximately 125 million in each eye and contain the light-sensitive pigments responsible for converting photons into chemical energy. Receptor cells are of two general varieties: *rods* and *cones.* The cones are responsible for the perception of color, and they function only in bright light. When the light is dim, only rods are sensitive enough to respond. Exposure to a single photon may result in a measurable increase in the membrane potential of a rod. This sensitivity is the result of a chemical cascade, similar in operation to the photo multiplier tube, in which a single photon generates a cascade of electrons. All rods use the same pigment, whereas three different pigments are found in three separate kinds of cones.

Examination of the retina with an otoscope reveals its gross topography. The yellow circular area occupying the central 5 degrees of the retina is called the *macula lutea,* within which a small circular pit called the *fovea* may be seen. Detailed vision occurs only in the fovea, where a dense concentration of cones provides visual acuity to the central 1 degree of the visual field.

On the inner layer of the retina one finds a layer of *ganglion cells,* whose axons make up the optic nerve, the output of the retina. They number approximately 1 million, or less than 1% of the number of receptor cells. Clearly, some data compression has occurred in the space between the receptors and the ganglion cells. Traversing this space are the *bipolar cells,* which run from the receptors through the retina to the ganglion cells. Bipolar cells exhibit the first level of information processing in the visual system; namely, their response to light on the retina demonstrates "center/surround" receptive fields. By this I mean that a small dot on the retina elicits a response, while the area surrounding the spot elicits the opposite response. If both the center and the surround are illuminated, the net result is no response. Thus bipolar cells respond only at the border between dark and light areas. Bipolar cells come in two varieties, on-center and off-center, with the center respectively brighter or darker than the surround.

The center response of bipolar cells results from direct contact with the receptors. The surround response is supplied by the *horizontal cells,* which run parallel to the surface of the retina between the receptor layer and the bipolar layer, allowing the surrounding area to oppose the influence of the center. The *amacrine cells,* a final cell type, also run parallel to the surface but in a different layer, between the bipolar cells and the ganglion cells, and are possibly involved in the detection of motion.

Ganglion cells, since they are triggered by bipolar cells, also have center/surround receptive fields and come in two types, on-center and off-center. On-center ganglion cells have a receptive field in which illumination of the center increases the firing rate and a surround where it decreases the rate. Off-center ganglion cells display the opposite behavior. Both types of ganglion cells produce little or no change in firing rate when the entire receptive field is illuminated, because the center and surround cancel each other. As in many other areas of the nervous system, the fibers of the optic nerve use frequency encoding to represent a scalar quantity.

Multiple ganglion cells may receive output from the same receptor, since many receptive fields overlap. However, this does not limit overall spatial resolution, which is maximum in the fovea, where two points separated by 0.5 minutes of arc may be discriminated. This separation corresponds to a distance on the retina of 2.5 μm, which is approximately the center-to-center spacing between cones. Spatial resolution falls off as one moves away from the fovea into the peripheral vision, where resolution is as low as 1 degree of arc.

Several aspects of this natural design deserve consideration. Why do we have center/surround receptive fields? The ganglion cells, whose axons make up the optic nerve, do not fire unless there is meaningful information, i.e., a border, falling within the receptive field. It is the edge of a shape we see rather than its interior. This represents a form of data compression. Center/surround receptive fields also allow for relative rather than absolute measurements of color and brightness. This is essential for analyzing the image independent of lighting conditions. Why do we have both on-center and off-center cells? Evidently, both light and dark are considered information. The same shape is detected whether it is lighter or darker than the background.

Optic Chiasm

The two optic nerves, from the left and right eyes, join at the optic chiasm, forming a *hemidecussation,* meaning that half the axons cross while the rest proceed uncrossed. The resulting two bundles of axons leaving the chiasm are called the *optic tracts.* The left optic tract contains only axons from the left half of each retina. Since the images are reversed by the lens, this represents light from the right side of the visual field. The division between the right and left optic tracts splits the retina down the middle, bisecting the fovea. The segregation of sensory information into the contralateral hemispheres corresponds to the general organization of sensory and motor centers in the brain.

Each optic tract has two major destinations on its side of the brain: (1) the superior colliculus and (2) the lateral geniculate nucleus (LGN). Although topographic mapping from the retina is scrambled within the optic tract, it is reestablished in both major destinations so that right, left, up, and down in the image correspond to specific directions within those anatomic structures.

Superior Colliculus

The *superior colliculus* is a small pair of bumps on the dorsal surface of the midbrain. Another pair, the *inferior colliculus,* is found just below it. Stimulation of the superior colliculus results in contralateral eye movement. Anatomically, output tracts from the superior colliculus run to areas that control eye and neck movement. Both the inferior and superior colliculi are apparently involved in locating sound. In the bat, the inferior colliculus is enormous, crucial to that animal's remarkable echolocation abilities. The superior colliculus processes information from the inferior colliculus, as well as from the retina, allowing the eyes to quickly find and follow targets based on visual and auditory cues.

Different types of eye movements have been classified. The *saccade* (French, for "jolt") is a quick motion of the eyes over a significant distance. The saccade is how the eyes explore an image, jumping from landmark to landmark, rarely stopping in featureless areas. *Nystagmus* is the smooth pursuit of a moving image, usually with periodic backward saccades to lock onto subsequent points as the image moves by. *Microsaccades* are small movements, several times per second, over 1 to 2 minutes of arc in a seemingly random direction. Microsaccades are necessary for sight; their stabilization leads to effective blindness.

LGN

The thalamus is often called "the gateway to the cortex" because it processes much of the sensory information reaching the brain. Within the thalamus, we find the *lateral geniculate nucleus* (LGN), a peanut-sized structure that contains a single synaptic stage in the major pathway of visual information to higher centers. The LGN also receives information back from the cortex, so-called reentrant connections, as well as from the nuclei in the brainstem that control attention and arousal.

The cells in the LGN are organized into three pairs of layers. Each pair contains two layers, one from each eye. The upper two pairs consist of parvocellular cells (*P cells*) that respond with preference to different colors. The remaining lower pair consists of magnocellular cells (*M cells*) with no color preference (Fig. 4.1). The topographic mapping is identical for all six layers; i.e., passing through the layers at a given point yields synapses responding to a single area of the retina. Axons from the LGN proceed to the primary visual cortex in broad bands, the *optic radiations*, preserving this topographic mapping and displaying the same center/surround response as the ganglion cells.

Area V1

The LGN contains approximately 1.5 million cells. By comparison, the *primary visual cortex*, or *striate cortex*, which receives the visual information from the LGN, contains 200 million cells. It consists of a thin (2-mm) layer of gray matter (neuronal cell bodies) over a thicker collection of white matter (myelinated axons) and occupies a few square inches of the occipital lobes. The primary visual cortex has been called *area 17* from the days when the cortical areas were first differentiated by their cytoarchitectonics (the microscopic architecture of their layered neurons). In modern terminology, the primary visual cortex is often called *visual area 1,* or simply *V1*.

Destroying any small piece of V1 eliminates a small area in the visual field, resulting in *scotoma*, a local blind spot. Clinical evidence has long been available that a scotoma may result from injury, stroke, or tumor in a local part of V1. Between neighboring cells in V1's gray matter, horizontal connections are at most 2 to 5 mm in length. Thus, at any given time, the image from the retina is analyzed piecemeal in V1. Topographic mapping from the retina is preserved in great detail. Such mapping is seen elsewhere in the brain, such as in the somatosensory cortex [Mountcastle, 1957]. Like all cortical surfaces, V1 is a highly convoluted sheet, with much of its area hidden within its

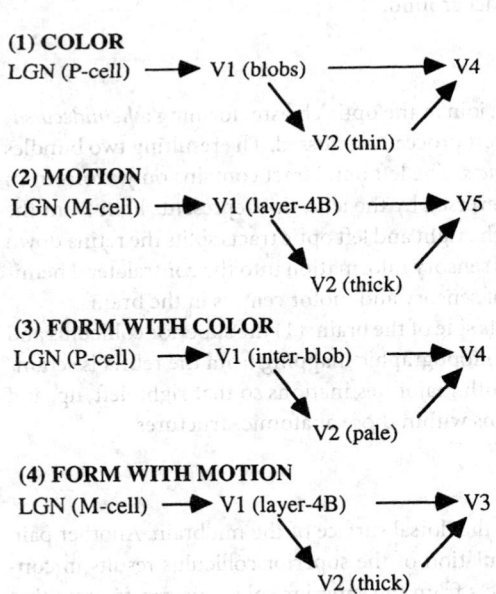

FIGURE 4.1 Visual pathways to cortical areas showing the separation of information by type. The lateral geniculate nucleus (LGN) and areas V1 and V2 act as gateways to more specialized higher areas.

folds. If unfolded, V1 would be roughly pear-shaped, with the top of the pear processing information from the fovea and the bottom of the pear processing the peripheral vision. Circling the pear at a given latitude would correspond roughly to circling the fovea at a fixed radius.

The primary visual cortex contains six layers, numbered 1 through 6. Distinct functional and anatomic types of cells are found in each layer. Layer 4 contains neurons that receive information from the LGN. Beyond the initial synapses, cells demonstrate progressively more complex responses. The outputs of V1 project to an area known as *visual area 2 (V2)*, which surrounds V1, and to higher visual areas in the occipital, temporal, and parietal lobes as well as to the superior colliculus. V1 also sends reentrant projections back to the LGN. Reentrant projections are present at almost every level of the visual system [Felleman and Essen, 1991; Edelman, 1978].

Cells in V1 have been studied extensively in animals by inserting small electrodes into the living brain (with surprisingly little damage) and monitoring the individual responses of neurons to visual stimuli. Various subpopulations of cortical cells have thus been identified. Some, termed *simple cells,* respond to illuminated edges or bars at specific locations and at specific angular orientations in the visual field. The angular orientation must be correct within 10 to 20 degrees for the particular cell to respond. All orientations are equally represented. Moving the electrode parallel to the surface yields a smooth rotation in the orientation of cell responses by about 10 degrees for each 50 μm that the electrode is advanced. This rotation is subject to reversals in direction, as well as "fractures," or sudden jumps in orientation.

Other cells, more common than simple cells, are termed *complex cells.* Complex cells respond to a set of closely spaced parallel edges within a particular receptive field. They may respond specifically to movement perpendicular to the orientation of the edge. Some prefer one direction of movement to the other. Some complex and simple cells are *end-stopped,* meaning they fire only if the illuminated bar or edge does not extend too far. Presumably, these cells detect corners, curves, or discontinuities in borders and lines. End-stopping takes place in layers 2 and 3 of the primary visual cortex. From the LGN through the simple cells and complex cells, there appears to be a sequential processing of the image. It is probable that simple cells combine the responses of adjacent LGN cells and that complex cells combine the responses of adjacent simple cells.

A remarkable feature in the organization of V1 is binocular convergence, in which a single neuron responds to identical receptive fields in both eyes, including location, orientation, and directional sensitivity to motion. It does not occur in the LGN, where axons from the left and right eyes are still segregated into different layers. Surprisingly, binocular connections to neurons are present in V1 at birth. Some binocular neurons are equally weighted in terms of responsiveness to both eyes, while others are more sensitive to one eye than to the other. One finds columns containing the latter type of cells in which one eye dominates, called *ocular dominance columns,* in uniform bands approximately 0.5 mm wide everywhere in V1. Ocular dominance columns occur in adjacent pairs, one for each eye, and are prominent in animals with forward-facing eyes, such as cats, chimpanzees, and humans. They are nearly absent in rodents and other animals whose eyes face outward.

The topography of orientation-specific cells and of ocular dominance columns is remarkably uniform throughout V1, which is surprising because the receptive fields near the fovea are 10 to 30 times smaller than those at the periphery. This phenomenon is called magnification. The fovea maps to a greater relative distance on the surface of V1 than does the peripheral retina, by as much as 36-fold [Daniel and Whitteridge, 1961]. In fact, the majority of V1 processes only the central 10 degrees of the visual field. Both simple and complex cells in the foveal portion can resolve bars as narrow as 2 minutes of arc. Toward the periphery, the resolution falls off to 1 degree of arc.

As an electrode is passed down through the cortex *perpendicular* to the surface, each layer demonstrates receptive fields of characteristic size, the smallest being a layer 4, the input layer. Receptive fields are larger in other layers due to lateral integration of information. Passing the electrode *parallel* to the surface of the cortex reveals another important uniformity to V1. For example, in layer 3, which sends output fibers to higher cortical centers, one must move the electrode approximately 2 mm to pass from one collection of receptive fields to another that does not overlap. An area approximately 2 mm across thus represents the smallest unit piece of V1, i.e., that which can completely process the visual information. Indeed, it is just the right size to contain a complete set of orientations and more than enough to contain information from both eyes. It receives a few tens of thousands of fibers from the LGN, produces perhaps 50,000 output fibers, and is fairly constant in cytoarchitectonics whether at the center of vision, where it processes approximately 30 minutes of arc, or at the far periphery, where it processes 7 to 8 degrees of arc.

The topographic mapping of the visual field onto the cortex suffers an abrupt discontinuity between the left and right hemispheres, and yet our perception of the visual scene suffers no obvious rift in the midline. This is due to the *corpus collousum,* an enormous tract containing at least 200 million axons, that connects the two hemispheres. The posterior portion of the corpus collousum connects the two halves of V1, linking cells that have similar orientations and whose receptive fields overlap in the vertical midline. Thus a perceptually seamless merging of left and right visual fields is achieved. Higher levels of the visual system are likewise connected across the corpus collousum. This is demonstrated, for example, by the clinical observation that cutting the corpus collousum prevents a subject from verbally describing objects in the left field of view (the right hemisphere). Speech, which normally involves the left hemisphere, cannot process visual objects from the right hemisphere without the corpus collousum.

By merging the information from both eyes, V1 is capable of analyzing the distance to an object. Many cues for depth are available to the visual system, including occlusion, parallax (detected by the convergence of the eyes), optical focusing of the lens, rotation of objects, expected size of objects, shape based on perspective, and shadow casting. Stereopsis, which uses the slight difference between images due to the parallax between the two eyes, was first enunciated in 1838 by Sir Charles Wheatstone and is probably the most important cue [Wheatstone, 1838]. Fixating on an object causes it to fall on the two foveas. Other objects that are nearer become outwardly displaced on the two retinas, while objects that are farther away become inwardly displaced. About 2 degrees of horizontal disparity is tolerated, with fusion by the visual system into a single object. Greater horizontal disparity results in double vision. Almost no vertical displacement (a few minutes of arc) is tolerated. Physiologic experiments have revealed a particular class of complex cells in V1 which are *disparity tuned.* They fall into three general classes. One class fires only when the object is at the fixation distance, another only when the object is nearer, and a third only when it is farther away [Poggio and Talbot, 1981]. Severing the corpus collousum leads to a loss of stereopsis in the vertical midline of the visual field.

When the inputs to the two retinas cannot be combined, one or the other image is rejected. This phenomenon is known as *retinal rivalry* and can occur in a piecewise manner or can even lead to blindness in one eye. The general term *amblyopia* refers to the partial or complete loss of eyesight not caused by abnormalities in the eye. The most common form of amblyopia is caused by *strabismus,* in which the eyes are not aimed in a parallel direction but rather are turned inward (cross-eyed) or outward (wall-eyed). This condition leads to habitual suppression of vision from one of the eyes and sometimes to blindness in that eye or to *alternation,* in which the subject maintains vision in both eyes by using only one eye at a time. Cutting selected ocular muscles in kittens causes strabismus, and the kittens respond by alternation, preserving functional vision in both eyes. However, the number of cells in the cortex displaying binocular responses is greatly reduced. In humans with long-standing alternating strabismus, surgical repair making the eyes parallel again does not bring back a sense of depth. Permanent damage has been caused by the subtle condition of the images on the two retinas not coinciding. This may be explained by the Hebb model for associative learning, in which temporal association between inputs strengthens synaptic connections [Hebb, 1961].

Further evidence that successful development of the visual system depends on proper input comes from clinical experience with children who have *cataracts* at birth. Cataracts constitute a clouding of the lens, permitting light, but not images, to reach the retina. If surgery to remove the cataracts is delayed until the child is several years old, the child remains blind even though images are restored to the retina. Kittens and monkeys whose eyelids are sown shut during a critical period of early development stay blind even when the eyes are opened. Physiologic studies in these animals show very few cells responding in the visual cortex. Other experiments depriving more specific elements of an image, such as certain orientations or motion in a certain direction, yield a cortex without the corresponding cell type.

Color

Cones, which dominate the fovea, can detect wavelengths between 400 and 700 nm. The population of cones in the retina can be divided into three categories, each containing a different pigment. This was established by direct microscopic illumination of the retina [Wald, 1974; Marks et al., 1964]. The pigments have a bandwidth on the order of 100 nm, with significant overlap, and with peak sensitivities at 560 nm (yellow-green), 530 nm (blue-green), and 430 nm (violet). These three classes are commonly known as red, green, and blue. Compared with the auditory system, whose array of cochlear sensors can discriminate thousands of different sonic frequencies, the visual system is relatively impoverished with only three frequency parameters. Instead, the retina expends most of its resolution on spatial information. Color vision is absent in many species, including cats, dogs, and some primates, as well as in most nocturnal animals, since cones are useless in low light.

By having three types of cones at a given locality on the retina, a simplified spectrum can be sensed and represented by three independent variables, a concept known as *trichromacy*. This model was developed by Thomas Young and Hermann von Helmholtz in the 19th century before neurobiology existed and does quite well at explaining the retina [Young, 1802; Helmholtz, 1889]. The model is also the underlying basis for red-green-blue (RGB) video monitors and color television [Ennes, 1981]. Rods do not help in discriminating color, even though the pigment in rods does add a fourth independent sensitivity peak.

Psychophysical experimentation yields a complex, redundant map between spectrum and perceived color, or *hue,* including not only the standard red, orange, yellow, green, and blue but hues such as pink, purple, brown, and olive green that are not themselves in the rainbow. Some of these may be achieved by introducing two more variables: *saturation,* which allows for mixing with white light, and *intensity,* which controls the level of color. Thus three variables are still involved: hue, saturation, and intensity.

Another model for color vision was put forth in the 19th century by Ewald Hering [Hering, 1864]. This theory also adheres to the concept of trichromacy, espousing three independent variables. However, unlike the Young-Helmholtz model, these variables are signed; they can be positive, negative, or zero. The resulting three axes are *red-green, yellow-blue,* and *black-white.* The Hering model is supported by the physiologic evidence for the center/surround response, which allows for positive as well as negative information. In fact, two populations of cells, activated and suppressed along the red-green and yellow-blue axes, have been found in monkey LGN. Yellow is apparently detected by a combination of red and green cones.

The Hering model explains, for example, the perception of the color brown, which results only when orange or yellow is surrounded by a brighter color. It also accounts for the phenomenon of color constancy, in which the perceived color of an object remains unchanged under differing ambient light conditions provided background colors are available for comparison. Research into color constancy was pioneered in the laboratory of Edwin Land [Land and McCann, 1971]. As David Hubel says, "We require color borders for color, just as we require luminance borders for black and white" [Hubel, 1988, p. 178]. As one might expect, when the corpus collousum is surgically severed, color constancy is absent across the midline.

Color processing in V1 is confined to small circular areas, known as *blobs,* in which *double-opponent cells* are found. They display a center/surround behavior based on the red-green and yellow-blue axes but lack orientation selectivity. The V1 blobs were first identified by their uptake of certain enzymes, and only later was their role in color vision discovered [Livingstone and Hubel, 1984]. The blobs are especially prominent in layers 2 and 3, which receive input from the P cells of the LGN.

Higher Cortical Centers

How are the primitive elements of image processing so far discussed united into an understanding of the image? Beyond V1 are many higher cortical centers for visual processing, at least 12 in the occipital lobe and others in the temporal and parietal lobes. Area V2 receives axons from both the blob and interblob areas of V1 and performs analytic functions such as filling in the missing segments of an edge. V2 contains three areas categorized by different kinds of stripes: *thick stripes* which process relative horizontal position and stereopsis, *thin stripes* which process color without orientations, and *pale stripes* which extend the processing of end-stopped orientation cells.

Beyond V2, higher centers have been labeled V3, V4, V5, etc. Four parallel systems have been delineated [Zeki, 1992], each system responsible for a different attribute of vision, as shown in Fig. 4.1. This is obviously an oversimplification of a tremendously complex system.

Corroborative clinical evidence supports this model. For example, lesions in V4 lead to *achromatopsia,* in which a patient can only see gray and cannot even recall colors. Conversely, a form of poisoning, *carbon monoxide chromatopsia,* results when the V1 blobs and V2 thin stripes selectively survive exposure to carbon monoxide thanks to their rich vasculature, leaving the patient with a sense of color but not of shape. A lesion in V5 leads to *akinetopsia,* in which moving objects disappear.

As depicted in Fig. 4.1, all visual information is processed through V1 and V2, although discrete channels within these areas keep different types of information separate. A total lesion of V1 results in the perception of total blindness. However, not all channels are shown in Fig. 4.1, and such a "totally blind" patient may perform better than randomly when forced to guess between colors or between motion in different directions. The patient with this condition, called *blindsight,* will deny being able to see anything [Weiskrantz, 1990].

Area V1 preserves retinal topographic mapping and shows small receptive fields, suggesting a piecewise analysis of the image, although a given area of V1 receives sequential information from disparate areas of the visual environment as the eyes move. V2 and higher visual centers show progressively larger receptive fields and less defined topographic mapping but more specialized responses. In the extreme of specialization, neurobiologists joke about the "grandmother cell," which would respond only to a particular face. No such cell has yet been found. However, cortical regions that respond to faces in general have been found in the temporal lobe. Rather than a "grandmother cell," it seems that face-selective neurons are members of ensembles for coding faces [Gross and Sergen, 1992].

Defining Terms

Binocular convergence: The response of a single neuron to the same location in the visual field of each eye.

Color constancy: The perception that the color of an object remains constant under different lighting conditions. Even though the spectrum reaching the eye from that object can be vastly different, other objects in the field of view are used to compare.

Cytoarchitectonics: The organization of neuron types into layers as seen by various staining techniques under the microscope. Electrophysiologic responses of individual cells can be correlated with their individual layer.

Magnification: The variation in amount of retinal area represented per unit area of V1 from the fovea to the peripheral vision. Even though the fovea takes up an inordinate percentage of V1 compared with the rest of the visual field, the scale of the cellular organization remains constant. Thus the image from the fovea is, in effect, magnified before processing.

Receptive field: The area in the visual field that evokes a response in a neuron. Receptive fields may respond to specific stimuli such as illuminated bars or edges with particular directions of motion, etc.

Stereopsis: The determination of distance to objects based on relative displacement on the two retinas because of parallax.

Topographic mapping: The one-to-one correspondence between location on the retina and location within a structure in the brain. Topographic mapping further implies that contiguous areas on the retina map to contiguous areas in the particular brain structure.

References

Belliveau JH, Kwong KK, et al. 1992. Magnetic resonance imaging mapping of brain function: Human visual cortex. Invest Radiol 27(suppl 2):S59.

Cohen MS, Bookheimer SY. 1994. Localization of brain function using magnetic resonance imaging. Trends Neurosci 17(7):268.

Daniel PM, Whitteridge D. 1961. The representation of the visual field on the cerebral cortex in monkeys. J Physiol 159:203.

Edelman GM. 1978. Group selection and phasic reentrant signalling: A theory of higher brain function. In GM Edelman and VB Mountcastle (eds), The Mindful Brain, pp 51–100. Cambridge, MIT Press.

Ennes HE. 1981. NTSC color fundamentals. In Television Broadcasting: Equipment, Systems, and Operating Fundamentals. Indianapolis, Howard W Sams & Co.

Felleman DJ, V Essen DC. 1991. Distributed hierarchical processing in the primate cerebral cortex. Cerebral Cortex 1(1):1.

Gross CG, Sergen J. 1992. Face recognition. Curr Opin Neurobiol 2(2):156.

Hebb DO. 1961. The Organization of Behavior. New York, Wiley.

Helmholtz H. 1889. Popular Scientific Lectures. London, Longmans.

Hering E. 1864. Outlines of a Theory of Light Sense. Cambridge, Harvard University Press.

Hubel DH. 1988. Eye, Brain, and Vision. New York, Scientific American Library.

Land EH, McCann JJ. 1971. Lightness and retinex theory. J Opt Soc Am 61:1.

Livingstone MS, Hubel DH. 1984. Anatomy and physiology of a color system in the primate visual cortex. J Neurosci 4:309.

Marks WB, Dobelle WH, MacNichol EF. 1964. Visual pigments of single primate cones. Science 143:1181.

Marr D. 1982. Vision. San Francisco, WH Freeman.

Mountcastle VB. 1957. Modality and topographic properties of single neurons of cat's somatic sensory cortex. J Neurophysiol 20(3):408.

Poggio GF, Talbot WH. 1981. Mechanisms of static and dynamic stereopsis in foveal cortex of the rhesus monkey. J Physiol 315:469.

Wald G. 1974. Proceedings: Visual pigments and photoreceptors—Review and outlook. Exp Eye Res 18(3):333.

Weiskrantz L. 1990. The Ferrier Lecture: Outlooks for blindsight: explicit methodologies for implicit processes. Proc R Soc Lond B239:247.

Wheatstone SC. 1838. Contribution to the physiology of vision. Philosoph Trans R Soc Lond

Young T. 1802. The Bakerian Lecture: On the theory of lights and colours. Philosoph Trans R Soc Lond 92:12.

Zeki S. 1992. The visual image in mind and brain. Sci Am, Sept. 1992, p 69.

Zeki S, Watson JD, Lueck CJ, et al. 1991. A direct demonstration of functional specialization in human visual cortex. J Neurosci 11(3):641.

Further Reading

An excellent introductory text about the visual system is *Eye, Brain, and Vision,* by Nobel laureate, David H. Hubel (1988, Scientific American Library, New York). A more recent general text with a thorough treatment of color vision, as well as the higher cortical centers, is *A Vision of the Brain,* by Semir Zeki (1993, Blackwell Scientific Publications, Oxford).

Other useful texts with greater detail about the nervous system are *From Neuron to Brain,* by Kuffler, Nicholls, and Martin (2nd ed., 1984, Sinauer Assoc., Sunderand Mass.), *The Synaptic Organization of the Brain,* by Shepherd (1979, Oxford Press, New York), and *Fundamental Neuroanatomy,* by Nauta and Feirtag (1986, Freeman, New York).

A classic text that laid the foundation of computer vision is *Vision,* by David Marr (1982, Freeman, New York). Other texts dealing with the mathematics of image processing and image analysis are *Digital Image Processing,* by Pratt (1991, Wiley, New York), and *Digital Image Processing and Computer Vision,* by Schalkoff (1989, Wiley, New York).

5

Auditory System

Ben M. Clopton
University of Washington

Francis A. Spelman
University of Washington

The auditory system can be divided into two large subsystems, peripheral and central. The peripheral auditory system converts the condensations and rarefactions that produce sound into neural codes that are interpreted by the central auditory system as specific sound tokens that may affect behavior.

The peripheral auditory system is subdivided into the external ear, the middle ear, and the inner ear (Fig. 5.1). The external ear collects sound energy as pressure waves which are converted to mechanical motion at the *eardrum*. This motion is transformed across the *middle ear* and transferred to the *inner ear*, where it is frequency analyzed and converted into neural codes that are carried by the eighth cranial nerve, or *auditory nerve*, to the central auditory system.

Sound information, encoded as discharges in an array of thousands of auditory nerve fibers, is processed in nuclei that make up the central auditory system. The major centers include the *cochlear nuclei* (CN), the *superior olivary complex* (SOC), the *nuclei of the lateral lemniscus* (NLL), the *inferior colliculi* (IC), the *medial geniculate body* (MGB) of the thalamus, and the *auditory cortex* (AC). The CN, SOC, and NLL are brainstem nuclei; the IC is at the midbrain level; and the MGB and AC constitute the auditory thalamocortical system.

While interesting data have been collected from groups other than mammals, this chapter will emphasize the mammalian auditory system. This chapter ignores the structure and function of the vestibular system. While a few specific references are included, most are general in order to provide a more introductory entry into topics.

5.1 Physical and Psychological Variables

Acoustics

Sound is produced by time-varying motion of the particles in air. The motions can be defined by their pressure variations or by their volume velocities. *Volume velocity* is defined as the average particle velocity produced across a cross-sectional area and is the acoustic analogue of electric current. *Pressure* is the acoustic analogue of voltage. *Acoustic intensity* is the average rate of the flow of

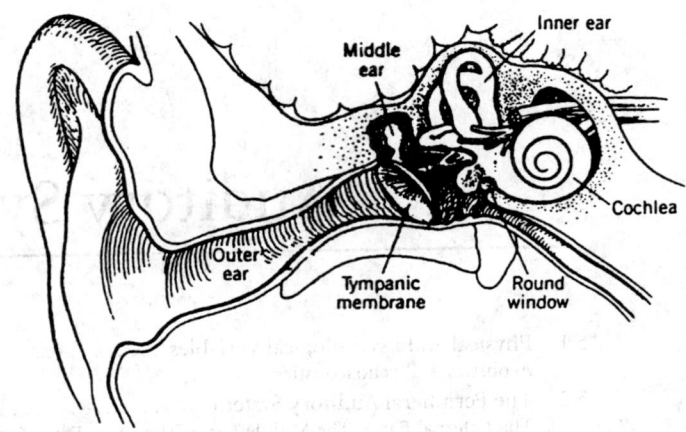

FIGURE 5.1   The peripheral auditory system showing the ear canal, tympanic membrane, middle ear and ossicles, and the inner ear consisting of the cochlea and semicircular canals of the vestibular system. Nerves
communicating with the brain are also shown.

energy through a unit area normal to the direction of the propagation of the sound wave. It is the
product of the acoustic pressure and the volume velocity and is analogous to electric power. *Acoustic
impedance,* the analogue of electrical impedance, is the complex ratio of acoustic pressure and volume velocity. Sound is often described in terms of either acoustic pressure or acoustic intensity
[Kinsler and Frey, 1962].

The auditory system has a wide dynamic range; i.e., it responds to several decades of change in
the magnitude of sound pressure. Because of this wide dynamic range, it is useful to describe the independent variables in terms of decibels, where acoustic intensity is described by $dB = 10 \log(I/I_0)$,
where I_0 is the reference intensity, or equivalently for acoustic pressure, $dB = 20 \log(P/P_0)$, where P_0
is the reference pressure.

Psychoacoustics

Physical variables, such as *frequency* and *intensity,* may have correlated psychological variables, such
as *pitch* and *loudness.* Relationships between acoustic and psychological variables, the subject of the
field of *psychoacoustics,* are generally not linear and may be very complex, but measurements of
human detection and discrimination can be made reliably. Humans without hearing loss detect
tonal frequencies from 20 Hz to 20 kHz. At 2 to 4 kHz their *dynamic range,* the span between threshold and pain, is approximately 120 dB. The minimum threshold for sound occurs between 2 and 5
kHz and is about 20 μPa. At the low end of the auditory spectrum, threshold is 80 dB higher, while
at the high end, it is 70 dB higher. Intensity differences of 1 dB can be detected, while frequency differences of 2 to 3 Hz can be detected at frequencies below about 3 kHz [Fay, 1988].

5.2 The Peripheral Auditory System

The External Ear

Ambient sounds are collected by the *pinna,* the visible portion of the external ear, and guided to the
middle ear by the *external auditory meatus,* or ear canal. The pinna acquires sounds selectively due to
its geometry and the sound shadowing effect produced by the head. In those species whose ears can be
moved voluntarily through large angles, selective scanning of the auditory environment is possible.

The ear canal serves as an acoustic waveguide that is open at one end and closed at the other. The
open end at the pinna approximates a short circuit (large volume velocity and small pressure vari-

ation), while that at the closed end is terminated by the *tympanic membrane* (eardrum). The tympanic membrane has a relatively high acoustic impedance compared with the characteristic impedance of the meatus and looks like an open circuit. Thus the ear canal can resonate at those frequencies for which its length is an odd number of quarter wavelengths. The first such frequency is at about 3 kHz in the human. The meatus is antiresonant for those frequencies for which its length is an integer number of half wavelengths. For a discussion of resonance and antiresonance in an acoustic waveguide, see a text on basic acoustics, e.g., Kinsler and Frey [1962].

The acoustic properties of the external ear produce differences between the sound pressure produced at the tympanic membrane and that at the opening of the ear canal. These differences are functions of frequency, with larger differences found at frequencies between 2 and 6 kHz than those below 2 kHz. These variations have an effect on the frequency selectivity of the overall auditory system.

The Middle Ear

Anatomy

Tracing the acoustic signal, the boundaries of the middle ear include the tympanic membrane at the input and the oval window at the output. The middle ear bones, the ossicles, lie between. Pressure relief for the tympanic membrane is provided by the eustachian tube. The middle ear is an air-filled cavity.

The Ossicles

The three bones that transfer sound from the tympanic membrane to the *oval window* are called the *malleus* (hammer), *incus* (anvil), and *stapes* (stirrup). The acoustic impedance of the atmospheric source is much less than that of the aqueous medium of the load. The ratio is 3700 in an open medium, or 36 dB [Kinsler and Frey, 1962]. The ossicles comprise an impedance transformer for sound, producing a mechanical advantage that allows the acoustic signal at the tympanic membrane to be transferred with low loss to the round window of the cochlea (inner ear). The air-based sound source produces an acoustic signal of low-pressure and high-volume velocity, while the mechanical properties of the inner ear demand a signal of high-pressure and low-volume velocity.

The impedance transformation is produced in two ways: The area of the tympanic membrane is greater than that of the footplate of the stapes, and the lengths of the malleus and incus produce a lever whose length is greater on the side of the tympanic membrane than it is on the side of the oval window. In the human, the mechanical advantage is about 22:1 [Dobie and Rubel, 1989] and the impedance ratio of the transformer is 480, 27 dB, changing the mismatch from 3700:1 to about 8:1.

This simplified discussion of the function of the ossicles holds at low frequencies, those below 2 kHz. First, the tympanic membrane does not behave as a piston at higher frequencies but can support modes of vibration. Second, the mass of the ossicles becomes significant. Third, the connections between the ossicles is not lossless, nor can the stiffness of these connections be ignored. Fourth, pressure variations in the middle ear cavity can change the stiffness of the tympanic membrane. Fifth, the cavity of the middle ear produces resonances at acoustic frequencies.

Pressure Relief

The eustachian tube is a bony channel that is lined with soft tissue. It extends from the middle ear to the nasopharynx and provides a means by which pressure can be equalized across the tympanic membrane. The function is clearly observed with changes in altitude or barometric pressure. A second function of the eustachian tube is to aerate the tissues of the middle ear.

The Inner Ear

The mammalian inner ear is a spiral structure, the *cochlea* (snail), consisting of three fluid-filled chambers, or scalae, the *scala vestibuli,* the *scala media,* and the *scala tympani* (Fig. 5.2). The stapes

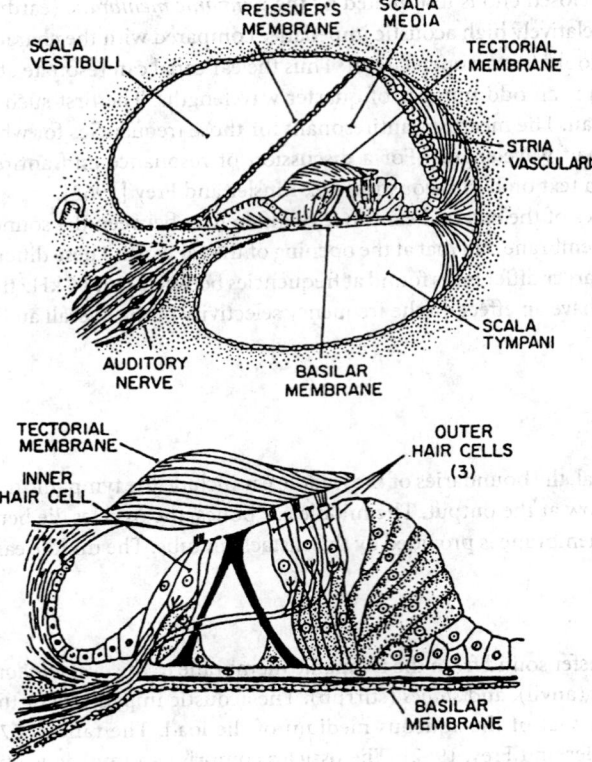

FIGURE 5.2   Cross section of one turn of the cochlea showing the scala vestibuli, scala media, and scala tympani. Reissner's membrane separates the SM and SV, while the basilar membrane and organ of Corti separate the SM and ST.

footplate introduces mechanical displacements into the scala vestibuli through the oval window at the *base* of the cochlea. At the other end of the spiral, the *apex* of the cochlea, the scala vestibuli and the scala tympani communicate by an opening, the *helicotrema*. Both are filled with an aqueous medium, the *perilymph*. The scala media spirals between them and is filled with *endolymph*, a medium that is high in K^+ and low in Na^+. The scala media is separated from the scala vestibuli by *Reissner's membrane*, which is impermeable to ions, and the scala media is separated from the scala tympani by the *basilar membrane* (BM) and *organ of Corti*. The organ of Corti contains the hair cells that transduce acoustic signals into neural signals, the cells that support the hair cells, and the tectorial membrane to which the outer hair cells are attached. The BM provides the primary filter function of the inner ear and is permeable so that the cell bodies of the hair cells are bathed in perilymph.

Fluid and tissue displacements travel from the footplate of the stapes along the cochlear spiral from base to apex. Pressure relief is provided for the incompressible fluids of the inner ear by the round window membrane; e.g., if a transient pressure increase at the stapes displaces its footplate inward, there will be a compensatory outward displacement of the round window membrane.

The Basilar Membrane

Physiology

The BM supports the hair cells and their supporting cells (see Fig. 5.2). Sound decomposition into its frequency components is a major role of the BM. A transient sound, such as a click, initiates a *traveling wave* of displacement in the BM, and this motion has frequency-dependent characteristics which arise from properties of the membrane and its surrounding structures [Bekesy, 1960]. The membrane's width varies as it traverses the cochlear duct: It is narrower at its basal end than at its apical end. It is stiffer at the base than at the apex, with stiffness varying by about two orders of magnitude [Dobie and Rubel, 1989]. The membrane is a distributed structure, which acts as a delay line, as suggested by the nature of the traveling wave [Lyon and Mead, 1989]. The combination of mechanical properties of the BM produces a structure that demonstrates a distance-dependent displacement when the ear is excited sinusoidally. The distance from the apex to the maximum displacement is logarithmically related to the frequency of a sinuoidal tone [LePage, 1991].

Tuning is quite sharp for sinusoidal signals. The slope of the tuning curve is much greater at the high-frequency edge than at the low-frequency edge, with slopes of more than 100 dB per octave at the high edge and about half that at the low edge [Lyon and Mead, 1989]. The filter is sharp, with a 10-dB bandwidth of 10 to 25% of the center frequency.

The auditory system includes both passive and active properties. The outer hair cells (see below) receive efferent output from the brain and actively modify the characteristics of the auditory system. The result is to produce a "cochlear amplifier," which sharpens the tuning of the BM [Lyon and Mead, 1989], as well as adding nonlinear properties to the system [Geisler, 1992; Cooper and Rhode, 1992], along with otoacoustic emissions [LePage, 1991].

The Organ of Corti

The organ of Corti is attached to the BM on the side of the aqueous fluid of the scala media. It is comprised of the supporting cells for the hair cells, the hair cells themselves, and the *tectorial membrane*. The cilia of the *inner hair cells* (IHCs) do not contact the tectorial membrane, while those of the *outer hair cells* (OHCs) do. Both IHCs and OHCs have precise patterns of stereocilia at one end which are held within the tectorial plate next to the overlying tectorial membrane. The IHCs synapse with *spiral ganglion cells,* the afferent neurons, while the OHCs synapse with efferent neurons. Both IHCs and OHCs are found along the length of the organ of Corti. The IHCs are found in a single line, numbering between about 3000 and 4000 in human. There are three lines of OHCs, numbering about 12,000 in human [Nadol, 1988].

Inner Hair Cells

The IHCs' stereocilia are of graded, decreasing length from one side of the cell where a kinocilium is positioned early in ontogeny. If the cilia are deflected in a direction toward this position, membrane channels are further opened to allow potassium to enter and depolarize the cell [Hudspeth, 1987]. Displacement in the other direction reduces channel opening and produces a relative hyperpolarization [Hudspeth and Corey, 1977]. These changes in intracellular potential modulate transmitter release at the base of the IHCs.

The IHCs are not attached to the tectorial membrane, so their response to motion of the membrane is proportional to the velocity of displacement rather than to displacement itself, since the cilia of the hair cells are bathed in endolymph. When the membrane vibrates selectively in response to a pure tone, the stereocilia are bent atop a small number of hair cells, which depolarize in response to the mechanical event. Thus the *tonotopic organization* of the BM is transferred to the hair cells and to the rest of the auditory system. The auditory system is organized tonotopically, i.e., in order of frequency, because the frequency ordering of the cochlea is mapped through successive levels of the system. While this organization is preserved throughout the system, it is much more complex than a huge set of finely tuned filters.

Hair cells in some species exhibit frequency tuning when isolated [Crawford and Fettiplace, 1985], but mammalian hair cells exhibit no tuning characteristics. The tuning of the mammalian auditory system depends on the mechanical characteristics of the BM as modified by the activity of the OHCs.

Outer Hair Cells

The OHCs have cilia that are attached to the tectorial membrane. Since their innervation is overwhelmingly efferent, they do not transfer information to the brain but are modulated in their mechanical action by the brain. There are several lines of evidence that lead to the conclusion that the OHCs play an active role in the processes of the inner ear. First, OHCs change their length in response to neurotransmitters [Dobie and Rubel, 1989]. Second, observation of the Henson's cells, passive cells that are intimately connected to OHCs, shows that spontaneous vibrations are produced by the Henson's cells in mammals and likely in the OHCs as well. These vibrations exhibit spectral peaks that are appropriate in frequency to their locations on the BM [Khanna et al., 1993]. Third, action of the OHCs as amplifiers leads to spontaneous otoacoustic emissions [Kim, 1984; Lyon and Mead, 1989] and to changes in the response of the auditory system [Lyon and Mead, 1989; Geisler, 1992]. Fourth, AC excitation of the OHCs of mammals produces changes in length [Cooke, 1993].

The OHCs appear to affect the response of the auditory system in several ways. They enhance the tuning characteristics of the system to sinusoidal stimuli, decreasing thresholds and narrowing the filter's bandwidth [Dobie and Rubel, 1989]. They likely influence the damping of the BM dynamically by actively changing its stiffness.

Spiral Ganglion Cells and the Auditory Nerve

Anatomy

The auditory nerve of the human contains about 30,000 fibers consisting of myelinated proximal processes of spiral ganglion cells (SGCs). The somas of spiral ganglion cells (SGCs) lie in *Rosenthal's canal*, which spirals medial to the three scalae of the cochlea. Most (93%) are large, heavily myelinated, *type I* SGCs whose distal processes synapse on IHCs. The rest are smaller *type II* SGCs, which are more lightly myelinated. Each IHC has, on average, a number of fibers that synapse with it, 8 in the human and 18 in the cat, although some fibers contact more than one IHC. In contrast, each type II SGC contacts OHCs at a rate of about 10 to 60 cells per fiber.

The auditory nerve collects in the center of the cochlea, its *modiolus*, as SGC fibers join it. Low-frequency fibers from the apex join first, and successively higher frequency fibers come to lie concentrically on the outer layers of the nerve in a spiraling fashion before it exits the modiolus to enter the internal auditory meatus of the temporal bone. A precise tonotopic organization is retrained in the concentrically wrapped fibers.

Physiology

Discharge spike patterns from neurons can be recorded extracellularly while repeating tone bursts are presented. A *threshold level* can be identified from the resulting *rate-level function* (RLF). In the absence of sound and at lower, subthreshold levels, a *spontaneous rate* of discharge is measured. In the nerve this ranges from 50 spikes per second to less than 10. As intensity is raised, the *threshold level* is encountered, where the evoked discharge rate significantly exceeds the spontaneous discharge rate. The plot of threshold levels as a function of frequency is the neuron's *threshold tuning curve*. The tuning curves for axons in the auditory nerve show a minimal threshold (maximum sensitivity) at a *characteristic frequency* (CF) with a narrow frequency range of responding for slightly more intense sounds. At high intensities, a large range of frequencies elicits spike discharges. RLFs for nerve fibers are *monotonic* (i.e., spike rate increases with stimulus intensity), and although a saturation rate is usually approached at high levels, the spike rate does not decline. Mechanical tuning curves for the BM and neural threshold tuning curves are highly similar (Fig. 5.3). Mechanical frequency analysis in the cochlea and the orderly projection of fibers through the nerve lead to correspondingly orderly maps for CFs in the nerve and the nuclei of the central pathways.

Sachs and Young [1979] found that the frequency content of lower intensity vowel sounds is represented as corresponding tonotopic rate peaks in nerve activity, but for higher intensities this rate code is lost as fibers tend toward equal discharge rates. At high intensities spike synchrony to fre-

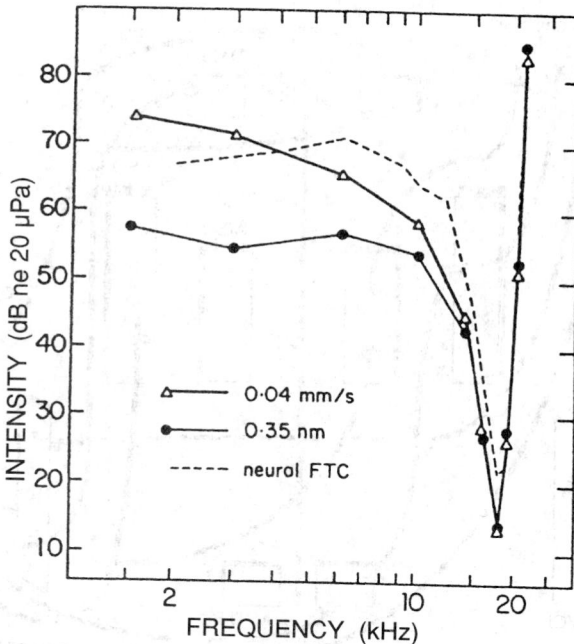

FIGURE 5.3 Mechanical and neural tuning curves from the BM and auditory nerve, respectively. The two mechanical curves show the intensity and frequency combinations for tones required to obtain a criterion displacement or velocity, while the neural curve shows the combinations needed to increase neural discharge rates a small amount over spontaneous rate.

quencies near CF continue to signal the relative spectral content of vowels, a temporal code. These results hold for *high-spontaneous-rate fibers* (over 15 spikes per second), which are numerous. Less common *low-spontaneous-rate fibers* (less than 15 spikes per second) appear to maintain the rate code at higher intensities, suggesting different coding roles for these two fiber populations.

5.3 The Central Auditory System

Overview

In ascending paths, obligatory synapses occur at the CN, IC, MGB, and AC, but a large number of alternative paths exist with ascending and descending internuclear paths and the shorter intranuclear connections between neighboring neurons and subdivisions within a major nuclear group. Each of the centers listed contains subpopulations of neurons that differ in aspects of their morphologies, discharge patterns to sounds, segregation in the nucleus, biochemistry, and synaptic connectivities. The arrangement of the major ascending auditory pathways is schematically illustrated in Fig. 5.4. For references, see Altschuler et al. [1991].

Neural Bases of Processing

The Cochlear Nuclei

Anatomy of the Cochlear Nuclei.   The CN can be subdivided into at least three distinct regions, the *anteroventral CN* (AVCN), the *posteroventral CN* (PVCN), and the *dorsal CN* (DCN). Each sub-

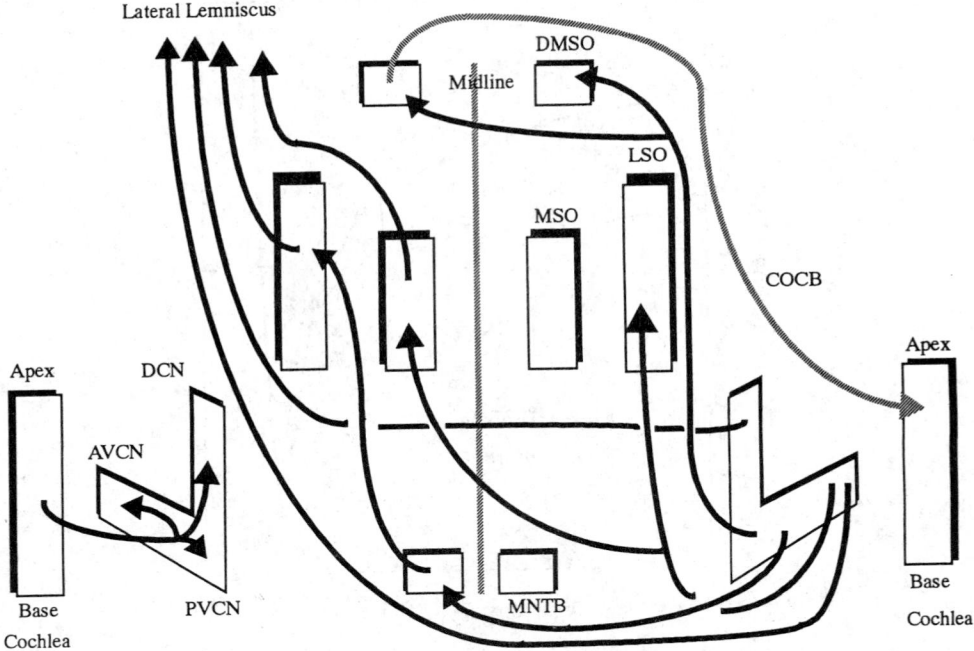

FIGURE 5.4   A schematic of major connections in the auditory brainstem discussed in the text. All structures and connections are bilaterally symmetrical, but connections have been shown on one side only for clarity. No cell types are indicated, but the subdivisions of origin are suggested in the CN. Note that the LSO and MSO receive inputs from both CN.

division has one or more distinctive neuron types and unique intra- and internuclear connections. The axon from each type I SGC in the nerve branches to reach each of the three divisions in an orderly manner so that tonotopic organization is maintained. Neurons with common morphologic classifications are found in all three divisions, especially *granule cells,* which tend to receive connections from type II spiral ganglion cells.

Morphologic classification of neurons based on the shapes of their dendritic trees and somas shows that the anterior part of the AVCN contains many *spherical bushy cells,* while in its posterior part both *globular bushy cells* and spherical bushy cells are found. Spherical bushy cells receive input from one type I ganglion cell through a large synapse formation containing end bulbs of Held, while the globular cells may receive inputs from a few afferent fibers. These endings cover a large part of the soma surface and parts of the proximal dendrite, especially in spherical bushy cells, and they have rounded vesicles presynaptically, indicating excitatory input to the bushy cells, while other synaptic endings of noncochlear origins tend to have flattened vesicles associated with inhibitory inputs. *Stellate cells* are found throughout the AVCN, as well as in the lower layers of the DCN. The AVCN is tonotopically organized, and neurons having similar CFs have been observed to lie in layers or laminae [Bourk et al., 1981]. *Isofrequency laminae* also have been indicated in other auditory nuclei.

The predominant neuron in the PVCN is the *octopus cell,* a label arising from its distinctive shape with asymmetrically placed dendrites. Octopus cells receive cochlear input from type I SGCs on their somas and proximal dendrites. Their dendrites cross the incoming array of cochlear fibers, and these often branch to follow the dendrite toward the soma.

The DCN is structurally the most intricate of the CN. In many species, four or five layers are noticeable, giving it a "cortical" structure, and its local circuitry has been compared with that of the cerebellum. *Fusiform cells* are the most common morphologic type. Their somas lie in the deeper layers of the DCN, and their dendrites extend toward the surface of the nucleus and receive primarily noncochlear inputs. Cochlear fibers pass deeply in the DCN and turn toward the surface to inner-vate fusiform and *giant cells* that lie in the deepest layer of the DCN. The axons of fusiform and giant cells project out of the DCN to the contralateral IC.

Intracellular recording in slice preparations is beginning to identify the membrane characteristics of neuronal types in the CN. The diversity of neuronal morphologic types, their participation in local circuits, and the emerging knowledge of their membrane biophysics are motivating detailed compartmental modeling [Arle and Kim, 1991].

Spike Discharge Patterns. Auditory nerve fibers and neurons in central nuclei may discharge only a few times during a brief tone burst, but if a histogram of spike events is synchronized to the onset of the tone burst, a *peristimulus time histogram* (PSTH) is obtained that is more representative of the neuron's response than any single one. The PSTH may be expressed in terms of spike counts, spike probability, or spike rate as a function of time, but all these retain the underlying temporal pattern of the response. PSTHs taken at the CF for a tone burst intensity roughly 40 dB above threshold have shapes that are distinctive to different nuclear subdivisions and even different morphologic types. They have been used for functionally classifying auditory neurons.

Figure 5.5 illustrates some of the major pattern types obtained from the auditory nerve and CN. Auditory nerve fibers and spherical bushy cells in AVCN have *primary-like* patterns in their PSTHs, an elevated spike rate after tone onset, falling to a slowly adapting level until the tone burst ends. Globular bushy cells may have primary-like, *pri-notch* (primary-like with a brief notch after onset), or chopper patterns. Stellate cells have non-primary-like patterns. *Onset* response patterns, one or a few brief peaks of discharge at onset with little or no discharges afterwards, are observed in the

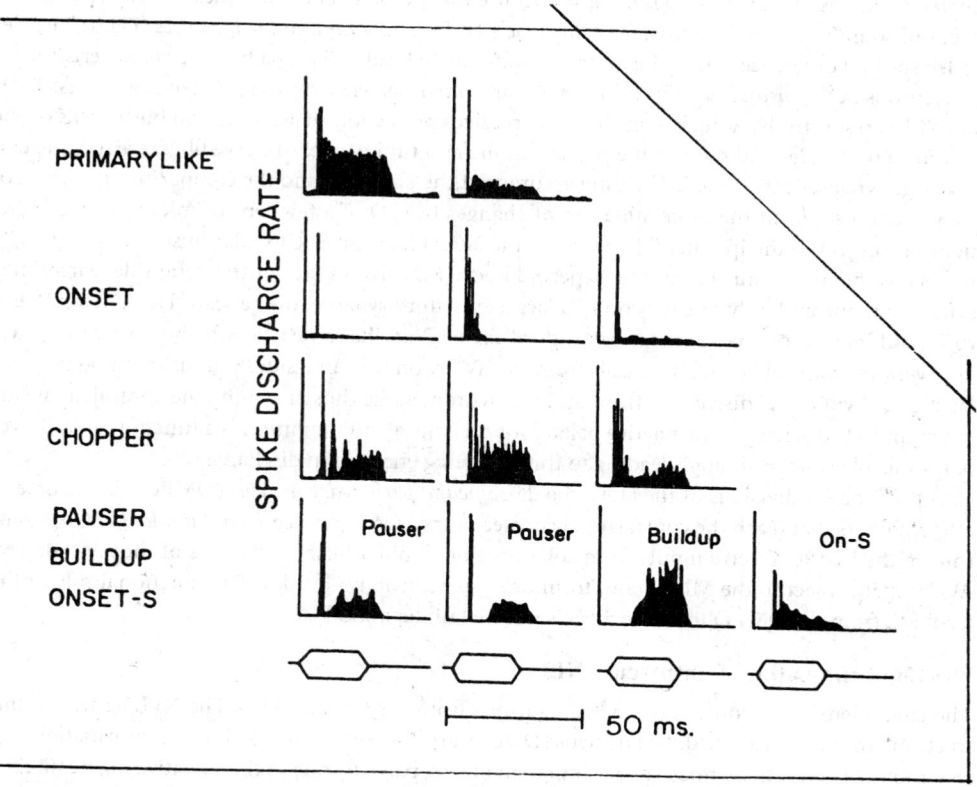

FIGURE 5.5 Peristimulus time histogram patterns obtained in the CN and nerve. Repeated presentations of a tone burst at CF are used to obtain these estimates of discharge rate during the stimulus. (Adapted from Young, 1984.)

PVCN from octopus cells. *Chopper, pauser,* and *buildup* patterns are observed in many cells of the DCN. For most neurons of the CN, these patterns are not necessarily stable over different stimulus intensities; a primary-like pattern may change to a pauser pattern and then to a chopper pattern as intensity is raised [Young, 1984].

Functional classification also has been based on the *response map,* a plot of a neuron's spike discharge rate as a function of tonal frequency and intensity. Fibers and neurons with primary-like PSTHs generally have response maps with only an *excitatory region* of elevated rate. The lower edges of this region approximate the threshold tuning curve. Octopus cells often have very broad tuning curves and extended response maps, as suggested by their frequency-spanning dendritic trees. More complex response maps are observed for some neurons, such as those in the DCN. Inhibitory regions alone, a frequency-intensity area of suppressed spontaneous discharge rates, or combinations of excitatory regions and inhibitory regions have been observed. Some neurons are excited only within islands of frequency-intensity combinations, demonstrating a CF but having no response to high-intensity sounds. In these cases, an RLF at CF would be *nonmonotonic;* i.e., spike rate decreases as the level is raised. Response maps in the DCN containing both excitatory and inhibitory regions have been shown to arise from a convergence of inputs from neurons with only excitatory or inhibitory regions in their maps [Young and Voigt, 1981].

Superior Olivary Complex (SOC)

The SOC contains 10 or more subdivisions in some species. It is the first site at which connections from the two ears converge and is therefore a center for binaural processing that underlies sound localization. There are large differences in the subdivisions between mammalian groups such as bats, primates, cetaceans, and burrowing rodents that utilize vastly different binaural cues. Binaural cues to the locus of sounds include *interaural level differences* (ILDs), *interaural time differences* (ITDs), and detailed spectral differences for multispectral sounds due to head and pinna filtering characteristics.

Neurons in the *medial superior olive* (MSO) and *lateral superior olive* (LSO) tend to process ITDs and ILDs, respectively. A neuron in the MSO receives projections from spherical bushy cells of the CN from both sides and thereby the precise timing and tuning cues of nerve fibers passed through the large synapses mentioned. The time accuracy of the pathways and the comparison precision of MSO neurons permit the discrimination of changes in ITD of a few tens of microseconds. MSO neurons project to the ipsilateral IC through the lateral lemniscus. Globular bushy cells of the CN project to the medial nucleus of the trapezoid body (MNTB) on the contralateral side, where they synapse on one and only one neuron in a large, excitatory synapse, the calyx of Held. MNTB neurons send inhibitory projections to neurons of the LSO on the same side, which also receives excitatory input from spherical bushy cells from the AVCN on the same side. Sounds reaching the ipsilateral side will excite discharges from an LSO neuron, while those reaching the contralateral side will inhibit its discharge. The relative balance of excitation and inhibition is a function of ILD over part of its physiological range, leading to this cue being encoded in discharge rate.

One of the subdivisions of the SOC, the *dorsomedial periolivary nucleus* (DMPO), is a source of efferent fibers that reach the contralateral cochlea in the *crossed olivocochlear bundle* (COCB). Neurons of the DMPO receive inputs from collaterals of globular bushy cell axons of the contralateral AVCN that project to the MNTB and from octopus cells on both sides. The functional role of the feedback from the DMPO to the cochlea is not well understood.

Nuclei of the Lateral Lemniscus (NLL)

The lateral lemniscus consists of ascending axons from the CN and LSO. The NLL lie within this tract, and some, such as the dorsal nucleus (DNLL), are known to process binaural information, but less is known about these nuclei as a group than others, partially due to their relative inaccessibility.

Inferior Colliculi (IC)

The IC are paired structures lying on the dorsal surface of the rostral brainstem. Each colliculus has a large *central nucleus* (ICC), a surface cortex, and paracentral nuclei. Each colliculus receives afferents from a number of lower brainstem nuclei, projects to the MGB through the *brachium*, and communicates with the other colliculus through a *commissure*. The ICC is the major division and has distinctive laminae in much of its volume. The laminae are formed from *disk-shaped cells* and afferent fibers. The disk-shaped cells, which make up about 80% of the ICC's neuronal population, have flattened dendritic fields that lie in the laminar plane. The terminal endings of afferents form fibrous layers between laminae. The remaining neurons in the ICC are *stellate cells* that have dendritic trees spanning laminae. Axons from these two cell types make up much of the ascending ICC output.

Tonotopic organization is preserved in the ICC's laminae, each corresponding to an *isofrequency lamina*. Both monaural and binaural information converges at the IC through direct projections from the CN and from the SOC and NLL. Crossed CN inputs and those from the ipsilateral MSO are excitatory. Inhibitory synapses in the ICC arise from the DNLL, mediated by gamma-aminobutyric acid (GABA), and from the ipsilateral LSO, mediated by glycine.

These connections provide an extensive base for identifying sound direction at this midbrain level, but due to their convergence, it is difficult to determine what binaural processing occurs at the IC as opposed to being passed from the SOC and NLL. Many neurons in the IC respond differently depending on binaural parameters. Varying ILDs for clicks or high-frequency tones often indicates that contralateral sound is excitatory. Ipsilateral sound may have no effect on responses to contralateral sound, classifying the cell as E0, or it may inhibit responses, in which case the neuron is classified as EI, or maximal excitation may occur for sound at both ears, classifying the neuron as EE. Neurons responding to lower frequencies are influenced by ITDs, specifically the phase difference between sinusoids at the ears. Spatial receptive fields for sounds are not well documented in the mammalian IC, but barn owls, who use the sounds of prey for hunting at night, have sound-based spatial maps in the homologous structure. The superior colliculus, situated just rostral to the IC, has spatial auditory receptive field maps for mammals and owl.

Auditory Thalamocortical System

Medial Geniculate Body (MGB).   The MGB and AC form the auditory thalamocortical system. As with other sensory systems, extensive projections to and from the cortical region exist in this system. The MGB has three divisions, the *ventral, dorsal* and *medial*. The ventral division is the largest and has the most precise tonotopic organization. Almost all its input is from the ipsilateral ICC through the brachium of the IC. Its large *bushy cells* have dendrites oriented so as to lie in isofrequency layers, and the axons of these neurons project to the AC, terminating in layers III and IV.

Auditory Cortex.   The auditory cortex (AC) consists of areas of the cerebral cortex that respond to sounds. In mammals, the AC is bilateral and has a primary area with surrounding secondary areas. In nonprimates, the AC is on the lateral surface of the cortex, but in most primates, it lies within the lateral fissure on the superior surface of the temporal lobe. Figure 5.6 reveals the area of the temporal lobe involved with auditory function in humans. Tonotopic mapping is usually evident in these areas as isofrequency surface lines. The primary AC responds most strongly and quickly to sounds. In echo-locating bats, the cortex has a large tonotopic area devoted to the frequency region of its emitted cries and cues related to its frequency modulation and returned Doppler shift [Aitkin, 1990].

The cytoarchitecture of the primary AC shows layers I (surface) through VI (next to white matter), with the largest neurons in layers V and VI. Columns with widths of 50 to 75 μm are evident from dendritic organization in layers III and IV, with fibers lying between the columns. A description of cell types is beyond this treatment.

Discharge patterns in the AC for sound stimuli are mainly of the onset type. Continuous stimuli often evoke later spikes, after the onset discharge, in unanesthetized animals. About half the neurons in the primary AC have monotonic RLFs, but the proportion of nonmonotonic RLFs in secondary areas is much higher. A number of studies have used complex sounds to study cortical responses. Neural responses to species-specific cries, speech, and other important sounds have proven to be labile and to a great extent dependent on the arousal level and behavioral set of the animal.

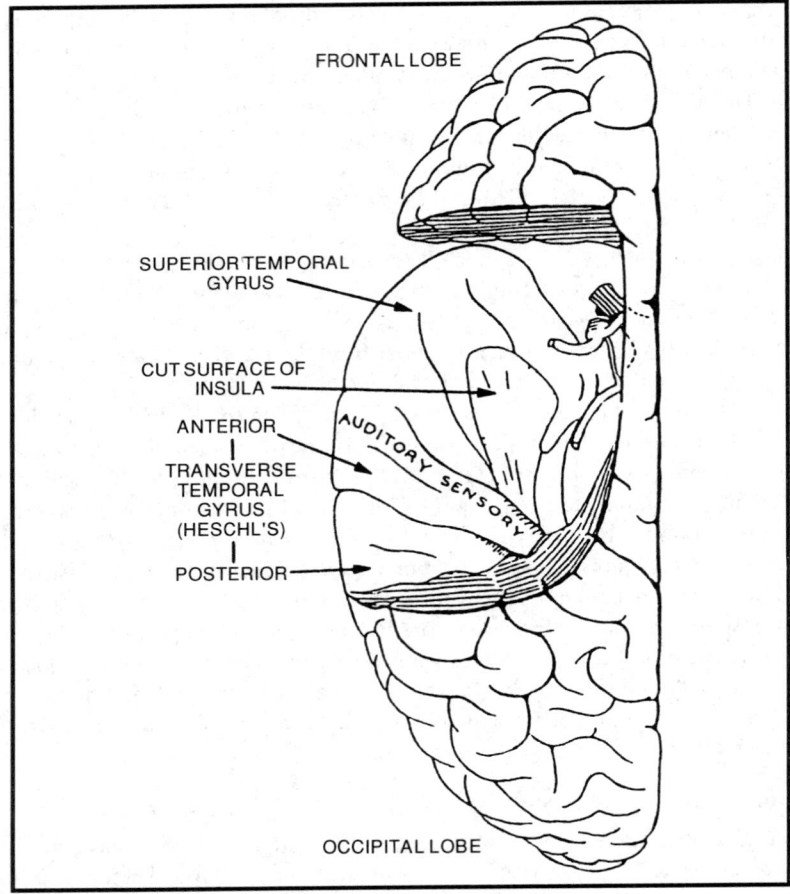

FRONTAL LOBE

SUPERIOR TEMPORAL
GYRUS

CUT SURFACE OF
INSULA

ANTERIOR

TRANSVERSE
TEMPORAL
GYRUS
(HESCHL'S)

POSTERIOR

AUDITORY SENSORY

OCCIPITAL LOBE

FIGURE 5.6 A view of the human cerebral cortex showing the auditory cortex on the superior surface of the left temporal lobe after removal of the overlying parietal cortex.

Cortical lesions in humans rarely produce deafness, although deficits in speech comprehension and generation may exist. Audiometric tests will generally indicate that sensitivity to tonal stimuli is retained. It has been known for some time that left-hemisphere lesions in the temporal region can disrupt comprehension (Wernicke's area) and in the region anterior to the precentral gyrus (Broca's area) can interfere with speech production. It is difficult to separate the effects of these areas because speech comprehension provides vital feedback for producing correct speech.

5.4 Pathologies

Hearing loss results from conductive and neural deficits. Conductive hearing loss due to attenuation in the outer or middle ear often can be alleviated by amplification provided by hearing aids and may be subject to surgical correction. Sensorineural loss due to the absence of IHCs results from genetic deficits, biochemical insult, exposure to intense sound, or aging (*presbycusis*). For some cases of sensorineural loss, partial hearing function can be restored with the cochlear prosthesis, electrical stimulation of remaining SGCs using small arrays of electrodes inserted into the scala tympani

[Miller and Spelman, 1990]. In a few patients having no auditory nerve, direct electrical stimulation of the CN has been used experimentally to provide auditory sensation. Lesions of the nerve and central structures occur due to trauma, tumor growth, and vascular accidents. These may be subject to surgical intervention to prevent further damage and promote functional recovery.

5.5 Models of Auditory Function

Hearing mechanisms have been modeled for many years at a phenomenologic level using psychophysical data. As physiologic and anatomic observations have provided detailed parameters for peripheral and central processing, models of auditory encoding and processing have become more quantitative and physically based. Compartmental models of single neurons, especially SGCs and neurons in the CN, having accurate morphometric geometries, electrical properties, membrane biophysics, and local circuitry are seeing increasing use.

References

Aitkin L. 1990. The Auditory Cortex: Structural and Functional Bases of Auditory Perception. London, Chapman and Hall.

Altschuler RA, Bobbin RP, Clopton BM, Hoffman DW (eds). 1991. Neurobiology of Hearing: The Central Auditory System. New York, Raven Press.

Arle JE, Kim DO. 1991. Neural modeling of intrinsic and spike-discharge properties of cochlear nucleus neurons. Biol Cybern 64:273.

Bekesy G von. 1960. Experiments in Hearing. New York, McGraw-Hill.

Bourk TR, Mielcarz JP, Norris BE. 1981. Tonotopic organization of the anteroventral cochlear nucleus of the cat. Hear Res 4:215.

Cooke M. 1993. Modelling Auditory Processing and Organisation. Cambridge, England, Cambridge University Press.

Cooper NP, Rhode WS. 1992. Basilar membrane mechanics in the hook region of cat and guinea-pig cochleae: Sharp tuning and nonlinearity in the absence of baseline position shifts. Hear Res 63:163.

Crawford AC, Fettiplace R. 1985. The mechanical properties of ciliary bundles of turtle cochlear hair cells. J Physiol 364:359.

Dobie RA, Rubel EW. 1989. The auditory system: Acoustics, psychoacoustics, and the periphery. In HD Patton et al (eds), Textbook of Physiology, vol 1: Excitable Cells and Neurophysiology, 21st ed. Philadelphia, Saunders.

Fay RR. 1988. Hearing in Vertebrates: A Psychophysics Databook. Winnetka, Hill-Fay Associates.

Geisler CD. 1992. Two-tone suppression by a saturating feedback model of the cochlear partition. Hear Res 63:203.

Hudspeth AJ. 1987. Mechanoelectrical transduction by hair cells in the acousticolateralis sensory system. Annu Rev Neurosci 6:187.

Hudspeth AJ, Corey DP. 1977. Sensitivity, polarity, and conductance change in the response of vertebrate hair cells to controlled mechanical stimuli. Proc Natl Acad Sci USA 74:2407.

Khanna SM, Keilson SE, Ulfendahl M, Teich MC. 1993. Spontaneous cellular vibrations in the guinea-pig temporal-bone preparation. Br J Audiol 27:79.

Kim DO. 1984. Functional roles of the inner- and outer-hair-cell subsystems in the cochlea and brainstem. In CI Berlin (ed), Hearing Science: Recent Advances. San Diego, Calif, College-Hill Press.

Kinsler LE, Frey AR. 1962. Fundamentals of Acoustics. New York, Wiley.

LePage EL. 1991. Helmholtz revisited: Direct mechanical data suggest a physical model for dynamic control of mapping frequency to place along the cochlear partition. In Lecture Notes in Biomechanics. New York, Springer-Verlag.

Lyon RF, Mead C. 1989. Electronic cochlea. In C Mead (ed), Analog VLSI and Neural Systems. Reading, Mass, Addison-Wesley.

Miller JM, Spelman FA (eds). 1990. Cochlear Implants: Models of the Electrically Stimulated Ear. New York, Springer-Verlag.

Nadol JB Jr. 1988. Comparative anatomy of the cochlea and auditory nerve in mammals. Hear Res 34:253.

Sachs MB, Young ED. 1979. Encoding of steady-state vowels in the auditory nerve: representation in terms of discharge rate. J Acoust Soc Am 66:470.

Young ED, Voigt HF. 1981. The internal organization of the dorsal cochlear nucleus. In J Syka and L Aitkin (eds), Neuronal Mechanisms in Hearing, pp 127–133. New York, Plenum Press.

Young ED. 1984. Response characteristics of neurons of the cochlear nuclei. In CI Berlin (ed), Hearing Science: Recent Advances. San Diego, Calif, College-Hill Press.

6

Gastrointestinal System

Berj L. Bardakjian
University of Toronto

The primary function of the gastrointestinal (GI) system (Fig. 6.1) is to supply the body with nutrients and water. The ingested food is moved along the alimentary canal at an appropriate rate for digestion, absorption, storage, and expulsion. To fulfill the various requirements of the system, each organ has adapted one or more functions. The esophagus acts as a conduit for the passage of food into the stomach for trituration and mixing. The ingested food is then emptied into the small intestine, which plays a major role in the digestion and absorption processes. The chyme is mixed thoroughly with secretions, and it is propelled distally (1) to allow further gastric emptying, (2) to allow for uniform exposure to the absorptive mucosal surface of the small intestine, and (3) to empty into the colon. The vigor of mixing and the rate of propulsion depend on the required contact time of chyme with enzymes and the mucosal surface for efficient performance of digestion and absorption. The colon absorbs water and electrolytes from the chyme, concentrating and collecting waste products that are expelled from the system at appropriate times. All these motor functions are performed by contractions of the muscle layers in the GI wall.

6.1 GI Electrical Oscillations

GI motility is governed by myogenic, neural, and chemical control systems (Fig. 6.2). The myogenic control system is manifested by periodic depolarizations of the smooth-muscle cells that constitute autonomous electrical oscillations called the *electrical control activity* (ECA) or *slow waves* [Daniel and Chapman, 1963]. The properties of this myogenic system and its electrical oscillations dictate to a large extent the contraction patterns in stomach, small intestine, and colon [Szurszewski, 1987]. The ECA controls the contractile excitability of smooth-muscle cells, since the cells may contract only when depolarization of the membrane voltage exceeds an excitation threshold. The normal spontaneous amplitude of ECA depolarization does not exceed this excitation threshold except when neural or chemical excitation is present. The myogenic system affects the frequency, the direction, and the velocity of the contractions. It also affects the coordination or lack of coordination

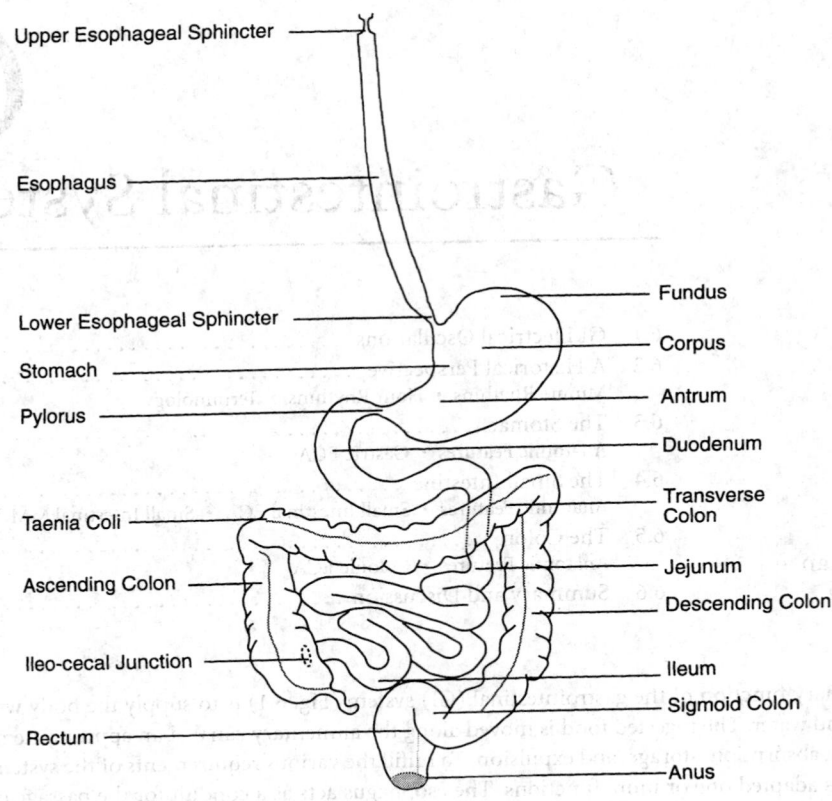

FIGURE 6.1   The GI tract.

between adjacent segments of the gut wall. Hence the electrical activities in the gut wall provide an electrical basis for GI motility.

In the distal stomach, small intestine, and colon, there are intermittent bursts of rapid electrical oscillations, called the *electrical response activity* (ERA) or *spike bursts*. The ERA occurs during the depolarization plateaus of the ECA if a cholinergic stimulus is present, and it is associated with muscular contractions (Fig. 6.3). Thus neural and chemical control systems determine whether contractions will occur or not, but when contractions are occurring, the *myogenic control system* (Fig. 6.4) determines the spatial and temporal patterns of contractions.

There is also a cyclic pattern of distally propagating ERA that appears in the small intestine during the fasted state [Szurszewski, 1969], called the *migrating motility complex* (MMC). This pattern consists of four phases [Code and Marlett, 1975]: Phase I has little or no ERA; phase II consists of irregular ERA bursts; phase III consists of intense, repetitive ERA bursts, where there is an ERA burst on each ECA cycle; and phase IV consists of irregular ERA bursts but is usually much shorter than phase II and may not be always present. The initiation and propagation of the MMC are controlled by enteric cholinergic neurons in the intestinal wall (see Fig. 6.2). The propagation of the MMC may be modulated by inputs from extrinsic nerves or circulating hormones [Sarna et al., 1981]. The MMC keeps the small intestine clean of residual food, debris, and desquamated cells.

6.2   A Historical Perspective

Minute Rhythms

Alvarez and Mahoney [1922] reported the presence of a rhythmic electrical activity (which they called "action currents") in the smooth-muscle layers of stomach, small intestine, and colon. Their

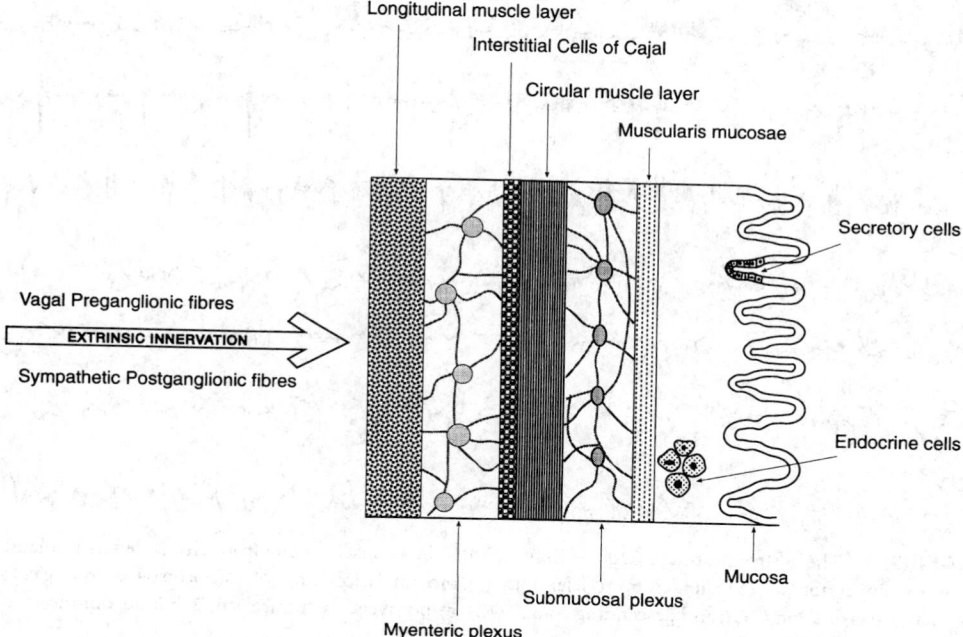

FIGURE 6.2 The layers of the GI wall.

data were acquired from cats (stomach, small intestine), dogs (stomach, small intestine, colon), and rabbits (small intestine, colon). They also demonstrated the existence of frequency gradients in excised stomach and bowel. Puestow [1933] confirmed the presence of a rhythmic electrical activity (which he called "waves of altered electrical potential") and a frequency gradient in isolated canine small intestinal segments. He also demonstrated the presence of an electrical spiking activity (associated with muscular contractions) superimposed on the rhythmic electrical activity. He implied that the rhythmic electrical activity persisted at all times, whereas the electrical spike activity was of an intermittent nature. Bozler [1938, 1939, 1941] confirmed the occurrence of an electrical spiking activity associated with muscular contractions both in vitro in isolated longitudinal muscle strips from guinea pigs (colon, small intestine) and rabbits (small intestine) and in situ in exposed loops

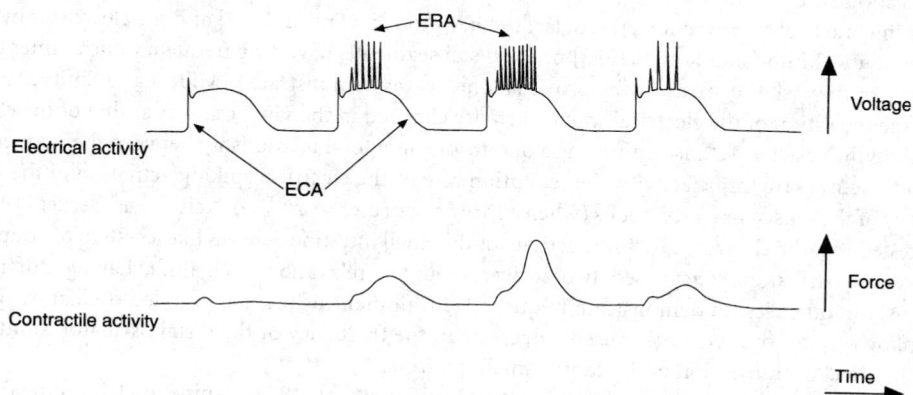

FIGURE 6.3 The relationships between ECA, ERA, and muscular contractions. The ERA occurs in the depolarized phase of the ECA. Muscular contractions are associated with the ERA, and their amplitude depends on the frequency of response potentials within an ERA burst.

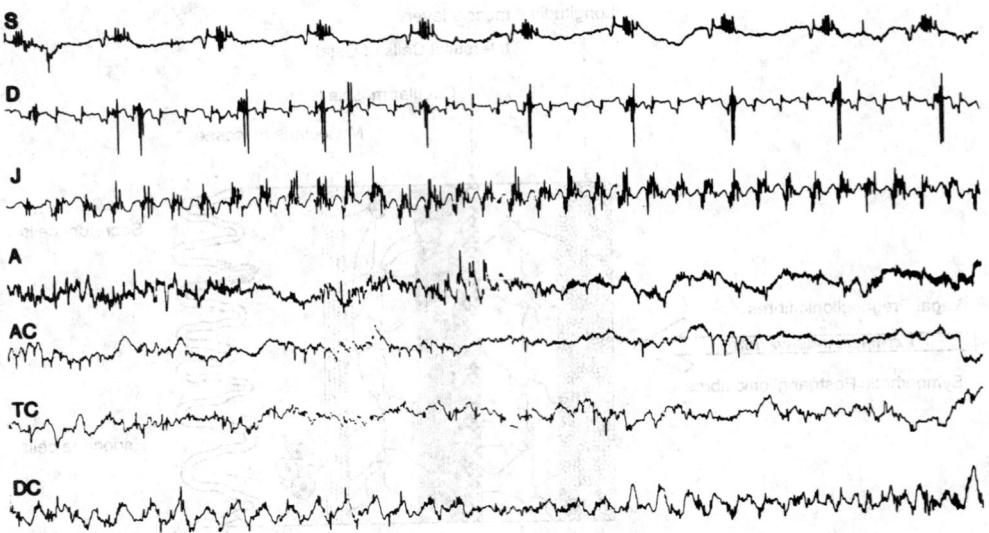

FIGURE 6.4   The gastrointestinal ECA and ERA recorded in a conscious dog from electrode sets implanted subserosally on stomach (*S*), duodenum (*D*), jejunum (*J*), proximal ascending colon (*A*), distal ascending colon (*AC*), transverse colon (*TC*), and descending colon (*DC*), respectively. Each trace is of 2-minute duration.

of small intestine of anesthetized cats, dogs, and rabbits, as well as in cat stomach. He also suggested that the strength of a spontaneous muscular contraction is proportional to the frequency and duration of the spikes associated with it.

The presence of two types of electrical activity in the smooth-muscle layers of the GI tract in several species had been established [Milton and Smith, 1956; Bulbring et al., 1958; Burnstock et al., 1963; Daniel and Chapman, 1963; Bass, 1965; Gillespie, 1962; Duthie, 1974; Christensen, 1975; Daniel, 1975; Sarna, 1975a]. The autonomous electrical rhythmic activity is an omnipresent myogenic activity [Burnstock et al., 1963] whose function is to control the appearance *in time and space* of the electrical spiking activity (an intermittent activity associated with muscular contractions) when neural and chemical factors are appropriate [Daniel and Chapman, 1963]. Neural and chemical factors determine whether contractions will occur or not, but when contractions are occurring, the myogenic control system determines the *spatial and temporal* patterns of contractions.

Isolation of a distal segment of canine small intestine from a proximal segment (using surgical transection or clamping) had been reported to produce a decrease in the frequency of both the rhythmic muscular contractions [Douglas, 1949; Milton and Smith, 1956] and the electrical rhythmic activity [Milton and Smith, 1956] of the distal segment, suggesting frequency entrainment or pulling of the distal segment by the proximal one. It was demonstrated [Milton and Smith, 1956] that the repetition of the electrical spiking activity changed in the same manner as that of the electrical rhythmic activity, thus confirming a one-to-one temporal relationship between the frequency of the electrical rhythmic activity, the repetition rate of the electrical spiking activity, and the frequency of the muscular contractions (when all are present at any one site). Nelson and Becker [1968] suggested that the electrical rhythmic activity of the small intestine behaves like a system of coupled relaxation oscillators. They used two forward-coupled relaxation oscillators, having different intrinsic frequencies, to demonstrate frequency entrainment of the two coupled oscillators. Uncoupling of the two oscillators caused a decrease in the frequency of the distal oscillator, simulating the effect of transection of the canine small intestine.

The electrical rhythmic activity in canine stomach [Sarna et al., 1972], canine small intestine [Nelson and Becker, 1968; Diamant et al., 1970; Sarna et al., 1971], human small intestine [Robertson-Dunn and Linkens, 1974], human colon [Bardakjian and Sarna, 1980], and human rectosigmoid

[Linkens et al., 1976] has been modeled by populations of coupled nonlinear oscillators. The interaction between coupled nonlinear oscillators is governed by both intrinsic oscillator properties and coupling mechanisms.

Hour Rhythms

The existence of periodic gastric activity in the fasted state in both dogs [Morat, 1882] and humans [Morat, 1893] has been reported. The occurrence of a periodic pattern of motor activity, comprising bursts of contractions alternating with "intervals of repose," in the GI tracts of fasted animals was noted early in the present century by Boldireff [1905]. He observed that (1) the bursts recurred with a periodicity of about 1.5 to 2.5 hours, (2) the amplitude of the gastric contractions during the bursts were larger than those seen postprandially, (3) the small bowel also was involved, and (4) with longer fasting periods, the bursts occurred less frequently and had a shorter duration. Periodic bursts of activity also were observed in (1) the lower esphageal sphincter [Cannon and Washburn, 1912] and (2) the pylorus [Wheelon and Thomas, 1921]. Further investigation of the fasting contractile activity in the upper small intestine was undertaken in the early 1920s, with particular emphasis on the coordination between the stomach and duodenum [Wheelon and Thomas, 1922; Alvarez and Mahoney, 1923]. More recently, evidence was obtained [Itoh et al., 1978] that the cyclic activity in the lower esophageal sphincter noted by Cannon and Washburn [1912] also was coordinated with that of the stomach and small intestine.

With the use of implanted strain gauges, it was possible to observe contractile activity over long periods of time, and it was demonstrated that the cyclic fasting pattern in the duodenum was altered by feeding [Jacoby et al., 1963]. The types of contractions observed during fasting and feeding were divided into four groups [Reinke et al., 1967; Carlson et al., 1972]. Three types of contractile patterns were observed in fasted animals: (1) quiescent interval, (2) a shorter interval of increasing activity, and (3) an interval of maximal activity. The fourth type was in fed animals, and it consisted of randomly occurring contractions of varying amplitudes.

With the use of implanted electrodes in the small intestine of fasted dogs, Szurszewski [1969] demonstrated that the cyclic appearance of electrical spiking activity at each electrode site was due to the migration of the cyclic pattern of quiescence, increasing activity and maximal electrical activity down the small intestine from the duodenum to the terminal ileum. He called this electrical pattern the *migrating myoelectric complex* (MMC). Grivel and Ruckebusch [1972] demonstrated that the mechanical correlate of this electrical pattern, which they called the *migrating motor complex*, occurs in other species such as sheep and rabbits. They also observed that the velocity of propagation of the maximal contractile activity was proportional to the length of the small intestine. Code and Marlett [1975] observed the electrical correlate of the cyclic activity in dog stomach that was reported by Morat [1882, 1893], and they demonstrated that the stomach MMC was coordinated with the duodenal MMC.

The MMC pattern has been demonstrated in other mammalian species [Ruckebusch and Fioramonti, 1975; Ruckebusch and Bueno, 1976], including humans. Bursts of distally propagating contractions had been noted in the GI tract of humans [Beck et al., 1965], and their cyclic nature was reported by Stanciu and Bennet [1975]. The MMC has been described in both normal volunteers [Vantrappen et al., 1977; Fleckenstein, 1978; Thompson et al., 1980; Kerlin and Phillips, 1982; Rees et al., 1982] and in patients [Vantrappen et al., 1977; Thompson et al., 1982; Summers et al., 1982].

Terminology

A nomenclature to describe the GI electrical activities has been proposed to describe the minute rhythm [Sarna, 1975b] and the hour rhythm [Carlson et al., 1972; Code and Marlett, 1975].

Control cycle is one depolarization and repolarization of the transmembrane voltage. *Control wave* (or *slow wave*) is the continuing rhythmic electrical activity recorded at any one site. It was assumed to be generated by the smooth-muscle cells behaving like a relaxation oscillator at that site. However, recent evidence [Hara et al., 1986; Suzuki et al., 1986; Barajas-Lopez et al., 1989; Serio et al., 1991] indicates that it is generated by a system of interstitial cells of Cajal (ICC) and smooth-muscle cells at that site. *Electrical control activity* (ECA) is the totality of the control waves recorded at one or several sites. *Response potentials* (or *spikes*) are the rapid oscillations of transmembrane voltage in the depolarized state of smooth-muscle cells. They are associated with muscular contraction, and their occurrence is assumed to be in response to a control cycle when acetylcholine is present. *Electrical response activity* (ERA) is the totality of the groups of response potentials at one or several sites.

   Migrating motility complex (MMC) is the entire cycle, which is composed of four phases. Initially, the electrical and mechanical patterns were referred to as the *migrating myoelectric complex* and the *migrating motor complex*, respectively. *Phase I* is the interval during which fewer than 5% of the ECA has associated ERA, and no or very few contractions are present. *Phase II* is the interval when 5 to 95% of the ECA has associated ERA, and intermittent contractions are present. *Phase III* is the interval when more than 95% of the ECA has associated ERA, and large cyclic contractions are present. *Phase IV* is a short and waning interval of intermittent ERA and contractions. Phases II and IV are not always present and are difficult to characterize, whereas phases I and III are always present. *MMC cycle time* is the interval from the end of one phase III to the end of a subsequent phase III at any one site. *Migration time* is the time taken for the MMC to migrate from the upper duodenum to the terminal ileum.

6.3 The Stomach

Anatomic Features

The stomach is somewhat pyriform in shape, with its large end directed upward at the lower esophageal sphincter and its small end bent to the right at the pylorus. It has two curvatures, the lesser curvature and the greater curvature, which is four to five times as long as the lesser curvature, and it consists of three regions, the fundus, corpus (or body), and antrum, respectively. It has three smooth-muscle layers. The outermost layer is the longitudinal muscle layer, the middle is the circular muscle layer, and the innermost is the oblique muscle layer. These layers thicken gradually in the distal stomach toward the pylorus, which is consistent with stomach function, since trituration occurs in the distal antrum. The size of the stomach varies considerably among subjects. In an adult male, its greatest length when distended is about 25 to 30 cm, and its widest diameter is about 10 to 12 cm [Pick and Howden, 1977].

   The structural relationships of nerve, muscle, and interstitial cells of Cajal (ICCs) in the canine corpus indicated a high density of gap junctions, suggesting very tight coupling between cells. Nerves in the corpus are not located close to circular muscle cells but are found exterior to the muscle bundles, whereas ICCs have gap junction contact with smooth-muscle cells and are closely innervated [Daniel and Sakai, 1984].

Gastric ECA

In the canine stomach, the fundus does not usually exhibit spontaneous electrical oscillations, but the corpus and antrum do exhibit such oscillations. In the intact stomach, the ECA is entrained to a frequency of about 5 cpm (about 3 cpm in humans) throughout the electrically active region, with phase lags in both the longitudinal and circumferential directions [Sarna et al., 1972]. The phase lags decrease distally from corpus to antrum.

   There is a marked intrinsic frequency gradient along the axis of the stomach and a slight intrinsic frequency gradient along the circumference. The intrinsic frequency of gastric ECA in isolated circular muscle of the orad and midcorpus is the highest (about 5 cpm) compared with about 3.5 cpm in the rest of the corpus and about 0.5 cpm in the antrum. Also, there is an orad to aborad intrinsic gradient in resting membrane potential, with the terminal antrum having the most negative resting membrane potential, about 30 mV more negative than the fundal regions [Szurszewski, 1987]. The relatively depolarized state of the fundal muscle may explain its electrical inactivity, since the voltage-sensitive ionic channels may be kept in a state of inactivation. Hyperpolarization of the fundus to a transmembrane voltage of −60 mV produces fundal control waves similar to those recorded from mid and orad corpus.

The ECA in the canine stomach was modeled [Sarna et al., 1972] using an array of 13 bidirectionally coupled relaxation oscillators. The model featured (1) an intrinsic frequency decline from corpus to pylorus and from greater curvature to lesser curvature, (2) entrainment of all coupled oscillators at a frequency close to the highest intrinsic frequency, and (3) distally decreasing phase lags between the entrained oscillators. A simulated circumferential transection caused the formation of another frequency plateau aboral to the transection. The frequency of the orad plateau remained unaffected, while that of the aborad plateau was decreased. This is consistent with the observed experimental data.

6.4 The Small Intestine

Anatomic Features

The small intestine is a long, hollow organ that consists of the duodenum, jejunum, and ileum, respectively. Its length is about 650 cm in humans and 300 cm in dogs. The duodenum extends from the pylorus to the ligament of Treitz (about 30 cm in humans and dogs). In humans, the duodenum forms a C-shaped pattern, with the ligament of Treitz near the corpus of the stomach. In dogs, the duodenum lies along the right side of the peritoneal cavity, with the ligament of Treitz in the pelvis. The duodenum receives pancreatic exocrine secretions and bile. In both humans and dogs, the jejunum consists of the next one-third, whereas the ileum consists of the remaining two-thirds of the intestine. The major differences between the jejunum and ileum are functional in nature, relating to their absorption characteristics and motor control. Most sugars, amino acids, lipids, electrolytes, and water are absorbed in the jejunum and proximal ileum, whereas bile acids and vitamin B_{12} are absorbed in the terminal ileum.

Small Intestinal ECA

In the canine small intestine, the ECA is not entrained throughout the entire length [Diamant and Bortoff, 1969a; Sarna et al., 1971]. However, the ECA exhibits a plateau of constant frequency in the proximal region whereby there is a distal increase in phase lag. The frequency plateau (of about 20 cpm) extends over the entire duodenum and part of the jejunum. There is a marked intrinsic frequency gradient in the longitudinal direction, with the highest intrinsic frequency being less than the plateau frequency. When the small intestine was transected in vivo into small segments (15 cm long), the intrinsic frequency of the ECA in adjacent segments tended to decrease aborally in an exponential manner [Sarna et al., 1971]. A single transection of the duodenum caused the formation of another frequency plateau aboral to the transection. The ECA frequency in the orad plateau was generally unaffected, while that in the aborad plateau was decreased [Diamant and Bortoff, 1969b; Sarna et al., 1971]. The frequency of the aborad plateau was either higher than or equal to the highest intrinsic frequency distal to the transection depending on whether the transection of the duodenum was either above or below the region of the bile duct [Diamant and Bortoff, 1969b].

The ECA in canine small intestine was modeled using a chain of 16 bidirectionally coupled relaxation oscillators [Sarna et al., 1971]. Coupling was not uniform along the chain, since the proximal oscillators were strongly coupled and the distal oscillators were weakly coupled. The model featured (1) an exponential intrinsic frequency decline along the chain, (2) a frequency plateau that was higher than the highest intrinsic frequency, and (3) a temporal variation of the frequencies distal to the frequency plateau region. A simulated transection in the frequency plateau region caused the formation of another frequency plateau aboral to the transection such that the frequency of the orad plateau was unchanged, whereas the frequency of the aborad plateau decreased.

The ECA in human small intestine was modeled using a chain of 100 bidirectionally coupled relaxation oscillators [Robertson-Dunn and Linkens, 1974]. Coupling was nonuniform and asymmetrical. The model featured (1) a piecewise linear decline in intrinsic frequency along the chain, (2) a piecewise linear decline in coupling similar to that of the intrinsic frequency, (3) forward coupling that was stronger than backward coupling, and (4) a frequency plateau in the proximal region that was higher than the highest intrinsic frequency in the region.

Small Intestinal MMC

The MMCs in canine small intestine have been observed in intrinsically isolated segments [Sarna et al., 1981, 1983], even after the isolated segment has been stripped of all extrinsic innervation [Sarr and Kelly, 1981] or removed in continuity with the remaining gut as a Thiry Vella loop [Itoh et al., 1981]. This intrinsic mechanism is able to function independently of extrinsic innervation because vagotomy [Weisbrodt et al., 1975; Ruckebusch and Bueno, 1977] does not hinder the initiation of the MMC. The initiation of the small intestinal MMC is controlled by integrative networks within the intrinsic plexuses using nicotinic and muscarinic cholinergic receptors [Ormsbee et al., 1979; El-Sharkawy et al., 1982].

When the canine small intestine was transected into four equal strips [Sarna et al., 1981, 1983], it was found that each strip was capable of generating an independent MMC that would appear to propagate from the proximal to the distal part of each segment. This suggested that the MMC can be modeled by a chain of coupled relaxation oscillators. The average intrinsic periods of the MMC for the four segments were reported to be 106.2, 66.8, 83.1, and 94.8 minutes, respectively. The segment containing the duodenum had the longest period, while the subsequent segment containing the jejunum had the shortest period. However, in the intact small intestine, the MMC starts in the duodenum and not the jejunum. Bardakjian and Sarna [1981] and Bardakjian et al. [1984] have demonstrated that both the intrinsic frequency gradients and resting level gradients have major roles in the entrainment of a chain of coupled oscillators. In modeling the small intestinal MMC with a chain of four coupled oscillators, it was necessary to include a gradient in the intrinsic resting levels of the MMC oscillators (with the proximal oscillator having the lowest resting level) in order to entrain the oscillators and allow the proximal oscillator to behave as the leading oscillator [Bardakjian and Ahmed, 1992].

6.5 The Colon

Anatomic Features

In humans, the colon is about 100 cm in length. The ileum joins the colon approximately 5 cm from its end, forming the cecum, which has a wormlike appendage, the appendix. The colon is sacculated, and the longitudinal smooth muscle is concentrated in three bands (the taeniae). It lies in front of the small intestine against the abdominal wall, and it consists of the ascending (on the right side), transverse (across the lower stomach), and descending (on the left side) colon. The descending colon becomes the sigmoid colon in the pelvis as it runs down and forward to the rectum. Major functions of the colon are (1) to absorb water, certain electrolytes, short-chain fatty acids, and bacterial metabolites, (2) to slowly propel its luminal contents in the caudad direction, (3) to store the residual matter in the distal region, and (4) to rapidly move its contents in the caudad direction during mass movements [Sarna, 1991].

In dogs, the colon is about 45 cm in length, and the cecum has no appendage. The colon is not sacculated, and the longitudinal smooth-muscle coat is continuous around the circumference

[Miller et al., 1968]. It lies posterior to the small intestine, and it consists mainly of ascending and descending segments with a small transverse segment. However, functionally, it is assumed to consist of three regions, each of about 15 cm in length, representing the ascending, transverse, and descending colon, respectively.

Colonic ECA

In the human colon, the ECA is almost completely phase unlocked between adjacent sites as close as 1 to 2 cm apart, and its frequency (about 3 to 15 cpm) and amplitude at each site vary with time [Sarna et al., 1980]. This results in short-duration contractions that are also disorganized in time and space. The disorganization of ECA and its associated contractions is consistent with the colonic function of extensive mixing, kneading, and slow net distal propulsion [Sarna, 1991]. In the canine colon, the reports about the intrinsic frequency gradient were conflicting [Vanasin et al., 1974; Shearin et al., 1978; El-Sharkawy, 1983].

The human colonic ECA was modeled [Bardakjian and Sarna, 1980] using a tubular structure of 99 bidirectionally coupled nonlinear oscillators arranged in 33 parallel rings, where each ring-contained 3 oscillators. Coupling was nonuniform, and it increased in the longitudinal direction. The model featured (1) no phase locking in the longitudinal or circumferential directions, (2) temporal and spatial variation of the frequency profile with large variations in the proximal and distal regions and small variations in the middle region, and (3) waxing and waning of the amplitudes of the ECA that was more pronounced in the proximal and distal regions. The model demonstrated that the "silent periods" occurred because of the interaction between oscillators, and they did not occur when the oscillators were uncoupled. The model was further refined [Bardakjian et al., 1990] such that when the ECA amplitude exceeded an excitation threshold, a burst of ERA was exhibited. The ERA bursts occurred in a seemingly random manner in adjacent sites because (1) the ECA was not phase locked, and (2) the ECA amplitudes and waveshapes varied in a seemingly random manner.

6.6 Summary and Discussion

The ECA in stomach, small intestine, and colon behaves like the outputs of a population of coupled nonlinear oscillators. The populations in the stomach and the proximal small intestine are entrained, whereas those in the distal small intestine and colon are not entrained. There are distinct intrinsic frequency gradients in the stomach and small intestine, but their profile in the colon is ambiguous.

Recently, the applicability of modeling of gastrointestinal ECA by coupled nonlinear oscillators was reconfirmed [Daniel et al., 1994]. Also, a novel nonlinear oscillator, the mapped clock oscillator, was proposed [Bardakjian and Diamant, 1994] for modeling the transmembrane electrical oscillations in excitable cells. The oscillator consists of a clock coupled to a transformer, and it has three different input portals to selectively change its frequency, amplitude, and entrainability. The clock may represent the interstitial cells of Cajal, and the transformer represents the smooth-muscle transmembrane ionic transport mechanisms [Skinner and Bardakjian, 1991]. Such a model accounts for the mounting evidence supporting the role of the interstitial cells of Cajal as a clock for the smooth-muscle transmembrane oscillations [Hara et al., 1986; Suzuki et al., 1986; Barajas-Lopez et al., 1989; Serio et al., 1991].

Modeling of the gastrointestinal ECA by populations of coupled nonlinear oscillators suggests that abnormal ECA can be normalized by (1) external pacing by electronic pacemakers, (2) localized removal of disrupting sites by surgical interventions, and (3) systemic stimulation by chemical interventions [Bardakjian, 1987]. Pacing has been demonstrated in canine stomach [Kelly and LaForce, 1972; Sarna and Daniel, 1973] and small intestine [Sarna and Daniel, 1975c; Becker et al., 1983]. Gastric and small intestinal pacing can be potentially effective treatments for disorders in GI motility.

Acknowledgments

The author would like to thank his colleagues Dr. Sharon Chung and Dr. Karen Hall for providing *biologic insight*.

References

Alvarez WC, Mahoney LJ. 1922. Action current in stomach and intestine. Am J Physiol 58:476.

Alvarez WC, Mahoney LJ. 1923. The relations between gastric and duodenal peristalsis. Am J Physiol 64:371.

Barajas-Lopez C, Berezin I, Daniel EE, Huizinga JD. 1989. Pacemaker activity recorded in interstitial cells of cajal of the gastrointestinal tract. Am J Physiol 257:C830.

Bardakjian BL, Sarna SK. 1980. A computer model of human colonic electrical control activity (ECA). IEEE Trans Biomed Eng 27:193.

Bardakjian BL, Sarna SK. 1981. Mathematical investigation of populations of coupled synthesized relaxation oscillators representing biological rhythms. IEEE Trans Biomed Eng 28:10.

Bardakjian BL, El-Sharkawy TY, Diamant NE. 1984. Interaction of coupled nonlinear oscillators having different intrinsic resting levels. J Theor Biol 106:9.

Bardakjian BL. 1987. Computer models of gastrointestinal myoelectric activity. Automedica 7:261.

Bardakjian BL, Sarna SK, Diamant NE. 1990. Composite synthesized relaxation oscillators: Application to modeling of colonic ECA and ERA. Gastrointest J Motil 2:109.

Bardakjian BL, Ahmed K. 1992. Is a peripheral pattern generator sufficient to produce both fasting and postprandial patterns of the migrating myoelectric complex (MMC)? Dig Dis Sci 37:986.

Bardakjian BL, Diamant NE. 1994. A mapped clock oscillator model for transmembrane electrical rhythmic activity in excitable cells. J Theor Biol 166:225.

Bass P. 1965. Electric activity of smooth muscle of the gastrointestinal tract. Gastroenterology 49:391.

Beck IT, McKenna RD, Peterfy G, et al. 1965. Pressure studies in the normal human jejunum. Am J Dig Dis 10:437.

Becker JM, Sava P, Kelly KA, Shturman L. 1983. Intestinal pacing for canine postgastrectomy dumping. Gastroenterology 84:383.

Boldireff WN. 1905. Le travail periodique de l'appareil digestif en dehors de la digestion. Arch Des Sci Biol 11:1.

Bozler E. 1938. Action potentials of visceral smooth muscle. Am J Physiol 124:502.

Bozler E. 1939. Electrophysiological studies on the motility of the gastrointestinal tract. Am J Physiol 127:301.

Bozler E. 1941. Action potentials and conduction of excitation in muscle. Biol Symp 3:95.

Bulbring E, Burnstock G, Holman ME. 1958. Excitation and conduction in the smooth muscle of the isolated taenia coli of the guinea pig. J Physiol 142:420.

Burnstock G, Holman ME, Prosser CL. 1963. Electrophysiology of smooth muscle. Physiol Rev 43:482.

Cannon WB, Washburn AL. 1912. An explanation of hunger. Am J Physiol 29:441.

Carlson GM, Bedi BS, Code CF. 1972. Mechanism of propagation of intestinal interdigestive myoelectric complex. Am J Physiol 222:1027.

Christensen J. 1975. Myoelectric control of the colon. Gastroenterology 68:601.

Code CF, Marlett JA. 1975. The interdigestive myoelectric complex of the stomach and small bowel of dogs. J Physiol 246:289.

Daniel EE, Chapman KM. 1963. Electrical activity of the gastrointestinal tract as an indication of mechanical activity. Am J Dig Dis 8:54.

Daniel EE. 1975. Electrophysiology of the colon. Gut 16:298.

Daniel EE, Sakai Y. 1984. Structural basis for function of circular muscle of canine corpus. Can J Physiol Pharmacol 62:1304.

Daniel EE, Bardakjian BL, Huizinga JD, Diamant NE. 1994. Relaxation oscillators and core conductor models are needed for understanding of GI electrical activities. Am J Physiol 266:G339.

Diamant NE, Bortoff A. 1969a. Nature of the intestinal slow wave frequency gradient. Am J Physiol 216:301.

Diamant NE, Bortoff A. 1969b. Effects of transection on the intestinal slow wave frequency gradient. Am J Physiol 216:734.

Diamant NE, Rose PK, Davison EJ. 1970. Computer simulation of intestinal slow-wave frequency gradient. Am J Physiol 219:1684.

Douglas DM. 1949. The decrease in frequency of contraction of the jejunum after transplantation to the ileum. J Physiol 110:66.

Duthie HL. 1974. Electrical activity of gastrointestinal smooth muscle. Gut 15:669.

El-Sharkawy TY, Markus H, Diamant NE. 1982. Neural control of the intestinal migrating myoelectric complex: A pharmacological analysis. Can J Physiol Pharmacol 60:794.

El-Sharkawy TY. 1983. Electrical activity of the muscle layers of the canine colon. J Physiol 342:67.

Fleckenstein P. 1978. Migrating electrical spike activity in the fasting human small intestine. Dig Dis Sci 23:769.

Gillespie JS. 1962. The electrical and mechanical responses of intestinal smooth muscle cells to stimulation of their extrinsic parasympathetic nerves. J Physiol 162:76.

Grivel ML, Ruckebusch Y. 1972. The propagation of segmental contractions along the small intestine. J Physiol 277:611.

Hara YM, Kubota M, Szurszewski JH. 1986. Electrophysiology of smooth muscle of the small intestine of some mammals. J Physiol 372:501.

Itoh Z, Honda R, Aizawa I, et al. 1978. Interdigestive motor activity of the lower esophageal sphincter in the conscious dog. Dig Dis Sci 23:239.

Itoh Z, Aizawa I, Takeuchi S. 1981. Neural regulation of interdigestive motor activity in canine jejunum. Am J Physiol 240:G324.

Jacoby HI, Bass P, Bennett DR. 1963. In vivo extraluminal contractile force transducer for gastrointestinal muscle. J Appl Physiol 18:658.

Kelly KA, LaForce RC. 1972. Pacing the canine stomach with electric stimulation. Am J Physiol 222:588.

Kerlin P, Phillips S. 1982. The variability of motility of the ileum and jejunum in healthy humans. Gastroenterology 82:694.

Linkens DA, Taylor I, Duthie HL. 1976. Mathematical modeling of the colorectal myoelectrical activity in humans. IEEE Trans Biomed Eng 23:101.

Milton GW, Smith AWM. 1956. The pacemaking area of the duodenum. J Physiol 132:100.

Miller ME, Christensen GC, Evans HE. 1968. Anatomy of the Dog. Philadelphia, Saunders.

Morat JP. 1882. Sur l'innervation motrice de l'estomac. Lyon Med 40:289.

Morat JP. 1893. Sur quelques particularites de l'innervation motrice de l'estomac et de l'intestin. Arch Physiol Norm Pathol 5:142.

Nelson TS, Becker JC. 1968. Simulation of the electrical and mechanical gradient of the small intestine. Am J Physiol 214:749.

Ormsbee HS, Telford GL, Mason GR. 1979. Required neural involvement in control of canine migrating motor complex. Am J Physiol 237:E451.

Pick TP, Howden R. 1977. Gray's Anatomy. New York, Bounty Books.

Puestow CB. 1933. Studies on the origins of the automaticity of the intestine: The action of certain drugs on isolated intestinal transplants. Am J Physiol 106:682.

Rees WDW, Malagelada JR, Miller LJ, Go VLW. 1982. Human interdigestive and postprandial gastrointestinal motor and gastrointestinal hormone patterns. Dig Dis Sci 27:321.

Reinke DA, Rosenbaum AH, Bennett DR. 1967. Patterns of dog gastrointestinal contractile activity monitored in vivo with extraluminal force transducers. Am J Dig Dis 12:113.

Robertson-Dunn B, Linkens DA. 1974. A mathematical model of the slow wave electrical activity of the human small intestine. Med Biol Eng 12:750.

Ruckebusch Y, Fioramonti S. 1975. Electrical spiking activity and propulsion in small intestine in fed and fasted states. Gastroenterology 68:1500.

Ruckebusch Y, Bueno L. 1976. The effects of feeding on the motility of the stomach and small intestine in the pig. Br J Nutr 35:397.

Ruckebusch Y, Bueno L. 1977. Migrating myoelectrical complex of the small intestine. Gastro-enterology 73:1309.

Shearin NL, Bowes KL, Kingma YJ. 1978. In vitro electrical activity in canine colon. Gut 20:780.

Sarna SK, Daniel EE, Kingma YJ. 1971. Simulation of slow wave electrical activity of small intestine. Am J Physiol 221:166.

Sarna SK, Daniel EE, Kingma YJ. 1972. Simulation of the electrical control activity of the stomach by an array of relaxation oscillators. Am J Dig Dis 17:299.

Sarna SK, Daniel EE. 1973. Electrical stimulation of gastric electrical control activity. Am J Physiol 225:125.

Sarna SK. 1975a. Models of smooth muscle electrical activity. In EE Daniel and DM Paton (eds), Methods in Pharmacology, pp 519–540. New York, Plenum Press.

Sarna SK. 1975b. Gastrointestinal electrical activity: Terminology. Gastroenterology 68:1631.

Sarna SK, Daniel EE. 1975c. Electrical stimulation of small intestinal electrical control activity. Gastroenterology 69:660.

Sarna SK, Bardakjian BL, Waterfall WE, Lind JF. 1980. Human colonic electrical control activity (ECA). Gastroenterology 78:1526.

Sarna SK, Stoddard C, Belbeck L, McWade D. 1981. Intrinsic nervous control of migrating myo-electric complexes. Am J Physiol 241:G16.

Sarna S, Condon RE, Cowles V. 1983. Enteric mechanisms of initiation of migrating myoelectric complexes in dogs. Gastroenterology 84:814.

Sarna SK. 1991. Physiology and pathophysiology of colonic motor activity. Dig Dis Sci 6:827.

Sarr MG, Kelly KA. 1981. Myoelectric activity of the autotransplanted canine jejunoileum. Gastroenterology 81:303.

Serio R, Barajas-Lopez C, Daniel EE, et al. 1991. Pacemaker activity in the colon: Role of interstitial cells of Cajal and smooth muscle cells. Am J Physiol 260:G636.

Stanciu C, Bennett JR. 1975. The general pattern of gastroduodenal motility: 24 hour recordings in normal subjects. Rev Med Chir Soc Med Nat Iasi 79:31.

Skinner FK, Bardakjian BL. 1991. A barrier kinetic mapping unit: Application to ionic transport in gastric smooth muscle. Gastrointest J Motil 3:213.

Summers RW, Anuras S, Green J. 1982. Jejunal motility patterns in normal subjects and sympto-matic patients with partial mechanical obstruction or pseudo-obstruction. In M Weinbeck (ed), Motility of the Digestive Tract, pp 467–470. New York, Raven Press.

Suzuki N, Prosser CL, Dahms V. 1986. Boundary cells between longitudinal and circular layers: Essential for electrical slow waves in cat intestine. Am J Physiol 280:G287.

Szurszewski JH. 1969. A migrating electric complex of the canine small intestine. Am J Physiol 217:1757.

Szurszewski JH. 1987. Electrical basis for gastrointestinal motility. In LR Johnson (ed), Physiology of the Gastrointestinal Tract, chap 12. New York, Raven Press.

Thompson DG, Wingate DL, Archer L, et al. 1980. Normal patterns of human upper small bowel motor activity recorded by prolonged radiotelemetry. Gut 21:500.

Vanasin B, Ustach TJ, Schuster MM. 1974. Electrical and motor activity of human and dog colon in vitro. Johns Hopkins Med J 134:201.

Vantrappen G, Janssens JJ, Hellemans J, Ghoos Y. 1977. The interdigestive motor complex of nor-mal subjects and patients with bacterial overgrowth of the small intestine. J Clin Invest 59:1158.

Weisbrodt NW, Copeland EM, Moore EP, et al. 1975. Effect of vagotomy on electrical activity of the small intestine of the dog. Am J Physiol 228:650.

Wheelon H, Thomas JE. 1921. Rhythmicity of the pyloric sphincter. Am J Physiol 54:460.

Wheelon H, Thomas JE. 1922. Observations on the motility of the duodenum and the relation of duodenal activity to that of the pars pylorica. Am J Physiol 59:72.

7

Respiratory System

Arthur T. Johnson
University of Maryland

Joseph D. Bronzino
*Trinity College/The Hartford
Graduate Center*

As functioning units, the lung and heart are usually considered a single complex organ, but because these organs contain essentially two compartments—one for blood and one for air—they are usually separated in terms of the tests conducted to evaluate heart or pulmonary function. This chapter focuses on some of the physiologic concepts responsible for normal function and specific measures of the lung's ability to supply tissue cells with enough oxygen while removing excess carbon dioxide.

7.1 Respiration Anatomy

The respiratory system consists of the lungs, conducting airways, pulmonary vasculature, respiratory muscles, and surrounding tissues and structures (Fig. 7.1). Each plays an important role in influencing respiratory responses.

Lungs

There are two lungs in the human chest; the right lung is composed of three incomplete divisions called *lobes*, and the left lung has two, leaving room for the heart. The right lung accounts for 55% of total gas volume and the left lung for 45%. Lung tissue is spongy because of the very small (200 to 300×10^{-6} m diameter in normal lungs at rest) gas-filled cavities called *alveoli*, which are the ultimate structures for gas exchange. There are 250 million to 350 million alveoli in the adult lung, with a total alveolar surface area of 50 to 100 m² depending on the degree of lung inflation [Johnson, 1991].

Conducting Airways

Air is transported from the atmosphere to the alveoli beginning with the oral and nasal cavities, through the pharynx (in the throat), past the glottal opening, and into the trachea or windpipe. Conduction of air begins at the larynx, or voice box, at the entrance to the trachea, which is a fibromuscular tube 10 to 12 cm in length and 1.4 to 2.0 cm in diameter [Kline, 1976]. At a location called the *carina*, the trachea terminates and divides into the left and right bronchi. Each bronchus has a dis-

0-8493-8346-3/95/$0.00+$.50

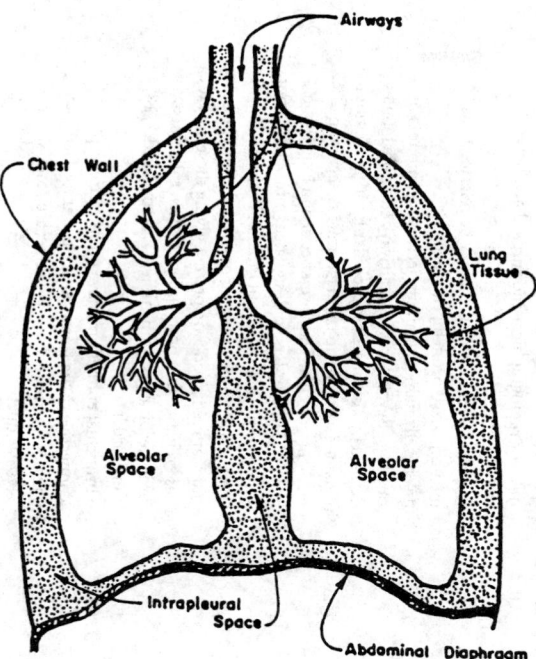

FIGURE 7.1 Schematic representation of the respiratory system.

continuous cartilaginous support in its wall. Muscle fibers capable of controlling airway diameter are incorporated into the walls of the bronchi, as well as in those of air passages closer to the alveoli. Smooth muscle is present throughout the respiratory bronchiolus and alveolar ducts but is absent in the last alveolar duct, which terminates in one to several alveoli. The alveolar walls are shared by other alveoli and are composed of highly pliable and collapsible squamous epithelium cells.

The bronchi subdivide into subbronchi, which further subdivide into bronchioli, which further subdivide, and so on, until finally reaching the alveolar level. Table 7.1 provides a description and dimensions of the airways of adult humans. A model of the geometric arrangement of these air passages is presented in Fig. 7.2. It will be noted that each airway is considered to branch into two sub-airways. In the adult human there are considered to be 23 such branchings, or generations, beginning at the trachea and ending in the alveoli.

Movement of gases in the respiratory airways occurs mainly by bulk flow (convection) throughout the region from the mouth to the nose to the fifteenth generation. Beyond the fifteenth generation, gas diffusion is relatively more important. With the low gas velocities that occur in diffusion, dimensions of the space over which diffusion occurs (alveolar space) must be small for adequate oxygen delivery into the walls; smaller alveoli are more efficient in the transfer of gas than are larger ones. Thus animals with high levels of oxygen consumption are found to have smaller-diameter alveoli compared with animals with low levels of oxygen consumption.

Alveoli

Alveoli are the structures through which gases diffuse to and from the body. To ensure gas exchange occurs efficiently, alveolar walls are extremely thin. For example, the total tissue thickness between the inside of the alveolus to pulmonary capillary blood plasma is only about 0.4×10^{-6} m. Consequently, the principal barrier to diffusion occurs at the plasma and red blood cell level, not at the alveolar membrane [Ruch and Patton, 1966].

TABLE 7.1 Classification and Approximate Dimensions of Airways of Adult Human Lung (Inflated to about 3/4 of TLC)*

Common Name	Numerical Order of Generation	Number of Each	Diameter, mm	Length, mm	Total Cross-Sectional Area, cm²	Description and Comment
Trachea	0	1	18	120	2.5	Main cartilaginous airway; partly in thorax.
Main bronchus	1	2	12	47.6	2.3	First branching of airway; one to each lung; in lung root; cartilage.
Lobar bronchus	2	4	8	19.0	2.1	Named for each lobe; cartilage.
Segmental bronchus	3	8	6	7.6	2.0	Named for radiographical and surgical anatomy; cartilage.
Subsegmental bronchus	4	16	4	12.7	2.4	Last generally named bronchi; may be referred to as medium-sized bronchi; cartilage.
Small bronchi	5–10	1,024†	1.3†	4.6†	13.4†	Not generally named; contain decreasing amounts of cartilage. Beyond this level airways enter the lobules as defined by a strong elastic lobular limiting membrane.
Bronchioles	11–13	8,192†	0.8†	2.7†	44.5†	Not named; contain no cartilage, mucus-secreting elements, or cilia. Tightly embedded in lung tissue.
Terminal bronchioles	14–15	32,768†	0.7†	2.0†	113.0†	Generally 2 or 3 orders so designated; morphology not significantly different from orders 11–13.
Respiratory bronchioles	16–18	262,144†	0.5†	1.2†	534.0†	Definite class; bronchiolar cuboidal epithelium present, but scattered alveoli are present giving these airways a gas exchange function. Order 16 often called first-order respiratory bronchiole; 17, second-order; 18, third-order.
Alveolar ducts	19–22	4,194,304†	0.4†	0.8†	5,880.0†	No bronchial epithelium; have no surface except connective tissue framework; open into alveoli.
Alveolar sacs	23	8,388,608	0.4	0.6	11,800.0	No reason to assign a special name; are really short alveolar ducts.
Alveoli	24	300,000,000	0.2			Pulmonary capillaries are in the septae that form the alveoli.

*The number of airways in each generation is based on regular dichotomous branching.

†Numbers refer to last generation in each group.

Source: Used with permission from Staub [1963] and Weibel [1963]; adapted by Comroe [1965].

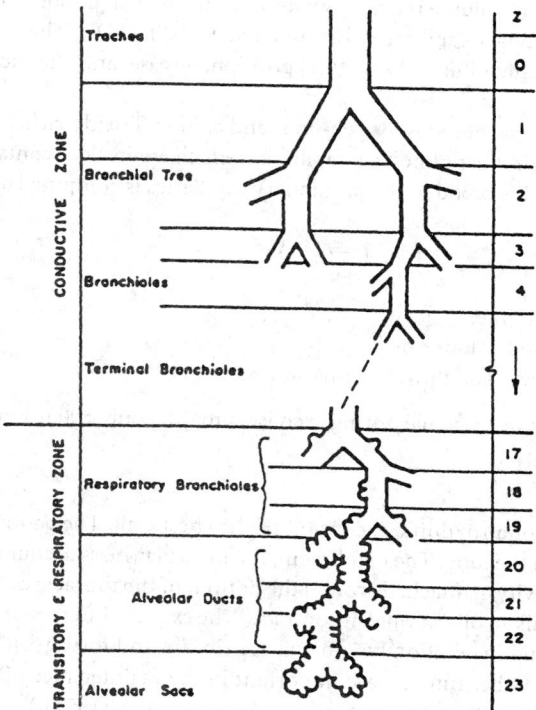

FIGURE 7.2 General architecture of conductive and transitory airways. (Used with permission from Weibel, 1963.) In the conductive zone air is conducted to and from the lungs while in the respiration zone, gas exchange occurs.

Molecular diffusion within the alveolar volume is responsible for mixing of the enclosed gas. Due to small alveolar dimensions, complete mixing probably occurs in less than 10 ms, fast enough that alveolar mixing time does not limit gaseous diffusion to or from the blood [Astrand and Rodahl, 1970].

Of particular importance to proper alveolar operation is a thin surface coating of surfactant. Without this material, large alveoli would tend to enlarge and small alveoli would collapse. It is the present view that surfactant acts like a detergent, changing the stress-strain relationship of the alveolar wall and thereby stabilizing the lung [Johnson, 1991].

Pulmonary Circulation

There is no true pulmonary analogue to the systemic arterioles, since the pulmonary circulation occurs under relatively low pressure [West, 1977]. Pulmonary blood vessels, especially capillaries and venules, are very thin walled and flexible. Unlike systemic capillaries, pulmonary capillaries increase in diameter, and pulmonary capillaries within alveolar walls separate adjacent alveoli with increases in blood pressure or decreases in alveolar pressure. Flow, therefore, is significantly influenced by elastic deformation. Although pulmonary circulation is largely unaffected by neural and chemical control, it does respond promptly to hypoxia.

There is also a high-pressure systemic blood delivery system to the bronchi that is completely independent of the pulmonary low-pressure ($\sim$3330 N/m^2) circulation in healthy individuals. In diseased states, however, bronchial arteries are reported to enlarge when pulmonary blood flow is reduced, and some arteriovenous shunts become prominent [West, 1977].

Total pulmonary blood volume is approximately 300 to 500 cm³ in normal adults, with about 60 to 100 cm³ in the pulmonary capillaries [Astrand and Rodahl, 1970]. This value, however, is quite variable, depending on such things as posture, position, disease, and chemical composition of the blood [Kline, 1976].

Since pulmonary arterial blood is oxygen-poor and carbon dioxide-rich, it exchanges excess carbon dioxide for oxygen in the pulmonary capillaries, which are in close contact with alveolar walls. At rest, the transit time for blood in the pulmonary capillaries is computed as

$$t = V_c / \dot{V}_c$$

where t = blood transit time, s
$\quad V_c$ = capillary blood volume, m³
$\quad \dot{V}_c$ = total capillary blood flow = cardiac output, m³/s

and is somewhat less than 1 s, while during exercise it may be only 500 ms or even less.

Respiratory Muscles

The lungs fill because of a rhythmic expansion of the chest wall. The action is indirect in that no muscle acts directly on the lung. The diaphragm, the muscular mass accounting for 75% of the expansion of the chest cavity, is attached around the bottom of the thoracic cage, arches over the liver, and moves downward like a piston when it contracts. The external intercostal muscles are positioned between the ribs and aid inspiration by moving the ribs up and forward. This, then, increases the volume of the thorax. Other muscles are important in the maintenance of thoracic shape during breathing. (For details, see Ruch and Patton [1966] and Johnson [1991].)

Quiet expiration is usually considered to be passive; i.e., pressure to force air from the lungs comes from elastic expansion of the lungs and chest wall. During moderate to severe exercise, the abdominal and internal intercostal muscles are very important in forcing air from the lungs much more quickly than would otherwise occur. Inspiration requires intimate contact between lung tissues, pleural tissues (the pleura is the membrane surrounding the lungs), and chest wall and diaphragm. This is accomplished by reduced intrathoracic pressure (which tends toward negative values) during inspiration.

Viewing the lungs as an entire unit, one can consider the lungs to be elastic sacs within an air-tight barrel—the thorax—which is bounded by the ribs and the diaphragm. Any movement of these two boundaries alters the volume of the lungs. The normal breathing cycle in humans is accomplished by the active contraction of the inspiratory muscles, which enlarges the thorax. This enlargement lowers intrathoracic and intrapleural pressure even further, pulls on the lungs, and enlarges the alveoli, alveolar ducts, and bronchioli, expanding the alveolar gas and decreasing its pressure below atmospheric. As a result, air at atmospheric pressure flows easily into the nose, mouth, and trachea.

7.2   Lung Volumes and Gas Exchange

Of primary importance to lung functioning is the movement and mixing of gases within the respiratory system. Depending on the anatomic level under consideration, gas movement is determined mainly by diffusion or convection.

Without the thoracic musculature and rib cage, as mentioned above, the barely inflated lungs would occupy a much smaller space than they occupy in situ. However, the thoracic cage holds them open. Conversely, the lungs exert an influence on the thorax, holding it smaller than should be the case without the lungs. Because the lungs and thorax are connected by tissue, the volume occupied by both together is between the extremes represented by relaxed lungs alone and thoracic cavity alone. The resting volume V_R, then, is that volume occupied by the lungs with glottis open and muscles relaxed.

Lung volumes greater than resting volume are achieved during inspiration. Maximum inspiration is represented by *inspiratory reserve volume* (IRV). IRV is the maximum additional volume that can be accommodated by the lung at the end of inspiration. Lung volumes less than resting volume do not normally occur at rest but do occur during exhalation while exercising (when exhalation is active). Maximum additional expiration, as measured from lung volume at the end of expiration, is called *expiratory reserve volume* (ERV). *Residual volume* is the amount of gas remaining in the lungs at the end of maximal expiration.

Tidal volume V_T is normally considered to be the volume of air entering the nose and mouth with each breath. Alveolar ventilation volume, the volume of fresh air that enters the alveoli during each breath, is always less than tidal volume. The extent of this difference in volume depends primarily on the *anatomic dead space,* the 150- to 160-ml internal volume of the conducting airway passages. The term *dead* is quite appropriate, since it represents wasted respiratory effort; i.e., no significant gas exchange occurs across the thick walls of the trachea, bronchi, and bronchiolus. Since normal tidal volume at rest is usually about 500 ml of air per breath, one can easily calculate that because of the presence of this dead space, about 340 to 350 ml of fresh air actually penetrates the alveoli and becomes involved in the gas exchange process. An additional 150 to 160 ml of stale air exhaled during the previous breath is also drawn into the alveoli.

The term *volume* is used for elemental differences of lung volume, whereas the term *capacity* is used for combination of lung volumes. Figure 7.3 illustrates the interrelationship between each of the following lung volumes and capacities:

1. *Total lung capacity* (TLC): The amount of gas contained in the lung at the end of maximal inspiration.
2. *Forced vital capacity* (FVC): The maximal volume of gas that can be forcefully expelled after maximal inspiration.
3. *Inspiratory capacity* (IC): The maximal volume of gas that can be inspired from the resting expiratory level.
4. *Functional residual capacity* (FRC): The volume of gas remaining after normal expiration. It will be noted that functional residual capacity (FRC) is the same as the resting volume. There is a small difference, however, between resting volume and FRC because FRC is measured while the patient breathes, whereas resting volume is measured with no breathing. FRC is properly defined only at end-expiration at rest and not during exercise.

These volumes and specific capacities, represented in Fig. 7.3, have led to the development of specific tests (that will be discussed below) to quantify the status of the pulmonary system. Typical values for these volumes and capacities are provided in Table 7.2.

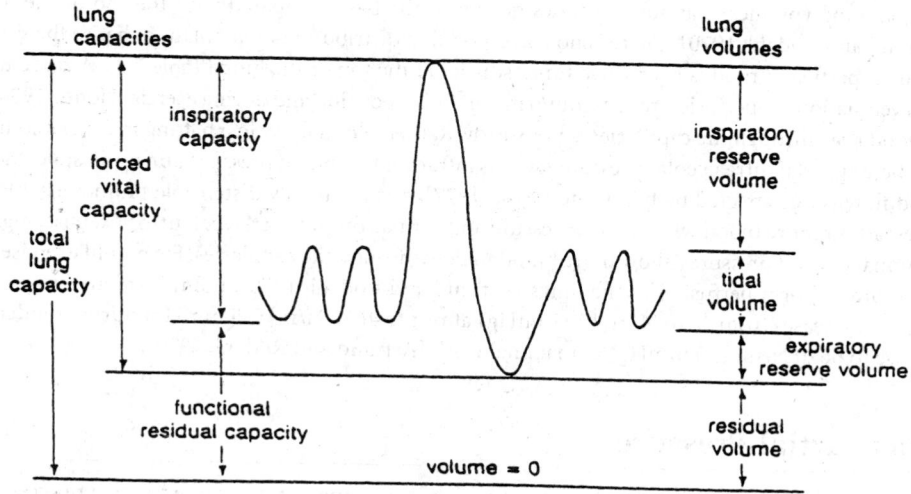

FIGURE 7.3 Lung capacities and lung volumes.

TABLE 7.2   Typical Lung Volumes for Normal, Healthy Males

Lung Volume		Normal Values
Total lung capacity (TLC)	$6.0 \times 10^{-3} m^3$	$(6,000\ cm^3)$
Residual volume (RV)	$1.2 \times 10^{-3}\ m^3$	$(1,200\ cm^3)$
Vital capacity (VC)	$4.8 \times 10^{-3}\ m^3$	$(4,800\ cm^3)$
Inspiratory reserve volume (IRV)	$3.6 \times 10^{-3}\ m^3$	$(3,600\ cm^3)$
Expiratory reserve volume (ERV)	$1.2 \times 10^{-3}\ m^3$	$(1,200\ cm^3)$
Functional residual capacity (FRC)	$2.4 \times 10^{-3}\ m^3$	$(2,400\ cm^3)$
Anatomic dead volume (V_D)	$1.5 \times 10^{-4}\ m^3$	$(150\ cm^3)$
Upper airways volume	$8.0 \times 10^{-5}\ m^3$	$(80\ cm^3)$
Lower airways volume	$7.0 \times 10^{-5}\ m^3$	$(70\ cm^3)$
Physiologic dead volume (V_D)	$1.8 \times 10^{-4}\ m^3$	$(180\ cm^3)$
Minute volume ($\dot{V}e$) at rest	$1.0 \times 10^{-4}\ m^3/s$	$(6,000\ cm^3/min)$
Respiratory period (T) at rest	$4\ s$	
Tidal volume (V_T) at rest	$4.0 \times 10^{-4}\ m^3$	$(400\ cm^3)$
Alveolar ventilation volume (V_A) at rest	$2.5 \times 10^{-4}\ m^3$	$(250\ cm^3)$
Minute volume during heavy exercise	$1.7 \times 10^{-3}\ m^3/s$	$(10,000\ cm^3/min)$
Respiratory period during heavy exercise	$1.2\ s$	
Tidal volume during heavy exercise	$2.0 \times 10^{-3}\ m^3$	$(2,000\ cm^3)$
Alveolar ventilation volume during exercise	$1.8 \times 10^{-3}\ m^3$	$(1,820\ cm^3)$

Source: Adapted and used with permission from Forster et al [1986].

7.3   Perfusion of the Lung

For gas exchange to occur properly in the lung, air must be delivered to the alveoli via the conducting airways, gas must diffuse from the alveoli to the capillaries through extremely thin walls, and the same gas must be removed to the cardiac atrium by blood flow. This three-step process involves (1) alveolar ventilation, (2) the process of diffusion, and (3) ventilatory perfusion, which involves pulmonary blood flow. Obviously, an alveolus that is ventilated but not perfused cannot exchange gas. Similarly, a perfused alveolus that is not properly ventilated cannot exchange gas. The most efficient gas exchange occurs when ventilation and perfusion are matched.

There is a wide range of ventilation-to-perfusion ratios that naturally occur in various regions of the lung [Johnson, 1991]. Blood flow is somewhat affected by posture because of the effects of gravity. In the upright position, there is a general reduction in the volume of blood in the thorax, allowing for larger lung volume. Gravity also influences the distribution of blood, such that the perfusion of equal lung volumes is about five times greater at the base compared with the top of the lung [Astrand and Rodahl, 1970]. There is no corresponding distribution of ventilation; hence the ventilation-to-perfusion ratio is nearly five times smaller at the top of the lung (Table 7.3). A more uniform ventilation-to-perfusion ratio is found in the supine position and during exercise [Jones, 1984b].

Blood flow through the capillaries is not steady. Rather, blood flows in a halting manner and may even be stopped if intraalveolar pressure exceeds intracapillary blood pressure during diastole. Mean blood flow is not affected by heart rate [West, 1977], but the highly distensible pulmonary blood vessels admit more blood when blood pressure and cardiac output increase. During exercise, higher pulmonary blood pressures allow more blood to flow through the capillaries. Even mild exercise favors more uniform perfusion of the lungs [Astrand and Rodahl, 1970]. Pulmonary artery systolic pressure increases from $2670\ N/m^2$ (20 mmHg) at rest to $4670\ N/m^2$ (35 mmHg) during moderate exercise to $6670\ N/m^2$ (50 mmHg) at maximal work [Astrand and Rodahl, 1970].

7.4   Gas Partial Pressure

The primary purpose of the respiratory system is gas exchange. In the gas-exchange process, gas must diffuse through the alveolar space, across tissue, and through plasma into the red blood cell,

TABLE 7.3   Ventilation-to-Perfusion Ratios from the Top to Bottom of the Lung of a Normal Man in the Sitting Position

Percent Lung Volume, %	Alveolar Ventilation Rate, cm³/s	Perfusion Rate, cm³/s	Ventilation-to-Perfusion Ratio
	Top		
7	4.0	1.2	3.3
8	5.5	3.2	1.8
10	7.0	5.5	1.3
11	8.7	8.3	1.0
12	9.8	11.0	0.90
13	11.2	13.8	0.80
13	12.0	16.3	0.73
13	13.0	19.2	0.68
	Bottom		
13	13.7	21.5	0.63
100	84.9	100.0	

Source: Used with permission from West [1962].

where it finally chemically joins to hemoglobin. A similar process occurs for carbon dioxide elimination.

As long as intermolecular interactions are small, most gases of physiologic significance can be considered to obey the ideal gas law:

$$pV = nRT$$

where p = pressure, N/m²
   V = volume of gas, m³
   n = number of moles, mol
   R = gas constant, (N × m)/(mol × K)
   T = absolute temperature, K

The ideal gas law can be applied without error up to atmospheric pressure; it can be applied to a mixture of gases, such as air, or to its constituents, such as oxygen or nitrogen. All individual gases in a mixture are considered to fill the total volume and have the same temperature but reduced pressures. The pressure exerted by each individual gas is called the *partial pressure* of the gas.

Dalton's law states that the total pressure is the sum of the partial pressures of the constituents of a mixture:

$$p = \sum_{i=1}^{N} p_i$$

where p_i = partial pressure of the ith constituent, N/m²
   N = total number of constituents

Dividing the ideal gas law for a constituent by that for the mixture gives

$$\frac{P_i V}{PV} = \frac{n_i R_i T}{nRT}$$

so that

$$\frac{p_i}{p} = \frac{n_i R_i}{nR}$$

which states that the partial pressure of a gas may be found if the total pressure, mole fraction, and ratio of gas constants are known. For most respiratory calculations, p will be considered to be the pressure of 1 atmosphere, 101 kN/m². Avogadro's principle states that different gases at the same temperature and pressure contain equal numbers of molecules:

$$\frac{V_1}{V_2} = \frac{nR_1}{nR_2} = \frac{R_1}{R_2}$$

Thus

$$\frac{p_i}{p} = \frac{V_i}{V}$$

where V_i/V is the volume fraction of a constituent in air and is therefore dimensionless. Table 7.4 provides individual gas constants, as well as volume fractions, of constituent gases of air.

Gas pressures and volumes can be measured for many different temperature and humidity conditions. Three of these are body temperature and pressure, saturated (BTPS); ambient temperature and pressure (ATP); and standard temperature and pressure, dry (STPD). To calculate constituent partial pressures at STPD, total pressure is taken as barometric pressure minus vapor pressure of water in the atmosphere:

$$p_i = (V_i/V)(p - pH_2O)$$

where p = total pressure, kN/m²
pH_2O = vapor pressure of water in atmosphere, kN/m²

and V_i/V as a ratio does not change in the conversion process.

Gas volume at STPD is converted from ambient condition volume as

$$V_i = V_{amb}[273/(273 + \Theta)][(p - pH_2O)/101.3]$$

where V_i = volume of gas i corrected to STPD, m³
V_{amb} = volume of gas i at ambient temperature and pressure, m³
Θ = ambient temperature, °C
p = ambient total pressure, kN/m²
pH_2O = vapor pressure of water in the air, kN/m²

Partial pressures and gas volumes may be expressed in BTPS conditions. In this case, gas partial pressures are usually known from other measurements. Gas volumes are converted from ambient conditions by

$$V_i = V_{amb}[310/(273 + \Theta)][(p - pH_2O)/p - 6.28]$$

Table 7.5 provides gas partial pressure throughout the respiratory and circulatory systems.

7.5 Pulmonary Mechanics

The respiratory system exhibits properties of resistance, compliance, and inertance analogous to the electrical properties of resistance, capacitance, and inductance. Of these, inertance is generally considered to be of less importance than the other two properties.

TABLE 7.4 Molecular Masses, Gas Constants, and Volume Fractions for Air and Constituents

Constituent	Molecular Mass, kg/mol	Gas Constant, N·m/(mol·K)	Volume Fraction in Air, m³/m³
Air	29.0	286.7	1.0000
Ammonia	17.0	489.1	0.0000
Argon	39.9	208.4	0.0093
Carbon dioxide	44.0	189.0	0.0003
Carbon monoxide	28.0	296.9	0.0000
Helium	4.0	2078.6	0.0000
Hydrogen	2.0	4157.2	0.0000
Nitrogen	28.0	296.9	0.7808
Oxygen	32.0	259.8	0.2095

Note: Universal gas constant is 8314.34 N·m/kg·mol·K.

Resistance is the ratio of pressure to flow:

$$R = p/V$$

where R = resistance, N × s/m⁵

p = pressure, N/m²

V = volume flow rate, m³/s

Resistance can be found in the conducting airways, in the lung tissue, and in the tissues of the chest wall. Airways exhalation resistance is usually higher than airways inhalation resistance because the surrounding lung tissue pulls the smaller, more distensible airways open when the lung is being inflated. Thus airways inhalation resistance is somewhat dependent on lung volume, and airways exhalation resistance can be very lung volume–dependent [Johnson, 1991].

Compliance is the ratio of lung volume to lung pressure:

$$C = V/p$$

where C = compliance, m⁵/N,

V = lung volume/m³

p = pressure, N/m²

As the lung is stretched, it acts as an expanded balloon that tends to push the air out and return to its normal size. The lung pressure-flow curve is S-shaped, indicating that compliance decreases at

TABLE 7.5 Gas Partial Pressures (kN/m²) Throughout the Respiratory and Circulatory Systems

Gas	Inspired Air*	Alveolar Air	Expired Air	Mixed Venous Blood	Arterial Blood	Muscle Tissue
H_2O	—	6.3	6.3	6.3	6.3	6.3
CO_2	0.04	5.3	4.2	6.1	5.3	6.7
O_2	21.2	14.0	15.5	5.3	13.3	4.0
N_2†	80.1	75.7	75.3	76.4	76.4	76.4
Total	101.3	101.3	101.3	94.1	101.3	93.4

*Inspired air considered dry for convenience

†Includes all other inert components.

Source: Used with permission from Astrand and Rodahl [1970].

extremes of lung volume. Airways, lung tissue, and chest wall also contribute to pulmonary system compliance [Johnson, 1991].

7.6   Respiratory Control

Control of respiration occurs in many different cerebral structures [Johnson, 1991] and regulates many things [Hornbein, 1981]. Respiration must be controlled to produce the respiratory rhythm, ensure adequate gas exchange, protect against inhalation of poisonous substances, assist in maintenance of body pH, remove irritations, and minimize energy cost. Respiratory control is more complex than cardiac control for at least three reasons:

1. Airways airflow occurs in both directions.
2. The respiratory system interfaces directly with the environment outside the body.
3. Parts of the respiratory system are used for other functions, such as swallowing and speaking.

As a result, respiratory muscular action must be exquisitely coordinated; it must be prepared to protect itself against environmental onslaught, and breathing must be temporarily suspended on demand.

All control systems require sensors, controllers, and effectors. Figure 7.4 presents the general scheme for respiratory control. There are mechanoreceptors throughout the respiratory system. For example, nasal receptors are important in sneezing, apnea (cessation of breathing), bronchodilation, bronchoconstriction, and the secretion of mucus. Laryngeal receptors are important in coughing, apnea, swallowing, bronchoconstriction, airway mucus secretion, and laryngeal constriction. Tracheobronchial receptors are important in coughing, pulmonary hypertension, bronchoconstriction, laryngeal constriction, and mucus production. Other mechanoreceptors are important in the generation of the respiratory pattern and are involved with respiratory sensation.

Respiratory chemoreceptors exist peripherally in the aortic arch and carotic bodies and centrally in the ventral medulla oblongata of the brain. These receptors are sensitive to partial pressures of CO_2 and O_2 and to blood pH.

The respiratory controller is located in several places in the brain. Each location appears to have its own function. Unlike the heart, the basic respiratory rhythm is not generated within the lungs but rather in the brain and is transmitted to the respiratory muscles by the phrenic nerve.

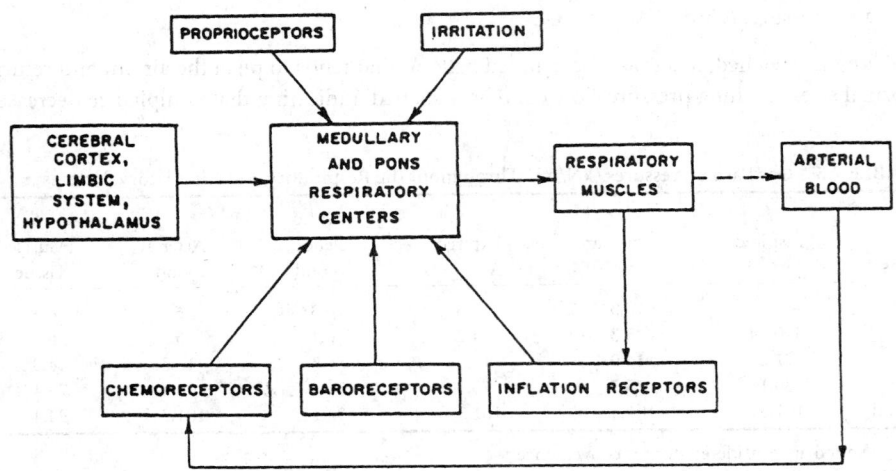

FIGURE 7.4   General scheme of respiratory control.

Effector organs are mainly the respiratory muscles, as described previously. Other effectors are muscles located in the airways and tissues for mucus secretion. Control of respiration appears to be based on two criteria: (1) removal of excess CO_2 and (2) minimization of energy expenditure. It is not the lack of oxygen that stimulates respiration but increased CO_2 partial pressure that acts as a powerful respiratory stimulus. Because of the buffering action of blood bicarbonate, blood pH usually falls as more CO_2 is produced in the working muscles. Lower blood pH also stimulates respiration.

A number of respiratory adjustments are made to reduce energy expenditure during exercise: Respiration rate increases, the ratio of inhalation time to exhalation time decreases, respiratory flow waveshapes become more trapezoidal, and expiratory reserve volume decreases. Other adjustments to reduce energy expenditure have been theorized but not proven [Johnson, 1991].

7.7 The Pulmonary Function Laboratory

The purpose of a pulmonary function laboratory is to obtain clinically useful data from patients with respiratory dysfunction. The pulmonary function tests (PFTs) within this laboratory fulfill a variety of functions. They permit (1) quantification of a patient's breathing deficiency, (2) diagnosis of different types of pulmonary diseases, (3) evaluation of a patient's response to therapy, and (4) preoperative screening to determine whether the presence of lung disease increases the risk of surgery.

Although PFTs can provide important information about a patient's condition, the limitations of these tests must be considered. First, they are nonspecific in that they cannot determine which portion of the lungs is diseased, only that the disease is present. Second, PFTs must be considered along with the medical history, physical examination, x-ray examination, and other diagnostic procedures to permit a complete evaluation. Finally, the major drawback to *some PFTs* is that they require full patient cooperation and for this reason cannot be conducted on critically ill patients. Consider some of the most widely used PFTs: spirometry, body plethysmography, and diffusing capacity.

Spirometry

The simplest PFT is the spirometry maneuver. In this test, the patient inhales to total lung capacity (TLC) and exhales forcefully to residual volume. The patient exhales into a displacement bell chamber that sits on a water seal. As the bell rises, a pen coupled to the bell chamber inscribes a tracing on a rotating drum. The spirometer offers very little resistance to breathing; therefore, the shape of the spirometry curve (Fig. 7.5) is purely a function of the patient's lung compliance, chest compliance, and airway resistance. At high lung volumes, a rise in intrapleural pressure results in greater expiratory flows. However, at intermediate and low lung volumes, the expiratory flow is independent of effort after a certain intrapleural pressure is reached.

Measurements made from the spirometry curve can determine the degree of a patient's ventilatory obstruction. Forced vital capacity (FVC), forced expiratory volumes (FEV), and forced expiratory flows (FEF) can be determined. The FEV indicates the volume that has been exhaled from TLC for a particular time interval. For example, $FEV_{0.5}$ is the volume exhaled during the first half-second of expiration, and $FEV_{1.0}$ is the volume exhaled during the first second of expiration; these are graphically represented in Fig. 7.5. Note that the more severe the ventilatory obstruction, the lower are the timed volumes ($FEV_{0.5}$ and $FEV_{1.0}$). The FEF is a measure of the average flow (volume/time) over specified portions of the spirometry curve and is represented by the slope of a straight line drawn between volume levels. The average flow over the first quarter of the forced expiration is the $FEF_{0-25\%}$, whereas the average flow over the middle 50% of the FVC is the $FEF_{25-75\%}$. These values are obtained directly from the spirometry curves. The less steep curves of obstructed patients would result in lower values of $FEF_{0-25\%}$ and $FEF_{25-75\%}$ compared with normal values, which are predicted on the basis of the patient's sex, age, and height. Equations for normal values are available from statistical analysis of data obtained from a normal population. Test results are then interpreted as a percentage of normal.

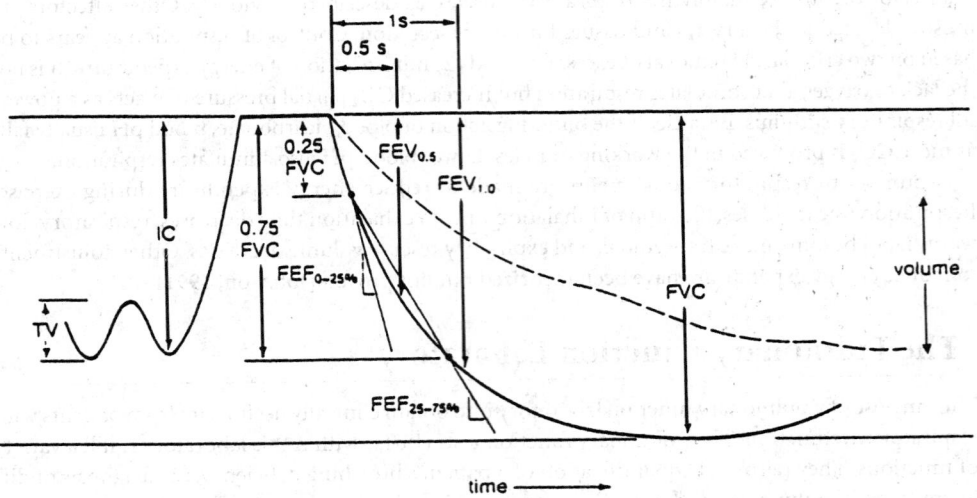

FIGURE 7.5 Typical spirometry tracing obtained during testing: inspiratory capacity (IC), tidal volume (TV), forced vital capacity (FVC), forced expiratory volume (FEV), and forced expiratory flows. Dashed line represents a patient with obstructive lung disease; solid line represents a normal, healthy individual.

Another way of presenting a spirometry curve is as a flow-volume curve. Figure 7.6 represents typical flow-volume curve. The expiratory flow is plotted against the exhaled volume, indicating the maximum flow that may be reached at each degree of lung inflation. Since there is no time axis, a timer must mark the $FEV_{0.5}$ and $FEV_{1.0}$ on the tracing. To obtain these flow-volume curves in the laboratory, the patient usually exhales through a *pneumotach*. The most widely used pneumotach measures a pressure drop across a flow-resistive element. The resistance to flow is constant over the measuring range of the device; therefore, the pressure drop is proportional to the flow through the tube. This signal, which is indicative of flow, is then integrated to determine the volume of gas that has passed through the tube.

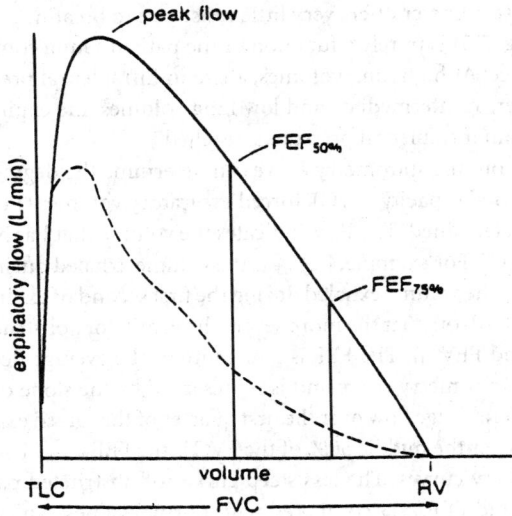

FIGURE 7.6 Flow-volume curve obtained from a spirometry maneuver. Solid line is a normal curve; dashed line represents a patient with obstructive lung disease.

Another type of pneumotach is the heated-element type. In this device, a small heated mass responds to airflow by cooling. As the element cools, a greater current is necessary to maintain a constant temperature. This current is proportional to the airflow through the tube. Again, to determine the volume that has passed through the tube, the flow signal is integrated.

The flow-volume loop in Fig. 7.7 is a dramatic representation displaying inspiratory and expiratory curves for both normal breathing and maximal breathing. The result is a graphic representation of the patient's reserve capacity in relation to normal breathing. For example, the normal patient's tidal breathing loop is small compared with the patient's maximum breathing loop. During these times of stress, this tidal breathing loop can be increased to the boundaries of the outer ventilatory loop. This increase in ventilation provides the greater gas exchange needed during the stressful situation. Compare this condition with that of the patient with obstructive lung disease. Not only is the tidal breathing loop larger than normal, but the maximal breathing loop is smaller than normal. The result is a decreased ventilatory reserve, limiting the individual's ability to move air in and out of the lungs. As the disease progresses, the outer loop becomes smaller, and the inner loop becomes larger.

The primary use of spirometry is in detection of obstructive lung disease that results from increased resistance to flow through the airways. This can occur in several ways:

1. Deterioration of the structure of the smaller airways that results in early airways closure.
2. Decreased airway diameters caused by bronchospasm or the presence of secretions increases the airway's resistance to airflow.
3. Partial blockage of a large airway by a tumor decreases airway diameter and causes turbulent flow.

Spirometry has its limitations, however. It can measure only ventilated volumes. It cannot measure lung capacities that contain the residual volume. Measurements of TLC, FRC, and RV have diagnostic value in defining lung overdistension or restrictive pulmonary disease; the body plethysmograph can determine these absolute lung volumes.

Body Plethysmography

In a typical body plethysmograph, the patient is put in an airtight enclosure and breathes through a pneumotach. The flow signal through the pneumotach is integrated and recorded as tidal breathing. At the end of a normal expiration (at FRC), an electronically operated shutter occludes the tube

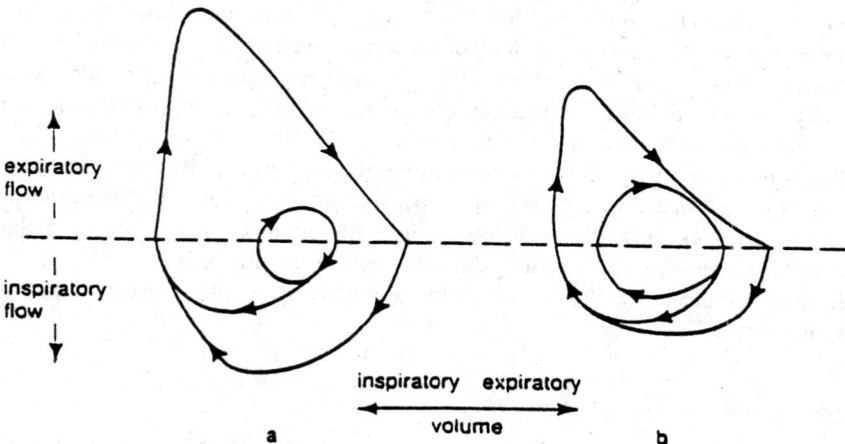

FIGURE 7.7 Typical flow-volume loops. (a) Normal flow-volume loop. (b) Flow-volume loop of patient with obstructive lung disease.

through which the patient is breathing. At this time the patient pants lightly against the occluded airway. Since there is no flow, pressure measured at the mouth must equal alveolar pressure. But movements of the chest that compress gas in the lung simultaneously rarify the air in the plethysmograph, and vice versa. The pressure change in the plethysmograph can be used to calculate the volume change in the plethysmograph, which is the same as the volume change in the chest. This leads directly to determination of FRC.

At the same time, alveolar pressure can be correlated to plethysmographic pressure. Therefore, when the shutter is again opened and flow rate is measured, airway resistance can be obtained as the ratio of alveolar pressure (obtainable from plethysmographic pressure) to flow rate [Carr and Brown, 1993]. Airway resistance is usually measured during panting, at a nominal lung volume of FRC and flow rate of ± 1 liter/s.

Airway resistance during inspiration is increased in patients with asthma, bronchitis, and upper respiratory tract infections. Expiratory resistance is elevated in patients with emphysema, since the causes of increased expiratory airway resistance are decreased driving pressures and the airway collapse. Airway resistance also may be used to determine the response of obstructed patients to bronchodilator medications.

Diffusing Capacity

So far the mechanical components of airflow through the lungs have been discussed. Another important parameter is the diffusing capacity of the lung, the rate at which oxygen or carbon dioxide travel from the alveoli to the blood (or vice versa for carbon dioxide) in the pulmonary capillaries. Diffusion of gas across a barrier is directly related to the surface area of the barrier and inversely related to the thickness. Also, diffusion is directly proportional to the solubility of the gas in the barrier material and inversely related to the molecular weight of the gas.

Lung diffusing capacity (D_L) is usually determined for carbon monoxide but can be related to oxygen diffusion. The popular method of measuring carbon monoxide diffusion utilizes a rebreathing technique in which the patient rebreathes rapidly in and out of a bag for approximately 30 s. Figure 7.8 illustrates the test apparatus. The patient begins breathing from a bag containing a known volume of gas consisting of 0.3% to 0.5% carbon monoxide made with heavy oxygen, 0.3% to 0.5% acetylene, 5% helium, 21% oxygen, and a balance of nitrogen. As the patient rebreathes the gas mixture in the bag, a modified mass spectrometer continuously analyzes it during both inspiration and expiration. During the rebreathing procedure, the carbon monoxide disappears from the patient-bag system; the rate at which this occurs is a function of the lung diffusing capacity.

The helium is inert and insoluble in lung tissue and blood and equilibrates quickly in unobstructed patients, indicating the dilution level of the test gas. Acetylene, on the other hand, is soluble in blood and is used to determine the blood flow through the pulmonary capillaries. Carbon monoxide is bound very tightly to hemoglobin and is used to obtain diffusing capacity at a constant pressure gradient across the alveolar-capillary membrane.

Decreased lung diffusing capacity can occur from the thickening of the alveolar membrane or the capillary membrane as well as the presence of interstitial fluid from edema. All these abnormalities increase the barrier thickness and cause a decrease in diffusing capacity. In addition, a characteristic of specific lung diseases is impaired lung diffusing capacity. For example, fibrotic lung tissue exhibits a decreased permeability to gas transfer, whereas pulmonary emphysema results in the loss of diffusion surface area.

Defining Terms

Alveoli: Respiratory airway terminals where most gas exchange with the pulmonary circulation takes place.

Diffusion: The process whereby a material moves from a region of higher concentration to a region of lower concentration.

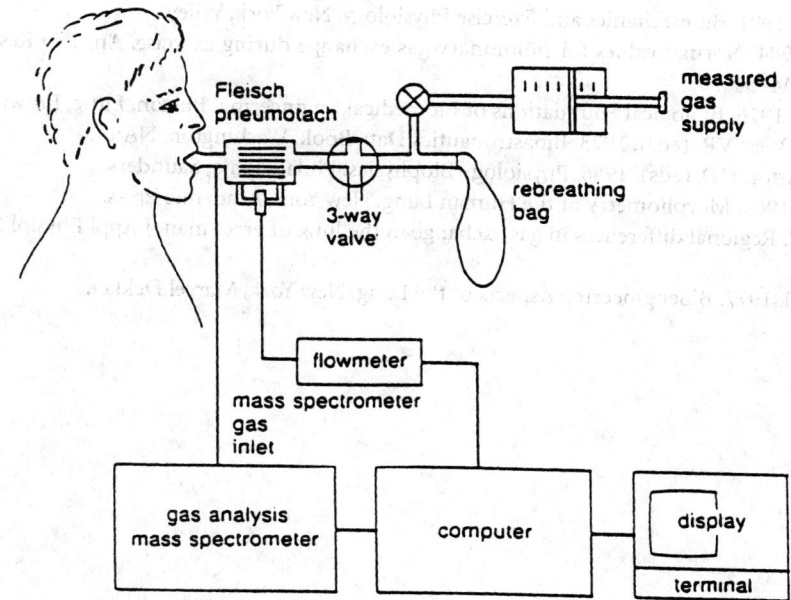

FIGURE 7.8 Typical system configuration for the measurement of rebreathing pulmonary diffusing capacity.

BTPS: Body temperature (37°C) and standard pressure (1 atm), saturated (6.28 kN/m²)

Chemoreceptors: Neural receptors sensitive to chemicals such as gas partial pressures.

Dead space: The portion of the respiratory system that does not take part in gas exchange with the blood.

Expiration: The breathing process whereby air is expelled from the mouth and nose. Also called *exhalation*.

Functional residual capacity: The lung volume at rest without breathing.

Inspiration: The breathing process whereby air is taken into the mouth and nose. Also called *inhalation*.

Mass spectrometer: A device that identifies relative concentrations of gases by means of mass-to-charge ratios of gas ions.

Mechanoreceptors: Neural receptors sensitive to mechanical inputs such as stretch, pressure, irritants, etc.

Partial pressure: The pressure that a gas would exert if it were the only constituent.

Perfusion: Blood flow to the lungs.

Plethysmography: Any measuring technique that depends on a volume change.

Pleura: The membrane surrounding the lung.

Pneumotach: A measuring device for airflow.

Pulmonary circulation: Blood flow from the right cardiac ventricle that perfuses the lung and is in intimate contact with alveolar membranes for effective gas exchange.

STPD: Standard temperature (0°C) and pressure (1 atm), dry (moisture removed)

Ventilation: Airflow to the lungs.

References

Astrand PO, Rodahl K. 1970. Textbook of Work Physiology. New York, McGraw-Hill.

Carr JJ, Brown JM. 1993. Introduction to Biomedical Equipment Technology. Englewood Cliffs, NJ, Prentice-Hall.

Hornbein TF (ed). 1981. Regulation of Breathing. New York, Marcel Dekker.

Johnson AT. 1991. Biomechanics and Exercise Physiology. New York, Wiley.

Jones NL. 1984. Normal values for pulmonary gas exchange during exercise. Am Rev Respir Dis 129:544–546.

Kline J (ed). 1976. Biological Foundations of Biomedical Engineering. Boston, Little, Brown.

Parker JF Jr, West VR. (eds). 1973. Bioastronautics Data Book. Washington, NASA.

Ruch TC, Patton HD. (eds). 1966. Physiology Biophysics. Philadelphia, Saunders.

Weibel, ER. 1963. Morphometry of the Human Lung. New York, Academic Press.

West J. 1962. Regional differences in gas exchange in the lung of erect man. J Appl Physiol 17:893–898.

West JB (ed). 1977. Bioengineering Aspects of the Lung. New York, Marcel Dekker.

Historical Perspectives 1
Cardiac Pacing—Historical Highlights

Leslie A. Geddes
Purdue University

The origin of modern cardiac pacing is accepted by many as the time when the first pacemaker was implanted without the need for opening the chest. This event was described by Parsonnet et al. [1962], who combined the implantable pacemaker created by Greatbatch and Chardack [1959] with the right-ventricular catheter electrode described by Furman et al. [1959]. However, the need for cardiac pacing was recognized much earlier, and many interesting investigations were reported. It is the objective of this short historical note to describe these studies and show how they provided the background knowledge for modern cardiac pacing.

Cardiac Arrest During Anesthesia

Gaseous anesthesia with ether entered medicine about 1850. Although a good anesthetic, induction was difficult because ether irritates the mucous membranes of the airway. In the search for other agents, chloroform was popularized in the late 1860s by Simpson in Scotland. However, when chloroform was used, occasional respiratory and cardiac arrest occurred. Although respirators were available, there was no way of restarting the heart.

Although Steiner [1871] in Germany investigated electrical cardiac pacing on animals, the chloroform-arrested heart in human subjects was paced noninvasively by Green in the United Kingdom [1872]. Pointing out that sudden disappearance of the pulse was an occasional complication of chloroform anesthesia, he resuscitated five of seven cases of cardiac arrest by intermittently applying the output of a 300-V battery using hand-held electrodes applied to the base of the neck and to the lower left chest. It is interesting to observe that the electrode applied to the lower left chest stimulated the ventricles. The other electrode applied to the base of the neck delivered current to the phrenic nerve and twitched the diaphragm, causing a brisk inspiratory motion. Thus Green applied electrical cardiopulmonary resuscitation and successfully recovered five of seven patients. He advocated that every operating room should have a galvanic battery "at the ready" at all times for such emergencies.

Ziemssen [1882] in Germany had the opportunity to apply cardiac pacing to Catherina Serafin, a 42-year-old woman (Fig. HP1.1a) who had a large defect in the anterior left chest wall following resection of an enchondroma. The heart was only covered by skin, on which Ziemssen placed electrodes; he also recorded radial artery pulses. Using induction-coil shocks, he paced the heart using a stimulus frequency higher than that of the normal heart rate; i.e., he achieved capture. Figure HP1.1b illustrates ventricular pacing (between the arrows) at 140, 120, and 180 beats per minute.

After performing many studies on animals with hearts arrested by chloroform, McWilliam in the United Kingdom proposed the routine use of closed-chest pacing. Writing in the *British Medical Journal* [1889], he recommended:

> In order that such excitation [of the heart] should be as effective as possible, it is probably best to send the stimulating shocks through the whole heart, so that the auricles may come directly under their influence as well as the ventricles. In order to do this in man one electrode should be applied in front over the area of cardiac impulse, and the other over the region of the fourth dorsal vertebra behind, so that the induction shocks may traverse the organ. The electrodes

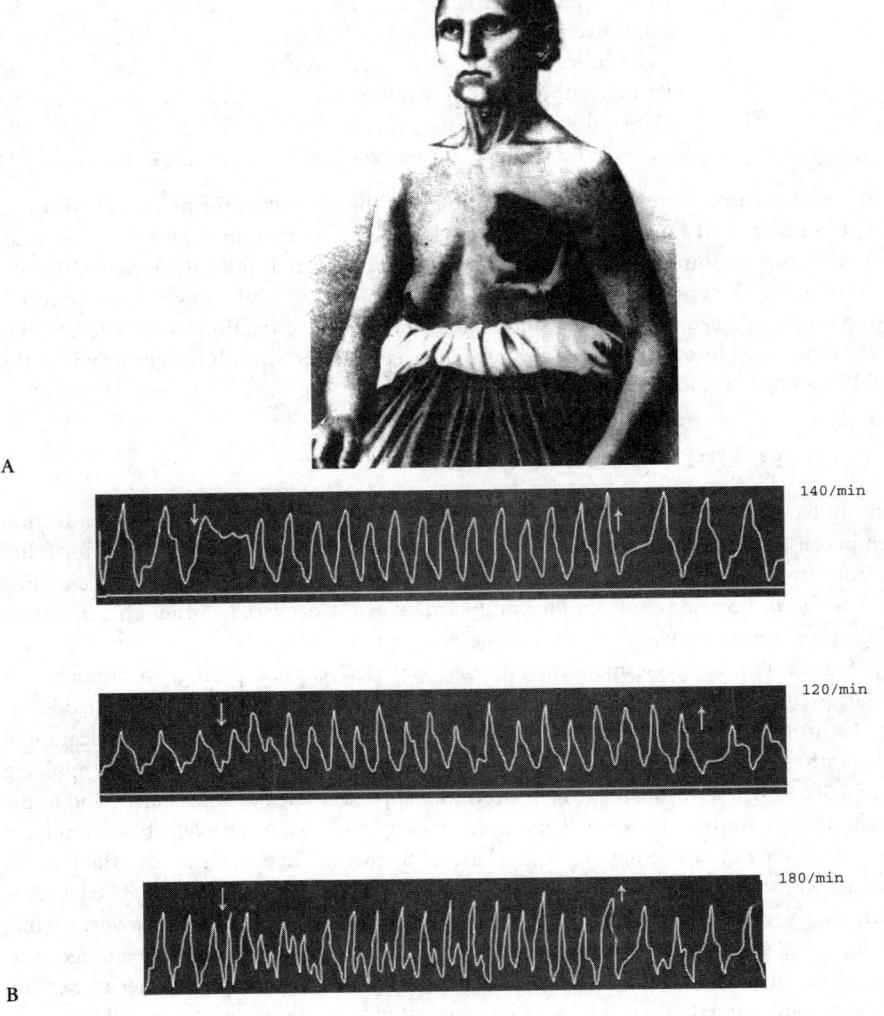

FIGURE HP1.1   Catherina Sarafin (*a*), a 42-year-old woman whose heart was paced by Ziemssen [1882] using induction-coil shocks. (*b*) The radial pulse, and between the arrows, pacing was carried out at the rates shown.

should be of considerable extent (for example, large sponge electrodes), and they and the skin should be well moistened with salt solution. The shocks employed should be strong, sufficient to excite powerful contraction in the voluntary muscles.

Such a method, it seems to me, is the only rational and effective one for stimulating by direct means the action of a heart which has been suddenly enfeebled or arrested in diastole by causes of a temporary and transient character. Of course, at the same time the expedient of artificial respiration must by no means be neglected, but on the contrary, most sedulously attended to.

Considerable time passed before the next cardiac pacing studies were reported. During that time, clinicians dealt with cardiac arrest by thrusting a hypodermic needle through the chest wall into the left ventricle and injecting epinephrine. Intentional cardiac pacing was not resumed until 1932, when Hyman [1932] in the United States pointed out that cardiac pacing could be practical clinically. He stated that Gould in Australia had stimulated a baby's heart using a chest electrode and a needle electrode thrust into the heart. Hyman stated that cardiac arrest was a common clinical event and that "random and badly executed procedures are used within the last minute in the hope of resuscitating the stopped heart." He called attention to the dubious value of injecting epinephrine directly into the left ventricle via a needle thrust into the thorax. He stated quite correctly (1) that it was the needle prick that evoked a ventricular contraction rather than the epinephrine, which obviously requires cardiac pumping to distribute it, and (2) the considerable danger of ventricular fibrillation from the needle stimulus and epinephrine, particularly in hypoxic hearts. Accordingly, he offered two solutions: (1) inject the epinephrine into an atrium and (2) apply rhythmic electrical stimuli to the needle thrust into an atrium. With the atrial injection of epinephrine, the risk of ventricular fibrillation is eliminated. It is unimportant if atrial fibrillation occurs, because the ventricles would be driven at a rapid rate and the epinephrine would be pumped through the circulatory system. The atrial fibrillation could be treated later with drugs. At that time there was no way of arresting ventricular fibrillation.

Hyman made a batteryless pacemaker for delivery of induction-shock stimuli (60 to 120 per minute) to the atria. His pacemaker (Fig. HP1.2) was powered by a hand-wound, spring-driven generator that provided 6 minutes of pacemaking without rewinding. He demonstrated the success of his portable, manually energized pacemaker by pacing guinea pig, rabbit, and (one) dog hearts that had been arrested by asphyxiation. He then used the pacemaker on a few human subjects. Unfortunately, there are no details of his clinical success, although he stated that the method of electrical cardiac pacemaking was gaining acceptance. However, this was a hope rather than a fact.

Closed-Chest Pacing for Stokes-Adams Disease

Interruption of the excitation from the atria to the ventricles (the main pumping chambers of the heart) is designated *atrioventricular (A-V) block*; Stokes-Adams disease causes A-V block. Although the ventricles have a low intrinsic rate, the A-V block does not develop immediately, and consciousness is usually lost at the onset of an attack. Even if the ventricles start to beat with their low intrinsic rate, cardiac output is seldom adequate. The application of rhythmic electrical stimuli to the ventricles provides adequate cardiac output.

Closed-chest ventricular pacing was introduced in the United States in 1952 when Zoll and colleagues [1952] reported successful cardiac pacemaking in 10 patients with A-V block. They first used needle electrodes inserted subcutaneously. A thyratron (capacitor-discharge) stimulator was employed which delivered 2-ms pulses. Later, Zoll [1955] used electrodes that were 3 in in diameter covered with a conducting paste, and these were found to be effective in a variety of electrode locations. The criterion for optimal location was pacing with the lower voltage. In one configuration, the negative electrode was located over the apex beat area and the other was on the right chest. Another location that appeared to produce less muscular twitching employed the negative electrode in the V_4–V_6 site for electrocardiography; the positive electrode was in the V_2–V_4 region. With either

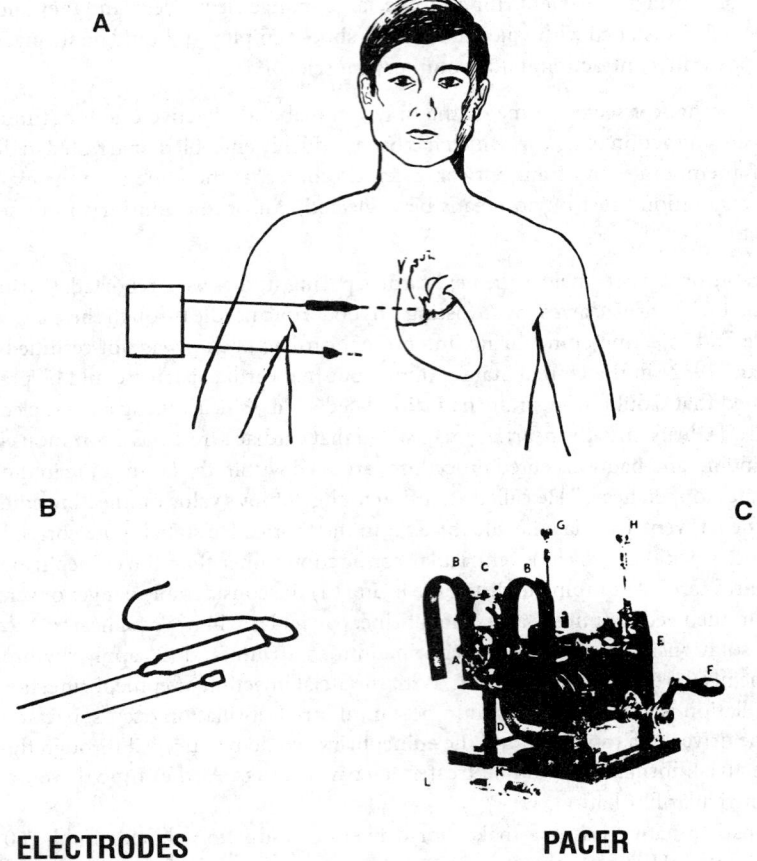

ELECTRODES   **PACER**

FIGURE HP1.2   Hyman's method of pacing the atria (*a*) using needle electrodes
(*b*). (*c*) His hand-wound pacemaker, which could provide 6 minutes of pacing.
(From Hyman AA. 1932. Arch Intern Med 50:283–305, by permission of AMA.)

location it was recommended that the spacing between the electrodes exceed 3 in. The stimulus voltage was 0 to 150 V, and the repetition rate was controllable from 30 to 180 per minute.

Zoll [1956] also introduced closed-chest ventricular defibrillation. Some of the early commercially available defibrillators also contained a pacemaker because following defibrillation the ventricles did not always start to beat. However, closed-chest pacing did not attract the attention of those who wished to pace conscious patients for prolonged periods. The muscle twitching and pain due to the strong, short-duration pacing stimuli made the method intolerable to many patients, albeit lifesaving. However, Zoll and his son, a physicist, found a way [1981] to reduce the pain considerably by using a long-duration pulse (40 ms) and high-impedance electrodes that employed a pad of a high-resistivity gel between the metal electrode and the skin. Use of this technique reduced the high current density under the perimeter of an electrode when placed directly on the skin. The muscle twitching was reduced by strategically locating the pacing electrodes on the chest. This technique is in use today.

Dawn of the Modern Era

In the early 1950s, cardiovascular surgery was becoming widespread because of the availability of the heart-lung machine and hypothermia. In some cases of heart surgery, an undesirable side effect was A-V block. To solve this problem, Weirich et al. [1958] demonstrated that direct heart stimulation in closed-chest patients could be achieved with surgically implanted slender-wire electrodes. In a series of experiments on animals, single and double electrodes were implanted in the ventricular myocardium at the time of surgery, and the leads were brought out through the chest wall. Complete control of ventricular rate (above the normal rate) was achieved. On January 30, 1957, the method was applied to the first human subjects, and Weirich et al. [1958] reported successful ventricular pacing in 18 patients with complete A-V block. One patient was paced for 21 days before the pacemaking could be discontinued. In these patients, a single myocardial electrode was implanted at the time of surgery. A chest electrode was used to complete the circuit. When pacing was to be discontinued, the myocardial electrode was withdrawn by a gentle pull. Such electrodes were frequently installed during cardiac surgery.

Aware of Zoll's [1952] precordial pacing and the use of myocardial wire electrodes by Weirich et al. [1958], but unaware of the catheter electrode used to stimulate the right atrium in dogs by Callaghan and Bigelow [1951], Furman and Schwedel [1959] used a monopolar catheter electrode for ventricular pacing in humans. The intracardiac electrode was mounted at the tip of a no. 6F catheter that was passed into the right ventricle via the median basilic vein. The indifferent electrode was a silver-plated copper wire implanted subcutaneously in the chest wall (Fig HP1.3*a*). The electrocardiogram and arterial pressure of one of these paced patients is shown in Fig. HP1.3*b,c*. The first patient was paced for 2 hours, and when pacing was stopped, asystole occurred and pacing had to be reinstated. Later, these authors found that it was possible to wean the patient from the pacemaker by reducing the pacing rate slowly from 60 beats per minute, being the rate adopted for pacing, following which the heart resumed its ventricular rhythm.

Furman and Schwedel's second patient was paced for more than 13 weeks. After about 2 weeks, they used the extracorporeal Electrodyne pacemaker, which incorporated the standby technique; i.e., the pacemaker turned on if more than a 5-second period of asystole was identified in the ECG being recorded on the patient monitor. The patient was ambulatory, and the energy to drive the pacemaker/monitor was derived from a long cord connected to the domestic power outlet. Thus,

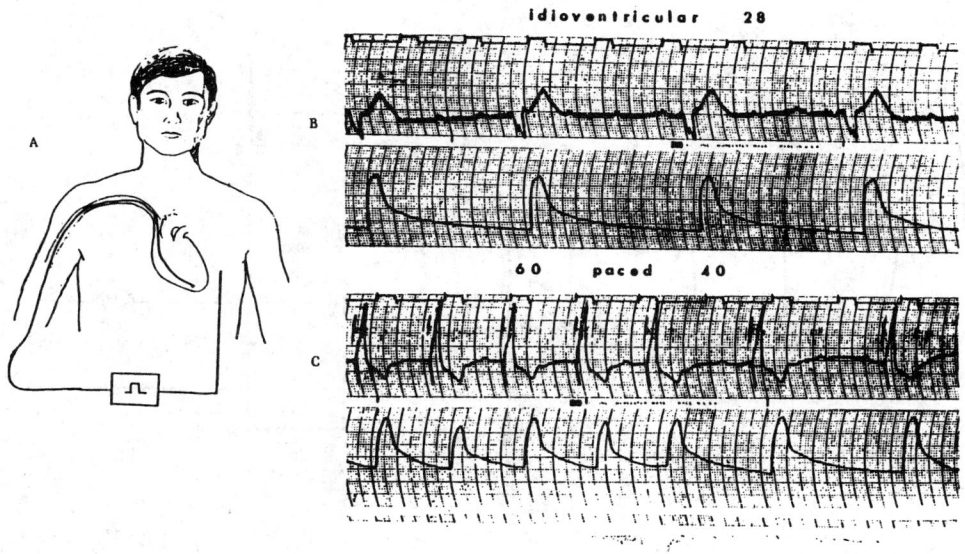

FIGURE HP1.3 (*a*) Method used in 1959 by Furman and Schwedel, who were the first to apply transvenous pacing to a human subject. (*b*) Record of the ECG and blood pressure of one of the first two patients showing complete A-V block with an idioventricular rate of 28/min. (*c*) The ECG and blood pressure of the same subject paced at 60/min (*left*) and 40/min (*right*). (Courtesy of S. Furman, M.D.)

when the patient walked around the ward, he pushed his pacemaker equipment with him on a small cart.

Furman and Schwedel clearly demonstrated that ventricular pacing could be instituted on an emergency basis by insertion of the catheter electrode into the right ventricle via a superficial vein. The threshold for pacing was low, amounting to only about 1.5 V at 0.75 mA. No muscular twitching or sensation was perceived by the patients, a fact that took some time for many to accept.

Implanted Pacemaker

It soon became obvious that portability was needed, and a leap in progress was made in 1959 when Greatbatch (a biomedical engineer) and Chardack (a surgeon) [1959] developed the first implantable pacemaker (Fig. HP1.4), which was first tested in dogs. Then Chardack and his team implanted it in human subjects. At that time, considerable surgery was needed for suturing the electrodes to the heart and implanting the pacemaker in the abdomen (Fig. HP1.4a). The implant (Fig. HP1.4b) consisted of a transistor oscillator and an amplifier energized by 10 mercury-zinc cells. The 10 cells and electronic circuitry were potted in epoxy and covered by a double shell of Silastic.

The Chardack-Greatbatch implantable pacemaker used the Hunter-Roth [1959, 1973] electrode (Fig. HP1.5a), which was about the size of a postage stamp. Implantation of the pacemaker and electrodes was a major surgical procedure. Breakage of electrode wires, short battery life, and the need for surgery for pacemaker and lead implantation were disadvantages in the early days of pacemakers. Because the heart beats over 35 million times each year, flexural strength of the lead wires was a major concern. A durable electrode wire made from the alloy that is used in the escapement springs of watches was described by Chardack [1961] and is shown in Fig. HP1.5b. Like its predecessor, it was sutured to the epicardium, and a thoracotomy was required.

Within a year, Lillehei et al. [1960] reported the use of right ventricular catheter electrodes with an external pacemaker to pace 66 patients. The pacemaker was built by Earl Bakken, a biomedical engineer who had founded Medtronic, Inc., in 1949, which soon became the pioneer pacemaker company that manufactured the Greatbatch-Chardack pacemaker.

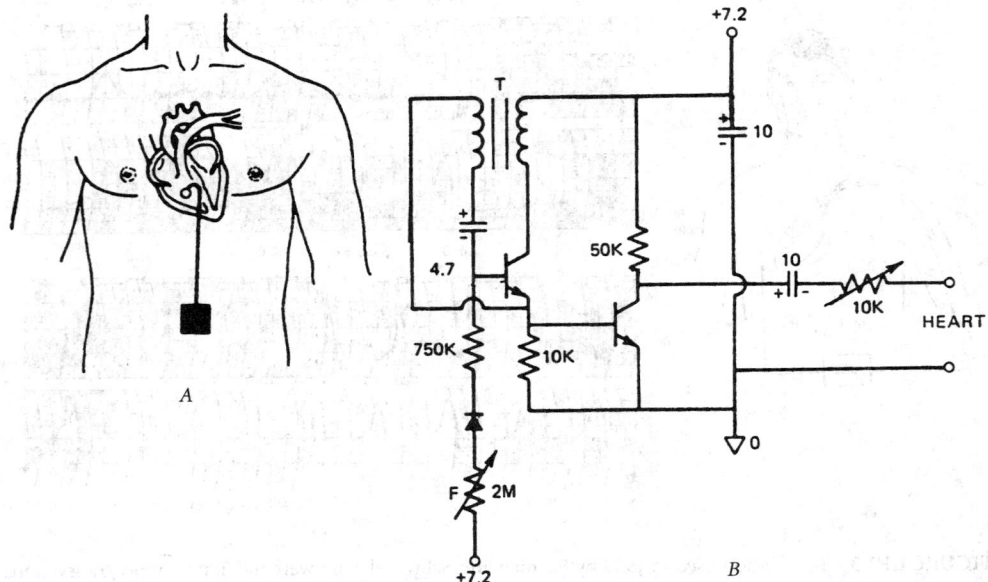

FIGURE HP1.4 Location for the first implanted pacemaker (a) and the circuit diagram (b) of the Greatbatch pacemaker. (Redrawn from Ann NY Acad Sci 1964, 111:1075.)

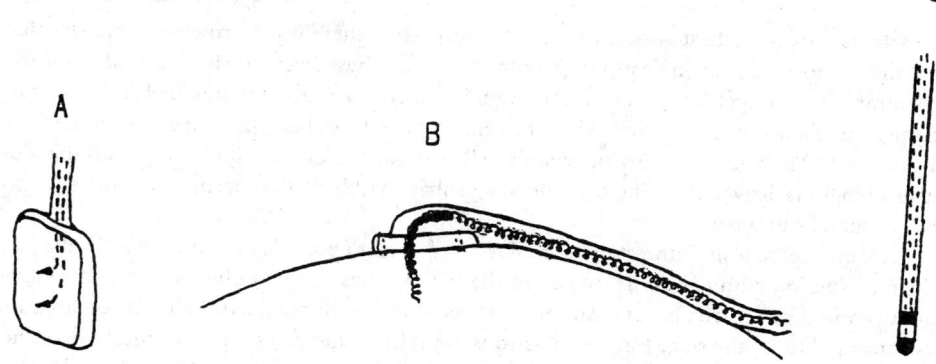

FIGURE HP1.5   Early pacing electrodes. (*a*) Hunter-Roth [1959]. (*b*) Chardack [1965]. (*c*) Catheter.

Pacemaker Batteries

Many were concerned about the short life of pacemaker batteries, as well as the gas produced by them. To solve the first problem, Elmqvist and Senning [1959] described an implantable pacemaker in which the batteries could be recharged by delivering the energy via a coil placed on the chest surface.

A few investigators described battery-less implanted pacemakers. The first of these was reported by Glenn et al. [1958], who developed a passive implanted receiver that was connected to ventricular electrodes. A body-surface transmitter broadcast the stimuli to the implant. A biomedical engineer (Hickman), working for the author, developed a similar pacer in 1961 and proved its effectiveness in dogs. Schuder, another biomedical engineer, and Stoeckle [1962] described an ingenious small passive implant that had protruding electrodes that allowed attachment of the tiny device directly to the ventricular surface. Bursts of radiofrequency energy were delivered through the chest wall into the implant to pace the ventricles.

Ingenious as the foregoing techniques were, the need for a chest-surface device to either recharge the batteries in the implanted pacemaker or to excite a passive implant proved to be unacceptable to clinicians and patients. The battery problem was solved in a different way.

Meanwhile, introduction of two different techniques conspired to extend pacemaker battery life. The first was employment of a short-duration pulse for the stimulus; the second was the use of small-area electrodes for stimulating. Both advances were introduced by Furman and colleagues [1966, 1971].

Pacing Without a Thoracotomy

Elimination of thoracotomy resulted from combining the implantable pacemaker with a catheter electrode that could be passed into the right ventricle via a superficial chest vein (Fig. HP1.6). Use of this technique was reported by Parsonnet et al. [1962].

Although monopolar and bipolar catheter electrodes (see Fig. HP1.5) had been around long before pacing, it was the new alloys that made them durable. When these new catheter electrodes were used, it was noted that the threshold for stimulation increased markedly if the electrode moved the slightest distance from the myocardium. The race soon started for electrode fixation techniques. Barbs, hooks, tynes, loops, and screens at the catheter tip all afforded a means for anchoring and providing a stable pacing threshold for a prolonged period.

Demand Pacemaker

In the early days of transchest and direct-ventricular pacing, there was a growing awareness that some of the unexpected sudden deaths in paced patients may have been due to ventricular fibrillation resulting from competitive pacing, a condition in which a pacemaker stimulus falls in the vulnerable period of a normally conducted beat or ventricular ectopic beat. In such a situation, fibrillation can result. The vulnerable period spans the T wave of the ECG, and if a single stimulus of adequate strength is delivered during this interval, ventricular fibrillation occurs immediately, and cardiac output falls to zero.

In the normal heart, a suprathreshold stimulus is required to precipitate ventricular fibrillation by vulnerable-period stimulation. However, in the hypoxic heart, a stimulus only slightly above threshold can induce ventricular fibrillation if delivered in the vulnerable period. Three circumstances conspired to set the stage for this disastrous event in pacing: (1) setting the intensity of the pacing pulse suprathreshold so that it will be effective when the threshold rises due to natural tissue encapsulation around the electrode, (2) an ectopic beat occurring during pacing, and (3) normally conducted beats breaking through the A-V node. To eliminate the danger of such competitive pacing, Lemberg and his team [1965], which included Berkovits, a biomedical engineer, introduced the demand concept first using a transchest pacemaker. In such a device, the ECG is monitored to determine if there is any ventricular electrical activity present; if so, the pacemaker is inhibited for a preset time. If A-V conduction returns, or if ventricular ectopic beats arise, the pacemaker is inhibited. If no such beats occur, the pacemaker operates in the fixed-rate mode.

The demand pacemaker made its point very well, for Parsonnet and his team, which included Myers, a biomedical engineer, soon reported clinical trials with the first implanted R-wave inhibited pacemaker [1966]. By this time, the pacing electrodes began to be used for R-wave sensing. This type of pacemaker is one of the most popular in use today because it solves the competitive pacing problem. Because it is only activated when pacing stimuli are needed, battery life is prolonged.

Activity-Responsive Pacemakers

In the early days of pacing, it was recognized that with a fixed-rate pacemaker, a subject would have a limited ability to tolerate exercise. Cardiac output does increase slightly when a subject with a

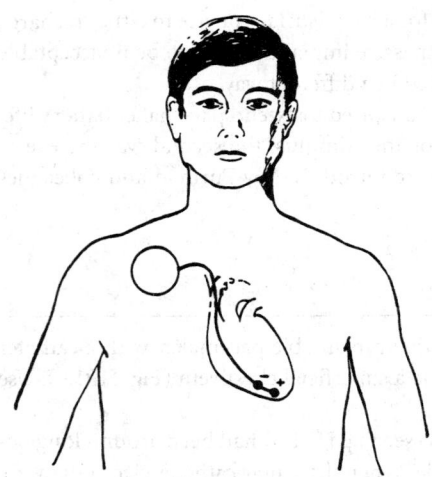

fixed-rate pacemaker exercises. The increase in cardiac output is due to the exercise-induced increase in venous return to the ventricles, thereby increasing the preload, which increases stroke volume via Starling's law. In addition, the increased sympathetic nervous drive to the ventricles contributes to increasing stroke volume. However, in a normal exercising subject, the same factors operate, but there is also an increase in heart rate; therefore, research was devoted to identifying strategies that would increase the rate of a pacemaker automatically with exercise.

In some situations of total A-V block, the atria are still beating; therefore, it was apparent that the P wave of the ECG could be used to develop a stimulus that could be delivered to ventricular electrodes. Even before pacing was popular in humans, Folkman and Watkins [1957] used a transistor amplifier to enlarge the atrial P waves and deliver them to the ventricles of dogs to evoke ventricular con-

FIGURE HP1.6 Combination of the implantable pacemaker and catheter electrode by Parsonnet et al. [1962] eliminated the need for a thoracotomy.

TABLE HP1.1 Activity Responsive Pacemakers

Sensed Quantity	Sensing Method	Principal Investigator and Year
Atrial excitation (P wave)	Apply delay and stimulate the right ventricle	Karlof (1975), Kapenberger (1981), Krause (1982)
Respiration rate	Impedance pneumograph	Krasner (1966, 1971)
Respiration rate	Diaphragm motion (by piezoelectric detector)	Ionescu (1980)
Respiration rate	Negative intrathoracic pressure transducer	Funke et al. (1975)
Respiration rate	Impedance RV to case	Rossi et al. (1983)
pH	RA venous blood with In-AgCl electrode	Cammilli (1979, 1980, 1981)
pH	In pacemaker pocket	Contini (1981)
Venous O_2 saturation	Catheter oximeter	Wirtzfeld (1980)
Arterial O_2 saturation	Electrodes on Hering's nerve	Bozal-Gonzalez (1980)
Ventricular cycle	Stimulus T-wave duration	Rickards (1981)
Core temperature	Temperature-sensitive capacitor in pacer	Fischell (1975)
Venous blood temperature	Thermistor RA, RV, PA	Griffin (1981)
Right-ventricular blood temperature	Thermistor	Jolgren (1983)
Body motion	Accelerometer	Anderson et al. (1984)

Source: From Geddes LA. 1984. Cardiovascular Devices. New York, Wiley.

tractions. The unit was carried in a backpack and was proven in dogs with surgically induced A-V block. Stephenson et al. [1959] created a P-wave–triggered stimulator with a built-in delay to simulate the A-V conduction time, and the unit was used successfully in dogs with A-V block. A similar pacemaker was reported by Kahn et al. [1960] and Nathan et al. [1963], whose team included Keller, a biomedical engineer.

In A-V block, use of the P wave of the ECG does indeed provide automatic control of the pacing rate based on bodily activity. However, in diseased hearts, there may be no P wave, or the atria may flutter or be in fibrillation. These cases must be handled differently. For example, if the P wave disappears, the pacemaker can revert to the fixed-rate mode. With flutter or fibrillation, it is necessary to prevent the pacemaker from following the electrical activity of the atria. Algorithms have been developed to limit the rate of the ventricular pacemaker in these situations.

The lack of a dependable P wave to trigger a ventricular pacemaker caused many to identify physiologic events that signal an increase in bodily activity; Table 1 presents a summary of most of them. Many of the methods shown in Table 1 have been embodied in commercially available pacemakers. Which method will turn out to be the best can only be identified by future clinical experience.

References

Anderson K, Humen D, Klein GJ, et al. 1983. A rate variable pacemaker which automatically adjusts for physical activity. PACE 6:A-12. U.S. patent 4,428,378, Jan 31, 1984.

Bozal-Gonzalez JL. 1980. Cardiac pacemaker. U.S. patent 4,201,219, May 4, 1980.

Callaghan JC, Bigelow WG. 1951. An electrical artificial pacemaker for standstill of the heart. Ann Surg 134:8.

Cammilli L. 1979. pH-triggered pacemaker. PACE 2,A6.

Cammilli L, Green GD, Ricci D, Risani R. 1980. pH-triggered pacemaker: Design and clinical results. In Proceedings of the 6th World Symposium on Cardiac Pacing, chap 19-8.

Cammilli L, Alcidi L, Bisi G. 1981. Results, problems and perspectives in the auto-regulating pacemaker. 2nd European Symposium on Cardiac Pacing, May–June 1981, PACE 4:A-36.

Chardack WM, Gage AA, Greatbatch W. 1960. A transistorized, self-contained, implantable pacemaker for long-term correction of complete heart block. Surgery 48:643.

Chardack WM, Gage AA, Greatbatch W. 1961. Corrections of complete heart block by a self-contained and subcutaneously implanted pacemaker. J Thorac Cardiovasc Surg 42:814.

Contini C, Papeschi G, Ricci D, et al. 1981. pH changes in chronic pacemaker pocket: A new means of increasing rate during exercise: preliminary results. PACE 2:366.

Elmqvist R, Senning A. 1960. Implantable pacemaker for the heart. In CN Smyth (ed), Medical Electronics: Proceedings of the Second International Conference on Medical Electronics, Paris, June 1959. London, Iliffe & Sons.

Fishell RR. 1975. Fixed-rate rechargeable cardiac pacemaker. U.S. patent 3,867,950.

Folkman MJ, Watkins E. 1957. An electrical conduction system for the management of experimental, complete heart block. Clin Cong Am Coll Surg 8:331.

Funke HD. 1975. Einherzschrittmacher mit beinstungsabhangiger frequenz-regulation. Biomed Tech 20:225.

Furman S, Schwedel JB. 1959. An intracardiac pacemaker for Stokes-Adams seizures. N Engl J Med 26:943.

Furman S, Denize A, Escher D, Schwedel JB. 1966. Energy considerations for cardiac stimulations a function of pulse duration. J Surg Res 8:441.

Furman S, Parker B, Escher D. 1971. Decreasing electrode size and increasing efficiency of cardiac stimulation. J Surg Res 11:105.

Glenn WWL, Mauro A, Longo E, et al. 1959. Remote stimulation of the heart by radiofrequency transmission. N Engl J Med 261 (18):948.

Greatbatch W, Chardack WM. 1959. Transistorized implantable pacemaker. Proc NEREM 1:8.

Green T. 1872. On death from chloroform; its prevention by galvanism. Br Med J 1:551.

Griffin JC, Tutzy KR, Claude JP, et al. 1981. Nonelectrographic indices of pacemaker rate. Proc AEMB 34:202.

Hickman DM, Geddes LA, Hoff HE, et al. 1961. A portable miniature transistorized radio-frequency coupled cardiac pacemaker. IRE PGBME Trans BME-8(4):258.

Hunter SW, Boldue L, Long V, Quattelbaum FW. 1973. A new myocardial pacemaker lead. Chest 63:430.

Hunter SW, Roth NA, Bernardez D, Noble JD. 1959. A bipolar myocardial electrode for complete heart block. Lancet 79:506.

Hyman AA. 1932. Resuscitation of the stopped heart by intracardiac therapy. Arch Intern Med 50:283.

Ionsecu VL. 1980. An "on demand" pacemaker responsive to respiratory rate. PACE 3:375.

Jolgren D, Fearnot NE, Geddes LA. 1983. A rate-responsive pacemaker controlled by right ventricular blood temperature, Proceedings of the 32nd Annual Science Session. Am Coll Cardiol J Acc 1(1):720.

Kahn M, Senderoff E, Shapiro J, et al. 1960. Bridging of interrupted A-V conduction in experimental heart block by electronic means. Am Heart J 59:548.

Kappenberger L, Turina M, Babotal J, 1981. Differentiated pacemaking therapy. Schweiz Med Wochenschr 111:45.

Karlof I. 1975. Hemodynamic effects of atrial-triggered versus fixed rate pacing at rest and during exercise in complete heart block. Acta Med Scand 197:195.

Krasner JL, Voukydis PC, Nardella PC. 1966. A physiologically controlled cardiac pacemaker. JAAMI 20.

Krasner JL, Nardella P. 1971. Physiologically controlled cardiac pacer. U.S. Patent 3,593,718.

Krause I, Arnman K, Conradson T, Ryden L. 1982. A comparison of the acute and long-term hemodynamic effects of ventricular inhibited and atrial synchronous-ventricular inhibited pacing. Circulation 65:846.

Lemberg L, Castellanos A, Berkovits BV. 1965. Pacemaking on demand in A-V block. JAMA 191:12.

Lillehei CW, Gott VL, Hodges PC, et al. 1960. Transistor pacemaker for treatment of complete atrioventricular dissociation. JAMA 172:2006.

McWilliam JA. 1889. Electrical stimulation of the heart in man. Br Med J 1:348.

Nathan DA, Center S, Wu CY, Keller W. 1963. An implantable synchronous pacemaker for the long-term correction of complete heart block. Circulation 27:682.

Parsonnet V, Zucker IR, Asa M. 1962. Preliminary investigation of a permanent implantable pacemaker utilizing an intracardiac dipolar catheter. Clin Res 10:391 (see also Am J Cardiol 10:261).

Parsonnet V, Zucker IR, Myers SH. 1966. Clinical use of an implanted standby pacemaker. JAMA 198:784.

Rickards AF. 1981. Physiologically adaptive cardiac pacemaker. U.S. patent 4,228,803.

Rickards AF, Norman J, Thalen A, et al. 1981. The use of stimulus-T interval to determine cardiac pacing rate. PACE 4:A68.

Rickards AF, Norman J. 1981. Relation between Q-T interval and heart rate. Br Heart J 45:56.

Rossi P, Plicchi G, Canducci GC, et al. 1983. The implantable respiratory dependent pacemaker. PACE 3:A-13.

Schuder JC, Stoeckle H. 1982. A micromodule pacemaker receiver for direct attachment to the ventricle. Trans Am Soc Artif Intern Organs 8:344.

Steiner F. 1871. Ueber die Electropunctur des Herzens als Wiederbelebungsmittel in der Chloroformsyncope. Arch Klin Chir 12:748.

Stephenson SE, Edwards WH, Jolly, et al. 1959. Physiologic P-wave cardiac stimulator. J Thorac Cardiovasc Surg 38:804.

Weirich WL, Paneth M, Gott VL, Lillehei CW. 1958. Control of complete heart block by use of an artificial pacemaker and a myocardial electrode. Circ Res 6:410.

Wirtzfield A. 1980. Cardiac pacemaker. U.S. patent 4,202,339.

Ziemssen H. 1882. Studien ubr die Bewegungsvorgange am mehschlichen Herzen. Deutch Arch Klin Med 30:270.

Zoll PM. 1952. Resuscitation of heart in ventricular standstill by external electric stimulation. N Engl J Med 247:768.

Zoll PM, Linenthal AJ, Gibson W, et al. 1956. Termination of ventricular fibrillation in man by externally applied electric countershock. N Engl J Med 254:727.

Zoll PM, Zoll RM, Belgard AH. 1981. External non-invasive electric stimulation of the heart. Crit Care Med 9:393.

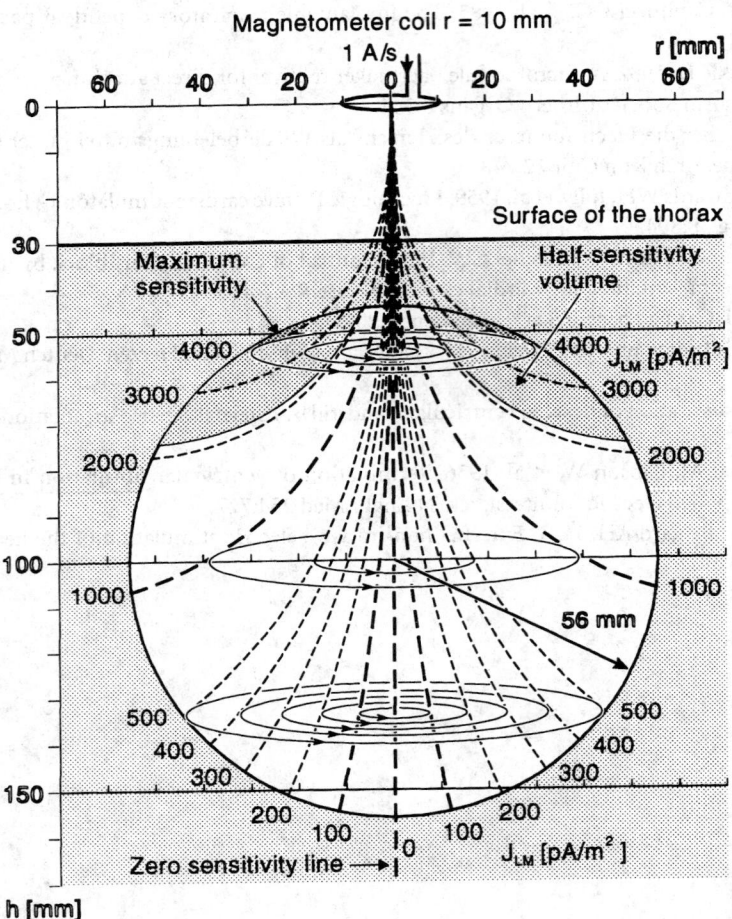

Sensitivity distributions in the measurement of the magnetic dipole of the heart.

II

Bioelectric Phenomena

Craig S. Henriquez
Duke University

T HE STUDY OF EXCITABLE CELLS and bioelectric processes in the body has had a significant impact on biomedical engineering. Clinical methods such as electroneurography, electromyography, electrocardiography, and electroencephalography all involve recording and interpreting bioelectric signals that arise from the propagation of action potentials, i.e., transient changes in potential across the cell membrane. The nature of the recorded signals depends on a number of factors, including the number of contributing cells, the geometry and electrical properties of the media through which the currents flow, and the distance of the recording electrode from the excitable tissue. All these factors must be accounted for when designing recording equipment and making proper interpretations.

The principles of bioelectricity also have resulted in the development and manufacture of a number of clinical devices capable of delivering currents to the body for the treatment or therapy of a variety of physical anomalies. Pacemakers and stimulators help to maintain or approximate proper electrical function of the heart, muscle, and nerve. Defibrillators are used to terminate potentially fatal arrhythmias. These devices have become increasingly sophisticated, with microprocessors capable of processing the bioelectric signals to help determine the appropriate action.

The study and use of bioelectric phenomena in biomedical technologies have advanced, in part, through careful experimentation and the development of increasingly accurate biophysical models and theoretical concepts. Continued progress in the techniques for diagnosis and treatment of derangements of electrical processes in the body will require that biomedical engineers are knowledgeable of the fundamentals of bioelectricity. This section focuses on these fundamentals and some of the clinical applications.

Chapter 8 presents a quantitative and qualitative overview of basic electrophysiology and membrane biophysics. Chapter 9 discusses how currents are supported in the body and how these currents set up potentials that can be measured with external electrodes. Chapter 10 reviews the electrical properties of various tissues. The ionic currents that give rise to action potentials of various tissues are currently being studied using modern patch-clamp techniques born out of the Nobel Prize–winning work of Hodgkin and Huxley. Descriptions of the techniques and some of the mathematical models that result from the experiments are discussed in Chapter 11. The theoretical advancements in bioelectric phenomena have led to a number of biophysical models that are used to interpret experimental and clinical observations. Some of the models are of such complexity that they can only be managed with the aid of a computer. The common numerical solution methods for bioelectric field problems are discussed in Chapter 12. The most common clinical applications of bioelectric phenomena, electromyography, electroencephelography, and electrocardiology, are discussed in Chapters 13 through 15. The flow of currents in the body also can give rise to magnetic fields that can be detected outside the body. The nature of biomagnetic fields and their clinical applications are discussed in Chapter 16. Finally, a number of devices have been developed to deliver current to the body. The fundamentals of electrical stimulation are presented in Chapter 17.

8

Basic Electrophysiology

Roger C. Barr
Duke University

This chapter serves as an overview of some widely accepted concepts of electrophysiology. Subsequent chapters in this section provide more specialized information for many of the particular topics mentioned here.

8.1 Membranes

Bioelectricity has its origin in the voltage differences present between the inside and outside of cells. These potentials arise from the specialized properties of the cell membrane, which separates the intracellular from the extracellular volume. Much of the membrane surface is made of a phospholipid bilayer, an electrically inert material [Byrne and Schultz, 1988]. Because the membrane is thin (about 75 Å), it has a high capacitance, about 1 μF/cm^2. (Membrane capacitance is less in nerve, except at nodes, because most of the membrane is myelinated, which makes it much thicker.)

Electrically active membrane also includes a number of *integral proteins* of different kinds. Integral proteins are compact but complex structures extending across the membrane. Each integral protein is composed of a large number of amino acids, often in a single long polypeptide chain, which folds into multiple domains. Each domain may span the membrane several times. The multiple crossings may build the functional structure, e.g., a *channel*, through which electrically charged ions may flow. The structure of integral proteins is loosely analogous to that of a length of thread passing back and forth across a fabric to form a buttonhole. As a buttonhole allows movement of a

0-8493-8346-3/95/$0.00+$.50
© 1995 by CRC Press, Inc.

button from one side of the fabric to the other, an integral protein may allow passage of ions from the exterior of a cell to the interior, or vice versa. In contrast to a buttonhole, an integral protein has active properties, e.g., the ability to open or close. Excellent drawings of channel structure and function are given by Watson et al. [1992].

Cell membrane possesses a number of active characteristics of marked importance to its bioelectric behavior, including these: (1) Some integral proteins functions as *pumps*. These pumps use energy to transport ions across membrane, working against a concentration gradient, a voltage gradient, or both. The most important pump moves sodium ions out of the intracellular volume and potassium ions in. (2) Other integral proteins function as *channels*, i.e., openings through the membrane that open and close over time. These channels can function selectively so that, for a particular kind of channel, only sodium ions may pass through. Another kind of channel may allow only potassium ions or calcium ions. (3) The activity of the membrane's integral proteins is modulated by signals specific to its particular function. For example, some channels open or close in response to photons or to odorants; thus they function as sensors for light or smell. Pumps respond to the concentrations of the ions they move. Rapid electrical impulse transmission in nerve and muscle is made possible by changes that respond to the transmembrane potential itself, forming a feedback mechanism. These active mechanisms provide ion-selective means of current crossing the membrane, both against the concentration or voltage gradients (pumps) or in response to them (channels). While the pumps build up the concentration differences (and thereby the potential energy) that allow events to occur, channels utilize this energy actively to create the fast changes in voltage and small intense current loops that constitute nerve signal transmission, initiate muscle contraction, and participate in other essential bioelectric phenomena.

8.2 Bioelectric Current Loops

Bioelectricity normally flows in current loops, as illustrated in Fig. 8.1.* A loop includes four segments: an outward traversal of the cell membrane (current I_m^1 at position $z = z_1$), an extracellular segment (current I_e, along a path outside a cell or cells), an inward traversal of the cell membrane (current I_m^2 at $z = z_2$), and an intracellular segment (current I_i, along a segment inside the cell membrane). Each of the segments has aspects that give it a unique importance to the current loop. Intense current loops often are contained within a millimeter or less, although loops of weaker intensity may extend throughout the whole body volume. The energy that supports the current flow arises from one or both of the segments of the loop that cross the membrane. Current loops involve potential differences of about 100 mV between extremes. The charge carriers are mobile ions. Especially important are ions of sodium, potassium, calcium, and chloride because some membranes allow one or more of these ion species to move across when others cannot.

Membrane Currents

Total membrane current I_m may be given mathematically as

$$I_m = I_c + I_{ion} \tag{8.1}$$

where each of these currents often is given per unit area, e.g., milliamperes per square centimeter.

The first component, I_c, corresponds to the charging or discharging of the membrane capacitance. Thus

$$I_c = C_m \partial V_m / \partial t \tag{8.2}$$

---

*For clarity, this chapter uses equations and examples describing flow in one dimension. Usually analogous equations based on the same principles have been developed for two and three dimensions.

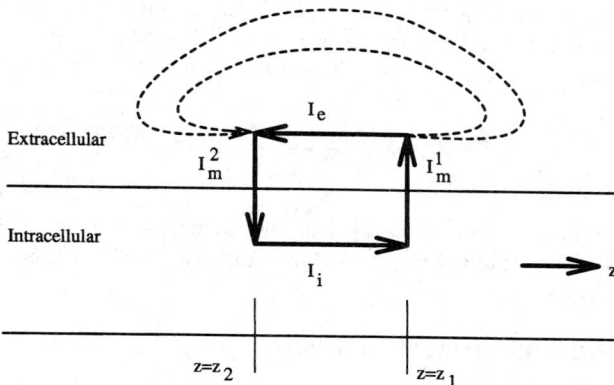

FIGURE 8.1 Bioelectric current loop, concept drawing. Current enters the membrane at $z = z_1$, flows intracellularly, and emerges at z_2. Flow in the extracellular volume may be along the membrane (*solid*) or throughout the surrounding volume conductor (*dashed*).

where C_m is the membrane capacitance per unit area, V_m is the transmembrane voltage, and t is time.

The second component, I_{ion}, corresponds to the current through the membrane carried by ions such as those of sodium, potassium, or calcium. It normally is found by summing each of the individual components, e.g.,

$$I_{ion} = I_K + I_{Na} + I_{Ca} \tag{8.3}$$

In turn, each of the component currents is often written in a form such as

$$I_K = g_K (V_m - E_K) \tag{8.4}$$

where E_K is the equilibrium potential for K (see below), a function of K concentrations, and g_K is the conductivity of the membrane to K ions. The conductivity g_K is not constant but rather varies markedly as a function of transmembrane voltage and time. More positive transmembrane voltages normally are associated with higher conductivities, at least transiently.

When a more detailed knowledge of channel structure is included, as in the DiFrancesco-Noble model for cardiac membrane, each of the individual ionic components, e.g., I_K, is found in turn as a sum of the currents through each kind of channel or pump through which that ion moves.

The total transmembrane current I_m contains the summed contributions from I_c and I_{ion}, as given by Eq. (8.1), but the effects of these components are quite different. At many membrane sites these components differ both in magnitude and in direction. Thinking in terms of the current loops that exist during membrane excitation, one often finds that current at the site of peak outward current is dominated by I_c. At the site of peak inward current, the total current I_m usually dominated by I_{ion} (see Propagation, below).

Conduction Along an Intracellular Path

Flow of electricity along a nerve or within a muscle occurs passively through the conducting medium inside the cell. The nature of the intracellular current path is closely related to the function of the current within that kind of cell. Nerve cells may have lengths of a meter or more, so intracellular currents can flow unimpeded and quickly throughout this length. Other cells, such as the muscle cells of the heart, are much smaller (about 100 µm in length). In cardiac cells, current flows intracellularly from cell to cell through specialized passages, called *junctions*, that occur in regions where the cell membranes fuse together. Thus intracellular regions may be connected over lengths of centimeters or more, even though each cell is much smaller. Mathematically, the intracellular current in a one-dimensional cable may be given as [Plonsey and Barr, 1988, p 109]

$$I_i = -\frac{1}{r_i}\frac{\partial \phi_i}{\partial z} \qquad (8.5)$$

where ϕ_i is the intracellular potential, z is the axial coordinate, r_i is the intracellular resistance per unit length, and I_i is the longitudinal axial current per unit cross-sectional area.

Conduction Along an Extracellular Path

Current flow outside of cells is not constrained to a particular path but rather flows throughout the whole surrounding conducting volume (the volume conductor), which may be the whole body. Current intensity is highest near the places where current enters or leaves cells through the membrane. (These sites are called *sinks* and *sources*, respectively, in view of their relation to the extracellular volume.) Current flow from bioelectric sources through the volume conductor generates small potential differences, usually with a magnitude of a millivolt or less, between different sites within the volume or on the body surface. (Current flow from artificial sources, such as stimulators or defibrillators, may generate much higher voltages.) The naturally occurring potential differences between points in the volume conductor, e.g., between the arms or across the head, are those commonly measured in the study of the heart (electrocardiography), the nerves and muscles (electromyography), and the brain (electroencephalography).

Mathematically, the extracellular current is easy to specify only in the special case where the extracellular current is confined to a small space surrounding a single fiber or nerve, as shown diagramatically by the solid I_e line in Fig. 8.1. In this special case, the extracellular current is equal in magnitude (but opposite in direction) to the intracellular current, that is, $I_e = -I_i$.

In most living systems, however, extracellular currents extend throughout a more extensive volume conductor, as suggested by the dashed lines for I_e in Fig. 8.1. Their direction and magnitude must be found as a solution to Poisson's equation in the extracellular medium, with the sources and sinks around the active medium used as boundary conditions. In this context, Poisson's equation becomes [Plonsey and Barr, 1988, p 22]

$$\nabla^2 \phi_e = -\frac{I_v}{\sigma_e} = -\frac{\nabla \cdot \vec{J}}{\sigma_e} \qquad (8.6)$$

where I_v is the volume density of the sources (sinks being negative sources), σ_e is the conductivity of the extracellular medium, and J is the current density. The fact that $\nabla \cdot \vec{J}$ takes on nonzero values appears at first to be physically unrealistic because it seems to violate the principle of conservation of charge. In fact, it only reflects the practice of solving for potentials and currents in the extracellular volume separately from those in the intracellular volume. Thus the nonzero divergence represents the movement of currents from the intracellular volume across the membrane and into the extracellular volume, where they appear from sources or disappear into sinks.

Duality

Note the duality between Eq. (8.6) and the form of Poisson's equation commonly used in problems in electrostatics. There, $\nabla^2 \phi = -\rho/\epsilon$, where ρ is the charge density, and ϵ is the permittivity. Recognition of this duality is useful not only in locating solution methods for bioelectric problems, since the mathematics is the same, but also in avoiding confusion between electrostatics and problems of extracellular current flow through a volume conductor. The problems obviously are physically quite different (e.g., permittivity ϵ is not conductivity σ_e).

8.3 Membrane Polarization

Ionic pumps within membranes operate, over time, to produce markedly different concentrations of ions in the intracellular and extracellular volumes around cells. In cardiac cells, the sodium-potassium pump produces concentrations* (millimoles per liter) for Purkinje cells as shown in Table 8.1.

A transmembrane voltage, or polarization, develops across the membrane because of the differences in concentrations across the membrane. In the steady state, the transmembrane potential for a two-ion system is, according to Goldman's equation [Plonsey and Barr, 1988, p. 51],

$$V_m = \frac{RT}{F} \ln\left(\frac{P_K[K]_e + P_{Na}[Na]_e}{P_K[K]_i + P_{Na}[Na]_i} \right) \tag{8.7}$$

where R is the gas constant, T is the temperature, and F is Faraday's constant ($RT/F \approx 25$ mV). P_K and P_{Na} are the permeabilities to potassium and sodium ions, respectively. [K] and [Na] are the concentrations of these ions, and the subscripts i and e indicate intracellular and extracellular, respectively. V_m is the transmembrane voltage at steady state.

Polarized State

At rest, P_{Na} is much smaller than P_K. Using Eq. (8.6), approximating $P_{Na} = P_K/100$, and using the concentrations in Table 8.1,

$$V_m \approx 25 \text{ mV} \times \ln\left[\frac{4 + (0.01 \times 140)}{140 + (0.01 \times 8)} \right] \approx -82 \text{ mV} \tag{8.8}$$

Cardiac Purkinje cells show a polarization at rest of about this amount. The negative sign indicates that the interior of the cell is negative with respect to the exterior.

One way to think about why this voltage exists at the steady state is as follows: In the steady state, diffusion tends to move K^+ from inside to outside because of the much higher concentration of K^+ intracellularly. This flow is offset, however, by a flow from outside to inside due to the potential gradient, with a higher potential outside, since K^+ is a positively charged ion. With the concentrations of Table 8.1, the effects of the diffusion gradient and potential gradient are almost equal and opposite when the potential intracellularly is about -82 mV with respect to the extracellular potential. The result is a steady state. Rather than a true equilibrium, this state has a small but nonzero flow of sodium ions, offset electrically by a sustained flow of potassium ions. Thus the membrane potential would run down over time were there no Na^+-K^+ pumps maintaining the transmembrane concentrations. (In the absence of such pumps, concentration differences diminish over a period of hours.)

TABLE 8.1 Ionic Concentrations (mmol/liter)

	Na^+	K^+
Intracellular	8	140
Extracellular	140	4

*Values taken from the program Heart, by Noble et al [1994], as restated in Cabo and Barr [1992].

Depolarized State

Suppose the permeabilities to sodium and potassium of Eq. (8.7) are changed from the values used for Eq. (8.8), which approximated membrane at rest (polarized). Instead, to approximate excited membrane, suppose that P_{Na} rises in comparison with P_K so that $P_K = P_{Na}/2$. Now,

$$V_m = 25 \text{ mV} \times \ln\left[\frac{4 + (2 \times 140)}{140 + (2 \times 8)}\right] \approx 15 \text{ mV} \tag{8.9}$$

Here the positive sign for V_m indicates that the interior of the membrane is positive with respect to the exterior. Because V_m is here more nearly zero in magnitude, this excited state is called *depolarized*.

8.4 Action Potentials

Membranes create *action potentials* by actively changing their permeabilities to ions such as sodium and potassium. A comparison of the results of Eqs. (8.8) and (8.9) shows a swing of about 100 mV between the resting and excited states (polarized to depolarized). The change of permeability from resting to excited values and then back again allows the membrane to generate an action potential.

Cardiac Action Potentials

Action potentials that characterize actual tissue have the roughly rectangular shape that is suggested by the preceding calculation, but only as an approximation. An action potential for the cardiac conduction system simulated with the DiFrancesco-Noble model is shown in Fig. 8.2. Initially, V_m has a baseline voltage (B) near −80mV. During excitation (E), the membrane permeabilities change, and V_m rises abruptly. After the peak overshoot at about +20 mV, the potential maintains a plateau voltage (P) near −20mV for nearly 300 ms and then recovers (R) rapidly to a baseline phase. The overall action potential duration is about 400 ms.

Nerve Action Potentials

For comparison, an action potential simulated with the Hodgkin-Huxley model for nerve is shown in Fig. 8.3. Corresponding baseline, excitation, plateau, and recovery phases may be identified, and

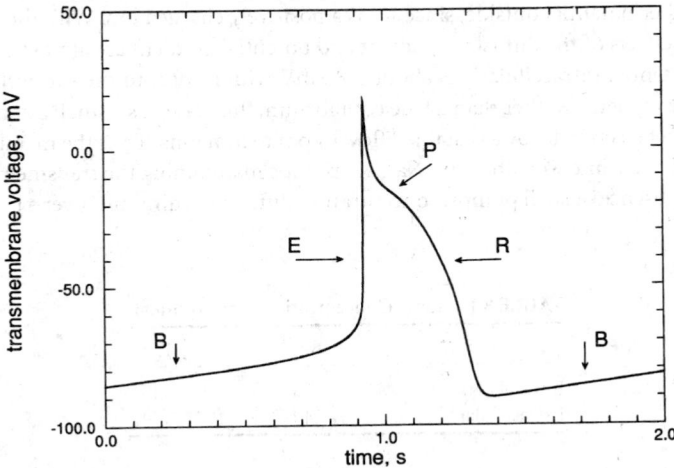

FIGURE 8.2   Cardiac action potential. Computed with the DiFrancesco-Noble membrane model for the cardiac conduction system (membrane patch). *B*, baseline; *E*, excitation; *P*, plateau; *R*, recovery (repolarization).

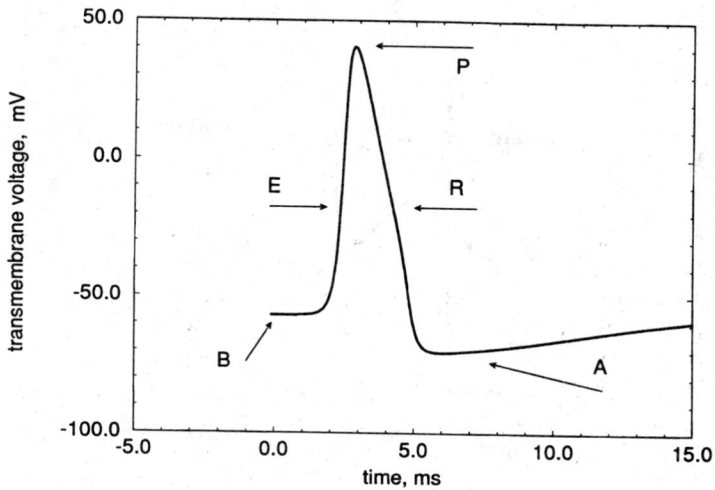

FIGURE 8.3 Nerve action potential. Computed with the Hodgkin-Huxley model for nerve membrane (membrane patch). *B*, baseline; *E*, excitation; *P*, plateau; *R*, recovery; *A*, afterpotential.

the voltage change between resting and excited states is again about 100 mV. The *plateau* phase is so short as to be virtually nonexistent, and the overall action potential duration is much shorter than that of Fig. 8.2, only about 4 ms.

Wave Shape and Function

All excitable membranes are characterized by their ability to change membrane permeabilities and to do so selectively. Both the cardiac action potential of Fig. 8.2 and the nerve action potential of Fig. 8.3 demonstrated rapid depolarization and a subsequent slower repolarization associated with membrane permeability changes and changes of about 100 mV in V_m amplitude. Conversely, the differences also have marked importance. Cardiac action potentials have a long duration that limits the shortest interval between heartbeats. This interval must be several hundred milliseconds long to allow time for movement of blood. The extended plateau of the cardiac action potential is associated with the movement of calcium ions, which is associated with muscle contraction. In contrast, nerve action potentials perform a signaling function. This function is supported by a shorter action potential duration, which allows more variability in the number of action potentials propagated per second, an important signaling variable. Conversely, nerves have no need for contraction and no need for a plateau period for calcium ion movement.

8.5 Initiation of Action Potentials

Action potentials of tissue with a specialized sensing function (e.g., for sight or smell) have membrane channels linked to receptors for the initiating agent [Watson et al., 1992, p 320]. In contrast, a large number of membrane channels are controlled by changes in transmembrane voltage. In particular, when the potential rises from its baseline value to a threshold level, the membrane initiates the sequence of permeability changes that create an action potential. The change of transmembrane voltage initiating the action potential normally comes from currents originating in adjacent tissue (see Propagation, below). Such currents also may come from artificial sources, such as stimulators.

Examples

Responses of a DiFrancesco-Noble membrane to transmembrane stimuli of three magnitudes are shown in Fig. 8.4. All three stimuli were 1 ms in duration. Stimulus *S1*, the largest, caused the trans-

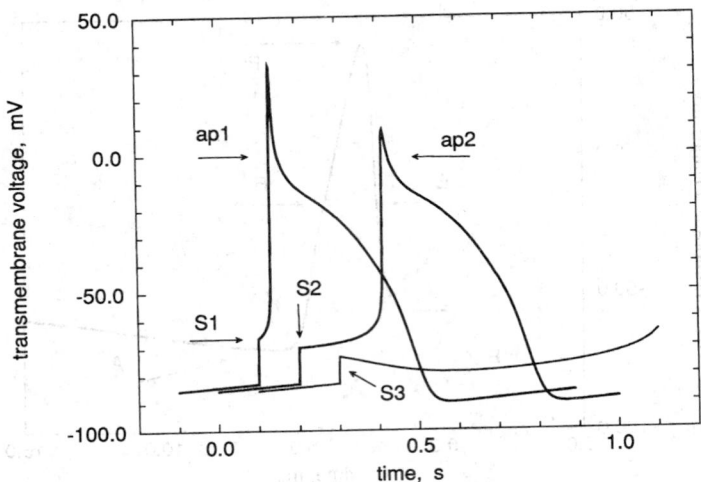

FIGURE 8.4 Variation in stimulus magnitude. In different trials, three stimuli (*S1, S2, S3*) of decreasing magnitude were applied. Action potentials followed the first two, but not the third.

membrane potential to rise from its baseline value to about −65 mV and initiated an action potential (*ap1*), which followed a few milliseconds after the stimulus. Stimulus *S2* had only 80% of the intensity of *S1*, and the stimulus itself caused a transmembrane voltage change that was proportionally smaller. As did *S1*, stimulus *S2* initiated an action potential (*ap2*), although there was a delay of about 200 ms before excitation occurred, and the action potential itself was somewhat diminished in amplitude. Stimulus *S3* had 80% of the magnitude of *S2* and caused a transmembrane voltage change that again was proportionally smaller. *S3*, however, produced no subsequent action potential.

Threshold

An important general result demonstrated in Fig. 8.4 is that action potential initiation has a threshold behavior. That is, stimuli producing transmembrane voltages above a threshold value initiate action potentials, while those below do not. This response is called "all or none," although (as Fig. 8.4 shows) there is a variation in response for near-threshold stimuli. The specific threshold value varies depends on factors such as the stimulus duration, the amount of membrane affected, and the intracellular potential gradient, which affects the rate of stimulus decay.

8.6 Propagation

Initiation of excitation at one end of a excitable fiber leads to an action potential there. Subsequently, action potentials may be observed at sites progressively further away.

Numerical Model

Use of a numerical model is extremely helpful in investigating the events of propagation, because a consistent picture can be obtained of temporal events at different sites and of spatial events at different times. For these reasons, such a model is used here. Consider the cylindrical fiber shown in Fig. 8.5, having radius $a = 75$ μm and a length of 10 mm. The fiber is surrounded by an extracellular volume extending $3a$ beyond the membrane. To establish a symmetric reference potential, the outside edge of the extracellular region was connected via resistances to a junction where $\phi_e = 0$. Intracellular specific resistance R_i was 250 $\Omega \cdot$ cm, and R_e was one-third of R_i. Solutions for intra-

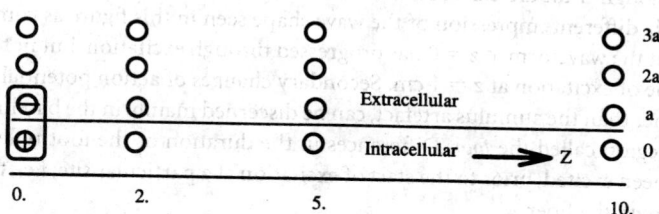

FIGURE 8.5 Geometry for numerical model. The model represented a fiber 10 mm in length. The cross section was a series of concentric bands. Nodes were space along the axial (z) dimension every 100 µm. These nodes are portrayed by the columns of circles drawn at four axial positions, although actually there were 101 columns. The innermost (*lower*) row of nodes, row 0, were sites where intracellular potentials were determined; four surrounding rows (rows 1 to 4), at increasing distances, were sites for extracellular potentials. The outermost boundary (*dashed line*) was assigned $\phi_e = 0$. Separation between all rows was the same as the fiber radius, $a = 75$ µm. Transmembrane stimuli were applied across the membrane at $z = 0$ (*nodes enclosed*).

cellular, extracellular, and transmembrane potentials were obtained through a process of numerical simulation. The structure of this example follows that of Spach et al. [1973], where cardiac Purkinje fibers were studied. Most of the examples below use the DiFrancesco-Noble model for Purkinje membrane [Noble et al., 1994].

Sequence of Action Potentials

Action potentials simulated for the cylindrical fiber are shown in Fig. 8.6. Waveforms are shown following a transmembrane stimulus at $z = 0$, where the first action potential originates, and also for

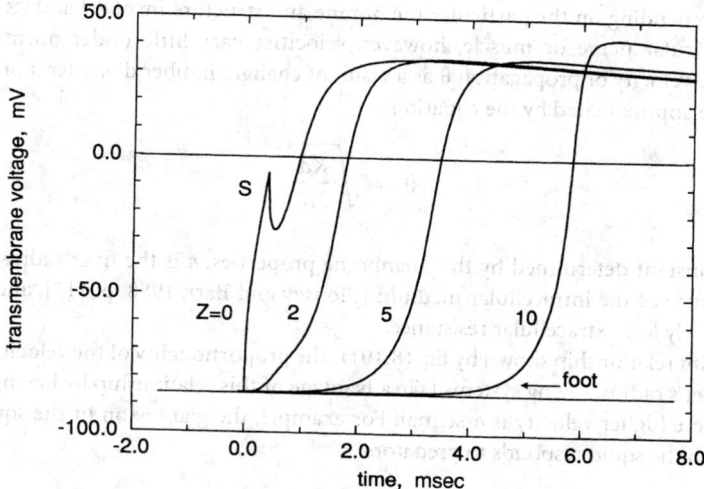

FIGURE 8.6 Action potentials for a 10-mm fiber. Transmembrane potentials $V_m(t)$ arising at z positions of 0, 2, 5, and 10 mm. The waveform at $z = 0$ shows a stimulus artefact S. $V_m(t)$ at $z = 10$ has a larger peak-to-peak rise because excitation terminates there, at the end of the fiber.

sites 2, 5, and 10 mm away. All the action potentials have similar wave shapes, differing mainly in their timing. Although these are cardiac waveforms simulated with the DiFrancesco-Noble model, note the markedly different impression of the wave shape seen in this figure as compared with Fig. 8.2. Note also that the waveform at $z = 0$ has progressed through excitation, but not into the plateau phase, by the time of excitation at $z = 1$ cm. Secondary changes of action potential wave shape as a function of z, other than the stimulus artefact, can be discerned mainly in the baseline as it rises into the upstroke, a region called the *foot*. Differences in the duration of the foot reflect the time that other tissue has been excited, prior to the start of excitation at a particular site; i.e., the foot is longer at sites further down the fiber.

Biophysical Basis

Although propagation in nerves and muscles often is compared to wave propagation of sound or light, to waves in the ocean, or to electrical waves in cables, bioelectric propagation does not have an analogous physical basis. In the former categories, energy used at the source creates a disturbance that propagates to the observer through an intervening passive medium. Propagation velocity depends on the properties of that medium. In bioelectric propagation, what is meant is that the source itself is moving down an excitable medium, the membrane, in a process more similar to setting off a chain of firecrackers. The velocities associated with bioelectric propagation relate to the magnitudes of transmembrane current passing through one site on the membrane and flowing to another and how fast the active responses of the membrane occur at the downstream sites. Although short intervals are required for passive propagation of the consequences of the active events through the surrounding tissue, these intervals are minuscule in comparison with the times required for the active changes. Consequently, most bioelectric events are analyzed as a sequence of "quasistatic" stages.

Velocity of Propagation

It is difficult to predict the velocity of propagation for a particular tissue structure prior to its measurement. Reported experimental velocities of propagation range from less than 0.01 m/s to more than 10 m/s, depending on the particular membrane and structure involved and its environment. Within a particular nerve or muscle, however, velocities vary little under normal conditions. Changes in the velocity of propagation θ as a result of changes in fiber diameter a or specific resistivity R_i can be approximated by the equation

$$\theta = \sqrt{\frac{Ka}{2R_i}} \tag{8.10}$$

Here K is a constant determined by the membrane properties, a is the fiber radius, and R_i is the specific resistance of the intracellular medium [Plonsey and Barr, 1988, p. 117], and the equation assumes relatively low extracellular resistance.

An important relationship shown by Eq. (8.10) is the proportionality of the velocity to the square root of the fiber's radius. Living systems take advantage of this relationship by having larger-diameter fibers where higher velocity is essential. For example, the giant axon of the squid carries the signal by which the squid responds to predators.

Transmembrane Current

The mathematical analysis of propagation is greatly aided by using the principle of conservation of charge to develop an equation for membrane current I_m that depends on the local distribution of intracellular potential rather than on currents through the membrane, as in Eq. (8.1). Conservation of current requires that current through the membrane at an axial position z be the difference between current coming to that site and current leaving that site (on one side, e.g., intracellularly). Because intracellular currents follow the first derivative of ϕ_i (Eq. 8.5), then for one-dimensional flow [Plonsey and Barr, 1988, p. 112],

$$I_m = \frac{1}{2\pi a r_i} \frac{\partial^2 \phi_i}{\partial z^2} \tag{8.11}$$

Here r_i is the axial resistance per unit length, a is the fiber radius, and ϕ_i is the intracellular potential. This result is used below, as well as in many mathematical analyses of propagation, because it provides a means (sometimes the sole means) of linking the membrane current at one site to electrical events at neighboring sites.

Movement of the Local Current Loop

Propagation occurs when a local current loop initiates an action potential in an adjacent region. The concept of how this occurs is illustrated in Fig. 8.7. At time t_1, a local current loop exists, as shown in Fig. 8.7a. This local loop produces outward current at site $z = z_1$. That there must be outward current at z_1 is shown by Fig. 8.7b, which plots $\phi_i(z)$ for time t_1. The gradient of ϕ_i between z_2 and z_1 is shown in Fig. 8.7b. This gradient produces intracellular current into z_1 from the left but not current out on the right (because the gradient is zero to the right). Current must therefore leave through the membrane at z_1. This positive membrane current is indicated by the upward arrow at z_1 in Fig. 8.7b. The positive membrane current at z_1 discharges the membrane capacitance there, so the potential at z_1 rises, producing a new voltage distribution. The change in the intracellular voltage distribution produces a shift in the site of the current loop; i.e., the loop propages to the right, as shown in Fig. 8.7c.

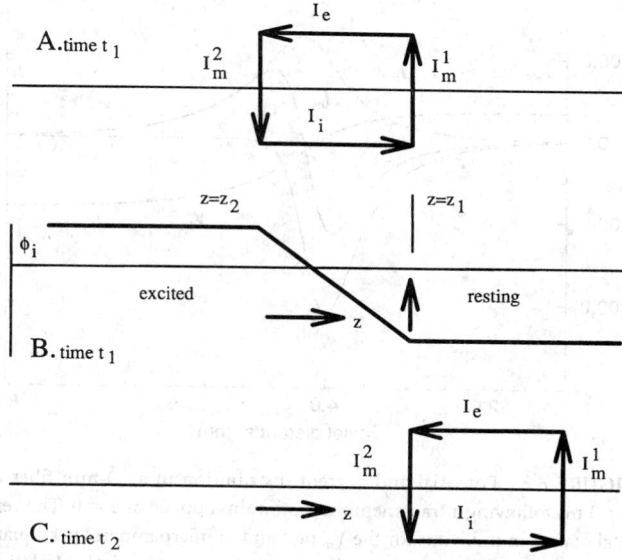

FIGURE 8.7 Propagation of a current loop, concept drawing. Panels *a* and *b* draw a hypothetical current loop as it might exist at time t_1. At this time, outward current is causing the potential to rise at $z = z_1$, as indicated by the upward arrow there, in panel *b*. The result is a shift in the distribution of intracellular potential ϕ_i. Thus the current loop moves to the position shown in panel *c*.

More mathematically, at z_1 at time t_1 the value of $\partial^2 \phi_i / \partial z^2$ is markedly positive, because ϕ_i changes slope there from negative to zero. Therefore, by Eq. (8.11), I_m is large and positive at $z = z_1$. Additionally, I_{ion} is relatively small at z_1 because the intracellular voltage is at its resting value, so (by Eq. 8.1) I_c must be large. By Eq. (8.2), if I_c is large and positive, then $\partial V_m / \partial t$ is large and positive. Thus the transmembrane potential at z_1 rises rapidly, and soon the current loop shown in Fig. 8.7c is achieved.

For comparison with the schematic drawings in Fig. 8.7, the distribution of voltages and currents in the 1-cm simulated fiber is shown in Fig. 8.8. The figure shows the transmembrane potential V_m and the total membrane current I_m. Both are shown as a function of axial distance z along the strand at time $t = 3$ ms after the stimulus. (This spatial plot came from the same simulation as the set of waveforms versus time shown in Fig. 8.6.) Because $V_m = \phi_i - \phi_e$, and because in this example the extracellular potentials ϕ_e are relatively small in magnitude (see below), V_m in Fig. 8.8 is a close approximation to ϕ_i in Fig. 8.7.

In Fig. 8.8, the total membrane current I_m is biphasic, with the outward current on the leading edge of the propagating waveform. Propagation is to the right, consistent with the direction of downward slope of V_m and consistent with the direction of movement of Fig. 8.7. The inward and outward currents of the distributed pattern in Fig. 8.8 are consistent with the concept of Fig. 8.7, where the distribution is lumped. (One might place $z_1 \approx 4.8$ mm in Fig. 8.8 and $z_2 \approx 4.0$ mm.) Figure 8.8 shows that the local current loop is more accurately described as a local current distribution, extending over a distance of a few millimeters (about 0.8 mm between the maximum and minimum of the I_m curve).

The composition of $I_m(z)$ can be evaluated by comparing I_m with its components, the ionic current I_{ion} and the membrane capacitative current I_c. At the outward current peak (the maximum of

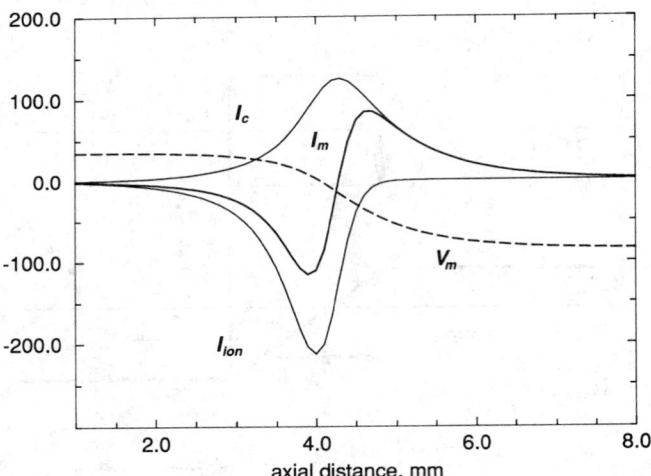

FIGURE 8.8 Potential and current distribution in a 10-mm fiber at $t = 3$ ms following a transmembrane stimulus applied at $z = 0$. The vertical scale is in millivolts for the V_m plot and in microamperes per square centimeter for the current plots. Results are from a numerical simulation using the geometry of Fig. 8.6. Transmembrane potential V_m at this moment is shown by the dashed line. Note the inward and outward peaks of the transmembrane current I_m near $z = 4$ and 4.8 mm. Plots for I_c and I_{ion}, the components of I_m, also are shown. They demonstrate that on the leading edge of the waveform (higher values of z), current I_c dominates. Compare the results with the concept drawing of Fig. 8.7.

I_m), the magnitude of the capacitive component I_c is greater than the magnitude of the ionic component I_{ion}. At the inward peak (the minimum of I_m), $|I_{ion}| > |I_c|$, although both magnitudes are significant. That is, the dominant components of I_m in Fig. 8.8 are consistent with the drawings in Fig. 8.7. In contrast to Fig. 8.7, however, the peak outward current occurs near where $V_m \approx -40$ mV rather than near the baseline value (≈ -85 mV). Consistent with Fig. 8.7, Fig. 8.8 shows that I_m is dominated by I_c at the peak outward I_m and increasingly more so as one moves forward on the leading edge.

8.7 Extracellular Waveforms

An understanding of the origin of extracellular waveforms is important because most electrophysiologic recordings, including those of most clinical studies, are observations of extracellular events rather than underlying transmembrane or intracellular events. The extracellular-intracellular relationship is not a simple one, however, because it involves distance from the membrane sources, and because a given extracellular site usually is affected by currents from many different excitable fibers.

Although extracellular waveforms $\phi_e(t)$ reflect the same current loops as the intracellular or transmembrane waveforms, their magnitude, wave shape, and timing usually are entirely different. (The greatest similarity occurs with a highly restricted extracellular volume.) With an extensive extracellular volume, the normal situation, waveforms such as those in Fig. 8.9 are seen. The three waveforms come from "electrodes" just outside the fiber at $z = 0$, $z = 5$, and $z = 10$ mm, or in other words at the site of the stimulus, the middle of the strand, and the end where excitation terminates. (For reference, the intracellular potential from the middle of the fiber also is shown, reduced to 2% of its true magnitude.) All three extracellular waveforms shown are small in comparison with transmembrane waveforms, less than 1 mV peak to peak. Their wave shapes differ: Near the stimulus (0), the wave shape has a negative deflection from the stimulus and continues to be negative thereafter. In the middle, the wave shape is biphasic. A positive deflection occurs as excitation approaches, and a negative deflection occurs once it goes past (compare the timing of the extracellular and intracellular waveforms, which are from the same axial position). At the terminating end (10), the extracellular wave shape is predominantly positive, showing also a long initial rise as excitation approaches.

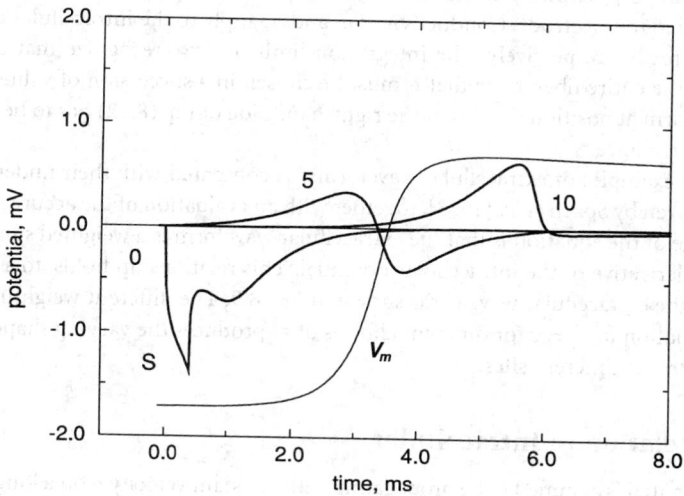

FIGURE 8.9 Extracellular waveforms from a 10-mm fiber. Extracellular potentials $\phi_e(t)$ are plotted for positions just outside the membrane at $z = 0$, 5, and 10 mm. The transmembrane stimulus at $z = 0$ affected the waveform there, as seen by stimulus artefact S. For reference, $V_m(t)$ at $z = 5$ mm also is drawn, reduced to 2% of its true amplitude.

It is interesting that these extracellular waveforms show such large changes in wave shape as a function of position, whereas their underlying transmembrane waveforms, at the same z values, show no such changes, as can be seen by comparison with the transmembrane waveforms shown in Fig. 8.6. The relative timing of the extracellular as compared with the transmembrane waveforms also is noteworthy: Close to the membrane, most of the major deflections of the extracellular waveforms are confined to the short time period when the transmembrane potential is undergoing excitation. During the hundreds of milliseconds thereafter, the intracellular potential is large but changing slowly (e.g., Fig. 8.2), so the transmembrane currents are small. These smaller currents are distributed and produce proportionally small deflections. As the recording site moves away from the membrane, however, the distributed recovery currents do not decline as rapidly with distance, so the potentials they produce become larger in relation to potentials produced by the currents of excitation. On the body surface, the voltages produced during recovery may have similar magnitudes and play a large role in waveform interpretation (e.g., the T wave of the electrocardiogram).

Biphasic waveforms are observed at most extracellular sites, because most sites are neither the origin or termination of excitation. Further, most real extracellular waveforms are more complicated and last longer than those shown in Fig. 8.9, because they show the composite effect from many different fibers rather than a single one in isolation.

Spatial Relation to Intracellular

Extracellular waveforms are created by the flow of current through the volume conductor surrounding the active membrane. An expression for the extracellular potential ϕ_e outside a cylindrical fiber with a large conducting volume was given by Spach et al. [1973] as

$$\phi_e(t_o, z) = \frac{a\sigma}{4\sigma} \int_{-\infty}^{\infty} \frac{(\partial^2 \phi_i/\partial z'^2)_{to}}{\sqrt{\left(\frac{d+a}{a}\right)^2 + \left[\frac{(z'-z)}{a}\right]^2}} \, dz' \tag{8.12}$$

where z is the axial coordinate of the fiber, t_o is the time when the spatial distribution was obtained, ϕ_i is the intracellular potential, a is the fiber radius, and d is the perpendicular distance from the fiber membrane to the electrode. Conductivities σ_i and σ_e apply to the intracellular and extracellular conducting media, respectively. The integration limits of $\pm\infty$ recognize that the integration should be over the entire fiber. Note that t_o must be chosen in a succession of values to generate a temporal waveform at position z and that the right-hand side of Eq. (8.12) has to be evaluated separately for each t_o choice.

A number of examples of extracellular waveforms, as compared with their underlying intracellular ones, are given by Spach et al. [1973], together with an evaluation of the accuracy of Eq. (8.12). A central feature of the equation is that the extracellular waveform is a weighted summation of the second spatial derivative of the intracellular potential. This relationship holds, to a good approximation, for all the extracellular waveforms shown in Fig. 8.9. The different weighting for different waveforms (variation in $z' - z$ for different choices of z) produces the varying shapes of the extracellular waveforms at different sites.

Temporal Relation to Intracellular

If an action potential is assumed to be propagating with constant velocity θ on a long fiber, then the spatial derivative in the preceding equation can be converted to a temporal derivative using $z = \theta t$ so that

$$\phi_e(t_o, z) = \frac{a\sigma}{4\theta} \int_{-\infty}^{\infty} \frac{(\partial^2 \phi_i/\partial z'^2)_{zo}}{\sqrt{\left(\frac{d+a}{a}\right)^2 + \left[\frac{\theta(t'-t)}{a}\right]^2}} \, dt' \tag{8.13}$$

where t is time, z_o is the axial coordinate of the position where the intracellular and extracellular "electrodes" are located, and θ is the velocity with which the action potential is moving along the z axis. The integration limits of $\pm\infty$ recognize that only in long fibers does the velocity remain approximately constant over a significant period of time.

Some of the limitations of Eq. (8.13) are apparent when considering the waveforms of Fig. 8.9. The equation would be suitable only for the extracellular waveform in the middle of the fiber ($z = 5$ mm). At either end, the equation would be unsuitable, because velocity is not constant through initiation or through termination of propagation.

8.8 Stimulation

The waveforms of Fig. 8.6 show that action potentials can be initiated and controlled by (artificially injected) transmembrane currents. Such transmembrane currents can be injected through use of penetrating microelectrodes. Some experimental studies use this method of initiating action potentials because the site of current injection is precisely localized. Most stimulation for clinical purposes and most experimental studies use extracellular electrodes, however, because positioning the electrodes outside the active tissue can be done more simply, usually without tissue damage.

Suppose two stimulating electrodes are placed just outside the 1-cm fiber, as identified in Fig. 8.10. Note that the anode is placed at $z = 10$ mm (encircled $+$), and the cathode is placed at $z = 0$ (encircled $-$). Both electrodes are extracellular. When current is injected through these electrodes, most of the current will flow along the extracellular path (thick flow line). Some current also will cross the resistive barrier formed by the membrane and flow intracellularly (thin flow line). Where the intracellular current emerges from the membrane, it will tend to depolarize the membrane. (Note the effects of the stimulus on potential differences: The region depolarized is the region where the intracellular potential becomes higher as compared with the extracellular potential directly across the membrane. In contrast, the region depolarized has a lower potential near the cathode as compared with the potential at the other end of the fiber, near the anode, in both the intracellular and extracellular volumes.) If the magnitude of the depolarization is large enough in relation to the size of the depolarized region, then the stimulus will initiate action potentials and propagation.

Transmembrane potential distributions following the extracellular stimulus are shown in Fig. 8.11. At time $t = 0$, the transmembrane potential (as a function of z) is flat, indicating that the membrane is uniformly in the resting state. Then a stimulus of 0.05 mA amplitude and 0.5 ms duration is applied to the stimulus electrodes, with the source-sink positioning that of Fig. 8.10. Figure 8.11

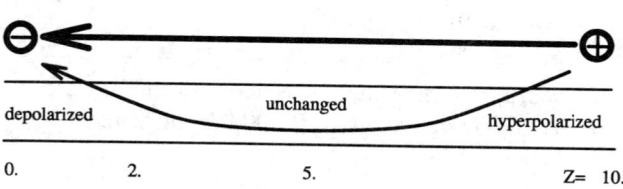

FIGURE 8.10   Extracellular stimulus currents, concept drawing. A stimulus is applied between an extracellular anode, at $z = 10$, and an extracellular cathode, at $z = 0$. Most current will flow in the extracellular volume (*thick line*). Some current will enter the intracellular volume (*thin line*). Current entering or leaving the membrane causes that portion of the membrane to become hyperpolarized (high z region) or depolarized (low z region).

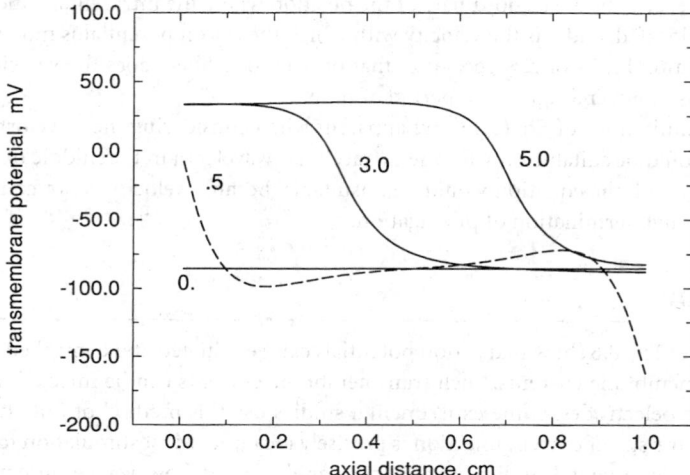

FIGURE 8.11 Transmembrane potentials following an extracellular stimulus. The simulation used the geometry of Fig. 8.5, except that the stimulus was applied to the row 2 nodes at $z = 0$ and $z = 10$ (similar to Fig. 8.10). Successive plots show the transmembrane potentials as a function of z at time 0 (just before the stimulus), 0.5 ms (end of the stimulus), 3.0 ms (propagation underway), and 5.0 ms. The potential distribution at 0.5 ms is consistent in its major features with the concept drawing of Fig. 8.10.

shows the distribution of transmembrane potentials at $t = 0.5$ ms, the time of the end of the stimulus. At $t = 0.5$ ms, the membrane is depolarized near the cathode (near $z = 0$) and is hyperpolarized near the anode (near $z = 10$). Interestingly, there is a small region of hyperpolarization beside the depolarized end (near $z = 2$ mm) and depolarization near the hyperpolarized end (near $z = 8$ mm), a predictable effect [Plonsey and Barr, 1995]. The transmembrane potentials along the central part of the fiber are much less affected by the stimulus than are the ends, even though the same magnitude of stimulus current flows along the entire length. This stimulus was large enough to produce action potentials, as can be seen by inspecting the transmembrane potentials for 3 ms. Figure 8.11 shows that the excitation wave that began near $z = 0$ has, by 3 ms, progressed about a third of the way down the fiber. Propagation to a further point is seen at 5.0 ms.

Many devices for medical stimulation have now come into routine use, e.g., cardiac pacemakers. Large artificial currents also are used to terminate action potentials in some cases, e.g., cardiac defibrillators.

8.9 Biomagnetism

Panofsky and Phillips [1962, p. 160] show the connection between the electric field **E** to the magnetic field **B** and current $\mathbf{j}_{true}$ by giving two (of the four) Maxwell's equations as

$$\nabla \times \mathbf{H} = -\mathbf{j}_{true} + \frac{\partial \mathbf{D}}{\partial t} \tag{8.14}$$

and

$$\nabla \times \mathbf{E} = -\frac{\partial \mathbf{B}}{\partial t} \tag{8.15}$$

together with the constituitive relations $\mathbf{H} = \mathbf{B}/\mu$ and $\mathbf{D} = \kappa\epsilon_o\mathbf{E}$, where μ, κ, and ϵ_o are constants for a given medium.

Both currents j_{true} and changing electric fields ($\mathbf{E}$ and thereby $\mathbf{D}$) are present naturally in and around excitable membranes, so Eq. (8.14) shows that corresponding magnetic fields are to be expected. These magnetic fields are small, however, even in comparison with the earth's magnetic field. They can nonetheless be precisely measured if careful attention is paid to the design of equipment and the surroundings, as demonstrated by Wikswo and Egeraat [1991]. At present, magnetic fields are not routinely measured for clinical purposes, but in principle, they offer some important advantages, including the absence of required electrode contact.

In a complementary way, rapidly changing magnetic fields induce electric fields (and thereby currents) in living tissue, as indicated by Eq. (8.15). Stimulation of nerves or muscles is thereby possible, either by design (see, e.g., Roth and Basser [1990]) or as a side effect of magnetic resonance imaging (MRI). Extensive consideration of biomagnetism has been presented by Malmivuo and Plonsey [1994].

Defining Terms

Action potential: The cycle of changes of transmembrane potential, negative to positive to negative again, that characterizes excitable tissue. This cycle also is described as resting to excited and returning to rest.

Excitation: The change of the membrane from resting to excited states, characterized by the movement of the transmembrane potential across a threshold.

Extracellular potentials: Potentials generated between two sites outside the membrane (external to active cells), e.g., between two sites on the skin, due to current flow in the volume conductor.

Intracellular (extracellular): Inside (outside) cells.

Membrane polarization: The sustained (and approximately constant) transmembrane potential of a cell at rest that arises due to different intracellular and extracellular ionic concentrations.

Propagation: Excitation of one region of tissue as a result of an action potential in an adjacent region.

Stimulation: Change in the transmembrane potential at a site due to an influence from another site. The term is used most frequently when current is applied through wires from an artificial current source.

Transmembrane potential: The potential inside a cell membrane minus the potential just outside the membrane.

Volume conductor: The electrically conductive interior region of the body surrounding electrically active membrane.

References

Byrne JH, Schultz SG. 1988. An Introduction to Membrane Transport and Bioelectricity. New York, Raven Press.

Cabo C, Barr RC. 1992. Propagation model using the DiFrancesco-Noble equations. Med Biol Eng Comput 30:292.

Malmivuo J, Plonsey R. 1995. Bioelectromagnetism: Principles and Applications of Bioelectric and Biomagnetic Fields. New York, Oxford University Press.

Noble D, DiFrancesco D, Noble S, et al. 1994. Oxsoft Heart Program Manual. Wellesley Hills, Mass, NB Datyner.

Panofsky WKH, Phillips M. 1962. Classical Electricity and Magnetism, 2nd ed. New York, Addison-Wesley.

Plonsey R, Barr RC. 1988. Bioelectricity: A Quantitative Approach. New York, Plenum Press.

Plonsey R, Barr RC. 1995. Electric field stimulation of excitable tissue. IEEE Transactions on Biomedical Engineering, to appear.

Roth BJ, Passer PJ. 1990. A model of the stimulation of a nerve fiber by electromagnetic stimulating. IEEE Trans BME 37:588–597.

Spach MS, Barr RC, Johnson EA, Kootsey JM. 1973. Cardiac extracellular potentials: Analysis of complex waveforms about the Purkinje network in dogs. Circ Res 31:465.

Watson JD, Gilman M, Witkowski J, Zoller M. 1992. Recombinant DNA, 2d ed. New York, Scientific American Books.

Wikswo JP Jr, van Egeraat JM. 1991. Cellular magnetic fields: Fundamental and applied measurements on nerve axons, peripheral nerve bundles, and skeletal muscle. J Clin Neurophysiol 8(2):170.

9

Volume Conductor
Theory

Robert Plonsey
Duke University

This chapter considers the properties of the volume conductor as it pertains to the evaluation of electric and magnetic fields arising therein. The sources of the aforementioned fields are described by $\vec{J}^i$, a function of position and time, which has the dimensions of current per unit area *or* dipole moment per unit volume. Such sources may arise from active endogenous electrophysiologic processes such as propagating action potentials, generator potentials, synaptic potentials, etc. Sources also may be established exogenously, as exemplified by electric or magnetic field stimulation. Details on how one may quantitatively evaluate a source function from an electrophysiologic process are found in other chapters. For our purposes here, we assume that such a source function $\vec{J}^i$ is known and, furthermore, that it has well-behaved mathematical properties. Given such a source, we focus attention here on a description of the volume conductor as it affects the electric and magnetic fields that are established in it. As a loose definition, we consider the *volume conductor* to be the contiguous passive conducting medium that surrounds the region occupied by the source $\vec{J}^i$. (This may include a portion of the excitable tissue itself that is sufficiently far from $\vec{J}^i$ to be described passively.)

9.1 Basic Relations in the Idealized Homogeneous Volume Conductor

Excitable tissue, when activated, will be found to generate currents both within itself and also in all surrounding conducting media. The latter passive region is characterized as a *volume conductor*. The adjective *volume* emphasizes that current flow is three-dimensional, in contrast to the confined one-dimensional flow within insulated wires. The volume conductor is usually assumed to be a mono-domain (whose meaning will be amplified later), isotropic, resistive, and (frequently) homogeneous. These are simplifying assumptions, as will be discussed subsequently. The permeability of biologic tissues is important when examining magnetic fields and is usually assumed to be that of free space. The permittivity is a more complicated property, but outside cell membranes (which have a high lipid content) it is also usually considered to be that of free space.

A general, mathematical description of a current source is specified by a function $\vec{J}^i(x, y, z, t)$, namely, a vector field of current density in say milliamperes per square centimeter that varies both

0-8493-8346-3/95/$0.00+$.50
© 1995 by CRC Press, Inc.

in space and time. A study of sources of physiologic origin shows that their temporal behavior lies in a low-frequency range. For example, currents generated by the heart have a power density spectrum that lies mainly under 1 kHz (in fact, clinical ECG instruments have upper frequency limits of 100 Hz), while most other electrophysiologic sources of interest (i.e., those underlying the EEG, EMG, EOG, etc.) are of even lower frequency. Examination of electromagnetic fields in regions with typical physiologic conductivities, with dimensions of under 1 m and frequencies less than 1 kHz, shows that *quasi-static* conditions apply. That is, at a given instant in time, source-field relationships correspond to those found under static conditions.* Thus, in effect, we are examining direct current (dc) flow in physiologic volume conductors, and these can be maintained only by the presence of a supply of energy (a "battery"). In fact, we may expect that wherever a physiologic current source $\vec{J}^i$ arises, we also can identify a (normally nonelectrical) energy source that generates this current. In electrophysiologic processes, the immediate repository of energy is the potential energy associated with the varying chemical compositions encountered (extracellular ionic concentrations that differ greatly from intracellular concentrations), but the long-term energy source is the adenosine triphosphate (ATP) that drives various pumps that create and maintain the aforementioned concentration gradients.

Based on the aforementioned assumptions, we consider a uniformly conducting medium of conductivity σ and of infinite extent within which a current source $\vec{J}^i$ lies. This, in turn, establishes an electric field $\vec{E}$ and, based on Ohm's law, a conduction current density $\sigma\vec{E}$. The total current density $\vec{J}$ is the sum of the aforementioned currents, namely,

$$\vec{J} = \sigma\vec{E} + \vec{J}^i \tag{9.1}$$

Now, by virtue of the quasi-static conditions, the electric field may be derived from a scalar potential Φ [Plonsey and Heppner, 1967] so that

$$\vec{E} = -\nabla\Phi \tag{9.2}$$

Since quasi–steady-state conditions apply, $\vec{J}$ must be solenoidal, and consequently, substituting Eq. (9.2) into Eq. (9.1) and then setting the divergence of Eq. (9.1) to zero show that Φ must satisfy Poisson's equation, namely,

$$\nabla^2\Phi = (1/\sigma)\nabla \cdot \vec{J}^i \tag{9.3}$$

An integral solution to Eq. (9.3) is [Plonsey and Collin, 1961]

$$\Phi_P(x', y', z') = -\frac{1}{4\pi\sigma}\int_v \frac{\nabla \cdot \vec{J}^i}{r}\, dv \tag{9.4}$$

where r in Eq. (9.4) is the distance from a field point $P(x', y', z')$ to an element of source at $dv(x, y, z)$, that is,

$$r = \sqrt{(x - x')^2 + (y - y')^2 + (z - z')^2} \tag{9.5}$$

Equation (9.4) may be transformed to an alternate form by employing the vector identity

$$\nabla \cdot [(1/r)\vec{J}^i] \equiv (1/r)\nabla \cdot \vec{J}^i + \nabla(1/r) \cdot \vec{J}^i \tag{9.6}$$

---

*Note that while, in effect, we consider relationships arising when $\partial/\partial t = 0$, all fields are actually assumed to vary in time synchronously with $\vec{J}^i$. Furthermore for the special case of magnetic field stimulation, the source of the primary electric field, $\partial\vec{A}/\partial t$, where $\vec{A}$ is the magnetic vector potential, must be retained.

Based on Eq. (9.6), we may substitute for the integrand in Eq. (9.4) the sum $\nabla \cdot [(1/r)\vec{J}^i] - \nabla(1/r) \cdot \vec{J}^i$, giving the following:

$$\Phi_P(x', y', z') = -\frac{1}{4\pi\sigma} \left\{ \int_v \nabla \cdot [(1/r)\vec{J}^i] \, dv - \int_v \nabla(1/r) \cdot \vec{J}^i \, dv \right\} \tag{9.7}$$

The first term on the right-hand side may be transformed using the divergence theorem as follows:

$$\int_v \nabla \cdot [(1/r)\vec{J}^i] \, dv = \int_s (1/r)\vec{J}^i \cdot d\vec{S} = 0 \tag{9.8}$$

The volume integral in Eq. (9.4) and (9.8) is defined simply to include all sources. Consequently, in Eq. (9.8), the surface S, which bounds V, necessarily lies away from $\vec{J}^i$. Since $\vec{J}^i$ thus is equal to zero on S, the expression in Eq. (9.8) must likewise equal zero. The result is that Eq. (9.4) also may be written as

$$\Phi_P(x', y', z') = -\frac{1}{4\pi\sigma} \int_v \frac{\nabla \cdot \vec{J}^i}{r} \, dv = \frac{1}{4\pi\sigma} \int_v \vec{J}^i \cdot \nabla(1/r) dv \tag{9.9}$$

We will derive the mathematical expressions for monopole and dipole fields in the next section, but based on those results, we can give a physical interpretation of the source terms in each of the integrals on the right-hand side of Eq. (9.9). In the first, we note that $-\nabla \cdot \vec{J}^i$ is a volume source density, akin to charge density in electrostatics. In the second integral of Eq. (9.9), $\vec{J}^i$ behaves with the dimensions of dipole moment per unit volume. This confirms an assertion, above, that $\vec{J}^i$ has a dual interpretation as a current density, as originally defined in Eq. (9.1), or a volume dipole density, as can be inferred from Eq. (9.9); in either case, its dimensions are mA/cm²/ = /mA · cm/cm³.

9.2 Monopole and Dipole Fields in the Uniform Volume of Infinite Extent

The monopole and dipole constitute the basic source elements in electrophysiology. We examine the fields produced by each in this section.

If one imagines an infinitely thin wire insulated over its extent except at its tip to be introducing a current into a uniform volume conductor of infinite extent, then we illustrate an idealized point source. Assuming the total applied current to be I_0 and located at the coordinate origin, then by symmetry the current density at a radius r must be given by the total current I_0 divided by the area of the spherical surface, or

$$\vec{J} = \frac{I_0}{4\pi r^2} \vec{a}_r \tag{9.10}$$

and $\vec{a}_r$ is a unit vector in the radial direction. This current source can be described by the nomenclature of the previous section as

$$\nabla \cdot \vec{J}^i = -I_0\delta(r) \tag{9.11}$$

where δ denotes a volume delta function.

One can apply Ohm's law to Eq. (9.10) and obtain an expression for the electric field, and if Eq. (9.2) is also applied, we get

$$\vec{E} = -\nabla\Phi = \frac{I_0}{4\pi\sigma r^2} \vec{a}_r \tag{9.12}$$

where σ is the conductivity of the volume conductor. Since the right-hand side of Eq. (9.12) is a function of r only, we can integrate to find Φ, which comes out

$$\Phi = \frac{I_0}{4\pi\sigma r} \qquad (9.13)$$

In obtaining Eq. (9.13), the constant of integration was set equal to zero so that the point at infinity has the usually chosen zero potential.

The dipole source consists of two monopoles of equal magnitude and opposite sign whose spacing approaches zero and whose magnitude during the limiting process increases such that the product of spacing and magnitude is constant. If we start out with both component monopoles at the origin, then the total source and field are zero. However, if we now displace the positive source in an arbitrary direction $\vec{d}$, then cancellation is no longer complete, and at a field point P we see simply the change in monopole field resulting from the displacement. For a very small displacement, this amounts to (i.e., we retain only the linear term in a Taylor series expansion)

$$\Phi_P = \frac{\partial}{\partial d}\left(\frac{I_0}{4\pi\sigma r}\right) d \qquad (9.14)$$

The partial derivative in Eq. (9.14) is called the *directional derivative*, and this can be evaluated by taking the dot product of the gradient of the expression enclosed in parentheses with the direction of d [that is, $\nabla(\ )\cdot\vec{a}_d$, where $\vec{a}_d$ is a unit vector in the $\vec{d}$ direction]. The result is

$$\Phi_P = \frac{I_0 d}{4\pi\sigma}\,\vec{a}_d \cdot \nabla(1/r) \qquad (9.15)$$

By definition, the dipole moment $\vec{m} = I_0\vec{d}$ in the limit as $d \to 0$; as noted, m remains finite. Thus, finally, the dipole field is given by [Plonsey, 1969]

$$\Phi_P = \frac{1}{4\pi\sigma}\,\vec{m} \cdot \nabla(1/r) \qquad (9.16)$$

9.3 Volume Conductor Properties of Passive Tissue

If one were considering an active single isolated fiber lying in an extensive volume conductor (e.g., an in vitro preparation in a Ringer's bath), then there is a clear separation between the excitable tissue and the surrounding volume conductor. However, consider in contrast activation proceeding in the in vivo heart. In this case, the source currents lie in only a portion of the heart (nominally where $\nabla V_m \neq 0$). The volume conductor now includes the remaining (passive) cardiac fibers along with an inhomogeneous torso containing a number of contiguous organs (internal to the heart are blood-filled cavities, while external are pericardium, lungs, skeletal muscle, bone, fat, skin, air, etc.).

The treatment of the surrounding multicellular cardiac tissue poses certain difficulties. A recently used and reasonable approximation is that the intracellular space, in view of the many intercellular junctions, can be represented as a continuum. A similar treatment can be extended to the interstitial space. This results in two domains that can be regarded as occupying the same physical space; each domain is separated from the other by the membrane. This view underlies the *bidomain* model [Plonsey, 1989]. To reflect the underlying fiber geometry, each domain is necessarily anisotropic, with the high conductivity axes defined by the fiber direction and with an approximate cross-fiber isotropy. A further simplification may be possible in a uniform tissue region that is sufficiently far from the sources, since beyond a few space constants transmembrane currents may become quite small and the tissue would therefore behave as a single domain (a *monodomain*). Such a tissue also would be substantially resistive. On the other hand, if the membranes behave passively and there is some degree of transmembrane current flow, then the tissue may still be approximated as a uniform monodomain, but it may be necessary to include some of the reactive properties introduced via the highly capacitive cell membranes. A classic study by Schwan and Kay [1957] of the macroscopic (averaged) properties of many tissues showed that the displacement current was normally negligible compared with the conduction current.

It is not always clear whether a bidomain model is appropriate to a particular tissue, and experimental measurements found in the literature are not always able to resolve this question. The problem is that if the experimenter believes the tissue under consideration to be, say, an isotropic monodomain, measurements are set up and interpreted that are consistent with this idea; the inherent inconsistencies may never come to light [Plonsey and Barr, 1986]. Thus one may find impedance data tabulated in the literature for a number of organs, but if the tissue is truly, say, an anisotropic bidomain, then the impedance tensor requires six numbers, and anything less is necessarily inadequate to some degree. For cardiac tissue, it is usually assumed that the impedance in the direction transverse to the fiber axis is isotropic. Consequently, only four numbers are needed. These values are given in Table 9.1 as obtained from, essentially, the only two experiments for which bidomain values were sought.

9.4 Effects of Volume Conductor Inhomogeneities: Secondary Sources and Images

In the preceding we have assumed that the volume conductor is homogeneous, and the evaluation of fields from the current sources given in Eq. (9.9) is based on this assumption. Consider what would happen if the volume conductor in which $\vec{J}^i$ lies is bounded by air, and the source is suddenly introduced. Equation (9.9) predicts an initial current flow into the boundary, but no current can escape into the nonconducting surrounding region. We must, consequently, have a transient during which charge piles up at the boundary, a process that continues until the field from the accumulating charges brings the net normal component of electric field to zero at the boundary. To characterize a steady-state condition with no further increase in charge requires satisfaction of the boundary condition that $\partial \Phi / \partial n = 0$ at the surface (within the tissue). The source that develops at the bounding surface is secondary to the initiation of the primary field; it is referred to as a *secondary source*. While the secondary source is essential for satisfaction of boundary conditions, it contributes to the total field everywhere else.

The preceding illustration is for a region bounded by air, but the same phenomena would arise if the region were simply bounded by one of different conductivity. In this case, when the source is first "turned on," since the primary electric field $\vec{E}_a$ is continuous across the interface between regions of different conductivity, the current flowing into such a boundary (e.g., $\sigma_1 \vec{E}_a$) is unequal to the current flowing away from that boundary (e.g., $\sigma_2 \vec{E}_a$). Again, this necessarily results in an accumulation of charge, and a secondary source will grow until the applied plus secondary field satisfies the required continuity of current density, namely,

$$-\sigma_1 \partial \Phi_1 / \partial n = -\sigma_2 \partial \Phi_2 / \partial n = J_n \tag{9.17}$$

TABLE 9.1 Conductivity Values for Cardiac Bidomain

S/mm	Clerc [1976]	Roberts [1982]
g_{ix}	1.74×10^{-4}	3.44×10^{-4}
g_{iy}	1.93×10^{-5}	5.96×10^{-5}
g_{ox}	6.25×10^{-4}	1.17×10^{-4}
g_{oy}	2.36×10^{-4}	8.02×10^{-5}

where the surface normal n is directed from region 1 to region 2. The accumulated single source density can be shown to be equal to the discontinuity of $\partial\Phi/\partial n$ in Eq. (9.17)[Plonsey, 1974], in particular, $K_s = J_n(1/\sigma_1 - 1/\sigma_2)\sigma$.

The magnitude of the steady-state secondary source also can be described as an *equivalent double layer*, the magnitude of which is [Plonsey, 1974]

$$\vec{K}_k^i = \Phi_k \, (\sigma_k'' - \sigma_k')\vec{n} \tag{9.18}$$

where the condition at the kth interface is described. In Eq. (9.18), the two abutting regions are designated with prime and double-prime superscripts, and $\vec{n}$ is directed from the primed to the double-primed region. Actually, Eq. (9.18) evaluates the double-layer source for the scalar function $\psi = \Phi\sigma$, its strength being given by the discontinuity in ψ at the interface [Plonsey, 1974] [the potential is necessarily continuous at the interface with the value Φ_k called for in Eq. (9.18)]. The (secondary) potential field generated by $\vec{K}_k^i$, since it constitutes a source for ψ with respect to which the medium is uniform and infinite in extent, can be found from Eq. (9.9) as

$$\psi_P^S = \sigma_P\Phi_P^S = \frac{1}{4\pi} \sum_k \int_k \Phi_k \, (\sigma_k'' - \sigma_k')\vec{n} \cdot \nabla(1/r) \, dS \tag{9.19}$$

where the superscript S denotes the secondary source/field component (alone). Solving Eq. (9.19) for Φ, we get

$$\Phi_P^S = \frac{1}{4\pi\sigma_P} \sum_k \int_k \Phi_k(\sigma_k'' - \sigma_k')\vec{n} \cdot \nabla(1/r) \, dS \tag{9.20}$$

where σ_P in Eqs. (9.19) and (9.20) takes on the conductivity at the field point. The total field is obtained from Eq. (9.20) by adding the primary field. Assuming that all applied currents lie in a region with conductivity σ_a, then we have

$$\Phi_P^S = \frac{1}{4\pi\sigma_a} \int \vec{J}^i \cdot \nabla(1/r)dv + \frac{1}{4\pi\sigma_P} \sum_k \int_k \Phi_k \, (\sigma_k'' - \sigma_k')\vec{n} \cdot \nabla(1/r) \, dS \tag{9.21}$$

[if the primary currents lie in several conductivity compartments, then each will yield a term similar to the first integral in Eq. (9.21)]. Note that in Eqs. (9.20) and (9.21) the secondary source field is similar in form to the field in a homogeneous medium of infinite extent, except that σ_P is piecewise constant and consequently introduces interfacial discontinuities. With regard to the potential, these just cancel the discontinuity introduced by the double layer itself so that Φ_k is appropriately continuous across each passive interface.

The primary and secondary source currents that generate the electrical potential in Eq. (9.21) also set up a magnetic field. The primary source, for example, is the forcing function in the Poisson equation for the vector potential $\vec{A}$ [Plonsey, 1981], namely,

$$\nabla^2 \vec{A} = -\vec{J}^i \tag{9.22}$$

From this it is not difficult to show that, due to Eq. (9.21) for Φ, we have the following expression for the magnetic field $\vec{H}$ [Plonsey, 1981]:

$$\vec{H} = \frac{1}{4\pi} \int \vec{J}^i \times \nabla(1/r) \, dv + \frac{1}{4\pi} \sum_k \int \Phi_k \, (\sigma_k'' - \sigma_k')\vec{n} \times \nabla(1/r) \, dS \tag{9.23}$$

A simple illustration of these ideas is found in the case of two semi-infinite regions of different conductivity, 1 and 2, with a unit point current source located in region 1 a distance h from the interface. Region 1, which we may think of as on the "left," has the conductivity σ_1, while region 2, on the "right," is at conductivity σ_2. The field in region 1 is that which arises from the actual point current source plus an image point source of magnitude $(\rho_2 - \rho_1)/(\rho_2 + \rho_1)$ located in region 2 at the mirror-image point [Schwan and Kay, 1957]. The field in region 2 arises from an equivalent point source located at the actual source point but of strength $[1 + (\rho_2 - \rho_1)/(\rho_2 + \rho_1)]$. One can confirm this by noting that all fields satisfy Poisson's equation and that at the interface Φ is continuous while the normal component of current density is also continuous (i.e., $\sigma_1 \partial \Phi_1 / \partial n = \sigma_2 \partial \Phi_2 / \partial n$).

The potential on the interface is constant along a circular path whose origin is the foot of the perpendicular from the point source. Calling this radius r and applying Eq. (9.13), we have for the surface potential Φ_S

$$\Phi_S = \frac{\rho_1}{4\pi \sqrt{h^2 + r^2}}\left(1 + \frac{\rho_2 - \rho_1}{\rho_2 + \rho_1}\right) \tag{9.24}$$

and consequently a secondary double-layer source $\vec{K}_S$ equals, according to Eq. (9.18),

$$\vec{K}_S = \frac{\rho_1}{4\pi\sqrt{h^2 + r^2}}\left(1 + \frac{\rho_2 - \rho_1}{\rho_2 + \rho_1}\right)(\sigma_2 - \sigma_1)\vec{n} \tag{9.25}$$

where $\vec{n}$ is directed from region 1 to region 2. The field from $\vec{K}_S$ in region 1 is exactly equal to that from a point source of strength $(\rho_2 - \rho_1)/(\rho_2 + \rho_1)$ at the mirror-image point, which can be verified by evaluating and showing the equality of the following:

$$\Phi_P = \frac{1}{4\pi\sigma_1}\int \vec{K}_S \cdot \nabla(1/r)\, dS = \frac{(\rho_2 - \rho_1)/(\rho_2 + \rho_1)}{4\pi\sigma_1 R} \tag{9.26}$$

where R in Eq. (9.26) is the distance from the mirror-image point to the field point P, and r in Eq. (9.26) is the distance from the surface integration point to the field point.

References

Clerc L. 1976. Directional differences of impulse spread in trabecular muscle from mammalian heart. J Physiol (Lond) 255:335.

Plonsey R. 1969. Bioelectric Phenomena. New York, McGraw-Hill.

Plonsey R. 1974. The formulation of bioelectric source-field relationship in terms of surface discontinuities. J Frank Inst 297:317.

Plonsey R. 1981. Generation of magnetic fields by the human body (theory). In S-N Erné, H-D Hahlbohm, H Lübbig (eds), Biomagnetism, pp 177–205. Berlin, W de Gruyter.

Plonsey R. 1989. The use of the bidomain model for the study of excitable media. Lect Math Life Sci 21:123.

Plonsey R, Barr RC. 1986. A critique of impedance measurements in cardiac tissue. Ann Biomed Eng 14:307.

Plonsey R, Collin RE. 1961. Principles and Applications of Electromagnetic Fields. New York, McGraw-Hill.

Plonsey R, Heppner D. 1967. Consideration of quasi-stationarity in electrophysiological systems. Bull Math Biophys 29:657.

Roberts D, Scher AM. 1982. Effect of tissue anisotropy on extracellular potential fields in canine myocardium in situ. Circ Res 50:342.

Schwan HP, Kay CF. 1957. The conductivity of living tissues. NY Acad Sci 65:1007.

10

The Electrical Properties
of Tissues

Bradley J. Roth
National Institute of Health

One of the most important problems in bioelectric theory is the calculation of the potential distribution Φ (V) throughout a **volume conductor**. The calculation of Φ is important in impedance imaging, cardiac pacing and defibrillation, electrocardiogram and electroencephalogram analysis, and functional electrical stimulation. In bioelectric problems, Φ often changes slowly enough that we can assume it to be **quasi-static** [Plonsey, 1969]; that is, we ignore capacitive and inductive effects and the finite speed of propagation of electromagnetic radiation. (For bioelectric phenomena, this approximation is usually valid for frequencies below roughly 100 kHz.) Under the quasi-static approximation, the continuity equation states that the divergence $\nabla\cdot$ of the current density $\mathbf{J}$ (A/m^2) is equal to the applied or endogenous source of electric current S (A/m^3):

$$\nabla \cdot \mathbf{J} = S \tag{10.1}$$

In regions of tissue where there are no such sources, S is zero. In these cases, the divergenceless of $\mathbf{J}$ is equivalent to the law of **conservation of current** that is often invoked when one is analyzing electric circuits. Another common property of a volume conductor is that the current density and the electric field $\mathbf{E}$ (V/m) are related linearly by **Ohm's law,**

$$\mathbf{J} = g\mathbf{E} \tag{10.2}$$

where g is the electrical **conductivity** (S/m). Finally, the relationship between the electric field and the gradient ∇ of the potential is, by definition,

$$\mathbf{E} = -\nabla\Phi \tag{10.3}$$

The purpose of this chapter is to characterize the electrical conductivity. This task is not easy because g is generally a macroscopic parameter (an "effective conductivity") that represents the electrical properties of the tissue averaged in space over many cells. The effective conductivity can be **anisotropic,** complex (containing real and imaginary parts), and can depend on both the temporal and spatial frequencies.

Before beginning our discussion of tissue conductivity, let us consider one of the simplest and most easily understood volume conductors: saline. The electrical conductivity of saline arises from

0-8493-8346-3/95/$0.00+$.50
© 1995 by CRC Press, Inc.

the motion of free ions in response to a steady electric field and is on the order of 1 S/m. Besides conductivity, another property of saline is its electrical permittivity ϵ (S · s/m). This property is related to the dielectric constant κ (dimensionless) by $\epsilon = \kappa\epsilon_0$, where ϵ_0 is the permittivity of free space, 8.854×10^{-12} S · s/m. (The permittivity is also related to the electric susceptibility χ by $\epsilon = \epsilon_0 + \chi$.) Dielectric properties arise from bound charge that is displaced by the electric field, creating a dipole. They also can arise if the applied electric field aligns molecular dipoles (such as the dipole moments of water molecules) that normally are oriented randomly. The direct current (dc) dielectric constant of saline is similar to that of water (about $\kappa = 80$).

Conductivity is produced by the movement of free charge, whereas permittivity is produced by stationary dipoles. In steady state, the distinction between the two is clear, but at higher frequencies, the concepts merge. In such a case, it is often useful to combine the electrical properties into a complex conductivity g':

$$g' = g + i\omega\epsilon \tag{10.4}$$

where ω (rad/s) is the angular frequency ($\omega = 2\pi f$, where f is the frequency in hertz), and i is equal to $\sqrt{-1}$. The real part of g' accounts for the movement of charge that is in phase with the electric field; the imaginary part accounts for out-of-phase motion. In general, both the real and imaginary parts of the complex conductivity depend on the frequency. For many bioelectric phenomena, the first term in Eq. (10.4) is much larger than the second, so the tissue can be represented as purely conductive [Plonsey, 1969]. (The imaginary part of the complex conductivity represents a capacitive effect and therefore technically violates our assumption of quasi-stationarity. This violation is the only exception we will make to our general rule of a quasi-static potential.)

10.1 Cell Suspensions

The earliest and simplest model describing the electrical properties of a biologic tissue is a suspension of cells in a saline solution [Cole, 1968]. Let us consider a suspension of spherical cells each of radius a (Fig. 10.1a). The saline surrounding the cells constitutes the interstitial space (conductivity σ_e), while the conducting fluid inside the cells constitutes the intracellular space (conductivity σ_i). (We shall follow Henriquez [1993] in denoting macroscopic effective conductivities by g and microscopic conductivities by σ.) The two spaces are separated by the cell membrane, represented as a thin layer having conductivity per unit area G_m (S/m²) and capacitance per unit area C_m (F/m²). One additional parameter, the intracellular volume fraction f (dimensionless) indicates how tightly the cells are packed together. The volume fraction can range from nearly zero (a dilute solution) to almost 1 (spherical cells cannot reach a volume fraction of 1, but tightly packed, nonspherical cells can). For irregularly shaped cells, the cell "radius" can be difficult to define. In these cases, it is often easier to specify the surface-to-volume ratio of the tissue (the ratio of the membrane surface to tissue volume). For spherical cells, the surface-to-volume ratio is $3f/a$.

The effective conductivity g of the cell suspension can be defined operationally by the following process (see Fig. 10.1a): Place the cell suspension in a cylindrical tube of length L and cross-sectional area A (be sure L and A are large enough that the volume contains many cells). Apply a dc potential difference V across the two ends of the cylinder (so that the electric field has strength V/L), and measure the total current I passing through the suspension. The effective conductivity is IL/VA.

Deriving an expression for the effective conductivity of a suspension of spheres in terms of microscopic parameters is an old and interesting problem in electromagnetic theory [Cole, 1968]. For dc fields, the effective conductivity g of a suspension of insulating spheres placed in a saline solution of conductivity σ_e is

$$g = \frac{2(1-f)}{2+f}\,\sigma_e \tag{10.5}$$

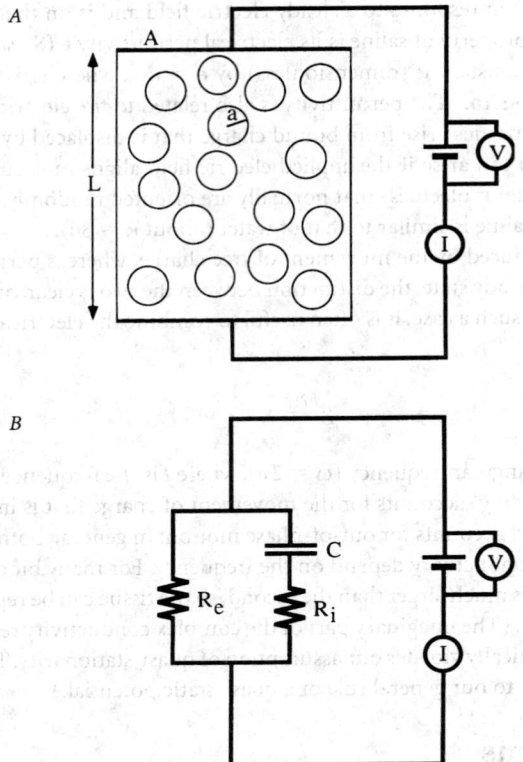

FIGURE 10.1 (*a*) A schematic diagram of a suspension of spherical cells; the effective conductivity of this suspension is *IL/VA*. (*b*) An electric circuit equivalent of the effective conductivity of this suspension.

For most cells, G_m is small enough that the membrane behaves essentially as an insulator at dc, in which case the assumption of insulating spheres is applicable. The net effect of the cells within the saline is to decrease the conductivity of the medium (the decrease can be substantial for tightly packed cells).

The cell membrane has a capacitance of about 0.01 F/m^2 (or, in traditional units, 1 μF/cm^2), which introduces a frequency dependence into the electrical conductivity. The suspension of cells can be represented by the electric circuit in Fig. 10.1*b*: R_e is the effective resistance to current passing entirely through the interstitial space; R_i is the effective resistance to current passing into the intracellular space; and C is the effective membrane capacitance. (The membrane conductance is usually small enough that it has little effect on the suspension behavior, regardless of the frequency.) At low frequencies, all the current is restricted to the interstitial space, and the electrical conductivity is given approximately by Eq. (10.5). At very large frequencies, C shunts current across the membrane so that the effective conductivity of the tissue is again entirely resistive (the complex conductivity is real):

$$g = \frac{2(1-f)\sigma_e + (1+2f)\sigma_i}{(2+f)\sigma_e + (1-f)\sigma_i}\,\sigma_e \tag{10.6}$$

At intermediate frequencies, the effective conductivity has both real and imaginary parts, because the membrane capacitance contributes significantly to the effective conductivity. In these cases, Eq. (10.6) still holds if σ_i is replaced by σ_i^*, where

$$\sigma_i^* = \frac{\sigma_i Y_m a}{\sigma_i + Y_m a} \quad \text{with } Y_m = G_m + i\omega C_m \tag{10.7}$$

Figure 10.2 shows the effective conductivity (magnitude and phase) as a function of frequency for a typical tissue. The rise in the phase of g at about 300 kHz is sometimes called the *beta dispersion*.

10.2 Fiber Suspensions

Some of the most interesting electrically active tissues, such as nerve and skeletal muscle, are better approximated as a suspension of fibers rather than as a suspension of spheres. This difference has profound implications, because it introduces the concept of anisotropy: The effective electrical conductivity depends on direction. Henceforth we must speak of the longitudinal effective conductivity parallel to the fibers g_L and the transverse effective conductivity perpendicular to the fibers g_T. (In theory, the conductivity could be different in three directions; however, we consider only the case in which the electrical properties in the two directions perpendicular to the fibers are the same.) In general, the conductivity is no longer a scalar quantity but is a tensor instead and must therefore be represented by a 3×3 symmetric matrix. If we choose our coordinate system axes along the principal directions of this matrix (invariably, the directions parallel to and perpendicular to the fibers), then the off-diagonal terms of the matrix are zero. If, however, we choose our coordinate axes differently, or if the fiber direction is curved so that the direction parallel to the fibers varies over space, we have to deal with tensor properties, including off-diagonal components.

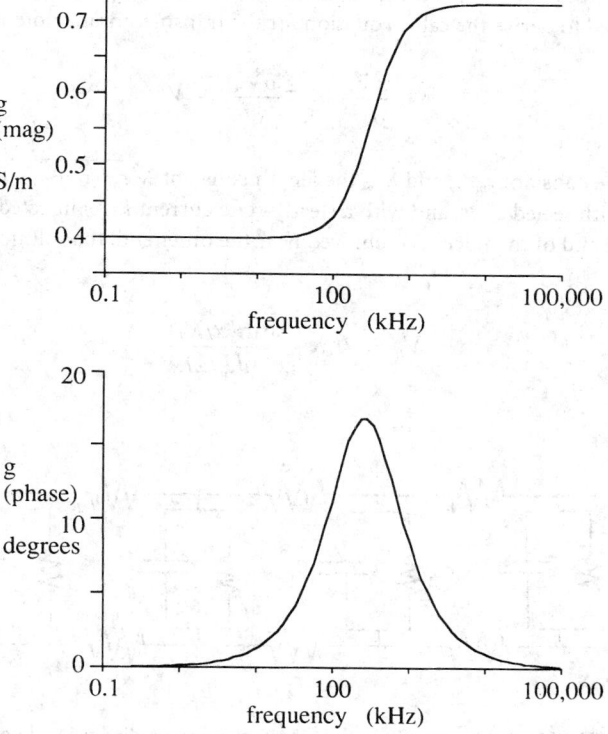

FIGURE 10.2 The magnitude and phase of the effective conductivity as a function of frequency for a suspension of spherical cells: $f = 0.5$, $a = 20\ \mu\text{m}$, $\sigma_e = 1$ S/m, $\sigma_i = 0.5$ S/m, $G_m = 0$, and $C_m = 0.01$ F/m^2.

When the electric field is applied perpendicular to the fiber direction, a suspension of fibers is similar to the suspension of cells described above (in Fig. 10.1*a*, we must now imagine that the circles represent cross sections of cylindrical fibers rather than cross sections of spherical cells). The expression for the effective transverse conductivity of a suspension of cylindrical cells, of radius *a* and intracellular conductivity σ_i, placed in a saline solution of conductivity σ_e, with intracellular volume fraction *f*, is [Cole, 1968]

$$g_T = \frac{(1-f)\sigma_e + (1+f)\sigma_i^*}{(1+f)\sigma_e + (1-f)\sigma_i^*} \, \sigma_e \qquad (10.8)$$

where σ_i^* is defined in Eq. (10.7). At dc (and assuming that $G_m = 0$), Eq. (10.8) reduces to

$$g_T = \frac{1-f}{1+f}\sigma_e \qquad (10.9)$$

When an electric field is applied parallel to the fiber direction, a new behavior arises that is fundamentally different than that observed for a suspension of spherical cells. Let us return for a moment to our operational definition of the dc effective conductivity. Surprisingly, the effective longitudinal conductivity of a suspension of fibers depends on the length *L* of the tissue sample used for the measurement. To understand this phenomenon, we must consider one-dimensional cable theory [Plonsey, 1969]. A single nerve or muscle fiber can be approximated by the circuit shown in Fig. 10.3. Adopting the traditional electrophysiology definitions, we denote the intracellular and extracellular resistances per unit length along the fiber by r_i and r_e (Ω/m), the membrane resistance times unit length by r_m ($\Omega \cdot$ m), and the capacitance per unit length by c_m (F/m). Standard cable analysis can be used to derive the cable equation for the transmembrane potential V_m:

$$\lambda^2 \frac{\partial^2 V_m}{\partial x^2} = \tau \frac{\partial V_m}{\partial t} + V_m \qquad (10.10)$$

where τ is the time constant $r_m c_m$, and λ is the length constant $\sqrt{r_m/(r_i + r_e)}$. For a truncated fiber of length *L* (m) with sealed ends, and with a steady-state current *I* (A) injected into the extracellular space near one end of the fiber and removed near the other end, the solution to the cable equation is

$$V_m = I r_e \lambda \, \frac{\sinh(x/\lambda)}{\cosh(L/2\lambda)} \qquad (10.11)$$

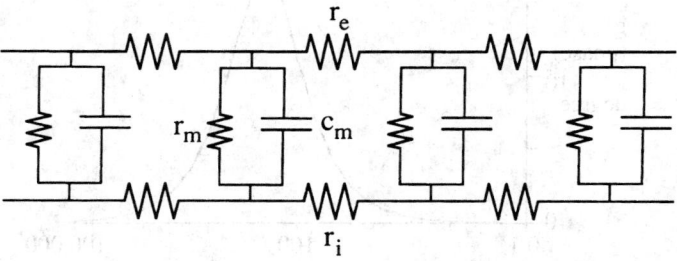

FIGURE 10.3   An electric circuit representing a one-dimensional nerve or muscle fiber; r_i and r_e are the intracellular and extracellular resistances per unit length (Ω/m); r_m is the membrane resistance times unit length ($\Omega \cdot$ m); and c_m is the membrane capacitance per unit length (F/m).

where the origin of the x axis is at the midpoint between electrodes. The extracellular potential V_e consists of two terms: One is proportional to x, and the other is $r_e/(r_i + r_e)$ times V_m. We can evaluate V_e at the two ends of the fiber to obtain the voltage drop between the electrodes ΔV_e:

$$\Delta V_e = \frac{r_i r_e}{r_i + r_e} I \left[L + \frac{r_e}{r_i} 2\lambda \tanh(L/2\lambda) \right] \tag{10.12}$$

Two limiting cases are of interest. If L is very large compared with λ, the extracellular voltage drop reduces to

$$\Delta V_e = \frac{r_i r_e}{r_i + r_e} LI \qquad L \gg \lambda \tag{10.13}$$

The leading factor is the parallel combination of the intracellular and extracellular resistances. If, on the other hand, L is very small compared with λ, the extracellular voltage drop becomes

$$\Delta V_e = r_e LI \qquad L \ll \lambda \tag{10.14}$$

In this case, the leading factor is simply the extracellular resistance. Physically, there is a redistribution of current into the intracellular space that occurs over a distance on the order of a length constant. If the tissue length is much longer than a length constant, the current is completely redistributed between the intracellular and extracellular spaces. If the tissue length is much smaller than a length constant, the current does not enter the fiber but instead is restricted to the extracellular space. If either of these two conditions is met, then the effective conductivity ($IL/A\Delta V_e$, where A is the cross-sectional area of the tissue strand) is independent of L. However, if L is comparable with λ, the effective conductivity depends on the size of the sample. A complete model of the effective conductivity of a suspension of fibers must take this behavior into account.

In order to avoid having the effective conductivity depend on the size of the sample used for the measurement, Roth et al. [1988] recast the expression for the effective longitudinal conductivity in terms of spatial frequency k (rad/m) rather than in terms of the sample length. There are two advantages to this approach. First, the temporal and spatial behaviors are both described using frequency analysis. Second, a parameter derived from a specific source geometry is not necessary: The spatial frequency dependence becomes a property of the tissue, not the source. The expression for the dc effective longitudinal conductivity is

$$g_L = \frac{(1-f)\sigma_e + f\sigma_i}{1 + \dfrac{f\sigma_i}{(1-f)\sigma_e} \dfrac{1}{1 + [1/(\lambda k)]^2}} \tag{10.15}$$

To relate the effective longitudinal conductivity to Eqs. (10.13) and (10.14), note that $1/k$ plays the same role as L. If $k\lambda \ll 1$, g_L reduces to $(1-f)\sigma_e + f\sigma_i$, which is equivalent to the parallel combination of resistances in Eq. (10.13). If $k\lambda \gg 1$, g_L becomes $(1-f)\sigma_e$, implying that the current is restricted to the interstitial space, as in Eq. (10.14). Equation (10.15) can be generalized to all temporal frequencies by defining λ in terms of Y_m instead of G_m [Roth et al., 1988]. Figure 10.4 shows the magnitude and phase of the longitudinal and transverse effective conductivities as functions of the temporal and spatial frequencies.

The measurement of effective conductivities is complicated by the traditionally used electrode geometry. Most often, a uniform electric field is not (or cannot be) applied parallel to the fibers and then perpendicular to them. A four-electrode technique is typically employed, in which current is injected through two point electrodes, and the potential is measured through two others (Fig. 10.5).

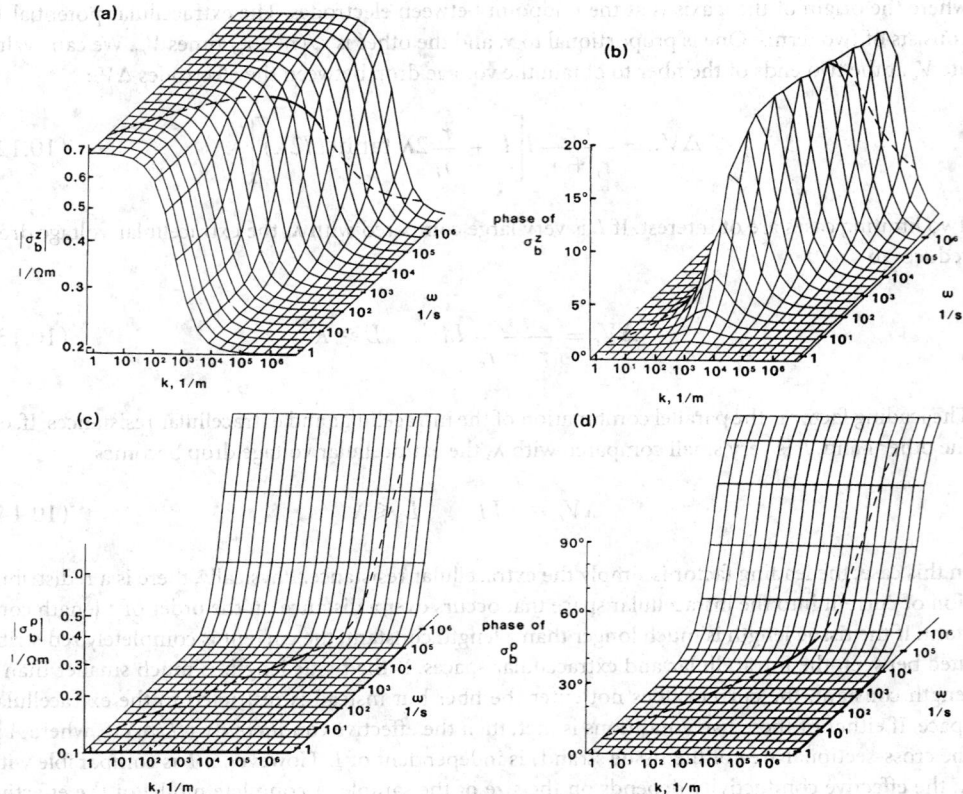

FIGURE 10.4 The magnitude (*a,c*) and phase (*b,d*) of the effective longitudinal (*a,b*) and transverse (*c,d*) effective conductivities calculated using the spatial *k* and temporal ω frequency model. The parameters used in this calculation are $G_m = 1$ S/m^2, $C_m = 0.01$ F/m^2, $f = 0.9$, $a = 20$ μm, $\sigma_i = 0.55$ S/m, and $\sigma_e = 2$ S/m. (*Source:* Roth BJ, Gielen FLH, Wikswo JP Jr. 1988. *Math Biosci* 88:159, with permission.)

Gielen et al. [1984] used this method to measure the electrical properties of skeletal muscle and found that the effective conductivity depended on the interelectrode distance. Roth [1989] reanalyzed the data of Gielen et al. using the spatial frequency–dependent model and found agreement with some of the more unexpected features of their data (Fig. 10.6). Typical values of skeletal muscle effective conductivities and microscopic tissue parameters are given in Table 10.1.

Altman and Plonsey [1988] have developed a model of a peripheral nerve as a suspension of one-dimensional axons, similar to the model described above for skeletal muscle. One limitation of this model was their assumption of identical fibers, because a peripheral nerve is known to be comprised of fibers having a wide range of diameters (and therefore different length constants). Roth and Altman [1992] have extended the peripheral nerve model to include the effects of a distribution of fiber diameters. Another complicating factor in the analysis of peripheral nerves

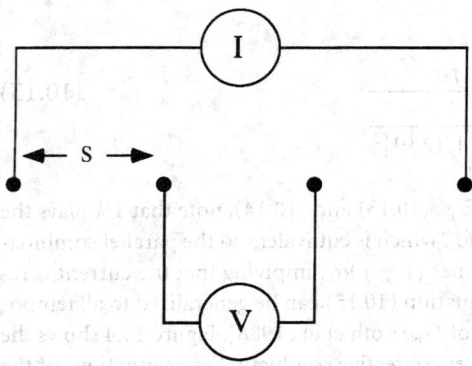

FIGURE 10.5 A schematic diagram of the four-electrode technique for measuring tissue conductivities. Current *I* is passed through the outer two electrodes, and the potential *V* is measured between the inner two. The interelectrode distance is *s*.

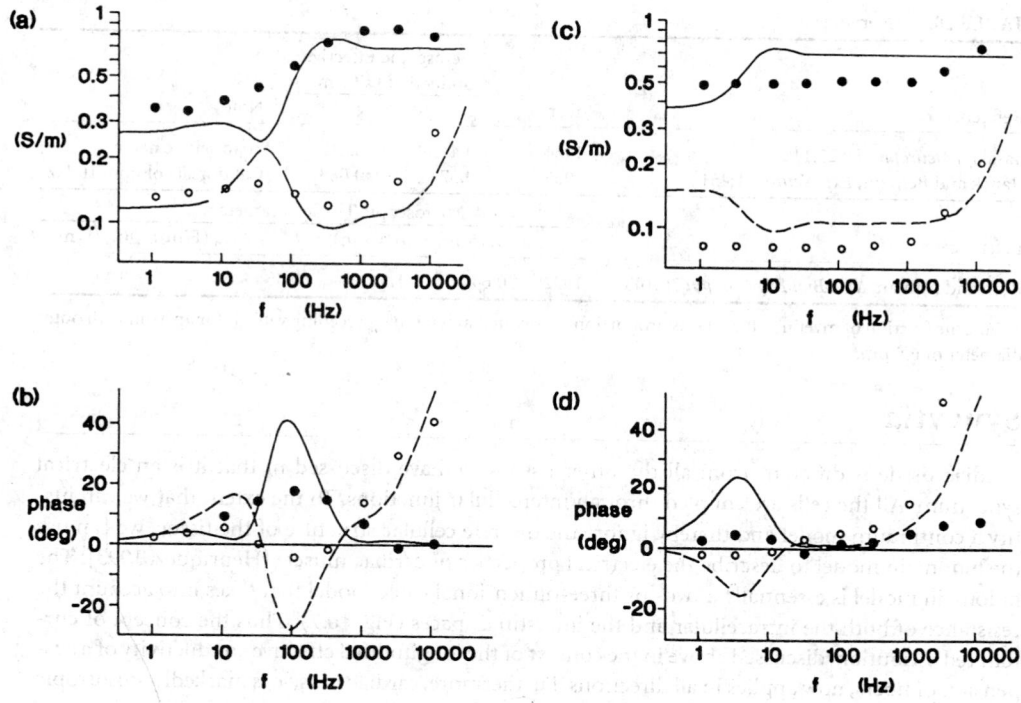

FIGURE 10.6   The calculated (*a*) amplitude and (*b*) phase of g_L (*solid*) and g_T (*dashed*) as a function of frequency for an interelectrode distance of 0.5 mm. (*c,d*) The quantities for an interelectrode distance of 3.0 mm. Circles represent experimental data; g_L (*filled*), g_T (*open*). (*Source:* Roth BJ. 1989. *Med Biol Eng Comput* 27:491, with permission.)

is that the high-resistance myelin sheath around each axon is interrupted periodically by nodes of Ranvier. Because the low-resistance path across the membrane is through a node, and because the spacing between nodes is proportional to axon diameter, the effective membrane conductance G_m is itself proportional to axon diameter [Roth and Altman, 1992]. Moreover, the myelin sheath is thick enough that it occupies a significant fraction of the nerve cross-sectional area; therefore, the sum of intracellular volume fraction and interstitial volume fraction is less than one. If high spatial frequencies contribute significantly to the potential distribution, the discrete structure of the nodes and myelin may become important. In such a case, a definition of an effective electrical conductivity may become impossible. Typical values of nerve effective conductivities are listed in Table 10.2.

TABLE 10.1   Skeletal Muscle

Reference	Year	Macroscopic Effective Conductivities (S/m)		Note
		g_L	g_T	
Gielen et al., *MBEC* 22:569	1984	0.35	0.086	10 Hz, IED = 3 mm
		0.20	0.092	10 Hz, IED = 0.5 mm
Epstein and Foster, *MBEC* 21:51	1983	0.52	0.076	20 Hz, IED = 17 mm
		0.70	0.32	100 kHz, IED = 17 mm
Rush et al., *Circ Res* 12:40	1963	0.67	0.040	0.1-s pulse

Reference		Microscopic Tissue Parameters				
		σ_i (S/m)	σ_e (S/m)	f	C_m (F/m²)	G_m (S/m²)
Gielen et al., *MBEC* 24:34	1986	0.55	2.4	0.9	0.01	1.0

IED = interelectrode distance; *MBEC* = *Med Biol Eng Comput.*

TABLE 10.2   Nerve

Reference	Year	Macroscopic Effective Conductivities (S/m)		Note
		g_L	g_T	
Tasaki, *J Neurophysiol* 27:1199	1964	0.41	0.01	Toad sciatic nerve
Ranck and BeMent, *Exp Neurol* 11:451	1965	0.57	0.083	Cat dorsal column, 10 Hz

Reference		Microscopic Tissue Parameters				
		σ_i (S/m)	σ_e (S/m)	f	C_m (F/m^2)	G_m (S/m^2)
Roth and Altman, *Med Biol Eng Comput* 30:103	1992	0.64	1.54	0.35	1	0.44

Volume fraction of myelin = 0.27; G_m is proportional to axon diameter; the preceding value is for an axon with outer diameter of 6.5 μm.

10.3 Syncytia

Cardiac tissue is different from all the other tissues we have discussed in that it is an electrical syncytium: All the cells are coupled through intercellular junctions. To the extent that we can justify a continuum model and thereby ignore the discrete cellular structure of the tissue, we can use the bidomain model to describe the electrical properties of cardiac muscle [Henriquez, 1993]. The bidomain model is essentially a two- or three-dimensional cable model that takes into account the resistance of both the intracellular and the interstitial spaces (Fig. 10.7). Thus the concept of current redistribution, discussed above in the context of the longitudinal effective conductivity of a suspension of fibers, now applies in all directions. Furthermore, cardiac muscle is markedly anisotropic

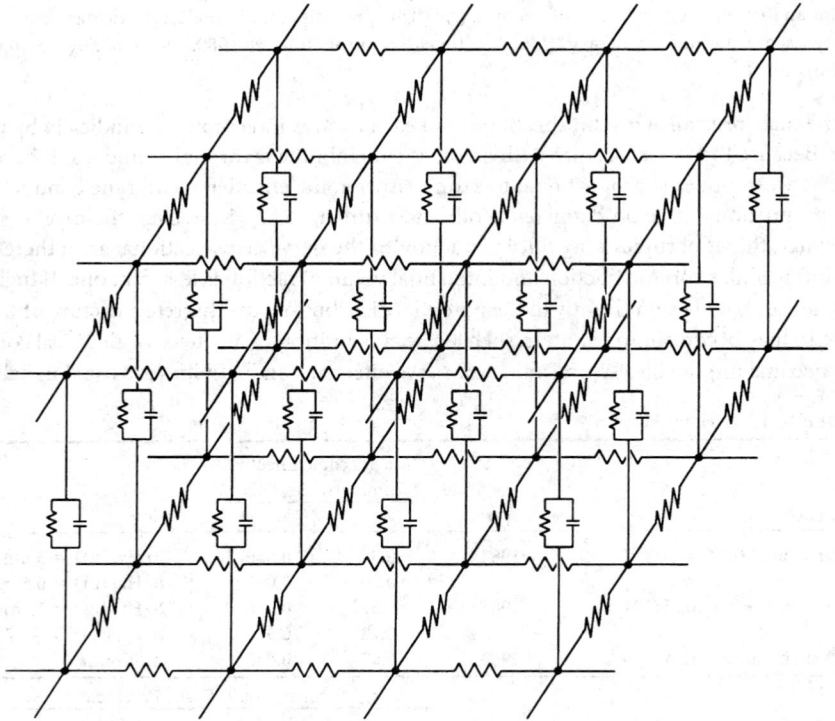

FIGURE 10.7   A circuit representing a two-dimensional syncytium (i.e., a bidomain). The lower array of resistors represents the intracellular space, the upper array represents the extracellular space, and the parallel resistors and capacitors represent the membrane.

due to the cylindrical geometry of the individual myocardial cells. These properties make imped- ance measurements of cardiac muscle difficult to interpret [Plonsey and Barr, 1986]. The situation is complicated further because the intracellular space is more anisotropic than is the interstitial space (in the jargon of bidomain modeling, this condition is known as *unequal anisotropy ratios*) [Henriquez, 1993]. Consequently, an expression for a single effective conductivity for cardiac mus- cle is difficult, if not impossible, to derive. In general, a pair of coupled partial differential equations must be solved simultaneously for the intracellular and interstitial potentials; for unequal anisotropy ratios, this solution is invariably found numerically.

The bidomain model characterizes the electrical properties of the tissue by four effective con- ductivities: $g_{iL}, g_{iT}, g_{eL},$ and g_{eT}, where i and e denote the intracellular and interstitial spaces, and L and T denote the directions parallel to and perpendicular to the myocardial fiber direction. We can re- late these parameters to the microscopic tissue properties by using an operational definition of an effective bidomain conductivity, similar to the operational definition given earlier. (The operational definition of a bidomain conductivity is most useful for thought experiments, since its actual im- plementation would be fraught with experimental difficulties.) To determine the interstitial con- ductivity, we first dissect a cylindrical tube of tissue of length L and cross-sectional area A (one must be sure that L and A are large enough so that the volume contains many cells and that a negligible amount of tissue is damaged during this dissection). Next, we apply a drug to the tissue that makes the membrane essentially insulating (i.e., the length constant is much longer than L). Finally, we apply a dc potential difference V across the two ends of the cylinder and measure the total current I passing through the tissue. The effective interstitial conductivity is then IL/VA. This procedure could be performed twice, once with the fibers parallel to the long axis of the cylinder and once with the fibers perpendicular to it. To determine the effective intracellular conductivities, the preceding procedure should be followed, except that the voltage difference must be applied to the intracellu- lar space instead of to the interstitial space. Although the procedure would be extraordinarily diffi- cult in practice, we can imagine two arrays of microelectrodes that impale the cells at both ends of the cylinder and that are used to maintain the potential at each end constant.

Expressions have been derived for the effective bidomain conductivities in terms of the micro- scopic tissue parameters [Roth, 1988; Henriquez, 1993; Neu and Krassowska, 1993]. The effective conductivities in the direction parallel to the fibers are easier to obtain. Imagine that the tissue is composed of long, straight fibers (like skeletal muscle) and that the intracellular space of these fibers occupies a fraction f of the tissue cross-sectional area. If the conductivity of the interstitial fluid is σ_e, then the effective interstitial conductivity parallel to the fibers g_{eL} is simply

$$g_{eL} = (1 - f)\sigma_e \tag{10.16}$$

If we neglect the resistance of the intercellular junctions, we obtain a similar expression for the effective intracellular conductivity parallel to the fibers in terms of the myoplasmic conductivity σ_i: $g_{iL} = f\sigma_i$. When the intercellular junctional resistance is not negligible compared with the myoplas- mic resistance, the expression for g_{iL} is more complicated:

$$g_{iL} = \frac{1}{1 + \dfrac{\pi a^2 \sigma_i}{bG}} f\sigma_i \tag{10.17}$$

where G is the junctional conductance between two cells (S), b is the cell length (m), and a is the cell radius (m). The effective interstitial conductivity perpendicular to the fibers is identical with the dc transverse effective conductivity for skeletal muscle given in Eq. (10.9):

$$g_{eT} = \frac{1 - f}{1 + f}\sigma_e \tag{10.18}$$

TABLE 10.3 Cardiac Muscle

Reference	Year	Macroscopic Effective Conductivities (Ventricular Muscle) (S/m)			
		g_{iL}	g_{iT}	g_{eL}	g_{eT}
Clerc, *J Physiol* 255:335	1976	0.17	0.019	0.62	0.24
Roberts et al., *Circ Res* 44:701	1979	0.28	0.026	0.22	0.13
Roberts and Scher, *Circ Res* 50:342	1982	0.34	0.060	0.12	0.080

Reference		Microscopic Tissue Parameters					
		σ_i (S/m)	σ_e (S/m)	f	a (µm)	b (µm)	G (µS)
Roth, *Ann Biomed Eng* 16:609	1988	1	1	0.7	100	10	3
Neu and Krassowska, *Crit Rev Biomed Eng* 21:137	1993	0.4	2	0.85	100	7.5	0.05

The effective intracellular conductivity perpendicular to the fibers is the most difficult to model, but a reasonable expression for g_{iT} is

$$g_{iT} = \frac{1}{1 + \dfrac{b\sigma_i}{G}} \, \sigma_i \tag{10.19}$$

Measured values of the bidomain conductivities are presented in Table 10.3. Typical values of the microscopic tissue parameters are also given, although some are quite uncertain (particularly G).

In our analysis of skeletal muscle, the redistribution of current between the intracellular and interstitial spaces was taken into account by the spatial and temporal frequency dependence of the effective conductivity. In the bidomain model, however, the current redistribution is accounted for by the pair of coupled equations that govern the intracellular and extracellular potentials. Thus the conductivities are simpler for cardiac muscle than for skeletal muscle (no temporal or spatial frequency dependence), but for cardiac muscle, two equations for the intracellular and extracellular potentials must now be solved instead of only one. Roth and Gielen [1987] have shown that, to a good approximation, the frequency-dependent conductivity model presented in Eq. (10.15) is equivalent to the bidomain model in the limit when $g_{iT} = 0$. Altman and Plonsey [1988] took advantage of this equivalence when using the bidomain model to study extracellular stimulation of a nerve.

If the intercellular junctions contribute significantly to the intracellular resistance, the bidomain model will only approximate the tissue behavior [Neu and Krassowska, 1993]. For sufficiently large junctional resistance, the discrete cellular properties become important, and the tissue is no longer well represented as a continuum. Interestingly, as the junctional resistance increases, cardiac tissue behaves less like a syncytium and more like a suspension of cells. Thus we have come full circle. We started by considering a suspension of cells, then examined suspensions of fibers, and finally generalized to syncytia. Yet, when the intercellular junctions in a syncytium are disrupted, we find ourselves again thinking of the tissue as a suspension of cells.

Defining Terms

Anisotropic: Having different properties in different directions.

Bidomain: A two- or three-dimensional cable model that takes into account the resistance of both the intracellular and the extracellular spaces.

Cable theory: Representation of a cylindrical fiber as two parallel rows of resistors (one each for the intracellular and extracellular spaces) connected in a ladder network by a parallel combination of resistors and capacitors (the cell membrane).

Conservation of current: A fundamental law of electrostatics stating that there is no *net* current entering or leaving at any point in a volume conductor.

Conductivity: A parameter g that measures how well a substance conducts electricity. The coefficient of proportionality between the electric field and the current density. The units of conductivity are siemens per meter (S/m). A siemens is an inverse ohm, sometimes called a *mho* in the older literature.

Interstitial space: The extracellular space between cells in a tissue.

Ohm's law: A linear relation between the electric field and current density vectors.

Permittivity: A parameter ϵ that measures the size of the dipole moment induced in a substance by an electric field. The units of permittivity are siemens second per meter (S · s/m).

Quasi-static: A potential distribution that changes slowly enough that we can accurately describe it by the equations of electrostatics (capacitive, inductive, and propagation effects are ignored).

Spatial frequency: A parameter governing how rapidly a function changes in space; $k = 1/(2\pi s)$, where s is the wavelength of a sinusoidally varying function.

Syncytium (pl., **syncytia**): A tissue in which the intracellular spaces of adjacent cells are coupled through intercellular channels so that current can pass between any two intracellular points without crossing the cell membrane.

Volume conductor: A three-dimensional region of space containing a material that passively conducts electrical current.

Acknowledgments

I thank Dr. Craig Henriquez for several suggestions and corrections, and Barry Bowman for carefully editing the manuscript.

References

Altman KW, Plonsey R. 1988. Development of a model for point source electrical fibre bundle stimulation. Med Biol Eng Comput 26:466.

Cole KS. 1968. Membranes, Ions, and Impulses. Berkeley, University of California Press.

Gielen FLH, Wallinga-de Jonge W, Boon KL. 1984. Electrical conductivity of skeletal muscle tissue: Experimental results from different muscles in vivo. Med Biol Eng Comput 22:569.

Henriquez CS. 1993. Simulating the electrical behavior of cardiac tissue using the bidomain model. Crit Rev Biomed Eng 21:1.

Neu JC, Krassowska W. 1993. Homogenization of syncytial tissues. Crit Rev Biomed Eng 21:137.

Plonsey R. 1969. Bioelectric Phenomena. New York, McGraw-Hill.

Plonsey R, Barr RC. 1986. A critique of impedance measurements in cardiac tissue. Ann Biomed Eng 14:307.

Roth BJ. 1988. The electrical potential produced by a strand of cardiac muscle: A bidomain analysis. Ann Biomed Eng 16:609.

Roth BJ. 1989. Interpretation of skeletal muscle four-electrode impedance measurements using spatial and temporal frequency-dependent conductivities. Med Biol Eng Comput 27:491.

Roth BJ, Gielen FLH. 1987. A comparison of two models for calculating the electrical potential in skeletal muscle. Ann Biomed Eng 15:591.

Roth BJ, Altman KW. 1992. Steady-state point-source stimulation of a nerve containing axons with an arbitrary distribution of diameters. Med Biol Eng Comput 30:103.

Roth BJ, Gielen FLH, Wikswo JP Jr. 1988. Spatial and temporal frequency-dependent conductivities in volume-conduction for skeletal muscle. Math Biosci 88:159.

Further Information

Mathematics and Physics

Jackson JD. Classical Electrodynamics. New York, Wiley, 1975. (*The classic graduate-level physics text.*)

Purcell EM. Electricity and Magnetism, Berkeley Physics Course, vol 2. New York, McGraw-Hill, 1963. (*An undergraduate physics text full of physical insight.*)

Schey HM. Div, Grad, Curl and All That. New York, Norton, 1973. (*An accessible and useful introduction to vector calculus.*)

Bioelectric Phenomena and Tissue Models

The texts by Cole and Plonsey, cited above, are classics in the field.

Geddes LA, Baker LE. 1967. The specific resistance of biologic material—A compendium of data for the biomedical engineer and physiologist. Med Biol Eng Comput 5:271. (*Measured conductivity values for a wide variety of tissues.*)

Plonsey R, Barr RC. Bioelectricity: A Quantitative Approach. New York, Plenum Press, 1988. (*An updated version of Plonsey's Bioelectric Phenomena.*)

Polk C, Postow E (eds). CRC Handbook of Biological Effects of Electromagnetic Fields. Boca Raton, Fla, CRC Press, 1986.

Journals: IEEE Transactions on Biomedical Engineering, Medical and Biological Engineering and Computing, Annals of Biomedical Engineering.

11

Membrane Models

Anthony Varghese
Johns Hopkins Medical School

The models discussed in this chapter involve the time behavior of electrochemical activity in animal cells. Thus these models are all systems of ordinary differential equations where the independent variable is time. The reader is advised that while a good understanding of linear circuit theory is useful in order to understand the works presented in this chapter, most of the phenomena of interest involve nonlinear circuits with time-varying components.

Electrical activity in plant and animal cells is caused by two main factors: First, there are differences in the concentrations of ions inside and outside the cell, and second, there are molecules embedded in the cell membrane that allow these ions to be transported across the membrane. The ion concentration differences and the presence of large membrane-impermeant anions inside the cell result in the existence of a polarity; the potential inside a cell is typically 50 to 100 mV lower than that in the external solution. It is important to note that almost all of this potential difference occurs across the membrane itself. The bulk solutions both inside and outside the cell are for the most part at a uniform potential. This transmembrane potential difference is in turn sensed by molecules in the membrane that control the flow of ions.

The lipid bilayer, which constitutes the majority of the cell membrane, acts as a capacitor with a specific capacitance that is typically $1\ \mu F/cm^2$. The rest of the membrane comprises large protein molecules that act as (1) ion channels, (2) ion pumps, or (3) ion exchangers. The flow of ions across the membrane causes changes in the transmembrane potential, which is typically the main observable quantity in experiments.

11.1 The Action Potential

The main behavior that will be examined in this chapter is the action potential. This is a term used to denote a temporal phenomenon exhibited by every electrically excitable cell. A schematic representation of an action potential is shown in Fig. 11.1. The transmembrane potential difference of most excitable cells usually stays at some negative potential called the *resting potential*. External current or voltage inputs can cause the potential of the cell to deviate in the positive direction, and if the input is large enough, the result is an action potential. An action potential is characterized by a depolarization, which typically results in an *overshoot* followed by repolarization. Some cells may actually hyperpolarize before returning to the resting potential.

A key concept in the modeling of excitable cells is the idea of ion channel selectivity. A particular ion channel will only allow one ionic species to pass through it. In most excitable cells at rest, the membrane is most permeable to potassium. This is so because only potassium channels (i.e., channels selective to potassium) are open at the resting potential. For a given stimulus to cause an action potential, the cell has to be brought to threshold. The upstroke of the action potential is caused by a large influx of sodium as sodium channels open (in some cells calcium is responsible for the upstroke, and in such cases, it is the calcium channels that are open during the upstroke) in response to a stimulus. This is followed by repolarization as potassium starts flowing out of the cell in response to the new potential gradient. While the responses of most cells to subthreshold inputs are usually linear and passive, the suprathreshold response—the action potential—is a nonlinear phenomenon. Unlike linear circuits and systems, where the principle of superposition holds, the nonlinear processes in cell membranes do not allow responses of two stimuli to be added. If an initial stimulus results in an action potential, a subsequent stimulus administered at the peak voltage will not necessarily produce an even larger action potential; instead, it may have no effect at all. Following an action potential, most cells have a refractory period, during which they are unable to respond to stimuli. Nonlinear features such as these make modeling of excitable cells a nontrivial task. In addition, the molecular behavior of channels is not completely known, and therefore, it is not possible to construct membrane models from first principles. The models in this chapter were all constructed using empirical data.

In 1952, Alan Hodgkin and Andrew Huxley published a paper showing how a nonlinear empirical model of the membrane processes could be constructed [Hodgkin and Huxley, 1952]. In the four decades since their work, the Hodgkin-Huxley (abbreviated HH) paradigm of modeling cell membranes has been enormously successful. It is now known that most of the passive transport of ions is accomplished by molecules called *channels* that allow certain ions to flow through them. In addition to constructing a nonlinear model, they also established a method to incorporate experimental data into a nonlinear membrane model.

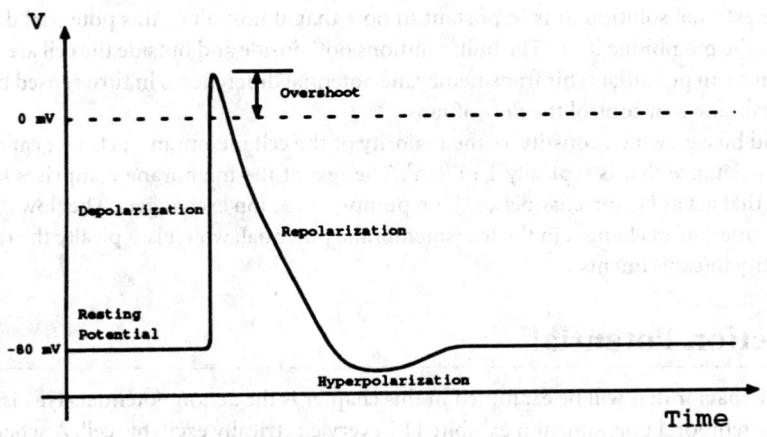

FIGURE 11.1 Schematic representation of an action potential in an excitable cell. The abscissa represents time, and the ordinate represents the transmembrane potential.

11.2 Voltage and Patch Clamp Data

The method of voltage clamping has been the main experimental tool used to reconstruct models of cell electrical activity. One electrode is inserted into the cell to keep the interior of the cell at a fixed potential, while a second electrode measures the potential of the external solution. This allows the current between the electrodes and hence the transmembrane current to be determined as well. An operational amplifier–based feedback circuit supplies enough current to keep the internal electrode at the desired potentials as pulses are applied. Voltage pulses are applied to the internal electrode, and data on the current flow are gathered. The time course of the transients and the steady-state currents at various pulse potentials are used to construct the nonlinear models. The reader is referred to Cole [1968] and Standen [1987] for further details.

The methods that are most often used today are called patch clamp methods [Hamill et al., 1981] and are shown schematically in Fig. 11.2. A glass pipette containing a solution that is close in ionic composition to the cytosolic fluid is brought down to the external surface of the cell, and a small amount of suction is applied to form at tight seal between the glass pipette and the membrane; this configuration is called the *on-cell* or *cell-attached state* (see Fig. 11.2a). A stronger suction can be applied to rupture the cell membrane and allow the fluid in the electrode to come in contact with the cytosol; this is called the *whole-cell voltage clamp* (see Fig. 11.2b). From the on-cell state, pulling the pipette away from the cell results in the patch of membrane under the pipette tearing away from the rest of the cell forming the *inside-out configuration*. Similarly, from the whole-cell state, pulling the electrode away results in the membrane surrounding the pipette tearing away from the cell and then joining together at the edges to form what is called the *outside-out patch*. These various configurations allow for a wide range of experiments to be performed and also allow the measurement of currents through single channels.

11.3 General Formulations of Membrane Currents

This section examines the various components common to membrane models. The section starts with the Nernst-Planck formulation of ion flow across a membrane. Although it is seldom used now, this equation is needed to derive other, more practical models such as the resistor-battery model or the Goldman-Hodgkin-Katz current model. Some preliminary remarks are in order before examining these models. At dilute concentrations, ions in aqueous solutions behave like gas molecules. This is why the *gas constant R* is ubiquitous in models of ion flow in cells. Similarly, the phenomenon of chemisorption of gas molecules is used as an analogue to study the binding of ions (and drug molecules) to receptors in the cell membrane. In chemisorption under equilibrium conditions, the fraction of gas molecules bound to fixed reaction sites is given by an expression of the form $[C]^n/(k + [C]^n)$, where $[C]$ is the concentration of gas, k is a constant, and n is typically a small positive number. This expression is also derived from Michaelis-Menten-type kinetic schemes. Similar terms arise in many membrane models, and these indicate that some fraction of the ionic species C is binding to receptor molecules on the surface of the cell membrane.

Nernst-Planck Equation

One of the most general descriptions of ion flow across a membrane is given by the Nernst-Planck equation. This is a partial differential equation where the independent variables represent space (x) and time (t). The main dependent variable is the concentration of the ion $[c(x,t)]$. The potential $u(x,t)$ is usually a fixed function but can be made a dependent variable, in which case an additional equation is required. The Nernst-Planck equations can be written as

$$\frac{\partial c(x,t)}{\partial t} = \frac{\partial}{\partial x} \frac{\mu(x,t)}{|z|} \left[\frac{RT}{F} \frac{\partial c(x,t)}{\partial x} + zc(x,t) \frac{\partial u}{\partial x}(x,t) \right] \qquad (11.1)$$

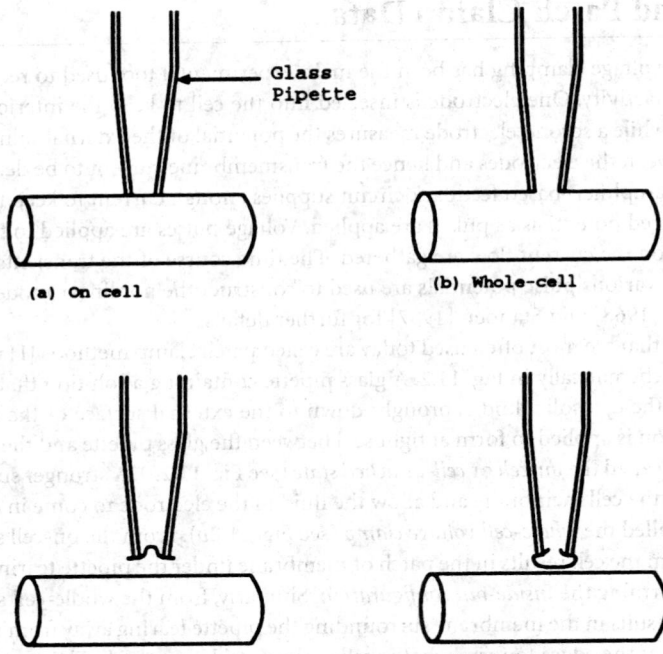

FIGURE 11.2   Schematic view of patch-clamp techniques.

where the symbols are defined as follows:

Variable	Description	Dimensions
R	Gas constant	8314.41 mJ/(mol · K)
T	Temperature	310 K
F	Faraday's constant	96485 C/mol
u	Potential	mV
c	Ion concentration	mol/liter
z	Valence of the ion	
E	Electric field force	mV/m
μ	Ion mobility	m²/(mV · s)

Note that μ can vary with both space and time depending on the type of ion channel or pump and its gating properties. Due to the complexity of this formulation, it is of limited use when examining behavior at the cellular level.

Hodgkin-Huxley Resistor Battery Model

This is the model that is employed most frequently to look at ions flowing through channels and is shown in terms of its circuit equivalent in Fig. 11.3. This models the passive flow of ions due to a potential gradient V and a concentration gradient (represented in the battery E_i) through a nonlinear membrane conductance. From the structure of the circuit, the equation for the current for ionic species i has the form

$$I_i = G_i m_i^p h_i^q (V - E_i) \tag{11.2}$$

where G_i represents the maximum value of the conductance of the membrane, and m_i and h_i are gating variables that vary in time and take values between 0 and 1. p and q are integers that depend on the characteristics of the membrane channel.

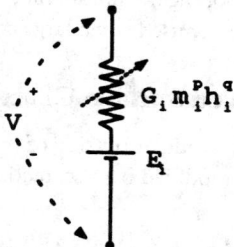

FIGURE 11.3 Circuit representation of membrane current.

The preceding expression can be derived from the Nernst-Planck equations with the assumption that concentration does not vary with time. In addition, the space dimension of Eq. (11.1) is reduced to a two-compartment—cell interior and exterior—model. Thus the steady state of Eq. (11.1) tells us that when there is no net current flow, the transmembrane potential will equal a quantity called the *Nernst potential*:

$$E_i = \frac{RT}{ZiF} \ln\left(\frac{[C_i]_o}{[C_i]_i} \right)$$

z_i is the valence of the ion, $[C_i]_o$ is the concentration of the ion on the outside, and $[C_i]_i$ is the concentration on the inside. Quantities such as the ion mobility are effectively lumped into the resistance ($G_i m_i^p h_i^q$) that is usually nonlinear and time-varying.

First-order differential equations are used to model the time behavior of m_i and h_i. For example, the equation for m_i will have the form

$$\frac{dm_i}{dt} = \alpha_m (1 - m_i) - \beta_m m_i \tag{11.3}$$

where the α_m and β_m are empirically determined functions of the membrane potential. This equation is also written as

$$\frac{dm_i}{dt} = \frac{m_{i\infty} - m_i}{\tau_i}$$

where $\quad m_{i\infty} = \dfrac{\alpha_m}{\alpha_m + \beta_m} \quad$ and $\quad \tau_i = \dfrac{1}{\alpha_m + \beta_m}$

Selectivity is automatically modeled by assuming that only one ionic species flows though a current branch. A number of such branches are connected in parallel to model the interaction of the various ion currents.

Goldman-Hodgkin-Katz (GHK) Constant Field Formulation

From Eq. (11.1), assuming that potential varies linearly across the membrane and that the ion flux is constant, an expression for current flow of the following form [Goldman, 1943] can be obtained:

$$I_i = P_i d_i^p f_i^q \frac{\dfrac{V}{RT/zF}}{1 - e^{-\frac{V}{RT/zF}}} \left([C_i]_i - [C_i]_o e^{-\frac{V}{RT/zF}} \right) \tag{11.4}$$

where P_i is the maximum permeability of the membrane, and d and f are gating variables like m and h in Eq. (11.2). This equation is frequently used when large concentration gradients are present.

GHK with Correction for Fixed Surface Charge

When surface charge is present on the inside or outside of the cell membrane, the effective potential gradient sensed by the channel is modified by a correction factor $V_{surface}$, and the current then has the form [Frankenhaeuser, 1960]

$$I_i = P_i d_i^p f_i^q \frac{\frac{V - V_{surface}}{RT/zF}}{1 - e^{-\frac{V - V_{surface}}{RT/zF}}} \left([C_i]_i - [C_i]_o e^{-\frac{V - V_{surface}}{RT/zF}}\right) \qquad (11.5)$$

Ion Pump

Ion pumps are membrane molecules that, unlike channels, require energy to function. While the workings of ion pumps can get quite complex, especially if the source of energy for these pumps needs to be modeled, most models assume a simplied form using Michaelis-Menten terms such as

$$I_p = I_{pmax} \frac{[X]_i}{[X]_i + k_x} \frac{[Y]_o}{[Y]_o + k_y} \qquad (11.6)$$

In this equation, I_{pmax} is the maximum pump current, $[X]_i$ is the concentration of the ionic species on the inside being pumped out, and $[Y]_o$ is the concentration of the ionic species on the outside being pumped in. k_x and k_y represent sensitivities of the pump to these ion concentrations.

Ion Exchangers

Ion exchangers use the concentration gradient of ion X to transport ion Y in the opposite direction. Examples of these currents are the cardiac Na-Ca exchanger, which uses the concentration gradient of sodium (high outside, low inside) to pump one calcium ion out of the cell for every three sodium ions allowed into the cell (see Appendix).

Synapses

Yamada and Zucker [1992] have tested various kinetic mechanisms to model calcium control of presynaptic release of transmitters. The classic model of postsynaptic response to a synaptic input is the so-called alpha function due to Rall [1967] and has the form

$$G(t) = \frac{t - t_0}{t_{peak}} e^{\frac{t - t_0}{t_{peak}}} \qquad (11.7)$$

where G is usually a conductance in a resistor-battery-type branch circuit. Although the alpha function is the one that is used most commonly, a more detailed model has been constructed [Destexhe et al., 1994] using a kinetic mechanism.

Calcium as a Second Messenger

Calcium entry into a cell frequently has a number of secondary effects such as initiation of contraction, release of neurotransmitters, and modulation of membrane ion channels. This is usually accomplished by the binding of calcium ions to calcium receptors inside the cell. Michaelis-Menten kinetic schemes with steady-state assumptions are used to model this binding, and therefore, expressions of the form

$$f = \frac{[Ca^{2+}]_i^n}{[Ca^{2+}]_i^n + K}$$

are frequently employed. Here, f is the fraction of receptor molecules that are bound to calcium, K is the dissociation constant for the reaction, and n is the number of calcium ions that bind to each receptor molecule.

11.4 Nerve Cells

Nerve cells typically have complex geometries with axons, branching dendrites, spines, and synapses. While the membranes in most of these units have nonlinear behavior, the membrane of the dendrites in many neurons can be modeled by simple linear resistor-capacitor circuits. In the following models, the presence of a capacitative current is always assumed. Since the Hodgkin-Huxley equation constitutes the basis for membrane modeling, the reader should be familiar with this model before examining the others.

Squid Axon: Hodgkin and Huxley. Most models of excitable cells are descendants of this model. The basic circuit equivalent of this model comprises a linear capacitance in parallel with three resistor-battery subcircuits (one each for sodium, potassium, and a third nonspecific leakage channel). The HH equations in their original form were

$$C_m \frac{dV}{dt} = -G_{Na} m^3 h (V - E_{Na}) - G_K n^4 (V - E_K) - G_l (V - E_l) \tag{11.8}$$

$$\frac{dm}{dt} = \alpha_m (1 - m) - \beta_m m$$

$$\frac{dh}{dt} = \alpha_h (1 - h) - \beta_h h$$

$$\frac{dn}{dt} = \alpha_n (1 - n) - \beta_n n$$

The rate constants were given originally as

$$\alpha_m = \frac{(V + 25)/10}{e^{(V+25)/10} - 1} \tag{11.9}$$

$$\beta_m = 4e^{V/18} \tag{11.10}$$

$$\alpha_h = 0.07 e^{V/20} \tag{11.11}$$

$$\beta_h = \frac{1}{e^{(V+30)/10} + 1} \tag{11.12}$$

$$\alpha_n = \frac{1}{10} \frac{(V + 10)/10}{e^{(V+10)/10} - 1} \tag{11.13}$$

$$\beta_n = \frac{e(V/80)}{8} \tag{11.14}$$

The physical constants used in these equations are $G_{Na} = 120$ mS/cm^2, $G_K = 36$ mS/cm^2, $G_l = 0.3$ mS/cm^2, $C_m = 1$ µF/cm^2, $E_{Na} = -115$ mV, $E_K = 12$ mV, and $E_l = -10.613$. The original equations as listed by Hodgkin and Huxley [1952] unfortunately used a sign convention that has not been followed since. Using the sign convention of today for the transmembrane potential, the rate constants can be rewritten by replacing all occurrences of V with $-(V_m + 60)$ and by recomputing the equilibrium potentials similarly.

The successes of this model include the ability to predict the velocity of action potential propagation when the spatial aspect is included, the continuous nature of the threshold of the nerve, and the repetitive firing behavior seen under the influence of a constant current. A couple of remarks should be made regarding this model that hold for other models as well. First, L'Hopital's rule allows us to compute the value of expressions of the form $x/(e^x - 1)$ at the point $x = 0$. Second, for temperatures other than 6.3°C, multiply each α and β by $\phi = 3^{(T - 6.3)/10}$, where T is given in degrees Celsius.

Gastropod Neuron.   The model of Connor and Stevens [1971] used an HH-type system of differential equations to model repetitive firing in isolated gastropod neurons. This was the first model to include an inactivating potassium current (the A-type current), which has since been used in a number of other cells.

Aplysia Abdominal Ganglion R15 cell.   The bursting behavior of *Aplysia* neurons has been studied extensively. The first model was that of Plant [1976], who extended the HH equations to include an inactivating potassium current, a slow potassium current, and a constant hyperpolarizing current due to the Na$^+$-K$^+$ pump. A review of bursting behavior in other molluscan neurons can be found in Benson and Adams [1989].

CA3 Hippocampal Pyramidal Neurons.   Traub et al. [1991] have constructed a multicompartment—soma and dendrites—model of hippocampal neurons with up to six membrane currents in each compartment: (1) a fast sodium current, (2) a calcium current, (3) a delayed rectifier potassium current, (4) an inactivating (A-type) potassium current, (5) a long-duration calcium-activated potassium current, and (6) a short-duration calcium-activated potassium current. Furthermore, calcium concentration changes in a restricted space beneath the membrane are modeled using a simplified linear buffering scheme.

CA1 Hippocampal Pyramidal Neurons.   A model that accurately predicts accommodation in CA1 neurons was recently constructed by Warman, Durand, and Yuen (1994). Using the previous work of Traub et al. (1991) and taking experimental data into consideration, they constructed a 16-compartment model with the following membrane currents: (1) a fast sodium current, (2) a calcium current, (3) a delayed rectifier potassium current, (4) an inactivating (A-type) potassium current, (5) a long-duration calcium dependent potassium current, (6) a short-duration calcium and voltage activated potassium current, (7) a persistent muscarinic potassium current, and (8) a leakage current. Unlike the model of Traub et al. (1991), separate pools of calcium were used to modulate the potassium currents. A linear buffering scheme was assumed for both internal calcium pools but the decay times were assumed to be different in each pool.

Stomatogastric Ganglion Neurons.   Epstein and Marder [1990] constructed an HH-type model of the lobster stomatogastric ganglion neuron with a fast sodium current, a delayed rectifier potassium current, a voltage-dependent calcium current, a calcium-dependent potassium current, and a linear leakage current in order to study the mechanism of bursting oscillations in these cells.

Retinal Ganglion Cells.   Fohlmeister et al. [1990] modeled the retinal ganglion cells using a fast inactivating sodium current, a calcium current, a noninactivating (delayed-rectifier) potassium current, an inactivating potassium current, and a calcium-activated potassium current. An important feature in this model is that it models the calcium concentration inside the cell using a simplified buffering scheme, and in this way, the authors are able to model the modulation of potassium currents by calcium.

Retinal Horizontal Cells. The model of Winslow and Knapp [1991] consisted of (1) a fast sodium current, (2) an inactivating (A-type) potassium current, (3) a noninactivating potassium current, (4) an anomalous rectifier potassium current, (5) a calcium-inactivated calcium current, and (6) a linear leakage current. In addition, calcium concentration changes in a restricted region beneath the membrane also were modeled.

Chopper Units in the Anteroventral Cochlear Nucleus. Banks and Sachs [1991] constructed an equivalent cylinder model of chopper units in the anteroventral cochlear nucleus. The model of the soma membrane included a fast sodium current, a delayed rectifier current, a linear leakage current, and inhibitory and excitatory synaptic currents using the Rall alpha-wave model.

Lamprey CNS Neurons. The model of Brodin et al. [1991] consisted of voltage-gated sodium, potassium, and calcium currents, a calcium-activated potassium current, and an NMDA receptor channel. The voltage-dependent magnesium block of the NMDA also was modeled in this paper. Two compartments were used to model calcium concentration changes inside the cells.

Sympathetic Neurons of the Superior Cervical Ganglia. Superior cervical ganglion neurons were modeled by Belluzzi and Sacchi [1991] using the following membrane currents: (1) sodium currents with fast and slow components, (2) a GHK-type calcium current, (3) a delayed rectifier potassium current, (4) an inactivating (A-type) potassium current, and (5) a calcium-activated potassium current. One drawback of this model is that the calcium activation of the potassium channels was modeled using a fixed time delay rather than by allowing the internal calcium concentration to change.

Thalamocortical Cells. Neurons in the thalamocortical system show various kinds of oscillatory behavior during sleep and wake cycles. It has been shown in the last decade that these neurons interact to produce a wide range of oscillatory activity. Huguenard and McCormick [1992] constructed a model of thalamic relay neurons with (1) a low-threshold transient calcium current, (2) an inactivating (A-type) potassium current, (3) a slowly inactivating potassium current, and (4) a hyperpolarization activated nonspecific current. McCormick and Huguenard [1992] extended their model to simulate the behavior of thalamocortical relay neurons by adding (1) a fast sodium current, (2) a persistent sodium current, (3) a high-threshold calcium current, (4) a calcium-activated potassium current, and (5) linear leakage currents. Destexhe et al. [1993a, 1993b] have examined similar models as well.

1.5 Skeletal Muscle Cells

Frog Sartorius Muscle Cell. Skeletal muscle cells have a significant amount of current flowing through the cell membrane in the T-tubules of the cells. For this reason, it becomes imperative to model the currents in the T-tubules along with the rest of the cell membrane. The Adrian-Peachey equations [Adrian and Peachey, 1973] are a system of coupled HH-type circuits and thus have a significant spatial component. The rate equations have the same structure as the Hodgkin-Huxley equations. Two models were suggested in the paper: If sodium and potassium channels are assumed to exist in the T-tubules, the usual HH formulation of the corresponding currents are used; otherwise, only a linear leakage current appears in the voltage equation.

Barnacle Muscle. Morris and Lecar [1981] sought to model the oscillatory activity in current-clamped barnacle muscle fibers using just two noninactivating currents: a fast calcium current and a potassium current. It should be kept in mind that their model does not take into account the presence of a calcium chelator (EGTA) inside the cells used to obtain experimental results. Their equations have the same general structure as the HH equations:

$$C_m \frac{dV}{dt} = -G_L(V - E_L) - G_{Ca}m(V - E_{Ca}) - G_K n(V - E_K) \tag{11.15}$$

$$\frac{dm}{dt} = \lambda_m(m_\infty - m) \tag{11.16}$$

$$\frac{dn}{dt} = \lambda_n(n_\infty - n) \tag{11.17}$$

where

$$m_\infty = \frac{1}{2}\left(\frac{1 + \tanh V - v_1}{v_2}\right) \tag{11.18}$$

$$\lambda_m = \overline{\lambda_m}\cosh\frac{V - v_1}{2v_2} \tag{11.19}$$

$$n_\infty = \frac{1}{2}\left(1 + \tanh\frac{V - v_3}{v_4}\right) \tag{11.20}$$

$$\lambda_n = \overline{\lambda_n}\cosh\frac{V - v_3}{2v_4} \tag{11.21}$$

Typical values of the parameters are $C_m = 20$ μF/cm^2, $G_L = 2$ mS/cm^2, $G_K = 8$ mS/cm^2, $G_{Ca} = 4$ mS/cm^2, $E_L = -50$ mV, $E_K = -70$ mV, $E_{Ca} = 100$ mV, $v_1 = 10$ mV, $v_2 = 15$ mV, $v_3 = 10$ mV, $v_4 = 14.5$ mV, $\lambda_m = 0.1$, and $\lambda_n = 1/15$. An alternative model of the calcium current also was proposed. Instead of the HH resistor-battery-type formulation, a GHK formulation was suggested:

$$I_{Ca} = G_{Ca}m \frac{V/12.5}{1 - e^{V/12.5}}\left[1 - \frac{[Ca^{2+}]_i}{[Ca^{2+}]_o} e^{V/12.5}\right] \tag{11.22}$$

where typical values of $[Ca^{2+}]_i$ and $[Ca^{2+}]_o$ were 0.001 mM and 100 mM, respectively.

11.6 Endocrine Cells

Pancreatic Beta Cells.   An interesting electrophysiologic phenomenon occurs in the islet of Langerhans of the pancreas: The release of insulin is controlled in these islets by trains of action potentials occurring in rapid bursts followed by periods of quiescence. This *bursting* behavior occurs only in intact islets; single cells do not display such bursting activity. Chay and Keizer [1983] were the first attempt to model this phenomenon quantitatively. Sherman et al. [1988] sought to explain the absence of bursting in single beta cells using the idea of *channel sharing*. Keizer [1988] modified this model by substituting an ATP- and ADP-dependent potassium channel instead of the calcium-dependent potassium channel. This model was then further improved by Keizer and Magnus [1989]. Sherman et al. [1990] constructed a domain model to examine the effect of calcium on calcium channel inactivation. Further refinements have been made by Keizer and Young [1993].

Pituitary Gonadotrophs   Li et al. [1994] have constructed a model of calcium release from the endoplasmic reticulum of rat pituitary gonadotrophs; although membrane fluxes have not yet been included in this model, they can be easily incorporated.

11.7 Cardiac Cells

Purkinje Fiber. Older models of the Purkinje fiber [Noble, 1960, 1962; Noble and Tsien, 1969; McAllister et al., 1975) failed to model the pacemaking currents correctly. Also, external and internal concentration changes were not modeled until the work of DiFrancesco and Noble [1985]. (The original paper contained a number of errors, and a corrected listing of the model equations is presented in the appendix to this chapter.) Despite the fact that the magnitude of the changes in calcium concentrations is at odds with recent experimental observations, this model has been very influential in directing modeling efforts. Most cardiac models being constructed now use the DiFrancesco-Noble structure.

Sinoatrial Node. As was the case with Purkinje fibers, the pacemaking mechanism was not modeled correctly in older models [Bristow and Clark, 1982; Yanagihara et al., 1980], and it was only after the Purkinje fiber model of DiFrancesco and Noble [1985] that accurate models of the sinoatrial node models could be constructed. An excellent summary of these modeling efforts can be found in Wilders et al. [1991], complete with listings of the equations. The most detailed model of sinoatrial node cells to date is that of Demir et al. (1994); this model includes a biophysically accurate description of internal calcium buffering and varying extracellular concentrations.

Atrial Muscle. The first detailed model of the excitation-contraction coupling mechanism in heart cells was constructed by Hilgemann and Noble [1987], and a single-cell model was completed by Earm and Noble [1990]. Since then, a number of other models with similar structure also have been formulated. The model of Earm et al. is considered the best model of single heart muscle cells available now. A listing of the model equations can be found in the appendix to this chapter; this version does not contain the equations that affect contractile properties of the cell.

Ventricular Muscle. The first model of ventricular cells (Beeler and Reuter, 1977) consisted of (1) a fast inward sodium current, (2) a slow inward calcium current, (3) an inward-rectifying potassium current, and (4) a voltage-dependent potassium current. A simple linear model of calcium buffering also was included. Drouhard and Roberge [1987] improved the Beeler-Reuter model by varying parameters and the equations for the rate constants for sodium activation and inactivation in order to match experimental results. Luo and Rudy [1991] brought further improvements by including a plateau potassium current and updating all the current characteristics to match data from whole-cell and patch-clamp experiments. A more detailed model with more accurate descriptions of internal calcium concentration changes also has been constructed [Luo and Rudy, 1994]. The main disadvantage of this latest effort is the formulation of the calcium release current: It depends on the time of the maximum rate of depolarization and activates with a time delay.

Noble et al. [1991] have completed a model of the guinea pig ventricular cell by varying parameters in equations for an atrial cell model. Nordin [1993] modified the DiFrancesco and Noble [1985] equations to model ventricular cells. His model included membrane calcium and potassium pumps and subcompartments inside the cell for sodium and calcium concentrations.

Amphibian Sinus Venosus and Atrial Cells. Rasmusson et al. [1990b] have constructed a detailed model of the bullfrog sinus venosus pacemaker cells that includes (1) a delayed rectifier potassium current, (2) a GHK-type calcium current, linear background (3) sodium and (4) calcium currents, (5) an Na^+-K^+ pump current, (6) an Na^+-Ca^+ exchanger current, and (7) a calcium pump current. Calcium binding to troponin, troponin-magnesium, and calmodulin also was included in the model. Furthermore, internal and external sodium, calcium, and potassium also were modeled as time-varying quantities. In addition to the features of the sinus venosus cell, the bullfrog atrial cell [Rasmusson et al., 1990a] includes a fast sodium current and an inward rectifying potassium current.

11.8 Smooth Muscle

Smooth-muscle cells, like many other kinds of cells, have significant currents carried by pumps and exchangers. While it should be possible to incorporate these components into a full model, this has yet to be done. A recent model of smooth-muscle cell membrane electrical activity is one constructed by Gonzalez-Fernandez and Ermentrout [1994]. This model has the same structure as the Morris-Lecar model of barnacle muscle fibers. Besides model parameter differences, the gating variable m is assumed to change fast enough that it is set at its steady-state value of m_∞; in addition, internal calcium is modeled as a time-varying quantity with a simple linear model of internal buffering.

11.9 Simplified Models

Hill.   The model constructed by Hill [1936] was one of the earliest differential equation models of nerve electrical activity. While the behavior of this model was compared with experimental observations in animal preparations, the model is a phenomenological one that only reproduced subthreshold responses. Hill's main focus was the modeling of accommodation, and he modeled this using a time-varying "threshold" U.

The basic model is a linear differential equation, with time being the independent variable and voltage V and threshold voltage U being the dependent variables:

$$\dot{V} = \frac{-1}{k}(V - V_o) + I(t)$$
$$\dot{U} = \frac{-1}{\lambda}(U - U_o) + \frac{1}{\beta}(V - V_o) \tag{11.23}$$

where V_o and U_o are some steady-state values of voltage and the threshold function and k, λ and β are relaxation time constants (k is a few milliseconds and λ and β are a few hundred milliseconds), and $I(t)$ is some time-varying current source. These equations can be solved using the variation of constants method, and Hill documented the responses of the model to various functions $I(t)$ and various parameter values. Such a model is of use only if one is not interested in suprathreshold behavior.

FitzHugh-Nagumo.   The FitzHugh-Nagumo equations are also called the *Bonhoeffer–Van der Pol equations* and have been used as a generic system that shows excitability and oscillatory activity. FitzHugh [1969] showed that much of the behavior of the Hodgkin-Huxley equations can be reproduced by a system of two differential equations:

$$\dot{V} = V - \frac{V^3}{3} - U + I(t)$$
$$\dot{U} = \phi(V - bU + a) \tag{11.24}$$

where a, b, and ϕ are positive constants (typical values are $a = 0.7$, $b = 0.8$, and $\phi = 0.08$). With no input current ($I = 0$), the system has a stable resting state, and at $I = 0.4$, the system exhibits oscillatory activity. This model reproduces excitability, threshold phenomena, and repetitive firing.

Hindmarsh-Rose models.   The first model of Hindmarsh and Rose [1982a] was an attempt to improve on the FitzHugh-Nagumo model without increasing the number of state variables. In most neurons undergoing repetitive firing, the time between action potentials is usually much greater than the duration of action potentials; however, the FHN model has an action potential duration that is roughly the same order of magnitude as the interspike interval. In addition, FHN does not yield a linear current-frequency relationship. These inadequacies were addressed by Hindmarsh and Rose, and in their model, the action potential duration and the interspike interval are closer to experimental recordings. Their model can be written as

$$\dot{V} = -a[f(V) - y - I]$$
$$\dot{y} = b[g(V) - y]$$

(11.25)

where the nonlinearities are defined to be $f(V) = cV^3 + dV^2 + eV + h$ and $g(V) = f(V) - qe^{rV} + s$. The constants used to model action potentials in snail visceral ganglion neurons were $a = 5400$ MΩ/s, $b = 30$ s^{-1}, $c = 0.00017$, $d = 0.001$, $e = 0.01$, $h = 0.1$, $q = 0.024$, $r = 0.088$, and $s = 0.046$.

A second model [Hindmarsh and Rose, 1982b] sought to include the phenomenon of bursting by adding a third variable. The model had the following form:

$$\dot{V} = -aV^3 + bV^2 + y - z + I$$
$$\dot{y} = c - dV^2 - y$$
$$\dot{z} = r[s(V - V_1) - z]$$

(11.26)

where $a = 1$, $b = 3$, $c = 1$, $d = 5$, $r = 0.001$, and $s = 1$ and setting $I = 1$ for a short period triggers the bursting response.

Defining Terms

Action potential: A phenomenon involving temporal changes in the transmembrane potential. An action potential is typically characterized by a fast depolarization followed by a slower repolarization and sometimes hyperpolarization as well.

Depolarization: Depolarization is a process that is said to occur whenever the transmembrane potential becomes more positive than some "resting" potential.

Hyperpolarization: A deviation of the transmembrane potential in the negative direction from a "resting" state is called *hyperpolarization*.

Ion channel: An ion channel is a protein molecule embedded in the cell membrane. It is thought to have the structure of a pipe with obstructions that gate the flow of ions into and out of the cell.

Ion exchanger: An ion exchanger molecule uses the potential energy in the electrochemical gradients to pump one ionic species into the cell and another species out.

Ion pump: An ion pump molecule uses energy (in the form of ATP molecules) to pump ions against their electrochemical gradients.

Refractory period: A period of time after an action potential during which the cell is unable to undergo another action potential in response to a stimulus.

Repolarization: Repolarization is a process that usually follows depolarization and causes the transmembrane potential to return to a polarized state.

Selectivity.   This is a property of ion channels where a certain type of channel only allows a specific ionic species to pass through it. Some channels are less specific than others and may allow more than one ionic species to pass through.

Threshold: There is no satisfactory definition or quantitative description of threshold that will work for all conditions. A working definition of threshold would be *the state the cell has to* *reach in order to produce an action potential.* It is usually characterized by the strength of an external stimulus required to bring the cell from some initial state to the threshold state. The problem with this definition is that the threshold stimulus will vary considerably depending on the initial state of the cell; the cell may be in a resting state, or it may be undergoing repolarization or depolarization.

Transmembrane potential difference: The potential difference between the inside and the outside of a cell manifests itself very close to the membrane. In many cases, the potential of the external fluid is taken to be the reference or ground potential, and the transmembrane potential difference is the same as the cell potential, otherwise also called the *membrane potential.*

Voltage clamp: This refers to the experimental procedure of using active electronic circuits to hold the transmembrane potential difference at a fixed value by pumping current into the cell.

References

Adrian RH, Peachey LD. 1973. Reconstruction of the action potential of frog sartorius muscle. J Physiol 235:103.

Banks MI, Sachs MB. 1991. Regularity analysis in a compartmental model of chopper units in the anteroventral cochlear nucleus. J Neurophysiol 65(3):606.

Beeler GW, Reuter H. 1977. Reconstruction of the action potential of ventricular myocardial fibres. Journal of Physiology (London) 268:177.

Belluzzi O, Sacchi O. 1991. A five-conductance model of the action potential in the rat sympathetic neurone. Prog Biophys Mol Biol 55:1.

Benson JA, Adams WB. 1989. Ionic mechanisms of endogenous activity in molluscan burster neurons. In JW Jacklet (ed), Neuronal and Cellular Oscillators, pp 87–120. New York, Marcel Dekker.

Bristow DG, Clark JW. 1982. A mathematical model of primary pacemaking cell in SA node of the heart. Am J Physiol 243:H207.

Brodin L, Traven HGC, Lansner A, et al. 1991. Computer simulations of *n*-methyl-D-aspartate receptor-induced membrane properties in a neuron model. J Neurophysiol 66(2):473.

Chay TR, Keizer J. 1983. Minimal model for membrane oscillations in the pancreatic β-cell. Biophys J 42:181.

Cole KS. 1968. Membranes, Ions and Impulses: A Chapter of Classical Biophysics, vol 1 of Biophysics Series. Berkeley, University of California Press.

Connor JA, Stevens CF. 1971. Prediction of repetitive firing behaviour from voltage clamp data on an isolated neurone soma. J Physiol 213:31.

Demir SS, Clark JW, Murphey CR, Giles WR. 1994. A mathematical model of a rabbit sinoatrial node cell. American Journal of Physiology 266:C832.

Destexhe A, Babloyantz A, Sejnowski TJ. 1993a. Ionic mechanisms for intrinsic slow oscillations in thalamic relay neurons. Biophys J 65(4):1538.

Destexhe A, Mainen ZF, Sejnowski TJ. 1994. An efficient method for computing synaptic conductances based on a kinetic model of receptor binding. Neural Comput 6:14.

Destexhe A, McCormick DA, Sejnowski TJ. 1993b. A model for 8–10 Hz spindling in interconnected thalamic relay and reticularis neurons. Biophys J 65(6):2473.

DiFrancesco D, Noble D. 1985. A model of cardiac electrical activity incorporating ionic pumps and concentration changes. Phil Trans R Soc Lond [B] 307:353.

Drouhard J-P, Roberge FA. 1987. Revised formulation of the Hodgkin-Huxley representation of the sodium current in cardiac cells. Comp Biomed Res 20:333.

Earm YE, Noble D. 1990. A model of the single atrial cell: Relation between calcium current and calcium release. Proc R Soc Lond [B] 240:83.

Epstein IR, Marder E. 1990. Multiple modes of a conditional neural oscillator. Biol Cybern 63:25.

FitzHugh R. 1969. Mathematical models of excitation and propagation in nerve. In HP Schwan (ed), Biological Engineering, chap 1, pp 1–85. New York, McGraw-Hill.

Fohlmeister JF, Coleman PA, Miller RF. 1990. Modeling the repetitive firing of retinal ganglion cells. Brain Res 510:343.

Frankenhaeuser B. 1960. Sodium permeability in toad nerve and in squid nerve. J Physiol 152:159.

Goldman DE. 1943. Potential, impedance, and rectification in membranes. J Gen Physiol 27:37.

Gonzalez-Fernandez JM, Ermentrout B. 1994. On the origin and dynamics of the vasomotion of small arteries. Math Biosci 119:127.

Hamill OP, Marty A, Neher E, et al. 1981. Improved patch-clamp techniques for high resolution current recording from cells and cell-free membrane patches. Pflugers Arch Ges Physiol 391:85.

Hilgemann DW, Noble D. 1987. Excitation-contraction coupling and extracellular calcium transients in rabbit atrium: Reconstruction of basic cellular mechanisms. Proc R Soc Lond [B] 230:163.

Hill AV. 1936. Excitation and accommodation in nerve. Proc R Soc Lond [B] 119:305.

Hindmarsh JL, Rose RM. 1982a. A model of the nerve impulse using two first-order differential equations. Nature 296:162.

Hindmarsh JL, Rose RM. 1982b. A model of the neuronal bursting using three coupled first order differential equations. Proc R Soc Lond [B] 221:87.

Hodgkin AL, Huxley AF. 1952. A quantitative description of membrane current and its application to conduction and excitation in nerve. J Physiol 117:500.

Huguenard JR, McCormick DA. 1992. Simulation of the currents involved in rhythmic oscillations in thalamic relay neurons. J Neurophysiol 68(4):1373.

Keizer J. 1988. Electrical activity and insulin release in pancreatic beta cells. Math Biosci 90:127.

Keizer J, Magnus G. 1989. ATP-sensitive potassium channel and bursting in the pancreatic beta cell: A theoretical study. Biophys J 89:229.

Keizer J, Young GWD. 1993. Effect of voltage-gated plasma membrane Ca^{2+} fluxes on IP_3-linked Ca^{2+} oscillations. Cell Calcium 14:397.

Li Y-X, Rinzel J, Keizer J, Stojilkovic SS. 1994. Calcium oscillations in pituitary gonadotrophs: Comparison of experiment and theory. Proc Natl Acad Sci USA 91:58.

Luo C, Rudy Y. 1991. A model of the ventricular cardiac action potential. Circ Res 68:1501.

Luo C, Rudy Y. 1994. A dynamic model of the cardiac ventricular action potential: I. Simulations of ionic currents and concentration changes. Circ Res 74:1071.

McAllister RE, Noble D, Tsien RW. 1975. Reconstruction of the electrical activity of cardiac Purkinje fibers. J Physiol 251:1.

McCormick DA, Huguenard JR. 1992. A model of the electrophysiological properties of thalamocortical relay neurons. J Neurophysiol 68(4):1373.

Morris C, Lecar H. 1981. Voltage oscillations in the barnacle giant muscle fiber. Biophys J 35:193.

Noble D. 1960. A description of cardiac pacemaker potentials based on the Hodgkin-Huxley equations. J Physiol 154:64P.

Noble D. 1962. A modification of the Hodgkin-Huxley equations applicable to Purkinje fiber action and pace-maker potentials. J Physiol 160:317.

Noble D, Noble SJ, Bett GCL et al. 1991. The role of sodium-calcium exchange during the cardiac action potential. Ann NY Acad Sci 639:334. Sodium-Calcium Exchange: Proceedings of the Second International Conference, Baltimore, Md, April 1991.

Noble D, Tsien RW. 1969. Reconstruction of the repolarization process in cardiac Purkinje fibers based on voltage clamp measurements of membrane current. J Physiol 200:205.

Nordin C. 1993. Computer model of membrane current and intracellular Ca^{2+} flux in the isolated guinea-pig ventricular myocyte. Am J Physiol 265:H2117.

Plant RE. 1976. Mathematical description of a bursting pacemaker neuron by a modification of the Hodgkin-Huxley equations. Biophys J 16:227.

Rall W. 1967. Distinguishing theoretical synaptic potentials computed for different soma-dendritic distributions of synaptic input. J Neurophysiol 30:1138.

Rasmusson RL, Clark JW, Giles WR, et al. 1990a. A mathematical model of electrophysiological activity in a bullfrog atrial cell. Am J Physiol 259:H370.

Rasmusson RL, Clark JW, Giles WR, et al. 1990b. A mathematical model of a bullfrog cardiac pacemaker cell. Am J Physiol 259:H352.

Sherman A, Keizer J, Rinzel J. 1990. Domain model for Ca^{2+}-inactivation of Ca^{2+} channels at low channel density. Biophys J 58:985.

Sherman A, Rinzel J, Keizer J. 1988. Emergence of organized bursting in clusters of pancreatic β-cells by channel sharing. Biophys J 54:411.

Standen NB. 1987. Microelectrode Techniques. Cambridge, The Company of Biologists.

Traub RD, Wong RKS, Miles R, Michelson H. 1991. A model of a CA3 hippocampal pyramidal neuron incorporating voltage-clamp data on intrinsic conductances. J Neurophysiol 66(2):635.

Warman EN, Durand DM, and Yuen GLF. 1994. Reconstruction of hippocampal CA1 pyramidal cell electrophysiology by computer simulation. Journal of Neurophysiology 71(6):2033.

Wilders R, Jongsma HJ, van Ginneken ACG. 1991. Pacemaker activity of the rabbit sinoatrial node: A comparison of mathematical models. Biophys J 60:1202.

Winslow RL, Knapp AG. 1991. Dynamic models of the retinal horizontal cell network. Prog Biophys Mol Biol 56:107.

Yamada WM, Zucker RS. 1992. Time course of transmitter release calculated from simulations of a calcium diffusion model. Biophys J 61:671.

Yanagihara K, Noma A, Irisawa H. 1980. Reconstruction of sinoatrial node pacemaker potential based on the voltage clamp experiments. Jpn J Physiol 30:841.

Appendix

The DiFrancesco-Noble Equations

Velocity Field Equations

$$\dot{V} = \frac{-1}{C_m} \left(I_{f\mathrm{K}} + I_{f\mathrm{Na}} + I_\mathrm{K} + I_{\mathrm{K}1} + I_{to} + I_{b\mathrm{Na}} + I_{\mathrm{NaK}} + I_{\mathrm{NaCa}} + I_\mathrm{Na} + I_{b\mathrm{Ca}} + I_{si\mathrm{Ca}} + I_{si\mathrm{K}} \right)$$

$$\dot{y} = 0.05e^{-0.067(V+42)}(1-y) - \frac{(V+42)}{1-e^{-0.2(V+42)}}y$$

$$\dot{x} = \frac{0.5e^{0.0826(V+50)}}{1+e^{0.057(V+50)}}(1-x) - \frac{1.3e^{-0.06(V+20)}}{1+e^{-0.04(V+20)}}x$$

$$\dot{r} = 0.033e^{-V/17}(1-r) - \frac{33}{1+e^{-(V+10)/8}}r$$

$$\dot{m} = \frac{200(V+41)}{1-e^{-0.1(V+41)}}(1-m) - 8000e^{-0.056(V+66)}m$$

$$\dot{h} = 20e^{-0.125(V+75)}(1-h) - \frac{2000}{1+320e^{-0.1(V+75)}}h$$

$$\dot{d} = \frac{30(V+19)}{1-e^{-(V+19)/4}}(1-d) - \frac{12(V+19)}{e^{(V+19)/10}-1}d$$

$$\dot{f} = \frac{6.25(V+34)}{e^{(V+34)/4}-1}(1-f) - \frac{50}{1+e^{-(V+34)/4}}f$$

$$\dot{f_2} = 5(1-f_2) - \frac{5}{k_{mf2}}[\mathrm{Ca}^{2+}]_i f_2$$

$$\dot{p} = \frac{0.625(V+34)}{e^{(V+34)/4}-1}(1-p) - \frac{5}{1+e^{-(V+34)/4}}p$$

$$[\dot{Na}^+]_i = \frac{-(I_{fNa} + I_{bNa} + 3I_{NaK} + \dfrac{n_{NaCa}}{(n_{NaCa} - 2)} I_{NaCa} + I_{Na})}{V_i F}$$

$$[\dot{K}^+]_i = \frac{-(I_{fK} + I_K + I_{K1} + I_{to} - 2I_{NaK} + I_{siK})}{V_i F}$$

$$[\dot{K}^+]_c = \frac{1}{V_i F}(I_{fK} + I_K + I_{K1} + I_{to} - 2I_{NaK} + I_{siK})$$
$$\qquad\qquad - D_{K^+}([K^+]_c - [K^+]_o)$$

$$[\dot{Ca}^{2+}]_i = \frac{-(I_{bCa} - \dfrac{2}{(n_{NaCa} - 2)} I_{NaCa} + I_{siCa} + I_{up} - I_{rel})}{2V_i F}$$

$$[\dot{Ca}^{2+}]_{up} = \frac{(I_{up} - I_{tr})}{2V_{up} F}$$

$$[\dot{Ca}^{2+}]_{rel} = \frac{(I_{tr} - I_{rel})}{2V_{rel} F}$$

Current Equations

$$I_{fK} = \frac{[K^+]_c}{[K^+]_c + k_{mf}} G_{fk}(V - E_K)y$$

$$I_{fNa} = \frac{[K^+]_c}{[K^+]_c + k_{mf}} G_{fNa}(V - E_{Na})y$$

$$I_K = \frac{I_{Kmax}}{140} ([K^+]_i - [K^+]_c e^{\frac{-V}{RT/F}})x$$

$$I_{K1} = G_{K1} \frac{[K^+]_c}{[K^+]_c + k_{mK1}} \left(\frac{V - E_K}{1 + e^{\frac{V - E_K + 10}{RT/2F}}} \right)$$

$$I_{to} = 0.28 \left(0.2 + \frac{[K^+]_c}{k_{mto} + [K^+]_c}\right) \frac{[Ca^{2+}]_i}{k_{act4} + [Ca^{2+}]_i} \left(\frac{V + 10}{1 - e^{-0.2(V+10)}} \right)$$
$$\qquad\qquad ([K^+]_i e^{0.02V} - [K^+]_c e^{-0.02V})r$$

$$I_{bNa} = G_{bNa}(V - E_{Na})$$

$$I_{Na} = G_{Na}(V - E_{mh})m^3 h$$

$$I_{bCa} = G_{bCa}(V - E_{Ca})$$

$$I_{siCa} = 4P_{Ca}dff_2 \frac{\dfrac{V - 50}{RT/F}}{1 - e^{\frac{-(V-50)}{RT/2}}} \left([Ca^{2+}]_i e^{\frac{50}{RT/2F}} - [Ca^{2+}]_o e^{\frac{-(V-50)}{RT/2F}} \right)$$

$$I_{siK} = P_{CaK} P_{Ca} df f_2 \frac{\dfrac{V - 50}{RT/F}}{1 - e^{\frac{-(V-50)}{RT/F}}}$$

$$\left([K^+]_i \, e^{\frac{50}{RT/F}} - [K^+]_c \, e^{\frac{-(V-50)}{RT/F}} \right)$$

Ion Pumps and Exchangers

$$I_{NaK} = I_{NaKmax} \frac{[K^+]_c}{[K^+]_c + k_{mk}} \frac{[Na^+]_i}{[Na^+]_i + k_{mNa}}$$

$$I_{NaCa} = k_{NaCa} \frac{e^{\gamma \frac{V}{RT/F}} [Na^+]_i^3 [Ca^{2+}]_o - e^{-(1-\gamma)\frac{V}{RT/F}} [Na^+]_o^3 [Ca^{2+}]_i}{1 + d_{NaCa} ([Ca^{2+}]_i [Na^+]_o^3 + [Ca^{2+}]_o [Na^+]_i^3)}$$

Calcium Sequestration

$$I_{up} = \alpha_{up} [Ca^{2+}]_i \left(\overline{[Ca^{2+}]}_{up} - [Ca^{2+}]_{up} \right)$$

$$I_{tr} = \alpha_{tr} p ([Ca^{2+}]_{up} - [Ca^{2+}]_{rel})$$

$$I_{rel} = \alpha_{rel} [Ca^{2+}]_{rel} \frac{[Ca^{2+}]_i^2}{[Ca^{2+}]_i^2 + k_{mca}}$$

Reversal Potentials

$$E_{Na} = \frac{RT}{F} \ln \left(\frac{[Na^+]_o}{[Na^+]_i} \right)$$

$$E_K = \frac{RT}{F} \ln \left(\frac{[K^+]_c}{[K^+]_i} \right)$$

$$E_{Ca} = \frac{RT}{2F} \ln \left(\frac{[Ca^{2+}]_o}{[Ca^{2+}]_i} \right)$$

$$E_{mh} = \frac{RT}{F} \ln \left(\frac{[Na^+]_o + 0.12 [K^+]_c}{[Na^+]_i + 0.12 [K^+]_i} \right)$$

Parameters

(Units: M = mol/liter; S = siemens; A = amperes; s = seconds; K = Kelvin.)

C_m	75 nF	k_{mto}	10 mM
k_{mf}	45 mM	k_{mf2}	1 μM
k_{mk1}	210 mM	k_{act4}	0.5 μM
k_{mk}	1 mM	k_{mCa}	$(10^{-3}$ m$M)^2$
k_{mNa}	40 mM	G_{Na}	750 μS

G_{fK}	3 μS	R	8314.41 mJ/(mol · K)
G_{fNa}	3 μS	T	310 K
G_{K1}	920 μS	V_{ecs}	0.1
G_{bNa}	0.18 μS	radius	50 μm
G_{bCa}	0.02 μS	length	2 mm
P_{Ca}	15 nA/mM	V_e	$V_{ecs} \pi$ radius^2 length
P_{CaK}	0.01	V_i	$(1 - V_{ecs}) \pi$ radius^2 length
I_{Kmax}	180 nA	V_{up}	0.05 V_i
I_{NaKmax}	125 nA	V_{rel}	0.02 V_i
$[K^+]_o$	4 mM	$[Ca^{2+}]_{up}$	5 mM
$[Na^+]_o$	140 mM		
$[Ca^{2+}]_o$	2 mM	α_{up}	$\dfrac{2V_iF}{\tau_{up}[Ca^{2+}]up}$
k_{NaCa}	0.02 nA		
d_{NaCa}	0.001		
γ	½	α_{tr}	$\dfrac{2V_{rel}F}{\tau_{rep}}$
n_{NaCa}	3		
τ_{up}	25 ms	α_{rel}	$\dfrac{2V_{rel}F}{\tau_{rep}}$
τ_{rep}	2 s		
τ_{rel}	50 ms	D_{K+}	0.7 s^{-1}
F	96485 C/mol		

The Earm-Hilgemann-Noble Equations for Cardiac Atrial Cells

Velocity Field Equations

$$\dot{V} = \frac{-1}{C_m} (I_{K1} + I_{to} + I_{siK} + I_{bK} + I_{NaK} + I_{Na} + I_{bNa} + I_{siNa}$$

$$+ I_{NaCa} + I_{siCa} + I_{bCa})$$

$$\dot{m} = \frac{200(V + 41)}{1 - e^{-0.1(V+41)}}(1 - m) - 8000e^{-0.056(V+66)}m$$

$$\dot{h} = 20e^{-0.125(V+75)}(1 - h) - \frac{2000}{1 + 320e^{-0.1(V+75)}}h$$

$$\dot{d} = \frac{90(V + 19)}{1 - e^{-(V+19)/4}}(1 - d) - \frac{36(V + 19)}{e^{(V+19)/10} - 1}d$$

$$\dot{f} = \frac{12}{1 + e^{-(V+34)/4}}\left(\frac{119\,[Ca^{2+}]_i}{k_{cachoff} + [Ca^{2+}]_i} + 1\right)(1 - f) - \frac{6.25(V + 34)}{e^{(V+34)/4} - 1}f$$

$$\dot{q} = 333\left(\frac{1}{1 + e^{-(V+4)/5}} - q\right)$$

$$\dot{r} = 0.033e^{-V/17}(1 - r) - \frac{33}{1 + e^{-(V+10)/8}}r$$

$$[\dot{Na^+}]_i = \frac{-1}{V_iF}(I_{Na} + I_{bNa} + 3I_{NaK} + 3I_{NaCa} + I_{siNa})$$

$$[\dot{K^+}]_i = \frac{-1}{V_iF}(I_{K1} + I_{siK} + I_{bK} + I_{to} - 2I_{NaK})$$

$$[\dot{Ca^{2+}}]_o = \frac{1}{2V_{cell}V_{ecs}F}(I_{siCa} + I_{bCa} - 2I_{NaCa}) - \text{Dif } f_{Ca}([Ca^{2+}]_o - [Ca^{2+}]_b)$$

$$[\dot{Ca}^{2+}]_i = \frac{-1}{2V_iF}(I_{siCa} + I_{bCa} - 2I_{NaCa}) - I_{up} + I_{rel}\frac{V_{SRup}V_{rel}}{V_iV_{up}}$$

$$- [\dot{Ca}^{2+}]_{calmod} - [\dot{Ca}^{2+}]_{troponin}$$

$$[\dot{Ca}^{2+}]_{up} = \frac{V_i}{V_{SRup}}I_{up} - I_{tr}$$

$$[\dot{Ca}^{2+}]_{rel} = \frac{V_{up}}{V_{rel}}I_{tr} - I_{rel}$$

$$[\dot{Ca}^{2+}]_{calmod} = 10^5(M_{trop} - [Ca^{2+}]_{calmod})\,[Ca^{2+}]_i - 50[Ca^{2+}]_{calmod}$$

$$[\dot{Ca}^{2+}]_{troponin} = 10^5(C_{trop} - [Ca^{2+}]_{troponin})\,[Ca^{2+}]_i - 200[Ca^{2+}]_{troponin}$$

$$\dot{f}_{activator} = (1 - f_{activator} - f_{product})[500\left(\frac{[Ca^{2+}]_i}{[Ca^{2+}]_i + k_{mCa}}\right)^2 + 600e^{(V-40)0.08}]$$

$$- f_{activator}[500\left(\frac{[Ca^{2+}]_i}{[Ca^{2+}]_i + k_{mCa}}\right)^2 + 60]$$

$$\dot{f}_{product} = f_{activator}[500\left(\frac{[Ca^{2+}]_i}{[Ca^{2+}]_i + k_{mCa}}\right)^2 + 60] - f_{product}$$

Membrane Current Equations

$$I_{K1} = G_{K1}\frac{[K^+]_o}{[K^+]_o + k_{mK1}}\left(\frac{V - E_K}{1 + e^{\frac{V - E_K - 10}{RT/2F}}}\right)$$

$$I_{to} = G_{to}(V - E_K)qr$$

$$I_{bK} = G_{bK}(V - E_K)$$

$$I_{Na} = G_{Na}(V - E_{mh})m^3h$$

$$I_{bNa} = G_{bNa}(V - E_{Na})\frac{[Na^+]_o}{140}$$

$$I_{siCa} = 4P_{Ca}d(1 - f)\frac{k_{cachoff}}{k_{cachoff} + [Ca^{2+}]_i}\frac{\frac{V - 50}{RT/F}}{1 - e^{\frac{-(V-50)}{RT/2F}}}\left([Ca^{2+}]_i e^{\frac{50}{RT/2F}} - [Ca^{2+}]_o e^{\frac{-(V-50)}{RT/2F}}\right)$$

$$I_{siK} = P_{CaK}P_{Ca}d(1 - f)\frac{k_{cachoff}}{k_{cachoff} + [Ca^{2+}]_i}\frac{\frac{V - 50}{RT/F}}{1 - e^{\frac{-(V-50)}{RT/F}}}\left([K+]_i e^{\frac{50}{RT/F}} - [K^+]_o e^{\frac{-(V-50)}{RT/F}}\right)$$

$$I_{siNa} = P_{CaNa}P_{Ca}d(1 - f)\frac{k_{cachoff}}{k_{cachoff} + [Ca^{2+}]_i}\frac{\frac{V - 50}{RT/F}}{1 - e^{\frac{-(V-50)}{RT/F}}}\left([Na^+]_i e^{\frac{50}{RT/F}} - [Na^+]_o e^{\frac{-(V-50)}{RT/F}}\right)$$

$$I_{bCa} = G_{bCa}(V - E_{Ca})$$

Pump/Exchanger Current Equations

$$I_{\text{NaK}} = I_{\text{NaKmax}} \frac{[K^+]_o}{[K^+]_o + k_{mK}} \frac{[Na^+]_i}{[Na^+]_i + k_{mNa}}$$

$$I_{\text{NaCa}} = k_{\text{NaCa}} \frac{e^{\gamma \frac{V}{RT/F}}[Na^+]_i^3[Ca^{2+}]_o - e^{-(1-\gamma)\frac{V}{RT/F}}[Na^+]_o^3[Ca^{2+}]_i}{1 + d_{\text{NaCa}}([Ca^{2+}]_i[Na^+]_o^3 + [Ca^{2+}]_o[Na^+]_i^3)}$$

Ca Sequestration Equations

$$I_{\text{up}} = \frac{3[Ca^{2+}]_i - 0.23 \, [Ca^{2+}]_{\text{up}} \dfrac{k_{cyCa}k_{xcs}}{k_{srCa}}}{[Ca^{2+}]_i + [Ca^{2+}]_{\text{up}} \dfrac{k_{cyCa}k_{xcs}}{k_{srCa}} + k_{cyCa}k_{xcs} + k_{cyCa}}$$

$$I_{\text{tr}} = 50([Ca^{2+}]_{\text{up}} - [Ca^{2+}]_{\text{rel}})$$

$$I_{\text{rel}} = \left(\frac{f_{\text{activator}}}{f_{\text{activator}} + 0.25}\right)^2 k_{mCa2} \, [Ca^{2+}]_{\text{rel}}$$

Reversal Potentials

$$E_{\text{Na}} = \frac{RT}{F} \ln\left(\frac{[Na^+]_o}{[Na^+]_i}\right)$$

$$E_{\text{K}} = \frac{RT}{F} \ln\left(\frac{[K^+]_o}{[K^+]_i}\right)$$

$$E_{\text{Ca}} = \frac{RT}{2F} \ln\left(\frac{[Ca^{2+}]_o}{[Ca^{2+}]_i}\right)$$

$$E_{\text{mh}} = \frac{RT}{F} \ln\left(\frac{[Na^+]_o + 0.12 \, [K^+]_o}{[Na^+]_i + 0.12 \, [K^+]_i}\right)$$

Parameters

(Units: M = mol/liter; S = siemens; A = amperes; s = seconds; K = Kelvin

C_m	$40(10)^{-6} \, \mu F$	Dif f_{Ca}	$5(10)^{-4} \, s^{-1}$
k_{cachoff}	$0.001 \, mM$	d_{NaCa}	10^{-4}
k_{mK1}	$10 \, mM$	γ	$\frac{1}{2}$
k_{mk}	$1 \, mM$	n_{NaCa}	3
k_{mNa}	$40 \, mM$	k_{cyCa}	$3(10)^{-4} \, mM$
k_{naCa}	$10^{-4} \, nA$	k_{xcs}	$0.4 \, mM$
k_{mCa}	$0.001 \, mM$	k_{srCa}	$0.5 \, mM$
		F	$96485 \, C/mol$
I_{NaKmax}	$0.14 \, nA$	R	$8314.41 \, mJ/(mol \cdot K)$
G_{Na}	$0.5 \, \mu S$	T	$310 \, K$
G_{to}	$0.01 \, \mu S$	V_{ecs}	0.4
G_{bK}	$.0017 \, \mu S$	radius	$10 \, \mu m$
G_{K1}	$0.017 \, \mu S$	length	$80 \, \mu m$
G_{bNa}	$.00012 \, \mu S$	V_{cell}	$10^{-9} \, \pi \, \text{radius}^2 \, \text{length} \, \mu l$

G_{bCa}	.00005 μS	V_i	$(1 - V_{ecs} - V_{up} - V_{rel})V_{cell}$ μl
P_{Ca}	0.05 nA/mM	V_{up}	0.01
P_{CaK}	0.002	V_{rel}	0.1
P_{CaNa}	0.002	V_{SRup}	$V_{cell}V_{up}$ μl
$[Ca^{2+}]_b$	2 mM	k_{mCa2}	250 nA/mM
$[K^+]_o$	4 mM	M_{trop}	0.02 mM
$[Na^+]_o$	140 mM	C_{trop}	0.15 mM

For Further Information

The best introduction to ion channels and excitable behavior in cells can be found in *Ionic Channels of Excitable Membranes* by Bertil Hille (Sunderland, Mass, Sinauer Associates, 1992). In the case of neurons, *Principles of Neural Science* by Kandel, Schwartz, and Jessell (New York, Elsevier, 1991) is the bible. Detailed discussions of cardiovascular cell membrane phenomena can be found in *The Heart and Cardiovascular System,* edited by Fozzard et al. (New York, Raven Press, 1992).

12

Numerical Methods for Bioelectric Field Problems

Christopher R.
Johnson
University of Utah

Computer modeling and simulation continue to grow more important to the field of bioengineering. The reasons for this growing importance are manyfold. First, mathematical modeling has been shown to be a substantial tool for the investigation of complex biophysical phenomena. Second, since the level of complexity one can model parallels existing hardware configurations, advances in computer architecture have made it feasible to apply the computational paradigm to complex biophysical systems. Hence, while biologic complexity continues to outstrip the capabilities of even the largest computational systems, the computational methodology has taken hold in bioengineering and has been used successfully to suggest physiologically and clinically important scenarios and results.

This chapter provides an overview of numerical techniques that can be applied to a class of bioelectric field problems. Bioelectric field problems are found in a wide variety of biomedical applications that range from single cells [1], to organs [2], up to models that incorporate partial to full human structures [3,4,5]. I describe some general modeling techniques that will be applicable, in part, to all the aforementioned problems. I focus this study on a class of bioelectric volume conductor problems that arise in electrocardiography and electroencephalography.

I begin by stating the mathematical formulation for a bioelectric volume conductor, continue by describing the model construction process, and follow with sections on numerical solutions and computational considerations. I conclude with a section on error analysis coupled with a brief introduction to adaptive methods.

0-8493-8346-3/95/$0.00+$.50
© 1995 by CRC Press, Inc.

12.1 Problem Formulation

As noted in Chap. 9, most bioelectric field problems can be formulated in terms of either the Poisson or the Laplace equation for electrical conduction. Since Laplace's equation is the homogeneous counterpart of the Poisson equation, I will develop the treatment for a general three-dimensional Poisson problem and discuss simplifications and special cases when necessary.

A *typical* bioelectric volume conductor can be posed as the following boundary value problem:

$$\nabla \cdot \sigma \nabla \Phi = -I_V \quad \text{in } \Omega \tag{12.1}$$

where Ω is the electrostatic potential, σ is the electrical conductivity tensor, and I_V is the current per unit volume defined within the solution domain, Ω. The associated boundary conditions depend on what type of problem one wishes to solve. There are generally considered to be two different types of direct and inverse volume conductor problems.

One type of problem deals with the interplay between the description of the bioelectric volume source currents and the resulting volume currents and volume and surface voltages. Here, the problem statement would be to solve Eq. (12.1) for Φ with a known description of I_V and the Neumann boundary condition:

$$\sigma \nabla \Phi \cdot \mathbf{n} = 0 \quad \text{on } \Gamma_T \tag{12.2}$$

which says that the normal component of the electric field is zero on the surface interfacing with air (here denoted by Γ_T). This problem can be used to solve two well-known problems in medicine, the direct EEG (electroencephalography) and ECG (electrocardiography) volume conductor problems. In the direct EEG problem, one usually discretizes the brain and surrounding tissue and skull. One then assumes a description of the bioelectric current source within the brain (this usually takes the form of dipoles or multipoles) and calculates the field within the brain and on the surface of the scalp. Similarly, in one version of the direct ECG problem, one utilizes descriptions of the current sources in the heart (either dipoles or membrane current source models such as the FitzHugh-Nagumo and Beeler-Reuter, among others) and calculates the currents and voltages within the volume conductor of the chest and voltages on the surface of the torso. The inverse problems associated with these direct problems involve estimating the current sources I_V within the volume conductor from measurements of voltages on the surface of either the head or body. Thus one would solve Eq. (12.1) with the boundary conditions

$$\Phi = \Phi_0 \quad \text{on } \Sigma \subseteq \Gamma_T \tag{12.3}$$

$$\sigma \nabla \Phi \cdot \mathbf{n} = 0 \quad \text{on } \Gamma_T \tag{12.4}$$

The first is the Dirichlet condition, which says that one has a set of discrete measurements of the voltage of a subset of the outer surface. The second is the natural Neumann condition. While it does not look much different than the formulation of the direct problem, the inverse formulations are ill-posed. The bioelectric inverse problem in terms of primary current sources does not have a unique solution, and the solution does not depend continuously on the data. Thus, to obtain *useful* solutions, one must try to restrict the solution domain (i.e., number of physiologically plausible solutions) [11] for the former case and apply so-called regularization techniques to attempt to restore the continuity of the solution on the data in the latter case.

Another bioelectric direct/inverse formulation poses both the problems in terms of scalar values at the surfaces. For the EEG problem, one would take the surface of the brain (cortex) as one bounded surface and the surface of the scalp as the other surface. The direct problem would involve making measurements of voltage of the surface of the cortex at discrete locations and then calculating the voltages on the surface of the scalp. Similarly, for the ECG problem, voltages could be measured on the surface of the heart and used to calculate the voltages at the surface of the torso, as well as within the volume conductor of the thorax. To formulate the inverse problems, one uses measurements on the surface of the scalp (torso) to calculate the voltages on the surface of the cortex (heart). Here, we solve Laplace's equation instead of Poisson's equation, because we are interested in the distributions of voltages on a surface instead of current sources within a volume. This leads to the following boundary value problem:

$$\nabla \cdot \sigma \nabla \Phi = 0 \qquad \text{in } \Omega \tag{12.5}$$

$$\Phi = \Phi_0 \qquad \text{on } \Sigma \subseteq \Gamma_T \tag{12.6}$$

$$\sigma \nabla \Phi \cdot \mathbf{n} = 0 \qquad \text{on } \Gamma_T \tag{12.7}$$

For this formulation, the solution to the inverse problem is unique [17]; however, there still exists the problem of continuity of the solution on the data. The linear algebra counterpart to the elliptic boundary value problem is often useful in discussing this problem of noncontinuity. The numerical solution to all elliptic boundary value problems (such as Poisson and Laplace problems) can be formulated in terms of a set of linear equations $A\Phi = \mathbf{b}$. For the solution of Laplace's equation, the system can be reformulated as

$$A\Phi_{\text{in}} = \Phi_{\text{out}}. \tag{12.8}$$

where Φ_{in} is the vector of data on the inner surface bounding the solution domain (the electrostatic potentials on the cortex or heart, for example), Φ_{out} is the vector of data that bound the outer surface (the subset of voltage values on the surface of the scalp or torso, for example), and A is the *transfer matrix* between Φ_{out} and Φ_{in}, which usually contains the geometry and physical properties (conductivities, dielectric constants, etc.) of the volume conductor. The direct problem is then simply (well) posed as solving Eq. (12.8) for Φ_{out} given Φ_{in}. Likewise, the inverse problem is to determine Φ_{in} given Φ_{out}.

A characteristic of A for ill-posed problems is that it has a very large condition number. In other words, the ill-conditioned matrix A is very near to being singular. Briefly, the condition number is defined as $\kappa(A) = \|A\| \cdot \|A^{-1}\|$ or the ratio of maximum to minimum singular values measured in the L_2 norm. The ideal problem conditioning occurs for orthogonal matrices which have $\kappa(A) \approx 1$, while an ill-conditioned matrix will have $\kappa(A) \gg 1$. When one inverts a matrix that has a very large condition number, the inversion process is unstable and is highly susceptible to errors. The condition of a matrix is relative. It is related to the precision level of computations and is a function of the size of the problem. For example, if the condition number exceeds a linear growth rate with respect to the size of the problem, the problem will become increasingly ill-conditioned. See [36] for more about the condition number of matrices.

A number of techniques have arisen to deal with ill-posed inverse problems. These techniques include truncated singular value decomposition (TSVD), generalized singular value decomposition (GSVD), maximum entropy, and a number of generalized least squares schemes, including Twomey and Tikhonov regularization methods. Since this chapter is concerned more with the numerical techniques for approximating bioelectric field problems, the reader is referred to [12–15] to further investigate the regularization of ill-posed problems. A particularly useful reference for discrete ill-posed problems is the Matlab package developed by Per Christian Hansen, which is available via netlib [16].

12.2 Model Construction and Mesh Generation

Once we have stated or derived the mathematical equations that define the physics of the system, we must figure out how to solve these equations for the particular domain we are interested in. Most numerical methods for solving boundary value problems require that the continuous domain be broken up into discrete elements, the so-called mesh or grid, which one can use to approximate the governing equation(s) using the particular numerical technique (finite element, boundary element, finite difference, or multigrid) best suited to the problem.

Because of the complex geometries often associated with bioelectric field problems, construction of the polygonal mesh can become one of the most time-consuming aspects of the modeling process. After deciding on the particular approximation method to use (and the most appropriate type of element), one needs to construct a mesh of the solution domain that matches the number of degrees of freedom of the fundamental element. For the sake of simplicity, we will assume that we will use linear elements, either tetrahedrons, which are usually used for modeling irregular three-dimensional domains, or hexahedrons, which are used for modeling regular, uniform domains.

There are several different strategies for discretizing the geometry into fundamental elements. For bioelectric field problems, two approaches to mesh generation have become standard: the *divide and conquer* (or subsequent subdivision) strategy and the *Delaunay triangulation* strategy.

In using the divide and conquer strategy, one starts with a set of points that define the bounding surface(s) in three dimensions (contours in two dimensions). The volume (surface) is repeatedly divided into smaller regions until a satisfactory discretization level has been achieved. Usually, the domain is broken up into eight-node cubic elements, which can then be subdivided into five (minimally) or six tetrahedral elements if so desired. This methodology has the advantage of being fairly easy to program; furthermore, commercial mesh generators exist for the divide and conquer method. For use in solving bioelectric field problems, its main disadvantage is that it allows elements to overlap interior boundaries. A single element may span two different conductive regions, for example, when part of an element represents muscle tissue (which could be anisotropic) and the other part of the element falls into a region representing fat tissue. It then becomes very difficult to assign unique conductivity parameters to each element and at the same time accurately represent the geometry.

A second method of mesh generation is the Delaunay triangulation strategy. Given a three-dimensional set of points that define the boundaries and interior regions of the domain to be modeled, one tessellates the point cloud into an optimal mesh of tetrahedra. For bioelectric field problems, the advantages and disadvantages tend to be exactly contrary to those arising from the divide and conquer strategy. The primary advantage is that one can create the mesh to fit any predefined geometry, including subsurfaces, by starting with points that define all the necessary surfaces and subsurfaces and then adding additional interior points to minimize the aspect ratio. For tetrahedra, the aspect ratio can be defined as $4\sqrt{3/2}\,(\rho_k/h_k)$, where ρ_k denotes the diameter of the sphere circumscribed about the tetrahedron, and h_k is the maximum distance between two vertices. These formulations yield a value of 1 for an equilateral tetrahedron and a value of 0 for a degenerate (flat) element [18]. The closer to the value of 1, the better. The Delaunay criterion is a method for minimizing the occurrence of obtuse angles in the mesh, yielding elements that have aspect ratios as close to 1 as possible, given the available point set. While the ideas behind Delaunay triangulation are straightforward, the programming is nontrivial and is the primary drawback to this method. Fortunately, there exist several public domain, two-dimensional versions, including one from netlib called sweep2.c from the directory Voronoi, as well as at least one three-dimensional package [41]. For more information on mesh generation and various aspects of biomedical modeling, see [19–27].

12.3 Numerical Methods

Because of the geometric complexity of and numerous inhomogeneities inherent in anatomic structures in physiologic models, solutions of bioelectric field problems are usually tractable (except in the most simplified of models) only when one employs a numerical approximation method such as the finite difference (FD), the finite element (FE), boundary element (BE), or the multigrid (MG) method to solve the governing field equation(s).

Approximation Techniques: The Galerkin Method

The problem posed in Eq. (12.1) can be solved using any of the aforementioned approximation schemes. One technique that addresses three of the previously mentioned techniques (FD, FE, and BE) can be derived by the Galerkin method. The Galerkin method is one of the most widely used methods for discretizing elliptic boundary value problems such as Eq. (12.1) and for treating the spatial portion of time-dependent parabolic problems, which are common in models of cardiac wave propagation. While the Galerkin technique is not essential to the application of any of the techniques, it provides for a unifying bridge between the various numerical methods. To express the problem in a Galerkin form, one begins by rewriting Eq. (12.1) as

$$A\Phi = -I_v \qquad (12.9)$$

where A is the differential operator, $A = \nabla \cdot (\sigma \nabla)$. An equivalent statement of Eq. (12.9) is, find Φ such that $(A\Phi + I_v, \bar{\Phi}) = 0$. Here, $\bar{\Phi}$ is an arbitrary *test function*, which can be thought of physically as a virtual potential field, and the notation $(\phi_1, \phi_2) \equiv \int_\Omega \phi_1 \phi_2 \, d\Omega$ denotes the inner product in $L_2(\Omega)$. Applying Green's theorem, one can equivalently write

$$(\sigma \nabla \Phi, \nabla \bar{\Phi}) - \left\langle \frac{\partial \Phi}{\partial n}, \bar{\Phi} \right\rangle = -(I_v, \bar{\Phi}) \qquad (12.10)$$

where the notation $\langle \phi_1, \phi_2 \rangle \equiv \int_s \phi_1 \phi_2 \, dS$ denotes the inner product on the boundary S. When the Dirichlet, $\Phi = \Phi_0$, and Neumann, $\sigma \nabla \Phi \cdot \mathbf{n} = 0$, boundary conditions are specified on S, one obtains the weak form of Eq. (12.1):

$$(\sigma \nabla \Phi, \nabla \bar{\Phi}) = -(I_v, \bar{\Phi}). \qquad (12.11)$$

It is understood that this equation must hold for all test functions $\bar{\Phi}$, which must vanish at the boundaries where $\Phi = \Phi_0$. The Galerkin approximation ϕ to the weak-form solution Φ in Eq. (12.11) can be expressed as

$$\phi(x) = \sum_{i=0}^{N} \phi_i \, \psi_i(x) \qquad (12.12)$$

The trial functions ψ_i, $i = 0, 1, \ldots, N$ form a basis for an $N + 1$ dimensional space $\mathscr{S}$. One can define the *Galerkin approximation* to be the element $\phi \in \mathscr{S}$ that satisfies

$$(\sigma \nabla \phi, \nabla \psi_j) = -(I_v, \psi_j) \qquad (\forall \psi_j \in \mathscr{S}) \qquad (12.13)$$

Since our differential operator A is positive definite and self adjoint [i.e., $(A\Phi, \Phi) \geq \alpha(\Phi, \Phi) > 0$ for some nonzero positive constant α and $(A\Phi, \bar{\Phi}) = (\Phi, A\bar{\Phi})$, respectively], then we can define a space E with an inner product defined as $(\Phi, \bar{\Phi})E = (A\Phi, \bar{\Phi}) \equiv a(\Phi, \bar{\Phi})$ and norm (the so-called energy norm) equal to

$$\|\Phi\|_E = \left\{ \int_\Omega (\nabla \Phi)^2 \, d\Omega \right\}^{\frac{1}{2}} = (\Phi, \Phi)_E^{\frac{1}{2}} \qquad (12.14)$$

The solution Φ of Eq. (12.9) satisfies

$$(A\Phi, \psi_i) = -(I_v, \psi_i) \qquad (\forall \psi_i \in \mathscr{S}) \qquad (12.15)$$

and the approximate Galerkin solution obtained by solving Eq. (12.13) satisfies

$$(A\phi, \psi_i) = -(I_v, \psi_i) \qquad (\forall \psi_i \in \mathcal{S}) \tag{12.16}$$

Subtracting Eq. (12.15) from Eq. (12.16) yields

$$(A(\phi - \Phi), \psi_i) = (\varphi - \bar{\varphi}, \psi_i)_E = 0 \qquad (\forall \psi_i \in \mathcal{S}) \tag{12.17}$$

The difference $\phi - \Phi$ denotes the error between the solution in the infinite dimensional space V and the $N + 1$ dimensional space $\mathcal{S}$. Equation (12.17) states that the error is orthogonal to all basis functions spanning the space of possible Galerkin solutions. Consequently, the error is orthogonal to all elements in $\mathcal{S}$ and must therefore be the minimum error. Thus the Galerkin approximation is an orthogonal projection of the true solution Φ onto the given finite dimensional space of possible approximate solutions. Therefore, the Galerkin approximation is the best approximation in the energy space E. Since the operator is positive definite, the approximate solution is unique. Assume for a moment that there are two solutions, ϕ_1 and ϕ_2, satisfying

$$(A\phi_1, \psi_i) = -(I_v, \psi_i) \qquad (A\phi_2, \psi_i) = -(I_v, \psi_i) \qquad (\forall \psi_i \in \mathcal{S}) \tag{12.18}$$

respectively. Then the difference yields

$$(A(\phi_1 - \phi_2), \psi_i) = 0 \qquad (\forall \psi_i \in \mathcal{S}) \tag{12.19}$$

The function arising from subtracting one member from another member in $\mathcal{S}$ also belongs in $\mathcal{S}$; hence the difference function can be expressed by the set of A orthogonal basis functions spanning $\mathcal{S}$:

$$\sum_{j=0}^{N} \Delta\phi_j (A(\psi_j, \psi_i)) = 0 \qquad (\forall \psi_i \in) \tag{12.20}$$

When $i \neq j$, the terms vanish due to the basis functions being orthogonal with respect to A. Since A is positive definite,

$$(A\Phi_i, \Phi_i) > 0 \qquad i = 0, \dots, N \tag{12.21}$$

Thus $\Delta\phi_i = 0$, $i = 0, \dots, N$, and by virtue of Eq. (12.20), $\delta\phi = 0$, such that $\phi_1 = \phi_2$. The identity contradicts the assumption of two distinct Galerkin solutions. This proves the solution is unique [28].

The Finite-Difference Method

Perhaps the most traditional way to solve Eq. (12.1) utilizes the finite-difference approach by discretizing the solution domain Ω using a grid of uniform hexahedral elements. The coordinates of a typical grid point are $x = lh$, $y = mh$, $z = nh$ ($l, m, n =$ integers), and the value of $\Phi(x, y, z)$ at a grid point is denoted by $\Phi_{l,m,n}$. Taylor's theorem can then be used to provide the difference equations. For example,

$$\Phi_{l+1,m,n} = (\Phi + h \frac{\partial \Phi}{\partial x} + \frac{1}{2}h^2 \frac{\partial^2 \Phi}{\partial x^2} + \frac{1}{6}h^3 \frac{\partial^3 \Phi}{\partial x^3} + \cdots)_{l,m,n} \tag{12.22}$$

with similar equations for $\Phi_{l-1,m,n}$, $\Phi_{l,m+1,n}$, $\Phi_{l,m-1,n}$,.... The finite-difference representation of Eq. (12.1) is

$$\frac{\Phi_{l+1,m,n} - 2\Phi_{l,m,n} + \Phi_{l-1,m,n}}{h^2} + \frac{\Phi_{l,m+1,n} - 2\Phi_{l,m,n} + \Phi_{l,m-1,n}}{h^2}$$

$$+ \frac{\Phi_{l,m,n+1} - 2\Phi_{l,m,n} + \Phi_{l,m,n-1}}{h^2} = -I_{l,m,n}(v) \tag{12.23}$$

or, equivalently,

$$\Phi_{l+1,m,n} + \Phi_{l-1,m,n} + \Phi_{l,m+1,n} + \Phi_{l,m-1,n} + \Phi_{l,m,n+1} + \Phi_{l,m,n-1}$$
$$- 6\Phi_{l,m,n} = -h^2 I_{l,m,n}(v) \tag{12.24}$$

If one defines the vector Φ to be $[\Phi_{1,1,1} \cdots \Phi_{1,1,N-1} \cdots \Phi_{1,N-1,1} \cdots \Phi_{N-1,N-1,N-1}]^T$ to designate the $(N-1)^3$ unknown grid values and pull out all the known information from (24), one can reformulate Eq. (12.1) by its finite-difference approximation in the form of the matrix equation $A\Phi = \mathbf{b}$, where $\mathbf{b}$ is a vector that contains the sources and modifications due to the Dirichlet boundary condition.

Unlike the traditional Taylor's series expansion method, the Galerkin approach utilizes basis functions, such as linear piecewise polynomials, to approximate the true solution. For example, the Galerkin approximation to sample problem (12.1) would require evaluating Eq. (12.13) for the specific grid formation and specific choice of basis function:

$$\int_\Omega \left(\sigma_x \frac{\partial \phi}{\partial x} \frac{\partial \psi_i}{\partial x} + \sigma_y \frac{\partial \phi}{\partial y} \frac{\partial \psi_i}{\partial y} + \sigma_z \frac{\partial \phi}{\partial z} \frac{\partial \psi_i}{\partial z} \right) d\Omega = -\int_\Omega I_v \, \psi_i \, d\Omega \tag{12.25}$$

Difference quotients are then used to approximate the derivatives in Eq. (12.25). Note that if linear basis functions are utilized in Eq. (12.25), one obtains a formulation that corresponds exactly with the standard finite-difference operator. Regardless of the difference scheme or order of basis function, the approximation results in a linear system of equations of the form $A\Phi = \mathbf{b}$, subject to the appropriate boundary conditions.

The Finite-Element Method

As seen earlier, in the classic numerical treatment for partial differential equations—the finite-difference method—the solution domain is approximated by a grid of uniformly spaced nodes. At each node, the governing differential equation is approximated by an algebraic expression that references adjacent grid points. A system of equations is obtained by evaluating the previous algebraic approximations for each node in the domain. Finally, the system is solved for each value of the dependent variable at each node. In the finite-element method, the solution domain can be discretized into a number of uniform or nonuniform finite elements that are connected via nodes. The change of the dependent variable with regard to location is approximated within each element by an interpolation function. The interpolation function is defined relative to the values of the variable at the nodes associated with each element. The original boundary value problem is then replaced with an equivalent integral formulation [such as Eq. (12.13)]. The interpolation functions are then substituted into the integral equation, integrated, and combined with the results from all other elements in the solution domain. The results of this procedure can be reformulated into a matrix equation of the form $A\Phi = \mathbf{b}$, which is subsequently solved for the unknown variable [20, 29].

The formulation of the finite-element approximation starts with the Galerkin approximation, $(\sigma\nabla\Phi, \nabla\bar{\Phi}) = -(I_v, \bar{\Phi})$, where $\bar{\Phi}$ is our test function. Now one can use the finite-element method to turn the continuous problems into a discrete formulation. First, one discretizes the solution domain,

$\Omega = \cup_{e=1}^{E}\Omega_e$, and defines a finite dimensional subspace, $V_h \subset V = \{\bar{\Phi} : \bar{\Phi}$ is continuous on Ω, $\nabla\bar{\Phi}$ is piecewise continuous on $\Omega\}$. One usually defines parameters of the function $\bar{\Phi} \in V_h$ at node points $\alpha_i = \bar{\Phi}(x_i), i = 0, 1, \ldots, N$. If one now defines the basis functions $\psi_i \in V_h$ as linear continuous piecewise functions that take the value 1 at node points and zero at other node points, then one can represent the function $\bar{\Phi} \in V_h$ as

$$\bar{\Phi}(x) = \sum_{i=0}^{N} d_i \psi_i(x) \tag{12.26}$$

such that each $\bar{\Phi} \in V_h$ can be written in a unique way as a linear combination of the basis functions $\Psi_i \in V_h$. Now the finite-element approximation of the original boundary value problem can be stated as

$$\text{Find } \Phi_h \in V_h \text{ such that } (\sigma\nabla\Phi_h, \nabla\bar{\Phi}) = -(I_v, \bar{\Phi}) \tag{12.27}$$

Furthermore, if $\Phi_h \in V_h$ satisfies problem (12.27), then we have $(\sigma\nabla\Phi_h, \nabla\Psi_i) = -(I_v, \Psi_i)$ [30]. Finally, since Φ_h itself can be expressed as the linear combination

$$\Phi_h = \sum_{i=0}^{N} \xi_i \Psi_i(x) \qquad \xi_i = \Phi_h(x_i) \tag{12.28}$$

one can then write problem (12.27) as

$$\sum_{i=0}^{N} \xi_i (\sigma_{ij}\nabla\Psi_i, \nabla\Psi_j) = -(I_v, \Psi_j) \qquad j = 0, \ldots, N \tag{12.29}$$

subject to the Dirichlet boundary condition. Then the finite-element approximation of Eq. (12.1) can equivalently be expressed as a system of N equations with N unknowns $\xi_i, \ldots, \xi_N$ (the electrostatic potentials, for example). In matrix form, the preceding system can be written as $A\xi = b$, where $A = (a_{ij})$ is called the *global stiffness matrix* and has elements $(a_{ij}) = (\sigma_{ij}\nabla\Psi_i, \nabla\Psi_j)$, while $b_i = -(I_v, \Psi_i)$ and is usually termed the *load vector*.

For volume conductor problems, A contains all the geometry and conductivity information of the model. The matrix A is symmetric and positive definite; thus it is nonsingular and has a unique solution. Because the basis function differs from zero for only a few intervals, A is sparse (only a few of its entries are nonzero).

Application of the FE Method for 3D Domains

Now let us illustrate the concepts of the finite-element method by considering the solution of Eq. (12.1) using linear three-dimensional elements. One starts with a 3D domain Ω that represents the geometry of our volume conductor and breaks it up into discrete elements to form a finite dimensional subspace Ω_h. For 3D domains, one has the choice of representing the function as either tetrahedra

$$\tilde{\Phi} = \alpha_1 + \alpha_2 x + \alpha_3 y + \alpha_4 z, \tag{12.30}$$

or hexahedra

$$\tilde{\Phi} = \alpha_1 + \alpha_2 x + \alpha_3 y + \alpha_4 z + \alpha_5 xy + \alpha_6 yz + \alpha_7 xz + \alpha_8 xyz \tag{12.31}$$

Because of space limitations, let us restrict the development to tetrahedra, knowing that it is easy to modify the formulas for hexahedra. Take out a specific tetrahedra from the finite dimensional subspace and apply the previous formulations for the four vertices:

$$\begin{pmatrix} \widetilde{\Phi}_1 \\ \widetilde{\Phi}_2 \\ \widetilde{\Phi}_3 \\ \widetilde{\Phi}_4 \end{pmatrix} = \begin{pmatrix} 1 & x_1 & y_1 & z_1 \\ 1 & x_2 & y_2 & z_2 \\ 1 & x_3 & y_3 & z_3 \\ 1 & x_4 & y_4 & z_4 \end{pmatrix} \begin{pmatrix} \alpha_1 \\ \alpha_2 \\ \alpha_3 \\ \alpha_4 \end{pmatrix} \tag{12.32}$$

or

$$\widetilde{\Phi}_i = \mathbf{C}\alpha \tag{12.33}$$

which define the coordinate vertices, and

$$\alpha = \mathbf{C}^{-1}\widetilde{\Phi}_i \tag{12.34}$$

which defines the coefficients. From Eqs. (12.30) and (12.34) one can express $\widetilde{\Phi}$ at any point within the tetrahedra,

$$\widetilde{\Phi} = [1, x, y, z]\alpha = \mathbf{S}\alpha = \mathbf{S}\mathbf{C}^{-1}\widetilde{\Phi}_i \tag{12.35}$$

or, most succinctly,

$$\widetilde{\Phi} = \sum_i N_i \widetilde{\Phi} \tag{12.36}$$

$\widetilde{\Phi}_i$ is the solution value at node i, and $\mathbf{N} = \mathbf{S}\mathbf{C}^{-1}$ is the local *shape function* or *basis function*. This can be expressed in a variety of ways in the literature (depending, usually, on whether you are reading engineering or mathematical treatments of finite element analysis):

$$\Phi_j (N_i) = N_i(x, y, z) = f_i(x, y, z) \equiv \frac{a_i + b_i x + c_i y + d_i z}{6V} \tag{12.37}$$

where

$$6V = \begin{vmatrix} 1 & x_1 & y_1 & z_1 \\ 1 & x_2 & y_2 & z_2 \\ 1 & x_3 & y_3 & z_3 \\ 1 & x_4 & y_4 & z_4 \end{vmatrix} \tag{12.38}$$

defines the volume of the tetrahedra V.

Now that a suitable set of basis functions is available, one can find the finite-element approximation to the 3D problem. The original problem can be formulated as

$$a(u, v) = (I_v, v) \qquad \forall v \in \Omega \tag{12.39}$$

where

$$a(u, v) = \int_\Omega \nabla u \cdot \nabla v d\Omega \tag{12.40}$$

and

$$(I_v, v) = \int_\Omega I_v \cdot v d\Omega \tag{12.41}$$

The finite-element approximation to the original boundary value problem is

$$a(u_h, v) = (I_v, v) \qquad \forall v \in \Omega_h \tag{12.42}$$

which has the equivalent form

$$\sum_{i=1}^{N} \xi_i a(\Phi_i, \Phi_j) = (I_v, \Phi_j) \qquad (12.43$$

where

$$a(\Phi_i, \Phi_j) = a(\Phi_i, (N_j), \Phi_j (N_i)) \qquad (12.44)$$

which can be expressed by the matrix and vector elements

$$(a_{ij}) = \int_{\Omega_E} \left(\frac{\partial N_i}{\partial x} \frac{\partial N_j}{\partial x} + \frac{\partial N_i}{\partial y} \frac{\partial N_j}{\partial y} + \frac{\partial N_i}{\partial z} \frac{\partial N_j}{\partial z} \right) d\Omega \qquad (12.45)$$

and

$$I_i = \int_{\Omega_E} N_i I_v \, d\Omega \qquad (12.46)$$

Fortunately, these quantities are easy to evaluate for linear tetrahedra. As a matter of fact, there are closed-form solutions for the matrix elements (a_{ij}):

$$\int_{\Omega_h} N_1^a N_2^b N_3^c N_4^d \, d\Omega = 6V \frac{a! b! c! d!}{(a + b + c + d + 3)!} \qquad (12.47)$$

Therefore,

$$(a_{ij}) = \int_{\Omega_E} \frac{b_i b_j + c_i c_j + d_i d_j}{6V^2} \, d\Omega = \frac{b_i b_j + c_i c_j + d_i d_j}{6V} \qquad (12.48)$$

and, for the right hand side, one has, assuming constant sources,

$$I_i = \int_{\Omega_E} \frac{a_i + b_i x + c_i y + d_i z}{6V} I_v \, d\Omega = \frac{V I_v}{4} \qquad (12.49)$$

which have the compact forms

$$a_{ij}^{(n)} = \frac{1}{6V} \left(b_i^{(n)} b_j^{(n)} + c_i^{(n)} c_j^{(n)} + d_i^{(n)} + d_j^{(n)} \right) \qquad (12.50)$$

and

$$I_i^{(n)} = \frac{V I_v}{4} \qquad \text{for constant sources} \qquad (12.51)$$

Now one adds up all the contributions from each element into a global matrix and global vector:

$$\sum_{n=1}^{N_{el}} (a_{ij}^{(n)}) (\xi_i) = (I_i^{(n)}) \qquad (12.52)$$

where N_{el} is equal to the total number of elements in the discretized solution domain, and i represents the node numbers (vertices). This yields a linear system of equations of the form $\mathbf{A}\Phi = \mathbf{b}$, where Φ is the solution vector of voltages, $\mathbf{A}$ represents the geometry and conductivity of the volume conductor, and $\mathbf{b}$ represents the contributions from the current sources and boundary conditions.

For the finite-difference method, it turns out that the Dirichlet boundary condition is easy to apply, while the Neumann condition takes a little extra effort. For the finite-element method, it is just the opposite. The Neumann boundary condition

$$\nabla \Phi \cdot \mathbf{n} = 0 \qquad (12.53)$$

is satisfied automatically within the Galerkin and variational formulations. This can be seen by using Green's divergence theorem,

$$\int_\Omega \nabla \cdot \mathbf{A}\, dx = \int_\Gamma \mathbf{A} \cdot \mathbf{n}\, dS \qquad (12.54)$$

and applying it to the left-hand side of the Galerkin finite-element formulation:

$$\int_\Omega \nabla v \cdot \nabla w\, d\Omega \equiv \int_\Omega \left(\frac{\partial v}{\partial x_1} \frac{\partial w}{\partial x_1} + \frac{\partial v}{\partial x_2} \frac{\partial w}{\partial x_2} \right) d\Omega$$

$$= \int_\Gamma \left(v \frac{\partial w}{\partial x_1}\, n_1 + v \frac{\partial w}{\partial x_2}\, n_2 \right) dS - \int_\Omega v \left(\frac{\partial^2 w}{\partial x_1^2} + \frac{\partial^2 w}{\partial x_2^2} \right) d\Omega$$

$$= \int_\Gamma v \frac{\partial w}{\partial n}\, dS - \int_\Omega v \nabla^2 w\, d\Omega \qquad (12.55)$$

If one multiplies the original differential equation, $\nabla^2 \Phi = -I_v$, by an arbitrary test function and integrates, one obtains

$$(I_v, v) = -\int_\Omega (\nabla^2 \Phi) v\, d\Omega = -\int_\Gamma \frac{\partial \Phi}{\partial n}\, v\, dS + \int_\Omega \nabla \Phi \cdot \nabla v\, d\Omega = a(\Phi, v) \qquad (12.56)$$

where the boundary integral term $\partial \Phi / \partial n$ vanishes, and one obtains the standard Galerkin finite-element formulation.

To apply the Dirichlet condition, one has to work a bit harder. To apply the Dirichlet boundary condition directly, one usually modifies the (a_{ij}) matrix and b_i vector such that one can use standard linear system solvers. This is accomplished by implementing the following steps. Assuming that the ith value of u_i is known,

1. Subtract from the ith member of the right-hand side the product of a_{ij} and the known value of Φ_i (call it $\bar{\Phi}_i$); this yields the new right-hand side, $\hat{b_i} = b_i - a_{ij}\bar{\Phi}_j$.
2. Zero the ith row and column of A: $\hat{a}_{ij} = \hat{a}_{ji} = 0$.
3. Assign $\hat{a}_{ii} = 1$.
4. Set the jth member of the right-hand side equal to Φ_i.
5. Continue for each Dirichlet condition.
6. Solve the augmented system $\hat{A}\Phi = \hat{b}_v$.

The Boundary-Element Method

For bioelectric field problems with isotropic domains (and few inhomogeneities), another technique, called the *boundary-element method,* may be used. This technique utilizes information only on the boundaries of interest and thus reduces the dimension of any field problem by one. For differential operators, the response at any given point to sources and boundary conditions depends only on the response at neighboring points. The FD and FE methods approximate differential operators defined on subregions (volume elements) in the domain; hence direct mutual influence (connectivity) exists only between neighboring elements, and the coefficient matrices generated by these methods have relatively few nonzero coefficients in any given matrix row. As is demonstrated by Maxwell's laws, equations in differential forms often can be replaced by equations in integral forms; e.g., the potential distribution in a domain is uniquely defined by the volume sources and the potential and current density on the boundary. The boundary-element method uses this fact by transforming the differential operators defined in the domain to integral operators defined on the boundary. In the boundary-element method [31–33], only the boundary is discretized; hence the mesh generation is considerably simpler for this method than for the volume methods. Boundary solutions are obtained directly by solving the set of linear equations; however, potentials and gradients in the domain can be evaluated only after the boundary solutions have been obtained. Since this method has a rich history in bioelectric field problems, the reader is referred to some of the classic references for further information regarding the application of the BE method to bioelectric field problems [6, 42–44].

Solution Methods and Computational Considerations

Application of each of the previous approximation methods to Eq. (12.1) yields a system of linear equations of the form $\mathbf{A}\Phi = \mathbf{b}$, which must be solved to obtain the final solution. There is a plethora of available techniques for the solutions of such systems. The solution techniques can be broadly categorized as *direct* and *iterative* solvers. Direct solvers include Gaussian elimination and LU decomposition, while iterative methods include Jacobi, Gauss-Seidel, successive overrelaxation (SOR), and conjugate gradient (CG) methods, among others. The choice of the particular solution method is highly dependent on the approximation technique employed to obtain the linear system, on the size of the resulting system, and on accessible computational resources. For example, the linear system resulting from the application of the FD or FE method will yield a matrix $\mathbf{A}$ that is symmetric, positive definite, and sparse. The matrix resulting from the FD method will have a specific band-diagonal structure that is dependent on the order of difference equations one uses to approximate the governing equation. The matrix resulting from the FE method will be exceedingly sparse and only a few of the off-diagonal elements will be nonzero. The application of the BE method, on the other hand, will yield a matrix $\mathbf{A}$ that is dense and nonsymmetric and thus requires a different choice of solver.

The choice of the optimal solver is further complicated by the size of the system versus access to computational resources. Sequential direct methods are usually confined to single workstations, and thus the size of the system should fit in memory for optimal performance. Sequential iterative methods can be employed when the size of the system exceeds the memory of the machine; however, one pays a price in terms of performance, since direct methods are usually much faster than iterative methods. In many cases, the size of the system exceeds the computational capability of a single workstation, and one must resort to the use of clusters of workstations and/or parallel computers.

While new and improved methods continue to appear in the numerical analysis literature, my studies comparing various solution techniques for direct and inverse bioelectric field problems have resulted in the conclusion that the preconditioned conjugate gradient methods and multigrid methods are the best overall performers for volume conductor problems computed on single workstations. Specifically, the incomplete Choleski conjugate gradient (ICCG) method works well for the FE method,[*] and the preconditioned biconjugate gradient (BCG) methods are often used for BE methods. When clusters of workstations and/or parallel architectures are considered, the choice is less clear. For use with some high-performance architectures that contain large amounts of memory, parallel direct methods such as LU decomposition become attractive; however, preconditioned conjugate gradient methods still perform well.

A discussion of parallel computing methods for the solution of biomedical field problems could fill an entire text. Thus the reader is directed to the following references on parallel scientific computing [45–47].

Comparison of Methods

Since there is not enough space to give a detailed, quantitative description of each of the previously mentioned methods, an abbreviated summary is given of the applicability of each method in solving different types of bioelectric field problems.

---

[*]This is specifically for the FE method applied to elliptic problems. Such problems yield a matrix that is symmetric and positive definite. The Choleski decomposition only exists for symmetric, positive-definite matrices.

As outlined earlier, the FD, FE, and BE methods can all be used to approximate the boundary value problems that arise in biomedical research problems. The choice depends on the nature of the problem. The FE and FD methods are similar in that the entire solution domain must be discretized, while with the BE method only the bounding surfaces must be discretized. For regular domains, the FD method is generally the easiest method to code and implement, but the FD method usually requires special modifications to define irregular boundaries, abrupt changes in material properties, and complex boundary conditions. While typically more difficult to implement, the BE and FE methods are preferred for problems with irregular, inhomogeneous domains and mixed boundary conditions. The FE method is superior to the BE method for representing nonlinearity and true anisotropy, while the BE method is superior to FE method for problems where only the boundary solution is of interest or where solutions are wanted in a set of highly irregularly spaced points in the domain. Because the computational mesh is simpler for the BE method than for the FE method, the BE program requires less bookkeeping than an FE program. For this reason, BE programs are often considered easier to develop than FE programs; however, the difficulties associated with singular integrals in the BE method are often highly underestimated. In general, the FE method is preferred for problems where the domain is highly heterogeneous, whereas the BE method is preferred for highly homogeneous domains.

12.4 Adaptive Methods

Thus far how one formulates the problem, discretizes the geometry, and finds an approximate solution have been discussed. Now one is faced with answering the difficult question pertaining to the accuracy of the solution. Without reference to experimental data, how can one judge the validity of the solutions? To give oneself an intuitive feel for the problem (and possible solution), consider the approximation of a two-dimensional region discretized into triangular elements. The finite-element method will be applied to solve Laplace's equation in the region.

First, consider the approximation of the potential field $\Phi(x, y)$ by a two-dimensional Taylor's series expansion about a point (x, y):

$$\Phi(x + h, y + k) = \Phi(x, y) + \left[h \frac{\partial \Phi(x, y)}{\partial x} + k \frac{\partial \Phi(x, y)}{\partial y}\right]$$
$$+ \frac{1}{2!} \left[h^2 \frac{\partial^2 \Phi(x, y)}{\partial^2 x} + 2hk \frac{\partial^2 \Phi(x, y)}{\partial x \partial y} + k^2 \frac{\partial^2 \Phi(x, y)}{\partial^2 y}\right] + \cdots \tag{12.57}$$

where h and k are the maximum x and y distances within an element. Using the first two terms (up to first-order terms) in the preceding Taylor's expansion, one can obtain the standard linear interpolation function for a triangle:

$$\frac{\partial \Phi(x_i, y_i)}{\partial x} = \frac{1}{2A} \left[\Phi_i(y_j - y_m) + \Phi_m (y_i - y_j) + \Phi_j (y_m - y_i)\right] \tag{12.58}$$

where A is the area of the triangle. Likewise, one could calculate the interpolant for the other two nodes and discover that

$$\frac{\partial \Phi(x_i, y_i)}{\partial x} = \frac{\partial \Phi(x_j, y_j)}{\partial x} = \frac{\partial \Phi(x_m, y_m)}{\partial x} \tag{12.59}$$

is constant over the triangle (and thus so is the gradient in y as well). Thus one can derive the standard linear interpolation formulas on a triangle that represents the first two terms of the Taylor's series expansion. This means that the error due to discretization (from using linear elements) is proportional to the third term of the Taylor's expansion:

$$\epsilon \approx \frac{1}{2!}\left[h^2 \frac{\partial^2 \Phi(x, y)}{\partial^2 x} + 2hk \frac{\partial^2 \Phi(x, y)}{\partial x \partial y} + k^2 \frac{\partial^2 \Phi(x, y)}{\partial^2 y}\right] \qquad (12.60)$$

where Φ is the exact solution. One can conjecture, then, that the error due to discretization for first-order linear elements is proportional to the second derivative. If Φ is a linear function over the element, then the first derivative is a constant and the second derivative is zero, and there is no error due to discretization. This implies that the gradient must be constant over each element. If the function is not linear or the gradient is not constant over an element, the second derivative will not be zero and is proportional to the error incurred due to "improper" discretization. Examining Eq. (12.60), one can easily see that one way to decrease the error is to decrease the size of h and k. As h and k go to zero, the error tends to zero as well. Thus decreasing the mesh size in places of high errors due to high gradients decreases the error. As an aside, note that if one divides Eq. (12.9) by hk, one also can express the error in terms of the elemental aspect ratio h/k, which is a measure of the relative shape of the element. It is easy to see that one must be careful to maintain an aspect ratio as close to unity as possible.

The problem with the preceding heuristic argument is that one has to know the exact solution a priori before one can estimate the error. This is certainly a drawback considering that one is trying to accurately approximate Φ.

Convergence of a Sequence of Approximate Solutions

Let's try to quantify the error a bit further. When one considers the preceding example, it seems to make sense that if one increases the number of degrees of freedom used to approximate the function, the accuracy must approach the true solution. That is, one would hope that the sequence of approximate solutions will *converge* to the exact solution as the number of degrees of freedom (DOF) increases indefinitely:

$$\|\Phi(x) - \tilde{\Phi}_n(x)\| \to 0 \qquad \text{as } n \to \infty \qquad (12.61)$$

This is a statement of *pointwise convergence*. It describes the approximate solution as approaching arbitrarily close to the exact solution at each point in the domain as the number of DOF increases.

Measures of convergence often depend on how the *closeness* of measuring the distance between functions is defined. Another common description of measuring convergence is *uniform convergence*, which requires that the maximum value of $\|\Phi(x) - \tilde{\Phi}_n(x)\|$ in the domain vanish as $N \to \infty$. This is stronger than pointwise convergence because it requires a uniform rate of convergence at every point in the domain. Two other commonly used measures are *convergence in energy* and *convergence in mean*, which involve measuring an *average* of a function of the pointwise error over the domain [40].

In general, proving pointwise convergence is very difficult except in the simplest cases, while proving the convergence of an averaged value, such as energy, is often easier. Of course, scientists and engineers are often much more interested in ensuring that their answers are accurate in a pointwise sense than in an energy sense because they typically want to know values of the solution $\Phi(x)$ and gradients $\nabla \Phi(x)$ at specific places.

One intermediate form of convergence is called the *Cauchy convergence*. Here, one requires the sequences of two different approximate solutions to approach arbitrarily close to each other:

$$\|\Phi_m(x) - \tilde{\Phi}_n(x)\| \to 0 \qquad \text{as } m, n \to \infty \qquad (12.62)$$

While the pointwise convergence expression would imply the preceding equation, it is important to note that the Cauchy convergence does not imply pointwise convergence, since the functions could converge to an answer other than the true solution.

While one cannot be assured of pointwise convergence of these functions for all but the simplest cases, there do exist theorems that ensure that a sequence of approximate solutions must converge to the exact solution (assuming no computational errors) if the basis functions satisfy certain conditions. The theorems can only ensure convergence in an average sense over the entire domain, but it is usually the case that if the solution converges in an average sense (energy, etc.), then it will converge in the pointwise sense as well.

Energy Norms

The error in energy, measured by the *energy norm,* is defined in general as [37–39]

$$\|e\| = \left(\int_\Omega e^T L e \, d\Omega \right)^{\frac{1}{2}} \tag{12.63}$$

where $e = \Phi(x) - \tilde{\Phi}_n(x)$, and L is the differential operator for the governing differential equation [i.e., it contains the derivatives operating on $\Phi(x)$ and any function multiplying $\Phi(x)$]. For physical problems, this is often associated with the energy density.

Another common measure of convergence utilizes the L_2 norm. This can be termed the *average error* and can be associated with errors in any quantity. The L_2 norm is defined as

$$\|e\|_{L2} = \left(\int_\Omega e^T e \, d\Omega \right)^{\frac{1}{2}} \tag{12.64}$$

While the norms given above are defined on the whole domain, one can note that the square of each can be obtained by summing element contributions:

$$\|e\|^2 = \sum_{i=1}^M \|e\|_i^2 \tag{12.65}$$

where i represents an element contribution and m the total element number. Often for an *optimal* finite-element mesh, one tries to make the contributions to this square of the norm equal for all elements.

While the absolute values given by the energy or L_2 norms have little value, one can construct a relative percentage error that can be more readily interpreted:

$$\eta = \frac{\|e\|}{\|\Phi\|} \times 100 \tag{12.66}$$

This quantity, in effect, represents a weighted RMS error. The analysis can be determined for the whole domain or for element subdomains. One can use it in an adaptive algorithm by checking element errors against some predefined tolerance η_0 and increasing the DOF only of those areas above the predefined tolerance.

Two other methods, the p and the hp methods, have been found, in most cases, to converge faster than the h method. The p method of refinement requires that one increase the order of the basis function that was used to represent the interpolation (i.e., linear to quadratic to cubic, etc.). The hp method is a combination of the h and p methods and has recently been shown to converge the fastest of the three methods (but, as you might imagine, it is the hardest to implement). To find out more about adaptive refinement methods, see [27, 30, 34, 35, 37, 40].

Acknowledgments

This work was supported in part by awards from the Whitaker Foundation, the NIH, and the NSF. I would like to thank K. Coles, J. Schmidt, and D. Weinstein for their helpful comments and suggestions. An expanded, educational case studies version of this chapter entitled, "Direct and Inverse Bioelectric Field Problems," may be found as part of the DOE-sponsored Computational Science Education Program (CSEP). The chapter is available freely via Mosaic at http://csep1.phy.ornl.gov/csep.html and contains exercises, projects, and C and Fortran computer codes.

References

1. Miller CE, Henriquez CS. Finite element analysis of bioelectric phenomena. Crit Rev Biomed Eng 18:181, 1990. *This represents the first review paper on the use of the finite-element method as applied to biomedical problems. As the authors note, bioengineers came to these methods only fairly recently as compared with other engineers. It contains a good survey of applications.*

2. Nenonen J, Rajala HM, Katilia T. Biomagnetic Localization and 3D Modelling. Report TKK-F-A689. Espoo, Finland, Helsinki University of Technology, 1992.

3. Johnson CR, MacLeod RS, Ershler PR. A computer model for the study of electrical current flow in the human thorax. Comput Biol Med 22(3):305, 1992. *This paper details the construction of a three-dimensional thorax model.*

4. Johnson CR, MacLeod RS, Matheson MA. Computer simulations reveal complexity of electrical activity in the human thorax. Comput Phys 6(3):230, 1992. *This paper deals with the computational and visualization aspects of the forward ECG problem.*

5. Kim Y, Fahy JB, Tupper BJ. Optimal electrode designs for electrosurgery. IEEE Trans Biomed Eng 33:845, 1986. *This paper discusses an example of the modeling of bioelectric fields for applications in surgery.*

6. Plonsey R. Bioelectric Phenomena. New York, McGraw-Hill, 1969. *This is the first text using physics, mathematics, and engineering principles to quantify bioelectric phenomena.*

7. Henriquez CS, Plonsey R. Simulation of propagation along a bundle of cardiac tissue. I. Mathematical formulation. IEEE Trans Biomed Eng 37:850, 1990. *This paper and the companion paper below describe the bidomain approach to the propagation of electrical signals through active cardiac tissue.*

8. Henriquez CS, Plonsey R. Simulation of propagation along a bundle of cardiac tissue: II. Results of simulation. IEEE Trans Biomed Eng 37:861, 1990.

9. Keener JP. Waves in excitable media. SIAM J Appl Math 46:1039, 1980. *This paper describes mathematical models for wave propagation in various excitable media. Both chemical and physiologic systems are addressed.*

10. Hadamard J. Sur les problemes aux derivees parielies et leur signification physique. Bull Univ Princeton, pp 49–52, 1902. *This is Hadamard's original paper describing the concepts of well- and ill-posedness, in French.*

11. Greensite F, Huiskamp G, van Oosterom A. New quantitative and qualitative approaches to the inverse problem of electrocardiology: Their theoretical relationship and experimental consistency. Med Phy 17(3):369, 1990. *This paper describes methods for constraining the inverse problem of electrocardiology in terms of sources. Methods are developed which put bounds on the space of acceptable solutions.*

12. Tikhonov A, Arsenin V. Solution of Ill-Posed Problems. Washington, Winston, 1977. *This is the book in which Tikhonov describes his method of regularization for ill-posed problems.*

13. Tikhonov AN, Goncharsky AV. Ill-Posed Problems in the Natural Sciences. Moscow, MIR Publishers, 1987. *This is a collection of research papers from physics, geophysics, optics, medicine, etc., which describe ill-posed problems and the solution techniques the authors have developed.*

14. Glasko VB. Inverse Problems of Mathematical Physics. New York, American Institute of Physics, 1984. *This book has several introductory chapters on the mathematics of ill-posed problems followed by several chapters on specific applications.*

15. Hansen PC. Analysis of discrete ill-posed problems by means of the *L*-curve. SIAM Rev 34(4):561, 1992. *This is an excellent review paper which describes the various techniques developed to solve ill-posed problems. Special attention is paid to the selection of the a priori approximation of the regularization parameter.*

16. Hansen PC. Regularization tools: A Matlab package for analysis and solution of discrete ill-posed problems. Available via netlib in the library numeralgo/no4. *This is an excellent set of tools for experimenting with and analyzing discrete ill-posed problems. The netlib library contains several Matlab routines as well as a postscript version of the accompanying technical report/manual.*

17. Yamashita Y. Theoretical studies on the inverse problem in electrocardiography and the uniqueness of the solution. IEEE Trans Biomed Eng 29:719, 1982. *The first paper to prove the uniqueness of the inverse problem in electrocardiography.*

18. Bertrand O. 3D finite element method in brain electrical activity studies. In J Nenonen, HM Rajala, T Katila (eds), Biomagnetic Localization and 3D Modeling, pp 154–171. Helsinki, Helsinki University of Technology, 1991. *This paper describes the inverse MEG problem using the finite-element method.*

19. Bowyer A. Computing Dirichlet tesselations. Comput J 24:162, 1981. *One of the first papers on the Delaunay triangulation in 3-space.*

20. Hoole SRH. Computer-Aided Analysis and Design of Electromagnetic Devices. New York, Elsevier, 1989. *While the title wouldn't make you think so, this is an excellent introductory text on the use of numerical techniques to solve boundary value problems in electrodynamics. The text also contains sections on mesh generation and solution methods. Furthermore, it provides pseudocode for most of the algorithms discussed throughout the text.*

21. MacLeod RS, Johnson CR, Matheson MA. Visualization tools for computational electrocardiography. In Visualization in Biomedical Computing, pp 433–444. 1992. *This paper and the paper which follows concern the modeling and visualization aspects of bioelectric field problems.*

22. MacLeod RS, Johnson CR, Matheson MA. Visualization of cardiac bioelectricity—A case study. IEEE Visualization 92:411, 1992.

23. Pilkington TC, Loftis B, Thompson JF, et al. High-Performance Computing in Biomedical Research. Boca Raton, Fla, CRC Press, 1993. *This edited collection of papers gives an overview of the state of the art in high-performance computing (as of 1993) as it pertains to biomedical research. While certainly not comprehensive, the text does showcase several interesting applications and methods.*

24. Thompson J, Weatherill NP. Structed and unstructed grid generation. In TC Pilkington, B Loftis, JF Thompson, et al. (ed), High-Performance Computing in Biomedical Research, pp 63–112. Boca Raton, Fla, CRC Press, 1993. *This paper contains some extensions of Thompson's classic textbook on numerical grid generation.*

25. George PL. Automatic Mesh Generation. New York, Wiley, 1991. *This is an excellent introduction to mesh generation. It contains a survey of all the major mesh generation schemes.*

26. Thompson JF, Warsi ZUA, Mastin CW. Numerical Grid Generation. New York, North-Holland, 1985. *This is the classic on mesh generation. The mathematical level is higher than that of George's book, and most of the applications are directed toward computational fluid dynamics.*

27. Schmidt JA, Johnson CR, Eason JC, MacLeod RS. Applications of automatic mesh generation and adaptive methods in computational medicine. In JE Flaherty and I Babuska (eds), Modeling, Mesh Generation, and Adaptive Methods for Partial Differential Equations. New York, Springer-Verlag, 1994. *This paper describes three-dimensional mesh generation techniques and adaptive methods for bioelectric field problems.*

28. Henriquez CS, Johnson CR, Henneberg KA, et al. Large scale biomedical modeling and simulation: From concept to results. In N Thakor (ed), Frontiers in Biomedical Computing. Philadelphia, IEEE Press, 1994. *This paper describes the process of large-scale modeling along with computational and visualization issues pertaining to bioelectric field problems.*

29. Akin JE. Finite Element Analysis for Undergraduates. New York, Academic Press, 1986. *This is an easy-to-read, self-contained text on the finite-element method aimed at undergraduate engineering students.*

30. Johnson C. Numerical Solution of Partial Differential Equations by the Finite Element Method. Cambridge, Cambridge University Press, 1990. *An excellent introductory book on the finite-element method. The text assumes mathematical background of a first-year graduate student in applied mathematics and computer science. An excellent introduction to the theory of adaptive methods.*

31. Brebbia CA, Dominguez J. Boundary Elements: An Introductory Course. New York, McGraw-Hill, 1989. *This is an introductory book on the boundary element method by one of the foremost experts on the subject.*

32. Jawson MA, Symm GT. Integral Equation Methods in Potential Theory and Elastostatics. London, Academic Press, 1977. *An introduction to the boundary integral method as applied to potential theory and elastostatics.*

33. Beer G, Watson JO. Introduction to Finite and Boundary Element Methods for Engineers. New York, Wiley, 1992. *This is an excellent first book for those wishing to learn about the practical aspects of the numerical solution of boundary value problems. The book covers not only finite and boundary element methods but also mesh generation and the solution of large systems.*

34. Johnson CR, MacLeod RS. Nonuniform spatial mesh adaption using a posteriori error estimates: Applications to forward and inverse problems. Appl Num Math 14:331, 1994. *This is a paper by the author which describes the application of the h-method of mesh refinement for large-scale two- and three-dimensional bioelectric field problems.*

35. Flaherty, JE. Adaptive Methods for Partial Differential Equations. Philadelphia, SIAM, 1989. *This is a collection of papers on adaptive methods, many by the founders in the field. Most of the papers are applied to adaptive methods for finite-element methods and deal with both theory and applications.*

36. Golub GH, Van Loan CF. Matrix Computations. Baltimore, Johns Hopkins, 1989. *This is a classic reference for matrix computations and is highly recommended.*

37. Zienkiewicz OC. The Finite Element Method in Engineering Science. New York, McGraw-Hill, 1971. *This is a classic text on the finite-element method. It is now in its fourth edition, 1991.*

38. Zienkiewicz OC, Zhu JZ. A simple error estimate and adaptive procedure for practical engineering analysis. Int J Num Meth Eng 24:337, 1987. *This is a classic paper which describes the use of the energy norm to globally refine the mesh based on a priori error estimates.*

39. Zienkiewicz OC, Zhu JZ. Adaptivity and mesh generation. Int J Num Meth Eng 32:783, 1991. *This is another good paper on adaptive methods which describes some more advanced methods than the 1987 paper.*

40. Burnett DS. Finite Element Method. Reading, Mass, Addison-Wesley, 1988. *This is an excellent introduction to the finite-element method. It covers all the basics and introduces more advanced concepts in a readily understandable context.*

41. Barber CB, Dobkin DP, Huhdanpaa H. The quickhull algorithm for convex hull. Geometry Center Technical Report GCG53. *A public domain two- and three-dimensional Delaunay mesh generation code. Available via anonymous ftp from geom.umn.edu:/pub/software/qhull.tar.Z. There is also a geometry viewer available from geom.umn.edu:/pub/software/geomview/geomview-sgi.tar.Z.*

42. Barr RC, Pilkington TC, Boineau JP, Spach MS. Determining surface potentials from current dipoles, with application to electrocardiography. IEEE Trans Biomed Eng 13:88, 1966. *This is the first paper on the application of the boundary-element method to problems in electrocardiography.*

43. Rudy Y, Messinger-Rapport BJ. The inverse solution in electrocardiography: Solutions in terms of epicardial potentials. CRC Crit Rev Biomed Eng 16:215, 1988. *An excellent overview on the inverse problem in electrocardiography as well as a section on the application of the boundary-element method to bioelectric field problems.*

44. Gulrajani RM, Roberge FA, Mailloux GE. The forward problem of electrocardiography. In PW Macfarlane and TD Lawrie (eds), Comprehensive Electrocardiology, pp 197–236. Oxford, England, Pergamon Press, 1989. *This contains a nice overview of the application of the boundary-element method to the direct ECG problem.*

45. Golub G, Ortega JM. Scientific Computing: An Introduction with Parallel Computing. New York, Academic Press, 1993. *An excellent introduction to scientific computing with sections on sequential and parallel direct and iterative solvers, including a short section on the multigrid method.*

46. Freeman TL, Phillips C. Parallel Numerical Algorithms. New York, Prentice-Hall, 1992. *A good introduction to parallel algorithms with emphasis on the use of BLAS subroutines.*

47. Van de Velde EF. Concurrent Scientific Computing. New York, Springer-Verlag, 1994. *This text contains an excellent introduction to parallel numerical algorithms including sections on the finite-difference and finite-element methods.*

13

Principles of Electrocardiography

Edward J. Berbari
Indiana University/Purdue
University at Indianapolis

The electrocardiogram (ECG) is the recording on the body surface of the electrical activity generated by heart. It was originally observed by Waller in 1889 [1] using his pet bulldog as the signal source and the capillary electrometer as the recording device. In 1903, Einthoven [2] enhanced the technology by employing the string galvanometer as the recording device and using human subjects with a variety of cardiac abnormalities. Einthoven is chiefly responsible for introducing some concepts still in use today, including the labeling of the various waves, defining some of the standard recording sites using the arms and legs, and developing the first theoretical construct whereby the heart is modeled as a single time-varying dipole. We also owe the *EKG* acronym to Einthoven's native Dutch language, where the root word *cardio* is spelled with a *k*.

In order to record an ECG waveform, a differential recording between two points on the body are made. Traditionally, each differential recording is referred to as a *lead*. Einthoven defined three leads numbered with the Roman numerals I, II, and III. They are defined as

$$I = V_{LA} - V_{RA}$$

$$II = V_{LL} - V_{RA}$$

$$III = V_{LL} - V_{LA}$$

where RA = right arm, LA = left arm, and LL = left leg. Because the body is assumed to be purely resistive at ECG frequencies, the four limbs can be thought of as wires attached to the torso. Hence lead I could be recorded from the respective shoulders without a loss of cardiac information. Note that these are not independent, and the following relationship holds: II = I + III.

The evolution of the ECG proceeded for 30 years when F. N. Wilson added concepts of a "unipolar" recording [3]. He created a reference point by tying the three limbs together and averaging their potentials so that individual recording sites on the limbs or chest surface would be differentially recorded with the same reference point. Wilson extended the biophysical models to include the concept of the cardiac source enclosed within the volume conductor of the body. He erroneously thought that the central terminal was a true zero potential. However, from the mid-1930s until today, the 12 leads composed of the 3 limb leads, 3 leads in which the limb potentials are referenced to a modified Wilson terminal (the augmented leads [4]), and 6 leads placed across the front of the chest and referenced to the Wilson terminal form the basis of the standard 12-lead ECG. Figure 13.1 summarizes the 12-lead set. These sites are historically based, have a built-in redundancy, and are not optimal for all cardiac events. The voltage difference from any two sites will record an ECG, but it is these standardized sites with the massive 90-year collection of empirical observations that have firmly established their role as the standard. Figure 13.2 is a typical or stylized ECG recording from lead II. Einthovin chose the letters of the alphabet from P to U to label the waves and to avoid conflict with other physiologic waves being studied at the turn of the century. The ECG signals are typically in the range of ± 2 mV and require a recording bandwidth of 0.05 to 150 Hz. Full technical specification for ECG equipment has been proposed by both the American Heart Association [5] and the Association for the Advancement of Medical Instrumentation [6].

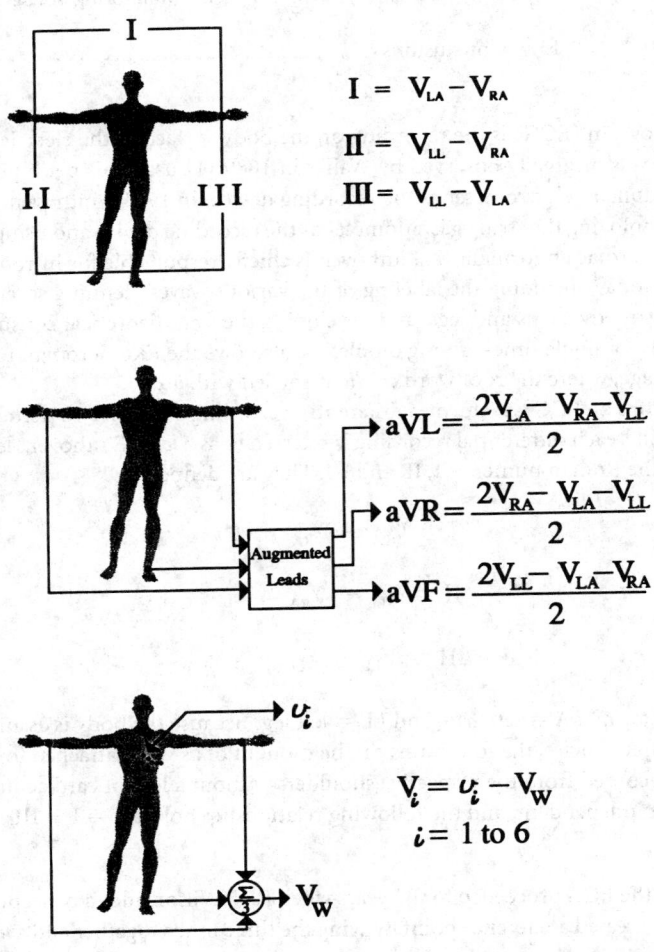

$$I = V_{LA} - V_{RA}$$
$$II = V_{LL} - V_{RA}$$
$$III = V_{LL} - V_{LA}$$

$$aVL = \frac{2V_{LA} - V_{RA} - V_{LL}}{2}$$
$$aVR = \frac{2V_{RA} - V_{LA} - V_{LL}}{2}$$
$$aVF = \frac{2V_{LL} - V_{LA} - V_{RA}}{2}$$

$$V_i = \upsilon_i - V_W$$
$$i = 1 \text{ to } 6$$

FIGURE 13.1 The 12-lead ECG is formed by the 3 bipolar surface leads: I, II, and III; the augmented Wilson terminal referenced limb leads: aV_R, aV_L, and aV_F; and the Wilson terminal referenced chest leads: V_1, V_2, V_3, V_4, V_5, and V_6.

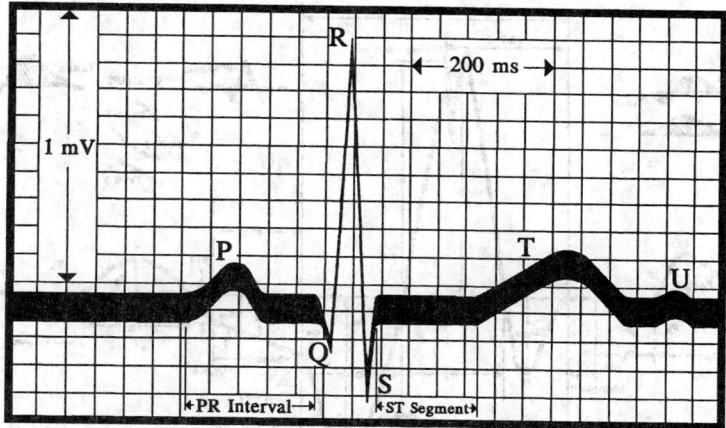

FIGURE 13.2 This is a stylized version of a normal lead II recording showing the P wave, QRS complex, and the T and U waves. The PR interval and the ST segment are significant time windows. The peak amplitude of the QRS is about 1 mV. The vertical scale is usually 1 mV/cm. The time scale is usually based on millimeters per second scales, with 25 mm/s being the standard form. The small boxes of the ECG are 1 × 1 mm.

There have been several attempts to change the approach for recording the ECG. The vectorcardiogram used a weighted set of recording sites to form an orthogonal *xyz* lead set. The advantage here was minimum lead set, but in practice it gained only a moderate degree of enthusiasm among physicians. *Body surface mapping* refers to the use of many recording sites (>64) arranged on the body so that isopotential surfaces could be computed and analyzed over time. This approach still has a role in research investigations. Other subsets of the 12-lead ECG are used in limited-mode recording situations such as the tape-recorded ambulatory ECG (usually 2 leads) or in intensive care monitoring at the bedside (usually 1 or 2 leads) or telemetered within regions of the hospital from patients who are not confined to bed (1 lead). The recording electronics of these ECG systems have followed the typical evolution of modern instrumentation, e.g., vacuum tubes, transistors, integrated chips, and microprocessors.

Application of computers to the ECG for machine interpretation was one of the earliest uses of computers in medicine [7]. Of primary interest in the computer-based systems was replacement of the human reader and elucidation of the standard waves and intervals. Originally this was performed by linking the ECG machine to a centralized computer via phone lines. The modern ECG machine is completely integrated with an analog front end, a 12- to 16-bit analog-to-digital (A/D) converter, a computational microprocessor, and dedicated input-output (I/O) processors. These systems compute a measurement matrix derived from the 12 lead signals and analyze this matrix with a set of rules to obtain the final set of interpretive statements [8]. Figure 13.3 shows the ECG of a heartbeat and the types of measurements that might be made on each of the component waves of the ECG and used for classifying each beat type and the subsequent cardiac rhythm. The depiction of the 12 analog signals and this set of interpretive statements form the final output, with an example shown in Fig. 13.4. The physician will overread each ECG and modify or correct those statements which are deemed inappropriate. The larger hospital-based system will record these corrections and maintain a large database of all ECGs accessible by any combination of parameters, e.g., all males, older than age 50, with an inferior myocardial infarction.

There are hundreds of interpretive statements from which a specific diagnosis is made for each ECG, but there are only about five or six major classification groups for which the ECG is used. The first step in analyzing an ECG requires determination of the rate and rhythm for the atria and

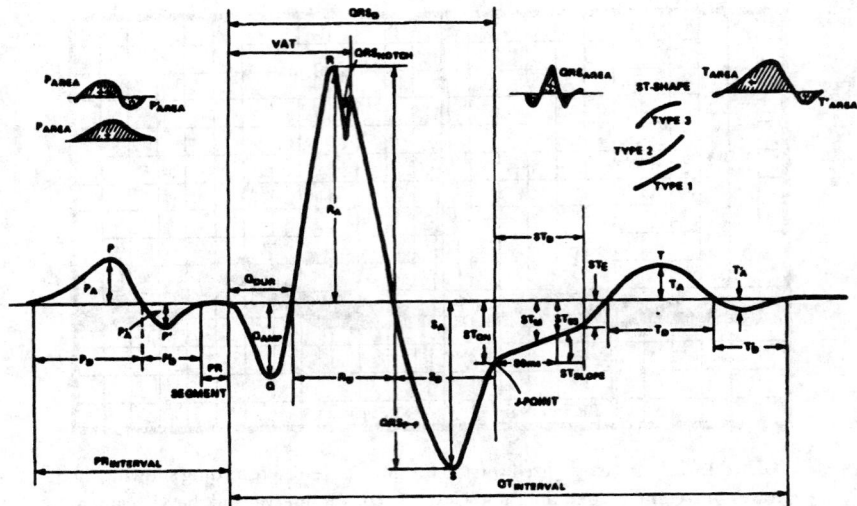

FIGURE 13.3 The ECG depicts numerous measurements that can be made with computer-based algorithms. These are primarily durations, amplitudes, and areas. (*Courtesy of Hewlett Packard Company, Palo Alto, Calif.*)

ventricles. Included here would be any conduction disturbances either in the relationship between the various chambers or within the chambers themselves. Then one would proceed to identify features that would relate to the presence or absence of scarring due to a myocardial infarction. There also may be evidence of acute events that would occur with ischemia or an evolving myocardial infarction. The ECG has been a primary tool for evaluating chamber size or enlargement, but one might argue that more accurate information in this area would be supplied by noninvasive imaging technologies.

More recently, the high-resolution ECG has been developed, whereby the digitized ECG is signal-averaged to reduce random noise [9,10]. This approach, coupled with postaveraging high-pass filtering, is used to detect and quantify low-level signals ($\sim$1.0 μV) not detectable with standard approaches. This computer-based approach has enabled the recording of events that are predictive of future life-threatening cardiac events [11,12].

13.1 Physiology

The heart has four chambers; the upper two chambers are called the *atria,* and the lower two chambers are called the *ventricles.* The atria are thin-walled, low-pressure pumps that receive blood from the venous circulation. Located in the top right atrium are a group of cells that act as the primary pacemaker of the heart. Through a complex change of ionic concentration across the cell membranes (the current source), an extracellular potential field is established which then excites neighboring cells, and a cell-to-cell propagation of electrical events occurs. Because the body acts as a purely resistive medium, these potential fields extend to the body surface [13]. The character of the body surface waves depends on the amount of tissue activating at one time and the relative speed and direction of the activation wavefront. Therefore, the pacemaker potentials that are generated by a small tissue mass are not seen on the ECG. As the activation wavefront encounters the increased mass of atrial muscle, the initiation of electrical activity is observed on the body surface, and the first ECG wave of the cardiac cycle is seen. This is the P wave, and it represents activation of the atria. Conduction of the cardiac impulse proceeds from the atria through a series of specialized cardiac cells (the A-V node and the His-Purkinje system) which again are too small in total mass to gener-

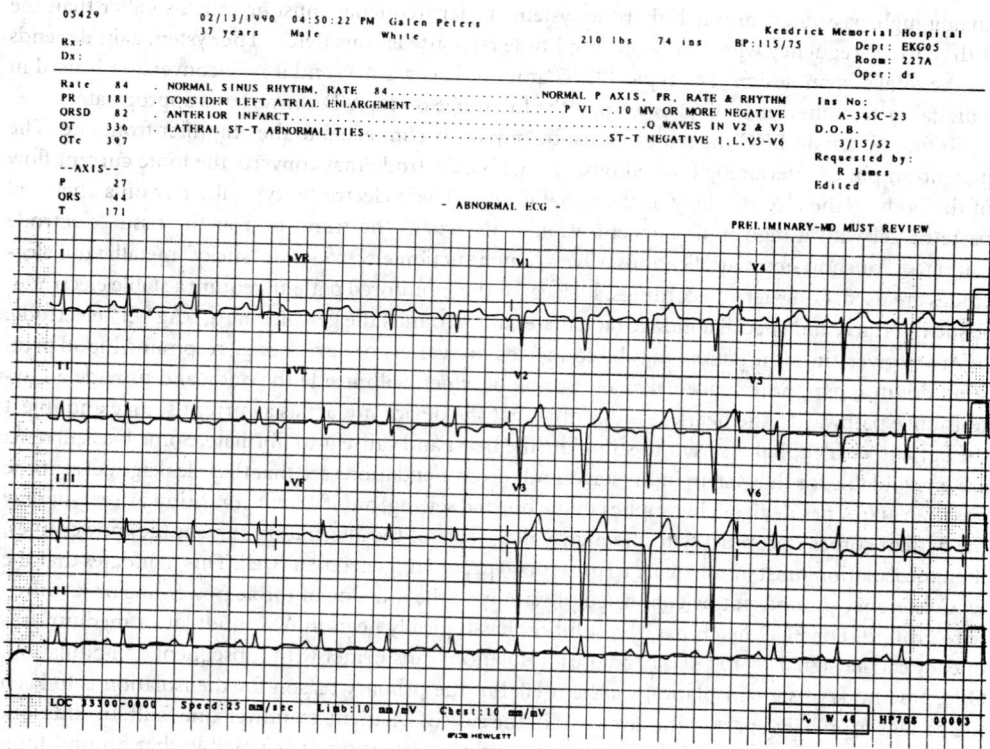

FIGURE 13.4   This is an example of an interpreted 12-lead ECG. A 2-1/2-s recording is shown for each of the 12 leads. The bottom trace is a continuous 10-s rhythm strip of lead II. Patient information is given in the top area, below which is printed the computerized interpretive statements. (*Courtesy of the Hewlett Packard Company, Palo Alto, Calif.*)

ate a signal large enough to be seen on the standard ECG. There is a short, relatively isoelectric segment following the P wave. Once the large muscle mass of the ventricles is excited, a rapid and large deflection is seen on the body surface. The excitation of the ventricles causes them to contract and provides the main force for circulating blood to the organs of the body. This large wave appears to have several components. The initial downward deflection is the Q wave, the initial upward deflection is the R wave, and the terminal downward deflection is the S wave. The polarity and actual presence of these three components depend on the position of the leads on the body as well as a multitude of abnormalities that may exist. In general, the large ventricular waveform is generically called the QRS complex regardless of its makeup. Following the QRS complex is another short relatively isoelectric segment. After this short segment, the ventricles return to their electrical resting state, and a wave of repolarization is seen as a low-frequency signal known as the T wave. In some individuals, a small peak occurs at the end or after the T wave and is the U wave. Its origin has never been fully established, but it is believed to be a repolarization potential.

13.2 Instrumentation

The general instrumentation requirements for the ECG have been addressed by professional societies through the years [5,6]. Briefly, they recommend a system bandwidth between 0.05 and 150 Hz. Of great importance in ECG diagnosis is the low-frequency response of the system, because shifts in some of the low-frequency regions, e.g., the ST segment, have critical diagnostic value. While the heart rate may only have a 1-Hz fundamental frequency, the phase responses of typical analog high-pass filters are such that the system corner frequency must be much smaller than the 3-dB corner frequency where only the amplitude response is considered. The system gain depends on the total system design. The typical ECG amplitude is ± 2 mV, and if A/D conversion is used in a digital system, then enough gain to span the full range of the A/D converter is appropriate.

To first obtain an ECG the patient must be physically connected to the amplifier front end. The patient-amplifier interface is formed by a special bioelectrode that converts the ionic current flow of the body to the electron flow of the metallic wire. These electrodes typically rely on a chemical paste or gel with a high ionic concentration. This acts as the transducer at the tissue-electrode interface. For short-term applications, silver-coated suction electrodes or "sticky" metallic foil electrodes are used. Long-term recordings, such as for the monitored patient, require a stable electrode-tissue interface, and special adhesive tape material surrounds the gel and an Ag^+/Ag^+Cl^- electrode.

At any given time, the patient may be connected to a variety of devices, e.g., respirator, blood pressure monitor, temporary pacemaker, etc., some of which will invade the body and provide a low-resistance pathway to the heart. It is essential that the device not act as a current source and inject the patient with enough current to stimulate the heart and cause it to fibrillate. Some bias currents are unavoidable for the system input stage, and recommendations are that these leakage currents be less than 10 μA per device. This applies to the normal setting, but if a fault condition arises whereby the patient comes in contact with the high-voltage side of the alternating current (ac) power lines, then the isolation must be adequate to prevent 10 μA of fault current as well. This mandates that the ECG reference ground not be connected physically to the low side of the ac power line or its third-wire ground. For ECG machines, the solution has typically been to AM modulate a medium frequency carrier signal (≈ 400 kHz) and use an isolation transformer with subsequent demodulation. Other methods of signal isolation can be used, but the primary reason for the isolation is to keep the patient from being part of the ac circuit in the case of a patient-to-power-line fault. In addition, with many devices connected in a patient monitoring situation, it is possible that ground loop currents will be generated. To obviate this potential hazard, a low-impedance ground buss is often installed in these rooms, and each device chassis will have an external ground wire connected to the buss. Another unique feature of these amplifiers is that they must be able to withstand the high-energy discharge of a cardiac defibrillator.

Older-style ECG machines recorded one lead at a time and then evolved to three simultaneous leads. This necessitated the use of switching circuits as well as analog weighting circuits to generate the various 12 leads. This is usually eliminated in modern digital systems by using an individual single-ended amplifier for each electrode on the body. Each potential signal is then digitally converted, and all the ECG leads can be formed mathematically in software. This would necessitate a 9-amplifier system. By performing some of the lead calculations with the analog differential amplifiers, this can be reduced to an 8-channel system. Thus only the individual chest leads V_1 through V_6 and any 2 of the limb leads, e.g., I and III, are needed to calculate the full 12-lead ECG. Figure 13.5 is a block diagram of a modern digital based ECG system. This system uses up to 13 single-ended amplifiers and a 16-bit A/D converter, all within a small lead wire manifold or amplifier lead stage. The digital signals are optically isolated and sent via a high-speed serial link to the main ECG instrument. Here the 32-bit CPU and DSP chip perform all the calculations, and a hard-copy report is generated (Fig. 13.4). Notice that each functional block has its own controller and that the system requires a real-time, multitasking operating system to coordinate all system functions. Concomitant with the data acquisition is the automatic interpretation of the ECG. These programs are quite sophisticated and are continually evolving. It is still a medical/legal requirement that these ECGs be overread by the physician.

13.3 Applications

Besides the standard 12-lead ECG, there are several other uses of ECG recording technology that rely on only a few leads. These applications have had a significant clinical and commercial impact.

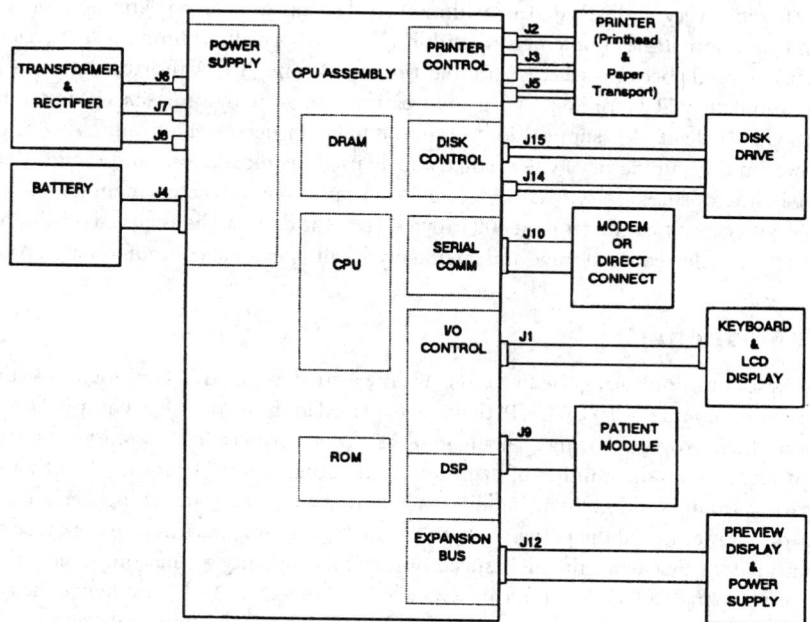

FIGURE 13.5 This is a block diagram of microprocessor-based ECG system. It includes all the elements of a personal computer class system, e.g., 80386 processor, 2 Mbytes of RAM, disk drive, 640 × 480 pixel LCD display, and battery operable. In addition, it includes a DSP56001 chip and multiple controllers which are managed with a real-time multitasking operating system. (*Courtesy of the Hewlett Packard Company, Palo Alto, Calif.*)

Following are brief descriptions of several ECG applications which are aimed at introducing the reader to some of the many uses of the ECG.

The Ambulatory ECG

The ambulatory or Holter ECG has an interesting history, and its evolution closely followed both technical and clinical progress. The original, analog, tape-based, portable ECG resembled a fully loaded backpack and was developed by Dr. Holter in the early 1960s [14]. It was soon followed by more compact devices that could be worn on the belt. The original large-scale clinical use of this technology was to identify patients who developed heart block transiently and could be treated by implanting a cardiac pacemaker. This required the secondary development of a device that could rapidly play back the 24 hours of tape-recorded ECG signals and present to the technician or physician a means of identifying periods of time where the patient's heart rate became abnormally low. The scanners had the circuitry not only to play back the ECG at speeds 30 to 60 times real time but also to detect the beats and display them in a superimposed mode on a CRT screen. In addition, an audible tachometer could be used to identify the periods of low heart rate. With this playback capability came numerous other observations, such as the identification of premature ventricular complexes (PVCs), which lead to the development of techniques to identify and quantify their number. Together with the development of antiarrhythmic drugs, a marriage was formed between pharmaceutical therapy and the diagnostic tool for quantifying PVCs. ECG tapes were recorded before and after drug administration, and drug efficacy was measured by the reduction of the number of PVCs. The scanner technology for detecting and quantifying these arrhythmias was originally implemented with analog hardware but soon advanced to computer technology as it became economically feasible. Very sophisticated algorithms were developed based on pattern-recognition techniques and were sometimes implemented with high-speed specialized numerical processors as the tape playback speeds became several hundred times real time [15]. Unfortunately, this approach using the ambulatory ECG for identifying and treating cardiac arrhythmias has been on the decline because the rationale of PVC suppression was found to be unsuccessful for improving cardiac mortality. However, the ambulatory ECG is still a widely used diagnostic tool, and modern units often have built-in microprocessors with considerable amounts of random access memory and even small disk drives with capacities greater than 400 Mbytes. Here the data can be analyzed on-line, with large segments of data selected for storage and later analysis with personal computer–based programs.

Patient Monitoring

The techniques for monitoring the ECG in real time were developed in conjunction with the concept of the coronary care unit (CCU). Patients were placed in these specialized hospital units to carefully observe their progress during an acute illness such as a myocardial infarction or after complex surgical procedures. As the number of beds increased in these units, it became clear that the highly trained medical staff could not continually watch a monitor screen, and computerized techniques were added that monitored the patient's rhythm. These programs were not unlike those developed for the ambulatory ECG, and the high-speed numerical capability of the computer was not taxed by monitoring a single ECG. The typical CCU would have 8 to 16 beds, and hence the computing power was taken to its limit by monitoring multiple beds. The modern units have the CPU distributed within the ECG module at the bedside, along with modules for measuring many other physiologic parameters. Each bedside monitor would be interconnected with a high-speed digital line, e.g., Ethernet, to a centralized computer used primarily to control communications and maintain a patient database.

High-Resolution ECG

High-resolution (HR) capability is now a standard feature on most digitally based ECG systems or as a stand-alone microprocessor-based unit [16]. The most common application of the HRECG is to record very low level ($\sim$1.0-μV) signals that occur after the QRS complex but are not evident on the standard ECG. These "late potentials" are generated from abnormal regions of the ventricles and have been strongly associated with the substrate responsible for a life-threatening rapid heart rate (ventricular tachycardia). The typical HRECG is derived from 3 bipolar leads configured in an anatomic xyz coordinate system. These 3 ECG signals are then digitized at a rate of 1000 to 2000 Hz per channel, time aligned via a real-time QRS correlator, and summated in the form of a signal average. Signal averaging will theoretically improve the signal-to-noise ratio by the square root of the number of beats averaged. The underlying assumptions are that the signals of interest do not vary, on a beat-to-beat basis, and that the noise is random. Figure 13.6 has four panels depicting the most common sequence for processing the HRECG to measure the late potentials. Panel a depicts a 3-second recording of the xyz leads close to normal resolution. Panel b was obtained after averaging 200 beats and with a sampling frequency of 10 times that shown in panel a. The gain is also 5 times greater. Panel c is the high-pass filtered signal using a partially time-reversed digital filter having a second-order Butterworth response and a 3-dB corner frequency of 40 Hz [12]. Note the appearance of the signals at the terminal portion of the QRS complex. A common method of analysis, but necessarily optimal, is to combine the filtered xyz leads into a vector magnitude, that is, $(X^2 + Y^2 + Z^2)^{1/2}$. This waveform is shown in panel d. From this waveform, several parameters have been derived such as total QRS duration (including late potentials), the RMS voltage value of the terminal 40 ms, and the low-amplitude signal (LAS) duration from the 40-μV level to the end of the late potentials. Abnormal values for these parameters are used to identify patients at high risk of ventricular tachycardia following a heart attack.

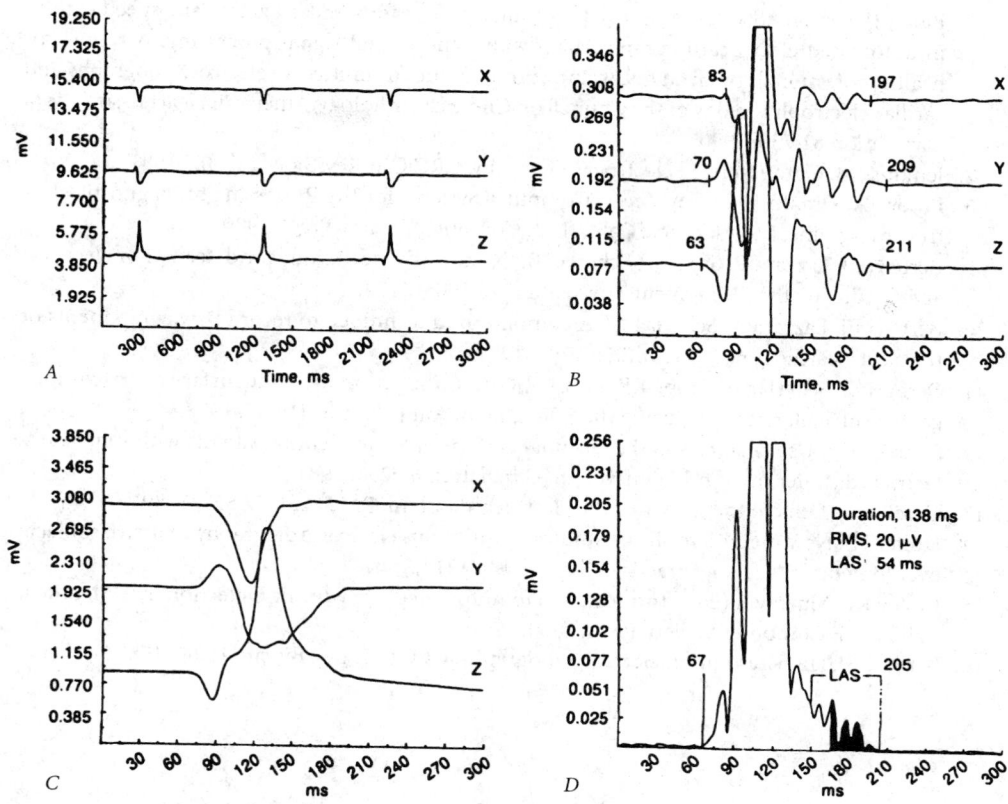

FIGURE 13.6 The signal-processing steps typically performed to obtain a high-resolution ECG are shown in panels A through D. See text for a full description.

13.4 Conclusions

The ECG is one of the oldest instrument-bound measurements in medicine. It has faithfully followed the progression of instrumentation technology. Its most recent evolutionary step, to the microprocessor-based system, has allowed patients to wear their computer monitor or has provided an enhanced, high-resolution ECG that has opened new vistas of ECG analysis and interpretation.

References

1. Waller AD. One the electromotive changes connected with the beat of the mammalian heart, and the human heart in particular. Phil Trans B 180:169, 1889.
2. Einthoven W. Die galvanometrische Registrirung des menschlichen Elektrokardiogramms, zugleich eine Beurtheilung der Anwendung des Capillar-Elecktrometers in der Physiologie. Pflugers Arch Ges Physiol 99:472, 1903.
3. Wilson FN, Johnston FS, Hill IGW. The interpretation of the falvanometric curves obtained when one electrode is distant from the heart and the other near or in contact with the ventricular surface. Am Heart J 10:176, 1934.
4. Goldberger E. A simple, indifferent, electrocardiographic electrode of zero potential and a technique of obtaining augmented, unipolar, extremity leads. Am Heart J 23:483, 1942.
5. Voluntary standard for diagnostic electrocardiographic devices. ANSI/AAMI EC11a. Arlington, Va: Association for the Advancement of Medical Instrumentation, 1984.

6. Bailey JJ, Berson AS, Garson A, et al. Recommendations for standardization and specifications in automated electrocardiography: bandwidth and digital signal processing: A report for health professionals by an ad hoc writing group of the committee on electrocardiography and cardiac electrophysiology of the Council on Clinical Cardiology, American Heart Association. Circulation 81:730, 1990.

7. Jenkins JM. Computerized electrocardiography. CRC Crit Rev Bioeng 6:307, 1981.

8. Pryor TA, Drazen E, Laks M (eds). Computer Systems for the Processing of diagnostic electrocardiograms. Los Alamitos, Calif, IEEE Computer Society Press, 1980.

9. Berbari EJ, Lazzara R, Samet P, Scherlag BJ. Noninvasive technique for detection of electrical activity during the PR segment. Circulation 48:1006, 1973.

10. Berbari EJ, Lazzara R, Scherlag BJ. A computerized technique to record new components of the electrocardiogram. Proc IEEE 65:799, 1977.

11. Berbari EJ, Scherlag BJ, Hope RR, Lazzara R. Recording from the body surface of arrhythmogenic ventricular activity during the ST segment. Am J Cardiol 41:697, 1978.

12. Simson MB. Use of signals in the terminal QRS complex to identify patients with ventricular tachycardia after myocardial infarction. Circulation 64:235, 1981.

13. Geselowitz DB. On the theory of the electrocardiogram. Proc IEEE 77:857, 1989.

14. Holter NJ. New method for heart studies: Continuous electrocardiography of active subjects over long periods is now practical. Science 134:1214, 1961.

15. Ripley KL, Murray A (eds). Introduction to Automated Arrhythmia Detection. Los Alamitos, Calif, IEEE Computer Society Press, 1980.

16. Berbari EJ. High-resolution electrocardiography. CRC Crit Rev Bioeng 16:67, 1988.

14

Principles of Electromyography

Kaj-Åge Henneberg
University of Montreal

Movement and position of limbs are controlled by electrical signals traveling back and forth between the muscles and the peripheral and central nervous system. When pathologic conditions arise in the motor system, whether in the spinal cord, the motor neurons, the muscle, or the neuromuscular junctions, the characteristics of the electrical signals in the muscle change. Careful registration and study of electrical signals in muscle (electromyograms) can thus be a valuable aid in discovering and diagnosing abnormalities not only in the muscles but also in the motor system as a whole. Electromyography (EMG) is the registration and interpretation of these muscle action potentials. Until recently, electromyograms were recorded primarily for exploratory or diagnostic purposes; however, with the advancement of bioelectric technology, electromyograms also have become a fundamental tool in achieving artificial control of limb movement, i.e., functional electrical stimulation (FES) and rehabilitation. This chapter will focus on the diagnostic application of electromyograms, while FES will be discussed in Chapter 17.

Since the rise of modern clinical EMG, the technical procedures used in recording and analyzing electromyograms have been dictated by the available technology. The concentric needle electrode introduced by Adrian and Bronk in 1929 provided an easy-to-use electrode with high mechanical qualities and stable, reproducible measurements. Replacement of galvanometers with high-gain amplifiers allowed smaller electrodes with higher impedances to be used and potentials of smaller amplitudes to be recorded. With these technical achievements, clinical EMG soon evolved into a highly specialized field where electromyographists with many years of experience read and interpreted long paper EMG records based on the visual appearance of the electromyograms. Slowly, a more quantitative approach emerged, where features such as potential duration, peak-to-peak amplitude, and number of phases were measured on the paper records and compared with a set of normal data gathered from healthy subjects of all ages. In the last decade, the general-purpose rack-mounted equipment of the past have been replaced by ergonomically designed EMG units with integrated computers. Electromyograms are digitized, processed, stored on removable media, and displayed on computer monitors with screen layouts that change in accordance with the type of recording and analysis chosen by the investigator.

With this in mind, this chapter provides an introduction to the basic concepts of clinical EMG, a review of basic anatomy, the origin of the electromyogram, and some of the main recording procedures and signal-analysis techniques in use.

8493-8346-3/95/$0.00+$.50
1995 by CRC Press, Inc.

14.1 The Structure and Function of Muscle

Muscles account for about 40% of the human mass, ranging from the small extraocular muscles that turn the eyeball in its socket to the large limb muscles that produce locomotion and control posture. The design of muscles varies depending on the range of motion and the force exerted (Fig. 14.1). In the most simple arrangement (*fusiform*), parallel fibers extend the full length of the muscle and attach to tendons at both ends. Muscles producing a large force have a more complicated structure in which many short muscle fibers attach to a flat tendon that extends over a large fraction of the muscle. This arrangement (*unipennate*) increases the cross-sectional area and thus the contractile force of the muscle. When muscle fibers fan out from both sides of the tendon, the muscle structure is referred to as *bipennate*.

A lipid bilayer (*sarcolemma*) encloses the muscle fiber and separates the intracellular myoplasma from the interstitial fluid. Between neighboring fibers runs a layer of connective tissue, the *endomysium*, composed mainly of collagen and elastin. Bundles of fibers, *fascicles*, are held together by a thicker layer of connective tissue called the *perimysium*. The whole muscle is wrapped in a layer of connective tissue called the *epimysium*. The connective tissue is continuous with the tendons attaching the muscle to the skeleton.

In the myoplasma, thin and thick filaments interdigitate and form short, serially connected identical units called *sarcomeres*. Numerous sarcomeres connect end to end, thereby forming longitudinal strands of myofibrils that extend the entire length of the muscle fiber. The total shortening of a muscle during contraction is the net effect of all sarcomeres shortening in series simultaneously. The individual sarcomeres shorten by forming cross-bridges between the thick and thin filaments. The cross-bridges pull the filaments toward each other, thereby increasing the amount of longitudinal overlap between the thick and thin filaments. The dense matrix of myofibrils is held in place by a structural framework of intermediate filaments composed of desmin, vimetin, and synemin [Squire, 1986].

At the site of the neuromuscular junction, each motor neuron forms collateral sprouts (Fig. 14.2) and innervates several muscle fibers distributed almost evenly within an elliptical or circular region ranging from 2 to 10 mm in diameter. The motor neuron and the muscle fibers it innervates constitute a functional unit, the motor unit. The cross section of muscle occupied by a motor unit is called the motor unit territory (MUT). A typical muscle fiber is only innervated at a single point,

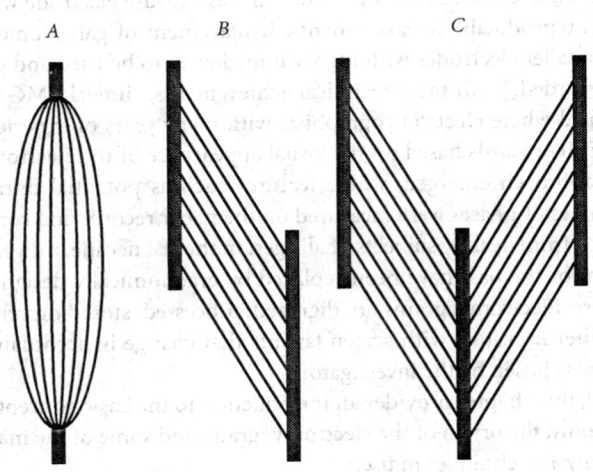

FIGURE 14.1 Schematic illustration of different types of muscles: (*a*) fusiform, (*b*) unipennate, and (*c*) bipennate.

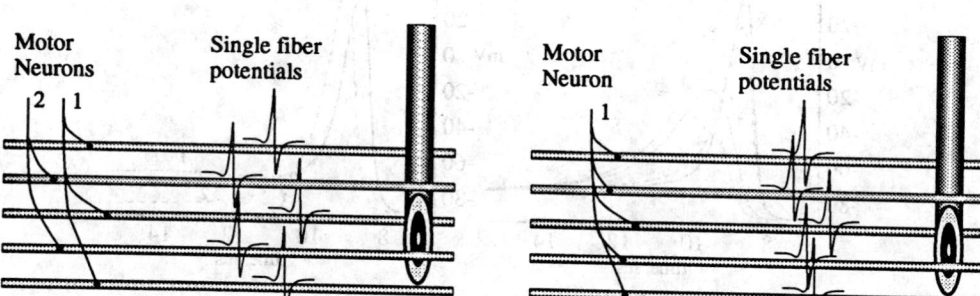

FIGURE 14.2 Innervation of muscle fibers. (*a*) Two normal motor units with intermingled muscle fibers. (*b*) Reinnervation of muscle fibers. The second and fourth muscle fibers have lost their motor neuron (2) and subsequently have become reinnervated by newly formed sprouts from the motor neuron (1) innervating adjacent muscle fibers. Not drawn to scale.

located within a cross-sectional band referred to as the *end-plate zone*. While the width of the end-plate zone is only a few millimeters, the zone itself may extend over a significant part of the muscle. The number of muscle fibers per motor neuron (i.e., the innervation ratio) ranges from 3:1 in extrinsic eye muscles where fine-graded contraction is required to 120:1 in some limb muscles with coarse movement [Kimura, 1981]. The fibers of one motor unit are intermingled with fibers of other motor units; thus several motor units reside within a given cross section. The fibers of the same motor unit are thought to be randomly or evenly distributed within the motor unit territory; however, reinnervation of denervated fibers often results in the formation of fiber clusters (see Fig. 14.2).

14.2 The Origin of Electromyograms

Unlike the myocardium, skeletal muscles do not contain pacemaker cells from which excitations arise and spread. Electrical excitation of skeletal muscle is initiated and regulated by the central and peripheral nervous systems. Motor neurons carry nerve impulses from the anterior horn cells of the spinal cord to the nerve endings, where the axonal action potential triggers the release of the neurotransmitter acetylcholine (Ach) into the narrow clefts separating the sarcolemma from the axon terminals. As Ach binds to the sarcolemma, Ach-sensitive sodium channels open, and miniature end-plate potentials arise in the sarcolemma. If sufficient Ach is released, the summation of miniature end-plate potentials, i.e., the end-plate potential, reaches the excitation threshold, and sarcolemmal action potentials propagate in opposite directions toward the tendons. As excitation propagates down the fiber, it spreads into a highly branched transverse network of tubules (T system) which interpenetrate the myofibrils. The effective radial conduction velocity (~4 cm/s) is about two orders of magnitude slower than the longitudinal conduction velocity (2 to 5 m/s). This is due to the fact that the main portion of the total membrane capacitance is located in the T system and that the lumen of the T system constitutes a higher electrical resistance than the myoplasma.

The slower tubular conduction velocity implies an increasingly delayed onset of tubular action potentials toward the center of the fiber relative to that of the sarcolemmal action potential (Fig. 14.3*a*). However, compared with the time course of the subsequent contraction, the spread of excitation along and within the muscle fiber is essentially instantaneous, thereby ensuring simultaneous release of calcium from the sarcoplasmic reticulum throughout the entire volume of the muscle. If calcium release were restricted to a small longitudinal section of the muscle fiber, only sarcomeres in this region would contract, and sarcomeres in the rest of the fiber would stretch

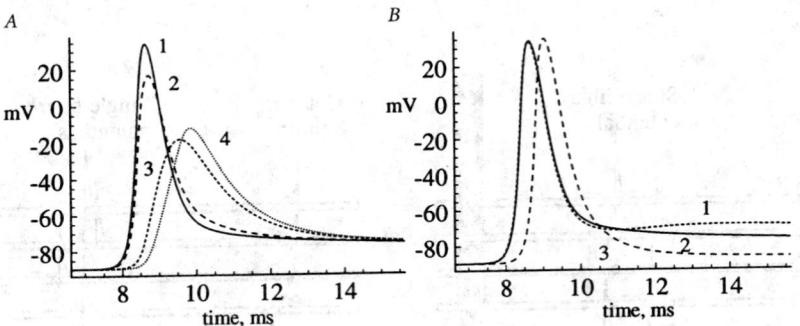

FIGURE 14.3 Simulated sarcolemmal and tubular action potentials of frog sartorius muscle fiber. (*a*) Temporal membrane action potentials calculated in a transverse plane 5 mm from the end-plate zone of a fiber with radius $a = 50$ μm. Curve 1: Sarcolemmal action potential; curves 2 to 4: action potentials in tubular membrane patches at $r = a$ (2), $r = a/2$ (3), and $r = a/20$ (4). (*b*) Sarcolemmal action potentials for fibers with radius 70 (1), 50 (2), and 30 (3) μm. The time axes have been expanded and truncated.

accordingly. Similarly, experiments in detubulated muscle fibers, i.e., fibers in which the continuation between the sarcolemmal and the tubular membrane has been disrupted, have demonstrated that only a thin layer of superficial myofibrils contracts when tubular action potentials fail to trigger calcium release deep in the muscle fiber.

It is well known that the shape of the skeletal muscle action potential differs from that of nerve action potentials with regard to the repolarization phase. In skeletal muscle, the falling phase of the action potential is interrupted by a long, slowly decaying potential known as the *afterpotential*. This late potential is caused by two opposing forces, the repolarization force due to the efflux of potassium through the sarcolemma and a depolarization force due to an influx of current from the interstitial space into the tubular lumen. The latter current is drawn in through the tubular openings by the repolarizing tubular membrane. Large muscle fibers have a higher tubular-sarcolemma area ratio; hence the inward surge of tubular current increases with fiber size. Figure 14.3*b* illustrates this by comparing sarcolemmal action potentials for fibers of increasing diameter. The small fiber has only a small amount of tubular membrane; hence the sarcolemmal potassium current has sufficient strength to rapidly repolarize the membrane. For the large fiber, inward tubular current actually depolarizes the sarcolemma slightly during repolarization of the tubular membrane system, thereby producing a small hump on the afterpotential. Since the hump on the afterpotential is influenced primarily by fiber size, this feature is more typical for large frog fibers than for smaller human fibers. Experiments have demonstrated that the sarcolemmal action potential of detubulated fibers hyperpolarizes in a manner similar to that of a nerve action potential.

In Fig. 14.4*a*, the time course of the sarcolemmal current density is compared with that of the current passing through the tubular mouth during the time course of the sarcolemmal action potential. The positive (outward) peak of the tubular current overlaps in time with the small capacitive sarcolemmal displacement current (initial positive peak) and the negative peak (inward sarcolemmal sodium current). As a result, the net current has a much larger positive peak than that of the sarcolemma alone, and the negative peak of the net current is only about half that of the sarcolemmal current. The outward sarcolemmal potassium current (late positive phase) is almost completely opposed by an antisymmetric inward tubular current, i.e., the current drawn into the tubular lumen by the repolarizing T system. The combined effect of the sarcolemmal and tubular interaction is a net current with an almost biphasic waveform and with similar amplitudes of the positive and negative peaks.

As the net current source propagates toward the tendon, an extracellular potential field arises and follows the action potential complex. At a given field point, this phenomenon is observed as a tem-

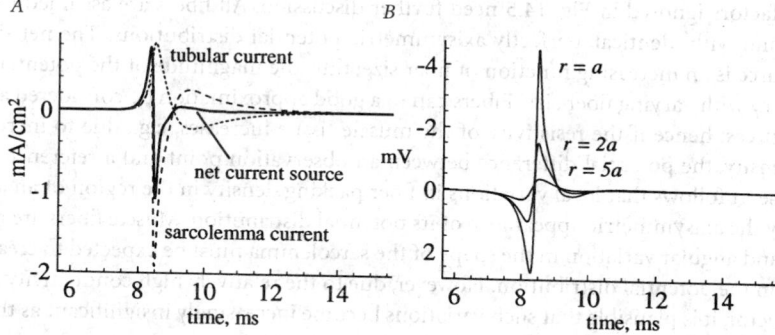

FIGURE 14.4 Simulated currents and extracellular potentials of frog sartorius muscle fiber (radius $a = 50$ μm). (*a*) The net fiber current density is the summation of the current density through the sarcolemma and that passing the tubular mouth. (*b*) Extracellular action potentials calculated at increasing radial distances (in units of fiber radius) using a bidomain volume conductor model and the net current source in panel *a*. The time axes have been expanded and truncated.

poral potential waveform (Fig. 14.4*b*); however, a more complete picture of the phenomenon is obtained by considering the spatial distribution of potentials in the cross section of the motor unit. Figure 14.5 shows schematically how the concentric isopotential lines of individual fibers overlap with those of other fibers in the same motor unit. In a typical healthy motor unit (Fig. 14.5*a*), the mean interfiber distance is on the order of a few hundred microns. Taking into account the steep radial decline of the potential amplitudes illustrated in Fig. 14.4*b*, it is evident that single-fiber action potential (SFAP) overlapping occurs between low-magnitude isopotential lines. Figure 14.5b illustrates how spatial overlapping between SFAPs might look like in a motor unit with extensive fiber grouping. In this case, higher-level isopotential lines overlap within the clusters, while regions with no fibers would appear as electrically silent.

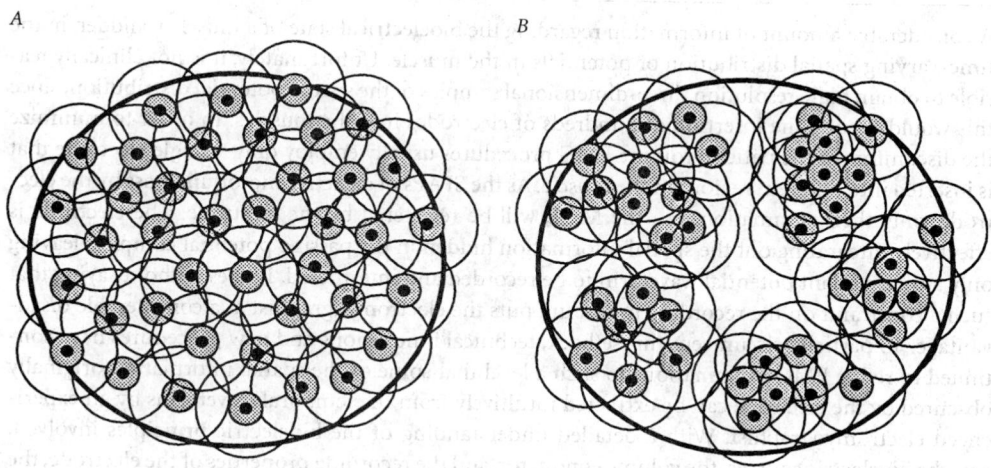

FIGURE 14.5 Schematic cross-sectional view of overlapping single-fiber action potential distributions in a normal (*a*) and reinnervated (*b*) motor unit. Muscle fibers are represented by filled black circles. Concentric rings represent axisymmetric isopotential lines of the individual single-fiber potentials at 2 (gray) and 5 radii from the fiber center, respectively. Compare with radial decline of extracellular potentials in Fig. 14.4. See text for discussion of simplifying assumptions.

Several factors ignored in Fig. 14.5 need further discussion. All fibers are assumed to be of the same size and with identical, perfectly axisymmetric potential distributions. The net single-fiber current source is an increasing function of fiber size; thus the magnitude of the potential distribution will vary with varying fiber size. Fibers can to a good approximation be considered as constant current sources; hence if the resistivity of the muscle tissue increases, e.g., due to increased fiber packing density, the potential difference between an observation point and a reference point also will increase. It follows that local variations in fiber packing density in the region of an active fiber will destroy the axisymmetric appearance of its potential distribution. Muscle fibers are not perfect cylinders, and angular variation in the shape of the sarcolemma must be expected to create angular variations in the potential distribution. However, due to the relatively high conductivity of the volume conductor, it is plausible that such variations become increasingly insignificant as the distance to the fiber is increased.

A very important factor not considered in Fig. 14.5 concerns the degree of longitudinal alignment of SFAPs in the motor unit. As illustrated in Fig. 14.2, SFAPs are usually dispersed along the motor unit axis, and their potential distributions do not sum up in a simple manner. SFAPs can be misaligned for several reasons. The end plates are not aligned; hence some SFAPs originate ahead of others. Variations in fiber size and packing density cause variations in conduction velocity; thus the dispersion of SFAPs may actually increase with increasing distance from the end-plate zone. Neuropathologic conditions can affect the alignment of SFAPs. Complete or partial failure of collateral nerve sprouts to conduct nerve action potentials can abolish or delay the onset of action potentials, and immature sprouts formed during reinnervation may cause significant variability (jitter) in the onset of muscle action potentials. Denervated muscle fibers shrink; hence a newly reinnervated muscle fiber is likely to have a slower conduction velocity. An increased dispersion of SFAPs creates a very complex and irregular spatial potential distribution. The superimposed temporal potential waveform in a fixed observation point, i.e., the motor unit potential (MUP), is therefore comprised of several peaks rather than a simple bi- or triphasic waveform. MUPs with five or more peaks are classified as *polyphasic*. A satellite potential is an SFAP that is so misaligned from the main potential complex that its waveform is completely separated from the MUP.

14.3 Electromyographic Recordings

A considerable amount of information regarding the bioelectrical state of a muscle is hidden in the time-varying spatial distribution of potentials in the muscle. Unfortunately, it is not clinically feasible to obtain high-resolution three-dimensional samples of the spatial potential distribution, since this would require the insertion of hundreds of electrodes into the muscles. In order to minimize the discomfort of the patient, routine EMG procedures usually employ only a single electrode that is inserted into different regions of the muscle. As the SFAPs of an active motor unit pass by the electrode, only their summation, i.e., the MUP, will be registered by the electrode. The electrode is effectively integrating out the spatial information hidden in the passing potential complex, leaving only a time-variant potential waveform to be recorded and interpreted. It goes without saying that such a constraint on the recording procedure puts the electromyographist at a considerable disadvantage. To partially circumvent this setback, technical innovations and new procedures have continued to refine EMG examinations to such a level that some of the spatial information originally obscured by the electrode can be extracted intuitively from the temporal waveforms by an experienced electromyographist. With a detailed understanding of the bioelectric principles involved, e.g., the bioelectric sources, the volume conductor, and the recording properties of the electrode, the electromyographist can quickly recognize and explain the waveform characteristics associated with various neuromuscular abnormalities.

To increase the amount of diagnostic information, several sets of EMG investigations may be performed using electrodes with different recording characteristics. Figure 14.6 illustrates three of the most popular EMG needle electrodes. The concentric and monopolar electrodes have an inter-

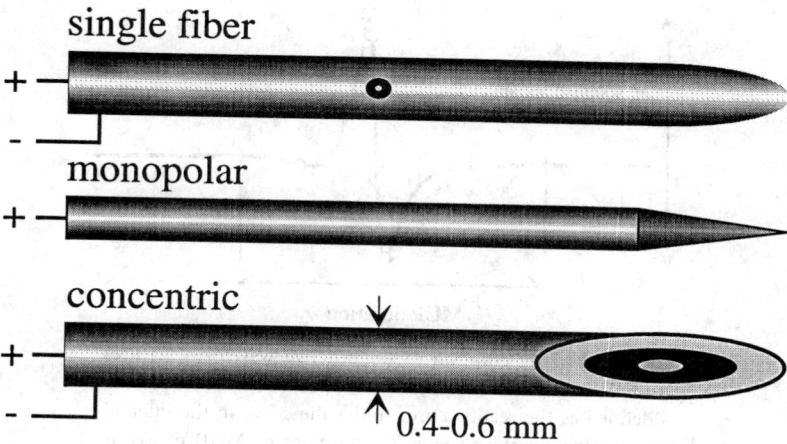

FIGURE 14.6   Needle electrodes for subcutaneous EMG recordings. For the single-fiber and concentric electrodes, the cannula of the hypodermic needle acts as reference electrode. The monopolar electrode is used with a remote reference electrode.

mediate pickup range and are used in conventional recordings. The single-fiber electrode is a more recent innovation. It has a very small pickup range and is used to obtain recordings from only one or two muscle fibers. The macro electrode, which is the cannula of either the concentric or single-fiber electrode in combination with a remote reference electrode, picks up potentials throughout the motor unit territory. This section will review these EMG electrodes, the waveforms they produce, and the signal analysis performed in each case.

Concentric Electrode EMG

Adrian and Bronk developed the concentric electrode (see Fig. 14.6) in order to obtain a pickup range that is smaller than that of wire electrodes. The modern version of the concentric electrode consists of a platinum or stainless steel wire located inside the lumen of a stainless steel cannula with an outer diameter of about 0.5 mm. The tip is beveled at 15 to 20 degrees, thereby exposing the central wire as an oblique elliptical surface of about 150×580 μm. The central wire is insulated from the cannula with araldite or epoxy.

The concentric electrode is connected to a differential amplifier; thus common-mode signals are effectively rejected, and a relatively stable baseline is achieved. The cannula cannot be regarded as an indifferent reference electrode because it is located within the potential distribution and thus will pick up potentials from active fibers. Simulation studies [Henneberg and Plonsey, 1993] have shown that the cannula shields the central wire from picking up potentials from fibers located behind the tip. The sensitivity of the concentric electrode is therefore largest in the hemisphere facing the oblique elliptical surface. Due to the asymmetric sensitivity function, the waveshape of the recorded potentials will vary if the electrode is rotated about its axis. This problem is not observed with the axisymmetric monopolar electrode; however, this electrode has a more unstable baseline due to the remote location of the reference electrode. Both the concentric and monopolar electrodes (see Fig. 14.6) are used in conventional EMG. Because of the differences in recording characteristics, however, concentric and monopolar recordings cannot be compared easily. A particular EMG laboratory therefore tends to use the one and not the other.

During the concentric needle examination, the investigator searches for abnormal insertional activity, spontaneous activity in relaxed muscles, and motor unit potentials with abnormal appearance. The waveshape of motor unit potentials is assessed on the basis of the quantitative waveform features defined in Fig. 14.7:

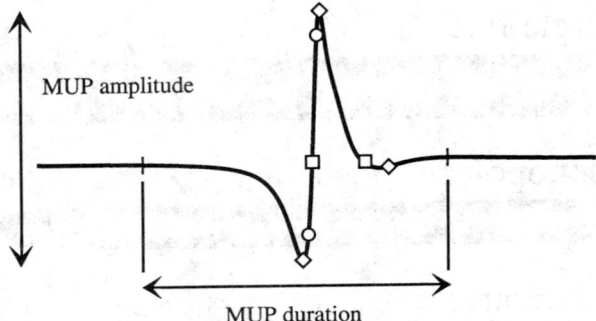

MUP amplitude

MUP duration

FIGURE 14.7 Definition of quantitative waveform features of MUPs recorded with a concentric EMG electrode. MUP area is defined as the rectified area under the curve in the interval between the onset and end. The number of MUP phases is defined as the number of baseline crossings (□) plus one. MUP turns are marked by a ◇. MUP rise time is the time interval between the 10% and 90% deflection (○) of the main negative-going slope. As by convention, negative voltage is displayed upward.

- *Amplitude* is determined by the presence of active fibers within the immediate vicinity of the electrode tip. Low-pass filtering by the volume conductor attenuates the high-frequency spikes of remote SFAPs; hence the MUP amplitude does not increase for a larger motor unit. However, MUP amplitude will increase if the tip of the electrode is located near a cluster of reinnervated fibers. Large MUP amplitudes are frequently observed in neurogenic diseases.
- *Rise time* is an increasing function of the distance between the electrode and the closest active muscle fiber. A short rise time in combination with a small MUP amplitude might therefore indicate that the amplitude is reduced due to fiber atrophy rather than to a large distance between the electrode and the closest fiber.
- *Number of phases* indicates the complexity of the MUP and the degree of misalignment between SFAPs. In neurogenic diseases, polyphasic MUPs arise due to slow conduction velocity in immature nerve sprouts or slow conduction velocity in reinnervated but still atrophied muscle fibers. Variation in muscle fiber size also causes polyphasic MUPs in myopathic diseases. To prevent noisy baseline fluctuations from affecting the count of MUP phases, a valid baseline crossing must exceed a minimum absolute amplitude criterion.
- *Duration* is the time interval between the first and last occurrence of the waveform exceeding a predefined amplitude threshold, e.g., 5 μV. The MUP onset and end are the summation of low-frequency components of SFAPs scattered over the entire pickup range of the electrode. As a result, the MUP duration provides information about the number of active fibers within the pickup range. However, since the motor unit territory can be larger than the pickup range of the electrode, MUP duration does not provide information about the total size of a large motor unit. MUP duration will increase if a motor unit has an increased number of fibers due to reinnervation. MUP duration is affected to a lesser degree by SFAP misalignment.
- *Area* indicates the number of fibers adjacent to the electrode; however, unlike MUP amplitude, MUP area depends on MUP duration and is therefore influenced by fibers in a larger region compared with that of MUP amplitude.
- *Turns* is a measure of the complexity of the MUP, much like the number of phases; however, since a valid turn does not require a baseline crossing like a valid phase, the number of turns

is more sensitive to changes in the MUP waveshape. In order to distinguish valid turns from signal noise, successive turns must be offset by a minimum amplitude difference.

Based on the complimentary information contained in the MUP features defined above, it is possible to infer about the number and density of fibers in a motor unit as well as the synchronicity of the SFAPs. However, the concentric electrode is not sufficiently selective to study individual fibers, nor is it sufficiently sensitive to measure the total size of a motor unit. The following two techniques were designed with these objectives in mind.

Single-Fiber EMG

The positive lead of the single-fiber electrode (see Fig. 14.6) is the end cap of a 25-μm wire exposed through a side port on the cannula of a steel needle. Due to the small size of the positive lead, bioelectric sources, which are located more than about 300 μm from the side port, will appear as common-mode signals and be suppressed by the differential amplifier. To further enhance the selectivity, the recorded signal is high-pass filtered at 500 Hz to remove low-frequency background activity from distant fibers.

Due to its very small pickup range, the single-fiber electrode rarely record potentials from more than one or two fibers from the same motor unit. Because of the close proximity of the fibers, potentials are of large amplitudes and with small rise times. When two potentials from the same motor unit are picked up, the slight variation in their *interpotential interval* (IPI) can be measured (Fig. 14.8). The mean IPI (**jitter**) is normally 5 to 50 μs but increases when neuromuscular transmission is disturbed. When the single-fiber electrode records potentials from an increased number of fibers, it usually indicates that the side port is close to either a cluster of fibers (reinnervation) or that the positive lead is close to fibers in the process of splitting.

Macro EMG

For this electrode, the cannula of a single-fiber or concentric electrode is used as the positive lead, while the reference electrode can be either a remote subcutaneous or remote surface electrode. Due to the large lead surface, this electrode picks up both near- and far-field activity. However, the signal has very small amplitude, and the macro electrode must therefore be coupled to an electronic averager. To ensure that only one and the same MUP is being averaged, the averager is triggered by a SFAP picked up from that motor unit by the side port wire of the single-fiber electrode or by the central wire of the concentric electrode. Since other MUPs are not time-locked to the triggering SFAP, they will appear as random background activity and become suppressed in the averaging pro-

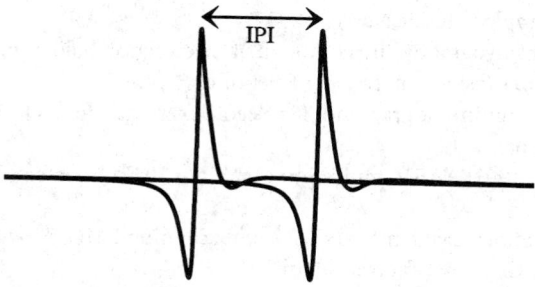

FIGURE 14.8 Measurement of interpotential interval (IPI) between single-fiber potentials recorded simultaneously from two fibers of the same motor unit.

cedure. Quantitative features of the macro MUP include the peak-to-peak amplitude, the rectified area under the curve, and the number of phases.

Defining Terms

Concentric electrode EMG: Registration and interpretation of motor unit potentials recorded with a concentric needle electrode.

Electromyograms (EMGs)   Bioelectric potentials recorded in muscles.

Jitter: Mean variation in interpotential interval between single-fiber action potentials of the same motor unit.

Macro EMG: The registration of motor unit potentials from the entire motor unit using the cannula of the single-fiber or concentric electrode.

Motor unit: The functional unit of an anterior horn cell, its axon, the neuromuscular junctions, and the muscle fibers innervated by the motor neuron.

Motor unit potential (MUP):   Spatial and temporal summation of all single-fiber potentials innervated by the same motor neuron. Also referred to as the *motor unit action potential* (MUAP).

Motor unit territory (MUT):   Cross-sectional region of muscle containing all fibers innervated by a single motor neuron.

Satellite potential: An isolated single-fiber action potential that is time-locked with the main MUP.

Single-fiber action potential (SFAP):   Extracellular potential generated by the extracellular current flow associated with the action potential of a single muscle fiber.

Single-fiber EMG (SFEMG):   Recording and analysis of single-fiber potentials with the single-fiber electrode.

References

Henneberg K, Plonsey R. 1993. Boundary element analysis of the directional sensitivity of the concentric EMG electrode. IEEE Trans Biomed Eng 40:621.

Kimura J. 1981. Electrodiagnosis in Diseases of Nerve and Muscle: Principles and Practice. Philadelphia, FA Davis.

Squire J. 1986. Muscle: Design, Diversity and Disease. Menlo Park, Calif, Benjamin/Cummings.

Further Information

Barry DT. 1991. AAEM minimonograph no. 36: Basic concepts of electricity and electronics in clinical electromyography. Muscle Nerve. 14:937.

Buchthal F. 1973. Electromyography. In Handbook of Electroencephalography and Clinical Neurophysiology, vol 16. Amsterdam, Elsevier Scientific.

Daube JR. 1991. AAEM minimonograph no. 11: Needle examination in clinical electromyography. Muscle Nerve 14:685.

Dumitru D, DeLisa JA. 1991. AAEM minimonograph no. 10: Volume conduction. Muscle Nerve 14:605.

Stålberg E. 1986. Single fiber EMG, macro EMG, and scanning EMG: New ways of looking at the motor unit. CRC Crit Rev Clin Neurobiol 2:125.

15
Principles of Electroencephalography

oseph D. Bronzino
*rinity College/The Hartford
;raduate Center

Electroencephalograms (EEGs) are recordings of the minute (generally less that 300 μV) electrical potentials produced by the brain. Since 1924, when Hans Berger reported the recording of rhythmic electrical activity from the human scalp, analysis of EEG activity has been conducted primarily in clinical settings to detect gross pathologies and epilepsies and in research facilities to quantify the central effects of new pharmacologic agents. As a result of these efforts, cortical EEG patterns have been shown to be modified by a wide range of variables, including biochemical, metabolic, circulatory, hormonal, neuroelectric, and behavioral factors. In the past, interpretation of the EEG was limited to visual inspection by an electroencephalographer, an individual trained to qualitatively distinguish normal EEG activity from localized or generalized abnormalities contained within relatively long EEG records. This approach left clinicians and researchers alike buried in a sea of EEG paper records. The advent of computers and the technologies associated with them has made it possible to effectively apply a host of methods to quantify EEG changes. With this in mind, this chapter provides a brief historical perspective followed by some insights regarding EEG recording procedures and an in-depth discussion of the quantitative techniques used to analyze alterations in the EEG.

15.1 Historical Perspective

In 1875, Richard Caton published the first account documenting the recording of spontaneous brain electrical activity from the cerebral cortex of an experimental animal. The amplitude of these electrical oscillations was so low (i.e., in the microvolt range) that Caton's discovery is all the more amazing because it was made 50 years before suitable electronic amplifiers became available. In 1924, Hans Berger, of the University of Jena in Austria, carried out the first human EEG recordings using metal strips pasted to the scalps of his subjects as electrodes and a sensitive galvanometer as the recording instrument. Berger was able to measure the irregular, relatively small electrical potentials (i.e., 50 to 100 μV) coming from the brain. By studying the successive positions of the moving element of the galvanometer recorded on a continuous roll of paper, he was able to observe the resultant patterns in these brain waves as they varied with time. From 1924 to 1938, Berger laid the foundation for many of the present applications of electroencephalography. He was the first to use the word *electro-*

encephalogram in describing these brain potentials in humans. Berger also noted that these brain waves were not entirely random but instead displayed certain periodicities and regularities. For example, he observed that although these brain waves were slow (i.e., exhibited a synchronized pattern of high amplitude and low frequency, <3 Hz) during sleep, they were faster (i.e., exhibited a desynchronized pattern of low amplitude and higher frequency, 15 to 25 Hz) during waking behaviors. He suggested, quite correctly, that the brain's activity changed in a consistent and recognizable fashion when the general status of the subject changed, as from relaxation to alertness. Berger also concluded that these brain waves could be greatly affected by certain pathologic conditions after noting a marked increase in the amplitude of these brain waves recorded during convulsive seizures. However, despite the insights provided by these studies, Berger's original paper, published in 1929, did not excite much attention. In essence, the efforts of this remarkable pioneer were largely ignored until similar investigations were carried out and verified by British investigators.

It was not until 1934, however, when Adrian and Matthews published their classic paper verifying Berger's findings, that the concept of "human brain waves" was truly accepted and the study of EEG activity was placed on a firm foundation. One of their primary contributions was the identification of certain rhythms in the EEG, e.g., a regular oscillation at approximately 10 to 12 Hz recorded from the occipital lobes of the cerebral cortex, which they termed the "alpha rhythm." This alpha rhythm was found to disappear when a subject displayed any type of attention or alertness or focused on objects in the visual field. The physiologic basis for these results, the "arousing influence" of external stimuli on the cortex, was not formulated until 1949, when Moruzzi and Magoun demonstrated the existence of pathways widely distributed through the central reticular core of the brainstem that were capable of exerting a diffuse activating influence on the cerebral cortex. This "reticular activating system" has been called the brain's response selector because it alerts the cortex to focus on certain pieces of incoming information while ignoring others. It is for this reason that a sleeping mother will immediately be awakened by her crying baby or the smell of smoke and yet ignore the traffic outside her window or the television playing in the next room. (*Note:* For the interested reader, an excellent historical review of this early era in brain research is provided in a fascinating text by Brazier [1968].)

15.2 EEG Recording Techniques

Scalp recordings of spontaneous neuronal activity in the brain, identified as the EEG, allow measurement of potential changes over time between a signal electrode and a reference electrode [Kondraski, 1986]. Compared with other biopotentials, such as the electrocardiogram, the EEG is extremely difficult for an untrained observer to interpret, partially as a result of the spatial mapping of functions onto different regions of the brain and electrode placement. Recognizing that some standardization was necessary, the International Federation in Electroencephalography and Clinical Neurophysiology adopted the 10–20 electrode placement system. In addition to the standard 10–20 scalp array, electrodes to monitor eye movement, ECG, and muscle activity are essential for discrimination of different vigilance or behavioral states.

Any EEG system consists of electrodes, amplifiers (with appropriate filters), and a recording device. Instrumentation required for recording EEG activity can be simple or elaborate. (*Note:* Although the discussion presented in this section is for a single-channel system, it can be extended to simultaneous multichannel recordings simply by multiplying the hardware by the number of channels required. In cases that do not require true simultaneous recordings, special electrode selector panels can minimize hardware requirements.)

Commonly used scalp electrodes consist of Ag-AgCl disks, 1 to 3 mm in diameter, with long flexible leads that can be plugged into an amplifier. Although a low-impedance contact is desirable at the electrode-skin interface (<10 kΩ), this objective is confounded by hair and the difficulty of mechanically stabilizing the electrodes. Conductive electrode paste helps obtain low impedance and keep the electrodes in place. Often a contact cement (collodion) is used to fix small patches of gauze over the electrodes for mechanical stability, and leads are usually taped to the subject to provide some strain relief. Slight abrasion of the skin is sometimes used to obtain lower electrode impedance, but this can cause slight irritation and sometimes infection (as well as pain in sensitive subjects).

For long-term recordings, as in seizure monitoring, electrodes present major problems. Needle electrodes, which must be inserted into the tissue between the surface of the scalp and the skull, are sometimes useful. However, the danger of infection increases significantly. Electrodes with self-contained miniature amplifiers are somewhat more tolerant because they provide a low-impedance source to interconnecting leads, but they are expensive. Despite numerous attempts to simplify the electrode application process and to guarantee long-term stability, no single method has been widely accepted.

Instruments are available for measuring impedance between electrode pairs. The procedure is recommended strongly as good practice, since high impedance leads to distortions that may be difficult to separate from actual EEG signals. In fact, electrode impedance monitors are built into some commercially available EEG devices. Note that standard dc ohmmeters should not be used, since they apply a polarizing current that can result in a buildup of noise at the skin-electrode interface.

From carefully applied electrodes, signal amplitudes of 1 to 10 μV can be obtained. Considerable amplification (gain $= 10^6$) is required to bring signal strength up to an acceptable level for input to recording devices. Because of the length of electrode leads and the electrically noisy environment where recordings commonly take place, differential amplifiers with inherently high input impedance and high common-mode rejection ratios are essential for high-quality EEG recordings.

In some facilities, special electrically shielded rooms minimize environmental electrical noise, particularly 60-Hz alternating current (ac) line noise. Since much of the information of interest in the EEG lies in frequency bands below 40 Hz, low-pass filters in the amplifier can be used to greatly reduce 60-Hz noise. For attenuating ac noise when the low-pass cutoff is above 60 Hz, many EEG amplifiers employ a notch filter specific only for frequencies in a narrow band centered around 60 Hz.

When trying to eliminate or minimize the effect of 60-Hz sources, it is sometimes useful to use a dummy source, such as a fixed 100-kΩ resistor attached to the electrodes. By employing a dummy source as one of the input signals, the output of the differential amplifier represents only contributions from interfering sources. If noise can be reduced to an acceptable level (at least by a factor of 10 less than EEG signals), it is likely that uncontaminated EEG records can be obtained.

Different types of recording instruments obtain a temporary or permanent record of the EEG. The most common recording device is a pen or chart recorder (usually multichannel), which is an integral part of most commercially available EEG instruments. Recordings are on a long sheet of continuous paper (from a folded stack) fed past the moving pen at one of several selectable constant speeds. Paper speed is selected according to the monitoring situation at hand: slow speed (10 mm/s) for observing the spiking characteristically associated with seizure activity and faster speeds (up to 120 mm/s) to identify the presence of individual frequency bands in the EEG.

In addition to (or instead of) a pen recorder, the EEG may be recorded on a multichannel frequency-modulated (FM) analog tape recorder. During such recordings, a visual output device such as an oscilloscope or video display is often used to allow visual monitoring of signals.

Sophisticated FM tape recording and playback systems allow clinicians to review long EEG recordings over a greatly reduced time compared with that required to flip through stacks of paper or to observe recordings in real time. Such systems take advantage of time-compensation schemes, whereby a signal recorded at one speed can be played back at a faster speed. The ratio of playback to recording speed is known, so the appropriate correction factor can be applied to played-back data generating a properly scaled video display. A standard ratio of 60:1 is often used. Thus a trained clinician can review each minute of real-time EEG in 1 s. The display is scrolled at a high rate horizontally across the display screen. Features of such instruments allow the clinician to freeze a segment of EEG on the display and to slow down or accelerate tape speed from the standard playback as needed. A vertical "tick" mark is usually displayed at periodic intervals by one channel as a time mark to provide a convenient timing reference.

Computers also can be used as recording devices. In such systems, one or more channels of analog EEG signal are repeatedly sampled at a fixed time interval (sampling interval), and each sample is converted into a digital representation by an analog-to-digital (A/D) converter. The A/D converter is interfaced to a computer system so that each sample can be saved in the computer's memory. The resolution of the A/D converter is determined by the smallest amplitude that can be sampled. This is determined by dividing the voltage range of the A/D converter by 2 raised to the power of the number of bits of the A/D converter. For example, an A/D converter with a range of ±5 V and 12-bit resolution can resolve sample amplitudes as small as ±2.4 mV. Appropriate matching of amplification and A/D converter sensitivity permits resolution of the smallest signal while preventing clipping of the largest signal amplitudes.

A set of such samples, acquired at a sufficient sampling rate (at least $2\times$ the highest frequency component of interest in the sampled signal), is sufficient to represent all the information in the waveform. To ensure that the signal is band-limited, a low-pass filter with a cutoff frequency equal to the highest frequency of interest is used. Since physically realizable filters do not have ideal characteristics, the sampling rate is usually set to $2\times$ the cutoff frequency of the filter or more. Furthermore, once converted to digital format, digital filtering techniques can be used.

On-line computer recordings are only practical for short-term recordings or for situations in which the EEG is immediately processed. This limitation is primarily due to storage requirements. For example, a typical sampling rate of 128 Hz yields 128 new points per second that require storage. For an 8-s sample, 1024 points are acquired per channel recorded. A 10-minute recording period yields 76,800 data points per channel. Assuming 12-bit resolution per sample, one can see that available computer memory quickly becomes a significant factor in determining the length (in terms of time) as well as the number of channels of EGG activity to be acquired in real time by the computer.

Further data processing can consist of compression for more efficient storage (with associated loss of total information content), as in the use of compressed spectral arrays, determination of a reduced features set including only data needed for quantification, as in evoked response recordings, or feature extraction and subsequent pattern recognition, as in automated spike detection during monitoring for epileptic seizure activity.

In addition to the information available from spontaneous EEG activity, the brain's electrical response to sensory stimulation is also important. Due to the relatively small amplitude of a stimulus-evoked potential compared with that of spontaneous EEG potentials, the technique of signal averaging is often used to enhance the characteristics of stimulus-evoked responses. Stimulus averaging takes advantage of the fact that the brain's electrical response is time locked to the onset of the stimulus, while nonevoked, background potential changes are randomly distributed in time. Consequently, the averaging of multiple stimulus-evoked responses results in the enhancement of the time-locked activity, while average random background activity approaches zero. The result is an evoked response that consists of a number of discrete and replicable peaks that occur, depending on the stimulus and recording parameters, at predictable latencies associated with the onset of stimulation.

15.3 Use of Amplitude Histographs to Quantify the EEG

In general, the EEG contains information regarding changes in the electrical potential of the brain obtained from a given set of recording electrodes. These data include the characteristic waveforms with accompanying variations in amplitude, frequency, phase, etc., as well as the brief occurrence of electrical patterns, such as spindles. *Any analysis procedure cannot simultaneously provide information regarding all these variables.* Consequently, the selection of any analytical technique will emphasize changes in one particular variable at the expense of the others. This observation is extremely important if one is to properly interpret the results obtained using a given technique.

In the computation of amplitude distributions of the EEG, for example, successive EEG amplitudes must be measured and ordered into specific amplitude classes, or *bins*. The amplitude histogram that results from this process is often a symmetrical, essentially gaussian distribution. The primary characteristics of the gaussian distribution are summarized simply by specifying its mean and standard deviation, since the higher control moments of the distribution, such as skewness and kurtosis, are equal to zero. However, in nongaussian distributions, the measures of skewness and kurtosis assume nonzero values and can be used to characterize that particular amplitude distribution. The four primary statistical measures used to characterize an EEG amplitude histogram include the mean, standard amplitude, skewness, and kurtosis.

Mean

Since the sum of (positive and negative) EEG potential is usually on the order of a few microvolts when the analysis time is not too short, the *mean* is essentially a constant, although of small value. Any shifts in values of the mean, therefore, are indicative of changes in potential that are of technical origin, such as amplifier drifts, etc.

Standard Amplitude

The variance of the EEG amplitude distribution is directly related to the total power of the EEG. For example, a flat EEG will provide low variance values, while a widely oscillating EEG will yield high variance values. To avoid confusion and use units that are more familiar to electroencephalographers, the term *standard amplitude* is often used.

Skewness

The degree of deviation from the symmetry of a normal or gaussian distribution is measured by *skewness*. This third central moment of the amplitude histogram has a value of zero when the distribution is completely symmetrical and assumes some nonzero value when the EEG waveforms are asymmetrical with respect to the baseline (as is the case in some characteristic sleep patterns, mu-rhythms, morphine spindles, barbiturate spiking, etc.). In general, a nonzero value of the skewness index reflects the presence of monophasic events in the waveform. The following methods can be used to obtain the measure of skewness.

Moment Coefficient of Skewness:

$$SK_{mc} = \frac{\sum\limits_{i=1}^{N} \dfrac{(x_i - \bar{x})^3}{N}}{\left[\sum\limits_{i=1}^{N} \dfrac{(x_i - \bar{x})^2}{N}\right]^{3/2}} \tag{15.1}$$

Pearson's Second Coefficient of Skewness:

$$SK_{2c} = \frac{3(\bar{x} \text{ median})}{SD} \tag{15.2}$$

Centile Index of Skewness:

$$SK_{cent} = \frac{(\text{number of points} > \bar{x})}{N} \tag{15.3}$$

Kurtosis

The *kurtosis* measure reveals the peakedness or flatness of a distribution. A kurtosis value greater than that of a normal distribution means that the distribution is leptokurtic, or simply more peaked than the normal curve. A value less than that of a normal distribution indicates a flatter distribution. In clinical electroencephalography, when analyzing EEGs with little frequency and amplitude modulation, one observes negative values of kurtosis. High positive values of kurtosis are present when the EEG contains transient spikes, isolated high-voltage wave groups, etc. The following methods can be used to obtain the measure of kurtosis.

Moment Coefficient of Kurtosis:

$$K_{mc} = \frac{\displaystyle\sum_{i=1}^{N} \frac{(x_i - \bar{x})^4}{N}}{\displaystyle\sum_{i=1}^{N} \left[\frac{(x_i - \bar{x})^2}{N} \right]^2} - 3 \tag{15.4}$$

Centile Index of Kurtosis:

$$K_{cent} = \frac{\text{number of patients such that } |x_i - \bar{x}| > \text{standard amplitude}}{N} \tag{15.5}$$

A normal distribution will have a value of 0.5 for this measure.

Figure 15.1 illustrates the sensitivity of these measures in analyzing the effect of systemic (IP) administration of morphine sulfate (30 mg/kg) on the cortical EEG. It will be noted that the skewness measure changes abruptly only immediately after the morphine injection, when the EEG was dominated by the appearance of spindles. However, the index of kurtosis characterizes the entire extent of the drug effect from onset to its return to baseline.

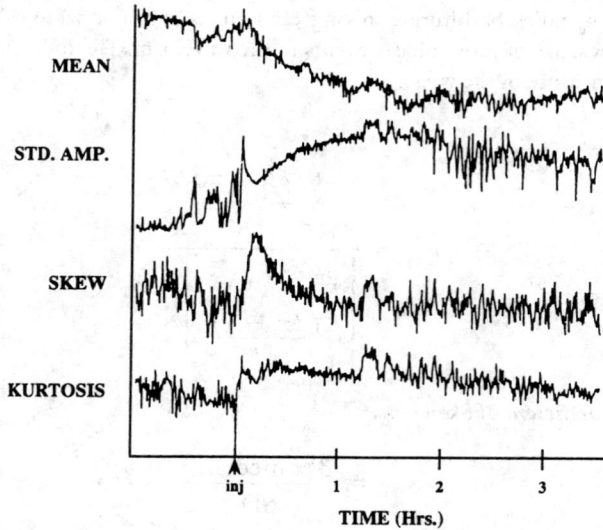

FIGURE 15.1 Plot of the indices of the amplitude distribution, i.e., the mean, standard amplitude, skewness, and kurtosis, of the EEG recorded from a rat prior to and for 3 hours following intraperitoneal injection of morphine sulfate (30 mg/kg). *Arrow (inj)* indicates time of injection.

The central moments of the EEG amplitude histogram, therefore, are capable of (1) characterizing the amplitude distributions of the EEG and (2) quantifying alterations in these electrical processes brought about by pharmacologic manipulations. In addition, use of the centile index for skewness and kurtosis provides a computer-efficient method for obtaining these measures in real-time.

15.4 Frequency Analysis of the EEG

In early attempts to correlate the EEG with behavior, analog frequency analyzers were used to examine single channels of EEG data. Although disappointing, these initial efforts did introduce the use of frequency analysis to the study of gross brain wave activity. Although power spectral analysis, i.e., the magnitude square of the Fourier transform, provides a quantitative measure of the frequency distribution of the EEG, it does so, as mentioned above, at the expense of other details in the EEG such as the amplitude distribution and information concerning the presence of specific EEG patterns.

The first systematic application of power spectral analysis by general-purpose computers was reported in 1963 by Walter; however, it was not until the introduction of the fast Fourier transform (FFT) by Cooley and Tukey in 1965 that machine computation of the EEG became commonplace. Although an individual FFT is ordinarily calculated for a short section of EEG data (e.g., from 1 to 8 s), such signal segmentation with subsequent averaging of individual modified periodograms has been shown to provide a consistent estimator of the power spectrum. An extension of this technique, the compressed spectral array, has been particularly useful for evaluating EEG spectra over long periods of time. A detailed review of the development and use of various methods to analyze the EEG is provided by Bronzino et al. [1984] and Givens and Remond [1987].

Figure 15.2 provides an overview of the computational processes involved in performing spectral analysis of the EEG, i.e., including computation of auto- and cross-spectra [Bronzino et al., 1984]. It is to be noted that the power spectrum is the *autocorrelellogram*, i.e., the correlation of the signal with itself. As a result, the power spectrum provides only magnitude information in the frequency domain; it does not provide any data regarding phase. The power spectrum is computed by

$$P(f) = R_e^2[X(f)] + I_m^2[X(f)] \qquad (15.6)$$

where $X(f)$ is the Fourier transform of the EEG signal.

Power spectral analysis not only provides a summary of the EEG in a convenient graphic form but also facilitates statistical analysis of EEG changes that may not be evident on simple inspection of the records. In addition to absolute power derived directly from the power spectrum, other measures calculated from absolute power have been demonstrated to be of value in quantifying various aspects of the EEG. Relative power expresses the percentage contribution of each frequency band to the total power and is calculated by dividing the power within a band by the total power across all bands. Relative power has the benefit of reducing the intersubject variance associated with absolute power that arises from intersubject differences in skull and scalp conductance. The disadvantage of relative power is that an increase in one frequency band will be reflected in the calculation by a de-

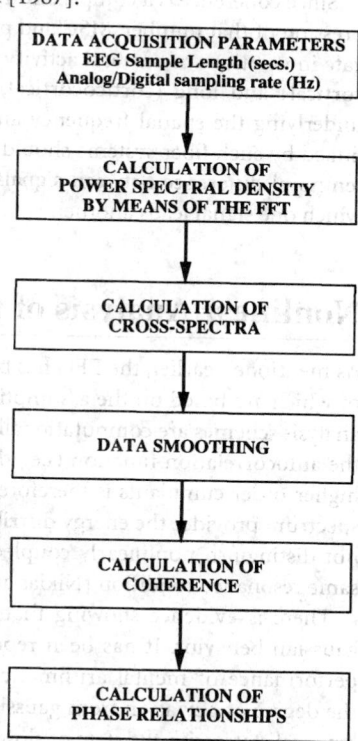

FIGURE 15.2 Block diagram illustrating the steps involved in conventional (linear) spectral analysis of EEG activity.

crease in other bands; for example, it has been reported that directional shifts between high and low frequencies are associated with changes in cerebral blood flow and metabolism. Power ratios between low (0 to 7 Hz) and high (10 to 20 Hz) frequency bands have been demonstrated to be an accurate estimator of changes in cerebral activity during these metabolic changes.

Although the power spectrum quantifies activity at each electrode, other variables derivable from the FFT offer a means of quantifying the relationships between signals recorded from multiple electrodes or sites. Coherence (which is a complex number), calculated from the cross-spectrum analysis of two signals, is similar to cross-correlation in the time domain.

The cross-spectrum is computed by

$$\text{Cross spectrum} = X(f)Y^*(f) \qquad (15.7)$$

where $X(f)$ and $Y(f)$ are Fourier transforms, and $*$ indicates the complex conjugate.

Coherence is calculated by

$$\text{Coherence} = \frac{\text{cross spectrum}}{\sqrt{PX(f) - PY(f)}} \qquad (15.8)$$

The magnitude squared coherence (MSC) values range from 1 to 0, indicating maximum and no synchrony, respectively. The temporal relationship between two signals is expressed by the phase angle, which is a measure of the lag between two signals of common frequency components or bands.

Since coherence is a complex number, the phase is simply the angle associated with the polar expression of that number. MSC and phase then represent measures that can be employed to investigate interactions of cerebral activity recorded from separate brain sites. For example, short (intracortical) and long (corticocortical) pathways have been proposed as the anatomic substrates underlying the spatial frequency and patterns of coherence. Therefore, discrete cortical regions linked by such fiber systems should demonstrate a relatively high degree of synchrony, while the temporal difference between signals, represented by the phase measure, quantifies the extent to which one signal leads another.

15.5 Nonlinear Analysis of the EEG

As mentioned earlier, the EEG has been studied extensively using signal-processing schemes, most of which are based on the assumption that the EEG is a linear, gaussian process. Although linear analysis schemes are computationally efficient and useful, they only utilize information retained in the autocorrelation function (i.e., the second-order cumulant). Additional information stored in higher-order cumulants is therefore ignored by linear analysis of the EEG. Thus, while the power spectrum provides the energy distribution of a stationary process in the frequency domain, it cannot distinguish nonlinearly coupled frequencies from spontaneously generated signals with the same resonance condition [Nikias and Raghvveer, 1987].

There is evidence showing that the amplitude distribution of the EEG often deviates from gaussian behavior. It has been reported, for example, that the EEG of humans involved in the performance of mental arithmetic task exhibits significant nongaussian behavior. In addition, the degree of deviation from gaussian behavior of the EEG has been shown to depend on the behavioral state, with the state of slow-wave sleep showing less gaussian behavior than quiet waking, which is less gaussian than rapid eye movement (REM) sleep [Ning and Bronzino, 1989a,b]. Nonlinear signal-processing algorithms such as bispectral analysis are therefore necessary to address nongaussian and nonlinear behavior of the EEG in order to better describe it in the frequency domain.

But what exactly is the bispectrum? For a zero-mean, stationary process $\{X(k)\}$, the bispectrum, by definition, is the Fourier transform of its third-order cumulant (TOC) sequence:

$$B(\omega_1, \omega_2) = \sum_{m=-\alpha}^{\alpha} \sum_{n=-\alpha}^{\alpha} C(m, n) \, e^{-j(w_1 m + w_2 n)} \qquad (15.9)$$

The TOC sequence $\{C(m, n)\}$ is defined as the expected value of the triple product

$$C(m, n) = E\{X(k) \, X(k + m) \, X(k + n)\} \qquad (15.10)$$

If process $X(k)$ is purely gaussian, then its third-order cumulant $C(m, n)$ is zero for each (m, n), and consequently, its Fourier transform, the bispectrum, $B(\omega_1, \omega_2)$ is also zero. This property makes the estimated bispectrum an immediate measure describing the degree of deviation from gaussian behavior. In our studies [Ning and Bronzino, 1989a,b], the sum of magnitude of the estimated bispectrum was used as a measure to describe the EEG's deviation from gaussian behavior, that is,

$$D = \sum_{(\omega_1 \omega_2)} |B(\omega_1, \omega_2)| \qquad (15.11)$$

Using bispectral analysis, the existence of significant quadratic phase coupling (QPC) in the hippocampal EEG obtained during REM sleep in the adult rat was demonstrated [Ning and Bronzino, 1989a,b, 1990]. The result of this nonlinear coupling is the appearance, in the frequency spectrum, of a small peak centered at approximately 13 to 14 Hz (beta range) that reflects the summation of the two theta frequency (i.e., in the 6- to 7-Hz range) waves (Fig. 15.3). Conventional power spectral (linear) approaches are incapable of distinguishing the fact that this peak results from the interaction of these two generators and is not intrinsic to either.

To examine the phase relationship between nonlinear signals collected at different sites, the *cross-bispectrum* is also a useful tool. For example, given three zero-mean, stationary processes $\{x_j(n) j = 1, 2, 3\}$, there are two conventional methods for determining the cross-bispectral relationship, *direct* and *indirect*. Both methods first divide these three processes into M segments of shorter but equal length. The direct method computes the Fourier transform of each segment for all three processes and then estimates the cross-bispectrum by taking the average of triple products of Fourier coefficients over M segments, that is,

$$B_{x_1 x_2 x_3}(\omega_1, \omega_2) = \frac{1}{M} \sum_{m=1}^{M} X_1^m(\omega_1) \, X_2^m(\omega_2) \, X_3^{m*}(\omega_1 + \omega_2) \qquad (15.12)$$

where $X_j^m(\omega)$ is the Fourier transform of the mth segment of $\{x_j(n)\}$, and $*$ indicates the complex conjugate.

The indirect method computes the third-order cross-cumulant sequence for all segments:

$$C_{x_1 x_2 x_3}^m(k, l) = \sum_{n \in \tau} x_1^m(n) \, x_2^m(n + k) \, x_3^m(n + l) \qquad (15.13)$$

where τ is the admissible set for argument n. The cross-cumulant sequences of all segments will be averaged to give a resultant estimate:

$$C_{x_1 x_2 x_3}(k, l) = \frac{1}{M} \sum_{m=1}^{M} C_{x_1 x_2 x_3}^m(k, l) \qquad (15.14)$$

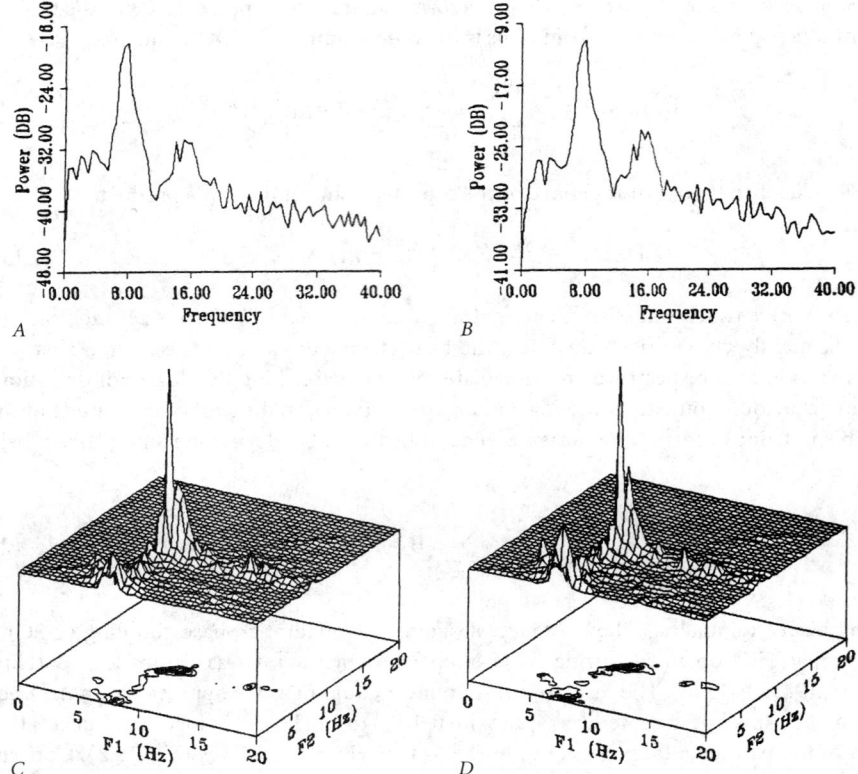

FIGURE 15.3 Plots *a* and *b* represent the averaged power spectra of sixteen 8-s epochs of REM sleep (digital sampling rate = 128 Hz) obtained from hippocampal subfields CA1 and the dentate gyrus, respectively. Note that both spectra exhibit clear power peaks at approximately 8 Hz (theta rhythm) and 16 Hz (beta activity). Plots *c* and *d* represent the bispectra of these same epochs, respectively. Computation of the bicoherence index at $f(1)$ = 8 Hz, $f(2)$ = 8 Hz showed significant quadratic phase coupling (QPC), indicating that the 16-Hz peak seen in the power spectra is not spontaneously generated but rather results from the summation of activity between the two recording sites.

The cross-bispectrum is then estimated by taking the Fourier transform of the third-order cross-cumulant sequence:

$$B_{x_1 x_2 x_3}(\omega_1, \omega_2) = \sum_{k=-\alpha}^{\alpha} \sum_{l=-\alpha}^{\alpha} C_{x_1 x_2 x_3}(k, l)^{-j(\omega_1 k + \omega_2 l)} \qquad (15.15)$$

Since the variance of the estimated cross-bispectrum is inversely proportional to the length of each segment, computation of the cross-bispectrum for processes of finite data length requires careful consideration of both the length of individual segments and the total number of segments to be used.

The cross-bispectrum can be applied to determine the level of cross-QPC occurring between $\{x_1(n)\}$ and $\{x_2(n)\}$ and its effects on $\{x_3(n)\}$. For example, a peak at $Bx_1x_2x_3(\omega_1, \omega_2)$ suggests that the energy component at frequency $\omega_1 + \omega_2$ of $\{x_3(n)\}$ is generated due to the QPC between frequency ω_1 of $\{x_1(n)\}$ and frequency ω_2 of $\{x_2(n)\}$. In theory, the absence of QPC will generate a flat cross-bispectrum. However, due to the finite data length encountered in practice, peaks may appear in the cross-bispectrum at locations where there is no significant cross-QPC. To avoid improper interpre-

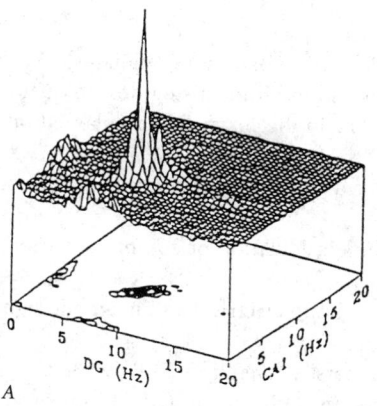
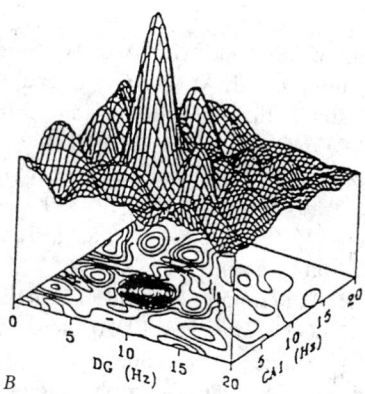

FIGURE 15.4 Cross-bispectral plots of $B_{CA1-DG-CA1}(\omega_1, \omega_2)$ computed using (*a*) the direct method and (*b*) the indirect method.

tation, the cross-bicoherence index, which indicates the significance level of cross-QPC, can be computed as follows:

$$bic_{x_1 x_2 x_3}(\omega_1, \omega_2) = \frac{B_{x_1 x_2 x_3}(\omega_1, \omega_2)}{\sqrt{P_{x_1}(\omega_1)P_{x_2}(\omega_2)P_{x_3}(\omega_1 + \omega_2)}} \qquad (15.16)$$

where $P_{xj}(\omega)$ is the power spectrum of process $\{x_j(n)\}$. The theoretical value of the bicoherence index ranges between 0 and 1, i.e., from nonsignificant to highly significant.

In situations where the interest is the presence of QPC and its effects on $\{x(n)\}$, the cross-bispectrum equations can be modified by replacing $\{x_1(n)\}$ and $\{x_3(n)\}$ with $\{x(n)\}$ and $\{x_2(n)\}$ with $\{y(n)\}$, that is,

$$B_{xyz}(\omega_1, \omega_2) = \frac{1}{M} \sum_{m=1}^{M} X^m(\omega_1)\, Y^m(\omega_2)\, X^{m\star}(\omega_1 + \omega_2) \qquad (15.17)$$

In theory, both methods will lead to the same cross-bispectrum when data length is infinite. However, with finite data records, direct and indirect methods generally lead to cross-bispectrum estimates with different shapes (Fig. 15.4). Therefore, like power spectrum estimation, users have to choose an appropriate method to extract the information desired.

Defining Terms

Bispectra: Computation of the frequency distribution of the EEG exhibiting nonlinear behavior.

Cross-spectra: Computation of the energy in the frequency distribution of two different electrical signals.

Electroencephalogram (EEG): Recordings of the electrical potentials produced by the brain.

Fast Fourier transform (FFT): Algorithms that permit rapid computation of the Fourier transform of an electrical signal, thereby representing it in the frequency domain.

Magnitude squared coherence (MSC): A measure of the degree of synchrony between two electrical signals at specified frequencies.

Power spectral analysis: Computation of the energy in the frequency distribution of an electrical signal.

Quadratic phase coupling (QPC): A measure of the degree to which specific frequencies interact to produce a third frequency.

References

Brazier M. 1968. Electrical Activity of the Nervous System, 3d ed. Baltimore, Williams & Wilkins.

Bronzino JD, Kelly M, Cordova C, et al. 1981. Utilization of amplitude histograms to quantify the EEG: Effects of systemic administration of morphine in the chronically implanted rat. IEEE Trans Biomed Eng 28(10):673.

Bronzino JD. 1984. Quantitative analysis of the EEG: General concepts and animal studies. IEEE Trans Biomed Eng 31(12):850.

Cooley JW, Tukey JS. 1965. An algorithm for the machine calculation of complex Fourier series. Math Comput 19:267.

Givens AS, Remond A (eds). 1987. Methods of analysis of brain electrical and magnetic signals. In EEG Handbook, vol 1. Amsterdam, Elsevier.

Kay SM, Maple SL. 1981. Spectrum analysis—A modern perspective. Proc IEEE 69:1380.

Kondraske GV. 1986. Neurophysiological measurements. In JD Bronzino (ed), Biomedical Engineering and Instrumentation, pp 138–179. Boston, PWS Publishing.

Nikias CL, Raghuveer MR. 1987. Bispectrum estimation: A digital signal processing framework. Proc IEEE 75:869.

Ning T, Bronzino JD. 1989a. Bispectral analysis of the rat EEG during different vigilance states. IEEE Trans Biomed Eng 36(4):497.

Ning T, Bronzino JD. 1989b. Bispectral analysis of the EEG in developing rats. In Proc Workshop Higher-Order Spectral Anal, Vail, CO, pp 235–238.

Ning T, Bronzino JD. 1990. Autoregressive and bispectral analysis techniques: EEG applications. Special Issue on Biomedical Signal Processing. IEEE Eng Med Biol Mag 9:47.

Smith JR. 1986. Automated analysis of sleep EEG data. In Clinical Applications of Computer Analysis of EEG and Other Neurophysiological Signals, EEG Handbook, revised series, vol 2, pp 93–130. Amsterdam, Elsevier.

Further Information

See *The Electroencephalogram: Its Patterns and Origins,* by J. S. Barlow (Cambridge, Mass., MIT Press, 1993). See also the journals, *IEEE Transactions in Biomedical Engineering* and *Electroencephalography and Clinical Neurophysiology.*

16

Biomagnetism

akko Malmivuo
gnar Granit Institute,
mpere University of
chnology

Since the first detection of the magnetocardiogram (MCG) in 1963 by Baule and McFee [Baule and McFee, 1963], new diagnostic information from biomagnetic signals has been widely anticipated. The first recording of the magnetoencephalogram (MEG) was made in 1968 by David Cohen [Cohen, 1968], but it was not possible to record biomagnetic signals with good signal quality before the invention of the superconducting quantum interference device (SQUID) in 1970 [Zimmerman et al., 1970].

16.1 Theoretical Background

Origin of Bioelectric and Biomagnetic Signals

In 1819, Hans Christian Örsted demonstrated that when an electric current flows in a conductor, it generates a magnetic field around it [Örsted, 1820]. This fundamental connection between electricity and magnetism was expressed in exact form by James Clerk Maxwell in 1864 [Maxwell, 1865]. In bioelectromagnetism, this means that when electrically active tissue produces a bioelectric field, it simultaneously produces a biomagnetic field as well. Thus the origin of both the bioelectric and the biomagnetic signals is the bioelectric activity of the tissue.

The following equations describe the electric potential field (16.1) and the magnetic field (16.2) of a volume source distribution $\bar{J}^i$ in an inhomogeneous volume conductor. The inhomogeneous volume conductor is represented by a piecewise homogeneous conductor where the regions of different conductivity σ are separated by surfaces S.

8493-8346-3/95/$0.00+$.50
1995 by CRC Press, Inc.

$$4\pi\sigma\Phi\,(r) = \int_{v} \bar{J}^{i} \cdot \nabla\left(\frac{1}{r}\right) dv + \sum_{j} \int_{S_j} (\sigma_j'' - \sigma_j') \Phi\nabla\left(\frac{1}{r}\right) d\bar{S}_j \qquad (16.1)$$

$$4\pi\bar{H}\,(r) = \int_{v} \bar{J}^{i} \times \nabla\left(\frac{1}{r}\right) dv + \sum_{j} \int_{S_j} (\sigma_j'' - \sigma_j') \Phi\nabla\left(\frac{1}{r}\right) d\bar{S}_j \qquad (16.2)$$

The first term on the right-hand side of Eqs. (16.1) and (16.2) describes the *contribution of the volume source,* and the second term describes the contribution of boundaries separating regions of different conductivity, i.e., the *contribution of the inhomogeneities* within the volume conductor. These equations were developed by David Geselowitz [Geselowitz, 1967, 1970].

Measurement of the Biomagnetic Signals

The amplitude of the biomagnetic signals is very low. The strongest of them is the MCG, having an amplitude on the order of 50 pT. This is roughly one-millionth of the static magnetic field of the earth. The amplitude of the MEG is roughly 1% of that of the MCG. This means that, in practice, the MEG can only be measured with the SQUID and that the measurements must be done in a magnetically shielded room. The MCG, instead, can be measured in the clinical environment without magnetic shielding.

Independence of Bioelectric and Biomagnetic Signals

The source of the biomagnetic signal is the *electric* activity of the tissue. Therefore, the most interesting and most important question in biomagnetism is whether the biomagnetic signals contain new information that cannot be obtained from bioelectric signals; in other words, whether the bioelectric and biomagnetic signals are fully independent or whether there is some interdependence. If the signals were fully independent, the biomagnetic measurement would possibly give about the same amount of new information as the bioelectric method. If there were some interdependence, the amount of new information would be reduced.

Helmholtz's theorem states that "A general vector field, that vanishes at infinity, can be completely represented as the sum of two independent vector fields, one that is irrotational (zero curl) and another that is solenoidal (zero divergence)" [Morse and Feshbach, 1953; Plonsey and Collin, 1961]. The impressed current density $\bar{J}^{i}$ is a vector field that vanishes at infinity and, according to the theorem, may be expressed as the sum of two components:

$$\bar{J}^{i} = \bar{J}^{i}_{F} + \bar{J}^{i}_{V} \qquad (16.3)$$

where the subscripts F and V denote *flow* and *vortex,* respectively. By definition, these vector fields satisfy $\nabla \times \bar{J}^{i}_{F} = 0$ and $\nabla \cdot \bar{J}^{i}_{V} = 0$. We first examine the independence of the electric and magnetic signals in the infinite homogeneous case, when the second term on the right-hand side of Eqs. (16.1) and (16.2), caused by inhomogeneities, is zero. The equation for the electric potential may be rewritten as

$$4\pi\sigma\Phi = \int_{v} \nabla\left(\frac{1}{r}\right) \cdot \bar{J}^{i}\, dv = \int_{v} \frac{\nabla \cdot \bar{J}^{i}}{r}\, dv \qquad (16.4)$$

and that for the magnetic field may be rewritten as

$$4\pi\bar{H} = -\int_{v} \nabla\left(\frac{1}{r}\right) \times \bar{J}^{i}\, dv = -\int_{v} \frac{\nabla \times \bar{J}^{i}}{r}\, dv \qquad (16.5)$$

Substituting Eq. (16.3) into Eqs. (16.4) and (16.5) shows that under homogeneous and unbounded conditions, the bioelectric field arises from $\nabla \cdot \bar{J}^i_v$, which is the *flow source*, and the biomagnetic field arises from $\nabla \times \bar{J}^i_v$, which is the *vortex source*. For this reason, in the early days of biomagnetic research it was generally believed that the bioelectric and biomagnetic signals were fully independent. However, it was soon recognized that this could not be the case. For example, when the heart beats, it produces an electric field recorded as the P, QRS, and T waves of the ECG, and it simultaneously produces the corresponding magnetic waves recorded as the MCG. Thus the ECG and MCG signals are not fully independent.

There have been several attempts to explain the independence/interdependence of bioelectric and biomagnetic signals. Usually these attempts discuss different detailed experiments and fail to give a satisfying general explanation. This important issue may be easily explained by considering the sensitivity distributions of the ECG and MCG lead systems, and this will be discussed in the next section.

16.2 Sensitivity Distribution of Dipolar Electric and Magnetic Leads

Concepts of Lead Vector and Lead Field

Lead Vector

Let us assume that two electrodes (or sets of electrodes) are placed on a volume conductor to form a lead. Let us further assume that inside the volume conductor in a certain location Q there is placed a unit dipole consecutively in the x, y, and z directions (Fig. 16.1a). Due to the sources, we measure from the lead the signals c_x, c_y, and c_z, respectively. Due to *linearity*, if instead of the unit dipoles we place in the source location dipoles that are p_x, p_y, and p_z times the unit vectors, we measure signals that are $c_x p_x$, $c_y p_y$, and $c_z p_z$, respectively.

If these dipoles are placed simultaneously to the source location, due to the principle of *superposition*, we measure from the lead a voltage that is

$$V = c_x p_x + c_y p_y + c_z p_z \tag{16.6}$$

These dipoles can be considered to be components of a dipole $\bar{p}$, that is, $\bar{p} = p_x \bar{i} + p_y \bar{j} + p_z \bar{k}$. We may understand the coefficients c_x, c_y, and c_z to be components of a vector $\bar{c}$, that is, $\bar{c} = c_x \bar{i} + c_y \bar{j} + c_z \bar{k}$. Now we may express the lead voltage Eq. (16.6) as the scalar product of the vector $\bar{c}$ and the dipole $\bar{p}$ as

$$V = \bar{c} \cdot \bar{p} \tag{16.7}$$

The vector $\bar{c}$ is a three-dimensional transfer coefficient that describes how a dipole source $\bar{p}$ at a fixed point Q inside a volume conductor influences the voltage measured from the lead and is called the *lead vector*.

The lead vector $\bar{c}$ describes what is the sensitivity of the lead to a source locating at the source location. It is self-evident that for another source location the sensitivity may have another value. Thus the sensitivity, i.e., the lead vector, varies as a function of the location, and we may say that it has a certain distribution in the volume conductor. This is called the *sensitivity distribution*.

Lead Field

We may define the value of the lead vector at every point in the volume conductor. If we then place the lead vectors to the points for which they are defined, we have a field of lead vectors throughout the volume conductor. This field of lead vectors is called the *lead field* $\bar{J}_L$. The lead field illustrates the

LINEARITY

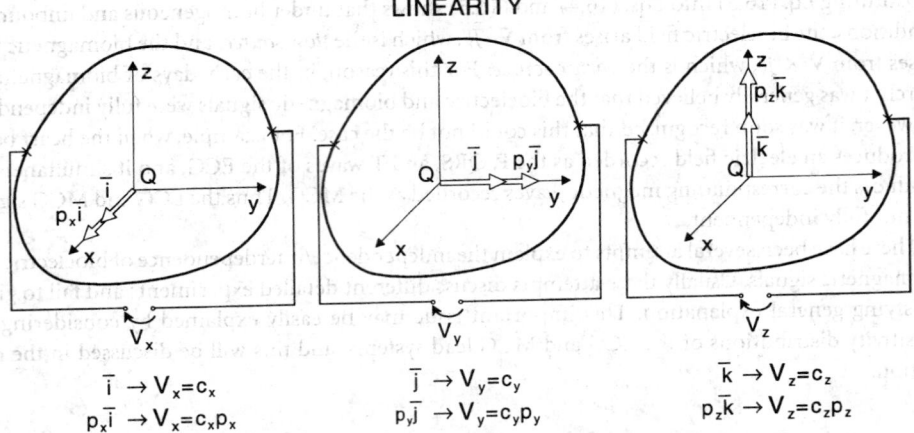

$$\bar{i} \rightarrow V_x = c_x$$
$$p_x\bar{i} \rightarrow V_x = c_x p_x$$

$$\bar{j} \rightarrow V_y = c_y$$
$$p_y\bar{j} \rightarrow V_y = c_y p_y$$

$$\bar{k} \rightarrow V_z = c_z$$
$$p_z\bar{k} \rightarrow V_z = c_z p_z$$

Because of linearity, in each case V is linearly proportional to the dipole magnitude.

SUPERPOSITION

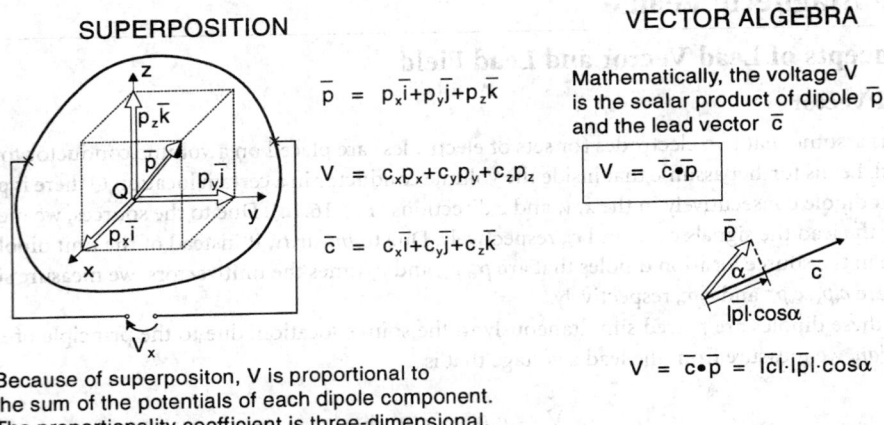

VECTOR ALGEBRA

$$\bar{p} = p_x\bar{i} + p_y\bar{j} + p_z\bar{k}$$

$$V = c_x p_x + c_y p_y + c_z p_z$$

$$\bar{c} = c_x\bar{i} + c_y\bar{j} + c_z\bar{k}$$

Mathematically, the voltage V
is the scalar product of dipole $\bar{p}$
and the lead vector $\bar{c}$

$$\boxed{V = \bar{c} \bullet \bar{p}}$$

$$V = \bar{c} \bullet \bar{p} = |\bar{c}| \cdot |\bar{p}| \cdot \cos\alpha$$

Because of superpositon, V is proportional to
the sum of the potentials of each dipole component.
The proportionality coefficient is three-dimensional.
It is the lead vector $\bar{c}$.

FIGURE 16.1   The concepts of (*a*) lead vector and (*b*) lead field. See the text for more details.

behavior of the sensitivity in the volume conductor and is a very powerful tool in analyzing the properties of electric and magnetic leads (see Fig. 16.1*b*).

It follows from the *principle of reciprocity*, described by Hermann von Helmholtz in 1853 [Helmholtz, 1853], that the lead field is identical to the electric current field that arises in the volume conductor if a unit current, called *reciprocal current* I_R, is fed to the lead.

When we know the lead field $\bar{J}_L$, we can determine the signal V_L in the lead due to the volume source distribution $\bar{J}^i$. For each source element the signal is, of course, proportional to the dot product of the source element and the lead field at the source location, as shown in Eq. (16.7). The contribution of the whole volume source is obtained by integrating this throughout the volume source. Thus the signal the volume source generates to the lead is

$$V_L = \int \frac{1}{\sigma} \bar{J}_L \cdot \bar{J}^i \, dv \qquad (16.8)$$

The lead field may be illustrated either with lead vectors in certain locations in the volume conductor or as the flow lines of the distribution of the reciprocal current in the volume conductor. This is called

FIELD OF LEAD VECTORS

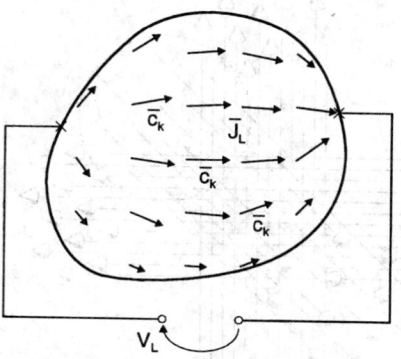

The field of the lead vectors $\bar{c}_k$ is the lead field $\bar{J}_L$

LEAD VOLTAGE

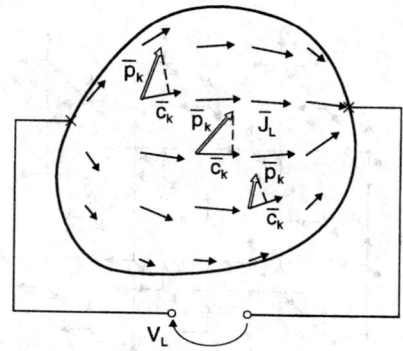

Each dipole element p_k contributes to the lead voltage by $V_k = \bar{c}_k \cdot \bar{p}_k$
The total lead voltage is the sum of the lead voltage elements $V_L = \sum_k \bar{c}_k \cdot \bar{p}_k$

RECIPROCITY

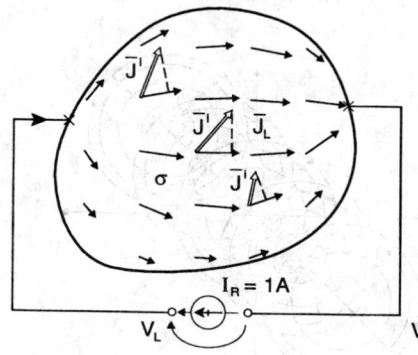

$$V_L = \int \frac{1}{\sigma} \bar{J}_L \cdot \bar{J}^i \, dv$$

Because of reciprocity, the field of lead vectors $\bar{J}_L$ is the same as the current field $\bar{J}_L$ raised by feeding a reciprocal current of 1A to the lead.

ALTERNATIVE ILLUSTRATION

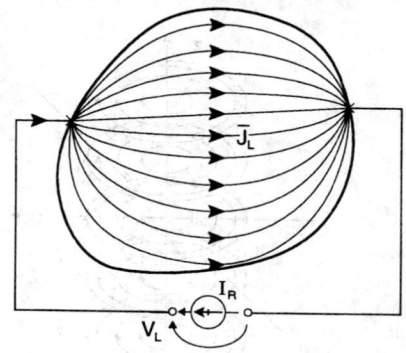

The lead field may also be illustrated with lead field current flow lines.

FIGURE 16.1 *(continued)*.

the *lead current field*. In the latter presentation, the lead field current flow lines are oriented in the direction of the sensitivity, and their density is proportional to the magnitude of the sensitivity.

Lead Fields of Leads Detecting the Electric and Magnetic Dipole Moments of a Volume Source

Electric Lead

The sensitivity of a lead system that detects the electric dipole moment of a volume source consists of three orthogonal components (Fig. 16.2a). Each of these is linear and homogeneous. In other words, one component of the electric dipole moment is detected when the corresponding component of all elements of the impressed current density $\bar{J}^i$ are detected with the same sensitivity throughout the source area.

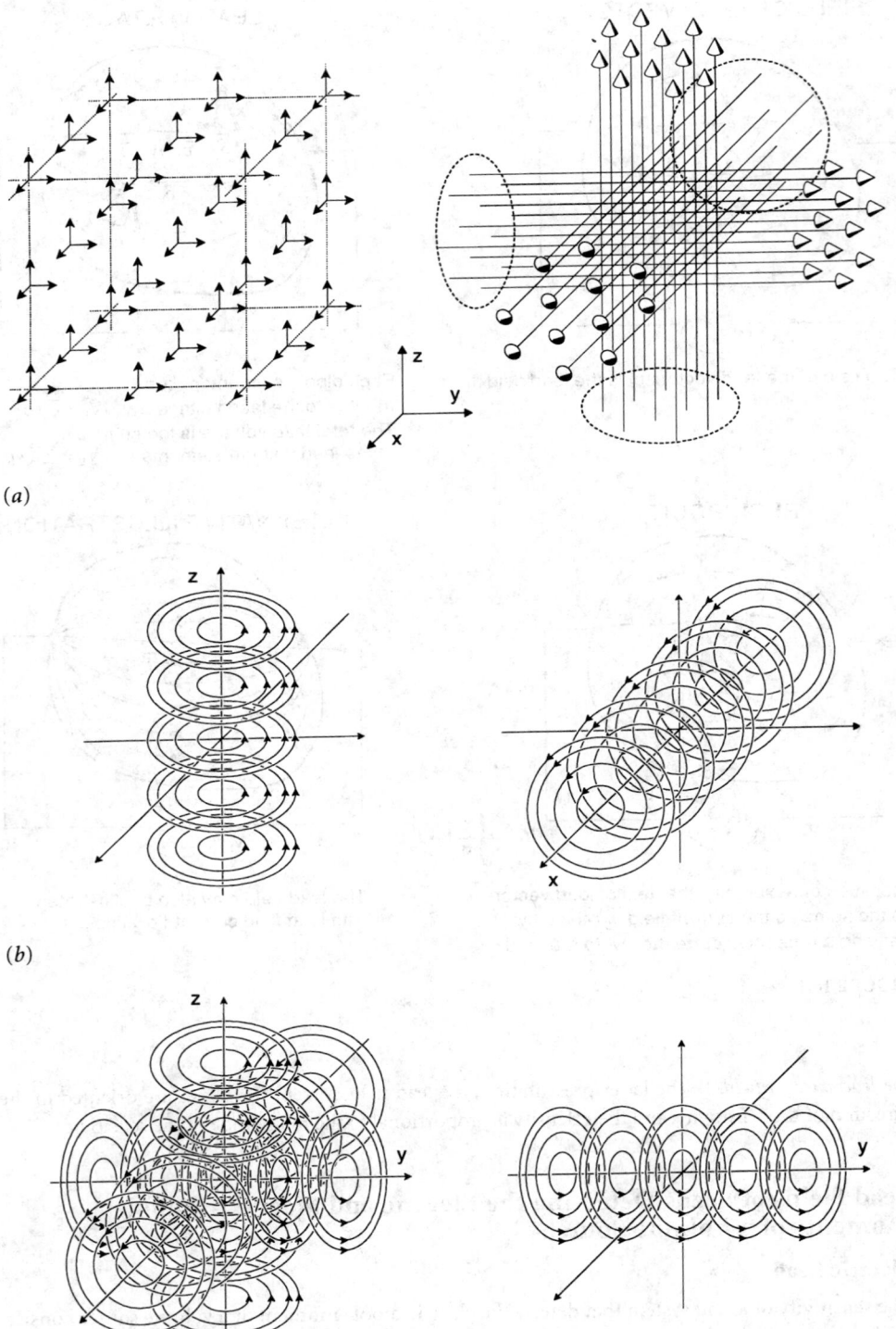

FIGURE 16.2 Sensitivity distributions, i.e., lead fields of lead systems detecting (*a*) electric and (*b*) magnetic dipole moments of a volume source. The lead field of the electric lead is shown both with vectors representing the magnitude and direction of the lead field (on the left) and with lead field current flow lines (on the right).

Magnetic Lead

The sensitivity distribution of a lead system that detects the magnetic dipole moment of a volume source also consists of three orthogonal components (Fig. 16.2b). Each of these has such a form that the sensitivity is always tangentially oriented around the symmetry axis (the coordinate axis). The magnitude of the sensitivity is proportional to the radial distance from the symmetry axis and is zero on the symmetry axis.

Independence of Dipolar Electric and Magnetic Leads

Electric Lead

The sensitivity distributions of the three components of the lead system detecting the electric dipole moment of a volume source are orthogonal. This means that none of them can be obtained as a linear combination of the two other ones. (Note that any fourth measurement having a similar linear sensitivity distribution would always be a linear combination of the three previous ones.) Thus the sensitivity distributions, i.e., the *leads,* are orthogonal and thus independent. However, because the three electric *signals* are only different aspects of the same volume source, they are not (fully) independent.

Magnetic Lead

The sensitivity distributions of the three components of the lead system detecting the magnetic dipole moment of a volume source are also orthogonal, meaning that no one of them can be obtained as a linear combination of the two other ones. Thus, similarly, as in measurement of the electric dipole moment, the sensitivity distributions, i.e., the *leads,* are orthogonal and thus independent. However, because the three magnetic *signals* are only different aspects of the same volume source, they are not (fully) independent.

   On the basis of the sensitivity distributions, we also can similarly explain the independence between the electric and magnetic signals. According to the Helmholtz's theorem, the electric leads are orthogonal to the three magnetic leads. This means that none of these six *leads* can be obtained as a linear combination of the other five. However, the six *signals,* which they measure, are not independent because they arise from the same electrically active volume source.

16.3 Magnetocardiography (MCG)

Selection of the Source Model for MCG

In ECG and MCG it is the clinical problem to solve the inverse problem, i.e., to solve the source of the detected signal in order to get information about the anatomy and physiology of the source. Although the actual clinical diagnostic procedure is based on measuring certain parameters, such as time intervals and amplitudes, from the detected signal and actually not to display the components of the source, the selection of the source model is very important from the point of view of available information.

   In clinical ECG, the source model is a dipole. This is the model for both the 12-lead ECG and vectorcardiography (VCG). In 12-lead ECG, the volume conductor (thorax) model is not considered, which causes considerable distortion of the leads. In VCG, only the form of the volume conductor is modeled. This decreases the distortion in the lead fields but does not eliminate it completely. Note that today the display systems used in these ECG and VCG systems do not play any role in the diagnostic procedure because the computerized diagnosis is always based on the signals, not on the display.

   In selection of the source model for MCG, it is logical, at least initially, to select the magnetic source model to be on the same theoretical level with the ECG. Only in this way is it possible to compare the diagnostic performance of these methods. It is clear, of course, that if the source model is more accurate, i.e., has more independent variables, the diagnostic performance is better, but when comparing ECG and MCG, the comparison is relevant only if their complexity is similar [Malmivuo and Plonsey, 1995].

Detection of the Equivalent Magnetic Dipole of the Heart

The basic detection method of the equivalent magnetic dipole moment of a volume source is to measure the magnetic field on each coordinate axis in the direction of that axis. To idealize the sensitivity distribution throughout the volume source, the measurements must be made at a distance that is large compared with the source dimensions. This, of course, decreases the signal amplitude. The quality of the measurement may be increased considerably if bipolar measurements are used; i.e., measurements are made on both sides of the source. Measurement of the magnetic field on each coordinate axis is, however, difficult to perform in MCG due to the geometry of the human body. It would require either six sequential measurements with one magnetometer (dewar) or six simultaneous measurements using six dewars (Fig. 16.3).

It has been shown [Malmivuo, 1976] that all three components of the magnetic dipole also can be measured from a single location. Applying this unipositional method symmetrically so that measurements are made on both the anterior and posterior sides of the thorax at the same distance from the heart, only two dewars are needed and a very high quality of lead fields is obtained. Figure 16.4 illustrates the sensitivity distributions in nonsymmetrical and symmetrical measurements [Malmivuo and Plonsey, 1995].

Diagnostic Performance of ECG and MCG

The diagnostic performances of ECG and MCG were compared in an extensive study made at the Ragnar Granit Institute [Oja, 1993]. The study was made using the asymmetrical unipositional lead

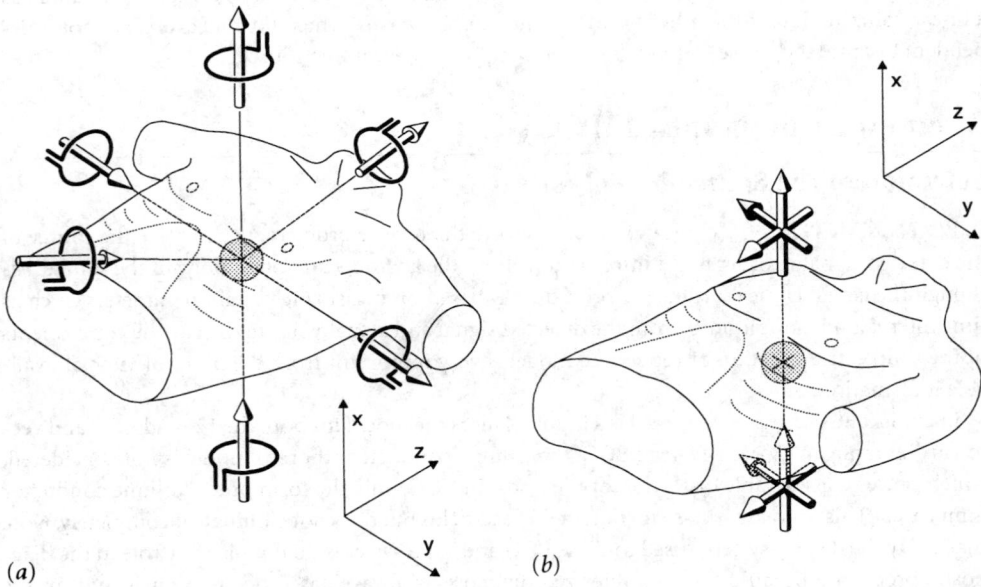

(a)   *(b)*

FIGURE 16.3   Measurement of the three orthogonal components of the magnetic dipole moment of the heart (*a*) on the coordinate axis (*xyz* lead system) and (*b*) at a single location over and under the chest (unipositional lead system).

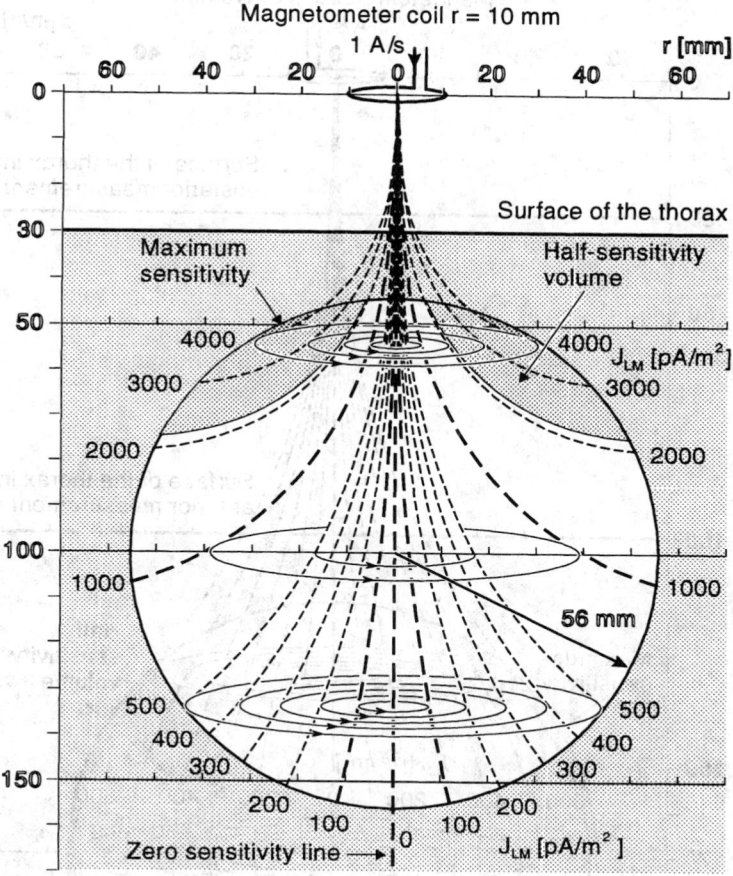

(a) h [mm]

FIGURE 16.4 Sensitivity distributions in the measurement of the magnetic dipole moment of the heart. (a) Nonsymmetrical and (b) symmetrical measurements of the x component. (c) Symmetrical measurement of the y and z components.

system, i.e., making measurements only on the anterior side of the thorax. The patient material was selected, however, so that myocardial changes were located dominantly on the anterior side.

This study consisted of 290 normal subjects and 259 patients with different myocardial disorders. It was found that the diagnostic performance of ECG and MCG is about the same (83%). Diagnostic parameters were then selected from both ECG and MCG. With this combined method, called *electromagnetocardiogram* (EMCG), a diagnostic performance of 90% was obtained. This improvement in diagnostic performance was obtained without increasing the number of parameters used in the diagnostic procedure. Moreover, this improvement is significant because it means that the number of incorrectly diagnosed patients was reduced by approximately 50%.

This important result may be explained as follows: The lead system recording the electric dipole moment of the volume source has three independent leads. (This is also the case in the 12-lead ECG system.) Similarly, the lead system detecting the magnetic dipole moment of the volume source has three independent leads. Therefore, the diagnostic performances of these methods are about the same. However, because the sensitivity distributions of electric and magnetic leads are different, the patient groups diagnosed correctly with both methods are not identical.

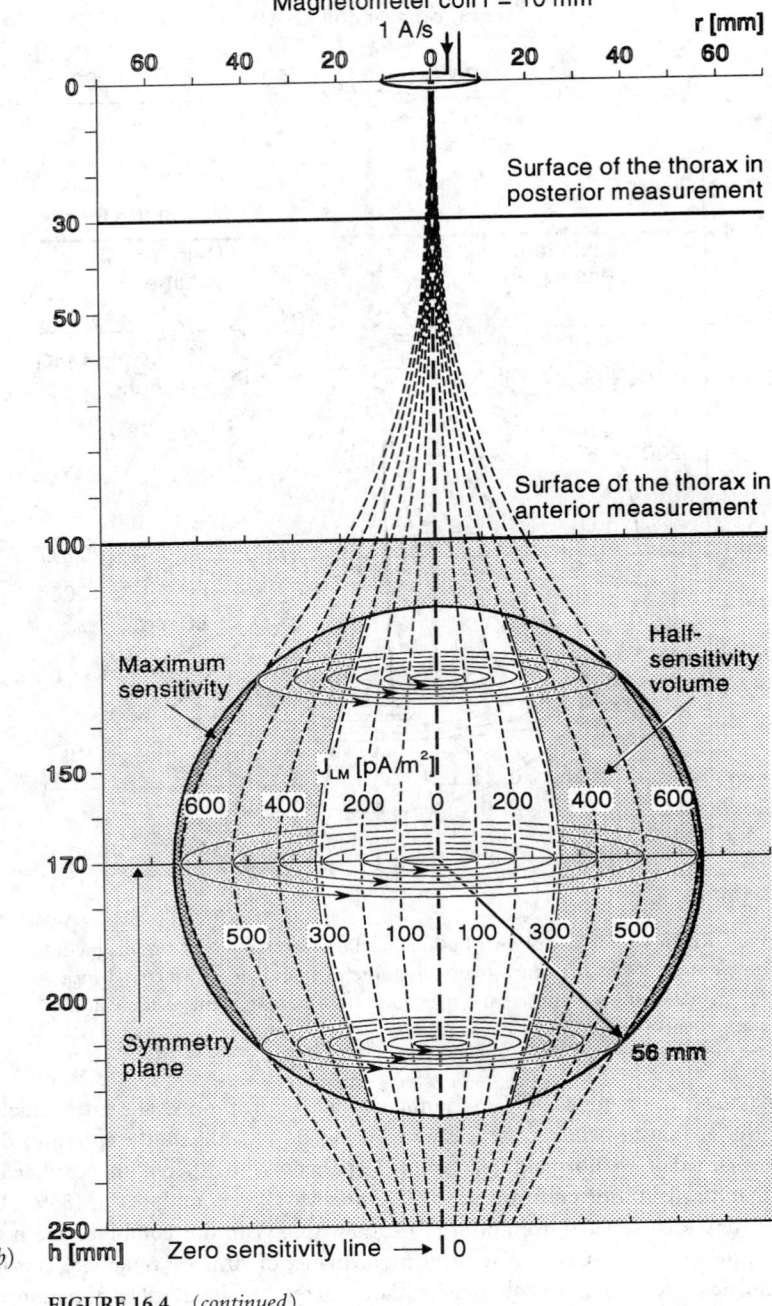

Magnetometer coil r = 10 mm

1 A/s

r [mm]

Surface of the thorax in posterior measurement

Surface of the thorax in anterior measurement

Maximum sensitivity

Half-sensitivity volume

J_{LM} [pA/m^2]

Symmetry plane

56 mm

Zero sensitivity line ⟶ ∣ 0

(b) h [mm]

FIGURE 16.4 (*continued*).

As stated before, the electric leads are independent of the magnetic leads. If the diagnostic procedure simultaneously uses both the ECG and the MCG leads, we obtain $3 + 3 = 6$ independent leads, and the correctly diagnosed patient groups may be combined. Thus the diagnostic performance of the combined method is better than that of either method alone. This is the first large-scale statistically relevant study of the clinical diagnostic performance of biomagnetism.

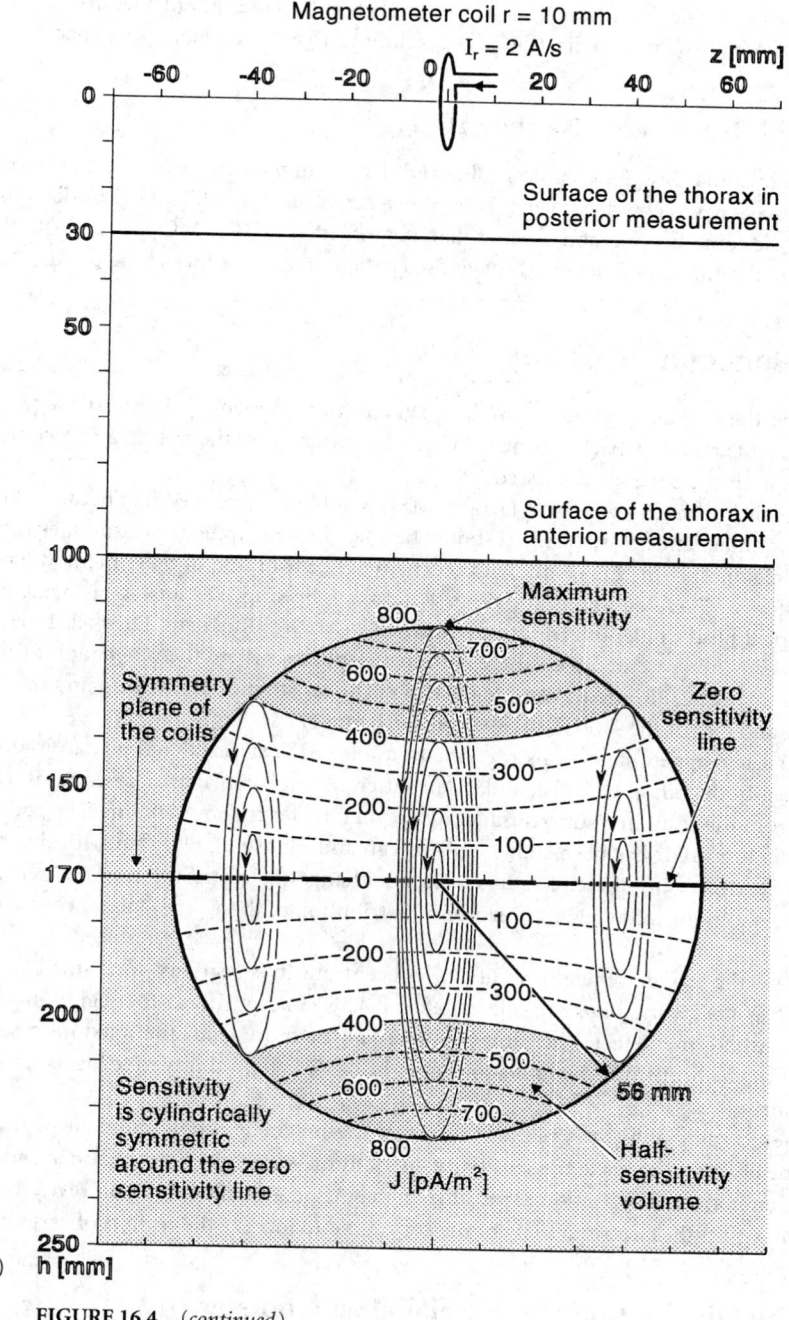

Magnetometer coil r = 10 mm

FIGURE 16.4 *(continued)*.

Technical Reasons to Use the MCG

The technical differences between ECG and MCG include the MCG's far better ability to record static sources, sources on the posterior side of the heart, monitor the fetal heart, and perform electrodeless recording. As a technical drawback, it should be mentioned that the MCG instrument costs 2 to 3 times more. An important feature of MCG is that, unlike the MEG instrument, it does not need a magnetically shielded room. This is very important because the shielded room is not only very expensive but also limits application of the technique to a certain laboratory space.

Theoretical Reasons to Use the MCG

It has been shown that MCG has clinical value and that it can be used either alone or in combination with ECG as a new technique called the *electromagnetocardiogram* (EMCG). The diagnostic performance of the combined method is better than that of either ECG or MCG alone. With the combined method, the number of incorrectly diagnosed patients may be reduced by approximately 50%.

16.4 Magnetoencephalography (MEG)

Similarly as in the cardiac applications, in the magnetic measurement of the electric activity of the brain, the benefits and drawbacks of the MEG can be divided into theoretical and technical ones. First, the theoretical aspects are discussed.

The two main theoretical aspects in favor of MEG are that it is believed that because the skull is transparent for magnetic fields, the MEG should be able to concentrate its measurement sensitivity in a smaller region than the EEG, and that the sensitivity distribution of these methods are fundamentally different. These questions are discussed in the following: The analysis is made using the classic spherical head model introduced by Rush and Driscoll [Rush and Driscoll, 1969]. In this model, the head is represented with three concentric spheres, where the outer radii of the scalp, skull, and brain are 92, 85, and 80 mm, respectively. The resistivities of the scalp and the brain are 2.22 $\Omega \cdot$ cm, and that of the skull is 80 times higher, being 177 $\Omega \cdot$ cm.

The two basic magnetometer constructions in use in MEG are axial and planar gradiometers. In the former, both coils are coaxial, and in the latter, they are coplanar. The minimum distance of the coil from the scalp in a superconducting magnetometer is about 20 mm. The coil radius is usually about 10 mm. It has been shown [Malmivuo and Plonsey, 1995] that with this measurement distance, decreasing the coil radius does not change the distribution of the sensitivity in the brain region. In the following the sensitivity distribution of these gradiometer constructions is discussed.

To indicate the magnetometer's ability to concentrate its sensitivity to a small region, the concept of *half-sensitivity volume* has been defined. This concept means the region in the source area (brain) where the detector sensitivity is one-half or more from the maximum sensitivity. The smaller the half-sensitivity volume, the better is the detector's ability to focus its sensitivity to a small region.

In magnetocardiography, it is relevant to detect the magnetic dipole moment of the volume source of the heart and to make the sensitivity distribution within the heart region as independent of the position in the axial direction as possible. In magnetoencephalography, however, the primary purpose is to detect the electric activity of the cortex and to localize the regions of certain activity.

Sensitivity Distribution of the Axial Magnetometer

In a cylindrically symmetrical volume conductor model, the lead field flow lines are concentric circles and do not cut the discontinuity boundaries. Therefore, the sensitivity distribution in the brain area of the spherical model equals that in an infinite, homogeneous volume conductor.

Figure 16.5 illustrates the sensitivity distribution of an axial magnetometer. The thin solid lines illustrate the lead field flow lines. The dashed lines join the points where the sensitivity has the same value, being thus so-called isosensitivity lines. The half-sensitivity volume is represented by the shaded region.

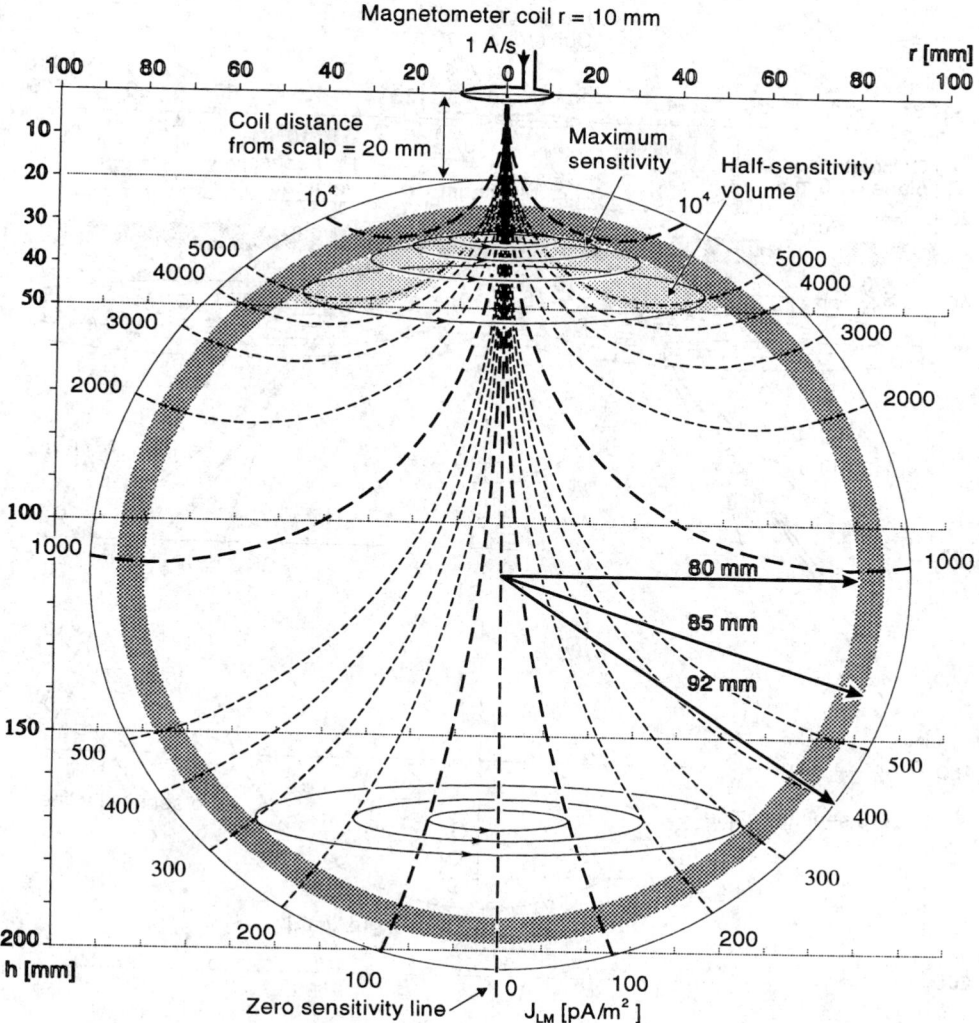

FIGURE 16.5 Sensitivity distribution of the axial magnetometer in measuring the MEG (spherical head model).

Sensitivity Distribution of the Planar Gradiometer

Figure 16.6 illustrates the sensitivity distribution of a planar gradiometer. Again, the thin solid lines illustrate the lead field flow lines, and the dashed lines represent the isosensitivity lines. The half-sensitivity volume is represented by the shaded region. The sensitivity of the planar gradiometer is concentrated under the center of the two coils and is mainly linearly oriented. Further, there exist two zero-sensitivity lines.

Half-Sensitivity Volumes of Electro- and Magnetoencephalography Leads

The half-sensitivity volumes for different EEG and MEG leads as a function of electrode distance and gradiometer baselines are shown in Fig. 16.7. The minimum half-sensitivity volume is, of course, achieved with the shortest distance/baseline. For three- and two-electrode EEG leads, the half-sensitivity volumes at 1 degree of electrode distance are 0.2 and 1.2 cm³, respectively. For

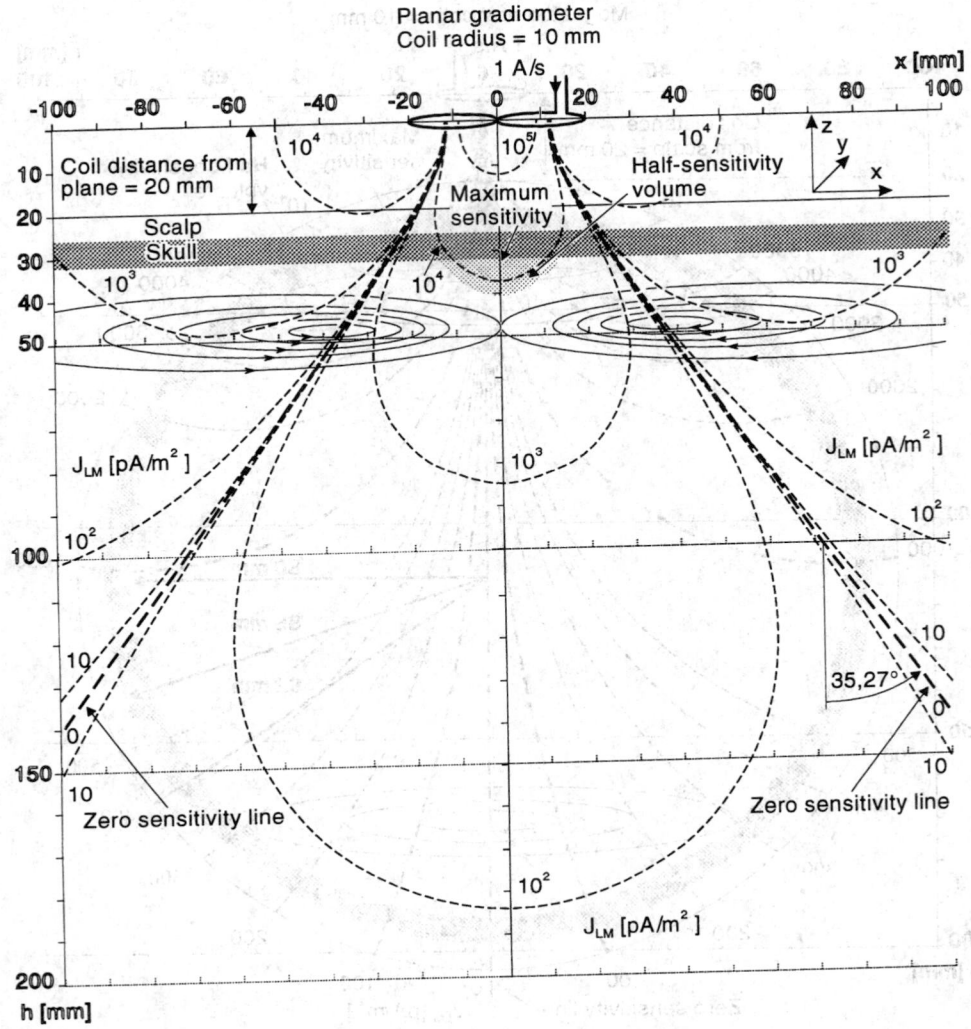

FIGURE 16.6 Sensitivity distribution of the planar gradiometer (half-space model).

10-mm-radius planar and axial gradiometer MEG leads, these volumes at 1 degree of coil separation (i.e., 1.6-mm baseline for axial gradiometer) are 3.4 and 21.8 cm^3, respectively.

The 20-mm coil distance from scalp and 10-mm coil radii are realistic for the helmet-like whole-head MEG detector. There exist, however, MEG devices for recording at a limited region where the coil distance and the coil radii are on the order of 1 mm. Therefore, the half-sensitivity volumes for planar gradiometers with 1-mm coil radius at 0- to 20-mm recording distances are also illustrated in Fig. 16.7. These curves show that when the recording distance is about 12 mm and the distance/baseline is 1 mm, such a planar gradiometer has about the same half-sensitivity volume as the two-electrode EEG.

Short separation will, of course, also decrease the signal amplitude. An optimal value is about 10 degrees of separation. Increasing the separation to 10 degrees increases the EEG and MEG signal amplitudes to approximately 70 to 80 % of their maximum value, but the half-sensitivity volumes do not increase considerably from their values at 1 degree of separation.

Thus, contrary to general belief, the EEG has a better ability to focus its sensitivity to a small region in the brain than the whole-head MEG. At about 20 to 30 degrees of separation, the two-

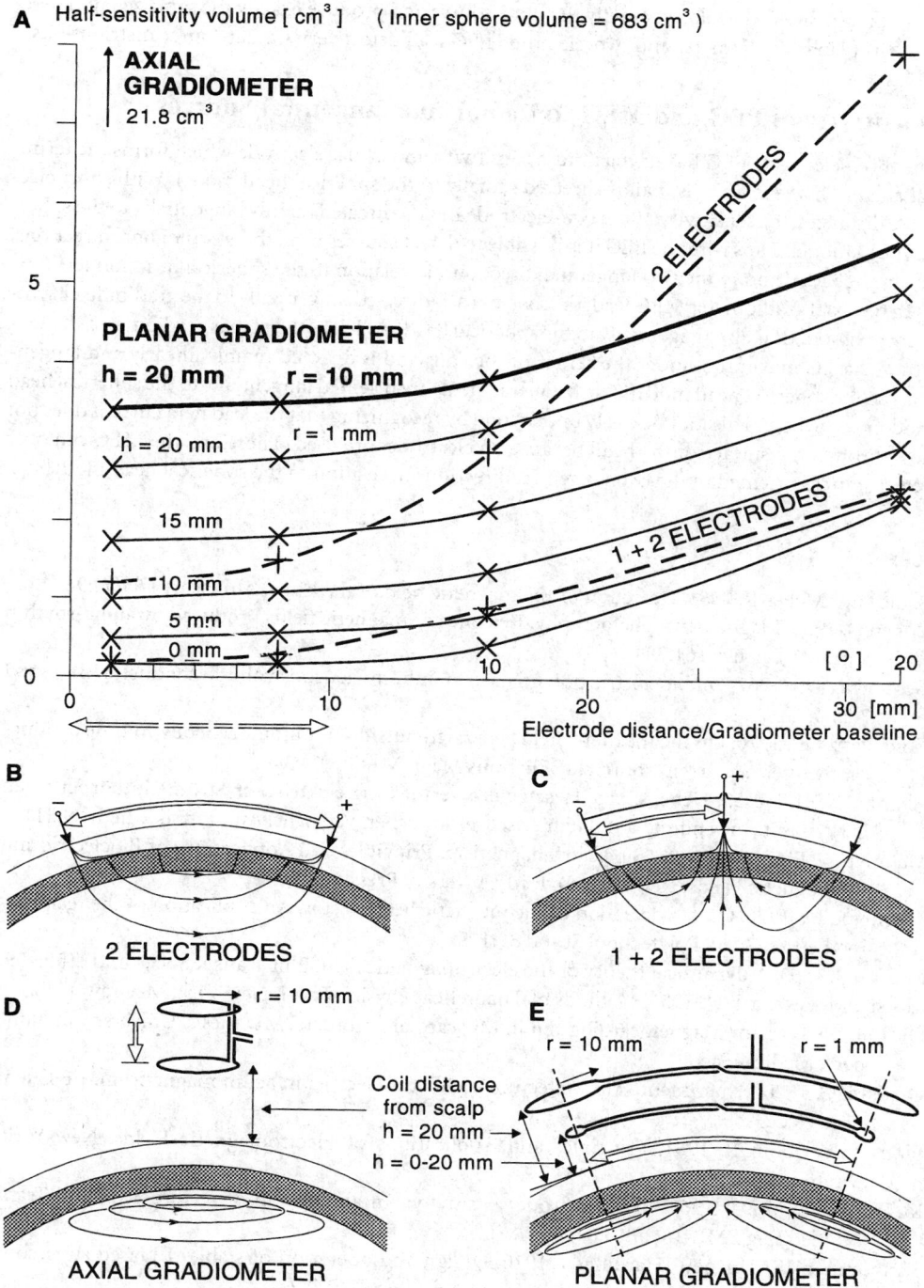

A Half-sensitivity volume [cm^3]   (Inner sphere volume = 683 cm^3)

AXIAL GRADIOMETER
21.8 cm^3

PLANAR GRADIOMETER

h = 20 mm   r = 10 mm

2 ELECTRODES

h = 20 mm   r = 1 mm

15 mm

1 + 2 ELECTRODES

10 mm

5 mm

0 mm

Electrode distance/Gradiometer baseline

B

2 ELECTRODES

C

1 + 2 ELECTRODES

D

r = 10 mm

AXIAL GRADIOMETER

E

r = 10 mm   r = 1 mm

Coil distance from scalp
h = 20 mm
h = 0-20 mm

PLANAR GRADIOMETER

FIGURE 16.7 Half-sensitivity volumes of different EEG leads (*dashed lines*) and MEG leads (*solid lines*) as a function of electrode distance and gradiometer baseline, respectively.

electrode EEG lead needs slightly smaller separation to achieve the same half-sensitivity volume as the planar gradiometer. The sensitivity distributions of these leads are, however, very similar. Note that if the sensitivity distributions of two different lead systems, whether they are electric or magnetic, are the same, they detect exactly the same source and produce exactly the same signal. Therefore, the planar gradiometer and two-electrode EEG lead detect very similar source distributions.

Sensitivity of EEG and MEG to Radial and Tangential Sources

The three-electrode EEG has its maximum sensitivity under that electrode which forms the terminal alone. This sensitivity is mainly directed radially to the spherical head model. With short electrode distances, the sensitivity of the two-electrode EEG is directed mainly tangentially to the spherical head model. Thus with the EEG it is possible to detect sources in all three orthogonal directions, i.e., in the radial and in the two tangential directions, in relation to the spherical head model.

In the axial gradiometer MEG lead, the sensitivity is directed tangentially to the gradiometer symmetry axis and thus also tangentially to the spherical head model. In the planar gradiometer, the sensitivity has its maximum under the center of the coils and is directed mainly linearly and tangentially to the spherical head model. The MEG lead fields are oriented tangentially to the spherical head model everywhere. This may be easily understood by recognizing that the lead field current does not flow through the surface of the head because no electrodes are used. Therefore, the MEG can only detect sources oriented in the two tangential directions in relation to the spherical head model.

References

Baule GM, McFee R. 1963. Detection of the magnetic field of the heart. Am Heart J 55(7):95.

Cohen D. 1968. Magnetoencephalography: Evidence of magnetic fields produced by alpha-rhythm currents. Science 161:784.

Geselowitz DB. 1967. On bioelectric potentials in an inhomogeneous volume conductor. Biophys J 7(1):1.

Geselowitz DB. 1970. On the magnetic field generated outside an inhomogeneous volume conductor by internal current sources. IEEE Trans Magn MAG-6(2):346.

Helmholtz HLF. 1853. Ueber einige Gesetze der Vertheilung elektrischer Ströme in körperlichen Leitern mit Anwendung auf die thierisch-elektrischen Versuche. Ann Physik Chem 89:211.

Malmivuo J, Plonsey R. 1995. Bioelectromagnetism: Principles and Applications of Bioelectric and Biomagnetic Fields. New York, Oxford University Press.

Malmivuo JA. 1976. On the detection of the magnetic heart vector: An application of the reciprocity theorem. Acta Polytechnol Scand 39:112.

Maxwell J. 1865. A dynamical theory of the electromagnetic field. Phil Trans R Soc (Lond) 155:459.

Morse PM, Feshbach H. 1953. Methods of Theoretical Physics, part I. New York, McGraw-Hill.

Oja OS. 1993. Vector Magnetocardiogram in Myocardial Disorders, MD thesis, University of Tampere, Medical Faculty.

Örsted HC. 1820. Experimenta circa effectum conflictus electrici in acum magneticam. J F Chem Phys 29:275.

Plonsey R, Collin R. 1961. Principles and Applications of Electromagnetic Fields. New York, McGraw-Hill.

Rush S, Driscoll DA. 1969. EEG-electrode sensitivity: An application of reciprocity. IEEE Trans Biomed Eng BME-16(1):15.

Zimmerman JE, Thiene P, Hardings J. 1970. Design and operation of stable rf biased superconducting point-contact quantum devices. J Appl Phys 41:1572.

17

Electric Stimulation of Excitable Tissue

Dominique M. Durand
Case Western Reserve University

17.1 Electric Stimulation of Neural Tissue

Functional electric stimulation (FES) of neural tissue provides a method to restore normal function to neurologically impaired individuals. By inserting electrodes inside or near nerves, it is possible to activate pathways to the brain or to muscles. *Functional nerve stimulation* (FNS) is often used to describe applications of electric stimulation in the peripheral nervous system. *Neural prostheses* refer to applications for which electric stimulation is used to replace a function previously lost or damaged.

Electric stimulation has been used to treat several types of neurologic dysfunction with varying amounts of success [see Hambrecht, 1979]. For example, electric stimulation of the auditory nerves to restore hearing in deaf patients has proved to be not only feasible but also clinically useful [Clark et al., 1990]. Similarly, the phrenic nerve of patients with high-level spinal cord injury can be stimulated to produce diaphragm contractions and restore ventilation [Glenn et al., 1984]. Electric stimulation of the visual cortex produces visual sensations called *phosphenes* [Brindley and Lewin, 1968], and a visual prosthesis for the blind is currently being tested. Electric stimulation in the peripheral

0-8493-8346-3/95/$0.00+$.50
© 1995 by CRC Press, Inc.

nerves of paralyzed patients can restore partial function of both the upper extremities for hand function [Peckham et al., 1977] and lower extremities for gait [Marsolais and Kobetic, 1988]. Several other attempts were not so successful. Electric stimulation of the cerebellum cortex for controlling epileptic seizures has been tried but was not reliable. However, a new method involving stimulation of the vagus nerve looks promising [Rutecki, 1990]. There are many other applications of electric stimulation of the nervous system and many problems associated with each one, but it is now clear that the potential and the limits of the technique have not yet been realized. Other excitable tissues such as cardiac muscle can also be excited by externally applied electric fields. The underlying principles are similar to those reviewed below for neural tissue.

Stimulation of the nervous system also can be achieved with magnetic fields [Chokroverty, 1990]. A coil is placed near the excitable tissue, and a capacitor is rapidly discharged into the coil. Large magnetic fluxes are generated, and the induced electric fields can generate excitation. Magnetic stimulation has several advantages over electric stimulation. Magnetic fields can easily penetrate low-conductivity tissues such as bone, and the stimulation is completely noninvasive. However, magnetic stimulation requires a large amount of energy, and the magnetic field is difficult to localize. Magnetic stimulation of excitable tissue shares many aspects with electric stimulation, since the electric field is, in both cases, the source of the stimulus [Roth and Basser, 1990]. However, there are several important differences [Durand et al., 1992; Nagarajan et al., 1993] that will not be reviewed below.

What is the basis for the effect of electric stimulation of the nervous system? Clearly, it comes from the fact that a propagated action potential can be triggered by applying a rapidly changing electric field near excitable tissue. This fact was demonstrated early in this century, and clinical experimental applications in the 1950s resulted in the highly successful cardiac pacemaker. Other clinical applications have been slow in coming for several reasons to be discussed below. One of the difficulties is that the fundamental principles of the interaction of electric fields and neurons is not completely understood. In order to understand how applied currents can generate excitation, it will necessary to describe the mechanisms underlying excitation (Sec. 17.2), the distribution of currents inside the volume conductor (Sec. 17.3), and the interaction between the axon and applied electric fields (Sec. 17.4).

Another difficulty lies at the interface between electrodes applying the current and neural tissue to be stimulated. Current in the wires to the electrodes is carried by electrons, whereas current in the volume conductor is carried by ions. Chemical reactions at the interface will take place, and these reactions are still poorly understood. The waveforms used to apply the current can significantly affect the threshold, the electrochemistry at the electrode site, and tissue damage. These issues will be reviewed in Sec. 17.5.

17.2 Physiology of Excitation

Electric stimulation of excitable tissue is mediated by artificially depolarizing membrane-containing channels capable of producing action potentials. Action potentials are normally elicited by synaptic currents, which in turn produce depolarization of the somatic membrane. The sodium channels are responsible for the generation of the depolarizing phase of the action potential and are sensitive to membrane voltage [Ferreira and Marshal, 1985]. Once initiated in the soma, the action potential is carried unattenuated along the axon to its intended target, such as another neuron or neuromuscular junction for muscle contraction (Fig. 17.1). Unmyelinated axons have ionic channels distributed throughout their membranes, and the action potential is carried smoothly along their length. The membranes of the axons containing the channels behave as resistive and capacitive elements, limiting the conduction velocity. Myelinated axons are surrounded by a insulation sheath of myelin that significantly decreases the membrane capacitance, thereby increasing the speed

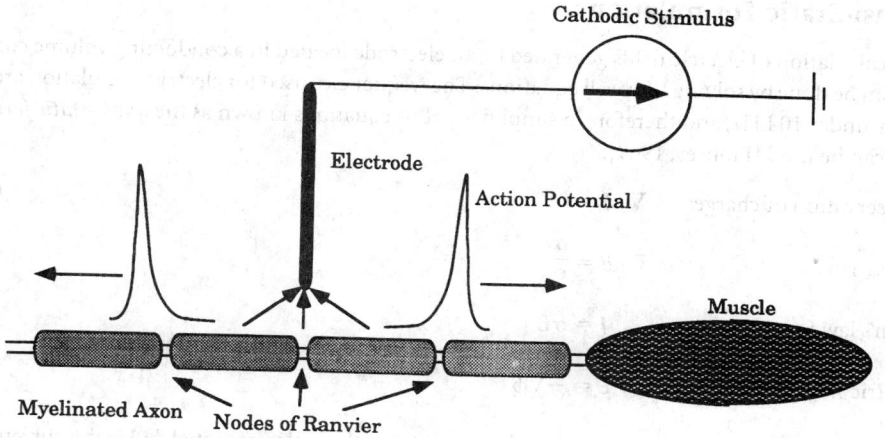

FIGURE 17.1 Electric stimulation of a myelinated fiber. An electrode is located near the axon, and a cathodic stimulus is applied to the electrode. The current flow in and around the axon is described in this chapter and causes depolarization of the membrane at the sites closest to the electrodes. Action potentials are generated underneath the electrode and propagate orthodromically and antidromically.

of propagation. Conduction of the action potential is no longer smooth but takes place in discrete steps (saltatory conduction). The myelin sheath is broken at regularly spaced intervals (nodes of Ranvier) to allow the current to flow through the membrane [Aidley, 1978].

Action potentials can be generated artificially by placing electrodes directly inside a cell. Current flowing from the inside to the outside will produce depolarization followed by excitation, provided that the current amplitude is large enough. This technique cannot be used for functional stimulation because we do not yet have the technology to interface electrodes with large numbers of single axons. Therefore, electrodes must be placed in the extracellular space near the tissue to be excited. It is then possible to activate many cells simultaneously. However, stimulation must be selective. *Selectivity* is defined as the ability of a stimulation system to activate any chosen set of axons. For example, the nervous system chooses to recruit small fibers connected to small motor units followed by large fibers connected to large motor units for smooth motor control. Applied current pulses activate first large fibers and then small fibers with increasing current (reverse recruitment) for reasons described in Sec. 17.4. The reverse recruitment order as well as our inability to recruit a chosen set of axons within a nerve bundle makes electric stimulation a powerful but difficult-to-control tool for activation of the nervous system.

17.3 Electric Fields in Volume Conductors

The excitable tissue to be stimulated (peripheral nerves, motor neurons, CNS neurons) are in all cases surrounded by an extracellular fluid with a relatively high conductivity (80 to 300 $\Omega \cdot$ cm). The electrodes used for electric stimulation are always placed in this "volume conductor," and it is essential to understand how the currents and the electric fields are distributed [Heringa et al., 1982]. The calculation of current density and electric fields can be done easily in simple cases such as a homogeneous (conductivity the same everywhere) and isotropic (conductivity the same in all directions) medium.

Quasi-Static Formulation

The calculation of electric fields generated by an electrode located in a conducting volume conductor can be done by solving Maxwell equations. The frequencies used for electric stimulation are generally under 10 kHz, and therefore, a simplified set of equations known as the *quasi-static formulation* can be used [Plonsey, 1969]:

Conservation of charge: $\nabla \cdot \mathbf{J} = 0$ (17.1)

Gauss' law: $\nabla \cdot \mathbf{E} = \dfrac{\rho}{\epsilon}$ (17.2)

Ohm's law for conductors: $\mathbf{J} = \sigma \mathbf{E}$ (17.3)

Electric field: $\mathbf{E} = -\nabla \phi$ (17.4)

where $\mathbf{E}$ is the electric field (V/m) defined as gradient of the scalar potential ϕ; $\mathbf{J}$ is the current density (defined as the current crossing a given surface, in A/m^2); σ is the conductivity (inverse of resistivity), in s/m; ρ is the charge density, in C/m^3; ϵ is the permittivity of the medium; and $\nabla \cdot \mathbf{A}$ is the divergence of vector $\mathbf{A}$.

Equivalence Between Dielectric and Conductive Media

Assuming an infinite homogeneous conducting medium with conductivity σ with a single point source as shown in Fig. 17.2a, the current density $\mathbf{J}$ at any point is the sum of a source term $\mathbf{J}_s$ and an ohmic term $\sigma\mathbf{E}$:

$$\mathbf{J} = \sigma\mathbf{E} + \mathbf{J}_s \qquad (17.5)$$

Using Eq. (17.1),

$$\nabla \cdot \mathbf{J} = \nabla \cdot \sigma\mathbf{E} + \nabla \cdot \mathbf{J}_s = 0 \qquad (17.6)$$

Since the volume conductor is homogeneous, $\nabla \cdot (\sigma\mathbf{E}) = \sigma\nabla \cdot \mathbf{E}$, and we then have

$$\sigma\nabla \cdot \mathbf{E} = -\nabla \cdot \mathbf{J}_s \qquad (17.7)$$

Since $\mathbf{E} = -\nabla\phi$ and $\nabla \cdot (\nabla\mathbf{A})$ is by definition the laplacian of $\mathbf{A}$, $\nabla^2\mathbf{A}$, we then have

$$\nabla^2\phi = \nabla \cdot \mathbf{J}_s/\sigma = -I_v/\sigma \qquad (17.8)$$

where I_v is a source term (in A/m^3). The source term I_v is zero everywhere except where the sources are located. This equation is nearly identical to the Poisson equation derived from Eq. (17.2) [Kraus and Carver, 1973]:

$$\nabla^2\phi = -\frac{\rho}{\epsilon} \qquad (17.9)$$

derived for dielectric media. Using the following equivalence,

$$\rho \rightarrow I_v$$

$$\epsilon \rightarrow \sigma$$

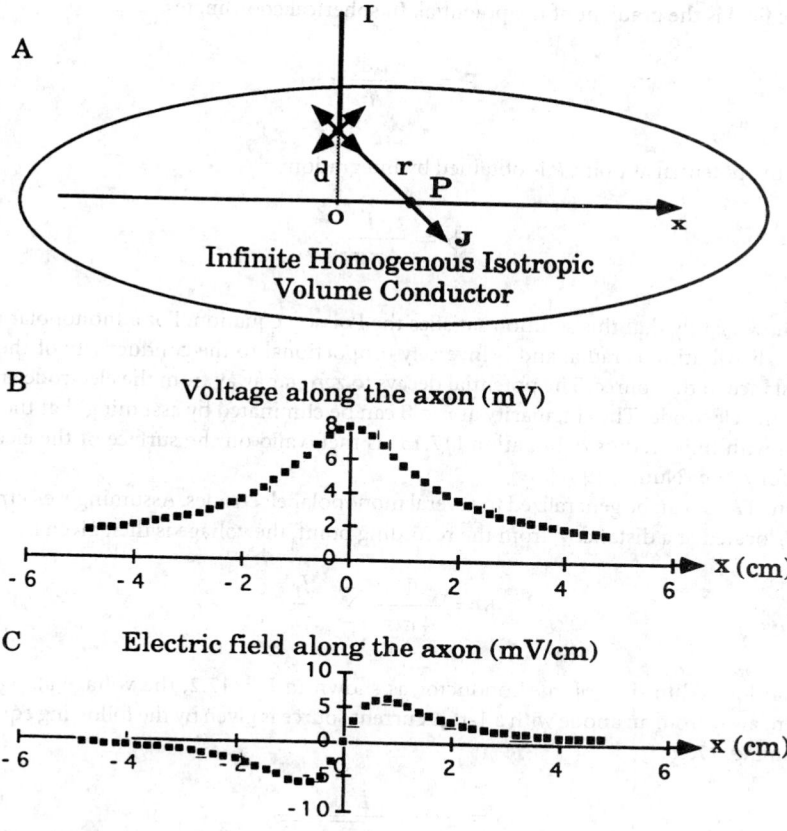

FIGURE 17.2   Voltage and electric field along an axon. (*a*) The current density **J** within an infinite, homogeneous, and isotropic volume conductor is radial and is inversely proportional to the square of the distance. (*b*) Voltage along an axon located 1 cm from an anode with 1 mA of current. (*c*) Electric field along the same axon.

the solution of the Poisson equation for dielectric problems can then be used for the solution of the current in volume conductors.

Potential from a Monopole Source

Given a point source (monopolar) in an infinite homogeneous and isotropic volume conductor connected to a current source *I*, the potential and currents anywhere can be derived easily. Using spherical symmetry, the current density **J** at a point *P* located at a distance *r* from the source is equal to the total current crossing a spherical surface with radius *r* (see Fig. 17.2):

$$\mathbf{J} = \frac{I}{4\pi r^2} \mathbf{u}_r \qquad (17.10)$$

where $\mathbf{u}_r$ is the unit radial vector, and *r* is the distance between the electrode and the measurement point. The electric field is then obtained from Eq. (17.3):

$$\mathbf{E} = \frac{I}{4\pi\sigma r^2} \mathbf{u}_r \qquad (17.11)$$

The electric field is the gradient of the potential. In spherical coordinates,

$$\mathbf{E} = -\frac{d\phi}{dr}\mathbf{u}_r \tag{17.12}$$

Therefore, the potential at point P is obtained by integration:

$$\phi = \frac{I}{4\pi\sigma r} \tag{17.13}$$

It can be shown easily that this solution satisfies the Poisson equation. For a monopolar electrode, the current distribution is radial and is inversely proportional to the conductivity of the medium and the distance to the source. The potential decays to zero far away from the electrode and goes to infinity on the electrode. The singularity at $r = 0$ can be eliminated by assuming that the electrode is spherical with finite radius a. Equation (17.13) is then valid on the surface of the electrode for $r = a$ and for $r > a$ [Nunez, 1981].

Equation (17.13) can be generalized to several monopolar electrodes. Assuming n electrodes with a current I_i located at a distance r_i from the recording point, the voltage is then given by

$$\phi = \frac{1}{4\pi\sigma} \sum_n \frac{I_i}{r_i} \tag{17.14}$$

For an axon located in the volume conductor as shown in Fig. 17.2, the voltage along the axon located 1 cm away from an anode with a 1-mA current source is given by the following equation and is plotted in Fig. 17.2b:

$$\phi = \frac{I}{4\pi\sigma\sqrt{d^2 + x^2}} \tag{17.15}$$

The electric field along the axon can be obtained by taking the spatial derivative of Eq. (17.15) and is plotted in Fig. 17.2c.

Potential from Bipolar Electrodes and Dipoles

In the derivation of the potential generated by a monopolar electrode, the current enters the volume conductor at the tip of the electrode and exits at infinity. However, in the following example (saltwater tank), a current is applied through two monopolar electrodes separated by a distance d as shown in Fig. 17.3a. The potential generated by this bipolar configuration can be calculated at point P (assuming that the voltage reference is at infinity) as follows:

$$\phi = \frac{I}{4\pi\sigma}\left(\frac{1}{r_1} - \frac{1}{r_2}\right) \tag{17.16}$$

When the distance d between the two electrodes is small compared with the distance r, the equation for the potential is given by the following dipole equation valid for $r \gg d$:

$$\phi = \frac{Id\cos\theta}{4\pi\sigma r^2} \tag{17.17}$$

where the angle θ is defined as in Fig. 17.3. The current distribution for a current dipole is no longer radial and is shown in Fig. 17.3b. The voltage along a line perpendicular to the axis of the dipole and

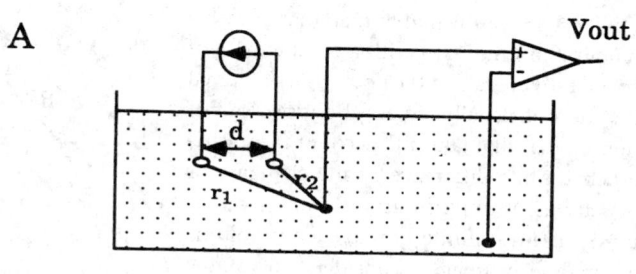

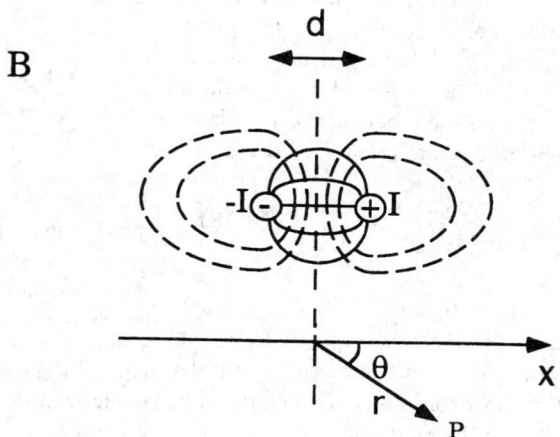

FIGURE 17.3 Voltage generated by bipolar electrodes. (*a*) Saltwater tank. Two electrodes are located within a large tank filled with a conduction solution. The voltage generated by the bipolar arrangement can be measured as shown provided that the reference electrode is located far away from the stimulation electrode. The effect of the stimulation electrode on the reference potential also can be taken into account. (*b*) Current lines and equipotential voltage distributions (*dashed lines*) for a dipole. The distance r between the observation P and the electrodes is much greater that the distance d between the electrodes.

passing through a point equidistant from the electrodes is zero. Therefore, an axon located in that region would not be excited regardless of the current amplitude. The potential generated by a dipole is inversely proportional to the square of the distance and therefore decays faster than the monopole. Therefore, the dipole configuration will have a more localized excitation region. However, the excitation thresholds are higher because most of the current flows around the electrode. For an observation point located at a distance r from a dipole or monopole with the same current, the ratio of the monopole voltage to that of the dipole voltage is proportional to r/d. Since r is assumed to be much larger than d, then the monopole voltage is much larger than the voltage generated by the dipole.

Inhomogeneous Volume Conductors

For practical applications of electric stimulation, electrodes are placed in various parts of the body. The volume conductors are clearly not homogeneous because we must consider the presence of bone with a conductivity significantly higher than that of extra-cellular space or even air above the skin with a conductivity of zero. How do those conductivities affect the potentials generated by the electrode? This question usually can only be answered numerically by computer models that take into account these various compartments such as finite-differences, finite-elements, or boundary-elements methods. A simple solution, however, can be obtained in the case of a semi-infinite homogeneous volume conductor using the method of images. Consider two volume conductors with conductivities σ_1 and σ_2 separated by an infinite plane as shown in Fig. 17.4. A monopolar stimulating electrode is placed in region 1. Potential recordings are made in that same region. It can be shown that the inhomogeneous volume conductor can be replaced by a homogeneous volume by adding another current source located on the other side of the plane (see Fig. 17.4) with an amplitude equal to [Nunez, 1981]

$$I' = \frac{\sigma_1 - \sigma_2}{\sigma_1 + \sigma_2} \, I \qquad (17.18)$$

The voltage at point P is then given by Eq. (17.14). The mirror-image theory is only applicable in simple cases but can be useful to obtain approximations when the distance between the recording electrode and the surface of discontinuity is small, thereby approximating an infinite surface [Durand et al., 1992].

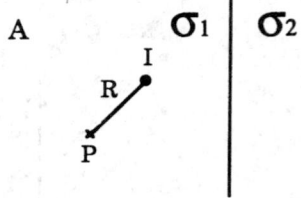

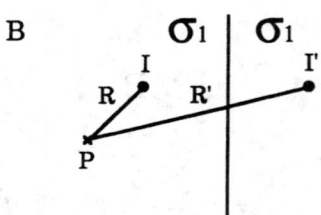

FIGURE 17.4   Method of images. The method of images can be used to calculate the voltage generated by an electrode in a homogeneous volume conductor. The two semi-infinite volume conductors with conductivities σ_1 and σ_2 (*a*) are replaced by a single infinite volume conductor with conductivity σ_1 and an additional image electrode (*b*).

17.4 Electric Field Interactions with Excitable Tissue

When axons are placed inside a volume conductor with a stimulation electrode, current flows according to equations derived in the preceding section. Some of the current lines enter and exit the axon at different locations and will produce excitation or inhibition. An example of this current distribution is shown in Fig. 17.5*a* for a monopolar anodic electrode. A length Δx of the axonal membrane can be modeled at rest by a capacitance C_m in parallel with a series combination of a battery (E_r) for the resting potential and a resistance R_m simulating the combined resistance at rest of all the membrane channels (see Fig. 17.5*b*). Nonlinear ionic channel conductances can be added in parallel with the membrane resistance and capacitance. Their contribution at rest is small and becomes significant only around threshold. Since we are interested here in how to drive the membrane potential toward threshold from resting values, their contribution is ignored. When current enters the membrane flowing from the outside to the inside, the membrane is hyperpolarized (moved closer to threshold), as illustrated in Fig. 17.5*c*. Similarly, when the current exits the membrane, depolarization is generated (the membrane voltage is moved closer to the threshold). In the case of an anodic electrode, illustrated in Fig. 17.5, stimulation should not take place directly underneath the electrode but further along the axon where the membrane is depolarized.

   A more quantitative approach to this problem can be obtained by modeling the interaction of the model with the applied current. The applied current I generates a voltage distribution in the extracellular space that can be calculated using Eq. (17.15) assuming a homogeneous and isotropic medium. An unmyelinated fiber is modeled as a one-dimensional network by linking together electrical models of the membrane with a resistance R_a to account for the internal resistance of the axon,

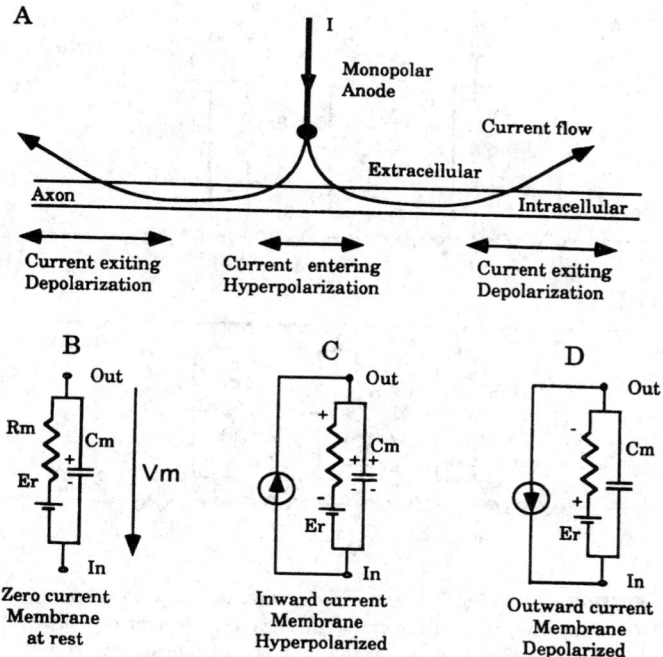

FIGURE 17.5 Effect of extracellular current on axon membrane polarization. (*a*) A monopolar anode is located near an axon, and current enters and exits the membrane. (*b*) At rest, the membrane can be modeled by a simple *RC* network. (*c*) When current enters the membrane, charge is added to the membrane capacitance, and additive membrane polarization is generated. Therefore, the membrane is hyperpolarized. (*d*) When current exits the axon, the membrane is depolarized.

as shown in Fig. 17.6*a*. The circuit can be simulated using numerical methods [Koch and Segev, 1989] or by using already available general software packages such as Pspice or neuronal simulation packages such as Neuron [Hines, 1984]. The variable of interest is the transmembrane potential V_m, since the sodium channels are sensitive to the voltage across the membrane. V_m is defined as the difference between the intracellular voltage V_i and the extracellular voltage V_e minus the resting potential E_r in order to the reflect the change from resting values. Stimulation of the fiber can occur when the extracellular voltage difference between two nodes is large enough to generate transmembrane voltage greater than the firing threshold. Applying Kirchoff's law at each node and taking the limit when the length of membrane Δx goes to zero, one obtains the following inhomogeneous cable equation [Rall, 1979; Clark and Plonsey, 1966; Altman and Plonsey, 1988; Rattay, 1989]:

$$\lambda^2 \frac{\partial^2 V_m}{\partial x^2} - \tau_m \frac{\partial V_m}{\partial t} - V_m = -\lambda^2 \frac{\partial^2 V_e}{\partial x^2} \qquad (17.19)$$

V_m and V_e are the transmembrane and extracellular voltages, respectively. λ is the space constant of the fiber and depends only on the geometric and electric properties of the axon:

$$\lambda = \frac{1}{2} \sqrt{\frac{R_m^s d}{R_a^s}} \qquad (17.20)$$

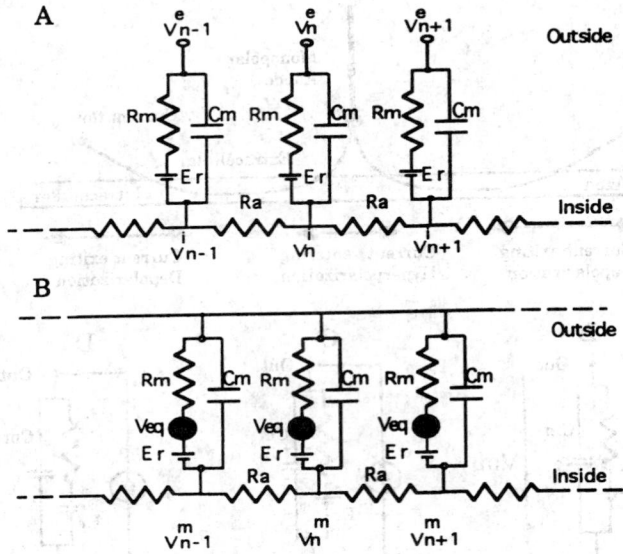

FIGURE 17.6 Model of extracellular voltage and axon interactions. (*a*) The effect of the extracellular voltage generated by the stimulating electrode on the axon can be modeled by directly connecting the membrane compartment to the extracellular source. The effect of the ion channels can be taken into account by adding nonlinear conductances and an equilibrium battery (not shown). (*b*) The axon with an extracellular voltage in *a* is equivalent to an axon inside an infinite conductance medium (zero voltage) and an equivalent voltage source inside the membrane.

where R_m^s is the specific membrane resistance, R_a^s is the axoplasmic-specific resistance, and d is the diameter of the axon. τ_m is the time constant of the axon and is given by

$$\tau_m = R_m C_m \tag{17.21}$$

The term on the right-hand side of the equation is called the *source term* or *forcing function* and is the product of the square of the space constant with the second spatial derivative of the extracellular voltage. In order to explain the significance of this term, it can be shown easily that the model in Fig. 17.6*a* is equivalent to a model in which the extracellular space with its electrode and voltage has been replaced by a set of equivalent voltage sources inside the nerve given by

$$V_{eq} = \lambda^2 \frac{\Delta^2 V_e}{\Delta x^2} = \lambda^2 \frac{d^2 V_e}{dx^2}\bigg|_{\Delta x \to 0} \tag{17.22}$$

The amplitude of the equivalent voltage sources is plotted in Fig. 17.7*a* for a 10-μm axon stimulated by a 1-mA anodic current located 1 cm away from the axon. A positive value for the equivalent voltage source indicates membrane depolarization, while a negative value indicates hyperpolarization. The peak value of the depolarization indicates the excitation site. Therefore, one would predict that for anodic stimulation, excitation would take place at the peak of the two depolarized regions, and two action potentials would propagate toward the ends of the axon away from the electrode. Note that the shape of V_{eq} calculated is similar to that predicted by simply examining the current flow in and out of the axon in Fig. 17.5. This analysis is valid only at the onset of the pulse, since during the pulse currents will be distributed throughout the cable and will affect the transmembrane

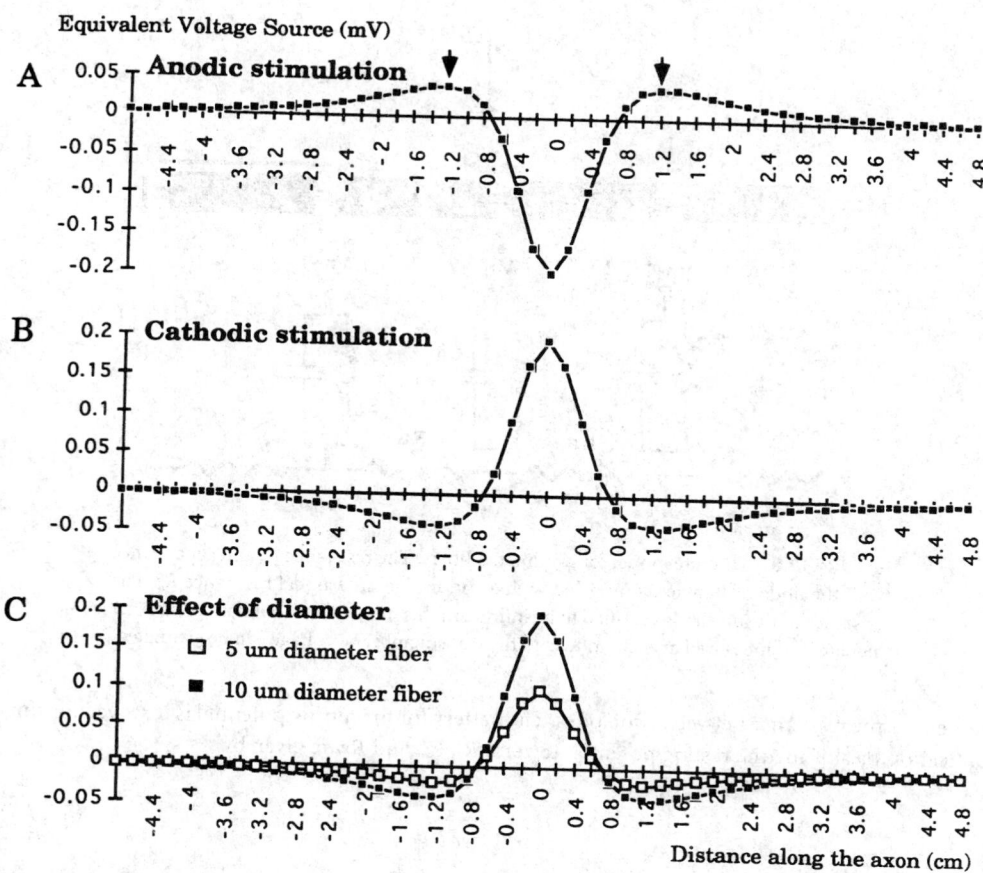

FIGURE 17.7 Equivalent source voltage (V_{eq}). A positive value of the V_{eq} indicates membrane depolarization, and a negative value indicates membrane hyperpolarization. (*a*) Equivalent source voltage plotted along the axon for an anodic stimulus. The peak value is negative, and therefore, the membrane is hyperpolarized underneath the electrode. Depolarization occurs at the sites of maximum value of V_{eq} (*arrows*). (*b*) Cathodic stimulation generates depolarization underneath the electrode, and the amplitude of V_{eq} is larger than for anodic stimulation. Therefore, a cathodic stimulus has a lower threshold than an anodic stimulus. (*c*) V_{eq} is larger for fibers with larger diameters; therefore, large-diameter fibers are recruited first.

potential [Warman et al., 1994]. However, it has been shown that for short pulses these effects are small, and the shape of the transmembrane voltage can be predicted using the source term of the cable equation.

Discrete Cable Equation for Myelinated Axons

Electric stimulation of myelinated fibers is significantly different from that of unmyelinated fibers because the presence of a myelin sheath around the axon forces the current to flow in and out of the membrane only at the nodes (see Fig. 17.1). The action potential propagates from one node to the next (saltatory conduction). The effect of an applied electric field on a myelinated fiber can be described using a discrete model of the axon and extracellular voltage [McNeal, 1976; Rattay, 1989]. Such a model is shown in Fig. 17.8, in which voltages are applied at each node. The resistance R_n represents the membrane resistance at the node of Ranvier only because the myelin resistance is considered very high for this model and is neglected. C_n is the capacitance at the node of Ranvier. R_a

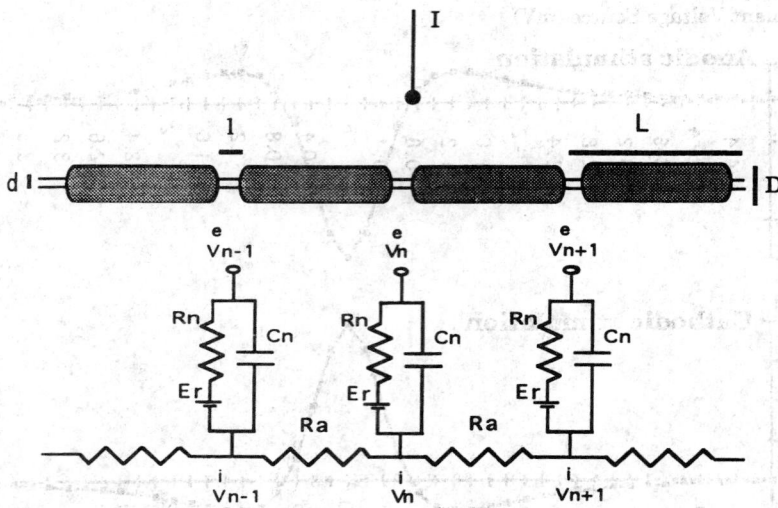

FIGURE 17.8 Discrete model for myelinated fibers. The resistance R_n and capacitance C_n of the node of Ranvier is modeled with an additional internodal resistance R_a. The resistance of the myelin is assumed to be infinite in this model. Extracellular voltages are calculated or measured at each node, and the transmembrane voltage can be estimated.

represents the resistance between two nodes. The battery for the resting potential is removed for simplification by shifting the resting potential to zero. R_n, C_n, and R_i are given by

$$R_n = \frac{R_n^s}{\pi d l} \tag{17.23}$$

$$R_a = \frac{4R_a^s L}{\pi d^2} \tag{17.24}$$

$$C_n = C_n^s \pi d l \tag{17.25}$$

where d is the inner fiber diameter, l is the width of the node, and L is the internodal distance (see Fig. 17.8). The cable equation for this model can be derived using Kirchoff's law:

$$\frac{R_n}{R_a} \Delta^2 V_m - R_n C_n \frac{\partial V_m}{\partial t} - V_m = -\frac{R_n}{R_a} \Delta^2 V_e \tag{17.26}$$

Δ^2 is the second difference operator: $\Delta^2 V = V_{n-1} - 2V_n + V_{n+1}$. Using Eqs. (17.23) to (17.25), one can show that $R_n C_n$ and R_n/R_a are independent of the diameter, since $L/D = 100$, $d/D = 0.7$ and l is constant. Therefore, the left side of Eq. (17.26) is independent of the diameter. The source term, however, does depend on the diameter but only implicitly. Since the distance between the node increases with the diameter of the fiber, the voltage across the nodes also increases, suggesting that fibers with larger diameters are more easily excitable because they "see" larger potentials along the nodes.

Equivalent Cable Equation for Myelinated Fibers

The diameter dependence of these fibers can be expressed explicitly by using an equivalent cable equation recently derived [Basser, 1993] and adapted here to take into effect the extracellular voltage:

$$\lambda_{my}^2 \frac{\partial^2 V_m}{\partial x^2} - \tau_{my} \frac{\partial V_m}{\partial t} - V_m = -\lambda_{my}^2 \frac{\partial^2 V_e}{\partial x^2} \qquad (17.27)$$

where λ_{my} is the equivalent space constant for the case of an axon with myelin sheath of infinite resistance and is defined as

$$\lambda_{my} = \frac{1}{2} \sqrt{\frac{R_n^s dL}{R_a^s l}} \qquad (17.28)$$

Unmyelinated/Myelinated Fibers

The equivalent cable equation for the myelinated fibers is similar to Eq. (17.20) derived for unmyelinated axons. The forcing function is also proportional to the first derivative of the extracellular electric field along the nerve. The dependence on the diameter can be observed directly by expressing the equivalent voltage source for myelinated fibers (V_{eqmy}) as function of the inner diameter d:

$$V_{eqmy} = 35.7 \frac{R_n^s}{R_a^s} \frac{d^2}{l} \frac{\partial^2 V_e}{\partial x^2} \qquad (17.29)$$

Equation (17.29) shows that V_{eqmy} is proportional to the square of the diameter of fiber d, while the equivalent voltage source for an unmyelinated fiber is proportional to its diameter (17.23). Therefore, the firing threshold for myelinated and unmyelinated fibers is proportional to d^2 and d respectively.

Anodic/Cathodic Stimulation

It has been demonstrated experimentally that in the case of electric stimulation of peripheral nerves, cathodic stimulation has a lower threshold (less current required) that anodic stimulation. This experimental result can be explained directly by plotting V_{eq} for a cathodic and an anodic electrode (1 mA) located 1 cm away from a 10-μm unmyelinated fiber (see Fig. 17.7). The maximum value of V_{eq} for anodic stimulation is 0.05 mV at the two sites indicated by the arrow. However, the maximum depolarization for the cathodic electrode is significantly larger at 0.2 mV, with the site of excitation located directly underneath the electrode. In special cases, such as an electrode located on the surface of a cortex, cathodic stimulation can have a higher threshold [Ranck, 1975].

Large/Small-Diameter Axons

The equivalent voltage source of the cable equation is proportional to the square of the space constant λ. λ^2 is proportional to the diameter of the fiber (17.20) for myelinated fibers and to the square of the diameter (17.29) for myelinated fibers. Therefore, in both cases, V_{eq} is higher for fibers with larger diameters (see Fig. 17.7c), and large-diameter fibers have a lower threshold. Since the physiologic recruitment order by the CNS is to first recruit the small fibers followed by large ones, electric stimulation produces a reverse recruitment order. However, techniques have been developed to recruit small fibers before large fibers by using a different stimulation waveform [Fang and Mortimer, 1991]. Since λ^2 is also dependent on the electrical properties of the axons, it is then possible to predict that fibers with a larger membrane resistance or lower axoplasmic resistance also will have lower thresholds.

Spatial Derivative of the Electric Field

The first spatial derivative (or the second spatial derivative of the voltage along the nerve) is responsible for electric excitation of the nerve. Therefore, an electric field with a nonzero second spatial derivative is required for excitation. An axon with a linearly decreasing voltage distribution would not be excited despite the presence of a large voltage difference along the axon. This is due to the fact that a linear voltage distribution gives a constant electric field, and therefore, the spatial derivative of the field is zero.

Activating Function

The second spatial derivative term of the equivalent voltage source is also known as the *activation function* [Rattay, 1990]:

$$f_{unmy} = \frac{d^2 V_e}{dx^2} \tag{17.30}$$

This function can be evaluated from knowledge of the extracellular voltage alone and can be used to predict the location of excitation. For unmyelinated fibers, the activation function does not contain any information about the axon to be stimulated. In the case of myelinated fibers, where the voltage is evaluated at the nodes of Ranvier, the activating function becomes

$$f_{my} = \frac{\Delta^2 V_e}{\Delta x^2} \tag{17.31}$$

The new function contains implicit information about the fiber diameter, since the distance L between the nodes of Ranvier is directly proportional to fiber diameter D ($L = 100 \times D$). The diameter dependence can be made explicit in Eq. (17.29).

Net Driving Function

The equivalent voltage source or the activating function represents only the source term in the electrical model of the axon (see Fig. 17.6). However, the transmembrane voltage is determined by a weighted sum of the currents flowing at all the nodes. A net driving function that takes into account both the source term at each node and the passive redistribution from sources at other nodes has been defined and found useful for accurate prediction of the excitation threshold for any applied field [Warman et al., 1994].

Current-Distance Relationship

The amount of current required to activate a fiber with a given diameter depends of its geometry but also on its distance from the electrode. The farther away the fiber, the lower is the voltage along the fiber (17.15); therefore, larger current will be required to reach threshold. This effect is illustrated in Fig. 17.9 for myelinated fibers. The distance as a function of current amplitude at threshold is plotted for several experiments [Ranck, 1975]. With a current of 1 mA, all fibers within 2 mm are activated. The calculated current-distance relationship for a 10-μm fiber has been shown to approximate well the experimental data (see dashed line in Fig. 17.9) [Rattay, 1989]. The current-distance relationship is linear only for small distances. For distances above 1 mm, doubling the distance will require four times the current amplitude.

Longitudinal/Transverse Field

The equivalent voltage source is also proportional to the second spatial derivative of the potential present at each point along the axon. It is important to note that it is the longitudinal component

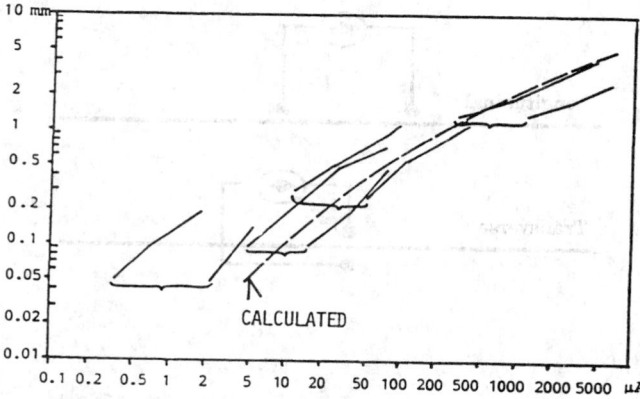

FIGURE 17.9 Current-distance relationship for monopolar cathodic stimulation of myelinated axons. The distance between the axon and the electrode is plotted as a function of current threshold amplitude for many experiments from several authors. The dashed line shows the current-distance relationship calculated for a 10-μm fiber stimulated with a 200-μs pulse. [From Rattay, 1989, with permission.]

of the electric field that is responsible for exciting the nerve. Therefore, electrodes placed longitudinally generate the most efficient stimulus, since this placement would produce a large longitudinal electric field component. Conversely, electrodes place transversely (on each side of the axon) require a much higher current, since the largest component of the field does not contribute to excitation of the nerve (Fig. 17.10a).

Anodal Surround Block

As shown by the current-distance relation, the current amplitudes required for excitation decrease with distance. This is not entirely true for cathodic stimulation. Cathodic stimulation produces membrane depolarization underneath the electrode and membrane hyperpolarization on both sides of the electrodes (see Fig. 17.7b). As the current amplitude is increased, the hyperpolarization also increases and can block propagation of the action potential along the axon. This effect is known as *anodal surround block* and is shown in Fig. 17.10b. It is possible to identify three regions around the electrode each giving different responses. There is a spherical region close to the electrode (I) in which no excitation will take place due to the surround block. Fibers located in the region (II) are excited, and fibers still further away (III) from the electrode are below threshold and are not excited.

Unidirectionally Propagated Action Potentials

Electric stimulation of nerves with electrodes normally depolarizes the membrane to threshold, producing two action potentials propagating in opposite directions, as shown in Fig. 17.1. Stimulation techniques have been developed to generate action potentials propagating in one direction only [Sweeney and Mortimer, 1986]. The techniques rely on the fact that bipolar stimulation generates depolarization under the cathode and hyperpolarization under the anode. By increasing the amount of hyperpolarization relative to the depolarization, the action potential generated underneath the cathode and traveling toward the anode can be blocked, while the action potential traveling in the other direction can escape.

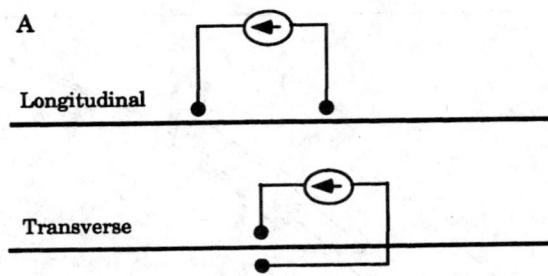

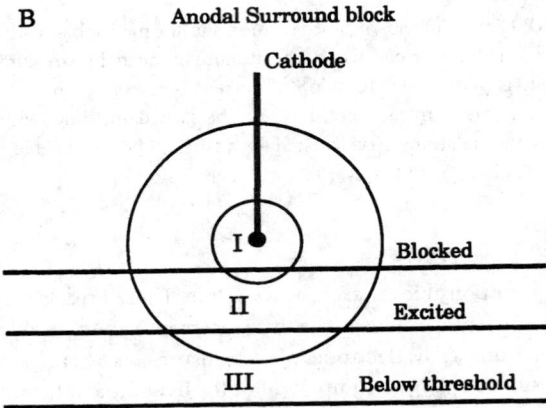

FIGURE 17.10 (*a*) Longitudinal/transverse electrode placement. (*b*) Anodal surround block.

17.5 Electrode-Tissue Interface

At the interface between the electrode and the tissue, the shape of the waveform can influence the threshold for activation as well as the corrosion of the electrode and the tissue damage generated.

Effect of Stimulation Waveform on Threshold

Strength-Duration Curve

It has been known for a long time that it is the time change in the applied current and not the continuous application of the external stimulus that can excite. Direct current (dc current) cannot excite and even in small amplitudes can cause significant tissue damage. It also has been observed experimentally that the relationship between the pulse width and the amplitude suggests that it is the total charge injected that is the important parameter. This relationship between the amplitude and the width of a pulse required to bring an excitable tissue to threshold is shown in Fig. 17.11*a*. The amplitude of the current threshold stimulus I_{th} decreases with increasing pulse width W and can be modeled by the following relationship derived experimentally [Lapicque, 1907]:

$$I_{th} = \frac{I_{rh}}{1 - \exp\left(-\dfrac{W}{T}\right)} \tag{17.32}$$

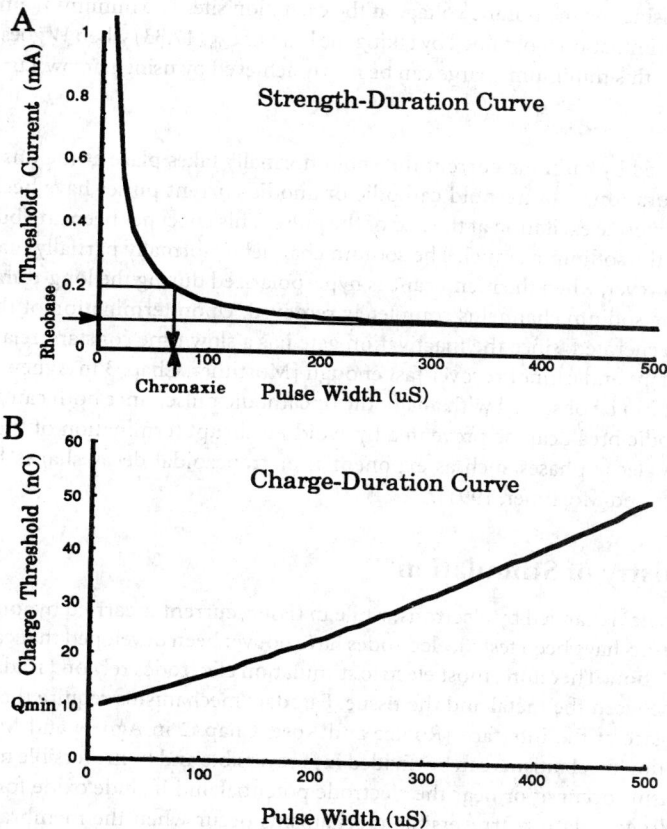

FIGURE 17.11 Effect of pulse width on excitation threshold. (*a*) Strength-duration curve. The amplitude of the current required to reach threshold decreases with width of the pulse. This effect can be derived theoretically by assuming that the charge on the cable at threshold is constant. (*b*) The threshold charge (amplitude times pulsewidth) injected into the tissue increases with the pulsewidth. Narrow pulses are recommended to minimize charge injection.

The smallest current amplitude required to cause excitation is known as the *rheobase current* I_{rh}. T is the membrane time constant of the axon if the axon is stimulated intracellularly. For extracellular stimulation, T is a time constant that takes into account the extracellular space resistance. The relationship between current amplitude and pulse width also can be derived theoretically using the cable equation by assuming that total charge on the cable for excitation is constant [Jack et al., 1983].

Charge Duration Curve

The threshold charge injected $Q_{th} = I_{th} \times W$ is plotted in Fig. 17.11*b* and increases as the pulse width increases:

$$Q_{th} = \frac{I_{rh}W}{1 - \exp\left(-\dfrac{W}{T}\right)} \tag{17.33}$$

The increase in the amount of charge required to fire the axon with increasing pulse width is due to the fact that for long pulse duration, the charge is distributed along the cable and does not participate directly in raising the membrane voltage at the excitation site. The minimum amount of charge Q_{min} required for stimulation is obtained by taking the limit of Q_{th} (17.33) when W goes to zero is equal to $I_{rh}T$. In practice, this minimum charge can be nearly achieved by using narrow, current pulses.

Anodic Break

Excitation generated by cathodic current threshold normally takes place at the onset of the pulse. However, long-duration, subthreshold cathodic or anodic current pulses have been observed experimentally to generate excitation at the end of the pulse. This effect has been attributed to the voltage sensitivity of the sodium channel. The sodium channel is normally partially inactivated at rest (see Chap. 1). However, when the membrane is hyperpolarized during the long-duration pulse, the inactivation of the sodium channel is completely removed. Upon termination of the pulse, an action potential is generated, since the inactivation gate has a slow time constant relative to the activation time constant and cannot recover fast enough [Mortimer, Chap. 3 in Agnew and McCreery, 1990]. This effect can be observed with an anodic or cathodic pulse, since both can generate hyperpolarization. Anodic break can be prevented by avoiding abrupt termination of the current. Pulse shapes with slow decay phases such as exponential or trapezoidal decay shapes have been used successfully [Fang and Mortimer, 1991].

Electrochemistry of Stimulation

Conduction in metal is carried by electrons, while in tissue, current is carried by ions. Although capacitive mechanisms have been tested, electrodes have not yet been developed that can store enough charge for stimulation. Therefore, most electric stimulation electrodes rely on faradaic mechanisms at the interface between the metal and the tissue. Faradaic mechanisms require that oxidation and reduction take place at the interface [Roblee and Rose, Chap. 2 in Agnew and McCreery, 1990]. Faradaic stimulation mechanisms can be divided into reversible and nonreversible mechanisms. Reversible mechanisms occur at or near the electrode potential and include oxide formation and reduction and hydrogen plating. Irreversible mechanisms occur when the membrane is driven far away from its equilibrium potential and include corrosion and hydrogen or oxygen evolution. These irreversible processes can cause damage to both the electrode and the tissue, since they alter the composition of the electrode surface and can generate toxic products with pH changes in the surrounding tissue. During charge injection, the electrode potential is modified by an amount related to the charge density (total charge divided by the surface area). In order to maintain the electrode potential within regions producing only minimal irreversible changes, this charge density must be kept below some values. The maximum charge density allowed depends on the metal used for the electrode, the stimulation waveform, the type of electrode used, and the location of the electrode within the body.

Stimulation of Brain Tissue

Electrodes can be placed on the surface of the brain and directly into the brain to activate CNS pathways. Experiments with stimulation of electrode arrays made of platinum and placed on the surface of the brain indicate that damage was produced for charge densities between 50 to 300 $\mu C/cm^2$ but that the total charge per phase also was an important factor and should be kept below 3 μC [Pudenz et al., 1975a, b]. Intracortical electrodes with small surface areas can tolerate a charge density as high as 1600 $\mu C/cm^2$, provided that the charge per phase remains below 0.0032 μC [Agnew et al., 1986].

Stimulation of the Peripheral Nerve

The electrodes used in the peripheral nerves are varied and include extraneural designs such as the spiral cuffs or helix electrodes [Naples et al., 1991] with electrode contacts directly on the surface of the nerve or intraneural designs placing electrodes contacts directly inside the nerve [Nannini and

Horch, 1991; Rutten et al., 1991]. Intraneural electrodes can cause significant damage, since electrodes are inserted directly into the nerve through the perineurium. However, these electrodes can display good selectivity. Extraneural electrodes are relatively safe because the newer designs such at the spiral or helix are self-sizing and allow for swelling without compression but display poor selectivity. New designs are aimed at producing selective stimulation by recruiting only small portions of the nerve and little damage [Veraart et al., 1990; Tyler and Durand, 1994]. Damage in peripheral nerve stimulation can be caused by the constriction of the nerve as well as by neuronal hyperactivity and irreversible reactions at the electrode [McCreery et al., 1992].

Stimulation of Muscle Tissue

Muscle tissue can best be excited by electrodes located on the nerve supplying the muscle [Popovic, 1991]. However, for some applications, electrodes can be placed directly on the surface of the skin (surface stimulation) [Myklebust et al., 1985], directly into the muscle (intramuscular electrode) [Caldwell and Reswick, 1975], or on the surface of the muscle (epimysial electrode) [Grandjean and Mortimer, 1985]. The current thresholds are higher when compared with nerve stimulation unless the electrode is carefully placed near the point of entry of the nerve [Mortimer, 1981]. Stainless steel is often used for these electrodes and is safe below 40 $\mu C/cm^2$ for coiled wire intramuscular electrodes [Mortimer et al., 1980].

Corrosion

Corrosion of the electrode is a major concern because it can cause electrode damage, metal dissolution, and tissue damage. However, corrosion occurs only during the anodic phase of the stimulation. Therefore, by using monophasic waveforms as shown in Fig. 17.12b, corrosion can be avoided. Conversely, the monophasic anodic waveform (Fig. 17.12a) must be avoided because it will cause corrosion. (This not true, however, for capacitive electrode metals such as tantalum, for which a dielectric layer of tantalum pentoxide is formed during the anodic phase and reduced during the cathodic phase.) For most applications, cathodic stimulation has a lower threshold than anodic stimulation. It appears, therefore, that monophasic cathodic waveforms (Fig. 17.11a) would be a preferred stimulation waveform, since it minimizes both the current to be injected and the corrosion. However, since the current only flows in one direction, the chemical reactions at the interface are not reversed, and the electrode is driven in the irreversible region.

Tissue Damage

Electrodes operating in the irreversible region can cause significant tissue damage because irreversible processes can modify the pH of the surrounding tissue and generate toxic products. Balanced biphasic waveforms are preferred because the second phase can completely reverse the charge injected into the tissue. Provided that the amplitude of the current is small, the electrode voltage can then be maintained within the reversible region. Waveforms that have the most unrecoverable charge are the most likely to induce tissue damage. Tissue damage also can be caused by generating a high rate of neural activity [Agnew et al., Chap. 6 in Agnew and McCreery, 1990]. The mechanisms underlying this effect are still unclear but could include damage to the blood-nerve barrier, ischemia, or a large metabolic demand on the tissue leading to changes in ionic concentration both intracellularly and extracellularly.

Biphasic Waveforms

Common biphasic waveforms for stainless steel or platinum use a cathodic pulse followed by an anodic phase. An example of a square balanced biphasic waveform is shown in Fig. 17.12c. Another commonly used biphasic waveform easily implemented with capacitor and switches is shown in

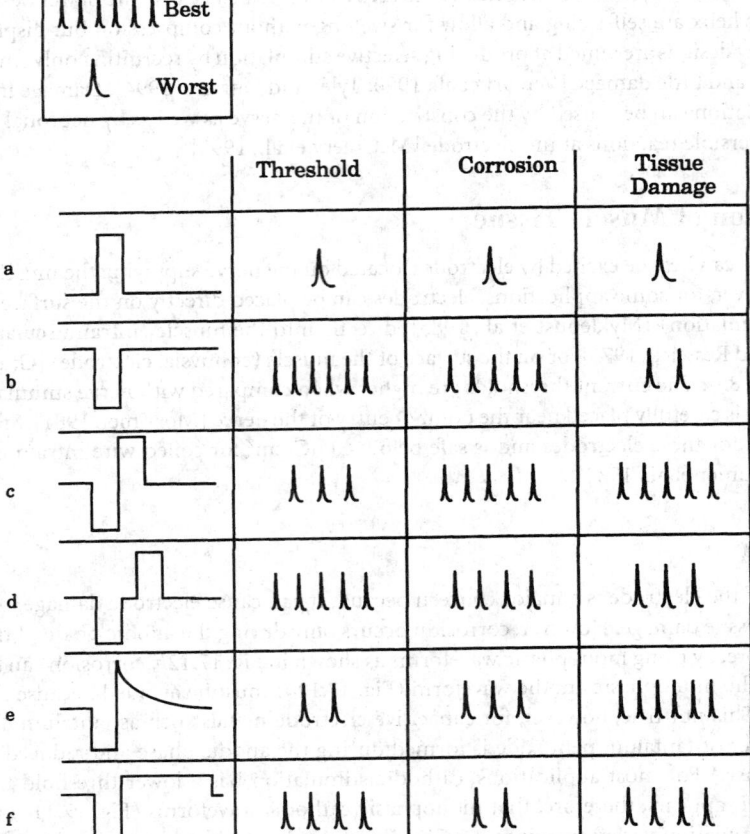

FIGURE 17.12 Comparison of stimulation waveforms. The waveforms are ranked for their ability to generate low threshold stimulation, low corrosion, and low tissue damage.

Fig. 17.12*e*. This waveform ensures that the charge is exactly balanced, since a capacitor is inserted in series with the tissue to be stimulated and the charge injected is then reversed by discharging the capacitor [Mortimer, 1981]. Biphasic cathodic-first waveforms have a higher threshold than monophasic waveforms because the maximum depolarization induced by the cathodic pulse is decreased by the following anodic pulse [Mortimer, Chap. 3 in Agnew and McCreery, 1990]. A delay can then be inserted between the cathodic and anodic phases, as shown in Fig. 17.12*d*. However, the time delay also can prevent adequate charge reversal and can be dangerous to the electrode and the tissue. An alternative method is to decrease the maximum amplitude of the anodic phase but increase its length as shown in Fig. 17.12*f*. However, this also can be damaging to the electrode because the charge is not reversed fast enough following the cathodic pulse. The various waveforms shown in Fig. 17.12 are ranked for their effect on tissue damage, corrosion, and threshold of activation.

17.6 Conclusion

Electric stimulation of excitable tissue has been used for over a century, and important discoveries have been made concerning the mechanisms underlying the interactions between the applied fields with the tissue and the electrochemistry at the electrode-tissue interface. It is now clear that electric stimulation is a powerful technique that could potentially activate any excitable tissue in the body and replace damaged functions. It is also clear, however, that if our goal is to provide intimate interfacing between excitable tissue and electrodes in order to reproduce the normal function of the nervous system, present technology is not adequate. The electrodes are too big and can only access either a few elements separately or a large number of elements simultaneously. Moreover, it is also clear that our understanding of the electrochemistry at the interface between the electrode and tissue is limited as well as the mechanisms underlying tissue damage. However, the substantial gains to be made are worth the efforts required to solve these problems.

Acknowledgment

I am grateful to Srikantan Nagarajan for critically reviewing this manuscript. Supported by NIH grant RO1 NS 32845-01.

References

Agnew WF, McCreery DB. 1990. Neural Prostheses: Fundamental Studies. Englewood Cliffs, NJ, Prentice-Hall.

Agnew WF, Yuen TGH, McCreery DB, Bullara LA. 1986. Histopathologic evaluation of prolonged intracortical electrical stimulation. Exp Neurol 92:162.

Aidley DJ. 1978. The Physiology of Excitable Cells. Cambridge, England, Cambridge University Press.

Altman KW, Plonsey R. 1988. Development of a model for point source electrical fibre bundle stimulation. Med Biol Eng Conmput 26:466.

Basser PJ. 1993. Cable equation for a myelinated axon derived from its microstructure, Med Biol Eng Comput 31:S87.

Brindley GS, Lewin WS. 1968. The sensations produced by electrical stimulation of the visual cortex. J Physiol 106:479.

Caldwell CW, Reswick JB. 1975. A percutaneous wire electrode for chronic research use. IEEE Trans Biomed Eng 22:429.

Chokroverty S. 1990. Magnetic Stimulation in Clinical Neurophysiology. London, Butterworth.

Clark GM, Tong YC, Patrick JF. 1990. Cochlear Prostheses. New York, Churchill-Linvinston.

Clark J, Plonsey R. 1966. A mathematical evaluation of the core conductor model. Biophys J 6:95.

Durand D, Ferguson ASF, Dalbasti T. 1992. Effects of surface boundary on neuronal magnetic stimulation. IEEE Trans Biomed Eng 37:588.

Fang ZP, Mortimer JT. 1991. A method to effect physiological recruitment order in electrically activated muscle. IEEE Trans Biomed Eng 38:175.

Ferreira HG, Marshal MW. 1985. The Biophysical Basis of Excitibility. Cambridge, England, Cambridge University Press.

Glenn WWL, Hogan JF, Loke JSO, et al. 1984. Ventilatory support by pacing of the conditioned diaphragm in quadraplegia. N Engl J Med 310:1150.

Grandjean PA, Mortimer JT. 1985. Recruitment properties of monopolar and bipolar epimysial electrodes. Ann Biomed Eng 14:429.

Hambrecht FT. 1979. Neural prostheses. Annu Rev Biophys Bioeng 8:239.

Heringa A, Stegeman DF, Uijen GJH, deWeerd JPC. 1982. Solution methods of electrical field in physiology. IEEE Trans Biomed Eng 29:34.

Hines M. 1984. Efficient computation of branched nerve equations. Int J Biol Med Comput 15:69.

Jack JJB, Noble D, Tsien RW. 1983. Electrical Current Flow in Excitable Cells. Oxford, Clarendon Press.

Koch C, Segev I. 1989. Methods in Neural Modeling. Cambridge, Mass, MIT Press.

Kraus JD, Carver KR. 1973. Electromagnetics. New York, McGraw-Hill.

Lapicque L. 1907. Recherches quantitatives sur l'excitation electrique des nerfs traites comme une polarization. J Physiol (Paris) 9:622.

Marsolais EB, Kobetic R. 1988. Development of a practical electrical stimulation system for restoring gait in the paralyzed patient. Clin Othrop 233:64.

McCreery DB, Agnew WF, Yuen TGH, Bullara LA. 1992. Damage in peripheral nerve from continuous electrical stimulation: Comparison of two stimulus waveforms. Med Biol Eng Comput 30:109.

McNeal DR. 1976. Analysis of a model for excitation of myelinated nerve. IEEE Trans Biomed Eng 23:329.

Mortimer JT, Kaufman D, Roessmann U. 1980. Coiled wire electrode intramuscular electrode: Tissue damage. Ann Biomed Eng 8:235.

Mortimer JT. 1981. Motor prostheses. In VB Brooks (ed), Handbook of Physiology—The Nervous System, vol 3, pp 155–187. New York, American Physiological Society.

Myklebust J, Cusick B, Sances A, Larson SLJ. 1985. Neural Stimulation. Boca Raton, Fla, CRC Press.

Nagarajan SS, Durand D, Warman EN. 1993. Effects of induced electric fields on finite neuronal structures: A simulation study. IEEE Trans Biomed Eng 40:1175.

Nannini N, Horch K. 1991. Muscle recruitment with intrafascicular electrodes. IEEE Trans Biomed Eng 38:769.

Naples et al. 1990. Overview of peripheral nerve electrode design and implementation. In WF Agnew and DB McCreery (eds), Neural Prostheses: Fundamental Studies. Englewood Cliffs, New Jersey, Prentice-Hall.

Nunez PL. 1981. Electric Fields in the Brain: The Neurophysics of EEG. Oxford, England, Oxford University Press.

Peckham PH, Keith MW, Freehofe AA. 1987. Restoration of functional control by electrical stimulation in the upper extremity of the quadriplegic patient. J Bone and Joint Surg. 70 A(1):144–148.

Plonsey R. 1969. Bioelectric Phenomena. New York, McGraw-Hill.

Popović D, Gordon T, ReeJuse VF, Prochazka A. 1991. Properties of implanted electrodes for functional electrical stimulation. Ann Biomed Eng 19:303–316.

Pudenz RHL, Bullara A, Dru D, Tallala A. 1975a. Electrical stimulation of the brain: II. Effects on the blood-brain barrier. Surg Neurol 4:2650.

Pudenz RH, Bullara LA, Jacques P, Hambrecht FT. 1975b. Electrical stimulation of the brain: III. The neural damage model. Surg Neurol 4:389.

Rall W. 1979. Core conductor theory and cable properties of neurons. In Handbook of Physiology—The Nervous System, vol 1, chap 3, pp 39–96. Bethesda,

Ranck JB. 1975. Which elements are excited in electrical stimulation of mammalian central nervous system: A review. Brain Res 98:417.

Rattay F. 1989. Analysis of models for extracellular fiber stimulation. IEEE Trans Biomed Eng 36:676.

Rattay F. 1990. Electrical Nerve Stimulation, Theory, Experiments and Applications. New York, Springer-Verlag.

Roth BJ. 1979. Core conductor theory and cable properties of neurons. In Handbook of Physiology: The Nervous System, vol 1, pp 39–96. Bethesda, Maryland, American Physiological Society.

Roth BJ, Basser PJ. 1990. A model for stimulation of a nerve fiber by electromagnetic induction. IEEE Trans Biomed Eng 37:588.

Rutecki P. 1990. Anatomical, physiological and theoretical basis for the antiepileptic effect of vagus nerve stimulation. Epilepsia 31:S1.

Rutten WLC, vanWier HJ, Put JJM. 1991. Sensitivity and selectivity of intraneural stimulation using a silicon electrode array. IEEE Trans Biomed Eng 38:192.

Sweeney JD, Mortimer JT. 1986. An asymmetric two electrode cuff for generation of unidirectionally propagated action potentials. IEEE Trans Biomed Eng 33:541.

Tyler DJ, Durand DM. 1994. Interfascicular electrical stimulation for selectively activating axons. IEEE Eng Med Biol. 13:575–583.

Veraart C, Grill WM, Mortimer JT. 1990. Selective control of muscle activation with a multipolar nerve cuff electrode. IEEE Trans Biomed Eng 37:688.

Warman NR, Durand DM, Yuen G. 1994. Reconstruction of hippocampal CA1 pyramidal cell electrophysiology by computer simulation. IEEE Trans Biomed Eng 39:1244.

Further Information

Information concerning functional electrical stimulation can be obtained from

FES Information Center
11000 Cedar Av.,
Cleveland, Ohio 44106-3052
Tel: 800 666 2353 or 216 231 3257

Articles concerning the latest research can be found mainly in the following journals:

IEEE Transactions in Biomedical Engineering
IEEE Transactions on Rehabilitation Engineering
Annals of Biomedical Engineering
Medical & Biological Engineering and Computing

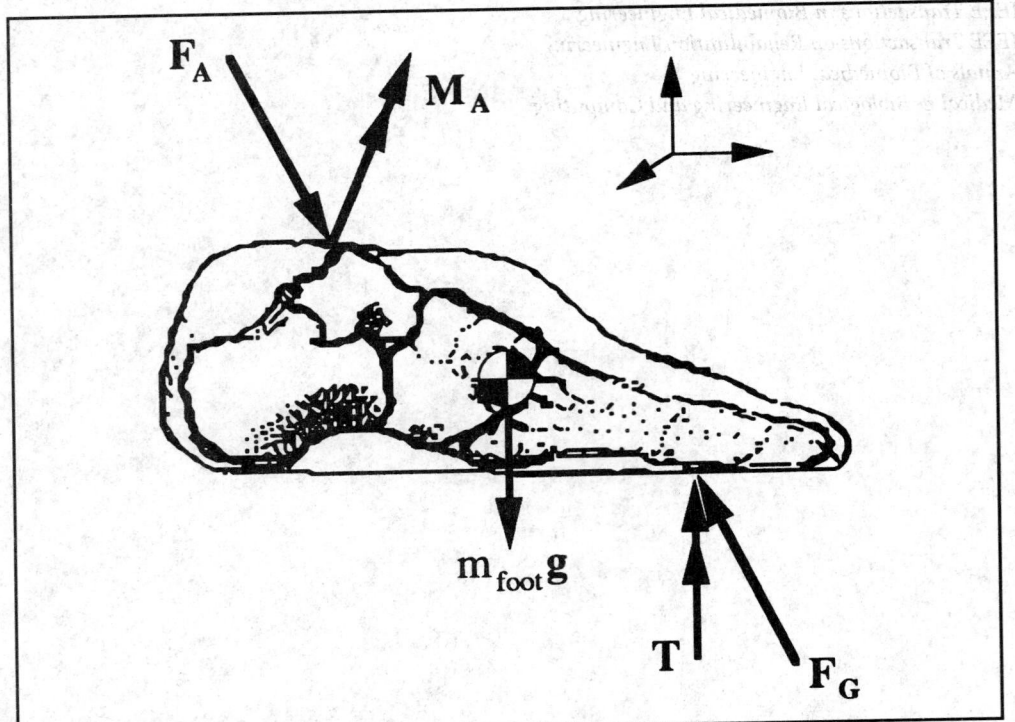

Free body diagram of the foot.

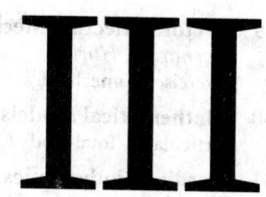

Biomechanics

Daniel J. Schneck
Virginia Polytechnic Institute and State University

MECHANICS IS THE ENGINEERING SCIENCE that deals with studying, defining, and mathematically quantifying "interactions" that take place among "things" in our universe. Our ability to perceive the physical manifestation of such interactions is embedded in the concept of a *force,* and the "things" that transmit forces among themselves are classified for purposes of analysis as being *solid, fluid,* or some combination of the two. The distinction between solid behavior and fluid behavior has to do with whether or not the "thing" involved has deformation-response characteristics that are time-rate-dependent. A constant force transmitted to a *solid* material will generally elicit a discrete, finite, time-independent deformation response, whereas the same force transmitted to a *fluid* will elicit a continuous, time-dependent response called *flow.* In general, whether or not a given material will behave as a solid or a fluid often depends on its thermodynamic state (i.e., its temperature, pressure, etc.). Moreover, for a given thermodynamic state, some "things" are solid-like when deformed at certain rates but show fluid behavior when disturbed at other rates, so they are appropriately called *viscoelastic,* which literally means, "fluid-solid." Thus a more technical definition of *mechanics* is the science that deals with the action of forces on solids, fluids, and viscoelastic materials. In Chapter 18, the first chapter of this section, Professor Scott Hendricks gives a brief outline of the basic concepts that define the subject of mechanics, and in Chapter 19, Professor Jafar Vossoughi addresses more specifically how the behavior of materials in general and biologic materials in particular is defined for purposes of mechanical analyses. Indeed, what makes mechanics *biomechanics* is the fact that *biomechanics* is the science that deals with the time and space response characteristics of *biologic* solids, fluids, and viscoelastic materials to imposed systems of internal and external forces.

As early as the fourth century B.C., we find in the works of Aristotle (384–322 B.C.) attempts to describe through geometric analysis the mechanical action of muscles in producing locomotion of parts or all of the animal body. Nearly two thousand years later, in his famous anatomic drawings, Leonardo da Vinci (A.D. 1452–1519) sought to describe the mechanics of standing, walking up and down hill, rising from a sitting position, and jumping, and Galileo (A.D. 1564–1643) followed a hundred years later with some of the earliest attempts to mathematically analyze physiologic function. Because of his pioneering efforts in defining the anatomic circulation of blood, William Harvey (A.D. 1578–1657) is credited by many as being the father of modern-day biofluid mechanics, and Alfonso Borelli (A.D. 1608–1679) shares the same honor for contemporary biosolid mechanics because of his efforts to explore the amount of force produced by various muscles and his theorization that bones serve as levers that are operated and controlled by muscles. The early work of these pioneers of biomechanics was followed up by the likes of Sir Isaac Newton (A.D. 1642–1727), Daniel Bernoulli (A.D. 1700–1782), Jean L. M. Poiseuille (A.D. 1799–1869), Thomas Young (A.D. 1773–1829), Euler (whose work was published in 1862), and others of equal fame. To enumerate all their individual contributions would take up much more space than is available in this short introduction, but there is a point to be made if one takes a closer look at the names involved.

In reviewing the preceding list of biomechanical scientists, it is interesting to observe that many of the earliest contributions to our ultimate understanding of the fundamental laws of *physics* and *engineering* (e.g., Bernoulli's equation of hydrodynamics, the famous Young's modulus in elasticity theory, Poiseuille flow, and so on) came from *physicians, physiologists,* and other health care practitioners seeking to study and explain *physiologic* structure and function. The irony in this is that as history has progressed, we have just about turned this situation completely around. That is, more recently, it has been *biomedical engineers* who have been making the greatest contributions to the advancement of the *medical* and *physiologic* sciences. These contributions will become more apparent in the chapters that follow in this section. The individual chapters address the subjects of *biosolid* mechanics and *biofluid* mechanics as they pertain to various subsystems of the human body.

Since the physiologic organism is 60 to 75% fluid, it is not surprising that the subject of biofluid mechanics should be so extensive, including—but not limited to—lubrication of human synovial joints (Chapter 23), cardiac biodynamics (Chapter 31), mechanics of heart valves (Chapter 32), arterial microcirculatory hemodynamics (Chapter 33), mechanics and transport in the microcirculation (Chapter 34), venous microcirculatory hemodynamics (Chapter 36), mechanics of the lymphatic system (Chapter 37), cochlear mechanics (Chapter 38), and vestibular mechanics (Chapter 39). The area of biosolid mechanics is somewhat more loosely defined—since all physiologic tissue is viscoelastic and not strictly solid in the engineering sense of the word. Also generally included under this heading are studies of the kinematics and kinetics of human posture and locomotion, i.e., *biodynamics,* so that under the generic section on biosolid mechanics in this *Handbook* you will find chapters addressing the mechanics of hard tissue (Chapter 20), the mechanics of blood vessels (Chapter 21) or, more generally, the mechanics of viscoelastic tissue, mechanics of joint articulating surface motion (Chapter 22), musculoskeletal soft tissue mechanics (Chapter 24), mechanics of the head/neck (Chapter 25), mechanics of the chest/abdomen (Chapter 26), the analysis of gait (Chapter 27), exercise physiology (Chapter 28), biomechanics and factors affecting mechanical work in humans (Chapter 29), mathematical models of human response to acceleration (Chapter 30), and mechanics and deformability of hematocytes (blood cells) (Chapter 35). In all cases, the ultimate objectives of the science of biomechanics are generally twofold. First, biomechanics aims to understand fundamental aspects of physiologic function for purely medical purposes, and second, it seeks to elucidate such function for mostly nonmedical applications.

In the first instance above, sophisticated techniques have been and continue to be developed to *monitor* physiologic function, to *process* the data thus accumulated, to formulate inductively *theories* that explain the data, and to extrapolate deductively, i.e., to *diagnose* why the human "engine" malfunctions as a result of disease (pathology), aging (gerontology), ordinary wear and tear from normal use (fatigue), and/or accidental impairment from extraordinary abuse (emergency medicine). However, the work does not stop there, for it goes on to provide as well the foundation for the development of technologies to treat and maintain (*therapy*) the human organism in response to malfunction, and this involves biomechanical analyses that have as their ultimate objective an improved health care delivery system. Such improvement includes, but is not limited to, a much healthier *lifestyle* (exercise physiology and sports biomechanics), the ability to *repair* and/or *rehabilitate* body parts, and a technology to *support* ailing physiologic organs (orthotics) and/or, if it should become necessary, to *replace* them completely (with prosthetic parts). Nonmedical applications of biomechanics exploit essentially the same methods and technologies as do those oriented toward the delivery of health care, but in the former case, they involve mostly studies to define the response of the body to "unusual" environments—such as subgravity conditions, the aerospace milieu, and extremes of temperature, humidity, altitude, pressure, acceleration, deceleration, impact, shock, and vibration, and so on. Additional applications include vehicular safety considerations, the mechanics of sports activities, and the expansion of the envelope of human performance capabilities—for whatever purpose! And so, with this very brief introduction, let us take a somewhat of a closer look at the subject of biomechanics.

18

Mechanics: Basic Concepts

Scott L. Hendricks
Virginia Polytechnic Institute
and State University

Mechanics is the science that studies how and why things move. Sir Isaac Newton and his contemporaries developed the basic understanding of motion using vector algebra. Later Joseph Louis Lagrange and Sir William Rowan Hamilton developed an approach to motion using scalar functions and generalized coordinates. Both approaches lead to the same mathematical description of motion. The mechanics of Newton, Lagrange, and Hamilton is called *classical mechanics* and is the subject of this chapter.

Einstein discovered that the ideas developed by Newton need to be modified when speeds approach the speed of light. We conclude from experiments that the speed of light is the same for all observers. This forces us to revise our view of motion so that we can enforce the constancy of the speed of light. The effects of Einstein's special theory of relativity are outside the range of classical mechanics and are not covered here.

Newtonian, Lagrangian, and Hamiltonian dynamics are based on concepts from calculus. Calculus assumes that the world is continuous. We can therefore define the limit of a ratio of two objects as both approach zero. In reality, the world is not continuous but comes in discrete chunks. When dealing with small objects (atomic or molecular), the dynamics must account for this discrete nature. The mechanics that accounts for this discontinuous nature is called *quantum mechanics* and is also outside the range of classical mechanics.

However, for the vast majority of engineering applications, the dynamics of Newton or Lagrange are perfectly adequate. This chapter will review the basic ideas of classical mechanics. Newton gives three laws of motion:

1. A body at rest stays at rest unless acted on by a force.
2. If there is an unbalanced force, then the force (a vector) is proportional to the product of mass (a scalar) and acceleration (a vector).
3. A force on body 1 due to interactions with body 2 is equal and opposite to the force on body 2 due to interactions with body 1.

Newton's first law defines an inertial reference frame that serves as a basis for the application of the second law, which is the fundamental equation of motion. The third law is valid for most but not all forces.

8493-8346-3/95/$0.00+$.50
1995 by CRC Press, Inc.

18.1 Particle Motion

Many problems in dynamics can be solved by modeling the system as a collection of particles. This model will be valid if the bodies in question translate without rotation and if the dimensions of the bodies are small compared with the motions in question.

Particle Kinematics

Kinematics is the study of motion without regard to whatever causes the motion. The simplest kind of motion for a particle is a bead that slides on a straight wire. The most important step in kinematics is to choose a fixed reference point on the wire. This point has to be fixed with respect to an inertial reference frame. The distance along the wire from this point is x. The following kinematic variables are defined by the process of differentiation:

$$\text{Distance:} \qquad x(t) \tag{18.1}$$

$$\text{Velocity:} \qquad v(t) = \frac{dx}{dt} \tag{18.2}$$

$$\text{Acceleration:} \qquad a(t) = \frac{d^2x}{dt^2} \tag{18.3}$$

If the bead moves in a plane (two dimensions), then one measures from some point fixed in an inertial frame. Two perpendicular lines are used to define the cartesian coordinates (distances) x and y. All the previous kinematical variables must then be presented as vectors:

$$\text{Distance:} \qquad \mathbf{R} = x\mathbf{i} + y\mathbf{j} \tag{18.4}$$

$$\text{Velocity:} \qquad \mathbf{V} = \frac{dx}{dt}\mathbf{i} + \frac{dy}{dt}\mathbf{j} \tag{18.5}$$

$$\text{Acceleration:} \qquad \mathbf{A} = \frac{d^2x}{dt^2}\mathbf{i} + \frac{d^2y}{dt^2}\mathbf{j} \tag{18.6}$$

Sometimes it is preferable to use path coordinates instead of cartesian coordinates. In path coordinates, we define the $\mathbf{t}$ unit vector to be in the direction of the velocity. Thus

$$\text{Velocity:} \qquad \mathbf{V} = v\mathbf{t} \tag{18.7}$$

$$\text{Acceleration:} \qquad \mathbf{A} = \frac{dv}{dt}\mathbf{t} + \frac{v^2}{\rho}\mathbf{n} \tag{18.8}$$

where ρ is the radius of curvature, and the unit vector $\mathbf{n}$ is perpendicular to the velocity, pointing to the center of curvature.

A final common method of describing motion is to use polar coordinates (r, θ). Using these variables, we have

$$\text{Distance:} \qquad \mathbf{R} = r\mathbf{r} \tag{18.9}$$

$$\text{Velocity:} \qquad \mathbf{V} = \frac{dr}{dt}\mathbf{r} + r\frac{d\theta}{dt}\boldsymbol{\theta} \tag{18.10}$$

Acceleration:
$$\mathbf{A} = \left[\frac{d^2r}{dt^2} - r\left(\frac{d\theta}{dt}\right)^2\right]\mathbf{r} + \left[r\frac{d^2\theta}{dt^2} + 2\frac{dr}{dt}\frac{d\theta}{dt}\right]\mathbf{\theta} \quad (18.11)$$

where $\mathbf{r}$ is a unit vector that points in the radial direction and $\mathbf{\theta}$ is a unit vector that points perpendicular to $\mathbf{r}$ in a direction given by increasing the angle θ.

When the motion occurs in three dimensions, we can use three cartesian coordinates (x, y, z), or we can use cylindrical coordinates (r, θ, z), which combine polar coordinates with one cartesian coordinate. Path coordinates can be extended to three dimensions by introducing the binormal direction. Spherical coordinates (r, θ, ϕ) are also commonly used.

Newtonian Particle Dynamics

The governing equation that describes particle motion is Newton's second law:

$$\mathbf{F} = m\mathbf{A} \quad (18.12)$$

This is a vector equation in either one, two, or three dimensions. To use this equation, it is necessary to clearly identify all the forces that act on a given body. Drawing a free-body diagram is the first step. It is important to put only real forces on this diagram.

There are two integrated forms of Newton's second law (18.12). These forms of the equation are useful if we are looking for relationships between velocity and location or between velocity and time.

If we integrate Eq. (18.12) with respect to distance along the path, then we derive the work-energy relationship:

$$T_1 + \int_1^2 \mathbf{F} \cdot d\mathbf{R} = T_2 \quad (18.13)$$

where T is the kinetic energy given by

$$T = \frac{1}{2}m\mathbf{V} \cdot \mathbf{V} \quad (18.14)$$

and the subscripts 1 and 2 represent two points along the path of the particle. The integral in Eq. (18.13) represents the work done on the particle as it moves from position 1 to position 2. This approach gives a relationship between velocity and position.

If we integrate Eq. (18.12) with respect to time, then we derive the impulse-momentum relationship:

$$m\mathbf{V}_1 + \int_1^2 \mathbf{F}\, dt = m\mathbf{V}_2 \quad (18.15)$$

The product of mass and velocity is called linear momentum. The integral in Eq. (18.15) is called the linear impulse. The subscripts in Eq. (18.15) represent two different times. The impulse-momentum equations give a relationship between velocity and time.

When a problem involves collisions, the only practical way to handle the problem is to use the impulse-momentum method. It is usually impossible to know the details of the forces during a collision; however, the change in momentum is easy to calculate if we have one experimentally determined parameter called the coefficient of restitution. This number, usually denoted by e, is used to find the ratio of the normal velocities after the collision to the normal velocities before the collision:

$$e\left(V_{Anb} - V_{Bnb}\right) = \left(V_{Bna} - V_{Ana}\right) \quad (18.16)$$

Here the subscripts A and B refer to the two bodies that collide, the subscript n means the normal component (perpendicular to the plane of collision), and the subscripts a and b refer to after and before the collision.

Lagrangian Particle Dynamics

Newton's approach can be cumbersome when the system consists of several particles. Lagrange developed an alternative approach using scalar functions. Lagrange's approach is based on a dynamic extension of the static principle of virtual work. In this approach, Newton's second law is applied only in those directions which are orthogonal to any constraint forces. This has the consequence of hiding the explicit effects of those constraint forces. The equations of motion involve only active forces. This is a big advantage if we want to study only the motion. This is a distinct disadvantage if we need to study the constraint forces between bodies. If we want a complete knowledge of all motion and all constraint forces, then we should use Newton's approach instead of Lagrange's approach.

Consider a system composed of N particles. If there are no constraints between the particles, then there are $3N$ degrees of freedom. For each constraint, we eliminate 1 degree of freedom. If there are m constraints, then we have $n = 3N - m$ degrees of freedom. We can now describe the motion in terms of n generalized coordinates ($q_1, q_2, \ldots, q_n$). These generalized coordinates can be distances, angles, expansion coefficients, or any other suitable set of coordinates. The Lagrangian machinery treats all coordinates the same way.

In the following scalar energy functions:

$$T = \sum_{i=1}^{i=N} \frac{1}{2} m_i \, \mathbf{V}_i \cdot \mathbf{V}_i \qquad V = \sum_{i=1}^{i=N} V_i \tag{18.17}$$

T represents the total kinetic energy of the system, and V represents the total potential energy of the system. A scalar potential energy is associated with every conservative force. The relationship between force and potential energy is

$$\mathbf{F}_i = -\nabla V_i \tag{18.18}$$

If there is viscous damping in the problem so that a force is proportional to velocity $\mathbf{F}_i = -c_i \mathbf{V}_i$, then we can define a scalar dissipation function

$$D = \sum_{i=1}^{i=N} \frac{1}{2} c_i \, \mathbf{V}_i \cdot \mathbf{V}_i \tag{18.19}$$

The equations of motion now follow by applying the following equation once for each generalized coordinate:

$$\frac{d}{dt} \left(\frac{\partial T}{\partial \dot{q}_j} \right) - \frac{\partial T}{\partial q_j} + \frac{\partial D}{\partial \dot{q}_j} + \frac{\partial V}{\partial q_j} = Q_j \tag{18.20}$$

Any forces that are conservative are accounted for in the term involving the potential energy V. Any viscous forces are included in the term involving the dissipation function D. If any other forces have not yet been accounted for, their effect must be included in the term Q_j, called the *generalized force:*

$$Q_j = \sum_{i=1}^{i=N} \mathbf{F}_i \cdot \frac{\partial \mathbf{R}_i}{\partial q_j} \tag{18.21}$$

18.2 Rigid-Body Motion

When a particle model is not adequate, we may model the system as a collection of rigid bodies. This model introduces rotation, rotational inertia, and significant complications.

Rigid-Body Kinematics

When analyzing a rigid body, it is necessary to know the rotational orientation in addition to the translational location. Although there is no such thing as a rotational position vector, we can define a rotational velocity vector called the *angular velocity vector* $\boldsymbol{\omega}$. The time derivative of the angular velocity vector is called the *angular acceleration vector* $\boldsymbol{\alpha}$. If A and B are two points on the same rigid body, then

$$\mathbf{V}_B = \mathbf{V}_A + \boldsymbol{\omega} \times \mathbf{AB} \tag{18.22}$$

$$\mathbf{A}_B = \mathbf{A}_A + \boldsymbol{\alpha} \times \mathbf{AB} + \boldsymbol{\omega} \times \boldsymbol{\omega} \times \mathbf{AB} \tag{18.23}$$

The vector $\mathbf{AB}$ is a position vector that starts at point A and ends at point B. These kinematic equations are commonly used to impose physical constraints on the system.

Newtonian Rigid-Body Dynamics

If the body is restricted to motion in a plane [translation only in the xy plane, and rotation only about a line perpendicular to the plane (z axis)], then newtonian dynamics are represented by the equations

$$\mathbf{F} = m\mathbf{A}_G \tag{18.24}$$

$$\mathbf{M}_G = I_G \boldsymbol{\alpha} \quad \text{or} \quad \mathbf{M}_{FP} = I_{FP}\, \boldsymbol{\alpha} \tag{18.25}$$

The subscript G means center of mass. Equation (18.24) says that the rigid body moves as if it were a particle with all the mass concentrated at a special point called the *center of mass*. This point is unique in that it is the only point for which Eq. (18.24) applies. In Eq. (18.25), $\mathbf{M}$ represents the moment of all forces applied to the body, and I represents the mass moment of inertia about the z axis (be careful not to use the area moment of inertia). Equation (18.25) only works if applied about the center of mass (G) or about a fixed point (FP). The rotational dynamics are significantly more complicated if it is applied about any point besides the center of mass or a fixed point.

If we allow the bodies to move so that they do not stay in a single plane of motion, then Eq. (18.24) still applies; however, Eq. (18.25) must be modified. Switching to matrix notation, Eq. (18.24) becomes

$$\begin{Bmatrix} M_1 \\ M_2 \\ M_3 \end{Bmatrix} = \begin{bmatrix} I_{11} & I_{12} & I_{13} \\ I_{12} & I_{22} & I_{23} \\ I_{13} & I_{23} & I_{33} \end{bmatrix} \begin{Bmatrix} \alpha_1 \\ \alpha_2 \\ \alpha_3 \end{Bmatrix} + \begin{bmatrix} 0 & -\omega_3 & \omega_2 \\ \omega_3 & 0 & -\omega_1 \\ -\omega_2 & \omega_1 & 0 \end{bmatrix} \begin{bmatrix} I_{11} & I_{12} & I_{13} \\ I_{12} & I_{22} & I_{23} \\ I_{13} & I_{23} & I_{33} \end{bmatrix} \begin{Bmatrix} \omega_1 \\ \omega_2 \\ \omega_3 \end{Bmatrix} \tag{18.26}$$

where M_i represents one of the components of the moment of the forces, I_{ij} represents one of the elements of the mass moment of inertia tensor, ω_i represents one of the components of the angular velocity vector, and α_i represents one of the components of angular acceleration. Equation (18.26) is only valid if we work around the center of mass or around a fixed point. The components of all vectors need to be calculated with respect to a set of body-fixed axes.

If the body-fixed axes are chosen in principal directions so that the off-diagonal terms in the inertia matrix are zero, then Eq. (18.26) becomes

$$M_1 = I_{11}\alpha_1 - (I_{22} - I_{33})\,\omega_2\,\omega_3$$
$$M_2 = I_{22}\alpha_2 - (I_{33} - I_{11})\,\omega_3\,\omega_1$$
$$M_3 = I_{33}\alpha_3 - (I_{11} - I_{22})\,\omega_1\,\omega_2 \tag{18.27}$$

Lagrangian Rigid-Body Dynamics

The machinery of lagrangian dynamics is the same for rigid bodies as it was for particles except that the kinetic energy is now given by

$$T = \sum \left(\frac{1}{2} m \mathbf{V}_G \cdot \mathbf{V}_G + \frac{1}{2} (\omega_1, \omega_2, \omega_3) \begin{bmatrix} I_{11} & I_{12} & I_{13} \\ I_{12} & I_{22} & I_{23} \\ I_{13} & I_{23} & I_{33} \end{bmatrix} \begin{Bmatrix} \omega_1 \\ \omega_2 \\ \omega_3 \end{Bmatrix} \right) \tag{18.28}$$

where G represents the center of mass or a fixed point, and the moments of inertia are calculated about the center of mass or the fixed point. The sum is over the number of rigid bodies.

The generalized force becomes

$$Q_j = \sum \left(\mathbf{F} \cdot \frac{\partial \mathbf{R}_A}{\partial q_j} + \mathbf{M}_A \cdot \frac{\partial \boldsymbol{\omega}}{\partial \mathbf{q}_j} \right) \tag{18.29}$$

where A represents any convenient point on the body and the summation is over the number of rigid bodies in the system.

Further Information

This chapter has reviewed basic mechanics ideas for particles and rigid bodies. The equations of motion are based on Newton's second law or equivalently on the developments of Lagrange and Hamilton. To use these equations properly, the kinematics must be based on an inertial reference system and the center of mass must be used in appropriate places.

A good basic introduction to particle rigid-body mechanics is contained in *Engineering Mechanics*, by J. L. Meriam and L. G. Kraige. For a more advanced treatment of rigid-body dynamics, see *Principles of Dynamics*, by Donald T. Greenwood. By far the most complete treatment on Lagrangian and Hamiltonian dynamics is contained in *Classical Mechanics*, by Herbert Goldstein.

The ideas presented in this chapter can be extended to apply to fluids (liquids or gases). A good overview of fluid mechanics can be found in *Fundamental Mechanics of Fluids*, by I. G. Currie. Vibrations are probably the most important application of mechanics. An excellent book that covers vibrations of rigid and flexible bodies is *Elements of Vibration Analysis*, by Leonard Meirovitch.

References

Currie IG. 1993. Fundamental Mechanics of Fluids, 2d ed. New York, McGraw-Hill.

Goldstein H. 1980. Classical Mechanics, 2d ed. Reading, Mass, Addison-Wesley.

Greenwood DT. 1988. Principles of Dynamics, 2d ed. Englewood Cliffs, NJ, Prentice-Hall.

Meirovitch L. 1986. Elements of Vibration Analysis, 2d ed. New York, McGraw-Hill.

Meriam JL, Kraige LG. 1992. Engineering Mechanics, 3d ed. New York, Wiley.

19

Constitutive Modeling of Biologic Materials

Jafar Vossoughi
Engineering Research Center,
University of the District
Columbia

Deformation of a body under known loading cannot be determined from the general physical laws alone; it is necessary to specify the material from which the body is made. Mathematically, such specification is known as *constitutive modeling* (equations or relations). Therefore, constitutive equations relate the stress tensor and the heat flux vector to deformation. The general principles are common to all media, and therefore, they are universal laws of nature, whereas the constitutive relations are tailored to specific media under restrictive conditions. For example, in classical theory of elasticity, it is assumed that the stress tensor is a linear function of deformation and is restrictive to liner materials undergoing infinitesimal deformations. Likewise, in classical theory of viscoelasticity, it is assumed that the stress tensor depends linearly on the deformation rate which is restrictive to linear viscous fluids. In fact, both these assumptions are not physically valid, but they are assumed for simplicity based on empirical facts obtained from numerous laboratory tests and observations. The assumptions are specific to ideal materials. They are also applied to materials as a continuum considered to be homogeneous on a macro scale. We know that assumption of homogeneity is not true for any material, especially biologic materials. Human-made materials, on the one hand, are more homogeneous than the biologic materials, and their degree of homogeneity can be improved in the process of manufacturing. Biologic materials, on the other hand, are nonuniformly inhomogeneous, and their homogeneity varies highly from specimen to specimen and tissue to tissue, not to mention from species to species. Homogeneity of the biologic materials cannot be improved, and in fact, the degree of inhomogeneity increases with metabolic actions, drugs, disease, environmental factors, aging, and so on. These arguments are purposely presented in the beginning of this chapter to emphasize the following: (1) many base assumptions regarding biologic materials are crude and therefore do not warrant the establishment of highly sophisticated constitutive formulations with many constitutive constants; (2) work in bioengineering is highly multidisciplinary, and therefore,

0-8493-8346-3/95/$0.00+$.50
© 1995 by CRC Press, Inc.

the constitutive formulation should be simple enough to be used and interpreted by the end users who may have problems even in using Hooke's law; and (3) since the constitutive constants should eventually be evaluated experimentally, the constitutive formulations should be simple enough to involve simple laboratory experiments in a quantitative determination of the constitutive constants.

19.1 Basic Principles of Mechanics

In applying the basic principles of mechanics, i.e., conservation of mass and energy and balance of momenta to a problem, no distinction needs to be made between different types of substances, e.g., elastic solids, fluids, gases, viscoelastic materials, and materials possessing different types of physical properties. The physical properties that are characteristic of materials are incorporated into the formulation through the appropriate constitutive equations for each particular material on a case-by-case basis. Since there are nearly an infinite number of materials, one should expect at least the same number of constitutive relations. However, in grouping certain materials in different categories, one can find that a single "form" of constitutive equation can characterize numerous materials in that category [9]. For example, most of the engineering materials around us can be characterized under certain restrictions with the simplest constitutive relations, i.e., Hooke's law, which states that the stress tensor σ_{ij} is linearly related to strain tensor e_{kl}, or

$$\sigma_{ij} = C_{ijkl} e_{kl} \qquad (19.1)$$

where C_{ijkl} are known as *constitutive constants,* or simply the *elastic moduli,* and are intrinsic material properties and independent of the coordinate system. In this restrictive category (linear elastic materials under infinitesimal deformations), C_{ijkl} are independent of stress and strain.

Similarly, a variety of nonviscous fluids can be characterized using the following simple constitutive relations:

$$\sigma_{ij} = -p\delta_{ij} \qquad (19.2)$$

where δ_{ij} is the Kronecker delta and p is a scalar called *pressure.* A variety of gases can be characterized mathematically using the following simple constitutive equation known as the *equation of state:*

$$p = \rho RT \qquad (19.3)$$

where p, ρ, and T represent the pressure, density, and temperature, respectively, and R is the gas constant.

For newtonian viscous fluids, the constitutive relations will take the following form:

$$\sigma_{ij} = -p\delta_{ij} + c_{ijkl} D_{kl} \qquad (19.4)$$

where D_{kl} is the strain rate tensor and c_{ijkl} is the viscosity coefficients tensor.

Although the preceding examples of the representative constitutive formulations are fairly *simple* and represent a large number of materials around us, if we incorporate other pertinent material behaviors such as thermal, viscoelastic, dynamic, chemical/biochemical, electrical, magnetic, and their combination, the problems can become fairly complicated and unmanageable mathematically as well as experimentally even for these simple groups. Furthermore, biologic materials such as soft tissues are highly nonlinear and capable of undergoing large deformations that prevent them from being characterized by a simple linear system such as Hooke's law even under physiologic conditions. Unfortunately, the superposition principle also cannot be used for nonlinear systems. All these problems make the development of constitutive formulations for biologic materials fairly difficult.

19.2 Axioms of Constitutive Theory

In adequate representation of materials by the constitutive relations, certain physical and mathematical requirements must be satisfied. The axioms of constitutive theory are listed below. Detailed information on the significance of the axioms is provided in any basic continuum mechanics textbook [9].

1. Axiom of admissibility
2. Axiom of causality
3. Axiom of determinism
4. Axiom of equipresence
5. Axiom of material invariance
6. Axiom of memory
7. Axiom of neighborhood
8. Axiom of objectivity

19.3 Determination of the Constitutive Relations

Constitutive equations (models) characterize the reactions of individual materials to the applied loads. These equations are called *constitutive* because they describe the macroscopic behavior resulting from the internal constitution of the material. The only way to determine constitutive relations for a material is through the interaction between the theory and experiment. Basically, one can write down the constitutive formulation using a series of open parameters (constitutive constants), simplify the formulation to represent the physical material behavior, and finally conduct appropriate experiments to evaluate the numerical values of the open parameters. The basic procedures for this three-phase process are explained in the following. Because of space limitations, most of the details are left out, and readers should consult the appropriate references, such as [9].

We are looking for a mathematical form or model (constitutive model) that relates stresses in the body to deformations (or strains or strain rates). There are three basic approaches: (1) purely theoretical, (2) experimental, and (3) guessing, i.e., trial and error. Most of the available work on constitutive relations for biologic tissues and materials has been obtained by guessing the form and selecting the best fit to the data. Here, however, because of the nature of this *Handbook*, a basic and systematic method based on theories of continuum mechanics is presented. The method is theoretical, and a general formulation (with open parameters) is first presented, and then, using appropriate experiments, the numerical values of the open parameters are evaluated.

The theoretical problem can be approached in two classic ways: (1) *Cauchy's method*, where stresses are expressed directly in terms of strains or deformation gradients, and (2) *Green's method*, where stresses are expressed in terms of the strain energy density function, which is a function of strains. Although Cauchy's method is more general, for simplicity, Green's method is often used because it involves less work and fewer constitutive constants. The second approach is based on the existence of the strain energy function. At least for adiabatic and isothermal deformations, it can be proven that such a strain energy density function exists.

19.4 Strain Energy Function

When the material or tissue is loaded externally, these external loads do work, and the work is stored in the body in the form of energy. Assuming the process is adiabatic, without internal dissipation, and with no other energy exchanges, the additional mechanical work due to external loading which is stored in the body as strain energy is available to do work when the deformation is allowed to recover. This stored energy is usually expressed per unit mass or volume, which is why it is called strain energy *density*. The strain energy for an elastic body is a function of the state of deformation only. The mathematical form of this strain energy is called the *strain energy density function*.

During the past three decades, a number of strain energy functions have been proposed by various investigators in describing the mechanical behavior of biologic materials and tissues. For solid biomaterials/tissues, most of the work is concentrated on blood vessels and myocardium. There is considerably less work on lung, skin, ligament, tendon, cartilage, and bone. Work on constitutive relations for biofluids is mostly limited to blood.

19.5 Constitutive Relations for Blood Vessels

The first mathematical/experimental treatment of biologic materials (blood vessels) in the context of large deformation and modern continuum mechanics is from Ticker and Sacks, 1964 and 1967 [33,34]. Later Tanaka and Fung [10, 32] proposed a constitutive relation for soft tissue in the form of exponential function for simple uniaxial state of stress-strain as

$$\sigma = (\sigma^* + \beta) \, e^{\alpha(\lambda - \lambda^*)} - \beta \tag{19.5}$$

where σ and λ are the stress and stretch ratio, σ^* and λ^* correspond to a point on the stress-strain curve, and β and α are the material constants. This information, however, is limited to a uniaxial state of stress-strain, and therefore, a more general multiaxial-based formulation is needed. A number of constitutive models are available that describe the passive material properties of blood vessels. If the material is linear and the deformation is limited to infinitesimal, then a simple linear relationship (Hooke's law) will be sufficient in describing the stress-strain relationship *uniquely*. For nonlinear materials capable of undergoing large deformations, the formulation *is not unique,* and in fact, any formulation that adequately relates stresses to strains (say, within the physiologic range) with sufficient accuracy is acceptable. Unfortunately, a simple constitutive model is yet to be discovered. Another problem frequently encountered is that one constitutive model may well represent one type of blood vessel but not the others, or a model may well approximate a portion of the stress-strain curve but not the entire space. All the functions presented are fairly complicated even to average engineers. Four such functions frequently used by various investigators are briefly summarized in the following.

Polynomial Form for the Strain Energy Function

A polynomial form for the strain energy density function is presented by Patel and Vaishnav [26] in the form of

$$\rho_o W = Aa^2 + Bab + Cb^2 + Da^3 + Ea^2b + Fab^2 + Gb^3 + \cdots \tag{19.6}$$

where ρ_o is the density of vascular wall, $A, B, \ldots, G, \ldots$ are material (constitutive) constants, and a and b are Green–St. Venant strains in circumferential and longitudinal directions, respectively [36]. Green–St. Venant strains are related to stretch ratios as

$$a = 1/2 \, (\lambda_\theta^2 - 1) \quad \text{and} \quad b = 1/2 \, (\lambda_z^2 - 1) \tag{19.7}$$

Having the strain energy density function W, one can evaluate the stresses by taking partial derivatives of W with respect to strains, which results in

$$S_\theta = \frac{\lambda_\theta}{\lambda_z \lambda_r} \frac{\partial W}{\partial a}$$

$$S_z = \frac{\lambda_z}{\lambda_\theta \lambda_r} \frac{\partial w}{\partial b} \tag{19.8}$$

Since the material of the artery is incompressible, the third strain (the radial strain) is related to a and b, and therefore, we started the expression for W as a function of a and b only. Also, for an incompressible material the stresses can be evaluated only within a hydrostatic pressure. Stress in the radial direction is simply the average of the pressure inside and outside the artery:

$$S_r = -\frac{p}{2} \tag{19.9}$$

where p is the intraluminal pressure. Since stresses in the circumferential and longitudinal directions are more important, the stress differences are calculated to eliminate the hydrostatic pressure. Using Eqs. (19.6) to (19.9), the stress differences can be evaluated as

$$
\begin{aligned}
S_\theta - S_r = {} & 2Aa + Bb + (4A + 3D)a^2 + (2B + 2E)ab + Fb^2 + (6D + 4H)a^3 \\
& + (4E + 3I)a^2b + (2F + 2J)ab^2 + Kb^3 + 8Ha^4 + 6Ia^3b + 4Ja^2b^2 + 2Kab^3
\end{aligned}
\tag{19.10}
$$

$$
\begin{aligned}
S_z - S_r = {} & Ba + 2Cb + Ea^2 + (2B + 2F)ab + (4C + 3G)b^2 + Ia^3 + (2E + 2J)a^2b \\
& + (4F + 3K) + ab^2 + (6G + 4L)b^3 + 2Ia^3b + 4Ja^2b^2 + 6Kab^3 + 8Lb^4
\end{aligned}
$$

These are stress-strain relations based on fourth-order strain energy density function (12-constant theory). Those for third and second order can be obtained from the preceding stress-strain relations by dropping the appropriate terms. For higher-order expressions for W, appropriate terms should be added to these equations. Patel and Vaishnav [26] have shown experimentally that the 7-constant theory is sufficient to represent the mechanical properties of canine thoracic aorta. A 3-constant theory also may be used to approximately represent the mechanical behavior of the arterial tissue. The type of experiment used was the inflation and extension of the arterial tube and measurement of the external diameter and axial extension. The constitutive constants for the 3- and 7-constant theories are shown in Table 19.1. Others also have used polynomial constitutive model for soft biologic tissues [3,6,7,11,12,26,36,40,41,43].

TABLE 19.1 Polynomial Form for Strain Energy Function

Three-Constant Theory
$W = Aa^2 + Bab + Cb^2$
$A = 0.372 \pm 0.030;\quad B = 0.219 \pm 0.019;\quad C = 0.288 \pm 0.038$
Seven-Constant Theory
$W = Aa^2 + Bab + Cb^2 + Da^3 + Ea^2b + Fab^2 + Gb^3$
$A = 0.412 \pm 0.066;\quad B = -0.067 \pm 0.131;\quad C = 0.191 \pm 0.059$
$D = -0.055 \pm 0.036;\quad E = 0.162 \pm 0.051;\quad F = 0.179 \pm 0.103$
$G = 0.099 \pm 0.087$
The values (average $\pm$ SEM) are in dyn/cm$^2 \times 10^6$

Exponential Form for the Strain Energy Function

The second type of strain energy density function frequently used is an exponential one [10–12] of the form

$$\rho_0 W = \frac{C}{2} [e^Q] \tag{19.11}$$

with
$$Q = a_1 (a^2 - a^{*2}) + a_2 (b^2 - b^{*2}) + 2a_4 (ab - a^* b^*)$$

where C (with unit of stress) and a_1, a_2, and a_4 (dimensionless) are material constants. Using inflation-extension tests on rabbit arteries, Fung et al. [12] experimentally evaluated the constitutive constants that are listed in Table 19.2. Both the polynomial and experimental models presented above have three problems: Both models are complicated and do not closely approximate the entire range of experimental data (from low stress to physiologic stress range), and the constants are highly different from vessel to vessel and from species to species. Perhaps there is no good solution to closely approximate all vessel types from all species within the physiologic range of stress-strain and beyond.

TABLE 19.2 Exponential Form for Strain Energy Function

$$W = \frac{C}{2} \{\exp [a_1 (a^2 - a^{*2}) + a_2 (b^2 - b^{*2}) + 2a_4 (ab - a^*b^*)]\}$$

$C = (2.9307 \pm 0.2730) \times 10^5 \text{ dyn/cm}^2; \quad a_1 = 2.5084 \pm 0.3485$
$a_2 = 0.4615 \pm 0.0710; \quad a_4 = 0.1764 \pm 0.0261$
All values, mean $\pm$ SEM

For more details and values of the constants for a variety of other arteries see Fung et al. [12].

Recently Fung et al. examined the *very low stress-strain range* [13] and concluded that linear (Hooke's law), exponential, and power law models all represent the experimental data very well. For the rest of the curve, none of the three forms is acceptable. In order to have one form well represent the entire stress-strain range, Fung et al. [13] proposed the following expression for strain energy (which is a combination of polynomial and exponential):

$$W = \frac{C}{2} (e^Q - Q - 1) + \frac{q}{2}$$

$$(19.12)$$

where

$$Q = a_1 a^2 + a_2 b^2 + 2a_4 ab$$

$$q = b_1 a^2 + b_2 b^2 + 2b_4 ab$$

Now there are seven constitutive constants. They have applied this new formulation to experiments on canine thoracic aorta and have evaluated the constitutive constants that are presented in Table 19.3.

TABLE 19.3 Combined Polynomial-Exponential Form for Strain Energy Function

$$W = \frac{C}{2} (e^Q - Q - 1) + \frac{q}{2}$$
$$Q = a_1 a^2 - a_2 b^2 + 2a_4 ab$$
$$q = b_1 a^2 + b_2 b^2 + 2b_4 ab$$

$C = 19.27 \pm 31.28$ kPa	$a_1 = 0.832 \pm 0.351$
$a_2 = 1.888 \pm 0.977$	$a_4 = -0.0344 \pm 0.0863$
$b_1 = 41.22 \pm 19.06$ kPa	$b_2 = 43.52 \pm 18.73$ kPa
$b_4 = 13.29 \pm 5.15$ kPa	

All values, mean $\pm$ SD, averaged for 6 canine thoracic aortas

Logarithmic Form for the Strain Energy Function

The third type of constitutive relations used (for arteries) is the logarithmic one [14,31] of the form

$$W = -C \ln (1 - \psi)$$
$$\psi = \frac{1}{2} a_1 a^2 + \frac{1}{2} a_2 b^2 + a_3 ab \tag{19.13}$$

where W, a, and b are the strain energy density function, circumferential strain, and longitudinal strain, respectively, and C, a_1, a_2, and a_3 are the constitutive constants. They [14,31] have applied the logarithmic form to the inflation extension experiments on dog common carotid arteries. The results are shown in Table 19.4. They also have applied polynomial and exponential forms to the same data and have concluded that the logarithmic form is far superior to the polynomial form and somewhat better than the exponential form [14]. It is also somewhat easier to attach physical meaning to the coefficients in the exponential and logarithmic forms compared with the polynomial form.

TABLE 19.4 Logarithmic Form for Strain Energy Function

$W = -C \ln (1 - \psi)$	
$\psi = \frac{1}{2} a_1 a^2 + \frac{1}{2} a_2 b^2 + a_3 ab$	
$C = 65.44 \pm 13.20$ kPa	$a_1 = 0.4532 \pm 0.1471$
$a_2 = 0.5982 \pm 0.2509$	$a_3 = 0.0710 \pm 0.0575$
All values, mean $\pm$ SD, averaged for 8 canine common carotid arteries	

Power Law Stress-Strain Model

The fourth type of constitutive relation used is the power law [28] of the form

$$T = KS^n \tag{19.14}$$

where T is the stress tensor, S is the strain or strain rate tensor, and K and n are the material constants. The significance of the power law constitutive form is its simplicity. The form involves only two material constants and can appropriately represent the experimental data, at least for the uniaxial case, from a variety of tissues fairly well [28,29]. Table 19.5 shows the values of the constants K and n when the power law is applied to the stress-strain data of various biologic tissues. For blood, the original power law representation, known as the *Walburn-Schneck power law*, is a classic [39].

For pseudo-strain-energy density function for the lung parenchyma, see Fung [11] and Lanir [22]. More than two dozen pseudoelastic constitutive models have been proposed to characterize the behavior of skin under stretch. For a complete review, see Lanir [23]. Other slightly different constitutive models are also used successfully for vascular and other tissues [2–8,17–27,30,36, 37,40–43].

TABLE 19.5 Power-Law Constitutive Modeling

$T = KS^n$		
$K = 1.8826 \times 10^5$ N/m^2	$n = 1.6$	for cardiac muscle
$K = 1.2580 \times 10^6$ N/m^2	$n = 2.66$	for smooth muscle
$K = 3.4870 \times 10^9$ N/m^2	$n = 3.226$	for fascia
$K = 9.5610 \times 10^9$ N/m^2	$n = 3.391$	for fibrocartilage
$K = 2.2580 \times 10^9$ N/m^2	$n = 0.638$	for human fibula bone

19.6 Biologic Residual Stress-Strain

Although residual stress in arteries was noticed a long time ago by Bergel [1], the first measurement of the residual strain in arteries was reported almost a decade ago [35]. Several researchers used the residual stress to correct the stress distribution across the thickness of the arteries (for comprehensive list of works on biologic residual stress-strain, see references in [38]). Theoretical solution of residually stressed bodies under large deformations already exists [15,16]. To date, no attempt has been made to rationally incorporate the values of the experimentally obtained biologic residual stress-strain into the constitutive relations in the framework of modern continuum mechanics.

19.7 Directions for Future Research in Constitutive Modeling of Biologic Materials/Tissues

The challenge of the next century is development of a highly simple constitutive formulation that (1) approximates all types of biologic tissues and materials with a reasonable accuracy over a wide range of deformations, (2) incorporates internal residual stresses inherent to the biologic tissues and organs, (3) includes the response of smooth muscle and active components (in terms of electrical, electromagnetic, and biochemical activities), (4) can predict the behavior of the tissues while the tissue is developing, growing, and undergoing remodeling due to drugs, aging, disease, and so on, (5) are sophisticated enough to predict the mechanical behavior of the organs and tissues up to and including failure, which is clinically relevant and has application in trauma; and finally, (6) has a certain degree of sophistication and flexibility so that the new formulation can be manipulated in a simple manner to cover mechanical behavior at organ, tissue, and cellular levels.

Acknowledgments

Support of the NSF Grant HRD-9104562 is greatly appreciated.

References

1. Bergel DH. 1960. The Viscoelastic Properties of the Arterial Wall, Ph.D thesis. University of London.
2. Bingham DN, Dehoff PH. 1979. A constitutive equation for the canine anterior cruciate ligament. J Biomech Eng 101:15.
3. Canfield TR, Dobrin PB. 1987. Static elastic properties of blood vessels. In R Skalak and S Chien (eds), Handbook of Bioengineering, chap 16. New York, McGraw-Hill.
4. Cowin, SC, Sadegh, AM, Luo GM. 1992. An evolutionary wolf's law for trabecular architecture. J Biomech Eng 114:129.
5. Cowin SC, Van Buskirk WC, Ashman RB. 1987. Properties of bone. In R Skalak and S Chien (eds), Handbook of Bioengineering, chap 2, New York, McGraw-Hill.
6. Dobrin PB. 1978. Mechanical properties of arteries. Physiol Rev 58:397.
7. Dobrin PB. 1983. Vascular mechanics. In JT Shepherd and F Abboud (eds) Handbook of Physiology, chap 3. Washington, DC, American Physiological Society.
8. Easthope PL, Brooks DE. 1980. A comparison of rheological constitutive functions for whole human blood. Biorheology 17:235.
9. Eringen AC. 1967. Mechanics of Continua. New York, Wiley.
10. Fung YC. 1967. Elasticity of soft tissues in simple elongation. Am J Physiol 213:1532.
11. Fung YC. 1990. Biomechanics: Motion, Flow Stress, and Growth. New York, Springer-Verlag.
12. Fung YC, Fronek K, Patitucci P. 1979. Pseudoelasticity of arteries and the choice of its mathematical expression. Am J Physiol 237(5):H620.

13. Fung YC, Liu SQ, Zhou JB. 1993. Remodeling of the constitutive equation while a blood vessel remodels itself under stress. J Biomech Eng 115:453.
14. Hayashi K. 1993. Experimental approach on measuring the mechanical properties and constitutive laws of arterial walls. J Biomech Eng 115:481.
15. Hoger A. 1986. On the determination of residual stress in an elastic bodies. J Elasticity 16:303.
16. Hoger A. 1994. On the determination of residual stress in biological materials. In J Vossoughi (ed), Biomedical Engineering/Recent Developments, pp 211–214, Washington, DC, University of the District of Columbia.
17. Humphrey JD, Yin FCP. 1987. A new constitutive formulation for characterizing the mechanical behavior of soft tissue. J Biophys 52:563.
18. Humphrey JD, Yin FCP. 1987. On constitutive relations and finite deformations of passive cardiac tissue: I. A pseudostrain-energy function. J Biomech Eng 109:298.
19. Humphrey JD, Strumpf RK, Yin FCP. 1989. A theoretically based experimental approach for identifying vascular constitutive relations. Biorheology 26:687.
20. Humphrey JD, Strumpf RK, Yin FCP. 1990. Determination of a constitutive relation for passive myocardium: II. Parameter estimation. J Biomech Eng 112:340.
21. Lai WM, Mow VC, Zhu W. 1993. Constitutive modelling of articular cartilage and biomacromolecular solutions. J Biomech Eng 115:464.
22. Lanir Y. 1983. Constitutive equation for lung tissue. J Biomech Eng 105:374.
23. Lanir Y. 1987. Skin mechanics. In R Skalak and S Chien (eds), Handbook of Bioengineering, chap 11, New York, McGraw-Hill.
24. Lin I-E, Taber LA. 1994. Mechanical effects of looping in the embryonic chick heart. J Biomech 27:311.
25. Mow VC, Kuei SC, Lai WM, Armstrong CG. 1980. Biphasic creep and stress relaxation of articular cartilage: Theory and experiment. J Biomech 102:73.
26. Patel DJ, Vaishnav RN. 1980. Basic Hemodynamics and Its Role in Disease Process. Baltimore, University Park Press.
27. Pinto JG. 1987. A constitutive description of contracting papillary muscle and its implications to the dynamics of the intact heart. J Biomech Eng 109:181.
28. Schneck DJ, Simanowith MC. 1994. Power-law modelling of the passive, nonlinear, time dependent constitutive behavior of physiologic tissue. In J Vossoughi (ed), Biomedical Engineering/Recent Developments, pp 325–328, Washington, DC, University of the District of Columbia.
29. Schneck DJ. 1992. Mechanics of Muscle, 2d ed, New York, New York University Press.
30. Skalak R, Tözeren A, Zarda RP, Chien S. 1973. Strain energy function of red blood cell membranes. Biophys 13:245.
31. Takamizawa K, Hayashi K. 1987. Strain energy density function and uniform strain hypothesis for arterial mechanics. J Biomech 20:7.
32. Tanaka TT, Fung YC. 1974. Elastic and inelastic properties of the canine aorta and their variation along the aortic tree. J Biomech 7:357.
33. Tickner EG, Sacks AH. 1964. Theoretical and experimental study of the elastic behavior of the human brachial and other human and canine arteries. Vidya Report no 162, Palo Alto, Calif.
34. Tickner EG, Sacks AH. 1967. A theory for the elastic behavior of blood vessels. Biorheology 4:151.
35. Vaishnav RN, Vossoughi J. 1983. Estimation of residual strain in aortic segment. In CW Hall (ed), Biomedical Engineering II. Recent Developments, pp 330–333. New York, Pergamon Press.
36. Vaishnav RN, Vossoughi J. 1984. Incremental formulation in vascular mechanics. J Biomech Eng 106:105.
37. Vito RP, Hickey J. 1980. The mechanical properties of soft tissue: II. The elastic response of arterial segments. J Biomech 13:951.

38. Vossoughi J. 1994. Biological residual stress and strain. In J Vossoughi (ed), Biomedical Engineering/Recent Developments, pp 200–206, Washington, DC, University of the District of Columbia.
39. Walburn FJ, Schneck DJ. 1976. A constitutive equation for whole human blood. J Biomech 13:201.
40. Weizsäcker HW, Lambert H, Pascale K. 1983. Analysis of the passive mechanical properties of rat carotid arteries. J Biomech 16:703.
41. Weizsäcker HW, Pinto JG. 1988. Isotropy and anisotrophy of the arterial wall. J Biomech 21:477.
42. Woo SL-Y, Johnson GA, Smith BA. 1983. Mathematical modelling of ligaments and tendons. J Biomech Eng 115: 473.
43. Wu SG, Lee GC, Tseng NT. 1984. Nonlinear elastic analysis of blood vessels. J Biomech Eng 106:376.

Nomenclature

σ_{ij}	Stress tensor
e_{ij}	Strain tensor
C	Material constitutive constant
p	Pressure
T	Stress tensor, temperature
S	Strain or strain rate tensor
K, n	Material constitutive constants
ρ, ρ_o	Density
R	Gas constant
$D_{\kappa l}$	Deformation rate tensor
σ	Stress
α, β	Material constitutive constants
λ	Stretch ratio
a, b	Circumferential and longitudinal Green–St. Venant strains
S_θ, S_z, S_r	Circumferential, longitudinal, and radial stresses
C_{ijkl}	Material constitutive constants (or moduli)
a_1, a_2, a_3, a_4	Material constitutive constant
b_1, b_2, b_3, b_4	Material constitutive constant
$A, B, \ldots$	Material constitutive constants
c_{ijkl}	Viscosity coefficient tensor
$\lambda_\theta, \lambda_z, \lambda_r$	Circumferential, longitudinal, and radial stretch ratios

20
Mechanics of Hard Tissue

Lawrence Katz
Department of Biomedical
Engineering, Case Western
Reserve University

Hard tissue, mineralized tissue, and *calcified tissue* are often used as synonyms for bone when describing the structure and properties of bone or tooth. The *hard* is self-evident in comparison with all other mammalian tissues, which often are referred to as *soft tissues.* Use of the terms *mineralized* and *calcified* arises from the fact that, in addition to the principle protein, collagen, and other proteins, glycoproteins, and protein-polysaccherides, comprising about 50% of the volume, the major constituent of bone is a calcium phosphate (thus the term *calcified*) in the form of a crystalline carbonate *apatite* (similar to naturally occurring minerals, thus the term *mineralized*). Irrespective of its biological function, bone is one of the most interesting materials known in terms of structure-property relationships. Bone is an anisotropic, heterogeneous, inhomogeneous, nonlinear, thermorheologically complex viscoelastic material. It exhibits electromechanical effects, presumed to be due to streaming potentials, both in vivo and in vitro when wet. In the dry state, bone exhibits piezoelectric properties. Because of the complexity of the structure-property relationships in bone, and the space limitation for this chapter, it is necessary to concentrate on one aspect of the mechanics. Currey [1984] states unequivocally that he thinks, "the most important feature of bone material is its stiffness." This is, of course, the premiere consideration for the weight-bearing long bones. Thus this chapter will concentrate on the elastic and viscoelastic properties of compact cortical bone as exemplar of mineralized tissue mechanics.

20.1 Structure of Bone

The complexity of bone's properties arises from the complexity in its structure. Thus it is important to have an understanding of the structure of mammalian bone in order to appreciate the related properties. Figure 20.1 is a diagram showing the structure of a human femur at different levels [Park, 1979]. For convenience, the structures shown in Fig. 20.1 will be grouped into four levels. A further subdivision of structural organization of mammalian bone is shown in Fig. 20.2 [Wainwright et al., 1982]. The individual figures within this diagram can be sorted into one of the appropriate levels of structure shown on Fig. 20.1 as described in the following. At the smallest unit of structure we have

-8493-8346-3/95/$0.00+$.50
1995 by CRC Press, Inc.

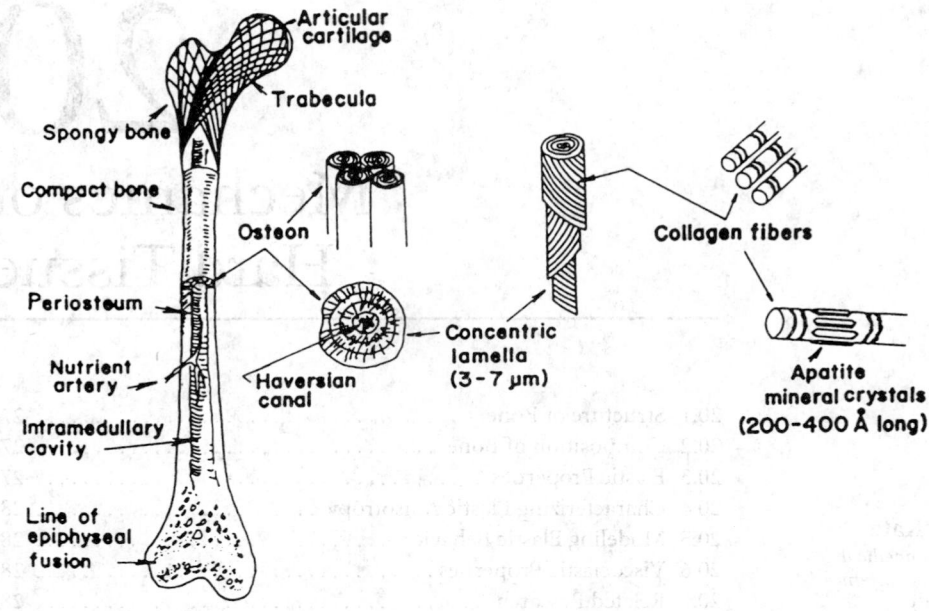

FIGURE 20.1   Hierarchical levels of structure in a human femur [Park, 1979] (Courtesy of Plenum Press and Dr. J.B. Park).

the *tropocollagen* molecule and the associated apatite crystallites (abbreviated Ap). The former is approximately 1.5 by 280 nm, made up of three individual left-handed helical polypeptide (alpha) chains coiled into a right-handed triple helix. Ap crystallites have been found to be carbonate-substituted hydroxyapatite, generally thought to be nonstoichiometric. The crystallites appear to be about $4 \times 20 \times 60$ nm in size. This level is denoted the *molecular*. The next level we denote the *ultrastructural*. Here, the collagen and Ap are intimately associated and assembled into a microfibrilar composite, several of which are then assembled into fibers from approximately 3 to 5 μm thick. At the next level, the *microstructural*, these fibers are either randomly arranged (woven bone) or organized into concentric lamellar groups (*osteons*) or linear lamellar groups (*plexiform bone*). This is the level of structure we usually mean when we talk about bone *tissue* properties. In addition to the differences in lamellar organization at this level, there are also two different types of architectural structure. The dense type of bone found, for example, in the shafts of long bone is known as compact or *cortical bone*. A more porous or spongy type of bone is found, for example, at the articulating ends of long bones. This is called *cancellous bone*. It is important to note that the material and structural organization of collagen-Ap making up osteonic or *haversian bone* and plexiform bone are the same as the material comprising cancellous bone.

Finally, we have the whole bone itself constructed of osteons and portions of older, partially destroyed osteons (called *interstitial lamellae*) in the case of humans or of osteons and/or plexiform bone in the case of mammals. This we denote the *macrostructural* level. The elastic properties of the whole bone results from the hierarchial contribution of each of these levels.

20.2 Composition of Bone

The composition of bone depends on a large number of factors: the species, which bone, the location from which the sample is taken, and the age, sex, and type of bone tissue, e.g., woven, cancellous, cortical. However, a rough estimate for overall composition by volume is one-third Ap, one-third collagen and other organic components, and one-third H_2O. Some data in the literature for the composition of adult human and bovine cortical bone are given in Table 20.1.

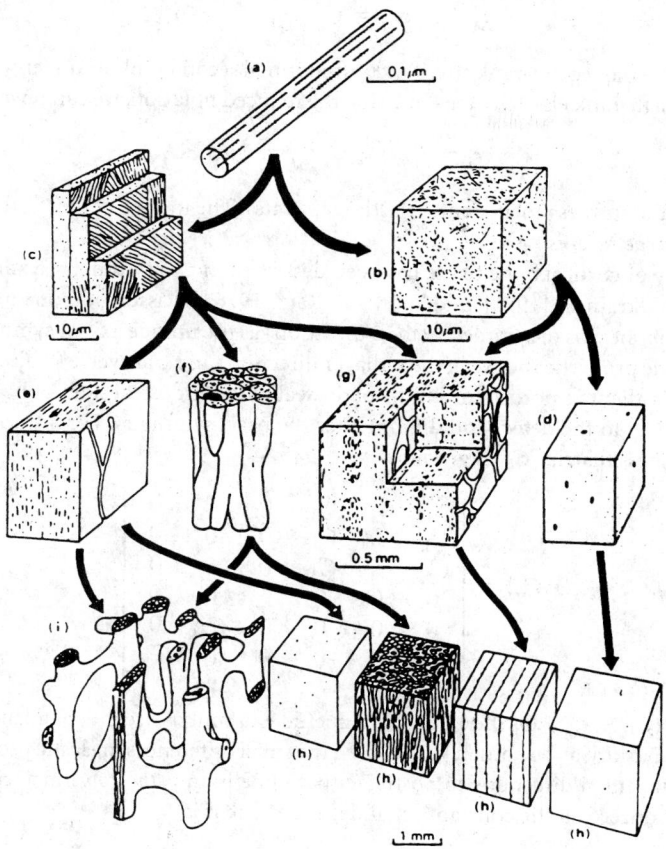

FIGURE 20.2   Diagram showing the structure of mammalian bone at different levels. Bone at the same level is drawn at the same magnification. The arrows show what types may contribute to structures at higher levels [Wainwright et al., 1982] (Courtesy Princeton University Press). (*a*) Collagen fibril with associated mineral crystals. (*b*) Woven bone. The collagen fibrils are arranged more or less randomly. Osteocytes are not shown. (*c*) Lamellar bone. There are separate lamellae, and the collagen fibrils are arranged in "domains" of preferred fibrillar orientation in each lamella. Osteocytes are not shown. (*d*) Woven bone. Blood channels are shown as large black spots. At this level woven bone is indicated by light dotting. (*e*) Primary lamellar bone. At this level lamellar bone is indicated by fine dashes. (*f*) Haversian bone. A collection of Haversian systems, each with concentric lamellae round a central blood channel. The large black area represents the cavity formed as a cylinder of bone is eroded away. It will be filled in with concentric lamellae and form a new Haversian system. (*g*) Laminar bone. Two blood channel networks are exposed. Note how layers of woven and lamellar bone alternate. (*h*) Compact bone of the types shown at the lower levels. (*i*) Cancellous bone.

20.3 Elastic Properties

Although bone is a viscoelastic material, at the quasi-static strain rates in mechanical testing and even at the ultrasonic frequencies used experimentally, it is a reasonable first approximation to model cortical bone as an anisotropic, linear elastic solid with Hooke's law as the appropriate constitutive equation. Tensor notation for the equation is written as:

$$\boldsymbol{\sigma}_{ij} = C_{ijkl} \, \boldsymbol{e}_{kl} \tag{20.1}$$

where σ_{ij} and ϵ_{kl} are the second-rank stress and infinitesimal second rank strain tensors, respectively, and C_{ijkl} is the fourth-rank elasticity tensor. Using the reduced notation, we can rewrite Eq. (20.1) as

$$\boldsymbol{\sigma}_i = C_{ij} \, \boldsymbol{\epsilon}_j \qquad i, j = 1 \text{ to } 6 \tag{20.2}$$

where the C_{ij} are the stiffness coefficients (elastic constants). The inverse of the C_{ij}, the S_{ij}, are known as the *compliance coefficients.*

The anisotropy of cortical bone tissue has been described in two symmetry arrangements. Lang [1969], Katz and Ukraincik [1971], and Yoon and Katz [1976a,b] assumed bone to be *transversely isotropic* with the bone axis of symmetry (the 3 direction) as the unique axis of symmetry. Any small difference in elastic properties between the radial (1 direction) and transverse (2 direction) axes, due to the apparent gradient in porosity from the periosteal to the endosteal sides of bone, was deemed to be due essentially to the defect and did not alter the basic symmetry. For a transverse isotropic material, the stiffness matrix $[C_{ij}]$ is given by

$$[C_{ij}] = \begin{bmatrix} C_{11} & C_{12} & C_{13} & 0 & 0 & 0 \\ C_{12} & C_{11} & C_{13} & 0 & 0 & 0 \\ C_{13} & C_{13} & C_{33} & 0 & 0 & 0 \\ 0 & 0 & 0 & C_{44} & 0 & 0 \\ 0 & 0 & 0 & 0 & C_{44} & 0 \\ 0 & 0 & 0 & 0 & 0 & C_{66} \end{bmatrix} \tag{20.3}$$

where $C_{66} = 1/2 \, (C_{11} - C_{12})$. Of the 12 nonzero coefficients, only 5 are independent.

However, Van Buskirk and Ashman [1981] used the small differences in elastic properties between the radial and tangential directions to postulate that bone is an *orthotropic* material; this requires that 9 of the 12 nonzero elastic constants be independent, that is,

$$[C_{ij}] = \begin{bmatrix} C_{11} & C_{12} & C_{13} & 0 & 0 & 0 \\ C_{12} & C_{22} & C_{23} & 0 & 0 & 0 \\ C_{13} & C_{23} & C_{33} & 0 & 0 & 0 \\ 0 & 0 & 0 & C_{44} & 0 & 0 \\ 0 & 0 & 0 & 0 & C_{55} & 0 \\ 0 & 0 & 0 & 0 & 0 & C_{66} \end{bmatrix} \tag{20.4}$$

Corresponding matrices can be written for the compliance coefficients, the S_{ij}, based on the inverse equation to Eq. (20.2):

$$\boldsymbol{\epsilon}_i = S_{ij} \, \boldsymbol{\sigma}_j \qquad i, j = 1 \text{ to } 6 \tag{20.5}$$

where the S_{ij}th compliance is obtained by dividing the $[C_{ij}]$ stiffness matrix, minus the ith row and jth column, by the full $[C_{ij}]$ matrix and vice versa to obtain the C_{ij} in terms of the S_{ij}. Thus, although

TABLE 20.1 Composition of Adult Human and Bovine Cortical Bone

Species	% H$_2$O	Ap	% Dry Weight Collagen	GAG*	Reference
Bovine	9.1	76.4	21.5	N.D[†]	Herring, 1977
Human	7.3	67.2	21.2	0.34	Pellagrino and Blitz, 1965; Vejlens, 1971

* Glycosaminoglycan
† Not determined

$S_{33} = 1/E_3$, where E_3 is Young's modulus in the bone axis direction, $E_3 \neq C_{33}$, since C_{33} and S_{33}, are not reciprocals of one another even for an isotropic material, let alone for transverse isotropy or orthotropic symmetry.

The relationship between the compliance matrix and the technical constants such as Young's modulus (Ei), shear modulus (Gi,) and Poisson's ratio (v_{ij}) measured in mechanical tests such as uniaxial or pure shear is expressed in Eq. (20.6).

$$[S_{ij}] = \begin{bmatrix} \dfrac{1}{E_1} & \dfrac{-v_{21}}{E_2} & \dfrac{-v_{31}}{E_3} & 0 & 0 & 0 \\[2mm] \dfrac{-v_{12}}{E_1} & \dfrac{1}{E_2} & \dfrac{-v_{32}}{E_3} & 0 & 0 & 0 \\[2mm] \dfrac{-v_{13}}{E_1} & \dfrac{-v_{23}}{E_2} & \dfrac{1}{E_3} & 0 & 0 & 0 \\[2mm] 0 & 0 & 0 & \dfrac{1}{G_{23}} & 0 & 0 \\[2mm] 0 & 0 & 0 & 0 & \dfrac{1}{G_{31}} & 0 \\[2mm] 0 & 0 & 0 & 0 & 0 & \dfrac{1}{G_{12}} \end{bmatrix} \tag{20.6}$$

Again, for an orthotropic material, only 9 of the above 12 nonzero terms are independent, due to the symmetry of the S_{ij} tensor:

$$\frac{v_{12}}{E_1} = \frac{v_{21}}{E_2} \qquad \frac{v_{13}}{E_1} = \frac{v_{31}}{E_3} \qquad \frac{v_{23}}{E_2} = \frac{v_{32}}{E_3} \tag{20.7}$$

For the transverse isotropic case, Eq. (20.5) reduces to only 5 independent coefficients, since

$$E_1 = E_2 \qquad v_{12} = v_{21} \qquad v_{31} = v_{32} = v_{13} = v_{23}$$

$$G_{23} = G_{31} \qquad G_{12} = \frac{E_1}{2(1 + v_{12})} \tag{20.8}$$

In addition to the mechanical tests cited above, ultrasonic wave propagation techniques have been used to measure the anisotropic elastic properties of bone [Lang, 1969; Yoon and Katz, 1976a,b; Van Buskirk and Ashman, 1981]. This is possible, since combining Hooke's law with Newton's second law results in a wave equation which yields the following relationship involving the stiffness matrix:

$$\rho V^2 \, U_m = C_{mrns} \, N_r \, N_s \, U_n \tag{20.9}$$

where ρ is the density of the medium, V is the wave speed, and **U** and **N** are unit vectors along the particle displacement and wave propagation directions, respectively, so that Um, Nr, etc. are direction cosines.

Thus to find the five transverse isotropic elastic constants, at least five independent measurements are required, e.g., a dilatational longitudinal wave in the 3 and 1(2) directions, a transverse wave in the 13 (23) and 12 planes, etc. The technical moduli must then be calculated from the full set of C_{ij}. For improved statistics, redundant measurements should be made. Correspondingly, for orthotropic symmetry, enough independent measurements must be made to obtain all 9 C_{ij}; again, redundancy in measurements is a suggested approach.

One major advantage of the ultrasonic measurements over mechanical testing is that the former can be done with specimens too small for the latter technique. Second, the reproducibility of measurements using the former technique is greater than for the latter. Still a third advantage is that the full set of either five or nine coefficients can be measured on one specimen, a procedure not possible with the latter techniques. Thus, at present, most of the studies of elastic anisotropy in both human and other mammalian bone are done using ultrasonic techniques. In addition to the bulk wave type measurements described above, it is possible to obtain Young's modulus directly. This is accomplished by using samples of small cross sections with transducers of low frequency so that the wavelength of the sound is much larger than the specimen size. In this case, an extensional longitudinal (bar) wave is propagated (which experimentally is analogous to a uniaxial mechanical test experiment), yielding

$$V^2 = \frac{E}{\rho} \tag{20.10}$$

This technique was used successfully to show that bovine plexiform bone was definitely orthotropic while bovine haversian bone could be treated as transversely isotropic [Lipson and Katz, 1984]. The results were subsequently confirmed using bulk wave propagation techniques with considerable redundancy [Maharidge, 1984].

Table 20.2 lists the C_{ij} (in GPa) for human (haversian) bone and bovine (both haversian and plexiform) bone. With the exception of Knets's [1978] measurements, which were made using quasi-static mechanical testing, all the other measurements were made using bulk ultrasonic wave propagation.

In Maharidge's study [1984], both types of tissue specimens, haversian and plexiform, were obtained from different aspects of the same level of an adult bovine femur. Thus the differences in C_{ij} reported between the two types of bone tissue are hypothesized to be due essentially to the differences in microstructural organization (Fig. 20.3.) [Wainwright et al., 1982]. The textural symmetry at this level of structure has dimensions comparable to those of the ultrasound wavelengths used in the experiment, and the molecular and ultrastructural levels of organization in both types

TABLE 20.2 Elastic Stiffness Coefficients for Various Human and Bovine Bones; All Measurements Made with Ultrasound except for Knets [1978] Mechanical Tests

Experiments (Bone Type)	C_{11} (GPa)	C_{22} (GPa)	C_{33} (GPa)	C_{44} (GPa)	C_{55} (GPa)	C_{66} (GPa)	C_{12} (GPa)	C_{13} (GPa)	C_{23} (GPa)
Van Buskirk and Ashman [1981] (bovine femur)	14.1	18.4	25.0	7.00	6.30	5.28	6.34	4.84	6.94
Knets [1978] (human tibia)	11.6	14.4	22.5	4.91	3.56	2.41	7.95	6.10	6.92
Van Buskirk and Ashman [1981] (human femur)	20.0	21.7	30.0	6.56	5.85	4.74	10.9	11.5	11.5
Maharidge [1984] (bovine femur haversian)	21.2	21.0	29.0	6.30	6.30	5.40	11.7	12.7	11.1
Maharidge [1984] (bovine femur plexiform)	22.4	25.0	35.0	8.20	7.10	6.10	14.0	15.8	13.6

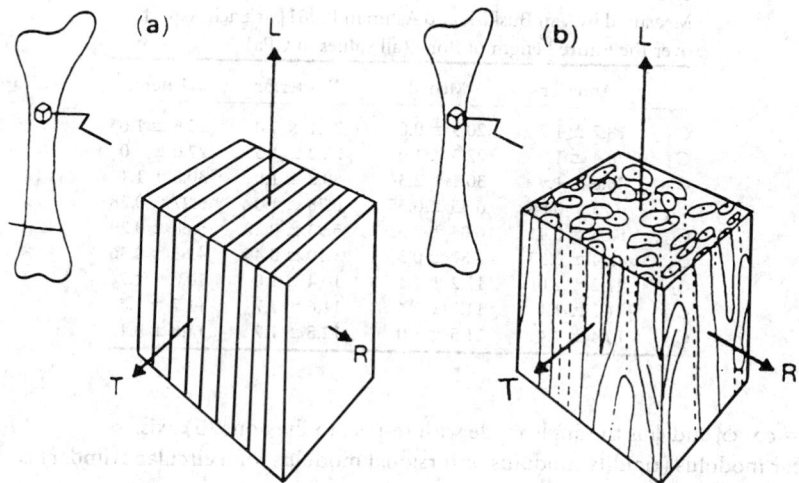

FIGURE 20.3 Diagram showing how laminar (plexiform) bone (*a*) differs more between radial and tangential directions (R and T) than does haversian bone (*b*). The arrows are vectors representing the various directions [Wainwright et al., 1982] (Courtesy Princeton University Press).

of tissues are essentially identical. Note that while C_{11} almost equals C_{22} and that C_{44} and C_{55} are equal for bovine haversian bone, C_{11} and C_{22} and C_{44} and C_{55} differ by 11.6 and 13.4%, respectively, for bovine plexiform bone. Similarly, although C_{66} and $\frac{1}{2}(C_{11} - C_{12})$ differ by 12.0% for the haversian bone, they differ by 31.1% for plexiform bone. Only the differences between C_{13} and C_{23} are somewhat comparable: 12.6% for haversian bone and 13.9% for plexiform. These results reinforce the importance of modeling bone as a hierarchical ensemble in order to understand the basis for bone's elastic properties as a composite material-structure system in which the collagen-Ap components define the material composite property. When this material property is entered into calculations based on the microtextural arrangement, the overall anisotropic elastic anisotropy can be modeled.

The human femur data [Van Buskirk and Ashman, 1981] support this description of bone tissue. Although they measured all nine individual C_{ij}, treating the femur as an orthotropic material, their results are consistent with a near transverse isotropic symmetry. However, their nine C_{ij} for bovine femoral bone clearly shows the influence of the orthotropic microtextural symmetry of the tissue's plexiform structure.

The data of Knets [1978] on human tibia are difficult to analyze. This could be due to the possibility of significant systematic errors due to mechanical testing on a large number of small specimens from a multitude of different positions in the tibia.

The variations in bone's elastic properties cited earlier above due to location is appropriately illustrated in Table 20.3, where the mean values and standard deviations (all in GPa) for all *g* orthotropic C_{ij} are given for bovine cortical bone at each aspect over the entire length of bone.

Since the C_{ij} are simply related to the "technical" elastic moduli, such as Young's modulus (E), shear modulus (G), bulk modulus (K), and others, it is possible to describe the moduli along any given direction. The full equations for the most general anisotropy are too long to present here. However, they can be found in Yoon and Katz [1976a]. Presented below are the simplified equations for the case of transverse isotropy. Young's modulus is

$$\frac{1}{E(\gamma_3)} = S'_{33} = (1 - \gamma_3^2)\, 2S_{11} + \gamma_3^4\, S_{33}$$
$$+ \gamma_3^2\, (1 - \gamma_3^2)\, (2S_{13} + S_{44}) \tag{20.11}$$

TABLE 20.3 Mean Values and Standard Deviations for the C_{ij} Measured by Van Buskirk and Ashman [1981] at Each Aspect over the Entire Length of Bone (all values in GPa)

	Anterior	Medial	Posterior	Lateral
C_{11}	18.7 ± 1.7	20.9 ± 0.8	20.1 ± 1.0	20.6 ± 1.6
C_{22}	20.4 ± 1.2	22.3 ± 1.0	22.2 ± 1.3	22.0 ± 1.0
C_{33}	28.6 ± 1.9	30.1 ± 2.3	30.8 ± 1.0	30.5 ± 1.1
C_{44}	6.73 ± 0.68	6.45 ± 0.35	6.78 ± 1.0	6.27 ± 0.28
C_{55}	5.55 ± 0.41	6.04 ± 0.51	5.93 ± 0.28	5.68 ± 0.29
C_{66}	4.34 ± 0.33	4.87 ± 0.35	5.10 ± 0.45	4.63 ± 0.36
C_{12}	11.2 ± 2.0	11.2 ± 1.1	10.4 ± 1.0	10.8 ± 1.7
C_{13}	11.2 ± 1.1	11.2 ± 2.4	11.6 ± 1.7	11.7 ± 1.8
C_{23}	10.4 ± 1.4	11.5 ± 1.0	12.5 ± 1.7	11.8 ± 1.1

where $\gamma_3 = \cos \phi$, and ϕ is the angle made with respect to the bone (3) axis.

The shear modulus (rigidity modulus or torsional modulus for a circular cylinder) is

$$\frac{1}{G(\gamma_3)} = \frac{1}{2}(S'_{44} + S'_{55}) = S_{44} + (S_{11} - S_{12}) - \frac{1}{2}S_{44}(1 - \gamma_3^2)$$
$$+ 2(S_{11} + S_{33} - 2S_{13} - S_{44})\gamma_3^2(1 - \gamma_3^2) \tag{20.12}$$

where, again, $\gamma_3 = \cos \phi$.

The bulk modulus (reciprocal of the volume compressibility) is

$$\frac{1}{K} = S_{33} + 2(S_{11} + S_{12} + 2S_{13}) = \frac{C_{11} + C_{12} + 2C_{33} - 4C_{13}}{C_{33}(C_{11} + C_{12}) - 2C_{13}^2} \tag{20.13}$$

Conversion of Eqs. (20.11) and (20.12) from S_{ij} to C_{ij} can be done by using the following transformation equations:

$$S_{11} = \frac{C_{22}C_{33} - C_{23}^2}{\Delta} \qquad S_{22} = \frac{C_{33}C_{11} - C_{13}^2}{\Delta}$$

$$S_{33} = \frac{C_{11}C_{22} - C_{12}^2}{\Delta} \qquad S_{12} = \frac{C_{13}C_{23} - C_{12}C_{33}}{\Delta}$$

$$S_{13} = \frac{C_{12}C_{23} - C_{13}C_{22}}{\Delta} \qquad S_{23} = \frac{C_{12}C_{13} - C_{23}C_{11}}{\Delta} \tag{20.14}$$

$$S_{44} = \frac{1}{C_{44}} \qquad S_{55} = \frac{1}{C_{55}} \qquad S_{66} = \frac{1}{C_{66}}$$

where

$$\Delta = \begin{bmatrix} C_{11} & C_{12} & C_{13} \\ C_{12} & C_{22} & C_{23} \\ C_{13} & C_{23} & C_{33} \end{bmatrix} = C_{11}C_{22}C_{33} + 2C_{12}C_{23}C_{13} - (C_{11}C_{23}^2 + C_{22}C_{13}^2 + C_{33}C_{12}^2) \tag{20.15}$$

20.4 Characterizing Elastic Anisotropy

Having a full set of five or nine C_{ij} does permit describing the anisotropy of that particular specimen of bone, but there is no simple way of comparing the relative anisotropy between different specimens of the same bone or between different species or between different experimenters' measurements by trying to relate individual C_{ij} between sets of measurements. Adapting a method from crystal physics [Chung and Buessem, 1968], Katz and Meunier [1987] presented a description for obtaining two scalar quantities defining the compressive and shear anisotropy for bone with transverse isotropic symmetry. Later, they developed a similar pair of scalar quantities for bone exhibiting orthotropic symmetry [Katz and Meunier, 1990]. For both cases, the percentage compressive (Ac^*) and shear (As^*) elastic anisotropy are given, respectively, by

$$Ac^* (\%) = 100 \frac{K^V - K_R}{K^V + K_R}$$

$$As^* (\%) = 100 \frac{G_V - G_R}{G^V + G_R} \tag{20.16}$$

where K^V and K_R are the Voigt (uniform strain across an interface) and Reuss (uniform stress across an interface) bulk moduli, respectively, and G^V and G_R are the Voigt and Reuss shear moduli, respectively. The equations for K^V, K_R, G^V, and G_R are provided for both transverse isotropy and orthotropic symmetry in App. 20A.

Table 20.4 lists the values of K^V, K_R, G^V, G_R, Ac^*, and As^* for the five experiments whose C_{ij} are given in Table 20.2.

It is interesting to note that haversian bones, whether human or bovine, have both their compressive and shear anisotropy factors considerably lower than the respective values for plexiform bone. Thus, not only is plexiform bone both stiffer and more rigid than haversian bone, it is also more anisotropic. The higher values of Ac^* and As^*, especially the latter at 7.88% for the Knets [1978] mechanical testing data on human haversian bone, supports the possibility of the systematic errors in such measurements suggested above.

20.5 Modeling Elastic Behavior

Currey [1964] first presented some preliminary ideas of modeling bone as a composite material composed of a simple linear superposition of collagen and Ap. He followed this later [1969] with an attempt to take into account the orientation of the Ap crystallites using a model proposed by Cox [1952] for fiber-reinforced composites. Katz [1971a] and Piekarski [1973] independently showed that the use of Voigt and Reuss or even Hashin-Shtrikman [1963] composite modeling showed the limitations of using linear combinations of either elastic moduli or elastic compliances. The failure of all these early models could be traced to the fact that they were based only on considerations of material properties. This is comparable to trying to determine the properties of an Eiffel Tower built using a composite material by simply modeling the composite material properties without considering void spaces and the interconnectivity of the structure [Lakes, 1993]. In neither case is the complexity of the structural organization involved. This consideration of hierarchical organization clearly must be introduced into the modeling.

TABLE 20.4 Values of K^V, K_R, G^V, and G_R, (all in GPa), and Ac^* and As^* (%) for the Bone Specimens Given in Table 20.2

Experiments (Bone Type)	K^V	K_R	G^V	G_R	Ac^*	As^*
Van Buskirk and Ashman [1981] (bovine femur)	10.4	9.87	6.34	6.07	2.68	2.19
Knets [1978] (human tibia)	10.1	9.52	4.01	3.43	2.68	7.88
Van Buskirk and Ashman [1981] (human femur)	15.5	15.0	5.95	5.74	1.59	1.82
Maharidge [1984] (bovine femur haversian)	15.8	15.5	5.98	5.82	1.11	1.37
Maharidge [1984] (bovine femur plexiform)	18.8	18.1	6.88	6.50	1.84	2.85

Katz in a number of papers [1971b, 1976] and meeting presentations put forth the hypothesis that haversian bone should be modeled as a hierarchical composite, eventually adapting a hollow fiber composite model by Hashin and Rosen [1964]. Bonfield and Grynpas [1977] used extensional (longitudinal) ultrasonic wave propagation in both wet and dry bovine femoral cortical bone specimens oriented at angles of 5, 10, 20, 40, 50, 70, 80, and 85 degrees with respect to the long bone axis. They compared their experimental results for Young's moduli with the theoretical curve predicted by Currey's model [1969]; this is shown in Fig. 20.4. The lack of agreement led them to "conclude, therefore that an alternative model is required to account for the dependence of Young's modulus on orientation" [Bonfield and Grynpas, 1977]. Katz [1980, 1981], applying his hierarchical material-structure composite model, showed that the data in Fig. 20.4 could be explained by considering different amounts of Ap crystallites aligned parallel to the long bone axis; this is shown in Fig. 20.5. This early attempt at hierarchical micromechanical modeling is now being extended with more sophisticated modeling using either finite-element micromechanical computations [Hogan, 1992] or homogenization theory [Crolet et al., 1993]. Further improvements will come by including more definitive information on the structural organization of collagen and Ap at the molecular-ultrastructural level [Wagner and Weiner, 1992; Weiner and Traub, 1989].

20.6 Viscoelastic Properties

As stated earlier, bone (along with all other biologic tissues) is a viscoelastic material. Clearly, for such materials, Hooke's law for linear elastic materials must be replaced by a constitutive equation which includes the time dependency of the material properties. The behavior of an anisotropic

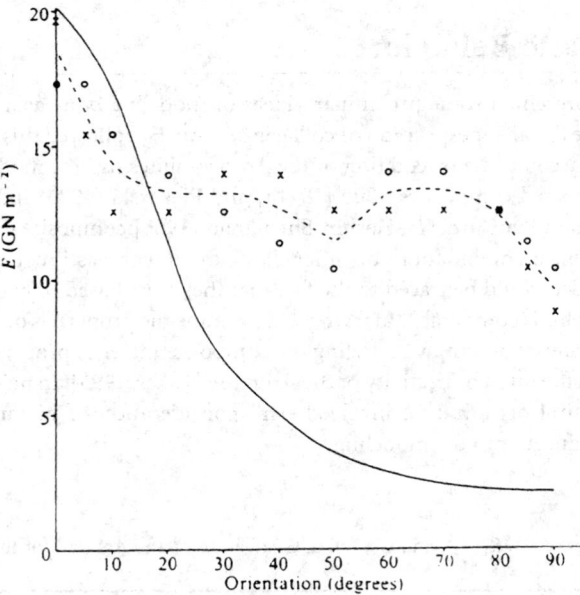

FIGURE 20.4 Variation in Young's modulus of bovine femur specimens (E) with the orientation of specimen axis to the long axis of the bone, for wet (o) and dry (x) conditions compared with the theoretical curve (————) predicted from a fibre-reinforced composite model [Bonfield and Grynpas, 1977] (Courtesy *Nature* 1977 270:453. © Macmillan Magazines Ltd.).

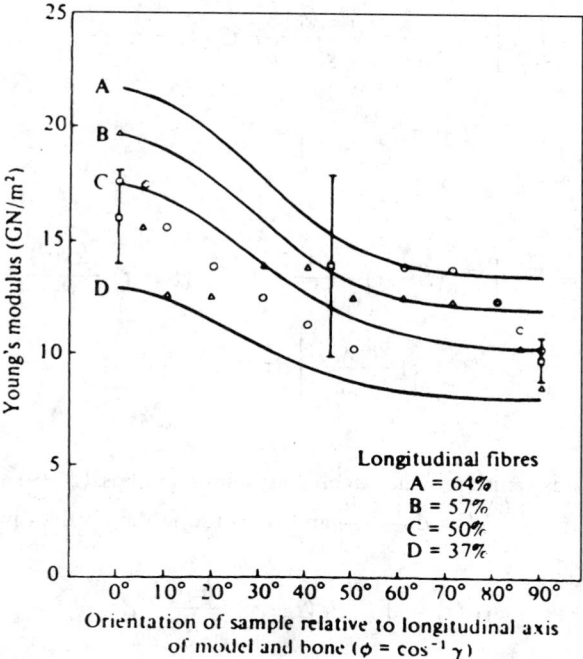

FIGURE 20.5 Comparison of predictions of Katz two-level composite model with the experimental data of Bonfield and Grynpas. Each curve represents a different lamellar configuration within a single osteon, with longitudinal fibers; A, 64%; B, 57%; C, 50%; D, 37%; and the rest of the fibers assumed horizontal. (From Katz JL, Mechanical Properties of Bone, AMD, Vol. 45, New York, American Society of Mechanical Engineers, 1981, with permission.)

linear viscoelastic material may be described by using the *Boltzmann superposition integral* as a constitutive equation:

$$\sigma_{ij}(t) = \int_{-\infty}^{t} C_{ijkl}\,(t - \tau)\,\frac{d\epsilon_{kl}(\tau)}{d\tau}\,d\tau \tag{20.17}$$

where $\sigma_{ij}(t)$ and $\epsilon_{kl}(\tau)$ are the time-dependent second rank stress and strain tensors, respectively, and $C_{ijkl}(t - \tau)$ is the fourth-rank relaxation modulus tensor. This tensor has 36 independent elements for the lowest symmetry case and 12 nonzero independent elements for an orthotropic solid. Again, as for linear elasticity, a reduced notation is used, i.e., $11 \rightarrow 1, 22 \rightarrow 2, 33 \rightarrow 3, 23 \rightarrow 4, 31 \rightarrow 5$, and $12 \rightarrow 6$. If we apply Eq. (20.17) to the case of an orthotropic material, e.g., plexiform bone, in uniaxial tension (compression) in the 1 direction [Lakes and Katz, 1974], in this case using the reduced notation, we obtain

$$\sigma_1(t) = \int_{-\infty}^{t} \left[C_{11}\,(t - \tau)\,\frac{d\epsilon_1(\tau)}{d\tau} + C_{12}\,(t - \tau)\,\frac{d\epsilon_2(\tau)}{d\tau} \right.$$

$$\left. + C_{13}\,(t - \tau)\,\frac{d\epsilon_3(\tau)}{d\tau} \right] d\tau \tag{20.18}$$

$$\sigma_2(t) = \int_{-\infty}^{t} \left[C_{21} \left(t - \tau \right) \frac{d\epsilon_1(\tau)}{d\tau} + C_{22} \left(t - \tau \right) \frac{d\epsilon_2(\tau)}{d\tau} \right. \tag{20.19}$$

$$\left. + C_{23} \left(t - \tau \right) \frac{d\epsilon_3(\tau)}{d\tau} \right] = 0$$

for all t, and

$$\sigma_3(t) = \int_{-\infty}^{t} \left[C_{31} \left(t - \tau \right) \frac{d\epsilon_1(\tau)}{d\tau} + C_{32} \left(t - \tau \right) \frac{d\epsilon_2(\tau)}{d\tau} \right. \tag{20.20}$$

$$\left. + C_{33} \left(t - \tau \right) \frac{d\epsilon_3(\tau)}{d\tau} \right] d\tau = 0$$

for all t.

Having the integrands vanish provides an obvious solution to Eqs. (20.19) and (20.20). Solving them simultaneously for $\frac{[d\epsilon_2^{(\tau)}]}{d\tau}$ and $\frac{[d\epsilon_3^{(\tau)}]}{d\tau}$ and substituting these values in Eq. (20.17) yields

$$\sigma_1(t) = \int_{-\infty}^{t} E_1 \left(t - \tau \right) \frac{d\epsilon_1(\tau)}{d\tau} \, d\tau \tag{20.21}$$

where, if for convenience we adopt the notation $C_{ij} \equiv C_{ij} \left(t - \tau \right)$, then Young's modulus is given by

$$E_1 \left(t - \tau \right) = C_{11} + C_{12} \frac{[C_{31} - (C_{21}C_{33}/C_{23})]}{[(C_{22}C_{33}/C_{23}) - C_{32}]} \tag{20.22}$$

$$+ C_{13} \frac{[C_{21} - (C_{31}C_{22}/C_{32})]}{[(C_{22}C_{33}/C_{32}) - C_{23}]}$$

In this case of uniaxial tension (compression), only nine independent orthotropic tensor components are involved, the three shear components being equal to zero. Still, this time-dependent Young's modulus is a rather complex function. As in the linear elastic case, the inverse form of the Boltzmann integral can be used; this would constitute the compliance formulation.

If we consider the bone being driven by a strain at a frequency ω, with a corresponding sinusoidal stress lagging by an angle δ, then the complex Young's modulus $E^*(\omega)$ may be expressed as

$$E^*(\omega) = E'(\omega) + iE''(\omega) \tag{20.23}$$

where $E'(\omega)$, which represents the stress-strain ratio in phase with the strain, is known as the *storage modulus*, and $E''(\omega)$, which represents the stress-strain ratio 90 degrees out of phase with the strain, is known as the *loss modulus*. The ratio of the loss modulus to the storage modulus is then equal to tan δ. Usually, data are presented by a graph of the storage modulus along with a graph of tan δ, both against frequency. For a more complete development of the values of $E'(\omega)$ and $E''(\omega)$, as well as for the derivation of other viscoelastic technical moduli, see Lakes and Katz [1974]; for a similar development of the shear storage and loss moduli, see Cowin [1989].

Thus, for a more complete understanding of bone's response to applied loads, it is important to know its rheologic properties. There have been a number of early studies of the viscoelastic properties of various long bones [Sedlin, 1965; Smith and Keiper, 1965; Laird and Kingsbury, 1973; Lugassy, 1968; Black and Korostoff, 1973]. However, none of these was performed over a wide enough range of frequency (or time) to completely define the viscoelastic properties measured, e.g., creep or stress relaxation. Thus it is not possible to mathematically transform one property into any other to compare results of three different experiments on different bones [Lakes and Katz, 1974].

In the first experiments over an extended frequency range, the biaxial viscoelastic as well as uniaxial viscoelastic properties of wet cortical human and bovine femoral bone were measured using both dynamic and stress relaxation techniques over eight decades of frequency (time) [Lakes et al., 1979]. The results of these experiments showed that bone was both nonlinear and thermorheologically complex, i.e., time-temperature superposition could not be used to extend the range of viscoelastic measurements. A nonlinear constitutive equation was developed based on these measurements [Lakes and Katz, 1979a]. In addition, relaxation spectrums for both human and bovine cortical bone were obtained; Fig. 20.6 shows the former [Lakes and Katz, 1979b]. The contributions of several mechanisms to the loss tangent of cortical bone is shown in Fig. 20.7 [Lakes and Katz, 1979b]. It is interesting to note that almost all the major loss mechanisms occur at frequencies (times) at or close to those in which there are "bumps," indicating possible strain energy dissipation, on the relaxation spectra shown on Fig. 20.6. An extensive review of the viscoelastic properties of bone can be found in the CRC publication *Natural and Living Biomaterials* [Lakes and Katz, 1984].

Following on Katz's [1976, 1980] adaptation of the Hashin-Rosen hollow fiber composite model [1964], Gottesman and Hashin [1979] presented a viscoelastic calculation using the same major assumptions.

20.7 Related Research

As stated earlier, this chapter has concentrated on the elastic and viscoelastic properties of mineralized tissues with special emphasis on the compact cortical bone found in the weight-bearing long bones. At present there is considerable research activity on the mechanical properties of cancellous bone with special interest in the changes in properties that occur due to pathologies and/or aging processes such as osteoarthritis and osteoporosis. Research on porous (spongy) bone is more complex than working with cortical bone for the following reasons. First, there is the intricate

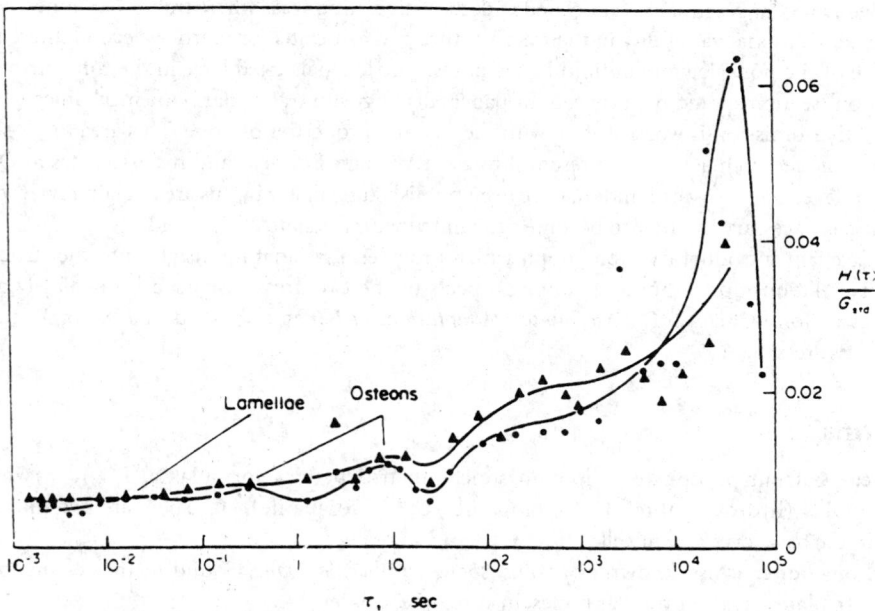

FIGURE 20.6 Comparison of relaxation spectra for wet human bone, specimens 5 and 6 [Lakes et al., 1979] in simple torsion; $T = 37°C$. First approximation from relaxation and dynamic data. ● Human tibial bone, specimen 6. ▲ Human tibial bone, specimen 5, $G_{std} = G(10 \text{ s})$. $G_{std}(5) = G(10 \text{ s})$. $G_{std}(5) = 0.590 \times 10^6$ lb/in². $G_{std}(6) \times 0.602 \times 10^6$ lb/in² (Courtesy *Journal of Biomechanics*, Pergamon Press).

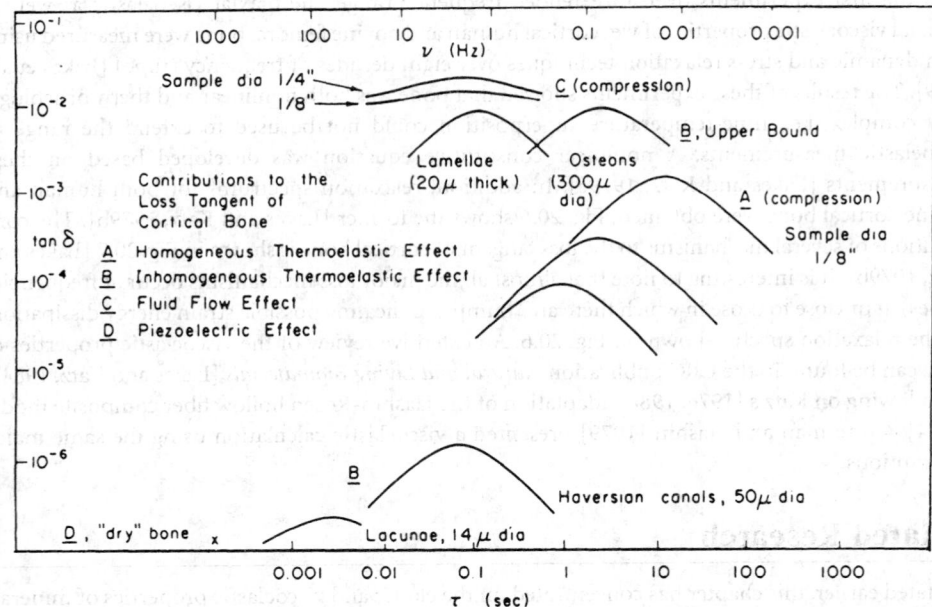

FIGURE 20.7 Contributions of several relaxation mechanisms to the loss tangent of cortical bone. *A:* Homogeneous thermoelastic effect. *B:* Inhomogeneous thermoelastic effect. *C:* Fluid flow effect. *D:* Piezoelectric effect [Lakes and Katz, 1984]. (Courtesy CRC Press)

microstructural organization which is difficult to describe in terms of symmetry and anisotropy. Moreover, the changes in shape associated with the articulating areas where trabecular bone is found introduce additional variability in the microtexture and associated properties. Second, there is the presence of the non-Newtonian fluid in the pores. The journals cited later in the for "Further Information" section should be reviewed for papers dealing with trabecular bone mechanics.

The other omission is work dealing with the fracture properties of bone. This area too is seeing considerable research activity at present. Professor William Bonfield and his associates at Queen Mary College, University of London, have been published regularly in this area. Again review of the literature is necessary in order to become acquainted with the state of this field.

An excellent introductory monograph which provides a fascinating insight into the structure-property relationships in bones including aspects of the two areas discussed immediately above is Professor John Currey's *The Mechanical Adaptations of Bones,* published in 1984 by Princeton University Press.

Defining Terms

Apatite: Calcium phosphate compound, stoichiometric chemical formula $Ca_5(PO_4)_3 \cdot X$, where X is OH^- (hydroxyapatite), F^- (fluorapatite), Cl^- (chlorapatite), etc. There are two molecules in the basic crystal unit cell.

Cancellous bone: Also known as *porous, spongy, trabecular bone.* Found in the regions of the articulating ends of tubular bones, in vertebrae, ribs, etc.

Cortical bone: The dense compact bone found throughout the shafts of long bones such as the femur, tibia, etc. also found in the outer portions of other bones in the body.

Haversian bone: Also called *osteonic.* The form of bone found in adult humans and mature mammals, consisting mainly of concentric lamellar structures, surrounding a central canal called the *haversian canal*, plus lamellar remnants of older haversian systems (osteons) called *interstitial lamellae.*

Interstitial lamellae: See **Haversian bone** above.

Orthotropic: The symmetrical arrangement of structure in which there are three distinct orthogonal axes of symmetry. In crystals this symmetry is called *orthothombic.*

Osteons: See **Haversian bone** above.

Plexiform: Also called *laminar.* The form of parallel lamellar bone found in younger, immature nonhuman mammals.

Transverse isotropy: The symmetrical arrangement of structure in which there is a unique axis perpendicular to a plane in which the other two axis are equivalent. The long bone direction is chosen as the unique axis. In crystals this symmetry is called *hexagonal.*

Further Information

Several societies both in the United States and abroad hold annual meetings during which a great many presentations deal with the mechanics of hard tissue. These societies include the Orthopaedic Research Society, the American Society of Mechanical Engineers, the Biomaterials Society, and the American Society of Biomechanics. In Europe there are annual meetings of the European Society for Biomechanics and the European Society for Biomaterials. Every four years there is a World Congress of Biomechanics; in 1990 it was in LaJolla, in 1994 in Amsterdam. All these meetings result in documented proceedings; some with extended papers in book form.

The two principal journals in which bone mechanics papers appear are the *Journal of Biomechanics* published by Pergamon Press and the *Journal of Biomechanical Engineering* published by the American Society of Mechanical Engineers. A third journal which periodically has papers in the field is the *Journal of Orthopaedic Research* published by Raven Press for the Orthopaedic Research Society.

The 1984 CRC volume, *Natural and Living Biomaterials* (G.W. Hastings and P. Ducheyne, eds.) provides a good introduction to the field. A more advanced book is *Bone Mechanics* [S.C. Cowin, 1989].

Many of the biomaterials journals and society meetings will have occasional papers dealing with hard tissue mechanics, especially those dealing with implant-bone interactions.

References

Black J, Korostoff E. 1973. Dynamic mechanical properties of viable human cortical bone. J Biomech 6:435.

Bonfield W, Grynpas MD. 1977. Anisotropy of Young's modulus of bone. Nature, London 270:453.

Chung DH, Buessem WR. 1968. In Anisotropy in Single-crystal Refractory Compounds, vol 2, p 217, FW Vahldiek and SA Mersol (eds) New York, Plenum Press.

Cowin SC. 1989. Bone Mechanics. Boca Raton, Fla, CRC Press.

Cox HL. 1952. The elasticity and strength of paper and other fibrous materials. British Appl Phys 3:72.

Crolet JM, Aoubiza B, Meunier A. 1993. Compact bone: Numerical simulation of mechanical characteristics. J Biomech 26:(6)677.

Currey JD. 1964. Three analogies to explain the mechanical properties of bone. Biorheology (2):1.

Currey, JD. 1969. The relationship between the stiffness and the mineral content of bone. J Biomech (2):477.

Currey, J. 1984. The Mechanical Adaptations of Bones. New Jersey, Princeton University Press.

Gottesman T, Hashin Z. 1979. Analysis of viscoelastic behavior of bones on the basis of microstructure. J Biomech 13:89.

Hashin Z, Rosen BW. 1964. The elastic moduli of fiber reinforced materials. J Appl Mech (31):223.

Hashin Z, Shtrikman S. 1963. A variational approach to the theory of elastic behavior of multiphase materials. J Mech Phys Solids (11):127.

Hastings GW, Ducheyne P (eds). 1984. Natural and Living Biomaterials, Boca Raton, Fla, CRC Press.

Herring GM. 1977. Methods for the study of the glycoproteins and proteoglycans of bone using bacterial collagenase. Determination of bone sialoprotein and chondroitin sulphate. Calcif Tiss Res (24):29.

Hogan HA. 1992. Micromechanics modeling of haversian cortical bone properties. J Biomech 25(5):549.

Katz JL. 1971a. Hard tissue as a composite material: I. Bounds on the elastic behavior. J Biomech 4:455.

Katz JL. 1971b. Elastic properties of calcified tissues. Isr J Med Sci 7:439.

Katz JL. 1976. Hierarchical modeling of compact haversian bone as a fiber reinforced material. In Mates, R.E. and Smith, CR (eds), Advances in Bioengineering, pp. 17–18. New York, American Society of Mechanical Engineers.

Katz JL. 1980. Anisotropy of Young's modulus of bone. Nature 283:106.

Katz JL. 1981. Composite material models for cortical bone. In Cowin SC (ed), Mechanical Properties of Bone vol 45, pp 171–184. New York, American Society of Mechanical Engineers.

Katz JL, Meunier A. 1987. The elastic anisotropy of bone. J Biomech 20:1063.

Katz JL, Meunier A. 1990. A generalized method for characterizing elastic anisotropy in solid living tissues. J Mat Sci Mater Med 1:1.

Katz JL, Ukraincik K. 1971. On the anisotropic elastic properties of hydroxyapatite. J Biomech 4:221.

Katz JL, Ukraincik K. 1972. A fiber-reinforced model for compact haversian bone. Program and Abstracts of the 16th Annual Meeting of the Biophysical Society, 28a FPM-C15, Toronto.

Knets IV. 1978. Mekhanika Polimerov 13:434.

Laird GW, Kingsbury HB. 1973. Complex viscoelastic moduli of bovine bone. J Biomech 6:59.

Lakes RS. 1993. Materials with structural hierarchy. Nature 361:511.

Lakes RS, Katz JL. 1974. Interrelationships among the viscoelastic function for anisotropic solids: Application to calcified tissues and related systems. J Biomech 7:259.

Lakes RS, Katz JL. 1979a. Viscoelastic properties and behavior of cortical bone. Part II. Relaxation mechanisms. J Biomech 12:679.

Lakes RS, Katz JL. 1979b. Viscoelastic properties of wet cortical bone: III. A nonlinear constitutive equation. J Biomech 12:689.

Lakes RS, Katz JL. 1984. Viscoelastic properties of bone. In GW Hastings and P Ducheyne (eds), Natural and Living Tissues, pp 1–87. Boca Raton, Fla, CRC Press.

Lakes RS, Katz, JL, Sternstein SS. 1979. Viscoelastic properties of wet cortical bone: I. Torsional and biaxial studies. J Biomech 12:657.

Lang SB. 1969. Elastic coefficients of animal bone. Science 165:287.

Lipson SF, Katz JL. 1984. The relationship between elastic properties and microstructure of bovine cortical bone. J Biomech 4:231.

Lugassy AA. 1968. Mechanical and Viscoelastic Properties of Bone and Dentin in Compression, thesis, Metallurgy and Materials Science, University of Pennsylvania.

Maharidge R. 1984. Ultrasonic properties and microstructure of bovine bone and Haversian bovine bone modeling. Thesis. Rensselaer Polytechnic Institute, Troy, NY.

Park JB. 1979. Biomaterials: An Introduction. New York, Plenum.

Pellegrino ED, Biltz RM. 1965. The composition of human bone in uremia. Medicine 44:397.

Piekarski K. 1973. Analysis of bone as a composite material. Int J Eng Sci 10:557.

Reuss A. 1929. Berechnung der fliessgrenze von mischkristallen auf grund der plastizitatsbedingung fur einkristalle, A. Zeitschrift fur Angewandte Mathematik und Mechanik 9:49–58.

Sedlin E. 1965. A rheological model for cortical bone. Acta Orthop Scand 36 (suppl 83).

Smith R, Keiper D. 1965. Dynamic measurement of viscoelastic properties of bone. Am J Med Elec 4:156.

Van Buskirk WC, Ashman RB. 1981. The elastic moduli of bone. In SC Cowin (ed), Mechanical Properties of Bone AMD vol 45, pp 131–143. New York, American Society of Mechanical Engineers.

Vejlens L. 1971. Glycosaminoglycans of human bone tissue: I. Pattern of compact bone in relation to age. Calcif Tiss Res 7:175.

Voigt W. 1966. Lehrbuch der Kristallphysik Teubner, Leipzig, 1910; reprinted (1928) with an additional appendix. Leipzig, Teubner. New York, Johnson Reprint.

Wagner HD, Weiner S. 1992. On the relationship between the microstructure of bone and its mechanical stiffness. J Biomech 25:1311.

Wainwright SA., Briggs WD, Currey JD, Gosline JM. 1982. Mechanical Design in Organisms. Princeton, N.J., Princeton University Press.

Weiner S, Traub W. 1989. Crystal size and organization in bone. Conn Tissue Res 21:259.

Yoon HS, Katz JL. 1976a. Ultrasonic wave propagation in human cortical bone: I. Theoretical considerations of hexagonal symmetry. J Biomech 9:407.

Yoon HS, Katz JL. 1976b. Ultrasonic wave propagation in human cortical bone: II. Measurements of elastic properties and microhardness. J Biomech 9:459.

Appendix

The Voigt and Reuss moduli for both transverse isotropic and orthotropic symmetry are given below:

Voigt Transverse Isotropic

$$K^V = \frac{2(C_{11} + C_{12}) + 4(C_{13} + C_{33})}{9}$$

$$G^V = \frac{(C_{11} + C_{12}) - 4C_{13} + 2C_{33} + 12(C_{44} + C_{66})}{30}$$

(20.A1)

Reuss Transverse Isotropic

$$K_R = \frac{C_{33}(C_{11} + C_{12}) - 2C_{13}^2}{(C_{11} + C_{12} - 4C_{13} + 2C_{33})}$$

$$G_R = \frac{5[C_{33}(C_{11} + C_{12}) - 2C_{13}^2]C_{44}C_{66}}{2\{[C_{33}(C_{11} + C_{12}) - 2C_{13}^2](C_{44} + C_{66}) + [C_{44}C_{66}(2C_{11} + C_{12}) + 4C_{13} + C_{33}]/3\}}$$

(20.A2)

Voigt Orthotropic

$$K^V = \frac{C_{11} + C_{22} + C_{33} + 2(C_{12} + C_{13} + C_{23})}{9}$$

$$G^V = \frac{[C_{11} + C_{22} + C_{33} + 3(C_{44} + C_{55} + C_{66}) - (C_{12} + C_{13} + C_{23})]}{15}$$

(20.A3)

Reuss Orthotropic

$$K_R = \frac{\Delta}{C_{11}C_{22} + C_{22}C_{33} + C_{33}C_{11}} - 2(C_{11}C_{23} + C_{22}C_{13} + C_{33}C_{12})$$
$$+ 2(C_{12}C_{23} + C_{23}C_{13} + C_{13}C_{12}) - (C_{12}^2 + C_{13}^2 + C_{23}^2)$$

$$G_R = 15/(4\{(C_{11}C_{22} + C_{22}C_{33} + C_{33}C_{11} + C_{11}C_{23} + C_{22}C_{13} + C_{33}C_{12})$$
$$- [C_{12}(C_{12} + C_{23}) + C_{23}(C_{23} + C_{13}) + C_{13}(C_{13} + C_{12})]\}/\Delta$$
$$+ 3(1/C_{44} + 1/C_{55} + 1/C_{66}))$$

(20.A4)

where Δ is given in Eq. (20.15).

21

Mechanics of Blood Vessels

Thomas R. Canfield
Argonne National Laboratory

Philip B. Dobrin
Hines VA Hospital and Loyola University Medical Center

21.1 Assumptions

This chapter is concerned with the mechanical behavior of blood vessels under static loading conditions and the methods required to analyze this behavior. The assumptions underlying this discussion are for *ideal* blood vessels that are at least regionally homogeneous, incompressible, elastic, and cylindrically orthotropic. Although physiologic systems are *nonideal*, much understanding of vascular mechanics has been gained through the use of methods based upon these ideal assumptions.

Homogeneity of the Vessel Wall

On visual inspection, blood vessels appear to be fairly homogeneous and distinct from surrounding connective tissue. The inhomogeneity of the vascular wall is realized when one examines the tissue under a low-power microscope, where one can easily identify two distinct structures: the media and adventitia. For this reason the assumption of vessel wall homogeneity is applied cautiously. Such an assumption may be valid only within distinct macroscopic structures. However, few investigators have incorporated macroscopic inhomogeneity into studies of vascular mechanics [17].

Incompressibility of the Vessel Wall

Experimental measurement of wall compressibility of 0.06% at 270 cm of H_2O indicates that the vessel can be considered incompressible when subjected to physiologic pressure and load [2]. In terms of the mechanical behavior of blood vessels, this is small relative to the large magnitude of the distortional strains that occur when blood vessels are deformed under the same conditions. Therefore, vascular compressibility may be important to understanding other physiologic processes related to blood vessels, such as the transport of interstitial fluid.

Work sponsored by the US Department of Energy order Contract W-31-109-Eng-38.

Inelasticity of the Vessel Wall

That blood vessel walls exhibit inelastic behavior such as length-tension and pressure-diameter hysteresis, stress relaxation, and creep has been reported extensively [1, 10]. However, blood vessels are able to maintain stability and contain the pressure and flow of blood under a variety of physiologic conditions. These conditions are dynamic but slowly varying with a large static component.

Residual Stress and Strain

Blood vessels are known to retract both longitudinally and circumferentially after excision. This retraction is caused by the relief of distending forces resulting from internal pressure and longitudinal tractions. The magnitude of retraction is influenced by several factors. Among these factors are growth, aging, and hypertension. Circumferential retraction of medium-caliber blood vessels, such as the carotid, iliac, and bracheal arteries, can exceed 70% following reduction of internal blood pressure to zero. In the case of the carotid artery, the amount of longitudinal retraction tends to increase during growth and to decrease in subsequent aging [5]. It would seem reasonable to assume that blood vessels are in a nearly stress-free state when they are fully retracted and free of external loads. This configuration also seems to be a reasonable choice for the reference configuration. However, this ignores residual stress and strain effects that have been the subject of current research [4, 11–14, 16].

Blood vessels are formed in a dynamic environment which gives rise to imbalances between the forces that tend to extend the diameter and length and the internal forces that tend to resist this extension. This imbalance is thought to stimulate the growth of elastin and collagen and to effectively reduce the stresses in the underlying tissue. Under these conditions it is not surprising that a residual stress state exists when the vessel is fully retracted and free of external tractions. This process has been called *remodeling* [11]. Striking evidence of this remodeling is found when a cylindrical slice of the fully retracted blood vessel is cut longitudinally through the wall. The cylinder springs open, releasing bending stresses kept in balance by the cylindrical geometry [16].

21.2 Vascular Anatomy

A blood vessel can be divided anatomically into three distinct cylindrical sections when viewed under the optical microscope. Starting at the inside of the vessel, they are the intima, the media, and the adventitia. These structures have distinct functions in terms of the blood vessel physiology and mechanical properties.

The intima consists of a thin monolayer of endothelial cells that line the inner surface of the blood vessel. The endothelial cells have little influence on blood vessel mechanics but do play an important role in hemodynamics and transport phenomena. Because of their anatomical location, these cells are subjected to large variations in stress and strain as a result of pulsatile changes in blood pressure and flow.

The media represents the major portion of the vessel wall and provides most of the mechanical strength necessary to sustain structural integrity. The media is organized into alternating layers of interconnected smooth muscle cells and elastic lamellae. There is evidence of collagen throughout the media. These small collagen fibers are found within the bands of smooth muscle and may participate in the transfer of forces between the smooth muscle cells and the elastic lamellae. The elastic lamellae are composed principally of the fiberous protein elastin. The number of elastic lamellae depends upon the wall thickness and the anatomical location [18]. In the case of the canine carotid, the elastic lamellae account for a major component of the static structural response of the blood vessel [6]. This response is modulated by the smooth-muscle cells, which have the ability to actively change the mechanical characteristics of the wall [7].

The adventitia consists of loose, more disorganized fiberous connective tissue, which may have less influence on mechanics.

21.3 Axisymmetric Deformation

In the following discussion we will concern ourselves with deformation of cylindrical tubes, see Fig. 21.1. Blood vessels tend to be nearly cylindrical in situ and tend to remain cylindrical when a cylindrical section is excised and studied in vitro. Only when the vessel is dissected further does the geometry begin to deviate from cylindrical. For this deformation there is a unique coordinate mapping

$$(R, \Theta, Z) \rightarrow (r, \theta, z) \tag{21.1}$$

where the undeformed coordinates are given by (R, Θ, Z) and the deformed coordinates are given by (r, θ, z). The deformation is given by a set of restricted functions

$$r = r(R) \tag{21.2}$$

$$\theta = \beta\Theta \tag{21.3}$$

$$z = \mu Z + c_1 \tag{21.4}$$

where the constants μ and β have been introduced to account for a uniform longitudinal strain and a symmetric residual strain that are both independent of the coordinate Θ.

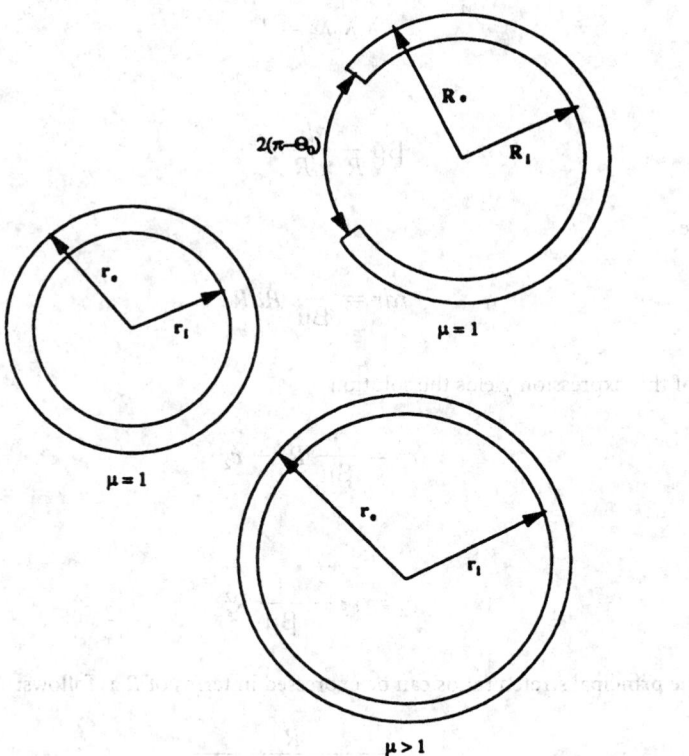

FIGURE 21.1 Cylindrical geometry of a blood vessel: *top:* stress-free reference configuration; *middle:* fully retracted vessel free of external traction; *bottom:* vessel in situ under longitudinal tether and internal pressurization.

If $\beta = 1$, there is no residual strain. If $\beta \neq 1$, residual stresses and strains are present. If $\beta > 1$, a longitudinal cut through the wall will cause the blood vessel to open up, and the new cross-section will form a *c*-shaped section of an annulus with larger internal and external radii. If $\beta < 1$, the cylindrical shape is unstable, but a thin section will tend to overlap itself. In Choung and Fung's formulation, $\beta = \pi/\Theta_o$, where the angle Θ_o is half the angle spanned by the open annular section [4].

For cylindrical blood vessels there are two assumed constraints. The first assumption is that the longitudinal strain is uniform through the wall and therefore

$$\lambda_z = \mu = \text{a constant} \tag{21.5}$$

for any cylindrical configuration. Given this, the principal stretch ratios are computed from the above functions as

$$\lambda_r = \frac{dr}{dR} \tag{21.6}$$

$$\lambda_\theta = \beta \frac{r}{R} \tag{21.7}$$

$$\lambda_z = \mu \tag{21.8}$$

The second assumption is wall incompressibility, which can be expressed by

$$\lambda_r \lambda_\theta \lambda_z \equiv 1 \tag{21.9}$$

or

$$\beta\mu \frac{r}{R} \frac{dr}{dR} = 1 \tag{21.10}$$

and therefore

$$r dr = \frac{1}{\beta\mu} R dR \tag{21.11}$$

Integration of this expression yields the solution

$$r^2 = \frac{1}{\beta\mu} R^2 + c_2 \tag{21.12}$$

where

$$c_2 = r_e^2 - \frac{1}{\beta\mu} R_e^2 \tag{21.13}$$

As a result, the principal stretch ratios can be expressed in terms of R as follows:

$$\lambda_r = \frac{R}{\sqrt{\beta\mu(R^2 + \beta\mu c_2)}} \tag{21.14}$$

$$\lambda_\theta = \sqrt{\frac{1}{\beta\mu} + \frac{c_2}{R^2}} \tag{21.15}$$

21.4 Experimental Measurements

The basic experimental setup required to measure the mechanical properties of blood vessels in vitro is described in [7]. It consists of a temperature-regulated bath of physiologic saline solution to maintain immersed cylindrical blood vessel segments, devices to measure diameter, an apparatus to hold the vessel at a constant longitudinal extension and to measure longitudinal distending force, and a system to deliver and control the internal pressure of the vessel with 100% oxygen. Typical data obtained from this type of experiment are shown in Figs. 21.2 and 21.3.

21.5 Equilibrium

When blood vessels are excised, they retract both longitudinally and circumferentially. Restoration to natural dimensions requires the application of internal pressure, p_i, and a longitudinal tether force, F_T. The internal pressure and longitudinal tether are balanced by the development of forces within the vessel wall. The internal pressure is balanced in the circumferential direction by a wall tension, T. The longitudinal tether force and pressure are balanced by the retractive force of the wall, F_R

$$T = p_i r_i \tag{21.16}$$

$$F_R = F_T + p_i \pi r_i^2 \tag{21.17}$$

The first equation is the familiar law of Laplace for a cylindrical tube with internal radius r_i. It indicates that the force due to internal pressure, p_i, must be balanced by a tensile force (per unit length), T, within the wall. This tension is the integral of the circumferentially directed force intensity (or stress, σ_θ) across the wall:

$$T = \int_{r_i}^{r_e} \sigma_\theta \, dr = \overline{\sigma}_\theta \, h \tag{21.18}$$

where $\overline{\sigma}_\theta$ is the mean value of the circumferential stress and h is the wall thickness. Similarly, the longitudinal tether force, F_T, and extending force due to internal pressure are balanced by a retractive internal force, F_R, due to axial stress, σ_z, in the blood vessel wall:

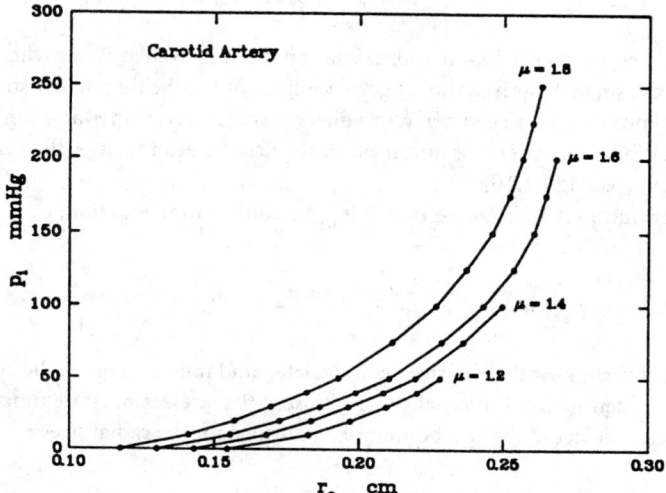

FIGURE 21.2 Pressure-radius curves for the canine carotid artery at various degrees of longitudinal extension.

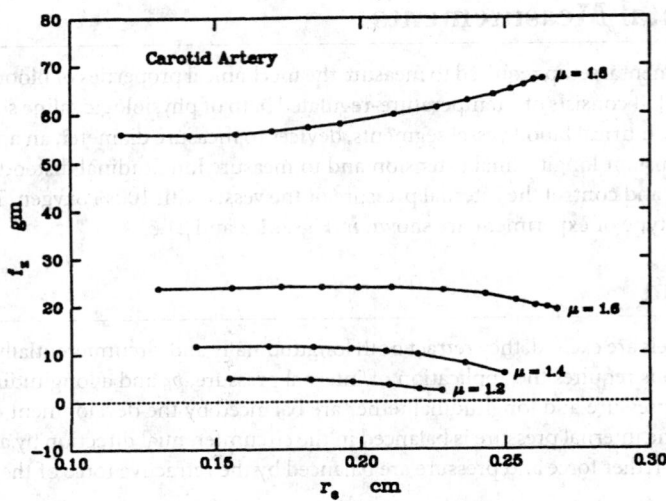

FIGURE 21.3   Longitudinal distending force as a function of radius at various degrees of longitudinal extension.

$$F_R = 2\pi \int_{r_i}^{r_e} \sigma_z r \, dr = \overline{\sigma}_z \pi h (r_e + r_i) \tag{21.19}$$

where $\overline{\sigma}_z$ is the mean value of this longitudinal stress. The mean stresses are calculated from the above equations as

$$\overline{\sigma}_\theta = p_i \frac{r_i}{h} \tag{21.20}$$

$$\overline{\sigma}_z = \frac{F_T}{\pi h (r_e + r_i)} + \frac{p_i}{2} \frac{r_i}{h} \tag{21.21}$$

The mean stresses are a fairly good approximation for thin-walled tubes where the variations through the wall are small. However, the range of applicability of the thin-wall assumption depends upon the material properties and geometry. In a linear elastic material, the variation in σ_θ is less than 5% for $r/h > 20$. When the material is nonlinear or the deformation is large, the variations in stress can be more severe (see Fig. 21.10).

The stress distribution is determined by solving the equilibrium equation,

$$\frac{1}{r} \frac{d}{dr}(r\sigma_r) - \frac{\sigma_\theta}{r} = 0 \tag{21.22}$$

This equation governs how the two stresses are related and must change in the cylindrical geometry. For uniform extension and internal pressurization, the stresses must be functions of a single radial coordinate, r, subject to the two boundary conditions for the radial stress:

$$\sigma_r(r_i, \mu) = -p_i \tag{21.23}$$

$$\sigma_r(r_e, \mu) = 0 \tag{21.24}$$

21.6 Strain Energy Density Functions

Blood vessels are able to maintain their structural stability and contain steady oscillating internal pressures. This property suggests a strong elastic component, which has been called the *pseudoelasticity* [10]. This elastic response can be characterized by a single potential function called the *strain energy density*. It is a scalar function of the strains that determines the amount of stored elastic energy per unit volume. In the case of a cylindrically orthotropic tube of incompressible material, the strain energy density can be written in the following functional form:

$$W = W^*(\lambda_r, \lambda_\theta, \lambda_z) + \lambda_r \lambda_\theta \lambda_z p, \tag{21.25}$$

where p is a scalar function of position, R. The stresses are computed from the strain energy by the following:

$$\sigma_i = \lambda_i \frac{\partial W^*}{\partial \lambda_i} + p \tag{21.26}$$

We make the following transformation [3]

$$\lambda = \frac{\beta r}{\sqrt{\beta \mu (r^2 - c_2)}} \tag{21.27}$$

which upon differentiation gives

$$r \frac{d\lambda}{dr} = \beta^{-1} (\beta \lambda - \mu \lambda^3) \tag{21.28}$$

After these expressions and the stresses in terms of the strain energy density function are introduced into the equilibrium equation, we obtain an ordinary differential equation for p

$$\frac{dp}{d\lambda} = \frac{\beta \ W^*_{,\lambda_\theta} - W^*_{,\lambda_r}}{\beta \lambda - \mu \lambda^3} - \frac{dW^*_{,\lambda_r}}{d\lambda} \tag{21.29}$$

subject to the boundary conditions

$$p(R_i) = p_i \tag{21.30}$$

$$p(R_e) = 0 \tag{21.31}$$

Isotropic Blood Vessels

A blood vessel generally exhibits anisotropic behavior when subjected to large variations in internal pressure and distending force. When the degree of anisotropy is small, the blood vessel may be treated as isotropic. For isotropic materials it is convenient to introduce the strain invariants:

$$I_1 = \lambda_r^2 + \lambda_\theta^2 + \lambda_z^2 \tag{21.32}$$

$$I_2 = \lambda_r^2 \lambda_\theta^2 + \lambda_\theta^2 \lambda_z^2 + \lambda_z^2 \lambda_r^2 \tag{21.33}$$

$$I_3 = \lambda_r^2 \lambda_\theta^2 \lambda_z^2 \tag{21.34}$$

These are measures of strain that are independent of the choice of coordinates. If the material is incompressible

$$I_3 = j^2 \equiv 1 \tag{21.35}$$

and the strain energy density is a function of the first two invariants, then

$$W = W(I_1, I_2). \tag{21.36}$$

The least complex form for an incompressible material is the first-order polynomial, which was first proposed by Mooney to characterize rubber:

$$W^\star = \frac{G}{2} \left[(I_1 - 3) + k(I_2 - 3) \right] \tag{21.37}$$

It involves only two elastic constants. A special case, where $k = 0$, is the neo-Hookean material, which can be derived from thermodynamics principles for a simple solid. Exact solutions can be obtained for the cylindrical deformation of a thick-walled tube. In the case where there is no residual strain, we have the following:

$$p = -G(1 + k\mu^2) \left[\frac{\log \lambda}{\mu} + \frac{1}{2\mu^2\lambda^2} \right] + c_0 \tag{21.38}$$

$$\sigma_r = G \left[\frac{1}{\lambda^2\mu^2} + k \left(\frac{1}{\mu^2} + \frac{1}{\lambda^2} \right) \right] + p \tag{21.39}$$

$$\sigma_\theta = G \left[\lambda^2 + k \left(\frac{1}{\mu^2} + \lambda^2\mu^2 \right) \right] + p \tag{21.40}$$

$$\sigma_z = G \left[\mu^2 + k \left(\lambda^2\mu^2 + \frac{1}{\lambda^2} \right) \right] + p \tag{21.41}$$

However, these equations predict stress softening for a vessel subjected to internal pressurization at fixed lengths, rather than the stress stiffening observed in experimental studies on arteries and veins (see Figs. 21.4 and 21.5).

An alternative isotropic strain energy density function which can predict the appropriate type of stress stiffening for blood vessels is an exponential where the argument is a polynomial of the strain invariants. The first-order form is given by

$$W^\star = \frac{G_0}{2k_1} \exp \left[k_1(I_1 - 3) + k_2(I_2 - 3) \right] \tag{21.42}$$

This requires the determination of only two independent elastic constants. The third, G_0, is introduced to facilitate scaling of the argument of the exponent (see Figs. 21.6 and 21.7). This exponential form is attractive for several reasons. It is a natural extension of the observation that biologic tissue stiffness is proportional to the load in simple elongation. This stress stiffening has been attributed to a statistical recruitment and alignment of tangled and disorganized long chains of proteins. The exponential forms resemble statistical distributions derived from these same arguments.

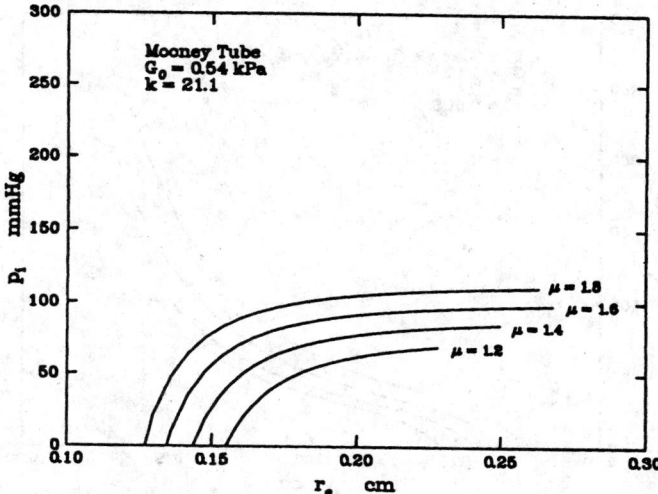

FIGURE 21.4 Pressure-radius curves for a Mooney-Rivlin tube with the approximate dimensions of the carotid.

Anisotropic Blood Vessels

Studies of the orthotropic behavior of blood vessels may employ polynomial or exponential strain energy density functions that include all strain terms or extension ratios. In particular, the strain energy density function can be of the form

$$W^* = q_n(\lambda_r, \lambda_\theta, \lambda_z) \tag{21.43}$$

or

$$W^* = e^{q_n(\lambda_r, \lambda_\theta, \lambda_z)} \tag{21.44}$$

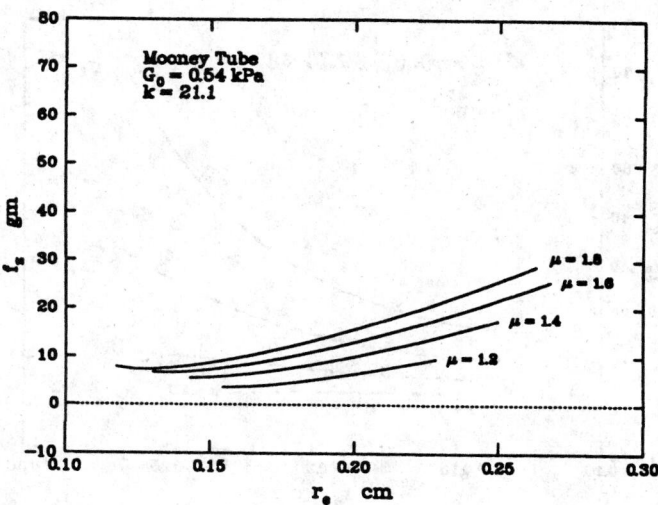

FIGURE 21.5 Longitudinal distending force as a function of radius for the Mooney-Rivlin tube.

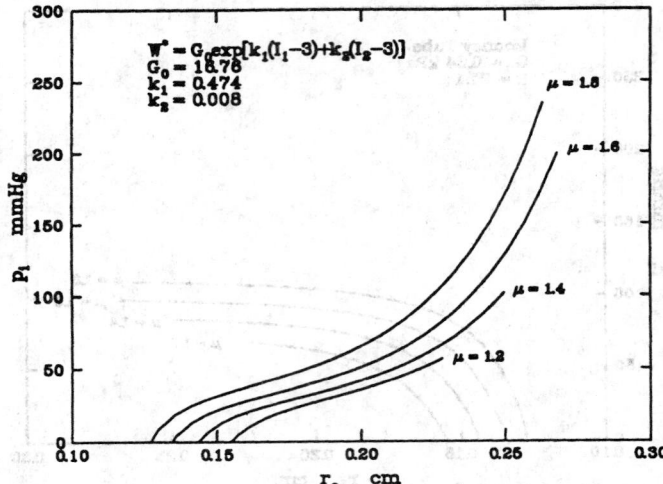

FIGURE 21.6 Pressure-radius curves for tube with the approximate dimensions of the carotid calculated using an isotropic exponential strain energy density function.

where q_n is a polynomial of order n. Since the material is incompressible, the explicit dependence upon λ_r can be eliminated either by substituting $\lambda_r = \lambda_\theta^{-1}\lambda_z^{-1}$ or by assuming that the wall is thin and hence that the contribution of these terms is small. Figures 21.8 and 21.9 illustrate how well the experimental data can be fitted to an exponential strain energy density function whose argument is a polynomial of order $n = 3$.

Care must be taken to formulate expressions that will lead to stresses that behave properly. For this reason it is convenient to formulate the strain energy density in terms of the lagrangian strains

$$e_i = 1/2(\lambda_i^2 - 1) \tag{21.45}$$

and in this case we can consider polynomials of the lagrangian strains, $q_n(e_r, e_\theta, e_z)$.

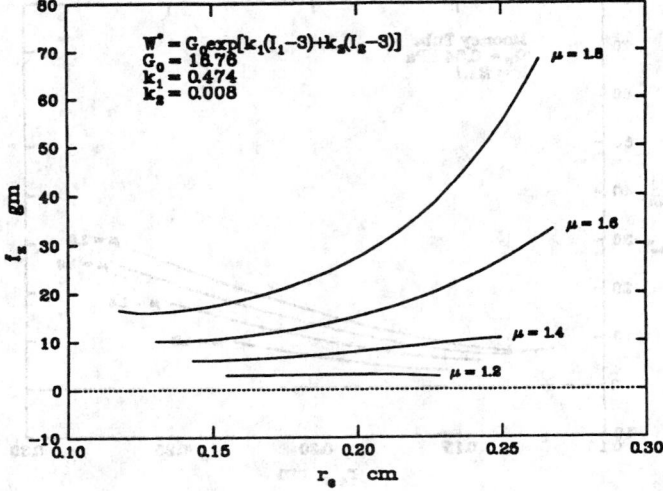

FIGURE 21.7 Longitudinal distending force as a function of radius for the isotropic tube.

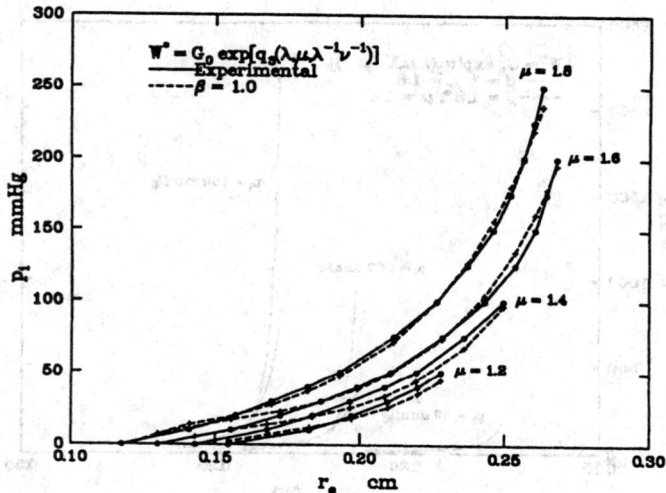

FIGURE 21.8 Pressure-radius curves for a fully orthotropic vessel calculated with an exponential strain energy density function.

Vaishnav et al. [15] proposed using a polynomial of the form

$$W^* = \sum_{i=2}^{n} \sum_{j=0}^{i} a_{ij-i} e_\theta^{i-j} e_z^j \tag{21.46}$$

to approximate the behavior of the canine aorta. They found better correlation with order-three polynomials over order-two, but order-four polynomials did not warrant the addition work.

Later, Fung et al. [10] found very good correlation with an expression of the form

$$W = \frac{C}{2} \exp \left[a_1 (e_\theta^2 - e_z^{*2}) + a_2 (e_z^2 - e_z^{*2}) + 2a_4 (e_\theta e_z - e_\theta^* e_z^*) \right] \tag{21.47}$$

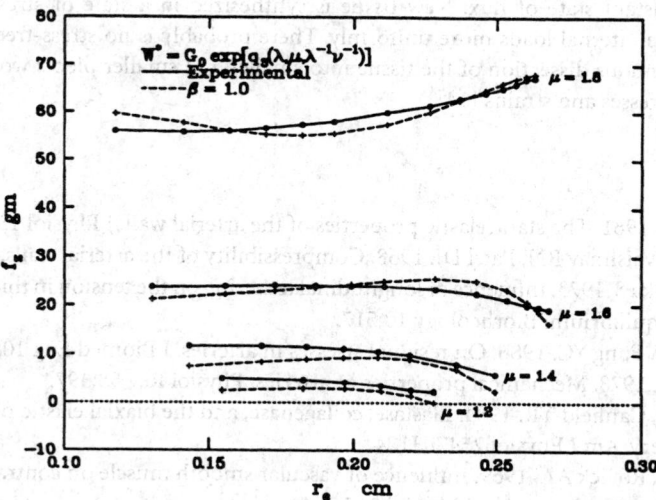

FIGURE 21.9 Longitudinal distending force as a function of radius for the orthotropic vessel.

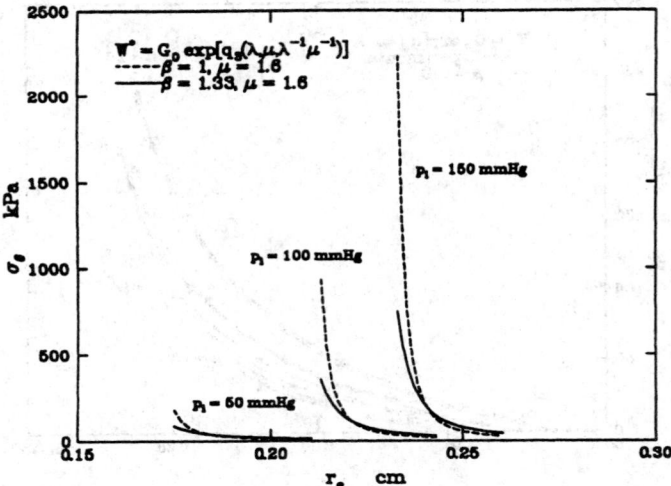

FIGURE 21.10 Stress distributions through the wall at various pressures for the orthotropic vessel.

for the canine carotid artery, where e_θ^* and e_z^* are the strains in a reference configuration at in situ length and pressure. Why should this work? One answer appears to be related to residual stresses and strains.

When residual stresses are ignored, large-deformation analysis of thick-walled blood vessels predicts steep distributions in σ_θ and σ_z through the vessel wall, with the highest stresses at the interior. This prediction is considered significant because high tensions in the inner wall could inhibit vascularization and oxygen transport to vascular tissue.

When residual stresses are considered, the stress distributions flatten considerably and become almost uniform at in situ length and pressure. Fig. 21.10 shows the radial stress distributions computed for a vessel with $\beta = 1$ and $\beta = 1.11$. Takamizawa and Hayashi have even considered the case where the strain distribution is uniform in situ [13]. The physiologic implications are that vascular tissue is in a constant state of flux. New tissue is synthesized in a state of stress that allows it to redistribute the internal loads more uniformly. There probably is no stress-free reference state [8, 11, 12]. Continuous dissection of the tissue into smaller and smaller pieces would continue to relieve residual stresses and strains [14].

References

1. Bergel DH. 1961. The static elastic properties of the arterial wall. J Physiol 156:445.
2. Carew TE, Vaishnav RN, Patel DJ. 1968. Compressibility of the arterial walls. Circ Res 23:61.
3. Chu BM, Oka S. 1973. Influence of longitudinal tethering on the tension in thick-walled blood vessels in equilibrium. Biorheology 10:517.
4. Choung CJ, Fung YC. 1986. On residual stresses in arteries. J Biomed Eng 108:189.
5. Dobrin PB. 1978. Mechanical properties of arteries. Physiol Rev 58:397.
6. Dobrin PB, Canfield TR. 1984. Elastase, collagenase, and the biaxial elastic properties of dog carotid artery. Am J Physiol 2547:H124.
7. Dobrin PB, Rovick AA. 1969. Influence of vascular smooth muscle on contractile mechanics and elasticity of arteries. Am J Physiol 217:1644.
8. Dobrin PD, Canfield T, Sinha S. 1975. Development of longitudinal retraction of carotid arteries in neonatal dogs. Experientia 31:1295.

9. Doyle JM, Dobrin PB. 1971. Finite deformation the relaxed and contracted dog carotid artery. Microvasc Res 3:400.

10. Fung YC, Fronek K, Patitucci P. 1979. Pseudoelasticity of arteries and the choice of its mathematical expression. Am J Physiol 237:H620.

11. Fung YC, Liu SQ, Zhou JB. 1993. Remodeling of the constitutive equation while a blood vessel remodels itself under strain. J Biomech Eng 115:453.

12. Rachev A, Greenwald S, Kane T, Moore J, Meister J-J. 1994. Effects of age-related changes in the residual strains on the stress distribution in the arterial wall. In J Vossoughi (ed), Proceedings of the Thirteenth Society of Biomedical Engineering Recent Developments, pp 409–412, Washington DC, University of District of Columbia.

13. Takamizawa K, Hayashi K. 1987. Strain energy density function and the uniform strain hypothesis for arterial mechanics. J Biomech 20:7.

14. Vassoughi J. 1992. Longitudinal residual strain in arteries. Proc of the 11th South Biomed Engrg Conf, Memphis, TN.

15. Vaishnav RN, Young JT, Janicki JS, Patel DJ. 1972. 'Nonlinear anisotropic elastic properties of the canine aorta. Biophys J 12:1008.

16. Vaishnav RN, Vassoughi J. 1983. Estimation of residual stresses in aortic segments. In CW Hall (ed), Biomedical Engineering II, Recent Developments, pp 330–333, New York, Pergamon Press.

17. Von Maltzahn W-W, Desdo D, Wiemier, W. 1981. Elastic properties of arteries: a nonlinear two-layer cylindrical model. J Biomech 4:389.

18. Wolinsky H, Glagov S. 1969. Comparison of abdominal and thoracic aortic media structure in mammals. Circ Res 25:677.

22

Joint-Articulating Surface Motion

Kenton R. Kaufman
Motion Analysis Laboratory,
Children's Hospital, San Diego

Kai-Nan An
Biomechanics Laboratory,
Mayo Clinic

Knowledge of joint-articulating surface motion is essential for design of prosthetic devices to restore function: assessment of joint wear, stability, and degeneration and determination of proper diagnosis and surgical treatment of joint disease. In general, kinematic analysis of human movement can be arranged into two separate categories: (1) gross movement of the limb segments interconnected by joints, or (2) detailed analysis of joint articulating surface motion which is described in this chapter. Gross movement is the relative three-dimensional joint rotation as described by adopting the Eulerian angle system. Movement of this type is described in Chapter 27: Analysis of Gait. In general, the three-dimensional unconstrained rotation and translation of an articulating joint can be described utilizing the concept of the screw displacement axis. The most commonly used analytic method for the description of 6-degree-of-freedom displacement of a rigid body is the screw displacement axis [Kinzel et al. 1972; Spoor & Veldpaus, 1980; Woltring et al. 1985].

Various degrees of simplification have been used for kinematic modeling of joints. A hinged joint is the simplest and most common model used to simulate an anatomic joint in planar motion about a single axis embedded in the fixed segment. Experimental methods have been developed for determination of the instantaneous center of rotation for planar motion. The *instantaneous center of*

0-8493-8346-3/95/$0.00+$.50

rotation is defined as the point of zero velocity. For a true hinged motion, the instantaneous center of rotation will be a fixed point throughout the movement. Otherwise, loci of the instantaneous center of rotation or centrodes will exist. The center of curvature has also been used to define joint anatomy. The *center of curvature* is defined as the geometric center of coordinates of the articulating surface.

For more general planar motion of an articulating surface, the terms *sliding, rolling,* and *spinning* are commonly used (Fig. 22.1). Sliding (gliding) motion is defined as the pure translation of a moving segment against the surface of a fixed segment. The contact point of the moving segment does not change, while the contact point of the fixed segment has a constantly changing contact point. If the surface of the fixed segment is flat, the instantaneous center of rotation is located at infinity. Otherwise, it is located at the center of curvature of the fixed surface. Spinning motion (rotation) is the exact opposite of sliding motion. In this case, the moving segment rotates, and the contact point on the fixed surface does not change. The instantaneous center of rotation is located at the center of curvature of the spinning body that is undergoing pure rotation. Rolling motion occurs between moving and fixed segments where the contact points in each surface are constantly changing and the arc lengths of contact are equal on each segment. The instantaneous center of rolling motion is located at the contact point. Most planar motion of anatomic joints can be described by using any two of these three basic descriptions.

In this chapter, various aspects of joint-articulating motion are covered. Topics include the anatomical characteristics, joint contact, and axes of rotation. Joints of both the upper and lower extremity are discussed.

22.1 Ankle

The ankle joint is composed of two joints: the talocrural (ankle) joint and the talocalcaneal (subtalar) joint. The talocrural joint is formed by the articulation of the distal tibia and fibula with the trochlea of the talus. The talocalcaneal joint is formed by the articulation of the talus with the calcaneus.

Geometry of the Articulating Surfaces

The upper articular surface of the talus is wedge-shaped, its width diminishing from front to back. The talus can be represented by a conical surface. The wedge shape of the talus is about 25% wider

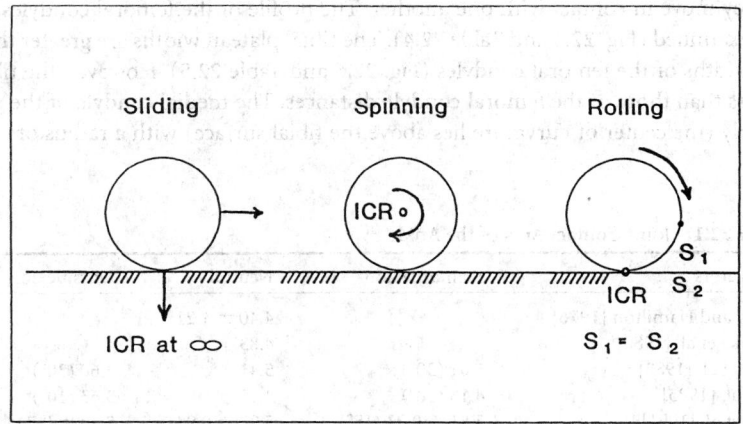

FIGURE 22.1 Three types of articulating surface motion in human joints.

in front than behind with an average difference of 2.4 mm ± 1.3 mm and a maximal difference of 6 mm [Inman, 1976].

Joint Contact

The talocrural joint contact area varies with flexion of the ankle (Table 22.1). During plantarflexion, such as would occur during the early stance phase of gait, the contact area is limited and the joint is incongruous. As the position of the joint progresses from neutral to dorsiflexion, as would occur during the midstance of gait, the contact area increases and the joint becomes more stable. The total contact area of the subtalar joint is 536 ± 137 mm² for the posterior facet and 131 ± 29 mm² for the anterior and middle facets [Sangeorzan et al., 1992]. The contact area/joint area ratio increases with increases in applied load (Fig. 22.2).

Axes of Rotation

Joint motion of the talocrural joint has been studied to define the axes of rotation and their location with respect to specific anatomic landmarks (Table 22.2). The axis of motion of the talocrural joint essentially passes through the inferior tibia at the fibular and tibial malleoli (Fig. 22.3). Three types of motion have been used to describe the axes of rotation: fixed, quasi-instantaneous, and instantaneous axes. The motion that occurs in the ankle joints consists of dorsiflexion and plantarflexion. Minimal or no transverse rotation takes place within the talocrural joint. The motion in the talocrural joint is intimately related to the motion in the talocalcaneal joint which is described next.

The motion axes of the talocalcaneal joint have been described by several authors (Table 22.3). The axis of motion in the talocalcaneal joint passes from the anterior medial superior aspect of the navicular bone to the posterior lateral inferior aspect of the calcaneus (Fig. 22.4). The motion that occurs in the talocalcaneal joint consists of inversion and eversion.

22.2 Knee

The knee is the intermediate joint of the lower limb. It is composed of the distal femur and proximal tibia. It is the largest and most complex joint in the body.

Geometry of the Articulating Surfaces

The shape of the articular surfaces of the proximal tibia and distal femur must fulfill the requirement that they move in contact with one another. The profile of the femoral condyles varies with the condyle examined (Fig. 22.5 and Table 22.4). The tibial plateau widths are greater than the corresponding widths of the femoral condyles (Fig. 22.6 and Table 22.5). However, the tibial plateau depths are less than those of the femoral condyle distances. The medial condyle of the tibia is concave superiorly (the center of curvature lies above the tibial surface) with a radius of curvature of

TABLE 22.1 Joint Contact Area of the Ankle

Investigators	Plantarflexion	Neutral	Dorsiflexion
Ramsey and Hamilton [1976]		4.40 ± 1.21	
Kimizuka et al. [1980]		4.83	
Libotte et al. [1982]	5.01 (30°)	5.41	3.60 (30°)
Paar et al. [1983]	4.15 (10°)	4.15	3.63 (10°)
Macko et al. [1991]	3.81 ± 0.93 (15°)	5.22 ± 0.94	5.40 ± 0.74 (10°)

Note: The contact area is expressed in square centimeters.

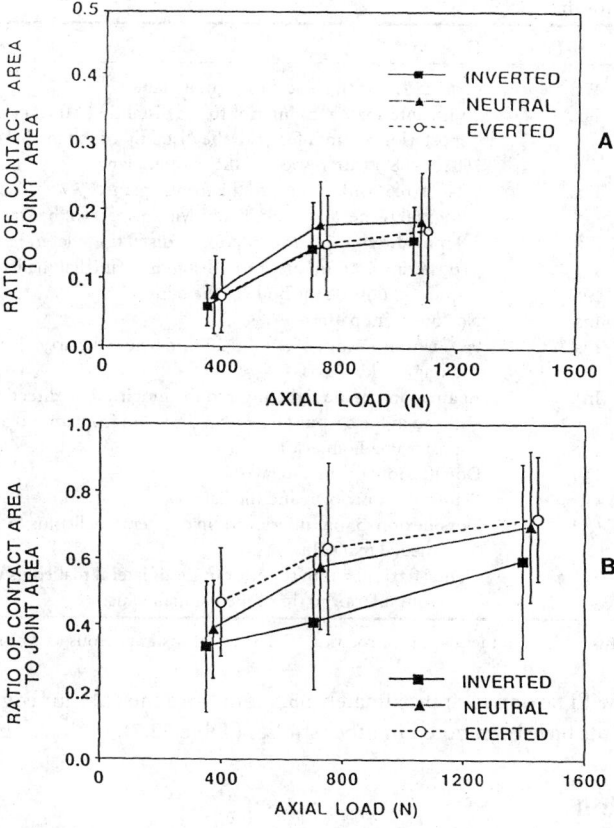

FIGURE 22.2 Ratio of total contact area to joint area in the (A) anterior/middle facet and (B) posterior facet as a function of applied axial load for three different positions of the foot. *Source:* Wagner UA, Sangeorzan BJ, Harrington RM, Tencer AF. 1992. Contact characteristics of the subtalar joint: load distribution between the anterior and posterior facets. J Orthop Res 10:535. With permission.

80 mm [Kapandji, 1987]. The lateral condyle is convex superiorly (the center of curvature lies below the tibial surface) with a radius of curvature of 70 mm [Kapandji, 1987]. The shape of the femoral surfaces is complementary to the shape of the tibial plateaus. The shape of the posterior femoral condyles may be approximated by spherical surfaces (Table 22.4).

Joint Contact

The mechanism of movement between the femur and tibia is a combination of rolling and gliding. Backward movement of the femur on the tibia during flexion has long been observed in the human knee. The magnitude of the rolling and gliding changes through the range of flexion. The tibial-femoral contact point has been shown to move posteriorly as the knee is flexed, reflecting the coupling of anterior/posterior motion with flexion/extension (Fig. 22.7). During flexion, the weight-bearing surfaces move backward on the tibial plateaus and become progressively smaller (Table 22.6).

It has been shown that in an intact knee at full extension the center of pressure is approximately 25 mm from the anterior edge of the knee joint line [Andriacchi et al., 1986]. This net contact point

TABLE 22.2 Axis of Rotation for the Ankle

Investigators	Axis*	Position
Elftman [1945]	Fix.	67.6° ± 7.4° with respect to sagittal plane
Isman and Inman [1969]	Fix.	8 mm anterior, 3 mm inferior to the distal tip of the lateral malleolus; 1 mm posterior, 5 mm inferior to the distal tip of the medial malleolus
Inman and Mann [1979]	Fix.	79° (68–88°) with respect to the sagittal plane
Allard et al. [1987]	Fix.	95.4° ± 6.6° with respect to the frontal plane, 77.7° ± 12.3° with respect to the sagittal plane, and 17.9° ± 4.5° with respect to the transverse plane
Singh et al. [1992]	Fix.	3.0 mm anterior, 2.5 mm inferior to distal tip of lateral malleolus, 2.2 mm posterior, 10 mm inferior to distal tip of medial malleolus
Sammarco et al. [1973]	Ins.	Inside and outside the body of the talus
D'Ambrosia et al. [1976]	Ins.	No consistent pattern
Parlasca et al. [1979]	Ins.	96% within 12 mm of a point 20 mm below the articular surface of the tibia along the long axis
Van Langelaan [1983]	Ins.	At an approximate right angle to the longitudinal direction of the foot, passing through the corpus tali, with a direction from anterolaterosuperior to posteromedioinferior
Barnett and Napier [1952]	Q-I	Dorsiflexion: down and lateral Plantarflexion: down and medial
Hicks [1953]	Q-I	Dorsiflexion: 5 mm inferior to tip of lateral malleolus to 15 mm anterior to tip of medial malleolus Plantarflexion: 5 mm superior to tip of lateral malleolus to 15 mm anterior, 10 mm inferior to tip of medial malleolus

* Fix. = fixed axis of rotation; Ins. = instantaneous axis of rotation; Q-I = quasi-instantaneous axis of rotation

moves posteriorly with flexion to approximately 38.5 mm from the anterior edge of the knee joint. Similar displacements have been noted in other studies (Table 22.7).

Axes of Rotation

The knee is mainly a joint with two degrees of freedom. The first degree of freedom allows movements of flexion and extension in the sagittal plane. The axis of rotation lies perpendicular to the

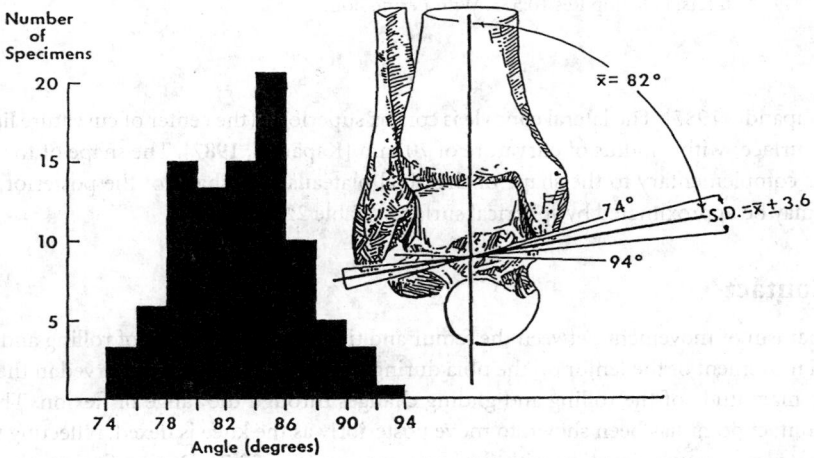

FIGURE 22.3 Variations in angle between middle of tibia and empirical axis of ankle. The histogram reveals a considerable spread of individual values. *Source:* Inman VT. 1976. The Joints of the Ankle, Baltimore, Williams and Wilkins. With permission.

TABLE 22.3 Axis of Rotation for the Talocalcaneal (Subtalar) Joint

Investigators	Axis*	Position
Manter [1941]	Fix.	16° (8–24°) with respect to sagittal plane, and 42° (29–47°) with respect to transverse plane
Shephard [1951]	Fix.	Tuberosity of the calcaneus to the neck of the talus
Hicks [1953]	Fix.	Posterolateral corner of the heel to superomedial aspect of the neck of the talus
Root et al. [1966]	Fix.	17° (8–29°) with respect to sagittal plane, and 41° (22–55°) with respect to transverse plane
Isman and Inman [1969]	Fix.	23° ± 11° with respect to sagittal plane, and 41° ± 9° with respect to transverse plane
Kirby [1947]	Fix.	Extends from the posterolateral heel, posteriorly, to the first intermetatarsal space, anteriorly
Rastegar et al. [1980]	Ins.	Instant centers of rotation pathways in posterolateral quadrant of the distal articulating tibial surface, varying with applied load
Van Langelaan [1983]	Ins.	A bundle of axes that make an acute angle with the longitudinal direction of the foot passing through the tarsal canal having a direction from antero-mediosuperior to posterolateroinferior
Engsberg [1987]	Ins.	A bundle of axes with a direction from anteromediosuperior to posterolateroinferior

* Fix. = fixed axis of rotation; Ins. = instantaneous axis of rotation

sagittal plane and intersects the femoral condyles. Both fixed axes and screw axes have been calculated (Fig. 22.8). In Fig. 22.8, the optimal axes are fixed axes, whereas the screw axes is an instantaneous axis. The symmetric optimal axis is constrained such that the axis is the same for both the right and left knee. The screw axis may sometimes coincide with the optimal axis but not always, depending upon the motions of the knee joint. The second degree of freedom is the axial rotation around the long axis of the tibia. Rotation of the leg around its long axis can only be performed with the knee flexed. There is also an automatic axial rotation which is involuntarily linked to flexion and extension. When the knee is flexed, the tibia internally rotates. Conversely, when the knee is extended, the tibia externally rotates.

22.3 Hip

The hip joint is composed of the head of the femur and the acetabulum of the pelvis. The hip joint is one of the most stable joints in the body. The stability is provided by the rigid ball-and-socket configuration.

Geometry of the Articulating Surfaces

The femoral head is spherical in its articular portion which forms two-thirds of a sphere. The diameter of the femoral head is smaller for females than for males (Table 22.8). In the normal hip, the center of the femoral head coincides exactly with the center of the acetabulum. The rounded part of the femoral head is spheroidal rather than spherical because the uppermost part is flattened slightly. This causes the load to be distributed in a ringlike pattern around the superior pole. The geometrical center of the femoral head is traversed by the three axes of the joint, the horizontal axes, the vertical axes, and the anterior/posterior axes. The head is supported by the neck of the femur, which joins the shaft. The axis of the femoral neck is obliquely set and runs superiorly, medially, and anteriorly. The angle of inclination of the femoral neck to the shaft in the frontal plane is the neck-shaft angle (Fig. 22.9). In most adults, this angle is about 130° (Table 22.8). An angle exceeding 130° is known as *coxa valga;* an angle less than 130° is known as *coxa vara.* The femoral neck forms an acute angle with the transverse axis of the femoral condyles. This angle faces medially and anteri-

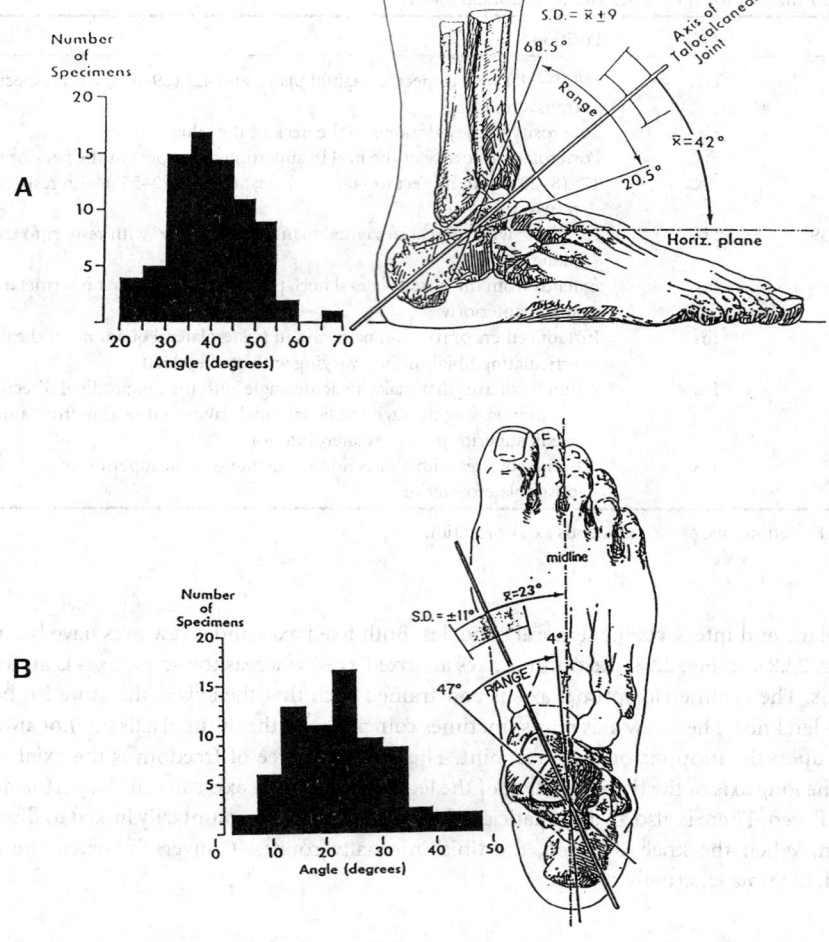

FIGURE 22.4 (A) Variations in inclination of axis of subtalar joint as projected upon the sagittal plane. The distribution of the measurements on the individual specimens is shown in the histogram. The single observation of an angle of almost 70° was present in a markedly cavus foot. (B) Variations in position of subtalar axis as projected onto the transverse plane. The angle was measured between the axis and the midline of the foot. The extent of individual variation is shown on the sketch and revealed in the histogram. *Source:* Inman VT. 1976. The Joints of the Ankle, Baltimore, Williams and Wilkins. With permission.

orly and is called the *angle of anteversion* (Fig. 22.10). In the adult, this angle averages about 7.5° (Table 22.8).

The acetabulum receives the femoral head and lies on the lateral aspect of the hip. The acetabulum of the adult is a hemispherical socket. Its cartilage area is approximately 16 cm² [Von Lanz & Wauchsmuth, 1938]. Together with the labrum, the acetabulum covers slightly more than 50% of the femoral head [Tönnis, 1987]. Only the sides of the acetabulum are lined by articular cartilage, which is interrupted inferiorly by the deep acetabular notch. The central part of the cavity is deeper than the articular cartilage and is nonarticular. This part is called the *acetabular fossae* and is separated from the interface of the pelvic bone by a thin plate of bone.

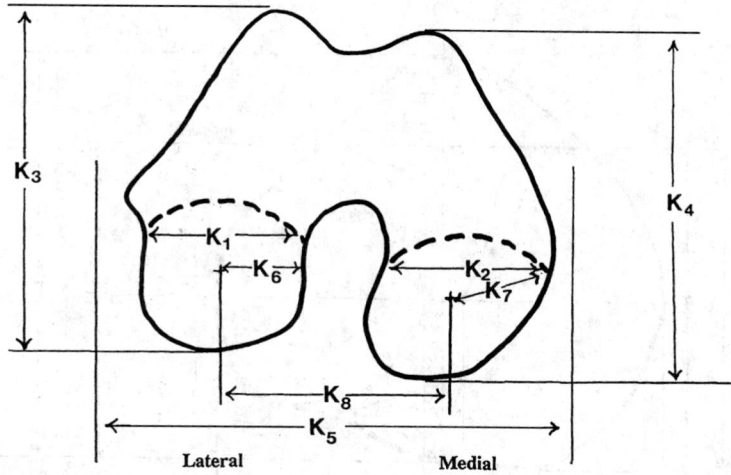

FIGURE 22.5   Geometry of distal femur. The distances are defined in Table 22.4.

Joint Contact

Miyanaga et al. [1984] studied the deformation of the hip joint under loading, the contact area between the articular surfaces, and the contact pressures. They found that at loads up to 1000 N, pressure was distributed largely to the anterior and posterior parts of the lunate surface with very little pressure applied to the central portion of the roof itself. As the load increased, the contact area enlarged to include the outer and inner edges of the lunate surface (Fig. 22.11). However, the highest pressures were still measured anteriorly and posteriorly. Of five hip joints studied, only one had a pressure maximum at the zenith or central part of the acetabulum.

Davy et al. [1989] utilized a telemetered total hip prosthesis to measure forces across the hip after total hip arthroplasty. The orientation of the resultant joint contact force varies over a relatively limited range during the weight-load–bearing portions of gait. Generally, the joint contact force on the

TABLE 22.4   Geometry of the Distal Femur

| | | Condyle | | | | |
| | Lateral | | Medial | | Overall | |
Parameter	Symbol	Distance (mm)	Symbol	Distance (mm)	Symbol	Distance (mm)
Medial/lateral distance	K1	31 ± 2.3 (male)	K2	32 ± 3.1 (male)		
		28 ± 1.8 (female)		27 ± 3.1 (female)		
Anterior/posterior distance	K3	72 ± 4.0 (male)	K4	70 ± 4.3 (male)		
		65 ± 3.7 (female)		63 ± 4.5 (female)		
Posterior femoral condyle spherical radii	K6	18.6 ± 0.56	K7	21.0 ± 0.3		
Epicondylar width					K5	90 ± 6 (male)
						80 ± 6 (female)
Medial/lateral spacing of center of spherical surfaces					K8	45.9 ± 3.4

Note: See Figure 22.5 for location of measurements.

Sources: Yoshioka Y, Siu D, Cooke TDV. 1987. The anatomy and functional axes of the femur. J Bone Joint Surg 69A(6):873–880.

   Kurosawa H, Walker PS, Abe S, Garg A, Hunter T. 1985. Geometry and motion of the knee for implant and orthotic design. J Biomech 18(7):487.

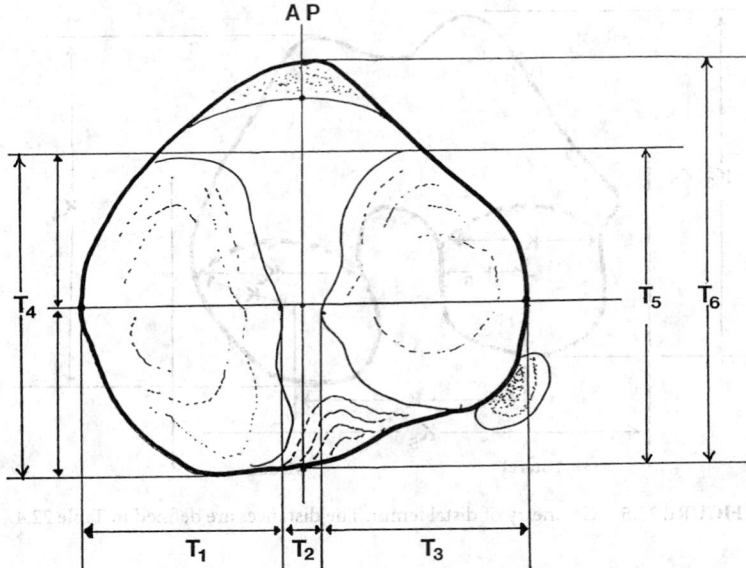

FIGURE 22.6 Contour of the tibial plateau (transverse plane). The distances are defined in Table 22.5.

TABLE 22.5 Geometry of the Proximal Tibia

Parameter	Symbols	All Limbs	Male	Female
Tibial plateau widths (mm)				
Medial plateau	T_1	32 ± 3.8	34 ± 3.9	30 ± 2.2
Lateral plateau	T_3	33 ± 2.6	35 ± 1.9	31 ± 1.7
Overall width	$T_1 + T_2 + T_3$	76 ± 6.2	81 ± 4.5	73 ± 4.5
Tibial plateau depths (mm)				
AP depth, medial	T_4	48 ± 5.0	52 ± 3.4	45 ± 4.1
AP depth, lateral	T_5	42 ± 3.7	45 ± 3.1	40 ± 2.3
Interspinous width (mm)	T_2	12 ± 1.7	12 ± 0.9	12 ± 2.2
Intercondylar depth (mm)	T_6	48 ± 5.9	52 ± 5.7	45 ± 3.9

Source: Yoshioka Y, Siu D, Scudamore RA, Cooke TDV. 1989. Tibial anatomy in functional axes. J Orthop Res 7:132.

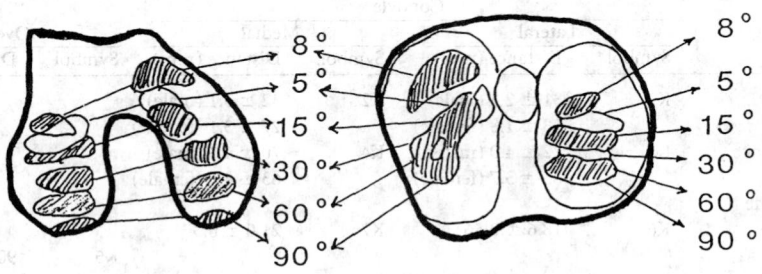

FIGURE 22.7 Tibio-femoral contact area as a function of knee flexion angle. *Source:* Iseki F, Tomatsu T. 1976. The biomechanics of the knee joint with special reference to the contact area. Keio J Med 25:37. With permission.

TABLE 22.6 Contact Area of the Knee Joint

Knee Flexion (deg)	Contact Area (cm²)
−5	20.2
5	19.8
15	19.2
25	18.2
35	14.0
45	13.4
55	11.8
65	13.6
75	11.4
85	12.1

Source: Maquet PG, Vandberg AJ, Simonet JC. 1975. Femorotibial weight bearing areas: Experimental determination. J Bone Joint Surg 57A(6): 766.

ball of the hip prosthesis is located in the anterior/superior region. A three-dimensional plot of the resultant joint force during the gait cycle, with crutches, is shown in Fig. 22.12.

Axes of Rotation

The human hip is a modified spherical (ball-and-socket) joint. Thus, the hip possesses three degrees of freedom of motion with three correspondingly arranged, mutually perpendicular axes that intersect at the geometric center of rotation of the spherical head. The transverse axis lies in the frontal plane and controls movements of flexion and extension. An anterior/posterior axis lies in the sagittal plane and controls movements of adduction and abduction. A vertical axis which coincides with the long axis of the limb when the hip joint is in the neutral position controls movements of internal and external rotation. Surface motion in the hip joint can be considered as spinning of the femoral head on the acetabulum. The pivoting of the bone socket in three planes around the center of rotation in the femoral head produces the spinning of the joint surfaces.

22.4 Shoulder

The shoulder represents the group of structures connecting the arm to the thorax. The combined movements of four distinct articulations—glenohumeral, acromioclavicular, sternoclavicular, and scapulothoracic—allow the arm to be positioned in space.

Geometry of the Articulating Surfaces

The articular surface of the humerus is approximately one-third of a sphere (Fig. 22.13). The articular surface is oriented with an upward tilt of approximately 45° and is retroverted approximately 30° with respect to the condylar line of the distal humerus [Morrey & An, 1990]. The average radius of curvature of the humeral head in the coronal plane is 24.0 ± 2.1 mm [Iannotti et al., 1992]. The humeral articulating surface is spherical in the center. However, the peripheral radius is 2 mm less in the axial plane than in the coronal plane. Thus the peripheral contour of the articular surface is elliptical with a ratio of 0.92 [Iannotti et al., 1992].

The glenoid fossa consists of a small, pear-shaped, cartilage-covered bony depression that measures 39.0 ± 3.5 mm in the superior/inferior direction and 29.0 ± 3.2 mm in the anterior/posterior direction [Iannotti et al., 1992]. The anterior/posterior dimension of the glenoid is pear-shaped with the lower half being larger than the top half. The ratio of the lower half to the top half is 1:0.80 ± 0.01 [Iannotti et al., 1992]. In the coronal plane the articular surface of the glenoid comprises an arc of approximately 75° and in the transverse plane the arc of curvature of the glenoid is about 50° [Morrey & An, 1990]. The glenoid has a slight upward tilt of about 5° [Basmajian & Bazant, 1959] with respect to the medial border of the scapula (Fig. 22.14) and is retroverted a mean of approximately 7° [Saha, 1971]. The re-

TABLE 22.7 Posterior Displacement of the Femur Relative to the Tibia

Authors	Condition	A/P Displacement (mm)
Kurosawa [1985]	In vitro	14.8
Andriacchi [1986]	In vitro	13.5
Draganich [1987]	In vitro	13.5
Nahass [1991]	In vivo (walking)	12.5
	In vivo (stairs)	13.9

LATERAL   POSTERIOR   MEDIAL

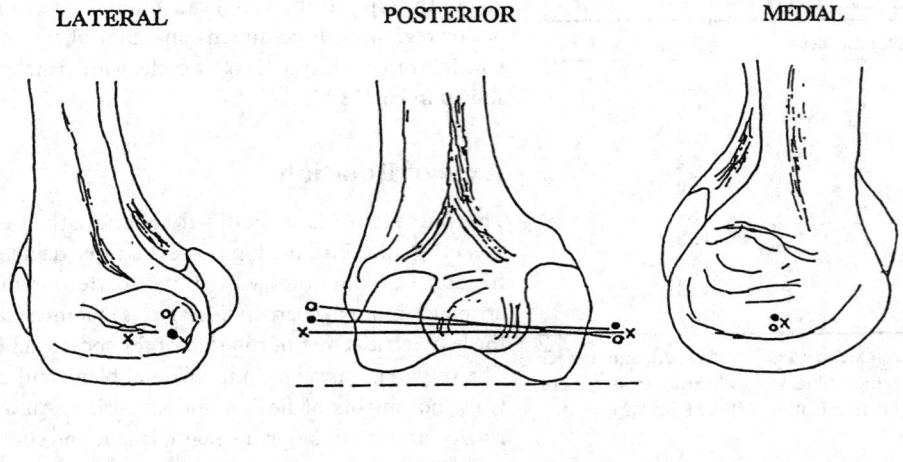

O NONSYMMETRICAL OPTIMAL AXIS

● SCREW AXIS

X SYMMETRICAL OPTIMAL AXIS

FIGURE 22.8 Approximate location of the optimal axis (case 1—nonsymmetric, case 3—symmetric), and the screw axis (case 2) on the medial and lateral condyles of the femur of a human subject for the range of motion of 0–90° flexion (standing to sitting, respectively). *Source:* Lewis JL, Lew WD. 1978. A method for locating an optimal "fixed" axis of rotation for the human knee joint. J Biomech Eng 100:187. With permission.

lationship of the dimension of the humeral head to the glenoid head is approximately 0.8 in the coronal plane and 0.6 in the horizontal or transverse plane [Saha, 1971]. The surface area of the glenoid fossa is only one-third to one-fourth that of the humeral head [Kent, 1971].

Joint Contact

Joint contact areas of the glenohumeral joint tend to be greater at mid-elevation positions than at either of the extremes of joint position (Table 22.9). These results suggest that the glenohumeral surface is maximum at these more functional positions, thus distributing joint load over a larger region in a more stable configuration. The contact point moves forward and inferior during internal rotation (Fig. 22.15). With external rotation, the contact is posterior/inferior. With elevation, the contact area moves superiorly.

Axes of Rotation

The shoulder complex consists of four distinct articulations: the glenohumeral joint, the acromioclavicular joint, the sternoclavicular joint, and the scapulothoracic articulation. The wide range of motion of the shoulder (exceeding a hemisphere) is the result of synchronous, simultaneous con-

TABLE 22.8 Geometry of the Proximal Femur

Parameter	Females	Males
Femoral head diameter (mm)	45.0 ± 3.0	52.0 ± 3.3
Neck shaft angle (degrees)	133 ± 6.6	129 ± 7.3
Anteversion (degrees)	8 ± 10	7.0 ± 6.8

Source: Yoshioka Y, Siu D, Cooke TDV. 1987. The anatomy and functional axes of the femur. J Bone Joint Surg 69A(6):873.

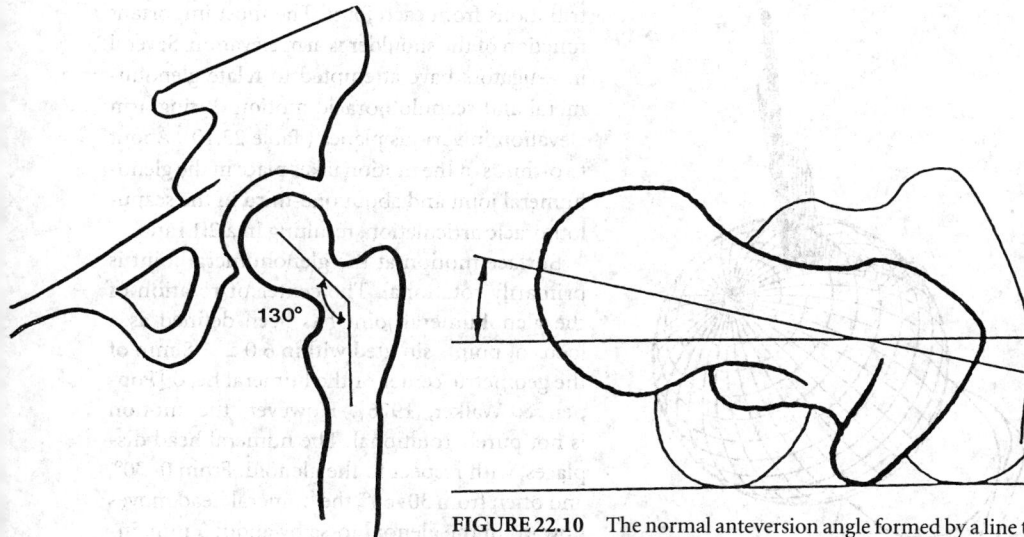

FIGURE 22.9 The neck-shaft angle.

FIGURE 22.10 The normal anteversion angle formed by a line tangent to the femoral condyles and the femoral neck axis, as displayed in the superior view.

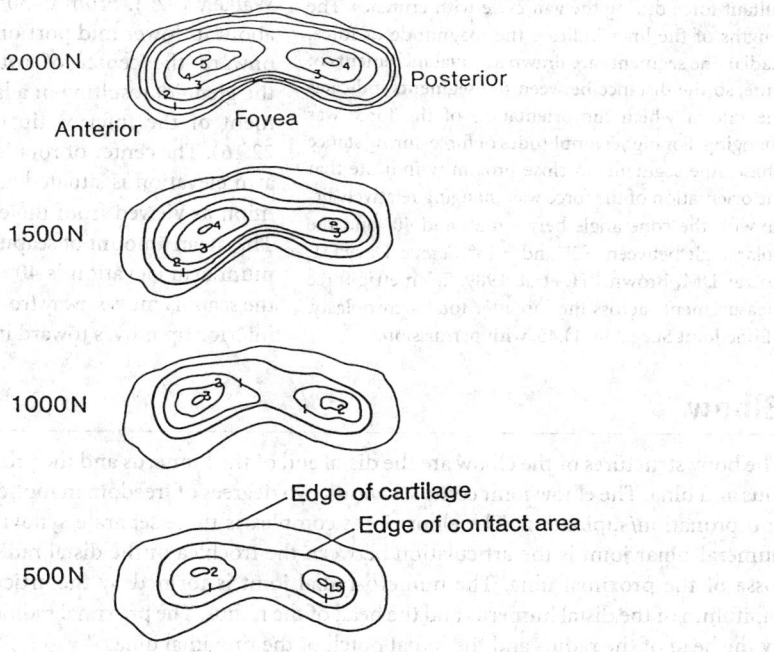

FIGURE 22.11 Pressure distribution and contact area of hip joint. The pressure is distributed largely to the anterior and posterior parts of the lunate surface. As the load increased, the contact area increased. *Source:* Miyanaga Y, Fukubayashi T, Kurosawa H. 1984. Contact study of the hip joint: Load deformation pattern, contact area, and contact pressure. Arch Orth Trauma Surg 103:13. With permission.

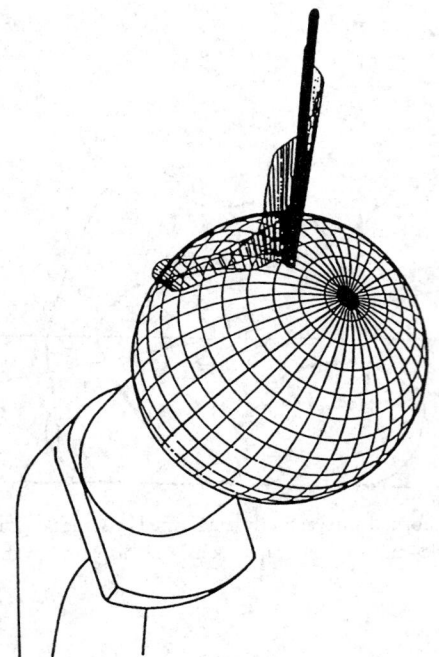

FIGURE 22.12 Scaled three-dimensional plot of resultant force during the gait cycle with crutches. The lengths of the lines indicate the magnitude of force. Radial line segments are drawn at equal increments of time, so the distance between the segments indicates the rate at which the orientation of the force was changing. For higher amplitudes of force during stance phase, line segments in close proximity indicate that the orientation of the force was changing relatively little with the cone angle between 30 and 40° and the polar angle between −25 and −15°. *Source:* Davy DT, Kotzar DM, Brown RH, et al. 1989. Telemetric force measurements across the hip after total arthroplasty. J Bone Joint Surg 70A(1):45, with permission.

tributions from each joint. The most important function of the shoulder is arm elevation. Several investigators have attempted to relate glenohumeral and scapulothoracic motion during arm elevation in various planes (Table 22.10). About two-thirds of the motion takes place in the glenohumeral joint and about one-third in the scapulothoracic articulation, resulting in a 2:1 ratio.

Surface motion at the glenohumeral joint is primarily rotational. The center of rotation of the glenohumeral joint has been defined as a locus of points situated within 6.0 ± 1.8 mm of the geometric center of the humeral head [Poppen & Walker, 1976]. However, the motion is not purely rotational. The humeral head displaces, with respect to the glenoid. From 0–30°, and often from 30–60°, the humeral head moves upward in the glenoid fossa by about 3 mm, indicating that rolling and/or gliding has taken place. Thereafter, the humeral head has only about 1 mm of additional excursion. During arm elevation in the scapular plane, the scapula moves in relation to the thorax [Poppen & Walker, 1976]. From 0–30° the scapula rotates about its lower mid portion, and then from 60° onward the center of rotation shifts toward the glenoid, resulting in a large lateral displacement of the inferior tip of the scapula (Fig. 22.16). The center of rotation of the scapula for arm elevation is situated at the tip of the acromion as viewed from the edge on (Fig. 22.17). The mean amount of scapular twisting at maximum arm elevation is 40°. The superior tip of the scapula moves away from the thorax, and the inferior tip moves toward it.

22.5 Elbow

The bony structures of the elbow are the distal end of the humerus and the proximal ends of the radius and ulna. The elbow joint complex allows two degrees of freedom in motion: flexion/extension and pronation/supination. The elbow joint complex is three separate synovial articulations. The humeral-ulnar joint is the articulation between the trochlea of the distal radius and the trochlear fossa of the proximal ulna. The humero-radial joint is formed by the articulation between the capitulum of the distal humerus and the head of the radius. The proximal radioulnar joint is formed by the head of the radius and the radial notch of the proximal ulna.

Geometry of the Articulating Surfaces

The curved, articulating portions of the trochlea and capitulum are approximately circular in a cross-section. The radius of the capitulum is larger than the central trochlear groove (Table 22.11). The centers of curvature of the trochlea and capitulum lie in a straight line located on a plane that slopes at 45–50° anterior and distal to the transepicondylar line and is inclined at 2.5° from the hor-

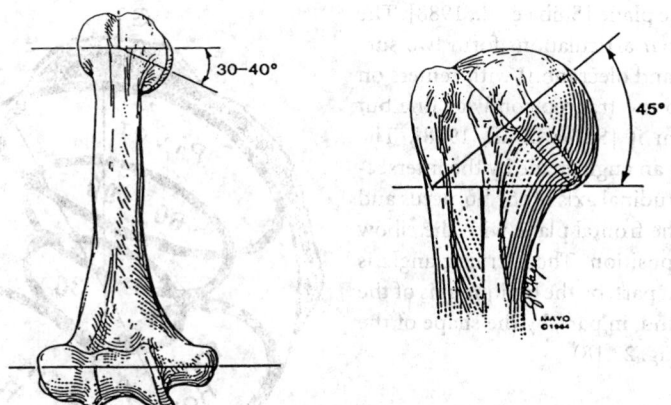

FIGURE 22.13 The two-dimensional orientation of the articular surface of the humerus with respect to the bicondylar axis. By permission of Mayo Foundation.

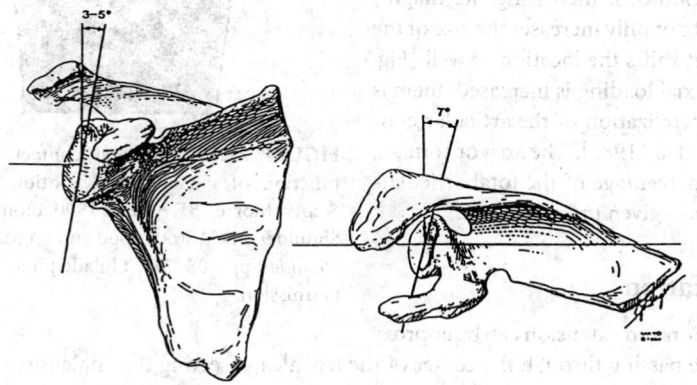

FIGURE 22.14 The glenoid faces slightly superior and posterior (retroverted) with respect to the body of the scapula. By permission of Mayo Foundation.

TABLE 22.9 Glenohumeral Contact Areas

Elevation angle (°)	Contact areas at SR (cm²)	Contact areas at 20° internal to SR (cm²)
0	0.87 ± 1.01	1.70 ± 1.68
30	2.09 ± 1.54	2.44 ± 2.15
60	3.48 ± 1.69	4.56 ± 1.84
90	4.95 ± 2.15	3.92 ± 2.10
120	5.07 ± 2.35	4.84 ± 1.84
150	3.52 ± 2.29	2.33 ± 1.47
180	2.59 ± 2.90	2.51 ± NA

SR = Starting external rotation which allowed the shoulder to reach maximal elevation in the scapular plane (≈40° ± 8°); NA = Not applicable

Source: Soslowsky LJ, Flatow EL, Bigliani LU, Pablak RJ, Mow VC, Athesian GA. 1992. Quantitation of in situ contact areas at the glenohumeral joint: A biomechanical study. J Orthop Res 10(4):524. With permission.

izontal transverse plane [Shiba et al., 1988]. The
curves of the ulnar articulations form two surfaces (coronoid and olecranon) with centers on
a line parallel to the transepicondylar line but
are distinct from it [Shiba et al., 1988]. The
carrying angle is an angle made by the intersection of the longitudinal axis of the humerus and
the forearm in the frontal plane with the elbow
in an extended position. The carrying angle is
contributed to, in part, by the oblique axis of the
distal humerus and, in part, by the shape of the
proximal ulna (Fig. 22.18).

Joint Contact

The contact area on the articular surfaces of the
elbow joint depends on the joint position and
the loading conditions. Increasing the magnitude of the load not only increases the size of the
contact area but shifts the location as well (Fig.
22.19). As the axial loading is increased, there is
an increased lateralization of the articular contact [Stormont et al., 1985]. The area of contact,
expressed as a percentage of the total articulating surface area, is given in Table 22.12.

Axes of Rotation

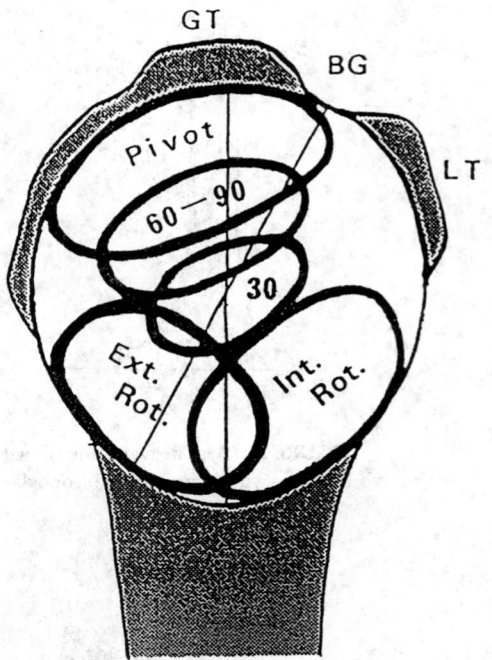

FIGURE 22.15 Humeral contact positions as a
function of glenohumeral motion and positions.
Source: Morrey BF, An KN. 1990. Biomechanics of the
Shoulder. In CA Rockwood and FA Matsen (eds), *The
Shoulder,* pp 208–245, Philadelphia, Saunders. With
permission.

The axes of flexion and extension can be approx-
imated by a line passing through the center of the trochlea, bisecting the angle formed by the longitudinal axes of the humerus and the ulna [Morrey & Chao, 1976]. The instant centers of flexion
and extension vary within 2–3 mm of this axis (Fig. 22.20). With the elbow fully extended and the
forearm fully supinated, the longitudinal axes of humerus and ulna normally intersect at a valgus
angle referred to as the *carrying angle.* In adults, this angle is usually 10–15° and normally is greater
on average in women [Zuckerman & Matsen, 1989]. As the elbow flexes, the carrying angle varies as
a function of flexion (Fig. 22.21). In extension there is a valgus angulation of 10°; at full flexion there
is a varus angulation of 8° [Morrey & Chao, 1976].

22.6 Wrist

The wrist functions by allowing changes of orientation of the hand relative to the forearm. The wrist
joint complex consists of multiple articulations of eight carpal bones with the distal radius, the
structures of the ulnocarpal space, the metacarpals, and each other. This collection of bones and soft
tissues is capable of a substantial arc of motion that augments hand and finger function.

Geometry of the Articulating Surfaces

The global geometry of the carpal bones has been quantified for grasp and active isometric contraction of the elbow flexors [Schuind et al., 1992]. During grasping there is a significant proximal
migration of the radius of 0.9 mm, apparent shortening of the capitate, a decrease in the carpal
height ratio, and an increase in the lunate uncovering index (Table 22.13). There is also a trend to-

TABLE 22.10 Arm Elevation: Glenohumeral-
Scapulothoracic Rotation

Investigator	Glenohumeral/Scapulothoracic Motion Ratio
Inman et al. [1994]	2:1
Freedman & Munro [1966]	1.35:1
Doody et al. [1970]	1.74:1
Poppen & Walker [1976]	4.3:1 (< 24° elevation)
	1.25:1 (> 24° elevation)
Saha, 1971	2.3:1 (30–135° elevation)

ward increase of the distal radioulnar joint with grasping. The addition of elbow flexion with concomitant grasping did not significantly change the global geometry, except for a significant decrease
in the forearm interosseous space [Schuind et al., 1992].

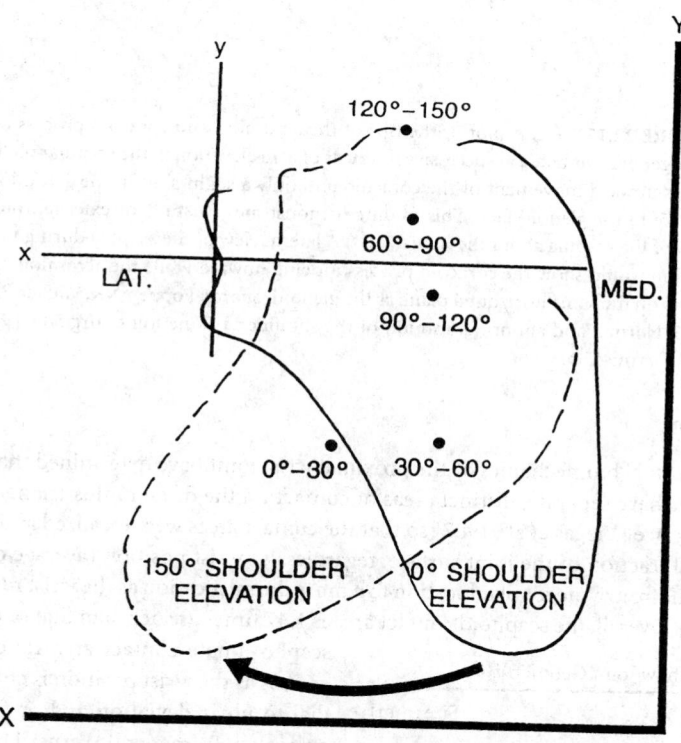

FIGURE 22.16 Rotation of the scapula on the thorax in the scapular plane.
Instant centers of rotation (solid dots) are shown for each 30° interval of motion during shoulder elevation in the scapular plane from zero to 150°. The
x and *y* axes are fixed in the scapula, whereas the *X* and *Y* axes are fixed in the
thorax. From zero to 30° in the scapula rotated about its lower midportion;
from 60° onward, rotation took place about the glenoid area, resulting in a
medial and upward displacement of the glenoid face and a large lateral displacement of the inferior tip of the scapula. *Source:* Poppen NK, Walker PS.
1976. Normal and abnormal motion of the shoulder. J Bone Joint Surg
58A:195. With permission.

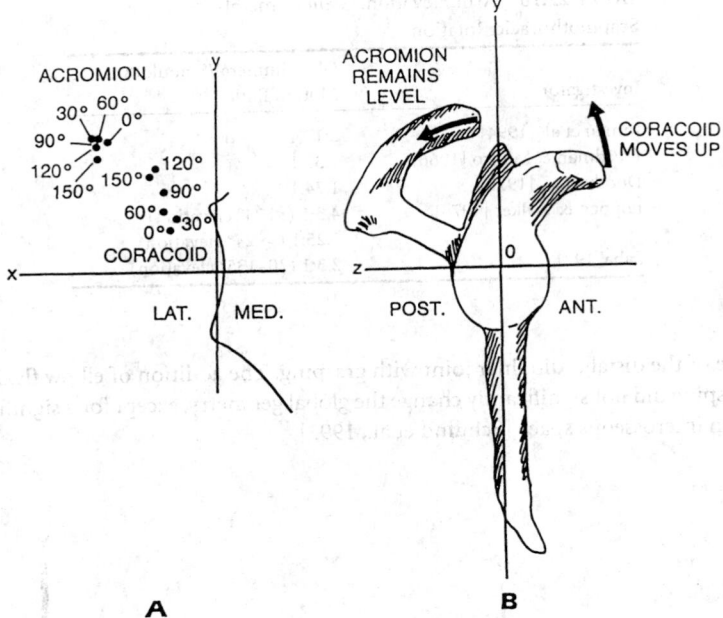

FIGURE 22.17 (A) A plot of the tips of the acromion and coracoid process on roentgenograms taken at successive intervals of arm elevation in the scapular plane shows upward movement of the coracoid and only a slight shift in the acromion relative to the glenoid face. This finding demonstrates twisting, or external rotation, of the scapula about the *x* axis.   (B) A lateral view of the scapula during this motion would show the coracoid process moving upward while the acromion remains on the same horizontal plane as the glenoid. *Source:* Poppen NK, Walker PS. 1976. Normal and abnormal motion of the shoulder. J Bone Joint Surg 58A:195. With permission.

Joint Contact

Studies of the normal biomechanics of the proximal wrist joint have determined that the scaphoid and lunate bones have separate, distinct areas of contact on the distal radius/triangular fibrocartilage complex surface [Viegas et al., 1987] so that the contact areas were localized and accounted for a relatively small fraction of the joint surface, regardless of wrist position (average of 20.6%). The contact areas shift from a more volar location to a more dorsal location as the wrist moves from flexion to extension. Overall, the scaphoid contact area is 1.47 times greater than that of the lunate. The scapho-lunate contact area ratio generally increases as the wrist position is changed from radial to ulnar deviation and/or from flexion to extension. Palmer and Werner [1984] also studied pressures in the proximal wrist joint and found that there are three distinct areas of contact: the ulno-lunate, radio-lunate, and radio-scaphoid. They determined that the peak articular pressure in the ulno-lunate fossa is 1.4 N/mm², in the radio-ulnate fossa is 3.0 N/mm², and in the radio-scaphoid fossa is 3.3 N/mm². Viegas et al. [1989] found a nonlinear relationship between increasing load and the joint con-

TABLE 22.11 Elbow Joint Geometry

Parameter	Size (mm)
Capitulum radius	10.6 ± 1.1
Lateral trochlear flange radius	10.8 ± 1.0
Central trochlear groove radius	8.8 ± 0.4
Medial trochlear groove radius	13.2 ± 1.4
Distal location of flexion/extension axis from transepicondylar line:	
Lateral	6.8 ± 0.2
Medial	8.7 ± 0.6

Source: Shiba R, Sorbie C, Siu DW, Bryant JT, Cooke TDV, Weavers HW. 1988. Geometry of the humeral-ulnar joint. J Orthop Res 6:897.

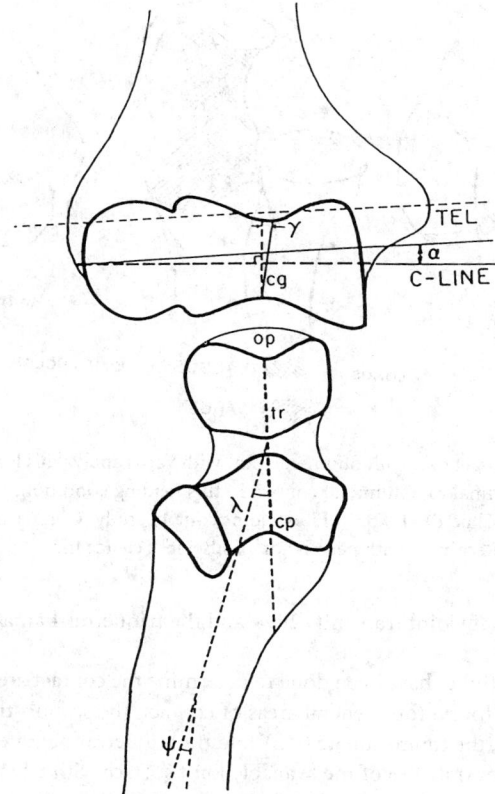

FIGURE 22.18 Components contributing to the carrying angles: $\alpha + \lambda + \psi$. Key: α, angle between C-line and TEL; γ, inclination of central groove (cg); λ, angle between trochlear notch (tn); ψ, reverse angulation of shaft of ulna; TLE, transepicondylar line; C-line, line joining centers of curvature of the trochlea and capitellum; cg, central groove; op, olecranon process; tr, trochlear ridge; cp, coronoid process. $\alpha = 2.5 \pm 0.0$; $\lambda = 17.5 \pm 5.0$ (females) and 12.0 ± 7.0 (males); $\psi = -6.5 \pm 0.7$ (females) and -9.5 ± 3.5 (males). *Source:* Shiba R, Sorbie C, Siu DW, Bryant JT, Cooke TDV, Weavers HW. 1988. Geometry of the humeral-ulnar joint. J Orthop Res 6:897. With permission.

tact area (Fig. 22.22). In general, the distribution of load between the scaphoid and lunate was consistent with all loads tested, with 60% of the total contact area involving the scaphoid and 40% involving the lunate. Loads greater than 46 lbs were found to not significantly increase the overall contact area. The overall contact area, even at the highest loads tested, was not more than 40% of the available joint surface.

Horii et al. [1990] calculated the total amount of force born by each joint with the intact wrist in the neutral position in the coronal plane and subjected to a total load of 143 N (Table 22.14). They found that 22% of the total force in the radio-ulno-carpal joint is dissipated through the ulna (14% through the ulno-lunate joint, and 18% through the ulno-triquetral joint) and 78% through the radius (46% through the scaphoid fossa and 32% through the lunate fossa). At the midcarpal joint, the scapho-trapezial joint transmits 31% of the total applied force, the scapho-capitate joint trans-

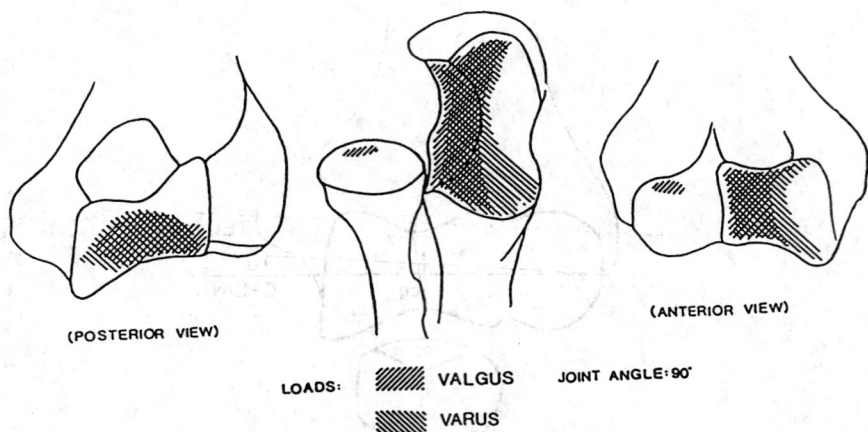

(POSTERIOR VIEW)   (ANTERIOR VIEW)

LOADS: ▨ VALGUS   JOINT ANGLE: 90°
        ▨ VARUS

FIGURE 22.19 Contact of the ulnohumeral joint with varus and valgus loads and the elbow at 90°. Notice only minimal radiohumeral contact in this loading condition. *Source:* Stormont TJ, An KN, Morrey BF, Chae EY. 1985. In Elbow joint contact study: Comparison of techniques. J Biomech 18(5):329. Reprinted with permission of Elsevier Science Inc.

mits 19%, the luno-capitate joint transmits 29%, and the triquetral-hamate joint transmits 21% of the load.

A limited amount of studies have been done to determine the contact areas in the midcarpal joint. Viegas et al. [1990] have found four general areas of contact: the scapho-trapezial-trapezoid (STT), the scapho-capitate (SC), the capito-lunate (CL), and the triquetral-hamate (TH). The high pressure contact area accounted for only 8% of the available joint surface with a load of 32 lbs and increased to a maximum of only 15% with a load of 118 lbs. The total contact area, expressed as a percentage of the total available joint area for each fossa was: STT = 1.3%, SC = 1.8%, CL = 3.1%, and TH = 1.8%.

Axes of Rotation

The complexity of joint motion at the wrist makes it difficult to calculate the instant center of motion. However, the trajectories of the hand during radioulnar deviation and flexion/extension, when they occur in a fixed plane, are circular, and the rotation in each plane takes place about a fixed axis. These axes are located within the head of the capitate and are not altered by the position of the hand in the plane of rotation [Youm et al., 1978]. During radioulnar deviation, the instant center of rotation lies at a point in the capitate situated distal to the proximal end of this bone by a distance equivalent to approximately one-quarter of its total length (Fig. 22.23). During flexion/extension, the instant center is close to the proximal cortex of the capitate, which is somewhat more proximal than the location for the instant center of radioulnar deviation.

TABLE 22.12 Elbow Joint Contact Area

Position	Total Articulating Surface Area of Ulna and Radial Head (mm²)	Contact Area (%)
Full extension	1598 ± 103	8.1 ± 2.7
90° flexion	1750 ± 123	10.8 ± 2.0
Full flexion	1594 ± 120	9.5 ± 2.1

Source: Goel VK, Singh D, Bijlani V. 1982. Contact areas in human elbow joints. J Biomech Eng 104:169.

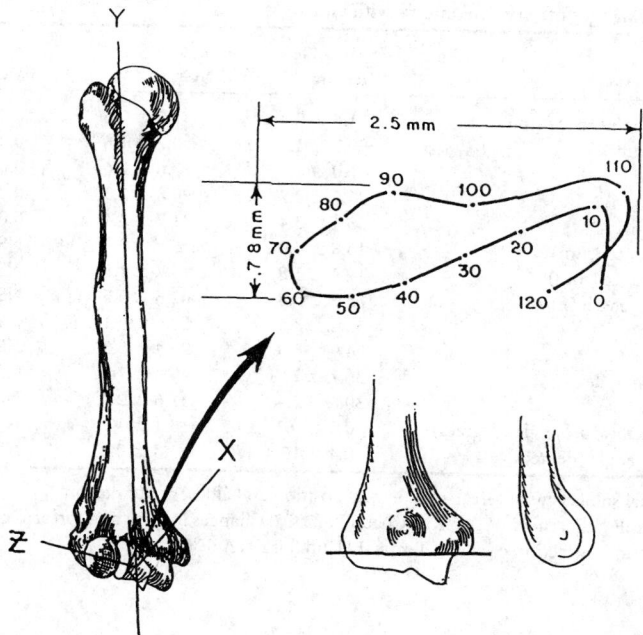

FIGURE 22.20 Very small locus of instant center of rotation for the elbow joint demonstrates that the axis may be replicated by a single line drawn from the inferior aspect of the medial epicondyle through the center of the lateral epicondyle, which is in the center of the lateral projected curvature of the trochlea and capitellum. *Source:* Modified from Morrey BF, Chao EYS. 1976. In Passive motion of the elbow joint: a biomechanical analysis. J Bone Joint Surg 58A(4):501. Reprinted with permission of the Journal of Bone and Joint Surgery.

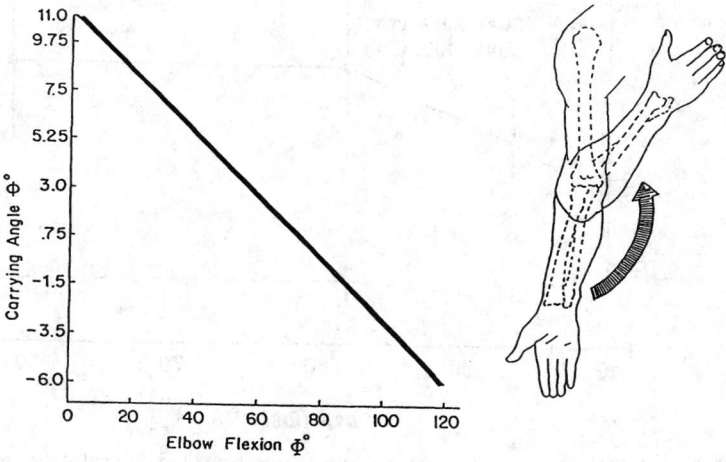

FIGURE 22.21 During elbow flexion and extension, a linear change in the carrying angle is demonstrated, typically going from valgus in extension to varus in flexion. *Source:* Morrey BF, Chao EYS. 1976. In Passive motion of the elbow joint: a biomechanical analysis. J Bone Joint Surg, 58A(4):501. Reprinted with permission of the Journal of Bone and Joint Surgery.

TABLE 22.13   Changes of Wrist Geometry with Grasp

	Resting	Grasp	Analysis of Variance (p = level)
Distal radioulnar joint space (mm)	1.6 ± 0.3	1.8 ± 0.6	0.06
Ulnar variance (mm)	−0.2 ± 1.6	0.7 ± 1.8	0.003
Lunate, uncovered length (mm)	6.0 ± 1.9	7.6 ± 2.6	0.0008
Capitate length (mm)	21.5 ± 2.2	20.8 ± 2.3	0.0002
Carpal height (mm)	33.4 ± 3.4	31.7 ± 3.4	0.0001
Carpal ulnar distance (mm)	15.8 ± 4.0	15.8 ± 3.0	NS
Carpal radial distance (mm)	19.4 ± 1.8	19.7 ± 1.8	NS
Third metacarpal length (mm)	63.8 ± 5.8	62.6 ± 5.5	NS
Carpal height ratio	52.4 ± 3.3	50.6 ± 4.1	0.02
Carpal ulnar ratio	24.9 ± 5.9	25.4 ± 5.3	NS
Lunate uncovering index	36.7 ± 12.1	45.3 ± 14.2	0.002
Carpal radial ratio	30.6 ± 2.4	31.6 ± 2.3	NS
Radius—third metacarpal angle (degrees)	−0.3 ± 9.2	−3.1 ± 12.8	NS
Radius—capitate angle (degrees)	0.4 ± 15.4	−3.8 ± 22.2	NS

Note: 15 normal subjects with forearm in neutral position and elbow at 90° flexion.
Source: Schuind FA, Linscheid RL, An KN, Chao EYS. 1992. Changes in wrist and forearm configuration with grasp and isometric contraction of elbow flexors. J Hand Surg 17A:698.

22.7 Hand

The hand is an extremely mobile organ that is capable of conforming to a large variety of object shapes and coordinating an infinite variety of movements in relation to each of its components. The mobility of this structure is possible through the unique arrangement of the bones in relation to one

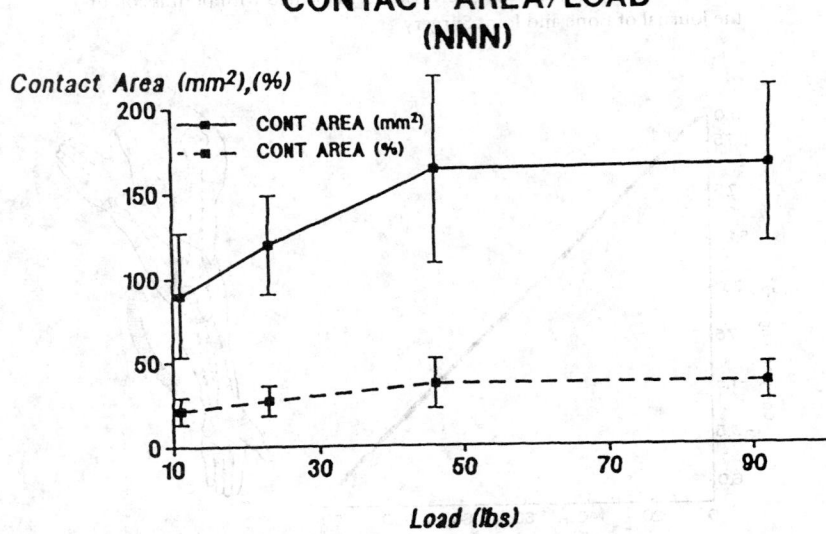

FIGURE 22.22   The nonlinear relation between the contact area and the load at the proximal wrist joint. The contact area was normalized as a percentage of the available joint surface. The load of 11, 23, 46, and 92 lbs. was applied at the position of neutral pronation/supination, neutral radioulnar deviation, and neutral flexion/extension. *Source:* Viegas SF, Patterson RM, Peterson PD, Roefs J, Tencer A, Choi S. 1989. The effects of various load paths and different loads on the load transfer characteristics of the wrist. J Hand Surg 14A(3):458. With permission.

TABLE 22.14 Force Transmission at the Intercarpal Joints

Joint	Force (N)
Radio-ulno-carpal	
Ulno-triquetral	12 ± 3
Ulno-lunate	23 ± 8
Radio-lunate	52 ± 8
Radio-scaphoid	74 ± 13
Midcarpal	
Triquetral-hamate	36 ± 6
Luno-capitate	51 ± 6
Scapho-capitate	32 ± 4
Scapho-trapezial	51 ± 8

Note: A total of 143 N axial force applied across the wrist.

Source: Horii E, Garcia-Elias M, An KN, Bishop AT, Cooney WP, Linscheid RL, Chao EY. 1990. Effect on force transmission across the carpus in procedures used to treat Kienböck's Disease. J Bone Joint Surg 15A(3):393.

another, the articular contours, and the actions of an intricate system of muscles.

Geometry of the Articulating Surfaces

Three-dimensional geometric models of the articular surfaces of the hand have been constructed. The sagittal contours of the metacarpal head and proximal phalanx grossly resemble the arc of a circle [Tamai et al., 1988]. The radius of curvature of a circle fitted to the entire proximal phalanx surface ranges from 11–13 mm, almost twice as much as that of the metacarpal head, which ranges from 6–7 mm (Table 22.15). The local centers of curvature along the sagittal contour of the metacarpal heads are not fixed. The locus of the center of curvature for the subchondral bony contour approximates the locus of the center for the acute curve of an ellipse (Fig. 22.24). However, the locus of center of curvature for the articular cartilage contour approximates the locus of the obtuse curve of an ellipse.

The surface geometry of the thumb carpometacarpal (CMC) joint has also been quantified [Athesian et al., 1992]. The surface area of the CMC joint is significantly greater for males than for females (Table 22.16). The minimum, maximum, and mean square curvature of these joints is reported in Table 22.16. The curvature of the surface is denoted by κ and the radius of curvature is $\rho = 1/\kappa$. The curvature is negative when the surface is concave and positive when the surface is convex.

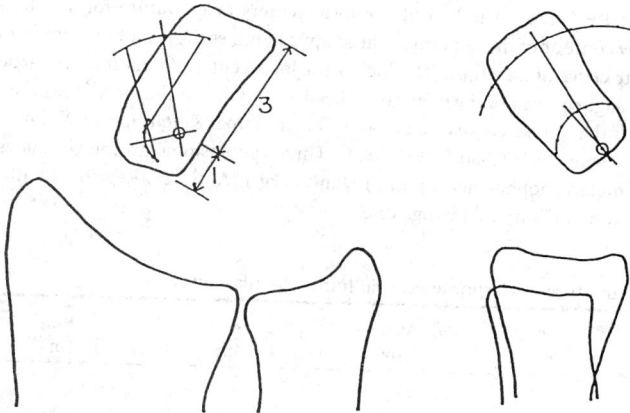

FIGURE 22.23 The location of the center of rotation during ulnar deviation (left) and extension (right), determined graphically using two metal markers embedded in the capitate. Note that during radial-ulnar deviation the center lies at a point in the capitate situated distal to the proximal end of this bone by a distance equivalent to approximately one-quarter of its total longitudinal length. During flexion-extension, the center of rotation is close to the proximal cortex of the capitate. *Source:* Youm Y, McMurty RY, Flatt AE, Gillespie TE. 1978. Kinematics of the wrist: an experimental study of radioulnar deviation and flexion/extension. J Bone Joint Surg 60A(4):423. With permission.

TABLE 22.15 Radius of Curvature of the Middle Sections of the Metacarpal Head and Proximal Phalanx Base

	Radius (mm)	
	Bony Contour	Cartilage Contour
MCH Index	6.42 ± 1.23	6.91 ± 1.03
Long	6.44 ± 1.08	6.66 ± 1.18
PPB Index	13.01 ± 4.09	12.07 ± 3.29
Long	11.46 ± 2.30	11.02 ± 2.48

Source: Tamai K, Ryu J, An KN, Linscheid RL, Cooney WP, Chao EYS. 1988. Three-dimensional geometric analysis of the metacarpophalangeal joint. J Hand Surg 13A(4):521.

Metacarpal Head

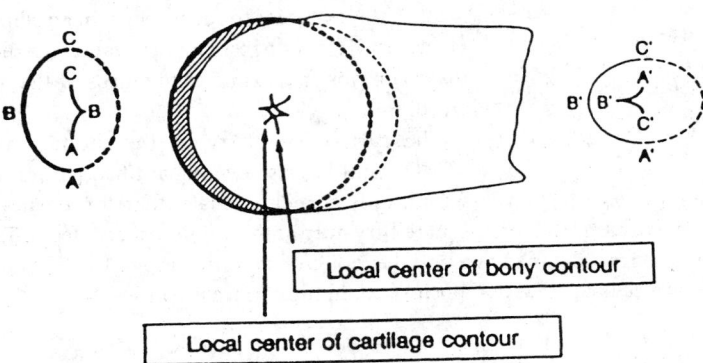

Local center of bony contour

Local center of cartilage contour

FIGURE 22.24 The loci of the local centers of curvature for subchondral bony contour of the metacarpal head approximates the loci of the center for the acute curve of an ellipse. The loci of the local center of curvature for articular cartilage contour of the metacarpal head approximates the loci of the bony center of the obtuse curve of an ellipse. *Source:* Tamai K, Ryu J, An KN, Linscheid RL, Cooney WP, Chao EYS. 1988. In Three-dimensional geometric analysis of the metacarpophalangeal joint. J Hand Surg 13A(4):521. Reprinted with permission of Churchill Livingstone.

TABLE 22.16 Curvature of Carpometacarpal Joint Articular Surfaces

	n	Area (cm²)	κ_{min} (m⁻¹)	κ_{max} (m⁻¹)	$\bar{\kappa}_{rms}$ (m⁻¹)
Trapezium					
Female	8	1.05 ± 0.21	−61 ± 22	190 ± 36	165 ± 32
Male	5	1.63 ± 0.18	−87 ± 17	114 ± 19	118 ± 6
Total	13	1.27 ± 0.35	−71 ± 24	161 ± 48	147 ± 34
Female versus male		$p \leq 0.01$	$p \leq 0.05$	$p \leq 0.01$	$p \leq 0.01$
Metacarpal					
Female	8	1.22 ± 0.36	−49 ± 10	175 ± 25	154 ± 20
Male	5	1.74 ± 0.21	−37 ± 11	131 ± 17	116 ± 8
Total	13	1.42 ± 0.40	−44 ± 12	158 ± 31	140 ± 25
Female versus male		$p \leq 0.01$	$p \leq 0.05$	$p \leq 0.01$	$p \leq 0.01$

Note: Radius of curvature: $\rho = 1/k$

Source: Athesian JA, Rosenwasser MP, Mow VC. 1992. Curvature characteristics and congruence of the thumb carpometacarpal joint: differences between female and male joints. J Biomech 25(6):591.

Joint Contact

The size and location of joint contact areas of the metacarpophalangeal (MCP) joint changes as a function of the joint flexion angle (Fig. 22.25). The radioulnar width of the contact area becomes narrow in the neutral position and expands in both the hyperextended and fully flexed positions [An & Cooney, 1991]. In the neutral position, the contact area occurs in the center of the phalangeal base, this area being slightly larger on the ulnar than on the radial side.

Axes of Rotation

Rolling and sliding actions of articulating surfaces exist during finger joint motion. The geometric shapes of the articular surfaces of the metacarpal head and proximal phalanx, as well as the inser-

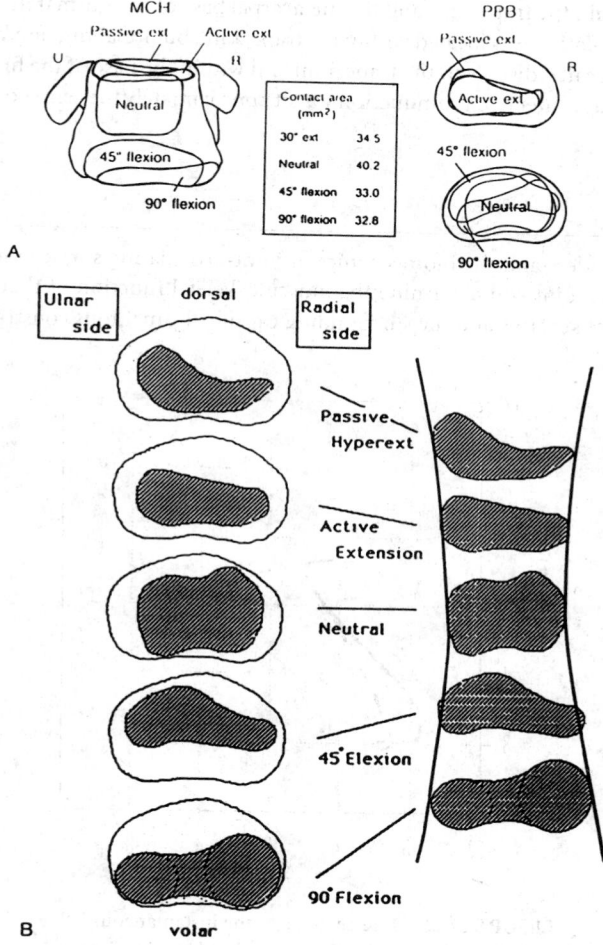

Contact area (mm²)	
30° ext	34 5
Neutral	40 2
45° flexion	33.0
90° flexion	32.8

FIGURE 22.25 (A) Contact area of the MCP joint in five joint positions. (B) End on view of the contact area on each of the proximal phalanx bases. The radioulnar width of the contact area becomes narrow in the neutral position and expands in both the hyperextended and fully flexed positions. *Source:* An KN, Cooney WP. 1991. Biomechanics, Section II. The hand and wrist. In BF Morrey (ed), Joint Replacement Arthroplasty, pp 137–146, New York, Churchill Livingstone, By permission of Mayo Foundation.

tion location of the collateral ligaments, significantly govern the articulating kinematics, and the center of rotation is not fixed but rather moves as a function of the angle of flexion [Pagowski & Piekarski, 1977]. The instant centers of rotation are within 3 mm of the center of the metacarpal head [Walker & Erhman, 1975]. Recently the axis of rotation of the MCP joint has been evaluated in vivo by Fioretti [1994]. The instantaneous helical axis of the MCP joint tends to be more palmar and tends to be displaced distally as flexion increases (Fig. 22.26).

The axes of rotation of the CMC joint have been described as being fixed [Hollister et al., 1992], but others believe that a polycentric center of rotation exists [Imaeda et al., 1994]. Hollister, et al. [1992] found the axes of the CMC joint are fixed and are not perpendicular to each other, or to the bones, and do not intersect. The flexion/extension axis is located in the trapezium, and the abduction/adduction axis is on the first metacarpal. In contrast, Imaeda et al. [1994] found that there was no single center of rotation, but rather the instantaneous motion occurred reciprocally between centers of rotations within the trapezium and the metacarpal base of the normal thumb. In flexion/extension, the axis of rotation was located within the trapezium, but for abduction/adduction the center of rotation was located distally to the trapezium and within the base of the first metacarpal. The average instantaneous center of circumduction was at approximately the center of the trapezial joint surface (Table 22.17).

22.8 Summary

It is important to understand the biomechanics of joint-articulating surface motion. The specific characteristics of the joint will determine the musculoskeletal function of that joint. The unique geometry of the joint surfaces and the surrounding capsule ligamentous constraints will guide the

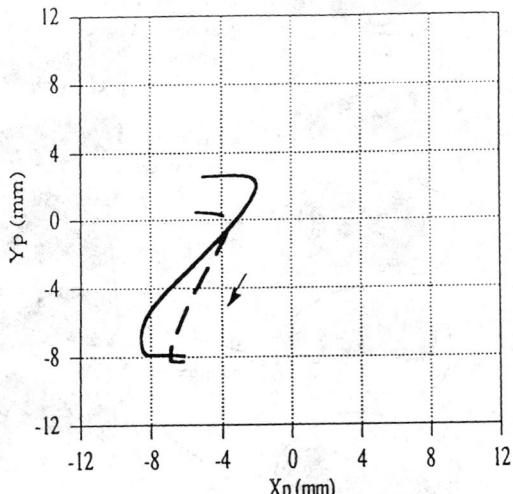

FIGURE 22.26 Intersections of the instantaneous helical angles with the metacarpal sagittal plane. They are relative to one subject tested twice in different days. The origin of the graph is coincident with the calibrated center of the metacarpal head. The arrow indicates the direction of flexion. *Source:* Fioretti S. 1994. Three-dimensional in-vivo kinematic analysis of finger movement. In F Schuind et al. (eds.), Advances in the Biomechanics of the Hand and Wrist, pp 363–375, New York, Plenum Press. With permission.

TABLE 22.17   Location of Center of Rotation
of Trapeziometacarpal Joint

	Mean ± SD (mm)
Circumduction	
X	0.1 ± 1.3
Y	−0.6 ± 1.3
Z	−0.5 ± 1.4
Flexion/Extension (in x–y plane)	
X	
Centroid	−4.2 ± 1.0
Radius	2.0 ± 0.5
Y	
Centroid	−0.4 ± 0.9
Radius	1.6 ± 0.5
Abduction/Adduction (in x–z plane)	
X	
Centroid	6.7 ± 1.7
Radius	4.6 ± 3.1
Z	
Centroid	−0.2 ± 0.7
Radius	1.7 ± 0.5

Note: The coordinate system is defined with the x axis
corresponding to internal/external rotation, the y axis corresponding to abduction/adduction, and the z axis corresponding to flexion/extension. The x axis is positive in the
distal direction, the y axis is positive in the dorsal direction
for the left hand and in the palmar direction for the right
hand, and the z axis is positive in the radial direction. The
origin of the coordinate system was at the intersection of a
line connecting the radial and ulnar prominences and a line
connecting the volar and dorsal tubercles.
Source: Imaeda T, Niebur G, Cooney WP, Linscheid RL,
An KN. 1994. Kinematics of the normal trapeziometacarpal
joint. J Orthop Res 12:197.

unique characteristics of the articulating surface motion. The range of joint motion, the stability of the joint, and the ultimate functional strength of the joint will depend on these specific characteristics. A congruent joint usually has a relatively limited range of motion but a high degree of stability, whereas a less congruent joint will have a relatively larger range of motion but less degree of stability. The characteristics of the joint-articulating surface will determine the pattern of joint contact and the axes of rotation. These characteristics will regulate the stresses on the joint surface which will influence the degree of degeneration of articular cartilage in an anatomic joint and the amount of wear of an artificial joint.

Acknowledgment

The authors thank Evelyn Grass for her careful preparation of the manuscript.

References

Allard P, Duhaime M, Labelle H, et al. 1987. Spatial reconstruction technique and kinematic mod-
eling of the ankle. IEEE Engr Med Biol 6:31.
An KN, Cooney WP. 1991. Biomechanics, Section II. The hand and wrist. In BF Morrey (ed), Joint
Replacement Arthroplasty, pp 137–146, New York, Churchill Livingstone.

Andriacchi TP, Stanwyck TS, Galante JO. 1986. Knee biomechanics in total knee replacement. J Arthroplasty 1(3):211.

Athesian JA, Rosenwasser MP, Mow VC. 1992. Curvature characteristics and congruence of the thumb carpometacarpal joint: differences between female and male joints. J Biomech 25(6): 591.

Barnett CH, Napier JR. 1952. The axis of rotation at the ankle joint in man. Its influence upon the form of the talus and the mobility of the fibula. J Anat 86:1.

Basmajian JV, Bazant FJ. 1959. Factors preventing downward dislocation of the adducted shoulder joint. An electromyographic and morphological study. J Bone Joint Surg 41A:1182.

D'Ambrosia RD, Shoji H, Van Meter J. 1976. Rotational axis of the ankle joint: Comparison of normal and pathological states. Surg Forum 27:507.

Davy DT, Kotzar DM, Brown RH, et al. 1989. Telemetric force measurements across the hip after total arthroplasty. J Bone Joint Surg 70A(1):45.

Doody SG, Freedman L, Waterland JC. 1970. Shoulder movements during abduction in the scapular plane. Arch Phys Med Rehabil 51:595.

Draganich LF, Andriacchi TP, Andersson GBJ. 1987. Interaction between intrinsic knee mechanics and the knee extensor mechanism. J Orthop Res 5:539.

Elftman H. 1945. The orientation of the joints of the lower extremity. Bull Hosp Joint Dis 6:139.

Engsberg JR. 1987. A biomechanical analysis of the talocalcaneal joint in vitro. J Biomech 20:429.

Fioretti S. 1994. Three-dimensional in-vivo kinematic analysis of finger movement. In F Schuind et al. (eds), Advances in the Biomechanics of the Hand and Wrist, pp 363–375, New York, Plenum.

Freedman L, Munro RR. 1966. Abduction of the arm in the scapular plane: scapular and glenohumeral movements. A roentgenographic study. J Bone Joint Surg 48A:1503.

Goel VK, Singh D, Bijlani V. 1982. Contact areas in human elbow joints. J Biomech Eng 104:169–175.

Hicks JH. 1953. The mechanics of the foot. The joints. J Anat 87:345–357.

Hollister A, Buford WL, Myers LM, et al. 1992. The axes of rotation of the thumb carpometacarpal joint. J Orthop Res 10:454.

Horii E, Garcia-Elias M, An KN, et al. 1990. Effect on force transmission across the carpus in procedures used to treat Kienböck's Disease. J Bone Joint Surg 15A(3):393.

Iannotti JP, Gabriel JP, Schneck SL, et al. 1992. The normal glenohumeral relationships: an anatomical study of 140 shoulders. J Bone Joint Surg 74A(4):491.

Imaeda T, Niebur G, Cooney WP, et al. 1994. Kinematics of the normal trapeziometacarpal joint. J Orthop Res 12:197.

Inman VT, Saunders JB deCM, Abbott LC. 1944. Observations on the function of the shoulder joint. J Bone Joint Surg 26A:1.

Inman VT. 1976. The Joints of the Ankle, Baltimore, Williams and Wilkins.

Inman VT, Mann RA. 1979. Biomechanics of the foot and ankle. In VT Inman (ed), DuVrie's Surgery of the Foot, St Louis, Mosby.

Iseki F, Tomatsu T. 1976. The biomechanics of the knee joint with special reference to the contact area. Keio J Med 25:37.

Isman RE, Inman VT. 1969. Anthropometric studies of the human foot and ankle. Pros Res 10–11:97.

Kapandji IA. 1987. The Physiology of the Joints, vol 2, Lower Limb, Edinburgh, Churchill-Livingstone, Edinburgh.

Kent BE. 1971. Functional anatomy of the shoulder complex. A review. Phys Ther 51:867.

Kimizuka M, Kurosawa H, Fukubayashi T. 1980. Load-bearing pattern of the ankle joint. Contact area and pressure distribution. Arch Orthop Trauma Surg 96:45–49.

Kinzel GL, Hall AL, Hillberry BM. 1972. Measurement of the total motion between two body segments: Part I. Analytic development. J Biomech 5:93.

Kirby KA. 1947. Methods for determination of positional variations in the subtalar and transverse tarsal joints. Anat Rec 80:397.

Kurosawa H, Walker PS, Abe S, et al. 1985. Geometry and motion of the knee for implant and orthotic design. J Biomech 18(7):487.

Lewis JL, Lew WD. 1978. A method for locating an optimal "fixed" axis of rotation for the human knee joint. J Biomech Eng 100:187.

Libotte M, Klein P, Colpaert H, et al. 1982. Contribution à l'étude biomécanique de la pince malléolaire. Rev Chir Orthop 68:299.

Macko VW, Matthews LS, Zwirkoski P, et al. 1991. The joint contact area of the ankle: the contribution of the posterior malleoli. J Bone Joint Surg 73A(3):347.

Manter JT. 1941. Movements of the subtalar and transverse tarsal joints. Anat Rec 80:397–402.

Maquet PG, Vandberg AJ, Simonet JC. 1975. Femorotibial weight bearing areas: Experimental determination. J Bone Joint Surg 57A(6):766–771.

Miyanaga Y, Fukubayashi T, Kurosawa H. 1984. Contact study of the hip joint: Load deformation pattern, contact area, and contact pressure. Arch Orth Trauma Surg, 103:13–17.

Morrey BF, An KN. 1990. Biomechanics of the Shoulder. In CA Rockwood and FA Matsen (eds), The Shoulder, pp 208–245, Philadelphia, Saunders.

Morrey BF, Chao EYS. 1976. Passive motion of the elbow joint: a biomechanical analysis. J Bone Joint Surg 58A(4):501.

Nahass BE, Madson MM, Walker PS. 1991. Motion of the knee after condylar resurfacing—an in vivo study. J Biomech 24(12):1107.

Paar O, Rieck B, Bernett P. 1983. Experimentelle untersuchungen über belastungsabhängige Druk- und Kontaktflächenverläufe an den Fussgelenken. Unfallheilkunde 85:531.

Pagowski S, Piekarski K. 1977. Biomechanics of metacarpophalangeal joint. J Biomech 10:205.

Palmer AK, Werner FW. 1984. Biomechanics of the distal radio-ulnar joint. Clin Orthop 187:26.

Parlasca R, Shoji H, D'Ambrosia RD. 1979. Effects of ligamentous injury on ankle and subtalar joints. A kinematic study. Clin Orthop 140:266.

Poppen NK, Walker PS. 1976. Normal and abnormal motion of the shoulder. J Bone Joint Surg 58A:195.

Ramsey PL, Hamilton W. 1976. Changes in tibiotalar area of contact caused by lateral talar shift. J Bone Joint Surg 58A:356.

Rastegar J, Miller N, Barmada R. 1980. An apparatus for measuring the load-displacement and load-dependent kinematic characteristics of articulating joints—application to the human ankle. J Biomech Eng 102:208.

Root ML, Weed JH, Sgarlato TE, Bluth DR. 1966. Axis of motion of the subtalar joint. J Am Podiatry Assoc 56:149.

Saha AK. 1971. Dynamic stability of the glenohumeral joint. Acta Orthop Scand 42:491.

Sammarco GJ, Burstein AH, Frankel VH. 1973. Biomechanics of the ankle: A kinematic study. Orthop Clin North Am, 4:75–96.

Sangeorzan BJ, Wagner UA, Karrington RM, et al. 1992. Contact characteristics of the subtalar joint: the effect of talar neck misalignment. J Orthop Res 10:544.

Schuind FA, Linscheid RL, An KN, et al. 1992. Changes in wrist and forearm configuration with grasp and isometric contraction of elbow flexors. J Hand Surg 17A:698.

Shephard E. 1951. Tarsal movements. J Bone Joint Surg 33B:258.

Shiba R, Sorbie C, Siu DW, et al. 1988. Geometry of the humeral-ulnar joint. J Orthop Res 6:897.

Singh AK, Starkweather KD, Hollister AM, et al. 1992. Kinematics of the ankle: A hinge axis model. Foot and Ankle 13(8):439.

Soslowsky LJ, Flatow EL, Bigliani LU, et al. 1992. Quantitation of in situ contact areas at the glenohumeral joint: A biomechanical study. J Orthop Res 10(4):524.

Spoor CW, Veldpaus FE. 1980. Rigid body motion calculated from spatial coordinates of markers. J Biomech 13:391.

Stormont TJ, An KA, Morrey BF, et al. 1985. Elbow joint contact study: comparison of techniques. J Biomech 18(5):329.

Tamai K, Ryu J, An KN, et al. 1988. Three-dimensional geometric analysis of the metacarpophalangeal joint. J Hand Surg 13A(4):521.

Tönnis D. 1987. Congenital Dysplasia and Dislocation of the Hip and Shoulder in Adults, pp 1–12, Berlin, Springer-Verlag.

Van Langelaan EJ. 1983. A kinematical analysis of the tarsal joints. An x-ray photogrammetric study. Acta Orthop Scand [Suppl] 204:211.

Viegas SF, Tencer AF, Cantrell J, et al. 1987. Load transfer characteristics of the wrist: Part I. The normal joint. J Hand Surg 12A(6):971.

Viegas SF, Patterson RM, Peterson PD, et al. 1989. The effects of various load paths and different loads on the load transfer characteristics of the wrist. J Hand Surg 14A(3):458.

Viegas SF, Patterson RM, Todd P, et al. October 7, 1990. Load transfer characteristics of the midcarpal joint. Presented at Wrist Biomechanics Symposium, Wrist Biomechanics Workshop, Mayo Clinic, Rochester, MN.

Von Lanz D, Wauchsmuth W. 1938. Das Hüftgelenk, Praktische Anatomie I Bd, pp 138–175, Teil 4: Bein und Statik, Berlin, Springer.

Wagner UA, Sangeorzan BJ, Harrington RM, et al. 1992. Contact characteristics of the subtalar joint: load distribution between the anterior and posterior facets. J Orthop Res 10:535.

Walker PS, Erhman MJ. 1975. Laboratory evaluation of a metaplastic type of metacarpophalangeal joint prosthesis. Clin Orthop 112:349.

Woltring HJ, Huiskes R, deLange A, Veldpaus FE. 1985. Finite centroid and helical axis estimation from noisy landmark measurements in the study of human joint kinematics. J Biomech 18:379.

Yoshioka Y, Siu D, Cooke TDV. 1987. The anatomy and functional axes of the femur. J Bone Joint Surg 69A(6):873.

Yoshioka Y, Siu D, Scudamore RA, et al. 1989. Tibial anatomy in functional axes. J Orthop Res 7:132.

Youm Y, McMurty RY, Flatt AE, et al. 1978. Kinematics of the wrist: an experimental study of radioulnar deviation and flexion/extension. J Bone Joint Surg 60A(4):423.

Zuckerman JD, Matsen FA: Biomechanics of the elbow. 1989. In M Nordine & VH Frankel (eds), Basic Biomechanics of the Musculoskeletal System, pp 249–260, Philadelphia, Lea & Febiger.

23

Joint Lubrication

Michael J. Furey
Department of Mechanical
Engineering, Virginia
Polytechnic Institute and
State University

The Fabric of the Joints in the Human Body is a subject so much the more entertaining, as it must strike every one that considers it attentively with an Idea of fine Mechanical Composition. Where-ever the Motion of one Bone upon another is requisite, there we find an excellent Apparatus for rendering that Motion safe and free: We see, for Instance, the Extremity of one Bone moulded into an orbicular Cavity, to receive the Head of another, in order to afford it an extensive Play. Both are covered with a smooth elastic Crust, to prevent mutual Abrasion; connected with strong Ligaments, to prevent Dislocation; and inclosed in a Bag that contains a proper Fluid Deposited there, for lubricating the Two contiguous Surfaces. So much in general.

The above is the opening paragraph of the classic paper by Sir William Hunter, surgeon, "Of the Structure and Diseases of Articulating Cartilages," which he read to a meeting of the Royal Society, June 2, 1743 [1]. Since then, a great deal of research has been carried out on the subject of synovial joint lubrication. However, the mechanisms involved are still unknown.

The purpose of this chapter is twofold, i.e., to introduce the reader to the subject of *tribology*—the study of friction, wear, and lubrication—and to extend this to the topic of *biotribology*, which includes the lubrication of natural synovial joints. This is not meant to be an exhaustive review of joint lubrication theories; space does not permit this. Instead, major concepts or principles will be discussed in light not only of what is known about synovial joint lubrication but, perhaps more important, in light of what is not known. Several references are given for those who wish to learn more about the topic. It is clear that synovial joints are by far the most complex and sophisticated tribological systems that exist. We shall see that although numerous theories have been put forth to attempt to explain joint lubrication, the mechanisms involved are still far from being understood. And when one begins to examine possible connections between tribology and degenerative joint disease or osteoarthritis, the picture is even more complex and controversial. Finally, this chapter does not treat the tribological behavior of artificial joints, partial joint replacements, or the possible use of elastic or poroplastic materials as artificial cartilage. That is a separate topic which would require detailed discussion and additional space.

23.1 Tribology

The word *tribology*, derived from the Greek τριβω "to rub," covers all frictional processes between solid bodies moving relative to one another in contact [2]. Thus tribology may be defined as the study of friction, wear, and lubrication.

Tribological processes are involved whenever one solid slides or rolls against another, as in bearings, cams, gears, piston rings and cylinders, machining and metalworking, grinding, rock drilling, sliding electrical contacts, frictional welding, brakes, the striking of a match, music from a cello, and articulation of human synovial joints (e.g., hip joints), machinery, and in numerous less obvious processes (e.g., walking, holding, stopping, writing and the use of fasteners such as nails, screws, and bolts).

Discovery and application of tribological principles can result in major advances in many areas, such as new alloys and materials, mechanical design, safety and reliability, energy, transportation, new products and manufacturing processes, advanced lubricants and biomedical systems. However, in spite of the importance of tribology, most engineers and scientists know little of this field. It is a multidisciplinary subject involving at least the areas of materials science, solid and surface mechanics, surface science and chemistry, rheology, engineering, mathematics, and even biology and biochemistry.

Although the word *tribology* is relatively new, interest in the phenomena of friction, wear, and lubrication is ancient. Unlike thermodynamics, there are no generally accepted "laws" in tribology. Tribology is an emerging science; thus, rather than seeking formulae or handbook data, it is important to learn how to approach the problems. It is perhaps as dangerous to find an equation which does not apply to a particular tribological problem and to believe the answers than to be entirely ignorant of developments in the field. This is important to understand in any study of lubrication and wear and even more so in a study of biotribology or biological lubrication phenomena.

Friction

Much of the early work in tribology was in the area of friction—possibly because frictional effects are more readily demonstrated and measured. In general, early theories of friction dealt with dry or unlubricated systems. The problem was often treated strictly from a mechanical viewpoint, with little or no regard for the environment, surface films, or chemistry.

In the first place, *friction may be defined as the tangential resistance which is offered to the sliding of one solid body over another.* Friction is the result of many factors and cannot be treated as something as singular as density or even viscosity. Unfortunately, there have been many attempts to explain friction between solid bodies on an all-or-nothing basis in which the resistance to motion is due solely or chiefly to one particular mechanism. Postulated sources of friction have included (1) the lifting of one asperity over another (increase in potential energy), (2) the interlocking of asperities followed by shear, (3) interlocking followed by plastic deformation or plowing, (4) adhesion followed by shear, (5) elastic hysteresis and waves of deformation, (6) adhesion or interlocking followed by tensile failure, (7) intermolecular attraction, (8) electrostatic effects, and (9) viscous drag.

Wear and Surface Damage

One definition of wear in a tribological sense is that it is the *progressive loss of substance from the operating surface of a body as a result of relative motion at the surface.* In comparison with friction, very little theoretical work has been done on the extremely important area of wear and surface damage. This is not too surprising in view of the complexity of wear and how little is known of the mechanisms by which it can occur. Variations in wear can be, and often are, enormous compared with variations in friction. For example, practically all the coefficients of sliding friction for diverse dry or lubricated systems fall within a relatively narrow range of 0.1–1. In some cases (e.g., certain regimes of hydrodynamic or "boundary" lubrication), the coefficient of friction may be <0.1 and as low as 0.01 or even 0.001. In other cases (e.g., very clean unlubricated metals in vacuum), friction coefficients may exceed 1. Reduction of friction by a factor of 2 through changes in design, materials, or lubricant would be a reasonable, although not always attainable, goal. However, it is not uncommon for wear rates to vary by a factor of a hundred, thousand, or even more.

For systems consisting of common materials (e.g., metals, polymers, ceramics), there are at least four main mechanisms by which wear and surface damage can occur between solids in relative motion: (1) abrasive wear, (2) adhesive wear, (3) fatigue wear, and (4) chemical or corrosive wear. For complex biological materials such as articular cartilage, it is likely that other mechanisms are involved.

Abrasive Wear

This is the type of wear which occurs when a hard solid, particle, or asperity rubs against a softer surface. Examples of abrasive wear include the smoothing of wood by sandpaper, the action of emery paper in polishing metals, grinding processes, and harmful effects of hard particles (e.g., sand, dirt, carbide or silica inclusions, oxides and work-hardened wear debris) in lubricated systems. Abrasive wear is a form of microcutting, involving a hard particle or shape which indents, grooves, and then cuts material out of the surface.

Adhesive Wear

This occurs when solids in contact adhere and the junction is stronger than one of the solids; wear arises from a shearing process. The basic idea is that there is an intermolecular attraction between solids. When two solids are placed together in contact under a load, the attraction or adhesion at the small regions of contact can be considerable. If the junction is weaker than either solid, shear will occur in the interface itself during sliding. However, if the junction is stronger than one of the solids, shearing will take place not at the interface but at some distance within the weaker material. The generally heavy surface damage and wear observed when similar materials slide together is the main reason for avoiding such combinations in sliding systems. According to the adhesion concept of wear, dissimilarity should be sought in choosing pairs of solids which will be in tribological contact. Thus, chrome alloy steel against polyethylene, as in an artificial hip joint, will function reasonably well whereas stainless steel on stainless steel would be a tribological disaster.

Fatigue Wear

This is the removal of particles detached by fatigue arising from cyclic stress variations in a tribological process. It is sometimes referred to as *surface fatigue* but involves subsurface layers as well. The number of loading cycles required to produce failure depends on the stress level. At high cyclical stress levels, fatigue failures occur more quickly. If the interaction of asperities during the sliding of one surface over another is considered, possible fatigue mechanisms leading to the failure of the asperities can be recognized. These mechanisms may involve momentary interlocking, adhesion, and elastic deformation of asperities, resulting eventually in removal of material to produce wear debris. Fatigue failure, which is initiated where the stress is highest, therefore often occurs below the surface. Cracks are produced by fatigue, and these lead to the removal of relatively large pieces of material.

Chemical or Corrosive Wear

This is a wear process in which chemical or electrochemical reactions with the environment predominate. For example, a chemical reaction between the rubbing solid and the environment (e.g., oxygen, water, acids from fuel combustion, chemical additives) can occur, followed by removal of corrosion products by tribological action. One example of corrosive wear is the wear observed between the piston rings and cylinders in internal combustion engines—particularly in low-temperature, cyclic, or stop-and-go operation. However, the presence of metal reaction products (e.g., iron oxides, chlorides, sulfates) does not necessarily prove that the process is one of corrosive wear; the particles could have been removed by mechanical action and then subsequently transformed chemically. In some cases, the formation of thicker surface films of oxides (e.g., iron oxides) may serve to reduce adhesive wear. The concept of oxidational wear—in which the high surface temperatures produced by friction in sliding steel systems lead to increased rates of iron oxide formation and removal—has also been proposed.

Fretting and Fretting Corrosion

There is another, more complex, form of wear which involves physical as well as chemical processes, i.e., fretting corrosion. *Fretting* is defined as wear occurring between two surfaces having oscillatory relative motion of small amplitude (e.g., from a few to a hundred μm). Fretting corrosion is defined as the type of fretting damage which occurs when the debris produced is a chemical reaction product between constituents of the surface and the environment; the reaction product may or may not be abrasive. Although various mechanisms have been proposed, fretting corrosion is not well understood. Fretting phenomena have been observed in human joints involving metallic pins, screws, or inserts.

23.2 Lubrication

Lubrication is a process of reducing friction and/or wear (or other forms of surface damage) between relatively moving surfaces by the application of a solid, liquid, or gaseous substance (i.e., a lubricant). Since friction and wear do not necessarily correlate with each other, the use of the word *and* in place of *and/or* in the above definition is a common mistake. A lubricant therefore is any substance which is used to reduce friction or wear or both between moving surfaces in contact. That is the primary function of a lubricant.

Examples of lubricants are wide and varied. They include automotive engine oils, wheel bearing greases, transmission fluids, electrical contact lubricants, rolling oils, cutting fluids, preservative oils, gear oils, jet fuels, instrument oils, turbine oils, textile lubricants, machine oils, jet engine lubricants, air, water, molten glass, liquid metals, oxide films, talcum powder, graphite, molybdenum disulfide, waxes, soaps, polymers, and the synovial fluid in human joints.

A few general principles of lubrication may be mentioned here:

1. The lubricant must be present at the place where it can function.
2. Almost any substance under carefully selected or special conditions can be shown to reduce friction or wear, but these substances are not necessarily lubricants.
3. Friction and wear do not necessarily go together. This is an extremely important principle which applies to nonlubricated (dry) as well as lubricated systems. It is particularly true under conditions of "boundary lubrication" to be discussed later. An additive may reduce friction and increase wear, reduce wear and increase friction, reduce both, or increase both. Although the reasons are not fully understood, this is an experimental observation. Thus, friction and wear should be thought of as separate phenomena—an important point when we discuss theories of synovial joint lubrication.
4. The effective or active lubricating film in a particular system may or may not consist of the original or bulk lubricant phase.

In a broad sense, the main function of a lubricant is to keep the surfaces apart so that interaction (e.g., adhesion, plowing, shear) between the solids cannot occur; thus friction and wear can be reduced or controlled.

In externally pressurized bearings, the two loaded solids are separated by a fluid film supplied to the interface from an external high-pressure source. The fluid may be a liquid or a gas. Such bearings, systems, or modes of lubrication are often called *hydrostatic* (for liquids, including oil as well as water) and *aerostatic* (for gases, including air). In these bearings, there is no required relative movement parallel or perpendicular to the surface (there may be movement in practice, but it is not an essential factor in the mode of operation).

The following regimes or types of lubrication may be considered in the order of increasing severity or decreasing lubricant film thickness (Fig. 23.1):

1. Hydrodynamic lubrication
2. Elastohydrodynamic lubrication
3. Transition from hydrodynamic and elastohydrodynamic lubrication to boundary lubrication
4. Boundary lubrication

A fifth regime—sometimes referred to as *dry* or *unlubricated*—may also be considered as an extreme or limit.

Hydrodynamic Lubrication Theories

In hydrodynamic lubrication, the load is supported by the pressure developed due to relative motion and the geometry of the system. In the regime of hydrodynamic or fluid film lubrication, there is no contact between the solids. The film thickness is governed by the bulk physical properties of the lubricants, the most important being viscosity; friction arises purely from shearing of viscous lubricant.

Contributions to our knowledge of hydrodynamic lubrication, with special focus on journal bearings, have been made by numerous investigators including Reynolds. The classic Reynolds treatment considered the equilibrium of a fluid element and the pressure and shear forces on this element. In this treatment, eight assumptions were made (e.g., surface curvature is large compared to lubricant film thickness, fluid is Newtonian, flow is laminar, viscosity is constant through film thickness). Velocity distributions due to relative motion and pressure buildup were developed and added together. The solution of the basic Reynolds equation for a particular bearing configuration results in a pressure distribution throughout the film as a function of viscosity, film shape and velocity.

The total load W and frictional (viscous) drag F can be calculated from this information. For rotating disks with parallel axes, the "simple" Reynolds equation yields

$$\frac{h_o}{R} = 4.9 \left[\frac{\eta U}{W} \right] \tag{23.1}$$

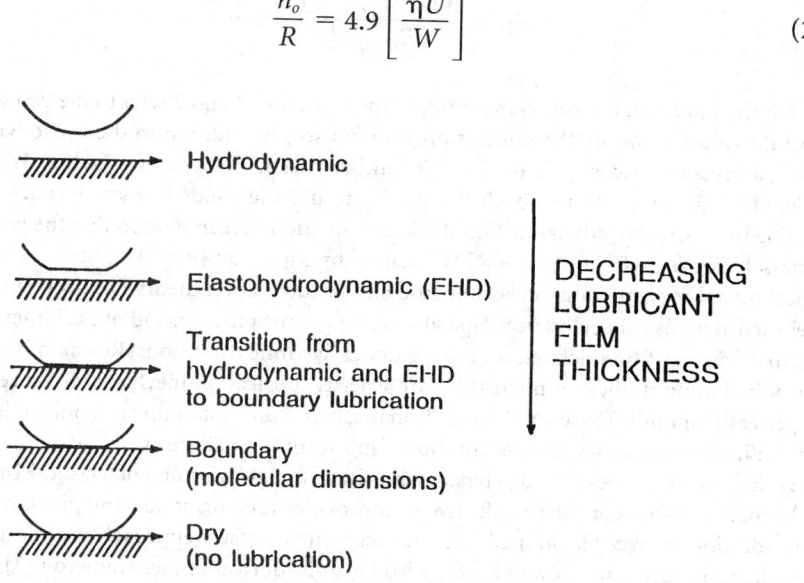

FIGURE 23.1 Regimes of lubrication.

where h_o is the minimum lubricant film thickness, η the absolute viscosity, U the average velocity $(U_1 + U_2)/2$, W the applied normal load per unit width of disk, and R the reduced radius of curvature $(1/R = 1/R_1 + 1/R_2)$.

The dimensionless term $(\eta U/W)$ is sometimes referred to as the hydrodynamic factor. It can be seen that doubling either the viscosity or velocity doubles the film thickness and that doubling the applied load halves the film thickness. This regime of lubrication is sometimes referred to as the *rigid isoviscous* or *classical Martin condition*, since the solid bodies are assumed to be perfectly rigid (nondeformable) and the fluid is assumed to have a constant viscosity.

At high loads with systems such as gears, ball bearings, and other high-contact-stress geometries, two additional factors have been considered in further developments of the hydrodynamic theory of lubrication. One of these is that the surfaces deform elastically; this leads to a localized change in geometry more favorable to lubrication. The second is that the lubricant becomes more viscous under the high pressure existing in the contact zone, according to relationships such as

$$\eta/\eta_o = \exp \alpha \, (p - p_o) \tag{23.2}$$

where η is the viscosity at pressure p, η_o the viscosity at atmospheric pressure p_o, and α the pressure-viscosity coefficient (e.g., in Pa^{-1}). In this concept, the lubricant pressures existing in the contact zone approximate those of dry contact Hertzian stress. This is the regime of elastohydrodynamic lubrication, sometimes abbreviated as EHL or EHD. It may also be described as the elastic-viscous type or mode of lubrication, since elastic deformation exists and the fluid viscosity is considerably greater due to the pressure effect.

The comparable Dowson-Higginson expression for minimum film thickness between cylinders or disks in contact with parallel axes is

$$\frac{h_o}{R} = 2.6 \left[\frac{\eta U}{W} \right]^{0.7} \left[\frac{\alpha W}{R} \right]^{0.54} \left[\frac{W}{RE'} \right]^{0.03} \tag{23.3}$$

The term E' represents the reduced modulus of elasticity:

$$\frac{1}{E'} = \frac{(1 - v_1^2)}{E_1} + \frac{(1 - v_2^2)}{E_2} \tag{23.4}$$

where E is the modulus, v is Poisson's ratio, and the subscripts 1 and 2 refer to the two solids in contact. All the other terms are the same as previously used. In addition to the hydrodynamic factor $(\eta U/W)$, a pressure-viscosity factor $(\alpha W/R)$ and an elastic deformation factor (W/RE') can be considered. Thus, properties of both the lubricant and the solids as materials are included. In examining the elastohydrodynamic film thickness equations, it can be seen that the velocity U is an important factor $(h_o \propto U^{0.7})$ but the load W is rather unimportant $(h_o \propto W^{-0.13})$.

Experimental confirmation of elastohydrodynamic lubrication theory has been obtained in certain selected systems using electrical capacitance, x-ray transmission, and optical interference techniques to determine film thickness and shape under dynamic conditions. Research is continuing in this area, including studies on micro-EHL or asperity lubrication mechanisms, since surfaces are never perfectly smooth. These studies may lead to a better understanding not only of lubricant film formation in high-contact-stress systems but of lubricant film failure as well.

Two other possible types of hydrodynamic lubrication, rigid-viscous and elastic-isoviscous, complete the matrix of four considering the two factors of elastic deformation and pressure-viscosity effects. In addition, *squeeze film* lubrication can occur when surfaces approach one another. For more information on hydrodynamic and elastohydrodynamic lubrication, see Cameron [3] and Dowson and Higginson [4].

Transition from Hydrodynamic to Boundary Lubrication

In spite of the fact that prevention of contact is probably the most important function of a lubricant, there is still much to be learned about the transition from hydrodynamic and elastohydrodynamic lubrication to boundary lubrication. This is the region in which lubrication goes from the desirable hydrodynamic condition of no contact to the less acceptable "boundary" condition, where increased contact usually leads to higher friction and wear. This regime is sometimes referred to as a condition of *mixed lubrication.*

Several examples of experimental approaches to thin-film lubrication have been reported. It is important in examining these techniques to make the distinction between methods which are used to determine lubricant film thickness under hydrodynamic or elastohydrodynamic conditions (e.g., optical interference, electrical capacitance, x-ray transmission) and methods which are used to determine the occurrence or frequency of contact.

Boundary Lubrication

Although there is no generally accepted definition of boundary lubrication, it is often described as a condition of lubrication in which the friction and wear between two surfaces in relative motion are determined by the surface properties.of the solids and the chemical nature of the lubricant rather than its viscosity. An example of the difficulty in defining boundary lubrication can be seen if the term *bulk viscosity* is used in place of viscosity in the preceding sentence—another frequent form. This opens the door to the inclusion of elastohydrodynamic effects which depend in part on the influence of pressure on viscosity. Increased friction under these circumstances could be attributed to increased viscous drag rather than solid-solid contact. According to another common definition, boundary lubrication occurs or exists when the surfaces of the bearing solids are separated by films of molecular thickness. That may be true, but it ignores the possibility that "boundary" layer surface films may indeed be very thick (i.e., 10, 20, or 100 molecular layers). The difficulty is that boundary lubrication is complex.

Although a considerable amount of research has been done on this topic, an understanding of the basic mechanisms and processes involved is by no means complete. Therefore, definitions of boundary lubrication tend to be nonoperational. This is an extremely important regime of lubrication because it involves more extensive solid-solid contact and interaction as well as generally greater friction, wear, and surface damage. In many practical systems, the occurrence of the boundary lubrication regime is unavoidable or at least quite common. The condition can be brought about by high loads, low relative sliding speeds (including zero for stop-and-go or reciprocating elements), and low lubricant viscosity—factors which are important in the transition from hydrodynamic to boundary lubrication.

The most important factor in boundary lubrication is the chemistry of the tribological system—the contacting solids and total environment including lubricants. More particularly, the surface chemistry and interactions occurring with and on the solid surfaces are important. This includes factors such as physisorption, chemisorption, intermolecular forces, surface chemical reactions, and the nature, structure, and properties of thin films on solid surfaces. It also includes many other effects brought on by the process of moving one solid over another, such as changes in topography and the area of contact, high surface temperatures, the generation of fresh reactive metal surfaces by the removal of oxide and other layers, catalysis, and electrical effects such as the emission of electrons and generation of electrical charges.

In examining the action of boundary lubricant compounds in reducing friction or wear or both between solids in sliding contact, it may be helpful to consider at least the following five modes of film formation on or protection of surfaces:

1. Physisorption
2. Chemisorption

3. Chemical reactions *with* the solid surface
4. Chemical reactions *on* the solid surface
5. Mere interposition of a solid or other material

Physisorption, or physical adsorption, is due to the operation of forces between the solid surface and the adsorbate molecules that are similar to the van der Waals forces between molecules. Physical adsorption is generally quite reversible, and the adsorption energies are low. There is also good evidence that physisorption can lead to adsorbed layers several molecules thick.

In contrast to physisorption, chemisorption is the result of much stronger binding forces, comparable with those leading to the formation of chemical compounds. The adsorption may be regarded as the formation of a kind of surface compound, with much higher energies of adsorption. Chemisorption is completed when a surface is covered by an adsorbed monolayer, and is seldom reversible.

Chemical reactions *with* surfaces (mode 3) is perhaps the one most commonly thought of in boundary lubrication and in mechanisms by which lubricant additives reduce friction or wear. One example is the concept of metal soap formation by fatty acids. Other examples include the formation of iron sulfides from sulfur-containing EP (extreme pressure) additives and the formation of iron chlorides from chlorine-containing additives. The important point to note is that the solid substrate in all the processes just described is a chemical part of the surface film; thus, removal of this film by wear, hydrolysis, or other processes means removal of the substrate.

The use of chemical reactions (mode 4) *on* the solid surface (not *with* the surface) to produce effective boundary lubrication—is rarely, if ever, considered in the literature on tribology. The distinction between this mode and chemical reactions with the solid surface is important, even though each involves a chemical reaction at the surfaces in contact. In film formation, the film is formed by a deposition process and may involve reactions such as decomposition or degradation, oxidation and polymerization. Physical adsorption may play a part in getting the molecules to the surface before reaction and in bonding the resulting products to the surface, but there is no chemical reaction with the solid surface. Thus, removal of such films by wear does not mean removal of the substrate.

The last mode of boundary lubrication discussed here, interposition of a solid or other material, involves the physical interposition of finely divided solids (e.g., graphite, molybdenum disulfide, polymers) dispersed in a carrier fluid such as a hydrocarbon. The dispersed solids can reduce the extent of interaction by generating sufficient film strength to prevent contact. Although adsorption on the rubbing solids could occur, it is not part of this mode of film formation. Rather, this is a mechanical, statistical concept which involves the probability of a solid particle being present where and when metallic contact occurs. Thus the concentrations required are generally much higher than those associated with soluble antiwear additives which react chemically at the regions of contact to form surface films (modes 3 and 4).

Solid materials such as graphite and molybdenum disulfide represent an important class of lubricants offering advantages for special applications, for example, under conditions of high vacuum, very low and very high temperatures, and unusual chemical environments. One common method of applying solid lubricants—bypassing the statistical dispersion problem discussed above—is to form in advance a solid, adherent, and often thick film on the surface using a variety of techniques (e.g., plasma spraying, applying solid lubricant and binder in a solvent, baking). Thus, contact is prevented. However, a serious disadvantage of this method is that the films wear off and are not replenished as in modes 3 and 4. The *in situ* surface polymerization concept proposed by the present author—the reduction of wear by the use of particular compounds capable of forming protective polymeric films directly on rubbing surfaces—is an example of a film-forming process which fits mode 4.

The beneficial effects that can be achieved by even minor concentrations of the proper antiwear or antifriction additive are often enormous in comparison with hydrodynamic and elastohydrodynamic effects. Thus, the surface and chemical properties of the solid materials used in tribological applications become especially important. One might expect that this would also be the case in biologic (e.g., human joint) lubrication.

23.3 Final Comments on Tribological Processes

It is important to recognize that friction and wear depend upon materials, design, operating conditions, and total environment (Fig. 23.2).

It is also pointed out that there are several examples of rather common myths, mistakes, and pitfalls in using laboratory tests to evaluate tribological systems (e.g., materials, surface films, lubricants). In the case of biologic systems such as synovial joints, the use of laboratory *in vitro* tests to study the tribological behavior of natural and artificial joints present considerable difficulties.

Last, but not least, it is emphasized once again that friction and wear are different phenomena. Low friction does not necessarily mean low wear. We will see examples of this common error in the discussion of joint lubrication research.

23.4 Synovial Joints

Examples of natural synovial or movable joints include the human hip, knee, elbow, ankle, finger, and shoulder. A simplified representation of a synovial joint is shown in Fig. 23.3. The bones are covered by a thin layer of articular cartilage bathed in synovial fluid confined by a synovial membrane. Synovial joints are truly remarkable systems—providing the basis of movement by allowing bones to articulate on one another with minimal friction and wear. Unfortunately, various joint diseases occur even among the young, causing pain, loss of freedom of movement, or instability.

Synovial joints are complex, sophisticated systems not yet fully understood. The loads are surprisingly high and the relative motion is complex. Articular cartilage has the deceptive appearance of simplicity and uniformity. But it is an extremely complex material with unusual properties. Basically, it consists of water (ca. 75%) enmeshed in a network of collagen fibers and high molecu-

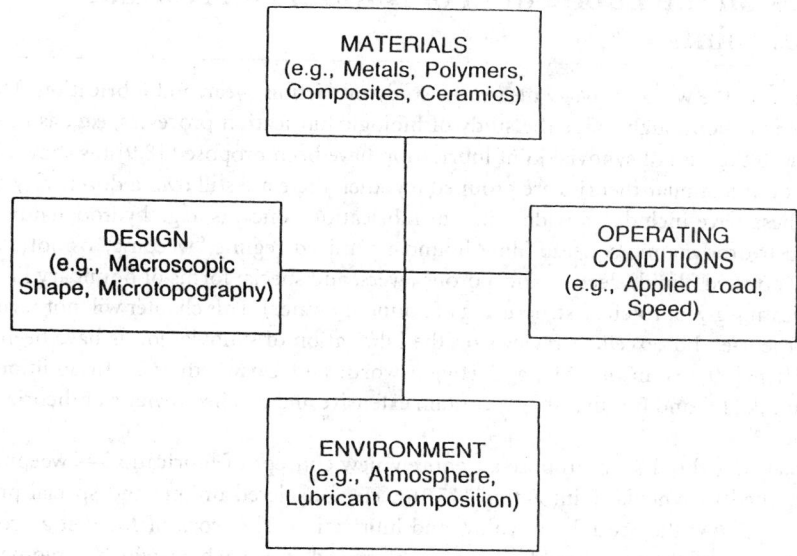

FIGURE 23.2 In any tribological system, friction, wear, and surface damage depend upon four interrelated factors.

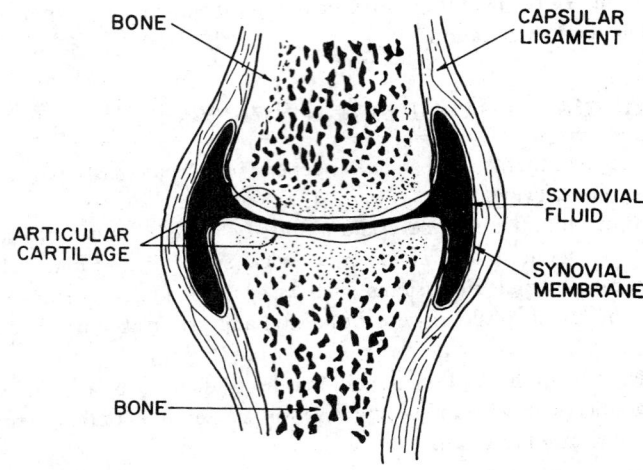

FIGURE 23.3   Representation of a synovial joint [9].

lar weight proteoglycans. In a way, cartilage could be considered as one of nature's composite materials. Articular cartilage also has no blood supply, no nerves, and very few cells (chondrocytes).

The other major component of an articular joint is *synovial fluid*, named by Paracelsus after "synovia" (egg white). It is essentially a dialysate of blood plasma with added hyaluronic acid. Synovial fluid contains complex proteins, polysaccharides, and other compounds. Its chief constituent is water (ca. 85%). Synovial fluid functions as a joint lubricant, nutrient for cartilage, and carrier for waste products.

For more information on the biochemistry, structure, and properties of articular cartilage, Freeman [5], Sokoloff [6], and Stockwell [7] are suggested.

23.5   Theories on the Lubrication of Natural and Normal Synovial Joints

As we have seen, the word *tribology* means the study of friction, wear, and lubrication. Therefore, *biotribology* may be thought of as the study of biologic lubrication processes, e.g., as in synovial joints. Over 30 theories of synovial joint lubrication have been proposed [8,9] (as shown in Table 23.1)! And even if similar theories are grouped together, there are still over a dozen very different theories. These have included a wide range of lubrication concepts, e.g., hydrodynamic, hydrostatic, elasto-hydrodynamic, squeeze-film, "boundary," mixed-regime, "weeping," osmotic, synovial mucin gel, "boosted," lipid, electrostatic, porous layers, and special forms of boundary lubrication (e.g., "lubricating glycoproteins," structuring of boundary water). This chapter will not review these numerous theories, but excellent reviews on the lubrication of synovial joints have been written by McCutchen [10], Swanson [11], and Higginsworth and Unsworth [12]. In addition, theses by Droogendijk [13] and Burkhardt [14] contain extensive and detailed reviews of theories of joint lubrication.

McCutchen was the first to propose an entirely new concept of lubrication—"weeping lubrication"—applied to synovial joint action [15,16]. He considered unique and special properties of cartilage and how they could affect flow and lubrication. The work of Mow et al. continued along a more complex, and possibly more sophisticated, approach in which a biomechanical model is proposed for the study of the dynamic interaction between synovial fluid and articular cartilage [17,18].

TABLE 23.1 More Than Two Dozen Theories Have Been Proposed To Explain Synovial Joint Lubrication—Examples of Proposed Mechanisms of Synovial Joint Lubrication

Mechanism	Author	Date
1. Hydrodynamic	MacConnail	1932
2. Boundary	Jones	1934
3. Hydrodynamic	Jones	1936
4. Boundary	Charnley	1959
5. Weeping	McCutchen	1959
6. Floating	Barnett and Cobbold	1962
7. Elastohydrodynamic	Tanner	1966
	Dowson	1967
8. Thixotropic/elastic fluid	Dintenfass	1963
9. Osmotic (boundary)	McCutchen	1966
10. Squeeze-film	Fein	1966
	Higginson et al.	1974
11. Synovial gel	Maroudas	1967
12. Thin-film	Faber et al.	1967
13. Combinations of hydrostatic, boundary, & EHL	Linn	1968
14. Boosted	Walker et al.	1968
15. Lipid	Little et al.	1969
16. Weeping + boundary	McCutchen and Wilkins	1969
	McCutchen	1969
17. Boundary	Caygill and West	1969
18. Fat (or mucin)	Freeman et al.	1970
19. Electrostatic	Roberts	1971
20. Boundary + fluid squeeze-film	Radin and Paul	1972
21. Mixed	Unsworth et al.	1974
22. Imbibe/exudate composite model	Ling	1974
23. Complex biomechanical model	Mow et al.	1974
24. Two porous layer model	Mansour and Mow	1977
	Dinnar	1974
25. Boundary	Reimann et al.	1975
26. Squeeze-film + fluid film + boundary	Unsworth, Dowson et al.	1975
27. Compliant bearing model	Rybicki	1977
28. Lubricating glycoproteins	Swann et al.	1977
29. Structuring of boundary water	Sokoloff et al.	1979
30. Surface flow	Kenyon	1980

Several additional studies have also been made of effects of porosity and compliance, including the behavior of elastic layers, in producing hydrodynamic and squeeze-film lubrication. One good review in this area was given by Unsworth, who discussed both human and artificial joints [19].

The following general observations are offered on the theories of synovial joint lubrication which have been proposed:

1. Most of the theories are strictly mechanical or rheological—involving such factors as deformation, pressure, and fluid flow.

2. There is a preoccupation with *friction,* which of course is very low for articular cartilage systems.

3. None of the theories consider *wear*—which is neither the same as friction nor simply related to it.

4. The detailed structure, biochemistry, complexity, and living nature of the total articular cartilage/synovial fluid system are generally ignored.

These are only general impressions. And although mechanical/rheological concepts seem dominant—with a focus on friction—wear and biochemistry are not completely ignored. For example,

Simon [20] abraded articular cartilage from human patellae and canine femoral heads with a stainless steel rotary file, measuring the depth of penetration with time and the amount of wear debris generated. Cartilage wear was also studied experimentally by Bloebaum and Wilson [21], Radin and Paul [22], and Lipshitz, Etheredge, and Glimcher [23–25]. The latter researchers carried out several *in vitro* studies of wear of articular cartilage using bovine cartilage plugs or specimens in sliding contact against stainless steel plates. They developed a means of measuring cartilage wear by determining the hydroxyproline content of both the lubricant and solid wear debris. Using this system and technique, effects of variables such as time, applied load, and chemical modification of articular cartilage on wear and profile changes were determined. This work is of particular importance in that they addressed the question of *cartilage wear and damage* rather than friction, recognizing that wear and friction are different phenomena.

Special note is also made of two researchers, Swann and Sokoloff, who considered biochemistry as an important factor in synovial joint lubrication. Swann et al. very carefully isolated fractions of bovine synovial fluid using sequential sedimentation techniques and gel permeation chromatography. They found a high molecular weight glycoprotein to be the major constituent in the "articular lubrication fraction" from bovine synovial fluid and called this *LGP-I* (from "lubricating glycoprotein"). This was based on friction measurements using cartilage in sliding contact against a glass disc. An excellent summary of this work with additional references is presented in a chapter by Swann in *The Joints and Synovial Fluid: I* [6].

Sokoloff et al. examined the "boundary lubricating ability" of several synovial fluids using a latex-glass test system and cartilage specimens obtained at necropsy from knees [26]. Measurements were made of friction. The research was extended to other *in vitro* friction tests using cartilage obtained from the nasal septum of cows and widely differing artificial surfaces [27]. As a result of this work, a new model of boundary lubrication by synovial fluid was proposed—the structuring of boundary water. The postulate involves adsorption of one part of a glycoprotein on a surface followed by the formation of hydration shells around the polar portions of the adsorbed glycoprotein; the net result is a thin layer of viscous "structured" water at the surface. This work is of particular interest in that it not only involves a specific and more detailed mechanism of boundary lubrication in synovial joints but also takes into account the possible importance of water in this system. The above summary of major synovial joint lubrication theories is taken from [9] as well as the thesis by Burkhardt [14].

Two more recent studies are of interest since cartilage wear was considered, although not as a part of a theory of joint lubrication. Stachowiak et al. [38] investigated the friction and wear characteristics of adult rat femur cartilage against a stainless steel plate using an environmental scanning electron microscope (ESEM) to examine damaged cartilage. One finding was evidence of a load limit to lubrication of cartilage, beyond which high friction and damage occurred. Another study, by Hayes et al. [39] on the influence of crystals on cartilage wear, is particularly interesting not only in the findings reported (e.g., certain crystals can increase cartilage wear) but also in the full description of the biochemical techniques used.

23.6 *In Vitro* Cartilage Wear Studies

During the 1983–84 academic year, the author carried out a sabbatical study in the Laboratory for the Study of Skeletal Disorders, The Children's Hospital Medical Center, Harvard Medical School in Boston. The laboratory is under the direction of Dr. Melvin Glimcher. One goal was to determine the effects, if any, of biochemical constituents of synovial fluid on cartilage wear using a modification of the device developed at Children's Hospital for this purpose—bovine articular cartilage specimens in oscillating contact against a highly polished stainless steel plate. This was made possible with the help of Dr. David Swann of the Shriners' Burns Medical Institute in Boston.

The thrust of this study as well as results obtained during that year and subsequently have been presented and summarized in several lectures and seminars and in Symposia of the European Society of Osteoarthrology in Finland [28], the former USSR [29], and The Netherlands [8].

The test conditions used in the cartilage wear studies carried out at The Children's Hospital Medical Center are summarized in Table 23.2. Cylindrical plugs (5.7 mm diam.) of bone and cartilage were cut from selected bovine medial femoral condyle sections approximately 50 × 50 mm in size. Four plugs were cut from each section using the procedure developed by Glimcher et al. These four plugs were then employed in a statistical design in which two plugs were used in wear tests with a reference fluid (a buffered saline solution) and two plugs with a test fluid.

Cartilage wear was determined by sampling the test fluid and determining the concentration of 4-hydroxyproline—a constituent of collagen. A typical plot of cartilage wear versus time under these conditions is shown in Fig. 23.4. It can be seen that over this period of 6 hours, the wear rate is linear with time. At the end of a test, the cartilage specimens are rinsed repeatedly and all fluids and washes collected for further treatment and hydroxyproline analysis.

Using this procedure, cartilage wear tests were carried out with several fluids prepared by David Swann. These included (1) a buffered saline reference fluid, (2) normal bovine synovial fluid, (3) the saline reference fluid plus hyaluronic acid, (4) the reference plus Swann's LGP-I (lubricating glycoprotein-I), and (5) the reference containing a protein complex isolated from bovine synovial fluid. In addition, some tests were also made with distilled water.

Figure 23.5 shows the average hydroxyproline contents of wear debris obtained from these *in vitro* experiments. These numbers are related to the cartilage wear which occurred. However, since the total quantities of collected fluids varied somewhat, the values shown in the bar graph should not be taken as exact or precise measures of fluid effects on cartilage wear.

The main conclusions drawn from Fig. 23.5 are these:

1. Normal bovine synovial fluid is very effective in reducing cartilage wear under these *in vitro* conditions as compared to the buffered saline reference fluid.
2. There is no significant difference in wear between the saline reference and distilled water.
3. The addition of hyaluronic acid to the reference fluid reduces wear, but its effect depends on the source.
4. Under these test conditions, Swann's LGP-I—known to be extremely effective in reducing friction in cartilage-on-glass tests—does not reduce cartilage wear.
5. However, a protein complex isolated by Swann is extremely effective in reducing wear—producing results similar to those obtained with synovial fluid. The detailed structure of this constituent is complex and has not yet been fully determined.
6. The lack of an added fluid in these experiments leads to extremely high wear and damage of the articular cartilage. The lower bar in Fig. 23.5 represents an inadvertent omission of test fluid. Initial oscillating contact proceeded normally for several minutes—very likely with the help of fluids exuded from the cartilage itself. But soon thereafter, the noise and severity of contact made it necessary to stop the test. The relative wear results determined are for a much shorter period of time but still very high.

TABLE 23.2 Test Conditions: *In Vitro* Cartilage Wear Experiments

Contact geometry	Flat-on-flat
Articular cartilage	Bovine (medial femoral condyle)
Cartilage plug diameter	5.7 mm
Applied load	53.4 N
Average pressure	2.10 MPa
Traverse	6.35 mm
Cycles/minute	40
Fluid temperature	25°C
Test duration	4 h
Total cycles	9600

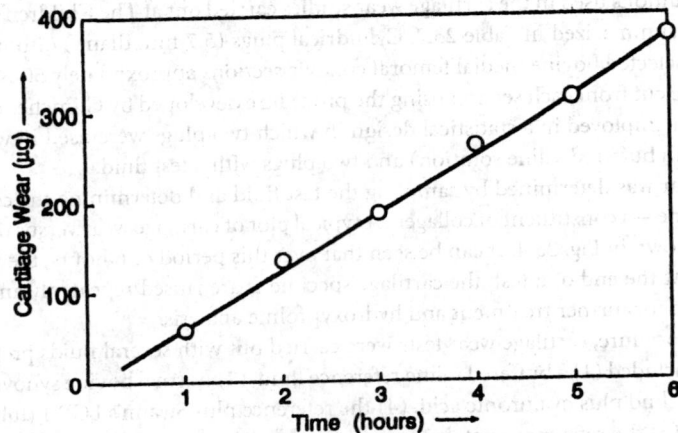

FIGURE 23.4 Cartilage wear versus time [9].

Scanning electron micrographs of the worn cartilage specimens were also made. This procedure was carried out by Karen Hodgens of Children's Hospital. The results of the SEM study showed three main things:

1. There is no question but that the action of sliding contact produces significant changes in the appearance of the cartilage surface structure; thus, the SEM results are not simply due to artifacts in the technique.
2. Each test fluid appears to create a characteristic or unique surface on the worn cartilage specimen.
3. In the case of the unlubricated cartilage specimen, the drastic damage and fissures that occurred are strikingly apparent.

In discussing the possible significance of these findings from a tribological point of view, it may be helpful first of all to emphasize once again that friction and wear are different phenomena. Furthermore, as suggested by Fig. 23.6, certain constituents of synovial fluid (e.g., Swann's lubricating glycoprotein) may act to reduce *friction* in synovial joints while other constituents (e.g., Swann's protein complex or hyaluronic acid) may act to reduce cartilage *wear*. In a sense, we may wish to distinguish between biochemical antifriction and antiwear compounds present in synovial fluid.

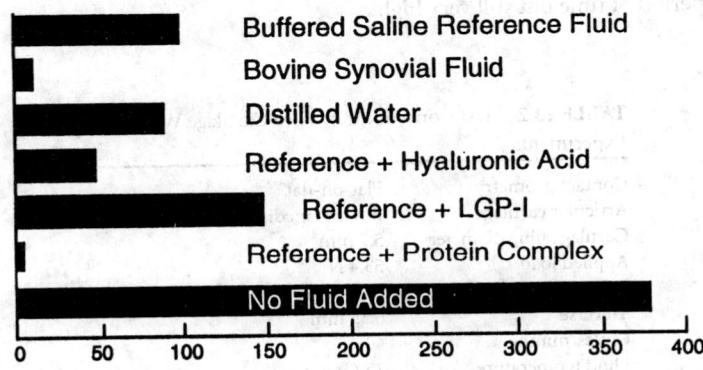

FIGURE 23.5 Relative cartilage wear based on hydroxyproline content of debris (*in vitro* cartilage on stainless steel) [9].

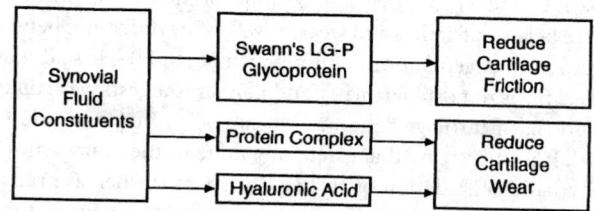

FIGURE 23.6 Friction and wear are different phenomena [9].

1. Has nature designed a special biochemical compound which has as its function to protect articular cartilage?
2. What is the mechanism (or mechanisms) by which biochemical constituents of synovial fluid can act to reduce wear of articular cartilage?
3. Does or can a lack of this biochemical constituent lead to increased cartilage wear and damage?

23.7 Biotribology and Arthritis: Are There Connections?

Arthritis is an umbrella term for more than 100 rheumatic diseases affecting joints and connective tissue. The two most common forms are osteoarthritis (OA) and rheumatoid arthritis (RA). Osteoarthritis—also referred to as *osteoarthrosis* or *degenerative joint disease*—is the most common form of arthritis. It is sometimes simplistically described as the "wear and tear" form of arthritis. The causes and progression of degenerative joint disease are still not understood. Rheumatoid arthritis is a chronic and often progressive disease of the synovial membrane leading to release of enzymes which attack, erode, and destroy articular cartilage. It is an inflammatory response involving the immune system and is more prevalent in females. Rheumatoid arthritis is extremely complex. And many of its causes are still unknown.

For more information on synovial joints and arthritis, the following books are suggested: *The Biology of Degenerative Joint Disease* by Leon Sokoloff [30], *Adult Articular Cartilage*, edited by Freeman [5], *The Joints and Synovial Fluid: I*, edited by Sokoloff [6], *Textbook of Rheumatology*, edited by Kelley et al. [31], *Osteoarthritis: Diagnosis and Management*, edited by Moskowitz et al. [32], *Degenerative Joints: Test Tubes, Tissues, Models, and Man*, edited by Verbruggen and Veyes [33], *Biology of the Articular Cartilage in Health and Disease*, Proceedings editor, Gastpar [34], and *Crystals and Joint Disease*, by Dieppe and Calvert [35].

Sokoloff defines degenerative joint disease as "an extremely common, noninflammatory, progressive disorder of movable joints, particularly weight-bearing joints, [which] is characterized pathologically by deterioration of articular cartilage and by formation of new bone in the subchondral areas and at the margins of the joint" [30]. As mentioned, osteoarthritis or osteoarthrosis is sometimes referred to as the wear-and-tear form of arthritis, but wear itself is rarely a simple process even in well-defined systems.

It has been noted by the author that tribological terms occasionally appear in hypotheses which describe the etiology of osteoarthritis, e.g., "reduced wear resistance of cartilage" or "poor lubricity of synovial fluid." It has also been noted that there is a general absence of hypotheses connecting normal synovial joint *lubrication* (or lack thereof) and synovial joint *degeneration*. Perhaps it is natural (and unhelpful) for a tribologist to imagine such a connection and that, for example, cartilage wear under certain circumstances might be due to or influenced by a lack of proper "boundary lubrication" by the synovial fluid. In this regard, it may be of interest to quote Swanson [36] who said in 1979 that "there exists at present no experimental evidence which certainly shows that a failure of lubrication is or is not a causative factor in the first stages of cartilage degeneration." A statement made by Professor Glimcher [37] may also be appropriate here. Glimcher fully recognized the fundamental difference between friction and wear as well as the difference between joint lubrication (one area of study) and joint degeneration (another area of study). He said that wearing or abrading cartilage with a steel file is not osteoarthritis, and neither is digesting cartilage in a test tube with an enzyme. But both forms of cartilage deterioration can occur in a living joint and in a way which is still not understood. It is interesting that essentially none of the many synovial joint lubrication theories consider enzymatic degradation of cartilage as a factor whereas practically all the models of the etiology of degenerative joint disease include this as an important factor.

It was stated earlier that there are at least two main areas to consider, i.e., (1) mechanisms of synovial joint lubrication and (2) the etiology of synovial joint degeneration (e.g., as in osteoarthrosis). Both areas are extremely complex. And the key questions as to what actually happens in each have yet to be answered (and perhaps asked). It would therefore be presumptuous of the present author to suggest possible connections between two areas which in themselves are still not fully understood.

Tribological processes in a movable joint involve not only the contacting surfaces (articular cartilage) but the surrounding medium (synovial fluid) as well. Each of these depends on the synthesis and transport of "necessary" biochemical constituents to the contact region or interface. As a result of relative motion (sliding, rubbing, rolling, impact) between the joint elements, friction and/or wear can occur.

It has already been shown and discussed—at least in some *in vitro* tests with articular cartilage—that compounds which reduce friction do not necessarily reduce wear; the latter was suggested as being more important [8,9]. It may be helpful first of all to emphasize once again that friction and wear are different phenomena. Furthermore, certain constituents of synovial fluid (e.g., Swann's lubricating glycoprotein) may act to reduce *friction* in synovial joints, whereas other constituents (e.g., Swann's protein complex or hyaluronic acid) may act to reduce cartilage *wear*.

A significant increase in joint friction could lead to a slight increase in local temperatures or possibly to reduced mobility. But the effects of cartilage wear would be expected to be more serious. When cartilage wear occurs, a very special material is lost, and the body is not capable of regenerating cartilage of the same quality nor at the desired rate. Thus, there are at least two major tribological dimensions involved—one concerning the nature of the synovial fluid and the other having to do with the properties of articular cartilage itself. Changes in *either* the synovial fluid or cartilage could conceivably lead to increased wear or damage (or friction) as shown in Figure 23.7.

In some cases, the body makes an unsuccessful attempt at repair, and bone growth may occur at the periphery of contact. This process and the generation of wear particles could lead to joint inflammation and the release of enzymes which further soften and degrade the articular cartilage. This softer, degraded cartilage does not possess the wear resistance of the original. Thus, there exists a feedback process in which the occurrence of cartilage wear can lead to even more damage. Degradative enzymes can also be released by trauma, shock, or injury to the joint. Ultimately, as the cartilage is progressively thinned and bony growth occurs, a condition of osteoarthritis or degenerative joint disease may exist. There are other pathways to the disease, pathways which may include

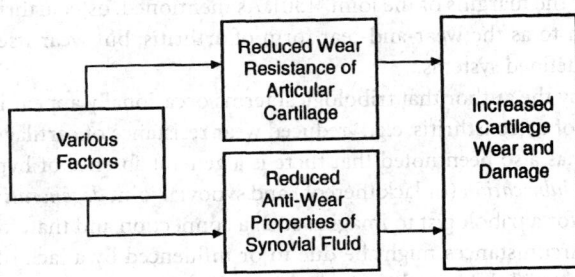

FIGURE 23.7 Two tribological aspects of synovial joint lubrication.

genetic factors. It is not argued that arthritis is a tribological problem. However, the inclusion of tribological processes in one set of pathways to osteoarthrosis would not seem strange or unusual, at least to this author.

23.8 Conclusions

The following main conclusions relating to the tribological behavior of natural, "normal" synovial joints are presented:

1. Over 30 different theories of joint lubrication have been proposed over the years! All the theories focus on friction, none deal with wear, many do not involve experimental studies with cartilage, and very few consider the complexity and detailed biochemistry of the synovial fluid/articular cartilage system.

2. It was shown by *in vitro* tests with bovine articular cartilage that the detailed biochemistry of synovial fluid has a significant effect on cartilage wear and damage. Normal bovine synovial fluid was found to provide excellent protection against wear. Various biochemical constituents isolated from bovine synovial fluid by Dr. David Swann of the Shriner's Burns Institute in Boston showed varying effects on cartilage wear when added back to a buffered saline reference fluid. This research demonstrates once again the importance of distinguishing between friction and wear.

3. It is suggested that these results could change significantly the way we look at mechanisms of synovial joint lubrication. Effects of biochemistry of the system on wear of articular cartilage are likely to be important; such effects may not be related to physical/rheological models of joint lubrication.

4. It is also suggested that connections between tribology/normal synovial joint lubrication and degenerative joint disease are not only possible but likely; however, such connections are undoubtedly complex. It is *not* argued that osteoarthritis is a tribological problem or that it is necessarily the result of a tribological deficiency. Ultimately, a better understanding of how normal synovial joints function from a tribological point of view could conceivably lead to advances in the prevention and treatment of osteoarthritis.

5. Last, the topic of synovial joint lubrication is far from being understood. It is a complex subject involving at least biophysics, biomechanics, biochemistry, and tribology. For a physical scientist or engineer, carrying out research in this area is a humbling experience.

Acknowledgments

The author wishes to acknowledge the Edward H. Lane and G. Harold and Leila Y. Mathers foundations for their support during a sabbatical study at The Children's Hospital Medical Center. He also wishes to thank Dr. David Swann for his invaluable help in providing the test fluids and carrying out the biochemical analyses as well as Ms. Karen Hodgens for conducting the scanning electron microscopy studies of worn cartilage specimens.

Last but certainly not least, I am indebted to the following researchers for their encouraging and stimulating discussions of this topic over the years and for teaching a tribologist something of the complexity of synovial joints, articular cartilage, and arthritis: Drs. Leon Sokoloff, Charles McCutchen, Melvin Glimcher, David Swann, Henry Mankin, Clement Sledge, Helen Muir, Heikki Helminen and colleagues, Paul Dieppe, E. T. Kornegay, Hugo Veit, and many others.

References

1. Hunter W. 1742–1743. Of the structure and diseases of articulating cartilages, Philosophical Transactions, vol 42, pp 514–521, London, The Royal Society of London.

2. Furey MJ. 1986. Tribology. In Encyclopedia of Materials Science and Engineering, pp 5145–5158, Oxford, Pergamon.

3. Cameron A. 1966. The Principles of Lubrication, London, Longmans Green.

4. Dowson D, Higginson GR. 1977. Elastohydrodynamic Lubrication, SI ed, Oxford, Pergamon.

5. Freeman MAR (ed). 1979. Adult Articular Cartilage, 2d ed, Tunbridge Wells, Kent, England, Pitman Medical Publishing.

6. Sokoloff L (ed.) 1978. The Joints and Synovial Fluid, vol. 1, New York, Academic Press.

7. Stockwell RA. 1979. Biology of Cartilage Cells, Cambridge, Cambridge Univ.

8. Furey MJ. 1992. Biochemical aspects of synovial joint lubrication and cartilage wear. European Society of Osteoarthrology Symp Joint Destruction in Arthritis and Osteoarthritis, Noordwijkerhout, The Netherlands, May 24–27.

9. Furey MJ. 1993. Biotribology: Cartilage lubrication and wear. Sixth International Congress on Tribology, EUROTRIB '93, Budapest, Hungary, Aug. 30–Sept. 2.

10. McCutchen CW. 1978. Lubrication of joints. In L Sokoloff (ed), The Joints and Synovial Fluid, vol. 1, pp 437–483, New York, Academic Press.

11. Swanson SAV. 1979. Friction, wear and lubrication. In MAR Freeman (ed), in Adult Articular Cartilage, 2d ed, pp 415–460, Tunbridge Wells, Kent, England, Pitman Medical Publishing.

12. Higginson GR, Unsworth T. 1981. The lubrication of natural joints, In J. H. Dumbleton (ed), Tribology of Natural and Artificial Joints, pp 47–73, Amsterdam and New York, Elsevier Scientific Publishing.

13. Droogendijk L. 1984. On the Lubrication of Synovial Joints, thesis, Twente University of Technology, The Netherlands.

14. Burkhardt BM. 1988. Development and Design of a Test Device for Cartilage Wear Studies, thesis, Mechanical Engineering, Virginia Polytechnic Institute & State University, Blacksburg, Virginia.

15. McCutchen CW. 1959. Mechanisms of animal joints: sponge-hydrostatic and weeping bearings. Nature 184:1284.

16. McCutchen CW. 1962. The frictional properties of animal joints. Wear 5(1):1.

17. Torzilli PA, Mow VC. 1976. On the fundamental fluid transport mechanisms through normal and pathological articular cartilage during friction: 1. The formulation. J Biomech 9:541.

18. Mansour JM, Mow VC. 1977. On the natural lubrication of synovial joints: normal and degenerated. Lubrication Technology April:163.

19. Unsworth A. 1991. Tribology of human and artificial joints. Proceedings, Institute of Mechanical Engineers, II: Engineering in Medicine. 205:163.

20. Simon WH. 1971. Wear properties of articular cartilage, in vitro. Rheumatic Diseases, Laboratory of Experimental Pathology, National Institute of Arthritis and Metabolic Diseases, National Institutes of Health, Bethesda, Md.

21. Bloebaum RD, Wilson AS. 1980. The morphology of the surface of articular cartilage in adult rats. J Anat 131:333.

22. Radin EL, Paul IL. 1971. Response of joints to impact loading: 1. "In vitro" wear tests. Arthritis Rheum 14(3):356–362.

23. Lipshitz H, Glimcher MJ. 1974. A technique for the preparation of plugs of articular cartilage and subchondral bone. J Biomech 7:293.

24. Lipshitz H, Etheredge R, III. 1975. "In vitro" wear of articular cartilage. J Bone Joint Surg 57-A:527.

25. Lipshitz H, Glimcher MJ. 1979. "In vitro" studies of wear of articular cartilage: II. Characteristics of the wear of articular cartilage when worn against stainless steel plates having characterized surfaces. Wear 52:297.

26. Sokoloff L, Davis WH, Lee SL. 1978. Boundary lubricating ability of synovial fluid in degenerative joint disease. Arthritis Rheum 21:754.

27. Sokoloff L, Davis WH, Lee SL. 1979. A proposed model of boundary lubrication by synovial fluid: structuring of boundary water. J Biomech Eng 101:185.

28. Furey MJ. 1986. Biotribology: An "in vitro" study of the effects of synovial fluid constituents on cartilage wear, Proc 15th Symp European Society of Osteoarthrology, Kuopio, Finland, June 25–27. Abstract in Scandinavian Journal of Rheumatology, Supplement.

29. Furey MJ. 1987. The influence of synovial fluid constituents on cartilage wear: A scanning electron microscope study. Conf Joint Destruction, 16th Symp European Society of Osteoarthrology, Sochi, USSR, Sept 28–Oct 3.

30. Sokoloff L. 1969. The Biology of Degenerative Joint Disease, Chicago, University of Chicago.

31. Kelley WN, Harris ED, Jr, Ruddy S, Sledge CB (eds). 1981. Textbook of Rheumatology, Philadelphia, Saunders.

32. Moskowitz RW, Howell DS, Goldberg VM et al (eds). 1984. Osteoarthritis: Diagnosis and Management, Philadelphia, Saunders.

33. Verbruggen G, Veyes EM (eds). 1980. Degenerative Joints: Test Tubes, Tissues, Models, and Man. Proc First Conf Degenerative Joint Diseases, Ghent, Oct 10–11; 1982. Amsterdam-Oxford-Princeton, Excerpta Medica.

34. Gastpar H (ed). 1979. Biology of the Articular Cartilage in Health and Disease, Proc Second Munich Symp Biology of Connective Tissue, Munich, July 23–24; 1980. Stuttgart-New York, F. K. Schattauer Verlag.

35. Dieppe P, Calvert P. 1983. Crystals and Joint Disease, London–New York, Chapman and Hall.

36. Swanson SAV. 1979. Friction, wear and lubrication. In MAR Freeman (ed), Adult Articular Cartilage, 2d ed, pp 415–460, Tunbridge Wells, Kent, England, Pitman Medical Publishing.

37. Discussions with M. J. Glimcher, The Children's Hospital Medical Center, Boston, Fall 1983.

38. Stachowiak GW, Batchelor AW, Griffiths LJ. 1994. Friction and wear changes in synovial joints. Wear 171:135.

39. Hayes A, Harris B, Dieppe PA et al. 1993. Wear of articular cartilage: The effect of crystals, Institute of Mechanical Engineers, pp 41–58.

24

Musculoskeletal Soft Tissue Mechanics

Richard L. Lieber
*University of California and
Veterans Administration
Medical Centers*

Thomas J. Burkholder
*University of California and
Veterans Administration
Medical Centers*

Skeletal muscles are length- and velocity-dependent force generators [Zajac, 1989]. Numerous extrinsic and intrinsic factors determine the magnitude of muscle force generated, maximum muscle contractile velocity and sensitivity of force generation to length and velocity. In this chapter, we provide a summary of experimental measurements of these factors. Such information is necessary to generate accurate and physiologically relevant musculoskeletal models. Since muscles transmit force to bones via tendons, quantification of tendon biomechanical properties is also of interest [Zajac, 1989].

24.1 Fundamentals of Soft Tissue Biomechanics

Maximum Muscle Stress

Muscles are anisotropic, with maximum active stress generated parallel to the fiber axis. The force a whole muscle can generate is proportional to the sum of the cross-sectional area of muscle fibers projected along the muscle's line of action. In practice, this is difficult to measure and so "physiologic" cross-sectional area (PCSA) has been defined for skeletal muscle as:

$$\text{PCSA (mm}^2) = \frac{M(g) \cdot \cos \theta}{\rho(g/mm^3) \cdot L_f(mm)} \tag{24.1}$$

where ρ = muscle density (1.056 g/cm³ in fresh tissue) and θ = surface pennation angle. (It should be noted that PCSA measured in this way is not necessarily related to any area measured in the anatomical planes; see Tables 24.1 and 24.2). PCSA is extremely dependent on the orientation, length, and number of muscle fibers within the tissue and must be experimentally determined for each muscle [Gans, 1982]. Given muscle PCSA, maximum force produced by a muscle can be predicted by multiplying this PCSA by specific tension (Table 24.3). Specific tension can also be calculated for isolated muscle fibers or motor units in which estimates of cross-sectional area have been made (Table 24.3).

0-8493-8346-3/95/$0.00+$.50
© 1995 by CRC Press, Inc.

TABLE 24.1 Architectural Properties of the Human Arm and Forearm*†

Muscle	Muscle Mass (g)	Muscle Length (mm)	Fiber Length (mm)	Pennation Angle (°)	Cross-Sectional Area (cm²)	FL/ML Ratio
BR (n = 8)	16.6 ± 2.8	175 ± 8.3	121 ± 8.3	2.4 ± 0.6	1.33 ± 0.22	0.69 ± 0.062
PT (n = 8)	15.9 ± 1.7	130 ± 4.7	36.4 ± 1.3	9.6 ± 0.8	4.13 ± 0.52	0.28 ± 0.012
PQ (n = 8)	5.21 ± 1.0	39.3 ± 2.3	23.3 ± 2.0	9.9 ± 0.3	2.07 ± 0.33	0.58 ± 0.021
EDC I (n = 8)	3.05 ± 0.45	114 ± 3.4	56.9 ± 3.6	3.1 ± 0.5	0.52 ± 0.08	0.49 ± 0.024
EDC M (n = 5)	6.13 ± 1.2	112 ± 4.7	58.8 ± 3.5	3.2 ± 1.0	1.02 ± 0.20	0.50 ± 0.014
EDC R (n = 7)	4.70 ± 0.75	125 ± 10.7	51.2 ± 1.8	3.2 ± 0.54	0.86 ± 0.13	0.42 ± 0.023
EDC S (n = 6)	2.23 ± 0.32	121 ± 8.0	52.9 ± 5.2	2.4 ± 0.7	0.40 ± 0.06	0.43 ± 0.029
EDQ (n = 7)	3.81 ± 0.70	152 ± 9.2	55.3 ± 3.7	2.6 ± 0.6	0.64 ± 0.10	0.36 ± 0.012
EIP (n = 6)	2.86 ± 0.61	105 ± 6.6	48.4 ± 2.3	6.3 ± 0.8	0.56 ± 0.11	0.46 ± 0.023
EPL (n = 7)	4.54 ± 0.68	138 ± 7.2	43.6 ± 2.6	5.6 ± 1.3	0.98 ± 0.13	0.31 ± 0.020
PL (n = 6)	3.78 ± 0.82	134 ± 11.5	52.3 ± 3.1	3.5 ± 1.2	0.69 ± 0.17	0.40 ± 0.032
FDS I(P) (n = 6)	6.0 ± 1.1	92.5 ± 8.4	31.6 ± 3.0	5.1 ± 0.2	1.81 ± 0.83	0.34 ± 0.022
FDS I(D) (n = 9)	6.6 ± 0.8	119 ± 6.1	37.9 ± 3.0	6.7 ± 0.3	1.63 ± 0.22	0.32 ± 0.013
FDS I(C) (n = 6)	12.4 ± 2.1	207 ± 10.7	67.6 ± 2.8	5.7 ± 0.2	1.71 ± 0.28	0.33 ± 0.025
FDS M (n = 9)	16.3 ± 2.2	183 ± 11.5	60.8 ± 3.9	6.9 ± 0.7	2.53 ± 0.34	0.34 ± 0.014
FDS R (n = 9)	10.2 ± 1.1	155 ± 7.7	60.1 ± 2.7	4.3 ± 0.6	1.61 ± 0.18	0.39 ± 0.023
FDS S (n = 9)	1.8 ± 0.3	103 ± 6.3	42.4 ± 2.2	4.9 ± 0.7	0.40 ± 0.05	0.42 ± 0.014
FDP I (n = 9)	11.7 ± 1.2	149 ± 3.8	61.4 ± 2.4	7.2 ± 0.7	1.77 ± 0.16	0.41 ± 0.018
FDP M (n = 9)	16.3 ± 1.7	200 ± 8.2	68.4 ± 2.7	5.7 ± 0.3	2.23 ± 0.22	0.34 ± 0.011
FDP R (n = 9)	11.9 ± 1.4	194 ± 7.0	64.6 ± 2.6	6.8 ± 0.5	1.72 ± 0.18	0.33 ± 0.009
FDP S (n = 9)	13.7 ± 1.5	150 ± 4.7	60.7 ± 3.9	7.8 ± 0.9	2.20 ± 0.30	0.40 ± 0.015
FPL (n = 9)	10.0 ± 1.1	168 ± 10.0	45.1 ± 2.1	6.9 ± 0.2	2.08 ± 0.22	0.24 ± 0.010

*Data from Lieber *et al.*, 1990, 1992.

†BR: brachioradialis; EDC I, EDC M, EDC R, and EDC S: extensor digitorum communis to the index, middle, ring, and small fingers, respectively; EDQ: extensor digiti quinti; EIP: extensor indicis proprious; EPL: extensor pollicis longus; FDP I, FDP M, FDP R, and FDP S: flexor digitorum profundus muscles; FDS I, FDS M, FDS R, and FDS S: flexor digitorum superficialis muscles; FDS I (P) and FDS I (D): proximal and distal bellies of the FDS I; FDS I (C): the combined properties of the two bellies as if they were a single muscle; FPL: flexor pollicis longus; PQ: pronator quadratus; PS: palmaris longus; PT: pronator teres.

Maximum Muscle Contraction Velocity

Muscle maximum contraction velocity is primarily dependent on the number of sarcomeres in series along the muscle fiber length [Gans, 1982]. This number has been experimentally determined for a number of skeletal muscles (Table 24.3). Maximum contraction velocity of a given muscle can thus be calculated based on a knowledge of the number of serial sarcomeres within the muscle multiplied by the maximum contraction velocity of an individual sarcomere (Tables 24.1 and 24.2).

Muscle Force-Velocity Relationship

Under conditions of constant contractile load the relationship between force and velocity is given by the Hill equation (Hill, 1938). The shortening force-velocity relation can be described by

$$(P + a)\,v = b\,(P_o - P) \tag{24.2}$$

whereas the lengthening relation can be described by

$$\frac{P}{P_o} = 1.8 - 0.8\,\frac{V_{max} + V}{V_{max} - 7.6\,V} \tag{24.3}$$

These dynamic parameters vary with species and fiber type (Table 24.4).

TABLE 24.2 Architectural Properties of Human Lower Limb*†

Muscle	Muscle Mass (g)	Muscle Length (mm)	Fiber Length (mm)	Pennation Angle (°)	Cross-Sectional Area (cm²)	FL/ML Ratio
RF (n = 3)	84.3 ± 14	316 ± 5.7	66.0 ± 1.5	5.0 ± 0.0	12.7 ± 1.9	0.209 ± 0.002
VL (n = 3)	220 ± 56	324 ± 14	65.7 ± 0.88	5.0 ± 0.0	30.6 ± 6.5	0.203 ± 0.007
VM (n = 3)	175 ± 41	335 ± 15	70.3 ± 3.3	5.0 ± 0.0	21.1 ± 4.3	0.210 ± 0.005
VI (n = 3)	160 ± 59	329 ± 15	68.3 ± 4.8	3.3 ± 1.7	22.3 ± 8.7	0.208 ± 0.007
SM (n = 3)	108 ± 13	262 ± 1.5	62.7 ± 4.7	15 ± 2.9	16.9 ± 1.5	0.239 ± 0.017
BF$_l$ (n = 3)	128 ± 28	342 ± 14	85.3 ± 5.0	0.0 ± 0.0	12.8 ± 2.8	0.251 ± 0.022
BF$_s$ (n = 3)		271 ± 11	139 ± 3.5	23 ± 0.9		0.517 ± 0.032
ST (n = 2)	76.9 ± 7.7	317 ± 4	158 ± 2.0	5.0 ± 0.0	5.4 ± 1.0	0.498 ± 0.0
SOL (n = 2)	215 (n = 1)	310 ± 1.5	19.5 ± 0.5	25 ± 5.0	58.0 (n = 1)	0.063 ± 0.002
MG (n = 3)	150 ± 14	248 ± 9.9	35.3 ± 2.0	16.7 ± 4.4	32.4 ± 3.1	0.143 ± 0.010
LG (n = 3)		217 ± 11	50.7 ± 5.6	8.3 ± 1.7		0.233 ± 0.016
PLT (n = 3)	5.30 ± 1.9	85.0 ± 15	39.3 ± 6.7	3.3 ± 1.7	1.2 ± 0.4	0.467 ± 0.031
FHL (n = 3)	21.5 ± 3.3	222 ± 5.0	34.0 ± 1.5	10.0 ± 2.9	5.3 ± 0.6	0.154 ± 0.010
FDL (n = 3)	16.3 ± 2.8	260 ± 15	27.0 ± 0.58	6.7 ± 1.7	5.1 ± 0.7	0.104 ± 0.004
PL (n = 3)	41.5 ± 8.5	286 ± 17	38.7 ± 3.2	10.0 ± 0.0	12.3 ± 2.9	0.136 ± 0.010
PB (n = 3)	17.3 ± 2.5	230 ± 13	39.3 ± 3.5	5.0 ± 0.0	5.7 ± 1.0	0.170 ± 0.006
TP (n = 3)	53.5 ± 7.3	254 ± 26	24.0 ± 4.0	11.7 ± 1.7	20.8 ± 3	0.095 ± 0.015
TA (n = 3)	65.7 ± 10	298 ± 12	77.3 ± 7.8	5.0 ± 0.0	9.9 ± 1.5	0.258 ± 0.015
EDL (n = 3)	35.2 ± 3.6	355 ± 13	80.3 ± 8.4	8.3 ± 1.7	5.6 ± 0.6	0.226 ± 0.024
EHL (n = 3)	12.9 ± 1.6	273 ± 2.4	87.0 ± 8.0	6.0 ± 1.0	1.8 ± 0.2	0.319 ± 0.030
SAR (n = 3)	61.7 ± 14	503 ± 27	455 ± 19	0.0 ± 0.0	1.7 ± 0.3	0.906 ± 0.017
GR (n = 3)	35.3 ± 7.4	335 ± 20	277 ± 12	3.3 ± 1.7	1.8 ± 0.3	0.828 ± 0.017
AM (n = 3)	229 ± 32	305 ± 12	115 ± 7.9	0.0 ± 0.0	18.2 ± 2.3	0.378 ± 0.013
AL (n = 3)	63.5 ± 16	229 ± 12	108 ± 2.0	6.0 ± 1.0	6.8 ± 1.9	0.475 ± 0.023
AB (n = 3)	43.8 ± 8.4	156 ± 12	103 ± 6.4	0.0 ± 0.0	4.7 ± 1.0	0.663 ± 0.036
PEC (n = 3)	26.4 ± 6.0	123 ± 4.5	104 ± 1.2	0.0 ± 0.0	2.9 ± 0.6	0.851 ± 0.040
POP (n = 2)	20.1 ± 2.4	108 ± 7.0	29.0 ± 7.0	0.0 ± 0.0	7.9 ± 1.4	0.265 ± 0.048

*Data from Wickiewicz *et al.*, (1982).

†AB, adductor brevis; AL, adductor longus; AM, adductor magnus; BF$_l$, biceps femoris, long head; BF$_s$, biceps femoris, short head; EDL, extensor digitorum longus; EHL, extensor hallucis longus; FDL, flexor digitorum longus; GR, gracilis; FHL, flexor hallucis longus; LG, lateral gastrocnemius; MG, medial gastrocnemius; PEC, pectineus; PB, peroneus brevis; PL, peroneus longus; PLT, plantaris; POP, popliteus; RF, rectus femoris; SAR, sartorius; SM, semimembranosus; SOL, soleus; ST, semitendinosus; TA, tibialis anterior; TP, tibialis posterior; VI, vastus intermedius; VL, vastus lateralis; VM, vastus medialis.

TABLE 24.3 Skeletal Muscle Specific Tension

Species	Muscle Type	Preparation	Specific Tension (kPa)	Reference
Rat	SO	Single fiber	134	Fitts et al [1991]
Human	Slow	Single fiber	133	Fitts et al [1991]
Rat	FOG	Single fiber	108	Fitts et al [1991]
Rat	FG	Single fiber	108	Fitts et al [1991]
Human	Fast	Single fiber	166	Fitts et al [1991]
Cat	1	Motor unit	59	Dum et al [1982]
Cat	S	Motor unit	172	Bodine et al [1987]
Cat	2A	Motor unit	284	Dum et al [1982]
Cat	FR	Motor unit	211	Bodine et al [1987]
Cat	2B + 2AB	Motor unit	343	Dum et al [1982]
Cat	FF/FI	Motor unit	249	Bodine et al [1987]
Human	Elbow	Whole muscle	230–420	Edgerton et al [1990]
Rat	TA	Whole muscle	272	Wells 1965
Rat	Soleus	Whole muscle	319	Wells 1965
Guinea pig	Hindlimb	Whole muscle	225	Powell et al [1984]
Guinea pig	Soleus	Whole muscle	154	Powell et al [1984]

Muscle Force-Length Relationship

Under conditions of constant length, muscle force generated is proportional to the magnitude of the interaction between the actin and myosin contractile filaments. Since myosin filament length in all species is approximately 1.6 μm and actin filament length varies (Table 24.5), optimal sarcomere length and maximum sarcomere length are calculated using these values. Optimal muscle length is then calculated by multiplying the number of serial sarcomeres within the muscle by the optimal sarcomere length.

Tendon Biomechanics

Tendons, like most biological structures, are highly nonlinear in their stress-strain properties. Tendons are more compliant at low loads and less compliant at high loads (Fig. 24-1). The highly nonlinear low load region has been referred to as the *toe* region and occurs up until approximately 3% strain [Butler et al, 1979; Zajac, 1989]. Typically tendons have linear properties from about 3% strain until ultimate strain which ranges from 9 to 10% (Table 24.6). Ultimate tensile stress reported for tendons is approximately 100 MPa (Table 24.6). Physiologically tendons appear to operate at a stress approximately 5 to 10 MPa (Table 24.6). Thus tendons operate with a safety factor of 10 to 20.

TABLE 24.4   Muscle Dynamic Properties

Species	Muscle Type	Preparation	V_{max}*	a/Po	b/V_{max}	Reference
Rat	SO	Single fiber	1.49 L/s			Fitts et al [1991]
Human	Slow	Single fiber	0.86 L/s			Fitts et al [1991]
Rat	FOG	Single fiber	4.91 L/s			Fitts et al [1991]
Rat	FG	Single fiber	8.05 L/s			Fitts et al [1991]
Human	Fast	Single fiber	4.85 L/s			Fitts et al [1991]
Mouse	Soleus	Whole muscle	31.7 μm/s			Close [1972]
Rat	Soleus	Whole muscle	18.2 μm/s			Close [1972]
Rat	Soleus	Whole muscle	5.4 cm/s	0.214	0.23	Wells [1965]
Cat	Soleus	Whole muscle	13 μm/s			Close [1972]
Mouse	EDL	Whole muscle	60.5 μm/s			Close [1972]
Rat	EDL	Whole muscle	42.7 μm/s			Close [1972]
Cat	EDL	Whole muscle	31 μm/s			Close [1972]
Rat	TA	Whole muscle	14.4 cm/s	0.356	0.38	Wells [1965]

*L/s, fiber or sarcomere lengths per second; μm/s, sarcomere velocity; cm/s, whole muscle velocity.

TABLE 24.5   Actin Filament Lengths

Species	1/2 actin filament length (μm)	Reference
Cat	1.12	Herzog et al [1992]
Rat	1.09	Herzog et al [1992]
Rabbit	1.09	Herzog et al [1992]
Frog	0.98	Page & Huxley [1963]
Monkey	1.16	Walker & Schrodt [1973]
Human	1.27	Walker & Schrodt [1973]
Hummingbird	1.75	Mathieu-Costello et al [1992]
Chicken	0.95	Page [1969]
Wild rabbit	1.12	Dimery [1985]
Carp	0.98	Sosnicki et al [1991]

TABLE 24.6   Tendon Biomechanical Properties

Tendon	Ultimate Stress	Ultimate Strain	Stress under Normal Loads	Strain under Normal Loads	Tangent Modulus	Reference
Wallaby			15–40 MPa		1.56 GPa	Bennett et al [1986]
Porpoise					1.53 GPa	Bennett et al [1986]
Dolphin					1.43 GPa	Bennett et al [1986]
Deer			28–74 MPa		1.59 GPa	Bennett et al [1986]
Sheep					1.65 GPa	Bennett et al [1986]
Donkey			22–44 MPa		1.25 GPa	Bennett et al [1986]
Human leg			53 MPa		1.0–1.2 GPa	Bennett et al [1986]
Cat leg					1.21 GPa	Bennett et al [1986]
Pig tail					0.9 GPa	Bennett et al [1986]
Rat tail					0.8–1.5 GPa	Bennett et al [1986]
Horse				4–10%		Ker et al [1988]
Dog leg			84 MPa			Ker et al [1988]
Camel ankle			18 MPa			Ker et al [1988]
Human limb (various)	60–120 MPa					McElhaney et al [1976]
Human calcaneal	55 MPa	9.5%				McElhaney et al [1976]
Human wrist	52–74 MPa	11–17%	3.2–3.3 MPa	1.5–3.5%		Loren & Lieber [1994]

References

Butler DL, Grood ES, Noyes FR et al. 1978. Biomechanics of ligaments and tendons. In RS Hutton (ed), Exercise and Sport Sciences Reviews, vol 6, pp 125–181, Franklin Institute Press.

Gans C. 1982. Fiber architecture and muscle function. Exer Sport Sci Rev 10:160.

Hill AV. 1938. The heat of shortening and the dynamic constants of muscle. Proc R Soc Lond [Biol] 126:136.

Lieber RL, Fazeli BM, Botte MJ. 1990. Architecture of selected wrist flexor and extensor muscles. J Hand Surg 15:244.

Lieber RL, Jacobson MD, Fazeli BM, et al. 1992. Architecture of selected muscles of the arm and forearm: Anatomy and implications for tendon transfer. J Hand Surg 17:787.

Wickiewicz TL, Roy RR, Powell PL, et al. 1983. Muscle architecture of the human lower limb. Clin Orthop Rel Res 179:275.

Zajac FE. 1989. Muscle and tendon: Properties, models, scaling and application to biomechanics and motor control. Crit Rev Biomed Eng 17:359.

25

Mechanics of Head/Neck

Albert I. King
Wayne State University

David C. Viano
Wayne State University

Injury is a major societal problem in the United States. Approximately 140,000 fatalities occur each year due to both intentional and unintentional injuries. Two-thirds of these are unintentional, and of these, about one-half are attributable to automotive-related injuries. In 1993, the estimated number of automotive-related fatalities dipped under 40,000 for the first time in the last three decades due to a continuing effort by both the industry and government to render vehicles safer in crash situations. However, for people under 40 years of age, automotive crashes, falls, and other unintentional injuries are the highest risks of fatality in the United States in comparison with all other causes.

The principal aim of impact biomechanics is the prevention of injury through environmental modification, such as the provision of an airbag for automotive occupants to protect them during a frontal crash. To achieve this aim effectively, it is necessary that workers in the field have a clear understanding of the *mechanisms of injury,* be able to describe the *mechanical response* of the tissues involved, have some basic information on *human tolerance* to impact, and be in possession of tools that can be used as *human surrogates* to assess a particular injury [Viano et al., 1989]. This chapter deals with the biomechanics of blunt impact injury to the head and neck.

25.1 Mechanisms of Injury

Head Injury Mechanisms

Among the more popular theories of brain injury due to blunt impact are changes in intracranial pressure and the development of shear strains in the brain. Positive pressure increases are found in the brain behind the site of impact on the skull. Rapid acceleration of the head, in-bending of the skull, and the propagation of a compressive pressure wave are proposed as mechanisms for the generation of intracranial compression that causes local contusion of brain tissue. At the contrecoup site, there is an opposite response in the form of a negative-pressure pulse that also causes bruising. It is not clear as to whether the injury is due to the negative pressure itself (tensile loading) or to a cavitation phenomenon similar to that seen on the surfaces of propellers of ships (compression load-

-8493-8346-3/95/$0.00+$.50
© 1995 by CRC Press, Inc.

ing). The pressure differential across the brain necessarily results in a pressure gradient that can give rise to shear strains developing within the deep structures of the brain. Furthermore, when the head is impacted, it not only translates but also rotates about the neck. It is postulated that the relative motion of the brain surface with respect to the rough inner surface of the skull results in surface contusions and the tearing of bridging veins between the brain and the dura mater, the principal membrane protecting the brain beneath the skull. Gennarelli [1983] has found that rotational acceleration of the head can cause a diffuse injury to the white matter of the brain in animal models, as evidenced by retraction balls developing along the axons of injured nerves. This injury was described by Strich [1961] as diffuse axonal injury (DAI) that she found in the white matter of autopsied human brains. Other researchers, including Lighthall et al. [1990], have been able to cause the development of DAI in the brain of an animal model (ferrets) by the application of direct impact to the brain without the associated head angular acceleration. Adams et al. [1986] indicated that DAI is the most important factor in severe head injury because it is irreversible and leads to incapacitation and dementia. It is postulated that DAI occurs as a result of the mechanical insult but cannot be detected by staining techniques at autopsy unless the patient survives the injury for at least several hours.

Neck Injury Mechanisms

The neck or the cervical spine is subjected to several forms of unique injuries that are not seen in the thoracolumbar spine. Injuries to the upper cervical spine, particularly at the atlanto-occipital joint, are considered to be more serious and life-threatening than those at the lower level. The atlanto-occipital joint can be dislocated either by an axial torsional load or a shear force applied in the anteroposterior direction, or vice versa. A large compression force can cause the arches of C1 to fracture, breaking it up into two or four sections. The odontoid process of C2 is also a vulnerable area. Extreme flexion of the neck is a common cause of odontoid fractures, and a large percentage of these injuries are related to automotive accidents [Pierce and Barr, 1983]. Fractures through the pars interarticularis of C2, commonly known as "hangman's fractures" in automotive collisions, are the result of a combined axial compression and extension (rearward bending) of the cervical spine. Impact of the forehead and face of unrestrained occupants with the windshield can result in this injury. Garfin and Rothman [1983] discussed this injury in relation to hanging and traced the history of this mode of execution. It was estimated by a British judiciary committee that the energy required to cause a hangman's fracture was 1708 N · m (1260 ft · lb).

In automotive-type accidents, the loading on the neck due to head contact forces is usually a combination of an axial or shear load with bending. Bending loads are almost always present, and the degree of axial or shear force depends on the location and direction of the contact force. For impacts near the crown of the head, compressive forces predominate. If the impact is principally in the transverse plane, there is less compression and more shear. Bending modes are infinite in number because the impact can come from any angle around the head. To limit the scope of the discussion, the following injury modes are considered: tension-flexion, tension-extension, compression-flexion and compression-extension in the midsagittal plane and lateral bending.

Tension-Flexion Injuries.   Forces resulting from inertial loading of the head-neck system can result in flexion of the cervical spine while it is being subjected to a tensile force. In experimental impacts of restrained subjects undergoing forward deceleration, Thomas and Jessop [1983] reported atlanto-occipital separation and C1–C2 separation occurring in subhuman primates at 120 *g*. Similar injuries in human cadavers were found at 34 to 38 *g* by Cheng et al. [1982], who used a preinflated driver airbag system that restrained the thorax but allowed the head and neck to rotate over the bag.

Tension-Extension Injuries.   The most common type of injury due to combined tension and extension of the cervical spine is the "whiplash" syndrome. However, a large majority of such injuries involve the soft tissues of the neck, and the pain is believed to reside in the joint capsules of the articular facets of the cervical vertebrae [Lord et al., 1993]. In severe cases, teardrop fractures of the anterosuperior aspect of the vertebral body can occur. Alternately, separation of the anterior aspect of the disk from the vertebral endplate is known to occur. More severe injuries occur when the chin impacts the instrument panel or when the forehead impacts the windshield. In both cases, the head rotates rearward and applies a tensile and bending load on the neck. In the case of windshield impact by the forehead, hangman's fracture of C2 can occur. Garfin and Rothman [1983] suggested that it is caused by spinal extension combined with compression on the lamina of C2, causing the pars to fracture.

Compression-Flexion Injuries. When a force is applied to the posterosuperior quadrant of the head or when a crown impact is administered while the head is in flexion, the neck is subjected to a combined load of axial compression and forward bending. Anterior wedge fractures of vertebral bodies are commonly seen, but with increased load, burst fractures and fracture-dislocations of the facets can result. The latter two conditions are unstable and tend to disrupt or injure the spinal cord, and the extent of the injury depends on the penetration of the vertebral body or its fragments into the spinal canal. Recent experiments by Pintar et al. [1989, 1990] indicate that burst fractures of lower cervical vertebrae can be reproduced in cadaveric specimens by a crown impact to a flexed cervical spine. A study by Nightingale et al. [1993] showed that fracture-dislocations of the cervical spine occur very early in the impact event (within the first 10 ms) and that the subsequent motion of the head or bending of the cervical spine cannot be used as a reliable indicator of the mechanism of injury.

Compression-Extension Injuries. Frontal impacts to the head with the neck in extension will cause compression-extension injuries. These involve the fracture of one or more spinous processes and, possibly, symmetrical lesions of the pedicles, facets, and laminae. If there is a fracture-dislocation, the inferior facet of the upper vertebra is displaced posteriorly and upward and appears to be more horizontal than normal on x-ray.

Injuries Involving Lateral Bending. If the applied force or inertial load on the head has a significant component out of the midsagittal plane, the neck will be subjected to lateral or oblique along with axial and shear loading. The injuries characteristic of lateral bending are lateral wedge fractures of the vertebral body and fractures to the posterior elements on one side of the vertebral column.

Whenever there is lateral or oblique bending, there is the possibility of twisting the neck. The associated torsional loads may be responsible for unilateral facet dislocations or unilateral locked facets [Moffat et al., 1978]. However, the authors postulated that pure torsional loads on the neck are rarely encountered in automotive accidents. It was shown by Wismans and Spenny [1983] that, in a purely lateral impact, the head rotated axially about the cervical axis while it translated laterally and vertically and rotated about an anteroposterior axis. These responses were obtained from lateral impact tests performed by the Naval Biodynamics Laboratory on human subjects who were fully restrained at and below the shoulders.

25.2 Mechanical Response

Mechanical Response of the Head

A large number of cadaveric studies on blunt head impact has been carried out over the past 50 years. The head was impacted by rigid and padded surfaces and by impactors of varying shapes to simulate flat surfaces and knobs encountered in the automotive environment. In general, the impact responses were described in terms of head acceleration or impact force. Both these responses are dependent on a variety of factors, including the inertial properties of the head and surface impacted by the head. In this section, the inertial properties of the head will be described, and response data for head impact against a flat, rigid surface will be provided. It should be noted that while response data against surfaces with a variety of shapes and stiffnesses are of interest, the only generally applicable and reproducible data are those of impacts to flat, rigid surfaces.

Inertial Properties of the Head.   There are several sources of data on the inertial properties of the human head. Mass data are shown in Table 25.1, while mass moment of inertial data can be found in Table 25.2. The data by Walker et al. [1973] shown in Table 25.1 were analyzed by Hubbard and McLeod [1974], who found that 16 of the 20 heads used by Walker et al. [1973] had dimensions that were close to those of the average male and provided the data for the average body and head mass. Similarly, Hubbard and McLeod [1974] analyzed the head-mass data of Hodgson and Thomas [1971] and Hodgson et al. [1972] for 11 heads, the dimensions of which were consistent with those of a fiftieth percentile male head and found an average value of 4.54 kg, as shown in Table 25.1. The data of Reynolds et al. [1975] were obtained from 6 cadavers that were of low body weight. The Human Mechanical Response Task Force (HMRTF) of the Society of Automotive Engineers (SAE) made an adjustment for the body and head mass, and the results are shown just below the original data of Reynolds et al. [1975] in Table 25.1. The data of Beier et al. [1980] are based on their original study. The studies of McConville et al. [1980] and Robbins [1983] were derived from anthropometric measurement of living subjects. In these studies, head mass was estimated from volumetric measurements and a previously determined value of the specific gravity of the head—1.097. For the average values of the mass moment of inertia, shown in Table 25.2, the origin of the coordinate axes is at the center of gravity (cg) of the head, and the x axis is in the posteroanterior direction, while the z axis is in the inferosuperior direction and the y axis is in a lateral direction. The adjustments made in Table 25.1 are applicable to Table 25.2 as well.

Cranial Impact Response.   Impact response of the head against a flat, rigid surface was obtained by Hodgson and Thomas [1973, 1975], who performed a series of drop tests using embalmed cadavers. The responses in terms of peak force and acceleration are shown in Figs. 25.1 and 25.2, respectively, as a function of an equivalent free-fall drop height. Details of adjustments made to the original data are described by Prasad et al. [1985]. It should be noted that the data shown were from the frontal, lateral, and occipital directions and that there was a large scatter in the peak values. For this reason, the data were pooled, and individual data points were not shown.

The difficulty with acceleration measurements in head impact is twofold. The head is not a rigid body, and accelerometers cannot be mounted at the center of gravity of the head. The center of gravity acceleration can be computed if head angular acceleration is measured, but the variation in skull stiffness cannot be corrected for easily. It is recommended that in all future head-impact studies, head angular acceleration be measured. Several methods for measuring this parameter have been

TABLE 25.1   Average Male Head Mass

Reference	No. of Subjects	Average Body Mass (kg)	Average Head Mass (kg)
Walker et al., 1973	16	67.1	4.49
Hubbard and McLeod, 1974	11		4.54
Reynolds et al., 1975	6	65.2	3.98
Adjusted per HMRTF	6	76.9	4.69
Beier et al., 1980	19	74.7	4.32
McConville et al., 1980	31	77.5	4.55*
Robbins, 1983	25	76.7	4.54†

*Based on adjusted head volume of 95% of the reported head volume (4396 cm³) and a head specific gravity of 1.097.

† Based on an estimated head volume of 4137 cm³ and a head specific gravity of 1.097.

TABLE 25.2 Average Mass Moments of Inertia* of the Male Head
$(\text{kg} \cdot \text{m}^2 \times 10^{-3})$

Reference	I_{xx}	I_{yy}	I_{zz}
Walker et al., 1973		23.3	
Hubbard and McLeod, 1974	17.4	16.4	20.3
Adjusted per HMRTF	22.6	21.3	26.3
Beier et al., 1980 (16 male subjects only)	20.7	22.6	14.9
McConville et al., 1980	20.4	23.2	15.1
Adjusted by sp. gr. 1.097	22.4	25.5	16.6
Robbins, 1983	20.0	22.2	14.5
Adjusted by sp. gr. 1.097	22.0	24.2	15.9

*The mass moments of inertia given are about the x, y, or z anatomic axes through the center of gravity of the head.

proposed. At present, the most reliable method appears to be that proposed by Padgaonkar et al. [1975] using an array of 9 linear accelerometers arranged in a 3-2-2-2 cluster.

The data presented in this section do not refer to the response of the brain during an injury-producing impact. For intact heads, the motion of the brain inside the skull has not been studied exhaustively. There is evidence that relative motion of the brain with respect to the skull occurs [Nusholtz et al., 1984], particularly during angular acceleration of the head. However, this motion does not fully explain injuries seen in the center of the brain and in the brainstem. More research is needed to explore the mechanical response of the brain to both linear and angular acceleration and to relate this response to observed injuries, such as diffuse axonal injury.

Mechanical Response of the Neck

The mechanical response of the cervical spine was studied by Mertz and Patrick [1967, 1971], Patrick and Chou [1976], Schneider et al. [1975], and Ewing et al. [1978]. Mertz et al. [1973] quantified the response in terms of rotation of the head relative to the torso as a function of bending moment at the occipital condyles. Loading corridors were obtained for flexion and extension, as shown in Figs. 25.3 and 25.4. An exacting definition of the impact environments to be used in evaluating dummy necks relative to the loading corridors illustrated in these figures is included in SAE J1460 [1985]. It should be noted that the primary basis for these curves is volunteer data and that the extension of these corridors to dummy tests in the injury-producing range is somewhat surprising. Static and dynamic lateral response data were provided by Patrick and Chou [1976]. A response envelope for lateral flexion is shown in Fig. 25.5. A limited amount of the voluminous data obtained by Ewing et al. [1978] (six runs) was analyzed by Wismans and Spenny [1983, 1984] for lateral and sagittal flexion. The rotations were represented in three dimensions by a rigid link of fixed length pivoted at T1 at the bottom and within the head at the top. In terms of torque at the occipital condyles and head rotation, the results fell within the corridor for forward and lateral flexion shown in Figs. 25.3 and 25.5, respectively.

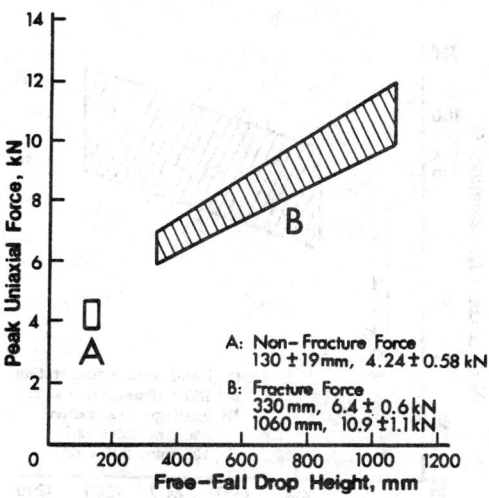

A: Non–Fracture Force
130 ±19mm, 4.24 ±0.58 kN

B: Fracture Force
330 mm, 6.4 ± 0.6kN
1060 mm, 10.9 ±1.1kN

FIGURE 25.1 Impact response of the head in terms of peak force.

25.3 Regional Tolerance of the Head and Neck to Blunt Impact

Regional Tolerance of the Head

The most commonly measured parameter for head injury is acceleration. It is therefore natural to express human tolerance to injury in terms of head acceleration. The first known tolerance criterion is the Wayne State Tolerance Curve, proposed by Lissner et al. [1960] and subsequently modified by Patrick et al. [1965] by the addition of animal and volunteer data to the original cadaveric data. The modified curve is shown in Fig. 25.6. The head can withstand higher accelerations for shorter durations, and any exposure above the curve is injurious. When this curve is plotted on logarithmic paper, it becomes a straight line with a slope of -2.5. This slope was used as an exponent by Gadd [1961] in his proposed severity index, now known as the *Gadd Severity Index (GSI)*:

$$ \text{GSI} = \int_0^T a^{2.5} \, dt $$

where a = instantaneous acceleration of the head
T = duration of the pulse

If the integrated value exceeds 1000, a severe injury will result. A modified form of the GSI, now known as the *Head Injury Criterion (HIC)*, was proposed by Versace [1970] to identify the most damaging part of the acceleration pulse by finding the maximum value of the following integral:

$$ \text{HIC} = (t_2 - t_1) \left[(t_2 - t_1)^{-1} \int_{t_1}^{t_2} a(t) \, dt \right]_{\max}^{2.5} $$

where $a(t)$ = resultant instantaneous acceleration of the head
$t_2 - t_1$ = time interval over which HIC is a maximum

A severe but not life-threatening injury would have occurred if the HIC reached or exceeded 1000. Subsequently, Prasad and Mertz [1985] proposed a probabilistic method of assessing head injury and developed the curve shown in Fig. 25.7. At an HIC of 1000, approximately 16% of the population would sustain a severe to fatal injury. It is apparent that this criterion is useful in automotive safety design and in the design of protective equipment for the head, such as football and bicycle helmets. However, there is another school of thought that believes in the injurious potential of angular acceleration in its ability to cause cerebral contusion of the brain surface and rupture of the parasagittal bridging veins between the brain and the dura mater. A proposed limit for angular acceleration is 4500 rad/s², based on a mathematical model developed by Lowenhielm [1974]. This limit has not received universal acceptance. Many other criteria have been proposed, but HIC is the current criterion for Federal Motor Vehicle Safety Standard (FMVSS) 214, and attempts to replace it have so far been unsuccessful.

Regional Tolerance of the Neck

Currently, there are no tolerance values for the neck for the various injury modes. This is not due to a lack of data but rather to the many in-

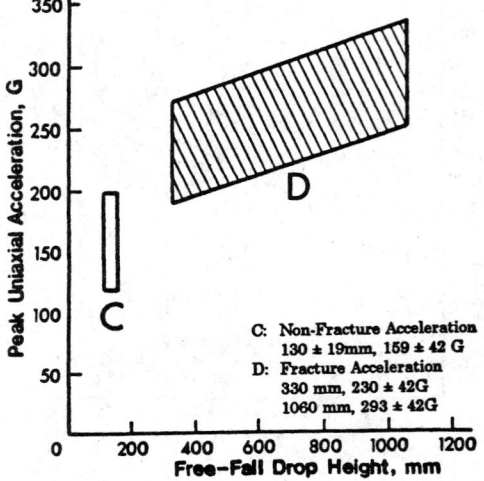

FIGURE 25.2   Impact response of the head in terms of peak acceleration.

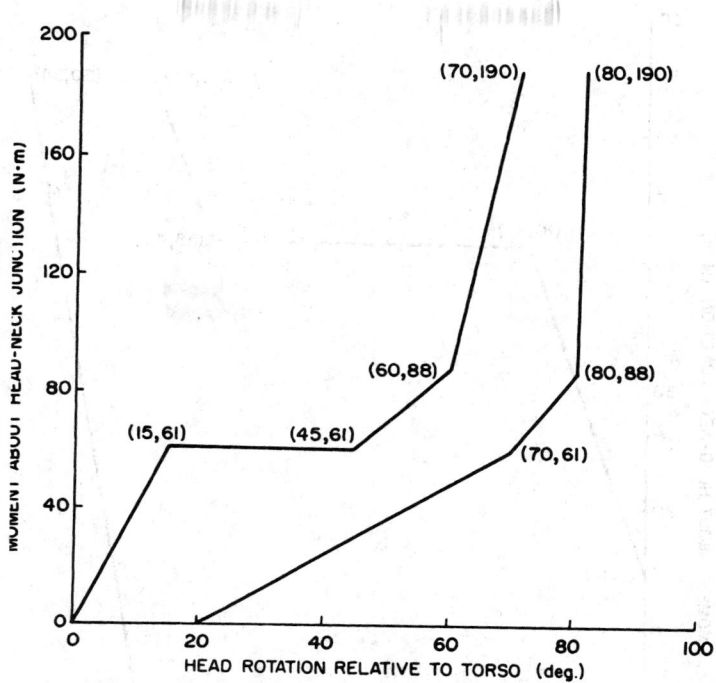

FIGURE 25.3 Loading corridor for neck flexion (forward bending).

jury mechanisms and several levels of injury severity, ranging from life-threatening injuries to the spinal cord to minor soft-tissue injuries that cannot be identified on radiographic or magnetic scans. It is likely that a combined criterion of axial load and bending moment about one or more axes will be adopted as a future FMVSS.

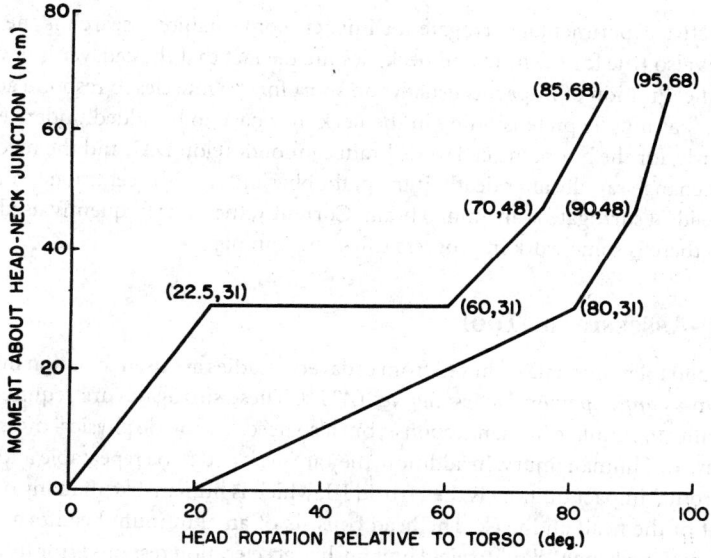

FIGURE 25.4 Loading corridor for neck extension (rearward bending).

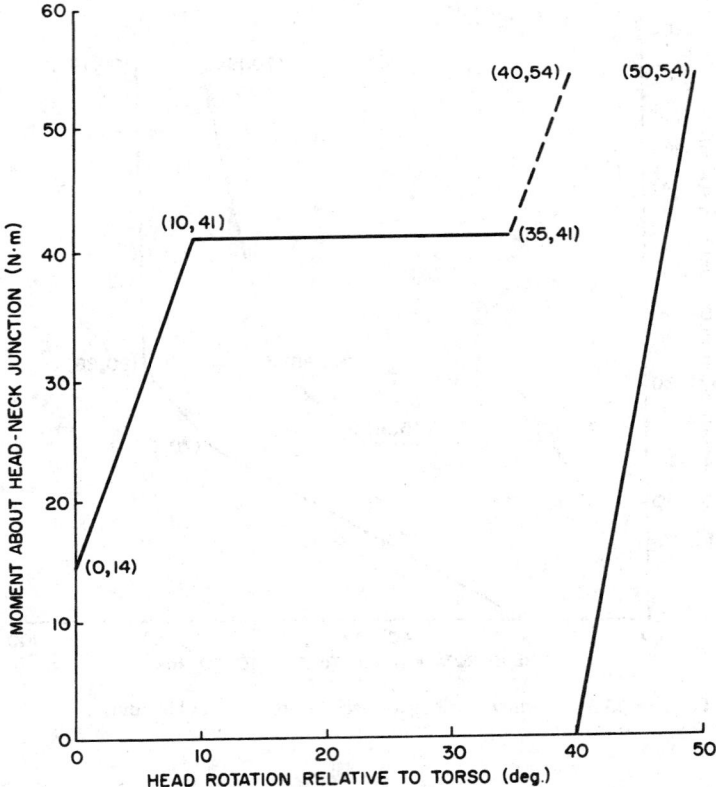

FIGURE 25.5   Lateral flexion response envelope.

25.4   Human Surrogates of the Head and Neck

The Experimental Surrogate

The most effective experimental surrogate for impact biomechanics research is the unembalmed cadaver. This is also true for the head and neck, despite the fact that the cadaver is devoid of muscle tone because the duration of impact is usually too short for the muscles to respond adequately. It is true, however, that muscle pretensioning in the neck may have to be added under certain circumstances. Similarly, for the brain, the cadaveric brain cannot develop DAI, and the mechanical properties of brain change rapidly after death. If the pathophysiology of the central nervous system is to be studied, the ideal surrogate is an animal brain. Currently, the rat is frequently used as the animal of choice, and there is some work in progress using the minipig.

The Injury-Assessment Tool

The response and tolerance data acquired from cadaveric studies are used to design human-like surrogates, known as *anthropomorphic test devices (ATD)*. These surrogates are required to have biofidelity, the ability to simulate human response, but also need to provide physical measurements that are representative of human injury. In addition, they are designed to be repeatable and reproducible. The current frontal impact dummy is the Hybrid III, which is human-like in many of its responses, including that of the head and neck. The head consists of an aluminum headform covered by an appropriately designed vinyl "skin" to yield human-like acceleration responses for frontal and lateral

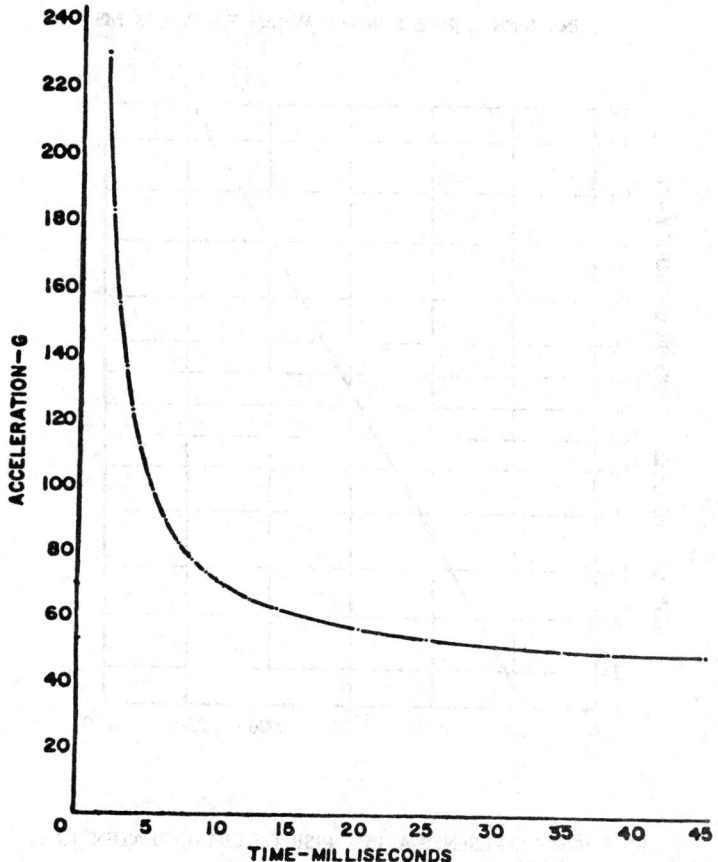

FIGURE 25.6   The Wayne State Tolerance Curve for head injury.

impacts against a flat, rigid surface. Two-dimensional physical models of the brain were proposed by Margulies et al. [1990] using a silicone gel in which preinscribed grid lines would deform under angular acceleration. No injury criterion is associated with this gel model.

The dummy neck was designed to yield responses in flexion and extension that would fit within the corridors shown in Figs. 25.3 and 25.4. The principal function of the dummy neck is to place the head in the approximate position of a human head in the same impact involving a human occupant.

Computer Models

Models of head impact first appeared over 50 years ago [Holbourn, 1943]. Extensive reviews of such models were made by King and Chou [1977] and Hardy et al. [1994]. The use of the finite-element method (FEM) to simulate the various components of the head appears to be the most effective and popular means of modeling brain response. Despite the large numbers of nodes and elements used, the models are still not detailed enough to predict the location of DAI development following a given impact. The research is also hampered by the limited amount of animal DAI data currently available.

A large number of neck and spinal models also have been developed over the past four decades. A recent paper by Kleinberger [1993] provides a brief and incomplete review of these models. However, the method of choice for modeling the response of the neck is the finite-element method, principally because of the complex geometry of the vertebral components and the interaction of several different materials. A fully validated model for impact response is still not available.

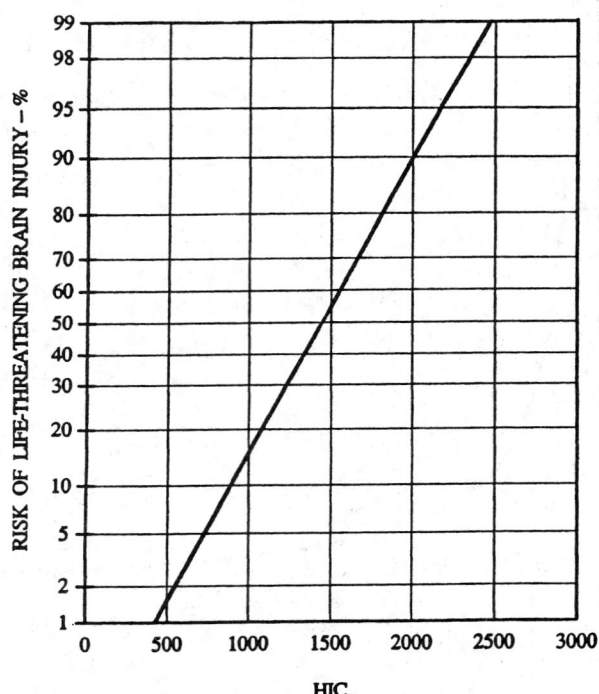

INJURY RISK CURVE FOR HIC WHEN $T_2 - T_1 \leq 15$ MS

FIGURE 25.7   Head injury risk curve based on HIC.

HIC = 1000 REPRESENTS A 15% RISK OF LIFE-THREATENING BRAIN INJURY IF $(T_2 - T_1) \leq 15$ MS.

References

Adams JH, Doyle D, Graham DI, et al. 1986. Gliding contusions in nonmissile head injury in humans. Arch Pathol Lab Med 110:485.

Beier G, Schuller E, Schuck M, et al. 1980. Center of gravity and moments of inertia of human head. In Proceedings of the 5th International Conference on the Biokinetics of Impacts, pp 218–228.

Cheng R, Yang KH, Levine RS, et al. 1982. Injuries to the cervical spine caused by a distributed frontal load to the chest. In Proceedings of the 26th Stapp Car Crash Conference, pp 1–40.

Ewing CL, Thomas DJ, Lustick L, et al. 1978. Effect of initial position on the human head and neck response to +Y impact acceleration. In Proceedings of the 22nd Stapp Car Crash Conference, pp 101–138.

Gadd CW. 1961. Criteria for injury potential. In Impact Acceleration Stress Symposium, National Research Council Publication No. 977, pp 141–144. Washington, National Academy of Sciences.

Garfin SR, Rothman RH. 1983. Traumatic spondylolisthesis of the axis (Hangman's fracture). In RW Baily (ed), The Cervical Spine, pp 223–232. Philadelphia, Lippincott.

Gennarelli TA. 1983. Head injuries in man and experimental animals: Clinical aspects. Acta Neurochir Suppl 32:1.

Hardy WN, Khalil TB, King AI. 1994. Literature review of head injury biomechanics. Int J Impact Engg 15:561–586.

Hodgson VR, Mason MW, Thomas LM. 1972. In Proceedings of the 16th Stapp Car Crash Conference, pp 1–13.

Hodgson VR, Thomas LM. 1971. Comparison of head acceleration injury indices in cadaver skull fracture. In Proceedings of 15th Stapp Car Crash Conference, pp 190–206.

Hodgson VR, Thomas LM. 1973. Breaking Strength of the Human Skull versus Impact Surface Curvature. Detroit, Wayne State University.

Hodgson VR, Thomas LM. 1975. Head Impact Response. Warrendale, Pa, Vehicle Research Institute, Society of Automotive Engineers.

Holbourn AHS. 1943. Mechanics of head injury. Lancet 2:438.

Hubbard RP, McLeod DG. 1974. Definition and development of a crash dummy head. In Proceedings of the 18th Stapp Car Crash Conference, pp 599–628.

King AI, Chou C. 1977. Mathematical modelling, simulation and experimental testing of biomechanical system crash response. J Biomech 9:310.

Kleinberger M. 1993. Application of finite element techniques to the study of cervical spine mechanics. In Proceedings of the 37th Stapp Car Crash Conference, pp 261–272.

Lighthall JW, Goshgarian HG, Pinderski CR. 1990. Characterization of axonal injury produced by controlled cortical impact. J Neurotrauma 7(2):65.

Lissner HR, Lebow M, Evans FG. 1960. Experimental studies on the relation between acceleration and intracranial pressure changes in man. Surg Gynecol Obstet 111:329.

Lord S, Barnsley L, Bogduk N. 1993. Cervical zygapophyseal joint pain in whiplash. In RW Teasell and AP Shapiro (eds), Cervical Flexion-Extension/Whiplash Injuries, pp 355–372. Philadelphia, Hanley & Belfus.

Lowenhielm P. 1975. Mathematical simulation of gliding contusions. J Biomech 8:351.

Margulies SS, Thibault LE, Gennarelli TA. 1990. Physical model simulation of brain injury in the primate. J Biomech 23:823.

McConville JT, Churchill TD, Kaleps I, et al. 1980. Anthropometric Relationships of Body and Body Segment Moments of Inertia, AMRL-TR-80-119. Wright-Patterson AFB, Ohio, Aerospace Medical Research Lab.

Mertz HJ, Patrick LM. 1967. Investigation of the kinematics and kinetics of whiplash. In Proceedings of the 11th Stapp Car Crash Conference, pp 267–317.

Mertz HJ, Patrick LM. 1971. Strength and response of the human neck. In Proceedings of the 15th Stapp Car Crash Conference, pp 207–255.

Mertz HJ, Neathery RF, Culver CC. 1973. Performance requirements and characteristics of mechanical necks. In WF King and HJ Mertz (eds), Human Impact Response: Measurement and Simulations, pp 263–288. New York, Plenum Press.

Moffat EA, Siegel AW, Huelke DF. 1978. The biomechanics of automotive cervical fractures. In Proceedings of the 22nd Conference of American Association for Automotive Medicine, pp 151–168.

Nightingale RW, McElhaney JH, Best TM, et al. 1993. In Proceedings of the 39th Meeting of the Orthopedic Research Society, p 233.

Nuscholtz G, Lux P, Kaiker P, Janicki MA. 1984. Head impact response: Skull deformation and angular accelerations. In Proceedings of the 28th Stapp Car Crash Conference, pp 41–74.

Padgaonkar AJ, Krieger KW, King AI. 1975. Measurement of angular acceleration of a rigid body using linear accelerometers. J Appl Mech 42:552.

Patrick LM, Lissner HR, Gurdjian ES. 1965. Survival by design: Head protection. In Proceedings of the 7th Stapp Car Crash Conference, pp 483–499.

Patrick LM, Chou C. 1976. Response of the Human Neck in Flexion, Extension, and Lateral Flexion, Vehicle Research Institute Report No. VRI-7-3. Warrendale, Pa, Society of Automotive Engineers.

Pierce DA, Barr JS. 1983. Fractures and dislocations at the base of the skull and upper spine. In RW Baily (ed), The Cervical Spine, pp 196–206. Philadelphia, Lippincott.

Pintar FA, Yoganandan N, Sances A Jr, et al. 1989. Kinematic and anatomical analysis of the human cervical spinal column under axial loading. In Proceedings of the 33rd Stapp Car Crash Conference, pp 191–214.

Pintar FA, Sances A Jr, Yoganandan N, et al. 1990. Biodynamics of the total human cadaveric spine. In Proceedings of the 34th Stapp Car Crash Conference, pp 55–72.

Prasad P, Melvin JW, Huelke DF, et al. 1985. Head. In Review of Biomechanical Impact Response and Injury in the Automotive Environment: Phase 1 Task B Report: Advanced Anthropomorphic Test Device Development Program, DOT Report No. DOT HS 807 042. Ann Arbor, University of Michigan.

Prasad P, Mertz HJ. 1985. The Position of the United States Delegation to the ISO Working Group 6 on the Use of HIC in the Automotive Environment, SAE Paper No. 851246. Warrendale, Pa, Society of Automotive Engineers.

Reynolds HM, Clauser CE, McConville J, et al. 1975. Mass Distribution Properties of the Male Cadaver, SAE Paper No. 750424. Warrendale, Pa, Society of Automotive Engineers.

Robbins DH. 1983. Development of Anthropometrically Based Design Specifications for an Advanced Adult Anthropomorphic Dummy Family, vol 2: Anthropometric Specifications for a Midsized Male Dummy, Report No. UMTRI 83-53-2. Ann Arbor, University of Michigan Transportation Research Institute.

Schneider LW, Foust DR, Bowman BM, et al. 1975. Biomechanical properties of the human neck in lateral flexion. In Proceedings of the 19th Stapp Car Crash Conference, pp. 455–486.

Society of Automotive Engineers, Human Mechanical Response Task Force. 1985. Human Mechanical Response Characteristics, SAE J1460. Warrendale, Pa, Society of Automotive Engineers.

Strich SJ. 1961. Shearing of nerve fibres as a cause of brain damage due to head injury. Lancet 2:443.

Thomas DJ, Jessop ME. 1983. Experimental head and neck injury. In CL Ewing et al. (eds), Impact Injury of the Head and Spine, pp 177–217. Springfield, Ill, Charles C Thomas.

Versace J. 1970. A review of the severity index. In Proceedings of the 15th Stapp Car Crash Conference, pp 771–796.

Viano DC, King AI, Melvin JW, Weber K. 1989. Injury biomechanics research: An essential element in the prevention of trauma. J Biomech 21:403.

Walker LB Jr, Harris EH, Pontius UR. 1973. Mass, volume, center of mass, and mass moment of inertia of head and neck of human body. In Proceedings of the 17th Stapp Car Crash Conference, pp 525–537.

Wismans J, Spenny DH. 1983. Performance requirements for mechanical necks in lateral flexion. In Proceedings of 27th Stapp Car Crash Conference, pp 137–148.

Wismans J, Spenny DH. 1984. Head-neck response in frontal flexion. In Proceedings of the 28th Stapp Car Crash Conference, pp 161–171.

26

Biomechanics of Chest and Abdomen Impact

David C. Viano
Wayne State University

Albert I. King
Wayne State University

Injury is caused by energy transfer to the body by an impacting object. It occurs when the body is struck by a blunt object, such as a vehicle instrument panel or side interior, and sufficient force is concentrated on the chest or abdomen. The risk of injury is influenced by the object's shape, stiffness, point of contact, and orientation. It can be reduced by energy-absorbing padding or crushable materials, which allow the surfaces in contact to deform, extend the duration of impact, and reduce loads. The torso is viscoelastic, so reaction force substantially increases with the speed of body deformation.

The biomechanical response of the body has three components: (1) inertial resistance by acceleration of body masses, (2) elastic resistance by compression of stiff structures and tissues, and (3) viscous resistance by rate-dependent properties of tissue. For low impact speeds, the elastic stiffness protects from crush injuries, whereas, for high rates of body deformation, the inertial and viscous properties determine the force developed and limit deformation. The risk of skeletal and internal organ injury relates to energy stored or absorbed by the elastic and viscous properties. The reaction load is related to these responses and inertial resistance of body masses that combine to resist deformation and prevent injury. When tissues are deformed beyond their recoverable limit, injuries result.

26.1 Chest and Abdomen Injury Mechanisms

The primary mechanism of chest and abdomen injury is compression of the body at high rates of loading. This causes deformation and stretching of internal organs and vessels. When the compression of the torso exceeds the ribcage tolerance, fractures occur and internal organs and vessels can be contused or ruptured. In some chest impacts, however, internal injury occurs without skeletal damage. This can happen during high-speed loading. It is due to the viscous or rate-sensitive nature of human tissue as biomechanical responses differ for low- and high-speed impact.

When organs or vessels are loaded slowly, the input energy is absorbed gradually through deformation, which is resisted by elastic properties and pressure buildup in tissue. When loaded rapidly, reaction force is proportional to the speed of tissue deformation as the viscous properties of the body resist deformation and provide a natural protection from impact. However, there is also a consider-

0-8493-8346-3/95/$0.00+$.50
© 1995 by CRC Press, Inc.

able inertial component to the reaction force. In this case, the body develops high internal pressure, and injuries can occur before the ribs deflect much. The ability of an organ or other biologic system to absorb impact energy without failure is called *tolerance*.

If an artery is stretched beyond its tensile strength, the tissue will tear. Organs and vessels can be stretched in different ways, which result in different types of injury. Motion of the heart during chest compression stretches the aorta along its axis from points of tethering in the body. This elongation generally leads to a transverse laceration when the strain limit is exceeded. In contrast, an increase in vascular pressure dilates the vessel and produces biaxial strain that is larger in the transverse than axial direction. If pressure rises beyond the vessel's limit, it will burst. For severe impacts, intraaortic pressure exceeds 500 to 1000 mmHg, which is a significant, nonphysiologic level but is tolerable for short durations. When laceration occurs, the predominant mode of aortic failure is axial, so the combined effects of stretch and internal pressure contribute to injury. Chest impact also compresses the ribcage, causing tensile strain on the outer surface of the ribs. As compression increases, the risk of rib fracture increases. In both cases, the mechanism of injury is tissue deformation.

The abdomen is more vulnerable to injury than the chest because there is little bony structure below the ribcage to protect internal organs in front and lateral impacts. Blunt impact of the upper abdomen can compress and injure the liver and spleen before significant whole-body motion occurs. In the liver, compression increases intrahepatic pressure and generates tensile or shear strains. If the tissue is sufficiently deformed, laceration of the major hepatic vessels can result in hemoperitoneum. Abdominal deformation also causes lobes of the liver to move relative to each other, stretching and shearing the vascular attachment at the hilar region.

Effective occupant restraints, safety systems, and protective equipment not only spread impact energy over the strongest body structures but also reduce contact velocity between the body and the impacted surface or object. The design of protective systems is aided by an understanding of injury mechanisms, quantification of human tolerance levels, and development of numerical relationships between measurable engineering parameters, such as force, acceleration, or deformation, and injury. These relationships are called *injury criteria*.

26.2 Injury Tolerance Criteria

Acceleration Injury

Stapp [1970] conducted rocket-sled experiments on belt-restraint systems and achieved a substantial human tolerance to long-duration, whole-body acceleration. Safety belts protected military personnel exposed to rapid but sustained acceleration. The experiments enabled Eiband [1959] to show in Fig. 26.1 that the tolerance to whole-body acceleration increased as the exposure duration decreased. This linked human tolerance and acceleration for exposures of 2- to 1000-ms duration. The tolerance data are based on average sled acceleration rather than the acceleration of the volunteer subject, which would be higher due to compliance of the restraint system. Even with this limitation, the data provide useful early guidelines for the development of military and civilian restraint systems.

More recent side impact tests have led to other tolerance formulas for chest injury. Morgan et al. [1986] evaluated rigid, side-wall cadaver tests and developed TTI, a thoracic trauma index, which is the average rib and spine acceleration. TTI limits human tolerance to 85 to 90g in vehicle crash tests. Better injury assessment was achieved by Cavanaugh [1993] using average spinal acceleration (ASA), which is the average slope of the integral of spinal acceleration. ASA is the rate of momentum transfer during side impact, and a value of 30g is proposed. In most cases, the torso can withstand 60 to 80g peak whole-body acceleration by a well-distributed load.

Force Injury

Whole-body tolerance is related to Newton's second law of motion, where acceleration of a rigid mass is proportional to the force acting on it, or $F = ma$. While the human body is not a rigid mass,

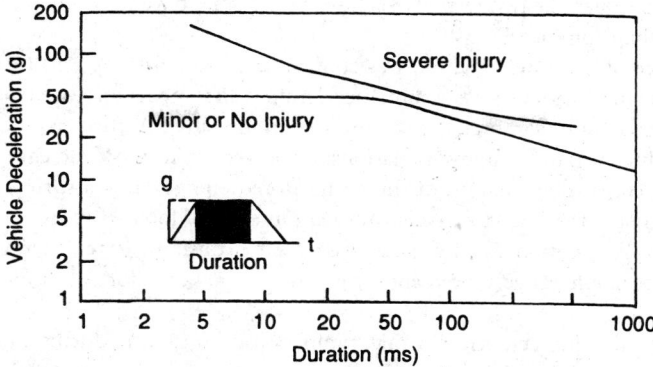

FIGURE 26.1 Whole-body human tolerance to vehicle acceleration based on impact duration. (Redrawn from Eiband [1959] and from Viano [1988], with permission.)

a well-distributed restraint system allows the torso to respond as though it were fairly rigid when load is applied through the shoulder and pelvis. The greater the acceleration, the greater is the force and risk of injury. For a high-speed frontal crash, a restrained occupant can experience 60g acceleration. For a body mass of 76 kg, the inertial load is 44.7 kN (10,000 lb) and is tolerable if distributed over strong skeletal elements.

The ability to withstand high acceleration for short durations implies that tolerance is related to momentum transfer, because an equivalent change in velocity can be achieved by increasing the acceleration and decreasing its duration, since $\Delta V = a\Delta t$. The implication for occupant protection systems is that the risk of injury can be decreased if the crash deceleration is extended over a greater period of time. For occupant restraint in 25 ms, a velocity change of 14.7 m/s (32.7 mi/h) occurs with 60g whole-body acceleration. This duration can be achieved by crushable vehicle structures and occupant restraints.

Prior to the widespread use of safety belts, safety engineers needed information on the tolerance of the chest to design energy-absorbing instrument panels and steering systems. The concept was to limit impact force below human tolerance by crushable materials and structures. Using the highest practical crush force, safety was extended to the greatest severity of vehicle crashes. GM Research and Wayne State University collaborated on the development of the first crash sled that was used to simulate progressively more severe frontal impacts. Embalmed human cadavers were exposed to head, chest, and knee impact on 15-cm-diameter (6-in) load cells until bone fracture was observed on x-ray. Patrick [1965] demonstrated that blunt chest loading of 3.3 kN (740 lb) could be tolerated with minimal risk of serious injury. This is a pressure of 187 kPa. Gadd and Patrick [1968] later found a tolerance of 8.0 kN (1800 lb) if the load was distributed over the shoulders and chest by a properly designed steering wheel and column. Cavanaugh [1993] found that side-impact tolerance is similar to frontal tolerance and that shoulder contact is also an important load path.

Compression Injury

High-speed films of cadaver impacts show that whole-body acceleration does not describe torso impact biomechanics. Tolerance of the chest and abdomen must consider body deformation. Force acting on the body causes two simultaneous responses: (1) compression of the compliant structures of the torso and (2) acceleration of body masses. The previously neglected mechanism of injury was compression, which causes the sternum to displace toward the spine as ribs bend and possibly fracture. Acceleration and force per se are not sufficient indicators of impact tolerance because they cannot discriminate between the two responses. Numerous studies have shown that acceleration is less related to injury than compression.

The importance of chest deformation was confirmed by Kroell [1971, 1974] in blunt thoracic impacts of unembalmed cadavers. Peak spinal acceleration and impact force were poorer injury predictors than the maximum compression of the chest, as measured by the percentage change in the anteroposterior thickness of the body. A relationship between injury risk and compression involves energy stored by elastic deformation of the body. Stored energy E_s by a spring representing the ribcage and soft tissues is related to the displacement integral of force: $E_s = \int F \, dx$. Force in a spring is proportional to deformation: $F = kx$, where k is a spring constant. Stored energy is $E_s = k\int x \, dx = 0.5kx^2$. Over a reasonable range, stored energy is proportional to deformation or compression, so $E_s \approx C$.

Tests with human volunteers showed that compression up to 20% during moderate-duration loading was fully reversible. Cadaver impacts with compression greater than 20% showed (Fig. 26.2a) an increase in rib fractures and internal organ injury as the compression increased to 40%. The deflection tolerance was originally set at 8.8 cm (3.5 in) for moderate but recoverable injury. This represents 39% compression. However, at this level of compression, multiple rib fractures and serious injury can occur, so a more conservative tolerance of 34% is used to avert the possibility of flail chest (Fig. 26.2b). This reduces the risk of direct loading on the heart, lungs, and internal organs by a loss of the protective function of the ribcage.

Viscous Injury

The velocity of body deformation is an important factor in impact injury. For example, when a fluid-filled organ is compressed slowly, energy can be absorbed by tissue deformation without damage. When loaded rapidly, the organ cannot deform fast enough, and rupture may occur without significant change in shape, even though the load is substantially higher than for the slow-loading condition.

The viscoelastic behavior of soft tissues is important when the velocity of deformation exceeds 3 m/s. For lower speeds, such as in slow crushing loads or for a belt-restrained occupant in a frontal crash, tissue compression is limited by elastic properties resisting skeletal and internal organ injury. For higher speeds of deformation, such as occupant loading by the door in a side impact or for an

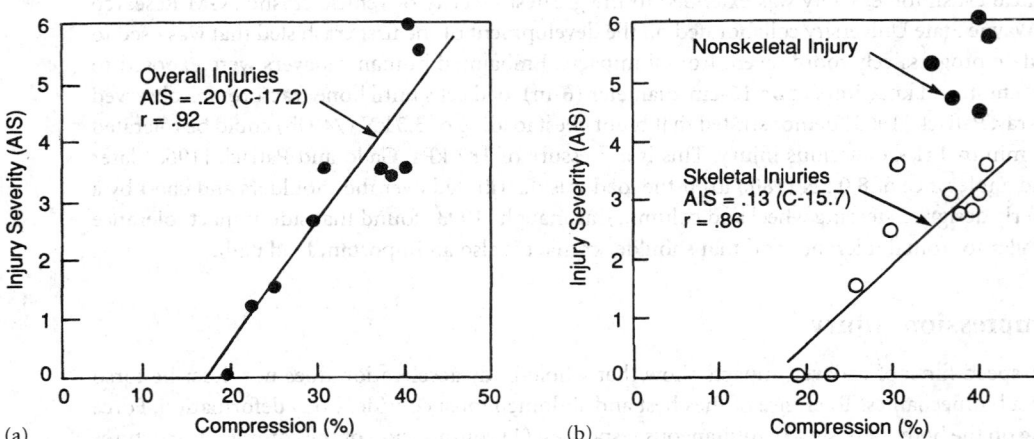

FIGURE 26.2   (*a*) Injury severity from blunt impact of human cadavers as a function of the maximum chest compression. (From Viano [1988], with permission.) (*b*) Severity of skeletal injury and incidence of internal organ injury as a function of maximum chest compression for blunt impacts of human cadavers. (From Viano [1988], with permission.)

unrestrained occupant or pedestrian, maximum compression does not adequately address the viscous and inertial properties of the torso, nor the time of greatest injury risk. In these conditions, the tolerance to compression is progressively lower as the speed of deformation increases, and the velocity of deformation becomes a dominant factor in injury.

Insight on a rate-dependent injury mechanism came from over 20 years of research by Clemedson and Jonsson [1979] on high-speed impact and blast-wave exposures. The studies confirmed that tolerable compression inversely varied with the velocity of impact. The concept was studied further in relation to the abdomen by Lau [1981] for frontal impacts in the range of 5 to 20 m/s (10 to 45 mi/h). The liver was the target organ. Using a maximum compression of 16%, the severity of injury increased with the speed of loading, including serious mutilation of the lobes and major vessels in the highest-speed impacts. While the compression was within limits of volunteer loading at low speeds, the exposure produced critical injury at higher speeds. Subsequent tests on other animals and target organs verified an interrelationship between body compression, deformation velocity, and injury.

The previous observations led Viano and Lau [1988] to propose a viscous injury mechanism for soft biologic tissues. The *viscous response VC* is defined as the product of velocity of deformation V and compression C, which is a time-varying function in an impact. The parameter has physical meaning to absorbed energy E_a by a viscous dashpot under impact loading. Absorbed energy is related to the displacement integral of force: $E_a = \int F\,dx$, and force in a dashpot is proportional to the velocity of deformation: $F = cV$, where c is a dashpot parameter. Absorbed energy is $E_a = c\int V\,dx$, or a time integral by substitution: $E_a = c\int V^2\,dt$. The integrand is composed of two responses, so $E_a = c[\int d(Vx) - \int ax\,dt]$, where a is acceleration across the dashpot. The first term is the viscous response, and the second is an inertial term related to the deceleration of fluid set in motion. Absorbed energy is given by $E_a = c(Vx - \int ax\,dt)$. The viscous response is proportional to absorbed energy, or $E_a \approx VC$, during the rapid phase of impact loading prior to peak compression.

Subsequent tests by Lau and Viano [1988, 1986] verified that serious injury occurred at the time of peak *VC*. For blunt chest impact, peak *VC* occurs in about half the time for maximum compression. Rib fractures also occur progressively with chest compression, as early as 9 to 14 ms—at peak *VC*—in a cadaver impact requiring 30 ms to reach peak compression. Upper abdominal injury by steering wheel contact also relates to viscous loading. Lau [1987] showed that limiting the viscous response by a self-aligning steering wheel reduced the risk of liver injury, as does force limiting an armrest in side impacts. Animal tests also have shown that *VC* is a good predictor of functional injury to the heart and respiratory systems. In these experiments, Stein [1982] found that the severity of cardiac arrhythmia and traumatic apnea was related to *VC*. This situation is important to baseball impact protection of children [Viano et al., 1992] and in the design of bulletproof protective vests [Quatros, 1994].

Figure 26.3 summarizes injury mechanisms associated with impact deformation. For low speeds of deformation, the limiting factor is crush injury from compression C of the body. This occurs at $C = 35$ to 40% depending on the contact area and orientation of loading. For deformation speeds above 3 m/s, injury is related to peak viscous response of $VC = 1.0$ m/s. In a particular situation, injury can occur by a compression or viscous responses, or both, since these responses occur at different times in an impact. At extreme rates of loading, such as in a blast-wave exposure, injury occurs with less than 10 to 15% compression by high energy transfer to viscous elements of the body.

26.3 Biomechanical Responses During Impact

The reaction force developed by the chest varies with the velocity of deformation, and biomechanics is best characterized by a family of force-deflection responses. Figure 26.4 summarizes frontal and lateral chest biomechanics for various impact speeds. The dynamic compliance is related to viscous, inertial, and elastic properties of the body. The initial rise in force is due to inertia as the sternal mass is rapidly accelerated to the impact speed. The plateau force is related to the viscous component, which is rate-dependent, and a superimposed elastic stiffness that increases force with chest compression. Unloading provides a hysteresis loop representing the energy absorbed by body deformation.

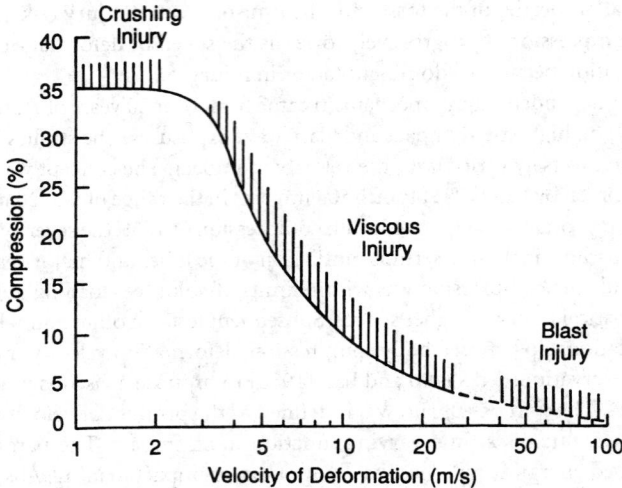

FIGURE 26.3 Biomechanics of chest injury by a crushing injury mechanism limited by tolerable compression at $C_{max} = 35\%$, a viscous injury mechanism limited by the product of velocity and extent of deformation at $VC_{max} = 1.0$ m/s, and a blast injury mechanism for shock-wave loading.

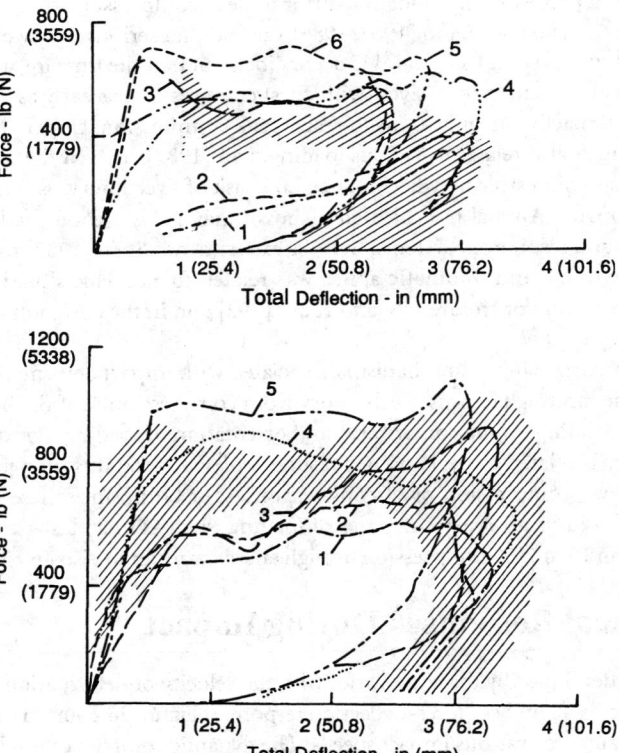

FIGURE 26.4 Frontal and lateral force-deflection response of the human cadaver chest at various speeds of blunt pendulum impact. The initial stiffness is followed by a plateau force until unloading. (From Kroell [1974] and Viano [1989], summarized by Cavanaugh [1993], with permission.)

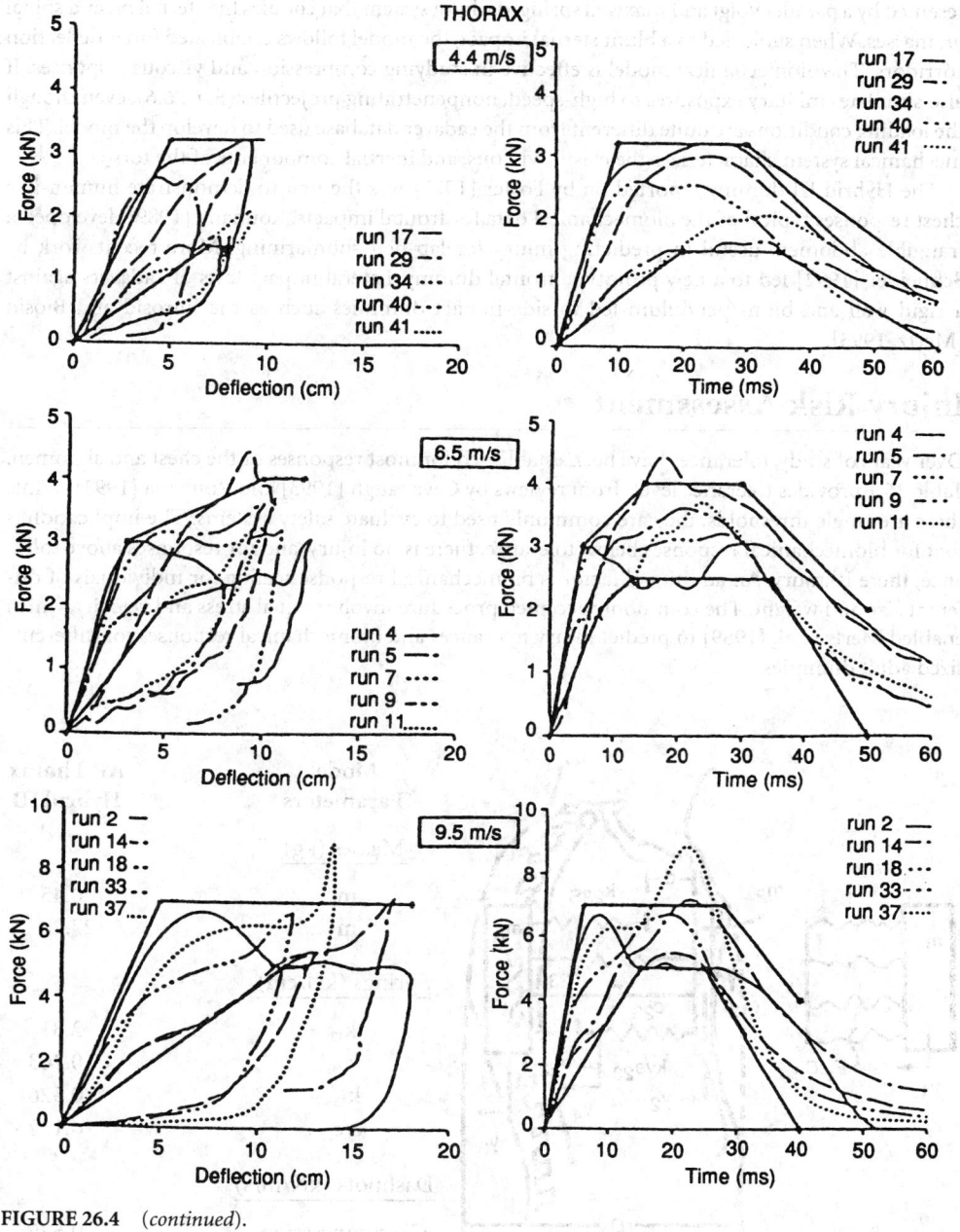

FIGURE 26.4 (*continued*).

Melvin [1988] analyzed frontal biomechanics and modeled the force-deflection response as an initial stiffness $A = 0.26 + 0.60(V - 1.3)$ and a plateau force $B = 1.0 + 0.75(V - 3.7)$, where A is in kN/cm, B is in kN, and V in m/s. The force B reasonably approximates the plateau level for lateral chest and abdominal impacts, but the initial stiffness is considerably lower at $A = 0.12(V - 1.2)$ for side loadings.

A simple, but relevant, lumped-mass model of the chest was developed by Lobdell [1973] and is shown in Fig. 26.5. The impacting mass is m_1, and skin compliance is represented by k_{12}. An energy-absorbing interface was added by Viano [1987] to evaluate protective padding. Chest structure is represented by a parallel Voigt and Maxwell spring-dashpot system that couples the sternal m_2 and spinal m_3 masses. When subjected to a blunt sternal impact, the model follows established force-deflection corridors. The biomechanical model is effective in studying compression and viscous responses. It also simulates military exposures to high-speed, nonpenetrating projectiles (Fig. 26.6), even though the loading conditions are quite different from the cadaver database used to develop the model. This mechanical system characterizes the elastic, viscous, and inertial components of the torso.

The Hybrid III dummy reported on by Foster [1977] was the first to demonstrate human-like chest responses typical of the biomechanical data for frontal impacts. Rouhana [1989] developed a frangible abdomen, useful in predicting injury for lap-belt submarining. More recent work by Schneider [1992] led to a new prototype frontal dummy. Lateral impact tests of cadavers against a rigid wall and blunt pendulum led to side-impact dummies such as the Eurosid and Biosid [Mertz, 1993].

26.4 Injury Risk Assessment

Over years of study, tolerances have been established for most responses of the chest and abdomen. Table 26.1 provides tolerance levels from reviews by Cavanaugh [1993] and Rouhana [1993]. While these are single thresholds, they are commonly used to evaluate safety systems. The implication is that for biomechanical responses below tolerance, there is no injury, and for responses above tolerance, there is injury. An additional factor is biomechanical response scaling for individuals of different size and weight. The commonly accepted procedure involves equal stress and velocity, which enabled Mertz et al. [1989] to predict injury tolerances and biomechanical responses for different-sized adult dummies.

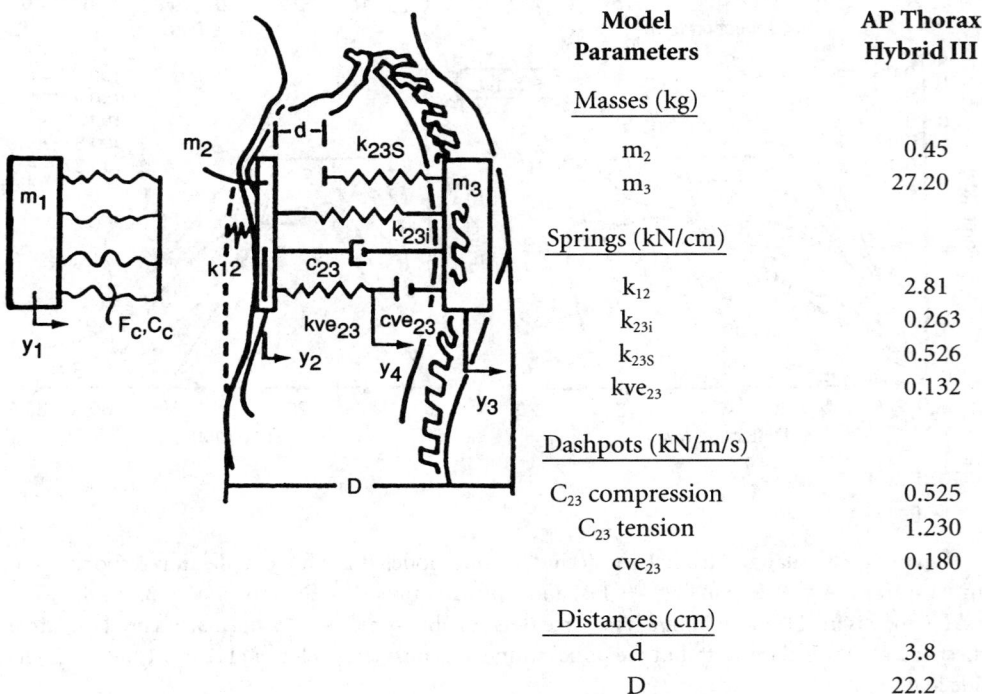

Model Parameters	AP Thorax Hybrid III
Masses (kg)	
m_2	0.45
m_3	27.20
Springs (kN/cm)	
k_{12}	2.81
k_{23i}	0.263
k_{23S}	0.526
kve_{23}	0.132
Dashpots (kN/m/s)	
C_{23} compression	0.525
C_{23} tension	1.230
cve_{23}	0.180
Distances (cm)	
d	3.8
D	22.2

FIGURE 26.5 Lumped-mass model of the human thorax with impacting mass and energy-absorbing material interface. The biomechanical parameters are given for mass, spring and damping characteristics of the chest in blunt frontal impact. (Modified from Lobdell [1973] by Viano [1987], with permission.)

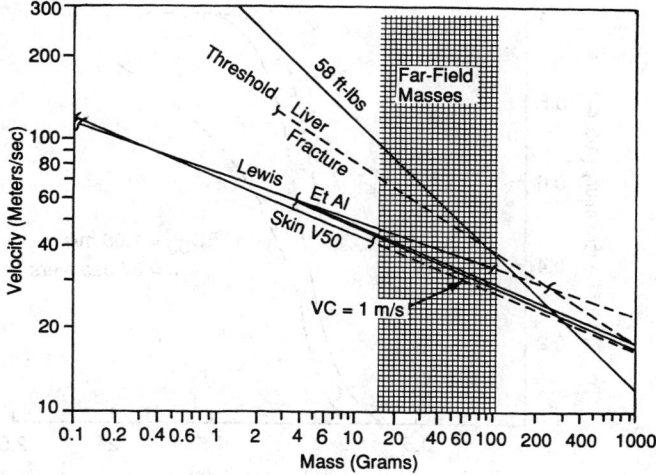

FIGURE 26.6 Tolerance levels for blunt loading as a function of impact mass and velocity. The plot includes information from automotive impact situations and from high-speed military projectile impacts. The Lobdell model is effective over the entire range of impact conditions. (Modified from Quatros [1993], with permission.)

Injury risk assessment is frequently used. It evaluates the probability of injury as a continuous function of a biomechanical response. A logist function relates injury probability p to a biomechanical response x by $p(x) = [1 + \exp(\alpha - \beta x)]^{-1}$, where α and β are parameters derived from statistical analysis of biomechanical data. This function provides a sigmoidal relationship with three distinct regions in Fig. 26.7. For low biomechanical response levels, there is a low probability of injury. Similarly, for very high levels, the risk asymptotes to 100%. The transition region between

TABLE 26.1 Human Tolerance for Chest and Abdomen Impact

	Chest		Abdomen		
Criteria	Frontal	Lateral	Frontal	Lateral	Criteria
Acceleration					Acceleration
3-ms limit	60*g*				
TTI		85–90*g*			
ASA		30*g*			
AIS 4+		45*g*		39*g*	AIS 4+
Force					Force
Sternum	3.3 kN				
Chest + shoulder	8.8 kN	10.2 kN			
AIS 3+			2.9 kN	3.1 kN	AIS 3+
AIS 4+		5.5 kN	3.8 kN	6.7 kN	AIS 4+
Pressure					Pressure
			166 kPa		AIS 3+
			216 kPa		AIS 4+
Compression					Compression
Rib fracture	20%				
Ribcage	32%		38%		AIS 3+
Flail chest	40%	38%	48%	44%	AIS 4+
Viscous					Viscous
AIS 3+	1.0 m/s				AIS 3+
AIS 4+	1.3 m/s	1.47 m/s	1.4 m/s	1.98 m/s	AIS 4+

Adapted from Cavanaugh [1993] and Rouhana [1993].

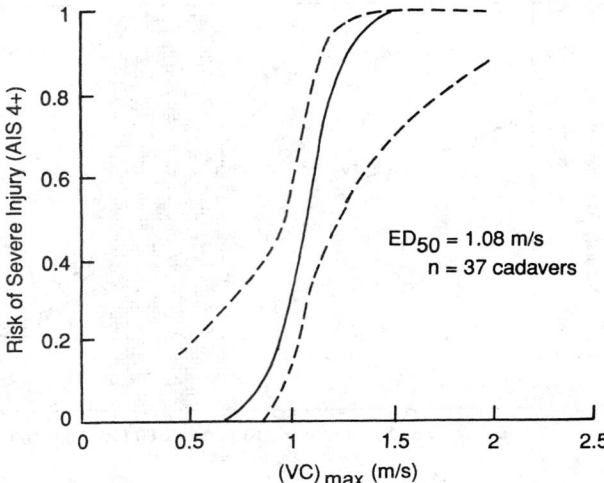

FIGURE 26.7   Typical logist injury-probability function relating the risk of serious injury to the viscous response of the chest. (From Viano [1988], with permission.)

TABLE 26.2   Injury Probability Functions for Blunt Impact (modified from Viano [1989])

Body Region	$ED_{25\%}$	α	β	X^2	p	R
			Frontal Impact			
Chest (AIS 4+)						
VC	1.0 m/s	11.42	11.56	25.6	0.000	0.68
C	34%	10.49	0.277	15.9	0.000	0.52
			Lateral Impact			
Chest (AIS 4+)						
VC	1.5 m/s	10.02	6.08	13.7	0.000	0.77
C	38%	31.22	0.79	13.5	0.000	0.76
Abdomen (AIS 4+)						
VC	2.0 m/s	8.64	3.81	6.1	0.013	0.60
C	47%	16.29	0.35	4.6	0.032	0.48
Pelvis (pubic ramus fracture)						
C	27%	84.02	3.07	11.5	0.001	0.91

the two extremes involves risk that is proportional to the biomechanical response. A sigmoidal function is typical of human tolerance because it represents the distribution in weak through strong subjects in a population exposed to impact. Table 26.2 summarizes available parameters for chest and abdominal injury risk assessment.

References

Cavanaugh JM. 1993. The biomechanics of thoracic trauma. In Nahum AM, Melvin JW (eds), Accidental Injury: Biomechanics and Prevention, pp 362–391. New York, Springer-Verlag.

Cavanaugh JM, Zhu Y, Huang Y, et al. 1993. Injury and response of the thorax in side impact cadaveric tests. In Proceedings of the 37th Stapp Car Crash Conference, pp 199–222, SAE Paper no. 933127. Warrendale, Pa, Society of Automotive Engineers.

Eiband AM. 1959. Human Tolerance to Rapidly Applied Acceleration: A Survey of the Literature, NASA Memo No. 5-19-59E. Washington, National Aeronautics and Space Administration.

Foster JK, Kortge JO, Wolanin MJ. 1977. Hybrid III—A biomechanically-based crash test dummy. In Proceedings of the Stapp Car Crash Conference, pp 975–1014, SAE Paper no. 770938. Warrendale, Pa, Society of Automotive Engineers.

Gadd CW, Patrick LM. 1968. Systems Versus Laboratory Impact Tests for Estimating Injury Hazards, SAE Paper no. 680053. Warrendale, Pa, Society of Automotive Engineers.

Jonsson A, Clemedson CJ, et al. 1979. Dynamic factors influencing the production of lung injury in rabbits subjected to blunt chest wall impact. Aviat Space Environ Med 50:325.

King Al. 1984. Regional tolerance to impact acceleration. In SP-622. Warrendale, Pa, Society of Automotive Engineers.

Kroell CK, Schneider DC, Nahum AM. 1971. Impact tolerance and response to the human thorax. In Proceedings of the 15th Stapp Car Crash Conference, pp 84–134, SAE Paper No. 710851. Warrendale, Pa, Society of Automotive Engineers.

Kroell CK, Schneider DC, Nahum AM. 1974. Impact tolerance and response to the human thorax II. In Proceedings of the 18th Stapp Car Crash Conference, pp 383–457, SAE Paper no. 741187. Warrendale Pa, Society of Automotive Engineers.

Lau IV, Viano DC. 1981. Influence of impact velocity on the severity of nonpenetrating hepatic injury. Trauma 21(2):115.

Lau IV, Viano DC. 1986. The viscous criterion—Bases and application of an injury severity index for soft tissue. In Proceedings of the 30th Stapp Car Crash Conference, pp 123–142, SAE Paper no. 861882. Warrendale, Pa, Society of Automotive Engineers.

Lau IV, Horsch JD, Andrzejak D, et al. 1987. Biomechanics of liver injury by steering wheel loading. Trauma 27:225.

Lau IV, Viano DC. 1988. How and when blunt injury occurs: Implications to frontal and side impact protection. In Proceedings of the 32nd Stapp Car Crash Conference, pp 81–100, SAE Paper no. 881714. Warrendale, Pa, Society of Automotive Engineers.

Lobdell TE, Kroell CK, Schneider DC, et al. 1973. Impact response of the human thorax. In King WF, Mertz HJ (eds), Human Impact Response Measurement and Simulation, pp 201–245. New York, Plenum Press.

Melvin JW, King Al, Alem NM. 1988. AATD system technical characteristics, design concepts, and trauma assessment criteria, AATD Task E-F Final Report, DOT-HS-807-224. Washington, U.S. Department of Transportation, National Highway Traffic Safety Administration.

Melvin JW, Weber K (eds). 1988. Review of biomechanical response and injury in the automotive environment, AATD Task B Final Report, DOT-HS-807-224. Washington, U.S. Department of Transportation, National Highway Traffic Safety Administration.

Mertz HJ, Gadd CW. 1971. Thoracic tolerance to whole-body deceleration. In Proceedings of the 15th Stapp Car Crash Conference, pp 135–157, SAE Paper no. 710852. Warrendale, Pa, Society of Automotive Engineers.

Mertz HJ, Irwin A, Melvin J, et al. 1989. Size, weight and biomechanical impact response requirements for adult size small female and large male dummies, SAE Paper no. 890756. Warrendale, Pa, Society of Automotive Engineers.

Mertz HJ. 1993. Anthropomorphic test devices. In Nahum AM, Melvin JW (eds), Accidental Injury: Biomechanics and Prevention, pp 66–84. New York, Springer-Verlag.

Morgan RM, Marcus JH, Eppinger RH. 1986. Side impact—The biofidelity of NHTSA's proposed ATD and efficacy of TTI. In Proceedings of the 30th Stapp Car Crash Conference, pp 27–40, SAE Paper no. 861877. Warrendale, Pa, Society of Automotive Engineers.

Patrick LM, Kroell CK, Mertz HJ. 1965. Forces on the human body in simulated crashes. In Proceedings of the 9th Stapp Car Crash Conference, pp 237–260. Warrendale, Pa, Society of Automotive Engineers.

Patrick LM, Mertz HJ, Kroell CK. 1967. Cadaver knee, chest, and head impact loads. In Proceedings of the 11th Stapp Car Crash Conference, pp 168–182, SAE Paper no. 670913. Warrendale, Pa, Society of Automotive Engineers.

Rouhana SW, Viano D, Jedrzejczak E, et al. 1989. Assessing submarining and abdominal injury risk in the Hybrid III family of dummies. In Proceedings of the 33rd Stapp Car Crash Conference, pp 257–279, SAE Paper no. 892440. Warrendale, Pa, Society of Automotive Engineers.

Rouhana SW. 1993. Biomechanics of abdominal trauma. In Nahum AM, Melvin JW (eds), Accidental Injury: Biomechanics and Prevention, pp 391–428. New York, Springer-Verlag.

Schneider LW, Haffner MP, et al. 1992. Development of an advanced ATD thorax for improved injury assessment in frontal crash environments. In Proceedings of the 36th Stapp Car Crash Conference, pp 129–156, SAE Paper no. 922520. Warrendale, Pa, Society of Automotive Engineers.

Society of Automotive Engineers. 1986. Human Tolerance to Impact Conditions as Related to Motor Vehicle Design, SAE J885. Warrendale, Pa, Society of Automotive Engineers.

Stalnaker RL, McElhaney JH, Roberts VL, Trollope ML. 1973. Human torso response to blunt trauma. In King WF, Mertz HJ (eds), Human Impact Response Measurement and Simulation, pp 181–199. New York, Plenum Press.

Stapp JP. 1970. Voluntary human tolerance levels. In Gurdjian ES, Lange WA, Patrick LM, Thomas LM (eds), Impact Injury and Crash Protection, pp 308–349. Springfield, Il, Charles C Thomas.

Stein PD, Sabbah HN, Viano D, et al. 1982. Response of the heart to nonpenetrating cardiac trauma. J Trauma 22(5):364.

Viano DC, King AI, Melvin J, et al. 1989. Injury biomechanics research: An essential element in the prevention of trauma. J Biomech 22:403.

Viano DC, Lau IV. 1988. A viscous tolerance criterion for soft tissue injury assessment. J Biomech 21:387.

Viano DC. 1988. Cause and control of automotive trauma. Bull NY Acad Med 64:376.

Viano DC. 1989. Biomechanical responses and injuries in blunt lateral impact. In Proceedings of the 33rd Stapp Car Crash Conference, pp 113–142, SAE Paper no. 892432. Warrendale, Pa, Society of Automotive Engineers.

Viano DC. 1987. Evaluation of the benefit of energy-absorbing materials for side impact protection. In Proceedings of the 31st Stapp Car Crash Conference, pp 185–224, SAE Paper no. 872213. Warrendale, Pa, Society of Automotive Engineers.

Viano DC, Andrzejak DV, Polley TZ, King AI. 1992. Mechanism of fatal chest injury by baseball impact: Development of an experimental model. Clin J Sports Med 2:166.

27

Analysis of Gait

Roy B. Davis
Gait Analysis Laboratory,
Department of Orthopaedics,
Newington Children's Hospital

Peter A. DeLuca
Gait Analysis Laboratory,
Department of Orthopaedics,
Newington Children's Hospital

Sylvia Õunpuu
Gait Analysis Laboratory,
Department of Orthopaedics,
Newington Children's Hospital

Gait analysis is the quantitative measurement and assessment of human locomotion including both walking and running. A number of different disciplines use gait analysis. Basic scientists seek a better understanding of the mechanisms that normal ambulators use to translate muscular contractions about articulating joints into functional accomplishment, e.g., level walking and stair climbing. Increasingly, researchers endeavor to better appreciate the relationship between the human motor control systems and gait dynamics. With respect to running, athletes and their coaches use gait analysis techniques in a ceaseless quest for meaningful improvements in performance while avoiding injury. Sports equipment manufacturers seek to quantify the perceived advantages of their products relative to a competitor's offering.

In the realm of clinical gait analysis, medical professionals apply an evolving knowledge base in the interpretation of the walking patterns of impaired ambulators for the planning of treatment protocols, e.g., orthotic prescription and surgical intervention. Clinical gait analysis is an evaluation tool that allows the clinician to determine the extent to which an individual's gait has been affected by an already diagnosed disorder [Brand & Crowninshield, 1981]. Examples of clinical pathologies currently served by gait analysis include amputation, cerebral palsy (CP), degenerative joint disease, poliomyelitis, multiple sclerosis, muscular dystrophy, myelodysplasia, rheumatoid arthritis, stroke, and traumatic brain injury.

Generally, gait analysis data collection protocols, measurement precision, and data reduction models have been developed to meet the requirements specific to the research, sport, or clinical setting. For example, gait measurement protocols in a research setting might include an extensive physical examination to characterize the anthropometrics of each subject. This time expenditure may not be possible in a clinical setting. Also, sport assessments generally require higher data acquisition rates because of increased velocity amplitudes relative to walking. The focus of this chapter is on the methods for the assessment of walking patterns of persons with locomotive impairment, i.e., clinical gait analysis. The discussion will include a description of the available measurement technology, the components of data collection and reduction, the type of gait information produced for clinical interpretation, and the strengths and limitations of clinical gait analysis.

0-8493-8346-3/95/$0.00+$.50

27.1 Fundamental Concepts

Clinical Gait Analysis Information

Gait is a cyclic activity for which certain discrete events have been defined as significant. Typically, the *gait cycle* is defined as the period of time from the point of initial contact (also referred to as *foot contact*) of the subject's foot with the ground to next point of initial contact for that same limb. Dividing the gait cycle in stance and swing phases is the point in the cycle where the stance limb leaves the ground, called *toe off* or *foot off*. Gait variables that change over time such as the patient's joint angular displacements are normally presented as a function of the individual's gait cycle for clinical analysis. This is done to facilitate the comparison of different walking trials and the use of a normative data base [Õunpuu et al., 1991]. Data that are currently provided for the clinical interpretation of gait include

- Static physical examination measures, such as passive joint range of motion, muscle strength and tone, and the presence and degree of bony deformity
- Stride and temporal parameters, such as step length and walking velocity
- Segment and joint angular displacements commonly referred to as *kinematics*
- The forces and torque applied to the subject's foot by the ground, or ground reaction forces
- The reactive joint moments produced about the lower extremity joints by active and passive soft tissue forces as well as the associated mechanical power of the joint moment, collectively referred to as *kinetics*
- Indications of muscle activity during gait, i.e., voltage potentials produced by contracting muscles, known as *dynamic electromyography* (EMG)
- A videotape of the individual's gait trial for qualitative review and quality control purposes

Data Collection Protocol

The steps involved in the gathering of data for the interpretation of gait pathologies usually include a complete physical examination, biplanar videotaping, and multiple walks of the "instrumented" subject along a walkway that is commonly both level and smooth. The time to complete these steps can range from three to five hours (Table 27.1). Although the standard for analysis is barefoot gait, subjects are tested in other conditions as well, e.g., lower extremity orthoses and crutches. Requirements and constraints associated with clinical gait data gathering include the following:

TABLE 27.1 Gait Data Collection Protocol Employed at the Newington Children's Hospital

Test Component	Estimated Time (minutes)
Pretest tasks: Test explanation to the adult subject or child and parent, system calibration	10
Videotaping: Brace, barefoot, close-up, standing	15–25
Clinical examination: Range of motion, muscle strength, etc.	30–45
Motion marker placement	15–20
Motion data collection: Subject calibration and multiple walks, per test condition (barefoot and orthosis)	30–60
Electromyography (surface electrodes and fine-wire electrodes)	20–60
Data reduction of all trials	30–90
Data interpretation	20–30
Report dictation, generation, and distribution	120–180

- The patient should not be intimidated or distracted by the testing environment.
- The measurement equipment and protocols should not alter the subject's gait.
- Patient preparation and testing time must be minimized, and rest (or play) intervals must be included in the process.
- Data collection techniques must be reasonably repeatable.
- Methodology must be sufficiently robust and flexible to allow the evaluation of a variety of pathological gait abnormalities where the dynamic range of motion and anatomy may be significantly different from normal.
- The collected data must be validated before the end of the test period, e.g., raw data fully processed before the patient leaves the facility.

Measurement Approaches and Systems

The purpose of this section is to provide an overview of the several technologies that are available to measure dynamic gait variables listed above, including stride and temporal parameters, kinematics, kinetics, and dynamic EMG. Methods of data reduction will be described in a section that follows.

Stride and Temporal Parameters

The timing of the gait cycle events of initial contact and toe off must be measured for the computation of the stride and temporal quantities. These measures may be obtained through a wide variety of approaches ranging from the use of simple tools such as a stop watch and tape measure to sophisticated arrays of photoelectric monitors. Foot switches may be applied to the plantar aspect of the subject's foot over the bony prominences of the heel and metatarsal heads in different configurations depending on the information desired. A typical configuration is the placement of a switch on the heel, first (and fifth) metatarsal heads and great toe. In a clinical population, foot switch placement is challenging because of the variability of foot deformities and foot-ground contact patterns. This switch placement difficulty is avoided through the use of either shoe insoles instrumented with one or two large foot switches or entire contact sensitive walkways. Alternatively, video cameras may be employed with video frame counters to determine the timing of initial contact and toe-off events. These gait events may also be measured using either the camera-based motion measurement systems or the force platform technology described below.

Motion Measurement

A number of alternative technologies are available for the measurement of body segment spatial position and orientation (Table 27.2). These include the use of electrogoniometry, high-speed photography, accelerometry, and video-based digitizers. These approaches are described below.

Electrogoniometry. A simple electrogoniometer consists of a rotary potentiometer with arms fixed to the shaft and base for attachment to the extremity across the joint of interest. The advantages of multiaxial goniometers (more appropriate for human joint motion measurement) include the capability for real-time display and rapid collection of single-joint information on many subjects. Electrogoniometers are limited to the measurement of relative angles and may be cumbersome in many typical clinical applications such as the simultaneous, bilateral assessment of hip, knee, and ankle motion.

Cinefilm. High-speed photography offers particular advantages in the assessment of activities such as sprinting that produce velocity and acceleration magnitudes greater than those realized in walking. This approach is not attractive for clinical use because it is labor intensive, e.g., each frame of data is digitized individually and requires an unacceptably long processing time.

TABLE 27.2   Sources for Gait Analysis Measurement Equipment and Systems

Motion Measurement Systems		
Elite	BTS Bioengineering Technology & Systems	
	747 Althouse Street, Woodmere, NY 11598	516-295-2721
ExpertVision	Motion Analysis Corporation	
	3650 North Laughlin Road, Santa Rosa, CA 95403	707-579-6500
Optotrak	Northern Digital, Inc.	
	403 Albert Street, Waterloo, Ontario N2L 3V2	519-884-5142
Peak Performance	Peak Performance Technologies	
	7388 South Revere Parkway, Suite 601, Englewood, CO 80112	303-799-8686
Selcon	Selspot Systems, Ltd.	
	21654 Melrose, Southfield, MI 48075	313-355-5900
Vicon	B & L Engineering	
	12309 East Florence Avenue, Santa Fe Springs, CA 90670	213-903-1221
Force Platforms		
AMTI	Advanced Mechanical Technology, Inc.	
	151 California Street, Newton, MA 02158	617-964-2042
Bertec	Bertec Corporation	
	819 Loch Lomond Lane, Worthington, OH 43085	614-436-9966
Kistler	Kistler Instrument Corporation	
	75 John Glenn Drive, Amherst, NY 14120	716-691-5100
EMG		
Biosentry	Biosentry Telemetry, Inc.	
	20720 Earl Street, Torrance, CA 90503	213-371-7535
Motion Lab Systems	Motion Lab Systems	
	7470 Highland Road, Baton Rouge, LA 70808-6611	504-767-2129
Foot Pressure Measurement		
AMTI	listed above	
EMED	Novel Electronics, Inc.	
	Suite 266, Box 82, 511 11th Avenue, South, Minneapolis, MN 55415	612-332-8606
Fscan	Tekscan, Inc.	
	4th floor, 451 D Street, Boston, MA 02210-1901	800-248-3669
Footswitches		
Motion Lab Systems	listed above	
B & L Engineering	listed above	

Accelerometry.   Multiaxis accelerometers can be employed to measure both linear and angular accelerations (if multiple transducers are properly configured). Velocity and position data may then be derived through numerical integration, although care must be taken with respect to the selection of initial conditions.

Videocamera-based Systems.   This approach to human motion measurement involves the use of external markers that are placed on the subject's body segments and aligned with specific bony landmarks. The marker trajectories produced by the subject's ambulation through a specific measurement volume are then monitored by a system of cameras (generally from two to seven) placed around the measurement volume. In a frame-by-frame analysis, stereophotogrammetric techniques are then used to produce the instantaneous three-dimensional (3-D) coordinates of each marker (relative to a fixed laboratory coordinate system) from the set of two-dimensional camera images. The processing of the 3-D marker coordinate data is described in a later section.

The videocamera-based systems employ either passive (retroreflective) or active (light-emitting diodes) markers. Passive marker camera systems use either strobe light sources (typically infrared light-emitting diodes (LEDs) configured in rings around the camera lens) or electronically shuttered cameras. The cameras then capture the light returned from the highly reflective markers (usually small spheres). Active marker camera systems record the light that is produced by small LED markers that are placed directly on the subject. Advantages and disadvantages are associated with each approach. For example, the anatomical location (or identity) of each marker used in an active marker system is immediately known because the markers are sequentially pulsed by the controlling computer. User interaction is required currently for marker identification in passive marker systems, although algorithms have been developed to expedite this process, i.e., automatic tracking. The system of cables required to power and control the LEDs of the active marker system may increase the possibility for subject distraction and gait alteration.

Ground Reaction Measurement

Force Platforms. The three components of the ground reaction force vector, the ground reaction torque (vertical), and the point of application of the ground reaction force vector (i.e., center of pressure) are measured with force platforms embedded in the walkway. Force plates with typical measurement surface dimensions of 0.5 × 0.5 m are comprised of several strain gauges or piezoelectric sensor arrays rigidly mounted together.

Foot Pressure Distributions. The dynamic distributed load that corresponds to the vertical ground reaction force can be evaluated with the use of a flat, two-dimensional array of small piezoresistive sensors. Overall resolution of the transducer is dictated by the size of the individual sensor "cell." Sensor arrays configured as shoe insole inserts and flat plates offer the clinical user two measurement alternatives. Although the currently available technology does afford the clinical practitioner better insight into the qualitative force distribution patterns across the plantar surface of the foot, its quantitative capability is limited because of the challenge of calibration and signal stability (e.g., temperature-dependent sensors).

Dynamic Electromyography (EMG)

Electrodes placed on the skin's surface and fine wires inserted into muscle are used to measure the voltage potentials produced by contracting muscles. The activity of the lower limb musculature is evaluated in this way with respect to the timing and the intensity of the contraction. Data collection variables that affect the quality of the EMG signal include the placement of and distance between recording electrodes, skin surface conditions, distance between electrode and target muscle, signal amplification and filtering, and the rate of data acquisition. The phasic characteristics of the muscle activity may be estimated from the raw EMG signal. The EMG data may also be presented as a rectified and/or integrated waveform. To evaluate the intensity of the contraction, the dynamic EMG amplitudes are typically normalized by a reference value, e.g., the EMG amplitude during a maximum voluntary contraction. This latter requirement is difficult to achieve consistently for patients who have limited isolated control of individual muscles, such as children with CP.

27.2 Gait Data Reduction

The predominant approach for the collection of clinical gait data involves the placement of external markers on the surface of body segments that are aligned with particular bony landmarks. These markers are commonly attached to the subject as either discrete units or in rigidly connected clusters (Fig. 27.1). As described briefly above, the products of the data acquisition process are arrays containing the 3-D coordinates (relative to an inertially fixed laboratory coordinate system) of the spatial trajectory of each marker over a gait cycle. If at least three markers or reference points are identified for each body segment, then the six degrees of freedom associated with the position of the segment may be determined. The following example illustrates this straightforward process.

Assume that a cluster of three markers has been attached to the thigh and shank of the test subject as shown in Fig. 27.2. A body-fixed coordinate system may be computed for each cluster. For example, for the thigh, the vector cross product of the unit vectors from markers B to A and B to C produces a vector that is perpendicular to the cluster plane. From these vectors, the unit vectors $\mathbf{T}_{Tx}$

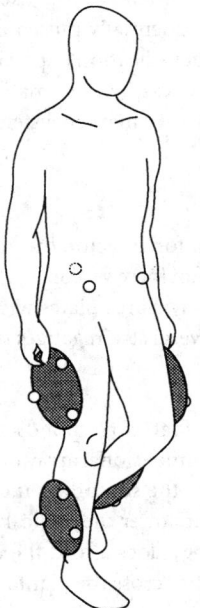

FIGURE 27.1 Videocamera-based motion measurement systems monitor the displacement of external markers that are placed on the subject's body segments and aligned with specific bony landmarks. These markers are commonly attached to the subject as either discrete units, e.g., the pelvis, or in rigidly connected clusters, e.g., on the thigh and shank.

and T_{TY} may be determined and used to compute the third orthogonal coordinate direction T_{TZ}. In a similar manner the marker-based, or technical, coordinate system may be calculated for the shank, i.e., S_{TX}, S_{TY}, and S_{TZ}. At this point, one might use these two technical coordinate systems to provide an estimate of the absolute orientation of the thigh or shank or the relative angles between the thigh and shank. This assumes that the technical coordinate systems reasonably approximate the anatomical axes of the body segments, e.g., that T_{TZ} approximates the long axis of the thigh. A more rigorous approach incorporates the use of a subject calibration procedure to relate technical coordinate systems with pertinent anatomical directions [Cappozzo, 1984].

In a subject calibration, usually performed with the subject standing, additional data are collected by the measurement system that connects the technical coordinate systems to the underlying anatomical structure. For example, as shown in Fig. 27.3, the medial and lateral femoral condyles and the medial and lateral malleoli may be used as anatomical references with the application of additional markers. With the hip center location estimated from markers placed on the pelvis [Bell et al., 1989], and knee and ankle center locations based on the additional markers, anatomical coordinate systems may be computed, e.g., $\{T_A\}$ and $\{S_A\}$. The relationship between the respective anatomical and technical coordinate system pairs as well as the location of the joint centers in terms of the appropriate technical coordinate system may be stored, to be recalled in the reduction of each frame of the walking data. In this way, the technical coordinate systems (shown in Fig. 27.3) are transformed into alignment with the anatomical coordinate systems.

Once anatomically aligned body-fixed coordinate systems have been computed for each body segment under investigation, one may compute the angular position of the joints and segments in a number of ways. The classical approach of Euler angles is commonly used in clinical gait analysis to describe the motion of the thigh relative to the pelvis (or hip angles), the motion of the shank relative to the thigh (or knee angles), the motion of the foot relative to the shank (or ankle angles), as well as the absolute orientation of the pelvis and foot in space [Grood & Suntay, 1983; Õunpuu et al., 1991]. The joint rotation sequence commonly used for the Euler angle computation is flexion-extension, adduction-abduction, and transverse plane rotation. Alternatively, joint motion has been described through the use of helical axes [Woltring et al, 1985].

The moments that soft tissue (e.g., muscle, ligaments, joint capsule) forces produce about approximate joint centers may be computed through the use of inverse dynamics, i.e., Newtonian mechanics. For example, the free body diagram of the foot shown in Fig. 27.4 shows the various external loads to the foot as well as the reactions produced at the ankle. The mass, mass moments of inertia, and location of the center of mass may be estimated from regression-based anthropometric relationships [Dempster et al., 1959], and linear and angular velocity and acceleration may be determined by numerical differentiation. If the ground reaction loads, F_G and T, are provided by a force platform, then the unknown ankle reaction force F_A may be solved for with Newton's second law. Euler's equations of motion may then be applied to compute the net ankle reaction moment, M_A.

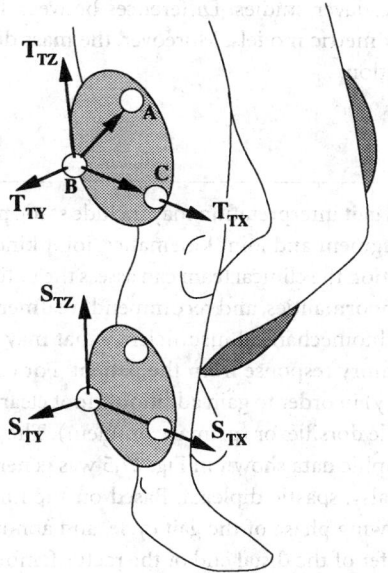

FIGURE 27.2 A body-fixed coordinate system may be computed for each cluster of three or more markers. On the thigh, for example, the vector cross product of the unit vectors from markers B to A and B to C produces a vector that is perpendicular to the cluster plane. From these vectors, the unit vectors T_{TX} and T_{TY} may be determined and used to compute the third orthogonal coordinate direction T_{TZ}.

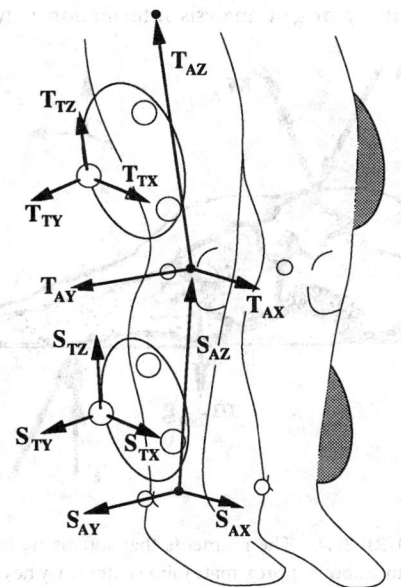

FIGURE 27.3 A subject calibration relates technical coordinate systems with anatomical coordinate systems, e.g., $\{T_T\}$ with $\{T_A\}$, through the identification of anatomical landmarks, e.g., the medial and lateral femoral condyles and medial and lateral malleoli.

In the application of Euler's equations of motion, care must be taken to perform the vector operations with all vectors transformed into the foot coordinate system which has been chosen to approximate the principle axes and located at the center of mass of the foot [Greenwood, 1965]. This process may then be repeated for the shank and thigh by using distal joint loads to solve for the proximal joint reactions. The mechanical power associated with a joint moment and the corresponding joint angular velocity may be computed from the vector dot product of the two vectors, e.g., ankle power is computed through $M_A \cdot \omega_A$ where ω_A is the angular velocity of the foot relative to the shank.

Although commonly referred to as *muscle moments* these net joint reaction moments are generated by several mechanisms, e.g., ligamentous forces, passive muscle and tendon force, and active muscle contractile force, in response to external loads. Currently, clinical muscle force evaluation is not possible because of the scarcity of data related to location of the instantaneous line of muscle force as well as the overall indeterminacy of the problem. The possibility of the cocontraction of opposing muscle groups also impacts the estimation of bone-on-bone force values, i.e., the magnitude of F_A found above reflects the *minimum* estimated value of the bone-on-bone force at the ankle.

With respect to the kinematic data reduction, the body segments are assumed to be rigid, e.g., soft-tissue movement relative to underlying bony structures is small. Consequently, marker or instrumentation attachment sites must be selected carefully, e.g., over tendonous structures of the distal shank as opposed to the more proximal muscle masses of the gastrocnemius and soleus. The models described above also assume that the joint center locations remain fixed relative to the respective segmental coordinate systems, e.g., the knee center is fixed relative to the thigh coordinate system. The measurement technology and associated protocols cannot currently produce data of sufficient quality for the reliable determination of instantaneous centers of rotation.

The additional assumptions associated with the gait kinetics model described above are related to the inertial properties of the body segments. Body segment mass and mass distribution, i.e., mass moments of inertia, are generally estimated from statistical relationships derived from cadaver studies. Differences between body types are not typically incorporated into these anthropometric models. Moreover, the mass distribution changes are assumed to be negligible during motion.

27.3 Illustrative Clinical Case

As indicated above, the information available for clinical gait interpretation may include static physical examination measures, stride and temporal data, segment and joint kinematics, joint kinetics, electromyograms, and a video record. With this information the clinical team can assess the patient's gait deviations, attempt to identify the etiology of the abnormalities, and recommend treatment alternatives. In this way, clinicians are able to isolate the biomechanical insufficiency that may produce a locomotive impairment and require a compensatory response from the patient. For example, a patient may excessively elevate a hip (compensatory) in order to gain additional foot clearance in swing which is perhaps inadequate due to a weak ankle dorsiflexor (primary problem). The knee kinematics and moments and associated electromyographic data shown in Fig. 27.5 was generated by an 11-year-old male with a diagnosis of cerebral palsy, spastic diplegia. Based on the limited knee range of motion, insufficient knee flexion in the swing phase of the gait cycle, and abnormal activity of the rectus femoris in the swing phase, a transfer of the distal end of the rectus femoris to the sartorius was recommended. Moreover, the excessive knee flexion at initial contact and throughout the stance phase due to overactivity of the hamstrings suggested intramuscular lengthenings of the medial and lateral hamstrings. Transverse plane deviations apparent from the gait analysis (not shown) lead to recommendations of derotational osteotomies of both the subject's femurs and tibias.

27.4 Gait Analysis: Current Status

As indicated in the modeling discussion above, the utility of gait analysis information may be limited by sources of error such as soft tissue displacement relative to bone, estimates of joint center locations, particularly the hip, approximations of the inertial properties of the body segments, and the numerical differentiation of noisy displacement data. Other errors associated with data collection alter the results as well, for example, a marker is improperly placed or a force platform is inadvertently contacted by the swing limb. The evaluation of small subjects weakens the data because intermarker distances are reduced, thereby reducing the precision of angular computations. It is essential that the potential adverse effects of these errors on the gait information be understood and appreciated by the clinician in the interpretation process.

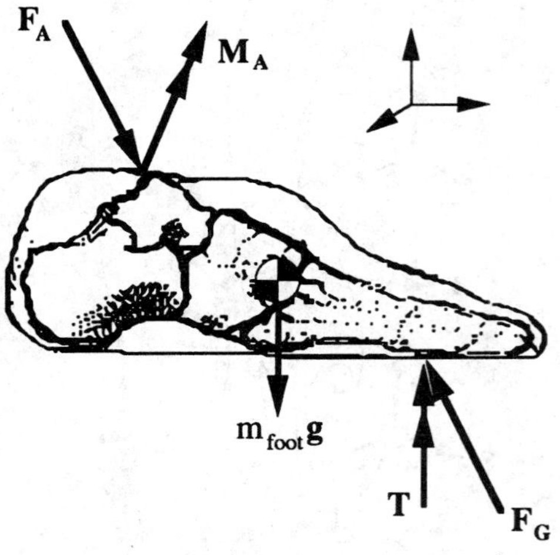

Controversies related to gait analysis techniques include the use of individually placed markers versus clusters of markers, the estimation of quasi-static, body-fixed locations of joint centers (as described above) versus the dynamic

FIGURE 27.4 The moments that soft-tissue forces produce about approximate joint centers may be computed through the use of Newtonian mechanics. This free-body diagram of the foot illustrates the external loads to the foot, e.g., the ground reaction loads, F_G and T, and the weight of the foot, $m_{foot}g$, as well as the unknown reactions produced at the ankle, F_A and M_A.

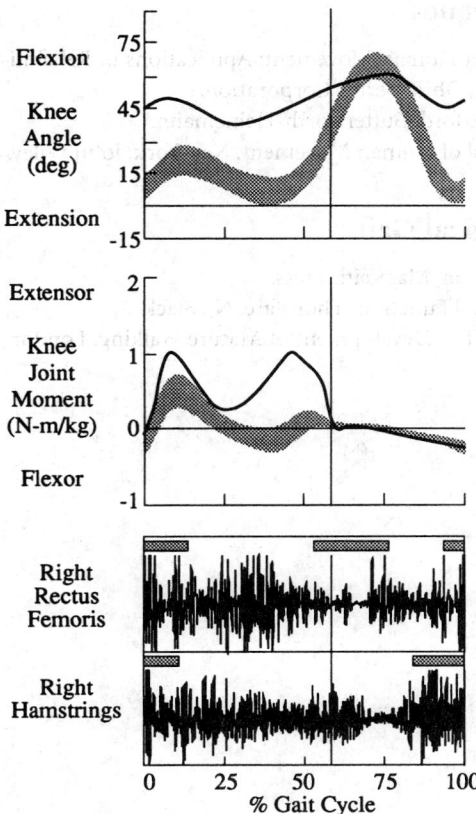

FIGURE 27.5 These are the knee kinematics and moments and associated electromyographic data for a representative subject with a diagnosis of cerebral palsy, spastic diplegia (including shaded bands/bars indicating one standard deviation about normal).

determination of the instantaneous locations, and the application of helical or screw axes versus the use of Euler angles. Additional research and development is needed to resolve these fundamental methodological issues.

Despite these limitations, gait analysis facilitates the systematic quantitative documentation of walking patterns. With the various gait data, the clinician has the opportunity to separate the primary causes of a gait abnormality from compensatory gait mechanisms. Apparent contradictions between the different types of gait information can result in a more carefully developed understanding of the gait deviations. It provides the clinical user the capability to more precisely (than observational gait analysis alone) plan complex multilevel surgeries and evaluate the efficacy of different surgical approaches or orthotic designs. Through gait analysis, movement in planes of motion not easily observed, such as about the long axes of the lower limb segments, may be quantified. Finally, quantities that cannot be observed may be assessed, e.g., muscular activity and joint kinetics. In the future, it is anticipated that our understanding of gait will be enhanced through the application of pattern recognition strategies, coupled dynamics, and the linkage of empirical results derived through inverse dynamics with the simulations provided by forward dynamics modeling.

References

Bell AL, Pederson DR, Brand RA. 1989. Prediction of hip joint center location from external landmarks. Human Movement Science 8:3.

Brand RA, Crowninshield RD. 1981. Comment on criteria for patient evaluation tools. J Biomech 14:655.

Cappozzo A. 1984. Gait analysis methodology. Human Movement Science 3:27.

Dempster WT, Gabel WC, Felts WJL. 1959. The anthropometry of manual work space for the seated subjects. Am J Phys Anthropometry 17:289.

Greenwood DT. 1965. Principles of Dynamics. Englewood Cliffs, NJ, Prentice-Hall.

Grood ES, Suntay WJ. 1983. A joint coordinate system for the clinical description of three-dimensional motions: Application to the knee. J Biomech Eng 105(2):136.

Õunpuu S, Gage JR, Davis RB. 1991. Three-dimensional lower extremity joint kinetics in normal pediatric gait. J Pediatr Orthop 11:341.

Woltring HJ, Huskies R, DeLange A. 1985. Finite centroid and helical axis estimation from noisy landmark measurement in the study of human joint kinematics. J Biomech 18:379.

Further Information on Gait Analysis Techniques

Berme N, Cappozzo A (eds). 1990. Biomechanics of Human Movement: Applications in Rehabilitation, Sports and Ergonomics. Worthington, Ohio, Bertec Corporation.

Whittle M. 1991. Gait Analysis: An Introduction. Oxford, Butterworth-Heinemann.

Winter DA. 1990. Biomechanics and Motor Control of Human Movement. New York, John Wiley.

Further Information on Normal and Pathological Gait

Gage JR. 1991. Gait Analysis in Cerebral Palsy. London, MacKeith Press.

Perry J. 1992. Gait Analysis: Normal and Pathological Function. Thorofare, NJ, Slack.

Sutherland DH, Olshen RA, Biden EN, et al. 1988. The Development of Mature Walking. London, MacKeith Press.

28

Exercise Physiology

Arthur T. Johnson
University of Maryland

Cathryn R. Dooly
University of Maryland

The study of exercise is important to medical and biological engineers. Cognizance of acute and chronic responses to exercise gives an understanding of the physiological stresses to which the body is subjected. To appreciate exercise responses requires a true systems approach to physiology, because during exercise all physiological responses become a highly integrated, total supportive mechanism for the performance of the physical stress of exercise. Unlike the study of pathology and disease, the study of exercise physiology leads to a wonderful understanding of the way the body is supposed to work while performing at its healthy best.

For exercise involving resistance, physiological and psychological adjustments begin even before the start of the exercise. The central nervous system (CNS) sizes up the task before it, assessing how much muscular force to apply and computing trial limb trajectories to accomplish the required movement. Heart rate may begin rising in anticipation of increased oxygen demands and respiration may also increase.

28.1 Muscle Energetics

Deep in muscle tissue, key components have been stored for this moment. Adenosine triphosphate (ATP), the fundamental energy source for muscle cells, is at maximal levels. Also stored are significant amounts of creatine phosphate and glycogen.

When the actinomyocin filaments of the muscles are caused to move in response to neural stimulation, ATP reserves are rapidly used, and ATP becomes adenosine diphosphate (ADP), a compound with much less energy density than ATP. Maximally contracting mammalian muscle uses approximately 1.7×10^{-5} mol of ATP per gram per second [White et al., 1959]. ATP stores in skeletal muscle tissue amount to 5×10^{-6} mole per gram of tissue, or enough to meet muscle energy demands for no more than 0.5 s.

Initial replenishment of ATP occurs through the transfer of creatine phosphate (CP) into creatine. The resting muscle contains 4 to 6 times as much CP as it does ATP, but the total supply of high-energy phosphate cannot sustain muscle activity for more than a few seconds.

Glycogen is a polysaccharide present in muscle tissues in large amounts. When required, glycogen is decomposed into glucose and pyruvic acid, which, in turn, becomes lactic acid. These reactions form ATP and proceed without oxygen. They are thus called *anaerobic*.

When sufficient oxygen is available (aerobic conditions), either in muscle tissue or elsewhere, these processes are reversed. ATP is reformed from ADP and AMP (adenosine monophosphate), CP is reformed from creatine and phosphate (P), and glycogen is reformed from glucose or lactic acid. Energy for these processes is derived from the complete oxidation of carbohydrates, fatty acids, or amino acids to form carbon dioxide and water. These reactions can be summarized by the following equations:

Anaerobic:

$$\text{ATP} \leftrightarrow \text{ADP} + \text{P} + \text{free energy} \qquad (28.1)$$

$$\text{CP} + \text{ADP} \leftrightarrow \text{creatine} + \text{ATP} \qquad (28.2)$$

$$\text{glycogen or glucose} + \text{P} + \text{ADP} \rightarrow \text{lactate} + \text{ATP} \qquad (28.3)$$

Aerobic:

$$\text{Glycogen or fatty acids} + \text{P} + \text{ADP} + O_2 \rightarrow CO_2 + H_2O + \text{ATP} \qquad (28.4)$$

All conditions:

$$2\text{ADP} \leftrightarrow \text{ATP} + \text{AMP} \qquad (28.5)$$

The most intense levels of exercise occur anaerobically [Molé, 1983] and can be maintained for only a minute or two (Fig. 28.1).

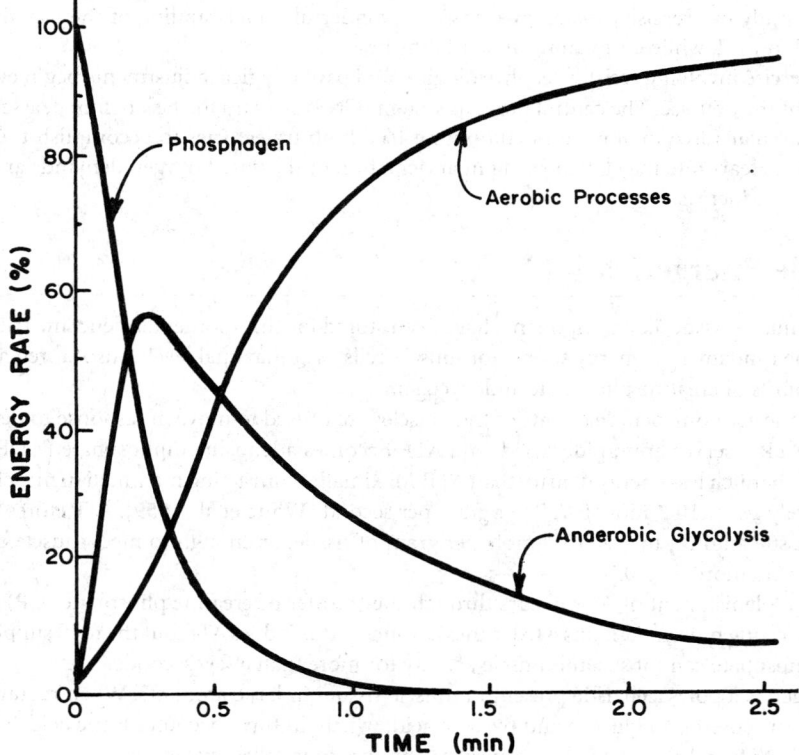

FIGURE 28.1 Muscle energy sources at the beginning of exercise. (Redrawn with permission from Molé, 1983)

28.2 Cardiovascular Adjustments

Mechanoreceptors in the muscles, tendons, and joints send information to the CNS that the muscles have begun movement, and this information is used by the CNS to increase heart rate via the sympathetic autonomic nervous system. Cardiac output, the rate of blood pumped by the heart, is the product of heart rate and stroke volume (amount of blood pumped per heart beat). Heart rate increases nearly exponentially at the beginning of exercise with a time constant of about 30 s. Stroke volume does not change immediately but lags a bit until the cardiac output completes the loop back to the heart.

During rest a large volume of blood is stored in the veins, especially in the extremities. When exercise begins, this blood is transferred from the venous side of the heart to the arterial side. Attempting to push extra blood flow through the resistance of the arteries causes a rise in both systolic (during heart ventricular contraction) and diastolic (during the pause between contractions) blood pressures. The increased blood pressures are sensed by baroreceptors located in the aortic arch and carotid sinus (Fig. 28.2).

As a consequence, small muscles encircling the entrance to the arterioles (small arteries) are caused to relax by the CNS. Since, by Poiseuille's Law:

$$R = \frac{8L\mu}{\pi r^4} \tag{28.6}$$

where

$$R = \text{resistance of a tube, N} \cdot \text{s/m}^5$$

$$L = \text{length of the tube, m}$$

$$\mu = \text{viscosity of the fluid, kg/(m} \cdot \text{s) or N} \cdot \text{s/m}^2$$

$$r = \text{radius of the tube lumen, m}$$

increasing the arteriole radius by 19% will decrease its resistance to one-half. Thus, systolic pressure returns to its resting value, and diastolic pressure may actually fall. Increased blood pressures are called *afterload* on the heart.

To meet the oxygen demand of the muscles, blood is redistributed from tissues and organs not directly involved with exercise performance. Thus, blood flows to the gastrointestinal tract and kidneys are reduced, whereas blood flows to skeletal muscle, cardiac muscle, and skin are increased.

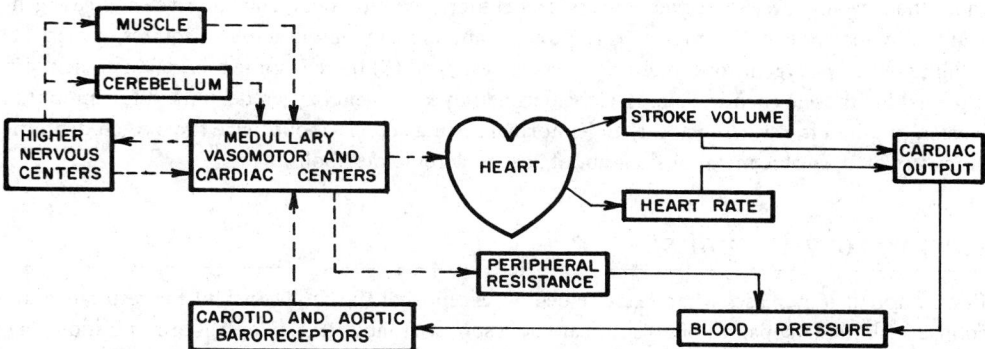

FIGURE 28.2 General scheme for blood pressure regulation. Dashed lines indicate neural communication, and solid lines indicate direct mechanical effect.

The heart is actually two pumping systems operated in series. The left heart pumps blood throughout the systemic blood vessels. The right heart pumps blood throughout the pulmonary system. Blood pressures in the systemic vessels are higher than blood pressures in the pulmonary system.

Two chambers comprise each heart. The atrium is like an assist device that produces some suction and collects blood from the veins. Its main purpose is to deliver blood to the ventricle, which is the more powerful chamber that develops blood pressure. The myocardium (heart muscle) of the left ventricle is larger and stronger than the myocardium of the right ventricle. With two hearts and four chambers in series, there could be a problem matching flow rates from each of them. If not properly matched, blood could easily accumulate downstream from the most powerful chamber and upstream from the weakest chamber.

Myocardial tissue exerts a more forceful contraction if it is stretched before contraction begins. This property (known as *Starling's law of the heart*) serves to equalize the flows between the two hearts by causing a more powerful ejection from the heart in which more blood accumulates during diastole. The amount of initial stretching of the cardiac muscle is known as *preload*.

28.3 Maximum Oxygen Uptake

The heart has been considered to be the limiting factor for delivery of oxygen to the tissues. As long as oxygen delivery is sufficient to meet demands of the working muscles, exercise is considered to be aerobic. If oxygen delivery is insufficient, anaerobic metabolism continues to supply muscular energy needs, but lactic acid accumulates in the blood. To remove lactic acid and reform glucose requires the presence of oxygen, which must usually be delayed until exercise ceases or exercise level is reduced.

Fitness of an individual is characterized by a mostly reproducible measurable quantity known as maximal oxygen uptake ($\dot{V}_{O_2 max}$) that indicates a person's capacity for aerobic energy transfer and the ability to sustain high-intensity exercise for longer than 4 or 5 minutes (Fig. 28.3). The more fit, the higher is $\dot{V}_{O_2 max}$. Typical values are 2.5 L/min for young male nonathletes, 5.0 L/min for well-trained male athletes; women have $\dot{V}_{O_2 max}$ values about 70–80% as large as males. Maximal oxygen uptake declines with age steadily at 1% per year.

Exercise levels higher than those that result in $\dot{V}_{O_2 max}$ can be sustained for various lengths of time. The accumulated difference between the oxygen equivalent of work and $\dot{V}_{O_2 max}$ is called the *oxygen deficit* incurred by an individual (Fig. 28.4). There is a maximum oxygen deficit that cannot be exceeded by an individual. Once this maximum deficit has been reached, the person must cease exercise.

The amount of oxygen used to repay the oxygen deficit is called the *excess postexercise oxygen consumption* (EPOC). EPOC is always larger than the oxygen deficit because: (1) elevated body temperature immediately following exercise increases bodily metabolism in general, which requires more than resting levels of oxygen to service, (2) increased blood epinephrine levels increase general bodily metabolism, (3) increased respiratory and cardiac muscle activity requires oxygen, (4) refilling of body oxygen stores requires excess oxygen, and (5) there is some thermal inefficiency in replenishing muscle chemical stores. Considering only lactic acid oxygen debt, the total amount of oxygen required to return the body to its normal resting state is about twice the oxygen debt; the efficiency of anaerobic metabolism is about 50% of aerobic metabolism.

28.4 Respiratory Responses

Respiration also increases when exercise begins, except that the time constant for respiratory response is about 45 s instead of 30 s for cardiac responses (Table 28.1). Control of respiration (Fig. 28.5) appears to begin with chemoreceptors located in the aortic arch, in the carotid bodies (in the neck), and in the ventral medula (in the brain). These receptors are sensitive to oxygen, carbon dioxide, and acidity levels but are most sensitive to carbon dioxide and acidity. Thus, the function of the respiratory system appears to be to remove excess carbon dioxide and, secondarily, to supply oxygen. Perhaps this is because excess CO_2 has narcotic effects, but insufficient oxygen does not produce severe reactions until oxygen levels in the inhaled air fall to one-half of normal. There is no well-established evidence that respiration limits oxygen delivery to the tissues in normal individuals.

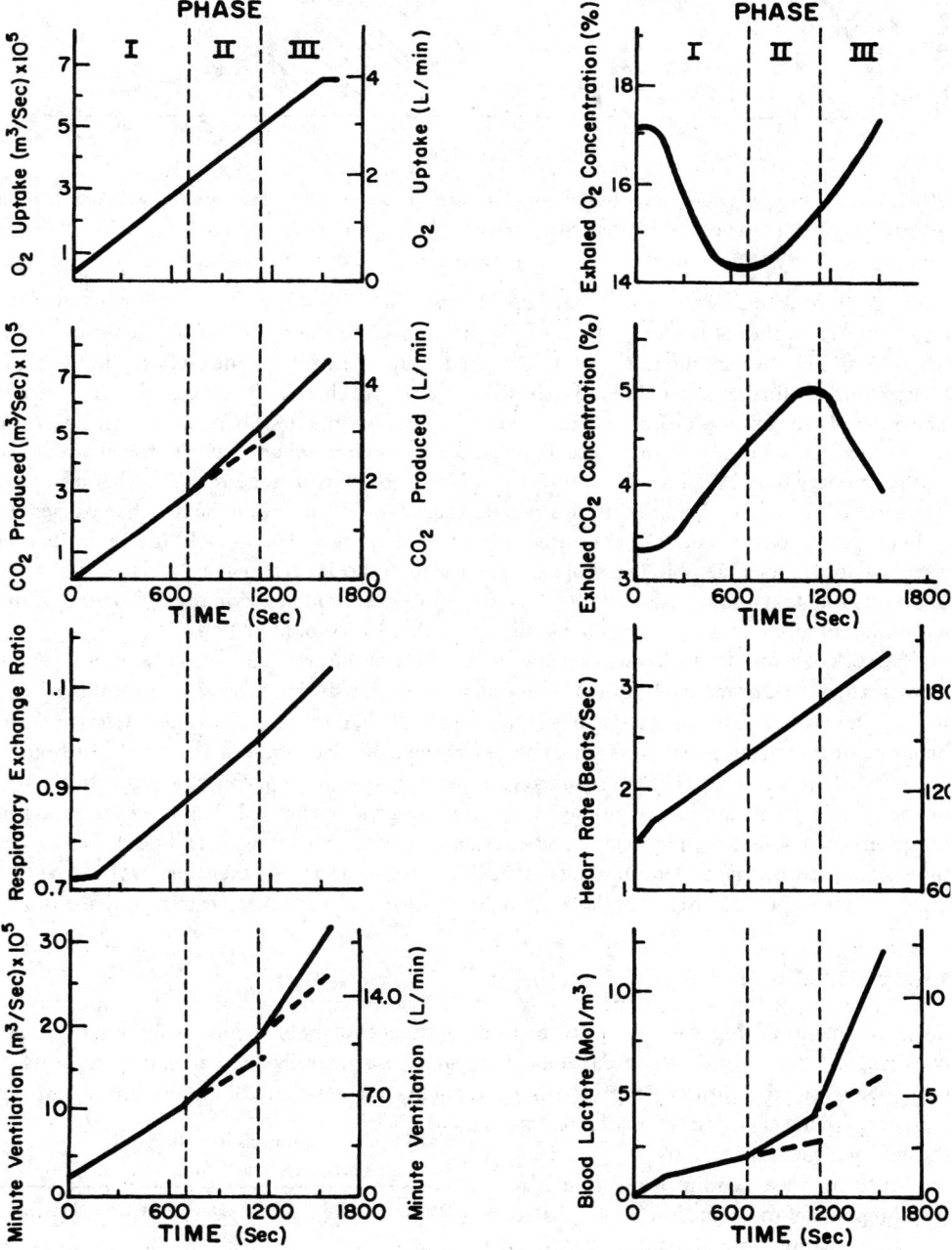

FIGURE 28.3 Concurrent typical changes in blood and respiratory parameters during exercise progressing from rest to maximum [adapted and redrawn from Skinner and McLellan (1980) by permission of the American Alliance for Health, Physical Education, Recreation and Dance].

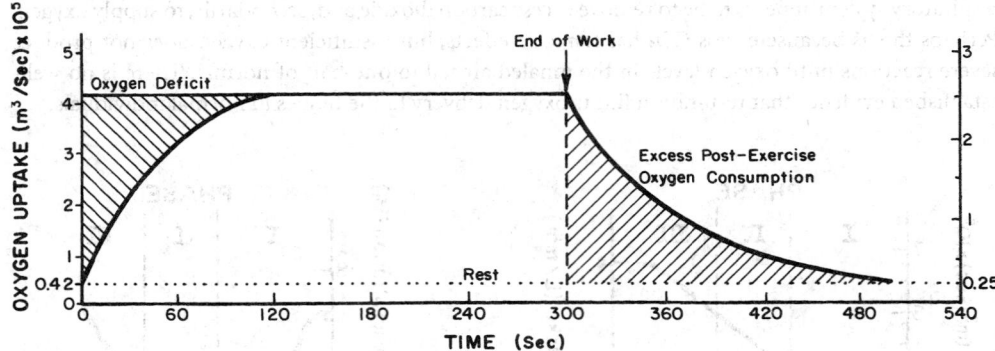

FIGURE 28.4 Oxygen uptake at the beginning of constant-load exercise increases gradually, accumulating an oxygen deficit that must be repaid at the end of exercise.

Oxygen is conveyed by convection in the upper airways and by diffusion in the lower airways to the alveoli (lower reaches of the lung where gas exchange with the blood occurs). Oxygen must diffuse from the alveoli, through the extremely thin alveolocapillary membrane into solution in the blood. Oxygen diffuses further into red blood cells where it is bound chemically to hemoglobin molecules. The order of each of these processes is reversed in the working muscles where the concentration gradient of oxygen is in the opposite direction. Complete equilibration of oxygen between alveolar air and pulmonary blood requires about 0.75 seconds. Carbon dioxide requires somewhat less, about 0.50 seconds. Thus, alveolar air more closely reflects levels of blood carbon dioxide than oxygen.

Both respiration rate and tidal volume (the amount of air moved per breath) increase with exercise, but above the anaerobic threshold the tidal volume no longer increases (remains at about 2–2.5 L). From that point, increases in ventilation require greater increases in respiration rate. A similar limitation occurs for stroke volume in the heart (limited to about 120 mL).

The work of respiration, representing only about 1–2% of the body's oxygen consumption at rest, increases to 8–10% or more of the body's oxygen consumption during exercise. Contributing greatly to this is the work to overcome resistance to movement of air, lung tissue, and chest wall tissue. Turbulent airflow in the upper airways (those nearest and including the mouth and nose) contributes a great deal of pressure drop. The lower airways are not as rigid as the upper airways and are influenced by the stretching and contraction of the lung surrounding them. High exhalation pressures external to the airways coupled with low static pressures inside (due to high flow rates inside) tend to close these airways somewhat and limit exhalation airflow rates. Resistance of these airways becomes very high, and the respiratory system appears like a flow source, but only during extreme exhalation.

28.5 Optimization

Energy demands during exercise are so great that optimal courses of action are followed for many physiological responses (Table 28.2). Walking occurs most naturally at a pace that represents the smallest energy expenditure; the transition from walking to running occurs when running expends less energy than walking; ejection of blood from the left ventricle appears to be optimized to minimize energy expenditure; respiratory rate, breathing waveforms, the ratio of inhalation time to exhalation time, airways resistance, tidal volume, and other respiratory parameters all appear to be regulated to minimize energy expenditure [Johnson, 1993].

TABLE 28.1 Comparison of Response Time Constants for Three Major Systems of the Body

System	Dominant Time Constant, s
Heart	30
Respiratory system	45
Oxygen uptake	49
Thermal system	3600

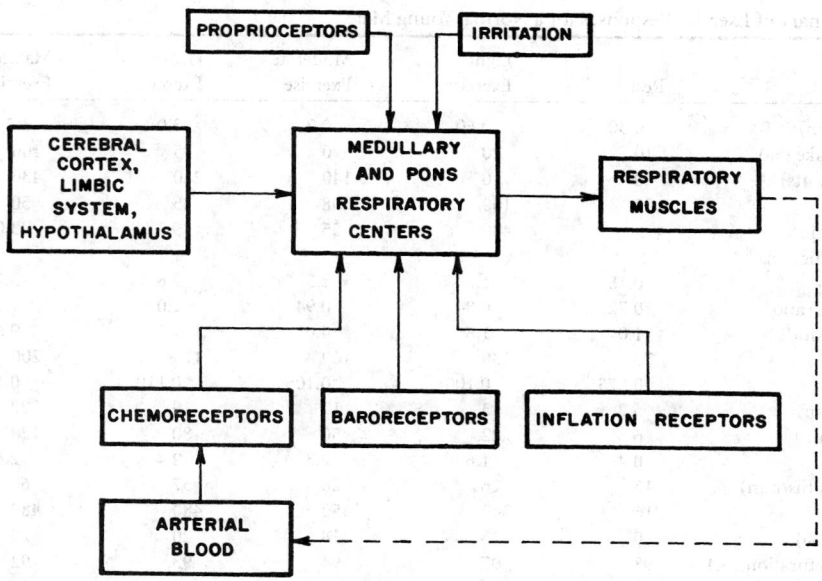

FIGURE 28.5 General scheme of respiratory control.

28.6 Thermal Responses

When exercise extends for a long enough time, heat begins to build up in the body. In order for heat accumulation to become important, exercise must be performed at a relatively low rate. Otherwise, performance time would not be long enough for significant amounts of heat to be stored.

Muscular activities are at most 20–25% efficient, and, in general, the smaller the muscle, the less efficient it is. Heat results from the other 75–80% of the energy supplied to the muscle.

Thermal challenges are met several ways. Blood sent to the limbs and blood returning from the limbs are normally conveyed by arteries and veins in close proximity deep inside the limb. This tends to conserve heat by countercurrent heat exchange between the arteries and veins. Thermal stress causes blood to return via surface veins rather than deep veins. Skin surface temperature increases and heat loss by convection and radiation also increases. In addition, vasodilation of cutaneous blood vessels augments surface heat loss but puts an additional burden on the heart to deliver added blood to the skin as well as the muscles. Heart rate increases as body temperature rises.

Sweating begins. Different areas of the body begin sweating earlier than others, but soon the whole body is involved. If sweat evaporation occurs on the skin surface, then the full cooling power of evaporating sweat ($670 \ W \cdot h/kg$) is felt. If the sweat is absorbed by clothing, then the full benefit of sweat evaporation is not realized at the skin. If the sweat falls from the skin, no benefit accrues.

Sweating for a long time causes loss of plasma volume (plasma shift), resulting in some hemoconcentration (2% or more). This increased concentration increases blood viscosity, and cardiac work becomes greater.

28.7 Applications

Knowledge of exercise physiology imparts to the medical or biological engineer the ability to design devices to be used with or by humans or animals, or to borrow ideas from human physiology to apply to other situations. There is need for engineers to design the many pieces of equipment used by sports and health enthusiasts, to modify prostheses or devices for the handicapped to allow for performance of greater than light levels of work and exercise, to alleviate physiological stresses

TABLE 28.2 Summary of Exercise Responses for a Normal Young Male.

	Rest	Light Exercise	Moderate Exercise	Heavy Exercise	Maximal Exercise
Oxygen uptake (L/min)	0.30	0.60	2.2	3.0	3.2
Maximal oxygen uptake (%)	10	20	70	95	100
Physical work rate (watts)	0	10	140	240	430
Aerobic fraction (%)	100	100	98	85	50
Performance time (min)	∞	480	55	9.3	3.0
Carbon dioxide production (L/min)	0.18	1.5	2.3	2.8	3.7
Respiratory exchange ratio	0.72	0.84	0.94	1.0	1.1
Blood lactic acid (mMol/L)	1.0	1.8	4.0	7.2	9.6
Heart rate (beats/min)	70	130	160	175	200
Stroke volume (L)	0.075	0.100	0.105	0.110	0.110
Cardiac output (L/min)	5.2	13	17	19	22
Minute volume (L/min)	6	22	50	80	120
Tidal volume (L)	0.4	1.6	2.3	2.4	2.4
Respiration rate (breaths/min)	15	26	28	57	60
Peak flow (L/min)	216	340	450	480	480
Muscular efficiency (%)	0	5	18	20	20
Aortic hemoglobin saturation (%)	98	97	94	93	92
Inhalation time (s)	1.5	1.25	1.0	0.7	0.5
Exhalation time (s)	3.0	2.0	1.1	0.75	0.5
Respiratory work rate (watts)	0.305	0.705	5.45	12.32	20.03
Cardiac work rate (watts)	1.89	4.67	9.61	11.81	14.30
Systolic pressure (mmHg)	120	134	140	162	172
Diastolic pressure (mmHg)	80	85	90	95	100
End-inspiratory lung volume (L)	2.8	3.2	4.6	4.6	4.6
End-expiratory lung volume (L)	2.4	2.2	2.1	2.1	2.1
Gas partial pressures (mmHg)					
Arterial pCO_2	40	41	45	48	50
pO_2	100	98	94	93	92
Venous pCO_2	44	57	64	70	72
pO_2	36	23	17	10	9
Alveolar pCO_2	32	40	28	20	10
pO_2	98	94	110	115	120
Skin conductance [watts/($m^2 \cdot °C$)]	5.3	7.9	12	13	13
Sweat rate (kg/s)	0.001	0.002	0.008	0.007	0.002
Walking/running speed (m/s)	0	1.0	2.2	6.7	7.1
Ventilation/perfusion of the lung	0.52	0.50	0.54	0.82	1.1
Respiratory evaporative water loss (L/min)	1.02×10^{-5}	4.41×10^{-5}	9.01×10^{-4}	1.35×10^{-3}	2.14×10^{-3}
Total body convective heat loss (watts)	24	131	142	149	151
Mean skin temperature (°C)	34	32	30.5	29	28
Heat production (watts)	105	190	640	960	1720
Equilibrium rectal temperature (°C)	36.7	38.5	39.3	39.7	500
Final rectal temperature (°C)	37.1	38.26	39.3	37.4	37

caused by personal protective equipment and other occupational ergonometric gear, to design human-powered machines that are compatible with the capabilities of the operators, and to invent systems to establish and maintain locally benign surroundings in otherwise harsh environments. Recipients of these efforts include athletes, the handicapped, laborers, firefighters, space explorers, military personnel, farmers, power-plant workers, and many others. The study of exercise physiology, especially in the language used by medical and biological engineers, can result in benefits to almost all of us.

Defining Terms

Anaerobic threshold: The transition between exercise levels that can be sustained through nearly complete aerobic metabolism and those that rely on at least partially anaerobic metabolism. Above the anaerobic threshold, blood lactate increases and the relationship between ventilation and oxygen uptake becomes nonlinear.

Maximum oxygen consumption: The maximum rate of oxygen use during exercise. The amount of maximum oxygen consumption is determined by age, sex, and physical condition.

Excess postexercise oxygen consumption (EPOC): The difference between resting oxygen consumption and the accumulated rate of oxygen consumption following exercise termination.

Oxygen deficit: The accumulated difference between actual oxygen consumption at the beginning of exercise and the rate of oxygen consumption that would exist if oxygen consumption rose immediately to its steady-state level corresponding to exercise level.

References

Johnson AT. 1993. How much work is expended for respiration? Front Med Biol Eng 5:265.

Molé PA. 1983. Exercise metabolism. In AA Bove and DT Lowenthal (eds), Exercise Medicine, pp 43–88. New York, Academic Press.

Skinner JS, McLellan TH. 1980. The transition from aerobic to anaerobic metabolism. Res Q Exerc Sport 51:234.

White A, Handler P, Smith EL, et al. 1959. Principles of Biochemistry. New York, McGraw-Hill.

Further Information

A comprehensive treatment of quantitative predictions in exercise physiology is presented in *Biomechanics and Exercise Physiology* by Arthur T. Johnson (John Wiley and Sons, 1991). There are a number of errors in the book, but an errata sheet is available from the author.

P.O. Astrand and K. Rodahl's *Textbook of Work Physiology* (McGraw-Hill, 1970) contains a great deal of exercise physiology and is probably considered to be the standard textbook on the subject.

Biological Foundations of Biomedical Engineering, edited by J. Kline (Little, Brown, Boston), is a very good textbook for physiology written for engineers.

29

Factors Affecting Mechanical Work in Humans

Arthur T. Johnson
University of Maryland

Bernard F. Hurley
University of Maryland

High technology has entered our diversions and leisure activities. Sports, exercise, and training are no longer just physical activities but include machines and techniques attuned to individual capabilities and needs. This chapter will consider several factors related to exercise and training that help in understanding human performance.

Physiological work performance is determined by energy transformations that begin with the process of photosynthesis and end with the production of biological work (Fig. 29.1). Energy in the form of nuclear transformations is converted to radiant energy, which then transforms the energy from carbon dioxide and water into oxygen and glucose through photosynthesis. In plants the glucose can also be converted to fats and proteins. Upon ingesting plants or other animals that eat plants, humans convert this energy through cellular respiration (the reverse of photosynthesis) to chemical energy in the form of adenosine triphosphate (ATP). The endergonic reactions (energy absorbed from the surroundings) that produce ATP are coupled with exergonic reactions (energy released to surroundings) that release energy from its breakdown to produce chemical and mechanical work in the human body. The steps involved in the synthesis and breakdown of carbohydrates, fats, and proteins produce chemical work and provide energy for the mechanical work produced from muscular contractions. The purpose of this chapter is to provide a brief summary of some factors that can affect mechanical work in humans.

29.1 Exercise Biomechanics

Equilibrium

Any body, including the human body, remains in stable equilibrium if the vectorial sum of all forces and torques acting on the body is zero. An unbalanced force results in linear acceleration, and an unbalanced torque results in rotational acceleration. Static equilibrium requires that:

0-8493-8346-3/95/$0.00+$.50
© 1995 by CRC Press, Inc.

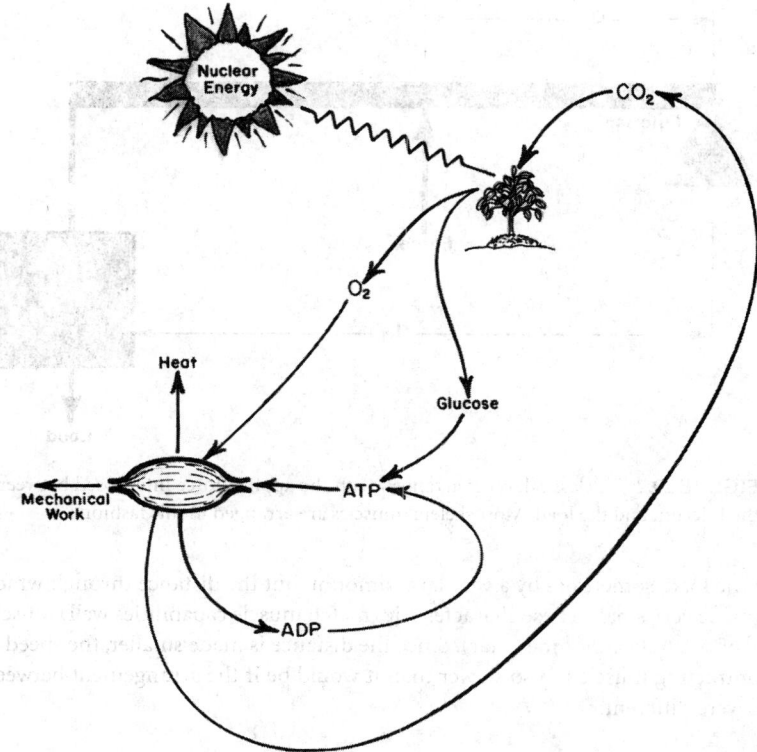

FIGURE 29.1 Schematic of energy transformations leading to muscular mechanical work.

$$\sum F = 0 \tag{29.1}$$

$$\sum T = 0 \tag{29.2}$$

where F = vectorial forces, N, and T = vectorial torques, N · m.

Some sport activities, such as wrestling, weightlifting, and fencing, require stability, whereas other activities, including running, jumping, and diving, cannot be performed unless there is managed instability. Shifting body position allows the proper control. The mass of the body is distributed as in Table 29.1, and center of mass is located at approximately 56% of a person's height and midway from side-to-side and front-to-back. The center of mass can be made to shift by extending the limbs or by bending the torso.

Muscular Movement

Mechanical movement results from contraction of muscles that are attached at each end to bones that can move relative to each other. The arrangement of this combination is commonly known as a class 3 lever (Fig. 29.2), where one joint acts as the fulcrum (Fig. 29.3), the other bone acts as the load, and the muscle provides the force interposed between fulcrum and load. This arrangement requires that the muscle force be

TABLE 29.1 Fraction of Body Weights for Various Parts of the Body

Body Part	Fraction
Head and neck	0.07
Trunk	0.43
Upper arms	0.07
Forearms and hands	0.06
Thighs	0.23
Lower legs and feet	0.14
	1.00

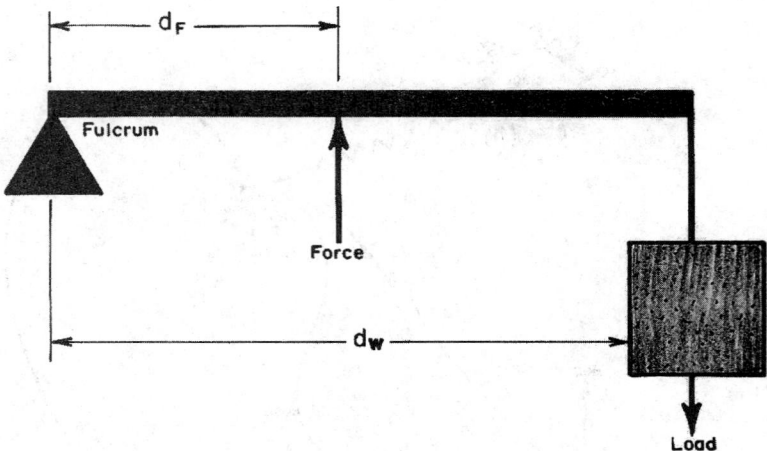

FIGURE 29.2   A class 3 lever is arranged with the applied force interposed between the fulcrum and the load. Most skeletal muscles are arranged in this fashion.

greater than the load, sometimes by a very large amount, but the distance through which the muscle moves is made very small. These characteristics match muscle capabilities well (muscles can produce 7×10^5 N/m², but cannot move far). Since the distance is made smaller, the speed of shortening of the contracting muscle is also slower than it would be if the arrangement between the force and the load were different:

$$\frac{S_L}{S_M} = \frac{d_L}{d_M}$$

(29.3)

where

$$S = \text{speed, m/s}$$
$$d = \text{distance from fulcrum, m}$$
$$L, M \text{ denote load and muscle}$$

Muscular Efficiency

Efficiency relates external, or physical, work produced to the total chemical energy consumed:

$$\eta = \frac{\text{External work produced}}{\text{Chemical energy consumed}}$$

(29.4)

Muscular efficiencies range from close to zero to about 20–25%. The larger numbers would be obtained for leg exercises that involve lifting body weight. In carpentry and foundry work, where both arms and legs are used, average mechanical efficiency is approximately 10% [Johnson, 1991]. For finer movements that require exquisite control, small muscles are often arranged in antagonistic fashion, that is, the final movement is produced as a result of the difference between two or more muscles working against each other. In this case, efficiencies approach zero. Isometric muscular contraction, where a force is produced but no movement results, has an efficiency of zero.

Muscles generally are able to exert the greatest force when the velocity of muscle contraction is zero. Power produced by this muscle would be zero. When the velocity of muscle contraction is

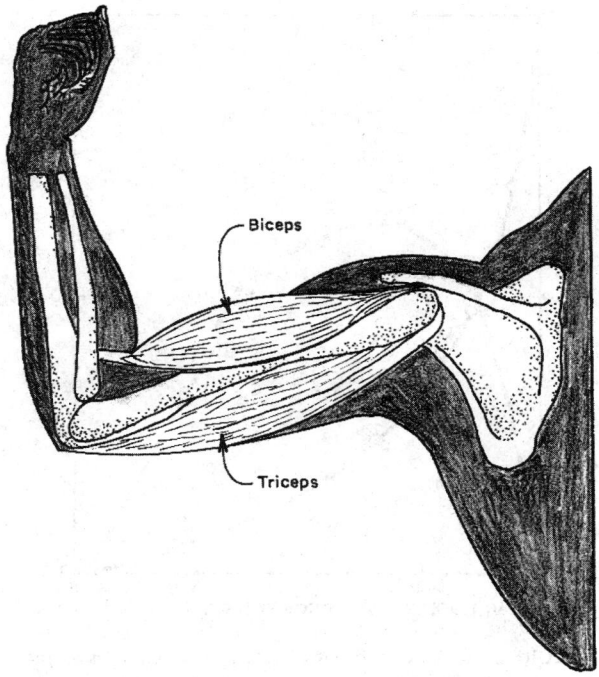

FIGURE 29.3 The biceps muscle of the arm is arranged as a class 3 lever. The load is located at the hand and the fulcrum at the elbow.

about 8 m/s, the force produced by the muscle becomes zero, and the power produced by this muscle again becomes zero. Somewhere between, the power produced, and the efficiency, becomes a maximum (Fig. 29.4).

The isometric length-tension relationship of a muscle shows that the maximum force developed by a muscle is exerted at its resting length (the length of a slightly stretched muscle attached by its tendons to the skeleton) and decreases to zero at twice its resting length. Maximum force also decreases to zero at the shortest possible muscular length. Since muscular contractile force depends on the length of the muscle and length changes during contraction, muscular efficiency is always changing (Fig. 29.5).

Negative (eccentric) work is produced by a muscle when it maintains a force against an external force tending to stretch the muscle. An example of negative work is found as the action of the leg muscle during a descent of a flight of stairs. Since the body is being lowered, external work is less than zero. The muscles are using physiological energy to control the descent and prevent the body from accumulating kinetic energy as it descends.

Muscular efficiencies for walking downhill approach −120% [McMahon, 1984]. Since heat produced by the muscle is the difference between 100% and the percent efficiency, heat produced by muscles walking downhill is about 220% of their energy expenditure. Energy expenditure of muscles undergoing negative work is about one-sixth that of a muscle doing positive work [Johnson, 1991], so a leg muscle going uphill produces about twice as much heat as a leg muscle going downhill.

Locomotion

The act of locomotion involves both positive and negative work. There are four successive stages of a walking stride. In the first stage, both feet are on the ground, with one foot ahead of the other. The trailing foot pushes forward, and the front foot is pushing backward. In the second stage the trail-

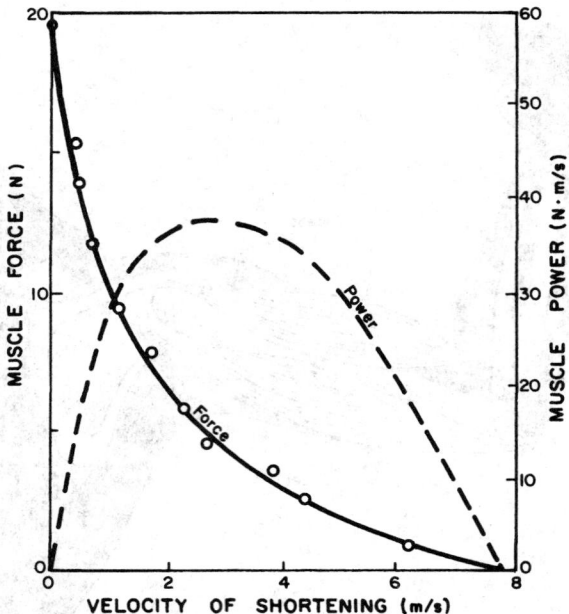

FIGURE 29.4   Force and power output of a muscle as a function of velocity. (Adapted and used with permission from Milsum, 1966)

ing foot leaves the ground and the front foot applies a braking force. The center of mass of the body begins to lift over the front foot. In the third stage the trailing foot is brought forward, and the supporting foot applies a vertical force. The body center of mass is at its highest point above the supporting foot. In the last stage, the body's center of mass is lowered, and the trailing foot provides an acceleration force.

This alternation of the raising and lowering of the body center of mass, along with the pushing and braking provided by the feet, makes walking a low-efficiency maneuver. Walking has been likened to alternately applying the brakes and accelerator while driving a car. Just as the fuel efficiency of the car would suffer from this mode of propulsion, so the energy efficiency of walking suffers from the way walking is performed.

There is an optimum speed of walking. Faster than this speed, additional muscular energy is required to propel the body forward. Moving slower than the optimal speed requires additional muscular energy to retard leg movement. Thus, the optimal speed is related to the rate at which the leg can swing forward. Simple analysis of the leg as a physical pendulum shows that the optimal walking speed is related to leg length:

$$S \propto \sqrt{L} \tag{29.5}$$

Unlike walking, there is a stage of running during which both feet leave the ground. The center of mass of the body does not rise and fall as much during running as during walking, so the efficiency for running can be greater than for walking.

At a speed of about 2.5 m/s, running appears to be more energy-efficient than walking, and the transition is usually made between these forms of locomotion (Fig. 29.6). Unlike walking, there does not appear to be a functional relationship between speed and leg length, so running power expenditure is linearly related to speed alone.

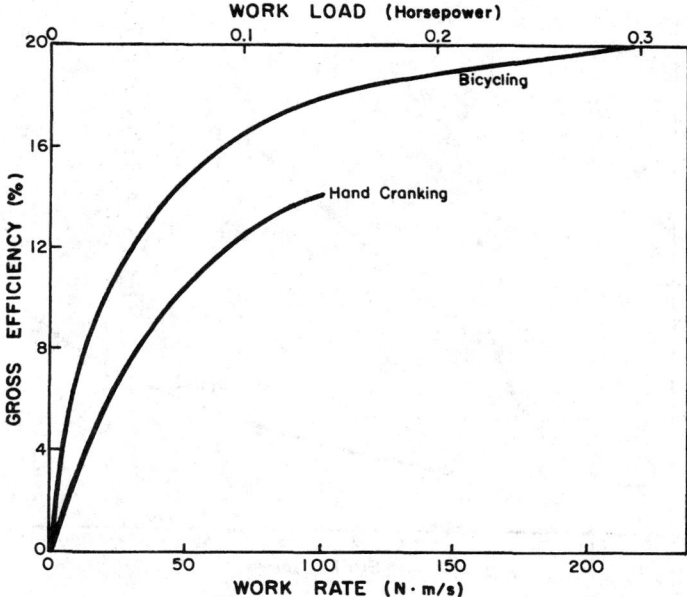

FIGURE 29.5 The gross efficiency for hand cranking or bicycling as a function of the rate of work [Goldman, 1978].

Why would anyone want to propel the extra weight of a bicycle in addition to body weight? On the surface it would appear that cycling would cost more energy than running or walking. However, the center of mass of the body does not move vertically as long as the cyclist sits on the seat. Without the positive and negative work associated with walking or running, cycling is a much more efficient form of locomotion than the other two (Fig. 29.6), and the cost of moving the additional weight of the bicycle can easily be supplied.

Many sports or leisure activities have a biomechanical basis. Understanding of the underlying biomechanical processes can lead to improved performance. Yet, there are limits to performance that cause frustrations for competitive athletes. Hence, additional ergogenic aids are sometimes employed to expand these limits. Following is a brief discussion of some of these factors.

29.2 Exercise Training

Many compensatory reactions allow the body to adapt to minor stresses, such as mild exercise, so that homeostasis (equilibrium) can be maintained. For example, the increased energy demands of exercise stimulate an increase in heart rate, respiration, blood flow, and many other reactions that allow the body to maintain homeostasis. As the intensity of exercise increases, it becomes more difficult for compensatory mechanisms to maintain homeostasis. After exceeding about 80% of an untrained person's maximal capacity, homeostasis can no longer be maintained for more than a few minutes before exhaustion results.

Exercising regularly (training) elevates the level that a single exercise session can be performed before disturbing homeostasis. It does this by elevating the maximal physiological capacity for homeostasis so that the same amount of exercise is a lower percentage of maximal capacity. In addition, training produces specific adaptations during submaximal exercise that permit greater and longer amounts of work before losing homeostasis. A good example of this is when blood lactate rises with increased intensity of exercise. Prior to training, blood lactate concentration rises substantially when the intensity of exercise exceeds about 75% of maximal oxygen consumption

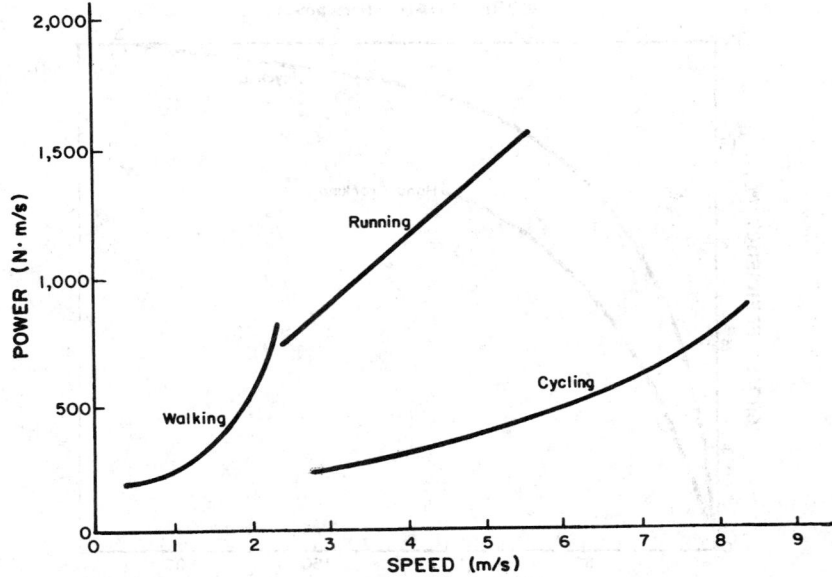

FIGURE 29.6 Power required for walking, running, and cycling by an adult male. Curves for walking and running interact at about 2.3 m/s and show that walking is more efficient below the intersection and running is more efficient above. (Redrawn with permission from Alexander, 1984)

($\dot{V}O_{2\,max}$). Following training, the same intensity of exercise results in a lower concentration of blood lactate, so exercise can now be performed at a higher fraction of $\dot{V}O_{2\,max}$ before blood lactate reaches the same level as before training [Hurley et al., 1984a]. Thus, exercise training allows an individual to perform a much greater amount of work before homeostasis is disturbed to the point at which muscular exhaustion results.

29.3 Age

It is well established that the maximal capacity to exercise declines with age. However, many factors that change with age also affect an individual's maximal capacity to exercise. These include a gain in body fat, a decrease in lean body mass, onset of disease, and a decline in the level of physical activity. For this reason it is difficult to determine exactly how much of the loss in capacity to exercise with age can really be attributed solely to the effects of aging. Maximal oxygen consumption starts to decline after the age of 25 to 30 years at about the rate of 10% per decade in healthy sedentary women and men. This rate of decline is only half as great (~5%) when people maintain their physical activity levels as they age. Thus, there is no doubt that maximal work capacity declines with advancing age, but regular exercise appears to reduce this decline substantially.

Cardiovascular fitness and muscular strength are substantially higher in men compared to women. The aerobic capacity in men is about 40 to 50% higher than women. In addition, upper body strength is about 50% higher, and lower body strength is about 30% higher in men [McArdle et al., 1994]. However, these differences are diminished substantially when body composition is taken into consideration. For example, when aerobic capacity is expressed with reference to body mass (ml 0_2/kg/min) this difference decreases to about 20% and to about 10% when differences in lean body mass are taken into consideration. Similar declines in the differences in muscular strength can be demonstrated when taking lean body mass differences into consideration. In fact, women may actually be stronger than men per amount of muscle tissue in the lower extremities. There do not appear to be any differences in responsiveness to training. Relative changes in aerobic capacity and muscular strength are approximately the same in women compared to men.

29.4 Ergogenic Aids

Anabolic Steroids

Anabolic steroids are drugs that function similar to the male sex hormone testosterone. Upon binding with specific receptor sites, these drugs contribute greatly to male secondary sex characteristics. These drugs have been used frequently by a large number of competitive athletes, particularly those involved in strength and power sports. Increases in muscular strength, total body mass, and lean body mass have been reported [ACSM, 1984]. It has been argued, however, that at least some of the increase in total body mass resulting from anabolic steroid use results from an increase in water retention [Casner et al., 1971]. Evidence indicates that many of these drugs act by decreasing muscle protein degradation rather than by enhancing protein synthesis [Hickson et al., 1990]. Hence, these drugs might be more appropriately named "anticatabolic" steroids. There is also some indication that these drugs work by increasing aggressive behavior and thereby promote a greater quantity and quality of training.

The factors that are responsible for transporting oxygen from the heart to skeletal muscle are enhanced following anabolic steroid administration through increases in blood volume, red blood cells (RBC), and hemoglobin. This would appear to improve cardiovascular fitness by increasing oxygen transport capacity. However, most studies show that anabolic steroids do not significantly increase cardiovascular fitness [Johnson et al., 1975]. This may be due to the increased blood viscosity resulting from the hemoconcentration effects of increasing RBCs and hemoglobin. Increases in blood viscosity may reduce blood flow to and from the heart and cause the heart to work harder in order to maintain cardiac output (Fig. 29.7).

It is clear that the use of anabolic steroids produces adverse effects on the liver and reproductive and cardiovascular systems. Effects on the liver include peliosis hepatitis (blood-filled cysts), impaired excretory function (jaundice), and liver tumors [Shapiro et al., 1977]. Cardiovascular effects include an increase in blood pressure, abnormal alterations in cardiac tissue, and abnormal lipoprotein-lipid profiles [Hurley et al., 1984b]. Males can experience a significant reduction in sperm production, testicular size, and testosterone and gonadotrophin production, and females often experience a deepening of voice, male pattern baldness, enlargement of the clitoris, a reduction in breast size, a disruption in their menstrual cycle, and an increase in facial hair. Most of these effects are irreversible even after the drugs are discontinued. There are also many psychological effects including an increase in aggressive behavior, an increase in anger and hostility, large deviations in mood, and sudden changes in libido.

Growth Hormone

Human growth hormone, also known as somatotropic hormone, is secreted from the pituitary gland and is involved in many anabolic processes in the body including normal growth and tissue synthesis. Athletes have become more interested in the use of growth hormone (GH) in recent years because of the many reports touting its benefits, the increased awareness of the dangers of anabolic steroids, and the reduced price due to the increased availability of synthetic forms. The appeal to athletes is that GH stimulates amino acid uptake and protein synthesis in skeletal muscle and a degradation of fat in adipose tissue. It has been shown to increase fat-free mass and reduce body fat independent of diet and exercise. Nevertheless, these benefits do not come without side effects, including acromegaly (enlargement of bony structures in the extremities) and impaired glucose tolerance.

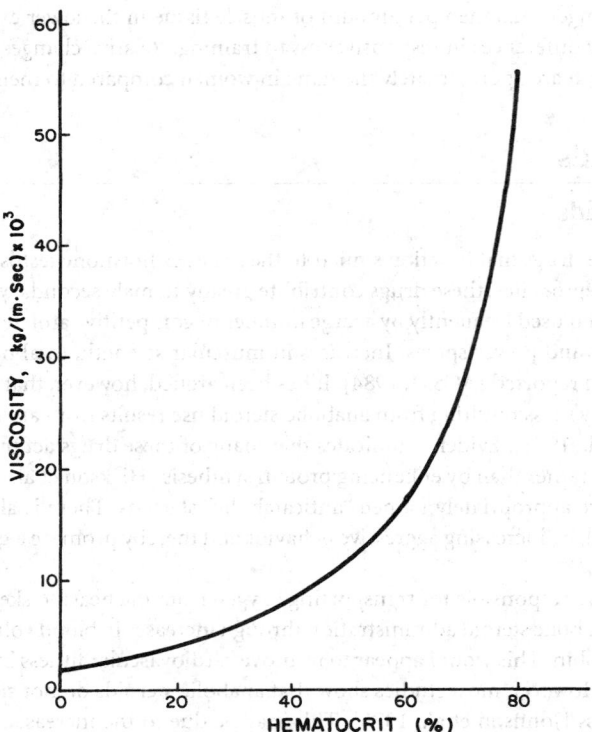

FIGURE 29.7 Blood viscosity related to blood hematocrit.

Blood Doping

This procedure is also called *red blood cell* (RBC) *reinfusion, induced erythrocythemia,* or *blood boost-ing.* It involves withdrawing between 1 and 4 units (1 unit = 450 ml of blood) of a person's blood and then separating the plasma (liquid portion) from the RBCs. The plasma portion is immediately reinfused, and the packed RBCs are frozen. Each unit of blood is withdrawn over a 3- to 8-week pe-riod to prevent sudden reduction in hematocrit (RBC concentration). The RBCs are then reinfused 1 to 7 days prior to an endurance event. This results in a 10 to 20% increase in RBC and hemoglo-bin levels as well as an increase in total blood volume. It is believed that blood doping enhances oxy-gen transport to the working muscles, and since oxygen transport is considered a limiting factor for increasing $\dot{V}O_{2\,max}$, this adaptation would appear to enhance cardiovascular endurance performance. Whether blood doping actually improves endurance performance depends on the balance between enhanced oxygen transport and increased viscosity of blood. The method of storing blood appears to be an important factor in determining the potential effects of blood doping on performance. When the proper procedures have been used it can increase $\dot{V}O_{2\,max}$ by 5 to 13% and reduce sub-maximal heart rate and blood lactate during a standard exercise test [McArdle et al., 1991].

Oxygen Inhalation

Inhaling high concentrations of oxygen gas mixtures prior to athletic competition or during rest pe-riods of sporting events are common observations. This practice is based on the notion that it will increase oxygen transport (more oxygen binding to hemoglobin), thereby increasing oxygen deliv-ery to the working muscle and resulting in a delay in the onset of fatigue. There are at least three problems with this belief. First, hemoglobin is already almost totally saturated with oxygen during normal breathing of ambient air at rest (95 to 98%). Hence, even if this practice allowed total oxygen saturation of hemoglobin it would only add a small amount of oxygen to the arterial blood leaving the lungs (10 ml of extra oxygen for every liter of whole blood). Second, for this practice to result in a delay of fatigue one must assume that oxygen transport and delivery is a limiting factor for the specific event or sport being performed. This assumption cannot be made for many of the power-type events in which oxygen inhalation is often used (e.g., football). Third, any enhancement of oxygen transport from this procedure is short-lived. Yet athletes are often observed inhaling oxygen on the sidelines for relatively long periods prior to participation. Thus, this practice does not appear to offer much more than psychological benefits when used prior to athletic competition or during prolonged rest periods.

However, breathing oxygen during prolonged steady rate exercise results in reduced heart rates, ventilation, and blood lactate levels. Apparently even small increases in oxygen saturation of hemoglobin and some added oxygen dissolved in plasma not bound to hemoglobin results in a substantial increase in oxygen availability under conditions that approach hypoxia. It may also increase oxygen diffusion capacity across muscle capillaries by elevating the partial pressure of oxygen in the blood. Nevertheless, the timing required for oxygen inhalation to be effective makes this procedure impractical to use for most athletic events, even if it were considered ethical and legal.

Defining Terms

Anabolic steroids: Synthetic forms of sex hormones (androgens) that possess both synthesizing and masculinizing characteristics.

Biceps muscle: The major muscle group in the upper arm responsible for flexion, joined by tendons at the shoulder and elbow. Two collaborating muscles are involved in the biceps.

Endergonic: An energy-absorbing process.

Ergogenic aids: Factors that affect human performance.

Exergonic: An energy-liberating process.

Hematocrit: The concentration of red blood cells.

Homeostasis: The tendency to maintain equilibrium.

Negative work: Work where the applied force and the direction of movement are opposite. **Positive work** involves an applied force in the same direction as the movement. Negative work is known as *eccentric work,* and positive work is known as *concentric* by biomechanists.

References

ACSM. 1984. The use of anabolic-androgenic steroids in sports. Sports Med Bull 19:13.

Alexander RM. 1984. Walking and running. Amer Sci.72:348.

Casner SW, Early RG, Carlson BR. 1971. Anabolic steroid effects on body composition in normal young men. J Sports Med Phys Fitness 11:98.

Goldman RF. 1978. Computer models in manual materials handling. In CG Drury (ed), Safety in Manual Materials Handling, pp 110–116, Cincinnati, Ohio, National Institute for Occupational Safety and Health (NIOSH).

Hickson RC, Czerwinski SM, Falduto MT, et al. 1990. Glucocorticoid antagonism by exercise and androgenic-anabolic steroids. Med Sci Sports Exerc 22:331.

Hurley BF, Hagberg JM, Allen WK, et al. 1984a. Effect of training on blood lactate levels during submaximal exercise. J Appl Physiol 56:1260.

Hurley BF, Seals DR, Hagberg JM, et al. 1984b. High-density-lipoprotein cholesterol in bodybuilders v powerlifters. JAMA 252:507.

Johnson AT. 1991. Biomechanics and Exercise Physiology, New York, John Wiley.

Johnson LC, Roundy ES, Allsen PE, et al. 1975. Effect of anabolic steroid treatment on endurance. Med Sci Sports Exerc 7:287.

McArdle WD, Katch FI, Katch VL. 1994. Training muscles to become stronger. In Essentials of Exercise Physiology, pp 373–397, Baltimore, Lea & Febiger.

McMahon TA. 1984. Muscles, Reflexes, and Locomotion, Princeton, NJ, Princeton University Press.

Milsum JH. 1966. Biological Control Systems Analysis, New York, McGraw-Hill.

Shapiro P, Ikedo RM, Ruebner BH, et al. 1977. Multiple hepatic tumors and peliosis hepatitis in Fanconi's anemia treated with androgens. Am J Dis Child 131:1104.

Further Information

A comprehensive treatment of quantitative predictions in exercise physiology and biomechanics is presented in *Biomechanics and Exercise Physiology* by A. T. Johnson (John Wiley and Sons, 1991). There are a number of errors in the book, but an errata sheet is available from the author.

Clear and simple explanations of the biomechanics of sports are given in *Physics in Biology and Medicine* by P. Davidovits (Prentice-Hall, 1975).

The book by Tom McMahon, *Muscles, Reflexes, and Locomotion* (Princeton University Press, 1984), is a classic not to be missed.

The article by McArdle and colleagues in *Essentials of Exercise Physiology* (Lea & Febiger, 1994) is an excellent source for a better understanding of physiological principles of work performance.

See D.A. Winter's *Biomechanics and Motor Control of Human Movement* (John Wiley, 1990) for a good in-depth explanation of more traditional biomechanics.

30

Mathematical Models of Human Response to Acceleration

Kennerly H. Digges

George Washington University

A principal impetus for the development of human mathematical models has been to simulate the dynamic response of a vehicle occupant in a crash. The U.S. federal government and private companies have sponsored extensive research to develop, validate, and apply human models that can be used to aid in the design of safety features for impact protection.

Two general-purpose models to simulate the gross motion of the occupant are presently in wide use. They are the articulated total-body (ATB) model and the MADYMO model. Although these models were developed to simulate vehicle occupants or pedestrians in a crash, they can be used to simulate the dynamics of many other systems of linked masses.

Each of these models incorporates a variety of alternatives for linking body masses to represent humans or crash dummies. The organizations that distribute the models have validated data sets for the crash dummies commonly used in testing.

The capabilities of both models include the representation of safety components including air bags, safety belts, and energy-absorbing surfaces. The accurate representation of these safety components requires component testing, model validation, and experience. Frequently, in developing safety systems that include air bags, it is desired to model characteristics of the system which are not easily incorporated in the ATB or MADYMO models. The DRISIM (*driver sim*ulation) and PASSIM (*passenger sim*ulation) models address this requirement. These models have simple occupants but detailed air bags and air bag inflation characteristics.

This chapter summarizes the characteristics of three occupant simulation models currently in wide use—ATB, MADYMO, and DRISIM/PASSIM. Numerous other special-purpose human simulation packages have been reported in the literature. The references at the end of the chapter provide additional information and source data on human models.

30.1 Articulated Total-Body (ATB) Model

ATB model version VI-3B, released in January 1994, is the current evolution of the Calspan three-dimensional (3-D) model and the crash victim simulator model (CVS) [Armstrong Aerospace Med-

8493-8346-3/95/$0.00+$.50
1995 by CRC Press, Inc.

ical Research Laboratory, 1994]. These models have been under development since 1970. The source code for the model is available. ATB version IV-3B runs a 486 PC or workstation. A typical simulation of a frontal crash takes less than 10 minutes.

The ATB model is a lumped-mass model for simulating the three-dimensional motion of sets of connected or disjointed rigid elements. The model uses a hybrid analytical formulation based on Newton's equations of motion with constraints but also including compatibility relationships based on Newton's third law. The various body segments are represented by lumped-mass elements connected by joints. Each rigid element is assigned the mass and inertia properties of the equivalent body segment. The body segments are visually represented by ellipsoids that are also the contact surfaces which demarcate the force interactions with the surrounding environment. The program can handle up to 60 segments. An 18-segment model of the Hybrid III dummy is shown in Fig. 30.1 [Armstrong Aerospace Medical Research Laboratory, 1988].

The joints are defined in such a way that they can be represented as follows: locked joint, single pin, a combination of pins connected together (Euler joint), ball and socket joint, slip joint (linear motion along one axis), null joint (allows multiple dummies or unconnected masses to be simulated). Joint characteristics are defined by functions of the type shown in Fig. 30.2. Five parameters are used in the specification: joint stop angle, energy-dissipation function, and the linear, square, and cubic torque coefficients. The joint-restoring torque may be specified as contours on a spherical joint surface. In addition, Coulomb friction and viscous damping coefficients can be specified.

External forces are applied to the body surfaces by contacts with planes, ellipsoids, and hyperellipsoids that represent external surfaces. Planes, specified by three coordinate points, are commonly used to represent contact surfaces. The method for determining the magnitude, direction, and location of ellipsoid-to-plane contact forces is illustrated in Fig. 30.3. A perpendicular from the plane to the point of maximum penetration of the ellipsoid defines the penetration function d. This d function is used to calculate the normal and frictional forces, based on force and displacement relationships provided in the input data set. The functions for energy dissipation and permanent deformation are based on d and its rate of change. Alternatively, hysteresis can be specified by R and G factors which produce penetration-dependent unloading and reloading characteristics. The contact-force relationships can be specified as constants, polynomials, tabular data, or combinations of the three. The point of application of the force can be specified by the user at any location along the perpendicular.

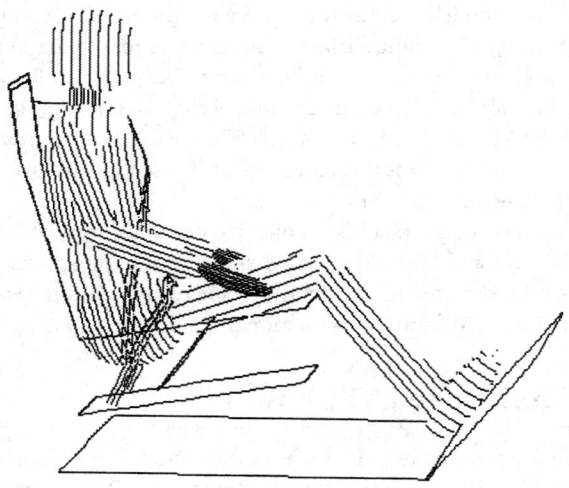

FIGURE 30.1 A Hybrid III dummy from VIEW postprocessor, ATB model.

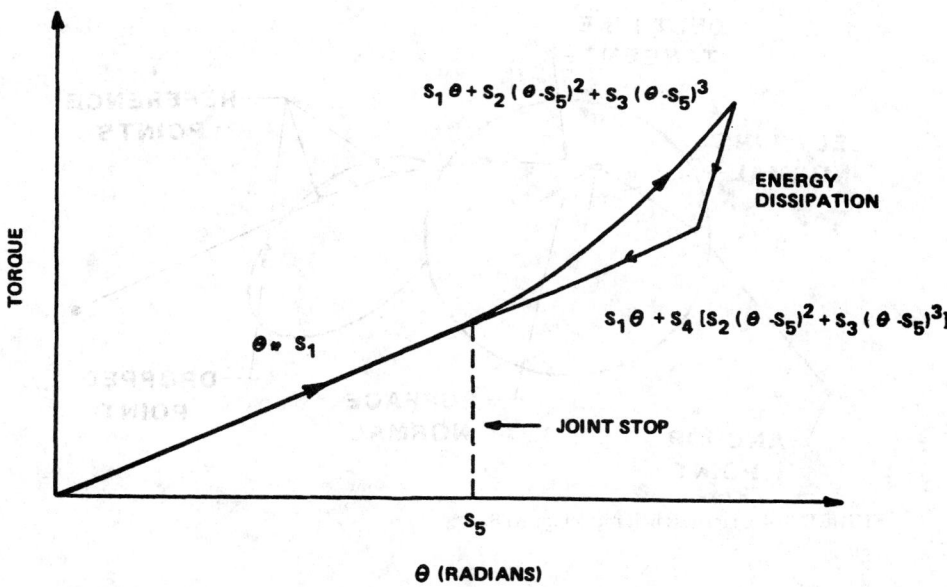

FIGURE 30.2 Joint torque model for ATB.

Narrow contact surfaces offer special problems when the perpendicular to the maximum penetration point of the ellipse falls outside the contact plane. This problem can be addressed by using an alternative "edge effects" calculation provided by the program or by representing the contact plane with an ellipsoid or hyperellipsoid.

The belt system, shown in Fig. 30.4, is represented by a stretched string that contacts a series of points on the surface of one or more body segment ellipsoids. For the simplest case (seat belt routine), these points are be rigidly attached to the body segment ellipsoid. For the more general case (harness belt routine), the points move across the surface as determined by anchor location, belt tension, belt physical properties, and the longitudinal and transverse friction coefficients. The belt

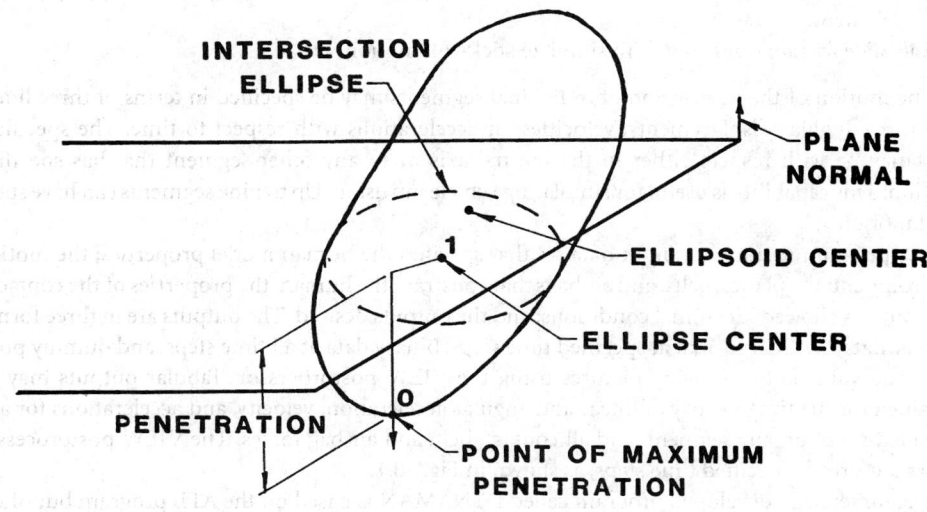

FIGURE 30.3 Plane-segment contact for ATB.

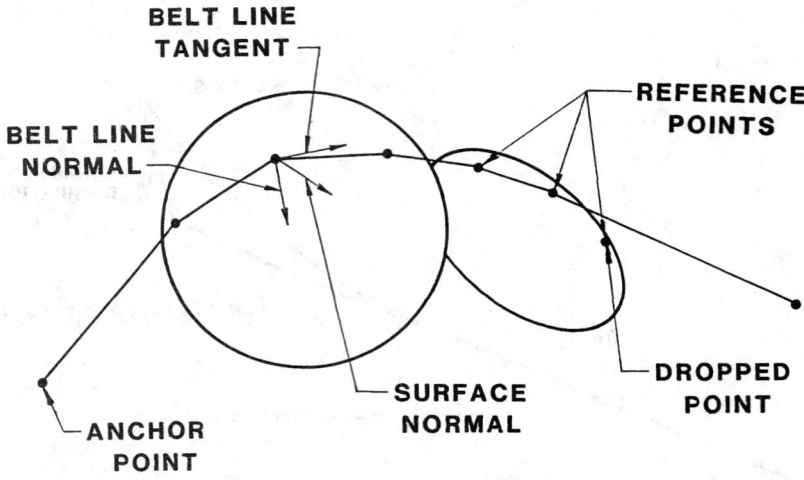

FIGURE 30.4   Harness belt model for ATB.

may penetrate the body surface, based on the physical properties of the body segment ellipsoid. The point locations are recalculated at each iteration and moved to maintain force equilibrium along the stretched belt.

The basic air bag system is represented by an ellipsoid anchored to a reaction surface. The base model is a stored gas inflator and an air bag with venting.

A number of special features are included in the program to address anticipated requirements of users. These include the following:

Tension element: Allows the transmission of tension only—to simulate muscle.
Flexible element: To simulate neck, spine elements.
Slip joint: To simulate elements like steering columns.
Spring-damper element: To simulate alternative connections.
Wind force application: To simulate aircraft ejections.
Force and torque application: To permit a time-dependent force or torque to be applied to any element.
Roll-slide friction constraints: To simulate stick-roll motion.

The motion of the vehicle and of individual segments may be specified in terms of three linear and three angular displacements, velocities, or accelerations with respect to time. The specification may be with respect either to the inertial axis or to any other segment that has specified motion. This capability is useful for simulating vehicle intrusion. Up to nine segments can have specified motion.

The program requires an input data set that specifies the human model properties; the motion environment; the planes, belts, and air bags that constrain the human; the properties of the contacts; the contacts allowed; the initial conditions; and the outputs desired. The outputs are in three forms: tabular data in ASCII format at specified time steps, binary data at all time steps, and dummy position data suitable for drawing pictures using the VIEW postprocessor. Tabular outputs may be obtained for the time history of linear and angular acceleration, velocity, and accelerations for any specified point on any segment, and all contact, belt, and air bag forces. The VIEW postprocessor offers pictures at specified time steps, as shown in Fig. 30.1.

A commercially developed program called DYNAMAN is based on the ATB program but offers enhancements, particularly in ease of use. The DYNAMAN program contains a preprocessor that greatly simplifies the development and modification of data sets. This preprocessor allows the user to view the configuration of the vehicle, dummy, and restraint systems as the modifications are made. The capability includes routines for positioning the dummy in equilibrium and for plotting the crash pulse and force deformation functions. The postprocessor provides tables and graphs of the time history of any of the output variables. Pictures and/or animations of occupant position with respect to time are also available from the postprocessor. The processor permits interactive translation, rotation, or zooming of each image.

Other enhancements offered by DYNAMAN include belt retractors with pretensioning, air bag shapes consisting of both cylindrical and ellipsoidal geometries that expand during inflation, and air bag inflation rates which can be specified from test data. The force-deformation functions have additional flexibility, permitting the force to be distributed in the contact area and allowing individual rather than combined contact properties.

The DYNAMAN model is available for PC or workstation. The current version is 3.0, released in February of 1993 [GESAC, 1993].

30.2 MADYMO Model

The MADYMO model, developed by TNO, Netherlands, has evolved since the early 1970s. The current version is 5.0, released in July of 1992 [TNO, 1992]. The source code is proprietary. The code runs on a workstation; a PC version is not available.

The code reportedly uses lagrangian methods for formulating the equations of motion for multiple tree structures composed of rigid bodies connected by joints. The segment and mass characteristics are generally similar to the ATB model. The number of bodies that the program can handle is 250, 15 of which can have specified motion.

The contact forces can be of the nonlinear spring, viscous damping, or frictional type. Hysteresis is specified by the unloading slope or by an alternative model that specifies an unloading curve used in conjunction with the unloading slope.

The programs input data set requires similar information to the ATB model but is structured to be more user friendly to develop and edit. To resolve the difficulty of achieving initial equilibrium of the dummy, the program adjusts the force-deformation curves so that equilibrium exists for the position of the dummy at time zero. This is a helpful feature, since a preprocessor to position the dummy is not provided.

The basic belt system is a string-type belt that attaches to fixed points on the dummy. A more advanced model that incorporates a finite-element belt is also offered.

Unique features that MADYMO contains include

Kelvin spring damper: A nonlinear spring in parallel with a damper with velocity-dependent damping coefficient.

Maxwell spring damper: A spring and damper in series.

Point-restraint element: Constrains motion to simulate elements like steering columns.

A 2-D semiempirical air bag: For simple air bag representation.

Finite-element air bag: A 3-node membrane element air bag with linear elastic isotropic material properties and simple gas dynamics. A preprocessor to assist in the mesh generation is available.

MADYMO postprocessors provide plots of time histories and cross-plots of force, acceleration, velocity, and displacement data. Alternative postprocessors provide wire frame or shaded pictures and animations of occupant motion. These processors are interactive, permitting rotation, translation, and zoom of each frame.

According to advertising literature, additional finite-element features are under development and may be expected in the next release.

30.3 DRISIM/PASSIM Models

The DRISIM and PASSIM models are oriented to the design of air bags. DRISIM and PASSIM evolved from DRACAR (driver air cushion—rotation) and PAC (passenger air cushion). The latter were government-sponsored programs dating from 1980. The current versions of these programs are DRISIM-PLUS and PASSIM-PLUS, released in April of 1992 [Fitzpatrick Engineering, 1992]. These programs run on a personal computer, typically in less than 5 minutes. The formulation and source codes for DRACAR and PAC are available. However, the current versions have been significantly improved and are proprietary.

The main features of these programs are simple human models but a detailed model of the air bag and air bag support systems. The human model is two-dimensional, represented by six masses. The air bag is a three-dimensional finite-element membrane. The inflation characteristics are determined by computing the rate of gas flow from the gas generator into the air bag based on data from standardized tests of inflators.

The program requires data of the same type as required by the ATB and MADYMO models. Libraries that contain the characteristics of small, large, and midsized dummies normally used for testing air bags are available from the program supplier. The input data are designed so that all physical properties data can be obtained from prescribed tests and measurements of components. The formulation uses lagrangian methods. Air bag forces include both pressure and bag tension forces during air bag deployment. PASSIM-PLUS also includes air bag inertia ("slap") forces from the unfolding bag.

The belt systems in the model are relatively simple, applying forces to the body at specified locations determined from analyses of test data.

The models contain preprocessors and postprocessors to assist in model operation. The preprocessor offers assistance in developing and modifying the input data set and viewing the resulting changes in the occupant, air bag, belt restraint, and vehicle. The preprocessor also aids in modeling the finite-element air bag, its tethers, and its venting. A wide variety of bag shapes are possible.

The postprocessor provides the capability of reviewing graphic and tabular results. The time histories of virtually all calculated variables are available. Output injury measures include head acceleration and HIC, femur force, neck forces and moments, and chest acceleration, deflection, and viscous response. The results of multiple runs can be stored and plotted together to examine trends. Occupant motion can be examined from pictures of the occupant and vehicle. The pictures can be sequenced rapidly to provide animation.

References

Armstrong Aerospace Medical Research Laboratory. 1994. Input Description for the Articulated Total Body Model, AAMRL Document. Wright Patterson AFB, Ohio, AAMRL.

Armstrong Aerospace Medical Research Laboratory. 1988. Measurement of Hybrid III Dummy Properties and Analytical Simulation Data Base Development, AAMRL-TR-88-005. Wright Patterson AFB, Ohio, AAMRL.

Chandler RG, Laananen DH. 1979. Seat/Occupant Crash Dynamic Analysis Verification Test Program, SAE Paper No 790590.

Digges K. 1988. Occupant/vehicle crash models and data bases maintained by the National Highway Traffic Safety Administration. In 1988 IRCOBI Conference Proceedings, pp 149–158. Bron, France, IRCOBI Secretariat.

Fitzpatrick Engineering. 1992. DRISIM-PLUS and PASSIM-PLUS Users Manuals. Duluth, Minn, Fitzpatrick Engineering.

GESAC. 1993. Dynaman User's Manual, Version 3.0. Kearneysville, WV, GESAC, Inc.

Huston RL, Hessel RE, Winget JM. 1977. Dynamics of a crash victim: A finite segment model. AIAA J 14(2):173.

Prasad P, Chou C. 1993. A review of mathematical occupant simulation models, pp 102–150. In AM Nahum, JW Melvin (eds), Accidental Injury. Berlin, Springer-Verlag.

TNO. 1992. MADYMO Users Manual 2D/3D, Version 5.0. Delft, The Netherlands, Department of Injury Prevention, TNO Road-Vehicle Institute.

Further Information

A number of other human models have been developed and applied to special problems. Two such models are

UCIN3D—a model composed of 12 body segments, developed in 1975 at the University of Cincinnati. It is described by Huston et al. [1976].

SOMLA—A 12-body-segment model developed by the Federal Aviation Administration in 1975. This model applies finite-element modeling to the seat in order to evaluate seating designs. The model is described by Chandler and Laananen [1979].

Additional information on these and other models may be found in *Accidental Injury,* edited by Nahum and Melvin (Berlin, Springer-Verlag). This reference also provides additional bibliography on validation and application of the models.

Data for the modeling humans and their interaction with the environment are available from a variety of databases. The Crash Analysis Center at The George Washington University, 20101 Academic Way, Ashburn, VA 22011-2604, maintains a film and data library of more than 15,000 crash tests conducted by the Department of Transportation. Other computer programs and databases to assist in developing input data were summarized by Digges [1988].

The science of vehicle and occupant modeling is currently expanding rapidly. Occupants represented by finite elements are now being incorporated into vehicle structural models, also represented by finite elements. Lumped-mass occupant models are being modified to include finite-element safety components. Ultimately, these models may include finite-element dummies. The sources of the present programs should be contacted for new developments. The sources are ATB, AL/CFBV, Bldg. 441, 2610 Seventh St., Wright Patterson AFB, Ohio, 45433; DYNAMAN, GESAC, Rt. 2, Box 339A, Kearneysville, WV 25430; MADYMO, TNO Crash Safety Research Centre, P.O. Box 6033, 2600 JA Delft, The Netherlands; and DRISIM/PASSIM, Fitzpatrick Engineering, 2411 Lakewood Rd., Duluth, MN 55804.

31

Cardiac Biomechanics

Andrew D. McCulloch

Institute for Biomedical Engineering, University of California at San Diego

The primary function of the heart, to pump blood through the circulatory system, is fundamentally mechanical. In this chapter, cardiac function is discussed in the context of the mechanics of the ventricular walls from the perspective of the determinants of myocardial stresses and strains (Table 31.1). Many physiologic, pathophysiologic, and clinical factors are directly or indirectly affected by myocardial stress and strain (Table 31.2). Of course, the factors in Tables 31.1 and 31.2 are closely interrelated—most of the factors affected by myocardial stress and strain in turn affect the stress and strain in the ventricular wall. For example, changes in wall stress due to altered hemodynamic load may cause ventricular remodeling, which in turn alters geometry, structure, and material properties. This chapter is organized around the governing determinants in Table 31.1, but mention is made where appropriate to some of the factors in Table 31.2.

31.1 Cardiac Geometry and Structure

The mammalian heart consists of four pumping chambers, the left and right atria and ventricles communicating through the atrioventricular (mitral and tricuspid) valves, which are structurally connected by chordae tendineae to papillary muscles that extend from the anterior and posterior aspects of the right and left ventricular lumens. The muscular cardiac wall is perfused via the coronary vessels that originate at the left and right coronary ostia located in the sinuses of Valsalva immediately distal to the aortic valve leaflets. Surrounding the whole heart is the collagenous parietal pericardium that fuses with the diaphragm and great vessels. These are the anatomical structures that are most commonly studied in the field of cardiac mechanics. Particular emphasis in this chapter is given to the ventricular walls, which are the most important for the pumping function of the heart. Most studies of cardiac mechanics have focused on the left ventricle, but many of the important conclusions apply equally to the right ventricle.

Ventricular Geometry

From the perspective of engineering mechanics, the ventricles are three-dimensional thick-walled pressure vessels with substantial variations in wall thickness and principal curvatures both regionally and temporally through the cardiac cycle. The ventricular walls in the normal heart are thickest at the equator and base of the left ventricle and thinnest at the left ventricular apex and right ventricular free wall. There are also variations in the principal dimensions of the left ventricle with species, age, phase of the cardiac cycle, and disease (Table 31.3). But, in general, the ratio of wall thickness to radius is too high to be treated accurately by all but the most sophisticated thick-wall shell theories [Taber, 1991].

Ventricular geometry has been studied in most quantitative detail in the dog heart [Nielsen et al., 1991; Streeter & Hanna, 1973]. Geometric models have been very useful in the analysis, especially the use of confocal and nonconfocal ellipses of revolution to describe the epicardial and endocardial surfaces of the left and right ventricular walls (Fig. 31.1). The canine left ventricle is reasonably modeled by a thick ellipsoid of revolution truncated at the base. The crescentic right ventricle occupies wraps about 180° around the heart wall circumferentially and extends longitudinally about two-thirds of the distance from the base to the apex. Using a truncated ellipsoidal model, left ventricular geometry in the dog can be defined by the major and minor radii of two surfaces, the left ventricular endocardium, and a surface defining the free wall epicardium and the septal endocardium of the right ventricle. Streeter and Hanna [1973] described the position of the basal plane using a truncation factor f_b defined as the ratio between the longitudinal distances from equator to base and equator to apex. Hence, the overall longitudinal distance from base to apex is $(1 + f_b)$ times the major radius of the ellipse. Since variations in f_b between diastole and systole are relatively small (0.45 to 0.51), the authors suggested a constant value of 0.5.

The focal length d of an ellipsoid is defined from the major and minor radii (a and b) by $d^2 = a^2 - b^2$ and varies only slightly in the dog from endocardium to epicardium between end-diastole (37.3

TABLE 31.1 Basic Determinants of Myocardial Stress and Strain

Geometry and structure	
3D shape	Wall thickness
	Curvature
	Stress-free and unloaded reference configurations
Tissue structure	Muscle fiber architecture
	Connective tissue organization
	Pericardium, epicardium, and endocardium
	Coronary vascular anatomy
Boundary/initial conditions	
Pressure	Filling pressure (preload)
	Arterial pressure (afterload)
	Direct and indirect ventricular interactions
	Thoracic and pericardial pressures
Constraints	Effects of inspiration and expiration
	Constraints due to the pericardium and its attachments
	Valves and fibrous valve annuli, chordae tendineae
	Great vessels, lungs
Material properties	
Resting or passive	Nonlinear finite elasticity
	Quasilinear viscoelasticity
	Anisotropy
	Biphasic poroelasticity
Active dynamic	Activation sequence
	Myofiber isometric and isotonic contractile dynamics
	Sarcomere length and length history
	Cellular calcium kinetics and metabolic energy supply

TABLE 31.2   Factors Affected by Myocardial Stress and Strain

Direct factors	Regional muscle work
	Myocardial oxygen demand and energetics
	Coronary blood flow
Electrophysiologic responses	Action potential duration (QT interval)
	Repolarization (T wave morphology)
	Excitability
	Risk of arrhythmia
Development and morphogenesis	Growth rate
	Cardiac looping and septation
	Valve formation
Vulnerability to injury	Ischemia
	Arrhythmia
	Cell dropout
	Aneurysm rupture
Remodeling, repair, and adaptation	Eccentric and concentric hypertrophy
	Fibrosis
	Scar formation
Progression of disease	Transition from hypertrophy to failure
	Ventricular dilation
	Infarct expansion
	Response to reperfusion
	Aneurysm formation

to 37.9 mm) and end-systole (37.7 to 37.1 mm) [Streeter & Hanna, 1973]. Hence, within the accuracy that the boundaries of left ventricular wall can be treated as ellipsoids of revolution, the assumption that the ellipsoids are confocal appears to be a good one. This has motivated the choice of prolate spheroidal (elliptic-hyperbolic-polar) coordinates (λ, μ, θ) as a system for economically representing ventricular geometries obtained postmortem or by noninvasive tomography [Nielsen et al., 1991; Young and Axel, 1992]. The Cartesian coordinates of a point are given in terms of its prolate spheroidal coordinates by

$$x_1 = d \cosh \lambda \cos \mu$$
$$x_2 = d \sinh \lambda \sin\mu \cos \theta \tag{31.1}$$
$$x_3 = d \sinh \lambda \sin \mu \sin \theta$$

Here, the focal length d defines a family of coordinate systems that vary from spherical polar when $d = 0$ to cylindrical polar in the limit when $d \to \infty$. A surface of constant transmural coordinate λ

TABLE 31.3   Representative Left Ventricular Minor-Axis Dimensions*

Species	Comments	Inner Radius (mm)	Outer Radius (mm)	Wall Thickness: Inner Radius
Dog (21 kg)	Unloaded diastole (0 mm Hg)	16	26	0.62
Dog	Normal diastole (2–12 mm Hg)	19	28	0.47
Dog	Dilated diastole (24–40 mm Hg)	22	30	0.36
Dog	Normal systole (1–9 mm Hg EDP)	14	26	0.86
Dog	Long axis, apex-equator (normal diastole)	42	47	0.12
Young rats	Unloaded diastole (0 mm Hg)	1.4	3.5	1.50
Mature rats	Unloaded diastole (0 mm Hg)	3.2	5.8	0.81
Human	Normal	24	32	0.34
Human	Compensated pressure overload	27	42	0.56
Human	Compensated volume overload	32	42	0.33

*Dog data from Ross et al. [1967] and Streeter and Hanna [1973]. Human data from Grossman et al. [1975, 1980]. Rat data are from unpublished observations in the author's laboratory.

(Fig. 31.1) is an ellipse of revolution with major radius $a = d \cosh \lambda$ and minor radius $b = d \sinh \lambda$. In an ellipsoidal model with a truncation factor of 0.5, the longitudinal coordinate μ varies from zero at the apex to 120° at the base. Integrating the Jacobian in prolate spheroidal coordinates gives the volume of the wall or cavity:

$$d^3 \int_0^{2\pi} \int_0^{\mu_2} \int_{\lambda_1}^{\lambda_2} ((\sinh^2\lambda + \sin^2\mu)\sinh\lambda \sin\mu) \, d\lambda \, d\mu \, d\theta$$
$$= \frac{2\pi d^3}{3} |(1 - \cos\mu_2)\cosh^3\lambda - (1 - \cos^3\mu_2) \cosh\lambda|_{\lambda_1}^{\lambda_2}$$

(31.2)

The scaling between heart mass M_H and body mass M within or between species is commonly described by the allometric formula

$$M_H = kM^\alpha$$

(31.3)

Using combined measurements from a variety of mammalian species with *M* expressed in kilograms, the coefficient *k* is 5.8 g and the power α is close to unity (0.98) [Stahl, 1967]. Within individual species, the ratio of heart weight to body weight is somewhat lower in mature rabbits and rats (about 2 g/kg) than in humans (5 g/kg) and higher in horses and dogs (8 g/kg) [Rakusan, 1984]. The rate α of heart growth with body weight decreases with age in most species but not humans. At birth, left and right ventricular weights are similar, but the left ventricle is substantially more massive than the right by adulthood.

Myofiber Architecture

The cardiac ventricles have a complex three-dimensional muscle fiber architecture [for a comprehensive review see Streeter (1979)]. Although the myocytes are relatively short, they are connected

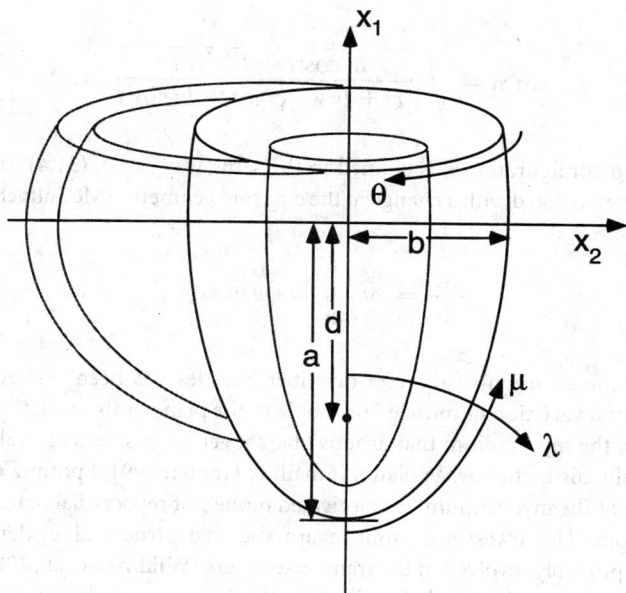

FIGURE 31.1 Truncated ellipsoid representation of ventricular geometry, showing major left ventricular radius (*a*), minor radius (*b*), focal length (*d*), and prolate spheroidal coordinates (λ, μ, θ).

such that at any point in the normal heart wall there is a clear predominant fiber axis that is approximately tangent with the wall (within 3–5° in most regions, except near the apex and papillary muscle insertions). Each ventricular myocyte is connected via gap junctions at intercalated disks to an average of 11.3 neighbors, 5.3 on the sides and 6.0 at the ends [Saffitz et al., 1994]. The classical anatomists dissected discrete bundles of fibrous swirls, but more modern histologic techniques have shown that in the plane of the wall, the muscle fiber angle makes a smooth transmural transition from epicardium to endocardium (Fig. 31.2). Similar patterns have been described for humans, dogs, baboons, macaques, pigs, guinea pigs, and rats. In the human or dog left ventricle, the muscle fiber angle typically varies continuously from about −60° (i.e., 60° clockwise from the circumferential axis) at the epicardium to about +70° at the endocardium. The rate of change of fiber angle is usually greatest at the epicardium—so that circumferential (0°) fibers are found in the outer half of the wall—and begins to slow approaching the inner third near the trabeculata-compacta interface.

Regional variations in ventricular myofiber orientations are generally smooth except at the junction between the right ventricular free wall and septum. A detailed study in the dog that mapped fiber angles throughout the entire right and left ventricles described the same general transmural pattern in all regions including the septum and right ventricular free wall, but with definite regional variations [Nielsen et al., 1991]. Transmural differences in fiber angle were about 120–140° in the left ventricular free wall, larger in the septum (160–180°), and smaller in the right ventricular free wall (100–120°). There are also small increases in fiber orientation from end-diastole to systole (7–19°), with greatest changes at the epicardium and apex [Streeter et al., 1969].

The locus of fiber orientations at a given depth in the ventricular wall has a spiral geometry that may be modeled as a general helix by simple differential geometry. The position vector $\mathbf{x}$ of a point on a helix inscribed on an ellipsoidal surface that is symmetric about the x_1 axis and has major and minor radii, a and b, is given by the parametric equation

$$\mathbf{x} = a \sin t\, \mathbf{e}_1 + b \cos t \sin wt\, \mathbf{e}_2 + b \cos t \cos wt\, \mathbf{e}_3 \qquad (31.4)$$

where the parameter is t, and the helix makes $w/4$ full turns between apex and equator. A positive w defines a left-handed helix with a positive pitch. The fiber angle or helix pitch angle η varies along the arc length:

$$\sin \eta = \sqrt{\frac{a^2 \cos^2 t + b^2 \sin^2 t}{(a^2 + b^2 w^2)\cos^2 t + b^2 \sin^2 t}} \qquad (31.5)$$

If another, deformed configuration $\hat{x}$ is defined in the same way as Eq. (31.4), the fiber segment extension ratio $d\hat{s}/ds$ associated with a change in the ellipsoid geometry [McCulloch et al., 1989] can be derived from

$$\frac{d\hat{s}}{ds} = \frac{d\hat{s}}{dt} \bigg/ \frac{ds}{dt} = \left|\frac{d\hat{\mathbf{x}}}{dt}\right| \bigg/ \left|\frac{d\mathbf{x}}{dt}\right| \qquad (31.6)$$

Although the traditional notion of discrete myofiber bundles has been revised in view of the continuous transmural variation of muscle fiber angle in the plane of the wall, there is a transverse laminar structure in the myocardium that groups fibers together in sheets several cells thick separated by histologically distinct cleavage planes [Smaill & Hunter, 1991; Spotnitz et al., 1974]. The fibrous architecture of the myocardium has motivated models of myocardial material symmetry as transversely isotropic. The transverse laminae are the first structural evidence for material orthotropy and are probably involved in the transverse shears [Waldman et al., 1985] and myofiber rearrangement [Spotnitz et al., 1974] described in the intact heart during systole. A detailed description of the morphogenesis of the muscle fiber system in the developing heart is not available, but there is evidence of an organized myofiber pattern by day 12 in the fetal mouse heart that is sim-

Epicardium

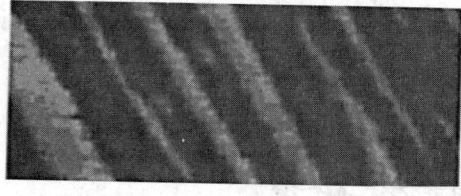

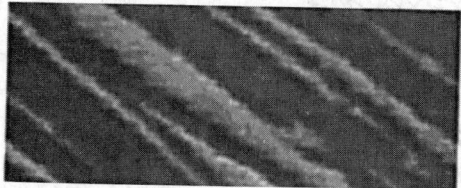

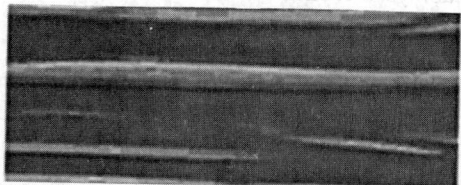

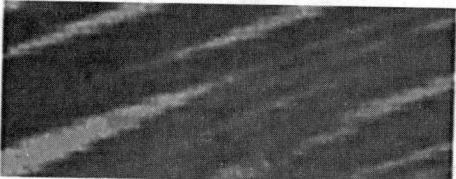

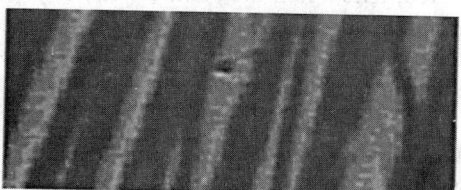

Endocardium

FIGURE 31.2 Cardiac muscle fiber orientations vary continuously through the left ventricular wall from a negative angle at the epicardium to near zero (circumferential) at the midwall and to increasing positive values toward the endocardium. (Micrographs of canine myocardium from the author's laboratory, courtesy Dr. Deidre MacKenna.)

ilar to that seen at birth (day 20) [McLean et al., 1989]. Abnormalities of cardiac muscle fiber patterns have been described in some disease conditions. In hypertrophic cardiomyopathy, which is often familial, there is substantial myofiber disarray, typically in the interventricular septum.

Extracellular Matrix Organization

The cardiac extracellular matrix consists primarily of the fibrillar collagens, types I (85%) and III (11%), synthesized by the cardiac fibroblasts, the most abundant cell type in the heart. Collagen is the major structural protein in connective tissues but only comprises 2–5% of the myocardium by weight, compared with the myocytes, which make up 90% [Weber, 1989]. The collagen matrix has a hierarchical organization (Fig. 31.3) and has been classified according to conventions established for skeletal muscle into endomysium, perimysium, epimysium [Caulfield & Borg, 1979; Robinson et al., 1983]. The endomysium is associated with individual cells and includes a fine weave surrounding the cell and transverse structural connections 120–150 nm long connecting adjacent myocytes, with attachments localized near the z-line of the sarcomere. The primary purpose of the endomysium is probably to maintain registration between adjacent cells. The perimysium groups cells together and includes the collagen fibers that wrap bundles of cells into the laminar sheets described above as well as large coiled fibers typically 1–3 μm in diameter composed of smaller collagen fibrils (40–50 nm) [Robinson et al., 1988]. The helix period of the coiled perimysial fibers is about 20 μm, and the convolution index (ratio of fiber arclength to midline length) is approximately 1.2 in the unloaded state of the ventricle. These perimysial fibers are most likely to be the major structural elements of the collagen extracellular matrix. Finally, a thick epimysial collagen sheath surrounds the entire myocardium forming the protective epicardium (visceral pericardium) and endocardium.

Collagen content, organization, and ratio of types I to III change with age and in various disease conditions including myocardial ischemia and infarction, hypertension, and hypertrophy. Changes in myocardial collagen content and organization coincide with alterations in diastolic myocardial stiffness. Hence the collagen matrix plays an important role in determining the elastic material properties of the resting ventricular myocardium.

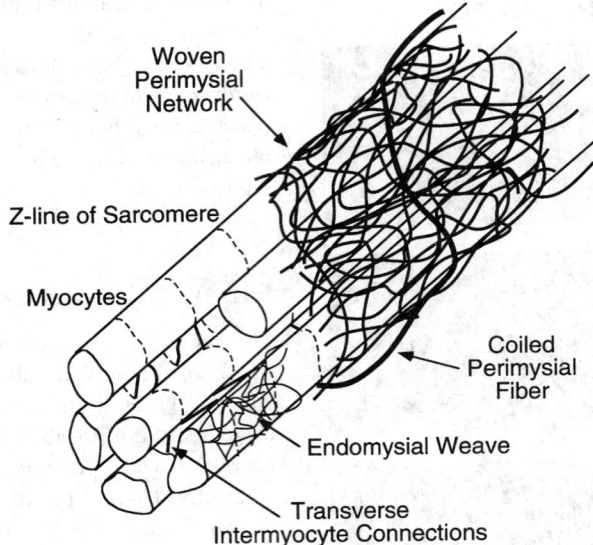

FIGURE 31.3 Schematic representation of cardiac tissue structure showing the association of endomysial and perimysial collagen fibers with cardiac myocytes. (Courtesy Dr. Deidre MacKenna.)

31.2 Cardiac Pump Function

Ventricular Hemodynamics

The most basic mechanical parameters of the cardiac pump are blood pressure and volume flow rate, especially in the major pumping chambers, the ventricles. From the point of view of wall mechanics, the ventricular pressure is the most important boundary condition. Schematic representations of the time-courses of pressure and volume in the left ventricle are shown in Fig. 31.4. Ventricular filling immediately following mitral valve opening (MVO) is initially rapid because the ventricle produces a diastolic suction as the relaxing myocardium recoils elastically from its compressed systolic configuration below the resting chamber volume. The later slow phase of ventricular filling (diastasis) is followed finally by atrial contraction. The deceleration of the inflowing blood reverses the pressure gradient across the valve leaflets and causes them to close (MVC). Valve closure may not, however, be completely passive, because the atrial side of the mitral valve leaflets, which, unlike the pulmonic and aortic valves, are cardiac in embryological origin, have muscle and nerve cells and are electrically coupled to atrial conduction [Sonnenblick et al., 1967].

Ventricular contraction is initiated by excitation, which is almost synchronous (the duration of the QRS complex of the ECG is only about 60 ms in the normal adult) and begins about 0.1 to 0.2 s after atrial depolarization. Pressure rises rapidly during the isovolumic contraction phase (about 50 ms in adult humans), and the aortic valve opens (AVO) when the developed pressure exceeds the aortic pressure (afterload). Most of the cardiac output is ejected within the first quarter of the ejection phase before the pressure has peaked. The aortic valve closes (AVC) 20–30 ms after AVO when the ventricular pressure falls below the aortic pressure owing to the deceleration of the ejecting blood. The dichrotic notch, a characteristic feature of the aortic pressure waveform and a useful marker of aortic valve closure, is caused by pulse wave reflections in the aorta. Since the pulmonary artery pressure against which the right ventricle pumps is much lower than the aortic pressure, the pulmonic valve opens before and closes after the aortic valve. The ventricular pressure falls during isovolumic relaxation, and the cycle continues. The rate of pressure decay from the value P_0 at the

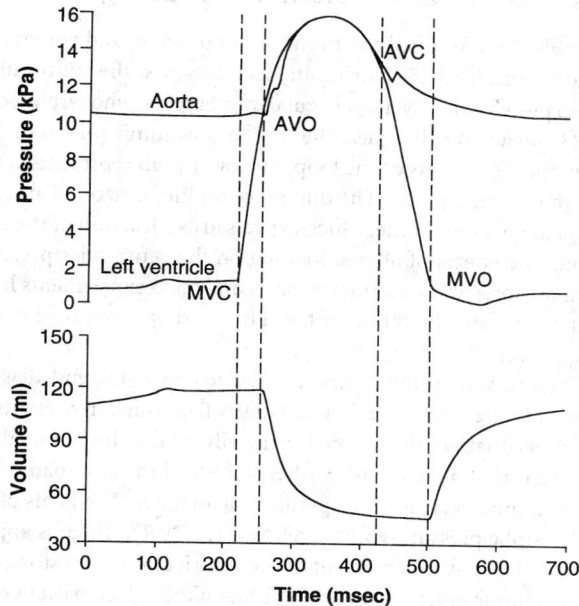

FIGURE 31.4 Left ventricular pressure, aortic pressure, and left ventricular volume during a single cardiac cycle showing the times of mitral valve closure (MVC), aortic valve opening (AVO), aortic valve closure (AVC), and mitral valve opening (MVO).

time of the peak rate of pressure fall until mitral valve opening is commonly characterized by a single exponential time constant, i.e.

$$P(t) = P_0 e^{-t/\tau} + P_\infty \qquad (31.7)$$

where P_∞ is the (negative) baseline pressure to which the ventricle would eventually relax if MVO were prevented [Yellin et al., 1986]. In dogs and humans, τ is normally about 40 ms, but it is increased by various factors including elevated afterload, asynchronous contraction associated with abnormal activation sequence or regional dysfunction, and slowed cytosolic calcium reuptake to the sarcoplasmic reticulum associated with cardiac hypertrophy and failure. The pressure and volume curves for the right ventricle look essentially the same; however, the right ventricular and pulmonary artery pressures are only about a fifth of the corresponding pressures on the left side of the heart. The intraventricular septum separates the right and left ventricles and can transmit forces from one to the other. An increase in right ventricular volume may increase the left ventricular pressure by deformation of the septum. This direct interaction is most significant during filling [Janicki & Weber, 1980].

The phases of the cardiac cycle are customarily divided into systole and diastole. The end of diastole—the start of systole—is generally defined as the time of mitral valve closure. Mechanical end-systole is usually defined as the end of ejection, but Brutsaert and colleagues proposed extending systole until the onset of diastasis [see the review by Brutsaert and Sys (1989)] since there remains considerable myofilament interaction and active tension during relaxation. The distinction is important from the point of view of cardiac muscle mechanics: The myocardium is still active for much of diastole and may never be fully relaxed at sufficiently high heart rates (over 150 beats per minute). Here, we will retain the traditional definition of diastole but consider the ventricular myocardium to be "passive" or "resting" only in the final slow-filling stage of diastole.

Ventricular Pressure—Volume Relations and Energetics

A useful alternative to Fig. 31.4 for displaying ventricular pressure and volume changes is the pressure-volume loop shown in Fig. 31.5. During the last 20 years, the ventricular pressure-volume relationship has been explored extensively, particularly by Sagawa, who wrote a comprehensive book on the approach [1988, Suga and colleagues, 1981]. The isovolumic phases of the cardiac cycle can be recognized as the vertical segments of the loop, the lower limb represents ventricular filling, and the upper segment is the ejection phase. The difference on the horizontal axis between the vertical isovolumic segments is the stroke volume, which expressed as a fraction of the end-diastolic volume is the ejection fraction. The effects of altered loading on the ventricular pressure-volume relation have been studied in many preparations, but the best controlled experiments have used the isolated cross-circulated canine heart in which the ventricle fills and ejects against a computer-controlled volume servo-pump.

Changes in the filling pressure of the ventricle (preload) move the end-diastolic point along the unique end-diastolic pressure-volume relation (EDPVR), which represents the passive filling mechanics of the chamber that are determined primarily by the thick-walled geometry and non-linear elasticity of the resting ventricular wall. Alternatively, if the afterload seen by the left ventricle is increased, stroke volume decreases in a predictable manner. The locus of end-ejection points (AVC) forms the end-systolic pressure-volume relation (ESPVR), which is approximately linear in a variety of conditions and largely independent of the ventricular load history. Hence, the ESPVR is almost the same for isovolumic beats as for ejecting beats, although consistent effects of ejection history have been well characterized [Hunter, 1989]. Connecting pressure-volume points at corresponding times in the cardiac cycle also results in a relatively linear relationship throughout systole with the intercept on the volume axis V_0 remaining nearly constant (Fig. 31.5b). This leads to the valuable approximation that the ventricular volume $V(t)$ at any instance during systole is simply proportional to the instantaneous pressure $P(t)$ through a time-varying elastance $E(t)$:

$$P(t) = E(t)[V(t) - V_0] \tag{31.8}$$

The maximum elastance E_{max}, the slope of the ESPVR, has acquired considerable significance as an index of cardiac contractility that is independent of ventricular loading conditions. As the inotropic state of the myocardium increases, for example with catecholamine infusion, E_{max} increases, and with a negative inotropic effect such as a reduction in coronary artery pressure, it decreases.

The area of the ventricular pressure-volume loop is the external work (EW) performed by the myocardium on the ejecting blood:

$$EW = \int_{EDV}^{ESV} P(t) \, dV \tag{31.9}$$

Plotting this stroke work against a suitable measure of preload gives a ventricular function curve, which illustrates the single most important intrinsic mechanical property of the heart pump. In 1914, Patterson and Starling [1914] performed detailed experiments on the canine heart-lung preparation, and Starling summarized their results with his famous "law of the heart," which states that the work output of the heart increases with ventricular filling. The so-called Frank-Starling mechanism is now well recognized to be an intrinsic mechanical property of cardiac muscle (see next section).

External stroke work is closely related to cardiac energy utilization. Since myocardial contraction is fueled by ATP, 90–95% of which is normally produced by oxidative phosphorylation, cardiac energy consumption is often studied in terms of myocardial oxygen consumption, V_{O_2} (ml $O_2 \cdot g^{-1} \cdot$ beat^{-1}). Since energy is also expended during nonworking contractions, Suga and colleagues [1981] defined the pressure-volume area PVA (J $\cdot g^{-1} \cdot$ beat^{-1}) as the loop area (external stroke work) plus

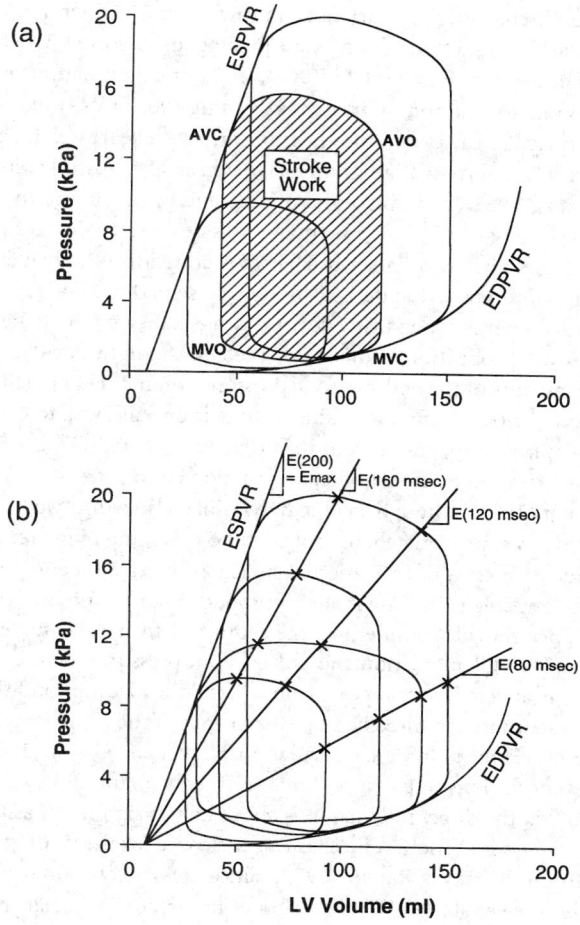

FIGURE 31.5 Schematic diagram of left ventricular pressure-volume loops: (*a*) End-systolic pressure-volume relation (ESPVR), end-diastolic pressure volume relation (EDPVR), and stroke work. The three P-V loops show the effects of changes in preload and afterload. (*b*) Time-varying elastance approximation of ventricular pump function (see text).

the end-systolic potential energy (internal work) which is the area under the ESPVR left of the isovolumic relaxation line (Fig. 31.5*a*),

$$PVA = EW + PE \tag{31.10}$$

The PVA has strong linear correlation with V_{O_2} independent of ejection history. Equation (31.11) has typical values for the dog heart:

$$V_{O_2} = 0.12(PVA) + 2.0 \times 10^{-4} \tag{31.11}$$

The intercept represents the sum of the oxygen consumption for basal metabolism and the energy associated with activation of the contractile apparatus, which is altered by calcium and other inotropic interventions [Suga et al., 1981].

In mammals, there are characteristic variations in cardiac function with heart size. In the power law relation for heart rate as a function of body mass [analogous to Eq. (31.3)], the coefficient k is 241 beats $\cdot$ min^{-1} and the power α is -0.25 [Stahl, 1967]. In the smallest mammals, like soricine shrews that weigh only a few grams, maximum heart rates exceeding 1000 beats $\cdot$ min^{-1} have been measured [Vornanen, 1992]. Ventricular cavity volume scales linearly with heart weight, and ejection fraction and blood pressure are reasonably invariant from rats to horses. Hence, stroke work also scales directly with heart size [Holt et al., 1962], and thus work rate and energy consumption would be expected to increase with decreased body size in the same manner as heart rate. However, careful studies have demonstrated only a 2-fold increase in myocardial heat production as body mass decreases in mammals ranging from humans to rats, despite a 4.6-fold increase in heart rate [Loiselle & Gibbs, 1979]. This suggests that cardiac energy expenditure does not scale in proportion to heart rate and that cardiac metabolism is a lower proportion of total body metabolism in the smaller species.

The primary determinants of the end-diastolic pressure-volume relation (EDPVR) are the material properties of resting myocardium, the chamber dimensions and wall thickness, and the boundary conditions at the epicardium, endocardium, and valve annulus [Gilbert & Glantz, 1989]. The EDPVR has been approximated by an exponential function of volume [see, for example, Chapter 9 in Gaasch and LeWinter (1994)], though a cubic polynomial also works well. Therefore, the passive chamber stiffness dP/dV is approximately proportional to the filling pressure. Important influences on the EDPVR include the extent of relaxation, ventricular interaction and pericardial constraints, and coronary vascular engorgement. The material properties and boundary conditions in the septum are important, since they determine how the septum deforms [Glantz et al., 1978; Glantz & Parmley, 1978]. Through septal interaction, the end-diastolic pressure-volume relationship of the left ventricle may be directly affected by changes the hemodynamic loading conditions of the right ventricle. The ventricles also interact indirectly, since the output of the right ventricle is returned as the input to the left ventricle via the pulmonary circulation. Slinker and Glantz [1986], using pulmonary artery and venae caval occlusions to produce direct (immediate) and indirect (delayed) interaction transients, concluded that the direct interaction is about half as significant as the indirect coupling. The pericardium provides a low-friction mechanical enclosure for the beating heart that constrains ventricular overextension [Mirsky & Rankin, 1979]. Since the pericardium has stiffer elastic properties than the ventricles [Lee et al., 1987], it contributes to direct ventricular interactions. The pericardium also augments the mechanical coupling between the atria and ventricles [Maruyama et al., 1982]. Increasing coronary perfusion pressure has been seen to increase the slope of the diastolic pressure-volume relation (an "erectile" effect) [May-Newman et al., 1994; Salisbury et al., 1960].

31.3 Myocardial Material Properties

Muscle Contractile Properties

Cardiac muscle mechanics testing is far more difficult than skeletal muscle testing mainly owing to the lack of ideal test specimens like the long single-fiber preparations that have been so valuable for studying the mechanisms of skeletal muscle mechanics. Moreover, under physiological conditions, cardiac muscle cannot be stimulated to produce sustained tetanic contractions due to the absolute refractory period of the myocyte cell membrane. Cardiac muscle also exhibits a mechanical property analogous to the relative refractory period of excitation. After a single isometric contraction, some recovery time is required before another contraction of equal amplitude can be activated. The time constant for this mechanical restitution property of cardiac muscle is about 1 second [Bers, 1991].

Unlike skeletal muscle, in which maximal active force generation occurs at a sarcomere length that optimizes myofilament overlap ($\sim$2.1 μm), the isometric twitch tension developed by isolated cardiac muscle continues to rise with increased sarcomere length in the physiological range (1.6–2.4 μm) (Fig. 31.6a). Early evidence for a descending limb of the cardiac muscle isometric length-tension curve was found to be caused by shortening in the central region of the isolated muscle at the expense of stretching at the damaged ends where specimen was tethered to the test apparatus. If muscle length is controlled so that sarcomere length in the undamaged part of the muscle is indeed constant, or if the developed tension is plotted against the instantaneous sarcomere length rather than the muscle length, the descending limb is eliminated [Ter Keurs et al., 1980b]. Thus, the increase with chamber volume of end-systolic pressure and stroke work is reflected in isolated muscle as a monotonic increase in peak isometric tension with sarcomere length (Fig. 31.6b). Note that the active tension shown in Fig. 31.6 is the total tension minus the resting tension which, unlike in skeletal muscle, becomes very significant at sarcomere lengths over 2.3 μm. The increase in slope of the ESPVR associated with increased contractility is mirrored by the effects of increased calcium concentration in the length-tension relation. The duration as well as the tension developed in the active cardiac twitch also increases substantially with sarcomere length (Fig. 31.6a).

The relationship between cytosolic calcium concentration and muscle tension is studied in skinned muscle. The myofilaments are activated in a graded manner by μM concentrations of calcium, which binds to troponin-C according to Michaelis-Menten kinetics [Rüegg, 1988]. Half-maximal tension in cardiac muscle is developed calcium concentrations of 10^{-6} to 10^{-5} M (the EC_{50}) depending on factors such as species and temperature [Bers, 1991]. Hence, relative isometric tension T_0/T_{max} may be modeled using [Tözeren, 1985]

$$\frac{T_0}{T_{max}} = \frac{[Ca]^n}{[Ca]^n + EC_{50}^n} \tag{31.12}$$

with a Hill coefficient n of 2. The steepness of the isometric length-tension relation (Fig. 31.6b) compared with that of skeletal muscle is due to length-dependent calcium sensitivity. That is, the EC_{50} increases with sarcomere length. The following approximation has been used for EC_{50} in μM [Guccione et al., 1993], based on experimental data from rat cardiac muscle

$$EC_{50} = \frac{4.35}{\sqrt{e^{4.75(L-1.58)} - 1}} \tag{31.13}$$

where L is the sarcomere length in μm.

The isotonic force-velocity relation of cardiac muscle is similar to that of skeletal muscle, and A.V. Hill's well-known hyperbolic relation is a good approximation except at larger forces greater than about 85% of the isometric value. The maximal (unloaded) velocity of shortening is essentially independent of preload but does change with time during the cardiac twitch and is affected by

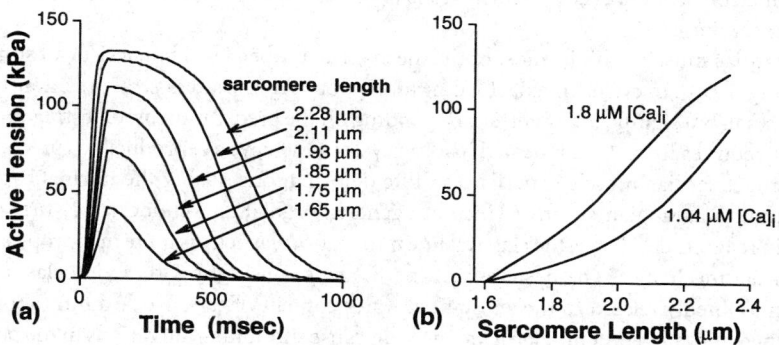

FIGURE 31.6 Cardiac muscle isometric twitch tension generated by a model of rat cardiac contraction (courtesy Dr. Julius Guccione): (a) Developed twitch tension as a function of time and sarcomere length; (b) Peak isometric twitch tension versus sarcomere length for low and high calcium concentration.

factors that affect contractile ATPase activity and hence crossbridge cycling rates. Cardiac muscle contraction also exhibits other significant length-history-dependent properties. An important example is "deactivation" associated with length transients. The isometric twitch tension redeveloped following a brief lengthening transient that dissociates crossbridges reaches the original isometric value when the transient is imposed early in the twitch before the peak tension is reached. But following transients applied at times after the peak twitch tension has occurred, the fraction of tension redeveloped declines progressively because cytoplasmic calcium has fallen below the level necessary for all crossbridges to reattach [Ter Keurs et al., 1980a]. Since the impulse response function of cardiac muscle thus varies in time, the fading memory of cardiac muscle cannot be considered linear as it can for skeletal muscle [Bergel & Hunter, 1979].

The many model formulations of cardiac muscle contractile mechanics are too numerous to summarize here. In essence they may be grouped into three categories: Time-varying elastance models include the essential dependence of cardiac active force development on muscle length and time. These models would seem to be well suited to the continuum analysis of whole heart mechanics [Arts et al., 1979; Chadwick, 1982; Taber, 1991] by virtue of the success of the time-varying elastance concept of ventricular function (see "Ventricular Pressure—Volume Relations and Energetics" above). In "Hill" models the active fiber stress development is modified by shortening or lengthening according to the force-velocity relation, so that fiber tension is reduced by increased shortening velocity [Arts et al., 1982; Nevo & Lanir, 1989]. Fully history-dependent models are more complex and are generally based on the crossbridge theory [Guccione et al., 1993; Panerai, 1980]. The appropriate choice of model will depend on the purpose of the analysis. For most models of global ventricular function, a time-varying elastance model will suffice, but for an analysis of sarcomere dynamics in isolated muscle or the ejecting heart, a history-dependent analysis is more appropriate.

Resting Myocardial Properties

Since, by the Frank-Starling mechanism, end-diastolic volume directly affects systolic ventricular work, the mechanics of resting myocardium also have fundamental physiologic significance. Most biomechanics studies of passive myocardial properties have been conducted in isolated, arrested whole heart or tissue preparations. Although Hill's basic assumption that resting and active muscle fiber tension are additive is axiomatic in one-dimensional tests of isolated cardiac mechanics, there remains almost no experimental information on how the passive and active material properties of myocardium superpose in two dimensions or three. Perhaps, the simplest assumption is that active stress is strictly one-dimensional and adds to the fiber component of the three-dimensional passive stress. However, even this addition will indirectly affect all the other components of the stress response, since myocardial elastic deformations are finite, nonlinear, and approximately isochoric (volume conserving).

Passive cardiac muscle exhibits most of the mechanical properties characteristic of soft tissues in general [Fung, 1993]. In cyclic uniaxial loading and unloading, the stress-strain relationship is nonlinear with small but significant hysteresis. Depending on the preparation used, resting cardiac muscle typically requires from 2–10 repeated loading cycles to achieve a reproducible (preconditioned) response. Intact cardiac muscle experiences finite deformations during the normal cardiac cycle, with maximum Lagrangian strains (which are generally radial and endocardial) that may easily exceed 0.5 in magnitude. Hence, the classical linear theory of elasticity is quite inappropriate for resting myocardial mechanics. The hysteresis of the tissue is consistent with a viscoelastic response, which is undoubtedly related to the substantial water content of the myocardium (about 80% by mass). Changes in water content, such as edema, can cause substantial alterations in the passive stiffness and viscoelastic properties of myocardium. The viscoelasticity of passive cardiac muscle has been characterized in creep and relaxation studies of papillary muscle from cat and rabbit. In both species, the tensile stress in response to a step in strain relaxes 30–40% in the first 10s [Pinto & Patitucci, 1977; Pinto & Patitucci, 1980]. The relaxation curves exhibit a short exponential time constant (<0.02 s) and a long one (about 1000 s) and are largely independent of the strain magnitude, which supports the approximation that myocardial viscoelasticity is quasilinear. Myocardial creep under isotonic loading is 2–3% of the original length after 100 s of isotonic loading and is also quasilinear with an exponential timecourse. There is also emerging evidence that passive ventricular muscle exhibits other anelastic properties such as "permanent" strain softening.

Since the hysteresis of passive cardiac muscle is small and only weakly affected by changes in strain rate, the assumption of pseudoelasticity [Fung, 1993] is often appropriate. That is, the resting myocardium is considered to be a finite elastic material with different elastic properties in loading versus unloading. Although various preparations have been used to study resting myocardial elasticity, the most detailed and complete information has come from biaxial and multiaxial tests of isolated sheets of cardiac tissue, mainly from the dog [Demer & Yin, 1983; Halperin et al., 1987; Humphrey et al., 1990a]. These experiments have shown that the arrested myocardium exhibits significant anisotropy with substantially greater stiffness in the muscle fiber direction than transversely. In equibiaxial tests of muscle sheets cut from planes parallel to the ventricular wall, fiber stress was greater than the transverse stress (Fig. 31.7) by an average factor of close to 2.0 [Yin et al., 1987]. Moreover, as suggested by the structural organization of the myocardium described in "Cardiac Geometry and Structure," there may also be significant anisotropy in the plane of the tissue transverse to the fiber axis.

The biaxial stress-strain properties of passive myocardium display some heterogeneity. Recently, Novak and colleagues [1994] measured regional variations of biaxial mechanics in the canine left ventricle. Specimens from the inner and outer thirds of the left ventricular free wall were stiffer than those from the midwall and interventricular septum, but the degree of anisotropy was similar in each region. Significant species variations in myocardial stiffness have also been described. Using measurements of two-dimensional regional strain during left ventricular inflation in the isolated whole heart, a parameter optimization approach showed that canine cardiac tissue was several times stiffer than that of the rat, though the nonlinearity and anisotropy were similar [Omens et al., 1993]. Biaxial testing of the collagenous parietal pericardium and epicardium have shown that these tissues have distinctly different properties than the myocardium being very compliant and isotropic at low

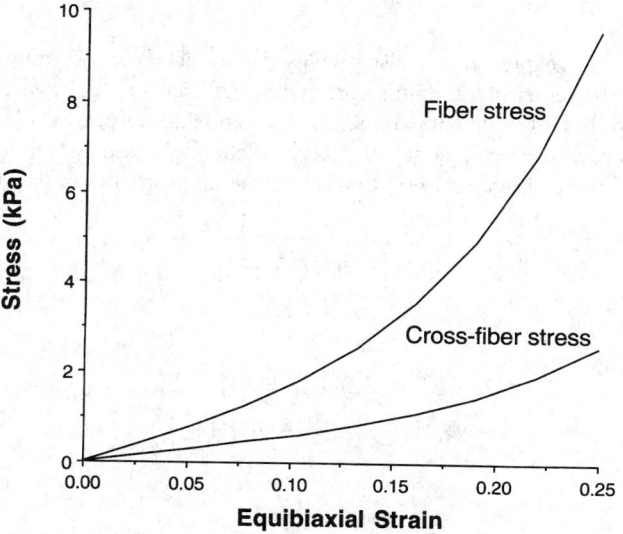

FIGURE 31.7 Representative stress-strain curves for passive rat myocardium computed using Eqs. (31.17) and (31.19). Fiber and crossfiber stress are shown for equibiaxial strain (courtesy, Dr. Jeffrey Omens).

biaxial strains (<0.1–0.15) but rapidly becoming very stiff and anisotropic as the strain is increased [Humphrey et al., 1990a; Lee et al., 1987].

Various constitutive models have been proposed for the elasticity of passive cardiac tissues. Because of the large deformations and nonlinearity of these materials, the most useful framework has been provided by the pseudostrain-energy formulation for hyperelasticity. For a detailed review of the material properties of passive myocardium and approaches to constitutive modeling, the reader is referred to Chapters 1–6 of Glass and colleagues [1991]. In hyperelasticity, the components of the second Piola-Kirchhoff stress P_{RS} are obtained from the strain energy W as a function of the Lagrangian (Green's) strain E_{RS}

$$P_{RS} = \frac{1}{2}\left(\frac{\partial W}{\partial E_{RS}} + \frac{\partial W}{\partial E_{SR}}\right) \tag{31.14}$$

The myocardium is generally assumed to be an incompressible material, which is a good approximation in the isolated tissue, although in the intact heart there can be significant redistributions of tissue volume associated with phasic changes in regional coronary blood volume. Incompressibility is included as a kinematic constraint in the finite elasticity analysis, which introduces a new pressure variable that is added as a Lagrange multiplier in the strain energy. The examples that follow are various strain-energy functions, with representative parameter values (for W in kPa, i.e., mJ $\cdot$ ml^{-1}), that have been suggested for cardiac tissues. For the two-dimensional properties of canine myocardium, Yin and colleagues [1987] obtained reasonable fits to experimental data with an exponential function

$$W = 0.47e^{\left(35E_{11}^{1.2}+20E_{22}^{1.2}\right)} \tag{31.15}$$

where E_{11} is the fiber strain and E_{22} is the crossfiber in-plane strain. Humphrey and Yin [1987] proposed a three-dimensional form for W as the sum of an isotropic exponential function of the first principal invariant I_1 of the right Cauchy-Green deformation tensor and another exponential function of the fiber stretch ratio λ_F:

$$W = 0.21\left(e^{9.4(I_1-3)} - 1\right) + 0.35\left(e^{66(\lambda_F-1)^2} - 1\right) \tag{31.16}$$

The isotropic part of this expression has also been used to model the myocardium of the embryonic chick heart during the ventricular looping stages, with coefficients of 0.02 kPa during diastole and 0.78 kPa at end-systole, and exponent parameters of 1.1 and 0.85, respectively [Lin & Taber, 1994]. Another, related transversely isotropic strain-energy function was used by Guccione and colleagues [1991] and Omens and colleagues [1991] to model material properties in the isolated mature rat and dog hearts:

$$W = 0.6\,(e^Q - 1) \tag{31.17}$$

where, in the dog

$$Q = 26.7E_{11}^2 + 2.0\left(E_{22}^2 + E_{33}^2 + E_{23}^2 + E_{32}^2\right) \\ + 14.7\left(E_{12}^2 + E_{21}^2 + E_{13}^2 + E_{31}^2\right) \tag{31.18}$$

and, in the rat

$$Q = 9.2E_{11}^2 + 2.0\left(E_{22}^2 + E_{33}^2 + E_{23}^2 + E_{32}^2\right) + 3.7\left(E_{12}^2 + E_{21}^2 + E_{13}^2 + E_{31}^2\right) \tag{31.19}$$

In Eqs. (31.18) and (31.19), normal and shear strain components involving the radial (x_3) axis are included. Humphrey and colleagues [1990b] determined a new polynomial form directly from biaxial tests. Novak and colleagues [1994] gave representative coefficients for canine myocardium from three layers of the left ventricular free wall. For the outer third, they obtained

$$W = 4.8(\lambda_F - 1)^2 + 3.4(\lambda_F - 1)^3 + 0.77(I_1 - 3)$$
$$- 6.1(I_1 - 3)(\lambda_F - 1) + 6.2(I_1 - 3)^2 \tag{31.20}$$

for the midwall region

$$W = 5.3(\lambda_F - 1)^2 + 7.5(\lambda_F - 1)^3 + 0.43(I_1 - 3)$$
$$- 7.7(I_1 - 3)(\lambda_F - 1) + 5.6(I_1 - 3)^2 \tag{31.21}$$

and for the inner layer of the wall

$$W = 0.51(\lambda_F - 1)^2 + 27.6(\lambda_F - 1)^3 + 0.74(I_1 - 3)$$
$$- 7.3(I_1 - 3)(\lambda_F - 1) + 7.0(I_1 - 3)^2 \tag{31.22}$$

Finally, a power law strain-energy function expressed in terms of circumferential, longitudinal, and transmural extension ratios (λ_1, λ_2, and λ_3) was recently used [Gupta et al., 1994] to describe the biaxial properties of sheep myocardium two weeks after experimental myocardial infarction, in the scarred infarct region:

$$W = 0.36\left(\frac{\lambda_1^{32}}{32} + \frac{\lambda_2^{30}}{30} + \frac{\lambda_3^{31}}{31} - 3\right) \tag{31.23}$$

and in the remote, nonischemic tissue:

$$W = 0.11\left(\frac{\lambda_1^{22}}{22} + \frac{\lambda_2^{26}}{26} + \frac{\lambda_3^{24}}{24} - 3\right) \tag{31.24}$$

The strain in the constitutive equation must generally be referred to the stress-free state of the tissue. However, the unloaded state of the passive left ventricle is not stress-free; residual stress exists in the intact, unloaded myocardium, as shown by Omens and Fung [1990]. Cross-sectional equatorial rings from potassium-arrested rat hearts spring open elastically when the left ventricular wall is resected radially. The average opening angle of the resulting curved arc is 45 ± 10° in the rat. Subsequent radial cuts produce no further change. Hence, a slice with one radial cut is considered to be stress-free, and there is a nonuniform distribution of residual strain across the intact wall, being compressive at the endocardium and tensile at the epicardium, with some regional differences. Stress analyses of the diastolic left ventricle have shown that residual stress acts to minimize the endocardial stress concentrations that would otherwise be associated with diastolic loading [Guccione et al., 1991]. An important physiological consequence of residual stress is that sarcomere length is nonuniform in the unloaded resting heart. Rodriguez and colleagues [1993] showed that sarcomere length is about 0.13 µm greater at epicardium than endocardium in the unloaded rat heart, and this gradient vanishes when residual stress is relieved. Residual stress and strain may have an important relationship to cardiac growth and remodeling. Theoretical studies have shown that residual stress in tissues can arise from growth fields that are kinematically incompatible [Rodriguez et al., 1994].

31.4 Regional Ventricular Mechanics: Stress and Strain

Although ventricular pressures and volumes are valuable for assessing the global pumping performance of the heart, myocardial stress and strain distributions are needed to characterize regional ventricular function, especially in pathological conditions, such as myocardial ischemia and infarction, where profound localized changes may occur. The measurement of stress in the intact myocardium involves resolving the local forces acting on defined planes in the heart wall. Attempts to measure local forces [Feigl et al., 1967; Huisman et al., 1980] have had limited success because of the large deformations of the myocardium and the uncertain nature of the mechanical coupling between the transducer elements and the tissue. Efforts to measure intramyocardial pressures using miniature implanted transducers have been more successful but have also raised controversy over the extent to which they accurately represent changes in interstitial fluid pressure. In all cases, these methods provide an incomplete description of three-dimensional wall stress distributions. Therefore, the most common approach for estimating myocardial stress distributions is the use of mathematical models based on the laws of continuum mechanics [Hunter & Smaill, 1989]. Although there is not room to review these analyses here, the important elements of such models are the geometry and structure, boundary conditions and material properties, described in the foregoing sections. An excellent review of ventricular wall stress analysis is given by Yin [1981]. The most versatile and powerful method for ventricular stress analysis is the finite element method, which has been used in cardiac mechanics for over 20 years [see (Yin, 1985)]. However, models must also be validated with experimental measurements. Since the measurement of myocardial stresses is not yet reliable, the best experimental data for model validation are measurements of strains in the ventricular wall.

The earliest myocardial strain gauges were mercury-in-rubber transducers sutured to the epicardium. These days, local segment length changes are routinely measured with various forms of the piezoelectric crystal sonomicrometer. However, since the ventricular myocardium is a three-dimensional continuum, the local strain is only fully defined by all the normal and shear components of the myocardial strain tensor. Villarreal and colleagues [1988] measured two-dimensional midwall strain components by arranging three piezoelectric crystals in a small triangle so that three segment lengths could be measured simultaneously. They showed that the principal axis of greatest shortening is not aligned with circumferential midwall fibers and that this axis changes with altered ventricular loading and contractility. Therefore, uniaxial segment measurements do not reveal the full extent of alterations in regional function caused by an experimental intervention. Another approach to measuring regional myocardial strains is the use of clinical imaging techniques, such as contrast ventriculography, high-speed x-ray tomography, magnetic resonance imaging (MRI), or two-dimensional echocardiography. But the conventional application of these techniques is not suitable for measuring regional strains because they cannot be used to identify the motion of distinct myocardial points. They only produce a profile or silhouette of a surface, except in the unusual circumstance when radiopaque markers are implanted in the myocardium during cardiac surgery or transplantation [Ingels et al., 1975]. Hunter and Zerhouni [1989] describe the prospects for noninvasive imaging of discrete points in the ventricular wall. The most promising method is the use of MRI tagging methods, which are now being used to map three-dimensional ventricular strain fields in conscious subjects [Young & Axel, 1992].

In experimental research, implantable radiopaque markers are used for tracking myocardial motions with high spatial and temporal resolution. Meier and coworkers [1980*a*; 1980*b*] placed triplets of metal markers 10–15 mm apart near the epicardium of the canine right ventricle and reconstructed their positions from biplane cinéradiographic recordings. By polar decomposition, they obtained the two principal epicardial strains, the principal angle, and the local rotation in the region. The use of radiopaque markers was extended to three dimensions by Waldman and colleagues [1985], who implanted three closely separated columns of 5–6 metal beads in the ventricular wall. With this technique, it is possible to find all six components of strain and all three rigid-body rotation angles at sites through the wall. For details of this method, see the review by Waldman in Chapter 7 of Glass and coworkers [1991]. An enhancement to this method uses high-order finite element interpolation of the marker positions to compute continuous transmural distributions of myocardial deformation [McCulloch & Omens, 1991].

Studies and models like these are producing an increasingly detailed picture of regional myocardial stress and strain distributions. Of the many interesting observations, there are some useful generalizations, particularly regarding the strain. Myocardial deformations are large and three-dimensional, and hence the nonlinear finite strain tensors are more appropriate measures than the linear infinitesimal Cauchy strain. During filling in the normal heart, the wall stretches biaxially but nonuniformly in the plane of the wall and thins in the transmural direction. During systole, shortening is also two-dimensional, and the wall thickens. There are substantial regional differences in the time course, magnitude, and pattern of myocardial deformations. In humans and dogs, in-plane systolic myocardial shortening and diastolic lengthening vary with longitudinal position on the left and right ventricular free walls generally increasing in magnitude from base to apex.

Both during systole and diastole, there are significant shear strains in the wall. In-plane (torsional) shears are negative during diastole, consistent with a small left-handed torsion of the left ventricle during filling, and positive as the ventricular twist reverses during ejection. Consequently, the principal axes of greatest diastolic segment lengthening and systolic shortening are not circumferential or longitudinal but at oblique axes that are typically rotated 10–60° clockwise from circumferential. There are circumferential variations in regional left ventricular strain. The principal axes of greatest diastolic lengthening and systolic shortening tend to be more longitudinal on the posterior wall and more circumferentially oriented on the anterior wall. Perhaps the most significant regional variations are transmural. In-plane and transmural, normal or principal strains, are usually significantly greater in magnitude at the endocardium than the epicardium both in filling and ejection. However, when the strain is resolved in the local muscle fiber direction, the transmural variation of fiber strain becomes insignificant. The combination of torsional deformation and the transmural variation in fiber direction means that systolic shortening and diastolic lengthening tend to be maximized in the fiber direction at the epicardium and minimized at the endocardium. Hence, whereas maximum shortening and lengthening are closely aligned with muscle fibers at the subepicardium, they are almost perpendicular to the fibers at the subendocardium. In the left ventricular wall there are also substantial transverse shear strains (i.e., in the circumferential-radial and longitudinal-radial planes) during systole, though during filling they are smaller. Their functional significance remains unclear, though they change substantially during acute myocardial ischemia or ventricular pacing and are very likely to be associated with the transverse laminae described earlier.

Sophisticated continuum mechanics models are needed to determine the stress distributions associated with these complex myocardial deformations. With modern finite element methods it is now possible to include in the analysis the three-dimensional geometry and fiber architecture, finite deformations, nonlinear material properties, and muscle contraction of the ventricular myocardium. Some models have included other factors such as viscoelasticity, poroelasticity, coronary perfusion, growth and remodeling, regional ischemia, and residual stress. To date, continuum models have provided some valuable insight into regional cardiac mechanics. These include the importance of muscle fiber orientation, torsional deformations and residual stress, and the substantial nonhomogeneities associated with regional variations in geometry and fiber angle or myocardial ischemia and infarction.

Acknowledgments

I am indebted to many colleagues and students, past and present, for their input and perspective of cardiac biomechanics. Owing to space constraints, I have relied on much of their work without adequate citation, especially in the final section. In roughly chronological order of association I wish to thank Drs. Peter Hunter, Bruce Smaill, Lew Waldman, Y-C Fung, Jeff Omens, Jim Covell, Wilbur Lew, Francisco Villarreal, Julius Guccione, Karen May-Newman, Jack Rogers, Anne Hoger, Ken Rodriguez, Deidre MacKenna, Sandra Van Leuven, Ian LeGrice, and Marc Courtemanche. I would also like to thank present students, Wolfgang Bluhm, Jeff Holmes, Ann Lee, Kevin Costa, Jeff Emery, and Jim Wilson.

References

Arts T, Reneman RS, Veenstra PC. 1979. A model of the mechanics of the left ventricle. Ann Biomed Eng 7:299.

Arts T, Veenstra PC, Reneman RS. 1982. Epicardial deformation and left ventricular wall mechanics during ejection in the dog. Am J Physiol 243:H379.

Bergel DA, Hunter PJ. 1979. The mechanics of the heart. In NHC Hwang, DR Gross, DJ Patel (eds), Quantitative Cardiovascular Studies, pp 151–213, Baltimore, University Park.

Bers DM. 1991. Excitation-Contraction Coupling and Cardiac Contractile Force. Kluwer, Dordrecht.

Brutsaert DL, Sys SU. 1989. Relaxation and diastole of the heart. Physiol Rev 69:1228.

Caulfield JB, Borg TK. 1979. The collagen network of the heart. Lab Invest 40:364.

Chadwick RS. 1982. Mechanics of the left ventricle. Biophys J 39:279.

Demer LL, Yin FCP. 1983. Passive biaxial mechanical properties of isolated canine myocardium. J Physiol 339:615.

Feigl EO, Simon GA, Fry DL. 1967. Auxotonic and isometric cardiac force transducers. J Appl Physiol 23:597.

Fung YC. 1993. Biomechanics: Mechanical Properties of Living Tissues. New York, Springer-Verlag.

Gaasch WH, LeWinter MM. 1994. Left Ventricular Diastolic Dysfunction and Heart Failure. Philadelphia, Lea & Febiger.

Gilbert JC, Glantz SA. 1989. Determinants of left ventricular filling and of the diastolic pressure-volume relation. Circ Res 64:827.

Glantz SA, Misbach GA, Moores WY, et al. 1978. The pericardium substantially affects the left ventricular diastolic pressure-volume relationship in the dog. Circ Res 42:433.

Glantz SA, Parmley WW. 1978. Factors which affect the diastolic pressure-volume curve. Circ Res 42:171.

Glass L, Hunter P, McCulloch A. 1991. Theory of Heart: Biomechanics, Biophysics and Nonlinear Dynamics of Cardiac Function. New York, Springer-Verlag.

Grossman W. 1980. Cardiac hypertrophy: Useful adaptation or pathologic process? Am J Med 69:576.

Grossman W, Jones D, McLaurin LP. 1975. Wall stress and patterns of hypertrophy in the human left ventricle. J Clin Invest 56:56.

Guccione JM, McCulloch AD, Waldman LK. 1991. Passive material properties of intact ventricular myocardium determined from a cylindrical model. ASME J Biomech Eng 113:42.

Guccione JM, Waldman LK, McCulloch AD. 1993. Mechanics of active contraction in cardiac muscle: II. Cylindrical models of the systolic left ventricle. ASME J Biomech Eng 115:82.

Gupta KB, Ratcliff MB, Fallert MA, et al. 1994. Changes in passive mechanical stiffness of myocardial tissue with aneurysm formation. Circ 89:2315.

Halperin HR, Chew PH, Weisfeldt ML, et al. 1987. Transverse stiffness: a method for estimation of myocardial wall stress. Circ Res 61:695.

Holt JP, Rhode EA, Peoples SA, et al. 1962. Left ventricular function in mammals of greatly different size. Circ Res 10:798.

Huisman RM, Elzinga G, Westerhof N, et al. 1980. Measurement of left ventricular wall stress. Cardiovasc Res 14:142.

Humphrey JD, Strumpf RK, Yin FCP. 1990a. Biaxial mechanical behavior of excised ventricular epicardium. Am J Physiol 259:H101.

Humphrey JD, Strumpf RK, Yin FCP. 1990b. Determination of a constitutive relation for passive myocardium: I. A new functional form. ASME J Biomech Eng 112:333.

Humphrey JD, Yin FCP. 1987. A new constitutive formulation for characterizing the mechanical behavior of soft tissues. Biophys J 52:563.

Hunter PJ, Smaill BH. 1989. The analysis of cardiac function: a continuum approach. Prog Biophys Mol Biol 52:101.

Hunter WC. 1989. End-systolic pressure as a balance between opposing effects of ejection. Circ Res 64: 265.

Hunter WC, Zerhouni EA. 1989. Imaging distinct points in left ventricular myocardium to study regional wall deformation. In JH Anderson (ed), Innovations in Diagnostic Radiology, pp 169–190, New York, Springer-Verlag.

Ingels NB Jr, Daughters GT II, Stinson EB, et al. 1975. Measurement of midwall myocardial dynamics in intact man by radiography of surgically implanted markers. Circulation 52:859.

Janicki JS, Weber KT. 1980. The pericardium and ventricular interaction, distensibility and function. Am J Physiol 238:H494.

Lee MC, Fung YC, Shabetai R., et al. 1987. Biaxial mechanical properties of human pericardium and canine comparisons. Am J Physiol 253:H75.

Lin I-E, Taber LA. 1994. Mechanical effects of looping in the embryonic chick heart. Biomech 27:311.

Loiselle DS, Gibbs CL. 1979. Species differences in cardiac energetics. Am J Physiol 237:H90.

Maruyama Y, Ashikawa K, Isoyama S, et al. 1982. Mechanical interactions between the four heart chambers with and without the pericardium in canine hearts. Circ Res 50:86.

May-Newman KD, Omens JH, Pavelec RS, et al. 1994. Three-dimensional transmural mechanical interaction between the coronary vasculature and passive myocardium in the dog. Circ Res 74:1166.

McCulloch AD, Omens JH. 1991. Non-homogeneous analysis of three-dimensional transmural finite deformations in canine ventricular myocardium. J Biomech 24:539.

McCulloch AD, Smaill BH, Hunter PJ. 1989. Regional left ventricular epicardial deformation in the passive dog heart. Circ Res 64:721.

McLean M, Ross MA, Prothero J. 1989. Three-dimensional reconstruction of the myofiber pattern in the fetal and neonatal mouse heart. Anat Rec 224:392.

Meier GD, Bove AA, Santamore WP, et al. 1980*a*. Contractile function in canine right ventricle. Am J Physiol 239:H794.

Meier GD, Ziskin MC, Santamore WP, et al. 1980*b*. Kinematics of the beating heart. IEEE Trans Biomed Eng BME-27:319.

Mirsky I, Rankin JS. 1979. The effects of geometry, elasticity, and external pressures on the diastolic pressure-volume and stiffness-stress relations: How important is the pericardium? Circ Res 44:601.

Nevo E, Lanir Y. 1989. Structural finite deformation model of the left ventricle during diastole and systole. J Biomech Eng 111:342.

Nielsen PMF, Le Grice IJ, Smaill BH, et al. 1991. Mathematical model of geometry and fibrous structure of the heart. Am J Physiol 260:H1365.

Novak VP, Yin FCP, Humphrey JD. 1994. Regional mechanical properties of passive myocardium. J Biomech 27:403.

Omens JH, Fung YC. 1990. Residual strain in rat left ventricle. Circ Res 66:37.

Omens JH, MacKenna DA, McCulloch AD. 1991. Measurement of two-dimensional strain and analysis of stress in the arrested rat left ventricle. Adv Bioeng BED-20:635.

Omens JH, MacKenna DA, McCulloch AD. 1993. Measurement of strain and analysis of stress in resting rat ventricular myocardium. J Biomech 26:665.

Panerai RB. 1980. A model of cardiac muscle mechanics and energetics. J Biomech 13:929.

Patterson SW, Starling EH. 1914. On the mechanical factors which determine the output of the ventricles. J Physiol 48:357.

Pinto JG, Patitucci PJ. 1977. Creep in cardiac muscle. Am J Physiol 232:H553.

Pinto JG, Patitucci PJ. 1980. Visco-elasticity of passive cardiac muscle. J Biomech Eng 102:57.

Rakusan K. 1984. Cardiac growth, maturation and aging. In R. Zak (ed), Growth of the Heart in Health and Disease, pp 131–164, New York, Raven Press.

Robinson TF, Cohen-Gould L, Factor SM. 1983. Skeletal framework of mammalian heart muscle: Arrangement of inter- and pericellular connective tissue structures. Lab Invest 49:482.

Robinson TF, Geraci MA, Sonnenblick EH, et al. 1988. Coiled perimysial fibers of papillary muscle in rat heart: morphology, distribution, and changes in configuration. Circ Res 63:577.

Rodriguez EK, Hoger A, McCulloch AD. 1994. Stress-dependent finite growth in soft elastic tissues. J Biomech 27:455.

Rodriguez EK, Omens JH, Waldman LK, et al. 1993. Effect of residual stress on transmural sarcomere length distributions in rat left ventricle. Am J Physiol 264:H1048.

Ross J Jr, Sonnenblick EH, Covell JW, et al. 1967. The architecture of the heart in systole and diastole: Technique of rapid fixation and analysis of left ventricular geometry. Circ Res 21:409.

Rüegg JC. 1988. Calcium in Muscle Activation. Berlin, Springer-Verlag.

Saffitz JE, Kanter HL, Green KG, et al. 1994. Tissue-specific determinants of anisotropic conduction velocity in canine atrial and ventricular myocardium. Circ Res 74:1065.

Sagawa K. 1988. Cardiac Contraction and the Pressure-Volume Relationship. New York, Oxford University Press.

Salisbury PF, Cross CE, Rieben PA. 1960. Influence of coronary artery pressure upon myocardial elasticity. Circ Res 8:794.

Slinker BK, Glantz SA. 1986. End-systolic and end-diastolic ventricular interaction. Am J Physiol 251:H1062.

Smaill BH, Hunter PJ. 1991. Structure and function of the diastolic heart. In L Glass, PJ Hunter, AD McCulloch (eds), Theory of Heart, New York, Springer-Verlag.

Sonnenblick EH, Napolitano LM, Daggett WM, et al. 1967. An intrinsic neuromuscular basis for mitral valve motion in the dog. Circ Res 21:9.

Spotnitz HM, Spotnitz WD, Cottrell TS, et al. 1974. Cellular basis for volume related wall thickness changes in the rat left ventricle. J Mol Cell Cardiol 6:317.

Stahl WR. 1967. Scaling of respiratory variable in mammals. J Appl Physiol 22:453.

Streeter DD Jr. 1979. Gross morphology and fiber geometry of the heart. In Berne RM (ed), Handbook of Physiology, Section 2: The Cardiovascular System, pp 61–112, Bethesda, MD, American Physiological Society.

Streeter DD Jr, Hanna WT. 1973. Engineering mechanics for successive states in canine left ventricular myocardium: I. Cavity and wall geometry. Circ Res 33:639.

Streeter DD Jr, Spotnitz HM, Patel DP, et al. 1969. Fiber orientation in the canine left ventricle during diastole and systole. Circ Res. 24:339.

Suga H, Hayashi T, Shirahata M. 1981. Ventricular systolic pressure-volume area as predictor of cardiac oxygen consumption. Am J Physiol 240:H39.

Taber LA. 1991. On a nonlinear theory for muscle shells: II. Application to the beating left ventricle. J Biomech Eng 113:63.

Ter Keurs, HEDJ, Rijnsburger WH, Van Heuningen R. 1980*a*. Restoring forces and relaxation of rat cardiac muscle. Eur Heart J 1:67.

Ter Keurs HEDJ, Rijnsburger WH, Van Heuningen R, et al. 1980*b*. Tension development and sarcomere length in rat cardiac trabeculae: Evidence of length-dependent activation. Circ Res 46:703.

Tözeren A. 1985. Continuum rheology of muscle contraction and its application to cardiac contractility. Biophys J 47:303.

Villarreal FJ, Waldman LK, Lew WYW. 1988. A technique for measuring regional two-dimensional finite strains in canine left ventricle. Circ Res 62:711.

Vornanen M. 1992. Maximum heart rate of sorcine shrews: correlation with contractile properties and myosin composition. Am J Physiol 31:R842.

Waldman LK, Fung YC, Covell JW. 1985. Transmural myocardial deformation in the canine left ventricle: Normal in vivo three-dimensional finite strains. Circ Res 57:152.

Weber KT. 1989. Cardiac interstituim in health and disease: The fibrillar collagen network. J Am Coll Cardiol 13:1637.

Yellin EL, Hori M, Yoran C, et al. 1986. Left ventricular relaxation in the filling and nonfilling intact canine heart. Am J Physiol 250:H620.

Yin FCP. 1981. Ventricular wall stress. Circ Res 49:829.

Yin FCP. 1985. Applications of the finite-element method to ventricular mechanics. Crit Rev Biomed Eng 12:311.

Yin FCP, Strumpf RK, Chew PH, et al. 1987. Quantification of the mechanical properties of non-contracting canine myocardium under simultaneous biaxial loading. J Biomech 20:577.

Young AA, Axel L. 1992. Three-dimensional motion and deformation of the heart wall—a model-based approach. Radiology 185:241.

32
Mechanics of Heart Valves

Ajit P. Yoganathan
Georgia Institute of Technology

Joanne Hopmeyer
Georgia Institute of Technology

Russell S. Heinrich
Georgia Institute of Technology

The heart has four valves which control the direction of blood flow through the heart. The aortic valve separates the left ventricle from the aorta. Its function is to prevent the blood pumped into the aorta from returning to the left ventricle. Similarly, the pulmonic valve is located between the right ventricle and pulmonary artery and ensures that blood flows in one direction only, away from the right ventricle and into the lungs. The mitral and tricuspid valves lie between the atria and ventricles of the left and right sides of the heart, respectively, and they prevent flow of blood back into the atria during ventricular contraction. The aortic and pulmonic valves open during systole when the ventricles are contracting and close during diastole when the ventricles are filling through the open mitral and tricuspid valves. During isovolumic contraction and relaxation, all four valves are closed, as illustrated in Fig. 32.1.

When closed, the aortic and pulmonic valves must withstand pressures of up to 100 mmHg and 30 mmHg, respectively, and the mitral and tricuspid valves close against pressures of 140 mmHg and 30 mmHg, respectively. Since diseases of the valves on the left side of the heart are more prevalent, most of this chapter will focus on the aortic and mitral valves. Where pertinent, reference will be made to the pulmonic and tricuspid valves.

32.1 Aortic and Pulmonic Valves

The aortic valve is composed of three semilunar cusps contained within a connective tissue sleeve. The valve cusps or leaflets are attached to a fibrous ring which is embedded in the fibers of the ventricular septum and the anterior leaflet of the mitral valve. Each of the leaflets is lined with endothelial cells and has a dense collagenous core adjacent to the high-pressure aortic side. The side adjacent to the aorta is termed the *fibrosa* and is the major fibrous layer within the belly of the leaflet. The layer covering the ventricular side of the valve is called the *ventricularis* and is composed of both collagen and elastin. The ventricularis is thinner than the fibrosa and presents a very smooth surface to the flow of blood [Christie, 1990]. The central portion of the valve, called the *spongiosa*, contains variable loose connective tissue and proteins and is normally not vascularized. The collagen fibers within the fibrosa and ventricularis are unorganized in the unstressed state, and when a stress

0-8493-8346-3/95/$0.00+$.50
© 1995 by CRC Press, Inc.

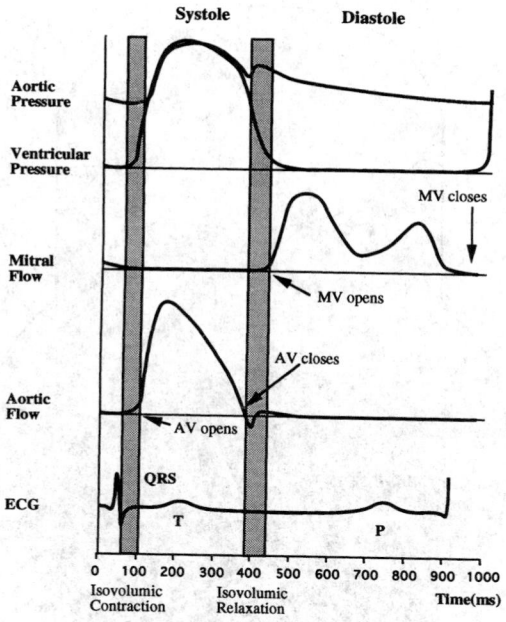

FIGURE 32.1 Typical pressure and flow curves for the aortic and mitral valves.

is applied, they become oriented primarily in the circumferential direction with a lower concentration of elastin and collagen in the radial direction [Christie, 1990; Thubrikar, 1990].

The fibrous annular ring of the aortic valve separates the aorta from the left ventricle, and superior to this ring is a structure called the *sinus of Valsalva* or *aortic sinus*. The aortic sinus comprises three bulges at the root of the aorta, with each bulge aligned with the belly or central part of the specific valve leaflet. Each valve cusp and corresponding sinus is named according to its anatomical location within the aorta. Two of these sinuses give rise to coronary arteries that branch off the aorta, providing the blood supply to the heart itself. The right coronary artery is based at the right or *right anterior sinus*, the left coronary artery exits the left or *left posterior sinus*, and the third sinus is called the *noncoronary* or *right posterior sinus*. Figure 32.2 shows the configuration of the normal aortic sinuses and valve in the closed position. When the valve is closed, because the length of the aortic valve cusps is greater than the annular radius, a small overlap of tissue from each leaflet protrudes and forms a coaptation surface within the aorta [Emery and Arom, 1991]. The overlapped tissue is called the *lunula*, and it may help to ensure that the valve is sealed during diastole. When the valve is open, the leaflets extend to the upper edge of the sinus of Valsalva. The anatomy of the pulmonic valve is similar to that of the aortic valve, but the surrounding structure is slightly different. The main differences are that the sinus are smaller in the pulmonary artery and that the pulmonic valve annulus is slightly larger than that of the aortic valve.

The dimensions of the aortic and pulmonic valves and their leaflets have been measured in a number of ways. Before noninvasive measurement techniques such as echocardiography became available, valve measurements were recorded from autopsy specimens. An examination of 160 pathologic specimens revealed the aortic valve diameter to be 23.2 ± 3.3 mm, and the diameter of the pulmonic valve was measured at 24.3 ± 3.0 mm [Westaby et al., 1984.] However, according to M-mode echocardiographic measurements, the aortic root diameter at end-systole was 35 ± 4.2 mm and 33.7 ± 4.4 mm at the end of diastole [Gramiak & Shah, 1970]. The differences in these measurements reflect the fact that the autopsy measurements were not performed under physiologic pressure conditions and that intrinsic differences in the measurement techniques exist.

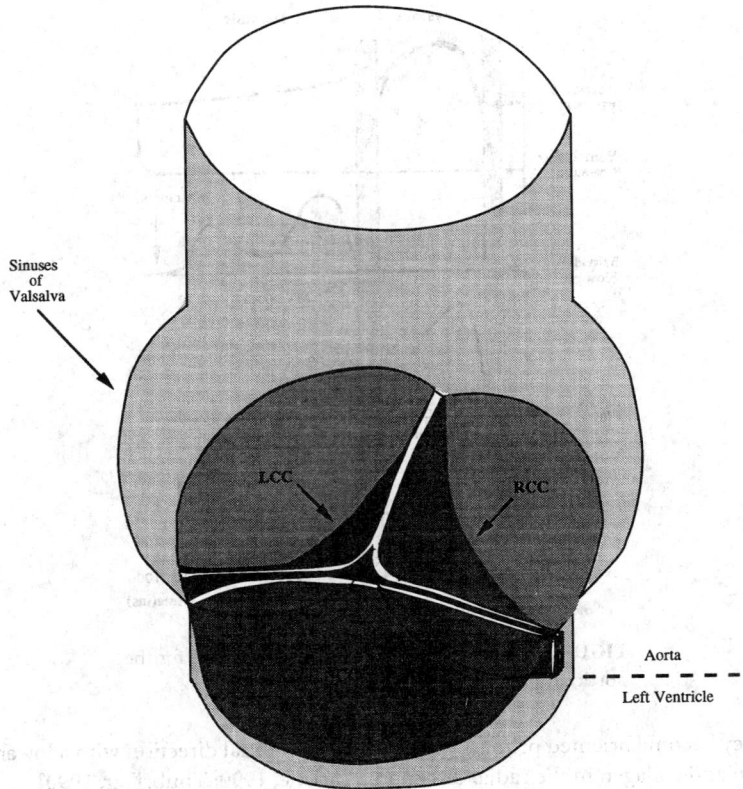

FIGURE 32.2   The aortic sinuses and valve in the closed position. The noncoronary cusp (NCC) is in front. The left and right coronary cusps (LCC and RCC) are positioned as marked. The aorta is above the closed valve in this orientation, and the left ventricle is below the dashed line.

Mechanical Properties

Due to the location and critical function of the aortic valve, it is difficult to obtain measurements of its mechanical properties in vivo; however, reports are available from a small number of animal studies. This section will reference the in vivo data whenever possible and defer to the in vitro data when necessary. Since little mathematical modeling of the aortic valve's material properties has been reported, it will be sufficient to describe the known mechanical properties of the valve. Like most biologic tissues, the aortic valve is anisotropic, inhomogeneous, and viscoelastic. The collagen fibers within each valve cusp are aligned along the circumferential direction. There are also elastin fibers, at a lesser concentration, that are oriented orthogonally to the collagen. It is this fiber structure that accounts for the anisotropic properties of the valve. The variation in thickness and composition across the leaflets is responsible for their inhomogeneous material properties. The valve's viscoelastic properties are actually dominated by the elastic component (over the range of in vitro testing) so that the viscous effects, largely responsible for energy losses, are small [Thubrikar, 1990].

Using marker fluoroscopy, in which the aortic valve leaflets were surgically tagged with radio-opaque markers and imaged with high-speed x rays, the leaflets have been shown to change length during the cardiac cycle [Thubrikar, 1990]. The cusps are longer during diastole than in systole in both the radial and circumferential direction. The variation in length is greatest in the radial direction in dogs, approximately 20%. The strain in the circumferential direction is about 10% of the normal systolic length. The difference in strain is due to the presence of the compliant elastin fibers aligned in this radial direction. The length change in both directions results in an increased valve surface area during diastole. The shortening of the valve leaflets helps to reduce obstruction of the aorta during the systolic ejection of blood. It should be noted that this change in area is by no means an active mechanism within the aortic valve; the valve simply reacts to the stresses it encounters in a passive manner.

In addition to this change in surface area, the aortic valve's leaflets also undergo bending in the circumferential direction during the cardiac cycle. In diastole when the valve is closed, each leaflet is convex toward the ventricular side. During systole when the valve is open, the curvature changes, and each leaflet is concave toward the ventricle. This bending is localized on the valve cusp near the wall of the aorta. This location is often thicker than the rest of the leaflet. The total diastolic stress in a valve leaflet has been estimated at 2.5×10^6 dynes/cm^2 for a strain of 15% [Thubrikar, 1990]. The stress in the circumferential direction was found to be the primary load-bearing element in the aortic valve. Due to the collagen fibers oriented circumferentially, the valve is relatively stiff in this direction. The strain that does occur circumferentially is primarily due to scissoring of the fibrous matrix and straightening of collagen fibers that are kinked or crimped in the presence of no external stress. However in the radial direction, because elastin is the primary element, the valve can undergo a great deal of strain, as high as 60% in tissue specimens [Christie, 1990]. In the closed position the radial stress levels are actually small compared to those in the circumferential direction. This demonstrates the importance of the lunula in ensuring that the valve seals tightly to prevent leakage. Because of their anatomical location, the lunula cause these high circumferential stress levels by enabling the aortic pressure to pull each leaflet in the circumferential direction towards the other leaflets.

Valve Dynamics

Since the aortic valve is a highly dynamic structure, discussion of its static material properties does not provide a complete understanding of its normal function. It is necessary to examine the dynamic function of the valve in the in vivo environment to fully understand its function. The aortic valve opens during systole when the ventricle is contracting and then closes during diastole as the ventricle relaxes and fills from the atrium. Systole lasts about one-third of the cardiac cycle and begins when the aortic valve opens, which typically takes only 20–30 ms [Bellhouse, 1969]. Blood rapidly accelerates through the valve and reaches a peak velocity after the leaflets have opened to their full extent and start to close again. Peak velocity is reached during the first third of systole, and the flow begins to decelerate rapidly after the peak is reached, albeit not as fast as its initial acceleration. The adverse pressure gradient that is developed affects the low-momentum fluid near the wall of the aorta more than that at the center; this causes reverse flow in the sinus region [Reul & Talukdar, 1979]. Figure 32.1 illustrates the pressure and flow relations across the aortic valve during the cardiac cycle. During systole, the pressure gradient required to drive the blood through the aortic valve is on the order of a few millimeters of mercury. Diastolic pressure gradients are much larger than systolic, the pressure usually being about 80 mmHg. The valve closes near the end of the deceleration phase of systole with very little reverse flow through the valve.

During the cardiac cycle the heart undergoes translation and rotation due to its own contraction pattern. As a result the base of the aortic valve varies in size and moves, mainly along the axis of the aorta. Using marker fluoroscopy to study the base of the aortic valve in dogs, it was found that the base perimeter is at its largest at end-diastole and decreases in size during systole [Thubrikar et al., 1993]. It reaches a minimum at the end of systole and then increases again during diastole. The range of this perimeter variation during the cardiac cycle was 22% for an aortic pressure variation of 120/80 mmHg. In addition the valve annulus also undergoes translation, primarily parallel to the aortic axis. The aortic annulus moves downward toward the ventricle during systole and then recoils back toward the aorta as the ventricle fills during diastole. The annulus also experiences a slight side-to-side translation with its magnitude approximately one-half the displacement along the aortic axis.

During systole, vortices develop in all three sinuses behind the leaflets of the aortic valve. The function of these vortices was first described by Leonardo da Vinci in 1513, and they have been researched extensively in this century, primarily using in vitro models [Bellhouse, 1969; Reul & Talukdar, 1979] It has been hypothesized that the vortices help to close the aortic valve so that blood is prevented from returning to the ventricle during the closing process. These vortices create a transverse pressure gradient that pushes the leaflets toward the center of the aorta and each other at the end of systole, thus minimizing any possible closing volume. However, as shown in vitro by Reul and Talukdar [1979], the axial pressure gradient alone is enough to close the valve. Without the vortices in the sinuses, the valve still closes, but its closure is not as quick as when the vortices are present. The adverse axial pressure gradient within the aorta causes the low inertia flow within the developing boundary layer along the aortic wall to decelerate first and to reverse direction. This forces the belly of the leaflets away from the aortic wall and toward the closed position. When this force is coupled with the vortices that push the leaflet tips toward the closed position, a very efficient and fast closure is obtained. As a result, only a very small amount of fluid reenters the left ventricle when the valve is closed. Closing volumes have been estimated at less than 5% of the forward flow [Bellhouse, 1969].

As shown in Fig. 32.1, during diastole there is a large pressure gradient between the aorta and the left ventricle which acts on the aortic valve. When this is coupled with the very low pressure gradient on the valve during systole, it is clear that the valve experiences extreme cyclic loading conditions during each cardiac cycle. For a person with an average heart rate of 70 beats per minute, the cyclic loading conditions occur approximately 40 million times per year. This is one reason that it is so difficult to design effective prosthetic valves—they are unable to endure the repeated stresses that a normal valve encounters with each heart beat.

The parameters that describe the normal blood flow through the aortic valve are the velocity profile, time course of the blood velocity or flow, and magnitude of the peak velocity. These are determined in part by the pressure gradient between the ventricle and aorta and by the geometry of the aortic valve complex. As seen in Fig. 32.3, the velocity profile at the level of the aortic valve annulus is relatively flat. However there is usually a slight skew toward the septal wall (less than 10% of the center-line velocity) which is caused by the orientation of the aortic valve relative to the long axis of the left ventricle. This skew in the velocity profile has been shown by many experimental techniques, including hot film anemometry, Doppler ultrasound, and MRI [Kilner et al., 1993; Paulsen & Hasenkam, 1983; Rossvol et al., 1991]. In healthy individuals, blood flows through the aortic valve at the beginning of systole and then rapidly accelerates to its peak value of 1.35 ± 0.3 m/s. For children this value is slightly higher at 1.5 ± 0.3 m/s [Hatle & Angelson, 1985]. At the end of systole there is a very short period of reverse flow that can be measured with Doppler ultrasound. This reverse flow is probably either a small closing volume or the velocity of the valve leaflets as they move toward their closed position. The flow patterns just downstream of the aortic valve are of particular interest because of their complexity and relation to arterial disease. Highly skewed velocity profiles and corresponding helical flow patterns have been observed in the human aortic arch using magnetic resonance phase velocity mapping [Kilner et al., 1993].

The pulmonic valve flow behaves similarly to that of the aortic valve, but the magnitude of the velocity is not as great. Typical peak velocities for healthy adults are 0.75 ± 0.15 m/s. Again these values are slightly higher for children at 0.9 ± 0.2 m/s [Weyman 1994]. As seen in Fig 32.4, a rotation of the peak velocity can be observed in the pulmonary artery velocity profile. During acceleration the peak velocity is observed inferiorly with the peak rotating counterclockwise throughout the remainder of the ejection phase [Sloth et al., 1994]. The mean spatial profile is relatively flat however, although there is a region of reversed flow that occurs in late systole which may

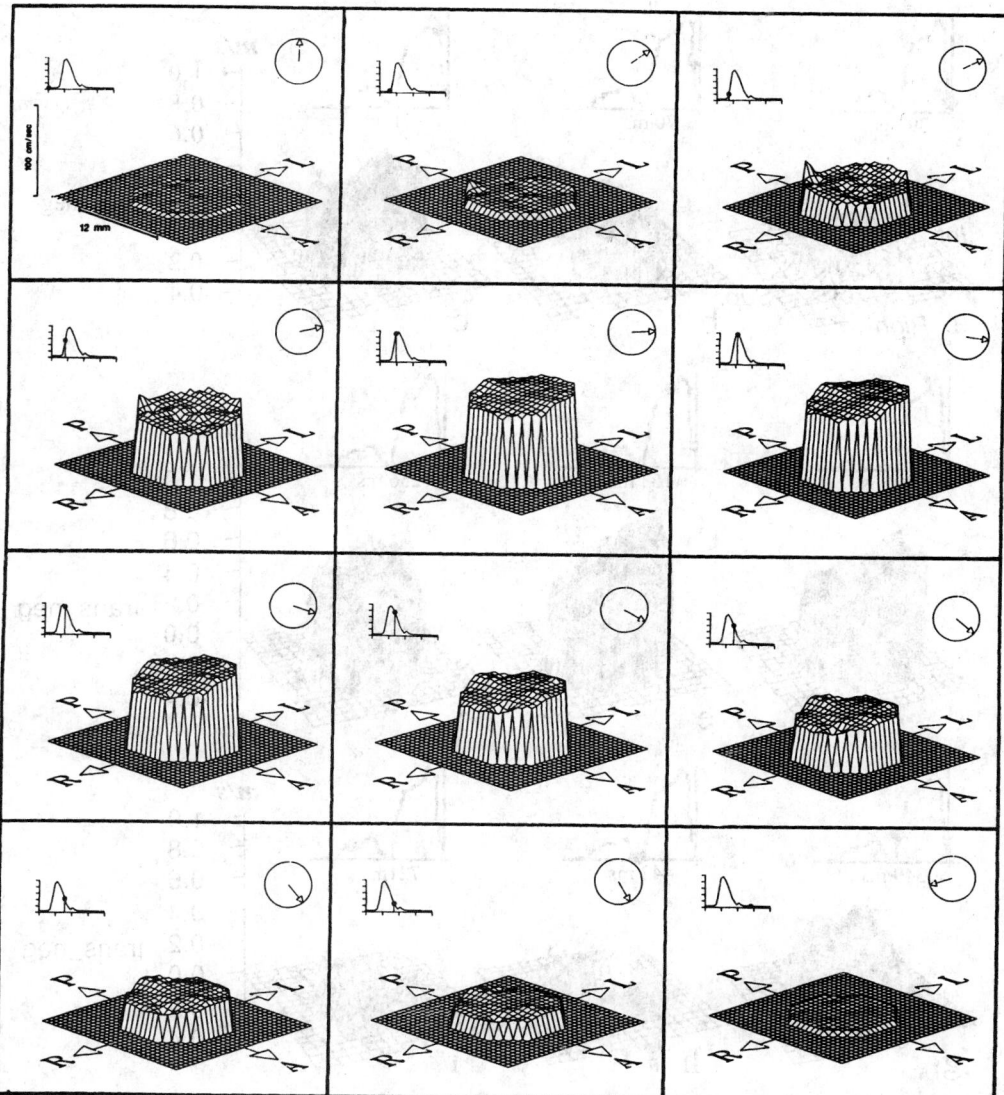

FIGURE 32.3 Velocity profiles measured 2 cm downstream of the aortic valve with hot film anemometry in dogs [Paulsen & Hasenkam, 1983]. The timing of the measurements during the cardiac cycle is shown by the marker on the aortic flow curve.

be representative of flow separation. Typically though, there is only a slight skew to the profile. The peak velocity is generally within 20% of the spatial mean throughout the cardiac cycle. Secondary flow patterns can also be observed in the pulmonary artery and its bifurcation. In vitro laser Doppler anemometry experiments have shown that these flow patterns are dependent on the valve geometry and thus can be used to evaluate function and fitness of the heart valve [Sung & Yoganathan, 1990].

The composition, properties, and dimensions of the aortic valve change with age and in the presence of certain diseases. The valve cusps become thicker, the lunula become fenestrated, or mesh-like, and in later stages the central portion of the valve may become calcified [Davies, 1980]. This thickening of the valve typically occurs on the ventricular side of the valve, in the region where the

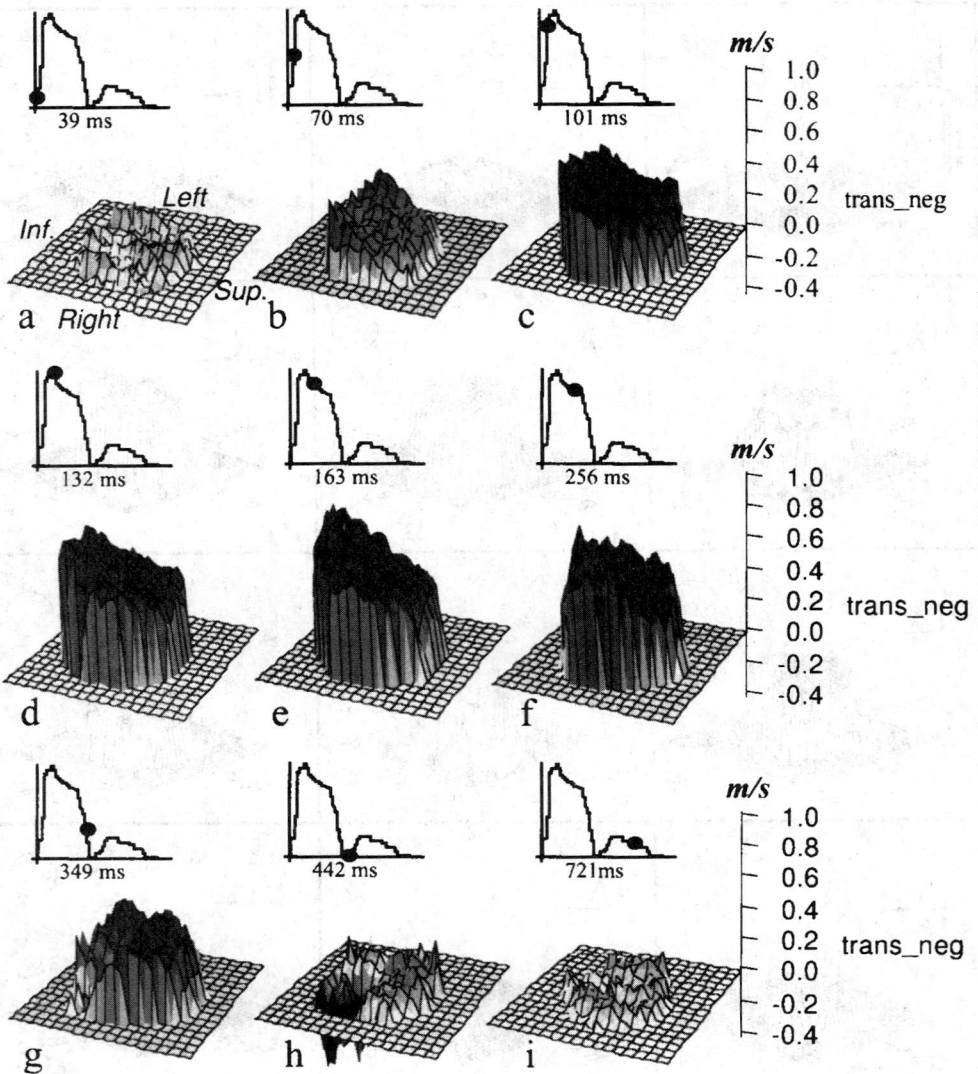

FIGURE 32.4 Velocity profiles downstream of the human pulmonary valve obtained with magnetic resonance phase velocity mapping [Sloth et al., 1994]. Again the timing of the measurements is shown by the marker on the flow curve.

tips of the leaflets come together. Another site of calcification and fibrosis is the point of maximum cusp flexion and is thought to be a response to fatigue in the normal valve tissue.

The aortic valve is prone to both acquired and congenital heart disease. Congenital bileaflet aortic valves occur in 1–2% of the population [Virmani et al., 1991]. Aortic regurgitation and stenosis can occur separately and in tandem and are often caused by calcification of the valve tissue. Aortic stenosis, which is more common, results in a reduced area for flow to leave the ventricle, because the aortic valve no longer opens to its full extent. High-velocity jets and large axial pressure gradients are subsequently developed. Aortic regurgitation occurs when the valve does not close properly or is damaged or punctured by congenital or acquired heart disease. This creates a channel between the high-pressure aorta and the low-pressure ventricle during diastole. As a result a high-velocity jet of blood enters the left ventricle. Knowing the large amount of stress and strain that the valve must undergo during its lifetime, it is amazing that aortic valvular disease is not more common.

32.2 Mitral and Tricuspid Valves

The mitral and tricuspid valves are similar in structure, and both valves are composed of four primary elements: the valve annulus, the valve leaflets, the papillary muscles, and the chordae tendineae, as shown in Fig. 32.5. The base of the mitral leaflets forms the mitral annulus. Collagen fibers extend from the annulus through the valve leaflets to form chordae tendineae which connect to papillary muscles, tethering the valve to the left ventricular wall. The normal function of the valvular apparatus requires a complex interplay between these components.

The mitral annulus is an elliptical ring which is composed of dense collagenous tissue surrounded by muscle. The circumference of the mitral annulus ranges from 8 to 12 cm during diastole. During systole, due to annular contraction, the annular circumference decreases. Recent observations have suggested that the mitral annulus is not planar but instead is saddle-shaped [Levine et al., 1987].

The mitral valve is a bileaflet valve and is comprised of an anterior leaflet and a posterior leaflet. The leaflet tissue is composed primarily of collagen-reinforced endothelium. However, striated muscle cells, nonmyelinated nerve fibers, and blood vessels are present in the mitral valve tissue, extending roughly two-thirds into the leaflet tissue towards the free edge. In addition, muscle fibers, which appear to originate from the atrium, are usually present on the anterior leaflet but are rarely observed on the posterior leaflet and may play a role in mitral valve function [Barlow, 1987]. The anterior and posterior leaflets of the mitral valve are actually one continuous piece of tissue, as shown in Fig. 32.6. The free edge of this tissue shows a number of indentations. Two of these indentations, the commissures, are regularly placed to permit the separation of the tissue into the anterior and posterior leaflets. The posterior leaflet encircles roughly two-thirds of the mitral annulus and is essentially an extension of the mural endocardium from the free walls of the left atrium. The anterior leaflet annulus is continuous with the wall of the ascending aorta, the aortic valve, and the ventricular and atrial septum. The anterior leaflet is slightly larger than the posterior leaflet and is roughly triangular in shape, as opposed to the posterior leaflet, which is more quadrangular in shape. The length of the anterior leaflet ranges from 2.4–4.5 cm and its height is 1.8–3.2 cm, roughly twice the height of the posterior leaflet. The posterior leaflet typically has indentations, called *scallops*, and thus can be divided into three regions: the medial scallop, the central scallop, and the lateral scallop. The combined surface area of both leaflets is approximately twice the area of the mitral orifice, which allows a large area of coaptation to permit the valve to close effectively [Barlow, 1987; Raganathan et al., 1970; Roberts, 1983; Silverman & Hurst, 1968].

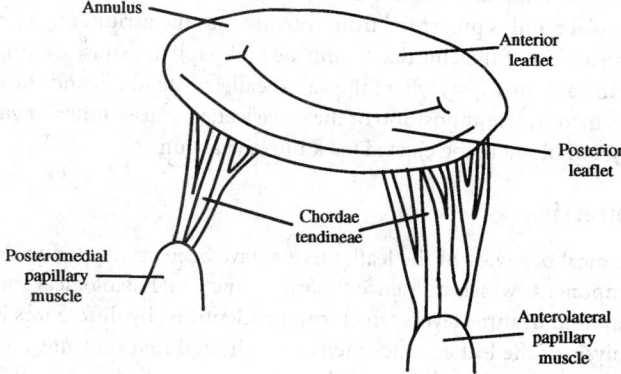

FIGURE 32.5 Schematic of the mitral valve showing the valve leaflets, papillary muscles, and chordae tendineae.

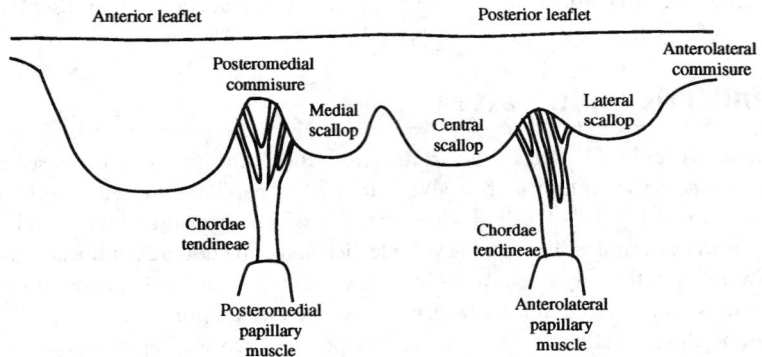

FIGURE 32.6   Diagram of the mitral valve as a continuous piece of tissue. The posterior and anterior leaflets are indicated, as are the scallops, chordae tendineae, and papillary muscles.

The mitral leaflet tissue can be divided into both a rough zone and a clear zone. The rough zone is the thicker part of the leaflet and is defined from the free edge of the valve to the valve's line of closure. This zone is rough and thick due to the insertion of the chordae tendineae at this location. The clear zone is thinner and translucent and extends from the line of closure to the annulus in the anterior leaflet and to the basal zone in the posterior leaflet. The basal zone on the posterior leaflet extends from the annulus to the clear zone and is usually a couple of millimeters wide. Unlike the mitral valve, the tricuspid valve has three leaflets: an anterior leaflet, a posterior leaflet with a variable number of scallops, and a septal leaflet. The tricuspid valve is larger and structurally more complicated than the mitral valve, and the separation of the valve tissue into distinct leaflets is less pronounced than with the mitral valve. The surface of the leaflets is similar to that of the mitral valve; however, the basal zone is present in all the leaflets [Silver et al., 1971].

In the mitral apparatus, chordae tendineae from both leaflets attach to the papillary muscles. The chordae tendineae consist of an inner core of collagen surrounded by loosely meshed elastin and collagen fibers with an outer layer of endothelial cells. On average, 12 primary chordae tendineae are attached to each papillary muscle, and the majority attach to the valve leaflets in the rough zone.

Two papillary muscles, called *anterolateral* and *posteromedial,* attach to the left ventricular free wall and tether the mitral valve in place. The tricuspid valve, however, has three papillary muscles. The largest one, the anterior papillary muscle, attaches to the valve at the commissure between the anterior and posterior leaflets. The posterior papillary muscle is located between the posterior and septal leaflets. The smallest papillary muscle, the septal muscle, is sometimes virtually absent. The mitral valve is held in place and is prevented from moving into the atrium during ventricular ejection by the restraining action of the chordae tendineae and papillary muscles. Improper tethering of the leaflets results in valve prolapse, where the valve leaflets extend beyond the annulus into the atrium during systole. Incomplete apposition of the valve leaflets causes mitral regurgitation, which is characterized by a jet of blood being ejected back into the atrium.

Mechanical Properties

Studies on the mechanical behavior of the leaflet tissue have been conducted to determine the key connective tissue components which influence the valve function. Histological studies have shown that the tissue is composed of three layers which can be identified by differences in cellularity and collagen density. Analysis of the leaflets under tension indicated that the anterior leaflet would be more capable of supporting larger tensile loads than the posterior leaflet. The differences between the mechanical properties between the two leaflets may require different material selection for repair or replacement of the individual leaflets [Kunzelman et al., 1993].

The chordae tendineae tension in dogs was monitored throughout the cardiac cycle by Salisbury and co-workers [1963]. They found that the chordae tendineae tension only paralleled the left ventricular pressure tracings during isovolumic contraction and that the chordae tendineae tracings and left ventricular pressure tracings were divergent during the rest of the cardiac cycle. Investigation of the tensile properties of the chordae tendineae at different strain rates by Lim and Bouchner [1975] found that the chordae had a nonlinear stress-strain relationship. They found that the size of the chordae had a more significant effect on the development of the tension than did the strain rate. The smaller chordae had a modulus of 2×10^9 dynes/cm^2, whereas larger chordae had a modulus of 1×10^9 dynes/cm^2.

The stresses sustained by the mitral valve were investigated by Ghista and Rao [1972], who determined that the stress in the mitral valve can reach as high as 2.2×10^6 dynes/cm^2 just prior to the opening of the aortic valve, when the pressure in the left ventricle reaches a maximum of up to 150 mmHg. A recently created model of the mechanics of the mitral valve incorporates the relationship between chordae tendineae tension, left ventricular pressure, and mitral valve geometry [Arts et al., 1983].

Valve Dynamics

The valve leaflets, chordae tendineae, and papillary muscles all participate in the normal functioning of the mitral valve. At the end of systole, when the pressure in the left atrium exceeds that of the left ventricle, the mitral valve cusps are forced open. Blood flows through the open mitral valve from the left atrium to the left ventricle during diastole. When the left ventricle distends, the mitral valve leaflets are pulled toward each other by the chordae tendineae of the stretched papillary muscles. Thus, the mitral velocity flow curve shows a peak in the flow curve, called the *E-wave,* for early filling. Peak E-wave velocities measured in patients using Doppler ultrasound both in healthy individuals [Samstad et al., 1989] and in pigs [Kim et al., 1994] are in the range of 50–80 cm/s at the mitral annulus. The velocity profiles at both the annulus and the mitral valve tips have been shown to be skewed, as shown in Fig. 32.7, and therefore are not flat as is commonly assumed. After the fluid acceleration in the E-wave, the fluid begins to decelerate, and the mitral valve undergoes partial closure. The atrial contraction then results in a second opening of the valve, and the fluid velocity then peaks again in the *A-wave.* The atrium contraction plays an important role in the filling of the ventricle during late diastole. In healthy individuals, velocities during the A-wave are typically lower than those of the E-wave. The fluid then decelerates before it closes completely. Thus, the diastolic filling of the left ventricle shows a peak in the flow, followed by a second peak due to the atrial contraction, with no flow through the normal mitral valve during systole.

The tricuspid flow profile is similar to that of the mitral valve. The velocities in the tricuspid valve are lower than those in the mitral valve because the tricuspid valve has a larger valve orifice. In addition, the timing of the valve openings is slightly different. The peak pressure in the right ventricle is less than that of the left ventricle. Thus, the time for the right ventricular pressure to fall below the right atrial pressure is less than the corresponding time period for the left side of the heart. This leads to a shorter right ventricular isovolumetric relaxation and, thus, an earlier tricuspid opening. Tricuspid closure occurs after mitral valve closure, since the activation of the left ventricle precedes the right ventricle [Weyman, 1994].

Attempts have been made in the past to explain the fluid mechanics of mitral valve function. A primary focus has been on understanding the closing mechanism of the mitral valve. Bellhouse [1972] first suggested the importance of ventricular vortices generated by ventricular filling in the early partial closure of the mitral valve. Bellhouse's in vitro model experiments suggested that without the strong vortices, the valve would remain open during ventricular contraction, thus resulting in a significant amount of mitral regurgitation before closing completely. However, while eliminating the vortices in the model experiments, the deceleration of the mitral flow was eliminated as were

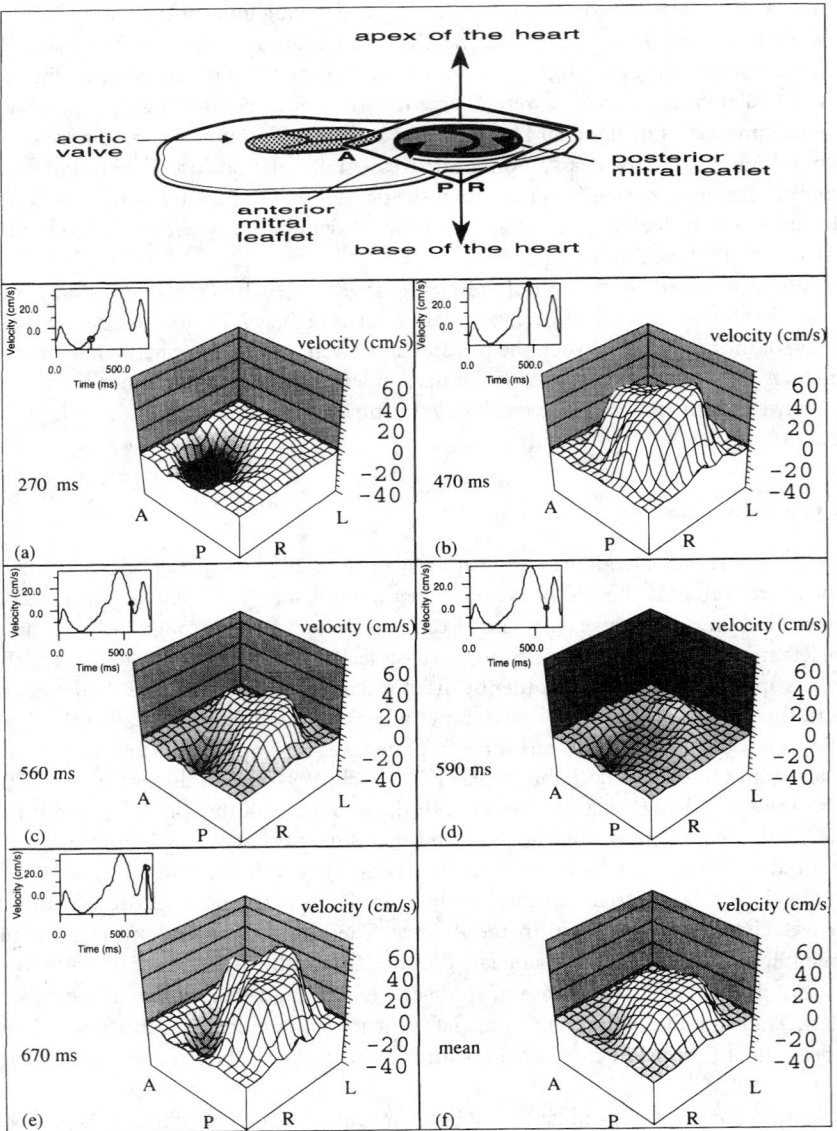

FIGURE 32.7 Two-dimensional transmitral velocity profiles recorded at the level of the mitral annulus in a pig [Kim et al., 1994]. (*a*) Systole; (*b*) peak E-wave; (*c*) deceleration phase of early diastole; (*d*) mid-diastolic period (diastasis); (*e*) peak A-wave; (*f*) time-averaged diastolic cross-sectional mitral velocity profile. Reprinted with permission from the American College of Cardiology (J Am Coll Cardiol 24:532–545).

the forces associated with this decelerating flow. Experiments were conducted in vitro by Reul and Talukdar [1979] in a model of the left ventricle made from silicone. Their results suggest that an adverse pressure gradient in mid-diastole could explain both the flow deceleration and the partial valve closure, even in the absence of a ventricular vortex. Thus, the studies by Reul and Talukdar [1979] suggest that the vortices may provide additional closing effects at the initial stage; however, the pressure forces are the dominant effects in valve closure. Animal experiments conducted by Yellin and colleagues [1979] suggested a more unified theory of valve closure including the importance of chordal tension, flow deceleration, and ventricular vortices, with chordal tension being a necessary condition for the other two. Their studies indicated that competent valve closure can occur even in the absence of vortices and flow deceleration. Recent studies using magnetic resonance imaging to visualize the three-dimensional flow field in the left ventricle in normal individuals showed that a large anterior vortex played a role in the initial partial closure of the valve. Following atrial contraction, the final closure was also associated with a ventricular vortex [Kim et al., submitted for publication]. Studies conducted in our laboratory using magnetic resonance imaging of healthy individuals clearly show the vortices in the left ventricle, as seen in Fig. 32.8. In addition to aiding in valve closure, studies in our laboratory suggest that the ventricular vortex plays an important role in storing kinetic energy during diastole in order to minimize the work required by the ventricle during ejection [Lefebvre et al., submitted for publication].

Another area of interest has been in the movement of the mitral valve. The heart moves throughout the cardiac cycle; similarly, the mitral apparatus moves and changes shape. Tsakiris and colleagues [1971] studied the movement of the mitral annulus in dogs. They looked at the difference in the size, shape, and position of the mitral annulus at different stages in the cardiac cycle. They noted an eccentric narrowing of the annulus during both atrial and ventricular contractions that reduced the mitral valve area by 10–36% from its peak diastolic area. This reduction in the annular area during systole is significant; thus, there is a much greater area of the leaflets available for coaptation. Similar experiments on the dynamic motion of the mitral annulus were conducted in humans by Ormiston and coworkers [1981], who used echocardiography to look at changes in the shape of the mitral valve annulus. They reconstructed the annular area at 12 different times during the cardiac cycle. In this study, the annuli were elliptical. The annuli were more circular in late diastole and were flatter in systole. They noted that it is important to be able to compare the area of the annulus in normal individuals to the area in patients with mitral valve disease to be able to predict the presence of mitral valve prolapse and regurgitation. The movement of the annulus toward the base has been suggested to play a role in ventricular filling. During ventricular contraction, there is a shortening of the left ventricular chamber along its longitudinal axis, and the mitral and tricuspid annuli move toward the apex. It has been suggested that the distance travelled by the mitral annulus is representative of the global function of the ventricle [Alam & Rosenhamer, 1992; Hammarström et al., 1991; Simonson & Schiller, 1989].

In addition to the importance of the mitral annular movement, the movement of the papillary muscles is important in maintaining proper mitral valve function. The papillary muscles play an important role in keeping the mitral valve in position. Abnormal strain on the papillary muscles could cause the chordae to rupture and result in mitral regurgitation. It is necessary for the papillary muscles to contract and shorten during systole to prevent mitral prolapse; therefore, the distance between the apex of the heart and the mitral apparatus is important. The distance from the papillary muscle tips to the annulus was measured in normal individuals during systole and was found to remain constant [Sanfilippo et al., 1992]. In patients with mitral valve prolapse, however, this distance decreased, corresponding to a superior displacement of the papillary muscle toward the annulus.

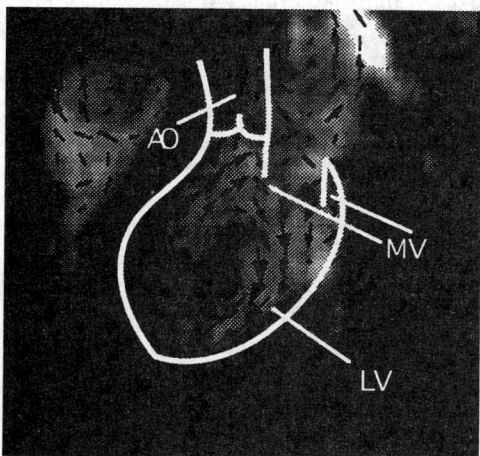

FIGURE 32.8 Magnetic resonance image of a healthy individual during diastole. An outline of the interior left ventricle (LV) is indicated in white as are the mitral valve leaflets (MV) and the aorta (AO). Velocity vectors were obtained from MRI phase velocity mapping and superimposed on the anatomical image. A large vortex can clearly be seen closing the valve.

The normal function of the mitral valve requires a balanced interplay between all the components of the mitral apparatus. The limited engineering studies of the mitral valve have provided insight into the mechanical properties and function of heart valves. Further fundamental and detailed engineering studies are needed to aid surgeons in repairing the diseased mitral valve and in understanding the changes in function due to mitral valve pathologies. In addition, further studies are needed to aid in the design of prosthetic valves that more closely replicate native valve function.

References

Arts T, Meerbaum S, Reneman R, et al. 1983. Stresses in the closed mitral valve: A model study. J Biomech 16:539.

Alam M, Rosenhamer G. 1992. Atrioventricular plane displacement and left ventricular function. J Am Soc Echocardiogr 5:427.

Barlow JB. 1987. Perspectives on the Mitral Valve. Philadelphia, FA Davis.

Bellhouse BJ. 1969. Velocity and pressure distributions in the aortic valve. J Fluid Mech 37:587.

Bellhouse BJ. 1972. The fluid mechanics of a model mitral valve and left ventricle. Cardiovasc Res 6:199.

Bellhouse BJ, Bellhouse F. 1969. Fluid mechanics of model normal and stenosed aortic valves. Circ Res 25:693.

Christie GW. 1992. Anatomy of aortic heart valve leaflets: The influence of glutaraldehyde fixation on function. Eur J Cardio-thorac Surg 6[supp 1]:S25.

Davies MJ. 1980. Pathology of Cardiac Valves. London-Boston, Butterworth.

Emery RW, Arom KV. 1991. The Aortic Valve. Philadelphia, Hanley & Belfus.

Ghista DN, Rao AP. 1972. Structural mechanics of the mitral valve: Stresses sustained by the valve; non-traumatic determination of the stiffness of the in vivo valve. J Biomech 5:295.

Gramiak R, Shah PM. 1970. Echocardiography of the normal and diseased aortic valve. Radiology 96:1.

Hammarström E, Wranne B, Pinto FJ, et al. 1991. Tricuspid annular motion. J Am Soc Echocardiogr 4:131.

Hatle L, Angelsen B. 1985. Doppler Ultrasound in Cardiology Physical Principals and Clinical Applications. Philadelphia, Lea and Febiger.

Kilner PJ, Yang GZ, Mohiaddin RH, et al. 1993. Helical and retrograde secondary flow patterns in the aortic arch studied by three-directional magnetic resonance velocity mapping. Circ 88[part I]:2235.

Kim WY, Bisgaard T, Nielsen SL, Poulsen JK, Pedersen EM, Hasenkam JM, Yoganathan AP. 1994. Two-dimensional mitral flow velocity profiles in pig models using epicardial Doppler echocardiography. J Am Coll Cardiol 24:532.

Kim WY, Walker PG, Pederson EM, et al. Submitted for pub. Left ventricular blood flow patterns in normal subjects: A quantitative analysis of three-dimensional magnetic resonance velocity mapping.

Kunzelman KS, Cochran RP, Murphee SS, et al. 1993. Differential collagen distribution in the mitral valve and its influence on biomechanical behaviour. J Heart Valve Dis 2:236.

Lefebvre XP, He S, Yoganathan AP, et al. Submitted for pub. Systolic anterior motion of the mitral valve in hypertrophic cardiomyopathy: An in-vitro pulsatile flow study.

Levine RA, Trivizi MO, Harrigan P, et al. 1987. The relationship of mitral annular shape to the diagnosis of mitral valve prolapse. Circ 75:756.

Lim KO, Bouchner DP. 1975. Mechanical properties of human mitral valve chordae tendineae: Variation with size and strain rate. Can J Physiol Pharmacol 53:330.

Mercer JL, Robotham K. 1992. A comparison between the inlet and outlet diameters of the normal aortic valve. J Biomech 25:1363.

Ormiston JA, Shah PM, Tei C, et al. 1981. Size and motion of the mitral valve annulus in man: A two-dimensional echocardiographic method and findings in normal subjects. Circ 64:113.

Paulsen PK, Hasenkam JM. 1983. Three-dimensional visualization of velocity profiles in the ascending aorta in dogs, measured with a hot film anemometer. J Biomech 16:201.

Raganathan N, Lam JHC, Wigle ED, et al. 1970. Morphology of the human mitral valve: The valve leaflets. Circ 41:459.

Reul H, Talukdar N. 1979. Heart valve mechanics. In NHC Hwang, DR Gross, DJ Patel (eds), Quantitative Cardiovascular Studies Clinical and Research Applications of Engineering Principles, pp 527–564, Baltimore, University Park Press.

Roberts WC. 1983. Morphologic features of the normal and abnormal mitral valve. Am J Cardiol 51:1005.

Rossvoll O, Samstad S, Torp HG, et al. 1991. The velocity distribution in the aortic annulus in normal subjects: A quantitative analysis of two-dimensional Doppler flow maps. J Am Soc Echocardiogr 4:367.

Salisbury PF, Cross CE, Rieben PA. 1963. Chordae tendinea tension. Am J Physiol 25:385.

Samstad O, Torp HG, Linker DT, et al. 1989. Cross sectional early mitral flow velocity profiles from colour Doppler. Br Heart J 62:177.

Sanfilippo AJ, Harrigan P, Popovic AD, et al. 1992. Papillary muscle traction in mitral valve prolapse: Quantitation by two-dimensional echocardiography. J Am Coll Cardiol 19:564.

Silver MD, Lam JHC, Raganathan N, et al. 1971. Morphology of the human tricuspid valve. Circ 43:333.

Silverman ME, Hurst JW. 1968. The mitral complex: Interaction of the anatomy, physiology, and pathology of the mitral annulus, mitral valve leaflets, chordae tendineae and papillary muscles. Am Heart J 76:399.

Simonson JS, Schiller NB. 1989. Descent of the base of the left ventricle: An echocardiographic index of left ventricular function. J Am Soc Echocardiogr 2:25.

Sloth E, Houlind KC, Oyre S, Kim WY, Pedersen EM, Jørgensen HS. 1994. Three-dimensional visualization of velocity profiles in the human pulmonary artery with magnetic resonance phase-velocity mapping. Am Heart J 128:1130.

Sung HW, Yoganathan AP. 1990. Axial flow velocity patterns in a normal human pulmonary artery model: Pulsatile in vitro studies. J Biomech 23(3):210.

Thubrikar M. 1990. The Aortic Valve. Boca Raton, Fla, CRC Press.

Thubrikar M, Heckman JL, Nolan SP. 1993. High speed cine-radiographic study of aortic valve leaflet motion. J Heart Valve Dis 2:653.

Titus JL, Edwards JE. 1991. The aortic root and valve. In RW Emery, KV Arom (eds), The Aortic Valve, Philadelphia, Hanley and Belfus.

Tsakiris AG, von Bernuth G, Rastelli GC, et al. 1971. Size and motion of the mitral valve annulus in anesthetized intact dogs. J Appl Physiol 30:611.

Virmani R, Atkinson J, Fenoglio J. 1991. Cardiovascular Pathology. Philadelphia, Saunders.

Westaby S, Karp RB, Blackstone EH, et al. 1984. Adult human valve dimensions and their surgical significance. Am J Cardiol 53:552.

Weyman, AE. 1994. Principles and Practices of Echocardiography. Philadelphia, Lea & Febiger.

Yellin EL, Peskin C, Yoran C, et al. 1981. Mechanisms of mitral valve motion during diastole. Am J Physiol 241:H389.

33

Arterial Macrocirculatory Hemodynamics

Robert E. Mates
SUNY University at Buffalo

The arterial circulation is a multiply branched network of compliant tubes. The geometry of the network is complex, and the vessels exhibit nonlinear *viscoelastic* behavior. Flow is pulsatile, and the blood flowing through the network is a suspension of red cells and other particles in plasma which exhibits complex *non-Newtonian* properties. Whereas the development of an exact biomechanical description of arterial hemodynamics is a formidable task, surprisingly useful results can be obtained with greatly simplified models.

The geometrical parameters of the canine *systemic* and *pulmonary* circulations are summarized in Table 33.1. Vessel diameters vary from a maximum of 19 mm in the proximal aorta to 0.008 mm (8 microns) in the capillaries. Because of the multiple branching, the total cross-sectional area increases from 2.8 cm² in the proximal aorta to 1357 cm² in the capillaries. Of the total blood volume, approximately 83% is in the systemic circulation, 12% is in the pulmonary circulation, and the remaining 5% is in the heart. Most of the systemic blood is in the venous circulation, where changes in compliance are used to control mean blood pressure. This chapter will be concerned with flow in the larger arteries, classes 1–5 in the systemic circulation and 1–3 in the pulmonary circulation in Table 33.1. Flow in the microcirculation is discussed in Chapter 34, and venous hemodynamics is covered in Chapter 36.

33.1 Blood Vessel Walls

The detailed properties of blood vessels were described earlier in this section, but a few general observations are made here to facilitate the following discussion. Blood vessels are composed of three layers, the intima, media, and adventitia. The inner layer, or intima, is composed primarily of *endothelial* cells, which line the vessel and are involved in control of vessel diameter. The media, composed of *elastin, collagen,* and smooth muscle, largely determines the elastic properties of the vessel. The outer layer, or adventitia, is composed mainly of connective tissue. Unlike in structures composed of passive elastic materials, vessel diameter and elastic modulus vary with smooth-muscle

0-8493-8346-3/95/$0.00+$.50

TABLE 33.1 Model of Vascular Dimensions in 20–kg dog

Class	Vessels	Mean Diam. (mm)	Number of Vessels	Mean Length (mm)	Total Cross-section (cm²)	Total Blood Volume (ml)	Percentage of Total Volume
			Systemic				
1	Aorta	(19–4.5)	1		(2.8–0.2)	60	
2	Arteries	4.000	40	150.0	5.0	75	
3	Arteries	1.300	500	45.0	6.6	30	
4	Arteries	0.450	6000	13.5	9.5	13	11%
5	Arteries	0.150	110,000	4.0	19.4	8	
6	Arterioles	0.050	2.8 × 10⁶	1.2	55.0	7	
7	Capillaries	0.008	2.7 × 10⁹	0.65	1357.0	88	5%
8	Venules	0.100	1.0 × 10⁷	1.6	785.4	126	
9	Veins	0.280	660,000	4.8	406.4	196	
10	Veins	0.700	40,000	13.5	154.0	208	
11	Veins	1.800	2,100	45.0	53.4	240	
12	Veins	4.500	110	150.0	17.5	263	67%
13	Venae cavae	(5–14)	2		(0.2–1.5)	92	
Total						1406	
			Pulmonary				
1	Main artery	1.600	1	28.0	2.0	6	
2	Arteries	4.000	20	10.0	2.5	25	3%
3	Arteries	1.000	1550	14.0	12.2	17	
4	Arterioles	0.100	1.5 × 10⁶	0.7	120.0	8	
5	Capillaries	0.008	2.7 × 10⁹	0.5	1357.0	68	4%
6	Venules	0.110	2.0 × 10⁶	0.7	190.0	13	
7	Veins	1.100	1650	14.0	15.7	22	
8	Veins	4.200	25	100.0		35	5%
9	Main veins	8.000	4	30.0		6	
Total						200	
			Heart				
	Atria		2			30	
	Ventricles		2			54	5%
Total						84	
Total circulation						1690	100%

Source: Milnor WR. 1989. Hemodynamics, 2d ed, p 45, Baltimore, Williams and Wilkins. With permission.

tone. Dilation in response to increases in flow and *myogenic* constriction in response to increases in pressure have been observed in some arteries. Smooth-muscle tone is also affected by circulating *vasoconstrictors* such as norepinephrine and *vasodilators* such as nitroprusside. Blood vessels, like other soft biological tissues, generally do not obey Hooke's law, becoming stiffer as pressure is increased. They also exhibit viscoelastic characteristics such as hysteresis and creep. Fortunately, for many purposes a linear elastic model of blood vessel behavior provides adequate results.

33.2 Flow Characteristics

Blood is a complex substance containing water, inorganic ions, proteins, and cells. Approximately 50% is plasma, a nearly Newtonian fluid consisting of water, ions, and proteins. The balance contains erythrocytes (red blood cells), leukocytes (white blood cells), and platelets. Whereas the behavior of blood in vessels smaller than approximately 100 µ exhibits significant non-Newtonian effects, flow in larger vessels can be described reasonably accurately using the Newtonian assumption. There is some recent evidence that wall shear stress distributions may differ somewhat from Newtonian values [Liepsch et al., 1991].

Flow in the arterial circulation is predominantly laminar with the possible exception of the aorta and main pulmonary artery. In steady flow, transition to turbulence occurs at Reynolds numbers (N_R) above approximately 2300, where

$$N_R = \frac{2rV}{v} \tag{33.1}$$

where

r = vessel radius, V = velocity, v = kinematic viscosity = viscosity/density.

Flow in the major systemic and pulmonary arteries is highly pulsatile. Peak-to-mean flow amplitudes as high as 6 to 1 have been reported in both human and dog [Milnor, 1989, p. 149]. Womersley's analysis of incompressible flow in rigid and elastic tubes [1957] showed that the importance of pulsatility in the velocity distributions depended on the parameter

$$N_W = r\sqrt{\frac{\omega}{v}} \tag{33.2}$$

where ω = frequency.

This is usually referred to as the *Womersley number* (N_w) or α-*parameter*. Womersley's original report is not readily available; however, Milnor provides a reasonably complete account [Milnor, 1989, pp. 106–121].

Mean and peak Reynolds numbers in human and dog are given in Table 33.2, which also includes mean, peak, and minimum velocities as well as the Womersley number. Mean Reynolds numbers in the entire systemic and pulmonary circulations are below 2300. Peak systolic Reynolds numbers exceed 2300 in the aorta and pulmonary artery, and some evidence of transition to turbulence has been reported. In dogs, disturbed flow occurs at Reynolds numbers as low as 1000, with higher Womersley numbers increasing the transition Reynolds number [Nerem & Seed, 1972]. The values in Table 33.2 are typical for individuals at rest. During exercise, cardiac output and hence Reynolds numbers can increase severalfold. The Womersley number also affects the shape of the instantaneous velocity profiles as discussed below.

TABLE 33.2 Normal Average Hemodynamic Values in Man and Dog

	Dog (20 kg)			Man (70 kg, 1.8 m²)		
	N_w	Velocity (cm/s)	N_R	N_w	Velocity (cm/s)	N_R
Systemic Vessels						
Ascending aorta	16	15.8 (89/0)*	870(4900)[†]	21	18 (112/0)*	1500 (9400)[†]
Abdominal aorta	9	12 (60/0)	370(1870)	12	14 (75/0)	640 (3600)
Renal artery	3	41 (74/26)	440 (800)	4	40 (73/26)	700 (1300)
Femoral artery	4	10 (42/1)	130 (580)	4	12 (52/2)	200 (860)
Femoral vein	5	5	92	7	4	104
Superior vena cava	10	8 (20/0)	320 (790)	15	9 (23/0)	550 (1400)
Inferior vena cava	11	19 (40/0)	800 (1800)	17	21 (46/0)	1400 (3000)
Pulmonary vessels						
Main artery	14	18 (72/0)	900 (3700)	20	19 (96/0)	1600 (7800)
Main vein‡	7	18 (30/9)	270 (800)	10	19 (38/10)	800 (2200)

* Mean (systolic/diastolic)
[†] Mean (peak)
‡ One of the usually four terminal pulmonary veins
Source: Milnor WR. 1989. Hemodynamics, 2d ed, p 148, Baltimore, Williams and Wilkins. With permission.

33.3 Wave Propagation

The elasticity of blood vessels affects the hemodynamics of arterial flow. The primary function of arterial elasticity is to store blood during systole so that forward flow continues when the aortic valve is closed. Elasticity also causes a finite wave propagation velocity, which is given approximately by the Moens-Korteweg relationship

$$c = \sqrt{\frac{Eh}{2\rho r}} \tag{33.3}$$

where E = wall elastic modulus, h = wall thickness, ρ = blood density.

Although Moens [1878] and Korteweg [1878] are credited with this formulation, Fung [1984, p. 107] has pointed out that the formula was first derived much earlier [Young, 1808]. Wave speeds in arterial blood vessels from several species are given in Table 33.3. In general, wave speeds increase toward the periphery as vessel radius decreases and are considerably lower in the main pulmonary artery than in the aorta owing primarily to the lower pressure and consequently greater elasticity.

Wave reflections occur at branches where there is not perfect *impedance* matching of parent and daughter vessels. The input impedance of a network of vessels is the ratio of pressure to flow. For rigid vessels with laminar flow and negligible inertial effects, the input impedance is simply the resistance and is independent of pressure and flow rate. For elastic vessels, the impedance is dependent on the frequency of the fluctuations in pressure and flow. The impedance can be described by a complex number expressing the amplitude ratio of pressure to flow oscillations and the phase difference between the peaks

$$\overline{Z}_i(\omega) = \frac{\overline{P}(\omega)}{\overline{Q}(\omega)}$$

$$|\overline{Z}_i(\omega)| = \left| \frac{\overline{P}(\omega)}{\overline{Q}(\omega)} \right| \tag{33.4}$$

$$\theta_i(\omega) = \theta[(\overline{P}(\omega))] - \theta[(\overline{Q}(\omega))]$$

where $\overline{Z}_i$ is the complex impedance, $|\overline{Z}_i|$ is the amplitude, and θ_i is the phase.

For an infinitely long straight tube with constant properties, input impedance will be independent of position in the tube and dependent only on vessel and fluid properties. The corresponding value of input impedance is called the *characteristic impedance* Z_o, given by

$$Z_0 = \frac{\rho c}{A} \tag{33.5}$$

where A = vessel cross-sectional area.

In general, the input impedance will vary from point to point in the network because of variations in vessel sizes and properties. If the network has the same impedance at each point (perfect impedance matching), there will be no wave reflections. Such a network will transmit

TABLE 33.3 Pressure Wave Velocities in Arteries[*],[†]

Artery	Species	Wave Velocity (cm/s)
Ascending Aorta	Man	440–520
	Dog	350–472
Thoracic aorta	Man	400–650
	Dog	400–700
Abdominal aorta	Man	500–620
	Dog	550–960
Iliac	Man	700–880
	Dog	700–800
Femoral	Man	800–1800
	Dog	800–1300
Popliteal	Dog	1220–1310
Tibial	Dog	1040–1430
Carotid	Man	680–830
	Dog	610–1240
Pulmonary	Man	168–182
	Dog	255–275
	Rabbit	100
	Pig	190

[*]All data are apparent pressure wave velocities (although the average of higher frequency harmonics approximates the true velocity in many cases), from relatively young subjects with normal cardiovascular systems, at approximately normal distending pressures.

[†]Ranges for each vessel and species taken from Table 9.1 of source.

Source: Milnor WR. 1989. Hemodynamics, 2d ed, p 235, Baltimore, Williams and Wilkins. With permission.

energy most efficiently. The reflection coefficient R, defined as the ratio of reflected to incident wave amplitude, is related to the relative characteristic impedance of the vessels at a junction. For a parent tube with characteristic impedance Z_0 branching into two daughter tubes with characteristic impedances Z_1 and Z_2, the reflection coefficient is given by

$$R = \frac{Z_0^{-1} - (Z_1^{-1} + Z_2^{-1})}{Z_0^{-1} + (Z_1^{-1} + Z_2^{-1})} \qquad (33.6)$$

and perfect impedance matching requires

$$\frac{1}{Z_0} = \frac{1}{Z_1} + \frac{1}{Z_2} \qquad (33.7)$$

The arterial circulation exhibits partial impedance matching; however, wave reflections do occur. At each branch point, local reflection coefficients typically are less than 0.2. However, global reflection coefficients, which account for all reflections distal to a given site, can be considerably higher [Milnor, 1989, p 217].

In the absence of wave reflections, the input impedance is equal to the characteristic impedance. Womersley's analysis predicts that impedance modulus will decrease monitonically with increasing frequency, whereas the phase angle is negative at low frequency and becomes progressively more positive with increasing frequency. Typical values calculated from Womersley's analysis are shown in Fig. 33.1. In the actual circulation, wave reflections cause oscillations in the modulus and phase. Figure 33.2 shows input impedance measured in the ascending aorta of a human. Measurements of input resistance, characteristic impedance, and the frequency of the first minimum in the input impedance are summarized in Table 33.4.

33.4 Velocity Profiles

Typical pressure and velocity fluctuations throughout the cardiac cycle in man are shown in Fig. 33.3. Although mean pressure decreases slightly toward the periphery due to viscous effects, peak pressure shows small increases in the distal aorta due to wave reflection and vessel taper. Velocity peaks during systole, with some backflow observed in the aorta early in diastole. Flow in the aorta is nearly zero through most of diastole; however, more peripheral arteries such as the iliac and renal show forward flow throughout the cardiac cycle. This is a result of capacitive discharge of the central arteries as arterial pressure decreases.

Velocity varies across the vessel due to viscous effects as mentioned earlier. The velocities in Fig. 33.3 were measured at one point in the artery. Velocity profiles are complex because the flow is pulsatile and vessels are elastic, curved, and tapered. Profiles measured in the thoracic aorta of a dog at normal arterial pressure and cardiac output are shown in Fig. 33.4. Backflow occurs during diastole, and profiles are flattened even during peak systolic flow. The shape of the profiles varies considerably with mean aortic pressure and cardiac output [Ling et al., 1973].

In more peripheral arteries the profiles are more parabolic as in fully developed laminar flow. The general features of these fully developed flow profiles can be modeled using Womersley's approach, although nonlinear effects may be important in some cases. The qualitative features of the profile depend on the Womersley number N_w. Unsteady effects become more important as N_w increases. Below a value of about 2 the instantaneous profiles are close to the steady parabolic shape. Profiles in the aortic arch are skewed due to curvature of the arch.

33.5 Pathology

Atherosclerosis is a disease of the arterial wall which appears to be strongly influenced by hemodynamics. The disease begins with a thickening of the intimal layer in locations which correlate with

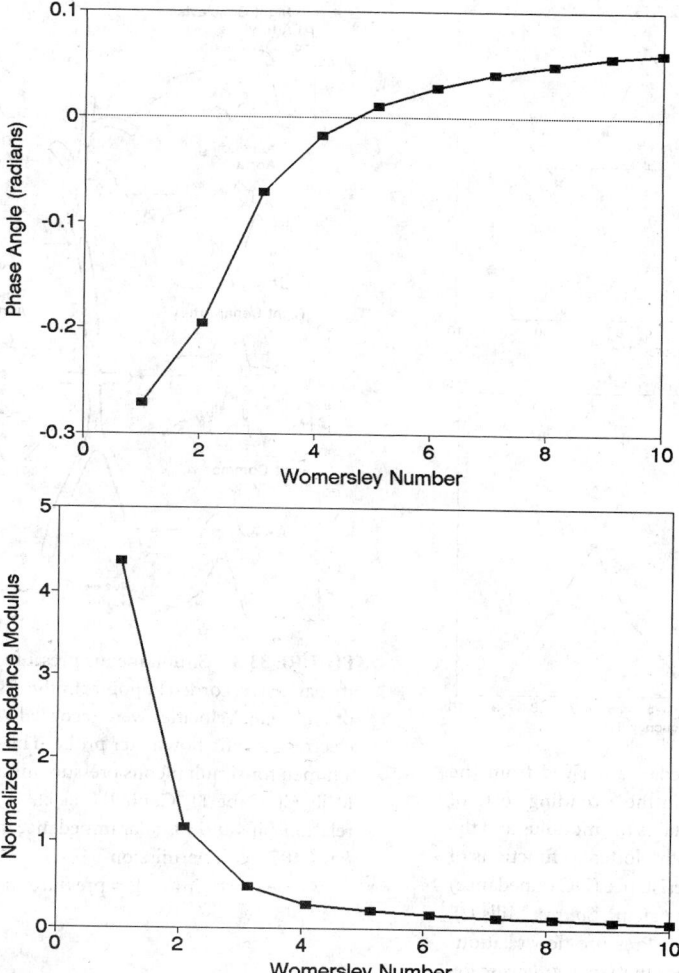

FIGURE 33.1 Characteristic impedance calculated from Womersley's analysis. The top panel contains the phase of the impedance and the bottom panel the modulus, both plotted as a function of the Womersley number N_w, which is promotional to frequency. The curves shown are for an unconstrained tube and include the effects of wall viscosity. The original figure has an error in the scale of the ordinate which has been corrected. *Source:* Milnor WR. 1989. Hemodynamics, 2d ed, p 172, Baltimore, Williams and Wilkins. With permission.

the shear stress distribution on the endothelial surface [Friedman et al., 1993]. Over time the lesion continues to grow until a significant portion of the vessel lumen is occluded. The peripheral circulation will dilate to compensate for the increase in resistance of the large vessels, compromising the ability of the system to respond to increases in demand during exercise. Eventually the circulation is completely dilated, and resting flow begins to decrease. A blood clot may form at the site or lodge in a narrowed segment, causing an acute loss of blood flow. The disease is particularly dangerous in the coronary and carotid arteries due to the critical oxygen requirements of the heart and brain.

In addition to intimal thickening, the arterial wall properties also change with age. Most measurements suggest that arterial elasticity decreases with age (hardening of the arteries); however, in some cases arteries appear to become more elastic [Learoyd & Taylor, 1966]. Local weakening of the

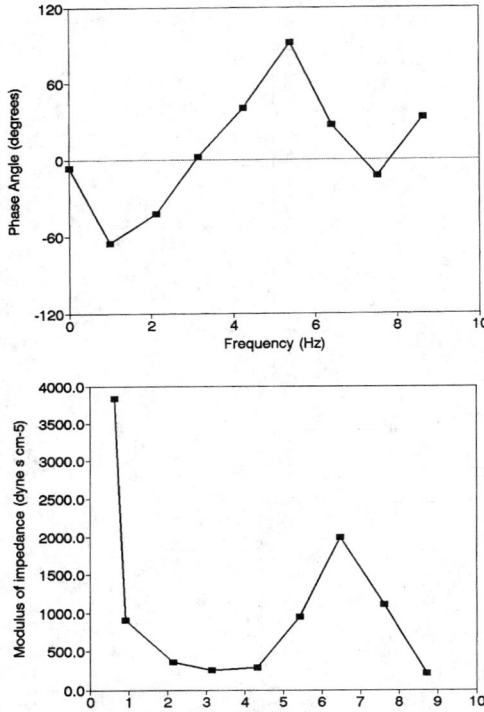

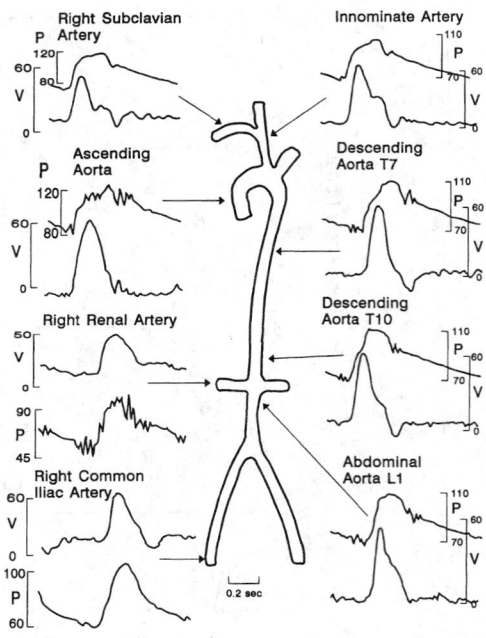

FIGURE 33.3 Simultaneous pressure and blood velocity patterns recorded at points in the systemic circulation of a human. Velocities were recorded with a catheter-tip electromagnetic flowmeter probe. The catheter included a lumen for simultaneous pressure measurement. *Source:* Mills CJ, Gabe IT, Gault JN, et al. 1970. Pressure-flow relationships and vascular impedance in man. *Cardiovasc Res* 4:405. With permission.

V = velocity (cm/s), P = pressure (mm/Hg)

FIGURE 33.2 Input impedance derived from the pressure and velocity data in the ascending aorta of Fig. 33.3. The top panel contains the modulus and the bottom panel the phase, both plotted as functions of frequency. The peripheral resistance (DC impedance) for this plot was 16470 dyne s/cm^5. *Source:* Mills CJ, Gabe IT, Gault JN, et al. 1970. Pressure-flow relationships and vascular impedance in man. *Cardiovasc Res* 4:405. With permission.

TABLE 33.4 Characteristic Arterial Impedances in Some Mammals: Average ($\pm$SE)[*,†]

Species	Artery	R_{in}	Z_o	f_{min}
Dog	Aorta	2809–6830	125–288	6–8
Dog	Pulmonary	536–807	132–295	2–3.5
Dog	Femoral	110–162[‡]	4.5–15.8[‡]	8–13
Dog	Carotid	69[‡]	7.0–9.4[‡]	8–11
Rabbit	Aorta	20–50[‡]	1.8–2.1[‡]	4.5–9.8
Rabbit	Pulmonary		1.1[‡]	3.0
Rat	Aorta	153[‡]	11.2[‡]	12

Abbreviations: R_{in}, input resistance (mean arterial pressure/flow) in dyn s/cm^5; Z_o, characteristic impedance, in dyn s/cm^5, estimated by averaging high-frequency input impedances in aorta and pulmonary artery; value at 5Hz for other arteries, f_{min}, frequency of first minimum of Z_i.

[*]Values estimated from published figures if averages were not reported.

[†]Ranges for each species and vessel taken from values in Table 7.2 of source.

[‡]10^3 dyn s/cm^5.

Source: Milnor WR. 1989. Hemodynamics, 2d ed, p 183, Baltimore, Williams and Wilkins. With permission.

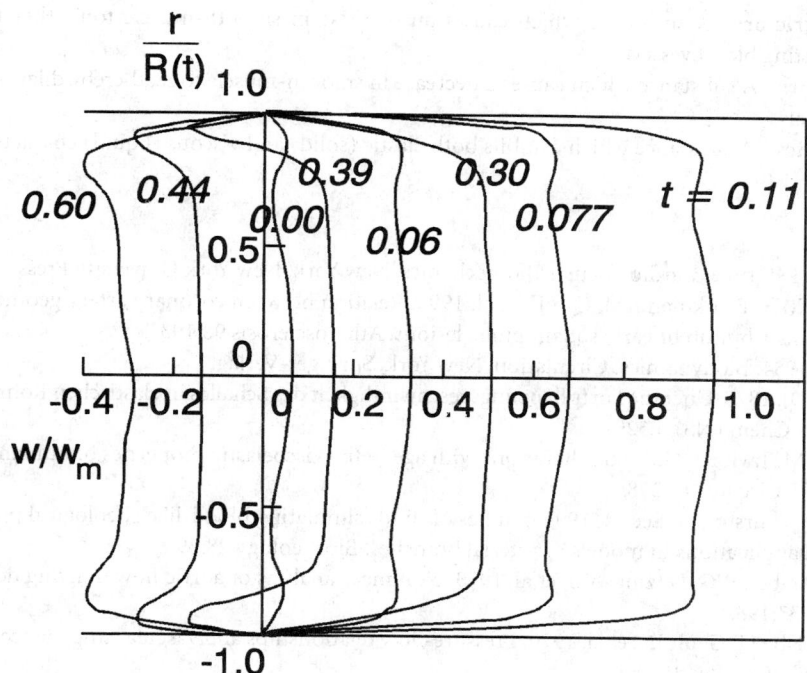

FIGURE 33.4 Velocity profiles obtained with a hot-film anemometer probe in the descending thoracic aorta of a dog at normal arterial pressure and cardiac output. The velocity at t = time/(cardiac period) is plotted as a function of radial position. Velocity w is normalized by the maximum velocity w_m and radial position at each time by the instantaneous vessel radius $R(t)$. The aortic valve opens at t = 0. Peak velocity occurs 11% of the cardiac period after aortic valve opening. *Source:* Ling SC, Atabek WG, Letzing WG, et al. 1973. Nonlinear analysis of aortic flow in living dogs. *Circ Res* 33:198. With permission.

wall may also occur, particularly in the descending aorta, giving rise to an *aneurism,* which, if it ruptures, can cause sudden death.

efining Terms

Aneurism: A ballooning of a blood vessel wall caused by weakening of the elastic material in the wall.

Atherosclerosis: A disease of the blood vessels characterized by thickening of the vessel wall and eventual occlusion of the vessel.

Collagen: A protein found in blood vessels which is much stiffer than elastin.

Elastin: A very elastic protein found in blood vessels.

Endothelial: The lining of blood vessels.

Impedance: A (generally) complex number expressing the ratio of pressure to flow.

Myogenic: A change in smooth-muscle tone due to stretch or relaxation, causing a blood vessel to resist changes in diameter.

Newtonian: A fluid whose stress–rate-of-strain relationship is linear, following Newton's law. The fluid will have a viscosity whose value is independent of rate of strain.

Pulmonary: The circulation which delivers blood to the lungs for reoxygenation and carbon dioxide removal.

Systemic: The circulation which supplies oxygenated blood to the tissues of the body.

Vasoconstrictor: A substance which causes an increase in smooth-muscle tone, thereby constricting blood vessels.

Vasodilator: A substance which causes a decrease in smooth-muscle tone, thereby dilating blood vessels.

Viscoelastic: A substance which exhibits both elastic (solid) and viscous (liquid) characteristics.

References

Chandran KB. 1992. Cardiovascular Biomechanics. New York, New York University Press.

Friedman MH, Brinkman AM, Qin JJ, et al. 1993. Relation between coronary artery geometry and the distribution of early sudanophilic lesions. Atherosclerosis 98:193.

Fung YC. 1984. Biodynamics: Circulation. New York, Springer-Verlag.

Korteweg DJ. 1878. Uber die Fortpflanzungsgeschwindigkeit des Schalles in elastischen Rohren. Ann Phys Chem (NS) 5:525.

Learoyd BM, Taylor MG. 1966. Alterations with age in the viscoelastic properties of human arterial walls. Circ Res 18:278.

Liepsch D, Thurston G, Lee M. 1991. Studies of fluids simulating blood-like rheological properties and applications in models of arterial branches. Biorheology 28:39.

Ling SC, Atabek WG, Letzing WG, et al. 1973. Nonlinear analysis of aortic flow in living dogs. Circ Res 33:198.

Mills CJ, Gabe IT, Gault JN, et al. 1970. Pressure-flow relationships and vascular impedance in man. Cardiovasc Res 4:405.

Milnor WR. 1989. Hemodynamics, 2d ed. Baltimore, Williams and Wilkins.

Moens AI. 1878. Die Pulskurve, Leiden.

Nerem RM, Seed WA. 1972. An in-vivo study of aortic flow disturbances. Cardiovasc Res 6:1.

Womersley JR. 1957. The mathematical analysis of the arterial circulation in a state of oscillatory motion. Wright Air Development Center Technical Report WADC-TR56-614.

Young T. 1808. Hydraulic investigations, subservient to an intended Croonian lecture on the motion of the blood. Phil Trans Roy Soc London 98:164.

Further Information

A good introduction to cardiovascular biomechanics, including arterial hemodynamics, is provided by K. B. Chandran in *Cardiovascular Biomechanics*. Y.C. Fung's *Biodynamics—Circulation* is also an excellent starting point, somewhat more mathematical than Chandran. Perhaps the most complete treatment of the subject is in *Hemodynamics* by W. R. Milnor, from which much of this chapter was taken. Milnor's book is quite mathematical and may be difficult for a novice to follow.

Current work in arterial hemodynamics is reported in a number of engineering and physiological journals, including the *Annals of Biomedical Engineering, Journal of Biomechanical Engineering, Circulation Research*, and *The American Journal of Physiology, Heart and Circulatory Physiology*. Symposia sponsored by the American Society of Mechanical Engineers, Biomedical Engineering Society, American Heart Association, and the American Physiological Society contain reports of current research.

34

Mechanics and Transport in the Microcirculation

Aleksander S. Popel
Department of Biomedical Engineering, School of Medicine, Johns Hopkins University,

Roland N. Pittman
Department of Physiology, Medical College of Virginia, Virginia Commonwealth University

The microcirculation comprises blood vessels (arterioles, capillaries, and venules) with diameters of less than approximately 150 μm. The importance of the microcirculation is underscored by the fact that most of the hydrodynamic resistance of the circulatory system lies in the microvessels (especially in arterioles), and most of the exchange of nutrients and waste products occurs at the level of the smallest microvessels. The subject of microcirculatory research is blood flow and molecular transport in microvessels, mechanical interactions and molecular exchange between these vessels and the surrounding tissue, and regulation of blood flow and molecular transport. Quantitative knowledge of microcirculatory mechanics and mass transport has been accumulated primarily in the past 25 years owing to significant innovations in methods and techniques to measure microcirculatory parameters and methods to analyze microcirculatory data. The development of these methods has required joint efforts of physiologists and biomedical engineers. Key innovations include significant improvements in intravital microscopy, the dual-slit method (Wayland-Johnson) for measuring velocity in microvessels, the servo-null method (Wiederhielm-Intaglietta) for measuring pressure in microvessels, the recessed oxygen microelectrode (Whalen) for polarographic measurements of partial pressure of oxygen, and the microspectrophotometric method (Pittman-Duling) for measuring oxyhemoglobin saturation in microvessels. The single-capillary cannulation method (Landis-Michel) has provided a powerful tool for studies of transport of water and solutes through the capillary endothelium. In the last decade, new experimental techniques have appeared, many adapted from cell biology and modified for in vivo studies, that are having a tremendous impact on the field. Examples include confocal microscopy for better three-dimensional resolution of microvascular structures, methods of optical imaging using fluorescent labels (e.g., labeling blood cells for velocity measurements) and fluorescent dyes (e.g., calcium-ion-sensitive dyes for measuring the dynamics of calcium ion concentration in arteriolar smooth muscle and endothelial cells in vivo), development of sensors (glass filaments, magnetic tweezers) for measuring forces in the

0-8493-8346-3/95/$0.00+$.50
© 1995 by CRC Press, Inc.

nanonewton range that are characteristic of cell-cell interactions, phosphorescence decay measurements as an indicator of oxygen tension, and methods of manipulating receptors on the surfaces of blood cells and endothelial cells. In addition to the dramatic developments in experimental techniques, quantitative knowledge and understanding of the microcirculation have been significantly enhanced by theoretical studies, perhaps having a larger impact than in other areas of physiology. Extensive theoretical work has been conducted on the mechanics of the red blood cell (RBC) and leukocyte, mechanics of blood flow in single microvessels and microvascular networks, oxygen (O_2) and carbon dioxide (CO_2) exchange between microvessels and surrounding tissue, and water and solute transport through capillary endothelium and the surrounding tissue. These theoretical studies not only aid in the interpretation of experimental data but in many cases also serve as a framework for quantitative testing of working hypotheses and as a guide in designing and conducting further experiments. The accumulated knowledge has led to significant progress in our understanding of mechanisms of regulation of blood flow and molecular exchange in the microcirculation in many organs and tissues under a variety of physiological and pathological conditions (e.g., hypoxia, hypertension, sickle cell anemia, diabetes, inflammation, sepsis, cancer).

The goal of this chapter is to give an overview of the current status of research on the systemic microcirculation. Issues of pulmonary microcirculation are not discussed. Because of space limitations, it is not possible to recognize numerous important contributions to the field of microcirculatory mechanics and mass transport. In most cases we refer to recent reviews, when available, and journal articles where earlier references can be found. We discuss experimental and theoretical findings and point out gaps in our understanding of microcirculatory flow phenomena.

34.1 Mechanics of Microvascular Blood Flow

Vessel dimensions in the microcirculation are small enough so that the effects of the particulate nature of blood are significant [Lipowsky, 1987]. Blood is a suspension of formed elements [red blood cells, white blood cells (leukocytes), and platelets] in plasma. Plasma is an aqueous solution of mostly proteins (albumins, globulins, and fibrinogen) and electrolytes. Under static conditions, human RBCs are biconcave discs with diameter ~7–9 μm. The chief function of the RBC is delivery of O_2 to tissue. Most of the O_2 carried by the blood is chemically bound to hemoglobin inside the RBCs. The mammalian RBC comprises a viscoelastic membrane filled with a viscous fluid, concentrated hemoglobin solution. The membrane consists of the plasma membrane and underlying cytoskeleton. The membrane can undergo deformations without changing its surface area, which is nearly conserved locally. RBCs are so easily deformable that they can flow through small pores with diameter <3 μm. Leukocytes (grouped into three categories: granulocytes, monocytes, and lymphocytes) are spherical cells with diameter ~10–20 μm. They are stiffer than RBCs. The main function of these cells is immunologic, i.e., protection of the body against microorganisms causing disease. In contrast to mammalian RBCs, leukocytes are nucleated and are endowed with an internal structural cytoskeleton. Leukocytes are capable of active ameboid motion, the property which allows their migration from the blood stream into the tissue. Platelets are disc-shaped blood elements with diameter ~2–3 μm. Platelets play a key role in thrombogenic processes and blood coagulation. The normal volume fraction of RBCs (hematocrit) in humans is 40–45%. The total volume of RBCs in blood is approximately 50 times greater than the volume of leukocytes and platelets. Rheological properties of blood in arterioles and venules and larger vessels are determined primarily by RBCs; however, leukocytes play an important mechanical role in capillaries and small venules.

Blood plasma is a newtonian fluid with viscosity of approximately 1.2 cP. The viscosity of whole blood in a rotational viscometer or a large-bore capillary viscometer exhibits shear-thinning behavior, i.e., decreases when shear rate increases. At shear rates >100 s^{-1} and a hematocrit of 40%, typical viscosity values are 3–4 cP. The dominant mechanism of the nonnewtonian behavior is RBC aggregation, and the secondary mechanism is RBC deformation under shear forces. The cross-sectional distribution of RBCs in vessels is nonuniform, with a core of concentrated RBC suspension and a cell-free or cell-depleted marginal layer, typically 2–5 µm thick, adjacent to the vessel wall. The nonuniform RBC distribution results in the *Fahraeus effect* (the microvessel hematocrit is smaller than the feed or discharge hematocrit) due to the fact that, on the average, RBCs move with a higher velocity than blood plasma, and the concomitant *Fahraeus-Lindqvist effect* (the apparent viscosity of blood is lower than the bulk viscosity measured with a rotational viscometer or a large-bore capillary viscometer at high shear rate). The *apparent viscosity* of a fluid flowing in a cylindrical vessel of radius R and length L under the influence of a pressure difference ΔP is defined as

$$\eta_a = \frac{\pi \Delta P R^4}{8QL} \tag{34.1}$$

where Q is the volumetric flow rate. For a newtonian fluid the apparent viscosity becomes the dynamic viscosity of the fluid, and the above equation represents *Poiseuille's law*. The apparent viscosity is a function of hematocrit, vessel radius, blood flow rate, and other parameters. In the microcirculation, blood flows through a complex branching network of arterioles, capillaries, and venules. Arterioles are typically 10–100 µm in diameter, capillaries are 4–8 µm, and venules are 10–150 µm. Now we will discuss vascular wall mechanics and blood flow in vessels of different size in more detail.

Mechanics of the Microvascular Wall

The wall of arterioles comprises the intima which contains a single layer of contiguous endothelial cells, the media which contains a single layer of smooth-muscle cells in terminal and medium-size arterioles or several layers in the larger arterioles, and the adventitia which contains collagen fibers with occasional fibroblasts and mast cells. Fibers situated between the endothelium and the smooth-muscle cells comprise the elastica lamina. The single layer of smooth-muscle cells terminates at the capillaries and reappears at the level of small venules; the capillary wall is devoid of smooth muscle cells. Venules typically have a larger diameter and smaller wall-thickness-to-diameter ratio than arterioles of the corresponding branching order.

 Most of our knowledge of the mechanics of the microvascular wall comes from in vivo or in vitro measurements of vessel diameter as a function of transmural pressure [Davis, 1993; Shoukas & Bohlen, 1990]. Development of isolated arteriole preparations has made it possible to precisely control the transmural pressure during experiments. In addition, these preparations allow one to separate the effects of metabolic factors and blood flow rate from the effect of pressure by controlling both the chemical environment and the flow rate through the vessel. Arterioles and venules exhibit vascular tone, i.e., their diameter is maximal when smooth muscle is completely relaxed (inactivated). When the vascular smooth muscle is constricted, small arterioles may even completely close their lumen to blood flow, presumably by buckling endothelial cells. Arterioles exhibit a *myogenic response* not observed in other blood vessels, with the exception of cerebral arteries: Within a certain physiological pressure range the vessels constrict in response to elevation of transmural pressure and dilate in response to reduction of transmural pressure; in other words, in a certain range of pressures the slope of the pressure-diameter relationship is negative. Arterioles of different size exhibit different degrees of myogenic responsiveness. This effect has been documented in many tissues both in vivo and in vitro (in isolated arterioles) and has been shown to play an important role in regulation of blood flow and capillary pressure (see the section below on regulation of blood flow).

 The stress-strain relationship for a thin-walled microvessel can be derived from the experimentally obtained pressure-diameter relationship using the law of Laplace. Stress in the vessel wall can be decomposed into passive and active components. The passive component corresponds to the state of complete vasodilation. The active component determines the vascular tone and the myogenic response. Steady-state stress-strain relationships are, generally, nonlinear. For arterioles, diameter variations of 50% or even 100% under physiological conditions are not unusual, so that finite deformations have to be considered in formulating the constitutive relationship for the wall (relationship between stress, strain, and their temporal derivatives). Pertinent to the question of microvascular mechanics is the mechanical interaction of a vessel with its environment that consists of connective tissue, parenchymal cells, and extracellular fluid. There is ultrastructural evidence that blood vessels are tethered to the surrounding tissue, so that mechanical forces can be generated when the vessels constrict or dilate or when the tissue is moving, e.g., in contracting striated muscle, myocardium, or intestine. Little quantitative information is currently available about the magnitude of these forces, chiefly because of the difficulty of such measurements. A recently reported technique, magnetic tweezers [Guilford & Gore, 1992], opens a new way of investigating the mechanics of the microvascular wall in vivo and its interaction with the surrounding tissue.

Under time-dependent conditions microvessels exhibit viscoelastic behavior. In response to a stepwise change in the transmural pressure, arterioles typically respond with a fast "passive" change in diameter followed by a slow "active" response with a characteristic time of the order of tens of seconds. For example, when the pressure is suddenly increased, the vessel diameter will quickly increase, with subsequent vasoconstriction which may result in a lower value of steady-state diameter than that prior to the increase in pressure. Therefore, to accurately describe the time-dependent vessel behavior, the constitutive relationship between stress and strain or pressure and diameter must also contain temporal derivatives of these variables. Theoretical analysis of the resulting nonlinear equations shows that such constitutive equations lead to predictions of spontaneous oscillations of vessel diameter (*vasomotion*) under certain conditions [Ursino & Fabbri, 1992]. It should be noted that there are mechanisms leading to spontaneous flow oscillations that are associated with blood rheology and not with vascular wall mechanics [Kiani et al., 1994]. Whether experimentally observed vasomotion and its effect on blood flow (flow motion) can be quantitatively described by the published theoretical studies remains to be established.

For most purposes, capillary compliance is not taken into account. However, in some situations, such as analysis of certain capillary water transport experiments or leukocyte flow in a capillary, this view is not adequate, and capillary compliance has to be accounted for. Since the capillary wall is devoid of smooth-muscle cells, much of this compliance is passive and its magnitude is small. However, the presence of contractile proteins in the cytoskeleton of capillary endothelial cells opens a possibility of active capillary constriction or dilation.

Capillary Blood Flow

Progress in this area is closely related to studies of mechanics of blood cells described elsewhere in this book. In narrow capillaries RBCs flow in single file, separated by gaps of plasma. They deform and assume a parachutelike shape, generally nonaxisymmetric, leaving a submicron plasma sleeve between the RBC and endothelium. In the smallest capillaries, the shape of RBCs is sausagelike. The hemoglobin solution inside an RBC is a newtonian fluid. The constitutive relationship for the membrane is expressed by the Evans-Skalak finite-deformations model. The coupled mechanical problem of membrane and fluid motion has been extensively investigated using both analytical and numerical approaches [Secomb, 1992; Skalak et al., 1989]. An important result of the theoretical studies is the prediction of the apparent viscosity of blood. Although these predictions are in good agreement with in vitro studies in glass tubes, they appear to underestimate a few available in vivo capillary measurements of apparent viscosity. In addition, in vivo capillary hematocrit in some tissues is lower than predicted from in vitro studies with tubes of the same size. To explain the low values of hematocrit, RBC interactions with the endothelial glycocalyx have been implicated [Desjardins and Duling, 1990]. A recent theoretical analysis of blood flow in microvascular networks, discussed in more detail below [Pries et al., 1990], suggests that the in vivo apparent viscosity of blood in capillaries may be higher than that measured in vitro or predicted theoretically based on the model of the capillary as a cylinder with smooth walls. Thus, there are fundamental questions in capillary flow mechanics that remain to be resolved.

The motion of leukocytes through blood capillaries has also been studied thoroughly in recent years. Because leukocytes are larger and stiffer than RBCs, under normal flow conditions an increase in capillary resistance caused by a single leukocyte may be 1000 times greater than that caused by a single RBC [Schmid-Schönbein et al., 1989]. Under certain conditions flow stoppage may be caused by leukocyte plugging. After a period of ischemia, leukocyte plugging may prevent tissue reperfusion [Schmid-Schönbein, 1993]. Chemical bonds between membrane-bound receptors and endothelial adhesion molecules play a crucial role in leukocyte-endothelium interactions. Methods of cell and molecular biology permit manipulation of the receptors and thus make it possible to study leukocyte microcirculatory mechanics at the molecular level. More generally, methods of cell and molecular biology open new and powerful ways to study cell micromechanics and cell-cell interactions [Chien, 1992].

Arteriolar and Venular Blood Flow

The cross-sectional distribution of RBCs in arterioles and venules is nonuniform. A concentrated suspension of RBCs forms a core surrounded by a cell-free or cell-depleted layer of plasma. This "lubrication" layer of lower viscosity fluid near the vessel wall results in lower values of the apparent viscosity of blood compared to its bulk viscosity, producing the Fahraeus-Lindqvist effect [Lipowsky, 1987]. There is experimental evidence that velocity profiles of RBCs are generally symmetric in arterioles (except very close to vascular bifurcations) but are generally asymmetric in venules; the profiles are blunted in vessels of both types [Ellsworth & Pittman, 1986; Tangelder et al., 1986]. Moreover, flow in the venules may be stratified as the result of converging blood streams that do not mix rapidly. The key to understanding the pattern of arteriolar and venular blood flow is the mechanics of flow at vascular bifurcations, diverging for arteriolar flow and converging for venular flow. A great deal of experimental and theoretical work has been done on arteriolar bifurcations [Enden & Popel, 1994]. In contrast, little quantitative information is available on venular flow in general and on venular bifurcations in particular. One of the main unresolved questions is under what physiological conditions does RBC aggregation affect venular velocity distribution and vascular resistance. Much is known about aggregation in vitro, but in vivo knowledge is incomplete.

Problems of leukocyte distribution in the microcirculation and leukocyte interaction with the microvascular endothelium have attracted considerable attention in recent years. Leukocyte rolling along the walls of venules, but not arterioles, has been demonstrated. This effect results from differences in the microvascular endothelium, not the flow conditions [Ley & Gaehtgens, 1991]. Platelet distribution in the lumen is important because of the role of platelets in blood coagulation. Detailed studies of platelet distribution in arterioles and venules show that the cross-sectional distribution of these disk-shaped blood elements depends on the blood flow rate and vessel hematocrit [Woldhuis et al., 1992].

To conclude, many important features of blood flow through arterioles and venules are qualitatively known and understood; however, a rigorous theoretical description of flow as a suspension of discrete particles is not available. Such description is necessary for a quantitative understanding of the mechanisms of the nonuniform distribution of blood cells in microvessels.

Blood Flow in Microvascular Networks

Microvascular networks in different organs and tissues differ in their appearance and structural organization. Methods have been developed to quantitatively describe network architectonics and hemodynamics [Popel, 1987]. Recently, methods of fractal analysis have been applied to interpret experimental data on blood flow distribution in the microcirculation; these methods explore the property of geometrical and flow similarity that exist at different scales in the network [Bassingthwaighte et al., 1994]. Microvascular hydraulic pressure varies systematically between consecutive branching orders, decreasing from the systemic values down to 20–25 mm Hg in the capillaries and decreasing further by 10–15 mm Hg in the venules. Mean microvascular blood flow rate in arterioles decreases toward the capillaries, in inverse proportion to the number of "parallel" vessels, and increases from capillaries through the venules. In addition to this longitudinal variation of blood flow and pressure among different branching orders, there are significant variations among vessels of the same branching order, referred to as *flow heterogeneity*. The heterogeneity of blood flow and RBC distribution in microvascular networks has been well documented in a variety of organs and tissues. This phenomenon may have important implications for tissue exchange processes, so significant efforts have been devoted to the quantitative analysis of blood flow in microvascular networks. A mathematical model of blood flow in a network can be formulated as follows. First, network topology or vessel interconnections have to be specified. Second, the diameter and length of every vascular segment has to be known. Alternatively, vessel diameter can be specified as a function of transmural pressure and perhaps some other parameters; these relationships are discussed in the preceding section on wall mechanics. Third, the apparent viscosity of blood has to be specified as a function of vessel diameter, local hematocrit, and shear rate. Fourth, a relationship between RBC flow rates and bulk blood flow rates at diverging bifurcations has to be specified; this relationship is often referred to as the *bifurcation law*. Finally, at the inlet vessel branches boundary conditions have to be specified: bulk flow rate as well as RBC flow rate or hematocrit; alternatively, pressure can be specified at both inlet and outlet branches. This set of generally nonlinear equations can be solved to yield pressure at each bifurcation, blood flow rate through each segment, and discharge or microvessel hematocrit in each segment. These equations also predict vessel diameters if vessel compliance is taken into account. The calculated variables can then be compared with experimental data. Such a detailed comparison was reported for rat mesentery [Pries et al., 1990]. The authors found a good agreement between theoretical and experimental data when histograms of parameter distributions were compared, but poor agreement, particularly for vessel hematocrit, when comparison was done on a vessel-by-vessel basis. In these calculations, the expression for apparent viscosity was taken from in vitro experiments. The agreement was improved when the apparent viscosity was increased substantially from its in vitro values, particularly in the smallest vessels. Thus, a working hypothesis was put forward that in vivo apparent viscosity in small vessels is higher than the corresponding in vitro viscosity in glass tubes. In vivo measurements of blood viscosity as well as further theoretical work delineating in vivo and in vitro differences is necessary.

34.2 Mass Transport in the Microcirculation

Transport of Oxygen and Carbon Dioxide

One of the most important functions of the microcirculation is the delivery of O_2 to tissue and the removal of waste products, particularly of CO_2, from tissue. O_2 is required for aerobic intracellular respiration for the production of adenosine triphosphate (ATP). CO_2 is produced as a by-product of these biochemical reactions. Tissue metabolic rate can change drastically, e.g., in aerobic muscle in the transition from rest to exercise, which necessitates commensurate changes in blood flow and O_2 delivery. One of the major issues studied is how O_2 delivery is matched to O_2 demand under different physiological and pathological conditions. This question arises for short-term or long-term regulation of O_2 delivery in an individual organism, organ, or tissue, as well as in the evolutionary sense, in phylogeny. The hypothesis of symmorphosis, a fundamental balance between structure and function, has been formulated for the respiratory and cardiovascular systems and tested successfully in a number of animal species [Weibel et al., 1992].

In the smallest exchange vessels (capillaries and small arterioles and venules), O_2 molecules are released from hemoglobin inside RBCs, diffuse through the plasma, and cross the endothelium, the extravascular space, and parenchymal cells until they reach mitochondria, where they are utilized in the process of oxidative phosphorylation. The nonlinear relationship between hemoglobin saturation with O_2 and the local O_2 tension (PO_2) is described by the *oxyhemoglobin dissociation curve*

(ODC). The theory of O_2 transport from capillaries to tissue was conceptually formulated by August Krogh in 1918, and it has dominated the thinking of physiologists for seven decades. The model he formulated considered a cylindrical tissue volume supplied by a single central capillary; this element was considered the building block for the entire tissue. A constant metabolic rate was assumed, and PO_2 at the capillary-tissue interface was specified. The solution to the corresponding transport equation is the Krogh-Erlang equation describing the radial variation of O_2 tension in tissue. Over the years, the *Krogh tissue cylinder model* has been modified by many investigators to include transport processes in the capillary and PO_2-dependent consumption. However, in the past few years new conceptual models of O_2 transport have emerged. First, it was discovered experimentally and subsequently corroborated by theoretical analysis that capillaries are not the only source of oxygen and that arterioles (*precapillary O_2 transport*) and to a smaller extent venules (*postcapillary O_2 transport*) also participate in tissue oxygenation; in fact, a complex pattern of O_2 exchange may exist between arterioles, venules, and adjacent capillary networks [Ellsworth et al., 1994]. Second, theoretical analysis of intracapillary transport suggested that a significant part of the resistance to O_2 transport, on the order of 50%, is located within the capillary, primarily due to poor diffusive conductance of the plasma gaps between the erythrocytes. Third, the role of *myoglobin-facilitated O_2 diffusion* in red muscle fibers and cardiac myocytes has been revealed. Experimental evidence is consistent with these theoretical predictions [Honig & Gayeski, 1993]. Fourth, geometric and hemodynamic heterogeneities in O_2 delivery have been quantified experimentally, and attempts have been made to model them. Discussion of these and other theoretical issues of O_2 transport can be found in Popel [1989].

Transport of CO_2 is coupled to O_2 through the Bohr effect (effect of CO_2 tension on the blood O_2 content) and the Haldane effect (effect of PO_2 on the blood CO_2 content). Diffusion of CO_2 is faster than that of O_2 because CO_2 solubility in tissue is higher; theoretical studies predict that countercurrent exchange of CO_2 between arterioles and venules is of major importance so that equilibration of CO_2 tension with surrounding tissue should occur before capillaries are reached. Experiments are needed to test these theoretical predictions.

Transport of Solutes and Water

The movement of solute molecules across the capillary wall occurs primarily by two mechanisms: diffusion and solvent drag. *Diffusion* is the passive mechanism of transport which rapidly and efficiently transports small solutes over the small distances (tens of microns) between the blood supply (capillaries) and tissue cells. *Solvent drag* refers to the movement of solute that is entrained in the bulk flow of fluid across the capillary wall and is generally negligible, except in cases of large molecules with small diffusivities and high transcapillary fluid flow.

The capillary wall is composed of a single layer of endothelial cells about 1 μm thick. Lipid soluble substances (e.g., O_2) can diffuse across the entire wall surface, whereas water soluble substances (e.g., glucose) are restricted to small aqueous pathways equivalent to cylindrical pores about 4 nm in diameter. Total pore area is about 0.02% of the surface area of a capillary. The permeability of the capillary wall to a particular substance depends upon the relative size of the substance and the pore ("restricted" diffusion). The efficiency of diffusive exchange can be increased by increasing the number of perfused capillaries (e.g., heart and muscle tissue from rest to exercise), since this increases the surface area available for exchange and decreases the distances across which molecules must diffuse.

The actual pathways through which small solutes traverse the capillary wall appear to be in the form of clefts between adjacent endothelial cells. Rather than being open slits, these porous channels appear to contain a matrix of small cylindrical fibers (perhaps glycosaminoglycans) that occupy about 5% of the volume of these pathways. The permeability properties of the capillary endothelium are modulated by a number of factors, among which are plasma protein concentration and composition, rearrangement of the endothelial cell glycocalyx, calcium influx into the endothelial cell, and endothelial cell membrane potential. Many of the studies that have established our current understanding of the endothelial exchange barrier have been carried out on single perfused capillaries of the frog mesentery; some recent investigations have examined these transport issues in mammalian tissues [Curry, 1994]. There could be, in addition to the porous pathways, nonporous pathways that involve selective uptake of solutes and subsequent transcellular transport. In order to study such pathways, one must try to minimize the contributions to transcapillary transport from solvent drag.

The processes whereby water passes back and forth across the capillary wall are called filtration and absorption. The flow of water depends upon the relative magnitude of hydraulic and osmotic pressures across the capillary wall and is described quantitatively by the Kedem-Katchalsky equations (the particular form of the equations applied to capillary water transport is referred to as *Starling's law*). Overall, in the steady state there is an approximate balance between hydraulic and osmotic pressures which leads to a small net flow of water. Generally, more fluid is filtered than is reabsorbed; the overflow is carried back to the vascular system by the lymphatic circulation. The lymphatic network is composed of a large number of small vessels, the terminal branches of which are closed. Flap valves (similar to those in veins) ensure unidirectional flow of lymph back to the central circulation. The smallest (terminal) vessels are very permeable, even to proteins which occasionally leak from systemic capillaries. Lymph flow is determined by interstitial fluid pressure and the lymphatic "pump" (one-way flap valves and skeletal muscle contraction). Control of interstitial fluid protein concentration is one of the most important functions of the lymphatic system. If more net fluid is filtered than can be pumped out by the lymphatics, the volume of interstitial fluid increases. This fluid accumulation is called *edema*. This circumstance is important clinically, since solute exchange (e.g., O_2) decreases due to the increased diffusion distances produced when the accumulated fluid pushes the capillaries, tethered to the interstitial matrix, away from each other.

34.3 Regulation of Blood Flow

The cardiovascular system controls blood flow to individual organs (1) by maintaining arterial pressure within narrow limits and (2) by allowing each organ to adjust its vascular resistance to blood flow so that each receives an appropriate fraction of the cardiac output. There are three major mechanisms that control the function of the cardiovascular system: local, neural, and humoral. The sympathetic nervous system and circulating hormones both provide overall vasoregulation, and thus coarse flow control, to all vascular beds. The local mechanisms provide finer regional control within a tissue, usually in response to local changes in tissue activity or local trauma. The three mechanisms can work independently of each other, but there are also interactions among them.

The classical view of blood flow control involved the action of vasomotor influences on a set of vessels called the "resistance vessels," generally arterioles and small arteries smaller than about 100 μm diameter, that controlled flow to and within an organ. The notion of "precapillary sphincters" that control flow in individual capillaries has been abandoned in favor of the current idea that the terminal arterioles control the flow in small capillary networks that branch off of these arterioles. In recent years, it has become clear that the resistance to blood flow is distributed over a wider range of vessel branching orders with diameters up to 500 μm. There are at least two mechanisms to be discussed below that are available for coordinating the actions of local control processes over wider regions.

Neurohumoral Regulation of Blood Flow

The role of neural influences on the vasculature varies greatly from organ to organ. Although all organs receive sympathetic innervation, regulation of blood flow in the cerebral and coronary vascular beds occurs mostly through intrinsic local (metabolic) mechanisms. The circulations in skeletal muscle, skin, and some other organs, however, are significantly affected by the sympathetic nerves. In general, the level of sympathetic discharge sets the state of vascular smooth-muscle contraction (basal vascular tone) and hence vascular resistance in organs. This basal tone is modulated by circulating and local vasoactive influences [e.g., EDRF (endothelium-derived relaxing factor), endothelin, vasoactive substances released from parenchymal cells and myogenic tone].

Local Regulation of Blood Flow

In addition to neural and humoral mechanisms for regulating the function of the cardiovascular system, mechanisms intrinsic to the various tissues can operate independently of neurohumoral influences. The site of local regulation is the microcirculation. Common examples of local control processes are autoregulation of blood flow, reactive hyperemia, and active (or functional) hyperemia. The two major theories of local regulation are (1) the myogenic hypothesis, which states, in essence, that vascular smooth muscle actively contracts in response to stretch, and (2) the metabolic hypothesis which states that there is a link between blood flow and tissue metabolism [Duling, 1991].

Cells have a continuous need for O_2 and continuously produce metabolic wastes, some of which are vasoactive (usually vasodilators). Under normal conditions there is a balance between O_2 supply and demand, but imbalances give rise to adjustments in blood flow that bring supply back into register with demand. Consider exercising skeletal muscle as an example. With the onset of exercise, metabolite production and O_2 requirements increase. The metabolites diffuse away from their sites of production and reach the vasculature. Vasodilation ensues, lowering resistance to blood flow. The resulting increase in blood flow increases the O_2 supply, and finally a new steady state is achieved in which O_2 supply and demand are matched. This scenario operates for other tissues in which metabolic activity changes.

The following O_2-linked metabolites have been implicated as potential chemical mediators in the metabolic hypothesis: adenosine (from ATP hydrolysis: ATP $\rightarrow$ ADP $\rightarrow$ AMP $\rightarrow$ adenosine), H^+, and lactate (from lactic acid generated by glycolysis). Their levels are increased when there is a reduction in O_2 supply relative to demand (i.e., tissue hypoxia). The production of more CO_2 as a result of increased tissue activity (leading to increased oxidative metabolism) leads to vasodilation through increased H^+ concentration. Increased potassium ion and interstitial fluid osmolarity (i.e., more osmotically active particles) transiently cause vasodilation under physiological conditions associated with increased tissue activity.

Some Functions of the Endothelium

Endothelial cells form the lining of all blood vessels. They provide a smooth, nonthrombogenic surface with which the blood is in intimate contact. In addition to their passive permeability barrier function, endothelial cells produce a number of important vasoactive substances, among which are: prostacyclin, a potent vascular smooth-muscle relaxant and inhibitor of platelet aggregation; endothelin, a potent vasoconstrictor peptide; and EDRF, a substance (nitric oxide, NO) that mediates the vasodilatory effect of a number of vasodilators (e.g., acetylcholine).

It has been observed in arteries and arterioles that increases in blood flow lead to vasodilation (flow-dependent dilation) [Smieško & Johnson, 1993]. This phenomenon appears to be mediated by EDRF release from the endothelium in those vessels. The sequence of events is: (1) blood flow increases; (2) shear stress at the vessel wall increases (thereby increasing the viscous drag on the endothelial lining of the vessel); (3) EDRF is released in response to the mechanical stimulus; and (4) vascular smooth-muscle relaxation (vasodilation) occurs.

Coordination of Vasomotor Responses

Communication between the two active cell types in the blood vessel wall, smooth-muscle and endothelial cells, appears to play an important role in coordinating the responses among resistance elements in the vascular network [Duling, 1991; Segal, 1992]. There is chemical and electrical coupling between the cells of the vessel wall, and this signal can travel along a vessel in either direction with a length constant of about 2 mm. There are two immediate consequences of this communication. A localized vasodilatory stimulus of metabolic origin will be propagated to contiguous vessels, thereby lowering the resistance to blood flow in a larger region. In addition, this more generalized vasodilation should increase the homogeneity of blood flow in response to the localized metabolic event. The increase in blood flow experienced as a result of this vasodilation will cause flow also to increase at upstream sites. The increased shear stress on the endothelium as a result of the flow increase will lead to vasodilation of these larger upstream vessels. Thus, the neurohumoral and local responses are linked in a complex control system that matches regional perfusion to the local metabolic needs.

Acknowledgments

This work supported by National Heart, Lung, and Blood Institute grants HL 18292 and HL 17421. The authors thank Tuhin Roy for useful comments.

Defining Terms

Apparent viscosity: The viscosity of a newtonian fluid that would require the same pressure difference to produce the same blood flow rate through a circular vessel as the blood.

Fahraeus effect: Microvessel hematocrit is smaller than hematocrit in the feed or discharge reservoir.

Fahraeus-Lindqvist effect: Apparent viscosity of blood in a microvessel is smaller than the bulk viscosity measured with a rotational viscometer or a large-bore capillary viscometer.

Krogh tissue cylinder model: A cylindrical volume of tissue supplied by a central cylindrical capillary.

Myogenic response: Vasoconstriction in response to elevated transmural pressure.

Myoglobin-facilitated O_2 diffusion: An increase of O_2 diffusive flux as a result of myoglobin molecules acting as a carrier for O_2 molecules.

Oxyhemoglobin dissociation curve: The equilibrium relationship between hemoglobin saturation and O_2 tension.

Poiseuille's law: The relationship between volumetric flow rate and pressure difference for steady flow of a newtonian fluid in a long circular tube.

Precapillary O_2 transport: O_2 diffusion from arterioles to the surrounding tissue.

Starling's law: The relationship between water flux through the endothelium and the difference between the hydraulic and osmotic transmural pressures.

Vasomotion: Spontaneous rhythmic variation of microvessel diameter.

References

Bassingthwaighte JB, Liebovitch LS, West BJ. 1994. Fractal Physiology. New York, London, Oxford University Press.

Chien S. 1992. Blood cell deformability and interactions: From molecules to micromechanics and microcirculation. Microvasc Res 44:243.

Curry F-RE. 1994. Regulation of water and solute exchange in microvessel endothelium: Studies in single perfused capillaries. Microcirculation 1:11.

Davis MJ. 1993. Myogenic response gradient in an arteriolar network. Am J Physiol (Heart Circ Physiol) 264:H2168.

Desjardins C, Duling BR. 1990. Heparinase treatment suggests a role for the endothelial cell glycocalyx in regulation of capillary hematocrit. Am J Physiol (Heart Circ Physiol) 258:H647.

Duling BR. 1991. Control of striated muscle blood flow. In RG Crystal, JB West (eds), The Lung: Scientific Foundations, pp 1497–1505, New York, Raven Press.

Ellsworth ML, Ellis CG, Popel AS, et al. 1994. Role of microvessels in oxygen supply to tissue. News Physiol Sci 9:119.

Ellsworth ML, Pittman RN. 1986. Evaluation of photometric methods for quantifying convective mass transport in microvessels. Am J Physiol (Heart Circ Physiol) 251:H869.

Enden G, Popel AS. 1994. A numerical study of plasma skimming in small vascular bifurcations. J Biomech Eng 116:79.

Guilford WH, Gore RW. 1992. A novel remote-sensing isometric force transducer for micromechanics studies. Am J Physiol (Cell Physiol) 263:C700.

Honig CR, Gayeski TEJ. 1993. Resistance to O_2 diffusion in anemic red muscle: Roles of flux density and cell PO_2. Am J Physiol (Heart Circ Physiol) 265:H868.

Kiani MF, Pries AR, Hsu LL, et al. 1994. Fluctuations in microvascular blood flow parameters caused by hemodynamic mechanisms. Am J Physiol (Heart Circ Physiol) 266:H1822.

Ley K, Gaehtgens P. 1991. Endothelial, not hemodynamic, differences are responsible for preferential leukocyte rolling in rat mesenteric venules. Circ Res 69:1034.

Lipowsky HH. 1987. Mechanics of blood flow in the microcirculation. In R Skalak, S Chien (eds), Handbook of Bioengineering, pp 18.1–18.25, New York, McGraw-Hill.

Popel AS. 1987. Network models of peripheral circulation. In R Skalak, S Chien (eds), Handbook of Bioengineering, pp 20.1–20.24, New York, McGraw-Hill.

Popel AS. 1989 Theory of oxygen transport to tissue. Crit Rev Biomed Eng 17:257.

Pries AR, Secomb TW, Gaehtgens P, et al. 1990. Blood flow in microvascular networks: Experiments and simulation. Circ Res 67:826.

Schmid-Schönbein GW. 1993. The damaging potential of leukocyte activation in the microcirculation. Angiology 44:45.

Schmid-Schönbein GW, Skalak TC, Sutton DW. 1989. Bioengineering analysis of blood flow in resting skeletal muscle. In J.-S. Lee and T.C. Skalak (eds), Microvascular Mechanics, pp 65–99, New York, Springer-Verlag.

Secomb TW. 1992. Red blood cell mechanics and capillary blood rheology. Cell Biophys 18:231.

Segal SS. 1992. Communication among endothelial and smooth muscle cells coordinates blood flow control during exercise. News Physiol Sci 7:152.

Shoukas AA, Bohlen HG. 1990. Rat venular pressure-diameter relationships are regulated by sympathetic activity. Am J Physiol (Heart Circ Physiol) 259:H674.

Skalak R, Özkaya N, Skalak TC. 1989. Biofluid mechanics. Ann Rev Fluid Mech 21:167.

Smieško V, Johnson PC. 1993. The arterial lumen is controlled by flow-related shear stress. News Physiol Sci 8:34.

Tangelder GJ, Slaaf DW, Muitjens AMM, et al. 1986. Velocity profiles in blood platelets and red blood cells flowing in arterioles of the rabbit mesentery. Circ Res 59:505.

Ursino M, Fabbri G. 1992. Role of the myogenic mechanism in the genesis of microvascular oscillations (vasomotion): Analysis with a mathematical model. Microvasc Res 43:156.

Weibel ER, Taylor CR, Hoppeler H. 1992. Variations in function and design: Testing symmorphosis in the respiratory system. Respir Physiol 87:325.

Woldhuis B, Tangelder G-J, Slaaf DW, et al. 1992. Concentration profile of blood platelets differs in arterioles and venules. Am J Physiol (Heart Circ Physiol) 262:H1217.

35

Mechanics and Deformability of Hematocytes

Richard E. Waugh
Department of Biophysics,
University of Rochester School
of Medicine and Dentistry

Robert M. Hochmuth
Department of Mechanical
Engineering and Materials
Science, Duke University

The term *hematocytes* refers to the circulating cells of the blood. These are divided into two main classes: erythrocytes, or red cells, and leukocytes, or white cells. In addition to these are specialized cell-like structures called *platelets*. The mechanical properties of these cells are of special interest because of their physiological role as circulating corpuscles in the flowing blood. The importance of the mechanical properties of these cells and their influence on blood flow is evident in a number of hematological pathologies. The properties of the two main types of hematocytes are distinctly different. The essential character of a red cell is that of an elastic bag enclosing a newtonian fluid of comparatively low viscosity. The essential behavior of white cells is that of a highly viscous fluid drop with a more or less constant cortical (surface) tension. Under the action of a given force, red cells deform much more readily than white cells. In this chapter we focus on descriptions of the behavior of the two cell types separately, concentrating on the viscoelastic characteristics of the red cell membrane and the fluid characteristics of the white cell cytosol.

35.1 Fundamentals

Stresses and Strains in Two Dimensions

The description of the mechanical deformation of the membrane is cast in terms of principal *force resultants* and principal *extension ratios* of the surface. The force resultants, like conventional three-dimensional strain, are generally expressed in terms of a tensorial quantity, the components of which depend on coordinate rotation. For the purposes of describing the constitutive behavior of the surface, it is convenient to express the surface resultants in terms of rotationally invariant quantities. These can be either the principal force resultants N_1 and N_2, or the isotropic resultant $\overline{N}$ and the maximum shear resultant N_s. The surface strain is also a tensorial quantity but may be expressed in

0-8493-8346-3/95/$0.00+$.50
© 1995 by CRC Press, Inc.

terms of the principal extension ratios of the surface λ_1 and λ_2. The rate of surface shear deformation [Evans & Skalak, 1979] is given by

$$V_s = \left(\frac{\lambda_2}{\lambda_1}\right)^{1/2} \frac{d}{dt}\left(\frac{\lambda_1}{\lambda_2}\right)^{1/2} \tag{35.1}$$

The membrane deformation is calculated from observed macroscopic changes in cell geometry, usually with the use of simple geometric shapes to approximate the cell shape. The membrane force resultants are calculated from force balance relationships. For example, in the determination of the *area expansivity modulus* of the red cell membrane or the *cortical tension* in neutrophils, the force resultants in the plane of the membrane of the red cell or the white cell are isotropic. In this case, as long as the membrane surface of the cell does not stick to the pipette, the membrane force resultant can be calculated from the law of Laplace:

$$\Delta P = 2\overline{N}\left(\frac{1}{R_p} - \frac{1}{R_c}\right) \tag{35.2}$$

where R_p is the radius of the pipette, R_c is the radius of the spherical portion of the cell outside the pipette, $\overline{N}$ is the isotropic force resultant (tension) in the membrane, and ΔP is the aspiration pressure in the pipette.

Basic Equations for Newtonian Fluid Flow

The constitutive relations for fluid flow in a sphere undergoing axisymmetric deformation can be written:

$$\sigma_{rr} = -p + 2\eta\frac{\partial V_r}{\partial r} \tag{35.3}$$

$$\sigma_{r\theta} = \eta\left[\frac{1}{r}\frac{\partial V_r}{\partial \theta} + r\frac{\partial}{\partial r}\left(\frac{V_\theta}{r}\right)\right] \tag{35.4}$$

where σ_{rr} and $\sigma_{r\theta}$ are components of the stress tensor, p is the hydrostatic pressure, r is the radial coordinate, θ is the angular coordinate in the direction of the axis of symmetry in spherical coordinates, and V_r and V_θ are components of the fluid velocity vector. These equations effectively define the material viscosity, η. In general, η may be a function of the strain rate. The second term in Eq. (35.3) contains the radial strain rate $\dot{\varepsilon}_{rr}$ and the bracketed term in Eq. (35.4) corresponds to $\dot{\varepsilon}_{r\theta}$. For the purposes of evaluating this dependence, it is convenient to define the mean shear rate $\dot{\gamma}_m$ averaged over the cell volume and duration of the deformation process t_e:

$$\dot{\gamma}_m = \left(\frac{3}{4}\frac{1}{t_e}\int_0^{t_e}\int_0^{R(t)}\int_0^\pi \frac{r^2}{R^3}(\dot{\varepsilon}_{ij}\dot{\varepsilon}_{ij})\sin\theta\,d\theta\,dr\,dt\right)^{\frac{1}{2}} \tag{35.5}$$

where repeated indices indicate summation.

35.2 Red Cells

Size and Shape

The normal red cell is a biconcave disk at rest. The average human cell is approximately 7.7 μm in diameter and varies in thickness from ∼2.8 μm at the rim to ∼1.4 μm at the center [Fung et al.,

1981]. However, red cells vary considerably in size even within a single individual. The mean surface area is $\sim$130 μm^2 and the mean volume is 98 μm^3 (Table 35.1), but the range of sizes within a population is gausian-distributed with standard deviations of $\sim$15.8 μm^2 for the area and $\sim$16.1 μm^3 for the volume [Fung et al., 1981]. Cells from different species vary enormously in size, and tables for different species have been tabulated elsewhere [Hawkey et al., 1991].

Red cell deformation takes place under two important constraints: fixed surface area and fixed volume. The constraint of fixed volume arises from the impermeability of the membrane to cations. Even though the membrane is highly permeable to water, the inability of salts to cross the membrane prevents significant water loss because of the requirement for colloidal osmotic equilibrium [Lew & Bookchin, 1986]. The constraint of fixed surface area arises from the large resistance of bilayer membranes to changes in area per molecule [Needham & Nunn, 1990]. These two constraints place strict limits on the kinds of deformations that the cell can undergo and the size of the aperture that the cell can negotiate. Thus, a major determinant of red cell deformability is its ratio of surface area to volume. One measure of this parameter is the *sphericity,* defined as the dimensionless ratio of the two-thirds power of the cell volume to the cell area times a constant that makes its maximum value 1.0:

$$S = \frac{4\pi}{(4\pi/3)^{2/3}} \cdot \frac{V^{2/3}}{A}. \tag{35.6}$$

The mean value of sphericity of a normal population of cells was measured by interference microscopy to be 0.79 with a standard deviation (SD) of 0.05 at room temperature [Fung et al., 1981]. Similar values were obtained using micropipettes: mean = 0.81, SD = 0.02 [Waugh & Agre, 1988]. The membrane area increases with temperature, and the membrane volume decreases with temperature, so the sphericity at physiological temperature is expected to be somewhat smaller. Based on measurements of the thermal area expansivity of 0.12%/°C [Waugh & Evans, 1979] and a change in volume of -0.14%/°C [Waugh & Evans, 1979], the mean sphericity at 37 °C is estimated to be 0.76–0.78. (See Table 35.1.)

Red Cell Cytosol

The interior of a red cell is a concentrated solution of hemoglobin, the oxygen-carrying protein, and it behaves as a newtonian fluid [Cokelet & Meiselman, 1968]. In a normal population of cells there is a distribution of hemoglobin concentrations in the range 29 to 39 g/dl. The viscosity of the cytosol depends on the hemoglobin concentration as well as temperature. (See Table 35.2.) Based on theoretical models [Ross & Minton, 1977], the temperature dependence of the cytosolic viscosity is expected to be the same as that of water, that is, the ratio of cytosolic viscosity at 37°C to the viscosity at 20°C is the same as the ratio of water viscosity at those same temperatures. In most cases, even in the most dense cells, the resistance to flow of the cytosol is small compared with the viscoelastic resistance of the membrane when membrane deformations are appreciable.

TABLE 35.1 Parameter Values for a Typical Red Blood Cell (37°C)

Area	132 μm^2
Volume	96 μm^3
Sphericity	0.77
Membrane area modulus	480 mN/m
Membrane shear modulus	0.006 mN/m
Membrane viscosity	0.00036 mN $\cdot$ s/m
Membrane bending stiffness	0.2×10^{-18} J
Thermal area expansivity	0.12%/°C
$\frac{1}{V}\frac{dV}{dT}$	-0.14%/°C

Membrane Area Dilation

The large resistance of the membrane to area dilation has been characterized in micromechanical experiments. The changes in surface area that can be produced in the membrane are small, and so they can be characterized in terms of a simple hookean elastic relationship between the isotropic force resultant $\overline{N}$ and the fractional change in surface area $\alpha = A/A_o - 1$:

$$\overline{N} = K\alpha. \tag{35.7}$$

TABLE 35.2 Viscosity of Red Cell Cytosol (37°C)

Hemoglobin Concentration, g/l	Measured Viscosity,* mPa·s	Best Fit Viscosity[†], mPa·s
290	4.1–5.0	4.2
310	5.2–6.6	5.3
330	6.6–9.2	6.7
350	8.5–13.0	8.9
370	10.8–17.1	12.1
390	15.0–23.9	17.2

*Data taken from Cokelet and Meiselman [1968] and Chien and coworkers [1970].
[†]Fitted curve from Ross and Minton [1977].

The proportionality constant K is called the *area compressibility modulus* or the *area expansivity modulus*. Early estimates placed its value at room temperature at ~450 mN/m [Evans & Waugh, 1977] and showed a dependence of the modulus on temperature, its value changing from ~300 mN/m at 45°C to a value of ~600 mN/m at 5°C [Waugh & Evans, 1979]. Subsequently it was shown that the measurement of this parameter using micropipettes is affected by extraneous electric fields, and the value at room temperature was corrected upward to ~500 mN/m [Katnik & Waugh, 1990]. The values in Table 35.3 are based on this measurement, and the fractional change in the modulus with temperature is based on the original micropipette measurements [Waugh & Evans, 1979].

Membrane Shear Deformation

The shear deformations of the red cell surface can be large, and so a simple linear relationship between force and extension is not adequate for describing the membrane behavior. The large resistance of the membrane composite to area dilation led early investigators to postulate that the membrane maintained constant surface density during shear deformation, that is, that the surface was two-dimensionally incompressible. Most of what exists in the literature about the shear deformation of the red cell membrane is based on this assumption. Only very recently has experimental evidence emerged that this assumption is an oversimplification of the true cellular behavior, and that deformation produces changes in the local surface density of the membrane elastic network [Mohandas & Evans, 1994]. Nevertheless, the older simpler relationships provide a relatively simple description of the cell behavior that can be useful for many applications, and so the properties of the cell defined under that assumption are summarized here.

TABLE 35.3 Temperature Dependence of Viscoelastic Coefficients of the Red Cell Membrane

Temperature (°C)	K (mN/m)*	μ_m (mN/m)[†]	η_m (mN · s/m)[‡]
5	670	0.0078	0.0021
15	580	0.0072	0.0014
25	500	0.0065	0.00074
37	400	0.0058	0.00036
45	330	0.0053	—

*Based on a value of the modulus at 25°C of 500 mN/m and the fractional change in modulus with temperature measured by Waugh and Evans [1979].
[†]Based on linear regression to the data of Waugh and Evans [1979].
[‡]Data from Hochmuth and colleagues [1980].

For a simple, two-dimensional, incompressible, hyperelastic material, the relationship between the membrane shear force resultant N_s and the material deformation [Evans & Skalak, 1979] is

$$N_s = \frac{\mu_m}{2} \left(\frac{\lambda_1}{\lambda_2} - \frac{\lambda_2}{\lambda_1} \right) + 2\eta_m V_s \qquad (35.8)$$

where λ_1 and λ_2 are the principal extension ratios for the deformation and V_s is the rate of surface shear deformation [Eq. (35.1)]. The *membrane shear modulus* μ_m and the *membrane viscosity* η_m are defined by this relationship. Values for these coefficients at different temperatures are given in Table 35.3.

Stress Relaxation and Strain Hardening

Subsequent to these original formulations a number of refinements to these relationships have been proposed. Observations of persistent deformations after micropipette aspiration for extended periods of time formed the basis for the development of a model for long-term stress relaxation [Markle et al., 1983]. The characteristic times for these relaxations were on the order of 1–2 h, and these times were thought to correlate with permanent rearrangements of the membrane elastic network.

Another type of stress relaxation is thought to occur over very short times (~0.1 s) after rapid deformation of the membrane either by micropipette [Chien et al., 1978] or in cell extension experiments (Waugh & Bisgrove, unpublished observations). This phenomenon is thought to be due to transient entanglements within the deforming network. Whether the phenomenon actually occurs remains controversial. The stresses relax rapidly, and it is difficult to account for inertial effects of the measuring system and to reliably assess the intrinsic cellular response.

Finally, there has been some evidence that the coefficient for shear elasticity may be a function of the surface extension, increasing with increasing deformation. This was first proposed by Fischer in an effort to resolve discrepancies between theoretical predictions and observed behavior of red cells undergoing dynamic deformations in fluid shear [Fischer et al., 1981]. Increasing elastic resistance with extension has also been proposed as an explanation for discrepancies between theoretical predictions based on a constant modulus and measurements of the length of a cell projection into a micropipette [Waugh & Marchesi, 1990]. However, due to the approximate nature of the mechanical analysis of cell deformation in shear flow, and the limits of optical resolution in micropipette experiments, the evidence for a dependence of the modulus on extension is not clear-cut, and this issue remains unresolved.

New Constitutive Relations for the Red Cell Membrane

The most modern picture of membrane deformation recognizes that the membrane is a composite of two layers with distinct mechanical behavior. The membrane bilayer, composed of phospholipids and integral membrane proteins, exhibits a large elastic resistance to area dilation but is fluid in surface shear. The membrane skeleton, composed of a network of structural proteins at the cytoplasmic surface of the bilayer, is locally compressible and exhibits an elastic resistance to surface shear. The assumption that the membrane skeleton is locally incompressible is no longer applied. This assumption had been challenged over the years on the basis of theoretical considerations, but only very recently has experimental evidence emerged that shows definitively that the membrane skeleton is compressible. This has led to a new constitutive model for membrane behavior [Mohandas & Evans, 1994]. The principal stress resultants in the membrane skeleton are related to the membrane deformation by

$$N_1 = \mu_N \left(\frac{\lambda_1}{\lambda_2} - 1 \right) + K_N \left(\lambda_1 \lambda_2 - \frac{1}{(\lambda_1 \lambda_2)^n} \right) \qquad (35.9)$$

and

$$N_2 = \mu_N\left(\frac{\lambda_2}{\lambda_1} - 1\right) + K_N\left(\lambda_1\lambda_2 - \frac{1}{(\lambda_1\lambda_2)^n}\right) \tag{35.10}$$

where μ_N and K_N are the shear and isotropic moduli of the membrane skeleton respectively, and n is a parameter to account for molecular crowding of the skeleton in compression. The original modulus based on the two-dimensionally incompressible case is related to these moduli by

$$\mu_m \approx \frac{\mu_N K_N}{\mu_N + K_N}. \tag{35.11}$$

Values for the coefficients determined from fluorescence measurements of skeletal density distributions during micropipette aspiration studies are $\mu_N \approx 6 \times 10^{-3}$ mN/m, and $K_N/\mu_N \approx 2$. The value for n is estimated to be ≥ 2 [Mohandas & Evans, 1994].

These new concepts for membrane constitutive behavior have only recently been introduced and have yet to be thoroughly explored. The temperature dependence of these moduli is unknown, and the implications such a model will have on interpretation of dynamic deformations of the membrane remain to be resolved.

Bending Elasticity

Even though the membrane is very thin, it has a high resistance to surface dilation. This property, coupled with the finite thickness of the membrane, gives the membrane a small but finite resistance to bending. This resistance is characterized in terms of the *membrane-bending modulus*. The bending resistance of biological membranes is inherently complex because of their lamellar structure. There is a local resistance to bending due to the inherent stiffness of the individual leaflets of the membrane bilayer. (Because the membrane skeleton is compressible, it is thought to contribute little if anything to the membrane-bending stiffness.) In addition to this local stiffness, there is a *nonlocal bending resistance* due to the net compression and expansion of the adjacent leaflets resulting from the curvature change. The nonlocal contribution is complicated by the fact that the leaflets may be redistributed laterally within the membrane capsule to equalize the area per molecule within each leaflet. The situation is further complicated by the likely possibility that molecules may exchange between leaflets to alleviate curvature-induced dilation/compression. Thus, the bending stiffness measured by different approaches probably reflects contributions from both local and nonlocal mechanisms, and the measured values may differ because of different contributions from the two mechanisms. Estimates based on buckling instabilities during micropipette aspiration give a value of $\sim0.18 \times 10^{-18}$ J [Evans, 1983]. Measurements based on the mechanical formation of lipid tubes from the cell surface give a value of $\sim0.25 \times 10^{-18}$ J [Waugh & Bauserman, 1995].

35.3 White Cells

Whereas red cells account for approximately 40% of the blood volume, white cells occupy less than 1% of the blood volume. Yet because white cells are less deformable, they can have a significant influence on blood flow, especially in the microvasculature. Unlike red cells, which are very similar to each other, as are platelets, there are several different kinds of white cells or *leukocytes*. In general, the white cells are classified into groups according to their appearance when viewed with the light microscope. Thus, there are *granulocytes, monocytes,* and *lymphocytes* [Alberts et al., 1989]. The granulocytes with their many internal granules are separated into *neutrophils, basophils,* and *eosinophils* according to the way each cell stains. The neutrophil, also called a *polymorphonuclear leukocyte* because of its segmented or multilobed nucleus, is the most common white cell in the blood. (See Table 35.4.)

TABLE 35.4   Size and Appearance of White Cells in the Circulation

	Occurrence,* % of WBCs	Cell Volume,[†] μm^3	Cell Diameter,[†] μm	Nucleus,[‡] % Cell Volume	Cortical Tension, mN/m
Granulocytes					
Neutrophils	50–70	300–310	8.2–8.4	21	0.024–0.035[§]
Basophils	0–1				
Eosinophils	1–3			18	
Monocytes	1–5	400	9.1	26	0.06[¶]
Lymphocytes	20–40	220	7.5	44	0.035[¶]

*Diggs et al. [1985].
[†]Ting-Beall et al. [1993]. (Diameter calculated from the volume of a sphere.)
[‡]Schmid-Schönbein et al. [1980].
[§]Evans and Yeung [1989], Needham and Hochmuth [1992], Tsai et al. [1993, 1994].
[¶]Preliminary data, Hochmuth, Zhelev, and Ting-Beall.

The lymphocytes, which constitute 20–40% of the white cells and which are further subdivided into *B lymphocytes* and *killer* and *helper T lymphocytes,* are the smallest of the white cells. The other types of leukocytes are found with much less frequency. Most of the geometric and mechanical studies of white cells reported below have focused on the neutrophil because it is the most common cell in the circulation, although the lymphocyte in now starting to receive more attention.

Size and Shape

White cells at rest are spherical. The surfaces of white cells contain many folds, projections, and "microvilli" to provide the cells with sufficient membrane area to deform as they enter capillaries with diameters much smaller than the resting diameter of the cell. (Without the reservoir of membrane area in these folds, the constraints of constant volume and membrane area would make a spherical cell essentially undeformable.) The excess surface area of the neutrophil, when measured in a wet preparation, is slightly more than twice the apparent surface area of a smooth sphere with the same diameter [Evans & Yeung, 1989; Ting-Beall et al., 1993]. It is interesting to note that each type of white cell has its own unique surface topography, which allows one to readily determine if a cell is, for example, either a neutrophil or monocyte or lymphocyte [Hochmuth et al., 1995].

The cell volumes listed in Table 35.4 were obtained with the light microscope, either by measuring the diameter of the spherical cell or by aspirating the cell into a small glass pipette with a known diameter and then measuring the resulting length of the cylindrically shaped cell. Other values for cell volume obtained using transmission electron microscopy are somewhat smaller, probably because of cell shrinkage due to fixation and drying prior to measurement [Schmid-Schönbein et al., 1980; Ting-Beall et al., 1995]. Although the absolute magnitude of the cell volume measured with the electron microscope may be erroneous, if it is assumed that all parts of the cell dehydrate equally when they are dried in preparation for viewing, then this approach can be used to determine the volume occupied by the nucleus (Table 35.4) and other organelles of various white cells. The volume occupied by the granules in the neutrophil and eosinophil (recall that both are granulocytes) is 15 and 23%, respectively, whereas the granular volume in monocytes and lymphocytes is less than a few percent.

Mechanical Behavior

The early observations of Bagge and colleagues [1977] led them to suggest that the neutrophil behaves as a simple viscoelastic solid with a Maxwell element (an elastic and viscous element in series) in parallel with an elastic element. This elastic element in the model was thought to pull the unstressed cell into its spherical shape. Subsequently, Evans and Kukan [1984] and Evans and Yeung [1989] showed that the cells flow continuously into a pipette, with no apparent approach to a static limit, when a constant suction pressure was applied. Thus, the cytoplasm of the neutrophil should be treated as a liquid rather than a solid, and its surface has a persistent *cortical tension* that causes the cell to assume a spherical shape.

Cortical Tension

Using a micropipet and a small suction pressure to aspirate a hemispherical projection from a cell body into the pipette, Evans and Yeung measured a value for the cortical tension of 0.035 mN/m. Needham and Hochmuth [1992] measured the cortical tension of individual cells that were driven down a tapered pipette in a series of equilibrium positions. In many cases the cortical tension increased as the cell moved further into the pipette, which means that the cell has an apparent area expansion modulus [Eq. (35.7)]. They obtained an average value of 0.04 mN/m for the expansion modulus and an extrapolated value for the cortical tension (at zero area dilation) in the resting state of 0.024 mN/m. The importance of the actin cytoskeleton in maintaining cortical tension was demonstrated by Tsai et al. [1994]. Treatment of the cells with a drug that disrupts actin filament structure (CTB = cytochalasin B) resulted in a decrease in cortical tension from 0.027 mN/m to 0.022 mN/m at a CTB concentration of 3 μM and to 0.014 mN/m at 30 μM.

Preliminary measurements in one of the authors' laboratories indicate that the value for the cortical tension of a monocyte is about double that for a granulocyte, that is, 0.06 mN/m, and the value for a lymphocyte is about 0.035 mN/m.

Bending Rigidity

The existence of a cortical tension suggests that there is a cortex—a relatively thick layer of F-actin filaments and myosin—that is capable of exerting a finite tension at the surface. If such a layer exists, it would have a finite thickness and bending rigidity. Zhelev and colleagues [1994] aspirated the surface of neutrophils into pipettes with increasingly smaller diameters and determined that the surface had a bending modulus of about 1 to 2 $\times$ 10^{-18} J, which is 5 to 50 times the bending moduli for erythrocyte or lipid bilayer membranes. The thickness of the cortex should be smaller than the radius of smallest pipette used in this study, which was 0.24 μm.

Apparent Viscosity

Using their model of the neutrophil as a newtonian liquid drop with a constant cortical tension and (as they showed) a negligible surface viscosity, Yeung and Evans [1989] analyzed the flow of neutrophils into a micropipette and obtained a value for the *cytoplasmic viscosity* of about 200 Pa·s. In their experiments, the aspiration pressures were on the order of 10 to 1000 Pa. Similar experiments by Needham and Hochmuth [1990] using the same newtonian model (with a negligible surface viscosity) but using higher aspiration pressures (ranging from 500 to 2000 Pa) gave an average value for the cytoplasmic viscosity of 135 Pa·s for 151 cells from five individuals. The apparent discrepancy between these two sets of experiments was resolved to a large extent by Tsai et al. [1993], who demonstrated that the neutrophil viscosity decreases with increasing rate of deformation. They proposed a model of the cytosol as a *power law fluid*:

$$\eta = \eta_c \left(\frac{\dot{\gamma}_m}{\dot{\gamma}_c} \right)^{-b} \tag{35.12}$$

where $b = 0.52$, $\dot{\gamma}_m$ is defined by Eq. (35.5), and η_c is a characteristic viscosity of 130 Pa·s when the characteristic mean shear rate, $\dot{\gamma}_c$, is 1 s^{-1}. These values are based on an approximate method for calculating the viscosity from measurements of the total time it takes for a cell to enter a micropipette. Because of different approximations used in the calculations, the values of viscosity reported by Tsai et al. [1993] tend to be somewhat smaller than those reported by Evans and coworkers or Hochmuth and coworkers. Nevertheless, the shear rate dependence of the viscosity is the same, regardless of the method of calculation. Values for the viscosity are given in Table 35.5.

In addition to the dependence of the viscosity on shear rate, there is also evidence that it depends on the extent of deformation. In micropipette experiments the initial rate at which the cell enters the pipette is significantly faster than predicted, even when the shear rate dependence of the viscosity is taken into account. In a separate approach, the cytosolic viscosity was estimated from observation of the time course of the cell's return to a spherical geometry after expulsion from a micropipette. When the cellular deformations were large, a viscosity of 150 Pa·s was estimated [Tran-Son-Tay et al., 1991], but when the deformation was small, the estimated viscosity was only 60 Pa·s [Hochmuth et al., 1993]. Thus, it appears that the viscosity is smaller when the magnitude of the deformation is small and increases as deformations become large.

An alternative attempt to account for the initial rapid entry of the cell into micropipettes involved the application of a *Maxwell fluid* model with a constant cortical tension. Dong and coworkers [1988] used this model to analyze both the shape recovery of neutrophils following small, complete deformations in pipettes and the small-deformation aspiration of neutrophils into pipettes. However, in another study by Dong and coworkers [1991], they used a finite-element, numerical approach and a Maxwell model with constant cortical tension to describe the continuous, finite-deformation flow of a neutrophil into a pipette. But in order to fit the theory to the data for the increase in length of the cell in the pipette with time, Dong and colleagues [1991] had to steadily increase both the elastic and viscous coefficients in their finite-deformation Maxwell model. This shows that even a Maxwell model is not adequate for describing the rheological properties of the neutrophil.

Although it is clear that the essential behavior of the cell is fluid, the simple fluid drop model with a constant and uniform viscosity does not match the observed time course of cell deformation in detail. Better agreement between theory and experiment is obtained if approximate account is taken for the shear rate dependence of the viscosity, but some discrepancies remain. A quantitative model that accounts for the dependence of viscosity on the magnitude of deformation has not yet been formulated, and a complete analysis in which the viscosity is made to vary in space and time according to the local shear rate and extent of deformation has not yet been performed. Nevertheless, the fluid drop model captures the essential behavior of the cell, and when it is applied consistently (that is, for similar rate and extent of deformation) it provides a sound basis for predicting cell behavior and comparing the behaviors of different types of cells.

Although the mechanical properties of the neutrophil have been studied extensively as discussed above, the other white cells have not been studied in depth. Preliminary unpublished results from Robert Hochmuth's laboratory indicate that monocytes are somewhat more viscous (from roughly 30% to a factor of 2) than neutrophils under similar conditions in both recovery experiments and experiments in which the monocyte flows into a pipette. A lymphocyte, when aspirated into a small pipette so that its relatively large nucleus is deformed, behaves as an elastic body in that the projec-

TABLE 35.5   Viscous Parameters of White Blood Cells

Cell Type	Range of Viscosities (Pa·s)*		Characteristic Viscosity (Pa·s)	Shear Rate Dependence (b)
	Min	Max		
Neutrophil	50	500	130†	0.52†
(30 M CTB)	41	52	54†	0.26†
Monocyte	70	1000		
HL60 (G1)			220‡	0.53‡
HL60 (S)			330‡	0.56‡

*Evans and Yeung [1989], Needham and Hochmuth [1992], Tsai et al. [1993, 1994].
†Tsai et al. [1993, 1994].
‡Tsai and Waugh (submitted).

tion length into the pipette increases linearly with the suction pressure. This elastic behavior appears to be due to the deformation of the nucleus, which has an apparent area elastic modulus of 2 mN/m. A lymphocyte recovers its shape somewhat more quickly than the neutrophil does, although this recovery process is driven both by the cortical tension and the elastic nucleus. These preliminary results are discussed by Tran-Son-Tay and coworkers [1994]. Finally, the properties of a human myeloid leukemic cell line (HL60) thought to resemble immature neutrophils of the bone marrow have also been characterized, as shown in Table 35.5. The apparent cytoplasmic viscosity varies both as a function of the cell cycle and during maturation toward a more neutrophillike cell. The characteristic viscosity ($\dot{\gamma}_c = 1\mathrm{s}^{-1}$) is 220 Pa·s for HL60 cells in the G1 stage of the cell cycle. This value increases to 400 Pa·s for cells in the S phase, but decreases with maturation, so that 7 days after induction the properties approach those of neutrophils (130 Pa·s) [Tsai & Waugh, manuscript in preparation].

It is important to note in closing that the characteristics described above apply to passive leukocytes. It is the nature of these cells to respond to environmental stimulation and engage in active movements and shape transformations. *White cell activation* produces significant heterogeneous changes in cell properties. The cell projections that form as a result of stimulation (called *pseudopodia*) are extremely rigid, whereas other regions of the cell may retain the characteristics of a passive cell. In addition, the cell may produce large protrusive or contractile forces. The changes in cellular mechanical properties that result from cellular activation are complex and only beginning to be formulated in terms of mechanical models. This is expected to be a major focus of research in the coming years.

Summary

Constitutive equations that capture the essential features of the responses of red blood cells and passive leukocytes have been formulated, and material parameters characterizing the cellular behavior have been measured. The red cell response is dominated by the cell membrane which can be described as a hyper-viscoelastic, two-dimensional continuum. The passive white cell behaves like a highly viscous fluid drop, and its response to external forces is dominated by the large viscosity of the cytosol. Refinements of these constitutive models and extension of mechanical analysis to activated white cells is anticipated as the ultrastructural events that occur during cellular deformation are delineated in increasing detail.

Defining Terms

Area expansivity modulus: A measure of the resistance of a membrane to area dilation. It is the proportionality between the isotropic force resultant in the membrane and the corresponding fractional change in membrane area. (Units: 1 mN/m = 1 dyn/cm)

Cortical tension: Analogous to surface tension of a liquid drop, it is a persistent contractile force per unit length at the surface of a white blood cell. (Units: 1 mN/m = 1 dyn/cm)

Cytoplasmic viscosity: A measure of the resistance of the cytosol to flow. (Units: 1 Pa·s = 10 poise)

Force resultant: The stress in a membrane integrated over the membrane thickness. It is the two-dimensional analog of stress with units of force/length. (Units: 1 mN/m = 1 dyn/cm)

Maxwell fluid: A constitutive model in which the response of the material to applied stress includes both an elastic and viscous response in series. In response to a constant applied force, the material will respond elastically at first, then flow. At fixed deformation, the stresses in the material will relax to zero.

Membrane-bending modulus: The intrinsic resistance of the membrane to changes in curvature. It is usually construed to exclude nonlocal contributions. It relates the moment resultants (force times length per unit length) in the membrane to the corresponding change in curvature (inverse length). (Units: 1 N·m = 1 joule = 10^7 erg)

Membrane shear modulus: A measure of the elastic resistance of the membrane to surface shear deformation; that is, changes in the shape of the surface at constant surface area [Eq. (35.8)]. (Units: 1 mN/ · m = 1 dyn/cm)

Membrane viscosity: A measure of the resistance of the membrane to surface shear flow, that is, to the rate of surface shear deformation [Eq. (35.8)]. (Units: 1 mN·s/m = 1 m$^{Pa·s}$ m = 1 dyn. s/cm = 1 surface poise)

Nonlocal bending resistance: A resistance to bending resulting from the differential expansion and compression of the two adjacent leaflets of a lipid bilayer. It is termed *nonlocal* because the leaflets can move laterally relative to one another to relieve local strains, such that the net resistance to bending depends on the integral of the change in curvature of the entire membrane capsule.

Power law fluid: A model to describe the dependence of the cytoplasmic viscosity on rate of deformation [Eq. (35.12)].

Principal extension ratios: The ratios of the deformed length and width of a rectangular material element (in principal coordinates) to the undeformed length and width.

Sphericity: A dimensionless ratio of the cell volume (to the 2/3 power) to the cell area. Its value ranges from near zero to one, the maximum value corresponding to a perfect sphere [Eq. (35.6)].

White cell activation: The response of a leukocyte to external stimuli that involves reorganization and polymerization of the cellular structures and is typically accompanied by changes in cell shape and cell movement.

References

Alberts B, Bray D, Lewis J, et al. 1989. Molecular Biology of the Cell, 2d ed. New York and London, Garland Publishing.

Bagge U, Skalak R, Attefors R. 1977. Granulocyte rheology. Adv Microcirc 7:29.

Chien S, Sung KLP, Skalak R, et al. 1978. Theoretical and experimental studies on viscoelastic properties of erythrocyte membrane. Biophys J 24:463.

Chien S, Usami S, Bertles JF. 1970. Abnormal rheology of oxygenated blood in sickle cell anemia. J Clin Invest 49:623.

Cokelet GR, Meiselman HJ. 1968. Rheological comparison of hemoglobin solutions and erythrocyte suspensions. Science 162:275.

Diggs LW, Sturm D, Bell A. 1985. The Morphology of Human Blood Cells, 5th ed. Abbott Park, Ill., Abbott Laboratories.

Dong C, Skalak R, Sung K-LP. 1991. Cytoplasmic rheology of passive neutrophils. Biorheology 28:557.

Dong C, Skalak R, Sung K-LP, et al. 1988. Passive deformation analysis of human leukocytes. J Biomech Eng 110:27.

Evans EA. 1983. Bending elastic modulus of red blood cell membrane derived from buckling instability in micropipet aspiration tests. Biophys J 43:27.

Evans E, Kukan B. 1984. Passive material behavior of granulocytes based on large deformation and recovery after deformation tests. Blood 64:1028.

Evans EA, Skalak R. 1979. Mechanics and thermodynamics of biomembrane. Crit Rev Bioeng 3:181.

Evans EA, Waugh R. 1977. Osmotic correction to elastic area compressibility measurements on red cell membrane. Biophys J 20:307.

Evans E, Yeung A. 1989. Apparent viscosity and cortical tension of blood granulocytes determined by micropipet aspiration. Biophys J 56:151.

Fischer TM, Haest CWM, Stohr-Liesen M, et al. 1981. The stress-free shape of the red blood cell membrane. Biophys J 34:409.

Fung YC, Tsang WCO, Patitucci P. 1981. High-resolution data on the geometry of red blood cells. Biorheology 18:369.

Hawkey CM, Bennett PM, Gascoyne SC, et al. 1991. Erythrocyte size, number and haemoglobin content in vertebrates. Brit J Haematol 77:392.

Hochmuth RM, Buxbaum KL, Evans EA. 1980. Temperature dependence of the viscoelastic recovery of red cell membrane. Biophys J 29:177.

Hochmuth RM, Ting-Beall HP, Beaty BB, et al. 1993. Viscosity of passive human neutrophils undergoing small deformations. Biophys J 64:1596.

Hochmuth RM, Ting-Beall HP, Zhelev DV. 1995. The mechanical properties of individual passive neutrophils in vitro. In DN Granger, GW Schmid-Schönbein (eds), Physiology and Pathophysiology of Leukocyte Adhesion, London, Oxford University Press, 83–96.

Katnik C, Waugh R. 1990. Alterations of the apparent area expansivity modulus of red blood cell membrane by electric fields. Biophys J 57:877.

Lew VL, Bookchin RM. 1986. Volume, pH and ion content regulation human red cells: Analysis of transient behavior with an integrated model. J Membr Biol 10:311.

Markle DR, Evans EA, Hochmuth RM. 1983. Force relaxation and permanent deformation of erythrocyte membrane. Biophys J 42:91.

Mohandas N, Evans E. 1994. Mechanical properties of the red cell membrane in relation to molecular structure and genetic defects. Annu Rev Biophys Biomol Struct 23:787.

Needham D, Hochmuth RM. 1990. Rapid flow of passive neutrophils into a 4 μm pipet and measurement of cytoplasmic viscosity. J Biomech Eng 112:269.

Needham D, Hochmuth RM. 1992. A sensitive measure of surface stress in the resting neutrophil. Biophys J 61:1664.

Needham D, Nunn RS. 1990. Elastic deformation and failure of lipid bilayer membranes containing cholesterol. Biophys J 58:997.

Ross PD, Minton AP. 1977. Hard quasispherical model for the viscosity of hemoglobin solutions. Biochem Biophys Res Commun 76:971.

Schmid-Schönbein GW, Shih YY, Chien S. 1980. Morphometry of human leukocytes. Blood 56(5):866.

Ting-Beall HP, Needham D, Hochmuth RM. 1993. Volume and osmotic properties of human neutrophils. Blood 81(10):2774.

Ting-Beall HP, Zhelev DV, Hochmuth RM. 1995. A comparison of different drying procedures for scanning electron microscopy using human leukocytes. Microscopy Res and Technique.

Ting-Beall HP, Zhelev DV, Needham D, et al. 1994b. The volume of white cells. Blood. To be submitted.

Tran-Son-Tay R, Kirk TF III, Zhelev DV, et al. 1994. Numerical simulation of the flow of highly viscous drops down a tapered tube. J Biomech Eng. 116:172.

Tran-Son-Tay R, Needham D, Yeung A, et al. 1991. Time-dependent recovery of passive neutrophils after large deformation. Biophys J 60:856.

Tsai MA, Frank RS, Waugh RE. 1993. Passive mechanical behavior of human neutrophils: Power-law fluid. Biophys J 65:2078.

Tsai MA, Frank RS, Waugh RE. 1994. Passive mechanical behavior of human neutrophils: Effect of Cytochalasin B. Biophys J. 66:2166.

Waugh RE, Agre P. 1988. Reductions of erythrocyte membrane viscoelastic coefficients reflect spectrin deficiencies in hereditary spherocytosis. J Clin Invest 81:133.

Waugh RE, Bauserman RG. 1995. Physical measurements of bilayer-skeletal separation forces. Annals Biomed Eng. In press.

Waugh R, Evans EA. 1979. Thermoelasticity of red blood cell membrane. Biophys J 26:115.

Waugh RE, Marchesi SL. 1990. Consequences of structural abnormalities on the mechanical properties of red blood cell membrane. In C. M. Cohen and J. Palek (eds), Cellular and Molecular Biology of Normal and Abnormal Erythrocyte Membranes, pp 185–199, New York, Alan R. Liss.

Yeung A, Evans E. 1989. Cortical shell-liquid core model for passive flow of liquid-like spherical cells into micropipets. Biophys J 56:139.

Zhelev DV, Needham D, Hochmuth RM. 1994. Role of the membrane cortex in neutrophil deformation in small pipets. Biophys J 67:696.

Further Information

Basic information on the mechanical analysis of biomembrane deformation can be found in Evans and Skalak [1979], which also appeared as a book under the same title (CRC Press, Boca Raton, Fla., 1980). A more recent work that focuses more closely on the structural basis of the membrane properties is Berk and colleagues, Chapter 15, pp. 423–454, in the book *Red Blood Cell Membranes: Structure, Function, Clinical Implications* edited by Peter Agre and John Parker (Marcel Dekker, New York, 1989). More detail about the membrane structure can be found in other chapters of that book.

Basic information about white blood cell biology can be found in the book by Alberts and coworkers [1989]. A more thorough review of white blood cell structure and response to stimulus can be found in two reviews by T. P. Stossel, one entitled, "The mechanical response of white blood cells," in the book *Inflammation: Basic Principles and Clinical Correlates*, edited by J. I. Galin and colleagues (Raven Press, New York, 1988), pp. 325–342, and the second entitled, "The molecular basis of white blood cell motility," in the book *The Molecular Basis of Blood Diseases*, edited by G. Stamatoyannopoulos and colleagues (W. B. Saunders, Philadelphia, 1994), pp. 541–562. The most recent advances in white cell rheology can be found in the book, *Cell Mechanics and Cellular Engineering*, edited by Van C. Mow and coworkers (Springer Verlag, New York, 1994).

36

The Venous System

Artin A. Shoukas
Johns Hopkins University

Carl F. Rothe
Indiana University

The venous system not only serves as a conduit for the return of blood from the capillaries to the heart but also provides a dynamic, variable blood storage compartment that influences cardiac output. The systemic (noncardiopulmonary) venous system contains more than 75% of the blood volume of the entire systemic circulation. Although the heart is the source of energy for propelling blood throughout the circulation, filling of the right heart before the subsequent beat is primarily passive. The subsequent amount of blood ejected is exquisitely sensitive to the transmural filling pressure. (For example, a change of right heart filling pressure of 1 cm water can cause the cardiac output to change by about 50%.)

Because the blood vessels are elastic and have smooth muscle in their walls, contraction or relaxation of the smooth muscle can quickly redistribute blood between the periphery and the heart to influence cardiac filling and thus cardiac output. Even though the right ventricle is not essential for life, its functioning acts to reduce the central venous pressure to facilitate venous return [1]. It largely determines the magnitude of the cardiac output by influencing the degree of filling of the left heart. Dynamic changes in venous tone, by redistributing blood volume, can thus, at rest, change cardiac output over a range of more than ±20%. The dimensions of the vasculature influence both blood flow—by way of their resistive properties—and contained blood volume—by way of their capacitive properties. The arteries have about 10 times the resistance of the veins, and the veins are more than 10 times as compliant as the arteries.

The conduit characteristics of the venous system primarily depend on the anatomy of the system. Valves in the veins of the limbs are crucial for reducing the pressure in dependent parts of the body. Even small movements from skeletal muscle activity tend to compress the veins and move blood toward the heart. A competent valve then blocks back flow, thus relieving the pressure when the movement stops. Even a few steps can reduce the transmural venous pressure in the ankle from as much as 100 mmHg to about 20 mmHg. Without this mechanism, transcapillary movement of fluid into the extravascular spaces results in edema. Varicose (swollen) veins and peripheral pooling of blood can result from damage to the venous valves. During exercise, the rhythmic contraction of the skeletal muscles, in conjunction with venous valves, provides an important mechanism—the skeletal muscle pump—aiding the large increases in blood flow through the muscles without excessive increases in capillary pressure and blood pooling in the veins of the muscles. Without this mechanism, the increase in venous return leading to the dramatic increases in cardiac output would be greatly limited.

36.1 Definitions

Capacitance

Capacitance is a general term that relates the magnitude of contained volume to the transmural pressure across the vessel walls and is defined by the pressure-volume relationship. In living blood vessels, the pressure-volume relationship is complex and nonlinear. At transmural pressures near zero, there is a finite volume within the vessels (see definition of *unstressed volume*). If this volume is then removed from the vessels, there is only a small decrease in transmural pressure as the vessel collapses from a circular cross-section to an elliptical one. This is especially true for superficial or isolated venous vessels. However, for vessels which are tethered or embedded in tissue a negative pressure may result without appreciably changing the shape of the vessels. With increases in contained volume, the vessel becomes distended, and there is a concomitant increase in transmural pressure. The incremental change in volume to incremental change in transmural pressure is often relatively constant. At very high transmural pressures vessels become stiffer, and the incremental volume change to transmural pressure change is small. Because all blood vessels exhibit these nonlinearities, no single parameter can describe capacitance; instead the entire pressure-volume relationship must be considered.

Compliance

Vascular compliance (C) is defined as the slope of the pressure-volume relationship. It is the ratio of the change in incremental volume (ΔV) to a change in incremental transmural pressure (ΔP). Thus $C = \Delta V/\Delta P$. Because the pressure-volume relationship is nonlinear, the slope of the relationship is not constant over its full range of pressures, and so the compliance should be specified at a given pressure. Units of compliance are those of volume divided by pressure, usually reported in ml/mmHg. Values are typically normalized to wet tissue weight or to total body weight. When the compliance is normalized by the total contained blood volume, it is termed the *vascular distensibility* and represents the fractional change in volume ($\Delta V/V$) per change in transmural pressure; $D = (\Delta V/V)/\Delta P$, where V is the volume at control or at zero transmural pressure.

Unstressed Volume

Unstressed volume (V_0) is the volume in the vascular system when the transmural pressure is zero. It is a calculated volume obtained by extrapolating the relatively linear segment of the pressure-volume relationship over the normal operating range to zero transmural pressure. Many studies have shown that reflexes and drugs have quantitatively more influence on V_0 than on the compliance.

Stressed Volume

The *stressed volume* (V_s) is the volume of blood in the vascular system that must be removed to change the computed transmural pressure from its prevailing value to zero transmural pressure. It is computed as the product of the vascular compliance and transmural distending pressure: $V_s = C \times P$. The total contained blood volume at a specific pressure (P) is the sum of stressed and unstressed volume. The unstressed volume is then computed as the total blood volume minus the stressed volume. Because of the marked nonlinearity around zero transmural pressure and the required extrapolation, both V_0 and V_s are virtual volumes.

Capacity

Capacity refers to the amount of blood volume contained in the blood vessel at a specific distending pressure. It is the sum of the unstressed volume and the stressed volume, $V = V_0 + V_s$.

Mean Filling Pressure

If the inflow and outflow of an organ are suddenly stopped, and blood volume is redistributed so that all pressures within the vasculature are the same, this pressure is the *mean filling pressure* [5]. This pressure can be measured for the systemic or pulmonary circuits or the body as a whole. The arterial pressure often does not equal the venous pressure as flow is reduced to zero, because blood must move from the distended arterial vessels to the venous beds during the measurement maneuver, and flow may stop before equilibrium occurs. This is because smooth-muscle activity in the arterial vessels, rheological properties of blood, or high interstitial pressures act to impede the flow. Thus corrections must often be made [4,5]. The experimentally measured mean filling pressure provides a good estimate of P_v, (the pressure in the minute venules), for estimating venous stressed volume.

Venous Resistance

Venous Resistance (R) refers to the hindrance to blood flow through the venous vasculature caused by friction of the moving blood along the venous vascular wall. By definition it is the ratio of the pressure gradient between the entrance of the venous circulation, namely the capillaries, and the venous outflow divided by the venous flow rate. Thus

$$R = \frac{(P_c - P_{ra})}{F} \qquad (36.1)$$

where R is the venous resistance, P_c is the capillary pressure, P_{ra} is the right atrial pressure, and F is the venous flow. As flow is decreased to zero, arterial closure may occur, leading to a positive perfusion pressure at zero flow. With partial collapse of veins, a Starling resistorlike condition is present in which an increase in outlet pressure has no influence on flow until the outlet pressure is greater than the "waterfall" pressure.

Venous Inertance

Venous inertance (I_v) is the opposition to a change in flow rate related to the mass of the bolus of blood that is accelerated or decelerated. The inertance I_v for a cylindrical tube with constant cross-sectional area is $I_v = L\rho/A$, where L is the length of the vessel, ρ is the density of the blood, and A is the cross-sectional area [9].

36.2 Methods to Measure Venous Characteristics

Our knowledge of the nature and role of the capacitance characteristics of the venous system has been limited by the difficulty of measuring the various variables needed to compute parameter values. State-of-the-art equipment is often needed because of the low pressures and many disturbing factors present. Many of the techniques that have been used to measure venous capacitance require numerous assumptions that may not be correct or are currently impossible to evaluate [4].

Resistance

For the estimate of vascular resistance, the upstream to outflow pressure gradient across the tissues must be estimated along with a measure of flow. Pressures in large vessels are measured with a catheter connected to a pressure transducer, which typically involves measurement of minute changes in resistance elements attached to a stiff diaphragm which flexes proportionally to the pressure. For the veins in tissue, the upstream pressure, just downstream from the capillaries, is much more difficult to measure because of the minute size (ca 15 μm) of the vessels. For this a servo-null micropipette technique may be used. A glass micropipette with a tip diameter of about 2 μm is filled with a 1–2 mol saline solution. When the pipette is inserted into a vein, the pressure tends to drive the lower conductance blood plasma into the pipette. The conductance is measured using an AC-driven bridge. A servosystem, driven by the imbalance signal, is used to develop a counter pressure to maintain the interface between the low-conductance filling solution and the plasma near the tip of the pipette. This counter pressure, which equals the intravascular pressure, is measured with a pressure transducer. Careful calibration is essential.

Another approach for estimating the upstream pressure in the veins is to measure the mean filling pressure of the organ (see above) and assume that this pressure is the upstream venous pressure. Because this venous pressure must be less than the capillary pressure and because most of the blood in an organ is in the small veins and venules, this assumption, though tenuous, is not unreasonable. To measure flow many approaches are available including electromagnetic, transit-time ultrasonic, or Doppler ultrasonic flowmeters. Usually the arterial inflow is measured with the assumption that the outflow is the same. Indicator dilution techniques are also used to estimate average flow. They are based on the principle that the reduction in concentration of infused indicator is inversely proportional to the rate of flow. Either a bolus injection or a continuous infusion may be used. Adequacy of mixing of indicator across the flow stream, lack of collateral flows, and adequately representative sampling must be considered [2].

Capacitance

For estimating the capacitance parameters of the veins, contained volume, rather then flow, and transmural pressure, rather then the longitudinal pressure gradient, must be measured. Pressures are measured as described above. For the desired pressure-volume relationship the total contained volume must be known.

Techniques used to measure total blood volume include *indicator dilution.* The ratio of the integral of indicator concentration time to that of concentration is used to compute the mean transit time (MTT) following the sudden injection of a bolus of indicator [2,4]. The active volume is the product of MTT and flow, with flow measured as outlined above. Scintigraphy provides an image of the distribution of radioactivity in tissues. A radioisotope, such as technicium 99 that is bound to red blood cells which in turn are contained within the vasculature, is injected and allowed to equilibrate. A camera, with many collimating channels sensitive to the emitted radiation, is placed over the tissue. The activity recorded is proportional to the volume of blood. Currently it is not possible to accurately calibrate the systems to provide measures of blood volume because of uncertain attenuation of radiation by the tissue and distance. Furthermore, delimiting a particular organ within the body and separating arterial and venous segments of the circulation are difficult.

Compliance

To estimate compliance, changes in volume are needed. This is generally easier than measuring the total blood volume. Using *plethysmography,* a rigid container is placed around the organ, and a servo system functions to change the fluid volume in the chamber to maintain the chamber pressure constant. The consequent volume change is measured and assumed to be primarily venous, because most of the vascular volume is venous. With a tight system and careful technique, at the end of the experiment both inflow and outflow blood vessels can be occluded and then the contained blood washed out and measured to provide a measure of the total blood volume [12].

Gravimetric Techniques

Gravimetric techniques can be used to measure changes in blood volume. If the organ can be isolated and weighed continuously with the blood vessels intact, changes in volume can be measured in response to drugs or reflexes. With an important modification, this approach can be applied to an organ or the systemic circulation; the tissues are perfused at a constant rate, and the outflow is emptied at a constant pressure into a reservoir. Because the reservoir is emptied at a constant rate for the perfusion, changes in reservoir volume reflect an opposite change in the perfused tissue blood volume [8]. To measure compliance, the outflow pressure is changed (2–5 mmHg) and the corresponding change in reservoir volume noted. With the inflow and outflow pressure held constant, the pressure gradients are assumed to be constant so that 100% of an outflow pressure change can be assumed to be transmitted to the primary capacitance vessels. Any reflex or drug-induced change in reservoir volume may be assumed to be inversely related to an active change in vascular volume [7,8,10]. If resistances are also changed by the reflex or drug, then corrections are needed and the interpretations are more complex.

Outflow Occlusion

If the outflow downstream from the venous catheter is suddenly occluded, the venous pressure increases, and its rate of increase is measured. The rate of inflow is also measured so that the compliance can be estimated as the ratio flow to rate of pressure rise: Compliance in ml/mmHg = (flow in ml/min)/(rate of venous pressure rise in mmHg/min). The method is predicated on the assumption that the inflow continues at a constant rate and that there is no pressure gradient between the pressure measuring point and the site of compliance for the first few seconds of occlusion when the rate of pressure rise is measured.

Integral of Inflow Minus Outflow

With this technique both inflow and outflow are measured and the difference integrated to provide the volume change during an experimental forcing. If there is a decrease in contained volume, the outflow will be transiently greater than the inflow. The volume change gives a measure of the response to drugs or reflexes. Following a change in venous pressure, the technique can be used to measure compliance. Accurate measures of flow are needed. Serious errors can result if the inflow is not measured but is only assumed to be constant during the experimental protocol. With all methods dependent on measured or controlled flow, small changes in zero offset, which is directly or indirectly integrated, leads to serious error after about 10 minutes, and so the methods are not useful for long-term or slow responses.

36.3 Typical Values

Cardiac output, the sine qua non of the cardiovascular system, averages about 100 ml/(min-kg). It is about 90 in humans, is over 110 ml/(min-kg) in dogs and cats, and is even higher on a body weight basis in small animals such as rats and mice. The mean arterial blood pressure in relaxed, resting, conscious mammals averages about 90 mmHg. The mean circulatory filling pressure averages about 7 mmHg, and the central venous pressure just outside the right heart about 2 mmHg. The blood volume of the body is about 75 ml/kg, but in humans it is about 10% less, and it is larger in small animals. It is difficult to measure accurately because the volume of distribution of the plasma is about 10% higher than that of the red blood cells.

Vascular compliance averages about 2 ml/(mmHg-kg body weight). The majority is in the venules and veins. Arterial compliance is only about 0.05 ml/(mmHg-kg). Skeletal muscle compliance is less than that of the body as a whole, whereas the vascular compliance of the liver is about 10 times that of other organs. The stressed volume is the product of compliance and mean filling pressure and so is about 15 ml/kg. By difference, the unstressed volume is about 60 ml/kg.

As flow is increased through a tissue, the contained volume increases even if the outflow pressure is held constant, because there is a finite pressure drop across the veins which is increased as flow increases. This increase in upstream distending pressure acts to increase the contained blood volume. The volume sensitivity to flow averages about 0.1 ml per 1 ml/min change in flow [6]. For the body as a whole, the sensitivity is about 0.25 ml per 1 ml/min with reflexes blocked, and with reflexes intact it averages about 0.4 ml per ml/min^3. Using similar techniques, it appears that the passive compensatory volume redistribution from the peripheral toward the heart during serious left heart failure is similar in magnitude to a reflex-engendered redistribution from activation of venous smooth muscle [6].

The high-pressure carotid sinus baroreceptor reflex system is capable of changing the venous capacitance [10]. Over the full operating range of the reflex it is capable of mobilizing up to 7.5 ml/kg of blood by primarily changing the unstressed vascular volume with little or no changes in venous compliance [7,8]. Although this represents only a 10% change in blood volume, it can cause nearly a 100% change in cardiac output. It is difficult to say with confidence what particular organ and/or tissue is contributing to this blood volume mobilization. Current evidence suggests that the splanchnic vascular bed contributes significantly to the capacitance change, but this also may vary between species [11].

Acknowledgments

This work was supported by National Heart Lung and Blood Institute grants HL 19039 and HL 07723.

References

1. Furey SAI, Zieske H, Levy MN. 1984. The essential function of the right heart. Am Heart J 107:404.
2. Lassen NA, Perl W. 1979. Tracer Kinetic Methods in Medical Physiology. New York, Raven Press.
3. Numao Y, Iriuchijima J. 1977. Effect of cardiac output on circulatory blood volume. Jpn J Physiol 27:145.
4. Rothe CF. 1983. Venous system: physiology of the capacitance vessels. In JT Shepherd, FM Abboud (eds), Handbook of Physiology: The Cardiovascular System, sec. 2, vol 3, pt 1, pp 397–452, Bethesda, MD, American Physiology Society.
5. Rothe CF. 1993. Mean circulatory filling pressure: its meaning and measurement. J Appl Physiol 74:499.
6. Rothe CF, Gaddis ML. 1990. Autoregulation of cardiac output by passive elastic characteristics of the vascular capacitance system. Circulation 81:360.
7. Shoukas AA, MacAnespie CL, Brunner MJ, et al. 1981. The importance of the spleen in blood volume shifts of the systemic vascular bed caused by the carotid sinus baroreceptor reflex in the dog. Circ Res 49:759.
8. Shoukas AA, Sagawa K. 1973. Control of total systemic vascular capacity by the carotid sinus baroreceptor reflex. Circ Res 33:22.
9. Rose W, Shoukas AA. 1993. Two-port analysis of systemic venous and arterial impedances. Am J Physiol 265 (Heart Circ Physiol 34):H1577.
10. Shoukas AA. 1993. Overall systems analysis of the carotid sinus baroreceptor reflex control of the circulation. Anesthesiol 79:1402.
11. Haase E, Shoukas AA. 1991. The role of the carotid sinus baroreceptor reflex on pressure and diameter relations of the microvasculature of the rat intestine. Am J Physiol 260:H752.
12. Zink J, Delaive J, Mazerall E, Greenway CV. 1976. An improved plethsmograph with servo control of hydrostatic pressure. J Appl Physiol 41(1):107.

37

Mechanics of Tissue/ Lymphatic Transport

Alan R. Hargens
*University of California
at San Diego*

J. Leonel Villavicencio
*Walter Reed Army and Bethesda
Naval Medical Centers*

Transport of fluid and metabolites from blood to tissue is critically important for maintaining the viability and function of cells within the body. Similarly, transport of fluid and waste products from tissue to the *lymphatic system* of vessels and nodes is also crucial to maintain tissue and organ health. Therefore, it is important to understand the mechanisms for transporting fluid containing micro- and macromolecules from blood to tissue and the drainage of this fluid into the lymphatic system. Because of the succinct nature of this chapter, readers are encouraged to consult more complete reviews of blood/tissue/lymphatic transport by Aukland and Reed [1993], Bert and Pearce [1984], Curry [1984], Hargens [1986], Jain [1987], Lai-Fook [1986], Levick [1984], Reddy [1986], Schmid-Schönbein [1990], Schmid-Schönbein and Zweifach [1994], Staub [1988], Staub and colleagues [1987], Taylor and Granger [1984], and Zweifach and Silverberg [1985].

Most previous studies of blood/tissue/lymphatic transport have used isolated organs or whole animals under general anesthesia. Under these conditions, transport of fluid and metabolites is artificially low in comparison to that of animals which are actively moving. In some cases, investigators employed passive motion by connecting an animal's limb to a motor in order to facilitate studies of blood to lymph transport and lymphatic flow. However, new methods and technology allow studies of physiologically active animals so that a better understanding of the importance of transport phenomena in moving tissues is now apparent. Therefore, this chapter emphasizes recent developments in the understanding of the mechanics of tissue/lymphatic transport and a summary of clinical problems related to this transport.

37.1 Basic Concepts of Tissue/Lymphatic Transport

Transcapillary Filtration

Because lymph is formed from fluid filtered from the blood, an understanding of transcapillary exchange must be considered first. Usually pressure parameters favor filtration of fluid across the *capillary* wall to the *interstitium* (J_c) according to the Starling-Landis equation (37.1):

$$J_c = L_pA\left[(P_c - P_t) - \sigma_p(\pi_c - \pi_t)\right] \tag{37.1}$$

where

J_c = net transcapillary fluid transport

L_p = hydraulic conductivity of capillary wall

A = capillary surface area

P_c = capillary blood pressure

P_t = interstitial fluid pressure

σ_p = reflection coefficient for protein

π_c = capillary blood colloid osmotic pressure

π_t = interstitial fluid colloid osmotic pressure

In many tissues, fluid transported out of the capillaries is passively drained by the initial lymphatic vessels so that

$$J_c = J_l \tag{37.2}$$

where J_l = lymph flow and pressure within the initial lymphatic vessels P_l depends on higher interstitial fluid pressure P_t for establishing lymph flow:

$$P_t \geq P_l \tag{37.3}$$

Starling Pressures and Edema Prevention

Hydrostatic and *colloid osmotic pressures* within the blood and interstitial fluid primarily govern transcapillary fluid shifts (Fig. 37.1). Although input arterial pressure averages about 100 mm Hg at heart level, capillary blood pressure P_c is significantly reduced due to resistance R, according to the Poiseuille equation

$$R = \frac{8\eta l}{\pi r^4} \tag{37.4}$$

where η = blood viscosity, l = vessel length between feed artery and capillary, and r = radius.

Therefore, normally at heart level, P_c is approximately 30 mm Hg. However, during upright posture, P_c at foot level is about 90 mm Hg and only about 25 mm Hg at head level [Parazynski et al., 1991]. Differences in P_c between capillaries of the head and feet are due to gravitational components of blood pressure according to $\rho g h$. For this reason, volumes of transcapillary filtration and lymph flows are generally higher in tissues of the lower body as compared to those of the upper body. Moreover, one might expect much more sparse distribution of lymphatic vessels in upper body tissues. In fact, tissues of the lower body of humans and other tall animals have efficient skeletal muscle pumps, prominent lymphatic systems, and noncompliant skin and fascial boundaries to prevent dependent *edema* [Aukland, 1994; Hargens et al., 1987].

Other pressure parameters in the Starling-Landis equation (37.1) such as P_t, π_c, and π_t are not as sensitive to changes in body posture as is P_c. Typical values for P_t range from -2 mm Hg to 10 mm Hg depending on the tissue or organ under investigation [Wiig, 1990]. However, during movement, P_t in skeletal muscle increases to 150 mm Hg or higher [Murthy et al., 1994], providing a mechanism to promote lymphatic flow and venous return via the skeletal muscle pump (Fig. 37.2). Blood colloid osmotic pressure π_c usually ranges 25–35 mm Hg and is the other major force for retaining

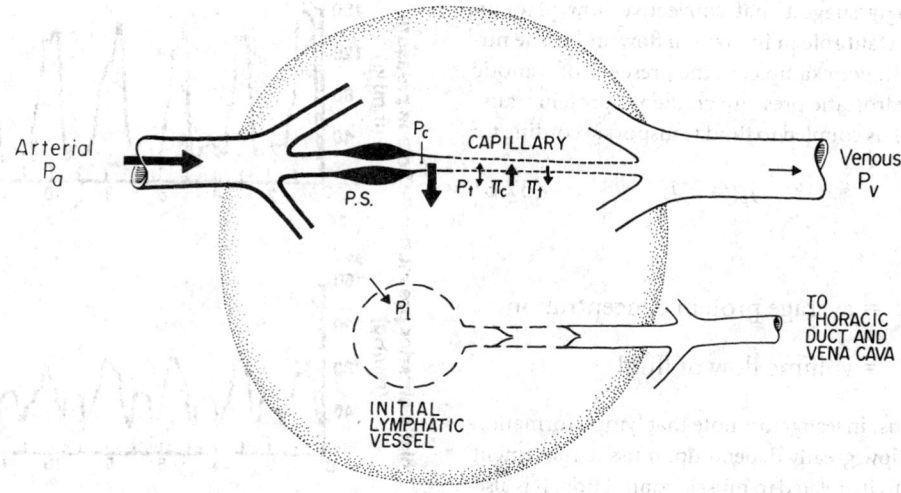

FIGURE 37.1 Starling pressures which regulate transcapillary fluid balance. Pressure parameters which determine direction and magnitude of transcapillary exchange include capillary blood pressure P_c, interstitial fluid pressure P_t (directed into capillary when positive or directed into tissue when negative), plasma colloid osmotic pressure π_c, and interstitial fluid colloid osmotic pressure π_t. Precapillary sphincters (PS) regulate P_c, capillary flow, and capillary surface area A. It is generally agreed that a hydrostatic pressure gradient ($P_t >$ lymph pressure P_l) drains off excess interstitial fluid under conditions of net filtration. Relative magnitudes of pressures are depicted by the size of arrows. *Source:* Hargens AR. 1986. Interstitial fluid pressure and lymph flow. In R. Skalak and S. Chien (eds), *Handbook of Bioengineering*, vol 19, pp 1–35, New York, McGraw-Hill. With permission.

plasma within the vascular system and preventing edema. Interstitial π_t depends on the reflection coefficient of the capillary wall (σ_p ranges from 0.5 to 0.9 for different tissues) as well as washout of interstitial proteins during high filtration rates [Aukland & Reed, 1993]. Typically π_t ranges between 8–15 mm Hg with higher values in upper-body tissues compared to those in the lower body [Aukland & Reed, 1993; Parazynski et al., 1991]. Precapillary sphincter activity (see Fig. 37.1) also decreases blood flow, decreases capillary filtration area A, and reduces P_c in dependent tissues of the body to help prevent edema during upright posture [Aratow et al., 1991].

Interstitial Flow and Lymph Formation

As stated in the introduction, many previous investigators were convinced that interstitial flow of proteins was limited by simple diffusion according to Fick's equation:

$$J_p = -D^{\partial cp/\partial x} \tag{37.5}$$

where

J_p = one-dimensional protein flux

D = diffusion coefficient

$\partial cp/\partial x$ = concentration gradient of protein through interstitium

However, recent experimental and theoretical understandings of the dependence of volume and solute flows on hydrostatic and osmotic pressures [Hammel, 1994; Hargens & Akeson, 1986]

strongly suggest that convective flow plays an important role in interstitial flow and tissue nutrition. For example, in the presence of osmotic or hydrostatic pressure gradients, protein transport J_p is coupled to fluid transport according to:

$$J_p = \bar{c}_p J_v \qquad (37.6)$$

where

$\bar{c}_p$ = average protein concentration

J_v = volume flow of fluid

Most investigators note that lymph formation and flow greatly depend upon tissue movement or activity related to muscle contraction. It is also generally agreed that formation of initial lymph depends mainly on the composition of nearby interstitial fluid and pressure gradients across the interstitial/lymphatic boundary [Hargens, 1986; Schmid-Schönbein & Zweifach, 1994; Zweifach & Lipowsky, 1984]. For this reason, lymph formation and flow can be quantified by measuring disappearance of isotope-labeled albumin from subcutis or skeletal muscle [Reed et al., 1985].

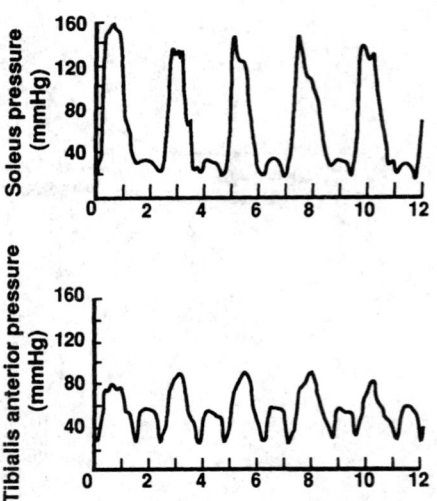

FIGURE 37.2 Simultaneous intramuscular pressure oscillations in the soleus (top panel) and the tibialis anterior (bottom panel) muscles during plantar- and dorsiflexion exercise. Soleus muscle is an integral part of the calf muscle pump. *Source:* Murthy G, Watenpaugh DE, Ballard RE, et al. 1994. Supine exercise during lower body negative pressure effectively simulates upright exercise in normal gravity. J Appl Physiol 76:2742. Modified with permission.

Lymphatic Transport

As shown in Fig. 37.1, the primary functions of the lymphatic system are to drain off excess fluid and metabolites from tissues and to return extravasated plasma proteins to the blood via the thoracic duct. These functions prevent buildup of interstitial proteins, maintain relatively low π_t, and importantly, prevent edema. After entry into the initial or terminal lymphatic vessels, lymph is mainly propelled by tissue motion, muscle contraction, and spontaneous contractions of smooth muscle which surrounds the lymphatic vessel [Hargens et al., 1987; McGeown et al., 1987; Ohhashi, 1987; Reed et al., 1985]. Pressures within the lymphatic system rise from slightly negative to ambient values in initial lymphatics up to 30 mm Hg or higher in large (200- to 300-μm) collecting vessels (Fig. 37.3). Depending on the contractile cycle of an initial lymphatic vessel, intraluminal pressures are negative (about −1 mm Hg) or positive (about +1 mm Hg) as determined by direct micropuncture [Hargens & Zweifach, 1976, 1977]. After entry into the 25- to 50-μm initial lymphatic vessel, intraluminal pressure increases downstream in each successive lymphatic segment (Fig. 37.3). Pressure increases in the downstream direction of lymph flow and is maintained by one-way valves which are prominent features of all mammalian lymphatic vessels.

In a normally functioning lymphatic segment, lymph flow is generated by an upstream contraction. This flow is associated with increased hydrostatic pressure in the segment and a progressive distension of the collecting lymphatic channel. After attaining a particular threshold pressure and corresponding diameter specific to that particular segment, the vessel contracts. During contraction, a further transient rise in pressure occurs, closing the upstream valve by a momentary retrograde or bidirectional flow and opening the downstream valve. As soon as the downstream valve opens, intraluminal pressure falls even though the contractile phase continues. As the contiguous, downstream segment contracts, pressure in the feeding segment falls to its minimum baseline value, and the valve separating the two segments closes. The whole cycle then repeats. As a result of the pressure-volume dynamics, a contractile wave propagates downstream from the initial lymphatic to the collecting lymphatic channels.

When intralymphatic pressure is reduced artificially by upstream occlusion or lymph withdrawal, spontaneous contractions are significantly decelerated to the point of quiescence. Because increased intraluminal pressure stretches the lymphatic wall, these results support the concept that contractions are induced by development of increased tension in smooth muscle which surrounds the vessel [Hargens & Zweifach, 1977]. Lymphatic wall tension T_l can be calculated from pressure-diameter results obtained during normal, artificially increased, and artificially decreased transmural pressures P_{tm} by use of the Laplace equation

$$T_l = P_{tm} \cdot r_l \qquad (37.7)$$

where r_l = internal radius of the lymphatic segment. Contraction frequency is a linear function of P_l through a frequency range of 1 to 12 Hz. Thus, a stretch or myogenic mechanism is a more plausible cause of lymphatic contraction than a neurogenic mechanism.

The next section of this chapter will proceed from the basic mechanics of tissue/lymphatic transport to clinical problems of the lymphatic system.

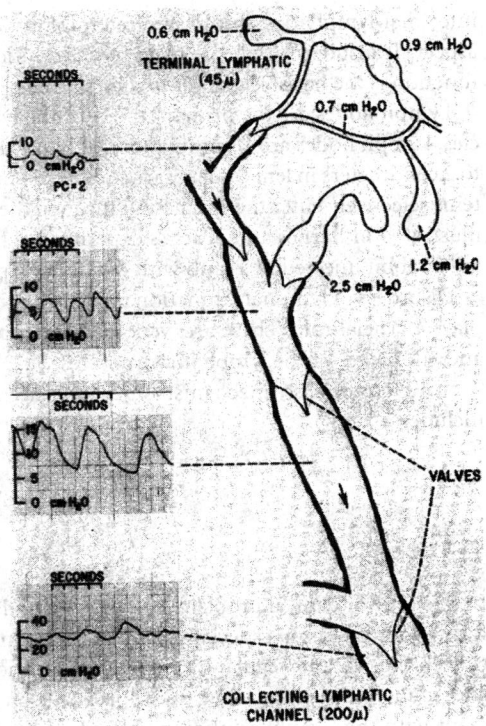

FIGURE 37.3 Intralymphatic pressures increase from initial ("terminal") lymphatic vessels, where lymph is formed to collecting lymphatic channels. Within a given intervalvular segment, pressures are equal. *Source:* Zweifach BW, Prather JW. 1975. Micromanipulation of pressure in terminal lymphatics of the mesentery. J Appl Physiol 228:1326. With permission.

7.2 Clinical Disorders of Tissue/Lymphatic Transport

Edema

Edema is the most common sign of derangement of the delicate balance between fluid production and fluid absorption in the microcirculation. Depending on the specific tissue, approximately 90% of the interstitial fluid is drained through venous capillary reabsorption and the remaining 10% through the lymphatic system. This system performs multiple functions: It eliminates macromolecules and toxic substances from the tissues and assists in clearing injured tissue debris. The system regulates tissue fluid volume, protecting the circulating blood volume against hypovolemia. Through the thoracic duct, an amount of lymph approximating the plasma volume returns to the circulation every 24 hours [Mayerson, 1963]. Along with proteins and other large molecules, lymphocytes and other cells enter the circulation via the lymphatic system. The different types of lymphatic cells are now identified largely by surface markers. Moretta and coworkers [1982] support the concept that lymphocytes derive from a specialized structure closely involved with the immunologic mechanism.

Chylomicrons and lipoproteins enter the circulation through the lymphatic network, contributing to form the stream of a system which handles large volumes of fluid, fat, protein, and cells. The intestinal lymphatics absorb cholesterol, fatty acids, and triglycerides which give chyle its milky aspect. Transudative exudate from serous cavities is continuously absorbed by the lymphatics. This function is the basis of *peritoneal dialysis.*

Lymph nodes are the primary filters of the lymphatic system, stopping bacterial and viral particles. Lymph nodes are accumulations of lymphatic tissue ranging in size from a few millimeters up to 2 centimeters in length. They are sites of important immunologic exchanges. Certain foreign proteins selectively enter the circulation through the lymphatics. Such is the case of some snake venoms illustrated in Barnes and Trueta's experiment [1941], where a lethal dose of snake venom failed to kill a rabbit injected in a limb with divided lymphatics.

Disorders of lymphatic function reflect prominently in a number of clinical entities where edema plays a crucial role. These are: venous disease, protein disorders, increased capillary permeability, and anomalies of the lymphatic structures.

In *venous disease,* mechanisms of microcirculatory derangement [see Eq. (37.1) for symbols] include

$$\uparrow P_c, P_c - P_t, \sigma_p, \pi_c, - \pi t, J_L$$

$$\downarrow L_p A, p_t \tag{37.8}$$

In this type of clinical problem, edema is secondary to increased venous pressure, which promotes formation of lymph, especially if there is retention of salt and plasma volume. In these cases, the existence of an autoregulatory increase in arteriolar resistance leading to a reduced arterial inflow and an increased lymph flow transport has been proposed [Folkow & Neil, 1971]. This is in agreement with the lymphoscintigraphic findings of increased and enhanced transport of lymph flow in patients with venous edema secondary to venous insufficiency and deep venous thrombosis [Stewart et al., 1985].

Protein Disorders

For practical purposes, all the protein passing from the capillaries to the circulation is returned via the lymphatic system. Protein accumulates in tissues and organs in cases of disordered lymphatic circulation producing at long range, thickening and fibrosis of the subcutaneous tissue. Edema results when there is a reduction in the capillary colloid osmotic pressure differential, which stimulates capillary filtration and lymph formation. In cases of protein-losing enteropathy, plasmapheresis, nephrotic syndrome, and severe nutritional disorders, there is

$$\uparrow \pi_c, \pi_c - \pi_t$$

$$\downarrow P_c, J_l \tag{37.9}$$

Reduced blood colloid pressure is a generalized phenomenon of which *anasarca* is a typical clinical presentation. Peritonitis, sepsis, histamine release, burns, and trauma, as well as allergic edemas are clinical manifestations of increased capillary permeability. In these cases, plasma leaks through the injured capillaries into the tissue spaces, modifying the pressure gradient [Perry et al., 1983]. Lymph is formed in large amounts containing most types of plasma protein including fibrinogen.

Lymphatic System Disorders

Figure 37.4 illustrates a normal lymphatic system with two inserts depicting hypoplasia and aplasia of the lymphatic system, conditions which are congenital in origin. Figure 37.5 shows a normal lymphatic system of the pelvis, abdomen, chest, and intestines. An insert illustrates intestinal hypoplasia of the lymphatic system, an anomaly which usually leads to chylus ascites early in life.

Primary and secondary abnormalities of the lymphatic system are manifested by lymphedema. Primary or congenital lymphedema most commonly affects the lower limbs. It may be present at birth (lymphedema congenita) or may appear at the time of puberty. When the swelling begins before the age of 35, the term *lymphedema praecox* is employed. *Lymphedema tarda* describes the disease which begins after the age of 35. Milroy's disease is a congenital form of lymphedema which appears at birth and is familial. There are some endocrine diseases in which lymphedema forms part of the syndrome (Turner's syndrome).

Secondary lymphedemas are due to trauma, infections, surgery for malignant disease, filariasis, and radiation. Lymphedema affecting the upper extremity is most often seen after radical mastectomy with removal of the axillary nodes with or without postoperative radiation. Excision of the lymphatic nodes in the course of surgery for malignant disease or congenital lymph node aplasia or hypoplasia leads to significant obstruction of the lymphatic flow with progressive stagnation of lymph in the tissue. Chronic venous insufficiency may result in impaired lymphatic function and lead to severe alterations of the lymphatic circulation. This condition has been carefully documented by Collins and associates [1989].

Investigation of the Lymphatic System

Visualization of the arterial and venous systems can be easily and successfully accomplished. Visualization of the lymphatic system has been technically challenging. Radionuclide scanning with isotope-labeled colloids allows visualization of the lymphatic system following an intradermal injection, thus eliminating the tradi-

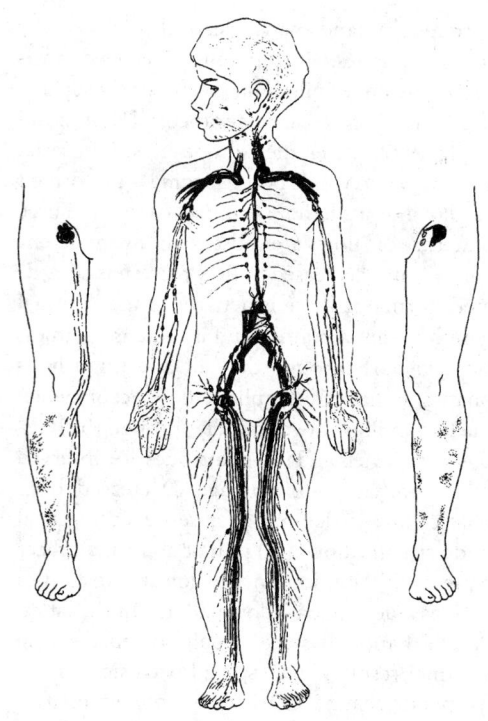

FIGURE 37.4 A normal lymphatic system is illustrated in the middle drawing. Eight to eleven lymphatic vessels are present in the lower extremity. Their number increases as they become more proximal. The number and size of the lymph nodes are important as in some cases they may be inflamed and obstruct the lymph flow. In the upper extremity, lymph vessels course along the main veins and have few epitrochlear nodes. Lymphatic hypoplasia is shown in the right insert. The number of lymph vessels is diminished and dermal backflow is observed when patent blue is injected in the web spaces. Aplasia of lymph nodes and vessels is represented in the left insert. Patent blue dye is seen in the dermal plexus as a sign of lymphatic obstruction. These abnormalities are of congenital origen. *Source:* Villavicencio JL. 1985. Direct operations on the lymphatics. In H Dudley, D Carter (eds), J DeWeese (guest ed), *Rob and Smith's Operative Surgery,* 4th ed, pp 365–376, London, Boston, Canada, Butterworths. With permission.

tional problems of lymphangiography, an invasive angiographic technique introduced by Kinmonth and coworkers [1957]. Even though the images obtained by lymphoscintigraphy do not have the anatomic definition obtained by lymphangiography, the method provides the investigator with a good tool to evaluate the function and dynamics of the lymphatic system. Many investigators [Cambria et al., 1993; Collins et al., 1989; McNeill et al., 1989] consider that whole body lymphangioscintigraphy should be the preferred method for the initial assessment of the lymphatic system. This technique consists of an intradermal injection of human serum albumin or antimony trisulfide colloid, labeled with technetium-99m. The isotope is injected in the interdigital web spaces of each foot or hand and is selectively picked up by the lymphatics. Technetium-99-labeled antimony trisulfide colloid has been extensively utilized in most research protocols [Hammond et al., 1991]. After the isotope injection, serial extremity and whole body imaging is performed employing a digital gamma camera. Three patterns of flow are observed: normal, enhanced, and decreased. A flow pattern is considered normal if there is activity in the inguinal lymph nodes at 30 min and if there is symmetric transport through the calf and thigh lymphatics. Enhanced lymphatic flow occurs when the lymph flow moves rapidly through the lymphatic channels and inguinal nodes are observed in the initial 10-min image. Decreased lymphatic flow is defined as absence of inguinal node visualization at 30 min or abnormal tracer pattern distribution in the lower extremities such as a dermal backflow pattern. In the latter, dermal lymphatics are visualized representing the final result of widespread occlusion of the lymphatic channels. Dermal lymphatic collaterals represent an alternative pathway of lymphatic obstruction, and their presence is not specific to any particular disease.

Cambria and associates [1993] described a method to semiquantify lymphoscintigraphy and obtain a transport index. In a group of 386 extremities, they scored five components of the lymphoscintigram: the time for the isotope to reach the regional nodes, the distribution pattern of the tracer, the transport kinetics, and the

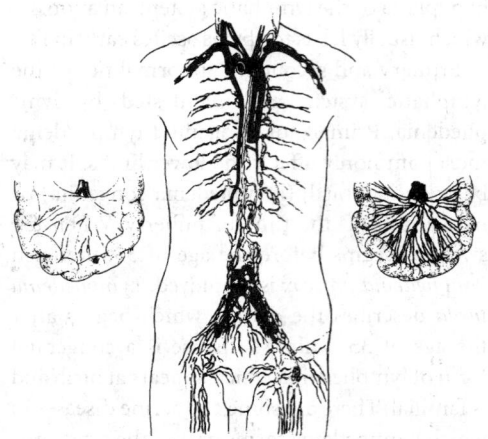

FIGURE 37.5 The large drawing represents a normal lymphatic system of thoracic and abdominal cavities. A number of trunks originating from the femoral and iliac regions drain lymph from the extremities and pelvis. The cysterna of Pecquet serves as collector of abdominal lymph and is the origin of the thoracic duct. The latter will drain about 3–4*l* of lymph in 24 h in a 70-kg man. The upper right insert shows normal intestinal lymphatics through which fatty acids, cholesterol, and other lipoproteins are absorbed and transported into the circulation. Hypoplasia of intestinal lymphatics is shown in the lower right insert. In these cases, chyle exudes from the intestinal wall, producing chylous ascites. *Source:* Villavicencio JL. 1985. Direct operations on the lymphatics. In H Dudley, D Carter (eds), J DeWeese (guest ed), *Rob and Smith's Operative Surgery*, 4th ed, pp 365–376, London, Boston, Canada, Butterworths. With permission.

appearance of the lymph vessels and lymphatic nodes. These five components were scored as illustrated in Table 37.1. The summation of the five components results in a transport index. The score could range from near 0 to 45, with higher numbers representing more severe abnormality. The lymphoscintigraphic data, together with a carefully taken clinical history and results of other diagnostic

TABLE 37.1 Transport Index Components

	Score			
	0	3	5	9
Transport kinetics	No delay	Mild delay	Extreme delay	No flow
Distribution pattern	Normal	Partial dermal	Diffuse dermal	No flow
Time Index = time in minutes for appearance of regional nodes × 0.04				
Lymph nodes	Normal	Visible, diminished	Barely visible	Not seen
Lymph vessels	Normal	Visible, diminished	Barely visible	Not seen

Source: Cambria RA, Gloviczki P, Naessens JM, et al. 1993. Noninvasive evaluation of the lymphatic system with lymphoscintigraphy: A prospective semiquantitative analysis of 386 extremities. *J Vasc Surg* 18:773. With permission.

examinations, were used to classify each patient as having primary or secondary lymphedema or swelling secondary to other causes. The transport index was a highly accurate indicator of lymphedema. Using a value of 5 as a cutoff point between normal and abnormal, the specificity of the test was 94% and the sensitivity 80%. Patients with lymphedema (primary or secondary) had a higher transport index than patients with other causes of limb swelling (23.1 ± 1.5 versus 1.9 ± 0.5; $p < 0.001$). All the component scores were also higher than those among patients with lymphedema. There was a marked difference in the transport index and all of its components between edematous extremities and normal limbs (16.0 ± 1.0 and 2.8 ± 0.5, respectively).

Magnetic resonance imaging (MRI), either alone or in combination with lymphoscintigraphy, has been utilized in the study of patients with lymphedema [Case et al., 1992]. MRI studies in patients with primary and secondary lymphedema clearly document the extent of the dermal and subcutaneous edema as well as the relative noninvolvement of the skeletal muscle compartment. Scintigraphy demonstrates dermal backflow of tracer, delayed transport, and delayed visualization or nonvisualization of regional nodes. The combination of these two new methods provides the necessary elements to differentiate lymphedema from all other causes of limb swelling and may be considered the studies of choice in the investigation of the swollen extremity.

Acknowledgments

We thank Karen Hutchinson for expert manuscript assistance. This work was supported by NASA grants 199-14-12-04 and 199-26-12-38.

Defining Terms

Anasarca: Generalized accumulation of fluid in the extravascular space.
Capillary: The smallest blood vessel of the body that provides oxygen and other nutrients to nearby cells and tissues.
Colloid osmotic pressure: A negative pressure which depends on protein concentration (mainly of albumin and globulins) and prevents excess filtration across the capillary wall.
Edema: Excess fluid or swelling within a given tissue.
Interstitium: The space between cells of various tissues of the body. Normally fluid and proteins within this space are transported from the capillary to the initial lymphatic vessel.
Lymphatic system: The clear network of vessels which return excess tissue fluid and proteins to the blood via the thoracic duct.
Lymphatic system disorders: Can be primary or secondary. Primary lymphedema comprises aplasia, hypoplasia, or excessive dilatation of lymphatic vessels. Absence or decreased number of lymph nodes may be present also. Secondary lymphedema occurs when there is damage to the normal lymphatic system (e.g., trauma, infection, surgical excision, burn, injury).
Peritoneal dialysis: An exchange of fluids occurring through catheters inserted in the peritoneal cavity to detoxify the blood. Its main indication is renal failure.
Protein disorders: In our context, it defines any pathologic entity where there is a decrease in the plasma protein content either because of excessive loss or deficient production.
Venous disease: Any pathologic process involving the venous system such as varicose veins, superficial and deep venous thrombosis, venous stasis, and venous leg ulcers.

References

Aratow M, Hargens AR, Meyer J-U, et al. 1991. Postural responses of head and foot cutaneous microvascular flow and their sensitivity to bed rest. Aviat Space Environ Med 62:246.
Aukland K. 1994. Why don't our feet swell in the upright posture? News in Physiol Sci 9:214.

Aukland K, Reed RK. 1993. Interstitial-lymphatic mechanisms in the control of extracellular fluid volume. Physiol Rev 73:1.

Barnes JM, Trueta J. 1941. Absorption of bacteria, toxins and snake venoms from tissues. Lancet 1:623.

Bert JL, Pearce RH. 1984. The interstitium and microvascular exchange. In E Renkin, CC Michel (eds), Handbook of Physiology: The Cardiovascular System: Microcirculation, sec 2, vol 4, pt 1, pp 521–547, Bethesda, Md, American Physiology Society.

Cambria RA, Gloviczki P. Naessens JM, et al. 1993. Noninvasive evaluation of the lymphatic system with lymphoscintigraphy: A prospective semiquantitative analysis in 386 extremities. J Vasc Surg 18:773.

Case TC, Witte CL, Witte MH, et al. 1992. Magnetic resonance imaging in human lymphedema: Comparison with lymphoscintigraphy. Magn Reson Imaging 10:549.

Collins PS, Villavicencio JL, Abreu SH, et al. 1989. Abnormalities of lymphatic drainage in lower extremities: A lymphoscintigraphic study. J Vasc Surg 9:145.

Curry F-RE. 1984. Mechanics and thermodynamics of transcapillary exchange. In E Renkin, CC Michel (eds), Handbook of Physiology: The Cardiovascular System: Microcirculation, sec 2, vol 4, pt 1, pp. 309–374, Bethesda, Md, American Physiology Society.

Folkow B, Neil E. 1971. The principles of vascular control. In E Renkin, CC Michel (eds), Circulation, pp 290–292, London, Oxford University Press.

Hammel HT. 1994. How solutes alter water in aqueous solutions. J Phys Chem 98:4196.

Hammond SL, Gomez ER, Coffey JA, et al. 1991. Involvement of the lymphatic system in chronic venous insufficiency. In JJ Bergan, JST Yao (eds), Venous Disorders, pp 333–343, Philadelphia, W.B. Saunders.

Hargens AR. 1986. Interstitial fluid pressure and lymph flow. In R Skalak, S Chien (eds), Handbook of Bioengineering, vol 19, pp 1–35, New York, McGraw-Hill.

Hargens AR, Akeson WH. 1986. Stress effects on tissue nutrition and viability. In AR Hargens (ed), Tissue Nutrition and Viability, pp 1–24, New York, Springer-Verlag.

Hargens AR, Millard RW, Pettersson K, et al. 1987. Gravitational haemodynamics and oedema prevention in the giraffe. Nature 329:59.

Hargens AR, Zweifach BW. 1976. Transport between blood and peripheral lymph in intestine. Microvasc Res 11:89.

Hargens AR, Zweifach BW. 1977. Contractile stimuli in collecting lymph vessels. Am J Physiol 233:H57.

Jain RK. 1987. Transport of molecules in the tumor interstitium: A review. Cancer Res 47:3039.

Kinmonth JB, Taylor GW, Tracy GD, et al. 1957. Primary lymphedema: Clinical lymphangiographic studies of a series of 107 patients in which the lower limbs were affected. Br J Surg 45:1.

Lai-Fook SJ. 1986. Mechanics of lung fluid balance. Crit Rev Biomed Eng 13:171.

Levick JR. 1984. Blood flow and mass transport in synovial joints. In E Renkin, CC Michel (eds), Handbook of Physiology: The Cardiovascular System: Microcirculation, sec 2, vol 4, pt 2, pp 917–947, Bethesda, Md, American Physiology Society.

Mayerson HS. 1963. The physiologic importance of lymph. In WF Hamilton, P Dow (eds), Handbook of Physiology, vol 2, pp 1035–1073, Washington, DC, American Physiology Society.

McGeown JG, McHale NG, Thornbury KD. 1987. The role of external compression and movement in lymph propulsion in the sheep hindlimb. J Physiol Lond 387:83.

McNeill GC, Witte MH, Witte ChL, et al. 1989. Whole-body lymphangioscintigraphy: Preferred method for initial assessment of the peripheral lymphatic system. Radiology 172:495.

Moretta L, Mingari MC, Moretta A, et al. 1982. Human lymphocyte surface markers. Hematology 19:273.

Murthy G, Watenpaugh DE, Ballard RE, et al. 1994. Supine exercise during lower body negative pressure effectively simulates upright exercise in normal gravity. J Appl Physiol 76:2742.

Ohhashi T. 1987. Regulation of motility of small collecting lymphatics. In NC Staub, JC Hogg, AR Hargens (eds), Interstitial-Lymphatic Liquid and Solute Movement, pp 171–183, Basel, Karger.

Parazynski SE, Hargens AR, Tucker B, et al. 1991. Transcapillary fluid shifts in tissues of the head and neck during and after simulated microgravity. J Appl Physiol 71:2469.

Perry MA, Benoit JN, Kvietys PR, et al. 1983. Restricted transport of cationic macromolecules across intestinal capillaries. Am J Physiol 245:G568.

Reddy NP. 1986. Lymph circulation: physiology, pharmacology, and biomechanics. Crit Rev Biomed Sci 14:45.

Reed RK, Johansen S, Noddeland H. 1985. Turnover rate of interstitial albumin in rat skin and skeletal muscle: Effects of limb movements and motor activity. Acta Physiol Scand 125:711.

Schmid-Schönbein GW. 1990. Microlymphatics and lymph flow. Physiol Rev 70:987.

Schmid-Schönbein GW, Zweifach BW. 1994. Fluid pump mechanisms in initial lymphatics. News in Physiol Sci 9:67.

Staub NC. 1988. New concepts about the pathophysiology of pulmonary edema. J Thorac Imaging 3:8.

Staub NC, Hogg JC, Hargens AR. 1987. Interstitial-Lymphatic Liquid and Solute Movement, pp 1–290, Basel, Karger.

Stewart G, Gaunt JI, Croft DN, et al. 1985. Isotope lymphography: A new method of investigating the role of lymphatics in chronic limb edema. Br J Surg 72:906.

Taylor AE, Granger DN. 1984. Exchange of macromolecules across the microcirculation. In E Renkin, CC Michel (eds), Handbook of Physiology: The Cardiovascular System: Microcirculation, sec 2, vol 4, pt 1, pp 467–520, Bethesda, Md, American Physiology Society.

Wiig H. 1990. Evaluation of methodologies for measurement of interstitial fluid pressure (Pi): Physiological implications of recent Pi data. Crit Rev Biomed Eng 18:27.

Zweifach BW, Lipowsky HH. 1984. Pressure-flow relations in blood and lymph microcirculation. In E Renkin, CC Michel (eds), Handbook of Physiology: The Cardiovascular System: Microcirculation, sec 2, vol 4, pt 1, pp 251–307, Bethesda, Md, American Physiology Society.

Zweifach BW, Prather, JW. 1975. Micromanipulation of pressure in terminal lymphatics of the mesentary. J Appl Physiol 228:1326.

Zweifach BW, Silverberg A. 1985. The interstitial-lymphatic flow system. In MG Johnston (ed), Experimental Biology of the Lymphatic Circulation, pp 45–79, Amsterdam, Elsevier.

Further Information

C.K. Drinker and J.M. Yoffey's *Lymphatics, Lymph and Lymphoid Tissue: Their Physiological and Clinical Significance* (Harvard University Press, Cambridge, Mass., 1941) is a classic treatise on the lymphatic circulation by two master pioneers in the field of lymphatic physiology. It is a delightful account of the experience of the investigators in the intricacies of the microcirculation involving the lymphatic system.

J.B. Kinmonth's *The Lymphatics: Surgery, Lymphography and Diseases of the Chyle and Lymph Systems* (Edward Arnold, London, 1982) is a comprehensive textbook on the lymphatic circulation and its pathophysiology written by a man who devoted his life to the study and treatment of patients with lymphatic disorders. Professor Kinmonth introduced the modern classification of lymphedemas and is the father of lymphography. This is a volume that deals with every aspect of the lymphatic system and can be considered the best book written on the subject.

S.A. Threefoot's article "Lymphatic circulation" (in H.L. Conn Jr., O. Horwitz (eds), *Cardiovascular Disease*, Lea & Febiger, Philadelphia, 1971) offers the reader a comprehensive insight into the basic aspects of the physiology and pathophysiology of the lymphatic circulation. It has numerous illustrations and an extensive list of pertinent references. It is a good review of lymph formation, ultrastructure, lymphodynamics, lymph pressure, and normal lympho-venous anastomosis.

J.H.N. Wolfe and J.W. Futrell's (in R.B. Rutherford (ed), *Vascular Surgery* chap 145, pp 1440–1449, W.B. Saunders, Philadelphia, 1984) and J.H.N. Wolfe's chapter "Diagnosis and classification of lymphedema" (in *Vascular Surgery*, pp 1450–1462) contain essential information on the pathophysiology, diagnosis, and management of lymphedema. The authors are recognized authorities in the field.

J.M. Yoffey and F.C. Courtice's *Lymphatics, Lymph and the Lymphomyeloid Complex* (Academic Press. London, New York, 1970) is a classic book by two investigators whose experience is rec-ognized worldwide in the field of lymphatic physiology and basic science concepts. The book contains a comprehensive review of pertinent literature and experimental physiology on the lymphatic system.

38

Cochlear Mechanics

Charles R. Steele
Stanford University

Gary J. Baker
Stanford University

Jason A. Tolomeo
Stanford University

Deborah E. Zetes
Stanford University

The inner ear is a transducer of mechanical force to appropriate neural excitation. The key element is the receptor cell, or hair cell, which has cilia on the apical surface and afferent (and sometimes efferent) neural synapses on the lateral walls and base. Generally for hair cells, mechanical displacement of the cilia in the forward direction toward the tallest cilia causes the generation of electrical impulses in the nerves, and backward displacement causes inhibition of spontaneous neural activity. Displacement in the lateral direction has no effect. For moderate frequencies of sinusoidal ciliary displacement (20–200 Hz), the neural impulses are in synchrony with the mechanical displacement. Such impulses are transmitted to the higher centers of the brain and can be perceived as sound. For lower frequencies, however, neural impulses in synchrony with the excitation are apparently confused with the spontaneous, random firing of the nerves. Consequently, three mechanical devices in the inner ear of vertebrates provide perception in the different frequency ranges. At zero frequency, i.e., linear acceleration, the otolith membrane provides a constant force acting on the cilia of hair cells. For low frequencies associated with rotation of the head, the semicircular canals provide the proper force on cilia. For frequencies in the hearing range, the cochlea provides the correct forcing of hair cell cilia. In nonmammalian vertebrates, the equivalent of the cochlea is a bent tube, and the upper frequency of hearing is around 7 kHz. For mammals, the upper frequency is considerably higher, 20 kHz for humans and extending to almost 200 kHz for toothed whales and some bats. Other creatures, such as certain insects, can perceive high frequencies but do not have a cochlea nor the frequency discrimination of vertebrates.

Auditory research is a broad field [Keidel & Neff, 1976]. This chapter presents a brief guide of a restricted view, focusing on the transfer of the input sound pressure into correct stimulation of hair cell cilia in the cochlea. In a general sense, the mechanical functions of the semicircular canals and the otoliths are clear, as are the functions of the outer ear and middle ear; however, the cochlea continues to elude a reasonably complete explanation. Substantial progress in cochlear research has been made in the past decade, triggered by several key discoveries, and there is a high level of excitement among workers in the area. It is evident that the normal function of the cochlea requires a full integration of mechanical, electrical, and chemical effects on the milli-, micro-, and nanometer

0-8493-8346-3/95/$0.00+$.50
© 1995 by CRC Press, Inc.

scales. Recent texts, which include details of the anatomy, are by Pickles [1988] and Gulick and coworkers [1989]. A summary of analysis and data related to the macromechanical aspect up to 1982 is given by Steele [1987], and more recent surveys specifically on the cochlea are by de Boer [1991], Dallos [1992], Hudspeth [1989], and Ruggero [1993].

38.1 Anatomy

The cochlea is a coiled tube in the shape of a snail shell (cochlea = schnecke = snail), with length about 35 mm and radius about 1 mm in humans. There is not a large size difference across species: the length is 60 mm in elephant and 7 mm in mouse. There are two and one-half turns of the coil in man and dolphin, and five turns in guinea pig. Despite the correlation of coiling with hearing capability of land animals [West, 1985], no significant effect of the coiling on the mechanical response has yet been identified.

Components

The cochlea is filled with fluid and divided along its length by two partitions. The main partition is at the center of the cross section and consists of three segments: on one side the *bony shelf* (or *primary spiral osseous lamina*), in the middle an elastic segment (*basilar membrane*) (shown in Fig. 38.1), and on the other side a thick support (*spiral ligament*). The second partition is *Reissner's membrane,* attached at one side above the edge of the bony shelf and attached at the other side to the wall of the cochlea. *Scala media,* the region between Reissner's membrane and the basilar membrane, is filled with *endolymphatic fluid.* This fluid has an ionic content similar to intracellular fluid, high in potassium and low in sodium but with a resting positive electrical potential of around +80 mV. The electrical potential is supplied by the *stria vascularis* on the wall in scala media. The region above Reissner's membrane is *scala vestibuli,* and the region below the main partition is *scala tympani.* Scala vestibuli and scala tympani are connected at the apical end of the cochlea by an opening in the bony shelf, the *helicotrema,* and are filled with *perilymphatic fluid.* This fluid is similar to extracellular fluid, low in potassium and high in sodium with zero electrical potential. Distributed along the scala media side of the basilar membrane is the sensory epithelium, the *organ of Corti.* This contains one row of *inner hair cells* and three rows of *outer hair cells.* In humans, each row contains about 4000 cells. Each of the inner hair cells has about twenty afferent synapses; these are considered to be the primary receptors. In comparison, the outer hair cells are sparsely innervated but have both afferent and efferent synapses.

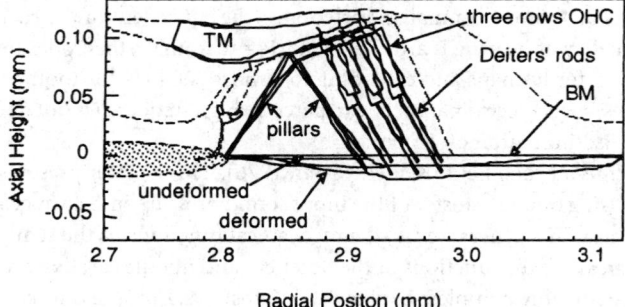

FIGURE 38.1   Finite element calculation for the deformation of the cochlear partition due to pressure on the basilar membrane (BM). Outer-hair-cell (OHC) stereocilia are sheared by the motion of the pillars of Corti and reticular lamina relative to the tectorial membrane (TM). The basilar membrane is supported on the left by the bony shelf and on the right by the spiral ligament.

The basilar membrane is divided into two sections. Connected to the edge of the bony shelf, on the left in Fig. 38.1, is the *arcuate zone,* consisting of a single layer of transverse fibers. Connected to the edge of the spiral ligament, on the right in Fig. 38.1, is the *pectinate zone,* consisting of a double layer of transverse fibers in an amorphous ground substance. The *arches of Corti* form a truss over the arcuate zone, which consist of two rows of *pillar cells.* The foot of the inner pillar is attached at the point of connection of the bony shelf to the arcuate zone, and the foot of the outer pillar cell is attached at the common border of the arcuate zone and pectinate zone. The heads of the inner and outer pillars are connected and form the support point for the *recticular lamina.* The other edge of the recticular lamina is attached to the top of *Henson cells,* which have bases connected to the basilar membrane. The inner hair cells are attached on the bony shelf side of the inner pillars, while the three rows of outer hair cells are attached to the recticular lamina. The region bounded by the inner pillar cells, the recticular lamina, the Henson cells, and the basilar membrane forms another fluid region. This fluid is considered to be perilymph, since it appears that ions can flow freely through the arcuate zone of the basilar membrane. The cilia of the hair cells protrude into the endolymph. Thus the outer hair cells are immersed in perilymph at 0 mV, have an intracellular potential of -70 mV, and have cilia at the upper surface immersed in endolymph at a potential of $+80$ mV. In some regions of the ears of some vertebrates [Freeman & Weiss, 1990], the cilia are freestanding. However, mammals have a *tectorial membrane,* originating near the edge of the bony shelf and overlying the rows of hair cells parallel to the recticular lamina. The tallest rows of cilia of the outer hair cells are attached to the tectorial membrane. Under the tectorial membrane and inside the inner hair cells is a fluid space, the *inner sulcus,* filled with endolymph. The cilia of the inner hair cells are not attached to the overlying tectorial membrane, so the motion of the fluid in the inner sulcus must provide the mechanical input to these primary receptor cells. Since the inner sulcus is found only in mammals, the fluid motion in this region generated by acoustic input may be crucial to high-frequency discrimination capability.

With a few exceptions of specialization, the dimensions of all the components in the cross-section of the mammalian cochlea change smoothly and slowly along the length, in a manner consistent with high stiffness at the base, or input end, and low stiffness at the apical end. For example, in the cat the basilar membrane width increases from 0.1 to 0.4 mm while the thickness decreases from 13 to 5 μm. The density of transverse fibers decreases more than the thickness, from about 6000 fibers per μm at the base to 500 per μm at the apex [Cabezudo, 1978].

Material Properties

Both perilymph and endolymph have the viscosity and density of water. The bone of the wall and the bony shelf appear to be similar to compact bone, with density approximately twice that of water. The remaining components of the cochlea are soft tissue with density near that of water. The stiffness of the components vary over a wide range, as indicated by the values of Young's modulus listed in Table 38.1. These values are taken directly or estimated from many sources, including the stiffness measurements in the cochlea by Békésy [1960], Gummer and coworkers [1981], Strelioff and Flock [1984], Miller [1985], Zwislocki and Cefaratti [1989], and Olson and Mountain [1994].

38.2 Passive Models

The anatomy of the cochlea is complex. By modeling, one attempts to isolate and understand the essential features. Following is an indication of proposition and controversy associated with a few such models.

Resonators

The ancient Greeks suggested that the ear consisted of a set of tuned resonant cavities. As each component in the cochlea was discovered subsequently, it was proposed to be the tuned resonator. The most well-known resonance theory is Helmholz's: According to this theory, the transverse fibers of

TABLE 38.1 Typical Values and Estimates for Young's Modulus *E*.

Compact bone	20	GPa
Keratin	3	GPa
Basilar membrane fibers	1.9	GPa
Microtubules	1.2	GPa
Collagen	1	GPa
Reissner's membrane	60	MPa
F-actin with Ca^{+2}	50	MPa
F-actin without Ca^{+2}	30	MPa
Red blood cell, extended (assuming thickness = 10 nm)	45	MPa
Rubber, elastin	4	MPa
Basilar membrane ground substance	200	kPa
Tectorial membrane	30	kPa
Jell-O	3	kPa
Henson's cells	1	kPa

the basilar membrane are under tension and respond like the strings of a piano. The short strings at the base respond to high frequencies and the long strings toward the apex respond to low frequencies. The important feature of the Helmholz theory is the *place principle,* according to which the receptor cells at a certain *place* along the cochlea are stimulated by a certain frequency. Thus the cochlea provides a real-time frequency separation (Fourier analysis) of any complex sound input. This aspect of the Helmholz theory has since been validated, since each of the some 30,000 fibers exiting the cochlea in the auditory nerve is sharply tuned to a particular frequency. A basic difficulty with such a resonance theory is that sharp tuning requires small damping, which is associated with a long ringing after the excitation ceases. Yet the cochlea is remarkable for combining sharp tuning with short time delay for the onset of reception and the same short time delay for the cessation of reception.

A particular problem with the Helmholtz theory arises from the equation for the resonant frequency for a string under tension

$$f = \frac{1}{2b} \sqrt{\frac{T}{\rho h}} \qquad (38.1)$$

in which *T* is the tensile force per unit width, ρ is the density, *b* is the length, and *h* is the thickness of the string. In humans the frequency range over which the cochlea operates is f = 200–20000 Hz, a factor of 100, whereas the change in length *b* is only a factor of 5 and the thickness of the basilar membrane *h* varies the wrong way by a factor of 2 or so. Thus to produce the necessary range of frequency, the tension *T* would have to vary by a factor of about 800. In fact, the spiral ligament, which would supply such tension, varies in area by a factor of only 10.

Traveling Waves

No theory anticipated the actual behavior found in the cochlea in 1928 by Békésy [1960]. He observed *traveling waves* moving along the cochlea from base toward apex which have a maximum amplitude at a certain place. The place depends on the frequency, as in the Helmholz theory, but the amplitude envelope is not very localized. In Békésy's experimental models, and in subsequent mathematical and experimental models, the anatomy of the cochlea is greatly simplified. The coiling, Reissner's membrane, and the organ of Corti are all ignored, so the cochlea is treated as a straight tube with a single partition. [An exception is in Fuhrmann and coworkers (1986)]. A gradient in the partition stiffness similar to that in the cochlea gives beautiful traveling waves in both experimental and mathematical models.

One-Dimensional Model

A majority of work has been based on the assumption that the fluid motion is one-dimensional. With this simplification the governing equations are similar to those for an electrical transmission line and for the long wave-length response of an elastic tube containing fluid. The equation for the pressure p in a tube with constant cross-sectional area A and with constant frequency of excitation is

$$\frac{d^2p}{dx^2} + \frac{2\rho\omega^2}{AK} p = 0 \tag{38.2}$$

in which x is the distance along the tube, ρ is the density of the fluid, ω is the frequency in radians per second, and K is the generalized partition stiffness, equal to the net pressure divided by the displaced area of the cross-section. The factor of 2 accounts for fluid on both sides of the elastic partition. Often K is represented in the form of a single-degree-of-freedom oscillator

$$K = k + i\omega d - m\omega^2 \tag{38.3}$$

in which k is the static stiffness, d is the damping, and m is the effective mass density

$$m = \rho_p h/b \tag{38.4}$$

in which ρ is the density of the plate, h is the thickness, and b is the width. A good approximation is to treat the pectinate zone of the basilar membrane as transverse beams with simply supported edges, for which

$$k = \frac{10\, Eh^3 c_f}{b^5} \tag{38.5}$$

in which E is the Young's modulus and c_f is the volume fraction of fibers. Thus for the moderate changes in the geometry along the cochlea as in the cat, h decreasing by a factor of 2, c_f decreasing by a factor of 12, and b increasing by a factor of 5, the stiffness k from Eq. (38.5) decreases by five orders of magnitude, which is ample for the required frequency range. Thus it is the bending stiffness of the basilar membrane pectinate zone and not the tension which governs the frequency response of the cochlea. The solution of Eq. (38.2) can be obtained by numerical or asymptotic (called *WKB* or *CLG*) methods. The result is traveling waves for which the amplitude of the basilar membrane displacement builds to a maximum and then rapidly diminishes. The parameters of K are adjusted to obtain agreement with measurements of the dynamic response in the cochlea. Often all the material of the organ of Corti is assumed to be rigidly attached to the basilar membrane so that h is relatively large and the effect of mass m is large. Then the maximum response is near the *in vacuo* resonance of the partition given by:

$$\omega^2 = \frac{b}{h}\frac{k}{\rho} \tag{38.6}$$

The following are objections to the one-dimensional (1-D) model [e.g., Siebert, 1974]: (1) The solutions of Eq. (38.2) show wavelengths of response in the region of maximum amplitude that are small in comparison with the size of the cross-section, violating the basic assumption of 1-D fluid flow. (2) In the drained cochlea, Békésy [1960] observed no resonance of the partition, so there is no significant partition mass. The significant mass is entirely from the fluid, and therefore Eq. (38.6) is not correct. This is consistent with the observations of experimental models. (3) In model studies by Békésy [1960] and others, the localization of response is independent of the area A of the cross-section. Thus Eq. (38.2) cannot govern the most interesting part of the response, the region near the maximum amplitude for a given frequency. (4) Mechanical and neural measurements in the cochlea show dispersion which is incompatible with the 1-D model [Lighthill, 1991]. (5) The 1-D model fails badly in comparison with experimental measurements in models for which the parameters of geometry, stiffness, viscosity, and density are known.

Nevertheless, the simplicity of Eq. (38.2) and the analogy with the transmission line have made the 1-D model popular. We note that there is interest in utilizing the principles in an analog model built on a silicon chip, because of the high performance of the actual cochlea. Watts [1993] reports on the first model with an electrical analog of two-dimensional (2-D) fluid in the scali. An interesting observation is that the transmission line hardware models are sensitive to failure of one component, but the 2-D model is not. In experimental models, Békésy found that a hole at one point in the membrane had little effect on the response at other points.

Two-Dimensional Model

The pioneering work with 2-D fluid motion was begun in 1931 by Ranke, as reported in Ranke [1950] and discussed by Siebert [1974]. Analysis of 2-D and 3-D fluid motion without the *a priori* assumption of long- or short-wave lengths and for physical values of all parameters is discussed by Steele [1987]. The significant features can be captured by a 2-D analysis of the fluid-partition interaction for infinite fluid depth, i.e., $A \to \infty$. For incompressible, inviscid fluid in the region $z \le 0$, the displacement potential may be written as:

$$\varphi(x, z) = e^{i(\omega t - \zeta)} \tag{38.7}$$

in which x is the distance along the cochlea, t is time, ω is frequency, and ζ is an analytic function of the complex number $x + iz$. The ratio of pressure p to the average displacement of the membrane $\overline{w}$ in the z-direction is:

$$\frac{p}{\overline{w}b} = \frac{\rho\omega^2\varphi}{g\varphi_{,z}} = \frac{\rho\omega^2}{-ig\zeta_{,z}} = \frac{\rho\omega^2}{g\zeta_{,x}} \tag{38.8}$$

in which b is the width of the membrane and g is the total width of the fluid duct. Thus the volume displacement of the membrane is equal to the net displacement of the fluid in the duct. The displacement of the fluid in the transverse y-direction is assumed to be negligible. The ratio in Eq. (38.8), multiplied by 2 to account for fluid above and below the membrane, must be equal to the membrane stiffness, which yields

$$\zeta_{,x} = \frac{2\rho\omega^2}{gK} \tag{38.9}$$

Thus, if the membrane stiffness K can be expressed as an analytic function of the distance x, the solution is exact, and ζ requires a single integration. For a physically realistic model, the mass of the membrane can be neglected and K written as

$$K = k(1 + i\epsilon) \tag{38.10}$$

in which k is the static stiffness. For many polymers, the material damping ϵ is nearly constant. If the damping comes from the viscous boundary layer of the fluid, then ϵ is approximated by

$$\epsilon \approx \zeta_{,x} \sqrt{\frac{\mu}{2\rho\omega}} \tag{38.11}$$

For water, ϵ is small with a value near 0.05 at the point of maximum amplitude.

The volume displacement of the partition is equal to the volume displacement of the input stapes. For constant duct width g, the membrane displacement can be integrated exactly, yielding the ratio of membrane to stapes displacement:

$$\frac{\overline{w}}{\delta_{st}} = i\,\frac{A_{st}}{b}\,\zeta_{,x}e^{i(\zeta_o - \zeta)} \tag{38.12}$$

where the stapes displacement and area are δ_{st} and A_{st}. The real part of ζ provides the phase of the traveling wave, and the imaginary part causes the rapid decay of amplitude past the peak. The integration of Eq. (38.9) is particularly easy for the exponential or power variation in stiffness. We note that, generally, the potential Eq. (38.7) is not bounded as $z \to -\infty$. However, it is exponentially small at a distance z from the membrane equal to the actual channel height.

The best verification of the mathematical model and calculation procedure comes from comparison with measurements in experimental models for which the parameters are known. Zhou and colleagues [1994] provide the first life-sized experimental model, designed to be similar to the human cochlea but with fluid viscosity 28 times that of water to facilitate optical imaging. Equation (38.12) gives reasonable agreement with the measurements.

Three-Dimensional Model

A further improvement in the agreement with experimental models can be obtained by adding the component of fluid motion in the direction across the membrane for a full 3-D model. The solution by direct numerical means is computationally intensive and has been carried out only by Raftenberg [1990], who reports a portion of his results for the fluid motion around the organ of Corti. The asymptotic WKB solution, however, can handle the 3-D motion easily [Steele, 1987] and provides excellent agreement with older measurements of the basilar membrane motion in the real cochlea. Before around 1980, it was thought that the processing may have two levels. First the basilar membrane and fluid provide the correct place for a given frequency (a purely mechanical "first filter"). Subsequently, the micromechanics and electrochemistry in the organ of Corti, with possible neural interactions, perform a further sharpening (a physiologically vulnerable "second filter").

38.3 The Active Process

A hint that the two-filter concept had difficulties was in the measurements of Rhode [1971], who found significant nonlinear behavior of basilar membrane in the region of the maximum amplitude at moderate amplitudes of tone intensity. Passive models cannot explain this, since the usual mechanical nonlinearities are significant only at very high intensities, i.e., at the threshold of pain. Russell and Sellick [1977] made the first in vivo mammalian intracellular hair cell recordings and found that the cells are as sharply tuned as the nerve fibers. Subsequently, improved measurement techniques in several laboratories found that the basilar membrane is actually as sharply tuned as the hair cells and the nerve fibers. Thus the sharp tuning occurs at the basilar membrane. No passive cochlear model, even with physically unreasonable parameters, has yielded amplitude and phase response similar to such measurements. Measurements in a damaged or dead cochlea show a response similar to that of a passive model. Further evidence for an active process comes from Kemp [1978], who discovered that sound pulses into the ear caused echoes coming from the cochlea at delay times corresponding to the travel time to the place for the frequency and back. Spontaneous emission of sound energy from the cochlea has now been measured in the external ear canal in all vertebrates [Probst, 1990]. Some of the emissions can be related to the hearing disability of tinnitus (ringing in the ear). The conclusion drawn from these discoveries is that normal hearing involves an active process in which the energy of the input sound is greatly enhanced. An accepted concept is that spontaneous emission of sound energy occurs when the local amplifiers are not functioning properly and enter some sort of limit cycle.

Outer-Hair-Cell Electromotility

Since the outer hair cells have sparse innervation, they have long been suspected of serving a basic motor function, perhaps beating and driving the subtectorial membrane fluid. It was surprising when Brownell and coworkers [1985] found that the outer hair cells have *electromotility:* The cell expands and contracts in an oscillating electric field, either extra- or intracellular. The electromotility exists at frequencies far higher than possible for normal contractile mechanisms [Ashmore, 1987]. The sensitivity is about 20 nm/mV (about 10^5 better than PZT-2, a widely used piezoelectric ceramic). It has not been determined if the electromotility can operate to the 200 kHz used by high-frequency mammals. However, a calculation of the cell as a pressure vessel with a fixed charge in the wall [Jen & Steele, 1987] indicates that, despite the small diameter (10 μm), the viscosity of the intra- and extracellular fluid is not a limitation to the frequency response. The motility appears to be due to a passive piezoelectric behavior of the cell plasma membrane [Kalinec et al., 1992]. Iwasa and Chadwick [1992] measured the deformation of a cell under pressure loading and voltage clamping and computed the elastic properties of the wall, assuming isotropy. It appears that for agreement with both the pressure and axial stiffness measurements, the cell wall must be orthotropic, similar to a filament-reinforced pressure vessel with close to the optimum filament angle of 52°. Note though that such a nanostructure in the cell membrane and cytoskeleton has not been found [Holley, 1990].

Hair-Cell Gating Channels

In 1984, Pickles and colleagues discovered tip links connecting the cilia of the hair cell, as shown in Fig. 38.2, that are necessary for the normal function of the cochlea. These links are about 6 nm in diameter and 200 nm long [Pickles, 1988]. Subsequent work by Hudspeth [1989] and Assad and Corey [1992] shows convincingly that there is a resting tension in the links. A displacement of the ciliary bundle in the excitatory direction increases the tension in the tip links, which causes an opening of ion channels in the cilia, which in turn decreases the intracellular potential. This depolarization causes neural excitation and in the piezoelectric outer hair cells a decrease of the cell length.

A purely mechanical analog model of the gating is in Steele [1992], in which the ion flow is replaced by viscous fluid flow and the intracellular pressure is analogous to the voltage. A constant flow-rate pump and leak channel at the base of the cell establish the steady-state condition of negative intracellular pressure, tension in the tip links, and a partially opened gate at the cilia through which there is an average magnitude of flow. The pressure drop of the flow through the gate has a nonlinear negative spring effect on the system. If the cilia are given a static displacement, the stiffness for small perturbation displacement depends on the amplitude of the initial displacement, as observed by Hudspeth [1989]. For oscillatory forcing of the cilia, the fluid analog shows that a gain in power is possible, as in an electrical or fluidic amplifier, and that a modest change in the parameters can lead to instability.

Thus it appears that amplification in the cochlea resides in the gating of the outer-hair-cell cilia, and the

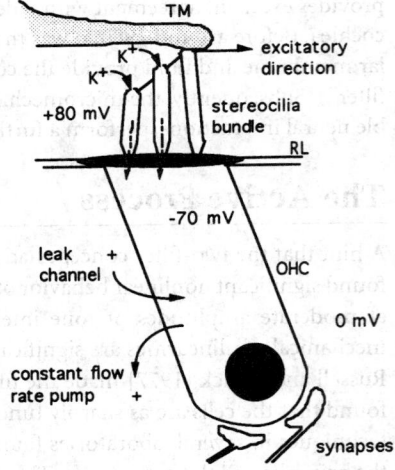

FIGURE 38.2 Model of outer hair cell. The normal pumping of ions produces negative intracellular electrical potential. Displacement of the cilia in the excitatory direction causes an increase in tension in the tip links, which opens the ion gates and decreases the intracellular potential, causing a piezoelectric contraction of the cell and excitation of the neural synapses. This can be modeled by a constant flow rate pump, leak channel, and spring-controlled gate. The mechanical effect of the flow on the gate is important.

motility is due to passive piezoelectric properties of the cell wall. The flow through the gate has significant nonlinearity at small amplitudes of displacement of the cilia (10 nm). Sufficiently high amplitudes of displacement of the cilia will cause the tip links to buckle. We estimate that this will occur at around 70 dB sound pressure level, thereby turning off the active process for higher sound intensity.

There may be a connection between the gating channels and the discovery by Canlon and coworkers [1988]. They find that acoustic stimulation of the wall of the isolated outer hair cell causes a tonic (DC) expansion of the cell over a narrow frequency band, which is related to the place for the cell along the cochlea. Khanna and colleagues [1989] observe a similar tonic displacement of the whole organ of Corti.

38.4 Active Models

Allen and Neely [1992], De Boer, [1991], Geisler [1993], and Hubbard [1993] discuss models in which the electromotility of the outer hair cells feeds energy into the basilar membrane. The partition stiffness K is expanded from Eq. (38.3) into a transfer function, containing a number of parameters and delay times. These are classed as phenomenological models for which the physiological basis of the parameters is not of primary concern. The displacement gain may be defined as the ratio of ciliary shearing displacement to cell expansion. For these models the gain used is larger by orders of magnitude than the maximum found in laboratory measurements.

Another approach, which is physiologically based, appears promising. The outer hair cells are inclined in the propagation direction. Thus the shearing of the cilia at the distance x causes a force from the hair cells acting on the basilar membrane at the distance $x + \Delta x$. This feed-forward law can be expressed in terms of the pressure as

$$p_c(x + \Delta x) = \alpha p(x) = \alpha \left[2p_f(x) + p_c(x) \right] \tag{38.13}$$

where p, the total pressure acting on the basilar membrane, consists of the effective pressure acting on the basilar membrane from the hair cells p_c and the pressure from the fluid p_f. The coefficient α is the force gain supplied by the outer hair cells. With this law, Eq. (38.9) is replaced by:

$$\zeta_{,x} \left(1 - \alpha e^{i\zeta_{,x}\Delta x} \right) = \frac{2\rho\omega^2}{gK} \tag{38.14}$$

from which the local wave number $\zeta_{,x}$ must be computed numerically. Only two new parameters are needed: the gain α and the spacing Δx. With physiologically reasonable gain $\alpha = 0.18$ and spacing $\Delta x = 20$ μm, the result is an increase of the response of the basilar membrane for higher frequencies by a factor of 100 in a narrow sector, apical to the passive peak. The simple feed-forward law Eq. (38.14) enhances a narrow band of wave lengths without a closed control loop. At this time, it appears that much of the elaborate structure of the organ of Corti is for the purpose of such a "feed forward." Some preliminary results are shown in Figs. 38.3 and 38.4.

38.5 Fluid Streaming?

Békésy [1960] and many others have observed significant fluid streaming in the actual cochlea and in experimental models. Particularly for the high frequencies, it is tempting to seek a component of steady streaming as the significant mechanical stimulation of the inner hair cells [Lighthill, 1992]. Passive models indicated that such streaming occurs only at high sound intensity. Among the many open questions is whether the enhancement of amplitude provided by the feed-forward of energy by the outer hair cells and the mechanical nonlinearity at low amplitudes of displacement provided by the ciliar gating can trigger significant streaming.

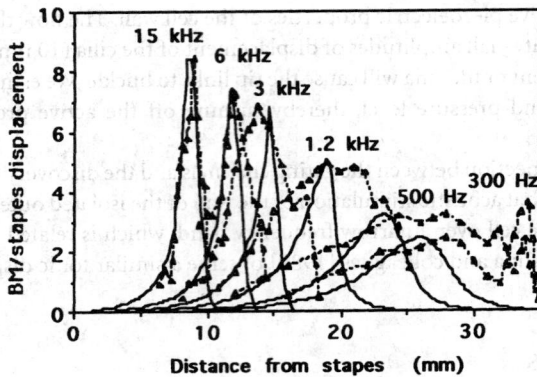

FIGURE 38.3 Comparison of 3-D model calculations (solid curves) with experimental results of Zhou et al. [1994] (dashed curves) for the amplitude envelopes for different frequencies. This is a life-size model, but with an isotropic BM and fluid viscosity 28 times that of water. The agreement is reasonable, except for the lower frequencies.

38.6 Clinical Possibilities

A better understanding of the cochlear mechanisms would be of clinical value. Auditory pathology related to the inner ear is discussed by Pickles [1988] and Gulick and coworkers [1989]. The spontaneous and stimulated emissions from the cochlea raise the possibility of diagnosing local inner ear

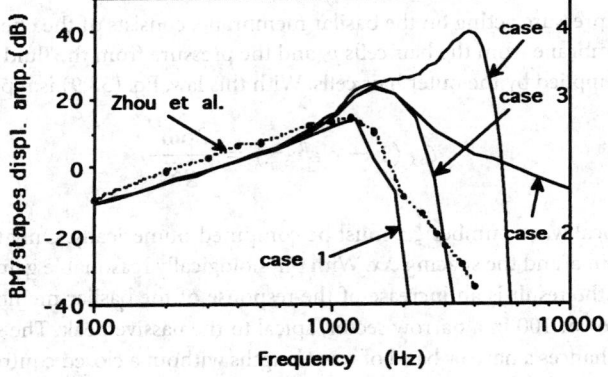

FIGURE 38.4 Comparison of 3-D model calculations with experimental results of Zhou et al. [1994] for amplitude at the place $x = 19$ mm as a function of frequency. The scales are logarithmic (20 dB is a factor of 10 in amplitude). Case 1 shows a direct comparison with the physical parameters of the experiment, with isotropic BM and viscosity 28 times that of water. Case 2 is computed for the viscosity reduced to that of water. Case 3 is computed for the BM made of transverse fibers. Case 4 shows the effect of active OHC feedforward, with the pressure gain $\alpha = 0.21$ and feed-forward distance $\Delta x = 25$ microns. Thus lower viscosity, BM orthotropy, and active feed-forward all contribute to higher amplitude and increased localization of the response.

problems, which is being pursued at various centers. The capability for more accurate, physically realistic modeling of the cochlea should assist in this process.

A patient with a completely nonfunctioning cochlea is referred to as having "nerve deafness." In fact, there is evidence that in many cases the nerves may be intact, but the receptor cells and organ of Corti are defective. For such patients, a goal is to restore hearing with cochlear electrode implants to directly stimulate the nerve endings. This goal is a great challenge, and significant progress has been made. However, despite electrode stimulation of nerves at the correct place along the cochlea for a high frequency, the perception of high frequency has not been achieved. So, although substantial advance in cochlear physiology has been made in the recent past, several such waves of progress may be needed to understand adequately the functioning of the cochlea.

References

Allen JB, Neely ST. 1992. Micromechanical models of the cochlea. Physics Today 45:40.

Ashmore JF. 1987. A fast motile response in guinea-pig outer hair cells: the cellular basis of the cochlear amplifier. J Physiol 388:323.

Assad JA, Corey DP. 1992. An active motor model for adaptation by vertebrate hair cells. J Neurosci 12(9):3291.

Békésy G von. 1960. Experiments in Hearing, New York, McGraw-Hill.

Brownell WE, Bader CR, Bertrand D, et al. 1985. Evoked mechanical responses of isolated cochlear outer hair cells. Science 227:194.

Canlon B, Brundlin L, Flock Å. 1988. Acoustic stimulation causes tonotopic alterations in the length of isolated outer hair cells from the guinea pig hearing organ. Proc Natl Acad Sci USA 85:7033.

Cabezudo LM. 1978. The ultrastructure of the basilar membrane in the cat. Acta Otolaryngol 86:160.

Dallos P. 1992. The active cochlea. J Neurosci 12(12):4575.

De Boer E. 1991. Auditory physics: III. Physical principles in hearing theory. Phys Rep 203(3):126.

Freeman DM, Weiss TF. 1990. Hydrodynamic analysis of a two-dimensional model for micromechanical resonance of free-standing hair bundles. Hear Res 48:37.

Fuhrmann E, Schneider W, Schultz M. 1987. Wave propagation in the cochlea (inner ear): Effects of Reissner's membrane and non-rectangular cross section. Acta Mechanica 70:15.

Geisler CD. 1993. A realizable cochlear model using feedback from motile outer hair cells. Hear Res 68:253.

Gulick WL, Gescheider GA, Fresina RD. 1989. Hearing: Physiological Acoustics, Neural Coding, and Psychoacoustics, London, Oxford University Press.

Gummer AW, Johnston BM, Armstrong NJ. 1981. Direct measurements of basilar membrane stiffness in the guinea pig. J Acoust Soc Am 70:1298.

Holley MD. 1990. Cell biology of hair cells. Seminars in the Neurosciences 2:41.

Hubbard, AE. 1993. A traveling wave-amplifier model of the cochlea. Science 259:68.

Hudspeth AJ. 1989. How the ear's works work. Nature 34:397.

Iwasa KH, Chadwick RS. 1992. Elasticity and active force generation of cochlear outer hair cells. J Acoust Soc Am 92:3169.

Jen DH, Steele CR. 1987. Electrokinetic model of cochlear hair cell motility. J Acoust Soc Am 82:1667.

Kalinec F, Holley MC, Iwasa KH, et al. 1992. A membrane-based force generation mechanism in auditory sensory cells. Proc Natl Acad Sci USA 89:8671.

Keidel WD, Neff WD. 1976. Handbook of Sensory Physiology, vol 5: Auditory System. Berlin, Springer-Verlag.

Kemp DT. 1978. Stimulated acoustic emissions from within the human auditory system. J Acoust Soc Am 64:1386.

Khanna SM, Flock Å, Ulfendahl, M. 1989. Comparison of the tuning of outer hair cells and the basilar membrane in the isolated cochlea. Acta Otolaryngol [Suppl] (Stockholm) 467:141.

Lighthill J. 1991. Biomechanics of hearing sensitivity. J Vibration and Acoustics 113:1.

Lighthill J. 1992. Acoustic streaming in the ear itself. J Fluid Mech 239:551.

Miller CE. 1985. Structural implications of basilar membrane compliance measurements. J Acoust Soc Am 77:1465.

Olson ES, Mountain DC. 1994. Mapping the cochlear partition's stiffness to its cellular architecture. J Acoust Soc Am 95(1):395.

Pickles JO. 1988. An Introduction to the Physiology of Hearing, 2d ed., London, Academic Press.

Probst R. 1990. Otoacoustic emissions: An overview. Adv Otorhinolaryngol 44:1.

Raftenberg MN. 1990. Flow of endolymph in the inner spiral sulcus and the subtectorial space. J Acoust Soc Am 87(6):2606.

Ranke OF. 1950. Theory of operation of the cochlea: A contribution to the hydrodynamics of the cochlea. J Acoust Soc Am 22:772.

Rhode WS. 1971. Observations of the vibration of the basilar membrane in squirrel monkeys using the Mössbauer technique. J Acoust Soc Am 49:1218.

Ruggero MA. 1993. Distortion in those good vibrations. Current Biology 3(11):755.

Russell IJ, Sellick PM. 1977. Tuning properties of cochlear hair cells. Nature 267:858.

Siebert WM. 1974. Ranke revisited—a simple short-wave cochlear model. J Acoust Soc Am 56(2):594.

Steele CR. 1987. Cochlear mechanics. In R Skalak, S Chien (eds), Handbook of Bioengineering, pp 30.11–30.22, New York, McGraw-Hill.

Steele CR. 1992. Electroelastic behavior of auditory receptor cells. Biomimetics 1(1):3.

Strelioff D, Flock Å. 1984. Stiffness of sensory-cell hair bundles in the isolated guinea pig cochlea. Hear Res 15:19.

Watts L. 1993. Cochlear Mechanics: Analysis and Analog VLSI, thesis, California Institute of Technology.

West CD. 1985. The relationship of the spiral turns of the cochlea and the length of the basilar membrane to the range of audible frequencies in ground dwelling mammals. J Acoust Soc Am 77(3):1091.

Zhou G, Bintz L, Anderson DZ, et al. 1994. A life-sized physical model of the human cochlea with optical holographic readout. J Acoust Soc Am 93(3):1516.

Zwislocki JJ, Cefaratti LK. 1989. Tectorial membrane: II. Stiffness measurements in vivo. Hear Res 42:211.

Further Information

The following are workshop proceedings that document most of the most recent developments on the subject.

Allen JB, Hall JL, Hubbard A, et al. (eds). 1985. Peripheral Auditory Mechanisms, Berlin, Springer.

Dallos P, Geisler CD, Matthews JW, et al. (eds). 1990. The Mechanics and Biophysics of Hearing, Berlin, Springer.

De Boer E, Viergever MA (eds). 1983. Mechanics of Hearing, The Hague, Nijhoff.

Duifhuis H, Horst JW, van Kijk P, et al. (eds). 1993. Biophysics of Hair Cell Sensory Systems, Singapore, World Scientific.

Wilson JP, Kemp DT (eds). 1988. Cochlear Mechanisms: Structure, Function, and Models, New York, Plenum.

39

Vestibular Mechanics

Wallace Grant
Virginia Polytechnic Institute
and State University

The vestibular system is responsible for sensing motion and gravity and using this information for control of postural and body motion. This sense is also used to control eyes position during head movement, allowing for a clear visual image. Vestibular function is rather inconspicuous and for this reason is frequently not recognized for its vital roll in maintaining balance and equilibrium and in controlling eye movements. Vestibular function is truly a sixth sense, different from the five originally defined by Greek physicians.

The vestibular system is named for its position within the vestibule of the temporal bone of the skull. It is located in the inner ear along with the auditory sense. The vestibular system has both central and peripheral components. This chapter deals with the mechanical sensory function of the peripheral end organ and its ability to measure linear and angular inertial motion of the skull over the frequency ranges encountered in normal activities.

39.1 Structure and Function

The vestibular system in each ear consists of the *otolith* and saccule (collectively called the *otolithic organs*) which are the linear motion sensors, and the three *semicircular canals* (SCCs) which sense rotational motion. The SCC are oriented in three nearly mutually perpendicular planes so that angular motion about any axis may be sensed. The otoliths and SCC consist of membranous structures which are situated in hollowed out sections of the temporal bone. This hollowed out section of the temporal bone is called the *bony labyrinth,* and the membranous labyrinth lies within this bony structure. The membranous labyrinth is filled with a fluid called *endolymph,* which is high in potassium, and the volume between the membranous and bony labyrinths is filled with a fluid called *perilymph*, which is similar to blood plasma.

The otolith sits in the utricle, and the saccule is located within membranous saccule. Each of these organs is rigidly attached to the temporal bone of the skull with connective tissue. The three semicircular canals terminate on the utricle forming a complete circular fluid path, and the membranous canals are also rigidly attached to the bony skull. This rigid attachment is vital to the roll of measuring inertial motion of the skull.

Each SCC has a bulge called the *ampulla* near one end, and inside the ampulla is the cupula, which is formed of saccharide gel. The capula forms a complete hermetic seal with the ampulla, and the cupula sits on top of the crista, which contains the sensory receptor cells called *hair cells.* These hair cells have small stereocilia (hairs) which extend into the cupula and sense its deformation. When the head is rotated the endolymph fluid, which fills the canal, tends to remain at rest due to its inertia, the relative flow of fluid in the canal deforms the cupula like a diaphragm, and the hair cells transduce the deformation into nerve signals.

The otolithic organs are flat layered structures covered above with endolymph. The top layer consists of calcium carbonate crystals called *otoconia* which are bound together by a saccharide gel. The middle layer consists of pure saccharide gel, and the bottom layer consists of receptor hair cells which have stereocilia that extend into the gel layer. When the head is accelerated, the dense otoconial crystals tend to remain at rest due to their inertia as the sensory layer tends to move away form the otoconial layer. This relative motion between the otoconial layer and the sensory layer deforms the gel layer. The hair cell stereocilia sense this deformation, and the receptor cells transduce this deformation into nerve signals. When the head is tilted, the weight acting on the otoconial layer also will deform the gel layer. The hair cell stereocilia also have directional sensitivity which allows them to determine the direction of the acceleration acting in the plane of the otolith and saccule. The planes of the two organs are arranged perpendicular to each other so that linear acceleration in any direction can be sensed. The vestibular nerve, which forms half of the VIII cranial nerve, innervates all the receptor cells of the vestibular apparatus.

39.2 Otolith Distributed Parameter Model

The otoliths are an overdamped second-order system whose structure is shown in Fig. 39.1. In this model the otoconial layer is assumed to be a rigid and nondeformable, the gel layer is a deformable layer of isotropic viscoelastic material, and the fluid endolymph is assumed to be a newtonian fluid. A small element of the layered structure with surface area dA is cut from the surface, and a vertical view of this surface element, of width dx, is shown in Fig. 39.2. To evaluate the forces that are pres-

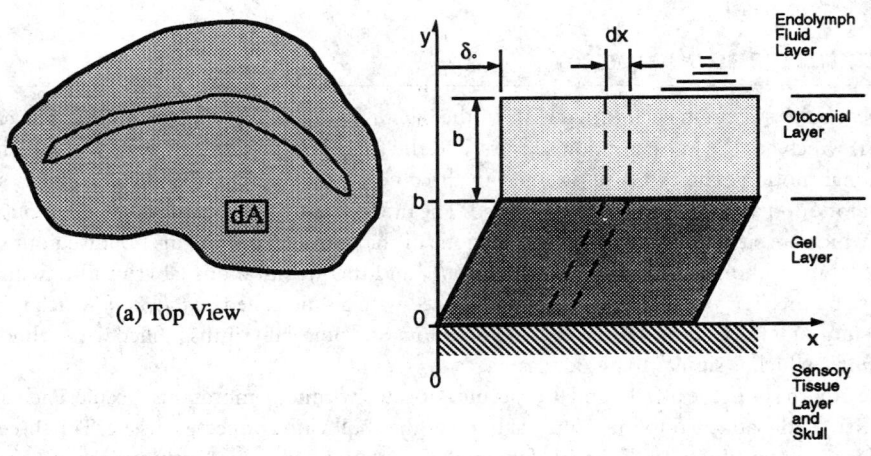

(a) Top View

(b) Cross-Section

FIGURE 39.1   Schematic of the otolith organ: (a) Top view showing the peripheral region with differential area dA where the model is developed. (b) Cross-section showing the layered structure where dx is the width of the differential area dA shown in the top view at the left.

Endolymph Fluid Layer The spatial coordinate in the vertical direction is y_f, and the velocity of the endolymph fluid is $u(y_f,t)$, a function of the fluid depth y_f and time t.

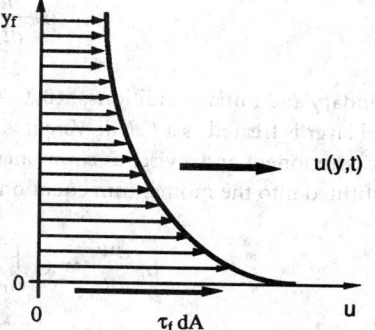

Otoconial Layer The otoconial layer with thickenss b and at a height b above the gel layer vertical coordinate origin. The velocity of the otoconial layer is $v(t)$, which is a function of time only.

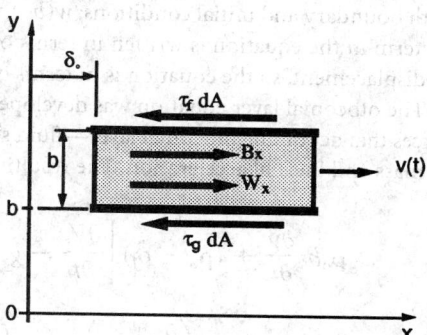

Gel Layer Gel layer of thickness c, vertical coordinate y_g, and horizontal coordinate δ_g the gel deflection. The gel deflection is a function of both y_g and time t. The velocity of the gel is $w(y_g, t)$, a function of y_g and t.

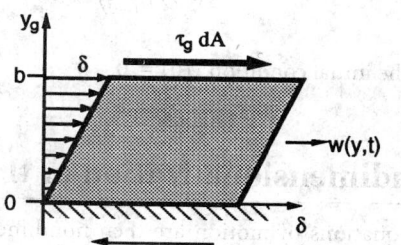

FIGURE 39.2 The free-body diagrams of each layer of the otolith with the forces that act on each layer. The interfaces are coupled by shear stresses of equal magnitude that act in opposite directions at each surface. The τ_g shear stress acts between the gel-otoconial layer, and the τ_f acts between the fluid-otoconial layer. The forces acting at these interfaces are the product of shear stress τ and area dA. The B_x and W_x forces are respectively the components of the buoyant and weight forces acting in the plane of the otoconial layer. See the nomenclature table for definitions of other variables.

ent, free-body diagrams are constructed of each elemental layer of the small differential strip. See the nomenclature table for a description of all variables used in the following formulas, and for derivation details see Grant and colleagues [1984, 1991].

In the equation of motion for the endolymph fluid, the force $\tau_f dA$ acts on the fluid at the fluid-otoconial layer interface. This shear stress τ_f is responsible for driving the fluid flow. The linear Navier-Stokes equations for an incompressible fluid are used to describe this endolymph flow. Expressions for the pressure gradient, the flow velocity of the fluid measured with respect to an inertial reference frame, and the force due to gravity (body force) are substituted into the Navier-Stokes equation for flow in the x-direction yielding

$$\rho_f \frac{\partial u}{\partial t} = \mu_f \frac{\partial^2 u}{\partial y_f^2} \tag{39.1}$$

with boundary and initial conditions: $u(0, t) = v(t)$; $u(\infty, t) = 0$; $u(y_f, 0) = 0$.

The gel layer is treated as a *Kelvin-Voight viscoelastic material* where the gel shear stress has both an elastic component and a viscous component acting in parallel. This viscoelastic material model was substituted into the momentum equation, and the resulting gel layer equation of motion is

$$\rho_f \frac{\partial w}{\partial t} = G \int_0^t \left(\frac{\partial^2 w}{\partial y_f^2} \right) dt + \mu_f \frac{\partial^2 w}{\partial y_f^2} \tag{39.2}$$

with boundary and initial conditions: $w(b,t) = v(t)$; $w(0,t) = 0$; $w(y_g,0) = 0$; $\delta_g(y_g,0) = 0$. The elastic term in the equation is written in terms of the integral of velocity with respect to time, instead of displacement, so the equation is in terms of a single dependent variable, the velocity.

The otoconial layer equation was developed using Newton's second law of motion, equating the forces that act on the otoconial layer—fluid shear, gel shear, buoyancy, and weight—to the product of mass and inertial acceleration. The resulting otoconial layer equation is

$$\rho_o b \frac{\partial v}{\partial t} + (\rho_o - \rho_f) \left[\frac{\partial V_s}{\partial t} - g_x \right]$$

$$= \mu_f \left(\frac{\partial u}{\partial y_f} \bigg|_{y_f=0} \right) - G \int_0^t \left(\frac{\partial w}{\partial y_g} \bigg|_{y_g=b} \right) dt + \mu_g \left(\frac{\partial w}{\partial y_g} \bigg|_{y_g=b} \right) \tag{39.3}$$

with the initial condition $v(0) = 0$.

39.3 Nondimensionalization of the Motion Equations

The equations of motion are then nondimensionalized to reduce the number of physical and dimensional parameters and combine them into some useful nondimensional numbers. The following nondimensional variables, which are indicated by overbars, are introduced into the motion equations:

$$\bar{y}_f = \frac{y_f}{b} \qquad \bar{y}_g = \frac{y_g}{b} \qquad \bar{t} = \left(\frac{\mu_f}{\rho_o b^2} \right) t \qquad \bar{u} = \frac{u}{V} \qquad \bar{v} = \frac{v}{V} \qquad \bar{w} = \frac{w}{V} \tag{39.4}$$

Several nondimensional parameters occur naturally as a part of the nondimensionalization process. These parameters are

$$R = \frac{\rho_f}{\rho_o} \qquad \epsilon = \frac{Gb^2\rho_o}{\mu_f^2} \qquad M = \frac{\mu_g}{\mu_f} \qquad \bar{g}_x = \left(\frac{\rho_o b^2}{V\mu_f} \right) g_x \tag{39.5}$$

These parameters represent the following: R is the density ratio, ϵ is a nondimensional elastic parameter, M is the viscosity ratio and represents a major portion of the system damping, and $\bar{g}_x$ is the nondimensional gravity.

The governing equations of motion in nondimensional form are then as follows. For the endolymph fluid layer

$$R\frac{\partial \overline{u}}{\partial \overline{t}} = \frac{\partial^2 \overline{u}}{\partial \overline{y}_f^2} \tag{39.6}$$

with boundary conditions of $\overline{u}(0,\overline{t}) = \overline{v}(\overline{t})$ and $\overline{u}(\infty,\overline{t}) = 0$ and initial conditions of $\overline{u}(\overline{y}_f, 0) = 0$. For the otoconial layer

$$\frac{\partial \overline{v}}{\partial \overline{t}} + (1 - R)\left[\frac{\partial \overline{V}_s}{\partial \overline{t}} - \overline{g}_x\right] = \left(\frac{\partial \overline{u}}{\partial \overline{y}_f}\Big|_0\right) - \epsilon \int_0^t \left(\frac{\partial \overline{w}}{\partial \overline{y}_g}\Big|_1\right) dt - M\left(\frac{\partial \overline{w}}{\partial \overline{y}_g}\Big|_1\right) \tag{39.7}$$

with an initial condition of $\overline{v}(0) = 0$. For the gel layer

$$R\frac{\partial \overline{w}}{\partial \overline{t}} = \epsilon \int_o^{\overline{t}} \left(\frac{\partial^2 \overline{w}}{\partial \overline{y}_g^2}\right) d\overline{t} + M\frac{\partial^2 \overline{w}}{\partial \overline{y}_g^2} \tag{39.8}$$

with boundary conditions of $\overline{w}(1,\overline{t}) = \overline{v}(\overline{t})$ and $\overline{w}(0,\overline{t}) = 0$ and initial conditions of $\overline{w}(\overline{y}_g, 0) = 0$ and $\overline{\delta}_g(\overline{y}_g, 0) = 0$.

These equations can be solved numerically for the case of a step change in velocity of the skull. This solution can be found in Grant and Cotton [1991].

39.4 Otolith Transfer Function

A transfer function of otoconial layer deflection related to skull acceleration can be obtained from the governing equations. For details of this derivation see Grant and colleagues [1994].

Starting with the nondimensional fluid and gel layer equations, taking the Laplace transform with respect to time, and using the initial conditions give two ordinary differential equations. These equations can then be solved, using the boundary conditions. Taking the Laplace transform of the otoconial layer motion equation, combining with the two differential equation solutions, and integrating otoconial layer velocity to get deflection produces the transfer function for displacement re acceleration

$$\frac{\delta_o}{A}(s) = \frac{(1 - R)}{s\left[s + \sqrt{Rs} + \left(\frac{\epsilon}{s} + M\right)\sqrt{\frac{Rs}{\frac{\epsilon}{s} + M}}\coth\left(\sqrt{\frac{Rs}{\frac{\epsilon}{s} + M}}\right)\right]} \tag{39.9}$$

where the overbars denoting nondimensional variables have been dropped, s is the Laplace transform variable, and a general acceleration term A is defined as

$$A = -\left(\frac{\partial V_s}{\partial t} - g_x\right) \tag{39.10}$$

39.5 Otolith Frequency Response

This transfer function can now be studied in the frequency domain. It should be noted that these are linear partial differential equations and that the process of frequency domain analysis is appropriate. The range of values of $\epsilon = 0.01$–0.2, $M = 5$–20, and $R = 0.75$ have been established by Grant and Cotton [1991] in a numerical finite difference solution of the governing equations. With these values established, the frequency response can be completed.

In order to construct a magnitude- and phase-versus-frequency plot of the transfer function, the nondimensional time will be converted back to real time for use on the frequency axis. For the conversion to real time the following physical variables will be used: $\rho_o = 1.35$ g/cm^3, $b = 15$ μm, $\mu_f = 0.85$ mPa · s. The general frequency response is shown in Fig. 39.3. The flat response form DC up to the first corner frequency establishes this system as an accelerometer. This is the range-of-motion frequencies encountered in normal motion environments where this transducer is expected to function.

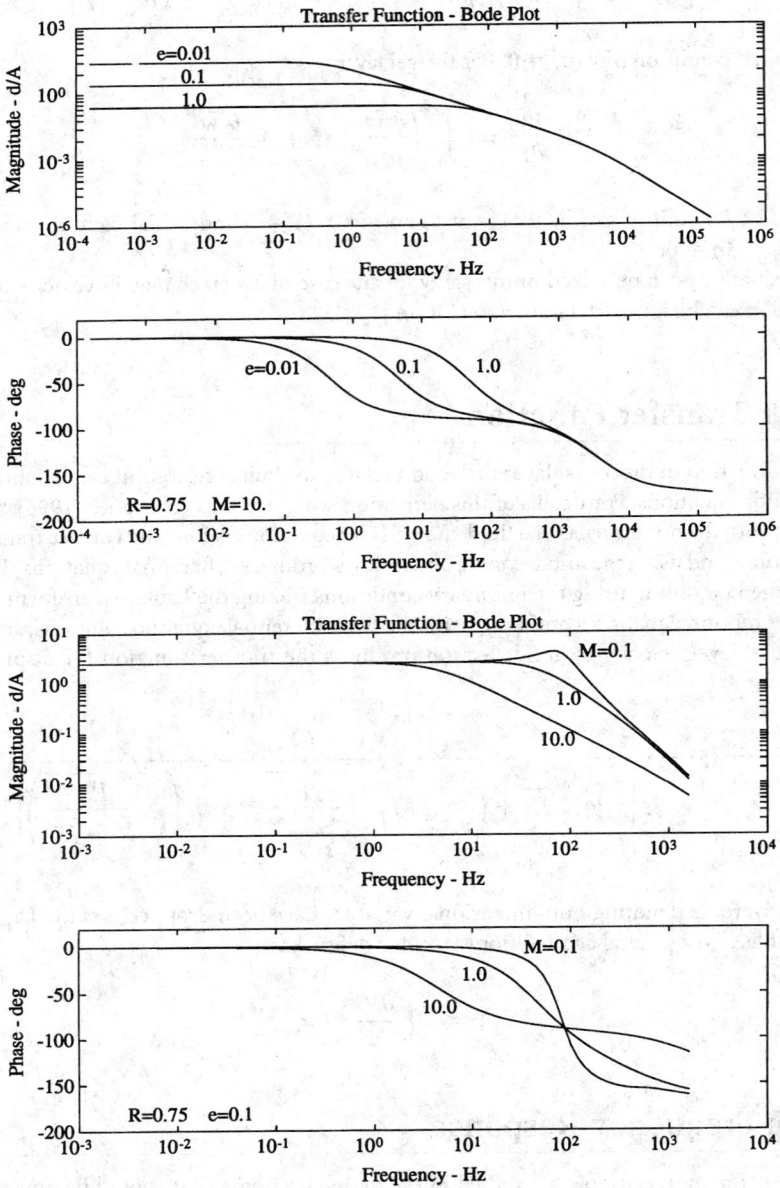

FIGURE 39.3 General performance of the otoconial layer transfer function shown for various values of the nondimensional elastic parameter ϵ and M. For these evaluations the other parameter was held constant and $R = 0.75$. The value of $M = 0.1$ shows an underdamped response which is entirely feasible with the model formulation, since no restriction was incorporated which limits the response to that of an overdamped system.

The range of flat response can be easily controlled with the two parameters ϵ and M. It is interesting to note that both the elastic term and the system damping are controlled by the gel layer, and thus an animal can easily control the system response by changing the parameters of this saccharide gel layer. The cross-linking of saccharide gels is extremely variable, yielding vastly different elastic and viscous properties of the resulting structure.

The otoconial layer transfer function can be compared to recent data from single-fiber neural recording. The only discrepancy between the experimental data and theoretical model is a low-frequency phase lead and accompanying amplitude reduction. This has been observed in most experimental single-fiber recordings and has been attributed to the hair cell.

39.6 Semicircular Canal Distributed Parameter Model

The membranous SCC duct is modeled as a section of a rigid torus filled with an incompressible newtonian fluid. The governing equations of motion for the fluid are developed from the Navier-Stokes equations. Refer to the nomenclature section for definition of all variables, and Fig. 39.4 for a cross-section of the SCC and utricle.

We are interested in the flow of endolymph fluid with respect to the duct wall, and this requires that the inertial motion of the duct wall $R\Omega$ be added to the fluid velocity u measured with respect to the duct wall. The curvature of the duct can be shown to be negligible since $a \ll R$, and no secondary flow is induced; thus the curve duct can be treated as straight. Pressure gradients arise from two sources in the duct: (1) the utricle, (2) the cupula. The cupula when deflected exerts a restoring force on the endolymph. The cupula can be modeled as a membrane with linear stiffness $K = \Delta p/\Delta V$, where Δp is the pressure difference across the cupula and ΔV is the volumetric displacement, where

$$\Delta V = 2\pi \int_0^t \int_0^a u\,(r,\,t)\,r dr\,dt \qquad (39.11)$$

If the angle subtended by the membranous duct is denoted by β, the pressure gradient in the duct produced by the cupula is

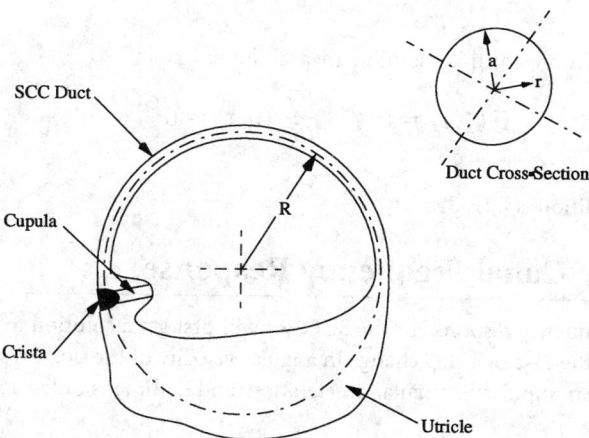

FIGURE 39.4 Schematic structure of the semicircular canal showing a cross-section through the canal duct and utricle. Also shown in the upper right corner is a cross-section of the duct. R is the radius of curvature of the semicircular canal, a is the inside radius to the duct wall, and r is the spatial coordinate in the radial direction of the duct.

$$\frac{\partial p}{\partial z} = \frac{K\Delta V}{\beta R} \qquad (39.12)$$

The utricle pressure gradient can be approximated [see Van Buskirk, 1977] by

$$\frac{\partial p}{\partial z} = \frac{(2\pi - \beta)}{\beta}\rho R\alpha \qquad (39.13)$$

When this information is substituted into the Navier-Stokes equation, the following governing equation for endolymph flow relative to the duct wall is obtained:

$$\frac{\partial u}{\partial t} + \left(\frac{2\pi}{\beta}\right)R\alpha = -\frac{2\pi K}{\rho\beta R}\int_0^t\int_0^a u\,(rdr)\,dt + v\frac{1}{r}\frac{\partial}{\partial r}\left(r\frac{\partial u}{\partial r}\right) \qquad (39.14)$$

This equation can be nondimensionalized using the following nondimensional variables denoted by overbars

$$\bar{r} = \frac{r}{a} \qquad \bar{t} = \left(\frac{v}{a^2}\right)t \qquad \bar{u} = \frac{u}{R\Omega} \qquad (39.15)$$

where Ω is a characteristic angular velocity of the canal. In terms of the nondimensional variables, the governing equation for endolymph flow velocity becomes

$$\frac{\partial\bar{u}}{\partial\bar{t}} + \left(\frac{2\pi}{\beta}\right)\alpha(\bar{t}) = -\epsilon\int_0^{\bar{t}}\int_0^1(\bar{u}\,\bar{r}d\bar{r})\,d\bar{t} + \frac{1}{\bar{r}}\frac{\partial}{\partial\bar{r}}\left(\bar{r}\frac{\partial\bar{u}}{\partial\bar{r}}\right) \qquad (39.16)$$

where the nondimensional parameter ϵ is defined by

$$\epsilon = \frac{2K\pi a^6}{\rho\beta Rv^2} \qquad (39.17)$$

The boundary conditions for this equation are as follows:

$$\bar{u}\,(1,\bar{t}) = 0 \qquad \frac{\partial\bar{u}}{\partial\bar{r}}\,(0,\bar{t}) = 0$$

and the initial condition is $\bar{u}\,(\bar{r},0) = 0$.

39.7 Semicircular Canal Frequency Response

To examine the frequency response of the SCC, we will first get a solution to the nondimensional canal equation for the case of a step change in angular velocity of the skull. A step in angular velocity corresponds to an impulse in angular acceleration, and in dimensionless form this impulse is

$$\alpha(t) = -\Omega\delta(t) \qquad (39.18)$$

where $\delta(t)$ is the unit impulse function and Ω is again a characteristic angular velocity of the canal. The nondimensional volumetric displacement is defined as

$$\phi = \int_0^{\bar{t}}\int_0^1(\bar{u}\,\bar{r}d\bar{r})\,d\bar{t} \qquad (39.19)$$

the dimensional volumetric displacement is given by $\Delta V = (4\pi R\Omega a^4/v)\phi$ and the solution (for $\epsilon \ll 1$) is given by

$$\phi = \sum_{n=1}^{\infty} \frac{2\,(2\pi/\beta)}{\lambda_n^4} \tag{39.20}$$

where λ_n represents the roots of the equation $J_0(x) = 0$, where J_0 is the Bessel function of zero order ($\lambda_1 = 2.405$, $\lambda_2 = 5.520$), and for infinite time $\phi = \pi/8\beta$. For details of the solution see Van Buskirk and Grant [1987] and Van Buskirk and coworkers [1978].

A transfer function can be developed from the previous solution for a step change in angular velocity of the canal. The transfer function of mean angular displacement of endolymph θ related to ω, the angular velocity of the head, is

$$\frac{\theta}{\omega}(s) = \left(s\frac{(2\pi/\beta)\lambda_1^2}{8}\right)\left(\frac{1}{\left(s + \dfrac{1}{\tau_L}\right)\left(s + \dfrac{1}{\tau_s}\right)}\right) \tag{39.21}$$

where $\tau_L = 8\rho v\beta R/K\pi a^4$, $\tau_s = a^2/\lambda_1^2 v$, and s is the Laplace transform variable.

The utility of the above transfer function is apparent when used to generate the frequency response of the system. The values for the various parameters are as follows: $a = 0.15$ mm, $R = 3.2$ mm, the dynamic viscosity of endolymph $\mu = 0.85$ mPa $\cdot$ s ($v = \mu/\rho$), $\rho = 1000$ kg/m³, $\beta = 1.4\pi$, and $K = 3.4$ GPa/m³. This produces values of the two time constants of $\tau_L = 20.8$ s and $\tau_s = 0.00385$ s. The frequency response of the system can be see in Fig. 39.5. The range of frequencies from

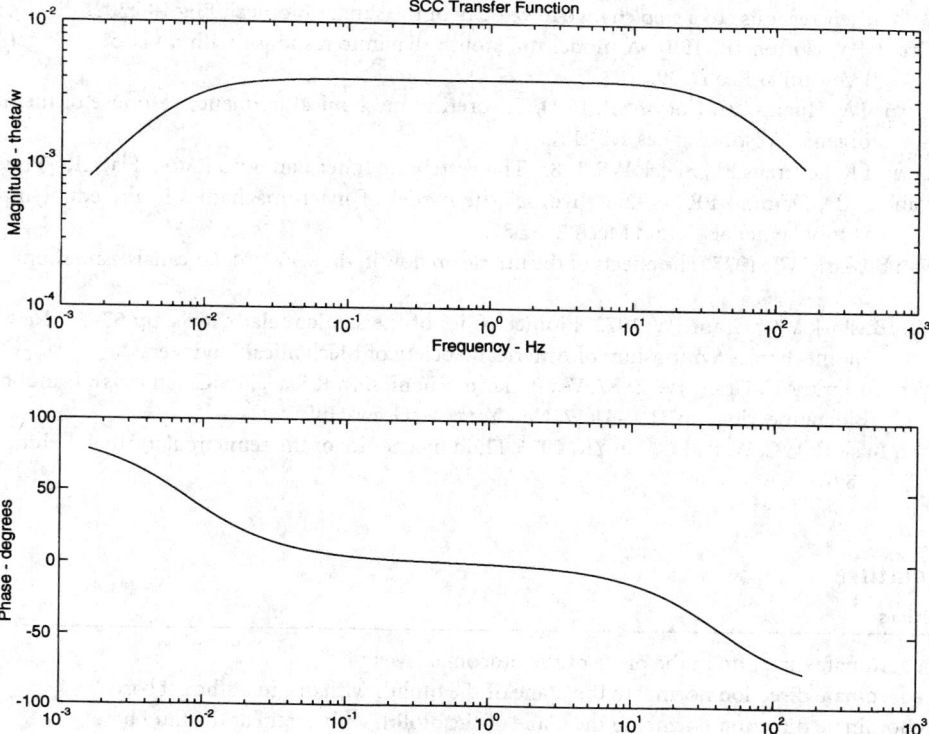

FIGURE 39.5 Frequency response of the human semicircular canals for the transfer function of mean angular displacement of endolymph fluid θ related to angular velocity of the head ω.

0.01 Hz to 30 Hz establishes the SCCs as angular velocity transducers of head motion. This range of frequencies is that encountered in everyday movement. Environments such as an aircraft flight can produce frequencies outside the linear range for these transducers.

Rabbit and Damino [1992] have modeled the flow of endolymph in the ampulla and its interaction with a cupula. This model indicates that the cupula in the mechanical system appears to add a high-frequency gain enhancement as well as phase lead over previous mechanical models. This is consistent with measurements of vestibular nerve recordings of gain and phase. Prior to this work this gain and phase enhancement were thought to be of hair cell origin.

Defining Terms

Endolymph: Fluid similar to intercellular fluid (high in potassium) which fills the membranous labyrinth, canals, utricle, and saccule.

Kelvin-Voight viscoelastic material: The simplest of solid materials which have both elastic and viscous responses to deformation. The viscous and elastic responses appear to act in parallel.

Otolith: Linear accelerometers of the vestibular system whose primary transduced signal is the sum of linear acceleration and gravity in the frequency range from DC (static) up to the maximum experienced by an animal.

Semicircular canals: Angular motion sensors of the vestibular system whose primary transduced signal is angular velocity in the frequency range of normal animal motion.

References

Grant JW, Best WA, Lonegro R. 1984. Governing equations of motion for the otolith organs and their response to a step change in velocity of the skull. J Biomech Eng 106:302.

Grant JW, Cotton JR. 1991. A model for otolith dynamic response with a viscoelastic gel layer. J Vestibular Res 1:139.

Grant JW, Huang CC, Cotton JR. 1994. Theoretical mechanical frequency response of the otolith organs. J Vestibular Res 4(2):137.

Lewis ER, Leverens EL, Bialek WS. 1985. The Vertebrate Inner Ear, Boca Raton, Fla, CRC Press.

Rabbit RD, Damino ER. 1992. A hydroelastic model of macromachanics in the ednolymphatic vestibular canal. J Fluid Mech 238:337.

Van Buskirk WC. 1977. The effects of the utricle on flow in the semicircular canals. Ann Biomed Eng 5:1.

Van Buskirk WC, Grant JW. 1973. Biomechanics of the semicircular canals, pp 53–54, New York, Biomechanics Symposium of American Society of Mechanical Engineers.

Van Buskirk WC, Grant JW. 1987. Vestibular mechanics. In R Skalak, S Chien (eds), Handbook of Bioengineering, pp 31.1–31.17, New York, McGraw-Hill.

Van Buskirk WC, Watts RG, Liu YK. 1976. Fluid mechanics of the semicircular canal. J Fluid Mech 78:87.

Nomenclature

Otolith Variables

x = coordinate direction in the plane of the otoconial layer
y_g = coordinate direction normal to the plane of the otolith with origin at the gel base
y_f = coordinate direction normal to the plane of the otolith with origin at the fluid base
t = time
$u(y_f,t)$ = velocity of the endolymph fluid measured with respect to the skull
$v(t)$ = velocity of the otoconial layer measured with respect to the skull

$w(y_g,t)$ = velocity of the gel layer measured with respect to the skull
$\delta_g(y_g,t)$ = displacement of the gel layer measured with respect to the skull
δ_o = displacement of the otoconial layer measured with respect to the skull
V_s = skull velocity in the x direction measured with respect to an inertial reference frame
V = a characteristic velocity of the skull in the problem (magnitude of a step change)
ρ_o = density of the otoconial layer
ρ_f = density of the endolymph fluid
τ_g = gel shear stress in the x direction
μ_g = viscosity of the gel material
μ_f = viscosity of the endolymph fluid
G = shear modulus of the gel material
b = gel layer and otoconial layer thickness (assumed equal)
g_x = gravity component in the x-direction

Semicircular Canal Variables

$u(r,t)$ = velocity of endolymph fluid measured with respect to the canal wall
r = radical coordinate of canal duct
a = inside radius of the canal duct
R = radius of curvature of semicircular canal
ρ = density of endolymph fluid
v = endolymph kinematic viscosity
ω = angular velocity of the canal wall measured with respect to an inertial frame
α = angular acceleration of the canal wall measured with respect to an inertial frame
K = pressure-volume modulus of the cupula = $\Delta p/\Delta V$
Δp = differential pressure across the cupula
ΔV = volumetric displacement of endolymph fluid
β = angle subtended by the canal in radians ($\beta = \pi$ for a true semicircular canal)
λ_n = roots of $J_o(x) = 0$, where J_o is Bessel's function of order 0 ($\lambda_1 = 2.405$, $\lambda_2 = 5.520$)

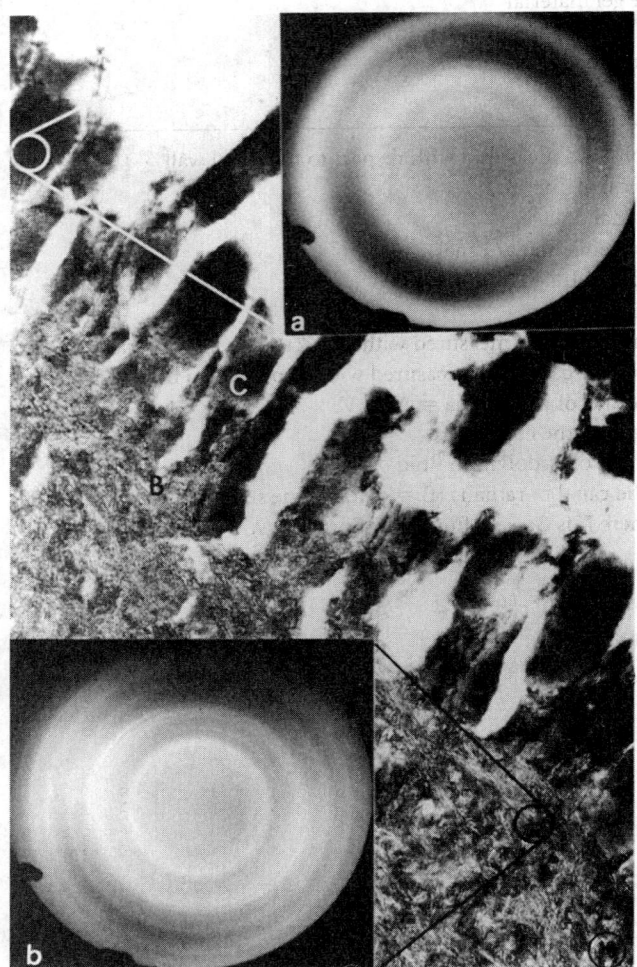

Transmission electron micrograph of well-mineralized bone.

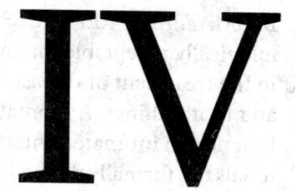

Biomaterials

Joon B. Park
University of Iowa

A BIOMATERIAL REPLACES A PART or a function of the body in a safe, reliable, economic, and physiologically acceptable manner [Hench & Ethridge, 1982]. A variety of devices and materials is used in the treatment of disease or injury. Common examples include sutures, needles, catheters, plates, and tooth fillings. A biomaterial is a synthetic material used to replace part of a living system or to function in intimate contact with living tissue. The Clemson University Advisory Board for Biomaterials has formally defined a *biomaterial* to be "a systemically and pharmacologically inert substance designed for implantation within or incorporation with living systems." Black [1992] defined a biomaterial as "a nonviable material used in a medical device, intended to interact with biological systems." Another definition is by Bruck [1980]: "materials of synthetic as well as of natural origin in contact with tissue, blood, and biological fluids, and intended for use for prosthetic, diagnostic, therapeutic, and storage applications without adversely affecting the living organism and its components." Still another definition of biomaterials is "any substance (other than drugs) or combination of substances synthetic or natural in origin, which can be used for any period of time, as a whole or as a part of a system which treats, arguments, or replaces any tissue, organ, or function of the body" [Williams, 1987]. By contrast, a *biological material* is a material such as skin or artery, produced by a biological system. Artificial materials which simply are in contact with the skin, such as hearing aids and wearable artificial limbs, are not included in our definition of biomaterials, since the skin acts as a barrier with the external world.

According to these definitions one must have a vast field of knowledge or collaborate with different specialties in order to develop and use biomaterials in medicine and dentistry, as Table IV.1 indicates. The uses of biomaterials, as indicated in Table IV.2, include replacing a body part which has lost function due to disease or trauma, to assisting in healing, improving function, and correcting abnormalities. The role of biomaterials has been influenced considerably by advances in many areas of biotechnology and science. For example, with the advent of antibiotics, infectious disease is less of a threat, so degenerative disease assumes a greater importance. Moreover, advances in surgical technique and instruments have permitted materials to be used in ways which were not possible previously. This section of the *Handbook* is intended to develop in the reader a familiarity both with the uses of materials in medicine and dentistry and with some rational basis for these applications.

The performance of materials in the body can be classified in many ways. First, we may consider biomaterials from the point of view of the problem area which is to be solved, as in Table IV.2. Second, we may consider the body on a tissue level, an organ level (Table IV.3), or a system level (Table IV.4). Third, we may consider the classification of materials as polymers, metals, ceramics, and composites as is done in Table IV.5. In that vein, the role of such materials as biomaterials is governed by the interaction between the material and the body, specifically, the effect of the body environment on the material and the effect of the material on the body [Black, 1992; Bruck, 1980; Greco, 1994; Hench & Ethridge, 1982; Park & Lakes, 1992; von Recum, 1986; Williams & Roaf, 1973]

It should be evident in any of these perspectives that most current applications of biomaterials involve structural functions even in those organs and systems which are not primarily structural in their nature or very simple chemical or electrical functions. Complex chemical functions such as

TABLE IV.1   Fields of Knowledge to Develop Biomaterials

Discipline	Examples
Science and engineering	Materials sciences: structure-property relationship of synthetic and biological materials including metals, ceramics, polymers, composites, tissues (blood and connective tissues), etc.
Biology and physiology	Cell and molecular biology, anatomy, animal and human physiology, histopathology, experimental surgery, immunology, etc.
Clinical sciences	All the clinical specialties: dentistry, maxillofacial, neurosurgery, obstetrics and gynecology, ophthalmology, orthopedics, otolaryngology, plastic and reconstructive surgery, thoracic and cardiovascular surgery, veterinary medicine and surgery, etc.

Source: Modified from von Recum [1994].

TABLE IV.2   Uses of Biomaterials

Problem Area	Examples
Replace diseased or damaged part	Artificial hip joint, kidney dialysis machine
Assist in healing	Sutures, bone plates and screws
Improve function	Cardiac pacemaker, intraocular lens
Correct functional abnormality	Cardiac pacemaker
Correct cosmetic problem	Augmentation mammoplasty, chin augmentation
Aid diagnosis	Probes and catheters
Aid treatment	Catheters, drains

those of the liver and complex electrical or electrochemical functions such as those of the brain and sense organs cannot be carried out by biomaterials at this time.

Historical Background

The use of biomaterials did not become practical until the advent of aseptic surgical technique developed by Dr. J. Lister in the 1860s. Earlier surgical procedures, whether they involve biomaterials or not, were generally unsuccessful as a result of infection. Problems of infection tend to be exacerbated in the presence of biomaterials, since the implant can provide a region inaccessible to the body's immunologically competent cells. The earliest successful implants, as well as a large fraction of modern ones, were in the skeletal system. Bone plates were introduced in the early 1900s to aid in the fixation of long bone fractures. Many of these early plates broke as a result of unsophisticated mechanical design: They were too thin and had stress-concentrating corners. Also, materials such as vanadium steel, which was chosen for its good mechanical properties, corroded rapidly in the body and caused adverse effect on the healing processes. Better designs and materials soon followed. Following the introduction of stainless steels and cobalt chromium alloys in the 1930s, greater success was achieved in fracture fixation, and the first joint replacement surgeries were performed. As for polymers, it was found that warplane pilots in World War II who were injured by fragments of plastic (polymethyl methacrylate) aircraft canopy did not suffer adverse chronic reactions from the presence of the fragments in the body. Polymethyl methacrylate (PMMA) became widely used after that time for corneal replacement and for replacements of sections of damaged skull bones. Following further advances in materials and in surgical technique, blood vessel replacements were tried in the 1950s and heart valve replacements and cemented joint replacements in the 1960s. Table IV.6 lists notable developments relating to implants. Recent years have seen many further advances.

Performance of Biomaterials

The success of a biomaterial in the body depends on factors such as the material properties, design, and *biocompatibility* of the material used, as well as other factors not under control of the engineer, including the technique used by the surgeon, the health and condition of the patient, and the activ-

TABLE IV.3   Biomaterials in Organs

Organ	Examples
Heart	Cardiac pacemaker, artificial heart valve, total artificial heart
Lung	Oxygenator machine
Eye	Contact lens, intraocular lens
Ear	Artificial stapes, cochlea implant
Bone	Bone plate, intramedullary rod
Kidney	Kidney dialysis machine
Bladder	Catheter and stent

TABLE IV.4 Biomaterials in Body Systems

System	Examples
Skeletal	Bone plate, total joint replacements
Muscular	Sutures, muscle stimulator
Circulatory	Artificial heart valves, blood vessels left ventircular assist device
Respiratory	Oxygenator machine
Integumentary	Sutures, burn dressings, artificial skin
Urinary	Catheters, stent, kidney dialysis machine
Nervous	Hydrocephalus drain, cardiac pacemaker, nerve stimulator
Endocrine	Microencapsulated pancreatic islet cells
Reproductive	Augmentation mammoplasty, other cosmetic replacements

ities of the patient. If we can assign a numerical value f to the probability of failure of an implant, then the *reliability, r,* can be expressed as

$$r = 1 - f \tag{IV.1}$$

If, as is usually the case, there are multiple modes of failure, the total reliability r_t is given by the product of the individual reliabilities $r_1 = (1 - f_1)$, and so on:

$$r_t = r_1 \cdot r_2 \cdots r_n \tag{IV.2}$$

Consequently, even if one failure mode such as implant fracture is perfectly controlled so that the corresponding reliability is unity, other failure modes such as infection could severely limit the utility represented by the total reliability of the implant. One mode of failure which can occur in a biomaterial but not in engineering materials used in other contexts is an attack by the body's immune system on the implant. Another such failure mode is an unwanted effect of the implant upon the body, for example, toxicity, inducing allergic reactions, or causing cancer. Consequently, biocompatibility is included as a material requirement in addition to those requirements associated directly with the function of the implant.

Biocompatibility involves the acceptance of an artificial implant by the surrounding tissues and by the body as a whole. Biocompatible materials do not irritate the surrounding structures, do not provoke an abnormal inflammatory response, do not incite allergic or immunologic reactions, and

TABLE IV.5 Materials for Use in the Body

Materials	Advantages	Disadvantages	Examples
Polymers (nylon, silicone rubber, polyester, polytetrafuoro-ethylene, etc.)	Resilient, easy to fabricate	Not strong, deforms with time, may degrade	Sutures, blood vessels, hip socket, ear, nose, other soft tissues
Metals (Ti and its alloys, Co-Cr alloys, stainless steels, Au, Ag, Pt, etc.)	Strong, tough, ductile	May corrode, dense, difficult to make	Joint replacements, bone plates and screws, dental root implants, pacer and suture wires
Ceramics (aluminum oxide, calcium phosphates including hydroxyapatite, carbon)	Very biocompatible, inert, strong in compression	Brittle, not resilient	Dental, joint replacements, coating of dental and orthopedic implants
Composites (carbon-carbon, wire or fiber reinforced bone cement)	Strong, tailor-made	Difficult to make	Joint implants, heart valves

TABLE IV.6 Notable Developments Relating to Implants

Year	Investigators	Development
Late 18th–19th century		Various metal devices to fix bone fractures; wires and pins from Fe, Au, Ag, and Pt.
1860–1870	J. Lister	Aseptic surgical techniques
1886	H. Hansmann	Ni-plated steel bone fracture plate
1893–1912	W.A. Lane	Steel screws and plates (Lane fracture plate)
1912	W.D. Sherman	Vanadium steel plates, first developed for medical use; lesser stress concentration and corrosion (Sherman plate)
1924	A.A. Zierold	Introduced Stellites (CoCrMo alloy)
1926	M.Z. Lange	Introduced 18-8sMo stainless steel, better than 18-8 stainless steel
1926	E.W. Hey-Goves	Used carpenter's screw for femoral neck fracture
1931	M.N. Sith-Petersen	First femoral neck fracture fixation device made of stainless steel
1936	C.S. Venable, W.G. Stuck	Introduced Vitallium (19-9 stainless steel), later changed the material to CoCr alloys
1938	P. Wiles	First total hip replacement prosthesis
1939	J.C. Burch, H.M Carney	Introduced tantalum (Ta)
1946	J. Judet, R. Judet	First biomechanically designed femoral head replacement prosthesis; first plastics (PMMA) used in joint replacements
1940s	M.J. Dorzee, A. Franceschetti	First used acrylics (PMMA) for corneal replacement
1947	J. Cotton	Introduced Ti and its alloys
1952	A.B. Voorhees, A. Jaretzta, A.B. Blackmore	First successful blood vessel replacement made of cloth for tissue ingrowth
1958	S. Furman, G. Robinson	First successful direct heart stimulation
1958	J. Charnley	First use of acrylic bone cement in total hip replacement on the advice of Dr. D. Smith
1960	A. Starr, M.L. Edwards	First commercial heart valves
1970s	W.J. Kolff	Total heart replacement

Source: Park [1984].

do not cause cancer. Other compatibility characteristics which may be important in the function of an implant device made of biomaterials include adequate mechanical properties such as strength, stiffness, and fatigue properties; appropriate optical properties if the material is to be used in the eye, skin, or tooth; appropriate density. Sterilizability, manufacturability, long-term storage, and appropriate engineering design are also to be considered.

The failure modes may differ in importance as time passes following the implant surgery. For example, consider the case of a total joint replacement in which infection is most likely soon after surgery, but loosening and implant fracture and wear become progressively more important as time goes on. Failure modes also depend on the type of implant and its location and function in the body. For example, an artificial blood vessel is more likely to cause problems by inducing a clot or becoming clogged with thrombus than by breaking or tearing mechanically.

Defining Terms

Biocompatibility: Acceptance of an artificial implant by the surrounding tissues and by the body as a whole.

Biological material: A material produced by a biological system.

Biomaterial: A synthetic material used to replace part of a living system or to function in intimate contact with living tissue.

References

Black J. 1992. Biological Performance of Materials: Fundamentals of Biocompatibility, 2d ed, p 6, New York, M. Dekker.

Bruck SD. 1980. Properties of Biomaterials in the Physiological Environment, p 1, Boca Raton, Fla., CRC Press.

Greco, RS (ed). 1994. Implantation Biology: The Host Response and Biomedical Devices, Boca Raton, Fla., CRC Press.

Hench LL, Ethridge EC. 1982. Biomaterials: An Interfacial Approach, p 1, New York, Academic Press.

Park JB. 1984. Biomaterials Science and Engineering, p 8, New York, Plenum.

Park JB, Lakes RS. 1992. Biomaterials: An Introduction 2d ed, pp 1–6, New York, Plenum.

Von Recum AF (ed.) 1986. Handbook of Biomaterials Evaluation, pp 97–158, 293–502, New York, Macmillan.

Von Recum AF. 1994. Biomaterials: Educational goals, Presidential Address, Society for Biomaterials, 20th Annual Meeting, Boston, MA.

Williams DF (ed). 1987. Definitions in biomaterials. Progress in Biomedical Engineering 4, p 67, Amsterdam, Elsevier.

Williams DF, Roaf R. 1973. Implants in Surgery, London, Saunders.

Further Information

Allgower M, Matter P, Perren SM, et al. 1973. The Dynamic Compression Plate, DCP, New York, Berlin, Springer-Verlag.

American Society for Testing and Materials, Yearly update. Annual Book of ASTM Standards, vol. 13, Medical Devices and Services, Philadelphia, ASTM.

Bechtol CO, Ferguson AB, Laing PG. 1959. Metals and Engineering in Bone and Joint Surgery, London, Balliere, Tindall and Cox.

Black J. 1992. Biological Performance of Materials, 2d ed, New York, M. Dekker.

Bloch B, Hastings GW. 1972. Plastic Materials in Surgery, 2d ed, Springfield, Ill., CC Thomas.

Bokros JC, Arkins RJ, Shim HS, et al. 1976. Carbon in prosthestic devices. In ML Deviney, TM O'Grady, (eds), Petroleum Derived Carbons, American Chemical Society Symposium, Series 21, Washington, DC, American Chemical Society.

Boretos JW. 1973. Concise Guide to Biomedical Polymers, Springfield, Ill., CC Thomas.

Boretos JW, Eden M (eds). 1984. Contemporary Biomaterials, Park Ridge, NJ, Noyes.

Brown PW, Constantz B. 1994. Hydroxyapatite and Related Materials, Boca Raton, Fla., CRC Press.

Bruck SD. 1974. Blood Compatible Synthetic Polymers: An Introduction, Springfield, Ill., CC Thomas.

Bruck SD. 1980. Properties of Biomaterials in the Physiological Environment, Boca Raton, Fla., CRC Press.

Chandran KB. 1992. Cardiovascular Biomechanics, New York, New York University.

Charnley J. 1970. Acrylic Cement in Orthopedic Surgery, Edinborough and London, Livingstone.

Cooney DO. 1976. Biomedical Engineering Principles, New York and Basel, M. Dekker.

Cranin AN (ed). 1970. Oral Implantology, Springfield, Ill., CC Thomas.

Dardik H (ed). 1978. Graft Materials in Vascular Surgery, Chicago, Year Book Medical Publishing.

De Groot K (ed). 1983. Bioceramics of Calcium Phosphate, Boca Raton, Fla., CRC Press.

Ducheyne P, Van der Perre G, Aubert AE (eds). 1984. Biomaterials and Biomechanics, Amsterdam, Elsevier Science.

Dumbleton JH, Black J. 1975. An Introduction to Orthopedic Materials, Springfield, Ill., CC Thomas.

Edwards WS. 1965. Plastic Arterial Grafts, Springfield, Ill., CC Thomas.

Eftekhar NS. 1978. Principles of Total Hip Arthroplasty, St. Louis, CV Mosby.

Frost HM. 1973. Orthopedic Biomechanics, Springfield, Ill., CC Thomas.

Fung YC. 1993. Biomechanics: Mechanical Properties of Living Tissues, 2d ed, New York, Berlin, Springer-Verlag.

Ghista DN, Roaf R (eds). 1978. Orthopedic Mechanics: Procedures and Devices, London, New York, Academic Press.

Goel VK, Weinstein JN (ed.) 1989. Biomechanics of Spine, Clinical and Surgical Perspective, Boca Raton, Fla., CRC Press.

Greco RS (ed). 1994. Implantation Biology, Boca Raton, Fla., CRC Press.

Guidelines for Blood-Material Interactions. Rev 1985. Report of the National Heart, Lung, and Blood Institute Working Group, Devices and Technology Branch, NHLBI, NIH Publication 80-2185.

Gyers GH, Parsonet V. 1969. Engineering in the Heart and Blood Vessels, New York, J. Wiley and Sons.

Hastings GW, Williams DF (eds). 1980. Mechanical Properties of Biomaterials, Chichester, New York, Brisbane, Toronto, J. Wiley.

Hench LL, Ethridge EC. 1982. Biomaterials: An Interfacial Approach, New York, Academic Press.

Heppenstall RB (ed). 1980. Fracture Treatment and Healing, Philadelphia, W.B. Saunders.

Homsy CA, Armeniades CD (eds). 1972. Biomaterials for skeletal and cardiovascular applications, Journal of Biomedical Materials Research Symposium, Res, no. 3, New York, John Wiley.

Hulbert SF, Young FA, Moyle DD (eds). 1972. Journal of Biomedical Materials Research Symposium, no 2, New York, John Wiley.

Kawahara H (ed). 1989. Oral Implantology and Biomaterials, Amsterdam, Elsevier.

Kronenthal RL, Oser Z (eds). 1975. Polymers in Medicine and Surgery, New York, Plenum Press.

Kuntscher G. 1947. The Practice of Intramedullary Nailing, Springfield, Ill., CC Thomas.

Lee H, Neville K. 1971. Handbook of Biomedical Plastics, Pasadena, Calif., Pasadena Technology Press.

Lee SM (ed). 1987. Advances in Biomaterials, Lancaster, Penn, Technomic Publishing AG.

Leinninger RI. 1972. Polymers as surgical implants. Crit Rev Bioeng 2:333.

Levine SN (ed). 1968. Materials in biomedical engineering. Ann N Y Acad Sci 146:.

Lynch W. 1982. Implants: Reconstructing Human Body, New York, Van Nostrand Reinhold.

Mears DC. 1979. Materials and Orthopedic Surgery, Baltimore, Williams & Wilkins.

Oonishi H, Aoki H, Sawai K (eds). 1989. Bioceramics, Tokyo, St. Louis, Ishiyaku EuroAmerica.

Park JB. 1979. Biomaterials: An Introduction, New York, London, Plenum.

Park JB. 1984. Biomaterials Science and Engineering, New York, London, Plenum.

Park JB, Lakes RS. 1992. Biomaterials: An Introduction, 2d ed, New York, London, Plenum.

Park K, Shalaby WSW, Park H. 1993. Biodegradable Hydrogels for Drug Delivery, Lancaster, Penn, Technomic Publishing.

Rubin LR (ed). 1983. Biomaterials in Reconstructive Surgery, St. Louis, CV Mosby.

Savastano AA (ed). 1980. Total Knee Replacement, New York, Appleton-Century-Crofts.

Sawyer PN, Kaplitt MH. 1978. Vascular Grafts, New York, Appleton-Century-Crofts.

Schaldach M, Hohmann D (eds). 1976. Advances in Artificial Hip and Knee Joint Technology, Berlin, Springer-Vergag.

Schnitman PA, Schulman LB (eds). 1980. Dental Implants: Benefits and Risk, A NIH-Harvard Consensus Development Conference, NIH Pub. No. 81-1531, U.S. Dept. Health and Human Services, Bethesda, Md.

Sharma CP, Szycher M (eds). 1991. Blood Compatible Materials and Devices, Lancaster, Penn, Technomic Publishing.

Stanley JC, Burkel WE, Lindenauer SM, et al. (eds). 1972. Biologic and Synthetic Vascular Prostheses, New York, Grune & Stratton.

Stark L, Agarwal G (eds). 1969. Biomaterials, New York, Plenum.

Swanson SAV, Freeman MAR (eds). 1977. The Scientific Basis of Joint Replacement, New York, Toronto, John Wiley and Sons.

Syrett BC, Acharya A (eds). 1979. Corrosion and Degradation of Implant Materials, ASTM STP 684, Philadelphia, American Society for Testing and Materials.

Szycher M (ed). 1991. High Performance Biomaterials, Lancaster, Penn, Technomic Publishing.

Szycher M, Robinson WJ (eds). 1990. Synthetic Biomedical Polymers, Concepts and Applications, Lancaster, Penn, Technomic Publishing.

Taylor AR. 1970. Endosseous Dental Implants, London, Butterworth.

Uhthoff HK (ed). 1980. Current Concepts of Internal Fixation of Fractures, Berlin, New York, Springer-Verlag.

Venable CS, Stuck WC. 1947. The Internal Fixation of Fractures, Springfield, Ill., CC Thomas.

Webster JG (ed). 1988. Encyclopedia of Medical Devices and Instrumentation, New York, John Wiley.

Williams DF (ed). 1976. Compatibility of Implant Materials, London, Sector Publishing.

Williams DF (ed). 1981. Fundamental Aspects of Biocompatibility, vols 1, 2, Boca Raton, Fla., CRC Press.

Williams DF (ed). 1981. Systemic Aspects of Blood Compatibility, Boca Raton, Fla., CRC Press.

Williams DF (ed). 1982. Biocompatibility in Clinical Practice, vols 1, 2, Boca Raton, Fla., CRC Press.

Wright V (ed). 1969. Lubrication and Wear in Joints, Philadelphia, Lippincott.

Yamamuro T, Hench LL, Wilson J (eds). 1990. CRC Handbook of Bioactive Ceramics, vols 1, 2, Boca Raton, Fla., CRC Press.

40

Metallic Biomaterials

Joon B. Park
University of Iowa

The first metal alloy developed specifically for human use was "vanadium steel," which was used to manufacture bone fracture plates (Sherman plates) and screws. Most metals such as iron (Fe), chromium (Cr), cobalt (Co), nickel (Ni), titanium (Ti), tantalum (Ta), molybdenum (Mo), and tungsten (W) used to make alloys for manufacturing implants can be tolerated by the body in minute amounts. Sometimes those metallic elements, in naturally occurring forms, are essential in cell functions (Fe) or synthesis of vitamin B_{12} (Co) but cannot be tolerated in large amounts in the body [Black, 1992]. The biocompatibility of the metallic implant is of considerable concern because these implants can corrode in an in vivo environment [Williams, 1982]. The consequences of corrosion are the disintegration of the implant material per se, which will weaken the implant, and the harmful effect of corrosion products which escape into the surrounding tissue.

40.1 Stainless Steels

The first stainless steel utilized for implant fabrication was 18-8 (type 302 in modern classification), which is stronger and more resistant to corrosion than the vanadium steel. Vanadium steel is no longer used in implants, since its corrosion resistance is inadequate in vivo. Later 18-8sMo stainless steel, which contains a small percentage of molybdenum to improve the corrosion resistance in salt water, was introduced. This alloy became known as *type 316 stainless steel*. In the 1950s, the carbon content of 316 stainless steel was reduced from 0.08% (all are weight percentages unless specified) to 0.03% maximum for better corrosion resistance to chloride solution and became known as type 316L stainless steel. The minimum effective concentration of chromium is 11% to impart corrosion resistance in stainless steels. Chromium is a reactive element, but it and its alloys can be *passivated* to give excellent corrosion resistance.

The *austenitic stainless steels*, especially types 316 and 316L, are most widely used for implant fabrication. These are *not* hardenable by heat treatment but can be hardened only by cold working. This group of stainless steels is nonmagnetic and possesses better corrosion resistance than any other. The inclusion of molybdenum enhances resistance to *pitting corrosion* in salt water. The American Soci-

0-8493-8346-3/95/$0.00+$.50
1995 by CRC Press, Inc.

ety of Testing and Materials (ASTM) recommends type 316L rather than 316 for implant fabrication. The specifications for 316L stainless steel are given in Table 40.1. The only difference in composition between the 316L and 316 stainless steel is the content of carbon, i.e. 0.03% maximum and 0.08%, respectively.

Nickel stabilizes the austenitic (γ) phase at room temperature and enhances corrosion resistance. The austenitic phase stability can be influenced by both the Ni and Cr contents as shown in Figure 40.1 for 0.10% carbon stainless steels.

Table 40.2 gives the mechanical properties of 316L stainless steel. A wide range of properties exists depending on the heat treatment (annealing to obtain softer materials) or cold working (for greater strength and hardness). Figure 40.2 shows the effect of cold working on the yield and

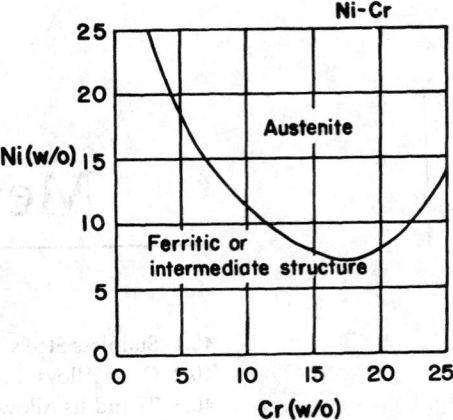

FIGURE 40.1 The effect of Ni and Cr contents on the austenitic phase of stainless steels containing 0.1% C [Keating, 1956].

ultimate tensile strength of 18-8 stainless steels. The designer must consequently be careful when selecting materials of this type. Even the 316L stainless steels may corrode inside the body under certain circumstances in a highly stressed and oxygen-depleted region such as the contacts under the screws of the fracture plate. Thus these stainless steels are suitable to use only in *temporary* implant devices such as fracture plates, screws, and hip nails.

TABLE 40.1 Compositions of 316L Stainless Steel

Element	Composition, %
Carbon	0.03 max
Manganese	2.00 max
Phosphorus*	0.03 max
Sulfur	0.03 max
Silicon	0.75 max
Chromium	17.00–20.00
Nickel	12.00–14.00
Molybdenum	2.00–4.00

American Society for Testing and Materials, 1992, F139-86, p 61.

*Slight variations are given (0.025 max) for special quality stainless steels.

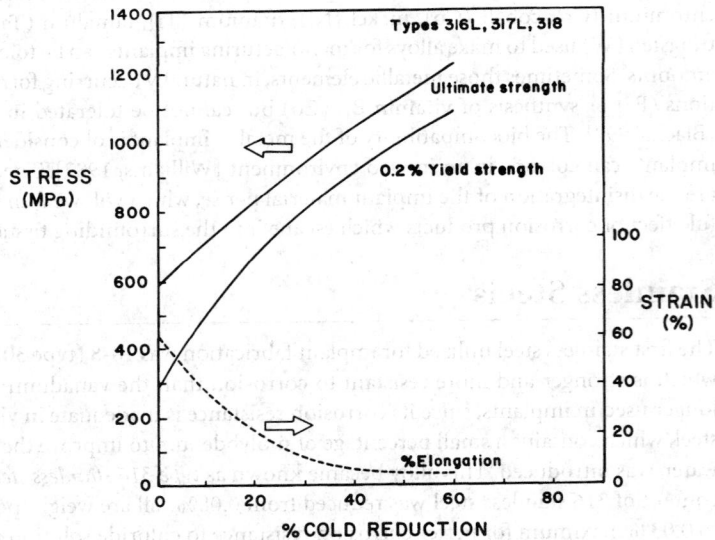

FIGURE 40.2 Effect of cold work on the yield and ultimate tensile strength of 18-8 stainless steel [American Society for Metal, 1978].

TABLE 40.2 Mechanical Properties of 316L Stainless Steel for Implants

Condition	Ultimate Tensile Strength, min (MPa)	Yield Strength (0.2% offset), min (MPa)	Elongation 2-in (50.8 mm) min%	Rockwell Hardness
Annealed	485	172	40	95 HRB
Cold-worked	860	690	12	—

American Society for Testing and Materials, 1992, F139-86, p 61.

40.2 CoCr Alloys

There are basically two types of cobalt-chromium alloys; one is the CoCrMo alloy which is usually used to *cast* a product and the other is CoNiCrMo alloy, which is usually *wrought* by (hot) *forging*. The castable CoCrMo alloy has been used for many decades in dentistry and, recently, in making artificial joints. The wrought CoNiCrMo alloy is a relative newcomer now used for making the stems of prostheses for heavily loaded joints such as the knee and hip.

ASTM lists four types of CoCr alloys which are recommended for surgical implant applications: (1) cast CoCrMo alloy (F75), (2) wrought CoCrWNi alloy (F90), (3) wrought CoNiCrMo alloy (F562), and (4) wrought CoNiCrMoWFe alloy (F563). Their chemical compositions are summarized in Table 40.3. At the present time only two of the four alloys are used extensively in implant fabrications, the castable CoCrMo and the wrought CoNiCrMo alloy. As can be noticed from Table 40.3, the compositions are quite different from one other.

The two basic elements of the CoCr alloys form a solid solution of up to 65% Co. The molybdenum is added to produce finer grains which results in higher strengths after casting or forging.

The CoNiCrMo alloy originally called MP35N (Standard Pressed Steel Co.) contains approximately 35% Co and Ni each. The alloy is highly corrosion resistant to seawater (containing chloride ions) under stress. Cold working can increase the strength of the alloy considerably as shown in Figure 40.3. However, there is considerable difficulty in cold working this alloy, especially when making large devices such as hip joint stems. Only hot-forging can be used to fabricate a large implant with the alloy.

The abrasive wear properties of the wrought CoNiCrMo alloy are similar to the cast CoCrMo alloy (about 0.14 mm/y in joint simulation test); however, the former is not recommended for the bearing surfaces of joint prosthesis because of its poor frictional properties with itself or other materials. The superior fatigue and ultimate tensile strength of the wrought CoNiCrMo alloy make it suitable for the applications which require long service life without fracture or stress fatigue. Such is the case for the stems of the hip joint prostheses. This advantage is better appreciated when the implant has to be replaced, since it is quite difficult to remove the failed piece of implant embedded deep in the femoral medullary canal. Furthermore, the revision arthroplasty is usually inferior to the original in terms of its function due to poorer fixation of the implant.

The mechanical properties required for CoCr alloys are given in Table 40.4. As with other alloys, the increased strength is accompanied by decreased ductility. Both the cast and wrought alloys have excellent corrosion resistance.

Experimental determination of the rate of nickel release from the CoNiCrMo alloy and 316L stainless steel in 37°C Ringer's solution showed an interesting result. Although the cobalt alloy has more initial release of nickel ions into the solution, the *rate* of release was about the same (3×10^{-10}

TABLE 40.3 Chemical Compositions of CoCr Alloys

Element	CoCrMo (F75)		CoCrWNi (F90)		CoNiCrMo (F562)		CoNiCrMoWFe (F563)	
	Minimum	Maximum	Minimum	Maximum	Minimum	Maximum	Minimum	Maximum
Cr	27.0	30.0	19.0	21.0	19.0	21.0	18.00	22.00
Mo	5.0	7.0	—	—	9.0	10.5	3.00	4.00
Ni	—	2.5	9.0	11.0	33.0	37.0	15.00	25.00
Fe	—	0.75	—	3.0	—	1.0	4.00	6.00
C	—	0.35	0.05	0.15	—	0.025	—	0.05
Si	—	1.00	—	1.00	—	0.15	—	0.50
Mn	—	1.00	—	2.00	—	0.15	—	1.00
W	—	—	14.0	16.0	—	—	3.00	4.00
	—	—	—	—	—	0.015	—	—
Ti	—	—	—	—	—	0.010	—	0.010
Co	—	—	Balance		—	1.0	0.50	3.50

Source: American Society for Testing and Materials, 1992, F75-87, p 42; F90-87, p 47; F562-84, p 150.

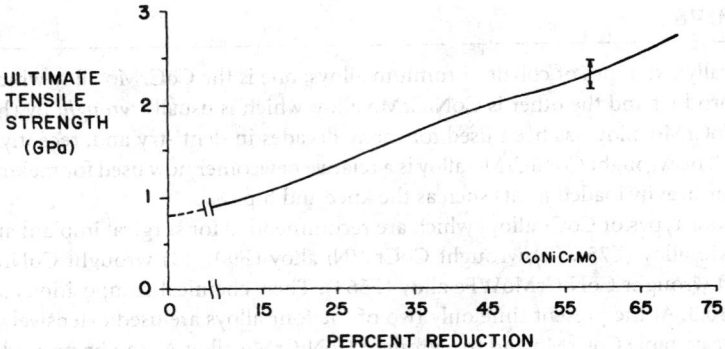

FIGURE 40.3   Relationship between ultimate tensile and the amount of cold work for CoNiCrMo alloy [Devine & Wulff, 1975].

$g/cm^2/d$) for both alloys [Richards Mfg. Co., 1980]. This is rather surprising since the nickel content of the CoNiCrMo alloy is about three times that of 316L stainless steel.

The modulus of elasticity for the CoCr alloys does not change with the changes in their ultimate tensile strength. The values range from 220 to 234 GPa, which are higher than other materials such as stainless steels. This may have some implications of different load transfer modes to the bone in artificial joint replacements, although the effect of the increased modulus on the fixation and longevity of implants is not clear.

40.3 Ti and Its Alloys

Attempts to use titanium for implant fabrication dates to the late 1930s. It was found that titanium was tolerated in cat femurs, as was stainless steel and Vitallium (CoCrMo alloy). Titanium's lightness (4.5 g/cm^3 compared to 7.9 g/cm^3 for 316 stainless steel, 8.3 g/cm^3 for cast CoCrMo, and 9.2 g/cm^3 for wrought CoNiCrMo alloys) and good mechanochemical properties are salient features for implant application.

There are four grades of unalloyed commercially pure (cp) titanium for surgical implant applications as given in Table 40.5. The impurity contents separate them; oxygen, iron, and nitrogen should be controlled carefully. Oxygen in particular has a great influence on the ductility and strength.

One titanium alloy (Ti6A14V) is widely used to manufacture implants, and its chemical requirements are given in Table 40.5. The main alloying elements of the alloy are aluminum (5.5–6.5%) and vanadium (3.5 ~ 4.5%).

TABLE 40.4   Mechanical Property Requirements of CoCr Alloys

Property	Cast CoCrMo (F75)	Wrought CoCrWNi (F90)	Wrought CoNiCrMo (F562) Solution Annealed	Wrought CoNiCrMo (F562) Cold Worked and Aged
Tensile strength, MPa	655	860	793–1000	1793 min
Yield strength (0.2% offset), MPa	450	310	240–655	1585
Elongation, %	8	10	50.0	8.0
Reduction of area, %	8		65.0	35.0
Fatigue strength, MPa*	310			

*From Semlitsch [Semlitsch, 1980]

Source: American Society for Testing and Materials, 1992, F75-87, p 42; F90-87, p 47; F562-84, p 150.

TABLE 40.5   Chemical Compositions of Titanium and Its Alloy

Element	Grade 1	Grade 2	Grade 3	Grade 4	Ti6Al4V*
Nitrogen	0.03	0.03	0.05	0.05	0.05
Carbon	0.10	0.10	0.10	0.10	0.08
Hydrogen	0.015	0.015	0.015	0.015	0.0125
Iron	0.20	0.30	0.30	0.50	0.25
Oxygen	0.18	0.25	0.35	0.40	0.13
Titanium			balance		

*Aluminum 6.00% (5.50–6.50), vanadium 4.00% (3.50–4.50), and other elements 0.1% maximum or 0.4% total.

Note: All are maximum allowable weight percent.

Source: American Society for Testing and Materials, 1992, F67-89, p 39; F136-84, p 55.

Titanium is an allotropic material which exists as a hexagonal close-packed structure (α-Ti) up to 882°C and as a body-centered cubic structure (β-Ti) above that temperature. The addition of alloying elements to titanium enables it to have a wide range of properties: (1) Aluminum tends to stabilize the α-phase, that is, to increase the transformation temperature from α- to β-phase (Figure 40.4). (2) Vanadium stabilizes the β-phase by lowering the temperature of the transformation from α to β.

The α-alloys have single-phase microstructure (Fig. 40.5*a*), which promotes good weldability. The stabilizing effect of the high aluminum content of these groups of alloys makes excellent strength characteristics and oxidation resistance at high temperature (300–600°C). These alloys cannot be heat-treated for strengthening since they are single-phased.

The addition of controlled amount of β-stabilizers causes the higher strength β-phase to persist below the transformation temperature which results in the two-phase system. The precipitates of β-phase will appear by heat treatment in the solid solution temperature and subsequent quenching, followed by aging at a somewhat lower temperature. The aging cycle causes the precipitation of some fine α particles from the metastable β, imparting α structure that is stronger than the annealed α-β structure (Figure 40.5*b*).

The higher percentage of β-stabilizing elements (13%V in Ti13V11Cr3Al alloy) results in a microstructure that is substantially β which can be strengthened by the heat treatment (Figure 40.5*c*). Another Ti alloy (Ti13Nb13Zr) with 13% niobium (Nb) and 13% Zirconium (Zr) showed *martensite* structure after it was water-quenched and aged, and this structure showed high corrosion resistance with low modulus (E = 79MPa) [Davidson et al., 1994].

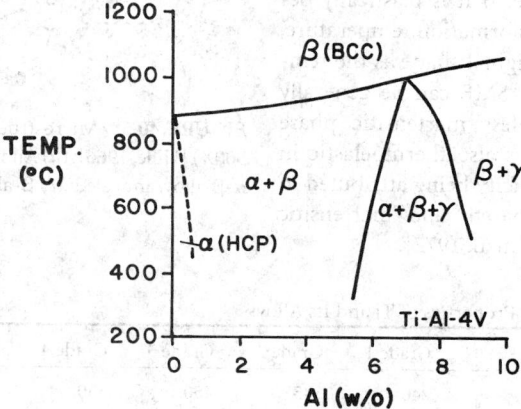

FIGURE 40.4   Part of phase-diagram of Ti-Al-V at 4 w/o V [Smith & Hughes, 1966].

The mechanical properties of the commercially pure titanium and its alloys are given in Table 40.6. The modulus of elasticity of these materials is about 110 GPa except 13Nb13Zr alloy, which is half the value of Co-Cr alloys. From Table 40.6 one can see that the higher impurity content of the cp-Ti leads to higher strength and reduced ductility. The strength of the material varies from a value much lower than that of 316 stainless steel or the CoCr alloys to a value about equal to that of annealed 316 stainless steel of the cast CoCrMo alloy. However, when compared by specific strength (strength per density), the titanium alloys excel any other implant materials, as shown in Figure 40.6. Titanium, nevertheless, has poor shear strength, making it less desirable for bone screws, plates, and similar applications. Titanium also tends to gall or seize when in sliding contact with itself or another metal.

Titanium derives its resistance to corrosion by the formation of a solid oxide layer. Under in vivo conditions the oxide (TiO_2) is the only stable reaction product. The oxide layer forms a thin adherent film and passivates the material. Corrosion-resistance mechanisms are discussed later.

The *titanium-nickel* alloy shows unusual properties, i.e., after it is deformed the material can snap back to its previous shape following heating of the material. This phenomenon is called *shape memory effect* (SME). The SME of TiNi alloy was first observed by Buehler and Wiley at the U.S. Naval Ordnance Laboratory [Buehler et al., 1963]. The equiatomic TiNi or NiTi alloy (Nitinol) exhibits an exceptional SME near room temperature: If it is plastically deformed below the transformation temperature, it reverts back to its original shape as the temperature is raised. The SME can be generally related to a diffusionless martensitic phase transformation which is also thermoelastic in nature, the thermoelasticity being attributed to the ordering in the parent and martensitic phases [Wayman & Shimizu, 1972].

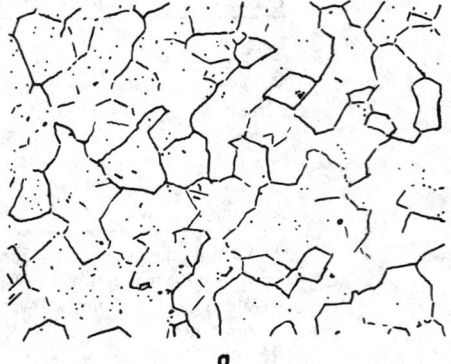

a

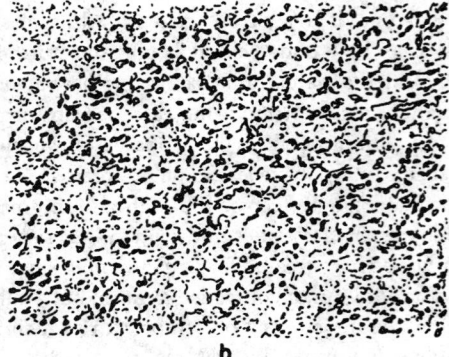

b

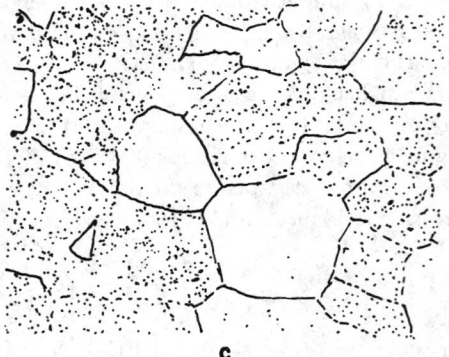

c

FIGURE 40.5   Microstructure of Ti alloys (all are 500X) [Hille, 1966]. (*a*) Annealed α-alloy; (*b*) Ti6Al4V, α-β alloy, annealed; (*c*) β-alloy, annealed.

TABLE 40.6   Mechanical Properties of Ti and Its Alloys

Properties	Grade 1	Grade 2	Grade 3	Grade 4	Ti6Al4V	Ti13Nb13Zr
Tensile strength, MPa	240	345	450	550	860	1030
Yield strength (0.2% offset), MPa	170	275	380	485	795	900
Elongation, %	24	20	18	15	10	15
Reduction of area, %	30	30	30	25	25	45

Source: American Society for Testing and Materials, 1994, F67-89, p 39; F136-84, p 55; and Davidson et al., 1994.

Some possible applications of shape memory alloys are orthodontic dental archwires, intracranial aneurysm clips, a vena cava filter, contractile artificial muscles for an artificial heart, and orthopedic implants. In order to develop such devices, it is necessary to understand fully the mechanical and thermal behavior associated with the martensitic phase transformation. A widely known NiTi alloy is 55-Nitinol (55 weight % or 50 atomic % Ni); it has a single phase and the mechanical memory plus other properties, including high acoustic damping, direct conversion of heat energy into mechanical energy, good fatigue properties, and low temperature ductility. Deviation from the 55-Nitinol (near stoichiometric NiTi) in the Ni-rich direction yields a second group of alloys which are also completely nonmagnetic but which differ from 55-Nitinol in their capability of being thermally hardened to higher hardness levels. Shape recovery capability decreases and heat treatability increases rapidly as the Ni content approaches 60%. Both 55- and 60-Nitinols have relatively low modulus of elasticity and can be tougher and more resilient than stainless steel, NiCr, or CoCr alloys.

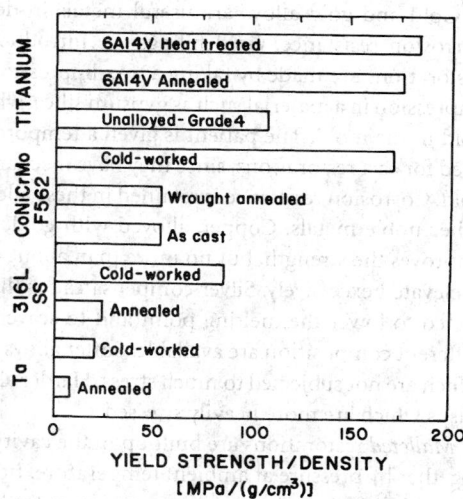

FIGURE 40.6 Yield-strength-to-density ratio of some implant materials [Hille, 1966].

Efficiency of 55-Nitinol shape recovery can be controlled by changing the final annealing temperatures during preparation of the alloy device [Lee et al., 1988]. For the most efficient recovery, the shape is fixed by constraining the specimen in a desired configuration and heating to between 482 and 510°C. If the annealed wire is deformed at a temperature below the shape recovery temperature, shape recovery will occur upon heating, provided the deformation has not exceeded crystallographic strain limits (~8% strain in tension). The NiTi alloys also exhibit good biocompatibility and corrosion resistance in vivo.

The mechanical properties of NiTi alloys are especially sensitive to the stoichiometry of composition (typical composition is given in Table 40.7) and the individual thermal and mechanical history. Although much is known about the processing, mechanical behavior, and properties relating to the shape memory effect, considerably less is known about the thermomechanical and physical metallurgy of the alloy.

40.4 Dental Metals

Dental *amalgam* is an alloy made of liquid mercury and other solid metal particulate alloy made of silver, tin, copper, etc. The solid alloy is mixed with (liquid) mercury in a mechanical vibrating mixer, and the resulting material is packed into the prepared cavity. One of the solid alloys is composed of at least 65% silver and not more than 29% tin, 6% copper, 2% zinc, and 3% mercury. The reaction during setting is thought to be

$$\gamma + Hg \rightarrow \gamma + \gamma_1 + \gamma_2 \qquad (40.1)$$

in which the γ phase is Ag_3Sn, the γ_1 phase is Ag_2Hg_3, and the γ_2 phase is Sn_7Hg. The phase diagram for the Ag-Sn-Hg system shows that over a wide compositional range all three phases are present. The final composition of dental amalgams typically contains 45 to 55% mercury, 35 to 45% silver, and about 15% tin after fully set in about one day.

TABLE 40.7 Chemical Composition of NiTi Alloy Wire

Element	Composition, %
Ni	54.01
Co	0.64
Cr	0.76
Mn	0.64
Fe	0.66
Ti	balance

Gold and gold alloys are useful metals in dentistry because of their durability, stability, and corrosion resistance. Gold fillings are introduced by two methods: casting and malleting. *Cast* restorations are made by taking a wax impression of the prepared cavity, making a mold from this impression in a material such as gypsum silica, which tolerates high temperature, and casting molten gold in the mold. The patient is given a temporary filling for the intervening time. Gold *alloys* are used for cast restorations, since they have mechanical properties which are superior to those of pure gold. Corrosion resistance is retained in these alloys provided they contain 75% or more of gold and other noble metals. Copper, alloyed with gold, significantly increases its strength. Platinum also improves the strength, but no more than about 4% can be added, or the melting point of the alloy is elevated excessively. Silver compensates for the color of copper. A small amount of zinc may be added to lower the melting point and to scavenge oxides formed during melting. Gold alloys of different composition are available. Softer alloys containing more than 83% gold are used for inlays which are not subjected to much stress. Harder alloys containing less gold are chosen for crowns and cusps which are more heavily stressed.

Malleted restorations are built up in the cavity from layers of *pure* gold foil. The foils are welded together by pressure at ambient temperature. In this type of welding, the metal layers are joined by thermal diffusion of atoms from one layer to the other. Since intimate contact is required in this procedure, it is particularly important to avoid contamination. The pure gold is relatively soft, so this type of restoration is limited to areas not subjected to much stress.

40.5 Other Metals

Several other metals have been used for a variety of specialized implant applications. *Tantalum* has been subjected to animal implant studies and has been shown to be very biocompatible. Due to its poor mechanical properties (Table 40.8) and its high density (16.6 g/cm^3) it is restricted to a few applications such as wire sutures for plastic surgeons and neurosurgeons and a radioisotope for bladder tumors.

Platinum and other noble metals in the platinum group are extremely corrosion resistant but have poor mechanical properties. They are mainly used as alloys for electrodes such as pacemaker tips because of their high resistance to corrosion and low threshold potentials.

Thermoseeds made of 70%Ni and 30%Cu have been produced which possess Curie points in the therapeutic hyperthermia range, approximately 40–50°C [Ferguson et al., 1992]. Upon the application of an alternating magnetic field, eddy currents are induced, which will provide a continuous heat source through resistive heating of the material. As the temperature of a ferromagnetic substance nears its Curie point, however, there is a loss of ferromagnetic properties and a resulting loss of heat output. Thus, self-regulation of temperature is achieved and can be used to deliver a constant hyperthermic temperature extracorporeally at any time and duration.

40.6 Corrosion of Metallic Implants

Corrosion is the unwanted chemical reaction of a metal with its environment, resulting in its continued degradation to oxides, hydroxides, or other compounds. Tissue fluid in the human body

TABLE 40.8 Mechanical Properties of Tantalum

Properties	Annealed	Cold-Worked
Tensile strength, MPa	207	517
Yield strength (0.2% offset), MPa	138	345
Elongation, %	20–30	2
Young's modulus, GPa	—	190

Source: American Society for Testing and Materials, F560-86, p 143, 1992].

contains water, dissolved oxygen, proteins, and various ions such as chloride and hydroxide. As a result, the human body presents a very aggressive environment to metals used for implantation. Corrosion resistance of a metallic implant material is consequently an important aspect of its biocompatibility.

Electrochemical Aspects

The lowest free energy state of many metals in an oxygenated and hydrated environment is that of the *oxide*. Corrosion occurs when metal atoms become ionized and go into solution or combine with oxygen or other species in solution to form a compound which flakes off or dissolves. The body environment is very aggressive in terms of corrosion, since the body is not only aqueous but also contains chloride ions and proteins. A variety of chemical reactions occur when a metal is exposed to an aqueous environment, as shown in Figure 40.7. The electrolyte, which contains ions in solution, serves to complete the electric circuit. In the human body the required ions are plentiful in the body fluids. Anions are negative ions which migrate toward the anode, and cations are positive ions which migrate toward the cathode. At the anode, or positive electrode, the metal oxidizes by losing valence electrons:

$$M \rightarrow M^{+n} + ne^- \qquad (40.2)$$

At the cathode, or negative electrode, the following reduction reactions are important.

$$M^{+n} + ne^- \rightarrow M \qquad (40.3)$$

$$M^{++} + OH^- + 2e^- \rightarrow MOH \qquad (40.4)$$

$$2H_3O^+ + 2e^- \rightarrow H_2\uparrow + 2H_2O \qquad (40.5)$$

$$1/2O_2 + H_2O + 2e^- \rightarrow 2OH^- \qquad (40.6)$$

The tendency of metals to corrode is expressed most simply in the standard electrochemical series of Nernst potentials, shown in Table 40.9. These potentials are obtained in electrochemical measurements in which one electrode is a standard hydrogen electrode formed by bubbling hydrogen through a layer of finely divided platinum black. The potential of this reference electrode is defined to be zero. Noble metals are those which have a potential higher than that of a standard hydrogen electrode; base metals have lower potentials.

If two dissimilar metals are present in the same environment, the one which is most negative in the galvanic series will become the anode, and bimetallic (or galvanic) corrosion will occur. Galvanic corrosion can be much more rapid than the corrosion of a single metal. Consequently, implantation of dissimilar metals (mixed metals) is to be avoided. Galvanic action can also result in corrosion within a single metal, if there is inhomogeneity in the metal or in its environment, as shown in Figure 40.8.

The potential difference E actually observed depends on the concentration of the metal ions in solution according to the Nernst equation

$$E = E_o + (RT/nF) \ln[M^{+n}] \qquad (40.7)$$

in which R is the gas constant, E_o is the standard electrochemical potential, T is the absolute temperature, F is Faraday's constant (96,487 C/mol), and n is the number of moles of ions.

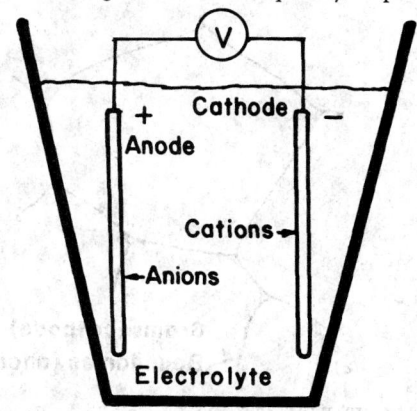

FIGURE 40.7 Electrochemical cell.

The order of nobility observed in actual practice may differ from that predicted thermodynamically. The reasons are that some metals become covered with a passivating film of reaction products which protects the metal from further attack. The dissolution reaction may be strongly irreversible so that a potential barrier must be overcome. In this case, corrosion may be inhibited even though it remains energetically favorable. The kinetics of corrosion reactions are not determined by the thermodynamics alone.

TABLE 40.9 Standard Electrochemical Series

Reaction	$\Delta E°$ (volts)
$Li \leftrightarrow (Li^+$	-3.05
$Na \leftrightarrow Na^+$	-2.71
$Al \leftrightarrow Al^{+++}$	-1.66
$Ti \leftrightarrow Ti^{+++}$	-1.63
$Cr \leftrightarrow Cr^{++}$	-0.56
$Fe \leftrightarrow Fe^{++}$	-0.44
$Cu \leftrightarrow Cu^{++}$	-0.34
$Co \leftrightarrow Co^{++}$	-0.28
$Ni \leftrightarrow Ni^{++}$	-0.23
$H_2 \leftrightarrow 2H^+$	0.00
$Ag \leftrightarrow Ag^+$	$+0.80$
$Au \leftrightarrow Au^+$	$+1.68$

Pourbaix Diagrams in Corrosion

The Pourbaix diagram is a plot of regions of *corrosion, passivity,* and *immunity* as they depend on electrode potential and pH [Pourbaix, 1974]. The Pourbaix diagrams are derived from the Nernst equation and from the solubility of the degradation products and the equilibrium constants of the reaction. For the sake of definition, the *corrosion region* is set arbitrarily at a concentration of greater than 10^{-6} gram atom per liter (molar) or more of metal in the solution at equilibrium. This corresponds to about 0.06 mg/l for metals such as iron and copper, and 0.03 mg/l for aluminum. *Immunity* is defined as equilibrium between metal and its ions at less than 10^{-6} molar. In the region of immunity, the corrosion is energetically impossible. Immunity is also referred to as *cathodic protection*. In the passivation domain, the stable solid constituent is an oxide, hydroxide, a hydride, or a salt of the metal. *Passivity* is defined as equilibrium between a metal and its reaction products (oxides, hydroxides, etc.) at a concentration of 10^{-6} molar or less. This situation is useful if reaction products are adherent. In the biomaterials setting, passivity may or may not be adequate: Disruption of a passive layer may cause an increase in corrosion. The equilibrium state may not occur if reaction products are removed by the tissue fluid. Materials differ in their propensity to reestablish a passive layer which has been damaged. This layer of material may protect the underlying metal if it is firmly adherent and nonporous; in that case further corrosion is prevented. Passivation can also result from a concentration polarization due to a buildup of ions near the electrodes. This is not likely to occur in the body, since the ions are continually replenished. Cathodic depolarization reactions can aid in the passivation of a metal by virtue of an energy barrier which hinders the kinetics. Equations (40.5) and (40.6) are examples.

There are two diagonal lines in the diagrams shown in Figure 40.9. The top "oxygen" line represents the upper limit of the stability of water and is associated with oxygen-rich solutions or electrolytes near oxidizing materials. In the region above this line, oxygen is evolved according to

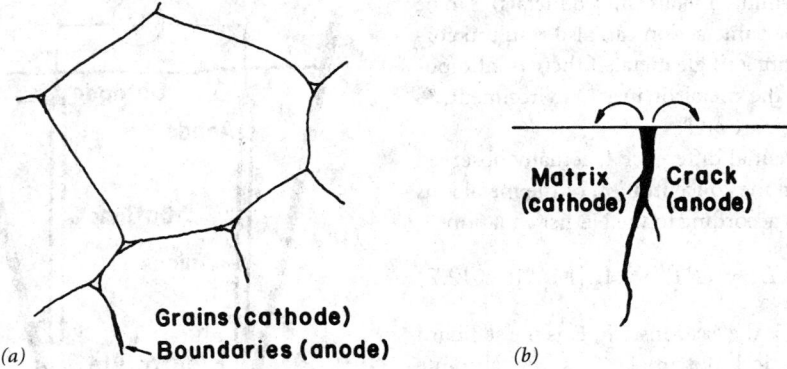

(a)   *(b)*

FIGURE 40.8 Microcorrosion cells. (*a*) Grain boundaries anodic with respect to the grain interior; (*b*) crevice corrosion due to oxygen-deficient zone in metal's environment.

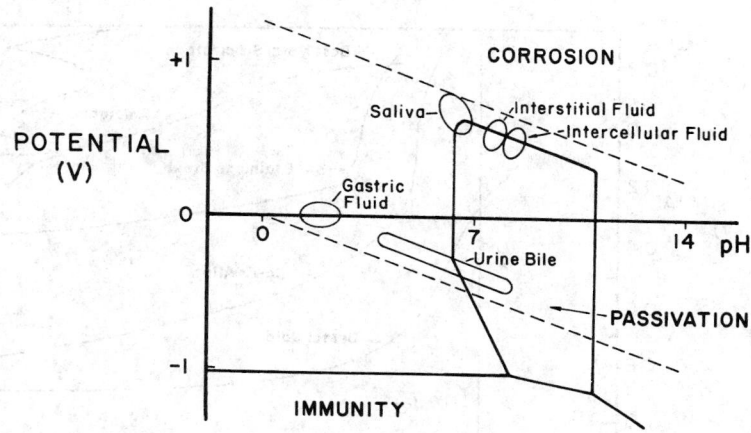

FIGURE 40.9 Pourbaix diagram for chromium, showing regions associated with various body fluids [modified from Black, 1992].

$2H_2O \rightarrow O_2\uparrow + 4H^+ + 4e^-$. In the human body, saliva, intracellular fluid, and interstitial fluid occupy regions near the oxygen line, since they are saturated with oxygen. The lower "hydrogen" diagonal line represents the lower limit of the stability of water. Hydrogen gas is evolved according to Equation (40.5). Aqueous corrosion occurs in the region between these diagonal lines on the Pourbaix diagram. In the human body, urine, bile, the lower gastrointestinal tract, and secretions of ductless glands occupy a region somewhat above the hydrogen line.

The significance of Pourbaix diagrams is as follows. Different parts of the body have different pH values and oxygen concentrations. Consequently a metal which performs well [is immune or passive] in one part of the body may suffer an unacceptable amount of corrosion in another part. Moreover, pH can change dramatically in tissue that has been injured or infected. In particular, normal tissue fluid has a pH of about 7.4, but in a wound it can be as low as 3.5, and in an infected wound the pH can increase to 9.0.

Pourbaix diagrams are useful but do not tell the whole story; there are some limitations. Diagrams are made considering equilibrium among metal, water, and reaction products. The presence of other ions, e.g., chloride, may result in very much different behavior, and large molecules in the body may also change the situation. Prediction of "passivity" may in some cases be optimistic, since reaction rates are not considered.

Rate of Corrosion and Polarization Curves

The regions in the Pourbaix diagram specify whether corrosion will take place, but they do not determine the rate. The rate, expressed as an electric current density [current per unit area] depends upon electrode potential as shown in the polarization curves shown in Figure 40.10. From such curves, it is possible to calculate the number of ions per unit time liberated into the tissue, as well as the depth of metal removed by corrosion in a given time. An alternative experiment is one in which the weight loss of a specimen of metal due to corrosion is measured as a function of time.

The rate of corrosion also depends on the presence of synergistic factors, such as those of mechanical origin. For example, in *fatigue corrosion*, repetitive deformation of a metal in a corrosive environment results in acceleration of both the corrosion and the fatigue microdamage. Since the body environment involves both repeated mechanical loading and a chemically aggressive environment, fatigue testing of implant materials should always be performed under physiological environmental conditions: under Ringer's solution at body temperature. In *fretting corrosion*, rubbing of one part on another disrupts the passivation layer, resulting in accelerated corrosion. In *pitting*, the corrosion rate is accelerated in a local region. Stainless steel is vulnerable to pitting. Localized corrosion can occur if there is inhomogeneity in the metal or in the environment. *Grain*

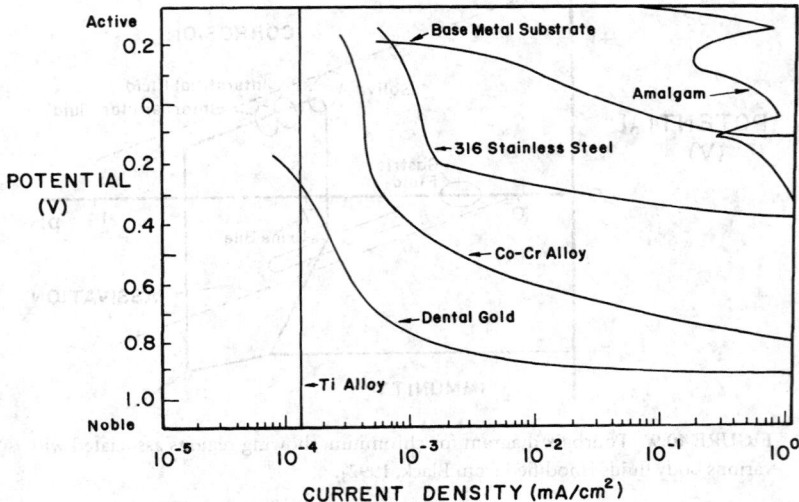

FIGURE 40.10 Potential-current density curves for some biomaterials [Greener et al., 1972].

boundaries in the metal may be susceptible to the initiation of corrosion, as a result of their higher energy level. *Crevices* are also vulnerable to corrosion, since the chemical environment in the crevice may differ from that in the surrounding medium. The area of contact between a screw and a bone plate, for example, can suffer crevice corrosion.

Corrosion of Available Metals

Choice of a metal for implantation should take into account the corrosion properties discussed above. Metals which are in current use as biomaterials include gold, cobalt chromium alloys, type 316 stainless steel, cp-titanium, titanium alloys, nickel-titanium alloys, and silver-tin-mercury amalgam.

The noble metals are immune to corrosion and would be ideal materials if corrosion resistance were the only concern. Gold is widely used in dental restorations, and in that setting it offers superior performance and longevity. Gold is not, however, used in orthopaedic applications as a result of its high density, insufficient strength, and high cost.

Titanium is a base metal in the context of the electrochemical series; however, it forms a robust passivating layer and remains passive under physiological conditions. Corrosion currents in normal saline are very low: 10^{-8} A/cm^2. Titanium implants remain virtually unchanged in appearance. Ti offers superior corrosion resistance but is not as stiff or strong as steel or CoCr alloys.

Cobalt-chromium alloys, like titanium, are passive in the human body. They are in wide use in orthopaedic applications. They do not exhibit pitting corrosion.

Stainless steels contain enough chromium to confer corrosion resistance by passivity. The passive layer is not as robust as in the case of titanium or the cobalt chrome alloys. Only the most corrosion resistant of the stainless steels are suitable for implants. These are the austentitic types 316, 316L, and 317, which contain molybdenum. Even these types of stainless steel are vulnerable to pitting and to crevice corrosion around screws.

The phases of dental amalgam are passive at neutral pH, and the transpassive potential for the γ_2 phase is easily exceeded, due to interphase galvanic couples or potentials due to differential aeration under dental plaque. Amalgam, therefore, often corrodes and is the most active (corrosion-prone) material used in dentistry.

Corrosion of an implant in the clinical setting can result in symptoms such as local pain and swelling in the region of the implant, with no evidence of infection; cracking or flaking of the implant as seen on x-ray films; and excretion of excess metal ions. At surgery, gray or black discoloration of the surrounding tissue may be seen, and flakes of metal may be found in the tissue. Corrosion also plays a role in the mechanical failures of orthopedic implants. Most of these failures are due to fatigue, and the presence of a saline environment certainly exacerbates fatigue. The extent to which corrosion influences fatigue in the body is not precisely known.

40.7 Manufacturing of Implants

Stainless Steels

The austenitic stainless steels work-harden very rapidly as shown in Figure 40.2 and therefore cannot be cold-worked without intermediate heat treatments. The heat treatments should not induce, however, the formation of chromium carbide (CCr_4) in the grain boundaries (sensitized); that may cause corrosion. For the same reason, the austenitic stainless steel implants are not usually welded.

The distortion of components by the heat treatments can occur, but this problem can be solved by controlling the uniformity of heating. Another undesirable effect of the heat treatment is the formation of surface oxide scales which have to be removed either chemically (acid) or mechanically (sand blasting). After the scales are removed, the surface of the component is polished to a mirror or matte finish. The surface is then cleaned, degreased, and passivated in nitric acid (ASTM Standard F86). The component is washed and cleaned again before packaging and sterilizing.

CoCr Alloys

The CoCrMo alloy is particularly susceptible to the work hardening so that the normal fabrication procedure used with other metals cannot be employed. Instead the alloy is cast by a lost wax (or investment casting) method which involves making a wax pattern of the desired component. The pattern is coated with a refractory material, first by a thin coating with a slurry (suspension of silica in ethyl silicate solution) followed by complete investing after drying. The wax is melted out in a furnace (100–150°C); the mold is heated to a high temperature, burning out any traces of wax or gas-forming materials; molten alloy is poured with gravitational or centrifugal force; and the mold is broken after cooling. The mold temperature is about 800–1000°C, and the alloy is at 1350–1400°C.

Controlling the mold temperature will have an effect on the grain size of the final cast; coarse ones are formed at higher temperatures which will decrease the strength. However, high processing temperature will result in larger carbide precipitates with greater distances between them resulting in a less brittle material. Again there is a complementary (trade-off) relationship between strength and ductility.

Ti and Its Alloys

Titanium is very reactive at high temperature and oxidizes readily in the presence of oxygen. Therefore, it requires an inert atmosphere for high-temperature processing or is processed by vacuum melting. Oxygen diffuses readily in titanium, and the dissolved oxygen embrittles the metal. As a result any hot working or forging operation should be carried out below 925°C. Machining at room temperature is not the solution to all the problems, since the material also tends to gall or seize the cutting tools. Very sharp tools with slow speeds and large feeds are used to minimize this effect. Electrochemical machining is an attractive means.

Defining Terms

Amalgam: An alloy obtained by mixing silver tin alloy with mercury.
Anode: Positive electrode in an electrochemical cell.
Cathode: Negative electrode in an electrochemical cell.

Corrosion: Unwanted reaction of metal with environment. In a Pourbaix diagram, it is the region in which the metal ions are present at a concentration of more than 10^{-6} molar.

Crevice corrosion: A form of localized corrosion in which concentration gradients around preexisting crevices in the material drive corrosion processes.

Curie temperature: Transition temperature of a material from ferromagnetic to paramagnetic.

Galvanic corrosion: Dissolution of metal driven by macroscopic differences in electrochemical potential, usually as a result of dissimilar metals in proximity.

Galvanic series: Table of electrochemical potentials (voltage) associated with the ionization of metal atoms. These are called *Nernst potentials.*

Hyperthermia: Application of high enough thermal energy (heat) to suppress the cancerous cell activities. Above 41.5°C (but below 60°C) is needed to have any effect.

Immunity: Resistance to corrosion by an energetic barrier. In a Pourbaix diagram, it is the region in which the metal is in equilibrium with its ions at a concentration of less than 10^{-6} molar. Noble metals resist corrosion by immunity.

Martensite: A metastable structure formed by quenching of austenite (g) structure in alloys such as steel, martensites are brittle and hard and therefore are further heat-treated to make them tougher.

Nernst potential: Standard electrochemical potential measured with respect to a standard hydrogen electrode.

Noble: Type of metal with a positive standard electrochemical potential.

Passivation: Production of corrosion resistance by a surface layer of reaction products (normally, oxide layer, which is impervious to gas and water).

Passivity: Resistance to corrosion by a surface layer of reaction products. In a Pourbaix diagram, it is the region in which the metal is in equilibrium with its reaction products at a concentration of less than 10^{-6} molar.

Pitting: A form of localized corrosion in which pits form on the metal surface.

Pourbaix diagram: Plot of electrical potential versus pH for a material in which the regions of corrosion, passivity, and immunity are identified.

Shape memory effect (SME):   Thermoelastic behavior of some alloys which can revert to their original shape when the temperature is greater than the phase transformation temperature of the alloy.

References

American Society for Metal. 1978. Source Book on Industrial Alloy and Engineering Data, p 223, Metal Park, Ohio.

American Society for Testing and Materials. 1992. Annual Book of ASTM Standards, vol 13, Medical Devices and Services, Philadelphia. American Society for Testing and Materials.

Black J. 1992. Biological Performance of Materials, 2d ed, p 43, New York, M. Dekker.

Buehler WJ, Gilfrich JV, Wiley RC. 1963. Effect of low-temperature phase changes on the mechanical properties of alloys near composition Ti-Ni. J Appl Phys 34:1475.

Davidson JA, Mishra AK, Kovacs P, et al. 1994. New surface hardened, low-modulus, corrosion-resistant Ti-13Nb-13Zr alloy for total hip arthroplasty. Biomed Mater Eng 4:231.

Devine TM, Wulff J. 1975. Cast vs. wrought cobalt-chromium surgical implant alloys. J Biomed Mater Res 9:151.

Ferguson SD, Paulus JA, Tucker RD, et al. 1992. Effect of thermal treatment on heating characteristics of Ni-Cu alloy for hyperthermie: Preliminary studies. J Appl Biomater 4:55.

Greener EH, Harcourt JK, Lautenschlager EP. 1972. Materials Science in Dentistry. Baltimore, Williams and Wilkins.

Hille GH. 1966. Titanium for surgical implants. J Mater 1:373.

Keating FH. 1956. Chromium-Nickel Austenitic Steels, London, Butterworth.

Lee JH, Park JB, Andreasen GF, et al. 1988. Thermomechanical study of Ni-Ti alloys. J Biomed Mater Res 22:573.

Pourbaix M. 1974. Atlas of Electrochemical Equilibria in Aqueous Solutions, 2d ed, Brussels, NACE, Houston/CEBELCOR.

Richards Manufacturing Company. 1980. Biophase Implant Material, Technical Information Pub. No. 3846, p 7, Memphis, Tenn.

Semlitsch M. 1980. Properties of wrought CoNiCrMo alloy Protasul-10, a highly corrosion and fatigue resistant implant material for joint endoprostheses. Eng Med 9:201.

Smith CJE, Hughes AN. 1966. The corrosion fatigue behavior of a titanium-6w/o aluminum-4w/o vanadium alloy. Eng Med 7:158.

Wayman CM, Shimizu K. 1972. The shape memory ('Marmem') effect in alloys. Metal Sci J 6:175.

Weinstein AM, Spires WP Jr, Klawitter JJ, et al. 1978. Orthopedic implant retrieval and analysis study. In BC Syrett, A Acharya (eds), Corrosion and Degradation of Implant Materials. ASTM STP 684, pp 245–258, Philadelphia, American Society for Testing and Materials.

Williams DF. 1982. Orthopedic implants: Fundamental principles and the significance of biocompatibility. In DF Williams (ed), Biocompatibility of Orthopedic Implants, vol 1, pp 1–50, Boca Raton, Fla, CRC Press.

Further Information

American Society for Testing and Materials. 1992. Annual Book of ASTM Standards, vol 13, Medical Devices and Services, Philadelphia, American Society for Testing and Materials.

Bardos DI. 1977. Stainless steels in medical devices. In D Peckner, IM Bernstein (eds), Handbook of Stainless Steels, pp 1–10, New York, McGraw-Hill.

Bechtol CO, Ferguson AB Jr, Laing PG. 1959. Metals and Engineering in Bone and Joint Surgery, Baltimore, Williams and Wilkins.

Comte TW. 1984. Metallurgical observations of biomaterials. In JW Boretos, M Eden (eds), Contemporary Biomaterials, pp 66–91, Park Ridge, NJ, Noyes.

Duerig TW, Melton KN, Stockel D, et al (eds). 1990. Engineering Aspects of Shape Memory Alloys, London, Boston, Butterworth-Heinemann.

Dumbleton JH, Black J. 1975. *An Introduction to Orthopaedic Materials,* Springfield, Ill, C Thomas.

Fontana MG, Greene NO. 1967. Corrosion Engineering, pp 163–168, New York, McGraw-Hill.

Greener EH, Harcourt JK, Lautenschlager EP. 1972. Materials Science in Dentistry, Baltimore, Williams and Wilkins.

Hildebrand HF, Champy M (eds). 1988. Biocompatibility of Co-Cr-Ni Alloys, New York, Plenum Press.

Levine SN (ed). 1968. Materials in Biomedical Engineering, Annals of New York Academy of Science, vol 146, New York.

Mears DC. 1979. Materials and Orthopaedic Surgery, chap 5, Baltimore, Williams and Wilkins.

Perkins J (ed). 1975. Shape Memory Effects in Alloys, New York, Plenum Press.

Puckering FB (ed). 1979. The Metallurgical Evolution of Stainless Steels, pp 1–42, Metals Park, Ohio, American Society for Metals and the Metals Society.

Weinstein A, Horowitz E, Ruff AW (eds). 1977. Retrieval and Analysis of Orthopaedic Implants, NBS, Washington, DC. US Department of Commerce.

Williams DF, Roaf R. 1973. Implants in Surgery, Chs 6, 8, London, WB Saunders.

41

Ceramic Biomaterials

Praphulla K. Bajpai
University of Dayton

William G. Billotte
Wright State University

Ceramics are defined as the art and science of making and using solid articles that have as their essential component inorganic nonmetallic materials [Kingery et al., 1976]. Ceramics are refractory, polycrystalline compounds, usually inorganic, including silicates, metallic oxides, carbides, and various refractory hydrides, sulfides, and selenides. Oxides such as Al_2O_3, MgO, SiO_2, and ZrO_2 contain metallic and nonmetallic elements and ionic salts, such as NaCl, CsCl, ZnS [Park & Lakes, 1992]. Exceptions to the preceding include covalently bonded ceramics such as diamond and carbonaceous structures such as graphite and pyrolized carbons [Park & Lakes, 1992].

Ceramics in the form of pottery have been used by humans for thousands of years. Until recently, their use was somewhat limited because of their inherent brittleness, susceptibility to notches or microcracks, low tensile strength, and low impact strength. However, within the last 100 years, innovative techniques for fabricating ceramics have led to their use as "high tech" materials. In recent years, humans have realized that ceramics and their composites also can be used to augment or replace various parts of the body, particularly bone. Thus the ceramics used for the latter purposes are classified as *bioceramics*. Their relative inertness to the body fluids, high compressive strength, and aesthetically pleasing appearance led to the use of ceramics in dentistry as dental crowns. Some carbons have found use as implants, especially for blood-interfacing applications, such as heart valves. Due to their high specific strength as fibers and their biocompatibility, ceramics are also being used as reinforcing components of composite implant materials and for tensile loading applications such as artificial tendon and ligaments [Park & Lakes, 1992].

Unlike metals and polymers, ceramics are difficult to shear plastically due to the (ionic) nature of the bonding and minimum number of slip systems. These characteristics make the ceramics nonductile and are responsible for almost zero creep at room temperature [Park & Lakes, 1992]. Consequently, ceramics are very susceptible to notches or microcracks because instead of undergoing plastic deformation (or yield), they will fracture elastically on initiation of a crack. At the crack tip, the stress could be many times higher than the stress in the material away from the tip, resulting in a *stress concentration* that weakens the material considerably. The latter makes it difficult to predict the tensile strength of the material (ceramic). This is also the reason ceramics have low tensile

0-8493-8346-3/95/$0.00+$.50
© 1995 by CRC Press, Inc.

strength compared with compressive strength. If a ceramic is flawless, it is very strong even when subjected to tension. Flawless glass fibers have twice the tensile strength of high-strength steel (~7 GPa) [Park & Lakes, 1992].

Ceramics are generally hard; in fact, the measurement of hardness is calibrated against ceramic materials. Diamond is the hardest, with a hardness index on Mohs scale of 10, and talc ($Mg_3Si_3O_{10}COH$) is the softest ceramic (Mohs hardness 1), while ceramics such as alumina (Al_2O_3, hardness 9), quartz (SiO_2, hardness 8), and apatite ($Ca_5P_3O_{12}F$, hardness 5) are in the middle range. Other characteristics of ceramic materials are their high melting temperatures and low conductivity of electricity and heat. These characteristics are due to the chemical bonding within ceramics.

In order to be classified as a bioceramic, the ceramic material must meet or exceed the properties listed in Table 41.1. The number of specific ceramics currently in use or under investigation cannot be accounted for in the space available for bioceramics in this book. Thus this chapter will focus on a general overview of the relatively bioinert, bioactive or surface-reactive ceramics, and biodegradable or resorbable bioceramics.

Ceramics used in fabricating implants can be classified as nonabsorbable (relatively inert), bioactive or surface reactive (semi-inert) [Hench, 1991, 1993], and biodegradable or resorbable (noninert) [Hentrich et al., 1971; Graves et al., 1972]. Alumina, zirconia, silicone nitrides, and carbons are inert bioceramics. Certain glass-ceramics and dense hydroxyapatites are semi-inert (bioreactive), and calcium phosphates and calcium aluminates are resorbable ceramics [Park & Lakes, 1992].

41.1 Nonabsorbable or Relatively Bioinert Bioceramics

Relatively Bioinert Ceramics

Relatively bioinert ceramics maintain their physical and mechanical properties while in the host. They resist corrosion and wear and have all the properties listed for bioceramics in Table 41.1. Examples of relatively bioinert ceramics are dense and porous aluminum oxides, zirconia ceramics, and single-phase calcium aluminates (Table 41.2). Relatively bioinert ceramics are typically used as structural-support implants. Some of these are bone plates, bone screws, and femoral heads (Table 41.3). Examples of non-structural-support uses are ventilation tubes, sterilization devices [Feenstra & de Groot, 1983], and drug delivery devices (see Table 41.3).

Alumina (Al_2O_3)

The main source of high-purity alumina (aluminum oxide, Al_2O_3) is bauxite and native corundum. The commonly available alumina (alpha, α) can be prepared by calcining alumina trihydrate. The chemical composition and density of commercially available "pure" calcined alumina are given in Table 41.4. The American Society for Testing and Materials (ASTM) specifies that alumina for implant use should contain 99.5% pure alumina and less than 0.1% combined SiO_2 and alkali oxides (mostly Na_2O) [F603-78].

Alpha alumina has a rhombohedral crystal structure ($a = 4.758$ Å and $c = 12.991$ Å). Natural alumina is known as sapphire or ruby depending on the types of impurities that give rise to color. The single-crystal form of alumina has been used successfully to make implants [Kawahara, 1989; Park, 1991]. Single-crystal alumina can be made by feeding fine alumina powders onto the surface

TABLE 41.1 Desired Properties of Implantable Bioceramics

1. Should be nontoxic.
2. Should be noncarcinogenic.
3. Should be nonallergic.
4. Should be noninflammatory.
5. Should be biocompatible.
6. Should be biofunctional for its lifetime in the host.

TABLE 41.2 Examples of Relatively Bioinert Bioceramics

Bioinert Ceramics	References
1. Pyrolitic carbon–coated devices	Adams and Williams, 1978
	Bokros et al., 1972
	Bokros, 1972
	Chandy and Sharma, 1991
	Dellsperger and Chandran, 1991
	Kaae, 1971
	More and Silver, 1990
	Shimm and Haubold, 1980
	Shobert, 1964
2. Dense and nonporous aluminum oxides	Hench, 1991
	Hentrich et al., 1971
	Krainess and Knapp, 1978
	Park, 1991
	Ritter et al., 1979
	Shackelford, 1988
3. Porous aluminum oxides	Hench, 1991
	Hentrich et al., 1971
	Park, 1991
	Ritter et al., 1979
	Shackelford, 1988
4. Zirconia ceramics	Barinov and Baschenko, 1992
	Drennan and Steele, 1991
	Hench, 1991
	Kumar et al., 1989
5. Dense hydroxyapatites	Bajpai, 1990
	Cotell et al., 1992
	Fulmer et al., 1992
	Huaxia et al., 1992
	Kijima and Tsutsumi, 1979
	Knowles et al., 1993
	Meenan et al., 1992
	Niwa et al., 1980
	Posner et al., 1958
	Schwartz et al., 1993
	Valiathan et al., 1993
	Whitehead et al., 1993
6. Calcium aluminates	Hammer et al., 1972
	Hentrich et al., 1971
	Hulbert and Klawitter, 1971

of a seed crystal which is slowly withdrawn from an electric arc or oxyhydrogen flame as the fused powder builds up. Single crystals of alumina up to 10 cm in diameter have been grown by this method [Park & Lakes, 1992].

The strength of polycrystalline alumina depends on its grain size and porosity. Generally, the smaller the grains, the lower the porosity and the higher the strength [Park & Lakes, 1992]. The ASTM standard (F603-78) requires a flexural strength greater than 400 MPa and an elastic modulus of 380 GPa (Table 41.5).

Aluminum oxide has been used in the area of orthopedics for more than a quarter of a century [Hench, 1991]. Single-crystal alumina has been used in orthopedics and dental surgery for almost 20 years. Alumina is usually a quite hard material, its hardness varying from 20 to 30 GPa. This high hardness permits its use as an abrasive (emery) and as bearings for watch movements [Park & Lakes, 1992]. Both polycrystalline and single-crystal alumina have been used clinically. The high hardness

TABLE 41.3 Uses of Bioinert Bioceramics

Bioinert Ceramics	References
1. In reconstruction of acetabular cavities	Boutin, 1981
	Dorlot et al., 1986
2. As bone plates and screws	Zimmermann et al., 1991
3. In the form of ceramic-ceramic composites	Boutin, 1981
	Chignier et al., 1987
	Sedel et al., 1991
	Terry et al., 1989
4. In the form of ceramic-polymer composites	Hulbert, 1992
5. As drug-delivery devices	Buykx et al., 1992
6. As femoral heads	Boutin, 1981
	Dörre, 1991
	Ohashi et al., 1988
	Oonishi, 1992
7. As middle ear ossicles	Grote, 1987
8. In the reconstruction of orbital rims	Heimke, 1992
9. As components of total and partial hips	Feenstra and de Groot, 1983
10. In the form of sterilization tubes	Feenstra and de Groot, 1983
11. As ventilation tubes	Feenstra and de Groot, 1983
12. In the repair of the cardiovascular area	Chignier et al., 1987
	Ely and Haubold, 1993

is accompanied by low friction and wear and inertness to the *in vivo* environment. These properties make alumina an ideal material for use in joint replacements [Park & Lakes, 1992]. Aluminum oxide implants in bones of rhesus monkeys have shown no signs of rejection or toxicity for 350 days [Graves et al., 1972; Hentrich et al., 1971]. One of the most popular uses for aluminum oxide is in total hip prostheses. Aluminum oxide hip prostheses with an ultra-high-molecular-weight polyethylene (UHMWPE) socket have been claimed to be a better device than a metal prostheses with a UHMWPE socket [Oonishi, 1992]. However, the key for success of any implant, besides the correct surgical implantation, is the highest possible quality control during fabrication of the material and the production of the implant [Hench, 1991].

Zirconia (ZrO$_2$)

Pure zirconia can be obtained from chemical conversion of zircon (ZrSiO$_4$), which is an abundant mineral deposit [Park & Lakes, 1992]. Zirconia has a high melting temperature (T_m = 2953 K) and chemical stability with a = 5.145 Å, b = 0.521 Å, c = 5.311 Å, and β = 99°14′ [Park & Lakes, 1992]. It undergoes a large volume change during phase changes at high temperature in pure form; therefore, a dopant oxide such as Y$_2$O$_3$ is used to stabilize the high-temperature (cubic) phase. We have used 6 mol% Y$_2$O$_3$ as dopant to make zirconia for implantation in bone [Hentrich et al., 1971].

Zirconia produced in this manner is referred to as *partially stabilized* zirconia [Drennan & Steele, 1991]. However, the physical properties of zirconia are somewhat inferior to that of alumina (Table 41.5).

High-density zirconia oxide showed excellent compatibility with autogenous rhesus monkey bone and was completely nonreactive to body environment for the duration of the 350-day study [Hentrich et al., 1971]. Zirconia has shown excellent biocompatibility and good wear and friction when combined with ultra-high-molecular-weight polyethylene (UHMWPE) [Kumar et al., 1989; Murakami & Ohtsuki, 1989].

TABLE 41.4 Chemical Composition of Calcined Alumina

Chemicals	Composition (weight %)
Al$_2$O$_3$	99.6
SiO$_2$	0.12
Fe$_2$O$_3$	0.03
Na$_2$O	0.04

Source: Park JB, Lakes RS. 1992. Ceramic implant materials. In Biomaterials: An Introduction, 2d ed, p 121. New York, Plenum Press.

Carbons

Carbons can be made in many allotropic forms: crystalline diamond, graphite, noncrystalline glassy carbon, and quasicrystalline pyrolitic carbon. Among these, only pyrolitic carbon is widely used for implant fabrication; it is normally used as a surface coating. It is also possible to coat surfaces with diamond. Although the techniques of coating with diamond have the potential to revolutionize medical device manufacturing, they are not yet commercially available [Park & Lakes, 1992].

TABLE 41.5 Physical Property Requirements of Alumina and Partially Stabilized Zirconia

Properties	Alumina	Zirconia
Elastic modulus (GPa)	380	190
Flexural strength (GPa)	>0.4	1.0
Hardness, Mohs	9	6.5
Density (g/cm³)	3.8–3.9	5.95
Grain size (μm)	4.0	0.6

Note: Both ceramics contain 3 mol% Y_2O_3.
Source: JB Park, personal communication, 1993.

The crystalline structure of carbon, as used in implants, is similar to the graphite structure shown in Fig. 41.1. The planar hexagonal arrays are formed by strong covalent bonds in which one of the valence electrons or atoms is free to move, resulting in high but anisotropic electric conductivity. Since the bonding between the layers is stronger than the van der Waals force, it has been suggested that the layers are *cross-linked.* However, the remarkable lubricating property of graphite cannot be attained unless the cross-links are eliminated [Park & Lakes, 1992].

The poorly crystalline carbons are thought to contain unassociated or unoriented carbon atoms. The hexagonal layers are not perfectly arranged, as shown in Fig. 41.2. Properties of individual crystallites seem to be highly anisotropic. However, if the crystallites are randomly dispersed, the aggregate becomes isotropic [Park & Lakes, 1992].

The mechanical properties of carbon, especially pyrolitic carbon, are largely dependent on its density, as shown in Figs. 41.3 and 41.4. The increased mechanical properties are directly related to increased density, which indicates that the properties of pyrolitic carbon depend mainly on the aggregate structure of the material [Park & Lakes, 1992].

Graphite and glassy carbon have much lower mechanical strength than pyrolitic carbon (Table 41.6). However, the average modulus of elasticity is almost the same for all carbons. The strength of pyrolitic carbon is quite high compared with graphite and glassy carbon. Again, this is due to the fewer number of flaws and unassociated carbons in the aggregate.

A composite carbon that is reinforced with carbon fiber has been considered for making implants. However, the carbon-carbon composite is highly anisotropic, and its density is in the range of 1.4 to 1.45 g/cm³ with a porosity of 35% to 38% (Table 41.7).

Carbons exhibit excellent compatibility with tissue. Compatibility of pyrolitic carbon–coated devices with blood have resulted in extensive use of these devices for repairing diseased heart valves and blood vessels [Park & Lakes, 1992].

Pyrolitic carbons can be deposited onto finished implants from hydrocarbon gas in a *fluidized bed* at a controlled temperature and pressure. The anisotropy, density, and crystallite size and structure of the deposited carbon can be controlled by temperature, composition of the fluidized gas, bed geometry, and residence time (velocity) of the gas molecules in the bed. The microstructure of deposited carbon should be highly controlled, since the formation of growth features associated with uneven crystallization can result in a weaker material (Fig. 41.5). It is also possible to introduce various elements into the fluidized gas and codeposit them with carbon. Usually, silicon (10 to 20 w/o) is codeposited (or alloyed) to increase hardness for applications requiring resistance to abrasion, such as heart valve disks.

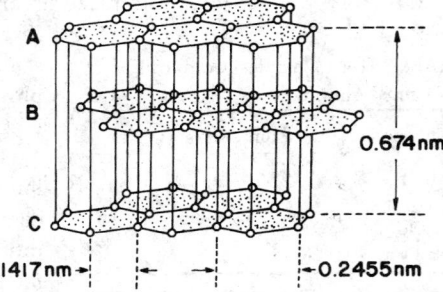

FIGURE 41.1 Crystal structure of graphite. (From Shobert EI II. 1964. Carbon and Graphite. New York, Academic Press.)

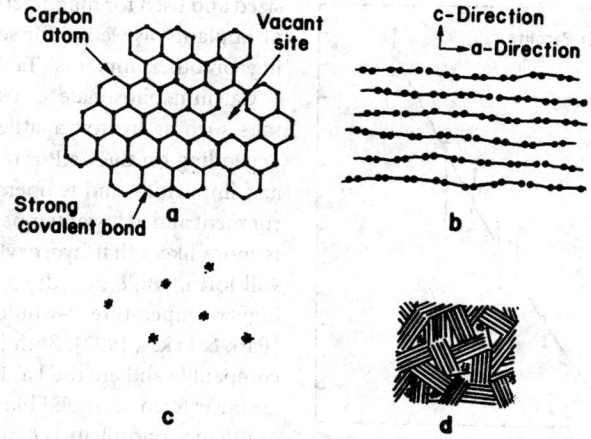

FIGURE 41.2 Schematic presentation of poorly crystalline carbon. (*a*) Single-layer plane. (*b*) Parallel layers in a crystallite. (*c*) Unassociated carbon. (*d*) An aggregate of crystallites, single layers, and unassociated carbon. (From Bokros JC. 1972. Deposition Structure and Properties of Pyrolitic Carbon. Chemistry and Physics of Carbon. 5, pp 70–81, New York, Marcel Dekker.)

Recently, success was achieved in depositing pyrolitic carbon onto the surfaces of blood vessel implants made of polymers. This type of carbon is called *ultra-low-temperature isotropic (ULTI) carbon* instead of low-temperature isotropic (LTI) carbon. The deposited carbon has excellent compatibility with blood and is thin enough not to interfere with the flexibility of the grafts [Park & Lakes, 1992].

The vitreous or glassy carbon is made by controlled pyrolysis of polymers such as phenolformaldehyde, Rayon (cellulose), and polyacrylnitrite at a high temperature in a controlled environment. This process is particularly useful for making carbon fibers and textiles which can be used alone or as components of composites.

41.2 Biodegradable or Resorbable Ceramics

Although Plaster of Paris was used in 1892 as a bone substitute [Peltier, 1961], the concept of using synthetic resorbable ceramics as bone substitutes was introduced in 1969 [Hentrich et al., 1969; Graves et al., 1972]. *Resorbable ceramics,* as the name implies, degrade on implantation in the host.

The resorbed material is replaced by endogenous tissues. The rate of degradation varies from material to material. Almost all bioresorbable ceramics except Biocoral and Plaster of Paris (calcium sulfate dihydrate) are variations of calcium phosphate (Table 41.8). Examples of resorbable ceramics are aluminum calcium phosphate, coralline, plaster of paris, hydroxyapatite, and tricalcium phosphate (see Table 41.8).

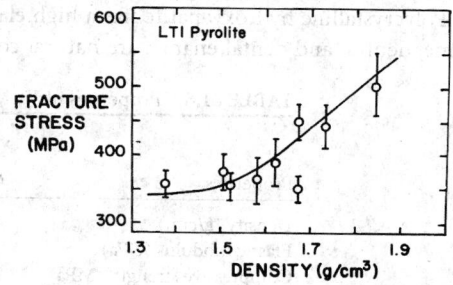

FIGURE 41.3 Fracture stress versus density for unalloyed LTI pyrolite carbons. (From Kaae JL. 1971. Structure and mechanical properties of isotropic pyrolytic carbon deposited below 1600°C. J Nucl Mater 38:42–50.)

Calcium Phosphate

Calcium phosphate has been used in the form of artificial bone. This material has been synthe-

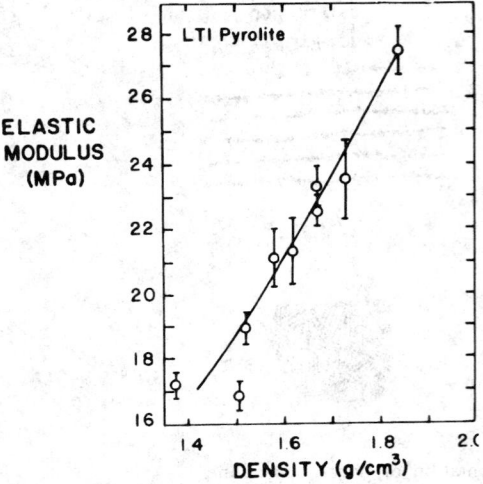

FIGURE 41.4   Elastic modulus versus density for unalloyed LTI pyrolite carbons. (From Kaae JL. 1971. Structure and mechanical properties of isotropic pyrolytic carbon deposited below 1600°C. J Nucl Mater 38:42–50.)

sized and used for manufacturing various forms of implants, as well as for solid or porous coatings on other implants (Table 41.9).

Calcium phosphate can be crystallized into salts such as hydroxyapatite and β-whitlockite depending on the Ca:P ratio, presence of water and impurities, and temperature. In a wet environment and at lower temperatures (<900°C), it is more likely that hydroxyl- or hydroxyapatite will form, while in a dry atmosphere and at a higher temperature, β-whitlockite will be formed [Park & Lakes, 1992]. Both forms are very tissue compatible and are used as bone substitutes in a granular form or a solid block. The apatite form of calcium phosphate is considered to be closely related to the mineral phase of bone and teeth.

The mineral part of bone and teeth is made of a crystalline form of calcium phosphate similar to hydroxyapatite $[Ca_{10}(PO_4)_6(OH)_2]$. The apatite family of mineral $[A_{10}(BO_4)_6X_2]$ crystallizes into hexagonal rhombic prisms and has unit-cell dimensions $a = 9.432$ Å and $c = 6.881$ Å.

The atomic structure of hydroxyapatite projected down on the c axis onto the basal plane is shown in Fig. 41.6. Note that the hydroxyl ions lie on the corners of the projected basal plane and occur at equidistant intervals (3.44 Å) along the columns perpendicular to the basal plane and parallel to the c axis. Six of the 10 calcium ions in the unit cell are associated with the hydroxyls in these columns, resulting in strong interactions among them [Park & Lakes, 1992].

The ideal Ca:P ratio of hydroxyapatite is 10:6, and the calculated density is 3.219 g/cm^3. Substitution of OH with fluoride gives the apatite greater chemical stability due to the closer coordination of fluoride (symmetrical shape) as compared with the hydroxyl (asymmetrical, two atoms) by the nearest calcium. This is why fluoridation of drinking water helps in resisting caries of the teeth [Park & Lakes, 1992].

The mechanical properties of synthetic calcium phosphates vary considerably (Table 41.10). The wide variations in properties of polycrystalline calcium phosphates are due to variations in the structure and manufacturing processes. Depending on the final firing conditions, the calcium phosphate can be calcium hydroxyapatite or β-whitlockite. In many instances, both types of structures exist in the same final product [Park & Lakes, 1992].

Polycrystalline hydroxyapatite has a high elastic modulus (40 to 117 GPa). Hard tissue such as bone, dentin, and dental enamel are natural composites that contain hydroxyapatite (or a similar

TABLE 41.6   Properties of Various Types of Carbon

	Types of Carbon		
Properties	Graphite	Glassy	Pyrolitic*
Density (g/cm₃)	1.5–1.9	1.5	1.5–2.0
Elastic modulus (GPa)	24	24	28
Compressive strength (MPa)	138	172	517 (575*)
Toughness (m · N/cm³)†	6.3	0.6	4.8

*1.0 w/o Si-alloyed pyrolitic carbon, Pyrolite (Carbomedics, Austin, TX).
†1 m · N/cm³ = 1.45 × 10⁻³ in · lb/in³.
Source: Park JB, Lakes RS. 1992. Ceramic implant materials. In Biomaterials: An Introduction, 2d ed, p 133. New York, Plenum Press.

TABLE 41.7 Mechanical Properties of Carbon Fiber–Reinforced Carbon

	Fiber Lay-up	
Property	Unidirectional	0–90° Crossply
Flexural modulus (GPa)		
Longitudinal	140	60
Transverse	7	60
Flexural strength (MPa)		
Longitudinal	1200	500
Transverse	15	500
Interlaminar shear strength (MPa)	18	18

Source: Adams D. and Williams DF. 1978. Carbon Fiber-Reinforced Carbon as a Potential Implant Material. J Biomed Mater Res 12:38.

mineral), as well as protein, other organic materials, and water. Enamel is the stiffest hard tissue, with an elastic modulus of 74 GPa, and contains the most mineral. Dentin ($E = 21$ GPa) and compact bone ($E = 12$ to 18 GPa) contain comparatively less mineral. The Poisson's ratio for the mineral or synthetic hydroxyapatite is about 0.27, which is close to that of bone (~0.3) [Park & Lakes, 1992].

Among the most important properties of hydroxyapatite as a biomaterial is its excellent biocompatability. Hydroxyapatite appears to form a direct chemical bond with hard tissues [Piattelli & Trisi, 1994]. On implantation of hydroxyapatite particles or porous blocks in bone, new lamellar cancellous bone forms within 4 to 8 weeks [Bajpai & Fuchs, 1985]. A scanning electron micrograph (500 ×) of a set and hardened hydroxyapatite-cysteine composite is shown in Fig. 41.7. The composite sets and hardens no addition of water.

Many different methods have been developed to make precipitates of hydroxyapatite from an aqueous solution of $Ca(NO_3)_2$ and NaH_2PO_4. We have successfully used a modification of Jarcho and coworkers' wet precipitation procedure for synthesizing hydroxyapatites for use as bone implants [Jarcho et al., 1979; Bajpai & Fuchs, 1985] and drug delivery devices [Abrams and Bajpai, 1994; Bajpai, 1992, 1994; Parker & Bajpai, 1993]. The dried filtered precipitate is placed in a high-temperature furnace and calcined at 1150°C for 1 hour. The calcined powder is then ground in a ball mill, and the particles are separated by an automatic sieve shaker and sieves. The sized particles are then pressed in a die and sintered at 1200°C for 36 hours for making drug delivery devices [Abrams & Bajpai, 1994; Bajpai, 1989, 1992]. Above 1250°C, hydroxyapatite shows a second precipitation phase along the grain boundaries [Park & Lakes, 1992].

Aluminum Calcium Phosphate (ALCAP) Ceramics

Initially, we fabricated a calcium aluminate ceramic containing phosphorous pentoxide [Hentrich et al., 1969, 1971; Graves et al., 1972]. Aluminum-calcium-phosphorous oxide ceramic (ALCAP) was developed later [Bajpai & Graves, 1980]. ALCAP has insulating dielectric properties but no magnetic or piezoelectric properties [Allaire et al., 1989]. ALCAP ceramics are unique because they provide a multipurpose crystallographic system wherein phase of the ceramic on implantation can be more rapidly resorbed than the others [Bajpai, 1983; Mattie & Bajpai, 1988; Wyatt et al., 1976]. ALCAP is prepared from stock powders of aluminum oxide, calcium oxide, and phosphorous pentoxide. A ratio of 50:34:16 by weight of AlO_2, CaO, and P_2O_5 is used to obtain the starting mixture for calcining at 1350°C in a high-temperature furnace for 12 hours. The calcined material is ground in a ball mill and sieved by an automatic siever to obtain particles of the desired size. The particulate powder is then pressed into solid blocks or hollow cylinders (green shape) and sintered at 1400°C for 36 hours to increase the mechanical strength. ALCAP ceramic implants have given excellent results in terms of biocompatibility and gradual replacement of the ceramic material with

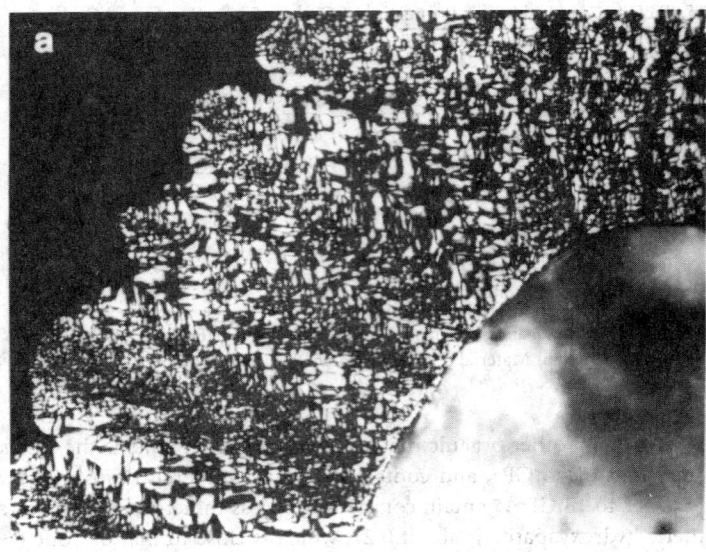

FIGURE 41.5   Microstructure of carbons deposited in a fluidized bed. (*a*) A granular carbon with distinct growth features. (*b*) An isotropic carbon without growth features. Both under polarized light; ×240. (From Bokros JC, LaGrange LD, Schoen GJ. 1972. Control of Structure of Carbon for Use in Bioengineering. Chemistry and Physics of Carbon 9, pp 103–171. New York, Marcel Dekker.)

endogenous bone [Bajpai, 1982; Mattie & Bajpai, 1988]. A scanning electron micrograph (1000×) of sintered porous ALCAP is shown in Fig. 41.8.

Coralline

Coral is a natural substance made by marine invertebrates. According to Holmes et al. [1984], the marine invertebrates live in the limestone exostructure, or coral. The porous structure of the coral

TABLE 41.8 Examples of Biodegradable Bioceramics

Biodegradable or Resorbable Bioceramic	References
1. Aluminum-calcium-phosphorous oxides	Bajpai et al., 1985
	Mattie and Bajpai, 1988
	Wyatt et al., 1976
2. Glass fibers and their composites	Alexander et al., 1987
	Zimmermann et al., 1991
3. Corals	Bajpai, 1983
	Guillemin et al., 1989
	Khavari and Bajpai, 1993
	Sartoris et al., 1986
	Wolford et al., 1987
4. Calcium sulfates, including plaster of paris	Bajpai, 1983
	Peltier, 1961
	Scheidler and Bajpai, 1992
5. Ferric-calcium-phosphorous oxides	Fuski et al., 1993
	Larrabee et al., 1993
	Stricker et al., 1992
6. Hydroxyapatites	Bajpai and Fuchs, 1985
	Bajpai, 1983
	Jenei et al., 1986
	Ricci et al., 1986
7. Tricalcium phosphate	Bajpai, 1983
	Bajpai et al., 1988
	Lemons et al., 1988
	Morris and Bajpai, 1989
8. Zinc-calcium-phosphorous oxides	Arar et al., 1989
	Bajpai, U.S. Patent No. 4778471
	Binzer and Bajpai, 1987
	Gromofsky et al., 1988
9. Zinc sulfate–calcium-phosphorous oxides	Scheidler and Bajpai, 1992

TABLE 41.9 Uses of Biodegradable Bioceramics

Biodegradable or Resorbable Ceramic	References
1. As drug-delivery devices	Abrams and Bajpai, 1994
	Bajpai, 1992
	Bajpai, 1994
	Benghuzzi et al., 1991
	Moldovan and Bajpai, 1994
	Nagy and Bajpai, 1994
2. For repairing damaged bone due to disease or trauma	Bajpai, 1990
	Gromofsky et al., 1988
	Khavari and Bajpai, 1993
	Morris and Bajpai, 1987
	Scheidler and Bajpai, 1992
3. For filling space vacated by bone screws, donor bone, excised tumors, and diseased bone loss	Bajpai and Fuchs, 1985
	Ricci et al., 1986
4. For repairing and fusion of spinal and lumbosacral vertebrae	Bajpai et al., 1984
	Yamamuro et al., 1988
5. For repairing herniated disks	Bajpai et al., 1984
6. For repairing maxillofacial and dental defects	Freeman et al., 1981
7. Hydroxyapatite ocular implants	De Potter et al., 1994
	Shields et al., 1993

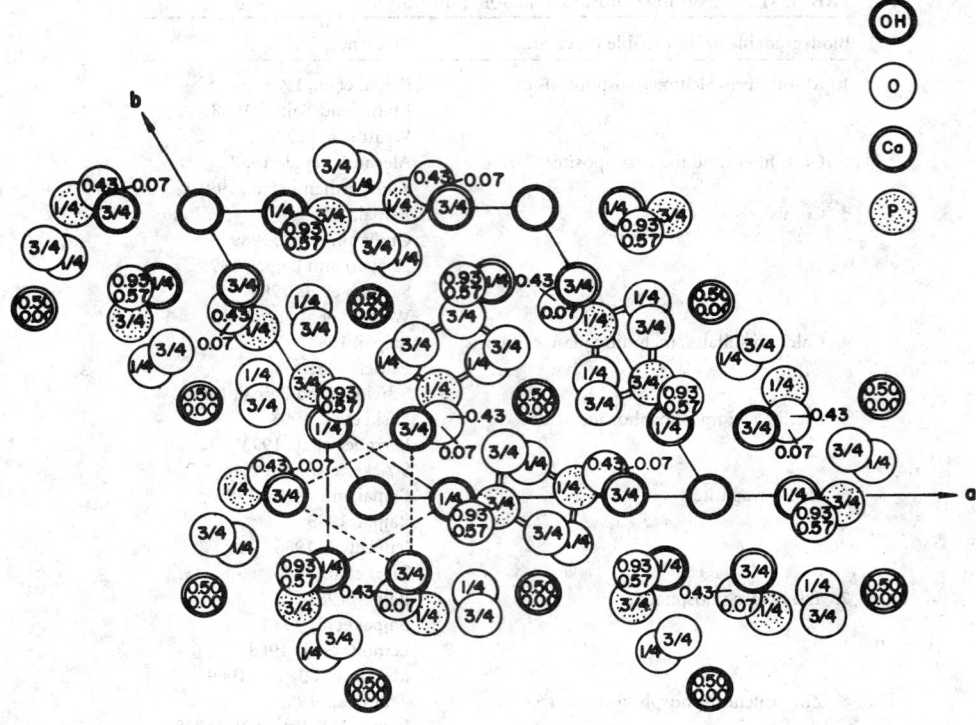

FIGURE 41.6   Hydroxyapatite structure projected down the *c* axis onto the basal plane. (From Posner AS, Perloff A, Diorio AD. 1958. Refinement of the Hydroxyapatite Structure. Acta Crystallogr 11:308–309.)

is unique for each species of marine invertebrate [Holmes et al., 1984]. Corals for use as bone implants are selected on the basis of structural similarity to bone [Holmes et al., 1984]. Coral provides an excellent structure for the ingrowth of bone, and the main component, calcium carbonate, is gradually resorbed by the body [Khavari & Bajpai, 1993]. Corals also can be converted to hydroxyapatite by a hydrothermal exchange process. Interpore 200, a coral hydroxyapatite, resembles cancellous bone [Sartoris et al., 1986]. Both pure coral (Biocoral) and coral transformed to hydroxyapatite are currently used to repair traumatized bone, replace diseased bone, and correct various bone defects.

Biocoral is composed of crystalline calcium carbonate or aragonite, the metastable form of calcium carbonate. The compressive strength of Biocoral varies from 26 (50% porous) to 395 MPa (dense) and depends on the porosity of the ceramic. Likewise, the modulus of elasticity (Young's modulus) of Biocoral varies from 8 (50% porous) to 100 GPa (dense) [Biocoral, 1989].

TABLE 41.10   Physical Properties of Calcium Phosphate

Properties	Values
Elastic modulus (GPa)	4.0–117
Compressive strength (MPa)	294
Bending strength (MPa)	147
Hardness (Vickers, GPa)	3.43
Poisson's ratio	0.27
Density (theoretical, g/cm^3)	3.16

Source: Park JB, Lakes RS. 1992. Ceramic implant materials. In Biomaterials: An Introduction, 2d ed, p 125. New York, Plenum Press.

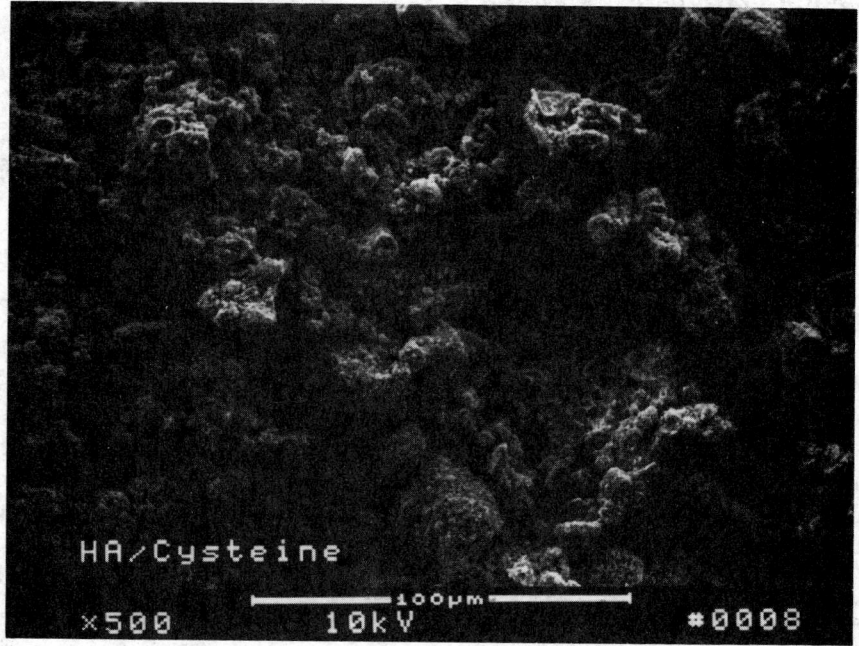

FIGURE 41.7 Scanning electron micrograph (×500) of a set and hardened hydroxyaptite (HA)–cysteine composite. The small white cysteine particles can be seen on the larger HA particles.

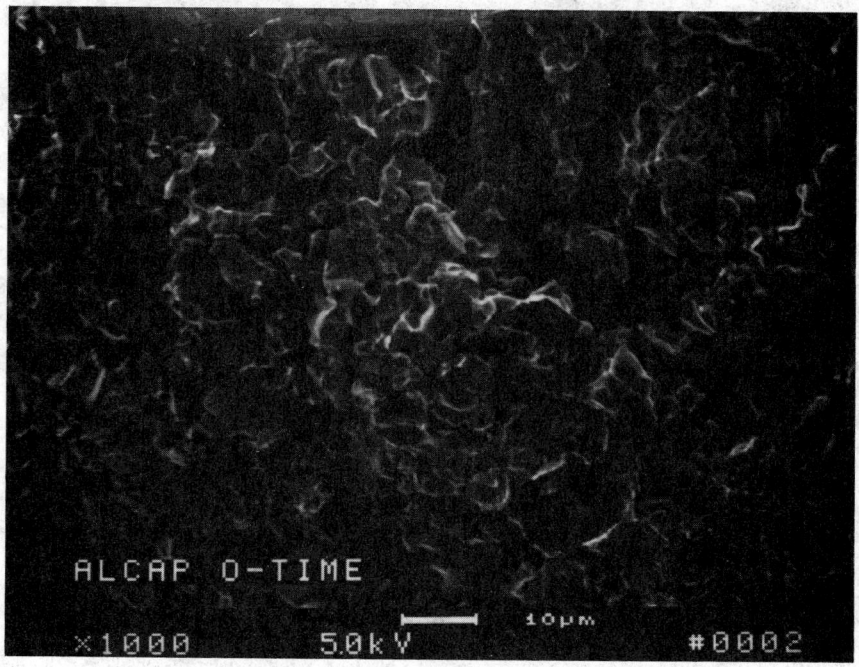

FIGURE 41.8 Scanning electron micrograph (×1000) of porous sintered ALCAP.

Tricalcium Phosphate (TCP) Ceramics

A multicrystalline porous form of β-tricalcium phosphate [β-CA$_3$(PO$_4$)$_2$] has been used success-fully to correct periodontal defects and augment bony contours [Metsger et al., 1982]. X-ray diffraction of β-tricalcium phosphate shows an average interconnected porosity of over 100 μm [Lemons et al., 1979]. Often tribasic calcium phosphate is mistaken for β-tricalcium phosphate. According to Metsger and coworkers [1982], tribasic calcium phosphate is a nonstoichiometric compound often bearing the formula of hydroxyapatite [Ca$_{10}$(PO$_4$)$_2$(OH)$_2$].

β-tricalcium phosphate is prepared by a wet precipitation procedure from an aqueous solution of Ca(NO$_3$)$_2$ and NaH$_2$PO$_4$ [Bajpai et al., 1988]. The precipitate is calcined at 1150°C for 1 hour, ground, and sieved to obtain the desired size particles for use as bone substitutes [Bajpai et al., 1988; Bajpai, 1990] and for making ceramic matrix drug delivery systems [Morris & Bajpai, 1989; Nagy & Bajpai, 1994; Moldovan & Bajpai, 1994]. These particles are used as such or pressed into cylindrical shapes and sintered at 1150 to 1200°C for 36 hours to achieve the appropriate mechanical strength for use as drug delivery devices [Bajpai, 1989, 1992, 1994; Benghuzzi et al., 1991]. A scanning elec-tron micrograph (500×) of a set and hardened TCP-cysteine composite is shown in Fig. 41.9. The composite sets and hardens on addition of water. TCP is usually more soluble than synthetic hydroxyapatite and, on implantation, allows good bone ingrowth and eventually is replaced by endogenous bone.

Zinc-Calcium-Phosphorous Oxide (ZCAP) Ceramics

Zinc is essential for human metabolism and is a component of at least 30 metalloenzymes [Pories & Strain, 1970]. In addition, zinc may also be involved in the process of wound healing [Pories & Strain, 1970]. Thus ZCAP ceramics were synthesized to repair bone defects and deliver drugs [Binzer & Bajpai, 1987; Bajpai, 1988, 1993; Arar & Bajpai, 1992]. Zinc-calcium-phosphorous oxide poly-

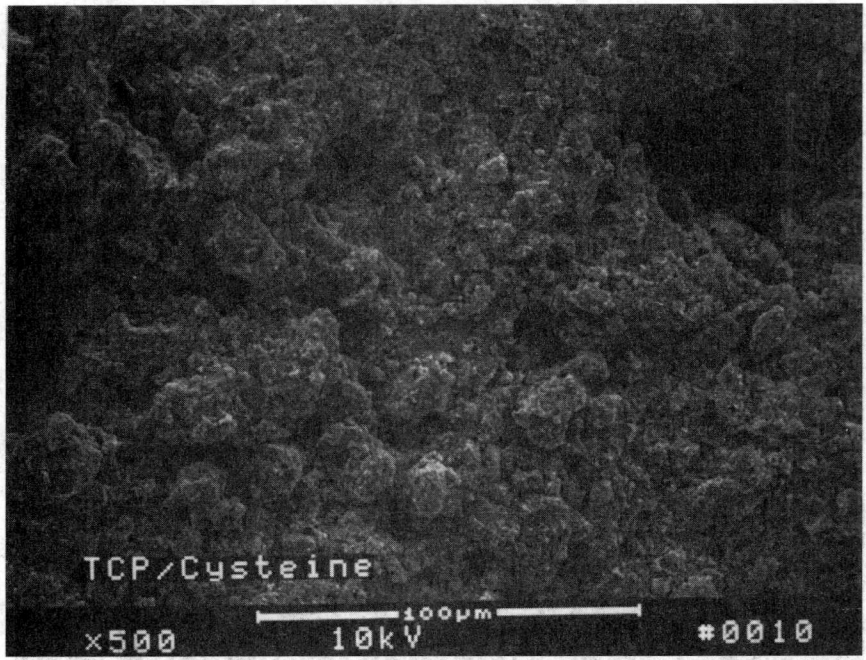

FIGURE 41.9 Scanning electron micrograph (×500) of a set and hardened TCP-cysteine composite. The small white cysteine particles can be seen on the larger TCP particles.

phasic (ZCAP) ceramic is prepared by a thermal mixing of zinc oxide, calcium oxide, and phosphorous pentoxide powders [Bajpai, 1988]. ZCAP, like ALCAP, has insulating dielectric properties but no magnetic or piezoelectric properties [Allaire et al., 1989]. Various ratios of these powders have been used to produce the desired material [Bajpai, 1988]. The oxide powders are mixed in a ball mill and subsequently calcined at 800°C for 24 hours. The calcined ceramic is then ground and sieved to obtain the desired size particles. A scanning electron micrograph (500×) of a set and hardened ZCAP-cysteine composite is shown in Fig. 41.10. The composite sets and hardens on addition of water. To date, ZCAP ceramics have been used to repair experimentally induced defects in bone and for delivering drugs [Binzer & Bajpai, 1987; Bajpai, 1993].

Zinc Sulfate–Calcium Phosphate (ZSCAP) Ceramics

Zinc sulfate–calcium phosphate polyphasic (ZSCAP) ceramic is prepared from stock powders of zinc sulfate, zinc oxide, calcium oxide, and phosphorous pentoxide [Bajpai, 1988]. A ratio of 15:30:30:25 by weight of $ZnSO_4$, ZnO, CaO, and P_2O_5 is mixed in a crucible and allowed to cool for 30 minutes after the exothermal reaction has subsided. The cooled mixture is calcined in a crucible at 650°C for 24 hours. The calcined ceramic is ground in a ball mill, and particles of the desired size are separated by sieving in an automatic siever. A scanning electron micrograph (2000×) of set and hardened ZSCAP particles (45 to 63 μm) is shown in Fig. 41.11. ZSCAP sets and hardens on addition of water. ZSCAP particles, on implantation in bone, set and harden on contact with blood and have been used to repair experimentally induced defects in bone [Scheidler & Bajpai, 1992].

Ferric Calcium Phosphorous Oxide (FECAP) Ceramics

Ferric calcium phosphorous oxide polyphasic ceramic is prepared from powders of ferric (III) oxide, calcium oxide, and phosphorous pentoxide [Fuski et al., 1993; Larrabee et al., 1993; Stricker et al.,

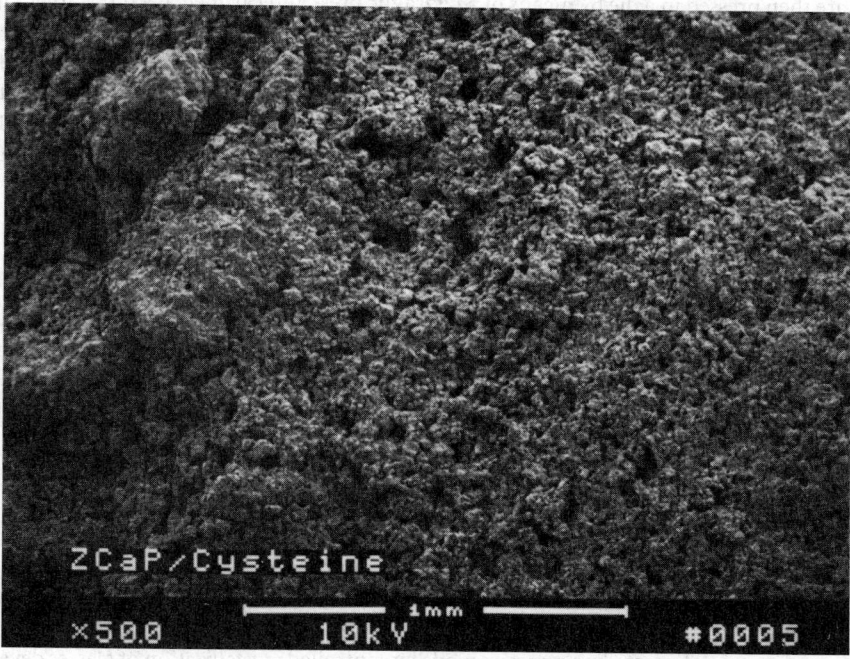

FIGURE 41.10 Scanning electron micrograph (×500) of a set and hardened ZCAP-cysteine composite. The small white cysteine particles have blended with the ZCAP particles.

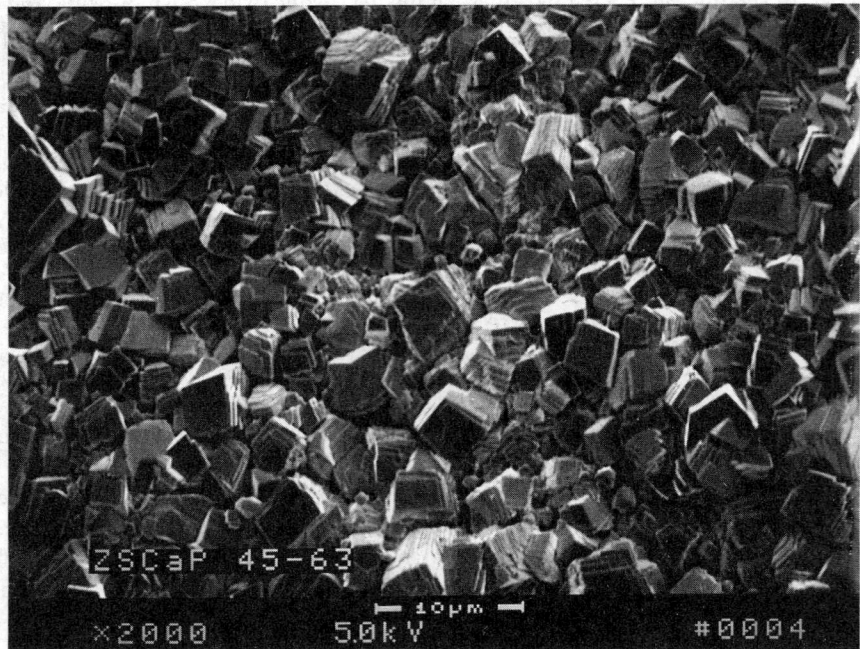

FIGURE 41.11 Scanning electron micrograph ($\times$2000) of a set and hardened ZSCAP particles (45 to 63 μm). Sulfate is hardly visible between the cube-shaped ZCAP particles.

1992]. The powders are combined in various ratios by weight and mixed in a blender. Blocks of the mixture are then pressed in a die by means of a hydraulic press and calcined at 1100°C for 12 hours. The calcined ceramic blocks are crushed and ground in a ball mill, and particles of the desired size are separated by sieving in an automatic siever. A scanning electron micrograph (1000$\times$) of a set and hardened ZCAP-α ketoglutaric acid composite is shown in Fig. 41.12. The composite sets and hardens on addition of water. Studies conducted to date suggest complete resorption of FECAP particles implanted in bone within 60 days [Larrabee et al., 1993]. This particular ceramic could be used in patients suffering from anemia and similar diseases [Fuski et al., 1993].

41.3 Bioactive or Surface-Reactive Ceramics

Upon implantation in the host, surface-reactive ceramics form strong bonds with adjacent tissue. Examples of surface reactive ceramics are the dense nonporous glasses Bioglass and Ceravital and hydroxyapatites (Table 41.11). One of their many uses is the coating of metal prostheses. This coating provides a stronger bonding to the adjacent tissues, which is very important for prostheses. A list of the uses of surface-reactive ceramics is shown in Table 41.12.

Glass-Ceramics

Several variations of bioglasses and Ceravital glass-ceramics have been used by various workers within the last decade. Glass-ceramics used for implantation are silicon oxide–based systems with or without phosphorous pentoxide.

Glass-ceramics are polycrystalline ceramics made by controlled crystallization of glasses developed by S.D. Stookey of Corning Glass Works in the early 1960s [Park & Lakes, 1992]. Glass-ceramics were first used in photosensitive glasses, in which small amounts of copper, silver, and gold are precipi-

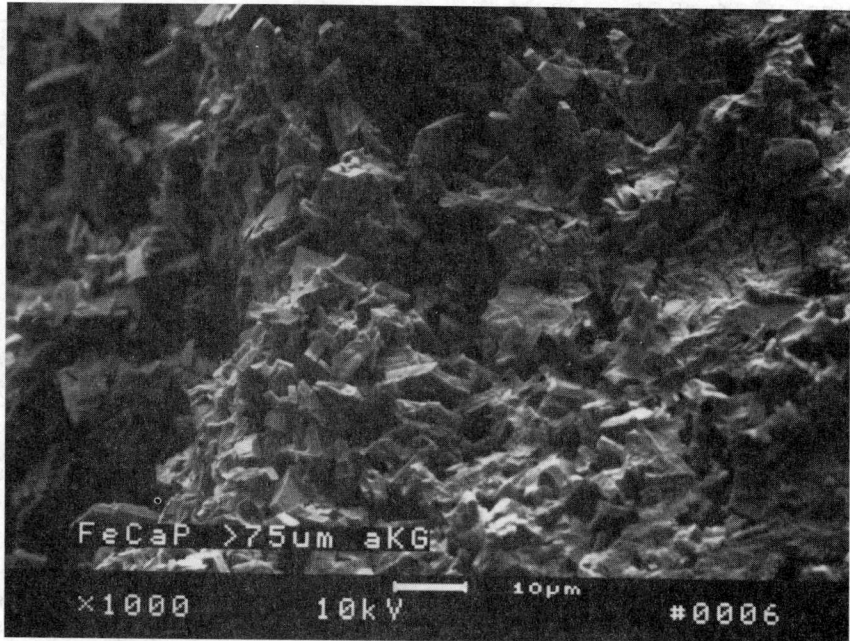

FIGURE 41.12 Scanning electron micrograph (×1000) of a set and hardened FECAP–α-ketoglutaric acid composite. Plate-shaped FECAP particles have been aggregated by the acid.

TABLE 41.11 Examples of Surface Reactive Bioceramics

Surface Reactive Bioceramic	References
1. Bioglasses and Ceravital	Ducheyne, 1985
	Gheyson et al., 1983
	Hench, 1991
	Hench, 1993
	Ogino et al., 1980
	Ritter et al., 1979
2. Dense and nonporous glasses	Andersson et al., 1992
	Blencke et al., 1978
	Li et al., 1991
	Ohtsuki et al., 1992
	Ohura et al., 1992
	Schepers et al., 1993
	Takatsuko et al., 1993
3. Hydroxyapatite	Bagambisa et al., 1993
	Bajpai, 1990
	Fredette et al., 1989
	Huaxia et al., 1992
	Knowles and Bonfield, 1993
	Niwa et al., 1980
	Park and Lakes, 1992
	Posner et al., 1958
	Schwartz et al., 1993
	Whitehead et al., 1993

TABLE 41.12   Uses of Surface Reactive Bioceramics

Surface Reactive Bioceramic	References
1. For coating of metal prostheses	Cotell et al., 1992
	Huaxia et al., 1992
	Ritter et al., 1979
	Takatsuko et al., 1993
	Whitehead et al., 1993
2. In reconstruction of dental defects	Gheysen et al., 1983
	Hulbert et al., 1987
	Schepers et al., 1988
	Schepers et al., 1989
3. For filling space vacated by bone screws, donor bone, excised tumors, and diseased bone loss	Hulbert et al., 1987
	Schepers et al., 1993
	Terry et al., 1989
4. As bone plates and screws	Doyle, 1990
	Ducheyne and McGuckin, 1990
	Yamamuro et al., 1988
5. As replacements of middle ear ossicles	Feenstra and de Groot, 1983
	Grote, 1987
	Hench, 1991
	Hench, 1993
	Reck et al., 1988
6. For lengthening of rami	Feenstra and de Groot, 1983
7. For correcting periodontal defects	Feenstra and de Groot, 1983
	Hulbert, 1992
8. In replacing subperiosteal teeth	Hulbert, 1992

tated by ultraviolet light irradiation. These metallic precipitates help to nucleate and crystallize the glass into a fine-grained ceramic that possesses excellent mechanical and thermal properties. Both Bioglass and Ceravital glass-ceramics have been used as implants [Yamamuro et al., 1990].

The formation of glass-ceramics is influenced by the nucleation and growth of small (<1 μm diameter) crystals as well as the size distribution of these crystals. It is estimated that about 10^{12} to 10^{15} nuclei per cubic centimeter are required to achieve such small crystals. In addition to the metallic agents already mentioned, Pt groups, TiO_2, ZrO_2, and P_2O_5 are widely used for nucleation and crystallization. The nucleation of glass is carried out at temperatures much lower than the melting temperature. During processing, the melt viscosity is kept in the range of 10^{11} and 10^{12} P for 1 to 2 hours. In order to obtain a larger fraction of the microcrystalline phase, the material is further heated to an appropriate temperature for maximum crystal growth. Deformation of the product, phase transformation within the crystalline phases, or redissolution of some of the phases should be avoided.

The crystallization is usually more than 90% complete, with grain sizes 0.1 to 1 μm. These grains are much smaller than those of conventional ceramics. Figure 41.13 shows a schematic representation of a temperature-time cycle for a glass-ceramic. [Park & Lakes, 1992]

The glass-ceramics developed for implantation are SiO_2-CaO-Na_2O-P_2O_5 and Li_2O-ZnO-SiO_2 systems. Two major groups are experimenting with the SiO_2-CaO-Na_2O-P_2O_5 glass-ceramic. One group varied the compositions (except for P_2O_5) in order to obtain the best glass-ceramic composition for inducing direct bonding with bone (Table 41.13). The bonding

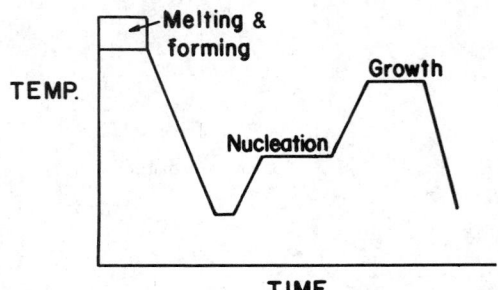

FIGURE 41.13   Temperature-time cycle for a glass-ceramic. (From Kingery WD, Bowen HK, Uhlmann DR. 1976. Introduction to Ceramics, 2nd ed, p 368. New York, J. Wiley and Sons.)

TABLE 41.13 Compositions of Bioglass and Ceravital Glass-Ceramics

Type	Code	SiO$_2$	CaO	Na$_2$O	P$_2$O$_5$	MgO	K$_2$O
Bioglass	42S5.6	42.1	29.0	26.3	2.6	—	—
	(45S5)46S5.2	46.1	26.9	24.4	2.6	—	—
	49S4.9	49.1	25.3	23.8	2.6	—	—
	52S4.6	52.1	23.8	21.5	2.6	—	—
	55S4.3	55.1	22.2	20.1	2.6	—	—
	60S3.8	60.1	19.6	17.7	2.6	—	—
Ceravital	Bioactive*	40–50	30–35	5–10	10–15	2.5–5	0.5–3
	Nonbioactive†	30–35	25–30	3.5–7.5	7.5–12	1–2.5	0.5–2

*The Ceravital composition is in wt%, while the Bioglass compositions are in mol%.
†In addition, Al$_2$O$_3$ (5.0–15.0), TiO$_2$(1.0–5.0), and Ta$_2$O$_5$ (5–15) are added.
Source: Park JB, Lakes RS. 1992. Ceramic implant materials. In Biomaterials: An Introduction, 2d ed, p 127. New York, Plenum Press.

to bone is related to the simultaneous formation of a calcium phosphate and SiO$_2$-rich film layer on the surface, as exhibited by the 46S5.2 type Bioglass. If an SiO$_2$-rich layer forms first and a calcium phosphate film develops later (46 to 55 mol% SiO$_2$ samples) or no phosphate film is formed (60 mol% SiO$_2$), then direct bonding with bone does not occur [Park & Lakes, 1992]. The approximate region of the SiO$_2$-CaO-Na$_2$O system for the tissue–glass-ceramic reaction is shown in Fig. 41.14. As can be seen, the best region (region *A*) for good tissue bonding is the composition given for 46S5.2 type Bioglass (see Table 41.13) [Park & Lakes, 1992].

Ceravital

The composition of Ceravital is similar to that of Bioglass in SiO$_2$ content but differs somewhat in other components (see Table 41.13). In order to control the dissolution rate, Al$_2$O$_3$, TiO$_2$, and Ta$_2$O$_5$ are added in Ceravital glass-ceramic. The mixtures, after melting in a platinum crucible at 1500°C for 3 hours, are annealed and cooled. The nucleation and crystallization temperatures are 680 and 750°C, respectively, for 24 hours each. When the size of crystallites reaches approximately 4 Å and the characteristic needle structure is not formed, the process is stopped to obtain a fine-grain structure [Park & Lakes, 1993].

Glass-ceramics have several desirable properties compared with glasses and ceramics. The thermal coefficient of expansion is very low, typically 10^{-7} to $10°C^{-1}$, and in some cases it can even be made negative. Due to the controlled grain size and improved resistance to surface damage, the tensile strength of these materials can be increased by at least a factor of 2 from about 100 to 200 MPa. The resistance to scratching and abrasion of glass-ceramics is similar to that of sapphire [Park & Lakes, 1992].

A transmission electron micrograph of Bioglass glass-ceramic implanted in the femur of rats for 6 weeks showed intimate contacts between the mineralized bone and the Bioglass (Fig. 41.15). The mechanical strength of the interfacial bond between bone and Bioglass ceramic is on the same order of magnitude as the strength of bulk glass-ceramic (850 kg/cm^2, or 83.3 MPa), which is about three-fourths that of the host bone strength [Park & Lakes, 1992].

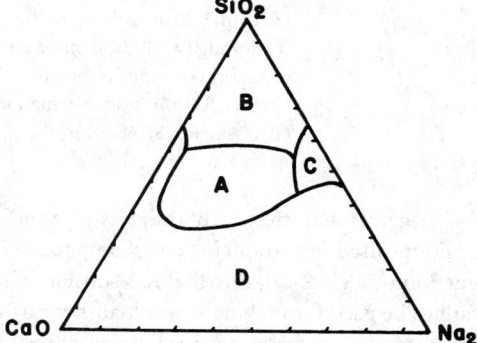

FIGURE 41.14 Approximate regions of the tissue-glass-ceramic bonding for the SiO$_2$-CaO-Na$_2$O system. (*A*) Bonding within 30 days. (*B*) Nonbonding; reactivity is too low. (*C*) Nonbonding; reactivity is too high. (*D*) Bonding does not form glass. (From Hench LL, Ethridge EC. 1982. Biomaterials: An Interfacial Approach, p. 147, New York, Academic Press.)

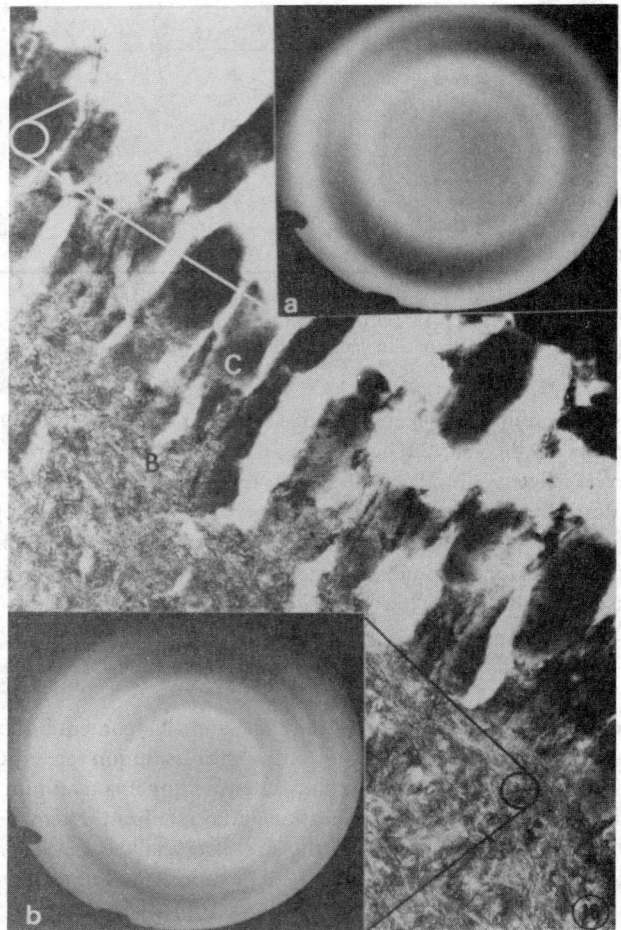

FIGURE 41.15 Transmission electron micrograph of well-mineralized bone (*b*) juxtaposed to the glass-ceramic (*c*) that fractured during sectioning (×51,500). Insert *a* is the diffraction pattern from ceramic area and *b* is from bone area. (From Beckham CA, Greenlee TK Jr, Crebo AR. 1971. Bone Formation at a Ceramic Implant Interface. Calcif Tissue Res 8:165–171.)

A negative characteristic of the glass-ceramic is its brittleness. In addition, limitations on the compositions used for producing a biocompatable (or osteoconductive) glass-ceramic hinder the production of a glass-ceramic that has substantially higher mechanical strength. Thus glass-ceramics cannot be used for making major load-bearing implants such as joint implants. However, they can be used as fillers for bone cement, dental restorative composites, and coating material (see Table 41.12). A glass-ceramic containing 36 wt% of magnetite in a β-wollastonite- and $CaOSiO_2$-based glassy matrix has been synthesized for treating bone tumors by hyperthermia [Kokubo et al., 1992].

41.4 Deterioration of Ceramics

It is of great interest to know whether the inert ceramics such as alumina undergo significant static or dynamic fatigue. Even for the biodegradable ceramics, the rate of degradation in vivo is of paramount importance. Controlled degradation of an implant with time on implantation is desirable. Above a critical stress level, the fatigue strength of alumina is reduced by the presence of water. This is due to the delayed crack growth, which is accelerated by the water molecules [Park & Lakes, 1992]. Reduction in strength occurs if water penetrates the ceramic. Decrease in strength was not observed in samples that did not show water marks on the fractured surface (Fig. 41.16). The presence of a small amount of silica in one sample lot may have contributed to the permeation of water molecules that is detrimental to the strength [Park & Lakes, 1992]. It is not clear whether a static fatigue mechanism operates in single-crystal alumina. It is reasonable to assume, however, that static fatigue will occur if the ceramic contains flaws or impurities, because these will act as the source of crack initiation and growth under stress. [Park & Lakes, 1992]

Study of the fatigue behavior of vapor-deposited pyrolitic carbon fibers (4000 to 5000 Å thick) onto stainless steel substrate showed that the film does not break unless the substrate undergoes plastic deformation at 1.3×10^{-2} strain and up to 1 million cycles of loading. Therefore, the fatigue is closely related to the substrate, as shown in Fig. 41.17. Similar substrate-carbon adherence is the basis for pyrolitic carbon–deposited polymer arterial grafts [Park & Lakes, 1992].

The fatigue life of ceramics can be predicted by assuming that the fatigue fracture is due to the slow growth of preexisting flaws. Generally, the strength distribution σ_i of ceramics in an inert environment can be correlated with the probability of failure F by the following equation:

$$"n"n(1/1 - F) = m"n(\sigma_i/\sigma_o)$$ (41.1)

Both m and σ_o are constants in the equation. Figure 41.18 shows a good fit for Bioglass-coated alumina [Park & Lakes, 1992].

A minimum service life t_{min} of a specimen can be predicted by means of a proof test wherein it is subjected to stresses that are greater than those expected in service. Proof tests also eliminate the weaker pieces. This minimum life can be predicted from the following equation:

$$t_{min} = B\sigma_p^{N-2} \sigma_a^{-N}$$ (41.2)

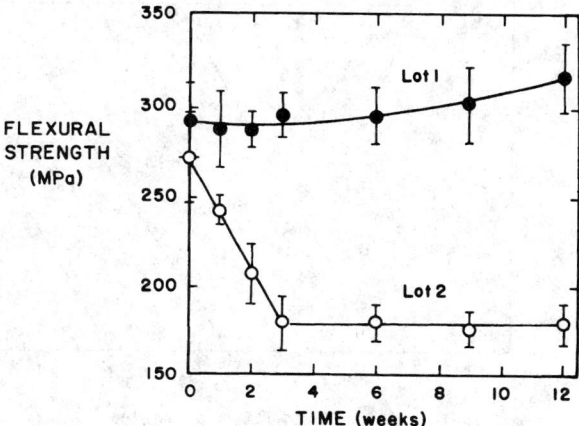

FIGURE 41.16 Flexural strength of dense alumina rods after aging under stress in Ringer's solution. Lots 1 and 2 are from different batches of production. (From Krainess FE, Knapp WJ. 1978. Strength of a dense alumina ceramic after aging *in vitro*. J Biomed Mater Res 12:245.)

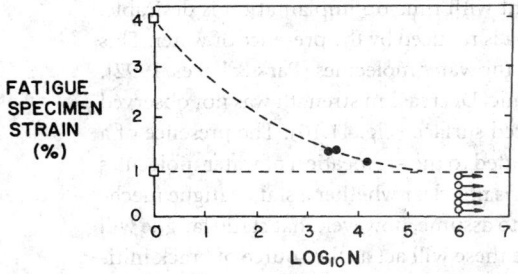

FIGURE 41.17   Strain versus number of cycles to failure (○ = absence of fatigue cracks in carbon film; ● = fracture of carbon film due to fatigue failure of substrates; □ = data from substrate determined in single-cycle tensile test). (From Shim HS, Haubold AD. 1980. The fatigue behavior of vapor deposited carbon films. Biomater Med Devices Artif Organs 8:333–334.)

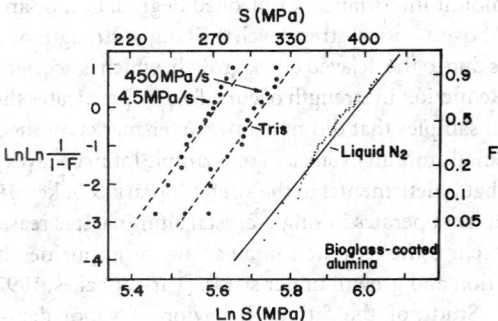

FIGURE 41.18   Plot of ln ln $[1/(1 - F)]$ versus ln S for Bioglass-coated alumina in a *tris*-hydroxyaminomethane buffer and liquid nitrogen. F is the probability of failure, and S is strength. (From Ritter JE Jr, Greenspan DC, Palmer RA, Hench LL. 1979. Use of fracture mechanics theory in lifetime predictions for alumina and bioglass-coated alumina. J Biomed Mater Res 13:260.)

Here σ_p is the proof-test stress, σ_a is the applied stress, and B and N are constants. Equation (41.2), after rearrangement, reads as follows:

$$t_{\min}\sigma_a^2 = B(\sigma_p/\sigma_a)^{N-2} \tag{41.3}$$

Figure 41.19 shows a plot of Eq. (41.3) for alumina on a logarithmic scale [Park & Lakes, 1992].

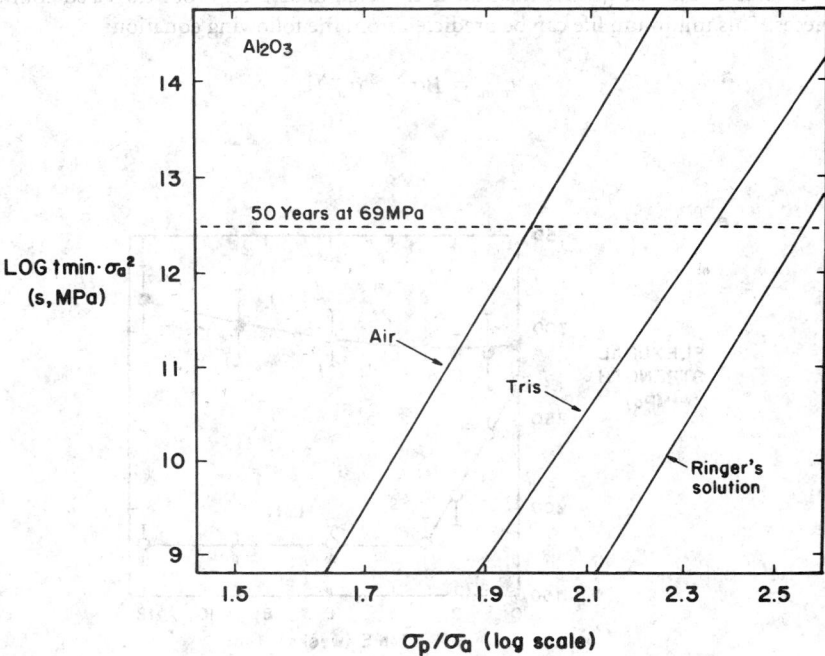

FIGURE 41.19   Plot of Eq. (41.3) for alumina after proof testing. $N = 43.85$, $m = 13.21$, and $\sigma_o = 55728$ psi. (From Ritter JE Jr, Greenspan DC, Palmer RA, Hench LL. 1979. Use of fracture mechanics theory in lifetime predictions for alumina and bioglass-coated alumina. J Biomed Mater Res 13:261.)

Acknowledgments

We are grateful to Dr. Joon B. Park for inviting us to write this chapter and providing the basic shell from his book to expand on.

Defining Terms

Alumina: Aluminum oxide (Al_2O_3), which is very hard (Mohs hardness 9) and strong. Single crystals are called sapphire or ruby depending on color. Alumina is used to fabricate hip joint socket components and dental root implants.

Calcium phosphate: A family of calcium phosphate ceramics including aluminum-calcium phosphate, ferric calcium phosphate, hydroxyapatite and tricalcium phosphate (TCP), and zinc-calcium phosphate which are used to substitute or augment bony structures and deliver drugs.

Glass-ceramics: A glass crystallized by heat treatment. Some of those have the ability to form chemical bonds with hard and soft tissues. Bioglass and Ceravital are well-known examples.

Hydroxyapatite: A calcium phosphate ceramic with a calcium-to-phosphorus ratio of 5:3 and nominal composition $Ca_{10}(PO_4)_6(OH)_2$. It has good mechanical properties and excellent biocompatibility. Hydroxyapatite is the mineral constituent of bone.

LTI carbon: A silicon-alloyed pyrolitic carbon deposited onto a substrate at low temperature with isotropic crystal morphology. It is highly compatible with blood and used for cardiovascular implant fabrication such as artificial heart valves.

Maximum radius ratio: The ratio of atomic radii computed by assuming the largest atom or ion which can be placed in a crystal's unit cell structure without deforming the structure.

Mohs scale: A hardness scale in which 10 (diamond) is the hardest and 1 (talc) is the softest.

References

Abrams L, Bajpai PK. 1994. Hydroxyapatite ceramics for continuous delivery of heparin. Biomed Sci Instrument 30:169.

Adams D, Williams DF. 1978. Carbon fiber-reinforced carbon as a potential implant material. J Biomed Mater Res 12:35.

Alexander H, Parsons JR, Ricci JL, et al. 1987. Calcium-based ceramics and composites in bone reconstruction. Crit Rev 4:43.

Allaire M, Reynolds D, Bajpai PK. 1989. Electrical properties of biocompatible ALCAP and ZCAP ceramics. Biomed Sci Instrument 25:163.

Andersson OH, Guizhi L, Kangasniemi K, Juhanoja J. 1992. Evaluation of the acceptance of glass in bone. J Mater Sci Mater Med 3:145.

Annual Book of ASTM Standards, part 46, F603-78. Philadelphia, American Society for Testing and Materials, 1980.

Arar HA, Bajpai PK. 1992. Insulin delivery by zinc calcium phosphate (ZCAP) ceramics. Biomed Sci Instrument 28:172.

Bagambisa FB, Joos U, Schilli W. 1993. Mechanisms and structure of the bond between bone and hydroxyapatite ceramics. J Biomed Mater Res 27:1047.

Bajpai PK. 1983. Biodegradable scaffolds in orthopedic, oral and maxillofacial surgery. In LR Rubin (ed), Biomaterials in Reconstructive Surgery, pp 312–328. St. Louis, Mosby.

Bajpai PK. 1988. ZCAP ceramics, US Patent No. 4778471.

Bajpai PK. 1989. Ceramic implantable drug delivery system. TIB & AO 3:203.

Bajpai PK. 1990. Ceramic amino acid composites for repairing traumatized hard tissues. In T Yamamuro, LL Hench, J Wilson-Hench (eds), Handbook of Bioactive Ceramics, vol II: Calcium Phosphate and Hydroxylapatite Ceramics, pp 255–270. Baton Raton, Fla, CRC Press.

Bajpai PK. 1992. Ceramics: A novel device for sustained long-term delivery of drugs. In JA Hulbert, SF Hulbert (eds), Bioceramics, vol 3, pp 87–99. Terre Haute, Ind, Rose-Hulman Institute of Technology.

Bajpai PK. 1993. Zinc-based ceramic cysteine composite for repairing vertebral defects. JIS 6:346.

Bajpai PK. 1994. Ceramic drug delivery systems. In Xingdong Zhang, Yoshito Ikada (eds), Biomedical Materials Research in the Far East, pp 41–42. Kyoto, Japan, Kobunshi Kankokai.

Bajpai PK, Fuchs CM. 1985. Development of a hydroxyapatite bone grout. In CW Hall (ed), Proceedings of the First Annual Scientific Session of the Academy of Surgical Research, pp 50–54. New York, Pergamon Press.

Bajpai PK, Fuchs CM, Strnat MAP. 1985. Development of alumino-calcium phosphorous oxide (ALCAP) ceramic cements. In MS Jackson (ed), Biomedical Engineering, vol IV: Recent Developments, pp 22–25. Proceedings of the Fourth Southern Biomedical Engineering Conference. New York, Pergamon Press.

Bajpai PK, Graves GA Jr. 1980. Porous ceramic carriers for controlled release of proteins, polypeptide hormones and other substances within human and/or mammalian species, US Patent No. 4218255.

Bajpai PK, Fuchs CM, McCullum DE. 1988. Development of tricalcium phosphate ceramic cements. In JE Lemons (ed), Quantitative Characterization and Performance of Porous Implants for Hard Tissue Applications, ASTM STP 953, pp 377–388. Philadelphia, American Society for Testing and Materials.

Bajpai PK, Graves GA Jr, Wilcox LG, Freeman MJ. 1984. Use of resorbable alumino-calcium-phosphorous-oxide ceramics (ALCAP) in health care. Trans Soc Biomater 7:353.

Barinov SM, Bashenko YuV. 1992. Application of ceramic composites as implants: Result and problem. In A Ravaglioli, A Krajewski (eds), Bioceramics and the Human Body, pp 206–210. London, Elsevier Applied Science.

Beckham CA, Greenlee TK Jr, Crebo AR. 1971. Bone formation at a ceramic implant interfaces. Calcif Tissue Res 8:165.

Benghuzzi HA, Giffin BF, Bajpai PK, England BG. 1991. Successful antidote of multiple lethal infections with sustained delivery of difluoromethylornithine by means of tricalcium phosphate drug delivery devices. Trans Soc Biomater 24:53.

Binzer TJ, Bajpai PK. 1987. The use of zinc-calcium-phosphorous oxide (ZCAP) ceramics in reconstructive bone surgery. In RC Eberhart (ed), Digest of Papers, Sixth Southern Biomedical Engineering Conference, Dallas, Texas, pp 182–185. Washington, McGregor and Werner.

Biocoral. 1989. From coral to Biocoral, p. 46. Paris, Innoteb.

Blencke BA, Bromer H, Deutscher KK. 1978. Compatibility and long-term stability of glass-ceramic implants. J Biomed Mater Res 12:307.

Bokros JC. 1972. Deposition structure and properties of pyrolitic carbon. Chem Phys Carbon 5:70.

Bokros JC, LaGrange LD, Schoen GJ. 1972. Control of structure of carbon for use in bioengineering. Chem Phys Carbon 9:103.

Boutin P. 1981. Using alumina-alumina sliding and a metallic stem: 1330 cases and an 11-year follow-up. In H Oonishi, HY Ooi (eds), Orthopaedic Ceramic Implants, vol 1. Tokyo, Japanese Society of Orthopaedic Ceramic Implants.

Buykx WJ, Drabarek E, Reeve KD, et al. 1992. Development of porous ceramics for drug release and other applications. In JE Hulbert, SF Hulbert (eds), Bioceramics, vol 3, pp 349–354. Terre Haute, Ind, Rose Hulman Institute of Technology.

Chandy T, Sharma CP. 1991. Biocompatibility and toxicological screening of materials. In CP Sharma, M Szycher (eds), Blood Compatible Materials and Devices, pp 153–166. Lancaster, Pa, Technomic Publishing Co.

Chignier E, Monties JR, Butazzoni B, et al. 1987. Haemocompatibility and biological course of carbonaceous composites for cardiovascular devices. Biomaterials 8:18.

Cotell CM, Chrisey DB, Grabowski KS, et al. 1992. Pulsed laser deposition of hydroxyapatite thin films on Ti-6AI-4V. J Appl Biomater 3:87.

de Groot K. 1983. Bioceramics of Calcium Phosphate. Boca Raton, Fla, CRC Press.

De Potter P, Shields CL, Shields JL, Singh AD. 1994. Use of the hydroxyapatite ocular implant in the pediatric population. Arch Opthalmol 112:208.

Dellsperger KC, Chandran KB. 1991. Prosthetic heart valves. In CP Sharma and M Szycher (eds), Blood Compatible Materials and Devices. Lancaster, Pa, Technomic Publishing Co.

Dorlot JM, Christel P, Meunier A. 1988. Alumina hip prostheses: Long-term behaviors. In H Oonishi, H Aoki, K Sawai (eds), Bioceramics: Proceedings of 1st International Symposium on Ceramics in Medicine, pp 236–301. Tokyo, Ishiyaku EuroAmerica.

Dörre E. 1991. Problems concerning the industrial production of alumina ceramic components for hip prostheses. In A Ravaglioli, A Krajewski (eds), Bioceramics and the Human Body, pp 454–460. New York, Elsevier Applied Science.

Doyle C. 1990. Composite bioactive ceramic-metal materials. In T Yamamuro, LL Hench, J Wilson (eds), Handbook of Bioactive Ceramics, pp 195–208. Boca Raton, Fla, CRC Press.

Drennan J, Steele BCH. 1991. Zirconia and hafnia. In RJ Brook (ed), Concise Encyclopedia of Advanced Ceramic Materials, pp 525–528, New York, Pergamon Press.

Ducheyne P, McGuckin JF Jr. 1990. Composite bioactive ceramic-metal materials. In T Yamamuro, LL Hench, J Wilson (eds), Handbook of Bioactive Ceramics, pp 75–86. Boca Raton, Fla, CRC Press.

Ducheyne P. 1985. Bioglass coatings and bioglass composites as implant materials. J Biomed Mater Res 19:273.

Ely JL, Haubald AO. 1993. Static fatigue and stress corrosion in pyrolitic carbon. In P Ducheyne, D Christiansen (eds), Bioceramics, vol 6, pp 199–204. Boston, Mass, Butterworth-Heinemann.

Feenstra L, de Groot K. 1983. Medical use of calcium phosphate ceramics. In K de Groot (ed), Bioceramics of Calcium Phosphate, pp 131–141. Boca Raton, Fla, CRC Press.

Freeman MJ, McCullum DE, Bajpai PK. 1981. Use of ALCAP ceramics for rebuilding maxillofacial defects. Trans Soc Biomater 4:109.

Fredette SA, Hanker JS, Terry BC, Beverly L. 1989. Comparison of dense versus porous hydroxy-apatite (HA) particles for rat mandibular defect repair. Mater Res Soc Symp Proc 110:233.

Fulmer MT, Martin RI, Brown PW. 1992. Formation of calcium-deficient hydroxyapatite at near-physiological temperature. J Mater Sci Mater Med 3:299.

Fuski MP, Larrabee RA, Bajpai PK. 1993. Effect of ferric calcium phosphorous oxide ceramic implant in bone on some parameters of blood. TIB AO 7:16.

Gheysen G, Ducheyne P, Hench LL, de Meester P. 1983. Bioglass composites: A potential material for dental application. Biomaterials 4:81.

Graves GA Jr, Hentrich RL Jr, Stein HG, Bajpai PK. 1972. Resorbable ceramic implants in bio-ceramics. In CW Hall, SF Hulbert, SN Levine, FA Young (eds), Engineering and Medicine, part I, pp 91–115. New York, Interscience Publishers.

Grenoble DE, Katz JL, Dunn KL, et al. 1972. The elastic properties of hard tissues and apatites. J Biomed Mater Res 6:221.

Gromofsky JR, Arar H, Bajpai PK. 1988. Development of zinc calcium phosphorous oxide ceramic–organic acid composites for repairing traumatized hard tissue. In DD Moyle (ed), Digest of Papers, Seventh Southern Biomedical Engineering Conference, Greenville, SC, pp 20–23. Washington, Mcgregor and Werner.

Grote JJ. 1987. Reconstruction of the ossicular chain with hydroxyapatite prostheses. Am J Otol 8:396.

Guillemin G, Meunier A, Dallant P, et al. 1989. Comparison of coral resorption and bone apposi-tion with two natural corals of different porosities. J Biomed Mater Res 23:765.

Hammer J III, Reed O, Greulich R. 1972. Ceramic root implantation in baboons. J Biomed Mater Res 6:1.

Heimke G. 1992. Use of alumina ceramics in medicine. In JE Hulbert SF Hulbert (eds), Bioceramics Volume, 3d ed., pp 19–30. Terre Haute, Ind, Rose Hulman Institute of Technology.

Hench LL. 1991. Bioceramics: From concept to clinic. J Am Ceramic Soc 74:1487.

Hench LL. 1993. Bioceramics: From concept to clinic. Am Ceramic Soc Bull 72:93.

Hench LL, Ethridge EC. 1982. Biomaterials: An Interfacial Approach, p 147. New York, Academic Press.

Hentrich RL Jr, Graves GA Jr, Stein HG, Bajpai PK. 1969. An evaluation of inert and resorbable ceramics for future clinical applications. Fall Meeting, Ceramics-Metals Systems, Division of the American Ceramic Society, Cleveland, Ohio.

Hentrich RL Jr, Graves GA Jr, Stein HG, Bajpai PK. 1971. An evaluation of inert and resorbable ceramics for future clinical applications. J Biomed Mater Res 5:25.

Holmes R, Mooney V, Bucholz R, Tencer A. 1984. A coralline hydroxyapatite bone graft substitute. Clin Orthop 188:252.

Huaxia JI, Ponton CB, Marquis PM. 1992. Microstructural characterization of hydroxyapatite coating on titanium. J Mater Sci Mater Med 3:283.

Hulbert SF. 1992. Use of ceramics in medicine. In JE Hulbert, SF Hulbert (eds), Bioceramics, vol 3, pp 1–18. Terre Haute, Ind, Rose Hulman Institute of Technology.

Hulbert SF, Klawitter JJ. 1971. Application of porous ceramics for the development of load-bearing internal orthopedic applications. Biomed Mater Symp 161.

Hulbert SF, Bokros JC, Hench LL, et al. 1987. Ceramics in clinical applications: Past, present, and future. In P Vincezini (ed), High Tech Ceramics, pp 189–213. Amsterdam, Elsevier.

Jarcho M, Salsbury RL, Thomas MB, Doremus RH. 1979. Synthesis and fabrication of β-tricalcium phosphate (whitlockite) ceramics for potential prosthetic applications. J Mater Sci 14:142.

Jenei SR, Bajpai PK, Salsbury RL. 1986. Resorbability of commercial hydroxyapatite in lactate buffer. In DN Powers (ed), Proceedings of the Second Annual Scientific Session of the Academy of Surgical Research, Clemson, SC, pp 13–16. Clemson, SC, Clemson University Press.

Kaae JL. 1971. Structure and mechanical properties of isotropic pyrolitic carbon deposited below 1600°C. J Nucl Mater 38:42.

Kawahara H (ed). 1989. Oral Implantology and Biomaterials. Amsterdam, Elsevier.

Khavari F, Bajpai PK. 1993. Coralline-sulfate bone substitutes. Biomed Sci Instrum 29:65.

Kijima T, Tsutsumi M. 1979. Preparation and thermal properties of dense polycrystalline oxyhydroxyapatite. J Am Ceramic Soc 62:954.

Kingery WD, Bowen HK, Uhlmann DR. 1976. Introduction to Ceramics, 2d ed, p 368. New York, Wiley.

Knowles JC, Bonfield W. 1993. Development of a glass reinforced hydroxyapatite with enhanced mechanical properties: The effect of glass composition on mechanical properties and its relationship to phase changes. J Biomed Mater Res 27:1591.

Kokubo T, Kushitani H, Ohtsuki C, et al. 1992. Chemical reaction of bioactive glass and glass-ceramics with a simulated body fluid. J Mater Sci Mater Med 3:79.

Krainess FE, Knapp WJ. 1978. Strength of a dense alumina ceramic after aging in vitro. J Biomed Mater Res 12:241.

Kumar P, Shimizu K, Oka M, et al. 1989. Biological reaction of zirconia ceramics. In H Oonishi, H Aoki, K Sawai (eds), Bioceramics: Proceedings of 1st International Symposium on Ceramics in Medicine, pp 341–346. Tokyo, Ishiyaku EuroAmerica.

Larrabee RA, Fuski MP, Bajpai PK. 1993. A ferric calcium phosphorous oxide ceramic for rebuilding bone. Biomed Sci Instrum 29:59.

Lemons JE, Bajpai PK, Patka P, et al. 1988. Significance of the porosity and physical chemistry of calcium phosphate ceramics for orthopaedic uses. In Bioceramics: Material Characteristics versus in Vivo Behavior, pp 190–197. New York, Academy of Sciences.

Lemons JE, Niemann KMW. 1979. Porous tricalcium phosphate ceramic for bone replacement. 25th Annual ORS Meetings, San Francisco, Calif, February 20–22.

Li R, Clark AE, Hench LL. 1991. An investigation of bioactive glass powders by Sol-Gel processing. J Appl Biomater 2:231.

Mattie DR, Bajpai PK. 1988. Analysis of the biocompatibility of ALCAP ceramics in rat femurs. J Biomed Maters Res 22:1101.

Meenen NM, Osborn JF, Dallek M, Donath K. 1992. Hydroxyapatite-ceramic for juxta-articular implantation. J Mater Sci Mater Med 3:345.

Metsger S, Driskell TD, Paulsrud JR. 1982. Tricalcium phosphate ceramic—A resorbable bone implant: Review and current status. J Am Dent Assoc 105:1035.

Moldovan K, Bajpai PK. 1994. A ceramic system for continuous release of aspirin. Biomed Sci Instrum 30:175.

More RB, Silver MD. 1990. Pyrolitic carbon prosthetic heart valve occluder wear: In vitro results for the Bjork-Shiley prosthesis. J Appl Biomater 1:267.

Morris LM, Bajpai PK. 1989. Development of a resorbable tricalcium phosphate (TCP) amine antibiotic composite. Mater Res Soc Symp 110:293.

Murakami T, Ohtsuki N. 1989. Friction and wear characteristics of sliding pairs of bioceramics and polyethylene. In H Oonishi, H Aoki, K Sawai (eds), Bioceramics: Proceedings of 1st International Symposium on Ceramics in Medicine, pp 225–230. Tokyo, Ishiyaku Euro-America.

Nagy EA, Bajpai PK. 1994. Development of a ceramic matrix system for continuous delivery of azidothymidine. Biomed Sci Instrum 30:181.

Niwa S, Sawai K, Takahashie S, et al. 1980. Experimental studies on the implantation of hydroxyapatite in the medullary canal of rabbits. Trans First World Biomaterials Congress, Baden, Austria, p 4.10.4.

Ogino M, Ohuchi F, Hench LL. 1980. Compositional dependence of the formation of calcium phosphate film on bioglass. J Biomed Mater Res 12:55.

Ohashi T, Inoue S, Kajikawa K, et al. 1988. The clinical wear rate of acetabular component accompanied with alumina ceramic head. In H Oonishi, H Aoki, K Sawai (eds), Bioceramics: Proceedings of 1st International Symposium on Ceramics in Medicine, pp 278–283. Tokyo, Ishiyaku EuroAmerica.

Ohtsuki C, Kokubo T, Yamamuro T. 1992. Compositional dependence of bioactivity of glasses in the system $CaO-SiO_2-Al_2O_3$: Its in vitro evaluation. J Mater Sci Mater Med 3:119.

Ohura K, Nakamura T, Yamamuro T, et al. 1992. Bioactivity of $CaO-SiO_2$ glasses added with various ions. J Mater Sci Mater Med 3:95.

Oonishi H. 1992. Bioceramic in orthopaedic surgery—Our clinical experiences. In JE Hulbert, SF Hulbert (eds), Bioceramics, vol 3, pp 31–42. Terre Haute, Ind, Rose Hulman Institute of Technology.

Park JB, Lakes RS. 1992. Biomaterials: An introduction, 2d ed. New York, Plenum Press.

Park JB. 1991. Aluminum oxides: Biomedical applications. In RJ Brook (ed), Concise Encyclopedia of Advanced Ceramic Materials, pp 13–16. New York, Pergamon Press.

Parker DR, Bajpai PK. 1993. Effect of locally delivered testosterone on bone healing. Trans Soc Biomater 26:293.

Peltier LF. 1961. The use of plaster of paris to fill defects in bone. Clin Orthop 21:1.

Piattelli A, Trisi P. 1994. A light and laser scanning microscopy study of bone/hydroxyapatite-coated titanium implants interface: Histochemical evidence of unmineralized material in humans. J Biomed Mater Res 28:529.

Pories WJ, Strain WH. 1970. Zinc and wound healing. In SA Prasad (ed), Zinc Metabolism, pp 378–394. Springfield, Ill, Charles C Thomas.

Posner AS, Perloff A, Diorio AD. 1958. Refinement of hydroxyapatite structure. Acta Cryst 11:308.

Reck R, Störkel S, Meyer A. 1988. Bioactive glass-ceramics in middle ear surgery: An 8-year review. In Bioceramics: Material Characteristics versus in Vivo Behavior, pp 100–106. New York, Academy of Sciences.

Ricci JL, Bajpai PK, Berkman A, et al. 1986. Development of a fast-setting ceramic based grout material for filling bone defects. In S Saha (ed), Biomedical Engineering: V. Recent Developments. Proceedings of the Fifth Southern Biomedical Engineering Conference, Shreveport, La, pp 475–481. New York, Pergamon Press.

Ritter JE Jr, Greenspan DC, Palmer RA, Hench LL. 1979. Use of fracture of an alumina and bioglass coated alumina. J Biomed Mater Res 13:251.

Sartoris DJ, Gershuni DH, Akeson WH, et al. 1986. Coralline hydroxyapatite bone graft substitutes: Preliminary report of radiographic evaluation. Radiology 159:133.

Scheidler PA, Bajpai PK. 1992. Zinc sulfate calcium phosphate (ZSCAP) composite for repairing traumatized bone. Biomed Sci Instrum 28:183.

Schepers E, Ducheyne P, De Clercq M. 1989. Interfacial analysis of fiber-reinforced bioactive dental root implants. J Biomed Mater Res 23:735.

Schepers E, De Clercq M, Ducheyne P. 1988. Interfacial behavior of bulk bioactive glass and fiber-reinforced bioactive glass dental root implants. Ann NY Acad Sci 523:178.

Schepers EJG, Ducheyne P, Barbier L, Schepers S. 1993. Bioactive glass particles of narrow size range: A new material for the repair of bone defects. Implant Dent 2:151.

Schwartz Z, Braun G, Kohave D, et al. 1993. Effects of hydroxyapatite implants on primary mineralization during rat tibial healing: Biochemical and morphometric analysis. J Biomed Mater Res 27:1029.

Sedel L, Meunier A, Nizard RS, Witvoet J. 1991. Ten-year survivorship of cemented ceramic-ceramic total hip replacement. In W Bonfield, GW Hastings, KE Tanner (eds), Bioceramics, vol 4: Proceedings of the 4th International Symposium on Ceramics in Medicine, pp 27–37. Boston, Butterworth-Heinemann.

Shackelford JF. 1988. Introduction to Materials Science for Engineers, 2d ed. New York, Macmillan.

Shimm HS, Haubold AD. 1980. The fatigue behavior of vapor deposited carbon films. Biomater Med Dev Artif Org 8:333.

Shields JA, Shields CL, De Potter P. 1993. Hydroxyapatite orbital implant after enucleation—Experience with 200 cases. Mayo Clin Proc 68:1191.

Shobert EI II. 1964. Carbon and Graphite. New York, Academic Press.

Stricker NJ, Larrabee RA, Bajpai PK. 1992. Biocompatibility of ferric calcium phosphorous oxide ceramics. Biomed Sci Instrum 28:123.

Takatsuko K, Yamamuro T, Kitsugi T, et al. 1993. A new bioactive glass-ceramic as a coating material on titanium alloy. J Appl Biomater 4:317.

Terry BC, Baker RD, Tucker MR, Hanker JS. 1989. Alveolar ridge augmentation with composite implants of hydroxylapatite and plaster for correction of bony defects, deficiencies and related contour abnormalities. Mater Res Soc Symp 110:187.

Valiathan A, Randhawa GS, Randhawa A. 1993. Biomaterial aspects of calcium hydroxyapatite. TIB AO 7:1.

Whitehead RY, Lacefield WR, Lucas LC. 1993. Structure and integrity of a plasma sprayed hydroxyapatite coating on titanium. J Biomed Mater Res 27:1501.

Wolford LM, Wardrop RW, Hartog JM. 1987. Coralline porous hydroxylapatite as a bone Graft substitute in orthognathic surgery. J Oral Maxillofac Surg 45:1034.

Wyatt DF, Bajpai PK, Graves GA Jr, Stull PA. 1976. Remodelling of calcium aluminate phosphorous pentoxide ceramic implants in bone. IRCS Med Sci 4:421.

Yamamuro T, Hench LL, Wilson J. 1990. Handbook of Bioactive Ceramics I and II. Boca Raton, Fla, CRC Press.

Yamamuro T, Shikata J, Kakutani Y, et al. 1988. Novel methods for clinical applications of bioactive ceramics. In Bioceramics: Material Characteristics versus in Vivo Behavior, pp 107–114. New York, Academy of Sciences.

Zimmerman MC, Alexander H, Parsons JR, Bajpai PK. 1991. The design and analysis of laminated degradable composite bone plates for fracture fixation. In TL Vigo, AF Turbak (eds), High-Tech Textiles, pp 132–148, ACS Symposium Series 457. Washington, American Chemical Society.

Further Information

Bajpai PK. 1988. ZCAP Ceramics, U.S. patent no. 4778471.

Bajpai PK. 1987. Surgical Cements, U.S. patent no. 4668295.

Bonfield W, Hastings GW, Tanner KE. 1991. Bioceramics, vol 4: Proceedings of the 4th International Symposium on Ceramics in Medicine. Boston, Butterworth-Heinemann.

Brook RJ. 1991. Concise Encyclopedia of Advanced Ceramic Materials. New York, Pergamon Press.

de Groot K. 1983. Bioceramics of Calcium Phosphate. Boca Raton, Fla, CRC Press.

Ducheyne P, Lemons JE. 1988. Bioceramics: Material characteristics versus in vivo behavior. New York, Academy of Sciences.

Ducheyne P, Christiansen D. 1993. Bioceramics, vol 6. Boston, Butterworth-Heinemann.

Filgueiras MRT, LaTorre G, Hench LL. 1993. Solution effects on the surface reactions of three bioactive glass compositions. J Biomed Mater Res 27:1485.

Frank RM, Wiedemann P, Hemmerle J, Freymann M. 1991. Pulp capping with synthetic hydroxyapatite in human premolars. J Appl Biomater 2:243.

Fulmer MT, Brown PW. 1993. Effects of Na_2HPO_4 and NaH_2PO_4 on hydroxyapatite formation. J Biomed Mater Res 27:1095.

Garcia R, Doremus RH. 1992. Electron microscopy of the bone-hydroxyapatite interface from a human dental implant. J Mater Sci Mater Med 3:154.

Hall CW, Hulbert SF, Levine SN, Young FA. 1972. Engineering and Medicine. New York, Interscience Publishers.

Hench LL. 1991. Bioceramics: From concept to clinic. J Am Ceramic Soc 74:1487.

Hench LL, Ethridge EC. 1982. Biomaterials: An Interfacial Approach. New York, Academic Press.

Hulbert JA, Hulbert SF. 1992. Bioceramics, vol 3: Proceedings of the 3rd International Symposium on Ceramics in Medicine. Terra Haute, Ind, Rose-Hulman Institute of Technology.

Kawahara H (ed). 1989. Oral Implantology and Biomaterials. Amsterdam, Elsevier.

Kingery WD, Bowen HK, Uhlmann DR. 1976. Introduction to Ceramics, 2d ed, p 368. New York, Wiley.

Lemons JE. 1988. Quantitative Characterization and Performance of Porous Implants for Hard Tissue Applications, ASTM STP 953. Philadelphia, Pa, American Society for Testing and Materials.

Mattie DR, Bajpai PK. 1986. Biocompatibility testing of ALCAP ceramics. IRCS Med Sci 14:641.

Neo M, Nakamura T, Ohtsuki C, et al. 1993. Apatite formation on three kinds of bioactive material at an early stage in vivo: A comparative study by transmission electron microscopy. J Biomed Mater Res 27:999.

Oonishi H, Aoki H, Sawai K. 1988. Bioceramics, vol 1: Proceedings of 1st International Symposium on Ceramics in Medicine. Tokyo, Ishiyaku EuroAmerica.

Oonishi H, Ooi Y. 1981. Orthopaedic Ceramic Implants, vol I. Tokyo, Japanese Society of Orthopaedic Ceramic Implants.

Park JB, Lakes RS. 1992. Biomaterials: An Introduction, 2d ed. New York, Plenum Press.

Ravaglioli A, Krajewski A. 1992. Bioceramics and the Human Body. Amsterdam, Elsevier Applied Science.

Rubin LR. 1983. Biomaterials in Reconstructive Surgery. St. Louis, Mosby.

Sharma CP, Szycher M. 1991. Blood Compatible Materials and Devices: Perspectives Toward the 21st Century. Lancaster, Pa, Technomic Publishing Co.

Signs SA, Pantano CG, Driskell TD, Bajpai PK. 1979. In vitro dissolution of synthos ceramics in an acellular physiological environment. Biomater Med Dev Artif Org 7:183.

Stea S, Tarabusi C, Ciapetti G, et al. 1992. Microhardness evaluations of the bone growing into porous implants. J Mater Sci Mater Med 3:252.

van Blitterswijk CA, Grote JJ. 1989. Biological performance of ceramics during inflammation and infection. Crit Rev Biocompat 5:13.

Wilson J, Low SB. 1992. Bioactive ceramics for periodontal treatment: Comparative studies in the patus monkey. J Appl Biomater 3:123.

Yamamuro T, Hench LL, Wilson J. 1990. Handbook of Bioactive Ceramics. Boca Raton, Fla, CRC Press.

Zhang X, Ikada Y. 1994. Biomedical Materials Research in the Far East (I). Kyoto, Japan, Kobunshi Kankokai.

42

Polymeric Biomaterials

Hae B. Lee
Korea Research Institute of Chemical Technology

Sung S. Kim
Korea Research Institute of Chemical Technology

Gilson Khang
Korea Research Institute of Chemical Technology

Synthetic polymeric materials have been widely used in medical disposable supplies, prosthetic materials, dental materials, implants, dressings, extracorporeal devices, encapsulants, polymeric drug delivery system, and orthopedic devices as that of metal and ceramics substituents [Lee, 1989]. The advantages of the polymeric biomaterials are ease of manufacturing into products with various shapes, ease of secondary processability, reasonable cost, and availability with desired mechanical and physical properties, e.g., latex, film, sheet, and fibers. The required properties of polymeric biomaterials are similar to other biomaterials, that is, biocompatibility, sterilizability, adequate mechanical and physical properties, and manufacturability as given in Table 42.1.

This chapter will discuss (1) basic chemical and physical properties of the synthetic polymers, (2) sterilization of the polymeric biomaterials, (3) importance of the surface treatment for improving biocompatibility, and (4) the application of the gradient surfaces for cell adhesions.

42.1 Polymerization and Basic Structure

Polymerization

In order to link the small molecules one has to force them to lose their electrons by the chemical processes of condensation and addition. By controlling the reaction temperature, pressure, and time in the presence of catalysts, the degree to which repeating units are put together into chains can be manipulated.

Condensation or Step Reaction Polymerization

During condensation polymerization a small molecule such as water will be condensed out by the chemical reaction

$$R\text{-}NH_2 \quad + \quad R'COOH \quad \rightarrow \quad R'CONHR \qquad (42.1)$$
$$\text{(amine)} \qquad\qquad \text{(carboxylic acid)} \quad \text{(amide)}$$

$$+ \; H_2O$$
$$\text{(condensation molecule)}$$

This particular process is used to make polyamides (nylons). First made in the 1930s, nylon was the first commercial polymer.

Some typical condensation polymers and their interunit linkages are given in Table 42.2. One major drawback of condensation polymerization is the tendency for the reaction to cease before the chains grow to sufficient length. This is due to the decreased mobility of the chains and reactant chemical species as polymerization progresses. This results in short chains. However, in the case of nylon, the chains are polymerized to a sufficiently large extent before this occurs, and the physical properties of the polymer are preserved.

Natural polymers, such as polysaccharides and proteins, are also made by condensation polymerization. The condensing molecule is always water (H_2O).

Addition or Free Radical Polymerization

Addition polymerization can be achieved by rearranging the bonds within each monomer. Since each "mer" has to share at least two covalent electrons with other mers, the monomer has to have at least one double bond. For example, in the case of ethylene:

$$\begin{array}{cccccc} H & H & H & H & H & H \\ n \; C = C & \rightarrow & -C-(C-C)_n-C- & & & \\ H & H & H & H & H & H \end{array} \qquad (42.2)$$

The breaking of a double bond can be made with an initiator. This is usually a free radical such as benzoyl peroxide ($C_6H_5COO\text{—}OOCC_6H_5$). The initiation can be activated by heat, ultraviolet light, and other chemicals. The free radicals (initiators) can react with monomers, and this free radical can react with another monomer, and the process can continue on. This process is called *propagation*. The propagation process can be terminated by combining two free radicals, by transfer, or by disproportionate processes. Some of the free radical polymers are given in Table 42.3. There are three more types of initiating species for addition polymerization beside free radicals: cations, anions, and coordination (stereospecific) catalysts. Some monomers can use two or more of the initiation processes, but others can use only one process as given in Table 42.3.

Basic Structure

Polymers have very long chain molecules which are formed by covalent bonding along the backbone chain. The long chains are held together either by secondary bonding forces such as van der Waals and hydrogen bonds or primary covalent bonding forces through crosslinks between chains. The long chains are very flexible and can be tangled easily. In addition, each chain can have side groups,

TABLE 42.1 Requirements for Biomedical Polymers

Properties	Description
Biocompatibility	Noncarcinogenesis, nonpyrogenicity, nontoxicity, nonallergic response
Sterilizability	Autoclave, dry heating, ethylenoxide gas, radiation
Physical property	Strength, elasticity, durability
Manufacturability	Machining, molding, extruding, fiber forming

Source: Modified from Ikada [1989].

branches, and copolymeric chains or blocks which can also interfere with the long-range ordering of chains. For example, paraffin wax has the same chemical formula as polyethylene [$(CH_2CH_2)_n$] but will crystallize almost completely because of its much shorter chain lengths. However, when the chains become extremely long [from 40 to 50 repeating units ($-CH_2CH_2-$) to several thousands as in linear polyethylene] they cannot be crystallized completely (up to 80–90% crystallization is possible). Also, branched polyethylene in which side chains are attached to the main backbone chain at positions where a hydrogen atom normally occupies will not crystallize easily due to the steric hindrance of side chains resulting in a more noncrystalline structure. The partially crystallized structure, called *semicrystalline*, is the most commonly occurring structure for linear polymers. The semicrystalline structure is represented by disordered noncrystalline regions and ordered crystalline regions which may contain folded chains as shown in Fig. 42.1.

TABLE 42.2 Typical Condensation Polymers

Type	Interunit Linkage
Polyester	$-\overset{\overset{\displaystyle O}{\|}}{C}-O-$
Polyamide	$-\overset{\overset{\displaystyle O}{\|\|}}{C}-\overset{\overset{\displaystyle H}{\|}}{N}-$
Polyurea	$-\overset{\overset{\displaystyle H}{\|}}{N}-\overset{\overset{\displaystyle O}{\|\|}}{C}-\overset{\overset{\displaystyle H}{\|}}{N}-$
Polyurethane	$-O-\overset{\overset{\displaystyle O}{\|\|}}{C}-\overset{\overset{\displaystyle H}{\|}}{N}-$
Polysiloxane	$-\overset{\overset{\displaystyle R}{\|}}{\underset{\underset{\displaystyle R}{\|}}{Si}}-O-$
Protein	$-\overset{\overset{\displaystyle O}{\|\|}}{C}-\overset{\overset{\displaystyle H}{\|}}{N}-$
Cellulose	$-C-O-C-$

The degree of polymerization (DP) is defined as average number of mers or repeating units per molecule, i.e., chain. Each chain may have a different number of mers depending on the condition of polymerization. Also the length of each chain may be different. Therefore, we deal with the average degree of polymerization or average molecular weight (MW). The relationship between molecular weight and degree of polymerization can be expressed as

$$\text{MW of polymer} = \text{DP} \times \text{MW of mer (or repeating unit)} \qquad (42.3)$$

The weight average molecular weight can be calculated according to the weight fraction (W_i) in each molecular weight fraction (M_{w_i})

$$M_w = \Sigma W_i \cdot \frac{M_{w_i}}{\Sigma W_i} = \Sigma W_i M_{w_i} \qquad (42.4)$$

since $\Sigma W_i = 1$. As the molecular chains become longer by the progress of polymerization, their relative mobility decreases. The chain mobility is also related to the physical properties of the final

TABLE 42.3 Monomers for Addition Polymerization and Suitable Processes

Monomer Name	Chemical Formula	Polymerization Mechanism			
		Radical	Cationic	Anionic	Coordination
Acrylonitrile	$CH_2{=}CH-CN$	+	−	+	+
Ethylene	$CH_2{=}CH_2$	+	+	−	−
Methylacrylate	$CH_2{=}CH-COOCH_3$	+	−	+	+
Methylmethacrylate	$CH_2{=}CCH_3$ $COOCH_3$	+	−	+	+
Propylene	$CH_2{=}CHCH_3$	−	−	−	+
Styrene	$CH_2{=}CH-C_6H_5$	+	+	+	+
Vinylchloride	$CH_2{=}CHCl$	+	−	−	+
Vinylidenechloride	$CH_2{=}CCl_2$	+	−	+	−

+: high polymer formed; −: no reaction or oligomers only
Source: Modified from Billmeyer [1984].

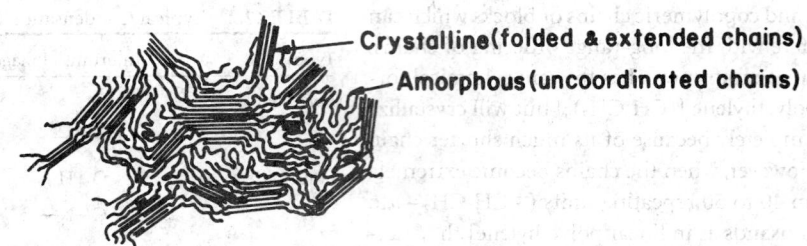

FIGURE 42.1   Fringed (micelle) model of a linear polymer with semicrystalline structure.

polymer. Generally, the higher the molecular weight, the lesser the mobility of chains which results in higher strength and greater thermal stability. The polymer chains can be arranged in three ways: linear, branched, and a crosslinked or three-dimensional network as shown in Fig. 42.2. Linear polymers such as polyvinyls, polyamides, and polyesters are much easier to crystallize than the crosslinked or branched polymers. However, these polymers cannot be crystallized 100% as with metals. Instead they become semicrystalline polymers. The arrangement of chains in crystalline regions is believed to be a combination of folded and extended chains. The chain folds, which are seemingly more difficult to form, are necessary to explain observed single-crystal structures in which the crystal thickness is too small to accommodate the length of the chain as determined by electron and x-ray diffraction studies. The classical "fringed micelle" model in which the amorphous and crystalline regions coexist has been modified to include chain folds in the crystalline regions. The crosslinked or three-dimensional network polymers such as polyphenolformaldehyde cannot be crystallized at all, and they become noncrystalline, amorphous polymers.

Vinyl polymers have a repeating unit —CH$_2$—CHX— where X is some monovalent side group. There are three possible arrangements of side groups (X): (1) atactic, (2) isotactic, and (3) syndiotactic. In atactic arrangements the side groups are randomly distributed; in syndiotactic and isotactic arrangements side groups are either in alternating positions or in one side of the main chain. If side groups are small like polyethylene (X=H) and the chains are linear, the polymer crystallizes easily. However, if the side groups are large as in polyvinyl chloride (X=Cl) and polystyrene (X=C$_6$H$_6$, benzene ring) and are randomly distributed along the chains (atactic), then a noncrystalline structure will be formed. The isotactic and syndiotactic polymers usually crystallize even when the side groups are large.

Copolymerization, in which two or more monomers (one type of repeating unit throughout its structure) are chemically combined, always disrupts the regularity of polymer chains, thus promoting the formation of noncrystalline structure. Possible arrangement of the different copolymerization is shown in Fig. 42.3. The addition of plasticizers to prevent crystallization by keeping the chains separated from one another will result in more flexible polymers, noncrystalline version of a polymer which normally crystallizes. An example is celluloid, which is made of normally crystalline nitrocellulose plasticized with camphor. Plasticizers are also used

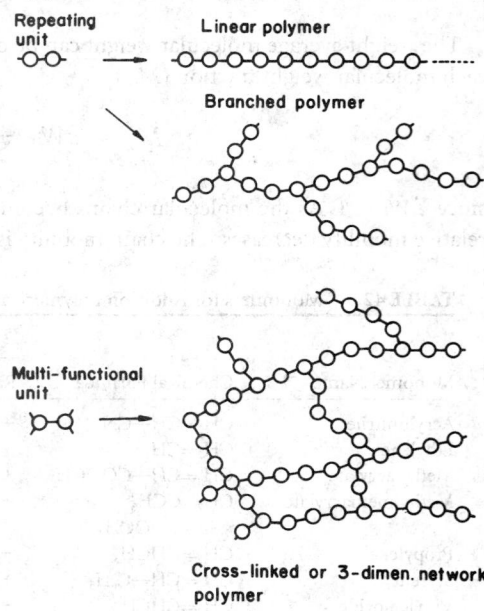

FIGURE 42.2   Arrangement of polymer chains into linear, branched, and network structure depending on the functionality of the repeating units.

to make rigid noncrystalline polymers such as polyvinylchloride (PVC) into a more flexible solid (a good example is Tygon tubing).

Elastomers or rubbers are polymers which exhibit large stretchability at room temperature and can snap back to their original dimensions when the load is released. The elastomers are noncrystalline polymers which have an intermediate structure consisting of long chain molecules in three-dimensional networks (see next section for more details). The chains also have "kinks" or "bends" in them which straighten when a load is applied. For example, the chains of *cis*-polyisoprene (natural rubber) are bent at the double bond due to the methyl group interfering with the neighboring hydrogen in the repeating unit $[-CH_2-C(CH_3)=CH-CH_2-]$. If the methyl group is on the opposite side of the hydrogen, then it becomes *trans*-polyisoprene, which will crystallize due to the absence of the steric hindrance present in the *cis* form. The resulting polymer is a very rigid solid called *gutta percha,* which is not an elastomer. Below the glass transition temperature (T_g, second-order transition temperature between viscous liquid

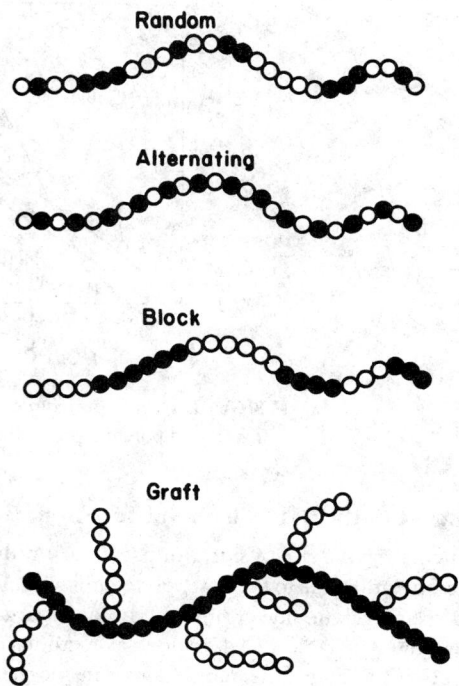

FIGURE 42.3 Possible arrangements of copolymers.

and solid), natural rubber loses its compliance and becomes a glasslike material. Therefore, to be flexible, all elastomers should have T_g well below room temperature. What makes the elastomers not behave like liquids above T_g is in fact the crosslinks between chains which act as pinning points. Without crosslinks the polymer would deform permanently. For example, latex behaves as a viscous liquid. Latex can be crosslinked with sulfur (vulcanization) by breaking double bonds (C=C) and forming C—S—S—C bonds between the chains. The more crosslinks are introduced, the more rigid the structure becomes. If all the chains are crosslinked together the material will become a three-dimensional rigid polymer.

Effect of Structural Modification on Properties

The physical properties of polymers can be affected in many ways. In particular, the chemical composition and arrangement of chains will have a great effect on the final properties. By such means we can tailor the polymers to meet the end use.

Effect of Molecular Weight and Composition

The molecular weight and its distribution have a great effect on the properties of a polymer, since its rigidity is primarily due to the immobilization or entanglement of the chains. This is because the chains are arranged like cooked spaghetti strands in a bowl. By increasing the molecular weight, the polymer chains become longer and less mobile, and a more rigid material results as shown in Fig. 42.4. Equally important is that all chains should be equal in length, since short chains will act as plasticizers. Another obvious way of changing properties is to change the chemical composition of the backbone or side chains. Substituting the backbone carbon of a polyethylene with divalent oxygen or sulfur will decrease the melting and glass transition temperatures, since the chain becomes more flexible due to the increased rotational freedom. However, if the backbone chains can be made more rigid, then a stiffer polymer will result.

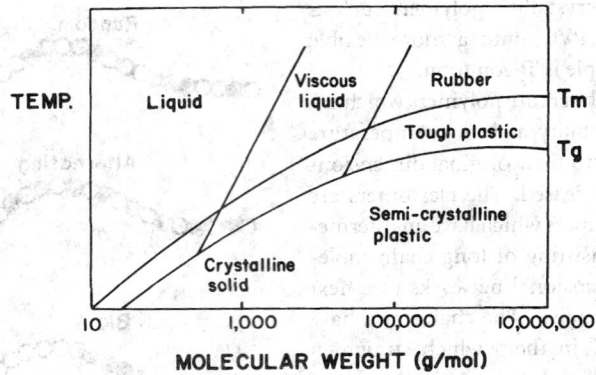

FIGURE 42.4   Approximate relations among molecular weight, T_g, T_m, and polymer properties.

Effect of the Side Chain Substitution, Crosslinking, and Branching

Increasing the size of side groups in linear polymers such as polyethylene will decrease the melting temperature due to the lesser perfection of molecular packing, i.e., decreased crystallinity. This effect is seen until the side group itself becomes large enough to hinder the movement of the main chain as shown in Table 42.4. Very long side groups can be thought of as branches.

Crosslinking of the main chains is in effect similar to the side-chain substitution with a small molecule, i.e., it lowers the melting temperature. This is due to the interference of the crosslinking, which causes lesser mobility of the chains resulting in further retardation of the crystallization rate. In fact, a large degree of crosslinking can prevent crystallization completely. However, when the crosslinking density increases for a rubber, the material becomes harder, and the glass transition temperature also increases.

Effect of Temperature on Properties

Amorphous polymers undergo a substantial change in their properties as a function of temperature. The glass transition temperature T_g is a demarcation between the glassy region of behavior in which the polymer is relatively stiff and the rubbery region in which it is very compliant. T_g can also be defined as the temperature at which the slope of volume change versus temperature has a discontinuity in slope as shown in Fig. 42.5. Since polymers are noncrystalline or at most semicrystalline, the value obtained in this measurement depends on how fast it is taken.

42.2 Polymers Used as Biomaterials

Although hundreds of polymers are easily synthesized and could be used as biomaterials, only ten to twenty polymers are mainly used in medical device fabrications from disposable to long-term implants as given in Table 42.5. In this section, the general information of the characteristics, properties, and applications of the most commonly used polymers will be discussed [Billmeyer, 1984; Brandrup & Immergut, 1989; Dumitriu, 1993; Leininger & Bigg, 1986; Park, 1984; Park & Lakes, 1992; Shalaby, 1988; Sharma & Szycher, 1991].

Polyvinylchloride (PVC)

PVC is an amorphous, rigid polymer due to the large side group (Cl) with a glass transition temperature of 75–105°C. PVC has a high melt viscosity; hence it is difficult to process. To prevent the thermal degradation of the polymer (HCl could be released), thermal stabilizers such as metallic soaps or salts are incorporated. Lubricants are formulated on PVC compounds to prevent adhesion to metal surfaces and facilitate the melt flow during processing. Plasticizers are used in the range of 10–100 parts per 100 parts of PVC resin to make it flexible. Di-2-ethylhexylphthalate (DEHP) is used in medical PVC formulation. However, the plasticizers of tri-octyltrimellitate (TOTM), polyester, azelate, and phosphate ester are also used to prevent extraction by blood, aqueous solution, and hot water during autoclaving sterilization.

PVC sheets and films are used in blood and solution bags and surgical packaging. PVC tubing is commonly used in IV administration, dialysis devices, catheters, and cannulae.

Polyethylene (PE)

PE is available commercially in five major grades: high density (HDPE), low density (LDPE), linear low density (LLDPE), very low density (VLDPE), and ultra high molecular weight (UHMWPE). HDPE is polymerized at a low temperature (60–80°C) and low pressure (~10kg/cm²) using metal catalysts. Highly crystalline, linear polymers with densities ranging from 0.94–0.965 g/cm³ are obtained. LDPE is derived from a high temperature (150–300°C) and pressures (1000–3000kg/cm²) using free radical initiators. A highly branched polymer with lower crystallinity and densities ranging from 0.915 to 0.935g/cm³ is obtained. LLDPE (density of 0.91–0.94g/cm³) and VLDPE (density of 0.88–0.89g/cm³), which are linear polymers, are polymerized under low pressures and temperatures using metal catalysts with comonomers such as 1-butene, 1-hexene, or 1-octene to obtain the desired physical properties and density ranges.

HDPE is used in the pharmaceutical bottle, nonwoven fabric, and caps. LDPE is found in flexible container application, nonwoven disposable and laminated or coextruded with paper, foil, and polymers for packaging. LLDPE is frequently employed in pouches and bags due to its excellent puncture resistance, and VLDPE is used in extruded tubes. UHMWPE (MW > 2 × 10⁶g/mol) has

TABLE 42.4 Effect of Side Chain Substitution on Melting Temperature in Polyethylene

Side Chain	$T_m(°C)$
—H	140
—CH_3	165
—CH_2CH_3	124
—$CH_2CH_2CH_3$	75
—$CH_2CH_2CH_2CH_3$	−55
—$CH_2CH\,CH_2CH_3$ CH_3	196
CH_3 —CH_2—C—CH_2CH_3 CH_3	350

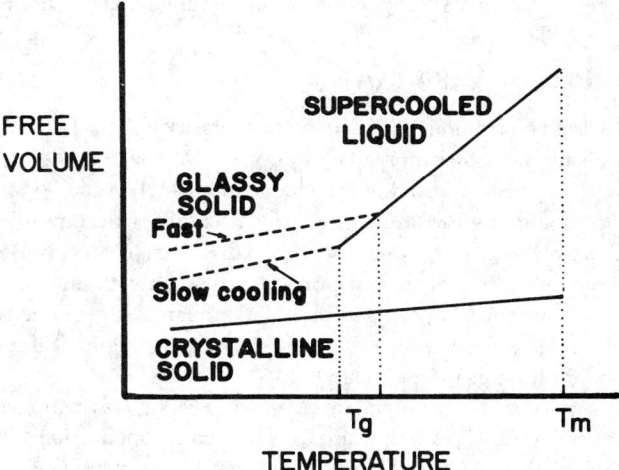

FIGURE 42.5 Change of volume versus temperature of a solid. The glass transition temperature (T_g) depends on the rate of cooling; below T_g the material behaves as a solid like a window glass.

TABLE 42.5 Biomedical Application of Polymeric Biomaterials

Synthetic polymers	Applications
Polyvinylchloride (PVC)	Blood and solution bag, surgical packaging, IV sets, dialysis devices, catheter bottles, connectors, and cannulae
Polyethylene (PE)	Pharmaceutical bottle, nonwoven fabric, catheter, pouch, flexible container, and orthopedic implants
Polypropylene (PP)	Disposable syringes, blood oxygenator membrane, suture, nonwoven fabric, and artificial vascular grafts
Polymethylmetacrylate (PMMA)	Blood pump and reservoirs, membrane for blood dialyzer, implantable ocular lens, and bone cement.
Polystyrene (PS)	Tissue culture flasks, roller bottles, and filterwares
Polyethylenterephthalate (PET)	Implantable suture, mesh, artificial vascular grafts, and heart valve
Polytetrafluoroethylene (PTFE)	Catheter and artificial vascular grafts
Polyurethane (PU)	Film, tubing, and components
Polyamide (nylon)	Packaging film, catheters, sutures, and mold parts

been used for orthopedic implant fabrications, especially for load-bearing applications such as acetabular cup of total hip of tibial plateau and patellar surface of knee joints. Biocompatability tests for PE are given by ASTM standards in F981, F639, and F755.

Polypropylene (PP)

PP can be polymerized by a Zeigler-Natta stereospecific catalyst which controls the isotactic position of the methyl group. Thermal (T_g: $-12°C$; T_m: $125–167°C$; density: $0.85–0.98$) and physical properties of PP are similar to PE. The average molecular weight of commercial PP ranges from $2.2–7.0 \times 10^5$g/mol, and PP has a wide molecular weight distribution (polydispersity) which is from 2.6 to 12. Additives for PP such as antioxidants, light stabilizer, nucleating agents, lubricants, mold release agents, and antiblock and slip agents are formulated to improve the physical properties and processability. PP has an exceptionally high flex life and excellent environment stress-cracking resistance, and hence it has been tried for finger joint prostheses with an integrally molded hinge design [Park, 1984]. The gas and water vapor permeability of PP are in between that of LDPE and HDPE. PP is used to make disposable hypothermic syringes, blood oxygenator membrane, packaging of devices, containers of solution and drug, suture, artificial vascular grafts, nonwoven fabrics, etc.

Polymethylmethacrylate (PMMA)

Commercial PMMA is an amorphous (T_g is $105°C$ and density is $1.15–1.195$) material with good resistance to dilute alkalis and other inorganic solution. PMMA is best known for its exceptional light transparency (92% transmission), high refractive index (1.49), good weathering properties, and its excellent biocompatibility. PMMA can be easily machined with conventional tools, molded, surface-coated, and plasma-etched with glow or corona discharge. PMMA is used broadly in medical applications such as blood pumps and reservoirs, IV systems, membranes for blood dialyzer, and in vitro diagnostics. It is also found in contact lenses and implantable ocular lenses due to excellent optical properties, dentures and maxillofacial prostheses due to good physical and coloring properties, and bone cement for joint prostheses fixation (ASTM standard F451).

Other acrylic polymers such as polymethylacrylate (PMA), polyhydroxyethyl-methacrylate (PHEMA), and polyacrylamide (PAAm) are also used in medical applications. PHEMA and PAAm are hydrogels, lightly crosslinked by ethyleneglycoldimethylacrylate (EGDM) to increase their mechanical strength. The extended-wear soft contact lenses are synthesized from PMMA and N-vinylpyrollidone or polyHEMA; these have high water content (above 70%) and high oxygen permeability.

Polystyrene (PS) and Its Copolymers

PS is polymerized by free radical polymerization and is usually atactic. Three grades are available, unmodified general purpose PS (GPPS) with a T_g of 100°C, high-impact PS (HIPS), and PS foam. GPPS has good transparency, lack of color, ease of fabrication, thermal stability, low specific gravity (1.04–1.12g/cm^3), and relatively high modulus. HIPS contains a rubbery modifier which forms chemical bonding with the growing PS chains. Hence the ductility and impact strength are increased and the resistance to environmental stress cracking is also improved. PS is mainly processed by injection molding at 180–250°C. To improve processability, additives such as stabilizers, lubricants, and mold releasing agent are formulated. GPPS is commonly used in tissue culture flasks, roller bottles, vacuum canisters, and filterware.

Acrylonitrile-butadiene-styrene (ABS) copolymers are produced by three monomers: acrylonitrile, butadiene, and styrene. The desired physical and chemical properties of ABS polymers with a wide range of functional characteristics can be controlled by changing the ratio of these monomers. They are resistant to the common inorganic solutions and have good surface properties and dimensional stability. ABS is used for IV sets, clamps, blood dialyzers, diagnostic test kits, and so on.

Polyesters

Polyesters such as polyethyleneterephthalate (PET), polycaprolactone, polyglycolide, polylactide, poly-p-dioxanone, and poly-β-hydroxy-butylate are frequently found in medical applications due to their unique chemical and physical properties. PET is by far the most important of this group of polymers in terms of biomedical applications such as artificial vascular graft, sutures, and meshes. PET is highly crystalline with high melting temperature (T_m is 265°C); PET is hydrophobic and resistant to hydrolysis in dilute acids. In addition, PET can be converted by conventional techniques into molded articles such as Luer filters, check valves, and catheter housing. Polycaprolactone is crystalline and has low melting temperature (T_m is 64°C). Its use as a soft matrix or coating for conventional polyester fibers was proposed by recent investigation [Leininger & Bigg, 1986]. Polyglycolide (with a T_m of 225–230°C), polylactide, poly-p-dioxanone (with a T_m of 107–112°C), and poly-β-hydroxybutylate are important polymers due to their usefulness in the production of biodegradable and absorbable implants. Polyglycolide can be melt-spun into fibers which can be converted into bioresorbable sutures, meshes, and surgical products. Poly-p-dioxanone is a bioabsorbable polymer which can be fabricated to flexible monofilament surgical sutures.

Polyamides (Nylons)

Polyamides are known as *nylons* and are designated by the number of carbon atoms in the repeating units. Nylons can be polymerized by step-reaction (or condensation) and ring-scission polymerization. They have excellent fiber-forming ability due to interchain hydrogen bonding and a high degree of crystallinity, which increases strength in the fiber direction.

The presence of —CONH— groups in polyamides attracts the chains strongly toward one another by hydrogen bonding. Since the hydrogen bond plays a major role in determining properties, the number and distribution of —CONH— groups are important factors. For example, the glass transition temperature can be decreased by decreasing the number of —CONH— groups. However, an increase in the number of —CONH— groups improves physical properties such as strength, and one can see that nylon 66 is stronger than nylon 610 and nylon 6 is stronger than nylon 11.

In addition to the higher nylons (610 and 11), there are aromatic polyamides named *aramids*. One of them is poly (p-phenylene terephthalate) commonly known as Kevlar, made by DuPont. This material can be made into fibers. The specific strength of such fibers is five times that of steel, and therefore it is most suitable for composites.

Nylons are hygroscopic and lose their strength *in vivo* when implanted. The water molecules serve as plasticizers which attack the amorphous region. Proteolytic enzymes also help to hydrolyze by attacking the amide group. This is probably due to the fact that the proteins also contain the amide group along their molecular chains which the proteolytic enzymes could attack.

Fluorocarbon Polymers

The best-known fluorocarbon polymer is polytetrafluoroethylene (PTFE), commonly known as Teflon (DuPont). Other polymers containing fluorine are polytrifluorochloroethylene (PTFCE), polyvinylfluoride (PVF), and fluorinated ethylene propylene (FEP). Only PTFE will be discussed here, since the others have rather inferior chemical and physical properties and are rarely used for implant fabrication.

PTFE is made from tetrafluoroethylene under pressure with a peroxide catalyst in the presence of excess water for removal of heat. The polymer is highly crystalline (over 94% crystallinity) with an average molecular weight of 0.5–5×10^6 g/mol. This polymer has a very high density (2.15–2.2 g/cm^3) and low modulus of elasticity (0.5 GPa) and tensile strength (14 MPa). It also has a very low surface tension (18.5 erg/cm^2) and friction coefficient (0.1).

Standard specifications for the implantable PTFE are given by ASTM F754. PTFE also has an unusual property of being able to expand on a microscopic scale into a microporous material which is an excellent thermal insulator. PTFE cannot be injection-molded or melt-extruded because of its very high melt viscosity, and it cannot be plasticized. Usually the powders are sintered to above 327°C under pressure to produce implants.

Rubbers

Silicone, natural, and synthetic rubbers have been used for the fabrication of implants. Natural rubber is made mostly from the latex of the Hevea brasiliensis tree, and the chemical formula is the same as that of *cis*-1,4 polyisoprene. Natural rubber was found to be compatible with blood in its pure form. Also, crosslinking by x-ray and organic peroxides produces rubber with superior blood compatibility compared with rubbers made by the conventional sulfur vulcanization.

Synthetic rubbers were developed to substitute for natural rubber. The Ziegler-Natta types of stereospecific polymerization techniques have made this variety possible. The synthetic rubbers have been used rarely to make implants. The physical properties vary widely due to the wide variations in preparation recipes of these rubbers.

Silicone rubber, developed by Dow Corning company, is one of the few polymers developed for medical use. The repeating unit is dimethyl siloxane, which is polymerized by a condensation polymerization. Low-molecular-weight polymers have low viscosity and can be crosslinked to make a higher-molecular-weight, rubberlike material. Medical-grade silicone rubbers contain stannous octate as a catalyst and can be mixed with base polymer at the time of implant fabrication.

Polyurethanes

Polyurethanes are usually thermosetting polymers. They are widely used to coat implants. Polyurethane rubbers are produced by reacting a prepared prepolymer chain with an aromatic diisocyanate to make very long chains possessing active isocyanate groups for crosslinking. The polyurethane rubber is quite strong and has good resistance to oil and chemicals.

Polyacetal, Polysulfone, and Polycarbonate

These polymers have excellent mechanical, thermal, and chemical properties due to their stiffened main backbone chains. Polyacetals and polysulfones are being tested as implant materials, and polycarbonates have found their applications in the heart/lung assist devices, food packaging, etc.

Polyacetals are produced by reacting formaldehyde. These are also sometimes called *polyoxymethylene* (POM) and are known widely as Delrin (DuPont). These polymers have a reasonably high molecular weight ($>2 \times 10^4$ g/mol) and have excellent mechanical properties. More important, they display an excellent resistance to most chemicals and to water over wide temperature ranges.

Polysulfones were developed by Union Carbide in the 1960s. These polymers have a high thermal stability due to the bulky side groups (therefore, they are amorphous) and rigid main backbone chains. They are also highly stable to most chemicals but are not so stable in the presence of polar organic solvents such as ketones and chlorinated hydrocarbons.

Polycarbonates are tough, amorphous, and transparent polymers made by reacting bisphenol A and diphenyl carbonate. Polycarbonate is noted for its excellent mechanical and thermal properties (a high T_g of 150°C), hydrophobicity, and antioxidative properties,

42.3 Sterilization

Sterilizability of biomedical polymers is an important aspect of their properties because polymers have lower thermal and chemical stability than other materials such as ceramics and metals; consequently, they are more difficult to sterilize using conventional techniques. Commonly used sterilization techniques are dry heat, autoclaving, radiation, and ethylene oxide gas [Block, 1977].

In dry heat sterilization, the temperature varies between 160 and 190°C. This is above the melting and softening temperatures of many linear polymers such as polyethylene and PMMA. In the case of polyamide (nylon), oxidation will occur at the dry sterilization temperature, although this is below its melting temperature. The only polymers which can safely be dry sterilized are PTFE and silicone rubber.

Steam sterilization (autoclaving) is performed under high steam pressure at relatively low temperature (125–130°C). However, if the polymer is subjected to attack by water vapor, this method cannot be employed. Polyvinylchlorides, polyacetals, polyethylenes (low-density variety), and polyamides belong to this category.

Chemical agents such as ethylene and propylene oxide gases [Glaser, 1979] and phenolic and hypochloride solutions are widely used for sterilizing polymers, since they can be used at low temperatures. Chemical agents sometimes cause polymer deterioration even when sterilization takes place at room temperature. However, the time of exposure is relatively short (overnight), and most polymeric implants can be sterilized with this method.

Radiation sterilization [Sato, 1983] using the isotopic ^{60}Co can also deteriorate polymers, since at high dosage the polymer chains can be dissociated and crosslinked according to the characteristics of the chemical structures as shown Table 42.6. Table 42.7 gives the safe level of the γ-radiation of

TABLE 42.6 Effect of Gamma Irradiation on Polymers Which Could Be Crosslinked or Degraded

Crosslinking polymers	Degradable polymers
Polyethylene	Polyisobutylene
Polypropylene	Poly-α-methylstyrene
Polystyrene	Polymethylmetacrylate
Polyarylates	Polymethacrylamide
Polyacrylamide	Polyvinylidenechloride
Polyvinylchloride	Cellulose and derivatives
Polyamides	Polytetrafluoroethylene
Polyesters	Polytrifluorochloroethylene
Polyvinylpyrrolidone	
Rubbers	
Polysiloxanes	
Polyvinylalcohol	
Polyacroleine	

TABLE 42.7 Safe Level of Gamma Radiation of Polymeric Biomaterials

Polymeric Biomaterials	Resistance for Gamma Radiation (Mrad)
Nylon	5–10
Polyethylene	100
Polystyrene	1000
Polypropylene	2.5–5.0
Polyvinylchloride	7–10
Polyvinylidenechloride	5
Polyester	100
Acrylonitrilbutadienestyrene (ABS)	5–10
Polytetrafluoroethylene	2.5
Silicone rubber	10
Neoprene rubber	10
Butyl rubber	2.5
Styrenebutadiene rubber	50
Polyurethane	100
Natural rubber	50
Epoxy resin	1000

1Mrad $=$ 10,000Gy

the polymeric biomaterials. In the case of polyethylene, at high dosage (above 10^6 Gy) it becomes a brittle and hard material. This is due to a combination of random chain scission crosslinking. Polypropylene articles will often discolor during irradiation, giving the product an undesirable color tint, but the more severe problem is the embrittlement resulting in flange breakage, luer cracking, and tip breakage. The physical properties continue to deteriorate with time following irradiation. These problems of coloration and changing of the physical properties are best resolved by avoiding the use of any additives which discolor at sterilizing dose of radiation. The *in vivo* effect on the polymer properties are not as severe as that of sterilization, but the long-term implantation may result in the similar deterioration as given in Table 42.8 for some selected polymers.

42.4 Surface Treatment for Improving Biocompatibility

Prevention of thrombus formation is important in clinical applications where blood is in contact such as hemodialysis membranes and tubes, artificial heart and heart-lung machine, prosthetic valve, and artificial vascular grafts. In spite of the use of anticoagulants, considerable platelet deposition and thrombus formation take place on the artificial surfaces [Branger et al., 1990].

Heparin, one of the complex carbohydrates known as mucopolysaccharides or glycosaminoglycan, is currently used to prevent formation of clots. In general, heparin is well tolerated and devoid

TABLE 42.8 Effect of Implantation on Polymers

Polymers	Effects of Implantation
Polyethylene	Low-density ones absorb some lipids and lose tensile strength; high-density ones are inert, and no deterioration occurs.
Polypropylene	Generally no deterioration.
Polyvinylchloride (rigid)	Tissue reaction, plasticizers may leach out and become brittle.
Polyethyleneterephthalate	Susceptible to hydrolysis and loss of tensile strength.
Polyamides (nylon)	Absorb water and irritate tissue, lose tensile strength rapidly.
Silicone rubber	No tissue reaction, very little deterioration.
Polytetrafluoroethylene	Solid specimens inert; if fragmented, irritation will occur.
Polymethylmethacrylate	Rigid form: crazing, abrasion, and loss of strength by heat sterilization. Cement form: high heat generation, unreacted monomers during and after polymerization may damage tissues.

Source: Bloch and Hastings [1972].

of serious consequences. However, it allows platelet adhesion to foreign surfaces and may cause hemorrhagic complications such as subdural hematoma, retroperitoneal hematoma, gastrointestinal bleeding, hemorrhage into joints, ocular and retinal bleeding, and bleeding at surgical sites [Lazarus, 1980]. These difficulties give rise to an interest in developing new methods of hemocompatible materials.

Many different groups have studied immobilization of heparin [Kim & Feijen, 1985] on the polymeric surfaces, heparin analogues, and heparin-prostaglandin or heparin-fibrinolytic enzyme conjugates [Jozefowicz & Jozefowicz, 1985]. The major drawback of these surfaces is that they are not stable in the blood environment. It has not been firmly established that a slow leakage of heparin is needed for it to be effective as an immobilized antithrombogenic agent; if not, its effectiveness could be hindered by being "coated over" with an adsorbed layer of more common proteins such as albumin and fibrinogen. Fibrinolytic enzymes, urokinase, and various prostaglandins have also been immobilized by themselves in order to take advantage of their unique fibrin dissolution or antiplatelet aggregation actions [Oshiro, 1983].

Albumin-coated surfaces have been studied because surfaces that resisted platelet adhesion *in vitro* were noted to adsorb albumin preferentially [Keogh et al., 1992]. Fibronectin coatings have been used in *in vitro* endothelial cell seeding to prepare a surface similar to the natural blood vessel lumen [Lee et al., 1989]. Also, algin-coated surfaces have been studied due to their good biocompatibility and biodegradability [Lee et al., 1990].

Recently plasma gas discharge and corona treatment with reactive groups introduced on the polymeric surfaces have been emerged as other ways to modify biomaterial surfaces [Lee et al., 1991; Lee et al., 1992].

Hydrophobic coatings composed of silicon- and fluorine-containing polymeric materials as well as polyurethanes have been studied because of the relatively good clinical performances of Silastic, Teflon, and polyurethane polymers in cardiovascular implants and devices. Polymeric fluorocarbon coatings deposited from a tetrafluoroethylene gas discharge have been found to greatly enhance resistance to both acute thrombotic occlusion and embolization in small-diameter Dacron grafts.

Hydrophilic coatings have also been popular because of their low interfacial tension in biologic environments [Hoffman, 1981]. Hydrogels as well as various combinations of hydrophilic and hydrophobic monomers have been studied on the premise that there will be an optimum polar–dispersion force ratio which could be matched to that on the surfaces of the most passivating proteins. The passive surface may induce less clot formation. Polyethylene oxide coated surfaces have been found to resist protein adsorption and cell adhesion and have therefore been proposed as potential "blood compatible" coatings [Lee et al., 1990].

Another way of making antithrombogenic surfaces is the saline perfusion method, which is designed to prevent direct contacts between blood and the surface of biomaterials by means of perfusing saline solution through the porous wall in contact with blood [Kim & Park, 1993; Park & Kim, 1993]. It has been demonstrated that the adhesion of the blood cells could be prevented by the saline perfusion through polyethylene, alumina, sulfonated/nonsulfonated PS/SBR, and ePTFE (expanded polytetrafluoroethylene) porous tubes.

42.5 Wettability Gradient Surfaces for Cell and Protein Interaction

The behavior of the adsorption and desorption of blood proteins or adhesion and proliferation of different types of mammalian cells on polymeric materials depend on the surface characteristics such as wettability (contact angle), hydrophilicity-hydrophobicity ratio, bulk chemistry, surface charge and charge distribution, surface roughness, and rigidity.

Many people have studied the effect of the surface wettability on the interactions of biological species with polymeric materials. Some have studied the interactions of different types of cultured cell or blood proteins with various polymers with different wettabilities to correlate the surface wettability and blood- or tissue-compatibility [Baier et al., 1984]. One problem encountered from the study using different kinds of polymers is that the surfaces are heterogeneous both chemically and physically (different surface chemistry, roughness, rigidity, crystallinity, etc.), which caused widely varying results. Some others have studied the interactions of different types of cells or proteins with a range of methacrylate copolymers that have different wettabilities and the same kind of chemistry but are still physically heterogeneous [van Wachem et al., 1985]. Another methodological problem is that such studies are often tedious, laborious, and time-consuming because a large number of samples must be prepared to characterize the complete range of the desired surface properties.

Many studies have been focused on the preparation of surfaces whose properties are changed gradually along the material length. Such gradient surfaces are of particular interest for basic studies of the interactions between biological species and synthetic materials surfaces, since the effect of a selected property can be examined in a single experiment on one surface preparation. A gradient of methyl groups was formed by diffusion of dimethyldichlorosilane through xylene on flat hydrophilic silicondioxide surfaces [Elwing et al., 1989]. The wettability gradient surfaces were made to investigate hydrophilicity-induced changes of adsorbed proteins. The wettability gradient surfaces have limitations, since they can be applied only to hydrophilic inorganic substrates.

Recently, a method for preparing wettability gradients on various polymer surfaces was developed [Lee et al., 1989, 1990]. The wettability gradients were produced via radio frequency (RF) plasma discharge treatment by exposing the polymer sheets continuously to the plasma [Lee et al., 1991]. The polymer surfaces oxidized gradually along the sample length with increasing plasma exposure time, and thus the wettability gradient was created. Another method for preparing a wettability gradient on polymer surfaces using corona discharge treatment has been developed [Lee et al., 1992]. The wettability gradient was produced by treating the polymer sheets with corona from a knife-type electrode whose power was changed gradually along the sample length. The polymer surface oxidized gradually with the increasing power, and the wettability gradient was created. This method of preparing a wettability gradient on polymer surfaces is simpler and more practical than the plasma treatment method, because the samples are discharged in air at atmospheric pressure, whereas they are discharged under vacuum in the plasma treatment method. Functional group gradient surfaces as —COOH, —CH$_2$OH, —CONH$_2$, and —CH$_2$NH$_2$ on the polyethylene were also produced on polymer surfaces by above corona treatment followed by vinyl monomer grafting and substitution reactions [Kim et al., 1993; Lee et al., 1994a, 1994b].

Fig. 42.6 shows carbon 1S core level spectra of the corona-treated PE gradient surface. The hydrophobic section of the gradient surface showed an alkyl carbon peak with a binding energy of 285eV. The corona-treated sections showed new peaks at higher binding energies, indicating the formation of carbon-oxygen functionalities, as labeled in Figure 42.6. The oxygen-based functional groups increased gradually along the sample length with increasing corona power. The Chinese hamster ovary (CHO) cells were adhered more onto the sections with moderate hydrophilicity of the gradient surface as shown in Figure 42.7. The maximum adhesion of the cells appeared at around a water contact angle of 50–55°. SEM observation also verified that the cells are adhered and spread more onto the sections with moderate hydro-

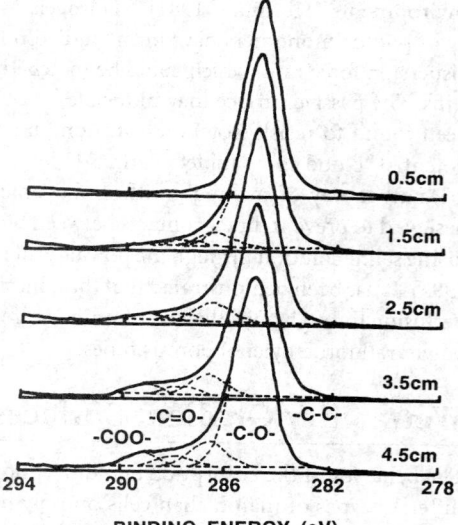

FIGURE 42.6 ESCA carbon 1S core spectra of corona-treated PE surface along the sample length. Numbers labeled on the spectra (0.5 to 4.5) represent the position from the untreated hydrophobic end of the gradient surface.

philicity. Cells attached on surfaces are spread only when they are compatible on the surfaces. It seems that surface wettability plays an important role for cell adhesion and spreading.

Defining Terms

Acetabulum: The socket portion of the hip joint.

Addition (or free radical) polymerization: Polymerization in which monomers are added to the growing chains, initiated by free radical agents.

Biocompatibility: Acceptance of an artificial implant by the surrounding tissues and by organism as a whole. The implant should be compatible with tissues in terms of mechanical, chemical, surface, and pharmacological properties.

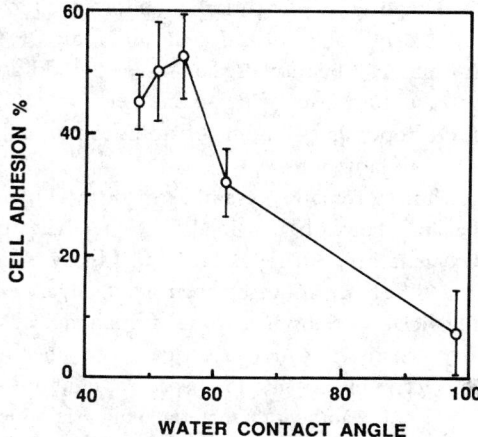

FIGURE 42.7 CHO cell adhesion on corona-treated PE surface (number of seeded cells, $4 \times 10^4/cm^2$, culture time, 2 h). Sample numbers, $n = 3$.

Biomaterials: Synthetic materials used to replace part of a living system or to function in intimate contact with living tissue.

Bone cement: Mixture of polymethylmethacrylate powder and methylmethacrylate monomer liquid to be used as a grouting material for the fixation of orthopedic implants.

Branching: Chains grown from the sides of the main backbone chains.

Condensation (step reaction) polymerization: Polymerization in which two or more chemicals are reacted to form a polymer by condensing out small molecules such as water and alcohol.

Copolymers: Polymers made from two or more monomers, which can be obtained by grafting, block, alternating, or random attachment of the other polymer segment.

Covalent bonding: Bonding of atoms or molecules by sharing valence electrons.

Dacron: Polyethyleneterephthalate polyester that is made into fiber. If the same polymer is made into a film, it is called Mylar.

Delrin: Polyacetal made by Union Carbide.

Elastomers: Rubbery materials. The restoring force comes from uncoiling or unkinking of coiled or kinked molecular chains. They can be highly stretched.

Embolus: Any foreign matter, such as a blood clot or air bubble, carried in the blood stream.

Fibrinogen: A plasma protein of high molecular weight that is converted to fibrin through the action of thrombin. This material is used to make (absorbable) tissue adhesives.

Filler: Materials added as a powder to a rubber to improve its mechanical properties.

Free volume: The difference in volume occupied by the crystalline state (minimum) and noncrystalline state of a material for a given temperature and a pressure.

Glass transition temperature: Glass transition temperature at which solidification without crystallization takes place from viscous liquid.

Gradient surface: The surface properties as wettability, surface charge, and hydrophilicity-hydrophobicity ratio are changed gradually along the material length.

Graft: A transplant.

Heparin: A substance found in various body tissues, especially in the liver, that prevents the clotting of blood.

Hydrogel: Polymer which can absorb water 30% or more of its weight.

Hydrogen bonding: A secondary bonding through dipole interactions in which hydrogen ion is one of the dipoles.

Hydroquinone: Chemical inhibitor added to the bone cement liquid monomer to prevent accidental polymerization during storage.

Initiator: Chemical used to initiate the addition polymerization by becoming a free radical which in turn reacts with a monomer.

Ionic bonding: Bonding of atoms or molecules through electrostatic interaction of positive and negative ions.

Kevlar: Aromatic polyamides made by DuPont.

Lexan: Polycarbonate made by General Electric.

Oxygenator: An apparatus by which oxygen is introduced into blood during circulation outside the body, as during open-heart surgery.

Plasticizer: Substance made of small molecules, mixed with (amorphous) polymers to make the chains slide more easily past each other, making the polymer less rigid.

Refractive index: Ratio of speed of light in vacuum to speed of light in a material. It is measure of the ability of a material a material to refract (bend) a beam of light.

Repeating unit: Basic molecular unit which can represent a polymer backbone chain. The average number of repeating unit is called the degree of polymerization.

Semicrystalline solid: Solid which contains both crystalline and noncrystalline regions and usually occurs in polymers due to their long chain molecules.

Side group: Chemical group attached to the main backbone chain. It is usually shorter than the branches and exists before polymerization.

Steric hindrance: Geometrical interference which restrains movements of molecular groups such as side chains and main chains of a polymer.

Suture: Material used in closing a wound with stitches.

Tacticity: Arrangement of asymmetrical side groups along the backbone chain of polymers; groups could be distributed at random (atactic), one side (isotactic), or alternating (syndiotactic).

Teflon: Polytetrafluoroethylene made by DuPont.

Thrombus: The fibrinous clot attached at the side of thrombosis.

Udel: Polysulfone made by General Electric.

Valence electrons: The outermost (shell) electrons of an atom.

Van der Waals bonding: A secondary bonding arising through the fluctuating dipole-dipole interactions.

Vinyl polymers: Thermoplastic linear polymers synthesized by free radical polymerization of vinyl monomers having a common structure of $CH_2{=}CHR$.

Vulcanization: Crosslinking of a (natural) rubber by adding sulfur.

Ziegler-Natta catalyst: Organometallic compounds which have the remarkable capacity of polymerizing a wide variety of monomers to linear and stereoregular polymers.

References

Baier RE, Meyer AE, Natiella JR, et al. 1984. Surface properties determine bioadhesive outcomes; Methods and results. J Biomed Mater Res 18:337.

Billmeyer FW Jr. 1984. Textbook of Polymer Science, 3d ed, New York, John Wiley & Sons.

Block SS (ed). 1977. Disinfection, Sterilization and Preservation, 2d ed, Philadelphia, Rea and Febiger.

Bloch B, Hastings GW. 1972. Plastic Materials in Surgery, 2d ed, Springfield, Ill, CC Thomas.

Brandrup J, Immergut EH (eds). 1989. Polymer Handbook, 3d ed, New York, Wiley-Interscience.

Branger B, Garreau M, Baudin G, et al. 1990. Biocompatibility of blood tubings. Int J Artif Organs 13(10):697.

Dumitriu S (ed). 1993. Polymeric Biomaterials, New York, Marcell Dekker.

Elwing E, Askendal A, Lundstorm I. 1989. Desorption of fibrinogen and γ-globulin from solid surfaces induced by a nonionic detergent. J Colloid Interface Sci 128:296.

Glaser ZR. 1979. Ethylene oxide: Toxicology review and field study results of hospital use. J Environ Pathol Toxic 2:173.

Hoffman AS. 1981. Radiation processing in biomaterials: A review. Radiat Phys Chem 18(1):323.

Ikada Y (ed). 1989. Bioresorbable fibers for medical use. In High Technology Fiber, Part B, New York, Marcel Dekker.

Jozefowicz M, Jozefowicz J. 1985. New approaches to anticoagulation: Heparin-like biomaterials. J Am Soc Art Intern Org 8:218.

Keogh JR, Valender FF, Eaton JW. 1992. Albumin-binding surfaces for implantable devices. J Biomed Mater Res 26:357.

Kim HG, Lee JH, Lee HB, et al. 1993. Dissociation behavior of surface-grafted poly(acrylic acid): Effects of surface density and counterion size. J Colloid Interface Sci 157(1):82.

Kim SW, Feijen J. 1985. Surface modification of polymers for improved blood biocompatibility. Crit Rev Biocompatibility 1(3):229.

Kim SS, Park JB. 1993. Prevention of blood cell adhesion in porous inner wall of double-layered tube by saline perfusion. Biomed Mater Eng 3:85.

Lazarus JM. 1980. Complications in hemodialysis: An Overview. Kidney Int 18:783.

Lee HB. 1989. Application of synthetic polymers in implants. In T Seagusa, T Higashimura, A Abe (eds), Frontiers of Macromolecular Science, pp 579–584, Oxford, Blackwell Scientific Publications.

Lee JH, Khang G, Park KH, et al. 1989. Polymer surfaces for cell adhesion: I. Surface modification of polymers and ESCA analysis. J Korean Soc Med Biolog Eng 10(1):43.

Lee JH, Khang G, Park JW, et al. 1990a. Plasma protein adsorption on polyethyleneoxide gradient surfaces. 33rd IUPAC International Symposium on Macromolecules, Montreal, Canada.

Lee JH, Shin BC, Khang G, et al. 1990b. Algin impregnated vascular graft: I. *in vitro* investigation. J Korean Soc Med Biolog Eng 11(1):97.

Lee JH, Park JW, Lee HB. 1991. Cell adhesion and growth on polymer surfaces with hydroxyl groups prepared by water vapor plasma treatment. Biomaterials 12:443.

Lee JH, Kim HG, Khang G, et al. 1992. Characterization of wettability gradient surfaces prepared by corona discharge treatment. J Colloid Interface Sci 151(2):563.

Lee JH, Kim HW, Pak PK, et al. 1994a. Preparation and characterization of functional group gradient surfaces. J Polym Sci, Part A, Polym Chem 32:1569.

Lee JH, Jung HW, Kang I-K, et al. 1994b. Cell behavior on polymer surfaces with different functional groups. Biomaterials 15: in press.

Leininger RI, Bigg DM. 1986. Polymers. In Handbook of Biomaterials Evaluation, pp 24–37, New York, Macmillan.

Oshiro T. 1983. Thrombosis, antithrombogenic characteristics of immobilized urokinase on synthetic polymers. In M Szycher (ed), Biocompatible Polymers, Metals, and Composites, pp 275–299, Lancaster, Penn, Technomic.

Park JB. 1984. Biomaterials Science and Engineering, New York, Plenum.

Park JB, Lakes R. 1992. Biomaterials: An Introduction, 2d ed, pp 141–168, New York, Plenum.

Park JB, Kim SS. 1993. Prevention of mural thrombus in porous inner tube of double-layered tube by saline perfusion. Biomed Mater Eng 3:101.

Sato K. 1983. Radiation sterilization of medical products. Radioisotopes 32:431.

Shalaby WS. 1988. Polymeric materials. In JG Webster (ed), Encyclopedia of Med. Dev. Instr., pp 2324–2335, New York, Wiley-Interscience.

Sharma CP, Szycher M, (eds). 1991. Blood Compatible Materials and Devices: Perspective Toward the 21st Century, Lancaster, Penn, Technomic.

Van Wachem PB, Beugeling T, Feijen J, et al. 1985. Interaction of cultured human endothelial cells with polymeric surfaces of different wettabilities, Biomaterials 6:403.

43

Composite Biomaterials

Roderic Lakes

Department of Biomedical Engineering, Department of Mechanical Engineering, and Center for Laser Science and Engineering, University of Iowa

Composite materials are solids that contain two or more distinct constituent materials or phases, on a scale larger than the atomic. The term *composite* is usually reserved for those materials in which the distinct phases are separated on a scale larger than the atomic and in which properties such as the elastic modulus are significantly altered in comparison with those of a homogeneous material. Accordingly, reinforced plastics such as fiberglass as well as bone are viewed as composite materials, but alloys such as brass are not. A foam is a composite in which one phase is empty space. Natural biological materials tend to be composites. Natural composites include bone, wood, dentin, cartilage, and skin. Natural foams include lung, cancellous bone, and wood. Natural composites often exhibit hierarchical structures in which particulate, porous, and fibrous structural features are seen on different microscales [Katz, 1980; Lakes, 1993]. In this segment, composite material fundamentals and applications in biomaterials [see, e.g., Park & Lakes, 1992] are explored. Composite materials offer a variety of advantages in comparison with homogeneous materials. These include the ability for the scientist or engineer to exercise considerable control over material properties. There is the potential for stiff, strong, lightweight materials as well as for highly resilient and compliant materials. In biomaterials, each constituent of the composite must be biocompatible. Moreover, the interface between constituents should not be degraded by the body environment. Some applications of composites in biomaterial applications are dental filling composites; reinforced methyl methacrylate bone cement and ultra-high-molecular-weight polyethylene; and orthopedic implants with porous surfaces.

43.1 Structure

The properties of composite materials depend very much upon *structure*. Composites differ from homogeneous materials in that considerable control can be exerted over the larger-scale structure and hence over the desired properties. In particular, the properties of a composite material depend upon the *shape* of the inhomogeneities, upon the *volume fraction* occupied by them, and upon the *interface* among the constituents. The shape of the inhomogeneities in a composite material is classified as follows: The principal inclusion shape categories are the particle, with no long dimension; the fiber, with one long dimension; and the platelet or lamina, with two long dimensions, as shown in Fig. 43.1. The inclusions may vary in size and shape within a category. For example, particulate

0-8493-8346-3/95/$0.00+$.50
© 1995 by CRC Press, Inc.

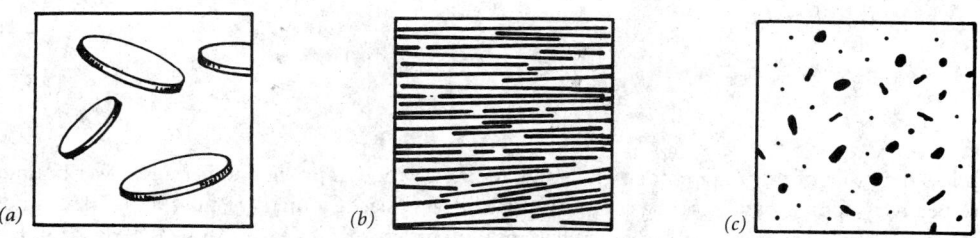

FIGURE 43.1 Morphology of basic composite inclusions: (*a*) platelet; (*b*) fiber; (*c*) particle.

inclusions may be spherical, ellipsoidal, polyhedral, or irregular. If one phase consists of voids, filled with air or liquid, the material is known as a *cellular solid*. If the cells are polygonal, the material is a honeycomb; if the cells are polyhedral, the material is a foam. It is necessary in the context of biomaterials to distinguish the above structural cells from biological cells, which occur only in living organisms. In each composite structure, we may moreover make the distinction between random orientation and preferred orientation.

43.2 Bounds on Properties

Mechanical properties in many composite materials depend on structure in a complex way; however, for some structures the prediction of properties is relatively simple. The simplest composite structures are the idealized Voigt and Reuss models, shown in Fig. 43.2. The dark and light areas in these diagrams represent the two constituent materials in the composite. In contrast to most composite structures, it is easy to calculate the stiffness of materials with the Voigt and Reuss structures, since in the Voigt structure the strain is the same in both constituents; in the Reuss structure the stress is the same. The Young's modulus *E* of the Voigt composite is

$$E = E_i V_i + E_m [1 - V_i] \tag{43.1}$$

in which E_i is the Young's modulus of the inclusions, V_i is the volume fraction of inclusions, and E_m is the Young's modulus of the matrix. The Voigt relation for the stiffness is referred to as the *rule of mixtures*.

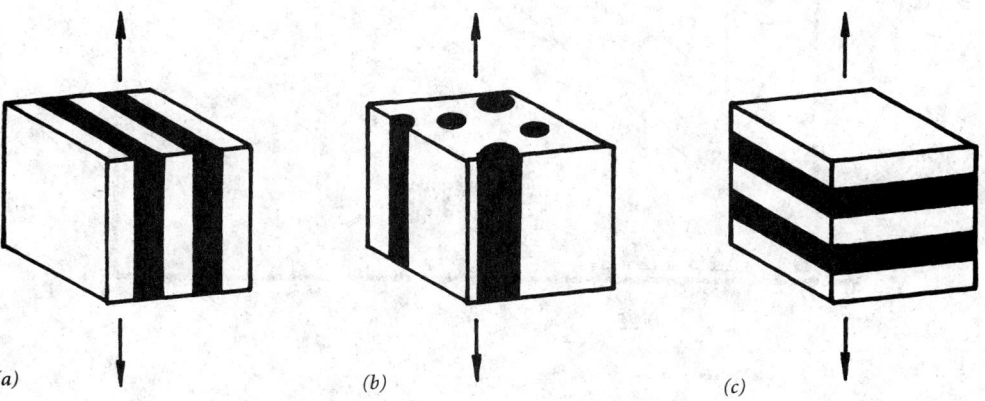

FIGURE 43.2 Voigt—(*a*) laminar, (*b*) fibrous—and Reuss (*c*) composite models, subjected to tension force indicated by arrows.

The Reuss stiffness E,

$$E = \left[\frac{V_i}{E_i} + \frac{(1 - V_i)}{E_m} \right]^{-1}$$

(43.2)

is less than that of the Voigt model. The Voigt and Reuss models provide upper and lower bounds respectively upon the stiffness of a composite of arbitrary phase geometry [Paul, 1960]. The bounds are far apart if, as is commonplace, the phase moduli differ a great deal, as shown in Fig. 43.3. For composite materials which are isotropic, the more complex relations of Hashin and Shtrickman [1963] provide tighter bounds upon the moduli; both the Young's and shear moduli must be known for each constituent.

43.3 Anisotropy of Composites

Observe that the Reuss laminate is identical to the Voigt laminate, except for a rotation with respect to the direction of load. Therefore, the stiffness of the laminate is *anisotropic*, that is, dependent on direction; see, for example, Agarwal and Broutman [1980], Nye [1976] and Lekhnitskii [1963]. Anisotropy is characteristic of composite materials. The relationship between stress σ_{ij} and strain ϵ_{kl} in anisotropic materials is given by the tensorial form of Hooke's law as follows:

$$\sigma_{ij} = \sum_{i,j=1}^{3} C_{ijkl} \epsilon_{kl}$$

(43.3)

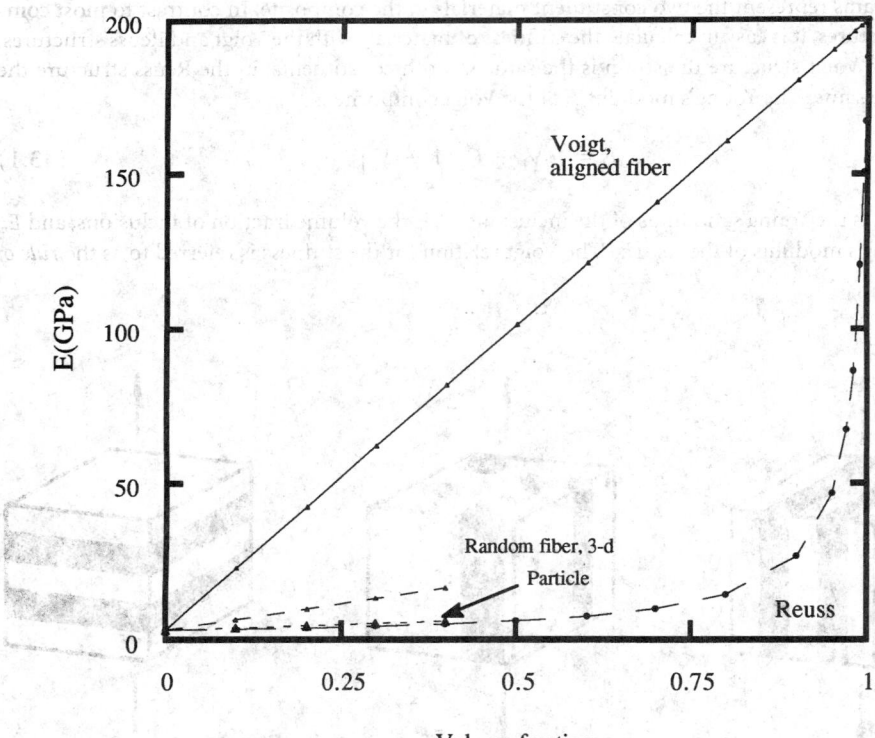

FIGURE 43.3 Stiffness vs volume fraction for Voigt and Reuss models, as well as for fibrous and particulate materials. Phase moduli are 200 GPa and 3 GPa.

Here C_{ijkl} is the elastic modulus tensor. It has $3^4 = 81$ elements; however, since the stress and strain are represented by symmetric matrices with six independent elements each, the number of independent modulus tensor elements is reduced to 36. An additional reduction to 21 is achieved by considering elastic materials for which a strain energy function exists. Physically, C_{2323} represents a shear modulus since it couples a shear stress with a shear strain. C_{1111} couples axial stress and strain in the 1 or *x* direction, but it is not the same as Young's modulus. The reason is that Young's modulus is measured with the lateral strains free to occur via the Poisson effect, whereas C_{1111} is the ratio of axial stress to strain when there is only one nonzero strain value; there is no lateral strain. A modulus tensor with 21 independent elements describes a *triclinic* crystal, which is the least symmetric crystal form. The unit cell has three different oblique angles and three different side lengths. A triclinic composite could be made with groups of fibers oriented in three different oblique directions. Triclinic modulus elements such as C_{2311}, known as *cross-coupling constants*, have the effect of producing a shear stress in response to a uniaxial strain; this is undesirable in many applications. An *orthorhombic* crystal or an *orthotropic* composite has a unit cell with orthogonal angles. There are nine elastic moduli. The associated engineering constants are three Young's moduli, three Poisson's ratio, and three shear moduli; the cross-coupling constants are zero when stresses are aligned to the symmetry directions. An example of such a composite is a unidirectional fibrous material with a rectangular pattern of fibers in the cross-section. Bovine bone, which has a laminated structure, exhibits orthotropic symmetry, as does wood. In *hexagonal* symmetry, there are five independent elastic constants out of the nine remaining *C* elements. For directions in the transverse plane, the elastic constants are the same, hence the alternative name *transverse isotropy*. A unidirectional fiber composite with a hexagonal or random fiber pattern has this symmetry, as does human haversian bone. In *cubic* symmetry, there are three independent elastic constants, a Young's modulus *E*, a shear modulus *G*, and an independent Poisson's ratio *v*. Cross-weave fabrics have cubic symmetry. Finally, an *isotropic* material has the same material properties in any direction. There are only two independent elastic constants, hence *E*, *G*, *v*, and the bulk modulus *B* are related in an isotropic material. Isotropic materials include amorphous solids, polycrystalline metals in which the grains are randomly oriented, and composite materials in which the constituents are randomly oriented.

Anisotropic composites offer superior strength and stiffness in comparison with isotropic ones. Material properties in one direction are gained at the expense of properties in other directions. It is sensible, therefore, to use anisotropic composite materials only if the direction of application of the stress is known in advance.

43.4 Particulate Composites

It is often convenient to stiffen or harden a material, commonly a polymer, by the incorporation of particulate inclusions. The shape of the particles is important [see, e.g., Christensen, 1979]. In isotropic systems, stiff platelet (or flake) inclusions are the most effective in creating a stiff composite, followed by fibers; and the least effective geometry for stiff inclusions is the spherical particle. A dilute concentration of spherical particulate inclusions of stiffness E_i and volume fraction V_i, in a matrix of Poisson's ratio $\frac{1}{2}$ denoted by the subscript *m*, gives rise to a composite with a stiffness *E*

$$E = \frac{5(E_i - E_m)V_i}{3 + 2E_i/E_m} + E_m \tag{43.4}$$

Even if the particles are perfectly rigid compared with the matrix, their stiffening effect at low concentrations is modest. Conversely, when the inclusions are more compliant than the matrix, spherical ones reduce the stiffness the least, and platelet ones reduce it the most. Indeed, platelets in this case are suggestive of cracklike defects. Soft platelets, therefore, result not only in a compliant composite but also in a weak one. Soft spherical inclusions are used intentionally as crack stoppers to enhance the toughness of polymers such as polystyrene (high-impact polystyrene), with a small sacrifice in stiffness.

Particle reinforcement has been used to improve the properties of bone cement. For example, inclusion of bone particles in PMMA cement somewhat improves the stiffness and improves the fatigue life considerably [Park et al., 1986]. Moreover, the bone particles at the interface with the patient's bone are ultimately resorbed and are replaced by ingrown new bone tissue. This approach is in the experimental stages.

Rubber used in catheters, rubber gloves, and the like is usually reinforced with very fine particles of silica (SiO_2) to make the rubber stronger and tougher.

Teeth with decayed regions have traditionally been restored with metals such as silver amalgam. Metallic restorations are not considered desirable for anterior teeth for cosmetic reasons. Acrylic resins and silicate cements had been used for anterior teeth, but their poor material properties led to short service life and clinical failures. Dental composite resins have virtually replaced these materials and are very commonly used to restore posterior teeth as well as anterior teeth [Cannon, 1988].

The composite resins consist of a polymer matrix and stiff inorganic inclusions [Craig, 1981]. A representative structure is shown in Fig. 43.4. The particles are very angular in shape. The inorganic inclusions confer a relatively high stiffness and high wear resistance on the material. Moreover, since they are translucent and their index of refraction is similar to that of dental enamel, they are cosmetically acceptable. Available dental composite resins use quartz, barium glass, and colloidal silica as fillers. Fillers have particle size from 0.04–13 µm and concentrations from 33–78% by weight. In view of the greater density of the inorganic filler phase, a 77% weight percent of filler corresponds to a volume percent of about 55%. The matrix consists of a polymer, typically BIS-GMA. In restoring a cavity, the dentist mixes several constituents, then places them in the prepared cavity to polymerize. For this procedure to be successful, the viscosity of the mixed paste must be sufficiently low and the polymerization must be controllable. Low-viscosity liquids such as triethylene glycol

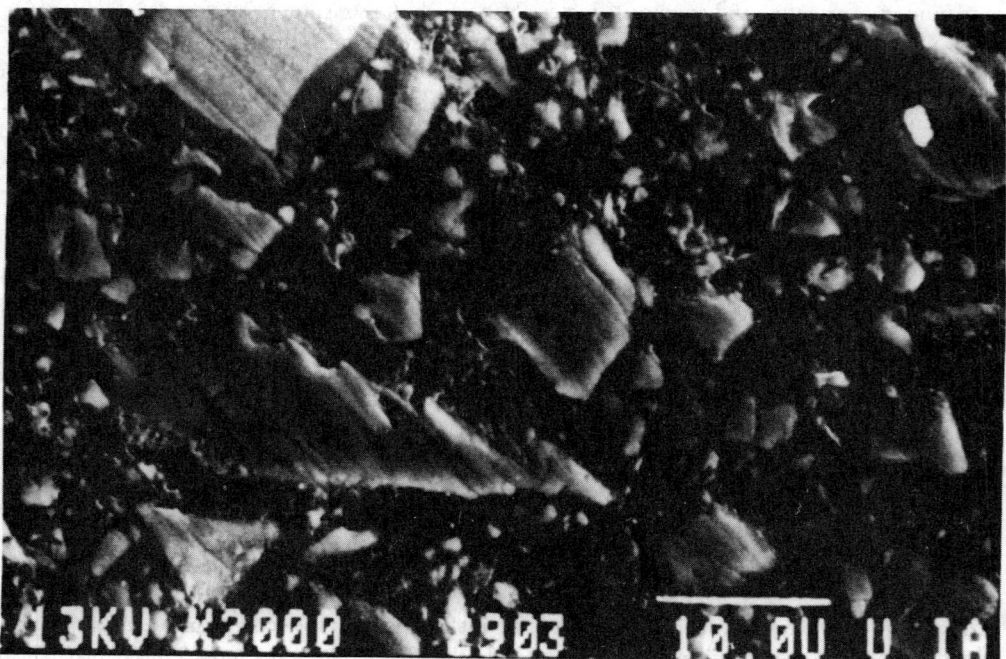

FIGURE 43.4   Microstructure of a dental composite. Miradapt (Johnson & Johnson) 50% by volume filler: barium glass and colloidal silica. From Park and Lakes [1992].

dimethacrylate are used to lower the viscosity, and inhibitors such as BHT (butylated trioxytoluene) are used to prevent premature polymerization. Polymerization can be initiated by a thermochemical initiator such as benzoyl peroxide or by a photochemical initiator (benzoin alkyl ether) which generates free radicals when subjected to ultraviolet light from a lamp used by the dentist.

The Young's modulus of dental composites may be in the range 10–16 GPa, and the compressive strength from 170–260 MPa [Cannon, 1988]. The thermal expansion of these materials, as with other dental materials, exceeds that of tooth structure. Moreover, there is a contraction during polymerization of 1.2–1.6%. These effects are thought to contribute to leakage of saliva, bacteria, and so on at the interface margins, which in some cases can cause further decay of the tooth. Use of colloidal silica in the so-called microfilled composites allows these resins to be polished, so that less wear occurs and less plaque accumulates. It is more difficult, however, to make these with a high fraction of filler, since the tendency for high viscosity of the unpolymerized paste must be counteracted. An excessively high viscosity is problematical, since it prevents the dentist from adequately packing the paste into the prepared cavity; the material will then fill in crevices less effectively. All the dental composites exhibit creep. The stiffness changes by a factor of from 2.5–4 (depending on the particular material) over a period from 10 seconds to 3 hours under steady load [Papadogianis et al., 1985]. This creep may result in indentation of the restoration, but wear seems to be a greater problem.

Dental composite resins have become established as restorative materials for both anterior and posterior teeth. The use of these materials is likely to increase as improved compositions are developed and in response to concern over long-term toxicity of silver-mercury amalgam fillings.

43.5 Fibrous Composites

Fibers incorporated in a polymer matrix increase the stiffness, strength, fatigue life, and other properties; see, for example, Agarwal and Broutman [1980]. Fibers are mechanically more effective in achieving a stiff, strong composite than are particles. Materials can be prepared in fiber form with very few defects which concentrate stress. Such fibers are very strong. The stiffness of a composite with aligned fibers, if it is loaded along the fibers, is equivalent to the Voigt upper bound, Eq. (43.1). Unidirectional fibrous composites, when loaded along the fibers, can have strengths and stiffnesses comparable to that of steel, but with much less weight. However if it is loaded transverse to the fibers, such a composite will be compliant, with a stiffness not much greater than that of the matrix alone. Although unidirectional fiber composites can be made very strong in the longitudinal direction, they are weaker than the matrix alone when loaded transversely, as a result of stress concentration around the fibers. If stiffness and strength are needed in all directions, the fibers may be oriented randomly. For such a three-dimensional isotropic composite,

$$E = \frac{E_i V_i}{6} + E_m \qquad (43.5)$$

so the stiffness is reduced by about a factor of six in comparison with an aligned composite. However if the fibers are aligned randomly in a plane, the reduction in stiffness is only a factor of 3. The degree of anisotropy in fibrous composites can be very well controlled by forming laminates consisting of layers of fibers embedded in matrix. Each layer can have fibers oriented in a different direction. Strength of composites depends on such particulars as the brittleness or ductility of the inclusions and the matrix. In fibrous composites failure may occur by fiber breakage, buckling, or pullout; matrix cracking; or debonding of fiber from matrix.

Short-fiber composites are used in many applications. They are not as strong as those with continuous fibers, but they can be formed economically by injection molding or by *in situ* polymerization. Choice of an optimal fiber length can result in improved toughness, due to the predominance of fiber pull-out as a fracture mechanism.

Carbon fibers have been incorporated in the high-density polyethylene used in total knee replacements (Fig. 43.5). The standard ultra-high-molecular-weight polyethylene (UHMWPE) used in these implants is considered adequate for most purposes for implantation in older patients. A longer wear-free implant lifetime is desirable for use in younger patients. It is considered desirable to improve the resistance to creep of the polymeric component, since excessive creep results in an indentation of that component after long-term use. Representative properties of carbon-reinforced ultra-high-molecular-weight polyethylene are shown in Fig. 43.6 [Sclippa & Piekarski, 1973]. Enhancements of various properties by a factor of 2 are feasible.

Polymethyl methacrylate (PMMA) used in bone cement is compliant and weak in comparison with bone. Therefore several reinforcement methods have been attempted. Metal wires have been used clinically as macroscopic "fibers" to reinforce PMMA cement used in spinal stabilization surgery [Fishbane & Pond, 1977]. The wires are made of a biocompatible alloy such as cobalt-chromium alloy or stainless steel. Such wires have not yet been in joint replacements owing to the limited space available. However, Kim and Park [1994] have found that reinforcement of bone ce-

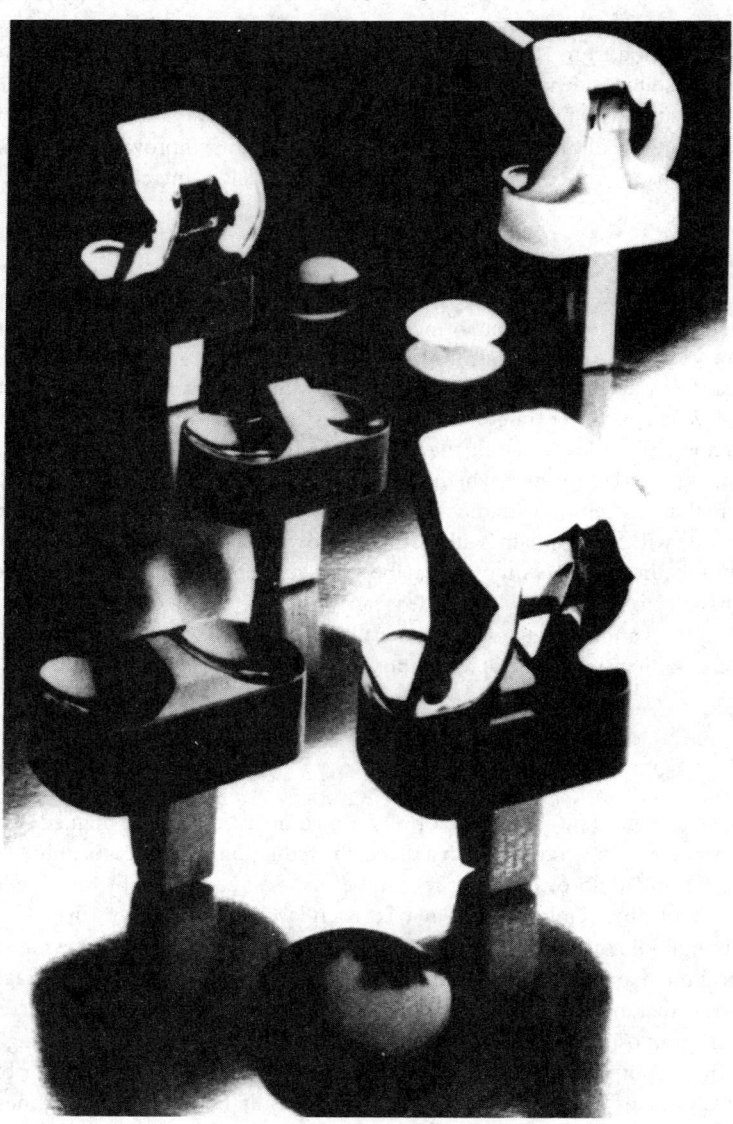

FIGURE 43.5   Knee prostheses with polyethylene tibial components reinforced with carbon fiber.

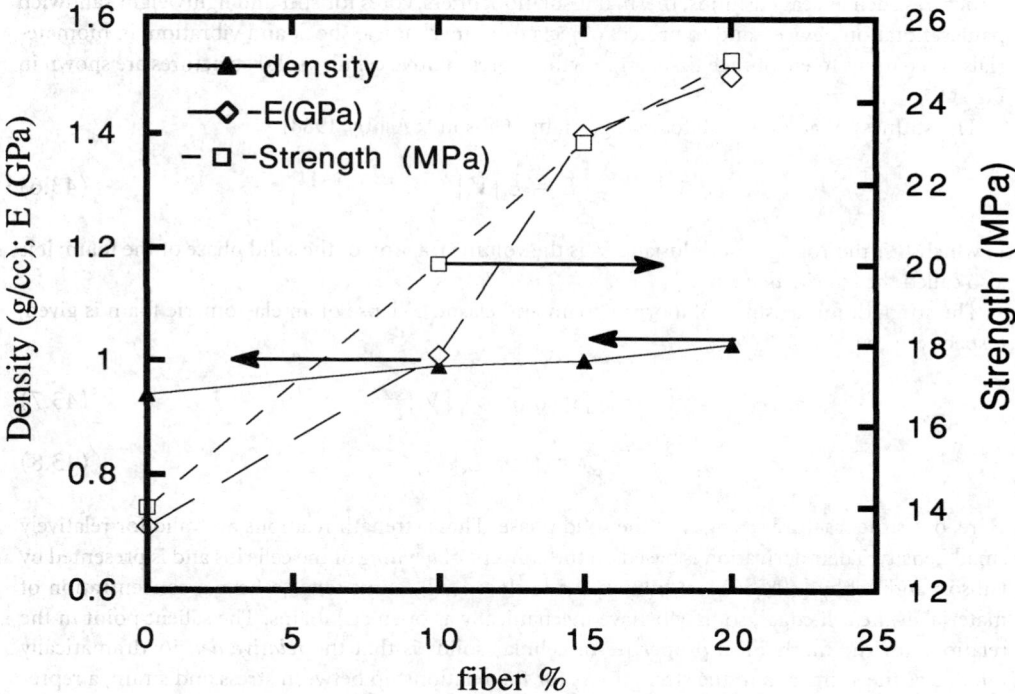

FIGURE 43.6 Properties of carbon-fiber-reinforced ultra-high-molecular-weight polyethylene. Replotted from Sclippa and Piekarski [1973].

ment by a coil of wire increases its strength in laboratory studies. Graphite fibers have been incorporated in bone cement [Knoell et al., 1975] on an experimental basis. Significant improvements in the mechanical properties can be achieved. Moreover the fibers have an added beneficial effect of reducing the rise in temperature which occurs during the polymerization of the PMMA in the body. Such high temperature can cause problems of necrosis of a portion of the bone into which it is implanted. Thin, short titanium fibers have been embedded in PMMA cement [Topoleski et al., 1992]; a toughness increase of 51% was observed with a 5% volumetric fiber content. Fiber reinforcement of PMMA cement has not found much acceptance, since the fibers also increase the viscosity of the unpolymerized material. It is consequently difficult to form and shape the polymerizing cement during the surgical procedure.

Metals are currently used in bone plates for immobilizing fractures and in the femoral component of total hip replacements. A problem with currently used implant metals is that they are much stiffer than bone, so they shield the nearby bone from mechanical stress. Stress shielding results in a kind of disuse atrophy: the bone resorbs. Therefore composite materials have been investigated as alternatives [Bradley et al., 1980; Skinner, 1988]. Fibrous composites can deform to higher strains without damage better than metals, an attractive characteristic for more flexible bone plates and femoral stems. Flexible composite bone plates are effective in promoting healing [Jockish et al., 1992]. Particulate debris from the plates gives rise to a foreign-body reaction similar to that caused by ultra-high-molecular-weight polyethylene. Fibrous composites have also been used in external medical devices such as knee braces [Yeaple 1989], in which biocompatibility is not a concern.

43.6 Porous Materials

The presence of voids in porous or cellular solids will reduce the stiffness of the material. For some purposes that is both acceptable and desirable. Porous solids are used for many purposes: flexible structures such as seat cushions, thermal insulation, filters, cores for stiff and lightweight sandwich panels, flotation devices, and to protect objects from mechanical shock and vibration; in biomaterials, as coatings to encourage tissue ingrowth. Representative cellular solid structures are shown in Fig. 43.7.

The stiffness of an open-cell foam is given by [Gibson & Ashby, 1988]

$$E = E_s[V_s]^2 \tag{43.6}$$

in which E_s is the Young's modulus and V_s is the volume fraction of the solid phase of the foam; it is also called the *relative density*.

The strength for crushing of a brittle foam and elastic collapse of an elastomeric foam is given, respectively, by

$$\sigma_{crush} = 0.65 \, \sigma_{f,s} \, [V_s]^{3/2} \tag{43.7}$$

$$\sigma_{coll} = 0.05 \, E_s[V_s]^2 \tag{43.8}$$

Here, $\sigma_{f,s}$ is the fracture strength of the solid phase. These strength relations are valid for relatively small density. Their derivation is based on the concept of *bending* of the cell ribs and is presented by Gibson and Ashby [1988]. Most human-made closed cell foams tend to have a concentration of material at the cell edges, so they behave mechanically as open cell foams. The salient point in the relations for the mechanical properties of cellular solids is that the *relative density* dramatically influences the stiffness and the strength. As for the relationship between stress and strain, a representative stress-strain curve is shown in Fig. 43.8. The physical mechanism for the deformation mode beyond the elastic limit depends on the material from which the foam is made. Trabecular

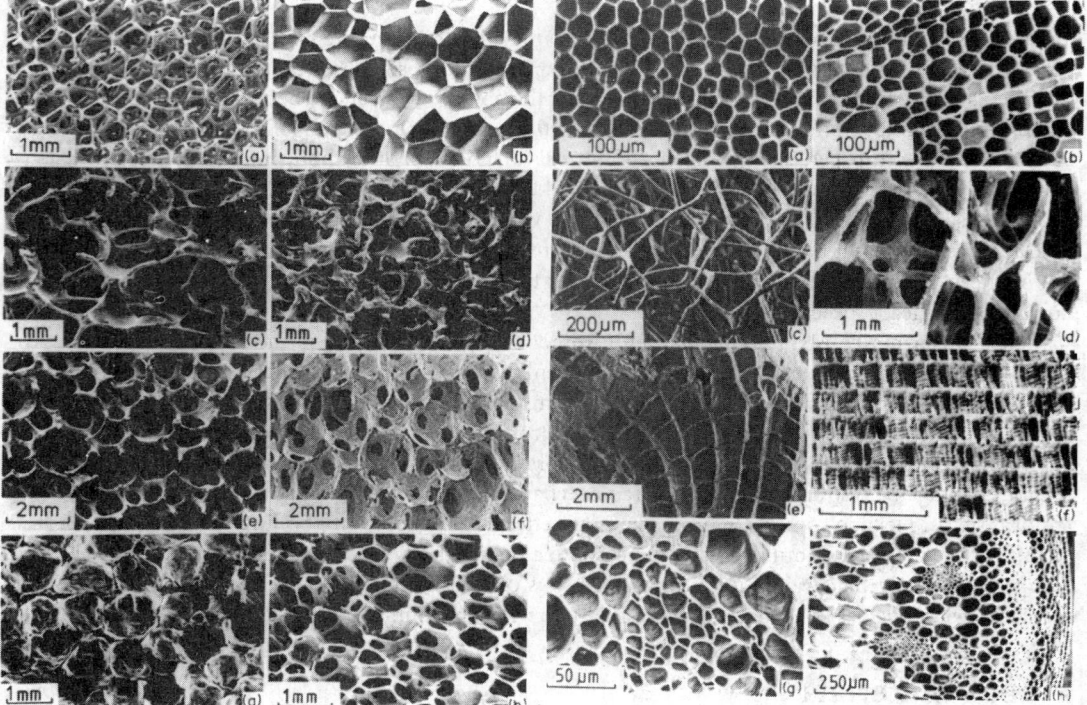

FIGURE 43.7   Cellular solids structures, after Gibson and Ashby [1988].

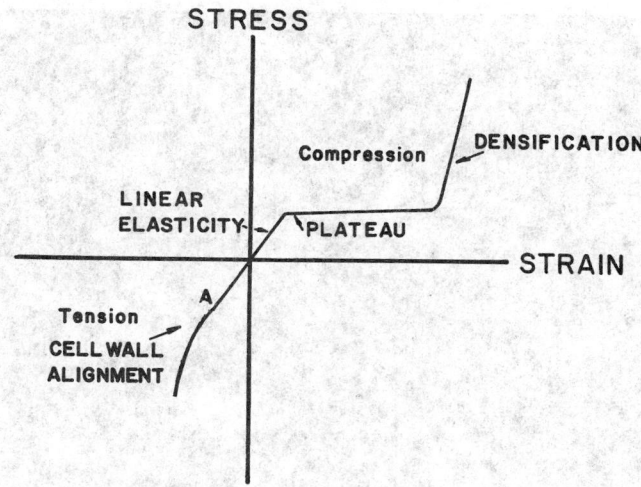

FIGURE 43.8 Representative stress-strain curve for a cellular solid. The plateau region for compression in the case of elastomeric foam (a rubbery polymer) represents elastic buckling; for an elastic-plastic foam (such as metallic foam), it represents plastic yield, and for an elastic-brittle foam (such as ceramic) it represents crushing. On the tension side, point *A* represents the transition between cell wall bending and cell wall alignment. In elastomeric foam, the alignment occurs elastically, in elastic plastic foam it occurs plastically, and an elastic-brittle foam fractures at *A*.

bone, for example, is a natural cellular solid, which tends to fail in compression by crushing. Many kinds of trabecular bone appear to behave mechanically as a normal open cell foam; however, different structures of trabecular bone may behave differently.

Porous materials have a high ratio of surface area to volume. When porous materials are used in biomaterial applications, the demands upon the inertness and biocompatibility are likely to be greater than for a homogeneous material.

Porous materials when used in implants allow tissue ingrowth [Spector et al., 1988]. The ingrowth is considered desirable in many contexts, since it allows a relatively permanent anchorage of the implant to the surrounding tissues. There are actually two composites to be considered in porous implants: the implant prior to ingrowth, in which the pores are filled with tissue fluid which is ordinarily of no mechanical consequence, and the implant filled with tissue. In the case of the implant prior to ingrowth, it must be recognized that the stiffness and strength of the porous solid are much less than in the case of the solid from which it is derived.

Porous layers are used on bone compatible implants to encourage bony ingrowth [Ducheyne, 1984; Galante et al., 1971]. The pore size of a cellular solid has no influence on its stiffness or strength (though it does influence the toughness); however, pore size can be of considerable biological importance. Specifically, in orthopedic implants with pores larger than about 150 μm, bony ingrowth into the pores occurs, and this is useful to anchor the implant. This minimum pore size is on the order of the diameter of osteons in normal haversian bone. It was found experimentally that pores smaller than 75 μm did not permit the ingrowth of bone tissue. Moreover, it was difficult to maintain fully viable osteons within pores in the 75–150 μm size range. Representative structure of such a porous surface layer is shown in Fig. 43.9. Porous coatings are also under study for application in anchoring the artificial roots of dental implants to the underlying jawbone. Porous hydroxyapatite has been studied for use in repairing large defects in bone [Holmes et al., 1986; Meffert et al., 1985]. Hydroxyapatite is the mineral constituent of bone, and it has the nominal composition

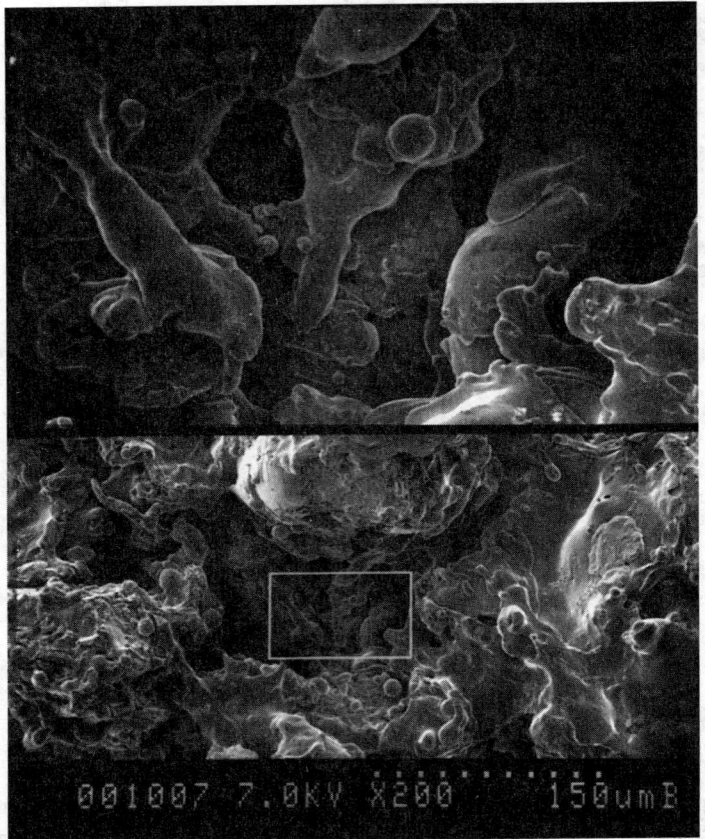

FIGURE 43.9 Irregular pore structure of porous coating in Ti5A14V alloy for bony ingrowth, from Park and Lakes [1992]. The top scanning electron microscopic picture is a 5× magnification of the rectangular region of the bottom picture (200×).

$Ca_{10}(PO_4)_6(OH)_2$. Implanted hydroxyapatite is slowly resorbed by the body over several years and replaced by bone. Tricalcium phosphate is resorbed more quickly and has been considered as an implant constituent to speed healing.

When a porous material is implanted in bone, the pores become filled first with blood which clots, then with osteoprogenitor mesenchymal cells, then, after about 4 weeks, bony trabeculae. The ingrown bones then become remodeled in response to mechanical stress. The bony ingrowth process depends on a degree of mechanical stability in the early stages. If too much motion occurs, the ingrown tissue will be collagenous scar tissue, not bone.

Porous materials used in soft-tissue applications include polyurethane, polyimide, and polyester velours used in percutaneous devices. Porous reconstituted collagen has been used in artificial skin, and braided polypropylene has been used in artificial ligaments. As in the case of bone implants, the porosity encourages tissue ingrowth, which anchors the device.

Blood vessel replacements are made with porous materials which encourage soft tissue to grow in, eventually forming a new lining, or neointima. The new lining consists of the patient's own cells. It is a natural nonthrombogenic surface resembling the lining of the original blood vessel. This is a further example of the biological role of porous materials as contrasted with the mechanical role.

Ingrowth of tissue into implant pores is not always desirable. For example, sponge (polyvinyl alcohol) implants used in early mammary augmentation surgery underwent ingrowth of fibrous tissue and contracture and calcification of that tissue, resulting in hardened, calcified breasts. Current mammary implants make use of a balloonlike nonporous silicone rubber layer enclosing silicone oil or gel, or perhaps a saline solution in water. A porous layer of polyester felt or velour attached to the balloon is provided at the back surface of the implant so that limited tissue ingrowth will anchor it to the chest wall and prevent it from migrating.

Porous materials are produced in a variety of ways. For example, in the case of bone compatible surfaces, porous materials are formed by sintering of beads or wires. Vascular and soft-tissue implants are produced by weaving or braiding fibers as well as by nonwoven "felting" methods. Protective foams for use outside the body are usually produced by use of a "blowing agent," which is a chemical which evolves gas during the polymerization of the foam. An interesting approach to producing microporous materials is the replication of structures found in biological materials: the *replamineform* process [White et al., 1976]. The rationale is that the unique structure of communicating pores is thought to offer advantages in the induction of tissue ingrowth. The skeletal structure of coral or echinoderms (such as sea urchins) is replicated by a casting process in metals and polymers; these have been tried in vascular and tracheal prostheses as well as in bone substitutes.

43.7 Summary

Composite materials are a relatively recent addition to the class of materials used in structural applications. In the biomaterials field, the ingress of composites has been even more recent. In view of their potential for high performance, composite materials are likely to find increasing use as biomaterials.

Defining Terms

Anisotropic: Dependent upon direction, referring to the material properties of composites.

Cellular solid: A composite material in which one phase consists of voids; also called a *porous material.* The voids may contain vacuum, air, or fluid.

Closed cell: A type of cellular solid in which a cell wall isolates the adjacent pores.

Composite: Composite materials are those which contain two or more distinct constituent materials or phases, on a microscopic or macroscopic scale.

Cubic: Anisotropic symmetry in which the unit cells are cube-shaped. There are three independent elastic constants.

Hexagonal: Anisotropic symmetry in which the unit cells are hexagonally shaped. There are five independent elastic constants. Transverse isotropy is mechanically equivalent to hexagonal symmetry.

Inclusion: Embedded phase of a composite.

Isotropic: Independent of direction, referring to material properties.

Matrix: The portion of the composite in which inclusions are embedded. The matrix is usually less stiff than the inclusions.

Neointima: New lining of a blood vessel. It is stimulated to form by fabric-type blood vessel replacements.

Open cell: A type of cellular solid in which there is no barrier between adjacent pores.

Orthotropic: Anisotropic symmetry in which the unit cells are shaped like rectangular parallelepipeds. In crystallography, this is called *orthorhombic.* There are nine independent elastic constants.

Porous ingrowth: Growth of tissue into the pores of an implanted porous biomaterial. Such ingrowth may or may not be desirable.

Replamineform: Cellular solid made using a biological material as a mold.

Transverse isotropy: See hexagonal.

Triclinic: Anisotropic symmetry in which the unit cells are oblique parallelepipeds with unequal sides and angles. There are 21 independent elastic constants.

References

Agarwal AG, Broutman LJ. 1980. Analysis and Performance of Fiber Composites, New York, Wiley.

Bradley JS, Hastings GW, Johnson-Hurse C. 1980. Carbon fibre reinforced epoxy as a high strength, low modulus material for internal fixation plates. Biomaterials 1:38.

Cannon ML. 1988. Composite resins. In JG Webster (ed), Encyclopedia of Medical Devices and Instrumentation, New York, Wiley.

Christensen RM. 1979. Mechanics of Composite Materials, New York, Wiley.

Craig R. 1981. Chemistry, composition, and properties of composite resins. In H Horn (ed), Dental Clinics of North America, Philadelphia, Saunders.

Ducheyne P. 1984. Biological fixation of implants. In GW Hastings, P Ducheyne (eds), Functional Behavior of Orthopaedic Biomaterials, Boca Raton, Fla, CRC Press.

Fishbane BM, Pond RB. 1977. Stainless steel fiber reinforcement of polymethylmethacrylate. Clin Orthop 128:490.

Galante J, Rostoker W, Lueck R, et al. 1971. Sintered fiber metal composites as a basis for attachment of implants to bone. J Bone Joint Surg 53A:101.

Gibson LJ, Ashby MF. 1988. Cellular Solids. Oxford, Pergamon Press.

Hashin Z, Shtrickman S. 1963. A variational approach to the theory of the elastic behavior of multiphase materials. J Mech Phys Solids 11:127.

Holmes DE, Bucholz RW, Mooney V. 1986. Porous hydroxyapatite as a bone graft substitute in metaphyseal defects. J Bone Joint Surg 68:904.

Jockish KA, Brown SA, Bauer TW, et al. 1992. Biological response to chopped carbon reinforced peek. J Biomed Mater Res 26:133.

Katz JL. 1980. Anisotropy of Young's modulus of bone. Nature 283:106.

Kim JK, Park JB. 1994. Reinforcement of bone cement around prostheses by pre-coated wire coil: A preliminary study. Biomed Mater and Eng 4:369.

Knoell A, Maxwell H, Bechtol C. 1975. Graphite fiber reinforced bone cement. Ann Biomed Eng 3:225.

Lakes RS. 1993. Materials with structural hierarchy. Nature 361:511.

Lekhnitskii SE. 1963. Elasticity of an Anisotropic Elastic Body, San Francisco, Holden Day.

Meffert RM, Thomas JR, Hamilton KM, et al. 1985. Hydroxylapatite as allopathic graft in the treatment of periodontal osseous defects. J Periodontol 56:63.

Nye JF. 1976. Physical Properties of Crystals, Oxford, Oxford University Press, 1976.

Papadogianis Y, Boyer DB, Lakes RS. 1985. Creep of posterior dental composites. J Biomed Mat Res 19:85.

Park HC, Liu YK, Lakes RS. 1986. The material properties of bone-particle impregnated PMMA. J Biomech Eng 108:141.

Park JB, Lakes RS. 1992. Biomaterials, New York, Plenum.

Paul B. 1960. Prediction of elastic constants of multiphase materials. Trans ASME 218:36.

Sclippa E, Piekarski K. 1973. Carbon fiber reinforced polyethylene for possible orthopaedic usage. J Biomed Mat Res 7:59.

Skinner HB. 1988. Composite technology for total hip arthroplasty. Clin Orthop 235:224.

Spector M, Heyligers I, Robertson JR. 1988a. Porous polymers for biological fixation. Clin Orthop 235:207.

Spector M, Miller M, Beals N. 1988b. Porous materials. In JG Webster (ed), Encyclopedia of Medical Devices and Instrumentation, New York, Wiley.

Topoleski LDT, Ducheyne P, Cackler JM. 1992. The fracture toughness of titanium fiber reinforced bone cement. J Biomed Mat Res 26:1599.

White RA, Weber JN, White EW. 1976. Replamineform: A new process for preparing porous ceramic, metal, and polymer prosthetic materials. Science 176:922.

Yeaple F. 1989. Composite knee brace returns stability to joint. Design News 46:116.

44

Biodegradable Polymeric Biomaterials: An Overview

Chih-Chang Chu

Fiber & Polymer Science Program, Department of Textiles & Apparel, Cornell University

The term *biodegradation* is frequently loosely associated with materials that could be broken down by nature either through hydrolytic mechanisms without the help of enzymes and/or enzymatic mechanism. Other terms such as *absorbable, erodible,* and *resorbable* have also been used in the literature to indicate biodegradation. The interest in biodegradable polymeric biomaterials for biomedical engineering use has increased dramatically during the past decade, because this class of biomaterials has two major advantages that nonbiodegradable biomaterials do not have. First, these biomaterials don't elicit permanent chronic foreign-body reaction due to the fact that they would be gradually absorbed by the human body, and they do not permanently retain trace of residual in the implantation sites. Second, some of them have recently been found to be able to regenerate tissues, so-called *tissue engineering*, through the interaction of their biodegradation with immunologic cells like macrophages. Hence, surgical implants made from biodegradable biomaterials could be used as temporary scaffold for tissue regeneration. This approach toward the reconstruction of injured, diseased, or aged tissues is one of the most promising fields for the next century.

Although the earliest and most commercially significant biodegradable polymeric biomaterials originated from linear aliphatic polyesters such as polyglycolide and polylactide from poly(α-hydroxyacetic acids), recent introduction of several new synthetic and natural biodegradable polymeric biomaterials extends the domain beyond this family of simple polyesters. These new commercially significant biodegradable polymeric biomaterials include poly(orthoesters), polyanhydrides, polysaccharides, poly(ester-amides), tyrosine-based polyarylates or polyiminocarbonates or polycarbonates, poly(D,L-lactide-urethane), poly(β-hydroxybutyrate), poly(ϵ-caprolactone), poly[bis(carboxylatophenoxy)phosphazene], poly(amino acids), pseudo-poly(amino acids), and copolymers derived from amino acids and nonamino acids.

All the above biodegradable polymeric biomaterials could be generally divided into eight groups based on their chemical origin: (1) biodegradable linear aliphatic polyesters (e.g., polyglycolide, polylactide, polycaprolactone, polyhydroxybutyrate) and their copolymers within the aliphatic polyester family such as poly(glycolide-L-lactide) copolymer, poly(glycolide-ϵ-caprolactone) copolymer; (2) biodegradable copolymers between linear aliphatic polyesters just mentioned and monomers other than linear aliphatic polyesters such as poly(glycolide-trimethylene carbonate) copolymer, poly(L-lactic acid-L-lysine) copolymer, Tyrosine-based polyarylates or polyiminocarbonates or polycarbonates, poly(D,L-lactide-urethane), and poly(ester-amide); (3) polyanhydrides; (4) poly(orthoesters); (5) poly(ester-ethers) like poly-p-dioxanone; (6) biodegradable polysaccharides such as hyaluronic acid, chitin, and chitson; (7) polyamino acids such as poly-L-glutamic acid and poly-L-lysine; (8) inorganic biodegradable polymers such as polyphosphazene and poly[bis(carboxylatophenoxy)phosphazene] which have nitrogen-phosphorus backbone instead of ester linkage. Recently, there is a new approach of making new biodegradable polymers through melt-blending of well-accepted biodegradable polymers like those of glycolide and lactide base[3] [Shalaby, 1994].

The earliest and most successful and frequent biomedical application of biodegradable polymeric biomaterials has been in wound closure. All biodegradable wound closure biomaterials are based upon the glycolide and lactide family. Examples include polyglycolide (Dexon from American Cyanamid), poly(glycolide-L-lactide) random copolymer with 90 to 10 molar ratio (Vicryl from Ethicon), poly(ester-ether) (PDS from Ethicon), poly(glycolide-trimethylene carbonate) random block copolymer (Maxon from American Cyanamid), and poly(glycolide-ϵ-caprolactone) copolymer (Monocryl from Ethicon). This class of biodegradable polymeric biomaterials is also the one most studied in terms of its chemical, physical, mechanical, morphological, and biological properties and their changes with degradation time and environment. Some of the above materials such as Vicryl have been commercially used as surgical meshes for hernia and body-wall repair.

The next largest biomedical application of biodegradable polymeric biomaterials that are commercially satisfactory is drug control/release devices. Some well-known examples in this application are polyanhydrides and poly(ortho-ester). Biodegradable polymeric biomaterials, particularly totally resorbable composites, have also been experimentally used in the field of orthopedics, mainly as components for internal bone fracture fixation such as PDS pins. However, use of these biomaterials in other parts of orthopedic implants may be limited due to their inherent mechanical properties and their biodegradation rate. Besides the commercial uses described above, biodegradable polymeric biomaterials have been experimented as vascular grafts, vascular stents, vascular couples for vessel anastomosis, nerve growth conduits, augmentations of defected bone, ligament/tendon prostheses, intramedullary plugs during total hip replacement, anastomosis rings for intestinal surgery, and stents in ureterostomies for accurate suture placement.

Due to space limitation, this chapter emphasizes those commercially most significant and successful biomedical biodegradable polymers based on linear aliphatic polyesters and a new theoretical approach to model the hydrolytic degradation of glycolide/lactide-based biodegradable polymers. The details of the applications of this family and other biodegradable polymeric biomaterials and their chemical, physical, mechanical, biological, and biodegradation properties can be found in other recent reviews [Barrows, 1986; Chu, in press; Kimura, 1993; Shalaby, 1994; Vert et al., 1992].

44.1 Glycolide/Lactide-Based Biodegradable Linear Aliphatic Polyesters

This class of biodegradable polymers is the most successful, important, and commercially widely used biodegradable biomaterial in surgery. It is also the class of biodegradable biomaterials that is most extensively studied in terms of degradation mechanisms and structure-property relationship.

Among biodegradable polymers, polyglycolide (PG), or polyglycolic acid (PGA), is the most important, because most other biodegradable polymers are derived from PG either through copolymerization, e.g., poly(glycolide-L-lactide) copolymer, or modified glycolide monomer, e.g., poly-p-dioxanone. Table 44.1 lists some important properties of this clas of biodegradable polymers.

Glycolide-Based Biodegradable Homopolymers Polyesters

PGA can be polymerized either directly or indirectly from glycolic acid. The direct polycondensation produces a polymer of M_n less than 10,000 because of the requirement of a very high degree of dehydration (99.28% up) and the absence of monofunctional impurities. For PGA of molecular weight higher than 10,000 it is necessary to proceed through the ring-opening polymerization of the cyclic dimers of glycolic acid. Numerous catalysts are available for this ring-opening polymerization. They include organometallic compounds and Lewis acids [Chujo et al., 1967b; Wise et al., 1979]. For biomedical applications, stannous chloride dihydrate or trialkyl aluminum are preferred. PGA was found to exhibit an orthorhombic unit cell with dimensions $a = 5.22$ Å, $b = 6.19$ Å, and c (fiber axis) = 7.02 Å. The planar zigzag-chain molecules form a sheet structure parallel to the ac plane and do not have the polyethylene-type arrangement [Chatani et al., 1968]. The molecules between two adjacent sheets orient in opposite directions. The tight molecular packing and the close approach of the ester groups might stabilize the crystal lattice and contribute to the high melting point, T_m, of PGA (224–230°C). The glass transition temperature, T_g, ranges from 36–40°C. The specific gravities of PGA are 1.707 for a perfect crystal and 1.50 in a completely amorphous state [Chujo et al., 1967b]. The heat of fusion of 100% crystallized PGA is reported to be 12 KJ/mol (45.7 cal/gram) [Brandrup et al., 1975]. A recent study of injection molded PGA disks reveals their IR spectroscopic characteristics [Chu et al., in press]. As shown in Fig. 44.1, the four bands at 850, 753, 713, and 560 cm^{-1} are associated with the amorphous regions of the PGA disks and could be used to assess the extends of hydrolysis. Peaks associated with the crystalline phase included those at 972, 901, 806, 627, and 590 cm^{-1}. Two broad intense peaks at 1142 and 1077 cm^{-1} can be assigned to C-O stretching modes in the ester and oxymethylene groups, respectively. These two peaks are associated mainly with ester and oxymethylene groups originating in the amorphous domains. Hydrolysis could cause both of these C-O stretching modes to substantially decrease in intensity.

Glycolide-Based Biodegradable Copolyesters Having Aliphatic-Polyester-Based Comonomers

Other commercially successful glycolide-based biodegradable polymeric biomaterials are the copolymers of glycolide with other monomers within linear aliphatic polyesters such as lactides, car-

TABLE 44.1 Properties of Synthetic Absorbable Polymers

Polymer	Crystallinity	T_m (°C)	T_g (°C)	T_{dec} (°C)	Fiber Strength MPa	Modulus GPa	Elongation (%)
PGA	High	230	36	260	890	8.4	30
PLLA	High	170	56	240	900	8.5	25
PLA	None	—	57	—	—	—	—
Polyglactin910*	High[†]	200	40	250	850	8.6	24
Polydioxanone	High	106	<20	190	490	2.1	35
Polyglyconate[‡]	High[†]	213	<20	260	550	2.4	45

*Glycolide per lactide = 9/1.
[†]Depending on the copolymer composition.
[‡]Glycolide per trimethylene carbonate = 9/1.

Source: Kimura Y. 1993, Biodegradable polymers. In T Tsuruta, T Hayashi, K Kataoka et al (eds), Biomedical Applications of Polymeric Materials, Boca Raton, Fla, CRC Press.

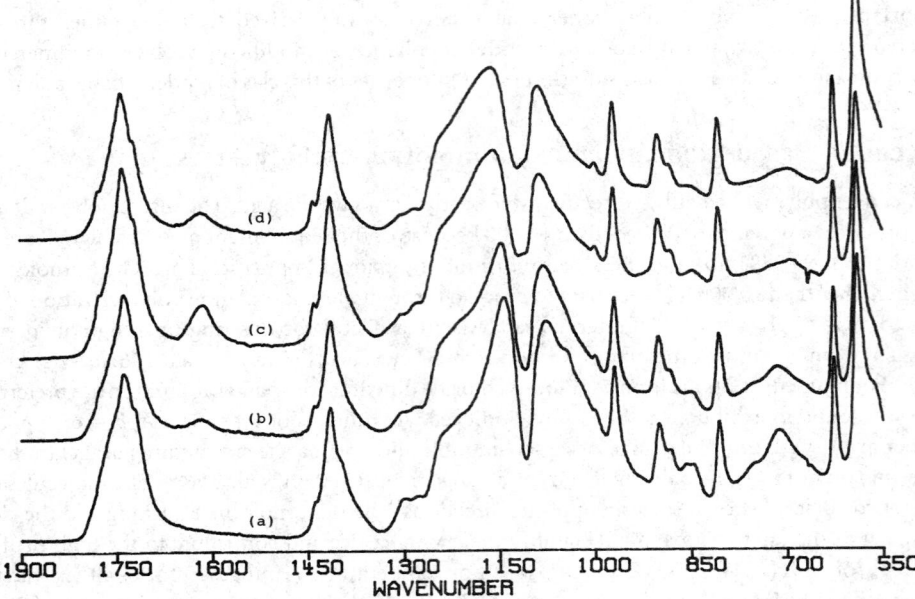

FIGURE 44.1   FTIR spectra of polyglycolic acid disks as a function of in vitro hydrolysis time in phosphate buffer of pH 7.44 at 37°C. (*a*) 0 day; (*b*) 55 hrs; (*c*) 7 days; (*d*) 21 days.

bonates, and ε-caprolactone. The glycolide-lactide random copolymers are the most studied and have a wide range of properties and applications, depending on the composition ratio of glycolide to lactide. Fig. 44.2 illustrates the dependence of biodegradation rate on the composition of glycolide to lactide in the copolymer. For wound closure purpose, a high concentration of glycolide monomer is required for proper mechanical and degradation properties. Vicryl sutures, sometimes called polyglactin 910, contain a 90/10 molar ratio of glycolic to L-lactide, and this molar ratio is important for the Vicryl suture to retain crystalline characteristics. For biomedical use, Lewis acid catalysts are preferred for the copolymers [Wise et al., 1979]. If DL- instead of L-lactide is used as the comonomer, the *U*-shape relationship between the level of crystallinity and glycolide composition disappears. This is because polylactide from 100% DL-lactide composition is totally amorphous. IR bands associated with Vicryl molecules in the amorphous domains are 560, 710, 850, and 888 cm^{-1}, whereas 590, 626, 808, 900, and 972 cm^{-1} are associated with the crystalline domains [Fredericks et al., 1984]. Like PGA, these IR bands could be used to assess the extent of hydrolysis.

A relatively new block copolymer of glycolide and carbonates, such as trimethylene carbonate, has been commercialized. Maxon is made from a block copolymer of glycolide and 1,3-dioxan-2-one (trimethylene carbonate or GTMC) and consists of 32.5% by weight (or 36 mol %) of trimethylene carbonate [Casey & Roby, 1984; Katz et al., 1985]. Maxon is a poly(ester-carbonate). The polymerization process of Maxon is divided into two stages. The first stage is the formation of middle block, which is a random copolymer of glycolide and 1,3-dioxan-2-one. Diethylene glycol is used as an initiator, and stannous chloride dihydrate (SnCl$_2$ · 2H$_2$O) serves as the catalyst. The polymerization is conducted at about 180°C. The weight ratio of glycolide to trimethylene carbonate in the middle block is 15:85. After the synthesis of the middle block, the temperature of the reactive bath is raised to about 220°C to prevent the crystallization of the copolymer, and additional glycolide monomers as the end blocks are added into the reaction bath to form the final triblock copolymer.

The latest glycolide-based copolymer that has become commercially successful is Monocryl suture. It is a segmented block copolymer consisting of both soft and hard segments. The purpose of having soft segments in the copolymer is to provide good handling property like pliability, while the hard segments are used to provide adequate strength. The generic copolymerization process between gly-

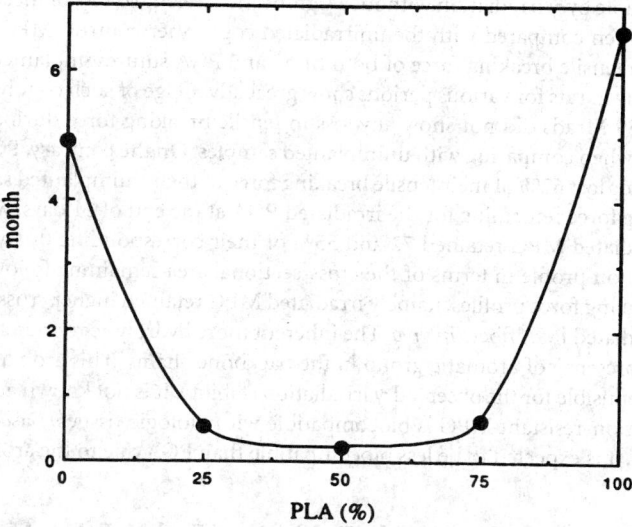

FIGURE 44.2 The effect of poly(L-lactide) composition in poly-glycolide on the time required for 50% mass loss implanted under the dorsal skin of rat. (*Source:* Miller RA, Brady JM, Cutright DE. 1977. Degradation rates of oral resorbable implants (polylactates and polyg-lycolates): Rate modification with changes in PLA/PGA copolymer ra-tios. J Biomed Mater Res 11(5):711. With permission.)

colic acid and ϵ-caprolactone was recently reported by Fukuzaki and coworkers in Japan [1989, 1991]. The resulting copolymers were low-molecular-weight biodegradable copolymers of glycolic acid and various lactones for potential drug delivery purpose. The composition of lactone ranged from as low as 15 to as high as 50 mol %, and the average molecular weight ranged from 4510 to 16,500. The glass transition temperature ranged from 18 to $-43°C$, depending on the copolymer composition and molecular weight. Monocryl is made from a two-stage polymerization process [Bezwada et al., 1993]. In the first stage, soft segments of prepolymer of glycolide and ϵ-caprolactone are made. This soft seg-mented prepolymer is further polymerized with glycolides to provide hard segments of polyglycol-ide. Monocryl has a composition of 75% glycolide and 25% ϵ-caprolactone and should have a higher molecular weight than those glycolide/ϵ-caprolactone copolymers reported by Fukuzaki and col-leagues for adequate mechanical properties required by sutures. The most unique aspect of Monocryl monofilament suture is its pliability as claimed by Ethicon [Bezwada et al., 1993]. The force required to bend a 2/0 suture is only about 2.8×10^4 lb-in^2 for Monocryl, whereas the same size PDSII and Maxon monofilament sutures require about 3.9 and 11.6×10^4 lb-in^2 force, respectively. This inher-ent pliability of Monocryl is due to the presence of soft segments and T_g resulting from the ϵ-capro-lactone comonomer unit. Its T_g is expected to be between 15 and $-36°C$.

Glycolide-Based Biodegradable Copolyesters with Nonaliphatic Polyester-Based Comonomers

In this category, the glycolide copolymer is the most important, consisting of poly(ethylene 1,4-phenylene-bis-oxyacetate) (PEPBO) [Jamiokowski & Shalaby, 1991]. The development of this type of glycolide-based copolymer grew out of the adverse effect of γ irradiation on the mechanical proper-ties of glycolide-based synthetic absorbable sutures. There is a great desire to develop γ-irradiation-sterilizable synthetic absorbable polymers to take the advantage of the highly convenient and reliable method of sterilization. Jamiokowski and Shalaby (1991) recently reported that the incorporation of about 10 mol% of a polymeric radiostabilizer like PEPBO into PGA backbone chains would make the copolymer sterilizable by γ irradiation without a significant accelerated loss of mechanical properties upon hydrolysis when compared with the unirradiated copolymer control (MPG). The copolymer control changes in tensile breaking force of both MPG and PGA sutures implanted intramuscularly and subcutaneously in rats for various periods show great advantage of such copolymers. MPG fibers γ-irradiated at 2.89 Mrads did not show any loss in tensile breaking force during the first 14 days postimplantation when comparing with unimplanted samples. On the contrary, PGA sutures γ-irradiated at 2.75 Mrads lost 62% of their tensile breaking force of their unimplanted samples. There was no tensile breaking force remaining for the irradiated PGA at the end of 21 days, whereas both 2.89- and 5-Mrads-irradiated MPG retained 72 and 55% of their corresponding 0-day controls, respectively. The absorption profile in terms of the cross-sectional area remaining followed the same pattern as tensile breaking force profiles, namely irradiated MPG retained higher cross-sectional area remaining than irradiated PGA fibers *in vivo*. The inherent more hydrolytic resistance of MPG must be attributed to the presence of aromatic group in the backbone chains. This aromatic polyester component is also responsible for the observed γ irradiation stability. It is not known at this time whether the new γ-irradiation-resistant MPG is biocompatible with biologic tissues. Based on the chemical structure of MPG, it is expected to be less biocompatible than PGA due to the aromatic ring.

Glycolide-Derived Biodegradable Polymers Having Ether Linkage

Poly-p-dioxanone (PDS) is derived from the glycolide family with better flexibility. It is polymerized from ether-containing lactones, 1,4-dioxane-2,5-dione (i.e., p-dioxanone) monomers with a hydroxylic initiator and tin catalyst [Shalaby, 1994]. The resulting polymer is semicrystalline with T_m about 106–115°C and T_g equal to -10 to 0°C. The improved flexibility of PDS relative to PGA, evidenced in its lower T_g, is due to the incorporation of ether segment in the repeating unit which reduces the density of ester linkages for intermolecular hydrogen bonds. Because of the less dense ester linkages in PDS when comparing with PGA or glycolide-L-lactide copolymers, PDS is expected and has been shown to degrade at a slower rate *in vitro* and *in vivo*. PDS's inherent viscosity of 2.0 dL/g in hexafluoroisopropanol is adequate for making monofilament sutures. Recently, an advanced version of PDS, PSDII, was introduced. PDSII was achieved by subjecting the melt-spun fibers to a high temperature (128°C) for a short period of time. This additional treatment partially melts the outermost surface layer of PDS fibers and leads to a distinctive skin-core morphology. The heat employed also results in larger crystallites in the core of the fiber than the untreated PDS fiber. The tensile strength loss profile of PDSII sutures is significantly better than PDS sutures.

A variety of copolymers with high molar ratios of PDS to other monomers within the same linear aliphatic polyester family have been reported for the purpose of improving the mechanical and biodegradation properties [Shalaby, 1994]. For examples, copolymer of PDS (80%) and PGA (up to 20%) has an absorption profile similar to Dexon and Vicryl sutures, but it has compliance similar to PDS. Copolymer of PDS (85%) and PLLA (up to 15%) results in a more compliant (low modulus) suture than homopolymer PDS but with similar absorption profiles as PDS [Bezwada et al., 1990].

Copolymer fibers made from PDS and monomers other than linear aliphatic polyester such as morpholine-2,5-dione (MD) exhibit rather interesting biodegradation properties. These copolymer fibers were absorbed 10–25% earlier than PDS; the copolymer, however, retained a tensile breaking strength profile similar to PDS with a slightly faster strength loss during the earlier stage, i.e., the first 14 days [Shalaby 1994]. This ability to break the inherent fiber structure-property relationship through copolymerization is a major improvement in biodegradation property of absorbable sutures. It is interesting to recognize that a small percentage (3%) of MD in the copolymer suture is sufficient to result in a faster mass loss profile without the expense of its tensile strength loss profile. The ability to achieve this ideal biodegradation property might be attributed to both an increasing hydrophilicity of the copolymer and the disruption of crystalline domains due to MD moeity. As described later, the loss of suture mass is mainly due to the destruction of crystalline domains, whereas the loss of tensile breaking strength is chiefly due to the scission of tie-chain segments located in the amorphous domains. The question is why MD-PDS copolymeric suture retains its strength loss similar to PDS. The possible explanation is that the amide functional groups in MD could form stronger intermolecular hydrogen bonds than ester functional groups. This stronger hydrogen bond contributes to the strength retention of the copolymer of PDS and MD during *in vivo* biodegradation. The incorporation of MD moeity into PDS also lowers the unknot and knot strength of unhydrolyzed specimens but increases elongation at break. This suggests that the copolymer of PDS and MD should have a lower level of crystallinity than PDS, which is consistent with its observed faster mass loss *in vivo*.

To improve γ-irradiation stability of PDS, radiostabilizers like PEPBO have been copolymerized with PDS to form segmented copolymers the same way as PEPBO with glycolide described above [Koelmel et al., 1991; Shabaly, 1994]. The incorporation of 5–10% of such stabilizer in PDS has been shown not only to improve γ-irradiation resistance considerably but also to increase the compliance of the material. For example, PEPBO-PDS copolymer retained 79, 72, and 57% of its original tensile breaking strength at 2, 3, and 4 weeks *in vivo* implantation, whereas PDS homopolymer retained only 43, 30, and 25% at the corresponding periods. It appeared that an increasing (CH_2) group between the two ester functional groups of the radiation stabilizers improved the copolymer resistance toward γ-irradiation.

Lactide Biodegradable Homopolymers and Copolymers

Polylactides, particularly poly-L-lactide (PLLA), and copolymers having greater than 50% L or DL-lactide have been explored for medical use even before the availability of PGA without much success mainly due to their much slower absorption and difficulty in melt processing. PLLAs are prepared in solid state through ring-opening polymerization due to their thermal instability and should be melt-processed at the lowest possible temperature [Shalaby, 1994]. Other methods like solution spinning, particularly for high molecular weight, and suspension polymerization have been reported as better alternatives. PLLA is a semicrystalline polymer with $T_m = 170°C$ and $T_g = 56°C$. This high T_g is mainly responsible for the observed extremely slow biodegradation rate at body temperature reported in the literature. The molecular weight of lactide-based biodegradable polymers suitable for medical use ranges from 1.5–5.0 dL/g inherent viscosity in chloroform. Ultra-high molecular weights of polylactides have recently been reported [Leenslag & Pennings, 1984; Tunc, 1983]. For example, an intrinsic viscosity as high as 13 dL/g was reported by Leenslag and Pennings. High-strength PLLA fibers from this ultra-high-molecular-weight polylactide was made by hot-drawing fibers from solutions of good solvents. The resulting fibers had tensile breaking strength close to 1.2 GPa [Gogolewski & Pennings, 1983]. Due to a dissymmetric nature of lactic acid, the polymer made from optically inactive racemic mixture of D and L enantiomers, poly-DL-lactide is an amorphous polymer.

Lactide-based copolymers having a high percentage of lactide have recently been reported, particularly those copolymerized with aliphatic polycarbonates like trimethylene carbonate (TMC) or 3,3-dimethyltrimethylene carbonate (DMTMC) [Shieh et al., 1990]. The major advantage of incorporating TMC or DMTMC units into lactide is that the degradation products from TMC or DMTMC are largely neutral pH and hence are considered to be advantageous. Both *in vitro* toxicity and *in vivo* nonspecific foreign-body reactions like sterile sinuses have been reported in orthopedic implants made from PGA and/or PLLA [Bostman et al., 1990; Daniels et al., 1992; Eitenmüller et al., 1989; Hofmann, 1992; Winet & Hollinger, 1993]. Several investigators indicated that the glycolic- or lactic-acid-rich degradation products have the potential to significantly lower the local pH in a closed and less body-fluid-buffered region surrounded by bone [Sugnuma et al., 1992]. This is particularly true if the degradation process proceeds with a burst mode (i.e., a sudden and rapid release of degradation products). This acidity tends to cause abnormal bone resorption and/or demineralization. The resulting environment may be cytotoxic [Daniels et al., 1992]. Indeed, inflammatory foreign-body reactions with a discharging sinus and osteolytic foci visible on x-ray have been encountered in clinical studies [Eitenmüller et al., 1989]. Winet and Hollinger (1993) recently confirmed the problem associated with PGA and/or PLLA orthopedic implants. They found that a rapid degradation of a 50:50 ratio of glycolide-lactide copolymer in bone chambers of rabbit tibias inhibited bone regeneration. However, they emphasized that the extrapolation of *in vitro* toxicity to in vivo biocompatibility must consider microcirculatory capacity. The increase in the local acidity due to a faster accumulation of highly acidic degradation products is also known to lead to an accelerated acid-catalyzed hydrolysis in the immediate vicinity of the biodegradable device. This acceleration in hydrolysis could lead to a faster loss of mechanical property of the device than we expect. This finding suggests the need to use components in totally biodegradable composites so that degradation products with less acidity would be released into the surrounding area. A controlled-slow rather than burst release of degradation products to the level that the surrounding tissue could timely metabolize would also be helpful in dealing with the acidity problem. Copolymers of composition ratio of 10DMTMC/90LLA or 10TMC/90LLA appear to be a promising absorbable orthopedic device. Other applications of this type of copolymers include nerve growth conduits, tendon prostheses, and coating materials for biodegradable devices.

Another unique example of L-lactide copolymer is the copolymer of L-lactide and 3-(S)[(alkyloxycarbonyl) methyl]-1,4-dioxane-2,5-dione, a cyclic diester [Kimura, 1993]. One unique aspect of this new biodegradable copolymer is the carboxyl acid pendant group, which obviously would make the new polymer not only more hydrophilic (hence encouraging faster biodegradation) but also more reactive toward future chemical modification through the pendant carboxyl group. The availability of these carboxyl reactive pendant sites could be used to chemically bond antimicrobial agents or other biochemicals such as growth factors, making future wound closure biomaterials with new and important biological functions. Unfortunately, no reported data evaluate the performance of these new absorbable polymers for biomedical engineering use.

Block copolymers of PLLA with poly(amino acids) have also been reported as potential controlled drug delivery systems [Nathan & Kohn, 1994]. This new class of copolymers consists of both ester and amide linkages in the backbone molecules and is sometimes referred to as poly(depsipeptides) or poly(estersamides). Poly(depsipeptides) could also be synthesized from ring-opening polymerization of morpholine-2,5-dione and its derivatives [Helder et al., 1986]. Barrows has also made a series of poly(ester-amides) from polyesterification of diols that contain preformed amide linkages, such as amidediols [Barrows, 1994]. The rationale for making poly(ester-amides) is to combine the well-known absorbability and biocompatibility of linear aliphatic polyesters with the high performance and the flexibility of potential chemical reactive sites of amide of polyamides. Poly(ester-amides) could be degraded either by enzyme or/and nonenzymatic mechanisms. There are no commercial uses of this class of copolymers at the present time.

Because of the characteristic of the very slow biodegradation rate of PLLA and the copolymers having a high composition ratio of PLLA, their biomedical applications have been limited to mainly orthopedic surgery, drug control/release devices, coating materials for suture, vascular grafts, and surgical meshes to facilitate wound healing after dental extraction.

44.2 Non-Glycolide/Lactide-Based Linear Aliphatic Polyesters

All glycolide/lactide-based linear aliphatic polyesters are based on poly(α-hydroxy acids). Two unique groups of linear aliphatic polyesters are based on poly(ω-hydroxy acids) and the most famous ones are poly(ϵ-caprolactone) [Kimura, 1993], poly(β-hydroxybutrate) (PHB), poly(β-hydroxyvalerate) (PHV), and the copolymers of PHB/PHV [Gross, 1994]. Poly(ϵ-caprolactone) has been used as a comonomer with a variety of glycolide/lactide-based linear aliphatic polyesters described earlier. PHB and PHV belong to the family of poly(hydroxyalkanoates) and are mainly produced by prokaryotic type of microorganisms such as *Pseudomonas olevorans* or *Alcaligenes eutrophus* through biotechnology. PHB and PHV are the principal energy and carbon storage compound for these microorganisms and are produced when there are excessive nutrients in the environment. These naturally produced PHB and PHV are stereochemically pure and are isotactic. They could also be synthesized in labs, but the characteristic of stereoregularity is lost. This family of biodegradable polyesters is considered to be environmentally friendly because they are produced from propionic acid and glucose and could be completely degraded to water, biogas, biomass, and humic materials [Gross, 1994]. Their biodegradation requires enzymes. Hence, PHB, PHV, and their copolymers are probably the most important biodegradable polymers for environmental use. However, the biodegradability of this class of linear aliphatic polyesters in human or animal tissues has been questionable. For example, high-molecular-weight PHB or PHB/PHV fibers do not degrade in tissues or simulated environment over periods of up to 6 months [Williams, 1990]. The degradability of PHB could be accelerated by γ-irradiation or copolymerization with PHV.

An interesting derivative of PHB, poly(β-malic acid) (PMA), has been synthesized from β-benzyl malolactonate followed by catalytic hydrogenolysis. PMA differs from PHB in that the β-(CH₃) substituent is replaced by -COOH[2] [Kimura, 1993]. The introduction of pendant carboxylic acid group would make PMA more hydrophilic and easier to be absorbed.

44.3 Non-Aliphatic-Polyester-Type Biodegradable Polymers

Aliphatic & Aromatic Polycarbonates

The most significant aliphatic polycarbonates are based upon DMTMC and TMC. They are made by the same ring-opening polymerization as glycolide-based biodegradable polymers. The homopolymers are biocompatible with a controllable rate of biodegradation. Pellets of poly(ethylene carbonate) were absorbed completely in 2 weeks in peritoneal cavity of rats. A slight variation of this polycarbonate, poly(propylene carbonate), however, did not show any sign of absorption after 2 months [Barrows, 1986]. Copolymers of DMTMC/ε-caprolactone and DMTMC/TMC have been reported to have adequate properties for wound closure, tendon prostheses, and vascular grafts. The most important advantage of aliphatic polycarbonates is the neutral pH of the degradation products.

Poly(BPA-carbonates) made from bisphenol A (BPA) and phosgene is nonbiodegradable, but analogs of poly(BPA-carbonate) like poly(iminocarbonates) have been shown to degrade in about 200 days [Barrows, 1986]. In general, this class of aromatic polycarbonates takes an undesirably long period to degrade presumably due to the presence of the aromatic ring which could protect adjacent ester bonds to be hydrolyzed by water or enzyme. Different types of degradation products of this polymer under different pH environment are produced. With pH > 7.0, degradation products of this polymer are BPA, ammonia, and CO_2, and insoluble poly(BPA-carbonate) oligomers were also produced with pH < 7.0 [Barrows, 1986]. The polymer had good mechanical properties and acceptable tissue biocompatibility. Unfortunately, there are no commercial uses of this class of polymer in surgery at the present time.

Poly(alkylene oxalates) and Copolymers

This class of high-crystalline biodegradable polymers was initially developed [Shalaby, 1994] for absorbable sutures and their coating. These polymers consist of [-ROOC-COO-]ₙ repeating unit where R is $(CH_2)_x$ with x ranging from 4 to 12. R could also be cyclic (1,4-trans-cyclohexanedimethanol) or aromatic (1,4-benzene, 1,3-benzene dimethanol) for achieving higher melting temperature. The biodegradation properties depend on the number of (CH_2) group, x, and the type of R group (i.e., acyclic versus cyclic or aromatic). In general, a higher number of methylene group and/or the incorporation of cyclic or aromatic R group would retard biodegradation rate and hence make the polymer be absorbed more slowly. For example, there was no mass of the polymer with $x = 4$ remaining *in vivo* (rats) after 28 days, whereas the polymer with $x = 6$ retained 80% of its mass after 42 days *in vivo*. An isomorphic copolyoxalate consisting of 80% cyclic R group, like 1,4-trans-cyclohexanedimethanol, and 20% with acyclic R group, like 1,6-hexanediol, retained 56%

of its original mass after 180 days *in vivo*. By varying the ratio of cyclic to acyclic monomers, co-polymers with a wide range of melting temperature could be made. For example, copolymer of 95/5 ratio of cyclic/acyclic (i.e., 1,4-trans-cyclohexanedimethanol/1,6-hexanediol) monomers had a $T_m = 210°C$, and the copolymer with 5/95 ratio had a $T_m = 69°C$. Poly(alkylene oxalates) with $x = 3$ or 6 had been experimented with as drug control/release devices. The tissue reaction to this class of biodegradable polymers has been minimal.

44.4 Theoretical Modeling of Biodegradation Properties of Synthetic Biodegradable Polymers

The reported biodegradation studies of a variety of biodegradable polymeric biomaterials have mainly focused on their tissue biocompatibility, the rate of drug release, or loss of strength and mass. Recent systematic research has looked at degradation mechanisms and the effects of intrinsic and extrinsic factors such as pH [Chu, 1981, 1982], enzymes [Chu & Williams, 1983; Williams, 1979; Williams & Mort, 1977; Williams & Chu, 1984; γ-irradiation [Chu et al., in press; Chu & Campbell, 1982, Chu & Williams, 1983, Chu & Louie, 1985; Williams & Chu, 1984; Campbell & Chu, 1984; Zhang et al., 1993], electrolytes [Pratt & Chu, 1993], cell medium [Chu et al, 1992], annealing treatment [Chu & Browning, 1988], plasma surface treatment [Loh et al., 1992], external stress [Chu & Louie, 1985; Miller et al., 1984], and polymer morphology [Chu & Kizil, 1989] and of a chemical means to examine the degradation of PGA fibers [Chu & Louie, 1985] have been systemically examined and the subject has been recently reviewed [Chu, 1985, 1991, in press]. Table 44.2 lists the structural factors of polymers that could control their degradation [Kimura, 1993]. Besides these series of experimental studies of a variety of factors that could affect the degradation of biodegradable polymeric biomaterials, Pratt and Chu have very recently reported the use of computational chemistry to theoretically model the effects of a variety of substituents which could exert either steric effect and/or inductive effect on the degradation properties of glycolide/lactide-based biodegradable polymers [Pratt & Chu, 1993, 1994].

This new approach could provide scientists with a better understanding of the relationship between chemical structure of biodegradable polymers and their degradation behavior at a molecular level. The approach also could help the future R/D of this class of polymers through the intelligent prediction of structure-property relationship. Among these theoretical research activities, [Pratt & Chu, 1993, 1994] the effect of various derivatives of linear aliphatic polyester (PGA) and a naturally occurring linear polysaccharide (hyaluronic acid) on their hydrolytic degradation phenomena and mechanisms were theoretically determined.

TABLE 44.2   Structural Factors to Control the Polymer Degradability

Factors	Methods of Control
Chemical structure of main chain and side groups	Selection of chemical bonds and functional groups
Aggregation state	Processing, copolymerization
Crystalline state	Polymer blend
Hydrophilic/hydrophobic balance	Copolymerization, introduction of functional groups
Surface area	Micropores
Shape and morphology	Fiber, film, composite

Source: Kimura Y. 1993. Biodegradable polymers. In T Tsuruta, T Hayashi, K Kataoka, Biomedical Applications of Polymeric Materials, pp 164–190, Boca Raton, Fla, CRC Press.

Steric Effect

Alkyl substituents on the glycolic esters cause an increase in activation enthalpies and a corresponding decrease in reaction rate, up to about three carbons, whereas bulkier alkyl substituents than isopropyl make the rate-determining elimination step more facile. As shown in Fig. 44.3, the calculated relative hydrolytic rate constants, $K_{rel} = exp(-\Delta\Delta H^{\dagger}/RT)$ determined by the rate-determining alkoxide elimination step, were examined as a function of the size of α substituent in both solvated and unsolvated conditions. The data show a decrease in the rate of hydrolysis by about a factor of 10^6 with isopropyl substituents but nearly a sixfold increase with t-butyl substituents. It therefore appears that polymers containing α isopropyl groups, or slightly larger linear alkyl groups, such as n-butyl and n-pentyl, will show a longer strength retention, given the same fiber morphology.

Inductive Effect

On the acyl portion of the molecule, halogen substituents would be expected to stabilize the negatively charged tetrahedral intermediate by their inductive effects, causing the reaction enthalpy of hydroxide attack to become more exothermic and increasing the endothermicity of the methoxide elimination. Fig. 44.3 summarizes the effect of halogen and amino substitution on the calculated relative hydrolytic rate constants, K_{rel}, for substitution at the α, β, and γ positions on the acyl portion of the molecule. K_{rel} decreased with increasing electronegativity of the substituent, indicating a stabilization of the tetrahedral intermediate relative to the transition state. A large unexpected difference, however, was noted in the elimination from the two diastereomeric F-substituted intermediates which cannot be explained by inductive effects alone. As expected, the effects of β substituents on the acyl portion of the ester were relatively small compared to α substituent effects. The observed effects appear to arise from a balance between the inductive effects and the conformational changes induced by the steric effects of the large halogen atoms; γ substitution on the acyl portion of the molecule tended to raise the activation barriers in the rate-determining elimination step by stabilization of the intermediate through relatively small inductive effects. A similar effect was observed in the activation enthalpies of hydroxide attack, but the largest effect was with Cl substitution, probably from a combination of its partial negative charge and its larger atomic size relative to fluorine.

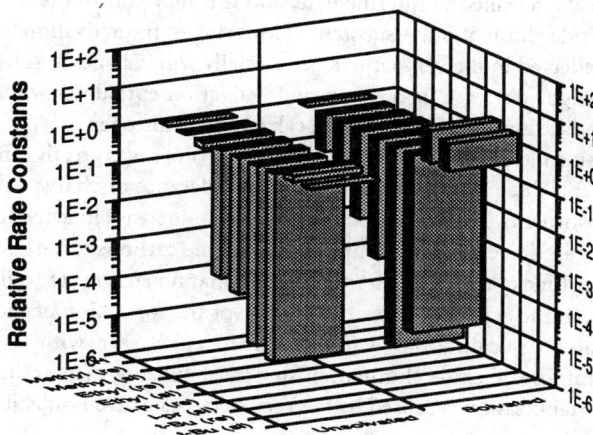

FIGURE 44.3 The steric effect of the α-substituted esters of glycolic acid on their calculated relative hydrolysis rate constant, K. (*Source*: Pratt L, Chu C. 1993. Hydrolytic degradation of alpha substituted polyglycolic acid: A semi-empirical computational study. J Computational Chemistry 14(7):809.)

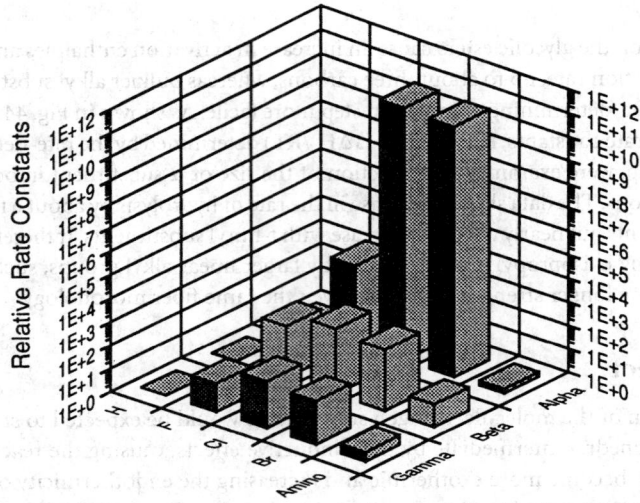

FIGURE 44.4 The inductive effect of the substituted esters on the alkyl portion of glycolic acid on their calculated relative hydrolysis rate constant, K. (*Source:* Pratt L, Chu CC. 1994. The effect of electron donating and electron withdrawing substituents on the degradation rate of bioabsorbable polymers: A semi-empirical computational study. J Mol Structure 304:213.)

On the alkyl portion of the ester, the effect of substituents was most noticeable in the rate-determining alkoxide elimination step, as the inductive effect greatly stabilized the negative charge on the leaving alkoxide ion. It was quite surprising that the effect of F was smaller than that of Cl or Br, where the elimination step actually became exothermic when the α position was substituted with either Cl or Br. Although fluorine is the most electronegative of the group, the larger size of the Cl and Br atoms may more effectively delocalize the negative charge. These larger atoms are also more sterically hindered in the tetrahedral intermediate, and this may contribute an additional driving force toward the alkoxide elimination. A substantial lowering of the activation barriers of this rate-determining step is reflected in the very large K_{rel}, especially with Cl and Br substitution, as shown in Fig. 44.3. Only a slight decrease in reaction and activation enthalpies was observed with the aminomethyl ester, indicating a slight charge delocalization by nitrogen.

Thus, Pratt and Chu concluded that the rate of ester hydrolysis was greatly affected by both alkyl and halogen substituents due primarily to either steric hindrance or charge delocalization. In the steric effect, alkyl substituents on the glycolic esters cause an increase in activation enthalpies, and a corresponding decrease in reaction rate, up to about three carbons, whereas bulkier alkyl substituents than isopropyl make the rate-determining elimination step more facile. In the inductive effect, α substituents on the acyl portion of the ester favor the formation of the tetrahedral intermediate through charge delocalization—with the largest effect seen with Cl substitution—but retard the rate-determining alkoxide elimination step by stabilizing the tetrahedral intermediate. The largest degree of stabilization is caused by the very electronegative F substituent.

Defining Terms

Biodegradation: Materials that could be broken down by nature through either hydrolytic mechanisms without the help of enzymes or enzymatic mechanism. It is loosely associated with *absorbable, eroidable, resorbable*.

Tissue engineering: The ability to regenerate tissue through the help of artificial materials and devices.

References

Barrows TH. 1986. Degradable implant materials: A review of synthetic absorbable polymers and their applications. Clin Materials 1:233.

Barrows TH. 1994. Bioabsorbable poly(ester-amides). In SW Shalaby (ed), Biomedical Polymers: Designed-to-Degrade Systems, chap 4, New York, Hanser.

Bezwada RS, Shalaby SW, Newman HD Jr, et al. 1990. Bioabsorbable copolymers of p-dioxanone and lactide for surgical devices. Trans Soc Biomater 8:194.

Bezwada RS, Jamiolkowski DD, Erneta M, et al. 1993. Monocryl, a new ultra-pliable absorbable monofilament suture derived from ε-caprolactone and glycolide. Somerville, NJ, Ethicon.

Bostman O, Hirvensalo E, Vainioupaa S, et al. 1990. Degradable polyglycolide rods for the internal fixation of displaced bimalleolar fractures. Int Orthop (Germany) 14(5):1–8.

Brandrup J, Immergut EH. 1975. Polymer Handbook, 2d ed, New York, Wiley.

Campbell ND, Chu CC. 1981. The effect of γ-irradiation on the biodegradation of polyglycolic acid synthetic sutures—tensile strength study, Twenty-Seventh International Symposium on Macromolecules, Abstracts of Communications, vol 2, pp 1348–1352, Strasbourg, France.

Casey DJ, Roby MS. 1984. Synthetic copolymer surgical articles and method of manufacturing the same. US Patent 4,429,080, American Cyanamid.

Chatani Y, Suehiro K, Okita Y, et al. 1968. Structural studies of polyesters: 1. Crystal structure of polyglycolide. Die Makromol Chemie 113:215.

Chu CC. 1981. The *in-vitro* degradation of poly(glycolic acid) sutures—effect of pH. J Biomed Mater Res 15:795.

Chu CC. 1982. The effect of pH on the *in vitro* degradation of poly(glycolide lactide) copolymer absorbable sutures. J Biomed Mater Res 16:117.

Chu CC. 1985a. Strain-accelerated hydrolytic degradation of synthetic absorbable sutures. In CW Hall (ed), Surgical Research Recent Development, San Antonio, Tex, Pergamon Press.

Chu CC. 1985b. The degradation and biocompatibility of suture materials. In DF Williams (ed-in-chief), CRC Critical Reviews in Biocompatibility, vol 1, issue 3, pp 261–322, Boca Raton, Fla, CRC Press.

Chu CC. 1991. Recent advancements in suture fibers for wound closure. In TL Vigo, AF Turbak (eds), High-Tech Fibrous Materials: Composites, Biomedical Materials, Protective Clothing and Geotextiles, pp 167–213, ACS Symposium Series #457, Washington, DC, American Chemical Society.

Chu CC. In press. Biodegradable suture materials: Intrinsic and extrinsic factors affecting bio-degradation phenomena. In DL Wise, DE Altobelli, ER Schwartz et al. (eds), Handbook of Biomaterials and Applications. New York, Marcel Dekker.

Chu CC, Browning A. 1988. The study of thermal and gross morphologic properties of polyglycolic acid upon annealing and degradation treatments. J Biomed Mater Res 22(8):699.

Chu CC, Campbell ND. 1982. Scanning electron microscope study of the hydrolytic degradation of poly(glycolic acid) suture. J Biomed Mater Res 16(4):417.

Chu CC, Hsu A, Appel M, et al. 1992. The effect of macrophage cell media on the in vitro hydrolytic degradation of synthetic absorbable sutures. Fourth World Biomaterials Congress, Berlin, Germany.

Chu CC, Kizil Z. 1989. The effect of polymer morphology on the hydrolytic degradation of synthetic absorbable sutures. Third International ITV Conference on Biomaterials—Medical Textiles, Stuttgart, W Germany.

Chu CC, Louie M. 1985. A chemical means to study the degradation phenomena of polyglycolic acid absorbable polymer. J Appl Polymer Sci 30:3133.

Chu CC, Williams DF. 1983. The effect of γ-irradiation on the enzymatic degradation of polyglycolic acid absorbable sutures. J Biomed Mater Res 17(6):1029.

Chu CC, Zhang L, Coyne L. In press. Effect of irradiation temperature on hydrolytic degradation properties of synthetic absorbable sutures and polymers. J Appl Polymeric Sci.

Chujo K, Kobayashi H, Suzuki J. et al. 1967a. Physical and chemical characteristics of polyglycolide. Die Makromol Chemie 100:267.

Chujo K, Kobayashi H, Suzuki J, et al. 1967b. Ring-opening polymerization of glycolide. Die Makromol Chemie 100:262.

Daniels AU, Taylor MS, Andriano KP, et al. 1992. Toxicity of absorbable polymers proposed for fracture fixation devices. Trans 38th Ann Mtg Orthop Res Soc 17:88.

Eitenmüller KL, Gerlach T, Schmickal et al. 1989. Die Versorgung von Sprung-gelenksfrakturen unter Verwendung von Platten und Schrauben aus resorbierbarem Polymer material. Presented at Jahrestagung der Deutschen Gesellschaft für Unfallheilkunde, Berlin.

Fredericks RJ, Melveger AJ, Dolegiewitz LJ. 1984. Morphological and structural changes in a copolymer of glycolide and lactide occurring as a result of hydrolysis. J Polymer Sci Phy Ed 22:57.

Fukuzaki H, Yoshida M, Asano M, et al. 1989. Direct copolymerization of glycolic acid with lactones in the absence of catalysts. Eur Polymer J 26:457.

Fukuzaki H, Yoshida M, Asano M, et al. 1991. A new biodegradable copolymer of glycolic acid and lactones with relatively low molecular weight prepared by direct copolycondensation in the absence of catalysts. J Biomed Mater Res 25:315.

Gogolewski S, Pennings AJ. 1983. Resorbable materials of poly(L-lactide): II. Fibres spun from solutions of poly(L-lactide) in good solvents. J Appl Polymer Sci 28:1045.

Gross RA. 1994. Bacterial polyesters: Structural variability in microbial synthesis. In SW Shalaby (ed), Biomedical Polymers: Designed-to-Degrade Systems, chap 7, New York, Hanser.

Helder J, Feijen J, Lee SJ, et al. 1986. Copolymers of DL-lactic acid and glycine. Makromol Chem Rapid Commun 7:193.

Hofmann GO, 1992. Biodegradable implants in orthopaedic surgery: A review of the state of the art. Clinical Materials 10(1&2):25.

Jamiokowski DD, Shalaby SW. 1991. A polymeric radiostabilizer for absorbable polyesters. In RL Clough, SW Shalaby (eds), Radiation Effect of Polymers, chap 18, pp 300–309. ACS Symposium Series #475, ACS, Washington, DC.

Katz A, Mukherjee DP, Kaganov AL, et al. 1985. A new synthetic monofilament absorbable suture made from polytrimethylene carbonate. Surg Gynecol Obstet 161:213.

Kimura Y. 1993. Biodegradable polymers. In T Tsuruta, T Hayashi, K Kataoka, K Ishihara, Y Kimura (eds), Biomedical Applications of Polymeric Materials, pp 164–190, Boca Raton, Fla, CRC Press.

Koelmel DF, Jamiokowski DD, Shalaby SW, et al. 1991. Low modulus radiation sterilizable monofilament sutures. Polymer Preparations 32(2):235.

Leenslag JW, Pennings AJ. 1984. Synthesis of high-molecular weight poly(L-lactide) initiated with tin 2-ethylhexanoate. Makromol Chem 188(8):1809.

Loh IH, Chu CC, Lin HL. 1992. Plasma surface modification of synthetic absorbable fibers for wound closure. J Appl Biomater 3(2):131.

Miller ND, Williams DF. 1984. The *in vivo* and *in vitro* degradation of poly (glycolic acid) suture material as a function of applied strain. Biomaterials 5:365–368.

Nathan A, Kohn J. 1994. Amino acid derived polymers. In SW Shalaby (ed), Biomedical Polymers: Designed-to-Degrade Systems, chap 5, New York, Hanser.

Pratt L, Chu A, Kim J, et al. 1993. The effect of electrolytes on the *in vitro* hydrolytic degradation of synthetic biodegradable polymers: Mechanical properties, thermodynamics and molecular modeling. J Polymer Sci Chem Ed 31:1759.

Pratt L, Chu C. 1993. Hydrolytic degradation of α substituted polyglycolic acid: A semi-empirical computational Study. J Computational Chemistry 14(7):809.

Pratt L, Chu CC. 1994*a*. A computational study of the hydrolysis of degradable polysaccharide biomaterials: Substituent effects on the hydrolytic mechanism. J Computational Chemistry 15:241.

Pratt L, Chu CC. 1994*b*. The effect of electron donating and electron withdrawing substituents on the degradation rate of bioabsorbable polymers: A semi-empirical computational study. J Mol Structure 304:213.

Shalaby SW. 1994. Biomedical Polymers: Designed-to-Degrade Systems, New York, Hanser.

Shieh SJ, Zimmerman MC, Parsons JR. 1990. Preliminary characterization of bioresorbable and nonresorbable synthetic fibers for the repair of soft tissue injuries. J Biomed Mater Res 24:789.

Sugnuma J, Alexander H, Traub J, et al. 1992. Biological response of intramedullary bone to poly-L-lactic acid. In LG Cima, ES Ron (eds), Tissue-Inducing Biomaterial vol. 252, p. 339. Pittsburgh, Materials Research Soc.

Tunc DC. 1983. A high strength absorbable polymer for internal bone fixation. Trans Soc Biomater 6:47.

Vert M, Feijen J, Albertsson A, et al. 1992. Biodegradable Polymers and Plastics, Cambridge, Royal Society of Chemists.

Williams DF. 1979. Some observations on the role of cellular enzymes in the in vivo degradation of polymers. ASTM Spec Tech Publ 684:61.

Williams DF. 1990. Biodegradation of medical polymers. In DF Williams (ed), Concise Encyclopedia of Medical & Dental Materials, pp 69–74, New York, Pergamon.

Williams DF, Mort E. 1977. Enzyme-accelerated hydrolysis of polyglycolic acid. J Bioeng 1:231.

Williams DF, Chu CC. 1984. The effects of enzymes and gamma irradiation on the tensile strength and morphology of poly(p-dioxanone) fibers. J Appl Polymer Sci 29:1865.

Winet H, Hollinger JO. 1993. Incorporation of polylactide-polyglycolide in a cortical defect: Neo-osteogenesis in a bone chamber. J Biomed Mater Res 27:667.

Wise DL, Fellmann TD, Sanderson JE, et al. 1979. Lactic/glycolic acid polymers. In G Gregoriadis (ed), Drug Carriers in Biology and Medicine, pp 237–270, New York, Academic.

Zhang L, Loh IH, Chu CC. 1993. A combined γ irradiation and plasma deposition treatment to achieve the ideal degradation properties of synthetic absorbable polymers. J Biomed Mater Res 27:1425.

Further Information

Several recent books have very comprehensive descriptions of a variety of biodegradable polymeric biomaterials, their synthesis and physical, chemical, mechanical, biodegradable, and biological properties:

Barrows TH. 1986. Degradable implant materials: A review of synthetic absorbable polymers and their applications. Clin Materials 1:233.

Chu CC. In press. Biodegradable suture materials: Intrinsic and extrinsic factors affecting biodegradation phenomena. In DL Wise, DE Altobelli, ER Schwartz, et al. (eds), Handbook of Biomaterials and Applications, New York, Marcel Dekker.

Kimura Y. 1993. Biodegradable polymers. In T Tsuruta, T Hayashi, K Kataoka, K Ishihara, Y Kimura (eds), Biomedical Applications of Polymeric Materials, pp 164–190, Boca Raton, Fla, CRC Press.

Shalaby SW. 1994. Biomedical Polymers: Designed-to-Degrade Systems, New York, Hanser.

Vert M, Feijen J, Albertsson A, et al. 1992. Biodegradable Polymers and Plastics, Cambridge, Royal Society of Chemists.

The review by Barrows is brief with an emphasis on applications and extensive lists of patents. The chapter by Kimura was an overview of the subject with some interesting new polymers. The chapter includes both enzymatically degradable natural polymers and nonenzymatically degradable synthetic polymers. Probably the most comprehensive coverage of biodegradable polymeric biomaterials is the very recent book edited by Shalaby. It has eight chapters and covers almost all commercially and experimentally available biodegradable polymers. The chapter by Chu focuses on the most successful use of biodegradable polymers in medicine, namely wound closure biomaterials such as sutures. It is so far the most comprehensive review of all aspects of biodegradable wound closure biomaterials with very detailed information in chemical, physical, mechanical, biodegradable, and biological information. The book edited by Vert and coworkers is based on the Proceedings of the Second International Scientific Workshop on Biodegradable Polymers and Plastics held in Montpellier, France, in November 1991. The book covers both medical and nonmedical applications of biodegradable polymers. It covers a broader aspect of biodegradable polymers with far more chapters than Shalaby's book. But its chapters are shorter and less comprehensive than those in Shalaby's book, which is far more focused on biomedical use.

Articles on biodegradable polymeric biomaterials can also be found in *Journal of Biomedical Materials Research, Journal of Applied Biomaterials, Biomaterials, Journal of Biomaterials Science, Polymer, Journal of Applied Polymer Science,* and *Journal of Materials Science.*

Biologic Biomaterials: Tissue-Derived Biomaterials (Collagen)

Shu-Tung Li
ReGen Biologics Inc.

45.1 Structure and Properties of Collagen and Collagen-Rich Tissues

Structure of Collagen

Collagen is a multifunctional family of proteins of unique structural characteristics. It is the most abundant and ubiquitous protein in the body, its functions ranging from serving crucial biomechanical functions in bone, skin, tendon, and ligament to controlling cellular gene expressions in development [Nimni & Harkness, 1988]. Collagen molecules like all proteins are formed in vivo by enzymatic regulated step-wise polymerization reaction between amino and carboxyl groups of amino acids, where R is a side group of an amino acid residue.

$$(-\overset{\overset{\textstyle O}{\|}}{C}-\overset{\overset{\textstyle H}{|}}{N}-\overset{\overset{\textstyle H}{|}}{\underset{\underset{\textstyle R}{|}}{C}}-)_n \tag{45.1}$$

The simplest amino acid is *glycine* (Gly) (R = H), where a hypothetical flat sheet organization of polyglycine molecules can form and be stabilized by intermolecular hydrogen bonds (Fig. 45.1*a*). However, when R is a large group as in most other amino acids, the stereochemical constraints frequently force the *polypeptide* chain to adapt a less constraining conformation by rotating the bulky R groups away from the crowded interactions, forming a helix, where the large R groups are directed toward the surface of the helix (Fig. 45.1*b*). The hydrogen bonds are allowed to form within a helix between the hydrogen attached to nitrogen in one amino acid residue and the oxygen attached to a second amino acid residue. Thus, the final conformation of a protein, which is directly related to its function, is governed primarily by the amino acid sequence of the particular protein.

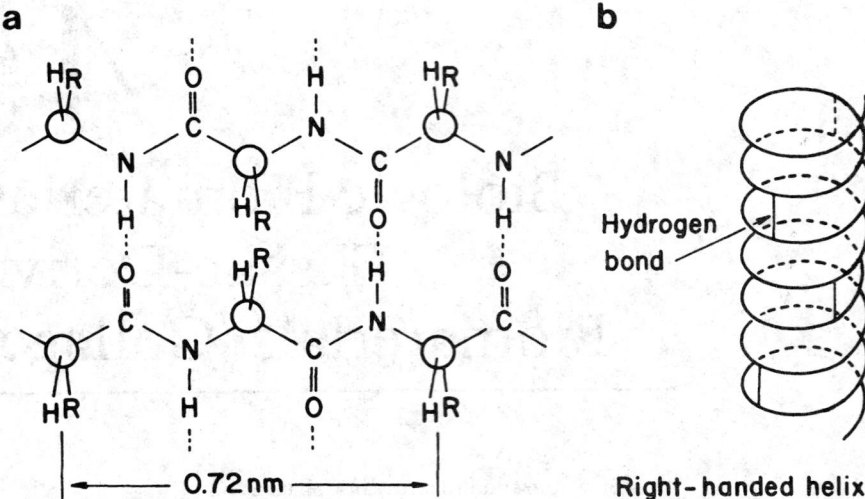

FIGURE 45.1   (*a*) Hypothetical flat sheet structure of a protein. (*b*) Helical arrangement of a protein chain.

Collagen is a protein comprised of three polypeptides (chains), each having a general amino acid sequence of (-Gly-*X*-*Y*-)$_n$, where *X* is any other amino acid and is frequently *proline* (Pro) and *Y* is any other amino acid and is frequently *hydroxyproline* (Hyp). A typical amino acid composition of collagen is shown in Table 45.1. The application of helical diffraction theory to high-angle collagen x-ray diffraction pattern [Rich & Crick, 1961] and the stereochemical constraints from the unusual amino acid composition [Eastoe, 1967] led to the initial triple-helical model and subsequent modified triple helix of the collagen molecule. Thus, collagen can be broadly defined as a protein which has a typical triple helix extending over the major part of the molecule. Within the triple helix, glycine must be present as every third amino acid, and proline and hydroxyproline are required to form and stabilize the triple helix.

To date, 14 proteins can be classified as collagen. Among the various collagens, type I collagen is the most abundant and is the major constituent of bone, skin, and tendon. Due to the abundance and ready accessibility of these tissues, they have been frequently used as a source for the preparation of collagen. This chapter will not review the details of the structure of the different collagens. The readers are referred to recent reviews for a more in-depth discussion of this subject [Nimni, 1988; van der Rest et al., 1990]. It is, however, of particular relevance to review some salient structural features of the type I collagen in order to facilitate the subsequent discussions of properties and its relation to biomedical applications.

TABLE 45.1   Amino Acid Content of Collagen

Amino Acids	Content, residues/1000 residues*
Gly	334
Pro	122
Hyp	96
Acid polar (Asp, Glu, Asn)	124
Basic polar (Lys, Arg, His)	91
Other	233

*Reported values are average values of 10 different determinations for tendon tissue.
Source: Eastoe [1967].

A type I collagen molecule (also referred to as *tropocollagen*) isolated from various tissues has a molecular weight of about 283,000 daltons. It is comprised of three left-handed helical polypeptide chains (Figure 45.2*a*) which are intertwined forming a right-handed helix around a central molecular axis (Figure 45.2*b*). Two of the polypeptide chains are identical (α_1) having 1056 amino acid residues, and the third polypeptide chain (α_2) has 1029 amino acid residues [Miller, 1984]. The triple-helical structure has a rise per residue of 0.286 nm and a unit twist of 108°, with 10 residues in three turns and a helical pitch (repeating distance within a single chain) of 30 residues or 8.68 nm [Fraser et al., 1983]. Over 95% of the amino acids have the sequence of Gly-*X*-*Y*. The remaining 5% of the molecule does not have the sequence of Gly-*X*-*Y* and is therefore not triple-helical. These non-helical portions of the molecule are located at the N- and C-terminal ends and are referred to as *telopeptides* (9~26 residues) [Miller, 1984]. The whole molecule has a length of about 280 nm and a diameter of about 1.5 nm and has a conformation similar to a rigid rod (Fig. 45.2*c*).

The triple-helical structure of a collagen molecule is stabilized by several factors (Fig. 45.3): (1) a tight fit of the amino acids within the triple-helix—this geometrical stabilization factor can be appreciated from a space-filling model constructed from a triple helix with (Gly-Pro-Hyp) sequence (Fig. 45.3); (2) the interchain hydrogen bond formation between the backbone carbonyl and amino hydrogen interactions; and (3) the contribution of water molecules to the interchain hydrogen bond formation.

The telopeptides are regions where *intermolecular crosslinks* are formed in vivo. A common intermolecular crosslink is formed between an *allysine* (the ϵ-amino group of lysine or hydroxylysine has been converted to an aldehyde) of one telopeptide of one molecule and an ϵ-amino group of a lysine or hydroxylysine in the triple helix of a second molecule. Thus the method commonly used to solubilize the collagen molecules from crosslinked fibrils with *proteolytic enzymes* such as *pepsin* removes the telopeptides (cleaves the intermolecular crosslinks) from the collagen molecule. The pepsin solubilized collagen is occasionally referred to as *atelocollagen* [Stenzl, 1974].

$$Pr-CH_2-CH_2-CH_2-CHO \quad + \quad H_2N-CH_2-\overset{\overset{\displaystyle OH}{|}}{CH}-CH_2-CH_2-Pr$$

$$\text{Allysine} \qquad\qquad\qquad \text{Hydroxylysine}$$

$$(45.2)$$

$$\rightarrow Pr-CH_2-CH_2-CH_2-CH{=}N-CH_2-\overset{\overset{\displaystyle OH}{|}}{CH}-CH_2-CH_2-Pr$$

$$\text{Dehydrohydroxylysinonorleucine}$$

Since the presence of hydroxyproline is unique in collagen (*elastin* contains a small amount), the determination of collagen content in a collagen-rich tissue is readily done by assaying the hydroxyproline content.

Collagen does not appear to exist as isolated molecules in the extracellular space in the body. Instead, collagens aggregate into *fibrils*. Depending on the tissue and age, a collagen fibril varies from about 50 nm to about 300 nm in diameter with indeterminate length and can be easily seen under electron microscopy (Fig. 45.4). The fibrils are important structural building units for large *fibers* (Fig. 45.5). Collagen molecules are arranged in specific orders both longitudinally and in cross-section, and the organization of collagen molecules in a fibril is tissue-specific [Katz and Li, 1972, 1973*b*]. The two-dimensional structure (the projection of a three-dimensional structure onto a two-dimensional plane) of a type I collagen fibril has been unequivocally defined both by an analysis of small-angle x-ray diffraction pattern along the meridian of a collagenous tissue [Bear, 1952] and by examination of the transmission electron micrographs of tissues stained with negative or positive stains [Hodge & Petruska, 1963]. In this structure (Fig. 45.2*d*), the collagen molecules are staggered

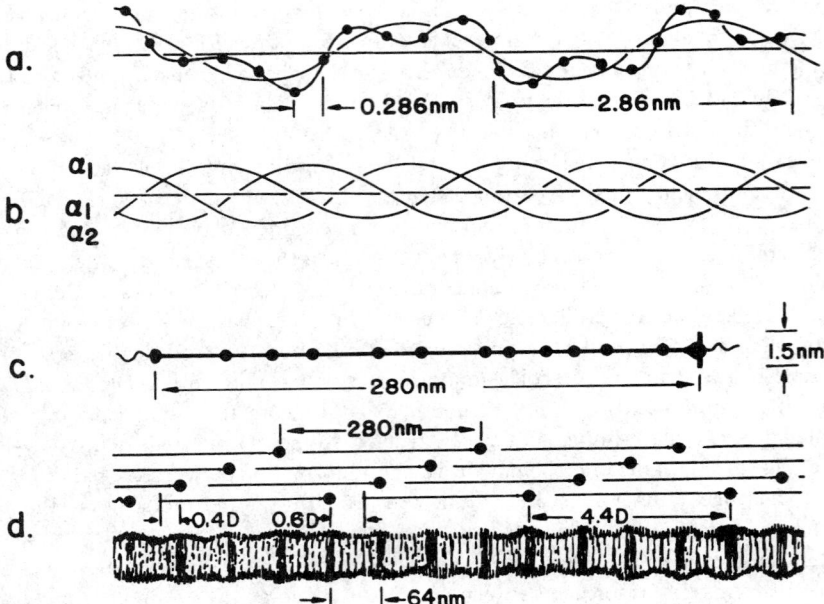

FIGURE 45.2 Diagram depicting the formation of collagen, which can be visualized as taking place in several steps: (*a*) single chain left-handed helix; (*b*) three single chains intertwined into a triple stranded helix; (*c*) a collagen (tropocollagen) molecule; (*d*) collagen molecules aligned in *D* staggered fashion in a fibril producing overlap and hole regions.

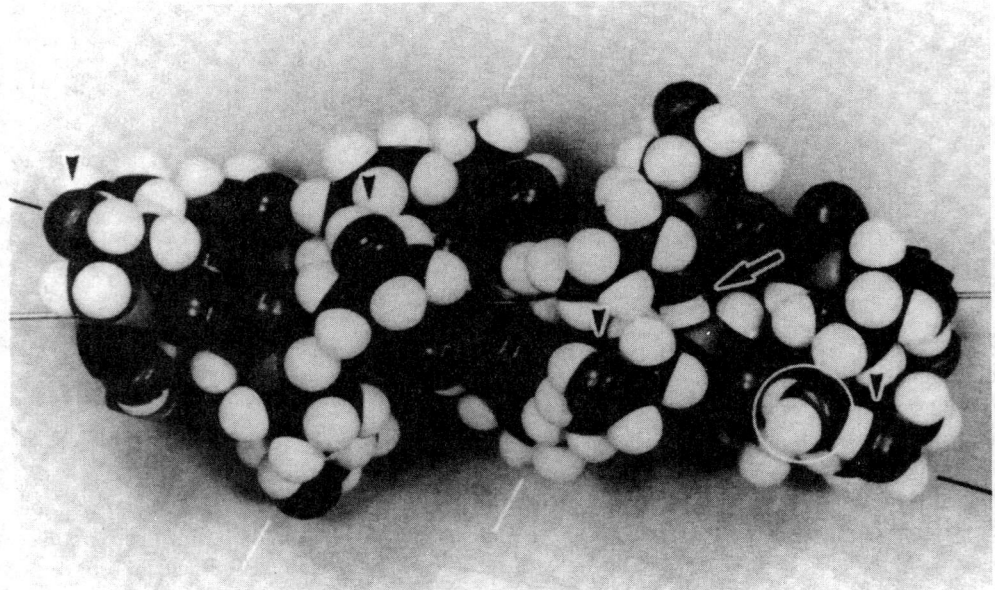

FIGURE 45.3 A space-filling model of the collagen triple helix, showing all the atoms in a ten-residue segment of repeating triplet sequence (Gly-Pro-Hyp)$_n$. The arrow shows an interchain hydrogen bond. The arrow heads identify the hydroxy groups of hydroxyproline in one chain. The circle shows a hydrogen-bonded water molecule. The short white lines identify the ridge of amino acid chains. The short black lines indicate the supercoil of one chain [Piez, 1984].

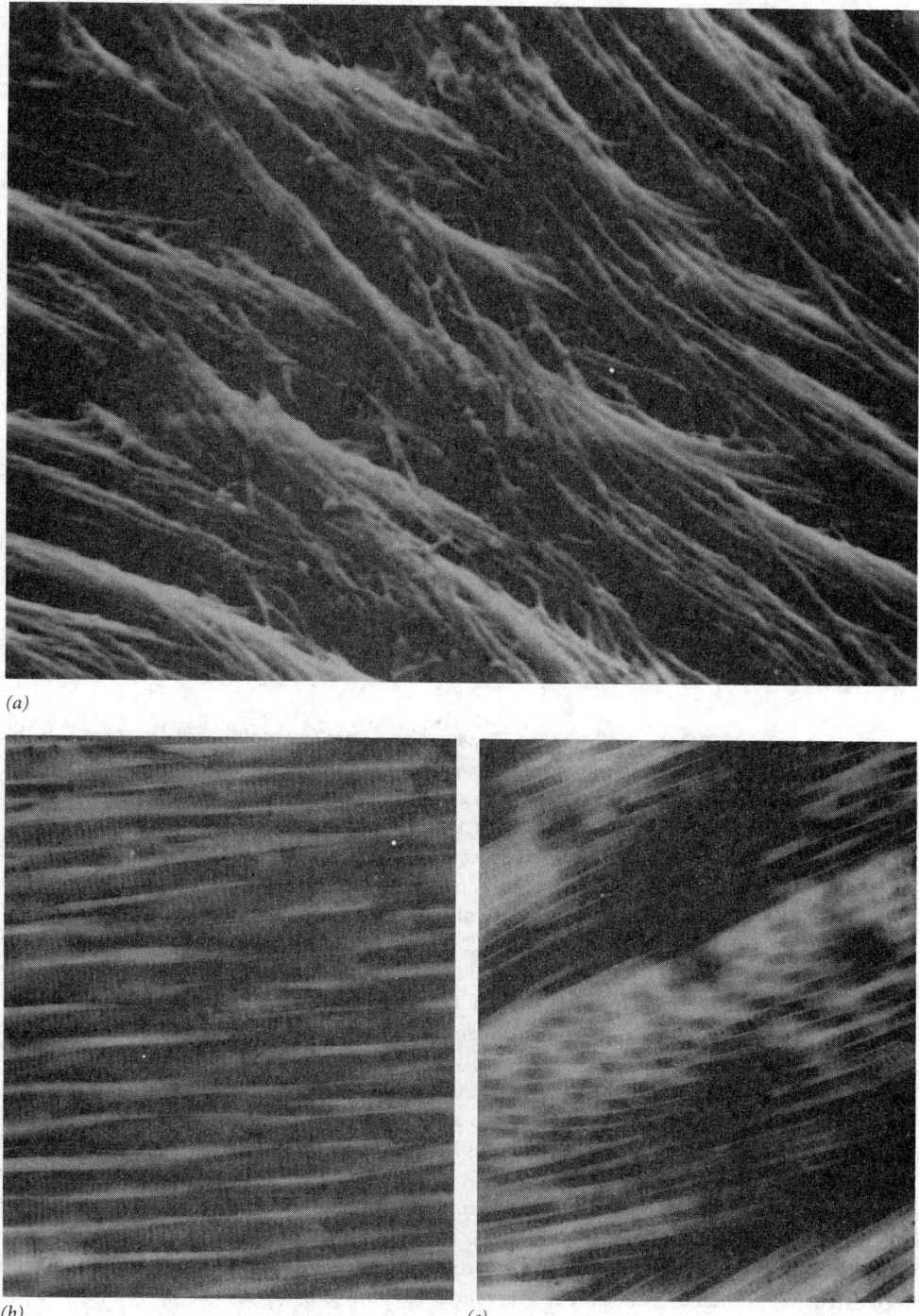

(a)

(b)   *(c)*

FIGURE 45.4 (*a*) Scanning electron micrograph of the surface of an adult rabbit bone matrix, showing how the collagen fibrils branch and interconnect in an intricate, woven pattern (×4800) [Tiffit, 1980]. (*b*) Transmission electron micrographs of (× 24,000) parallel collagen fibrils in tendon, [Fung, 1992]. (*c*) Transmission electron micrographs of (× 24,000) mesh work of fibrils in skin [Fung, 1993].

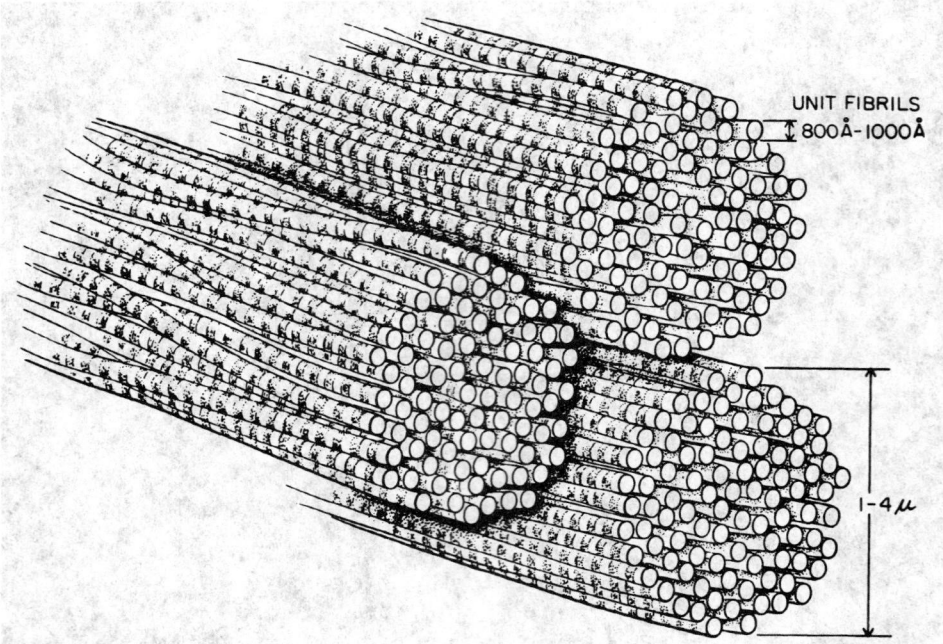

UNIT FIBRILS
800Å-1000Å

1-4 μ

FIGURE 45.5   Diagram showing the collagen fibers of the connective tissue in general which are composed of unit collagen fibrils.

with respect to one another by a distance of D (64 nm to 67 nm) or multiple of D, where D is the fundamental repeat distance seen in the small-angle x-ray diffraction pattern, or the repeating distance seen in the electron micrographs. This staggering of collagen molecules creates overlap regions of about $0.4D$ and hole or defect regions of about $0.6D$.

One interesting and important structural aspect of collagen is its approximate equal number of acidic (*aspartic* and *glutamic* acids) and basic (lysines and *arginines*) side groups. Since these groups are charged under physiological conditions, the collagen is essentially electrically neutral [Li & Katz, 1976]. The packing of collagen molecules with a D staggering results in clusters of regions where the charged groups are located [Hofmann & Kuhn, 1981]. These groups therefore are in close proximity to form intra- and intermolecular hydrogen-bonded *salt-linkages* of the form (Pr-COO$^-$ $^+$H$_3$N-Pr) [Li et al., 1975]. In addition, the side groups of many amino acids are nonpolar [*alanine* (Ala), *valine* (Val), *leucine* (Leu), *isoleucine* (Ile), *proline* (Pro), and *phenolalanine* (Phe)] in character and hence *hydrophobic;* therefore, chains with these amino acids avoid contact with water molecules and seek interactions with the nonpolar chains of amino acids. In fact, the result of molecular packing of collagen in a fibril is such that the nonpolar groups are also clustered, forming hydrophobic regions within collagen fibrils [Hofmann & Kuhn, 1981]. Indeed, the packing of the collagen molecules in various tissues is believed to be a result of intermolecular interactions involving both the electrostatic and hydrophobic interactions [Hofmann & Kuhn, 1981; Katz and Li, 1981; Li et al., 1975].

The three-dimensional organization of type I collagen molecules within a fibril has been the subject of extensive research over the past 40 years [Fraser et al., 1983; Katz and Li, 1972, 1973*a*, 1973*b*, 1981; Miller, 1976; Ramachandran, 1967; Yamuchi et al., 1986]. Many structural models have been proposed based on an analysis of equatorial and off-equatorial x-ray diffraction patterns of rat-tail-tendon collagen [Miller, 1976; North et al., 1954], *intrafibrillar volume* determination of various collagenous tissues [Katz and Li, 1972, 1973*a*, 1973*b*], intermolecular side chain interactions [Hofmann & Kuhn, 1981; Katz and Li, 1981; Li et al., 1981], and intermolecular crosslinking patterns studies [Yamuchi et al., 1986]. The general understanding of the three-dimensional molecular packing in type I collagen fibrils is that the collagen molecules are arranged in hexagonal or near hexagonal arrays [Katz & Li, 1972, 1981; Miller, 1976]. Depending on the tissue, the intermolecular distance varies from about 0.15 nm in rat tail tendon to as large as 0.18 nm in bone and dentin [Katz & Li, 1973*b*]. The axial staggering of the molecules by $1{\sim}4D$ with respect to one another is tissue-specific and has not yet been fully elucidated.

There are very few interspecies differences in the structure of type I collagen molecule. The extensive homology of the structure of type I collagen may explain why this collagen obtained from animal species is acceptable as a material for human implantation.

Properties of Collagen-Rich Tissue

The function of collagenous tissue is related to its structure and properties. This section reviews some important properties of collagen-rich tissues.

Physical and Biomechanical Properties

The physical properties of tissues vary according to the amount and structural variations of the collagen fibers. In general, a collagen-rich tissue contains about 75–90% of collagen on a dry weight basis. Table 45.2 is a typical composition of a collagen-rich soft tissue such as skin. Collagen fibers (bundles of collagen fibrils) are arranged in different configurations in different tissues for their respective functions at specific anatomic sites. For example, collagen fibers are arranged in parallel in tendon [Fig. 45.4*b*] and ligament for their high-tensile strength requirements, whereas collagen fibers in skin are arranged in random arrays [Fig. 45.4*c*] to provide the resiliency of the tissue under stress. Other structure-supporting functions of collagen such as transparency for the lens of the eye and shaping of the ear or tip of the nose can also be provided by the collagen fibers. Thus, an important physical property of collagen is the three-dimensional organization of the collagen fibers.

The collagen-rich tissues can be thought of as a composite polymeric material in which the highly oriented crystalline collagen fibrils are embedded in the amorphous ground substance of noncollagenous *polysaccharides, glycoproteins,* and elastin. When the tissue is heated, its specific volume increases, exhibiting a glass transition at about 40°C and a melting of the crystalline collagen fibrils at about 56°C. The melting temperature of crystalline collagen fibrils is referred to as the *denaturation temperature* of collagenous tissues.

The stress-strain curves of a collagenous tissue such as tendon exhibit nonlinear behavior (Fig. 45.6). This nonlinear behavior of stress-strain of tendon collagen is similar to that observed in synthetic fibers. The initial toe region represents alignment of fibers in the direction of stress. The steep rise in slope represents the majority of fibers stretched along their long axes. The decrease in slope following the steep rise may represent the breaking of individual fibers prior to the final catastrophic failure. Table 45.3 summarizes some mechanical properties of collagen and elastic fibers. The difference in biomechanical properties between collagen and elastin is a good example of the requirements for these proteins to serve their specific functions in the body.

Unlike tendon or ligament, skin consists of collagen fibers randomly arranged in layers or lamellae. Thus skin tissues show mechanical anisotropy (Fig. 45.7). Another feature of the stress-strain curve of the skin is its extensibility under small load as compared to tendon. At small load the fibers

TABLE 45.2 Composition of Collagen-Rich Soft Tissues

Component	Composition, %
Collagen	75 (dry), 30 (wet)
Proteoglycans and polysaccharides	20 (dry)
Elastin and glycoproteins	< 5 (dry)
Water	60–70

Source: Park and Lakes [1992].

are straightened and aligned rather than stretched. Upon further stretching the fibrous lamellae align with respect to each other and resist further extension. When the skin is highly stretched the modulus of elasticity approaches that of tendon as expected of the aligned collagen fibers.

Cartilage is another collagen-rich tissue which has two main physiological functions. One is the maintenance of shape (ear, tip of nose, and rings around the trachea), and the other is to provide bearing surfaces at joints. It contains very large and diffuse proteoglycan (protein-polysaccharide) molecules which form a gel in which the collagen-rich molecules are entangled. They can affect the mechanical properties of the collagen by hindering the movements through the interstices of the collagenous matrix network.

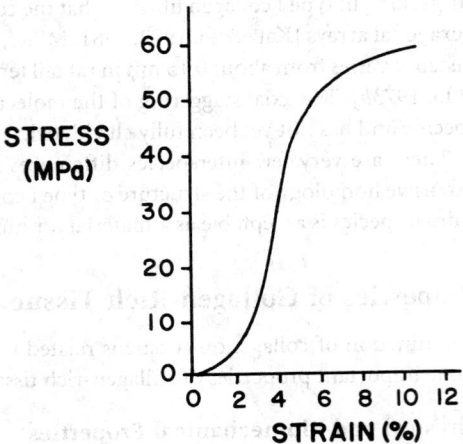

FIGURE 45.6 A typical stress-strain curve for tendon [Rigby et al., 1959].

The joint cartilage has a very low coefficient of friction (< 0.01). This is largely attributed to the squeeze-film effect between cartilage and synovial fluid. The synovial fluid can be squeezed out through highly fenestrated cartilage upon compressive loading, and the reverse action will take place in tension. The lubricating function is carried out in conjunction with *glycosaminoglycans* (GAG), especially *chondroitin sulfates*. The modulus of elasticity (10.3~20.7 MPa) and tensile strength (3.4 MPa) are quite low. However, wherever high stress is required the cartilage is replaced by purely collagenous tissue. Mechanical properties of some collagen-rich tissues are given in Table 45.4 as a reference.

Physiochemical Properties

Electrostatic Properties. A collagen molecule has a total of approximately 240 ϵ-amino and guanidino groups of lysines and arginines and 230 carboxyl groups of aspartic and glutamic acids. These groups are charged under physiological conditions. In a native fibril, most of these groups interact either intra- or intermolecularly forming salt-linkages providing significant stabilization energy to the collagen fibril [Li et al., 1975]. Only a small number of charged groups is free. However, the electrostatic state within a collagen fibril can be altered by changing the pH of the environment. Since the pK for an amino group is about 10 and about 4 for a carboxyl group, the electrostatic interactions are significantly perturbed at a pH below 4 and above 10. The net result of the pH change is a weakening of the intra- and intermolecular electrostatic interactions, resulting in a swelling of the fibrils. The fibril swelling can be prevented by chemically introducing covalent intermolecular crosslinks. Any bifunctional reagent which reacts with amino, carboxyl, and hydroxyl groups can serve as a crosslinking agent. The introduction of covalent intermolecular crosslinks fixes the physical state of the fibrillar structure and balances the swelling pressures obtained from any pH changes.

TABLE 45.3 Elastic Properties of Collagen and Elastic Fibers

Fibers	Modulus of Elasticity, MPa	Tensile Strength, MPa	Ultimate Elongation, %
Collagen	1000	50–100	10
Elastin	0.6	1	100

Source: Park and Lakes [1992].

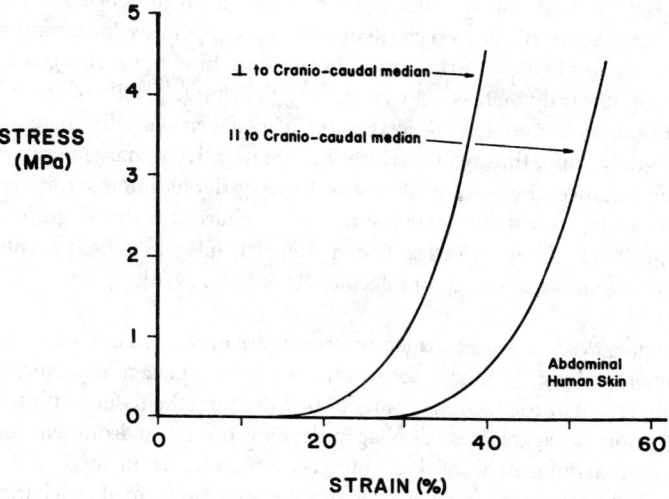

FIGURE 45.7 Stress-strain curves of human abdominal skin [Daly, 1966].

Another way of altering the electrostatic state of a collagen fibril is by chemically modifying the electrostatic side groups. For example, the positively charged ε-amino groups of lysine and hydroxylysine can be chemically modified with acetic anhydride, which converts the ε-amino groups to a neutral acetyl group [Green et al., 1953]. The result of this modification increases the number of the net negative charges of the fibril. Conversely, the negatively charged carboxyl groups of aspartic and glutamic acid can be chemically modified to a neutral group by methylation [Fraenkel-Conrat, 1945]. Thus, by adjusting the pH of the solution and applying chemical modification methods, a range of electrostatic properties of collagen can be obtained.

Ion and Macromolecular Binding Properties. In the native state and under physiological conditions, a collagen molecule has only about 60 free carboxyl groups [Li et al., 1975]. These groups have the capability of binding cations such as calcium with a free energy of formation for the protein-$COO\text{-}Ca^{++}$ of about 1.2 Kcal/mol. This energy is not large enough to compete for the hydrogen bonded salt-linkage interactions, which have a free energy of formation of about ~1.6 Kcal/mol. The extent of ion binding, however, can be enhanced in the presence of lyotropic salts such as KCNS,

TABLE 45.4 Mechanical Properties of Some Nonmineralized Human Tissues

Tissues	Tensile Strength, MPa	Ultimate Elongation, %
Skin	7.6	78.0
Tendon	53.0	9.4
Elastic cartilage	3.0	30.0
Heart valves (aortic)		
Radial	0.45	15.3
Circumferential	2.6	10.0
Aorta		
Transverse	1.1	77.0
Longitudinal	0.07	81.0

Source: Park and Lakes [1992].

which breaks the salt-linkages, or by shifting the pH away from the *isoelectric point* of collagen. Macromolecules can bind to collagen via covalent bonding, cooperative ionic binding, entrapment, entanglement, and a combination of the above. In addition, binding of charged ions and macromolecules can be significantly increased by modifying the charge profile of collagen as described previously. For example, a complete N-acetylation of collagen will eliminate all the positively charged ϵ-amino groups and, thus, will increase the free negatively charged groups. The resulting acetylated collagen enhances the binding of positively charged ions and macromolecules. However, the methylation of collagen will eliminate the negatively charged carboxyl groups and, thus, will increase the free positively charge moieties. The methylated collagen, therefore, enhances the binding of negatively charged ions and macromolecules [Li & Katz, 1976].

Fiber-Forming Properties.   Native collagen molecules are organized in tissues in specific orders. *Polymorphic* forms of collagen can be reconstituted from the collagen molecules, obtained either from enzymatic digestion of collagenous tissues or by extracting the tissues with salt solutions. The formation of polymorphic aggregates of collagen depends on the environment for reconstitution [Piez, 1984]. Native arrangement of the collagen molecules is formed under physiological conditions. Various polymorphic molecular aggregates may be formed by changing the state of intermolecular interactions. For example, when collagen molecules are aggregated under high concentrations of a neutral salt or under nonaqueous conditions, the collagen molecules associate into random arrays having no specific regularities detectable by electron microscopy. The collagen molecules can be induced to aggregate into other polymorphic forms such as the *segment-long-spacing* (SLS) form where all heads are aligned in parallel and the *fibrous-long-spacing* (FLS) form where the molecules are randomly aligned in either a head-to-tail, tail-to-tail, or head-to-head orientation.

Biologic Properties

Hemostatic Properties.   Native collagen aggregates are intrinsically hemostatic. The mechanism of collagen-induced hemostasis has been the subject of numerous investigations [Jaffe & Deykin, 1974; Wang et al., 1978; Wilner et al., 1968]. The general conclusion from these studies is that *platelets* first adhere to a collagen surface. This induces the release of platelet contents, followed by platelet aggregation, leading to the eventual hemostatic plug. The hemostatic activity of collagen is dependent on the size of the collagen aggregate and the native organization of the molecules [Wang et al., 1978]. Denatured collagen (*gelatin*) is not effective in inducing hemostasis [Guidoin et al., 1987].

Cell Interaction Properties.   Collagen forms the essential framework of the tissues and organs. Many cells, such as epithelial and endothelial cells, are found resting on the collagenous surfaces or within a collagenous matrix such as that of many connective tissue cells. Collagen-cell interactions are essential features during the development stage and during wound healing and tissue remodeling in adults [Kleinman et al., 1981]. Studying collagen-cell interactions is useful in developing simulated tissue and organ structures and in investigating cell behavior in the in vitro simulated systems. Numerous studies have aimed at developing viable tissues and organs in vitro for transplantation applications [Bell et al., 1981; Montesano et al., 1983; Silbermann, 1990].

Immunologic Properties.   Soluble collagen has long been known to be a poor immunogen [Timpl, 1982]. A significant level of antibodies cannot be raised without the use of Freund's complete adjuvant (a mixture of mineral oil and heat-killed *mycobacteria*) which augments antibody response. Insoluble collagen is even less immunogenic. Thus, xenogeneic collagenous tissue devices such as porcine and bovine pericardial heart valves are acceptable for long-term implantation in humans. The reasons for the low antibody response against collagen are not known. It may be related to the homology of the collagen structure from different species (low level of foreignness) or to certain structural features associated with collagen [Timpl, 1982].

45.2 Biotechnology of Collagen

Isolation and Purification of Collagen

There are two distinct ways of isolating and purifying collagen material. One is the molecular technology and the other is the fibrillar technology. These two technologies are briefly reviewed here.

Isolation and Purification of Soluble Collagen Molecules

The isolation and purification of soluble collagen molecules from a collagenous tissue is achieved by using a proteolytic enzyme such as pepsin to cleave the telopeptides. Since telopeptides are the natural crosslinking sites of collagen, the removal of telopeptides renders the collagen molecules and small collagen aggregates soluble in an aqueous solution. The pepsin-solubilized collagen can be purified by repetitive precipitation with a neutral salt. Pepsin-solubilized collagen in monomeric form is generally soluble in a buffer solution at low temperature. The collagen molecules may be reconstituted into fibrils of various polymorphisms. However, the reconstitution of the pepsin-solubilized collagen into fibrils of native molecular packing is not as efficient as the intact molecules, since the telopeptides facilitate fibril formation [Comper & Veis, 1977].

Isolation and Purification of Fibrillar Collagen

The isolation and purification of collagen fibers relies on the removal of noncollagenous materials from the collagenous tissue. Salt extraction removes the newly synthesized collagen molecules that have not been covalently incorporated into the collagen fibrils. Salt also removes the noncollagenous materials that are soluble in aqueous conditions and are bound to collagen fibrils by nonspecific interactions. *Lipids* are removed by low-molecular-weight organic solvents such as low-molecular-weight ethers and alcohols. Acid extraction facilitates the removal of acidic proteins and glycosaminoglycans due to weakening of the interactions between the acidic proteins and collagen fibrils. Alkaline extraction weakens the interaction between the basic proteins and collagen fibrils and thus facilitates the removal of basic proteins. In addition, various enzymes other than collagenase can be used to facilitate the removal of the small amounts of glycoproteins, proteoglycans, and elastins from the tissue. Purified collagen fibers can be obtained through these sequential extractions and enzymatic digestions from the collagen-rich tissues.

Matrix Fabrication Technology

The purified collagen materials obtained from either the molecular technology or from the fibrillar technology are subjected to additional processing to fabricate the materials into useful devices for specific medical applications. The different matrices and their medical applications are summarized in Table 45.5. The technology in fabricating these matrices is briefly outlined below.

TABLE 45.5 Summary of Different Collagen Matrices and Their Medical Applications

Matrix Form	Medical Application
Membrane (film, sheet)	Oral tissue repair; wound dressings; dura repair; patches
Porous (sponge, felt, fibers)	Hemostats; wound dressings; cartilage repair; soft-tissue augmentation
Gel	Drug and biologically active macromolecule delivery; soft- and hard-tissue augmentation
Solution	Soft-tissue augmentation; drug delivery
Filament	Tendon and ligament repair; sutures
Tubular (membrane, sponge)	Nerve repair; vascular repair
Composite	
Collagen/synthetic polymer	Vascular repair; skin repair; wound dressings
Collagen/biological polymer	Soft-tissue augmentation; skin repair
Collagen/ceramic	Hard-tissue repair

Membranous Matrix

Collagen membranes can be produced by drying a collagen solution or a fibrillar collagen dispersion cast on a nonadhesive surface. The thickness of the membrane is governed by the concentration and the initial thickness of the cast solution or dispersion. In general, membrane thickness of up to 0.5 mm can be easily obtained by air drying a cast collagen material. Additional chemical crosslinking is required to stabilize the membrane from dissolution or dissociation. The membrane produced by casting and air drying does not permit manipulation of the pore structure. Generally, the structure of a cast membrane is dense and amorphous with minimal *permeability* to macromolecules [Li et al., 1991]. Porous membranes may be obtained by freeze-drying a cast solution or dispersion of a predetermined density or by partially compressing a preformed porous matrix to a predetermined density and pore structure.

Porous Matrix

Porous collagen matrices are generally obtained by freeze-drying an aqueous volume of collagen solution or dispersion. The freeze-dried porous matrix requires chemical crosslinking to stabilize the structure. A convenient way to stabilize the porous matrix is to crosslink the matrix by vapor using a volatile crosslinking agent such as formaldehyde. The pore structure of the matrix depends, to a large extent, on the concentration of the collagen in the solution or dispersion. Other factors that contribute to the pore structure include the rate of freezing, the size of fibers in the dispersion, and the presence and absence of other macromolecules. *Apparent densities* from 0.05 to 0.3 gram matrix per cubic centimeter matrix volume can be obtained. These porous matrices generally have pores from about 50 μm to as large as 1500 μm.

Gel Matrix

A *gel matrix* may be defined as a homogeneous phase between a liquid and a solid. As such, a gel may vary from a simple viscous fluid to a highly concentrated puttylike material. Collagen gels may be formed by shifting the pH of a dispersion away from its isoelectric point. Alternatively, the collagen material may be subjected to a chemical modification procedure to change its charge profile to a net positively charged or a net negatively charged protein before hydrating the material to form a gel matrix. For example, native fibers dispersed in water at pH 7 will be in the form of two phases. The dispersed fibers become gel when the pH changes from 7 to 3. Succinylating the primary amino groups of collagen, which converts the positively charged amino groups to negatively charged carboxyl groups, changes the isoelectric point of collagen from about 7 to about 4.5. Such a collagen material swells to a gel at a pH of 7.

Solution Matrix

A collagen solution is obtained by dissolving the collagen molecules in an aqueous solution. Collagen molecules are obtained by digesting the insoluble tissue with pepsin to cleave the crosslinking sites of collagen (telopeptides) as previously described. The solubility of collagen depends on the pH, the temperature, the ionic strength of the solution, and the molecular weight. Generally, collagen is more soluble in the cold. Collagen molecules aggregate into fibrils when the temperature of the solution increases to the body temperature, and pH plays an important role in solubilizing collagen. Collagen is more soluble at a pH away from the isoelectric point of the protein. Collagen is less soluble at higher ionic strength of a solution. The solubility of collagen decreases with increasing the size of molecular aggregates. Thus, collagen becomes increasingly less soluble with increasing the extent of crosslinking [Bailey & Rhodes, 1964].

Filamentous Matrix

Collagen filaments can be produced by extrusion techniques [Li & Stone, 1993; Schimpf & Rodriquez, 1976]. A collagen dispersion having a concentration in the range of 1–4% (w/v) is first prepared. Collagen is extruded into a coacervation bath containing a high concentration of a salt or into an aqueous solution at a pH of the isoelectric point of the collagen. Tensile strength of 30 MPa has been obtained for the reconstituted filaments.

Tubular Matrix

Tubular matrices may be formed by extrusion through a coaxial cylinder [Stenzl et al., 1974], or by coating collagen onto a mandrel [Li, 1990]. Different properties of the tubular membranes can be obtained by controlling the drying procedures.

Composite Matrix

Collagen can form a variety of homogeneous composites with other water-soluble materials. Ions, peptides, proteins, and polysaccharides can all be uniformly incorporated into a collagen matrix. The methods of homogeneous composite formation include ionic and covalent bonding, entrapment, entanglement, and coprecipitation. A heterogeneous composite can be formed between collagen, ceramics, and synthetic polymers that have distinct properties for medical applications [Li, 1988].

45.3 Design of a Resorbable Collagen-Based Medical Implant

Designing a medical implant for tissue or organ repair requires a thorough understanding of the structure and function of the tissue and organ to be repaired, the structure and properties of the materials used for repair, and the design requirements. There are at present two schools of thought regarding the design of an implant, namely the permanent implant and the *resorbable implant*. The permanent implants are intended to permanently replace the damaged tissues or organs and are fabricated from various materials including metals and natural or synthetic polymers. For example, most of the weight-bearing orthopedic and oral implants are made of metals or alloys. Non-weight-bearing tissues and organs are generally replaced with implants that are fabricated either from synthetic or natural materials. Implants for blood vessel, heart valve, and most soft tissue repair fall into this class. Permanent implants, particularly those made of synthetic and biological materials, frequently suffer from the long-term effects of material degradation. Material degradation can result from biological processes such as enzymatic degradation or environmentally induced degradation from mechanical, metal-catalyzed oxidation and from the permeation of body fluids into the polymeric devices [Bruck, 1991]. The material degradation is particularly manifested in applications where there is repetitive stress-strain on the implant, such as artificial blood vessels and heart valves.

As a result of the lack of suitable materials for long-term implantation, the concept of using a resorbable template to induce host tissue regeneration (guided tissue regeneration) has received vigorous attention in recent years. This area of research can be categorized into synthetic and biological templates. *Polyglycolic acid* (PGA), *polylactic acid* (PLA), polyglycolic-polylactic acid copolymers, and *polydioxanone* are among the polymers most selected for resorbable medical implant development. Among the biological materials used for resorbable medical implant development, *resorbable collagen* has been one of the most popular materials in this category. Collagen-based templates have been developed for skin [Yannas & Burke, 1981], peripheral nerve [Li et al., 1990; Yannas et al., 1985], oral tissue [Altman & Li, 1990; Blumenthal, 1988], meniscus [Li et al., 1994], and a variety of other tissue repair and regeneration applications [Goldstein et al., 1989; Ma et al., 1990].

The following discussion is useful in designing a template for tissue repair and regeneration applications. By way of an example, the design parameters listed below are specifically applied to the development of a resorbable collagen template for meniscal tissue repair and regeneration in the knee joint.

A *meniscus* is a semilunar fibrocartilage that is anatomically located between the femoral condyles and tibial plateau, providing stability, weight bearing, and shock absorption and assisting in lubrication of the knee joint. A major portion of the meniscal tissue is avascular except the peripheral rim, which comprises about 10–30% of the total width of the structure and is nourished by the peripheral vasculature [Arnoczky & Warren, 1982]. Collagen is the major matrix material of the meniscus, and the fibers are oriented primarily in the circumferential direction in the line of stress for mechanical function. Repair of damaged meniscal tissue in the peripheral vascular rim can be accomplished with sutures. However, in cases where the injured site is in the avascular region, partial or total removal of the meniscal tissue is often indicated. This is primarily due to the inadequacy of the *fibrochondrocytes* alone to self-repair the damaged meniscal tissue. Studies in animals and humans have shown that removal of the meniscus is a prelude to degenerative knees manifested by the development of *osteoarthritis* [Shapiro & Glimcher, 1980]. At present there is no suitable permanent substitute for meniscal tissue.

Biocompatibility

Biocompatibility of the materials and their degraded products is a prerequisite for resorbable implant development. Purified collagen materials either have been used as implants or have been extensively tested in clinical studies as implants without adverse effects. The meniscus template can be fabricated from insoluble matrix of purified collagen fibers that are further crosslinked chemically to increase the stability and reduce the immunogenicity in vivo. In addition, small amounts of noncollagenous materials such as glycosaminoglycans and growth factors can be incorporated into the collagen matrix to improve the osmotic properties as well as the rate of tissue ingrowth.

Despite the safety record of collagen materials for implantation, during the process of preparing the collagen template, small amounts of unwanted noncollagenous materials could be incorporated into the device such as salts and crosslinking agent. Therefore, a series of biocompatibility testing must be conducted to ensure the residuals of these materials do not cause any safety issues. The FDA has published a guideline for biocompatibility testing of implantable devices [Tripartite Guidance for Medical Devices, 1986].

Since the primary structure of a collagen molecule from bovine is homologous to human collagen [Miller, 1984], the in vivo degradation of bovine collagen implant should be similar to the normal host tissue remodeling process during wound healing. For a resorbable collagen template, the matrix is slowly degraded by the host over time. It is known that a number of cell types such as *polymorphonuclear leukocytes, fibroblasts,* and *macrophages* are capable, during the wound healing period, of secreting enzyme collagenases which cleave a collagen molecule at 1/4 position from the C-terminal end of the molecule [Woolley, 1984]. The enzyme first reduces a collagen molecule to two smaller triple helices which are not stable at body temperature and are subsequently denatured to random coiled polypeptides. These polypeptides are further degraded by proteases into amino acids and short peptides that are metabolized through normal metabolic pathways [Nimni & Harkness, 1988].

Physical Dimension

The physical dimension of a template defines the boundary of regeneration. Thus, the size of the collagen template should match the tissue defect to be repaired. A properly sized meniscal substitute has been found to function better than a substitute which mismatches the physical dimension of the host meniscus [Sommerlath et al., 1991]. For a porous, elastic matrix such as the one designed from collagen for meniscal tissue repair, the shape of the meniscus is further defined in vivo by the space available between the femoral condyles and tibial plateau within the synovial joint.

Apparent Density

The apparent density is defined as the weight of the dry matrix in a unit volume of matrix. Thus, the apparent density is a direct measure of the empty space which is not occupied by the matrix material per se in the dry state. For example, for a collagen matrix of an apparent density 0.2 g/cm^3, the empty space would be 0.86 cm^3 for a 1 cm^3 total space occupied by the matrix, taking the density of collagen to be 1.41 g/cm^3. The apparent density is also directly related to the mechanical strength of a matrix. In weight-bearing applications, the apparent density has to be optimized such that the mechanical properties are not compromised for the intended function of the implant as described in the mechanical properties section.

Pore Structure

The dimension of a mammalian fibrogenic cell body is in the order of 10–50 μm, depending on the substrate to which the cell adheres [Folkman & Moscona, 1978]. In order for cells to infiltrate into the interstitial space of a matrix, the majority of the pores must be significantly larger than the dimension of a cell such that both the cell and its cellular processes can easily enter the interstitial space. In a number of studies using collagen-based matrices for tissue regeneration, it has been found that pore size plays an important role in the effectiveness of the collagen matrix to induce host tissue regeneration [Chvapil, 1982; Dagalailis et al., 1980]. It was suggested that pore size in the range of 100–400 μm was optimal for tissue regeneration. Similar observations were also found to be true for porous metal implants in total hip replacement [Cook et al., 1991]. The question of interconnecting pores may not be a critical issue in a collagen template as collagenases are synthesized by most *inflammatory cells* during wound healing and remodeling processes. The interporous membranes which exist in the noninterconnecting pores should be digested as part of resorption and wound healing processes.

Mechanical Property

In designing a resorbable collagen implant for weight-bearing applications, not only the initial mechanical strength is important, but the gradual strength reduction of the partially resorbed template has to be compensated by the strength increase from the regenerated tissue such that at any given time the total mechanical properties of the template are maintained. In order to accomplish this goal, one must first be certain that the initial mechanical properties are adequate for supporting the weight-bearing application. For example, compressing the implant with multiple body weights should not cause fraying of the collagen matrix material. It is also of particular importance to design an implant having an adequate and consistent suture pullout strength in order to reduce the incidence of detachment of the implant from the host tissue. The suture pullout strength is also important during surgical procedures as the lack of suture pull strength may result in retrieval and reimplantation of the template. In meniscal tissue repair the suture pullout strength of 1 kg has been found to be adequate for arthroscopically assisted surgery in simulated placement procedures in human cadaver knees, and this suture pullout strength should be maintained as the minimal strength required for this particular application.

Hydrophilicity

Hydration of an implant facilitates nutrient diffusion. The extent of hydration would also provide information on the space available for tissue ingrowth. The porous collagen matrix is highly hydrophilic and therefore facilitates cellular ingrowth. The biomechanical properties of the hydrophilic collagen matrix such as fluid outflow under stress, fluid inflow in the absence of stress, and the resiliency for shock absorption are the properties also found in the weight-bearing cartilagenous tissues.

Permeability

The permeability of ions and macromolecules is of primary importance in tissues that do not rely on vascular transport of nutrients to the end organs. The diffusion of nutrients into the interstitial space ensures the survival of the cells and their continued ability of growth and synthesis of tissue specific extracellular matrix. Generally, the permeability of a macromolecule the size of bovine serum albumin (MW 67,000) can be used as a guideline for probing accessibility of the interstitial space of a collagen template [Li et al., 1994].

In Vivo Stability

As stated above, the rate of template resorption and the rate of new tissue regeneration have to be balanced so that the adequate mechanical properties are maintained at all times. The rate of in vivo resorption of a collagen-based implant can be controlled by controlling the density of the implant and the extent of intermolecular crosslinking. The lower the density, the greater the interstitial space and generally the larger the pores for cell infiltration, leading to a higher rate of matrix degradation. Control of intermolecular crosslinking can be accomplished by using bifunctional crosslinking agents under conditions that do not denature the collagen. Glutaraldehyde, formaldehyde, adipyl chloride, hexamethylene diisocyanate, and carbodiimides are among the many agents used in crosslinking the collagen-based implants. Crosslinking can also be achieved through vapor phase of a crosslinking agent. The vapor phase crosslinking is effective using crosslinking agents of high vapor pressures such as formaldehyde. The vapor crosslinking is particularly useful for thick implants of vapor permeable dense fibers where crosslinking in solution produces nonuniform crosslinking. The shrinkage temperature of the crosslinked matrix has been used as a guide for in vivo stability of a collagen implant [Li, 1988]. The temperature of shrinkage of collagen fibers measures the transition of the collagen molecules from the triple helix to a random coil conformation. This temperature depends on the number of intermolecular crosslinks formed by chemical means. Generally, the higher the number of intermolecular crosslinks, the higher the thermal shrinkage temperature and more stable the material in vivo.

Another method that has been frequently used in assessing the in vivo stability of a collagen-based implant is to conduct an in vitro collagenase digestion of a collagen implant. Bacterial collagenase is generally used in this application. The action of bacterial collagenase on collagen is different from that of mammalian collagenase [Woolley, 1984]. In addition, the enzymatic activity used in in vitro studies is arbitrarily defined. Thus, the data generated from the bacterial collagenase should be viewed with caution. The bacterial collagenase digestion studies, however, are useful in comparing a prototype with a collagen material of known rate of in vivo resorption.

Each of the above parameters should be considered in designing a resorbable implant. The interdependency of the parameters must also be balanced for maximal efficacy of the implant.

In summary, biomedical applications of collagen have entered a new era in the past decade. The potential use of collagen materials in medicine has increasingly been appreciated as the science and technology advances. To date, collagen-based materials have been used for many tissue and organ repair and regeneration applications. A complete historical survey of all potential medical applications of collagen is a formidable task, but a selected survey of collagen-based medical products and the research and development activities are summarized in Table 45.6 as a reference.

Defining Terms

Alanine (Ala):   One of the amino acids in collagen molecules.

Allysine: The ϵ-amino group of lysine has been enzymatically modified to an aldehyde group.

Apparent density: Calculated as the weight of the dry collagen matrix per unit volume of matrix.

Arginine (Arg):   One of the amino acids in collagen molecules.

Aspartic acid (Asp):   One of the amino acids in collagen molecules.

Atelocollagen: A collagen molecule without the telopeptides.

Chondroitin sulfate: Sulfated polysaccharide commonly found in cartilages, bone, corea, tendon and skin.

Collagen: A family of fibrous insoluble proteins having a triple helical conformation extending over a major part of the molecule. Glycine is present at every third amino acid in the triple helix and proline and hydroxyproline are required in the triple helix.

Collagenase: A proteolytic enzyme that specifically catalyzes the degradation of collagen molecules.

Dehydrohydroxylysinonorleucine (deH-HLNL):   A covalently crosslinked product between an allysine and a hydroxylysine residues in collagen fibrils.

D spacing: The repeat distance observed in collagen fibrils by electron microscopic and x-ray diffraction methods.

TABLE 45.6 Survey of Collagen-Based Medical Products and Research and Development Activities

Applications	Comments
Hemostasis	Commercial products: Sponge, fiber, and felt forms are used in cardiovascular [Abbott & Austin, 1975]; neurosurgical [Rybock & Long, 1977]; dermatological [Larson, 1988]; ob/gyn [Correll et al., 1985]; orthopedic [Blanche & Chaux, 1988]; oral surgical applications [Stein et al., 1985].
Dermatology	Commercial products: Injectable collagen for soft-tissue augmentation [Webster et al., 1984]. Research and development: Collagen-based wound dressings [Armstrong et al., 1986]; collagen-based artificial skins [Bell et al., 1981; Yannas & Burke, 1981].
Cardiovascular surgery	Commercial products: Collagen-coated and gelatin-coated vascular grafts [JGuidoin et al., 1987; Li 1988]; chemically processed human vein graft [Dardik et al., 1974]; bovine arterial grafts [Sawyer et al., 1977]; porcine heart valves [Angell et al., 1982]; bovine pericardial heart valves [Walker et al., 1983].
Neurosurgery	Research and development: Guiding peripheral nerve regeneration [Archibald et al., 1991; Yannas et al., 1985]; dura replacement material [Collins et al., 1991].
Periodontal and oral surgery	Research and development: Collagen membranes for periodontal ligament regeneration [Blumenthal, 1988]; resorbable oral tissue wound dressings [Ceravalo & Li, 1988]; collagen/hydroxyapatite for augmentation of alveolor ridge [Gongloff & Montgomery, 1985].
Ophthalmology	Commercial products: Collagen corneal shield to facilitate epithelial healing [Ruffini et al., 1989]. Research and development: Collagen shield for drug delivery to the eye [Reidy et al., 1990].
Orthopaedic surgery	Commercial products: Collagen with hydroxyapatite and autogenous bone marrow for bone repair [Hollinger et al., 1989]. Research and development: Collagen matrix for meniscus regeneration [Li et al., 1994]; collagenous material for replacement and regeneration of Achilles tendon [Kato et al., 1991].
Other applications	Research and development: Drug delivery support [Sorensen et al., 1990]; delivery vehicles for growth factors and bioactive macromolecules [Deatherage & Miller, 1987]; collagenous matrix for delivery of cells for tissue and organ regeneration [Bell et al., 1981].

Elastin: One of the proteins in connective tissue. It is highly stable at high temperatures and in chemicals. It also has rubberlike properties.

Fiber: A bundled group of collagen fibrils.

Fibril: A self-assembled group of collagen molecules.

Fibroblast: Any cell from which connective tissue is developed.

Fibrochondrocyte: Type of cells that are associated with special type of cartilage tissues such as meniscus of the knee and intervertebral disc of the spine.

Fibrous long spacing (FLS): One of the polymorphic forms of collagen where the collagen molecules are randomly aligned in either head-to-tail, tail-to-tail, or head-to-head orientation.

Gelatin: A random coiled form (denatured form) of collagen molecules.

Glutamic acid (Glu): One of the amino acids in collagen molecules.

Glycine (Gly): One of the amino acids in collagen molecules having the simplest structure.

Glycoprotein: A compound consisting of a carbohydrate and protein. The carbohydrate is generally hexosamine, an amino sugar.

Glycosaminoglycan (GAG): A polymerized sugar (see polysaccharide) commonly found in various connective tissues.

Helical pitch: Repeating distance within a single polypeptide chain in a collagen molecule.

Hemostat: Device or medicine which arrests the flow of blood.

Hydrophilicity: The tendency to attract and hold water.

Hydrophobicity: The tendency to repel or avoid contact with water. Substances generally are nonpolar in character, such as lipids and nonpolar amino acids.

Hydroxylysine (Hyl): One of the amino acids in collagen molecules.

Hydroxyproline (Hyp): One of the amino acids uniquely present in collagen molecules.

Inflammatory cell: Cells associated with the succession of changes which occur in living tissue when it is injured. These include macrophages, polymorphonuclear leukocytes, and lymphocytes.

Intermolecular crosslink: Covalent bonds formed in vivo between a side group of one molecule and a side group of another molecule; covalent bonds formed between a side group of one molecule and one end of a bifunctional agent and between a side group of a second molecule and the other end of a bifunctional agent.

Intrafibrillar volume: The volume of a fibril excluding the volume occupied by the collagen molecule.

In vitro: In glass, as in a test tube. An in vitro test is one done in the laboratory, usually involving isolated tissues, organs, or cells.

In vivo: In the living body or organism. A test performed in a living organism.

Isoelectric point: Generally used to refer to a particular pH of a protein solution. At this pH, there is no net electric charge on the molecule.

Isoleucine (Ile):   One of the amino acids in collagen molecules.

Leucine (Leu):   One of the amino acids in collagen molecules.

Lipid: Any one of a group of fats or fat-like substances, characterized by their insolubility in water and solubility in fat solvents such as alcohol, ether, and chloroform.

Lysine (Lys):   One of the amino acids in collagen molecules.

Meniscus: A C-shaped fibrocartilage anatomically located between the femoral condyles and tibial plateau providing stability and shock absorption and assisting in lubrication of the knee joint.

Macrophage: Cells of the reticuloendothelial system having the ability to phagocytose particulate substances and to store vital dyes and other colloidal substances. They are found in loose connective tissues and various organs of the body.

Mycobacterium: A genus of acid-fast organisms belonging to the Mycobacteriaceae which includes the causative organisms of tuberculosis and leprosy. They are slender, nonmotile, gram-positive rods and do not produce spores or capsules.

Osteoarthritis: A chronic disease involving the joint, especially those bearing the weight, characterized by destruction of articular cartilage, overgrown of bone with impaired function.

Permeability: The space within a collagen matrix, excluding the space occupied by collagen molecules, which is accessible to a given size of molecule.

Pepsin: A proteolytic enzyme commonly found in the gastric juice. It is formed by the chief cells of gastric glands and produces maximum activity at a pH of 1.5–2.0.

Phenolalanine (Phe):   One of the amino acids in collagen molecules.

Platelet: A round or oval disk, 2 to 4 μm in diameter, found in the blood of vertebrates. Platelets contain no hemoglobin.

Polydioxanone: A synthetic polymer formed from dioxanone monomers which degrades by hydrolysis.

Polyglycolic acid (PGA):   A synthetic polymer formed from glycolic acid monomers which degrades by hydrolysis.

Polylactic acid (PLA):   A synthetic polymer formed from lactic acid monomers which degrades by hydrolysis.

Polymorphism: Different types of aggregated states of the collagen molecules.

Polymorphonuclear leukocyte: A white blood cell which possesses a nucleus composed of two or more lobes or parts; a granulocyte (neutrophil, eosinophil, basophil).

Polypeptide: Polymerized amino acid molecules formed by enzymatically regulated stepwise polymerization in vivo between the carboxyl group of one amino acid and the amino group of a second amino acid.

Polysaccharide: Polymerized sugar molecules found in tissues as lubricant (synovial fluid) or cement (between osteons, tooth root attachment) or complexed with proteins such as glycoproteins or proteoglycans.

Proline (Pro):   One of the amino acids commonly occurring in collagen molecules.

Proteolytic enzyme: Enzymes which catalyze the breakdown of native proteins.

Resorbable collagen: Collagen which can be biodegraded in vivo.

Salt-linkage: An electrostatic bond formed between a negative charge group and a positive charge group in collagen molecules and fibrils.

Segment-long-spacing (SLS):   One of the polymorphic forms of collagen where all heads of collagen molecules are aligned in parallel.

Soluble collagen: Collagen molecules that can be extracted with salts and dilute acids. Soluble collagen molecules contain the telopeptides.

Telopeptide: The two short nontriple helical peptide segments located at the ends of collagen molecules.

Valine (Val):   One of the amino acids in collagen molecules.

References

Abbott WM, Austin WG. 1975. Surgery 78:723.

Altman R, Li ST. 1990. Int J Oral Implantol 7:75.

Angell WW, Angell JD, Kosek JC. 1982. 83:493.

Archibald SJ, Krarup C, Shefner J, et al. 1991. J Comp Neurol 306:685.

Armstrong RB, Nichols J, Pachance J. 1986. Arch Dermatol 122:546.

Arnoczky SP, Warren RF. 1982. Am J Sports Med 10:90.

Baily AJ, Rhodes DN. 1964. Radiation Res 22:606–621.

Bear RS. 1952. Adv Prot Chem 7:69–160.

Bell E, Ehrlich HP, Buttle DJ, et al. 1981. Science 211:1042.

Blanche C, Chaux A. 1988. Int Surg 73:42.

Blumenthal NM. 1988. J Periodontol 59:830.

Bruck SD. 1991. J Long-Term Effects of Med. Implants 1:89.

Ceravolo F, Li ST. 1988. Int J Oral Implantol 4:15.

Chvapil M. 1982. J Biomed Mater Res 16:245.

Collins RL, Christiansen D, Zazanis GA, et al. 1991. J Biomed Mater Res 25:267.

Comper WD, Veis A. 1977. Biopolymers 16:2134.

Cook SD, Thomas KA, Dalton JE, et al. 1991. Trans Orthop Res Soc 16:550.

Correll JT, Prentice HR, Wise RC. 1985. Surg Gynecol Obstet 81:585.

Dagalailis N, Flink J, Stasikalis P, et al. 1980. J Biomed Mater Res 14:511.

Daly CH. 1966. The Biomechanical Characteristics of Human Skin, Ph.D. thesis, University of Strathclyde, Scotland.

Dardik H, Veith FJ, Spreyregen S, et al. 1974. Ann Surg 180:144.

Deatherage JR, Miller EJ. 1987. Collagen Rel Res 7:225.

Eastoe JE. 1967. Composition of collagen and allied proteins. In GN Ramachadran (ed), Treatise on Collagen, pp1–72, New York, Academic Press.

Folkman J, Moscona A. 1978. Nature 273:345.

Fraenkel-Conrat H, Olcott HS. 1945. J Biol Chem 161:259.

Fraser RDB, MacRae TP, Miller A, et al. 1983. J Mol Biol 167:497.

Fung YC. 1993. Biomechanics, Mechanical Properties of Living Tissues, 2d ed, Berlin, New York, Springer-Verlag.

Goldstein JD, Tria AJ, Zawadsky JP, et al. 1989. J Bone Joint Surg 71A:1183.

Gongloff RK, Montgomery CK. 1985. J Oral Maxillofac Surg 43:570.

Green RW, Ang KP, Lam LC. 1953. Biochem J 54:181.

Guidon R, Marcean D, Rao TJ, et al. 1987. Biomaterials 8:433–441.

Hodge AJ, Petruska JA. 1963. Recent studies with the electron microscope on the ordered aggregates of the tropocollagen molecule. In GN Ramachandran (ed), Aspects of Proteins Structure, pp 289–300, New York, Academic Press.

Hofmann H, Kuhn K. 1981. Statistical analysis of collagen sequences with regard to fibril assembly and evolution. In M Balaban, JL Sussman, W Traub, et al. (eds), Structural Aspects of Recognition and Assembly in Biological Macromolecules, pp 403–425, Malabann ISS, PA.

Hollinger J, Mark DE, Bach DE, et al. 1989. J Oral Maxillofac Surg 47:1182.

Jaffe R, Deykin DJ. 1974. Clin Invest 53:875.

Kato YP, Dunn MG, Zawadsky JP, et al. 1991. J Bone Joint Surg 73A:561.

Katz EP, Li ST. 1972. Biochem Biophys Res Commun 3:1368.

Katz EP, Li ST. 1973a. J Mol Biol 73:351.

Katz EP, Li ST. 1973b. J Mol Biol 80:1.

Katz EP, Li ST. 1981. The molecular packing of type I collagen fibrils. In A Veis (ed), The Chemistry and Biology of Mineralized Connective Tissues, pp 101–105, North Holland, Elsevier.

Kleinman HK, Klebe RJ, Martin GR. 1981. J Cell Biol 88:473.

Larson PO. 1988. J Dermatol Surg Oncol 14:23.

Li ST. 1988. Collagen and vascular prosthesis. In ME Nimni (ed), Collagen, vol 3, pp 253–271, Boca Raton, Fla, CRC Press.

Li, ST. 1990. U.S. Patent 4,963,146.

Li ST, Archibald SJ, Krarup C, et al. 1990. Poly Mater Sci Eng 62:575. 582.

Li ST, Archibald SJ, Krarup C, et al. 1991. The development of collagen nerve guiding conduits that promote peripheral nerve regeneration. In CG Gebelein (ed), Biotechnology and Polymers, pp 282–293, New York, Plenum Press.

Li ST, Golub E, Katz EP. 1975. J Mol Biol 98:835.

Li ST, Katz EP. 1976. Biopolymers 15:1439.

Li ST, Stone KR. 1993. U.S. Patent 5,263,984.

Li ST, Sullman S, Katz EP. 1981. In A Veis (ed), The Chemistry and Biology of Mineralized Tissues, pp 123–127, North Holland, Elsevier.

Li ST, Yuen D, Li PC, et al. 1994. Mat Res Soc Symp Proc 331:25.

Ma S, Chen G, Reddi AH. 1990. Ann NY Acad Sci 580:524.

Miller A. 1976. In GN Ramachandran, H Reddi (eds), Biochemistry of Collagen, pp 85–136, New York, Plenum Press.

Miller EJ. 1984. Chemistry of the collagens and their distribution. In KA Piez, AH Reddi (eds), Extracellular Matrix Biochemistry, pp 41–82, New York, Elsevier.

Montesano R, Mouron P, Amherdt M, et al. 1983. J Cell Biol 97:935.

Nimni ME (ed). 1988. The Collagen, vols 1, 2, 3, Boca Raton, Fla, CRC Press.

Nimni ME, Harkness RD. 1988. Molecular structures and functions of collagen. In ME Nimni (ed), Collagen, vol 1, pp 1–78, Boca Raton, Fla, CRC Press.

Park JB, Lakes RS. 1992. Biomaterials: An Introduction, 2d ed, New York, London, Plenum.

Piez KA. 1984. Molecular and aggregate structures of the collagens. In KA Piez, AH Reddy (eds), Extracellular Matrix Biochemistry, pp 1–35, New York, Elsevier.

Ramachandran GN. 1967. Structure of collagen at the molecular level. In GN Ramachandran (ed), Treatise on Collagen, vol 1, pp 103–183, New York, Academic Press.

Reidy JJ, Limberg M, Kaufman HE. 1990. Am Acad Ophthal 97:1201.

Rich A, Crick FHC. 1961. J Mol Biol 3:483.

Rigby BJ, Hiraci N, Spikes JD, et al. 1959. J Gen Physiol 43:265.

Ruffini JJ, Aquavella JV, LoCascio JA. 1989. Ophthal Surg 20:21.

Rybock JD, Long DM. 1977. J Neurosurg 46:501.

Sawyer PN, Stanczewski B, Kirschenbaum D. 1977. Artif Organs 1:83.

Schimpf WC, Rodriquez F. 1976. Ind Eng Chem Prod Res Rev 16:90.

Shapiro F, Glimcher MJ. 1980. Clin Orthop 147:287.

Silbermann M. 1990. Biomaterials 11:47.

Sommerlath K, Gallino M, Gillquist J. 1991. Trans Ortop Res Soc 16:375.

Sorensen TS, Sorensen AI, Merser S. 1990. Acta Orthop Scand 61:353.

Stein MD, Salkin LM, Freedman AL, et al. 1985. J Periodontol 56:35.

Stenzl KH, Miyata T, Rubin AL. 1974. Annu Rev Biophys Bioeng 3:231.

Tiffit JT. 1980. The organic matrix of bone tissue. In MR Urist (ed), Fundamental and Clinical Bone Physiology, chap 3, Philadelphia, Lippincott.

Timpl R. 1982. Methods Enzymol 82:472.

Tripartite Sub-committee on Medical Devices. 1986. Tripartite guidance for medical devices. Department of Health and Human Resources,

Van der Rest M, Dublet B, Champliaud MF. 1990. Biomaterials 11:28.

Walker WE, Duncan JM, Frazier OH, et al. 1983. J Thorac Cardiovasc Surg 86:570.

Wang C-L, Miyata T, Weksler B, et al. 1978. Biochem Biophys Acta 544:568.

Webster RC, Kattner, MD, Smith RC. 1984. Arch Otolaryngol 110:652.

Wilner GD, Nossel HL, Leroy EC. 1968. J Clin Invest 47:2608.

Woolley DE. 1984. Mammalian collagenases. In KA Piez, AH Reddi (eds), Extracellular Matrix Biochemistry, New York, Elsevier.

Yamuchi M, Katz EP, Mechanic GL. 1986. Am Chem Soc 25:4907.

Yannas IV, Burke JF. 1981. J Biomed Mater Res 14:65.

Yannas IV, Orgill DP, Silver J, et al. 1985. Poly Mater Sci Eng 53:216.

46

Soft Tissue Replacements

K. B. Chandran
University of Iowa

S. W. Shalaby
Clemson University

46.1 Blood-Interfacing Implants

K. B. Chandran

Blood comes in contact with foreign materials for a short term in extracorporeal devices such as *dialysers, blood oxygenators,* ventricular assist devices, and *catheters.* Long-term vascular implants include heart valve prostheses, *vascular grafts,* and *cardiac pacemakers.* In this chapter, we will be concerned with development of biomaterials for long-term implants, specifically for heart valve prostheses, total artificial heart (TAH), and vascular grafts. The primary requirements for biomaterials for long-term implants are biocompatibility, nontoxicity, and durability. Furthermore, the material should be nonirritating to the tissue, resistant to *platelet* and *thrombus* deposition, and nondegradable in the physiological environment and must neither absorb blood constituents nor release foreign substances into the blood stream [Shim & Lenker, 1988]. In addition, design considerations include that the implant should mimic the function of the organ that it replaces without interfering with the surrounding anatomical structures and must be of suitable size and weight. The biomaterials chosen must be easily available, inexpensive, easily machinable, and sterilizable and must have a long storage life. The selection of material will also be dictated by the strength requirement for the implant being made. For example, an artificial heart valve prosthesis must open and close on an average once every second. The biomaterial chosen must be such that the valve is durable and will not fail under *fatigue stress* after implantation in a patient. As sophisticated measurement techniques and detailed computational analyses become available with the advent of supercomputers, our knowledge about the complex dynamics of the functioning of the implants is increasing. Improvements in design based on such knowledge and improvements in selection and manufacture of biomaterials will minimize problems associated with blood-interfacing implants and significantly improve the quality of life of patients with implants. We will discuss the development of biomaterials for the blood-interfacing implants, problems associated with the same, and future directions on the development of such implants.

Heart Valve Prostheses

Attempts at replacing diseased natural human valves with prostheses began more than three decades ago. The details of the development of heart valve prostheses, design considerations, in vitro functional testing, and durability testing of valve prototypes can be found in several monographs [Chandran, 1992; Shim & Lenker, 1988]. The heart valve prostheses can be broadly classified into *mechanical prostheses* (made out of nonbiologic material) and *bioprostheses* (made out of biologic tissue). Currently available mechanical and tissue heart valve prostheses in the United States are listed in Table 46.1.

Mechanical Heart Valves

Lefrak and Starr [1970] describe the early history of mechanical valve development. The initial designs of mechanical valves were of centrally occluding caged ball or caged disc type. The Starr-Edwards caged ball prostheses, commercially available at the present time, were successfully implanted in the mitral position in 1961. The caged ball prosthesis is made of a polished CoCr alloy (*Stellite 21*) cage and a silicone rubber ball (Silastic®) which contains 2 percent by weight barium sulfate for *radiopacity* (Fig. 46.1). The valve *sewing rings* use a silicone rubber insert under a knitted composite polytetrafluorethylene (PTFE -*Teflon*) and *polypropylene* cloth. Even though these valves have proven to be durable, the centrally occluding design of the valve results in a larger pressure drop in flow across the valve and higher *turbulent stresses* distal to the valve compared to other designs of mechanical valve prostheses [Chandran et al., 1983; Yoganathan et al., 1979a, 1979b, 1986]. The relatively large profile design of caged ball or disc construction also increases the possibility of interference with anatomic structures after implantation. The *tilting disc valves,* with improved hemodynamic characteristics, were introduced in late 1960s. The initial design consisted of a polyacetal (*Delrin*) disc with a Teflon sewing ring. Delrin acetal resins are thermoplastic polymers manufactured by the polymerization of *formaldehyde* [Shim & Lenker, 1988]. Even though Delrin exhibited excellent wear resistance and mechanical strength with satisfactory performance after more than 20 years of implantation, it also swelled when exposed to humid environment such as *autoclaving* and blood contact. To avoid design and manufacturing difficulties due to the swelling phenomenon, the Delrin disc was soon replaced by a *pyrolytic carbon* disc, which has become the preferred material for mechanical valve prostheses occluders to date. Pyrolytic carbons are formed in a fluidized bed by pyrolysis of a gaseous hydrocarbon in the range of 1000–2400°C. For biomedical applications, carbon is deposited onto performed polycrystalline graphite substrate at temperatures below 1500°C (low-temperature isotropic pyrolytic carbon, *LTI* Pyrolite). Increase in strength and wear resistance are obtained by codepositing silicone (up to 10% by weight) with carbon in applications for heart valve prostheses. The pyrolytic carbon discs exhibit excellent blood compatibil-

TABLE 46.1 Heart Valve Prostheses Developed and Currently Available in the United States

Type	Name	Manufacturer
Caged ball	Starr-Edwards, Irvine, CA	Baxter Health Care, Irvine, CA
Double caged ball	Smelloff-Cutter	Sutter Biomedical, San Diego, CA
Tilting disc	Medtronic-Hall	Medtronic Blood Systems, Minneapolis, MN
	Lillehei-Kaster, Omni-Science	Medical Inc., Inner Grove Heights, MN
Bileaflet	St. Jude Medical	St. Jude Medical, Inc., St. Paul, MN
	Carbomedics	Carbomedics, Austin, TX
	Edwards-Tekna*	Baxter Health Care, Irvine, CA
Porcine bioprostheses	Carpentier-Edwards Standard	Baxter Health Care, Irvine, CA
	Hancock Standard, Hancock modified orifice, Hancock I	Medtronic Blood Systems, Santa Ana, CA
Pericardial bioprostheses	Carpentier-Edwards	Baxter Health Care, Irvine, CA

*FDA approval pending.

ity as well as wear and fatigue resistance. The guiding *struts* of tilting disc valves are made of *titanium* or CoCr alloy (*Haynes 25* and Stellite 21). The CoCr-based alloys and pure titanium and its alloy (Ti6A14V) exhibit excellent mechanical properties as well as resistance to corrosion and thrombus deposition. Tilting disc valve prostheses with leaflet made of carbon and Delrin composite (Jomed Implantate—Fig. 46.2*a*) and *ultra-high-molecular-weight polyethylene* (Chitra valve—Fig. 46.2*b*) are also currently undergoing clinical trials in Europe and India, respectively. The advantages of *leaflets* with relatively more flexibility compared to pyrolytic carbon leaflets are discussed in Chandran et al. [1994*a*].

In the late 1970s, a bileaflet design was introduced for mechanical valve prostheses, and several different bileaflet models are being intro duced into the market today. The leaflets and the housing of the bileaflet valves are made of pyrolytic carbon, and the bileaflet valves show im-

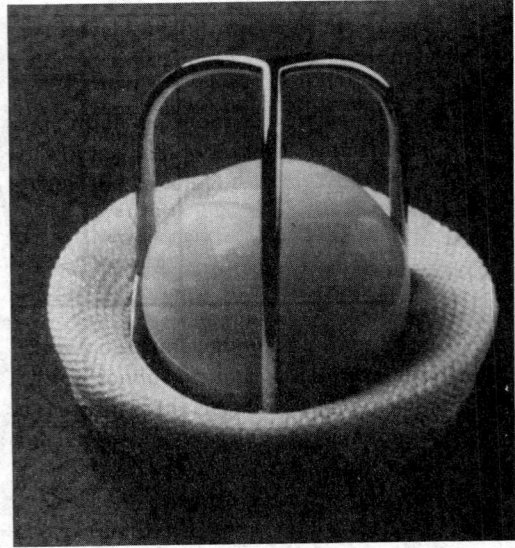

FIGURE 46.1 A caged-ball heart valve prosthesis (courtesy of Baxter Health Care, Irvine, CA).

proved hemodynamic characteristics especially in smaller sizes compared to tilting disc valves. A typical bileaflet valve is shown in Fig. 46.3. The biomaterials used in commercially available mechanical and bioprosthetic heart valves are included in Table 46.2.

In spite of the desirable characteristics of the biomaterials used in the heart valve prostheses, problems with *thromboembolic* complications are significant with implanted valves, and patients

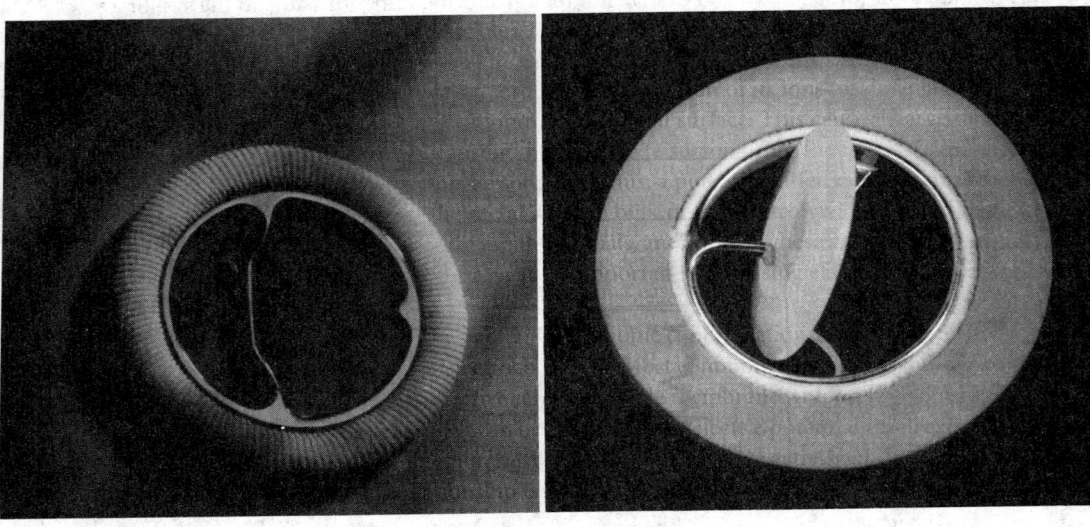

(a)   *(b)*

FIGURE 46.2 Photographs of typical tilting disc valve prostheses with leaflets made of novel biomaterial: (*a*) Jomed Implantate prosthesis with the occluder made of carbon/Delrin composite (courtesy of Jomed Implanatate, Hechingen, Germany); (*b*) Chitra tilting disc valve prosthesis with the occluder made of ultra-high-molecular-weight polyethylene (courtesy of Sree Chitra Tirunal Institute for Medical Sciences and Technology, India).

with mechanical valves are under long-term anticoagulant therapy. The mechanical stresses induced by the flow of blood across the valve prostheses have been linked to the lysis and activation of *formed elements in blood* (red blood cells, white blood cells, and platelets) resulting in the deposition of thrombi in regions with relative stasis in the vicinity of the prostheses. Numerous in vitro studies with mechanical valves in pulse duplicators simulating physiologic flow have been reported in the literature and have been reviewed by Chandran [1988] and Dellsperger and Chandran [1991]. Such studies have included measurement of velocity profiles and turbulent stresses distal to the valve due to flow across the valve. The aim of these studies has been the correlation of regions prone to thrombus deposition and tissue overgrowth with explanted valves and the experimentally

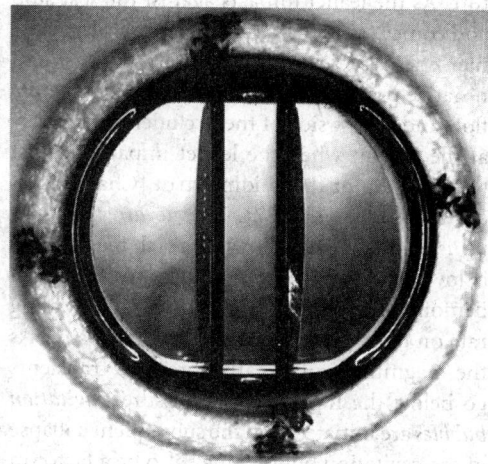

FIGURE 46.3 A St. Jude Medical bileaflet valve with pyrolytic carbon leaflets and housing (courtesy of St. Jude Medical, Inc., St. Paul, MN).

measured bulk turbulent shear stresses as well as regions of relative stasis. Despite improvements in design of the prostheses to afford a centralized flow with minimal flow disturbances and fluid mechanical stresses, the problems with thrombus deposition remain significant.

Reports of strut failure, material *erosion,* and leaflet escapes as well as *pitting* and erosion of valve leaflets and housing have resulted in numerous investigations of the *closing dynamics* of mechanical valves. The dynamics of the leaflet motion and its impact with the valve housing or seat stop is very complex, and a number of experimental and numerical studies have appeared recently in the litera-

TABLE 46.2 Biomaterial Used in Heart Valve Prostheses

Type	Component	Biomaterial
Caged ball	Ball/occluder	Hollow Stellite 21/silastic
	Cage	Stellite 21/titanium
	Suture ring	Silicone rubber insert under knitted composite Teflon/polypropylene cloth
Tilting disc	Leaflet	Delrin; pyrolytic carbon (carbon deposited on graphite substrate); carbon/Delrin composite; ultra-high-molecular polyethylene (UHMPE)
	Housing/strut	Haynes 25/Titanium
	Suture ring	Teflon/Dacron
Bileaflet	Leaflets	Pyrolytic carbon
	Housing	Pyrolytic carbon
	Suture ring	Double-velour Dacron
Porcine bioprostheses	Leaflets	Porcine aortic valve fixed by stabilized gluteraldehyde
	Stents	Polypropylene stent covered with Dacron; lightweight Elgiloy wire covered with porous knitted Teflon cloth
	Suture ring	Dacron; soft silicone rubber insert covered with porous, seamless Teflon cloth
Pericardial bioprostheses	Leaflets	Porcine pericardial tissue fixed by stabilized gluteraldehyde before leaflets are sewn to the valve stents
	Stents	Polypropylene stent covered with Dacron; Elgiloy wire and nylon support band covered with polyester and Teflon cloth
	Suture ring	PTFE fabric over silicone rubber filter

Source: Dellsperger and Chandran [1988], Shim and Lenker [1988].

ture. As the leaflet impacts against the seat stop and comes to rest instantaneously, a water hammer effect is the result with high positive and negative pressure transients present on the outflow and inflow side of the occluder respectively at the instant when the leaflet impacts against the seat stop or the guiding strut [Chandran et al., 1994a; Leuer, 1987]. The *negative pressure transients* have been shown to reach magnitudes below the *liquid vapor pressure* and have been demonstrated to be a function of the loading rate on the leaflet inducing the valve closure. As the magnitudes of negative pressure transients go below the liquid vapor pressure, *cavitation bubbles* are initiated, and the subsequent collapse of the cavitation bubbles may also be a factor in the lysis of red blood cells, platelets, and *valvular structures* [Chandran et al., 1994a; Lee et al., 1994]. Typical cavitation bubbles visualized in an in vitro study with tilting disc and bileaflet valves are shown in Fig. 46.4. A correlation is also observed between the region where cavitation bubbles are present, even though for a period of time less than a millisecond after valve closure, and sites of pitting and erosion reported in the pyrolytic carbon material in the valve housing and on the leaflets with explanted valves [Kafesjian, 1994] as well as those used in total artificial hearts [Leuer, 1987]. An electron micrograph of pitting and erosion observed in the pyrolytic carbon valve housing of an explanted bileaflet mechanical valve is shown in Fig. 46.5. The pressure transients at valve closure are substantially smaller in mechanical valves with a flexible occluder, and leaflets made of ultra-high-molecular-weight polyethylene (Fig. 46.2b) may prove to be advantageous based on the closing dynamic analysis [Chandran et al., 1994a]. Detailed analysis of the complex closing dynamics of the leaflets may also be exploited in improving the design of the mechanical valves to minimize problems with structural failure [Cheon & Chandran, 1994].

The pressure distribution on the leaflets and impact forces between the leaflets and guiding struts are also being experimentally measured in order to understand the causes for strut failure [Chandran et al., 1994b, 1994c]. The flow through the clearance between the leaflet and the housing at the instant of valve closure [Lee & Chandran, 1994a, 1994b] and in the fully closed

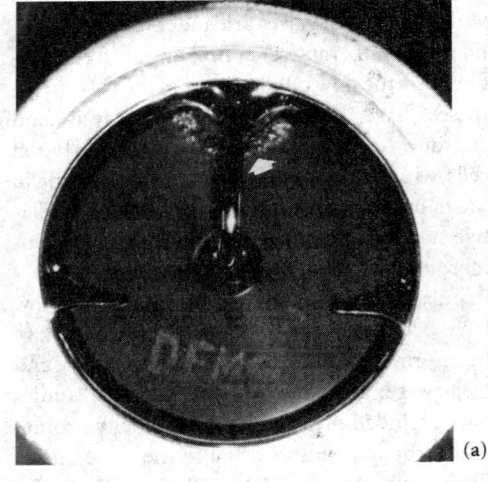

(a)

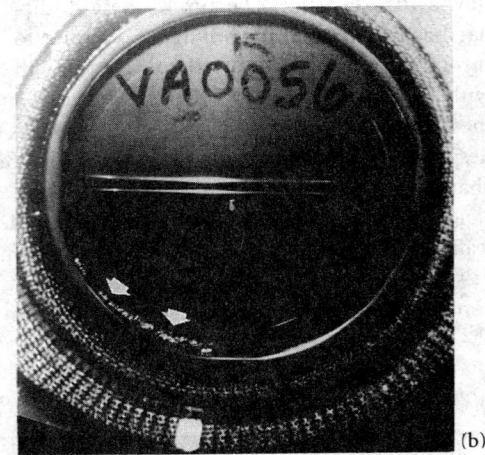

(b)

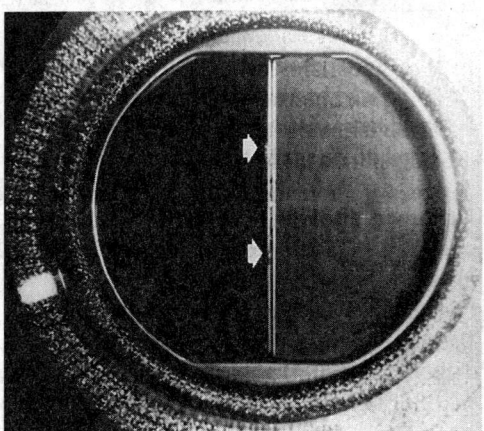

FIGURE 46.4 Cavitation bubbles visualized on the inflow side of the valves *in vitro* [Chandran et al., 1994a]: (a) Medtronic Hall tilting disc valve; (b) Edwards-Duromedics bileaflet valve; (c) Carbomedics bileaflet valve.

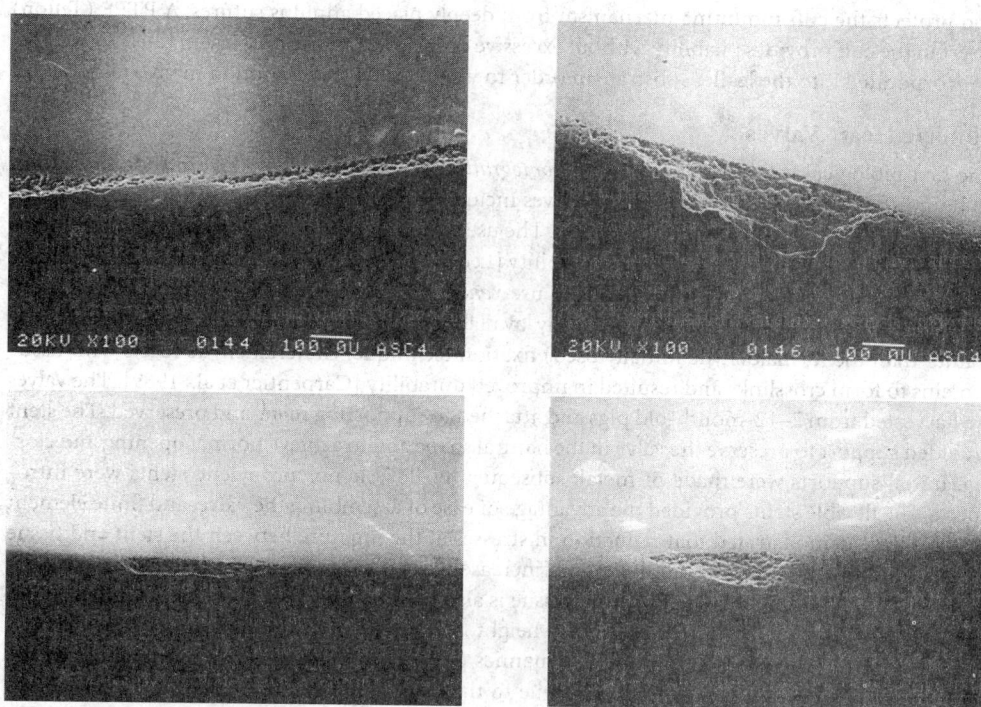

FIGURE 46.5 Photographs showing pitting on pyrolytic carbon surface of a mechanical heart valve (courtesy of Baxter Health Care, Irvine, CA).

position [Reif, 1991], and the resulting wall shear stresses within the clearance are also being suggested as responsible for clinically significant hemolysis and thrombus initiation. Further improvements in the design of the valves based on the closing dynamics as well as improvements in material may result in minimizing thromboembolic complications as well as occasional structural failure with implanted mechanical valves. A recent improvement in the design of mechanical valves that reduces thromboembolic complications is the *ATS valve* (Fig. 46.6) which is of a bileaflet design. An open pivot area in this valve, as opposed to the recessed pivot areas in the previous bileaflet valve designs, shows promise of reduced thrombus deposition in preliminary clinical studies. Further detailed studies on such design changes on the local flow dynamics and valve closing dynamics may prove to be valuable in design improvements aimed at reducing complications with thrombus deposition with implanted valves. The cuff of the ATS valve is made of double polyester (Dacron) velour material to encourage rapid and controlled tissue ingrowth. The cuff is mounted on a rotation ring which surrounds the orifice ring

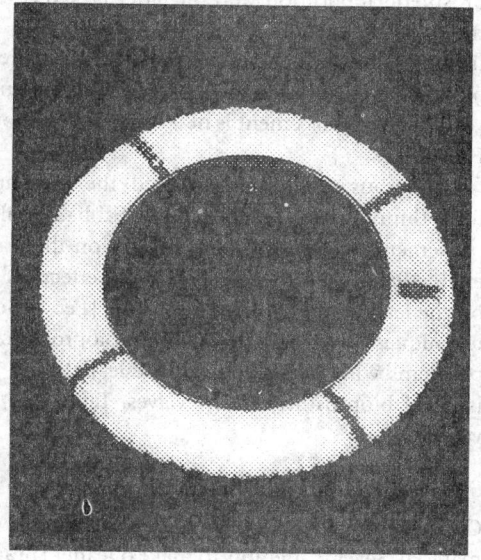

FIGURE 46.6 Photograph of an ATS bileaflet valve with an open pivot design (courtesy of ATS Medical, Inc., St. Paul, MN).

and protects the cuff mounting mechanism from deeply placed annulus sutures. A PTFE (Teflon) insert in the cuff provides pliability without excessive drag on the sutures. Tungsten (20% by weight) is incorporated into the leaflet substrate in order to visualize the leaflet motion in vivo.

Biologic Heart Valves

The first biological valves implanted were *homografts* with valves explanted from cadavers within 48 hours after death. Preservation of the valves included various techniques of sterilization, freeze drying, and immersing in antibiotic solution. The use of homografts is not popular due to problems with long-term durability and limited availability [Lee & Boughner, 1991; Shim & Lenker, 1988]. Attempts were also made in the early 1960s to use *xenografts* (valves made from animal tissue), and porcine bioprostheses became commercially available after the introduction of gluteraldehyde (rather than the formaldehyde initially used) fixation technique. Gluteraldehyde reacts with tissue proteins to form crosslinks and resulted in improved durability [Carpentier et al., 1969]. The valves are harvested from 7–12-month-old pigs and attached to supporting *stents* and preserved. The stent provided support to preserve the valve in the natural shape and to achieve normal opening and closing. Initial supports were made of metal; subsequently, flexible polypropylene stents were introduced. The flexible stents provided the advantage of ease of assembling the valve, and finite element analyses have demonstrated that reduction in stresses at the juncture between the stent and tissue leaflets resulting in increased durability and increased leaflet coaptation area [Hamid et al., 1985; Reis et al., 1971]. Fixed bovine pericardial tissue is also used to construct heart valves in which design characteristics such as orifice area, valve height, and degree of coaptation can be specified and controlled. Thus, the geometry and flow dynamics past *pericardial prostheses* mimic those of the natural human aortic valves more closely. Due to the low-profile design of pericardial prostheses and increased orifice area, these valves are less stenotic compared to porcine bioprostheses especially in smaller sizes [Chandran et al., 1984]. In the currently available bioprostheses, the stents are constructed from polypropylene, *Acetol* homopolymer or copolymer, Elgiloy wire, or titanium. A stainless steel radiopaque marker is also introduced to visualize the valve in vivo. Other biomaterials which have been employed in making the bioprostheses include *fascia lata* tissue as well as human *dura mater* tissue. The former was prone to deterioration and hence unsuitable for bioprosthetic application, and the latter lacked commercial availability. The advantage with bioprostheses is the freedom from thromboembolism and hence avoidance of long-term anticoagulant therapy. These prostheses are preferable in patients who do not tolerate anticoagulants. However, bioprosthetic valves are prone to *calcification* and leaflet tear with an average lifetime of about 10 years before replacement is necessary. Typical porcine and pericardial bioprostheses are included in Fig. 46.7.

Numerous studies have linked the mechanical stresses on the leaflets with calcification, focal thinning, and leaflet failure [Sabbah et al., 1985; Thubrikar et al., 1982*b*], and design improvements to minimize the stresses on the leaflets have been reported in literature [Thubrikar et al., 1982*a*] . Further details on the effects of tissue fixation and mechanical effects of fixation on the leaflets are reported elsewhere [Lee & Boughner, 1991]. Further improvements in fixation techniques as well as in design of the bioprostheses are continually being made in order to minimize problems with calcification of the leaflets and improve the durability and functional characteristics of bioprosthetic heart valves. Table 46.3 summarized the problems associated with heart valves.

Synthetic Heart Valves

Concurrently, efforts are also being made in the development of valve prostheses made of synthetic material. Several attempts to make bileaflet [Braunwald et al., 1960] and trileaflet valves [Gerring et al., 1974; Ghista & Reul, 1977; Hufnagel, 1977; Roe et al., 1958] made of polyurethanes, polyester fabrics, and silicone rubber were not successful due to problems with durability of relatively thin

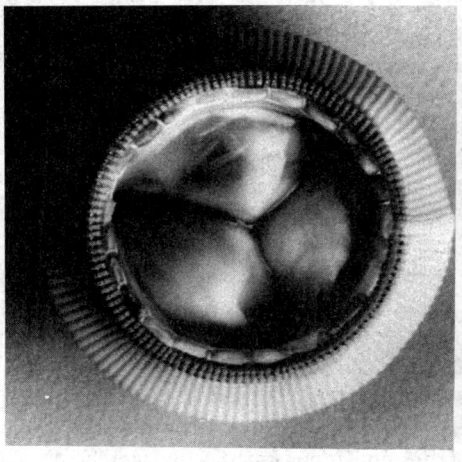
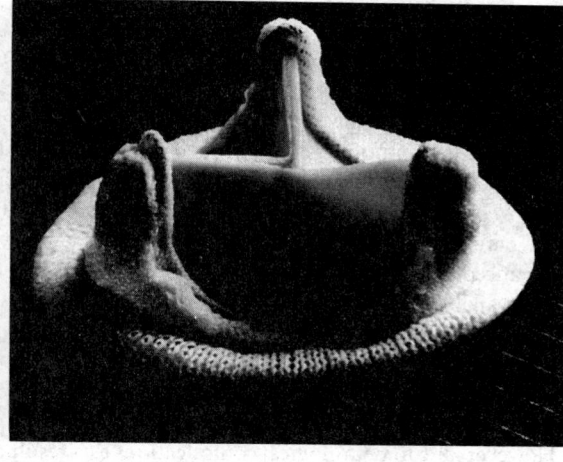

(a)   (b)

FIGURE 46.7 Typical bioprostheses: (*a*) Hancock procine bioprosthesis (courtesy of Medtronic, Inc, Minneapolis, MN); (*b*) Edwards pericardial prosthesis (courtesy of Baxter Health Care, Irvine, CA).

leaflets made of synthetic material. With the advent of the total artificial hearts (TAHs) and *left ventricular assist devices* (LVADs) in the 1980s, an additional impetus to the development of synthetic valves is present. Due to problems with thrombus deposition in the vicinity of the mechanical valves used in the TAH and subsequent stroke episodes in patients with permanent implants, the use of the device is currently restricted as a bridge to transplantation. In such temporary use before a donor heart becomes available (on an average of several weeks), the four mechanical prostheses used in the TAH results in substantial cost. Hence, efforts are being made to replace the mechanical valves with those made with synthetic material. With *vacuum-forming* or *solution-casting* techniques, synthetic valves can be made at a fraction of the cost of mechanical valves, provided their function in a TAH environment for several weeks will be satisfactory. Implantation of synthetic trileaflet valves [Harold et al., 1987; Russel et al., 1980], even more recently, have resulted in limited success due to leaflet failure and calcification. Hemodynamic comparison of vacuum-formed and solution-cast trileaflet valves to currently available bioprostheses have produced satisfactory results [Chandran et al., 1989*a*, 1989*b*]. *Finite element analysis* of synthetic valves can be exploited in design improvements similar to those reported for bioprostheses [Chandran et al., 1991*a*].

TABLE 46.3 Common Problems with Implanted Prosthetic Heart Valves

Mechanical valves
    Thromboembolism
    Structural failure
    Red blood cell and platelet destruction
    Tissue overgrowth
    Damage to endothelial lining
    Paravalvular/perivalvular leakage
    Tearing of sutures
    Infection
Bioprosthetic valves
    Tissue calcification
    Leaflet rupture
    Paravalvular/perivalvular leakage
    Infection

Source: Chandran [1992], Shim and Lenker [1988], Yoganathan et al. [1979*a*].

Total Artificial Hearts (TAHs)

Artificial circulatory support can be broadly classified into two categories. In the first category are those patients who undergo open heart surgery to correct *valvular disorders,* ventricular *aneurysm,* or coronary *artery* disease. In several cases, the heart may not recover sufficiently after surgery to take over the pumping action. In such patients ventricular assist devices are used as extracarporeal devices to maintain circulation until the heart recovers. Other ventricular assist devices include *intra-aortic balloon pumps* as well as *cardiopulmonary* bypass. Within several days or weeks, when the natural heart recovers, these devices will be removed. In the second category are patients with advanced stages of cardiomyopathy who are subjects for heart transplantation. Due to problems in the availability of suitable donor hearts, not all patients with a failed heart are candidates for heart transplantation. For those patients not selected for transplantation, the concept of replacing the natural heart with a total artificial heart has gained attention in the recent years [Akutsu & Kolff, 1958; DeVries & Joyce, 1983; Jarvick, 1981; Kambic & Nose, 1991; Unger, 1989]. A number of attempts at permanent implantation of TAHs with pneumatically powered units were attempted in the 1980s. However, due to neurological complications as a result of thromboembolism, infection, and hematological and renal complications, permanent implantations currently are suspended. If a suitable donor heart is not readily available, TAHs can be used as "bridge to transplantation" for several weeks until a donor heart becomes available.

Electrically driven blood pumps, which can afford tether-free operation within the body unlike pneumatically powered pumps, are currently at various stages of development for long-term use (of more than 2 years). Typical designs of pneumatically driven and electrically powered total artificial hearts under development for long-term implantation are shown in Fig. 46.8. The components of such devices include the blood pump in direct contact with blood, energy converter (from electrical to mechanical energy), variable column compensator, implantable batteries, transcutaneous energy transmission system, and external batteries. The blood pump configuration in these devices ranges from sac, diaphragm, and *pusher plate devices.* Materials used in blood-contacting surfaces in these devices are synthetic polymers (polyurethanes, segmented polyurethanes, *Biomer,* and others). Segmented polyurethane elastomer used in prosthetic ventricles with a thromboresistant additive modifying the polymeric surface have resulted in improved blood compatibility and reduced thromboembolic risk in animal trials [Farrar et al., 1988]. Design considerations include reduction of regions of stagnation of blood within the blood chamber and minimizing the mechanical stresses induced on the formed elements in blood. Apart from the characteristics of these material to withstand repetitive high mechanical stresses and minimize failure due to fatigue, surface interactions with blood is also another crucial factor.

Due to significant problems with thromboembolic complications and subsequent neurological problems with long-term implantation of TAHs in humans, attention has focused on minimizing factors responsible for thrombus deposition. To eliminate crevices formed with the quick connect system, valves sutured in place at the inflow and outflow orifices were offered as an alternative in the Philadelphia heart [Wurzel et al., 1988]. An alternative quick connect system using precision machined components has been demonstrated to reduce valve and connector-associated thrombus formation substantially [Holfert et al., 1987]. Several in vitro studies have been reported in the literature that assess the effect of fluid dynamic stresses on thrombus deposition [Baldwin et al., 1988; Jarvis et al., 1991; Phillips et al., 1979; Tarbell et al., 1986]. These have included flow visualization and laser Doppler anemometry velocity and turbulence measurements within the ventricular chamber as well as in the vicinity of the inflow and outflow orifices. The results of such studies indicate that the flow within the chamber generally has a smooth washout of blood in each pulsatile flow cycle with relatively large turbulent stresses and regions of stasis found near the valves. The thrombus deposition found with implanted TAH in the vicinity of the inflow valves also indicates that the major problems with the working of these devices are still with the flow dynamics across the mechanical valves. Computational flow dynamic analysis within the ventricular chamber may also be exploited to improve the design of the valve chambers and the mechanical valves in order to reduce

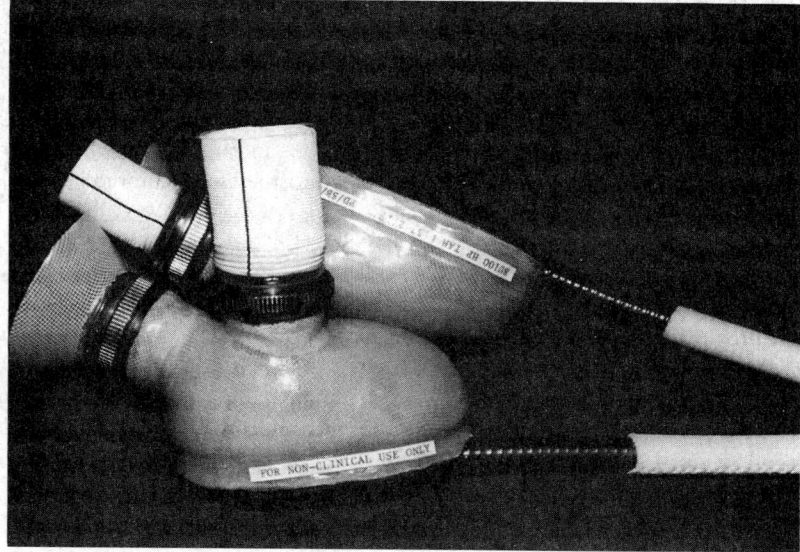

(a)

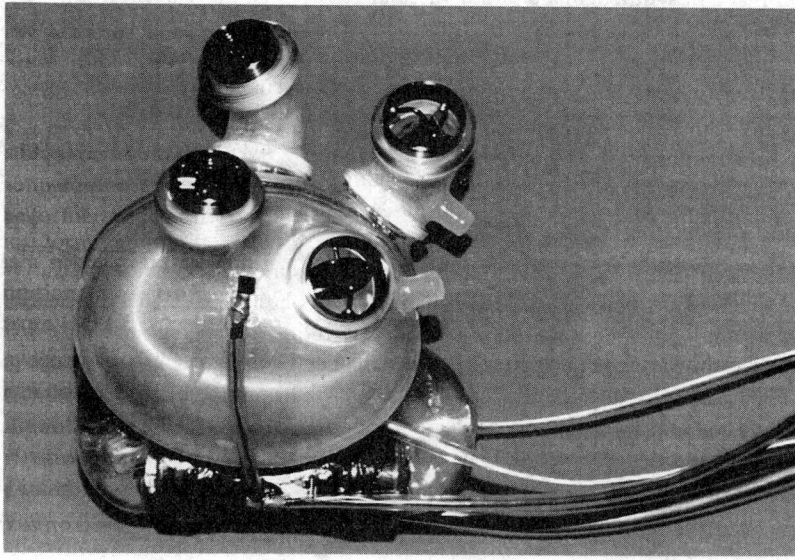

(b)

FIGURE 46.8 Typical prototype designs of total artificial hearts: (*a*) pneumatically powered TAH; (*b*) electrohydraulic blood pump (courtesy of George Pantalos, University of Utah).

the turbulent stresses near the vicinity of the inflow and outflow orifices [Kim et al., 1992]. Structural failure of the mechanical valves initially reported with the TAH may have been the result of increased load on the valves during closure due to the relatively large dp/dt (p is pressure, t is time) at which the TAH was operated. Attempts at reducing the dp/dt during closure of the inflow valves have also been reported with modified designs of the artificial heart driver [Wurzel et al., 1988]. Due to the relatively large dp/dt at which TAHs are operated, there is increased possibility of cavitation bubbles initiation, and subsequent collapse of the bubbles may also be another important reason for thrombus deposition near the mechanical valve at the inflow orifice. Introducing flexible valve chambers and synthetic valves to replace the mechanical valves [Chandran et al., 1991*b*] may prove to be advantageous with respect to cavitation initiation and minimizing thrombus formation.

Vascular Prostheses

In advanced stages of vascular diseases such as *atherosclerosis* and aneurysms, when other treatment modalities fail, replacement of diseased segments with prostheses is a common practice. Vascular prostheses can be classified as given in Table 46.4.

Biological Grafts

Arterial homografts, even though initially used in large scale, resulted in aneurysm formation especially in the proximal suture line [Strandness & Sumner, 1975]. Still a viable alternative is to use the saphenous vein graft from the same patient. Vein grafts have a failure rate of about 20% in 1 year and up to 30% in 5 years after implantation. Vein grafts from the same patients are also unavailable or unsuitable in about 10–30% of the patients [Abbott & Bouchier-Hayes, 1978]. Modified *bovine heterograft* and gluteraldehyde-treated *umbilical cord vein grafts* have also been employed as vascular prostheses with less success compared to autologous vein grafts.

Synthetic Grafts

Prostheses made of synthetic material for vascular replacement have been used for over 40 years. Polymeric materials currently used as implants include *nylon,* polyester, *polytetrafluoroethylene (PTFE),* polypropylene, polyacrylonitrile, and silicone rubber [Park & Lakes, 1992]. However, Dacron (polyethylene terephthalate) and PTFE are more common vascular prostheses material currently available. These materials exhibit the essential qualities for implants—they are being biocompatible, resilient, flexible, durable, and resistant to sterilization and biodegradation. Detailed discussion of the properties, manufacturing techniques, and testing of Dacron prostheses are included in Guidoin and Couture [1991]. Figure 46.9 shows typical vascular grafts currently available for implantation.

Synthetic vascular grafts implanted as large-vessel replacement have achieved a reasonable degree of success. However, in medium- and small-diameter prostheses (less than 6 mm in diameter), loss of *patency* within several months after implantation is more acute. Graft failure due to thrombosis or intimal hyperplasia with thrombosis is primarily responsible in failures within 30 days after implantation, and intimal hyperplasia formation is the reason for failures within 6 months after surgery. Soon after implantation, a layer of *fibrin* and fibrous tissue covers the intimal and outer surface of the prosthesis respectively. A layer of *fibroblasts* replaces the fibrin and is referred to as *neointima.* In the latter stages, *neointimal hyperplasia* formation occurs and ultimately results in the occlusion of the vessels in small-diameter vascular grafts. Attempts are being made to suitably modify the surface characteristics of the prostheses in order to reduce the problems with loss of patency. Studies are also being performed to understand the mechanical stresses induced at the anastomotic

TABLE 46.4   Classification of Vascular Grafts

Grafts	Comments
Biological grafts	
Autograft	Venous (e.g. saphenous vein graft) arterial graft
Allograft (homograft)	Gluteraldehyde treated umbilical cord vein graft
Xenograft (heterograft)	Modified bovine heterograft
Synthetic grafts	
Dacron	Woven, knitted
PTFE	Knitted, expanded
Other	Nylon, etc.

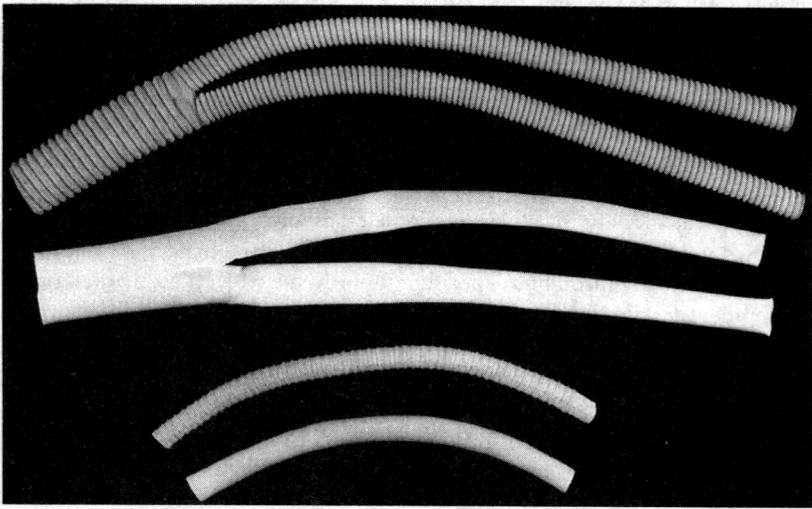

FIGURE 46.9 Photograph of typical vascular grafts made of knitted crimped Dacron (first and third) and PTFE. The top two are bifurcation grafts (courtesy of John Corson, University of Iowa).

region which may result in deposits in the intimal surface and occlusion of the vessels [Chandran & Kim, 1994]. The alterations in mechanical stresses with the implantation of vascular prostheses in the arterial circulation may include changes in the deformation and stress concentrations at the anastomotic site. Altered fluid shear stresses at the intimal surface in the vicinity of the anastomosis have also been identified as important, particularly since the loss of patency is present more often at the distal anastomosis. The vascular prostheses should have the same dynamic response after implantation as the host artery in order to reduce the effect of abnormal mechanical stresses at the junction. For a replacement graft of the same size as the host artery, mismatch in *compliance* may be the most important factor resulting in graft failure [Abbott & Bouchier-Hayes, 1978]. In implanting the prostheses, *end-to-end* configuration is common in the reconstruction of peripheral arteries. *End-to-side configuration* is common in coronary artery bypass, where blood will flow from the host artery (aorta) to the prosthesis branching out at the anastomotic site. At the other end, the graft is attached distally to the occlusion in the host (coronary) vessel to enable perfusion of the vascular bed downstream from the occlusion. Numerous studies analyzing the abnormal flow dynamics within the anastomotic geometry and stress distribution within the vascular material at the junction to the prostheses have been reported in delineating the causes for intimal hyperplasia formation and loss of patency [Chandran et al., 1992; Keynton et al., 1991; Kim & Chandran, 1993; Kim et al., 1993; Ojha et al., 1990; Rhee and Tarbell, 1994; Rodgers et al. 1987] and a detailed discussion on the mechanical aspects of vascular prostheses can be found in Chandran and Kim [1994]. Improvements in the blood-surface interactions are also being attempted in order to improve the functioning capability of vascular grafts. Attempts at seeding the grafts with *endothelial cells* [Hunter et al., 1983], modifying the graft material properties by removing the *crimping* and heat fusing a coil of bendable and dimensionally stable polypropylene at the outer surface to make it kink resistant [Guidoin et al., 1983], employing a compliant and biodegradable graft which will promote regeneration of arterial wall in small-caliber vessels [Van der Lei et al., 1985, 1986] are a few examples of such improvements.

Conclusions

In the last four decades, we have observed significant advances in the development of biocompatible materials to be used in blood-interfacing implants. In the case of mechanical heart valve prostheses, pyrolytic carbon has become the material of choice for the occluder and the housing. The pyrolytic carbon is chemically inert and exhibits very little wear even after more than 20 years of use. However, thromboembolic complications remain significant with mechanical valve implantation. The complex dynamics of valve function and the resulting mechanical stresses on the formed elements of blood appear to be the main cause for initiation of thrombus. More recent reports of structural failure with implanted mechanical valves and pitting and erosion observed on the pyrolytic carbon surfaces have resulted in investigations of cavitation bubble formation during valve closure. Along with further improvements in biomaterials for heart valves, detailed analysis of the closing dynamics and design improvements to minimize the adverse effects of mechanical stresses may be the key to reducing thrombus deposition. Improvements with mechanical heart valves or further developments on durable synthetic leaflet valves may also be vital for the development of TAHs for long-term implantation without neurologic complications.

   In the case of vascular grafts, the mismatch of material properties (compliance) between the host artery and the graft as well as geometric considerations in end-to-side anastomoses appear to be important for the loss of patency within several months after implantation particularly with medium- and small-diameter arterial replacement. Most of the vascular grafts are stiffer than the host artery, and it has been suggested that the mechanical stresses resulting from the discontinuity at the junction is the major cause for neointimal hyperplasia formation and subsequent occlusion of the conduit. Developments with more compliant grafts and in modifying the surface interaction of the graft with blood (endothelialization or other treatment of the graft material) may result in reducing the problems with loss of patency.

Defining Terms

Acetol: Product of the addition of two moles of alcohol to one of an aldehyde.

Aneurysms: Abnormal bulging or dilatation of a segment of a blood vessel or myocardium.

Artery: Blood vessel transporting blood in a direction away from the heart.

Atherosclerosis: Lipid deposits in the intima of arteries.

ATS valve: A bileaflet mechanical valve made by ATS (Advancing the Standard) Inc.

Autoclaving: Sterilizing by steam under pressure.

Biomer: Segmented polyurethane elastomer made by Ethicon, Inc.

Bioprostheses: Prosthetic heart valves made of biological tissue.

Blood oxygenators: Extracarporeal devices to oxygenate blood during heart bypass surgery.

Bovine heterograft: Graft material (arterial) transplanted from bovine species.

Calcification: Deposition of insoluble salts of calcium.

Cardiac pacemakers: Prostheses implanted to stimulate cardiac muscles to contract.

Cardiopulmonary bypass: Connectors bypassing circulation to the heart and the lungs.

Catheters: Hollow cylindrical tubing to be passed through the blood vessels or other canals.

Cavitation bubbles (vapor cavitation):   Formation of vapor bubbles due to transient reduction in pressure to below the liquid vapor pressure.

Closing dynamics: Dynamics during the closing phase of heart valves.

Compliance: A measure of ease with which a structure can be deformed: ratio of volumetric strain to increase in unit pressure.

Crimping: Creasing of the synthetic vascular grafts in the longitudinal direction to accommodate the large intermittent flow of blood.

Delrin: Polyacetal made by Union Carbide.

Dialysers: Devices to filter the blood of waste products taking over the function of the kidney.

dp/dt: Slope of the pressure versus time curve of the ventricles.

Dura mater: A tough fibrous membrane forming the outer cover of the brain and the spinal cord.

Electrohydraulic blood pump: Blood pump energized by the conversion of electric to hydraulic energy.

End-to-end configuration: End of the vascular graft anastamosed to the end of the host artery.

End-to-side configuration: End of the vascular graft anastamosed to the side of the host.

Endothelial cells: A layer of flat cells lining the intimal surface of blood vessels.

Erosion: A state of being worn away.

Fascia lata: A sheet of fibrous tissue enveloping the muscles of the thigh.

Fatigue stress: Level of stress below which the material would not undergo fatigue failure (10^7 cycles used as the normal limit).

Fibrin: An elastic filamentous protein derived from fibrinogen in coagulation of the blood.

Fibroblasts: An elongated cell with cytoplasmic processes present in connective tissue capable of forming collagen fibers.

Finite element analysis: A structural analysis done with the aid of computer by dividing the structure into finite elements and applying the laws of mechanics on each element.

Formaldehyde: Formic aldehyde, methyl aldehyde—a pungent gas used as antiseptic.

Formed elements in blood: Red blood cells, white blood cells, platelets, and other cells in whole blood.

Haynes 25: CoCr alloy.

Homografts: Transplants (heart valves, arterial segments, etc.) from the same species.

Intra-aortic balloon pumps: A balloon catheter inserted in the descending aorta and alternately inflated and deflated timed to the EKG in order to assist the ventricular pumping.

Laser Doppler anemometry: A velocity measurement device using the principle of Doppler-shifted frequency of laser light by particles moving with the fluid.

Leaflets: Occluders on valves which open and close to aid blood flow in one direction.

Left ventricular assist devices: Prosthetic devices to assist the left ventricle in pumping blood.

Liquid vapor pressure: Pressure at which liquid vaporizes.

LTI: Low-temperature (below 1500°C) isotropic pyrolytic carbon.

Mechanical prostheses: Prostheses made of nonbiologic material.

Negative pressure transients: Reduction in pressure for a short duration.

Neointima: Newly formed intimal surface.

Neointimal hyperplasia: Growth of new intimal surface formed by fibroblasts.

Nylon: Synthetic polymer with condensation polymerization.

Patency: State of being freely open.

Pericardial prostheses: Heart valve prosthesis made with fixed bovine pericardial tissue.

Pitting: Depression or indent on a surface.

Platelet: One of the formed elements of blood responsible for blood coagulation.

Polypropylene: Vinyl polymer with good flex life and good environmental stress crack resistance.

Polytetrafluoroethylene (PTFE): A fluorocarbon polymer known as Teflon made by Dupont.

Pusher plate devices: Artificial heart devices working with pusher plates moving the blood.

Pyrolytic carbon: Carbon deposited onto performed polycrystalline graphite substrate.

Radiopacity: The state of being opaque to x ray.

Sewing rings: Rings surrounding the housing of artificial heart valves used to sew the valve to the tissue orifice with suture.

Solution casting: Casting by pouring molten material on dyes to form a structure.

Stellite 21: CoCr alloy.

Stent: A device used to maintain the bodily orifice or cavity.

Strut: A projection in the structure such as guiding struts in heart valves used to guide the leaflets during opening and closing.

TAH: Total artificial heart replacing failed natural heart.

Teflon: See *PTFE*.

Thromboembolic complications: Complications due to breaking away (emboli) of thrombus blocking the distal blood vessels.

Thrombus: A clot in the blood vessels or in the cavities of the heart formed from the constituents of blood.

Tilting disc valves: Valves with a single leaflet tilting open and shut.

Titanium: Highly reactive metal having low density, good mechanical properties, and biocompatibility due to tenacious oxide layer formation.

Turbulent stresses: Stresses generated in the fluid due to agitated random motion of particles.

Ultra-high-molecular-weight polyethylene: Linear thermoplastics with very high molecular weight ($>2 \times 10^6$ g/mol) used for orthopedic devices such as acetabular cups for hip joint replacement.

Umbilical cord vein grafts: Vascular graft made from umbilical cord veins.

Vacuum forming: A manufacturing technique for thermoplastic polymer in which a sheet is heated and formed over a mold while a vacuum is present under the sheet.

Valvular disorders: Diseased states of valves such as stenosis.

Valvular structures: Components of valves such as leaflets and struts.

Vascular grafts: Grafts to replace segments of diseased vessel.

Xenografts: Grafts obtained from species other than that of the recipient.

References

Abbott WM, Bouchier-Hayes DJ. 1978. The role of mechanical properties in graft design. In H Dardick (ed), Graft Materials in Vascular Surgery, pp 59–78, Chicago, Year Book Medical Publishers.

Akutsu T, Kolff WJ. 1958. Permanent substitutes for valves and hearts. Trans Amer Soc Art Intern Organs 4:230.

Baldwin JT, Tarbell JM, Deutsch S, et al. 1988. Hot-film wall shear probe measurements inside a ventricular assist device. J Biomech Eng 110:326.

Braunwald NS, Cooper T, Morrow AG. 1960. Complete replacement of the mitral valve: Successful application of a flexible polyurethane prosthesis. J Thorac Cardiovasc Surg 40:1.

Carpentier A, Lamaigre CG, Robert L, et al. 1969. Biological factors affecting long-term results of valvular heterografts. J Thorac Cardiovasc Surg 58:467.

Chandran KB. 1988. Heart valve prostheses: In vitro flow dynamics. In JG Webster (ed), Encyclopedia of Medical Devices and Instrumentation, vol 3, pp 1475–1483, New York, Wiley Interscience.

Chandran KB. 1992. Cardiovascular Biomechanics. New York, New York University Press.

Chandran KB, Cabell GN, Khalighi B, et al. 1983. Laser anemometry measurements of pulsatile flow past aortic valve prostheses. J Biomech 16:865.

Chandran KB, Cabell GN, Khalighi B, et al. 1984. Pulsatile flow past aortic valve bioprostheses in a model human aorta. J Biomech 17:609.

Chandran KB, Fatemi R, Schoephoerster R, et al. 1989a. In vitro comparison of velocity profiles and turbulent shear distal to polyurethane trileaflet and pericardial prosthetic valves. Artif Org 13:148.

Chandran KB, Schoephoerster RT, Wurzel D, et al. 1989b. Hemodynamic comparison of polyurethane trileaflet and bioprosthetic heart valves. Trans Amer Soc Art Intern Organs 35:132.

Chandran KB, Gao D, Han G, et al. 1992. Finite element analysis of arterial anastomosis with vein, Dacron and PTFE grafts. Med Biol Eng Comp 30:413.

Chandran KB, Kim YH. 1994. Mechanical aspects of vascular graft-host artery anastomoses. Eng Med Bio Aug/Sep, 517.

Chandran KB, Kim S-H, Han G. 1991a. Stress distribution on the cusps of a polyurethane trileaflet heart valve prosthesis in the closed position. J Biomech 24:385.

Chandran KB, Lee CS, Shipkowitz T, et al. 1991b. In vitro hemodynamic analysis of flexible artificial ventricle. Artif Org 15:420.

Chandran KB, Lee CS, Chen LD. 1994*a*. Pressure field in the vicinity of mechanical valve occluders at the instant of valve closure: Correlation with cavitation initiation. J Heart Valve Dis 3: S65–S76.

Chandran KB, Lee CS, Aluri S, et al. 1994*b*. Pressure distribution near the occluders and impact forces on the outlet struts of Björk-Shiley convexo-concave valves during closing. Proceedings of the Second World Congress of Biomechanics, vol 2, 199.

Chandran KB, Schreck S, Lee CS, et al. 1994*c*. Effect of wedging on the closing dynamics of Björk-Shiley convexo-concave tilting disc valves in the mitral position. Proceedings of the 8th International Conference on Biomedical Engineering, in press.

Cheon GJ, Chandran KB. 1994. Transient behavior analysis of a mechanical monoleaflet heart valve prosthesis in the closing phase. J Biomech Eng 116:452.

Dellsperger KC, Chandran KB. 1991. Prosthetic heart valves. In P Sharma, M Szycher (eds), Blood Compatible Materials and Devices: Perspectives towards the 21st Century, *M.* chap 9, pp 153–165, Lancaster, Penn, Technomic Publishing.

DeVries WC, Joyce LD. 1983. The artificial heart. CIBA Clinical Symposia, 35(6):1–32.

Farrar DJ, Litwak P, Lawson JH., et al. 1988. In vivo evaluations of a new thromboresistant polyurethane for artificial heart blood pumps. J Thorac Cardiovasc Surg 95:191.

Gerring EL, Bellhouse BJ, Bellhouse FH, et al. 1974. Long term animal trials of the Oxford aortic/pulmonary valve prosthesis without anticoagulants. Trans. ASAIO 20:703.

Ghista DN, Reul H. 1977. Optimal prosthetic aortic leaflet valve: Design, parametric and longevity analysis: Development of the avcothane-51 leaflet valve based on the optimal design analysis. J Biomech 10:313.

Guidoin R, Couture J. 1991. Polyester prostheses: The outlook for the future. In CP Sharma, M Szycher (eds), Blood Compatible Materials and Devices: Perspectives towards the 21st Century, chap 9, pp 153–165, Lancaster, Penn, Technomic Publishing.

Guidoin R, Gosselin C, Martin L, et al. 1983. Polyester prostheses as substitutes in the thoracic aorta of dogs: I. Evaluation of commercial prostheses. J Biomed Mat Res 17:1049.

Hamid MS, Sabbah HN, Stein PD. 1985. Finite element evaluation of stresses on closed leaflets of bioprosthetic heart valves with flexible stents. Finite Elem Analysis Des 1:213.

Harold M, Lo HB, Reul H, et al. 1987. The Helmholtz Institute tri-leaflet polyurethane heart valve prosthesis: Design, manufacturing, and first *in vitro* and *in vivo* results. In H Planck, I Syre, M Dauner (eds), Polyurethanes in Biomedical Engineering II. pp 321–356, Amsterdam, Elsevier.

Holfert JW, Reibman JB, Dew PA, et al. 1987. A new connector system for total artificial hearts: Preliminary results. Trans ASAIO 10:151.

Hufnagel CA. 1977. Reflections on the development of valvular prostheses. Med Instrum 11:74.

Hunter GC, Schmidt SP, Sharp WV, et al. 1983. Controlled flow studies in 4 mm endothelialized Dacron® grafts. Trans ASAIO 29:177.

Jarvick RK. 1981. The total artificial heart. Scientific American 244:66.

Jarvis P, Tarbell JM, Frangos JA. 1991. An *in vitro* evaluation of an artificial heart. Trans ASAIO 37:27.

Kafesjian R, Howanec M, Ward GD, et al. 1994. Cavitation damage of pyrolytic carbon in mechanical heart valves. J Heart Valve Dis 3 (suppl. 1):S2.

Kambic HE, Nose Y. 1991. Biomaterials for blood pumps. In CP Sharma, M Szycher (eds), Blood Compatible Materials and Devices: Perspectives towards the 21st Century, chap 8, pp 141–151, Lancaster, Penn, Technomic.

Keynton RS, Rittgers SE, Shu MCS. 1991. The effect of angle and flow rate upon hemodynamics in distal vascular graft anastomoses: An *in vitro* model study. J Biomech Eng 113:458.

Kim SH, Chandran KB, Chen CJ. 1992. Numerical simulation of steady flow in a two-dimensional total artificial heart model. J Biomech Eng 114:497.

Kim SH, Chandran KB. 1993. Steady flow analysis in the vicinity of an end-to-end anastomosis. Biorheology 30:117.

Kim SH, Chandran KB, Bower TJ, et al. 1993. Flow dynamics across end-to-end vascular bypass graft anastomoses. Ann Biomed Eng 21:311.

Lee CS, Chandran KB. 1994*a*. Instantaneous backflow through peripheral clearance of Medtronic Hall valve at the moment of closure. Ann Biomed Eng, in press.

Lee CS, Chandran KB. 1994*b*. Numerical simulation of instantaneous backflow through central clearance of bileaflet mechanical heart valves at the moment of closure: Shear stress and pressure fields within the clearance. Med Biol Eng Comp, in press.

Lee CS, Chandran KB, Chen LD. 1994. Cavitation dynamics of mechanical heart valve prostheses. Artif Org, in press.

Lee JM, Boughner DR. 1991. Bioprosthetic heart valves: Tissue mechanics and implications for design. In CP Sharma, M Szycher (eds), Blood Compatible Materials and Devices: Perspectives towards the 21st Century, chap 10, pp 167–188, Lancaster, Penn, Technomic.

Lefrak EA, Starr A (eds). 1970. Cardiac Valve Prostheses. New York, Appleton-Century-Crofts.

Leuer L. 1987. Dynamics of mechanical valves in the artificial heart. Proc 40th Ann Conf Eng Med Biol 82.

Ojha M, Ethier CR, Johnston KW, et al. 1990. Steady and pulsatile flow fields in an end-to-side arterial anastomosis model. J Vasc Surg 12:747.

Park JB, Lakes RS. 1992. Biomaterials: An Introduction, 2d ed, New York, Plenum Press.

Phillips WM, Brighton JA, Pierce WS. 1979. Laser Doppler anemometer studies in unsteady ventricular flows. Trans ASAIO 25:56.

Reif TH. 1991. A numerical analysis of the back flow between the leaflets of a St. Jude Medical cardiac valve prosthesis. J Biomech 24:733.

Reis RL, Hancock WD, Yarbrough JW, et al. 1971. The flexible stent. J Thorac Cardiovasc Surg 62:683.

Rhee K, Tarbell JM. 1994. A study of wall shear rate distribution near the end-to-end anastomosis of a rigid graft and a compliant artery. J Biomech 27:329.

Rodgers VGJ, Teodori MF, Borovetz HS. 1987. Experimental determination of mechanical shear stress about an anastomotic junction. J Biomech 20:795.

Roe BB, Owsley JW, Boudoures PC. 1958. Experimental results with a prosthetic aortic valve. J Thorac Cardiovasc Surg 36:563.

Russel FB, Lederman DM, Singh PI, et al. 1980. Development of seamless trileaflet valves. Trans ASAIO 26:66.

Sabbah HN, Hamid MS, Stein PD. 1985. Estimation of mechanical stresses on closed cusps of porcine bioprosthetic valves: Effect of stiffening, focal calcium and focal thinning. Am J Cardiol 55:1091.

Shim HS, Lenker JA. 1988. Heart valve prostheses. In JG Webster (ed), Encyclopedia of Medical Devices and Instrumentation, vol 3, pp 1457–1474,

Strandness DE, Sumner DS. 1975. Grafts and grafting. In Hemodynamics for Surgeons, pp 342–395, New York, Grune and Stratton.

Tarbell JM, Gunishan JP, Geselowitz DB, et al. 1986. Pulsed ultrasonic Doppler velocity measurements inside a left ventricular assist device. J Biomech Eng 108:232.

Thubrikar MJ, Skinner JR, Eppink TR, et al. 1982*a*. Stress analysis of porcine bioprosthetic heart valves *in vivo*. J Biomed Mat Res 16:811.

Thubrikar MJ, Skinner JR, Nolan SP. 1982*b*. Design and stress analysis of bioprosthetic valves *in vivo*. In LH Colin, V Gallucci (eds), Cardiac Bioprostheses, pp 445–455, New York, Yorke Medical Books.

Unger F. 1989. Assisted Circulation, vol. 3, Berlin, Springer-Verlag.

Van der Lei B, Wildevuur CRH, Nieuwenhuis P. 1986. Compliance and biodegradation of vascular grafts stimulate the regeneration of elastic laminae in neoarterial tissue: An experimental study in rats. Surg 99:45.

Van der Lei B, Wildevuur CRH, Niewenhuis P, et al. 1985. Regeneration of the arterial wall in microporous, compliant, biodegradable vascular grafts after implantation into the rat abdominal aorta. Cell Tissue Res 242:569.

Wurzel D, Kolff J, Missfeldt W, et al. 1988. Development of the Philadelphia heart system. Artif Org 12:410.

Yoganathan AP, Corcoran WH, Harrison EC. 1979a. In vitro velocity measurements in the vicinity of aortic prostheses. J Biomech 12:135.

Yoganathan AP, Corcoran WH, Harrison EC. 1979b. Pressure drops across prosthetic aortic heart valves under steady and pulsatile flow—*in vitro* measurements. J Biomech 12:153.

Yoganathan AP, Woo YR, Sung HW. 1986. Turbulent shear stress measurements in the vicinity of aortic heart valve prostheses. J Biomech 19:433.

46.2 Non-Blood-Interfacing Implants for Soft Tissues

S. W. Shalaby

Practically all tissues other than bone and cartilage are of the soft category. With the exception of those used in blood-contracting mode, primarily in the cardiovascular systems, known implants do not interface directly with blood. These implants are used to augment, replace natural tissues, or redirect specific biological functions. On one hand, the implants can be transient, that is, of short-term function and thus made of absorbable materials. On the other hand, long-term implants, which are expected to have prolonged functions, are made of nonabsorbable materials.

Toward the successful development of a new biomedical device or implant, including those used for soft tissues, a number of milestones must be achieved which entail (1) acquiring certain biologic and biomechanic data about the implant site and its function to aid in the selection of materials and engineering design of such an implant, to meet carefully developed product requirements; (2) constructing a prototype and evaluating its physical and biologic properties both in vitro and in vivo, using the appropriate animal model; and (3) conducting a clinical study following a successful battery of animal safety studies depending on intended application and availability of historical safety and clinical data on the material or design. Extent of the studies associated with any specific milestone can vary considerably. Even though different applications require different materials with specific properties, minimum requirements for soft-tissue implants should be met. These typically include (1) exhibiting physical properties (e.g., flexibility and texture) which are equivalent or comparable to those called for in the product profile; (2) maintaining the expected physical properties after implantation for a specific period; (3) eliciting no adverse tissue reaction; (4) displaying no carcinogenic, toxic, allergenic, and/or immunogenic effect; and (5) achieving assured sterility without compromising the physicochemical properties. In addition to these criteria, a product of potentially broad applications is expected to (1) be easily mass produced at a reasonable cost; (2) have acceptable aesthetic quality; (3) be enclosed in durable, properly labeled, easy-access packaging; and (4) have adequate shelf stability.

The most common type of soft-tissue implants are (1) sutures and allied augmentation devices; (2) percutaneous and cutaneous systems, (3) maxillofacial devices, (4) ear and eye protheses, (5) space-filling articles, and (6) fluid transfer devices.

Sutures and Allied Augmentation Devices

Sutures and staples are the most common types of augmentation devices. In recent years, interest in using tapes and adhesives has increased and may continue to do so, should new efficacious systems be developed.

Sutures

Sutures are usually packaged as a thread attached to a metallic needle. Although almost all needles are made of stainless steel alloys, the thread component can be made of different materials, and the type used determines the class of the entire suture. In fact, it is common to refer to the thread as the suture. Presently, most needles are drilled (mechanically or by laser beam) at one end for thread insertion. Securing the thread in the needle hole can be achieved by crimping or adhesive attachment. Among the critical physical properties of sutures are their diameter, in vitro knot strength, needle-holding strength, needle penetration force, ease of knotting, knot security, and in vitro strength retention profile.

Two types of threads are used in suture manufacturing and are distinguished according to the retention of their properties in the biologic environments, namely, absorbable and nonabsorbable sutures. These may also be classified according to their source of raw materials, that is, natural (catgut, silk, and cotton), synthetic (nylon, polypropylene, polyethylene terephthalate, and polyglycolide and its copolymers), and metallic sutures (stainless steel and tantalum). Sutures may also be classified according to their physical form, that is, monofilament and braided multifilament (or, simply, braids).

The first known suture, the absorbable catgut, is made primarily of collagen derived from sheep intestinal submucosa. It is usually treated with a chromic salt to increase its in vivo strength retention and through imparted crosslinking that retards absorption. Such treatment extends the functional performance of catgut suture from 1–2 weeks up to about 3 weeks. The catgut sutures are packaged in a specially formulated fluid to prevent drying and maintain necessary compliance for surgical handling and knot formation.

For the past two decades, the use of synthetic absorbable sutures exceeded that of catgut. This was attributed to many factors including (1) higher initial breaking strength and superior handling characteristics; (2) availability of sutures with a broad range of in vivo strength retention profiles; (3) considerably milder tissue reactions and no immunogenic response; and (4) reproducible properties and highly predictable in vivo performance. Polyglycolide (PG) was the first synthetic absorbable suture to be introduced, about three decades ago. Because of the high modulus of oriented fibers, PG is made mostly in the braided form. A typical PG suture braid absorbs in about 4 months and retains some in vivo strength at 3 weeks. However, braids made of the 90/10 glycolide/1-lactide copolymer were shown to have a comparable or improved strength retention profile and faster absorption rate relative to PG. The copolymeric sutures absorb in about 3 months and have gained wide acceptance by the surgical community. Like any braided suture, the use of the appropriate absorbable coating to improve suture handling and knot formation has been a common feature in absorbable braids. To minimize the risk of infection and tissue drag that are sometimes associated with braided sutures, three types of monofilament sutures have been commercialized. To approach the engineering compliance of braided sutures, materials used in the production of absorbable monofilaments were characterized by having low modulus, e.g., polydioxanone and copolymers of glycolide with caprolactone or trimethylene carbonate.

Members of the nonabsorbable family of sutures include braided silk (a natural protein), nylon (e.g., Nylon 66), and polyethylene terephthalate (PET). These braids are used as coated sutures. Although silk sutures have retained wide acceptance by surgeons, nylon and, particularly, PET sutures are used for critical procedures where high strength and predictable long-term performance are emphasized. Meanwhile, the use of cotton sutures is decreasing constantly, because of their low strength and occasional tissue reactivity due to contaminants. Monofilaments are important forms of nonabsorbable sutures and are made primarily of polypropylene, nylon (e.g., Nylons 6 and 66), and stainless steel. The polypropylene sutures exhibit not only the desirable properties of monofilaments but also the biologic inertness reflected in the minimal tissue reactions associated with their use in almost all surgical sites. With the exception of its natural tendency to undergo hydrolytic degradation and, hence, continued loss of mechanical strength postoperatively, nylon monofilament has similar attributes to those of polypropylene. Because of their exceptionally high modulus, stainless steel sutures are not used in soft-tissue repair—they can tear these tissues. With the exception of sutures made of synthetic absorbable polymers, polypropylene sutures and cotton, which are sterilized by ethylene oxide, all sutures can be sterilized by gamma radiation. An interesting application of monofilament sutures is illustrated in the use of polypropylene loops (or haptics) for intraocular lenses.

Nonsuture Fibrous and Microporous Implants

Woven PET and polypropylene fabrics are commonly used as surgical meshes for abdominal wall repair and similar surgical procedures where surgical "patching" is required. Braid forms and similar construction made of multifilament PET yarns have been used for repairing tendons and ligaments. Microporous foams of polytetrafluoroethylene (PTFE) are used as pledgets (to aid in anchoring sutures to soft tissues) and in repair of tendons and ligaments. Microporous collagen-based foams are used in wound repair to accelerate healing.

Clips, Staples, and Pins

Ligating clips are most commonly used for temporary or long-term management of the flow in tubular tissues. Titanium clips are among the oldest and still-versatile types of clips. Thermoplastic polymers such as nylon can be injection-molded into different forms of ligating clips. These are normally designed to have a latch and living hinge. Absorbable polymers made of lactide/glycolide copolymers and polydioxanone have been successfully converted to ligating clips with different design features for a broad range of applications.

Metallic staples were introduced about three decades ago as strong competitors to sutures for wound augmentation; their use has grown considerably over the past ten years for everything from skin closure procedures to a multiplicity of internal surgical applications. Major advantages associated with the use of staples are ease of application and minimal tissue trauma. Metallic staples can be made of tantalum, stainless steel, or titanium-nickel alloys. Staples are widely used to facilitate closure of large incisions produced in procedures such as Caesarean sections and intestinal surgery. Most interesting applications of small staples have been in the ophthalmic area and endoscopic procedures, a fast-growing area of minimally invasive surgery.

Thermoplastic materials based on lactide/glycolide copolymers have been used to produce absorbable staples for use in skin and internal would closures. These staples consist primarily of two interlocking components, a fastener and receiver.

A new form of ligating device is the subcutaneous pin. This is designed with a unique applicator to introduce the pin parallel to the axis of the wound. During its application, the linear pin acquires a zig-zag-like configuration for stabilized tissue anchoring. The available forms of these pins are made of lactide/glycolide polymers.

Surgical Tapes

Surgical tapes are intended to offer a means of minimizing necrosis, scar tissue formation, problems of stitch abscesses, and weakened tissues. The problems with surgical tapes are similar to those experienced with traditional skin tapes: These include (1) misaligned wound edges, (2) poor adhesion due to moisture or dirty wounds, and (3) late separation of tapes when hematoma or wound drainage occur.

Wound strength and scar formation in skin may depend on the type of incision made. If the subcutaneous muscles in the fatty tissue are cut and the overlying skin is closed with tape, then the muscles retract. This, in turn, increases the scar area, resulting in poor cosmetic appearance when compared to a suture closure. Tapes have been also used successfully for assembling scraps of donor skin for skin graft.

Tissue Adhesives

The constant call for tissue adhesives is particularly justified on the basis of certain biomechanical principles, when dealing with the repair of exceptionally soft tissues. Such tissues cannot be easily approximated by sutures, for they inflict substantial mechanical damage following the traditional knotting scheme and associated shear stresses. However, the variable biological environments about soft tissues and their regenerative capacity make the development of an ideal tissue adhesive a difficult task. Experience indicates that an ideal tissue adhesive should (1) be able to wet and bond to tissues, (2) be capable of onsite formation by the rapid polymerization of a liquid monomer without producing excessive heat or toxic byproducts, (3) be absorbable, (4) not interfere with the normal healing process, and (5) be easily applied during surgery. The two common types of tissue adhesives are based on alkyl-α-cyanoacrylates and fibrin. The latter is a natural adhesive derived from fibrinogen, which is one of the clotting components of blood. Although fibrin is useful in Europe, its use in the United States has not been approved to eliminate the risk of its contamination with hepatitis and/or immune disease viruses. Due to its limited mechanical strength (tensile strength and elastic modulus of 0.1 and 0.15 MPa, respectively), fibrin is used mostly as a sealant and for adjoining delicate tissues as in nerve anastomoses. Meanwhile, two members of the cyanoacrylate family of adhesives, namely n-butyl- and iso-butyl-cyano-acrylates, are used in a number of countries as sealants and adhesives, as well as blocking agents. They are yet to be approved for use in the United States because of the lack of sufficient safety data. Due to a fast rate of polymerization and some limited manageability in localizing the adhesive to the specific surgical site, the in vivo performance of cyanoacrulates is not highly predictable. Because of the low strength of the adhesive joints or sealant films produced upon in vivo polymerization of these cyanoacrylates, their applications are limited mostly to use in traumatized fragile tissues such as spleen, liver, and kidney as well as after extensive surgery on soft lung tissues. A major concern over the safety of these alkyl-cyanoacrylates is related to their being nonabsorbable. Hence, a number of investigators have directed their attention to certain alkoxy-alkyl cyanoacrylates which can be converted to polymeric adhesives with acceptable absorbable profiles and rheological properties.

Percutaneous and Skin Implants

The need for percutaneous (*trans* or through the skin) implants has been accelerated by the advent of artificial kidneys and hearts and the need for prolonged injection of drugs and nutrients. Artificial skin is urgently needed to maintain the body temperature of severely burned patients. Actual permanent replacement of skin by biomaterials is still a great clinical challenge.

Percutaneous Devices

The problem of obtaining a functional and viable interface between the tissue (skin) and an implant (percutaneous device) is primarily due to the following factors. First, although initial attachment of the tissue into the interstices of the implant surface occurs, attachment cannot be maintained for a long period, since the dermal tissue cells turn over continuously. Downgrowth of epithelium around the implant or overgrowth on the implant leads to extrusion or invagination, respectively. Second, any opening about the implant that is large enough for bacteria to penetrate may result in infection, even though initially there may be a tight seal between skin and implant. Several factors are involved in the development of percutaneous devices: (1) type of end use—this may deal with transmission of information (biopotentials, temperature, pressure, blood flow rate), energy (electrical stimulation, power for heart-assist devices), transfer of matter (cannula for blood), and load (attachment of a prosthesis); (2) engineering factors—these may address materials selection (polymers, ceramics, metals, and composites), design variation (button, tube with and without skirt, porous or smooth surface), and mechanical stresses (soft and hard interface, porous or smooth interface); (3) biologic factors—these are determined by the implant host (human, dog, hog, rabbit, sheep), and implant location (abdominal, dorsal, forearm); and (4) human factors—these can pertain to post-surgical care, implantation technique, and esthetic outlook.

No percutaneous devices are completely satisfactory. Nevertheless, some researchers believe that hydroxyapatite may be part of a successful approach. In one experimental trial, a hydroxyapatite-based percutaneous device was associated with relatively less epidermal downgrowth (1 mm after 17 months versus 4.6 mm after 3 months) when compared with a silicone rubber control specimen in the dorsal skin of canines.

Artificial Skins

Artificial skin is another example of a percutaneous implant, and the problems are similar to those described above. Most needed for this application is a material which can adhere to a large (burned) surface and thus prevent the loss of fluids, electrolytes, and other biomolecules until the wound has healed. Although a permanent skin implant is needed, it is a long way from being realized for the same reasons given in the case of percutaneous implants proper. At present, autografting and homografting (skin transplants) are the only practical methods available.

In one study on wound-covering materials with controlled physicochemical properties, an artificial skin was designed to consist of a crosslinked collagen-polysaccharide (chondroitin 6-sulfate) composite membrane. This was particularly designed to have controlled porosity (5–150 μm in diameter), flexibility (by varying crosslink density), and moisture flux rate.

Several polymeric materials and reconstituted collagen have also been examined as burn dressings. Among the synthetic ones are the copolymers of vinyl chloride and vinyl acetate and polymethyl cyanoacrylate (applied as a fast-polymerizing monomer). The latter polymer and/or its monomer were found to be too brittle and histotoxic for use as a burn dressing. The ingrowth of tissue into the pores of polyvinyl alcohol sponges and woven fabric (nylon and silicone rubber velour) was also attempted without much success.

Rapid epithelial layer growth by culturing cells *in vitro* from the skin of the burn patient for covering the wound area may offer a practical solution.

Maxillofacial Implants

There are two types of maxillofacial implants: extraoral and intraoral. The former deals with the use of artificial substitutes for reconstructing defective regions in the maxilla, mandible, and face. Useful polymeric materials for extraoral implants require: (1) match of color and texture with those of the patient; (2) mechanical and chemical stability, i.e., material should not creep or change color or irritate skin; (3) ease of fabrication. Copolymers of vinyl chloride and vinyl acetate (with 5–20% acetate), polymethyl methacrylate, silicones, and polyurethane rubbers are currently used. Intraoral implants are used for repairing maxilla, mandibular, and facial bone defects. Material requirements for the intraoral implants are similar to those of the extraoral ones. For the latter group of implants, metallic materials such as tantalum, titanium, and CoCr alloys are commonly used. For soft tissues such as gum and chin, polymers such as silicone rubber and polymethylmethacrylate are used for augmentation.

Ear and Eye Implants

Implants can be used to restore conductive hearing loss from otosclerosis (a hereditary defect which involves a change in the bony tissue of the ear) and chronic otitis media (the inflammation of the middle ear which may cause partial or complete impairment of the ossicular chain). A number of prostheses are available for correcting these defects. The porous polyethylene total ossicular implant is used to achieve a firm fixation by tissue ingrowth. The tilt-top implant is designed to retard tissue ingrowth into the section of the shaft which may diminish sound conduction. Materials used in fabricating these implants include polymethyl methacrylate, polytetrafluoroethylene, polyethylene, silicone rubber, stainless steel, and tantalum. More recently, polytetrafluoroethylene-carbon composites, porous polyethylene, and pyrolytic carbon have been described as suitable materials for cochlear (inner ear) implants.

Artificial ear implants capable of processing speech have been developed with electrodes to stimulate cochlear nerve cells. Cochlear implants also have a speech processor which transforms sound waves into electrical impulses that can be conducted through coupled external and internal coils. The electrical impulses can be transmitted directly by means of a percutaneous device.

Eye implants are used to restore the functionality of damaged or diseased corneas and lenses. Usually the cornea is transplanted from a suitable donor. In cataracts, eye lenses become cloudy and can be removed surgically. Intraocular lenses (IOL) are implanted surgically to replace the original eye lens and to restore function. Intraocular lenses are made from transparent acrylics, particularly polymethyl methacrylate, which has excellent optical properties. Infection and fixation of the lens to the tissues are frequent concerns, and a number of measures are being used to address them.

Space-Filling Implants

Breast implants are common space-filling implants. At one time, the enlargement of breasts was done with various materials such as paraffin wax and silicone fluids, by direct injection or by enclosure in a rubber balloon. Several problems have been associated with directly injected implants, including progressive instability and ultimate loss of original shape and texture as well as infection and pain. One of the early efforts in breast augmentation was to implant sponge made of polyvinyl alcohol. However, soft tissues grew into the pores and then calcified with time, and the so-called marble breast resulted. Although the enlargement or replacement of breasts for cosmetic reasons alone is not recommended, prostheses have been developed for patients who have undergone radical mastectomy or who have nonsymmetrical deformities. A silicone rubber bag filled with silicone gel and backed with polyester mesh to permit tissue ingrowth for fixation is a widely used prosthesis, primarily for psychological reasons. The artificial penis, testicles, and vagina fall into the same category as breast implants, in that they make use of silicones and are implanted for psychological reasons rather than to improve physical health.

Fluid Transfer Implants

Fluid transfer implants are required for cases such as hydrocephalus, urinary incontinence, and chronic ear infection. Hydrocephalus, caused by abnormally high pressure of the cerebrospinal fluid in the brain, can be treated by draining the fluid (essentially an ultrafiltrate of blood) through a cannula. Earlier shunts had 2 one-way valves at either end. However, the more recent Ames shunt has simple slits at the discharging end, which opens when enough fluid pressure is exerted. The Ames shunt empties the fluid in the peritoneum while others drain into the blood stream through the right internal jugular vein or right atrium of the heart. The simpler peritoneal shunt shows less incidence of infection.

The use of implants for correcting the urinary system has not been successful because of the difficulty of adjoining a prosthesis to the living system for achieving fluid tightness. In addition, blockage of the passage by deposits from urine and constant danger of infection are major concerns. Several materials have been used, with limited long-term success, for producing these implants; these include glass, rubber, silver, tantalum, Vitallium, prolyethylene, Dacron, Teflon, and polyvinyl alcohol. The drainage tubes, which are impermanent implants for chronic ear infection, can be made from polytetrafluoroethylene (Teflon).

Further Information

Chvapil M. 1982. Considerations on manufacturing principles of a synthetic burn dressing: A review. J Biomed Mater Res 16:245.

Gantz BJ. 1987. Cochlear implants: An overview. Acta Otolaryng Head Neck Surg 1:171.

Kablitz C, Kessler T, Dew PA, et al. 1979. Subcutaneous peritoneal catheter: 1½ years experience. Artif Org 3:210.

Lynch W. 1982. Implants: Reconstructing the Human Body. New York, Cincinnati, Van Nostrand Reinhold.

Park JB, Lakes RS. 1992. Biomaterials Science and Engineering, 2d ed, New York, Plenum Press.

Postlethwait RW, Schaube JF, Dillan ML, et al. 1959. An evaluation of surgical suture material. Surg Gyn Obstet 108:555.

Shalaby SW. 1985. Fibrous materials for biomedical applications. In M Lewin, J Preston (eds), High Technology Fibers: Part A. New York, Dekker.

Shalaby SW. 1988. Bioabsorbable polymers. In JC Boylan, J Swarbrick (eds), Encyclopedia of Pharmaceutical Technology, vol 1, New York, Dekker.

Shalaby SW (ed). 1994. Biomedical Polymers Designed to Degrade Systems, New York, Hanser.

VonRecum AG, Park JB. 1979. Percutaneous devices. Crit Rev Bioeng 5:37.

Yannas IV, Burke JF. 1980. Design of an artificial skin:1. Basic design principles. J Biomed Mater Res 14:107.

47

Hard Tissue Replacements

S-H. Park
University of Southern California

A. Llinás
Javeriana University

V. K. Goel
University of Iowa

J. C. Keller
University of Iowa

47.1 Bone Repair and Joint Implants

S-H. Park, A. Llinás, and V. K. Goel

The use of biomaterials to restore the function of traumatized or degenerated connective tissues and thus improve the quality of life of a patient has become widespread. In the past, implants were designed with insufficient cognizance of biomechanics. Accordingly, the clinical results were not very encouraging. An upsurge of research activities into the mechanics of joints and materials has resulted in better designs with better *in vivo* performance. The improving long-term success of total joint replacements for the lower limb is a testimony to this. As a result, researchers and surgeons have developed and used fixation devices for other joints, including artificial spine discs. A large number of devices are also available for the repair of the bone tissue. This chapter provides an overview of the contemporary scientific work related to the use of biomaterials for the repair of bone (e.g., fracture) and joint replacements ranging from a hip joint to a spine.

Long Bone Repair

The principal functions of the skeleton are to provide a frame to support the organ systems, and to determine the direction and range of body movements. Bone provides an anchoring point (insertion) for most skeletal muscles and ligaments. When the muscles contract, long bones act as levers, with the joints functioning as pivots, to cause body movement.

0-8493-8346-3/95/$0.00+$.50
© 1995 by CRC Press, Inc.

Bone is able to undergo regeneration and to remodel its micro- and macrostructure. This is accomplished through a delicate balance between an *osteogenic* (bone-forming) and *osteoclastic* (bone-removing) process [Brighton, 1984]. Bone can adapt to a new mechanical environment by changing the equilibrium between osteogenesis and osteoclasis. These processes will respond to changes in the static and dynamic stress applied to bone; that is, if more stress than the normal physiological level is applied, the equilibrium tilts toward more osteogenic activity. Conversely, if less stress is applied, the equilibrium tilts toward osteoclastic activity (this is known as Wolff's law of bone remodeling) [Wolff, 1986].

Nature provides different types of mechanisms to repair fractures in order to be able to cope with different mechanical environments surrounding a fracture [Hulth, 1989; Schenk, 1992]. For example, incomplete fractures (cracks) which only allow micromotion between the fracture fragments heal with or without a small amount of fracture-line *callus*, known as primary healing. In contrast, complete fractures which are unstable and therefore generate macromotion heal with a voluminous callus stemming from the sides of the bone, known as secondary healing [Brighton, 1984; Hulth, 1989].

The goals of fracture treatment are obtaining rapid healing, restoring function, and preserving cosmesis, without general or local complications. Implicit to the selection of the treatment method is the need to avoid potentially deleterious conditions, for example, the presence of excessive motion between bone fragments which may delay or prevent fracture healing [Brand & Rubin, 1987; Brighton, 1984].

Each fracture pattern and location results in a unique combination of characteristics ("fracture personality") that require specific treatment methods. The treatments can be nonsurgical or surgical. Examples of nonsurgical treatments are immobilization with cast (plaster or resin) or with plastic brace. The surgical treatments are divided into an external fracture fixation, which does not require opening the fracture site, and internal fracture fixation, which requires opening the fracture site.

With external fracture fixation, the bone fragments are held in alignment by pins placed through the skin onto the skeleton, structurally supported by external bars. With internal fracture fixation, the bone fragment are held by wires, screws, plates, and/or intramedullary devices. Figure 47.1 (*a* and *b*) shows radiographs of externally and internally fixed fractures.

All the internal fixation devices should meet the general requirement of biomaterials, that is, biocompatability, sufficient strength within dimensional constrains, and corrosion resistance. In addition, the device should provide a suitable mechanical environment for fracture healing. From this perspective, stainless steel, cobalt-chrome alloys, and titanium alloys are most suitable for internal fixation. Detailed mechanical properties of the metallic alloys are discussed in the chapter on metallic biomaterials. Most internal fixation devices remain in the body after the fracture has healed, often causing discomfort and requiring removal. Recently, biodegradable polymers, e.g., polylactic acid (PLA) and polyglycolic acid (PGA), have been used to treat minimally loaded fractures, thereby eliminating the need for a second surgery for implant removal. A summary of the basic application of biomaterials in internal fixation is presented in Table 47.1. A description of the principal failure modes of internal fixation devices is presented in Table 47.2.

Wires

Surgical wires are used to reattach large fragments of bone, like the greater trochanter, which is often detached during total hip replacement. Wires are also used to provide additional stability in long-oblique or spiral fractures of long bones which have already been stabilized by other means (Fig. 47.1b). Similar approaches based on the use of wires have been employed to restore stability in the lower cervical spine region and in the lumbar segment as well (Fig. 47.1c).

Twisting and knotting is unavoidable when fastening wires to bone; however, doing so can reduce the strength of the wire by 25% or more due to stress concentration [Tencer et al., 1993]. This can be partially overcome by using a thicker wire, since its strength increases directly proportional to its diameter squared. The deformed regions of the wire are more prone to corrosion than the

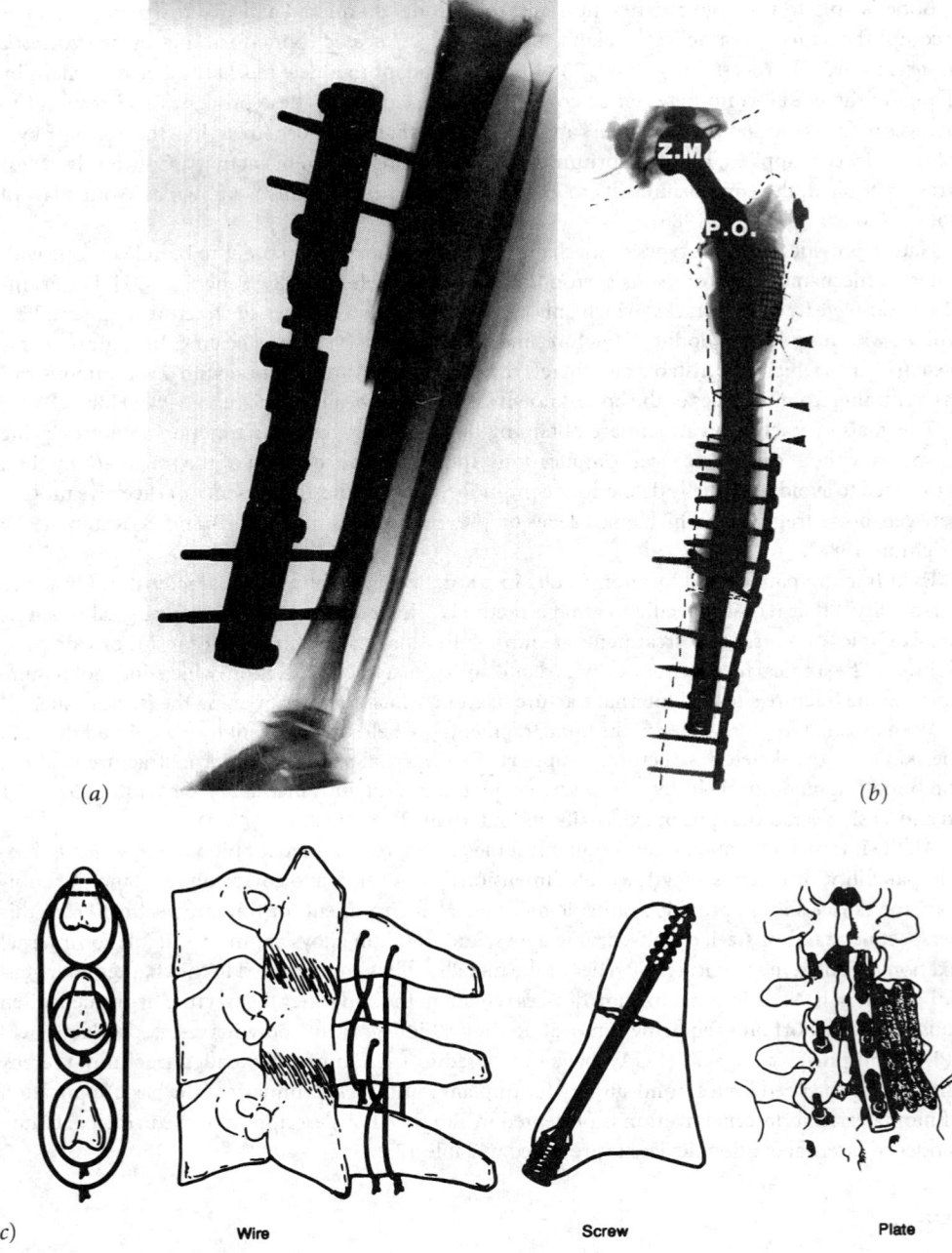

(a)

(b)

(c)   Wire   Screw   Plate

FIGURE 47.1   Radiographs of (*a*) tibial fracture fixed with four pins and an external bar; (*b*) a total hip joint replacement implanted in a patient who later sustained a femoral fracture and was treated with double bone plates, screws, and surgical wire (arrows); (*c*) applications of wires, screws, and plates in the spine.

undeformed, because of the higher strain energy. To decrease this problem and increase ease of handling during surgery, most wires are annealed to increase the ductility.

Braided multistrain (multifilament) wire is an attractive alternative, because it has similar tensile strength as a monofilament wire of equal diameter but more flexibility and higher fatigue strength [Taitsman & Saha, 1977]. However, bone often grows into the grooves of the braided multistrain

TABLE 47.1 Biomaterials Applications in Internal Fixation

Materials	Properties	Application
Stainless steel [316L]	Low cost, easy fabrication	Surgical wire (annealed)
		Pin, plate, screw
		IM nail
Ti alloy	High cost	Surgical wire
	Low density and modulus	Plate, screws, IM nails
	Excellent osseointegration	
CoCr alloys (wrought)	High cost	Surgical wire
	High density and modulus	IM nails
	Difficult to fabricate	
Polylactic acid or polyglycolic acid	Resorbable	Pin, screw
	Low strength	
Nylon	Nonresorbable plastic	Cerclage band

wire, making it exceedingly difficult to remove, since it prevents the wire from sliding when pulled. When a wire is used with other metallic implants, the metal alloys should be matched to prevent galvanic corrosion [Park & Lakes, 1992].

Pins

Straight wires are called Steinmann pins; however, if the pin diameter is less than 2.38 mm, it is called Kirschner wire. These pins are widely used, primarily to hold fragments of bones together provisionally or permanently and to guide large screws during insertion. To facilitate implantation, the pins have different tip designs which have been optimized for different types of bone (Fig. 47.2). The trochar tip, which has three cutting faces, is the most efficient in cutting; hence it is often used for cortical bone.

The holding power of the pin comes from elastic deformation of surrounding bone. In order to increase the holding power to bone, threaded pins are used. Most pins are made of 316L stainless steel; however, recently, biodegradable pins made of polylactic or polyglycolic acid have been employed for the treatment of minimally loaded fractures.

The pins can be used as part of elaborate frames designed for external fracture fixation (Fig. 47.1*a*). In this application, several pins are placed above and below the fracture but away from it. After the fracture fragments are manually approximated (reduced) to resemble the intact bone, the pins are attached to various bars, which upon assembly will provide stability to the fracture.

TABLE 47.2 Failure Modes of Internal Fixation Devices

Failure Mode	Failure Location	Reasons of Failure
Overload	Bone fracture site	Small-size implant
	Implant screw hole	Unstable reduction
	Screw thread	Early weight bearing
Fatigue	Bone fracture site	Early weight bearing
	Implant screw hole	Small-size implant
	Screw thread	Unstable reduction, fracture nonunion
Corrosion	Screw head-plate hole	Mismatch of implant alloys
	Bent area	Overtightening screw
		Misalignment of screw
		Over bent
		Scratches during insertion
Loosening	Screw	Motion
		Wrong choice of screw type
		Osteoporotic bone

Screws

Screws are the most widely used devices for fixation of bone fragments. There are two types of
bone screws: (1) cortical bone screws, which
have small threads, and, (2) cancellous screws,
which have large threads, to get more thread-to-
bone contact. Screws may have either *V* or buttress threads (Fig. 47.3). The cortical screws are
subclassified further according to their ability to
purchase onto bone: self-tapping and non-self-
tapping (Fig. 47.3). The self-tapping screws have
cutting flutes which thread the pilot drill-hole
during insertion; in contrast, the non-self-tapping screws require a tapped pilot drill-hole for
insertion.

The holding power of screws can be affected
by the size of the pilot drill-hole, the depth of
screw engagement, the outside diameter of the
screw, and quality of the bone [Cochran, 1982;
DeCoster et al., 1990]. Therefore, the selection of
the screw type should be based on the assessment
of the quality of the bone at time of insertion.
Under identical conditions, self-tapping screws
provide a slightly greater holding power than
non-self-tapping screws [Tencer et al., 1993].

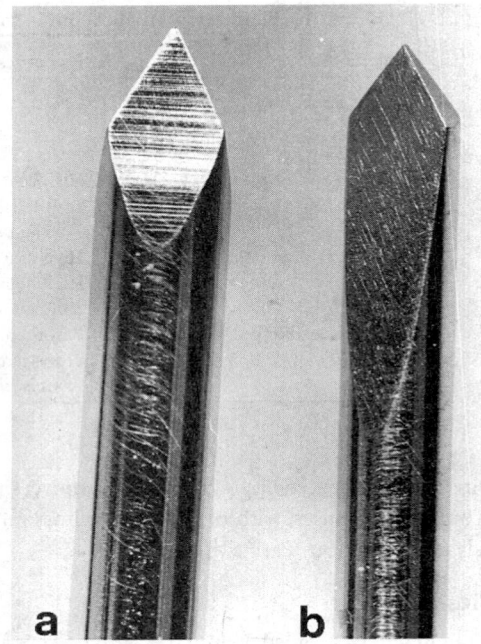

FIGURE 47.2   Pin tips: (*a*) Trocher end, and (*b*) diamond end.

Screw pullout strength varies with time after insertion *in vivo*, and it depends on the growth of
bone into the screw threads and/or resorption of the surrounding bone [Schatzker et al., 1975]. The
bone immediately adjacent to the screw often undergoes *necrosis* initially, but if the screw is firmly
fixed, when the bone revascularizes, permanent secure fixation may be achieved. This is particularly
true for titanium alloy screws or screws with a roughened thread surface, with which bone ongrowth
results in an increase in removal torque [Hutzschenreuter & Brümmer, 1980]. When the screw is

subject to micro- or macromovement, the contacting bone is replaced by a fibrous membrane,
the purchase is diminished, and the screw
loosens.

The two principal applications of bone screws
are: (1) as interfragmentary fixation devices to
"lag" or fasten bone fragments together, or (2) to
attach a metallic plate to bone. Interfragmentary
fixation is used in most fractures involving cancellous bone and in those oblique fractures in
cortical bone. In order to lag the fracture fragments, the head of the screw must engage the
cortex on the side of insertion without gripping
the bone, while the threads engage cancellous
bone and/or the cortex on the opposite side.
When screws are employed for bone plate fixation, the bone screw threads must engage both
cortices. Screws (ordinary or compression type)
are also used for the fixation of spinal fractures
(Fig. 47.1*c*).

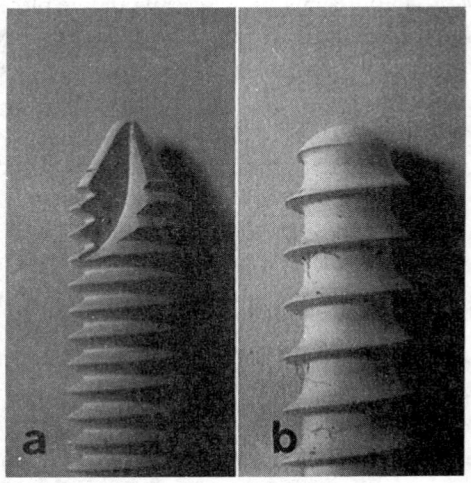

FIGURE 47.3   Bone screws: (*a*) self-tapping *V*-
threaded screw, and (*b*) a non-self-tapping, buttress-
threaded screw.

Plates

Plates are available in a wide variety of shapes and are intended to facilitate fixation of bone fragments. They range from the very rigid, intended to produce primary bone healing, to the relatively flexible, intended to facilitate physiological loading of bone.

The rigidity and strength of a plate in bending depend on the cross-sectional shape (mostly thickness) and material of which it is made. Consequently, the weakest region in the plate is the screw hole, especially if the screw hole is left empty, due to a reduction of the cross-sectional area in this region. The effect of the material on the rigidity of the plate is defined by the elastic modulus of the material for bending and by the shear modulus for twisting [Cochran, 1982]. Thus, given the same dimensions, a titanium alloy plate will be less rigid than a stainless steel plate, since the elastic modulus of each alloy is 110 GPa and 200 GPa, respectively.

Stiff plates often shield the underlying bone from the physiological loads necessary for its healthful existence [O'Slullivan et al., 1989; Perren et al., 1988]. Similarly, flat plates closely applied to the bone prevent blood vessels from nourishing the outer layers of the bone [Perren et al., 1988]. For these reasons, the current clinical trend is to use more flexible plates to allow micromotion and low-contact plates (LCP) to allow restoration of vascularity to the bone [Uhthoff & Finnegan, 1984; Claes, 1989]. The underlying goals of this change are to increase the fracture healing rate, to decrease the loss of bone mass in the region shielded by the plate, and, consequently, to decrease the incidence of refractures which may occur following plate removal.

The interaction of bone and plate is extremely important, since the two are combined into a composite structure. The stability of the plate-bone composite and the service life of the plate depend upon accurate fracture reduction. The plate is most resistant in tension; therefore, in fractures of long bones, the plate is placed along the side of the bone that is typically loaded in tension. Having excellent apposition of the bone fragments, as well as developing compression between them, is critical in maintaining the stability of the fixation and preventing the plate from repetitive bending and fatigue failure. Interfragmentary compression also creates friction at the fracture surface, increasing resistance to torsional loads [Perren, 1991; Tencer et al., 1993].

Compression between the fracture fragments can be achieved with a special type of plate called a *dynamic compression plate* (DCP). The dynamic compression plate has elliptic shape screw holes with its long axis oriented parallel to that of the plate. The screw hole has a sliding ramp to the long axis of the plate. Figure 47.4 explains the principle of the dynamic compression plate.

Bone plates are often contoured in the operating room to conform to an irregular bone shape and thus to achieve maximum contact of the fracture fragments. However, excessive bending decreases the service life of the plate. The most common failure modes of a bone plate–screw fixation are screw loosening and plate failure. The latter typically occurs through a screw hole, due to fatigue and/or crevice corrosion [Weinstein et al., 1979].

In the vicinity of the joints, where the diameter of long bones is wider, the cortex thinner, and cancellous bone abundant, plates are often used as a buttress or as a retaining wall. A buttress plate

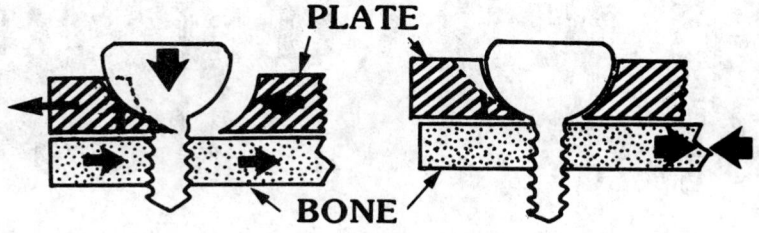

FIGURE 47.4 Principle of a dynamic compression plate for fracture fixation: During tightening, the screw head will slide down on a ramp in a plate screw hole. This will displace the plate away from the fracture and compress the fracture fragments.

applies force to the bone perpendicular to the surface of the plate and prevents shearing or sliding at the fracture site. Buttress plates are designed to fit specific anatomic locations and often incorporate other methods of fixation besides cortical or cancellous screws, for example, a large lag screw or an I-beam. Figure 47.5 illustrates variety types of bone plates.

For the fusion of vertebral bodies following diskectomy, spinal plates are used along with bone grafts. These plates are secured to the vertebral bodies using screws (Fig. 47.1c). Similar approaches have been employed to restore stability in the thoracolumbar and cervical spine regions as well.

Intramedullary Nails

Intramedullary devices (IM nails) are used as internal struts to stabilize long bone fractures. Intramedullary nails are also used for fixation of femoral neck or intertrochanteric bone fractures; however, this application requires the addition of screws. A gamut of designs are available, going from solid to cylindrical, with shapes such as cloverleaf, diamond, and C (slotted cylinders). Figure 47.6 shows variety of intramedullary devices.

Compared to plates, IM nails are better positioned to resist multidirectional bending, since they are located in the center of the bone. However, their torsional resistance is less than that of the plate [Cochran, 1982]. Therefore, when designing or selecting an intramedullary nail, a high polar moment of inertia is desirable to improve torsional rigidity and strength.

The torsional rigidity is proportional to the elastic modulus and the moment of inertia. For nails with a circular cross-section, torsional stiffness is proportional to the fourth power of the nail's radius. The wall thickness of the nail also affects the stiffness. A slotted, open-section nail is more flexible in torsion and bending, allowing for easy insertion into a curved medullary canal, for example, that of the femur [Tencer et al., 1993]. However, in bending, a slot is asymmetrical with respect to rigidity and strength. For example, a slotted nail is strongest when bending is applied so that the slot is near the neutral plane; the nail is weakest when oriented so that the slot is under tension.

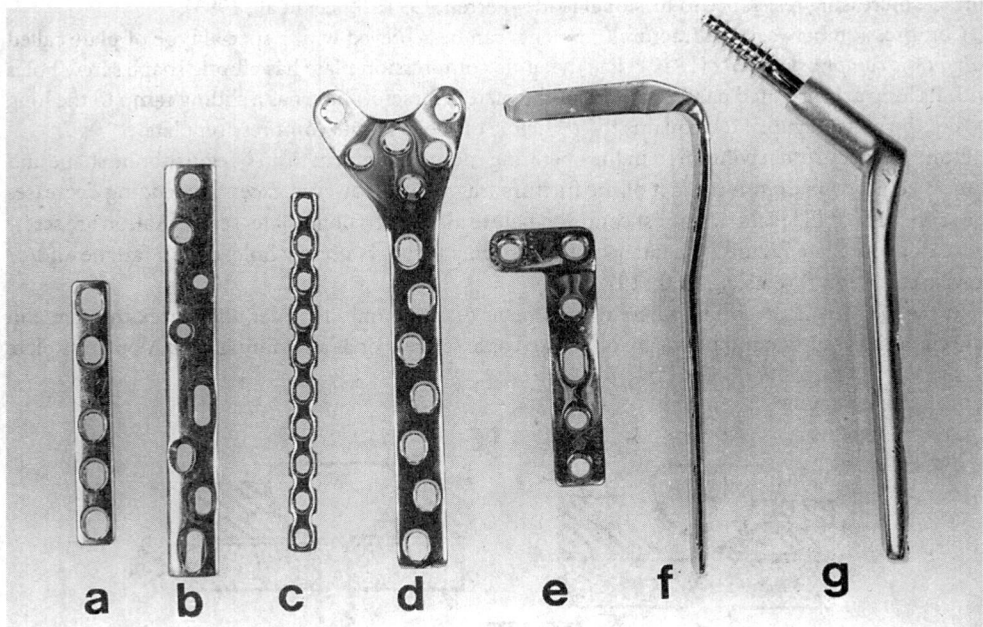

FIGURE 47.5 Bone plates: (*a*) Dynamic compression plate, (*b*) hybrid plate (lower part has dynamic compression screw holes), (*c*) reconstruction bone plate (easy contouring), (*d*) buttress bone plate, (*e*) L-shaped buttress plate, (*f*) nail plate (for condylar fracture), and (*g*) dynamic compression hip screw.

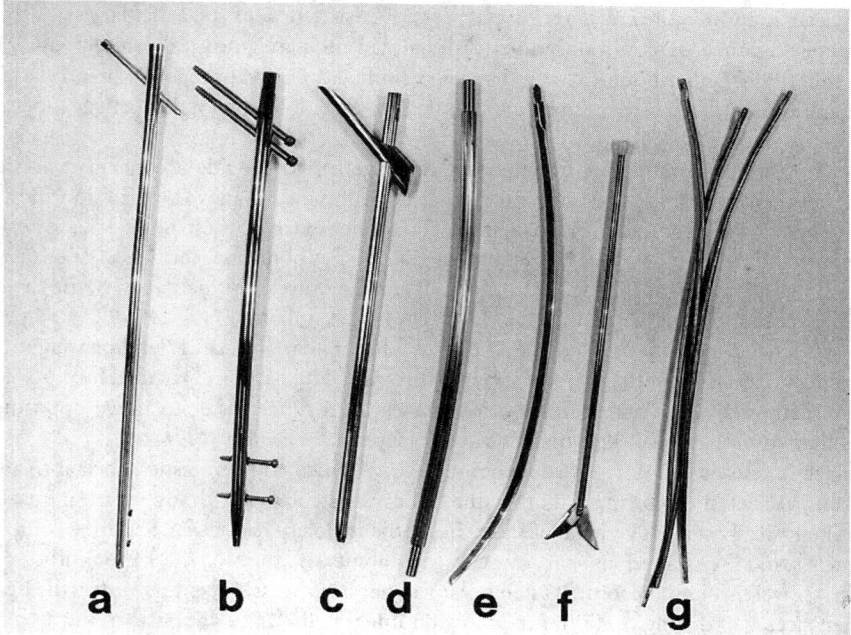

FIGURE 47.6 Intramedullary (IM) devices: (*a*) Gross-Kempf (slotted), (*b*) Uniflex (Ti alloy, slotted), (*c*) Kuntscher, (*d*) Samson, (*e*) Harris, (*f*) Brooker-Wills distal locking pin, and (*g*) Enders pins.

In addition to the need to resist bending and torsion, it is vital for an IM nail to have a large contact area with the internal cortex of the bone to permit torsional loads to be transmitted and resisted by shear stress. Two different concepts are used to develop shear stress: (1) a three-point, high-pressure contact, achieved with the insertion of curved pins, and (2) a positive interlocking between the nail and intramedullary canal, to produce a unified structure. Positive interlocking can be enhanced by reaming the intramedullary canal. Reaming permits a larger, longer, nail-bone contact area and allows the use of a larger nail with increased rigidity and strength [Kessler et al., 1986].

The addition of screws through the bone and nail, proximal and distal to the fracture, known as *interlocking,* increases torsional stability and prevents shortening of the bone, especially in unstable fractures [Perren, 1989]. The IM nail which has not been interlocked allows interfragmentary compressive force, due to its low resistance to axial load. Another advantage of the intramedullary nails is that they do not require opening the fracture site, since they can be inserted through a small skin incision, typically located in one extreme of the bone. The insertion of an IM nail, especially one that requires reaming of the medullary canal, destroys the intramedullary vessels which supply two thirds of the cortex. However, this is not of clinical significance because revascularization occurs rapidly [Kessler et al., 1986; O'Sullivan et al., 1989].

Joint Replacements

Our ability to replace damaged joints with prosthetic implants has brought relief to millions of patients who would otherwise have been severely limited in their most basic activities and doomed to a life in pain. It is estimated that about 16 million people in the United States are affected by osteoarthritis, one of the various conditions that may cause joint degeneration and may lead a patient to a total joint replacement.

Joint degeneration is the end stage of a process of destruction of the articular cartilage, which results in severe pain, loss of motion, and, occasionally, in angular deformity of the extremity [Buckwalter et al., 1993]. Unlike bone, cartilage has a very limited capacity for repair [Salter, 1988]. Therefore, when exposed to a severe mechanical, chemical, or metabolic injury, the damage is permanent and often progressive.

Under normal conditions, the functions of cartilage are to provide a congruent articulation surfaces between bones, to transmit load across the joint, and to allow low-friction movements between opposing joint surfaces. The sophisticated manner in which these functions are performed becomes evident from some of the mechanical characteristics of normal cartilage. For example, due to the leverage geometry of the muscles and the dynamic nature of human activity, the cartilage of the hip is exposed to about eight times body weight in fast walking [Paul, 1976]. Over a period of 10 years, an active person may subject the cartilage of the hip to more than 17 million weight-bearing cycles [Jeffery, 1994]. From the point of view of the optimal lubrication provided by synovial fluid, cartilage's extremely low frictional resistance makes it 15 times easier to move opposing joint surfaces than to move an ice-skate on ice [Mow & Hayes, 1991; Jeffery, 1994].

Cartilage functions as a unit with subchondral bone, which contributes to shock absorption by undergoing viscoelastic deformation of its fine trabecular structure. Although some joints, like the hip, are intrinsically stable by virtue of their shape, the majority require an elaborate combination of ligaments, meniscus, tendons, and muscles for stability. Because of the large multidirectional forces that travel through the joint, its stability is a dynamic process. Receptors within the ligaments fire, when stretched during motion, producing an integrated muscular contraction that provides stability for that specific displacement. Therefore, the ligaments are not passive joint restraints as once believed. The extreme complexity and high level of performance of biologic joints determine the standard to be met by artificial implants.

Total joint replacements are permanent implants, unlike those used to treat fractures, and the extensive bone and cartilage removed during implantation makes this procedure irreversible. Therefore, when faced with prosthesis failure and the impossibility to reimplant, the patient will face severe shortening of the extremity, instability or total rigidity of the joint, and difficulty in ambulation and often will be wheelchair-ridden.

The design of an implant for joint replacement should be based on the kinematics and dynamic load transfer characteristic of the joint. The material properties, shape, and methods used for fixation of the implant to the patient determine the load transfer characteristics. This is one of the most important elements that determines long-term survival of the implant, since bone responds to changes in load transfer with remodelling, mentioned earlier as Wolff's law. Overloading the implant-bone interface or shielding it from load transfer may result in bone resorption and subsequent loosening of the implant [Sarmiento et al., 1990]. The articulating surfaces of the joint should function with minimum friction and produce the least amount of wear products [Charnley, 1979]. The implant should be securely fixed to the body as early as possible (ideally immediately after implantation); however, removal of the implant should not require destruction of large amount of surrounding tissues. Loss of tissue, especially of bone, makes reimplantation difficult and often shortens the life span of the second joint replacement [Dupont & Charnley, 1972].

Decades of basic and clinical experimentation have resulted in a vast number of prosthetic designs and material combinations (Tables 47.3 and 47.4.) [Griss, 1984]. In the following section, the most relevant achievements in fixation methods and prosthetic design for different joints will be discussed at a conceptual level. Most joints can undergo partial replacement (hemiarthroplasty), that is, reconstruction of only one side of the joint while retaining the other. This is indicated in selected conditions when global joint degeneration has not taken place. This section will focus on total joint replacement, since this allows for a broader discussion of the biomaterials used.

Implant Fixation Method[1]

The development of a permanent fixation mechanism of implants to bone has been one of the most formidable challenges in the evolution of joint replacement. There are three types of methods of fix-

[1]See also Chapter 48.

TABLE 47.3 Biomaterials for Total Joint Replacements

Materials	Applications	Properties
CoCr alloy (cast or wrought)	Stem, head (ball)	Heavy, hard, stiff
	Cup, porous coating	High wear resistance
	Metal backing for UHMWPE	
Ti alloy	Stem, porous coating	Low stiffness
	Metal backing for UHMWPE	Low wear resistance
Pure titanium	Porous coating	Excellent osseointegration
Calcium hydroxyapatite	Surface coating	Fast osseointegration
		Long-term degradation
		Brittle
Alumina	Head, cup	Hard, brittle
		High wear resistance
Zirconia	Head	Heavy and high toughness
		High wear resistance
UHMWPE	Cup, tibial plateau	Low friction
		Low creep resistance
PMMA	Bone cement fixation	Brittle, weak in tension
		Low fatigue strength

Note: Stem: femoral hip stem/chondylar knee stem; head: femoral head of the hip stem; cup: acetabular cup of the hip.

ation: First, by means of mechanical interlock, which is achieved by press-fitting the implant [Cameron, 1994a], by using polymethylmethacrylate as a grouting agent [Charnley, 1979], or by using threaded components [Albrektsson et al., 1994]; second, by means of biological fixation, which is achieved by using textured or porous surfaces which allow bone to grow into the interstices [Cameron, 1994b]; third, by means of direct chemical bonding between implant and bone, for example, by coating the implant with calcium hydroxyapatite, which has a similar mineral structure to bone [Morscher, 1992]. Recently, direct bonding with bone was observed with bioglass, a glass-ceramic, through selective dissolution of the surface film [Hench, 1994]; however, its clinical application is still under investigation.

Each of the fixation mechanisms has an idiosyncratic behavior, and their load transfer characteristics as well as the failure mechanisms are different. Further complexity arises from prostheses that combine two or more of the fixation mechanisms in different regions of the implant. Multiple mechanisms of fixation are used in an effort to customize load transfer to requirements of different regions of bone, in an effort to preserve bone mass. Loosening, unlocking, or debonding between implant and bone constitute some of the most important mechanisms of prosthetic failure.

Bone Cement Fixation. Fixation of implants with polymethylmethacrylate (bone cement) provides immediate stability, allowing patients to bear all their weight on the extremity at once. In contrast, implants which depend on bone ingrowth require the patient to wait about 12 weeks to bear full weight.

TABLE 47.4 Types of Total Joint Replacement

Joint	Types
Hip	Ball and socket
Knee	Hinged, semiconstrained, surface replacement: unicompartment or bicompartment
Shoulder	Ball and socket
Ankle	Surface replacement
Elbow	Hinged, semiconstrained surface, surface replacement
Wrist	Ball and socket, space filler
Finger	Hinged, space filler

Source: Modified from Griss [1984].

Bone cement functions as a grouting material; consequently, its anchoring power depends on its ability to penetrate between bone trabeculae during the insertion of the prosthesis [Charnley, 1979]. Being a viscoelastic polymer, it has the ability to function as a shock absorber. It allows loads to be transmitted uniformly between the implant and bone, reducing localized high-contact stress.

Fixation with bone cement creates bone-cement and cement-implant interfaces, and loosening may occur at either one. The mechanisms to enhance the stability of the metal-cement interface constitute an area of controversy in joint replacement. Some investigators have focused their efforts in increasing the bond between metal and cement by roughening the implant, or precoating it with polymethylmethacrylate to prevent sinking of the prosthesis within the mantle, and circulation of debris within the interface [Park et al., 1978; Barb et al., 1982; Harris & Davies, 1988]. In contrast, others polish the implant surfaces and favor wedge-shaped designs which encourage sinking of the prosthesis within the cement, to profit from the viscoelastic deformation of the mantle by loading the cement in compression [Ling, 1992].

The problems with bone-cement interface may arise from intrinsic factors such as the properties of the polymethylmethacrylate and bone, as well as extrinsic factors such as the cementing technique. Refinements in the cementing technique, such as pulsatile lavage of the medullary canal, optimal hemostasis of the cancellous bone, and drying of medullary canal and pressurized insertion of the prosthesis, can result in a cement-bone interface free of gaps, with maximal interdigitation with cancellous bone [Harris & Davies, 1988]. Despite optimal cementing technique, a thin fibrous membrane may appear in various regions of the interface, due to various factors, for example, to the toxic effect of free methylmethacrylate monomer, to necrosis of the bone resulting from high polymerization temperatures, or to devascularization during preparation of the canal [Goldring et al., 1983]. Although a fibrous membrane between bone and cement interface may be present in a well-functioning implant, it may also increase in width over time (most probably as a result of the accumulation of polyethylene debris from the bearing couple) and may result in macromotion, bone loss, and eventual loosening [Ebramzadeh et al., 1994]. Finally, the cement itself may be improved by mixing monomer and polymer under vacuum and/or centrifuging it [Harris & Davies, 1988]. During implantation, various devices are used to guarantee uniform thickness of the mantle to minimize risk of fatigue failure of the cement [Oh et al., 1978].

Porous Ingrowth Fixation. Bone ingrowth can occur with biocompatible implants which provide pores larger than 75 microns in diameter, which is the size required to accommodate an osteon. The optimum pore size range in clinical practice is 100–350 microns [Cameron, 1994*b*]. Implant motion inhibits bony ingrowth, and a large bone-metal gap prolongs or prevents the *osseointegration* time [Curtis et al., 1992]. Therefore, precise surgical implantation and prevention of postoperative weight bearing for about 12 weeks are required for implant fixation.

The porous coated implants require active participation of the bone in the fixation of the implant, in contrast to cementation where the bone has a passive role. Therefore, porous coated implants are best indicated in conditions where the bone mass is near normal. The implant design should allow ingrown bone to be subjected to continuous loading within a physiologic range in order to prevent loss of bone mass due to stress shielding. Porous ingrowth prostheses are notoriously difficult to remove, and substantial bone damage often results during the removal process. For this reason, they should be optimized to provide predictable ingrowth with a minimal area of surgically accessible porous coated surface.

Commercially pure titanium, titanium alloy, and calcium hydroxyapatite (HA) are used for porous coating materials. With pure titanium, three different types of porosity can be achieved: plasma spray coating, and sintering of wire mesh or beads, on an implant surface (Fig. 47.7) [Morscher, 1992]. Thermal processing of the porous coating may weaken the underlying metal (implant). Additional problems may result from flaking of the porous coating materials, since loosened metal particles may cause severe wear when they migrate into the articulation site (bearing couple) [Agins et al., 1988].

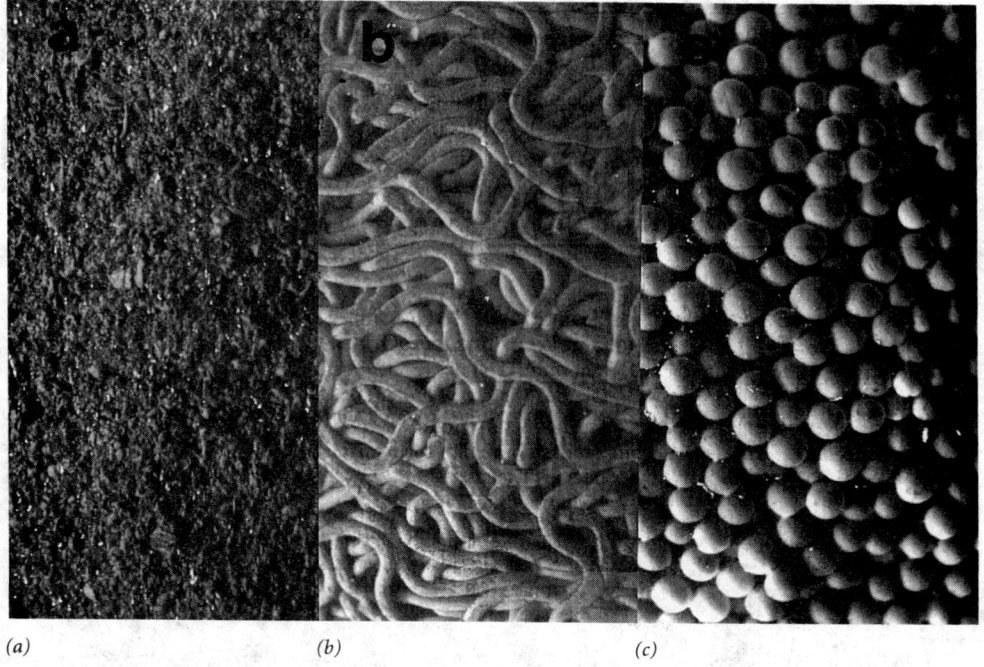

(a) *(b)* *(c)*

FIGURE 47.7 Scanning electron micrographs of three different types of porous coating: (*a*) plasma sprayed, (*b*) sintered wire mesh, and (*c*) sintered beads.

A thin calcium hydroxyapatite coating over the porous titanium surface has been used in an effort to enhance osseointegration; however, this coating improves only early-stage interfacial strength [Friedman, 1992; Capello & Bauer, 1994]. The long-term degradation and/or resorption of hydroxyapatite is still under investigation.

Total Joint Replacements

Hip Joint Replacement.   The prosthesis for total hip replacement consists of a femoral component and an acetabular component (Fig. 47.8*a*). The femoral stem is divided into head, neck, and shaft. The femoral stem is made of Ti alloy or CoCr alloy (316L stainless steel was used earlier) and is fixed into a reamed medullary canal by cementation or press fitting. Femoral head is made of CoCr alloy, alumina, or zirconia. Although Ti alloy heads function well under clean articulating conditions, they have fallen into disuse because of their low resistance to third-body wear.

The prostheses can be monolithic when they consist of one part or modular when they consist of two or more parts and require assembly during surgery. Monolithic components are often less expensive and less prone to corrosion or disassembly. However, modular components allow customizing of the implant intraoperatively and during future revision surgeries, for example, modifying the length of an extremity by using a different femoral neck length after the stem has been cemented in place or exchanging a worn polyethylene bearing surface for a new one without removing the metallic part of the prosthesis from the bone. In modular implants (Fig. 47.8*b*), the femoral head is fitted to the femoral neck with a Morse taper, which allows changes in head material and diameter and neck length. Table 47.5 illustrates the most frequently used combinations of material in total hip replacement.

When the acetabular component is monolithic, it is made of ultra-high-molecular-weight polyethylene (UHMWPE); when it is modular, it consists of a metallic shell and an UHMWPE insert. The metallic shell seeks to decrease the microdeformation of the UHMWPE and to provide a porous surface for fixation of the cup [Skinner, 1992]. The metallic shell allows worn polyethylene liners to

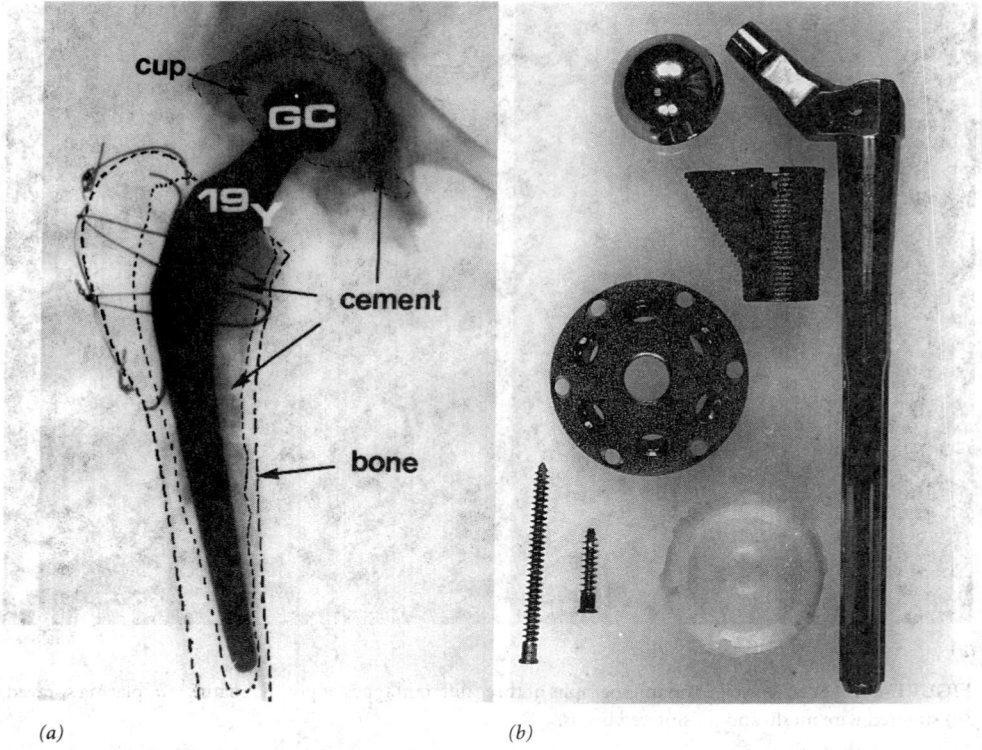

(a)   *(b)*

FIGURE 47.8   (*a*) Radiograph of a cemented Charnley hip prosthesis (monolithic femoral and ac- etabular component, 15-year follow-up). (*b*) Modular total hip systems: head, stem, porous coated proximal sleeve, porous coated metal backing, UHMWPE cup, and fixation screws.

be exchanged. In cases of repetitive dislocation of the hip after surgery, the metallic shell allows replacing the old liner with a more constrained one to provide additional stability. Great effort has been placed on developing an effective retaining system for the insert as well as on maximizing the congruity between insert and metallic shell (Fig. 47.8*b*). Dislodgement of the insert results in dislocation of the hip and damage of the femoral head, since it contacts the metallic shell directly. Micromotion between insert and shell produces additional polyethylene debris which can eventually contribute to bone loss [Friedman et al., 1994].

The hip joint is a ball-and-socket joint, which derives its stability from congruity of the implants, pelvic muscles, and capsule. The prosthetic hip components are optimized to provide a wide range of motion without impingement of the neck of the prosthesis on the rim of the acetabular cup to prevent dislocation. The design characteristics must enable implants to support loads that may reach more than 8 times body weight [Paul, 1976]. Proper femoral neck length and correct restoration of the center of motion and femoral offset decrease the bending stress on the prosthesis-bone inter- face. High stress concentration or stress shielding may result in bone resorption around the implant. For example, if the femoral stem is designed with sharp corners (diamond-shaped in a cross- section), the bone in contact with the corners of the implant may necrose and resorb.

Load bearing and motion of the prosthesis produce wear debris from the articulating surface and from the interfaces where there is micromotion. The principal source of wear under normal con- ditions is the UHMWPE-bearing surface in the cup. Several hundred thousands of particles are generated with each step, and a large proportion of these particles are smaller then one micron [McKellop et al., 1995]. Cells from the immune system of the host are able to identify the polyeth- ylene particles as foreign and initiate a complex inflammatory response. This response may lead to

TABLE 47.5 Possible Combinations of Total Hip Replacements

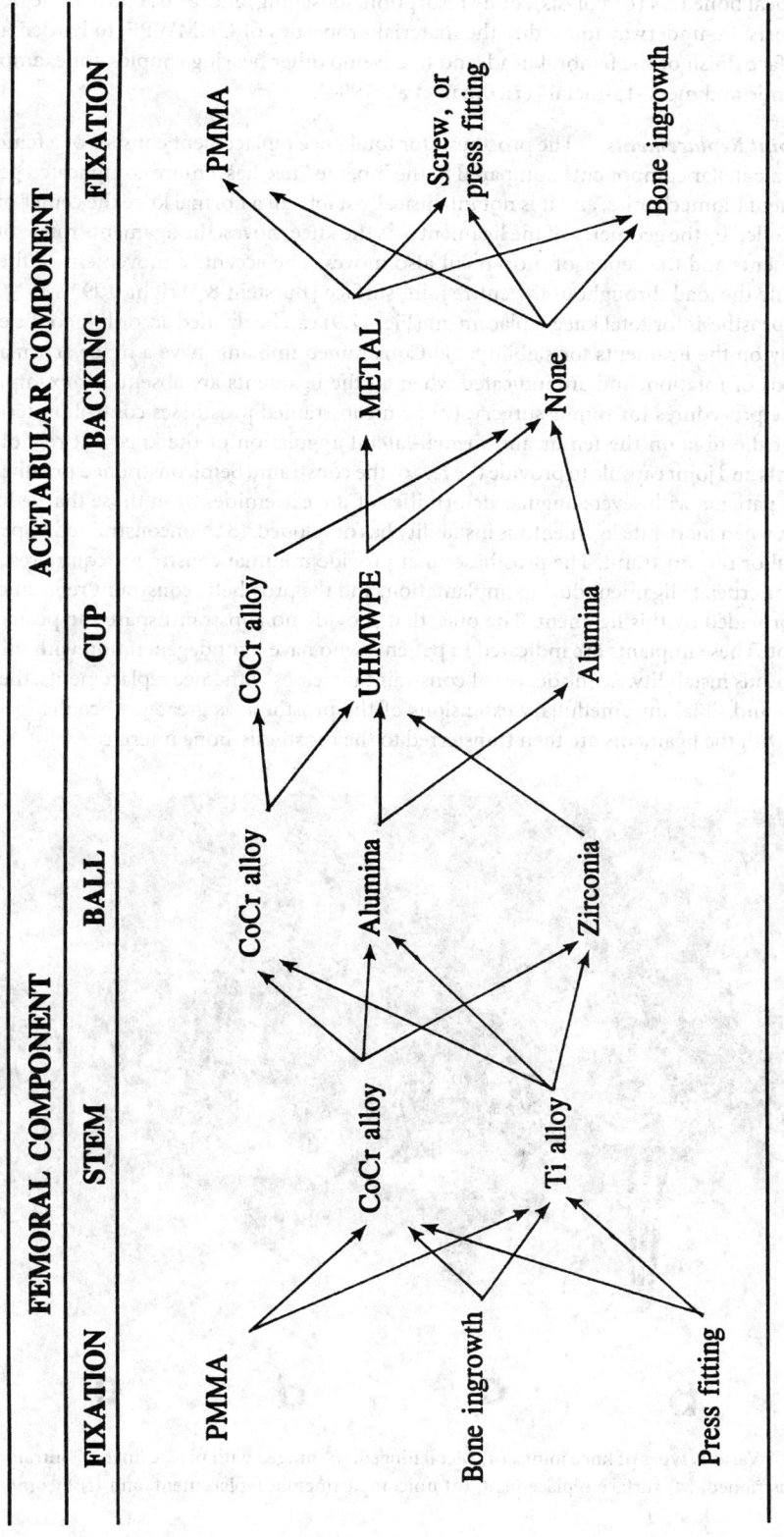

rapid focal bone loss (osteolysis), bone resorption, loosening, and/or fracture of the bone. Numerous efforts are underway to modify the material properties of UHMWPE, to harden and improve the surface finish of the femoral head, and to develop other bearing couples, for example, ceramic-to-ceramic and metal-to-metal [Friedman et al., 1994].

Knee Joint Replacements.   The prosthesis for total knee replacement consists of a femoral, a tibial, and/or a patellar component. Compared to the hip, the knee has a more complicated geometry and movement biomechanics, and it is not intrinsically stable. In a normal knee the center of movement is controlled by the geometry of the ligaments. As the knee moves, the ligaments rotate on their bony attachments and the center of movement also moves. The eccentric movement of the knee helps distribute the load throughout the entire joint surface [Burstein & Wright, 1993].

The prosthesis for total knee replacement (Fig. 47.9) can be divided according to the extent which they rely on the ligaments for stability: (1) Constrained implants have a hinge articulation, with a fixed axis of rotation, and are indicated when all the ligaments are absent, for example, in reconstructive procedures for tumor surgery. (2) Semiconstrained prostheses control posterior displacement of the tibia on the femur and medial-lateral angulation of the knee but rely on remaining ligaments and joint capsule to provide the rest of the constraint. Semiconstrained prostheses are often used in patients with severe angular deformities of the extremities or in those that require revision surgery, when moderate ligamentous instability has developed. (3) Nonconstrained implants provide minimal or no constraint. The prostheses that provide minimal constraint require resection of the posterior cruciate ligament during implantation, and the prosthetic constraint reproduces that normally provided by this ligament. The ones that provide no constraint spare the posterior cruciate ligament. These implants are indicated in patients who have joint degeneration with minimal or no ligamentous instability. As the degree of constraint increases with knee replacements, the need to use femoral and tibial intramedullary extensions of the prosthesis is greater, since the loads normally shared with the ligaments are then transferred to the prosthesis-bone interface.

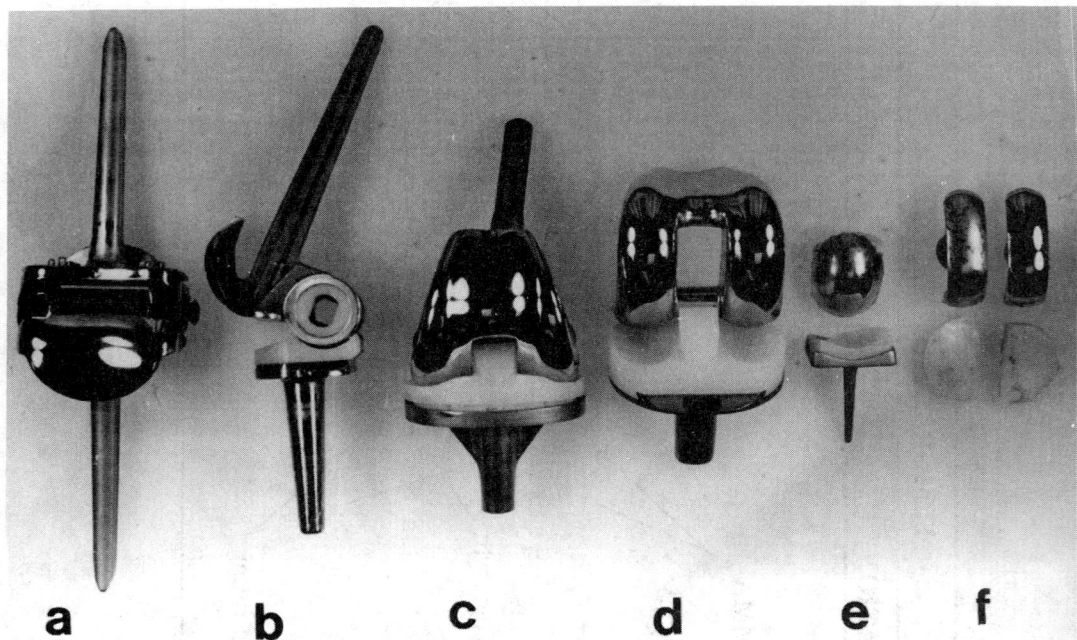

FIGURE 47.9   Various types of knee joints: (*a*) Metal hinged, (*b*) hinged with plastic liner, (*c*) intramedullary fixed semiconstrained, (*d*) surface replacement, (*e*) unicompartmental replacement, and (*f*) bicompartment replacement.

Total knee replacements can be implanted with cement or without cement, the latter relying on porous coating for fixation. The femoral components are typically made of CoCr or titanium alloy and the tibial components of UHMWPE. In modular components, the tibial polyethylene component assembles onto a metallic tibial tray. The patellar component is made of UHMWP, and a metal back is added to components designed for uncemented use.

The wear characteristic of the surface of tibial plateaus differs from acetabular components. The point contact stress and sliding motion of the components result in delamination and fatigue wear of the UHMWPE [Walker, 1993]. Presumably because of the relatively larger particle size of polyethylene debris, osteolysis around a total knee joint is less frequent than in a total hip replacement.

The relatively small size of the patellar component compared to the forces that travel through the extensor mechanism and the small area of bone available for anchorage of the prosthesis make the patella vulnerable.

Ankle Joint Replacement.   Total ankle replacements have not met with as much success as total hip and knee replacements, and they typically loosen within a few years of service [Claridge et al., 1991]. This is mainly due to the high load transfer demand over the relatively small ankle surface area and the need to replace three articulating surfaces (tibial, talar, and fibular). The joint configurations that have been used are cylindrical, reverse cylindrical, and spherical. The materials used to construct ankle joints are usually CoCr alloy and UHMWPE. Degeneration of the ankle joint is currently treated with fusion of the joint, since prostheses for total ankle replacement are considered to be still under initial development. Figure 47.10 shows ankle and other total joint replacements.

Shoulder Joint Replacements.   The prostheses for total shoulder replacement consist of a humeral and a glenoid component. Like the femoral stem, the humeral component can be divided into head, neck, and shaft. Variations in the length of the neck result in changes in the length of the extremity. However, since the patient's perception of length of the upper extremity is not as accurate as that of

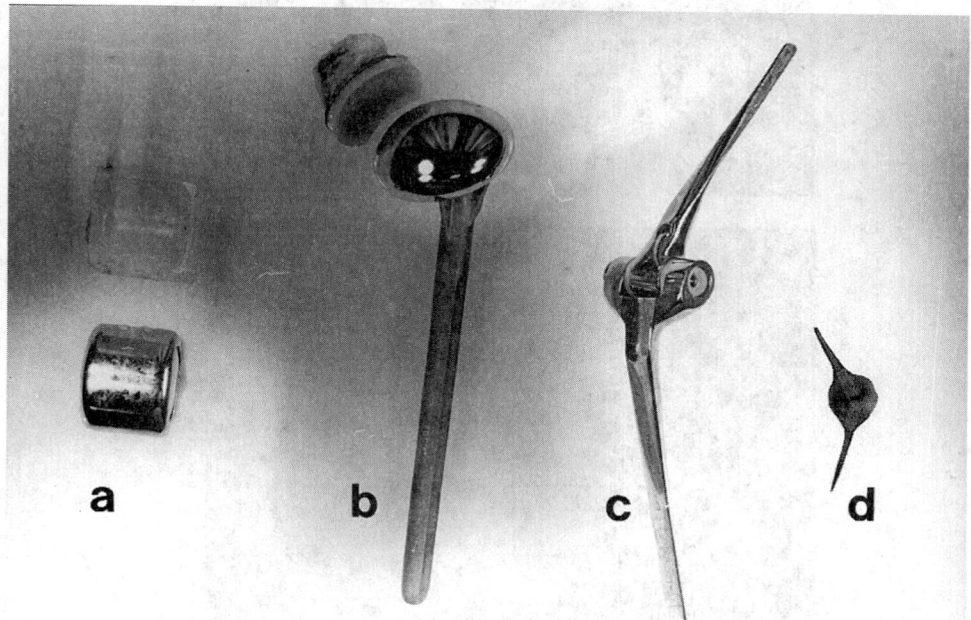

FIGURE 47.10   Miscellaneous examples of prosthesis for total joint replacements: (*a*) Ankle, (*b*) socket-ball shoulder joint, (*c*) hinged elbow joint, and (*d*) encapsulated finger joint.

the lower, the various neck lengths are used to fine-tune the tension of the soft tissues, to obtain maximal stability, and range of motion.

The shoulder has the largest range of motion in a body, which results from a shallow ball and socket joint that allows a combination of rotation and sliding motions between the joint surfaces. To compensate for the compromise in congruity, the shoulder has an elaborate capsular and ligamentous structure, which provides the basic stabilization; however, the muscle girdle of the shoulder provides additional dynamic stability. A decrease in the radius of curvature of the implant to compensate for soft-tissue instability will result in a decrease in the range of motion [Neer, 1990].

Elbow Joint Replacements.   The elbow joint is a hinge-type joint allowing mostly flexion and extension but having a polycentric motion [Goel & Blair, 1985]. The elbow joint implants are hinged, semiconstrained, or unconstrained. These implants, like those of the ankle, have a high failure rate and are not used commonly. The high loosening rate is the result of high rotational moments, limited bone stock for fixation, and minimal ligamentous support [Morrey, 1993]. In contrast to fusions of the ankle which function well, fusions of the elbow result in a moderate degree of incapacitation.

Finger Joint Replacements.   Finger joint replacements are divided into three types: (1) hinge, (2) polycentric, and (3) space filler. The most widely used are the space-filler type. These are made of high-performance silicone rubber (polydimethylsiloxane) and are stabilized with a passive fixa-

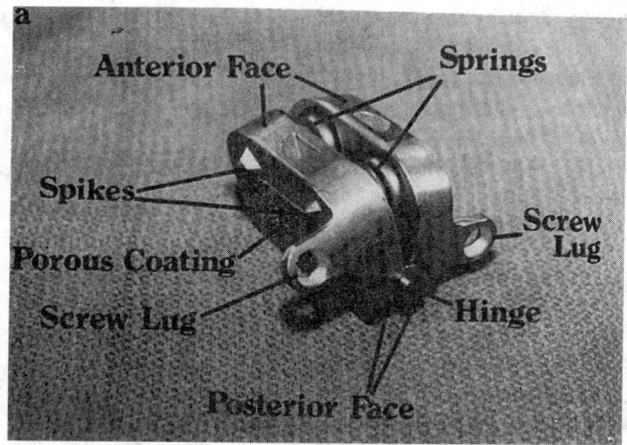

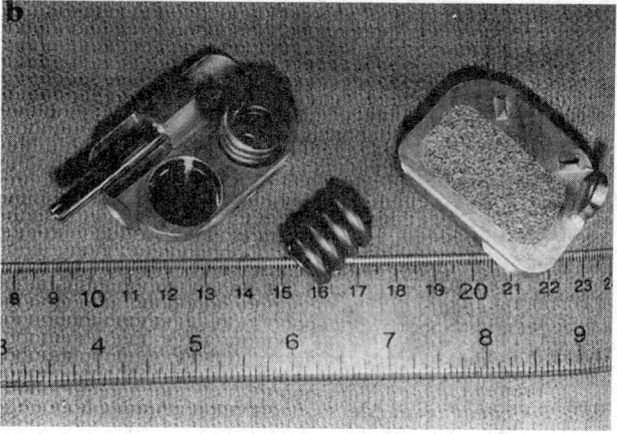

FIGURE 47.11   Experimental artificial disc "used" to restore function of the degenerated spine disc.

tion method. This method depends on the development of a thin, fibrous membrane between implant and bone. This fixation can provide only minimal rigidity of the joint [Swanson, 1973]. Implant wear and cold flow associated with erosive cystic changes of adjacent bone have been reported with silicone implant [Carter et al., 1986; Maistrelli, 1994].

Prosthetic Intervertebral Disc.   Fusion of a spinal motion segment in degenerative disc disease increases (1) the stiffness across the stabilized segment, and (2) stress on adjacent levels. The results of spinal fusion have been unpredictable. It can lead to further degeneration of the adjacent spinal levels, among other complications. In order to reduce the adverse effects of the fusion process, artificial disc prostheses, similar in concept to the total joint replacements presented in the above sections, have been developed (Fig. 47.11). These designs, although in infancy, range from flexible polymer inserts to ball-and-socket or hinge-type designs [Hedman et al., 1991].

fining Terms

Bone resorption: A type of bone loss due to the greater osteoclastic activity than osteogenic activity.

Callus: Unorganized meshwork of woven bone which is formed following fracture of bone to achieve an early stability of the fracture.

Fibrous membrane: Thin layer of soft tissue which covers an implant to isolate it from the body.

Necrosis: Cell death caused by enzymes or heat.

Osseointegration: Direct contact of bone tissues to an implant surface without fibrous membrane.

Osteoclastic: Activity of bone destruction or removal of old bone by bone cells called *osteoclasts*.

Osteogenic: Activity for bone formation in growth or repair of bone. Bone cells for the osteogenic activity are called *osteoblasts*.

Primary healing: Bone healing in which union occurs directly without forming callus.

Secondary healing: Bone union with a callus formation.

ferences

Agins HJ, Alcock NW, Bansal M, et al. 1988. Metallic wear in failed Titanium-alloy total hip replacements. A histological and quantitative analysis. J Bone Joint Surg 70A(3): 347.

Albrektsson T, Carlsson LV, Morberg P, et al. 1994. Directly bone-anchored implants. In R Hurley (ed), Bone Implant Interface, pp 97–120, St. Louis, Mosby.

Barb W, Park JB, von Recum AF, et al. 1982. Intramedullary fixation of artificial hip joints with bone cement precoated implants: I. Interfacial strengths. J Biomed Mater Res 16:447.

Brand RA, Rubin CT. 1987. Fracture healing. In J Albert, R Brand (eds), Scientific Basis of Orthopaedics, 2d ed, pp 325–340, Norwalk, Conn, Appleton & Lange.

Brighton CT. 1984. Principle of fracture healing. Instructional Course Lectures, American Academy of Orthopaedic Surgeons.

Buckwalter JA, Woo S, et al. 1993. Soft-tissue aging and musculoskeletal function. J Bone Joint Surg 75A(10):1533.

Burstein AH, Wright TH. 1993. Biomechanics. In J Insall, R Windsor, W Scott, et al. (eds). Surgery of the Knee, 2d ed, vol 7, pp 43–62, New York, Churchill Livingstone.

Cameron HU. 1994*a*. Smooth metal-bone interface. In R Hurley (ed), Bone Implant Interface, pp 121–144, St. Louis, Mosby.

Cameron HU. 1994*b*. The implant-bone interface: porous metals. In R Hurley (ed), Bone Implant Interface, pp 145–168, St. Louis, Mosby.

Capello WN, Bauer TW. 1994. Hydroxyapatite in orthopaedic surgery. In R Hurley (ed), Bone Implant Interface, pp 191–202, St. Louis, Mosby.

Carter P, Benton L, Dysert P. 1986. Silicone rubber carpal implants: A study of the incidence of late osseous complications. J Hand Surg 11(5):639.

Charnley J. 1979. Low Friction Arthroplasty of the Hip. Berlin, Springer-Verlag.

Claes L. 1989. The mechanical and morphological properties of bone beneath internal fixation plates of differing rigidity. J Orthop Res 7:170.

Claridge RJ, Hart MB, Jones RA, et al. 1991. Replacement arthroplasties of the ankle and foot. In M Jahss (ed), Disorder of the Foot & Ankle, 2d ed, pp 2647–2664, Philadelphia, Saunders.

Cochran GVB. 1982. Biomechanics of orthopaedic structures. In Primer in Orthopaedic Biomechanics, pp 143–215, New York, Churchill Livingstone.

Curtis MJ, Jinnah RH, Wilson VD, et al. 1992. The initial stability of uncemented acetabular components. J Bone Joint Surg 74B(3):372.

DeCoster TA, Heetderks DB, Downey DJ, et al. 1990. Optimizing bone screw pullout force. J Orthop Trauma 4(2):169.

Dupont JA, Charnley J. 1972. Low-friction arthroplasty of the hip for the failures of previous operations. J Bone Joint Surg 54B(1):77.

Ebramzadeh E, Sarmiento A, McKellop HA, et al. 1994. The cement mantle in total hip arthroplasty: Analysis of long-term radiographic results. J Bone Joint Surg 76A(1):77.

Friedman RJ, Black J, Galante JO, et al. 1994. Current concepts in orthopaedic biomaterials and implant fixation. Instructional Course Lectures, American Academy of Orthopaedic Surgeons 43:233.

Friedman RJ. 1992. Advance in biomaterials and factors affecting implant fixation. Instructional Course Lectures. American Academy of Orthopaedic Surgeons 41:127.

Goel VK, Blair W. 1985. Biomechanics of the elbow joint. Automedica 6:119.

Goldring SR, Schiller AL, Roelke M, et al. 1983. The synovial-like membrane at the bone-cement interface in loose total hip replacements and its proposed role in bone lysis. J Bone Joint Surg 65A(5):575.

Griss P. 1984. Assessment of clinical status of total joint replacement. In P Ducheyne, GW Hastings (eds), Functional Behavior of Orthopaedic Biomaterials, pp 21–48, Boca Raton, Fla, CRC Press.

Harris WH, Davies JP. 1988. Modern use of modern cement for total hip replacement. Orthop Clin North Am 19(3):581.

Hedman TP, Kostuik JP, Fernie GR, et al. 1991. Design of an intervertebral disc prosthesis. Spine 16:256.

Hench LL. 1994. Bioactive glasses, ceramics and composites. In R Hurley (ed), Bone Implant Interface, pp 181–190, St. Louis, Mosby.

Hulth A. 1989. Current concepts of fracture healing. Clin Orthop 249:265.

Hutzschenreuter P, Brümmer H. 1980. Screw design and stability. In H Uhthoff (ed), Current Concepts of Internal Fixation, pp 244–250, Berlin, Springer-Verlag.

Insall JN. 1993. Surgery of the Knee, 2d ed. Insall J. Windsor, R., Scott, W., Kelly, M., and Aglietti, P. New York, Churchill Livingstone.

Jeffery AK. 1994. Articular cartilage and the orthopaedic surgeon. Part 1: Structure and function. Cur Orthop 8:38.

Kessler SB, Hallfeldt KK, Perren SM, et al. 1986. The effects of reaming and intramedullary nailing on fracture healing. Clin Orthop 212:18.

Ling RS. 1992. The use of a collar and precoating on cemented femoral stems is unnecessary and detrimental. Clin Orthop 285:73.

Maistrelli GL. 1994. Polymers in orthopaedic surgery. In R Hurley (ed), Bone Implant Interface, pp 169–190, St. Louis, Mosby.

McKellop HA, Campbell P, Park SH, et al. 1995. The origin of submicron polyethylene wear debris in total hip arthroplasty. Clin Orthop 311:3.

Morrey BF. 1993. The Elbow and Its Disorders, 2d ed, Philadelphia. Saunders.

Morscher EW. 1992. Current status of acetabular fixation in primary total hip arthroplasty. Clin Orthop 274:172.

Mow VC, Hayes WC. 1991. Basic Orthopaedic Biomechanics, New York, Raven Press.

Neer CS. 1990. Shoulder Reconstruction, Philadelphia, Saunders.

Oh I, Carlson CE, Tomford WW, et al. 1978. Improved fixation of the femoral component after total hip replacement using a methacrylate intramedullary plug. J Bone Joint Surg 60A(5):608.

O'Sullivan ME, Chao EYS, Kelly PJ. 1989. Current concepts review: The effects of fixation on fracture healing. J Bone Joint Surg 71A(2):306.

Park JB, Lakes RS. 1992. Biomaterials: An Introduction, 2d ed, New York, London, Plenum.

Park JB, Malstrom CS, von Recum AF. 1978. Intramedullary fixation of implants precoated with bone cement: A preliminary study. Biomater Med Dev Artif Org 6(4):361.

Paul, JP. 1976. Loading on normal hip and knee joints and joint replacement. In S Mchaldach, D Hohmann (eds.), Advances in Hip and Knee Joint Technology, p. 53–77, Berlin, Springer-Verlag.

Perren SM. 1989. The biomechanics and biology of internal fixation using plates and nails. Orthopaedics, 12(1):21.

Perren SM. 1991. Basic aspects of internal fixation. In M Müller, M Allgöwer, R Schneider, H Willenegger (eds), Manual of Internal Fixation, 3d ed, pp 1–112, Berlin, Springer-Verlag.

Perren SM, Cordey J, Rahn BA. 1988. Early temporary porosis of bone induced by internal fixation implants: A reaction to necrosis, not to stress protection? Clin Orthop 232:139.

Salter RB. 1988. The biologic concept of continuous passive motion of synovial joints. The first 18 years of basic research and its clinical application. Clin Orthop 242:12.

Sarmiento A. Ebramzadeh E, Gogan WJ, et al. 1990. Cup containment and orientation in cemented total hip arthroplasties. J Bone Joint Surg 72B(6):996.

Schatzker J, Sanderson R, Murnaghan JP. 1975. The holding power of orthopaedic screws in vivo. Clin Orthop 108:115.

Schenk RK. 1992. Biology of fracture repair. In B Browner, J Jupitor, A Levine, et al (eds), Skeletal Trauma, pp 31–75, Philadelphia, Saunders.

Skinner HB. 1992. Current biomaterial problems in implants. Instructional Course Lectures, American Academy of Orthopaedic Surgeons 41:137.

Swanson AB. 1973. Concepts of flexible implant design. In A Swanson (ed), Flexible Implant Reconstruction Arthroplasty in the Hand and Extremities, pp 47–59, St. Louis, Mosby.

Taitsman JP, Saha S. 1977. Tensile strength of wire-reinforced bone cement and twisted stainless-steel wire. J Bone Joint Surg 59A: 419.

Tencer AF, Johnson KD, Kely RF, et al. 1993. Biomechanics of fractures and fracture fixation. Instructional Course Lectures, American Academy of Orthopaedic Surgeons 42:19.

Uhthoff HK, Finnegan MA. 1984. The role of rigidity in fracture fixation. Arch Orthop Trauma Surg 102:163.

Walker PS. 1993. Design of total knee arthroplasy. In J Insall, R Windsor, W Scott et al. (eds), Surgery of the Knee, 2d ed, pp 723–738, New York, Churchill Livingstone.

Weinstein AM, Spires WP Jr, Klawitter JJ, et al. 1979. Orthopedic implant retrieval and analysis study. In BC Syrett, A Acharya (eds), Corrosion and Degradation of Implant Materials, pp 212–228, Philadelphia, American Society for Testing and Materials Tech. Pub. No. 684.

Wolff J. 1986. The Law of Bone Remodelling, R Maquet, R Furlong (trans), Berlin, Springer-Verlag.

47.2 Dental Implants: The Relationship of Materials Characteristic to Biologic Properties

J. C. Keller

As dental implants have become an accepted treatment modality for partially and fully edentulous patients, it has become increasingly apparent that the interaction of the host tissue with the underlying implant surface is of critical importance for long-term prognosis [Smith, 1993; Young, 1988]. From the anatomical viewpoint, it is generally accepted that dental implants must contact and become integrated with several types of host tissues. Due largely to the work of Branemark and his colleagues [Albrektsson et al., 1983; Branemark, 1983], the importance of developing and maintaining a substantial bone-implant interface for mechanical retention and transmission of occlusal forces was realized. Despite documented long-term success of dental implants, longer-term implant failures are noted due to poor integration of connective and epithelial tissues and subsequent failure to develop a permucosal seal akin to that with natural tooth structures. From a biologic point of view, the characteristics of the implant substrate which permit hard and soft tissue integration and prevent adhesion of bacteria and plaque need to be further understood. It is likely that as a more complete understanding of the basic biologic responses of host tissues becomes known, refinements in the currently employed materials as well as new and improved materials will become available for use in the dental implant field.

It is important to realize that the overall biologic response of host tissue to dental implants can be divided into two distinct but interrelated phases (as given in Table 47.6). Phase I consists of the tissue responses which occur during the clinical healing phase immediately following implantation of dental implants. During this healing phase, the initial biologic processes of protein and molecular deposition on the implant surface are followed by cellular attachment, migration, and differentiation [Stanford & Keller, 1991]. It is therefore important to understand the characteristics of the implant material which affect the initial formation of the host tissue–implant interface. These characteristics include materials selection and the physical and chemical properties of the implant surface. These initial tissue responses lead to the cellular expression and maturation of extracellular matrix and ultimately to the development of bony interfaces with the implant material. After the initial healing phase is complete, usually between 3–6 months according to the two-stage Branemark implant design, the bone interface remodels under the occlusal forces placed on the implant during the Phase II functional period [Brunski, 1992; Skalak, 1985]. The overall bioresponses including bone remodeling during the functional phase of implant service life are then strongly influenced by the characteristics of loading and distribution of stress at the interface [Brunski, 1992]. The ability of the maturing interface to "remodel" as stresses are placed on the implant thus depend in large part on the original degree of tissue–implant surface interaction.

This chapter will focus on the factors concerning dental implants which affect biologic properties of currently available dental implant materials. As pertains to each major topic, the influence of the materials properties on biologic responses will be emphasized.

TABLE 47.6   Correlation Between the Clinical Phases of Implant Service Life with Biologic Events and Important Implant Materials Characteristics

Clinical Phase	Biological Events	Influential Materials Characteristics
I (healing)	Protein deposition	Materials selection
	Cell attachment	Metals
	Cell migration	Ceramics
	Development of extracellular matrix	Chemical and physical characteristics
	Bone deposition	Topography
		Micro
		Macro
		Surface chemistry
		Inert
		Dissolution
II (functional)	Matrix and bone remodeling	

Effects of Materials Selection

Metals and Alloys

Previously, dental implants have been fabricated from several metallic systems, including stainless steel and cobalt-chrome alloys as well as from the titanium family of metals. Several studies have reported on the ability of host bone tissues to "integrate" with various metal implant surfaces [Albrektsson et al., 1983; Johansson et al., 1989; Katsikeris et al., 1987]. In current paradigms, the term *osseointegration* refers to the ability of host tissues to form a functional interface with implant surfaces without an intervening layer of connective tissue akin to a foreign body tissue capsule observable at the light microscopic level [Albrektsson et al., 1983; Branemark, 1983]. By this definition, it becomes apparent that several biomedical materials including Ti and Ti alloy fulfill this general criterion. Ultrastructural investigations using transmission electron microscopy (TEM) approaches have further refined descriptions of the tissue implant interface, and the early work by Albrektsson and colleagues [1983] has become the descriptive standard by which other materials interfaces are compared. When bone was allowed to grow on Ti, a partially calcified amorphous ground substance was deposited in immediate contact with the implant, followed by a collagenous fibril-based extracellular matrix, osteoblast cell processes, and a more highly calcified matrix generally 200–300 Å from the implant surface.

However, other metallic materials have fallen from favor for use as dental implants due to widely differing mechanical properties compared to bone (Table 47.7), which can result in a phenomenon termed *stress shielding* [Brunski, 1992; Slalak, 1985], and the propensity for formation of potentially toxic corrosion products due to insufficient corrosion resistance properties [Lucas et al., 1987; Van Orden, 1985]. Ultrastructurally, the interface between bone and 316L stainless steel was described as consisting of a multiple-cell layer separating the bone from metal. Inflammatory cells were prominent in this layer, and a thick proteoglycan noncollagenous coating was present. This histologic appearance resembled that of a typical foreign body reaction and typifies a nonosseointegration-type response. The poor biologic response to stainless steel alloys has been reconfirmed by recently conducted in vitro studies which related the inability of host tissue to attach to the metal surface to the toxicity associated with metal ion release [Vrouwenvelder et al., 1993].

Due in large measure to the introduction and overall clinical success of the Branemark system, the range of metallic materials utilized for dental implants has become limited largely to commercially pure titanium (cpTi > 99.5%) and its major alloy, Ti-6A1-4V [De Porter et al., 1986; Keller et al., 1987]. Controversy remains, largely due to commercial advertising interests, as to which material provides a more suitable surface for tissue integration. Early work by Johansson and coworkers [1989] reported that sputtercoated Ti alloy surfaces resulted in wide (5000 Å) *amorphous zones* devoid of collagen filaments, compared to the thinner 200–400 Å collagen-free amorphous zone surrounding cpTi surfaces. Subsequent studies revealed differences in the oxide characteristics between

TABLE 47.7 Approximate Room Temperature Mechanical Properties of Selected Implant Materials Compared to Bone

	Elastic Modulus (MPa x 10^3)	Proportional Limit (MPa)	Ultimate Tensile Strength (MPa)	Percent Elongation
316L SS				
Annealed	200	240	550	50
Cold worked	200	790	965	20
CoCrMo(ASTM-F75)	240	500	700	10
Ti (ASTM-F67)	100	520	620	18
Ti-6Al-4V(ASTM-F136)	110	840	900	12
Cortical bone	18	130	140	1

Source: Keller and Lautenshlager [1986].

these sputtercoated cpTi and Ti alloy surfaces used for histologic and ultrastructural interfacial analyses. Significant surface contamination and the presence of V was observed in the Ti alloy surface, which led to an overall woven bone interface compared to the cpTi surface which had a more compact bone interface. Orr and colleagues [1992] demonstrated a similar ultrastructural morphology for interfaces of bone to Ti and Ti alloy, respectively. In each case an afibrillar matrix with calcified globular accretions, similar in appearance to cement lines in haversian systems, were observed in intimate contact with the oxide surface. Any slight differences in morphology were attributed to minor differences in surface topography or microtexture rather than chemical differences between the two surface oxides.

This is an area that is still under investigation, although recent research indicates that the stable oxide of cpTi and Ti alloy provide suitable surfaces for biologic integration [Keller et al., 1994]. Studies involving comprehensive surface analyses of prepared bulk cpTi and Ti alloy indicated that although the oxide on Ti alloy is somewhat thicker following standard surface preparations (polishing, cleaning, and acid passivation), the overall topography, the chemical characteristics, including presence and concentration of contaminants, and surface energetics were virtually identical for both materials as given in Table 47.8. In vitro experiments confirmed that the inherently clean condition of these oxides supports significant osteoblast cell attachment and migration and provides a hospitable surface to allow in vitro mineralization processes to occur [Orr et al., 1992].

In vitro experiments designed to study the ultrastructural details of bone-implant interfaces made from cpTi and Ti alloy may provide additional clues as to the histologic and ultrastructural differences which have been observed with these materials. Since clinical implants made from both materials appear to be successful [Branemark, 1983; De Porter et al., 1986], it is possible that because of the difference in mechanical properties between unalloyed and Ti alloy material, the longer-term tissue interface results from differences in bone remodelling due to the local biomechanical environment surrounding these materials [Brunski, 1992]. This hypothesis requires continued investigation for more definitive answers.

Ceramics and Ceramic Coatings

The use of single crystal sapphire or Al_2O_3 ceramic implants has remained an important component in the dental implant field [Driskell et al., 1973]. Although this material demonstrates excellent biologic compatibility, implants fabricated from Al_2O_3 have not reached a high degree of popularity in the United States. Morphologic analyses of the soft tissue interface with Al_2O_3 revealed a hemidesmosomal external lamina attachment adjacent to the *junctional epithelium*–implant interface [Steflik et al., 1984]. This ultrastructural description is often used for comparison purposes when determining the extent of soft-tissue interaction with dental implants. Similarly, in vivo studies

TABLE 47.8 Surface Characterizations of CpTi and Ti Alloy (means ± standard deviations)

	CpTi	Ti-6Al-4V
Surface roughness (Ra) (μm)		
Sandblasted	0.9 ± 0.2	0.7 ± 0.03
600 grit polish	0.2 ± 0.02	0.1 ± 0.02
Smooth, 1 μm polish	0.04 ± 0.01	0.03 ± 0.01
Atomic ratios to Ti		
C	1.5 ± 0.2	1.2 ± 0.1
O	2.8 ± 0.1	3.1 ± 0.2
N	0.08 ± 0.01	0.05 ± 0.01
Al	—	0.2 ± 0.04
V*	—	(0.02)*
Oxide thickness (Å)	32 ± 8	83 ± 12
Wetting angles (°)	52 ± 2	56 ± 4

*One specimen

of the bone–Al$_2$O$_3$ implant interface reveal high levels of bone-to-implant contact, with areas of intervening fibrous connective tissue. Although fibrous tissue was present at the interface, the implant remained immobile, and the interface was consistent with a dynamic support system. More recent ultrastructural studies have demonstrated a mineralized matrix in immediate apposition to the Al$_2$O$_3$ implants similar to that described for Ti implants [Steflik et al., 1993].

An approach to enhancing tissue responses at dental implant interfaces has been the introduction of ceramiclike, *calcium-phosphate-containing (CP) materials* as implant devices. The use of calcium-phosphatelike materials, in bulk or particulate form or as coatings on metal substrates has taken a predominant position in the biomedical implant area and has been the focus of several recent reviews [Kay, 1992; Koeneman et al., 1990]. One of the most important uses of CP materials has been as a coating on metallic (cp Ti and Ti alloy) substrates. This approach has taken advantage of thin-film-coating technology to apply thin coatings of hydroxyapatite (HA) and tricalcium phosphate (TCP) materials to the substrate in order to enhance bone responses at implant sites. The most popular method of coating has been the *plasma spray* process [Herman, 1988]; although this process has some advantages, there are reports of nonuniform coatings, interfacial porosity, and vaporization of elements in the powder [Cook et al., 1991; Kay, 1992].

The use of this class of materials is based on the premise that a more natural hydroxyapatitelike surface (HA-like) surface could act as a scaffold for enhanced bone response—osseointegration—and thereby minimize the long-term healing periods currently required for uncoated metal implants.

Numerous in vivo investigations have clearly demonstrated that HA-like coatings can enhance bone responses at implant interfaces [Cook et al., 1991; Jarcho et al., 1977], although the mechanisms responsible for the development of the interface between hard tissue and these ceramic coatings are not well understood [Jansen et al., 1993]. Histologically, the overall bone-coating interface is similar in appearance and chronologic development to that reported for uncoated implant surfaces. Initially, an immature, trabecular, woven bone interface is formed followed by more dense, compact lamellar supporting bone structure. Ultrastructurally, the interface is reported to consist of a globular, afibrillar matrix directly on the HA surface, an electron-dense, proteoglycan rich layer (20–60 nm thick) and the presence of a mineralized collagenous matrix [De Bruijn et al., 1993]. Although the morphologic descriptions of the HA and Ti interfaces are similar, numerous studies have shown that the bone response to HA coatings is more rapid than with uncoated Ti surfaces, requiring approximately one-third to one-half the time to establish a firm osseous bed as uncoated Ti. Likewise, the extent of the bone response to HA coatings is superior and, according to some studies, leads to a several-fold increase in interfacial strength compared to uncoated Ti [Cook et al., 1991].

The cellular events which take place and lead to the interfacial ultrastructure with bone tissue and ceramic surfaces are under current investigation. Based upon preliminary findings, the advantageous biologic properties of HA coatings do not appear to be related to recruitment of additional cells during the early attachment phase of healing. Although recent work indicated that bone cells and tissue form normal cellular focal contacts during attachment to HA coatings, the level of initial in vitro attachment generally only approximates that observed with Ti [Keller et al., 1992; Puleo et al., 1991]. Rather, the mechanisms for the enhanced in vitro cell responses appears to be related, to a certain degree, to the degradation properties and release of Ca^{+2} and PO$_4$$^{-3}$ ions into the biologic milieu. This surface corrosion is associated with highly degradable amorphous components of the coating and leads to surface irregularities which may enhance the quality of cell adhesion to these roughened materials [Bowers et al., 1992; Chehroudi et al., 1992]. Cellular events which occur following attachment may be influenced by the nature of the ceramic surface. Emerging evidence from a number of laboratories suggests that cellular-mediated events, including proliferation, matrix expression, and bone formation are enhanced following attachment to HA coatings and appear to be related to the gene expression of osteoblasts when cultured on different ceramic materials. These early cellular events lead to histologic and ultrastructural descriptions of bone healing which take place on these surfaces and are very similar to those reported from in vivo studies [Orr et al., 1992; Steflik et al., 1993].

As determined from in vitro dissolution studies, there is general agreement that the biodegradation properties of the pertinent CP materials can be summarized as α-TCP > β-TCP >>> HA, whereas amorphous HA is more prone to biodegradation than crystalline HA [Koeneman et al., 1990]. Considerable attempts to investigate the effects of coating composition (relative percentages of HA, TCP) on bone integration have been undertaken. Using an orthopedic canine total hip model, Jasty and coworkers (1992) reported that by 3 weeks, a TCP/HA mixed coating resulted in significantly more woven bone apposition to the implants than uncoated implants. As determined by x-ray diffraction, the mixed coating consisted of 60% TCP, 20% crystalline HA, and 20% unknown Ca-PO$_4$ materials. Jansen and colleagues [1993] reported that, using HA-coated implants (90% HA, 10% amorphous CP), bony apposition was extensive in a rabbit tibia model by 12 weeks. However, significant loss of the coating occurred as early as 6 weeks after implantation. Most recently, Maxian and coworkers [1993] reported that poorly crystallized HA (60% crystalline) coatings demonstrated significant degradation and poor bone apposition in vivo compared to amorphous coatings. Both these reports suggest that although considerable bioresorption of the coating occurred in the cortical bone, there was significant bone apposition (81 $\pm$ 2% for amorphous HA at 12 weeks, 77% for crystalline HA, respectively) which was not significantly affected by bioresorption.

From these in vivo reports, it is clear that HA coatings with relatively low levels of crystallinity are capable of significant bone apposition. However, as reported in a 1990 workshop report, the FDA is strongly urging commercial implant manufacturers to use techniques to increase the postdeposition crystallinity and to provide adequate adhesion of the coating to the implant substrate [Filiaggi et al., 1993]. Although the biologic responses to HA coatings are encouraging, other factors regarding HA coatings continue to lead to clinical questions regarding their efficacy. Although the overall bone response to HA-coated implants occurs more rapidly than with uncoated devices, with time an equivalent bone contact area is formed for both materials [Jasty et al., 1992]. These results have questioned the true need for HA-coated implants, especially when there are a number of disadvantages associated with the coating concept. Clinical difficulties have arisen due to failures within the coating itself and with continued dissolution of the coating, and to catastrophic failure at the coating-substrate interface [Koeneman et al., 1988].

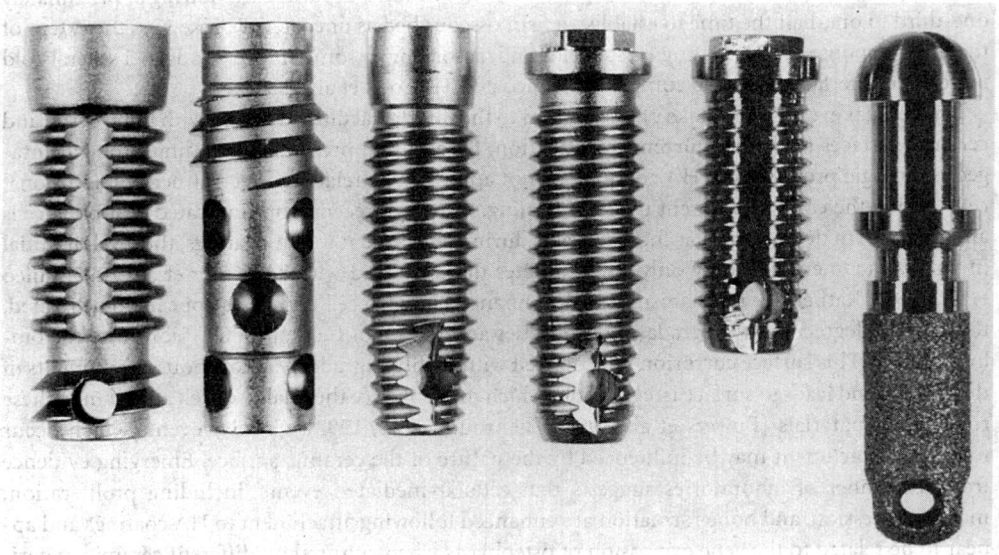

FIGURE 47.12 Examples of current dental implant designs, illustrating the variety of macroscopic topographies which are used to encourage tissue ingrowth. Left to right: Microvent, Corevent, Screw-vent, Swedevent, Branemark, IMZ implants.

Recent progress is reported in terms of the improvements in coating technology. Postdeposition heat treatments are often utilized to control the crystallinity (and therefore the dissolution characteristics) of the coatings, although there is still debate as to the relationship between compositional variations associated with differing crystallinity and optimization of biologic responses. Additional coating-related properties are also under investigation in regard to their effects on bone. These include coating thickness, level of acceptable porosity in the coating, and adherence of the coating to the underlying substrate. However, until answers concerning these variables have been more firmly established, HA coatings used for dental implants will remain an area of controversy and interest.

Effects of Surface Properties

Surface Topography

The effects of surface topography are different than the overall three-dimensional design or geometry of the implant, which is related to the interaction of the host tissues with the implant on a macroscopic scale as shown in Fig. 47.12. This important consideration in overall biologic response to implants is discussed later in this chapter. In this discussion the concept of *surface topography* refers to the surface texture on a microlevel. It is on this microscopic level that the intimate cell and tissue interactions leading to osseointegration are based as shown in Fig. 47.13.

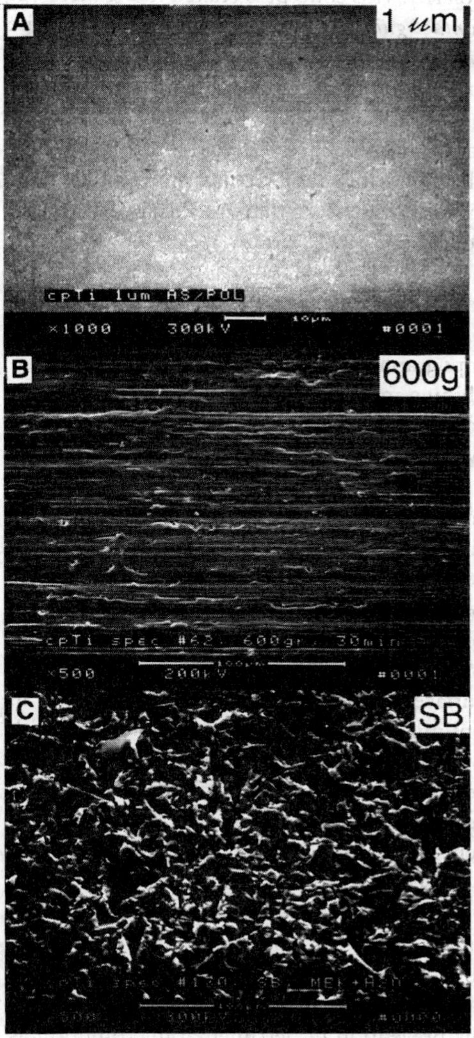

The effects of surface topography on in vitro and in vivo cell and tissue responses have been a field of intense study in recent years. The overall goal of these studies is to identify surface topographies which mimic the natural substrata

FIGURE 47.13 Laboratory-prepared cpTi surfaces with (*a–c*, top to bottom) smooth (1 μm polish), grooved (600 grit polish), and rough (sandblasted) surfaces.

in order to permit tissue integration and improve clinical fixation of the implant. In terms of cell attachment, the in vitro work by Bowers and colleagues [1992] established that levels of short-term osteoblast cell attachment were higher on rough compared to smooth surfaces and cell morphology was directly related to the nature of the underlying substrate. After initial attachment, in many cases, cells of various origin often take on the morphology of the substrate as shown in Fig. 47.14. Increased surface roughness, produced by such techniques as sand or grit blasting or by rough polishing, provided the rugosity necessary for optimum cell behavior.

Work in progress in several laboratories is attempting to relate the nature of the implant surface to cell morphology, intracellular cytoskeletal organization, and extracellular matrix development. Pioneering work by Chehroudi and coworkers [1992] suggests that microtextured surfaces (via micromachining or other techniques) could help orchestrate cellular activity and osteoblast mineralization by several mechanisms including proper orientation of collagen bundles and cell shape and polarity. This concept is related to the theory of *contact guidance* and the belief that cell shape will dictate cell differentiation through gene expression. In Chehroudi's work, both tapered pitted and grooved surfaces (with specific orientation and sequence patterns) supported mineralization with ultrastructural morphology similar in appearance to that observed by Davies and colleagues [1990]. However, mineralization was not observed on smooth surfaces in which osteoblastlike cells did not have a preferred growth orientation. Thus the control of surface microtopography by such procedures as micromachining may prove to be a valuable technology for the control and perhaps optimization of bone formation on implant surfaces.

It is apparent that macroscopic as well as microscopic topography may affect osteoblast differentiation and mineralization. In a recent study by Groessner-Schrieber and Tuan [1992], osteoblast growth, differentiation, and synthesis of matrix and mineralized nodules was observed on rough, textured, or porous coated titanium surface. It may be possible therefore, not only to optimize the interactions of host tissues with implant surfaces during the Phase I tissue responses but also to influence the overall bone responses to biomechanical forces during the remodeling phase (Phase II) of tissue responses.

Based on these concepts, current implant designs employ microtopographically roughened surfaces with macroscopic grooves, threads, or porous surfaces to provide sufficient bone ingrowth for mechanical stabilization and the prevention of detrimental micromotion as shown in Figs. 47.15 and 47.16 [Brunski, 1992; De Porter et al., 1986; Keller et al., 1987; Pilliar et al., 1991].

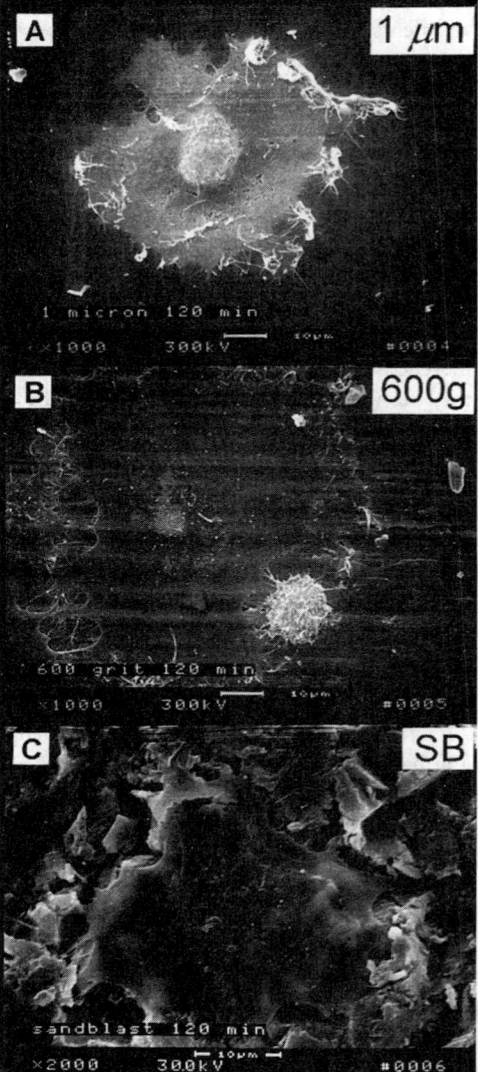

FIGURE 47.14 Osteoblastlike cell morphology after 2 hours' attachment on (*a–c*, top to bottom) smooth, grooved, and rough cpTi surfaces.

Surface Chemistry

Considerable attention has focused on the properties of the oxide found on titanium implant surfaces following surface preparation. Sterilization procedures are especially important and are known to affect not only the oxide condition but also the subsequent in vitro [Stanford et al., 1994; Swart et al., 1992] and in vivo [Hartman et al., 1989] biologic responses. Interfacial surface analyses and determinations of surface energetics strongly suggest that steam autoclaving is especially damaging to titanium oxide surfaces. Depending upon the purity of the autoclave water, contaminants have been observed on the metal oxide and are correlated with poor tissue responses on a cellular [Keller et al., 1990, 1994] and tissue [Baier et al., 1984; Hartman et al., 1989; Meenaghan et al., 1979] level.

The role of multiple sterilization regimens on the practice of implant utilization is also under scrutiny. Many implants and especially bone plate systems are designed for repackaging if the kit is not exhausted. However, early evidence indicates that this practice is faulty and, depending on the method of sterilization, may affect the integrity of the metal oxide surface chemistry [Vezeau et al., 1991]. In vitro experiments have verified that multiple-steam-autoclaved and ethylene-oxide-treated implant surfaces adversely affected cellular and morphologic integration. However, the effects of these treatments on long-term biological responses including in vivo situations remain to be clarified.

Other more recently introduced techniques such as radiofrequency argon plasma cleaning treatments have succeeded in altering metal oxide chemistry and structure [Baier et al., 1984; Swart et al., 1992]. Numerous studies have demonstrated that PC treatments produce a relatively contaminant-free surface with improved surface energy (wettability), but conflicting biologic results have been reported with these surfaces. Recent in vitro studies have demonstrated that these highly energetic surfaces do not necessarily improve cellular responses such as attachment and cell expression. This has been confirmed by in vivo studies which indicate that the overall histologic and ultrastructural morphology of the bone-implant interface is similar for plasma-cleaned and dry-heat-sterilized implant surfaces [Albrektsson et al., 1983]. Another promising technique for the sterilization of implant materials is the exposure of the implant surface to ultraviolet light [Singh & Schaff, 1989] or gamma irradiation [Keller et al., 1994]. Both these methods of sterilization produce a relatively contaminant-free thin oxide layer which fosters high levels of cell attachment [Keller et

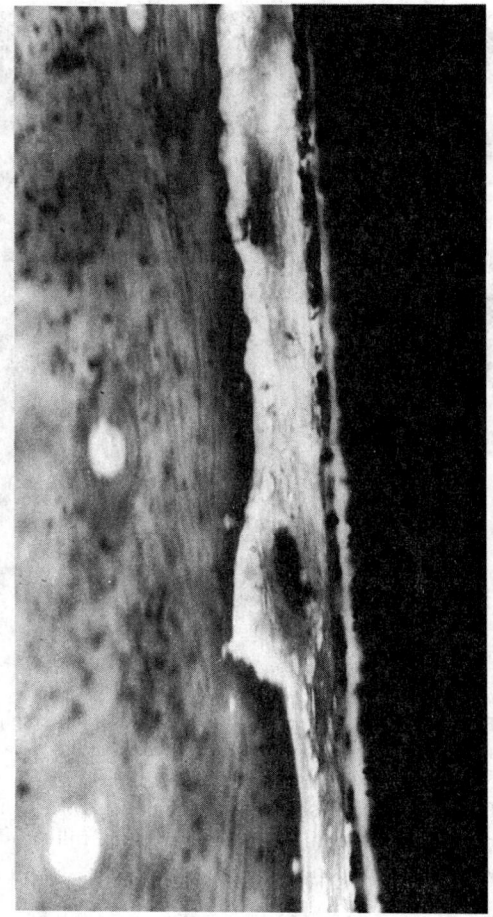

FIGURE 47.15 Light microscopic photomicrograph of a bone–smooth cpTi interface with intervening layer of soft connective tissue. This implant was mobile in the surgical site due to lack of tissue ingrowth. (Original magnification = 50×.)

al., 1994] and inflammatory-free long-term in vivo responses [Hartman et al., 1989]. Currently, gamma irradiation procedures are widely used for the sterilization of metallic dental implant devices.

Metallic Corrosion

Throughout the history of the use of metals for biomedical implant applications, electrochemical corrosion with subsequent metal release has been problematic [Galante et al., 1991]. Of the biomedical metal systems available today, Ti and its major medical alloy, Ti-6A1-4V, are thought to be the most corrosion resistant; however, Ti metals are not totally inert in vivo [Woodman et al., 1984]. Release of Ti ions from Ti oxides can occur under relatively passive conditions [Ducheyne, 1988]. Whereas other factors such as positioning of the implant and subsequent biomechanical forces may play important roles in the overall tissue response to implants, it is not unreasonable to predict that electrochemical interactions between the implant surface and host tissue may affect the overall response of host bone [Blumenthal & Cosma, 1989]. For example, it has been shown by several groups [De Porter et al., 1986; Keller et al., 1987] that the percentages of intimate bony contact with the implant is inconsistent, at best, and generally averages approximately 50% over a 5-year period.

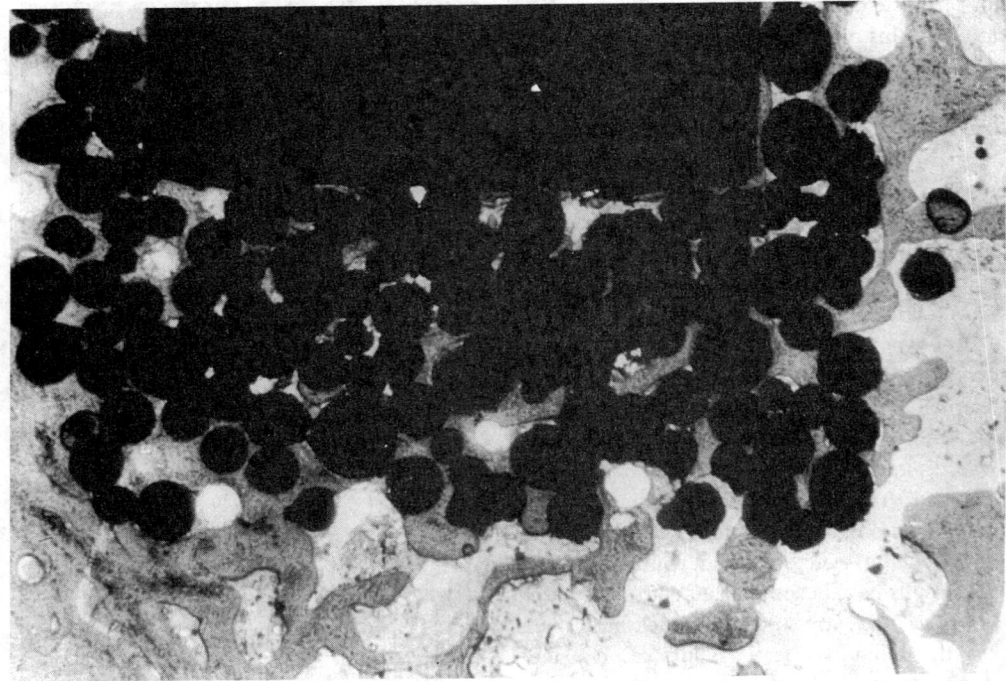

FIGURE 47.16 Light microscopic photomicrograph of a bone–porous Ti allow implant interface. Note significant bone ingrowth in open porosity at the apical end of the implant. (Original magnification = 10×.)

Continued studies involving the effects of dissolution products on both local and systemic host responses are required in order to more fully understand the consequences of biologic interaction with metal implants.

Future Considerations for Implant Surfaces

It is clear that future efforts to improve the host tissue responses to implant materials will focus, in large part, on controlling cell and tissue responses at implant interfaces. This goal will require continued acquisition of fundamental knowledge of cell behavior and cell response to specific materials' characteristics. It is likely that a better understanding of the cellular-derived extracellular matrix-implant interface will offer a mechanism by which biologic response modifiers such as growth and attachment factors or hormones may be incorporated. Advancements of this type will likely shift the focus of future research from implant surfaces which are osseoconductive (permissive) to those which are osseoinductive (bioactive).

Defining Terms

Amorphous zone: A region of the tissue-implant interface immediately adjacent to the implant substrate. This zone is of variable thickness (usually < 1000 Å), is free of collagen, and is comprised of proteoglycans of unknown composition.

Calcium phosphate: A family of calcium- and phosphate-containing materials of synthetic or natural origin which are utilized for implants and bone augmentation purposes. The most prominent materials are the tricalcium-phosphate- and hydroxyapatite-based materials, although most synthetic implants are a mixture of the various compositions.

Contact guidance: The theory by which cells attach to and migrate on substrates of specific microstructure and topographic orientation. The ability of the cell to attach and migrate on a substrate is related to the cytoskeletal and attachment molecules present on the cell membrane.

Junctional epithelium: The epithelial attachment mechanism which occurs with teeth, and has been observed infrequently with implants by some researchers. Less than 10 cell layers thick, the hemidesmosomal attachments of the basal cells to the implant surface provide a mechanical attachment for epithelium and prevent bacterial penetration into the sulcular area.

Osseointegration: A phrase developed by P.I. Branemark and his colleagues indicating the ability of host bone tissues to form a functional, mechanically immobile interface with the implant. Originally described for titanium only, several other materials are capable of forming this interface, which presumes a lack of connective tissue (foreign body) layer.

Plasma spray: A high-temperature process by which calcium-phosphate-containing materials are coated onto a suitable implant substrate. Although the target material may be of high purity, the high-temperature softening process can dramatically affect and alter the resultant composition of the coating.

References

Albrektsson T, Branemark PI, Hansson HA, et al. 1983. The interface zone of inorganic implants *in vivo:* titanium implants in bone. Ann Biomed Eng 11:1.

Albrektsson T, Hansson HA, Ivarsson B. 1985. Interface analysis of titanium and zirconium bone implants. Biomaterials 6:97.

Baier RE, Meyer AE, Natiella JR, et al. 1984. Surface properties determine bioadhesive outcomes. J Biomed Mater Res 18:337.

Blumenthal NC, Cosma V. 1989. Inhibition of appetite formation by titanium and vanadium ions. J Biomed Mater Res 23(A1):13.

Bowers KT, Keller JC, Michaels CM, et al. 1992. Optimization of surface micromorphology for enhanced osteoblast responses *in vitro.* Int J Oral Maxillofac Implants 7:302.

Branemark PI. 1983. Osseointegration and its experimental background. J Pros Dent 50(3):399.

Brunski JB. 1992. Biomechanical factors affecting the bone-dental implant interface. Clin Mater 10:153.

Chehroudi B, Ratkay J, Brunette DM. 1992. The role of implant surface geometry on mineralization *in vivo* and *in vitro:* A transmission and scanning electron microscopic study. Cells Materials 2(2):89–104.

Cook SD, Kay JF, Thomas KA, et al. 1987. Interface mechanics and histology of titanium and hydroxylapatite coated titanium for dental implant applications. Int J Oral Maxillofac Implants 2(1):15.

Cook SD, Thomas KA, Kay JF. 1991. Experimental coating defects in hydroxylapatite coated implants. Clin Orthop Rel Res 265:280.

Davies JE, Lowenberg B, Shiga A. 1990. The bone-titanium interface *in vitro.* J Biomed Mater Res 24:1289–1306.

De Bruijn JD, Flach JS, deGroot K, et al. 1993. Analysis of the bony interface with various types of hydroxyapatite *in vitro.* Cells Mater 3(2):115.

De Porter DA, Watson PA, Pilliar RM et al. 1986. A histological assessment of the initial healing response adjacent to porous-surfaced, titanium alloy dental implants in dogs. J Dent Res 65(8):1064.

Driskell TD, Spungenberg HD, Tennery VJ, et al. 1973. Current status of high density alumina ceramic tooth roof structures. J Dent Res 52:123.

Ducheyne P. 1988. Titanium and calcium phosphate ceramic dental implants, surfaces, coatings and interfaces. J Oral Implantol 19(3):325.

Filiaggi MJ, Pilliar RM, Coombs NA. 1993. Post-plasma spraying heat treatment of the HA coating/Ti-6A1-4V implant system. J Biomed Mater Res 27:191.

Galante JO, Lemons J, Spector M, et al. 1991. The biologic effects of implant materials. J Orthop Res 9:760.

Groessner-Schreiber B, Tuan RS. 1992. Enhanced extracellular matrix production and mineralization by osteoblasts cultured on titanium surfaces *in vitro*. J Cell Sci 101:209.

Hartman LC, Meenaghan MA, Schaaf NG, et al. 1989. Effects of pretreatment sterilization and cleaning methods on materials properties and osseoinductivity of a threaded implant. Int J Oral Maxillofac Implants 4:11.

Herman H. 1988. Plasma spray deposition processes. Mater Res Soc Bull 13:60.

Jansen JA, van der Waerden JPCM, Wolke JGC. 1993. Histological and histomorphometrical evaluation of the bone reaction to three different titanium alloy and hydroxyapatite coated implants. J Appl Biomater 4:213.

Jarcho M, Kay JF, Gumaer KI, et al. 1977. Tissue, cellular and subcellular events at a bone-ceramic hydroxylapatite interface. J Bioeng 1:79.

Jasty M, Rubash HE, Paiemont GD, et al. 1992. Porous coated uncemented components in experimental total hip arthroplasty in dogs. Clin Orthop Rel Res 280:300.

Johansson CB, Lausman J, Ask M, et al. 1989. Ultrastructural differences of the interface zone between bone and Ti-6A1-4V or commercially pure titanium. J Biomed Eng 11:3.

Katsikeris N, Listrom RD, Symington JM. 1987. Interface between titanium 6-A1-4V alloy implants and bone. Int J Oral Maxillofac Surg 16:473.

Kay JF. 1992. Calcium phosphate coatings for dental implants. Dent Clinics N Amer 36(1):1.

Keller JC, Draughn RA, Wightman JP, et al. 1990. Characterization of sterilized cp titanium implant surfaces. Int J Oral Maxillofac Implants 5:360.

Keller JC, Lautenschlager EP. 1986. Metals and alloys. In A Von Recon (ed), *Handbook of Biomaterials Evaluation*, pp 3–23, New York, Macmillan.

Keller JC, Niederaurer GG, Lacefield WR, et al. 1992. Interaction of osteoblast-like cells with calcium phosphate ceramic materials. Trans Acad Dent Mater 5(3):107.

Keller JC, Stanford CM, Wightman JP, et al. 1994. Characterization of titanium implant surfaces. J Biomed Mater Res.

Keller JC, Young FA, Natiella JR. 1987. Quantitative bone remodeling resulting from the use of porous dental implants. J Biomed Mater Res 21:305.

Koeneman J, Lemons JE, Ducheyne P, et al. 1990. Workshop of characterization of calcium phosphate materials. J Appl Biomater 1:79.

Lucas LC, Lemons JE, Lee J, et al. 1987. In vivo corrosion characteristics of Co-Cr-Mu/Ti-6A1-4V-Ti alloys. In JE Lemons (ed), *Quantitative Characterization and Performance of Porous Alloys for Hard Tissue Applications*, pp 124–136, Philadelphia, ASTM.

Maxian SH, Zawadsky JP, Durin MG. 1993. Mechanical and histological evaluation of amorphous calcium phosphate and poorly crystallized hydroxylapatite coatings on titanium implants. J Biomed Mater Res 27:717.

Meenaghan MA, Natiella JR, Moresi JC, et al. 1979. Tissue response to surface treated tantalum implants: Preliminary observations in primates. J Biomed Mater Res 13:631.

Orr RD, de Bruijn JD, Davies JE. 1992. Scanning electron microscopy of the bone interface with titanium, titanium alloy and hydroxyapatite. Cells Mater 2(3):241.

Pilliar RM, DePorter DA, Watson PA, et al. 1991. Dental implant design—effect on bone remodeling. J Biomed Mater Res 25:467.

Puleo DA, Holleran LA, Doremus RH, et al. 1991. Osteoblast responses to orthopedic implant materials *in vitro*. J Biomed Mater Res 25:711.

Singh S, Schaaf NG. 1989. Dynamic sterilization of titanium implants with ultraviolet light. Int J Oral Maxillofac Implants 4:139.

Skalak R. 1985. Aspects of biomechanical considerations. In PI Branemark, G Zarb, T Albrektsson (eds), *Tissue Integrated Prostheses*, pp 117–128, Chicago, Quintessence.

Smith DC. 1993. Dental implants: Materials and design considerations. Int J Prosth 6(2):106.

Stanford CM, Keller JC. 1991. Osseointegration and matrix production at the implant surface. CRC Crit Rev Oral Bio Med 2:83.

Stanford CM, Keller JC, Solursh M. 1994. Bone cell expression on titanium surfaces is altered by sterilization treatments. J Dent Res.

Steflik DE, McKinney RV, Koth DL, et al. 1984. Biomaterial-tissue interface: A morphological study utilizing conventional and alternative ultrastructural modalities. Scanning Electron Microscopy 2:547.

Steflik DE, Sisk AL, Parr GR, et al. 1993. Osteogenesis at the dental implant interface: High voltage electron microscopic and conventional transmission electric microscopic observations. J Biomed Mater Res 27:791.

Swart KM, Keller JC, Wightman JP, et al. 1992. Short term plasma cleaning treatments enhance *in vitro* osteoblast attachment to titanium. J Oral Implant 18(2):130.

Van Orden A. 1985. Corrosive response of the interface tissue to 316L stainless steel, Ti-based alloy and cobalt-based alloys. In: R McKinney, J.E. Lemons (eds), The Dental Implant, pp 1–25, Littleton, PSG.

Vezeau PJ, Keller JC, Koorbusch GF. 1991. Effect of multiple sterilization regimens on fibroblast attachment to titanium. J Dent Res 70:530.

Vrouwenvelder WCA, Groot CG Groot, K. 1993. Histological and biochemical evaluation of osteoblasts cultured on bioactive glass, hydroxylapatite, titanium alloy and stainless steel. J Biomed Mater Res 27:465–475.

Woodman JL, Jacobs JJ, Galante JO, et al. Metal ion release from titanium-based prosthetic segmental replacements of long bones in baboons: A long term study. J Orthop Res 1:421–430.

Young FA. 1988. Future directions in dental implant materials research. J Dent Ed 52(12):770.

48

Orthopedic Prosthesis Fixation

Joon B. Park
University of Iowa

Ever since the introduction of bone cement for the fixation of artificial hip joints by Dr. John Charnley on the advice of Dr. Dennis Smith in the late 1950s, the procedure has been adopted throughout the world [Charnley, 1970, 1972; Charnley & Cupic, 1973; Wroblewski, 1986]. The initial success of the procedure in the total hip arthroplasties (THA) has been extended to the total knee arthroplasties (TKA), but success has been tempered by problems related not only to bone cement but also to the implants per se [Brand, 1987; Eftekhar, 1978, 1987; Mears, 1979; Morscher, 1984; Williams and Roaf, 1973]. One of the inherent problems of orthopedic joint prosthesis implantation is the fixation and the maintenance of a stable interface between the device and the host tissue at the cellular and organ levels [Freeman & Tennant, 1992]. The fixation can be classified into several categories as given in Table 48.1.

The most frequent fixation problems are related to infection, wear and wear particulate, failure of implants, and loosening, of which the long-term loosening of the implant is especially important [Ducheyne, 1988]. Many factors such as mismatch of the physical properties between tissues and implant, biocompatibility of the implant, deterioration of physical properties of implant materials, and problems with surgical techniques, design of the implant, selection of patients, and postsurgical care are related to the (late) loosening [Crowninshield, 1988; Gruen et al., 1979; Harris & McGann, 1984]. Various fixation techniques and some possible solutions as they relate to the total (hip and knee) joint arthroplasty will be presented in this section.

48.1 Mechanical Fixation

Early designs of total hip prosthesis used bolts and nuts to fix the femoral component to the femur, and metal pegs were used to fix acetabular component with metal to metal-bearing surfaces [Bechtol et al., 1959]. This technique of fixation and bearing surface were abandoned due to the massive tissue reaction by the wear particles released by the metal-on-metal friction between the cup and femoral head and destabilization of the femoral stem fixation. It is also possible that the stress concentration around the holes would have resulted in the failure of the fixation.

0-8493-8346-3/95/$0.00+$.50
© 1995 by CRC Press, Inc.

TABLE 48.1 Summary of Various Methods of Prosthesis Fixation

Methods of Fixation	Notes
Mechanical fixation	
Active—use of screws, bolts, nuts, wires, etc.	Pre-Charnley implants [Williams & Roaf, 1973]
Passive—interference fit and noninterference fit	Moore [1952], Mittlemeier [1975, 1976]
Bone cement fixation	
Pure cement	Charnley [1970, 1972], Charnley and Cupic [1973]
Modified cement—composite cement, resorbable particle impregnated cement	Dai et al. [1991], Liu et al. [1987], Park et al. [1986], Park [1993]
Biological Fixation	
Porous ingrowth	Klawitter and Hulbert [1972], Sauer et al. [1974], Hirshhorn et al. [1972], Homsy et al. [1972], Smith [1962]
Modified porous ingrowth—electrical and pulsed electromagnetic field (PEMF) stimulation	Park [1983b], Park and Kenner [1975], Weinstein et al. [1976]
Direct (Chemical) Bonding Fixation	
Osteogenic/inductive—glass-ceramics	Hench and Paschall [1973], Blencke et al. [1978]
Osteoconductive—hydroxyapatite	Kay [1988], de Groot [1983]

The *passive* mechanical fixation has been applied, in limited circumstances, to hip and finger joint prostheses. Due to the nature of the loading (mostly compressive and some shear) and shape (wedged or tapered), an interference or press fit can be used to fix the femoral stem of a hip joint. This passive fixation technique was largely used for ceramic stems, since the large size of the stem (it must be large due to failure unpredictability of brittle materials such as alumina ceramic) can distribute the stresses over a large area, thus minimizing stress necrosis of bone [Mittlemeier, 1975, 1976]. Also, Moore [1952] type hemiarthroplastic stems can be fixed by the passive fixation. The passive fixation often results in induced collagenous membrane formation at the interface between bone and implant unless there is a negligible relative motion between them [Kim et al., 1991]. It is also conceivable that under constant loading by the body, continuous sinking of the implant may take place throughout the life of the implant. However, passive fixation could provide a sufficient mechanical restraint for the femoral prosthesis to function through the lifetime of the prosthesis itself without undue sinking of the prosthesis down to the medullary canal.

The acetabular cup of the hip and tibial prosthesis of the knee use a similar fixation technique due to the similarity of loading, i.e., mostly compressive with some shear load. In this case, screws or pegs are used to stabilize the implant either with or without bone cement for tissue ingrowth where the surface of the implant should be deeply grooved or porous to accommodate interdigitation of bone cement or tissues for cementless fixation. Hemiarthroplastic and condylar prosthesis use similar techniques of fixation, i.e., either tissue ingrowth or use of grouting material such as bone cement.

Materials used to make implants could play an important role in the fixation of prosthesis [Crowninshield, 1988]. For example the modulus of the femoral stem can dictate the viability of ingrown tissues in the porous (biologic) fixation due to the bone remodeling according to Wolff's law [Wolff, 1986]. If the modulus is too high then osteoporosis may develop in the bone proper as well as desorption of the ingrown bony tissues in the interstices of pores due to the "stress shielding" effect. If the modulus is too low, then the implant itself may not be able to withstand the physiologic loading, and tissues can not be ingrown to begin with for the fixation due to the excessive strain experienced by the bony tissue. Some of the materials widely used to fabricate implants and their properties along with the bone are given in Table 48.2 for comparison.

48.2 Bone Cement Fixation

Basic Properties of Bone Cement

Bone cement is primarily made of poly(methylmethacrylate) (PMMA) powder and methylmethacrylate (MMA) monomer liquid as given in Table 48.3. Hydroquinone is added to prevent

TABLE 48.2 Physical properties of materials used for joint prosthesis and bone [Park and Lakes, 1992]

Materials	Young's Modulus, GPa	UTS,* MPa	Elongation, %	Density, g/cm³
Metals				
316L S.S. (wrought)	200	1000	9	7.9
CoCrMo (cast)	230	660	8	8.3
CoNiCrMo (wrought)	230	1800	8	9.2
Ti6Al4V	110	900	10	4.5
Ceramics				
Alumina (Al₂O₃, polycrystalline)	400	260	<0.1†	3.9
Glass-ceramic(Bioglass)	200	200	~0.1†	2.5†
Calcium phosphate (Dense hydroxyapatite)	120	200	~0.1†	3.2
Polymers				
PMMA (solid)‡	3.0	65	5	1.18
PMMA bone cement	2.0	30	3	1.10
UHMW polyethylene¶	1.0	30	200	0.94
Polysulfone	2.5	70	50	1.24
Silicone rubber	<0.01	6	>350	1.12
Fibers and wires				
Aramid (Kevlar)	130	2700	2	1.45
Carbon	400	2500	1	2.00
Nylon	5	500	10	1.07
Steel (piano wire)	200	2450	1.2	7.80
Bone				
Femur (compact), long axis	17.0	130	3.0	2.0
Femur (compact), tangential	12.0	60	1.0	2.0
Spongy bone	0.1	2	2.5	1.0

*UTS: ultimate tensile strength, for ceramics the Young's modulus and UTS are for the flexural modulus and bending strength respectively.

†Estimated values.

‡PMMA: poly(methylmethacrylate)

¶UHMW: ultra high molecular weight (>2 × 10⁶ g/mole)

premature polymerization of the monomer which may occur under certain conditions, for example, exposure to light or elevated temperatures. N,N-dimethyl-p-toluidine is added to promote or accelerate (cold) curing of the polymerizing compound. The name *cold curing* is used here to distinguish cold curing from the high-temperature and -pressure (hot) molding technique used to make articles in dental laboratories.

TABLE 48.3 Bone Cement Components and Their Roles*

Components	Role	Amount
Liquid		20ml
Methyl methacrylate (monomer)	Wetting PMMA particles	97.4 v/o
N,N,-dimethyl-p-toluidine	Polymerization accelerator	2.6 v/o
Hydroquinone	Polymerization inhibitor	75 ± 15 ppm
Solid powder		40g
Polymethyl methacrylate	Matrix material	15.0 w/o
Methyl methacrylate-styrene-copolymer	Matrix material	75.0 w/o
Barium sulfate (BaSO₄), USP	Radiopacifying agent	10.0 w/o
Dibenzoyl peroxide	Polymerization initiator	0.75 w/o†

Note: v/o: % by volume; w/o: % by weight.

*Surgical Simplex P Radiopaque Bone Cement (Howmedica, Inc. Rutherford, NJ).

†From other bone cement, 1980. Low viscosity bone cement, Bone Cement Topics, Warsaw, Ind, Zimmer USA.

When the powder and liquid are mixed together, the monomer liquid is polymerized by the free radical (addition) polymerization process. An activator (also called an *initiator*) dibenzoyl peroxide is free radicalized during mixing and reacts with a monomer to form an initiator-monomer radical which will then attack another monomer to form an initiator-dimer radical. The process will continue until long chain molecules are produced as given in the following sequence:

$$C_6H_5COO\text{-}OOC_6H_5 \rightarrow 2C_6H_5 \ (R\cdot) + 2CO_2 \tag{48.1}$$

$$R\cdot + M \rightarrow RM\cdot + \text{Heat} \tag{48.2}$$

$$RM\cdot + M \rightarrow RMM\cdot + \text{Heat} \tag{48.3}$$

$$COOCH_3$$

where M is the MMA monomer $\{CH_2\!=\!CCH_3\}$, and $R\cdot$ is the initiator free radical. The polymerization reaction is exothermic (about 130 cal/ml of monomer) and continues until all the monomers are consumed and the free radicals disappear through the termination either by combination of free radicals of growing chains or by disproportionate termination.

The monomer liquid will wet the polymer powder particle surfaces and link them by the polymerization, becoming a dough state which is injected into the prepared intramedurally cavity. The prosthesis is subsequently placed over the cement as shown in Fig. 48.1. The ASTM standard (F451)

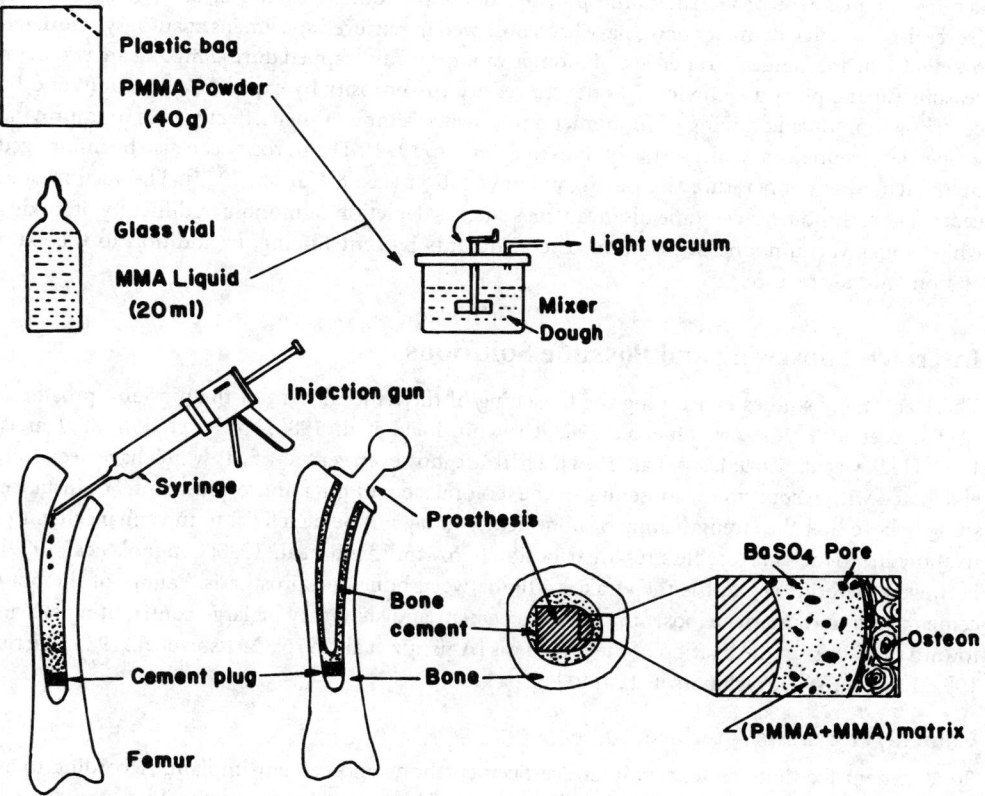

FIGURE 48.1 Schematic diagram of the bone cement mixing and injecting into intramedullary cavity and seating of a femoral prosthesis. Also, cross-sectional view of the prosthesis/cement/bone is shown.

TABLE 48.4 Requirements for Powder and Liquid Mixture of Bone Cement

Maximum Dough Time (min)	Setting Time Range (min)	Maximum Exotherm (°C)	Minimum Intrusion (mm)
5.0	5 ~ 15	90	2.0

Source: ASTM Standards, F451.

TABLE 48.5 Requirements for Bone Cement after Curing

Minimum Compressive Strength, MPa	Maximum Indentation, mm	Minimum Recovery, %	Maximum Water Sorption, mg/cm^2	Maximum Water Solubility, mg/cm^2
70	0.14	60	0.7	0.05

Source: ASTM Standards, F451.

specifies the characteristics of the powder-liquid mixture and cured polymer after setting as given in Tables 48.4 and 48.5.

Polymerization during curing obviously increases the degree of polymerization, that is, increases in molecular weight as given in Table 48.6. However, the molecular weight distribution does not change significantly after curing. The properties of cured bone cement are compared with those of commercial acrylic resins in Table 48.7. Studies show that bone cement properties can be affected by the intrinsic and extrinsic factors listed in Table 48.8. The most important factor controlling the acrylic bone cement properties is the porosity developed during curing or setting. Large pores (several-millimeter-diameter pores have been observed in retrieved specimens at autopsy) are detrimental to the mechanical properties. Monomer vapors and air trapped during mixing are two main reasons for the porosity. Obviously, one can reduce the porosity by exposure to vacuum and by centrifugation during mixing of monomer and powder, although their effectiveness in improving properties is somewhat controversial [Hansen & Jensen, 1992]. The porosity can also be minimized by reducing the temperature rise during polymerization [Lee & Turner, 1977]. The vacuum and centrifuge techniques have some disadvantages such as depletion of monomer, difficulty of mixing while under vacuum, and segregation of constituents by centrifuging, in addition to the extra equipment they require.

Interface Loosening and Possible Solutions

There are many studies concerning the loosening of the femoral stem of the hip joint prosthesis [Amstutz et al., 1976; Carlsson et al., 1983; Crowninshield et al., 1980; Fowler et al., 1988; Harris, 1992; Hedley et al., 1979; Jasty et al., 1991]. There are, however, very few facts which have been fully elucidated with respect to the loosening of the femoral stem of hip joint replacement. For instance, some believe that the strengthening of bone cement may not be beneficial to the enhancement of fixation due to the unfavorable stress distribution [Crowninshield, et al., 1980; Crugnola et al, 1979]. However, the bone cement is the weakest link between bone and prosthesis. Failure of the bone cement itself and interface loosening between cement and stem may be large contributing factors toward the failure of the fixation of the prosthesis [Amstutz et al., 1976; Carlsson et al., 1983; Harris, 1992; Lu et al., 1993; Wykman et al., 1991].

Cement/Prosthesis Interface

Bone cement fixation creates two interfaces: cement-bone and cement-implant. According to an earlier report [Amstutz et al., 1976] the incidence of loosening for the femoral prostheses were evenly divided at about 10% and 11% for cement-bone and cement-implant interfaces, respectively. The cement-implant interface loosening can be minimized by precoating with bone cement or

TABLE 48.6 Molecular Weight of Bone Cement

Type of MW, g/mol	Monomer	Powder	Cured
M_n (number average)	100	44,000	51,000
M_w (weight average)	100	198,000	242,000

Source: Haas SS, Brauer GM, Dickson G. 1975. A characterization of PMMA bone cement. J Bone Joint Surg 57A:280.

TABLE 48.7 Physical Properties of Bone Cement and Commercial Acrylic Resins

Properties	Radiopaque Bone Cement*	Commercial Acrylic Resins[†]
Tensile strength, MPa	28.9 ± 1.6	55 ~ 76
Compressive strength, MPa	91.7 ± 2.5	76 ~ 131
Young's modulus compressive loading, MPa	2,200 ± 60	2,960 ~ 3,280
Endurance limit[‡]	0.3 uts[¶]	0.3 uts[¶]
Density, g/cm³	1.10 ~ 1.23	1.18
Water sorption, %	0.5	0.3 ~ 0.4
Shrinkage after setting, %	2.75 ~ 5	—

*Haas SS, Brauer GM, Dickson G. 1975. A characterization of PMMA bone cement, J Bone Joint Surg 57A:280.

[†]Modern Plastics Encyclopedia. 1980. New York, McGraw-Hill, p. 533.

[‡]Kusy RP. 1978. Characterization of self-curing acrylic bone cements. J Biomed Mater Res 12:271.

[¶]Ultimate tensile strength.

polymethylmethacrylate polymer. Precoating can achieve a good bonding between the cement and prosthesis during the manufacturing process. During surgery, the freshly doughed cement adheres well to the precoated cement [Ahmed et al., 1984; Barb et al., 1982, Park et al., 1978, 1979, 1982a, 1982b; Raab et al., 1982].

The high strains or stresses on the cement at the tip of the prosthesis are strong indications that the location is a likely site for the initial event of failure [O'Connor et al., 1991]. Others reported that high strains at the proximal and distal tip of the prosthesis appeared to cause debonding between the stem and cement and was associated with radial crack initiation at the debonded surface of the pores in the cement surrounding the areas of debonding [Harrigan et al., 1992]. These radial cracks seemed to be due to stress changes secondary to debonding.

The cement-prosthesis interface strength could be enhanced by placing reinforcing material around the stem to resist the radial and hoop stress caused by body loading [Park, 1993]. It is also critical that the cement is reinforced to counteract the hoop stress and to a lesser extent the radial stress created by the prosthesis when it is loaded [Ahmed et al., 1984; Mann et al., 1991]. Therefore, a coil or mesh or wire conforming to the contours of the prosthesis could be placed prior to bone cement injection during surgery as shown in Fig. 48.2. Wire could also be prefabricated around the

TABLE 48.8 Factors Affecting Bone Cement Properties

Intrinsic factors
  Chemical composition of monomer and powder
  Powder particle size, shape, and distribution
  Powder degree of polymerization
  Liquid/powder ratio
Extrinsic factors
  Mixing environment: temperature, humidity, type of container
  Mixing technique: rate and number of beating with spatula, Use of vacuum, centrifuge
  Curing environment: temperature, humidity, pressure, contacting surface (tissue, air, water, prosthesis, etc.)

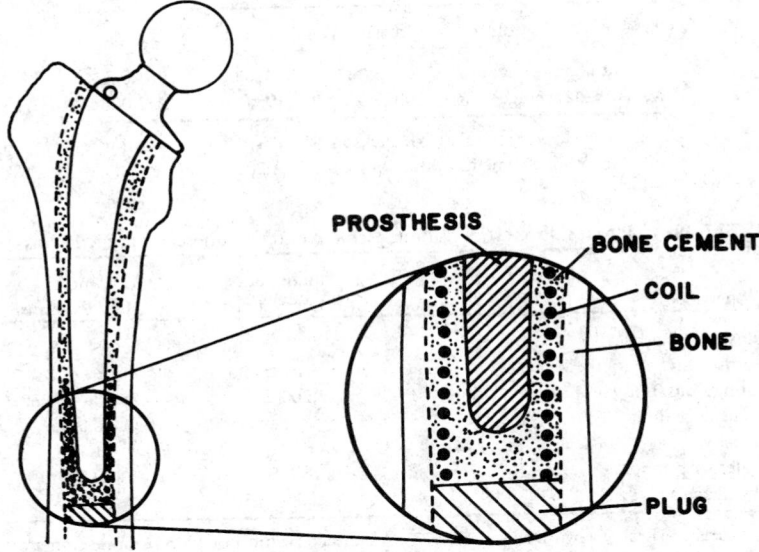

FIGURE 48.2 Illustration of the reinforcement of the bone cement around the prosthesis to resist radial and hoop stress on the cement mantle by incorporating a wire coil conforming to the contours of the stem of the prosthesis which can be placed during surgery or prefabricated during manufacturing of the implant [Kim & Park, 1994].

prosthesis. Also, some people advocate the use of a mesh reinforcement around a prosthesis which can be fixed with fresh bone cement at the time of surgery; this is similar to the coil but more difficult to incorporate [Davidson, 1988; Willert et al., 1991]. The simple wire coil would resist the hoop stress developed by the prosthesis which in turn will decrease the stress on the bone cement beyond the wire coil toward the bone.

The decreased radial and hoop stresses and strains on the cement will result in:

1. Decreased stress and strain in the bone-cement interface. This will also decrease the large strain developed in the distal end of the cemented femoral prosthesis.
2. Decreased microcrack development in the cement. This would make the cement mantle stronger and more fatigue resistant, i.e., a tougher composite structure.
3. Better adherence of the precoated wire coil to the bone cement. This will minimize the problem of poor cement adherence with the metal surface during surgery.
4. Decreased creep of the bone cement. The metal wire coil or mesh would not creep plastically unlike the "viscoelastic" cement. An in vivo canine model study showed the interfacial strength decreased continuously with time, indicating creep behavior of the interface between the cement and stem [Park et al., 1982].

However, the coil placement would have these unfavorable results:

1. Increased surgical time.
2. More difficult to remove the cement mantle for a revision surgery. However, it may help to remove the cement *en block* instead of in pieces, since the cement is held together by the wire.

The mechanical property changes of the bone cement produced by reinforcing the cement with a wire coil in a simulated stem loading condition has been tried [Kim & Park, 1994] instead of the traditional reinforcement by adding wires, fibers, etc. into the bone cement [Saha & Pal, 1984]. The coils were made from 20 gage 302/304 stainless steel wire as given in Tables 48.9 and 48.10, since they are easy to fabricate and insert and could directly counteract the radial- and hoop-stress as

TABLE 48.9 Some Physical Characteristics and Curing Conditions of the Coil and Specimens

Characteristics	Gauge	Wire Diameter, mm	Wire Length, mm	ID of Coil, mm	Height of Coil, mm	No. of Turns	Curing Time, day
Value	20	0.8	607	17.9	19.0	9	7&5

TABLE 48.10 Push-out Specimen Characteristics and Their Densities

Specimen Type	No of Specimen	Coil Weight, g	Specimen Weight, g	Cement Net Weight, g	Density, g/ml
Control	19		7.090 ± 0.066	7.090	1.119 ± 0.011
Wire reinforced	6	2.397 ± 0.009	9.138 ± 0.045	6.741	1.117 ± 0.007

mentioned previously. The specimens (2.54-in. outside diameter, top diameter of 5/8 in. tapered to 1.51 degree and height of 3/4 in) were cast in a split mold as shown in Fig. 48.3. (The 24-gage wire specimens were fabricated and tested but not discussed here since the results are similar to the

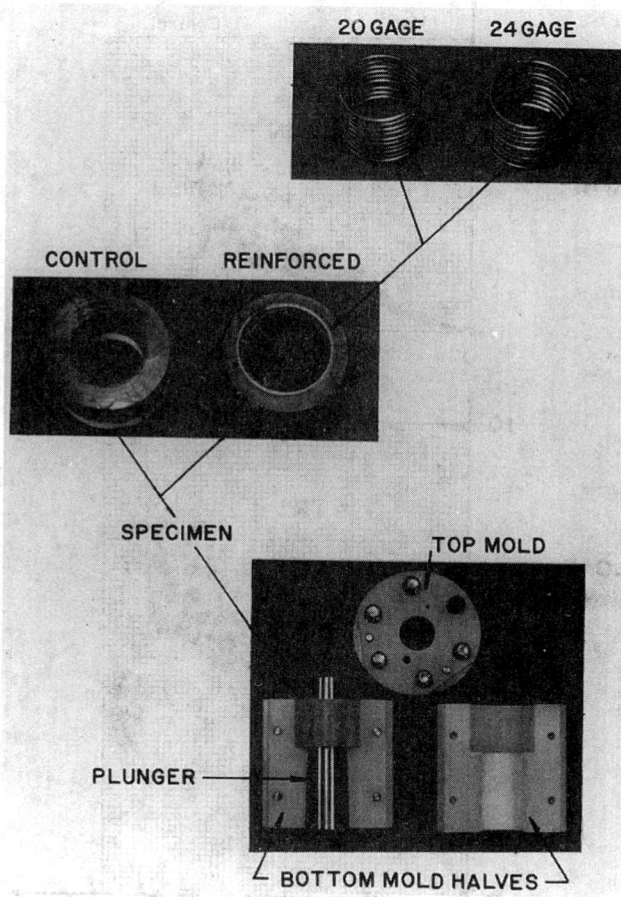

FIGURE 48.3 Mechanical test specimen fabrication with and without coil by using a split mold. The holes in the top mold are for the injection of bone cement and bleeding of trapped air (smaller hole) [Kim & Park, 1994]. The metal plunger in the middle of the bottom halves is tapered 1.51 degrees, simulating tapered prosthesis [Mann et al., 1991].

20-gage specimens. See Kim and Park [1994].) Typical load-displacement curves are shown in Fig. 48.4 for the control (pure cement) and wire-reinforced bone cement specimen. These curves show the characteristic slip-stick between the metal surface (plunger substituting the prosthesis) and the cement which was also observed by others [Mann et al., 1991]. The results of mechanical property measurements are summarized in Table 48.11. Table 48.12 gives the percentage changes of all measured parameters, and Table 48.13 gives some statistical analyses of the results. The cement densities were about the same for the reinforced and control specimens. The magnitude of the ultimate load of the control specimens (3.70 ± 1.13kN) is similar to those obtained by Mann and colleagues (~ 32kN), whose specimen was 8 times longer than that used in the present study [Mann et al., 1991]. If we extrapolate the ultimate load of the wire-reinforced specimens to that of Mann's work (which is closer to the in vivo condition), the load to fracture would be about 72kN, well above the normal loading on the prosthesis even in dynamic loading (6 ~ 8 times body weight; 4kN) [Paul, 1973]. The percentage increases of improvements in mechanical properties are similar or higher than other studies, although the increases are not as high as predicted by the composite theory [Taitsman & Saha, 1977; Topoleski et al., 1990].

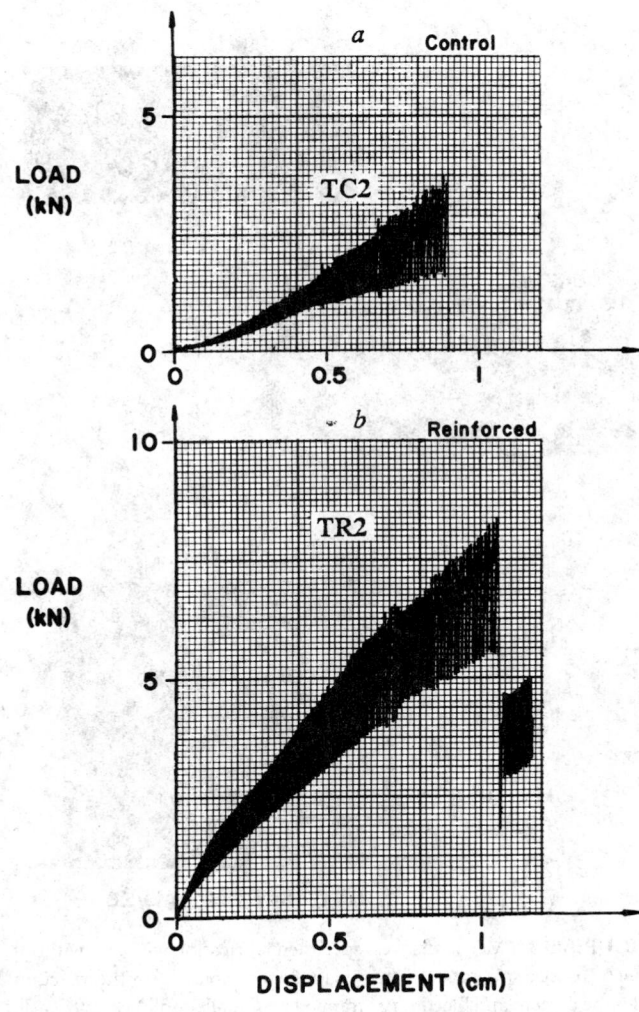

FIGURE 48.4   Typical load displacement curves for the control and reinforced specimens: (*a*) control and (*b*) reinforced [Kim & Park, 1994].

TABLE 48.11 Summary of the Mechanical Property Measurements

Specimen Type	Maximum Strain, %	Maximum Load, kN	Stiffness, GNm/m	Toughness, Nm/m
Control	2.6 ± 0.5	3.70 ± 1.13	1.73 ± 0.39	49.33 ± 18.63
Wire reinforced	3.2 ± 0.9	7.68 ± 2.33	4.17 ± 1.16	129.48 ± 65.3

TABLE 48.12 Percentage Changes of the Measured Variables over Control

Density	Strain	Load	Stiffness	Toughness
−0.2	+22.7	+107.6	+141.0	+162.5

All measured mechanical properties show that the wire coil reinforcement significantly enhanced the strength, fracture strain, stiffness, and toughness over the control. The most significant increases were the toughness, indicating that the coil-reinforced cement mantle will resist the load much more than the nonreinforced control. This may result in a prolonged fixation life of the prosthesis which is the ultimate goal of all arthroplasties.

Cement/Bone Interface

The problems at the bone-cement interface cannot be easily overcome, since these problems arise from the intrinsic properties of the bone cement as well as extrinsic factors such as cementing technique. The toxicity of the monomer, inherent weakness of the cement as a material (see Table 48.1), inevitable inclusion of the pores, and blood and tissue debris mixed during surgery can contribute to the problem of loosening at the bone-cement interface [Park, 1983a].

The bone-cement interface strength may be enhanced by growing bone into the cement after fixation. Bone cement can be used for immediate fixation yet provide tissue ingrowth space later by incorporating resorbable particles (such as inorganic bone particles) as shown conceptually in Fig. 48.5. Recent studies [Dai et al., 1991; Henrich, et al., 1993; Liu et al., 1987; Park et al., 1986] indicate that the concept can be used effectively at least for rabbit and canine models. In one study the bone-particle-impregnated bone cement was used to fix femoral stem prosthesis in femora of dogs (one side was experimental, the other was control), and after a predetermined time, the femora were harvested and sectioned into disks for the push-out test to measure the interfacial strength between the bone and cement interface [Dai et al., 1991]. The results as shown in Fig. 48.6 indicate that the experimental side increased its strength up to 5 months, and the control side decreased slightly. The histology also showed the integration of tissues into the spaces of the dissolved particles. Of course, care should be taken to control the amount of particles to balance out the increased viscosity and decreased strength. Table 48.14 illustrates the relationship between the number of resorbable particles (inorganic bone particles, 100–300μm) and the porosity and pore size [Kim et al., 1994]. As more particles were incorporated onto the bone cement, a lesser amount of porosity resulted but the average pore size increased. As mentioned earlier, the tensile strength decreased with increased number of bone particles. Fatigue properties improved with higher particle inclusion; however, it was found that about 30% (by weight) of bone particles can provide sufficient interconnected porosity for bony ingrowth and yet give reasonable compromises to other parameters

TABLE 48.13 The t-Statistics among Measured Variables for Each Group of Samples

Variables	Density	Strain	Load	Stiffness	Toughness
t values	0.752	0.031*	0.000*	0.000*	0.000*

* Statistically significant versus control ($p < 0.05$).

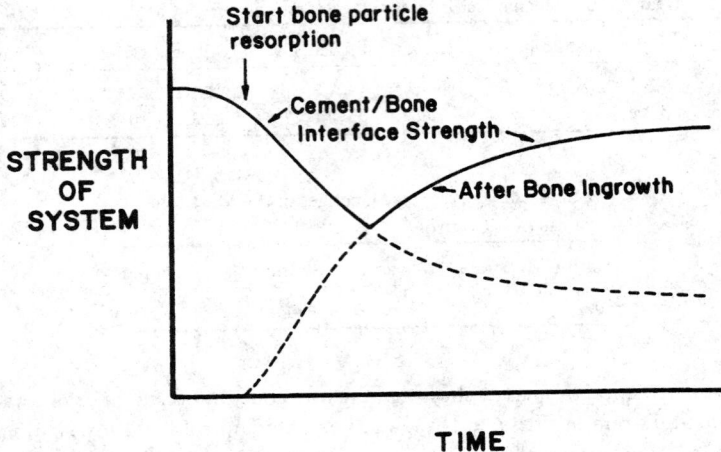

FIGURE 48.5   Basic concept of the bone cement with resorbable particle fixation. Immediate fixation is achieved as in the ordinary bone cement with the enhanced biological fixation to be achieved later for a prolonged stabilization of the implant [Park, 1992].

[Liu et al., 1987]. The bone-particle-impregnated bone cement has been used clinically, but its long-term success remains to be proven [Dai, 1991].

48.3 Porous Ingrowth (Biologic) Fixation

Efforts to develop a viable interface between the tissue and implants have been made ever since Moore [1952] designed a femoral prosthesis which had a fenestrated large hole in the proximal

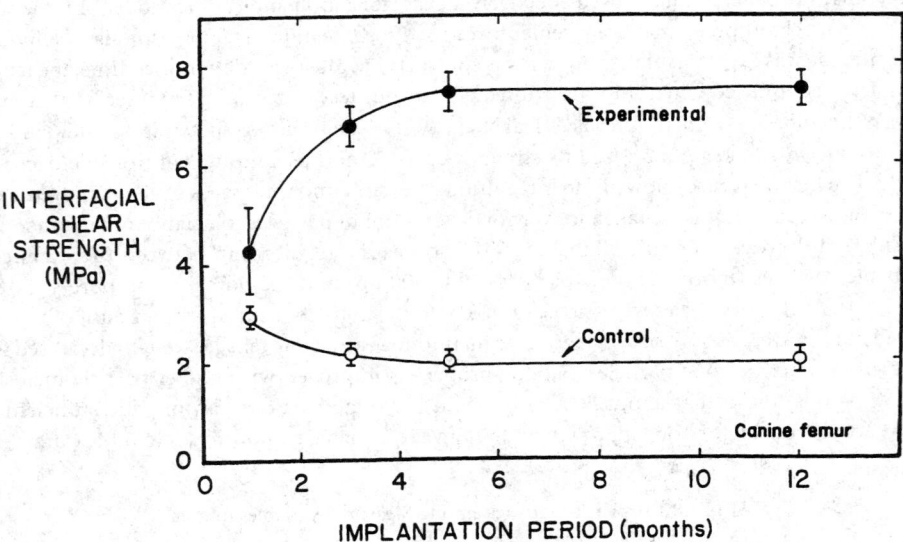

FIGURE 48.6   Maximum interfacial shear strength between bone and bone cement versus implant period when the femoral stems were implanted with ordinary bone cement and cement with bone particles. In both cases the interfacial strength was stabilized after 5 months for this canine model [Dai et al., 1991].

TABLE 48.14 Effect of Inorganic Bone Particle Mixed with Acrylic Bone Cement on the Pore Size, Porosity, and Tensile Strength

Particle Amount, %	Pore size, μm	Porosity, %	Tensile Strength, MPa
0	154.7 ± 72	7.2 ± 2.5	23.2 ± 2.3
10	160.6 ± 68	5.0 ± 1.7*	22.6 ± 2.0*
20	172.9 ± 52*	4.9 ± 1.5*	20.1 ± 1.1*
30	218.0 ± 92*	2.4 ± 0.7*	19.7 ± 1.1*

* Statistically significant versus control ($p < 0.05$)
Note: 15 specimens for each group.
Source: Kim et al. [1994].

region. Ironically the fixation itself is by the passive mechanical fixation technique as discussed earlier. Smith [1963] tried to develop a bone substitute with porous aluminate ceramic impregnated with an epoxy resin called Cerocium. Although the material demonstrated a good adherence to the tissues, the pore size (average 18 μm diameter) was too small to allow any bony tissue ingrowth. Later, ceramics [Klawitter & Hulbert, 1972; Oonishi et al., 1989; Predecki et al., 1972], metals [Hirshhorn et al., 1972; Niles & Lapitsky, 1975], and polymers [Sauer et al., 1974] were used to test the ingrowth idea. Basically, any biocompatible material will allow bony tissues to grow into any spaces large enough to accommodate osteons. However, to be continuously viable the space must be large enough (more than 75 μm diameter for the bony tissues) and contiguous to the surface of bone matrix [Heimke, 1990]. In addition, Wolff's law dictates that the ingrown tissues should be subjected to bodily loading in order to prevent resorption, even after the initial ingrowth has taken place. The same principle also makes it difficult to have a uniform tissue ingrowth throughout the implant surface. This is why the tissue ingrowth takes place where the stress transfer occurs, e.g., in the distal lateral region of the femoral stem of the artificial hip joint.

Figure 48.7 shows the general trends of the fixation (interfacial) strength variation with implantation period in animals up to 6 months for metallic implants (CoCr alloys, Ti and its alloys, and

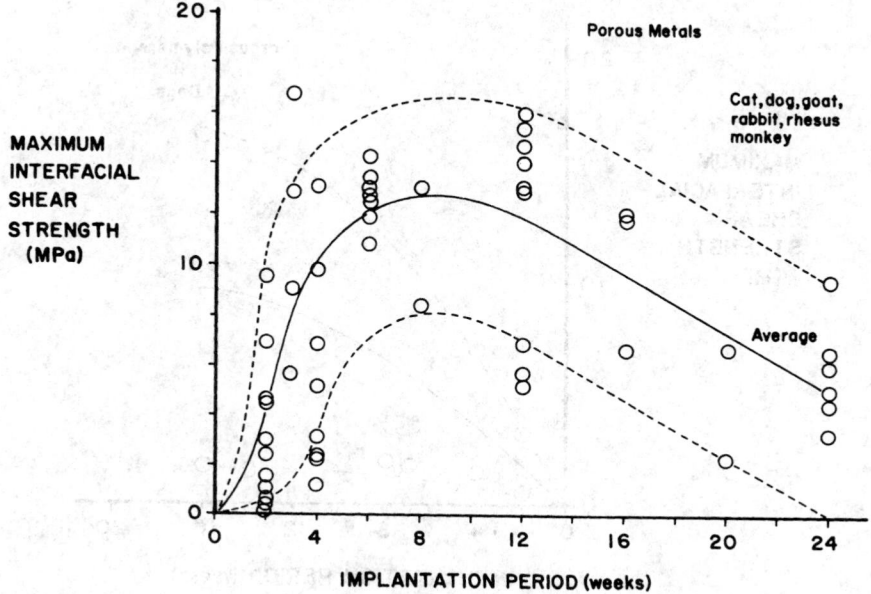

FIGURE 48.7 Maximum interfacial shear strength between bone and porous metal implants versus implant of various metals and animals, data from Spector [1982b].

stainless steel). A few remarks can be made from these data. First, the maximum interfacial shear strength between bone and porous implant peaked at about 12~13 MPa in about 6~8 weeks regardless of the implant material, animal type, or location of the implants (i.e., cortical or cancellous bone and transcortical or intramedullary canal). Second, the data are widely scattered. [The original data showed wide variations; therefore, they are not distinguished among the variables]. The *decrease* in interfacial strength with time after peak for the metallic implants is somewhat distressing, since this may also be true with human patients. This may be caused by two factors. The first is that of bone resorption from the initially ingrown area due to the stress shielding. The second is the release of a large number of metal ions due to the increased surface area resulting from making the implant porous. Porous polymers did not have the decreasing trends as shown in Fig. 48.8 [Spector, 1982a]. This may be interpreted as the lack of stress shielding (after bone is ingrown into the pores) due to the low modulus of the polymers. However, not enough data are available to come to a definitive conclusion [Keet & Runne, 1989; Sadr & Arden, 1987; Spector, 1982b; Tullos et al., 1984].

Further problems with biologic fixation are: the unforgiving nature of the surgery, the long immobilization time for tissue ingrowth, the unpredictable time to ambulate, and the difficulty in eradicating infection. In addition, once the interface is destroyed by an accidental overloading, it cannot be regrown with certainty. Moreover, the porous coating may weaken the underlying prosthesis itself, and, in the case of metals, there is an increased danger of corrosion fatigue metal ions released due to the increased surface area [Brien, Salvat, Betts, et al., 1992; Brand, 1987; Morscher, 1984]. Due to these problems and clinical results of porous fixation, some investigators have insisted that the bone-cement-fixation technique is still the gold standard at this time [Johnston, 1987].

In order to alleviate these problems several modifications have been tried, including the following.

Precoating Metallic Porous Surface with Ceramics or Carbons

This method has been tried with limited success [Cranin et al., 1972; Thomas et al., 1985]. The problem of coating deep in the pores and the thermal expansion difference between the metal and ceramic materials make a uniform and good adherent coating very difficult. An attractive material

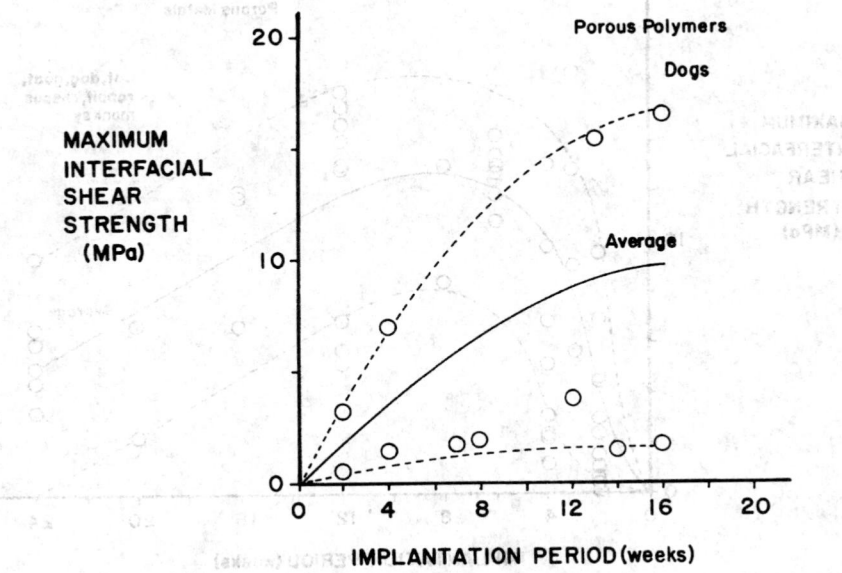

FIGURE 48.8 Maximum interfacial shear strength between bone and porous polymeric implants versus implant, data from Spector [1982a].

for coating is hydroxyapatite [$Ca_{10}(PO_4)_6(OH)_2$] ceramic which is similar to bone mineral. It is not yet conclusive that this material is more beneficial than other ceramics. Some preliminary studies in our laboratory indicate that during the early period of fixation, the bioactive hydroxyapatite coating may be more beneficial but the effect may diminish after 3 weeks as shown in Fig. 48.9. The result is for the simple cortical bone plug experiment performed on canine femora [Park, 1988]. Others have shown promising results with the same material system used on rabbits instead of canines as in our study [Oonishi et al., 1989].

Precoating with Porous Polymeric Materials on Metal Stem

Theoretically, this method has two distinct advantages over ceramics or carbon coating method discussed above [Homsy, 1972; Keet & Runne, 1989; Sadr & Arden, 1987; Spector, 1982a; Tullos et al., 1984]. First, the low modulus polymeric material could transfer the load from the implant to the bone more gradually and evenly and thus prevent stress-shielding effects on the ingrown tissues. Second, this method would prevent the metallic surface ion release, i.e., less corrosion of the metal. One major problem with this technique is the weak interfacial strength between the polymer and metallic stem especially in dynamic loading conditions in vivo.

Enhancement of Porous Ingrowth with Electrical or Electromagnetic Stimulation

This technique combines the porous ingrowth with the stimulating effects of electrical and/or electromagnetic stimulation [Park & Kenner, 1975; Weinstein et al., 1976]. Direct current stimulation can indeed accelerate tissue ingrowth in the early stages of healing, but its effect diminishes over time [Weinstein et al., 1976]. Direct current stimulation has one distinct problem: the invasive nature of the power source. The pulsed electromagnetic field stimulation is a better method, since the stimulation can be carried out extracorporeally. A preliminary study using canine femur indicates that it can be effective as shown in Fig. 48.10 [Park, 1983b]. More studies are needed to lend further support.

Porous Ingrowth with the Use of Filling Materials

There has been some effort to use filling materials around the porous implant, since it is very difficult to prepare the tissue bed with the exact shape of the prosthesis to eliminate the micromovement

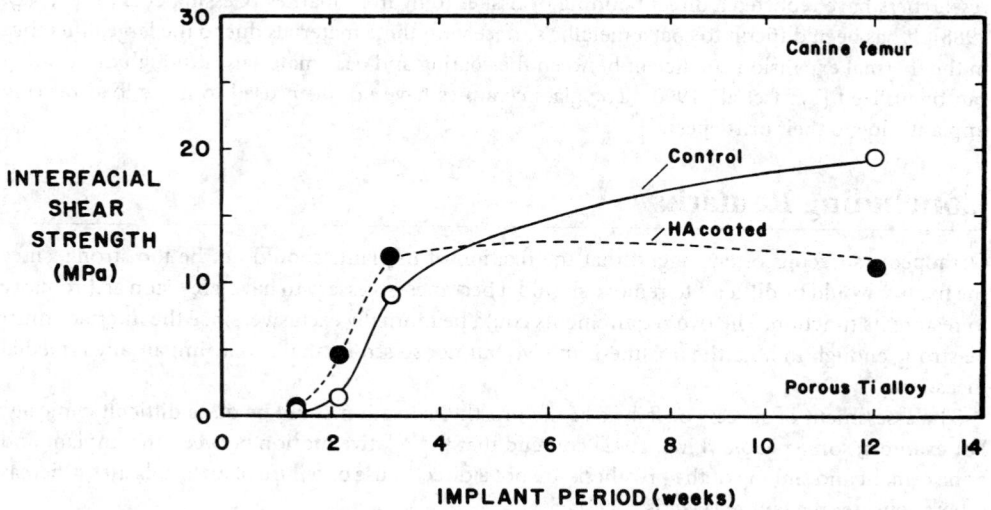

FIGURE 48.9 Maximum interfacial shear strength between bone and bioactive ceramic coated porous plug implants versus implant period when the plugs with and without (control) coating were implanted in the cortices of canine femora [Park, 1988].

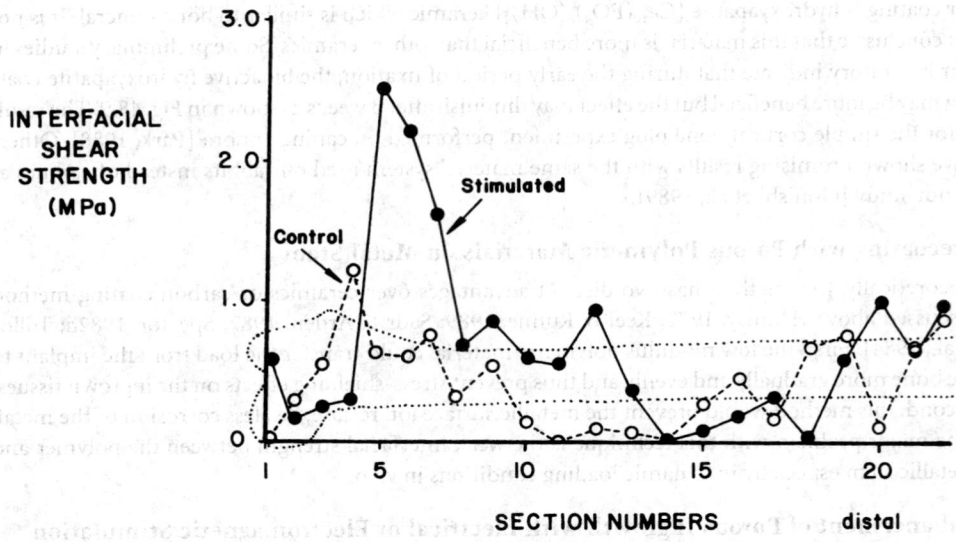

FIGURE 48.10 Maximum interfacial shear strength between bone and porous metallic intramedullary implant with and without (control) pulsed electromagnetic field stimulation. The porous implants were implanted in the medullary canals of canine femora (one side was control, the other was experimental) [Park, 1983*b*].

of the prosthesis after implantation. Bone matrix proteins (BMP) or demineralized bone and hydroxyapatite crystals can be used for this purpose [Parsons et al., 1987]. The success of this technique has not been fully documented.

48.4 Direct Bonding of Implant and Bone

Some glass ceramics tend to achieve direct bonding with the bone through a selective dissolution of the surface film [Blencke et al., 1978; Hench & Paschall, 1973; Yamamuro et al., 1990]. Some researchers have reported a direct bonding of tissues to hydroxyapatites [Gessink et al., 1987; Kay, 1988]. It has been difficult to coat a metallic surface with these materials due to the large difference in the thermal expansion coefficient between the coating and base materials, although dip-coating can be utilized [West et al., 1990]. The glass ceramics have not been used to make load-bearing implants due to their brittleness.

48.5 Concluding Remarks

Orthopedic surgeons often suggest that the fixation of implants should not be too strong, since the fixative would be difficult to remove should it becomes necessary to have a revision arthroplasty to restore its function. The two requirements could be mutually exclusive, since the interface must be strong enough to hold the prosthesis in vivo but not so strong that it may impair any remedial measures.

The assessment of success or failure of the prosthesis fixation could be quite difficult clinically. For example, some people [Ling, 1992] contend that the relative motion between the implant and bone cement and sinking of the prosthesis are not a direct cause of failure of arthroplasties, whereas others consider it a failure [Harris, 1992].

Another problem is related to the increasing use of the implants for younger patients, which requires firmer fixation and longer implant life. The original expectation of cementless porous ingrowth fixation for the young is tempered somewhat, and we need to explore a method of fixation that lasts longer [Callaghan, 1992].

Defining Terms

ASTM Standard: The American Society for Testing and Materials sets the standards for testing and materials' properties to make any products including medical products. It publishes all the standards annually in many volumes.

Biological fixation: A method of using tissue ingrowth into the pores of implant to stabilize implants. Large pores ($>75\mu m$ in diameter) and interconnecting porosity are needed for maintaining a viable interface between bone and prosthesis.

Bone cement: A general term referring to a material which could be used to hold the prosthesis in place. Usually refers to the acrylic-based polymer powder and monomer liquid system which are mixed together at the time of surgery and used to seat the prosthesis. It is generally believed that the acrylic bone cement acts as a grouting medium rather than adhesive in nature, although the name *cement* implies an adhesive.

Bone morphogenetic protein (BMP): Demineralized bone having osteogenetic capacity when implanted. First extracted by M. Urist of UCLA; the real nature of the BMP is not fully understood.

Bone remodeling: Due to the alterations in the stress or loading on the bone, bone changes in mass according to the loading the bone experiences. Reduced loading may result in osteoporosis and increased loading may result in hypertrophy of the bone in long bones such as femur and tibia.

Cerocium: An aluminate ceramic and epoxy polymer matrix composite material developed to induce bony tissues into the pores of the implant.

Charnley prosthesis: Originally designed by Sir John Charnley by using high-density polyethylene (HDPE) acetabular cup and small size head femoral hip prosthesis which showed low friction due to smaller contact area. The implants are fixed by acrylic bone cement.

Degree of polymerization: Defined as the average number of monomer or repeating unit in a polymer chain or molecule. Some can be very large such as ultra-high-molecular-weight polyethylene (UHMWPE), which could reach 6,000,000 g/mol.

Free radical (addition) polymerization: A chemical reaction to make a long chain molecules of polymers (plastics) in which an initiator and a catalyst are used to make a free radical which in turn attacks a monomer to make another free radical. The propagation of the chains terminate after consuming the monomers resulting in long chain molecules. Vinyl polymers such as acrylics, polyolefins, and polystyrene are made by this process.

Glass ceramic: A class of ceramics made by first quenching from molten state into glass state and subsequently crystallizing into ceramic state. Controlling the grain size can increase its strength many folds; it has low thermal expansion coefficient. The ceramic could be made incorporating calcium and phosphorous, for example, Bioglass and Ceravital, making direct bonding to bone possible.

Hoop stress: Stress developed in the cement and bone by the loading of implant in the tangential direction perpendicular to the longitudinal axis of bone.

Hydroxyapatite: One of the apatite ceramic materials composed of calcium and phosphorous, $[Ca_{10}(PO_4)_6(OH)_2]$ which is similar to the mineral phase of bone.

Loosening: Related to the relative motion between implant and bone for direct fixation and among implant, bone cement, and bone in case of cemented fixation. It may lead to the failure of total hip and total knee arthroplasty.

Osteon: A bone cell or osteocyte made of haversian canal in the middle with concentric layers of collagen laminae embedded with hydroxyapatitelike mineral crystals discretely. Only highly developed animals have this structure. (Rabbit is the smallest animal having the osteons.)

Precoating: The coating of prosthesis usually by the manufacturer with bone-cement-like material such as polymethylmethacrylate to prevent the debonding of the interface between prosthesis and bone cement.

Push-out test: A mechanical test to obtain the interfacial strength between two materials such as interface between bone cement and prosthesis or between bone and porous surfaced implant.

Absolute values are hard to obtain with this, test since the test is very sensitive to the thickness of the specimen, clearance and alignment of the plunger. One should use this test for comparison between control and experimental specimens by making sure that all the test protocols are the same.

Radial stress: Stress developed in the cement and bone in the radial direction by the loading of implant.

Stress concentration: Higher stresses due to material inhomogeneity such as in pores and design such as sharp corners and holes, which lead to failure of the (implant) materials faster.

Stress shielding effect: Bones may displace their mass where the stress is shielded such as under the fracture plate and cortices of the (stiff) femoral prostheses, resulting in bone resorption, i.e., osteoporosis.

Wolff's law: The rule that remodeling of bone takes place in response to the mechanical loading such that the new structure becomes better adapted to the load.

References

Ahmed AM, Raab S, Miller JE. 1984. Metal/cement interface strength in cemented stem fixation. J Orthop Res 2:105.

Amstutz H, Markolf KL, McNeice GM, et al. 1976. Loosening of total hip components: Cause and prevention. In The Hip, pp 102–116, St. Louis, Mosby.

Barb W, Park JB, Von Recum, AF, et al. 1982. Intramedullary fixation of artificial hip joints with bone cement precoated implants: I. Interfacial strengths. J Biomed Mater Res 16:447.

Bechtol CO, Ferguson AB, Laing PG. 1959. Metals and Engineering in Bone and Joint Surgery, London, Balliere, Tindall and Cox.

Blencke BA, Bromer H, Deutscher KK. 1978. Compatibility and long-term stability of glass ceramic implants. J Biomed Mater Res 12:307.

Brand RA (ed). 1987. The Hip: Non-Cemented Hip Implants, St. Louis, Mosby.

Brien WW, Salvat EA, Betts F, et al. 1992. Metal levels in cemented total hip arthroplasty: A comparison of well-fixed and loose implants. Clin Orthop Rel Res 276:66.

Callaghan JJ. 1992. Total hip arthroplasty: A clinical perspective. Clin Orthop Rel Res 276:33.

Carlsson AS, Gentz C-F, Lindberg HO. 1983. Thirty-two noninfected total hip arthroplasties revised due to stem loosening. Clin Orthop Rel Res 181:196.

Charnley J. 1970. Acrylic Cement in Orthopedic Surgery, pp 213–358, Baltimore, Williams and Wilkins.

Charnley J. 1972. The long-term results of low-friction arthroplasty of the hip, performed as a primary intervention. J Bone Joint Surg 54B:61.

Charnley J, Cupic Z. 1973. The nine and ten year results of the low-friction arthroplasty of the hip. Clin Orthop Rel Res 95:9.

Cranin AN, Schnitman PA, Rabkin M, et al. 1972. Alumina and zirconia coated Vitallium oral endosteal implants. J Biomed Mater Res Symp (6):257.

Crowninshield R. 1988. An overview of prosthetic materials for fixation. Clin Orthop Rel Res 235:166.

Crowninshield RD, Brand RA, Johnston RC, et al. 1980. An analysis of femoral component stem design in total hip arthroplasty. J Bone Joint Surg 62A:68.

Crugnola A, Ellis EJ, Radin EL, et al. 1979. A second generation of acrylic cements. Trans Soc Biomat 3:91.

Dai KR. 1991. Personnal communication.

Dai KR, Liu YK, Park JB, et al. 1991. Bone particle impregnated bone cement: An *in vivo* weight-bearing study. J Biomed Mater Res 25:141.

Davidson JA. April 5, 1988. Bone cement reinforcement and method. US patent no. 4,735,625.

De Groot K. 1983. Bioceramics of Calcium Phosphate, pp 99–114, Boca Raton, Fla, CRC Press.

Ducheyne P. 1988. Prosthesis fixation for orthopedics. In JG Webster (ed), Encyclopedia of Medical Devices and Instrumentation, pp 2146–2154, New York, Wiley-Interscience.

Eftekhar NS. 1978. Principles of Total Hip Arthroplasty, pp 125–148, St. Louis, Mosby.

Eftekhar NS. 1987. Long-term results of cemented total hip arthroplasty. Clin Orthop Rel Res 225:207.

Fowler JL, Gie GA, Lee AJC, et al. 1988. Experience with Exeter total hip replacement since 1970. Orthop Clin N Am 19:477.

Freeman MAR, Tennant R. 1992. The scientific basis of cement versus cementless fixation. Clin Orthop Rel Res 276:19.

Gessink RG, deGroot K, Klein C. 1987. Chemical implant fixation using hydroxyaptite coatings. Clinic Orthop Rel Res 226:147.

Gruen TS, McNeice GM, Amstutz HA. 1979. "Modes of failure" of cemented stem-type femoral components. Clin Orthop Rel Res 141:17.

Haas SS, Brauer GM, Dickson G. 1975. A characterization of PMMA bone cement. J Bone Joint Surg 57A:280.

Hansen D, Jensen JS. 1992. Mixing does not improve mechanical properties of all bone cements. Manual and centrifugation-vacuum mixing compared for 10 cement brands. Acta Orthop Scand 63(1):13.

Harrigan TP, Kareh JA, O'Connor DO, et al. 1992. A finite element study of the initiation of failure of fixation in cemented femoral total hip components. J Orthop Res 10:134.

Harris WH. 1992. Is it advantageous to strengthen the cement-metal interface and use a collar for cemented femoral components of total hip replacements? Clin Orthop Rel Res 285:67.

Harris WH, McGann WA. 1984. Loosening of the femoral component after use of the medullary-plug cementing technique. J Bone Joint Surg 67B:222.

Hedley AK, Moreland J, Bloebaum RD, et al. 1979. Press-fit, cemented, and bone ingrowth surface replacement-canine fixation model. Trans Orthop Res Soc 4:163.

Heimke G(ed). 1990. Osseo-Integrated Implants, vols 1, 2, Boca Raton, Fla, CRC Press.

Hench LL, Paschall HA. 1973. Direct chemical bond of bioactive glass-ceramic materials to bone and muscle. J Biomed Mater Res Symp (4):25.

Henrich DE, Cram AE, Park JB, et al. 1993. Inorganic bone and bone morphogenetic protein impregnated bone cement: A preliminary *in vivo* study. J Biomed Mater Res 27:277.

Hirshhorn JS, McBeath AA, Dustoor MR. 1972. Porous titanium surgical implant materials. J Biomed Mater Res Symp (2):49.

Homsy CA, Cain TE, Kessler FB, et al. 1972. Porous implant systems for prosthetic stabilization. Clinic Orthop Rel Res 89:220.

Jasty M, Maloney WJ, Bragdon CR, et al. 1991. The initiation of failure in cemented femoral components of hip arthroplasties. J Bone Joint Surg 73B:551.

Johnston RC. 1987. The case for cemented hips. In RA Brand (ed), The Hip, pp 351–358, St. Louis, Mosby.

Kay JF. 1988. Bioactive surface coatings: Cause for encouragement and caution. J Oral Implant 16:43.

Keet GGM, Runne WC. 1989. The anaform endoprosthesis: A proplast-coated femoral endopros-thesis. Orthopedics 12:1185.

Kim KJ, Greis P, Wilson SC, et al. 1991. Histological and biological comparison of membranes from titanium, cobalt-chromium, and polyethylene hip prosthesis. Trans Orthopedic Res Soc 16:191.

Kim YS, Kang YH, Kim JK, et al. 1994. Effect of bone mineral particles on the porosity of bone cement. Biomed Mater Eng 4(1):1.

Kim JK, Park JB. 1994. Reinforcement of bone cement around prostheses by pre-coated wire coil: A preliminary study. Biomed Mater Eng.

Klawitter JJ, Hulbert SF. 1972. Application of porous ceramics for the attachment of load bearing internal orthopaedic applications. J Biomed Mater Res Symp (2) (Part 1):161.

Kusy RP. 1978. Characterization of self-curing acrylic bone cements. J Biomed Mater Res 12:271.

Lee HB, Turner DT. 1977. Temperature control of a bone cement by addition of a crystalline monomer. J Biomed Mater Res 11:671.

Ling RSM. 1992. The use of a collar and precoating on cemented femoral stems is unnecessary and detrimental. Clin Orthop Rel Res 285:73.

Liu YK, Park JB, Njus GO, et al. 1987. Bone particle impregnated bone cement I. *In vitro* study. J Biomed Mater Res 21:247.

Lu Z, Ebramzadeh E, Sarmiento A. 1993. The effect of failure of the cement interfaces on gross loosening of cemented total hip femoral components. Trans Orthop Res Soc 18:519.

Mann KA, Bartel DL, Wright TM, et al. 1991. Mechanical characteristics of stem-cement interface. J Orthop Res 9:798–808.

Mears DC. 1979. Materials and Orthopedic Surgery, pp. 602–603, Baltimore, Williams and Wilkins.

Mittelmeier H. 1975. New development of wear-resistant ceramic and metal composite prostheses with ribbed support shafts for cement-free implantation. Hefte zur Unfallheilkunde: Beihefe zue Monatsschrift fur Unfallheilkunde, Verischerings, Versorgungs und Verkehrsmedizin, 126:333.

Mittelmeier H. 1976. Anchoring hip endoprosthesis without bone cement. In M Schaldach, D Hohmann (eds), Advances in Artificial Hip and Knee Joint Technology, pp. 387–402, Berlin, Springer-Verlag.

Modern Plastics Encyclopedia. 1980. New York, McGraw-Hill.

Moore AT. 1952. Metal hip joint: A new self-locking Vitallium prosthesis. South Med J 45:10.

Morscher E (ed). 1984. The Cementless Fixation of Hip Endoprosthesis, Heidelberg, Springer-Verlag.

Niles JL, Lapitsky M. 1975. Biomechanical investigations of bone-porous carbon and metal inter-faces. J Biomed Mater Res Symp (4):63.

O'Connor DO, Burke DW, Sedlacek RC, et al. 1991. Peak cement strains in cemented femoral total hip. Trans Orthop Res Soc 16:220.

Oonishi H, Yamamoto M, Ishimaru H, et al. 1989. Comparisons of bone ingrowth into porous Ti-6Al-4V beads uncoated and coated with hydroxyapatite. In H Ooonoishi, H Aoki, K Sawai (eds), Bioceramics, pp 400–405, Tokyo, St. Louis. Ishiyaku EuroAmerica.

Park JB. 1983*a*. Acrylic bone cement; *In vitro* and *in vivo* property-structure relationship—a selective review. Ann Biomed Eng 11:297.

Park JB. 1983*b*. Implant fixation by pulsed electromagnetic field stimulation. Unpublished study, Iowa City, University of Iowa.

Park JB. 1984. Biomaterials Science and Engineering, pp 282–288, New York, Plenum.

Park JB. 1988. *In vivo* evaluation of resorbable surface bone implant. Unpublished study, Iowa City, University of Iowa.

Park JB. 1992. Orthopedic prosthesis fixation. Ann Biomed Eng 20:583.

Park JB. October 13, 1993. Reinforcement of bone cement around prosthesis by pre-coated wire coil/wire mesh. Invention disclosure, Iowa City, University of Iowa.

Park JB, Barb W, Davies JP. 1982. Long-term evaluation of precoated canine femoral prosthesis. In S Saha (ed), Biomedical Engineering I: Recent Developments, pp. 295–298, New York, Perga-mon.

Park JB, Barb W, Kenner GH, et al. 1982. Intramedullary fixation of artificial hip joints with bone cement precoated implants: II. Density and histological study. J Biomed Mater Res 16:459.

Park JB, Choi WW, Liu YK, et al. 1986. Bone particle impregnated polymethylmethacrylate: *In vitro* and *in vivo* study. In D Steenberghe (ed), Tissue Integration in Oral and Facial Reconstruc-tion, pp 118–124, Amsterdam, Excerptu Medica.

Park JB, Kenner GH. 1975. Effect of electrical stimulation on the tensile strength of the porous implant and bone interface. Biomater Med Dev Artif Org 3:233.

Park JB, Lakes RS. 1992. Biomaterials: An Introduction, 2d ed, New York, Plenum.

Park JB, Malstrom CS, von Recum AF. 1978. Intramedullary fixation of implants precoated with bone cement: A preliminary study. Biomater Med Dev Artif Org 6:361.

Park JB, von Recum AF, Gratzick GE. 1979. Pre-coated orthopedic implants with bone cement. Biomater Med Dev Artif Org 7:41.

Parsons JR, Ricci JL, Liebrecht P, et al. 1987. Enhanced stabilization of orthopaedic implants with spherical hydroxylapatite particulate. Dublin, Calif, OrthoMatrix.

Paul JP. 1973. Design aspects of endoprostheses for the lower limb. In RM Kenedi (ed), Perspectives in Biomedical Engineering, pp 91–94, New York, McMillan.

Predecki P, Stephan JE, Auslander BE, et al. 1972. Kinetics of bone growth into cylindrical channels in aluminum oxide and titanium. J Biomed Mater Res 6:375.

Raab S, Ahmed AM, Provan JW. 1982. Thin film PMMA precoating for improved implant bone-cement fixation. J Biomed Mater Res 16:679.

Sadr B, Arden GP. 1987. A comparison of the stability of proplast-coated and cemented Thompson prosthesis in the treatment of subcapital femoral fractures. Injury 8:234.

Saha S, Pal S. 1984. Mechanical properties of bone cement: A review. J Biomed Mater Res 18:435.

Sauer BW, Weinstein AM, Klawitter JJ, et al. 1974. The role of porous polymeric materials in prosthesis attachment. J Biomed Mater Res Symp (5):145.

Smith L. 1963. Ceramic-plastic material as a bone substitute. Arch Surg 87:653.

Spector M. 1982a. Bone ingrowth into porous polymers. In DF Williams (ed), Biocompatibility of Orthopedic Implants, vol 2, pp 89–128, Boca Raton, Fla, CRC Press.

Spector M. 1982b. Bone ingrowth into porous metals. In DF Williams (ed), Biocompatibility of Orthopedic Implants, Vol 2, pp 55–88, Boca Raton, Fla, CRC Press.

Taitsman JP, Saha S. 1977. Tensile strength of wire-reinforced bone cement and twisted stainless-steel wire. J Bone Joint Surg 59A:419.

Thomas KA, Cook SD, Renz EA, et al. 1985. The effect of surface treatments on the interface mechanics of LTI pyrolytic carbon implants. J Biomed Mater Res 19:145.

Topoleski LDT, Ducheyne P, Cuckler JM. 1990. The fracture toughness of short-titanium-fiber reinforced bone cement. Trans Soc Biomat 13:107.

Tullos HS, McCaskill BL, Dickey R, et al. 1984. Total hip arthroplasty with a low-modulus porous-coated femoral component. J Bone Joint Surg 66A:888.

Weinstein AM, Klawitter JJ, Cleveland TW, et al. 1976. Electrical stimulation of bone growth into porous Al_2O_3. J Biomed Mater Res 10:231.

West JK, Clark AE, Hall MB, et al. 1990. In vivo bone-bonding study of Bioglass®-coated titanium alloy. In T Yamamuro, LL Hench, J Wilson (eds), RC Handbook of Bioactive Ceramics, vol 1, Bioactive Glasses and Glass-Ceramics J, pp 161–166, Boca Raton, Fla, CRC Press.

Willert HG, Koch R, Burgi M. July 30, 1991. Reinforcement for a bone cement bed. US patent no. 5,035,714.

Williams DF, Roaf R. 1973. Implants in Surgery. London, Saunders.

Wroblewski BM. 1986. 15–21 year results of the Charnley low-fiction arthroplasty. Clin Orthop Rel Res 211:30.

Wykman A, Olsson E, Axdorph G, et al. 1991. Total hip arthroplasty: A comparison between cemented and press-fit noncemented fixation. J Arthoplasty 6:19.

Yamamuro T, Hench LL, Wilson J (eds). 1990. CRC Handbook of Bioactive Ceramics, vol 1, Bioactive Glasses and Glass-Ceramics, vol 2, Calcium Phosphate and Hydroxylapatite Ceramics, Boca Raton, Fla, CRC Press.

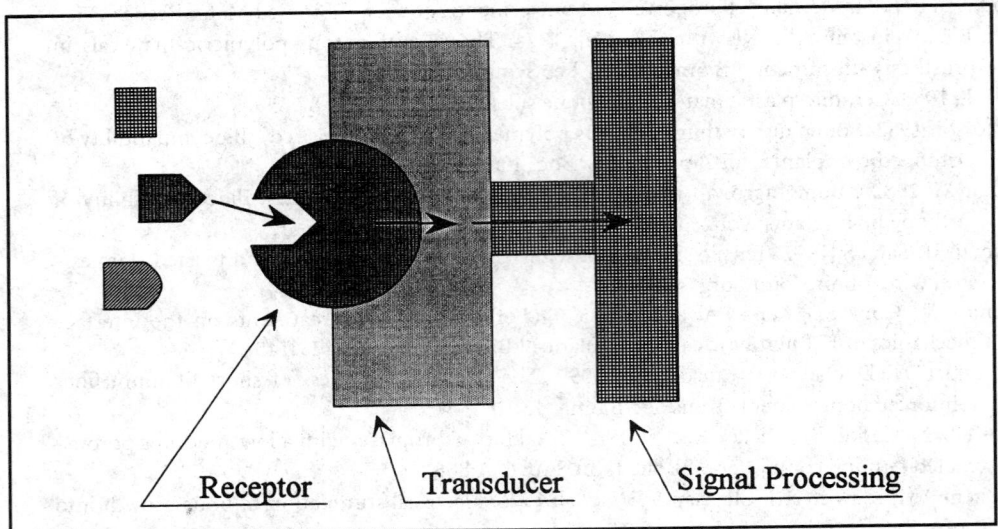

Generic bioanalytical analyzer.

V

Biomedical Sensors

Michael R. Neuman
Case Western Reserve University

SENSORS CONVERT SIGNALS OF ONE type of quantity such as hydrostatic fluid pressure into an equivalent signal of another type of quantity, for example, an electrical signal. Biomedical sensors take signals representing biomedical variables and convert them into what is usually an electrical signal. As such, the biomedical sensor serves as the interface between a biologic and an electronic system and must function in such a way as to not adversely affect either of these systems. In considering biomedical sensors, it is necessary to consider both sides of the interface: the biologic and the electronic, since both biologic and electronic factors play an important role in sensor performance.

Many different types of sensors can be used in biomedical applications. Table V.1 gives a general classification of these sensors. It is possible to categorize all sensors as being either physical or chemical. In the case of physical sensors, quantities such as geometric, mechanical, thermal, and hydraulic variables are measured. In biomedical applications these can include things such as muscle displacement, blood pressure, core body temperature, blood flow, cerebrospinal fluid pressure, and bone growth. Two types of physical sensors deserve special mention with regard to their biomedical application: Sensors of electrical phenomena in the body, usually known as electrodes, play a special role as a result of their diagnostic and therapeutic applications. The most familiar of these are sensors used to pick up the electrocardiogram, an electrical signal produced by the heart. The other type of physical sensor that finds many applications in biology and medicine is the optical sensor. These sensors can use light to collect information, and, in the case of fiber optic sensors, light is the transmission medium as well.

TABLE V.1   Classifications of Biomedical Sensors

Physical sensors
   Geometric
   Mechanical
   Thermal
   Hydraulic
   Electric
   Optical
Chemical
   Gas
   Electrochemical
   Photometric
   Other physical chemical methods
   Bioanalytic

The second major classification of sensing devices is chemical sensors. In this case the sensors are concerned with measuring chemical quantities such as identifying the presence of particular chemical compounds, detecting the concentrations of various chemical species, and monitoring chemical activities in the body for diagnostic and therapeutic applications. A wide variety of chemical sensors can be classified in many ways. One such classification scheme is illustrated in Table V.1 and is based upon the methods used to detect the chemical components being measured. Chemical compositions can be measured in the gas phase using several techniques, and these methods are especially useful in biomedical measurements associated with the pulmonary system. Electrochemical sensors measure chemical concentrations or, more precisely, activities, based upon chemical reactions that interact with electrical systems. Photometric chemical sensors are optical devices that detect chemical concentrations based upon changes in light transmission, reflection, or color. The familiar litmus test is an example of an optical change that can be used to measure the acidity or alkalinity of a solution. Other types of physical chemical sensors such as the mass spectrometer use various physical methods to detect and quantify chemicals associated with biologic systems.

Although they are essentially chemical sensors, bioanalytic sensors are often classified as a separate major sensor category. These devices incorporate biologic recognition reactions such as enzyme-substrate, antigen-antibody, or ligand-receptor to identify complex biochemical molecules. The use of biologic reactions gives bioanalytic sensors high sensitivity and specificity in identifying and quantifying biochemical substances.

One can also look at biomedical sensors from the standpoint of their applications. These can be generally divided according to whether a sensor is used for diagnostic or therapeutic purposes in clinical medicine and for data collection in biomedical research. Sensors for clinical studies such as those carried out in the clinical chemistry laboratory must be standardized in such a way that errors that could result in an incorrect diagnosis or inappropriate therapy are kept to an absolute minimum. Thus these sensors must not only be reliable themselves, but appropriate methods must exist for testing the sensors that are a part of the routine use of the sensors for making biomedical measurements.

One can also look at biomedical sensors from the standpoint of how they are applied to the patient or research subject. Table V.2 shows the range of general approaches to attaching biomedical sensors. At the top of the list we have the method that involves the least interaction with the biologic object being studied; the bottom of the list includes sensors that interact to the greatest extent. Clearly if a measurement can be made equally well by a sensor that does not contact the subject being measured and by one that must be surgically implanted, the former is by far the most desirable. However, a sensor that is used to provide information to help control a device surgically placed in the body to replace or assist a failing organ should be implanted, since this is the best way to communicate with the internal device.

You will notice in reading this section that the majority of biomedical sensors are essentially the same as sensors used in other applications. The unique part about biomedical sensors is their application. There are, however, special problems that are encountered by biomedical sensors that are unique to

TABLE V.2 Types of Sensor-Subject Interfaces

Noncontacting (noninvasive)
Skin surface (contacting)
Indwelling (minimally invasive)
Implantable (invasive)

them. These problems relate to the interface between the sensor and the biologic system being measured. The presence of foreign materials, especially implanted materials, can affect the biologic environment in which they are located. Many biologic systems are designed to deal with foreign materials by making a major effort to eliminate them. The rejection reaction that is often discussed with regard to implanted materials or transplanted tissues is an example of this. Thus, in considering biomedical sensors, one must worry about this rejection phenomenon and how it will affect the performance of the sensor. If the rejection phenomenon changes the local biology around the sensor, this can result in the sensor measuring phenomena associated with the reaction that it has produced as opposed to phenomena characteristic of the biologic system being studied.

Biologic systems can also affect sensor performance. This is especially true for indwelling and implanted sensors. Biologic tissue represents a hostile environment which can degrade sensor performance. In addition to many corrosive ions, body fluids contain enzymes that break down complex molecules as a part of the body's effort to rid itself of foreign and toxic materials. These can attack the materials that make up the sensor and its package, causing the sensor to lose calibration or fail.

Sensor packaging is an especially important problem. The package must not only protect the sensor from the corrosive environment of the body, but it must allow that portion of the sensor that performs the actual measurement to communicate with the biologic system. Furthermore, because it is frequently desirable to have sensors be as small as possible, especially those that are implanted and indwelling, it is important that the packaging function be carried out without significantly increasing the size of the sensor structure. Although there have been many improvements in sensor packaging, this remains a major problem in biomedical sensor research. High-quality packaging materials that do not elicit major foreign body responses from the biologic system are still being sought.

Another problem that is associated with implanted sensors is that once they are implanted, access to them is very limited. This requires that these sensors be highly reliable so that there is no need to repair or replace them. It is also important that these sensors be highly stable, since in most applications it is not possible to calibrate the sensor *in vivo*. Thus, sensors must maintain their calibration once they are implanted, and for applications such as organ replacement, this can represent a potentially long time, the remainder of the patient's life.

In the following sections we will look at some of the sensors described above in more detail. We will consider physical sensors with special sections on biopotential electrodes and optical sensors. We will also look at chemical sensors, including bioanalytic sensing systems. Although it is not possible to cover the field in extensive detail in a handbook such as this, it is hoped that these sections can serve as an introduction to this important aspect of biomedical engineering and instrumentation.

49

Physical Measurements

Michael R. Neuman
Case Western Reserve
University

Physical variables associated with biomedical systems are measured by a group of sensors known as physical sensors. Although many specific physical variables can be measured in biomedical systems, these can be categorized into a simple list as shown in Table 49.1. Sensors for these variables, whether they are measuring biomedical systems or other systems, are essentially the same. Thus, sensors of linear displacement can frequently be used equally well for measuring the displacement of the heart muscle during the cardiac cycle or the movement of a robot arm. There is, however, one notable exception regarding the similarity of these sensors: the packaging of the sensor and attachment to the system being measured. Although physical sensors used in nonbiomedical applications need to be packaged so as to be protected from their environment, few of these sensors have to deal with the harsh environment of biologic tissue, especially with the mechanisms inherent in this tissue for trying to eliminate the sensor as a foreign body. Another notable exception to the similarity of sensors for measuring physical quantities in biologic and nonbiologic systems are the sensors used for fluidic measurements such as pressure and flow. Special needs for these measurements in biologic systems have resulted in special sensors and instrumentation systems for these measurements that can be quite different from systems for measuring pressure and flow in nonbiologic environments.

In this chapter we will attempt to review various examples of sensors used for physical measurements in biologic systems. Although it would be beyond the scope of this chapter to cover all these in detail, the principal sensors applied for biologic measurements will be described. Each section will include a brief description of the principle of operation of the sensor and the underlying physical principles, examples of some of the more common forms of these sensors for application in biologic systems, methods of signal processing for these sensors where appropriate, and important considerations for when the sensor is applied.

49.1 Description of Sensors

Linear and Angular Displacement Sensors

A comparison of various characteristics of displacement sensors described in detail below is outlined in Table 49.2.

0-8493-8346-3/95/$0.00+$.50
© 1995 by CRC Press, Inc.

TABLE 49.1 Physical Variables and Sensors

Physical Quantity	Sensor	Variable Sensed
Geometric	Strain gauge	Strain
	LVDT	Displacement
	Ultrasonic transit time	Displacement
Kinematic	Velocimeter	Velocity
	Accelerometer	Acceleration
Force-Torque	Load cell	Applied force or torque
Fluidic	Pressure transducer	Pressure
	Flow meter	Flow
Thermal	Thermometer	Temperature
	Thermal flux sensor	Heat flux

Variable Resistance Sensor

One of the simplest sensors for measuring displacement is a variable resistor similar to the volume control on an audio electronic device [1]. The resistance between two terminals on this device is related to the linear or angular displacement of a sliding tap along a resistance element. Precision devices are available that have a reproducible, linear relationship between resistance and displacement. These devices can be connected in circuits that measure resistance such as an ohmmeter or bridge, or they can be used as a part of a circuit that provides a voltage that is proportional to the displacement. Such circuits include the voltage divider (as illustrated in Fig. 49.1a) or driving a known constant current through the resistance and measuring the resulting voltage across it. This sensor is simple and inexpensive and can be used for measuring relatively large displacements.

Strain Gauge

Another displacement sensor based on an electrical resistance change is the strain gauge [2]. If a long narrow electrical conductor such as a piece of metal foil or a fine gauge wire is stretched within its elastic limit, it will increase in length and decrease in cross-sectional area. Because the electric resistance between both ends of this foil or wire can be given by

$$R = \rho \frac{l}{A} \tag{49.1}$$

TABLE 49.2 Comparison of Displacement Sensors

Sensor	Electrical Variable	Measurement Circuit	Sensitivity	Precision	Range
Variable resistor	Resistance	Voltage divider, ohmmeter, bridge, current source	High	Moderate	Large
Foil strain gauge	Resistance	Bridge	Low	Moderate	Small
Liquid metal strain gauge	Resistance	Ohmmeter, bridge	Moderate	Moderate	Large
Silicon strain gauge	Resistance	Bridge	High	Moderate	Small
Mutual inductance coils	Inductance	Impedance bridge, inductance meter	Moderate to high	Moderate to Low	Moderate to large
Variable reluctance	Inductance	Impedance bridge, inductance meter	High	Moderate	Large
LVDT	Inductance	Voltmeter	High	High	High
Parallel plate capacitor	Capacitance	Impedance bridge, capacitance meter	Moderate to high	Moderate	Moderate to large
Sonic/ultrasonic	Time	Timer circuit	High	High	Large

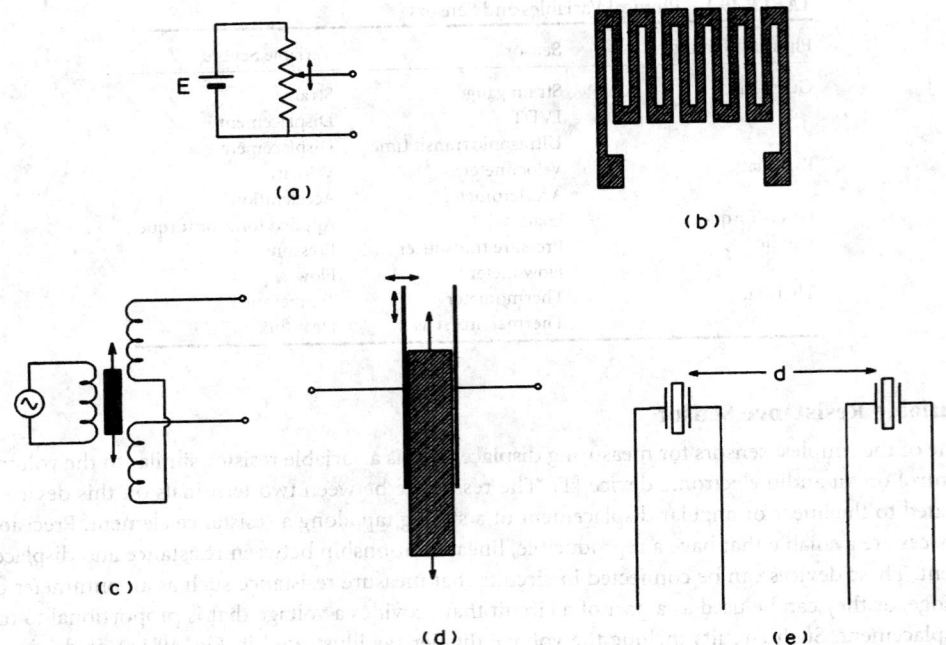

FIGURE 49.1   Examples of displacement sensors: (*a*) variable resistance sensor, (*b*) foil strain gauge, (*c*) linear variable differential transformer (LVDT), (*d*) parallel plate capacitive sensor, and (*e*) ultrasonic transit time displacement sensor.

where ρ is the electrical resistivity of the foil or wire material, *l* is its length, and *A* is its cross-sectional area, this stretching will result in an increase in resistance. The change in length can only be very small for the foil to remain within its elastic limit, so the change in electric resistance will also be small. The relative sensitivity of this device is given by its gauge factor, γ, which is defined as

$$\gamma = \frac{\Delta R/R}{\Delta l/l} \tag{49.2}$$

where ΔR is the change in resistance when the structure is stretched by an amount Δl. Foil strain gauges are the most frequently applied and consist of a structure such as shown in Fig. 49.1*b*. A piece of metal foil that is attached to an insulating polymeric film such as polyimide that has a much greater compliance than the foil itself is chemically etched into the pattern shown in Fig. 49.1*b*. When a strain is applied in the sensitive direction, the direction of the individual elements of the strain gauge, the length of the gauge will be slightly increased, and this will result in an increase in the electrical resistance seen between the terminals. Since the displacement or strain that this structure can measure is quite small for it to remain within its elastic limit, it can only be used to measure small displacements such as occur as loads are applied to structural beams. If one wants to increase the range of a foil strain gauge, one has to attach it to some sort of a mechanical impedance converter such as a cantilever beam. If the strain gauge is attached to one surface of the beam as shown in Fig. 49.2, a fairly large displacement at the unsupported end of the beam can be translated to a relatively small displacement on the beam's surface. It would be possible for this structure to be used to measure larger displacements at the cantilever beam tip using a strain gauge on the beam.

Because the electric resistance changes for a strain gauge are quite small, the measurement of this resistance change can be challenging. Generally, Wheatstone bridge circuits are used. It is important to note, however, that changes in temperature can also result in electric resistance changes that are

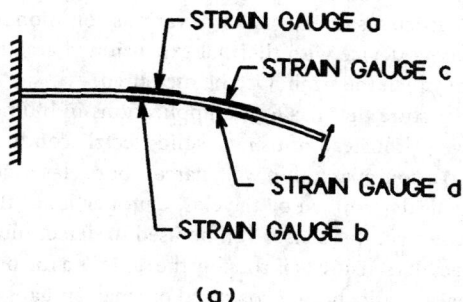

(a)

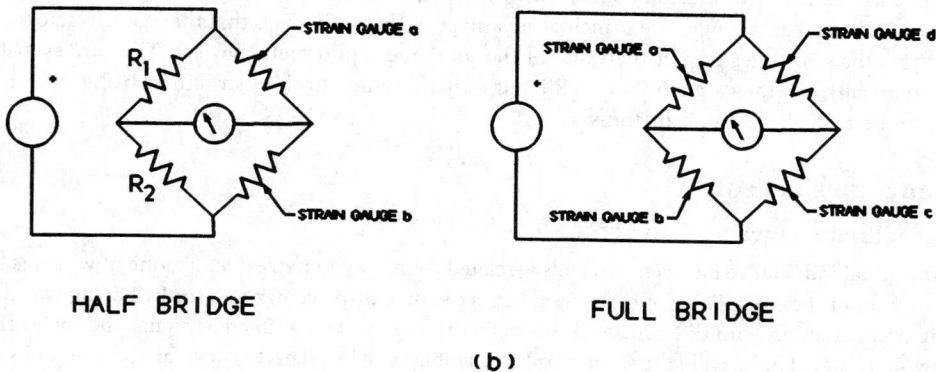

HALF BRIDGE   FULL BRIDGE

(b)

FIGURE 49.2 Strain gauges on a cantilever structure to provide temperature compensation: (*a*) cross-sectional view of the cantilever and (*b*) placement of the strain gauges in a half bridge or full bridge for temperature compensation and enhanced sensitivity.

of the same order of magnitude or even larger than the electric resistance changes due to the strain. Thus, it is important to temperature-compensate strain gauges in most applications. A simple method of temperature compensation is to use a double or quadruple strain gauge and a bridge circuit for measuring the resistance change. This is illustrated in Fig. 49.2. If one can use the strain gauge in an application such as the cantilever beam application described above, one can place one or two of the strain gauge structures on the concave side of the beam and the other one or two on the convex side of the beam. Thus, as the beam deflects, the strain gauge on the convex side will experience tension, and that on the concave side will experience compression. By putting these gauges in adjacent arms of the Wheatstone bridge, their effects can double the sensitivity of the circuit in the case of the double strain gauge and quadruple it in the case where the entire bridge is made up of strain gauges on a cantilever.

In some applications it is not possible to place strain gauges so that one gauge is undergoing tension while the other is undergoing compression. In this case, the second strain gauge used for temperature compensation can be oriented such that its sensitive axis is in a direction where strain is minimal. Thus, it is still possible to have the temperature compensation by having two identical strain gauges at the same temperature in adjacent arms of the bridge circuit, but the sensitivity improvement described in the previous paragraph is not seen.

Another constraint imposed by temperature is that the material to which the strain gauge is attached and the strain gauge both have temperature coefficients of expansion. Thus, even if a gauge is attached to a structure under conditions of no strain, if the temperature is changed the strain gauge could experience some strain due to the different expansion that it will have compared to the structure to which it is attached. To avoid this problem, strain gauges have been developed that have identical temperature coefficients of expansion to various common materials. In selecting a strain gauge, one should choose a device with thermal expansion characteristics as close as possible to those of the object upon which the strain is to be measured.

A more compliant structure that has found applications in biomedical instrumentation is the liquid metal strain gauge [3]. Instead of using a solid electric conductor such as the wire or metal foil, mercury confined to a compliant, thin wall, narrow bore elastomeric tube is used. The compliance of this strain gauge is determined by the elastic properties of the tube. Since only the elastic limit of the tube is of concern, this sensor can be used to detect much larger displacements than conventional strain gauges. Its sensitivity is roughly the same as a foil or wire strain gauge, but it is not as reliable. The mercury can easily become oxidized or small air gaps can occur in the mercury column. These effects make the sensor's characteristics noisy and sometimes results in complete failure.

Another variation on the strain gauge is the semiconductor strain gauge. These devices are frequently made out of pieces of silicon with strain gauge patterns formed using semiconductor microelectronic technology. The principal advantage of these devices is that their gauge factors can be more than 50 times greater than that of the solid and liquid metal devices. They are available commercially, but they are a bit more difficult to handle and attach to structures being measured due to their small size and brittleness.

Inductance Sensors

Mutual Inductance

The mutual inductance between two coils is related to many geometric factors, one of which is the separation of the coils. Thus, one can create a very simple displacement sensor by having two coils that are coaxial but with different separation. By driving one coil with an ac signal and measuring the voltage signal induced in the second coil, this voltage will be related to how far apart the coils are from one another. When the coils are close together, the mutual inductance will be high, and so a higher voltage will be induced in the second coil; when the coils are more widely separated, the mutual inductance will be lower as will the induced voltage. The relationship between voltage and separation will be determined by specific geometry of the coils and in general will not be a linear relationship with separation unless the change of displacement is relatively small. Nevertheless, this is a simple method of measuring separation that works reasonably well provided the coils remain coaxial. If there is movement of the coils transverse to their axes, it is difficult to separate transverse displacement from displacement along the axis.

Variable Reluctance

A variation on this sensor is the variable reluctance sensor wherein a single coil or two coils remain fixed on a form which allows a high reluctance slug to move into or out of the coil or coils along their axis. Since the position of this core material determines the number of flux linkages through the coil or coils, this can affect the self-inductance or mutual inductance of the coils. In the case of the mutual inductance, this can be measured using the technique described in the previous paragraph, whereas self-inductance changes can be measured using various instrumentation circuits used for measuring inductance. This method is also a simple method for measuring displacements, but the characteristics are generally nonlinear, and the sensor generally has only moderate precision.

Linear Variable Differential Transformer

By far the most frequently applied displacement transducer based upon inductance is the linear variable differential transformer (LVDT) [4]. This device is illustrated in Fig. 49.1c and is essentially a three-coil variable reluctance transducer. The two secondary coils are situated symmetrically about the primary coil and connected such that the induced voltages in each secondary oppose each other. When the core is located in the center of the structure equidistant from each secondary coil, the voltage induced in each secondary will be the same. Since these voltages oppose one another, the output voltage from the device will be zero. As the core is moved closer to one or the other secondary coils, the voltages in each coil will no longer be equal, and there will be an output voltage proportional to the displacement of the core from the central, zero-voltage position. Because of the symmetry of the structure, this voltage is linearly related to the core displacement. When the core passes through the central, zero point, the phase of the output voltage from the sensor changes by 180 degrees. Thus, by measuring the phase angle as well as the voltage, one can determine the position of the core. The circuit associated with the LVDT not only measures the voltage but often measures the phase angle as well.

LVDTs are available commercially in many sizes and shapes. Depending on the configuration of the coils, they can measure displacements ranging from tens of micrometers through centimeters.

Capacitive Sensors

Displacement sensors can be based upon measurements of capacitance as well as inductance. The fundamental principle of operation is the capacitance of a parallel plate capacitor as given by

$$c = \epsilon \frac{A}{d} \tag{49.3}$$

where ϵ is the dielectric constant of the medium between the plates, d is the separation between the plates, and A is the cross-sectional area of the plates. Each of the quantities in Eq. (49.3) can be varied to form a displacement transducer as shown in Fig. 49.1c. By moving one of the plates with respect to the other, Eq. (49.3) shows us that the capacitance will vary inversely with respect to the plate separation. This will give a hyperbolic capacitance-displacement characteristic. However, if the plate separation is maintained at a constant value and the plates are displaced laterally with respect to one another so that the area of overlap changes, this can produce a capacitance-displacement characteristic that can be linear, depending on the shape of the actual plates.

The third way that a variable capacitance transducer can measure displacement is by having a fixed parallel plate capacitor with a slab of dielectric material having a dielectric constant different from that of air that can slide between the plates. The effective dielectric constant for the capacitor will depend on how much of the slab is between the plates and how much of the region between the plates is occupied only by air. This, also, can yield a transducer with linear characteristics.

The electronic circuitry used with variable capacitance transducers is essentially the same as any other circuitry used to measure capacitance. As with the inductance transducers, this circuit can take the form of a bridge circuit or specific circuits that measure capacitive reactance.

Sonic and Ultrasonic Sensors

If the velocity of sound in a medium is constant, the time it takes a short burst of that sound energy to propagate from a source to a receiver will be proportional to the displacement between the two transducers. This is given by

$$d = cT \tag{49.4}$$

where c is the velocity of sound in the medium, T is the transit time, and d is the displacement. A simple system for making such a measurement is shown in Fig. 49.1e [5]. A brief sonic or ultrasonic pulse is generated at the transmitting transducer and propagates through the medium. It is detected by the receiving transducer at time T after the burst was initiated. The displacement can then be determined by applying Eq. (49.4).

In practice, this method is best used with ultrasound, since the wavelength is shorter, and the device will neither produce annoying sounds nor respond to extraneous sounds in the environment. Small piezoelectric transducers to generate and receive ultrasonic pulses are readily available. The electronic circuit used with this instrument carries out three functions: (1) generation of the sonic or ultrasonic burst, (2) detection of the received burst, and (3) measurement of the time of propagation of the ultrasound. An advantage of this system is that the two transducers are coupled to one another only sonically. There is no physical connection as was the case for the other sensors described in this section.

Velocity Measurement

Velocity is the time derivative of displacement, and so all the displacement transducers mentioned above can be used to measure velocity if their signals are processed by passing them through a differentiator circuit. There are, however, two additional methods that can be applied to measure velocity directly.

Magnetic Induction

If a magnetic field that passes through a conducting coil varies with time, a voltage is induced in that coil that is proportional to the time-varying magnetic field. This relationship is given by

$$v = N \frac{d\phi}{dt} \tag{49.5}$$

where v is the voltage induced in the coil, N is the number of turns in the coil, and ϕ is the total magnetic flux passing through the coil (the product of flux density and area within the coil). Thus a simple way to apply this principle is to attach a small permanent magnet to an object whose velocity is to be determined, and attach a coil to a nearby structure that will serve as the reference against which the velocity is to be measured. A voltage will be induced in this coil whenever the structure containing the permanent magnet moves, and this voltage will be related to the velocity of that movement. The exact relationship will be determined by the field distribution for the particular magnet and the orientation of the magnet with respect to the coil.

Doppler Ultrasound

When the receiver of a signal in the form of a wave such as electromagnetic radiation or sound is moving at a nonzero velocity with respect to the emitter of that wave, the frequency of the wave perceived by the receiver will be different than the frequency of the transmitter. This frequency difference, known as the Doppler shift, is determined by the relative velocity of the receiver with respect to the emitter and is given by

$$f_d = \frac{f_o u}{c} \tag{49.6}$$

where f_d is the Doppler frequency shift, f_o is the frequency of the transmitted wave, u is the relative velocity between the transmitter and receiver, and c is the velocity of sound in the medium. This principle can be applied in biomedical applications as a Doppler velocimeter. A piezoelectric transducer can be used as the ultrasound source with a similar transducer as the receiver. When there is no relative movement between the two transducers, the frequency of the signal at the receiver will be the same as that at the emitter, but when there is relative motion, the frequency at the receiver will be shifted according to Eq. (49.6).

The ultrasonic velocimeter can be applied in the same way that the ultrasonic displacement sensor is used. In this case the electronic circuit produces a continuous ultrasonic wave and, instead of detecting the transit time of the signal, now detects the frequency difference between the transmitted and received signals. This frequency difference can then be converted into a signal proportional to the relative velocity between the two transducers.

Accelerometers

Acceleration is the time derivative of velocity and the second derivative with respect to time of displacement. Thus, sensors of displacement and velocity can be used to determine acceleration when their signals are appropriately processed through differentiator circuits. In addition, there are direct sensors of acceleration based upon Newton's second law and Hook's law. The fundamental structure of an accelerometer is shown in Fig. 49.3. A known seismic mass is attached to the housing by an elastic element. As the structure is accelerated in the sensitive direction of the elastic element, a force is applied to that element according to Newton's second law. This force causes the elastic element to be distorted according to Hook's law, which results in a displacement of the mass with respect to the accelerometer housing. This displacement is measured by a displacement sensor. The relationship between the displacement and the acceleration is found by combining Newton's second law and Hook's law

$$a = \frac{k}{m} x \qquad (49.7)$$

where x is the measured displacement, m is the known mass, k is the spring constant of the elastic element, and a is the acceleration. Any of the displacement sensors described above can be used in an accelerometer. The most frequently used displacement sensors are strain gauges or the LVDT. One type of accelerometer uses a piezoelectric sensor as both the displacement sensor and the elastic element. A piezoelectric sensor generates an electric signal that is related to the dynamic change in shape of the piezoelectric material as the force is applied. Thus, piezoelectric materials can only directly measure time varying forces. A piezoelectric accelerometer is, therefore, better for measuring changes in acceleration than for measuring constant accelerations. A principal advantage of piezoelectric accelerometers is that they can be made very small, which is useful in many biomedical applications.

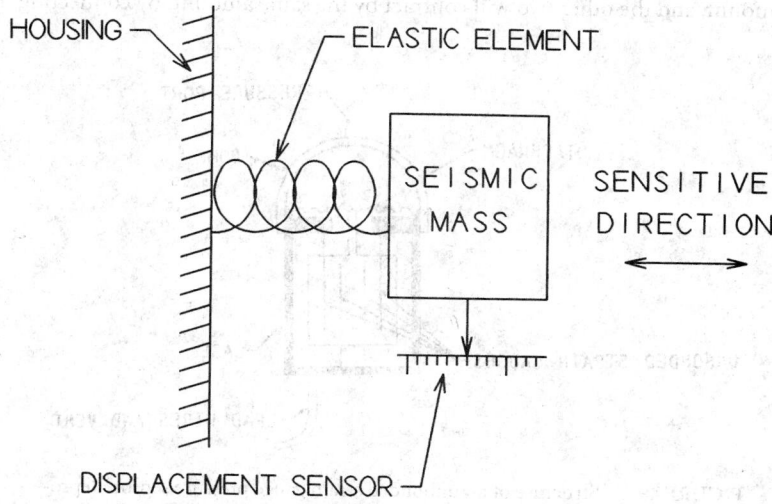

FIGURE 49.3 Fundamental structure of an accelerometer.

Force

Force is measured by converting the force to a displacement and measuring the displacement with a displacement sensor. The conversion takes place as a result of the elastic properties of a material. Applying a force to the material distorts the material's shape, and this distortion can be determined by a displacement sensor. For example, the cantilever structure shown in Fig. 49.2a could be a force sensor. Applying a vertical force at the tip of the beam will cause the beam to deflect according to its elastic properties. This deflection can be detected using a displacement sensor such as a strain gauge as described previously.

A common form of force sensor is the load cell. This consists of a block of material with known elastic properties that has strain gauges attached to it. Applying a force to the load cell stresses the material, resulting in a strain that can be measured by the strain gauge. Applying Hook's law, one finds that the strain is proportional to the applied force. The strain gauges on a load cell are usually in a half-bridge or full-bridge configuration to minimize the temperature sensitivity of the device. Load cells come in various sizes and configurations, and they can measure a wide range of forces.

Measurement of Fluid Dynamic Variables

The measurement of the fluid variables of pressure and flow in both liquids and gases is important in many biomedical applications. These two variables, however, often are the most difficult variables to measure in biologic applications because of interactions with the biologic system and stability problems. Some of the most frequently applied sensors for these measurements are described in the following paragraphs.

Pressure Measurement

Sensors of pressure for biomedical measurements such as blood pressure [7] consist of a structure such as shown in Fig. 49.4. In this case a fluid coupled to the fluid to be measured is housed in a chamber with a flexible diaphragm making up a portion of the wall, with the other side of the diaphragm at atmospheric pressure. When a pressure exists across the diaphragm, it will cause the diaphragm to deflect. This deflection is then measured by a displacement sensor. In the example in Fig. 49.4, the displacement transducer consists of four fine-gauge wires drawn between a structure attached to the diaphragm and the housing of the sensor so that these wires serve as strain gauges. When pressure causes the diaphragm to deflect, two of the fine-wire strain gauges will be extended by a small amount, and the other two will contract by the same amount. By connecting these wires

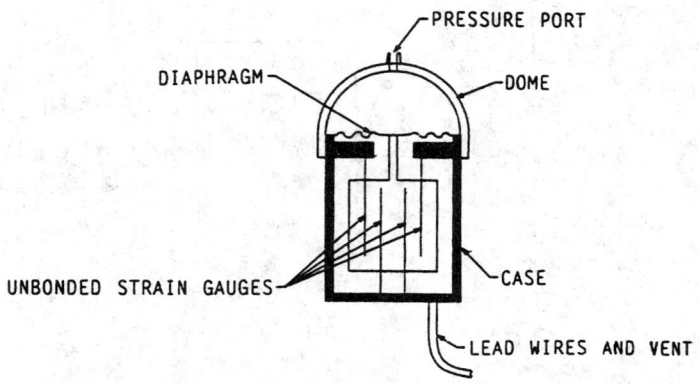

FIGURE 49.4 Structure of an unbonded strain gauge pressure sensor. Reproduced with permission from Neuman MR. 1993. Biomedical sensors. In RC Dorf (ed), The Electrical Engineering Handbook, Boca Raton, Fla, CRC Press.

into a bridge circuit, a voltage proportional to the deflection of the diaphragm and hence the pressure can be obtained.

Semiconductor technology has been applied to the design of pressure transducers such that the entire structure can be fabricated from silicon. A portion of a silicon chip can be formed into a diaphragm and semiconductor strain gauges incorporated directly into that diaphragm to produce a small, inexpensive, and sensitive pressure sensor. Such sensors can be used as disposable, single-use devices for measuring blood pressure without the need for sterilization before being used on the next patient. This minimizes the risk of transmitting blood-borne infections in cases where the transducer is coupled directly to the patient's blood for direct blood pressure measurement.

In using this type of sensor to measure blood pressure, it is necessary to couple the chamber containing the diaphragm to the blood or other fluids being measured. This is usually done using a small, flexible plastic tube, known as a catheter, that can have one end placed in an artery of the subject while the other is connected to the pressure sensor. This catheter is filled with a physiologic saline solution so that the arterial blood pressure is coupled to the diaphragm. This external direct blood-pressure-measurement method is used quite frequently in the clinic and research laboratory, but it has the limitation that the properties of the fluid in the catheter and the catheter itself can affect the measurement. For example, both ends of the catheter must be at the same vertical level to avoid a pressure offset due to hydrostatic effects. Also, the compliance of the tube will affect the frequency response of the pressure measurement. Air bubbles in the catheter or obstructions due to clotted blood or other materials can introduce distortion of the waveform due to resonance and damping. These problems can be minimized by utilizing a miniature semiconductor pressure transducer that is located at the tip of a catheter and can be placed in the blood vessel rather than being positioned external to the body. Such internal pressure sensors are available commercially and have the advantages of a much broader frequency response, no hydrostatic pressure error, and generally clearer signals than the external system.

Although it is possible to measure blood pressure using the techniques described above, this remains one of the major problems in biomedical sensor technology. Long-term stability of pressure transducers is not very good. This is especially true for pressure measurements of venous blood, cerebrospinal fluid, or fluids in the gastrointestinal tract, where pressures are relatively low. Long-term changes in baseline pressure for most pressure sensors require that they be frequently adjusted to be certain of zero pressure. Although this can be done relatively easily when the pressure transducer is located external to the body, this can be a major problem for indwelling pressure transducers. Thus, these transducers must be extremely stable and have low baseline drift to be useful in long-term applications. The packaging of the pressure transducer is also a problem that needs to be addressed, especially when the transducer is in contact with blood for long periods. Not only must the package be biocompatible, but it also must allow the appropriate pressure to be transmitted from the biologic fluid to the diaphragm. Thus, a material that is mechanically stable under corrosive and aqueous environments in the body is needed.

Measurement of Flow

The measurement of true volummetric flow in the body represents one of the most difficult problems in biomedical sensing [8]. The sensors that have been developed measure velocity rather than volume, and they can only be used to measure flow if the velocity is measured for a tube of known cross-section. Thus, most flow sensors constrain the vessel to have a specific cross-sectional area.

The most frequently used flow sensor in biomedical systems is the electromagnetic flow meter illustrated in Fig. 49.5. This device consists of a means of generating a magnetic field transverse to the flow vector in a vessel. A pair of very small biopotential electrodes are attached to the wall of the vessel such that the vessel diameter between them is at right angles to the direction of the magnetic field. As the blood flows in the structure, ions in the blood deflect in the direction of one or the other electrodes due to the magnetic field, and the voltage across the electrodes is given by

$$v = Blu \tag{49.8}$$

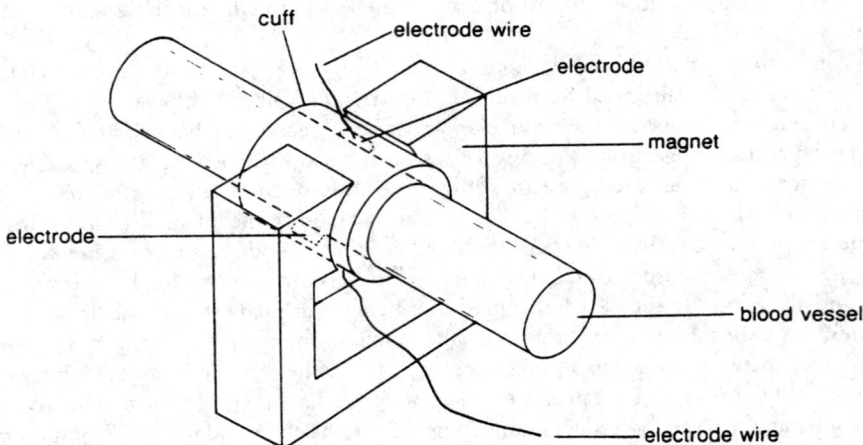

FIGURE 49.5 Fundamental structure of an electromagnetic flowmeter. Reproduced with permission from Neuman MR. 1986. Biosensors: Transducers, electrodes, and physiologic systems. In JD Bronzino (ed), Biomedical Engineering and Instrumentation: Basic Concepts and Applications, Boston, PWS Publishers.

where B is the magnetic field, l is the distance between the electrodes, and u is the average instantaneous velocity of the fluid across the vessel. If the sensor constrains the blood vessel to have a specific diameter, then its cross-sectional area will be known, and multiplying this area by the velocity will give the volume flow.

Although dc flow sensors have been developed and are available commercially, the most desirable method is to use ac excitation of the magnetic field so that offset potential effects from the biopotential electrodes do not generate errors in this measurement.

Small ultrasonic transducers can also be attached to a blood vessel to measure flow as illustrated in Fig. 49.6. In this case the transducers are oriented such that one transmits a continuous ultrasound signal that illuminates the blood. Cells within the blood reflect this signal in the direction of the second sensor so that the received signal undergoes a Doppler shift in frequency that is proportional to the velocity of the blood. By measuring the frequency shift and knowing the cross-sectional area of the vessel, it is possible to determine the flow.

Another method of measuring flow that has had biomedical application is the measurement of cooling of a heated object by convection. The object is usually a thermistor (see section on temperature measurement, below) placed either in a blood vessel or in tissue, and the thermistor serves as both the heating element and the temperature sensor. In one mode of operation, the amount of power required to maintain the thermistor at a temperature slightly above that of the blood upstream is measured. As the flow around the thermistor increases, more heat is removed from the thermistor by convection, and so more power is required to keep it at a constant temperature. Relative flow is then measured by determining the amount of power supplied to the thermistor.

In a second approach the thermistor is heated by applying a current pulse and then measuring the cooling curve of the thermistor as the blood flows across it. The thermistor will cool more quickly as the blood flow increases. Both these methods are relatively simple to achieve electronically, but both also have severe limitations. They are essentially qualitative measures and strongly depend on how the thermistor probe is positioned in the vessel being measured. If the probe is closer to the periphery or even in contact with the vessel wall, the measured flow will be different than if the sensor is in the center of the vessel.

Temperature

There are many different sensors of temperature [9], but three find particularly wide application to biomedical problems. Table 49.3 summarizes the properties of various temperature sensors, and

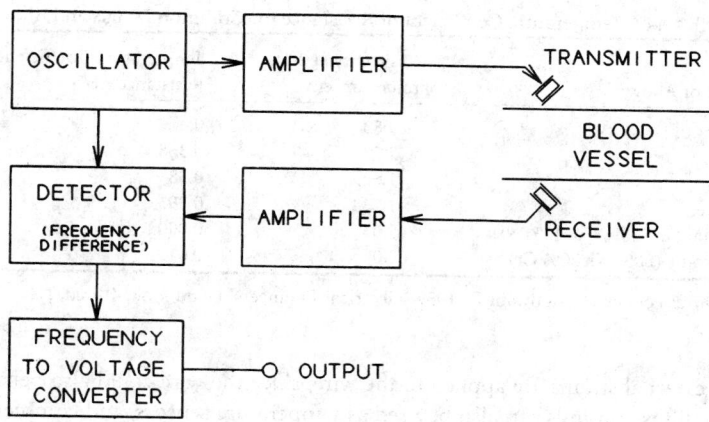

FIGURE 49.6 Structure of an ultrasonic Doppler flowmeter with the major blocks of the electronic signal processing system. The oscillator generates a signal that, after amplification, drives the transmitting transducer. The oscillator frequency is usually in the range of 1–10 MHz. The reflected ultrasound from the blood is sensed by the receiving transducer and amplified before being processed by a detector circuit. This block generates the frequency difference between the transmitted and received ultrasonic signals. This difference frequency can be converted into a voltage proportional to frequency, and hence flow velocity, by the frequency to voltage converter circuit.

these three, including metallic resistance thermometers, thermistors, and thermocouples, are described in the following paragraphs.

Metallic Resistance Thermometers

The electric resistance of a piece of metal or wire generally increases as the temperature of that electric conductor increases. A linear approximation to this relationship is given by

$$R = R_0[1 + \alpha(T - T_0)] \tag{49.9}$$

where R_0 is the resistance at temperature T_0, α is the temperature coefficient of resistance, and T is the temperature at which the resistance is being measured. Most metals have temperature coefficients of resistance of the order of 0.1–0.4%/°C, as indicated in Table 49.4. The noble metals are preferred for resistance thermometers, since they do not corrode easily and, when drawn into fine wires, their cross-section will remain constant, thus avoiding drift in the resistance over time which could result in an unstable sensor. It is also seen from Table 49.4 that the noble metals of gold and platinum have some of the highest temperature coefficients of resistance of the common metals.

Metal resistance thermometers are often fabricated from fine-gauge insulated wire that is wound into a small coil. It is important in doing so to make certain that there are not other sources of resistance change that could affect the sensor. For example, the structure should be utilized in such

TABLE 49.3 Properties of Temperature Sensors

Sensor	Form	Sensitivity	Stability	Range
Metal resistance thermometer	Coil of fine platinum wire	Low	High	−100–700°C
Thermistor	Bead, disk, or rod	High	Moderate	−50–100°C
Thermocouple	Pair of wires	Low	High	−100–>1000°C
Mercury in glass thermometer	Column of Hg in glass capillary	Moderate	High	−50–400°C
Silicon p-n diode	Electronic component	Moderate	High	−50–150°C

TABLE 49.4 Temperature Coefficient of Resistance for Common Metals and Alloys

Metal or Alloy	Resistivity at 20°C, microhm-cm	Temperature Coefficient of Resistance, %/°C
Platinum	9.83	0.3
Gold	2.22	0.368
Silver	1.629	0.38
Copper	1.724	0.393
Constantan (60% Cu, 40% Ni)	49.0	0.0002
Nichrome (80% Ni, 20% Cr)	108.0	0.013

Source: Pender H, McIlwain K. 1957. Electrical Engineers' Handbook, 4th ed, New York, Wiley.

a way that no external strains are applied to the wire, since the wire could also behave as a strain gauge. Metallic films and foils can also be used as temperature sensors, and commercial products are available in the wire, foil, or film forms. The electric circuits used to measure resistance, and hence the temperature, are similar to those used with the wire or foil strain gauges. A bridge circuit is the most desirable, although ohmmeter circuits can also be used. It is important to make sure that the electronic circuit does not pass a large current through the resistance thermometer to provide self-heating due to the Joule conversion of electric energy to heat.

Thermistors

Unlike metals, semiconductor materials have an inverse relationship between resistance and temperature. This characteristic is very nonlinear and cannot be characterized by a linear equation such as for the metals. The thermistor is a semiconductor temperature sensor. Its resistance as a function of temperature is given by

$$R = R_0 e^{\beta \left[\frac{1}{T} - \frac{1}{T_0} \right]} \tag{49.10}$$

where β is a constant determined by the materials that make up the thermistor. Thermistors can take a variety of forms and cover a large range of resistances. The most common forms used in biomedical applications are the bead, disk, or rod forms of the sensor as illustrated in Fig. 49.7. These structures can be formed from a variety of different semiconductors ranging from elements such as silicon and germanium to mixtures of various semiconducting metallic oxides. Most commercially available thermistors are manufactured from the latter materials, and the specific materials as well as the processes for fabricating them are closely held industrial secrets. These materials are chosen not only to have high sensitivity but also to have the greatest stability, since thermistors are generally not as stable as the metallic resistance thermometers. However, thermistors are close to an order of magnitude more sensitive.

Thermocouples

When different regions of an electric conductor or semiconductor are at different temperatures, there is an electric potential between these regions that is directly related to the temperature difference. This phenomenon, known as the Seebeck effect, can be used to produce a temperature sensor known as a *thermocouple* by taking a wire of metal or alloy A and another wire of metal or alloy B and connecting them as shown in Fig. 49.8. One of the junctions is known as the sensing junction, and the other is the reference junction. When these junctions are at different temperatures, a voltage proportional to the temperature difference will be seen at the voltmeter when metals A and B have different Seebeck effects. This voltage is roughly proportional to the temperature difference and can be represented over the relatively small temperature differences encountered in biomedical applications by the linear equation

$$V = S_{AB} (T_s - T_r) \quad (49.11)$$

where S_{AB} is the Seebeck coefficient for the thermocouple made up of metals A and B. Although
this equation is a reasonable approximation,
more accurate data are usually found in tables of
actual voltages of the function of temperature
difference. In some applications the voltmeter is
located at the reference junction, and one uses
some independent means such as a mercury in
glass thermometer to measure the reference
junction temperature. Where precision measurements are made, the reference junction is
often placed in an environment of known temperatures such as an ice bath. Electronic measurement of reference junction temperature can
also be carried out and used to compensate for
the reference junction temperature so that the
voltmeter reads a signal equivalent to what
would be seen if the reference junction were at
0°C. This electronic reference junction compensation is usually carried out using a metal
resistance temperature sensor to determine
reference junction temperature.

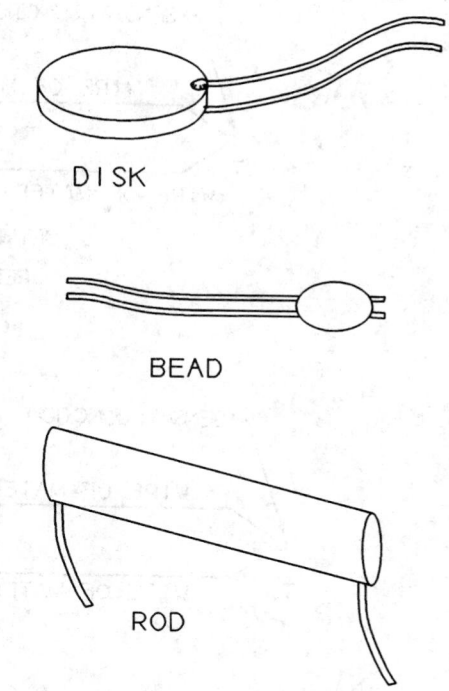

FIGURE 49.7   Common forms of thermistors.

The voltages generated by thermocouples
used for temperature measurement are generally quite small being on the order of tens of microvolts per degree C. Thus, for most biomedical measurements where there is only a small difference
in temperature between the sensing and reference junction, very sensitive amplifiers must be used
to measure these potentials. Thermocouples have been used in industry for temperature measurement for many years. Several standard alloys to provide optimal sensitivity and stability of these sensors have evolved. Table 49.5 lists these common alloys, the Seebeck coefficient for thermocouples
of these materials at room temperature, and the full range of temperatures over which these thermocouples can be used.

Thermocouples can be fabricated in many different ways depending on their applications. They
are especially suitable for measuring temperature differences between two structures, since the sensing junction can be placed on one while the other has the reference junction. Higher-output thermocouples or thermopiles can be produced by connecting several thermocouples in series.
Thermocouples can be made from very fine wires that can be implanted in biologic tissues for
temperature measurements, and it is also possible to place these fine-wire thermocouples within the
lumen of a hypodermic needle to make short-term temperature measurements in tissue.

49.2 Biomedical Applications of Physical Sensors

Just as it is not possible to cover the full range of physical sensors in this chapter, it is also impossible to consider the many biomedical applications that have been reported for these sensors. Instead,
some representative examples will be given. These are summarized in Table 49.6 and will be briefly
described in the following paragraphs.

Liquid metal strain gauges are especially useful in biomedical applications, because they are
mechanically compliant and provide a better impedance match to most biomedical tissues than
other types of strain gauges. By wrapping one of these strain gauges around a circumference of the

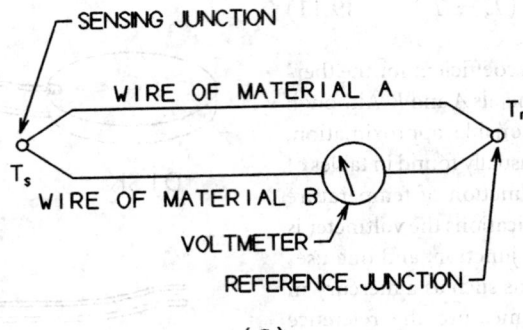

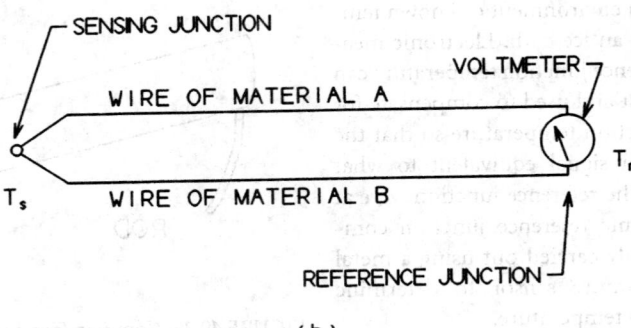

FIGURE 49.8 Circuit arrangement for a thermocouple showing the voltage-measuring device, the voltmeter, interrupting one of the thermocouple wires (*a*) and at the cold junction (*b*).

abdomen, it will stretch and contract with the abdominal breathing movements. The signal from the strain gauge can then be used to monitor breathing in patients or experimental animals. The advantage of this sensor is its compliance so that it does not interfere with the breathing movements or substantially increase the required breathing effort.

One of the original applications of the liquid metal strain gauge was in limb plethysmography [3]. One or more of these sensors are wrapped around an arm or leg at various points and can be used to measure changes in circumference that are related to the cross-sectional area and hence the volume of the limb at those points. If the venous drainage from the limb is occluded, the limb volume will increase as it fills with blood. Releasing the occlusion allows the volume to return to normal. The rate of this decrease in volume can be monitored using the liquid metal strain gauges, and this can be used to identify venous blockage when this return to baseline volume is too slow.

Breathing movements, although not volume, can be seen using a simple magnetic velocity detector. By placing a small permanent magnet on the anterior side of the chest or abdomen and a flat, large-area coil on the posterior side opposite from the magnet, voltages are induced in the coil as the

TABLE 49.5 Common Thermocouples

Type	Materials	Seebeck Coefficient, $\mu V/^\circ C$	Temperature Range
S	Platinum/platinum 10% rhodium	6	$0-1700^\circ C$
T	Copper/constantan	50	$-190-400^\circ C$
K	Chromel/alumel	41	$-200-1370^\circ C$
J	Iron/constantan	53	$-200-760^\circ C$
E	Chromel/constantan	78	$-200-970^\circ C$

TABLE 49.6 Examples of Biomedical Applications of Physical Sensors

Sensor	Application	Signal Range	Reference
Liquid metal strain gauge	Breathing movement	0–0.05	
	Limb plethysmography	0–0.02	3
Magnetic displacement sensor	Breathing movement	0–10 mm	10
LVDT	Muscle contraction	0–20 mm	
	Uterine contraction sensor	0–5 mm	11
Load cell	Electronic scale	0–440 lbs (0–200 kg)	12
Accelerometer	Subject activity	0–20 m/s^2	13
Miniature silicon pressure sensor	Intra-arterial blood pressure	0–50 Pa (0–350 mm Hg)	
	Urinary bladder pressure	0–10 Pa (0–70 mm Hg)	
	Intrauterine pressure	0–15 Pa (0–100 mm Hg)	14
Electromagnetic flow sensor	Cardiac output (with integrator)	0–500 ml/min	
	Organ blood flow	0–100 ml/min	15

chest of abdomen moves during breathing. The voltage itself can be used to detect the presence of breathing movements, or it can be electronically integrated to give a signal related to displacement.

The LVDT is a displacement sensor that can be used for more precise applications. For example, it can be used in studies of muscle physiology where one wants to measure the displacement of a muscle or where one is measuring the isometric force generated by the muscle (using a load cell) and must ensure that there is no muscle movement. It can also be incorporated into other physical sensors such as a pressure sensor or a tocodynamometer, a sensor used to electronically "feel" uterine contractions of patients in labor or those at risk of premature labor and delivery.

In addition to studying muscle forces, load cells can be used in various types of electronic scales for weighing patients or study animals. The simplest electronic scale consists of a platform placed on top of a load cell. The weight of any object placed on the platform will produce a force that can be sensed by the load cell. In some critical care situations in the hospital, it is important to carefully monitor the weight of a patient. For example, this is important in watching water balance in patients receiving fluid therapy. The electronic scale concept can be extended by placing a load cell under each leg of the patient's bed and summing the forces seen by each load cell to get the total weight of the patient and the bed. Since the bed weight remains fixed, weight changes seen will reflect changes in patient weight.

Accelerometers can be used to measure patient or research subject activity. By attaching a small accelerometer to the individual being studied, any movements can be detected. This can be useful in sleep studies where movement can help to determine the sleep state. Miniature accelerometers and recording devices can also be worn by patients to study activity patterns and determine effects of disease or treatments on patient activity [13].

Miniature silicon pressure sensors are used for the indwelling measurement of fluid pressure in most body cavities. The measurement of intra-arterial blood pressure is the most frequent application, but pressures in other cavities such as the urinary bladder and the uterus are also measured. The small size of these sensors and the resulting ease of introduction of the sensor into the cavity make these sensors important for these applications.

The electromagnetic flow sensor has been a standard method in use in the physiology laboratory for many years. Its primary application has been for measurement of cardiac output and blood flow to specific organs in research animals. New miniature inverted electromagnetic flow sensors make it possible to temporarily introduce a flow probe into an artery through its lumen to make clinical measurements.

The measurement of body temperature using instruments employing thermistors as the sensor has greatly increased in recent years. Rapid response times of these low-mass sensors make it possible to quickly assess patients' body temperatures so that more patients can be evaluated in a given period. This can then help to reduce health care costs. The rapid response time of low-mass thermistors makes them a simple sensor to be used for sensing breathing. By placing small thermistors near the nose and mouth, the elevated temperature of exhaled air can be sensed to document a breath.

The potential applications of physical sensors in medicine and biology are almost limitless. To be able to use these devices, however, scientists must first be familiar with the underlying sensing principles. It is then possible to apply these in a form that addresses the problems at hand.

References

1. Doebelin EO. 1990. Measurement Systems: Application and Design, New York, McGraw-Hill.
2. Dechow PC. 1988. Strain Gauges. In J Webster (ed), Encyclopedia of Medical Devices and Instrumentation, pp 2715–2721, New York, Wiley.
3. Whitney RJ. 1949. The measurement of changes in human limb-volume by means of a mercury-in-rubber strain gauge. J Physiol 109:5p.
4. Schaevitz H. 1947. The linear variable differential transformer. Proc Soc Stress Anal 4:79.
5. Stegall HF, Kardon MB, Stone HL, et al. 1967. A portable simple sonomicrometer. J Appl Physiol 23:289.
6. Angelsen BA, Brubakk AO. 1976. Transcutaneous measurement of blood flow velocity in the human aorta. Cardiovasc Res 10:368.
7. Geddes LA. 1970. The Direct and Indirect Measurement of Blood Pressure, Chicago, Year Book.
8. Roberts VC. 1972. Blood Flow Measurements, Baltimore, Williams & Wilkins.
9. Herzfeld CM (ed). 1962. Temperature: Its Measurement and Control in Science and Industry, New York, Reinhold.
10. Rolfe P. 1971. A magnetometer respiration monitor for use with premature babies. Biomed Eng 6:402.
11. Reddy NP, Kesavan SK. 1988. Linear variable differential transformers. In J Webster (ed), Encyclopedia of Medical Devices and Instrumentation, pp 1800–1806, New York, Wiley.
12. Roe FC. 1966. New equipment for metabolic studies. Nurs Clin N Am 1:621.
13. Patterson SM, Krantz DS, Montgomery LC, et al. 1993. Automated physical activity monitoring: Validation and comparison with physiological and self-report measures. Psychophysiology 30:296.
14. Fleming DG, Ko WH, Neuman MR (eds). 1977. Indwelling and Implantable Pressure Transducers, Cleveland, CRC Press.
15. Wyatt DG. 1971. Electromagnetic blood flow measurements. In BW Watson (ed), IEE Medical Electronics Monographs, London, Peregrinus.

Further Information

Good overviews of physical sensors are found in these books: Doebelin EO. 1990. Measurement Systems: Application and Design, 4th ed, New York, McGraw-Hill; Harvey, GF (ed). 1969. Transducer Compendium, 2d ed, New York, Plenum. One can also find good descriptions of physical sensors in chapters of two works edited by John Webster. Chapters 2, 7, and 8 of his textbook (1992) Medical Instrumentation: Application and Design, 2d ed, Boston, Houghton Mifflin, and several articles in his Encyclopedia on Medical Devices and Instrumentation, published by Wiley in 1988, cover topics on physical sensors.

Although a bit old, the text Transducers for Biomedical Measurements (New York, J. Wiley, 1974) by Richard S. C. Cobbold, remains one of the best descriptions of biomedical sensors available. By supplementing the material in this book with recent manufacturers' literature, the reader can obtain a wealth of information on physical (and for that matter chemical) sensors for biomedical application.

The journals *IEEE Transactions on Biomedical Engineering* and *Medical and Biological Engineering and Computing* are good sources of recent research on biomedical applications of physical sensors. The journal *Sensors and Actuators* is also a good source for this material.

50

Biopotential Electrodes

Michael R. Neuman
Case Western Reserve
University

Biologic systems frequently have electric activity associated with them. This activity can be a constant dc electric field, a constant flux of charge-carrying particles or current, or a time-varying electric field or current associated with some time-dependent biologic or biochemical phenomenon. Bioelectric phenomena are associated with the distribution of ions or charged molecules in a biologic structure and the changes in this distribution resulting from specific processes. These changes can occur as a result of biochemical reactions, or they can emanate from phenomena that alter local anatomy.

One can find bioelectric phenomena associated with just about every organ system in the body. Nevertheless, a large proportion of these signals are associated with phenomena that are at the present time not especially useful in clinical medicine and represent time-invariant, low-level signals that are not easily measured in practice. There are, however, several signals that are of diagnostic significance or that provide a means of electronic assessment to aid in understanding biologic systems. These signals, their usual abbreviations, and the systems they measure are listed in Table 50.1. Of these, the most familiar is the electrocardiogram, a signal derived from the electric activity of the heart. This signal is widely used in diagnosing disturbances in cardiac rhythm, signal conduction through the heart, and damage due to cardiac ischemia and infarction. The electromyogram is used for diagnosing neuromuscular diseases, and the electroencephalogram is important in identifying brain dysfunction and evaluating sleep. The other signals listed in Table 50.1 are currently of lesser diagnostic significance but are, nevertheless, used for studies of the associated organ systems.

Although Table 50.1 and the above discussion are concerned with bioelectric phenomena in animals and these techniques are used primarily in studying mammals, bioelectric signals also arise from plants [1]. These signals are generally steady-state or slowly changing, as opposed to the time-varying signals listed in Table 50.1. An extensive literature exists on the origins of bioelectric signals, and the interested reviewer is referred to the text by Plonsey and Barr for a general overview of this area [2].

50.1 Sensing Bioelectric Signals

The mechanism of electric conductivity in the body involves ions as charge carriers. Thus, picking up bioelectric signals involves interacting with these ionic charge carriers and transducing ionic cur-

TABLE 50.1 Bioelectric Signals Sensed by Biopotential Electrodes and Their Sources

Bioelectric Signal	Abbreviation	Biologic Source
Electrocardiogram	ECG	Heart—as seen from body surface
Cardiac electrogram	—	Heart—as seen from within
Electromyogram	EMG	Muscle
Electroencephalogram	EEG	Brain
Electrooptigram	EOG	Eye dipole field
Electroretinogram	ERG	Eye retina
Action potential	—	Nerve or muscle
Electrogastrogram	EGG	Stomach
Galvanic skin reflex	GSR	Skin

rents into electric currents required by wires and electronic instrumentation. This transducing function is carried out by electrodes that consist of electrical conductors in contact with the aqueous ionic solutions of the body. The interaction between electrons in the electrodes and ions in the body can greatly affect the performance of these sensors and requires that specific considerations be made in their application.

At the interface between an electrode and an ionic solution redox (oxidation-reduction), reactions need to occur for charge to be transferred between the electrode and the solution. These reactions can be represented in general by the following equations:

$$C \rightleftharpoons C^{n+} + ne^-$$ (50.1)

$$A^{m-} \rightleftharpoons A + me^-$$ (50.2)

where n is the valence of cation material C, and m is the valence of anion material A. For most electrode systems, the cations in solution and the metal of the electrodes are the same, so the atoms C are oxidized when they give up electrons and go into solution as positively charged ions. These ions are reduced when the process occurs in the reverse direction. In the case of the anion reaction, Eq. (50.2), the directions for oxidation and reduction are reversed. For best operation of the electrodes, these two reactions should be reversible, that is, it should be just as easy for them to occur in one direction as the other.

The interaction between a metal in contact with a solution of its ions produces a local change in the concentration of the ions in solution near the metal surface. This causes charge neutrality not to be maintained in this region, causing the electrolyte surrounding the metal to be at a different electrical potential from the rest of the solution. Thus, a potential difference known as the *half-cell potential* is established between the metal and the bulk of the electrolyte. It is found that different characteristic potentials occur for different materials, and some of these potentials are summarized in Table 50.2. These half-cell potentials can be important when using electrodes for low frequency or dc measurements.

The relationship between electric potential and ionic concentrations or, more precisely, ionic activities is frequently considered in electrochemistry. Most commonly two ionic solutions of different activity are separated by an ion-selective semipermeable membrane which allows one type of ion to pass freely through the membrane. It can be shown that an electric potential E will exist between the solutions on either side of the membrane, based upon the relative activity of the permeable ions in each of these solutions. This relationship is known as the Nernst equation

$$E = -\frac{RT}{nF} \ln \left(\frac{a_1}{a_2} \right)$$ (50.3)

where a_1 and a_2 are the activities of the ions on either side of the membrane, R is the universal gas constant, T is the absolute temperature, n is the valence of the ions, and F is the Faraday constant. More detail on this relationship can be found in Chapter 51.

When no electric current flows between an electrode and the solution of its ions or across an ion-permeable membrane, the potential observed should be the half-cell potential or the Nernst potential, respectively. If, however, there is a current, these potentials can be altered. The difference between the potential at zero current and the measured potentials while current is passing is known as the *over voltage* and is the result of an alteration in the charge distribution in the solution in contact with the electrodes or the ion-selective membrane. This effect is known as polarization and can result in diminished electrode performance, especially under conditions of motion. There are three basic components to the polarization over potential: the ohmic, the concentration, and the activation over potentials. Of these, the activation over potential is of greatest concern in bioelectric measurements. More details on these over potentials can be found in electrochemistry or biomedical instrumentation texts [4].

TABLE 50.2 Half-cell Potentials for Materials and Reactions Encountered in Biopotential Measurement

Metal and Reaction	Half-cell Potential, V
$Al \rightarrow Al^{3+} + 3e^-$	-1.706
$Ni \rightarrow Ni^{2+} + 2e^-$	-0.230
$H_2 \rightarrow 2H^+ + 2e^-$	0.000 (by definition)
$Ag + Cl^- \rightarrow AgCl + e^-$	$+0.223$
$Ag \rightarrow Ag^+ + e^-$	$+0.799$
$Au \rightarrow Au^+ + e^-$	$+1.680$

Perfectly polarizable electrodes pass a current between the electrode and the electrolytic solution by changing the charge distribution within the solution near the electrode. Thus, no actual current crosses the electrode-electrolyte interface. Nonpolarized electrodes, however, allow the current to pass freely across the electrode-electrolyte interface without changing the charge distribution in the electrolytic solution adjacent to the electrode. Although these types of electrodes can be described theoretically, neither can be fabricated in practice. It is possible, however, to come up with electrode structures that closely approximate their characteristics.

Electrodes made from noble metals such as platinum are often highly polarizable. A charge distribution different from that of the bulk electrolytic solution is found in the solution close to the electrode surface. Such a distribution can create serious limitations when movement is present and the measurement involves low frequency or even dc signals. If the electrode moves with respect to the electrolytic solution, the charge distribution in the solution adjacent to the electrode surface will change, and this will induce a voltage change in the electrode which will appear as motion artifact in the measurement. Thus, for most biomedical measurements, nonpolarizable electrodes are preferred to those that are polarizable.

The silver–silver chloride electrode is one that has characteristics similar to a perfectly nonpolarizable electrode and is practical for use in many biomedical applications. The electrode (Fig. 50.1*a*) consists of a silver base structure that is coated with a layer of the ionic compound silver chloride. Some of the silver chloride when exposed to light is reduced to metallic silver, so a typical silver–silver chloride electrode has finely divided metallic silver within a matrix of silver chloride on its surface. Since the silver chloride is relatively insoluble in aqueous solutions, this surface remains stable. Because there is minimal polarization associated with this electrode, motion artifact is reduced compared to polarizable electrodes such as the platinum electrode. Furthermore, due to the reduction in polarization, there is also a smaller effect of frequency on electrode impedance, especially at low frequencies.

Silver–silver chloride electrodes of this type can be fabricated by starting with a silver base and electrolytically growing the silver chloride layer on its surface [4]. Although an electrode produced in this way can be used for most biomedical measurements, it is not a robust structure, and pieces of the silver chloride film can be chipped away after repeated use of the structure. A structure with greater mechanical stability is the sintered silver–silver chloride electrode shown in Fig. 50.1*b*. This electrode consists of a silver lead wire surrounded by a sintered cylinder made up of finely divided silver and silver-chloride powder pressed together.

In addition to its nonpolarizable behavior, the silver–silver chloride electrode exhibits less electrical noise than the equivalent polarizable electrodes. This is especially true at low frequencies, and so silver–silver chloride electrodes are recommended for measurements involving very low voltages

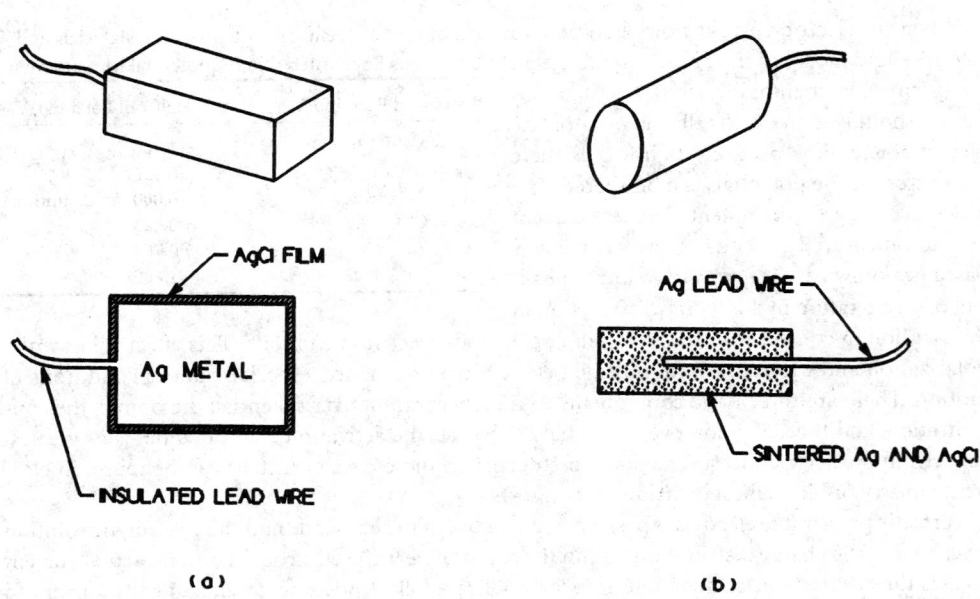

FIGURE 50.1 Silver–silver chloride electrodes for biopotential measurements: (*a*) metallic silver with a silver chloride surface layer and (*b*) sintered electrode structure. The lower views show the electrodes in cross-section.

for signals that are made up primarily of low frequencies. A more detailed description of silver–silver chloride electrodes and methods to fabricate these devices can be found in Janz and Ives [5] and biomedical instrumentation textbooks [4].

50.2 Electric Characteristics

The electric characteristics of biopotential electrodes are generally nonlinear and a function of the current density at their surface. Thus, having the devices represented by linear models requires that they be operated at low potentials and currents. Under these idealized conditions, electrodes can be represented by an equivalent circuit of the form shown in Fig. 50.2. In this circuit R_d and C_d are components that represent the impedance associated with the electrode-electrolyte interface and polarization at this interface. R_s is the series resistance associated with interfacial effects and the resistance of the electrode materials themselves. The battery E_{hc} represents the half-cell potential described above. It is seen that the impedance of this electrode will be frequency dependent, as illustrated in Fig. 50.3. At low frequencies the impedance is dominated by the series combination of R_s and R_d,

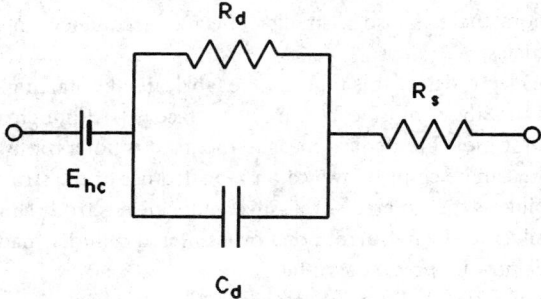

FIGURE 50.2 The equivalent circuit for a biopotential electrode.

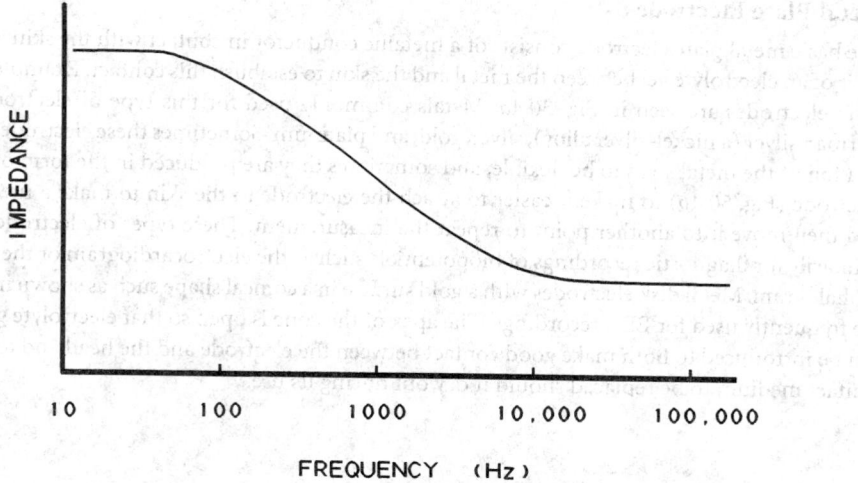

FIGURE 50.3 An example of biopotential electrode impedance as a function of frequency. Characteristic frequencies will be somewhat different for different electrode geometries and materials.

whereas at higher frequencies C_d bypasses the effect of R_d so that the impedance is now close to R_s. Thus, by measuring the impedance of an electrode at high and low frequencies, it is possible to determine the component values for the equivalent circuit for that electrode.

The electrical characteristics of electrodes are affected by many physical properties of these electrodes. Table 50.3 lists some of the more common physical properties of electrodes and qualitatively indicates how these can affect electrode impedance.

50.3 Practical Electrodes for Biomedical Measurements

Many different forms of electrodes have been developed for different types of biomedical measurements. To describe each of these would go beyond the constraints of this article, but some of the more commonly used electrodes are presented in this section. The reader is referred to the monograph by Geddes for more details and a wider selection of practical electrodes [6].

Body-Surface Biopotential Electrodes

This category includes electrodes that can be placed on the body surface for recording bioelectric signals. The integrity of the skin is not compromised when these electrodes are applied, and they can be used for short-term diagnostic recording such as taking a clinical electrocardiogram or long-term chronic recording such as occurs in cardiac monitoring.

TABLE 50.3 The Effect of Electrode Properties on Electrode Impedance

Property	Change in Property	Change in Electrode Impedance
Surface area	↑	↓
Polarization	↑	↑ At low frequencies
Surface roughness	↑	↓
Radius of curvature	↑	↓
Surface contamination	↑	↑

Metal Plate Electrodes

The basic metal plate electrode consists of a metallic conductor in contact with the skin with a thin layer of an electrolyte gel between the metal and the skin to establish this contact. Examples of metal plate electrodes are seen in Fig. 50.4*a*. Metals commonly used for this type of electrode include German silver (a nickel-silver alloy), silver, gold, and platinum. Sometimes these electrodes are made of a foil of the metal so as to be flexible, and sometimes they are produced in the form of a suction electrode (Fig. 50.4*b*) to make it easier to attach the electrode to the skin to make a measurement and then move it to another point to repeat the measurement. These types of electrodes are used primarily for diagnostic recordings of biopotentials such as the electrocardiogram or the electroencephalogram. Metal disk electrodes with a gold surface in a conical shape such as shown in Fig. 50.4*c* are frequently used for EEG recordings. The apex of the cone is open so that electrolyte gel or paste can be introduced to both make good contact between the electrode and the head and to allow this contact medium to be replaced should it dry out during its use.

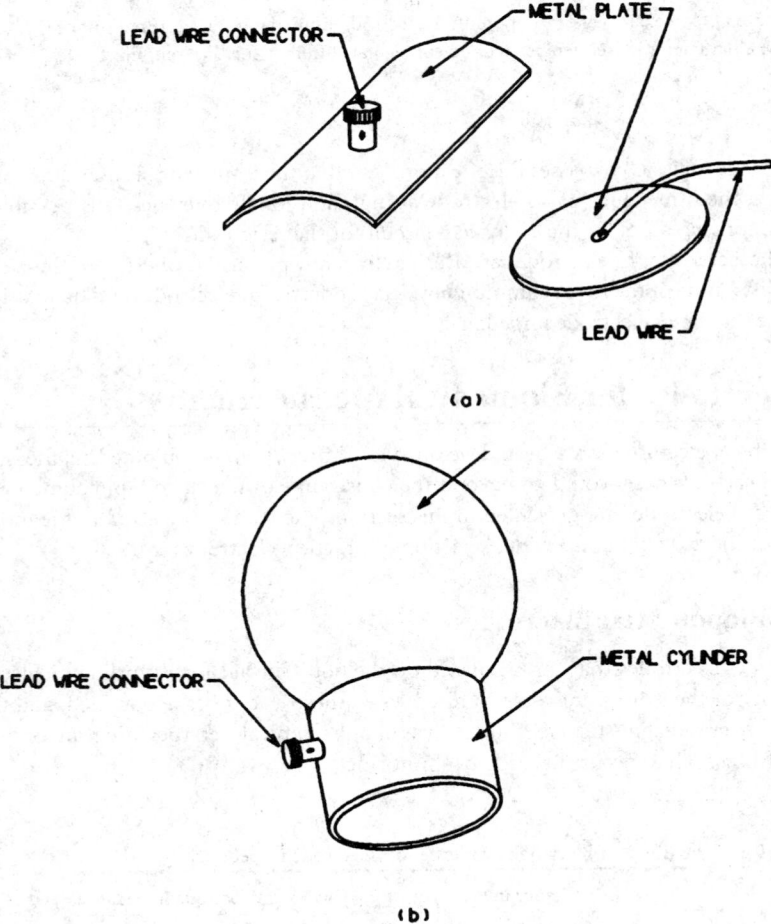

FIGURE 50.4 Examples of different skin electrodes: (*a*) metal plate electrodes, (*b*) suction electrode for ECG, (*c*) metal cup EEG electrode, (*d*) recessed electrode, (*e*) disposable electrode with electrolyte-impregnated sponge (shown in cross-section), (*f*) disposable hydrogel electrode (shown in cross-section), (*g*) thin-film electrode for use with neonates (shown in cross-section), (*h*) carbon-filled elastomer dry electrode.

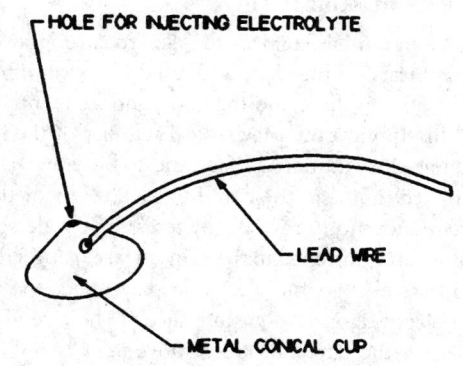

(c)

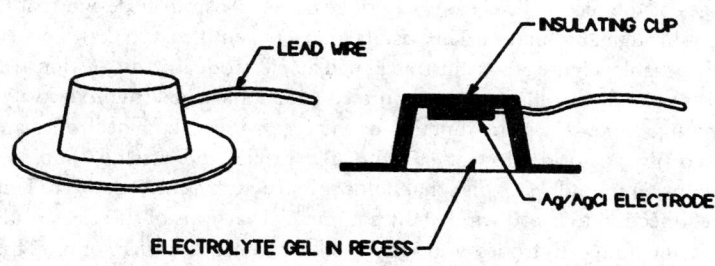

(d)

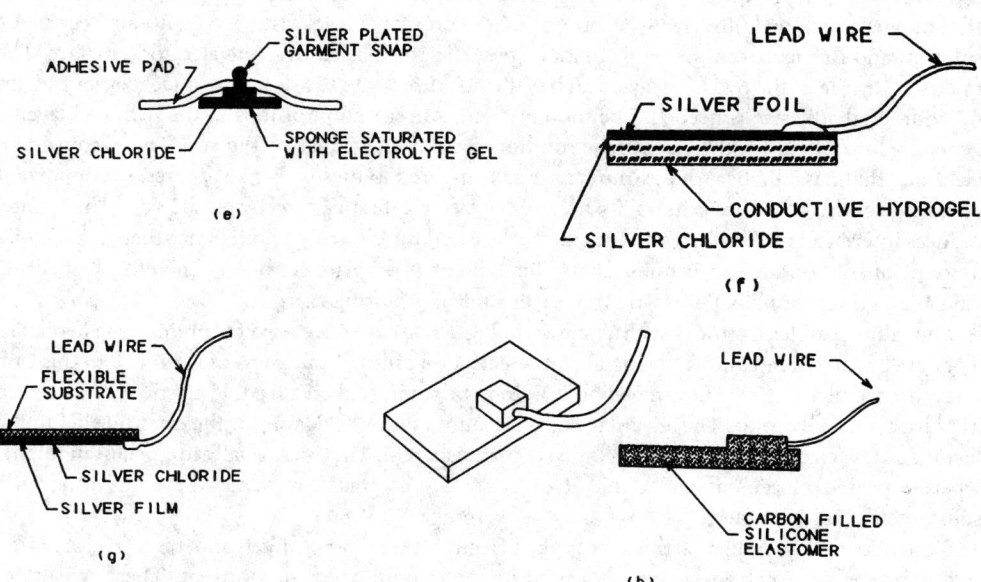

FIGURE 50.4 *(continued)*

Electrodes for Chronic Patient Monitoring

Long-term monitoring of biopotentials such as the electrocardiogram as performed by cardiac monitors places special constraints on the electrodes used to pick up the signals. These electrodes must have a stable interface between them and the body, and frequently nonpolarizable electrodes are, therefore, the best for this application. Mechanical stability of the interface between the electrode and the skin can help to reduce motion artifact, and so there are various approaches to reduce interfacial motion between electrode and the coupling electrolyte or the skin. Figure 50.4d is an example of one approach to reduce motion artifact by recessing the electrode in a cup of electrolytic fluid or gel. The cup is then securely fastened to the skin surface using a double-sided adhesive ring. Movement of the skin with respect to the electrode may affect the electrolyte near the skin-electrolyte interface, but the electrode-electrolyte interface can be several millimeters away from this location, since it is recessed in the cup. The fluid movement is unlikely to affect the recessed electrode-electrolyte interface as compared to what would happen if the electrode was separated from the skin by just a thin layer of electrolyte.

The advantages of the recessed electrode can be realized in a simpler design that lends itself to mass production through automation. This results in low per-unit cost so that these electrodes can be considered disposable. Figure 50.4e illustrates such an electrode in cross section. The electrolyte layer now consists of an open-celled sponge saturated with a thickened (high-viscosity) electrolytic solution. The sponge serves the same function as the recess in the cup electrodes and is coupled directly to a silver–silver chloride electrode. Frequently, the electrode itself is coupled to a clothing snap through an insulating-adhesive disk that holds the structure against the skin. This snap serves as the point of connection to a lead wire. Many commercial versions of these electrodes in various sizes are available, including electrodes with a silver–silver chloride interface or ones that use metallic silver as the electrode material.

A recently developed modification of this basic monitoring electrode structure is shown in Fig. 50.4f. In this case the metal electrode is a silver foil with a surface coating of silver chloride. The foil gives the electrode increased flexibility to fit more closely over body contours. Instead of using the sponge, a hydrogel film (really a sponge on a microscopic level) saturated with an electrolytic solution and formed from materials that are very sticky is placed over the electrode surface. The opposite surface of the hydrogel layer can be attached directly to the skin, and since it is very sticky, no additional adhesive is needed. The mobility and concentration of ions in the hydrogel layer is generally lower than for the electrolytic solution used in the sponge or the cup. This results in an electrode that has a higher source impedance as compared to these other structures. An important advantage of this structure is its ability to have the electrolyte stick directly on the skin. This greatly reduces interfacial motion between the skin surface and the electrolyte, and hence there is a smaller amount of motion artifact in the signal. This type of hydrogel electrode is, therefore, especially valuable in monitoring patients who move a great deal or during exercise.

Thin-film flexible electrodes such as shown in Fig. 50.4g have been used for monitoring neonates. They are basically the same as the metal plate electrodes; only the thickness of the metal in this case is less than a micrometer. These metal films need to be supported on a flexible plastic substrate such as polyester or polyimide. The advantage of using only a thin metal layer for the electrode lies in the fact that these electrodes will then become x-ray transparent. This is especially important in infants where repeated placement and removal of electrodes so that x-rays may be taken can cause substantial skin irritation.

Electrodes that do not use artificially applied electrolyte solutions or gels and, therefore, are often referred to as dry electrodes have been used in some monitoring applications. These sensors as illustrated in Fig. 50.4h can be placed on the skin and held in position by an elastic band or tape. They are made up of a graphite or metal-filled polymer such as silicone. The conducting particles are ground into a fine powder, and this is added to the silicone elastomer before it cures so to produce a conductive material with physical properties similar to that of the elastomer. When held against the skin surface, these electrodes establish contact with the skin without the need for an electrolytic fluid or gel. In actuality such a layer is formed by sweat under the electrode surface. For this reason these electrodes tend to perform better after they have been left in place for an hour or two so that this layer forms. Some investigators have found that placing a drop of physiologic saline solution on the skin before applying the electrode accelerates this process. This type of electrode has found wide application in home infant cardiorespiratory monitoring because of the ease with which it can be applied by untrained caregivers.

Intracavitary and Intratissue Electrodes

Electrodes can be placed within the body for biopotential measurements. These electrodes are generally smaller than skin surface electrodes and do not require special electrolytic coupling fluid, since natural body fluids serve this function. There are many different designs for these internal electrodes, and only a few examples are given in the following paragraphs. Basically these electrodes can be classified as needle electrodes, which can be used to penetrate the skin and tissue to reach the point where the measurement is to be made, or they are electrodes that can be placed in a natural cavity or surgically produced cavity in tissue. Figure 50.5 illustrates some of these internal electrodes.

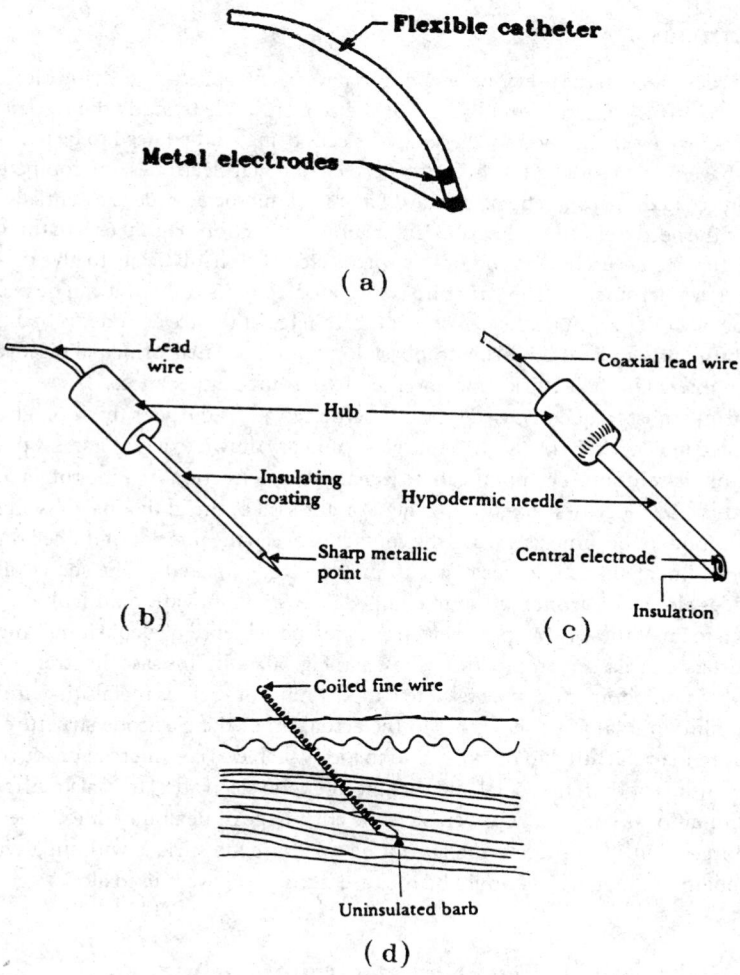

FIGURE 50.5 Examples of different internal electrodes: (*a*) catheter or probe electrode, (*b*) needle electrode, (*c*) coaxial needle electrode, (*d*) coiled wire electrode. (Reprinted with permission from Webster JG (ed). 1992. Medical Instrumentation: Application and Design, Houghton Mifflin, Boston.)

A catheter tip or probe electrode is placed in a naturally occurring cavity in the body such as in the gastrointestinal system. A metal tip or segment on a catheter makes up the electrode. The catheter or, in the case where there is no hollow lumen, probe, is inserted into the cavity so that the metal electrode makes contact with the tissue. A lead wire down the lumen of the catheter or down the center of the probe connects the electrode to the external circuitry.

The basic needle electrode shown in Fig. 50.5b consists of a solid needle, usually made of stainless steel, with a sharp point. An insulating material coats the shank of the needle up to a millimeter or two of the tip so that the very tip of the needle remains exposed. When this structure is placed in tissue such as skeletal muscle, electrical signals can be picked up by the exposed tip. One can also make needle electrodes by running one or more insulated wires down the lumen of a standard hypodermic needle. The electrode as shown in Fig. 50.5c is shielded by the metal of the needle and can be used to pick up very localized signals in tissue.

Fine wires can also be introduced into tissue using a hypodermic needle, which is then withdrawn. This wire can remain in tissue for acute or chronic measurements. Caldwell and Reswick have used fine coiled wire electrodes in skeletal muscle for several years without adverse effects [7].

Microelectrodes

The electrodes described in the previous paragraphs have been applied to studying bioelectric signals at the organism, organ, or tissue level but not at the cellular level. To study the electric behavior of cells, electrodes that are themselves smaller than the cells being studied need to be used. Three types of electrodes have been described for this purpose: etched metal electrodes, micropipette electrodes, and metal-film-coated micropipette electrodes. The metal microelectrode is essentially a subminiature version of the needle electrode described in the previous section (Fig. 50.6a). In this case, a strong metal such as tungsten is used. One end of this wire is etched electrolytically to give tip diameters of the order of a few micrometers. The structure is insulated up to its tip, and it can be passed through the membrane of a cell to contact the cytosol. The advantage of these electrodes is that they are both small and robust and can be used for neurophysiologic studies. Their principal disadvantage is the difficulty encountered in their fabrication and their high source impedance.

The second and most frequently used type of microelectrode is the glass micropipette. This structure as illustrated in Fig. 50.6b consists of a fine glass capillary drawn to a very narrow point and filled with an electrolytic solution. The point can be as narrow as a fraction of a micrometer, and the dimensions of this electrode are strongly dependent on the skill of the individual drawing the tip. The electrolytic solution in the lumen serves as the contact between the interior of the cell through which the tip has been impaled and a larger conventional electrode located in the shank of the pipette. These electrodes also suffer from high source impedances and fabrication difficulty.

A combined form of these two types of electrodes can be achieved by depositing a metal film over the outside surface of a glass micropipette as shown in Fig. 50.6c. In this case the strength and smaller dimensions of the micropipette can be used to support films of various metals that are insulated by an additional film up to a point very close to the actual tip of the electrode structure. These electrodes have been manufactured in quantity and made available as commercial products. Since they combine the features of both the metal and the micropipette electrodes, they also suffer from many of the same limitations. They do, however, have the advantage of flexibility due to the capability of being able to make films of different metals on the micropipette surface without having to worry about the strength of the metal, as would be the case if the metal were used alone.

Electrodes Fabricated Using Microelectronic Technology

Modern microelectronic technology can be used to fabricate many different types of electrodes for specific biomedical applications. For example, dry electrodes with high source resistances or

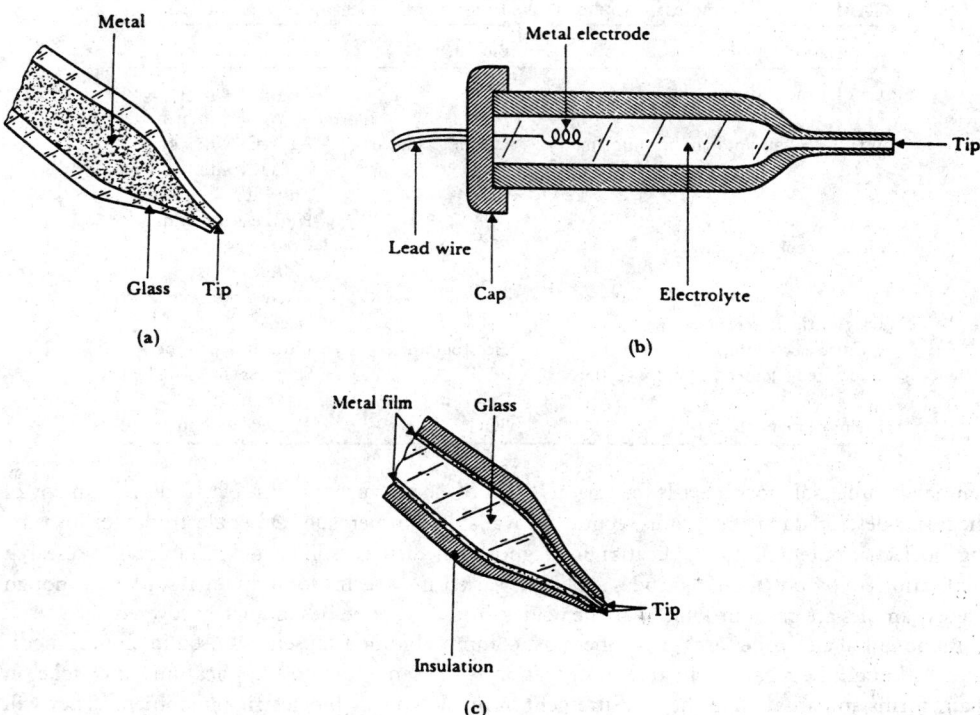

FIGURE 50.6   Microelectrodes: (*a*) metal, (*b*) micropipette, (*c*) thin metal film on micropipette. (Reprinted with permission from Webster JG (ed). 1992. Medical Instrumentation: Application and Design, Houghton Mifflin, Boston.)

microelectrodes with similar characteristics can be improved by incorporating a microelectronic amplifier for impedance conversion right on the electrode itself. In the case of the conventional-sized electrodes, a metal disk 5–10 mm in diameter can have a high input impedance microelectronic amplifier configured as a follower integrated into the back of the electrode so that localized processing of the high source impedance signal can produce one of lower, more practical impedance for signal transmission [8]. Single- and multiple-element electrodes can be made from thin-film or silicon technology. Mastrototaro and colleagues have demonstrated probes for measuring intramyocardial potentials using thin, patterned gold films on polyimide or oxidised molybdenum substrates [9]. When electrodes are made from pieces of micromachined silicon, it is possible to integrate such an amplifier directly into the electrode [10]. Multichannel amplifiers or multiplexers can be used with multiple electrodes on the same probe. Electrodes for contact with individual nerve fibers can be fabricated using micromachined holes in a silicon chip that are just big enough to pass a single growing axon. Electrical contacts on the sides of these holes can then be used to pick up electrical activity from these nerves [11]. These examples are just a few of the many possibilities that can be realized using microelectronics and three-dimensional micromachining technology to fabricate specialized electrodes.

50.4 Biomedical Applications

Electrodes can be used to perform a wide variety of measurements of bioelectric signals. An extensive review of this would be beyond the scope of this chapter, but some typical examples of applications are highlighted in Table 50.4. The most popular application for biopotential electrodes is in obtaining the electrocardiogram for diagnostic and patient-monitoring applications. A sub-

TABLE 50.4   Examples of Applications of Biopotential Electrodes

Application	Biopotential	Type of Electrode
Cardiac monitoring	ECG	Ag/AgCl with sponge
		Ag/AgCl with hydrogel
Infant cardiopulmonary monitoring	ECG impedance	Ag/AgCl with sponge
		Ag/AgCl with hydrogel
		Thin-film
		Filled elastomer dry
Sleep encephalography	EEG	Gold cups
		Ag/AgCl cups
		Active electrodes
Diagnostic muscle activity	EMG	Needle
Cardiac electrograms	Electrogram	Intracardiac probe
Implanted telemetry of biopotentials	ECG	Stainless steel wire loops
	EMG	Platinum disks
Eye movement	EOG	Ag/AgCl with hydrogel

stantial commercial market exists for various types of electrocardiographic electrodes, and many of the forms described in the previous section are available commercially. Other electrodes for measuring bioelectric potentials for application in diagnostic medicine are indicated in Table 50.4. Research applications of biopotential electrodes are highly varied and specific for individual studies. Although a few examples are given in Table 50.4, the field is far too broad to be completely covered here.

Biopotential electrodes are one of the most common biomedical sensors used in clinical medicine. Although their basic principle of operation is the same for most applications, they take on many forms and are used in the measurement of many types of bioelectric phenomena. They will continue to play an important role in biomedical instrumentation systems.

References

1. Yoshida T, Hayashi K, Toko K. 1988. The effect of anoxia on the spatial pattern of electric potential formed along the root. Ann Bot 62(5):497.
2. Plonsey R, Barr RC. 1988. Bioelectricity, New York, Plenum.
3. Weast RC (ed). 1974. Handbook of Chemistry and Physics, 55th ed, Boca Raton, Fla, CRC Press.
4. Webster JG (ed). 1992. Medical Instrumentation: Application and Design, Boston, Houghton Mifflin.
5. Janz GJ, Ives DJG. 1968. Silver–silver chloride electrodes. Ann N Y Acad Sci 148:210.
6. Geddes LA. 1972. Electrodes and the Measurement of Bioelectric Events, New York, Wiley.
7. Caldwell CW, Reswick JB. 1975. A percutaneous wire electrode for chronic research use. IEEE Trans Biomed Eng 22:429.
8. Ko WH, Hynecek J. 1974. Dry electrodes and electrode amplifiers. In HA Miller, Harrison DC (eds), Biomedical Electrode Technology, pp 169–181, New York, Academic Press.
9. Mastrototaro JJ, Massoud HZ, Pilkington PC, et al. 1992. Rigid and flexible thin-film microelectrode arrays for transmural cardiac recording. IEEE Trans Biomed Eng 39(3):271.
10. Wise KD, Najafi K, Ji J, et al. 1990. Micromachined silicon microprobes for CNS recording and stimulation. Proc Ann Conf IEEE Eng Med Biol Soc 12:2334.
11. Edell DJ. 1986. A peripheral nerve information transducer for amputees: Long-term multichannel recordings from rabbit peripheral nerves. IEEE Trans Biomed Eng 33:203.

Further Information

Good overviews of biopotential electrodes are found in Geddes LA. 1972. *Electrodes and the Measurement of Bioelectric Events*, New York, Wiley; and Ferris CD. 1974. *Introduction to*

Bioelectrodes, New York, Plenum. Even though these references are more than 20 years old, they clearly cover the field, and little has changed since these books were written.

Overviews of biopotential electrodes are found in chapters of two works edited by John Webster. Chapter 5 of his textbook, Medical Instrumentation: Application and Design, covers the material of this chapter in more detail, and there is a section on "Bioelectrodes" in his *Encyclopedia on Medical Devices and Instrumentation*, published by Wiley in 1988.

The journals *IEEE Transactions on Biomedical Engineering* and *Medical and Biological Engineering and Computing* are good sources of recent research on biopotential electrodes.

51
Electrochemical Sensors

Chung-Chiun Liu

*Electronics Design Center and
Edison Sensor Technology
Center, Case Western Reserve
University*

Electrochemical sensors have been used extensively either as a whole or an integral part of a chemical and biomedical sensing element. For instance, blood gas (PO2, PCO2, and pH) sensing can be accomplished entirely by electrochemical means. Many important biomedical enzymatic sensors, including glucose sensors, incorporate an enzymatic catalyst and an electrochemical sensing element. The Clark type of oxygen sensor [Clark, 1956] is a well-known practical biomedical sensor based on electrochemical principles, an amperometric device. Electrochemical sensors generally can be categorized as conductivity/capacitance, potentiometric, amperometric, and voltammetric sensors. The amperometric and voltammetric sensors are characterized by their current-potential relationship with the electrochemical system and are less well-defined. Amperometric sensors can also be viewed as a subclass of voltammetric sensors.

Electrochemical sensors are essentially an electrochemical cell which employs a two or three-electrode arrangement. Electrochemical sensor measurements can be made at steady-state or transient. The applied current or potential for electrochemical sensors may vary according to the mode of operation, and the selection of the mode is often intended to enhance the sensitivity and selectivity of a particular sensor. The general principles of electrochemical sensors have been extensively discussed in many electroanalytic references. However, many electroanalytic methods are not practical in biomedical sensing applications. For instance, dropping mercury electrode polarography is a well-established electroanalytic method, yet its usefulness in biomedical sensor development, particularly for potential in vivo sensing, is rather limited. In this chapter, we shall focus on the electrochemical methodologies which are useful in biomedical sensor development.

51.1 Conductivity/Capacitance Electrochemical Sensors

Measurement of the conductivity of an electrochemical cell can be the basis for an electrochemical sensor. This differs from an electrical (physical) measurement, for the electrochemical sensor measures the conductivity change of the system in the presence of a given solute concentration. This solute is often the sensing species of interest. Electrochemical sensors may also involve a capacitative impedance resulting from the polarization of the electrodes and the faradaic or charge transfer processes.

It has been established that the conductance of a homogeneous solution is directly proportional to the cross-sectional area perpendicular to the electrical field and inversely proportional to the

0-8493-8346-3/95/$0.00+$.50

segment of solution along the electrical field. Thus, the conductance of this solution (electrolyte), $G \ (\Omega^{-1})$, can be expressed as

$$G = \sigma A/L \tag{51.1}$$

where A is the cross-sectional area (in cm^2), L is the segment of the solution along the electrical field (in cm), and σ (in $\Omega^{-1} \ cm^{-1}$) is the specific conductivity of the electrolyte and is related quantitatively to the concentration and the magnitude of the charges of the ionic species. For a practical conductivity sensor, A is the surface area of the electrode, and L is the distance between the two electrodes.

Equivalent and molar conductivities are commonly used to express the conductivity of the electrolyte. Equivalent conductance depends on the concentration of the solution. If the solution is a strong electrolyte, it will completely dissociate the components in the solution to ionic forms. Kohlrauch [MacInnes, 1939] found that the equivalent conductance of a strong electrolyte was proportional to the square root of its concentration. However, if the solution is a weak electrolyte which does not completely dissociate the components in the solution to respective ions, the above observation by Kohlrauch is not applicable.

The formation of ions leads to consideration of their contribution to the overall conductance of the electrolyte. The equivalent conductance of a strong electrolyte approaches a constant limiting value at infinite dilution, namely,

$$\Lambda_o = \Lambda_{\lim \to o} = \lambda_o^+ + \lambda_o^- \tag{51.2}$$

where Λ_o is the equivalent conductance of the electrolyte at infinite dilution and λ_o^+ and λ_o^- are the ionic equivalent conductance of cations and anions at infinite dilution, respectively.

Kohlrauch also established the law of independent mobilities of ions at infinite dilution. This implies that Λ_o at infinite dilution is a constant at a given temperature and will not be affected by the presence of other ions in the electrolyte. This provides a practical estimation of the value of Λ_o from the values of λ_o^+ and λ_o^-. As mentioned, the conductance of an electrolyte is influenced by its concentration. Kohlrausch stated that the equivalent conductance of the electrolyte at any concentration C in mol/l or any other convenient units can be expressed as

$$\Lambda = \Lambda_o - \beta C^{0.5} \tag{51.3}$$

where β is a constant depending on the electrolyte.

In general, electrolytes can be classified as weak electrolytes, strong electrolytes, and ion-pair electrolytes. Weak electrolytes only dissociate to their component ions to a limited extent, and the degree of the dissociation is temperature dependent. However, strong electrolytes dissociate completely, and Eq. (51.3) is applicable to evaluate its equivalent conductance. Ion-pair electrolytes can be characterized by their tendency to form ion pairs. The dissociation of ion pairs is similar to that of a weak electrolyte and is affected by ionic activities. The conductivity of ion-pair electrolytes is often nonlinear related to its concentration.

The electrolytic conductance measurement technique, in principle, is relatively straightforward. However, the conductivity measurement of an electrolyte is often complicated by the polarization of the electrodes at the operating potential. Faradaic or charge transfer processes occur at the electrode surface, complicating the conductance measurement of the system. Thus, if possible, the conductivity electrochemical sensor should operate at a potential where no faradaic processes occur. Also, another important consideration is the formation of the double layer adjacent to each electrode surface when a potential is imposed on the electrochemical sensor. The effect of the double layer complicates the interpretation of the conductivity measurement and is usually described by the Warburg impedance. Thus, even in the absence of faradaic processes, the potential effect of the double layer on the conductance of the electrolyte must be carefully assessed. The influence of a faradaic process can be minimized by maintaining a high center constant, L/A, of the electrochemical conductivity sensor, so that the cell resistance lies in the region of 1–50 kΩ. This implies the desirable feature of a small electrode surface area and a relatively large distance between the two electrodes. Yet, a large electrode surface area enhances the accuracy of the measurement, since a large deviation from the null point facilitates the balance of the Wheatstone bridge, resulting in improvement of sensor sensitivity. These opposing features can be resolved by using a multiple-sensing electrode configuration in which the surface area of each electrode element is small compared to the distance between the electrodes. The multiple electrodes are connected in parallel, and the output of the sensor represents the total sum of the current through each pair of electrodes. In this mode of measurement, the effect of the double layer is included in the conductance measurement. The effects of both the double layers and the faradaic processes can be minimized by using a high-frequency, low-amplitude alternating current. The higher the frequency and the lower the amplitude of the imposed alternating current, the closer the measured value is to the true conductance of the electrolyte.

51.2 Potentiometric Sensors

When a redox reaction, Ox + Ze = Red, takes place at an electrode surface in an electrochemical cell, a potential may develop at the electrode-electrolyte interface. This potential may then be used to quantify the activity (on concentration) of the species involved in the reaction forming the fundamental of potentiometric sensors.

The above reduction reaction occurs at the surface of the cathode and is defined as a *half-cell reaction*. At thermodynamic equilibrium, the Nernst equation is applicable and can be expressed as:

$$E = E^\circ + \frac{RT}{ZF} \ln \left(\frac{a_{ox}}{a_{red}} \right) \tag{51.4}$$

where E and E° are the measured electrode potential and the electrode potential at standard state, respectively; a_{ox} and a_{red} are the activities of Ox (reactant in this case) and Red (product in this case), respectively; Z is the number of electrons transferred, F the Faraday constant, R the gas constant, and T the operating temperature in absolute scale. In the electrochemical cell, two half-cell reactions will take place simultaneously. However, for sensing purposes, only one of the two half-cell reactions should involve the species of interest, and the other half-cell reaction is preferably reversible and noninterfering. As indicated in Eq. (51.4), a linear relation exists between the measured potential E and the natural logarithm of the ratio of the activities of the reactant and product. If the number of electrons transferred Z is one, at ambient temperature (25°C or 298°K) the slope is approximately 60 mV. This slope value governs the sensitivity of the potentiometric sensor.

Potentiometric sensors can be classified based on whether the electrode is inert or active. An inert electrode does not participate in the half-cell reaction and merely provides the surface for the electron transfer or provides a catalytic surface for the reaction. However, an active electrode is either an ion donor or acceptor in the reaction. In general, there are three types of active electrodes: the metal/metal ion, the metal/insoluble salt or oxide, and metal/metal chelate electrodes.

Noble metals such as platinum and gold, graphite, and glassy carbon are commonly used as inert electrodes on which the half-cell reaction of interest takes place. To complete the circuitry for the potentiometric sensor, the other electrode is usually a reference electrode on which a noninterference half-cell reaction occurs. Silver–silver chloride and calomel electrodes are the most commonly used reference electrodes. Calomel electrode consists of $Hg/HgCl_2$ and is less desirable for biomedical systems in terms of safety.

An active electrode may incorporate chemical or biocatalysts and is involved as either an ion donor or acceptor in the half-cell reaction. The other half-cell reaction takes place on the reference electrode and should also be noninterference.

If more than a single type of ion contributes to the measured potential in Eq. (51.4), the potential can no longer be used to quantify the ions of interest. This is the interference in a potentiometric sensor. Thus, in many cases, the surface of the active electrode often incorporates with a specific functional membrane which may be ion-selective, ion-permeable, or ion-exchange properties. These membranes tend to selectively permit the ions of interest to diffuse or migrate through. This minimizes the ionic interference.

Potentiometric sensors operate at thermodynamic equilibrium conditions. Thus, in practical potentiometric sensing, the potential measurement needs to be made under zero-current conditions. Consequently, a high-input impedance electrometer is often used for measurements. Also, the response time for a potentiometric sensor to reach equilibrium condition in order to obtain a meaningful reading can be quite long. These considerations are essential in the design and selection of potentiometric sensors for biomedical applications.

51.3 Voltammetric Sensors

The current potential relationship of an electrochemical cell provides the basis for voltammetric sensors. Amperometric sensors, which are also based on the current potential relationship of the electrochemical cell, can be considered a subclass of voltammetric sensors. In amperometric sensors, a fixed potential is applied to the electrochemical cell, and a corresponding current, due to a reduction or oxidation reaction, is then obtained. This current can be used to quantify the species involved in the reaction. The key consideration of an amperometric sensors is that it operates at a fixed potential. However, a voltammetric sensor can operate in other modes such as linear or cyclic voltammetric modes. Consequently, the respective current potential response for each mode will be different.

In general, voltammetric sensors examine the concentration effect of the detecting species on the current potential characteristics of the reduction or oxidation reaction involved.

The mass transfer rate of the detecting species in the reaction onto the electrode surface and the kinetics of the faradaic or charge transfer reaction at the electrode surface directly affect the current-potential characteristics. This mass transfer can be accomplished through (*a*) an ionic migration as a result of an electric potential gradient, (*b*) a diffusion under a chemical potential difference or concentration gradient, and (*c*) a bulk transfer by natural or forced convection. The electrode reaction kinetics and the mass transfer processes contribute to the rate of the faradaic process in an electrochemical cell. This provides the basis for the operation of the voltammetric sensor. However, assessment of the simultaneous mass transfer and kinetic mechanism is rather complicated. Thus, the system is usually operated under definitive hydrodynamic conditions. Various techniques to control either the potential or current are used to simplify the analysis of the voltammetric measurement. A description of these techniques and their corresponding mathematical analyses are well documented in many texts on electrochemistry or electroanalysis [Adams, 1969; Bard & Faulkner, 1980; Lingane, 1958; Macdonald, 1977; Murray & Reilley 1966].

A preferred mass transfer condition is total diffusion, which can be described by Fick's law of diffusion. Under this condition, the cell current, a measure of the rate of the faradaic process at an electrode, usually increases with increases in the electrode potential. This current approaches a limiting value when the rate of the faradaic process at the electrode surface reaches its maximum mass transfer rate. Under this condition, the concentration of the detecting species at the electrode surface is considered as zero and is diffusional mass transfer. Consequently, the limiting current and the bulk concentration of the detecting species can be related by

$$i = ZFkmC^*$$ (51.5)

where km is the mass transfer coefficient and C^* is the bulk concentration of the detecting species. At the other extreme, when the electrode kinetics is slow compared with the mass transfer rate, the electrochemical system is operated in the reaction kinetic control regime. This usually corresponds to a small overpotential. The limiting current and the bulk concentration of the detecting species can be related as

$$i = ZFkcC^*\qquad\qquad(51.6)$$

where kc is the kinetic rate constant for the electrode process. Both equations (51.5) and (51.6) show the linear relationship between the limiting current and the bulk concentration of the detecting species. In many cases, the current does not tend to a limiting value with an increase in the electrode potential. This is because other faradaic or nonfaradaic processes become active, and the cell current represents the cumulative rates of all active electrode processes. The relative rates of these processes, expressing current efficiency, depend on the current density of the electrode. Assessment of such a system is rather complicated, and the limiting current technique may become ineffective.

When a voltammetric sensor operates with a small overpotential, the rate of faradaic reaction is also small; consequently, a high-precision instrument for the measurement is needed. An amperometric sensor is usually operated under limiting current or relatively small overpotential conditions. Amperometric sensors operate under an imposed fixed electrode potential. Under this condition, the cell current can be correlated with the bulk concentration of the detecting species (the solute). This operating mode is commonly classified as amperometric in most sensor work, but it also is referred to as the *chronosuperometric* method, since time is involved.

Voltammetric sensors can be operated in a linear or cyclic sweep mode. Linear sweep voltammetry involves an increase in the imposed potential linearly at a constant scanning rate from an initial potential to a defined upper potential limit. This is the so-called potential window. The current-potential curve usually shows a peak at a potential where the oxidation or reduction reaction occurs. The height of the peak current can be used for the quantification of the concentration of the oxidation or reduction species. Cyclic voltammetry is similar to the linear sweep voltammetry except that the electrode potential returns to its initial value at a fixed scanning rate. The cyclic sweep normally generates the current peaks corresponding to the oxidation and reduction reactions. Under these circumstances, the peak current value can relate to the corresponding oxidation or reduction reaction. However, the voltammogram can be very complicated for a system involving adsorption (nonfaradaic processes) and charge processes (faradaic processes). The potential scanning rate, diffusivity of the reactant, and operating temperature are essential parameters for sensor operation, similar to the effects of these parameters for linear sweep voltammograms. The peak current may be used to quantify the concentration of the reactant of interest, provided that the effect of concentration on the diffusivity is negligible. The potential at which the peak current occurs can be used in some cases to identify the reaction, or the reactant. This identification is based on the half-cell potential of the electrochemical reactions, either oxidation or reduction. The values of these half-cell reactions are listed extensively in handbooks and references.

The described voltammetric and amperometric sensors can be used very effectively to carry out qualitative and quantitative analyses of chemical and biochemical species. The fundamentals of this sensing technique are well established, and the critical issue is the applicability of the technique to a complex, practical environment, such as in whole blood or other biologic fluids. This is also the exciting challenge of designing a biosensor using voltammetric and amperometric principles.

51.4 Reference Electrodes

Potentiometric, voltammetric, and amperometric sensors employ a reference electrode. The reference electrode in the case of potentiometric and amperometric sensors serves as a counter electrode to complete the circuitry. In either case, the reaction of interest takes place at the surface of the working electrode, and this reaction is either oxidation or reduction reaction. Consequently, the reaction at the counter electrode, i.e., the reference electrode, is a separate reduction or oxidation reaction, respectively. It is necessary that the reaction occurring at the reference electrode does not interfere with the reaction at the working electrode. For practical applications, the reaction occurring at the reference electrode should be highly reversible and, as stated, does not contribute to the reaction at the working electrode. In electrochemistry, the hydrogen electrode is universally accepted as the primary standard with which other electrodes are compared. Consequently, the hydrogen electrode serves extensively as a standard reference. A hydrogen reference electrode is relatively simple to prepare. However, for practical applications hydrogen reference electrodes are too cumbersome to be meaningful.

A class of electrode called the *electrode of the second kind,* which forms from a metal and its sparingly soluble metal salt, finds use as the reference electrode. The most common electrode of this type includes the calomel electrode, $Hg/HgCl_2$, and the silver–silver chloride electrode, $Ag/AgCl$. In biomedical applications, particularly in in vivo applications, $Ag/AgCl$ is more suitable as a reference electrode.

An $Ag/AgCl$ electrode can be small, compact, and relatively simple to fabricate. As a reference electrode, the stability and reproducibility of an $Ag/AgCl$ electrode is very important. Contributing factors to instability and poor reproducibility of $Ag/AgCl$ electrodes include the purity of the materials used, the aging effect of the electrode, the light effect, and so on. When in use, the electrode and the electrolyte interface contribute to the stability of the reference electrode. It is necessary that a sufficient quantity of Cl^- ions exists in the electrolyte when the $Ag/AgCl$ electrode serves as a reference. Therefore, other silver–silver halides such as $Ag/AgBr$ or Ag/AgI electrodes are used in cases where suitable halide ions are present in the electrolyte.

In a voltammetric sensor, the reference electrode serves as a true reference for the working electrode, and no current flows between the working and reference electrodes. Nevertheless, the stability of the reference electrode remains essential for a voltammetric sensor.

51.5 Summary

Electrochemical sensors are used extensively in many biomedical applications including blood gas sensors, PO_2, PCO_2, and pH electrodes. Many practical enzymatic sensors, including glucose and lactate sensors, also employ electrochemical sensors as sensing elements. Electrochemically based biomedical sensors have found in vivo and in vitro applications. We believe that electrochemical sensors will continue to be an important aspect of biomedical sensor development.

References

Adams RN. 1969. Electrochemistry at Solid Electrodes, New York, Marcel Dekker.

Bard A, Faulkner LR. 1980. Electrochemical Methods, New York, Wiley.

Clark LC Jr. 1956. Monitor and control of blood and tissue oxygen tissues. Trans Am Soc Artif Organs 2:41.

Lingane JJ. 1958. Electroanalytical Chemistry, New York, London, Interscience.

Macdonald DD. 1977. Transient Techniques in Electrochemistry, New York, Plenum.

MacInnes DA. 1939. The Principles of Electrochemistry, New York, Reinhold.

Murray RW, Reilley CN. 1966. Electroanalytical Principles, New York–London, Interscience.

52
Optical Sensors

Yitzhak Mendelson
Worcester Polytechnic Institute

Optical methods are among the oldest and best-established techniques for sensing biochemical analytes. Instrumentation for optical measurements generally consists of a light source, a number of optical components to generate a light beam with specific characteristics and to direct this light to some modulating agent, and a photodetector for processing the optical signal. The central part of an optical sensor is the modulating component, and a major part of this chapter will focus on how to exploit the interaction of an analyte with optical radiation in order to obtain essential biochemical information.

The number of publications in the field of optical sensors for biomedical applications has grown significantly during the past two decades. Numerous scientific reviews and historical perspectives have been published, and the reader interested in this rapidly growing field is advised to consult these sources for additional details. This chapter will emphasize the basic concept of typical optical sensors intended for continuous in vivo monitoring of biochemical variables, concentrating on those sensors which have generally progressed beyond the initial feasibility stage and reached the promising stage of practical development or commercialization.

Optical sensors are usually based on optical fibers or on planar waveguides. Generally, there are three distinctive methods for quantitative optical sensing at surfaces:

1. The analyte directly affects the optical properties of a waveguide, such as evanescent waves (electromagnetic waves generated in the medium outside the optical waveguide when light is reflected from within) or surface plasmons (resonances induced by an evanescent wave in a thin film deposited on a waveguide surface).

2. An optical fiber is used as a plain transducer to guide light to a remote sample and return light from the sample to the detection system. Changes in the intrinsic optical properties of the medium itself are sensed by an external spectrophotometer.

3. An indicator or chemical reagent placed inside, or on, a polymeric support near the tip of the optical fiber is used as a mediator to produce an observable optical signal. Typically, conventional techniques, such as absorption spectroscopy and fluorimetry, are employed to measure changes in the optical signal.

0-8493-8346-3/95/$0.00+$.50
© 1995 by CRC Press, Inc.

52.1 Instrumentation

The actual implementation of instrumentation designed to interface with optical sensors will vary greatly depending on the type of optical sensor used and its intended application. A block diagram of a generic instrument is illustrated in Fig. 52.1. The basic building blocks of such an instrument are the light source, various optical elements, and photodetectors.

Light Source

A wide selection of light sources are available for optical sensor applications. These include: highly coherent gas and semiconductor diode lasers, broad spectral band incandescent lamps, and narrow-band, solid-state, light-emitting diodes (LEDs). The important requirement of a light source is obviously good stability. In certain applications, for example in portable instrumentation, LEDs have significant advantages over other light sources because they are small and inexpensive, consume low power, produce selective wavelengths, and are easy to work with. In contrast, tungsten lamps produce a broader range of wavelengths, higher intensity, and better stability but require a sizable power supply and can cause heating problems inside the apparatus.

Optical Elements

Various optical elements are used routinely to manipulate light in optical instrumentation. These include lenses, mirrors, light choppers, beam splitters, and couplers for directing the light from the light source into the small aperture of a fiber optic sensor or a specific area on a waveguide surface and collecting the light from the sensor before it is processed by the photodetector. For wavelength selection, optical filters, prisms, and diffraction gratings are the most common components used to provide a narrow bandwidth of excitation when a broadwidth light source is utilized.

Photodetectors

In choosing photodetectors for optical sensors, a number of factors must be considered. These include sensitivity, detectivity, noise, spectral response, and response time. Photomultipliers and

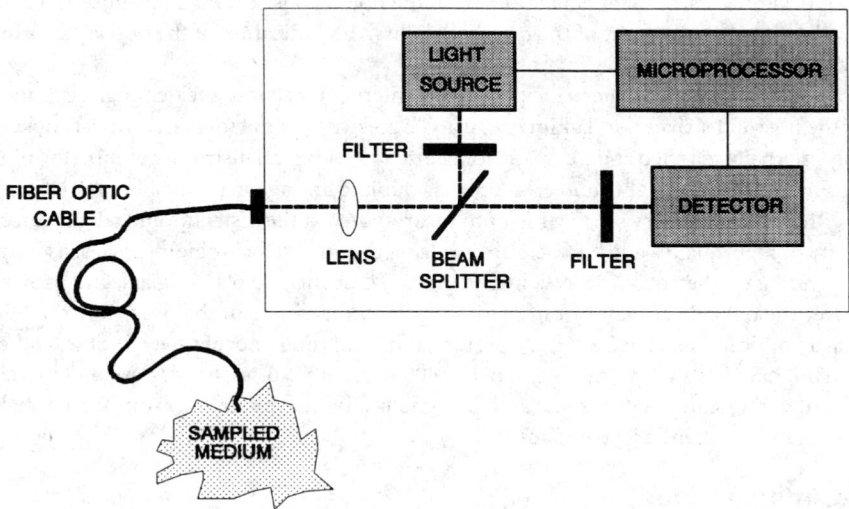

FIGURE 52.1 General diagram representing the basic building blocks of an optical instrument for optical sensor applications.

semiconductor quantum photodetectors, such as photoconductors and photodiodes, are both suitable. The choice, however, is somewhat dependent on the wavelength region of interest. Generally, both give adequate performance. Photodiodes are usually more attractive because of the compactness and simplicity of the circuitry involved.

Typically, two photodetectors are used in optical instrumentation because it is often necessary to include a separate reference detector to track fluctuations in source intensity and temperature. By taking a ratio between the two detector readings, whereby a part of the light that is not affected by the measurement variable is used for correcting any optical variations in the measurement system, a more accurate and stable measurement can be obtained.

Signal Processing

Typically, the signal obtained from a photodetector provides a voltage or a current proportional to the measured light intensity. Therefore, either simple analog computing circuitry (e.g., a current-to-voltage converter) or direct connection to a programmable gain voltage stage is appropriate. Usually, the output from a photodetector is connected directly to a preamplifier before it is applied to sampling and analog-to-digital conversion circuitry residing inside a computer.

Quite often two different wavelengths of light are utilized to perform a specific measurement. One wavelength is usually sensitive to changes in the species being measured, and the other wavelength is unaffected by changes in the analyte concentration. In this manner, the unaffected wavelength is used as a reference to compensate for fluctuations in instrumentation over time. In other applications, additional discriminations, such as pulse excitation or electronic background subtraction utilizing synchronized lock-in amplifier detection, are useful, allowing improved selectivity and enhanced signal-to-noise ratio.

52.2 Optical Fibers

Several types of biomedical measurements can be made by using either plain optical fibers as a remote device for detecting changes in the spectral properties of tissue and blood or optical fibers tightly coupled to various indicator-mediated transducers. The measurement relies either on direct illumination of a sample through the endface of the fiber or by excitation of a coating on the side wall surface through evanescent wave coupling. In both cases, sensing takes place in a region outside the optical fiber itself. Light emanating from the fiber end is scattered or fluoresced back into the fiber, allowing measurement of the returning light as an indication of the optical absorption or fluorescence of the sample at the fiber optic tip.

Optical fibers are based on the principle of total internal reflection. Incident light is transmitted through the fiber if it strikes the cladding at an angle greater than the so-called critical angle, so that it is totally internally reflected at the core/cladding interface. A typical instrument for performing fiber optic sensing consists of a light source, an optical coupling arrangement, the fiber optic light guide with or without the necessary sensing medium incorporated at the distal tip, and a light detector.

A variety of high-quality optical fibers are available commercially for biomedical sensor applications, depending on the analytic wavelength desired. These include plastic, glass, and quartz fibers which cover the optical spectrum from the UV through the visible to the near IR region. On one hand, plastic optical fibers have a larger aperture and are strong, inexpensive, flexible, and easy to work with but have poor UV transmission below 400 nm. On the other hand, glass and quartz fibers have low attenuation and better transmission in the UV but have small apertures, are fragile, and present a potential risk in in vivo applications.

Probe Configurations

There are many different ways to implement fiber optic sensors. Most fiber optic chemical sensors employ either a single-fiber configuration, where light travels to and from the sensing tip in one fiber, or a double-fiber configuration, where separate optical fibers are used for illumination and detection. A single fiber optic configuration offers the most compact and potentially least expensive implementation. However, additional challenges in instrumentation are involved in separating the illuminating signal from the composite signal returning for processing.

The design of intravascular catheters require special considerations related to the sterility and biocompatibility of the sensor. For example, intravascular fiberoptic sensors must be sterilizable and their material nonthrombogenic and resistant to platelet and protein deposition. Therefore, these catheters are typically made of materials covalently bound with heparin or antiplatelet agents. The catheter is normally introduced into the jugular vein via a peripheral cut-down and a slow heparin flush is maintained until it is removed from the blood.

Optical Fiber Sensors

Advantages cited for fiber optic sensors include their small size and low cost. In contrast to electrical measurements, where the difference of two absolute potentials must be measured, fiber optics are self-contained and do not require an external reference signal. Because the signal is optical, there is no electrical risk to the patient, and there is no direct interference from surrounding electric or magnetic fields. Chemical analysis can be performed in real-time with almost an instantaneous response. Furthermore, versatile sensors can be developed that respond to multiple analytes by utilizing multiwavelength measurements.

Despite these advantages, optical fiber sensors exhibit several shortcomings. Sensors with immobilized dyes and other indicators have limited long-term stability, and their shelf life degrades over time. Moreover, ambient light can interfere with the optical measurement unless optical shielding or special time-synchronous gating is performed.

Indicator-Mediated Transducers

Only a limited number of biochemical analytes have an intrinsic optical absorption that can be measured with sufficient selectivity directly by spectroscopic methods. Other species, particularly hydrogen, oxygen, carbon dioxide, and glucose, which are of primary interest in diagnostic applications, are not susceptible to direct photometry. Therefore, indicator-mediated sensors have been developed using specific reagents that are properly immobilized on the surface of an optical sensor.

The most difficult aspect of developing an optical biosensor is the coupling of light to the specific recognition element so that the sensor can respond selectively and reversibly to a change in the concentration of a particular analyte. In fiber-optic-based sensors, light travels efficiently to the end of the fiber where it exits and interacts with a specific chemical or biologic recognition element that is immobilized at the tip of the fiber optic. These transducers may include indicators and ionophores (i.e., ion-binding compounds) as well as a wide variety of selective polymeric materials. After the light interacts with the sample, the light returns through the same or a different optical fiber to a detector which correlates the degree of change with the analyte concentration.

Typical indicator-mediated fiber-optic-sensor configurations are shown schematically in Fig. 52.2. In (*a*) the indicator is immobilized directly on a membrane positioned at the end of a fiber. An indicator in the form of a powder can be either glued directly onto a membrane, as shown in (*b*), or physically retained in position at the end of the fiber by a special permeable membrane (*c*), a tubular capillary/membrane (*d*), or a hollow capillary tube (*e*).

52.3 General Principles of Optical Sensing

Two major optical techniques are commonly available to sense optical changes at sensor interfaces. These are usually based on evanescent wave and surface plasmon resonance principles.

Evanescent Wave Spectroscopy

When light propagates along an optical fiber, it is not confined to the core region but penetrates to some extent into the surrounding cladding region. In this case, an electromagnetic component of the light penetrates a characteristic distance (on the order of one wavelength) beyond the reflecting surface into the less optically dense medium where it is attenuated exponentially according to Beer-Lambert's law (Fig. 52.3).

The evanescent wave depends on the angle of incidence and the incident wavelength. This phenomenon has been widely exploited to construct different types of optical sensors for biomedical applications. Because of the short penetration depth and the exponential decay of the intensity, the evanescent wave is absorbed mainly by absorbing compounds very close to the surface. In the case of particularly weak absorbing analytes, sensitivity can be enhanced by combining the evanescent wave principle with multiple internal

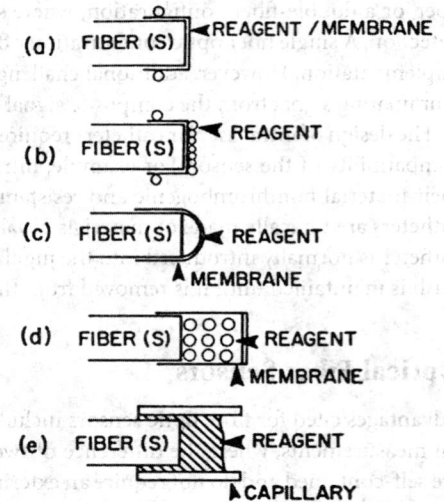

FIGURE 52.2 Typical configuration of different indicator-mediated fiber optic sensor tips (from Otto S. Wolfbeis, Fiber Optic Chemical Sensors and Biosensors, vol. 1, CRC Press, Boca Raton, 1990).

reflections along the sides of an unclad portion of a fiber optic tip.

Instead of an absorbing species, a fluorophore can also be used. Light is absorbed by the fluorophore emitting detectable fluorescent light at a higher wavelength, thus providing improved sensitivity. Evanescent wave sensors have been applied successfully to measure the fluorescence of indicators in solution, for pH measurement, and in immunodiagnostics.

Surface Plasmon Resonance

Instead of the dielectric/dielectric interface used in evanescent wave sensors, it is possible to arrange a dielectric/metal/dielectric sandwich layer such that when monochromatic polarized light (e.g., from a laser source) impinges on a transparent medium having a metallized (e.g., Ag or Au) surface, light is absorbed within the plasma formed by the conduction electrons of the metal. This results in a phenomenon known as *surface plasmon resonance* (SPR). When SPR is induced, the effect is

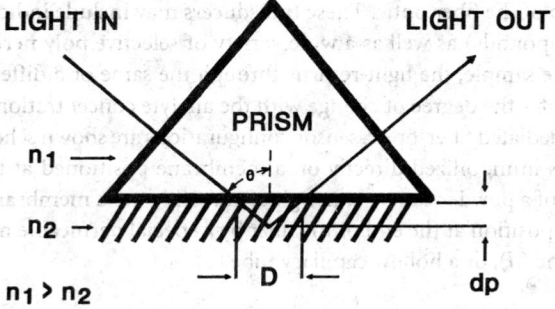

FIGURE 52.3 Schematic diagram of the path of a light ray at the interface of two different optical materials with index of refraction n_1 and n_2. The ray penetrates a fraction of a wavelength (dp) beyond the interface into the medium with the smaller refractive index.

observed as a minimum in the intensity of the light reflected off the metal surface.

As is the case with the evanescent wave, an SPR is exponentially decaying into solution with a penetration depth of about 20 nm. The resonance between the incident light and the plasma wave depends on the angle, wavelength, and polarization state of the incident light and the refractive indices of the metal film and the materials on either side of the metal film. A change in the dielectric constant or the refractive index at the surface causes the resonance angle to shift, thus providing a highly sensitive means of monitoring surface reactions.

The method of SPR is generally used for sensitive measurement of variations in the refractive index of the medium immediately surrounding the metal film. For example, if an antibody is bound to or absorbed into the metal surface, a noticeable change in the resonance angle can be readily observed because of the change of the refraction index at the surface, assuming all other parameters are kept constant (Fig. 52.4). The advantage of this concept is the improved ability to detect the direct interaction between antibody and antigen as an interfacial measurement.

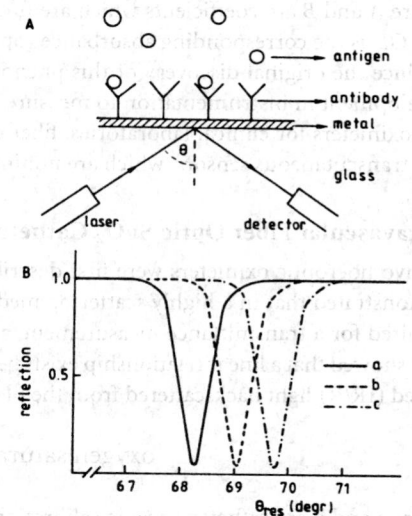

FIGURE 52.4 Surface plasmon resonance at the interface between a thin metallic surface and a liquid (A). A sharp decrease in the reflected light intensity can be observed in (B). The location of the resonance angle is dependent on the refractive index of the material present at the interface.

SPR has been used to analyze immunochemicals and to detect gases. The main limitations of SPR, however, is that the sensitivity depends on the optical thickness of the adsorbed layer, and, therefore, small molecules cannot be measured in very low concentrations.

52.4 Applications

Oximetry

Oximetry refers to the colorimetric measurement of the degree of oxygen saturation, that is, the relative amount of oxygen carried by the hemoglobin in the erythrocytes, by recording the variation in the color of deoxyhemoglobin (Hb) and oxyhemoglobin (HbO_2). A quantitative method for measuring blood oxygenation is of great importance in assessing the circulatory and respiratory status of a patient.

Various optical methods for measuring the oxygen saturation of arterial (SaO_2) and mixed venous (SvO_2) blood have been developed, all based on light transmission through, or reflecting from, tissue and blood. The measurement is performed at two specific wavelengths: λ_1, where there is a large difference in light absorbance between Hb and HbO_2 (e.g., 660 nm red light), and λ_2, which can be an isobestic wavelength (e.g., 805 nm infrared light), where the absorbance of light is independent of blood oxygenation, or a different wavelength in the infrared region > 805 nm, where the absorbance of Hb is slightly smaller than that of HbO_2.

Assuming for simplicity that a hemolyzed blood sample consists of a two-component homogeneous mixture of Hb and HbO_2, and that light absorbance by the mixture of these two components is additive, a simple quantitative relationship can be derived for computing the oxygen saturation of blood:

$$\text{Oxygen saturation} = A - B \left[\frac{OD(\lambda_1)}{OD(\lambda_2)} \right]$$

where A and B are coefficients which are functions of the specific absorptivities of Hb and HbO_2, and OD is the corresponding absorbance (optical density) of the blood.

Since the original discovery of this phenomenon over 50 years ago, there has been progressive development in instrumentation to measure oxygen saturation along three different paths: bench-top oximeters for clinical laboratories, fiber optic catheters for invasive intravascular monitoring, and transcutaneous sensors, which are noninvasive devices placed against the skin.

Intravascular Fiber Optic SvO_2 Catheters

In vivo fiberoptic oximeters were first described in the early 1960s by Polanyi and Heir [1]. They demonstrated that in a highly scattering medium such as blood, where a very short path length is required for a transmittance measurement, a reflectance measurement was practical. Accordingly, they showed that a linear relationship exists between oxygen saturation and the ratio of the infrared-to-red (IR/R) light backscattered from the blood

$$\text{oxygen saturation} = \mathbf{a} - \mathbf{b}(\text{IR/R})$$

where $\mathbf{a}$ and $\mathbf{b}$ are catheter-specific calibration coefficients.

Fiber optic SvO_2 catheters consist of two separate optical fibers. One fiber is used for transmitting the light to the flowing blood, and a second fiber directs the backscattered light to a photodetector. In some commercial instruments (e.g., Oximetrix), automatic compensation for hematocrit is employed utilizing three, rather than two, infrared reference wavelengths. Bornzin and coworkers [2] and Mendelson and coworkers [3] described a 5-lumen, 7.5F thermodilution catheter that is comprised of three unequally spaced optical fibers, each fiber 250 μm in diameter, and provides continuous SvO_2 reading with automatic corrections for hematocrit variations (Fig. 52.5).

Intravenous fiberoptic catheters are utilized in monitoring SvO_2 in the pulmonary artery and can be used to indicate the effectiveness of the cardiopulmonary system during cardiac surgery and in the ICU. Several problems limit the wide clinical application of intravascular fiberoptic oximeters. These include the dependence of the individual red and infrared backscattered light intensities and their ratio on hematocrit (especially for SvO_2 below 80%), blood flow, motion artifacts due to catheter tip "whipping" against the blood vessel wall, blood temperature, and pH.

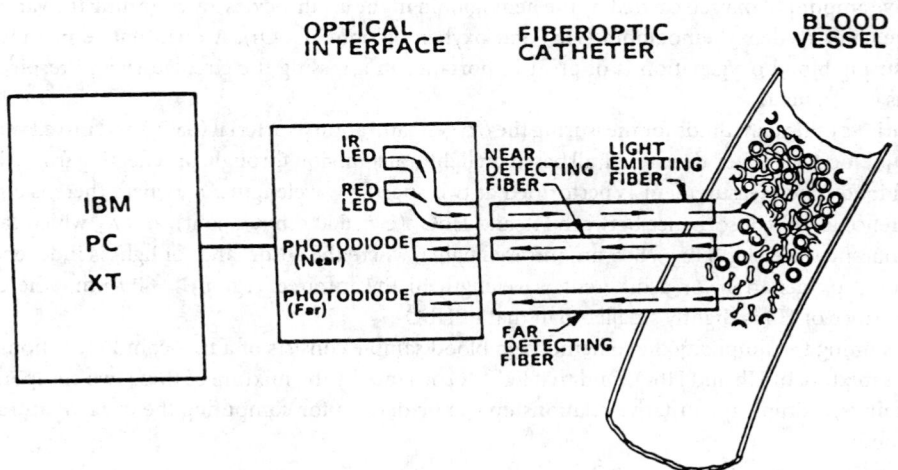

FIGURE 52.5   Principle of a three-fiber optical catheter for SvO_2/HCT measurement [2].

Noninvasive Pulse Oximetry

Noninvasive monitoring of SaO_2 by pulse oximetry is a rapidly growing practice in many fields of clinical medicine [4]. The most important advantage of this technique is the capability to provide continuous, safe, and effective monitoring of blood oxygenation at the patient's bedside without the need to calibrate the instrument before each use.

Pulse oximetry, which was first suggested by Aoyagi and colleagues [5] and Yoshiya and colleagues [6], relies on the detection of the time-variant photoplethysmographic signal, caused by changes in arterial blood volume associated with cardiac contraction. SaO_2 is derived by analyzing only the time-variant changes in absorbance caused by the pulsating arterial blood at the same red and infrared wavelengths used in conventional invasive type oximeters. A normalization process is commonly performed by which the pulsatile (*ac*) component at each wavelength, which results from the expansion and relaxation of the arterial bed, is divided by the corresponding nonpulsatile (*dc*) component of the photoplethysmogram, which is composed of the light absorbed by the blood-less tissue and the nonpulsatile portion of the blood compartment. This effective scaling process results in a normalized red/infrared ratio which is dependent on SaO_2 but is largely independent of the incident light intensity, skin pigmentation, skin thickness, and tissue vasculature.

Pulse oximeter sensors consist of a pair of small and inexpensive red and infrared LEDs and a single, highly sensitive, silicone photodetector. These components are mounted inside a reusable rigid spring-loaded clip, a flexible probe, or a disposable adhesive wrap (Fig. 52.6). The majority of the commercially available sensors are of the transmittance type in which the pulsatile arterial bed, e.g., ear lobe, fingertip, or toe, is positioned between the LEDs and the photodetector. Other probes are available for reflectance (backscatter) measurement where both the LEDs and photodetector are mounted side-by-side facing the skin [7, 8].

Noninvasive Cerebral Oximetry

Another substance whose optical absorption in the near infrared changes corresponding to its reduced and oxidized state is cytochrome aa3, the terminal member of the respiratory chain. Although the concentration of cytochrome aa3 is considerably lower than that of hemoglobin, advanced instrumentation including time-resolved spectroscopy and differential measurements is being used successfully to obtain noninvasive measurements of hemoglobin saturation and cytochrome aa3 by transilluminating areas of the neonatal brain [9–11].

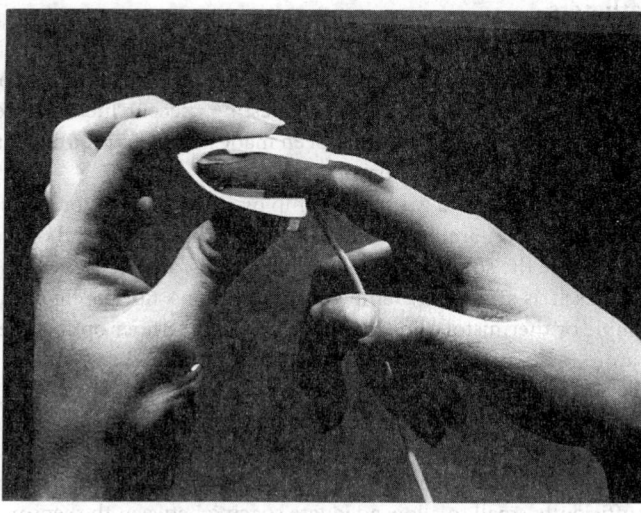

FIGURE 52.6 Disposable finger probe of a noninvasive pulse oximeter.

Blood Gases

Frequent measurement of blood gases, i.e., oxygen partial pressure (pO_2), carbon dioxide partial pressure (pCO_2), and pH, is essential to clinical diagnosis and management of respiratory and metabolic problems in the operating room and the ICU. Considerable effort has been devoted over the last two decades to developing disposable extracorporeal and in particular intravascular fiber optic sensors which can be used to provide continuous information on the acid-base status of a patient.

In the early 1970s, Lubbers and Opitz [12] originated what they called *optodes* (from the Greek, *optical path*) for measurements of important physiologic gases in fluids and in gases. The principle upon which these sensors was designed was a closed cell containing a fluorescent indicator in solution, with a membrane permeable to the analyte of interest (either ions or gases) constituting one of the cell walls. The cell was coupled by optical fibers to a system that measured the fluorescence in the cell. The cell solution would equilibrate with the pO_2 or pCO_2 of the medium placed against it, and the fluorescence of an indicator reagent in the solution would correspond to the partial pressure of the measured gas.

Extracorporeal Measurement

Following the initial feasibility studies of Lubbers and Opitz, Cardiovascular Devices (CDI, USA) developed a GasStat extracorporeal system suitable for continuous online monitoring of blood gases ex vivo during cardiopulmonary bypass operations. The system consists of a disposable plastic sensor connected inline with a blood loop through a fiber optic cable. Permeable membranes separate the flowing blood from the sensor chemistry. The CO_2-sensitive indicator consists of a fine emulsion of a bicarbonate buffer in a two-component silicone. The pH-sensitive indicator is a cellulose material to which hydroxypyrene trisulfonate (HPTS) is bonded covalently. The O_2-sensitive chemistry is composed of a solution of oxygen-quenching decacyclene in a one-component silicone covered with a thin layer of black PTFE for optical isolation and to render the measurement insensitive to the halothane anesthetic.

The extracorporeal device has two channels, one for arterial blood and the other for venous blood, and is capable of recording the temperature of the blood for correcting the measurements to 37°C. Several studies have been conducted comparing the specifications of the GasStat with that of intermittent blood samples analyzed on bench-top blood gas analyzers [13–15].

Intravascular Catheters

During the past decade, numerous efforts have been made to develop integrated fiber optic sensors for intravascular monitoring of blood gases. A few commercial systems for monitoring blood gases and pH are currently undergoing extensive clinical testing. Recent literature reports of sensor performance show that considerable progress has been made mainly in improving the accuracy and reliability of these intravascular blood gas sensors [16–19].

Most fiber optic intravascular blood gas sensors employ either a single- or a double-fiber configuration. Typically, the matrix containing the indicator is attached to the end of the optical fiber as illustrated in Fig. 52.7. Since the solubility of O_2 and CO_2 gases, as well as the optical properties of the sensing chemistry itself, is affected by temperature variations, fiber optic intravascular sensors include a thermocouple or thermistor wire running alongside the fiber optic cable to monitor and correct for temperature fluctuations near the sensor tip. A nonlinear response is characteristic of most chemical indicator sensors, so they are designed to match the concentration region of the intended application. Also, the response time of the optode is somewhat slower compared to electrochemical sensors.

Intravascular fiber optic blood gas sensors are normally placed inside a standard 20-gauge catheter, which is sufficiently small to allow adequate spacing between the sensor and the catheter wall. The resulting lumen is large enough to permit the withdrawal of blood samples, introduction

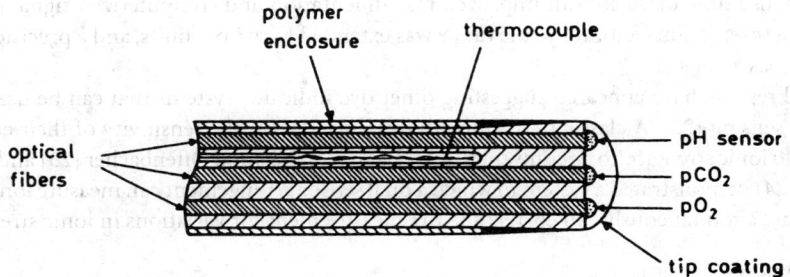

FIGURE 52.7 Principle diagram of an integrated fiber optic blood gas catheter (from Otto S. Wolfbeis, Fiber Optic Chemical Sensors and Biosensors, vol. 2, CRC Press, Boca Raton, 1990).

of a continuous heparin flush, and the recording of a blood pressure waveform. In addition, the optical fibers are encased in a protective tubing to contain any fiber fragments in case they break off.

pH Sensors

In 1976, Peterson and coworkers [20] originated the development of the first fiber optic chemical sensor for physiological pH measurement. The basic idea was to contain a reversible color-changing indicator at the end of a pair of optical fibers. The indicator, phenol red, was covalently bound to a hydrophilic polymer in the form of water-permeable microbeads. This technique stabilized the indicator concentration. The indicator beads were contained in a sealed hydrogen-ion-permeable envelope made out of a hollow cellulose tubing. In effect, this formed a miniature spectrophotometric cell at the end of the fibers and represented an early prototype of a fiber optic chemical sensor.

The phenol red dye indicator is a weak organic acid, and the acid form (un-ionized) and base form (ionized) are present in a concentration ratio determined by the ionization constant of the acid and the pH of the medium according to the familiar Henderson-Hasselbalch equation. The two forms of the dye have different optical absorption spectra, so the relative concentration of one of the forms, which varies as a function of pH, can be measured optically and related to variations in pH. In the pH sensor, green (560 nm) and red (longer than 600 nm) light emerging form the end of one fiber passes through the dye and is reflected back into the other fiber by light-scattering particles. The green light is absorbed by the base form of the indicator. The red light is not absorbed by the indicator and is used as an optical reference. The ratio of green to red light is measured and is related to pH by an S-shaped curve with an approximate high-sensitivity linear region where the equilibrium constant (pK) of the indicator matches the pH of the solution.

The same principle can also be used with a reversible fluorescent indicator, in which case the concentration of one of the indicator forms is measured by its fluorescence rather than absorbance intensity. Light in the blue or UV wavelength region excites the fluorescent dye to emit longer wavelength light, and the two forms of the dye may have different excitation or emission spectra to allow their distinction.

The original instrument design for a pH measurement was very simple and consisted of a tungsten lamp for fiber illumination, a rotating filter wheel to select the green and red light returning from the fiber optic sensor, and signal processing instrumentation to give a pH output based on the green-to-red ratio. This system was capable of measuring pH in the physiologic range between 7.0–7.4 with an accuracy and precision of 0.01 pH units. The sensor was susceptible to ionic strength variation in the order of 0.01 pH unit per 11% change in ionic strength.

Further development of the pH probe for practical use was continued by Markle and colleagues [21]. They designed the fiber optic probe in the form of a 25-gauge (0.5 mm o.d.) hypodermic needle, with an ion-permeable side window, using 75-mm-diameter plastic optical fibers. The sensor had a

90% response time of 30 s. With improved instrumentation and computerized signal processing, and with a three-point calibration, the range was extended to ± 3 pH units, and a precision of 0.001 pH units was achieved.

Several reports have appeared suggesting other dye indicator systems that can be used for fiber optic pH sensing [22]. A classic problem with dye indicators is the sensitivity of their equilibrium constant to ionic strength. To circumvent this problem, Wolfbeis and Offenbacher [23] and Opitz and Lubbers [24] demonstrated a system in which a dual sensor arrangement can measure ionic strength and pH and simultaneously can correct the pH measurement for variations in ionic strength.

pCO₂ Sensors

The pCO_2 of a sample is typically determined by measuring changes in the pH of a bicarbonate solution which is isolated from the sample by a CO_2-permeable membrane but remains in equilibrium with the CO_2. The bicarbonate and CO_2, as carbonic acid, form a pH buffer system, and, by the Henderson-Hasselbalch equation, hydrogen ion concentration is proportional to the pCO_2 in the sample. This measurement is done with either a pH electrode or a dye indicator in solution.

Vurek [25] demonstrated that the same techniques can be used also with a fiber optic sensor. In his design, one plastic fiber carries light to the transducer, which is made of a silicone rubber tubing about 0.6 mm in diameter and 1.0 mm long, filled with a phenol red solution in a 35-mM bicarbonate. Ambient pCO_2 controls the pH of the solution which changes the optical absorption of the phenol red dye. The CO_2 permeates through the rubber to equilibrate with the indicator solution. A second optical fiber carries the transmitted signal to a photodetector for analysis. The design by Zhujun and Seitz [26] uses a pCO_2 sensor based on a pair of membranes separated from a bifurcated optical fiber by a cavity filled with bicarbonate buffer. The external membrane is made of silicone, and the internal membrane is HPTS immobilized on an ion-exchange membrane.

pO₂ Sensors

The development of an indicator system for fiber optic pO_2 sensing is challenging because there are very few known ways to measure pO_2 optically. Although a color-changing indicator would have been desirable, the development of a sufficiently stable indicator has been difficult. The only principle applicable to fiber optics appears to be the quenching effect of oxygen on fluorescence.

Fluorescence quenching is a general property of aromatic molecules, dyes containing them, and some other substances. In brief, when light is absorbed by a molecule, the absorbed energy is held as an excited electronic state of the molecule. It is then lost by coupling to the mechanical movement of the molecule (heat), reradiated from the molecule in a mean time of about 10 ns (fluorescence), or converted into another excited state with much longer mean lifetime and then reradiated (phosphorescence). Quenching reduces the intensity of fluorescence and is related to the concentration of the quenching molecules, such as O_2.

A fiber optic sensor for measuring pO_2 using the principle of fluorescence quenching was developed by Peterson and colleagues [27]. The dye is excited at around 470 nm (blue) and fluoresces at about 515 nm (green) with an intensity that depends on the pO_2. The optical information is derived from the ratio of green fluorescence to the blue excitation light, which serves as an internal reference signal. The system was chosen for visible light excitation, because plastic optical fibers block light transmission at wavelengths shorter than 450 nm, and glass fibers were not considered acceptable for biomedical use.

The sensor was similar in design to the pH probe continuing the basic idea of an indicator packing in a permeable container at the end of a pair of optical fibers. A dye perylene dibutyrate, absorbed on a macroreticular polystyrene adsorbent, is contained in a oxygen-permeable porous polystyrene envelope. The ratio of green to blue intensity was processed according to the Stren-Volmer equation

$$\frac{I_0}{I} = 1 + K\,pO_2$$

where I and I_0 are the fluorescence emission intensities in the presence and absence of quencher, respectively, and K is the Stern-Volmer quenching coefficient. This provides a nearly linear readout of pO_2 over the range of 0–150 mmHg (0–20 kPa), with a precision of 1 mm Hg (0.13 kPa). The original sensor was 0.5 mm in diameter, but it can be made much smaller. Although its response time in a gas mixture is a fraction of a second, it is slower in an aqueous system, about 1.5 min for 90% response.

Wolfbeis and coworkers [28] designed a system for measuring the widely used halothane anesthetic which interferes with the measurement of oxygen. This dual-sensor combination had two semipermeable membranes (one of which blocked halothane) so that the probe could measure both oxygen and halothane simultaneously. The response time of their sensor, 15–20 s for halothane and 10–15 s for oxygen, is considered short enough to allow gas analysis in the breathing circuit. Potential applications of this device include the continuous monitoring of halothane in breathing circuits and in the blood.

Glucose Sensors

Another important principle that can be used in fiber optic sensors for measurements of high sensitivity and specificity is the concept of competitive binding. This was first described by Schultz, Mansouri, and Goldstein [29] to construct a glucose sensor. In their unique sensor, the analyte (glucose) competes for binding sites on a substrate (the lectin concanavalin A) with a fluorescent indicator-tagged polymer [fluorescein isothiocyanate (FITC)-dextran]. The sensor, which is illustrated in Fig. 52.8, is arranged so that the substrate is fixed in a position out of the optical path of the fiber end. The substrate is bound to the inner wall of a glucose-permeable hollow fiber tubing (300 μ O.D.$\times$200 μ I.D.) and fastened to the end of an optical fiber. The hollow fiber acts as the container and is impermeable to the large molecules of the fluorescent indicator. The light beam that extends from the fiber "sees" only the unbound indicator in solution inside the hollow fiber but not the indicator bound on the container wall. Excitation light passes through the fiber and into the solution, fluorescing the unbound indicator, and the fluorescent light passes back along the same fiber to a measuring system. The fluorescent indicator and the glucose are in competitive binding equilibrium with the substrate. The interior glucose concentration equilibrates with its concentration exterior to the probe. If the glucose concentration increases, the indicator is driven off the substrate to increase the concentration of the indicator. Thus, fluorescence intensity as seen by the optical fiber follows the glucose concentration.

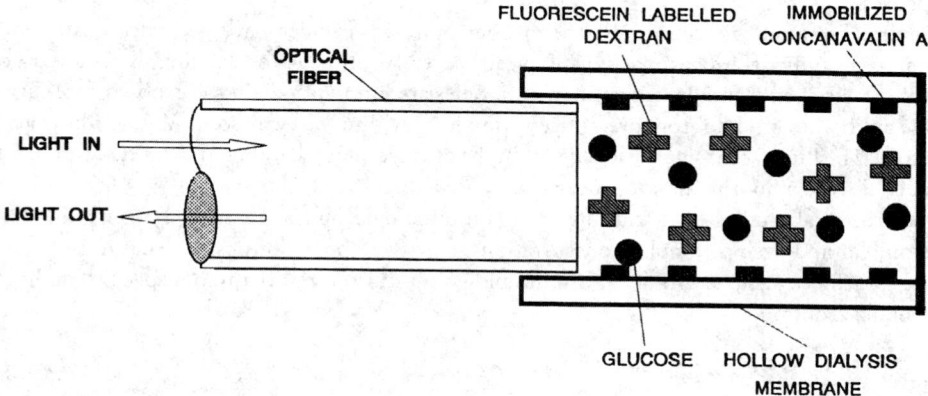

FIGURE 52.8 Schematic diagram of a competitive binding fluorescence affinity sensor for glucose measurement [29].

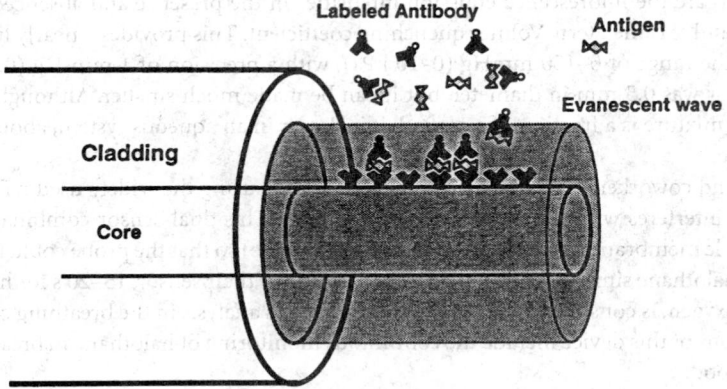

FIGURE 52.9   Basic principle of a fiber optic antigen-antibody sensor [33].

The response time of the sensor was found to be about 5 min. In vivo studies demonstrated fairly close correspondence between the sensor output and actual blood glucose levels. A time lag of about 5 min was found and is believed to be due to the diffusion of glucose across the hollow fiber membrane and the diffusion of FTIC-dextran within the tubing.

In principle, the concept of competitive binding can be applied to any analysis for which a specific reaction can be devised. However, long-term stability of these sensors remains the major limiting factor that needs to be solved.

Immunosensors

Immunologic techniques offer outstanding selectivity and sensitivity through the process of antibody-antigen interaction. This is the primary recognition mechanism by which the immune system detects and fights foreign matter and has therefore allowed the measurement of many important compounds at trace levels in complex biologic samples.

In principle, it is possible to design competitive binding optical sensors utilizing immobilized antibodies as selective reagents and detecting the displacement of a labeled antigen by the analyte. Therefore, antibody-based immunologic optical sensors have been the subject of considerable research in the past few years [30–34]. In practice, however, the strong binding of antigens to antibodies and vice versa causes difficulties in constructing reversible sensors with fast dynamic responses.

Several immunologic sensors based on fiber optic waveguides have been demonstrated for monitoring antibody-antigen reactions. Typically, several centimeters of cladding are removed along the fiber's distal end, and the recognition antibodies are immobilized on the exposed core surface. These antibodies bind fluorophore-antigen complexes within the evanescent wave as illustrated in Fig. 52.9. The fluorescent signal excited within the evanescent wave is then transmitted through the cladded fiber to a fluorimeter for processing.

Experimental studies have indicated that immunologic optical sensors can generally detect micromolar and even picomolar concentrations. However, the major obstacle that must be overcome to achieve high sensitivity in immunologic optical sensors is the nonspecific binding of immobilized antibodies.

References

1. Polanyi ML, Heir RM. 1962. In vivo oximeter with fast dynamic response. Rev Sci Instrum 33:1050.

2. Bornzin GA, Mendelson Y, Moran BL, et al. 1987. Measuring oxygen saturation and hematocrit using a fiberoptic catheter. Proc 9th Ann Conf Eng Med Bio Soc 807–809.

3. Mendelson Y, Galvin JJ, Wang Y. 1990. In vitro evaluation of a dual oxygen saturation/hematocrit intravascular fiberoptic catheter. Biomed Instrum Tech 24:199.

4. Mendelson Y. 1992. Pulse oximetry: Theory and applications for noninvasive monitoring. Clin Chem 28(9): 1601.

5. Aoyagi T, Kishi M, Yamaguchi K, et al. 1974. Improvement of the earpiece oximeter. Jpn Soc Med Electron Biomed Eng 90–91.

6. Yoshiya I, Shimada Y, Tanaka K. 1980. Spectrophotometric monitoring of arterial oxygen saturation in the fingertip. Med Biol Eng Comput 18:27.

7. Mendelson Y, Solomita MV. 1992. The feasibility of spectrophotometric measurements of arterial oxygen saturation from the scalp utilizing noninvasive skin reflectance pulse oximetry. Biomed Instrum Technol 26:215.

8. Mendelson Y, McGinn MJ. 1991. Skin reflectance pulse oximetry: In vivo measurements from the forearm and calf. J Clin Monit 7:7.

9. Chance B, Leigh H, Miyake H, et al. 1988. Comparison of time resolved and un-resolved measurements of deoxyhemoglobin in brain. Proc Nat Acad Sci 85:4971.

10. Jobsis FF, Keizer JH, LaManna JC, et al. 1977. Reflection spectrophotometry of cytochrome aa3 in vivo. Appl Physiol: Respirat Environ Excerc Physiol 43(5): 858.

11. Kurth CD, Steven IM, Benaron D, et al. 1993. Near-infrared monitoring of the cerebral circulation. J Clin Monit 9:163.

12. Lubbers DW, Opitz N. 1975. The pCO_2/pO_2-optode: A new probe for measurement of pCO_2 or pO_2 in fluids and gases. Z Naturforsch C: Biosci 30C:532.

13. Clark CL, O'Brien J, McCulloch J, et al. 1986. Early clinical experience with GasStat. J Extra Corporeal Technol 18:185.

14. Hill AG, Groom RC, Vinansky RP, et al. 1985. On-line or off-line blood gas analysis: Cost vs. time vs. accuracy. Proc Am Acad Cardiovasc Perfusion 6:148.

15. Siggaard-Andersen O, Gothgen IH, Wimberley, et al. 1988. Evaluation of the GasStat fluorescence sensors for continuous measurement of pH, pCO_2 and pO_2 during CPB and hypothermia. Scand J Clin Lab Invest 48 (Suppl. 189):77.

16. Zimmerman JL, Dellinger RP. 1993. Initial evaluation of a new intra-arterial blood gas system in humans. Crit Care Med 21(4):495.

17. Gottlieb A. 1992. The optical measurement of blood gases—approaches, problems and trends: Fiber optic medical and fluorescent sensors and applications. Proc SPIE 1648:4.

18. Barker SL, Hyatt J. 1991. Continuous measurement of intraarterial pHa, $PaCO_2$, and PaO_2 in the operation room. Anesth Analg 73:43.

19. Larson CP, Divers GA, Riccitelli SD. 1991. Continuous monitoring of PaO_2 and $PaCO_2$ in surgical patients. Abstr Crit Care Med 19:525.

20. Peterson JI, Goldstein SR, Fitzgerald RV. 1980. Fiber optic pH probe for physiological use. Anal Chem 52:864.

21. Markle DR, McGuire DA, Goldstein SR, et al. 1981. A pH measurement system for use in tissue and blood, employing miniature fiber optic probes, In DC Viano (ed), Advances in Bioengineering, p 123, New York, American Society of Mechanical Engineers.

22. Wolfbeis OS, Furlinger E, Kroneis H, et al. 1983. Fluorimetric analysis: 1. A study on fluorescent indicators for measuring near neutral (physiological) pH values. Fresenius' Z Anal Chem 314:119.

23. Wolfbeis OS, Offenbacher H. 1986. Fluorescence sensor for monitoring ionic strength and physiological pH values. Sens Actuators 9:85.

24. Opitz N, Lubbers DW. 1983. New fluorescence photomatrical techniques for simultaneous and continuous measurements of ionic strength and hydrogen ion activities. Sens Actuators 4:473.

25. Vurek GG, Feustel PJ, Severinghaus JW. 1983. A fiber optic pCO$_2$ sensor. Ann Biomed Eng 11:499.

26. Zhujun Z, Seitz WR. 1984. A carbon dioxide sensor based on fluorescence. Anal Chim Acta 160:305.

27. Peterson JI, Fitzgerald RV, Buckhold DK. 1984. Fiber-optic probe for in vivo measurement of oxygen partial pressure. Anal Chem 56:62.

28. Wolfbeis OS, Posch HE, Kroneis HW. 1985. Fiber optical fluorosensor for determination of halothane and/or oxygen. Anal Chem 57:2556.

29. Schultz JS, Mansouri S, Goldstein IJ. 1982. Affinity sensor: A new technique for developing implantable sensors for glucose and other metabolites. Diabetes Care 5:245.

30. Andrade JD, Vanwagenen RA, Gregonis DE, et al. 1985. Remote fiber optic biosensors based on evanescent-excited fluoro-immunoassay: Concept and progress. IEEE Trans Electron Devices ED-32: 1175.

31. Sutherland RM, Daehne C, Place JF, et al. 1984. Optical detection of antibody-antigen reactions at a glass-liquid interface. Clin Chem 30:1533.

32. Hirschfeld TE, Block MJ. 1984. Fluorescent immunoassay employing optical fiber in a capillary tube. US Patent No. 4,447,546.

33. Anderson GP, Golden JP, Ligler FS. 1994. An evanescent wave biosensor: Part I. Fluorescent signal acquisition from step-etched fiber optic probes. IEEE Trans Biomes Eng 41(6):578.

34. Golden JP, Anderson GP, Rabbany SY, et al. 1994. An evanescent wave biosensor: Part II. Fluorescent signal acquisition from tapered fiber optic probes. IEEE Trans Biomed Eng 41(6):585.

53

Bioanalytic Sensors

Richard P. Buck
University of North Carolina

53.1 Classification of Biochemical Reactions in the Context of Sensor Design and Development

Introduction and Definitions

Since sensors generate a measurable material property, they belong in some grouping of transducer devices. Sensors specifically contain a recognition process that is characteristic of a material sample at the molecular-chemical level, and a sensor incorporates a transduction process (step) to create a useful signal. Biomedical sensors include a whole range of devices that may be chemical sensors, physical sensors, or some kind of mixed sensor.

Chemical sensors use chemical processes in the recognition and transduction steps. Biosensors are also chemical sensors, but they use particular classes of biological recognition/transduction processes. A pure physical sensor generates and transduces a parameter that does not depend on the chemistry per se but is a result of the sensor responding as an aggregate of point masses or charges. All these when used in a biologic system (biomatrix) may be considered *bioanalytic* sensors without regard to the chemical, biochemical, or physical distinctions. They provide an "analytic signal of the biologic system" for some further use.

The chemical recognition process focuses on some molecular-level chemical entity, usually a kind of chemical structure. In classical analysis this structure may be a simple functional group: SiO^- in a glass electrode surface, a chromophore in an indicator dye, or a metallic surface structure, such as silver metal that recognizes Ag^+ in solution. In recent times, the biologic recognition processes have been better understood, and the general concept of recognition by *receptor* or *chemoreceptor* has come into fashion. Although these are often large molecules bound to cell membranes, they contain specific structures that permit a wide variety of different molecular recognition steps including recognition of large and small species and of charged and uncharged species. Thus, *chemoreceptor* appears in the sensor literature as a generic term for the principal entity doing the recognition. For a history and examples, see references [1–6].

8493-8346-3/95/$0.00+$.50
1995 by CRC Press, Inc.

Biorecognition in biosensors has especially stressed "receptors" and their categories. Historically, application of receptors has not necessarily meant measurement directly of the receptor. Usually there are coupled chemical reactions, and the transduction has used measurement of the subsidiary products: change of pH, change of dissolved O_2, generation of H_2O_2, changes of conductivity, changes of optical adsorption, and changes of temperature. Principal receptors are enzymes because of their extraordinary selectivity. Other receptors can be the more subtle species of biochemistry: antibodies, organelles, microbes, and tissue slices, not to mention the trace level "receptors" that guide ants such as pheromones and other unusual species. A sketch of a generic bioanalytic sensor is shown in Fig. 53.1.

Classification of Recognition Reactions and Receptor Processes

The concept of *recognition* in chemistry is universal. It almost goes without saying that all chemical reactions involved recognition and selection on the basis of size, shape, and charge. For the purpose of constructing sensors, general recognition based on these factors is not usually enough. Frequently in inorganic chemistry a given ion will react indiscriminantly with similar ions of the same size and charge. Changes in charge from unity to two, for example, do change the driving forces of some ionic reactions. By control of dielectric constant of phases, heterogeneous reactions can often be "tailored" to select divalent ions over monovalent ions and to select small versus large ions or vice versa.

Shape, however, has more special possibilities, and natural synthetic methods permit product control. Nature manages to use shape together with charge to build organic molecules, called enzymes, that have acquired remarkable selectivity. It is in the realm of biochemistry that these natural constructions are investigated and catalogued. Biochemistry books list large numbers of enzymes and other selective materials that direct chemical reactions. Many of these have been tried as the basis of selective sensors for bioanalytic and biomedical purposes. The list in Table 53.1 shows how some of these materials can be grouped into lists according to function and to analytic substrate, both organic and inorganic. The principles seem general, so there is no reason to discriminate against the inorganic substrates in favor or the organic substrates. All can be used in biomedical analysis.

53.2 Classification of Transduction Processes—Detection Methods

Some years ago, the engineering community addressed the topic of sensor classification—Richard M. White in IEEE Trans. Ultra., Ferro., Freq. Control (UFFC), UFFC-34 (1987) 124, and Wen E. Ko in IEEE/EMBS Symposium Abstract T.1.1 84CH2068-5 (1984). It is interesting because the physical

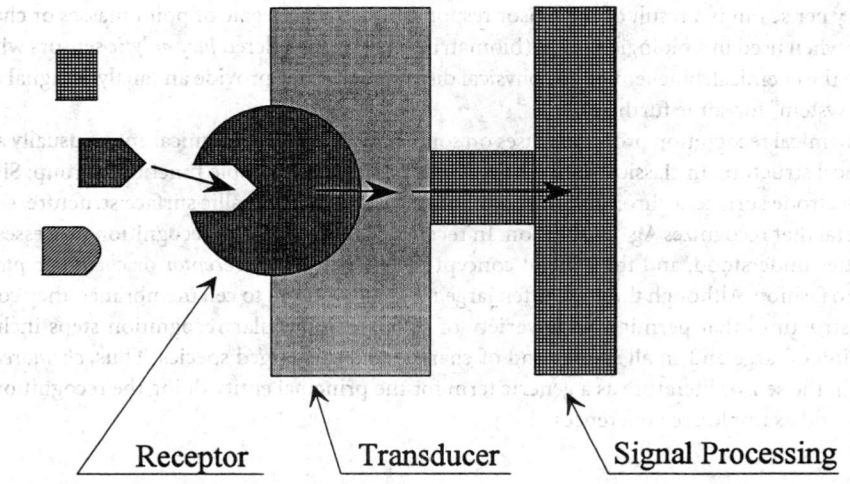

FIGURE 53.1   Generic bioanalytic sensor.

TABLE 53.1   Recognition Reactions and Receptor Processes

1. Insoluble salt-based sensors
   a. $$S^+ + R^- \rightleftharpoons \text{(insoluble salt)}$$
   Ion exchange with crystalline SR (homogeneous or heterogeneous crystals)

chemical signal S^{+n}	receptor R^{-n}
inorganic cations	inorganic anions
examples: $Ag^+, Hg_2^{2+}, Pb^{2+}, Cd^{2+}, Cu^{2+}$	$S^=, Se^{2=}, SCN^-, I^-, Br^-, Cl^-$

   b. $$S^{-n} + R^{+n} \rightleftharpoons SR \text{ (insoluble salt)}$$
   Ion exchange with crystalline SR (homogeneous or heterogeneous crystals)

chemical signal S^{-n}	receptor R^{+n}
inorganic anions	inorganic cations
examples: $F^-, S^=, Se^{2=}, SCN^-, I^-, Br^-, Cl^-$	$LaF_2^+, Ag^+, Hg_2^{2+}, Pb^{2+}, Cd^{2+}, Cu^{2+}$

2. Solid ion exchangers
   a. $$S^{+n} + R^{-n} \text{ (sites)} \rightleftharpoons S^{+n}R^{-n} = SR \text{ (in ion exchanger phase)}$$
   Ion exchange with synthetic ion exchangers containing negative fixed sites (homogeneous or heterogeneous, inorganic or organic materials)

chemical signal S^{+n}	receptor R^{-n}
inorganic and organic ions	inorganic and organic ion sites
examples: H^+, Na^+, K^+	silicate glass $Si\text{-}0^-$
H^+, Na^+, K^+, other M^{+n}	synthetic sulfonated, phosphorylated, EDTA-substituted polystyrenes

   b. $$S^{-n} + R^{+n} \text{(sites)} \rightleftharpoons S^{-n}R^{+n} = SR \text{ (in ion exchanger phase)}$$
   Ion exchange with synthetic ion exchangers containing positive fixed sites (homogeneous or heterogeneous, inorganic or organic materials)

chemical signal S^{-n}	receptor R^{+n}
organic and inorganic ions	organic and inorganic ion sites
examples: hydrophobic anions	quaternized polystyrene

3. Liquid ion exchanger sensors with electrostatic selection
   a. $$S^{+n} + R^{-n} \text{(sites)} \rightleftharpoons S^{+n}R^{-n} = SR \text{ (in ion exchanger phase)}$$
   Plasticized, passive membranes containing mobile, trapped negative fixed sites (homogeneous or heterogeneous, inorganic or organic materials)

chemical signal S^{+n}	receptor R^{-n}
inorganic and organic ions	inorganic and organic ion sites
examples: Ca^{2+}	diester of phosphoric acid or monoester of a phosphonic acid
M^{+n}	dinonylnaphthalene sulfonate and other organic, hydrophobic anions
$R_1R_2R_3R_4N^+$ and bis-Quaternary Cations cationic drugs tetrasubstituted arsonium$^+$	tetraphenylborate anion or substituted derivatives

   b. $$S^{-n} + R^{+n} \text{(sites)} \rightleftharpoons S^{-n}R^{+n} = SR \text{ (in ion exchanger phase)}$$
   Plasticized, passive membranes containing mobile, trapped negative fixed sites (homogeneous or heterogeneous, inorganic or organic materials)

chemical signal S^{-n}	receptor R^{+n}
inorganic and organic ions	inorganic and organic ion sites
examples: anions, simple Cl^-, Br^-, ClO_4^-	quaternary ammonium cations: e.g. tridodecylmethyl-ammonium
anions, complex, drugs	quaternary ammonium cations: e.g. tridodecylmethyl-ammonium

4. Liquid ion exchanger sensors with neutral (or charged) carrier selection
   a. $$S^{+n} + X \text{ and } R^{-n} \text{(sites)} \rightleftharpoons S^{+n}X\,R^{-n} = SXR \text{ (in ion exchanger phase)}$$
   Plasticized, passive membranes containing mobile, trapped negative fixed sites (homogeneous or heterogeneous, inorganic or organic materials)

chemical signal S^{+n}	receptor R^{-n}
inorganic and organic ions	inorganic and organic ion sites
examples: Ca^{2+}	X = synthetic ionophore complexing agent selective to Ca^{2+}
	R^{-n} usually a substituted tetra phenylborate salt
Na^+, K^+, H^+	X = selective ionophore complexing agent

(continued)

TABLE 53.1   Recognition Reactions and Receptor Processes *(continued)*

b. $S^{-n} + X$ and R^{+n}(sites) $\rightleftharpoons$ $S^{-n}X\ R^{+n}$ = SXR (in ion exchanger phase)

Plasticized, passive membranes containing mobile, trapped negative fixed sites (homogeneous or heterogeneous, inorganic or organic materials)

chemical signal S^{-n}	receptor R^{+n}
inorganic and organic ions	inorganic and organic ion sites
examples: $HPO_4^{2=}$	R^{+n} = quaternary ammonium salt
	X = synthetic ionophore complexing agent: aryl organotin compound or suggested cyclic polyamido-polyamines
HCO_3^{-}	X = synthetic ionophore: trifluoro acetophenone
Cl^{-}	X = aliphatic organotin compound

5. Bioaffinity sensors based on change of local electron densities

$$S + R \rightleftharpoons SR$$

chemical signal S	receptor R
protein	dyes
saccharide	lectin
glycoprotein	
substrate	enzyme
inhibitor	
	Transferases
	Hydrolases (peptidases, esterases, etc.)
	Lyases
	Isomerases
	Ligases
prosthetic group	apoenzyme
antigen	antibody
hormone	"receptor"
sustrate analogue	transport system

6. Metabolism sensors based on substrate consumption and product formation

$$S + R \rightleftharpoons SR \rightarrow P + R$$

chemical signal S	receptor R
substrate	enzyme
examples: lactate (SH_2)	hydrogenases catalyze hydrogen transfer from S to acceptor A (not molecular oxygen!) reversibly
$SH_2 + A \rightleftharpoons S + AH_2$	pyruvate + NADH + H^+ using lactate
lactate + NAD^+	dehydrogenase
glucose (SH_2)	oxidases catalyze hydrogen transfer to molecular oxygen using glucose oxidase
$SH_2 + \frac{1}{2} O_2 \rightleftharpoons S + H_2O$ or	
$SH_2 + O_2 \rightleftharpoons S + H_2O_2$	
glucose + $O_2 \rightleftharpoons$ gluconolactone + H_2O_2	
reducing agents (S)	peroxidases catalyze oxidation of a substrate by H_2O_2
$2S + 2H^+ + H_2O_2 \rightleftharpoons 2S^+ + 2H_2O$	using horseradish peroxidase
$Fe^{2+} + H_2O_2 + 2H^+ \rightleftharpoons Fe^{3+} + 2H_2O$	
reducing agents	oxygenases catalyze substrate oxidations by molecular O_2
L-lactate + $O_2 \rightleftharpoons$ acetate + CO_2 + H_2O	
cofactor	organelle
inhibitor	microbe
activator	tissue slice
enzyme activity	

7. Coupled and hybrid systems using sequences, competition, anti-interference and amplification concepts and reactions

8. Biomimetic sensors

chemical signal S	receptor R
sound	carrier-enzyme
stress	
light	

Source: Adapted from [2, 6].

and chemical properties are given equal weight. There are many ideas given here that remain without embodiment. This list is reproduced as Table 53.2. Of particular interest in this section are "detection means used in sensors" and "sensor conversion phenomena." At present the principle transduction schemes use electrochemical, optical, and thermal detection effects and principles.

Calorimetric, Thermometric, and Pyroelectric Transducers

Especially useful for enzymatic reactions, the generation of heat (enthalpy change) can be used easily and generally. The enzyme provides the selectivity and the reaction enthalpy cannot be confused with other reactions from species in a typical biologic mixture. The ideal aim is to measure total evolved heat, i.e., to perform a calorimetric measurement. In real systems there is always heat loss, i.e., heat is conducted away by the sample and sample container so that the process cannot be adiabatic as required for a total heat evolution measurement. As a result, temperature difference before and after evolution is measured most often. It has to be assumed that the heat capacity of the specimen and container is constant over the small temperature range usually measured.

The simplest transducer is a thermometer coated with the enzyme that permits the selected reaction to proceed. Thermistors are used rather than thermometers or thermocouples. The change of resistance of certain oxides is much greater than the change of length of a mercury column or the microvolt changes of thermocouple junctions.

TABLE 53.2 Detection Means and Conversion Phenomena Used in Sensors

Detection means
Biologic
Chemical
Electric, magnetic, or electromagnetic wave
Heat, temperature
Mechanical displacement of wave
Radioactivity, radiation
Other
Conversion phenomena
Biologic
Biochemical transformation
Physical transformation
Effect on test organism
Spectroscopy
Other
Chemical
Chemical transformation
Physical transformation
Electrochemical process
Spectroscopy
Other
Physical
Thermoelectric
Photoelectric
Photomagnetic
Magnetoelectric
Elastomagnetic
Thermoelastic
Elastoelectric
Thermomagnetic
Thermooptic
Photoelastic
Other

Pyroelectric heat flow transducers are relatively new. Heat flows from a heated region to a lower temperature region, controlled to occur in one dimension. The lower temperature side can be coated with an enzyme. When the substrate is converted, the lower temperature side is warmed. The pyroelectric material is from a category of materials that develops a spontaneous voltage difference in a thermal gradient. If the gradient is disturbed by evolution or adsorption of heat, the voltage temporarily changes.

In biomedical sensing, some of the solid-state devices based on thermal sensing cannot be used effectively. The reason is that the sensor itself has to be heated or is heated quite hot by catalytic surface reactions. Thus pellistors (oxides with catalytic surfaces and embedded platinum wire thermometer), chemiresistors, and "Figaro" sensor "smoke" detectors have not found many biologic applications.

Optical, Optoelectronic Transducers

Most optical detection systems for sensors are small, i.e., they occupy a small region of space because the sample size and volume are themselves small. This means that common absorption spectrophotometers and photofluorometers are not used with their conventional sample-containing cells or with their conventional beam-handling systems. Instead light-conducting *optical fibers* are used to connect the sample with the more remote monochromator and optical readout system. The techniques still remain absorption spectrophotometry, fluorimetry including fluorescence quenching, and reflectometry.

The most widely published optical sensors use a miniature reagent contained or immobilized at the tip of an optical fiber. In most systems a permselective membrane coating allows the detected species to penetrate the dye region. The corresponding absorption change, usually at a sensitive externally preset wavelength, is changed and correlated with the sample concentration. Similarly, fluorescence can be stimulated by the higher-frequency external light source and the lower-frequency emission detected. Some configurations are illustrated in references [1, 2]. Fluorimetric detection of coenzyme A, NAD$^+$/NADH, is involved in many so-called pyridine-linked enzyme systems. The fluorescence of NADH contained or immobilized can be a convenient way to follow these reactions. Optodes, miniature encapsulated dyes, can be placed in vivo. Their fluorescence can be enhanced or quenched and used to detect acidity, oxygen, and other species.

A subtle form of optical transduction uses the "peeled" optical fiber as a multiple reflectance cell. The normal fiber core glass has a refractive index greater than that of the exterior coating; there is a range of angles of entry to the fiber so that *all* the light beam remains inside the core. If the coating is removed and materials of lower index of refraction are coated on the exterior surface, there can be absorption by multiple reflections, since the evanescent wave can peretrate the coating. Chemical reagent can be added externally to create selective layers on the optical fiber.

Ellipsometry is a reflectance technique that depends on the optical constants and thickness of surface layer. For colorless layers, a polarized light beam will change its plane of polarization upon reflection by the surface film. The thickness can sometimes be determined when optical constants are known or approximated by constants of the bulk material. Antibody-antigen surface reaction can be detected this way.

Piezoelectric Transducers

Cut quartz crystals have characteristic modes of vibration that can be induced by painting electrodes on the opposite surfaces and applying a megaHertz ac voltage. The frequency is searched until the crystal goes into a resonance. The resonant frequency is very stable. It is a property of the material and maintains a value to a few parts per hundred million. When the surface is coated with a stiff mass, the frequency is altered. The shift in frequency is directly related to the surface mass for thin, stiff layers. The reaction of a substrate with this layer changes the constants of the film and further shifts the resonant frequency. These devices can be used in air, in vacuum, or in electrolyte solutions.

Electrochemical Transducers

Electrochemical transducers are commonly used in the sensor field. The main forms of electrochemistry used are potentiometry [zero-current cell voltage (potential difference measurements)], amperometry (current measurement at constant applied voltage at the working electrode), and ac conductivity of a cell.

Potentiometric Transduction

The classical generation of an activity-sensitive voltage is spontaneous in a solution containing both nonredox ions and redox ions. Classical electrodes of types 1, 2, and 3 respond by ion exchange directly or indirectly to ions of the same material as the electrode. Inert metal electrodes (sometimes called *type 0*)—Pt, Ir, Rh, and occasionally carbon C—respond by electron exchange from redox pairs in solution. Potential differences are interfacial and reflect ratios of activities of oxidized to reduced forms.

Amperometric Transduction

For dissolved species that can exchange electrons with an inert electrode, it is possible to force the transfer in one direction by applying a voltage very oxidizing (anodic) or reducing (cathodic). When the voltage is fixed, the species will be, by definition, out of equilibrium with the electrode at its present applied voltage. Locally, the species (regardless of charge) will oxidize or reduce by moving from bulk solution to the electrode surface where they react. Ions do not move like electrons. Rather they diffuse from high to low concentration and do not usually move by drift or migration. The reason is that the electrolytes in solutions are at high concentrations, and the electric field is virtually eliminated from the bulk. The field drops through the first 1000 Angstroms at the electrode surface. The concentration of the moving species is from high concentration in bulk to zero at the electrode surface where it reacts. This process is called *concentration polarization*. The current flowing is limited by mass transport and so is proportional to the bulk concentration.

Conductometric Transducers

Ac conductivity (impedance) can be purely resistive when the frequency is picked to be about 1000 to 10,000 Hz. In this range the transport of ions is sufficiently slow that they never lose their uniform concentration. They simply quiver in space and carry current forward and backward each half cycle. In the lower and higher frequencies, the cell capacitance can become involved, but this effect is to be avoided.

3.3 Tables of Sensors from the Literature

The longest and most consistently complete references to the chemical sensor field is the review issue of *Analytical Chemistry Journal.* In the 1970s and 1980s these appeared in the April issue, but more recently they appear in the June issue. The editors are Jiri Janata and various colleagues [7–10]. Not all possible or imaginable sensors have been made according to the list in Table 53.2. A more realistic table can be constructed from the existing literature that describes actual devices. This list is Table 53.3. Book references are listed in Table 53.4 in reverse time order to about 1986. This list covers

TABLE 53.3 Chemical Sensors and Properties Documented in the Literature

I.   General topics including items II-V: selectivity, fabrication, data processing
II.   Thermal sensors
III.   Mass sensors
Gas sensors
Liquid sensors
IV.   Electrochemical sensors
Potentiometric sensors
References electrodes
Biomedical electrodes
Applications to cations, anions
Coated wire/hybrids
ISFETs and related
Biosensors
Gas sensors
Amperometric sensors
Modified electrodes
Gas sensors
Biosensors
Direct electron transfer
Mediated electron transfer
Biomedical
Conductimetric sensors
Semiconducting oxide sensors
Zinc oxide-based
Chemiresistors
Dielectrometers
V.   Optical sensors
Liquid sensors
Biosensors
Gas sensors

most of the major source books and many of the symposium proceedings volumes. The reviews [7–10] are a principal source of references to the published research literature.

53.4 Applications of Microelectronics in Sensor Fabrication

The reviews of sensors since 1988 cover fabrication papers and microfabrication methods and examples [7–10]. A recent review by two of the few *chemical* sensor scientists (chemical engineers) who

TABLE 53.4   Books and Long Reviews Keyed to Items in Table 53.3
(Reviewed since 1988 in reverse time sequence)

I. Yamauchi S (ed). 1992. Chemical Sensor Technology, vol 4, Tokyo, Kodansha Ltd.

    Flores JR, Lorenzo E. 1992. Amperometric Biosensors, In MR Smyth, JG Vos (eds), Comprehensive Analytical Chemistry Amsterdam, Elsevier.

    Vaihinger S, Goepel W. 1991. Multicomponent analysis in chemical sensing. In W Goepel, J Hesse, J Zemel (eds), Sensors vol 2 Part 1, pp 191–237, Weinheim, Germany, VCH Publishers.

    Wise DL (ed). 1991. Bioinstrumentation and Biosensors, New York, Marcel Dekker.

    Scheller F, Schubert F. 1989. Biosensors, Basel, Switzerland, Birkhauser Verlag, see also [2].

    Madou M, Morrison SR. 1989. Chemical Sensing with Solid State Devices, New York, Academic Press.

    Janata J. 1989. Principles of Chemical Sensors, New York, Plenum Press.

    Edmonds TE (ed). 1988. Chemical Sensors, Glasgow, Blackie.

    Yoda K. 1988. Immobilized enzyme cells. Methods Enzymology, 137:61.

    Turner APF, Karube I, Wilson GS eds. 1987. Biosensors: Fundamentals and Applications, Oxford, Oxford University Press.

    Seiyama T (ed). 1986. Chemical Sensor Technology, Tokyo, Kodansha Ltd.

II. Thermal Sensor

    There are extensive research and application papers and these are mentioned in books listed under I. However, the up-to-date lists of papers are given in references 7–10.

III. Mass Sensors

    There are extensive research and application papers and these are mentioned in books listed under I. However, the up-to-date lists of papers are given in references 7–10. Fundamentals of this rapidly expanding field are recently reviewed:

    Buttry DA, Ward MD. 1992. Measurement of Interfacial processes at Electrode Surfaces with the Electrochemical Quartz Crystal Microbalance, Chemical Reviews 92:1355.

    Grate JW, Martin SJ, White RM. 1993. Acoustic Wave Microsensors, part 1, Analyt Chem 65:940A; part 2, Analyt Chem 65:987A.

    Ricco AT. 1994. SAW Chemical Sensors, The Electrochemical Society Interface Winter: 38–44.

IVA. Electrochemical Sensors—Liquid Samples

    Scheller F, Schmid RD (eds). 1992. Biosensors: Fundamentals, Technologies and Applications, GBF Monograph Series, New York, VCH Publishers.

    Erbach R, Vogel A, Hoffmann B. 1992. Ion-sensitive field-effect structures with Langmuir-Blodgett membranes, In F Scheller, RD Schmid (eds). Biosensors: Fundamentals, Technologies, and Applications, GBF Monograph 17, pp 353–357, New York, VCH Publishers.

    Ho May YK, Rechnitz GA. 1992. An Introduction to Biosensors, In RM Nakamura, Y Kasahara, GA Rechnitz (eds), Immunochemical Assays and Biosensors Technology, pp 275–291, Washington DC, American Society Microbiology.

    Mattiasson B, Haakanson H. Immunochemically-based assays for process control, 1992. Advances in Biochemical Engineering and Biotechnology 46:81.

    Maas AH, Sprokholt R. 1990. Proposed IFCC Recommendations for electrolyte measurements with ISEs in clinical chemistry, In A Ivaska, A Lewenstam, R Sara (eds), Contemporary Electroanalytical Chemistry, Proceedings of the ElectroFinnAnalysis International Conference on Electroanalytical Chemistry, pp 311–315, New York, Plenum.

    Vanrolleghem P, Dries D, Verstreate W. RODTOX: Biosensor for rapid determination of the biochemical oxygen demand, 1990. In C Christiansen, L Munck, J Villadsen, (eds), Proceedings of the 5th European Congress Biotechnology, vol 1, pp 161–164, Copenhagen, Denmark, Munksgaard.

    Cronenberg C, Van den Heuvel H, Van den Hauw M, Van Groen B. Development of glucose microelectrodes for measurements in biofilms, 1990. In C Christiansen, L Munck, J Villadsen J, (eds), Proceedings of the 5th European Congress Biotechnology, vol 1, pp 548–551, Copenhagen, Denmark, Munksgaard.

    Wise DL (ed). 1989. Bioinstrumentation Research, Development and Applications, Boston, MA, Butterworth-Heinemann.

Pungor E (ed). 1989. Ion-Selective Electrodes—Proceedings of the 5th Symposium (Matrafured, Hungary 1988), Oxford, Pergamon.

Wang J (ed). 1988. Electrochemical Techniques in Clinical Chemistry and Laboratory Medicine, New York, VCH Publishers.

Evans A. 1987. Potentiometry and Ion-selective Electrodes, New York, Wiley.

Ngo TT (ed) 1987. Electrochemical Sensors in Immunological Analysis, New York, Plenum.

IVB. Electrochemical Sensors—Gas Samples

Sberveglieri G (ed). 1992. Gas Sensors, Dordrecht , The Netherlands, Kluwer.

Moseley PT, Norris JOW, Williams DE. 1991. Technology and Mechanisms of Gas Sensors, Bristol, U.K., Hilger.

Moseley PT, Tofield BD (eds). 1989. Solid State Gas Sensors, Philadelphia, Taylor and Francis, Publishers.

V. Optical Sensors

Coulet PR, Blum LJ. Luminescence in Biosensor Design, 1991. In DL Wise, LB Wingard, Jr (eds). Biosensors with Fiberoptics, pp 293–324, Clifton, N.J., Humana.

Wolfbeis OS. 1991. Spectroscopic Techniques, In OS Wolfbeis (ed). Fiber Optic Chemical Sensors and Biosensors, vol 1, pp 25–60. Boca Raton, Fla, CRC Press.

Wolfbeis OS. 1987. Fibre-optic sensors for chemical parameters of interest in biotechnology, In RD Schmidt (ed). GBF (Gesellschaft fur Biotechnologische Forschung) Monogr. Series, vol 10, pp 197–206, New York, VCH Publishers.

also operate a microfabrication laboratory is C. C. Liu, Z.-R. Zhang. 1992. Research and development of chemical sensors using microfabrication techniques. Selective Electrode Rev 14:147.

References

1. Janata J. 1989. Principles of Chemical Sensors, New York, Plenum.
2. Scheller F, Schubert F. 1989. Biosensors, #18 in Advances in Research Technologies (Beitrage zur Forschungstechnologie), Berlin, Akademie-Verlag, Amsterdam, Elsevier (English translation).
3. Turner APF, Karube I, Wilson GS. 1987. Biosensors: Fundamentals and Applications, Oxford, Oxford University Press.
4. Hall EAH. 1990. Biosensors, Milton Keynes, England, Open University Press.
5. Eddoes MJ. 1990. Theoretical Methods for Analyzing Biosensor Performance. In AEG Cass (ed), Biosensor—A Practical Approach, Oxford, IRL Press at Oxford University Ch. 9 pp 211–262.
6. Cosofret VV, Buck RP. 1992. Pharmaceutical Applications of Membrane Sensors, Boca Raton, Fla, CRC Press.
7. Janata J, Bezegh A. 1988. Chemical sensors, Analyt Chem 60:62R.
8. Janata J. 1990. Chemical sensors, Analyt Chem 62:33R.
9. Janata J. 1992. Chemical sensors, Analyt Chem 66:196R.
10. Janata J, Josowicz M, DeVaney M. 1994. Chemical Sensors, Analyt Chem 66:207R.

Historical Perspectives 2
The Electrocardiograph

Leslie A. Geddes
Purdue University

Recording and display of bioelectric events occupied a long time and required the development and adaptation of a variety of primitive instruments, not all of which were electronic. The first bioelectric recorder was the rheoscopic frog, consisting of a sciatic nerve and its innervated gastrocnemius muscle. So sensitive was the nerve that it could be stimulated by the beating heart or a contracting muscle; both events contracted the gastrocnemius muscle. However, such a response provided no information on the time course of these bioelectric events. Sensitive and rapidly responding indicators of current were essential for this purpose.

As Etienne Jules Marey [1885], champion of the graphic method, stated:

> In effect, in the field of rigorous experimentation all the sciences give a hand. Whatever is the object of these studies, that which measures a force or movement, an electrical state or a temperature, whether he be a physician, chemist or physiologist, he has recourse to the same method and employs the same instruments.

Development of the galvanometer and the electric telegraph provided design concepts and instruments that could be adapted to the measurement of bioelectric events. For example, Thomson's reflecting telegraphic galvanometer was used by Caton [1875] to display the first electroencephalogram. Ader's telegraphic string galvanometer [1897] was modified by Einthoven [1903] to create the instrument that introduced clinical electrocardiography. Gasser and Erlanger [1922] adapted the Braun cathode-ray tube to enable recording of short-duration nerve action potentials. Garceau [1935] used the Western Union telegraphic recorder, called the Undulator, to create the first direct-inking electroencephalograph. However, in the early days of bioelectricity, ingenious electrophysiologists appropriated many devices from physics and engineering to establish the existence of bioelectric phenomena.

The First Electrocardiogram

The electrical activity accompanying the heartbeat was discovered with the rheoscopic frog by Kolliker and Mueller [1856]. When these investigators laid the nerve over the beating ventricle of a frog heart, the muscle twitched once and sometimes twice. Stimulation of the nerve obviously occurred with depolarization and repolarization of the ventricles. Because at that time there were no rapidly

0-8493-8346-3/95/$0.00+$.50
© 1995 by CRC Press, Inc.

responding galvanometers, Donders [1872] recorded the twitches of the rheoscope to provide a graphic demonstration of the existence of an electrocardiographic signal.

Capillary Electrometer Record

The capillary electrometer was created especially for recording the electrocardiogram. The principle underlying its operation was being investigated by Lippmann, a colleague of Marey in France. The phenomenon of electrocapillarity is the change in contour of a drop of mercury in dilute sulfuric acid when a current is passed through the mercury–sulfuric acid interface. This phenomenon was put to practical use by Marey [1876], who placed the interface in a capillary tube, transilluminated it, and recorded the contour change on a moving (falling) photographic plate. The two wires from the electrometer were connected to electrodes placed against the exposed tortoise ventricle. Figure HP2.1a illustrates the capillary electrometer, and Fig. HP2.1b is a reproduction of the tortoise ventricular electrogram showing what we now call the R and T waves.

Rheotome Record

Probably unaware that Marey had recorded the cardiac electrogram with the capillary electrometer, Burdon-Sanderson [1879] in England used a slow-speed, d'Arsonval-type galvanometer, the rheotome [see Hoff and Geddes, 1957], and induction-coil stimulator [see Geddes et al., 1989] to reconstruct the ventricular electrogram of the frog heart; Fig. HP2.2 illustrates his reconstruction, showing the R and T waves; note their similarity with those obtained by Marey in Fig. HP2.1b.

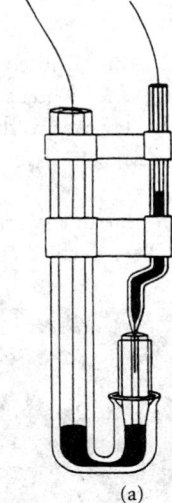

(a)

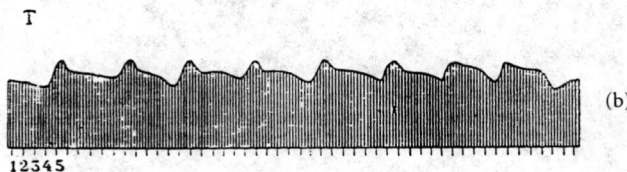

(b)

T

12345

FIGURE HP2.1   The capillary electrometer (a) used by Marey and Lippmann in 1876 and a tortoise ventricular electrogram (b) made with it. This is the first cardiac electrogram from a spontaneously beating heart.

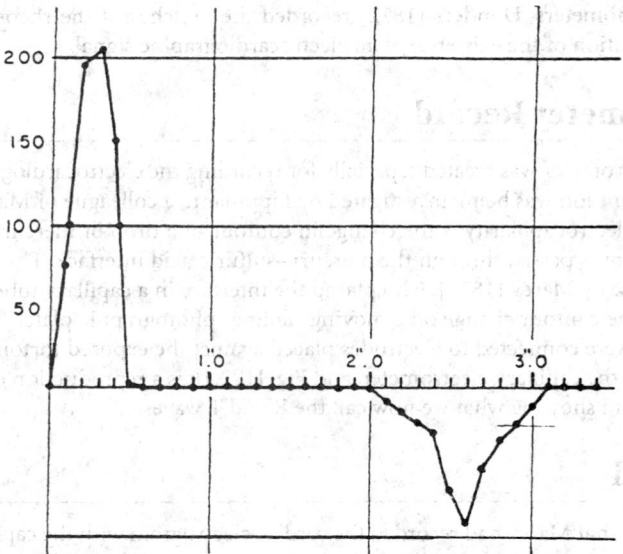

FIGURE HP2.2   Burdon-Sanderson's plot of the frog cardiac electrogram. Thirty-five points were determined to make the reconstruction. [Burdon-Sanderson and Page, 1879.]

Mammalian Electrocardiograms

When news of the capillary electrometer reached the United Kingdom, many investigators fabricated their own instruments. One of these was Waller, who used it to record the electrocardiogram of a patient whom he called Jimmy. In 1910, Waller revealed the identity of Jimmy, his pet bulldog, shown in Fig. HP2.3 having his ECG recorded with a forepaw and hindpaw in glass vessels containing saline and metal electrodes.

Waller [1887] obtained the first ECGs from human subjects; Fig. HP2.4*a* is one of his records, which displays the apex cardiogram and the capillary electrometer record, showing the R and T waves.

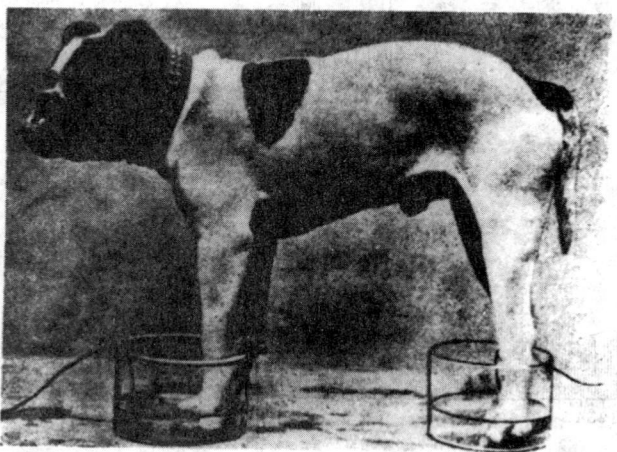

FIGURE HP2.3   Waller's patient Jimmy having his ECG recorded with the capillary electrometer. (From Waller AD, Hitchcock Lectures, University of London, 1910.)

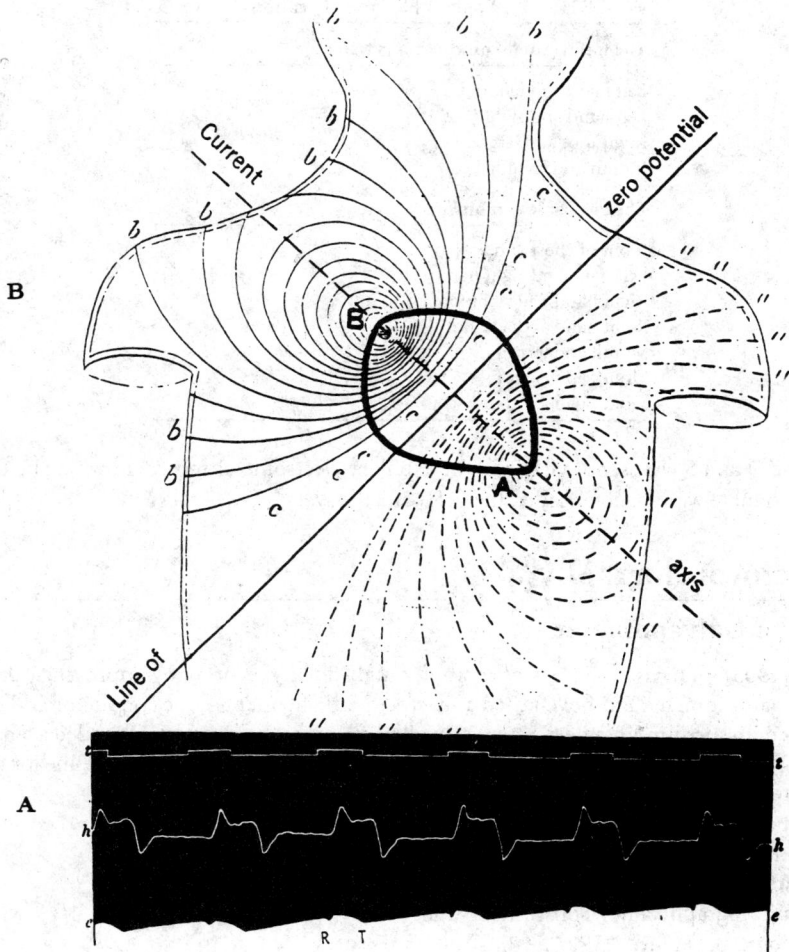

FIGURE HP2.4   First human apex cardiogram and capillary electrometer ECG (*a*) and the dipole map for the heart (*b*). (*a* from Waller [1887]; *b* from Waller [1889].)

At that time there were no standard sites for electrode placement. Using the extremities, Waller experimented with different sites, discovering that there were favorable and unfavorable sites, i.e., sites where the amplitude was large or small; Table HP2.1 summarizes his findings. From recordings made with these electrodes, Waller [1887] proposed that the heart could be represented as a dipole, as shown in Fig. HP2.4*b*.

Corrected Capillary Electrometer Records

By the 1890s, it was known that the response of the capillary electrometer was slow, and methods were developed to correct recordings to obtain a true voltage-time record. Burch [1892] in the United Kingdom developed a geometric method that used the tangent at each point along the recording. Figure HP2.5 is an illustration showing a capillary electrometer record (dark hump) and the true voltage-time record (biphasic waveform).

One who was very dissatisfied with capillary-electrometer records was Einthoven in the Netherlands. He obtained a capillary electrometer record from a subject (Fig. HP2.6*a*) and applied the correction method to create the ECG shown in Fig. HP2.6*b*, revealing the intimate details of what

TABLE HP2.1   Waller's Electrode Locations

The unfavorable combinations were:

Left hand and left foot
Left hand and right foot
Right foot and left foot
Mouth and right hand

The favorable combinations were:

Front of chest and back of chest
Left hand and right hand
Right hand and right foot
Right hand and left foot
Mouth and left hand
Mouth and right foot
Mouth and left foot

he called the Q and S waves, not visible in the capillary electrometer record, in which he used A, B, and C to designate what he later called the P, R, and T waves.

Clinical Electrocardiography

The String Galvanometer

Einthoven [1903] set himself the task of creating a high-fidelity recorder by improving Ader's string telegraphic galvanometer. Einthoven used a silvered quartz filament as the conductor and increased the field strength surrounding the filament by using a strong electromagnet. He added a lens to focus the image of the filament onto a moving photographic surface. Thus the thick baseline for the string galvanometer recording was the image of the "string" (quartz filament). Electrocardiac current caused the silvered filament to be deflected, and its excursions, when magnified optically and recorded photographically, constituted the electrocardiogram. Figure HP2.7a illustrates Einthoven's string galvanometer, and Fig. HP2.7b shows a patient in hospital clothing having his ECG recorded. Measurement of calibration records published by Einthoven reveals a response time (10% to 90%) of 20 ms. The corresponding sinusoidal frequency response is 0 to 25 Hz (30% attenuation).

Figure HP2.8 illustrates one of Einthoven's electromagnets (lower left) and one of his early cameras (center) and string galvanometers (right). Above the bench supporting these are mounted a bow and arrow, which were used by Einthoven to provide the tension on the quartz rod while it was being heated to the melting point, after which the arrow left the bow and extruded the rod to a long slender filament, which was later silvered to make it conducting.

Einthoven borrowed handsomely from previous work; he used Marey's recording chart speed (25 mm/s) and Waller's bucket electrodes, as well as some of his leads. With the string gal-

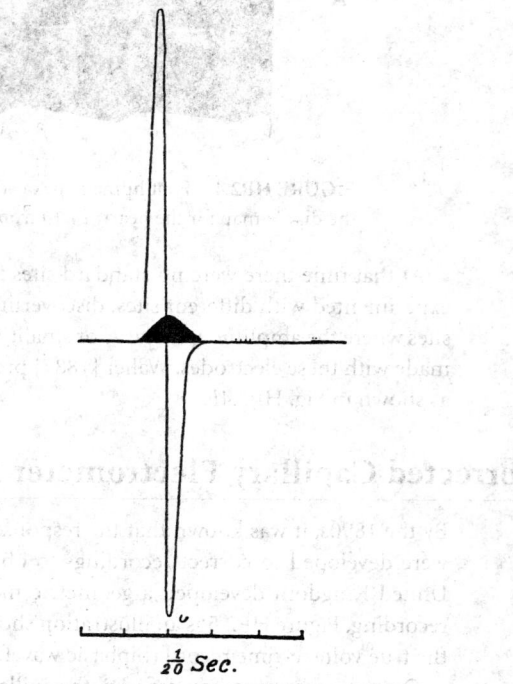

$\frac{1}{20}$ *Sec.*

FIGURE HP2.5   Capillary electrometer record (*dark hump*) and the corrected voltage-time record (*biphasic wave*).

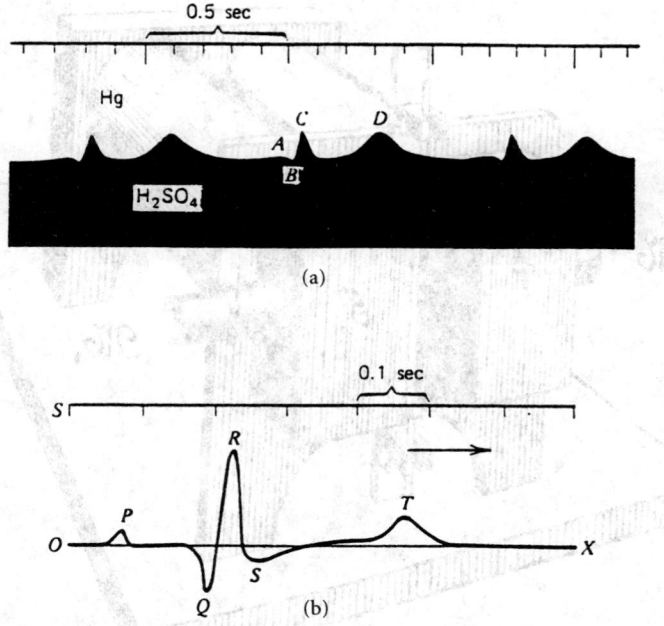

FIGURE HP2.6 A capillary electrometer record (*a*) and its corrected version (*b*) presented by Eithoven to show the inadequacy of the capillary electrometer in displaying rapidly changing waveforms. (From FA Willius. 1941. TE Keys, Cardiac Classics. St. Louis, Mosby.)

vanometer, Einthoven ushered in clinical electrocardiography in the early 1900s; soon the string galvanometer was used worldwide. The first string galvanometer appeared in the United States in 1912, when it was used at the Rockefeller Institute Hospital until 1959. This instrument, which is now in the Smithsonian Institution, was designed by Horatio B. Williams, professor of physiology at the College of Physicians and Surgeons at Columbia University. Williams had spent some time with Einthoven in Leiden in 1910 and 1911. On his return to New York, Williams had Charles F. Hindle, a machinist at Columbia, construct the first American string galvanometer. Soon thereafter, the Cambridge Instrument Company took over manufacture of the Hindle instrument and made them available for sale in the United States.

Although it is clear that the concept of an electrical axis, i.e., a cardiac vector, was demonstrated by Waller's studies, it remained for Einthoven [1913] to make practical use of the concept. Einthoven postulated that the heart was at the center of an equilateral triangle, the apices of which were the right and left shoulders and the point where both legs joined the trunk. In his early studies, Einthoven used the right and left arms and both feet in saline-filled buckets as the three electrodes. Soon he found that the electrocardiogram was negligibly altered if the right foot was removed from the bucket electrode. Thus he adopted three standard leads: right and left arms and left leg (foot). He postulated that if the amplitudes of the electrocardiographic waves are plotted on this triaxial reference frame, it is possible to calculate the magnitude and direction of an electric vector that produces these same voltages in leads I, II, and III, corresponding to the limb electrodes. He further stated that the arithmetic sum of the amplitudes in lead I plus lead III equals the amplitude in lead II. This is *Einthoven's law*, and the relationship is true only for an equilateral triangle reference frame [Valentinuzzi et al., 1970].

Vacuum-Tube Electrocardiograph

Not long after Einthoven described his string galvanometer, efforts were begun in the United States to create an electrocardiograph that used vacuum tubes. At that time, there were rapidly responding mirror galvanometers, as well as a limited number of vacuum tubes, despite the fact that they

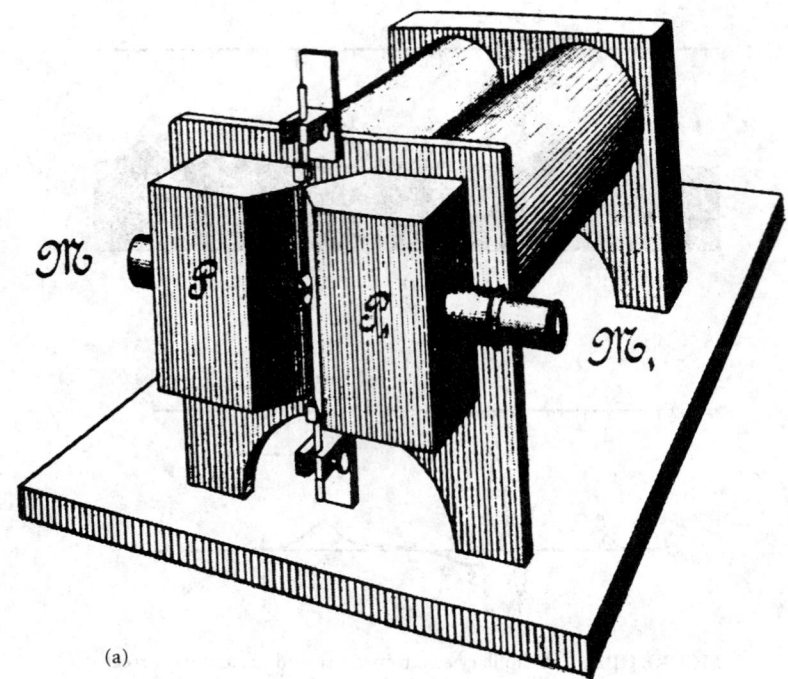

(a)

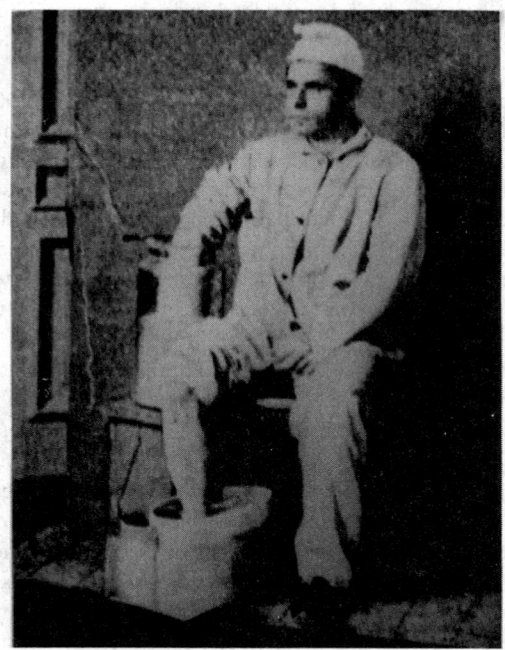

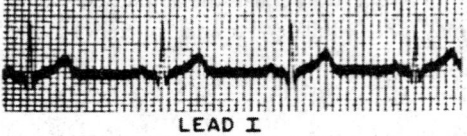

LEAD I

(b)

FIGURE HP2.7 Einthoven's string galvanmeter (*a*) and a patient having his ECG (lead 1) recorded (*b*).

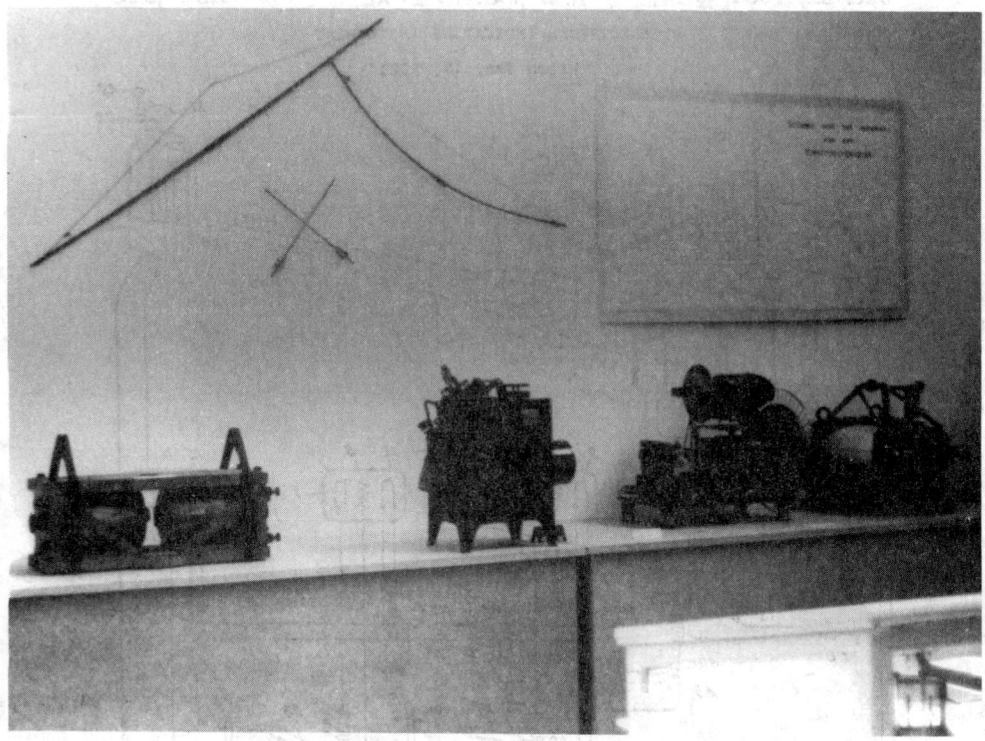

FIGURE HP2.8 Some of Einthoven's early equipment. On the bench (*left*) is an electromagnet. In the center is a camera, and on the right is a string galvanometer. On the wall are a bow and arrow; the latter was used to apply force to a quartz rod which was heated, and when pulled by the arrow, created the quartz filament which was later silvered.

had been patented only a few years earlier [1907] by DeForest. According to Marvin [1954], the first discussions relative to such an instrument were held in 1917 between Steinmetz, Neuman, and Robinson of the General Electric Engineering Laboratory. The task of establishing feasibility fell to W. R. G. Baker, who assembled a unit and demonstrated its operation to those just identified. However, because of urgent wartime priorities, the project was shelved.

In 1921, General Electric reopened the issue of a vacuum-tube ECG. A second prototype was built and demonstrated to the Schenectady County Medical Association some time in 1924 by Robinson and Marvin. The instrument was used by Drs. Neuman, Pardee, Mann, and Oppenheim, all physicians in New York City. Subsequently, six commercial models were made. One instrument was sent to each of the four physicians just identified; the fifth was sent to the General Electric Company Hospital; and the sixth was sent to the AMA Convention in Atlantic City in 1925. This latter instrument became a prototype for future models provided by the General Electric X-Ray Division. A U.S. patent application was filed on January 15, 1925, and the instrument was described by Mann [1930].

On December 22, 1931, a patent on the General Electric vacuum-tube ECG was granted to Marvin and Leibing; Fig. HP2.9 shows the circuit diagram of the instrument, including a specimen record (*lower left,* Fig. HP2.9). The instrument used three triode vacuum tubes in a single-sided, resistance-capacitance-coupled amplifier. It was battery operated, and a unique feature was a viewing screen that allowed the operator to see the motion of the galvanometer beam as it was being recorded by the camera.

Between introduction of the string galvanometer and the hot-stylus recorder for ECG, attempts were made to create direct-inking ECG recorders. In a review of scientific instruments, Brian

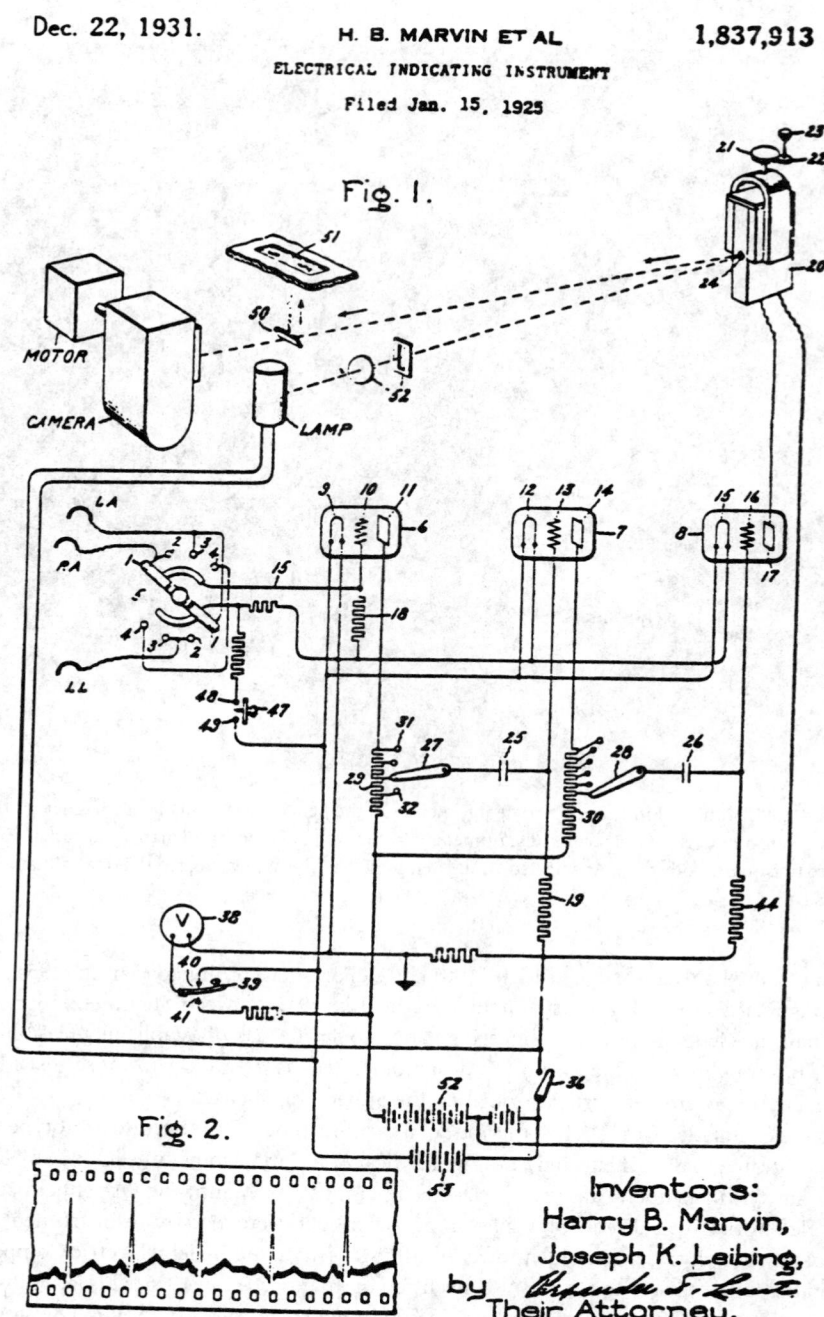

Dec. 22, 1931.   H. B. MARVIN ET AL   1,837,913
                              ELECTRICAL INDICATING INSTRUMENT
                                   Filed Jan. 15, 1925

Fig. 1.

Fig. 2.

Inventors:
Harry B. Marvin,
Joseph K. Leibing,
by
Their Attorney.

FIGURE HP2.9   Circuit diagram of the first vacuum-tube ECG, patented on December 12, 1931.

Matthews [1935] reported

There are two ink-writing electrocardiographs available, the author's and that of Drs. Duschel and Luthi. Both utilize a moving-iron driving unit with oil damping, a tubular pen writing on moving paper. The former has a battery-coupled amplifier. The latter gives in effect D.C.

amplification; the potentials to be recorded are interrupted about 500 times per second by a special type of buzzer, after amplification by resistance capacity coupled valves the interrupted output is rectified by the output valve; the amplifier achieves in effect what can be done with a battery-coupled amplifier and obviates the coupling batteries. At present the speed of these direct-recording instruments is barely adequate to show the finer details of the electrocardiogram, but they enable its main features to be recorded instantly.

Despite the instant availability of inked recordings of the ECG, those produced by the string galvanometer were superior, and it took some time for a competitor to appear. Such an instrument did appear in the form of the hot-stylus recorder.

Hot-Stylus Recorder

The final step toward modern electrocardiography was introduction of the hot-stylus recorder by Haynes [1936] of the Bell Telephone Laboratories (New York). Prior to that time, there was colored, wax-coated recording paper, the wax being scraped off by a recording stylus, exposing the colored paper. Referring to the scraping method, Haynes wrote

> However, the method is not adaptable to many types of recording instruments because of the large amount of friction between the recording stylus and paper arising from the pressure necessary to engrave the wax.
>
> This pressure can be removed and the friction largely eliminated by the use of a special stylus consisting essentially of a small electric heating coil situated close to the end of a pointed rod in such a way that the temperature of the pont may be raised to about 80°C. The point is then capable of melting the wax and engraving its surface with only a very small fraction of the pressure before necessary.
>
> The described stylus, when used with waxed recording paper, will provide a means of obtaining a permanent record without the use of pen and ink which is adaptable to the most sensitive recording instruments.

Following the end of World War II, vacuum-tube electrocardiographs with heated-stylus recorders became very popular; they are still in use today. However, the heritage of a thick baseline, derived from the string-galvanometer days, had to be preserved for some time because clinicians objected to a thin baseline. It took many years for the hot-stylus baseline to be narrowed without protest.

References

Ader M. 1897. Sur un nouvel appareil enregistreur pour cables sousmarins. C R Acad Sci 124:1440.

Burch GJ. 1892. On the time relations of the excursions of the capillary electrometer. Philos Trans R Soc (Lond) 83A:81.

Burch GJ. 1892. On a method of determining the value of rapid variations of potential by means of the capillary electrometer communicated by J. B. Sanderson. Proc R Soc (Lond) 48:89.

Burdon-Sanderson JS, Page FJM. 1879. On the time relations of the excitatory process of the ventricle of the heart of the frog. J Physiol (Lond) 2:384.

Caton R. 1875. The electric currents of the brain. Br Med 2:278.

DeForest L. U.S. patents 841,387 (1907) and 879,532 (1908).

Donders FC. 1872. De secondaire contracties order den involed der systolen van het hart, met en zonder vagus-prikkfung. Oncerszoek ged in h physiol Lab d Utrecht Hoogesch, Bd. 1, S. 256, Derde reeks TI p 246 bis 255.

Einthoven W. 1903. Ein neues Galvanometer. Ann Phys 12 (suppl 4):1059.

Einthoven W, Fahr G, de Waart A. 1913. Uber die Richtung und die manifeste Grosse der Potential schwankunzen in menschlichen Herzen. Pflugers Arch 150:275.

Garceau EL, Davis H. 1935. An ink-writing electroencephalograph. Arch Neurol Psychiatry 34:1292.

Gasser HS, Erlanger J. 1922. A study of the action currents of nerve with the cathode ray oscillograph. Am Physiol 62:496.

Gasser HS, Newcomer HS. 1921. Physiological action currents in the phrenic nerve. Am Physiol 57(1):1.

Geddes LA, Foster KS, Senior J, Kahfeld A. 1989. The Inductorium: The stimulator associated with discovery. Med Instrum 23(4):308.

Haynes JR. 1936. Heated stylus for use with waxed recording paper. Rev Sci Instrsum 7:108.

Hoff HE, Geddes LA. 1957. The rheotome and its prehistory: A study in the historical interrelation of electrophysiology and electromechanics. Bull Hist Med 31(3):212.

Kolliker RA, Muller J. 1856. Nachweiss der negativen Schwankung des Muskelstromsnaturlich sic contrakinenden Muskel: Verhandl. Phys Med Ges Wurzburg 6:528.

Mann H. 1930–31. A light weight portable EKG. Am Heart J 7:796.

Marey EJ. 1885. Methode Graphique, 2d ed. Paris, Masosn.

Marey EJ. 1876. Des variations electriques des muscles du coeur en particulier etudiee au moyen de l'ectrometre d M. Lippmann. C R Acad Sci 82:975.

Marvin HB, et al. 1925. U.S. patent 1,817,913.

Matthews BHC. 1935. Recent developments in electrical instruments for biological and medical purposes. J Sci Instrum 12(7):209.

Valentinuzzi ME, Geddes LA, Hoff HE, Bourland JD. 1970. Properties of the 30° hexaxial (Einthoven-Goldberger) system of vectorcardiography. Cardiovasc Res Cent Bull 9(2):64.

Waller AD. 1887. A demonstration on man of electromotive changes accompanying the heart's beat. J Physiol (Lond) 8:229.

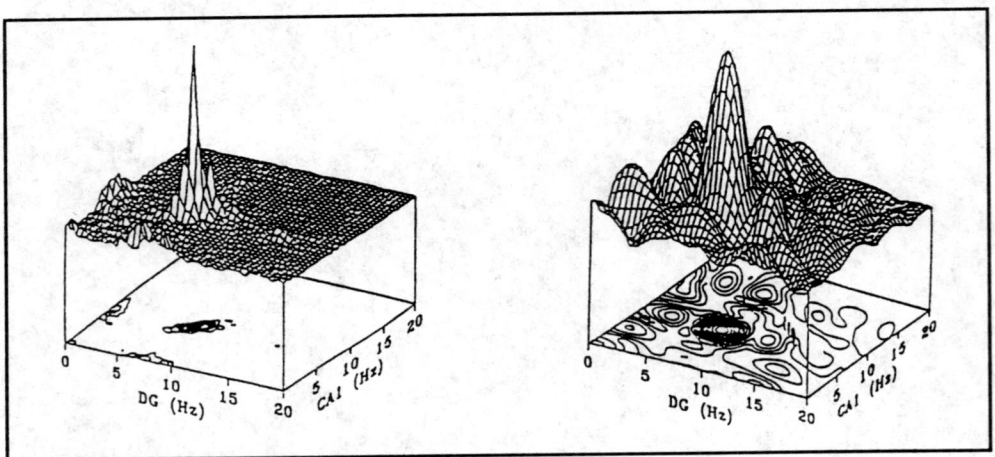

Cross-biospectral plots of hippocampal EEG.

VI

Biomedical Signal Analysis

Banu Onaral
Drexel University

B IOMEDICAL SIGNAL ANALYSIS CENTERS ON the acquisition and processing of information-bearing signals that emanate from living systems. These vital signals permit us to probe the state of the underlying biologic and physiologic structures and dynamics. Therefore, their interpretation has significant diagnostic value for clinicians and researchers.

The detected signals are commonly corrupted with noise. Often, the information cannot be readily extracted from the raw signal, which must be processed in order to yield useful results. Signals and systems engineering knowledge and, in particular, signal-processing expertise are therefore critical in all phases of signal collection and analysis.

Biomedical engineers are called on to conceive and implement processing schemes suitable for biomedical signals. They also play a key role in the design and development of biomedical monitoring devices and systems that match advances in signal processing and instrumentation technologies with biomedical needs and requirements.

This section is organized in two main parts. In the first part, contributing authors review contemporary methods in biomedical signal processing. The second part is devoted to emerging methods that hold the promise for major enhancements in our ability to extract information from vital signals.

The success of signal-processing applications strongly depends on the knowledge about the origin and the nature of the signal. Biomedical signals possess many special properties and hence require special treatment. Also, the need for noninvasive measurements presents unique challenges that demand a clear understanding of biomedical signal characteristics. In the lead chapter, entitled, "Biomedical Signals: Origin and Dynamic Characteristics; Frequency-Domain Analysis," Arnon Cohen provides a general classification of biomedical signals and discusses basics of frequency domain methods.

The advent of digital computing coupled with fast progress in discrete-time signal processing has led to efficient and flexible methods to acquire and treat biomedical data in digital form. The chapter entitled, "Digital Biomedical Signal Acquisition and Processing," by Luca T. Mainardi, Anna M. Bianchi, and Sergio Cerutti, presents basic elements of signal acquisition and processing in the special context of biomedical signals.

Especially in the case of long-term monitoring, digital biomedical signal-processing applications generate vast amounts of data that strain transmission and storage resources. The creation of multipatient reference signal bases also places severe demands on storage. Data compression methods overcome these obstacles by eliminating signal redundancies while retaining clinically significant information. A. Enis Cetin and Hayrettin Köymen provide a comparative overview of a range of approaches from conventional to modern compression techniques suitable for biomedical signals. Futuristic applications involving long-term and ambulatory recording systems, and remote diagnosis opportunities will be made possible by breakthroughs in biomedical data compression. This chapter serves well as a point of departure.

Constraints such as stationarity (and time invariance), gaussianity (and minimum phaseness), and the assumption of a characteristic scale in time and space have constituted the basic, and by now implicit, assumptions upon which the conventional signals and systems theories have been founded.

However, investigators engaged in the study of biomedical processes have long known that they did not hold under most realistic situations and hence could not sustain the test of practice.

Rejecting or at least relaxing restrictive assumptions always opens new avenues for research and yields fruitful results. Liberating forces in signals and systems theories have conspired in recent years to create research fronts that target long-standing constraints in the established wisdom (dogma?) of classic signal processing and system analysis. The emergence of new fields in signals and system theories that address these shortcomings and aim to relax these restrictions has been motivated by scientists who, rather than mold natural behavior into artificial models, seek methods inherently suited to represent reality. Biomedical scientists and engineers are inspired by insights gained from a deeper appreciation for the dynamic richness displayed by biomedical phenomena; hence, more than their counterparts in other disciplines, they more forcefully embrace innovations in signal processing.

One of these novel directions is concerned with time-frequency representations tailored for nonstationary and transient signals. Faye Boudreaux-Bartels and Robin Murray address this issue, provide an introduction to concepts and tools of time-frequency analysis, and point out candidate applications.

Many physiologic structures and dynamics defy the concept of a characteristic spatial and temporal scale and must be dealt with employing methods compatible with their multiscale nature. Judging from the recent success of biomedical signal-processing applications based on time-scale analysis and wavelet transforms, the resolution of many outstanding processing issues may be at hand. The chapter entitled, "Time-Scale Analysis and Wavelets in Biomedical Signals," by Nitish V. Thakor, familiarizes the reader with fundamental concepts and methods of wavelet analysis and suggests fruitful directions in biomedical signal processing.

The presence of nonlinearities and statistics that do not comply with the gaussianity assumption and the desire for phase reconstruction have been the moving forces behind investigations of higher-order statistics and polyspectra in signal-processing and system-identification fields. An introduction to the topic and potential uses in biomedical signal-processing applications are presented by Athina Petropulu in the chapter entitled, "Higher-Order Spectra in Biomedical Signal Processing."

Neural networks derive their cue from biologic systems and, in turn, mimic many of the functions of the nervous system. Simple networks can filter, recall, switch, amplify, and recognize patterns and hence serve well many signal-processing purposes. In the chapter entitled, "Neural Networks in Biomedical Signal Processing," Evangelia Tzanakou helps the reader explore the power of the approach while stressing how biomedical signal-processing applications benefit from incorporating neural-network principles.

The dichotomy between order and disorder is now perceived as a ubiquitous property inherent to the unfolding of many natural complex phenomena. In the last decade, it has become clear that the common thread shared by natural forms and functions are the "physics of disorder" and the "scaling order," the hallmark of broad classes of fractal entities. Biomedical signals are the global observables of underlying complex physical and physiologic processes. "Complexity" theories therefore hold the potential to provide mathematical tools that describe and possibly shed light on the internal workings of physiologic systems. In the next to last chapter in this section, Banu Onaral and Joseph P. Cammarota introduce the reader to basic tenets of complexity theories and the attendant scaling concepts with hopes to facilitate their integration into the biomedical engineering practice.

The section concludes with a brief chapter on the visions of the future when biomedical signal processing will merge with the rising technologies in telecommunication and multimedia computing, and eventually with virtual reality, to enable remote monitoring, diagnosis, and intervention. The impact of this development on the delivery of health care and the quality of life will no doubt be profound. The promise of biomedical signal analysis will then be fulfilled.

54

Biomedical Signals: Origin and Dynamic Characteristics; Frequency-Domain Analysis

Arnon Cohen
Ben-Gurion University

A *signal* is a phenomenon that conveys information. Biomedical signals are signals, used in biomedical fields, mainly for extracting information on a biologic system under investigation. The complete process of information extraction may be as simple as a physician estimating the patient's mean heart rate by feeling, with the fingertips, the blood pressure pulse or as complex as analyzing the structure of internal soft tissues by means of a complex CT machine.

Most often in biomedical applications (as in many other applications), the acquisition of the signal is not sufficient. It is required to process the acquired signal to get the relevant information "buried" in it. This may be due to the fact that the signal is noisy and thus must be "cleaned" (or in more professional terminology, the signal has to be enhanced) or due to the fact that the relevant information is not "visible" in the signal. In the latter case, we usually apply some transformation to enhance the required information.

The processing of biomedical signals poses some unique problems. The reason for this is mainly the complexity of the underlying system and the need to perform indirect, noninvasive measurements. A large number of processing methods and algorithms is available. In order to apply the best method, the user must know the goal of the processing, the test conditions, and the characteristics of the underlying signal. In this chapter, the characteristics of biomedical signals will be discussed [Cohen, 1986]. Biomedical signals will be divided into characteristic classes, requiring different classes of processing methods. Also in this chapter, the basics of frequency-domain processing methods will be presented.

54.1 Origin of Biomedical Signals

From the broad definition of the biomedical signal presented in the preceding section, it is clear that biomedical signals differ from other signals only in terms of the application—signals that are used in the biomedical field. As such, biomedical signals originate from a variety of sources. The following is a brief description of these sources:

- *Bioelectric signals.* The bioelectric signal is unique to biomedical systems. It is generated by nerve cells and muscle cells. Its source is the membrane potential, which under certain conditions may be excited to generate an action potential. In single cell measurements, where specific microelectrodes are used as sensors, the action potential itself is the biomedical signal. In more gross measurements, where, for example, surface electrodes are used as sensors, the electric field generated by the action of many cells, distributed in the electrode's vicinity, constitutes the bioelectric signal. Bioelectric signals are probably the most important biosignals. The fact that most important biosystems use excitable cells makes it possible to use biosignals to study and monitor the main functions of the systems. The electric field propagates through the biologic medium, and thus the potential may be acquired at relatively convenient locations on the surface, eliminating the need to invade the system. The bioelectric signal requires a relatively simple transducer for its acquisition. A transducer is needed because the electric conduction in the biomedical medium is done by means of ions, while the conduction in the measurement system is by electrons. All these lead to the fact that the bioelectric signal is widely used in most fields of biomedicine.

- *Bioimpedance signals.* The impedance of the tissue contains important information concerning its composition, blood volume, blood distribution, endocrine activity, automatic nervous system activity, and more. The bioimpedance signal is usually generated by injecting into the tissue under test sinusoidal currents (frequency range of 50 kHz to 1 MHz, with low current densities of the order of 20 μA to 20 mA). The frequency range is chosen to minimize electrode polarization problems, and the low current densities are chosen to avoid tissue damage mainly due to heating effects. Bioimpedance measurements are usually performed with four electrodes. Two source electrodes are connected to a current source and are used to inject the current into the tissue. The two measurement electrodes are placed on the tissue under investigation and are used to measure the voltage drop generated by the current and the tissue impedance.

- *Bioacoustic signals.* Many biomedical phenomena create acoustic noise. The measurement of this acoustic noise provides information about the underlying phenomenon. The flow of blood in the heart, through the heart's valves, or through blood vessels generates typical acoustic noise. The flow of air through the upper and lower airways and in the lungs creates acoustic sounds. These sounds, known as coughs, snores, and chest and lung sounds, are used extensively in medicine. Sounds are also generated in the digestive tract and in the joints. It also has been observed that the contracting muscle produces an acoustic noise (muscle noise). Since the acoustic energy propagates through the biologic medium, the bioacoustic signal may be conveniently acquired on the surface, using acoustic transducers (microphones or accelerometers).

- *Biomagnetic signals.* Various organs, such as the brain, heart, and lungs, produce extremely weak magnetic fields. The measurement of these fields provides information not included in other biosignals (such as bioelectric signals). Due to the low level of the magnetic fields to be measured, biomagnetic signals are usually of very low signal-to-noise ratio. Extreme caution must be taken in designing the acquisition system of these signals.
- *Biomechanical signals.* The term *biomechanical signals* includes all signals used in the biomedicine fields that originate from some mechanical function of the biologic system. These signals include motion and displacement signals, pressure and tension and flow signals, and others. The measurement of biomechanical signals requires a variety of transducers, not always simple and inexpensive. The mechanical phenomenon does not propagate, as do the electric, magnetic, and acoustic fields. The measurement therefore usually has to be performed at the exact site. This very often complicates the measurement and forces it to be an invasive one.
- *Biochemical signals.* Biochemical signals are the result of chemical measurements from the living tissue or from samples analyzed in the clinical laboratory. Measuring the concentration of various ions inside and in the vicinity of a cell by means of specific ion electrodes is an example of such a signal. Partial pressures of oxygen (pO_2) and of carbon dioxide (pCO_2) in the blood or respiratory system are other examples. Biochemical signals are most often very low frequency signals. Most biochemical signals are actually dc signals.
- *Biooptical signals.* Biooptical signals are the result of optical functions of the biologic system, occurring naturally or induced by the measurement. Blood oxygenation may be estimated by measuring the transmitted and backscattered light from a tissue (in vivo or in vitro) in several wavelengths. Important information about the fetus may be acquired by measuring fluorescence characteristics of the amniotic fluid. Estimation of the heart output may be performed by the dye dilution method, which requires the monitoring of the appearance of recirculated dye in the bloodstream. The development of fiberoptic technology has opened vast applications of biooptical signals.

Table 54.1 lists some of the more common biomedical signals with some of their characteristics.

54.2 Classification of Biosignals

Biosignals may be classified in many ways. The following is a brief discussion of some of the most important classifications.

- *Classification according to source.* Biosignals may be classified according to their source or physical nature. This classification was described in the preceding section. This classification may be used when the basic physical characteristics of the underlying process is of interest, e.g., when a model for the signal is desired.
- *Classification according to biomedical application.* The biomedical signal is acquired and processed with some diagnostic, monitoring, or other goal in mind. Classification may be constructed according to the field of application, e.g., cardiology or neurology. Such classification may be of interest when the goal is, for example, the study of physiologic systems.
- *Classification according to signal characteristics.* From point of view of signal analysis, this is the most relevant classification method. When the main goal is processing, it is not relevant what is the source of the signal or to which biomedical system it belongs; what matters are the signal characteristics.

We recognize two broad classes of signals: *continuous signals* and *discrete signals*. Continuous signals are described by a continuous function $s(t)$ which provides information about the signal at any given time. Discrete signals are described by a *sequence* $s(m)$ which provides information at a given discrete point on the time axis. Most of the biomedical signals are continuous. Since current tech-

TABLE 54.1 Biomedical Signals

Classification	Acquisition	Frequency Range	Dynamic Range	Comments
Bioelectric				
Action potential	Microelectrodes	100 Hz–2 kHz	10 μV–100 mV	Invasive measurement of cell membrane potential
Electroneurogram (ENG)	Needle electrode	100 Hz–1 kHz	5 μV–10 mV	Potential of a nerve bundle
Electroretinogram (ERG)	Microelectrode	0.2–200 Hz	0.5 μV–1 mV	Evoked flash potential
Electro-oculogram (EOG)	Surface electrodes	dc–100 Hz	10 μV–5 mV	Steady corneal-retinal potential
Electroencephalogram (EEG)				
Surface	Surface electrodes	0.5–100 Hz	2–100 μV	Multichannel (6–32) scalp potential
Delta range		0.5–4 Hz		Young children, deep sleep and pathologies
Theta range		4–8 Hz		Temporal and central areas during alert states
Alpha range		8–13 Hz		Awake, relaxed, closed eyes
Beta range		13–22 Hz		
Sleep spindles		6–15 Hz	50–100 μV	Bursts of about 0.2 to 0.6 s
K-complexes		12–14 Hz	100–200 μV	Bursts during moderate and deep sleep
Evoked potentials (EP)	Surface electrodes		0.1–20 μV	Response of brain potential to stimulus
Visual (VEP)		1–300 Hz	1–20 μV	Occipital lobe recordings, 200-ms duration
Somatosensory (SEP)		2 Hz–3 kHz		Sensory cortex
Auditory (AEP)		100 Hz–3 kHz	0.5–10 μV	Vertex recordings
Electrocorticogram	Needle electrodes	100 Hz–5kHz		Recordings from exposed surface of brain
Electromyography (EMG)				
Single-fiber (SFEMG)	Needle electrode	500 Hz–10 kHz	1–10 mV	Action potentials from single muscle fiber
Motor unit action Potential (MUAP)	Needle electrode	5 Hz–10 kHz	100 μV–2 mV	
Surface EMG (SEMG)	Surface electrodes			
Skeletal muscle		2–500 Hz	50 μV–5 mV	
Smooth muscle		0.01–1 Hz		
Electrocardiogram (ECG)	Surface electrodes	0.05–100 Hz	1–10 mV	
High-Frequency ECG	Surface electrodes	100 Hz–1 kHz	100 μV–2 mV	Notchs and slus waveforms super-imposed on the ECG.

nology provides powerful tools for discrete signal processing, we most often transform a continuous signal into a discrete one by a process known as *sampling*. A given signal $s(t)$ is sampled into the sequence $s(m)$ by

$$s(m) = s(t)|_{t=mT_s} \qquad m = \ldots, -1, 0, 1, \ldots \qquad (54.1)$$

where T_s is the sampling interval and $f_s = (2\pi/T_s)$ is the sampling frequency. Further characteristic classification, which applies to continuous as well as discrete signals, is described in Fig. 54.1.

We divide signals into two main groups: *deterministic* and *stochastic* signals. Deterministic signals are signals that can be exactly described mathematically or graphically. If a signal is deterministic and its mathematical description is given, it conveys no information. Real-world signals are never deterministic. There is always some unknown and unpredictable noise added, some unpredictable change in the parameters and the underlying characteristics of the signal that render it nondeterministic. It is, however, very often convenient to approximate or model the signal by means of a deterministic function.

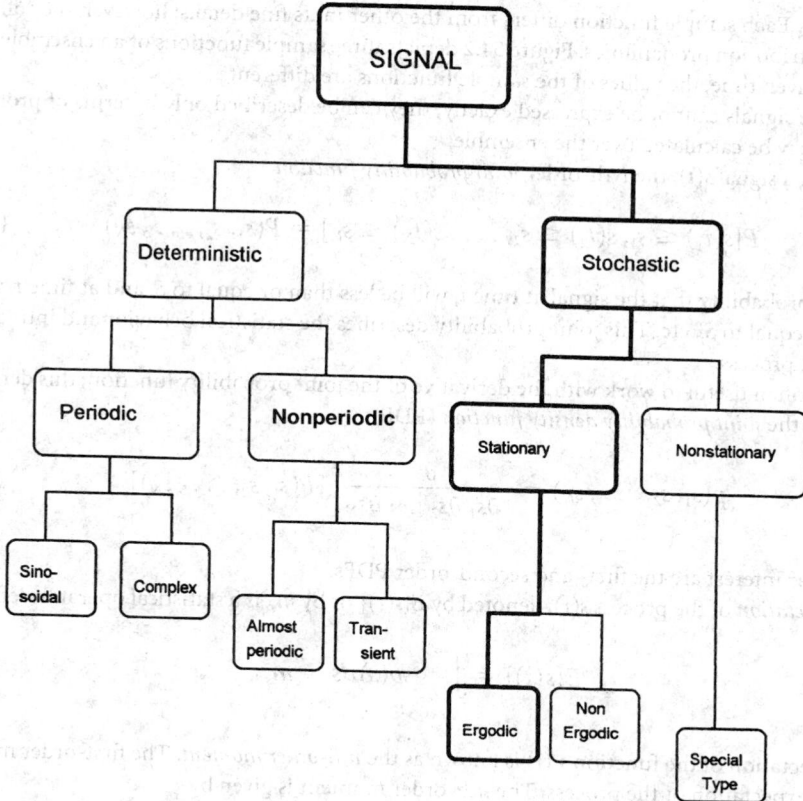

FIGURE 54.1 Classification of signals according to characteristics.

An important family of deterministic signals is the periodic family. A *periodic signal* is a deterministic signal that may be expressed by

$$s(t) = s(t + nT) \qquad (54.2)$$

where n is an integer, and T is the period. The periodic signal consists of a basic wave shape with a duration of T seconds. The basic wave shape repeats itself an infinite number of times on the time axis. The simplest periodic signal is the sinusoidal signal. Complex periodic signals have more elaborate wave shapes. Under some conditions, the blood pressure signal may be modeled by a complex periodic signal, with the heart rate as its period and the blood pressure wave shape as its basic wave shape. This is, of course, a very rough and inaccurate model.

Most deterministic functions are nonperiodic. It is sometimes worthwhile to consider an "almost periodic" type of signal. The ECG signal can sometimes be considered "almost periodic." The ECG's RR interval is never constant; in addition, the PQRST complex of one heartbeat is never exactly the same as that of another beat. The signal is definitely nonperiodic. Under certain conditions, however, the RR interval is almost constant, and one PQRST is almost the same as the other. The ECG may thus sometimes be modeled as "almost periodic."

54.3 Stochastic Signals

The most important class of signals is the *stochastic* class. A stochastic signal is a sample function of a stochastic process. The process produces sample functions, the infinite collection of which is called the *ensemble*. Each sample function differs from the other in its fine details; however, they all share the same distribution probabilities. Figure 54.2 depicts three sample functions of an ensemble. Note that at any given time, the values of the sample functions are different.

Stochastic signals cannot be expressed exactly; they can be described only in terms of probabilities which may be calculated over the ensemble.

Assuming a signal $s(t)$, the Nth-order *joint probability function*

$$P[s(t_1) \leq s_1, s(t_2) \leq s_2, \ldots, s(t_N) \leq s_N] = P(s_1, s_2, \ldots, s_N) \qquad (54.3)$$

is the joint probability that the signal at time t_i will be less than or equal to S_i and at time t_j will be less than or equal to S_j, etc. This joint probability describes the statistical behavior and intradependence of the process.

It is very often useful to work with the derivative of the joint probability function; this derivative is known as the *joint probability density function* (PDF):

$$p(s_1, s_2, \ldots, s_N) = \frac{\partial^N}{\partial s_1 \, \partial s_2 \cdots \partial s_N} [P(s_1, s_2, \ldots, s_N)] \qquad (54.4)$$

Of particular interest are the first- and second-order PDFs.

The *expectation* of the process $s(t)$, denoted by $E\{s(t)\}$ or by m_s, is a statistical operator defined as

$$E\{s(t)\} = \int_{-\infty}^{\infty} sp(s) \, ds = m_s \qquad (54.5)$$

The expectation of the function $s^n(t)$ is known as the *nth-order moment*. The first-order moment is thus the expectation of the process. The nth-order moment is given by

$$E\{s^n(t)\} = \int_{-\infty}^{\infty} s^n p(s) \, ds \qquad (54.6)$$

Another important statistical operator is the *nth central moment*:

$$\mu_n = E\{(s - m_s)^n\} = \int_{-\infty}^{\infty} (s - m_s)^n p(s) \, ds \qquad (54.7)$$

The second central moment is known as the *variance* (the square root of which is the *standard deviation*). The variance is denoted by σ^2:

$$\sigma^2 = \mu_2 = E\{(s - m_s)^2\} = \int_{-\infty}^{\infty} (s - m_s)^2 p(s) \, ds \qquad (54.8)$$

The second-order joint moment is defined by the joint PDF. Of particular interest is the *autocorrelation function* r_{ss}:

$$r_{ss}(t_1, t_2) = E\{s(t_1)s(t_2)\} = \int_{-\infty}^{\infty} \int_{-\infty}^{\infty} s(t_1)s(t_2)p(s_1, s_2) \, ds_1 \, ds_2 \qquad (54.9)$$

The *cross-correlation function* is defined as the second joint moment of the signal s at time t_1, $s(t_1)$, and the signal y at time t_2, $y(t_2)$:

$$r_{sy}(t_1, t_2) = E\{s(t_1)y(t_2)\} = \int_{-\infty}^{\infty} \int_{-\infty}^{\infty} s(t_1)y(t_2)p(s_1, y_2) \, ds_1 \, dy_2 \qquad (54.10)$$

Stationary stochastic processes are processes whose statistics do not change in time. The expectation and the variance (as with any other statistical mean) of a stationary process will be time-independent. The autocorrelation function, for example, of a stationary process will thus be a function of the time difference $\tau = t_2 - t_1$ (one-dimensional function) rather than a function of t_2 and t_1 (two-dimensional function).

Ergodic stationary processes possess an important characteristic: Their statistical probability distributions (along the ensemble) equal those of their time distributions (along the time axis of any one of its sample functions). For example, the correlation function of an ergodic process may be calculated by its definition (along the ensemble) or along the time axis of any one of its sample functions:

$$r_{ss}(\tau) = E\{s(t)s(t-\tau)\}$$

$$= \lim_{T \to \infty} \frac{1}{2T} \int_{-T}^{T} s(t)s(t-\tau)\, dt \qquad (54.11)$$

The right side of Eq. (54.11) is the *time autocorrelation function*.

Ergodic processes are nice because one does not need the ensemble for calculating the distributions; a single sample function is sufficient.

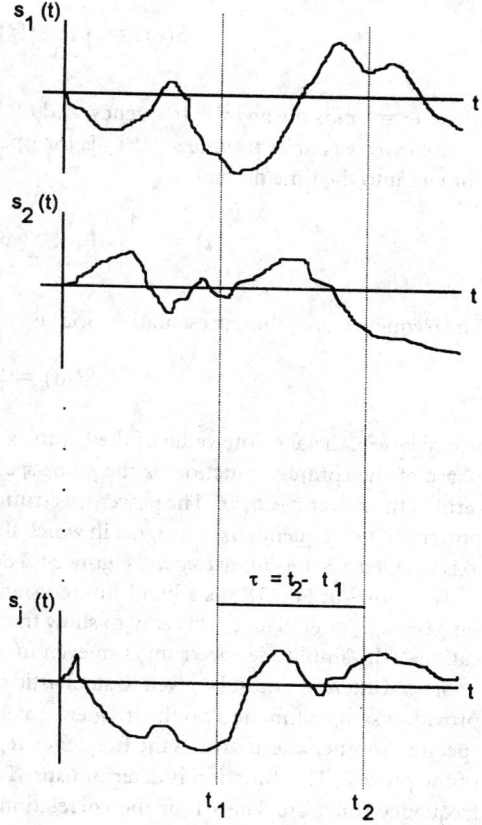

FIGURE 54.2 The ensemble of the stochastic process $s(t)$.

From the point of view of processing, it is desirable to model the signal as an ergodic one. Unfortunately, almost all signals are nonstationary (and hence nonergodic). One must therefore use nonstationary processing methods (such as, for example, wavelet transformation) which are relatively complex or cut the signals into short-duration segments in such a way that each may be considered stationary.

The sleep EEG signal, for example, is a nonstationary signal. We may consider segments of the signal, in which the subject was at a given sleep state, as stationary. In order to describe the signal, we need to estimate its probability distributions. However, the ensemble is unavailable. If we further assume that the process is ergodic, the distributions may be estimated along the time axis of the given sample function. Most of the standard processing techniques assume the signal to be stationary and ergodic.

54.4 Frequency-Domain Analysis

Until now we have dealt with signals represented in the time domain, that is to say, we have described the signal by means of its value on the time axis. It is possible to use another representation for the same signal: that of the frequency domain. Any signal may be described as a continuum of sine waves having different amplitudes and phases. The frequency representation describes the signals by means of the amplitudes and phases of the sine waves. The transformation between the two representations is given by the *Fourier transform* (FT):

$$S(\omega) = \int_{-\infty}^{\infty} s(t)e^{-j\omega t}\, dt = F\{s(t)\} \qquad (54.12)$$

where $\omega = 2\pi f$ is the angular frequency, and $F\{*\}$ is the Fourier operator.

The *inverse Fourier transform* (IFT) is the operator that transforms a signal from the frequency domain into the time domain:

$$s(t) = \frac{1}{2\pi} \int_{-\infty}^{\infty} S(\omega)e^{j\omega t}\, dw = F^{-1}\{S(\omega)\} \qquad (54.13)$$

The frequency domain representation $S(\omega)$ is complex; hence

$$S(\omega) = |S(\omega)|e^{j\theta(\omega)} \qquad (54.14)$$

where $|S(\omega)|$, the absolute value of the complex function, is the *amplitude spectrum,* and $\theta(\omega)$, the phase of the complex function, is the *phase spectrum*. The square of the absolute value, $|S(\omega)|^2$, is termed the *power spectrum*. The power spectrum of a signal describes the distribution of the signal's power on the frequency axis. A signal in which the power is limited to a finite range of the frequency axis is called a *band-limited signal*. Figure 54.3 depicts an example of such a signal.

The signal in Fig. 54.3 is a band-limited signal; its power spectrum is limited to the frequency range $-\omega_{max} \le \omega \le \omega_{max}$. It is easy to show that if $s(t)$ is real (which is the case in almost all applications), the amplitude spectrum is an even function and the phase spectrum is an odd function.

Special attention must be given to stochastic signals. Applying the FT to a sample function would provide a sample function on the frequency axis. The process may be described by the ensemble of spectra. Another alternative to the frequency representation is to consider the correlation function of the process. This function is deterministic. The FT may be applied to it, yielding a deterministic frequency function. The FT of the correlation function is defined as the *power spectral density function* (PSD):

$$\text{PSD}\,[s(t)] = S_{ss}(\omega) = F\{r_{ss}(\tau)\} = \int_{-\infty}^{\infty} r_{ss}(\tau)e^{-j\omega\tau}d\tau \qquad (54.15)$$

The PSD is used to describe stochastic signals; it describes the density of power on the frequency axis. Note that since the autocorrelation function is an even function, the PSD is real; hence no phase spectrum is required.

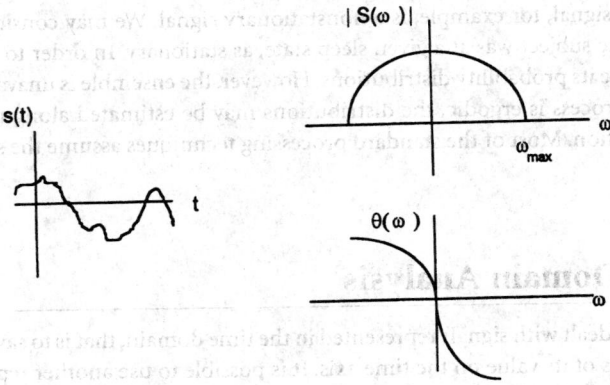

FIGURE 54.3 Example of a signal described in the time and frequency domains.

The EEG signal may serve as an example of the importance of the PSD in signal processing. When processing the EEG, it is very helpful to use the PSD. It turns out that the power distribution of the EEG changes according to the physiologic and psychological states of the subject. The PSD may thus serve as a tool for the analysis and recognition of such states.

Very often we are interested in the relationship between two processes. This may be the case, for example, when two sides of the brain are investigated by means of EEG signals. The time-domain expression of such relationships is given by the cross-correlation function (Eq. 54.10). The frequency-domain representation of this is given by the FT of the cross-correlation function, which is called the *cross-power spectral density function* (C-PSD) or the *cross-spectrum*:

$$S_{sy}(\omega) = F\{r_{sy}(\tau)\} = |S_{sy}(\omega)|e^{j\theta_{sy}(\omega)} \tag{54.16}$$

Note that we have assumed the signals $s(t)$ and $y(t)$ are stationary; hence the cross-correlation function is not a function of time but of the time difference τ. Note also that unlike the autocorrelation function, $r_{sy}(\tau)$ is not even; hence its FT is not real. Both absolute value and phase are required.

It can be shown that the absolute value of the C-PSD is bounded:

$$|S_{sy}(\omega)|^2 \leq S_{ss}(\omega)S_{yy}(\omega) \tag{54.17}$$

The absolute value information of the C-PSD may thus be normalized to provide the *coherence function*:

$$\gamma^2_{sy} = \frac{|S_{sy}(\omega)|^2}{S_{ss}(\omega)S_{yy}(\omega)} \leq 1 \tag{54.18}$$

The coherence function is used in a variety of biomedical applications. It has been used, for example, in EEG analysis to investigate brain asymmetry.

54.5 Discrete Signals

Assume now that the signal $s(t)$ of Fig. 54.3 was sampled using a sampling frequency of $f_s = \omega_s/(2\pi) = (2\pi)/T_s$. The sampled signal is the sequence $s(m)$. The representation of the sampled signal in the frequency domain is given by applying the Fourier operator:

$$S_s(\omega) = F\{s(m)\} = |S_s(\omega)|e^{j\theta_s(\omega)} \tag{54.19}$$

The amplitude spectrum of the sampled signal is depicted in Fig. 54.4. It can easily be proven that the spectrum of the sampled signal is the spectrum of the original signal repeated infinite times at frequencies of $n\omega_s$. The spectrum of a sampled signal is thus a periodic signal in the frequency domain. It can be observed, in Fig. 54.4, that provided the sampling frequency is large enough, the wave shapes of the spectrum do not overlap. In such a case, the original (continuous) signal may be extracted from the sampled signal by low-pass filtering. A low-pass filter with a cutoff frequency of ω_{max} will yield at its output only the first period of the spectrum, which is exactly the continuous signal. If, however, the sampling frequency is low, the wave shapes overlap, and it will be impossible to regain the continuous signal.

The sampling frequency must obey the inequality

$$\omega_s \geq 2\omega_{max} \tag{54.20}$$

Equation (54.20) is known as the *sampling theorem*, and the lowest allowable sampling frequency is called the *Nyquist frequency*. When overlapping does occur, there are errors between the sampled and

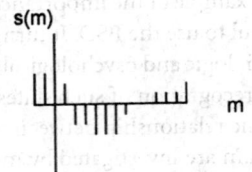

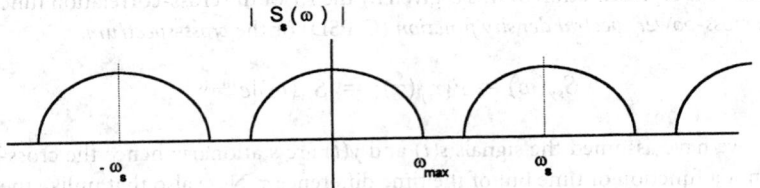

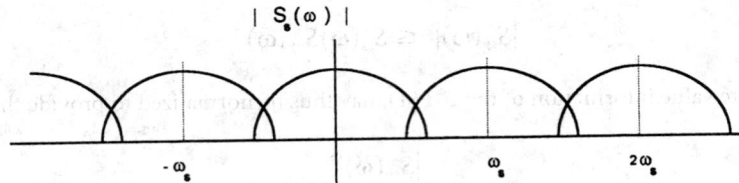

FIGURE 54.4 Amplitude spectrum of a sampled signal with sampling frequency above the Nyquist frequency (*upper trace*) and below the Nyquist frequency (*lower trace*).

original signals. These errors are known as *aliasing errors*. In practical applications, the signal does not possess a finite bandwidth; we therefore limit its bandwidth by an *antialiasing filter* prior to sampling.

The *discrete Fourier transform* (DFT) [Proakis & Manolakis, 1988] is an important operator that maps a finite sequence $s(m)$, $m = 0, 1, \ldots, N-1$, into another finite sequence $S(k)$, $k = 0, 1, \ldots, N-1$. The DFT is defined as

$$S(k) = \text{DFT}\{s(m)\} = \sum_{m=0}^{N-1} s(m)e^{-jkm} \tag{54.21}$$

An inverse operator, the *inverse discrete Fourier transform* (IDFT), is an operator that transforms the sequence $S(k)$ back into the sequence $s(m)$. It is given by

$$s(m) = \text{IDFT}\{S(k)\} = \frac{1}{N} \sum_{k=0}^{N-1} S(k)e^{jkm} \tag{54.22}$$

It can be shown that if the sequence $s(m)$ is the samples of the band-limited signal $s(t)$, sampled under Nyquist conditions with sampling interval of T_s, the DFT sequence $S(k)$ (neglecting windowing effects) is the samples of the FT of the original signal:

$$S(k) = S_s(\omega)\big|_{\omega=k\frac{\omega_s}{N}} \qquad k = 0, 1, \ldots, N-1 \tag{54.23}$$

Figure 54.5 depicts the DFT and its relations to the FT. Note that the N samples of the DFT span the frequency range one period. Since the amplitude spectrum is even, only half the DFT samples carry the information; the other half is composed of the complex conjugates of the first half.

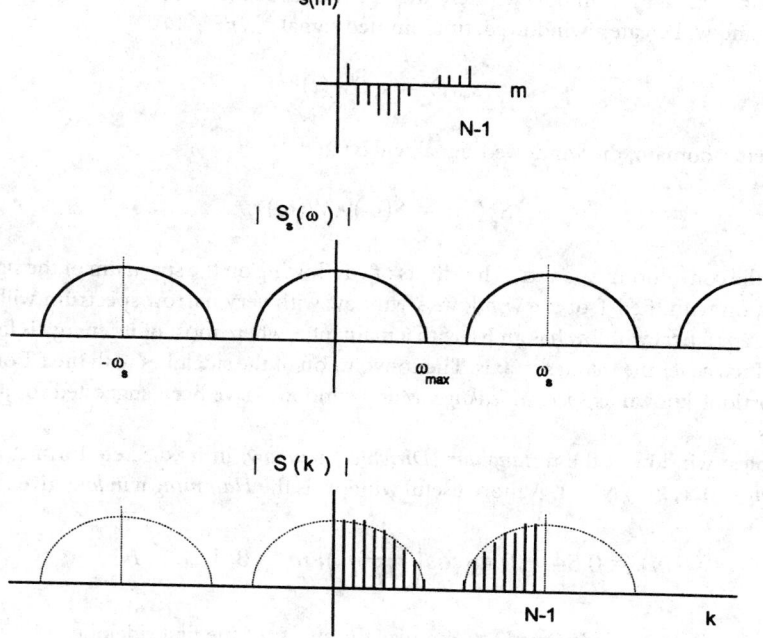

FIGURE 54.5 The sampled signal $s(m)$ and its DFT.

The DFT may be calculated very efficiently by means of the *fast (discrete) Fourier transform* (FFT) algorithm. It is this fact that makes the DFT an attractive means for FT estimation. The DFT provides an estimate for the FT with frequency resolution of

$$\Delta f = \frac{2\pi f_s}{N} = \frac{2\pi}{T} \qquad (54.24)$$

where T is the duration of the data window. The resolution may be improved by using a longer window. In cases where it is not possible to have a longer data window, e.g., because the signal is not stationary, *zero padding* may be used. The sequence may be augmented with zeroes:

$$s_A(m) = \{s(0), s(1), \ldots, s(N-1), 0, \ldots, 0\} \qquad (54.25)$$

The zero padded sequence $s_A(m)$, $m = 0, 1, \ldots, L-1$, contains N elements of the original sequence and $L-N$ zeroes. It can be shown that its DFT is the samples of the FT with an increased resolution of $\Delta f = 2\pi f_s L^{-1}$.

54.6 Data Windows

Calculation of the various functions previously defined, such as the correlation function, requires knowledge of the signal from minus infinity to infinity. This is, of course, impractical because the signal is not available for long durations and the results of the calculations are expected at a reasonable time. We therefore do not use the signal itself but the *windowed signal*.

A *window* $w(t)$ is defined as a real and even function that is also time-limited:

$$w(t) = 0 \qquad \forall |t| > T/2$$

The FT of a window $W(\omega)$ is thus real and even and is not band-limited.

Multiplying a signal by a window will zero the signal outside the window duration (the observation period) and will create a windowed, time-limited signal $s_w(t)$:

$$s_w(t) = s(t)w(t) \tag{54.26}$$

In the frequency domain, the windowed signal will be

$$S_w(\omega) = S(\omega) * W(\omega) \tag{54.27}$$

where $(*)$ is the convolution operator. The effects of windowing on the spectrum of the signal is thus the convolution with the FT of the window. A window with very narrow spectrum will cause low distortions. A practical window has an FT with a main lobe, where most of its energy is located, and sidelobes, which cover the frequency axis. The convolution of the sidelobes with the FT of the signal causes distortions known as *spectral leakage*. Many windows have been suggested for a variety of applications.

The simplest window is the *rectangular (Dirichlet) window;* in its discrete form it is given by $w(m) = 1, m = 0, 1, \ldots, N - 1$. A more useful window is the *Hamming window,* given by

$$w(m) = 0.54 - 0.46\cos\left(\frac{2\pi}{N}m\right); m = 0, 1, \ldots, N - 1 \tag{54.28}$$

The Hamming window was designed to minimize the effects of the first sidelobe.

54.7 Short-Time Fourier Transform (STFT)

The Fourier analysis discussed in preceding sections assumed that the signal is stationary. Unfortunately, most signals are nonstationary. A relatively simple way to deal with the problem is to divide the signal into short segments. The segments are chosen such that each one by itself can be considered a windowed sample of a stationary process. The duration of the segments have to be determined either by having some a priori information about the signal or by examining its local characteristics. Depending on the signal and the application, the segments may be of equal or different duration.

We want to represent such a segmented signal in the frequency domain. We define the *short-time Fourier transform* (STFT):

$$\text{STFT}_s(\omega, \tau) = F\{s(t)w(t - \tau)\} = \int_{-\infty}^{\infty} s(t)w(t - \tau)e^{-j\omega t}\, dt \tag{54.29}$$

The window is shifted on the time axis to $t = \tau$ so that the FT is performed on a windowed segment in the range $\tau - (T/2) \le t \le \tau + (T/2)$. The STFT describes the amplitude and phase-frequency distributions of the signal in the vicinity of $t = \tau$.

In general, the STFT is a two-dimensional, time-frequency function. The resolution of the STFT on the time axis depends on the duration T of the window. The narrower the window, the better is the time resolution. Unfortunately, choosing a short-duration window means a wider-band window. The wider the window in the frequency domain, the larger is the spectral leakage and hence the deterioration of the frequency resolution. One of the main drawbacks of the STFT method is the fact that the time and frequency resolutions are linked together. Other methods, such as the *wavelet transform,* are able to better deal with the problem.

In highly nonstationary signals, such as speech signals, equal-duration windows are used. Window duration is on the order of 10 to 20 ms. In other signals, such as the EEG, variable-duration windows are used. In the EEG, windows on the order of 5 to 30 s are often used.

A common way for representing the two-dimensional STFT function is by means of the *spectrogram*. In the spectrogram, the time and frequency axes are plotted, and the STFT PSD value is given by the gray-scale code or by a color code. Figure 54.6 depicts a simple spectrogram. The time axis is quantized to the window duration *T*. The gray scale codes the PSD such that black denotes maximum power and white denotes zero power. In Figure 54.6, the PSD is quantized into only four levels of gray. The spectrogram shows a signal that is nonstationary in the time range 0 to 8*T*. In this time range, the PSD possesses a peak that is shifted from about $0.6f_s$ to about $0.1f_s$ at time 0.7*T*. From time 0.8*T*, the signal becomes stationary with a PSD peak power in the low-frequency range and the high-frequency range.

54.8 Spectral Estimation

The PSD is a very useful tool in biomedical signal processing. It is, however, impossible to calculate, since it requires infinite integration time. Estimation methods must be used to acquire an estimate of the PSD from a given finite sample of the process under investigation. Many algorithms for spectral estimation are available in the literature [Kay, 1988], each with its advantages and drawbacks. One method may be suitable for processes with sharp spectral peaks, while another will perform best for broad, smoothed spectra. An a priori knowledge on the type of PSD one is investigating helps in choosing the proper spectral estimation method. Some of the PSD estimation methods will be discussed here.

The Blackman-Tukey Method

This method estimates the PSD directly from its definition (Eq. 54.15) but uses finite integration time and an estimate rather than the true correlation function. In its discrete form, the PSD estimation is

$$\hat{S}_{xx}(\omega) = T_s \sum_{m=-M}^{M} \hat{r}_{xx}(m) e^{-j\omega m T_s}$$

$$\hat{r}_{xx}(m) = \frac{1}{N} \sum_{i=0}^{N-i-1} x(m+i)x(i)$$

(54.30)

where *N* is the number of samples used for the estimation of the correlation coefficients, and *M* is the number of correlation coefficients used for estimation of the PSD. Note that a biased estimation of the correlation is employed. Note also that once the correlations have been estimated, the PSD may be calculated by applying the FFT to the correlation sequence.

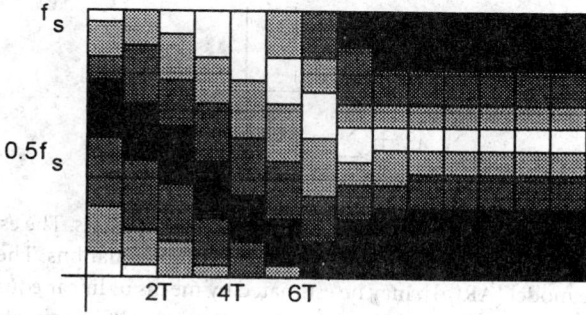

FIGURE 54.6 A spectrogram.

The Periodogram

The periodogram estimates the PSD directly from the signal without the need to first estimate the correlation. It can be shown that

$$S_{xx}(\omega) = \lim_{T \to \infty} E\left\{ \frac{1}{2T} \left| \int_{-T}^{T} x(t)e^{-j\omega t}\, dt \right|^2 \right\} \tag{54.31}$$

The PSD presented in Eq. (54.31) requires infinite integration time. The periodogram estimates the PSD from a finite observation time by dropping the lim operator. It can be shown that in its discrete form, the periodogram estimator is given by

$$\hat{S}_{xx}(\omega) = \frac{T_s}{N} |\text{DFT}\{x(m)\}|^2 \tag{54.32}$$

The great advantage of the periodogram is that the DFT operator can very efficiently be calculated by the FFT algorithm.

A modification to the periodogram is *weighted overlapped segment averaging* (WOSA). Rather than use one segment of N samples, we divide the observation segment into shorter subsegments, perform a periodogram for each one, and then average all periodograms. The WOSA method provides a smoother estimate of the PSD.

Time-Series Analysis Methods

Time-series analysis methods model the signal as an output of a linear system driven by a white source. Figure 54.7 depicts this model in its discrete form. Since the input is a white noise process (with zero mean and unity variance), the PSD of the signal is given by

$$S_{ss}(\omega) = |H(\omega)|^2 \tag{54.33}$$

The PSD of the signal may thus be represented by the system's transfer function. Consider a general pole-zero system with p poles and q zeroes [ARMA(p, q)]:

$$H(z) = \frac{\displaystyle\sum_{i=0}^{q} b_i z^{-i}}{1 + \displaystyle\sum_{i=1}^{p} a_i z^{-i}} \tag{54.34}$$

Its absolute value evaluated on the frequency axis is

$$|H(\omega)|^2 = \frac{\left| \displaystyle\sum_{i=0}^{q} b_i z^{-i} \right|^2}{\left| 1 + \displaystyle\sum_{i=1}^{p} a_i z^{-i} \right|^2} \Bigg|_{z = e^{-j\omega T_s}} \tag{54.35}$$

Several algorithms are available for the estimation of the model's coefficients. The estimation of the ARMA model parameters requires the solution of a nonlinear set of equations. The special case of $q = 0$, namely, an all-pole model [AR(p)], may be estimated by means of linear equations. Efficient AR estimation algorithms are available, making it a popular means for PSD estimation. Figure 54.8 shows the estimation of EMG PSD using several estimation methods.

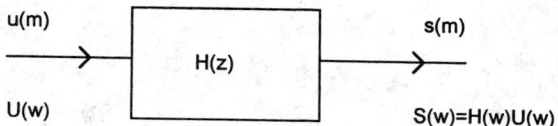

FIGURE 54.7 Time-series model for the signal $s(m)$.

54.9 Signal Enhancement

The biomedical signal is very often a weak signal contaminated by noise. Consider, for example, the problem of monitoring the ECG signal. The signal is acquired by surface electrodes that pick up the electric potential generated by the heart muscle. In addition, the electrodes pick up potentials from other active muscles. When the subject is at rest, this type of noise may be very small, but when the subject is an athlete performing some exercise, the muscle noise may become dominant. Additional noise may enter the system from electrodes motion, from the power lines, and from other sources. The first task of processing is usually to enhance the signal by "cleaning" the noise without (if possible) distorting the signal.

Assume a simple case where the measured signal $x(t)$ is given by

$$x(t) = s(t) + n(t) \qquad X(\omega) = S(\omega) + N(\omega) \qquad (54.36)$$

where $s(t)$ is the desired signal and $n(t)$ is the additive noise. For simplicity, we assume that both the signal and noise are band-limited, namely, for the signal, $S(\omega) = 0$, for $\omega_{max} \le \omega$, $\omega_{min} \ge \omega$. Figure 54.9 depicts the PSD of the signal in two cases, the first where the PSD of the signal and noise do not overlap and the second where they do overlap (for the sake of simplicity, only the positive frequency axis was plotted). We want to enhance the signal by means of linear filtering. The problem is to design the linear filter that will provide best enhancement. Assuming we have the filter, its output, the enhanced signal, is given by

$$y(t) = x(t) * h(t) \qquad Y(\omega) = X(\omega)H(\omega) \qquad (54.37)$$

where $y(t) = \hat{s}(t) + n_o(t)$ is the enhanced output, and $h(t)$ is the impulse response of the filter. The solution for the first case is trivial; we need an ideal bandpass filter whose transfer function $H(\omega)$ is

$$H(\omega) = \begin{cases} 1 & \omega_{min} < \omega < \omega_{max} \\ 0 & \text{otherwise} \end{cases} \qquad (54.38)$$

Such a filter and its output are depicted in Fig. 54.10.

As is clearly seen in Fig. 54.10, the desired signal $s(t)$ was completely recovered from the given noisy signal $x(t)$. Practically, we do not have ideal filters, so some distortions and some noise contamination will always appear at the output. With the correct design, we can approximate the ideal filter so that the distortions and noise may be as small as we desire. The enhancement of overlapping noisy signals is far from being trivial.

54.10 Optimal Filtering

When the PSD of signal and noise overlap, complete, undistorted recovery of the signal is impossible. Optimal processing is required, with the first task being definition of the optimality criterion. Different criteria will result in different solutions to the problem. Two approaches will be presented here: the *Wiener filter* and the *matched filter*.

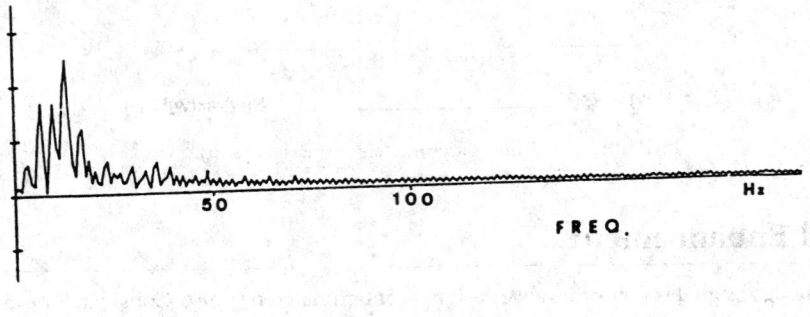

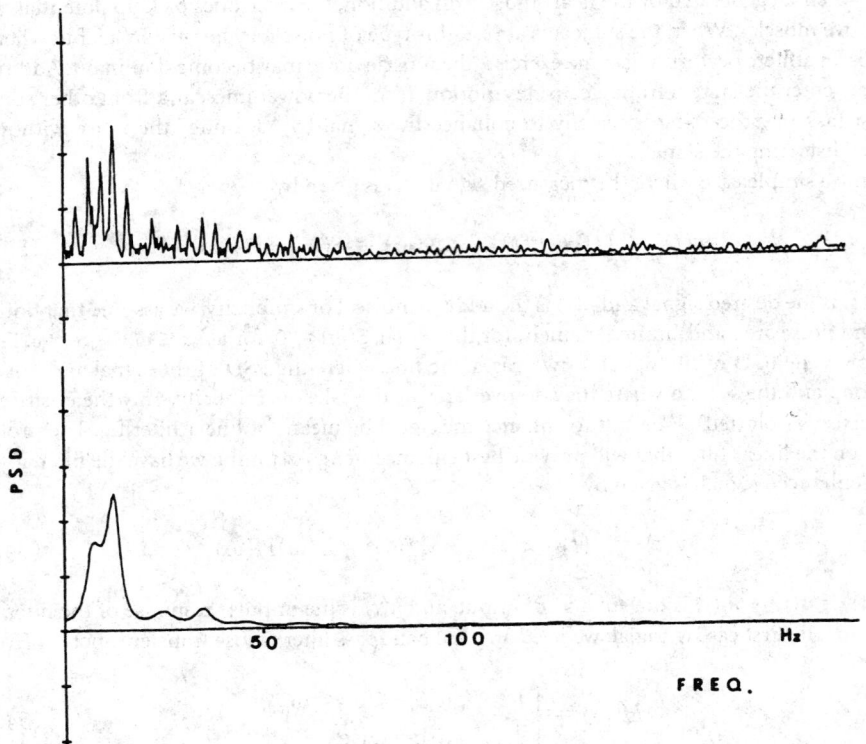

FIGURE 54.8   PSD of surface EMG. (*Upper trace*) Blackman-Tukey (256 correlation coefficients and 256 padding zeroes). (*Middle trace*) Periodogram (512 samples and 512 padding zeroes). (*Lower trace*) AR model ($p = 40$).

Minimization of Mean Squared Error: The Wiener Filter

Assume that our goal is to estimate, at time $t + \xi$, the value of the signal $s(t + \xi)$, based on the observations $x(t)$. The case $\xi = 0$ is known as *smoothing*, while the case $\xi > 0$ is called *prediction*.

We define an *output error* $\epsilon(t)$ as the error between the filter's output and the desired output. The expectation of the square of the error is given by

$$
\begin{aligned}
E\{\epsilon^2(t)\} &= E\{[s(t + \xi) - y(t + \xi)]^2\} \\
&= E\{[s(t + \xi) - \int_{-\infty}^{\infty} h(\tau)x(t - \tau)\, d\tau]^2\}
\end{aligned}
\tag{54.39}
$$

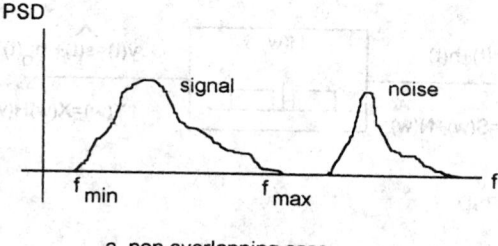

a. non overlapping case

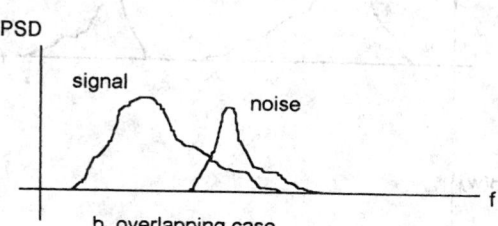

b. overlapping case

FIGURE 54.9 Noisy signal in the frequency domain.

The integral term on the right side of Eq. (54.39) is the convolution integral expressing the output of the filter.

The minimization of Eq. (54.39) with respect of $h(t)$ yields the optimal filter (in the sense of minimum squared error). The minimization yields the *Wiener-Hopf equation*:

$$r_{sx}(\tau + \xi) = \int_{-\infty}^{\infty} h(\eta) r_{xx}(\tau - \eta)\, d\eta \tag{54.40}$$

In the frequency domain, this equation becomes

$$S_{sx}(\omega) e^{j\omega\xi} = H_{opt}(\omega) S_{xx}(\omega) \tag{54.41}$$

from which the optimal filter $H_{opt}(\omega)$ can be calculated:

$$H_{opt}(\omega) = \frac{S_{sx}(\omega)}{S_{xx}(\omega)}\, e^{j\omega\xi} = \frac{S_{sx}(\omega)}{S_{ss}(\omega) + S_{nn}(\omega)}\, e^{j\omega\xi} \tag{54.42}$$

If the signal and noise are uncorrelated and either the signal or the noise has zero mean, the last equation becomes

$$H_{opt}(\omega) = \frac{S_{ss}(\omega)}{S_{ss}(\omega) + S_{nn}(\omega)}\, e^{j\omega\xi} \tag{54.43}$$

The optimal filter requires a priori knowledge of the PSD of noise and signal. These are very often not available and must be estimated from the available signal. The optimal filter given in Eqs. (54.42) and (54.43) is not necessarily realizable. In performing the minimization, we have not introduced a constraint that will ensure that the filter is causal. This can be done, yielding the realizable optimal filter.

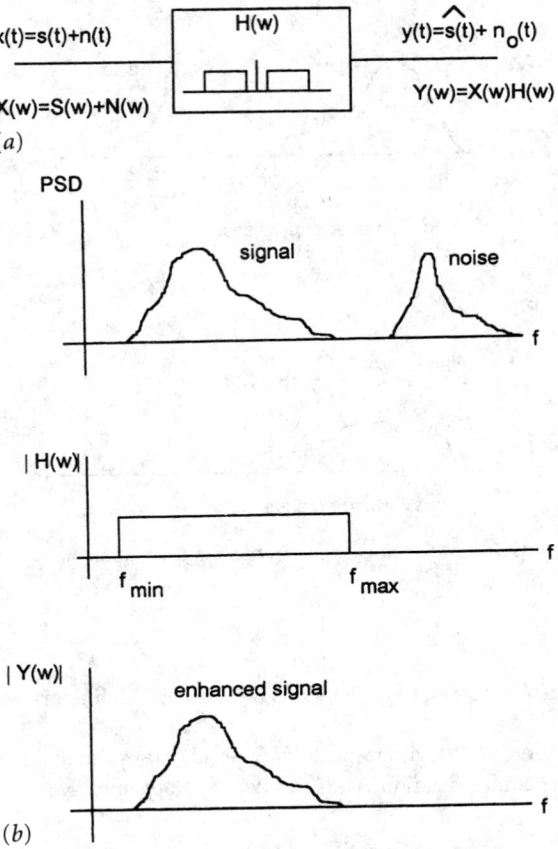

FIGURE 54.10 (*a*) An ideal bandpass filter. (*b*) Enhancement of a nonoverlapping noisy signal by an ideal bandpass filter.

Maximization of the Signal-to-Noise Ratio: The Matched Filter

The Wiener filter was optimally designed to yield an output as close as possible to the signal. In many cases we are not interested in the fine details of the signal but only in the question whether the signal exists at a particular observation or not. Consider, for example, the case of determining the heart rate of a subject under noisy conditions. We need to detect the presence of the R wave in the ECG. The exact shape of the wave is not important. For this case, the optimality criterion used in the last section is not suitable. To find a more suitable criterion, we define the output signal-to-noise ratio: Let us assume that the signal $s(t)$ is a deterministic function. The response of the filter, $\hat{s}(t) = s(t) * h(t)$, to the signal is also deterministic. We shall define the output signal-to-noise ratio

$$\text{SNR}_o(t) = \frac{\hat{s}(t)}{E\{n_o^2(t)\}} \tag{54.44}$$

as the optimality criterion. The optimal filter will be the filter that maximizes the output SNR at a certain given time $t = t_o$. The maximization yields the following integral equation:

$$\int_0^T h(\xi) r_{nn}(\tau - \xi)\, d\xi = \alpha s(t_o - \tau) \qquad o \le \tau \le T \tag{54.45}$$

where T is the observation time and α is any constant. This equation has to be solved for any given noise and signal.

A special important case is the case where the noise is a white noise so that its autocorrelation function is a delta function. In this case, the solution of Eq. (54.45) is

$$h(\tau) = \frac{1}{N} s(t_o - \tau) \tag{54.46}$$

where N is the noise power. For this special case, the impulse response of the optimal filter has the form of the signal run backward, shifted to the time t_o. This type of filter is called a *matched filter*.

54.11 Adaptive Filtering

The optimal filters discussed in the preceding section assumed the signals to be stationary with known PSD. Both assumptions rarely occur in reality. In most biomedical applications, the signals are nonstationary with unknown PSD. To enhance such signals, we require a filter that will continuously adjust itself to perform optimally under the changing circumstances. Such a filter is called an *adaptive filter* [Widrow & Stearns 1985].

The general description of an adaptive filter is depicted in Fig. 54.11. The signal $s(t)$ is to be corrected according to the specific application. The correction may be enhancement or some reshaping. The signal is given in terms of the noisy observation signal $x(t)$. The main part of the system is a filter, and the parameters (gain, poles, and zeroes) are controllable by the adaptive algorithm. The adaptive algorithm has some a priori information on the signal and the noise (the amount and type of information depend on the application). It also has a correction criterion, according to which the system is operating. The adaptive algorithm also gets the input and output signals of the filter so that its performance can be analyzed continuously.

The adaptive filter requires a correction algorithm. This can best be implemented digitally. Most adaptive filters therefore are implemented by means of computers or special digital processing chips.

An important class of adaptive filters requires a *reference signal*. The knowledge on the noise required by this type of adaptive filter is a reference signal that is correlated with the noise. The filter thus has two inputs: the noisy signal $x(t) = s(t) + n(t)$ and the reference signal $n_R(t)$. The adaptive

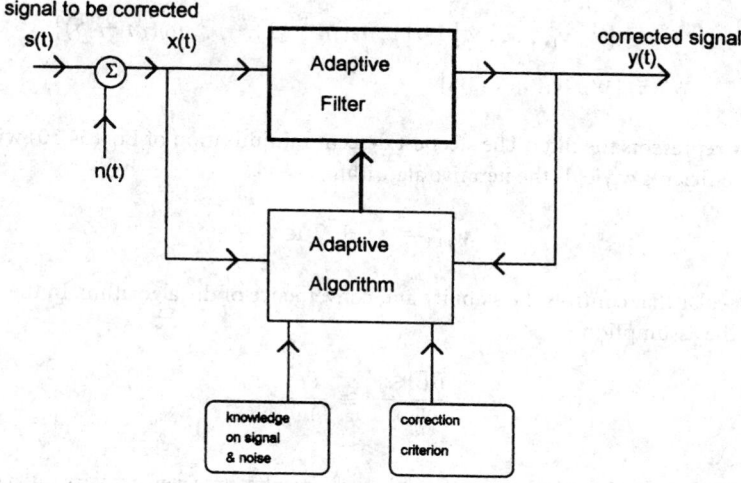

FIGURE 54.11 Adaptive filter, general scheme.

filter, functioning as a *noise canceler*, estimates the noise $n(t)$ and, by subtracting it from the given noisy input, gets an estimate for the signal. Hence

$$y(t) = x(t) - \hat{n}(t) = s(t) + [n(t) - \hat{n}(t)] = \hat{s}(t) \tag{54.47}$$

The output of the filter is the enhanced signal. Since the reference signal is correlated with the noise, the following relationship exists:

$$N_R(\omega) = G(\omega)N(\omega) \tag{54.48}$$

which means that the reference noise may be represented as the output of an unknown filter $G(\omega)$. The adaptive filter estimates the inverse of this unknown noise filter and from it estimates the noise:

$$\hat{n}(t) = F^{-1}\{\hat{G}^{-1}(\omega)N_R(\omega)\} \tag{54.49}$$

The estimation of the inverse filter is done by the minimization of some performance criterion. There are two dominant algorithms for the optimization: the *recursive least squares* (RLS) and the *least mean squares* (LMS). The LMS algorithm will be discussed here.

Consider the mean square error:

$$E\{\varepsilon^2(t)\} = E\{y^2(t)\} = E\{(s(t) + [n(t) - \hat{n}(t)])^2\}$$
$$= E\{s^2(t)\} + E\{[n(t) - \hat{n}(t)]^2\} \tag{54.50}$$

The right side of Eq. (54.50) is correct, assuming that the signal and noise are uncorrelated. We are searching for the estimate $\hat{G}^{-1}(\omega)$ that will minimize the mean square error: $E\{[n(t) - \hat{n}(t)]^2\}$. Since the estimated filter affects only the estimated noise, the minimization of the noise error is equivalent to the minimization of Eq. (54.50). The implementation of the LMS filter will be presented in its discrete form (see Fig. 54.12).

The estimated noise is

$$\hat{n}_R(m) = \sum_{i=0}^{p} v_i w_i = v_m^T w \tag{54.51}$$

where
$$v_m^T = [v_0, v_1, \ldots, v_p] = [1, n_R(m-1), \ldots, n_R(m-p)]$$
$$w^T = [w_0, w_1, \ldots, w_p] \tag{54.52}$$

The vector w represents the filter. The steepest descent minimization of Eq. (54.50) with respect to the filter's coefficients w yields the iterative algorithm

$$w_{j+1} = w_j + 2\mu\epsilon_j v_j \tag{54.53}$$

where μ is a scalar that controls the stability and convergence of the algorithm. In the evaluation of Eq. (54.53), the assumption

$$\frac{\partial E\{\epsilon_j^2\}}{\partial w_k} \cong \frac{\partial \epsilon_j^2}{\partial w_k} \tag{54.54}$$

was made. This is indeed a drastic approximation; the results, however, are very satisfactory. Figure 54.12 depicts the block diagram of the LMS adaptive noise canceler.

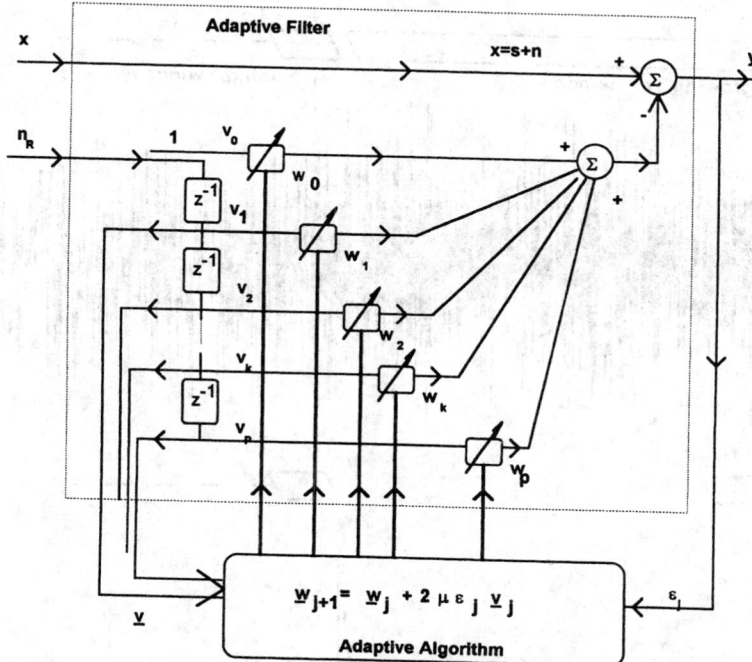

FIGURE 54.12 Block diagram of LMS adaptive noise canceler.

The LMS adaptive noise canceler has been applied to many biomedical problems, among them cancellation of power-line interferences, elimination of electrosurgical interferences, enhancement of fetal ECG, noise reduction for the hearing impaired, and enhancement of evoked potentials.

54.12 Segmentation of Nonstationary Signals

Most biomedical signals are nonstationary, yet the common processing techniques (such as the FT) deal with stationary signals. The STFT is one method of processing nonstationary signals, but it does require, however, the segmentation of the signal into "almost" stationary segments. The signal is thus represented as a piecewise-stationary signal.

An important problem in biomedical signal processing is efficient segmentation. In very highly nonstationary signals, such as the speech signal, short, constant-duration (of the order of 15 ms) segments are used. The segmentation processing in such a case is simple and inexpensive. In other cases, such as, for example, the monitoring of nocturnal EEG, a more elaborate segmentation procedure is called for because the signal may consist of "stationary" segments with very wide duration range. Segmentation into a priori fixed-duration segments will be very inefficient in such cases.

Several adaptive segmentation algorithms have been suggested. Figure 54.13 demonstrates the basic idea of these algorithms. A fixed reference window is used to define an initial segment of the signal. The duration of the reference window is determined such that it is long enough to allow a reliable PSD estimate yet short enough so that the segment may still be considered stationary. Some a priori information about the signal will help in determining the reference window duration. A second, sliding window is shifted along the signal. The PSD of the segment defined by the sliding window is estimated at each window position. The two spectra are compared using some spectral distance measure. As long as this distance measure remains below a certain decision threshold, the reference segment and the sliding segment are considered close enough and are related to the same stationary segment. Once the

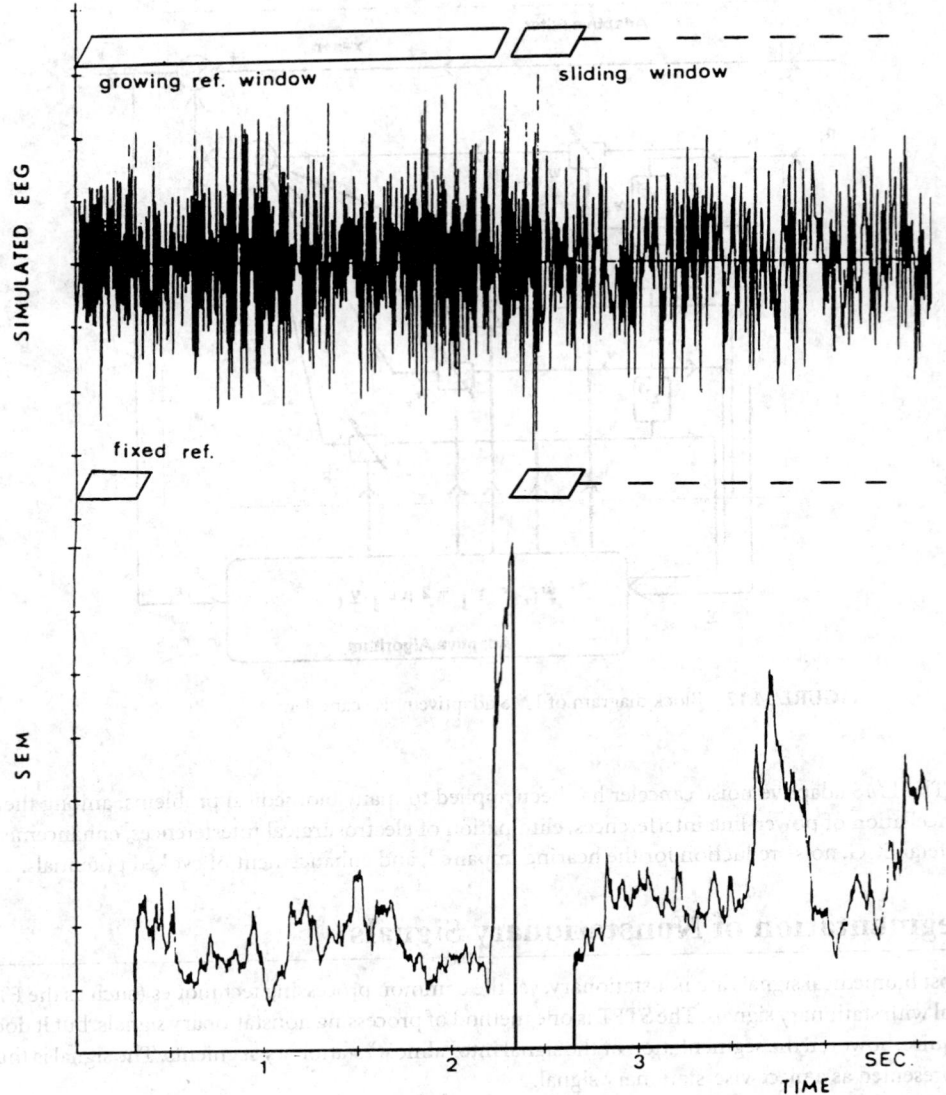

FIGURE 54.13 Adaptive segmentation of simulated EEG. First 2.5 seconds and last 2.5 seconds were simulated by means of different AR models. (*Lower trace*) SEM calculated with fixed reference window. A new segment has been detected at $t = 2.5$. [From Cohen, 1986, with permission.]

distance measure exceeds the decision threshold, a new segment is defined. The process continues by defining the last sliding window as the reference window of the new segment.

Let us define a relative spectral distance measure

$$D_t(\omega) = \int_{\omega_M}^{\omega_M} \left(\frac{S_R(\omega) - S_t(\omega)}{S_R(\omega)} \right)^2 d\omega \tag{54.55}$$

where $S_R(\omega)$ and $S_t(\omega)$ are the PSD estimates of the reference and sliding segments, respectively, and ω_M is the bandwidth of the signal. A normalized spectral measure was chosen, since we are interested in differences in the shape of the PSD and not in the gain.

Some of the segmentation algorithms use growing reference windows rather than fixed ones. This is depicted in the upper part of Fig. 54.13. The various segmentation methods differ in the way the PSDs are estimated. Two of the more known segmentation methods are the *auto-correlation measure method* (ACM) and the *spectral error measure* (SEM).

References

Cohen A. 1986. Biomedical Signal Processing. Boca Raton, Fla, CRC Press.

Kay SM. 1988. Modern Spectral Estimation: Theory and Application. Englewood Cliffs, NJ, Prentice-Hall.

Proakis JG, Manolakis DG. 1988. Introduction to Digital Signal Processing. New York, Macmillan.

Weitkunat R (ed). 1991. Digital Biosignal Processing. Amsterdam, Elsevier.

Widrow B, Stearns SD. 1985. Adaptive Signal Processing. Englewood Cliffs, NJ, Prentice-Hall.

55

Digital Biomedical Signal Acquisition and Processing

Luca T. Mainardi
Polytechnic University, Milan

Anna M. Bianchi
St. Raffaele Hospital, Milan

Sergio Cerutti
Polytechnic University, Milan

Biologic signals carry information that is useful for comprehension of the complex pathophysiologic mechanisms underlying the behavior of living systems. Nevertheless, such information cannot be available directly from the raw recorded signals; it can be masked by other biologic signals contemporaneously detected (endogenous effects) or buried in some additive noise (exogenous effects). For such reasons, some additional processing is usually required to enhance the relevant information and to extract from it parameters that quantify the behavior of the system under study, mainly for physiologic studies, or that define the degree of pathology for routine clinical procedures (diagnosis, therapy, or rehabilitation).

Several processing techniques can be used for such purposes (they are also called *preprocessing techniques*): time- or frequency-domain methods including filtering, averaging, spectral estimation, and others. Even if it is possible to deal with continuous time waveforms, it is usually convenient to convert them into a numerical form before processing. The recent progress of digital technology, in terms of both hardware and software, makes more efficient and flexible digital rather than analog processing. Digital techniques have several advantages: Their performance is generally powerful, being able to easily implement even complex algorithms, and accuracy depends only on the truncation and round-off errors, whose effects can be predicted and controlled by the designer and are largely unaffected by other unpredictable variables such as component aging and temperature, which can degrade the performances of analog devices. Moreover, design parameters can be more easily changed because they involve software rather than hardware modifications.

A few basic elements of signal acquisition and processing will be presented in the following; our aim is to stress mainly the aspects connected with acquisition and analysis of biologic signals, leaving to the cited literature a deeper insight into the various subjects for both the fundamentals of digital signal processing and the applications.

55.1 Acquisition

A schematic representation of a general acquisition system is shown in Fig. 55.1. Several physical magnitudes are usually measured from biologic systems. They include electromagnetic quantities

0-8493-8346-3/95/$0.00+$.50
© 1995 by CRC Press, Inc.

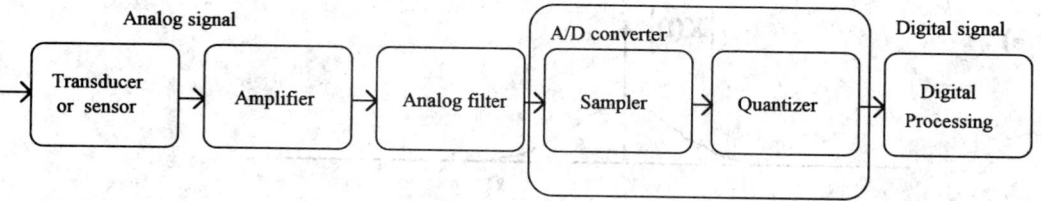

FIGURE 55.1 General block diagram of the acquisition procedure of a digital signal.

(currents, potential differences, field strengths, etc.), as well as mechanical, chemical, or generally nonelectrical variables (pressure, temperature, movements, etc.). Electric signals are detected by *sensors* (mainly electrodes), while nonelectric magnitudes are first converted by *transducers* into electric signals that can be easily treated, transmitted, and stored. Several books of biomedical instrumentation give detailed descriptions of the various transducers and the hardware requirements associated with the acquisition of the different biologic signals [Cobbold, 1988; Tompkins & Webster, 1981; Webster, 1992].

An analog preprocessing block is usually required to amplify and filter the signal (in order to make it satisfy the requirements of the following hardware such as the dynamic of the analog-to-digital converter), to compensate some unwanted sensor characteristics, or to reduce the portion of undesired noise. Moreover, the continuous-time signal should be bandlimited before analog-to-digital (A/D) conversion. Such an operation is needed to reduce the effect of aliasing induced by sampling, as will be described in the next section. Here it is important to remember that the acquisition procedure should preserve the information contained in the original signal waveform. This is a crucial point when recording biologic signals, whose characteristics often may be considered by physicians as indices of some underlying pathologies (i.e., the ST-segment displacement on an ECG signal can be considered a marker of ischemia, the peak-and-wave pattern on an EEG tracing can be a sign of epilepsy, and so on). Thus the acquisition system should not introduce any form of distortion that can be misleading or can destroy real pathologic alterations. For this reason, the analog prefiltering block should be designed with *constant modulus* and *linear phase* (or zero-phase) frequency response, at least in the passband, over the frequencies of interest. Such requirements make the signal arrive undistorted up to the A/D converter.

The analog waveform is then A/D converted into a digital signal; i.e., it is transformed into a series of numbers discretized both in time and amplitude that can be easily managed by digital processors. The A/D conversion ideally can be divided in two steps, as shown in Fig. 55.1: the *sampling* process, which converts the continuous signal in a discrete-time series and whose elements are named *samples*, and a *quantization* procedure, which assigns the amplitude value of each sample within a set of determined discrete values. Both processes modify the characteristics of the signal, and their effects will be discussed in the following sections.

The Sampling Theorem

The advantages of processing a digital series instead of an analog signal have been reported previously. Furthermore, the basic property when using a sampled series instead of its continuous waveform lies in the fact that the former, under certain hypotheses, is completely representative of the latter. When this happens, the continuous waveform can be perfectly reconstructed just from the series of sampled values. This is known as the *sampling theorem* (or *Shannon theorem*) [Shannon, 1949]. It states that a continuous-time signal can be completely recovered from its samples if, and only if, the sampling rate is greater than twice the signal bandwidth.

In order to understand the assumptions of the theorem, let us consider a continuous band-limited signal $x(t)$ (up to f_b) whose Fourier transform $X(f)$ is shown in Fig. 55.2a and suppose to uni-

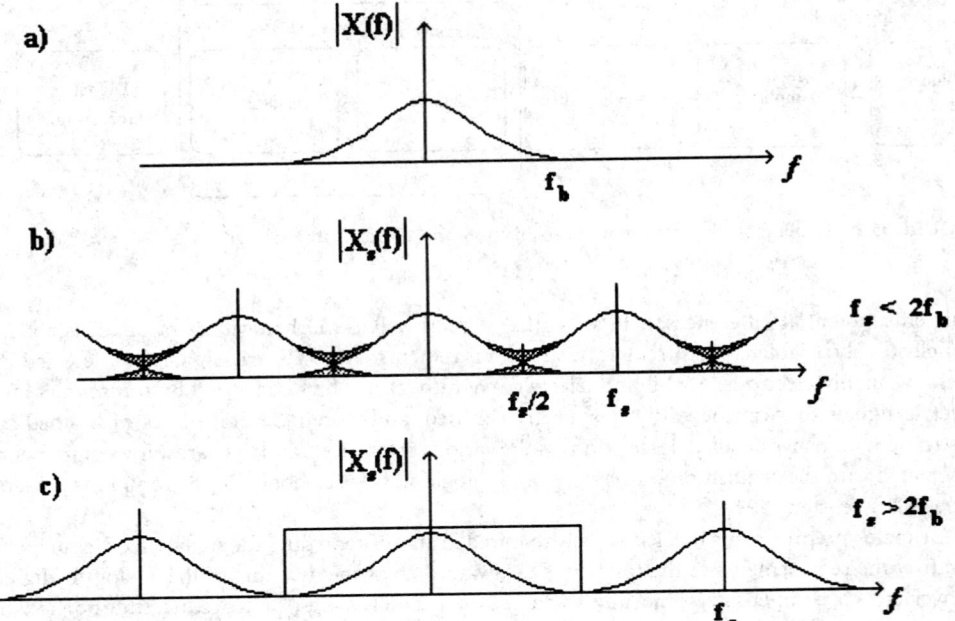

FIGURE 55.2 Effect of sampling frequency (f_s) on a band-limited signal (up to frequency f_b). Fourier transform of the original time signal (a), of the sampled signal when $f_s < 2f_b$ (b), and when $f_s > 2f_b$ (c). The dark areas in part b indicate the aliased frequencies.

formly sample it. The sampling procedure can be modeled by the multiplication of $x(t)$ with an impulse train

$$i(t) = \sum_{k=-\infty,\infty} \delta(t - kT_s) \tag{55.1}$$

where $\delta(t)$ is the delta (Dirac) function, k is an integer, and T_s is the sampling interval. The sampled signal becomes

$$x_s(t) = x(t) \cdot i(t) = \sum_{k=-\infty,\infty} x(t) \cdot \delta(t - kT_s) \tag{55.2}$$

Taking into account that multiplication in time domain implies convolution in frequency domain, we obtain

$$X_s(f) = X(f) * I(f) = X(f) * \frac{1}{T_s} \sum_{k=-\infty,\infty} \delta(f - kf_s) = \frac{1}{T_s} \sum_{k=-\infty,\infty} X(f - kf_s) \tag{55.3}$$

where $f_s = 1/T_s$ is the sampling frequency.

Thus $X_s(f)$, i.e., the Fourier transform of the sampled signal, is periodic and consists of a series of identical repeats of $X(f)$ centered around multiples of the sampling frequency, as depicted in Fig. 55.2b,c. It is worth noting in Fig. 55.2b that the frequency components of $X(f)$ placed above $f_s/2$ appears, when $f_s < 2f_b$, as folded back, summing up to the lower-frequency components. This phenomenon is known as *aliasing* (higher components look "alias" lower components). When aliasing occurs, the original information (Fig. 55.2a) cannot be recovered because the frequency components of the original signal are irreversibly corrupted by the overlaps of the shifted versions of $X(f)$.

A visual inspection of Fig. 55.2 allows one to observe that such frequency contamination can be avoided when the original signal is bandlimited [$X(f) = 0$ for $f > f_b$] and sampled at a frequency $f_s \geq 2f_b$. In this case, shown in Fig. 55.2c, no overlaps exist between adjacent replay of $X(f)$, and the original waveform can be retrieved by low-pass filtering the sampled signal [Oppenheim & Schafer, 1975]. Such observations are the basis of the sampling theorem previously reported.

The hypothesis of a bandlimited signal is hardly verified in practice, due to the signal characteristics or to the effect of superimposed wideband noise. It is worth noting that filtering before sampling is always needed even if we assume the incoming signal to be bandlimited. Let us consider the following example of an EEG signal whose frequency content of interest ranges between 0 and 40 Hz (the usual diagnostic bands are δ, 0 to 3.5 Hz; ϑ, 4 to 7 Hz; α, 8 to 13 Hz; β, 14 to 40 Hz). We may decide to sample it at 80 Hz, thus literarily respecting the Shannon theorem. If we do it without prefiltering, we could find some unpleasant results. Typically, the 50-Hz mains noise will replicate itself in the signal band (30 Hz, i.e., the β band), thus corrupting irreversibly the information, which is of great interest from a physiologic and clinical point of view. The effect is shown in Fig. 55.3a (before sampling) and Fig. 55.3b (after sampling). Generally, it is advisable to sample at a frequency greater than $2f_b$ [Gardenhire, 1964] in order to take into account the nonideal behaviour of the filter or the other preprocessing devices. Therefore, the prefiltering block of Fig. 55.1 is always required to bandlimit the signal before sampling and to avoid aliasing errors.

The Quantization Effects

The quantization produces a discrete signal, whose samples can assume only certain values according to the way they are coded. Typical step functions for a uniform quantizer are reported in Fig. 55.4a,b, where the quantization interval Δ between two quantization levels is evidenced in two cases: rounding and truncation, respectively.

Quantization is a heavily nonlinear procedure, but fortunately, its effects can be statistically modeled. Figure 55.4c,d shows it; the nonlinear quantization block is substituted by a statistical model in which the error induced by quantization is treated as an additive noise $e(n)$ (**quantization error**) to the signal $x(n)$. The following hypotheses are considered in order to deal with a simple mathematical problem:

1. $e(n)$ is supposed to be a white noise with uniform distribution.
2. $e(n)$ and $x(n)$ are uncorrelated.

First of all, it should be noted that the probability density of $e(n)$ changes according to the adopted coding procedure. If we decide to round the real sample to the nearest quantization level, we have

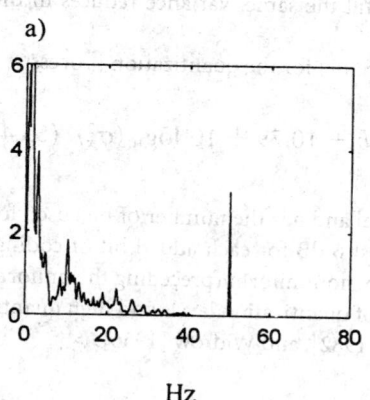
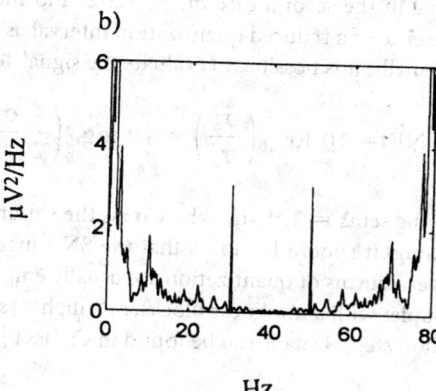

a)

b)

FIGURE 55.3   Power spectrum of an EEG signal (originally bandlimited up to 40 Hz). The presence of 50-Hz mains noise (*a*) causes aliasing error in the 30-Hz component (i.e., in the β diagnostic band) in the sampled signal (*b*) if $f_s = 80$ Hz.

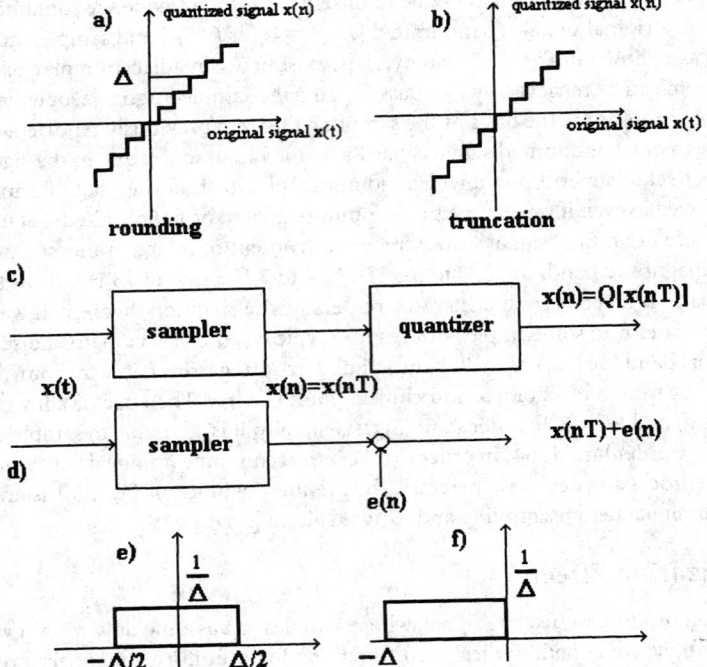

FIGURE 55.4 Nonlinear relationships for rounding (*a*) and truncation (*b*) quantization procedures. Description of quantization block (*c*) by a statistical model (*d*) and probability densities for the quantization noise $e(n)$ for rounding (*e*) and truncation (*f*). Δ is the quantization interval.

$-\Delta/2 \leq e(n) < \Delta/2$, while if we decide to truncate the sample amplitude, we have $-\Delta \leq e(n) < 0$. The two probability densities are plotted in Fig. 55.4*e,f*.

The two ways of coding yield processes with different statistical properties. In the first case the mean and variance value of $e(n)$ are

$$m_e = 0 \qquad \sigma_e^2 = \Delta^2/12$$

while in the second case $m_e = -\Delta/2$, and the variance is still the same. Variance reduces in the presence of a reduced quantization interval as expected.

Finally, it is possible to evaluate the signal-to-noise ratio (SNR) for the quantization process:

$$\text{SNR} = 10 \log_{10}\left(\frac{\sigma_x^2}{\sigma_e^2}\right) = 10 \log_{10}\left(\frac{\sigma_x^2}{2^{-2b}/12}\right) = 6.02b + 10.79 + 10 \log_{10}(\sigma_x^2) \quad (55.4)$$

having set $\Delta = 2^{-2b}$ and where σ_x^2 is the variance of the signal and b is the number of bits used for coding. It should be noted that the SNR increases by almost 6 dB for each added bit of coding. Several forms of quantization are usually employed: uniform, nonuniform (preceding the uniform sampler with a nonlinear block), or roughly (small number of quantization levels and high quantization step). Details can be found in Carassa [1983], Jaeger [1982], and Widrow [1956].

55.2 Signal Processing

A brief review of different signal-processing techniques will be given in this section. They include traditional filtering, averaging techniques, and spectral estimators.

Only the main concepts of analysis and design of digital filters are presented, and a few examples are illustrated in the processing of the ECG signal. Averaging techniques will then be described briefly and their usefulness evidenced when noise and signal have similar frequency contents but different statistical properties; an example for evoked potentials enhancement from EEG background noise is illustrated. Finally, different spectral estimators will be considered and some applications shown in the analysis of RR fluctuations [i.e., the heart rate variability (HRV) signal].

Digital Filters

A *digital filter* is a discrete-time system that operates some transformation on a digital input signal $x(n)$ generating an output sequence $y(n)$, as schematically shown by the block diagram in Fig. 55.5. The characteristics of transformation $T[\cdot]$ identify the filter. The filter will be *time-variant* if $T[\cdot]$ is a function of time or *time-invariant* otherwise, while is said to be *linear* if, and only if, having $x_1(n)$ and $x_2(n)$ as inputs producing $y_1(n)$ and $y_2(n)$, respectively, we have

$$T[ax_1 + bx_2] = aT[x_1] + bT[x_2] = ay_1 + by_2. \tag{55.5}$$

In the following, only linear, time-invariant filters will be considered, even if several interesting applications of nonlinear [Glaser & Ruchkin, 1976; Tompkins, 1993] or time-variant [Cohen, 1983; Huta & Webster, 1973; Thakor, 1987; Widrow et al., 1975] filters have been proposed in the literature for the analysis of biologic signals.

The behavior of a filter is usually described in terms of input-output relationships. They are usually assessed by exciting the filter with different inputs and evaluating which is the response (output) of the system. In particular, if the input is the impulse sequence $\delta(n)$, the resulting output, the impulse response, has a relevant role in describing the characteristic of the filter. Such a response can be used to determine the response to more complicated input sequences. In fact, let us consider a generic input sequence $x(n)$ as a sum of weighed and delayed impulses

$$x(n) = \sum_{k=-\infty,\infty} x(k) \cdot \delta(n-k) \tag{55.6}$$

and let us identify the response to $\delta(n-k)$ as $h(n-k)$. If the filter is time-invariant, each delayed impulse will produce the same response, but time-shifted; due to the linearity property, such responses will be summed at the output:

$$y(n) = \sum_{k=-\infty,\infty} x(k) \cdot h(n-k). \tag{55.7}$$

This convolution product links input and output and defines the property of the filter. Two of them should be recalled: *stability* and *causality*. The former ensures that bounded (finite) inputs will

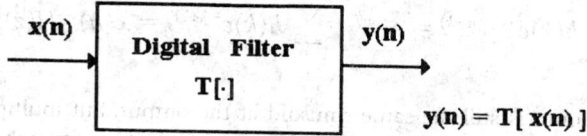

FIGURE 55.5 General block diagram of a digital filter. The output digital signal $y(n)$ is obtained from the input $x(n)$ by means of a transformation $T[\cdot]$ which identifies the filter.

produce bounded outputs. Such a property can be deduced by the impulse response; it can be proved that the filter is stable if and only if

$$\sum_{k=-\infty,\infty} |h(k)| < \infty \qquad (55.8)$$

Causality means that the filter will not respond to an input before the input is applied. This is in agreement with our physical concept of a system, but it is not strictly required for a digital filter that can be implemented in a noncausal form. A filter is causal if and only if

$$h(k) = 0 \qquad \text{for } k < 0$$

Even if relation (55.7) completely describes the properties of the filter, most often it is necessary to express the input-output relationships of linear discrete-time systems under the form of the *z*-transform operator, which allows one to express relation (55.7) in a more useful, operative, and simpler form.

The z-Transform

The *z*-transform of a sequence $x(n)$ is defined by [Rainer et al., 1972]

$$X(z) = \sum_{k=-\infty,\infty} x(k) \cdot z^{-k} \qquad (55.9)$$

where z is a complex variable. This series will converge or diverge for different z values. The set of z values which makes Eq. (55.9) converge is the region of convergence, and it depends on the series $x(n)$ considered.

Among the properties of the *z*-transform, we recall

- The delay (shift) property:
  If $\quad w(n) = x(n - T) \quad$ then $\quad W(z) = X(z) \cdot z^{-T}$
- The product of convolution:
  If $\quad w(n) = \sum_{k=-\infty,\infty} x(k) \cdot y(n - k) \quad$ then $\quad W(z) = X(z) \cdot Y(z)$

The Transfer Function in the z-Domain

Thanks to the previous property, we can express Eq. (55.7) in the *z*-domain as a simple multiplication:

$$Y(z) = H(z) \cdot X(z) \qquad (55.10)$$

where $H(z)$, known as *transfer function* of the filter, is the *z*-transform of the impulse response. $H(z)$ plays a relevant role in the analysis and design of digital filters. The response to input sinusoids can be evaluated as follows: Assume a complex sinusoid $x(n) = e^{j\omega nT_s}$ as input, the correspondent filter output will be

$$y(n) = \sum_{k=0,\infty} h(k)e^{j\omega T_s(n-k)} = e^{j\omega nT_s} \sum_{k=0,\infty} h(k)e^{-j\omega kT_s} = x(n) \cdot H(z)|_{z=e^{j\omega T_s}} \quad (55.11)$$

Then a sinusoid in input is still the same sinusoid at the output, but multiplied by a complex quantity $H(\omega)$. Such complex function defines the response of the filter for each sinusoid of ω pulse in input, and it is known as the frequency response of the filter. It is evaluated in the complex z plane by computing $H(z)$ for $z = e^{j\omega T_s}$, namely, on the point locus that describes the unitary circle on the z plane ($|e^{j\omega T_s}| = 1$). As a complex function, $H(\omega)$ will be defined by its module $|H(\omega)|$ and by its phase $\angle H(\omega)$ functions, as shown in Fig. 55.6 for a moving average filter of order 5. The figure indicates that the lower-frequency components will come through the filter almost unaffected, while the higher-frequency components will be drastically reduced. It is usual to express the horizontal axis of frequency response from 0 to π. This is obtained because only pulse frequencies up to $\omega_s/2$ are reconstructable (due to the Shannon theorem), and therefore, in the horizontal axis, the value of ωT_s is reported which goes from 0 to π. Furthermore, Fig. 55.6b demonstrates that the phase is piecewise linear, and in correspondence with the zeroes of $|H(\omega)|$, there is a change in phase of π value. According to their frequency response, the filters are usually classified as (1) low-pass, (2) high-pass, (3) bandpass, or (4) bandstop filters. Figure 55.7 shows the ideal frequency response for such filters with the proper low- and high-frequency cutoffs.

For a large class of linear, time-invariant systems, $H(z)$ can be expressed in the following general form:

$$H(z) = \frac{\sum_{m=0,M} b_m z^{-m}}{1 + \sum_{k=1,N} a_k z^{-k}} \quad (55.12)$$

which describes in the z domain the following *difference equation* in the discrete time domain:

$$y(n) = -\sum_{k=1,N} a_k y(n-k) + \sum_{m=0,M} b_m x(n-m) \quad (55.13)$$

a)

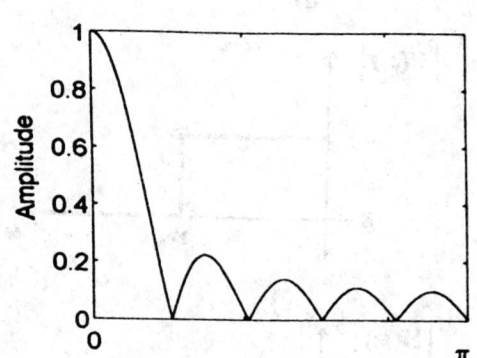

b)

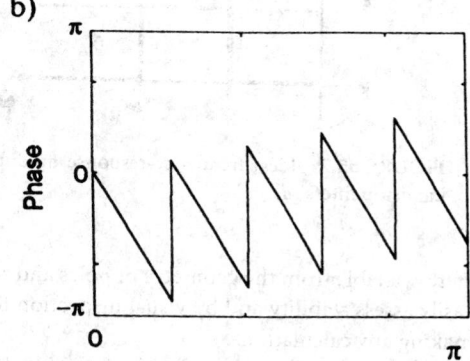

FIGURE 55.6 Modulus (*a*) and phase (*b*) diagrams of the frequency response of a moving average filter of order 5. Note that the frequency plots are depicted up to π. In fact, taking into account that we are dealing with a sampled signal whose frequency information is up to $f_s/2$, we have $\omega_{max} = 2\pi f_s/2 = \pi f_s$ or $\omega_{max} = \pi$ if normalized with respect to the sampling rate.

When at least one of the a_k coefficient is different from zero, some output values contribute to the current output. The filter contains some feedback, and it is said to be implemented in a *recursive* form. On the other hand, when the a_k values are all zero, the filter output is obtained only from the current or previous inputs, and the filter is said to be implemented in a *nonrecursive* form.

The transfer function can be expressed in a more useful form by finding the roots of both numerator and denominator:

$$H(z) = \frac{b_0 z^{N-M} \Pi_{m=1,M} (z - z_m)}{\Pi_{k=1,N} (z - p_k)} \quad (55.14)$$

where z_m are the zeroes and p_k are the poles. It is worth nothing that $H(z)$ presents $N - M$ zeros in correspondence with the origin of the z plane and M zeroes elsewhere (N zeroes totally) and N poles. The pole-zero form of $H(z)$ is of great interest because several properties of the filter are immedi-

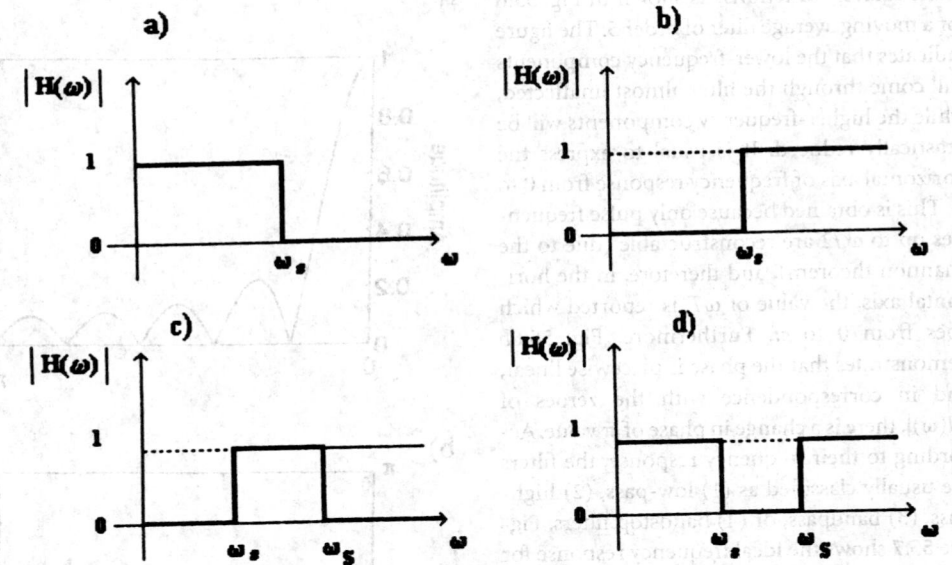

FIGURE 55.7 Ideal frequency-response moduli for low-pass (*a*), high-pass (*b*), bandpass (*c*), and bandstop filters (*d*).

ately available from the geometry of poles and zeroes in the complex *z* plane. In fact, it is possible to easily assess stability and by visual inspection to roughly estimate the frequency response without making any calculations.

Stability is verified when all poles lie inside the unitary circle, as can be proved by considering the relationships between the *z*-transform and the Laplace *s*-transform and by observing that the left side of the *s* plane is mapped inside the unitary circle [Jackson, 1986; Oppenheim & Schafer, 1975].

The frequency response can be estimated by noting that $(z - z_m)|_{z=e^{j\omega T_s}}$ is a vector joining the *m*th zero with the point on the unitary circle identified by the angle ωT_s. Defining

$$\vec{B}_m = (z - z_m)|_{z=e^{j\omega T_s}}$$
$$\vec{A}_k = (z - p_k)|_{z=e^{j\omega T_s}} \tag{55.15}$$

we obtain

$$|H(\omega)| = \frac{b_0 \Pi_{m=1,M} |\vec{B}_m|}{\Pi_{k=1,N} |\vec{A}_k|} \tag{55.16}$$

$$\angle H(\omega) = \sum_{m=1,M} \angle \vec{B}_m - \sum_{k=1,N} \angle \vec{A}_k + (N - M)\omega T_s.$$

Thus the modulus of $H(\omega)$ can be evaluated at any frequency $\omega°$ by computing the distances between poles and zeroes and the point on the unitary circle corresponding to $\omega = \omega°$, as evidenced by Fig. 55.8, where a filter with two pairs of complex poles and three zeros is considered.

To obtain the estimate of $H(\omega)$, we move around the unitary circle and roughly evaluate the effect of poles and zeroes by keeping in mind a few rules [Challis & Kitney, 1982]: (1) when we are close to a zero, $|H(\omega)|$ will approach zero, and a positive phase shift will appear in $\angle H(\omega)$ as the vector from the zero reverses its angle; (2) when we are close to a pole, $|H(\omega)|$ will tend to peak, and a negative phase change is found in $\angle H(\omega)$ (the closer the pole to unitary circle, the sharper is the peak until it reaches infinite and the filter becomes unstable); and (3) near a closer pole-zero pair, the response modulus will tends to zero or infinity if the zero or the pole is closer, while far from this pair, the modulus can be considered unitary. As an example, it is possible to compare the modulus and phase diagram of Fig. 55.8*b,c* with the relative geometry of poles and zeroes of Fig. 55.8*a*.

FIR and IIR Filters

A common way of classifying digital filters is based on the characteristics of their impulse response. For finite impulse response (FIR) filters, $h(n)$ is composed of a finite number of nonzero values, while for infinite impulse response (IIR) filters, $h(n)$ oscillates up to infinity with nonzero values. It is clearly evident that in order to obtain an infinite response to an impulse in input, the IIR filter must contain some feedback that sustains the output as the input vanishes. The presence of feedback paths requires to put particular attention to the filter stability.

Even if FIR filters are usually implemented in a nonrecursive form and IIR filters in a recursive form, the two ways of classification are not coincident. In fact, as shown by the following example, a FIR filter can be expressed in a recursive form

$$H(z) = \sum_{k=0,N-1} z^{-k} = \sum_{k=0,N-1} z^{-k} \frac{(1 - z^{-1})}{(1 - z^{-1})} = \frac{1 - z^{-N}}{1 - z^{-1}} \tag{55.17}$$

for a more convenient computational implementation.

As shown previously, two important requirements for filters are stability and linear phase response. FIR filters can be easily designed to fulfill such requirements; they are always stable (having no poles outside the origin), and the linear phase response is obtained by constraining the impulse response coefficients to have symmetry around their midpoint. Such constrain implies

$$b_m = \pm b_{M-m}^* \tag{55.18}$$

where the b_m are the M coefficients of an FIR filter. The sign $+$ or $-$ stays in accordance with the symmetry (even or odd) and M value (even or odd). This is a necessary and sufficient condition for FIR filters to have linear phase response. Two cases of impulse response that yield a linear phase filter are shown in Fig. 55.9.

It should be noted that condition (55.18) imposes geometric constrains to the zero locus of $H(z)$. Taking into account Eq. (55.12), we have

$$z^M H(z) = H\left(\frac{1}{z^*}\right) \tag{55.19}$$

Thus, both z_m and $1/z_m^*$ must be zeros of $H(z)$. Then the zeroes of linear phase FIR filters must lie on the unitary circle, or they must appear in pairs and with inverse moduli.

Design Criteria

In many cases, the filter is designed in order to satisfy some requirements, usually on the frequency response, which depend on the characteristic of the particular application the filter is intended for. It is known that ideal filters, like those reported in Fig. 55.7, are not physically realizable (they would require an infinite number of coefficients of impulse response); thus we can design FIR or IIR filters that can only mimic, with an acceptable error, the ideal response. Figure 55.10 shows a frequency response of a not ideal low-pass filter. Here, there are ripples in passband and in stopband, and there is a transition band from passband to stopband, defined by the interval $\omega_s - \omega_p$.

Several design techniques are available, and some of them require heavy computational tasks, which are capable of developing filters with defined specific requirements. They include window tech-

nique, frequency-sampling method, or equiripple design for FIR filters. Butterworth, Cheby-
chev, elliptical design, and impulse-invariant or
bilinear transformation are instead employed
for IIR filters. For detailed analysis of digital filter techniques, see Antoniou [1979], Cerutti
[1983], and Oppenheim and Schafer [1975].

Examples

A few examples of different kinds of filters will
be presented in the following, showing some applications on ECG signal processing. It is known
that the ECG contains relevant information
over a wide range of frequencies; the lower-
frequency contents should be preserved for
correct measurement of the slow ST displacements, while higher-frequency contents are
needed to correctly estimate amplitude and
duration of the faster contributions, mainly at
the level of the QRS complex. Unfortunately,
several sources of noise are present in the same
frequency band, such as, for example, higher-
frequency noise due to muscle contraction
(EMG noise), the lower-frequency noise due to
motion artifacts (baseline wandering), the effect
of respiration or the low-frequency noise in the
skin-electrode interface, and others.

In the first example, the effect of two different low-pass filters will be considered. An ECG
signal corrupted by an EMG noise (Fig. 55.11a)
is low-pass filtered by two different low-pass filters whose frequency responses are shown in
Fig. 55.11b,c. The two FIR filters have cutoff frequencies at 40 and 20 Hz, respectively, and were
designed through window techniques (Weber-
Cappellini window, filter length = 256 points)
[Cappellini et al., 1978].

The output signals are shown in Fig. 55.11d,e.
Filtering drastically reduces the superimposed
noise but at the same time alters the original
ECG waveform. In particular, the R wave amplitude is progressively reduced by decreasing the
cutoff frequency, and the QRS width is progressively increased as well. On the other hand, P
waves appears almost unaffected, having frequency components generally lower than 20 to
30 Hz. At this point, it is worth noting that an
increase in QRS duration is generally associated

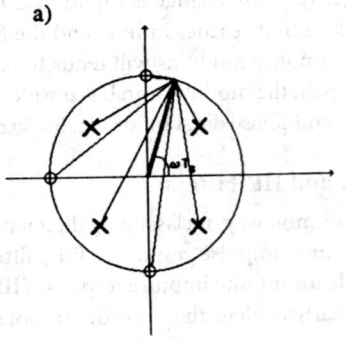

a)

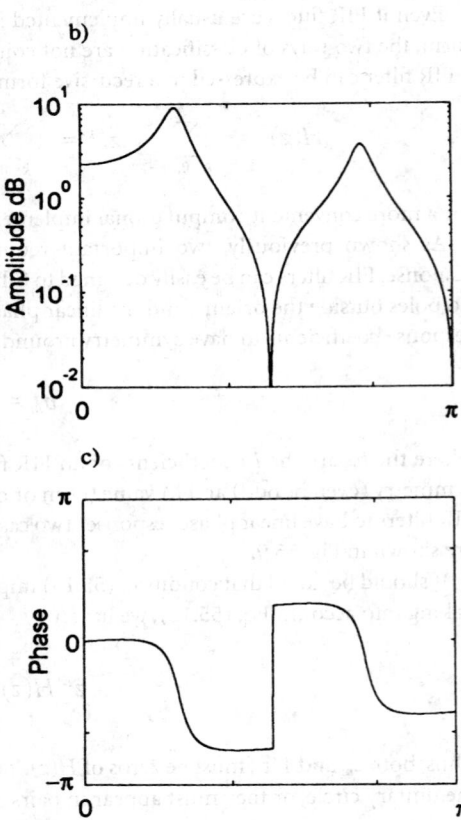

b)

c)

FIGURE 55.8 Poles and zeroes geometry (*a*) and
relative frequency response modulus (*b*) and phase (*c*)
characteristics. Moving around the unitary circle a
rough estimation of $|H(\omega)|$ and $\angle H(\omega)$ can be ob-
tained. Note the zeros' effects at π and $\pi/2$ and modulus rising in proximity of the poles. Phase shifts are
cleary evident in part *c* closer to zeros and poles.

with various pathologies, such as ventricular hypertrophy or bundle-branch block. It is therefore
necessary to check that an excessive band limitation does not introduce a false-positive indication
in the diagnosis of the ECG signal.

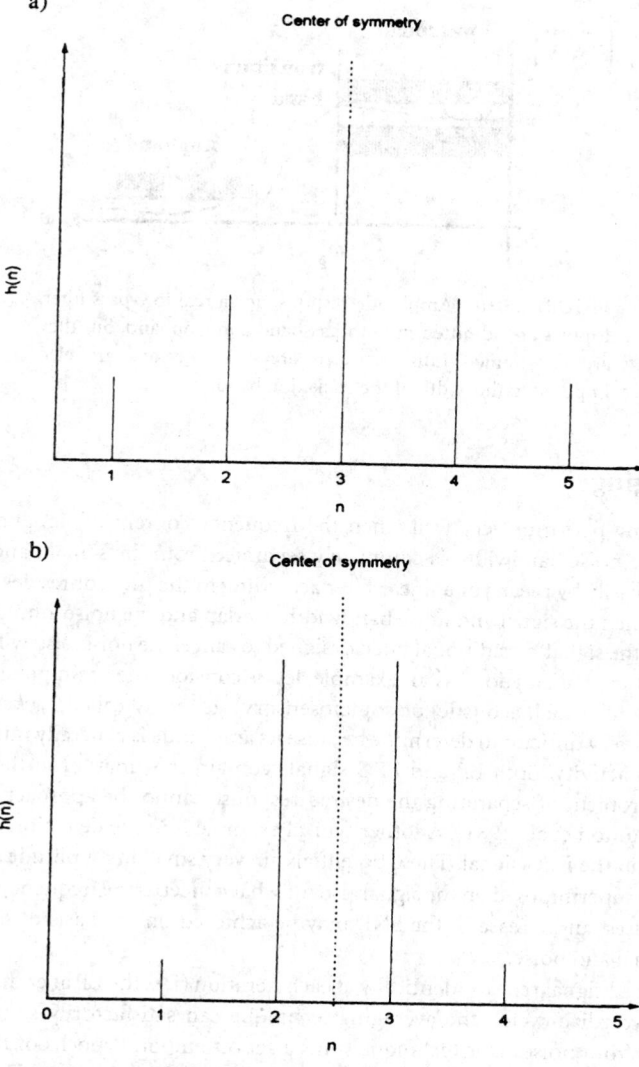

FIGURE 55.9 Examples of impulse response for linear phase FIR filters: odd (*a*) and even (*b*) number of coefficients.

An example of an application for stopband filters (notch filters) is presented in Fig. 55.12. It is used to reduce the 50-Hz mains noise on the ECG signal, and it was designed by placing a zero in correspondence of the frequency we want to suppress.

Finally, an example of a high-pass filter is shown for the detection of the QRS complex. Detecting the time occurrence of a fiducial point in the QRS complex is indeed the first task usually performed in ECG signal analysis. The QRS complex usually contains the higher-frequency components with respect to the other ECG waves, and thus such components will be enhanced by a high-pass filter. Figure 55.13 shows how QRS complexes (Fig. 55.13*a*) can be identified by a derivative high-pass filter with a cutoff frequency to decrease the effect of the noise contributions at high frequencies (Fig. 55.13*b*). The filtered signal (Fig. 55.13*c*) presents sharp and well-defined peaks that are easily recognized by a threshold value.

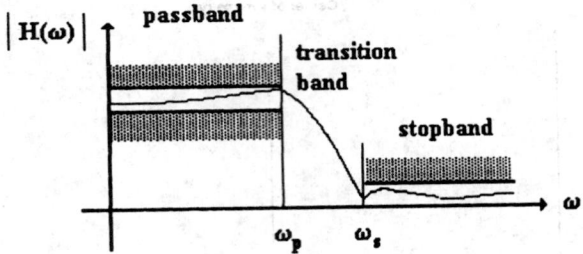

FIGURE 55.10 Amplitude response for a real low-pass filter. Ripples are admitted in both passband and stopband, but they are constrained into restricted areas. Limitations are also imposed to the width of the transition band.

Signal Averaging

Traditional filtering performs very well when the frequency content of signal and noise do not overlap. When the noise bandwidth is completely separated from the signal bandwidth, the noise can be decreased easily by means of a linear filter according to the procedures described earlier. On the other hand, when the signal and noise bandwidth overlap and the noise amplitude is enough to seriously corrupt the signal, a traditional filter, designed to cancel the noise, also will introduce signal cancellation or, at least, distortion. As an example, let us consider the brain potentials evoked by a sensory stimulation (visual, acoustic, or somatosensory) generally called *evoked potentials* (EP). Such a response is very difficult to determine because its amplitude is generally much lower than the background EEG activity. Both EP and EEG signals contain information in the same frequency range; thus the problem of separating the desired response cannot be approached via traditional digital filtering [Aunon et al., 1981]. Another typical example is in the detection of ventricular late potentials (VLP) in the ECG signal. These potentials are very small in amplitude and are comparable with the noise superimposed on the signal also for what concerns the frequency content [Simson, 1981]. In such cases, an increase in the SNR may be achieved on the basis of different statistical properties of signal and noise.

When the desired signal repeats identically at each iteration (i.e., the EP at each sensory stimulus, the VLP at each cardiac cycle), the averaging technique can satisfactorily solve the problem of separating signal from noise. This technique sums a set of temporal epochs of the signal together with the superimposed noise. If the time epochs are properly aligned, through efficient trigger-point recognition, the signal waveforms directly sum together. If the signal and the noise are characterized by the following statistical properties:

1. All the signal epochs contain a deterministic signal component $x(n)$ that does not vary for all the epochs.
2. The superimposed noise $w(n)$ is a broadband stationary process with zero mean and variance σ^2 so that

$$E[w(n)] = 0$$
$$E[w^2(n)] = \sigma^2 \tag{55.20}$$

3. Signal $x(n)$ and noise $w(n)$ are uncorrelated so that the recorded signal $y(n)$ at the *i*th iteration can be expressed as

$$y(n)_i = x(n) + w_i(n), \tag{55.21}$$

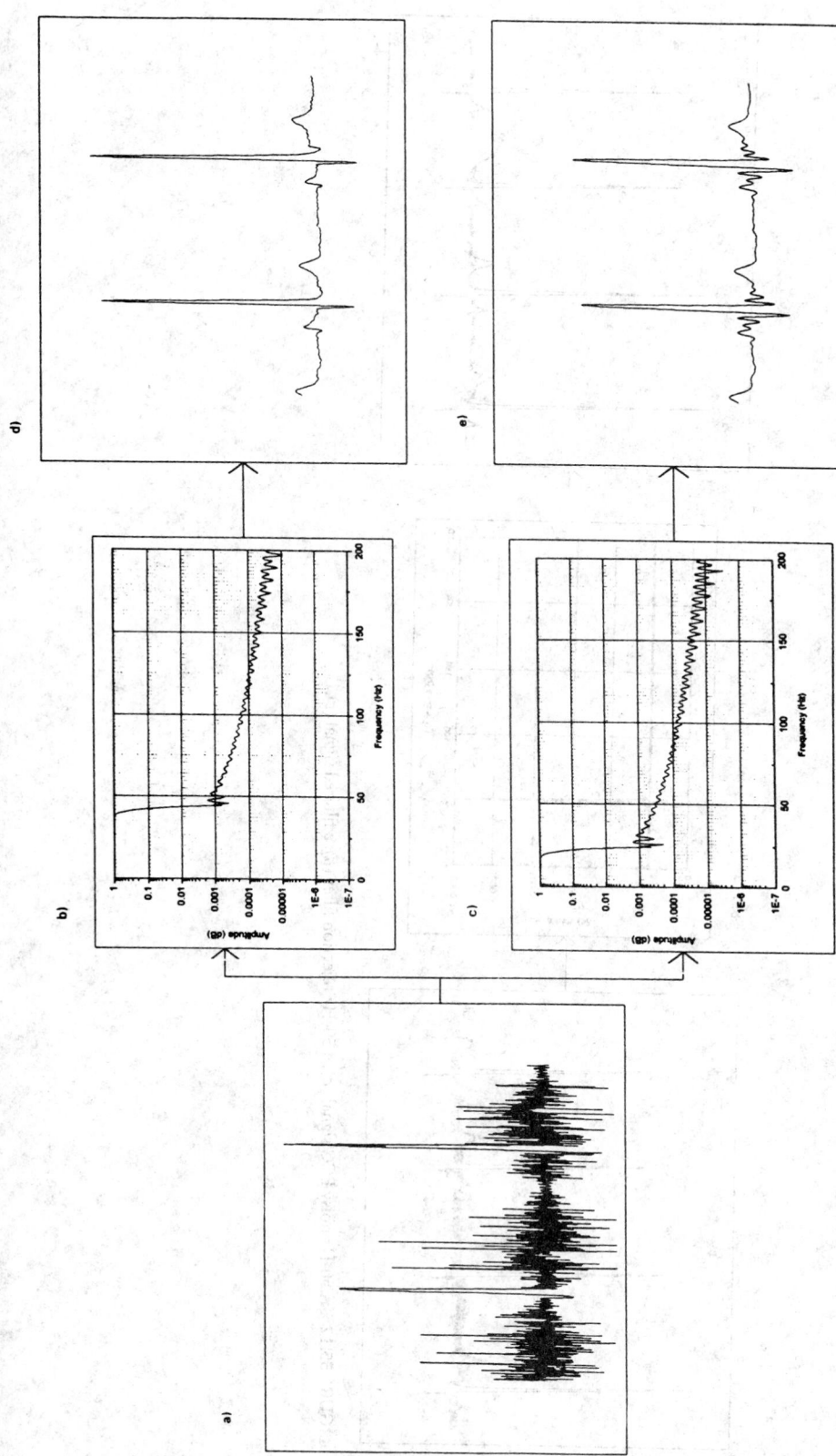

FIGURE 55.11 Effects of two different low-pass filters (*b*) and (*c*) on an ECG trace (*a*) corrupted by EMG noise. Both amplitude reduction and variation in the QRS width induced by too drastic lowpass filtering are evidenced.

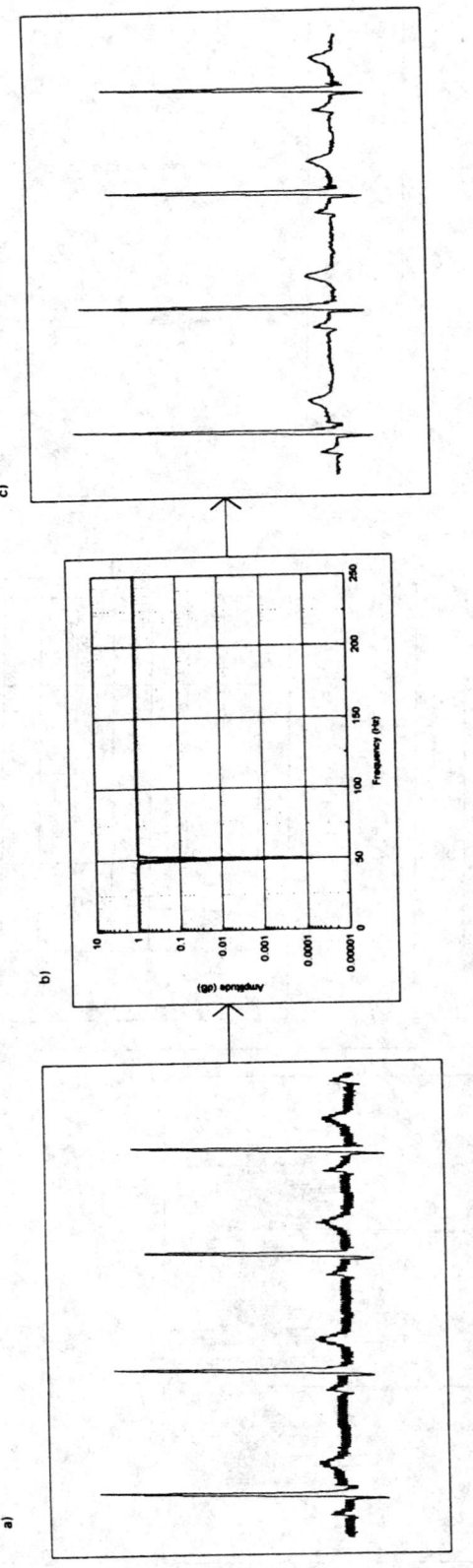

FIGURE 55.12 A 50-Hz noisy ECG signal (*a*); a 50-Hz rejection filter (*b*); a filtered signal (*c*).

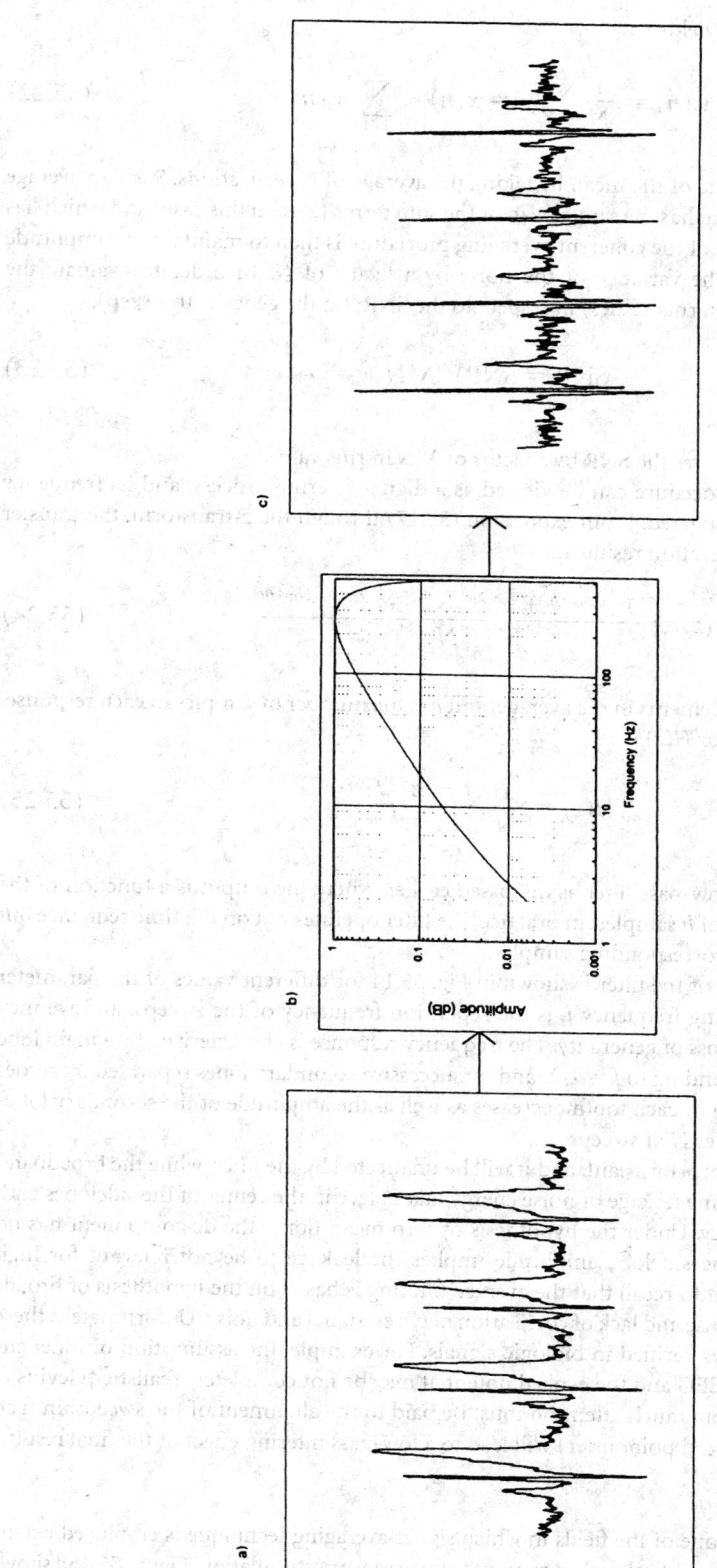

FIGURE 55.13 Effect of a derivative high-pass filter (*b*) on an ECG lead (*a*). (*c*) The output of the filter.

Then the averaging process yields y_t:

$$y_t(n) = \frac{1}{N} \sum_{i=1}^{N} y_i = x(n) + \sum_{i=1}^{N} w_i(n) \tag{55.22}$$

The noise term is an estimate of the mean by taking the average of N realizations. Such an average is a new random variable that has the same mean of the sum terms (zero in this case) and which has variance of σ^2/N. The effect of the coherent averaging procedure is then to maintain the amplitude of the signal and reduce the variance of the noise by a factor of N. In order to evaluate the improvement in the SNR (in rms values) in respect to the SNR; (at the generic ith sweep):

$$SNR = SNR_i \cdot \sqrt{N} \tag{55.23}$$

Thus signal averaging improves the SNR by a factor of $\sqrt{N}$ in rms value.

A coherent averaging procedure can be viewed as a digital filtering process, and its frequency characteristics can be investigated. From expression (55.17) through the z-transform, the transfer function of the filtering operation results in

$$H(z) = \frac{1 + z^{-h} + z^{-2h} + \cdots + z^{-(N-1)h}}{N} \tag{55.24}$$

where N is the number of elements in the average, and h is the number of samples in each response. An alternative expression for $H(z)$ is

$$H(z) = \frac{1}{N} \frac{1 - z^{-Nh}}{1 - z^h} \tag{55.25}$$

This is a moving average low-pass filter as discussed earlier, where the output is a function of the preceding value with a lag of h samples; in practice, the filter operates not on the time sequence but in the sweep sequence on corresponding samples.

The frequency response of the filter is shown in Fig. 55.14 for different values of the parameter N. In this case, the sampling frequency f_s is the repetition frequency of the sweeps, and we may assume it to be 1 without loss of generality. The frequency response is characterized by a main lobe with the first zero corresponding to $f = 1/N$ and by successive secondary lobes separated by zeroes at intervals $1/N$. The width of each tooth decreases as well as the amplitude of the secondary lobes when increasing the number N of sweeps.

The desired signal is sweep-invariant, and it will be unaffected by the filter, while the broadband noise will be decreased. Some leakage of noise energy takes place in the center of the sidelobes and, of course, at zero frequency. Under the hypothesis of zero mean noise, the dc component has no effect, and the diminishing sidelobe amplitude implies the leakage to be not relevant for high frequencies. It is important to recall that the average filtering is based on the hypothesis of broadband distribution of the noise and lack of correlation between signal and noise. Unfortunately, these assumptions are not always verified in biologic signals. For example, the assumption of independence of the background EEG and the evoked potential may be not completely realistic [Gevins & Remond, 1987]. In addition, much attention must be paid to the alignment of the sweeps; in fact, slight misalignments (fiducial point jitter) will lead to a low-pass filtering effect of the final result.

Example

As mentioned previously, one of the fields in which signal-averaging technique is employed extensively is in the evaluation of cerebral evoked response after a sensory stimulation. Figure 55.15a shows

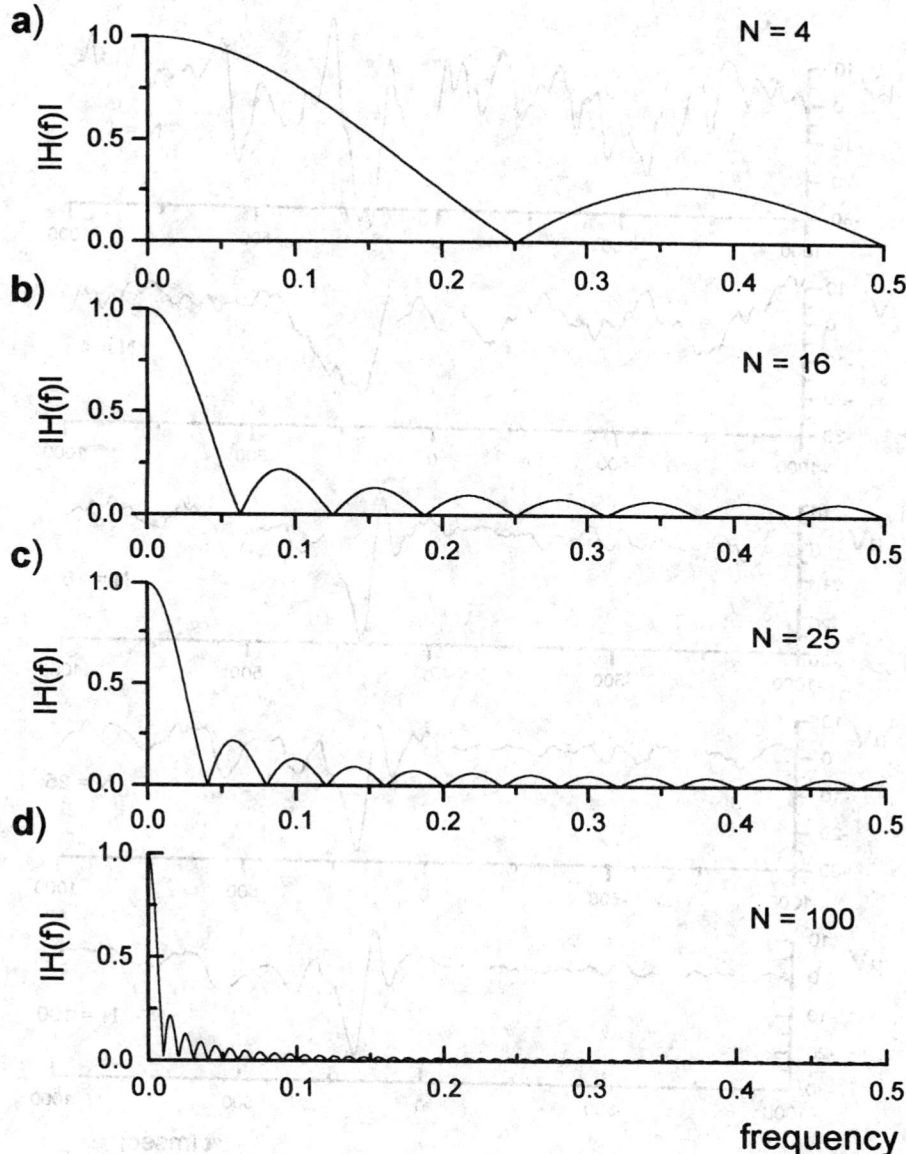

FIGURE 55.14 Equivalent frequency response for the signal-averaging procedure for different values of N (see text).

the EEG recorded from the scalp of a normal subject after a somatosensory stimulation released at time $t = 0$. The evoked potential ($N = 1$) is not visible because it is buried in the background EEG (upper panel). In the successive panels there is the same evoked potential after averaging different numbers of sweeps corresponding to the frequency responses shown in Fig. 55.14. As N increases, the SNR is improved by a factor $\sqrt{N}$ (in rms value), and the morphology of the evoked potential becomes more recognizable while the EEG contribution is markedly diminished. In this way it is easy to evaluate the quantitative indices of clinical interest, such as the amplitude and the latency of the relevant waves.

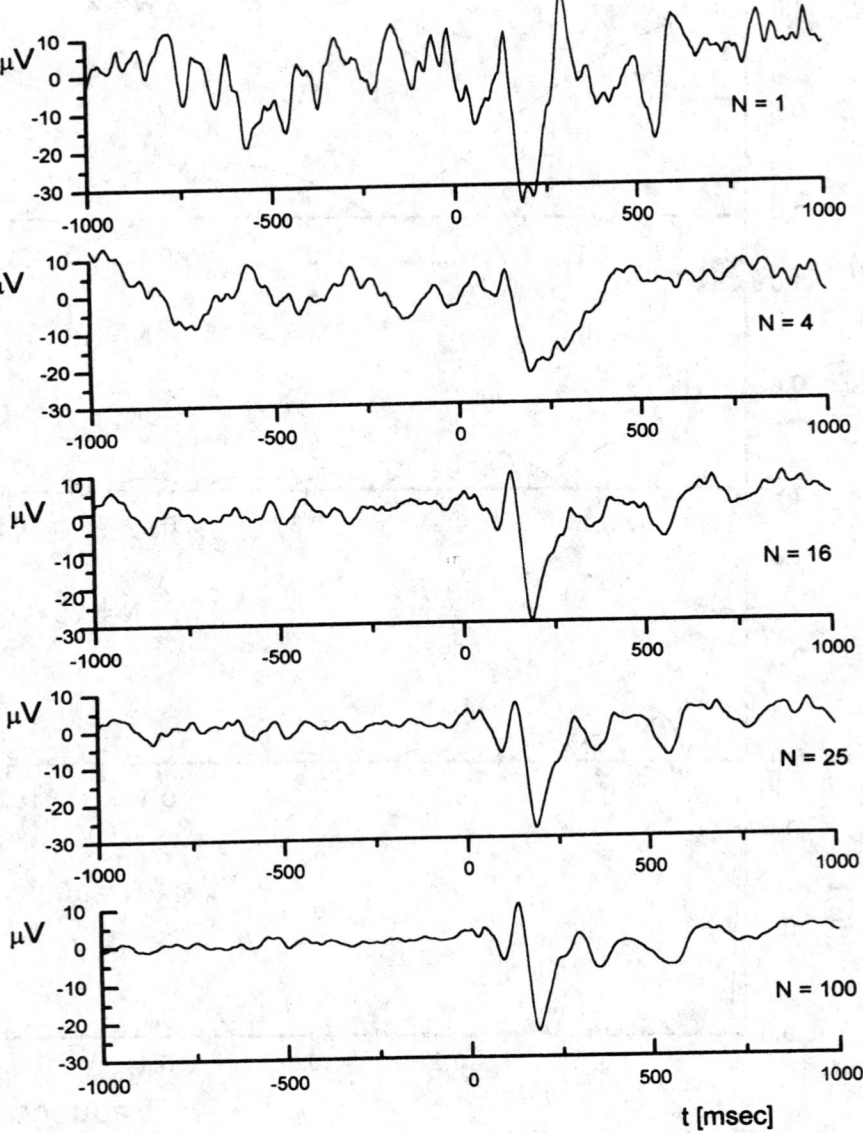

FIGURE 55.15 Enhancement of evoked potential (EP) by means of averaging technique. The EEG noise is progressively reduced, and the EP morphology becomes more recognizable as the number of averaged sweeps (*N*) is increased.

Spectral Analysis

The various methods to estimate the power spectrum density (PSD) of a signal may be classified as *nonparametric* and *parametric*.

Nonparametric Estimators of PSD

This is a traditional method of frequency analysis based on the Fourier transform that can be evaluated easily through the fast Fourier transform (FFT) algorithm [Marple, 1987]. The expression of the PSD as a function of the frequency $P(f)$ can be obtained directly from the time series $y(n)$ by using the periodogram expression

$$P(f) = \frac{1}{T_s} \left| T_s \sum_{k=0}^{N-1} y(k)e^{-j2\pi fkT_s} \right|^2 = \frac{1}{NT_s} |Y(f)|^2 \qquad (55.26)$$

where T_s is the sampling period, N is the number of samples, and $Y(f)$ is the discrete time Fourier transform of $y(n)$.

On the basis of the Wiener-Khintchin theorem, PSD is also obtainable in two steps from the FFT of the autocorrelation function $R_{yy}(k)$ of the signal, where $R_{yy}(k)$ is estimated by means of the following expression:

$$\hat{R}_{yy}(k) = \frac{1}{N} \sum_{i=0}^{N-k-1} y(i)y^*(i+k) \qquad (55.27)$$

where * denotes the complex conjugate. Thus the PSD is expressed as

$$P(f) = T_s \cdot \sum_{k=-N}^{N} \hat{R}_{yy}(k)e^{-j2\pi fkT_s} \qquad (55.28)$$

based on the available lag estimates $\hat{R}_{yy}(k)$, where $-(1/2T_s) \leq f \leq (1/2T_s)$

FFT-based methods are widely diffused, for their easy applicability, computational speed, and direct interpretation of the results. Quantitative parameters are obtained by evaluating the power contribution at different frequency bands. This is achieved by dividing the frequency axis in ranges of interest and by integrating the PSD on such intervals. The area under this portion of the spectrum is the fraction of the total signal variance due to the specific frequencies. However, autocorrelation function and Fourier transform are theoretically defined on infinite data sequences. Thus errors are introduced by the need to operate on finite data records in order to obtain estimators of the true functions. In addition, for the finite data set it is necessary to make assumptions, sometimes not realistic, about the data outside the recording window; commonly they are considered to be zero. This implicit rectangular windowing of the data results in a spectral leakage in the PSD. Different windows that smoothly connect the side samples to zero are most often used in order to solve this problem, even if they may introduce a reduction in the frequency resolution [Harris, 1978]. Furthermore, the estimators of the signal PSD are not statistically consistent, and various techniques are needed to improve their statistical performances. Various methods are mentioned in the literature; the methods of Dariell [1946], Bartlett [1948], and Welch [1970] are the most diffused ones. Of course, all these procedures cause a further reduction in frequency resolution.

Parametric Estimators

Parametric approaches assume the time series under analysis to be the output of a given mathematical model, and no drastic assumptions are made about the data outside the recording window. The PSD is calculated as a function of the model parameters according to appropriate expressions. A critical point in this approach is the choice of an adequate model to represent the data sequence. The model is completely independent of the physiologic, anatomic, and physical characteristics of the biologic system but provides simply the input-output relationships of the process in the so-called black-box approach.

Among the numerous possibilities of modeling, linear models, characterized by a rational transfer function, are able to describe a wide number of different processes. In the most general case, they are represented by the following linear equation that relates the input-driving signal $w(k)$ and the output of an autoregressive moving average (ARMA) process:

$$y(k) = -\sum_{i=1}^{p} a_i y(k-i) + \sum_{j=1}^{q} b_j w(k-j) + w(k) \qquad (55.29)$$

where $w(k)$ is the input white noise with zero mean value and variance λ^2, p and q are the orders of AR and MA parts, respectively, and a_i and b_j are the proper coefficients.

The ARMA model may be reformulated as an AR or an MA if the coefficients b_j or a_i are, respectively, set to zero. Since the estimation of the AR parameters results in linear equations, AR models are usually employed in place of ARMA or MA models, also on the basis of the Wold decomposition theorem [Marple, 1987] that establishes that any stationary ARMA or MA process of finite variance can be represented as a unique AR model of appropriate order, even infinite; likewise, any ARMA or AR process can be represented by an MA model of sufficiently high order.

The AR PSD is then obtained from the following expression:

$$P(f) = \frac{\lambda^2 T_s}{\left|1 + \sum_{i=1}^{p} a_i z^{-i}\right|^2_{z=\exp(j2\pi f T_s)}} = \frac{\lambda^2 T_s}{\left|\prod_{l=1}^{p} (z - z_l)\right|^2_{z=\exp(j2\pi f T_s)}} \qquad (55.30)$$

The right side of the relation puts into evidence the poles of the transfer function that can be plotted in the z-transform plane. Figure 55.16b shows the PSD function of the HRV signal depicted in Fig. 55.16a, while Fig. 55.16c displays the corresponding pole diagram obtained according to the procedure described in the preceding section.

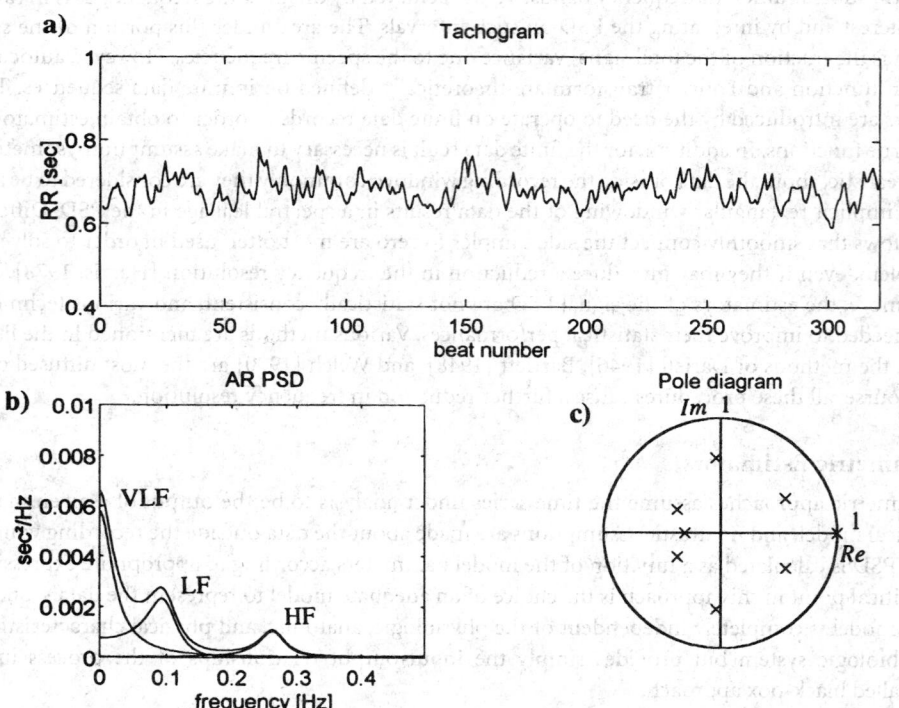

FIGURE 55.16   (*a*) Interval tachogram obtained from an ECG recording as the sequence of the RR time intervals expressed in seconds as a function of the beat number. (*b*) PSD of the signal (*a*) evaluated by means of an AR model (see text). (*c*) Pole diagram of the PSD shown in (*b*).

Parametric methods are methodologically and computationally more complex than the nonparametric ones, since they require an a priori choice of the structure and of the order of the model of the signal-generation mechanism. Some tests are required a posteriori to verify the whiteness of the prediction error, such as the Anderson test (autocorrelation test) [Box & Jenkins, 1976] in order to test the reliability of the estimation. Postprocessing of the spectra can be performed as well as for nonparametric approaches by integrating the $P(f)$ function in predefined frequency ranges; however, the AR modeling has the advantage of allowing a spectral decomposition for a direct and automatic calculation of the power and frequency of each spectral component. In the z-transform domain, the autocorrelation function (ACF) $R(k)$ and the $P(z)$ of the signal are related by the following expression:

$$R(k) = \frac{1}{2\pi j} \int_{|z|=1} P(z)z^{k-1}dz \qquad (55.31)$$

If the integral is calculated by means of the residual method, the ACF is decomposed into a sum of dumped sinusoids, each one related to a pair of complex conjugate poles, and of dumped exponential functions, related to the real poles [Zetterberg, 1969]. The Fourier transform of each one of these terms gives the expression of each spectral component that fits the component related to the relevant pole or pole pair. The argument of the pole gives the central frequency of the component, while the ith spectral component power is the residual γ_i in case of real poles and $2Re(\gamma_i)$ in case of conjugate pole pairs. γ_i is computed from the following expression:

$$\gamma_i = z^{-1}(z - z_i)P(z)\big|_{z=z_i} \qquad (55.32)$$

It is advisable to point out the basic characteristics of the two approaches that have been described above: the nonparametric and the parametric. The latter (parametric) has evident advantages with respect to the former, which can be summarized in the following:

- It has a more statistical consistency even on short segments of data; i.e., under certain assumptions, a spectrum estimated through autoregressive modeling is a maximum entropy spectrum (MES).
- The spectrum is more easily interpretable with an "implicit" filtering of what is considered random noise.
- An easy and more reliable calculation of the spectral parameters (postprocessing of the spectrum), through the spectral decomposition procedure, is possible. Such parameters are directly interpretable from a physiologic point of view.
- There is no need to window the data in order to decrease the spectral leakage.
- The frequency resolution does not depend on the number of data.

On the other hand, the parametric approach

- Is more complex from a methodologic and computational point of view.
- Requires an a priori definition of the kind of the model (AR, MA, ARMA, or other) to be fitted and mainly its complexity defined (i.e., the number of parameters).

Some figures of merit introduced in literature may be of help in determining their value [Akaike, 1974]. Still, this procedure may be difficult in some cases.

Example

As an example, let us consider the frequency analysis of the heart rate variability (HRV) signal. In Fig. 55.16a, the time sequence of the RR intervals obtained from an ECG recording is shown. The RR intervals are expressed in seconds as a function of the beat number in the so-called interval tachogram. It is worth noting that the RR series is not constant but is characterized by oscillations of up to the 10% of its mean value. These oscillations are not casual but are the effect of the action of the autonomic nervous system in controlling heart rate. In particular, the frequency analysis of such a signal (Fig. 55.16*b* shows the PSD obtained by mean of an AR model) has evidenced three principal contributions in the overall variability of the HRV signal. A very low frequency (VLF) component is due to the long-term regulation mechanisms that cannot be resolved by analyzing a few minutes of signal (3 to 5 minutes are generally studied in the traditional spectral analysis of the HRV signal). Other techniques are needed for a complete understanding of such mechanisms. The low-frequency (LF) component is centered around 0.1 Hz, in a range between 0.03 and 0.15 Hz. An increase in its power has always been observed in relation to sympathetic activations. Finally, the high-frequency (HF) component, in synchrony with the respiration rate, is due to the respiration activity mediated by the vagus nerve; thus it can be a marker of vagal activity. In particular, LF and HF power, both in absolute and in normalized units (i.e., as percentage value on the total power without the VLF contribution), and their ratio LF/HF are quantitative indices widely employed for the quantification of the sympathovagal balance in controlling heart rate [Malliani et al., 1991].

55.3 Conclusion

The basic aspects of signal acquisition and processing have been illustrated, intended as fundamental tools for the treatment of biologic signals. A few examples also were reported relative to the ECG signal, as well as EEG signals and EPs. Particular processing algorithms have been described that use digital filtering techniques, coherent averaging, and power spectrum analysis as reference examples on how traditional or innovative techniques of digital signal processing may impact the phase of informative parameter extraction from biologic signals. They may improve the knowledge of many physiologic systems as well as help clinicians in dealing with new quantitative parameters that could better discriminate between normal and pathologic cases.

Defining Terms

Aliasing: Phenomenon that takes place when, in A/D conversion, the sampling frequency f_s is lower than twice the frequency content f_b of the signal; frequency components above $f_s/2$ are folded back and are summed to the lower-frequency components, distorting the signal.

Averaging: Filtering technique based on the summation of N stationary waveforms buried in casual broadband noise. The SNR is improved by a factor of $\sqrt{N}$.

Frequency response: A complex quantity that, multiplied by a sinusoid input of a linear filter, gives the output sinusoid. It completely characterizes the filter and is the Fourier transform of the impulse response.

Impulse response: Output of a digital filter when the input is the impulse sequence $\delta(n)$. It completely characterizes linear filters and is used for evaluating the output corresponding to different kinds of inputs.

Notch filter: A stopband filter whose stopped band is very sharp and narrow.

Parametric methods: Spectral estimation methods based on the identification of a signal generating model. The power spectral density is a function of the model *parameters*.

Quantization error: Error added to the signal, during the A/D procedure, due to the fact that the analog signal is represented by a digital signal that can assume only a limited and predefined set of values.

Region of convergence: In the *z*-transform plane, the ensemble containing the *z*-complex points that makes a series converge to a finite value.

References

Akaike H. 1974. A new look at the statistical model identification. IEEE Trans Autom Contr (AC-19):716.

Antoniou A. 1979. Digital Filters: Analysis and Design. New York, McGraw-Hill.

Aunon JL, McGillim CD, Childers DG. 1981. Signal processing in evoked potential research: Averaging and modeling. CRC Crit Rev Bioing 5:323.

Bartlett MS. 1948. Smoothing priodograms from time series with continuous spectra. Nature 61:686.

Box GEP, Jenkins GM. 1976. Time Series Analysis: Forecasting and Control. San Francisco, Holden-Day.

Cappellini V, Constantinides AG, Emiliani P. 1978. Digital Filters and Their Applications. London, Academic Press.

Carassa F. 1983. Comunicazioni Elettriche. Torino, Boringhieri.

Cerutti S. 1983. Filtri numerici per l'eleborazione di segnali biologici. Milano, CLUP.

Challis RE, Kitney RI. 1982. The design of digital filters for biomedical signal processing: 1. Basic concepts. J Biomed Eng 5:267.

Cobbold RSC. 1988. Transducers for Biomedical Measurements. New York, Wiley.

Cohen A. 1983. Biomedical Signal Processing: Time and Frequency Domains Analysis. Boca Raton, Fla, CRC Press.

Dariell PJ. 1946. On the theoretical specification and sampling properties of autocorrelated time-series (discussion). JR Stat Soc 8:88.

Gardenhire LW. 1964. Selecting sample rate. ISA J 4:59.

Gevins AS, Remond A (eds). 1987. Handbook of Electrophysiology and Clinical Neurophysiology. Amsterdam, Elsevier.

Glaser EM, Ruchkin DS. 1976. Principles of Neurophysiological Signal Processing. New York, Academic Press.

Harris FJ, 1978. On the use of windows for harmonic analysis with the discrete Fourier transform. Proc IEEE 64(1):51.

Huta K, Webster JG. 1973. 60-Hz interference in electrocardiography. IEEE Trans Biomed Eng 20(2):91.

Jackson LB. 1986. Digital Signal Processing. Hingham, Mass, Kluer Academic.

Jaeger RC. 1982. Tutorial: Analog data acquisition technology: II. Analog to digital conversion. IEEE Micro 8:46.

Malliani A, Pagani M, Lombardi F, Cerutti S. 1991. Cardiovascular neural regulation explored in the frequency domain. Circulation 84:482.

Marple SL. 1987. Digital Spectral Analysis with Applications. Englewood Cliff, NJ, Prentice-Hall.

Oppenheim AV, Schafer RW. 1975. Digital Signal Processing. Englewood Cliffs, NJ, Prentice-Hall.

Rainer LR, Cooley JW, Helms HD, et al. 1972. Terminology in digital signal processing. IEEE Trans Audio Electroac AU-20:322.

Shannon CE. 1949. Communication in presence of noise. Proc IRE 37:10.

Simson MB. 1981. Use of signals in the terminal QRS complex to identify patients with ventricular tachycardia after myocardial infarction. Circulation 64:235.

Thakor NV. 1987. Adaptive filtering of evoked potential. IEEE Trans Biomed Eng 34:1706.

Tompkins WJ (ed). 1993. Biomedical Digital Signal Processing. Englewood Cliffs, NJ, Prentice-Hall.

Tompkins WJ, Webster JG (eds). 1981. Design of Microcomputer-Based Medical Instrumentation. Englewood Cliffs, NJ, Prentice-Hall.

Webster JG (ed). 1992. Medical Instrumentation, 2d ed. Boston, Houghton-Mufflin.

Welch DP. 1970. The use of fast Fourier transform for the estimation of power spectra: A method based on time averaging over short modified periodograms. IEEE Trans Acoust AU-15:70.

Widrow B. 1956. A study of rough amplitude quantization by means of Nyquist sampling theory. IRE Trans Cric Theory 3:266.

Widrow B, Glover JRJ, Kaunitz J, et al. 1975. Adaptive noise cancelling: Principles and applications. Proc IEEE 63(12):1692.

Zetterberg LH. 1969. Estimation of parameters for a linear difference equation with application to EEG analysis. Math Biosci 5:227.

Further Information

A book that provides a general overview of basic concepts in biomedical signal processing is *Digital Biosignal Processing,* by Rolf Weitkunat (ed) (Elsevier Science Publishers, Amsterdam, 1991). Contributions by different authors provide descriptions of several processing techniques and many applicative examples on biologic signal analysis. A deeper and more specific insight of actual knowledge and future perspectives on ECG analysis can be found in *Electrocardiography: Past and Future,* by Philippe Coumel and Oscar B. Garfein (eds) (Annals of the New York Academy Press, vol 601, 1990). Advances in signal processing are monthly published in the journal *IEEE Transactions on Signal Processing,* while the *IEEE Transaction on Biomedical Engineering* provides examples of applications in biomedical engineering fields.

56

Compression of Digital Biomedical Signals

A. Enis Çetin
Bilkent University and
Koç University

Hayrettin Köymen
Bilkent University and
Koç University

Computerized electrocardiographic (ECG), electroencephalographic (EEG), and magnetoencephalographic (MEG) processing systems have been used widely in clinical practice [1]. These digital devices are capable of recording and processing long records of biomedical signals. Digital recording of biomedical signals (1) enables the construction of large signal databases for subsequent evaluation and comparison, (2) makes the transmission of biomedical information feasible over telecommunication networks in real time or off-line, and (3) increases the capabilities of ambulatory recording systems such as the Holter recorders for ECG signals. Despite the great advances in VLSI memory technology, the amount of data generated by digital systems may become excessive quickly. For example, a Holter recorder needs more than 200 Mbits/day of memory space to store two-channel ECG signals sampled at a rate of 200 samples per second with 10 bit per sample resolution. The storage problem can be overcome by the use of data compression techniques, which have been used successfully in speech, image, and video signals [2].

The aim of any biomedical signal compression scheme is to minimize the storage space without loosing any clinically significant information. This can be achieved by eliminating redundancies in the signal. Clearly, samples of a typical biomedical signal are related to each other, and consequitive samples are statistically dependent. Data compression methods reduce the amount of data by taking advantage of this dependency.

Signal compression methods can be classified into two categories: *lossless* and *lossy* coding methods. In lossless data compression, the signal samples are considered to be realizations of a random variable, and they are stored by assigning shorter (longer) codewords to sample values with higher (lower) probabilities. In this way, savings in the memory volume are obtained. Entropy of the source signal determines the lowest compression ratio that can be achieved. In lossless coding, the source signal can be perfectly reconstructed by reversing the codebook assignment. For typical biomedical signals, lossless (reversible) compression methods can only achieve compression ratios* (CRs) on

---

*CR is defined as the ratio of the total number of bits used to represent the digital signal before and after compression.

the order of 2:1, whereas lossy (irreversible) techniques may produce CR results of 10:1 without introducing any clinically significant degradation. The CR levels of 2:1 are too low for most practical applications. Therefore, lossy coding methods that introduce small reconstruction errors are preferred. In fact, most of the available biomedical signal coding methods are lossy methods. The next section will review irreversible biomedical data compression methods.

56.1 Time-Domain Coding of Biomedical Signals

Biomedical waveform coding methods can be classified as time-domain and frequency-domain methods. The following subsection will review the time-domain techniques, which are also the earlier approaches to biomedical signal compression.

Data Compression by DPCM

Differential pulse-code modulation (DPCM) is a well-known data coding technique in which the main idea is to decorrelate the input signal samples by linear prediction. Current signal sample $x(n)$ is estimated from the past samples by using either a fixed or adaptive linear predictor:

$$\hat{x}(n) = \sum_{k=1}^{N} a_k x(n - k) \tag{56.1}$$

where $\hat{x}(n)$ is the estimate of $x(n)$ at discrete time instant n, and $\{a_k\}$ are the predictor weights.* The estimation error sequence

$$e(n) = x(n) - \hat{x}(n) \tag{56.2}$$

not only has less correlation but also less variance than the original signal $x(n)$. The error sequence is quantized by using a nonuniform quantizer, and quantizer outputs are entropy coded by assigning variable-length codewords to the quantized error sequence according to the frequency of occurrence. The variable-length codebook is constructed by Huffman coding, which assigns shorter (longer) codewords to values occurring with higher (lower) probabilities. Huffman coding method approaches the entropy of the quantized error sequence arbitrarily closely. If the quantization step is removed, then the resulting DPCM coder becomes lossless.

The highest ECG compression ratio (CR = 7.8) has been reported in Ruttiman and Pipberger [6] for an ECG signal recorded at a rate of 500 Hz with 8 bit/sample resolution. The CR is given by

$$CR = \frac{\text{total number of bits used before compression}}{\text{total number of bits used after compression}} \tag{56.3}$$

In this case, the percent root mean square difference (PRD = 3.5%), which is a measure of reconstruction error, is defined as

$$PRD = \sqrt{\frac{\sum_{n=0}^{N-1} [x(n) - x_{\text{rec}}(n)]^2}{\sum_{n=0}^{N-1} x^2(n)}} \times 100 \tag{56.4}$$

---

*In practical DPCM implementation, instead of $x(n - k)$ in the linear predictor of Eq. (56.1), quantized past samples of the signal are used [2].

where N is the total number of samples in the ECG signal $x(n)$, and $x_{rec}(n)$ is the reconstructed ECG signal.

AZTEC ECG Compression Method

The amplitude zone time epoch coding (AZTEC) method is one of the earliest ECG coding methods. It was developed by Cox et al. [17] as a preprocessing software for real-time monitoring of ECGs. It was observed to be useful for automatic analysis of ECGs such as QRS detection, but it is inadequate for visual presentation of the ECG signal because the reconstructed signal has a staircase appearance.

In this method, the ECG signal is considered to consist of flat regions and "slopes." If the signal value stays within a predetermined constant for more than three consecutive samples, then that region is assumed to be constant and is stored by its duration (number of samples) and a fixed amplitude value. Otherwise, the signal is assumed to have a slope. A slope is stored by its duration and the amplitude of the last sample point. Linear interpolation is used to reconstruct the coded ECG signal. As a result, the resulting signal has a discontinuous nature, as shown in Fig. 56.1.

Even though AZTEC produces a high compression ratio (CR = 10:1, for 500-Hz sampled data with 12 bit/sample resolution), the quality of the reconstructed signal is very low, and it is not acceptable to the cardiologists.

Various modified versions of AZTEC are proposed in the literature [3]. One notable example is the CORTES technique [18]. The CORTES technique is a hybrid of the AZTEC and the turning point method, which is described in the next subsection.

Turning Point ECG Compression Method

The turning point data reduction method [19] is basically an adaptive downsampling method developed especially for ECGs. It reduces the sampling frequency of an ECG signal by a factor of 2.

The method is based on the trends of the signal samples. It processes three input samples at a time. Let $x(n)$ be the current sample at discrete time instant n. Among the two consecutive input samples $x(n + 1)$ and $x(n + 2)$, the one producing the highest slope (in magnitude) is retained, and the other sample is dropped. In this way, the overall sampling rate is reduced to one-half the original sampling rate. No other coding is carried out. Therefore, the resulting CR is 2:1. In Mueller [19], a PRD of 5.3% is reported for an ECG signal sampled at 200 Hz with 12 bit/sample resolution. In practice, the CR value actually may be lower than 2 because the retained samples may not be equally spaced and some extra bits may be needed for timing determination.

ECG Compression via Parameter Extraction

In this method, the signal is analyzed and some important features such as typical cycles, extreme locations, etc. are determined. These features are properly stored. Reconstruction is carried out by using appropriate interpolation schemes.

The location of the extrema or peaks in an ECG signal is important in diagnosis because they basically determine the shape of each ECG period. The ECG compression techniques described in Imai et al. [20] take advantage of this feature and record only the maxima, minima, slope changes, zero-crossing intervals, etc. of the signal. During reconstruction, various interpo-

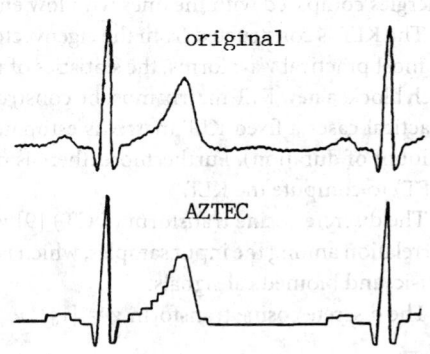

FIGURE 56.1 AZTEC representation of an ECG waveform.

lation schemes such as polynomial fitting spline functions are used. In Imai et al. [20], the performance of the extrema-based methods was compared with that of the AZTEC method, and it was reported that for a given CR, the RMS error is half that of AZTEC method.

Other parameter extraction methods include those of Jalaleddine et al. [4] and Hamilton and Tompkins [16], where ECG signals are analyzed in a cycle-synchronous manner. In Angelidou et al. [21], an AR model is fitted to the MEG signal, and parameters of the AR model are stored.

Review of some other time-domain ECG data compression methods can be found in Jalaleddine et al. [3].

56.2 Frequency-Domain Data Compression Methods

Transform coding (TC) and subband coding (SBC) are the two most important frequency-domain digital waveform compression methods [2]. Both methods are general waveform coding methods that have been applied to the compression of biomedical signals. The key idea is to divide the signal into frequency components and judiciously allocate bits in the frequency domain. The next three subsections will review TC and SBC methods and describe a hybrid transform domain multichannel ECG coding method.

Transform Coding (TC)

In this method, the input signal is divided into blocks, and each block is linearly transformed into the "frequency" domain. Compression is carried out in the frequency domain by nonuniformly allocating the bits to the "frequency components."

Let $\mathbf{x} = [x_0 \quad x_1 \quad \cdots \quad x_{N-1}]^T$ be a vector obtained from a block of N input samples. The transform domain coefficients $y_i, i = 0, 1, \ldots, N - 1$, are given by

$$\mathbf{v} = A\mathbf{x} \tag{56.5}$$

where $\mathbf{v} = [v_0 \quad v_1 \quad \cdots \quad v_{N-1}]^T$, and A is the $N \times N$ transform matrix representing the linear transform. Many transform matrices including the discrete Fourier transform (DFT) matrix are used in digital waveform coding [2]. In this subsection, the Karhunen-Loeve transform (KLT) and the discrete cosine transform, which are the most widely used ones, are reviewed.

If the input signal is a wide-sense stationary random process, then the so-called optimum linear transform KLT is well defined, and it decorrelates the entries of the input vector. This is equivalent to removing all the unnecessary information contained in the vector $\mathbf{x}$. Therefore, by coding the entries of the $\mathbf{y}$ vector, only the useful information is stored. Usually, different quantizers are used to quantize the entries of the $\mathbf{y}$ vector. More bits are allocated to those entries which have high energies compared with the ones with low energies.

The KLT is constructed from the eigenvectors of the autocovariance matrix of the input vector $\mathbf{x}$. In most practical waveforms, the statistics of the input vector change from block to block. Thus, for each block, a new KLT matrix must be constructed. This is computationally very expensive (in some practical cases a fixed KLT matrix is estimated, and it is assumed to be constant for a reasonable amount of duration). Furthermore, there is no fast algorithm similar to the fast Fourier transform (FFT) to compute the KLT.

The discrete cosine transform (DCT) [9] was developed to approximate the KLT if there is high correlation among the input samples, which is the case in many digital waveforms, including speech, music, and biomedical signals.

The discrete cosine transform $\mathbf{v} = [v_0 \quad v_1 \quad \cdots \quad v_{n-1}]^T$ of the vector $\mathbf{x}$ is defined as

$$v_0 = \frac{1}{\sqrt{N}} \sum_{n=0}^{N-1} x_n \tag{56.6}$$

$$v_k = \sqrt{\frac{2}{N}} \sum_{n=0}^{N-1} x_n \cos \frac{(2n+1)k\pi}{2N} \qquad k = 1, 2, \dots, N-1 \qquad (56.7)$$

where v_k is the kth DCT coefficient. The inverse discrete cosine transform (IDCT) of **v** is given as

$$x_n = \frac{1}{\sqrt{N}} v_0 + \sqrt{\frac{2}{N}} \sum_{k=1}^{N-1} v_k \cos \frac{(2n+1)k\pi}{2N} \qquad n = 0, 1, 2, \dots, N-1 \qquad (56.8)$$

There exist fast algorithms, order $(N \log N)$, to compute the DCT [9]. Thus it is computationally more efficient to implement the DCT than the KLT, which requires order (N^2) multiplications. Two recent image and video coding standards, JPEG and MPEG, use DCT as the main building block.

In Ahmed et al. [11], a CR of 3:1 for a single-channel ECG is reported by using DCT- and KLT-based coders. For multilead systems, two-dimensional (2-D) transform–based methods can be used. A CR of 12:1 was reported in Womble et al. [22] for a three-lead system by using a 2-D KLT.

Recently, Philips [23] developed a new transform using time-warped polynomials and obtained a CR of 26.9. In this case, a DCT-based coding procedure produced a CR of 24.3.

Subband Coding and Wavelet Transform

In a subband coding (SBC) structure, the basic building block is a digital filter bank which consists of a low-pass and a high-pass filter. In the ideal case, the passband (stopband) of the low-pass filter is $[0, \pi/2]$ ($[\pi/2, \pi]$). Let $H_l(e^{j\omega})$ $[H_u(e^{j\omega})]$ be the frequency response of the low-pass [high-pass] filter. In SBC, the input signal, which is sampled at the rate of f_s, is filtered by $H_l(e^{j\omega})$ and $H_u(e^{j\omega})$ parallelly, and the filter outputs are downsampled by a factor of 2 (every other sample is dropped) in order to maintain the overall sampling rate equal to the original rate. In this way, two subsignals $x_l(n)$ and $x_u(n)$ which both have a sampling rate of $f_s/2$ are obtained. The block diagram of a two-level SBC structure is shown in Fig. 56.1.

The subsignal $x_l(n)$ $[x_u(n)]$ contains the low-pass [high-pass] frequency-domain information of the original signal. The subsignals $x_l(n)$ and $x_u(n)$ can be further divided into their frequency components in a similar manner. This SB division process can be repeated until the frequency domain is divided in a sufficient manner. In Aydin et al. [7], the two-level subband structure of Fig. 56.2,

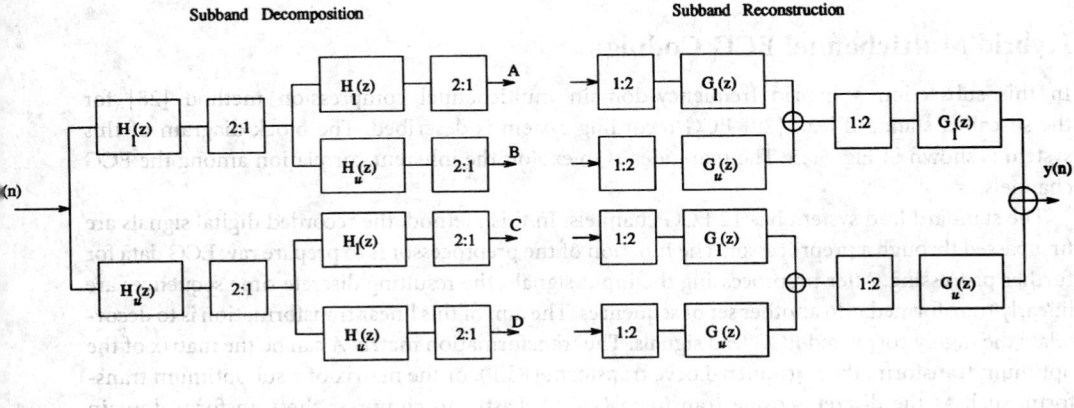

2:1 : Downsampler by a factor of 2   1:2 : Upsampler by a factor of 2

FIGURE 56.2 Two-level (four-branch) subband coder structure. This structure divides the frequency domain into four regions.

which divides the frequency domain into four regions, $(k\pi/4, (k + 1)\pi/4), k = 0, 1, 2, 3$, is used to code a single-channel ECG signal. The resultant subsignals can be represented by various coding methods, including DPCM, entropy coding, and transform coding. These coders should be designed to exploit the special nature of the subsignals to achieve the best possible CR for each band.

The signal reconstruction from the coded subsignals is carried out by using a filter bank consisting of two filters, $G_l(e^{j\omega})$ and $G_u(e^{j\omega})$. In this case, the subsignal $x_l(n)$ $[x_u(n)]$ is first upsampled by inserting a zero between every other sample and filtered by $G_l(e^{j\omega})$ $[G_u(e^{j\omega})]$. The reconstructed signal $y(n)$ is the sum of the outputs of these two filters. The signal $y(n)$ is related to $x(n)$ via the z-transform relation

$$Y(z) = \frac{1}{2} X(z)[H_l(z)G_l(z) + H_u(z)G_u(z)]$$

$$+ \frac{1}{2} X(-z)[H_l(-z)G_l(z) + H_u(-z)G_u(z)] \tag{56.9}$$

where $Y(z)$ and $X(z)$ are the z-transforms of the signals $y(n)$ and $x(n)$, respectively, and $H_l(z), H_u(z)$, $G_l(z)$, and $G_u(z)$ are the transfer functions of the filters of the SBC structure.

By properly selecting the filters $H_l(z)$, $H_u(z)$, $G_l(z)$, and $G_u(z)$, the so-called aliasing term $[H_l(-z)G_l(z) + H_u(-z)G_u(z)]$ can be made equal to zero and the signal term $[H_l(z)G_l(z) + H_u(z)G_u(z)] = z^{-K}$, which is just a delay. Such an SBC structure is called a *perfect reconstruction* (PR) filter bank. There are many ways of designing PR filter banks [24]. Therefore, in the absence of coding errors, perfect reconstruction is possible, i.e.,

$$y(n) = x(n - K) \tag{56.10}$$

In other words, filtering and downsampling operations in the SB decomposition structure do not introduce any loss.

In Aydin et al. [7], a CR of 5.22 corresponding to a PRD of 5.94% is reported for an ECG signal sampled at 500 Hz with 12 bit/sample resolution.

Recently, wavelet transforms (WT) also have been applied to ECG coding [25,26,27]. WT and SBC are very closely related to each other. In fact, the implementation of WTs is carried out by using SB filter banks. For this reason, WT-based coding methods are essentially similar to the SBC-based methods.

Hybrid Multichannel ECG Coding

In this subsection a hybrid frequency-domain multichannel compression method [28] for the so-called standard lead [29] ECG recording system is described. The block diagram of this system is shown in Fig. 56.3. The main idea is to exploit the inherent correlation among the ECG channels.

The standard lead system has 12 ECG channels. In this method, the recorded digital signals are first passed through a preprocessor. The function of the preprocessor is to prepare raw ECG data for further processing. After preprocessing the input signals, the resulting discrete time sequences are linearly transformed into another set of sequences. The aim of this linear transformation is to decorrelate the highly correlated ECG lead signals. The transformation matrix A can be the matrix of the optimum transform, the Karhunen-Loève transform (KLT), or the matrix of a suboptimum transform, such as the discrete cosine transform (DCT). Lastly, to compress the transform domain signals, various coding schemes that exploit their special nature are used.

In the paragraphs that follow, detailed descriptions of the subblocks of the multichannel ECG compression method are given.

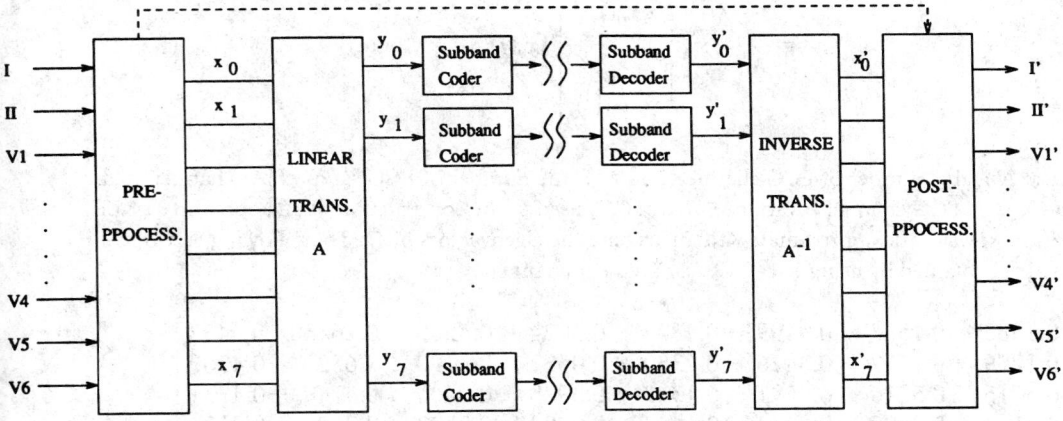

FIGURE 56.3 Block diagram of the multichannel ECG data compression scheme.

Preprocessor

The standard lead ECG recording configuration consists of 12 ECG leads: I, II, III, aV_R, aV_L, aV_F, V_1, V_2, ..., V_6. The leads III, aV_R, aV_L, and aV_F are linearly related to leads I and II. Therefore, only 8 channels are enough to represent the standard 12-channel ECG recording system.

The preprocessor discards the redundant channels, leads III, aV_R, aV_L, and aV_F, and rearranges the order of the ECG channels in order to bring correlated channels close to each other. The six precordial (chest) leads, V_1 to V_6, represent variations of the electrical heart vector amplitude with respect to time from six different narrow angles. During a cardiac cycle, it is natural to expect high correlation among precordial leads, so the channels V_1 to V_6 are selected as the first six signals, i.e., $x_{i-1} = V_i$, $i = 1, 2, \ldots, 6$. The two horizontal lead waveforms (I and II, which have relatively less energy contents with respect to precordial ECG lead waveforms) are chosen as the seventh, $x_6 = $ I, and eighth channels, $x_7 = $ II. A typical set of standard ECG lead waveforms x_i, $i = 0, 1, \ldots, 7$, are shown in Fig. 56.4.

The aim of reordering the ECG channels is to increase the efficiency of the linear transformation operation that is described in the next subsection.

Linear Transformer

The outputs of the preprocessor block x_i, $i = 0, 1, \ldots, 7$, are fed to the linear transformer. In this block, the ECG channels are linearly transformed to another domain, and 8 new transform domain signals y_i, $i = 0, 1, \ldots, 7$, which are significantly less correlated (ideally uncorrelated) than the ECG signal set x_i, $i = 0, 1, \ldots, 7$, are obtained.

Let $x_k(m)$, $k = 0, 1, \ldots, N - 1$ (N is equal to 8 in our case), be the reordered ECG signal samples at discrete time instant m; the transform-domain samples at time instant m are given as follows:

$$Y_m = A \cdot X_m \qquad (56.11)$$

where $Y_m = [y_0(m), \ldots, y_{N-1}(m)]^T$, $X_m = [x_0(m), \ldots, x_{N-1}(m)]^T$, and A is the $N \times N$ transform matrix.

The optimum linear transform, the discrete Karhunen-Loève transform (KLT), can be properly defined for stationary random processes, and the entries of the transform matrix A_{KLT} depend on the statistics of the random processes. For slowly varying nonstationary signals, an approximate KLT matrix also can be defined. Although ECG signals cannot be considered to be wide-sense stationary random processes, a covariance matrix $\hat{C}_x$ of the ECG channels is estimated as follows:

$$\hat{C}_X = \frac{1}{M} \sum_{i=0}^{M-1} \begin{bmatrix} x_0(i) \\ \vdots \\ x_{N-1}(i) \end{bmatrix} [x_0(i) \ \cdots \ x_{N-1}(i)] \tag{56.12}$$

where N is the number of ECG channels and M is the number of ECG samples per channel used. The $N \times N$ ECG channel covariance matrix $\hat{C}_x$ is used in the construction of an approximate KLT matrix. Rows of the approximate KLT matrix are the eigenvectors of $\hat{C}_x$. The following 8×8 KLT matrix is obtained by using 1024 ECG samples per channel:

$$A_{KLT} = \begin{bmatrix} 0.1883 & 0.1568 & 0.4199 & 0.4874 & 0.5024 & 0.4509 & 0.2615 & 0.0452 \\ -0.1779 & -0.1707 & -0.3426 & -0.2350 & -0.0552 & 0.3290 & 0.6821 & 0.4360 \\ 0.3715 & 0.5210 & 0.0591 & -0.1347 & -0.3928 & -0.0400 & 0.4749 & -0.4331 \\ -0.2164 & 0.7699 & -0.4322 & 0.1633 & 0.0982 & 0.0392 & -0.2231 & 0.2934 \\ -0.8073 & 0.0066 & 0.0553 & 0.1945 & -0.0723 & 0.1165 & 0.1529 & -0.5149 \\ -0.2528 & 0.2391 & 0.4301 & -0.4758 & 0.4233 & -0.4700 & 0.2042 & 0.1609 \\ -0.1722 & 0.0805 & 0.5204 & 0.2431 & -0.6256 & -0.0420 & -0.0233 & 0.4902 \\ 0.0522 & -0.1359 & -0.2392 & 0.5823 & 0.0699 & -0.6702 & 0.3543 & 0.0544 \end{bmatrix} \tag{56.13}$$

Although there is no fast algorithm to compute the KLT, the computational burden is not high because N is only equal to 8.

The (DCT) also can be used as a linear transformer because it approximates the KLT if there is high correlation between the entries of the input vector [9].

Compression of the Transform-Domain Signals

In this subsection, the compression of the uncorrelated transform domain signals $y_k, k = 0, 1, \ldots, 7$, is described. In Fig. 56.5, a typical set of uncorrelated signals $y_k, k = 0, 1, \ldots, 7$, is shown. The signals in Fig. 56.5 are obtained by KL transforming the ECG signals $x_k, k = 0, 1, \ldots, 7$, shown in Fig. 56.4

Transform-domain signals $y_k, k = 0, 1, \ldots, 7$, are divided into two classes according to their energy contents. The first class of signals, $y_0, y_1, \ldots, y_4$, have higher energy than the second class of signals, $y_5, y_6,$ and y_7. More bits should be allocated to the high-energy signals $y_0, y_1, \ldots, y_4$ compared with the low-energy signals $y_5, y_6,$ and y_7 in coding.

Subband (SB) Coder

High-energy signals $y_0(n), y_1(n), \ldots, y_4(n)$ contain more information than the low-energy signals $y_5(n), y_6(n),$ and $y_7(n)$. Therefore, the high-energy signals $y_0(n), \ldots, y_4(n)$ should be compressed very accurately. In Aydin et al. [7], an SB coder for ECG signals is developed. In this SB coding scheme, reconstructed ECG signals are visually almost indistinguishable from the original signals. Hence the use of this SB coder is decided to compress the signals $y_0(n), \ldots, y_4(n)$.

The block diagram of the SB coder is shown in Fig. 56.2. The input signal is decomposed into four subsignals by using a quadrature mirror filter (QMF) bank in a tree-structured manner. The SB decomposition structure of Fig. 56.2 splits the signal y_i into four consecutive bands $[l\pi/4, (l+1)\pi/4], l = 0, 1, 2, 3,$ in the frequency domain [2]. For example, $y_{i,0,0}$ (the subsignal at branch A of Fig. 56.2) comes from the low-pass frequency band $[0, \pi/4]$ of the signal y_i. In the coding of the subband signals $y_{i,j,k}, j = 0, 1, k = 0, 1,$ one takes advantage of the nonuniform distribution of energy in the frequency domain to judiciously allocate the bits. The number of bits used to encode each frequency band can be different, so the encoding accuracy is always maintained at the required frequency bands [2].

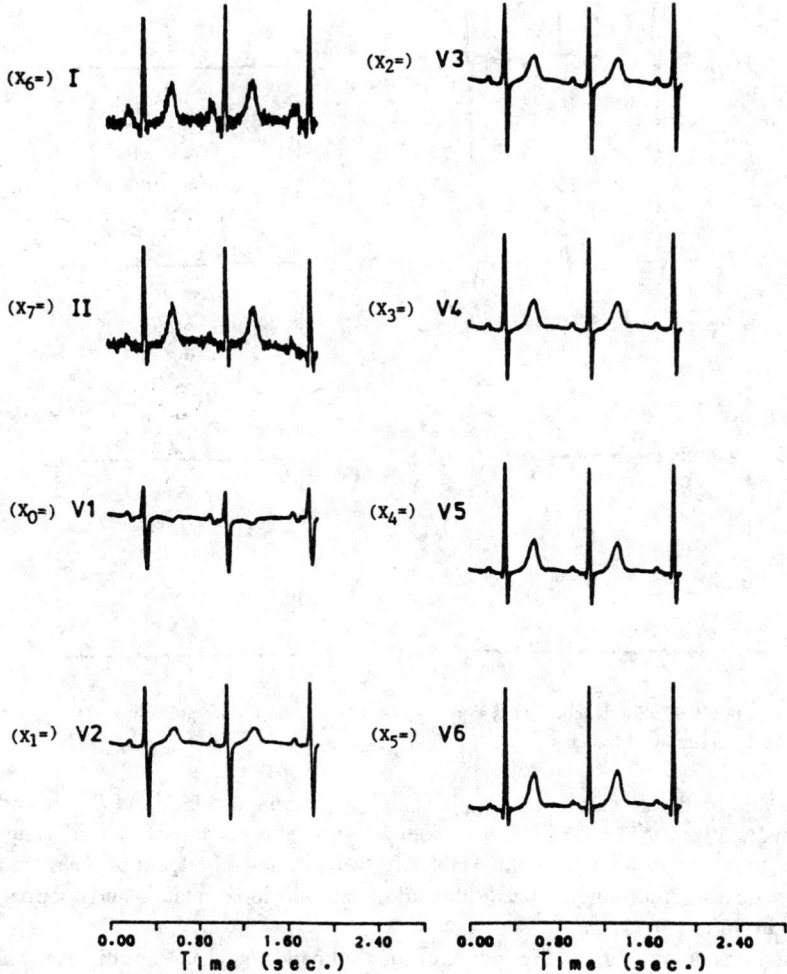

FIGURE 56.4 A typical set of standard ECG lead waveforms x_i, $i = 0, 1, \ldots, 7$.

It is observed that the energy of the signal y_i is mainly concentrated in the lowest-frequency band $[0, \pi/4]$. Because of this, the low-band subsignal $y_{i,0,0}$ has to be carefully coded. High correlation among neighboring samples of $y_{i,0,0}$ makes this signal a good candidate for efficient predictive or transform coding. In this method, a DCT-based scheme is also chosen to compress $y_{i,0,0}$. After the application of DCT with a block size of 64 samples to the low-band subsignal $y_{i,0,0}$, the transform-domain coefficients $G_{i,0,0}(k)$, $k = 0, 1, \ldots, 63$, are obtained.

DCT coefficients $G_{i,0,0}(k)$ are thresholded and quantized. The coefficients whose magnitudes are above a preselected threshold β are retained, and the other coefficients are discarded. Thresholding squeezes the dynamic range of the amplitude values. This operation is followed by quantization of the thresholded DCT coefficients. Thresholded and quantized nonzero coefficients are variable-length coded by using an amplitude table, and the zero values are run-length coded. The amplitude and run-length lookup tables are Huffman coding tables, which are obtained according to the histograms of the DCT coefficients.

In practice, ECG recording levels do not change from one recording to another one. If drastic variations occur, one can first scale the input by a factor α and then apply DCT.

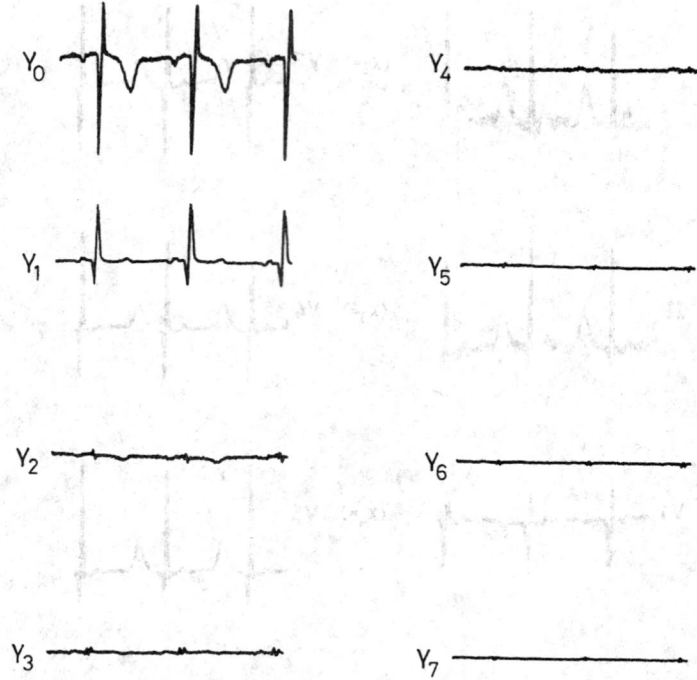

FIGURE 56.5   Uncorrelated signals y_i, $i = 0, 1, 2, \ldots, 7$, corresponding to the ECG signals shown in Fig. 56.4.

Bandpass and high-pass subsignals $y_{i,0,1}$, $y_{i,1,0}$, and $y_{i,1,1}$ (branches B, C, and D) are coded using nonuniform quantizers. After quantization, a code assignment procedure is realized using variable-length amplitude and run-length lookup tables for zero values. The lookup tables are obtained according to the histograms of quantized subband signals. The lookup tables and quantizers can be found in Aydin [8].

The bit streams obtained from the coding of four subband signals are multiplexed and stored. Appropriate decoders are assigned to each branch to convert the bit streams into time-domain samples, and the four-branch synthesis QMF bank performs the reconstruction [7].

The low-energy signals $y_5(n)$, $y_6(n)$, and $y_7(n)$ are also coded by using the SB coder described earlier. However, it is observed that all the subsignals except the subsignal at branch A of Fig. 56.2 contain very little information when QMF subband decomposition is applied to the signals $y_5(n)$, $y_6(n)$, and $y_7(n)$. Because of this, only the subsignals at branch A (low-band signals) are processed. The other branches are discarded. Although the three high-frequency branches of the SB coder are discarded, it is observed experimentally that the reconstruction error for the signals $y_5(n)$, $y_6(n)$, and $y_7(n)$ is very close to the SB coding results.

Original and reconstructed ECG waveforms are shown in Fig. 56.6 for CR = 6.17 (CR = 7.98) with PRD = 6.19% when DCT (KLT) is used as the linear transformer. Recorded ECG signals are sampled at 500 Hz with 12 bit/sample resolution. Also, the raw ECG signals are filtered to attenuate the high-frequency noise with a 33-tap equiripple Parks-McClellan FIR filter whose cutoff frequency is equal to 125 Hz. In this case, a CR = 9.41 is obtained for a PRD = 5.94%.

The effect of compressing the data on diagnostic computer analysis results is tested on a Cardionics program derived from the Mount Sinai program developed by Pordy et al. in conjunction with CRO-MED Bionics Company [15]. Morphologic measurements include intervals PR, QRS, and QT; widths Q, R, S, R', S', T, and P; amplitudes P, Q, R, R', S, S', T, and JJ; and areas of QRS and QRST. There was no difference in the measurement results of both the compressed and the original data.

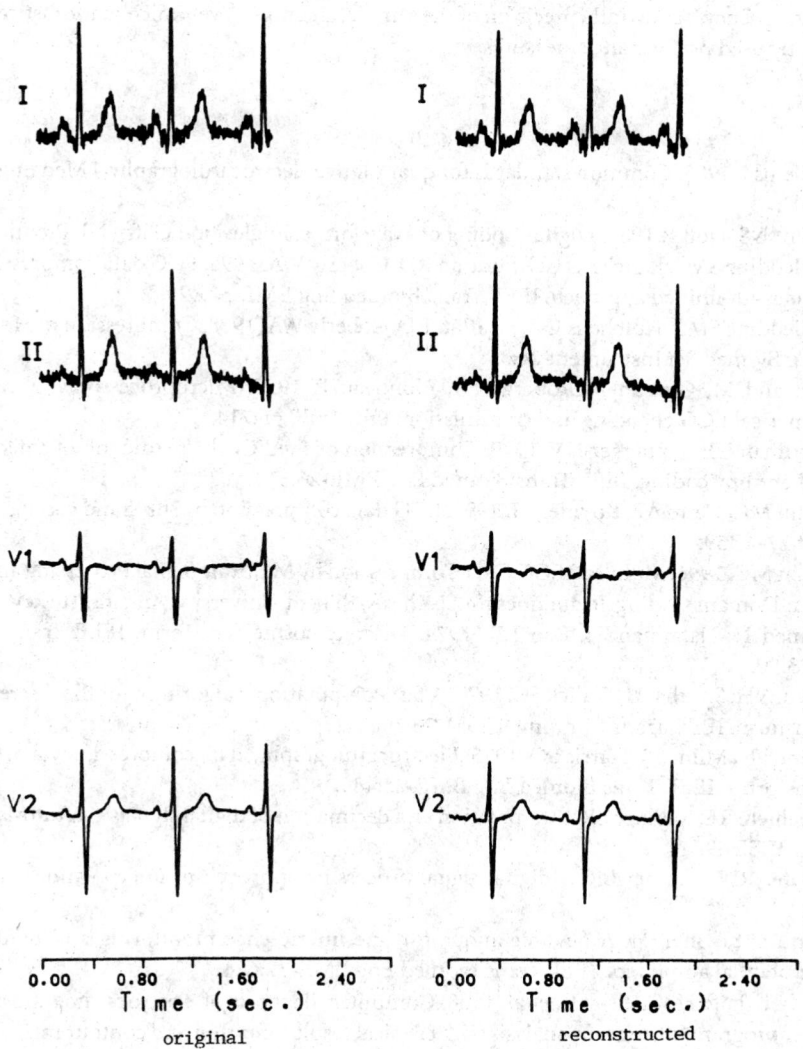

FIGURE 56.6 The original and reconstructed ECG lead signals I, II, V_1, and V_2 (CR = 6.17, APRD = 6).

It is observed experimentally that the multichannel technique produces better compression results than single-channel schemes. Also, the computational complexity of the multichannel scheme is comparable with single-channel ECG coding schemes, and the algorithm can be implemented by using a digital signal processor for real-time applications, such as transmission of ECG signals over telephone lines.

56.3 Conclusion

In this chapter biomedical signal compression methods were reviewed. Most of the biomedical data compression methods have been developed for ECG signals. However, these methods can be applied to other biomedical signals with some modifications.

It is very difficult to compare biomedical data compression schemes because coding results of various data compression schemes are obtained under different recording conditions such as sampling frequency, bandwidth, precision of the sample, and noise level which may drastically affect the currently used performance measures.

References

1. Willems J. 1985. Common standards for quantitative electrocardiography. J Med Eng Technol 9:209.
2. Jayant NS, Noll P. 1984. Digital Coding of Waveforms. Englewood Cliffs, NJ, Prentice-Hall.
3. Jalaleddine SMS, Hutchens CG, Strattan RD, Coberly WA. 1990. ECG data compression techniques—A unified approach. IEEE Trans Biomed Eng BME-37:329.
4. Jalaleddine SMS, Hutchens CG, Strattan RD, Coberly WA. 1988. Compression of Holter ECG data. Biomed Sci Instrument 24:35.
5. Bertrand M, Guardo R, Roberge FA, Blondeau P. 1977. Microprocessor application for numerical ECG encoding and transmission. Proc IEEE 65:714.
6. Ruttiman UE, Pipberger HV. 1979. Compression of the ECG by prediction or interpolation and entropy coding. IEEE Trans Biomed Eng BME-26:613.
7. Aydin MC, Çetin AE, Köymen H. 1991. ECG data compression by sub-band coding. Electron Lett 27-4:359.
8. Aydin MC. 1991. Multilead ECG Data Compression by Multirate Signal Processing and Transform Domain Coding Techniques. M.Sc. thesis, Bilkent University, Ankara, Turkey.
9. Ahmed N, Natarajan TJ, Rao KR. 1974. Discrete cosine transform. IEEE Trans Comput C-23:90.
10. Chen WH, Smith CH, Fralick SC. 1977. A fast computational algorithm for the discrete cosine transform. IEEE Trans Commun COM-25:1004.
11. Ahmed N, Milne PJ, Harris SG. 1975. Electrocardiographic data compression via orthogonal transforms. IEEE Trans Biomed Eng BME-22:484.
12. Crochiere RE, Rabiner LR. Interpolation and decimation of digital signals—A tutorial review. Proc IEEE 69.
13. Schafer RW, Rabiner LR. A digital signal processing approach to interpolation. Proc IEEE 61:692.
14. Ider YZ, Koymen H. A new technique for line interference monitoring and reduction in biopotential amplifiers. IEEE Trans Biomed Eng BME-37:624.
15. Pordy L, Jaffe H, Chelsky K, et al. 1968. Computer diagnosis of electrocardiograms: A computer program for contour analysis with classical results of rythm and contour interpretation. Comput Biomed Res 1:408.
16. Hamilton PS, Tompkins WJ. 1991. Compression of the ambulatory ECG by average beat subtraction and residual differencing. IEEE Trans Biomed Eng BME-38:253.
17. Cox JR, et al. 1968. AZTEC, a preprocessing program for real-time ECG rhythm analysis. IEEE Trans Biomed Eng BME-15:128.
18. Abenstein JP, Tompkins WJ. 1982. New data reduction algorithm for real-time ECG analysis. IEEE Trans Biomed Eng BME-29:43.
19. Mueller WC. 1978. Arrhythmia detection program for an ambulatory ECG monitor. Biomed Sci Instrument 14:81.
20. Imai H, Kimura N, Yoshida Y. 1985. An efficient encoding method for ECG using spline functions. Syst Comput Japan 16:85.
21. Angelidou A, et al. 1992. On AR modeling for MEG spectral estimation, data compression and classification. Comput Biol Med 22:379.
22. Womble ME, et al. 1977. Data compression for storing and transmitting ECGs/VCGs. Proc IEEE 65:702.
23. Philips W. 1993. ECG data compression with time-warped polynomials. IEEE Trans Biomed Eng BME-40:1095.

24. Akansu AN. 1992. Multiresolution Signal Decomposition: Transforms, Subbands, and Wavelets. New York, Academic Press.
25. Crowe JA, et al. 1992. Wavelet transform as a potential tool for ECG analysis and compression. Biomed Eng 14:268.
26. Tai SC. 1992. 6-Band subband coder on ECG waveforms. Med Biol Eng Comput 30:187.
27. Thakor NV, et al. 1993. Multiwave: A wavelet-based ECG data compression algorithm. IEICE Trans Inf Systems E76-D:1462–1469.
28. Çetin AE, Köymen H, Aydin MC. 1993. Multichannel ECG data compression by multirate signal processing and transform coding techniques. IEEE Trans Biomed Eng BME-40:495.
29. Wyngaarden JB, Smith LH. 1985. Textbook of Medicine. Philadelphia, Saunders.

Further Information

Biomedical signal compression is a current research area, and most of the research articles describing the advances in biomedical data compression appear in the journals *IEEE Transactions on Biomedical Engineering, Journal of Biomedical Engineering,* and *Medical and Biological Engineering and Computing.*

57

Time-Frequency Signal Representations for Biomedical Signals

**G. Faye Boudreaux-
Bartels**
University of Rhode Island

Robin Murray
University of Rhode Island

The Fourier transform of a signal $x(t)$

$$X(f) = \int x(t)e^{-j2\pi ft}dt \tag{57.1}$$

is a useful tool for analyzing the spectral content of a stationary signal and for transforming difficult operations such as convolution, differentiation, and integration into very simple algebraic operations in the Fourier dual domain. The inverse Fourier transform equation

$$x(t) = \int X(f)e^{j2\pi ft}df \tag{57.2}$$

is a linear combination of complex sinusoids of infinite duration which implicitly assumes that each sinusoidal component is present at all times and, hence, that the spectral content of the signal does not change with time. However, many signals in bioengineering are produced by biologic systems whose spectral characteristics can change rapidly with time. To analyze these rapid spectral changes, one needs a two-dimensional, mixed time-frequency signal representation (TFR) that is analogous to a musical score with time represented along one axis and frequency along the other, indicating which frequency components (notes) are present at each time instant.

The first purpose of this chapter is to review several TFRs defined in Table 57.1 and to describe many of the desirable properties listed in Table 57.2 that an ideal TFR should satisfy. TFRs will be grouped into classes satisfying similar properties to provide a more intuitive understanding of their similarities, advantages, and disadvantages. Further, each TFR within a given class is completely characterized by a unique set of kernels that provide valuable insight into whether or not a given TFR (1) satisfies other ideal TFR properties, (2) is easy to compute, and (3) reduces nonlinear cross-

0-8493-8346-3/95/$0.00+$.50
© 1995 by CRC Press, Inc.

BLE 57.1   List of Time-Frequency Representations (TFR) of a Signal $x(t)$ Whose Fourier Transform is $X(f)$.

kroyd distribution:
$$ACK_x(t,f) = Re\{x^*(t)X(f)e^{j2\pi ft}\}$$

fine Wigner distribution:
$$AWD_x(t,f;G,F) = \int G\left(\frac{\nu}{f}\right)X\left(fF\left(\frac{\nu}{f}\right)+\frac{\nu}{2}\right)X^*\left(fF\left(\frac{\nu}{f}\right)-\frac{\nu}{2}\right)e^{j2\pi t\nu}\,d\nu$$

tes-Marinovic distribution:
$$AM_x(t,f) = |f|\left|\int X(fe^{u/2})X^*(fe^{-u/2})e^{j2\pi tfu}\,du\right| = |f|\int\int WAF_x(\tau,e^\beta)e^{j2\pi(tf\beta-f\tau)}\,d\tau\,d\beta$$

arrowband) ambiguity function:
$$AF_x(\tau,\nu) = \int x\left(t+\frac{\tau}{2}\right)x^*\left(t-\frac{\tau}{2}\right)e^{-j2\pi\nu t}\,dt = \int X\left(f+\frac{\nu}{2}\right)X^*\left(f-\frac{\nu}{2}\right)e^{j2\pi\tau f}\,df$$

drieux et al. distribution:
$$AND_x(t,f) = \int\int \frac{1}{\sigma_{(t-t')}\sigma_{(f-f')}}\exp\left[-\left(\frac{(t-t')^2}{2\sigma^2_{(t-t')}}+\frac{(f-b_{(t-t')}(t-t'))^2}{2\sigma^2_{(f-f')}}\right)\right]$$
$$WD_x(t',f')\,dt'\,df'$$

where for $x(t) = e^{j2\pi\varphi(t)}$, then $b_t = \dfrac{d^2}{dt^2}\varphi(t)$, $\sigma_t = \left|\dfrac{d^3}{dt^3}\varphi(t)\right|^{-1/3}$, and $2\pi\sigma_t\sigma_f = \dfrac{1}{2}$.

itocorrelation function:

Temporal:
$$act_x(\tau) = \int x^*(t)x(t+\tau)\,dt = \int |X(f)|^2 e^{j2\pi f\tau}\,df$$

Spectral:
$$ACF_X(\nu) = \int X^*(f)X(f+\nu)\,df = \int |x(t)|^2 e^{-j2\pi t\nu}\,dt$$

ertrand P_k distribution:
$$BkD_x(t,f;\mu_k) = |f|\int X(f\lambda_k(u))X^*(f\lambda_k(-u))\mu_k(u)e^{j2\pi tf(\lambda k(u)-\lambda k(-u))}\,du$$

with $\lambda_0(u) = \dfrac{u/2e^{u/2}}{\sinh(u/2)}$, $\lambda_1(u) = \exp\left[\dfrac{1+ue^{-u}}{e^{-u}-1}\right]$, $\lambda_k(u) = \left[k\,\dfrac{e^u-1}{e^{-ku}-1}\right]^{\frac{1}{k-1}}$ $k \neq 0,1, \mu_k(u) = \mu_k(-u) > 0$

orn-Jordan distribution:
$$BJD_x(t,f) = \int \frac{1}{\tau}\left[\int_{t-|\tau|/2}^{t+|\tau|/2} x\left(t'+\frac{\tau}{2}\right)x^*\left(t'-\frac{\tau}{2}\right)dt'\right]e^{-j2\pi f\tau}\,d\tau$$

utterworth distribution:
$$BUD_x(t,f) = \int\int\left(1+\left(\frac{\tau}{\tau_0}\right)^{2M}\left(\frac{\nu}{\nu_0}\right)^{2N}\right)^{-1}AF_x(\tau,\nu)e^{j2\pi(t\nu-f\tau)}\,d\tau\,d\nu$$

hoi-Williams exponential distribution:
$$CWD_x(t,f) = \int\int\sqrt{\frac{\sigma}{4\pi}}\,\frac{1}{|\tau|}\exp\left[-\frac{\sigma}{4}\left(\frac{t-t'}{\tau}\right)^2\right]x\left(t'+\frac{\tau}{2}\right)x^*\left(t'-\frac{\tau}{2}\right)e^{-j2\pi f\tau}\,dt'\,d\tau$$

ohen's nonnegative distribution:
$$CND_x(t,f) = \frac{|x(t)|^2\,|X(f)|^2}{E_x}\,[1+c\rho\,(\xi_x(t),\eta_x(f))]$$

with $\xi_x(t) = \dfrac{1}{E_x}\int_{-\infty}^{t}\left|x(\tau)\right|^2 d\tau$, $\eta_x(f) = \dfrac{1}{E_x}\int_{-\infty}^{f}\left|X(f')\right|^2 df'$, $E_x = \int\left|x(t)\right|^2 dt$

one-Kernel distribution:
$$CKD_x(t,f) = \int g(\tau)\left[\int_{t-|\tau|/2}^{t+|\tau|/2} x\left(t'+\frac{\tau}{2}\right)x^*\left(t'-\frac{\tau}{2}\right)dt'\right]e^{-j2\pi f\tau}\,d\tau$$

umulative attack spectrum:
$$CAS_x(t,f) = \left|\int_{-\infty}^{t} x(\tau)e^{-j2\pi f\tau}\,d\tau\right|^2$$

umulative decay spectrum:
$$CDS_x(t,f) = \left|\int_{t}^{\infty} x(\tau)e^{-j2\pi f\tau}\,d\tau\right|^2$$

landrin D-distribution:
$$FD_X(t,f) = |f|\int X\left(f\left[1+\frac{u}{4}\right]^2\right)X^*\left(f\left[1-\frac{u}{4}\right]^2\right)\left[1-\left(\frac{u}{4}\right)^2\right]e^{j2\pi tfu}\,du$$

(continued)

TABLE 57.1   *(continued)*

Gabor expansion, $GE_x(n, k; g)$:

$$x(t) = \sum_n \sum_k GE_x(n, k; g) g(t - n\Delta T) e^{j2\pi(k\Delta F)t}$$

Generalized Altes distribution:

$$GAM_X(t, f; \alpha) = |f| \int e^{-\alpha u} X\left(fe^{\left(\frac{1}{2} - \alpha\right)u}\right) X^*\left(fe^{-\left(\frac{1}{2} + \alpha\right)u}\right) e^{j2\pi t f u} \, du$$

Generalized exponential distribution:

$$GED_x(t, f) = \iint \exp\left[-\left(\frac{\tau}{\tau_0}\right)^{2M}\left(\frac{\nu}{\nu_0}\right)^{2N}\right] AF_x(\tau, \nu) e^{j2\pi(t\nu - f\tau)} \, d\tau \, d\nu$$

Generalized Wigner distribution:

$$GWD_x(t, f; \tilde{\alpha}) = \int x\left(t + \left(\frac{1}{2} + \tilde{\alpha}\right)\tau\right) x^*\left(t - \left(\frac{1}{2} - \tilde{\alpha}\right)\tau\right) e^{-j2\pi f\tau} \, d\tau$$

Hyperbolic ambiguity function:

$$HAF_X(\zeta, \beta) = \int_0^\infty X\left(fe^{\beta/2}\right) X^*\left(fe^{-\beta/2}\right) e^{j2\pi\zeta \ln(f/f_r)} \, df$$

Hyperbolic wavelet transform:

$$HWT_x(t, f; \Gamma) = \sqrt{\frac{f_r}{f}} \int_0^\infty X(\xi) \Gamma^*\left(\frac{f_r}{f}\xi\right) e^{j2\pi t f \ln(\xi/f_r)} \, d\xi$$

Hyperbologram:

$$HYP_x(t, f; \Gamma) = \left|\sqrt{\frac{f_r}{f}} \int_0^\infty X(\xi) \Gamma^*\left(\frac{f_r}{f}\xi\right) e^{j2\pi t f \ln(\xi/f_r)} \, d\xi\right|^2 = |HWT_x(t, f; \Gamma)|^2$$

Levin distribution:

$$LD_x(t, f) = -\frac{d}{dt} \left|\int_t^\infty x(\tau) e^{-j2\pi f\tau} \, d\tau\right|^2$$

Margineau-Hill distribution:

$$MH_x(t, f) = Re\{x(t)X^*(f)e^{-j2\pi ft}\}$$

Multiform, Tiltable distributions:

Let $\tilde{\mu}(\tilde{\tau}, \tilde{\nu}; \alpha, r, \beta, \gamma) = ((\tilde{\tau})^2 ((\tilde{\nu})^2)^\alpha + ((\tilde{\tau})^2)^\alpha (\tilde{\nu})^2 + 2r ((\tilde{\tau}\tilde{\nu})^\beta)^\gamma)$

    Butterworth:

$$MTBD_x(t, f) = \iint \left[1 + \tilde{\mu}^{2\lambda}\left(\frac{\tau}{\tau_0}, \frac{\nu}{\nu_0}; \alpha, r, \beta, \gamma\right)\right]^{-1} AF_x(\tau, \nu) e^{j2\pi(t\nu - f\tau)} \, d\tau \, d\nu$$

    Exponential:

$$MTED_x(t, f) = \iint \exp\left\{-\pi\tilde{\mu}^{2\lambda}\left(\frac{\tau}{\tau_0}, \frac{\nu}{\nu_0}; \alpha, r, \beta, \gamma\right)\right\} AF_x(\tau, \nu) e^{j2\pi(t\nu - f\tau)} \, d\tau \, d\nu$$

    (Inverse) Chebyshev:

$$MT(I)C_x(t, f) = \iint \left[1 + \epsilon^2 C_\lambda^{\pm 2}\left(\tilde{\mu}\left(\frac{\tau}{\tau_0}, \frac{\nu}{\nu_0}; \alpha, r, \beta, \gamma\right)^{\pm 1}\right)\right]^{-1} AF_x(\tau, \nu) e^{j2\pi(t\nu - f\tau)} \, d\tau \, d\nu$$

where $C_\lambda(a)$ is a Chebyshev polynomial of order λ

Nutall-Griffin distribution:

$$ND_x(t, f) = \iint \exp\left\{-\pi\left[\left(\frac{\tau}{\tau_0}\right)^2 + \left(\frac{\nu}{\nu_0}\right)^2 + 2r\left(\frac{\tau\nu}{\tau_0\nu_0}\right)\right]\right\} AF_x(\tau, \nu) e^{j2\pi(t\nu - f\tau)} \, d\tau \, d\nu$$

Page distribution:

$$PD_x(t, f) = \frac{d}{dt} \left|\int_{-\infty}^t x(\tau) e^{-j2\pi f\tau} \, d\tau\right|^2$$

κth power

    Ambiguity function:

$$B_X^{(\kappa)}(\zeta, \beta) = AF_{W_\kappa X}\left(\frac{\zeta}{f_r}, f_r\beta\right), \quad (W_\kappa X)(f) = \frac{1}{\sqrt{f_r|\tau_\kappa(f_r\xi_\kappa^{-1}(f/f_r))|}} X\left(f_r\xi_\kappa^{-1}\left(\frac{f}{f_r}\right)\right)$$

    Central member:

$$AM_X^{(\kappa)}(t, f) = WD_{W_\kappa X}\left(\frac{t}{f_r\tau_\kappa(f)}, f_r\xi_\kappa\left(\frac{f}{f_r}\right)\right), \quad \tau_\kappa(f) = \frac{d}{df} \xi_\kappa\left(\frac{f}{f_r}\right)$$

where $\xi_\kappa(b) = \begin{cases} sgn(b)|b|^\kappa, & b \in \mathcal{R} \text{ for } \kappa \neq 0 \\ \ln(b), & b > 0 \text{ for } \kappa = 0 \end{cases}$ and $\xi_\kappa^{-1}(b) = \begin{cases} sgn(b)|b|^{1/\kappa}, & b \in \mathcal{R}, \kappa \neq 0 \\ e^b, & b > 0, \kappa = 0 \end{cases}$

Power spectral density:

$$PSD_x(f) = |X(f)|^2 = \int act_x(\tau) e^{-j2\pi f\tau} \, d\tau$$

(continued)

ABLE 57.1 *(continued)*

Pseudo-Altes distribution:
$$PAD_X(t, f; \Gamma) = f_r \int_0^\infty AM_\Gamma\left(0, f_r \frac{f}{f'}\right) AM_X\left(\frac{tf}{f'}, f'\right) \frac{df'}{f'}$$

Pseudo-Wigner distribution:
$$PWD_x(t, f; \eta) = \int x\left(t + \frac{\tau}{2}\right) x^*\left(t - \frac{\tau}{2}\right) \eta\left(\frac{\tau}{2}\right) \eta^*\left(-\frac{\tau}{2}\right) e^{-j2\pi f\tau} d\tau$$

Radially adaptive Gaussian distribution:
$$RAGD_x(t, f) = \int\int \exp\left[-\frac{(\tau/\tau_0)^2 + (\nu/\nu_0)^2}{2\sigma_x^2(\theta)}\right] AF_x(\tau, \nu) e^{j2\pi(t\nu - f\tau)} d\tau d\nu$$

$$\text{where } \theta = \arctan\left[\frac{\nu/\nu_0}{\tau/\tau_0}\right]$$

Real generalized Wigner distribution:
$$RGWD_x(t, f; \tilde{\alpha}) = Re\left\{\int x\left(t + \left(\frac{1}{2} + \tilde{\alpha}\right)\tau\right)^x\left(t - \left(\frac{1}{2} - \tilde{\alpha}\right)\tau\right) e^{-j2\pi f\tau} d\tau\right\}$$

Reduced interference distribution:
$$RID_x(t, f; s_{RID}) = \int\int \frac{1}{|\tau|} s_{RID}\left(\frac{t - t'}{\tau}\right) x\left(t' + \frac{\tau}{2}\right) x^*\left(t' - \frac{\tau}{2}\right) e^{-j2\pi f\tau} dt' d\tau$$

with $S_{RID}(\beta) \in \mathcal{R}$, $S_{RID}(0) = 1$, $\left\{\frac{d}{d\beta} S_{RID}(\beta)\Big|_{\beta=0} = 0\right\}$, $\left\{s_{RID}(\alpha) = 0 \text{ for } |\alpha| > \frac{1}{2}\right\}$

Rihaczek distribution:
$$RD_x(t, f) = x(t)X^*(f)e^{-j2\pi tf}$$

Running spectrum, past and future:
$$RSP_x(t, f) = \int_{-\infty}^t x(u)e^{-j2\pi fu} du, \quad RSF_x(t, f) = \int_t^\infty x(u)e^{-j2\pi fu} du$$

Scalogram:
$$SCAL_x(t, f; \gamma) = \left|\int x(\tau) \sqrt{\left|\frac{f}{f_r}\right|} \gamma^*\left(\frac{f}{f_r}(\tau - t)\right) d\tau\right|^2 = |WT_x(t, f; \gamma)|^2$$

Short-time Fourier transform:
$$STFT_x(t, f; \gamma) = \int x(\tau)\gamma^*(\tau - t)e^{-j2\pi f\tau} d\tau = e^{-j2\pi tf} \int X(f')\Gamma^*(f' - f)e^{j2\pi tf'} df'$$

Smoothed Pseudo-Altes distribution:
$$SPAD_X(t, f; \Gamma, g) = \int g(tf - c) PAD_X\left(\frac{c}{f}, f; \Gamma\right) dc$$

Smoothed Pseudo-Wigner distribution:
$$SPWD_x(t, f; \gamma, \eta) = \int\int \gamma(t - t')\eta\left(\frac{\tau}{2}\right)\eta^*\left(-\frac{\tau}{2}\right) x\left(t' + \frac{\tau}{2}\right) x^*\left(t' - \frac{\tau}{2}\right) e^{-j2\pi f_r} dt' d\tau$$

Spectrogram:
$$SPEC_x(t, f; \gamma) = \left|\int x(\tau)\,\gamma^*(\tau - t)e^{-j2\pi f\tau} d\tau\right|^2 = |STFT_x(t, f; \gamma)|^2$$

Unterberger active distribution:
$$UAD_X(t, f) = f \int_0^\infty X(fu)X^*(f/u)[1 + u^{-2}]\, e^{j2\pi tf(u - 1/u)} du$$

Unterberger passive distribution:
$$UPD_X(t, f) = 2f \int_0^\infty X(fu)X^*(f/u)[u^{-1}]\, e^{j2\pi tf(u - 1/u)} du$$

Wavelet transform:
$$WT_x(t, f; \gamma) = \int x(\tau) \sqrt{\left|\frac{f}{f_r}\right|} \gamma^*\left(\frac{f}{f_r}(\tau - t)\right) d\tau = \int X(f') \sqrt{\left|\frac{f_r}{f}\right|} \Gamma^*\left(\frac{f_r}{f} f'\right) e^{j2\pi tf'} df'$$

Wideband ambiguity function:
$$WAF_X(\tau, \alpha) = \int_0^\infty X(f\sqrt{\alpha})X^*(f\sqrt{\alpha})e^{j2\pi\tau f} df$$

Wigner distribution:
$$WD_x(t, f) = \int x\left(t + \frac{\tau}{2}\right) x^*\left(t - \frac{\tau}{2}\right) e^{-j2\pi f\tau} d\tau = \int X\left(f + \frac{\nu}{2}\right) X^*\left(f - \frac{\nu}{2}\right) e^{j2\pi t\nu} d\nu$$

TABLE 57.2   List of Desirable Properties for Time-Frequency Representations and Their Corresponding Kernel Constraints

Property Name	TFR Property	Kernel Constraints for Cohen's Class	Kernel Constraints for Hyperbolic Class
P_1: Frequency-shift covariant	$T_y(t,f) = T_x(t, f - f_0)$ for $y(t) = x(t)e^{j2\pi f_0 t}$	Always satisfied	$\Psi_{H_1}(\zeta, \beta) = B_H(\beta)e^{-j2\pi\zeta \ln G(\beta)}$
P_2: Time-shift covariant	$T_y(t,f) = T_x(t - t_0, f)$ for $y(t) = x(t - t_0)$	Always satisfied	with $G(\beta) = \dfrac{\beta/2}{\sinh(\beta/2)}$
P_3: Scale covariant	$T_y(t,f) = T_x(at, f/a)$ for $y(t) = \sqrt{\lvert a\rvert}x(at)$		Always satisfied
P_4: Hyperbolic time shift	$T_y(t,f) = T_x(t - c/f, f)$ if $Y(f) = \exp(-j2\pi c \ln \frac{f}{f_r})X(f)$	$\Psi_C(\tau, \nu) = S_C(\tau\nu)$	Always satisfied
P_5: Convolution covariant	$T_y(t,f) = \int T_h(t - \tau, f)T_x(\tau, f)\,d\tau$ for $y(t) = \int h(t - \tau)x(\tau)\,d\tau$	$\Psi_C(\tau, \nu) = e^{\tau P_C(\nu)}$	$\Phi_H(b_1, \beta)\Phi_H(b_2, \beta) = e^{b_1}\Phi_H(b_1, \beta)\delta(b_1 - b_2)$
P_6: Modulation covariant	$T_y(t,f) = \int T_h(t, f - f')T_x(t, f')\,df'$ for $y(t) = h(t)x(t)$	$\Psi_C(\tau, \nu) = e^{\nu P_C(\tau)}$	
P_7: Real-valued	$T_x^*(t,f) = T_x(t,f)$	$\Psi_C^*(-\tau, -\nu) = \Psi_C(\tau, \nu)$	$\Psi_H^*(-\zeta, -\beta) = \Psi_H(\zeta, \beta)$
P_8: Positivity	$T_x(t,f) \geq 0$	$\Psi_C(\tau, \nu) = AF\gamma(-\tau, -\nu)$	$\Psi_H(\zeta, \beta) = HAF_\Gamma(-\zeta, -\beta)$
P_9: Time marginal	$\int T_x(t,f)\,df = \lvert x(t)\rvert^2$	$\Psi_C(0, \nu) = 1$	
P_{10}: Frequency marginal	$\int T_x(t,f)\,dt = \lvert X(f)\rvert^2$	$\Psi_C(\tau, 0) = 1$	$\Psi_H(0, \beta) = 1$
P_{11}: Energy distribution	$\iint T_x(t,f)\,dt\,df = \int \lvert X(f)\rvert^2\,df$	$\Psi_C(0, 0) = 1$	$\Psi_H(0, 0) = 1$
P_{12}: Time moments	$\iint t^n T_x(t,f)\,dt\,df = \int t^n\lvert x(t)\rvert^2\,dt$	$\Psi_C(0, \nu) = 1$	
P_{13}: Frequency moments	$\iint f^n T_x(t,f)\,dt\,df = \int f^n\lvert X(f)\rvert^2\,df$	$\Psi_C(\tau, 0) = 1$	

Property	Definition	Condition (C)	Condition (H)
P_{14}: Finite time support	$T_x(t,f) = 0$ for $t \notin (t_1, t_2)$ if $x(t) = 0$ for $t \notin (t_1, t_2)$	$\varphi_C(t, \tau) = 0,\ \left\|\dfrac{t}{\tau}\right\| > \dfrac{1}{2}$	
P_{15}: Finite frequency support	$T_x(t,f) = 0$ for $f \notin (f_1, f_2)$ if $X(f) = 0$ for $f \notin (f_1, f_2)$	$\Phi_C(f, \nu) = 0,\ \left\|\dfrac{f}{\nu}\right\| > \dfrac{1}{2}$	$\Phi_H(G, \zeta) = 0,\ \left\|\dfrac{c}{\zeta}\right\| > \dfrac{1}{2}$
P_{16}: Instantaneous frequency	$\dfrac{\int f T_x(t,f)\,df}{\int T_x(t,f)\,df} = \dfrac{1}{2\pi}\dfrac{d}{dt}\,arg\{x(t)\}$	$\Psi_C(0, \nu) = 1$ and $\dfrac{\partial}{\partial \tau}\Psi_C(\tau, \nu)\big\|_{\tau=0} = 0$	
P_{17}: Group delay	$\dfrac{\int t T_x(t,f)\,dt}{\int T_x(t,f)\,dt} = -\dfrac{1}{2\pi}\dfrac{d}{df}\,arg\{X(f)\}$	$\Psi_C(\tau, 0) = 1$ and $\dfrac{\partial}{\partial \nu}\Psi_C(\tau, \nu)\big\|_{\nu=0} = 0$	$\Psi_H(\zeta, 0) = 1$ and $\dfrac{\partial}{\partial \beta}\Psi_H(\zeta, \beta)\big\|_{\beta=0} = 0$
P_{18}: Fourier transform	$T_y(t,f) = T_x(-f, t)$ for $y(t) = X(t)$	$\Psi_C(-\nu, \tau) = \Psi_C(\tau, \nu)$	

Property	Definition	Condition (C)	Condition (H)
P_{19}: Frequency localization	$T_x(t,f) = \delta(f - f_0)$ for $X(f) = \delta(f - f_0)$	$\Psi_C(\tau, 0) = 1$	
P_{20}: Time localization	$T_x(t,f) = \delta(t - t_0)$ for $x(t) = \delta(t - t_0)$	$\Psi_C(0, \nu) = 1$	
P_{21}: Linear chirp localization	$T_x(t,f) = \delta(t - cf)$ for $X(f) = e^{-j\pi c f^2}$	$\Psi_C(\tau, \nu) = 1$	
P_{22}: Hyperbolic localization	$T_x(t,f) = \dfrac{1}{f}\delta\left(t - \dfrac{c}{f}\right), f > 0$ if $X_c(f) = \dfrac{1}{\sqrt{f}} e^{-j2\pi c \ln \frac{f}{f_r}}, f > 0$		$\Psi_H(0, \beta) = 1$
P_{23}: Chirp convolution	$T_y(t,f) = T_x(t - f|c, f)$ for $y(t) = \int x(t - \tau)\sqrt{\|c\|}e^{j\pi c \tau^2}\,d\tau$	$\Psi_C\left(\tau - \dfrac{\nu}{c}, \nu\right) = \Psi_C(\tau, \nu)$	
P_{24}: Chirp multiplication	$T_y(t,f) = T_x(t, f - ct)$ for $y(t) = x(t)e^{j\pi ct^2}$	$\Psi_C(\tau, \nu - c\tau) = \Psi_C(\tau, \nu)$	

Property	Definition	Condition (C)	Condition (H)
P_{25}: Moyal's formula	$\iint T_x(t,f) T_y^*(t,f)\,dt\,df = \left\|\int x(t)y^*(t)\,dt\right\|^2$	$\|\Psi_C(\tau, \nu)\| = 1$	$\|\Psi_H(\zeta, \beta)\| = 1$

terms. The second goal of this chapter is to discuss applications of TFRs to signal analysis and detection problems in bioengineering. Unfortunately, none of the current TFRs is ideal; some give erroneous information when the signal's spectra are rapidly time-varying. Researchers often analyze several TFRs side by side, keeping in mind the relative strengths and weaknesses of each TFR before drawing any conclusions.

57.1 One-Dimensional Signal Representations

The instantaneous frequency and the group delay of a signal are one-dimensional representations that attempt to represent temporal and spectral signal characteristics simultaneously. The instantaneous frequency of the signal

$$f_x(t) = \frac{1}{2\pi} \frac{d}{dt} \, arg\{x(t)\} \tag{57.3}$$

has been used in communication theory to characterize the time-varying frequency content of narrowband, frequency-modulated signals. It is a generalization of the fact that the frequency f_0 of a complex sinusoidal signal $x(t) = \exp(j2\pi f_0 t)$ is proportional to the derivative of the signal's phase. A dual concept used in filter analysis is the group delay

$$\tau_H(f) = -\frac{1}{2\pi} \frac{d}{df} \, arg\{H(f)\} \tag{57.4}$$

which can be interpreted as the time delay or distortion introduced by the filter's frequency response $H(f)$ at each frequency. Group delay is a generalization of the fact that time translations are coded in the derivative of the phase of the Fourier transform. Unfortunately, if the signal contains several signal components that overlap in time or frequency, then $f_x(t)$ or $\tau_H(f)$ only provides average spectral characteristics, which are not very useful.

57.2 Desirable Properties of Time-Frequency Representations

Mixed time-frequency representations (TFRs) map a one-dimensional signal into a two-dimensional function of time and frequency in order to analyze the time-varying spectral content of the signal. Before discussing any particular TFR in Table 57.1, it is helpful to first investigate what types of properties an "ideal" time-frequency representation should satisfy. The list of desirable TFR properties in Table 57.2 can be broken up conceptually into the following categories: covariance, statistical, signal analysis, localization, and inner products [Boashash, 1991; Claasen & Mecklenbräuker, 1980; Cohen, 1989; Flandrin, 1993; Hlawatsch & Boudreaux-Bartels, 1992]. The covariance properties P_1 to P_6 basically state that certain operations on the signal, such as translations, dilations, or convolution, should be preserved, i.e., produce exactly the same operation on the signal's TFR. The second category of properties originates from the desire to generalize the concepts of the one-dimensional instantaneous signal energy $|x(t)|^2$ and power spectral density $|X(f)|^2$ into a two-dimensional statistical energy distribution $T_x(t_0, f_0)$ that provides a measure of the local signal energy or the probability that a signal contains a sinusoidal component of frequency f_0 at time t_0. Properties P_7 to P_{13} state that such an energy-distribution TFR should be real and nonnegative, have its marginal distributions equal to the signal's temporal and spectral energy densities $|x(t)|^2$ and $|X(f)|^2$, respectively, and preserve the signal energy, mean, variance, and other higher-order moments of the instantaneous signal energy and power spectral density. The next category of properties, P_{14} to P_{18}, arises from signal-processing considerations. A TFR should have the same duration and bandwidth as the signal under analysis. At any given time t, the average frequency should equal the instantaneous frequency of the signal, while the average or center of gravity in the time direction should equal the group delay of the signal. These two properties have been used to analyze the distortion of audio systems and the complex FM sonar signals used by bats and whales for echolocation. Property P_{18} is the TFR equivalent of the duality property of Fourier transforms. The group of properties P_{19} to P_{24} constitutes ideal TFR localization properties that are desirable for high resolution capabilities. Here, $\delta(a)$ is the Dirac function. These properties state that if a signal is perfectly concentrated in time or frequency, i.e., an impulse or a sinusoid, then its TFR also should be perfectly concentrated at the same time or frequency. Properties P_{21} and P_{22} state that the TFRs of linear or hyperbolic spectral FM chirp signals should be perfectly concentrated along the chirp signal's group delay. Property P_{24} states that a signal modulated by a linear FM chirp should have a TFR whose instantaneous frequency has been sheared by an amount equal to the linear instantaneous frequency of the chirp. The last property, known as *Moyal's formula* or the *unitarity property,* states that TFRs should preserve the signal projections, inner products, and orthonormal signal basis functions that are used frequently in signal detection, synthesis, and approximation theory. Table 57.3 indicates which properties are satisfied by the TFRs listed in Table 57.1.

A TFR should be relatively easy to compute and interpret. Interpretation is greatly simplified if the TFR is linear, i.e.,

$$T_y(t, f) = \sum_{n=1}^{N} T_{x_n}(t, f) \qquad \text{for } y(t) = \sum_{n=1}^{N} x_n(t) \tag{57.5}$$

However, energy is a quadratic function of the signal, and hence so too are many of the TFRs in Table 57.1. The nonlinear nature of TFRs gives rise to troublesome cross-terms. If $y(t)$ contains N signal components or *auto-terms* $x_n(t)$ in Eq. (57.5), then a quadratic TFR of $y(t)$ can have as many nonzero cross-terms as there are unique pairs of autoterms, i.e., $N(N - 1)/2$. For many TFRs, these cross-terms are oscillatory and overlap with autoterms, obscuring visual analysis of TFRs.

Two common methods used to reduce the number of cross-terms are to reduce any redundancy in the signal representation and to use local smoothing or averaging to reduce oscillating cross-terms. TFR analysis of real, bandpass signals should be carried out using the analytic signal representation, i.e., the signal added to $\sqrt{-1}$ times its Hilbert transform, in order to remove cross-terms between the positive- and negative-frequency axis components of the signal's Fourier transform. As we will see in upcoming sections, cross-term reduction by smoothing is often achieved at the expense of significant autoterm distortion and loss of desirable TFR properties.

57.3 TFR Classes

This section will briefly review Cohen's class of shift covariant TFRs, the Affine class of affine covariant TFRs, the Hyperbolic class (developed for signals with hyperbolic group delay), and the Power class (which is useful for signals with polynomial group delay). Each class is formed by grouping TFRs that satisfy two properties. They provide very helpful insight as to which types of TFRs will work best in different situations. Within a class, each TFR is completely characterized by a unique set of TFR-dependent kernels which can be compared against a class-dependent list of kernel constraints in Tables 57.2 and 57.6 to quickly determine which properties the TFR satisfies.

Cohen's Class of TFRs

Cohen's class consists of all quadratic TFRs that satisfy the frequency-shift and time-shift covariance properties, i.e., those TFRs with a check in the first two property rows in Table 57.3 [Claasen & Mecklenbräuker, 1980; Cohen, 1989; Flandrin, 1993; Hlawatsch & Boudreaux-Bartels, 1992]. Time- and frequency-shift covariances are very useful properties in the analysis of speech, narrowband Doppler systems, and multipath environments. Any TFR in Cohen's class can be written in one of the four equivalent "normal forms":

TABLE 57.3 List of Desirable Properties Satisfied by Time-Frequency Representations

Property	TFR (c,a)	BJD (c,a)	BUD (c,a)	CKD (c,a)	CWD (c,a)	CADS (c)	GADM (c,a)	GEWD (c,a)	HYP (h)	LMH (c,a)	MTED (c)	NPDD (c)	APMκ (c,p)	APWD (c,p)	PWD (c)	PRID (c,a)	RID (c,a)	SCAL (a,h)	SPADL (a)	SPWD (c)	SPEC (c)	UACD (a)	UAPD (a)	WD (c,a)
1 Frequency shift	√	√	√	√	√	√	√	√		√	√	√	√	√	√	√	√			√	√		√	√
2 Time shift	√	√	√	√	√	√	√	√	√	√	√	√	√	√	√	√	√	√	√	√	√	√	√	√
3 Scale covariance	√	√	√	√	√	√	√1	√1	√	√	√9	√	√	√	√	√	√	√	√	√	√	√	√	√
4 Hyperbolic time shift		√							√				√					√				√	√	
5 Convolution							√6				√10				√									√
6 Modulation							√7			√	√10	√			√									√
7 Real-valued	√	√	√	√4	√	√	√	√	√	√	√		√	√	√	√	√	√17	√18	√	√			√
8 Positivity		√		√					√									√			√			
9 Time marginal	√	√	√	√	√	√	√		√11	√	√11	√	√	√13		√	√							√
10 Frequency marginal	√	√	√	√	√	√	√		√11	√	√11	√	√	√13		√	√							√
11 Energy distribution	√	√	√	√	√	√	√	√8	√	√	√	√	√12	√12/√13		√16	√	√19	√	√20			√	√
12 Time moments	√	√	√	√	√	√	√		√11	√	√11	√	√	√13			√							√
13 Frequency moments	√	√	√	√	√	√	√		√11	√	√11	√	√				√							√
14 Finite time support	√	√	√	√	√		√5	√5		√		√	√	√		√	√							√
15 Finite frequency support	√	√	√	√	√	√	√5	√5		√		√	√			√	√							√
16 Instantaneous frequency	√	√2	√	√	√	√	√2		√11	√	√11	√	√	√14		√	√				√			√
17 Group delay	√	√3	√	√	√	√	√3		√11	√	√11	√	√	√14		√	√				√			√
18 Fourier transform	√	√1	√	√	√	√	√1	√1		√	√9	√	√		√15		√						√	√
19 Frequency localization	√	√	√	√	√	√	√		√11	√	√11	√	√	√13		√	√				√			√
20 Time localization	√		√	√	√	√	√		√11	√	√11	√	√	√13		√	√				√			√
21 Linear chirp localization	√						√										√							√
22 Hyperbolic localization		√							√													√	√	
23 Chirp convolution		√										√												
24 Chirp multiplication		√					√					√											√	
25 Moyal's formula	√	√	√	√	√	√	√					√	√										√	√

A √ indicates that the TFR can be shown to satisfy the given property. A number following the √ indicates that additional constraints are needed to satisfy the property. The constraints are as follows: (1): $M = N$; (2): $M > 1/2$; (3): $N > 1/2$; (4): $g(\tau)$ even; (5): $|\alpha| < 1/2$; (6): $M = 1/2$; (7): $N = 1/2$; (8): $\int_0^\infty |\Gamma(f)|^2 df = 1$; (9): $\alpha = 1$; (10): $r = 0, \alpha = 1, \gamma = 1/4$; (11): $\alpha \neq 1$; (12): $|\rho_\Gamma(0)|^2 = 1$; (13): $\eta(0) = \dfrac{1}{\tilde{f}}$; (14): $\eta(0) = 1$; (15): $s_{WD}(\beta)$ even; (16): $\int |\Gamma(b)|^2 db|b| = 1$; (17): $g(c) \in$ Real; (18): $\gamma(t) \in$ Real; (19): $\Gamma(0)\eta(0)|^2 = 1$; (20): $\int |\gamma(t)|^2 dt = 1$. In the second row, the letters c, a, h, and p indicate that the corresponding TFR is a member of the Cohen, Affine, Hyperbolic and Power class, respectively.

$$C_x(t, f; \Psi_C) = \int \int \varphi_C(t - t', \tau) \, x\left(t' + \frac{\tau}{2}\right) x^*\left(t' - \frac{\tau}{2}\right) e^{-j2\pi f\tau} dt' \, d\tau \quad (57.6)$$

$$= \int \int \Phi_C(f - f', v) \, X\left(f' + \frac{v}{2}\right) X^*\left(f' - \frac{v}{2}\right) e^{j2\pi tv} df' \, dv \quad (57.7)$$

$$= \int \int \psi_C(t - t', f - f') \, WD_x(t', f') \, dt' \, df' \quad (57.8)$$

$$= \int \int \Psi_C(\tau, v) \, AF_x(\tau, v) e^{j2\pi(tv - f\tau)} d\tau \, dv. \quad (57.9)$$

Each normal form is characterized by one of the four kernels $\varphi_C(t, \tau), \Phi_C(f, v), \psi_C(t, f)$, and $\Psi_C(\tau, v)$ which are interrelated by the following Fourier transforms:

$$\varphi_C(t, \tau) = \int \int \Phi_C(f, v) e^{j2\pi(f\tau + vt)} df \, dv = \int \Psi_C(\tau, v) e^{j2\pi vt} dv \quad (57.10)$$

$$\psi_C(t, f) = \int \int \Psi_C(\tau, v) e^{j2\pi(vt - f\tau)} d\tau \, dv = \int \Phi_C(f, v) e^{j2\pi vt} dv. \quad (57.11)$$

The kernels for the TFRs in Cohen's class are given in Table 57.4.

The four normal forms offer various computational and analysis advantages. For example, the first two normal forms can be computed directly from the signal $x(t)$ or its Fourier transform $X(f)$ via a one-dimensional convolution with $\varphi_C(t, \tau)$ or $\Phi_C(f, v)$. If $\varphi_C(t, \tau)$ is of fairly short duration, then it may be possible to implement Eq. (57.6) on a digital computer in real time using only a small number of signal samples. The third normal form indicates that any TFR in Cohen's shift covariant class can be computed by convolving the TFR-dependent kernel $\psi_C(t, f)$ with the Wigner distribution (WD) of the signal, defined in Table 57.1. Hence the WD is one of the key members of Cohen's class, and many TFRs correspond to smoothed WDs, as can be seen in the top of Table 57.5. Equation (57.11) and the fourth normal form in Eq. (57.9) indicate that the two-dimensional convolution in Eq. (57.8) transforms to multiplication of the Fourier transform of the kernel $\psi_C(t, f)$ with the Fourier transform of the WD, which is the ambiguity function (AF) in Table 57.1. This last normal form provides an intuitive interpretation that the "AF domain" kernel $\Psi_C(\tau, v)$ can be thought of as the frequency response of a two-dimensional filter.

The kernels in Eqs. (57.6) to (57.11) are signal-independent and provide valuable insight into the performance of each Cohen class TFR, regardless of the input signal. For good cross-term reduction and little autoterm distortion, each TFR kernel $\Psi_C(\tau, v)$ given in Table 57.4 should be as close as possible to an ideal low-pass filter. If these kernels satisfy the constraints in the third column of Table 57.2, then the TFR properties in the first column are guaranteed to always hold [Claasen & Mecklenbräuker, 1980; Hlawatsch & Boudreaux-Bartels, 1992]. For example, the last row of Table 57.2 indicates that Moyal's formula is satisfied by any TFR whose AF domain kernel, listed in the third column of Table 57.4, has unit modulus, e.g., the Rihaczek distribution. Since the AF domain kernel of the WD is equal to 1, i.e., $\Psi_{WD}(\tau, v) = 1$, then the WD automatically satisfies the kernel constraints in Table 57.2 for properties P_9 to P_{13} and P_{16} to P_{21} as well as Moyal's formula. However, it also acts as an all-pass filter, passing all cross-terms. The Choi-Williams Gaussian kernel in Table 57.4 was formulated to satisfy the marginal property constraints of having an AF domain kernel equal to 1 along the axes and to be a low-pass filter that reduces cross-terms.

Affine Class of TFRs

TFRs that are covariant to scale changes and time translations, i.e., properties P_2 and P_3 in Tables 57.2 and 57.3, are members of the *Affine class* [Bertrand chapter in Boashash, 1991; Flandrin, 1993].

TABLE 57.4　Kernels of Cohen's Shift-Invariant Class of Time-Frequency Representations (TFR)

TFR	$\psi_C(t,f)$	$\Psi_C(\tau,\nu)$	$\varphi_C(t,\tau)$	$\Phi_C(f,\nu)$
ACK	$2\cos(4\pi tf)$	$\cos(\pi\tau\nu)$	$\dfrac{\delta(t+\tau/2)+\delta(t-\tau/2)}{2}$	$\dfrac{\delta(f-\nu/2)+\delta(f+\nu/2)}{2}$
BJD		$\dfrac{\sin(\pi\tau\nu)}{\pi\tau\nu}$	$\begin{cases}\dfrac{1}{\lvert\tau\rvert}, & \lvert t/\tau\rvert < 1/2 \\ 0, & \lvert t/\tau\rvert > 1/2\end{cases}$	$\begin{cases}\dfrac{1}{\lvert\nu\rvert}, & \lvert f/\nu\rvert < 1/2 \\ 0, & \lvert f/\nu\rvert > 1/2\end{cases}$
BUD		$\left(1+\left(\dfrac{\tau}{\tau_0}\right)^{2M}\left(\dfrac{\nu}{\nu_0}\right)^{2N}\right)^{-1}$		
CWD		$e^{-(2\pi\tau\nu)^2/\sigma}$	$\sqrt{\dfrac{\sigma}{4\pi}}\dfrac{1}{\lvert\tau\rvert}\exp\left[-\dfrac{\sigma}{4}\left(\dfrac{t}{\tau}\right)^2\right]$	$\sqrt{\dfrac{\sigma}{4\pi}}\dfrac{1}{\lvert\nu\rvert}\exp\left[-\dfrac{\sigma}{4}\left(\dfrac{f}{\nu}\right)^2\right]$
CKD		$g(\tau)\lvert\tau\rvert\dfrac{\sin(\pi\tau\nu)}{\pi\tau\nu}$	$\begin{cases}g(\tau), & \lvert t/\tau\rvert < 1/2 \\ 0, & \lvert t/\tau\rvert > 1/2\end{cases}$	
CAS		$\left[\dfrac{1}{2}\delta(\nu)+\dfrac{1}{j\nu}\right]e^{-j\pi\lvert\tau\rvert\nu}$		
CDS		$\left[\dfrac{1}{2}\delta(-\nu)-\dfrac{1}{j\nu}\right]e^{j\pi\lvert\tau\rvert\nu}$		
GED^2		$\exp\left[-\left(\dfrac{\tau}{\tau_0}\right)^{2M}\left(\dfrac{\nu}{\nu_0}\right)^{2N}\right]$	$\dfrac{\nu_0}{2\sqrt{\pi}}\left\lvert\dfrac{\tau_0}{\tau}\right\rvert^{M}\exp\left[\dfrac{-\nu_0^2\tau_0^{2M}t^2}{4\tau^{2M}}\right]$ $N=1$ *only*	$\dfrac{\tau_0}{2\sqrt{\pi}}\left\lvert\dfrac{\nu_0}{\nu}\right\rvert^{N}\exp\left[\dfrac{-\tau_0^2\nu_0^{2N}f^2}{4\nu^{2N}}\right]$ $M=1$ *only*
GRD		$\begin{cases}1, & \lvert\tau\rvert^{M/N}\lvert\nu\rvert/r < 1 \\ 0, & \lvert\tau\rvert^{M/N}\lvert\nu\rvert/r > 1\end{cases}$	$\dfrac{\sin(2\pi\lvert r\rvert t/\lvert\tau\rvert^{M/N})}{\pi t}$	
GWD	$\dfrac{1}{\lvert\tilde{\alpha}\rvert}e^{j2\pi tf/\tilde{\alpha}}$	$e^{j2\pi\tilde{\alpha}\tau\nu}$	$\delta(t+\tilde{\alpha}\tau)$	$\delta(f-\tilde{\alpha}\nu)$
LD		$e^{j\pi\lvert\tau\rvert\nu}$	$\delta(t+\lvert\tau\rvert/2)$	
MH		$\cos(\pi\tau\nu)$	$\dfrac{\delta(t+\tau/2)+\delta(t-\tau/2)}{2}$	$\dfrac{\delta(f-\nu/2)+\delta(f+\nu/2)}{2}$
MTBD		$\left[1+\bar{\mu}^{2\lambda}\left(\dfrac{\tau}{\tau_0},\dfrac{\nu}{\nu_0};\alpha,r,\beta,\gamma\right)\right]^{-1}$		
MTC		$\left[1+\epsilon_p^2 C_\lambda^2\left(\bar{\mu}\left(\dfrac{\tau}{\tau_0},\dfrac{\nu}{\nu_0};\alpha,r,\beta,\gamma\right)\right)\right]^{-1}$		
MTED		$\exp\left[-\pi\bar{\mu}^{2\lambda}\left(\dfrac{\tau}{\tau_0},\dfrac{\nu}{\nu_0};\alpha,r,\beta,\gamma\right)\right]$		
MTIC		$\left[1+\epsilon_s^2 C_\lambda^{-2}\left(\bar{\mu}^{-1}\left(\dfrac{\tau}{\tau_0},\dfrac{\nu}{\nu_0};\alpha,r,\beta,\gamma\right)\right)\right]^{-1}$		
ND		$\exp\left[-\pi\bar{\mu}\left(\dfrac{\tau}{\tau_0},\dfrac{\nu}{\nu_0};0,r,1,1\right)\right]$		
PD		$e^{-j\pi\lvert\tau\rvert\nu}$	$\delta(t-\lvert\tau\rvert/2)$	
PWD	$\delta(t)WD_\eta(0,f)$	$\eta(\tau/2)\eta^*(-\tau/2)$	$\delta(t)\eta(\tau/2)\eta^*(-\tau/2)$	$WD_\eta(0,f)$
RGWD	$\dfrac{1}{\lvert\tilde{\alpha}\rvert}\cos(2\pi tf/\tilde{\alpha})$	$\cos(2\pi\tilde{\alpha}\tau\nu)$	$\dfrac{\delta(t+\tilde{\alpha}\tau)+\delta(t-\tilde{\alpha}\tau)}{2}$	$\dfrac{\delta(f-\tilde{\alpha}\nu)+\delta(f+\tilde{\alpha}\nu)}{2}$
RID	$\displaystyle\int\dfrac{1}{\lvert\tau\rvert}S_{RID}\left(\dfrac{t}{\tau}\right),$	$S_{RID}(\tau\nu),$	$\dfrac{1}{\lvert\tau\rvert}S_{RID}\left(\dfrac{t}{\tau}\right),$	$\dfrac{1}{\lvert\nu\rvert}S_{RID}\left(-\dfrac{f}{\nu}\right),$
	$e^{-j2\pi f\tau}d\tau$	$S_{RID}(\beta)\epsilon Real,\ S_{RID}(0)=1$	$s_{RID}(\alpha)=0,\lvert\alpha\rvert>\dfrac{1}{2}$	$s_{RID}(\alpha)=0,\lvert\alpha\rvert>\dfrac{1}{2}$

(continued)

ABLE 57.4 *(continued)*

FR	$\psi_C(t,f)$	$\Psi_C(\tau,\nu)$	$\varphi_C(t,\tau)$	$\Phi_C(f,\nu)$
D	$2e^{-j4\pi tf}$	$e^{-j\pi\tau\nu}$	$\delta(t-\tau/2)$	$\delta(f+\nu/2)$
PWD	$\gamma(t)WD_\eta(0,f)$	$\eta\left(\dfrac{\tau}{2}\right)\eta^*\left(-\dfrac{\tau}{2}\right)\Gamma(\nu)$	$\gamma(t)\eta\left(\dfrac{\tau}{2}\right)\eta^*\left(-\dfrac{\tau}{2}\right)$	$\Gamma(\nu)WD_\eta(0,f)$
PEC	$WD_\gamma(-t,-f)$	$AF_\gamma(-\tau,-\nu)$	$\gamma\left(-t-\dfrac{\tau}{2}\right)\gamma^*\left(-t+\dfrac{\tau}{2}\right)$	$\Gamma\left(f-\dfrac{\nu}{2}\right)\Gamma^*\left(-f+\dfrac{\nu}{2}\right)$
D	$\delta(t)\delta(f)$	1	$\delta(t)$	$\delta(f)$

Here, $\tilde{\mu}(\tilde{\tau},\tilde{\nu};\alpha,r,\beta,\gamma)=((\tilde{\tau})^2\,((\tilde{\nu})^2)^\alpha+((\tilde{\tau})^2)^\alpha(\tilde{\nu})^2+2r((\tilde{\tau}\,\tilde{\nu})^\beta)^\gamma)$ and $C_\lambda(a)$ is a Chebyshev polynomial of order λ. Functions ith lowercase and uppercase letters, e.g. $\gamma(t)$ and $\Gamma(f)$, indicate Fourier transform pairs.

The scale covariance property P_3 is useful when analyzing wideband Doppler systems, signals with fractal structure, octave-band systems such as the cochlea of the inner ear, and detecting short-duration "transients." Any Affine class TFR can be written in four "normal form" equations similar to those of Cohen's class:

$$A_x(t,f;\Psi_A)=|f|\int\int \varphi_A(f(t'-t),f\tau)x(t+\tau/2)x^*(t-\tau/2)\,dt'\,d\tau \qquad (57.12)$$

$$=\frac{1}{|f|}\int\int \Phi_A\left(\frac{f'}{f},\frac{\nu}{f}\right)X(f'+\nu/2)X^*(f'-\nu/2)e^{j2\pi t\nu}\,df'\,d\nu \qquad (57.13)$$

TABLE 57.5 Many TFRs Are Equivalent to Smoothed or Warped Wigner Distributions

TFR name	TFR formulation
Cohen's class TFR	$C_x(t,f;\psi_C)=\int\int\psi_C(t-t',f-f')WD_x(t',f')\,dt'\,df'$
Pseudo-Wigner distribution	$PWD_x(t,f;\eta)=\int WD_\eta(0,f-f')WD_x(t,f')\,df'$
Scalogram	$SCAL_x(t,f;\gamma)=\int\int WD_\gamma\left(\dfrac{f}{f_r}\,(t'-t),f_r\dfrac{f'}{f}\right)WD_x(t',f')\,dt'\,df'$
Smoothed Pseudo-Wigner distribution	$SPWD_x(t,f;\gamma,\eta)=\int\int\gamma(t-t')WD_\eta(0,f-f')\,WD_x(t',f')\,dt'\,df'$
Spectrogram	$SPEC_x(t,f;\gamma)=\int\int WD_\gamma(t'-t,f'-f)\,WD_x(t',f')\,dt'df'$
Altes distribution	$AM_X(t,f)=WD_{\mathcal{W}X}\left(\dfrac{tf}{f_r},f_r\ln\dfrac{f}{f_r}\right)$
κth Power Altes distribution	$AM_X^{(\kappa)}(t,f)=WD_{\mathcal{W}_\kappa X}\left(\dfrac{t}{\kappa|f/f_r|^{\kappa-1}},f_r sgn(f)|f/f_r|^\kappa\right),\kappa\neq0$
Hyperbologram	$HYP_X(t,f;\Gamma)=\displaystyle\int_{-\infty}^{\infty}\int_0^{\infty}WD_{\mathcal{W}\Gamma}\left(t'-\dfrac{tf}{f_r},f'-f_r\ln\dfrac{f}{f_r}\right)WD_{\mathcal{W}X}(t',f')\,dt'\,df'$
Pseudo-Altes distribution	$PAD_X(t,f;\Gamma)=f_r\displaystyle\int_0^{\infty}WD_{\mathcal{W}\Gamma}\left(0,f_r\ln\dfrac{f}{f'}\right)WD_{\mathcal{W}X}\left(\dfrac{tf}{f_r},f_r\ln\dfrac{f'}{f_r}\right)\dfrac{df'}{f'}$
Smoothed Pseudo-Altes distribution	$SPAD_X(t,f;\Gamma,g)=f_r\displaystyle\int_{-\infty}^{\infty}\int_0^{\infty}g(tf-c)WD_{\mathcal{W}\Gamma}\left(0,f_r\ln\dfrac{f}{f'}\right)WD_{\mathcal{W}X}\left(\dfrac{c}{f_r},f_r\ln\dfrac{f'}{f_r}\right)\dfrac{df'}{f'}\,dc$

Where $f_r>0$ is a positive reference frequency, $(\mathcal{W}H)(f)=\sqrt{e^{f/f_r}}H(f_r e^{f/f_r})$, $(\mathcal{W}_\kappa H)(f)=|\kappa|f_r/f|^{(\kappa-1)/\kappa}|^{-1/2}H(f_r sgn(f)|f/f_r|^{1/\kappa})$, $\kappa\neq0$, and $sgn(f)=\begin{cases}1, & f>0\\ -1, & f<0\end{cases}$

$$= \int\int \psi_A\left(f(t - t'), \frac{f'}{f}\right) W D_x(t', f')\, dt'\, df' \tag{57.14}$$

$$= \int\int \Psi_A\left(f\tau, \frac{\nu}{f}\right) AF_x(\tau, \nu)e^{j2\pi t\nu}\, d\tau\, d\nu. \tag{57.15}$$

The Affine class kernels are interrelated by the same Fourier transforms given in Eqs. (57.10) and (57.11). Note that the third normal form of the Affine class involves an Affine smoothing of the WD. Well-known members of the Affine class are the Bertrands' P_0 distribution, the scalogram, and the Unterberger distributions. All are defined in Table 57.1, and their kernel forms and TFR property constraints are listed in Table 57.6. Because of the scale covariance property, many TFRs in the Affine class exhibit constant-Q behavior, permitting multiresolution analysis.

TABLE 57.6 Affine Class Kernels and Constraints

TFR	$\Psi_A(\zeta, \beta)$	$\Phi_A(b, \beta)$
BOD	$\dfrac{\beta/2}{\sinh \beta/2}\, e^{-j2\pi\zeta\left[\frac{\beta}{2}\coth\frac{\beta}{2}\right]}$	$\dfrac{\beta/2}{\sinh \beta/2}\, \delta\left(b - \left[\frac{\beta}{2}\coth\frac{\beta}{2}\right]\right)$
FD	$\left[1 - \left(\frac{\beta}{4}\right)^2\right]e^{-j2\pi\zeta\left[1 + (\beta/4)^2\right]}$	$\left[1 - \left(\frac{\beta}{4}\right)^2\right]\delta(b - [1 + (\beta/4)^2])$
GWD	$e^{-j2\pi\zeta[1 - \tilde{\zeta}\beta]}$	$\delta(b - [1 - \tilde{\zeta}\beta])$
SCAL	$AF_\gamma(-\zeta/f_r, -f_r\beta)$	$f_r\Gamma(f_r(b - \beta/2))\Gamma^*(f_r(b + \beta/2))$
UAD	$e^{-j2\pi\zeta\sqrt{1 + \beta^2/4}}$	$\delta(b - \sqrt{1 + \beta^2/4})$
UPD	$[1 + \beta^2/4]^{-1/2}e^{-j2\pi\zeta\sqrt{1 + \beta^2/4}}$	$[1 + \beta^2/4]^{-1/2}\delta(b - \sqrt{1 + \beta^2/4})$
WD	$e^{-j2\pi\zeta}$	$\delta(b - 1)$

Property	Constraint on Kernel
P_1: Frequency shift	$\psi_A(\alpha_0 a, (b - 1)/\alpha_0 + 1) = \psi_A(a, b)$
P_2: Time shift	Always satisfied
P_3: Scale covariance	Always satisfied
P_4: Hyperbolic time shift	$\Phi_A(b, \beta) = G_A(\beta)\delta\left(b - \frac{\beta}{2}\coth\frac{\beta}{2}\right)$
P_5: Convolution	$\Psi_A(\zeta, \beta) = e^{\zeta P_A(\beta)}$
P_7: Real-valued	$\Psi_A(\zeta, \beta) = \Psi_A^*(-\zeta, -\beta)$
P_9: Time marginal	$\int \Phi_A(b, -2b)\, \dfrac{db}{|b|} = 1$
P_{10}: Frequency marginal	$\Phi_A(b, 0) = \delta(b - 1)$
P_{11}: Energy distribution	$\int \Phi_A(b, 0)\, \dfrac{db}{|b|} = 1$
P_{14}: Finite time support	$\varphi_A(a, \zeta) = 0, \left|\dfrac{a}{\zeta}\right| > \dfrac{1}{2}$
P_{15}: Finite frequency support	$\Phi_A(b, \beta) = 0, \left|\dfrac{b - 1}{\beta}\right| > \dfrac{1}{2}$
P_{17}: Group delay	$\Phi_A(b, 0) = \delta(b - 1)$ and $\left.\dfrac{\partial}{\partial\beta}\Phi_A(b, \beta)\right|_{\beta=0} = 0$
P_{19}: Frequency localization	$\Phi_A(b, 0) = \delta(b - 1)$
P_{25}: Moyal's formula	$\int \Phi_A^*(b\beta, \bar{\eta}\beta)\Phi_A(\beta, \bar{\eta}\beta)\, d\beta = \delta(b - 1), \forall \bar{\eta}$

Hyperbolic Class of TFRs

The Hyperbolic class of TFRs consists of all TFRs that are covariant to scale changes and hyperbolic time shifts, i.e., properties P_3 and P_4 in Table 57.2 [Papandreou et al., 1993]. They can be analyzed using the following four normal forms:

$$H_X(t, f; \Psi_H) = \int\int \varphi_H(tf - c, \zeta)\, v_X(c, \zeta) e^{-j2\pi[\ln(f/f_r)]\zeta}\, dc\, d\zeta \tag{57.16}$$

$$= \int\int \Phi_H(\ln\frac{f}{f_r} - b, \beta) f_r e^b X(f_r e^{b+\beta/2}) X^*(f_r e^{b-\beta/2}) e^{j2\pi tf\beta}\, db\, d\beta \tag{57.17}$$

$$= \int_{-\infty}^{\infty}\int_0^{\infty} \psi_H\left(tf - t'f', \ln\frac{f}{f'}\right) AM_X(t', f')\, dt'\, df' \tag{57.18}$$

$$= \int\int \Psi_H(\zeta, \beta)\, HAF_X(\zeta, \beta) e^{j2\pi(tf\beta - [\ln(f/f_r)]\zeta)}\, d\zeta\, d\beta \tag{57.19}$$

where $AM_X(t, f)$ is the Altes distribution and $HAF_X(\zeta, \beta)$ is the hyperbolic ambiguity function defined in Table 57.1, $v_X(c, \zeta)$ is defined in Table 57.7, $(\mathcal{W}X)(f) = \sqrt{e^{f/f_r}}\, X(f_r e^{f/f_r})$ is a unitary warping on the frequency axis of the signal, and the kernels are interrelated via the Fourier transforms in Eqs. (57.10) and (57.11).

Table 57.3 reveals that the Altes-Marinovic, the Bertrands' P_0, and the hyperbologram distributions are members of the Hyperbolic class. Their kernels are given in Table 57.7, and kernel property constraints are given in Table 57.2. The hyperbolic TFRs give highly concentrated TFR representations for signals with hyperbolic group delay. Each Hyperbolic class TFR, kernel, and property corresponds to a warped version of a Cohen's class TFR, kernel, and property, respectively. For example, Table 57.5 shows that the Altes distribution is equal to the WD after both the signal and the time-frequency axes are warped appropriately. The WD's perfect localization of linear FM chirps (P_{21}) corresponds to the Altes distribution's perfect localization for hyperbolic FM chirps (P_{22}). This one-to-one correspondence between the Cohen and Hyperbolic classes greatly facilitates their analysis and gives alternative methods for calculating various TFRs.

TABLE 57.7   Kernels of the Hyperbolic Class of Time-Frequency Representations

TFR	$\psi_H(c, b)$	$\Psi_H(\zeta, \beta)$	$\varphi_H(c, \zeta)$	$\Phi_H(b, \beta)$
AM	$\delta(c)\delta(b)$	1	$\delta(c)$	$\delta(b)$
B0D	$\int \delta(b + \ln\lambda(\beta)) e^{j2\pi c\beta}\, d\beta$	$e^{-j2\pi\zeta\ln\lambda(\beta)}$	$\int e^{j2\pi(c\beta - \zeta\ln\lambda(\beta))}\, d\beta$	$\delta(b + \ln\lambda(\beta))$
GAM	$\dfrac{1}{\lvert\tilde{\alpha}\rvert}\, e^{j2\pi cb/\tilde{\alpha}}$	$e^{j2\pi\tilde{\alpha}\zeta\beta}$	$\delta(c + \tilde{\alpha}\zeta)$	$\delta(b - \tilde{\alpha}\beta)$
HYP	$AM_\Gamma\!\left(\dfrac{-c}{f_r e^{-b}}, f_r e^{-b}\right)$	$HAF_\Gamma(-\zeta, -\beta)$	$v_\Gamma(-c, -\zeta)$	$V_\Gamma(-b, -\beta)$
PAD	$f_r\, AM_\Gamma(0, f_r e^b)$	$f_r\, \delta(c)\, AM_\Gamma(0, f_r e^b)$	$f_r\, v_\Gamma(0, \zeta)$	$f_r\, \delta(c)\, v_\Gamma(0, \zeta)$
SPAD	$f_r\, g(c)\, AM_\Gamma(0, f_r e^b)$	$f_r\, G(\beta)\, v_\Gamma(0, \zeta)$	$f_r\, g(c)\, v_\Gamma(0, \zeta)$	$f_r\, G(\beta)\, AM_\Gamma(0, f_r e^b)$

Here, $\lambda(\beta) = \dfrac{\beta/2}{\sinh\beta/2}$, $V_\Gamma(b, \beta) = f_r e^b \Gamma(f_r e^{b+\beta/2})\, \Gamma^*(f_r e^{b-\beta/2})$, $v_\Gamma(c, \zeta) = \rho_\Gamma(c + \zeta/2)\rho_\Gamma^*(c - \zeta/2)$, and

$$\rho_\Gamma(c) = \int_0^{\infty} \Gamma(f)\left(\frac{f}{f_r}\right)^{j2\pi c}\frac{df}{\sqrt{f}}.$$

κth Power Class

The Power class of TFRs consists of all TFRs that are scale covariant and power time-shift covariant, i.e.,

$$PC_Y^{(\kappa)}(t, f) = PC_X^{(\kappa)}\left(t - c\frac{d}{df}\xi(f/f_r), f\right) \qquad \text{for } Y(f) = e^{-j2\pi c\xi_\kappa(f/f_r)}X(f) \qquad (57.20)$$

where $\xi_\kappa(f) = \text{sgn}(f)|f|^\kappa$, for $\kappa \neq 0$ [Hlawatsch et al., 1993]. Consequently, the κth Power class perfectly represents group delay changes in the signal that are powers of frequency. When $\kappa = 1$, the Power class is equivalent to the Affine class. The central member, $AM^{(\kappa)}$ in Table 57.1, is the Power class equivalent to the Altes-Marinovic distribution.

57.4 Common TFRs and Their Use in Biomedical Applications

This section will briefly review some of the TFRs commonly used in biomedical analysis and summarize their relative advantages and disadvantages.

Wigner Distribution

One of the oldest TFRs in Table 57.1 is the Wigner distribution (WD), which Wigner proposed in quantum mechanics as a two-dimensional statistical distribution relating the Fourier transform pairs of position and momentum of a particle. Table 57.3 reveals that the WD satisfies a large number of desirable TFR properties, P_1 to P_3, P_5 to P_7, P_9 to P_{21}, and P_{23} to P_{25}. It is a member of both the Cohen and the Affine classes. The WD is a high-resolution TFR for linear FM chirps, sinusoids, and impulses. Since the WD satisfies Moyal's formula, it has been used to design optimal signal-detection and synthesis algorithms. The drawbacks of the WD are that it can be negative, it requires the signal to be known for all time, and it is a quadratic TFR with no implicit smoothing to remove cross-terms.

Smoothed Wigner Distributions

Many TFRs are related to the WD by either smoothing or a warping; e.g., see Eqs. (57.8) and (57.18) and Table 57.5. An intuitive understanding of the effects of cross-terms on quadratic TFRs can be obtained by analyzing the WD of a multicomponent signal $y(t)$ in Eq. (57.5) under the assumption that each signal component is a shifted version of a basic envelope, i.e., $x_n(t) = x(t - t_n)e^{j2\pi f_n t}$:

$$WD_y(t, f) = \sum_{n=1}^{N} WD_x(t - t_n, f - f_n)$$

$$+ 2\sum_{k=1}^{N-1}\sum_{q=k+1}^{N} WD_x(t - \bar{t}_{k,q}, f - \bar{f}_{k,q})\cos(2\pi[\Delta f_{k,q}(t - \Delta t_{k,q}) \quad (57.21)$$

$$- \Delta t_{k,q}(f - \Delta f_{k,q}) + \Delta f_{k,q}\Delta t_{k,q}])$$

where $\Delta f_{k,q} = f_k - f_q$ is the difference or "beat" frequency and $\bar{f}_{k,q} = (f_k + f_q)/2$ is the average frequency between the kth and qth signal components. Similarly, $\Delta t_{k,q}$ is the difference time and $\bar{t}_{k,q}$ is the average time. The auto-WD terms in the first summation properly reflect the fact that the WD is a member of Cohen's shift covariant class. Unfortunately, the cross-WD terms in the second summation occur midway in the time-frequency plane between each pair of signal components and oscillate with a spatial frequency proportional to the distance between them. The Pseudo-WD (PWD) and the smoothed Pseudo-WD (SPWD) defined in Table 57.1 use low-pass smoothing windows $\eta(\tau)$ and $\gamma(t)$ to reduce oscillatory cross-components. However, Table 57.5 reveals that the Pseudo-WD performs smoothing only in the frequency direction. Short smoothing windows greatly reduce the limit of integration in the Pseudo-WD and SPWD formulations and hence reduce computation time. However, Table 57.3 reveals that smoothing the WD reduces the number of desirable properties it satisfies from 18 to 7 for the Pseudo-WD and to only 3 for the SPWD.

Spectrogram

One of the most commonly used TFRs for slowly time-varying or quasi-stationary signals is the spectrogram, defined in Tables 57.1 and 57.5 [Rabiner & Schafer, 1978]. It is equal to the squared magnitude of the short-time Fourier transform, performing a local or "short-time" Fourier analysis by using a sliding analysis window $\gamma(t)$ to segment the signal into short sections centered near the output time t before computing a Fourier transformation. The spectrogram is easy to compute, using either FFTs or a parallel bank of filters, and it is often easy to interpret. The quadratic spectrogram smooths away all cross-terms except those which occur when two signal components overlap. This smoothing also distorts auto-terms. The spectrogram does a poor job representing rapidly changing spectral characteristics or resolving two closely spaced components because there is an inherent trade-off between good time resolution, which requires a short analysis window, and good frequency resolution, which requires a long analysis window. The spectrogram satisfies only three TFR properties listed in Tables 57.2 and 57.3; i.e., it is a nonnegative member of Cohen's shift invariant class.

Choi-Williams Exponential and Reduced Interference Distributions

The Choi-Williams exponential distribution (CWD) and the reduced interference distribution (RID) in Table 57.1 are often used as a compromise between the high-resolution but cluttered WD versus the smeared but easy to interpret spectrogram [Jeong & Williams, 1992; Williams & Jeong, 1991]. Since they are members of both Cohen's class and the Affine class, their AF domain kernels in Table 57.4 have a very special form, i.e. $\Psi_C(\tau, \nu) = S_c(\tau\nu)$, called a *product kernel,* which is a one-dimensional kernel evaluated at the product of its time-frequency variables [Hlawatsch & Boudreaux-Bartels, 1992]. The CWD uses a Gaussian product kernel in the AF plane to reduce cross-terms, while the RID typically uses a classic window function that is time-limited and normalized to automatically satisfy many desirable TFR properties (see Table 57.3). The CWD has one scaling factor σ that allows the user to select either good cross-term reduction or good auto-term preservation but, unfortunately, not always both. The generalized exponential distribution in Table 57.1 is an extension of the CWD that permits both [Hlawatsch & Boudreaux-Bartels, 1992]. Because the CWD and RID product kernels have hyperbolic isocontours in the AF plane, they always pass cross-terms between signal components that occur at either the same time or frequency, and they can distort auto-terms of linear FM chirp signals whose instantaneous frequency has a slope close to 1. The multiform tiltable exponential distribution (MTED) [Costa & Boudreaux-Bartels, 1994], another extension of the CWD, works works well for any linear FM chirp.

Scalogram or Wavelet Transform Squared Magnitude

The scalogram [Flandrin, 1993], defined in Tables 57.1 and 57.5, is the squared magnitude of the recently introduced wavelet transform (WT) [Daubechies, 1992; Meyer, 1993] and is a member of the Affine class. It uses a special sliding analysis window $\gamma(t)$, called the *mother wavelet,* to analyze local spectral information of the signal $x(t)$. The mother wavelet is either compressed or dilated to give a multiresolution signal representation. The scalogram can be thought of as the multiresolution output of a parallel bank of octave-band filters. High-frequency regions of the WT domain have very good time resolution, whereas low-frequency regions of the WT domain have very good spectral resolution. The WT has been used to model the middle- to high-frequency range operation of the cochlea, to track transients such as speech pitch and the onset of the QRS complex in ECG signals, and to analyze fractal and chaotic signals. One drawback of the scalogram is its poor temporal resolution at low-frequency regions of the time-frequency plane and poor spectral resolution at high frequencies. Moreover, many "classic" windows do not satisfy the conditions needed for a mother wavelet. The scalogram cannot remove cross-terms when signal components overlap. Further, many discrete WT implementations do not preserve the important time-shift covariance property.

Biomedical Applications

The electrocardiogram (ECG) signal is a recording of the time-varying electric rhythm of the heart. The short-duration QRS complex is the most predominant feature of the normal ECG signal. Abnormal heart rhythms can be identified on the ECG by detecting the QRS complex from one cycle to the next. The transient detection capability of the wavelet transform (WT) has been exploited for detection of the QRS complex by Kadambe et al. [1992] and Li and Zheng [1993]. The WT exhibits local maxima which align across successive (dyadic) scales at the location of transient components, such as QRS complexes. The advantage of using the WT is that it is robust both to noise and to nonstationarities in the QRS complex.

Other pathologic features in the heart's electrical rhythm that appear only in high-resolution signal-averaged ECG signals are ventricular late potentials (VLPs). VLPs are small-amplitude, short-duration components that occur after the QRS complex and are precursors of dangerous, life-threatening cardiac arrhythmias. Tuteur [1989] used the peak of the WT at a fixed scale to identify simulated VLPs. More recently, Jones et al. [1992] compared different time-frequency techniques, such as the spectrogram, short-time spectral estimators, the smoothed WD, and the WT, in their ability to discriminate between normal patients and patients susceptible to dangerous arrhythmias. Morlet et al. [1993] used the transient detection capability of the WT to identify VLPs.

The WT also has been applied to the ECG signal in the context of ECG analysis and compression by Crowe et al. [1992]. Furthermore, Crowe et al. [1992] exploited the capability of the WT to analyze fractal-like signals to study heart rate variability (HRV) data, which have been described as having fractal-like properties.

The recording of heart sounds, or phonocardiogram (PCG) signal, has been analyzed using many time-frequency techniques. Bulgrin et al. [1993] compared the short-time Fourier transform and the WT for the analysis of abnormal PCGs. Picard et al. [1991] analyzed the sounds produced by different prosthetic valves using the spectrogram. The binomial RID, which is a fast approximation to the CWD, was used to analyze the short-time, narrow-bandwidth features of first heart sound in mongrel dogs by Wood et al. [1992].

TFRs also have been applied to nonstationary brain wave signals, including the electrocardiogram (EEG), the electrocorticogram (ECoG), and evoked potentials (EPs). Zaveri et al. [1992] used the spectrogram, the WD, and the CWD to characterize the nonstationary behavior of the ECoG of epileptic patients. Of the three techniques, the CWD exhibited superior results. The WT was used to identify the onset of epileptic seizures in the EEG by Schiff and Milton [1993], to extract a single EP by Bartnik et al. [1992], and to characterize changes in somatosensory EPs due to brain injury caused by oxygen deprivation by Thakor et al. [1993].

Crackles are lung sounds indicative of pathologic conditions. Verreault [1989] used AR models of slices of the WD to discriminate crackles from normal lung sounds.

The electrogastrogram (EGG) is a noninvasive measure of the time-varying electrical activity of the stomach. Promising results regarding abnormal EGG rhythms and the frequency of the EGG slow wave were obtained using the CWD by Lin and Chen [1994].

Widmalm et al. [1991] analyzed temporomandibular joint (TMJ) clicking using the spectrogram, the WD, and the RID. The RID allowed for better time-frequency resolution of the TMJ sounds than the spectrogram while reducing the cross-terms associated with the WD. TMJ signals also were modeled using nonorthogonal Gabor logons by Brown et al. [1994]. The primary advantage of this technique, which optimizes the location and support of each Gabor log-on, is that only a few such logons were needed to represent the TMJ clicks.

Auditory applications of TFRs are intuitively appealing because the cochlea exhibits constant-bandwidth behavior at low frequencies and constant-Q behavior at middle to high frequencies. Applications include a wavelet-based model of the early stages of acoustic signal processing in the auditory system [Yang et al., 1992], a comparison of the WD and Rihaczek distribution on the response of auditory neurons to wideband noise stimulation [Eggermont & Smith, 1990], and spectrotemporal analysis of dorsal cochlear neurons in the guinea pig [Backoff & Clopton, 1992].

The importance of mammography, x-ray examination of the breast, lies in the early identification of tumors. Kaewlium and Longbotham [1993] used the spectrogram with a Gabor window as a texture discriminator to identify breast masses. Recently, a mammographic feature-enhancement technique using the WT was proposed by Laine et al. [1993]. The wavelet coefficients of the image are modified and then reconstructed to the desired resolution. This technique enhanced the visualization of mammographic features of interest without additional cost or radiation.

Magnetic resonance imaging (MRI) allows for the imaging of the soft tissues in the body. Weaver et al. [1992] reduced the long processing time of traditional phase encoding of MRI images by WT encoding. Moreover, unlike phase-encoded images, Gibb's ringing phenomena and motion artifacts are localized in WT encoded images.

The Doppler ultrasound signal is the reflection of an ultrasonic beam due to moving red blood cells and provides information regarding blood vessels and heart chambers. Doppler ultrasound signals in patients with narrowing of the aortic valve were analyzed using the spectrogram by Cloutier et al. [1991]. Guo and colleagues [1994] examined and compared the application of five different time-frequency representations (the spectrogram, short-time AR model, CWD, RID, and Bessel distributions) with simulated Doppler ultrasound signals of the femoral artery. Promising results were obtained from the Bessel distribution, the CWD, and the short-time AR model.

Another focus of bioengineering applications of TFRs has concerned the analysis of biologic signals of interest, including the sounds generated by marine mammals, such as dolphins and whales, and the sonar echolocation systems used by bats to locate and identify their prey. The RID was applied to sperm whale acoustic signals by Williams and Jeong [1991] and revealed an intricate time-frequency structure that was not apparent in the original time-series data. The complicated time-frequency characteristics of dolphin whistles were analyzed by Tyack et al. [1992] using the spectrogram, the WD, and the RID, with the RID giving the best results. Flandrin [1988] analyzed the time-frequency structure of the different signals emitted by bats during hunting, navigation, and identifying prey using the smoothed Pseudo-WD. In addition, the instantaneous frequency of the various signals was estimated using time-frequency representations. Saillant et al. [1993] proposed a model of the bat's echolocation system using the spectrogram. The most common application of the spectrogram is the analysis and modification of quasi-stationary speech signals [Rabiner & Schafer, 1978].

Acknowledgments

The authors would like to acknowledge the use of the personal notes of Franz Hlawatsch and Antonia Papandreou on TFR kernel constraints as well as the help given by Antonia Papandreou in critiquing the article and its tables.

References

Backoff PM, Clopton BM. 1991. A spectrotemporal analysis of DCN single unit responses to wideband noise in guinea pig. Hear Res 53:28.

Bartnik EA, Blinowska KJ, Durka PJ. 1992. Single evoked potential reconstruction by means of a wavelet transform. Biol Cybernet 67:175.

Boashash B (ed). 1991. Time-Frequency Signal Analysis-Methods and Applications. Melbourne, Australia, Longman-Chesire.

Brown ML, Williams WJ, Hero AO. 1994. Non-orthogonal Gabor representation for biological signals. In Proc Intl Conf ASSP, Australia, pp 305–308.

Bulgrin JR, Rubal BJ, Thompson CR, Moody JM. 1993. Comparison of short-time Fourier transform, wavelet and time-domain analyses of intracardiac sounds. Biol Sci Instrum 29:465.

Cloutier G, Lemire F, Durand L, et al. 1991. Change in amplitude distributions of Doppler spectrograms recorded below the aortic valve in patients with a valvular aortic stenosis. IEEE Trans Biomed Eng 39:502.

Cohen L. 1989. Time-frequency distributions—A review. Proc IEEE 77:941.

Claasen TACM, Mecklenbräuker WFG. 1980. The Wigner distribution: A tool for time-frequency signal analysis, parts I–III. Philips J Res 35:217, 35:276, 35:372.

Costa A, Boudreaux-Bartels GF. 1994. Design of time-frequency representations using multiform, tiltable kernels. In Proc IEEE-SP Intl Symp T-F and T-S Anal (Pacific Grove, CA).

Crowe JA, Gibson NM, Woolfson MS, Somekh MG. 1992. Wavelet transform as a potential tool for ECG analysis and compression. J Biomed Eng 14:268.

Daubechies I. 1992. Ten Lectures on Wavelets. Montpelier, Vt, Capital City Press.

Eggermont JJ, Smith GM. 1990. Characterizing auditory neurons using the Wigner and Rihacek distributions: A comparison. JASA 87:246.

Flandrin P. 1993. Temps-Fréquence. Hermes, Paris, France.

Flandrin P. 1988. Time-frequency processing of bat sonar signals. In Nachtigall PE, Moore PWB, (eds), Animal Sonar: Processes and Performance, pp 797–802. New York, Plenum Press.

Guo Z, Durand LG, Lee HC. 1994. Comparison of time-frequency distribution techniques for analysis of simulated Doppler ultrasound signals of the femoral artery. IEEE Trans Biomed Eng 41:332.

Hlawatsch F, Boudreaux-Bartels GF. 1992. Linear and quadratic time-frequency signal representations. IEEE Sig Proc Mag March:21.

Hlawatsch F, Papandreou A, Boudreaux-Bartels GF. 1993. Time-frequency representations: A generalization of the Affine and Hyperbolic classes. In Proc 26th Ann Asil Conf Sig Syst Comput (Pacific Grove, CA).

Jeong J, Williams WJ. 1992. Kernel design for reduced interference distributions. IEEE Trans SP 40:402.

Jones DL, Tovannas JS, Lander P, Albert DE. 1992. Advanced time-frequency methods for signal averaged ECG analysis. J Electrocardiol 25(suppl):188.

Kadambe S, Murray R, Boudreaux-Bartels GF. 1992. The dyadic wavelet transform based QRS detector. In Proc 26th Ann Asil Conf Sig Syst Comput (Pacific Grove, CA).

Kaewlium A, Longbotham H. 1993. Application of Gabor transform as texture discriminator of masses in digital mammograms. Biol Sci Instrum 29:183.

Laine A, Schuler S, Fan J. 1993. Mammographic feature enhancement by multiscale analysis. Submitted to IEEE Trans Med Imaging.

Li C, Zheng C. 1993. QRS detection by wavelet transform. In Proc Ann Intl Conf IEEE EMBS, pp 330–331.

Lin ZY, Chen JDZ. 1994. Time-frequency representation of the electrogastrogram: Application of the exponential distribution. IEEE Trans Biomed Eng 41:267.

Meyer Y. 1993. Wavelets—Algorithms and Applications. Philadephia, SIAM.

Morlet D, Peyrin F, Desseigne P, et al. 1993. Wavelet analysis of high resolution signal averaged ECGs in postinfarction patients. J Electrocardiol 26:311.

Murray R. 1994. Summary of biomedical applications of time-frequency representations. Technical report no. 0195-0001, Univ. of Rhode Island.

Papandreou A, Hlawatsch F, Boudreaux-Bartels GF. 1993. The Hyperbolic class of quadratic time-frequency representations: I. Constant-Q warping, the hyperbolic paradigm, properties, and members. IEEE Trans SP 41:3425.

Picard D, Charara J, Guidoin F, et al. 1991. Phonocardiogram spectral analysis simulator of mitral valve prostheses. J Med Eng Technol 15:222.

Porat B. 1994. Digital Processing of Random Signals: Theory and Methods. Englewood Cliffs, NJ, Prentice-Hall.

Rabiner LR, Schafer RW. 1978. Digital Processing of Speech Signals. Englewood Cliffs, NJ, Prentice-Hall.

Rioul O, Vetterli M. 1991. Wavelets and signal processing. IEEE Sig Proc Mag October:14.

Saillant PA, Simmons JA, Dear SP. 1993. A computational model of echo processing and acoustic imaging in frequency modulated echo-locating bats: The spectrogram correlation and transformation receiver. JASA 94:2691.

Schiff SJ, Milton JG. 1993. Wavelet transforms for electroencephalographic spike and seizure detection. In Proc SPIE—Intl Soc Opt Eng, pp 50–56.

Tuteur FB. 1989. Wavelet transformations in signal detection. In Proc Intl Conf ASSP, pp 1435–1438.

Tyack PL, Williams WJ, Cunningham G. 1992. Time-frequency fine structure of dolphin whistles. In Proc IEEE—SP Intl Symp T-F and T-S Anal (Victoria, BC, Canada), pp 17–20.

Verreault E. 1989. Détection et Caractérisation des Rales Crépitants (French). PhD thesis, l'Université Laval, Faculte des Sciences et de Genie.

Weaver JB, Xu Y, Healy DM, Driscoll JR. 1992. Wavelet encoded MR imaging. Magnet Reson Med 24:275.

Widmalm WE, Williams WJ, Zheng C. 1991. Reduced interference time-frequency distributions. In Boashash B (ed), Time frequency distributions of TMJ sounds. J Oral Rehabil 18:403.

Williams WJ, Jeong J. 1991. Time-Frequency Signal Analysis—Methods and Applications, pp 878–881. Chesire, England, Longman.

Yang X, Wang K, Shamma S. 1992. Auditory representations of acoustic signals. IEEE Trans Info Theory 38:824.

Zaveri HP, Williams WJ, Iasemidis LD, Sackellares JC. 1992. Time-frequency representations of electrocorticograms in temporal lobe epilepsy. IEEE Trans Biomed Eng 39:502.

urther Information

Several TFR tutorials exist on the Cohen class [Boashash, 1991; Cohen, 1989; Flandrin, 1993; Hlawatsch & Boudreaux-Bartels, 1992], Affine class [Bertrand chapter in Boashash, 1991; Flandrin, 1993], hyperbolic class [Papandreou et al., 1993], and power class [Hlawatsch et al., 1993]. Several special conferences or issues of IEEE journals devoted to TFRs and the WT include *Proc. of the IEEE-SP Time-Frequency and Time-Scale Workshop*, 1992, IEEE Sig. Proc. Soc.; Special issue on wavelet transforms and multiresolution signal analysis, *IEEE Trans. Info. Theory*, 1992; and Special issue on wavelets and signal processing, *IEEE Trans. SP*, 1993. An extended list of references on the application of TFRs to problems in biomedical or bio-engineering can be found in Murray [1994].

58

Wavelet (Time-Scale) Analysis in Biomedical Signal Processing

Nitish V. Thakor
Johns Hopkins University

David Sherman
Johns Hopkins University

Digital signal processing uses sophisticated mathematical analysis and algorithms to extract information hidden in signals derived from sensors. In biomedical applications, these sensors, such as electrodes, accelerometers, optical imagers, etc., record signals from biologic tissue with the goal of revealing their health and well-being in clinical and research settings. Refining these signal-processing algorithms for biologic applications requires building suitable signal models to capture signal features and components that are of diagnostic importance. Since most signals of a biologic origin are time-varying, there is a special need for capturing transient phenomena in both healthy and chronically ill states.

A critical feature of many biologic signals is frequency-domain parameters. Time localization of these changes is an issue for biomedical researchers who need to understand subtle frequency content changes over time. Certainly signals marking the transition from severe normative to diseased states of an organism sometimes undergo severe changes that can easily be detected using methods such as the short-time Fourier transform (STFT) for deterministic or energy signals and its companion, the spectrogram, for power signals. The basis function for the STFT is the complex sinusoid $e^{j2\pi ft}$, which is suitable for stationary analyses of narrowband signals. For signals of a biologic origin, the sinusoid may not be a suitable analysis signal. Biologic signals are often spread out over wide areas of the frequency spectrum. Also, as Rioul and Vetterli [1] point out, when the frequency content of a signal changes in a rapid fashion, the frequency content becomes smeared over the entire frequency spectrum, as it does in the case of the onset of seizure spikes in epilepsy or a fibrillating heartbeat as revealed on an ECG. The use of a narrowband basis function does not accurately represent wideband signals. We would prefer that our basis functions be similar to the signal under study. In fact, for a compact representation using as few basis functions as possible, it is desirable to

0-8493-8346-3/95/$0.00+$.50
© 1995 by CRC Press, Inc.

use basis functions that have a wider frequency spread, as most biologic signals do. Wavelet theory, which provides for wideband representation of signals, is therefore a natural choice for biomedical engineers involved in signal processing and is currently under intense study [2].

58.1 The Wavelet Transform: Variable Time and Frequency Resolution

A decomposition of a signal based on a wider frequency mapping and consequently better time resolution is possible with the wavelet transform. The *continuous wavelet transform* (CWT) is defined as follows for a continuous signal $x(t)$:

$$\text{CWT}_x(\tau, a) = \frac{1}{\sqrt{a}} \int x(t) g^* \left(\frac{t - \tau}{a} \right) dt \tag{58.1a}$$

or with change of variable as

$$\text{CWT}_x(\tau, a) = \sqrt{a} \int x(at) g^* \left(t - \frac{\tau}{a} \right) dt \tag{58.1b}$$

where $g(t)$ is the *mother* or *basic wavelet* [3], and a is the scale factor. Typically, $g(t)$ is a bandpass function centered around some center frequency f_0. Scale allows the compression or expansion of $g(t)$ [1,3]. A larger scale factor generates the same function compressed in time, whereas a smaller scale factor generates the opposite. When the analyzing signal is contracted in time, similar signal features or changes that occur over a smaller time window can be studied. For the wavelet transform, the same basic wavelet is employed, with alterations in this signal arising only from scale changes. Likewise, a smaller scale function enables larger time translations or delays in the basic signal.

The notion of scale is a critical feature of the wavelet transform because of time and frequency domain reciprocity. When the scale factor a is enlarged, the effect on frequency is compression, as the analysis window in the frequency domain is contracted by the amount $1/a$ [3]. This equal and opposite frequency-domain scaling effect can be put to advantageous use for frequency localization. Since we are using bandpass filter functions, a center frequency change at a given scale yields wider or narrower frequency-response changes depending on size of the center frequency. This is the same in analog or digital filtering theory as *constant-Q* or *quality* factor analysis [1,3,4]. At a given Q or scale factor, frequency translates are accompanied by proportional bandwidth or resolution changes. In this regard, wavelet transforms are often written with the scale factor rendered as

$$a = \frac{f}{f_0} \tag{58.2}$$

or

$$\text{CWT}_x \left(\tau, a = \frac{f}{f_0} \right) = \frac{1}{\sqrt{f/f_0}} \int x(t) g^* \left(\frac{t - \tau}{f/f_0} \right) dt \tag{58.3}$$

This is the equivalent to logarithmic scaling of the filter bandwidth or octave scaling of the filter bandwidth for power-of-two growth in center frequencies. Larger center frequency entails a larger bandwidth, and vice versa.

Another representation, *Morlet's wavelet*, is often used because it can be used to scale time and select center frequency independently. Morlet's wavelet [4] is defined as

$$g(t) = e^{j2\pi f_0 t} e^{-(t^2/2)} \tag{58.4}$$

with its scaled version written as

$$g\left(\frac{t}{a}\right) = e^{j(2\pi f_0/a)t}\, e^{-(t^2/2a^2)} \tag{58.5}$$

Morlet's wavelet ensures that the time-scale representation can be viewed as a time-frequency one. A gaussian window is modulated to the desired center frequency and scaled accordingly. It has the best representation in both time and frequency because it is based on the gaussian window. This is the best compromise for a simultaneous localization in both time and frequency, since the gaussian function's Fourier transform is simply a scaled version of its time-domain function. Also, the Morlet wavelet is defined by an explicit function and leads to a quasi-continuous discrete version [4]. A modified version of Morlet's wavelet leads to fixed center frequency f_0 with width parameter σ:

$$g(\sigma, t) = e^{j2\pi f_0 t}\, e^{-(t^2/2\sigma^2)} \tag{58.6}$$

Once again, time-frequency reciprocity determines the degree of resolution available in time and frequency domains. Choosing a small window size σ in the time domain yields poor frequency resolution while offering excellent time resolution, and vice versa.

The STFT has the same frequency-time resolution as observed regardless of frequency translations. The STFT can be written as

$$\text{STFT}(\tau, f) = \int_{-\infty}^{\infty} x(t)g^*(t - \tau)e^{-2\pi j f t}\, dt \tag{58.7}$$

where $g(t)$ is the time window that selects the time interval for analysis, otherwise known as the *spectrum localized in time*. Figure 58.1 shows comparative frequency resolution of both the STFT and the wavelet transform. The STFT is often thought to be analogous to a bank of bandpass filters each shifted by a certain modulation frequency f_0. In fact, the Fourier transform of a signal can be interpreted as passing the signal through multiple bandpass filters with impulse response $g(t)e^{j2\pi f t}$ and then using complex demodulation to downshift the filter output. Ultimately, the STFT as bandpass filter rendition simply translates the same low-pass filter function through the operation of modulation. The characteristics of the filter stays the same even though the frequency is shifted.

Unlike the STFT, the wavelet transform implementation is not frequency-independent, so higher frequencies are studied with analysis filters with wider bandwidths. Scale changes are not equivalent

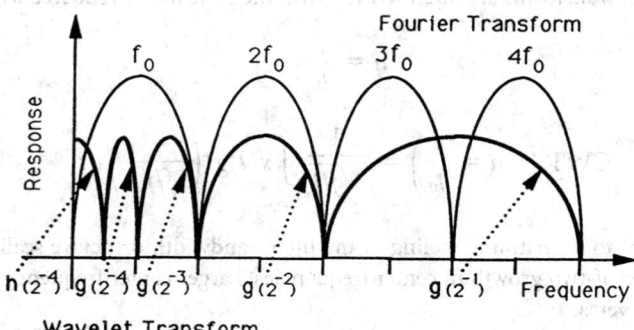

FIGURE 58.1 Comparative frequency resolution for short-time Fourier transform (STFT) and wavelet transform (WT). Note that frequency resolution of the STFT is constant across frequency spectrum. The WT has a frequency resolution that is proportional to the center frequency of the bandpass filter.

to varying modulation frequencies that the STFT uses. The dilations and contractions of the basis function allow for variation of time and frequency resolution instead of uniform resolution of the Fourier transform.

Both the wavelet and Fourier transforms are linear TFRs (time-frequency representation) and the rules of superposition or linearity apply [3]. This is advantageous in cases of two or more separate signal constituents. Linearity means that cross-terms are not generated in applying either the linear time-frequency or time-scale operations. Aside from linear TFRs, there are quadratic time-frequency representations that are quite useful in displaying energy and correlation-domain information. These techniques are described elsewhere in this volume, including the Wigner-Ville distribution (W-VD), smoothed W-V, the reduced inference distribution (RID), etc. One example of the smoothed Wigner-Ville distribution is

$$W(t, f) = \int s^*\left(t - \frac{1}{2}\tau\right) e^{-j\tau 2\pi f} s\left(^*t + \frac{1}{2}\tau\right) h\left(\frac{\tau}{2}\right) d\tau \qquad (58.8)$$

where $h(t)$ is a smoothing function. In this case, the smoothing kernel for the generalized or Cohen's class of time-frequency representations is

$$\phi(t, \tau) = h\left(\frac{\tau}{2}\right)\delta(t)$$

These methods display joint time-frequency information in such a fashion as to display rapid changes of energy over the entire frequency spectrum. They are not subject to variations due to window selection, as in the case of the STFT. A problematic area for these cases is the elimination of those cross-terms which are the result of the embedded correlation.

It is to be noted that the scalogram or scaled energy representation for wavelets can be represented as a Wigner-Ville distribution [1] as

$$|\text{CWT}_x(\tau, a)|^2 = \iint W_x(u, n) W_g^*\left(\frac{u - t}{a}, an\right) du \, dn \qquad (58.9)$$

where

$$W_x(t, f) = \int x^*\left(t - \frac{1}{2}\tau\right) e^{-j\tau 2\pi f} x^*\left(t + \frac{1}{2}\tau\right) d\tau$$

58.2 The Discrete Wavelet Transform

In discrete time, scale changes themselves are discrete. Scaling for the discrete wavelet transform involves sampling rate changes. A larger scale corresponds to subsampling the signal. For a given number of samples, a larger time swath is covered for a larger scale. This is the basis of signal compression schemes as well [5]. Typically, a dyadic or binary scaling system is employed so that given a discrete wavelet function $\psi(t)$ is scaled by values that are binary. Thus

$$\psi_{2j}(t) = 2^j \psi(2^j t)$$

where j is the scaling index and $j = 0, -1, -2, \ldots$. In a dyadic scheme, subsampling is always decimation-in-time by a power of 2. Translations in time will be proportionally larger as well as for a more sizable scale.

It is for discrete time signals that scale and resolution are related. When the scale is increased, resolution is lowered. Resolution is strongly related to frequency. Subsampling means lowered frequency content. Rioul and Vetterli [1] use the microscope analogy to point out that smaller scale (higher resolution) helps us to explore fine details of a signal. This higher resolution is apparent with samples taken at *smaller* time intervals.

58.3 A Multiresolution Theory: Decomposition of Signals Using Orthogonal Wavelets

One key result of the wavelet theory is that signals can be decomposed in a series of orthogonal wavelets. This is similar to the notion of decomposing a signal in terms of discrete Fourier transform components or Walsh or Haar functions. Orthogonality ensures a unique and complete representation of the signal. Likewise, the orthogonal complement provides some measure of the error in the representation. The difference in terms of wavelets is that the each of the orthogonal vector spaces offers component signals with varying levels of resolution and scale. This is why Mallat [6] named his algorithm *multiresolution signal decomposition*. Each stage of the algorithm generates wavelets with sequentially finer representations of signal content. To achieve an orthogonal wavelet representation, a given wavelet function $\phi(t)$ at a scaling index level equal to zero is first dilated by the scale coefficient 2^j, and then translating it by $2^{-j}n$ and normalizing by $\sqrt{2^{-j}}$ gives

$$\sqrt{2^{-j}}\phi_{2^j}(t - 2^{-j}n) \tag{58.10}$$

The algorithm begins with an operator A_{2^j} for discrete signals that takes the projections of a signal $f(t)$ onto the orthonormal basis $\mathbf{V}_{2^j}$:

$$A_{2^j}f(t) = 2^{-j}\sum_{n=-\infty}^{\infty}\langle f(u), \phi_{2^j}(u - 2^{-j}n)\rangle\phi_{2^j}(t - 2^{-j}n) \tag{58.11}$$

where 2^j defines the level of resolution, and A_{2^j} is defined as the multiresolution operator that approximates a signal at a resolution 2^j. Signals at successively lower resolutions can be obtained by repeated application of the operator $A_{2^j}(-J \leq j \leq -1)$, where $-J$ specifies the minimum resolution, such that $A_{2^j}f(x)$ is the closest approximation of function $f(x)$ at resolution 2^j. Here we note that $< >$ is simply a convolution defined as follows:

$$\langle f(u), \phi_{2^j}(u - 2^{-j}n)\rangle = \int_{-\infty}^{\infty} f(u)\phi(u - 2^{-j}n)\,du \tag{58.12}$$

Here $\phi(t)$ is the impulse response of the scaling function. The Fourier transforms of the these functions are low-pass filter functions with successively smaller halfband low-pass filters as in Fig. 58.2b. This convolution synthesizes the coarse signal at a resolution/scaling level j:

$$C_{2^j}f = \langle f(t), \phi_{2^j}(t - 2^{-j}n)\rangle \tag{58.13}$$

Each level j generates new basis functions of the particular orthonormal basis with a given discrete approximation. In this case, larger j values provide for decreasing resolution and increasing the scale in proportional fashion for each level of the orthonormal basis. Likewise, each sequentially larger j provides for time shift in accordance with scale changes, as mentioned above, and the convolution or inner-product operation generates the set of coefficients for the particular basis function. A set of scaling functions at decreasing levels of resolution, $j = 0, -1, -2, \ldots, -6$, is shown in Fig. 58.2a.

The next step in the algorithm is the expression of the basis function of one level of resolution ϕ_{2^j} by a higher resolution $\phi_{2^{j+1}}$. In the same fashion as above, an orthogonal representation of the basis $\mathbf{V}_{2^j}$ in terms of $\mathbf{V}_{2^{j+1}}$ is possible, or

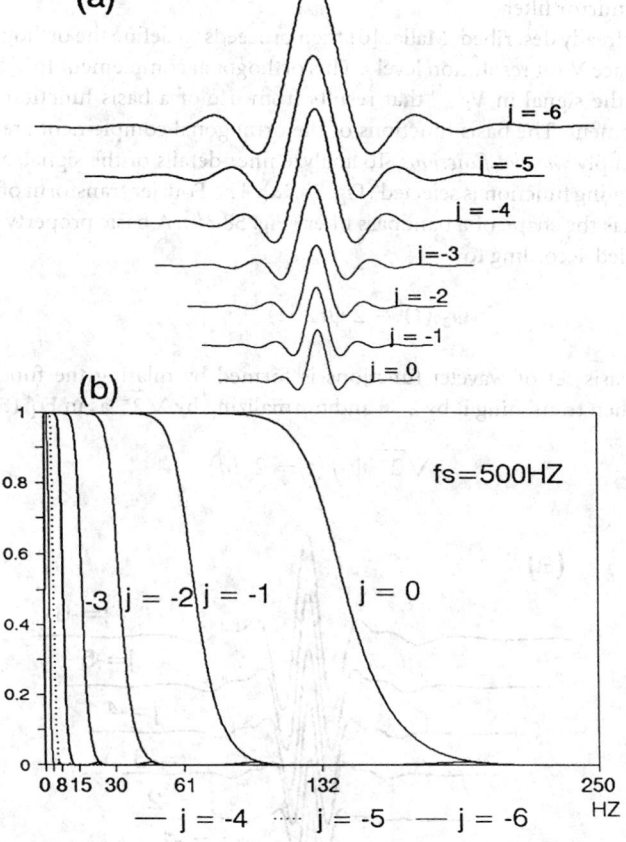

FIGURE 58.2 (*a*) Scaling functions $\phi(x)$ at various decreasing resolutions ($j = 0, -1, -2, \ldots, -6$). (*b*) Respective Fourier transforms of wavelet functions.

$$\phi_{2^j}(t - 2^{-j}n) = 2^{-j-1} \sum_{k=-\infty}^{\infty} \langle \phi_{2^j}(u - 2^{-j}n),$$

$$\phi_{2^{j+1}}(u - 2^{-j-1}k) \rangle \phi_{2^{j+1}}(t - 2^{-j-1}k) \tag{58.14}$$

Here, the coefficients are once again the inner products between the two basis functions. A means of translation is possible for converting the coefficients of one basis function to the coefficients of the basis function at a higher resolution:

$$C_{2^j}f = \langle f(u), \phi_{2^j}(t - 2^{-j}n) \rangle = 2^{-j-1} \sum_{k=-\infty}^{\infty} \langle \phi_{2^j}(u - 2^{-j}n),$$

$$\phi_{2^{j+1}}(u - 2^{-j-1}k) \rangle \langle f(u), \phi_{2^{j+1}}(t - 2^{-j-1}k) \rangle \tag{58.15}$$

Mallat [6] also conceives of the filter function $h(n)$ whose impulse response provides this conversion, namely,

$$C_{2^j}f = \langle f(u), \phi_{2^j}(t - 2^{-j}n) \rangle$$

$$= 2^{-j-1} \sum_{k=-\infty}^{\infty} \tilde{h}(2n - k) \langle f(u), \phi_{2^{j+1}}(t - 2^{-j-1}k) \rangle \tag{58.16}$$

where $h(n) = 2^{-j-1}\langle \phi_{2j}(u - 2^{-j}n), \phi_{2j+1}(u - 2^{-j-1}k)\rangle$ and $\widetilde{h}(n) = h(-n)$ are the impulse responses of the appropriate mirror filter.

Using the tools already described, Mallat [6] then proceeds to define the orthogonal complement O_{2j} to the vector space V_{2j} at resolution level j. This orthogonal complement to V_{2j} is the error in the approximation of the signal in V_2^{j+1} that results from use of a basis function belonging to the orthogonal complement. The basis functions of the orthogonal complement are called *orthogonal wavelets* $\psi(x)$ or simply *wavelet functions*. To analyze finer details of the signal, a wavelet function derived from the scaling function is selected (Fig. 58.3a). The Fourier transform of the wavelet function in Fig. 58.3a has the shape of a bandpass filter (Fig. 58.3b). A basic property of the function ψ is that it can be scaled according to

$$\psi_{2j}(t) = 2^j \psi(2^j \cdot t)$$

An orthonormal basis set of wavelet functions is formed by dilating the function $\psi(x)$ with a coefficient 2^j and then translating it by $2^{-j}n$ and normalizing by $\sqrt{2^{-j}}$ as in Eq. (58.10):

$$\sqrt{2^{-j}}\psi_{2j}(t - 2^{-j}n)$$

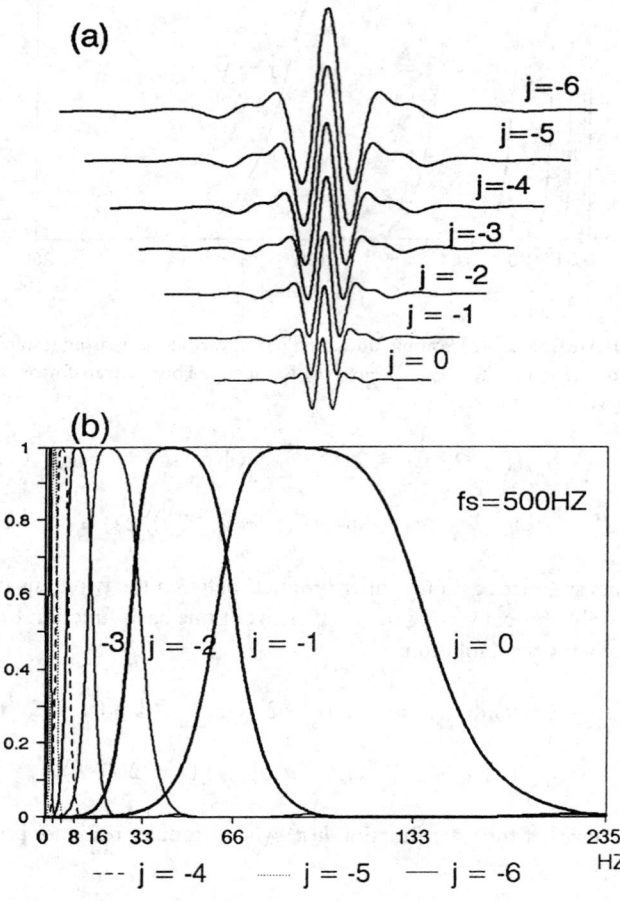

FIGURE 58.3 (a) Wavelet functions $\psi(x)$ at various decreasing resolutions ($j = 0, -1, -2, \ldots, -6$). (b) Respective Fourier transforms of wavelet functions.

They are formed by the operation of convolving the scale function with the quadrature mirror filter:

$$\psi(\omega) = G\left(\frac{\omega}{2}\right)\phi\left(\frac{\omega}{2}\right)$$

where $G(\omega) = e^{-j\omega}\overline{H}(\omega + \pi)$ is the quadrature mirror filter transfer response, and $g(n) = (-1)^{1-n}h(1 - n)$ is the corresponding impulse response function.

The set of scaling and wavelet functions presented here forms a duality, together resolving the temporal signal into coarse and fine details, respectively. For a given level j, then this detail signal can once again be represented as a set of inner products as

$$D_{2j}f = \langle f(t),\psi_{2j}(x - 2^{-j}n)\rangle \tag{58.17}$$

For a specific signal $f(x)$, we can employ the projection operator as before to generate the approximation to this signal on the orthogonal complement. As before, the detail signal can be decomposed using the higher-resolution basis function:

$$
\begin{aligned}
D_{2j}f &= \langle f(u),\psi_{2j}(t - 2^{-j}n)\rangle \\
&= 2^{-j-1}\sum_{k=-\infty}^{\infty} \langle \psi_{2j}(t - 2^{-j}n), \phi_{2j+1}(u - 2^{-j-1}k)\rangle\langle f(u), \phi_{2j+1}(t - 2^{-j-1}k)\rangle
\end{aligned}
\tag{58.18}
$$

or in terms of the synthesis filter response for the orthogonal wavelet:

$$D_{2j}f = \langle f(u),\psi_{2j}(t - 2^{-j}n)\rangle = 2^{-j-1}\sum_{k=-\infty}^{\infty} \tilde{g}(2n - k)\langle f(u),\phi_{2j+1}(t - 2^{-j-1}k)\rangle \tag{58.19}$$

At this point we have the tools necessary for decomposition of a signal in terms of wavelet components, coarse, and detail signals. Multiresolution wavelet description provides for the analysis of a signal into low-pass components at each level of resolution called *coarse signals* through the C operators. At the same time, the detail components through the D operator provide information regarding bandpass components. With each decreasing resolution level, different signal approximations are made to capture unique signal features. Procedural details for realizing this algorithm follow.

58.4 Implementation of the Multiresolution Wavelet Transform: Analysis and Synthesis Algorithms

A diagram of the algorithm for multiresolution wavelet decomposition is shown in Fig. 58.4. A step-by-step rendition of the analysis is as follows:

1. Start with N samples original signal $x(t)$ at resolution level $j = 0$.
2. Convolve the signal with the original scaling function $\phi(t)$ to find $C_1 f$ as in Eq. (58.13) with $j = 0$.
3. Find the coarse signal at successive resolution levels, $j = -1, -2, \ldots, -J$, through Eq. (58.16); keep every other sample of the output.
4. Find the detail signal at successive resolution levels, $j = -1, -2, \ldots, -J$, through Eq. (58.19); keep every other sample of the output.
5. Decrease j and repeat steps 3 through 5 until $j = -J$.

Signal reconstruction details are presented in Mallat [6] and Thakor et al. [7].

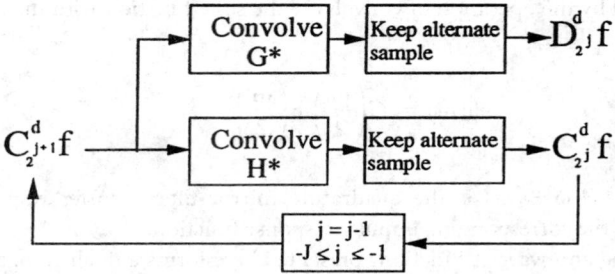

FIGURE 58.4 Flowchart of multiresolution algorithm showing how successive coarse and detail components of resolution level *j* are generated from higher-resolution level *j* + 1.

58.5 Applications

Cardiac Signal Processing

Signals from the heart, especially the ECG, are well suited for analysis by joint time-frequency and time-scale analysis. That is so because the ECG signal has a very characteristic time-varying morphology, identified as the P-QRS-T complex. Throughout this complex, the signal frequencies are distributed: low-frequency P and T waves, middle- to high-frequency QRS complex [8]. When an ischemic injury occurs, the Q wave and the ST segment of the complex show characteristic changes; when the heart is reperfused after injury, the same ST segment is restored and the frequency spectra of the QRS complex are altered. Late in the ECG cycle, when high-frequency events occur, these are identified as *late potentials* [9]. Late potentials have been shown to be predictive of arrhythmias of the heart. When arrhythmias, such as premature ventricular contractions (PVCs) and tachycardia, do occur, the P-QRS-T complex undergoes a significant morphologic change; in particular, the QRS complex may widen and sometimes invert with PVCs. As the QRS complex widens, its power spectrum shows diminished contributions at higher frequencies, and these are spread out over a wider body of the signal. This empirical description of the time-domain features of the ECG signal lends itself particularly well to analysis by time-frequency and time-scale techniques. Two examples are presented below.

Analysis of the QRS Complex

When the heart muscle becomes ischemic or infarcted, characteristic changes are seen in the form of elevation or depression of the ST segment. Detection of these changes requires an extension of the signal bandwidth to frequencies down to 0.05 Hz and less, making the measurements susceptible to motion artifact errors. Detection of ischemia-related changes in the QRS complex is less well known, and interpretation of the QRS complex would be less susceptible to artifactual errors. Thus time-frequency or time-scale analysis would serve a useful function in localizing the ischemia-related changes within the QRS complex, but would be somewhat independent of the artifactual errors. In experimental animals, we studied the response of the heart to coronary artery occlusion and then reperfusion. The left coronary artery was temporarily occluded for 20 minutes. Subsequent to that, the occlusion was removed, and resulting reperfusion more or less restored the ECG signal after 20 minutes. The coronary artery was occluded a second time for 60 minutes, and once again, occlusion was removed and blood flow was restored. Single ECG cycles were analyzed using the continuous wavelet transform [10]. Figure 58.5 shows the time-scale plots for the ECG cycles for each of the five stages of this experiment. The three-dimensional plots give time in the P-QRS-T complex on one axis, the scale (or equivalent frequency) on another axis, and the normalized magnitude on the third axis. First, occlusion results in a localized alteration around 100 ms and the midscale which shows

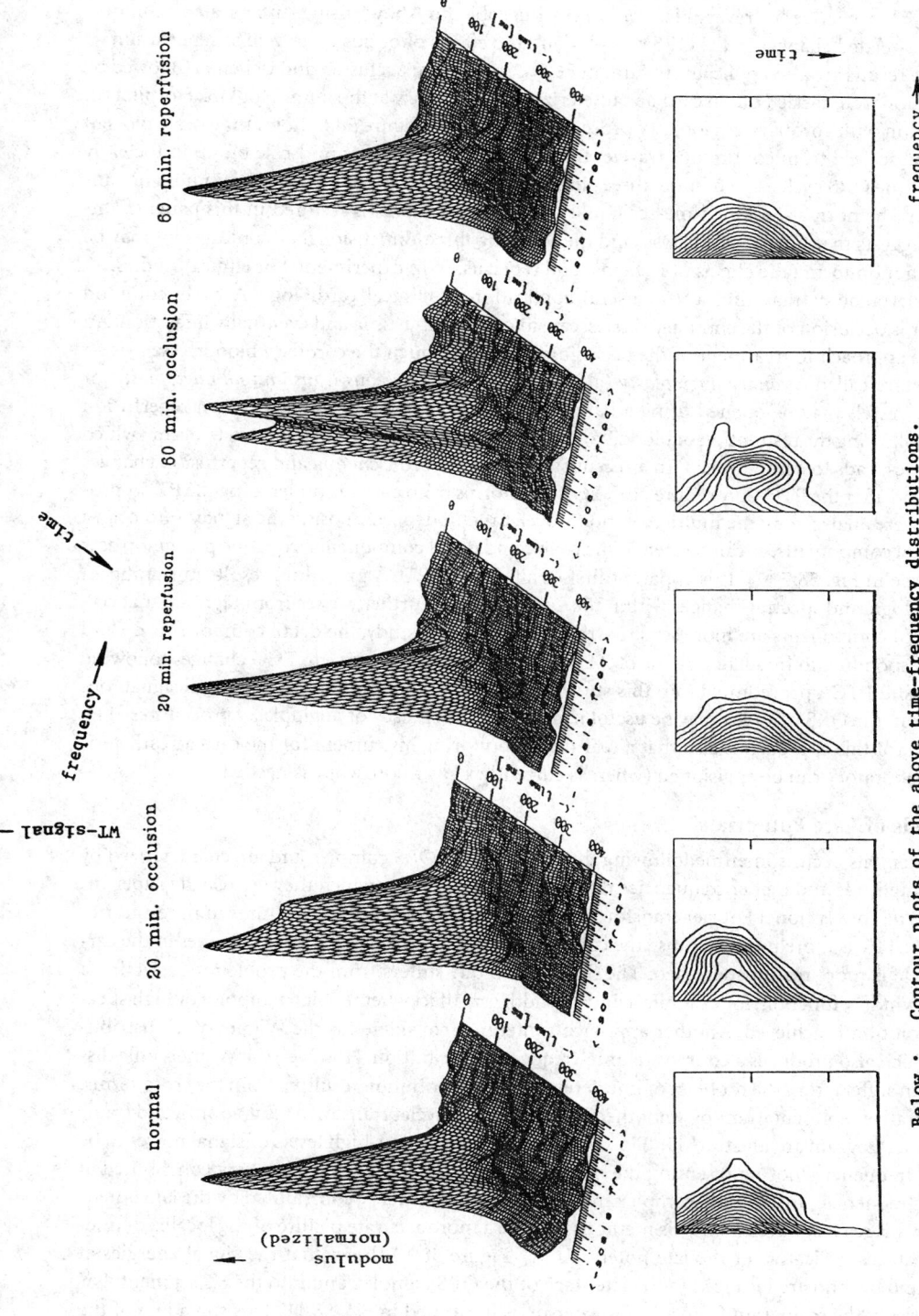

Below :   Contour plots of the above time-frequency distributions.

FIGURE 58.5   Time-frequency distributions of the vector magnitude of two ECG leads during five stages of a controlled animal experiment. The frequency scale is logarithmic, 16 to 200 Hz. The z axis represents the modulus (normalized) of the complex wavelet-transformed signal.

up as a bump in the three-dimensional plot or a broadening in the contour plot. Upon reperfusion, the time-scale plot returns to the preocclusion state. The second occlusion brings about a far more significant change in the time-scale plot, with increased response in the 0- to 200-ms and midscale ranges. This change is reversible. We were thus able to show, using time-scale technique, ischemia-related changes in the QRS complex and the effects of occlusion as well as reperfusion.

These results are also applicable to human ECGs. Short-term occlusion and ischemia followed by reperfusion were carried out in cardiac catheterization laboratory at the Johns Hopkins Hospital (in connection with coronary angioplasty procedure; see below). Figure 58.6 shows time-scale plots of a patient derived from continuous wavelet transform. A characteristic midscale bump in the early stages of the QRS cycle is seen in the three-dimensional time-scale plot. Then, 60 minutes after angioplasty, the normal-looking time-scale plot of the QRS complex is restored in this patient. This study suggests that time-scale analysis and the resulting three-dimensional or contour plot may be usable in monitoring the effects of ischemia and reperfusion in experimental or clinical studies.

Wavelet analysis may find a very useful application in clinical cardiology. A fairly common disorder is occlusion of the coronary vessels, causing cardiac ischemia and eventually infarction. An effective approach to treatment of the occlusion injury is to open the coronary blood vessels using a procedure called *coronary angioplasty* (also known as *percutaneous transluminal angioplasty,* or PTCA). Vessels may be opened using a balloon-type or a laser-based catheter. When reperfusion occurs following the restoration of blood flow, initially a reperfusion injury is known to occur (which sometimes leads to arrhythmias). In a recent study, we analyzed ischemia and reperfusion changes before and after the PTCA procedure [10]. ECG waveforms from patients undergoing the PTCA procedure were analyzed by the multiresolution wavelet method, decomposing the signals into coarse and detail components, as can be seen in the coarse and detail components from one preangioplasty ECG cycle in Fig. 58.7 [7]. It is apparent first of all that the PTCA procedure results in significant morphologic and spectral changes within the QRS complex. Further, we see from Fig. 58.8 that certain detail components are more sensitive than others; in our study, the detail components d6 and d5 corresponding to frequency bands of 2.2 to 8.3 Hz are most sensitive to ECG changes following a successful PTCA procedure. From this study we concluded that monitoring the detail signals derived from the QRS complex may be useful in assessing the efficacy of angioplasty procedures [11]. A benefit of this approach is also that a real-time monitoring instrument for the cardiac catheterization laboratory can be envisioned (whereas currently x-ray fluoroscopy is needed).

Analysis of Late Potentials

Late potentials occur sometime following the S wave of the QRS complex and are characterized by small amplitude and higher frequencies than the ST segment over which they are usually superimposed. The conventional Fourier transform does not readily localize these features in time and frequency. STFT is more useful because the concentration of signal energy at various times in the cardiac cycle is more readily identified. The STFT technique suffers from the problem of selecting a proper window function; for example, window width can affect whether high temporal or high spectral resolution is achieved. Another approach sometimes considered is the Wigner-Ville distribution, which also produces a composite time-frequency distribution. However, the Wigner-Ville distribution suffers from the problem of interference in the distribution resulting from the cross-terms. Comparative representations by smoothed Wigner-Ville, wavelet transform (scalogram), and traditional spectrogram are illustrated in Fig. 58.9. This problem causes high levels of signal power to be seen at frequencies not representing the original signal; for example, signal energy contributed at certain frequencies by the QRS complex may mask the signal energy contributed by the late potentials. In this regard, wavelet analysis methods provide a more accurate picture of the localized time-scale features indicative of the late potentials [4]. Figure 58.10 shows that the signal energies at 60 Hz and beyond are localized in the late stage of the QRS complex and into the ST segment. For comparison, the scalogram from a healthy person is illustrated in Fig. 58.11. This spreading of the high frequencies into the late cycle stages of the QRS-T complex is a hallmark of the late potentials.

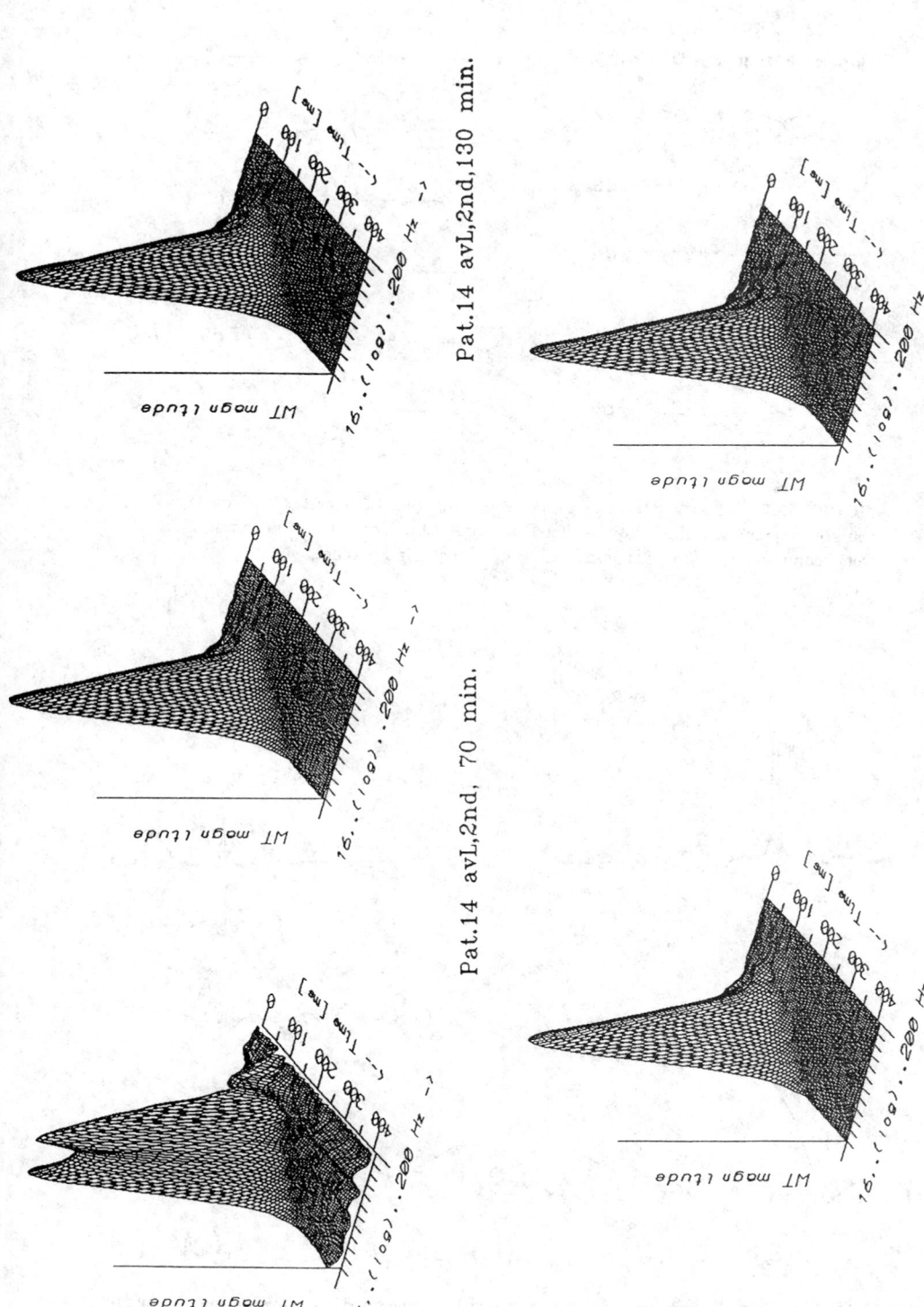

FIGURE 58.6 Contour plots of human ECG study using WT. Preangioplasty contour plot shows characteristic second hump. This disappears, as indicated by plots taken after two angioplasty treatments.

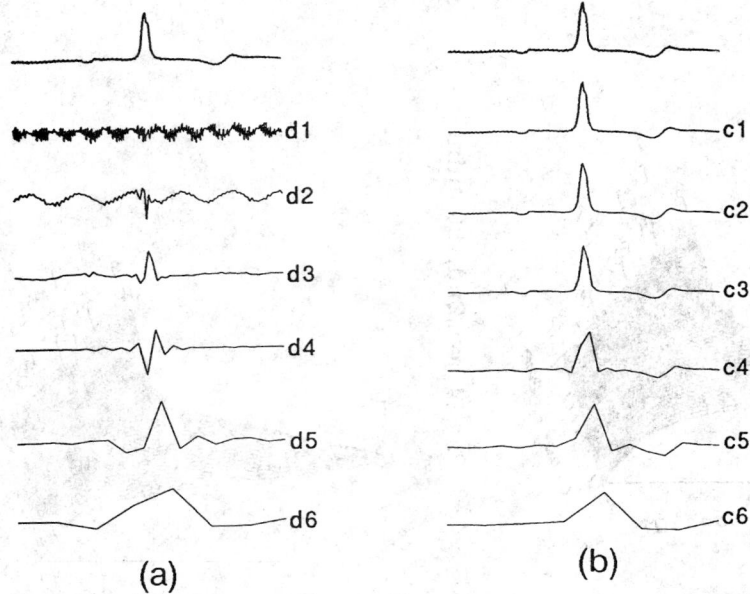

FIGURE 58.7 Detail and coarse components from one ECG cycle. The coarse components represent the low-pass-filtered versions of the signal at successive scales. Detail components d1 and d2 consist mainly of electrical interference.

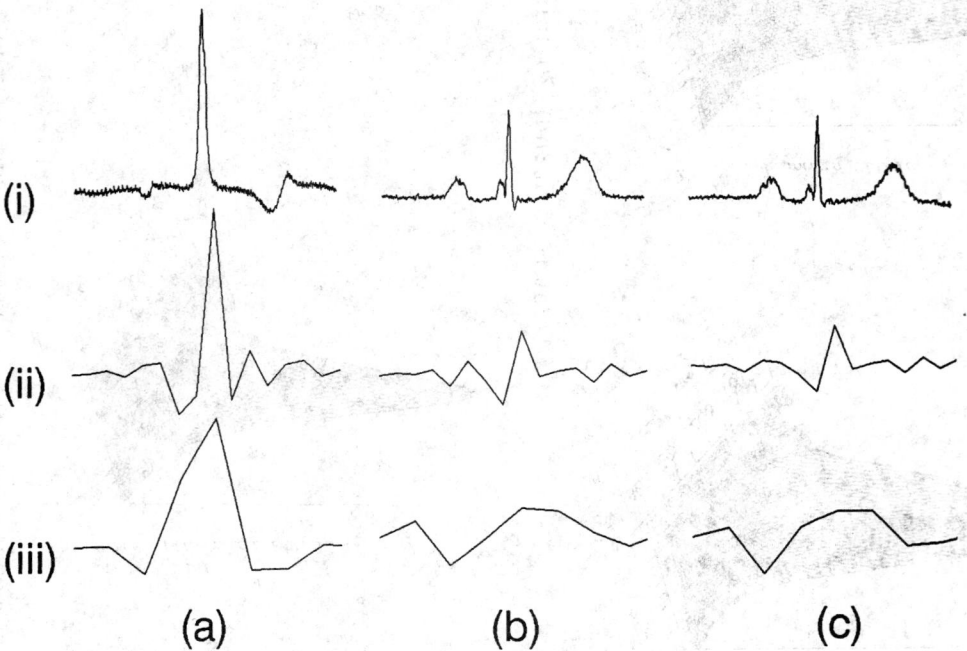

FIGURE 58.8 Certain detail components are more sensitive to changes in ECG following angioplasty procedure. Shown are detail components d5 and d6 before angioplasty and 60 and 120 minutes after angioplasty.

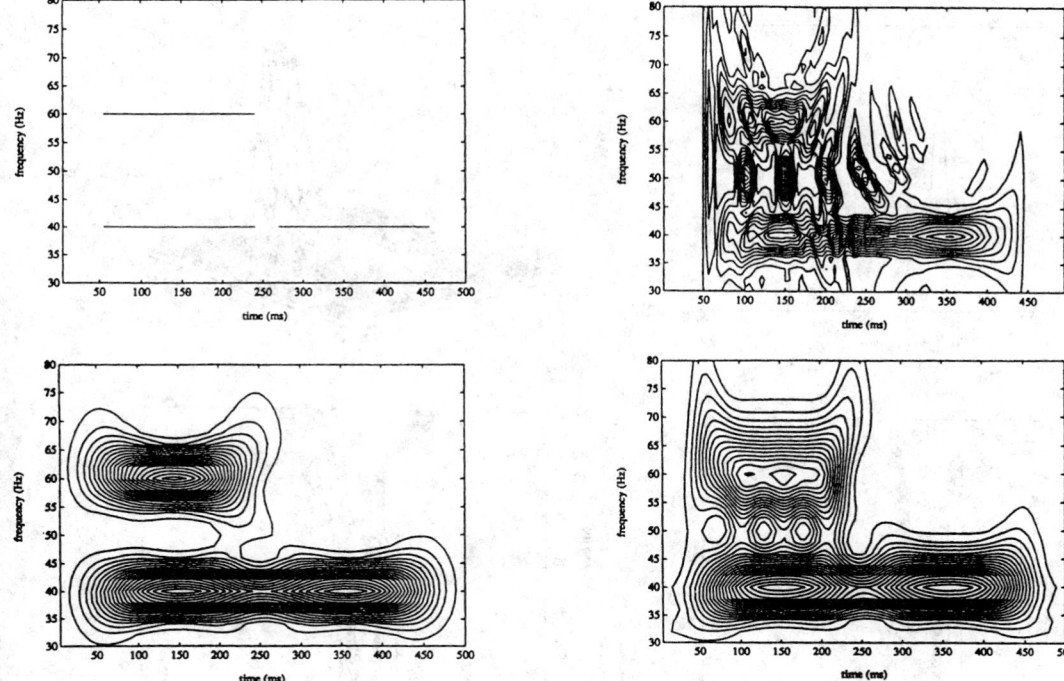

FIGURE 58.9 Comparison of time-frequency representations of sinusoids with specific on-off times. (*a*) True time-frequency representation of 40- and 60-Hz sinusoids. (*b*) Representation of smoothed Wigner-Ville transform. (*c*) Spectrogram representation. (*d*) Wavelet transform version of signal.

The presence of late potentials may indicate underlying dispersion of electrical activity of the cells in the heart and therefore may provide a substrate for production of arrhythmias. Time-scale analysis of late potential may therefore serve as a noninvasive diagnostic tool for ischemic heart disease and for predicting the likelihood of arrhythmias in the heart.

Neurologic Signal Processing

Evoked Potentials

Evoked potentials are the signals recorded from the brain in response to external stimulation. Evoked responses can be elicited by electrical stimulation (somatosensory evoked response), visual stimulation (visual evoked response), or auditory stimulation (brainstem auditory evoked response). Usually, the signals are small, while the background noise, mostly the background EEG activity, is quite large. The low signal-to-noise ratio (SNR) necessitates use of ensemble averaging, sometimes signal averaging as many as one thousand responses [12]. After enhancing the SNR, one obtains a characteristic wave pattern that includes the stimulus artifact and an undulating pattern characterized by one or more peaks at specific latencies beyond the stimulus. Conventionally, the amplitude and the latency of the signal peaks are used in arriving at a clinical diagnosis. However, when the signals have a complex morphology, simple amplitude and latency analysis does not adequately describe all the complex changes that may occur as a result of brain injury or disease. Time-frequency and wavelet analysis have been shown to be useful in identifying the features localized within the waveform that are most indicative of the brain's response [13].

In one recent experimental study, we evaluated the somatosensory evoked response from experimental animals in whom injury was caused by oxygen deprivation. The evoked response signal was

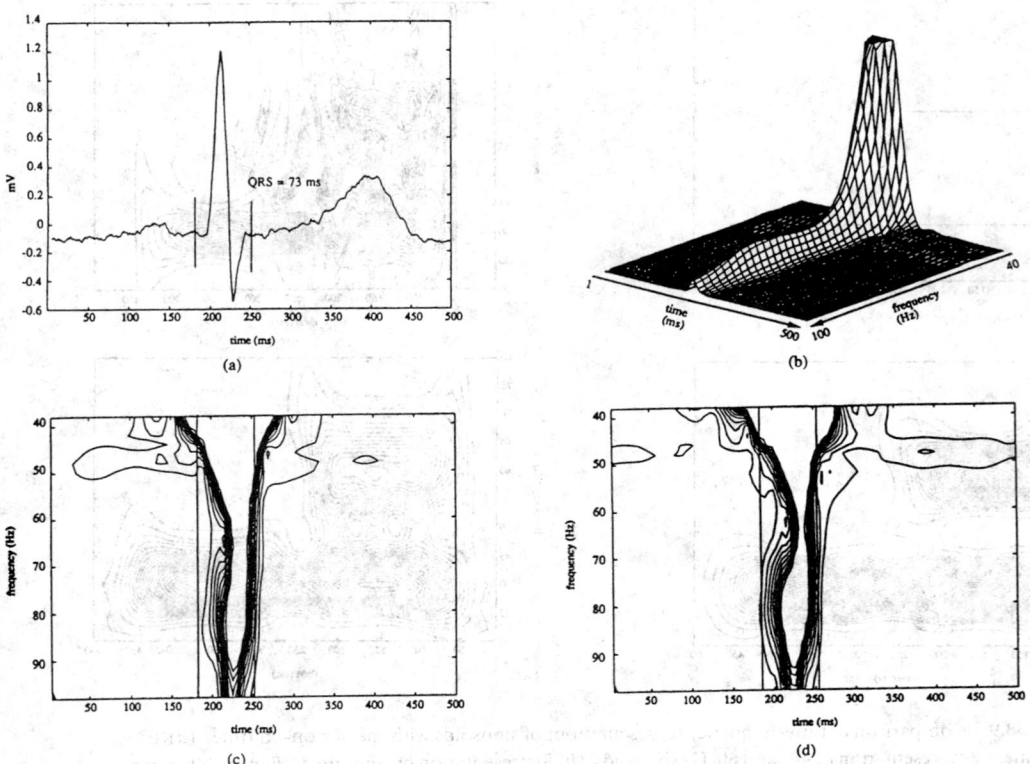

FIGURE 58.10 Patient with ventricular tachycardia diagnosis. (*a*) First beat. (*b*) 3-D representation of the modified WT for the first beat. (*c*) Contour plot of the modified WT for the first beat. (*d*) Contour plot of the modified WT for the second beat.

decomposed into its coarse and detail components with the aid of multiresolution wavelet analysis techniques [14] (Fig. 58.12). The magnitude of the detail components was observed to be sensitive to the cerebral hypoxia during its early stages. Figure 58.13 shows a time trend of the magnitude of the detail components along with the trend of the amplitude and the latency of the primary peak of the somatosensory evoked response. The experimental animal was initially challenged by nitrous oxide gas mixed with 100% oxygen (a non-injury-causing event) and later by inspired air with 7% to 8% oxygen. As expected, the amplitude trend shows an initial rise because of the 100% oxygen and later a gradual decline in response to hypoxia. The magnitude of the detail component shows a trend more responsive to injury; while there is not a significant change in response to the non-injury-causing event, the magnitude of the detail component d4 drops quite rapidly when the brain becomes hypoxic. These data suggest that detail components of the evoked response may serve as an indicator of early stages of brain injury. Evoked response monitoring can be useful in patient monitoring during surgery and in neurologic critical care [15,16]. Other applications include study of cognitive or event-related potentials in human patients for normal cognitive function evaluation or for assessment of clinical situations such as response in Alzheimer's disease [17]. Proper characterization of evoked responses from multiple-channel recordings facilitates localization of the source using dipole localization theory [18].

EEG and Seizures

Electroencephalographic signals are usually analyzed by spectrum analysis techniques, dividing the EEG signal into various arbitrary frequency bands (α, β, θ, δ). Conventional spectrum analysis is

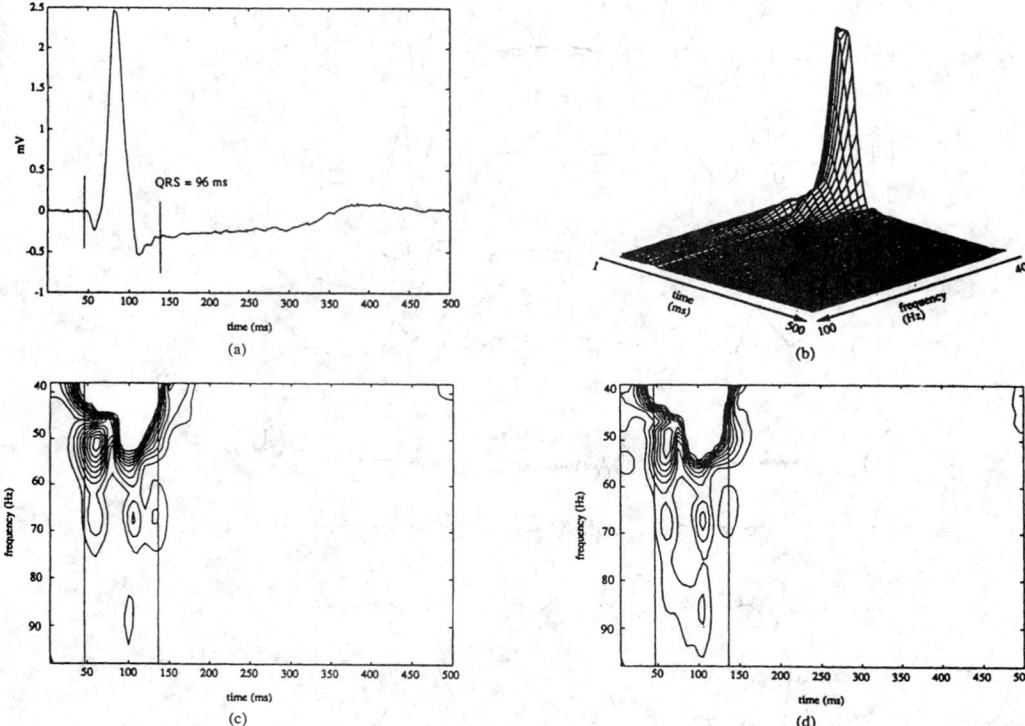

FIGURE 58.11 Healthy person. (*a*) First recorded beat. (*b*) 3-D representation of the modified WT for the first beat. (*c*) Contour plot of the modified WT for the first beat. (*d*) Contour plot of the modified WT for the second beat.

useful when these events are slowly unfolding, for example, when a person goes to sleep, or when the power in the EEG shifts from higher- to lower-frequency bands. However, when transient events such as epileptic seizures occur, there are often sharp spikes or bursting series of events in the recorded waveform. This form of the signal, which is temporally well localized and has a spectrum that is distinctive from normal or ongoing events, lends itself to wavelet analysis. A patient's EEG recorded over an extended period preceding and following the seizure was recorded and analyzed. Figure 58.14 shows a short segment of the EEG signal with a seizure burst. Multiresolution wavelet analysis technique was employed to identify the initiation of the seizure burst. Figure 58.15 shows a sudden burst onset in the magnitude of the detail components when the seizure event starts. The bursting subsides at the end of the seizure, as seen by a significant drop in the magnitude of the detail components. Wavelet analysis thus may be employed for the detection of onset and termination of seizures. Further possibilities exist in the use of this technique for discriminating interictal spikes and classifying them [19]. Certain seizures, such as petit mal and grand mal epilepsy, have very characteristic morphology (e.g., spike and dome pattern). These waveforms would be expected to lend themselves very well to wavelet analysis.

Other Applications

Wavelet, or time-scale, analysis is applicable to problems in which signals have characteristic morphology or equivalently differing spectral signatures attributed to different parts of the waveform, and the events of diagnostic interest are well localized in time and scale. The examples of such situations and applications are many.

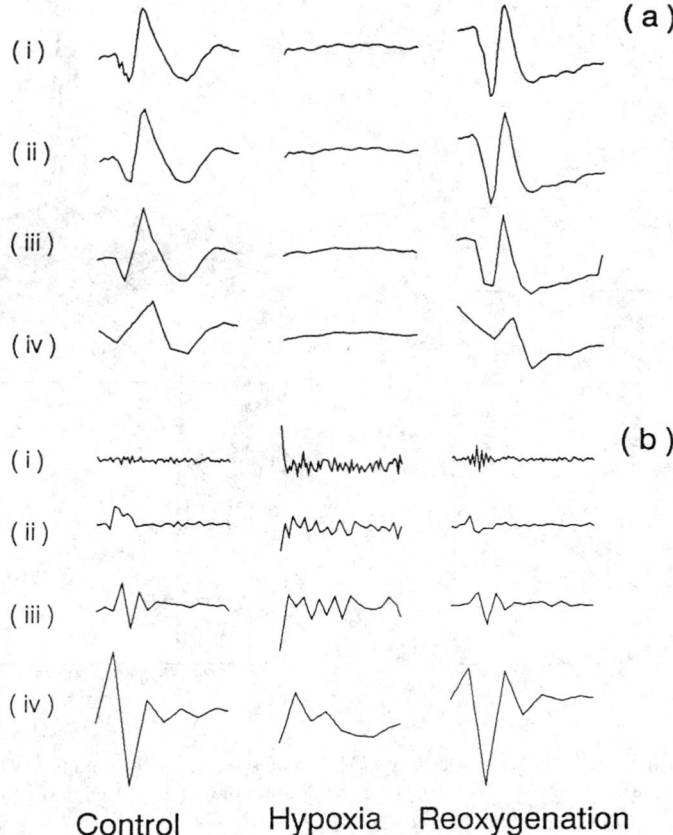

FIGURE 58.12   Coarse (*a*) and detail (*b*) components from somatosensory evoked potentials during normal, hypoxic, and reoxygenation phases of experiment.

In cardiac signal processing, there are several potential applications. Well-localized features of ECG signals, such as the P-QRS-T complex, lend themselves well to wavelet analysis [20]. We illustrated above the application of wavelet analysis to ischemia-reperfusion injury changes and the late potentials. This idea has been extended to the study of body surface maps recorded using numerous electrodes placed on the chest. In a preliminary study [21], spatiotemporal maps could be constructed and interpreted using time-scale analysis techniques. Further applications to the generalized field of arrhythmia classification can be envisioned [22]. Abnormal beats, such as premature ventricular contractions (PVCs), have different time-scale signatures than normal beats. A more challenging problem is to distinguish multiform PVCs. In experimental situations, noise and artifacts result in inaccurate detection of the QRS complex. Wavelet analysis may prove to be helpful in removal of electric interference from ECG signals [23]. A more challenging application would be in distinguishing artifact from signal. Since wavelet analysis naturally decomposes the signals at different scales at well-localized times, the artifactual events can be localized and eliminated. Fast computational methods may prove to be useful in real-time monitoring of ECG signals at a bedside or in analysis of signals recorded by Holter monitors.

Other cardiovascular signals, such as heart sounds, may be analyzed by time-frequency or time-scale analysis techniques. Characteristic responses to various normal and abnormal conditions, along with sounds that are well localized in time and scale, make these signals good candidates for

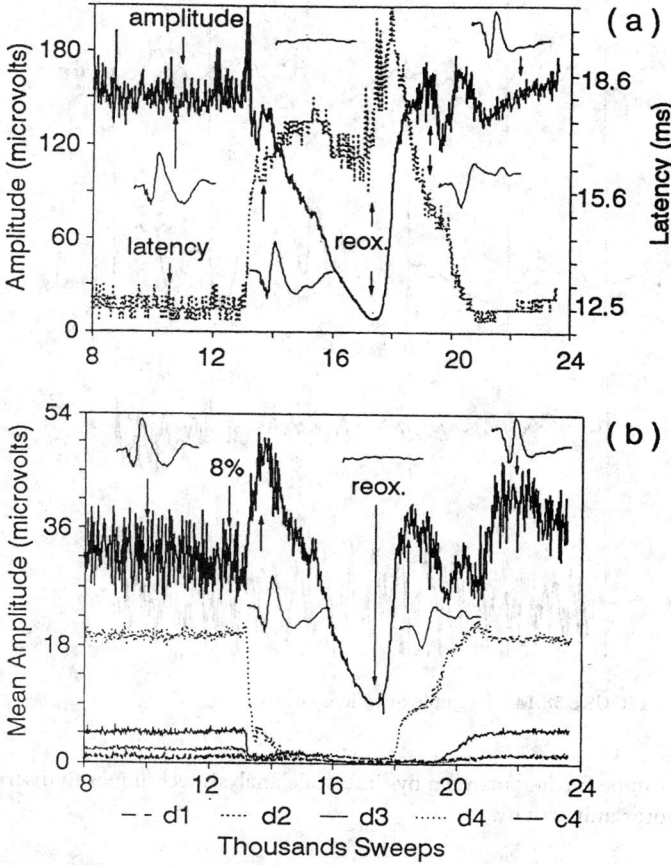

FIGURE 58.13 (a) Amplitude and latency of major evoked potential peak during control, hypoxic, and reoxygenation portions of experiment. (b) Mean amplitude of respective detail components during phases of experiment.

wavelet analysis [24]. Normal sound patterns from pathologic sound patterns may be discriminated, or sounds from various blood vessels can be identified [25]. Blood pressure waveform similarly has a characteristic pattern amenable to time-scale analysis. The dicrotic notch of the pressure waveform results from blood flow through the valves, whose opening and closing affects the pressure signal pattern. The dicrotic notch can be detected by wavelet analysis [26]. Sounds from the chest indicative of respiratory patterns are being investigated using wavelet techniques. Applications include analysis of respiratory patterns of infants [27] and respiration during sleep [28].

Two applications in neurologic signal processing, evoked response and seizure detection, were described earlier. Other potential applications include detection and interpretation of signals from multiple neurons obtained using microelectrodes [29]. Since waveforms (called *spikes*) from individual neurons (called *units*) have different patterns because of their separation and orientation with respect to the recording microelectrode, multiunit spike analysis becomes a challenging problem. Time-scale analysis techniques may be employed to localize and analyze the responses of individual units and from that derive the overall activity and interrelation among these units so as to understand the behavior of neural networks. An analogous problem is that of detecting and discriminating signals from "motor units," i.e., the muscle cells and fibers [30]. Signals from motor units are obtained by using small microelectrodes or needle electrodes, and characteristic spikes trains are

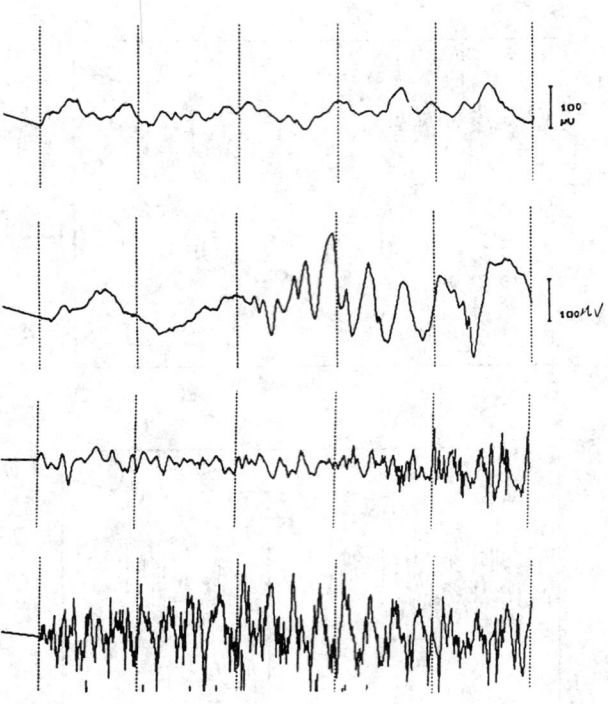

FIGURE 58.14   Example of epilepsy burst.

obtained, which can be further analyzed by time-scale analysis techniques to discriminate normal and abnormal motor unit activity.

58.6 Discussion and Conclusions

Biologic signals with their time-varying nature and characteristic morphologies and spectral signatures are particularly well suited for analysis and interpretation using time-frequency and time-scale analysis techniques. For example, the P-QRS-T complex of the ECG signal shows localized low frequencies in the P and ST segments and high frequencies in the QRS complex. In time-scale frame, the ischemia-related changes are seen in certain detail components of the QRS complex. The late segment of the QRS cycle exhibits the so-called late potentials more easily localized by means of time-scale analysis. Other cardiovascular signals, such as pressure waves, heart sounds, and blood flow, are being analyzed by the newly developed wavelet analysis algorithms. Other examples of time-scale analysis include neurologic signals with potential applications in the analysis of single and multiunit recordings from neurons, evoked response, EEG, and epileptic spikes and seizures.

The desirable requirements of successful application of time-scale analysis to biomedical signals is that events are well localized in time and exhibit morphologic and spectral variations within these localized events. Objectively viewing the signal at different scales should provide meaningful new information. For example, are there fine features of signal that are observable only at scales that pick out the detail components? Are there features of the signal that span a significant portion of the waveform so that they are best studied at a coarse scale? The signal analysis should be able to optimize the tradeoff between time and scale, i.e., distinguish short-lasting events and long-lasting events.

For these reasons, the signals described in this chapter have been found to be particularly useful models for data analysis. However, one needs to be cautious in using any newly developed tools and technologies. Most important questions to be addressed before proceeding with a new application

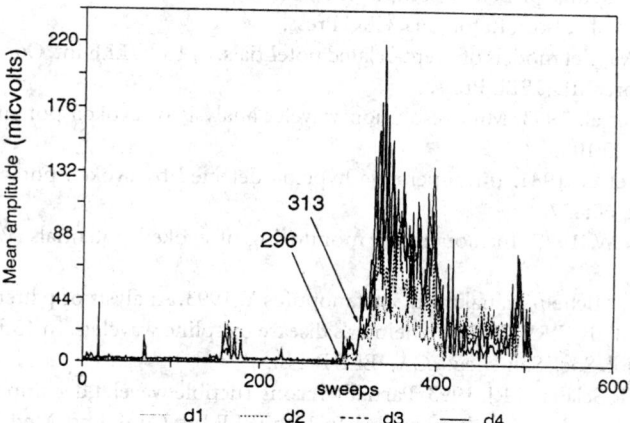

FIGURE 58.15 Localization of burst example with wavelet detail components.

are: Is the signal well suited to the tool, and in applying the tool, are any errors inadvertently introduced? Does the analysis provide new and more useful interpretation of the data and assist in the discovery of new diagnostic information?

Wavelet analysis techniques appear to have robust theoretical properties allowing novel interpretation of biomedical data. As new algorithms emerge, they are likely to find application in the analysis of more diverse biomedical signals. Analogously, the problems faced in the biomedical signal acquisition and processing world will hopefully stimulate development of new algorithms.

References

1. Rioul O, Vetterli M. 1991. Wavelets and signal processing. IEEE Sig Proc Mag October:14.
2. Raghuveer M, Samar V, Swartz KP, et al. 1992. Wavelet decomposition of event related potentials: Toward the definition of biologically natural components. In Sixth SSAP Workshop on Statistical Signal and Array Processing. Victoria, BC, IEEE Press.
3. Hlawatsch F, Bourdeaux-Bartels GF. 1992. Linear and quadratic time-frequency signal representations. IEEE Sig Proc Mag April:21.
4. Meste O, et al. 1994. Detection of late potentials by means of wavelet transform. IEEE Trans Biomed Eng 41:625.
5. Thakor NV, et al. 1993. Multiwave: A wavelet-based ECG data compression algorithm. IEICE Trans Inf Syst E76-D:1462.
6. Mallat S. 1989. A theory for multiresolution signal decomposition: The wavelet representation. IEEE Trans Pattern Ana Mach Intell 11:674.
7. Thakor NV, et al. 1993. Multiresolution wavelet analysis of ECG during ischemia and reperfusion. In Comput Cardiol London: IEEE Compu Soc Press.
8. Thakor NV, Webster JG, Tompkins WJ. 1984. Estimation of QRS complex power spectra for design of QRS filter. IEEE Trans Biomed Eng 31:702.
9. Berbari EJ. 1987. Critical review of late potential recordings. J Electrocardiol 20:125.
10. Gramatikov B, Thakor NV. 1993. Wavelet analysis of coronary artery occlusion related changes in dogs. In 15th Ann Intl Conf IEEE Eng Med Biol Soc. San Diego, IEEE.
11. Gramatikov B, Yi-chun S, Rix H, et al. 1994. Multiresolution wavelet analysis of the body surface ECG before and after angioplasty. Ann Biomed Eng (accepted).

12. Aunon JI, McGillem CD, Childers DG (eds). 1981. Signal processing in evoked potential research: Averaging, principal components, modeling. In Critical Reviews in Biomedical Engineering, Vol 5. Boca Raton, Fla, CRC Press.

13. Raz J. 1994. Wavelet models of event-related potentials. In 16th IEEE Int. Conf. Eng. Med. Biol. Soc., Baltimore, MD, IEEE Press.

14. Thakor NV, et al. 1993. Multiresolution wavelet analysis of evoked potentials. IEEE Trans Biomed Eng 40:1085.

15. Grundy BL, et al. 1981. Intraoperative hypoxia detected by evoked potential monitoring. Anasth Analg 60:437.

16. McPherson RW. 1987. Intraoperative monitoring of evoked potentials. Prog Neurol Surg 12:146.

17. Ademoglu A, Micheli-Tzanakou E, Istefanopulos Y. 1993. Analysis of pattern reversal visual evoked potentials (PRVEP) in Alzheimer's disease by spline wavelets. In 15th IEEE Int. Conf. Eng. Med. Biol. Soc., San Diego, CA, IEEE Press.

18. Sun M, Tsui F, Sclabassi RJ. 1993. Partially reconstructible wavelet decomposition of evoked potentials for dipole source localization. In 15th IEEE Int. Conf. Eng. Med. Biol., San Diego, CA, IEEE Press.

19. Schiff J. 1994. Wavelet transforms for epileptic spike and seizure detection. In 16th IEEE Int. Conf. Eng. Med. Biol. Soc., Baltimore, MD, IEEE Press.

20. Li C, Zheng C. 1993. QRS detection by wavelet transform. In 15th IEEE Int. Conf. Eng. Med. Biol. Soc., San Diego, CA, IEEE Press.

21. Brooks DH, et al. 1994. Spatio-temporal wavelet analysis of body surface maps during PTCA-induced ischemia. In 16th IEEE Int. Conf. Eng. Med. Biol. Soc., Baltimore, MD, IEEE Press.

22. Jouney I, Hamilton P, Kanapathipillai M. 1994. Adaptive wavelet representation and classification of ECG signals. In 16th IEEE Int. Conf. Eng. Med. Biol. Soc., Baltimore, MD, IEEE Press.

23. Karrakchou M. 1994. New structures for multirate adaptive filtering: Application to intereference canceling in biomedical engineering. In 16th IEEE Int. Conf. Eng. Med. Biol. Soc., Baltimore, MD, IEEE Press.

24. Bentley PM, McDonnel JTE. 1994. Analysis of heart sounds using the wavelet transform. In 16th IEEE Int. Conf. Eng. Med. Biol. Soc., Baltimore, MD, IEEE Press.

25. Akay M, et al. 1994. Investigating the effects of vasodilator drugs on the turbulent sound caused by femoral artery using short term Fourier and wavelet transform methods. IEEE Trans Biomed Eng

26. Antonelli L. 1994. Dicrotic notch detection using wavelet transform analysis. In 16th IEEE Int. Conf. Eng. Med. Biol. Soc., Baltimore, MD, IEEE Press.

27. Ademovic E, Charbonneau G, Pesquet J-C. 1994. Segmentation of infant respiratory sounds with Mallat's wavelets. In 16th IEEE Int. Conf. Eng. Med. Biol. Soc., Baltimore, MD, IEEE Press.

28. Sartene R, et al. 1994. Using wavelet transform to analyze cardiorespiratory and electroencephalographic signals during sleep. In 16th IEEE Int. Conf. Eng. Med. Biol. Soc., Baltimore, MD, IEEE Press.

29. Akay YM, Micheli-Tzanakou E. 1993. Wavelet analysis of the multiple single unit recordings in the optic tectum of the frog. In 15th IEEE Int. Conf. Eng. Med. Biol. Soc., San Diego, CA, IEEE Press.

30. Pattichis M, Pattichis CS. 1993. Fast wavelet transform in motor unit action potential analysis. In 15th IEEE Int. Conf. Eng. Med. Biol. Soc., San Diego, CA, IEEE Press.

59
Higher-Order Spectra in Biomedical Signal Processing

Athina P. Petropulu
Drexel University

The past 20 years have witnessed an expansion of power spectrum estimation techniques, which have proved essential in many applications, such as communications, sonar, radar, speech/image processing, geophysics, and biomedical signal processing [Kay, 1988; Haykin, 1983; Marple, 1987]. In power spectrum estimation, the process under consideration is treated as a superposition of statistically uncorrelated harmonic components. The distribution of power among these frequency components is the power spectrum. As such, phase relations between frequency components are suppressed. The information in the power spectrum is essentially present in the autocorrelation sequence, which would suffice for the complete statistical description of a gaussian process of known mean. However, there are applications where one would need to obtain information regarding deviations from the gaussianity assumption and presence of nonlinearities. In these cases, power spectrum is of little help, and one would have to look beyond the power spectrum or autocorrelation domain. Higher-order spectra (HOS) (of order greater that 2), which are defined in terms of higher-order cumulants of the data, do contain such information [Nikias and Petropulu, 1993]. The third-order spectrum is commonly referred to as *bispectrum*, the fourth-order one as *trispectrum*, and in fact, the power spectrum is also a member of the higher-order spectral class; it is the second-order spectrum.

HOS consist of higher-order moment spectra, which are defined for deterministic signals, and cumulant spectra, which are defined for random processes. In general, there are three motivations behind the use of HOS analysis in signal processing:

- To suppress gaussian noise of unknown mean and variance in detection and parameter estimation problems. This motivation is based on the property that gaussian processes have zero higher-order spectra (of order greater than 2). Due to this property, HOS are high signal-to-noise ratio domains, in which one can perform detection, parameter estimation, or even signal reconstruction.

- To reconstruct the phase as well as the magnitude response of signals or systems. Unlike power spectrum, HOS preserve the Fourier phase of signals. In the modeling of time series, second-order statistics (autocorrelation) have been heavily used because they are the result of least-squares optimization criteria. However, an accurate phase reconstruction in the autocorrelation domain can be achieved only if the signal is minimum phase. Non-minimum-phase signal reconstruction can be achieved only in the HOS domain, due to the HOS ability to preserve phase.

- To detect and characterize nonlinearities in the data. HOS, being nonlinear functions of the data, are quite natural tools for detection of nonlinearities in time series.

The organization of this chapter is as follows: First, the definitions and properties of higher-order statistics and higher-order spectra are presented. Then, procedures for their estimation from finite-length data are discussed. Then some important results from the application of HOS in signal processing are discussed briefly. Finally, potential uses of HOS in biomedical signal processing are pointed out.

59.1 Definitions and Properties of HOS

This chapter will consider only random one-dimensional signals. The definitions can be easily extended to the two-dimensional case [Mendel, 1991]. For a stationary discrete-time random process $X(k)$ (k denotes discrete time), the *moments* of order n are given by

$$m_n^x(\tau_1, \tau_2, \ldots, \tau_{n-1}) = E\{X(k)X(k + \tau_1) \cdots X(k + \tau_{n-1})\} \qquad (59.1)$$

where $E\{\cdot\}$ denotes expectation. The nth-order *cumulants* are functions of the moments of order up to n, i.e., first-order cumulants:

$$c_1^x = m_1^x = E\{X(k)\} \qquad \text{(mean)} \qquad (59.2)$$

second-order cumulants:

$$c_2^x(\tau_1) = m_2^x(\tau_1) - (m_1^x)^2 \qquad \text{(covariance)} \qquad (59.3)$$

third-order cumulants:

$$c_3^x(\tau_1, \tau_2) = m_3^x(\tau_1, \tau_2) - (m_1^x)[m_2^x(\tau_1) + m_2^x(\tau_2) + m_2^x(\tau_2 - \tau_1)] + 2(m_1^x)^3 \qquad (59.4)$$

and fourth-order cumulants:

$$\begin{aligned}
c_4^x(\tau_1, \tau_2, \tau_3) = {} & m_4^x(\tau_1, \tau_2, \tau_3) - m_2^x(\tau_1)m_2^x(\tau_3 - \tau_2) - m_2^x(\tau_2)m_2^x(\tau_3 - \tau_1) \\
& - m_2^x(\tau_3)m_2^x(\tau_2 - \tau_1) - m_1^x[m_3^x(\tau_2 - \tau_1, \tau_3 - \tau_1) \\
& + m_3^x(\tau_2, \tau_3) + m_3^x(\tau_2, \tau_4) + m_3^x(\tau_1, \tau_2)] + (m_2^x)^2[m_2^x(\tau_1) \\
& + m_2^x(\tau_2) + m_2^x(\tau_3) + m_2^x(\tau_3 - \tau_1) + m_2^x(\tau_3 - \tau_2) \\
& + m_2^x(\tau_2 - \tau_1)] - 6(m_1^x)^4
\end{aligned} \qquad (59.5)$$

where $m_3^x(\tau_1, \tau_2)$ is the third-order moment sequence, $m_2^x(\tau_1)$ is the second-order moment, and m_1^x is the mean. The general relationship between cumulants and moments is given in Nikias and Petropulu [1993].

Some important properties of cumulants and their practical implications are discussed next:

C1. If $X(k)$ is gaussian, the $c_n^x(\tau_1, \tau_2, \ldots, \tau_{n-1}) = 0$ for $n > 2$. In other words, all the information about a gaussian process is contained in its first- and second-order cumulants. This property can be used to suppress gaussian noise or as a measure for nongaussianity in time series.

C2. If $X(k)$ is symmetrically distributed, then $c_3^x(\tau_1, \tau_2) = 0$. Third-order cumulants suppress not only gaussian processes but also all symmetrically distributed processes, such as uniform, Laplace, and Bernoulli-gaussian.

C3. For cumulants, additivity holds. If $X(k) = S(k) + W(k)$, where $S(k)$ and $W(k)$ are stationary and statistically independent random processes, then $c_n^x(\tau_1, \tau_2, \ldots, \tau_{n-1}) = c_n^s(\tau_1, \tau_2, \ldots, \tau_{n-1}) + c_n^w(\tau_1, \tau_2, \ldots, \tau_{n-1})$. It is important to note that additivity does not hold for moments. If $W(k)$ is gaussian, representing noise that corrupts the signal of interest $S(k)$, then by means of C1 and C3, $c_n^x(\tau_1, \tau_2, \ldots, \tau_{n-1}) = c_n^s(\tau_1, \tau_2, \ldots, \tau_{n-1})$, for $n > 2$. In other words, in the higher-order cumulants domain, the signal of interest propagates noise-free. This property can be used as a measure of statistical dependence of two processes.

C4. If $X(k)$ has zero mean, then $c_n^x(\tau_1, \ldots, \tau_{n-1}) = m_n^s(\tau_1, \ldots, \tau_{n-1})$, for $n \leq 3$.

C5. If $X(k)$ is white, independent, and identically distributed (i.i.d.), then $c_n^x(\tau_1, \tau_2, \ldots, \tau_{n-1}) = \gamma_n^x \delta(\tau_1, \tau_2, \ldots, \tau_{n-1})$, where γ_n^x is a scalar and $\delta(\tau_1, \tau_2, \ldots, \tau_{n-1})$ represents an impulse at the origin of the $(\tau_1, \tau_2, \ldots, \tau_{n-1})$ plane.

Assuming that the nth-order cumulant sequence is absolutely summable, the nth-order *cumulant spectrum* of $X(k)$, $C_n^x(\omega_1, \omega_2, \ldots, \omega_{n-1})$, exists and is defined to be the $(n - 1)$-dimensional Fourier transform of the the nth-order cumulant sequence. In general, $C_n^x(\omega_1, \omega_2, \ldots, \omega_{n-1})$ is complex, i.e., it has magnitude and phase.

If a process $X(k)$ is generated by exciting a linear time-invariant (LTI) system with frequency response $H(\omega)$ with a white i.i.d. process $V(k)$, then its higher-order spectrum can be written as

$$C_n^x(\omega_1, \omega_2, \ldots, \omega_{n-1}) = \gamma_n^v H(\omega_1) \cdots H(\omega_{n-1}) H^*(\omega_1 + \cdots + \omega_{n-1}) \quad (59.6)$$

where γ_n^v is a scalar constant and equals the nth-order spectrum of $V(k)$. For a linear nongaussian random process $X(k)$, the nth-order spectrum can be factorized as in Eq. (59.6) for every order n, while for a nonlinear process such a factorization might be valid for some orders only (it is always valid for $n = 2$).

59.2 HOS Computation from Real Data

The definitions of cumulants presented in the preceding section are based on expectation operations, and they assume infinite length data. In practice, we always deal with data of finite length; therefore, the cumulants can only be approximated. Two methods for cumulants and spectra estimation are presented next for the third-order case.

Indirect Method

Let $X(k), k = 1, \ldots, N$ be the available data.

1. Segment the data into K records of M samples each. Let $X^i(k), k = 1, \ldots, M$, represent the ith record.
2. Subtract the mean of each record.
3. Estimate the moments of each segment $X^i(k)$ as follows:

$$m_3^{x_i}(\tau_1, \tau_2) = \frac{1}{M} \sum_{l=l_1}^{l_2} X^i(l)X^i(l + \tau_1)X^i(l + \tau_2)$$

$$l_1 = \max(0, -\tau_1, -\tau_2)$$

$$l_2 = \min(M - 1, M - 2) \qquad |\tau_1| < L, |\tau_2| < L \tag{59.7}$$

$$i = 1, 2, \ldots, K$$

Since each segment has zero mean, its third-order moments and cumulants are identical, i.e., $c_3^{x_i}(\tau_1, \tau_2) = m_3^{x_i}(\tau_1, \tau_2)$.

4. Compute the average cumulants as

$$\hat{c}_3^x(\tau_1, \tau_2) = \frac{1}{K} \sum_{i=1}^{K} m_3^{x_i}(\tau_1, \tau_2) \tag{59.8}$$

5. Obtain the third-order spectrum (bispectrum) estimate as

$$\hat{C}_3^x(\omega_1, \omega_2) = \sum_{\tau_1=-L}^{L} \sum_{\tau_2=-L}^{L} \hat{c}_3^x(\tau_1, \tau_2)e^{-j(\omega_1\tau_1 + \omega_2\tau_2)}W(\tau_1, \tau_2) \tag{59.9}$$

where $L < M - 1$, and $W(\tau_1, \tau_2)$ is a two-dimensional window of bounded support, introduced to smooth out edge effects. A complete description of appropriate windows and their properties can be found in Nikias and Petropulu [1993]. The bandwidth of the final bispectrum estimate is $\Delta = 1/L$.

Direct Method

Let $X(k), k = 1, \ldots, N$, be the available data and T the sampling period.

1. Segment the data into K records of M samples each. Let $X^i(k), k = 1, \ldots, M$, represent the ith record.
2. Subtract the mean of each record.
3. Compute the Fourier transform $Y^i(f)$ of each segment, based on M points, i.e.,

$$Y^i(f) = \sum_{k=0}^{M-1} X^i(k)e^{-j2\pi fk} \qquad f = \frac{n}{M} \tag{59.10}$$

$$n = 0, 1, \ldots, M - 1 \qquad i = 1, 2, \ldots, K$$

4. The third-order spectrum of each segment is obtained as

$$C_3^{x_i}(f_1, f_2) = \frac{1}{M} Y^i(f_1)Y^i(f_2)Y^{i*}(f_1 + f_2) \qquad i = 1, \ldots, K \tag{59.11}$$

Due to the bispectrum symmetry properties, $\hat{C}_3^{x_i}(f_1, f_2)$ needs to be computed only in the triangular region $0 \leq f_2 \leq f_1, f_1 + f_2 < 1/2T$.

5. In order to reduce the variance of the estimate, additional smoothing over a rectangular window of size $(M_3 \times M_3)$ can be performed around each frequency, assuming that the third-order spectrum is smooth enough, i.e.,

$$\hat{C}_3^{x_i}(f_1, f_2) = \frac{1}{M_3^2} \sum_{n_1=-M_3/2}^{M_3/2-1} \sum_{n_1=-M_3/2}^{M_3/2-1} C_3^{x_i}(f_1 + n_1/M, f_2 + n_2/M) \tag{59.12}$$

6. Finally, the third-order spectrum is given as the average over all $C_3^{x_i}(f_1, f_2)$ obtained above, i.e.,

$$\hat{C}_3^x(f_1, f_2) = \frac{1}{K} \sum_{i=1}^{K} C_3^{x_i}(f_1, f_2) \tag{59.13}$$

The final bandwidth of this bispectrum estimate is $\Delta = M_3/M$, and this is the spacing between frequency samples in the bispectrum domain.

For large N, and as long as

$$\Delta \to 0 \quad \text{and} \quad \Delta^2 N \to \infty \tag{59.14}$$

[Subba Rao & Gabr, 1984], both the direct and the indirect methods produce asymptotically unbiased and consistent bispectrum estimates, with real and imaginary part variances:

$$\text{var}\,\{Re[\hat{C}_3^x(\omega_1, \omega_2)]\} = \text{var}\,\{Im[\hat{C}_3^x(\omega_1, \omega_2)]\}$$

$$= \frac{1}{\Delta^2 N} C_2^x(\omega_1)\, C_2^x(\omega_2)\, C_2^x(\omega_1 + \omega_2)$$

$$= \begin{cases} \dfrac{VL^2}{MK} C_2^x(\omega_1)\, C_2^x(\omega_2)\, C_2^x(\omega_1 + \omega_2) & \text{indirect} \\[2ex] \dfrac{M}{KM_3^2} C_2^x(\omega_1)\, C_2^x(\omega_2)\, C_2^x(\omega_1 + \omega_2) & \text{direct} \end{cases} \tag{59.15}$$

where V is the energy of the bispectrum window used in Eq. (59.9). The parameters $M, K, L,$ and M_3 must be chosen appropriately so that Eq. (59.14) holds.

59.3 Parametric Modeling of Time Series

A linear process $X(k)$ can be modeled as the output of a linear system, generally nonminimum phase, excited by white i.i.d. noise. If $H(\omega)$ is the frequency response of the filter, and assuming that the input noise is nongaussian, Eq. (59.6) holds for the nth-order cumulants of $X(k)$. While for $n = 2$ Eq. (59.6) leads to reconstruction of only the minimum phase equivalent of the system, for $n \geq 3$ it can lead to the true system response $H(\omega)$ (within a linear phase and a scalar constant) or to its time-domain equivalent $h(k)$ (within a time delay and scalar constant). A significant amount of research has been devoted to the estimation of $h(k)$ from the third- or fourth-order cumulants of the process [Mendel, 1991, and references therein; Pan & Nikias, 1988]. Also, a lot of effort has been devoted to estimation of the ARMA parameters of the systems transfer function [Giannakis & Swami, 1990; Nikias & Chiang, 1988; Pan & Nikias, 1988; Swami & Mendel, 1990; Tugnait, 1987]:

$$H(z) = \frac{B(z)}{A(z)}$$

$$= \frac{\sum_{j=0}^{q} b(j) z^{-j}}{\sum_{i=0}^{p} a(i) z^{-i}} \tag{59.16}$$

where $a(i)$ and $b(j)$ represent the AR and MA parameters of the system. It is well established in the literature that identification of nonminimum-phase noncausal ARMA models is possible only by using higher-order cumulants of the observation process. An excellent review of the existing parameter estimation methods can be found in Mendel [1991].

59.4 Quadratic Phase Coupling

A nonlinear process can be modeled as the output of a nonlinear filter excited by random input. For certain types of nonlinearities, the parameters of the Volterra series expansion of the nonlinear filter can be estimated using higher-order cross-correlations of the input and output sequences [Schetzen, 1989].

An interesting phenomenon caused by a second-order nonlinearity is quadratic phase coupling. There are situations where nonlinear interactions between two harmonic components of a process contribute to the power of the sum and/or difference frequencies. Quadratic phase coupling can arise only among harmonically related components. Three frequencies are harmonically related when one of them is the sum or difference of the other two. Sometimes it is important to find out if peaks at harmonically related positions in the power spectrum are in fact phase-coupled. Due to phase suppression, the power spectrum is unable to provide an answer to this problem. For example, consider the process [Raghuveer & Nikias, 1985]

$$X(k) = \sum_{i=1}^{6} \cos(\lambda_i k + \phi_i) \tag{59.17}$$

where $\lambda_1 > \lambda_2 > 0, \lambda_4 + \lambda_5 > 0, \lambda_3 = \lambda_1 + \lambda_2, \lambda_6 = \lambda_4 + \lambda_5, \phi_1, \ldots, \phi_5$ are all independent, uniformly distributed random variables over $(0, 2\pi)$ and $\phi_6 = \phi_4 + \phi_5$. Among the six frequencies, $(\lambda_1, \lambda_2, \lambda_3)$ and $(\lambda_4, \lambda_5, \lambda_6)$ are harmonically related; however, only λ_6 is the result of phase coupling between λ_4 and λ_5. The power spectrum of this process consists of six impulses at $\lambda_i, i = 1, \ldots, 6$ (Fig. 59.1a), offering no indication whether each frequency component is independent or the result of frequency coupling. On the other hand, the bispectrum of $X(k)$, $C_3^x(\omega_1, \omega_2)$ (evaluated in its principal region), is zero everywhere except at point (λ_4, λ_5) of the (ω_1, ω_2) plane, where it exhibits an impulse (see Fig. 59.1b). The peak indicates that only λ_4 and λ_5 are phase-coupled.

In practical situations where bispectral estimates must be obtained, the bicoherence index, defined as

$$P_3^x(\omega_1, \omega_2) = \frac{C_3^x(\omega_1, \omega_2)}{\sqrt{C_2^x(\omega_1)\, C_2^x(\omega_2)\, C_2^x(\omega_1 + \omega_2)}} \tag{59.18}$$

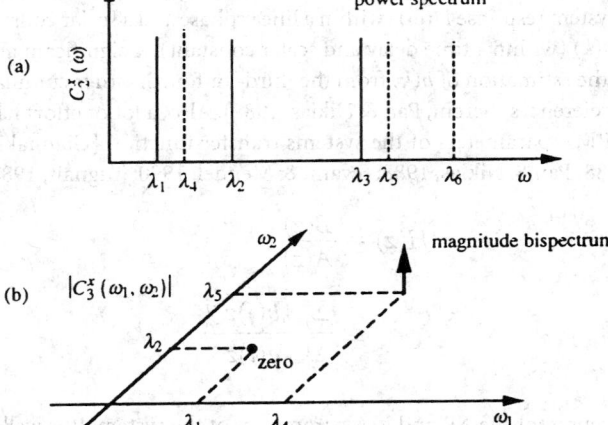

FIGURE 59.1.   The effect of the phase coupling in (*a*) the power spectrum and (*b*) the magnitude bispectrum.

has been used extensively [Kim & Powers, 1978] for the detection and quantification of quadratic phase coupling. The value of the bicoherence index at each frequency pair indicates the degree of coupling among the frequencies of that pair. Almost all bispectral estimators can be used in Eq. (59.18). However, estimates obtained based on parametric modeling of the bispectrum have been shown to yield superior resolution [Raghuveer & Nikias, 1985, 1986].

59.5 Blind Deconvolution Using HOS

A blind deconvolution method for the reconstruction of a nonwhite nongaussian random process (target) based on two filtered (distorted) and noisy versions of it was proposed by Petropulu and Nikias [1993]. The proposed algorithm processes the available data (observations) using higher-order spectra and the theory of signal reconstruction from phase only, identifies the distortion associated with each observation, and reconstructs the target signal. The algorithm is briefly described next. Let

$$y_i(k) = f(k) * h_i(k) + w_i(k) \qquad k = 1, \dots, N \qquad i = 1, 2 \qquad (59.19)$$

represent two filtered and noisy version of $f(k)$, where $f(k)$ is a stationary, nongaussian, nonwhite random process; $h_i(k)$ and $w_i(k)$ correspond to distortion and noise, respectively; $f(k)$ and $w_i(k)$ are statistically independent; $*$ denotes convolution, and N is the data length.

Assuming that the noises have a symmetrical probability density function, in the bispectrum domain Eq. (59.19) becomes

$$C_3^{y_i}(\omega_1, \omega_2) = C_3^f(\omega_1, \omega_2)H_i(\omega_1)H_i(\omega_2)H_i^*(\omega_1 + \omega_2) \qquad i = 1, 2 \qquad (59.20)$$

where $C_3^f(\omega_1, \omega_2)$ is the third-order moment spectrum of $f(k)$. Taking the logarithm of the third-order moment spectrum, followed by an inverse Fourier transform, we get to the bispectrum domain, i.e.,

$$c_3^{y_i}(k_1, k_2) = c_3^f(k_1, k_2) + c_3^{h_i}(k_1, k_2) \qquad (59.21)$$

where $c_3^f(k_1, k_2)$ and $c_3^{h_i}(k_1, k_2)$ are the bispectra of $f(k)$ and $h_i(n)$, respectively.

Let

$$D_+(k) = \begin{cases} -(j/2)[c_3^{y_1}(k, 0) - c_3^{y_2}(k, 0)] & k > 0 \\ 0 & k = 0 \\ (j/2)[c_3^{y_1}(-k, 0) - c_3^{y_2}(-k, 0)] & k < 0 \end{cases} \qquad (59.22)$$

and

$$D_-(k) = \begin{cases} -(j/2)[c_3^{y_1}(-k, 0) - c_3^{y_2}(-k, 0)] & k > 0 \\ 0 & k = 0 \\ (j/2)[c_3^{y_1}(k, 0) - c_3^{y_2}(k, 0)] & k < 0 \end{cases} \qquad (59.23)$$

It was shown in Petropulu and Nikias [1992] that the Fourier transform of $D_+(k)$ equals the Fourier phase $\phi_{min}(\omega)$ of the sequence

$$h_{min}(n) \triangleq Z^{-1}\{H_1^{min}(z^{-1})[H_2^{min}(z^{-1})]^*\} \qquad (59.24)$$

where $Z^{-1}\{\cdot\}$ denotes inverse Z-transform, and $H_i^{min}(z^{-1})$, $i = 1, 2$, are the minimum-phase components of the distortions $h_i(n)$, $i = 1, 2$, respectively. Similarly, the Fourier transform $D_-(k)$ equals the Fourier phase $\phi_{max}(\omega)$, of the sequence

$$h_{max}(n) \triangleq Z^{-1}\{[H_1^{max}(z)]^* H_2^{max}(z)^*\} \qquad (59.25)$$

where $H_i^{max}(z)$, $i = 1, 2$, are the maximum-phase components of the distortion $h_i(n)$, $i = 1, 2$, respectively.

Under mild assumptions on $h_1(n)$ and $h_2(n)$ (e.g., the two distortions do not have common convolutional components) and due to their special structure, $h_{min}(n)$ and $h_{max}(n)$ can be reconstructed from their Fourier phases $\phi_{min}(\omega)$ and $\phi_{max}(\omega)$ only [Hayes et al., 1980; Petropulu & Nikias, 1992]. Once $h_{min}(n)$ has been reconstructed, its minimum- and maximum-phase parts, which are directly related to the minimum-phase parts of $h_1(n)$ and $h_2(n)$, can be reconstructed. Similarly, $h_{max}(n)$ leads to reconstruction of the maximum-phase parts of the two distortions. Finally, the distortions can be composed (within a linear phase and a scalar) from the minimum- and maximum-phase parts as follows:

$$H_i(z) = H_i^{min}(z^{-1}) H_i^{max}(z) \qquad i = 1, 2 \qquad (59.26)$$

After the distorting systems have been estimated, the signal $f(k)$ can be reconstructed via inverse filtering.

The same deconvolution procedure holds even if the target signal is not the same in both observations, as long as it has the same statistics; in other words, Eq. (59.19) can be modified as

$$y_i(k) = f_i(k) * h_i(k) + w_i(k) \qquad k = 1, \ldots, N \qquad i = 1, 2, \qquad (59.27)$$

where $f_1(k)$ and $f_2(k)$ are stationary processes with the same statistics (i.e., same third-order cumulants).

59.6 Potential Uses of HOS in Biomedical Signal Processing

Modeling of Speckle in Ultrasound Images

The speckle in ultrasound (US) images has been modeled assuming that it follows a gaussian distribution. Cohen [1992] modeled speckle by a noncausal gaussian Markov random field. The method appeared to capture the speckle structure well, and the model parameters provided the basis for statistical tests to detect targets embedded in the speckle image. Based on tests conducted on real US images, we concluded that the speckle is not gaussian. For the RF image (128×128) that consists of speckle only (Fig. 59.2a), we estimated its bispectrum ($16 \times 16 \times 16 \times 16$) using the indirect

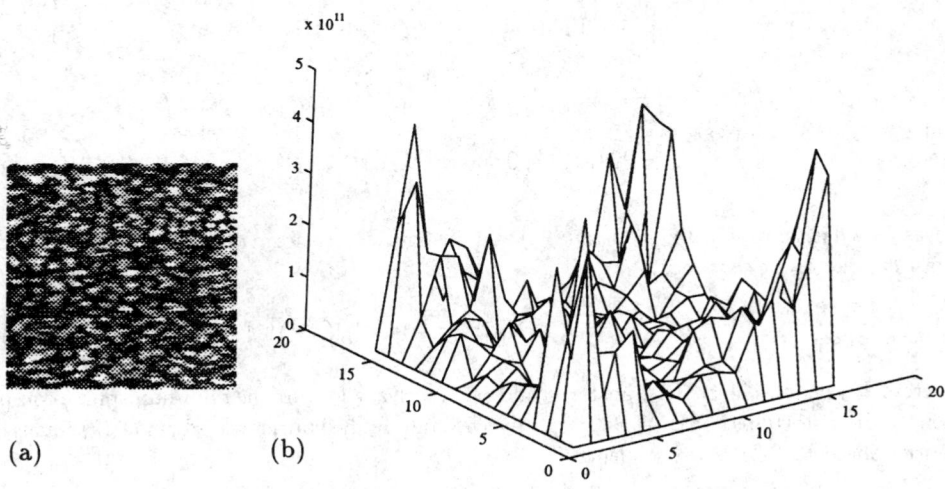

(a)   (b)

FIGURE 59.2.   (*a*) Speckle only image. (*b*) A slice of the bispectrum of the image in part *a*.

method on (16×16) image segments. One slice of the resulting bispectrum is shown in Fig. 59.2*b*. The clearly nonzero structure of the bispectrum indicates deviation of the speckle image from the gaussianity assumption.

Parametric modeling of data using HOS assumes no information about the statistical description of the data. Therefore, if we perform parametric modeling of speckle using higher-order statistics, we will get a more accurate modeling of speckle, and as a result the obtained parameters would lead to more robust target detection schemes.

Studying the Frequency Content of Signals

Analysis of quadratic phase coupling (QPC) has provided insight on the formation and nature of frequencies present in signals. The bispectrum has already been applied in EEG signals of the rat during various vigilance states [Ning & Bronzino, 1989], where quadratic phase coupling (QPC) between specific frequencies was observed. QPC changes in auditory evoked potentials of healthy subjects and subjects with Alzheimer's dementia were reported in Samar et al. [1993]. QPC also was observed in the EEG of humans [Barnet et al., 1971; Huber et al., 1971].

Improving the Resolution of US Images

The blind deconvolution algorithm presented earlier can be applied directly to improving the resolution of medical US images. During an ultrasonic investigation, a pulsed pressure field is emitted into the tissue. The field interacts with the tissue and eventually is reflected and scattered back to the transducer. It has been shown [Jensen, 1992] that the received pressure field can be expressed as the two-dimensional convolution of a term that accounts for inhomogeneities in the tissue (tissue response) and a time and spatially varying kernel that combines the effect of the transducer geometry and the spatial extend of the scattered field (ultrasonic system response). Additive noise is also assumed present in the received signal, to account for measurement noise and for physical effects not explained by the convolution model. The quantity of interest is the tissue response. Due to the convolution operation, however, we are only able to measure a spatially and time-smoothed version of it, which obscures the fine details in the image. The algorithm presented earlier can be applied on US data obtained through different imaging systems (e.g., transducers with differently sized or shaped apertures) to identify the effect of the US system on the measured signal and, at least partially, cancel it [Abeyratne & Petropolou, 1994; Abeyratne & Petropolou, 1994, 1995].

59.7 Conclusions

Higher-order spectra were introduced over 30 years ago; however, due to their complexity, they had not been widely used. With the current technology, complexity is not a critical issue, and HOS can proven to be very powerful tools in modeling and characterizing biomedical signals, as they have been in other signal processing applications.

Acknowledgments

Support for this work came from US Army Medical Research under grant DAMD17-94-J-4362 and from Drexel University.

References

Abeyratne U, Petropulu AP, Reid JM. 1994. Blind deconvolution of ultrasound images. In SPIE International Symposium on Optics, Imaging and Instrumentation. San Diego.

Abeyratne V, Petropolou AP, Reid JM. 1995. On modeling the tissue response from ultrasound B-scan images. IEEE Trans Medical Imaging, submitted.

Abeyratne V, Petropolou AP, Reid JM. 1994. Higher-order spectra based deconvolution of ultrasound images. IEEE Trans Ultrasonics, Ferroelectrics, and Frequency Control, submitted.

Barnett TP, Johnson LC, et al. 1971. Bispectrum analysis of electroencephalogram signals during waking and sleeping. Science 172:401.

Cohen F. 1992. Modeling of ultrasound speckle with applications in flaw detection in metals. IEEE Trans Signal Processing 40(3):624.

Giannakis GB, Swami A. 1990. On estimating noncausal nonminimum phase ARMA models of non-gaussian processes. IEEE Trans Acoustics, Speech, Signal Processing 38(3):478.

Hayes MH, Lim JS, Oppenheim AV. 1980. Signal reconstruction from the phase or magnitude. IEEE Trans Acoustics, Speech, Signal Processing 28:672.

Haykin S. 1983. Nonlinear Methods of Spectral Analysis, 2d ed. Berlin, Springer-Verlag.

Huber PJ, Kleiner B, et al. 1971. Statistical methods for investigating phase relations in stochastic processes. IEEE Trans Audio Electroacoustics Au-19(1):78.

Jensen JA. 1992. Deconvolution of ultrasound images. Ultrasonic Imaging 14:1.

Kay SM. 1988. Modern Spectral Estimation. Englewood Cliffs, NJ, Prentice-Hall.

Kim YC, Powers EJ. 1978. Digital bispectral analysis of self-excited fluctuation spectral. Phys Fluids 21(8):1452.

Marple SL Jr. 1987. Digital Spectral Analysis with Applications. Englewood Cliffs, NJ, Prentice-Hall.

Mendel JM. 1991. Tutorial on higher-order statistics (spectra) in signal processing and system theory: Theoretical results and some applications. IEEE Proc 79:278.

Nikias CL, Chiang H-H. 1988. Higher-order spectrum estimation via noncausal autoregressive modeling and deconvolution. IEEE Trans Acoustics, Speech, Signal Processing 36(12):1911.

Nikias CL, Pan R. 1987. Non-minimum phase system identification via spectrum modeling of higher-order moments. Proc ICASSP-87, 980–983, Dallas, TX.

Nikias CL, Petropulu AP. 1993. Higher-Order Spectra Analysis: A Nonlinear Signal Processing Framework. Englewood Cliffs, NJ, Prentice-Hall.

Ning T, Bronzino JD. 1989. Bispectral analysis of the EEG during various vigilance states. IEEE Trans Biomed Eng 36(4):497.

Pan R, Nikias CL. 1988. The complex cepstrum of higher order cumulants and nonminimum phase system identification. IEEE Trans Acoustics, Speech, Signal Processing 36(2):186.

Petropulu AP, Nikias CL. 1992. Signal reconstruction from the phase of the bispectrum. IEEE Trans Signal Processing 40(3):601.

Petropulu AP, Nikias CL. 1993a. Blind deconvolution of stochastic signals using higher order cepstra operations. IEEE Proc 140(6):356.

Petropulu AP, Nikias CL. 1993b. Blind deconvolution using reconstruction from partial higher order spectral information. IEEE Trans Signal Processing 41(6):2088.

Raghuveer MR, Nikias CL. 1985. Bispectrum estimation: A parametric approach. IEEE Trans Acoustics, Speech, Signal Processing 33(5):1213.

Raghuveer MR, Nikias CL. 1986. Bispectrum estimation via AR modeling. Signal Processing 10:35.

Subba Rao T, Gabr MM. 1984. An introduction to bispectral analysis and bilinear time series models. In Lecture Notes in Statistics. New York, Springer-Verlag.

Samar VJ, Swartz KP, Raghuveer MR, et al. 1993. Quadratic phase coupling in auditory evoked potentials from healthy old subjects and subjects with Alzheimer's dementia. In IEEE Signal Processing Workshop on Higher-Order Statistics, pp 361–365.

Schetzen M. 1989. The Volterra and Wiener Theories on Nonlinear System. Malabar, Fla, Krieger.

Swami A, Mendel JM. 1990. ARMA parameter estimation using only output cumulants. IEEE Trans Acoustics, Speech, Signal Processing 38:1257.

Tugnait J. 1987a. Fitting non-causal AR signal plus noise models to noisy non-gaussian linear processes. IEEE Trans Automat Control 32:547.

Tugnait J. 1987b. Identification of linear stochastic systems via second- and fourth-order cumulant matching. IEEE Trans Inform Theory 33:393.

60

Neural Networks in Biomedical Signal Processing

Computing with neural networks (NNs) is one of the fastest growing fields in the history of artificial intelligence (AI), largely because NNs can be trained to identify nonlinear patterns between input and output values and can solve complex problems much faster than digital computers. Owing to their wide range of applicability and their ability to learn complex and nonlinear relationships—including noisy or less precise information—NNs are very well suited to solving problems in biomedical engineering and, in particular, in analyzing biomedical signals.

NNs have made strong advances in continuous speech recognition and synthesis, pattern recognition, classification of noisy data, nonlinear feature detection, and other fields. By their nature, NNs are capable of high-speed parallel signal processing in real time. They have an advantage over conventional technologies because they can solve problems that are too complex—problems that do not have an algorithmic solution or for which an algorithmic solution is too complex to be found. NNs are trained by example instead of rules and are automated. When used in medical diagnosis, they are not affected by factors such as human fatigue, emotional states, and habituation. They are capable of rapid identification, analysis of conditions, and diagnosis in real time.

The most widely used architecture of an NN is that of a multilayer perceptron (MLP) trained by an algorithm called *backpropagation* (BP). Backpropagation is a gradient-decent algorithm that tries to minimize the average squared error of the network. In real applications, the network is not a simple one-dimensional system, and the error curve is not a smooth, bowl-shaped curve. Instead, it is a highly complex, multidimensional curve with hills and valleys (for a mathematical description of the algorithm, see Chapter 184).

BP was first developed by P. Werbos in 1974 [1], rediscovered by Parker in 1982 [2], and popularized later by Rummelhart et al. in 1986 [3]. There exist many variations of this algorithm, especially trying to improve its speed and performance in avoiding getting stuck into local minima—one of its main drawbacks.

In my work, I use the ALOPEX algorithm developed by my colleagues and myself (see Chapter 184) [4–10], and my colleagues and I have applied it in a variety of world problems of considerable

0-8493-8346-3/95/$0.00+$.50
© 1995 by CRC Press, Inc.

complexity. This chapter will examine several applications of NNs in biomedical signal processing. One- and two-dimensional signals are examined.

60.1 Neural Networks in Sensory Waveform Analysis

Mathematical analysis of the equations describing the processes in NNs can establish any dependencies between quantitative network characteristics, the information capacity of the network, and the probabilities of recognition and retention of information. It has been proposed that electromyographic (EMG) patterns can be analyzed and classified by NNs [11] where the standard BP algorithm is used for decomposing surface EMG signals into their constituent action potentials (APs) and their firing patterns [12]. A system such as this may help a physician in diagnosing time-behavior changes in the EMG.

The need for a knowledge-based system using NNs for evoked potential recognition was described in a paper by Bruha and Madhavan [13]. In this paper, the authors used syntax pattern-recognition algorithms as a first step, while a second step included a two-layer perceptron to process the list of numerical features produced by the first step.

Myoelectric signals (MES) also have been analyzed by NNs [14]. A discrete Hopfield network was used to calculate the time-series parameters for a moving-average MES. It was demonstrated that this network was capable of producing the same time-series parameters as those produced by a conventional sequential least-squares algorithm. In the same paper, a second implementation of a two-layered perceptron was used for comparison. The features used were a time-series parameter and the signal power in order to train the perceptron on four separate arm functions, and again, the network performed well.

Moving averages have been simulated for nonlinear processes by the use of NNs [15]. The results obtained were comparable with those of linear adaptive techniques.

Moody and colleagues [16] used an adaptive approach in analyzing visual evoked potentials. This method is based on spectral analysis that results in spectral peaks of uniform width in the frequency domain. Tunable data windows were used. Specifically, the modified Bessel functions $I_o - \sin h$, the gaus-sian, and the cosine-taper windows are compared. The modified Bessel function window proved to be superior in classifying normal and abnormal populations.

Pulse-transmission NNs—networks that consist of neurons that communicate with other neurons via pulses rather than numbers—also have been modeled [7,17]. This kind of network is much more realistic, since, in biologic systems, action potentials are the means of neuronal communication. Dayhoff [18] has developed a pulse-transmission network that can temporally integrate arriving signals and also display some resistance to temporal noise.

Another method is optimal filtering, which is a variation of the traditional matched filter in noise [19]. This has the advantage of separating even overlapping waveforms. It also carries the disadvantage that the needed knowledge of the noise power spectral density and the Fourier transform of the spikes might not be always available.

Principal-components analysis also has been used. Here the incoming spike waveforms are represented by templates given by eigenvectors from their average autocorrelation functions [20]. The authors found that two to three eigenvectors are enough to account for 90% of the total energy of the signal. This way each spike can be represented by the coordinates of its projection onto the eigenvector space. These coordinates are the only information needed for spike classification, which is further done by clustering techniques.

Multineuronal Activity Analysis

When dealing with single- or multineuron activities, the practice is to determine how many neurons (or units) are involved in the "spike train" evoked by some sensory stimulation. Each spike in a spike train represents an action potential elicited by a neuron in close proximity to the recording electrode. These action potentials have different amplitudes, latencies, and shape configurations and, when superimposed on each other, create a complex waveform—a composite spike. The dilemma that many scientists face is how to decompose these composite potentials into their constituents and how to assess the question of how many neurons their electrode is recording from. One of the most widely used methods is window discrimination, in which different thresholds are set, above which the activity of any given neuron is assigned, according to amplitude. Peak detection techniques also have been used [21]. These methods perform well if the number of neurons is very small and the spikes are well separated. Statistical methods of different complexity also have been used [22–24] involving the time intervals between spikes. Each spike is assigned a unique instant of time so that a spike train can be described by a process of time points corresponding to the times where the action potential had occurred. Processes such as these are called *point* processes, since they are characterized by only one number. Given this, a spike train can be treated as a stochastic point process that may or may not be stationary. In the former case, its statistics do not vary in the time of observation [25]. In the second case, when nonstationarity is assumed, any kind of statistical analysis becomes formidable.

Correlations between spike trains of neurons can be found because of many factors, but mostly because of excitatory or inhibitory interactions between them or due to a common input to both. Simulations on each possibility have been conducted in the past [26]. In our research, when recording from the optic tectum of the frog, the problem is the reversed situation of the one given above. That is, we have the recorded signal with noise superimposed, and we have to decompose it to its constituents so that we can make inferences on the neuronal circuitry involved. What one might do would be to set the minimal requirements on a neural network, which could behave the same way as the vast number of neurons that could have resulted in a neural spike train similar to the one recorded.

This is a very difficult problem to attack with no unique solution. A method that has attracted attention is the one developed by Gerstein et al. [22,27]. This technique detects various functional groups in the recorded data by the use of the so-called gravitational clustering method. Although promising, the analysis becomes cumbersome due to the many possible subgroups of neurons firing in synchrony. Temporal patterns of neuronal activity also have been studied with great interest. Some computational methods have been developed for the detection of favored temporal patterns [28–31]. My group also has been involved in the analysis of complex waveforms by the development of a novel method, the ST-scan method [32]. This method is based on well-known tomographic techniques, statistical analysis, and template matching. The method proved to be very sensitive to even small variations of the waveforms due to the fact that many orientations of them are considered, as it is done in tomographic imaging. Each histogram represents the number of times a stroke vector at a specific orientation is cutting the composite waveform positioned at the center of the window. These histograms were then fed to a NN for categorization. The histograms are statistical representations of individual action potentials. The NN therefore must be able to learn to recognize histograms by categorizing them with the action potential waveform that they represent. The NN also must be able to recognize any histogram as belonging to one of the "learned" patterns or not belonging to any of them [33]. In analyzing the ST-histograms, the NN must act as an "adaptive demultiplexer." That is, given a set of inputs, the network must determine the correspondingly correct output. This is a categorization procedure performed by a perceptron, originally described by Rosenblatt [34]. In analyzing the ST-histograms, the preprocessing is done by a perceptron, and the error is found either by an LMS algorithm [35] or by an ALOPEX algorithm [36,39,40].

Visual Evoked Potentials

Visual evoked potentials (VEPs) have been used in the clinical environment as a diagnostic tool for many decades. Stochastic analysis of experimental recordings of VEPs may yield useful information that is not well understood in its original form. Such information may provide a good diagnostic criterion in differentiating normal subjects from subjects with neurologic diseases as well as provide an index of the progress of diseases.

These potentials are embedded in noise. Averaging is then used in order to improve the signal-to-noise (S/N) ratio. When analyzing these potentials, several methods have been used, such as spectral analysis of their properties [42], adaptive filtering techniques [43,44], and some signal enhancers, again based on adaptive processes [45]. In this latter method, no a priori knowledge of the signal is needed. The adaptive signal enhancer consists of a bank of adaptive filters, the output of which is shown to be a minimum mean-square error estimate of the signal.

If we assume that the VEP represents a composite of many action potentials and that each one of these action potentials propagates to the point of the VEP recording, the only difference between the various action potentials is their amplitudes and time delays. The conformational changes observed in the VEP waveforms of normal individuals and defected subjects can then be attributed to an asynchrony in the arrival of these action potentials at a focal point (integration site) in the visual cortex [36]. One can simulate this process by simulating action potentials and trying to fit them to normal and abnormal VEPs with NNs.

Action potentials were simulated using methods similar to those of Moore and Ramon [37] and Bell and Cook [38]. Briefly, preprocessing of the VEP waveforms is done first by smoothing a five-point filter that performs a weighted averaging over its neighboring points:

$$S(n) = [F(n - 2) + 2F(n - 1) + 3F(n) + 2F(n + 1) + F(n + 2)]/9 \quad (60.1)$$

The individual signals v_j are modulated so that at the VEP recording site each v_j has been changed in amplitude $am(j)$ and in phase $ph(j)$. The amplitude change represents the propagation decay, and the phases represent the propagation delays of signals according to the equation

$$v_j(i) = am(j) \cdot AP[i - ph(j)] \quad (60.2)$$

For a specific choice of $am(j)$ and $ph(j), j = 1, 2, \ldots, N$, the simulated VEP can be found by

$$VEP = b + k \sum_{j=1}^{N} v_j^{\alpha} \quad (60.3)$$

where k is a scaling factor, b is a dc component, and α a constant [39,40].

The ALOPEX process was used again, here in order to adjust the parameters (amplitude and phase) so that the cost function reaches a minimum and therefore the calculated waveform coincides with the experimental one.

The modified ALOPEX equation is given by

$$p_i(n) = p_i(n - 1) + \gamma \Delta p_i(n) \, \Delta R(n) + \mu r_i(n) \quad (60.4)$$

where $p_i(n)$ are the parameters at iteration n, and γ and μ are scaling factors of the deterministic and random components, respectively, which are adjusted so that at the beginning γ is small and μ is large. As the number of iterations increases, γ increases while μ decreases. The cost function R is monitored until convergence has been achieved at least 80% or until a preset number of iterations has been covered.

The results obtained show a good separation between normal and abnormal VEPs. This separation is based on an index λ, which is defined as the ratio of two summations, namely, the summation of amplitudes whose $ph(i)$ is less than 256 ms and the summation of amplitudes whose $ph(i)$ is greater than 256 ms. A large value of λ indicates an abnormal VEP, while a small λ indicates a normal VEP.

The convergences of the process for a normal and an abnormal VEP are shown in Figs. 60.1 and 60.2, respectively, at different iteration numbers. The main assumption here is that in normal individuals, the action potentials all arrive at a focal point in the cortex in resonance, while in abnormal

(a)

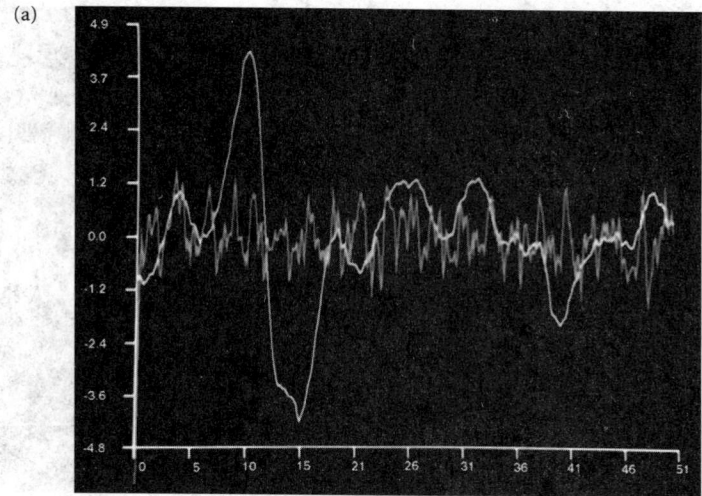

(b)

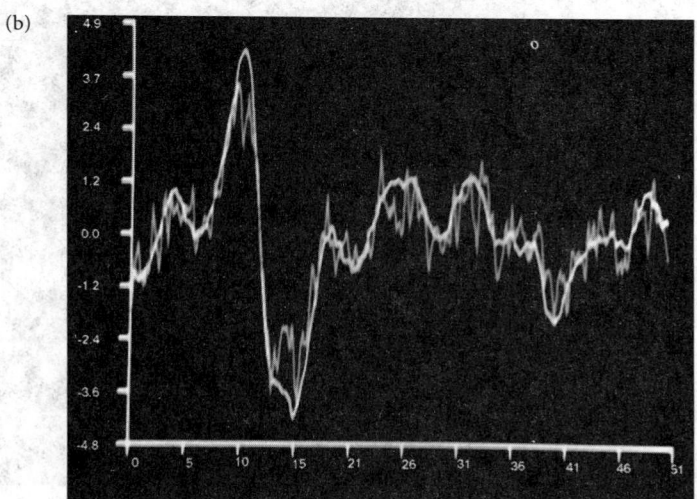

(c)

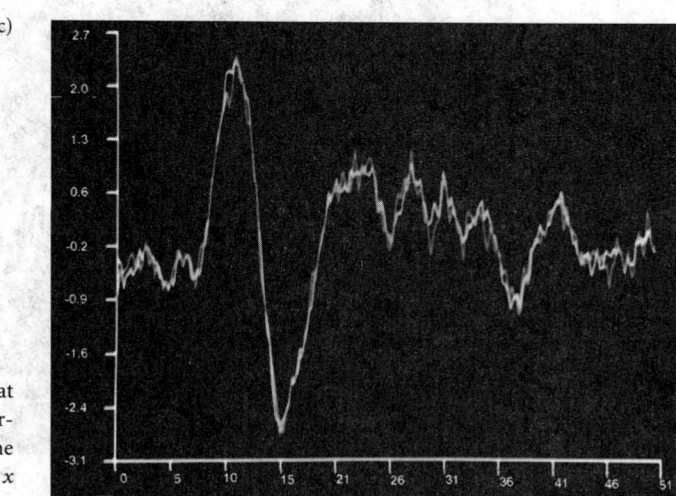

FIGURE 60.1 Normal VEP. (*a*) The fitting at the beginning of the process, (*b*) after 500 iterations, and (*c*) after 1000 iterations. Only one action potential is repeated 1000 times. The *x* axis is ×10 ms; the *y* axis is millivolts.

(a)

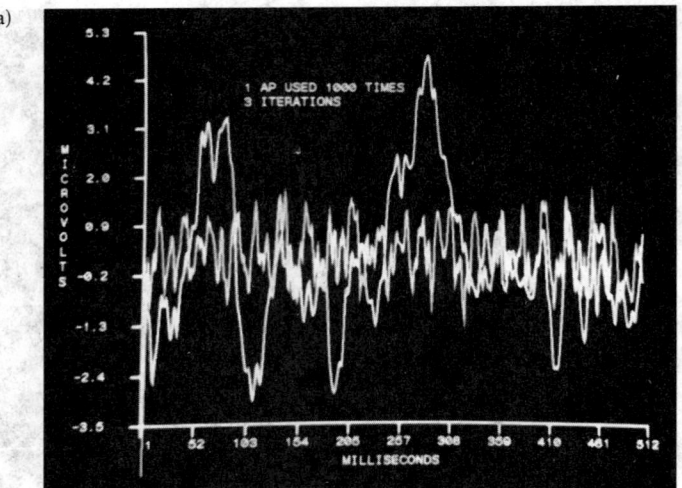

(b)

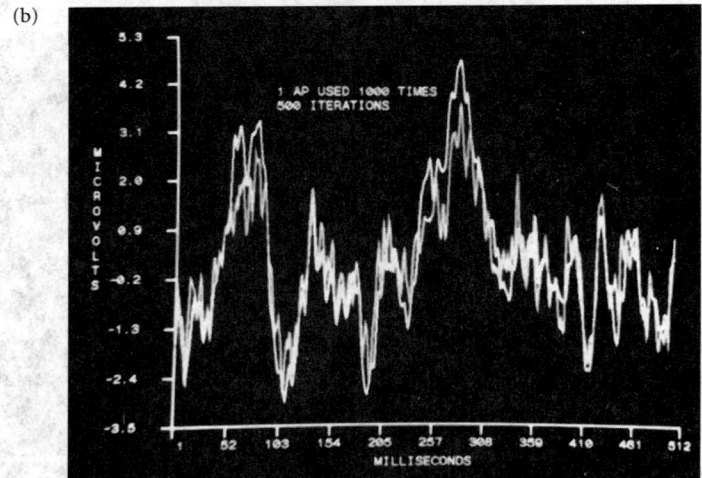

(c)

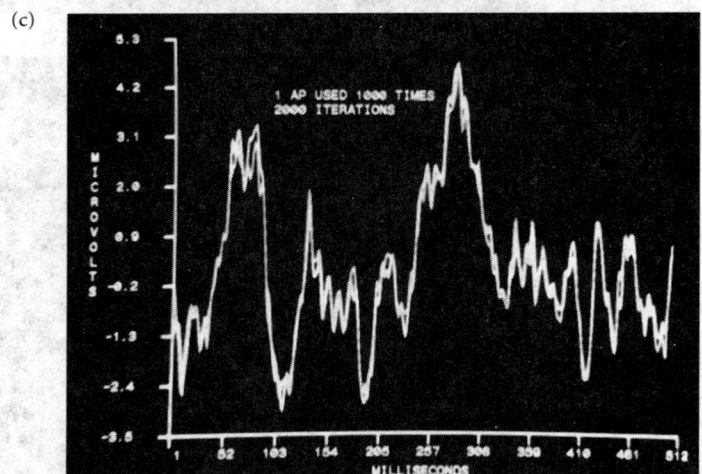

FIGURE 60.2   Abnormal VEP. (*a*) Fitting at *t* = 3 iterations, (*b*) after
500 iterations, and (*c*) after 2000 iterations. One action potential was
used 1000 times.

subjects there exists an asynchrony of the arrival times. Maier and colleagues [41] noted the importance of source localization of VEPs in humans in studying the perceptual behavior in humans. The optimization procedure used in this section can help that task, since individual neuronal responses are optimally isolated. One of the interesting points here is that signals (action potentials) with different delay times result in composite signals of different forms. Thus the reverse solution of this problem, i.e., extracting individual signals from a composite measurement, can help resolve the problem of signal source localization. The multiunit recordings presented in the early sections of this paper fall in the same category with that of decomposing VEPs. This analysis might provide insights as to how neurons communicate.

60.2 Neural Networks in Speech Recognition

Another place where NNs find wide applications is in speech recognition. Tebelski et al. [46] have studied the performance of linked predictive NNs (LPNNs) for large-vocabulary, continuous-speech recognition. The authors used a six-state phoneme topology, and without any other optimization, the LPNN achieved an average of 90%, 58%, and 39% accuracy on tasks with perplexity of 5, 11, and 402, respectively, which is better than the performance of several other simpler NNs tested. These results show that the main advantages of predictive networks are mainly that they produce nonbinary distortion measures in a simple way and that they can model dynamic properties such as those found in speech. Their weakness is that they show poor discrimination, which may be corrected by corrective training and function work modeling.

Allen and Kanam [47] designed an NN architecture that locates word boundaries and identifies words from phoneme sequences. They tested the model in three different regimes with a highly redundant corpus and a restricted vocabulary, and the NN was trained with a limited number of phonemic variations for the words in the corpus. These tests yielded a very low error rate. In a second experiment, the network was trained to identify words from expert transcriptions of speech. The error rate for correct simultaneous identification of words and word boundaries was 18%. Finally, they tested the use of the output of a phoneme classifier as the input to the word and word boundary identification network. The error rate increased almost exponentially to 49%.

The best discrimination came from hybrid systems such as the use of an MLP and a hidden Markov model (HMM). These systems incorporate multiple sources of evidence such as features and temporal context without any restrictive assumptions of distributions or statistical independence. Bourland et al. [48] used MLPs as linear predictions for autoregressive HMMs. This approach, although more compatible with the HMM formalism, still suffers from several limitations. Although these authors generalized their approach to take into account time correlations between successive observations without any restrictive assumptions about the driving noise, the reputed results show that many of the tricks used to improve standard HMMs are also valid for this hybrid approach.

In another study, Intrator [49] used an unsupervised NN for dimensionality reduction that seeks directions emphasizing multimodality and derived a new statistical insight to the synaptic modification equations governing learning as in the Bienenstock, Cooper, and Munro (BCM) neurons [50]. The speech data consisted of 20 consecutive time windows of 32 ms with 30-ms overlap aligned at the beginning of the time. For each window, a set of 22 energy levels was computed corresponding to the Zwicker critical-band filters [51]. The classification results were compared with those of a backpropagation network. These results showed that the backpropagation network does well in finding structures useful for classification of the trained data, but these structures are more sensitive to voicing. Classification results using a BCM network, on the other hand, suggest that for the specified task, structures that are more sensitive to voicing can be extracted, even though voicing imposes several effects on the speech signal. These features are more speaker-invariant.

Phan et al. [52] have attempted to solve the "cocktail party effect," which describes phenomena in which humans can selectively focus attention on one sound source among competing sound sources. This is an ability that is hampered for the hearing-impaired. A system was developed that successfully identifies a speaker in the presence of competing speakers for short utterances. Features used for identification are monaural, whose feature space represent a 90% data reduction from the original data. This system is presently used off-line and also has been applied successfully to intraspeaker speech recognition. The features used in the preprocessing were obtained by wavelet analysis. This multiresolution analysis decomposes a signal into a hierarchical system of subspaces that are one-dimensional and are square integrable. Each subspace is spanned by basis functions that have scaling characteristics of either dilation or compression depending on the resolution. The implementation of these basis functions is incorporated in a recursive pyramidal algorithm in which the discrete approximation of a current resolution is convolved with quadrature mirror filters in the subsequent resolution [53]. After preprocessing, speech waveform is analyzed by the wavelet transform. Analysis is limited to four octaves. For pattern-recognition input configuration, the wavelet coefficients are mapped to a vector and used as inputs to a neural network trained by the ALOPEX algorithm. White noise was superimposed on the features as well in order to establish a threshold of robustness of the algorithm.

60.3 Neural Networks in Cardiology

Two-dimensional echocardiography is an important noninvasive clinical tool for cardiac imaging. The endocardial and epicardial boundaries of the left ventricle (LV) are very useful quantitative measures of various functions of the heart. Cardiac structures detection in ECG images are also very important in recognizing the image parts.

A lot of research in the last couple of years has taken place around these issues and the application of neural networks in solving them. Hunter et al. [54] have used NNs in detecting echocardiographic LV boundaries and the center of the LV cavity. The points detected are then linked by a "snake" energy-minimizing function to give the epicardial and endocardial boundaries. A *snake* is an energy-minimizing deformable curve [55] fined by an internal energy that is the controller of the differential properties in terms of its curvature and its metrics. The most robust results were obtained by a 9×9 square input vector with a resolution reduction of 32:1. Energy minimization is carried out by simulated annealing. The minimum energy solution was obtained after 1000 iterations over the entire snake. The use of NNs as edge detectors allows the classification of points to be done by their probability of being edges rather than by their edge strength, a very important factor for echocardiographic images due to their wide variations in edge strength.

A complex area in electrocardiography is the differentiation of wide QRS tachycardias in ventricular (VT) and supraventricular tachycardia (SVT). A set of criteria for this differentiation has been proposed recently by Brugada et al. [56]. One important aspect of applying NNs in interpreting ECGs is to use parameters that not only make sense but are also meaningful for diagnosis. Dassen et al. [57] developed an induction algorithm that further improved the criteria set by Brugada et al., also using NNs.

Nadal and deBossan [58] used principal-components analysis (PCA) and the relative R-wave to R-wave intervals of P-QRS complexes to evaluate arrhythmias. Arrhythmias are one of the risks of sudden cardiac arrest in coronary care units. In this study, the authors used the first 10 PCA coefficients (PCCs) to reduce the data of each P-QRS complex and a feedforward NN classifier that splits the vector space generated by the PCCs into regions that separate the different classes of beats in an efficient way. They obtained better classification than using other methods, with correct classification of 98.5% for normal beats, 98.5% for ventricular premature beats, and 93.5% for fusion beats, using only the first two PCCs. When 4 PCCs were used, these classifications improved to 99.2%, 99.1%, and 94.1%, respectively. These results are better than those obtained by logistic regression when the input space is composed of more than two classes of beats. The difficulties encountered include the elimination of redundant data in order not to overestimate the importance of normal beat detection by the classifier.

In another work, Silipo et al. [59] used an NN as an autoassociator. In previous work they had proved that NNs had better performances than the traditional clustering and statistical methods.

They considered beat features derived from both morphologic and prematurity information. Their classification is adequate for ventricular ectopic beats, but the criteria used were not reliable enough to characterize the supraventricular ectopic beat.

A lot of studies also have used NNs for characterization of myocardial infarction (MI). Myocardial infarction is one of the leading causes of death in the United States. The currently available techniques for diagnosis are accurate enough, but they suffer from certain drawbacks, such as accurate quantitative measure of severity, extent, and precise location of the infarction. Since the acoustic properties in the involved region are mostly changing, one can study them by the use of ultrasound.

Baxt [60] used an NN to identify MI in patients presented to an emergency department with anterior chest pain. An NN was trained on clinical pattern sets retrospectively derived from patients hospitalized with a high likelihood of having MI, and the ability of the NN was compared with that of physicians caring for the same patients. The network performed with a sensitivity of 92% and a specificity of 96%. These figures were better than the physicians, with a sensitivity of 88% and a specificity of 71%, or any other computer technology (88% sensitivity, 74% specificity) [61].

Diagnosis of inferior MI with NNs was studied by Hedén et al. [62] with sensitivity of 84% and a specificity of 97%, findings that are similar to those of Pahlm et al. [63].

Yi et al. [64] used intensity changes in an echocardiogram to detect MI. Once an echocardiogram is obtained, it is digitized and saved in a file as a gray-scale image (512 × 400) (Fig. 60.3). A window of the region of interest is then selected between the systole and diastole of the cardiac cycle and saved in a different file. The window can be either of a constant size or it can be adaptive (varying) in size. This new file can be enlarged (zoom) for examination of finer details in the image. All image artifacts are filtered out, and contrast enhancement is performed. This new image is then saved and serves as input to the NN. A traditional three-layer NN with 300 input nodes (one node for each pixel intensity in the input file), a varying number of hidden nodes, and two output nodes was used. The output node indicates the status of the patient under testing. A "one" indicates normal and a "zero" an abnormal case.

The weights of the connections were calculated using the optimization algorithms of ALOPEX. One sub-ALOPEX was used for the weights between hidden nodes and input nodes, and a second sub-ALOPEX was used for those from the output to the hidden layer.

The network was trained with a population of 256 patients, some with scars and some normal. These patients were used to obtain "templates" for each category. These templates were then used for comparison with the test images. None of these testing images was included in the training set.

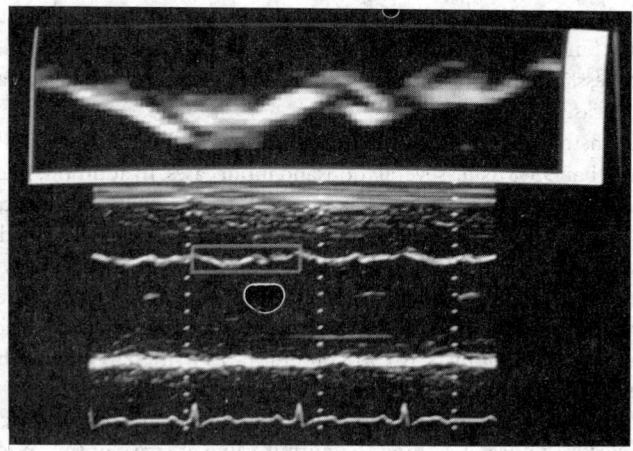

FIGURE 60.3   Selection of region of interest. The intensity pattern in the box is used as input to the NN.

The cost function used for the process was the least-squares rule, which, although slow, produces reliable results.

A similar process is used for the output layer. The noise was made adaptable. The intensities of the images are normalized before being submitted to the NN. A cutoff of 0.2 was used. Therefore, anything above 0.8 is normal, below 0.2 is scar, and all the in-between values are classified as unknown. Due to the fact that the scar training set was very small compared with the normals, a better classification of normals than scars was observed. A study was made as to how the number of hidden nodes influences the results for the same standard deviation of noise.

In another study, Kostis et al. [65] used NNs in estimating the prognosis of acute MI. Patients who survive the acute phase of an MI have an increased risk of mortality persisting up to 10 years or more. Estimation of the probability of being alive at a given time in the future is important to the patients and their physicians and is usually ascertained by the use of statistical methods. The purpose of the investigation was to use an NN to estimate future mortality of patients with acute MI. The existence of a large database (Myocardial Infarction Data Acquisition Systems, or MIDAS) that includes MI occurring in the state of New Jersey and has long-term follow-up allows the development and testing of such a computer algorithm. Since the information included in the database does not allow the exact prediction of vital status (dead or alive) in all patients with 100% accuracy, the NN should be able to categorize patients according to the probability of dying within a given period of time.

Because information included in the database is not sufficient to allow the exact prediction of vital status (dead or alive) in all patients with 100% accuracy, we developed an NN able to categorize patients according to the probability of dying within a given period of time rather than predicting categorically whether a patient will be dead or alive at a given time in the future. It was observed that there were many instances where two or more patients had identical input characteristics while some were dead and some alive at the end of the study period. For this reason, it is difficult to train a standard NN. Since there is no unique output value for all input cases, the network had difficulty converging to a unique set of solutions. To alleviate this problem, a conflict-resolution algorithm was developed. The algorithm takes templates with identical input vectors and averages each of their input characteristics to produce a single case. Their output values of vital status are averaged, producing, in effect, a percentage probability of mortality for the particular set of input characteristics. As each new subject template is read into the program, its input characteristics are compared with those of all previous templates. If no match is found, its input values and corresponding output value are accepted. If a match is found, the output value is brought together with the stored output value (percentage probability of mortality and the number of templates on which it is based), and a new output value is calculated, representing the percentage average mortality of the entire characteristic group. Since each member of the group is an identical input case, no input characteristic averaging is necessary, thus preserving the statistical significance of the average mortality with respect to that exact case.

This new algorithm, using the two-hidden-layer perceptron optimized by ALOPEX, seems to have converged to greater than 98% using several thousand input cases. In addition, 10 output nodes were used in the final layer, each corresponding to a range of percent chance or mortality (e.g., node 1: 0% to 10%; node 2: 10% to 20%; etc.). The outputs of the network are designed to maximize one of the 10 potential output "binds," each corresponding to a decile of mortality between 0% and 100%. The output node containing the correct probability value was set to a value of 1.0; the others to 0.0. In this manner, the network should be able to provide percentage probability of mortality and also to resolve input-case conflicts. An SAS program was written to present the predicted probability of mortality separately in patients who are dead or alive at the end of the follow-up period. The NNs constructed as described above were able to be trained and evaluated according to several definitions of network response: matching the output value at every output node, identifying the correct location of which node was to contain the peak output value, and matching the output value at the peak output location.

The network was tested on known and then on unknown cases. A correspondence of the observed to the predicted probability of being alive at a given time was observed. The categorical classifications (dead or alive) yielded an overall accuracy of 74%. A reciprocal relationship between sensitivity and specificity of the rules for determination of vital status was observed.

60.4 Neural Networks in Neurology

Lately, NNs found application in neurology as well and, in particular, in characterizing memory defects, as are apparent in diseases such as Parkinson's and Alzheimer's. Both diseases exhibit devastating effects and disrupt the lives of those affected.

For several decades, in an attempt to further understand brain functions, computational neuroscientists have addressed the issue by modeling biologic neural network structure with computer simulations. A recent article by Stern et al. [66] reports on an important relationship of Alzheimer's disease expression and levels of education. A similar inverse relationship was earlier reported by Zhang et al. [67] in a Chinese population. This inverse relationship was attributed to a protective role of the brain reserve capacity [68]. Such a capacity becomes important, since in an educated person's brain more synapses exist, which might protect the individual in the expression of symptoms of the disease. It is not argued, however, that the disease will not be acquired; rather, that it will be delayed. Zahner et al. [69] have employed a three-layer feedforward NN trained with ALOPEX to simulate the effects of education in dementia, age-related changes, and in general, brain damage. Our results show that the higher level of training of the NN, 50%, 60%, 70%, 80%, etc., the slower is the damage on the "brain." Damage was simulated by systematically adding noise on the weights of the network. Noise had a gaussian distribution with varying standard deviations and mean of zero. Figure 60.4 shows the results of these simulations as recognition rate versus standard

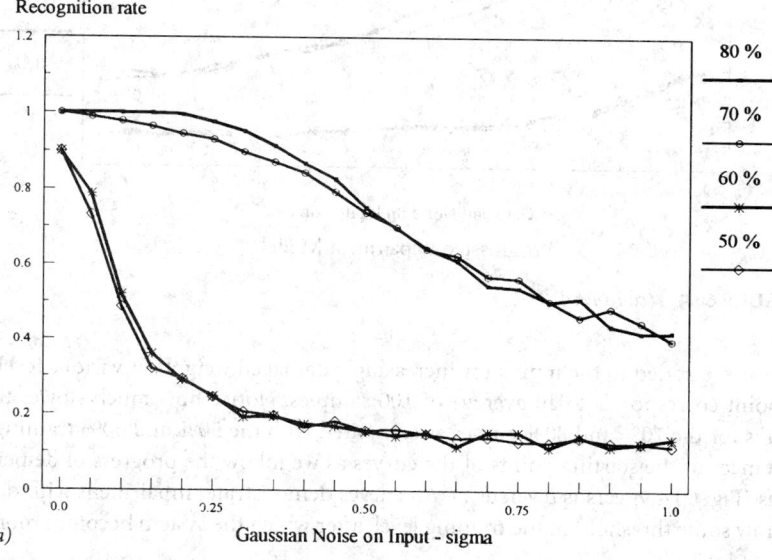

FIGURE 60.4 Recognition rate versus standardization of noise added to the inputs. Different curves correspond to various learning levels with damaged weights. (*a*) Noise added only to the inputs. (*b*) Noise added to the weights to mimic "brain damage," $\sigma = 0.05$. (*c*) Noise on the weights with $\sigma = 0.1$. Notice how much more robust the "brain" is to noise with higher levels of education.

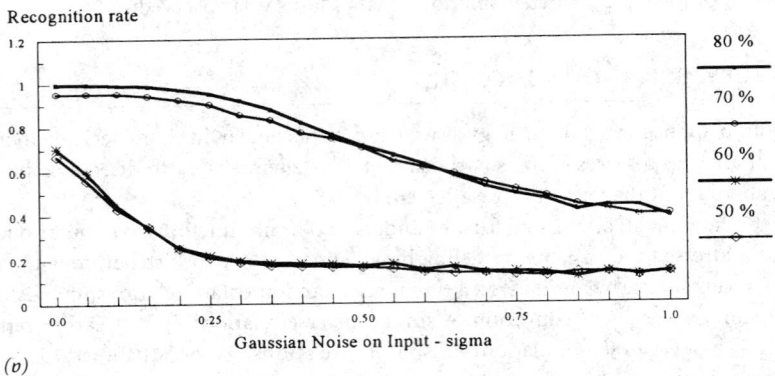

(v)

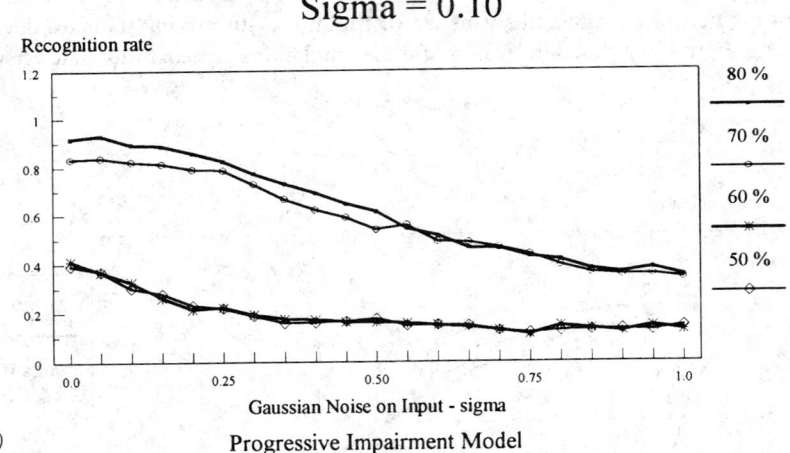

(c)   Progressive Impairment Model

FIGURE 60.4   *(continued)*

deviation of noise added to the inputs for increasingly damaged weights at various levels of training. Each point corresponds to an average of 100 samples. Notice how much slower the drop in recognition is for the 70% and 80% curves as compared with the 50% and 60% training. Also notice the distances of the starting points of the curves as we follow the progress of dementia at different stages (Fig. 60.4, *a* versus *b* versus *c*). All curves demonstrate impairment with damage, but they also show some threshold in the training level, after which the system becomes more robust.

60.5 Discussion

Neural networks provide a powerful tool for analysis of biosignals. This chapter has reviewed applications of NNs in cardiology, neurology, speech processing, and brain waveforms. The literature is vast, and this chapter is by no means exhaustive. In the last 5 years, NNs have been used more and more extensively in a variety of fields, and biomedical engineering is not short of it. Besides the applications, a lot of research is still going on in order to find optimal algorithms and optimal values for the parameters used in these algorithms. In industry, an explosion of VLSI chip designs on NNs has been observed. The parallel character of NNs makes them very desirable solutions to computational bottlenecks.

References

1. Werbos P. 1974. Beyond Regression: New Tools for Prediction and Analysis in the Behavioral Sciences. Ph.D. thesis, Harvard University, Cambridge, Mass.
2. Parker DB. 1985. Learning logic, S-81-64, file 1, Office of Technology Licensing, Stanford University, Stanford, Calif.
3. Rumelhart DE, Hinuton GE, Williams RJ. 1986. Learning internal representations by error propagation. In DE Rumelhart, JL McClelland (eds), Parallel Distributed Processing, vol 2: Foundations. Cambridge, Mass, MIT Press.
4. Harth E, Tzanakou E. 1974. A stochastic method for determining visual receptive fields. Vision Res 14:1475.
5. Tzanakou E, Michalak R, Harth E. 1984. The ALOPEX process: Visual receptive fields with response feedback. Biol Cybernet 51:53.
6. Micheli-Tzanakou E. 1984. Nonlinear characteristics in the frog's visual system. Biol Cybernet 51:53.
7. Deutsch S, Micheli-Tzanakou E. 1987. Neuroelectric Systems. New York, NYU Press.
8. Marsic I, Micheli-Tzanakou E. 1990. Distributed optimization with the ALOPEX algorithms. In Proceedings of the 12th Annual International Conference of the IEEE/EMBS 12:1415.
9. Dasey TJ, Micheli-Tzanakou E. 1989. A pattern recognition application of the ALOPEX process with hexagonal arrays. In International Joint Conference on Neural Networks 12:119.
10. Xiao L-T., Micheli-Tzanakou E, Dasey TJ. 1990. Analysis of composite neuronal waveforms into their constituents. In Proceedings of the 12th Annual International Conference of the IEEE/EMBS 12(3):1433.
11. Hiraiwa A, Shimohara K, Tokunaga Y. 1989. EMG pattern analysis and classification by Neural Networks. In IEEE International Conference on Systems, Man and Cybernetics, part 3, pp 1113–1115.
12. Huang Q, Graupe D, Huang Y-F, Liu RW. 1989. Identification of firing patterns of neuronal signals. In Proceedings of the 28th IEEE Conference on Decision and Control, vol 1, pp 266–271.
13. Bruha I, Madhavan GP. 1989. Need for a knowledge-based subsystem in evoked potential neural-net recognition system. In Proceedings of the 11th Annual International Conference of the IEEE/EMBS, vol 11, part 6, pp 2042–2043.
14. Kelly MF, Parker PA, Scott RN. 1990. Applications of neural networks to myoelectric signal analysis: A preliminary study. IEEE Trans Biomed Eng 37(3):221.
15. Ramamoorthy PA, Govid G, Iyer VK. 1988. Signal modeling and prediction using neural networks. Neural Networks 1(1):461.
16. Moody EB Jr, Micheli-Tzanakou E, Chokroverty S. 1989. An adaptive approach to spectral analysis of pattern-reversal visual evoked potentials. IEEE Trans Biomed Eng 36(4):439.
17. Dayhoff JE. 1990. Regularity properties in pulse transmission networks. Proc IJCNN 3:621.
18. Dayhoff JE. 1990. A pulse transmission (PT) neural network architecture that recognizes patterns and temporally integrates. Proc IJCNN 2:A-979.
19. Roberts WM, Hartile DK. 1975. Separation of multi-unit nerve impulse trains by the multi-channel linear filter algorithm. Brain Res 94:141.
20. Abeles M, Goldstein MH. 1977. Multiple spike train analysis. Proc IEEE 65:762.

21. Wiemer W, Kaack D, Kezdi P. 1975. Comparative evaluation of methods for quantification of neural activity. Med Biol Eng 358.

22. Perkel DH, Gerstein GL, Moore GP. 1967. Neuronal spike trains and stochastic point processes: I. The single spike train. Biophys J 7:391.

23. Perkel DH, Gerstein GL, Moore GP. 1967. Neuronal spike trains and stochastic point processes: II. Simultaneous spike trains. Biophys J 7:419.

24. Gerstein GL, Perkel DH, Subramanian KN. 1978. Identification of functionally related neuronal assemblies. Brain Res 140:43.

25. Papoulis A. 1984. Probability, Random Variables and Stochastic Processes, 2d ed. New York, McGraw-Hill.

26. Moore GP, Segundo JP, Perkel DH, Levitan H. 1970. Statistical signs of synaptic interactions in neurons. Biophys J 10:876.

27. Gerstein GL, Perkel DH, Dayhoff JE. 1985. Cooperative firing activity in simultaneously recorded populations of neurons: detection and measurement. J Neurosci 5:881.

28. Dayhoff JE, Gerstein GL. 1983. Favored patterns in nerve spike trains: I. Detection. J Neurophysiol 49(6):1334.

29. Dayhoff JE, Gerstein GL. 1983. Favored patterns in nerve spike trains: II. Application. J Neurophysiol 49(6):1349.

30. Abeles M, Gerstein GL. 1988. Detecting spatiotemporal firing patterns among simultaneously recorded single neurons. J Neurophysiol 60(3):909.

31. Frostig RD, Gerstein GL. 1990. Recurring discharge patterns in multispike trains. Biol Cybernet 62:487.

32. Micheli-Tzanakou E, Iezzi R. 1985. Spike recognition by stroke density function calculation. In Proceedings of the 11th Northeast Bioengineering Conference, pp 309–312.

33. Iezzi R, Micheli-Tzanakou E. 1990. Neural network analysis of neuronal spike-trains. In Annual International Conference of the IEEE/EMBS, vol 12, no 3, pp 1435–1436.

34. Rosenblatt F. 1962. Principles of Neurodynamics. Washington, Spartan Books.

35. Davilla CE, Welch AJ, Rylander HG. 1986. Adaptive estimation of single evoked potentials. In Proceedings of the 8th IEEE EMBS Annual Conference, pp 406–409.

36. Wang J-Z, Micheli-Tzanakou E. 1990. The use of the ALOPEX process in extracting normal and abnormal visual evoked potentials. IEEE/EMBS Mag 9(1):44.

37. Moore J, Ramon F. 1974. On numerical integration of the Hodgkin and Huxley equations for a membrane action potential. J Theor Biol 45:249.

38. Bell J, Cook LP. 1979. A model of the nerve action potential. Math Biosci 46:11.

39. Micheli-Tzanakou E, O'Malley KG. 1985. Harmonic context of patterns and their correlations to VEP waveforms. In Proceedings of IEEE, 9th Annual Conference EMBS, pp 426–430.

40. Micheli-Tzanakou E. 1990. A neural network approach of decomposing brain waveforms to their constituents. In Proceedings of the IASTED International Symposium on Computers and Advanced Technology in Medicine, Healthcare and Bioengineering, pp 56–60.

41. Maier J, Dagnelie G, Spekreijse H, Van Duk W. 1987. Principal component analysis for source localization of VEPs in man. Vis Res 27:165.

42. Nahamura M, Nishida S, Shibasaki H. 1989. Spectral properties of signal averaging and a novel technique for improving the signal to noise ration. J Biomed Eng 2(1):72.

43. Orfanidis S, Aafif F, Micheli-Tzanakou E. 1987. Visual evoked potentials extraction by adaptive filtering. In Proceedings of the IEEE/EMBS International Conference, vol 2, pp 968–969.

44. Doncarli C, Goerig I. 1988. Adaptive smoothing of evoked potentials: A new approach. In Proceedings of the Annual International Conference of the IEEE/EMBS, part 3(of 4), pp 1152–1153

45. Davilla E, Welch AJ, Rylander HG. 1986. Adaptive estimation of single evoked potentials. In Proceedings of the 8th IEEE/EMBS Annual International Conference, pp 406–409.

46. Tebelski J, Waibel A, Bojan P, Schmidbauer O. 1991. Continuous speech recognition by linked predictive neural networks. In PR Lippman, JE Moody, DS Touretzky (eds), Advances in Neural Information Processing Systems 3, pp 199–205. San Mateo, Calif, Morgan Kauffman.

47. Allen RB, Kanam CA. 1991. A recurrent neural network for word identification from continuous phonemena strings. In PR Lippman, JE Moody, DS Touretzky (eds), Advances in Neural Information Processing Systems 3, pp 206–212. San Mateo, Calif, Morgan Kauffman.

48. Bourland H, Morgan N, Wooters C. 1991. Connectionist approaches to the use of Markov models for speech recognition. In PR Lippman, JE Moody, DS Touretzky (eds), Advances in Neural Information Processing Systems 3, pp 213–219. San Mateo, Calif, Morgan Kauffman.

49. Intrator N. 1991. Exploratory feature extraction in speech signals. In PR Lippman, JE Moody, DS Touretzky (eds), Advances in Neural Information Processing Systems 3, pp 241–247. San Mateo, Calif, Morgan Kauffman.

50. Bienenstock EL, Cooper LN, Munro PW. 1992. Theory for the development of neuron selectivity: Orientation specificity and binocular interaction in visual cortex. J Neurosci 2:32.

51. Zwicker E. 1961. Sudivision of the audible frequency range into critical bands (frequenagruppen). J Acoust Soc Am 33:248.

52. Phan F, Zahner D, Micheli-Tzanakou E, Sideman S. 1994. Speaker identification through wavelet multiresolution decomposition and Alopex. In Proceedings of the 1994 Long Island Conference on Artificial Intelligence and Computer Graphics, pp 53–68.

53. Mallat SG. 1989. A theory of multiresolution signal decomposition: The wavelet representation. IEEE Trans Pattern Anal Mach Int 11:674.

54. Hunter IA, Soraghan JJ, Christie J, Durani TS. 1993. Detection of echocardiographic left ventricle boundaries using neural networks. Comput Cardiol 201.

55. Cohen LD. 1991. On active contour models and balloons. CVGIP Image Understanding 53(92):211.

56. Brugada P, Brugada T, Mont L, et al. 1991. A new approach to the differential diagnosis of a regular tachycardia with a wide QRS complex. Circulation 83(5):1649.

57. Dassen WRM, Mulleneers RGA, Den Dulk K, et al. 1993. Further improvement of classical criteria for differentiation of wide-QRS tachycardia in SUT and VT using artificial neural network techniques. Comput Cardiol 337.

58. Nadal J, deBossan MC. 1993. Classification of cardiac arrhythmias based on principal components analysis and feedforward neural networks. Comput Cardiol 341.

59. Silipo R, Gori M, Marchesi C. 1993. Autoassociator structured neural network for rhythm classification of long-term electrocardiogram. Comput Cardiol 349.

60. Baxt WB. 1991. Use of an artificial neural network for the diagnosis of myocardial infarction. Ann Intern Med 115(II):843.

61. Goldman L, Cook SF, Brand DA, et al. 1988. A computer protocol to predict myocardial infarction in emergency department patients with chest pain. N Engl J Med 18:797.

62. Hedén B, Edenbrandt L, Haisty WK Jr, Pahlm O. 1993. Neural networks for ECG diagnosis of inferior myocardial infarction. Comput Cardiol 345.

63. Pahlm O, Case D, Howard G, et al. 1990. Decision rules for the ECK diagnosis of inferior myocardial infarction. Comput Biomed Res 23:332.

64. Yi C, Micheli-Tzanakou E, Shindler D, Kostis JB. 1993. A new neural network algorithm to study myocardial ultrasound for tissue characterization. In 19th Northeastern Bioengineering Conference, NJIT, pp 109–110.

65. Kostis WJ, Yi C, Micheli-Tzanakou E. 1993. Estimation of long-term mortality of myocardial infarction using a neural network based on the ALOPEX algorithm. In ME Cohen and DL Hudson (eds), Comparative Approaches in Medical Reasoning.

66. Stern Y, Gurland B, Tatemichi TK, et al. 1994. Influence of education and occupation on the incidence of Alzheimer's disease. JAMA 271:1004.

67. Zhang M, Katzman R, Salmon D, et al. 1990. The prevalence of dementia and Alzheimer's disease in Shanghai, China: Impact of age, gender and education. Ann Neurol 27:428.

68. Satz P. 1993. Brain reserve capacity on symptom onset after brain injury: A formulation and review of evidence for threshold theory. Neurophysiology 7(3):723.

69. Zahner DA, Micheli-Tzanakou E, Powell A, et al. 1994. Protective effects of learning on a progressively impaired neural network model of memory. In Proceedings of the 16th IEEE/EMBS Annual International Conference, Baltimore, Md. vol 2, pp 1065–1066.

61

Complexity, Scaling, and Fractals in Biomedical Signals

Banu Onaral
Drexel University

Joseph P. Cammarota
Naval Air Warfare Center,
Aircraft Division

Complexity, a contemporary theme embraced by physical as well as social sciences, is concerned with the collective behavior observed in composite systems in which long-range order is induced by short-range interactions of the constituent parts. Complex forms and functions abound in nature. Particularly in biology and physiology, branched, nested, granular, or otherwise richly packed, ir-regular, or disordered objects are the rule rather than the exception. Similarly ubiquitous are dis-tributed, broad-band phenomena that appear to fluctuate randomly. The rising science of com-plexity holds the promise to lead to powerful tools to analyze, model, process, and control the global behavior of complex biomedical systems.

   The basic tenets of the complexity theory rest on the revelation that large classes of complex sys-tems (composed of a multitude of richly interacting components) are reducible to simple rules. In particular, the structure and dynamics of complex systems invariably exist or evolve over a multi-tude of spatial and temporal scales. Moreover, they exhibit a systematic relationship between scales. From the biomedical engineering standpoint, the worthwhile outcome is the ability to characterize these intricate objects and processes in terms of straightforward scaling and fractal concepts and measures that often can be translated into simple iterative rules. In this sense, the set of concepts and tools, emerging under the rubric of complexity, complements the prediction made by the chaos theory that simple (low-order deterministic) systems may generate complex behavior.

   In their many incarnations, the concepts of complexity and scaling are playing a refreshingly uni-fying role among diverse scientific pursuits; therein lie compelling opportunities for scientific dis-coveries and technical innovations. Since these advances span a host of disciplines, hence different scientific languages, cultures, and dissemination media, finding one's path has become confusing. One of the aims of this presentation is to serve as a resource for key literature. We hope to guide the

-8493-8346-3/95/$0.00+$.50

reader toward substantial contributions and away from figments of fascination in the popular press that have tended to stretch emerging concepts ahead of the rigorous examination of evidence and the scientific verification of facts.

This chapter is organized in three main parts. The first part is intended to serve as a primer for the fundamental aspects of the complexity theory. An overview of the attendant notions of scaling theories constitutes the core of the second part. In the third part, we illustrate the potential of the complexity approach by presenting an application to predict acceleration-induced loss of consciousness in pilots.

61.1 Complex Dynamics

There exists a class of systems in which very complex spatial and temporal behavior is produced through the rich interactions among a large number of local subsystems. Complexity theory is concerned with systems that have many degrees of freedom (composite systems), are spatially extended (systems with both spatial and temporal degrees of freedom), and are dissipative as well as nonlinear due to the interplay among local components (agents). In general, such systems exhibit emergent global behavior. This means that macroscopic characteristics cannot be deduced from the microscopic characteristics of the elementary components considered in isolation. The global behavior emerges from the interactions of the local dynamics.

Complexity theories draw their power from recognition that the behavior of a complex dynamic system does not, in general, depend on the physical particulars of the local elements but rather on how they interact to collectively (cooperatively or competitively) produce the globally observable behavior. The local agents of a complex dynamic system interact with their neighbors through a set of usually (very) simple rules.

The emergent global organization that occurs through the interplay of the local agents arises without the intervention of a central controller. That is, there is self-organization, a spontaneous emergence of global order. Long-range correlations between local elements are not explicitly defined in such models, but they are induced though local interactions. The global organization also may exert a top-down influence on the local elements, providing feedback between the macroscopic and microscopic structures [Forrest, 1990] (Fig. 61.1).

Overcoming the Limits of Newtonian Mathematics

Linearity, as well as the inherent predictive ability, was an important factor in the success of newtonian mechanics. If a linear system is perturbed by a small amount, then the system response will

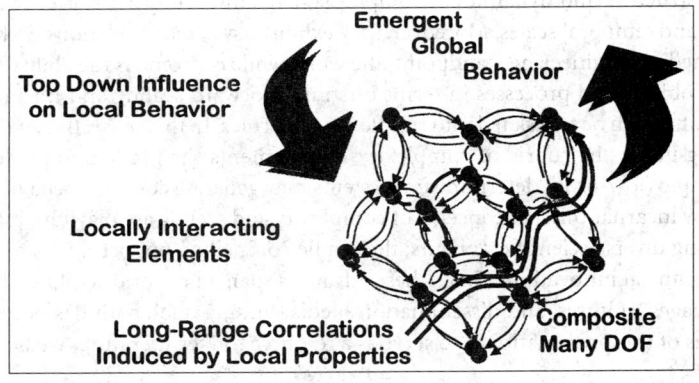

FIGURE 61.1 A complex dynamic system.

change by a proportionally small amount. In nonlinear systems, however, if the system is perturbed by a small amount, the response could be no change, a small change, a large change, oscillations (limit cycle), or *chaotic* behavior. The response depends on the state of the system at the time it was perturbed. Since most of nature is nonlinear, the key to success in understanding nature lies in embracing this nonlinearity.

Another feature found in linear systems is the property of superposition. *Superposition* means that the whole is equal to the sum of the parts. All the properties of a linear system can be understood through the analysis of each of its parts. This is not the case for complex systems, where the interaction among simple local elements can produce complex emergent global behavior.

Complexity theory stands in stark contrast to a purely reductionist approach that would seek to explain global behavior by breaking down the system into its most elementary components. The reductionist approach is not guaranteed to generate knowledge about the behavior of a complex system, since it is likely that the information about the local interactions (which determine the global behavior) will not be revealed in such an analysis. For example, knowing everything there is to know about a single ant will reveal nothing about why an ant colony is capable of such complex behaviors as waging war, farming, husbandry, and the ability to quickly adapt to changing environmental conditions. The approach that complexity theory proposes is to look at the system as a whole and not merely as a collection of irreducible parts.

Complexity research depends on digital computers for simulation of interactions. Cellular automata (one of the principal tools of complexity) have been constructed to model sand piles, earthquakes, traffic patterns, satellite communication networks, evolution, molecular autocatalysis, forest fires, and species interactions (among others) [Toffoli & Margoulis, 1987]. We note here that complexity is building on, and in some cases unifying, developments made in the fields of chaotic dynamics [Devaney, 1992], critical phenomena, phase transitions, renormalization [Wilson, 1983], percolation [Stauffer & Aharony, 1992], neural networks [Harvey, 1994; Simpson, 1990], genetic algorithms [Goldberg, 1989], and artificial life [Langton, 1989; Langton et al., 1992].

Critical Phenomena: Phase Transitions

For the purpose of this discussion, a *phase transition* can be defined as any abrupt change between the physical and/or dynamic states of a system. The most familiar examples of phase transitions are between the fundamental states of matter: solid, liquid, gas, and plasma. Phase transitions are also used to define other changes in matter, such as changes in the crystalline structure or state of magnetism. There are also phase transitions in the dynamics of systems from ordered (fixed-point and limit-cycle stability) to disordered (chaos). Determining the state of matter is not always straightforward. Sometimes the apparent state of matter changes when the scale of the observation (macroscopic versus microscopic) is changed. A *critical point* is a special case of phase transitions where order and disorder are intermixed at all scales [Wilson, 1983]. At criticality, all spatial and temporal features become scale invariant or self-similar. Magnetism is a good example of this phenomenon.

An Illustration of Critical Phenomena: Magnetism

The atoms of a ferromagnetic substance have more electrons with spins in one direction than in the other, resulting in a net magnetic field for the atom as a whole. The individual magnetic fields of the atoms tend to line up in one direction, with the result that there is a measurable level of magnetism in the material. At a temperature of absolute zero, all the atomic dipoles are perfectly aligned. At normal room temperature, however, some of the atoms are not aligned to the global magnetic field due to thermal fluctuations. This creates small regions that are nonmagnetic, although the substance is still magnetic. *Spatial renormalization,* or coarse graining, is the process of averaging the microscopic properties of the substance over a specified range in order to replace the multiple elements with a single equivalent element.

If measurements of the magnetic property were taken at a very fine resolution (without renor-malization), there would be some measurements that detect small pockets of nonmagnetism, al-though most measurements would indicate that the substance was magnetic. As the scale of the mea-surements is increased, i.e., spatially renormalized, the small pockets of nonmagnetism would be averaged out and would not be measurable. Therefore, measurements at the larger scale would in-dicate that the substance is magnetic, thereby decreasing its apparent temperature and making the apparent magnetic state dependent on the resolution of the measurements. The situation is similar (but reversed) at high temperatures. That is, spatial renormalization results in apparently higher temperatures, since microscopic islands of magnetism are missed because of the large areas of dis-order in the material.

At the Curie temperature there is long-range correlation in both the magnetic and nonmagnetic regions. The distribution of magnetic and nonmagnetic regions is invariant under the spatial re-normalization transform. These results are independent of the scale at which the measurement is taken, and the apparent temperature does not change under the renormalization transform. This scale invariance (self-similarity) occurs at only three temperatures: absolute zero, infinity, and the Curie temperature. The Curie temperature represents a critical point (criticality) in the tuning parameter (temperature) that governs the phase transition from a magnetic to a nonmagnetic state [Pietgen & Richter, 1986].

A Model for Phase Transitions: Percolation

A percolation model is created by using a simple regular geometric framework and by establishing simple interaction rules among the elements on the grid. Yet these models give rise to very complex structures and relationships that can be described by using scaling concepts such as fractals and power laws. A percolation model can be constructed on any regular infinite n-dimensional lattice [Stauffer & Aharony, 1992]. For simplicity, the example discussed here will use a two-dimensional finite square grid. In site percolation, each node in the grid has only two states, occupied or vacant. The nodes in the lattice are populated-based on a uniform probability distribution, independent of the state of any other node. The probability of a node being occupied is p (and thus the proba-bility of a node being vacant is $1 - p$). Nodes that are neighbors on the grid link together to form clusters (Fig. 61.2).

Clusters represent connections between nodes in the lattice. Anything associated with the cluster can therefore travel (flow) to any node that belongs to the cluster. Percolation can describe the abil-ity of water to flow through a porous medium such as igneous rock, oil fields, or finely ground Colombian coffee. As the occupation probability increases, the clusters of the percolation network grow from local connectedness to global connectedness [Feder, 1988]. At the critical occupation probability, a cluster that spans the entire lattice emerges. It is easy to see how percolation could be used to describe such phenomena as phase transitions by viewing occupied nodes as ordered mat-ter, with vacant nodes representing disordered matter. Percolation networks have been used to model magnetism, forest fires, and the permeability of ion channels in cell membranes.

Self-Organized Criticality

The concept of self-organized criticality has been introduced as a possible underlying principle of complexity [Bak et al., 1988; Bak & Chen, 1991]. The class of self-organized critical systems is spa-tially extended, composite, and dissipative with many locally interacting degrees of freedom. These systems have the capability to naturally evolve (i.e., there is no explicit tuning parameter such as temperature or pressure) toward a critical state.

Self-organized criticality is best illustrated by a sand pile. Start with a flat plate. Begin to add sand one grain at a time. The mound will continue to grow until criticality is reached. This criticality is dependent only on the local interactions among the grains of sand. The local slope determines what

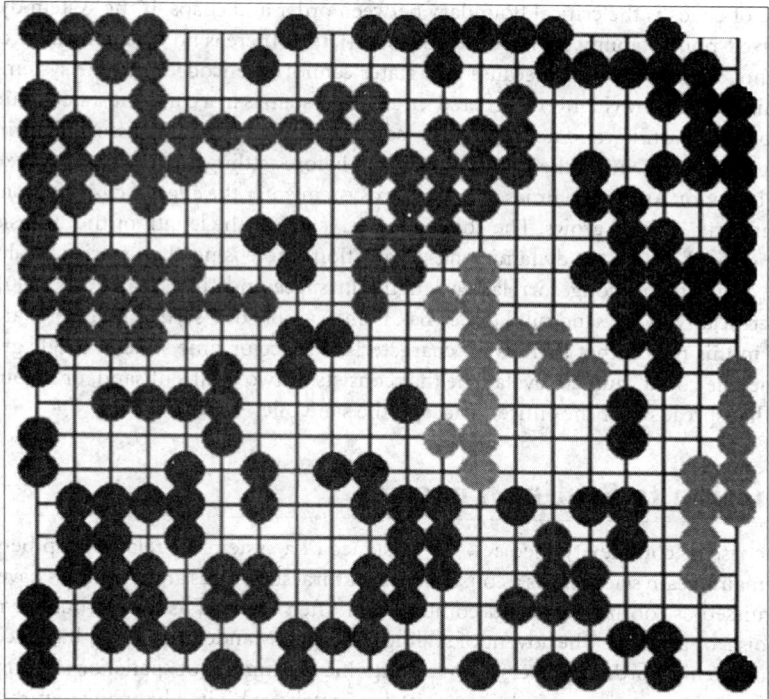

FIGURE 61.2 A percolation network.

will happen if another grain of sand is added. If the local slope is below the criticality (i.e., flat) the new grain of sand will stay put and increase the local slope. If the local slope is at the criticality, then adding the new grain of sand will increase the slope beyond the criticality, causing it to collapse. The collapsing grains of sand spread to adjoining areas. If those areas are at the criticality, then the avalanche will continue until local areas with slopes below the criticality are reached. Long-range correlations (up to the length of the sand pile) may emerge from the interactions of the local elements. Small avalanches are very common, while large avalanches are rare. The size (and duration) of the avalanche plotted against the frequency of occurrence of the avalanche can be described by a power law [Bak et al., 1988]. The sand pile seeks the criticality on its own. The slope in the sand pile will remain constant regardless of even the largest avalanches. These same power laws are observed in traffic patterns, earthquakes, and many other complex phenomena.

Dynamics at the Edge of Chaos

The dynamics of systems can be divided into several categories. Dynamic systems that exhibit *a fixed-point stability* will return to their initial state after being perturbed. A periodic evolution of states will result from a system that exhibits *a limit-cycle stability*. Either of these systems may display a transient evolution of states before the stable regions are reached. Dynamic systems also may exhibit *chaotic* behavior. The evolution of states associated with chaotic behavior is aperiodic, well-bounded, and very sensitive to initial conditions and resembles noise but is completely deterministic [Tsonis & Tsonis, 1989].

The criticality that lies between highly ordered and highly disordered dynamics has been referred to as the *edge of chaos* [Langton, 1990] and is analogous to a phase transition between states of matter, where the highly ordered system can be thought of as a solid and the highly disordered system a liquid.

The edge of chaos is the critical boundary between order and chaos. If the system dynamics are stagnant (fixed-point stability, highly ordered system), then there is no mechanism for change. The system cannot adapt and evolve because new states cannot be encoded into the system. If the system dynamics are chaotic (highly disordered), then the system is in a constant state of flux, and there is no memory, no learning, and no adaptation (some of the main qualities associated with life). Systems may exhibit transients in the evolution of states before settling down into either fixed-point or limit-cycle behavior. As the dynamics of a complex system enter the edge of chaos region, the length of these transients quickly grows. The chaotic region is where the length of the "transient" is infinite. At the edge of chaos (the dynamic phase transition) there is no characteristic scale due to the emergence of arbitrarily long correlation lengths in space and time [Langton, 1990]. The self-organized criticality in the sand piles of Per Bak is an example of a system that exists at the edge of chaos. It is in this region that there is no characteristic space or time scale. A single grain of sand added to the pile could cause an avalanche that consists of two grains of sand, or it could cause an avalanche that spreads over the entire surface of the sand pile.

61.2 Introduction to Scaling Theories

Prior to the rise of complexity theories, the existence of a systematic relationship between scales eluded the mainstream sciences. As a consequence, natural structures and dynamics have been commonly dismissed as too irregular and complex and often rejected as monstrous formations, intractable noise, or artifacts. The advent of scaling concepts [Mandelbrot, 1983] has uncovered a remarkable hierarchical order that persists over a significant number of spatial or temporal scales.

Scaling theories capitalize on scale-invariant symmetries exhibited by many natural broadband (i.e. multiscale) phenomena. According to the theory of self-organized criticality (see Section 61.1), this scaling order is a manifestation of dilation (compression) symmetries that define the organization inherent to complex systems which naturally evolve toward a critical state while dissipating energies on broad ranges of space and time scales. Long overlooked, this symmetry is now added to the repertoire of mathematical modeling concepts, which had included approaches based largely on displacement invariances under translation and/or rotation.

Many natural forms and functions maintain some form of exact or statistical invariance under transformations of scale and thus belong in the scaling category. Objects and processes that remain invariant under ordinary geometric similarity constitute the self-similar subset in this class.

Methods to capture scaling information in the form of simple rules that relate features on different scales are actively developed in many scientific fields [Barnsley, 1993]. Engineers are coping with scaling nature of forms and functions by investigating multiscale system theory [Basseville et al., 1992], multiresolution and multirate signal processing [Akansu & Hadad, 1992; Vaidyanathan, 1993], subband coding, wavelets, and filter banks [Meyer, 1993], and fractal compression [Barnsley & Hurd, 1993].

These emerging tools empower engineers to reexamine old data and to re-formulate the question at the root of many unresolved inverse problems—What can small patterns say about large patterns, and vice versa? They also offer the possibility to establish cause-effect relationships between a given physical (spatial) medium and the monitored dynamic (temporal) behavior that constitutes the primary preoccupation of diagnostic scientists.

Fractal Preliminaries

In the broadest sense, the noun or adjective *fractal* refers to physical objects or dynamic processes that reveal new details on space or time magnification. A staple of a truly fractal object or process is therefore the lack of characteristic scale in time or space. Most structures in nature are broadband over a finite range, covering at least a number of frequency decades in space or time. Scaling fractals often consist of a hierarchy or heterarchy of spatial or temporal structures in cascade and are often accomplished through recursive replication of patterns at finer scales. If the replication rule preserves scale invariance throughout the entity, such fractals are recognized as *self-similar* in either an exact or a statistical sense.

A prominent feature of fractals is their ability to pack structure with economy of resources, whether energy, space, or whatever other real estate. Fitting nearly infinite networks into finite spaces is just one such achievement. These types of fractals are pervasive in physiology, i.e., the branching patterns of the bronchi, the cardiovascular tree, and the nervous tissue [West and Goldberger, 1987], which have the additional feature of being "fault tolerant" [West, 1990].

Despite expectations heightened by the colorful publicity campaign mounted by promoters of fractal concepts, it is advisable to view fractals only as a starting approximation in analyzing scaling shapes and fluctuations in nature. Fractal concepts are usually descriptive at a phenomenologic level without pretense to reveal the exact nature of the underlying elementary processes. They do not offer, for that matter, conclusive evidence of whatever particular collective, coupled, or isolated repetitive mechanism that created the fractal object.

In many situations, the power of invoking fractal concepts resides in the fact that they bring the logic of constraints, whether in the form of asymmetry of motion caused by defects, traps, energy barriers, residual memories, irreversibility, or any other appropriate interaction or coupling mechanisms that hinder free random behavior. As discussed earlier, the spontaneous or forced organization and the ensuing divergence in correlations and coherences that emerges out of random behavior are presumably responsible for the irregular structures pervasive throughout the physical world.

More important, the versatility of fractal concepts as a magnifying tool is rooted in the facility to account for scale hierarchies and/or scale invariances in an exact or statistical sense. In the role of a scale microscope, they suggest a fresh look, with due respect to all scales of significance, at many structural and dynamic problems deemed thus far anomalous or insoluble.

Mathematical and Natural Fractals

The history of mathematics is rife with "pathologic" constructions of the iterated kind which defy the euclidian dimension concepts. The collection once included an assortment of anomalous dust sets, lines, surfaces, volumes, and other mathematical miscellenia mostly born out of the continuous yet nondifferentiable category of functions such as the Weierstrass series.

The feature unifying these mathematical creations with natural fractals is the fractional or integer dimensions distinct from the euclidian definition. Simply stated, a fractional dimension positions an object in between two integer dimensions in the euclidian sense, best articulated by the critical dimension in the Hausdorff-Besicovith derivation [Feder, 1988]. When this notion of dimension is pursued to the extreme and the dimension reaches an integer value, one is confronted with the counterintuitive reality of space-filling curves, volume-filling planes, etc. These objects can be seen readily to share intrinsic scaling properties with the nearly infinite networks accomplished by the branching patterns of bronchi and blood vessels and the intricate folding of the cortex.

A rewarding outcome afforded by the advent of scaling concepts is the ability to characterize such structures in terms of straightforward "scaling" or "dimension" measures. From these, simple iterative rules may be deduced to yield models with maximum economy (or minimum number) or parameters [Barnsley, 1993]. This principle is suspected to underlie the succinct coding adopted by nature in order to store extensive information needed to create complex shapes and forms.

Fractal Measures

The measure most often used in the diagnosis of a fractal is the basic *fractal dimension*, which, in the true spirit of fractals, has eluded a rigorous definition embracing the entire family of fractal objects. The guiding factor in the choice of the appropriate measures is the recognition that most fractal objects scale self-similarly; in other words, they can be characterized by a measure expressed in the form of a power factor, or scaling exponent ∂, that links the change in the observed dependent quantity V to the independent variable x as $V(x) \approx x^{\partial}$ [Falconer, 1990, p 36]. Clearly, ∂ is proportional to the ratio of the logarithm of $V(x)$ and x, i.e., $\partial = \log V(x)/\log x$. In the case of fractal objects, ∂ is the scaling exponent in the fractal sense and may have a fractional value. In the final analysis, most scaling relationships can be cast into some form of a logarithmic dependence on the independent variable with respect to which a scaling property is analyzed, the latter also expressed on the logarithmic scale. A number of dimension formulas have been developed based on this observation, and comprehensive compilations are now available [Falconer, 1990; Feder, 1988].

One approach to formalize the concept of scale invariance utilizes the *homogeneity* or the *renormalization* principle given by $f(\mu) = f(a\mu)/b$, where a and b are constants and μ is the independent variable [West & Goldberger, 1987]. The function f that satisfies this relationship is referred as a *scaling function*. The power-law function $f(\mu) \approx \mu^{\beta}$ is a prominent example in this category provided $\beta = \log b/\log a$. The usefulness of this particular scaling function has been proven many times over in many areas of science, including the thermodynamics of phase transitions and the threshold behavior of percolation networks [Schroeder, 1991; Stauffer & Aharony, 1992; Wilson, 1983].

Power Law and 1/f Processes

The revived interest in power-law behavior largely stems from the recognition that a large class of noisy signals exhibits spectra that attenuate with a fractional power dependence on frequency [West & Shlesinger, 1989; Wornell, 1993]. Such behavior is often viewed as a manifestation of the interplay of a multitude of local processes evolving on a spectrum of time scales that collectively give rise to the so-called $1/f^{\beta}$ or, more generally, the $1/f$-type behavior. As in the case of spatial fractals that lack a characteristic length scale, $1/f$ processes such as the fractional brownian motion cannot be described adequately within the confines of a "characteristic" time scale and hence exhibit the "fractal time" property [Mandelbrot, 1967].

Distributed Relaxation Processes

Since the later part of the nineteenth century, the fractional power function dependence of the frequency spectrum also has been recognized as a macroscopic dynamic property manifested by strongly interacting dielectric, viscoelastic, and magnetic materials and interfaces between different conducting materials [Daniel, 1967]. More recently, the $1/f$-type dynamic behavior has been observed in percolating networks composed of random mixtures of conductors and insulators and layered wave propagation in heterogeneous media [Orbach, 1986]. In immittance (impedance or admittance) studies, this frequency dispersion has been analyzed conventionally to distinguish a broad class of the so-called anomalous, i.e. nonexponential, relaxation/dispersion systems from those which can be described by the "ideal" single exponential form due to Debye [Daniel, 1967].

The fractal time or the multiplicity of time scales prevalent in distributed relaxation systems necessarily translates into fractional constitutive models amenable to analysis by fractional calculus [Ross, 1977] and fractional state-space methods [Bagley & Calico, 1991]. This corresponds to logarithmic distribution functions ranging in symmetry from the log-normal with even center symmetry at one extreme to single-sided hyperbolic distributions with diverging moments at the other. The realization that systems that do not possess a characteristic time can be described in terms of distributions renewed the interest in the field of dispersion/relaxation analysis. Logarithmic distribution functions have been used conventionally as means to characterize such complexity [West, 1994].

Multifractals

Fractal objects and processes in nature are rarely strictly homogeneous in their scaling properties and often display a distribution of scaling exponents that echos the structural heterogeneities occurring at a myriad of length or time scales. In systems with spectra that attenuate following a pure power law over extended frequency scales, as in the case of Davidson-Cole dispersion [Daniel, 1967], the corresponding distribution of relaxation times is logarithmic and single-tailed. In many natural relaxation systems, however, the spectral dimension exhibits a gradual dependence on frequency, as in phenomena conventionally modeled by the Cole-Cole type dispersion. The equivalent distribution functions exhibit double-sided symmetries on the logarithmic relaxation time scale ranging from the even symmetry of the log-normal through intermediate symmetries down to strictly one-sided functions.

The concept that a fractal structure can be composed of fractal subsets with uniform scaling property within the subset has gained popularity in recent years [Feder, 1988]. From this perspective, one may view a complicated fractal object, say, the strange attractor of a chaotic process, as a superposition of simple fractal subsystems. The idea has been formalized under the term *multifractal*. It follows that each individual member contributes to the overall scaling behavior according to a spectrum of scaling exponents or dimensions. The latter function is called the *multifractal spectrum* and summarizes the global scaling information of the complete set.

61.3 An Example of the Use of Complexity Theory in the Development of a Model of the Central Nervous System

Consciousness can be viewed as an emergent behavior arising from the interactions among a very large number of local agents, which, in this case, range from electrons through neurons and glial cells to networks of neurons. The hierarchical organization of the brain [Churchland & Sejnowski, 1992; Newell, 1990], which exists and evolves on a multitude of spatial and temporal scales, is a good example of the scaling characteristics found in many complex dynamic systems. There is no master controller for this emergent behavior, which results from the intricate interactions among a very large number of local agents.

A model that duplicates the global dynamics of the induction of unconsciousness in humans due to cerebral ischemia produced by linear acceleration stress (G-LOC) was constructed using some of the tenets of complexity [Cammarota, 1994]. It was an attempt to provide a theory that could both replicate historical human acceleration tolerance data and present a possible underlying mechanism. The model coupled the realization that an abrupt loss of consciousness could be thought of as a phase transition from consciousness to unconsciousness with the proposed neurophysiologic theory of G-LOC [Whinnery, 1989]. This phase transition was modeled using a percolation network to evaluate the connectivity of neural pathways within the central nervous system.

In order to construct the model, several hypotheses had to be formulated to account for the unobservable interplay among the local elements of the central nervous system. The inspiration for the characteristics of the locally interacting elements (the nodes of the percolation lattice) was provided by the physiologic mechanism of arousal (the all-or-nothing aspect of consciousness), the utilization of oxygen in neural tissue during ischemia, and the response of neural cells to metabolic threats. The neurophysiologic theory of acceleration tolerance views unconsciousness as an active protective mechanism that is triggered by a metabolic threat which in this case is acceleration-induced ischemia. The interplay among the local systems is determined by using a percolation network that models the connectivity of the arousal mechanism (the reticular activating system). When normal neuronal function is suppressed due to local cerebral ischemia, the corresponding node is removed from the percolation network. The configuration of the percolation network varies as a function of time. When the network is no longer able to support arousal, unconsciousness results.

The model simulated a wide range of human data with a high degree of fidelity. It duplicated the population response (measured as the time it took to lose consciousness) over a range of stresses that varied from a simulation of the acute arrest of cerebral circulation to a gradual application of acceleration stress. Moreover, the model was able to offer a possible unified explanation for apparently contradictory historical data. An analysis of the parameters responsible for the determination of the time of LOC indicated that there is a phase transition in the dynamics that was not explicitly incorporated into the construction of the model. The model spontaneously captured an interplay of the cardiovascular and neurologic systems that could not have been predicted based on existing data.

The keys to the model's success are the reasonable assumptions that were made about the characteristics and interaction of the local dynamic subsystems through the integration of a wide range of human and animal physiologic data in the design of the model. None of the local parameters was explicitly tuned to produce the global (input-output) behavior. By successfully duplicating the observed global behavior of humans under acceleration stress, however, this model provided insight into some (currently) unobservable inner dynamics of the central nervous system. Furthermore, the model suggests new experimental protocols specifically aimed at exploring further the microscopic interplay responsible for the macroscopic (observable) behavior.

Defining Terms

1/f process: Signals or systems that exhibit spectra which attenuate following a fractional power dependence on frequency.

Cellular automata: Composite discrete-time and discrete-space dynamic systems defined on a regular lattice. Neighborhood rules determine the state transitions of the individual local elements (cells).

Chaos: A state that produces a signal that resembles noise and is aperiodic, well-bounded, and very sensitive to initial conditions but is governed by a low-order deterministic differential or difference equation.

Complexity: Complexity theory is concerned with systems that have many degrees of freedom (composite systems), are spatially extended (systems with both spatial and temporal degrees of freedom), and are dissipative as well as nonlinear due to the rich interactions among the local components (agents). Some of the terms associated with such systems are emergent global behavior, collective behavior, cooperative behavior, self-organization, critical phenomena, and scale invariance.

Criticality: A state of a system where spatial and/or temporal characteristics are scale invariant.

Emergent global behavior: The observable behavior of a system that cannot be deduced from the properties of constituent components considered in isolation and results from the collective (cooperative or competitive) evolution of local events.

Fractal: Refers to physical objects or dynamic processes that reveal new details on space or time magnification. Fractals lack a characteristic scale.

Fractional brownian motion: A generalization of the random function created by the record of the motion of a "brownian particle" executing random walk. Brownian motion is commonly used to model diffusion in constraint-free media. Fractional brownian motion is often used to model diffusion of particles in constrained environments or anomalous diffusion.

Percolation: A simple mathematical construct commonly used to measure the extent of connectedness in a partially occupied (site percolation) or connected (bond percolation) lattice structure.

Phase transition: Any abrupt change between the physical and/or the dynamic states of a system, usually between ordered and disordered organization or behavior.

Renormalization: Changing the characteristic scale of a measurement though a process of systematic averaging applied to the microscopic elements of a system (also referred to as *coarse graining*).

Scaling: Structures or dynamics that maintain some form of exact or statistical invariance under transformations of scale.

Self-organization: The spontaneous emergence of order. This occurs without the direction of a global controller.

Self-similarity: A subset of objects and processes in the scaling category that remain invariant under ordinary geometric similarity.

References

Akansu AN, Haddad RA. 1992. Multiresolution Signal Decomposition: Transforms, Subbands, and Wavelets. New York, Academic Press.

Bagley R, Calico R. 1991. Fractional order state equations for the control of viscoelastic damped structures. J Guidance 14(2):304.

Bak P, Tang C, Wiesenfeld K. 1988. Self-organized criticality. Phys Rev A 38(1):364.

Bak P, Chen K. 1991. Self-organized criticality. Sci Am Jan:45.

Barnsley MF. 1993. Fractals Everywhere, 2d ed. New York, Academic Press.

Barnsley MF, Hurd LP. 1993. Fractal Image Compression. Wellesley, Mass, AK Peters.

Basseville M, Benveniste A, Chou KC, et al. 1992. Modeling and estimation of multiresolution stochastic processes. IEEE Trans Information Theory 38(2):766.

Cammarota JP. 1994. A Dynamic Percolation Model of the Central Nervous System under Acceleration (+Gz) Induced Ischemic/Hypoxic Stress. Ph.D. thesis, Drexel University, Philadelphia.

Churchland PS, Sejnowski TJ. 1992. The Computational Brain. Cambridge, Mass, MIT Press.

Daniel V. 1967. Dielectric Relaxation. New York, Academic Press.

Devaney RL. 1992. A First Course in Chaotic Dynamical Systems: Theory and Experiment. Reading, Mass, Addison-Wesley.

Falconer K. 1990. Fractal Geometry: Mathematical Foundations and Applications. New York, Wiley.

Feder J. 1988. Fractals. New York, Plenum Press.

Forrest S. 1990. Emergent computation: Self-organization, collective, and cooperative phenomena in natural and artificial computing networks. Physica D 42:1.

Goldberg DE. 1989. Genetic Algorithms in Search, Optimization, and Machine Learning. Reading, Mass, Addison-Wesley.

Harvey RL. 1994. Neural Network Principles. Englewood Cliffs, NJ, Prentice-Hall.

Langton CG. 1989. Artificial Life: Proceedings of on Interdisciplinary Workshop on the Synthesis and Simulation of Living Systems, September 1987, Los Alamos, New Mexico. Redwood City, Calif, Addison-Wesley.

Langton CG. 1990. Computation at the edge of chaos: Phase transitions and emergent computation. Physica D 42:12.

Langton CG, Taylor C, Farmer JD, Rasmussen S. 1992. Artificial Life II: Proceedings of the Workshop on Artificial Life, February 1990, Sante Fe, New Mexico. Redwood City, Calif, Addison-Wesley.

Mandelbrot B. 1967. Some noises with 1/f spectrum, a bridge between direct current and white noise. IEEE Trans Information Theory IT-13(2):289.

Mandelbrot B. 1983. The Fractal Geometry of Nature. New York, WH Freeman.

Meyer Y. 1993. Wavelets: Algorithms and Applications. Philadelphia, SIAM.

Newell A. 1990. Unified Theories of Cognition. Cambridge, Mass, Harvard University Press.

Orbach R. 1986. Dynamics of fractal networks. Science 231:814.

Peitgen HO, Richter PH. 1986. The Beauty of Fractals. New York, Springer-Verlag.

Ross B. 1977. Fractional calculus. Math Mag 50(3):115.

Shroeder M. 1990. Fractals, Chaos, Power Laws. New York, WH Freeman.

Simpson PK. 1990. Artificial Neural Systems: Foundations, Paradigms, Applications, and Implementations. New York, Pergamon Press.

Stauffer D, Aharony A. 1992. Introduction to Percolation, 2d ed. London, Taylor & Francis.

Toffoli T, Margolus N. 1987. Cellular Automata Machines: A New Environment for Modeling. Cambridge, Mass, MIT Press.

Tsonis PA, Tsonis AA. 1989. Chaos: Principles and implications in biology. Comput Appl Biosci 5(1):27.

Vaidyanathan PP. 1993. Multi-rate Systems and Filter Banks. Englewood Cliffs, NJ, Prentice-Hall.

West BJ. 1990. Physiology in fractal dimensions: Error tolerance. Ann Biomed Eng 18:135.

West BJ. 1994. Scaling statistics in biomedical phenomena. In Proceedings of the IFAC Conference on Modeling and Control in Biomedical Systems, Galveston, Texas.

West BJ, Goldberger A. 1987. Physiology in fractal dimensions. Am Scientist 75:354.

West BJ, Shlesinger M. 1989. On the ubiquity of $1/f$ noise. Int J Mod Phys 3(6):795.

Whinnery JE. 1989. Observations on the neurophysiologic theory of acceleration (+Gz) induced loss of consciousness. Aviat Space Environ Med 60:589.

Wilson KG. 1983. The renormalization group and critical phenomena. Rev Mod Phys 55(3):583.

Wornell GW. 1993. Wavelet-based representations for the $1/f$ family of fractal processes. IEEE Proc 81(10):1428.

62

Future Directions: Biomedical Signal Processing and Networked Multimedia Communications

Banu Onaral
Drexel University

The long anticipated "information age" is taking shape at the cross-section of multimedia signal processing and telecommunications-based networking. By defying the traditional concepts of space and time, these emerging technologies promise to affect all facets of our lives in a pervasive and profound manner [Mayo, 1992]. The physical constraints of location have naturally led, over the centuries, to the creation of the conventional patient care services and facilities. As the "information superhighway" is laid down with branches spanning the nation, and eventually the world, via wired and wireless communication channels, we will come closer to a bold new era in health care delivery, namely, the era of remote monitoring, diagnosis, and intervention.

Forward-looking medical industries are engaging in research and development efforts to capitalize on the emerging technologies. Medical institutions in particular recognize the transforming power of the impending revolution. A number of hospitals are undertaking pilot projects to experiment with the potentials of the new communication and interaction media that will constitute the foundations of futuristic health care systems. There is consensus among health care administrators that the agility and effectiveness with which an institution positions itself to fully embrace the new medical lifestyle will decide its viability in the next millennium.

Although multimedia communications is yet in its infancy, recent developments foretell a bright future. Many agree that multimedia networking is becoming a reality thanks to advances in digital signal-processing research and development. Trends toward implementation of algorithms by fewer components are leading to decreasing hardware complexity while increasing processing functionality [Andrews, 1994]. The vast and vibrant industry producing multimedia hardware and software ranging from application-specific digital signal processors and video chip sets to videophones and multimedia terminals heavily relies on digital signal processing know-how.

As in the case of generic digital signal processing, biomedical signal processing is expected to play a key role in mainstreaming patient care at a distance. Earlier in this section, emerging methods in biomedical signal analysis that promise major enhancements in our ability to extract information from vital signals were introduced. This chapter provides a glimpse of the future—when biomedical signals will be integrated with other patient information and transmitted via networked multimedia—by examining trends in key communications technologies, namely, public switched-network protocols, wireless communications, photonics, and virtual reality.

62.1 Public Switched Network and ATM

The public switched network already can accommodate a wide array of networked multimedia communications. The introduction of new standards such as the asynchronous transfer mode (ATM) is a strong sign that the network will evolve to handle an array of novel communication services.

ATM is a technology based on a switched network that uses dedicated media connections [ATM Networking, 1994]. Each connection between users is physically established by setting up a path or virtual channel through a series of integrated circuits in the switch. In conventional shared media networks, connections are made by breaking the information into packets labeled with their destination; these packets then share bandwidth until they reach their destination. In switched networks, instead of sharing bandwidth, connections can be run in parallel, since each connection has its own pathway. This approach prevents degradation of the response time despite increased number of users who are running intensive applications on the network, such as videoconferencing. Therefore, ATM offers consistently high performance to all users on the network, particularly in real-time networked multimedia applications which often encounter severe response time degradation on shared media networks. Also, the ATM standards for both local area networks (LANs) and wide area networks (WANs) are the same; this allows for seamless integration of LANs and WANs.

Small-scale experiments based on ATM-based multimedia communications are already launched in a number of medical centers. Early examples involve departments where doctors and staff can remotely work on chest x-rays, CT exams, and MRI images around the hospital over an ATM switched network. Since ATM integrates LANs and WANs, collaborating institutions will be able to access the same information in the future. Similar patient multimedia information-sharing efforts are underway which integrate all vital information including physiologic signals and sounds, images, and video and patient data and make them available remotely. In some recent experiments, the access is accomplished in real time such that medical conferencing, and hence remote diagnosis, becomes a possibility.

62.2 Wireless Communication

Wireless communication is the fastest growing sector of the telecommunications industry [Wittman, 1994]. Wireless networking technology is rapidly coming of age with the recent passage of initial standards, widespread performance improvements, and the introduction of personal communications networks (PCNs). Pocket-sized portable "smart" terminals are combined with wireless communication to free users from the constraints of wired connection to networks. The progress in this direction is closely monitored by the health care community because the technology holds the potential to liberate ambulatory patients who require long-term monitoring and processing of biomedical signals for timely intervention. Wireless and interactive access by medical personnel to physiologic multimedia information will no doubt be a stable of the future distributed health care delivery systems.

62.3 Photonics

Photonics, or lightwave, is an evolving technology with the capacity to support a wide range of high-bandwidth multimedia applications. In current practice, photonics plays a complementary role to electronics in the hybrid technology referred to as *electro-optics*. Optical fibers are widely used for transmission of signals, from long-distance links to undersea cables to local loops linking customers with the central switching office. The trend in photonics is to move beyond functions limited to transmission toward logic operations. Recent advances in photonic logic devices suggest that optical computers may present characteristics more desirable than electronics in many biomedical processing applications requiring parallel tasks. A case in point is on-line pattern recognition, which may bring a new dimension to remote diagnosis.

62.4 Virtual Reality

Virtual reality—the ultimate networked multimedia service—is a simulated environment that enables one to remotely experience an event or a place in all dimensions. Virtual reality makes telepresence possible. The nascent technology builds on the capabilities of interactive telecommunications and is expected to become a consumer reality early in the next century. Applications in the field of endoscopic surgery are being developed. Demonstration projects in remote surgery are underway, paving the way to remote medical intervention.

Acknowledgment

Contributions by Prabhakar R. Chitrapu, Dialogic Corporation, to material on networked multimedia communications in this chapter are gratefully acknowledged.

Defining Terms

ATM (asynchronous transfer mode): Technology based on a switched network that uses dedicated media connections.

CT: Computer tomography.

MRI: Magnetic resonance imaging.

Multimedia: Technology to integrate sights, sounds, and data. The media may include audio signals such as speech, music, biomedical sounds, images, animation, and video signals, as well as text, graphics, and fax. One key feature is the common linkage, synchronization, and control of the various media that contribute to the overall multimedia signal. In general, multimedia services and products are interactive, hence real-time, as in the case of collaborative computing and videoconferencing.

Photonics: Switching, computing, and communications technologies based on lightwave.

Virtual reality: Technology that creates a simulated environment enabling one to remotely experience an event or a place in all dimensions.

Wireless network: Technology based on communication between nodes such as stationary desktops, laptops, or personal digital assistants (PDAs) and the LAN hub or access point using a wireless adapter with radio circuitry and an antenna. The LAN hub has a LAN attachment on one interface and one or more antennas on another.

References

Andrews D. 1994. Digital signal processing: The engine to make multimedia mainstream. Byte 22.

ATM Networking: Increasing performance on the network. HEPC Syllabus 3(7):12, 1994.

Mayo JS. 1992. The promise of networked multimedia communications. Bear Stearns Sixth Annual Media and Communications Conference, Coronado, Calif.

Wittmann A. 1994. Will wireless win the war? Network Computing 58.

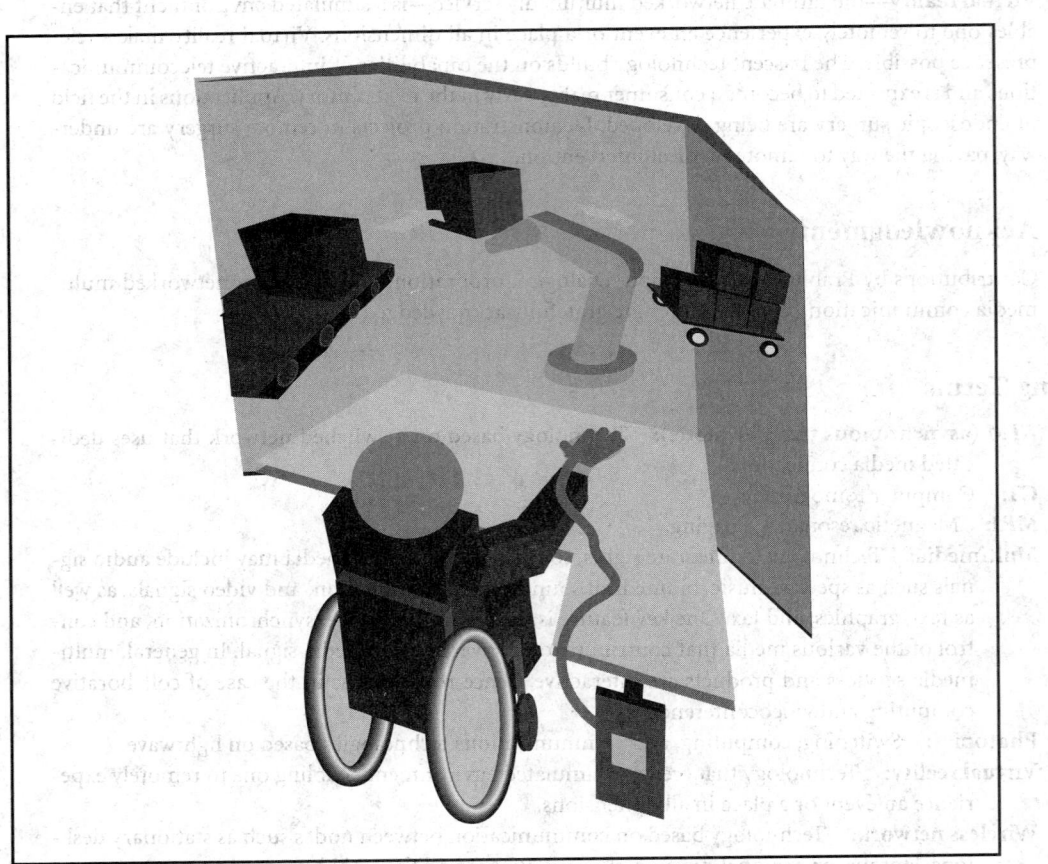

VR system used by the disabled.

VII

Imaging

Karen M. Mudry
The Whitaker Foundation

T HE FIELD OF MEDICAL IMAGING has experienced phenomenal growth within the last century. Whereas imaging was the prerogative of the defense and the space science communities in the past, with the advent of powerful, less-expensive computers, new and expanded imaging systems have found their way into the medical field. Systems range from those devoted to planar imaging using x-rays to technologies that are just emerging, such as virtual reality. Some of the systems, such as ultrasound, are relatively inexpensive, while others, such as positron emission tomography (PET) facilities, cost millions of dollars for the hardware and the employment of Ph.D.-level personnel to operate them. Systems that make use of x-rays have been designed to image anatomic structures, while others that make use of radioisotopes provide functional information. The fields of view that can be imaged range from the whole body obtained with nuclear medicine bone scans to images of cellular components using magnetic resonance (MR) microscopy. The design of transducers for the imaging devices to the postprocessing of the data to allow easier interpretation of the images by medical personnel are all aspects of the medical imaging devices field.

Even with the sophisticated systems now available, challenges remain in the medical imaging field. With the increasing emphasis on health care costs, and with medical imaging systems often cited as an example of the investment that health care providers must make and, consequently, recover that is involved in escalating costs, there is increasing emphasis on lowering the costs of new systems. Researchers, for example, are trying to find alternatives to the high-cost superconducting magnets used for magnetic resonance systems. With the decreasing cost of the powerful computers that are currently contained within most imaging systems and with the intense competition among imaging companies, prices for these systems are bound to fall. Other challenges entail presentation of the imaging data. Often multiple modalities are used during a clinical evaluation. If both anatomic and functional information are required, methods to combine and present these data for medical interpretation need to be achieved. The use of medical image data to more effectively execute surgery is a field that is only starting to be explored. How can anatomic data obtained with a tomographic scan be correlated with the surgical field, given that movement of tissues and organs occurs during surgery? Virtual reality is likely to play an important role in this integration of imaging information with surgery. There also are imaging modalities that are just beginning to be intensively explored, such as the detection of impedance and magnetic field data or the use of optical sources and detectors.

Engineers and physical scientists are involved throughout the medical imaging field. They are employed by both large and small companies. The names of the medical imaging giants, such as General Electric, Siemens, Picker, and Acuson, are familiar to most. Small startup companies are prevalent. In addition to the medical imaging companies, Ph.D.-trained engineers and scientists are employed by departments of engineering, physics, and chemistry in universities and more and more by radiology departments of research-oriented medical centers. Whereas only a few years ago researchers working in the medical imaging field would submit papers to general scientific journals, such as the *IEEE Transactions on Biomedical Engineering*, now there is a journal, *IEEE Transactions on Medical Imaging*, devoted to the medical imaging field and journals dedicated to certain modalities, such as *Magnetic Resonance in Medicine* and *Journal of Computer Assisted Tomography*. Large scientific meetings for medical imaging, such as the Radiological Society of North America's annual meeting with over 20,000 attendees, are held each year. Modality-specific meetings, such as that of the Society for Magnetic Resonance in Imaging, have thousands of attendees.

Although entire books have been written on each of the medical imaging modalities, this section will provide an overview of the main medical imaging devices and also highlight a few emerging systems. Chapter 63 describes x-ray systems, the backbone of the medical imaging field. X-ray systems are still quite important because of their relatively low system acquisition cost, the low cost of the diagnostic procedures, and the speed with which results are obtained. Chapter 64 describes computed tomographic (CT) systems. This technology became available in the 1970s, with current improvements focused on acquisition speed and data presentations. Chapter 65 highlights magnetic resonance imaging (MRI), a technology that first became available in the 1980s. The technology is rapidly evolving, with major advances recently in the areas of functional and spectroscopic MRI. Nuclear medicine, the subject of Chapter 66, covers both planar and single-photon emission computed tomography (SPECT) systems. Chapter 67 covers ultrasound, the technology that is widely used for obstetrical imaging and vascular flow evaluation. The latest research on linear and two-dimensional transducers, which will be able to provide real-time three-dimensional ultrasound images, is also covered in this chapter. Less prevalent technologies are presented in Chapters 68 to 71.

These include the field of MR microscopy, which requires high-field-strength magnets; position emission tomography (PET), which has a tremendous potential for functional imaging; impedance tomography, which is aimed at constructing images based on difference in conductivity between different body tissues; and virtual reality, which provides an overview of the high-tech field of interactive imaging that is bound to become increasingly important as computing power increases.

63
X-Ray

Robert E. Shroy, Jr.
Picker International

Michael S. Van Lysel
University of Wisconsin

Martin J. Yaffe
University of Toronto

63.1 X-Ray Equipment

Robert E. Shroy, Jr.

Conventional x-ray radiography produces images of anatomy that are shadowgrams based on x-ray absorption. The x-rays are produced in a region that is nearly a point source and then are directed on the anatomy to be imaged. The x-rays emerging from the anatomy are detected to form a two-dimensional image, where each point in the image has a brightness related to the intensity of the x-rays at that point. Image production relies on the fact that significant numbers of x-rays penetrate through the anatomy and that different parts of the anatomy absorb different amounts of x-rays. In cases where the anatomy of interest does not absorb x-rays differently from surrounding regions, contrast may be increased by introducing strong x-ray absorbers. For example, barium is often used to image the gastrointestinal tract.

X-rays are electromagnetic waves (like light) having an energy in the general range of approximately 1 to several hundred kiloelectronvolts (keV). In medical x-ray imaging, the x-ray energy typically lies between 5 and 150 keV, with the energy adjusted to the anatomic thickness and the type of study being performed.

X-rays striking an object may either pass through unaffected or may undergo an interaction. These interactions usually involve either the photoelectric effect (where the x-ray is absorbed) or scattering (where the x-ray is deflected to the side with a loss of some energy). X-rays that have been scattered may undergo deflection through a small angle and still reach the image detector; in this case they reduce image contrast and thus degrade the image. This degradation can be reduced by the use of an air gap between the anatomy and the image receptor or by use of an antiscatter grid.

Because of health effects, the doses in radiography are kept as low as possible. However, x-ray quantum noise becomes more apparent in the image as the dose is lowered. This noise is due to the fact that there is an unavoidable random variation in the number of x-rays reaching a point on an image detector. The quantum noise depends on the average number of x-rays striking the image detector and is a fundamental limit to radiographic image quality.

The equipment of conventional x-ray radiography mostly deals with the creation of a desirable beam of x-rays and with the detection of a high-quality image of the transmitted x-rays. These are discussed in the following sections.

Production of X-Rays

X-Ray Tube

The standard device for production of x-rays is the rotating anode x-ray tube, as illustrated in Fig. 63.1. The x-rays are produced from electrons that have been accelerated in vacuum from the cathode to the anode. The electrons are emitted from a filament mounted within a groove in the cathode. Emission occurs when the filament is heated by passing a current through it. When the filament is hot enough, some electrons obtain a thermal energy sufficient to overcome the energy binding the electron to the metal of the filament. Once the electrons have "boiled off" from the filament, they are accelerated by a voltage difference applied from the cathode to the anode. This voltage is supplied by a generator (see below).

After the electrons have been accelerated to the anode, they will be stopped in a short distance. Most of the electrons' energy is converted into heating of the anode, but a small percentage is converted to x-rays by two main methods. One method of x-ray production relies on the fact that deceleration of a charged particle results in emission of electromagnetic radiation, called *bremmstralung radiation*. These x-rays will have a wide, continuous distribution of energies, with the maximum being the total energy the electron had when reaching the anode. The number of x-rays is relatively small at higher energies and increases for lower energies.

A second method of x-ray production occurs when an accelerated electron strikes an atom in the anode and removes an inner electron from this atom. The vacant electron orbital will be filled by a neighboring electron, and an x-ray may be emitted whose energy matches the energy change of the electron. The result is production of large numbers of x-rays at a few discrete energies. Since the en-

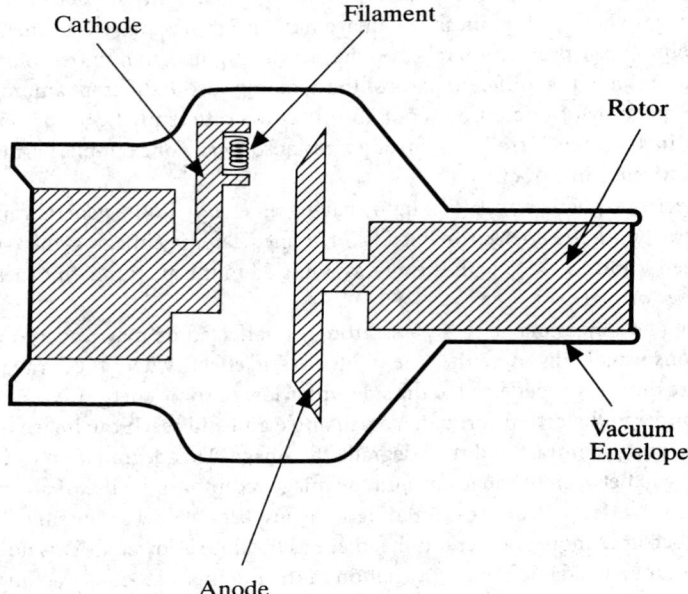

FIGURE 63.1   X-ray tube.

ergy of these characteristic x-rays depends on the material on the surface of the anode, materials are chosen partially to produce x-rays with desired energies. For example, molybdenum is frequently used in anodes of mammography x-ray tubes because of its 20-keV characteristic x-rays.

Low-energy x-rays are undesirable because they increase dose to the patient but do not contribute to the final image because they are almost totally absorbed. Therefore, the number of low-energy x-rays is usually reduced by use of a layer of absorber that preferentially absorbs them. The extent to which low-energy x-rays have been removed can be quantified by the half-value layer of the x-ray beam.

It is ideal to create x-rays from a point source because any increase in source size will result in blurring of the final image. Quantitatively, the effects of the blurring are described by the focal spot's contribution to the system modulation transfer function (MTF). The blurring has its main effect on edges and small objects, which correspond to the higher frequencies. The effect of this blurring depends on the geometry of the imaging and is worse for larger distances between the object and the image receptor (which corresponds to larger geometric magnifications).

To avoid this blurring, the electrons must be focused to strike a small spot of the anode. The focusing is achieved by electric fields determined by the exact shape of the cathode. However, there is a limit to the size of this focal spot because the anode material will melt if too much power is deposited into too small an area. This limit is improved by use of a rotating anode, where the anode target material is rotated about a central axis and new (cooler) anode material is constantly being rotated into place at the focal spot. To further increase the power limit, the anode is made with an angled surface. This allows the heat to be deposited in a relatively large spot while the apparent spot size at the detector will be smaller by a factor of the sine of the anode angle. Unfortunately, this angle cannot be made too small because it limits the area that can be covered with x-rays. In practice, tubes are usually supplied with two (or more) focal spots of differing sizes, allowing choice of a smaller (sharper, lower-power) spot or a larger (more blurry, higher-power) spot.

The x-ray tube also limits the total number of x-rays that can be used in an exposure because the anode will melt if too much total energy is deposited in it. This limit can be increased by using a more massive anode.

Generator

The voltages and currents in an x-ray tube are supplied by an x-ray generator. This controls the cathode-anode voltage, which partially defines the number of x-rays made because the number of x-rays produced increases with voltage. The voltage is also chosen to produce x-rays with desired energies: Higher voltages make x-rays that generally are more penetrating but give a lower contrast image. The generator also determines the number of x-rays created by controlling the amount of current flowing from the cathode to anode and by controlling the length of time this current flows. This points out the two major parameters that describe an x-ray exposure: the peak kilovolts (peak kilovolts from the anode to the cathode during the exposure) and the milliampere-seconds (the product of the current in milliamperes and the exposure time in seconds).

The peak kilovolts and milliampere-seconds for an exposure may be set manually by an operator based on estimates of the anatomy. Some generators use manual entry of kilovolts and milliamperes but determine the exposure time automatically. This involves sampling the radiation either before or after the image sensor and is referred to as *phototiming*.

The anode-cathode voltage (often 15 to 150 kV) can be produced by a transformer that converts 120 or 220 V ac to higher voltages. This output is then rectified and filtered. Use of three-phase transformers gives voltages that are more nearly constant than those from single-phase transformers, thus avoiding low kilovoltages that produce undesired low-energy x-rays. In a variation of this method, the transformer output can be controlled at a constant voltage by electron tubes. This gives practically constant voltages and, further, allows the voltage to be turned on and off so quickly that millisecond exposure times can be achieved. In a third approach, an ac input can be rectified and filtered to produce a nearly dc voltage, which is then sent to a solid-state inverter that can turn on and off thousands of times a second. This higher-frequency ac voltage can be converted more easily to a high voltage by a transformer. Equipment operating on this principle is referred to as *midfrequency* or *high-frequency generators.*

Image Detection: Screen Film Combinations

Special properties are needed for image detection in radiographic applications, where a few high-quality images are made in a study. Because decisions are not immediately made from the images, it is not necessary to display them instantly (although it may be desirable).

The most commonly used method of detecting such a radiographic x-ray image uses light-sensitive negative film as a medium. Because high-quality film has a poor response to x-rays, it must used together with x-ray–sensitive screens. Such screens are usually made with $CaWO_2$ or phosphors using rare earth elements such as doped Gd_2O_2S or LaOBr. The film is enclosed in a light-tight cassette in contact with an x-ray screen or in between two x-ray screens. When an x-ray image strikes the cassette, the x-rays are absorbed by the screens with high efficiency, and their energy is converted to visible light. The light then exposes a negative image on the film, which is in close contact with the screen.

Several properties have been found to be important in describing the relative performance of different films. One critical property is the *contrast,* which describes the amount of additional darkening caused by an additional amount of light when working near the center of a film's exposure range. Another property, the *latitude* of a film, describes the film's ability to create a usable image with a wide range in input light levels. Generally, latitude and contrast are competing properties, and a film with a large latitude will have a low contrast. Additionally, the modulation transfer function (MTF) of a film is an important property. MTF is most degraded at higher frequencies; this high-frequency MTF also is described by the film's *resolution,* its ability to image small objects.

X-ray screens also have several key performance parameters. It is essential that screens detect and use a large percentage of the x-rays striking them, which is measured as the screen's quantum detection efficiency. Currently used screens may detect 30% of x-rays for images at higher peak kilovolts and as much 60% for lower peak kilovolt images. Such efficiencies lead to the use of two screens (one on each side of the film) for improved x-ray utilization. As with films, a good high-frequency MTF is needed to give good visibility of small structures and edges. Some MTF degradation is associated with blurring that occurs when light spreads as it travels through the screen and to the film. This leads to a compromise on thickness; screens must be thick enough for good quantum detection efficiency but thin enough to avoid excess blurring.

For a film/screen system, a certain amount of radiation will be required to produce a usable amount of film darkening. The ability of the film/screen system to make an image with a small amount of radiation is referred to as its *speed.* The speed depends on a number of parameters: the quantum detection efficiency of the screen, the efficiency with which the screen converts x-ray energy to light, the match between the color emitted by the screen and the colors to which the film is sensitive, and the amount of film darkening for a given amount of light. The number of x-rays used in producing a radiographic image will be chosen to give a viewable amount of exposure to the film. Therefore, patient dose will be reduced by the use of a high-speed screen/film system. However, high-speed film/screen combinations give a "noisier" image because of the smaller number of x-rays detected in its creation.

Image Detection: X-Ray Image Intensifiers with Televisions

Although screen-film systems are excellent for radiography, they are not usable for fluoroscopy, where lower x-ray levels are produced continuously and many images must be presented almost immediately. Fluoroscopic images are not used for diagnosis but rather as an aid in performing tasks such as placement of catheters in blood vessels during angiography. For fluoroscopy, x-ray image intensifiers are used in conjunction with television cameras. An x-ray image intensifier detects the x-ray image and converts it to a small, bright image of visible light. This visible image is then transferred by lenses to a television camera for final display on a monitor.

The basic structure of an x-ray image intensifier is shown in Fig. 63.2. The components are held in a vacuum by an enclosure made of glass and/or metal. The x-rays enter through a low-absorption window and then strike an input phosphor usually made of doped CsI. As in the x-ray screens described above, the x-rays are converted to light in the CsI. On top of the CsI layer is a photoemitter, which absorbs the light and emits a number of low-energy electrons that initially spread in various directions. The photoelectrons are accelerated and steered by a set of grids that have voltages applied to them. The electrons strike an output phosphor structure that converts their energy to the final output image made of light. This light then travels through an output window to a lens system. The grid voltages serve to add energy to the electrons so that the output image is brighter. Grid voltages and shapes are also chosen so that the x-ray image is converted to a light image with minimal distortion. Further, the grids must be designed to take photoelectrons that are spreading from a point on the photoemitter and focus them back together at a point on the output phosphor.

It is possible to adjust grid voltages on an image intensifier so that it has different fields of coverage. Either the whole input area can be imaged on the output phosphor, or smaller parts of the input can be imaged on the whole output. Use of smaller parts of the input is advantageous when only smaller parts of anatomy need to be imaged with maximum resolution and a large display. For example, an image intensifier that could cover a 12-in-diameter input also might be operated so that a 9-in-diameter or 6-in-diameter input covers all the output phosphor.

X-ray image intensifiers can be described by a set of performance parameters not unlike those of screen/film combinations. It is important that x-rays be detected and used with a high efficiency; current image intensifiers have quantum detection efficiencies of 60% to 70% for 59-keV x-rays. As with film/screens, a good high-frequency MTF is needed to image small objects and sharp edges without blurring. However, low-frequency MTF also must be controlled carefully in image intensifiers, since it can be degraded by internal scattering of x-rays, photoelectrons, and light over rela-

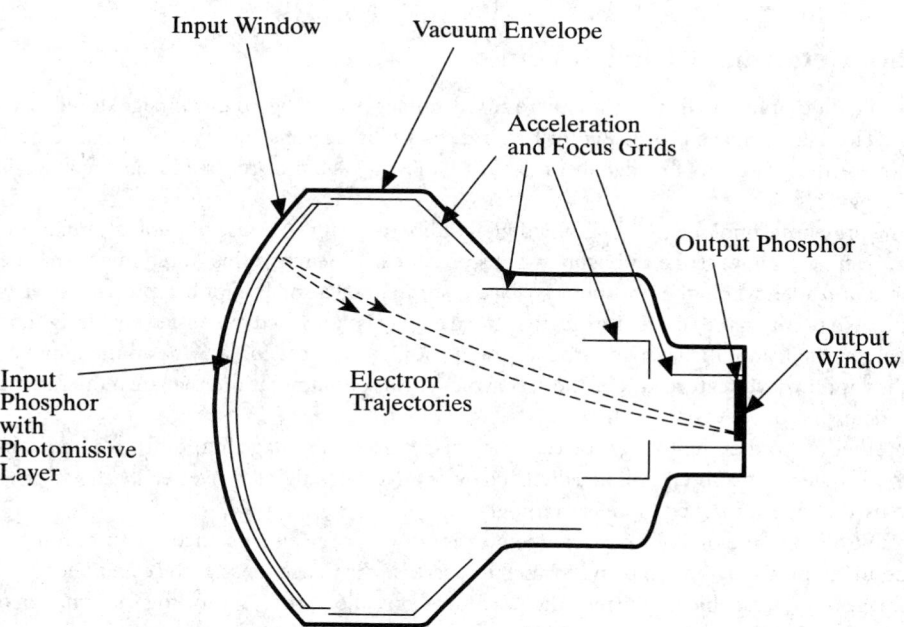

FIGURE 63.2   X-ray image intensifier.

tively large distances. The amount of intensification depends on brightness and size of the output image for a given x-ray input. This is described either by the gain (specified relative to a standard x-ray screen) or by conversion efficiency [a light output per radiation input measured in $(cd/m^2)/(mR/min)$]. Note that producing a smaller output image is as important as making a light image with more photons because the small image can be handled more efficiently by the lenses that follow. Especially when imaging the full input area, image intensifiers introduce a pincushion distortion into the output image. Thus a square object placed off-center will produce an image that is stretched in the direction away from the center.

Although an image intensifier output could be viewed directly with a lens system, there is more flexibility when the image intensifier is viewed with a television camera and the output is displayed on a monitor. Televisions are currently used with pickup tubes and with CCD sensors.

When a television tube is used, the image is focused on a charged photoconducting material at the tube's input. A number of materials are used, including SbS_3, PbO, and $SeTeAs$. The light image discharges regions of the photoconductor, converting the image to a charge distribution on the back of the photoconducting layer. Next, the charge distribution is read by scanning a small beam of electrons across the surface, which recharges the photoconductor. The recharging current is proportional to the light intensity at the point being scanned; this current is amplified and then used to produce an image on a monitor. The tube target is generally scanned in an interlaced mode in order to be consistent with broadcast television and allow use of standard equipment.

In fluoroscopy, it is desirable to use the same detected dose for all studies so that the image noise is approximately constant. This is usually achieved by monitoring the image brightness in a central part of the image intensifier's output, since brightness generally increases with dose. The brightness may be monitored by a photomultiplier tube that samples it directly or by analyzing signal levels in the television. However, maintaining a constant detected dose would lead to high patient doses in the case of very absorptive anatomy. To avoid problems here, systems are generally required by federal regulations to have a limit on the maximum patient dose. In those cases where the dose limit prevents the image intensifier from receiving the usual dose, the output image becomes darker. To compensate for this, television systems are often operated with automatic gain control that gives an image on the monitor of a constant brightness no matter what the brightness from the image intensifier.

Image Detection: Digital Systems

In both radiography and fluoroscopy, there are advantages to having a digital image stored in a computer. This allows image processing for better displayed images, use of lower doses in some cases, and opens the possibility for digital storage with a PACS system or remote image viewing via teleradiology.

One present technology for obtaining digital radiographs involves use of photostimulable phosphors. Here the x-rays strike a phosphor that stores the x-ray energy; this stored image can then be taken to a reader, where the phosphor surface is scanned by a small light beam of a proper wavelength. As a point on the surface is read, the stored energy is converted to emitted visible light, which is then detected, amplified, and digitized. A range of image processing may be applied. In particular, the window/level feature may let the user avoid repeats of examinations that are moderately over- or underexposed.

Another method of digitizing medical x-ray images uses the voltage output from a image-intensifier/TV system. This voltage may be digitized by an analog-to-digital converter at rates fast enough to be used with fluoroscopy as well as radiography.

In fluoroscopy, the digital image can be processed with edge enhancement or smoothing. Also, frame-to-frame averaging can be performed to decrease the image noise at the expense of blurring the image of moving objects. Further, digital fluoroscopy allows the TV tube to be scanned in other formats than standard interlaced; the image can always be displayed with an interlaced or other high-quality format. When fluoroscopy is ended, the digital image is not allowed to go black, but a repeated display of the last image is shown. This last image hold significantly reduces dose in those cases where the radiologist needs to see an image for evaluation but does not necessarily need a continuously updated image.

The processing of digital systems additionally allows the use of pulsed fluoroscopy, where the x-rays are produced in a short, intense burst instead of continuously. In this method, brief pulses of x-rays are made either by biasing the x-ray tube filament or by quickly turning on and off the anode-cathode voltage. This has the advantage of making sharper images of objects that are moving. Usually there is one x-ray pulse per television frame, but there is also the ability to obtain dose reduction by not turning on an x-ray pulse for every television frame. With this reduced exposure rate, doses can be reduced a factor of two or four by only making x-rays every second or fourth frame. For those frames with no x-ray pulse, the system repeats a display of the previous frame.

The image-intensifier/TV system also can be used to produce digital radiographic images. Such digital radiography can be used with significant dose reductions in common applications such as gastrointestinal studies. In radiography, the image from the image intensifier is much brighter than in fluoroscopy, which leads to use of a smaller iris in the lens system at the television's input. Higher x-ray fluxes give better image signal-to-noise ratios, which puts tight limits on television electronic noise; signal-to-noise ratios of over 1000:1 are common for televisions in this application. A full range of image processing is available, and the immediate availability of images is useful in evaluating the quality of a study or in making decisions about further studies.

Digital radiographs from image intensifier/TVs are especially useful in angiography, where iodine dye is usually injected into arteries in order to make them visible in x-ray images. In such an application, digital images will be taken before dye is injected and as the dye flows through the arteries. Images from before injection are subtracted from images with dye, thus removing overlaying anatomy and giving images of just the arteries. In order to avoid having the arteries change brightness as they pass over structures of different x-ray absorption, logarithmic processing is applied to images before subtraction. If there is patient motion between the dye and mask frames, the mask frame can be digitally reregistered.

Defining Terms

Antiscatter grid: A thin structure made of alternating strips of lead and material transmissive to x-rays. Strips are oriented so that most scattered x-rays go through lead sections and are preferentially absorbed, while unscattered x-rays go through transmissive sections.

Focal spot: The small area on the anode of an x-ray tube from where x-rays are emitted. It is the place where the accelerated electron beam is focused.

Half-value layer (HVL):   The thickness of a material (often aluminum) needed to absorb half the x-rays in a beam.

keV: A unit of energy useful with x-rays. It is equal to the energy supplied to an electron when accelerated through 1 kilovolt.

Modulation transfer function (MTF):   The ratio of the contrast in the output image of a system to the contrast in the object, specified for sine waves of various frequencies. Describes blurring (loss of contrast) in an imaging system for different-sized objects.

Quantum detection efficiency: The percentage of incident x-rays effectively used to create an image.

References

Bushberg JT, Seibert JA, Leidholdt EM, Boone JM. 1994. The Essential Physics of Medical Imaging. Baltimore, Williams & Wilkins.

Curry TS, Dowdey JE, Murry RC. 1984. Christensen's Introduction to the Physics of Diagnostic Radiology. Philadelphia, Lea & Febiger.

Hendee WR, Ritenour R. 1992. Medical Imaging Physics. St. Louis, Mosby–Year Book.

Ter-Pogossian MM. 1969. The Physical Aspects of Diagnostic Radiology. New York, Harper & Row.

Further Information

Medical Physics is a monthly scientific and informational journal published for the American Association of Physicists in Medicine. Papers here generally cover evaluation of existing medical equipment and development of new systems. For more information, contact the American Association of Physicists in Medicine, One Physics Ellipse, College Park, MD 20740-3846.

The Society of Photo-Optical Instrumentation Engineers (SPIE) sponsors numerous conferences and publishes their proceedings. Especially relevant is the annual conference on Medical Imaging. Contact SPIE, P.O. Box 10, Bellham, WA 98227-0010.

Several corporations active in medical imaging work together under the National Electrical Manufacturers Association to develop definitions and testing standards for equipment used in the field. Information can be obtained from NEMA, 2101 L Street N.W., Washington, DC 20037.

Critical aspects of medical x-ray imaging are covered by rules of the Food and Drug Administration, part of the Department of Health and Human Services. These are listed in the *Code of Federal Regulations*, Title 21. Copies are for sale by the Superintendent of Documents, U.S. Government Printing Office, Washington, DC 20402.

63.2 X-Ray Projection Angiography

Michael S. Van Lysel

Angiography is a diagnostic and, increasingly, therapeutic modality concerned with diseases of the circulatory system. While many imaging modalities (ultrasound, computed tomography, magnetic resonance imaging, angioscopy) are now available, either clinically or for research, to study vascular structures, this section will focus on the clinical angiographic workhouse, projection radiography. In this method, the vessel of interest is opacified by injection of a radiopaque contrast agent. Serial radiographs of the contrast material flowing through the vessel are then acquired. This examination is performed in an angiographic suite, a special procedures laboratory, or a cardiac catheterization laboratory.

Contrast material is needed to opacify vascular structures because the radiographic contrast of blood is essentially the same as that of soft tissue. Contrast material consists of an iodine-containing ($Z = 53$) compound, with maximum iodine concentrations of about 350 mg/cm^3. Contrast material is injected through a catheter ranging in diameter roughly from 1 to 3 mm, depending on the injection flow rate to be used. Radiographic images of the contrast-filled vessels are recorded using either film or video.

The most important change in angiography during the last decade has been the rapid adoption of digital imaging technology to the acquisition and storage of angiographic images. The most important application of digital imaging is digital subtraction angiography (DSA). Temporal subtraction is a DSA mode in which a preinjection image (the mask) is acquired, the injection of contrast agent is then performed, and then sequential images of the opacified vessel(s) are acquired and subtracted from the mask. The result, ideally, is that the fixed anatomy is canceled, allowing contrast enhancement (similar to computed tomographic windowing and leveling) to provide increased contrast sensitivity.

Introduced in the early 1980s, DSA was first used to perform intravenous DSA (IV-DSA), in which the contrast agent is injected into the venous side of the circulation (usually the vena cava or right atrium). The allure of IV-DSA was the belief that injection into the venous system, as opposed to the more conventional direct arterial injection, was less invasive and therefore resulted in less risk and less discomfort to the patient. IV injection is not practical without the contrast enhancement of DSA (film subtraction also allows contrast enhancement but is considerably more cumbersome and provides less contrast sensitivity than digital subtraction) because of the 10× to 20× dilution of the contrast agent at the arterial site of interest. However, several factors have greatly reduced the enthusiasm for IV-DSA, including sensitivity to artifacts resulting from patient motion, low signal-to-noise ratio, higher patient contrast load, and vessel superposition. The majority of angiography today, while still performed via DSA, uses direct injection of the contrast agent into the arterial side of the circulatory system.

An increasingly important facet of the angiographic procedure is the use of transluminal interventional techniques to effect a therapeutic result. These techniques, including angioplasty, atherectomy, laser ablation, and intraluminal stents, rely on digital angiographic imaging technology to facilitate the precise catheter manipulations necessary for a successful result. In fact, digital enhancement, storage, and retrieval of fluoroscopic images have become mandatory capabilities for digital angiographic systems.

Figure 63.3 is a schematic representation of an angiographic imaging system. The basic components include an x-ray tube and generator, image intensifier, video camera, cine camera (for cine), digital image processor (optional), and a film changer (optional).

X-Ray Generation

Angiographic systems require a high-power, sophisticated x-ray generation system in order to produce the short, intense x-ray pulses needed to produce clear images of moving vessels. Required exposure times range from 100 to 200 ms for cerebral studies to 1 to 10 ms for cardiac studies. Angiographic systems use either a three-phase 12-pulse x-ray generator, a constant potential generator, or, increasingly, a medium/high-frequency inverter generator. Power ratings for angiographic generators are generally greater than or equal to 80 kW at 100 kW and must be capable of producing reasonably square x-ray pulses. In most cases (pediatric cardiology being an exception), pulse widths of 5 ms or greater are necessary to keep the x-ray tube potential in the desirable, high-contrast range of 70 to 90 kVp.

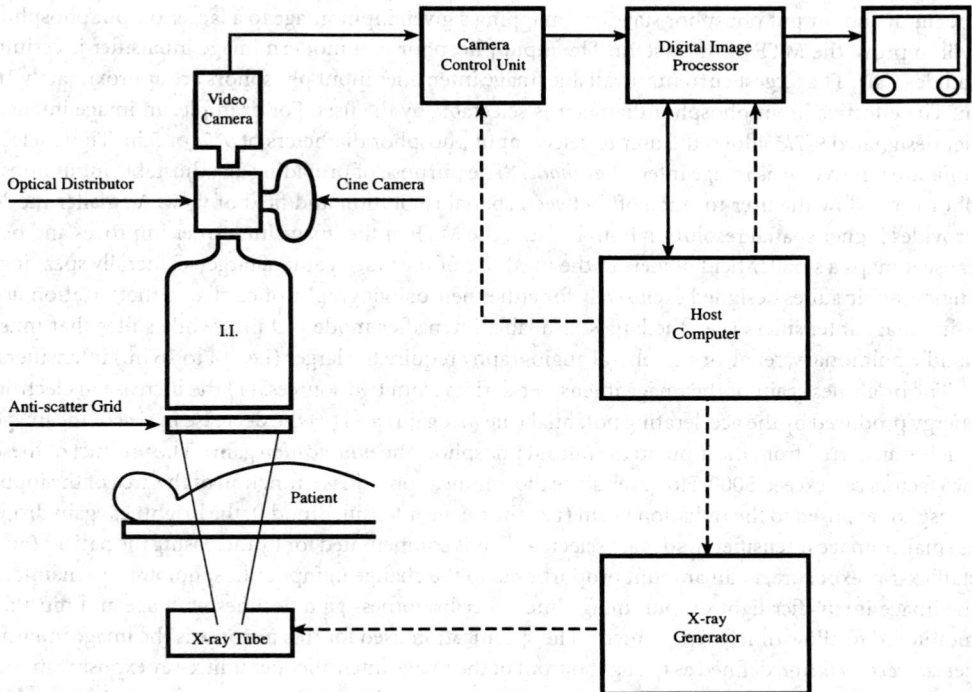

FIGURE 63.3 Schematic diagram of an image intensifier–based digital angiographic and cine imaging system. Solid arrows indicate image signals, and dotted arrows indicate control signals.

The x-ray tube is of the rotating-anode variety. Serial runs of high-intensity x-ray pulses result in high heat loads. Anode heat storage capacities of 1 mega-heat units (MHU) or greater are desirable, especially in the case of cine angiography. Electronic "heat computers," which calculate and display the current heat load of the x-ray tube, are very useful in preventing damage to the x-ray tube. In a high-throughput angiographic suite, forced liquid cooling of the x-ray tube housing is essential. Angiographic x-ray tubes are of multifocal design, with the focal spot sizes tailored for the intended use. A 0.6-mm (50-kW loading), 1.2-mm (100-kW loading) bifocal insert is common. The specified heat loads for a given focal spot are for single exposures. When serial angiographic exposures are performed, the focal spot load limit must be derated (reduced) to account for the accumulation of heat in the focal spot target track during the run. Larger focal spots (e.g., 1.8 mm) can be obtained for high-load procedures. A smaller focal spot [e.g., 0.3 and 0.1 mm (bias)] is needed for magnification studies. Small focal spots have become increasingly desirable for high-resolution fluoroscopic interventional studies performed with 1000-line video systems.

Image Formation

Image Intensifier

The image intensifier (II) is fundamental to the modern angiographic procedure. The purpose of the image intensifier is (1) to produce a light image with sufficient brightness to allow the use of video and film cameras and (2) to produce an output image of small enough size to allow convenient coupling to video and film cameras. The image intensifier provides both real-time imaging capability (fluoroscopy), which allows patient positioning and catheter manipulation, and recording of the angiographic injection (digital angiography, analog video recording, photospot, cine).

Image intensifier output phosphors are approximately 25 mm in diameter, although large (e.g., 50 to 60 mm) output phosphor image intensifiers have been developed to increase spatial resolution. The modulation transfer function (MTF) of the image intensifier is determined primarily by the input and output phosphor stages, so mapping a given input image to a larger output phosphor will improve the MTF of the system. The input phosphor of a modern image intensifier is cesium iodide (CsI). The largest currently available image intensifier input phosphors are approximately 16 in. The effective input phosphor diameter is selectable by the user. For example, an image intensifier designated 9/7/5 allows the user to select input phosphor diameters of 9, 7, or 5 in. These selections are referred to as image intensifier *modes*. The purpose of providing an adjustable input phosphor is to allow the user to trade off between spatial resolution and field of view. A smaller mode provides higher spatial resolution both because the MTF of the image intensifier improves and because it maps a smaller field of view to the fixed size of the video camera target. Generally speaking, angiographic suites designed exclusively for either neuroangiography or cardiac catheterization use 9-in. image intensifiers (i.e., the largest available intensifier mode is 9 in.), while suites that must handle pulmonary, renal, or peripheral angiography require the larger (i.e., 14 to 16 in.) intensifiers.

The brightness gain of the image intensifier derives from two sources: (1) the increase in electron energy produced by the accelerating potential (the *flux* gain) and (2) the decrease in size of the image as it is transferred from the input to the output phosphor (the *minification* gain). The product of these two factors can exceed 5000. However, since the minification gain is a function of the area of the input phosphor exposed to the radiation beam (i.e., the image intensifier mode), the brightness gain drops as smaller image intensifier modes are selected. This is compensated for by increasing the patient (and staff) x-ray exposure, in an amount proportional to the change in input phosphor area, to maintain the image intensifier light output. Image intensifier brightness gain declines with age and must be monitored to allow timely replacement. The specification used for this purpose is the image intensifier *conversion factor,* defined as the light output of the image intensifier per unit x-ray exposure input. Modern image intensifiers have a conversion factor of 100 cd/m^2/mR/s or more for the 9-in. mode.

With the increasing emergence of digital angiography as the primary angiographic imaging modality, image intensifier performance has become increasingly important. In the field, the high-spatial-frequency response of an image intensifier is assessed by determining the limiting resolution [in the neighborhood of 4 to 5 line-pairs/mm (lp/mm) in the 9-in. mode], while the low-spatial-frequency response is assessed using the contrast ratio (in the neighborhood of 15:1 to 30:1). The National Electrical Manufacturers Association (NEMA) has defined test procedures for measuring the contrast ratio [NEMA, 1992]. The *detective quantum efficiency* (DQE), which is a measure of the efficiency with which the image intensifier utilizes the x-ray energy incident on it, is in the neighborhood of 65%. A tabulation of the specifications of several commercially available image intensifiers has been published by Siedband [Siedband, 1994].

Optical Distributor

The image present at the image intensifier output phosphor is coupled to the video camera, and any film camera present (e.g., cine), by the optical distributor. The components of the distributor are shown in Fig. 63.4. There is an aperture for each camera to allow the light intensity presented to each camera to be adjusted independently. The video camera aperture is usually a motor-driven variable iris, while the film camera aperture is usually fixed. It is important to realize that while the aperture does ensure that the proper light level is presented to the camera, more fundamentally, the aperture determines the x-ray exposure input to the image intensifier. As a result, both the patient exposure and the level of quantum noise in the image are set by the aperture. The noise amplitude in a fluoroscopic or digital angiographic image is inversely proportional to the f-number of the optical system. Because the *quantum sink* of a properly adjusted fluorographic system is at the input of the image in-

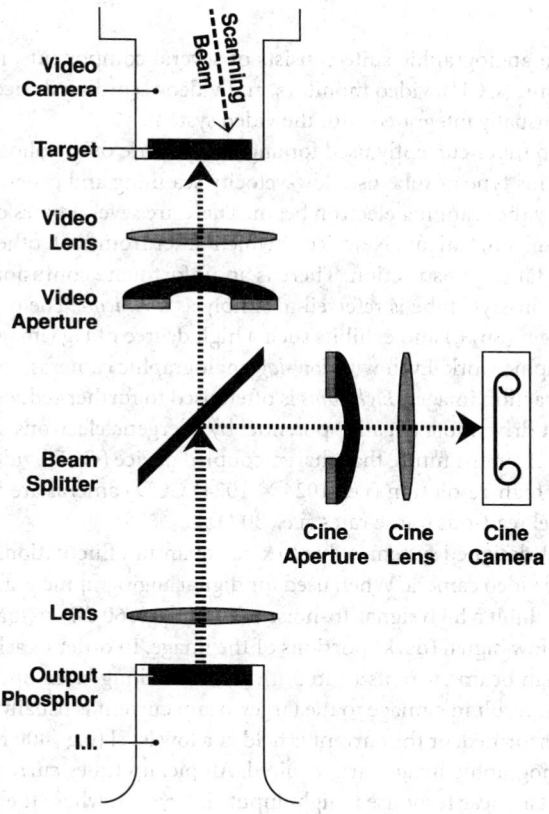

FIGURE 63.4 Schematic diagram of the optical distributor used to couple the image intensifier (I.I.) output phosphor to a video and cine camera. (From Van Lysel MS. (In press). Digital angiography. In S Baum (ed), Abrams' Angiography, 4th ed. Boston, Little, Brown, with permission.)

tensifier, the aperture diameter is set, for a given type of examination, to provide the desired level of quantum mottle present in the image. The x-ray exposure factors are then adjusted for each patient, by an *automatic exposure control* (AEC) system, to produce the proper postaperture light level. However, some video systems do provide for increasing the video camera aperture during fluoroscopy when the maximum entrance exposure does not provide adequate light levels on a large patient.

The beam-splitting mirror was originally meant to provide a moderate-quality video image simultaneous with cine recording in order to monitor the contrast injection during cardiac studies. More recently, as the importance of digital angiography has mushroomed, precision-quality mirrors with higher transmission have been used in order to provide simultaneous diagnostic-quality cine and video. The latest development has been the introduction of *cine-less* digital cardiac systems, in which the video image is the sole recording means. The introduction of these systems has sometimes been accompanied by the claim that a cine-less system requires less patient exposure due to the fact that light does not have to be provided to the cine camera. However, a conventional cine system operates with an excess of light (i.e., the cine camera aperture is stopped down). Because the image intensifier input is the quantum sink of the system, exposure is determined by the need to limit quantum mottle, not to maintain a given light level at the image intensifier output. Therefore, the validity of this claim is dubious. It should be noted, however, that because of the difference in spatial resolution capabilities of cine and video, the noise power spectrum of images acquired with equal exposure will be different. It is possible that observers accept a lower exposure in a video image than in the higher-resolution film image.

Video System

The video system in an angiographic suite consists of several components, including the camera head, camera control unit (CCU), video monitors, and video recording devices. In addition, a digital image processor is usually integrated with the video system.

Video camera pickup tubes currently used for angiography are of the photoconductive *vidicon-style* of construction. This type of tube uses low-velocity scanning and generates a signal from the recharge of the target by the scanning electron beam. There are several types of vidicon-style tubes in use (Plumbicon, Primicon, Saticon, Newvicon) which differ from each other in the material and configuration used for target construction. There is an unfortunate confusion in terminology because the original vidicon-style tube is referred to simply as a *vidicon*. The original vidicon has an antimony trisulfide target (Sb_2S_3) and exhibits such a high degree of lag (image retention) that it is not useful for angiographic work. Even with *low-lag* angiographic cameras, the residual lag can result in artifacts in subtraction images. *Light bias* is often used to further reduce lag by ensuring that the target surface is not driven to a negative potential by energetic electrons in the scanning beam [Sandrik, 1984]. It is likely in the future that charge-coupled device (CCD) video cameras will eliminate this problem, but high-resolution (i.e., 1024×1024) CCD cameras are not yet available with sufficient single-channel read-out frame rates (i.e., 30 Hz).

Image noise in a well-designed system is due to x-ray quantum fluctuations and noise related to signal generation in the video camera. When used for digital angiographic purposes, it is important that the video camera exhibit a high signal-to-noise ratio (at least 60 dB) so that video camera noise does not dominate the low-signal (dark) portions of the image. In order to achieve this, the pickup tube must be run at high beam currents (2 to 3 μA). Because long-term operation of the tube at these beam currents can result in damage to the target, beam current is usually either blanked when imaging is not being performed, or the current is held at a low level (e.g., 400 nA) and boosted only when high-quality angiographic images are required. All pickup tubes currently in use for angiographic imaging exhibit a linear response to light input (i.e., $\gamma = 1$, where the relationship between signal current I and image brightness B is described by a relationship of the form $I/I_o = (B/B_o)^\gamma$). This has the disadvantage that the range in image brightness presented to the camera often exceeds the camera's dynamic range when a highly transmissive portion of the patient's anatomy (e.g., lung) or unattenuated radiation is included in the image field. A camera with $\gamma < 1$, such as the Sb_2S_3 vidicon, has the desirable property of reduced sensitivity at high light levels, but when $\gamma = 1$, either the highlights saturate or the rest of the image is forced to a low signal level (or both). To deal with this problem, it is necessary for the operator to mechanically bolus the bright area with metal filters, saline bags, etc. Specially constructed filters are available for commonly encountered problems, such as the transmissive region between the patient's legs during *runoff* studies of the legs, and most vendors provide a controllable metal filter in the x-ray collimator that the operator can position over bright spots with a joystick.

In addition to mechanical bolusing performed by the laboratory staff, most system vendors have incorporated some form of *gamma curve modification* into their systems. Usually performed using analog processing in the CCU, the technique applies a nonlinear transfer curve to the originally linear data. There are two advantages to this technique. First, the CRT of the display monitor has reduced gain at low signal, so imposing a transfer function with $\gamma \approx 0.5$ via gamma-curve modification provides a better match between the video signal and the display monitor. Second, if the modification is performed prior to digitization, a $\gamma < 1$ results in a more constant ratio between the ADC step size and the image noise amplitude across the full range of the video signal. This results in less contouring in the dark portions of the digital image, especially in images that have been spatially filtered. It is important to note, however, that, contrary to some reports, gamma-curve modification does not eliminate the desirable effects of mechanically bolusing the image field prior to image acquisition. This is so because bolusing allows more photon flux to be selectively applied to the more attenuating regions of the patient, which decreases both quantum and video noise in those regions. Bolusing is especially important for subtraction imaging.

The video system characteristic most apparent to the user is the method employed in scanning the image. Prior to the advent of digital angiography, EIA RS-170 video (525-line, 30-Hz frames, 2:1 interlace) was the predominate standard used for fluoroscopic systems in the United States. However, this method of scanning has definite disadvantages for angiography, including low resolution and image artifacts related to the interlaced format. The inclusion of a digital image processor in the imaging chain, functioning as an image buffer, allows the scanning mode to be tailored to the angiographic procedure. Many of the important video scanning modes used for angiographic work are dependent on the ability of image processors to perform *scan conversion* operations. Two typical scan conversion operations are progressive-to-interlaced conversion and upscanning. Progressive-to-interlaced scan conversion allows progressive scanning (also referred to as *sequential scanning*) to be used for image acquisition and interlaced scanning for image display. Progressive scanning is a noninterlaced scan mode in which all the lines are read out in a single vertical scan. Progressive scanning is especially necessary when imaging moving arteries, such as during coronary angiography [Seibert et al., 1984]. In noncardiac work, progressive scan acquisition is usually combined with beam blanking. *Beam blanking* refers to the condition in which the pickup tube beam current is blanked (turned off) for one or more integer number of frames. This mode is used in order to allow the image to integrate on the camera target prior to readout (Fig. 63.5). In this way, x-ray pulses shorter than one frame period can be acquired without scanning artifacts, and x-ray pulses longer than one frame period can be used in order to increase the x-ray quantum statistics of an image.

Upscanning refers to the acquisition of data at a low line rate (e.g., 525 lines) and the display of that data at a higher line rate (e.g., 1023 lines) [Holmes et al., 1989]. The extra lines are produced by either replication of the actual data or, more commonly, by interpolation (either linear or spline). Upscanning also can be performed in the horizontal direction as well, but this is less typical. The motivation for upscanning (discussed below in more detail) is that while the MTF of many video cameras does not support the full improvement one would expect from doubling the number of lines, the increase in lines definitely improves image display, increasing display contrast and decreasing perception of the raster pattern. Thus upscanning is used to decrease the demands on the video camera, system bandwidth, and digital storage requirements.

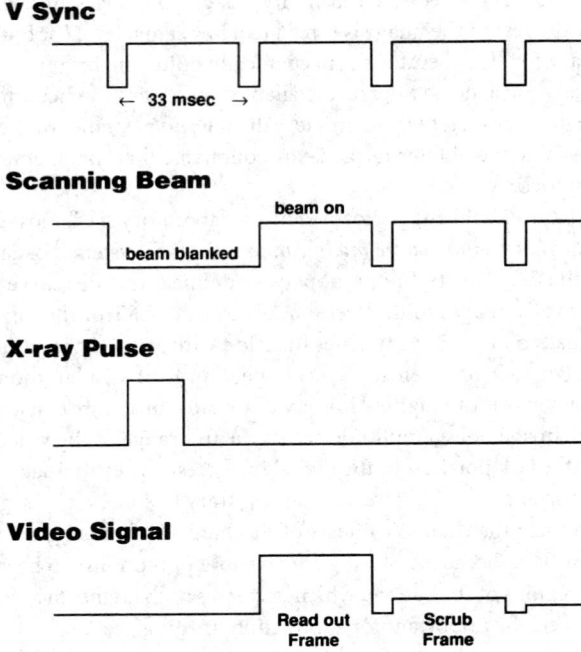

FIGURE 63.5   Timing diagram for image acquisition using the pulsed-progressive mode. (From Van Lysel MS. (In press.) Digital angiography. In S Baum (ed), Abrams' Angiography, 4th ed. Boston, Little, Brown, with permission.)

The image buffering capability of a digital system can provide several operations aimed at reducing patient exposure. If fluoroscopy is performed with pulsed rather than continuous x-rays, then the operator has the freedom to choose the frame rate. During pulsed-progressive fluoroscopy, the digital system provides for display refresh without flicker. Frame rates of less than 30 frames per second can result in lower patient exposure, though; because of the phenomenon of eye integration, the x-ray exposure per pulse must be increased as the frame rate drops in order to maintain low contrast detectability [Aufrichtig et al., 1994]. *Last image hold,* which stores and displays the last acquired fluoroscopic frame, also can result in an exposure reduction. Combining last image hold with graphic overlays allows collimator shutters and bolus filters to be positioned with the x-rays turned off.

Film/Screen

Film/screen angiography is quickly being replaced by digital angiography. Film does have some advantages with respect to digital, primarily higher spatial resolution (≥ 5 lp/mm versus 2 lp/mm). The susceptibility of DSA to motion artifacts is often listed as another advantage in favor of film, but this ignores the fact that digital angiography can provide high-quality nonsubtraction images.

Nonetheless, because of its high spatial resolution, many angiographers consider high-resolution film/screen angiography to be necessary for particular studies, including pulmonary examinations and locating gastrointestinal bleeding sites. In addition, peripheral angiography is still commonly performed with film (sophisticated digital runoff equipment is only now becoming available). An increasingly popular strategy for providing film capability is to equip the digital laboratory with a serial film changer integrated with the image intensifier rather than purchase a stand-based changer. The film changer is mounted on the image intensifier gantry (e.g., the C-arm) and is brought into place in front of the image intensifier when needed. Because the fields of view of the image intensifier and film changer are coaxial, film positioning is facilitated by this approach.

Digital Angiography

Digital imaging technology has quickly replaced film-based recording for most angiographic procedures. The advantages afforded by digital image processing provide the ability to manipulate the contrast and spatial-frequency characteristics of the angiographic image, as well as providing immediate access to the image data during the procedure.

The rapid application of digital imaging technology to the angiographic procedure was facilitated by the fact that the image intensifier and video camera imaging chain was already in use when digital imaging appeared. It is a relatively simple matter to digitize the video camera output. Theoretically, additional noise is added to the image due to quantitization errors associated with the digitization process. This additional noise can be kept insignificantly small by using a sufficient number of digital levels so that the amplitude of one digital level is approximately equal to the amplitude of the standard deviation in image values associated with the noise (x-ray quantum and electronic noise) in the image prior to digitization [Kruger et al., 1981]. To meet this condition, most digital angiographic systems employ a 10-bit (1024-level) analog-to-digital convertor (ADC). Those systems which are designed to digitize high-noise (i.e., low x-ray exposure) images exclusively can employ an 8-bit (256-level) ADC. Such systems include those designed for cardiac and fluoroscopic applications.

The spatial resolution of a digital angiographic image is determined by several factors, including the size of the x-ray tube focal spot, the modulation transfer function of the image intensifier–video camera chain, and the size of the pixel matrix. Typical image matrix dimensions for digital angiographic images are 512×512 and 1024×1024. Sampling rates required to digitize 512^2 and 1024^2 matrices in the 33-ms frame period of conventional video are 10 and 40 MHz, respectively. Figure 63.6 shows an example of the detector MTF of a digital angiographic system. The product of the image intensifier and video system MTF constitute the *presampling MTF* [Fujita et al., 1985]. It is seen that the effect of sampling with a 512-pixel matrix is to truncate the high-frequency tail of the presampling MTF, while a 1024-pixel matrix imposes little additional limitations beyond that associated with the analog components (especially for small image intensifier modes) [Verhoeven, 1985]. However, a 1024^2 matrix is associated with a significant increase in cost for image storage, as well as additional noise due to the necessary increase in system bandwidth. Because of the limitations imposed by the presampling MTF, as well as limitations due to focal spot blurring (Fig. 63.7), only objects with high intrinsic contrast will benefit from the higher sampling matrix. However, clinically,

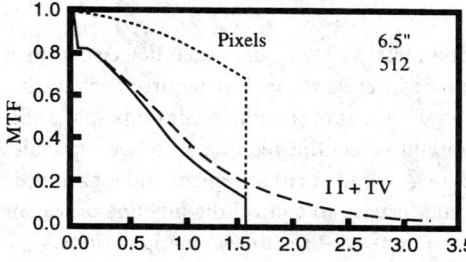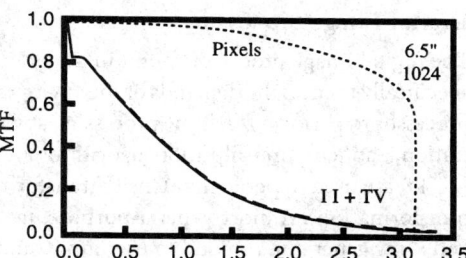

spatial frequency (mm⁻¹)

FIGURE 63.6 Detector modulation transfer function, including limits due to the image intensifier (II), video camera (TV), and sampling, including the antialiasing filter (pixels). Figures are for the 6.5-in image intensifier mode for 512- and 1024-pixel matrices. In both cases, the total detector MTF if given by the solid line. Data used for this figure from Verhoeven [1985].

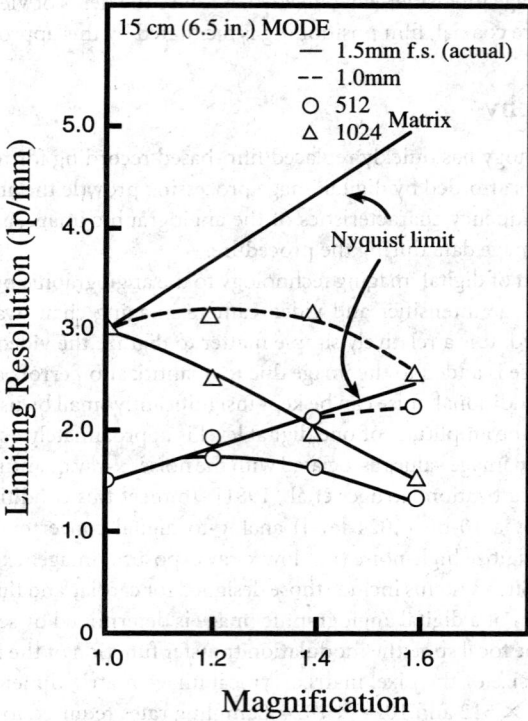

FIGURE 63.7 Experimental determination of the limiting resolution (high-contrast object and high x-ray exposure) for 512- and 1024-pixel matrices, focal spots of actual dimensions 1.0 and 1.5 mm, and a 6.5-in image intensifier mode, as a function of geometric magnification. (From Mistretta CA, Peppler WW. 1988. Digital cardiac x-ray imaging: Fundamental principles. Am J Cardiac Imaging 2:26, with permission.)

most small objects are of low contrast and will thus not be passed by the system MTF. This is the logic behind using an upscanned 512 system.

Digital Image Processor

The digital image processor found in a modern angiographic suite is a dedicated device designed specifically to meet the demands of the angiographic procedure. Hardware is structured as a pipeline processor to perform real-time processing at video rates. Image-subtraction, integration, spatial-filtration, and temporal-filtration algorithms are hardwired to meet this requirement. Lookup tables (LUTs) are used to perform intensity transformations (e.g., contrast enhancement and logarithmic transformation). A more general-purpose *host* computer is used to control the pipeline processor and x-ray generator, respond to user input, and perform non-real-time image manipulations.

The most clinically important image-processing algorithm is temporal subtraction (DSA). Subtraction imaging is used for most vascular studies. Subtraction allows approximately a factor of 2 reduction in the amount of injected contrast material. As a result, DSA studies can be performed with less contrast load and with smaller catheters than film/screen angiography. The primary limitation of DSA is a susceptibility to misregistration artifacts resulting from patient motion. Some procedures that are particularly susceptible to motion artifacts are routinely performed in a nonsubtracted mode. Unsubtracted digital angiographic studies are usually performed with the same amount of contrast material as film/screen studies. Cardiac angiography is one procedure that is generally performed without subtraction, although in any particular study, if patient and respiratory motion are absent, it is possible to obtain high-quality time subtractions using phase-matched mask subtractions in which the preinjection mask and postinjection contrast images are matched with respect to cardiac phase. In order to do this efficiently, it is necessary to digitize the ECG signal along with the image data.

Additional examples of unsubtracted digital angiographic studies are those in uncooperative patients (e.g., trauma) and digital runoff studies of the vessels in the leg. In a digital runoff study it is necessary to follow the bolus down the legs by moving the patient (or the image gantry). This motion causes difficulties with both mask registration and uniform exposure intensities between the mask and contrast images. The high contrast sensitivity of DSA is valuable for runoff studies, however, because the small vessels and slow flow in the lower extremities can make vessel visualization difficult. Recently, making use of programmed table (or gantry) motion and pixel-shifting strategies, x-ray vendors have begun to offer a viable digital subtraction runoff mode.

In addition to subtraction angiography, two filtration algorithms have become clinically important. The first is high-pass spatial filtration for the purposes of providing edge enhancement. Real-time edge enhancement of fluoroscopy is especially important for interventional procedures, such as angioplasty, where the task requires visualization of high-frequency objects such as vessel edges and guidewires. The need for spatial filtration has made the inclusion of a digital system mandatory in the cardiac catheterization laboratory, even though cardiac temporal subtraction has proven to be of little use. Because increasing the degree of edge enhancement also increases image noise, operator control of the degree of enhancement (accomplished by adjusting the size and weighting of the convolution kernel) is an important feature.

The second filtration algorithm often available from a digital angiographic system is low-pass temporal filtration (recursive filtering) [Rowlands, 1992]. Temporal filtration is used to reduce quantum noise levels in fluoroscopic images without increasing patient exposure. Recursive filtering is a more desirable method than simple image integration because it requires only two memory planes and because it is a simple matter to turn the filtering algorithm off, on a pixel-by-pixel basis, when motion is detected. Motion-detection circuits monitor the frame-to-frame change in pixel values and assume that an object has moved into or out of the pixel if the change exceeds a preset threshold.

Image Storage

Storage strategies for images generated by a digital angiographic system must provide both online and archival storage. Online storage is provided by real-time (i.e., video rate) digital disks. Real-time recording capability is achieved by the use of parallel-head drives, disk arrays, and data compression.

The immediate access to images provided by real-time disk technology is one of the major advantages of digital angiography over film. Not only is it unnecessary to wait for film to be developed, but review of the image data after the patient's procedure is completed is facilitated by directories and specialized review software. For example, a popular image menu feature is the presentation to users of a low-resolution collage of available images from which they may select a single image or entire run for full-resolution display.

While online storage of recent studies is a strength of digital angiography, long-term (archival) storage is a weakness. Archival devices provided by vendors are generally proprietary devices that make use of various recording media. There is an established communications protocol (ACR-NEMA) [NEMA, 1993] for network transfer of images. For the time being, while large institutions and teaching hospitals are investing in sophisticated digital picture archiving and communications systems (PACS), archival needs at most institutions are met by storage of hardcopy films generated from the digital images. Hardcopy devices include multiformat cameras (laser or video) and video thermal printers. Laser cameras, using either an analog or a digital interface to the digital angiographic unit, can provide diagnostic-quality, large-format, high-contrast, high-resolution films. Multiformat video cameras, which expose the film with a CRT, are a less expensive method of generating diagnostic-quality images but are also more susceptible to drift and geometric distortions. Thermal printer images are generally used as a convenient method to generate temporary hardcopy images.

The archiving problems related to speed, capacity, and intersystem compatibility are most acute for cardiac studies. While the cost of providing noncardiac systems with real-time disk recording is reasonably modest, cardiac requirements can stretch budgets. Cardiac angiographic frame rates are generally 30 frames per second per plane for adults (60 frames per second per plane for pediatrics). The use of biplane imaging, which is required for pediatrics, doubles the required recording rate. A standard adult catheterization procedure usually results in about 1 minute of imaging time per plane, so the number of images per study is at least 1800 images per patient per plane. A busy cardiac catheterization laboratory may study 10 patients in a day. While it is desirable to have enough digital storage to record one entire day's worth of studies, this is quite expensive. Real-time disk storage for more than 1 day is not cost-effective.

Various devices have been produced by x-ray vendors to archive digital cardiac studies, including SMPTE D-2 digital video, digital streamer tape cassettes, digital optical disks, and even analog optical disks. The major limitation of all these schemes is that compatibility between institutions—and even between generations of equipment from the same vendor at a given institution—does not exist. Compare this with 35-mm cine film, where film recorded years ago at a different institution may be viewed easily when the patient presents with new symptoms. An additional problem is confronted by slow devices, such as digital optical disks. While recording onto the disk can be performed conveniently in a background mode, review of the images at a later date requires a significant delay while data are loaded from the archive to a real-time disk or RAM that can provide high-speed replay. Another issue that remains to be resolved, including the potential legal questions, is the acceptability of lossy data compression algorithms. Until these issues are settled, many cardiac catheterization laboratories are employing a method referred to as **parallel cine,** in which both digital and cine images are recorded simultaneously by use of the semitransparent mirror in the image intensifier optical distributor.

Cine

While digital imaging has replaced film for most angiographic procedures, cardiac imaging retains a significant dependence on film. Cineangiography is performed with a 35-mm motion picture camera optically coupled to the image intensifier output phosphor. The primary clinical application is coronary angiography and ventriculography. During cineangiography, x-ray pulses are synchronized both with the cine camera shutter and the vertical retrace of the video camera. To limit motion blurring, it is desirable to keep the x-ray pulses as short as possible, but no longer than 10 ms.

Imaging runs generally last from 5 to 10 s at a frame rate of 30 or 60 frames per second (fps). Sixty frames per second is generally used for pediatric studies, where higher heart rates are encountered, while 30 fps is more typical for adult studies. The high frame rates are used to accurately record the cardiac cycle, although for ventriculography 15 fps may be adequate [Bove et al., 1970] and 7.5 fps may be adequate for coronary arteries. Some cineangiographic installations provide biplane imaging, in which two independent imaging chains can acquire orthogonal images of the injection sequence. The eccentricity of coronary lesions and the asymmetric nature of cardiac contraction abnormalities require that multiple x-ray projections be acquired. Biplane systems allow this to be done with a smaller patient contrast load. For this reason, biplane systems are considered a requirement for pediatric catheterization labs. They are relatively uncommon for adult catheterization labs, however, where the less complicated positioning of a single-plane system is often valued over the reduced number of injections possible with a biplane system. The anteroposterior and lateral planes of a biplane system are energized out of phase, which results in the potential for image degradation due to detection of the radiation scattered from the opposite plane. Image intensifier blanking, which shuts down the accelerating voltage of the nonimaging plane, is used to eliminate this problem.

As discussed earlier, while cine film retains a prominent role in cardiac imaging, digital angiography has now become fully integrated into the cardiac catheterization procedure. In fact, while there are some labs that have eliminated cine in favor of digital, a cine-only lab is considered obsolete. Currently, the most common configuration is simultaneous digital and cine acquisition, and it is becoming common for the primary diagnosis to be made off the digital monitor. It is expected by many in the field that as systems and standards are developed to deal with the archive and transfer of digital cardiac images, cine film will eventually be eliminated.

Summary

For decades, x-ray projection film/screen angiography was the only invasive modality available for the diagnosis of vascular disease. Now several imaging modalities are available to study the cardiovascular system, most of which are less invasive than x-ray projection angiography. However, conventional angiography also has changed dramatically during the last decade. Digital angiography has replaced film/screen angiography in most applications. In addition, the use and capabilities of transluminal interventional techniques have mushroomed, and digital angiographic processor modes have expanded significantly in support of these interventional procedures. As a consequence, while it is possible that less invasive technologies, such as MR angiography, may make inroads into conventional angiography's diagnostic applications, it is likely that x-ray projection angiography will remain an important clinical modality for many years to come.

Defining Terms

Bolus: This term has two, independent definitions: (1) material placed in a portion of the x-ray beam to reduce the scene dynamic range and (2) the injected contrast material.

Digital subtraction angiography (DSA): Methodology in which digitized angiographic images are subtracted in order to provide contrast enhancement of the opacified vasculature. Clinically, temporal subtraction is the algorithm used, though energy subtraction methods also fall under the generic term DSA.

Parallel cine: The simultaneous recording of digital and cine-film images during cardiac angiography. In this mode, digital image acquisition provides diagnostic-quality images (as compared with the previously employed method of simultaneously videotaping cardiac injections).

Picture archiving and communications systems (PACS): Digital system or network for the electronic storage and retrieval of patient images and data.

Progressive scanning: Video raster scan method in which all horizontal lines are read out in a single vertical scan of the video camera target.

Pulsed-progressive fluoroscopy: Method of acquiring fluoroscopic images in which x-rays are produced in discrete pulses coincident with the vertical retrace period of the video camera. The video camera is then read out using progressive scanning. This compares with the older fluoroscopic method of producing x-rays continuously, coupled with interlaced video camera scanning.

Temporal subtraction: Also known as *time subtraction* or *mask-mode subtraction*. A subtraction mode in which an unopacified image (the mask, usually acquired prior to injection) is subtracted from an opacified image.

Upscanning: Scan conversion method in which the number of pixels or video lines displayed is higher (usually by a factor of 2) than those actually acquired from the video camera. Extra display data are produced by either replication or interpolation of the acquired data.

References

Aufrichtig R, Xue P, Thomas CW, et al. 1994. Perceptual comparison of pulsed and continuous fluoroscopy. Med Phys 21(2):245.

Bove AA, Ziskin MC, Freeman E, et al. 1970. Selection of optimum cineradiographic frame rate: Relation to accuracy of cardiac measurements. Invest Radiol 5:329.

Fujita H, Doi K, Lissak Giger M. 1985. Investigation of basic imaging properties in digital radiography: 6. MTFs of II-TV digital imaging systems. Med Phys 12(6):713.

Holmes DR Jr, Wondrow MA, Reeder GS, et al. 1989. Optimal display of the coronary arterial tree with an upscan 1023-line video display system. Cathet Cardiovasc Diagn 18(3):175.

Kruger RA, Mistretta CA, Riederer SJ. 1981. Physical and technical considerations of computerized fluoroscopy difference imaging. IEEE Trans Nucl Sci 28:205.

National Electrical Manufacturers Association. 1992. Test Standard for the Determination of the System Contrast Ratio and System Veiling Glare Index of an X-Ray Image Intensifier System, NEMA Standards Publication No. XR 16. Washington, National Electrical Manufacturers Association.

National Electrical Manufacturers Association. 1993. Digital Imaging and Communications in Medicine (DICOM), NEMA Standards Publication PS3.0(1993). Washington, National Electrical Manufacturers Association.

Rowlands JA. 1992. Real-time digital processing of video image sequences for videofluoroscopy. SPIE Proc 1652:294.

Sandrik JM. 1984. The video camera for medical imaging. In GD Fullerton, WR Hendee, JC Lasher, et al. (eds): Electronic Imaging in Medicine, pp 145–183. New York, American Institute of Physics.

Seibert JA, Barr DH, Borger DJ, et al. 1984. Interlaced versus progressive readout of television cameras for digital radiographic acquisitions. Med Phys 11:703.

Siedband MP. 1994. Image intensification and television. In JM Taveras, JT Ferrucci (eds), Radiology: Diagnosis-Imaging-Intervention, Chap 10. Philadelphia, JB Lippincott.

Verhoeven LAJ. 1985. DSA imaging: Some physical and technical aspects. Medicamundi 30:46.

Further Information

Abrams HL (ed). 1983. Abrams Angiography: Vascular and Interventional Angiography, 3d ed. Boston, Little, Brown. A fourth edition of this classic text is currently in preparation.

Thompson TT. 1985. A Practical Approach to Modern Imaging Equipment, 2d ed. Boston, Little, Brown.

Moore RJ. 1990. Imaging Principles of Cardiac Angiography. Rockville, Md, Aspen Publishers.

Report of the Inter-Society Commission for Heart Disease Resources. 1983. Optimal resources for examination of the heart and lungs: Cardiac catheterization and radiographic facilities. Circulation 68(4):889A.

63.3 Mammography

Martin J. Yaffe

Mammography is an x-ray imaging procedure for examination of the breast. It is used primarily for the detection and diagnosis of breast cancer but also for preoperative localization of suspicious areas and in the guidance of needle biopsies.

Breast cancer is a major killer of women [Boring et al., 1992]. Approximately 182,000 women were diagnosed with breast cancer in the United States in 1993, and 46,000 women died of this disease. Its cause is not currently known; however, it has been demonstrated that survival is greatly improved if disease is detected at an *early stage* [Smart et al., 1993; Tabar et al., 1993]. Mammography is at present the most effective means of detecting early-stage breast cancer. It is used both for investigating symptomatic patients (diagnostic mammography) and for screening of asymptomatic women in selected age groups.

Breast cancer is detected on the basis of four types of signs on the mammogram:

1. The characteristic morphology of a tumor mass
2. Certain presentations of mineral deposits as specks called *microcalcifications*
3. Architectural distortion of normal tissue patterns caused by the disease
4. Asymmetry between images of the left and right breasts

Principles of Mammography

The mammogram is an x-ray shadowgram formed when x-rays from a quasi-point source irradiate the breast and the transmitted x-rays are recorded by an image receptor. Because of the spreading of the x-rays from the source, structures are magnified as they are projected onto the image receptor. The signal is a result of differential attenuation of x-rays along paths passing through the structures of the breast.

The essential features of image quality are summarized in Fig. 63.8. This is a one-dimensional profile of x-ray transmission through a simplified computer model of the breast [Fahrig et al., 1992], illustrated in Fig. 63.9. A region of reduced transmission corresponding to a structure of interest such as a tumor, a calcification, or normal fibroglandular tissue is shown. The imaging system must have sufficient *spatial resolution* to delineate the edges of fine structures in the breast. Structural detail as small as 50 μm must be resolved adequately. Variation in x-ray attenuation gives rise to *contrast*. The detectability of structures providing subtle contrast is impaired, however, by an overall random fluctuation in the profile, referred to as *mottle* or *noise*. Because the breast is sensitive to ionizing radiation, which at least for high doses is known to cause breast cancer, it is desirable to use the lowest radiation dose compatible with excellent image quality. The components of the imaging system will be described and their design will be related to the imaging performance factors discussed in this section.

Production of the Mammogram

Physics of Image Formation

In the model of Fig. 63.9, an "average" breast composed of 50% adipose tissue and 50% fibroglandular tissue is considered. For the simplified case of monoenergetic x-rays of energy E, the number of x-rays recorded in a fixed area of the image is proportional to

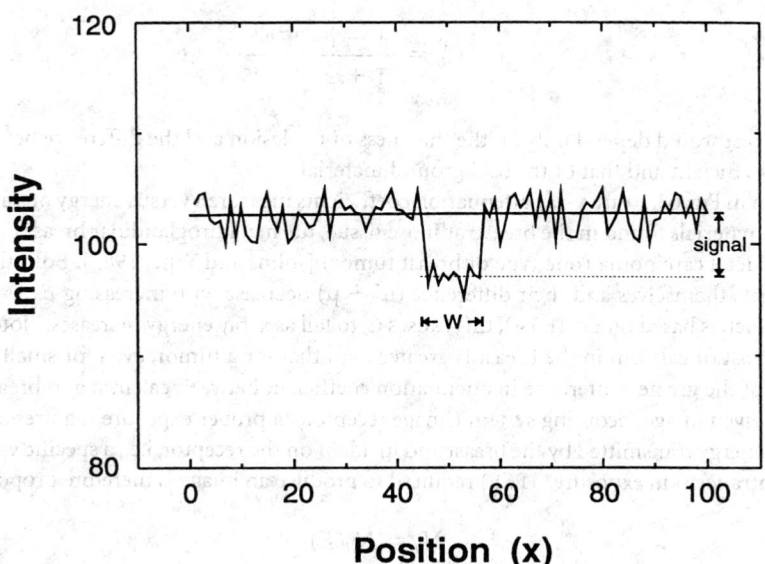

FIGURE 63.8   Profile of a simple x-ray projection image illustrating the role of contrast, spatial resolution, and noise in mammographic image quality.

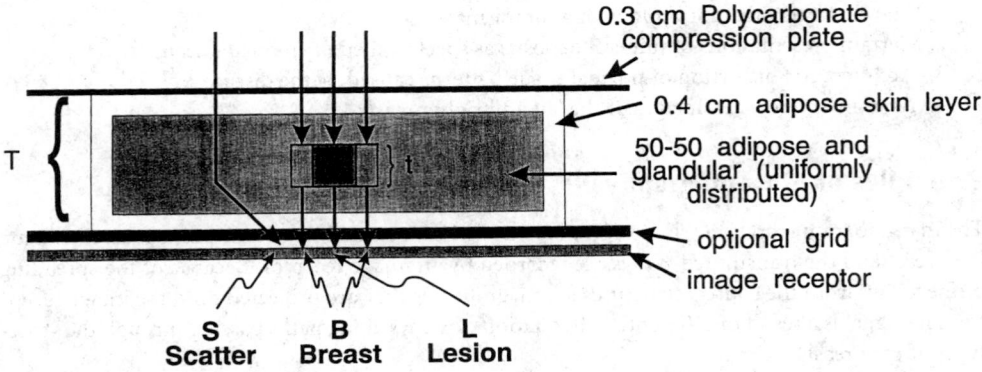

FIGURE 63.9   Simplified computer model of the mammographic image acquisition process.

$$N_B = N_0(E)e^{-\mu T} \tag{63.1}$$

in the "background" and

$$N_L = N_0(E)e^{-[\mu(T-t) + \mu't]} \tag{63.2}$$

in the shadow of the lesion or other structure of interest. In Eqs. (63.1) and (63.2), $N_0(E)$ is the number of x-rays that would be recorded in the absence of tissue in the beam, μ and μ' are the attenuation coefficients of the breast tissue and the lesion, respectively, T is the thickness of the breast, and t is the thickness of the lesion.

The difference in x-ray transmission gives rise to *subject contrast*, which can be defined as

$$C_0 = \frac{N_B - N_L}{N_B + N_L} \tag{63.3}$$

For monoenergetic x-rays and temporarily ignoring scattered radiation,

$$C_0 = \frac{1 - e^{-(\mu'-\mu)t}}{1 + e^{-(\mu'-\mu)t}} \tag{63.4}$$

i.e., contrast would depend only on the thickness of the lesion and the difference between its attenuation coefficient and that of the background material.

Shown in Fig. 63.10 are x-ray attenuation coefficients measured versus energy on samples of three types of materials found in the breast: adipose tissue, normal fibroglandular breast tissue, and infiltrating ductal carcinoma (one type of breast tumor) [Johns and Yaffe, 1987]. Both the attenuation coefficients themselves and their difference $(\mu' - \mu)$ decrease with increasing E. As shown in Fig. 63.11, which is based on Eq. (63.4), this causes C_s to fall as x-ray energy increases. Note that the subject contrast of calcium in the breast is greater than that for a tumor, even for small calcifications, because of the greater difference in attenuation coefficient between calcium and breast tissue.

For a given image recording system (image receptor), a proper exposure requires a specific value of x-ray energy transmitted by the breast and incident on the receptor, i.e., a specific value of N_B. The breast entrance skin exposure* (ESE) required to produce an image is therefore proportional to

$$N_0 = N_B(E)e^{+\mu T} \tag{63.5}$$

---

*Exposure is expressed in roentgens (R) (which is not a SI unit) or in coulombs of ionization collected per kilogram of air).

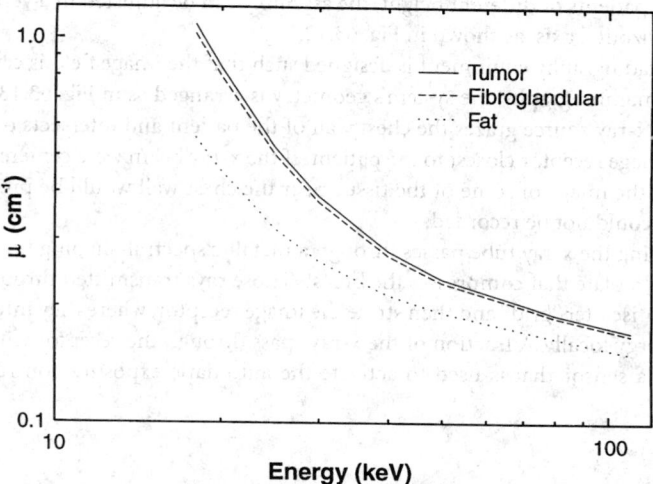

FIGURE 63.10 Measured x-ray linear attenuation coefficients of breast fibroglandular tissue, breast fat, and infiltrating ductal carcinoma plotted versus x-ray energy.

Because μ decreases with energy, the required exposure for constant signal at the image receptor N_B will increase if E is reduced to improve image contrast. A better measure of the risk of radiation-induced breast cancer than ESE is the mean glandular dose (MGD) [BEIR V, 1990]. MGD is calculated as the product of the ESE and a factor, obtained experimentally or by Monte Carlo radiation transport calculations, that converts from incident exposure to dose [Wu et al., 1991]. The conversion factor increases with E so that MGD does not fall as quickly with energy as does entrance exposure. The tradeoff between image contrast and radiation dose necessitates important compromises in establishing mammographic operating conditions.

Equipment

The mammography unit consists of an x-ray tube and an image receptor mounted on opposite sides of a mechanical assembly or gantry. Because the breast must be imaged from different aspects, and

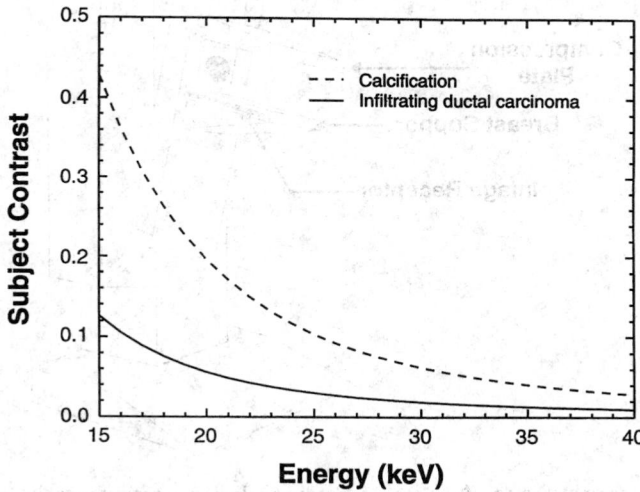

FIGURE 63.11 Dependence of mammographic subject contrast on x-ray energy.

to accommodate patients of different height, the assembly can be adjusted in a vertical axis and rotated about a horizontal axis, as shown in Fig. 63.12.

Most general radiography equipment is designed such that the image field is centered below the x-ray source. In mammography, the system's geometry is arranged as in Fig. 63.13a, where a vertical line from the x-ray source grazes the chest wall of the patient and intersects orthogonally with the edge of the image receptor closest to the patient. If the x-ray beam were centered over the breast as in Fig. 63.13b, the image of some of the tissue near the chest wall would be projected inside the patient, where it could not be recorded.

Radiation leaving the x-ray tube passes through a metallic spectral-shaping filter, a beam-defining aperture, and a plate that compresses the breast. Those rays transmitted through the breast are incident on an antiscatter "grid" and then strike the image receptor, where they interact and deposit most of their energy locally. A fraction of the x-rays pass through the receptor without interaction and impinge on a sensor that is used to activate the automatic exposure-control mechanism of the unit.

X-Ray Source

Practical monoenergetic x-ray sources are not available, and the x-rays used in mammography arise from bombardment of a metal target by electrons in a hot-cathode vacuum tube. The x-rays are emitted from the target over a spectrum of energies ranging up to the peak kilovoltage applied to the x-ray tube. Typically, the x-ray tube employs a rotating-anode design, in which electrons from the cathode strike the anode *target* material at a small angle (0 to 16 degrees) from normal incidence (Fig. 63.14). Over 99% of the energy from the electrons is dissipated as heat in the anode. The angled surface and the distribution of the electron bombardment along the circumference of the anode disk allow the energy to be spread over a larger area of target material while presenting a much

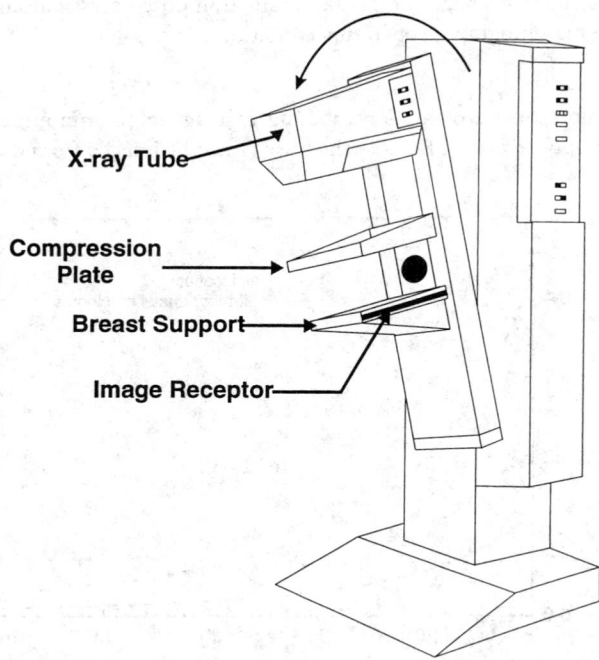

FIGURE 63.12   Schematic diagram of a dedicated mammography machine.

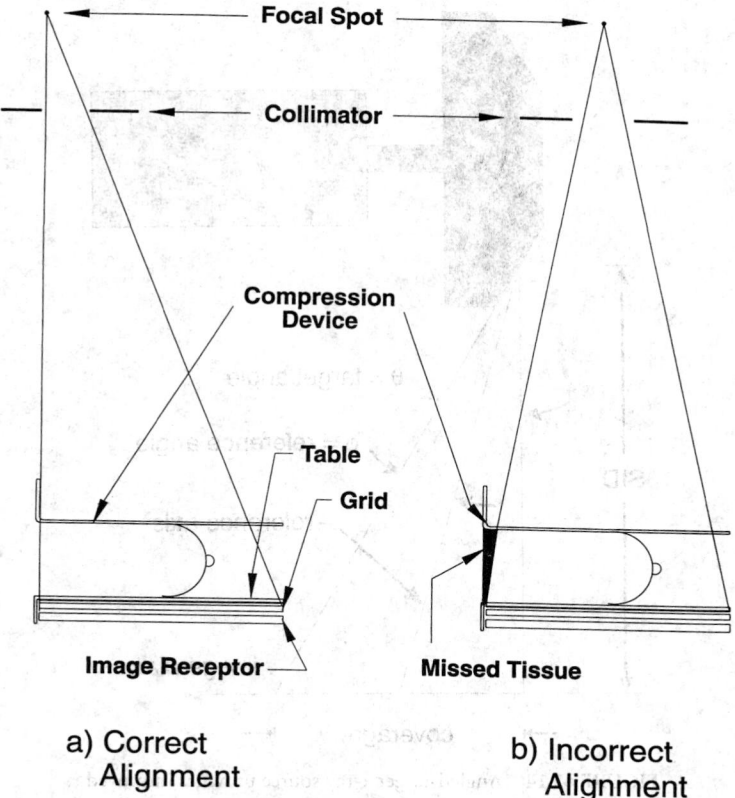

FIGURE 63.13 Geometric arrangement of system components in mammography. (*a*) Correct alignment provides good tissue coverage. (*b*) Incorrect alignment causes tissue near the chest wall not to be imaged.

smaller effective focal spot as viewed from the imaging plane. On modern equipment, the typical "nominal" focal spot size for normal contact mammography is 0.3 mm, while the smaller spot used primarily for magnification is 0.1 mm. The specifications for x-ray focal spot size tolerance, established by the National Electrical Manufacturers Association (NEMA) or the International Electrotechnical Commission (IEC), allow the *effective focal spot size* to be considerably larger than these nominal sizes. For example, the NEMA specification allows the effective focal spot size to be 0.45 mm in width and 0.65 mm in length for a nominal 0.3-mm spot and 0.15 mm in each dimension for a nominal 0.1-mm spot.

The nominal focal spot size is defined relative to the effective spot size at a "reference axis." As shown in Fig. 63.14, this reference axis, which may vary from manufacturer to manufacturer, is normally specified at some midpoint in the image. The effective size of the focal spot will increase monotonically from the anode side to the cathode side of the imaging field. Normally, x-ray tubes are arranged such that the cathode side of the tube is adjacent to the patient's chest wall, since the highest intensity of x-rays is available at the cathode side, and the attenuation of x-rays by the patient is generally greater near the chest wall of the image.

The spatial-resolution capability of the imaging system is partially determined by the effective size of the focal spot and by the degree of magnification of the anatomy at any plane in the breast. This is illustrated in Fig. 63.15, where, by similar triangles, the unsharpness region due to the finite size of the focal spot is linearly related to the effective size of the spot and to the ratio of OID to SOD, where SOD is the source-object distance and OID is the object–image receptor distance. Since the

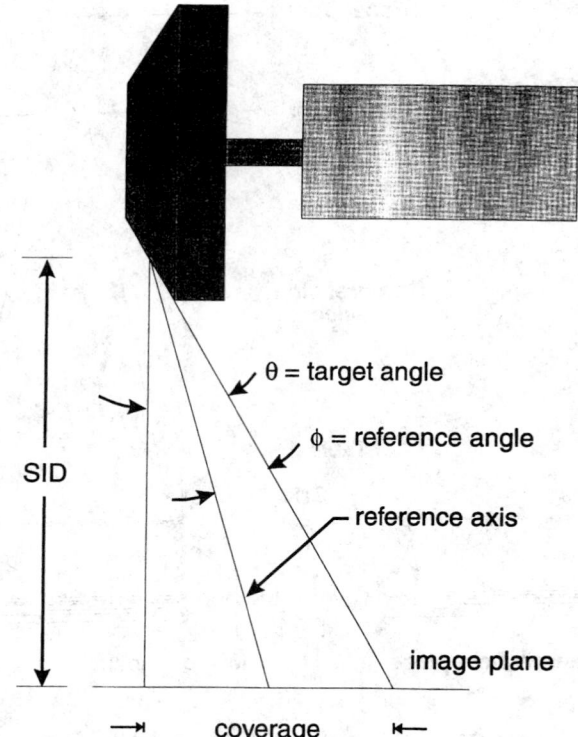

FIGURE 63.14 Angled-target x-ray source provides improved heat loading but causes effective focal spot size to vary across the image.

breast is a three-dimensional structure, this ratio, and therefore, the unsharpness, will vary for different planes within the breast.

The size of the focal spot determines the heat-loading capability of the x-ray tube target. For smaller focal spots, the current through the x-ray tube must be reduced, necessitating increased exposure times and the possibility of loss of resolution due to motion of anatomic structures. Loss of geometric resolution can be controlled in part by minimizing OID/SOD, i.e., by designing the equipment with greater source-breast distances, by minimizing space between the breast and the image receptor, and by compressing the breast to reduce its overall thickness.

Magnification is often used intentionally to improve the signal-to-noise ratio of the image. This is accomplished by elevating the breast above the image receptor, in effect reducing SOD and increasing OID. Under these conditions, resolution is invariably limited by focal spot size, and use of a small spot is critical.

Since monoenergetic x-rays are not available, one attempts to define a spectrum providing energies that give a reasonable compromise between radiation dose and image contrast. The spectral shape can be controlled by adjustment of the kilovoltage, choice of the target material, and the type and thickness of metallic filter placed between the x-ray tube and the breast.

Based on models of the imaging problem in mammography, it has been suggested that the optimal energy for imaging lies between 18 and 23 keV, depending on the thickness and composition of the breast [Beaman and Lillicrap, 1982]. It has been found that for the breast of typical thickness and composition, the characteristic x-rays from molybdenum at 17.4 and 19.6 keV provide good imaging performance. For this reason, molybdenum target x-ray tubes are used on the vast majority of mammography machines.

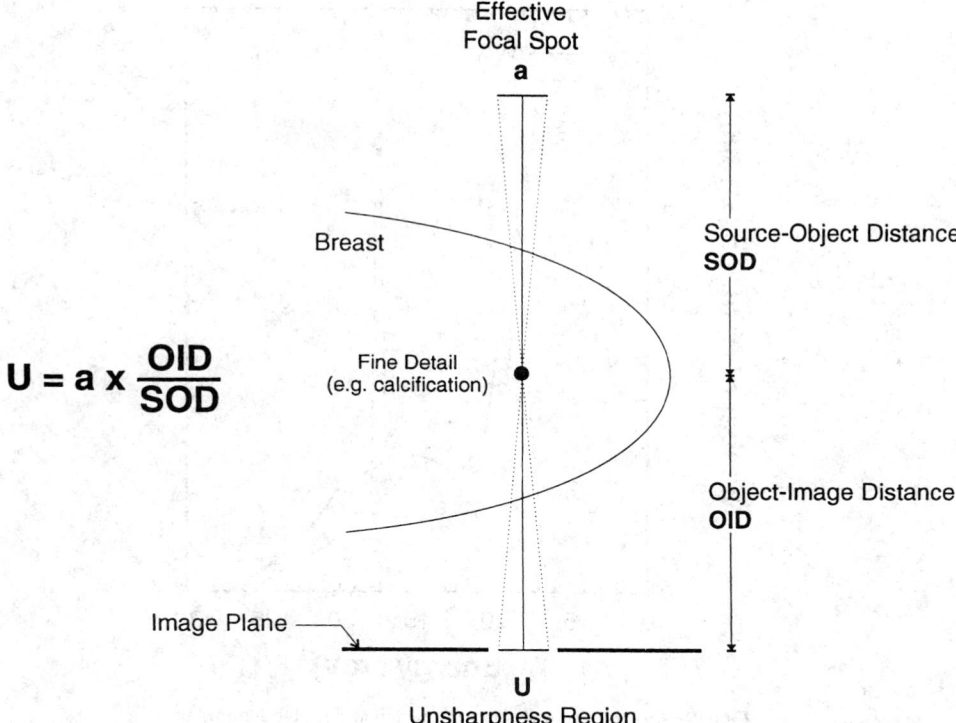

Effective
Focal Spot
a

Breast

Source-Object Distance
SOD

$$U = a \times \frac{OID}{SOD}$$

Fine Detail
(e.g. calcification)

Object-Image Distance
OID

Image Plane

U
Unsharpness Region

FIGURE 63.15   Dependence of focal spot unsharpness on focal spot size and magnification factor.

Most mammography tubes use beryllium exit windows between the evacuated tube and the outside world because glass or other metals used in general-purpose tubes would provide excessive attenuation of the useful energies for mammography. Figure 63.16 compares tungsten target and molybdenum target spectra for beryllium window x-ray tubes. Under some conditions, tungsten may provide appropriate image quality for mammography; however, it is essential that the intense emission of L radiation from tungsten be filtered from the beam before it is incident on the breast, since extremely high doses to the skin would result from this radiation without useful contribution to the mammogram.

Filtration of the X-Ray Beam

In conventional radiology, filters made of aluminum or copper are used to provide selective removal of low x-ray energies from the beam before it is incident on the patient. In mammography, particularly when a molybdenum anode x-ray tube is employed, a molybdenum filter 20 to 35 μm thick is generally used. This filter attenuates x-rays both at low energies and at those above its own K-absorption edge, allowing the molybdenum characteristic x-rays from the target to pass through the filter with relatively high efficiency. As illustrated in Fig. 63.17, this K-edge filtration results in a spectrum enriched with x-ray energies in the range of 17 to 20 keV.

Although this spectrum is relatively well suited for imaging the breast of average attenuation slightly higher energies are desirable for imaging dense, thicker breasts. Because the molybdenum target spectrum is so heavily influenced by the characteristic x-rays, an increase in the kilovoltage does not substantially change the shape of the spectrum.

To optimize imaging performance, it would be desirable to "tune" the effective spectral energy by use of other target materials in combination with appropriate K-edge filters [Jennings et al., 1993]. A system employing a combination molybdenum-rhodium target x-ray tube where the elec-

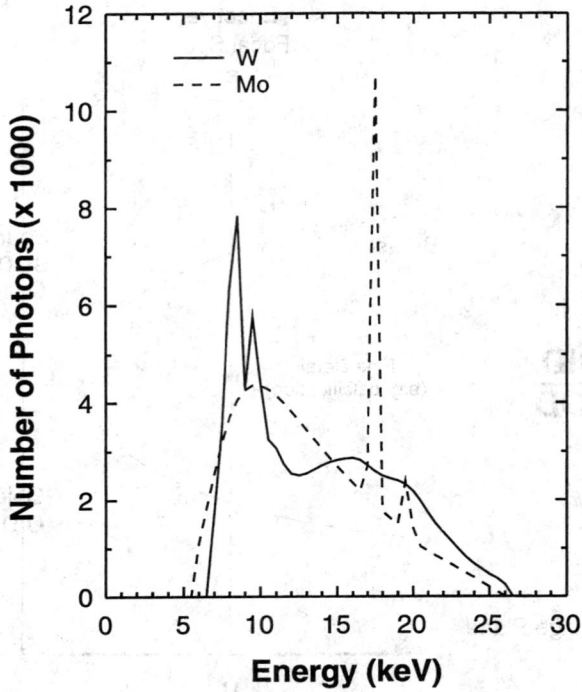

FIGURE 63.16 Comparison of tungsten and molybdenum target x-ray spectra.

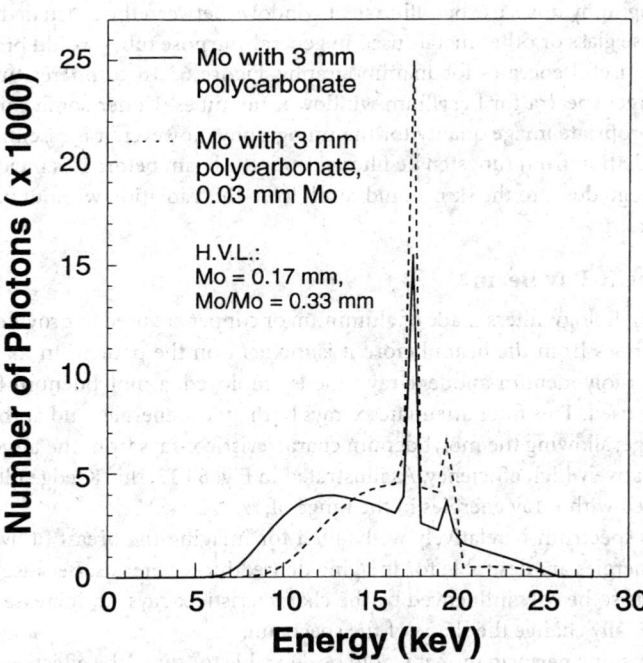

FIGURE 63.17 Molybdenum target spectrum filtered by 0.03-mm Mo foil.

tron beam can be directed toward one or the other of these materials has been recently introduced [Heidsieck et al., 1991]. On this system, the filter material (rhodium, molybdenum, etc.) can be varied to suit the target that has been selected. Similarly, work has been reported on K-edge filtration of tungsten spectra [Desponds et al., 1991], where the lack of pronounced K-characteristic peaks provides more flexibility in spectral shaping with filters.

Compression Device

There are several reasons for applying firm (but not necessarily painful) compression to the breast during the examination. Compression causes the different tissues to be spread out, minimizing superposition from different planes and thereby improving conspicuity of structures. As will be discussed later, scattered radiation can degrade contrast in the mammogram. The use of compression decreases the ratio of scattered to directly transmitted radiation reaching the image receptor. Compression also decreases the distance from any plane within the breast to the image receptor (i.e., OID) and in this way reduces geometric unsharpness. The compressed breast provides lower overall attenuation to the incident x-ray beam, allowing radiation dose to be reduced. The compressed breast also provides more uniform attenuation over the image. This reduces the exposure range that must be recorded by the imaging system, allowing more flexibility in choice of films to be used. Finally, compression provides a clamping action, which reduces anatomic motion during the exposure, reducing this source of image unsharpness.

It is important that the compression plate allows the breast to be compressed parallel to the image receptor and that the edge of the plate at the chest wall be straight and aligned with both the focal spot and image receptor to maximize the amount of breast tissue that is included in the image (see Fig. 63.13).

Antiscatter Grid

Lower x-ray energies are used for mammography than for other radiologic examinations. At these energies, the probability of photoelectric interactions within the breast is significant. Nevertheless, the probability of Compton scattering of x-rays within the breast is still quite high. Scattered radiation recorded by the image receptor has the effect of creating a quasi-uniform haze on the image and causes the subject contrast to be reduced to

$$C_S = \frac{C_0}{1 + \text{SPR}} \qquad (63.6)$$

where C_0 is the contrast in the absence of scattered radiation, given by Eq. (63.4), and SPR is the scatter-to-primary (directly transmitted) x-ray ratio at the location of interest in the image. In the absence of an antiscatter device, 37% to 50% of the total radiation incident on the image receptor would have experienced a scattering interaction within the breast; i.e., the scatter-to-primary ratio would be 0.6 to 1.0. In addition to contrast reduction, the recording of scattered radiation uses up part of the dynamic range of the image receptor and adds statistical noise to the image.

Antiscatter grids have been designed for mammography. These are composed of linear lead (Pb) septa separated by a rigid interspace material. Generally, the grid septa are not strictly parallel but are focused (toward the x-ray source). Because the primary x-rays all travel along direct lines from the x-ray source to the image receptor while the scatter diverges from points within the breasts, the grid presents a smaller acceptance aperture to scattered radiation than to primary and thereby discriminates against scattered radiation. Grids are characterized by their *grid ratio* (ratio of the path length through the interspace material to the interseptal width), which typically ranges from 3.5:1 to 5:1. When a grid is used, the SPR typically is reduced by a factor of about 5, leading in most cases to a substantial improvement in image contrast [Wagner, 1991].

On modern mammography equipment, the grid is an integral part of the system and, during x-ray exposure, is moved to blur the image of the grid septa to avoid a distracting pattern in the mammogram. It is important that this motion be uniform and of sufficient amplitude to avoid nonuniformities in the image, particularly for short exposures that occur when the breast is relatively lucent.

Because of absorption of primary radiation by the septa and by the interspace material, part of the primary radiation transmitted by the patient does not arrive at the image receptor. In addition, by removing some of the scattered radiation, the grid causes the overall radiation fluence to be reduced from that which would be obtained in its absence. To obtain a radiograph of proper optical density, the entrance exposure to the patient must be increased by a factor known as the *Bucky factor* to compensate for these losses. Typical Bucky factors are in the range of 2 to 3.

Image Receptor

Fluorescent Screens

When first introduced, mammography was carried out using direct-exposure radiographic film in order to obtain the high spatial resolution required. Since the mid-1970s, high-resolution fluorescent screens have been used to convert the x-ray pattern from the breast into an optical image. These screens are used in conjunction with single-coated radiographic film, and the configuration is shown in Fig. 63.18. With this arrangement, the x-rays pass through the cover of a light-tight cassette and the film to impinge on the screen. Absorption is exponential, so a large fraction of the x-rays is absorbed near the entrance surface of the screen. These produce light in an isotropic distribution. Because the film emulsion is pressed tightly against the entrance surface of the screen, the majority of the light quanta have only a short distance to travel to reach the film. Light quanta traveling longer distances have an opportunity to spread laterally (see graph in Fig. 63.18) and in this way degrade the spatial resolution. To discriminate against light quanta that travel along these longer, oblique paths, the phosphor material of the screen is generally treated with a dye that absorbs much of this light, giving rise to a sharper image. A typical phosphor used for mammography is gadolinium oxysulphide (Gd_2O_2S). Although the K-absorption edge of gadolinium occurs at too

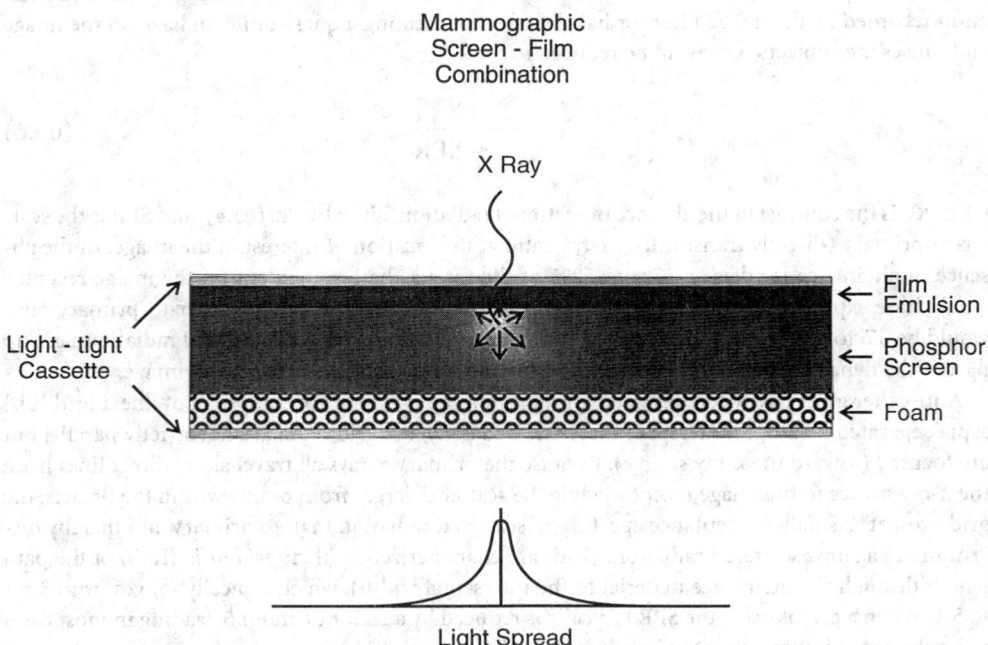

FIGURE 63.18   Design of a screen/film image receptor for mammography.

high an energy to be useful in mammography, the phosphor material is dense (7.44 g/cm³) so that the quantum efficiency (the fraction of incident x-rays that interact with the screen) is good (about 60%). Also, the conversion efficiency of this phosphor (fraction of the absorbed x-ray energy converted to light) is relatively high. The light emitted from the fluorescent screen is essentially linearly dependent on the total amount of energy deposited by x-rays within the screen.

Film

The photographic film emulsion for mammography is designed with a characteristic curve such as that shown in Fig. 63.19, which is a plot of the optical density (blackness) provided by the processed film versus the logarithm of the x-ray exposure to the screen. Film provides nonlinear input-output transfer characteristics. The local gradient of this curve controls the display contrast presented to the radiologist. Where the curve is of shallow gradient, a given increment of radiation exposure provides little change in optical density, rendering structures imaged in this part of the curve difficult to visualize. Where the curve is steep, the film provides excellent image contrast. The range of exposures over which contrast is appreciable is referred to as the *latitude* of the film. Because the film is constrained between two optical density values—the *base plus fog* density of the film, where no intentional x-ray exposure has resulted, and the maximum density provided by the emulsion—there is a compromise between maximum gradient of the film and the latitude which it provides. For this reason, some regions of the mammogram will generally be underexposed or overexposed, i.e., rendered with suboptimal contrast.

Noise

Noise in mammography results primarily from two sources: the random absorption of x-rays in the detector and the granularity associated with the film emulsion. The first, commonly known as *quan-*

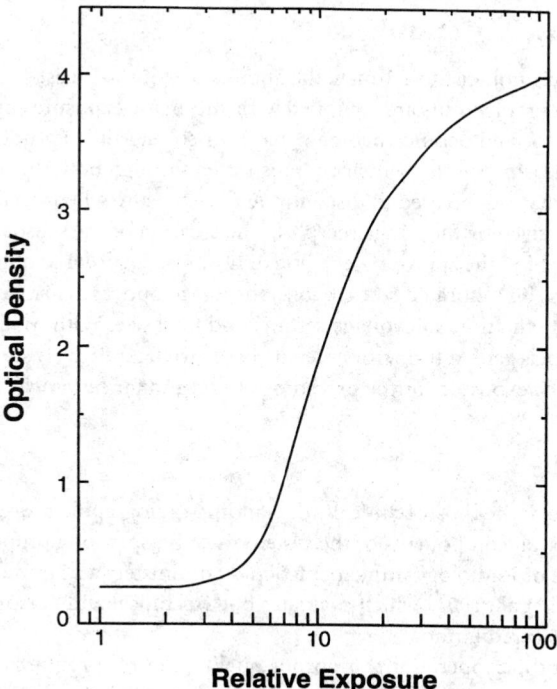

FIGURE 63.19 Characteristic curve of a mammographic screen/film image receptor.

tum noise, is governed by a Poisson distribution such that for a given area of image the standard deviation in the number of x-rays recorded is equal to the square root of the mean number recorded. In other words, the noise in the image is dependent on both the amount of radiation that strikes the imaging system per unit area and the quantum efficiency of the imaging system. The quantum efficiency is related to the attenuation coefficient of the phosphor material and the thickness of the screen. In order to maintain high spatial resolution, the screen must be relatively thin to avoid lateral diffusion of light. The desirability of maintaining a relatively low quantum noise level in the image mandates that the conversion efficiency of the screen material and the sensitivity of the film not be excessively high. With very high conversion efficiency, the image could be produced at low dose but with an inadequate number of quanta contributing to the image. Similarly, film granularity increases as more sensitive films are used so that, again, film speed must be limited to maintain high image quality. For current high-quality mammographic imaging employing an antiscatter grid, with films exposed to a mean optical density of at least 1.35, the mean glandular dose to a 5-cm-thick compressed breast consisting of 50% fibroglandular and 50% adipose tissue is in the range of 1 to 2 mGy [Conway et al., 1992].

Film Processing

Mammography film is processed in an automatic processor similar to that used for general radiographic films. It is important that the development temperature, time, and rate of replenishment of the developer chemistry be compatible with the type of film emulsion used and be designed to maintain good contrast of the film. Currently, there are two methods for processing mammography film: normal cycle, in which the immersion time in the developer is approximately 25 s, and extended cycle, where the development time is increased to about 45 s. Extended processing provides increased sensitivity and contrast; however, image noise levels are increased because fewer x-rays are used to produce the image.

Automatic Exposure Control

It is difficult for the technologist to estimate the attenuation of the breast by inspection, and therefore, modern mammography units are equipped with automatic exposure control (AEC). The AEC radiation sensors are located behind the image receptor so that they do not cast a shadow on the image. The sensors measure the x-ray fluence transmitted through both the breast and the receptor and provide a signal that can be used to discontinue the exposure when a certain preset amount of radiation has been received by the image receptor. The location of the sensor must be adjustable so that it can be placed behind the appropriate region of the breast in order to obtain proper image density. AEC devices must be calibrated so that constant image optical density results independent of variations in breast attenuation, kilovoltage setting, and field size. With modern equipment, automatic exposure control is generally microprocessor-based so that relatively sophisticated corrections can be made during the exposure for the preceding effects and for *reciprocity law failure* of the film.

Quality Control

Mammography is one of the most technically demanding radiographic procedures, and in order to obtain optimal results, all components of the system must be operating properly. Recognizing this, the American College of Radiology implemented and administers a Mammography Accreditation Program [McClelland et al., 1991] which evaluates both technical and personnel-related factors in facilities applying for accreditation.

In order to verify proper operation, a rigorous quality-control program should be in effect. In fact, the U.S. Mammography Quality Standards Act stipulates that a quality-control program must be in place in all facilities performing mammography. A program of tests (summarized in Table

63.1) and methods for performing them are contained in the quality-control manuals for mammography published by the American College of Radiology [Hendrick et al., 1994].

Stereotactic Biopsy Devices

Stereoscopic x-ray imaging techniques are currently used for the guidance of needle "core" biopsies. These procedures can be used to investigate suspicious mammographic or clinical findings without the need for surgical excisional biopsies, resulting in reduced patient risk, discomfort, and cost. In these stereotactic biopsies, the gantry of a mammography machine is modified to allow angulated views of the breast (typically ±15 degrees from normal incidence) to be achieved. From measurements obtained from these images, the three-dimensional location of a suspicious lesion is determined, and a needle equipped with a spring-loaded cutting device can be accurately placed in the breast to obtain tissue samples. While this procedure can be performed on an upright mammography unit, special dedicated systems have recently been introduced to allow its performance with the patient lying prone on a table. The accuracy of sampling the appropriate tissue depends critically on the alignment of the system components and the quality of the images produced. A thorough review of stereotactic imaging, including recommended quality-control procedures, is given by Hendrick and Parker [1994].

Digital Mammography

There are several technical factors associated with screen/film mammography which limit the ability to display the finest or most subtle details and produce images with the most efficient use of radiation dose to the patient. In screen/film mammography, the film must act as an image acquisition detector as well as a storage and display device. Because of its sigmoidal shape, the range of x-ray exposures over which the film display gradient is significant, i.e., the image latitude, is limited. If a

TABLE 63.1 Mammographic Quality Control Minimum Test Frequencies

Test	Performed by	Minimum Frequency
Darkroom cleanliness	Radiologic technologist	Daily
Processor quality control		Daily
Screen cleanliness		Weekly
Viewboxes and viewing conditions		Weekly
Phantom images		Monthly
Visual checklist		Monthly
Repeat analysis		Quarterly
Analysis of fixer retention in film		Quarterly
Darkroom fog		Semiannually
Screen/film contact		Semiannually
Compression		Semiannually
Mammographic unit assembly evaluation	Medical physicist	Annually
Collimation assessment		Annually
Focal spot size performance		Annually
kVp accuracy/reproducibility		Annually
Beam quality assessment (half-value-layer)		Annually
Automatic exposure control (AEC) system performance assessment		Annually
Uniformity of screen speed		Annually
Breast entrance exposure and mean glandular dose		Annually
Phantom evaluation of image quality		Annually
Artifact assessment		Annually

Source: Hendrick, et al. 1994. Mammography Quality Control Manuals (Radiologist, Radiologic Technologist, Medical Physicist). Reston, Va, American College of Radiology, with permission.

tumor is located in either a relatively lucent or more opaque region of the breast, then the contrast displayed to the radiologist may be inadequate because of the limited gradient of the film. This is particularly a concern in patients whose breasts contain large amounts of fibroglandular tissue, the so-called dense breast.

Another limitation of film mammography is the effect of structural noise due to the granularity of the film emulsion used to record the image. This impairs the detectibility of microcalcifications and other fine structures within the breast. While Poisson quantum noise is unavoidable, it should be possible to virtually eliminate structural noise by technical improvements. Existing screen/film mammography also suffers because of the inefficiency of grids in removing the effects of scattered radiation and because of compromises in spatial resolution versus quantum efficiency inherent in the screen/film image receptor.

Many of the limitations of conventional mammography can be effectively overcome with a *digital mammography* imaging system (Fig. 63.20), in which image acquisition, display, and storage are performed independently, allowing optimization of each. For example, acquisition can be performed with low-noise, highly linear x-ray detectors, while since the image is stored digitally, it can be displayed with contrast independent of the detector properties and defined by the needs of the radiologist. Whatever image-processing techniques are found useful, ranging from simple contrast enhancement to histogram modification and spatial frequency filtering, could conveniently be applied.

The challenges in creating a digital mammography system with improved performance are mainly related to the x-ray detector and the display device. There is active development of high-resolution display monitors and hardcopy devices to meet the demanding requirements (number of pixels, luminance, speed, multi-image capacity) of displaying digital mammography images, and suitable systems for this purpose should be available in the near future. The detector should have the following characteristics:

1. Efficient absorption of the incident radiation beam
2. Linear response over a wide range of incident radiation intensity

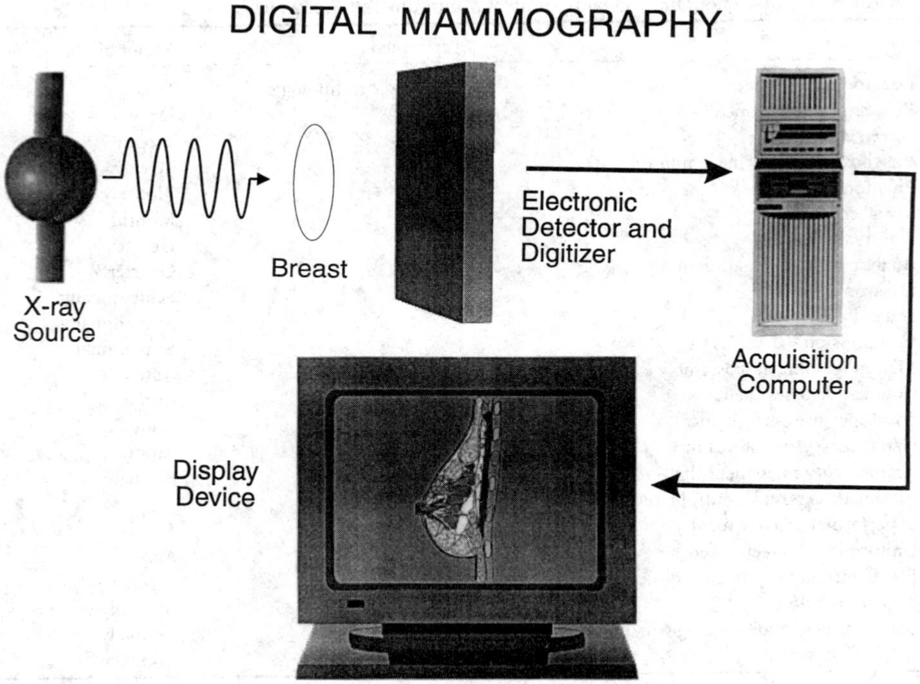

DIGITAL MAMMOGRAPHY

FIGURE 63.20   Schematic representation of a digital mammography system.

3. Low intrinsic noise
4. Spatial resolution on the order of 10 cycles/mm (50-μm sampling)
5. Can accommodate at least an 18 × 24 cm and preferably a 24 × 30 cm field size
6. Acceptable imaging time and heat loading of the x-ray tube

Two main approaches have been taken in detector development: area detectors and slot detectors. In the former, the entire image is acquired simultaneously, while in the latter only a portion of the image is acquired at one time and the full image is obtained by scanning the x-ray beam and detector across the breast. Area detectors offer convenient fast image acquisition and could be used with conventional x-ray machines but may still require a grid, while slot systems are slower, require a scanning x-ray beam, but use relatively simple detectors and have excellent intrinsic efficiency at scatter rejection. At the time of this writing, no clinical digital mammography system is in use for full breast imaging, although systems that produce small area (5 × 5 cm) digital images [Karellas et al., 1990] have recently been introduced commercially [Lorad, Fischer] in imaging devices to facilitate stereotactic breast biopsy. These use a lens or a fiberoptic taper to couple a phosphor to a CCD whose format is approximately square and typically provide 1K × 1K images with 50-μm pixels. Adjustment of display contrast enhances the localization of the lesion, while the immediate display of images (no film processing is required) greatly accelerates the clinical procedure.

Various detector technologies are being developed and evaluated for use in digital mammography. These include large-area CCDs, photostimulable phosphors, amorphous silicon coupled to scintillators, amorphous selenium, and other solid-state devices. A review of the field of digital mammography is given in Yaffe [1994].

Summary

Mammography is a technically demanding imaging procedure that can help reduce mortality from breast cancer. To be successful at this purpose, both the technology and the technique used for imaging must be optimized. This requires careful system design and attention to quality-control procedures. Imaging systems for mammography are still evolving and will, in the future, make greater use of computer imaging methods.

Defining Terms

Conversion efficiency: The efficiency of converting the energy from x-rays absorbed in a phosphor material into that of emitted light quanta.

Fibroglandular tissue: A mixture of tissues within the breast composed of the functional glandular tissue and the fibrous supporting structures.

Focal spot: The area of the anode of an x-ray tube from which the useful beam of x-rays is emitted. Also known as the *target*.

Grid: A device consisting of evenly spaced lead strips which functions like a venetian blind in preferentially allowing x-rays traveling directly from the focal spot without interaction in the patient to pass through, while those whose direction has been diverted by scattering in the patient strike the slats of the grid and are rejected. Grids improve the contrast of radiographic images at the price of increased dose to the patient.

Image receptor: A device that records the distribution of x-rays to form an image. In mammography, the image receptor is generally composed of a light-tight cassette containing a fluorescent screen, which absorbs x-rays and produces light, coupled to a sheet of photographic film.

References

Beaman SA, Lillicrap SC. 1982. Optimum x-ray spectra for mammography. Phys Med Biol 27:1209.

Health Effects of Exposure to Low Levels of Ionizing Radiation (BEIR V). 1990. Washington, National Academy Press. 163–170.

Boring CC, Squires TS, Tong T. 1992. Cancer statistics. CA 42:19.

Conway BJ, Suleiman OH, Rueter FG, et al. 1992. Does credentialing make a difference in mammography? Radiology 185(P):250.

Desponds L, Depeursinge C, Grecescu M, et al. 1991. Image of anode and filter material on image quality and glandular dose for screen-film mammography. Phys Med Biol 36:1165.

Fahrig R, Maidment ADA, Yaffe MJ. 1992. Optimization of peak kilovoltage and spectral shape for digital mammography. Proc SPIE 1651:74.

Heidsieck R, Laurencin G, Ponchin A, et al. 1991. Dual target x-ray tubes for mammographic examinations: Dose reduction with image quality equivalent to that with standard mammographic tubes. Radiology 181(P):311.

Hendrick RE, Bassett LW, Botsco MA et al. 1992. Mammography Quality Control Manuals (Radiologist, Radiologic Technologist, Medical Physicist). Reston, Va, American College of Radiology.

Hendrick RE, Parker SH. 1994. Stereotaxic imaging. In AG Haus, MJ Yaffe (eds), A Categorical Course in Physics: Technical Aspects of Breast Imaging, pp 263–274. Oak Brook, Ill, RSNA Publications.

Jennings RJ, Quinn PW, Gagne RM, Fewell TR. 1993. Evaluation of x-ray sources for mammography. Proc SPIE 1896:259.

Johns PC, Yaffe MJ. 1987. X-ray characterization of normal and neoplastic breast tissues. Phys Med Biol 32:675.

Karellas A, Harris LJ, D'Orsi CJ. 1990. Small field digital mammography with a 2048×2048 pixel charge-coupled device. Radiology 177:288.

Lorad Medical Systems, Danbury, Connecticut, and Fischer Imaging Corp., Denver Colorado.

McClelland R, Hendrick RE, Zinninger MD, Wilcox PW. 1991. The American College of Radiology Mammographic Accreditation Program. AJR. 157:473.

Nishikawa RM, Yaffe MJ. 1985. Signal-to-noise properties of mammography filmscreen systems. Med Phys 12:32.

Smart CR, Hartmann WH, Beahrs OH, et al. 1993. Insights into breast cancer screening of younger women: Evidence from the 14-year follow-up of the Breast Cancer Detection Demonstration Project. Cancer 72:1449.

Tabar L, Duffy SW, Burhenne LW. 1993. New Swedish breast cancer detection results for women aged 40–49. Cancer (Suppl) 72:1437.

Wagner AJ. 1991. Contrast and grid performance in mammography. In GT Barnes, GD Frey (eds), Screen Film Mammography: Imaging Considerations and Medical Physics Responsibilities, pp 115–134. Madison, Wisc, Medical Physics Publishing.

Wu X, Barnes GT, Tucker DM. 1991. Spectral dependence of glandular tissue dose in screen-film mammography. Radiology 179:143.

Yaffe MJ. 1994. Digital mammography. In AG Haus, MJ Yaffe (eds), A Categorical Course in Physics: Technical Aspects of Breast Imaging, pp 275–286. Oak Brook, Ill, RSNA Publications.

Further Information

Barnes GT, Frey GD (eds). 1991. Screen Film Mammography: Imaging Considerations and Medical Physics Responsibilities. Madison, Wisc, Medical Physics Publishing. Considerable practical information related to obtaining and maintaining high quality mammography is provided here.

Haus AG (ed). 1993. Film Processing in Medical Imaging Madison, Wisc, Medical Physics Publishing. This book deals with all aspects of medical film processing with particular emphasis on mammography.

Haus AG, Yaffe MJ. 1994. A Categorical Course in Physics: Technical Aspects of Breast Imaging. Oak Brook, Ill, RSNA Publications. In this syllabus to a course presented at the Radiological Society of North America, all technical aspects of mammography are addressed by experts, and a clinical overview is presented in language understandable by the physicist or biomedical engineer.

Yaffe MJ, et al. 1993. Recommended Specifications for New Mammography Equipment, ACR-CDC Cooperative Agreement for Quality Assurance Activities in Mammography. Reston, Va, ACR Publications.

64

Computed Tomography

Ian A. Cunningham
Victoria Hospital, the John P.
Robarts Research Institute, and
the University of Western
Ontario

Philip F. Judy
Brigham and Women's Hospital
and Harvard Medical School

64.1 Instrumentation

Ian A. Cunningham

The development of computed tomography (CT) in the early 1970s revolutionized medical radiology. For the first time, physicians were able to obtain high-quality tomographic (cross-sectional) images of internal structures of the body. Over the next 10 years, 18 manufacturers competed for the exploding world CT market. Technical sophistication increased dramatically, and even today, CT continues to mature, with new capabilities being researched and developed.

Computed tomographic images are reconstructed from a large number of measurements of x-ray transmission through the patient (called projection data). The resulting images are tomographic "maps" of the x-ray linear attenuation coefficient. The mathematical methods used to reconstruct CT images from projection data are discussed in the next section. In this section, the hardware and instrumentation in a modern scanner are described.

The first practical CT instrument was developed in 1971 by Dr. G. N. Hounsfield in England and was used to image the brain [Hounsfield, 1980]. The projection data were acquired in approximately 5 minutes, and the tomographic image was reconstructed in approximately 20 minutes. Since then, CT technology has developed dramatically, and CT has become a standard imaging procedure for virtually all parts of the body in thousands of facilities throughout the world. Projection data are typically acquired in approximately 1 second, and the image is reconstructed in 3 to 5 seconds. One special-purpose scanner described below acquires the projection data for one tomographic image in 50 ms. A typical modern CT scanner is shown in Fig. 64.1, and typical CT images are shown in Fig. 64.2.

The fundamental task of CT systems is to make an extremely large number (approximately 500,000) of highly accurate measurements of x-ray transmission through the patient in a precisely controlled geometry. A basic system generally consists of a gantry, a patient table, a control console, and a computer. The gantry contains the x-ray source, x-ray detectors, and the data-acquisition system (DAS).

Data-Acquisition Geometries

Projection data may be acquired in one of several possible geometries described below, based on the scanning configuration, scanning motions, and detector arrangement. The evolution of these

0-8493-8346-3/95/$0.00+$.50
© 1995 by CRC Press, Inc.

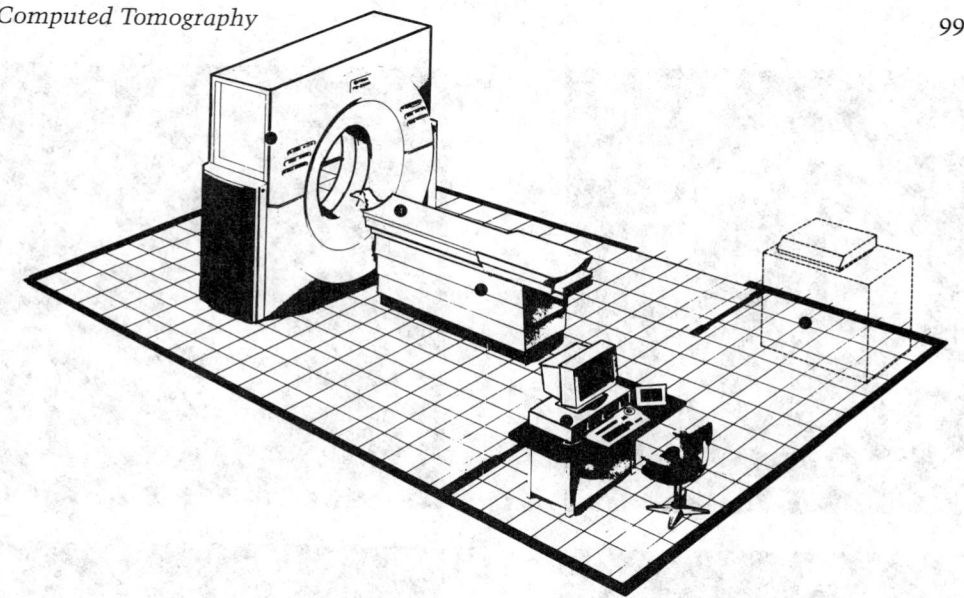

FIGURE 64.1 Schematic drawing of a typical CT scanner installation, consisting of (1) control console, (2) gantry stand, (3) patient table, (4) head holder, and (5) laser imager. (Courtesy of Picker International, Inc.)

geometries is described in terms of "generations," as illustrated in Fig. 64.3, and reflects the historical development [Newton and Potts, 1981; Seeram, 1994]. Current CT scanners use either third-, fourth-, or fifth-generation geometries, each having their own pros and cons.

First Generation: Parallel-Beam Geometry

Parallel-beam geometry is the simplest technically and the easiest with which to understand the important CT principles. Multiple measurements of x-ray transmission are obtained using a single highly collimated x-ray pencil beam and detector. The beam is translated in a linear motion across the patient to obtain a projection profile. The source and detector are then rotated about the patient isocenter by approximately 1 degree, and another projection profile is obtained. This translate-rotate scanning motion is repeated until the source and detector have been rotated by 180 degrees. The highly collimated beam provides excellent rejection of radiation scattered in the patient; however, the complex scanning motion results in long (approximately 5-minute) scan times. This geometry was used by Hounsfield in his original experiments [Hounsfield, 1980] but is not used in modern scanners.

Second Generation: Fan Beam, Multiple Detectors

Scan times were reduced to approximately 30 s with the use of a fan beam of x-rays and a linear detector array. A translate-rotate scanning motion was still employed; however, a larger rotate increment could be used, which resulted in shorter scan times. The reconstruction algorithms are slightly more complicated than those for first-generation algorithms because they must handle fan-beam projection data.

Third Generation: Fan Beam, Rotating Detectors

Third-generation scanners were introduced in 1976. A fan beam of x-rays is rotated 360 degrees around the isocenter. No translation motion is used; however, the fan beam must be wide enough to completely contain the patient. A curved detector array consisting of several hundred independent detectors is mechanically coupled to the x-ray source, and both rotate together. As a result, these rotate-only motions acquire projection data for a single image in as little as 1 s. Third-generation designs have the advantage that thin tungsten septa can be placed between each detector in the array and focused on the x-ray source to reject scattered radiation.

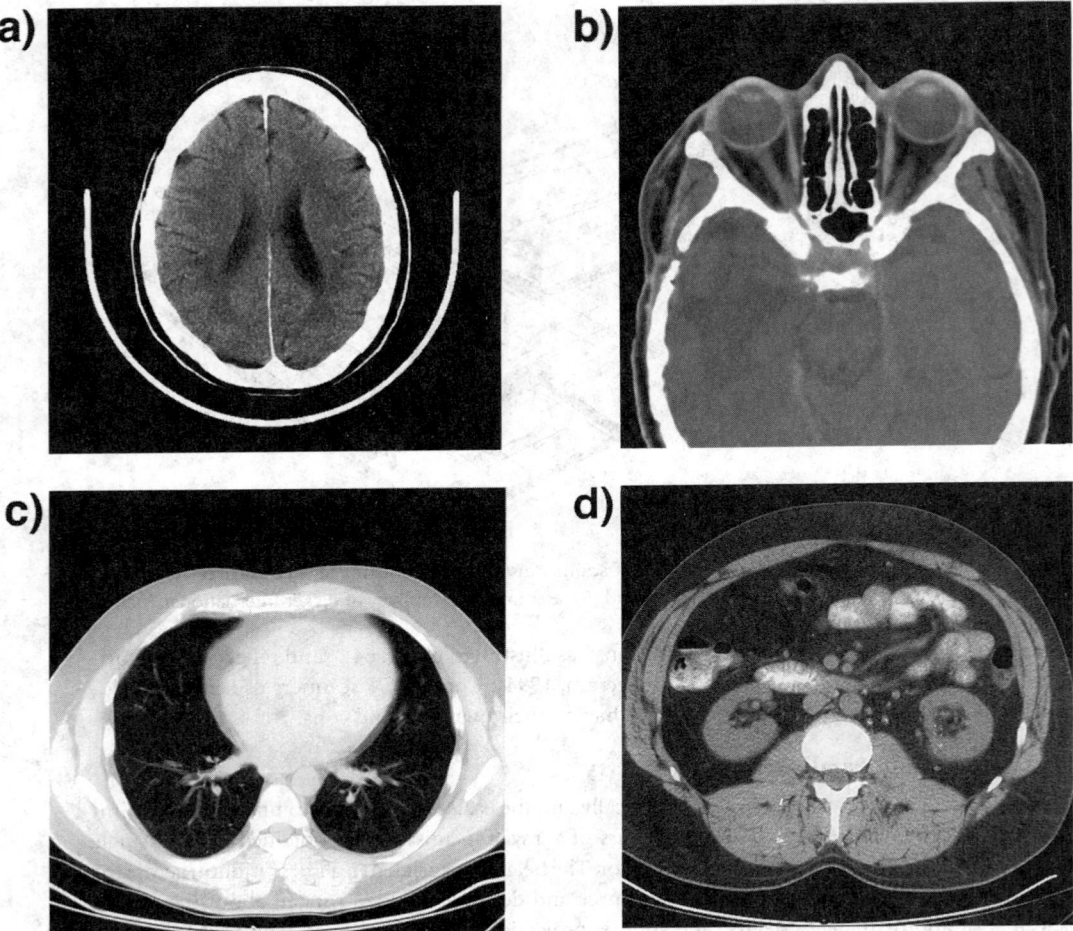

FIGURE 64.2 Typical CT images of (*a*) brain, (*b*) head showing orbits, (*c*) chest showing lungs, and (*d*) abdomen.

Fourth Generation: Fan Beam, Fixed Detectors

In a fourth-generation scanner, the x-ray source and fan beam rotate about the isocenter, while the detector array remains stationary. The detector array consists of 600 to 4800 (depending on the manufacturer) independent detectors in a circle that completely surrounds the patient. Scan times are similar to those of third-generation scanners. The detectors are no longer coupled to the x-ray source and hence cannot make use of focused septa to reject scattered radiation. However, detectors are calibrated twice during each rotation of the x-ray source, providing a self-calibrating system. Third-generation systems are calibrated only once every few hours.

Two detector geometries are currently used for fourth-generation systems: (1) a rotating x-ray source inside a fixed detector array and (2) a rotating x-ray source outside a nutating detector array. Figure 64.4 shows the major components in the gantry of a typical fourth-generation system using a fixed-detector array. Both third- and fourth-generation systems are commercially available, and both have been highly successful clinically. Neither can be considered an overall superior design.

Fifth Generation: Scanning Electron Beam

Fifth-generation scanners are unique in that the x-ray source becomes an integral part of the system design. The detector array remains stationary, while a high-energy electron beam is electroni-

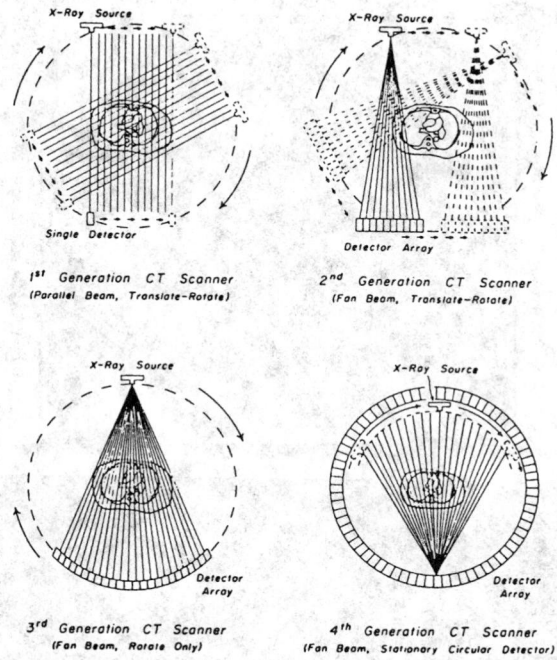

FIGURE 64.3 Four generations of CT scanners illustrating the parallel- and fan-beam geometries [Robb, 1982].

cally swept along a semicircular tungsten strip anode, as illustrated in Fig. 64.5. X-rays are produced at the point where the electron beam hits the anode, resulting in a source of x-rays that rotates about the patient with no moving parts [Boyd et al., 1979]. Projection data can be acquired in approximately 50 ms, which is fast enough to image the beating heart without significant motion artifacts [Boyd and Lipton, 1983].

An alternative fifth-generation design, called the *dynamic spatial reconstructor (DSR) scanner,* is in use at the Mayo Clinic [Ritman, 1980, 1990]. This machine is a research prototype and is not available commercially. It consists of 14 x-ray tubes, scintillation screens, and video cameras. Volume CT images can be produced in as little as 10 ms.

Spiral/Helical Scanning

The requirement for faster scan times, and in particular for fast multiple scans for three-dimensional imaging, has resulted in the development of spiral (helical) scanning systems [Kalendar et al., 1990]. Both third- and fourth-generation systems achieve this using self-lubricating slip-ring technology (Fig. 64.6) to make the electrical connections with rotating components. This removes the need for power and signal cables which would otherwise have to be rewound between scans and allows for a continuous rotating motion of the x-ray fan beam. Multiple images are acquired while the patient is translated through the gantry in a smooth continuous motion rather than stopping for each image. Projection data for multiple images covering a volume of the patient can be acquired in a single breath hold at rates of approximately one slice per second. The reconstruction algorithms are more sophisticated because they must accommodate the spiral or helical path traced by the x-ray source around the patient, as illustrated in Fig. 64.7.

X-Ray System

The x-ray system consists of the x-ray source, detectors, and a data-acquisition system.

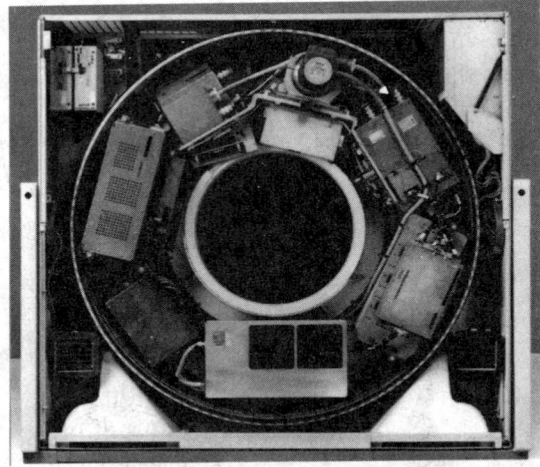

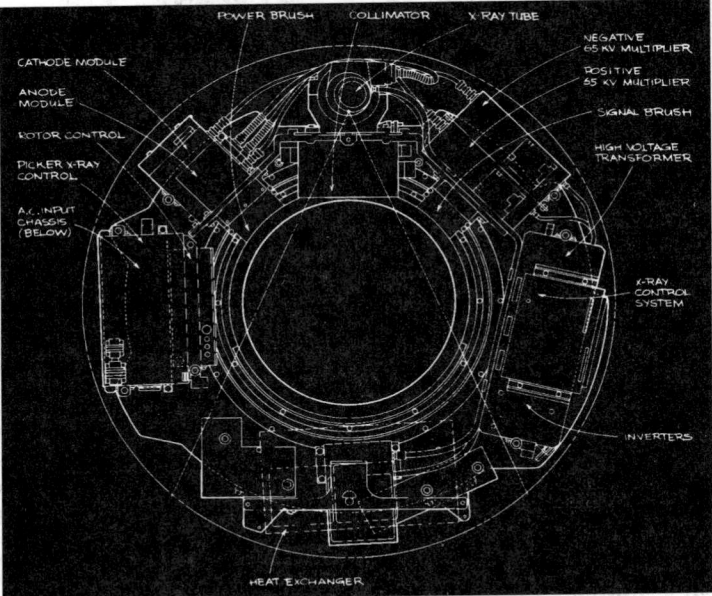

FIGURE 64.4 The major internal components of a fourth-generation CT gantry are shown in a photograph with the gantry cover removed (upper) and identified in the line drawing (lower). (Courtesy of Picker International, Inc.)

X-Ray Source

With the exception of one fifth-generation system described above, all CT scanners use bremsstrahlung x-ray tubes as the source of radiation. These tubes are typical of those used in diagnostic imaging and produce x-rays by accelerating a beam of electrons onto a target anode. The anode area from which x-rays are emitted, projected along the direction of the beam, is called the focal spot. Most systems have two possible focal spot sizes, approximately 0.5 × 1.5 mm and 1.0 × 2.5 mm. A collimator assembly is used to control the width of the fan beam between 1.0 and 10 mm, which in turn controls the width of the imaged slice.

The power requirements of these tubes are typically 120 kV at 200 to 500 mA, producing x-rays with an energy spectrum ranging between approximately 30 and 120 keV. All modern systems use high-frequency generators, typically operating between 5 and 50 kHz [Brunnett et al., 1990]. Some spiral systems use a stationary generator in the gantry, requiring high-voltage (120-kV) slip rings,

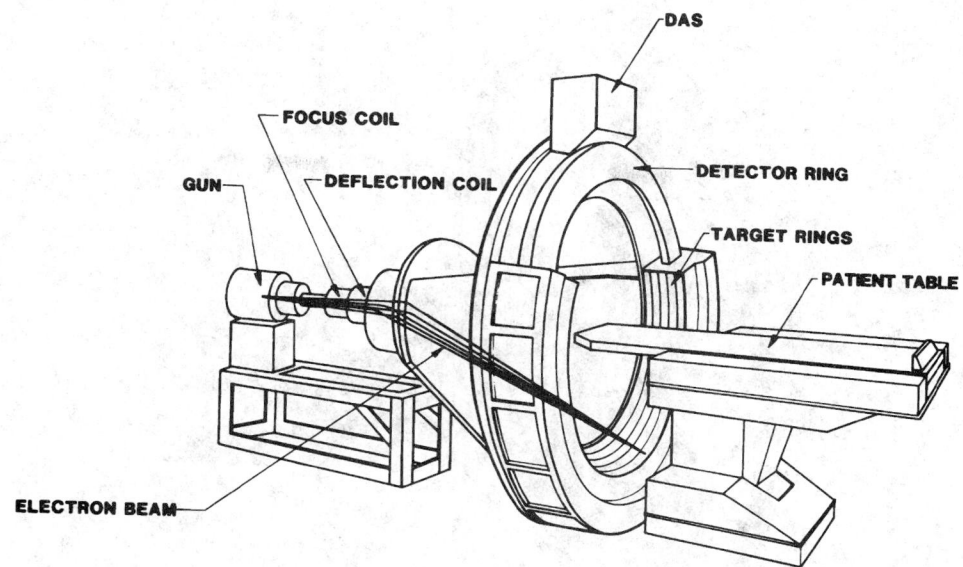

FIGURE 64.5 Schematic illustration of a fifth-generation ultrafast CT system. Image data are acquired in as little as 50 ms, as an electron beam is swept over the strip anode electronically. (Courtesy of Imatron, Inc.)

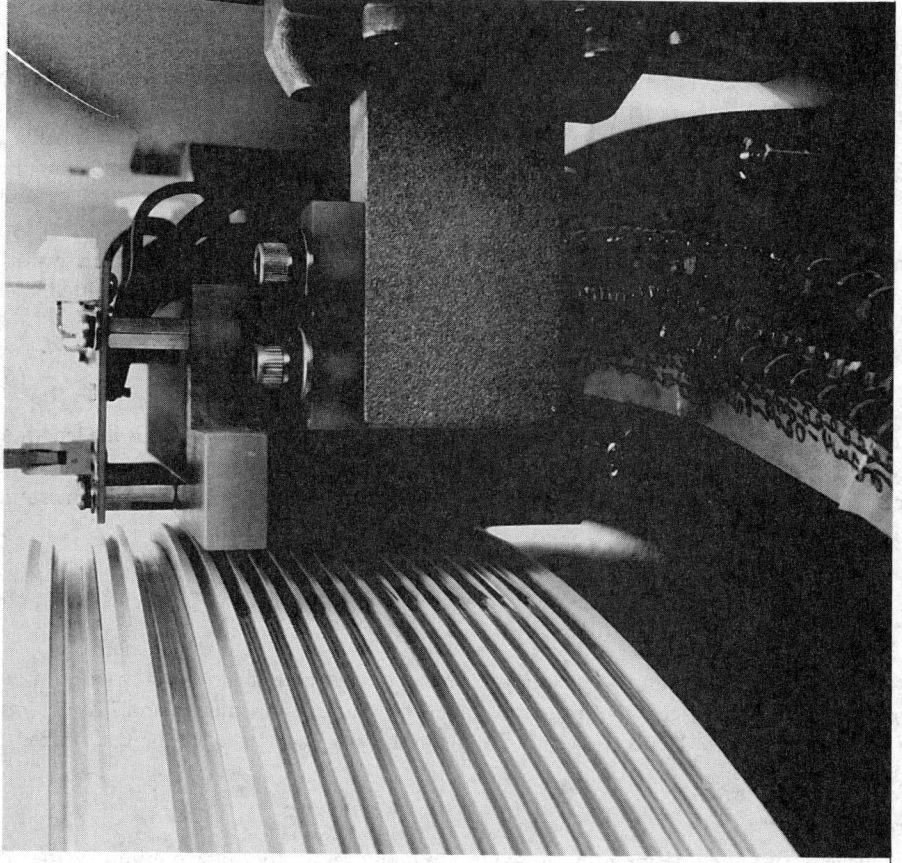

FIGURE 64.6 Photograph of the slip rings used to pass power and control signals to the rotating gantry. (Courtesy of Picker International, Inc.)

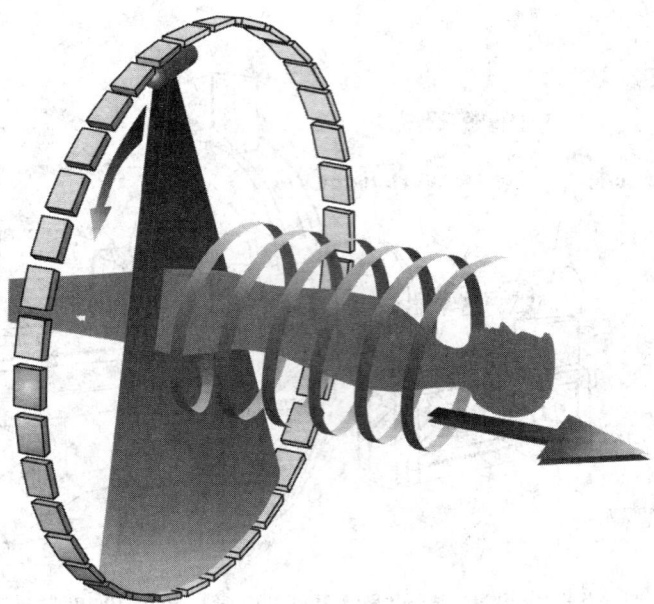

FIGURE 64.7 Spiral scanning causes the focal spot to follow a spiral path around the patient as indicated. (Courtesy of Picker International, Inc..)

while others use a rotating generator with lower-voltage (480-V) slip rings. Production of x-rays in bremsstrahlung tubes is an inefficient process, and hence most of the power delivered to the tubes results in heating of the anode. A heat exchanger on the rotating gantry is used to cool the tube. Spiral scanning, in particular, places heavy demands on the heat-storage capacity and cooling rate of the x-ray tube.

The intensity of the x-ray beam is attenuated by absorption and scattering processes as it passes through the patient. The degree of attenuation depends on the energy spectrum of the x-rays as well as on the average atomic number and mass density of the patient tissues. The transmitted intensity is given by

$$I_t = I_o e^{-\int_0^L \mu(x)\,dx} \tag{64.1}$$

where I_o and I_t are the incident and transmitted beam intensities, respectively; L is the length of the x-ray path; and $\mu(x)$ is the x-ray linear attenuation coefficient, which varies with tissue type and hence is a function of the distance x through the patient. The integral of the attenuation coefficient is therefore given by

$$\int_0^L \mu(x)\,dx = -\frac{1}{L}\ln\,(I_t/I_o) \tag{64.2}$$

The reconstruction algorithm requires measurements of this integral along many paths in the fan beam at each of many angles about the isocenter. The value of L is known, and I_o is determined by a system calibration. Hence values of the integral along each path can be determined from measurements of I_t.

X-Ray Detectors

X-ray detectors used in CT systems must (a) have a high overall efficiency to minimize the patient radiation dose, have a large dynamic range, (b) be very stable with time, and (c) be insensitive to temperature variations within the gantry. Three important factors contributing to the detector efficiency are geometric efficiency, quantum (also called *capture*) efficiency, and conversion efficiency [Villafanaet al., 1987]. *Geometric efficiency* refers to the area of the detectors sensitive to radiation as a fraction of the total exposed area. Thin septa between detector elements to remove scattered radiation, or other insensitive regions, will degrade this value. *Quantum efficiency* refers to the fraction of incident x-rays on the detector that are absorbed and contribute to the measured signal. *Conversion efficiency* refers to the ability to accurately convert the absorbed x-ray signal into an electrical signal (but is not the same as the energy conversion efficiency). *Overall efficiency* is the product of the three, and it generally lies between 0.45 and 0.85. A value of less than 1 indicates a nonideal detector system and results in a required increase in patient radiation dose if image quality is to be maintained. The term *dose efficiency* sometimes has been used to indicate overall efficiency.

Modern commercial systems use one of two detector types: solid-state or gas ionization detectors.

Solid-State Detectors. Solid-state detectors consist of an array of scintillating crystals and photodiodes, as illustrated in Fig. 64.8. The scintillators generally are either cadmium tungstate ($CdWO_4$) or a ceramic material made of rare earth oxides, although previous scanners have used bismuth germanate crystals with photomultiplier tubes. Solid-state detectors generally have very high quantum and conversion efficiencies and a large dynamic range.

Gas Ionization Detectors. Gas ionization detectors, as illustrated in Fig. 64.9, consist of an array of chambers containing compressed gas (usually xenon at up to 30 atm pressure). A high voltage is applied to tungsten septa between chambers to collect ions produced by the radiation. These detectors have excellent stability and a large dynamic range; however, they generally have a lower quantum efficiency than solid-state detectors.

Data-Acquisition System

The transmitted fraction I_t/I_o in Eq. (64.2) through an obese patient can be less than 10^{-4}. Thus it is the task of the data-acquisition system (DAS) to accurately measure I_t over a dynamic range of more than 10^4, encode the results into digital values, and transmit the values to the system computer for reconstruction. Some manufacturers use the approach illustrated in Fig. 64.10, consisting of precision preamplifiers, current-to-voltage converters, analog integrators, multiplexers, and analog-to-digital converters. Alternatively, some manufacturers use the preamplifier to control a synchronous voltage-to-frequency converter (SVFC), replacing the need for the integrators, multiplexers, and analog-to-digital converters [Brunnett et al., 1990]. The logarithmic conversion required in Eq. (64.2) is performed with either an analog logarithmic amplifier or a digital lookup table, depending on the manufacturer.

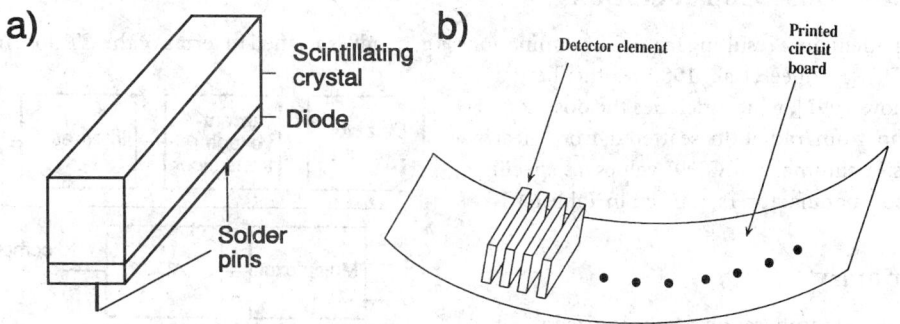

FIGURE 64.8 (*a*) A solid-state detector consists of a scintillating crystal and photodiode combination. (*b*) Many such detectors are placed side by side to form a detector array that may contain up to 4800 detectors.

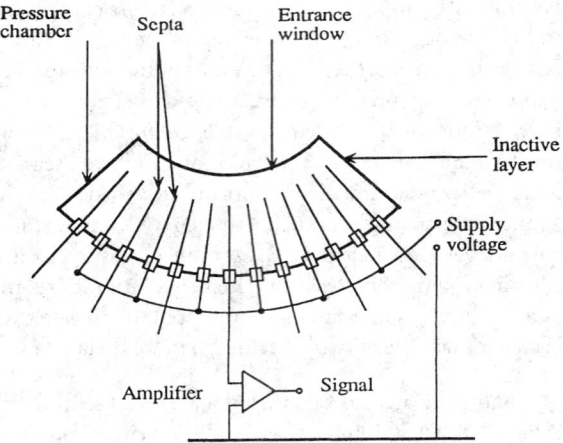

FIGURE 64.9 Gas ionization detector arrays consist of high-pressure gas in multiple chambers separated by thin septa. A voltage is applied between alternating septa. The septa also act as electrodes and collect the ions created by the radiation, converting them into an electrical signal.

Sustained data transfer rates to the computer are as high as 10 Mbytes/s for some scanners. This can be accomplished with a direct connection for systems having a fixed detector array. However, third-generation slip-ring systems must use more sophisticated techniques. At least one manufacturer uses optical transmitters on the rotating gantry to send data to fixed optical receivers [Siemens, 1989].

Computer System

Various computer systems are used by manufacturers to control system hardware, acquire the projection data, and reconstruct, display, and manipulate the tomographic images. A typical system is illustrated in Fig. 64.11, which uses 12 independent processors connected by a 40-Mbyte/s multibus. Multiple custom array processors are used to achieve a combined computational speed of 200 MFLOPS (million floating-point operations per second) and a reconstruction time of approximately 5 s to produce an image on a 1024 × 1024 pixel display. A simplified UNIX operating system is used to provide a multitasking, multiuser environment to coordinate tasks.

Patient Dose Considerations

The patient dose resulting from CT examinations is generally specified in terms of the CT dose index (CTDI) [Felmlee et al., 1989; Rothenberg and Pentlow, 1992], which includes the dose contribution from radiation scattered from nearby slices. A summary of CTDI values, as specified by four manufacturers, is given in Table 64.1.

Summary

Computed tomography revolutionized medical radiology in the early 1970s. Since that time, CT technology has developed dramatically, taking advantage of developments in computer hard-

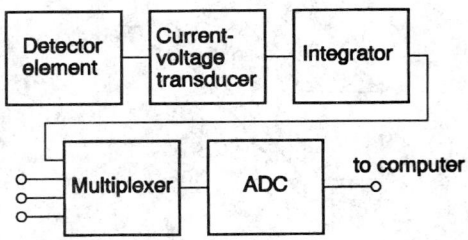

FIGURE 64.10 The data-acquisition system converts the electrical signal produced by each detector to a digital value for the computer.

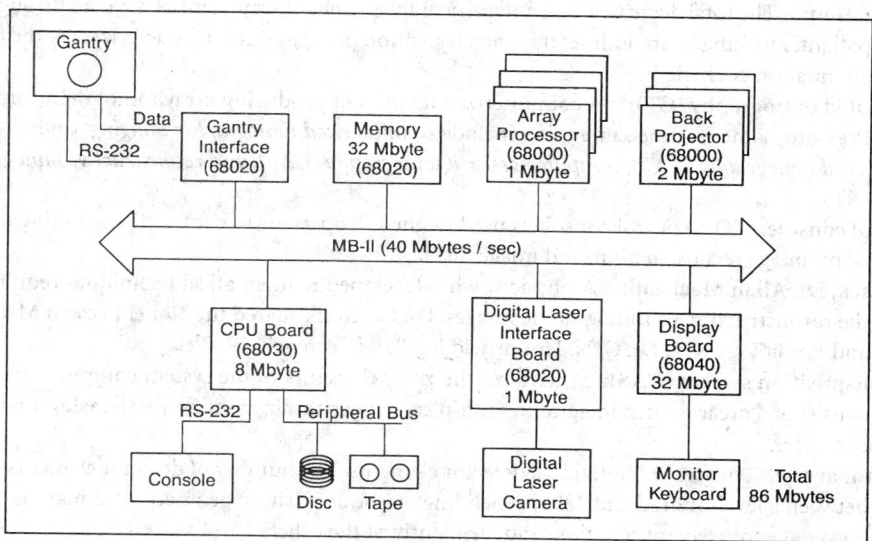

FIGURE 64.11 The computer system controls the gantry motions, acquires the x-ray transmission measurements, and reconstructs the final image. The system shown here uses 12 68000-family CPUs. (Courtesy of Picker International, Inc.)

TABLE 64.1 Summary of the CT Dose Index (CTDI) Values at Two Positions (Center of the Patient and Near the Skin) as Specified by Four CT Manufacturers for Standard Head and Body Scans.

Manufacturer	Detector	kVp	mA	Scan Time (s)	CTDI, center (mGy)	CTDI, skin (mGy)
A, head	Xexon	120	170	2	50	48
A, body	Xexon	120	170	2	14	25
A, head	Solid state	120	170	2	40	40
A, body	Solid state	120	170	2	11	20
B, head	Solid state	130	80	2	37	41
B, body	Solid state	130	80	2	15	34
C, head	Solid state	120	500	2	39	50
C, body	Solid state	120	290	1	12	28
D, head	Solid state	120	200	2	78	78
D, body	Solid state	120	200	2	9	16

ware and detector technology. Modern systems acquire the projection data required for one tomographic image in approximately 1 s and present the reconstructed image on a 1024 × 1024 matrix display within a few seconds. The images are high-quality tomographic "maps" of the x-ray linear attenuation coefficient of the patient tissues.

Defining Terms

Absorption: Some of the incident x-ray energy is absorbed in patient tissues and hence does not contribute to the transmitted beam.

Anode: A tungsten target bombarded by a beam of electrons to produce x-rays. In all but one fifth-generation system, the anode rotates to distribute the resulting heat around the perimeter. The anode heat-storage capacity and maximum cooling rate often limit the maximum scanning rates of CT systems.

Attenuation: The total decrease in the intensity of the primary x-ray beam as it passes through the patient, resulting from both scatter and absorption processes. It is characterized by the linear attenuation coefficient.

Computed tomography (CT):   A computerized method of producing x-ray tomographic images. Previous names for the same thing include *computerized tomographic imaging, computerized axial tomography (CAT), computer-assisted tomography (CAT),* and *reconstructive tomography (RT).*

Control console: The control console is used by the CT operator to control the scanning operations, image reconstruction, and image display.

Cormack, Dr. Allan MacLeod: A physicist who developed mathematical techniques required in the reconstruction of tomographic images. Dr. Cormack shared the Nobel Prize in Medicine and Physiology with Dr. G. N. Hounsfield in 1979 [Cormack, 1980].

Data-acquisition system (DAS):   Interfaces the x-ray detectors to the system computer and may consist of a preamplifier, integrator, multiplexer, logarithmic amplifier, and analog-to-digital converter.

Detector array: An array of individual detector elements. The number of detector elements varies between a few hundred and 4800, depending on the acquisition geometry and manufacturer. Each detector element functions independently of the others.

Fan beam: The x-ray beam is generated at the focal spot and so diverges as it passes through the patient to the detector array. The thickness of the beam is generally selectable between 1.0 and 10 mm and defines the slice thickness.

Focal spot: The region on the anode where x-rays are generated.

Focused septa: Thin metal plates between detector elements which are aligned with the focal spot so that the primary beam passes unattenuated to the detector elements, while scattered x-rays which normally travel in an altered direction are blocked.

Gantry: The largest component of the CT installation, containing the x-ray tube, collimators, detector array, DAS, other control electronics, and the mechanical components required for the scanning motions.

Helical scanning: The scanning motions in which the x-ray tube rotates continuously around the patient while the patient is continuously translated through the fan beam. The focal spot therefore traces a helix around the patient. Projection data are obtained which allow the reconstruction of multiple contiguous images. This operation is sometimes called *spiral, volume,* or *three-dimensional* CT scanning.

Hounsfield, Dr. Godfrey Newbold: An engineer who developed the first practical CT instrument in 1971. Dr. Hounsfield received the McRobert Award in 1972 and shared the Nobel Prize in Medicine and Physiology with Dr. A. M. Cormack in 1979 for this invention [Hounsfield, 1980].

Image plane: The plane through the patient that is imaged. In practice, this plane (also called a *slice*) has a selectable thickness between 1.0 and 10 mm centered on the image plane.

Pencil beam: A narrow, well-collimated beam of x-rays.

Projection data: The set of transmission measurements used to reconstruct the image.

Reconstruct: The mathematical operation of generating the tomographic image from the projection data.

Scan time: The time required to acquire the projection data for one image, typically 1.0 s.

Scattered radiation: Radiation that is removed from the primary beam by a scattering process. This radiation is not absorbed but continues along a path in an altered direction.

Slice: See Image plane.

Spiral scanning: See Helical scanning.

Three-dimensional imaging: See Helical scanning.

Tomography: A technique of imaging a cross-sectional slice.

Volume CT: See Helical scanning.

X-ray detector: A device that absorbs radiation and converts some or all of the absorbed energy into a small electrical signal.

X-ray linear attenuation coefficient μ: Expresses the relative rate of attenuation of a radiation beam as it passes through a material. The value of μ depends on the density and atomic number of the material and on the x-ray energy. The units of μ are cm^{-1}.

X-ray source: The device that generates the x-ray beam. All CT scanners use rotating-anode bremsstrahlung x-ray tubes except one fifth-generation system, which uses a unique scanned electron beam and a strip anode.

X-ray transmission: The fraction of the x-ray beam intensity that is transmitted through the patient without being scattered or absorbed. It is equal to I_t/I_o in Eq. (64.2), can be determined by measuring the beam intensity both with (I_t) and without (I_o) the patient present, and is expressed as a fraction. As a rule of thumb, n^2 independent transmission measurements are required to reconstruct an image with an $n \times n$ sized pixel matrix.

References

Boyd DP, et al. 1979. A proposed dynamic cardiac 3D densitometer for early detection and evaluation of heart disease. IEEE Trans Nucl Sci 2724.

Boyd DP, Lipton MJ. 1983. Cardiac computed tomography. Proc IEEE 198.

Brunnett CJ, Heuscher DJ, Mattson RA, Vrettos CJ. 1990. CT Design Considerations and Specifications. Picker International, CT Engineering Department, Ohio.

Cormack AM. 1980. Nobel Award Address: Early two-dimensional reconstruction and recent topics stemming from it. Med Phys 7(4):277.

Felmlee JP, Gray JE, Leetzow ML, Price JC. 1989. Estimated fetal radiation dose from multislice CT studies. Am Roent Ray Soc 154:185.

Hounsfield GN. 1980. Nobel Award Address: Computed medical imaging. Med Phys 7(4):283.

Kalendar WA, Seissler W, Klotz E, et al. 1990. Spiral volumetric CT with single-breath-hold technique, continous transport, and continous scanner rotation. Radiology 176:181.

Newton TH, Potts DG (eds). 1981. Radiology of the Skull and Brain: Technical Aspects of Computed Tomography. St. Louis, Mosby.

Picker. 1990. Computed Dose Index PQ2000 CT Scanner. Picker International, Ohio.

Ritman EL. 1980. Physical and technical considerations in the design of the DSR, and high temporal resolution volume scanner. AJR 134:369.

Ritman EL. 1990. Fast computed tomography for quantitative cardiac analysis—State of the art and future perspectives. Mayo Clin Proc 65:1336.

Robb RA. 1982. X-ray computed tomography: An engineering synthesis of multiscientific principles. CRC Crit Rev Biomed Eng 7:265.

Rothenberg LN, Pentlow KS. 1992. Radiation dose in CT. RadioGraphics 12:1225.

Seeram E. 1994. Computed Tomography: Physical Principles, Clinical Applications and Quality Control. Philadelphia, Saunders.

Siemens. 1989. The Technology and Performance of the Somatom Plus. Siemens Aktiengesellschaft, Medical Engineering Group, Erlangen, Germany.

Villafana T, Lee SH, Rao KCVG (eds). 1987. Cranial Computed Tomography. New York, McGraw-Hill.

Further Information

A recent summary of CT instrumentation and concepts is given by E. Seeram in *Computed Tomography: Physical Principles, Clinical Applications and Quality Control.* The author summarizes CT from the perspective of the nonmedical, nonspecialist user. A summary of average CT patient doses is described by Rothenberg and Pentlow [1992] in *Radiation Dose in CT.* Research papers on both fundamental and practical aspects of CT physics and instrumentation are published in numerous journals, including *Medical Physics, Physics in Medicine and Biology, Journal of Computer Assisted Tomography, Radiology, British Journal of Radiology,* and the IEEE Press. A comparison of technical specifications of CT systems provided by the manufacturers is available from ECRI to help orient the new purchaser in a selection process. Their *Product Comparison System* includes a table of basic specifications for all the major international manufacturers.

64.2 Reconstruction Principles

Philip F. Judy

Computed tomography (CT) is a two-step process: (1) the transmission of an x-ray beam is measured through all possible straight-line paths in a plane of an object, and (2) the attenuation of x-ray beam is estimated at points in the object. Initially, the transmission measurements will be assumed to be the results of an experiment performed with a narrow monoenergetic beam of x-rays that are confined to a plane. The designs of devices that attempt to realize these measurements are described in the preceding section. One formal consequence of these assumptions is that the logarithmic transformation of the measured x-ray intensity is proportional the line integral of attenuation coefficients. In order to satisfy this assumption, computer processing procedures on the measurements of x-ray intensity are necessary even before image reconstruction is performed. These linearization procedures will reviewed after background.

Both analytical and iterative estimations of linear x-ray attenuation have been used for transmission CT reconstruction. Iterative procedures are of historic interest because an iterative reconstruction procedure was used in the first commercially successful CT scanner [EMI, Mark I, Hounsfield, 1973]. They also permit easy incorporation of physical processes that cause deviations from the linearity. Their practical usefulness is limited. The first EMI scanner required 20 minutes to finish its reconstruction. Using the identical hardware and employing an analytical calculation, the estimation of attenuation values was performed during the 4.5-minute data acquisition and was made on a 160 × 160 matrix. The original iterative procedure reconstructed the attenuation values on an 80 × 80 matrix and consequently failed to exploit all the spatial information inherent in transmission data.

Analytical estimation, or direct reconstruction, uses a numerical approximation of the inverse Radon transform [Radon, 1917]. The direct reconstruction technique (convolution-backprojection) presently used in x-ray CT was initially applied in other areas such as radio astronomy [Bracewell and Riddle, 1967] and electron microscopy [Crowther et al., 1970; Ramachandran and Lakshminarayana, 1971]. These investigations demonstrated that the reconstructions from discrete spatial sampling of bandlimited data led to full recovery of the cross-sectional attenuation. The random variation (noise) in x-ray transmission measurements may not be bandlimited. Subsequent investigators [e.g., Chesler and Riederer, 1975; Herman and Roland, 1973; Shepp and Logan, 1974] have suggested various bandlimiting windows that reduce the propagation and amplification of noise by the reconstruction. These issues have been investigated by simulation, and investigators continue to pursue these issues using a computer phantom [e.g., Guedon and Bizais, 1994, and references therein] described by Shepp and Logan. The subsequent investigations of the details of choice of reconstruction parameters has had limited practical impact because real variation of transmission data is bandlimited by the finite size of the focal spot and radiation detector, a straightforward design question, and because random variation of the transmission tends to be uncorrelated. Consequently, the classic precedures suffice.

Image Processing: Artifact and Reconstruction Error

An *artifact* is a reconstruction defect that is obviously visible in the image. The classification of an image feature as an artifact involves some visual criterion. The effect must produce an image feature that is greater than the random variation in image caused by the intrinsic variation in transmission measurements. An artifact not recognized by the physician observer as an artifact may be reported as a lesion. Such false-positive reports could lead to an unnecessary medical procedure, e.g., surgery to remove an imaginary tumor. A *reconstruction error* is a deviation of the reconstruction value from its expected value. Reconstruction errors are significant if the application involves a quantitative measurement, not a common medical application. The reconstruction errors are characterized by identical material at different points in the object leading to different reconstructed attenuation values in the image which are not visible in the medical image.

Investigators have used computer simulation to investigate artifact [Herman, 1980] because image noise limits the visibility of their visibility. One important issue investigated was required spatial sampling of transmission slice plane [Crawford and Kak, 1979; Parker et al., 1982]. These simulations provided a useful guideline in design. In practice, these aliasing artifacts are overwhelmed by random noise, and designers tend to oversample in the slice plane. A second issue that was understood by computer stimulation was the partial volume artifact [Glover and Pelc, 1980]. This artifact would occur even for mononergetic beams and finite beam size, particularly in the axial dimension. The axial dimension of the beams tend to be greater (about 10 mm) than their dimensions in the slice plane (about 1 mm). The artifact is created when the variation of transmission within the beam varies considerably, and the exponential variation within the beam is summed by the radiation detector. The logarithm transformation of the detected signal produces a nonlinear effect that is propagated throughout the image by the reconstruction process. Simulation was useful in demonstrating that isolated features in the same cross-section act together to produce streak artifacts. Simulations have been useful to illustrate the effects of patient motion during the data-acquisition streaks off high-contrast objects.

Projection Data to Image: Calibrations

Processing of transmission data is necessary to obtain high-quality images. In general, optimization of the projection data will optimize the reconstructed image. Reconstruction is a process that removes the spatial correlation of attenuation effects in the transmitted image by taking advantage of completely sampling the possible transmissions. Two distinct calibrations are required: registration of beams with the reconstruction matrix and linearization of the measured signal.

Without loss of generalization, a projection will be considered a set of transmissions made along parallel lines in the slice plane of the CT scanner. *Without loss of generalization* means that essential aspects of all calibration and reconstruction procedures required for fan-beam geometries are captured by the calibration and reconstruction procedures described for parallel projections. One line of each projection is assumed to pass through the center of rotation of data collection. Shepp et al. [1979] showed that errors in the assignment of that center-of-rotation point in the projections could lead to considerable distinctive artifacts and that small errors (0.05 mm) would produce these effects. The consequences of these errors have been generalized to fan-beam collection schemes, and images reconstructed from 180-degree projection sets were compared with images reconstructed from 360-degree data sets [Kijewski and Judy, 1983]. A simple misregistration of the center of rotation was found to produce blurring of image without the artifact. These differences may explain the empirical observation that most commercial CT scanners collect a full 360-degree data set even though 180 degrees of data will suffice.

The data-acquisition scheme that was designed to overcome the limited sampling inherent in third-generation fan-beam systems by shifting detectors a quarter sampling distance while opposite 180-degree projection is measured has particularly stringent registration requirements. Also, the fourth-generation scanner does not link the motion of the x-ray tube and the detector; consequently, the center of rotation is determined as part of a calibration procedure, and unsystematic effects lead to artifacts that mimic noise besides blurring the image.

Misregistration artifacts also can be mitigated by *feathering*. This procedure requires collection of redundant projection data at the end of the scan. A single data set is produce by linearly weighting the redundant data at the beginning and end of the data collection [Parker et al., 1982]. These procedures have be useful in reducing artifacts from gated data collections [Moore et al., 1987].

The other processing necessary before reconstruction of project data is *linearization*. The formal requirement for reconstruction is that the line integrals of some variable be available; it is this variable that ultimately is reconstructed. The logarithm of x-ray transmission approximates this requirement. There are physical effects in real x-ray transmissions that cause deviations from this assumption. X-ray beams of sufficient intensity are composed of photons of different energies. Some photons in the beam interact with objects and are scattered rather than absorbed. The spectrum of x-ray photons of different attenuation coefficients means the logarithm of the transmission measurement will not be proportional to the line integral of the attenuation coefficient along that path, because an attenuation coefficient cannot even be defined. An effective attenuation coefficient can only be defined uniquely for a spectrum for a small mass of material that alters that intensity. It has to be small enough not to alter the spectrum [McCullough, 1979].

A straightforward approach to this nonunique attenuation coefficient error, called *hardening*, is to assume that the energy dependence of the attenuation coefficient is constant and that differences in attenuation are related to a generalized density factor that multiplies the spectral dependence of attenuation. The transmission of a x-ray beam then can be estimated for a standard material, typically water, as a function of thickness. This assumption is that attenuations of materials in the object, the human body, differ because specific gravities of the materials differ. Direct measurements of the transmission of an actual x-ray beam may provide initial estimates that can be parameterized. The inverse of this function provides the projection variable that is reconstructed. The parameters of the function are usually modified as part of a calibration to make the CT image of a uniform water phantom flat.

Such a calibration procedure does not deal completely with the hardening effects. The spectral dependence of bone differs considerably from that of water. This is particularly critical in imaging of the brain, which is contained within the skull. Without additional correction, the attenuation values of brain are lower in the center than near the skull.

The detection of scattered energy means that the reconstructed attenuation coefficient will differ from the attenuation coefficient estimated with careful narrow-beam measurements. The x-rays appear more penetrating because scattered x-rays are detected. The zero-order scatter, a decrease in the attenuation coefficient by some constant amount, is dealt with automatically by the calibration that treats hardening. First-order scattering leads to a widening of the x-ray beam and can be dealt with by a modification of the reconstruction kernel.

Projection Data to Image: Reconstruction

The impact of CT created considerable interest in the formal aspects of reconstruction. There are many detailed descriptions of direct reconstruction procedures. Some are presented in textbooks used in graduate courses for medical imaging [Barrett and Swindell, 1981; Cho et al., 1993]. Herman [1980] published a textbook that was based on a two-semester course that dealt exclusively with reconstruction principles, demonstrating the reconstruction principles with simulation.

The standard reconstruction method is called *convolution-backprojection*. The first step in the procedure is to convolve the projection, a set of transmissions made along parallel lines in the slice plane, with a reconstruction kernel derived from the inverse Radon transform. The choice of kernel is dictated by bandlimiting issues [Chesler and Riederer, 1975; Herman and Roland, 1973; Shepp and Logan, 1974]. It can be modified to deal with the physical aperture of the CT system [Bracewell, 1977], which might include the effects of scatter. The convolved projection is then backprojected onto a two-dimensional image matrix. Backprojection is the opposite of projection; the value of the projection is added to each point along the line of the projection. This procedure makes sense in the continuous description, but in the discrete world of the computer, the summation is done over the image matrix.

Consider a point of the image matrix; very few, possibly no lines of the discrete projection data intersect the point. Consequently, to estimate the projection value to be added to that point, the procedure must interpolate between two values of sampled convolve projection. The linear interpolation scheme is a significant improvement over nearest project nearest to the point. More complex schemes get confounded with choices of reconstruction kernel, which are designed to accomplish standard image processing in the image, e.g., edge enhancement.

Scanners have been developed to acquire a three-dimensional set of projection data [Kalender et al., 1990]. The motion of the source defines a spiral motion relative to the patient. The spiral motion defines an axis. Consequently, only one projection is available for reconstruction of the attenuation values in the plane. This is the back-projection problem just discussed; no correct projection value is available from the discrete projection data set. The solution is identical: a projection value is interpolated from the existing projection values to estimate the necessary projections for each plane to be reconstructed. This procedure has the advantage that overlapping slices can be reconstructed without additional exposure, and this eliminates the risk that a small lesion will be missed because it straddles adjacent slices. This data-collection scheme is possible because systems that continuously rotate have been developed. The spiral scan motion is realized by moving the patient through the gantry. Spiral CT scanners have made possible the acquisition of an entire data set in a single breath hold.

References

Barrett H.H, Swindell W. 1981. Radiological Imaging: The Theory and Image Formation, Detection, and Processing, vol 2. New York, Academic Press.

Bracewell RN, Riddle AC. 1976. Inversion of fan-beam scans in radio astronomy. The Astrophysical Journal 150:427–434.

Chesler DA, Riederer SJ. 1975. Ripple suppression during reconstruction in transverse tomography. Phys Med Biol 20(4):632–636.

Cho Z, Jones JP, Singh M. 1993. Foundations of medical imaging. New York, Wiley & Sons, Inc.

Crawford CR, Kak AC. 1979. Aliasing artifacts in computerized tomography. Applied Optics 18:3704–3711.

Glover GH, Pelc NJ. 1980. Nonlinear partial volume artifacts in x-ray computed tomography. Med Phys 7:238–248.

Guedon J-P, Bizais. 1994. Bandlimited and harr filtered back-projection reconstruction. IEEE Trans Medical Imaging 13(3):430–440.

Herman GT, Rowland SW. 1973. Three methods for reconstruction objects for x-rays—a comparative study. Comp Graph Imag Process 2:151–178.

Herman GT. 1980. Image Reconstruction from Projection: The Fundamentals of Computerized Tomography. New York, New York Academic Press.

Hounsfield, GN. 1973. Computerized transverse axial scanning (tomography): Part I. Brit J Radiol 46:1016–1022.

Kalender WA, Weissler, Klotz E, et al. 1990. Spiral volumetric CT with single-breath-hold techique, continuous transport, and continuous scanner rotation. Radiology 176:181–183.

Kijewski MF, Judy PF. 1983. The effect of misregistration of the projections on spatial resolution of CT scanners. Med Phys 10:169–175.

McCullough EC. 1979. Specifying and evaluating the performance of computed tomographic (CT) scanners. Med Phys 7:291–296.

Moore SC, Judy PF, Garnic JD, et al. 1983. The effect of misregistration of the projections on spatial resolution of CT scanners. Med Phys 10:169–175.

65

Magnetic Resonance Imaging

Steven Conolly
Stanford University

Albert Macovski
Stanford University

John Pauly
Stanford University

John Schenck
General Electric Corporate Research and Development Center

Kenneth K. Kwong
Massachusetts General Hospital and Harvard University Medical School

David A. Chesler
Massachusetts General Hospital and Harvard University Medical School

Xiaoping Hu
Center for Magnetic Resonance Research and the University of Minnesota Medical School

Wei Chen
Center for Magnetic Resonance Research and the University of Minnesota Medical School

Maqbool Patel
Center for Magnetic Resonance Research and the University of Minnesota Medical School

Kamil Ugurbil
Center for Magnetic Resonance Research and the University of Minnesota Medical School

65.1 Acquisition and Processing

Steven Conolly, Albert Macovski, and John Pauly

Magnetic resonance imaging (MRI) is a clinically important medical imaging modality due to its exceptional soft-tissue contrast. MRI was invented in the early 1970s [1]. The first commercial scanners appeared about 10 years later. Noninvasive MRI studies are now supplanting many conventional invasive procedures. A 1990 study [2] found that the principal applications for MRI are examinations of the head (40%), spine (33%), bone and joints (17%), and the body (10%). The percentage of bone and joint studies was growing in 1990.

Although typical imaging studies range from 1 to 10 minutes, new fast imaging techniques acquire images in less than 50 ms. MRI research involves fundamental tradeoffs between resolution, imaging time, and signal-to-noise ratio (SNR). It also depends heavily on both gradient and receiver coil hardware innovations.

In this section we provide a brief synopsis of basic nuclear magnetic resonance (NMR) physics. We then derive the k-space analysis of MRI, which interprets the received signal as a scan of the Fourier transform of the

0-8493-8346-3/95/$0.00+$.50
© 1995 by CRC Press, Inc.

image. This powerful formalism is used to analyze the most important imaging sequences. Finally, we discuss the fundamental contrast mechanisms for MRI.

Fundamentals of MRI

Magnetic resonance imaging exploits the existence of induced nuclear magnetism in the patient. Materials with an odd number of protons or neutrons possess a weak but observable nuclear magnetic moment. Most commonly protons (^{1}H) are imaged, although carbon (^{13}C), phosphorous (^{31}P), sodium (^{23}Na), and fluorine (^{19}F) are also of significant interest. The nuclear moments are normally randomly oriented, but they align when placed in a strong magnetic field. Typical field strengths for imaging range between 0.2 and 1.5 T, although spectroscopic and functional imaging work is often performed with higher field strengths. The nuclear magnetization is very weak; the ratio of the induced magnetization to the applied field is only 4×10^{-9}. The collection of nuclear moments is often referred to as magnetization or spins.

The static nuclear moment is far too weak to be measured when it is aligned with the strong static magnetic field. Physicists in the 1940s developed resonance techniques that permit this weak moment to be measured. The key idea is to measure the moment while it oscillates in a plane perpendicular to the static field [3,4]. First one must tip the moment away from the static field. When perpendicular to the static field, the moment feels a torque proportional to the strength of the static magnetic field. The torque always points perpendicular to the magnetization and causes the spins to oscillate or precess in a plane perpendicular to the static field. The frequency of the rotation ω_0 is proportional to the field:

$$\omega_0 = -\gamma B_0$$

where γ, the gyromagnetic ratio, is a constant specific to the nucleus, and B_0 is the magnetic field strength. The direction of B_0 defines the z axis. The precession frequency is called the Larmor frequency. The negative sign indicates the direction of the precession.

Since the precessing moments constitute a time-varying flux, they produce a measurable voltage in a loop antenna arranged to receive the x and y components of induction. It is remarkable that in MRI we are able to directly measure induction from the precessing nuclear moments of water protons.

Recall that to observe this precession, we first need to tip the magnetization away from the static field. This is accomplished with a weak rotating radiofrequency (RF) field. It can be shown that a rotating RF field introduces a fictitious field in the z direction of strength ω/γ. By tuning the frequency of the RF field to ω_0, we effectively delete the B_0 field. The RF slowly nutates the magnetization away from the z axis. The Larmor relation still holds in this "rotating frame," so the frequency of the nutation is γB_1, where B_1 is the amplitude of the RF field. Since the coils receive x and y (transverse) components of induction, the signal is maximized by tipping the spins completely into the transverse plane. This is accomplished by a $\pi/2$ RF pulse, which requires $\gamma B_1 \tau = \pi/2$, where τ is the duration of the RF pulse. Another useful RF pulse rotates spins by π radians. This can be used to invert spins. It also can be used to refocus transverse spins that have dephased due to B_0 field inhomogeneity. This is called a spin echo and is widely used in imaging.

NMR has been used for decades in chemistry. A complex molecule is placed in a strong, highly uniform magnetic field. Electronic shielding produces microscopic field variations within the molecule so that geometrically isolated nuclei rotate about distinct fields. Each distinct magnetic environment produces a peak in the spectra of the received signal. The relative size of the spectral peaks gives the ratio of nuclei in each magnetic environment. Hence the NMR spectrum is extremely useful for elucidating molecular structure.

The NMR signal from a human is due predominantly to water protons. Since these protons exist in identical magnetic environments, they all resonate at the same frequency. Hence the NMR signal is simply proportional to the volume of the water. The key innovation for MRI is to impose spatial variations on the magnetic field to distinguish spins by their location. Applying a magnetic field gradient causes each region of the volume to oscillate at a distinct frequency. The most effective nonuniform field is a linear gradient where the field and the resulting frequencies vary linearly with distance along the object being studied. Fourier analysis of the signal obtains a map of the spatial distribution of spins. This argument is formalized below, where we derive the powerful k-space analysis of MRI [5,6].

k-Space Analysis of Data Acquisition

In MRI, we receive a volume integral from an array of oscillators. By ensuring that the phase "signature" of each oscillator is unique, one can assign a unique location to each spin and thereby reconstruct an image. During signal reception, the applied magnetic field points in the z direction. Spins precess in the xy plane at the Larmor frequency. Hence a spin at position $\mathbf{r} = (x,y,z)$ has a unique phase θ that describes its angle relative to the y axis in the xy plane:

$$\theta(\mathbf{r},t) = -\gamma \int_0^t B_z(\mathbf{r},\tau)\, d\tau \tag{65.1}$$

where $B_z(\mathbf{r},t)$ is the z component of the instantaneous, local magnetic flux density. This formula assumes there are no x and y field components.

A coil large enough to receive a time-varying flux uniformly from the entire volume produces an EMF proportional to

$$s(t) \propto \frac{d}{dt} \int_V M(\mathbf{r}) e^{-i\theta(\mathbf{r},t)}\, dr \tag{65.2}$$

where $M(\mathbf{r})$ represents the equilibrium moment density at each point $\mathbf{r}$.

The key idea for imaging is to superimpose a linear field gradient on the static field B_0. This field points in the direction z, and its magnitude varies linearly with a coordinate direction. For example, an x gradient points in the z direction and varies along the coordinate x. This is described by the vector field $xG_x\hat{\mathbf{z}}$, where $\hat{\mathbf{z}}$ is the unit vector in the z direction. In general, the gradient is $(xG_x + yG_y + zG_z)\,\hat{\mathbf{z}}$, which can be written compactly as the dot product $\mathbf{G} \cdot \mathbf{r}\,\hat{\mathbf{z}}$. These gradient field components can vary with time, so the total z field is

$$B_z(\mathbf{r},t) = B_0 + \mathbf{G}(t) \cdot \mathbf{r} \tag{65.3}$$

In the presence of this general time-varying gradient, the received signal is

$$s(t) \propto \frac{d}{dt} \int_V e^{-i\gamma B_0 t} M(\mathbf{r}) e^{-i\gamma \int_0^t \mathbf{G}(\tau) \cdot \mathbf{r}\, d\tau}\, dr \tag{65.4}$$

The center frequency γB_0 is always much larger than the bandwidth of the signal. Hence the derivative operation is approximately equivalent to multiplication by $-i\omega_0$. The signal is demodulated by the waveform $e^{i\gamma B_0 t}$ to obtain the "baseband" signal:

$$S(t) \propto -i\omega_0 \int_V M(\mathbf{r}) e^{-i\gamma \int_0^t \mathbf{G}(\tau) \cdot \mathbf{r}\, d\tau}\, dr \tag{65.5}$$

It will be helpful to define the term $\mathbf{k}(t)$:

$$\mathbf{k}(t) = \gamma \int_0^t \mathbf{G}(\tau)\, d\tau \tag{65.6}$$

Then we can rewrite the received baseband signal as

$$S(t) \propto \int_V M(\mathbf{r})e^{-i\mathbf{k}(t)\cdot\mathbf{r}}\,dr \tag{65.7}$$

which we can now identify as *the spatial Fourier transform of $M(\mathbf{r})$ evaluated at $\mathbf{k}(t)$*. That is, $S(t)$ scans the spatial frequencies of the function $M(\mathbf{r})$. This can be written explicitly as

$$S(t) \propto \mathscr{M}(\mathbf{k}(t)) \tag{65.8}$$

where $\mathscr{M}(\mathbf{k})$ is the three-dimensional Fourier transform of the object distribution $M(\mathbf{r})$. Thus we can view MRI with linear gradients as a "scan" of k-space or the spatial Fourier transform of the image. After the desired portion of k-space is scanned, the image $M(\mathbf{r})$ is reconstructed using an inverse Fourier transform.

2D Imaging. Many different gradient waveforms can be used to scan k-space and to obtain a desired image. The most common approach, called *two-dimensional Fourier transform imaging* (**2D FT**), is to scan through k-space along several horizontal lines covering a rectilinear grid in 2D k-space. See Fig. 65.1 for a schematic of the k-space traversal. The horizontal grid lines are acquired using 128 to 256 excitations separated by a time TR, which is determined by the desired contrast, RF flip angle, and the T_1 of the desired components of the image. The horizontal-line scans through k-space are offset in k_y by a variable area y-gradient pulse, which happens before data acquisition starts. These variable offsets in k_y are called *phase encodes* because they affect the phase of the signal rather than the frequency. Then for each k_y phase encode, signal is acquired while scanning horizontally with a constant x gradient.

Resolution and Field of View. The fundamental image characteristics of resolution and field of view (FOV) are completely determined by the characteristics of the k-space scan. The extent of the

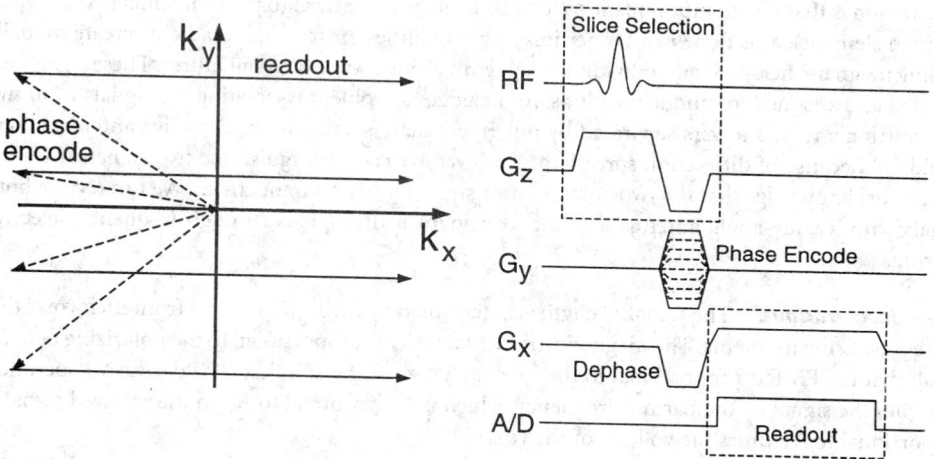

FIGURE 65.1 The drawing on the left illustrates the scanning pattern of the 2D Fourier transform imaging sequence. On the right is a plot of the gradient and RF waveforms that produce this pattern. Only four of the N_y horizontal k-space lines are shown. The phase-encode period initiates each acquisition at a different k_y and at $-k_x(\text{max})$. Data are collected during the horizontal traversals. After all N_y k-space lines have been acquired, a 2D FFT reconstructs the image. Usually 128 or 256 k_y lines are collected, each with 256 samples along k_x. The RF pulse and the z gradient waveform together restrict the image to a particular slice through the subject.

coverage of k-space determines the resolution of the reconstructed image. The resolution is inversely proportional to the highest spatial frequency acquired:

$$\frac{1}{\Delta x} = \frac{k_x(\text{max})}{\pi} = \frac{\gamma G_x T}{2\pi} \tag{65.9}$$

$$\frac{1}{\Delta y} = \frac{k_y(\text{max})}{\pi} = \frac{\gamma G_y T_{\text{phase}}}{\pi} \tag{65.10}$$

where G_x is the readout gradient amplitude and T is the readout duration. The time T_{phase} is the duration of the phase-encode gradient G_y. For proton imaging on a 1.5-T imaging system, a typical gradient strength is $G_x = 1$ G/cm. The signal is usually read for about 8 ms. For water protons, $\gamma = 26{,}751$ rad/s/G, so the maximum excursion in k_x is about 21 rad/mm. Hence we cannot resolve an object smaller than 0.3 mm in width. From this one might be tempted to improve the resolution dramatically using very strong gradients or very long readouts. But there are severe practical obstacles, since higher resolution increases the scan time and also degrades the image SNR.

In the phase-encode direction, the k-space data are sampled discretely. This discrete sampling in k-space introduces replication in the image domain [7]. If the sampling in k-space is finer than 1/FOV, then the image of the object will not fold back on itself. When the k-space sampling is coarser than 1/FOV, the image of the object does fold back over itself. This is termed *aliasing*. Aliasing is prevented in the readout direction by the sampling filter.

Perspective.   For most imaging systems, diffraction limits the resolution. That is, the resolution is limited to the wavelength divided by the angle subtended by the receiver aperture, which means that the ultimate resolution is approximately the wavelength itself. This is true for imaging systems based on optics, ultrasound, and x-rays (although there are other important factors, such as quantum noise, in x-ray).

MRI is the only imaging system for which the resolution is independent of the wavelength. In MRI, the wavelength is often many meters, yet submillimeter resolution is routinely achieved. The basic reason is that no attempt is made to focus the radiation pattern to the individual pixel or voxel (volume element), as is done in all other imaging modalities. Instead, the gradients create spatially varying magnetic fields so that individual pixels emit unique waveform signatures. These signals are decoded and assigned to unique positions. An analogous problem is isolating the signals from two transmitting antenna towers separated by much less than a wavelength. Directive antenna arrays would fail because of diffraction spreading. However, we can distinguish the two signals if we use the a priori knowledge that the two antennas transmit at different frequencies. We can receive both signals with a wide-angle antenna and then distinguish the signals through frequency-selective filtering.

SNR Considerations.   The signal strength is determined by the EMF induced from each voxel due to the processing moments. The magnetic moment density is proportional to the polarizing field B_0. Recall that the EMF is proportional to the rate of change of the coil flux. The derivative operation multiples the signal by the Larmor frequency, which is proportional to B_0, so the received signal is proportional to B_0^2 times the volume of the voxel V_v.

In a well-designed MRI system, the dominant noise source is due to thermally generated currents within the conductive tissues of the body. These currents create a time-varying flux which induces noise voltages in the receiver coil. Other noise sources include the thermal noise from the antenna and from the first amplifier. These subsystems are designed so that the noise is negligible compared with the noise from the patient. The noise received is determined by the total volume seen by the antenna pattern V_n and the effective resistivity and temperature of the conductive tissue. One can show [8] that the standard deviation of the noise from conductive tissue varies linearly with B_0. The noise is filtered by an integration over the total acquisition time T_{acq}, which effectively attenuates the noise standard deviation by $\sqrt{T_{acq}}$. Therefore, the SNR varies as

$$\text{SNR} \propto \frac{B_0^2 V_v}{B_0 V_n / \sqrt{T_{acq}}} = B_0 \sqrt{T_{acq}}\,(V_v/V_n) \tag{65.11}$$

The noise volume V_n is the effective volume based on the distribution of thermally generated currents. For example, when imaging a spherical object of radius r, the noise standard deviation varies as $r^{5/2}$ [9]. The effective resistance depends strongly on the radius because currents near the outer radius contribute more to the noise flux seen by the receiver coil.

To significantly improve the SNR, most systems use *surface coils*, which are simply small coils that are just big enough to see the desired region of the body. Such a coil effectively maximizes the voxel-volume to noise-volume ratio. The noise is significantly reduced because these coils are sensitive to currents from a smaller part of the body. However, the field of view is somewhat limited, so "phased arrays" of small coils are now being offered by the major manufacturers [10]. In the phased array, each coil sees a small noise volume, while the combined responses provide the wide coverage at a greatly improved SNR.

Fast Imaging. The 2D FT scan of k-space has the disadvantage that the scan time is proportional to the number of phase encodes. It is often advantageous to trade off SNR for a shorter scan time. This is especially true when motion artifacts dominate thermal noise. To allow for a flexible trade-off of SNR for imaging time, more than a single line in k-space must be covered in a single excitation. The most popular approach, called *echo-planar imaging* (EPI), traverses k-space back and forth on a single excitation pulse. The k-space trajectory is drawn in Fig. 65.2.

It is important that the tradeoff be flexible so that you can maximize the imaging time given the motion constraints. For example, patients can hold their breath for about 12 seconds. So a scan of 12 seconds' duration gives the best SNR given the breath-hold constraint. The EPI trajectory can be *interleaved* to take full advantage of the breath-hold interval. If each acquisition takes about a second, 12 interleaves can be collected. Each interleaf acquires every twelfth line in k-space.

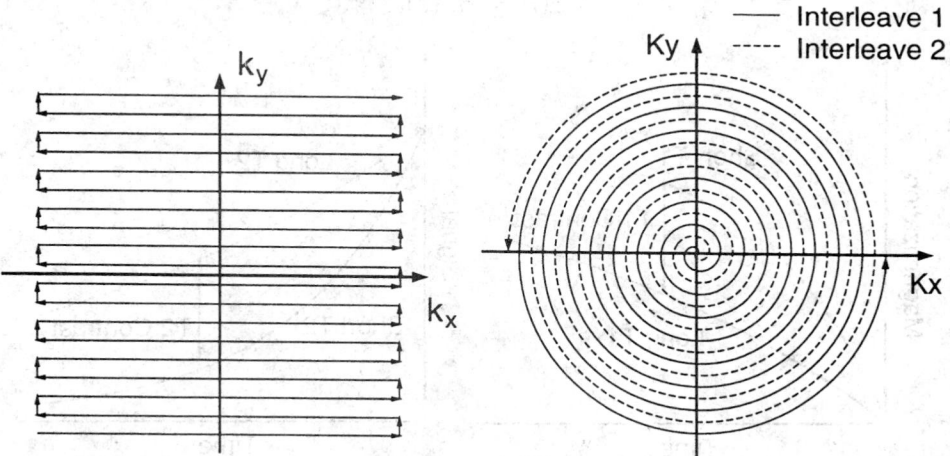

FIGURE 65.2 Alternative methods for the rapid traversal of k space. On the left is the echo planar trajectory. Data are collected during the horizontal traversals. When all N_y horizontal lines in k space have been acquired, the data are sent to a 2D FFT to reconstruct the image. On the right is an interleaved spiral trajectory. The data are interpolated to a 2D rectilinear grid and then Fourier transformed to reconstruct the image. These scanning techniques allow for imaging within a breathhold.

Another trajectory that allows for a flexible tradeoff between scan time and SNR is the spiral trajectory. Here the trajectory starts at the origin in *k*-space and spirals outward. Interleaving is accomplished by rotating the spirals. Figure 65.2 shows two interleaves in a spiral format. Interleaving is very helpful for reducing the hardware requirements (peak amplitude, peak slew rate, average dissipation, etc.) for the gradient amplifiers. For reconstruction, the data are interpolated to a 2D rectilinear grid and then Fourier-transformed. Our group has found spiral imaging to be very useful for imaging coronary arteries within a breath-hold scan [11]. The spiral trajectory is relatively immune to artifacts due to the motion of blood.

Contrast Mechanisms

The tremendous clinical utility of MRI is due to the great variety of mechanisms that can be exploited to create image contrast. If magnetic resonance images were restricted to water density, MRI would be considerably less useful, since most tissues would appear identical. Fortunately, many different MRI contrast mechanisms can be employed to distinguish different tissues and disease processes.

The primary contrast mechanisms exploit *relaxation* of the magnetization. The two types of relaxations are termed spin-lattice relaxation, characterized by a relaxation time T_1, and spin-spin relaxation, characterized by a relaxation time T_2.

Spin-lattice relaxation describes the rate of recovery of the z component of magnetization toward equilibrium after it has been disturbed by RF pulses. The recovery is given by

$$M_z(t) = M_0(1 - e^{-t/T_1}) + M_z(0)e^{-t/T_1} \qquad (65.12)$$

where M_0 is the equilibrium magnetization. Differences in the T_1 time constant can be used to produce image contrast by exciting all magnetization and then imaging before full recovery has been achieved. This is illustrated on the left in Fig. 65.3. An initial $\pi/2$ RF pulse destroys all the longitudinal magnetization. The plots show the recovery of two different T_1 components. The short T_1 component recovers faster and produces more signal. This gives a T_1-weighted image.

Spin-spin relaxation describes the rate at which the NMR signal decays after it has been created. The signal is proportional to the transverse magnetization and is given by

$$M_{xy}(t) = M_{xy}(0)e^{-t/T_2} \qquad (65.13)$$

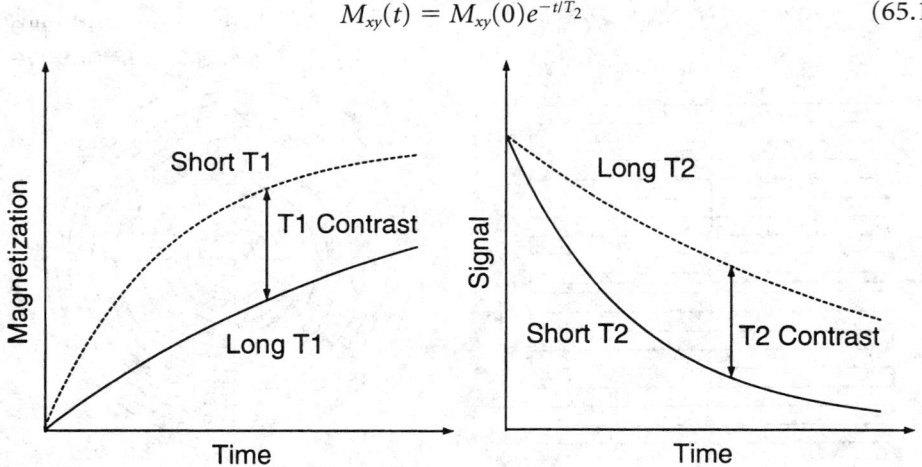

FIGURE 65.3 The two primary MRI contrast mechanisms, T_1 and T_2. T_1, illustrated on the left, describes the rate at which the equilibrium M_{zk} magnetization is restored after it has been disturbed. T_1 contrast is produced by imaging before full recovery has been obtained. T_2, illustrated on the right, describes the rate at which the MRI signal decays after it has been created. T_2 contrast is produced by delaying data acquisition, so shorter T_2 components produce less signal.

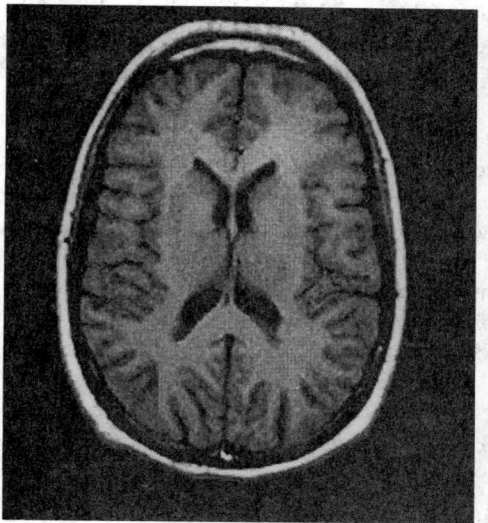 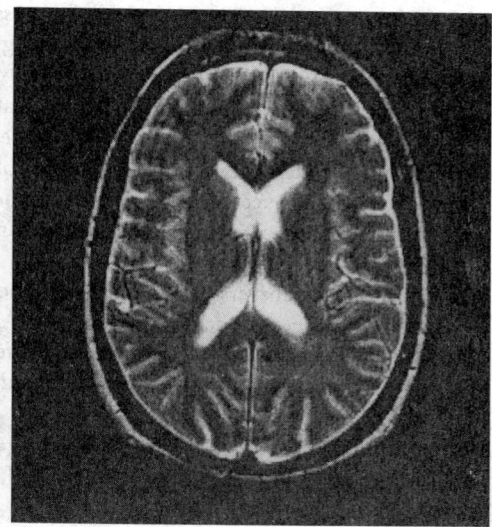

FIGURE 65.4 Example images of a normal volunteer demonstrating T_1 contrast on the left and T_2 contrast on the right.

Image contrast is produced by delaying the data acquisition. The decay of two different T_2 species is plotted on the right in Fig. 65.3. The signal from the shorter T_2 component decays more rapidly, while that of the longer T_2 component persists. At the time of data collection, the longer T_2 component produces more signal. This produces a T_2-weighted image.

Figure 65.4 shows examples of these two basic types of contrast. These images are of identical axial sections through the brain of a normal volunteer. The image on the left was acquired with an imaging method that produces T_1 contrast. The very bright ring of subcutaneous fat is due to its relatively short T_1. White matter has a shorter T_1 than gray matter, so it shows up brighter in this image. The image on the right was acquired with an imaging method that produces T_2 contrast. Here the cerebrospinal fluid in the ventricles is bright due to its long T_2. White matter has a shorter T_2 than gray matter, so it is darker in this image.

There are many other contrast mechanisms that are important in MRI. Different chemical species have slightly different resonant frequencies, and this can be used to image one particular component. It is possible to design RF and gradient waveforms so that the image shows only moving spins. This is of great utility in MR angiography, allowing the noninvasive depiction of the vascular system. Another contrast mechanism is called T_2^*. This relaxation parameter is useful for functional imaging. It occurs when there is a significant spread of Larmor frequencies within a voxel. The superposition signal is attenuated faster than T_2 due to destructive interference between the different frequencies.

In addition to the intrinsic tissue contrast, artificial MRI contrast agents also can be introduced. These are usually administered intravenously or orally. Many different contrast mechanisms can be exploited, but the most popular agents decrease both T_1 and T_2. One agent approved for clinical use is gadolinium DPTA. Decreasing T_1 causes faster signal recovery and a higher signal on a T_1-weighted image. The contrast-enhanced regions then show up bright relative to the rest of the image.

Defining Terms

Gyromagnetic ratio γ: An intrinsic property of a nucleus. It determines the Larmor frequency through the relation $\omega_0 = -\gamma B_0$.

***k*-space:**   The reciprocal of object space, *k*-space describes MRI data acquisition in the spatial Fourier transform coordinate system.

Larmor frequency ω_0: The frequency of precession of the spins. It depends on the product of the applied flux density B_0 and on the gyromagnetic ratio γ. The Larmor frequency is $\omega_0 = -\gamma B_0$.

Magnetization M: The macroscopic ensemble of nuclear moments. The moments are induced by an applied magnetic field. At body temperatures, the amount of magnetization is linearly proportional ($M_0 = 4 \times 10^{-9} H_0$) to the applied magnetic field.

Precession: The term used to describe the motion of the magnetization about an applied magnetic field. The vector locus traverses a cone. The precession frequency is the frequency of the magnetization components perpendicular to the applied field. The precession frequency is also called the *Larmor frequency ω_0*.

Spin echo: The transverse magnetization response to a π RF pulse. The effects of field inhomogeneity are refocused at the middle of the spin echo.

Spin-lattice relaxation T_1: The exponential rate constant describing the decay of the z component of magnetization toward the equilibrium magnetization. Typical values in the body are between 300 and 3000 ms.

Spin-spin relaxation T_2: The exponential rate constant describing the decay of the transverse components of magnetization (M_x and M_y).

Spins M: Another name for magnetization.

2D FT: A rectilinear trajectory through k-space. This popular acquisition scheme requires several (usually 128 to 256) excitations separated by a time *TR*, which is determined by the desired contrast, RF flip angle, and the T_1 of the desired components of the image.

References

1. Lauterbur PC. 1973. Nature 242:190.
2. Evens RG, Evens JRG. 1991. AJR 157:603.
3. Bloch F, Hansen WW, Packard ME. 1946. Phys Rev 70:474.
4. Bloch F. 1946. Phys Rev 70:460.
5. Twieg DB. 1983. Med Phys 10:610.
6. Ljunggren S. 1983. J Magnet Reson 54:338.
7. Bracewell RN. 1978. The Fourier Transform and Its Applications. New York, McGraw-Hill.
8. Hoult DI, Lauterbur PC. 1979. J Magnet Reson 34:425.
9. Chen CN, Hoult D. 1989. Biomedical Magnetic Resonance Technology. New York, Adam Hilger.
10. Roemer PB, Edelstein WA, Hayes CE, et al. 1990. Magn Reson Med 16:192.
11. Meyer CH, Hu BS, Nishimura DG, Macovski A. 1992. Magn Reson Med 28(2):202.

65.2 Hardware/Instrumentation

John Schenck

This section describes the basic components and the operating principles of MRI scanners. Although scanners capable of making diagnostic images of the human internal anatomy through the use of magnetic resonance imaging (MRI) are now ubiquitous devices in the radiology departments of hospitals in the United States and around the world, as recently as 1980 such scanners were available only in a handful of research institutions. However, by 1991, more than 2800 of these instruments were in clinical operation worldwide, and more than 6 million diagnostic scans were performed annually. MRI scanners use the technique of nuclear magnetic resonance (NMR) to induce and detect a very weak radiofrequency signal that is a manifestation of nuclear magnetism. The term *nuclear magnetism* refers to weak magnetic properties that are exhibited by some materials as a consequence of the nuclear spin that is associated with their atomic nuclei. In particular, the proton, which is the nucleus of the hydrogen atom, possesses a nonzero nuclear spin and is an excellent source of NMR signals. The human body contains enormous numbers of hydrogen atoms—especially in water (H_2O) and lipid molecules. Although biologically significant NMR signals can be obtained from other chemical elements in the body, such as phosphorous and sodium, the great majority of clinical MRI studies are based on signals originating from protons that are present in the lipid and water molecules within the patient's body.

The patient to be imaged must be placed in an environment in which several different magnetic fields can be simultaneously or sequentially applied to elicit the desired NMR signal. Every MRI scanner utilizes a strong static field magnet in conjunction with a sophisticated set of gradient coils and radiofrequency coils. The gradients and the radiofrequency components are switched on and off in a precisely timed pattern, or pulse sequence. Different pulse sequences are used to extract different types of data from the patient. MR images are characterized by excellent contrast between the various forms of soft tissues within the body. For patients who have no ferromagnetic foreign bodies within them, MRI scanning appears to be perfectly safe and can be repeated as often as necessary without danger [Shellock and Kanal, 1994]. This provides one of the major advantages of MRI over conventional x-ray and computed tomographic (CT) scanners. The NMR signal is not blocked at all by regions of air or bone within the body, which provides a significant advantage over ultrasound imaging. Also, unlike the case of nuclear medicine scanning, it is not necessary to add radioactive tracer materials to the patient.

Fundamentals of MRI Instrumentation

Three types of magnetic fields—main fields or static fields (B_0), gradient fields, and radiofrequency (RF) fields (B_1)—are required in MRI scanners. In practice, it is also usually necessary to use coils or magnets that produce shimming fields to enhance the spatial uniformity of the static field B_0. Most MRI hardware engineering is concerned with producing and controlling these various forms of magnetic fields. The ability to construct NMR instruments capable of examining test tube–sized samples has been available since shortly after World War II. The special challenge associated with the design and construction of medical scanners was to develop a practical means of scaling these devices up to sizes capable of safely and comfortably accommodating an entire human patient. Instruments capable of human scanning first became available in the late 1970s. The successful implementation of MRI requires a two-way flow of information between analog and digital formats (Fig. 65.5). The main magnet, the gradient and RF coils, and the gradient and RF power supplies operate in the analog domain. The digital domain is centered on a general-purpose computer

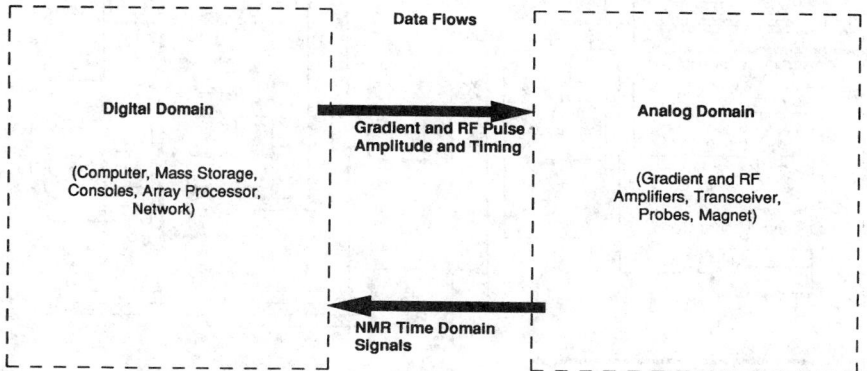

FIGURE 65.5 Digital and analog domains for MRI imaging. MRI involves the flow of data and system commands between these two domains. (Courtesy of WM Leue. Reprinted, by permission, from Schenck and Leue, 1991.)

(Fig. 65.6) that is used to provide control information (signal timing and amplitude) to the gradient and RF amplifiers, to process time-domain MRI signal data returning from the receiver, and to drive image display and storage systems. The computer also provides miscellaneous control functions, such as permitting the operator to control the position of the patient table.

Static Field Magnets

The main field magnet [Thomas, 1993] is required to produce an intense, static magnetic field over the entire region to be imaged. To be useful for imaging purposes, this field must be extremely uniform in space and constant in time. In practice, the spatial variation of the main field of a whole-body scanner must be less than about 1 to 10 parts per million (ppm) over a region approximately 40 cm in diameter. To achieve these high levels of homogeneity requires careful attention to magnet design and to manufacturing tolerances. The temporal drift of the field strength is normally required to be less than 0.1 ppm/h.

Two units of magnetic field strength are now in common use. The gauss (G) has a long historical usage and is firmly embedded in the older scientific literature. The tesla (T) is a more recently adopted unit, but it is a part of the SI system of units and, for this reason, is generally preferred. The tesla is a much larger unit than the gauss—1 tesla corresponds to 10,000 gauss. The magnitude of the earth's magnetic field is about .05 mT (0.5 G), and the field of a fairly powerful permanent magnet is about 0.5 T (5000 G). The static magnetic fields of modern MRI scanners are most commonly in the range from 0.5 to 1.5 T; useful scanners, however, have been built using the entire range from 0.02 to 4 T. The signal-to-noise ratio (SNR) is the ratio of the NMR signal voltage to the ever-present noise voltages that arise within the patient and within the electronic components of the receiving system. The SNR is one of the key parameters that determine the performance capabilities of a scanner. The maximum available SNR increases linearly with field strength. The improvement

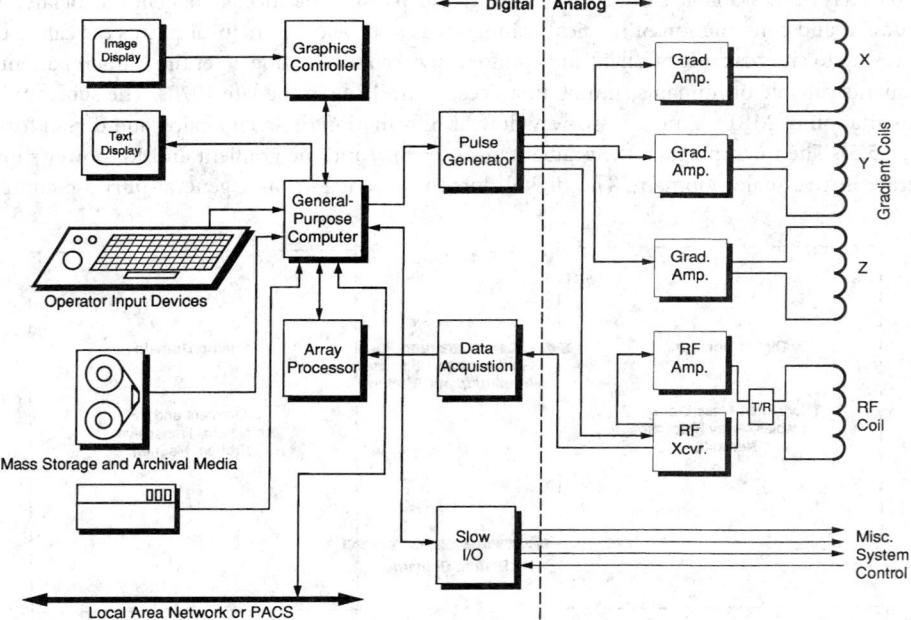

FIGURE 65.6 Block diagram for an MRI scanner. A general-purpose computer is used to generate the commands that control the pulse sequence and to process data during MR scanning. (Courtesy of WM Leue. Reprinted, by permission, from Schenck and Leue, 1991.)

in SNR as the field strength is increased is the major reason that so much effort has gone into producing high-field magnets for MRI systems.

Magnetic fields can be produced by using either electric currents or permanently magnetized materials as sources. In either case, the field strength falls off rapidly away from the source, and it is not possible to create a highly uniform magnetic field on the outside of a set of sources. Consequently, to produce the highly uniform field required for MRI, it is necessary to more or less surround the patient with a magnet. The main field magnet must be large enough, therefore, to effectively surround the patient; in addition, it must meet other stringent performance requirements. For these reasons, the main field magnet is the most important determinant of the cost, performance, and appearance of an MRI scanner. Four different classes of main magnets—permanent magnets, electromagnets, resistive magnets, and superconducting magnets—have been used in MR scanners.

Permanent Magnets and Electromagnets. Both these magnet types use magnetized materials to produce the field that is applied to the patient. In a permanent magnet, the patient is placed in the gap between a pair of permanently magnetized pole faces. Electromagnets use a similar configuration, but the pole faces are made of soft magnetic materials which become magnetized only when subjected to the influence of electric current coils that are wound around them. Electromagnets, but not permanent magnets, require the use of an external power supply. For both types of magnets, the magnetic circuit is completed by use of a soft iron yoke connecting the pole faces to one another (Fig. 65.7). The gap between the pole faces must be large enough to contain the patient as well as the gradient and RF coils.

The permanent magnet materials available for use in MRI scanners include high-carbon iron, alloys such as Alnico, ceramics such as barium ferrite, and rare earth alloys such as samarium cobalt.

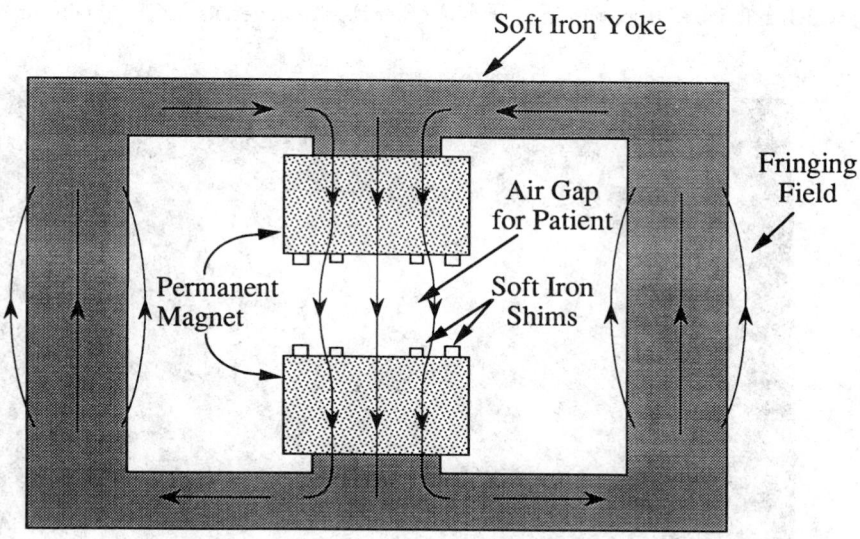

Permanent Magnet Schematic Cross Section

FIGURE 65.7 Permanent magnet. The figure shows a schematic cross-section of a typical permanent magnet configuration. Electromagnets have a similar construction but are energized by current-carrying coils wound around the iron yoke. Soft magnetic shims are used to enhance the homogeneity of the field. (Reprinted, by permission, from Schenck and Leue, 1991.)

Permanent magnet scanners have some advantages: They produce a relatively small fringing field and do not require power supplies. However, they tend to be very heavy (up to 100 tons) and can produce only relatively low fields—on the order of 0.3 T or less. They are also subject to temporal field drift caused by temperature changes. If the pole faces are made from an electrically conducting material, eddy currents induced in the pole faces by the pulsed gradient fields also can limit performance. A recently introduced alloy of neodymium, boron, and iron (usually referred to as *neodymium iron*) has been used to make lighter-weight permanent magnet scanners.

Resistive Magnets.   The first whole-body scanners, manufactured in the late 1970s and early 1980s, used four to six large coils of copper or aluminum wire surrounding the patient. These coils are energized by powerful (40 to 100 kW) direct-current (dc) power supplies. The electrical resistance of the coils leads to substantial joule heating, and the use of cooling water flowing through the coils is necessary to prevent overheating. The heat dissipation increases rapidly with field strength, and it is not feasible to build resistive magnets operating at fields much higher than 0.15 to 0.3 T. At present, resistive magnets are seldom used except for very low field strength (0.02 to 0.06 T) applications.

Superconducting Magnets.   Since the early 1980s, the use of cryogenically cooled superconducting magnets [Wilson, 1983] has been the most satisfactory solution to the problem of producing the static magnet field for MRI scanners. The property of exhibiting absolutely no electrical resistance near absolute zero has been known as an exotic property of some materials since 1911. Unfortunately, the most common of these materials, such as lead, tin, and mercury, exhibit a phase change back to the normal state at relatively low magnetic field strengths and cannot be used to produce powerful magnetic fields. In the 1950s, a new class of materials (type II superconductors) was discovered. These materials retain the ability to carry loss-free electric currents in very high fields. One such material, an alloy of niobium and titanium, has been used in most of the thousands of superconducting whole-body magnets that have been constructed for use in MRI scanners (Fig. 65.8). The widely publicized discovery in 1986 of another class of materials which remain superconduct-

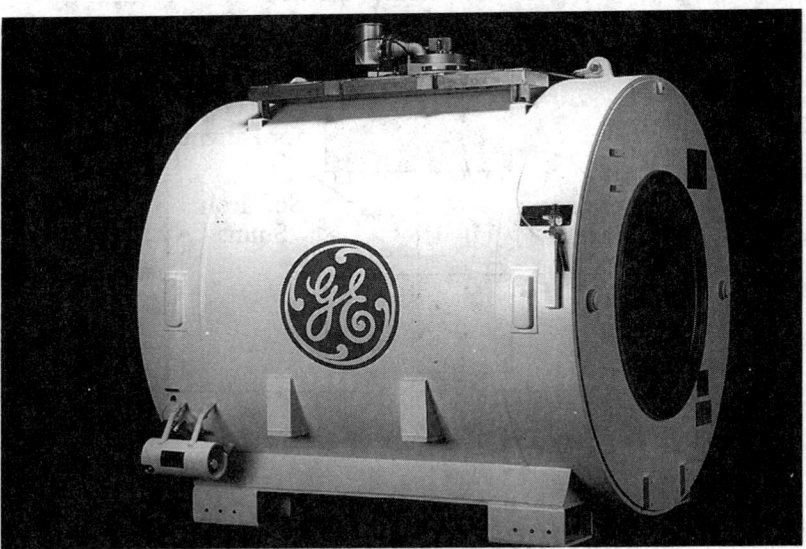

FIGURE 65.8   Superconducting magnet. This figure shows a 1.5-T whole-body superconducting magnet. The nominal warm bore diameter is 1 m. The patient to be imaged, as well as the RF and gradient coils, are located within this bore. (Courtesy of General Electric Medical Systems. Reprinted, by permission, from Schenck and Leue, 1991.)

ing at much higher temperatures than any previously known material has not yet lead to any material capable of carrying sufficient current to be useful in MRI scanners.

Figure 65.9 illustrates the construction of a typical superconducting whole-body magnet. In this case, six coils of superconducting wire are connected in series and carry an intense current—on the order of 200 A—to produce the 1.5-T magnetic field at the magnet's center. The diameter of the coils is about 1.3 m, and the total length of wire is about 65 km (40 mi). The entire length of this wire must be without any flaws—such as imperfect welds—that would interrupt the superconducting properties. If the magnet wire has no such flaws, the magnet can be operated in the persistent mode—that is, once the current is established, the terminals may be connected together, and a constant persistent current will flow indefinitely so long as the temperature of the coils is maintained below the superconducting transition temperature. This temperature is about 10 K for niobium-titanium wire. The coils are kept at this low temperature by encasing them in a double-walled cryostat (analogous to a Thermos bottle) that permits them to be immersed in liquid helium at a temperature of 4.2 K. The gradual boiling of liquid helium caused by inevitable heat leaks into the cryostat requires that the helium be replaced on a regular schedule. Many magnets now make use of cryogenic refrigerators that reduce or eliminate the need for refilling the liquid helium reservoir. The temporal stability of superconducting magnets operating in the persistent mode is truly remarkable—magnets have operated for years completely disconnected from power supplies and maintained their magnetic field constant to within a few parts per million. Because of their ability to achieve very strong and stable magnetic field strengths without undue power consumption, superconducting magnets have become the most widely used source of the main magnetic fields for MRI scanners.

Magnetic Field Homogeneity. The necessary degree of spatial uniformity of the field can be achieved only by carefully placing the coils at specific spatial locations. It is well known that a single loop of wire will produce, on its axis, a field that is directed along the coil axis and that can be ex-

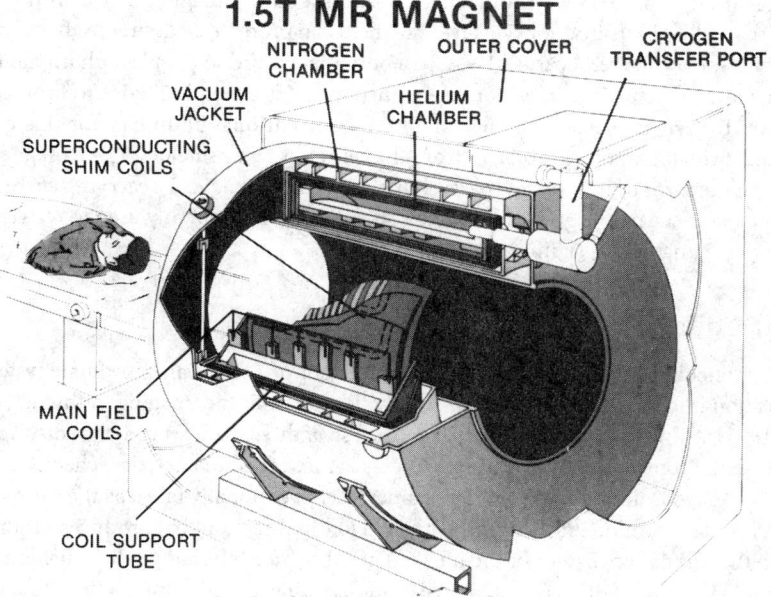

1.5T MR MAGNET

FIGURE 65.9 Schematic drawing of a superconducting magnet. The main magnet coils and the superconducting shim coils are maintained at liquid helium temperature. A computer-controlled table is used to advance the patient into the region of imaging. (Reprinted, by permission, from Schenck and Leue, 1991.)

pressed as a sum of spherical harmonic fields. The first term in this sum is constant in space and represents the desired field that is completely independent of position. The higher-order terms represent contaminating field inhomogeneities that spoil the field uniformity. More than a century ago, a two-coil magnet system—known as the *Helmholtz pair*—was developed that produced a much more homogeneous field at its center than is produced by a single current loop. This design is based on the mathematical finding that when two coaxial coils of the same radius are separated by a distance equal to their radius, the first nonzero contaminating term in the harmonic expansion is of the fourth order. This results in an increased region of field homogeneity which, although it is useful in many applications, is far too small to be useful in MRI scanners. However, the principle of eliminating low-order harmonic fields can be extended by using additional coils. This is the method now used to increase the volume of field homogeneity to values that are useful for MRI. For example, in the commonly used six-coil system, it is possible to eliminate all the error fields through the twelfth order.

In practice, manufacturing tolerances and field perturbations caused by extraneous magnetic field sources—such as steel girders in the building surrounding the magnet—produce additional inhomogeneity in the imaging region. These field imperfections are reduced by the use of shimming fields. One approach—*active shimming*—uses additional coils (either resistive coils, superconducting coils, or some of each) which are designed to produce a magnetic field corresponding to a particular term in the spherical harmonic expansion. When the magnet is installed, the magnetic field is carefully mapped, and the currents in the shim coils are adjusted to cancel out the terms in the harmonic expansion to some prescribed high order. The alternative approach—*passive shimming*—utilizes small permanent magnets that are placed at the proper locations along the inner walls of the magnet bore to cancel out contaminating fields. If a large object containing magnetic materials—such as a power supply—is moved in the vicinity of superconducting magnets, it may be necessary to reset the shimming currents or magnet locations to account for the changed pattern of field inhomogeneity.

Fringing Fields. A large, powerful magnet produces a strong magnetic field in the region surrounding it as well as in its interior. This fringing field can produce undesirable effects such as erasing magnetic tapes (and credit cards). It is also a potential hazard to people with implanted medical devices such as cardiac pacemakers. For safety purposes, it is general practice to limit access to the region where the fringing field becomes intense. A conventional boundary for this region is the "5-gauss line," which is about 10 to 12 m from the center of an unshielded 1.5-T magnet. Magnetic shielding—in the form of iron plates (passive shielding) or external coils carrying current in the direction opposite to the main coil current (active shielding)—is frequently used to restrict the region in which the fringing field is significant.

Gradient Coils

Three gradient fields, one each for the *x, y,* and *z* directions of a cartesian coordinate system, are used to code position information into the MRI signal and to permit the imaging of thin anatomic slices [Thomas, 1993]. Along with their larger size, it is the use of these gradient coils that distinguishes MRI scanners from the conventional NMR systems such as those used in analytical chemistry. The direction of the static field, along the axis of the scanner, is conventionally taken as the *z* direction, and it is only the cartesian component of the gradient field in this direction that produces a significant contribution to the resonant behavior of the nuclei. Thus the three relevant gradient fields are $B_z = G_x x$, $B_z = G_y y$, and $B_z = G_z z$. MRI scans are carried out by subjecting the spin system to a sequence of pulsed gradient and RF fields. Therefore, it is necessary to have three separate coils—one for each of the relevant gradient fields—each with its own power supply and under independent computer control. Ordinarily, the most practical method for constructing the gradient coils is to wind them on a cylindrical coil form that surrounds the patient and is located inside the warm bore of the magnet.

The z gradient field can be produced by sets of circular coils wound around the cylinder with the current direction reversed for coils on the opposite sides of the magnet center ($z = 0$). To reduce deviations from a perfectly linear B_z gradient field, a spiral winding can be used with the direction of the turns reversed at $z = 0$ and the spacing between windings decreasing away from the coil center (Fig. 65.10). A more complex current pattern is required to produce the transverse (x and y) gradients. As indicated in Fig. 65.11, transverse gradient fields are produced by windings which utilize a four-quadrant current pattern.

The generation of MR images requires that a rapid sequence of time-dependent gradient fields (on all three axes) be applied to the patient. For example, the commonly used technique of spin-warp imaging [Edelstein et al., 1980] utilizes a slice-selection gradient pulse to select the spins in a thin (3 to 10 mm) slice of the patient and then applies readout and phase-encoding gradients in the two orthogonal directions to encode two-dimensional spatial information into the NMR signal. This, in turn, requires that the currents in the three gradient coils can be rapidly switched by computer-controlled power supples. The rate at which gradient currents can be switched is an important determinant of the imaging capabilities of a scanner. In typical scanners, the gradient coils have an electrical resistance of about 1 Ω and an inductance L of about 1 mH, and the gradient fields can be switched from 0 to 10 mT/m (1 G/cm) in about 0.5 ms. The current I must be switched from 0 to about 100 A in this interval, and the instantaneous voltage on the coils, $L\, dI/dt$, is on the order of 200 V. The power dissipation during the switching interval is about 20 kW. In many pulse sequences, the switching duty cycle is relatively low, and coil heating is not significant. However, fast-scanning protocols use very rapidly switched gradients at a high duty cycle . This places very strong demands on the power supplies, and it is often necessary to use water cooling to prevent overheating the gradient coils.

Radiofrequency Coils

Radiofrequency (RF) coils are components of every scanner and are used for two essential purposes—transmitting and receiving signals at the resonant frequency of the protons within the pa-

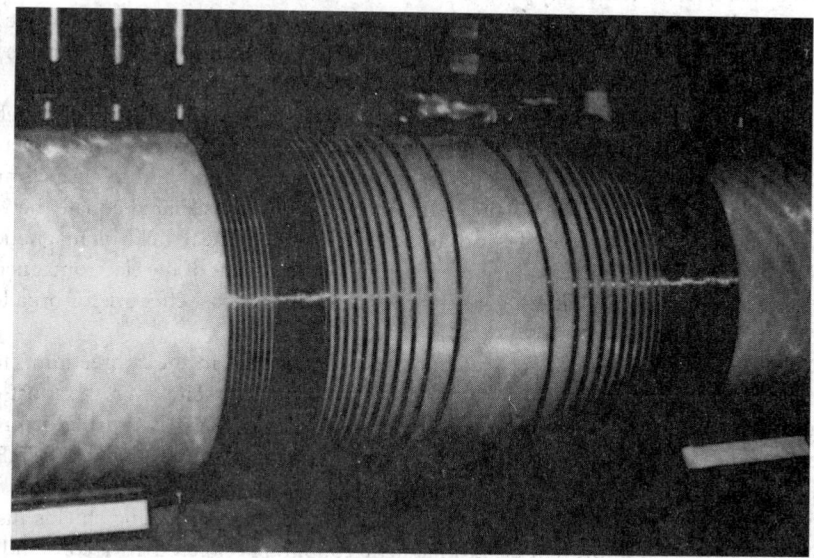

FIGURE 65.10   *Z*-gradient coil. The photograph shows a spiral coil wound on a cylindrical surface with an overwinding near the end of the coil. (Courtesy of RJ Dobberstein, General Electric Medical Systems. Reprinted, by permission, from Schenck and Leue, 1991.)

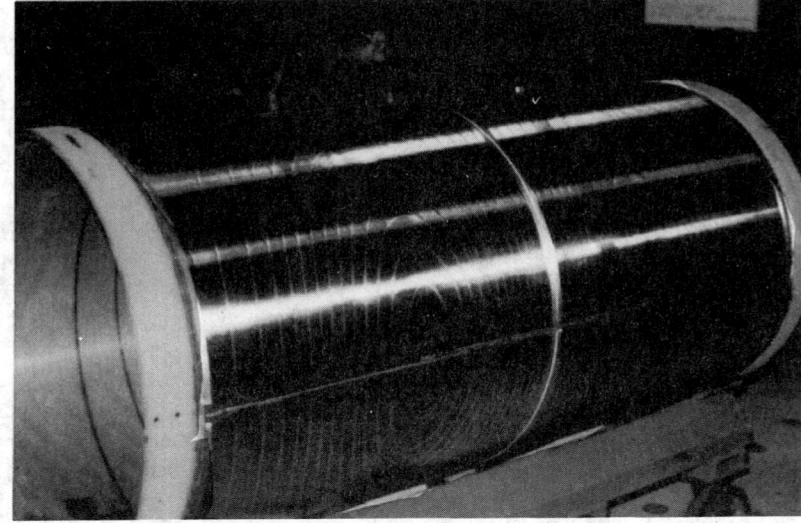

FIGURE 65.11 Transverse gradient coil. The photograph shows the outer coil pattern of an actively shielded transverse gradient coil. (Courtesy of RJ Dobberstein, General Electric Medical Systems. Reprinted, by permission, from Schenck and Leue, 1991.)

tient [Schenck, 1993]. The precession occurs at the Larmor frequency of the protons, which is proportional to the static magnetic field. At 1 T this frequency is 42.58 MHz. Thus, in the range of field strengths currently used in whole-body scanners, 0.02 to 4 T, the operating frequency ranges from 0.85 to 170.3 MHz. For the commonly used 1.5-T scanners, the operating frequency is 63.86 MHz. The frequency of MRI scanners overlaps the spectral region used for radio and television broadcasting. As an example, the frequency of a 1.5-T scanner is within the frequency band 60 to 66 MHz, which is allocated to television channel 3. Therefore, it is not surprising that the electronic components in MRI transmitter and receiver chains closely resemble corresponding components in radio and television circuitry. An important difference between MRI scanners and broadcasting systems is that the transmitting and receiving antennas of broadcast systems operate in the far field of the electromagnetic wave. These antennas are separated by many wavelengths. On the other hand, MRI systems operate in the near field, and the spatial separation of the sources and receivers is much less than a wavelength. In far-field systems, the electromagnetic energy is shared equally between the electric and magnetic components of the wave. However, in the near field of magnetic dipole sources, the field energy is almost entirely in the magnetic component of the electromagnetic wave. This difference accounts for the differing geometries that are most cost effective for broadcast and MRI antenna structures.

Ideally, the RF field is perpendicular to the static field, which is in the z direction. Therefore, the RF field can be linearly polarized in either the x or y direction. However, the most efficient RF field results from quadrature excitation, which requires a coil that is capable of producing simultaneous x and y fields with a 90-degree phase shift between them. Three classes of RF coils—body coils, head coils, and surface coils—are commonly used in MRI scanners. These coils are located in the space between the patient and the gradient coils. Conducting shields just inside the gradient coils are used to prevent electromagnetic coupling between the RF coils and the rest of the scanner. Head and body coils are large enough to surround the region being imaged and are designed to produce an RF magnetic field that is uniform across the region to be imaged. Body coils are usually constructed on cylindrical coil forms and have a large enough diameter (50 to

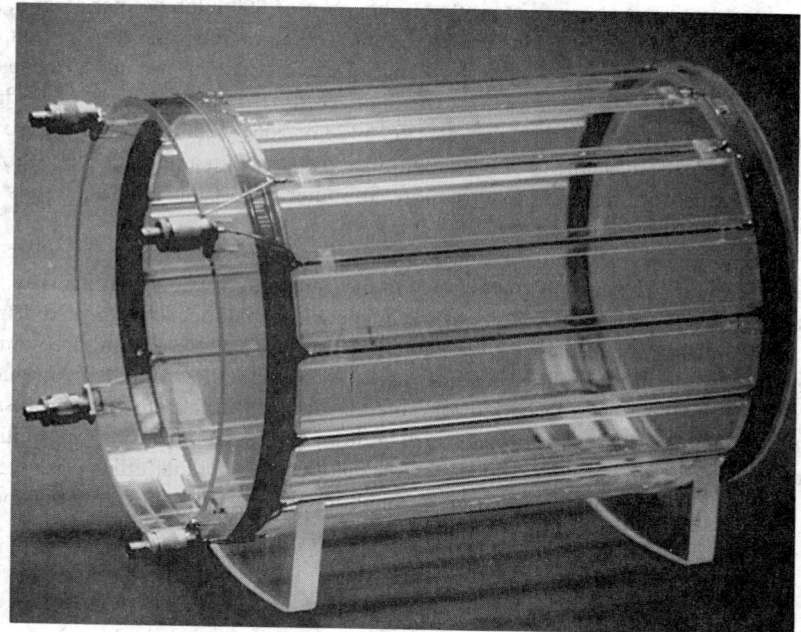

FIGURE 65.12 Birdcage resonator. This is a head coil designed to operate in a 4-T scanner at 170 MHz. Quadrature excitation and receiver performance are achieved by using two adjacent ports with a 90-degree phase shift between them. (Reprinted, by permission, from Schenck and Leue, 1991.)

60 cm) to entirely surround the patient's body. Coils designed only for head imaging (Fig. 65.12) have a smaller diameter (typically 28 cm). Surface coils are smaller coils designed to image a restricted region of the patient's anatomy. They come in a wide variety of shapes and sizes. Because they can be closely applied to the region of interest, surface coils can provide SNR advantages over head and body coils for localized regions, but because of their asymmetric design, they do not have uniform sensitivity.

A common practice is to use separate coils for the transmitter and receiver functions. This permits the use of a large coil—such as the body coil—with a uniform excitation pattern as the transmitter and a small surface coil optimized to the anatomic region—such as the spine—being imaged. When this two-coil approach is used, it is important to provide for electronically decoupling of the two coils because they are tuned at the same frequency and will tend to have harmful mutual interactions otherwise.

Digital Data Processing

A typical scan protocol calls for a sequence of tailored RF and gradient pulses with duration controlled in steps of 0.1 μs. To achieve sufficient dynamic range in control of pulse amplitudes, 12- to 16-bit digital-to-analog converters are used. The RF signal at the Larmor frequency (usually in the range from 1 to 200 MHz) is mixed with a local oscillator to produce a baseband signal which typically has a bandwidth of 16 to 32 kHz. The data-acquisition system must digitize the baseband signal at the Nyquist rate, which requires sampling the detected RF signal at a rate one digital data point every 5 to 20 μs. Again, it is necessary to provide sufficient dynamic range. Analog-to-digital converters with 16 to 18 bits are used to produce the desired digitized signal data. During the data acquisition, information is acquired at a rate on the order of 800 kilobytes per second, and each image can contain up to a megabyte of digital data. The array processor (AP) is a specialized computer that is designed for the rapid performance of specific algorithms, such as the fast Fourier transform (FFT), which are used to convert the digitized time-domain data to image data. Two-dimensional images are typically displayed as 256×128 or 256×256 or 512×512 pixel arrays. The images can be made available for viewing within about 1 second after data acquisition. Three-dimensional imaging data, however, require more computer processing, and this results in longer delays between acquisition and display.

A brightness number, typically containing 16 bits of gray-scale information, is calculated for each pixel element of the image, and this corresponds to the signal intensity originating in each voxel of the object. To make the most effective use of the imaging information, sophisticated display techniques, such as multi-image displays, rapid sequential displays (cine loop), and three-dimensional renderings of anatomic surfaces, are frequently used. These techniques are often computationally intensive and require the use of specialized computer hardware. Interfaces to microprocessor-based workstations are frequently used to provide such additional display and analysis capabilities. MRI images are available as digital data, and therefore, there is considerable utilization of local area networks (LANs) to distribute information throughout the hospital, and long-distance digital transmission of the images can be used for purposes of teleradiology.

Current Trends in MRI

At present, there is a substantial effort directed at enhancing the capabilities and cost-effectiveness of MR imagers. The activities include efforts to reduce the cost of these scanners, to improve image quality, to reduce scan times, and to increase the number of useful clinical applications. Three specific examples of these efforts are the continuing drive to reduce the time necessary to acquire a complete MR image, the development of high-field scanners, and the advent of MRI-guided therapy. Conventional spin-warp images typically require several minutes to acquire. The fast spin echo (FSE) technique can reduce this to the order of 20 s, and gradient-echo techniques can reduce this time to a few seconds. The echo-planar technique (EPI) [Cohen and Weisskoff, 1991; Wehrli, 1990] requires substantially increased gradient power and receiver bandwidth but can produce images in 40 to 60 ms. Scanners with improved gradient hardware that are capable of handling higher data-acquisition rates are now available.

For most of the 1980s, the highest field strength commonly used in MRI scanners was 1.5 T. To achieve better SNRs, higher-field scanners, operating at fields up to 4 T, were studied experimentally. The need for very high-field scanners has been enhanced by the development of functional brain MRI. This technique utilizes magnetization differences between oxygenated and deoxygenated hemoglobin, and this difference is enhanced at higher field strengths. It has now become possible to construct 3- and 4-T scanners of the same physical size as the 1.5-T systems, and this is resulting in a considerable increase in the use of high-field systems.

For the first decade or so after their introduction, MRI scanners were used almost entirely to provide diagnostic information. However, there is now considerable interest in systems capable of performing image-guided, invasive surgical procedures. Because MRI is capable of providing excellent soft-tissue contrast and has the potential for providing excellent positional information with sub-millimeter accuracy, it can be used for guiding biopsies and stereotactic surgery. The full capabilities of MRI-guided procedures can only be achieved if it is possible to provide surgical access to the patient simultaneously with the MRI scanning. This has lead to the development of new system designs, including the introduction of a scanner with a radically modified superconducting magnet system that permits the surgeon to operate at the patient's side within the scanner (Fig. 65.13). These systems have lead to the introduction of magnetic field–compatible surgical instruments, anesthesia stations, and patient monitoring equipment.

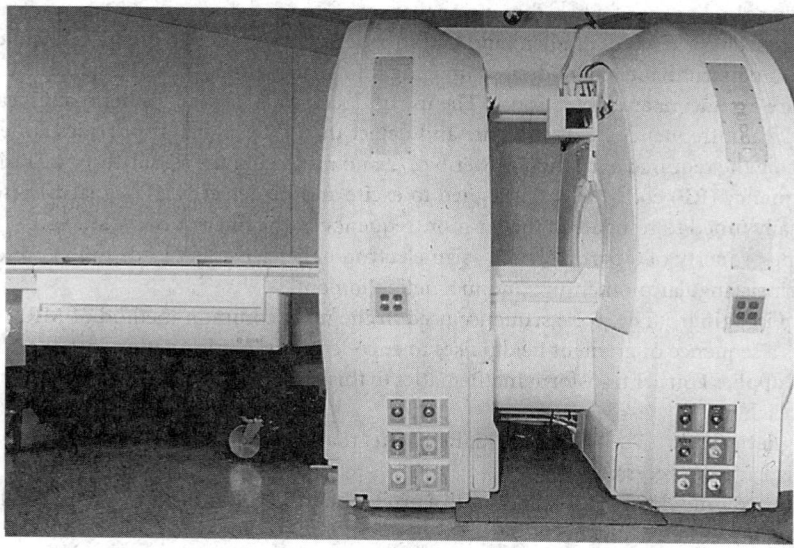

FIGURE 65.13   Open magnet for MRI-guided therapy. This open-geometry supercon-ducting magnet provides a surgeon with direct patient access and the ability to interac-tively control the MRI scanner. This permits imaging to be performed simultaneously with surgical interventions.

Defining Terms

Bandwidth: The narrow frequency range, approximately 32 kHz, over which the MRI signal is transmitted. The bandwidth is proportional to the strength of the readout gradient field.

Echo-planar imaging (EPI):   A pulse sequence used to produce very fast MRI scans. EPI imaging times can be as short as 50 ms.

Fast Fourier transform (FFT):   A mathematical technique used to convert data sampled from the MRI signal into image data. This version of the Fourier transform can be performed with par-ticular efficiency on modern array processors.

Gradient coil: A coil designed to produce a magnetic field for which the field component B_z varies linearly with position. Three gradient coils, one each for the x, y, and z directions, are required in MRI. These coils are used to permit slice selection and to encode position information into the MRI signal.

Larmor frequency: The rate at which the magnetic dipole moment of a particle precesses in an applied magnetic field. It is proportional to the field strength and is 42.58 MHz for protons in a 1-T field.

Magnetic resonance imaging (MRI):   A technique for obtaining images of the internal anatomy based on the use of nuclear magnetic resonance signals. During the 1980s, it became a major modality for medical diagnostic imaging.

Nuclear magnetic resonance (NMR):   A technique for observing and studying nuclear magnet-ism. It is based on partially aligning the nuclear spins by use of a strong, static magnetic field, stimulating these spins with a radiofrequency field oscillating at the Larmor frequency, and detecting the signal that is induced at this frequency.

Nuclear magnetism: The magnetic properties arising from the small magnetic dipole moments possessed by the atomic nuclei of some materials. This form of magnetism is much weaker than the more familiar form that originates from the magnetic dipole moments of the atomic electrons.

Pixel: A single element of a two-dimensional array of image data.

Pulse sequence: A series of gradient and radiofrequency pulses used to organize the nuclear spins into a pattern that encodes desired imaging information into the NMR signal.

Quadrature excitation and detection: The use of circularly polarized, rather than linearly polarized, radiofrequency fields to excite and detect the NMR signal. It provides a means of reducing the required excitation power by 1/2 and increasing the signal-to-noise ratio by $\sqrt{2}$.

Radiofrequency (RF) coil: A coil designed to excite and/or detect NMR signals. These coils are usually tuned to resonate at the Larmor frequency of the nucleus being studied.

Spin: The property of a particle, such as an electron or nucleus, that leads to the presence of an intrinsic angular momentum and magnetic moment.

Spin-warp imaging: The pulse sequence used in the most common method of MRI imaging. It uses a sequence of gradient field pulses to encode position information into the NMR signal and applies Fourier transform mathematics to this signal to calculate the image intensity value for each pixel.

Static magnetic field: The field of the main magnet that is used to magnetize the spins and to drive their Larmor precession.

Voxel: The volume element associated with a pixel. The voxel volume is equal to the pixel area multiplied by the slice thickness.

References

Cohen MS, Weisskoff RM. 1991. Ultra-fast imaging. Magn Reson Imaging 9:1.

Edelstein WA, Hutchinson JMS, Johnson G, Redpath TW. 1980. Spin-warp NMR imaging and applications to human whole-body imaging. Phys Med Biol 25:751.

Schenck JF, Leue WM. 1991. Instrumentation: Magnets coils and hardware. In SW Atlas (ed), Magnetic Resonance Imaging of the Brain and Spine, pp 1–22. New York, Raven Press.

Schenck JF. 1993. Radiofrequency coils: Types and characteristics. In MJ Bronskill, P Sprawls (eds), The Physics of MRI, Medical Physics Monograph No. 21, pp 98–134. Woodbury, NY, American Institute of Physics.

Shellock FG, Kanal E. 1994. Magnetic Resonance: Bioeffects, Safety and Patient Management. New York, Raven Press.

Thomas SR. 1993. Magnets and gradient coils: Types and characteristics. In MJ Bronskill, P Sprawls (eds), The Physics of MRI, Medical Physics Monograph No. 21, pp 56–97. Woodbury, NY, American Institute of Physics.

Wehrli FW. 1990. Fast scan magnetic resonance: principles and applications. Magn Reson Q 6:165.

Wilson MN. 1983. Superconducting Magnets. Oxford, Clarendon Press.

Further Information

There are several journals devoted entirely to MR imaging. These include *Magnetic Resonance Imaging* (Elsevier Publishing, 660 White Plains Road, Tarrytown, NY 10591), *Magnetic Resonance in Medicine* (Williams & Wilkins, 428 E. Preston Street, Baltimore, MD 21202), and *JMRI—Journal of Magnetic Resonance Imaging* (Society of Magnetic Resonance, 213 W. Institute Place, Suite 501, Chicago, IL 60610). In addition, the clinical aspects of MRI are covered extensively in *Radiology* (Radiological Society of North America, 1991 Northampton St., Easton, PA 18042), the *American Journal of Radiology* (American Roentgen Ray Society, 1891 Preston White Drive, Reston, VA 22091), and several other journals devoted to the practice of radiology. There is a professional society, now known as the Society of Magnetic Resonance, devoted to the medical aspects of magnetic resonance. The main offices of this society are at 2118 Milvia, Suite 201, Berkeley, CA 94704. This society holds an annual meeting that includes displays of equipment and the presentation of about 1500 technical papers on new developments in the field. The annual *Book of Abstracts* of this meeting provides an excellent summary of current activities in the field. Similarly, the annual meeting of the Radiological Society of North America (RSNA) provides extensive coverage of MRI that is particularly strong on the clinical applications. The RSNA is located at 2021 Spring Road, Suite 600, Oak Brook, IL 60521.

Several book-length accounts of MRI instrumentation and techniques are available. *Biomedical Magnetic Resonance Technology* (Adam Hilger, Bristol, 1989) by C.-N. Chen and D. I. Hoult, and *The Physics of MRI* (Medical Physics Monograph 21, American Institute of Physics, Woodbury, NY, 1993), edited by M. J. Bronskill and P. Sprawls, both contain thorough accounts of instrumentation and the physical aspects of MRI. There are many books that cover the clinical aspects of MRI. Of particular interest are *Magnetic Resonance Imaging,* 2nd edition (Mosby, St. Louis, 1992), edited by D. D. Stark and W. G. Bradley, Jr., and *Magnetic Resonance Imaging of the Brain and Spine,* 2d ed. (Raven Press, New York, in press), edited by S. W. Atlas.

65.3 Functional MRI

Kenneth K. Kwong and David A. Chesler

Functional magnetic resonance imaging (fMRI), a technique that images intrinsic blood signal change with magnetic resonance (MR) imagers, has in the last 3 years become one of the most successful tools used to study blood flow and perfusion in the brain. Since changes in neuronal activity are accompanied by focal changes in cerebral blood flow (CBF), blood volume (CBV), blood oxygenation, and metabolism, these physiologic changes can be used to produce functional maps of mental operations.

There are two basic but completely different techniques used in fMRI to measure CBF. The first one is a classic steady-state perfusion technique first proposed by Detre et al. [1], who suggested the use of saturation or inversion of incoming blood signal to quantify absolute blood flow [1–5]. By focusing on blood flow *change* and not just steady-state blood flow, Kwong et al. [6] were successful in imaging brain visual functions associated with quantitative perfusion change. There are many advantages in studying blood flow change because many common baseline artifacts associated with MRI absolute flow techniques can be subtracted out when we are interested only in changes. And one obtains adequate information in most functional neuroimaging studies with information on flow change alone.

The second technique also looks at change of a blood parameter—blood oxygenation *change* during neuronal activity. The utility of the change of blood oxygenation characteristics was strongly evident in Turner's work [7] with cats with induced hypoxia. Turner et al. found that with hypoxia, the MRI signal from the cats' brains went down as the level of deoxyhemoglobin rose, a result that was an extension of an earlier study by Ogawa et al. [8,9] of the effect of deoxyhemoglobin on MRI signals in animals' veins. Turner's new observation was that when oxygen was restored, the cats' brain signals climbed up and went *above* their baseline levels. This was the suggestion that the vascular system overcompensated by bringing more oxygen, and with more oxygen in the blood, the MRI signal would rise beyond the baseline.

Based on Turner's observation and the perfusion method suggested by Detre et al., movies of human visual cortex activation utilizing both the perfusion and blood oxygenation techniques were successfully acquired in May of 1991 (Fig. 65.14) at the Massachusetts General Hospital with a specially equipped superfast 1.5-T system known as an *echo-planar imaging* (EPI) MRI system [10]. fMRI results using intrinsic blood contrast were first presented in public at the Tenth Annual Meeting of the Society of Magnetic Resonance in Medicine in August of 1991 [6,11]. The visual cortex activation work was carried out with flickering goggles, a photic stimulation protocol employed by Belliveau et al. [12] earlier to acquire the MRI functional imaging of the visual cortex with the injection of the contrast agent gadolinium-DTPA. The use of an external contrast agent allows the study of change in blood volume. The intrinsic blood contrast technique, sensitive to blood flow and blood oxygenation, uses no external contrast material. Early model calculation showed that signal due to blood perfusion change would only be around 1% above baseline, and the signal due to blood oxygenation change also was quite small. It was quite a pleasant surprise that fMRI results turned out to be so robust and easily detectable.

The blood oxygenation–sensitive MRI signal change, coined *blood oxygenation level dependent* (BOLD) by Ogawa et al. [8,9,13], is in general much larger than the MRI perfusion signal change during brain activation. Also, while the first intrinsic blood contrast fMRI technique was demonstrated with a superfast EPI MRI system, most centers doing fMRI today are only equipped with conventional MRI systems, which are really not capable of applying Detre's perfusion method. Instead, the explosive growth of MR functional neuroimaging [14–33] in the last three years relies mainly on the measurement of blood oxygenation change, utilizing a MR parameter called T_2^*. Both high speed echo planar (EPI) and conventional MR have now been successfully employed for functional imaging in MRI systems with magnet field strength ranging from 1.5 to 4.0 T.

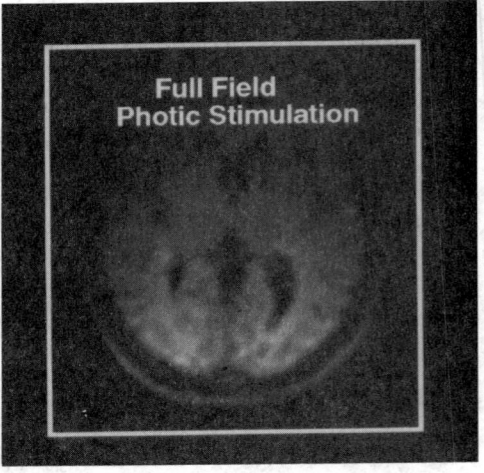

FIGURE 65.14 Functional MR image demonstrating activation of the primary visual cortex (V1). Image acquired on May 9, 1991 with a blood oxygenation–sensitive MRI gradient-echo (GE) technique.

Advances in Functional Brain Mapping

The popularity of fMRI is based on many factors. It is safe and totally noninvasive. It can be acquired in single subjects for a scanning duration of several minutes, and it can be repeated on the same subjects as many times as necessary. The implementation of the blood oxygenation sensitive MR technique is universally available. Early neuroimaging work focused on time-resolved MR topographic mapping of human primary visual (V1) (Figs. 65.15, 65.16), motor (MI), somatosensory (S1), and auditory (A1) cortices during task activation. Today, with BOLD technique combined with EPI, one can acquire 20 or more contiguous brain slices covering the whole head (3 × 3 mm in plane and 5 mm slice thickness) every 3 seconds for a total duration of several minutes. Conventional scanners can only acquire a couple of slices at a time. The benefits of whole-head imaging are many. Not only can researchers identify and test their hypotheses on known brain activation centers, they can also search for previous unknown or unsuspected sites. High resolution work done with EPI has a resolution of 1.5 × 1.5 mm in plane and a slice thickness of 3 mm. Higher spatial resolution has been reported in conventional 1.5-T MR systems (34).

Of note with Fig. 65.16 is that with blood oxygenation–sensitive MR technique, one observes an undershoot [6,15,35] in signal in V1 when the light stimulus is turned off. The physiologic mechanism underlying the undershoot is still not well understood.

The data collected in the last 3 years have demonstrated that fMRI maps of the visual cortex correlate well with known retinotopic organization [24,36]. Higher visual regions such as V5/MT [37] and motor-cortex organization [6,14,27,38] have been explored successfully. Preoperative planning work (Fig. 65.17) using motor stimulation [21,39,40] has helped neurosurgeons who attempt to preserve primary areas from tumors to be resected. For higher cognitive functions, several fMRI language studies have already demonstrated known language-associated regions [25,26,41,42] (Fig. 65.18). There is more detailed modeling work on the mechanism of functional brain mapping by blood-oxygenation change [43–46]. Postprocessing techniques that would help to alleviate the serious problem of motion/displacement artifacts are available [47].

Mechanism

Flow-sensitive images show increased perfusion with stimulation, while blood oxygenation–sensitive images show changes consistent with an increase in venous blood oxygenation. Although the

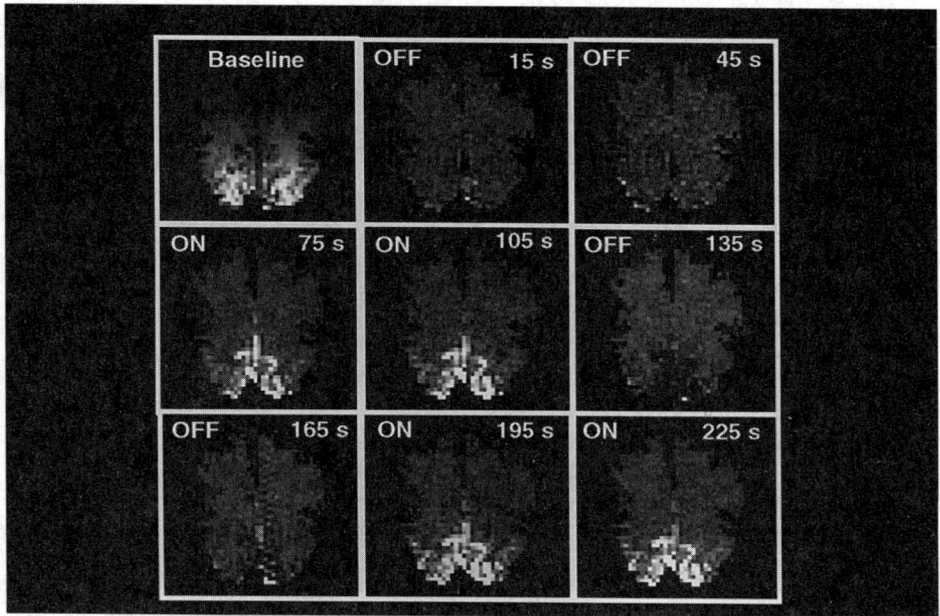

FIGURE 65.15   Movie of fMRI mapping of primary visual cortex (V1) activation during visual stimulation. Images are obliquely aligned along the calcarie fissures with the occipital pole at the bottom. Images were acquired at 3-s intervals using a blood oxygenation–sensitive MRI sequence (80 images total). A baseline image acquired during darkness (*upper left*) was subtracted from subsequent images. Eight of these subtraction images are displayed, chosen when the image intensities reached a steady-state signal level during darkness (OFF) and during 8-Hz photic stimulation (ON). During stimulation, local increases in signal intensity are detected in the posteromedial regions of the occipital lobes along the calcarine fissures.

precise biophysical mechanisms responsible for the signal changes have yet to be determined, good hypotheses exist to account for our observations.

Two fundamental MRI relaxation rates, T_1 and T_2^*, are used to describe the fMRI signal. T_1 is the rate at which the nuclei approach thermal equilibrium, and perfusion change can be considered as an additional T_1 change. T_2^* represents the rate of the decay of MRI signal due to magnetic field inhomogeneities, and the change of T_2^* is used to measure blood-oxygenation change.

T_2^* changes reflect the interplay between changes in cerebral blood flow, volume, and oxygenation. As hemoglobin becomes deoxygenated, it becomes more paramagnetic than the surrounding tissue [48] and thus creates a magnetically inhomogeneous environment. The observed *increased* signal on T_2^*-weighted images during activation reflects a decrease in deoxyhemoglobin content, i.e., an increase in venous blood oxygenation. Oxygen delivery, cerebral blood flow, and cerebral blood volume all increase with neuronal activation. Because CBF (and hence oxygen-delivery) changes exceed CBV changes by 2 to 4 times [49], while blood-oxygen extraction increases only slightly [50,51], the total paramagnetic blood deoxyhemoglobin content within brain tissue voxels will decrease with brain activation. The resulting decrease in the tissue-blood magnetic susceptibility difference leads to less intravoxel dephasing within brain tissue voxels and hence *increased* signal on T_2^*-weighted images [6,14,15,17]. These results independently confirm PET observations that activation-induced changes in blood flow and volume are accompanied by little or no increases in tissue oxygen consumption [50,51,52]

Since the effect of volume susceptibility difference $\Delta\chi$ is more pronounced at high field strength [53], higher-field imaging magnets [17] will increase the observed T_2^* changes.

Signal changes can also be observed on T_1-weighted MR images. The relationship between T_1 and regional blood flow was characterized by Detre et al. [1]:

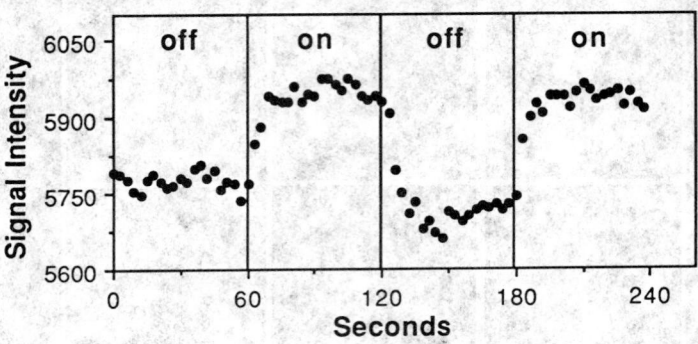

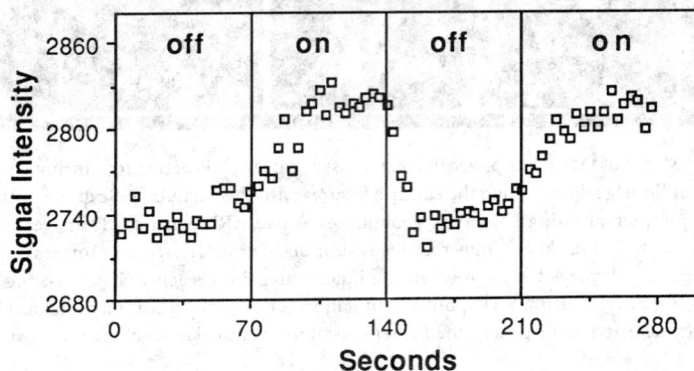

FIGURE 65.16 Signal intensity changes for a region of interest (~60 mm²) within the visual cortex during darkness and during 8-Hz photic stimulation. Results using oxygenation-sensitive (*top graph*) and flow-sensitive (*bottom graph*) techniques are shown. The flow-sensitive data were collected once every 3.5 s, and the oxygenation-sensitive data were collected once every 3 s. Upon termination of photic stimulation, an undershoot in the oxygenation-sensitive signal intensity is observed.

$$\frac{dM}{dt} = \frac{M_0 - M}{T_1} + fM_b - \frac{f}{\lambda}M \qquad (65.14)$$

where M is tissue magnetization and M_b is incoming blood signal. M_0 is proton density, f is the flow in ml/gm/unit time, and λ is the brain-blood partition coefficient of water (~0.95 ml/gm). From this equation, the brain tissue magnetization M relaxes with an apparent T_1 time constant $T_{1\,app}$ given by

$$\frac{f}{\lambda} = \frac{1}{T_{1\,app}} - \frac{1}{T_1} \qquad (65.15)$$

where the $T_{1\,app}$ is the observed (apparent) longitudinal relaxation time with flow effects included. T_1 is the true tissue longitudinal relaxation time in the absence of flow. If we assume that the true tissue T_1 remains constant with stimulation, a change in blood flow Δf will lead to a change in the observed $T_{1\,app}$:

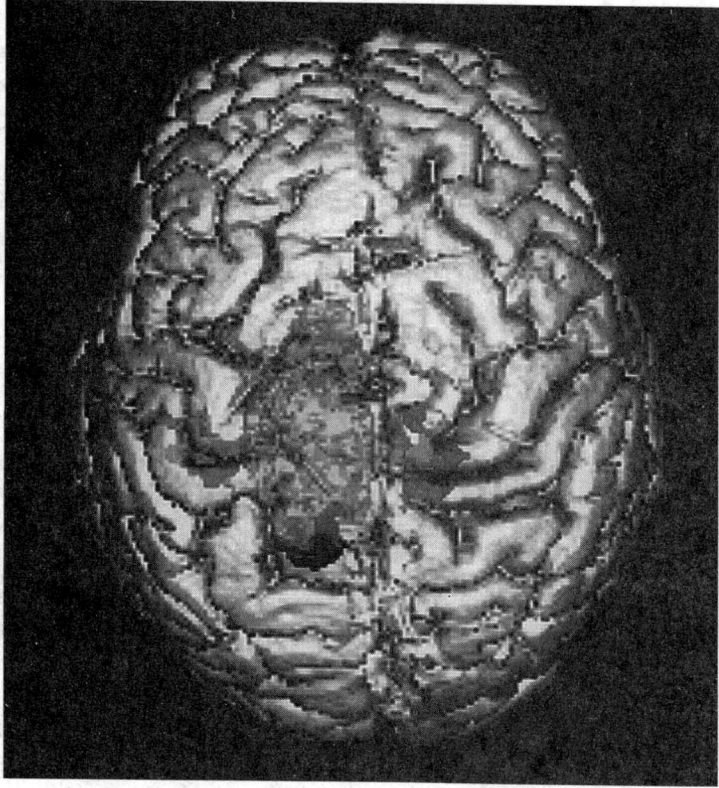

FIGURE 65.17 Functional MRI mapping of motor cortex for preoperative planning. This three-dimensional rendering of the brain represents fusion of functional and structural anatomy. Brain is viewed from the top. A tumor is shown in the left hemisphere, near the midline. The other areas depict sites of functional activation during movement of the right hand, right foot, and left foot. The right foot cortical representation is displaced by tumor mass effect from its usual location. (Courtesy of Dr. Brad Buchbinder.)

$$\Delta \frac{1}{T_{1\,app}} = \Delta \frac{f}{\lambda} \qquad (65.16)$$

Thus the MRI signal change can be used to estimate the change in blood flow.

From Eq. (65.14), if the magnetization of blood and tissue always undergoes a similar T_1 relaxation, the flow effect would be minimized. This is a condition that can be approximated by using a flow-nonsensitive T_1 technique inverting *all* the blood coming into the imaged slice of interest. This flow-nonsensitive sequence can be subtracted from a flow-sensitive T_1 technique to provide an index of CBF without the need of external stimulation [54,55] (Fig. 65.19). Initial results with tumor patients show that such flow-mapping techniques are useful for mapping out blood flow of tumor regions [55].

Other flow techniques under investigation include the continuous inversion of incoming blood at the carotid level [1] or the use of a single inversion pulse at the carotid level (EPIstar) inverting the incoming blood [56,57]. Compared with the flow-nonsensitive and flow-sensitive methods, the blood-tagging techniques at the carotid level are basically similar concepts except that the MRI signal of tagged blood is expected to be smaller by a factor that depends on the time it takes blood to

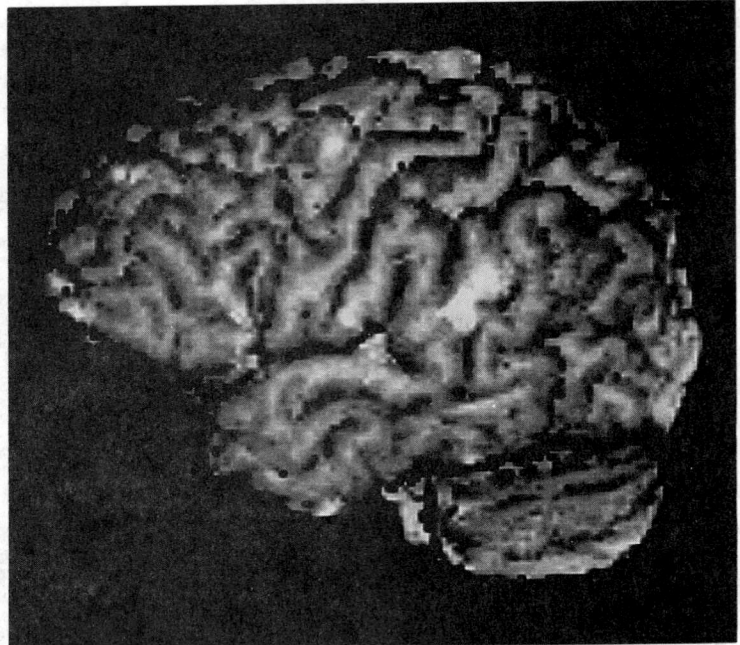

FIGURE 65.18   Left hemisphere surface rendering of functional data (EPI, gradient-echo, 10 oblique coronal slices extending to posterior sylvian fissure) and high-resolution anatomic image obtained on a subject (age 33 years) during performance of a same-different (visual matching) task of pairs of words or nonwords (false font strings). Foci of greatest activation for this study are located in dominant perisylvian cortex, i.e., inferior frontal gyrus (Broca's area), superior temporal gyrus (Wernicke's area), and inferior parietal lobule (angular gyrus). Also active in this task are sensorimotor cortex and prefrontal cortex. The perisylvian sites of activation are known to be key nodes in a left hemisphere language network. Prefrontal cortex probably plays a more general, modulatory role on attentional aspects of the task. Sensorimotor activation is observed in most language studies despite the absence of overt vocalization. (Courtesy of Dr. Randall Benson.)

travel from the tagged site to the imaged slice of interest [55]. The continuous-inversion technique also has a significant problem of magnetization transfer [1] that contaminates the flow signal with a magnetization transfer signal that is several times larger. On the other hand, the advantage of the continuous inversion is that it can under optimal conditions provide a flow contrast larger than all the other methods by a factor of e [55].

Problem and Artifacts in fMRI: The Brain-Vein Problem? The Brain-Inflow Problem?

The artifacts arising from large vessels pose serious problems to the interpretation of oxygenation sensitive fMRI data. It is generally believed that microvascular changes are specific to the underlying region of neuronal activation. However, MRI gradient echo (GE) is sensitive to vessels of all dimensions [46,58], and there is concern that macrovascular changes distal to the site of neuronal activity can be induced [20]. This has been known as the *brain-vein problem.* For laboratories not equipped with EPI, gradient echo (GE) sensitive to variations in T_2^* and magnetic susceptibility are the only realistic sequences available for fMRI acquisition, so the problem is particularly acute.

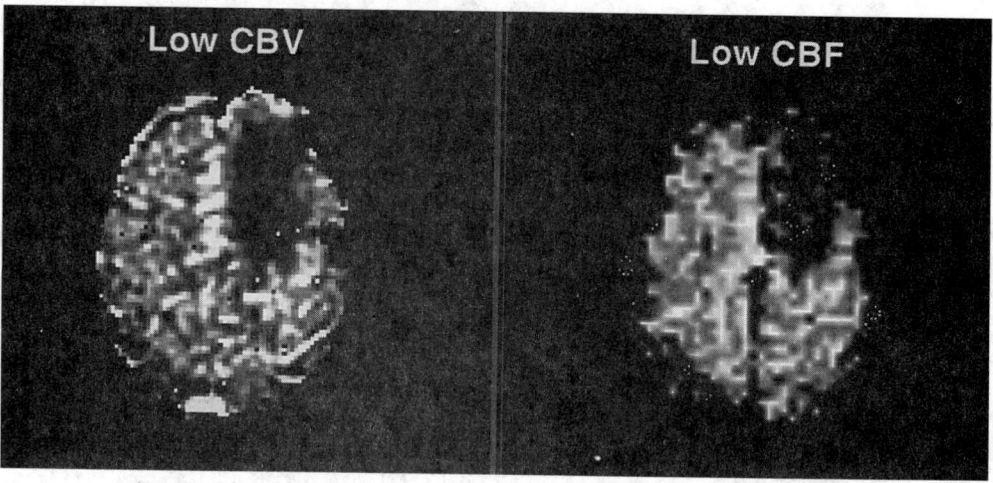

FIGURE 65.19 Functional MRI cerebral blood flow (CBF) index (*right*) of a low-flow brain tumor (dark region right of the midline) generated by the subtraction of a flow-nonsensitive image from a flow-sensitive image. This low-flow region matches well with a cerebral blood volume (CBV) map (*left*) of the tumor region generated by the injection of a bolus of MRI contrast agent Gd-DTPA, a completely different and established method to measure hemodynamics with MRI.

In addition, there is a non-deoxhemoglobin-related problem, especially acute in conventional MRI. This is the inflow problem of fresh blood that can be time-locked to stimulation [28,29,59]. Such nonparenchymal and macrovascular responses can introduce error in the estimate of activated volumes.

Techniques to Reduce the Large Vessel Problems

In dealing with the inflow problems, EPI has special advantages over conventional scanners. The use of long repetition times (2 to 3 s) in EPI significantly reduces the brain-inflow problem. Small-flip-angle methods in conventional MRI scanners can be used to reduce inflow effect [59]. Based on inflow modeling, one observes that at an angle smaller than the Ernst angle [60], the inflow effect drops much faster than the tissue signal response to activation. Thus one can effectively remove the inflow artifacts with small-flip-angle techniques.

A new exciting possibility is to add small additional velocity-dephasing gradients to suppress slow in-plane vessel flow [60,61]. Basically, moving spins lose signals, while stationary spins are unaffected. The addition of these velocity-dephasing gradients drops the overall MRI signal (Fig. 65.20). The hypothesis that large vessel signals are suppressed while tissue signals remain intact is a subject of ongoing research.

Another advantage with EPI is that another oxygenation-sensitive method such as the EPI T_2-weighted spin-echo (T2SE) is also available. T2SE methods are sensitive to the MRI parameter T_2, which is affected by microscopic susceptibility and hence blood oxygenation. Theoretically, T2SE methods are far less sensitive to large vessel signals [1,6,46,58]. For conventional scanners, T2SE methods take too long to perform and therefore are not practical options.

The flow model [1] based on T_1-weighted sequences and independent of deoxyhemoglobin is also not so prone to larger vessel artifacts, since the T_1 model is a model of perfusion at the tissue level.

Based on the study of volunteers, the average T_2^*-weighted GE signal percentage change at V1 was $2.5 \pm 0.8\%$. The average oxygenation-weighted T2SE signal percentage change was $0.7 \pm 0.3\%$. The average perfusion-weighted and T_1-weighted MRI signal percentage change was $1.5 \pm 0.5\%$. These results demonstrate that T2SE and T_1 methods, despite their ability to suppress large vessels, are not

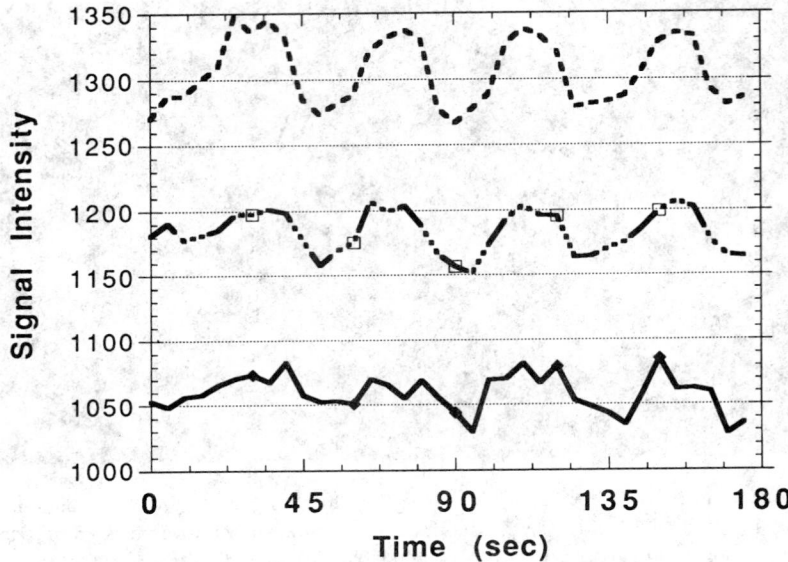

FIGURE 65.20 The curves represent time courses of MRI response to photic stimulation (off-on-off-on $\cdots$) with different levels of velocity-dephasing gradients turned on to remove MRI signals coming from the flowing blood of large vessels. The top curve had no velocity-dephasing gradients turned on. The bottom curve was obtained with such strong velocity-dephasing gradients turned on that all large vessel signals were supposed to have been eliminated. The middle curve represents a moderate amount of velocity-dephasing gradients, a tradeoff between removing large vessel signals and retaining a reasonable amount of MRI signal to noise.

competitive with T_2^* effect at 1.5 T. However, since the microscopic effect detected by T2SE scales up with field strength [62], we expect the T2SE to be a useful sequence at high field strength such as 3 or 4 T. Advancing field strength also should benefit T_1 studies due to better signal-to-noise and to the fact that T_1 gets longer at higher field strength.

While gradient-echo sequence has a certain ambiguity when it comes to tissue versus vessels, its sensitivity at current clinical field strength makes it an extremely attractive technique to identify activation sites. By using careful paradigms that rule out possible links between the primary activation site and secondary sites, one can circumvent many of the worries of "signal from the primary site draining down to secondary sites." A good example is as follows: Photic stimulation activates both the primary visual cortex and the extrastriates. To show that the extrastriates are not just a drainage from the primary cortex, one can utilize paradigms that activate the primary visual cortex but not the extrastriate, and vice versa. There are many permutations of this [37]. This allows us to study the higher-order functions unambiguously even if we are using gradient-echo sequences.

The continuous advance of MRI mapping techniques utilizing intrinsic blood-tissue contrast promises the development of a functional human neuroanatomy of unprecedented spatial and temporal resolution.

References

1. Detre J, Leigh J, Williams D, Koretsky A. 1992. Magn Reson Med 23:37.
2. Williams DS, Detre JA, Leigh JS, Koretsky AP. 1992. Proc Natl Acad Sci USA 89:212.
3. Zhang W, Williams DS, Detre JA. 1992. Magn Reson Med 25:362.

4. Zhang W, Williams DS, Koretsky AP. 1993 Magn Reson Med 29:416.

5. Dixon WT, Du LN, Faul D, et al. 1986. Magn Reson Med 3:454.

6. Kwong KK, Belliveau JW, Chesler DA, et al. 1992. Proc Natl Acad Sci USA 89:5675.

7. Turner R, Le Bihan D, Moonen CT, et al. 1991. Magn Reson Med 22:159.

8. Ogawa S, Lee TM, Kay AR, Tank DW. 1990. Proc Natl Acad Sci USA 87:9868.

9. Ogawa S, Lee TM. 1990. Magn Reson Med 16:9.

10. Cohen MS, Weisskoff RM. 1991. Magn Reson Imaging 9:1.

11. Brady TJ, Society of Magnetic Resonance in Medicine, San Francisco, CA 2, 1991.

12. Belliveau JW, Kennedy DN Jr, McKinstry RC, et al. 1991. Science 254:716.

13. Ogawa S, Lee TM, Nayak AS, Glynn P. 1990. Magn Reson Med 14:68.

14. Bandettini PA, Wong EC, Hinks RS, et al. 1992. Magn Reson Med 25:390.

15. Ogawa S, Tank DW, Menon R, et al. 1992. Proc Natl Acad Sci USA 89:5951.

16. Frahm J, Bruhn H, Merboldt K, Hanicke W. 1992. J Magn Reson Imaging 2:501.

17. Turner R, Jezzard P, Wen H, et al. 1992. Society of Magnetic Resonance in Medicine Eleventh Annual Meeting, Berlin.

18. Blamire A, Ogawa S, Ugurbil K, et al. 1992. Proc Natl Acad Sci USA 89:11069.

19. Menon R, Ogawa S, Tank D, Ugurbil K. 1993. Magn Reson Med 30:380.

20. Lai S, Hopkins A, Haacke E, et al. 1993. Magn Reson Med 30:387.

21. Cao Y, Towle VL, Levin DN, et al. 1993. Society of Magnetic Resonance in Medicine Meeting.

22. Connelly A, Jackson GD, Frackowiak RSJ, et al. 1993. Radiology 125.

23. Kim SG, Ashe J, Georgopouplos AP, et al. 1993. J Neurophys 69:297.

24. Schneider W, Noll DC, Cohen JD. 1993. Nature 365:150.

25. Hinke RM, Hu X, Stillman AE, et al. 1993. Neurol Rep 4:675.

26. Binder JR, Rao SM, Hammeke TA, et al. 1993. Neurology (suppl 2):189.

27. Rao SM, Binder JR, Bandettini PA, et al. 1993. Neurology 43:2311.

28. Gomiscek G, Beisteiner R, Hittmair K, et al. 1993. MAGMA 1:109.

29. Duyn J, Moonen C, de Boer R, et al. 1993. Society of Magnetic Resonance in Medicine, 12th Annual Meeting, New York, New York.

30. Hajnal JV, Collins AG, White SJ, et al. 1993. Magn Reson Med 30:650.

31. Hennig J, Ernst T, Speck O, et al. 1994. Magn Reson Med 31:85.

32. Constable RT, Kennan RP, Puce A, et al. 1994. Magn Res Med 31:686.

33. Binder JR, Rao SM, Hammeke TA, et al. 1994. Ann Neurol 35:662.

34. Frahm J, Merboldt K, Hänicke W. 1993. Magn Reson Med 29:139.

35. Stern CE, Kwong KK, Belliveau JW, et al. 1992. Society of Magnetic Resonance in Medicine Annual Meeting, Berlin, Germany.

36. Belliveau JW, Kwong KK, Baker JR, et al. 1992. Society of Magnetic Resonance in Medicine Annual Meeting, Berlin, Germany.

37. Tootell RBH, Kwong KK, Belliveau JW, et al. 1993. Investigative Opthalmology and Visual Science, p 813.

38. Kim S-G, Ashe J, Hendrich K, et al. 1993. Science 261:615.

39. Buchbinder BR, Jiang HJ, Cosgrove GR, et al. 1994. ASNR 162.

40. Jack CR, Thompson RM, Butts RK, et al. 1994. Radiology 190:85.

41. Benson RR, Kwong KK, Belliveau JW, et al. 1993. Soc Neurosci.

42. Benson RR, Kwong KK, Buchbinder BR, et al. 1994. Society of Magnetic Resonance, San Francisco.

43. Ogawa S, Menon R, Tank D, et al. 1993. Biophys J 64:803.

44. Ogawa S, Lee TM, Barrere B. 1993. Magn Reson Med 29:205.

45. Kennan RP, Zhong J, Gore JC. 1994. Magn Reson Med 31:9.

46. Weisskoff RM, Zuo CS, Boxerman JL, Rosen BR. 1994. Magn Res Med 31:601.

47. Bandettini PA, Jesmanowicz A, Wong EC, Hyde JS. 1993. Magn Reson Med 30:161.

48. Thulborn KR, Waterton JC, Matthews PM, Radda GK. 1982. Biochim Biophys Acta 714:265.

49. Grubb RL, Raichle ME, Eichling JO, Ter-Pogossian MM. 1974. Stroke 5:630.

50. Fox PT, Raichle ME. 1986. Proc Natl Acad Sci USA 83:1140.

51. Fox PT, Raichle ME, Mintun MA, Dence C. 1988. Science 241:462.

52. Prichard J, Rothman D, Novotny E, et al. 1991. Proc Natl Acad Sci USA 88:5829.

53. Brooks RA, Di Chiro G. 1987. Med Phys 14:903.

54. Kwong K, Chesler D, Zuo C, et al. 1993. Society of Magnetic Resonance in Medicine, 12th Annual Meeting, New York, New York, p 172.

55. Kwong KK, Chesler DA, Weisskoff RM, Rosen BR. 1994. Society of Magnetic Resonance, San Francisco.

56. Edelman R, Sievert B, Wielopolski P, et al. 1994. JMRI 4(P).

57. Warach S, Sievert B, Darby D, et al. 1994. JMRI 4(**P**):S8.

58. Fisel CR, Ackerman JL, Buxton RB, et al. 1991. Magn Reson Med 17:336.

59. Frahm J, Merboldt K, Hanicke W. 1993. Society of Magnetic Resonance in Medicine, 12th Annual Meeting, New York, New York, p 1427.

60. Kwong KK, Chesler DA, Boxerman JL, et al. 1994. Society of Magnetic Resonance, San Francisco.

61. Song W, Bandettini P, Wong E, Hyde J. 1994. Personal communication.

62. Zuo C, Boxerman J, Weisskoff R. 1992. Society of Magnetic Resonance in Medicine, 11th Annual Meeting, Berlin, p 866.

65.4 Chemical-Shift Imaging: An Introduction to Its Theory and Practice

Xiaoping Hu, Wei Chen, Maqbool Patel, and Kamil Ugurbil

Over the past two decades, there has been a great deal of development in the application of nuclear magnetic resonance (NMR) to biomedical research and clinical medicine. Along with the development of magnetic resonance imaging [1], in vivo magnetic resonance spectroscopy (MRS) is becoming a research tool for biochemical studies of humans as well as a potentially more specific diagnostic tool, since it provides specific information on individual chemical species in living systems. Experimental studies in animals and humans have demonstrated that MRS can be used to study the biochemical basis of disease and to follow the treatment of disease.

Since biologic subjects (e.g., humans) are heterogeneous, it is necessary to spatially localize the spectroscopic signals to a well-defined volume or region of interest (VOI or ROI, respectively) in the intact body. Toward this goal, various localization techniques have been developed (see ref. [2] for a recent review). Among these techniques, chemical-shift imaging (CSI) or spectroscopic imaging [3–6] is an attractive technique, since it is capable of producing images reflecting the spatial distribution of various chemical species of interest. Since the initial development of CSI in 1982 [3], further developments have been made to provide better spatial localization and sensitivity, and the technique has been applied to numerous biomedical problems.

In this section we will first present a qualitative description of the basic principles of chemical-shift imaging and subsequently present some practical examples to illustrate the technique. Finally, a summary is provided in the last subsection.

General Methodology

In an NMR experiment, the subject is placed in a static magnetic field B_0. Under the equilibrium condition, nuclear spins with nonzero magnetic moment are aligned along B_0, giving rise to an induced bulk magnetization. To observe the bulk magnetization, it is tipped to a direction perpendicular to B_0 (transverse plane) with a radiofrequency (RF) pulse that has a frequency corresponding to the resonance frequency of the nuclei. The resonance frequency is determined by the product of the gyromagnetic ratio of the nucleus γ and the strength of the static field, i.e., γB_0, and is called the *Larmor frequency.* The Larmor frequency also depends on the chemical environment of the nuclei, and this dependency gives rise to chemical shifts that allow one to identify different chemical species in an NMR spectrum. Upon excitation, the magnetization in the transverse plane (perpendicular to the main B_0 field direction) oscillates with the Larmor frequencies of all the different chemical species and induces a signal in a receiving RF coil; the signal is also termed the *free induction decay (FID).* The FID can be Fourier transformed with respect to time to produce a spectrum in frequency domain.

In order to localize an NMR signal from an intact subject, spatially selective excitation and/or spatial encoding are usually utilized. Selective excitation is achieved as follows: In the excitation, an RF pulse with a finite bandwidth is applied in the presence of a linear static magnetic field gradient. With the application of the gradient, the Larmor frequency of spins depends linearly on the spatial location along the direction of the gradient. Consequently, only the spins in a slice whose resonance frequency falls into the bandwidth of the RF pulse are excited.

The RF excitation rotates all or a portion of the magnetization to the transverse plane, which can be detected by a receiving RF coil. Without spatial encoding, the signal detected is the integral of the signals over the entire excited volume. In CSI based on Fourier imaging, spatial discrimination is achieved by phase encoding. Phase encoding is accomplished by applying a gradient pulse after the excitation and before the data acquisition. During the gradient pulse, spins precess at Larmor frequencies that vary linearly along the direction of the gradient and accrue a phase proportional to the position along the phase-encoding gradient as well as the strength and the duration of the gradient pulse. This acquired spatially encoded phase is typically expressed as $\vec{k} \cdot \vec{r} = \int \gamma \vec{g}(t) \cdot \vec{r}\, dt$, where γ is the gyromagnetic ratio; $\vec{r}$ is the vector designating spatial location; $\vec{g}(t)$ defines the magnitude, the direction, and the time dependence of the magnetic field gradient applied during the phase-encoding gradient; and the integration is performed over time when the phase-encoding gradient is on. Thus, in one-dimensional phase encoding, if the phase encoding is along, for example, the y axis, the phase acquired becomes $k \times y = \int \gamma g_y(t) \times y\, dt$. The acquired signal $S(t)$ is the integral of the spatially distributed signals modulated by a spatially dependent phase, given by the equation

$$S(t) = \int \rho(\vec{r},t)e^{(i\vec{k} \cdot \vec{r})}d^3r \qquad (65.17)$$

where ρ is a function that describes the spatial density and the time evolution of the transverse magnetization of all the chemical species in the sample. This signal mathematically corresponds to a sample of the Fourier transform along the direction of the gradient. The excitation and detection process is repeated with various phase-encoding gradients to obtain many phase-encoded signals that can be inversely Fourier-transformed to resolve an equal number of pixels along this direction. Taking the example of one-dimensional phase encoding along the y axis to obtain a one-dimensional image along this direction of n pixels, the phase-encoding gradient is incremented n times so that n FIDs are acquired, each of which is described as

$$S(t,n) = \int \rho^\star(y,t)e^{(ink_0 y)}\, dy \qquad (65.18)$$

where $\rho^\star$ is r already integrated over the x and z directions, and k_0 is the phase-encoding increment; the latter is decided on using the criteria that the full field of view undergo a 360-degree phase difference when $n = 1$, as dictated by the sampling theorem. The time required for each repetition (TR), which is dictated by the longitudinal relaxation time, is usually on the order of seconds.

In CSI, phase encoding is applied in one, two, or three dimensions to provide spatial localization. Meanwhile, selective excitation also can be utilized in one or more dimensions to restrict the volume to be resolved with the phase encodings. For example, with selective excitation in two dimensions, CSI in one spatial dimension can resolve voxels within the selected column. In multidimensional CSI, all the phase-encoding steps along one dimension need to be repeated for all the steps along the others. Thus, for three dimensions with M, N, and L number of phase encoding steps, one must acquire $M \times N \times L$ number of FIDs:

$$S(t,m,n,l) = \int \rho(\vec{r},t) e^{i(mkx_0 x + nky_0 y + lkz_0 z)} \, d^3\vec{r} \qquad (65.19)$$

where m, n, and l must step through M, N, and L in integer steps, respectively. As a result, the time needed for acquiring a chemical-shift image is proportional to the number of pixels desired and may be very long. In practice, due to the time limitation as well as the signal-to-noise ratio (SNR) limitation, chemical-shift imaging is usually performed with relatively few spatial encoding steps, such as 16×16 or 32×32 in a two-dimensional experiment.

The data acquired with the CSI sequence need to be properly processed before the metabolite information can be visualized and quantitated. The processing consists of spatial reconstruction and spectral processing. Spatial reconstruction is achieved by performing discrete inverse Fourier transformation, for each of the spatial dimensions, with respect to the phase-encoding steps. The spatial Fourier transform is applied for all the points of the acquired FID. For example, for a data set from a CSI in two spatial dimensions with 32×32 phase-encoding steps and 1024 sampled data points for each FID, a 32×32 two-dimensional inverse Fourier transform is applied to each of the 1024 data points. Although the nominal spatial resolution achieved by the spatial reconstruction is determined by the number of phase-encoding steps and the field of view (FOV), it is important to note that due to the limited number of phase-encoding steps used in most CSI experiments, the spatial resolution is severely degraded by the truncation artifacts, which results in signal "bleeding" between pixels. Various methods have been developed to reduce this problem [7–14].

The localized FIDs derived from the spatial reconstruction are to be further processed by spectral analysis. Standard procedures include Fourier transformation, filtering, zero-filling, and phasing. The localized spectra can be subsequently presented for visualization or further processed to produce quantitative metabolite information. The presentation of the localized spectra in CSI is not a straightforward task because there can be thousands of spectra. In one-dimensional experiments, localized spectra are usually presented in a stack plot. In two-dimensional experiments, localized spectra are plotted in small boxes representing the extent of the pixels, and the plots can be overlaid on corresponding anatomic image for reference. Spectra from three-dimensional CSI experiments are usually presented slice by slice, each displaying the spectra as in the two-dimensional case.

To derive metabolite maps, peaks corresponding to the metabolites of interest need to be quantified. In principle, the peaks can be quantified using the standard methods developed for spectral quantification [15–17]. The most straightforward technique is to calculate the peak areas by integrating the spectra over the peak of interest if it does not overlap with other peaks significantly. In integrating all the localized spectra, spectral shift due to B_0 inhomogeneity should be taken into account. A more robust approach is to utilize spectral fitting programs to each spectrum to obtain various parameters of each peak. The fitted area for the peak of interest can then be used to represent the metabolite signal. The peak areas are then used to generate metabolite maps, which are images with intensities proportional to the localized peak area. The metabolite map can be displayed by itself as a gray-scale image or color-coded image or overlaid on the reference anatomic image.

Practical Examples

To illustrate the practical utility of CSI, we present two representative CSI studies in detail in this section. The sequence for the first study is shown in Fig. 65.21. This is a three-dimensional sequence in which phase encoding is applied in all three directions and no slice selection is used. Such a

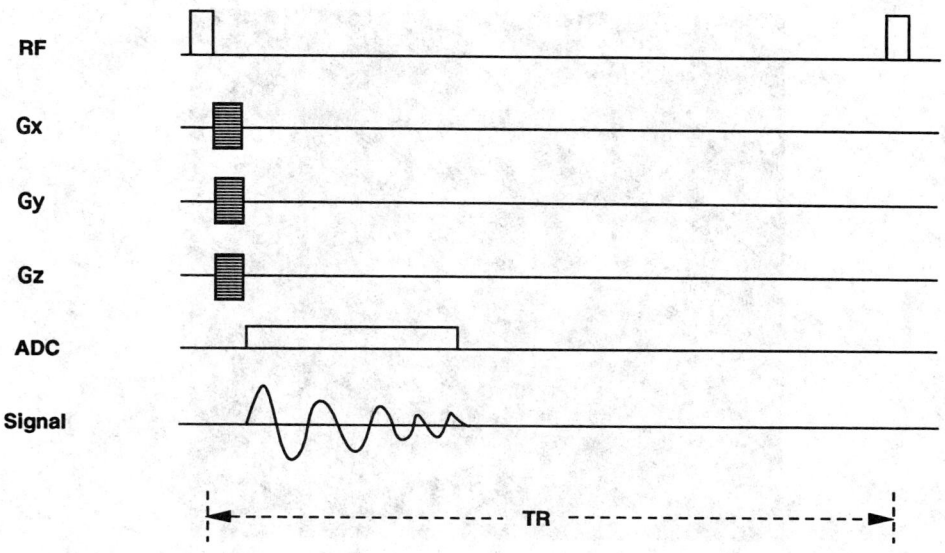

FIGURE 65.21 Sequence diagram for a three-dimensional chemical shift imaging sequence using a nonselective RF pulse.

sequence is usually used with a surface RF coil whose spatial extent of sensitivity defines the field of view. In this sequence, the FID is acquired immediately after application of the phase-encoding gradient to minimize the decay of the transverse magnetization, and the sequence is suitable for imaging metabolites with short transverse relaxation time (e.g., ATP).

With the sequence shown in Fig. 65.21, a phosphorus-31 CSI study of the human brain was conducted using a quadrature surface coil. A nonselective RF pulse with an Ernest angle (40 degrees) optimized for the repetition time was used for the excitation. Phase-encoding gradients were applied for a duration of 500 μs; the phase-encoding gradients were incremented according to a FOV of $25 \times 25 \times 20$ cm^3. Phase-encoded FIDs were acquired with 1024 complex data points over a sampling window of 204.8 ms; the corresponding spectral width was 5000 Hz. To reduce intervoxel signal contamination, a technique that utilizes variable data averaging to introduce spatial filtering during the data acquisition for optimal signal-to-noise ratio is employed [7–10], resulting in spherical voxels with diameter of 3 cm (15 cc volume). The data were acquired with a *TR* of 1 s, and the total acquisition time was approximately 28 minutes.

The acquired data were processed to generate three-dimensional voxels, each containing a localized phosphorus spectrum, in a $17 \times 13 \times 17$ matrix. In Fig. 65.22*a–c*, spectra in three slices of the three-dimensional CSI are presented; these spectra are overlaid on the corresponding anatomic images obtained with a T_1-weighted imaging sequence. One representative spectrum of the brain is illustrated in Fig. 65.22*d*, where the peaks corresponding to various metabolites are labeled. It is evident that the localized phosphorus spectra contain a wealth of information about several metabolites of interest, including adenosine triphosphate (ATP), phosphocreatine (PCr), phosphomonoester (PME), inorganic phosphate (P_i), and phosphodiester (PDE). In pathologic cases, focal abnormalities in phosphorus metabolites have been detected in patients with tumor, epilepsy, and other diseases [18–25].

The second study described below is performed with the sequence depicted in Fig. 65.23. This is a two-dimensional spin-echo sequence in which a slice is selectively excited by a 90-degree excitation pulse. The 180-degree refocusing pulse is selective with a slightly broader slice profile. Here the phase-encoding gradients are applied before the refocusing pulse; they also can be placed after the

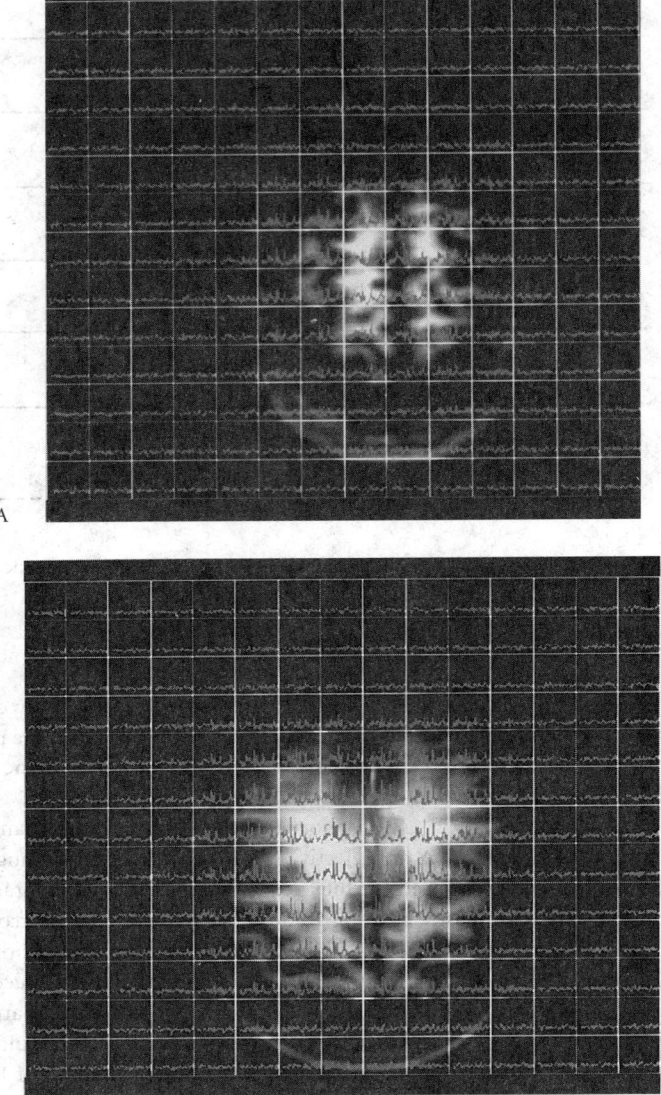

FIGURE 65.22   (A–C) Boxed plot of spectra in three slices from the three-dimensional ^{31}P CSI experiment overlaid on corresponding anatomic images. The spectral extent displayed is from 10 to −20 ppm. A 20-Hz line broadening is applied to all the spectra. (D) Representative spectrum from the three-dimensional ^{31}P CSI shown in (B). Metabolite peaks are labeled.

180-degree pulse or split to both sides of the 180-degree pulse. This sequence was used for a proton CSI experiment. In proton CSI, a major problem arises from the strong water signal that overwhelms that of the metabolites. In order to suppress the water signal, many techniques have been devised [26–29]. In this study, a three-pulse CHESS [26] technique was applied before application of the excitation pulse as shown in Fig. 65.23. The CSI experiment was performed on a 1.4-cm slice with 32×32 phase encodings over a 22×22 cm^2 FOV. The second half of the spin-echo was acquired with 512 complex data points over a sampling window of 256 ms, corresponding to a spectral width of 2000 Hz. Each phase-encoding FID was acquired twice for data averaging. The repetition time

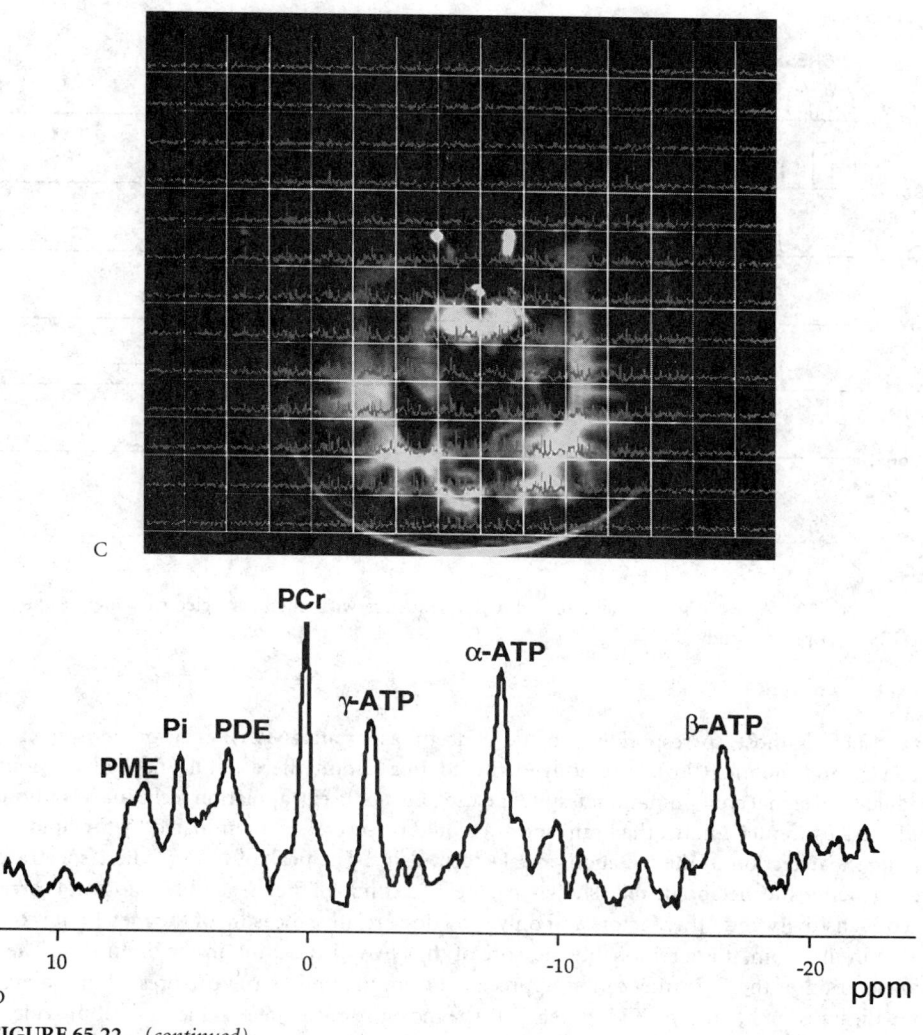

C

D

FIGURE 65.22   (*continued*)

(*TR*) and the echo time (*TE*) used were 1.2 s and 136 ms, respectively. The total acquisition time was approximately 40 minutes.

Another major problem in proton CSI study of the brain is that the signal from the subcutaneous lipid usually is much stronger than those of the metabolites, and this strong signal leaks into pixels within the brain due to truncation artifacts. To avoid lipid signal contamination, many proton CSI studies of the brain are performed within a selected region of interest excluding the subcutaneous fat [30–34]. Recently, several techniques have been proposed to suppress the lipid signal and consequently suppress the lipid signal contamination. These include the use of WEFT [27] and the use of outer-volume signal suppression [34]. In the example described below, we used a technique that utilizes the spatial location of the lipid to extrapolate data in the *k*-space to reduce the signal contamination due to truncation [35].

In Fig. 65.24, the results from the proton CSI study are presented. In panel (*a*), the localized spectra are displayed. Note that the spectra in the subcutaneous lipid are ignored because they are all off the scale. The nominal spatial resolution is approximately 0.66 cc. A spectrum from an individual pixel in this study is presented in Fig. 65.24*b* with metabolite peaks indicated. Several metabolite

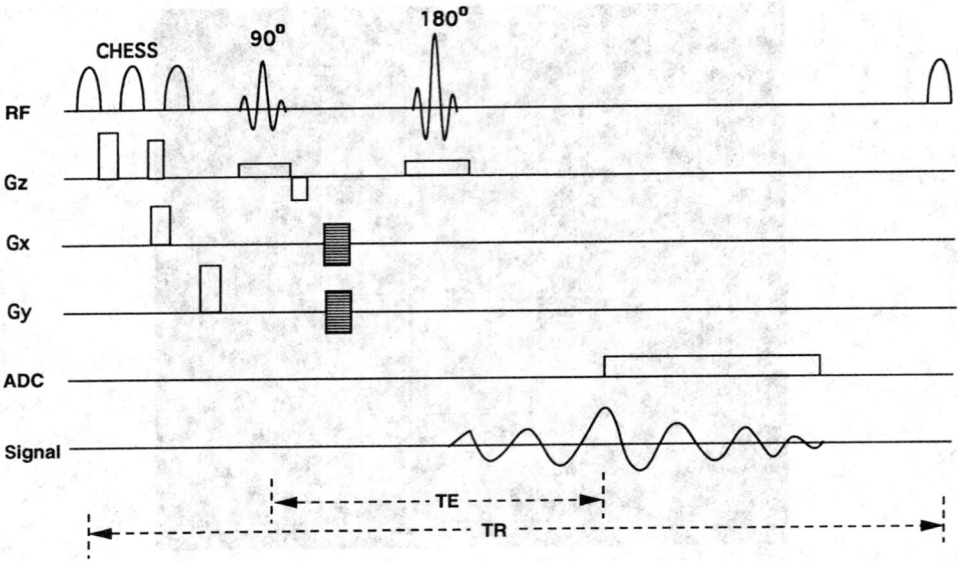

FIGURE 65.23 A two-dimensional spin-echo CSI sequence with chemical selective water suppression (CHESS) for proton study.

peaks, such as those corresponding to the *N*-acetyl aspartate (NAA), creatine/phosphocreatine (Cr/PCr), and choline (Cho), are readily identified. In addition, there is still a negligible amount of residual lipid signal contamination despite the use of the data extrapolation technique. Without the lipid suppression technique, the brain spectra would be severely contaminated by the lipid signal, making the detection of the metabolite peaks formidable. The peak of NAA in these spectra is fitted to generate the metabolite map shown in panel (*c*). Although the metabolite map is not corrected for coil sensitivity and other factors and only provides a relative measure of the metabolite concentration in the brain, it is a reasonable measure of the NAA distribution in the brain slice. The spatial resolution of the CSI study can be appreciated from the brain structure present in the map. In biomedical research, proton CSI is potentially the most promising technique, since it provides best sensitivity and spatial resolution. Various in vivo applications of proton spectroscopy can be found in the literature [36].

Summary

CSI is a technique for generating localized spectra that provide a wealth of biochemical information that can be used to study the metabolic activity of living system and to detect disease associated biochemical changes. This section provides an introduction to the technique and illustrates it by two representative examples. More specific topics concerning various aspects of CSI can be found in the literature.

Acknowledgments

The authors would like to thank Dr. Xiao-Hong Zhu for assisting data acquisition and Mr. Gregory Adriany for hardware support. The studies presented here are supported by the National Institutes of Health (RR08079).

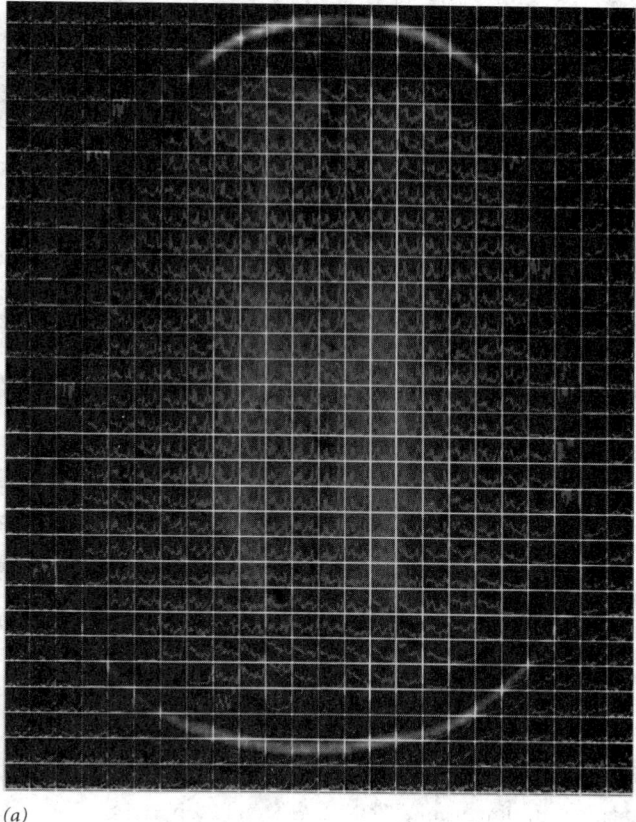

(a)

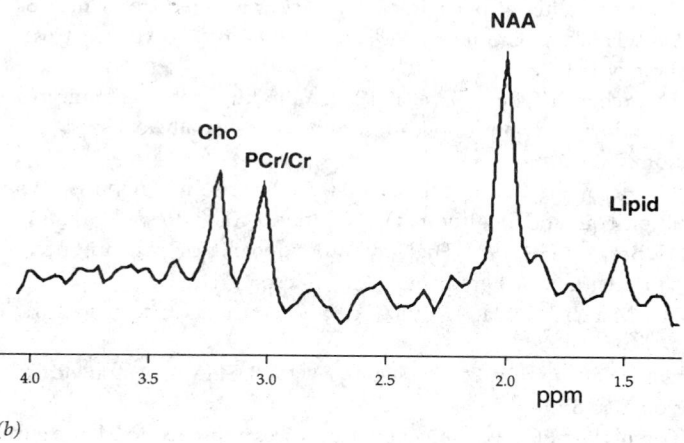

(b)

FIGURE 65.24 (a) Boxed plot of spectra for the two-dimensional proton study overlaid on the anatomic image. A spectral range of 1.7 to 3.5 ppm is used in the plot to show Cho, PCr/Cr, and NAA. A 5-Hz line broadening is applied in the spectral processing. (b) A representative spectrum from the two-dimensional CSI in panel (a). Peaks corresponding to Cho, PCr/Cr, and NAA are indicated. (c) A map of the area under the NAA peak obtained by spectral fitting. The anatomic image is presented along with the metabolite map for reference. The spatial resolution of the metabolite image can be appreciated from the similarities between the two images. The lipid suppression technique has successfully eliminated the signal contamination from the lipid in the skull.

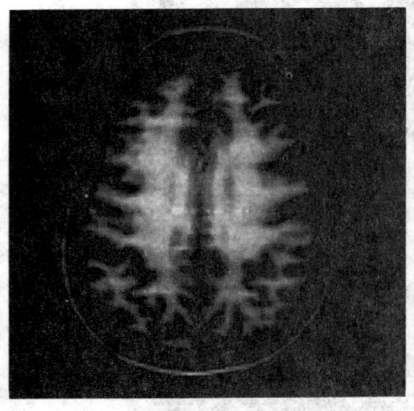 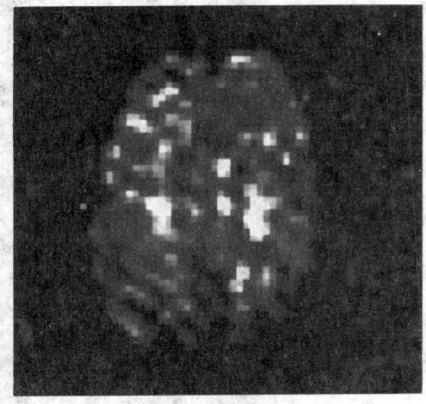

(c)

FIGURE 65.24   *(continued)*

References

1. Lauterbur PC. 1973. Image formation by induced local interactions: Examples employing nuclear magnetic resonance. Nature 242:190.
2. Alger JR. 1994. Spatial localization for in vivo magnetic resonance spectroscopy: Concepts and commentary. In RJ Gillies (ed), NMR in Physiology and Biomedicine, pp 151–168. San Diego, Calif, Academic Press.
3. Brown TR, Kincaid MB, Ugurbil K. 1982. NMR chemical shift imaging in three dimensions. Proc Natl Acad Sci USA 79:3523.
4. Maudsley AA, Hilal SK, Simon HE, Perman WH. 1983. Spatially resolved high resolution spectroscopy by "four dimensional" NMR. J Magn Reson 51:147.
5. Haselgrove JC, Subramanian VH, Leigh JS Jr, et al. 1983. In vivo one-dimensional imaging of phosphorus metabolites by phosphorus-31 nuclear magnetic resonance. Science 220:1170.
6. Maudsley AA, Hilal SK, Simon HE, Wittekoek S. 1984. In vivo MR spectroscopic imaging with P-31. Radiology 153:745.
7. Garwood M, Schleich T, Ross BD, et al. 1985. A modified rotating frame experiment based on a Fourier window function: Application to in vivo spatially localized NMR spectroscopy. J Magn Reson 65:239.
8. Garwood M, Robitalle PM, Ugurbil K. 1987. Fourier series windows on and off resonance using multiple coils and longitudinal modulation. J Magn Reson 75:244.
9. Mareci TH, Brooker HR. 1984. High-resolution magnetic resonance spectra from a sensitive region defined with pulsed gradients. J Magn Reson 57:157.
10. Brooker HR, Mareci TH, Mao JT. 1987. Selective Fourier transform localization. Magn Reson Med 5:417.
11. Hu X, Levin DN, Lauterbur PC, Spraggins TA. 1988. SLIM: Spectral localization by imaging. Magn Reson Med 8:314.
12. Liang ZP, Lauterbur PC. 1991. A generalized series approach to MR spectroscopic imaging. IEEE Trans Med Imag MI-10:132.
13. Hu X, Stillman AE. 1991. Technique for reduction of truncation artifact in chemical shift images. IEEE Trans Med Imag MI-10(3):290.
14. Hu X, Patel MS, Ugurbil K. 1993. A new strategy for chemical shift imaging. J Magn Reson B103:30.
15. van den Boogaart A, Ala-Korpela M, Jokisaari J, Griffiths JR. 1994. Time and frequency domain analysis of NMR data compared: An application to 1D ^1H spectra of lipoproteins. Magn Reson Med 31:347.

16. Ernst T, Kreis R, Ross B. 1993. Absolute quantification of water and metabolites in human brain: I. Compartments and water. J Magn Reson 102:1.

17. Kreis R, Ernst T, Ross B. 1993. Absolute quantification of water and metabolites in human brain: II. Metabolite concentration. J Magn Reson 102:9.

18. Lenkinski RE, Holland GA, Allman T, et al. 1988. Integrated MR imaging and spectroscopy with chemical shift imaging of P-31 at 1.5 T: Initial clinical experience. Radiology 169:201.

19. Hugg JW, Matson GB, Twieg DB, et al. 1992. ^{31}P MR spectroscopic imaging of normal and pathological human brains. Magn Reson Imaging 10:227.

20. Vigneron DB, Nelson SJ, Murphy-Boesch J, et al. 1990. Chemical shift imaging of human brain: Axial, sagittal, and coronal ^{31}P metabolite images. Radiology 177:643.

21. Hugg JW, Laxer KD, Matson GB, et al. 1992. Lateralization of human focal epilepsy by ^{31}P magnetic resonance spectroscopic imaging. Neurology 42:2011.

22. Meyerhoff DJ, Maudsley AA, Schaefer S, Weiner MW. 1992. Phosphorus-31 magnetic resonance metabolite imaging in the human body. Magn Reson Imaging 10:245.

23. Bottomley PA, Hardy C, Boemer P. 1990. Phosphate metabolite imaging and concentration measurements in human heart by nuclear magnetic resonance. Magn Reson Med 14:425.

24. Robitaille PM, Lew B, Merkle H, et al. 1990. Transmural high energy phosphate distribution and response to alterations in workload in the normal canine myocardium as studied with spatially localized ^{31}P NMR spectroscopy. Magn Reson Med 16:91.

25. Ugurbil K, Garwood M, Merkle H, et al. 1989. Metabolic consequences of coronary stenosis: Transmurally heterogeneous myocardial ischemia studied by spatially localized ^{31}P NMR spectroscopy. NMR Biomed 2:317.

26. Hasse A, Frahm J, Hanicker H, Mataei D. 1985. ^{1}H NMR chemical shift selective (CHESS) imaging. Phys Med Biol 30(4):341.

27. Patt SL, Sykes BD. 1972. T_1 water eliminated Fourier transform NMR spectroscopy. Chem Phys 56:3182.

28. Moonen CTW, van Zijl PCM. 1990. Highly effective water suppression for in vivo proton NMR spectroscopy (DRYSTEAM). J Magn Reson 88:28.

29. Ogg R, Kingsley P, Taylor JS. 1994. WET: A T_1 and B_1 insensitive water suppression method for in vivo localized ^{1}H NMR spectroscopy. B104:1.

30. Lampman DA, Murdoch JB, Paley M. 1991. In vivo proton metabolite maps using MESA 3D technique. Magn Reson Med 18:169.

31. Luyten PR, Marien AJH, Heindel W, et al. 1990. Metabolic imaging of patients with intracranial tumors: ^{1}H MR spectroscopic imaging and PET. Radiology 176:791.

32. Arnold DL, Matthews PM, Francis GF, et al. 1992. Proton magnetic resonance spectroscopic imaging for metabolite characterization of demyelinating plaque. Ann Neurol 31:319.

33. Duijin JH, Matson GB, Maudsley AA, et al. 1992. Human brain infarction: Proton MR spectroscopy. Radiology 183:711.

34. Duyn JH, Gillen J, Sobering G, et al. 1993. Multisection proton MR spectroscopic imaging of the brain. Radiology 188:277.

35. Patel MS, Hu X. 1994. Selective data extrapolation for chemical shift imaging. Soc Magn Reson Abstr 3:1168.

36. Rothman DL. 1994. ^{1}H NMR studies of human brain metabolism and physiology. In RJ Gillies (ed), NMR in Physiology and Biomedicine, pp 353–372. San Diego, Calif, Academic Press.

Nuclear Medicine

Barbara Y. Croft
University of Virginia

Benjamin M.W. Tsui
*University of North
Carolina at Chapel Hill*

66.1 Instrumentation

Barbara Y. Croft

Nuclear medicine can be defined as the practice of making patients radioactive for diagnostic and therapeutic purposes. The radioactivity is injected intravenously, rebreathed, or ingested. It is the internal circulation of radioactive material that distinguishes nuclear medicine from diagnostic radiology and radiation oncology in most of its forms. This section will examine only the diagnostic use and will concentrate on methods for detecting the radioactivity from outside the body without trauma to the patient. Diagnostic nuclear medicine is successful for two main reasons: (1) It can rely on the use of very small amounts of materials (picomolar concentrations in chemical terms) thus usually not having any effect on the processes being studied, and (2) The radionuclides being used can penetrate tissue and be detected outside the patient. Thus the materials can trace processes or "opacify" organs without affecting their function.

Parameters for Choices in Nuclear Medicine

Of the various kinds of emanations from radioactive materials, photons alone have a range in tissue great enough to escape so that they can be detected externally. Electrons or beta-minus particles of high energy can create bremsstrahlung in interactions with tissue, but the radiation emanates from the site of the interaction, not the site of the beta ray's production. Positrons or beta-plus particles annihilate with electrons to create gamma rays so that they can be detected (see Chap. 69). For certain radionuclides, the emanation being detected is x-rays, in the 50- to 100-KeV energy range.

The half-lives of materials in use in nuclear medicine range from a few minutes to weeks. The half-life must be chosen with two major points in mind: the time course of the process being studied and the radiation dose to the target organ, i.e., that organ with the highest concentration over the longest time (the cumulated activity or area underneath the activity versus time curve). In general, it is desired to stay under 5 rad to the target organ.

The choice of the best energy range to use is also based on two major criteria: the energy that will penetrate tissue but can be channeled by heavy metal shielding and collimation and that which will

0-8493-8346-3/95/$0.00+$.50
© 1995 by CRC Press, Inc.

interact in the detector to produce a pulse. Thus the ideal energy is dependent on the detector being used and the kind of examination being performed. Table 66.1 describes the kinds of gamma-ray detection, the activity and energy ranges, and an example of the kind of information to be gained. The lesser amounts of activity are used in situations of lesser spatial resolution and/or of greater sensitivity. Positron imaging is omitted because it is treated elsewhere.

Radiation dose is affected by all the emanations of a radionuclide, not just the desirable ones, thus constricting the choice of nuclide further. There can be no alpha radiation used in diagnosis; the use of materials with primary beta radiation should be avoided because the beta radiation confers a radiation dose without adding to the information being gained. For imaging, in addition, even if there is a primary gamma ray in the correct energy window for the detector, there should be no large amount of radiation, either of primary radiation of higher energy, because it interferes with the image collimation, or of secondary radiation of a very similar-energy, because it interferes with the perception of the primary radiation emanating from the site of interest.

For imaging using heavy-metal collimation, the energy range is constrained to be that which will emanate from the human body and which the collimation can contain, or about 50 to 500 keV.

Detectors must be made from materials that exhibit some detectable change when ionizing radiation is absorbed and that are of a high enough atomic number and density to make possible stopping large percentages of those gamma rays emanating (high sensitivity). In addition, because the primary gamma rays are not the only rays emanating from the source—a human body and therefore a distributed source accompanied by an absorber—there must be energy discrimination in the instrument to prevent the formation of an image of the scattered radiation. To achieve pulse size proportional to energy, and therefore to achieve identification of the energy and source of the energy, the detector must be a proportional detector. This means that Geiger-Muller detection, operating in an all-or-none fashion, is not acceptable.

Gaseous detectors are not practical because their density is not great enough. Liquid detectors (in which any component is liquid) are not practical because the liquid can spill when the detector is positioned; this problem can be compensated for if absolutely necessary, but it is better to consider it from the outset. Another property of a good detector is its ability to detect large numbers of gamma rays per time unit. With detection capabilities to separate 100,000 counts per second or a dead time of 2 μs, the system is still only detecting perhaps 1000 counts per square centimeter per second over a 10 $\times$ 10 cm area. The precision of the information is governed by Poisson statistics, so the imprecision in information collected for 1 s in a square centimeter is $\pm3\%$ at the 1 standard deviation level. Since we would hope for better spatial resolution than 1 cm^2, the precision is obviously worse than this. This points to the need for fast detectors, in addition to the aforementioned sensitivity. The more detector that surrounds the patient, the more sensitive the system will be. Table 66.2 lists in order from least sensitive to most sensitive some of the geometries used for imaging in nuclear medicine. This generally is also a listing from the older methods to the more recent.

For the purposes of this section, we shall consider that the problems of counting patient and other samples and of detecting the time course of activity changes in extended areas with probes are not

TABLE 66.1 Gamma Ray Detection

Type of Sample	Activity	Energy	Type of Instrument
Patient samples, e.g., blood, urine	0.001 μCi	20–5000 keV	Gamma counter with annular NaI(Tl) detector, 1 or 2 PMTs, external Pb shielding
Small organ function <30 cm field of view at 60 cm distance	5–200 μCi	20–1500 keV	2–4-in. NaI(Tl) detector with flared Pb collimator
Static image of body part, e.g., liver, lung	0.2–30 mCi	50–650 keV	Rectilinear scanner with focused Pb collimator
Dynamic image of body part, e.g., xenon in airways	2–30 mCi	80–300 keV	Anger camera and parallel-hole Pb collimator
Static tomographic image of body part	See Sec. 66.1		

TABLE 66.2   Ways of Imaging Using Lead Collimation

Moving probe: rectilinear scanner
Array of multiple crystals: autofluoroscope, "fly-eye" camera
Two moving probes: dual-head rectilinear scanner
Large single-crystal system: Anger camera
Two crystals on opposite sides of patient for two views using Anger logic
Large multiple-crystal systems using Anger logic: SPECT
Other possibilities

our topic and confine ourselves to the attempts made to image distributions of gamma-emitting radionuclides in patients and research subjects. The previous section treats the three-dimensional imaging of these distributions; this section will treat detection of the distribution in a planar fashion or the image of the projection of the distribution onto a planar detector.

Detection of Photon Radiation

Gamma rays are detected when atoms in a detector are ionized and the ions are collected either directly as in gaseous or semiconductor systems or by first conversion of the ionized electrons to light and subsequent conversion of the light to electrons in a photomultiplier tube (P-M-tube or PMT). In all cases there is a voltage applied across some distance that causes a pulse to be created when a photon is absorbed.

The gamma rays are emitted according to Poisson statistics because each decaying nucleus is independent of the others and has an equal probability of decaying per unit time. Because the uncertainty in the production of gamma rays is therefore on the order of magnitude of the square root of the number of gamma rays, the more gamma rays that are detected, the less the proportional uncertainty will be. Thus sensitivity is a very important issue for the creation of images, since the rays will be detected by area. To get better resolution, one must have the numbers of counts and the apparatus to resolve them spatially. Having the large numbers of counts also means the apparatus must resolve them temporally.

The need for energy resolution carries its own burden. Depending on the detector, the energy resolution may be easily achieved or not (Table 66.3). In any case, the attenuation and scattering inside the body mean that there will be a range of gamma rays emitted, and it will be difficult to tell those scattered through very small angles from those not scattered at all. This affects the spatial resolution of the instrument.

The current practice of nuclear medicine has defined the limits of the amount of activity that can be administered to a patient by the amount of radiation dose. Since planar imaging with one detector allows only 2 pi detection at best and generally a view of somewhat less because the source is in the patient and the lead collimation means that only rays that are directed from the decay toward the crystal will be detected, it is of utmost importance to detect every ray possible. To the extent that

TABLE 66.3   Detector Substances and Size Considerations, Atomic Number of the Attenuator, Energy Resolution Capability

PMT connected
NaI(Tl): up to 50 cm across; 53; 5–10%
Plastic scintillators: unlimited; 6; only Compton absorption for gamma rays used in imaging
CsI(Tl): <3 cm × 3 cm; 53, 55; poorer than NaI(Tl)
BiGermanate: < 3 cm × 3 cm; 83; poorer than NaI(Tl)
Semiconductors: Liquid nitrogen operation and liquid nitrogen storage
GeLi: <3 cm × 3 cm; 32; <1%
SiLi: <3 cm × 3 cm; 14; <1%

no one is ever satisfied with the resolution of any system and always wishes for better, there is the need to be able to get spatial resolution better than the intrinsic 2 mm currently achievable. Some better collimation system, such as envisioned in a coincidence detection system like that used in PET, might make it possible to avoid stopping so many of the rays with the collimator.

We have now seen that energy resolution, sensitivity, and resolving time of the detector are all bound up together to produce the spatial resolution of the instrument as well as the more obvious temporal resolution. The need to collimate to create an image rather than a blush greatly decreases the numbers of counts and makes Poisson statistics a major determinant of the appearance of nuclear medical images.

Table 66.4 shows a calculation for the NaI(TI)-based Anger camera showing 0.06% efficiency for the detection system. Thus the number of counts per second is not high and so is well within the temporal resolving capabilities of the detector system. The problem is the 0.06% efficiency, which is the effect of both the crystal thickness being optimized for imaging rather than for stopping all the gamma rays, and the lead collimation. Improvements in nuclear medicine imaging resolution can only come if both these factors are addressed.

Various Detector Configurations

The detectors in clinical nuclear medicine are NaI(TI) crystals. In research applications, other substances are employed, but the engineering considerations for the use of other detectors are more complex and have been less thoroughly explored (see Table 66.3).

The possibilities for configuring the detectors have been increasing, although the older methods tend to be discarded as the new ones are exploited (see Table 66.2). This is in part because each laboratory cannot afford to have one of every kind of instrument, although there are tasks for which each one is ideally suited.

The first instruments possible for plane-projection imaging consisted of a moving single crystal probe, called a *rectilinear scanner*. The probe consisted of a detector [beginning with NaI(TI) but later incorporating small semiconductors] that was collimated by a focused lead collimator of appreciable thickness (often 2 in. of lead or more) with hole sizes and thicknesses of septa consonant with the intended energy and organ size and depth to be imaged. The collimated detector was caused to move across the patient at a constant speed; the pulses from the detector were converted to visible signals either by virtue of markings on a sheet or of light flashes exposing a film. This detector could see only one spot at a time, so only slow temporal changes in activity could be appreciated. A small organ such as the thyroid could be imaged in this fashion very satisfactorily. Bone imaging also could be done with the later versions of this instrument.

TABLE 66.4   Calculation of Number of Counts Achieved with Anger Camera

	cpm	cps
Activity	0.001	
mCi/cm^3		
counts/sec		3.7×10^7
counts/min	2.22×10^9	
2π geometry	1.11×10^9	1.85×10^7
Attenuated by tissue of 0.12/cm attenuation		
and 3 cm thick	7.44×10^8	1.29×10^7
X Camera efficiency of 0.0006	4.64×10^5	7744
Good uptake in liver = 5 mCi/1000 g =		
0.005 mCi/g	2.32×10^6	3.8×10^4
Thyroid uptake of Tc-99m = (2 mCi/37 g) *		
2% = 0.001 mCi/g	4.6×10^5	7.7×10^3

To enlarge the size of the detector, several probes, each with its own photomultiplier tube and collimator, could be used. Versions of this idea were used to create dual-probe instruments to image both side of the patient simultaneously, bars of probes to sweep down the patient and create a combined image, etc.

To go further with the multiple crystals to create yet larger fields of view, the autofluoroscope (Fig. 66.1) combined crystals in a rectangular array. For each to have its own photomultiplier tube required too many PMTs, so the instrument was designed with a light pipe to connect each crystal with a PMT to indicate its row and a second one to indicate its column. The crystals are separated by lead septa to prevent scattered photons from one crystal affecting the next. Because of the large number of crystals and PMTs, the instrument is very fast, but because of the size of the crystals, the resolution is coarse. To improve the resolution, the collimator is often jittered so that each crystal is made to see more than one field of view to create a better resolved image. For those dynamic examinations in which temporal resolution is more important than spatial resolution, the system has a clear advantage. It has not been very popular for general use, however. In its commercial realization, the field of view was not large enough to image either lungs or livers or bones in any single image fashion.

As larger NaI(TI) crystals became a reality, new ways to use them were conceived. The Anger camera (Fig. 66.2) is one of the older of these methods. The idea is to use a single crystal of diameter large enough to image a significant part of the human body and to back the crystal by an array of photomultiplier tubes to give positional sensitivity. Each PMT is assigned coordinates (Fig. 66.3). When a photon is absorbed by the crystal, a number of PMTs receive light and therefore emit signals. The X and Y signal values for the emanation are determined by the strength of the signal from each of the tubes and its x and y position, and the energy of the emanation (which determines if it will be used to create the image) is the sum of all the signals (the Z pulse). If the discriminator passes the Z pulse, then the X and Y signals are sent to whatever device is recording the image, be it an oscilloscope and film recording system or the analog-to-digital (A/D) converters of a computer system. More recently, the A/D conversion is done earlier in the system so that the X and Y signals are themselves digital. The Anger camera is the major instrument in use in nuclear medicine today. It has been optimized for use with the 140-keV radiation from Tc-99m, although collimators have been designed for lower and higher energies, as well as optimized for higher sensitivity and higher resolution. The early systems used circular crystals, while the current configuration is likely to be rectangular or square.

A combination of the Anger positional logic and the focused collimator in a scanner produced the PhoCon instrument, which, because of the design of its collimators, had planar tomographic capabilities (the instrument could partially resolve activity in different planes, parallel to the direction of movement of the detector).

Ancillary Electronic Equipment for Detection

The detectors use in nuclear medicine are attached to preamplifiers, amplifiers, and pulse shapers to form a signal that can be examined for information about the energy of the detected photon (Fig. 66.4). The energy discriminator has lower and upper windows that are set with reference radionuclides so that typically the particular nuclide in use can be dialed in along with the width of the energy window. A photon with an energy that falls in the selected range will cause the creation of a pulse of a voltage that falls in between the levels; all other photon energies will cause voltages either too high or too low. If only gross features are being recorded, any of the instruments may be used as probe detectors and the results recorded on strip-chart recordings of activity versus time.

The PMT "multiplies" photons (Fig. 66.5) because it has a quartz entrance window which is coated to release electrons when it absorbs a light photon and there is a voltage drop; the number of electrons released is proportional to the amount of light that hits the coating. The electrons are guided through a hole and caused to hit the first dynode, which is coated with a special substance to allow it to release electrons when it is hit by an electron. There are a series of dynodes each with

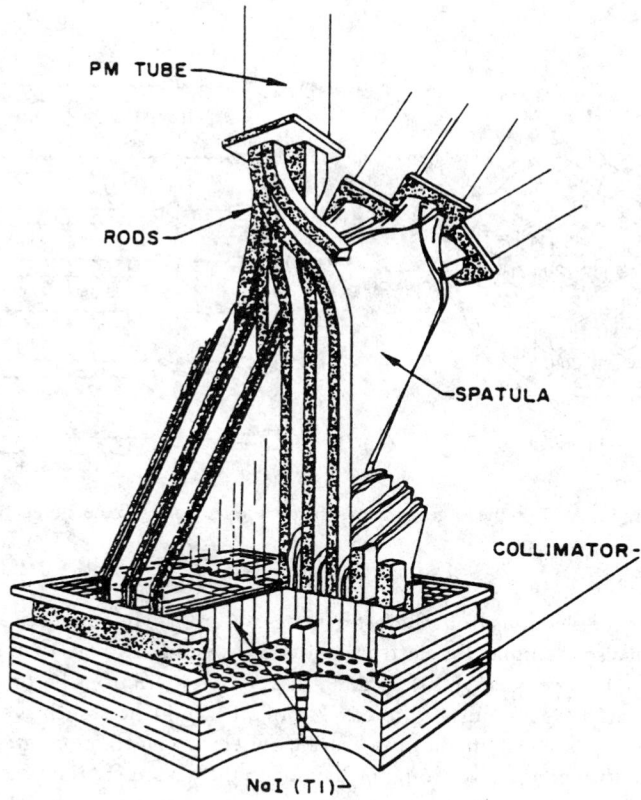

FIGURE 66.1 The Bender-Blau autofluoroscope is a multicrystal imager with a rectangular array of crystals connected to PMTs by plastic light guides. There is a PMT for each row of crystals and a PMT for each column of crystals, so an *N* by *M* array would have (*N* + *M*) PMTs.

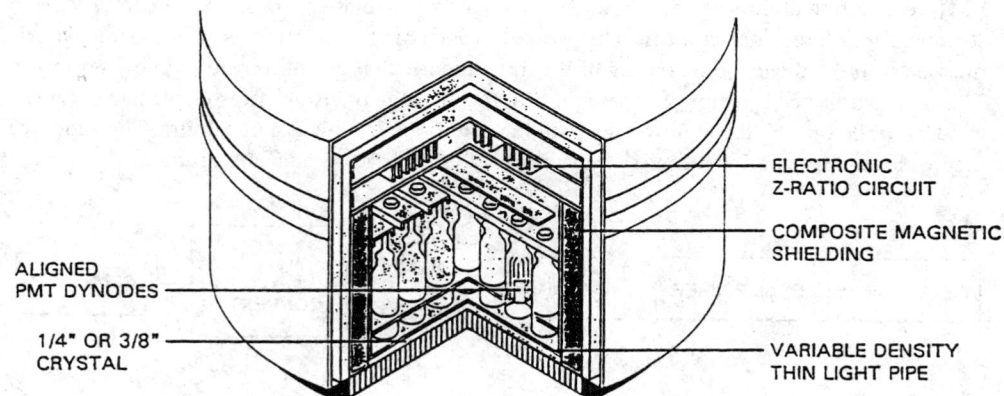

FIGURE 66.2 Anger camera detector design. This figure shows a cross section through the camera head. The active surface is pointed down. Shielding surrounds the assembly on the sides and top.

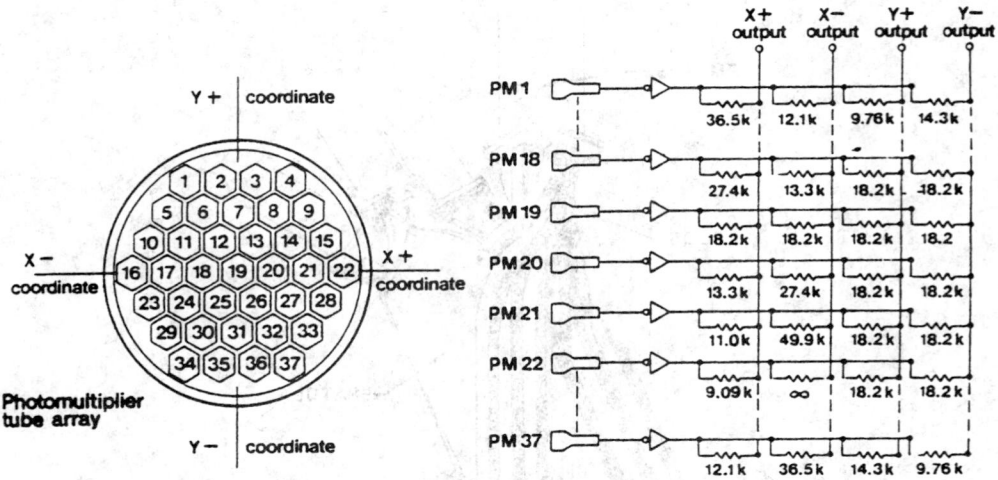

FIGURE 66.3 An array of PMTs in the Anger camera showing the geometric connection between the PMTs and the *X* and *Y* output.

a voltage that pulls the electrons from the last dynodes toward it. The surface coating not only releases electrons but also multiplies the electron shower. In a cascade through 10 to 12 dynodes, there is a multiplication of approximately 10^6, so that pulses of a few electrons become currents of the order of 10^{-12} amps. The PMTs must be protected from other influences, such as stray radioactivity or strong magnetic fields, which might cause extraneous electron formation or curves in the electron path. Without the voltage drop from one dynode to the next, there is no cascade of electrons and no counting.

For imaging, the *x* and *y* positions of those photons in the correct energy range will be recorded in the image because they have a *Z* pulse. Once the pulse has been accepted and the position determined, that position may be recorded to make an image either in analog or digital fashion; a spot may be made on an oscilloscope screen and recorded on film or paper, or the position may be digitized and stored in a computer file for later imaging on an oscilloscope screen and/or for photography. In general, the computers required are very similar to those used for other imaging modalities, except for the hardware that allows the acceptance of the pulse. The software is usually specifically created for nuclear medicine because of the unique needs for determination of function.

The calibration of the systems follows a similar pattern, no matter how simple or complex the instrument. Most probe detectors must be "peaked," which means that the energy of the radioactivity must be connected with some setting of the instrument, often meant to read in kiloelectronvolts. This is accomplished by counting a sample with the instrument, using a reasonably narrow energy window, while varying the high voltage until the count rate reading is a maximum. The window is then widened for counting samples to encompass all the energy peak being counted. The detector

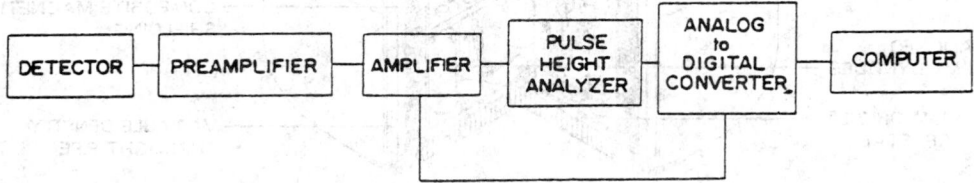

FIGURE 66.4 Schematic drawing of a generalized detector system. There would be a high-voltage power supply for the detector in an NaI(Tl)-PMT detector system.

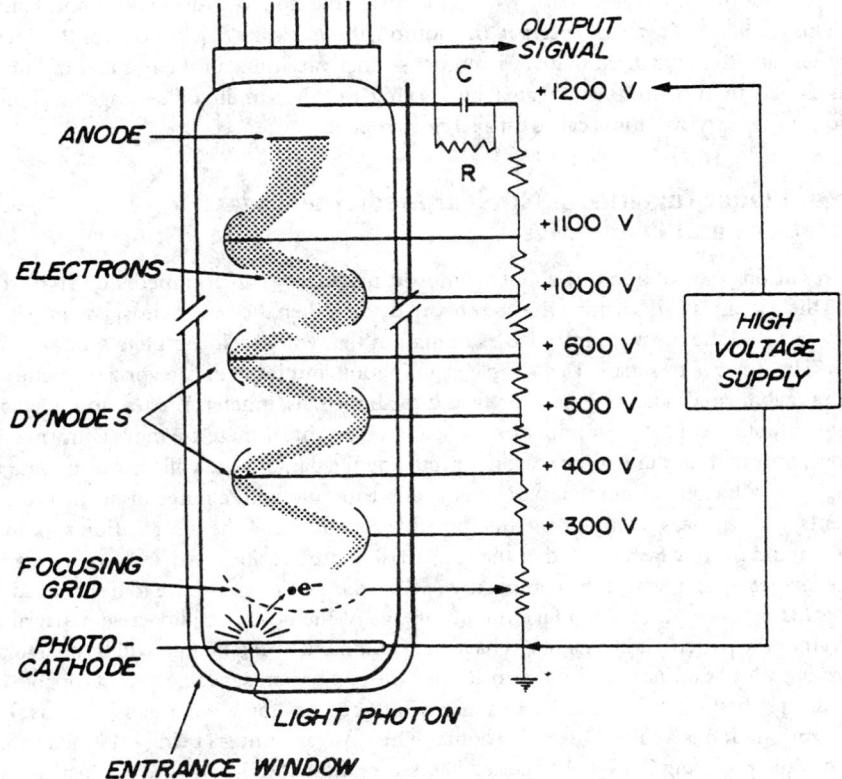

FIGURE 66.5 Schematic drawing of a photomultiplier tube (PMT). Each of the dynodes and the anode is connected to a separate pin in the tube socket. The inside of the tube is evacuated of all gas. Dynodes are typically copper with a special oxidized coating for electron multiplication.

is said to be linear if it can be set with one energy and another energy can be found where it should be on the kiloelectronvolt scale.

To ensure that the images of the radioactivity accurately depict the distribution in the object being imaged, the system must be initialized correctly and tested at intervals. The several properties that must be calibrated and corrected are sensitivity, uniformity, energy pulse shape, and linearity.

These issues are addressed in several ways. The first is that all the PMTs used in an imaging system must be chosen to have matched sensitivities and energy spectra. Next, during manufacture, and at intervals during maintenance, the PMTs' response to voltage is matched so that the voltage from the power supply causes all the tubes to have maximum counts at the same voltage. The sensitivities of all the tubes are also matched during periodic maintenance. Prior to operation, usually at the start of each working day, the user will check the radioactive peak and then present the instrument with a source of activity to give an even exposure over the whole crystal. This uniform "flood" is recorded. The image may be used by the instrument for calibration; recalibration is usually performed at weekly intervals. The number of counts needed depends on the use the instrument is to be put to, but generally the instrument must be tested and calibrated with numbers of counts at least equal to those being emitted by the patients and other objects being imaged.

Because the PMT placement means that placement of the x and y locations is not perfect over the face of the crystal but has the effect of creating wiggly lines that may be closer together over the center of the PMT and farther apart at the interstices between tubes, the image may suffer from spatial nonlinearity. This can be corrected for by presenting the system with a lead pattern in straight-line bars or holes in rows and using a hard-wired or software method to position the *X* and *Y* signals correctly. This is called a *linearity correction*. In addition, there may be adjustments of the energy spectra of each tube to make them match each other so that variations in the number of kiloelectron-volts included in the window (created by varying the discriminator settings) will not create variations in sensitivity. This is called an *energy correction*.

Place of Planar Imaging in Nuclear Medicine Today: Applications and Economics

There are various ways of thinking about diagnostic imaging and nuclear medicine. If the reason for imaging the patient is to determine the presence of disease, then there are at least two possible strategies. One is to do the most complicated examination that will give a complete set of results on all patients. The other is to start with a simple examination and hope to categorize patients, perhaps into certain abnormals and all others, or even into abnormals, indeterminates, and normals. Then a subsequent, more complex examination is used to determine if there are more abnormals, or perhaps how abnormal they are. If the reason for imaging the patient is to collect a set of data that will be compared with results from that patient at a later time and with a range of normal results from all patients, then the least complex method possible for collecting the information should be used in a regular and routine fashion so that the comparisons are possible.

In the former setting, where the complexity of the examination may have to be changed after the initial results are seen, in order to take full advantage of the dose of radioactive material that has been given to the patient, it is sensible to have the equipment available that will be able to perform the more complex examination and not to confine the equipment available to that capable of doing only the simple first examination. For this reason and because for some organs, such as the brain, the first examination is a SPECT examination, the new Anger cameras being sold today are mostly capable of doing rotating SPECT. The added necessities that SPECT brings to the instrument specifications are of degree: better stability, uniformity, and resolution. Thus they do not obviate the use of the equipment for planar imaging but rather enhance it. In the setting of performing only the examination necessary to define the disease, the Anger SPECT camera can be used for plane projection imaging and afterward for SPECT to further refine the examination. There are settings in which a planar camera will be purchased because of the simplicity of all the examinations (as in a very large laboratory that can have specialized instruments, a thyroid practice, or in the developing countries), but in the small- to medium-sized nuclear medicine practice, the new cameras being purchased are all SPECT-capable.

Nuclear medicine studies are generally less expensive than x-ray computed tomography or magnetic resonance imaging and more so than planar x-ray or ultrasound imaging. The general conduct of a nuclear medicine laboratory is more complex than these others because of the radioactive materials and the accompanying regulations. The specialty is practiced both in clinics and in hospitals, but again, the complication imposed by the presence of radioactive materials tips the balance of the practices toward the hospital. In that setting the practitioners may be imagers with a broad range of studies offered or cardiologists with a concentration on cardiac studies. Thus the setting also will determine what kind of instrument is most suitable.

Defining Terms

Energy resolution: Full width at half maximum of graph of detected counts versus energy, expressed as a percentage of the energy.

Poisson statistics: Expresses probability in situations of equal probability for an event per unit time, such as radioactive decay or cosmic-ray appearance. The standard deviation of a mean number of counts is the square root of the mean number of counts, which is decreasing fraction of the number of counts when expressed as a fraction of the number of counts.

rad: The unit of radiation energy absorption (dose) in matter, defined as the absorption of 100 ergs per gram of irradiated material. The unit is being replaced by the gray, an SI unit, where 1 gray (Gy) = 100 rad.

Further Information

A good introduction to nuclear medicine, written as a text for technologists, is *Nuclear Medicine Technology and Techniques,* edited by D. R. Bernier, J. K. Langan, and L. D. Wells. A treatment of many of the nuclear medicine physics issues is given in L. E. Williams' *Nuclear Medicine Physics,* published in three volumes. Journals that publish nuclear medicine articles include the monthly *Journal of Nuclear Medicine,* the *European Journal of Nuclear Medicine, Clinical Nuclear Medicine, IEEE Transactions in Nuclear Science, IEEE Transactions in Medical Imaging,* and *Medical Physics.* Quarterly and annual publications include *Seminars in Nuclear Medicine, Yearbook of Nuclear Medicine,* and *Nuclear Medicine Annual.*

The Society of Nuclear Medicine holds an annual scientific meeting that includes scientific papers, continuing education which could give the novice a broad introduction, poster sessions, and a large equipment exhibition. Another large meeting, devoted to many radiologic specialties is the Radiologic Society of North America's annual meeting, held just after Thanksgiving.

66.2 SPECT (Single-Photon Emission Computed Tomography)

Benjamin M.W. Tsui

During the last three decades, there has been much excitement in the development of diagnostic radiology. The development is fueled by inventions and advances made in a number of exciting new medical imaging modalities, including ultrasound (US), x-ray CT (computed tomography), PET (positron emission tomography), SPECT (single-photon emission computed tomography), and MRI (magnetic resonance imaging). These new imaging modalities have revolutionized the practice of diagnostic radiology, resulting in substantial improvement in patient care.

Single-photon emission computed tomography (SPECT) is a medical imaging modality that combines conventional nuclear medicine (NM) imaging technique and CT methods. Different from x-ray CT, SPECT uses radioactive-labeled pharmaceuticals, i.e., radiopharmaceuticals, that distribute in different internal tissues or organs instead of an external x-ray source. The spatial and uptake distributions of the radiopharmaceuticals depend on the biokinetic properties of the pharmaceuticals and the normal or abnormal state of the patient. The gamma photons emitted from the radioactive source are detected by radiation detectors similar to those used in conventional nuclear medicine. The CT method requires projection (or planar) image data to be acquired from different views around the patient. These projection data are subsequently reconstructed using image reconstruction methods that generate cross-sectional images of the internally distributed radiopharmaceuticals. The SPECT images provide much improved contrast and detailed information about the radiopharmaceutical distribution as compared with the planar images obtained from conventional nuclear medicine methods.

As an emission computed tomographic (ECT) method, SPECT differs from PET in the types of radionuclides used. PET uses radionuclides such as C-11, N-13, O-15, and F-18 that emit positrons with subsequent emission of two coincident 511-keV annihilation photons. These radionuclides allow studies of biophysiologic functions that cannot be obtained from other means. However, they have very short half-lives, often requiring an on-site cyclotron for their production. Also, detection of the annihilation photons requires expensive imaging systems. SPECT uses standard radionuclides normally found in nuclear medicine clinics and which emit individual gamma-ray photons with energies that are much lower than 511 keV. Typical examples are the 140-keV photons from Tc-99m and the ~70-keV photons from Tl-201. Subsequently, the costs of SPECT instrumentation and of performing SPECT are substantially less than PET.

Furthermore, substantial advances have been made in the development of new radiopharmaceuticals, instrumentation, and image processing and reconstruction methods for SPECT. The results are much improved quality and quantitative accuracy of SPECT images. These advances, combined with the relatively lower costs, have propelled SPECT to become an increasingly more important diagnostic tool in nuclear medicine clinics.

This section will present the basic principles of SPECT and the instrumentation and image processing and reconstruction methods that are necessary to reconstruct SPECT images. Finally, recent advances and future development that will continue to improve the diagnostic capability of SPECT will be discussed.

Basic Principles of SPECT

Single-photon emission computed tomography (SPECT) is a medical imaging technique that is based on the conventional nuclear medicine imaging technique and tomographic reconstruction methods. General review of the basic principles, instrumentation, and reconstruction technique for SPECT can be found in a few review articles [Barrett, 1986; Jaszczak et al., 1980; Jaszczak and Coleman, 1985a; Jaszczak and Tsui, 1994].

The SPECT Imaging Process

The imaging process of SPECT can be simply depicted as in Fig. 66.6. Gamma-ray photons emitted from the internal distributed radiopharmaceutical penetrate through the patient's body and are detected by a single or a set of collimated radiation detectors. The emitted photons experience interactions with the intervening tissues through basic interactions of radiation with matter [Evans, 1955]. The photoelectric effect absorbs all the energy of the photons and stops their emergence from the patient's body. The other major interaction is Compton interaction, which transfer part of the

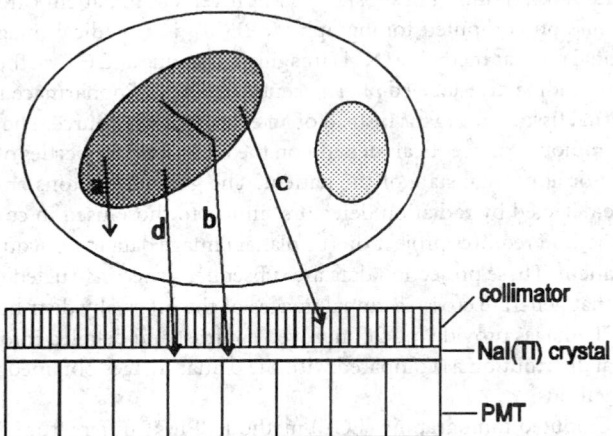

FIGURE 66.6   The conventional nuclear medicine imaging process. Gamma-ray photons emitted from the internally distributed radioactivity may experience photoelectric (*a*) or scatter (*b*) interactions. Photons that are not traveling in the direction within the acceptance analog of the collimator (*c*) will be intercepted by the lead collimator. Photons that experience no interaction and travel within the acceptance angle of the collimator will be detected (*d*).

photon energy to free electrons. The original photon is scattered into a new direction with reduced energy that is dependent on the scatter angle. Photons that escape from the patient's body include those that have not experienced any interactions and those which have experienced Compton scattering. For the primary photons from the commonly used radionuclides in SPECT, e.g., 140-keV of Tc-99m and ~70-keV of Tl-201, the probability of pair production is zero.

Most of the radiation detectors used in current SPECT systems are based on a single or multiple NaI(Tl) scintillation detectors. The most significant development in nuclear medicine is the scintillation camera (or Anger camera) that is based on a large-area (typically 40 cm in diameter) NaI(Tl) crystal [Anger, 1958, 1964]. An array of photomultipier tubes (PMTs) is placed at the back of the scintillation crystal. When a photon hits and interacts with the crystal, the scintillation generated will be detected by the array of PMTs. An electronic circuitry evaluates the relative signals from the PMTs and determines the location of interaction of the incident photon in the scintillation crystal. In addition, the scintillation cameras have built-in energy discrimination electronic circuitry with finite energy resolution that provides selection of the photons that have not been scattered or been scattered within a small scattered angle. The scintillation cameras are commonly used in commercial SPECT systems.

Analogous to the lens in an optical imaging system, a scintillation camera system consists of a collimator placed in front of the NaI(Tl) crystal for the imaging purpose. The commonly used collimator is made of a large number of parallel holes separated by lead septa [Anger, 1964; Keller, 1968; Tsui, 1988]. The geometric dimensions, i.e., length, size, and shape of the collimator apertures, determine the directions of photons that will be detected by the scintillation crystals or the geometric response of the collimator. The width of the geometric response function increases (or the spatial resolution worsens) as the source distance from the collimator increases. Photons that do not pass through the collimator holes properly will be intercepted and absorbed by the lead septal walls of the collimator. In general, the detection efficiency is approximately proportional to the square of the width of the geometric response function of the collimator. This tradeoff between detection efficiency and spatial resolution is a fundamental property of a typical SPECT system using conventional collimators.

The amount of radioactivity that is used in SPECT is restricted by the allowable radiation dose to the patient. Combined with photon attenuation within the patient, the practical limit on imaging time, and the tradeoff between detection efficiency and spatial resolution of the collimator, the number of photons that are collected by a SPECT system is limited. These limitations resulted in SPECT images with relatively poor spatial resolution and high statistical noise fluctuations as compared with other medical imaging modalities. For example, currently a typical brain SPECT image has a total of about 500K counts per image slice and a spatial resolution in the order of approximately 8 mm. A typical myocardial SPECT study using Tl-201 has about 150K total count per image slice and a spatial resolution of approximately 15 mm.

In SPECT, projection data are acquired from different views around the patient. Similar to x-ray CT, image processing and reconstruction methods are used to obtain transaxial or cross-sectional images from the multiple projection data. These methods consist of preprocessing and calibration procedures before further processing, mathematical algorithms for reconstruction from projections, and compensation methods for image degradation due to photon attenuation, scatter, and detector response.

The biokinetics of the radiopharmaceutical used, anatomy of the patient, instrumentation for data acquisition, preprocessing methods, image reconstruction techniques, and compensation methods have important effects on the quality and quantitative accuracy of the final SPECT images. A full understanding of SPECT cannot be accomplished without clear understanding of these factors. The biokinetics of radiopharmaceuticals and conventional radiation detectors have been described in the previous section on conventional nuclear medicine. The following subsections will present the major physical factors that affect SPECT and a summary review of the instrumentation, image reconstruction techniques, and compensation methods that are important technological and engineering aspects in the practice of SPECT.

Physical and Instrumentation Factors that Affect SPECT Images

There are several important physical and instrumentation factors that affect the measured data and subsequently the SPECT images. The characteristics and effects of these factors can be found in a few review articles [Jaszczak et al., 1981; Jaszczak and Tsui, 1994; Tsui et al., 1994a, 1994b]. As described earlier, gamma-ray photons that emit from an internal source may experience photoelectric absorption within the patient without contributing to the acquired data, Compton scattering with change in direction and loss of energy, or no interaction before exiting the patient's body. The exiting photons will be further selected by the geometric response of the collimator-detector. The photoelectric and Compton interactions and the characteristics of the collimator-detector have significant effects on both the quality and quantitative accuracy of SPECT image.

Photon attenuation is defined as the effect due to photoelectric and Compton interactions resulting in a reduced number of photons that would have been detected without them. The degree of attenuation is determined by the linear attenuation coefficient, which is a function of photon energy and the amount and types of materials contained in the attenuating medium. For example, the attenuation coefficient for the 140-keV photon emitted from the commonly used Tc-99m in water or soft tissue is 0.15 cm^{-1}. This gives rise to a half-valued-layer, the thickness of material that attenuates half the incident photons, or 4.5 cm H_2O for the 140-keV photon. Attenuation is the most important factor that affects the quantitative accuracy of SPECT images.

Attenuation effect is complicated by the fact that within the patient the attenuation coefficient can be quite different in various organs. The effect is most prominent in the thorax, where the attenuation coefficients range from as low as 0.05 cm^{-1} in the lung to as high as 0.18 cm^{-1} in the compact bone for the 140-keV photons. In x-ray CT, the attenuation coefficient distribution is the target for image reconstruction. In SPECT, however, the wide range of attenuation coefficient values and the variations of attenuation coefficient distributions among patients are major difficulties in obtaining quantitative accurate SPECT images. Therefore, compensation for attenuation is important to ensure good image quality and quantitatively high accuracy in SPECT. Review of different attenuation methods that have been used in SPECT is a subject of discussion later in this chapter.

Photons that have been scattered before reaching the radiation detector provide misplaced spatial information about the origin of the radioactive source. The results are inaccurate quantitative information and poor contrast in the SPECT images. For radiation detectors with perfect energy discrimination, scattered photons can be completely rejected. In a typical scintillation camera system, however, the energy resolution is in the order of 10% at 140 keV. With this energy resolution, the ratio of scattered to scattered total photons detected by a typical scintillation detector is about 20% to 30% in brain and about 30% to 40% in cardiac and body SPECT studies for 140-keV photons. Furthermore, the effect of scatter depends on the distribution of the radiopharmaceutical, the proximity of the source organ to the target organ, and the energy window used in addition to the photon energy and the energy resolution of the scintillation detector. The compensation of scatter is another important aspect of SPECT to ensure good image quality and quantitative accuracy.

The advances in SPECT can be attributed to simultaneous development of new radiopharmaceuticals, instrumentation, reconstruction methods, and clinical applications. Most radiopharmaceuticals that are developed for conventional nuclear medicine can readily be used in SPECT, and review of these development is beyond the scope of this chapter. Recent advances include new agents that are labeled with iodine and technetium for blood perfusion for brain and cardiac studies. Also, the use of receptor agents and labeled antibodies is also being investigated. These developments have resulted in radiopharmaceuticals with improved uptake distributions, biokinetics properties, and potentially new clinical applications. The following subsections will concentrate on the development of instrumentation and image reconstruction methods that have made substantial impact on SPECT.

SPECT Instrumentation

Review of the advances in SPECT instrumentation can be found in several recent articles [Jaszczak et al., 1980; Rogers and Ackermann, 1992; Jaszczak and Tsui, 1994]. A typical SPECT system consists of a single or multiple units of radiation detectors arranged in a specific geometric configuration and a mechanism for moving the radiation detector(s) or specially designed collimators to acquire data from different projection views. In general, SPECT instrumentation can be divided into three general categories: (1) arrays of multiple scintillation detectors, (2) one or more scintillation cameras, and (3) hybrid scintillation detectors combining the first two approaches. In addition, special collimator designs have been proposed for SPECT for specific purposes and clinical applications. The following is a brief review of these SPECT systems and special collimators.

Multidetector SPECT System

The first fully functional SPECT imaging acquisition system was designed and constructed by Kuhl and Edwards [Kuhl and Edwards, 1963, 1964, 1968] in the 1960s, well before the conception of x-ray CT. As shown in Fig. 66.7a, the MARK IV brain SPECT system consisted of four linear arrays of eight discrete NaI(Tl) scintillation detectors assembled in a square arrangement. Projection data were obtained by rotating the square detector array around the patient's head. Although images from the pioneer MARK IV SPECT system were unimpressive without the use of proper reconstruction methods that were developed in later years, the multidetector design has been the theme of several other SPECT systems that were developed. An example is the Gammatom-1 developed by Cho et al. [1982]. The design concept also was used in a dynamic SPECT system [Stokely et al., 1980] and commercial multidetector SPECT systems marketed by Medimatic, A/S (Tomomatic-32). Recently, the system design was extended to a multislice SPECT system with the Tomomatic-896, consisting of 8 layers of 96 scintillation detectors. Also, the system allows both body and brain SPECT imaging by varying the aperture size.

Variations of the multiple-detectors arrangement have been proposed for SPECT system designs. Figure 66.7b shows the Headtome-II system by Shimadzu Corporation [Hirose et al., 1982], which consists of a stationary array of scintillation detectors arranged in a circular ring. Projection data are obtained by a set of collimator vanes that swings in front of the discrete detectors. A unique Cleon brain SPECT system (see Fig. 66.7c), originally developed by Union Carbide Corporation in the 1970s, consists of 12 detectors that scan both radially and tangentially [Stoddart and Stoddart, 1979]. Images from the original system were unimpressive due to inadequate sampling, poor axial resolution, and a reconstruction algorithm that did not take full advantage of the unique system de-

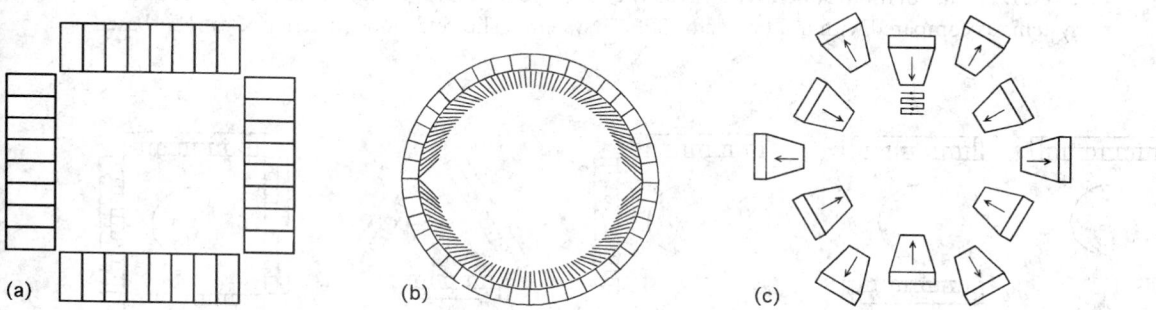

FIGURE 66.7 Examples of multidetector-based SPECT systems. (*a*) The MARK IV system consists of four arrays of eight individual NaI(Tl) detectors arranged in a square configuration. (*b*) The Headtome-II system consists of a circular ring of detectors. A set of collimator vanes that swings in front of the discrete detector is used to collect projection data from different views. (*c*) A unique Cleon brain SPECT system consists of 12 detectors that scan both radially and tangentially.

sign and data acquisition strategy. A much improved version of the system with a new reconstruction method [Moore et al., 1984] is currently marketed by Strichman Corporation.

The advantage of multidetector SPECT systems are their high sensitivity per image slice and high counting rate capability resulting from the array of multidetectors fully surrounding the patient. However, disadvantages of multidetector SPECT include their ability to provide only one or a few noncontiguous cross-sectional image slices. Also, these systems are relatively more expensive compared with camera-based SPECT systems described in the next subsection. With the advance of multicamera SPECT systems, the disadvantages of multidetector SPECT systems outweigh their advantages. As a result, they are less often found in nuclear medicine clinics.

Camera-Based SPECT Systems

The most popular SPECT systems are based on a single or multiple scintillation cameras mounted on a rotating gantry. The successful design was developed almost simultaneously by three separate groups [Budinger and Gullberg, 1977; Jaszczak et al., 1977; Keyes et al., 1977]. In 1981, General Electric Medical Systems offered the first commercial SPECT system based on a single rotating camera and brought SPECT to clinical use. Today, there are over 10 manufacturers (e.g., ADAC, Elscint, General Electric, Hitachi, Picker, Siemens, Sopha, Toshiba, Trionix) offering an array of commercial SPECT systems in the marketplace.

An advantage of camera-based SPECT systems is their use of off-the-shelf scintillation cameras that have been widely used in conventional nuclear medicine. These systems usually can be used in both conventional planar and SPECT imaging. Also, camera-based SPECT systems allow truly three-dimensional (3D) imaging by providing a large set of contiguous transaxial images that cover the entire organ of interest. They are easily adaptable for SPECT imaging of the brain or body by simply changing the radius of rotation of the camera.

A disadvantage of camera-based SPECT system is its relatively low counting rate capability. The dead time of a typical state-of-the-art scintillation camera gives rise to a loss of 20% of its true counts at about 80K counts per second. A few special high-count-rate systems give the same count rate loss at about 150K counts per second. For SPECT systems using a single scintillation camera, the sensitivity per image slice is relative low compared with a typical multidetector SPECT system.

Recently, SPECT systems based on multiple cameras became increasingly more popular. Systems with two [Jaszczak et al., 1979a], three [Lim et al., 1980, 1985], and four cameras provide increased sensitivity per image slice that is proportional to the number of cameras. Figure 66.3 shows the system configurations of these camera-based SPECT systems. The dual-camera systems with two opposing cameras (Fig. 66.8b) can be used for both whole-body scanning and SPECT, and those with two right-angled cameras (Fig. 66.8c) are especially useful for 180-degree acquisition in cardiac SPECT. The use of multicameras has virtually eliminated the disadvantages of camera-based SPECT systems as compared with multidetector SPECT systems. The detection efficiency of camera-based

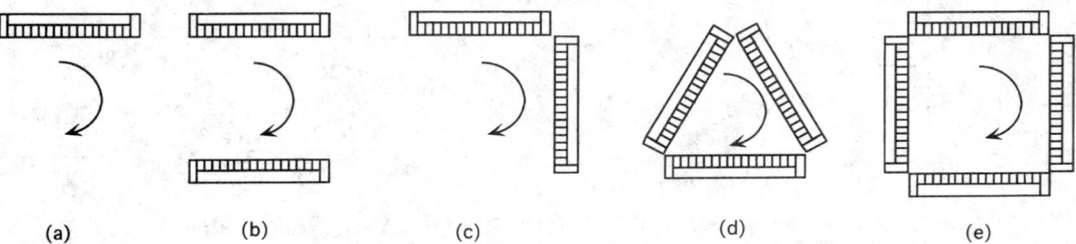

FIGURE 66.8 Examples of camera-based SPECT systems. (*a*) Single-camera system. (*b*) Dual-camera system with the two cameras placed at opposing sides of patient during rotation. (*c*) Dual-cameral system with the two cameras placed at right angles. (*d*) Triple-camera system. (*e*) Quadruple-camera system.

SPECT systems can be further increased by using converging-hole collimators such as fan, cone, and astigmatic collimators at the cost of a smaller field of view. The use of converging-hole collimators in SPECT will be described in a later subsection.

Novel SPECT System Designs

There are several special SPECT systems designs that do not fit into the preceding two general categories. The commercially available CERESPECT (formerly known as ASPECT) [Genna and Smith, 1988] is a dedicated brain SPECT system. As shown in Fig. 66.9a, it consists of a single fixed annular NaI(T1) crystal that completely surrounds the patient's head. Similar to a scintillation camera, an array of PMTs and electronics circuitry are placed behind the crystal to provide positional and energy information about photons that interact with the crystal. Projection data are obtained by rotating a segmented annular collimator with parallel holes that fits inside the stationary detector. A similar system is also being developed by Larsson et al. [1991] in Sweden.

Several unique SPECT systems are currently being developed in research laboratories. They consist of modules of small scintillation cameras that surround the patient. The hybrid designs combine the advantage of multidetector and camera-based SPECT systems with added flexibility in system configuration. An example is the SPRINT II brain SPECT system developed at the University of Michigan [Rogers et al., 1988]. As shown in Fig. 66.4b, the system consists of 11 detector modules arranged in a circular ring around the patient's head. Each detector module consists of 44 one-dimensional bar NaI(T1) scintillation cameras. Projection data are required through a series of narrow slit openings on a rotating lead ring that fits inside the circular detector assemblies. A similar system is developed at the University of Iowa [Chang et al., 1990] with 22 detector modules, each consisting of 4 bar detectors. A set of rotating focused collimators is used to acquired projection data necessary for image reconstruction. At the University of Arizona, a novel SPECT system is being developed that consists of 20 small modular scintillation cameras [Milster et al., 1990] arranged in a hemispherical shell surrounding the patient's head [Rowe et al., 1992]. Projection data are acquired through a stationary hemispherical array of pinholes that are fitted inside the camera array. Without moving parts, the system allows acquisition of dynamic 3D SPECT data.

Special Collimator Designs for SPECT Systems

Similar to conventional nuclear medicine imaging, parallel-hole collimators (Fig. 66.10a) are commonly used in camera-based SPECT systems. As described earlier, the tradeoff between detection efficiency and spatial resolution of parallel-hole collimator is a limiting factor for SPECT. A means to improve SPECT system performance is to improve the tradeoff imposed by the parallel-hole collimation.

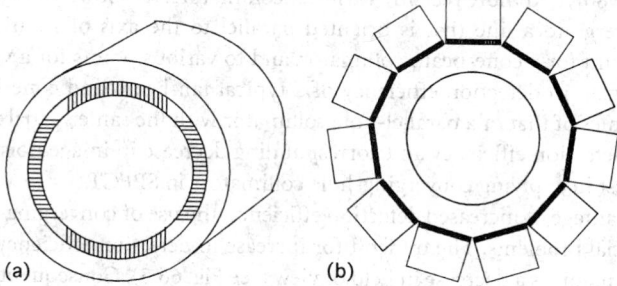

FIGURE 66.9 Examples of novel SPECT system designs. (a) The CERESPECT brain SPECT system consists of a single fixed annular NaI(Tl) crystal and a rotating segmented annular collimator. (b) The SPRINT II brain SPECT system consists of 11 detector modules and a rotating lead ring with slit opening.

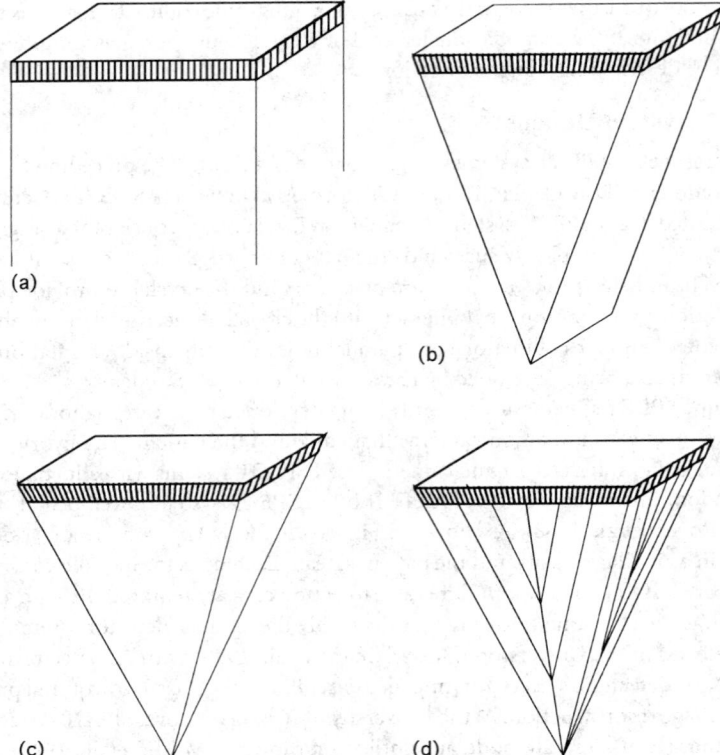

FIGURE 66.10   Collimator designs used in camera-based SPECT systems. (*a*) The commonly used parallel-hole collimator. (*b*) The fan-beam collimator, where the collimator holes are converged to a line that is parallel to the axis of rotation. (*c*) The cone-beam collimator, where the collimator holes are converged to a point. (*d*) A varifocal collimator, where the collimator holes are converged to various focal points.

   To achieve this goal, converging-hole collimator designs that increase the angle of acceptance of incoming photons without sacrificing spatial resolution have been developed. Examples are fan-beam [Jaszczak et al., 1979b; Tsui et al., 1986], cone-beam [Jaszczak et al., 1987], astigmatic [Hawman and Hsieh, 1986], and more recently varifocal collimators. As shown in Fig. 66.5b–d, the collimator holes converge to a line that is oriented parallel to the axis of rotation for a fan-beam collimator, to a point for a cone-beam collimator, and to various points for a varifocal collimator, respectively. The gain in detection efficiency of a typical fan-beam and cone-beam collimator is about 1.5 and 2 times of that of a parallel-hole collimator with the same spatial resolution. The anticipated gain in detection efficiency and corresponding decrease in image noise are the main reasons for the interest in applying converging-hole collimators in SPECT.

   Despite the advantage of increased detection efficiency, the use of converging-hole collimators in SPECT poses special problems. The tradeoff for increase in detection efficiency as compared with parallel-hole collimators is a decrease in field of view (see Fig. 66.5). Consequently, converging-hole collimators are restricted to imaging small organs or body parts such as the head [Jaszczak et al., 1979b; Tsui et al., 1986] and heart [Gullberg et al., 1991]. In addition, the use of converging-hole collimators requires special data-acquisition strategies and image reconstruction algorithms. For example, for cone-beam tomography using a conventional single planar orbit, the acquired projection data become increasingly insufficient for reconstructing transaxial image sections that are farther away from the central plane of the cone-beam geometry. Active research is underway to study special rotational orbits for sufficient projection data acquisition and 3D image reconstruction methods specific for cone-beam SPECT.

Reconstruction Methods

As discussed earlier, SPECT combines conventional nuclear medicine image techniques and methods for image reconstruction from projections. Aside from radiopharmaceuticals and instrumentation, image reconstruction methods are another important engineering and technological aspect of the SPECT imaging technique.

In x-ray CT, accurate transaxial images can be obtained through the use of standard algorithms for image reconstruction from projections. The results are images of attenuation coefficient distribution of various organs within the patient's body. In SPECT, the goal of image reconstruction is to determine the distribution of administered radiopharmaceutical in the patient. However, the presence of photon attenuation affects the measured projection data. If conventional reconstruction algorithms are used without proper compensation for the attenuation effects, inaccurate reconstructed images will be obtained. Effects of scatter and the finite collimator-detector response impose additional difficulties on image reconstruction in SPECT.

In order to achieve quantitatively accurate images, special reconstruction methods are required for SPECT. Quantitatively accurate image reconstruction methods for SPECT consist of two major components. They are the standard algorithms for image reconstruction from projections and methods that compensate for the image-degrading effects described earlier. Often, image reconstruction algorithms are inseparable from the compensation methods, resulting in a new breed of reconstruction method not found in other tomographic medical imaging modalities. The following subsections will present the reconstruction problem and a brief review of conventional algorithms for image reconstruction from projections. Then quantitative SPECT reconstruction methods that include additional compensation methods will be described.

Image Reconstruction Problem

Figure 66.11 shows a schematic diagram of the two-dimensional (2D) image reconstruction problem. Let $f(x, y)$ represent a 2D object distribution that is to be determined. A one-dimension (1D) detector array is oriented at an angle θ with respect to the x axis of the laboratory coordinates system (x, y). The data collected into each detector element at location t, called the *projection data* $p(t, \theta)$, is equal to the sum of $f(x, y)$ along a ray that is perpendicular to the detector array and intersects the detector at position t; that is,

$$p(t, \theta) = c \int_{-\alpha}^{\alpha} f(x, y)\, ds \qquad (66.1)$$

where (s, t) represent a coordinate system with s along the direction of the ray sum and t parallel to the 1D detector array, and c is the gain factor of the detection system. The angle between the s and x axes is θ. The relationship between the

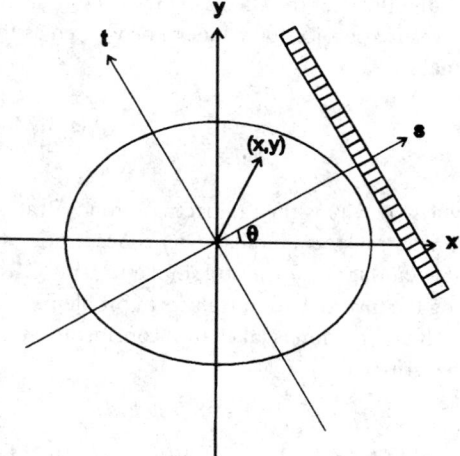

FIGURE 66.11 Schematic diagram of the two-dimensional image reconstruction problem. The projection data are line integrals of the object distribution along rays that are perpendicular to the detector. A source point (x, y) is projected onto a point $p(t, \theta)$, where t is a position along the projection and θ is the projection angle.

source position (x, y), the projection angle θ, and the position of detection on the 1D detector array is given by

$$t = y \cos \theta - x \sin \theta \qquad (66.2)$$

In 2D tomographic imaging, the 1D detector array rotates around the object distribution $f(x, y)$ and collects projection data from various projection data from various projection angles θ. The integral transform of the object distribution to its projections given by Eq. (66.1) is called the *Radon transform* [Radon, 1917]. The goal of image reconstruction is to solve the inverse Radon transform. The solution is the reconstructed image estimate $\hat{f}(x, y)$ of the object distribution $f(x, y)$.

In x-ray CT, the measured projection data is given by

$$p'(t, \theta) = c_t I_o \exp \left[-\int_{-\alpha}^{+\alpha} \mu(x, y) \, ds \right] \qquad (66.3)$$

where I_o is the intensity of the incident x-ray, $\mu(x, y)$ is the 2D attenuation coefficient, and c_t is the gain factor which transforms x-ray intensity to detected signals. The reconstruction problem can be rewritten as

$$p(t, \theta) = \ln \left[\frac{I_o}{p'(t, \theta)} \right] = \int_{-\alpha}^{+\alpha} \mu(x, y) \, ds \qquad (66.4)$$

with the goal to solve for the attenuation coefficient distribution $\mu(x, y)$. Also, in x-ray CT, if parallel rays are used, the projection data at opposing views are the same, i.e., $p(t, \theta) = p(t, \theta + \pi)$, and projection data acquired over 180 degrees will be sufficient for reconstruction. The number of linear samples along the 1D projection array and angular samples, i.e., the number of projection views, over 180 degrees must be chosen carefully to avoid aliasing error and resolution loss in the reconstructed images.

In SPECT, if the effects of attenuation, scatter, and collimator-detector response are ignored, the measured projection data can be written as the integral of radioactivity along the projection rays; that is,

$$p(t, \theta) = c_e \int_{-\alpha}^{+\alpha} \rho(x, y) \, ds \qquad (66.5)$$

where $\rho(x, y)$ is the radioactivity concentration distribution of the object, and c_e is the gain factor which transform radioactivity concentration to detected signals. Equation (66.5) fits in the form of the Radon transform, and similar to x-ray CT, the radioactivity distribution can be obtained by solving the inverse Radon transform problem.

If attenuation is taken into consideration, the attenuated Radon transform [Gullberg, 1979] can be written as

$$p(t, \theta_i) = c_e \int_{-\alpha}^{+\alpha} \rho(x, y) \exp \left[-\int_{(x,y)}^{+\alpha} \mu(u, v) \, ds' \right] ds \qquad (66.6)$$

where $\mu(u, v)$ is the 2D attenuation coefficient distribution, and $\int_{(x,y)}^{+\alpha} \mu(u,v) \, ds$ is the attenuation factor for photons that originate from (x, y), travel along the direction perpendicular to the detector array, and are detected by the collimator-detector. A major difficulty in SPECT image reconstruction lies in the attenuation factor, which makes the inverse problem given by Eq. (66.6) difficult to solve analytically. However, the solution is important in cardiac SPECT, where the widely different attenuation coefficients are found in various organs within the thorax. Also, due to the attenuation factor, the projection views at opposing angles are different. Hence full 360-degree projection data are usually necessary for image reconstruction in SPECT.

Different from x-ray CT, small differences in attenuation coefficient are not as important in SPECT. When the attenuation coefficient in the body region can be considered constant, the attenuated Radon transform given by Eq. (66.6) can be written as [Tretiak and Metz, 1980]

$$p(t, \theta) = c_e \int_{-\alpha}^{+\alpha} \rho(x, y) \exp \left[-\mu l(x, y)\right] ds \qquad (66.7)$$

where μ is the constant attenuation coefficient in the body region, and $l(x, y)$ is the path length between the point (x, y) and the edge of the attenuator (or patient's body) along the direction of the projection ray. The solution of the inverse problem with constant attenuator has been a subject of several investigations. It forms the basis for analytical methods for compensation of uniform attenuation described later in this chapter.

When scatter and collimator-detector response are taken into consideration, the assumption that the projection data can be represented by line integrals given by Eqs. (66.1) to (66.7) will no longer be exactly correct. Instead, the integration will have to include a wider region covering the field of view of the collimator-detector (or the collimator-detector response function). The image reconstruction problem is further complicated by the nonstationary properties of the collimator-detector and scatter response functions and their dependence on the size and composition of the patient's body.

Algorithms for Image Reconstruction from Projections

The application of methods for image reconstruction from projections was a major component in the development of x-ray CT in the 1970s. The goal was to solve for the inverse Radon transform problem given in Eq. (66.1). There is an extensive literature on these reconstruction algorithms. Reviews of the application of these algorithms to SPECT can be found in several articles [Barrett, 1986; Brooks and Di Chiro, 1975, 1976; Budinger and Gullberg, 1974].

Simple Backprojection. An intuitive image reconstruction method is *simple backprojection*. Here, the reconstructed image is formed simply by spreading the values of the measured projection data uniformly along the projection ray into the reconstructed image array. By backprojecting the measured projection data from all projection views, an estimate of the object distribution can be obtained. Mathematically, the simple backproject operation is given by

$$\hat{f}(x, y) = \sum_{j=1}^{m} p(y \cos \theta_j - x \sin \theta_j, \theta_j) \, \Delta\theta \qquad (66.8)$$

where θ_j is the jth projection angle, m is the number of projection views, and $\Delta\theta$ is the angular spacing between adjacent projections. The simple backprojected image $\hat{f}(x, y)$ is a poor approximation of the true objection distribution $f(x, y)$. It is equivalent to the true object distribution blurred by a blurring function in the form of $1/r$.

There are two approaches for accurate image reconstruction, and both have been applied to SPECT. The first approach is based on direct analytical methods and is widely used in commercial SPECT systems. The second approach is based on statistical criteria and iterative algorithms. They have been found useful in reconstruction methods that include compensation for the image-degrading effects.

Analytical Reconstruction Algorithms: Filtered Backprojection. The most widely used analytical image-reconstruction algorithm is the *filtered backprojection* (FBP) method, which involves backprojecting the filtered projections [Bracewell and Riddle, 1967; Ramachandran and Lakshminarayanan, 1971]. The algorithm consists of two major steps:

1. Filter the measured projection data at different projection angles with a special function.
2. Backproject the filtered projection data to form the reconstructed image.

The first step of the filtered backprojection method can be implemented in two different ways. In the spatial domain, the filter operation is equivalent to convolving the measured projection data using a special convolving function $h(t)$; that is,

$$p'(t, \theta) = p(t, \theta) \circledast h(t) \tag{66.8}$$

where $\circledast$ is the convolution operation. With the advance of fast Fourier transform (FFT) methods, the convolution operation can be replaced by a more efficient multiplication in the spatial frequency domain. The equivalent operation consists of three steps:

1. Fourier-transform the measured projection data into spatial frequency domain using the FFT method, i.e., $P(v, \theta) = \text{FT}\{p(t, \theta)\}$, where FT is the Fourier transform operation.
2. Multiply the Fourier-transformed projection data with a special function that is equal to the Fourier transform of the special function used in the convolution operation described above, i.e., $P'(v, \theta) = P(v, \theta) \cdot H(v)$, where $H(v) = \text{FT}\{h(x)\}$ is the Fourier transform of $h(x)$.
3. Inverse Fourier transform the product $P'(v, \theta)$ into spatial domain.

Again, the filtered projections from different projection angles are backprojected to form the reconstructed image.

The solution of the inverse Radon transform given in Eq. (66.1) specifies the form of the special function. In the spatial domain, the special function $h(x)$ used in the convolution operation in Eq. (66.8) is given by

$$h(x) = \frac{1}{2(\Delta x)^2}\left\{\text{sinc}\left[\frac{x}{(\Delta x)}\right]\right\} - \frac{1}{4(\Delta x)^2}\left\{\text{sinc}^2\left[\frac{x}{2(\Delta x)}\right]\right\} \tag{66.9}$$

where Δx is the linear sampling interval, and $\text{sinc}(z) = [\sin(z)]/z$. The function $h(x)$ consists of a narrow central peak with high magnitude and small negative side lobes. It removes the blurring from the $1/r$ function found in the simple backprojected images.

In the frequency domain, the special function $H(v)$ is equivalent to the Fourier transform of $h(x)$ and is a truncated ramp function given by

$$H(v) = |v| \cdot \text{rect}(v) \tag{66.10}$$

where $|v|$ is the ramp function, and

$$\text{rect}(v) = \begin{cases} 1 & |v| \le 0.5 \\ 0 & |v| < 0.5 \end{cases} \tag{66.11}$$

that is, the rectangular function $\text{rect}(v)$ has a value of 1 when the absolute value of v is less than the Nyquist frequency at 0.5 cycles per pixel.

For noisy projection data, the ramp function tends to amplify the high-frequency noise. In these situations, an additional smoothing filter is often applied to smoothly roll off the high-frequency response of the ramp function. Examples are Hann and Butterworth filters [Huesman et al., 1977]. Also, deconvolution filters also have been used to provide partial compensation of spatial resolution loss due to the collimator-detection response and noise smoothing. Examples are the Metz and Wiener filters (see below).

Iterative Reconstruction Algorithms.   Another approach to image reconstruction is based on statistical criteria and iterative algorithms. They were investigated for application in SPECT before the development of analytical image reconstruction methods [Gilbert, 1972; Goitein, 1972; Gordon et al., 1970; Kuhl and Edwards, 1968]. The major drawbacks of iterative reconstruction algorithms are the extensive computations and long processing time required. For these reasons, the analytical reconstruction methods have gained widespread acceptance in clinical SPECT systems. In recent years, there has been renewed interest in the use of iterative reconstruction algorithms in SPECT to achieve accurate quantitation by compensating for the image-degrading effects.

A typical iterative reconstruction algorithm starts with an initial estimate of the object source distribution. A set of projection data is estimated from the initial estimate using a projector that models the imaging process. The estimated projection data are compared with the measured projection data at the same projection angles, and their differences are calculated. Using an algorithm derived from specific statistical criteria, the differences are used to update the initial image estimate. The updated image estimate is then used to recalculate a new set of estimated projection data that are again compared with the measured projection data. The procedure is repeated until the differences between the estimated and measured projection data are smaller than a preselected small value. Statistical criteria that have been used in formulating iterative reconstruction algorithms include the minimum mean squares error (MMSE) [Budinger and Gullberg, 1977], weighted least squares (WLS) [Huesman et al., 1977], maximum entropy (ME) [Minerbo, 1979], maximum likelihood (ML) [Shepp and Vardi, 1982], and maximum a posteriori approaches [Barrett, 1986; Geman and McClure, 1985; Johnson et al., 1991; Levitan and Herman, 1987; Liang and Hart, 1987]. Iterative algorithms that have been used in estimating the reconstructed images include the conjugate gradient (CG) [Huesman et al., 1977] and expectation maximization (EM) [Lange and Carson, 1984].

Recently, interest in the application of iterative reconstruction algorithms in SPECT has been revitalized. The interest is sparked by the need to compensate for the spatially variant and/or nonstationary image-degrading factors in the SPECT imaging process. The compensation can be achieved by modeling the imaging process that includes the image-degrading factors in the projection and backprojection operations of the iterative steps. The development is aided by advances made in computer technology and custom-dedicated processors. The drawback of long processing time in using these algorithms is substantially reduced. Discussion of the application of iterative reconstruction algorithm in SPECT will be presented in a later subsection.

Compensation Methods

For a typical SPECT system, the measured projection data are severely affected by attenuation, scatter, and collimator-detector response. Direct reconstruction of the measured projection data without compensation of these effects produces images with artifacts, distortions, and inaccurate quantitation. In recent years, substantial efforts have been made to develop compensation methods for these image-degrading effects. This development has produced much improved quality and quantitatively accurate reconstructed images. The following subsections will present a brief review of some of these compensation methods.

Compensation for Attenuation.   Methods for attenuation compensation can be grouped into two categories: (1) methods that assume the attenuation coefficient is uniform over the body region, and (2) methods that address situations of nonuniform attenuation coefficient distribution. The assumption of uniform attenuation can be applied to SPECT imaging of the head and abdomen regions. The compensation methods seek to solve for the inverse of the attenuated Radon transform given in Eq. (66.7). For cardiac and lung SPECT imaging, nonuniform attenuation compensation methods must be used due to the very different attenuation coefficient values in various organs in the thorax. Here, the goal is to solve the more complicated problem of the inverse of the attenuated Radon transform in Eq. (66.6).

There are several approximate methods for compensating uniform attenuation. They include methods that preprocess the projection data or postprocess the reconstructed image. The typical preprocess methods are those which use the geometric or arithmetic mean [Sorenson, 1974] of projections from opposing views. These compensation methods are easy to implement and work well with a single, isolated source. However, they are relatively inaccurate for more complicated source configurations. Another method achieves uniform attenuation compensation by processing the Fourier transform of the sinogram [Bellini et al., 1979]. The method provides accurate compensation even for complicated source configurations.

A popular compensation method for uniform attenuation is that proposed by Chang [1978]. The method requires knowledge of the body contour. The information is used in calculating the average attenuation factor at each image point from all projection views. The array of attenuation factors is used to multiply the reconstructed image obtained without attenuation compensation. The result is the attenuation-compensated image. An iterative scheme also can be implemented for improved accuracy. In general, the Chang method performs well for uniform attenuation situations. However, the noise level in the reconstructed images increases with iteration number. Also, certain image features tend to fluctuate as a function of iteration. For these reasons, no more than one or two iterations are recommended.

Another class of methods for uniform attenuation compensation is based on analytical solution of the inverse of the attenuation Radon transform given in Eq. (66.7) for a convex-shaped medium [Gullberg and Budinger, 1981; Tretiak and Metz, 1980]. The resultant compensation method involves multiplying the projection data by an exponential function. Then the FBP algorithm is used in the image reconstruction except that the ramp filter is modified such that its value is zero in the frequency range between 0 and $\mu/2\pi$, where μ is the constant attenuation coefficient. The compensation method is easy to implement and provides good quantitative accuracy. However, it tends to amplify noise in the resulting image, and smoothing is required to obtain acceptable image quality [Gullberg and Budinger, 1981].

An analytical solution for the more complicated inverse attenuated Radon transform with nonuniform attenuation distribution [Eq. (66.6)] has been found difficult [Gullberg, 1979]. Instead, iterative approaches have been used to estimate a solution of the problem. The application is especially important in cardiac and lung SPECT studies. The iterative methods model the attenuation distribution in the projection and backprojection operations [Manglos et al., 1987; Tsui et al., 1989]. The ML criterion with the EM algorithm [Lange and Carson, 1984] has been used with success [Tsui et al., 1989]. The compensation method requires information about the attenuation distribution of the region to be imaged. Recently, transmission CT methods are being developed using existing SPECT systems to obtain attenuation distribution from the patient. The accurate attenuation compensation of cardiac SPECT promises to provide much improved quality and quantitative accuracy in cardiac SPECT images [Tsui et al., 1989, 1994a].

Compensation for Scatter. As described earlier in this chapter, scattered photons carry misplaced positional information about the source distribution resulting in lower image contrast and inaccurate quantitation in SPECT images. Compensation for scatter will improve image contrast for better image quality and images that will more accurately represent the true object distribution. Much research has been devoted to develop scatter compensation methods that can be grouped into two general approaches. In the first approach, various methods have been developed to estimate the scatter contribution in the measured data. The scatter component is then subtracted from the measured data or from the reconstructed images to obtain scatter-free reconstructed images. The compensation method based on this approach tends to increase noise level in the compensated images.

One method estimates the scatter contribution as a convolution of the measured projection data with an empirically derived function [Axelsson et al., 1984]. Another method models the scatter component as the convolution of the primary (or unscattered) component of the projection data with an exponential function [Floyd et al., 1985]. The convolution method is extended to 3D by estimating the 2D scatter component [Yanch et al., 1988]. These convolution methods assume that the scatter response function is stationary, which is only an approximation.

The scatter component also has been estimated using two energy windows acquisition methods.

One method estimates the scatter component in the primary energy window from the measured data obtained from a lower and adjacent energy window [Jaszczak et al., 1984, 1985b]. In a dual photopeak window (DPW) method, two nonoverlapping windows spanning the primary photopeak window are used [King et al., 1992]. This method provides more accurate estimation of the scatter response function.

Multiple energy windows also have been used to estimate the scatter component. One method uses two satellite energy windows that are placed directly above and below the photopeak window to estimate the scatter component in the center window [Ogawa et al., 1991]. In another method, the energy spectrum detected at each image pixel is used to predict the scatter contribution [Koral et al., 1988]. An energy-weighted acquisition (EWA) technique acquires data from multiple energy windows. The images reconstructed from these data are weighted with energy-dependent factors to minimize scatter contribution to the weighted image [DeVito et al., 1989; DeVito and Hamill, 1991]. Finally, the holospectral imaging method [Gagnon et al., 1989] estimates the scatter contribution from a series of eigenimages derived from images reconstructed from data obtained from a series of multiple energy windows.

In the second approach, the scatter photons are utilized in estimating the true object distribu-tion. Without subtracting the scatter component, the compensated images are less noisy than those obtained from the first approach. In one method, an average scatter response function can be combined with the geometric response of the collimator-detector to form the total response of the imaging system [Gilland et al., 1988; Tsui et al., 1994a]. The total response function is then use to generate a restoration filter for an approximate geometric and scatter response compensation (see below).

Another class of methods characterizes the exact scatter response function and incorporates it into iterative reconstruction algorithms for accurate compensation for scatter [Floyd et al., 1985; Frey and Tsui, 1992]. Since the exact scatter response functions are nonstationary and are asymmetric in shape, implementation of the methods requires extensive computations. However, efforts are being made to parameterize the scatter response function and to optimize the algorithm for substantial reduction in processing time [Frey et al., 1993; Frey and Tsui, 1991].

Compensation for Collimator-Detector Response. As described earlier, for a typical collimator-detector, the response function broadens as the distance from the collimator face increases. The effect of the collimator-detector response is loss of spatial resolution and blurring of fine detail in SPECT images. Also, the spatially variant detector response function will cause nonisotropic point response in SPECT images [Knesaurek et al., 1989; Maniawski et al., 1991]. The spatially variant collimator-detector response is a major difficulty in its exact compensation.

By assuming an average and stationary collimator-detector response function, restoration filters can be used to provide partial and approximate compensation for the effects of the collimator-detector. Examples are the Metz [King et al., 1984, 1986] and Wiener [Penney et al., 1990] filters, where the inverse of the average collimator-detector response function is used in the design of the restoration filters. Two-dimensional (2D) compensation is achieved by applying the 1D restoration filters to the 1D projection data, and 3D compensation by applying the 2D filters to the 2D projection images [Tsui et al., 1994b].

Analytical methods have been developed for compensation of the spatially variant detector response. A spatially variant filtering method has been proposed which is based on the frequency distance principle (FDP) [Edholm et al., 1986; Lewitt et al., 1989]. The method has been shown to provide an isotropic point response function in phantom SPECT images [Glick et al., 1993].

Iterative reconstruction methods also have been used to accurately compensate for both nonuniform attenuation and collimator-detector response by modeling the attenuation distribution and spatially variant detector response function in the projection and backprojection steps. The compensation methods have been applied in 2D reconstruction [Formiconi et al., 1990; Tsui et al., 1988], and more recently in 3D reconstruction [Tsui et al., 1994b; Zeng et al., 1991]. It has been found that the iterative reconstruction methods provide better image quality and more accurate quantitation when compared with the conventional restoration filtering techniques. Furthermore, 3D compensation outperforms 2D compensation at the expense of more extensive computations [Tsui et al., 1994*b*].

Sample SPECT Images

This subsection presents sample SPECT images to demonstrate the performance of various reconstruction and compensation methods. Two data sets were used. The first data set was acquired from a 3D physical phantom that mimics a human brain perfusion study. The phantom study provided knowledge of the true radioactivity distribution for evaluation purposes. The second data set was obtained from a patient myocardial SPECT study using thallium-201.

Figure 66.12*a* shows the radioactivity distribution from a selected slice of a 3D brain phantom manufactured by the Data Spectrum Corporation. The phantom design was based on PET images from a normal patient to simulate cerebral blood flow [Hoffman et al., 1990]. The phantom was filled with water containing 74 mBq of Tc-99m. A single-camera-based GE 400AC/T SPECT system fitted with a high-resolution collimator was used for data collection. The projection data were acquired into 128×128 matrices at 128 views over 360 degrees. Figure 66.12*b* shows the reconstructed image obtained from the FBP algorithm without any compensation. The poor image quality is due to statistical noise fluctuations, effects of attenuation (especially at the central portion of the image), loss of spatial resolution due to the collimator-detector response, and loss of contrast due to scatter.

Figure 66.12*c* shows the reconstructed image obtained with the application of a noise-smoothing filter and compensation for the uniform attenuation and scatter. The resulting image has lower noise level, reduced attenuation effect, and higher contrast as compared with the image shown in Fig. 66.12*b*. Figure 66.12*d* is similar to Fig. 66.12*c* except for an additional application of a Metz filter to partially compensate for the collimator-detector blurring. Figure 66.12*e* shows the reconstructed image obtained from the iterative ML-EM algorithm that accurately modeled the attenuation and spatially variant detector response. The much superior image quality is apparent.

Figure 66.13*a* shows a selected FBP reconstructed transaxial image slice from a typical patient myocardial SPECT study using thallium-201. Figure 66.13*b* shows the reconstructed image obtained from the Chang algorithm for approximate nonuniform attenuation compensation and 2D processing using a Metz filter for approximate compensation for collimator-detector response. Figure 66.13*c* shows the reconstructed image obtained from the iterative ML-EM algorithm using a measured transmission CT image for accurate attenuation compensation and a 2D model of the collimator-detector response for accurate collimator-detector response compensation. The reconstructed image in Fig. 66.13*d* is similar to that in Fig. 66.13*b* except that the Metz filter was implemented in 3D. Finally, the reconstructed image in Fig. 66.13*e* is similar to that in Fig. 66.13*c* except that a 3D model of the collimator-detector response is used. The superior image quality obtained from using an accurate 3D model of the imaging process is evident.

Discussion

The development of SPECT has been a combination of advances in radiopharmaceuticals, instrumentation, image processing and reconstruction methods, and clinical applications. Although substantial progress has been made during the last decade, there are many opportunities for contributions from biomedical engineering in the future.

The future SPECT instrumentation will consist of more detector area to fully surround the patient for high detection efficiency and multiple contiguous transaxial slice capability. Multicamera SPECT systems will continue to dominate the commercial market. The use of new radiation detector materials and detector systems with high spatial resolution will receive increased attention. Continued research is needed to investigate special converging-hole collimator design geometries, fully 3D reconstruction algorithms, and their clinical applications.

To improve image quality and to achieve quantitatively accurate SPECT images will continue to be the goals of image processing and image reconstruction methods for SPECT. An important direction of research in analytical reconstruction methods will involve solving the inverse Radon

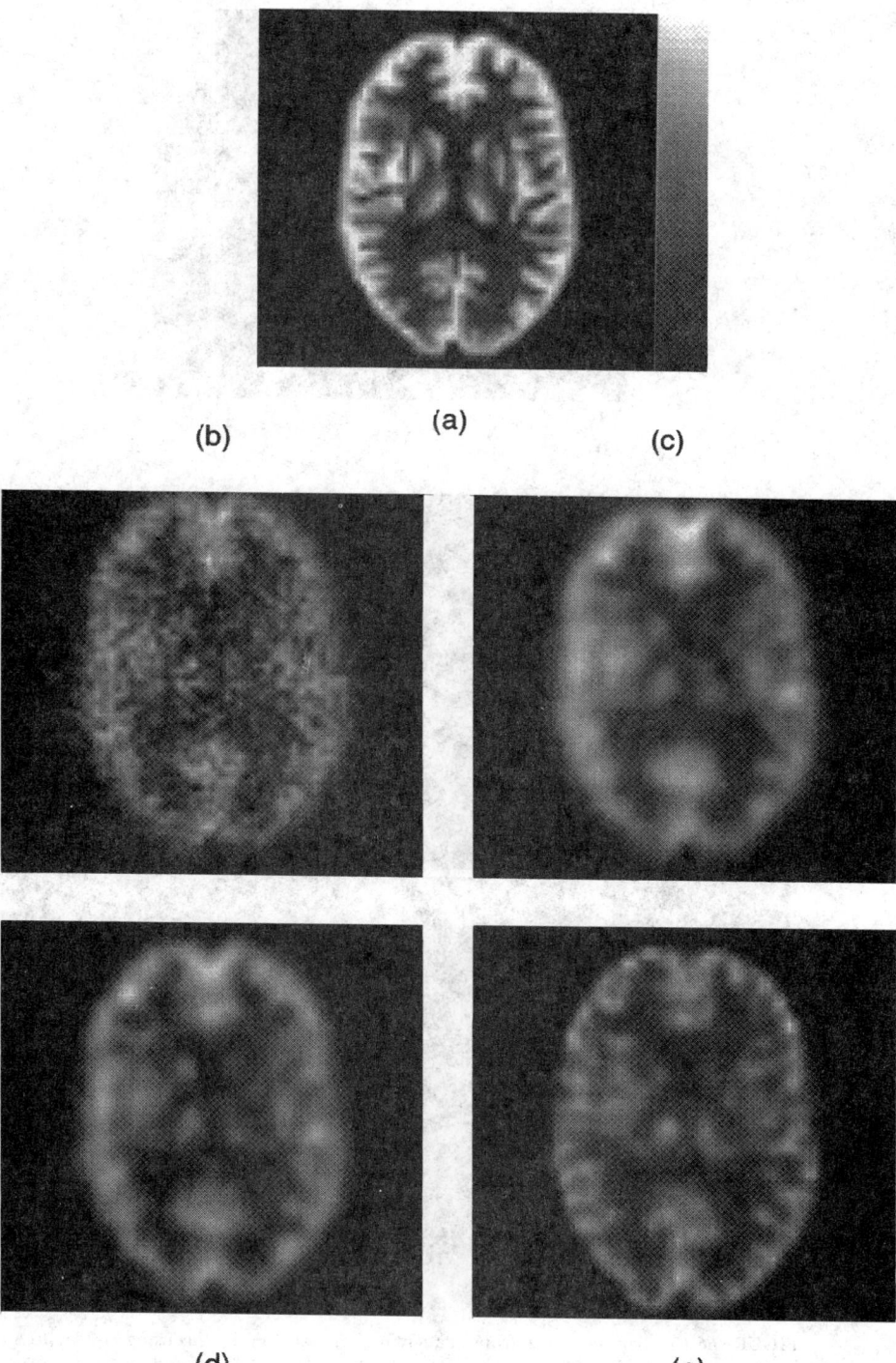

(b)   **(a)**   **(c)**

(d)   **(e)**

FIGURE 66.12   Sample images from a phantom SPECT study. (*a*) Radioactivity distribution from a selected slice of a 3D brain phantom. (*b*) Reconstructed image obtained from the FBP algorithm without any compensation. (*c*) Reconstructed image obtained with the application of noise-smoothing filter and compensation for uniform attenuation and scatter. (*d*) Similar to (*c*) except for an additional application of a Metz filter to partially compensate for the collimator-detector blurring. (*e*) Reconstructed image similar to that obtained from the iterative ML-EM algorithm that accurately models the attenuation and spatially variant detector response. (From Tsui BMW, Frey EC, Zhao X-D, et al. 1994. Reprinted with permission.)

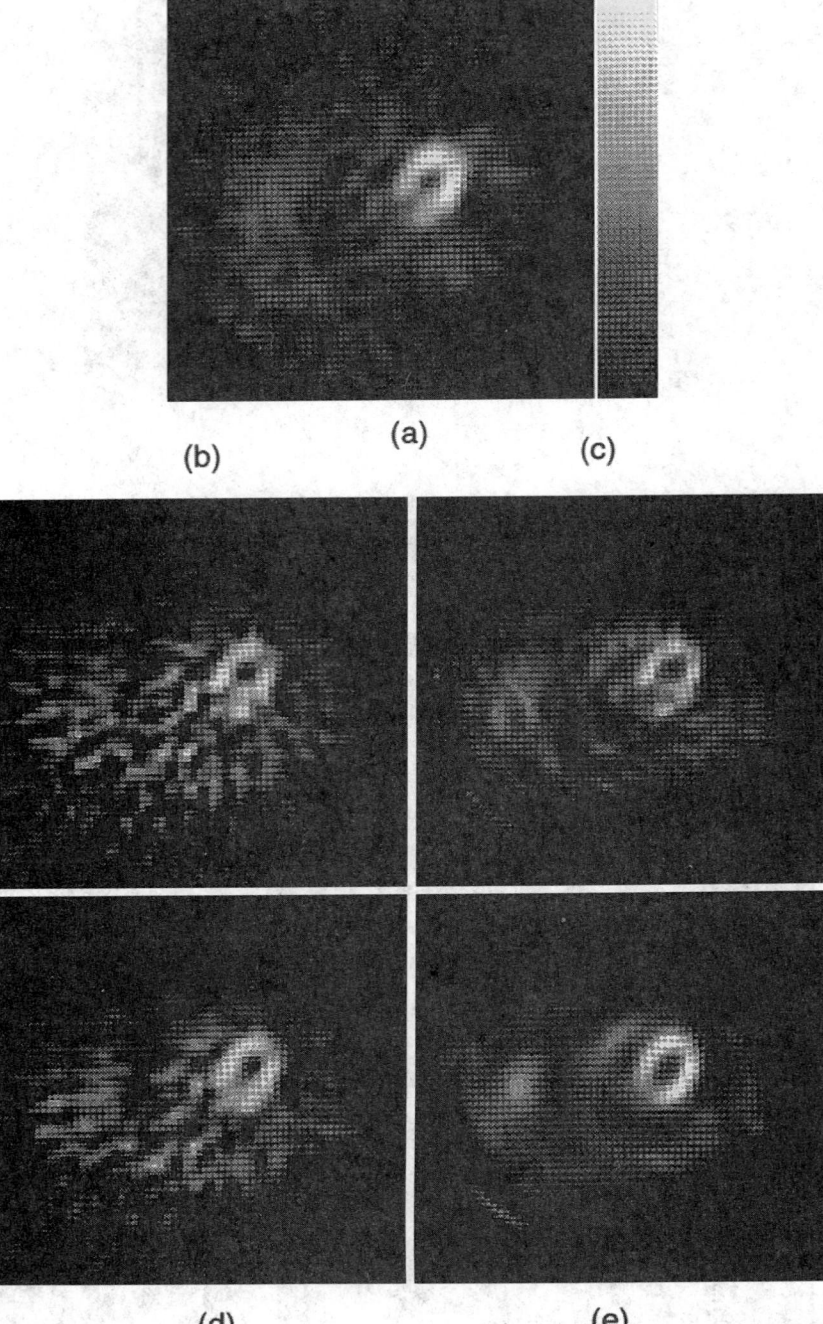

FIGURE 66.13 Sample images from a patient myocardial SPECT study using Tl-201. (*a*) A selected transaxial image slice from a typical patient myocardial SPECT study using Tl-201. The reconstructed image was obtained with the FBP algorithm without any compensation. (*b*) Reconstructed image obtained from the Chang algorithm for approximate nonuniform attenuation compensation and 2D processing using a Metz filter for approximate compensation for collimator-detector response. (*c*) Reconstructed image obtained from the iterative ML-EM algorithm using a measured transmission CT image for accurate attenuation compensation and 2D model of the collimator-detector response for accurate collimator-detector response compensation. (*d*) Similar to (*b*) except that the Metz filter was implemented in 3D. (*e*) Similar to (*c*) except that a 3D model of the collimator-detector response is used.

transform, which includes the effects of attenuation, the spatially variant collimator-detector response function, and scatter. The development of iterative reconstruction methods will require more accurate models of the complex SPECT imaging process, faster and more stable iterative algorithms, and more powerful computer and special computational hardware.

These improvements in SPECT instrumentation and image reconstruction methods, combined with newly developed radiopharmaceuticals, will bring SPECT images with increasingly higher quality and more accurate quantitation to nuclear medicine clinics for improved diagnosis and patient care.

References

Anger HO. 1958. Scintillation camera. Rev Sci Instrum 29:27.

Anger HO. 1964. Scintillation camera with multichannel collimators. J Nucl Med 5:515.

Axelsson B, Msaki P, Israelsson A. 1984. Subtraction of Compton-scattered photons in single-photon emission computed tomography. J Nucl Med 25:490.

Barrett HH. 1986. Perspectives on SPECT. SPIE 671:178.

Bellini S, Piacentini M, Cafforio C, et al. 1979. Compensation of tissue absorption in emission tomography. IEEE Trans Acoust Speech Signal Processing ASSP-27:213.

Bracewell RN, Riddle AC. 1967. Inversion of fan-beam scans in radio astronomy. Astrophys J 150:427.

Brooks RA, Di Chiro G. 1975. Theory of image reconstruction in computed tomography. Radiology 117:561.

Brooks RA, Di Chiro G. 1976. Principles of computer assisted tomography (CAT) in radiographic and radioisotopic imaging. Phys Med Biol 21:689.

Budinger TF, Gullberg GT. 1974. Three-dimensional reconstruction in nuclear medicine emission imaging. IEEE Trans Nucl Sci NS-21:2.

Budinger TF, Gullberg GT. 1977. Transverse section reconstruction of gamma-ray emitting radionuclides in patients. In MM Ter-Pogossian, ME Phelps, GL Brownell, et al. (eds), Reconstruction Tomography in Diagnostic Radiology and Nuclear Medicine. Baltimore, University Park Press.

Chang LT. 1978. A method for attenuation correction in radionuclide computed tomography. IEEE Trans Nucl Sci NS-25:638.

Chang W, Huang G, Wang L. 1990. A multi-detector cylindrical SPECT system for phantom imaging. In Conference Record of the 1990 Nuclear Science Symposium, vol 2, pp 1208–1211. Piscataway, NJ, IEEE.

Cho ZH, Yi W, Jung KJ, et al. 1982. Performance of single photon tomographic system-Gammatom-1. IEEE Trans Nucl Sci NS-29:484.

DeVito RP, Hamill JJ. 1991. Determination of weighting functions for energy-weighted acquisition. J Nucl Med 32:343.

DeVito RP, Hamill JJ, Treffert JD, Stoub EW. 1989. Energy-weighted acquisition of scintigraphic images using finite spatial filters. J Nucl Med 30:2029.

Edholm PR, Lewitt RM, Lindholm B. 1986. Novel properties of the Fourier decomposition of the sinogram. Proc SPIE 671:8.

Evans RD. 1955. The Atomic Nucleus. Malabar, Fla, Robert E. Krieger.

Floyd CE, Jaszczak RJ, Greer KL, Coleman RE. 1985. Deconvolution of Compton scatter in SPECT. J Nucl Med 26:403.

Formiconi AR, Pupi A, Passeri A. 1990. Compensation of spatial system response in SPECT with conjugate gradient reconstruction technique. Phys Med Biol 34:69.

Frey EC, Ju Z-W, Tsui BMW. 1993. A fast projector-backprojector pair modeling the asymmetric, spatially varying scatter response function for scatter compensation in SPECT imaging. IEEE Trans Nucl Sci NS-40(4):1192.

Frey EC, Tsui BMW. 1991 Spatial properties of the scatter response function in SPECT. IEEE Trans Nucl Sci NS-38:789.

Frey EC, Tsui BMW. 1992. A comparison of scatter compensation methods in SPECT: Subtraction-based techniques versus iterative reconstruction with an accurate scatter model. In Conference Record of the 1992 Nuclear Science Symposium and the Medical Imaging Conference, October 27–31, Orlando, Fla, pp 1035–1037.

Gagnon D, Todd-Pokropek A, Arsenault A, Dupros G. 1989. Introduction to holospectral imaging in nuclear medicine for scatter subtraction. IEEE Trans Med Imag 8:245.

Geman S, McClure DE. 1985. Bayesian image analysis: An application to single photon emission tomography. In Proceedings of the Statistical Computing Section. Washington, American Statistical Association.

Genna S, Smith A. 1988. The development of ASPECT, an annular single crystal brain camera for high efficiency SPECT. IEEE Trans Nucl Sci NS-35:654.

Gilland DR, Tsui BMW, Perry JR, et al. 1988. Optimum filter function for SPECT imaging. J Nucl Med 29:643.

Gilbert P. 1972. Iterative methods for the three-dimensional reconstruction of an object from projections. J Theor Biol 36:105.

Glick SJ, Penney BC, King MA, Byrne CL. 1993. Non-iterative compensation for the distance-dependent detector response and photon attenuation in SPECT imaging. IEEE Trans Med Imaging 13(2):363.

Goitein M. 1972. Three-dimensional density reconstruction from a series of two-dimensional projections. Nucl Instrum Methods 101:509.

Gordon R. 1974. A tutorial on ART (Algebraic reconstruction techniques). IEEE Trans Nucl Sci 21:78.

Gordon R, Bender R, Herman GT. 1970. Algebraic reconstruction techniques (ART) for three-dimensional electron microscopy and x-ray photography. J Theor Biol 29:471.

Gullberg GT. 1979. The attenuated Radon transform: Theory and application in medicine and biology. Ph.D. dissertation, University of California at Berkeley.

Gullberg GT, Budinger TF. 1981. The use of filtering methods to compensate for constant attenuation in single-photon emission computed tomography. IEEE Trans Biomed Eng BME-28:142.

Gullberg GT, Christian PE, Zeng GL, et al. 1991. Cone beam tomography of the heart using single-photon emission-computed tomography. Invest Radiol 26:681.

Hawman EG, Hsieh J. 1986. An astigmatic collimator for high sensitivity SPECT of the brain. J Nucl Med 27:930.

Hirose Y, Ikeda Y, Higashi Y, et al. 1982. A hybrid emission CT-HEADTOME II. IEEE Trans Nucl Sci NS-29:520.

Hoffman EJ, Cutler PD, Kigby WM, Mazziotta JC. 1990. 3-D phantom to simulate cerebral blood flow and metabolic images for PET. IEEE Trans Nucl Sci NS-37:616.

Huesman RH, Gullberg GT, Greenberg WL, Budinger TF. 1977. RECLBL Library Users Manual, Donner Algorithms for Reconstruction Tomography. Lawrence Berkeley Laboratory, University of California.

Jaszczak RJ, Chang LT, Murphy PH. 1979. Single photon emission computed tomography using multi-slice fan beam collimators. IEEE Trans Nucl Sci NS-26:610.

Jaszczak RJ, Chang LT, Stein NA, Moore FE. 1979. Whole-body single-photon emission computed tomography using dual, large-field-of-view scintillation cameras. Phys Med Biol 24:1123.

Jaszczak RJ, Coleman RE. 1985. Single photon emission computed tomography (SPECT) principles and instrumentation. Invest Radiol 20:897.

Jaszczak RJ, Coleman RE, Lim CB. 1980. SPECT: Single photon emission computed tomography. IEEE Trans Nucl Sci NS-27:1137.

Jaszczak RJ, Coleman RE, Whitehead FR. 1981. Physical factors affecting quantitative measurements using camera-based single photon emission computed tomography (SPECT). IEEE Trans Nucl Sci NS-28:69.

Jaszczak RJ, Floyd CE, Coleman RE. 1985. Scatter compensation techniques for SPECT. IEEE Trans Nucl Sci NS-32:786.

Jaszczak RJ, Floyd CE, Manglos SM, et al. 1987. Cone beam collimation for single photon emission computed tomography: Analysis, simulation, and image reconstruction using filtered back-projection. Med Phys 13:484.

Jaszczak RJ, Greer KL, Floyd, CE, et al. 1984. Improved SPECT quantification using compensation for scattered photons. J Nucl Med 25:893.

Jaszczak RJ, Murphy PH, Huard D, Burdine JA. 1977. Radionuclide emission computed tomography of the head with ^{99m}Tc and a scintillation camera. J Nucl Med 18:373.

Jaszczak RJ, Tsui BMW. 1994. Single photon emission computed tomography. In HN Wagner and Z Szabo (eds), Principles of Nuclear Medicine, 2d ed. Philadelphia, Saunders.

Johnson VE, Wong WH, Hu X, Chen CT. 1991. Image restoration using Gibbs priors: Boundary modeling, treatment of blurring, and selection of hyperparameters. IEEE Trans Pat 13:413.

Keller EL. 1968. Optimum dimensions of parallel-hole, multiaperture collimators for gamma-ray camera. J Nucl Med 9:233.

Keyes JW Jr, Orlandea N, Heetderks WJ, et al. 1977. The humogotron—A scintillation-camera transaxial tomography. J Nucl Med 18:381.

King MA, Hademenos G, Glick SJ. 1992. A dual photopeak window method for scatter correction. J Nucl Med 33:605.

King MA, Schwinger RB, Doherty PW, Penney BC. 1984. Two-dimensional filtering of SPECT images using the Metz and Wiener filters. J Nucl Med 25:1234.

King MA, Schwinger RB, Penney BC. 1986. Variation of the count-dependent Metz filter with imaging system modulation transfer function. Med Phys 25:139.

Knesaurek K, King MA, Glick SJ, et al. 1989. Investigation of causes of geometric distortion in 180 degree and 360 degree angular sampling in SPECT. J Nucl Med 30:1666.

Koral KF, Wang X, Rogers WL, Clinthorne NH. 1988. SPECT Compton-scattering correction by analysis of energy spectra. J Nucl Med 29:195.

Kuhl DE, Edwards RQ. 1963. Image separation radioisotope scanning. Radiology 80:653.

Kuhl DE, Edwards RQ. 1964. Cylindrical and section radioisotope scanning of the liver and brain. Radiology 83:926.

Kuhl DE, Edwards RQ. 1968. Reorganizing data from transverse section scans of the brain using digital processing. Radiology 91:975.

Lange K, Carson R. 1984. EM reconstruction algorithms for emission and transmission tomography. J Comput Assist Tomogr 8:306.

Levitan E, Herman GT. 1987. A maximum a posteriori probability expectation maximization algorithm for image reconstruction in emission tomography. IEEE Trans Med Imag MI-6:185.

Liang Z, Hart H. 1987. Bayesian image processing of data from constrained source distribution: I. Nonvalued, uncorrelated and correlated constraints. Bull Math Biol 49:51.

Larsson SA, Hohm C, Carnebrink T, et al. 1991. A new cylindrical SPECT Anger camera with a de-centralized transputer based data acquisition system. IEEE Trans Nucl Sci NS-38:654.

Lassen NA, Sveinsdottir E, Kanno I, et al. 1978. A fast moving single photon emission tomograph for regional cerebral blood flow studies in man. J Comput Assist Tomog 2:661.

Lewitt RM, Edholm PR, Xia W. 1989. Fourier method for correction of depth dependent collimator blurring. SPIE Proc 1092:232.

Lim CB, Chang LT, Jaszczak RJ. 1980. Performance analysis of three camera configurations for single photon emission computed tomography. IEEE Trans Nucl Sci NS-27:559.

Lim CB, Gottschalk S, Walker R, et al. 1985. Tri-angular SPECT system for 3-D total organ volume imaging: Design concept and preliminary imaging results. IEEE Trans Nucl Sci NS-32:741.

Manglos SH, Jaszczak RJ, Floyd CE, et al. 1987. Nonisotropic attenuation in SPECT: Phantom test of quantitative effects and compensation techniques. J Nucl Med 28:1584.

Maniawski PJ, Morgan HT, Wackers FJT. 1991. Orbit-related variations in spatial resolution as a source of artifactual defects in thallium-201 SPECT. J Nucl Med 32:871.

Milster TD, Aarsvold JN, Barrett HH, et al. 1990. A full-field modular gamma camera. J Nucl Med 31:632.

Minerbo G. 1979. Maximum entropy reconstruction from cone-beam projection data. Comput Biol Med 9:29.

M ore SC, Doherty MD, Zimmerman RE, Holman BL. 1984. Improved performance from modifications to the multidetector SPECT brain scanner. J Nucl Med 25:688.

Ogawa K, Harata Y, Ichihara T, et al. 1991. A practical method for position-dependent Compton scatter correction in SPECT. IEEE Trans Med Imaging 10:408.

Penney BC, Glick SJ, and King MA. 1990. Relative importance of the errors sources in Wiener restoration of scintigrams. IEEE Trans Med Imaging 9:60.

Radon J. 1917. Uber die bestimmung von funktionen durch ihre integral-werte langs gewisser mannigfaltigkeiten. Ber Verh Sachs Akad Wiss 67:26.

Ramachandran GN, Lakshminarayanan AV. 1971. Three-dimensional reconstruction from radiographs and electron micrographs: Application of convolutions instead of Fourier transforms. Proc Natl Acad Sci USA 68:2236.

Rogers WL, Ackermann RJ. 1992. SPECT Instrumentation. Am J Physiol Imaging 314:105.

Rogers WL, Clinthorne NH, Shao L, et al. 1988. SPRINT II: A second-generation single photon ring tomograph. IEEE Trans Med Imaging 7:291.

Rowe RK, Aarsvold JN, Barrett HH, et al. 1992. A stationary, hemispherical SPECT imager for 3D brain imaging. J Nucl Med 34:474.

Sorenson JA. 1974. Quantitative measurement of radiation in vivo by whole body counting. In GH Hine and JA Sorenson (eds), Instrumentation in Nuclear Medicine, vol 2, pp 311–348. New York, Academic Press.

Shepp LA, Vardi Y. 1982. Maximum likelihood reconstruction for emission tomography. IEEE Trans Med Imaging MI-1:113.

Stoddart HF, Stoddart HA. 1979. A new development in single gamma transaxial tomography Union Carbide focused collimator scanner. IEEE Trans Nucl Sci NS-26:2710.

Stokely EM, Sveinsdottir E, Lassen NA, Rommer P. 1980. A single photon dynamic computer assisted tomography (DCAT) for imaging brain function in multiple cross-sections. J Comput Assist Tomogr 4:230.

Tretiak OJ, Metz CE. 1980. The exponential Radon transform. SIAM J Appl Math 39:341.

Tsui BMW. 1988. Collimator design, properties and characteristics. Chapter 2. In GH Simmons (ed), The Scintillaion Camera, pp 17–45. New York, The Society of Nuclear Medicine.

Tsui BMW, Frey EC, Zhao X-D, et al. 1994. The importance and implementation of accurate 3D compensation methods for quantitative SPECT. Phys Med Biol 39:509.

Tsui BMW, Gullberg GT, Edgerton ER, et al. 1986. The design and clinical utility of a fan beam collimator for a SPECT system. J Nucl Med 247:810.

Tsui BMW, Gullberg GT, Edgerton ER, et al. 1989. Correction of nonuniform attenuation in cardiac SPECT imaging. J Nucl Med 30:497.

Tsui BMW, Hu HB, Gilland DR, Gullberg GT. 1988. Implementation of simultaneous attenuation and detector response correction in SPECT. IEEE Trans Nucl Sci NS-35:778.

Tsui BMW, Zhao X-D, Frey EC, McCartney WH. 1994. Quantitative single-photon emission computed tomography: Basics and clinical considerations. Semin Nucl Med 24(1):38.

Yanch JC, Flower MA, Webb S. 1988. Comparison of deconvolution and windowed subtraction techniques for scatter compensation in SPECT. IEEE Trans Med Imaging 7:13.

Zeng GL, Gullberg GT, Tsui BMW, Terry JA. 1991. Three-dimensional iterative reconstruction algorithms with attenuation and geometric point response correction. IEEE Trans Nucl Sci NS-38:693.

67

Ultrasound

Richard L. Goldberg
University of North Carolina

Stephen W. Smith
Duke University

Jack G. Mottley
University of Rochester

K. Whittaker Ferrara
Riverside Research Institute

67.1 Transducers

Richard L. Goldberg and Stephen W. Smith

An ultrasound transducer generates acoustic waves by converting magnetic, thermal, or electrical energy into mechanical energy. The most efficient technique for medical ultrasound uses the piezoelectric effect, which was first demonstrated in 1880 by Jacques and Pierre Curie [Curie and Curie, 1880]. They applied a stress to a quartz crystal and detected an electrical potential across opposite faces of the material. The Curies also discovered the inverse piezoelectric effect by applying an electric field across the crystal to induce a mechanical deformation. In this manner, a piezoelectric transducer converts an oscillating electric signal into an acoustic wave, and vice versa.

Many significant advances in ultrasound imaging have resulted from innovations in transducer technology. One such instance was the development of linear-array transducers. Previously, ultrasound systems had made an image by manually moving the transducer across the region of interest. Even the faster scanners had required several seconds to generate an ultrasound image, and as a result, only static targets could be scanned. On the other hand, if the acoustic beam could be scanned rapidly, clinicians could visualize moving targets such as a beating heart. In addition, real-time imaging would provide instantaneous feedback to the clinician of the transducer position and system settings.

To implement real-time imaging, researchers developed new types of transducers that rapidly steer the acoustic beam. Piston-shaped transducers were designed to wobble or rotate about a fixed axis to *mechanically* steer the beam through a sector-shaped region. Linear sequential arrays were designed to *electronically* focus the beam in a rectangular image region. Linear phased-array transducers were designed to *electronically* steer and focus the beam at high speed in a sector image format.

This section describes the application of piezoelectric ceramics to transducer arrays for medical ultrasound. Background is presented on transducer materials and beam steering with phased arrays. Array performance is described, and the design of an idealized array is presented.

8493-8346-3/95/$0.00+$.50
1995 by CRC Press, Inc.

Transducer Materials

Ferroelectric materials strongly exhibit the piezoelectric effect, and they are ideal materials for medical ultrasound. For many years, the ferroelectric ceramic lead-zirconate-titanate (PZT) has been the standard transducer material for medical ultrasound, in part because of its high electromechanical conversion efficiency and low intrinsic losses. The properties of PZT can be adjusted by modifying the ratio of zirconium to titanium and introducing small amounts of other substances, such as lanthanum [Berlincourt, 1971]. Table 67.1 shows the material properties of linear-array elements made from PZT-5H.

PZT has a high dielectric constant compared with many piezoelectric materials, resulting in favorable electrical characteristics. The ceramic is mechanically strong, and it can be machined to various shapes and sizes. PZT can operate at temperatures up to 100°C or higher, and it is stable over long periods of time.

The disadvantages of PZT include its high acoustic impedance ($Z = 30$ MRayls) compared with body tissue ($Z = 1.5$ MRayls) and the presence of lateral modes in array elements. One or more acoustic matching layers can largely compensate for the acoustic impedance mismatch. The effect of lateral modes can be diminished by choosing the appropriate element dimensions or by subdicing the elements.

Other piezoelectric materials are used for various applications. Composites are made from PZT interspersed in an epoxy matrix [Smith, 1992]. Lateral modes are reduced in a composite because of its inhomogeneous structure. By combining the PZT and epoxy in different ratios and spatial distributions, one can tailor the composite's properties for different applications. Polyvinylidene difluoride (PVDF) is a ferroelectric polymer that has been used effectively in high-frequency transducers [Sherar and Foster, 1989]. The copolymer of PVDF with trifluoroethylene has an improved electromechanical conversion efficiency. Relaxor ferroelectric materials, such as lead-magnesium-niobate (PMN), become piezoelectric when a large direct-current (dc) bias voltage is applied [Takeuchi et al., 1990]. They have a very large dielectric constant ($\varepsilon > 20,000\varepsilon_0$), resulting in higher transducer capacitance and a lower electrical impedance.

Scanning with Array Transducers

Array transducers use the same principles as acoustic lenses to focus an acoustic beam. In both cases, variable delays are applied across the transducer aperture. With a sequential or phased array, however, the delays are electronically controlled and can be changed instantaneously to focus the beam in different regions. Linear arrays were first developed for radar, sonar, and radio astronomy [Allen, 1964; Bobber, 1970], and they were implemented in a medical ultrasound system by Somer in 1968 [Somer, 1968].

Linear-array transducers have increased versatility over piston transducers. Electronic scanning involves no moving parts, and the focal point can be changed dynamically to any location in the scanning plane. The system can generate a wide variety of scan formats, and it can process the received echoes for other applications, such as dynamic receive focusing [von Ramm and Thurstone,

TABLE 67.1   Material Properties of Linear-Array Elements Made of PZT-5H

Parameter	Symbol	Value	Units
Density	ρ	7500	kg/m^3
Speed of sound	c	3970	m/s
Acoustic impedance	Z	29.75	MRayls
Relative dielectric constant	$\varepsilon/\varepsilon_0$	1475	None
Electromechanical coupling coefficient	k	0.698	None
Mechanical loss tangent	$\tan \delta_m$	0.015	None
Electrical loss tangent	$\tan \delta_e$	0.02	None

1976], correction for phase aberrations [Flax and O'Donnell, 1988; Trahey et al., 1990], and synthetic aperture imaging [Nock and Trahey, 1992].

The disadvantages of linear arrays are due to the increased complexity and higher cost of the transducers and scanners. For high-quality ultrasound images, many identical array elements are required (currently 128 and rising). The array elements are typically less than a millimeter on one side, and each has a separate connection to its own transmitter and receiver electronics.

The widespread use of array transducers for many applications indicates that the advantages often outweigh the disadvantages. In addition, improvements in transducer fabrication techniques and integrated circuit technology have led to more advanced array transducers and scanners.

Focusing and Steering with Phased Arrays

This subsection describes how a phased-array transducer can focus and steer an acoustic beam along a specific direction. An ultrasound image is formed by repeating this process over 100 times to interrogate a two- (2D) or three-dimensional (3D) region of the medium.

Figure 67.1*a* illustrates a simple example of a six-element linear array focusing the transmitted beam. One can assume that each array element is a point source that radiates a spherically shaped wavefront into the medium. Since the top element is farthest from the focus in this example, it is excited first. The remaining elements are excited at the appropriate time intervals so that the acoustic signals from all the elements reach the focal point at the same time. According to Huygens' principle, the net acoustic signal is the sum of the signals that have arrived from each source. At the focal point, the contributions from every element add in phase to produce a peak in the acoustic signal. Elsewhere, at least some of the contributions add out of phase, reducing the signal relative to the peak.

For receiving an ultrasound echo, the phased array works in reverse. Fig. 67.1*b* shows an echo originating from focus 1. The echo is incident on each array element at a different time interval. The received signals are electronically delayed so that the delayed signals add in phase for an echo orig-

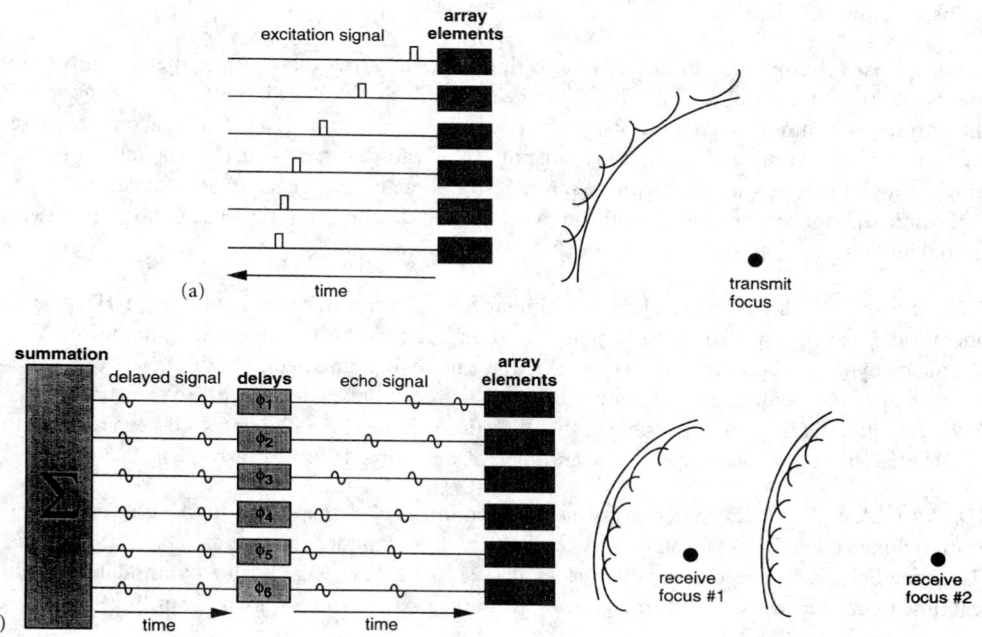

FIGURE 67.1 Focusing and steering an acoustic beam using a phased array. A 6-element linear array is shown (*a*) in the transmit mode and (*b*) in the receive mode. Dynamic focusing in receive allows the scanner focus to track the range of returning echoes.

inating at the focal point. For echoes originating elsewhere, at least some of the delayed signals will add out of phase, reducing the receive signal relative to the peak at the focus.

In the receive mode, the focal point can be dynamically adjusted so that it coincides with the range of returning echoes. After transmission of an acoustic pulse, the initial echoes return from targets near the transducer. Therefore, the scanner focuses the phased array on these targets, located at focus 1 in Fig. 67.1b. As echoes return from more distant targets, the scanner focuses at a greater depth (focus 2 in the figure). Focal zones are established with adequate depth of field so that the targets are always in focus in receive. This process is called *dynamic receive focusing* and was first implemented by von Ramm and Thurstone in 1976 [von Ramm and Thurstone, 1976].

Array-Element Configurations

An ultrasound image is formed by repeating the preceding process many times to scan a 2D or 3D region of tissue. For a 2D image, the scanning plane is the **azimuth dimension;** the **elevation dimension** is perpendicular to the azimuth scanning plane. The shape of the region scanned is determined by the array-element configuration, described in the paragraphs below.

Linear Sequential Arrays. Sequential linear arrays have as many as 512 elements in current commercial scanners. A subaperture of up to 128 elements is selected to operate at a given time. As shown in Fig. 67.2a, the scanning lines are directed perpendicular to the face of the transducer; the acoustic beam is focused but not steered. The advantage of this scheme is that the array elements have high sensitivity when the beam is directed straight ahead. The disadvantage is that the field of view is limited to the rectangular region directly in front of the transducer. Linear-array transducers have a large footprint to obtain an adequate field of view.

Curvilinear Arrays. Curvilinear or convex arrays have a different shape than sequential linear arrays, but they operate in the same manner. In both cases, the scan lines are directed perpendicular to the transducer face. A curvilinear array, however, scans a wider field of view because of its convex shape, as shown in Fig. 67.2b.

Linear Phased Arrays. The more advanced linear phased arrays have 128 elements. All the elements are used to transmit and receive each line of data. As shown in Fig. 67.2c, the scanner steers the ultrasound beam through a sector-shaped region in the azimuth plane. Phased arrays scan a region that is significantly wider than the footprint of the transducer, making them suitable for scanning through restricted acoustic windows. As a result, these transducers are ideal for cardiac imaging, where the transducer must scan through a small window to avoid the obstructions of the ribs (bone) and lungs (air).

1.5D Arrays. The so-called 1.5D array is similar to a 2D array in construction but a 1D array in operation. The 1.5D array contains elements along both the azimuth and elevation dimensions. Features such dynamic focusing and phase correction can be implemented in both dimensions to improve image quality. Since a 1.5D array contains a limited number of elements in elevation (e.g., 3 to 9 elements), steering is not possible in that direction. Figure 67.2d illustrates a B-scan made with a 1.5D phased array. Linear sequential scanning is also possible with 1.5D arrays.

2D Phased Arrays. A 2D phased-array has a large number of elements in both the azimuth and elevation dimensions. Therefore, 2D arrays can focus and steer the acoustic beam in both dimensions. Using parallel receive processing [Shattuck et al., 1984], a 2D array can scan a pyramidal region in real time to produce a volumetric image, as shown in Fig. 67.2e [von Ramm and Smith, 1990].

Linear-Array Transducer Performance

Designing an ultrasound transducer array involves many compromises. Ideally, a transducer has high sensitivity or SNR, good spatial resolution, and no artifacts. The individual array elements

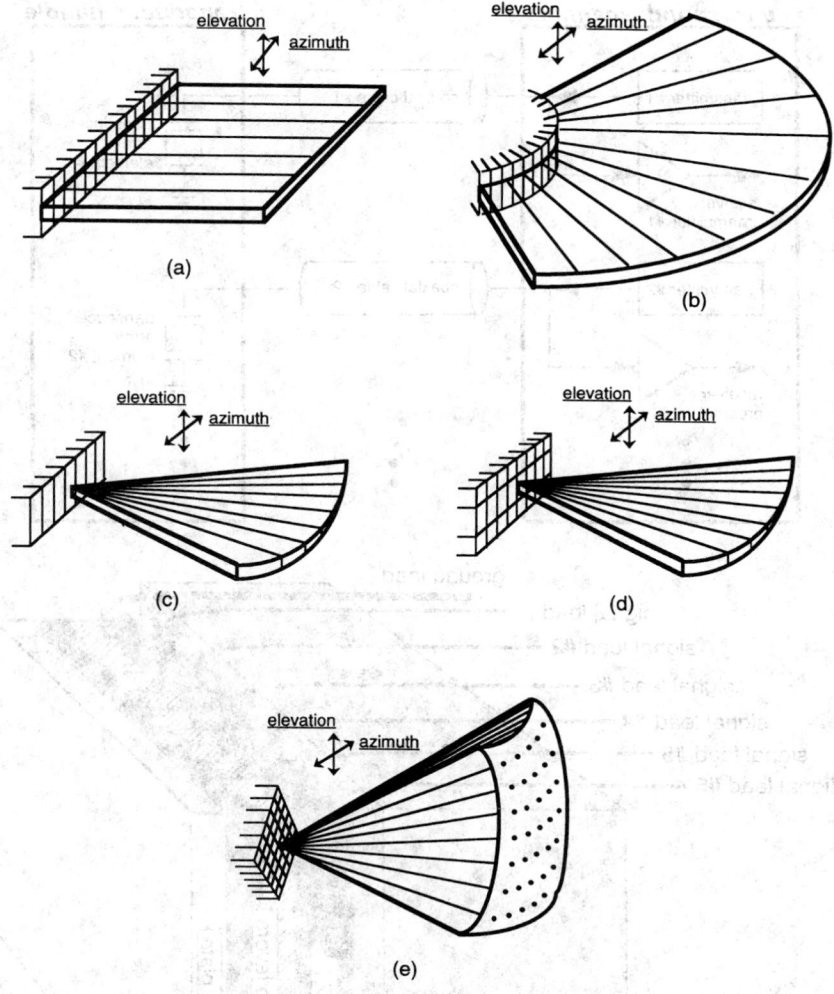

FIGURE 67.2 Array-element configurations and the region scanned by the acoustic beam. (*a*) A sequential linear array scans a rectangular region; (*b*) a curvilinear array scans a sector-shaped region; (*c*) a linear phased array scans a sector-shaped region; (*d*) a 1.5D array scans a sector-shaped region; (*e*) a 2D array scans a pyramidal-shaped region.

should have wide angular response in the steering dimensions, low cross-coupling, and an electrical impedance matched to the transmitter.

Figure 67.3*a* illustrates the connections to the transducer assembly. The transmitter and receiver circuits are located in the ultrasound scanner and are connected to the array elements through 1 to 2 m of coaxial cable. Electrical matching networks can be added to tune out the capacitance of the coaxial cable and/or the transducer element and increase the signal-to-noise ratio (SNR).

A more detailed picture of six-transducer elements is shown in Fig. 67.3*b*. Electrical leads connect to the ground and signal electrodes of the piezoelectric material. Acoustically, the array elements are loaded on the front side by one or two quarter-wave matching layers and the tissue medium. The matching layers may be made from glass or epoxy. A backing material, such as epoxy, loads the back side of the array elements. The faceplate protects the transducer assembly and also may act as an acoustic lens. Faceplates are often made from silicone or polyurethane.

The following subsections describe several important characteristics of an array transducer. Figure 67.3*c* shows a six-element array and its dimensions. The element thickness, width, and length

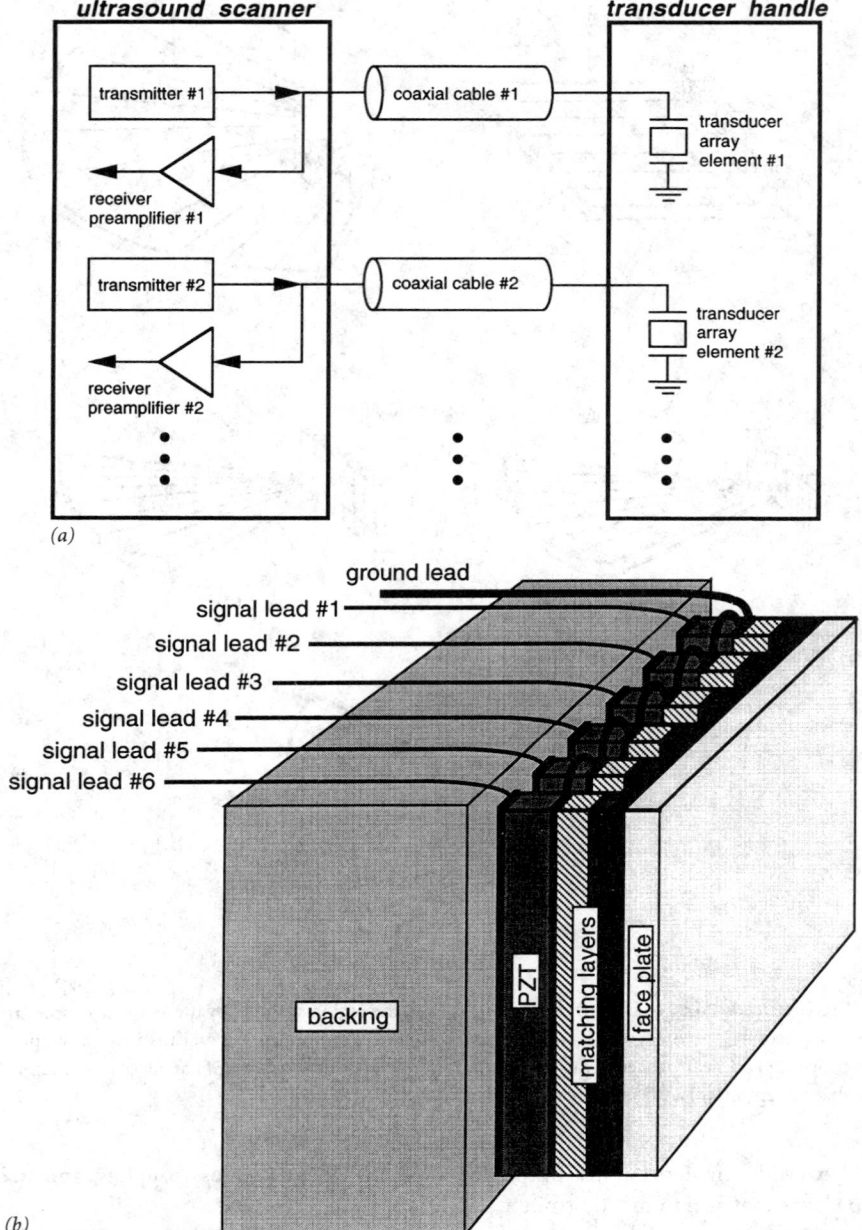

FIGURE 67.3 (*a*) The connections between the ultrasound scanner and the transducer assembly for two elements of an array. (*b*) A more detailed picture the transducer assembly for six elements of an array. (*c*) Coordinate system and labeling used to describe an array transducer.

are labeled as *t, a,* and *b,* respectively. The interelement spacing is *d,* and the total aperture size is *D* in azimuth. The acoustic wavelength in the load medium, usually human tissue, is designated as λ, while the wavelength in the transducer material is λ_t.

Examples are given below for a 128-element linear array operating at 5 MHz. The array is made of PZT-5H with element dimensions of 0.1 $\times$ 5 $\times$ 0.3 mm. The interelement spacing is *d* = 0.15

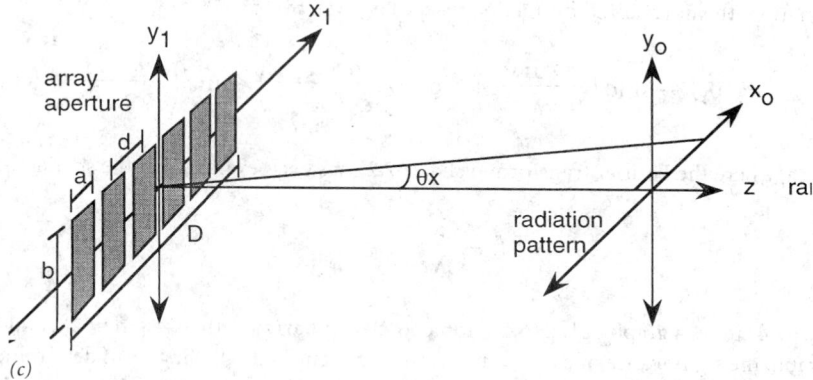

(c)

FIGURE 67.3   *(continued)*

mm in azimuth, and the total aperture is $D = 128 \cdot 0.15$ mm $= 19.3$ mm. See Table 67.1 for the piezoelectric material characteristics. The elements have an epoxy backing of $Z = 3.25$ MRayls. For simplicity, the example array does not contain a $\lambda/4$ matching layer.

Axial Resolution

Axial resolution determines the ability to distinguish between targets aligned in the axial direction (the direction of acoustic propagation). In pulse-echo imagining, the echoes off of two targets separated by $r/2$ have a path length difference of r. If the acoustic pulse length is r, then echoes off the two targets are just distinguishable. As a result, the axial resolution is often defined as one-half the pulse length [Christensen, 1988]. A transducer with a high resonant frequency and a broad bandwidth has a short acoustic pulse and good axial resolution.

Radiation Pattern

The radiation pattern of a transducer determines the insonified region of tissue. For good lateral resolution and sensitivity, the acoustic energy should be concentrated in a small region. The radiation pattern for a narrow-band or continuous-wave (CW) transducer is described by the Rayleigh-Sommerfeld diffraction formula [Goodman, 1986]. For a pulse-echo imaging system, this diffraction formula is not exact due to the broadband acoustic waves used. Nevertheless, the Rayleigh-Sommerfeld formula is a reasonable first-order approximation to the actual radiation pattern.

The following analysis considers only the azimuth scanning dimension. Near the focal point or in the far field, the Fraunhofer approximation reduces the diffraction formula to a Fourier transform formula. For a circular or rectangular aperture, the far field is at a range of

$$z > \frac{D^2}{4\lambda} \tag{67.1}$$

Figure 67.3c shows the coordinate system used to label the array aperture and its radiation pattern. The array aperture is described by

$$\text{Array}\,(x_1) = \text{rect}\left(\frac{x_1}{a}\right) * \text{comb}\left(\frac{x_1}{d}\right) \cdot \text{rect}\left(\frac{x_1}{D}\right) \tag{67.2}$$

where the rect(x) function is a rectangular pulse of width x, and the comb(x) function is a delta function repeated at intervals of x. The diffraction pattern is evaluated in the x_0 plane at a distance z from the transducer, and θ_x is the angle of the point x_0 from the normal axis. With the Fraunhofer approximation, the normalized diffraction pattern is given by

$$P_x(\theta_x) = \text{sinc}\left(\frac{a \sin \theta_x}{\lambda}\right) \cdot \text{comb}\left(\frac{d \sin \theta_x}{\lambda}\right) * \text{sinc}\left(\frac{D \sin \theta_x}{\lambda}\right) \tag{67.3}$$

in azimuth, where the Fourier transform of Eq. (67.2) has been evaluated at the spatial frequency

$$f_x = \frac{x_0}{\lambda z} = \frac{\sin \theta_x}{\lambda} \tag{67.4}$$

Figure 67.4 shows a graph of Eq. (67.3) for a 16-element array with $a = \lambda, d = 2\lambda$, and $D = 32\lambda$. In the graph, the significance of each term is easily distinguished. The first term determines the angular response weighting, the second term determines the location of grating lobes off-axis, and the third term determines the shape of the main lobe and the grating lobes. The significance of **lateral resolution, angular response,** and **grating lobes** is seen from the CW diffraction pattern.

Lateral resolution determines the ability to distinguish between targets in the azimuth and elevation dimensions. According to the Rayleigh criterion [Goodman, 1986], the *lateral resolution* can be defined by the first null in the main lobe, which is determined from the third term of Eq. (67.3).

$$\theta_x = \sin^{-1}\frac{\lambda}{D} \tag{67.5}$$

in the azimuth dimension. A larger aperture results in a more narrow main lobe and better resolution.

A broad angular response is desired to maintain sensitivity while steering off-axis. The first term of Eq. (67.3) determines the one-way angular response. The element is usually surrounded by a soft

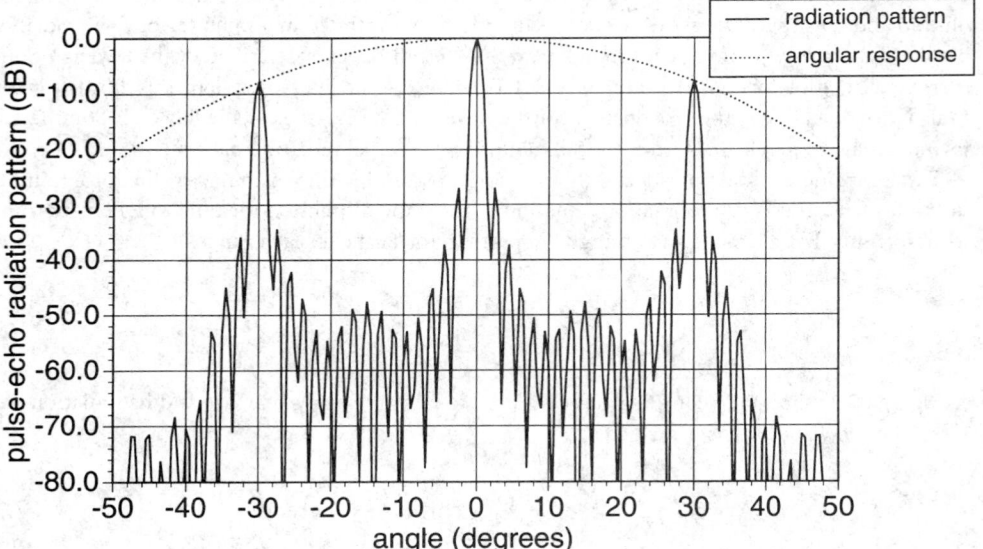

FIGURE 67.4 Radiation pattern of Eq. (67.3) for a 16-element array with $a = \lambda, d = 2\lambda$, and $D = 32\lambda$. The angular response, the first term of Eq. (67.3), is also shown as a dashed line.

baffle, such as air, resulting in an additional cosine factor in the radiation pattern [Selfridge et al., 1980]. Assuming transmit/receive reciprocity, the pulse-echo angular response for a single element is

$$P_x(\theta_x) = \frac{\sin^2(\pi a/\lambda \cdot \sin \theta_x)}{(\pi a/\lambda \cdot \sin \theta_x)^2} \cdot \cos^2 \theta_x \qquad (67.6)$$

in the azimuth dimension. As the aperture size becomes smaller, the element more closely resembles a point source, and the angular response becomes more broad. Another useful indicator is the −6-dB angular response, defined as the full-width half-maximum of the angular response graph.

Grating lobes are produced at a location where the path length difference to adjacent array elements is a multiple of a wavelength (the main lobe is located where the path length difference is zero). The acoustic contributions from the elements constructively interfere, producing off-axis peaks. The term *grating lobe* was originally used to describe the optical peaks produced by a diffraction grating. In ultrasound, grating lobes are undesirable because they represent acoustic energy steered away from the main lobe. From the Comb function in Eq. (67.3), the grating lobes are located at

$$\theta_x = \sin^{-1} \frac{i\lambda}{d} \qquad i = 1, 2, 3, \ldots \qquad (67.7)$$

in azimuth.

If d is a wavelength, then grating lobes are centered at ±90 degrees from the steering direction in that dimension. Grating lobes at such large angles are less significant because the array elements have poor angular response in those regions. If the main lobe is steered at a large angle, however, the grating lobes are brought toward the front of the array. In this case, the angular response weighting produces a relatively weak main lobe and a relatively strong grating lobe. To eliminate grating lobes at all steering angles, the interelement spacing is set to $\lambda/2$ or less [Steinberg, 1976].

Figure 67.5 shows the theoretical radiation pattern of the 128-element example. For this graph, the angular response weighting of Eq. (67.6) was substituted into Eq. (67.3). The lateral resolution,

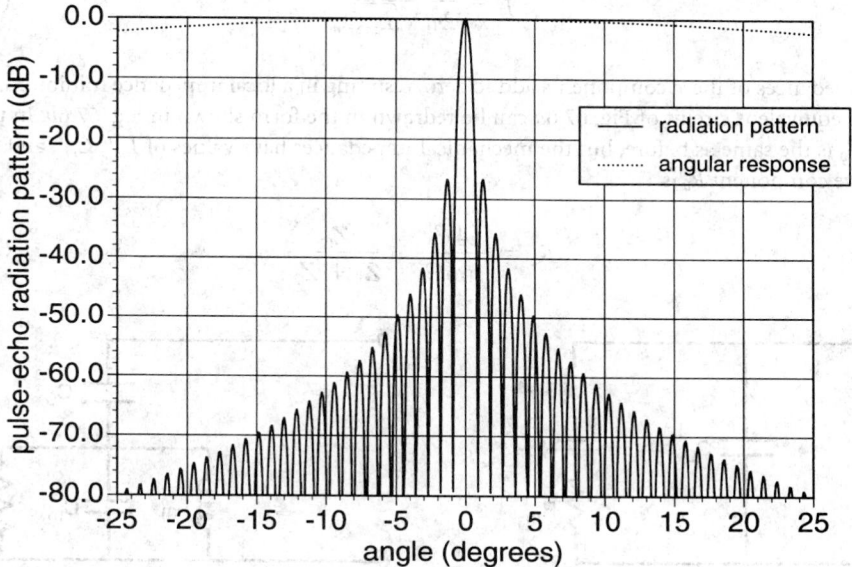

FIGURE 67.5 Radiation pattern of the example array element with $a = 0.1$ mm, $d = 0.15$ mm, $D = 19.2$ mm, and $\lambda = 0.3$ mm. The angular response of Eq. (67.6) was substituted into Eq. (67.3) for this graph.

as defined by Eq. (67.5), is $\theta_x = 0.9$ degree at the focal point. The -6-dB angular response is ± 40 degrees from Eq. (67.6).

Electrical Impedance

The electrical impedance of an element relative to the electrical loads has a significant impact on transducer signal-to-noise ratio (SNR). At frequencies away from resonance, the transducer has electrical characteristics of a capacitor. The construction of the transducer is a parallel-plate capacitor with clamped capacitance of

$$C_0 = \varepsilon^S \frac{ab}{t} \qquad (67.8)$$

where ε^S is the clamped dielectric constant.

Near resonance, equivalent circuits help to explain the impedance behavior of a transducer. The simplified circuit of Fig. 67.6a is valid for transducers operating at series resonance without losses and with low acoustic impedance loads [Kino, 1987]. The mechanical resistance R_m represents the acoustic loads as seen from the electrical terminals:

$$R_m = \frac{\pi}{4k^2 \omega C_0} \cdot \frac{Z_1 + Z_2}{Z_C} \qquad (67.9)$$

where k is the electromechanical coupling coefficient of the piezoelectric material, Z_C is the acoustic impedance of the piezoelectric material, Z_1 is the acoustic impedance of the transducer backing, and Z_2 is the acoustic impedance of the load medium (body tissue). The power dissipated through R_m corresponds to the acoustic output power from the transducer.

The mechanical inductance L_m and mechanical capacitance C_m are analogous to the inductance and capacitance of a mass-spring system. At the series resonant frequency of

$$f_s = \frac{1}{2\pi\sqrt{L_m C_m}} \qquad (67.10)$$

the impedances of these components add to zero, resulting in a local impedance minimum.

The equivalent circuit of Fig. 67.6a can be redrawn in the form shown in Fig. 67.6b. In this circuit, C_0 is the same as before, but the mechanical impedances have values of $L_m{}'$, $C_m{}'$, and R_a. The resistive component R_a is

$$R_a = \frac{4k^2}{\pi \omega C_0} \cdot \frac{Z_C}{Z_1 + Z_2} \qquad (67.11)$$

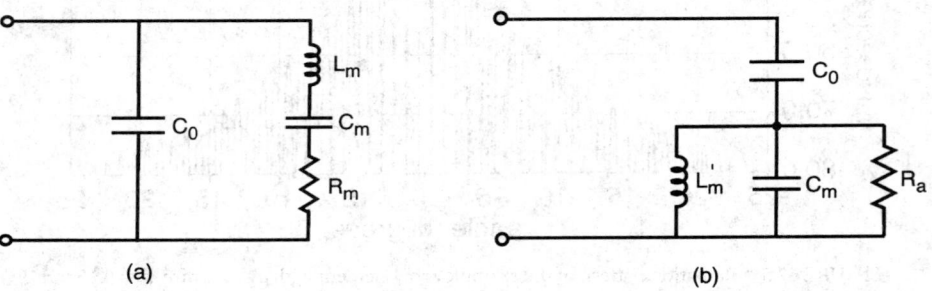

(a)   (b)

FIGURE 67.6 Simplified equivalent circuits for a piezoelectric transducer: (a) near-series resonance and (b) near-parallel resonance.

The inductor and capacitor combine to form an open circuit at the parallel resonant frequency of

$$f_p = \frac{1}{2\pi\sqrt{L_m'C_m'}} \tag{67.12}$$

The parallel resonance, which is at a slightly higher frequency than the series resonance, is indicated by a local impedance maximum.

Figure 67.7 shows a simulated plot of magnitude and phase versus frequency for the example array element described at the beginning of this subsection. The series resonant frequency is immediately identified at 5.0 MHz with an impedance minimum of $|Z| = 350\ \Omega$. Parallel resonance occurs at 6.7 MHz with an impedance maximum of $|Z| = 4000\ \Omega$. Note the capacitive behavior (approximately -90-degree phase) at frequencies far from resonance.

Designing a Phased-Array Transducer

In this subsection the design of an idealized phased-array transducer is considered in terms of the performance characteristics described above. Criteria are described for selecting array dimensions, acoustic backing and matching layers, and electrical matching networks.

Choosing Array Dimensions

The array element thickness is determined by the parallel resonant frequency. For $\lambda/2$ resonance, the thickness is

$$t = \frac{\lambda_t}{2} = \frac{c_t}{2f_p} \tag{67.13}$$

where c_t is the longitudinal speed of sound in the transducer material.

There are three constraints for choosing the element width and length: (1) a nearly square cross-section should be avoided so that lateral vibrations are not coupled to the thickness vibration; as a rule of thumb [Kino and DeSilets, 1979],

$$a/t \le 0.6 \quad\quad \text{or} \quad\quad a/t \ge 10 \tag{67.14}$$

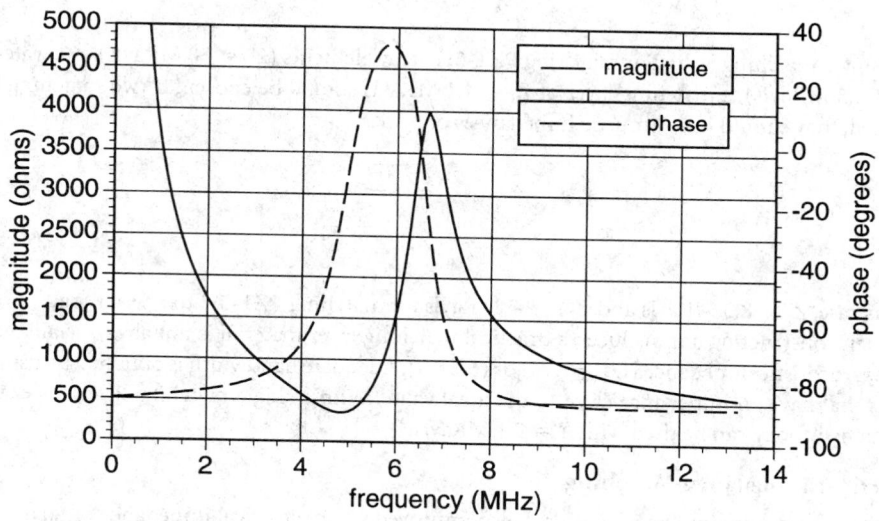

FIGURE 67.7 Complex electrical impedance of the example array element. Series resonance is located at 5.0 MHz, and parallel resonance is located at 6.7 MHz.

(2) a small width and length are also desirable for a wide angular response weighting function; and
(3) an interelement spacing of $\lambda/2$ or less is necessary to eliminate grating lobes.

Fortunately, these requirements are consistent for PZT array elements. For all forms of PZT, $c_t > 2c$, where c is the speed of sound in body tissue (an average of 1540 m/s). At a given frequency, then $\lambda_t > 2\lambda$. Also, Eq. (67.13) states that $\lambda_t = 2t$ at a frequency of f_p. By combining these equations, $t > \lambda$ for PZT array elements operating at a frequency of f_p. If $d = \lambda/2$, then $a < \lambda/2$ because of the finite kerf width that separates the elements. Given this observation, then $a < t/2$. This is consistent with Eq. (67.14) to reduce lateral modes.

An element having $d = \lambda/2$ also has adequate angular response. For illustrative purposes, one can assume a zero kerf width so that $a = \lambda/2$. In this case, the -6-dB angular response is $\theta_x = \pm 35$ degrees according to Eq. (67.6).

The array dimensions determine the transducer's lateral resolution. In the azimuth dimension, if $d = \lambda/2$, then the transducer aperture is $D = n\lambda/2$, where n is the number of elements in a fully sampled array. From Eq. (67.5), the lateral resolution in azimuth is

$$\theta_x = \sin^{-1}\frac{2}{n} \tag{67.15}$$

Therefore, the lateral resolution is independent of frequency in a fully sampled array with $d = \lambda/2$. For this configuration, the lateral resolution is improved by increasing the number of elements.

Acoustic Backing and Matching Layers

The backing and matching layers affect the transducer bandwidth and sensitivity. While a lossy, matched backing improves bandwidth, it also dissipates acoustic energy that could otherwise be transmitted into the tissue medium. Therefore, a low-impedance acoustic backing is preferred because it reflects the acoustic pulses toward the front side of the transducer. In this case, adequate bandwidth is maintained by acoustically matching the transducer to the tissue medium using matching layers.

Matching layers are designed with a thickness of $\lambda/4$ at the center frequency and an acoustic impedance between those of the transducer Z_T and the load medium Z_L. The ideal acoustic impedances can be determined from several different models [Hunt et al., 1983]. Using the KLM equivalent circuit model [Desilets et al., 1978], the ideal acoustic impedance is

$$Z_1 = \sqrt[3]{Z_T Z_L^2} \tag{67.16}$$

for a single matching layer. For matching PZT-5H array elements ($Z_T = 30$ MRayls) to a water load ($Z_L = 1.5$ MRayls), a matching layer of $Z_1 = 4.1$ MRayls should be chosen. If two matching layers are used, they should have acoustic impedances of

$$Z_1 = \sqrt[7]{Z_T^4 Z_L^3} \tag{67.17a}$$

$$Z_2 = \sqrt[7]{Z_T Z_L^6} \tag{67.17b}$$

In this case, $Z_1 = 8.3$ MRayls and $Z_2 = 2.3$ MRayls for matching PZT-5H to a water load.

When constructing a transducer, a practical matching layer material is not always available with the ideal acoustic impedance [Eq. (67.16) or (67.17)]. Adequate bandwidth is obtained by using materials that have an impedance close to the ideal value. With a single matching layer, for example, conductive epoxy can be used with $Z = 5.1$ MRayls.

Electrical Impedance Matching

Signal-to-noise ratio and bandwidth are also improved when electrical impedance of an array element is matched to that of the transmit circuitry. Consider the simplified circuit in Fig. 67.8 with a

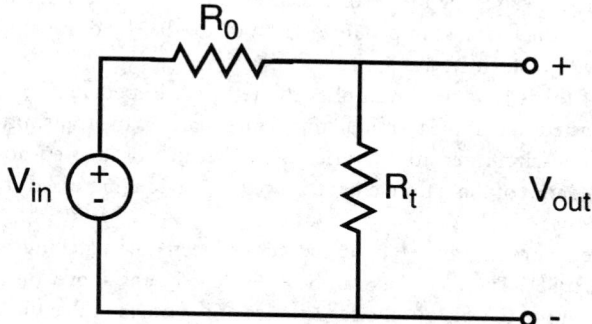

FIGURE 67.8 A transducer of real impedance R_t being excited by a transmitter with source impedance R_0 and source voltage V_{in}.

transmitter of impedance R_0 and a transducer of real impedance R_t. The power output is proportional to the power dissipated in R_t, expressed as

$$P_{out} = \frac{V_{out}^2}{R_t} \quad \text{where } V_{out} = \frac{R_t}{R_0 + R_t} V_{in} \tag{67.18}$$

The power available from the transmitter is

$$P_{in} = \frac{(V_{in}/2)^2}{R_0} \tag{67.19}$$

into a matched load. From the two previous equations, the power efficiency is

$$\frac{P_{out}}{P_{in}} = \frac{4R_0R_t}{(R_0 + R_t)^2} \tag{67.20}$$

For a fixed-source impedance, the maximum efficiency is obtained by taking the derivative of Eq. (67.20) with respect to R_t and setting it to zero. Maximum efficiency occurs when the source impedance is matched to the transducer impedance, $R_0 = R_t$.

In practice, the transducer has a complex impedance of R_m in parallel with C_0 (see Fig. 67.6), which is excited by a transmitter with a real impedance of 50 Ω. The transducer has a maximum efficiency when the imaginary component is tuned out and the real component is 50 Ω. This can be accomplished with electrical matching networks.

The capacitance C_0 is tuned out in the frequency range near ω_0 using an inductor of

$$L_0 = \frac{1}{\omega_0^2 C_0} \tag{67.21}$$

for an inductor in shunt, or

$$L_1 = \frac{1}{\omega_0^2 C_0 + 1/R_m^2 C_0} \tag{67.22}$$

for an inductor in series. The example array elements described in the preceding subsection have $C_0 = 22$ pF and $R_m = 340$ Ω at series resonance of 5.0 MHz. Therefore, tuning inductors of $L_0 = 46$ μH or $L_1 = 2.4$ μH should be used.

A shunt inductor also raises the impedance of the transducer, as seen from the scanner, while a series inductor lowers the terminal impedance [Hunt et al., 1983]. For more significant changes in terminal impedance, transformers are used.

A transformer of turns ratio $1:N$ multiplies the terminal impedance by $1/N^2$. In the transmit mode, N can be adjusted so that the terminal impedance matches the transmitter impedance. In the receive mode, the open-circuit sensitivity varies as $1/N$ because of the step-down transformer. The lower terminal impedance of the array element, however, provides increased ability to drive an electrical load.

More complicated circuits can be used for better electrical matching across a wide bandwidth [Hunt et al., 1983]. These circuits can be either passive, as above, or active. Inductors also can be used in the scanner to tune out the capacitance of the coaxial cable that loads the transducer on receive.

Another alternative for electrical matching is to use multilayer piezoelectric ceramics [Goldberg and Smith, 1994]. Figure 67.9 shows an example of a single layer and a five-layer array element with the same overall dimensions of a, b, and t. Since the layers are connected electrically in parallel, the clamped capacitance of a multilayer ceramic (MLC) element is

$$C_0 = N \cdot \varepsilon^S \cdot \frac{ab}{t/N} = N^2 \cdot C_{\text{single}} \tag{67.23}$$

where C_{single} is the capacitance of the single-layer element (Eq. 67.8). As a result, the MLC impedance is reduced by a factor of N^2. Acoustically, the layers of the MLC are in series so the $\lambda/2$ resonant thickness is t, the stack thickness.

To a first order, an N-layer ceramic has identical performance compared with a $1:N$ transformer, but the impedance is transformed within the ceramic. MLCs also can be fabricated in large quantities more easily than hand-wound transformers. While MLCs do not tune out the reactive impedance, they make it easier to tune a low capacitance array element. By lowering the terminal impedance of an array element, MLCs significantly improve transducer SNR.

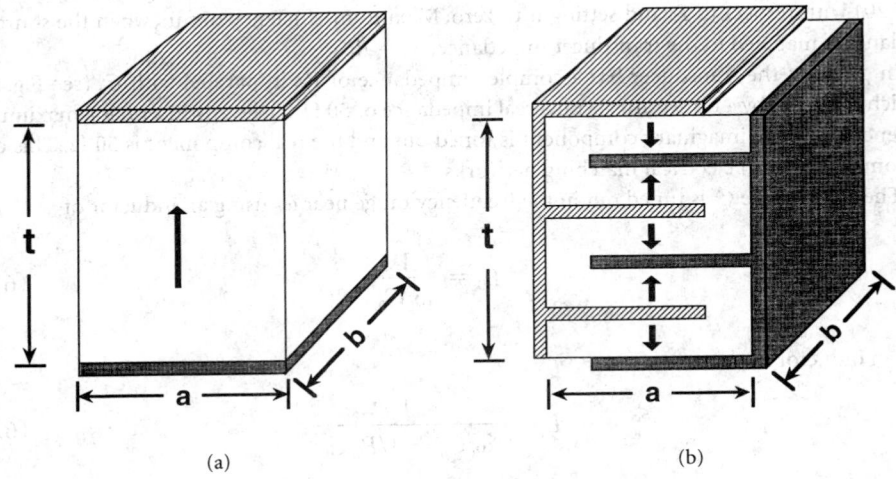

(a)   (b)

FIGURE 67.9 (*a*) Conventional single-layer ceramic; (*b*) five-layer ceramic of the same overall dimensions. The layers are electrically in parallel and acoustically in series. The arrows indicate the piezoelectric poling directions of each layer.

Summary

The piezoelectric transducer is an important component in the ultrasound imaging system. The transducer often consists of a linear array that can electronically focus an acoustic beam. Depending on the configuration of array elements, the region scanned may be sector shaped or rectangular in two dimensions or pyramidal shaped in three dimensions.

The transducer performance largely determines the resolution and the signal-to-noise ratio of the resulting ultrasound image. The design of an array involves many compromises in choosing operating frequency and array-element dimensions. Electrical matching networks and quarter-wave matching layers may be added to improve transducer performance.

Further improvements in transducer performance may result from several areas of research. Newer materials, such as composites, are gaining widespread use in medical ultrasound. In addition, 1.5D arrays or 2D arrays may be employed to control the acoustic beam in both azimuth and elevation. Problems in fabrication and electrical impedance matching must be overcome to implement these arrays in an ultrasound system.

Defining Terms

Acoustic impedance: In an analogy to transmission line impedance, the acoustic impedance is the ratio of pressure to particle velocity in a medium; more commonly, it is defined as $Z = \rho c$, where ρ = density and c = speed of sound in a medium [the units are kg/(m$^2 \cdot$ sec) or Rayls].

Angular response: The radiation pattern versus angle for a single element of an array.

Axial resolution: The ability to distinguish between targets aligned in the axial direction (the direction of acoustic propagation).

Azimuth dimension: The lateral dimension that is along the scanning plane for an array transducer.

Electrical matching networks: Active or passive networks designed to tune out reactive components of the transducer and/or match the transducer impedance to the source and receiver impedance.

Elevation dimension: The lateral dimension that is perpendicular to the scanning plane for an array transducer.

Grating lobes: Undesirable artifacts in the radiation pattern of a transducer; they are produced at a location where the path length difference to adjacent array elements is a multiple of a wavelength.

Lateral modes: Transducer vibrations that occur in the lateral dimensions when the transducer is excited in the thickness dimension.

Lateral resolution: The ability to distinguish between targets in the azimuth and elevation dimensions (perpendicular to the axial dimension).

Quarter-wave matching layers: One or more layers of material placed between the transducer and the load medium (water or human tissue); they effectively match the acoustic impedance of the transducer to the load medium to improve the transducer bandwidth and signal-to-noise ratio.

References

Allen JL. 1964. Array antennas: New applications for an old technique. IEEE Spect 1:115.

Berlincourt D. 1971. Piezoelectric crystals and ceramics. In OE Mattiat (ed), Ultrasonic Transducer Materials. New York, Plenum Press.

Bobber RJ. 1970. Underwater Electroacoustic Measurements. Washington, Naval Research Laboratory.

Christensen DA. 1988. Ultrasonic Bioinstrumentation. New York, Wiley.

Curie P, Curie J. 1880. Developpement par pression de l'electricite polaire dans les cristaux hemiedres a faces enclinees. Comp Rend 91:383.

Desilets CS, Fraser JD, Kino GS. 1978. The design of efficient broad-band piezoelectric transducers. IEEE Trans Son Ultrason SU-25:115.

Flax SW, O'Donnell M. 1988. Phase aberration correction using signals from point reflectors and diffuse scatters: Basic principles. IEEE Trans Ultrason Ferroelec Freq Contr 35:758.

Goldberg RL, Smith SW. 1994. Multi-layer piezoelectric ceramics for two-dimensional array transducers. IEEE Trans Ultrason Ferroelec Freq Contr

Goodman W. 1986. Introduction to Fourier Optics. New York, McGraw-Hill.

Hunt JW, Arditi M, Foster FS. 1983. Ultrasound transducers for pulse-echo medical imaging. IEEE Trans Biomed Eng 30:453.

Kino GS. 1987 Acoustic Waves. Englewood Cliffs, NJ, Prentice-Hall.

Kino GS, DeSilets CS. 1979. Design of slotted transducer arrays with matched backings. Ultrason Imag 1:189.

Nock LF, Trahey GE. 1992. Synthetic receive aperture imaging with phase correction for motion and for tissue inhomogeneities: I. Basic principles. IEEE Trans Ultrason Ferroelec Freq Contr 39:489.

Selfridge AR, Kino GS, Khuri-Yahub BT. 1980. A theory for the radiation pattern of a narrow strip acoustic transducer. Appl Phys Lett 37:35.

Shattuck DP, Weinshenker MD, Smith SW, von Ramm OT. 1984. Explososcan: A parallel processing technique for high speed ultrasound imaging with linear phased arrays. J Acoust Soc Am 75:1273.

Sherar MD, Foster FS. 1989. The design and fabrication of high frequency poly(vinylidene fluoride) transducers. Ultrason Imag 11:75.

Smith WA. 1992. New opportunities in ultrasonic transducers emerging from innovations in piezoelectric materials. In FL Lizzi (ed), New Developments in Ultrasonic Transducers and Transducer Systems, 3–26. New York, SPIE.

Somer JC. 1968. Electronic sector scanning for ultrasonic diagnosis. Ultrasonics 153.

Steinberg BD. 1976. Principles of Aperture and Array System Design. New York, Wiley.

Takeuchi H, Masuzawa H, Nakaya C, Ito Y. 1990. Relaxor ferroelectric transducers. Proc IEEE Ultrasonics Symposium, IEEE cat no 90CH2938-9, pp 697–705.

Trahey GE, Zhao D, Miglin JA, Smith SW. 1990. Experimental results with a real-time adaptive ultrasonic imaging system for viewing through distorting media. IEEE Trans Ultrason Ferroelec Freq Contr 37:418.

von Ramm OT, Smith SW. 1990. Real time volumetric ultrasound imaging system. In SPIE Medical Imaging IV: Image Formation, vol 1231, pp 15–22. New York, SPIE.

von Ramm OT, Thurstone FL. 1976. Cardiac imaging using a phased array ultrasound system: I. System design. Circulation 53:258.

Further Information

A good overview of linear array design and performance is contained in von O.T. Ramm and S.W. Smith (1983), Beam steering with linear arrays, *IEEE Trans Biomed Eng* 30:438. The same issue contains a more general article on transducer design and performance: J.W. Hunt, M. Arditi, and F.S. Foster (1983), Ultrasound transducers for pulse-echo medical imaging, *IEEE Trans Biomed Eng* 30:453.

The journal *IEEE Transactions on Ultrasonics, Ferroelectrics, and Frequency Control* frequently contains articles on medical ultrasound transducers. For subscription information, contact IEEE Service Center, 445 Hoes Lane, P.O. Box 1331, Piscataway, NJ 08855-1331, phone (800) 678-IEEE.

Another good source is the proceedings of the IEEE Ultrasonics Symposium, published each year. Also, the proceedings from *New Developments in Ultrasonic Transducers and Transducer Systems*, edited by F.L. Lizzi, was published by SPIE, Vol. 1733, in 1992.

67.2 Ultrasonic Imaging

Jack G. Mottley

It was recognized long ago that the tissues of the body are inhomogeneous and that signals sent into them, like pulses of high-frequency sound, are reflected and scattered by those tissues. Scattering, or redirection of some of an incident energy signal to other directions by small particles, is why we see the beam of a spotlight in fog or smoke. That part of the scattered energy that returns to the transmitter is called the backscatter.

Ultrasonic imaging of the soft tissues of the body really began in the early 1970s. At that time, the technologies began to become available to capture and display the echoes backscattered by structures within the body as images, at first as static compound images and later as real-time moving images. The development followed much the same sequence (and borrowed much of the terminology) as did radar and sonar, from initial crude single-line-of-sight displays (A-mode) to recording these side by side to build up recordings over time to show motion (M-mode), to finally sweeping the transducer either mechanically or electronically over many directions and building up two-dimensional views (B-mode or 2D).

Since this technology was intended for civilian use, applications had to wait for the development of inexpensive data handling, storage, and display technologies. A-mode was usually shown on oscilloscopes, M-modes were printed onto specially treated light-sensitive thermal paper, and B-mode was initially built up as a static image in analog scan converters and shown on television monitors. Now all modes are produced in real time in proprietary scan converters, shown on television monitors, and recorded either on commercially available videotape recorders (for organs or studies in which motion is a part of the diagnostic information) or as still frames on photographic film (for those cases in which organ dimensions and appearance are useful, but motion is not important).

Using commercial videotape reduces expenses and greatly simplifies the review of cases for quality control and training, since review stations can be set up in offices or conference rooms with commonly available monitors and videocassette recorders, and tapes from any imaging system can be played back. Also, the tapes are immediately available and do not have to be chemically processed.

Since the earliest systems were mostly capable of showing motion, the first applications were in studying the heart, which must move to carry out its function. A-mode and M-mode displays (see Figs. 67.10 through 67.12) were able to demonstrate the motion of valves, thickening of heart chamber walls, relationships between heart motion and pressure, and other parameters that enabled diagnoses of heart problems that had been difficult or impossible before. For some valvular diseases, the preferred display format for diagnosis is still the M-mode, on which the speed of valve motions can be measured and the relations of valve motions to the electrocardiogram (ECG) are easily seen.

Later, as 2D displays became available, ultrasound was applied more and more to imaging of the soft abdominal organs and in obstetrics (Fig. 67.13). In this format, organ dimensions and structural relations are seen more easily, and since the images are now made in real time, motions of organs such as the heart are still well appreciated. These images are used in a wide variety of areas from obstetrics and gynecology to ophthalmology to measure the dimensions of organs or tissue masses and have been widely accepted as a safe and convenient imaging modality.

Fundamentals

Strictly speaking, ultrasound is simply any sound wave whose frequency is above the limit of human hearing, which is usually taken to be 20 kHz. In the context of imaging of the human body, since frequency and wavelength (and therefore resolution) are inversely related, the lowest frequency of sound commonly used is around 1 MHz, with a constant trend toward higher frequencies in order to obtain better resolution. Axial resolution is approximately one wavelength, and at 1 MHz, the wavelength is 1.5 mm in most soft tissues, so one must go to 1.5 MHz to achieve 1-mm resolution.

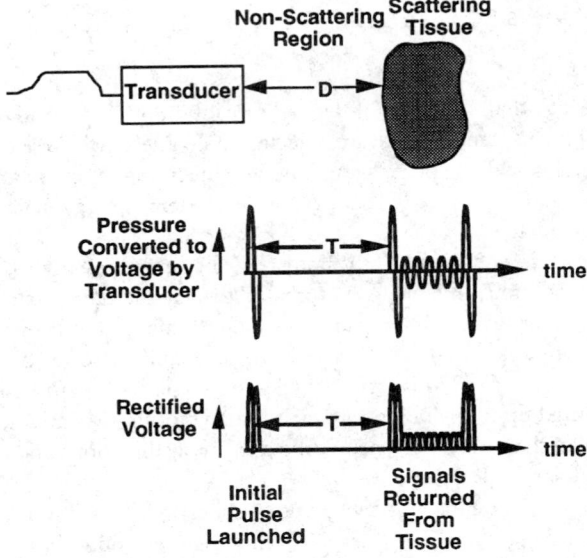

FIGURE 67.10 Schematic representation of the signal received from along a single line of sight in a tissue. The rectified voltage signals are displayed for A-mode.

Attenuation of ultrasonic signals increases with frequency in soft tissues, and so a tradeoff must be made between the depth of penetration that must be achieved for a particular application and the highest frequency that can be used. Applications that require deep penetration (e.g., cardiology, abdominal, obstetrics) typically use frequencies in the 2- to 5-MHz range, while those applications which only require shallow penetration but high resolution (e.g., ophthalmology, peripheral vascular, testicular) use frequencies up to around 20 MHz. Intraarterial imaging systems, requiring submillimeter resolution, use even higher frequencies of 20 to 50 MHz, and laboratory applications of ultrasonic microscopy use frequencies up to 100 or even 200 MHz to examine structures within individual cells.

There are two basic equations used in ultrasonic imaging. One relates the (one-way) distance d of an object that caused an echo from the transducer to the (round-trip) time delay t and speed of sound in the medium c:

$$d = \frac{1}{2}tc \tag{67.24}$$

The speed of sound in soft body tissues lies in a fairly narrow range from 1450 to 1520 m/s. For rough estimates of time of flight, one often uses 1500 m/s, which can be converted to 1.5 mm/μs, a more convenient set of units. This leads to delay times for the longest-range measurements (20 cm) of 270 μs. To allow echoes and reverberations to die out, one needs to wait several of these periods before launching the next interrogating pulse, so pulse repetition frequencies of about a kilohertz are possible.

The other equation relates the received signal strength $S(t)$ to the transmitted signal $T(t)$, the transducer's properties $B(t)$, the attenuation of the signal path to and from the scatterer $A(t)$, and the strength of the scatterer $\eta(t)$:

$$S(t) = T(t) \otimes B(t) \otimes A(t) \otimes \eta(t) \tag{67.25}$$

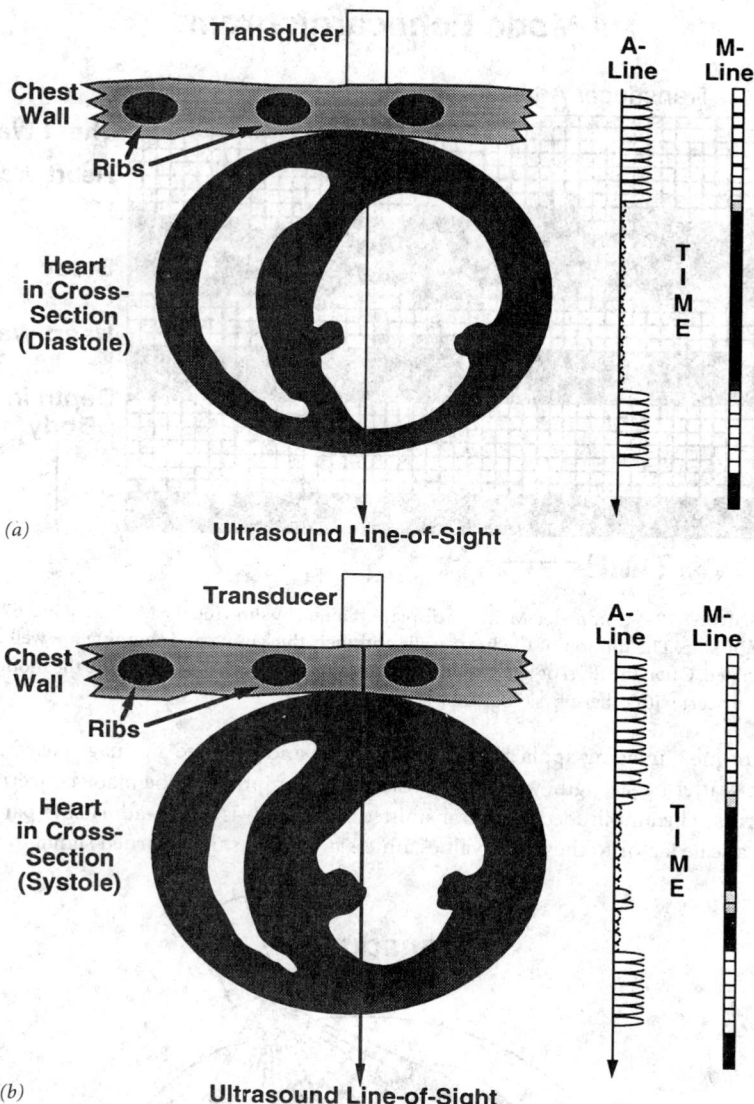

FIGURE 67.11 Example of M-mode imaging of a heart at two points during the cardiac cycle. (a) Upper panel shows heart during diastole (relaxation) with a line of sight through it and the corresponding A-line converted to an M-line. (b) The lower panel shows the same heart during systole (contraction) and the A- and M-lines. Note the thicker walls and smaller ventricular cross-section during systole.

where $\otimes$ denotes time-domain convolution. Using the property of Fourier transforms that a convolution in the time domain is a multiplication in the frequency domain, this is more often written in the frequency domain as

$$S(f) = T(f)B(f)A(f)\eta(f) \qquad (67.26)$$

where each term is the Fourier transform of the corresponding term in the time-domain expression (67.25) and is written as a function of frequency f.

M-Mode Echocardiogram

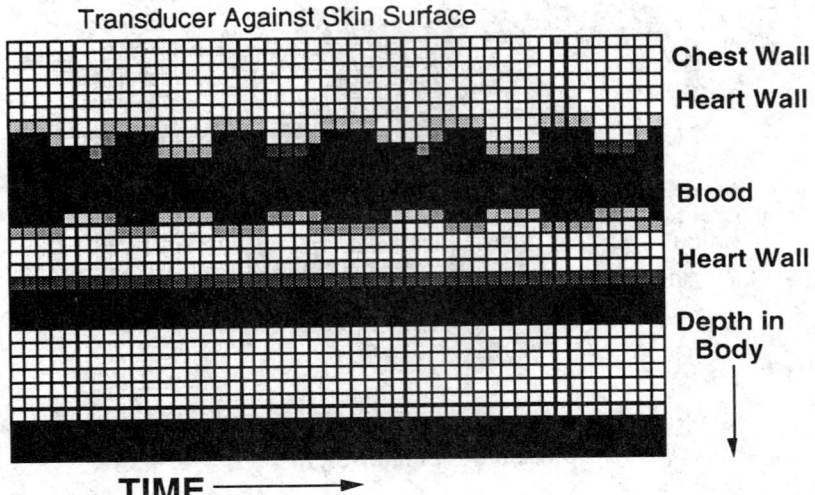

FIGURE 67.12 Completed M-mode display obtained by showing the M-lines of Fig. 67.11 side by side. The motion of the heart walls and their thickening and thinning are well appreciated. Often the ECG or heart sounds are also shown in order to coordinate the motions of the heart with other physiologic markers.

The goal of most imaging applications is to measure and produce an image based on the local values of the scattering strength, which requires some assumptions to be made concerning each of the other terms. The amplitude of the transmitted signal $T(f)$ is a user-adjustable parameter that simply adds a scale factor to the image values, unless it increases the returned signal to the point of

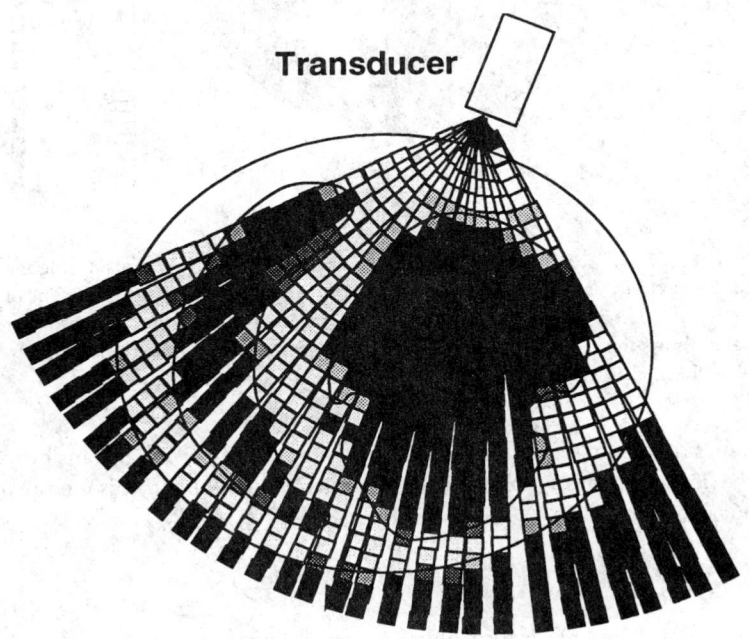

FIGURE 67.13 Schematic representation of a heart and how a 2D image is constructed by scanning the transducer.

saturating the receiver amplifier. Increasing the transmit power increases the strength of return from distant or faint echoes simply by increasing the power that illuminates them, like using a more powerful flashlight lets you see farther at night. Some care must be taken to not turn the transmit power up too high, since very high power levels are capable of causing acoustic cavitation or local heating of tissues, both of which can cause cellular damage. Advances in both electronics and transducers make it possible to transmit more and more power. For this reason, new ultrasonic imaging systems are required to display an index value that indicates the transmitted power. If the index exceeds established thresholds, it is possible that damage may occur, and the examiner should limit the time of exposure.

Most imaging systems are fairly narrow band, so the transducer properties $B(f)$ are constant and produce only a scale factor to the image values. On phased-array systems it is possible to change the depth of focus on both transmit and receive. This improves image quality and detection of lesions by matching the focusing characteristics of the transducer to best image the object in question, like focusing a pair of binoculars on a particular object.

As the ultrasonic energy travels along the path from transmitter to scatterer and back, attenuation causes the signal to decrease with distance. This builds up as a line integral from time 0 to time t as

$$A(f,t) = e^{-\int_0^t \alpha(f)c\,dt'}$$

An average value of attenuation can be corrected for electronically by increasing the gain of the imaging system as a function of time [variously called time gain compensation (TGC) or depth gain compensation (DGC)]. In addition, some systems allow for lateral portions of the image region to have different attenuation by adding a lateral gain compensation in which the gain is increased to either side of the center region of the image.

Time gain compensation is usually set to give a uniform gray level to the scattering along the center of the image. Most operators develop a "usual" setting on each machine, and if it becomes necessary to change those settings to obtain acceptable images on a patient, then that indicates that the patient has a higher attenuation or that there is a problem with the electronics, transducer, or acoustic coupling.

Applications and Example Calculations

As an example of calculating the time of flight of an ultrasonic image, consider the following.

Example 1. A tissue has a speed of sound $c = 1460$ m/s, and a given feature is 10 cm deep within. Calculate the time it will take an ultrasonic signal to travel from the surface to the feature and back.

Answer. $t = 2 \times (10\text{ cm})/(1460\text{ m/s}) = 137$ μs, where the factor of 2 is to account for the round trip the signal has to make (i.e., go in and back out.)

Example 2. Typical soft tissues attenuate ultrasonic signals at a rate of 0.5 dB/cm/MHz. How much attenuation would be suffered by a 3-MHz signal going through 5 cm of tissue and returning?

Answer. $a = 3\text{ MHz} \times (0.5\text{ dB/cm/MHz}) / (8.686\text{ dB/neper}) = 0.173$ neper/cm, $A(3\text{ MHz}, 5\text{ cm}) = e^{(-0.173\text{ neper/cm}) \times (5\text{ cm}) \times 2} = 0.177$.

Economics

Ultrasonic imaging has many economic advantages over other imaging modalities. The imaging systems are typically much less expensive than those used for other modalities and do not require special preparations of facilities such as shielding for x-rays or uniformity of magnetic field for MRI.

Most ultrasonic imaging systems can be rolled easily from one location to another, so one system can be shared among technicians or examining rooms or even taken to patients' rooms for critically ill patients.

There are minimal expendables used in ultrasonic examinations, mostly the coupling gel used to couple the transducer to the skin and videotape or film for recording. Transducers are reusable and amortized over many examinations. These low costs make ultrasonic imaging one of the least expensive modalities, far preferred over others when indicated. The low cost also means these systems can be a part of private practices and used only occasionally.

As an indication of the interest in ultrasonic imaging as an alternative to other modalities, in 1993, the *Wall Street Journal* reported that spending in the United States on MRI units was approximately $520 million, on CT units $800 million, and on ultrasonic imaging systems $1000 million, and that sales of ultrasound systems was growing at 15% annually [1].

Defining Terms

A-mode: The original display of ultrasound measurements, in which the amplitude of the returned echoes along a single line is displayed on an oscilloscope.

Attenuation: The reduction is signal amplitude that occurs per unit distance traveled. Some attenuation occurs in homogeneous media such as water due to viscous heating and other phenomena, but that is very small and is usually taken to be negligible over the 10- to 20-cm distances typical of imaging systems. In inhomogeneous media such as soft tissues, the attenuation is much higher and increases with frequency. The values reported for most soft tissues lie around 0.5 dB/cm/MHz.

Backscatter: That part of a scattered signal that goes back toward the transmitter of the energy.

B-mode or 2D: The current display mode of choice. This is produced by sweeping the transducer from side to side and displaying the strength of the returned echoes as bright spots in their geometrically correct direction and distance.

Compound images: Images built up by adding, or compounding, data obtained from a single transducer or multiple transducers swept through arcs. Often these transducers were not fixed to a single point of rotation but could be swept over a surface of the body like the abdomen in order to build up a picture of the underlying organs such as the liver. This required an elaborate position-sensing apparatus attached to the patient's bed or the scanner and that the organ in question be held very still throughout the scanning process, or else the image was blurred.

M-mode: Followed A-mode by recording the strength of the echoes as dark spots on moving light-sensitive paper. Objects that move, such as the heart, caused standard patterns of motion to be displayed, and a lot of diagnostic information such as valve closure rates, whether valves opened or closed completely, and wall thickness could be obtained from M-mode recordings.

Real-time images: Images currently made on ultrasound imaging systems by rapidly sweeping the transducer through an arc either mechanically or electronically. Typical images might have 120 scan lines in each image, each 20 cm long. Since each line has a time of flight of 267 µs, a single frame takes 120 × 267 µs = 32 ms. It is therefore possible to produce images at standard video frame rates (30 frames/sec, or 33.3 msec/frame).

Reflection: Occurs at interfaces between large regions (much larger than a wavelength) of media with differing acoustic properties such as density or compressibility. This is similar to the reflection of light at interfaces and can be either *total*, like a mirror, or *partial*, like a half-silvered mirror or the ghostlike reflection seen in a sheet of glass.

Scattering: Occurs when there are irregularities or inhomogeneities in the acoustic properties of a medium over distances comparable with or smaller than the wavelength of the sound. Scattering from objects much smaller than a wavelength typically increases with frequency (the blue-sky law in optics), while that from an object comparable to a wavelength is constant with frequency (why clouds appear white).

Reference

1. Naj AK. 1993. Industry focus: Big medical equipment makers try ultrasound market; cost-cutting pressures prompt shift away from more expensive devices. Wall Street Journal, November 30, p B-4.

Further Information

There are many textbooks that contain good introductions to ultrasonic imaging. *Physical Principles of Ultrasonic Diagnosis*, by P. N. Wells, is a classic, and there is a new edition of another classic, *Diagnostic Ultrasound: Principles, Instruments and Exercises*, 4th ed., by Frederick Kremkau. Books on medical imaging that contain introductions to ultrasonic imaging include *Medical Imaging Systems*, by Albert Macovski; *Principles of Medical Imaging*, by Kirk Shung, Michael Smith, and Benjamin Tsui; and *Foundations of Medical Imaging*, by Zang-Hee Cho, Joie P. Jones, and Manbir Singh.

The monthly journals *IEEE Transactions on Ultrasonics, Ferroelectrics, and Frequency Control* and *IEEE Transactions on Biomedical Engineering* often contain information and research reports on ultrasonic imaging. For subscription information, contact IEEE Service Center, 445 Hoes Lane, P.O. Box 1331, Piscataway, NJ 08855-1331, phone (800) 678-4333. Another journal that often contains articles on ultrasonic imaging is the *Journal of the Acoustical Society of America*. For subscription information, contact AIP Circulation and Fulfillment Division, 500 Sunnyside Blvd., Woodbury, NY 11797-2999, phone (800) 344-6908; e-mail: elecprod\@pinet.aip.org.

There are many journals that deal with medical ultrasonic imaging exclusively. These include *Ultrasonic Imaging*, the *Journal of Ultrasound in Medicine*, American Institute of Ultrasound in Medicine (AIUM), 14750 Switzer Lane, Suite 100, Laurel, MD 20707-5906, and the *Journal of Ultrasound in Medicine and Biology*, Elsevier Science, Inc., 660 White Plains Road, Tarrytown, NY 10591-5153, e-mail: esuk.usa@elsevier.com.

There are also specialty journals for particular medical areas, e.g., the *Journal of the American Society of Echocardiography*, that are available through medical libraries and are indexed in Index Medicus, Current Contents, Science Citation Index, and other databases.

67.3 Blood Flow Measurement Using Ultrasound

K. Whittaker Ferrara

In order to introduce the fundamental challenges of blood velocity estimation, a brief description of the unique operating environment produced by the ultrasonic system, intervening tissue, and the scattering of ultrasound by blood is provided. In providing an overview of the parameters that differentiate this problem from radar and sonar target estimation problems, an introduction to the fluid dynamics of the cardiovascular system is presented, and the requirements of specific clinical applications are summarized. An overview of blood flow estimation systems and their performance limitations is then presented. Next, an overview of the theory of moving target estimation, with its roots in radar and sonar signal processing, is provided. The application of this theory to blood velocity estimation is then reviewed, and a number of signal processing strategies that have been applied to this problem are considered. Areas of new research including three-dimensional (3D) velocity estimation and the use of ultrasonic contrast agents are described in the final section.

Fundamental Concepts

In blood velocity estimation, the goal is not simply to estimate the mean target position and mean target velocity. The goal instead is to measure the velocity profile over the smallest region possible and to repeat this measurement quickly and accurately over the entire target. Therefore, the joint optimization of spatial, velocity, and temporal resolution is critical. In addition to the mean velocity, diagnostically useful information is contained in the volume of blood flowing through various vessels, spatial variations in the velocity profile, and the presence of turbulence. While current methods have proven extremely valuable in the assessment of the velocity profile over an entire vessel, improved *spatial resolution* is required in several diagnostic situations. Improved *velocity resolution* is also desirable for a number of clinical applications. Blood velocity estimation algorithms implemented in current systems also suffer from a velocity ambiguity due to aliasing.

Unique Features of the Operating Environment

A number of features make blood flow estimation distinct from typical radar and sonar target estimation situations. The combination of factors associated with the beam formation system, properties of the intervening medium, and properties of the target medium lead to a difficult and unique operating environment. Figure 67.14 summarizes the operating environment of an ultrasonic blood velocity estimation system, and Table 67.2 summarizes the key parameters.

Beam Formation–Data Acquisition System. *The transducer bandwidth is limited.* Most current transducers are limited to a 50% to 75% fractional bandwidth due to their finite dimensions and a variety of electrical and mechanical properties. This limits the form of the transmitted signal. The transmitted pulse is typically a short pulse with a carrier frequency, which is the center frequency in the spectrum of the transmitted signal.

Federal agencies monitor four distinct intensity levels. These levels are *TASA, TASP, TPSA,* and *TPSP,* where *T* represents temporal, *S* represents spatial, *A* represents average, and *P* represents peak. Therefore, the use of long bursts requires a proportionate reduction in the transmitted peak power. This may limit the signal-to-noise ratio (SNR) obtained with a long transmitted burst due to the weak reflections from the complex set of targets within the body.

Intervening Medium. Acoustic windows, which are locations for placement of a transducer to successfully interrogate particular organs, are limited in number and size. Due to the presence of bone and air, the number of usable acoustic windows is extremely limited. The reflection of acoustic energy from bone is only 3 dB below that of a perfect reflector [Wells, 1977]. Therefore, transducers cannot typically surround a desired imaging site. In many cases, it is difficult to find a single small access window. This limits the use of inverse techniques.

Intervening tissue produces acoustic refraction and reflection. Energy is reflected at unpredictable angles.

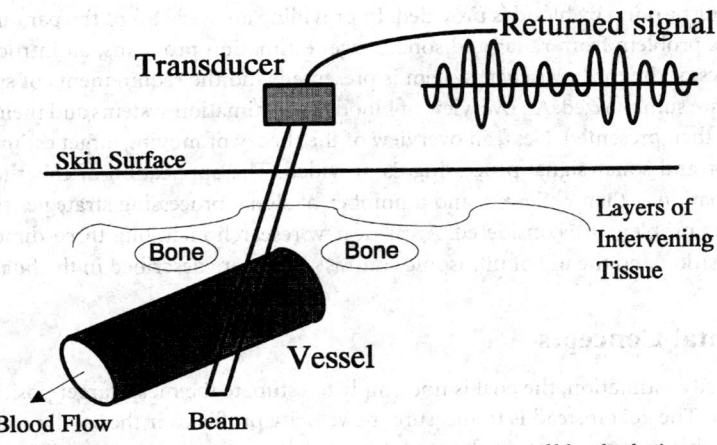

FIGURE 67.14 Operating environment for the estimation of blood velocity.

TABLE 67.2   Important Parameters

Typical transducer center frequency	2–10MHz
Maximum transducer fractional bandwidth	50–75%
Speed of sound c	1500–1600 m/s
Acoustic wavelength ($c = 1540$)	0.154–1.54 mm
Phased-array size	$>32 \cdot$ wavelength
Sample volume size	mm^3
Blood velocity	Normal: up to 1 m/s
	Pathological: up to 8 m/s
Vessel wall echo/blood echo	20–40 dB
Diameter of a red blood cell	8.5 μm
Thickness of a red blood cell	2.4 μm
Volume of a red blood cell	$87 \pm 6 \; \mu m^3$
Volume concentration of cells (hematocrit)	45%
Maximum concentration without cell deformation	58%

The clutter-to-signal ratio is very high. Clutter is the returned signal from stationary or slowly moving tissue, which can be 40 dB above the returned signal from blood. Movement of the vessel walls and valves during the cardiac cycle introduces a high-amplitude, low-frequency signal. This is typically considered to be unwanted noise, and a high-pass filter is used to eliminate the estimated wall frequencies.

The sampling rate is restricted. The speed of sound in tissue is low (approximately 1540 m/s), and each transmitted pulse must reach the target and return before the returned signal is recorded. Thus the sampling rate is restricted, and the aliasing limit is often exceeded.

The total observation time is limited (due to low acoustic velocity). In order to estimate the velocity of blood in all locations in a 2D field in real time, the estimate for each region must be based on the return from a limited number of pulses because of the low speed of sound.

Frequency-dependent attenuation affects the signal. Tissue acts as a low-pass transmission filter; the scattering functions as a high-pass filter. The received signal is therefore a distorted version of the transmitted signal. In order to estimate the effective filter function, the type and extent of each tissue type encountered by the wave must be known. Also, extension of the bandwidth of the transmitted signal to higher frequencies increases absorption, requiring higher power levels that can increase health concerns.

Target Scattering Medium (Red Blood Cells).   Multiple groups of scatterers are present. The target medium consists of multiple volumes of diffuse moving scatterers with velocity vectors that vary in magnitude and direction. The target medium is spread in space and velocity. The goal is to estimate the velocity over the smallest region possible.

There is a limited period of statistical stationarity. The underlying cardiac process can only be considered to be stationary for a limited time. This time was estimated to be 10 ms for the arterial system by Hatle and Angelsen [1985]. If an observation interval greater than this period is used, the average scatterer velocity cannot be considered to be constant.

Overview of Ultrasonic Flow Estimation Systems

Current ultrasonic imaging systems operate in a pulse-echo (PE) or continuous-wave (CW) intensity mapping mode. In pulse-echo mode, a very short pulse is transmitted, and the reflected signal is analyzed. For a continuous-wave system, a lower-intensity signal is continuously transmitted into the body, and the reflected energy is analyzed. In both types of systems, an acoustic wave is launched along a specific path into the body, and the return from this wave is processed as a function of time. The return is due to reflected waves from structures along the line of sight, combined with unwanted noise. Spatial selectivity is provided by beam formation performed on burst transmission and reception. Steering of the beam to a particular angle and creating a narrow beam width at the depth of interest are accomplished by an effective lens applied to the ultrasonic transducer. This lens may be produced by a contoured material, or it may be simulated by phased pulses applied to a transducer array. The spatial weighting pattern will ultimately be the product of the effective lens on transmission and reception. The returned signal from the formed beam can be used to map the backscattered intensity into a two-dimensional gray-scale image, or to estimate target velocity. *We shall focus on the use of this information to estimate the velocity of red blood cells moving through the body.*

Single Sample Volume Doppler Instruments.   One type of system uses the Doppler effect to estimate velocity in a single volume of blood, known as the sample volume, which is designated by the system operator. The Doppler shift frequency from a moving target can be shown to equal $2f_cv/c$, where f_c is the transducer center frequency in Hertz, c is the speed of sound within tissue, and v is the velocity component of the blood cells toward or away from the transducer. These "Doppler" systems transmit a train of long pulses with a well-defined carrier frequency and measure the Doppler shift in the returned signal. The spectrum of Doppler frequencies is proportional to the distribution of velocities present in the sample volume. The sample volume is on a cubic millimeter scale for typical pulse-echo systems operating in the frequency range of 2 to 10 MHz. Therefore, a thorough cardiac or peripheral vascular examination requires a long period. In these systems, 64 to 128 temporal samples are acquired for each estimate. The spectrum of these samples is typically computed using a fast Fourier transform (FFT) technique [Kay and Marple, 1981]. The range of velocities present within the sample volume can then be estimated. The spectrum is scaled to represent velocity and plotted on the vertical axis. Subsequent spectral estimates are then calculated and plotted vertically adjacent to the first estimate.

Color Flow Mapping.   In color flow mapping, a pseudo-color velocity display is overlaid on a 2D gray-scale image. Simultaneous amplitude and velocity information is thus available for a 2D sector area of the body. The clinical advantage is a reduction in the examination time and the ability to visualize the velocity profile as a 2D map. Figure 67.15 shows a typical color flow map of ovarian blood flow combined with the Doppler spectrum of the region indicated by the small graphic sample volume. The color flow map shows color-encoded velocities superimposed on the gray-scale image with the velocity magnitude indicated by the color bar on the side of the image. Motion toward the transducer is shown in yellow and red, and motion away from the transducer is shown in blue and green, with the range of colors representing a range of velocities to a maximum of 6 cm/s in each direction. Velocities above this limit would produce aliasing for the parameters used in optimizing the instrument for the display of ovarian flow. A velocity of 0 m/s would be indicated by

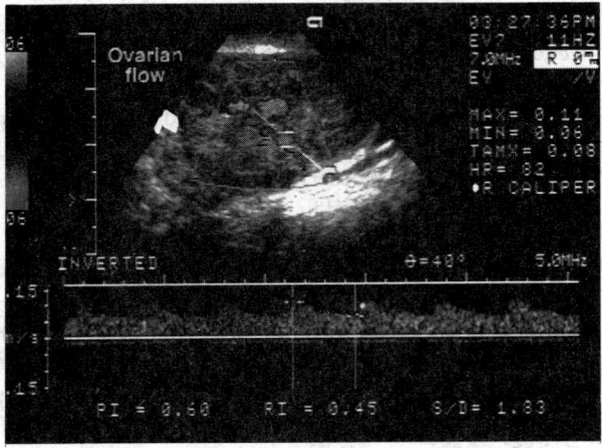

FIGURE 67.15 Flow map and Doppler spectrum for ovarian blood flow.

black, as shown at the center of the color bar. Early discussions of the implementation of color flow mapping systems can be found in Curry and White [1978] and Nowicki and Reid [1981].

The lower portion of the image presents an intensity-modulated display of instantaneous Doppler components along the vertical axis. As time progresses, the display is translated along the horizontal axis to generate a Doppler time history for the selected region of interest [provided by Acuson Corporation, Mountain View, Calif.].

Limitations of color flow instruments result in part from the transmission of a narrowband (long) pulse that is needed for velocity estimation but degrades spatial resolution and prevents mapping of the spatial-velocity profile. Due to the velocity gradient in each blood vessel, the transmission of a long pulse also degrades the velocity resolution. This is caused by the simultaneous examination of blood cells moving at different velocities and the resulting mixing of regions of the scattering medium, which can be distinctly resolved on a conventional B-mode image. Since the limited speed of acoustic propagation velocity limits the sampling rate, a second problem is aliasing of the Doppler frequency. Third, information regarding the presence of velocity gradients and turbulence is desired and is not currently available. Finally, estimation of blood velocity based on the Doppler shift provides only an estimate of the axial velocity, which is the movement toward or away from the transducer, and cannot be used to estimate movement across the transducer beam. It is the 3D velocity magnitude that is of clinical interest.

For a color flow map, the velocity estimation technique is based on estimation of the mean Doppler shift using signal-processing techniques optimized for rapid (real-time) estimation of velocity in each region of the image. The transmitted pulse is typically a burst of 4 to 8 cycles of the carrier frequency. Data acquisition for use in velocity estimation is interleaved with the acquisition of information for the gray-scale image. Each frame of acquired data samples is used to generate one update of the image display. An azimuthal line is a line that describes the direction of the beam from the transducer to the target. A typical 2D ultrasound scanner uses 128 azimuthal lines per frame and 30 frames per second to generate a gray-scale image. Data acquisition for the velocity estimator used in color flow imaging requires an additional 4 to 18 transducer firings per azimuthal line and therefore reduces both the number of azimuthal lines and the number of frames per second. If the number of lines per frame is decreased, spatial undersampling or a reduced examination area results. If the number of frames per second is decreased, temporal undersampling results, and the display becomes difficult to interpret.

The number of data samples available for each color flow velocity estimate is reduced to 4 to 18 in comparison with the 64 to 128 data samples available to estimate velocity in a single sample volume Doppler mode. This reduction, required to estimate velocity over the 2D image, produces a large increase in the estimator variance.

Fluid Dynamics and the Cardiovascular System

In order to predict and adequately assess blood flow profiles within the body, the fluid dynamics of the cardiovascular system will be briefly reviewed. The idealized case known as *Poiseuille flow* will be considered first, followed by a summary of the factors that disturb Poiseuille flow.

A Poiseuille flow model is appropriate in a long rigid circular pipe at a large distance from the entrance. The velocity in this case is described by the equation $v/v_0 = 1 - (r/a)^2$, where v represents the velocity parallel to the wall, v_0 represents the center-line velocity, r is the radial distance variable, and a is the radius of the tube. In this case, the mean velocity is half the center-line velocity, and the volume flow rate is given by the mean velocity multiplied by the cross-sectional area of the vessel.

For the actual conditions within the arterial system, Poiseuille flow is only an approximation. The actual arterial geometry is tortuous and individualistic, and the resulting flow is perturbed by entrance effects and reflections. Reflections are produced by vascular branches and the geometric taper of the arterial diameter. In addition, spatial variations in vessel elasticity influence the amplitude and wave velocity of the arterial pulse. Several parameters can be used to characterize the velocity profile, including the Reynolds number, the Womersly number, the pulsatility index, and the resistive index. The pulsatility and resistive indices are frequently estimated during a clinical examination.

The Reynolds number is denoted Re and measures the ratio of fluid inertia to the viscous forces acting on the fluid. The Reynolds number is defined by $\text{Re} = Dv'/\mu_k$, where v' is the average cross-sectional velocity, μ_k is the kinematic viscosity, and D is the vessel diameter. *Kinematic viscosity* is defined as the fluid viscosity divided by the fluid density. When the Reynolds number is high, fluid inertia dominates. This is true in the aorta and larger arteries, and bursts of turbulence are possible. When the number is low, viscous effects dominate.

The Womersly number is used to describe the effect introduced by the unsteady, pulsatile nature of the flow. This parameter, defined by $a(\omega/\mu_k)^{1/2}$, where ω represents radian frequency of the wave, governs propagation along an elastic, fluid-filled tube. When the Womersly number is small, the instantaneous profile will be parabolic in shape, the flow is viscous dominated, and the profile is oscillatory and Poiseuille in nature. When the Womersly number is large, the flow will be blunt, inviscid, and have thin wall layers [Nichols and O'Rourke, 1990].

The pulsatility index represents the ratio of the unsteady and steady velocity components of the flow. This shows the magnitude of the velocity changes that occur during acceleration and deceleration of blood constituents. Since the arterial pulse decreases in magnitude as it travels, this index is maximum in the aorta. The pulsatility index is given by the difference between the peak systolic and minimum diastolic values divided by the average value over one cardiac cycle. The Pourcelot, or resistance, index is the peak-to-peak swing in velocity from systole to diastole divided by the peak systolic value [Nichols and O'Rourke, 1990].

Blood Velocity Profiles. Specific factors that influence the blood velocity profile include the entrance effect, vessel curvature, skewing, stenosis, acceleration, secondary flows, and turbulence. These effects are briefly introduced in this subsection.

The entrance effect is a result of fluid flow passing from a large tube or chamber into a smaller tube. The velocity distribution at the entrance becomes blunt. At a distance known as the *entry length,* the fully developed parabolic profile is restored, where the entry length is given by 0.06Re · (2a) [Nerem, 1985]. Distal to this point the profile is independent of distance.

If the vessel is curved, there will also be an entrance effect. The blunt profile in this case is skewed, with the peak velocity closer to the inner wall of curvature. When the fully developed profile occurs downstream, the distribution will again be skewed, with the maximal velocity toward the outer wall of curvature. Skewing also occurs at a bifurcation where proximal flow divides into daughter vessels. The higher-velocity components, which occurred at the center of the parent vessel, are then closer to the flow divider, and the velocity distribution in the daughter vessels is skewed toward the divider.

Stenosis, a localized narrowing of the vessel diameter, dampens the pulsatility of the flow and pressure waveforms. The downstream flow profile depends on the shape and degree of stenosis. Acceleration adds a flat component to the velocity profile. It is responsible for the flat profile during systole, as well as the negative flat component near the walls in the deceleration phase.

Secondary flows are swirling components which are superimposed on the main velocity profile. These occur at bends and branches, although regions of secondary flow can break away from the vessel wall and are then known as *separated flow*. These regions reattach to the wall at a point downstream.

One definition of turbulent flow is flow that demonstrates a random fluctuation in the magnitude and direction of velocity as a function of space and time. The intensity of turbulence is calculated using the magnitude of the fluctuating velocities. The relative intensity of turbulence is given by $I_t = u_{rms}/u_{mean}$, where u_{rms} represents the root-mean-square value of the fluctuating portion of the velocity, and u_{mean} represents the nonfluctuating mean velocity [Hinze, 1975].

Clinical Applications and Their Requirements

Blood flow measurement with ultrasound is used in estimating the velocity and volume of flow within the heart and peripheral arteries and veins. Normal blood vessels vary in diameter up to a maximum of 2 cm, although most vessels examined with ultrasound have a diameter of 1 to 10 mm. Motion of the vessel wall results in a diameter change of 5% to 10% during a cardiac cycle.

Carotid Arteries (Common, Internal, External). The evaluation of flow in the carotid arteries is of great clinical interest due to their importance in supplying blood to the brain, their proximity to the skin, and the wealth of experience that has been developed in characterizing vascular pathology through an evaluation of flow. The size of the carotid arteries is moderate; they narrow quickly from a maximum diameter of 0.8 cm. The shape of carotid flow waveforms over the cardiac cycle can be related to the pathophysiology of the circulation. Numerous attempts have been made to characterize the parameters of carotid waveforms and to compare these parameters in normal and stenotic cases. A number of indices have been used to summarize the information contained in these waveforms. The normal range of the Pourcelot index is 0.55 to 0.75. Many researchers have shown that accurate detection of a minor stenosis requires accurate quantitation of the entire Doppler spectrum and remains very difficult with current technology. The presence of a stenosis causes spectral broadening with the introduction of lower frequency or velocity components.

Cardiology. Blood velocity measurement in cardiology requires analysis of information at depths up to 18 cm. A relatively low center frequency (e.g., 2.5 to 3.5 MHz) typically is used in order to reduce attenuation. Areas commonly studied and the maximum rate of flow include the following [Hatle, 1985]:

Normal Adult Maximal Velocity (m/s)

Mitral flow	0.9
Tricuspid flow	0.5
Pulmonary artery	0.75
Left ventricle	0.9

Aorta. Aortic flow exhibits a blunt profile with entrance region characteristics. The entrance length is approximately 30 cm. The vessel diameter is approximately 2 cm. The mean Reynolds number is 2500 [Nerem, 1985], although the peak Reynolds number in the ascending aorta can range from 4300 to 8900, and the peak Reynolds number in the abdominal aorta is in the range of 400 to 1100 [Nichols and O'Rourke, 1990]. The maximal velocity is on the order of 1.35 m/s. The flow is skewed in the aortic arch with a higher velocity at the inner wall. The flow is unsteady and laminar with possible turbulent bursts at peak systole.

Peripheral Arteries [Hatsukami et al., 1992]. The peak systolic velocity in centimeters per second and standard deviation of the velocity measurement technique are provided below for selected arteries.

Artery	Peak Systolic Velocity (cm/s)	Standard Deviation
Proximal external iliac	99	22
Distal external iliac	96	13
Proximal common femoral	89	16
Distal common femoral	71	15
Proximal popliteal	53	9
Distal popliteal	53	24
Proximal peroneal	46	14
Distal peroneal	44	12

Nearly all the vessels above normally show some flow reversal during early diastole. A value of the pulsatility index of 5 or more in a limb artery is considered to be normal.

Velocity Estimation Techniques

Prior to the basic overview of theoretical approaches to target velocity estimation, it is necessary to understand a few basic features of the received signal from blood scatterers. It is the statistical correlation of the received signal in space and time that provides the opportunity to use a variety of velocity estimation strategies. Velocity estimation based on analysis of the frequency shift or the temporal correlation can be justified by these statistical properties.

Blood velocity mapping has unique features due to the substantial viscosity of blood and the spatial limitations imposed by the vessel walls. Because of these properties, groups of red blood cells can be tracked over a significant distance. Blood consists of a viscous incompressible fluid containing an average volume concentration of red blood cells of 45%, although this concentration varies randomly through the blood medium. The red blood cells are primarily responsible for producing the scattered wave, due to the difference in their acoustic properties in comparison with plasma. Recent research into the characteristics of blood has led to stochastic models for its properties as a function of time and space [Angelson, 1980; Atkinson and Berry, 1974; Mo and Cobbold, 1986; Shung et al., 1976, 1992]. The scattered signal from an insonified spatial volume is a random process that varies with the fluctuations in the density of scatterers in the insonified area, the shear rate within the vessel, and the hematocrit [Atkinson and Berry, 1974; Ferrara and Algazi, 1994a, 1994b; Mo and Cobbold, 1986].

Since the concentration of cells varies randomly through the vessel, the magnitude of the returned signal varies when the group of scatterers being insonified changes. The returned amplitude from one spatial region is independent of the amplitude of the signal from adjacent spatial areas. As blood flows through a vessel, it transports cells whose backscattered signals can be tracked to estimate flow velocities.

Between the transmission of one pulse and the next, the scatterers move a small distance within the vessel. As shown in Fig. 67.16, a group of cells with a particular concentration which are originally located at depth D_1 at time T_1 move to depth D_2 at time T_2. The resulting change in axial depth produces a change in the delay of the signal returning to the transducer from each group of scatter-

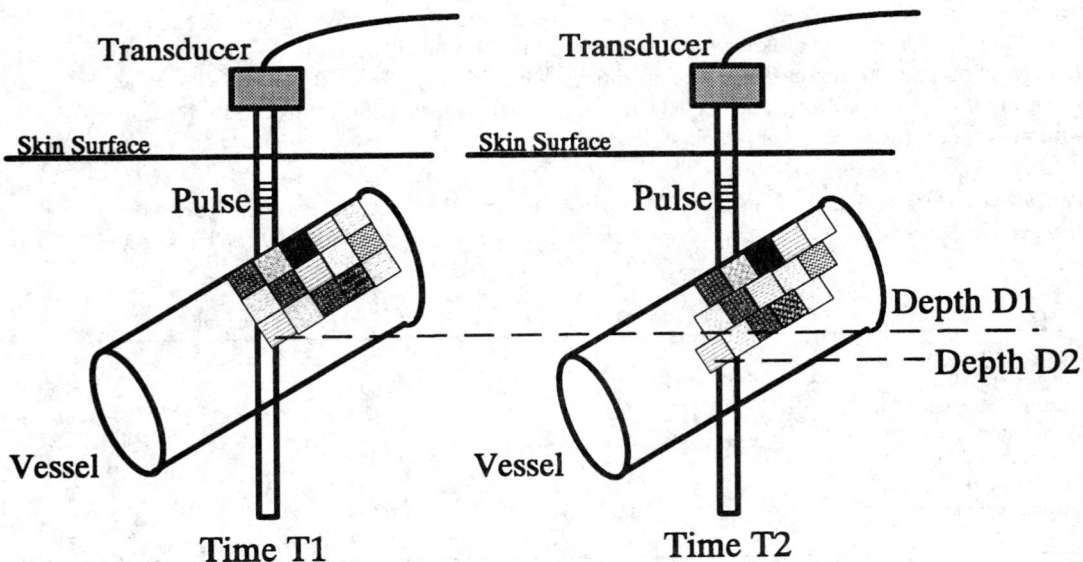

FIGURE 67.16   Random concentration of red blood cells within a vessel at times T_1 and T_2, where the change in depth from $D_{;1}$ to D_2 would be used to estimate velocity.

ers. This change in delay of the radiofrequency (RF) signal can be estimated in several ways. As shown in Fig. 67.17, the returned signal from a set of sequential pulses then shows a random amplitude that can be used to estimate the velocity. Motion is detected using signal-processing techniques that estimate the shift of the signal between pulses.

Clutter. In addition to the desired signal from the blood scatterers, the received signal contains clutter echoes returned from the surrounding tissue. An important component of this clutter signal arises from slowly moving vessel walls. The wall motion produces Doppler frequency shifts typically below 1 kHz, while the desired information from the blood cells exists in frequencies up to 15 kHz. Due to the smooth structure of the walls, energy is scattered coherently, and the clutter signal can be 40 dB above the scattered signal from blood. High-pass filters have been developed to remove the unwanted signal from the surrounding vessel walls.

Classic Theory of Velocity Estimation. Most current commercial ultrasound systems transmit a train of long pulses with a carrier frequency of 2 to 10 MHz and estimate velocity using the Doppler shift of the reflected signal. The transmission of a train of short pulses and new signal-processing strategies may improve the spatial resolution and quality of the resulting velocity estimate. In order to provide a basis for discussion and comparison of these techniques, the problem of blood velocity estimation is considered in this subsection from the view of classic velocity estimation theory typically applied to radar and sonar problems.

Important differences exist between classic detection and estimation for radar and sonar and the application of such techniques to medical ultrasound. The Van Trees [1971] approach is based on joint estimation of the Doppler shift and position over the entire target. In medical ultrasound, the velocity is estimated in small regions of a large target, where the target position is assumed to be known. While classic theories have been developed for estimation of all velocities within a large target by Van Trees and others, such techniques require a model for the velocity in each spatial region of interest. For the case of blood velocity estimation, the spatial variation in the velocity profile is complex, and it is difficult to postulate a model that can be used to derive a high-quality estimate.

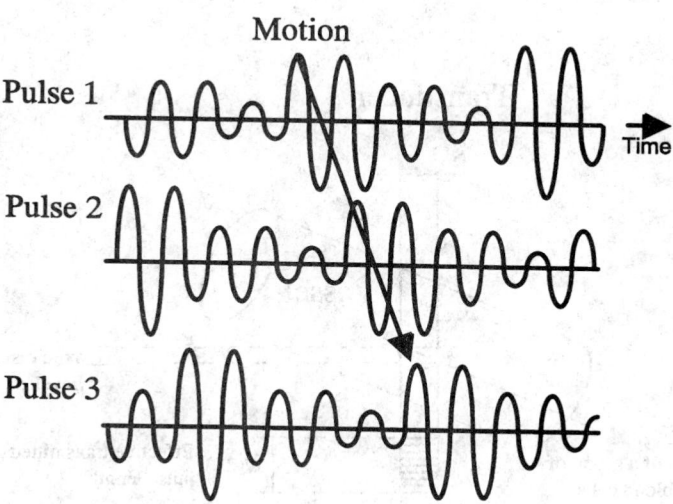

FIGURE 67.17 Received RF signal from three transmitted pulses, with a random amplitude which can be used to estimate the axial movement of blood between pulses. Motion is shown by the shift in the signal with a recognizable amplitude.

The theory of velocity estimation in the presence of spread targets is also discussed by Kennedy [1969] and Price [1968] as it applies to radar astronomy and dispersive communication channels.

It is the desire to improve the spatial and velocity resolution of the estimate of blood velocity that has motivated the evaluation of alternative wideband estimation techniques. Narrowband velocity estimation techniques use the Doppler frequency shift produced by the moving cells with a sample volume that is fixed in space. Wideband estimation techniques incorporate the change in delay of the returned pulse due to the motion of the moving cells. Within the classification of narrowband techniques are a number of estimation strategies to be detailed below. These include the fast Fourier transform (FFT), finite derivative estimation, the autocorrelator, and modern spectral estimation techniques, including autoregressive strategies. Within the classification of wideband techniques are cross-correlation strategies and the wideband maximum likelihood estimator (WMLE).

For improving the spatial mapping of blood velocity within the body, the transmission of short pulses is desirable. Therefore, it is of interest to assess the quality of velocity estimates made using narrowband and wideband estimators with transmitted signals of varying lengths. If $(2v/c)BT \ll 1$, where v represents the axial velocity of the target, c represents the speed of the wave in tissue, B represents the transmitted signal bandwidth, and T represents the total time interval used in estimating velocity within an individual region, then the change in delay produced by the motion of the red blood cells can be ignored [Van Trees, 1971].

This inequality is interpreted for the physical conditions of medical ultrasound in Fig. 67.18. As shown in Fig. 67.18, the value vT represents the axial distance traveled by the target while it is observed by the transducer beam, and $c/(2B)$ represents the effective length of the signal that is used to observe the moving cells. If $vT \ll c/(2B)$, the shift in the position of a group of red blood cells during their travel though the ultrasonic beam is not a detectable fraction of the signal length. This leads to two important restrictions on estimation techniques. First, under the "narrowband" condition of transmission of a long (narrowband) pulse, motion of a group of cells through the beam can only be estimated using the Doppler frequency shift. Second, if the inequality is not satisfied and therefore the transmitted signal is short (wideband), faster-moving red blood cells leave the region of interest, and the use of a narrowband estimation technique produces a biased velocity estimate. Thus two strategies can be used to estimate velocity. A long (narrowband) pulse can be transmitted, and the signal from a fixed depth then can be used to estimate velocity. Alternatively, a short (wide-

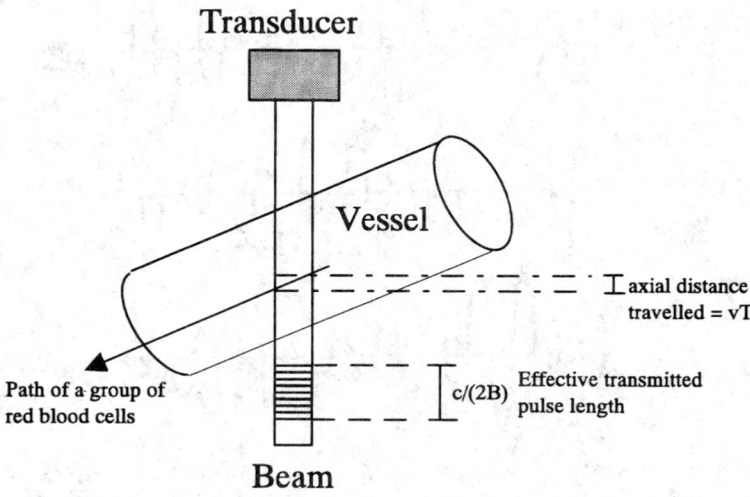

FIGURE 67.18   Comparison of the axial distance traveled and the effective length of the transmitted pulse.

band) signal can be transmitted in order to improve spatial resolution, and the estimator used to determine the velocity must move along with the red blood cells.

The inequality is now evaluated for typical parameters. When the angle between the axis of the beam and the axis of the vessel is 45 degrees, the axial distance traveled by the red blood cells while they cross the beam is equivalent to the lateral beam width. Using an axial distance vT of 0.75 mm, which is a reasonable lateral beam width, and an acoustic velocity of 1540 m/s, the bandwidth of the transmitted pulse must be much less than 1.026 MHz for the narrowband approximation to be valid.

Due to practical advantages in the implementation of the smaller bandwidth required by baseband signals, the center frequency of the signal is often removed before velocity estimation. The processing required for the extraction of the baseband signal is shown in Fig. 67.19. The returned signal from the transducer is amplified and coherently demodulated, through multiplication by the carrier frequency, and then a low-pass filter is applied to remove the signal sideband frequencies and noise. The remaining signal is the complex envelope. A high-pass filter is then applied to the signal from each fixed depth to remove the unwanted echoes from stationary tissue. The output of this processing is denoted as $I_k(t)$ for the in-phase signal from the kth pulse as a function of time and $Q_k(t)$ for the quadrature signal from the kth pulse.

Narrowband Estimation

Narrowband estimation techniques that estimate velocity for blood at a fixed depth are described in this subsection. Both the classic Doppler technique, which frequently is used in single-sample volume systems, and the autocorrelator, which frequently is used in color flow mapping systems, are included, as well as a finite derivative estimator and an autoregressive estimator, which have been the subject of previous research. The autocorrelator is used in real-time color flow mapping systems due to the ease of implementation and the relatively small bias and variance.

Classic Doppler Estimation. If the carrier frequency is removed by coherently demodulating the signal, the change in delay of the RF signal becomes a change in the phase of the baseband signal. The Doppler shift frequency from a moving target equals $2f_cv/c$. With a center frequency of 5 MHz, sound velocity of 1540 m/s, and blood velocity of 1 m/s, the resulting frequency shift is 6493.5 Hz. For the estimation of blood velocity, the Doppler shift is not detectable using a single short pulse, and therefore, the signal from a fixed depth and a train of pulses is acquired.

A pulse-echo Doppler processing block diagram is shown in Fig. 67.20. The baseband signal, from Fig. 67.19, is shown as the input to this processing block. The received signal from each pulse is multiplied by a time window that is typically equal to the length of the transmitted pulse and integrated to produce a single data sample from each pulse. The set of data samples from a train of pulses is then Fourier-transformed, with the resulting frequency spectrum related to the axial velocity using the Doppler relationship.

Estimation of velocity using the Fourier transform of the signal from a fixed depth suffers from the limitations of all narrowband estimators, in that the variance of the estimate increases when a

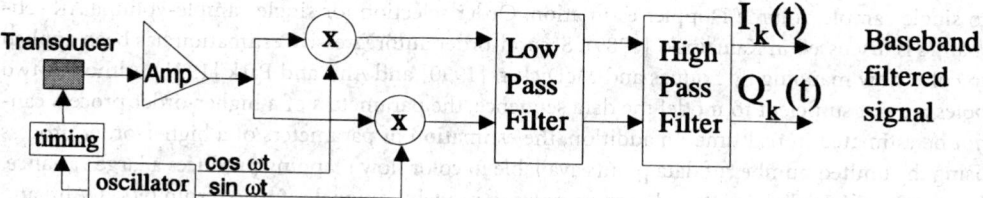

FIGURE 67.19 Block diagram of the system architecture required to generate the baseband signal used by several estimation techniques.

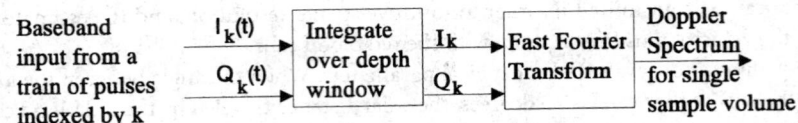

FIGURE 67.20   Block diagram of the system architecture required to estimate the Doppler spectrum from a set of baseband samples from a fixed depth.

short pulse is transmitted. In addition, the velocity resolution produced using the Fourier transform is inversely proportional to the length of the data window. Therefore, if 64 pulses with a pulse repetition frequency of 5 kHz are used in the spectral estimate, the frequency resolution is on the order of 78.125 Hz (5000/64). The velocity resolution for a carrier frequency of 5 MHz and speed of sound of 1540 m/s is then on the order of 1.2 cm/s, determined from the Doppler relationship. Increasing the data window only improves the velocity resolution if the majority of the red blood cells have not left the sample volume and the flow conditions have not produced a decorrelation of the signal. It is this relationship between the data window and velocity resolution, a fundamental feature of Fourier transform techniques, that has motivated the use of autoregressive estimators. The frequency and velocity resolution are not fundamentally constrained by the data window using these modern spectral estimators introduced below.

Autoregressive Estimation (AR).   In addition to the classic techniques discussed previously, higher-order modern spectral estimation techniques have been used in an attempt to improve the velocity resolution of the estimate. These techniques are again narrowband estimation techniques, since the data samples used in computing the estimate are obtained from a fixed depth. The challenges encountered in applying such techniques to blood velocity estimation include the selection of an appropriate order which adequately models the data sequence while providing the opportunity for real-time velocity estimation and determination of the length of the data sequence to be used in the estimation process.

The goal in autoregressive velocity estimation is to model the frequency content of the received signal by a set of coefficients which could be used to reconstruct the signal spectrum. The coefficients $a(m)$ represent the AR parameters of the $AR(p)$ process, where p is the number of poles in the model for the signal. Estimation of the AR parameters has been accomplished using the Burg and Levinson-Durban recursion methods. The spectrum $P(f)$ is then estimated using the following equation:

$$P(f) = k \left| 1 + \sum_{m=1}^{p} a(m) \exp\left[-i2\pi mf\right] \right|^{-2}$$

The poles of the AR transfer function which lie within the unit circle can then be determined based on these parameters, and the velocity associated with each pole is determined by the Doppler equation.

Both autoregressive and autoregressive moving-average estimation techniques have been applied to single-sample-volume Doppler estimation. Order selection for single-sample-volume AR estimators is discussed in Kaluzinski [1989]. Second-order autoregressive estimation has been applied to color flow mapping by Loupas and McDicken [1990] and Ahn and Park [1991]. Although two poles are not sufficient to model the data sequence, the parameters of a higher-order process cannot be estimated in real time. In addition, the estimation of parameters of a higher-order process using the limited number of data points available in color flow mapping produces a large variance. Loupas and McDicken have used the two poles to model the signal returned from blood. Ahn and Park have used one pole to model the received signal from blood and the second pole to model the stationary signal from the surrounding tissue.

While AR techniques are useful in modeling the stationary tissue and blood and in providing a high-resolution estimate of multiple velocity components, several problems have been encountered in the practical application to blood velocity estimation. First, the order required to adequately model any region of the vessel can change when stationary tissue is present in the sample volume or when the range of velocity components in the sample volume increases. In addition, the performance of an AR estimate degrades rapidly in the presence of white noise, particularly with a small number of data samples.

Autocorrelator. Kasai et al. [1985] and Barber et al. [1985] discussed a narrowband *mean* velocity estimation structure for use in color flow mapping. The phase of the signal correlation at a lag of one transmitted period is estimated and used in an inverse tangent calculation of the estimated mean Doppler shift f_{mean} of the returned signal. A block diagram of the autocorrelator is shown in Fig. 67.21. The baseband signal is first integrated over a short depth window. The phase of the correlation at a lag of one pulse period is then estimated as the inverse tangent of the imaginary part of the correlation divided by the real part of the correlation. The estimated mean velocity v_{mean} of the scattering medium is then determined by scaling the estimated Doppler shift by several factors, including the expected center frequency of the returned signal.

The autocorrelator structure can be derived from the definition of instantaneous frequency, from the phase of the correlation at a lag of one period, or as the first-order autoregressive estimate of the mean frequency of a baseband signal. The contributions of uncorrelated noise should average to zero in both the numerator and denominator of the autocorrelator. This is an advantage because the autocorrelation estimate is unbiased when the input signal includes the desired flow signal and noise. Alternatively, in the absence of a moving target, the input to the autocorrelator may consist only of white noise. Under these conditions, both the numerator and denominator can average to values near zero, and the resulting output of the autocorrelator has a very large variance. This estimation structure must therefore be used with a power threshold that can determine the presence or absence of a signal from blood flow and set the output of the estimator to zero when this motion is absent.

The variance of the autocorrelation estimate increases with the transmitted bandwidth, and therefore, the performance is degraded by transmitting a short pulse.

Finite Derivative Estimator (FDE). A second approach to mean velocity or frequency estimation is based on a finite implementation of a derivative operator. The *finite derivative* estimator is derived based on the first and second moments of the spectrum. The basis for this estimator comes from the definition of the spectral centroid:

$$v_{mean} = \frac{\int \omega S(\omega)\, d\omega}{\int S(\omega)\, d\omega} \tag{67.27}$$

The mean velocity is given by v_{mean}, which is a scaled version of the mean frequency, where the scaling constant is given by k', and $S(\omega)$ represents the power spectral density. Letting $R_r(\cdot)$ represent the complex signal correlation and τ represent the difference between the two times used in the correlation estimate, Eq. (67.27) is equivalent to

$$v_{mean} = k' \frac{\left[\dfrac{\partial}{\partial \tau} R_r(\tau) \Big|_{\tau=0} \right]}{R_r(0)} \tag{67.28}$$

Writing the baseband signal as the sum $I(t) + jQ(t)$ and letting E indicate the statistical expectation, Brody and Meindl [1974] have shown that the mean velocity estimate can be rewritten as

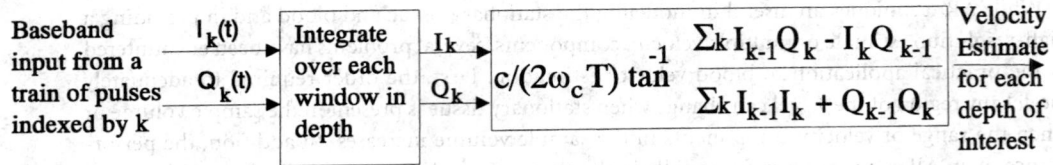

Baseband input from a train of pulses indexed by k → $I_k(t)$, $Q_k(t)$ → **Integrate over each window in depth** → I_k, Q_k → $c/(2\omega_c T)\,\tan^{-1}\dfrac{\sum_k I_{k-1}Q_k - I_k Q_{k-1}}{\sum_k I_{k-1}I_k + Q_{k-1}Q_k}$ → **Velocity Estimate for each depth of interest**

FIGURE 67.21 Block diagram of the system architecture required to estimate the mean Doppler shift for each depth location using the autocorrelator.

$$v_{mean} = \frac{k'\, E\left\{\frac{\partial}{\partial t}[I(t)]Q(t) - \frac{\partial}{\partial t}[Q(t)]I(t)\right\}}{E[I^2(t) + Q^2(t)]} \tag{67.29}$$

The estimate of this quantity requires estimation of the derivative of the in-phase portion $I(t)$ and quadrature portion $Q(t)$ of the signal. For an analog, continuous-time implementation, the bias and variance were evaluated by Brody and Meindl [1974]. The discrete case has been studied by Kristoffersen [1986]. The differentiation has been implemented in the discrete case as a finite difference or as a finite impulse response differentiation filter. The estimator is biased by noise, since the denominator represents power in the returned signal. Therefore, for nonzero noise power, the averaged noise power in the denominator will not be zero mean and will constitute a bias. The variance of the finite derivative estimator depends on the shape and bandwidth of the Doppler spectrum, as well as on the observation interval.

Wideband Estimation Techniques

It is desirable to transmit a short ultrasonic pulse in order to examine blood flow in small regions individually. For these short pulses, the narrowband approximation is not valid, and the estimation techniques used should track the motion of the red blood cells as they move to a new position over time. Estimation techniques that track the motion of the red blood cells are known as *wideband estimation techniques* and include cross-correlation techniques, the wideband maximum likelihood estimator, and high time bandwidth estimation techniques. A thorough review of time-domain estimation techniques to estimate tissue motion is presented in Hein and O'Brien [1993].

Cross-Correlation Estimator.   The use of time shift to estimate signal parameters has been studied extensively in radar. If the transmitted signal is known, a maximum likelihood (ML) solution for the estimation of delay has been discussed by Van Trees [1971] and others. If the signal shape is not known, the use of cross-correlation for delay estimation has been discussed by Helstrom [1968] and Knapp and Carter [1976]. If information regarding the statistics of the signal and noise are available, an MLE based on cross-correlation has been proposed by Knapp and Carter [1976] known as the *generalized correlation method for the estimation of time delay.*

Several researchers have applied cross-correlation analysis to medical ultrasound. Bonnefous and Pesque [1986], Embree and O'Brien [1986], Foster et al. [1990], and Trahey et al. [1987] have studied the estimation of mean velocity based on the change in delay due to target movement. This analysis has assumed the shape of the transmitted signal to be unknown, and a cross-correlation technique has been used to estimate the difference in delay between successive pulses. This differential delay has then been used to estimate target velocity, where the velocity estimate is now based on the change in delay of the signal over an axial window, by maximizing the cross-correlation of the returned signal over all possible target velocities. Cross-correlation processing is typically performed on the radiofrequency (RF) signal, and a typical cross-correlation block diagram is shown in Fig. 67.22. A high-pass filter is first applied to the signal from a fixed depth to remove the

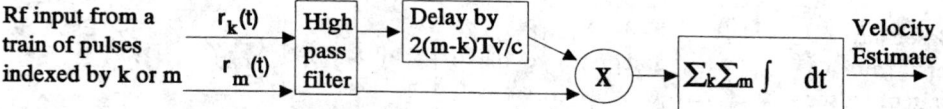

FIGURE 67.22 Block diagram of the system architecture required to estimate the velocity at each depth using a cross-correlation estimator.

unwanted return from stationary tissue. One advantage of this strategy is that the variance is now inversely proportional to bandwidth of the transmitted signal rather than proportional.

Wideband Maximum Likelihood Estimator (WMLE). Wideband maximum likelihood estimation is a baseband strategy with performance properties that are similar to cross-correlation. The estimate of the velocity of the blood cells is jointly based on the shift in the signal envelope and the shift in the carrier frequency of the returned signal. This estimator can be derived using a model for the signal that is expected to be reflected from the moving blood medium after the signal passes through intervening tissue. The processing of the signal can be interpreted as a filter matched to the expected signal. A diagram of the processing required for the wideband maximum likelihood estimator is shown in Fig. 67.23 [Ferrara and Algazi, 1991]. Assume that P pulses were transmitted. Required processing involves the delay of the signal from the $(P - k)$th pulse by an amount equal to $2v/ckT$, which corresponds to the movement of the cells between pulses for a specific v, followed by multiplication by a frequency which corresponds to the expected Doppler shift frequency of the baseband returned signal. The result of this multiplication is summed for all pulses, and the maximum likelihood velocity is then the velocity which produces the largest output from this estimator structure.

Estimation Using High-Time-Bandwidth Signals. Several researchers have also investigated the use of long wideband signals including "chirp" modulated signals and pseudo-random noise for the estimation of blood velocity. These signals are transmitted continuously (or with a short "flyback" time). Since these signals require continual transmission, the instantaneous power level must be reduced in order to achieve safe average power levels.

Bertram [1979] concluded that transmission of a "chirp" appears to give inferior precision for range measurement and inferior resolution of closely spaced multiple targets than a conventional pulse-echo system applied to a similar transducer. Multiple targets confuse the analysis. Using a simple sawtooth waveform, it is not possible to differentiate a stationary target at one range from a moving target at a different range. This problem could possibly be overcome with increasing and decreasing frequency intervals. Axial resolution is independent of the modulation rate, dependent only on the spectral frequency range (which is limited).

The limitations of systems that have transmitted a long pulse of random noise and correlated the return with the transmitted signal include reverberations from outside the sample volume which degrade the signal-to-noise ratio (the federally required reduction in peak transmitted power also reduces SNR), limited signal bandwidth due to frequency-dependent attenuation in tissue, and the finite transducer bandwidth [Bendick and Newhouse, 1974; Cooper and McGillem, 1972].

New Directions

Areas of research interest, including estimation of the 3D velocity magnitude, volume flow estimation, the use of high-frequency catheter-based transducers, mapping blood flow within malignant tumors, a new display mode known as *color Doppler energy,* and the use of contrast agents, are summarized in this subsection.

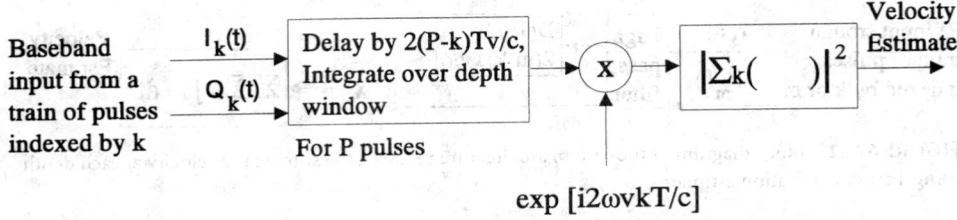

FIGURE 67.23   Block diagram of the system architecture required to estimate the velocity at each depth using the wideband MLE.

Estimation of the 3D Velocity Magnitude and Beam Vessel Angle.   Continued research designed to provide an estimate of the 3D magnitude of the flow velocity includes the use of crossed-beam Doppler systems [Overbeck et al., 1992; Wang and Yao, 1982] and tracking of speckle in two and three dimensions [Trahey et al., 1987]. Mapping of the velocity estimate in two and three dimensions, resulting in a 3D color flow map has been described by Carson et al. [1992], Picot et al. [1993], and Cosgrove et al. [1990].

Volume Flow Estimation.   Along with the peak velocity, instantaneous velocity profile, and velocity indices, a parameter of clinical interest is the volume of flow through vessels as a function of time. Estimation strategies for the determination of the volume of flow through a vessel have been described by Embree and O'Brien [1990], Gill [1979], Hottinger and Meindl [1979], and Uematsu [1981].

Intravascular Ultrasound.   It has been shown that intravascular ultrasonic imaging can provide information about the composition of healthy tissue and atheroma as well as anatomic data. A number of researchers have now shown that using frequencies of 30 MHz or above, individual layers and tissue types can be differentiated [de Kroon et al., 1991a, 1991b; Lockwood et al., 1991]. Although obvious changes in the vessel wall, such as dense fibrosis and calcification, have been identified with lower-frequency transducers, more subtle changes have been difficult to detect. Recent research has indicated that the character of plaque may be a more reliable predictor of subsequent cerebrovascular symptoms than the degree of vessel narrowing or the presence of ulceration [Merritt et al., 1992]. Therefore, the recognition of subtle differences in tissue type may be extremely valuable. One signal-processing challenge in imaging the vascular wall at frequencies of 30 MHz or above is the removal of the unwanted echo from red blood cells, which is a strong interfering signal at high frequencies.

Vascular Changes Associated with Tumors.   Three-dimensional color flow mapping of the vascular structure is proposed to provide new information for the differentiation of benign and malignant masses. Judah Folkman and associates first recognized the importance of tumor vascularity in 1971 [Folkman et al., 1971]. They hypothesized that the increased cell population required for the growth of a malignant tumor must be preceded by the production of new vessels. Subsequent work has shown that the walls of these vessels are deficient in muscular elements, and this deficiency results in a low impedance to flow [Gammill et al., 1976]. This change can be detected by an increase in diastolic flow and a change in the resistive index.

More recently, Less et al. [1991] have shown that the vascular architecture of solid mammary tumors has several distinct differences from normal tissues, at least in the microvasculature. A type of network exists that exhibits fluctuations in both the diameter and length of the vessel with increasing branch order. Current color flow mapping systems with a center frequency of 5 MHz or above have been able to detect abnormal flow with varying degrees of clinical sensitivity from 40% to 82%

[Balu-Maestro et al., 1991; Belcaro et al., 1988; Luska et al., 1992]. Researchers using traditional Doppler systems also have reported a range of clinical sensitivity, with a general reporting of high sensitivity but moderate to low specificity. Burns et al. [1982] studied the signal from benign and malignant masses with 10-MHz CW Doppler. They hypothesized, and confirmed through angiography, that the tumors under study were fed by multiple small arteries, with a mean flow velocity below 10 cm/s. Carson et al. [1992] compared 10-MHz CW Doppler to 5- and 7.5-MHz color flow mapping and concluded that while 3D reconstruction of the vasculature could provide significant additional information, color flow mapping systems must increase their ability to detect slow flow in small vessels in order to effectively map the vasculature.

Ultrasound Contrast Agents. The introduction of substances that enhance the ultrasonic echo signal from blood primarily through the production of microbubbles is of growing interest in ultrasonic flow measurement. The increased echo power may have a significant impact in contrast echocardiography, where acquisition of the signal from the coronary arteries has been difficult. In addition, such agents have been used to increase the backscattered signal from small vessels in masses that are suspected to be malignant. Contrast agents have been developed using sonicated albumen, saccharide microbubbles, and gelatin-encapsulated microbubbles.

Research to improve the sensitivity of flow measurement systems to low-velocity flow and small volumes of flow, with the goal of mapping the vasculature architecture, includes the use of ultrasonic contrast agents with conventional Doppler signal processing [Hartley et al., 1993], as well as the detection of the second harmonic of the transducer center frequency [Shrope and Newhouse, 1993].

Color Doppler Energy. During 1993, a new format for the presentation of the returned signal from the blood scattering medium was introduced and termed *color Doppler energy (CDE)* or *color power imaging (CPI).* In this format, the backscattered signal is filtered to remove the signal from stationary tissue, and the remaining energy in the backscattered signal is color encoded and displayed as an overlay on the gray-scale image. The advantage of this signal-processing technique is the sensitivity to very low flow velocities.

Defining Terms

Baseband signal: The received signal after the center frequency component (carrier frequency) has been removed by demodulation.

Carrier frequency: The center frequency in the spectrum of the transmitted signal.

Clutter: An unwanted fixed signal component generated by stationary targets typically outside the region of interest (such as vessel walls).

Complex envelope: A signal expressed by the product of the carrier, a high-frequency component, and other lower-frequency components that comprise the envelope. The envelope is usually expressed in complex form.

Maximum likelihood: A statistical estimation technique that maximizes the probability of the occurrence of an event to estimate a parameter. ML estimate is the minimum variance, unbiased estimate.

References

Ahn Y, Park S. 1991. Estimation of mean frequency and variance of ultrasonic Doppler signal by using second-order autoregressive model. IEEE Trans Ultrason Ferroelec Freq Cont 38(3): 172.

Angelson B. 1980. Theoretical study of the scattering of ultrasound from blood. IEEE Trans Biomed Eng 27(2):61.

Atkinson P, Berry MV. 1974. Random noise in ultrasonic echoes diffracted by blood. J Phys A Math Nucl Gen 7(11):1293.

Balu-Maestro C, Bruneton JN, Giudicelli T, et al. 1991. Color Doppler in breast tumor pathology. J Radiol 72(11):579.

Barber W, Eberhard JW, Karr S. 1985. A new time domain technique for velocity measurements using Doppler ultrasound. IEEE Trans Biomed Eng 32(3):213.

Belcaro G, Laurora G, Ricci A, et al. 1988. Evaluation of flow in nodular tumors of the breast by Doppler and duplex scanning. Acta Chir Belg 88(5):323.

Bertram CD. 1979. Distance resolution with the FM-CW ultrasonic echo-ranging system. Ultrasound Med Biol (5):61.

Bonnefous O, Pesque P. 1986. Time domain formulation of pulse-Doppler ultrasound and blood velocity estimators by cross correlation. Ultrasonic Imaging 8:73.

Brody W, Meindl J. 1974. Theoretical analysis of the CW Doppler ultrasonic flowmeter. IEEE Trans Biomed Eng 21(3):183.

Burns PN, Halliwell M, Wells PNT, Webb AJ. 1982 Ultrasonic Doppler studies of the breast. Ultrasound Med Biol 8(2):127.

Carson PL, Adler DD, Fowlkes JB, et al. 1992. Enhanced color flow imaging of breast cancer vasculature: continuous wave Doppler and three-dimensional display. J Ultrasound Med 11(8):77.

Cosgrove DO, Bamber JC, Davey JB, et al. 1990. Color Doppler signals from breast tumors: Work in progress. Radiology 176(1):175.

Curry GR, White DN. 1978. Color coded ultrasonic differential velocity arterial scanner. Ultrasound Med Biol 4:27.

de Kroon MGM, Slager CJ, Gussenhoven WJ, et al. 1991. Cyclic changes of blood echogenicity in high-frequency ultrasound. Ultrasound Med Biol 17(7):723.

de Kroon MGM, van der Wal LF, Gussenhoven WJ, et al. 1991. Backscatter directivity and integrated backscatter power of arterial tissue. Int J Cardiac Imaging 6:265.

Embree PM, O'Brien WD Jr. 1990. Volumetric blood flow via time-domain correlation: Experimental verification. IEEE Trans Ultrason Ferroelec Freq Cont 37(3):176.

Ferrara KW, Algazi VR. 1994*a*. A statistical analysis of the received signal from blood during laminar flow. IEEE Trans Ultrason Ferroelec Freq Cont 41(2):185.

Ferrara KW, Algazi VR. 1994*b*. A theoretical and experimental analysis of the received signal from disturbed blood flow. IEEE Trans Ultrason Ferroelec Freq Cont 41(2):172.

Ferrara KW, Algazi VR. 1991. A new wideband spread target maximum likelihood estimator for blood velocity estimation: I. Theory. IEEE Trans Ultrason Ferroelec Freq Cont 38(1):1.

Folkman J, Nerler E, Abernathy C, Williams G. 1971. Isolation of a tumor factor responsible for angiogenesis. J Exp Med 33:275.

Foster SG, Embree PM, O'Brien WD Jr. 1990. Flow velocity profile via time-domain correlation: Error analysis and computer simulation. IEEE Trans Ultrason Ferroelec Freq Cont 37(3):164.

Gammill SL, Stapkey KB, Himmellarb EH. 1976. Roenigenology—Pathology correlative study of neovascularay. AJR 126:376.

Gill RW. 1979. Pulsed Doppler with B-mode imaging for quantitative blood flow measurement. Ultrasound Med Biol 5:223.

Hartley CJ, Cheirif J, Collier KR, Bravenec JS. 1993. Doppler quantification of echo-contrast injections in vivo. Ultrasound Med Biol 19(4):269.

Hatle L, Angelsen B. 1985. Doppler Ultrasound in Cardiology, 3d ed. Philadelphia, Lea and Febiger.

Hatsukami TS, Primozich J, Zierler RE, Strandness DE. 1992. Color Doppler characteristics in normal lower extremity arteries. Ultrasound Med Biol 18(2):167.

Hein I, O'Brien W. 1993. Current time domain methods for assessing tissue motion. IEEE Trans Ultrason Ferroelec Freq Cont 40(2):84.

Helstrom CW. 1968. Statistical Theory of Signal Detection. London, Pergamon Press.

Hinze JO. 1975. Turbulence. New York, McGraw-Hill.

Hottinger CF, Meindl JD. 1979. Blood flow measurement using the attenuation compensated volume flowmeter. Ultrasonic Imaging (1)1:1.

Kaluzinski K. 1989. Order selection in Doppler blood flow signal spectral analysis using autoregressive modelling. Med Biol Eng Com 27:89.

Kasai C, Namekawa K, Koyano A, Omoto R. 1985. Real-time two-dimensional blood flow imaging using an autocorrelation technique. IEEE Trans Sonics Ultrason 32(3).

Kay S, Marple SL. 1981. Spectrum analysis. A modern perspective. Proc IEEE 69(11):1380.

Kennedy RS. 1969. Fading Dispersive Channel Theory. New York, Wiley Interscience.

Knapp CH, Carter GC. 1976. The generalized correlation method for estimation of time delay. IEEE Trans Acoustics Speech Signal Proc 24(4):320.

Kristoffersen K, Angelsen BJ. 1985. A comparison between mean frequency estimators for multigated Doppler systems with serial signal processing. IEEE Trans Biomed Eng 32(9):645.

Less JR, Skalak TC, Sevick EM, Jain RK. 1991. Microvascular architecture in a mammary carcinoma: Branching patterns and vessel dimensions. Cancer Res 51(1):265.

Lockwood GR, Ryan LK, Hunt JW, Foster FS. 1991. Measurement of the ultrasonic properties of vascular tissues and blood from 35–65 MHz. Ultrasound Med Biol 17(7):653.

Loupas T, McDicken WN. 1990. Low-order AR models for mean and maximum frequency estimation in the context of Doppler color flow mapping. IEEE Trans Ultrason Ferroelec Freq Cont 37(6):590.

Luska G, Lott D, Risch U, von Boetticher H. 1992. The findings of color Doppler sonography in breast tumors. Rofo Forts auf dem Gebiete der Rontgens und der Neuen Bildg Verf 156(2):142.

Merritt C, Bluth E. 1992. The future of carotid sonography. AJR 158:37.

Mo L, Cobbold R. 1986. A stochastic model of the backscattered Doppler ultrasound from blood. IEEE Trans Biomed Eng 33(1):20.

Nerem RM. 1985. Fluid dynamic considerations in the application of ultrasound flowmetry. In SA Altobelli, WF Voyles, ER Greene (eds), Cardiovascular Ultrasonic Flowmetry. New York, Elsevier.

Nichols WW, O'Rourke MF. 1990. McDonald's Blood Flow in Arteries: Theoretic, Experimental and Clinical principles. Philadelphia, Lea and Febiger.

Nowicki A, Reid JM. 1981. An infinite gate pulse Doppler. Ultrasound Med Biol 7:1.

Overbeck JR, Beach KW, Strandness DE Jr. 1992. Vector Doppler: Accurate measurement of blood velocity in two dimensions. Ultrasound Med Biol 18(1):19.

Picot PA, Rickey DW, Mitchell R, et al. 1993. Three dimensional color Doppler mapping. Ultrasound Med Biol 19(2):95.

Price R. 1968. Detectors for radar astronomy. In J Evans, T Hagfors (eds), Radar Astronomy. New York, McGraw-Hill.

Schrope BA, Newhouse VL. 1993. Second harmonic ultrasonic blood perfusion measurement. Ultrasound Med Biol 19(7):567.

Shung KK, Sigelman RA, Reid JM. 1976. Scattering of ultrasound by blood. IEEE Trans Biomed Eng 23(6):460.

Shung KK, Cloutier G, Lim CC. 1992. The effects of hematocrit, shear rate, and turbulence on ultrasonic Doppler spectrum from blood. IEEE Trans Biomed Eng 39(5):462.

Trahey GE, Allison JW, Von Ramm OT. 1987. Angle independent ultrasonic detection of blood flow. IEEE Trans Biomed Eng 34(12):964.

Uematsu S. 1981. Determination of volume of arterial blood flow by an ultrasonic device. J Clin Ultrason 9:209.

Van Trees HL. 1971. Detection, Estimation and Modulation Theory, Part III. New York, Wiley.

Wang W, Yao L. 1982. A double beam Doppler ultrasound method for quantitative blood flow velocity measurement. Ultrasound Med Biol (8)421.

Wells PNT. 1977. Biomedical Ultrasonics. London, Academic Press.

Further Information

The bimonthly journal *IEEE Transactions on Ultrasonics Ferroelectrics and Frequency Control* reports engineering advances in the area of ultrasonic flow measurement. For subscription information, contact IEEE Service Center, 445 Hoes Lane, P.O. Box 1331, Piscataway, NJ 08855-1331. Phone (800) 678-IEEE. The journal and the yearly conference proceedings of the IEEE Ultrasonics Symposium are published by the IEEE Ultrasonics Ferroelectrics and Frequency Control Society. Membership information can be obtained from the IEEE address above or from K. Ferrara, Riverside Research Institute, 330 West 42nd Street, New York, NY 10036.

The journal *Ultrasound in Medicine and Biology*, published 10 times per year, includes new developments in ultrasound signal processing and the clinical application of these developments. For subscription information, contact Pergamon Press, Inc., 660 White Plains Road, Tarrytown, NY 10591-5153. The American Institute of Ultrasound in Medicine sponsors a yearly meeting which reviews new developments in ultrasound instrumentation and the clinical applications. For information, please contact American Institute of Ultrasound in Medicine, 11200 Rockville Pike, Suite 205, Rockville, MD 20852-3139; phone: (800) 638-5352.

68

Magnetic Resonance Microscopy

Xiaohong Zhou
Duke University Medical Center

G. Allan Johnson
Duke University Medical Center

Visualization of internal structures of opaque biologic objects is essential in many biomedical studies. Limited by the penetration depth of the probing sources (photons and electrons) and the lack of endogenous contrast, conventional forms of microscopy such as optical microscopy and electron microscopy require tissues to be sectioned into thin slices and stained with organic chemicals or heavy-metal compounds prior to examination. These invasive and destructive procedures, as well as the harmful radiation in the case of electron microscopy, make it difficult to obtain three-dimensional information and virtually impossible to study biologic tissues in vivo.

Magnetic resonance (MR) microscopy is a new form of microscopy that overcomes the aforementioned limitations. Operating in the radiofrequency (RF) range, MR microscopy allows biologic samples to be examined in the living state without bleaching or damage by ionizing radiation and in fresh and fixed specimens after minimal preparation. It also can use a number of endogenous contrast mechanisms that are directly related to tissue biochemistry, physiology, and pathology. Additionally, MR microscopy is digital and three-dimensional; internal structures of opaque tissues can be quantitatively mapped out in three dimensions to accurately reveal their histopathologic status. These unique properties provide new opportunities for biomedical scientists to attack problems that have been difficult to investigate using conventional techniques.

Conceptually, MR microscopy is an extension of magnetic resonance imaging (MRI) to the microscopic domain, generating images with spatial resolution better than 100 μm [Lauterbur, 1984]. As such, MR microscopy is challenged by a new set of theoretical and technical problems [Johnson et al., 1992]. For example, to improve isotropic resolution from 1 mm to 10 μm, signal-to-noise ratio (SNR) per voxel must be increased by a million times to maintain the same image quality. In order to do so, almost every component of hardware must be optimized to the fullest extent, pulse sequences have to be carefully designed to minimize any potential signal loss, and special software and dedicated computation facilities must be involved to handle large image arrays (e.g., 256^3). Over the past decade, development of MR microscopy has focused mainly on these issues. Persistent efforts by many researchers have recently lead to images with isotropic resolution of the order of ~ 10 μm. [Cho et al., 1992; Jacobs and Fraser, 1994; Johnson et al., 1992; Zhou and Lauterbur, 1992]. The sig-

0-8493-8346-3/95/$0.00+$.50
© 1995 by CRC Press, Inc.

nificant resolution improvement opens up a broad range of applications, from histology to cancer biology and from toxicology to plant biology [Johnson et al., 1992]. In this chapter we will first discuss the basic principles of MR microscopy, with special attention to such issues as resolution limits and sensitivity improvements. Then we will give an overview of the instrumentation. Finally, we will provide some examples to demonstrate the applications.

68.1 Basic Principles

Spatial Encoding and Decoding

Any digital imaging systems involve two processes. First, spatially resolved information must be encoded into a measurable signal, and second, the spatially encoded signal must be decoded to produce an image. In MR microscopy, the spatial encoding process is accomplished by acquiring nuclear magnetic resonance (NMR) signals under the influence of three orthogonal magnetic field gradients. There are many ways that a gradient can interact with a spin system. If the gradient is applied during a frequency-selective RF pulse, then the NMR signal arises only from a thin slab along the gradient direction. Thus a slice is selected from a three-dimensional (3D) object. If the gradient is applied during the acquisition of an NMR signal, the signal will consist of a range of spatially dependent frequencies given by

$$\omega(\vec{r}) = \gamma B_0 + \gamma \vec{G} \cdot \vec{r} \tag{68.1}$$

where γ is gyromagnetic ratio, B_0 is the static magnetic field, $\vec{G}$ is the magnetic field gradient, and $\vec{r}$ is the spatial variable. In this way, the spatial information along $\vec{G}$ direction is encoded into the signal as frequency variations. This method of encoding is called *frequency encoding,* and the gradient is referred to as a *frequency-encoding gradient* (or *read-out gradient*). If the gradient is applied for a fixed amount of time t_{pe} before the signal acquisition, then the phase of the signal, instead of the frequency, becomes spatially dependent, as given by

$$\phi(\vec{r}) = \int_0^{t_{pe}} \omega(\vec{r})\, dt = \phi_0 + \int_0^{t_{pe}} \gamma \vec{G} \cdot \vec{r}\, dt \tag{68.2}$$

where ϕ_0 is the phase originated from the static magnetic field. This encoding method is known as *phase encoding,* and the gradient is called a *phase-encoding gradient.*

Based on the three basic spatial encoding approaches, many imaging schemes can be synthesized. For two-dimensional (2D) imaging, a slice-selection gradient is first applied to confine the NMR signal in a slice. Spatial encoding within the slice is then accomplished by frequency encoding and/or by phase encoding. For 3D imaging, the slice-selection gradient is replaced by either a frequency-encoding or a phase-encoding gradient. If all spatial directions are frequency-encoded, the encoding scheme is called *projection acquisition,* and the corresponding decoding method is called *projection reconstruction* [Lai and Lauterbur, 1981; Lauterbur, 1973]. If one of the spatial dimensions is frequency encoded while the rest are phase encoded, the method is known as *Fourier imaging,* and the image can be reconstructed simply by a multidimensional Fourier transform [Edelstein et al., 1980; Kumar et al., 1975]. Although other methods do exist, projection reconstruction and Fourier imaging are the two most popular in MR microscopy.

Projection reconstruction is particularly useful for spin systems with short apparent T_2 values, such as protons in lung and liver. Since the T_2 of most tissues decreases as static magnetic field increases, the advantage of projection reconstruction is more obvious at high magnetic fields. Another advantage of projection reconstruction is its superior SNR to Fourier imaging. This advantage has been theoretically analyzed and experimentally demonstrated in a number of independent studies

[Callaghan and Eccles, 1987; Gewalt et al., 1993; Zhou and Lauterbur, 1992]. Recently, it also has been shown that projection reconstruction is less sensitive to motion, and motion artifacts can be effectively reduced using sinograms [Glover and Noll, 1993; Glover and Pauly, 1992; Gmitro and Alexander, 1993]. Unlike projection reconstruction, data acquisition in Fourier imaging generates Fourier coefficients of the image in a cartesian coordinate. Since multidimensional fast Fourier transform algorithms can be applied directly to the raw data, Fourier imaging is computationally more efficient than projection reconstruction. This advantage is most evident when reconstructing 3D images with large arrays (e.g., 256^3). In addition, Fourier transform imaging is less prone to image artifacts arising from various off-resonance effects and is more robust in applications such as chemical shift imaging [Brown et al., 1982] and flow imaging [Moran, 1982].

Image Contrast

A variety of contrast mechanisms can be exploited in MR microscopy, including spin density (ρ), spin-spin relaxation time (T_1), spin-lattice relaxation time (T_2), apparent T_2 relaxation time (T_2^*), diffusion coefficient (D), flow, and chemical shift (δ). One of the contrasts can be highlighted by varying data-acquisition parameters or by choosing different pulse sequences. Table 68.1 summarizes the pulse sequences and data-acquisition parameters to obtain each of the preceding contrasts.

In high-field MR microscopy (>1.5 T), T_2 and diffusion contrast are strongly coupled together. An increasing number of evidences indicate that the apparent T_2 contrast observed in high-field MR microscopy is largely due to microscopic magnetic susceptibility variations [Majumdar and Gore, 1988; Zhong and Gore, 1991]. The magnetic susceptibility difference produces strong local magnetic field gradients. Molecular diffusion through the induced gradients causes significant signal loss. In addition, the large external magnetic field gradients required for spatial encoding further increase the diffusion-induced signal loss. Since the signal loss has similar dependence on echo time (TE) to T_2-related loss, the diffusion contrast mechanism is involved in virtually all T_2-weighted images. This unique contrast mechanism provides a direct means to probe the microscopic tissue heterogeneities and forms the basis for many histopathologic studies [Benveniste et al., 1992; Zhou et al., 1994].

Chemical shift is another unique contrast mechanism. Changes in chemical shift can directly reveal tissue metabolic and histopathologic stages. This mechanism exists in many spin systems such as ^1H, ^{31}P, and ^{13}C. Recently, Lean et al. [1993] showed that based on proton chemical shifts, MR microscopy can detect tissue pathologic changes with superior sensitivity to optical microscopy in a number of tumor models. A major limitation for chemical-shift MR microscopy is the rather poor spatial resolution, since most spin species other than water protons are of considerably low concentration and/or sensitivity. In addition, the long data-acquisition time required to resolve both spatial and spectral information also appears as an obstacle.

TABLE 68.1   Choice of Acquisition Parameters for Different Image Contrasts

Contrast	TR[#]	TE[#]	Pulse Sequences[§]
ρ	3–5 $T_{1,max}$	$\ll T_{2,min}$	SE, GE
T_1	$\sim T_{1,avg}$	$\ll T_{2,min}$	SE, GE
T_2	3–5 $T_{1,max}$	$\sim T_{2,avg}$	SE, FSE
T_2^*	3–5 $T_{1,max}$	$\sim T_{2,avg}^*$	GE
$D^\dagger$	3–5 $T_{1,max}$	$\ll T_{2,min}$	diffusion-weighted SE, GE, or FSE

[§]SE: spin echo; GE: gradient echo; FSE: fast spin echo.

[#]Subscripts *min, max* and *avg* stand for minimum, maximum and average values, respectively.

[†]A pair of diffusion weighting gradients must be used.

68.2 Resolution Limits

Intrinsic Resolution Limit

Intrinsic resolution is defined as the width of the point-spread function originated from physics laws. In MR microscopy, the intrinsic resolution arises from two sources: natural linewidth broadening and diffusion [Callaghan and Eccles, 1988; Cho et al., 1988; House, 1984].

In most conventional pulse sequences, natural linewidth broadening affects the resolution limit only in the frequency-encoding direction. In some special cases, such as fast spin echo [Hennig et al., 1986] and echo planar imaging [Mansfield and Maudsley, 1977], natural linewidth broadening also imposes resolution limits in the phase-encoding direction [Zhou et al., 1993]. The natural linewidth resolution limit, defined by

$$\Delta r_{\text{n.l.w.}} = \frac{2}{\gamma G T_2} \tag{68.3}$$

is determined by the T_2 relaxation time and can be improved using a stronger gradient G. To obtain 1-μm resolution from a specimen with $T_2 = 50$ ms, the gradient should be at least 14.9 G/cm. This gradient requirement is well within the range of most MR microscopes.

Molecular diffusion affects the spatial resolution in a number of ways. The bounded diffusion is responsible for many interesting phenomena known as *edge enhancements* [Callaghan et al., 1993; Hills et al., 1990; Hyslop and Lauterbur, 1991; Putz et al., 1991]. They are observable only at the microscopic resolution and are potentially useful to detect microscopic boundaries. The unbounded diffusion, on the other hand, causes signal attenuation, line broadening, and phase misregistration. All these effects originate from an incoherent and irreversible phase dispersion. The root-mean-square value of the phase dispersion is

$$\sigma = \gamma \left\{ 2D \int_0^t [\int_{t'}^t G(t'') \, dt'']^2 \, dt' \right\}^{1/2} \tag{68.4}$$

where t' and t are pulse-sequence-dependent time variables defined by Ahn and Cho [1989]. Because of the phase uncertainty, an intrinsic resolution limit along the phase encoding direction arises:

$$\Delta r_{pe} = \frac{\sigma}{\gamma \int_0^t G_{pe}(t') \, dt'} \tag{68.5}$$

For a rectangularly shaped phase-encoding gradient, the preceding equation can be reduced to a very simple form:

$$\Delta r_{pe} = \sqrt{\frac{2}{3} D t_{pe}} \tag{68.6}$$

This simple result indicates that the diffusion resolution limit in the phase-encoded direction is determined only by the phase-encoding time t_{pe} (D is a constant for a chosen sample). This is so because the phase uncertainty is introduced only during the phase-encoding period. Once the spins are phase-encoded, they always carry the same spatial information no matter where they diffuse to. In the frequency-encoding direction, diffusion imposes resolution limits by broadening the point-spread function. Unlike natural linewidth broadening, broadening caused by diffusion is pulse-sequence-dependent. For the simplest pulse sequence, a 3D projection acquisition using free induction decays, the full width at half maximum [Callaghan and Eccles, 1988; McFarland, 1992; Zhou, 1992] is

$$\Delta r_{fr} = 8 \left[\frac{D(\ln 2)^2}{3\gamma G_{fr}} \right]^{1/3}$$

(68.7)

Compared with the case of the natural linewidth broadening (Eq. 68.3), the resolution limit caused by diffusion varies slowly with the frequency-encoding gradient G_{fr}. Therefore, to improve resolution by a same factor, a much larger gradient is required. With the currently achievable gradient strength, the diffusion resolution limit is estimated to be 5 to 10 μm.

Digital Resolution Limit

When the requirements imposed by intrinsic resolution limits are satisfied, image resolution is largely determined by the voxel size, provided that SNR is sufficient and the amplitude of physiologic motion is limited to a voxel. The voxel size, also known as *digital resolution*, can be calculated from the following equations:

Frequency-encoding direction: $\quad \Delta x \equiv \dfrac{L_x}{N_x} = \dfrac{\Delta v}{2\pi\gamma G_x N_x}$ (68.8)

Phase-encoding direction: $\quad \Delta y \equiv \dfrac{L_y}{N_y} = \dfrac{\Delta\phi}{\gamma G_y t_{pe}}$ (68.9)

where L is the field of view, N is the number of data points or the linear matrix size, G is the gradient strength, Δv is the receiver bandwidth, $\Delta\phi$ is the phase range of the phase-encoding data (e.g., if the data cover a phase range from $-\pi$ to $+\pi$, then $\Delta\phi = 2\pi$), and the subscripts x and y represent frequency- and phase-encoding directions, respectively. To obtain a high digital resolution, L should be kept minimal, while N maximal. In practice, the minimal field of view and the maximal data points are constrained by other experimental parameters. In the frequency-encoding direction, decreasing field of view results in an increase in gradient amplitude at a constant receiver bandwidth or a decrease in the bandwidth for a constant gradient (Eq. 68.8). Since the receiver bandwidth must be large enough to keep the acquisition of NMR signals within a certain time window, the largest available gradient strength thus imposes the digital resolution limit. In the phase-encoding direction, $\Delta\phi$ is fixed at 2π in most experiments, and the maximum t_{pe} value is refrained by the echo time. Thus digital resolution is also determined by the maximum available gradient, as indicated by Eq. (68.9). It has been estimated that in order to achieve 1-μm resolution with a phase-encoding time of 4 ms, the required gradient strength is as high as 587 G/cm. This gradient requirement is beyond the range of current MR microscopes. Fortunately, the requirement is fully relaxed in projection acquisition where no phase encoding is involved.

Practical Resolution Limit

The intrinsic resolution limits predict that MR microscopy can theoretically reach the micron regime. To realize the resolution, one must overcome several technical obstacles. These obstacles, or practical resolution limits, include insufficient SNR, long data-acquisition times, and physiologic motion. At the current stage of development, these practical limitations are considerably more important than other resolution limits discussed earlier and actually determine the true image resolution.

SNR is of paramount importance in MR microscopy. As resolution improves, the total number of spins per voxel decreases drastically, resulting in a cubic decrease in signal intensity. When the voxel signal intensity becomes comparable with noise level, structures become unresolvable even if the digital resolution and intrinsic resolution are adequate.

SNR in a voxel depends on many factors. The relationship between SNR and common experimental variables is given by

$$\text{SNR} \propto \frac{B_1 B_0^2 \sqrt{n}}{\sqrt{4kT\Delta\nu(R_{\text{coil}} + R_{\text{sample}})}} \tag{68.10}$$

where B_1 is the RF magnetic field, B_0 is the static magnetic field, n is the number of average, T is the temperature, $\Delta\nu$ is the bandwidth, k is the Boltzmann constant, and R_{coil} and R_{sample} are the coil and sample resistance, respectively. When small RF coils are used, R_{sample} is negligible. Since R_{coil} is proportional to $\sqrt{B_0}$ due to skin effects, the overall SNR increases as $B_0^{7/4}$. This result strongly suggests that MR microscopy be performed at high magnetic field. Another way to improve SNR is to increase the B_1 field. This is accomplished by reducing the size of RF coils [McFarland and Mortara, 1992; Peck et al., 1990; Schoeniger et al., 1991; Zhou and Lauterbur, 1992]. Although increasing B_0 and B_1 is the most common approach to attacking the SNR problem, other methods such as signal averaging, pulse-sequence optimization, and post data processing are also useful in MR microscopy. For example, diffusion-induced signal loss can be effectively minimized using diffusion-reduced-gradient (DRG) echo pulse sequences [Cho et al., 1992]. Various forms of projection acquisition techniques [Gewalt et al., 1993; Hedges, 1984; McFarland and Mortara, 1992; Zhou and Lauterbur, 1992], as well as new k-space sampling schemes [Zhou et al., 1993], also have proved useful in SNR improvements. Recently, Black et al. used high-temperature superconducting materials for coil fabrication to simultaneously reduce coil resistance R_{coil} and coil temperature T [Black et al., 1993]. This novel approach can provide up to 70-fold SNR increase, equivalent to the SNR gain by increasing the magnetic field strength 11 times.

Long data-acquisition time is another practical limitation. Large image arrays, long repetition times (TR), and signal averaging all contribute to the overall acquisition time. For instance, a T_2-weighted image with a 256^3 image array requires a total acquisition time of more than 18 hours (assuming $TR = 500$ ms and $n = 2$). Such a long acquisition time is unacceptable for most applications. To reduce the acquisition time while still maintaining the desired contrast, fast-imaging pulse sequences such as echo-planar imaging (EPI) [Mansfield and Maudsley, 1977], driven equilibrium Fourier transform (DEFT) [Maki et al., 1988], fast low angle shot (FLASH) [Haase et al., 1986], gradient refocused acquisition at steady state (GRASS) [Karis et al., 1987], and rapid acquisition with relaxation enhancement (RARE) [Hennig et al., 1986] have been developed and applied to MR microscopy. The RARE pulse sequence, or fast spin-echo (FSE) [Mulkern et al., 1990], is particularly useful in high-field MR microscopy because of its insensitivity to magnetic susceptibility effects as well as the reduced diffusion loss [Zhou et al., 1993]. Using fast spin-echo techniques, a 256^3 image has been acquired in less than 2 hours [Zhou et al., 1993].

For in vivo studies, the true image resolution is also limited by physiologic motion [Hedges, 1984; Wood and Henkelman, 1985]. Techniques to minimize the motion effects have been largely focused on pulse sequences and post data processing algorithms, including navigator echoes [Ehman and Felmlee, 1989], motion compensation using even echo or moment nulling gradients, projection acquisition [Glover and Noll, 1993], and various kinds of ghost-image decomposition techniques [Xiang and Henkelman, 1991]. It should be noted, however, that by refining animal handling techniques and using synchronized data acquisition, physiologic motion effects can be effectively avoided and very high quality images can be obtained [Hedlund et al., 1986; Johnson et al., 1992].

68.3 Instrumentation

An MR microscope consists of a high-field magnet (>1.5 T), a set of gradient coils, an RF coil (or RF coils), and the associated RF systems, gradient power supplies, and computers. Among these components, RF coils and gradient coils are often customized for specific applications in order to achieve optimal performance. Some general guidelines to design customized RF coils and gradient coils are presented below.

Radiofrequency Coils

Many types of RF coils can be used in MR microscopy (Fig. 68.1). The choice of a particular coil configuration is determined by specific task and specimen size. If possible, the smallest coil size should always be chosen in order to obtain the highest SNR. For ex vivo studies of tissue specimens, solenoid coils are common choice because of their superior B_1 field homogeneity, high sensitivity, as well as simplicity in fabrication. Using a 2.9-mm solenoid coil (5 turn), Zhou and Lauterbur [1992] have achieved the highest ever reported spatial resolution at 6.4 μm^3. Solenoid coil configurations are also used by others to obtain images with similar resolution ($\sim$10 μm) [Cho et al., 1988; Hedges, 1984; McFarland and Mortara, 1992; Schoeniger et al., 1991]. Recently, several researchers began to develop microscopic solenoid coils with a size of a few hundred microns [McFarland and Mortara, 1992; Peck et al., 1990]. Fabrication of these microcoils often requires special techniques, such as light lithography and electron-beam lithography.

The direction of the B_1 field generated by a solenoid coil prevents the coil from being coaxially placed in the magnet. Thus accessing and positioning samples are difficult. To solve this problem, Banson et al. [1992] devised a unique Helmholtz coil that consists of two separate loops. Each loop is made from a microwave laminate with a dielectric material sandwiched between two copper foils. By making use of the distributed capacitance, the coil can be tuned to a desired frequency. Since the two loops of the coil are mechanically separated, samples can be easily slid into the gap between the loops without any obstruction. Under certain circumstances, the Helmholtz coil can outperform an optimally designed solenoid coil with similar dimensions.

For in vivo studies, although volume coils such as solenoid coils and birdcage coils can be employed, most high-resolution experiments are carried out using local RF coils, including surface coils [Banson et al., 1992; Rudin, 1987] and implanted coils [Farmer et al., 1989; Hollett et al., 1987; Zhou et al., 1994]. Surface coils can effectively reduce coil size and simultaneously limit the field of view to a small region of interest. They can be easily adaptable to the shape of samples and provide high sensitivity in the surface region. The problem of inhomogeneous B_1 field can be minimized using composite pulses [Hetherington et al., 1986] or adiabatic pulses [Ugurbil et al., 1987]. To obtain high-resolution images from regions distant from the surface, surgically implantable coils become the method of choice. These coils not only give better SNR than optimized surface coils [Zhou et al., 1992] but also provide accurate and consistent localization. The latter advantage is particularly useful for time-course studies on dynamic processes such as the development of pathology and monitoring the effects of therapeutic drugs.

The recent advent of high-temperature superconducting (HTS) RF coils has brought new excitement to MR microscopy [Black et al., 1993]. The substantial improvement, as discussed earlier, makes signal averaging unnecessary. Using these coils, the total imaging time will be solely determined by the efficiency to traverse the k space. Although much research is yet to be done in this new area, combination of the HTS coils with fast-imaging algorithms will most likely provide a unique way to fully realize the potential of MR microscopy and eventually bring the technique into routine use.

Magnetic Field Gradient Coils

As discussed previously, high spatial resolution requires strong magnetic field gradients. The gradient strength increases proportional to the coil current and inversely proportional to the coil size. Since increasing current generates many undesirable effects (overheating, mechanical vibrations, eddy current, etc.), strong magnetic field gradient is almost exclusively achieved by reducing the coil diameter.

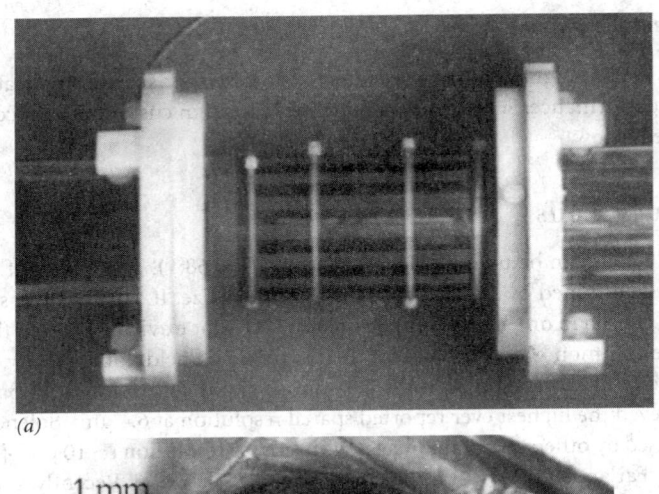

(a)

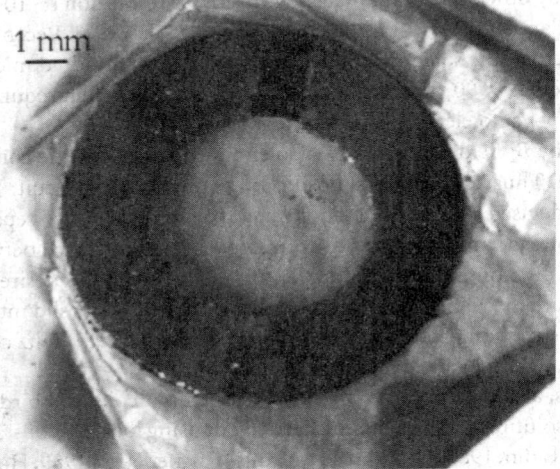

1 mm

(b)

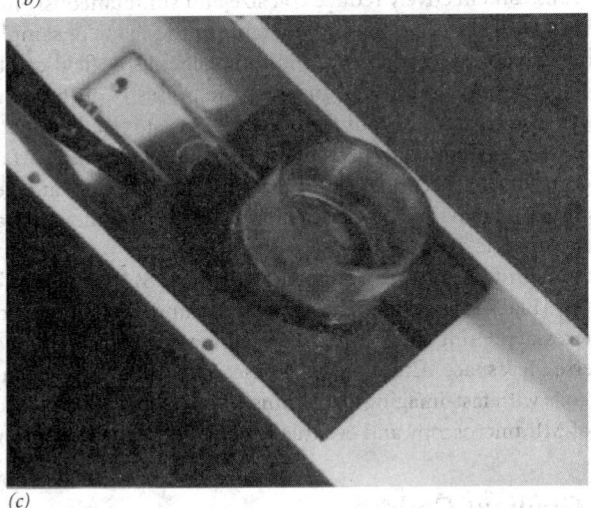

(c)

FIGURE 68.1 A range of radiofrequency coils are used in MR microscopy. (*a*) A quadrature birdcage coil scaled to the appropriate diameter for rats (6 cm) is used for whole-body imaging. (*b*) Resonant coils have been constructed on microwave substrate that can be surgically implanted to provide both localization and improved SNR. (*c*) MR microscopy of specimens is accomplished with a modified Helmholz coil providing good filling factors, high B_1 homogeneity, and ease of access.

Design of magnetic field gradient coils for MR microscopy is a classic problem. Based on Maxwell equations, ideal surface current density can be calculated for a chosen geometry of the conducting surface. Two conducting surfaces are mostly used: a cylindrical surface parallel to the axis of the magnet and a cylindrical surface perpendicular to the axis. The ideal surface current density distributions for these two geometries are illustrated in Fig. 68.2 [Suits and Wilken, 1989]. After the ideal surface current density distribution is obtained, design of gradient coils is reduced to a problem of using discrete conductors with a finite length to approximate the continuous current distribution function. The error in the approximation determines the gradient linearity. Recent advancements in computer-based fabrication and etching techniques have made it feasible to produce complicated current density distributions. Using these techniques, nonlinear terms up to the eleventh order can be eliminated over a predefined cylindrical volume.

Another issue in gradient coil design involves minimizing the gradient rise time so that fast-imaging techniques can be implemented successfully and short echo times can be achieved to minimize signal loss for short T_2 specimens. The gradient rise time relies on three factors: the inductance over resistance ratio of the gradient coil, the time constant of the feedback circuit of the gradient power supply, and the decay rate of eddy current triggered by gradient switching. The time constant attributed to inductive resistance (L/R) is relatively short (<100 μs) for most microscopy gradient coils, and the inductive resistance from the power supply can be easily adjusted to match the time constant of the coil. However, considering the high magnetic field gradient strength used

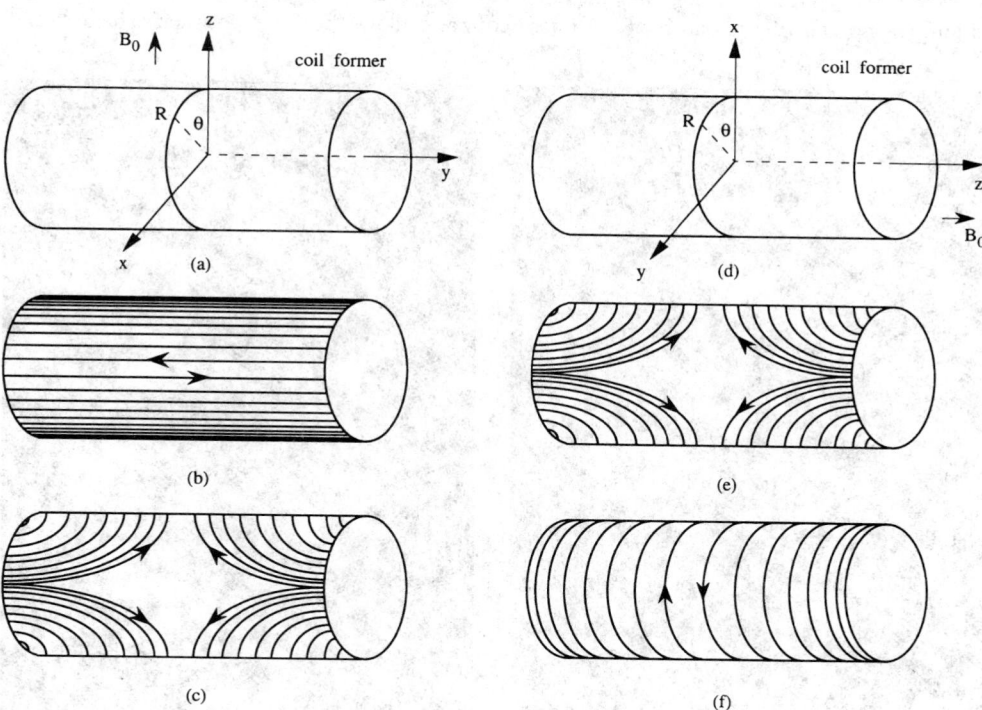

FIGURE 68.2 (*Left*) Ideal surface current distributions to generate linear magnetic field gradients when the gradient coil former is parallel to the magnet bore: (*b*) for x gradient and (*c*) for z gradient. The analytical expressions for the current density distribution functions are $J_x = KG_x[R \cos \theta(\sin \theta i - \cos \theta j) - z\sin \theta k]$ and $J_z = KG_z z[\sin \theta i - \cos \theta j]$. The y gradient can be obtained by rotating J_x 90 degrees. (*Right*) Ideal surface current distributions to generate linear magnetic field gradients when the gradient coil former is perpendicular to the magnet bore: (*e* for x gradient and (*f*) for y gradient. The analytical expressions for the current density distribution functions are: $J_x = KG_x R(\sin 2\theta j)$ and $J_y = KG_y(-R \cos^2\theta i + y \sin j + 0.5R \sin 2\theta k)$. The z gradient can be obtained by rotating J_x 45 degrees. (The graphs are adapted based on Suits and Wilken [1989].)

in MR microscopy, eddy currents can be a serious problem. This problem is even worsened when the gradient coils are closely placed in a narrow magnet bore. To minimize the eddy currents, modern design on gradient coils uses an extra set of coils so that the eddy currents can be actively canceled [Mansfield and Chapman, 1986]. Under close to optimal conditions, a rise time of <150 μs can be achieved with a maximum gradient of 82 G/cm in a set of 8-cm coils [Johnson et al., 1992].

Although the majority of microscopic MR images are obtained using cylindrical gradient coils, surface gradient coils have been used recently in several studies [Cho et al., 1992]. Similar to surface RF coils, surface gradient coils can be easily adapted to the shape of samples and are capable of producing strong magnetic field gradient in limited areas. The surface gradient coils also provide more free space in the magnet, allowing easy access to samples. A major problem with surface gradient coils is the gradient nonlinearity. But when the region of interest is small, high-quality images can still be obtained with negligible distortions.

68.4 Applications

MR microscopy has a broad range of applications. We include here several examples. Figure 68.3 illustrates an application of MR microscopy in ex vivo histology. In this study, a fixed sheep heart with experimentally-induced infarct is imaged at 2 T using 3D fast-spin-echo techniques with T_1 (Fig. 68.3a) and T_2 (Fig. 68.3b) contrasts. The infarct region is clearly detected in both images. The region of infarct can be segmented from the rest of the tissue and its volume can be accurately measured. Since the image is three-dimensional, the tissue pathology can be examined in any arbitrary orientation. The nondestructive nature of MR microscopy also allows the same specimen to be restudied

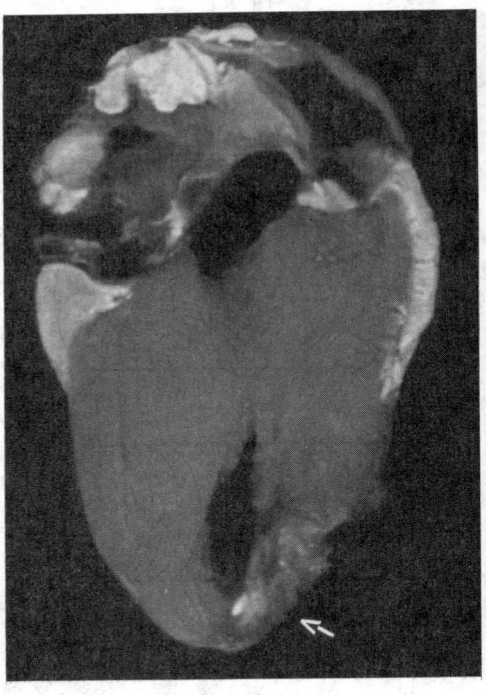
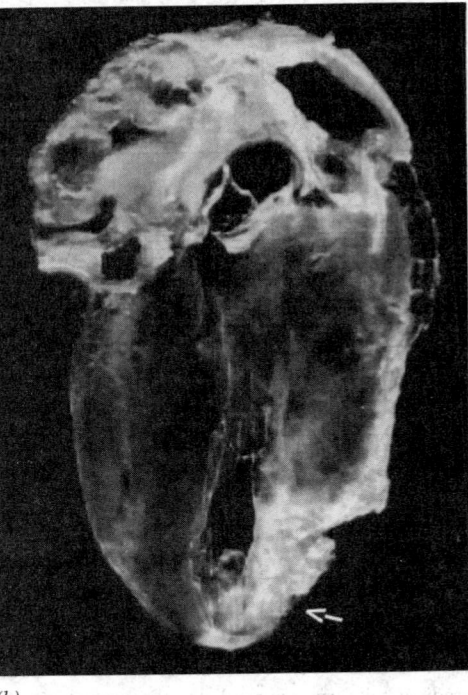

(a)   (b)

FIGURE 68.3   Selected sections of 3D isotropic images of a sheep heart with experimentally induced infarct show the utility of MRM in pathology studies. A 3D FSE sequence has been designed to allow rapid acquisition of either (a) T_1-weighted or (b) T_2-weighted images giving two separate "stains" for the pathology. Arrows indicate areas of necrosis.

using other techniques as well as using other contrast mechanisms of MR microscopy. Obtaining this dimension of information from conventional histologic studies would be virtually impossible.

The in vivo capability of MR microscopy for toxicologic studies is illustrated in Fig. 68.4. In this study [Farmer et al., 1989], the effect of mercuric chloride in rat kidney is monitored in a single animal. Therefore, development of tissue pathology over a time period is directly observed without the unnecessary interference arising from interanimal variabilities. Since the kidney was the only region of interest in this study, a surgically implanted coil was chosen to optimize SNR and to obtain consistent localization. Figure 68.4 shows four images obtained from the same animal at different time points to show the progression and regression of the HgCl2-induced renal pathology. Tissue damage is first observed 24 hours after the animal was treated by the chemical, as evident by the blurring between the cortex and the outer medulla. The degree of damage is greater in the image obtained at 48 hours. Finally, at 360 hours, the blurred boundary between the two tissue regions completely disappeared, indicating full recovery of the organ. The capability to monitor tissue pathologic changes in vivo, as illustrated in this example, bodes well for a broad range of applications in pharmacology, toxicology, and pathology.

Development biology is another area where MR microscopy has found an increasing number of applications. Jacobs and Fraser [1994] used MR microscopy to follow cell movements and lineages

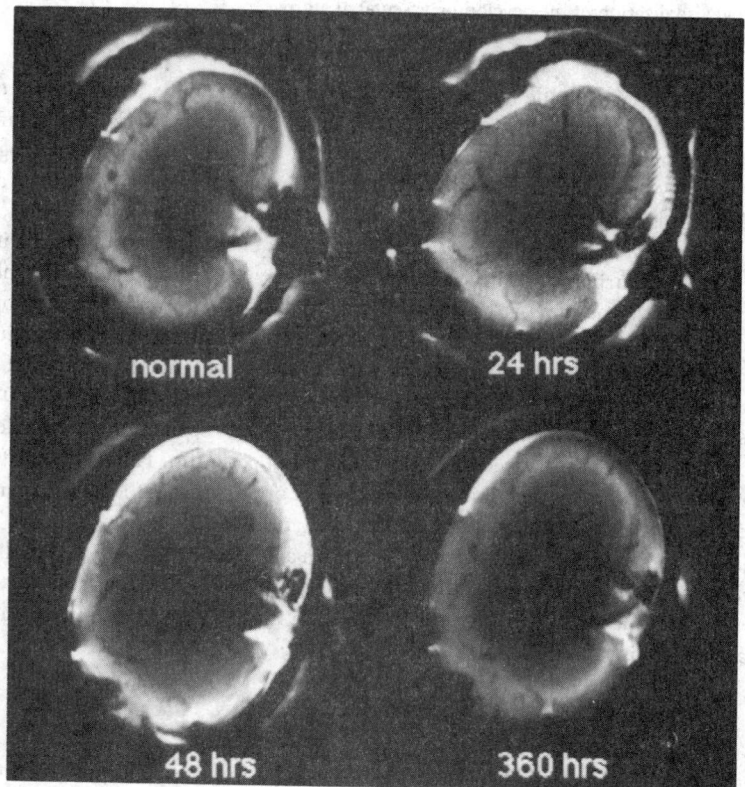

FIGURE 68.4 Implanted RF coils allow in vivo studies of deep structures with much higher spatial resolution by limiting the field of view during excitation and by increasing the SNR over volume coils. An added benefit is the ability to accurately localize the same region during a time course study. Shown here is the same region of a kidney at four different time points following exposure to mercuric chloride. Note the description of boundaries between the several zones of the kidney in the early part of the study followed by regeneration of the boundaries upon repair.

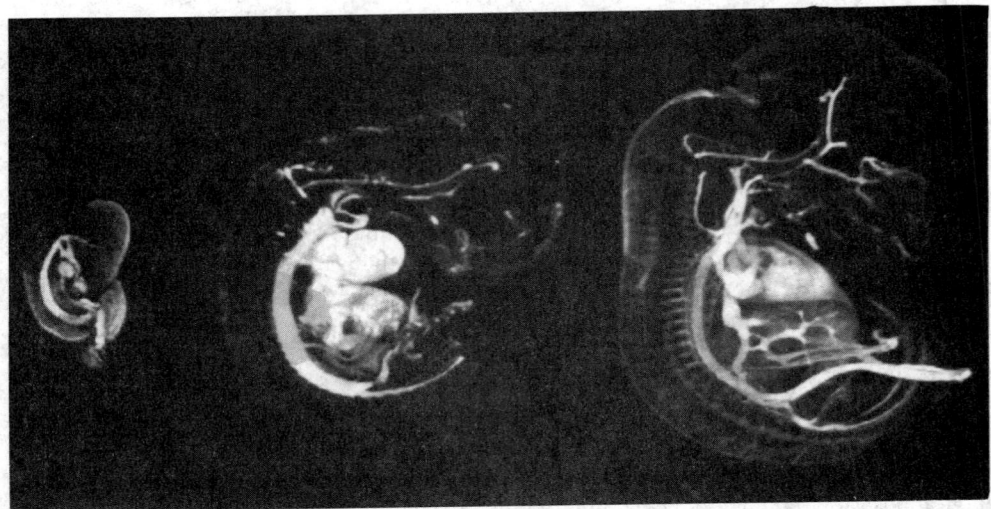

FIGURE 68.5   Isotropic 3D images of fixed mouse embryos at three stages of development have been volume rendered to allow visualization of the developing vascular anatomy.

in developing frog embryos. In their study, 3D images of the developing embryo were obtained on a time scale faster than the cell division time and analyzed forward and backward in time to reconstruct full cell divisions and cell movements. By labeling a 16-cell embryo with an exogenous contrast agent (Gd-DTPA), they successfully followed the progression from early cleavage and blastula stage through gastrulation, neurulation, and finally to tail bud stage. More important, they found that external ectodermal and internal mesodermal tissues extend at different rates during amphibian gastrulation and neurulation. This and many other key events in vertebrate embryogenesis would be very difficult to observe with optical microscopy. Another example in developmental biology is given in Fig. 68.5. Using 3D high-field (9.4-T) MR microscopy with large image arrays (256^3), Smith et al. [1993] studied the early development of the circulatory system of mouse embryos. With the aid of a T_1 contrast agent made from bovine serum albumin and Gd-DTPA, vasculature such as ventricles, atria, aorta, cardinal sinuses, basilar arteries, and thoracic arteries are clearly identified in mouse embryos at between 9.5 and 12.5 days of gestation. The ability to study embryonic development in a noninvasive fashion provided great opportunities to explore many problems in transgenic studies, gene targeting, and in situ hybridization.

In less than 10 years, MR microscopy has grown from a scientific curiosity to a tool with a wide range of applications. Although many theoretical and experimental problems still exist at the present time, there is no doubt that MR microscopy will soon make a significant impact in many areas of basic research and clinical diagnosis.

References

Ahn CB, Cho ZH. 1989. A generalized formulation of diffusion effects in μm resolution nuclear magnetic resonance imaging. Med Phys 16:22.

Banson MB, Cofer GP, Black RD, Johnson GA. 1992. A probe for specimen magnetic resonance microscopy. Invest Radiol 27:157.

Banson ML, Cofer GP, Hedlund LW, Johnson GA. 1992. Surface coil imaging of rat spine at 7.0 T. Magn Reson Imaging 10:929.

Benveniste H, Hedlund LW, Johnson GA. 1992. Mechanism of detection of acute cerebral ischemia in rats by diffusion-weighted magnetic resonance microscopy. Stroke 23:746.

Black RD, Early TA, Roemer PB, et al. 1993. A high-temperature superconducting receiver for NMR microscopy. Science 259:793.

Brown TR, Kincaid BM, Ugurbil K. 1982. NMR chemical shift imaging in three dimensions. Proc Natl Acad Sci USA 79:3523.

Callaghan PT, Coy A, Forde LC, Rofe CJ. 1993. Diffusive relaxation and edge enhancement in NMR microscopy. J Magn Reson Series A 101:347.

Callaghan PT, Eccles CD. 1987. Sensitivity and resolution in NMR imaging. J Magn Reson 71:426.

Callaghan PT, Eccles CD. 1988. Diffusion-limited resolution in nuclear magnetic resonance microscopy. J Magn Reson 78:1.

Cho ZH, Ahn CB, Juh SC, et al. 1988. Nuclear magnetic resonance microscopy with 4 μm resolution: Theoretical study and experimental results. Med Phys 15(6):815.

Cho ZH, Yi JH, Friedenberg RM. 1992. NMR microscopy and ultra-high resolution NMR imaging. Rev Magn Reson Med 4:221.

Edelstein WA, Hutchison JMS, Johnson G, Redpath T. 1980. Spin warp NMR imaging and applications to human whole-body imaging. Phys Med Biol 25:751.

Ehman RL, Felmlee JP. 1989. Adaptive technique for high-definition MR imaging of moving structures. Radiology 173:255.

Farmer THR, Johnson GA, Cofer GP, et al. 1989. Implanted coil MR microscopy of renal pathology. Magn Reson Med 10:310.

Gewalt SL, Glover GH, MacFall JR, et al. 1993. MR microscopy of the rat lung using projection reconstruction. Magn Reson Med 29:99.

Glover GH, Noll DC. 1993. Consistent projection reconstruction techniques for MRI. Magn Reson Med 29:345.

Glover GH, Pauly JM. 1992. Projection reconstruction techniques for suppression of motion artifacts. Magn Reson Med 28:275.

Gmitro A, Alexander AL. 1993. Use of a projection reconstruction method to decrease motion sensitivity in diffusion-weighted MRI. Magn Reson Med 29:835.

Haase A, Frahm J, Matthaei D, et al. 1986. FLASH imaging: Rapid NMR imaging using low flip angle pulses. J Magn Reson 67:258.

Hedges HK. 1984. Nuclear magnetic resonance microscopy. Ph.D. dissertation, State University of New York at Stony Brook.

Hedlund LW, Deitz J, Nassar R, et al. 1986. A ventilator for magnetic resonance imaging. Invest Radiol 21:18.

Hennig J, Nauerth A, Friedburg H. 1986. RARE imaging: A fast imaging method for clinical MR. Magn Reson Med 3:823.

Hetherington HP, Wishart D, Fitzpatrick SM, et al. 1986. The application of composite pulses to surface coil NMR. J Magn Reson 66:313.

Hills BP, Wright KM, Belton PS. 1990. The effects of restricted diffusion in nuclear magnetic resonance microscopy. Magn Reson Imaging 8:755.

Hollett MD, Cofer GP, Johnson GA. 1987. In situ magnetic resonance microscopy. Invest Radiol 22:965.

House WV. 1984. NMR microscopy. IEEE Trans Nucl Sci NS-31:570.

Hyslop WB, Lauterbur PC. 1991. Effects of restricted diffusion on microscopic NMR imaging. J Magn Reson 94:501.

Jacobs RE, Fraser SE. 1994. Magnetic resonance microscopy of embryonic cell lineages and movements. Science 263:681.

Johnson GA, Hedlund LW, Cofer GP, Suddarth SA. 1992. Magnetic resonance microscopy in the life sciences. Rev Magn Reson Med 4:187.

Karis JP, Johnson GA, Glover GH. 1987. Signal to noise improvements in three dimensional NMR microscopy using limited angle excitation. J Magn Reson 71:24.

Kumar A, Welti D, Ernst RR. 1975. NMR Fourier zeugmatography. J Magn Reson 18:69.

Lai CM, Lauterbur PC. 1981. True three-dimensional image reconstruction by nuclear magnetic resonance zeugmatography. Phys Med Biol 26:851.

Lauterbur PC. 1984. New direction in NMR imaging. IEEE Trans Nucl Sci NS-31:1010.

Lauterbur PC. 1973. Image formation by induced local interactions: Examples employing nuclear magnetic resonance. Nature 242:190.

Lean CL, Russell P, Delbridge L, et al. 1993. Metastatic follicular thyroid diagnosed by ^{1}H MRS. Proc Soc Magn Reson Med 1:71.

Majumdar S, Gore JC. 1988. Studies of diffusion in random fields produced by variations in susceptibility. J Magn Reson 78:41.

Maki JH, Johnson GA, Cofer GP, MacFall JR. 1988. SNR improvement in NMR microscopy using DEFT. J Magn Reson 80:482.

Mansfield P, Chapman B. 1986. Active magnetic screening of gradient coils in NMR imaging. J Magn Reson 66:573.

Mansfield P, Maudsley AA. 1977. Planar spin imaging by NMR. J Magn Reson 27:129.

McFarland EW. 1992. Time independent point-spread function for MR microscopy. Magn Reson Imaging 10:269.

McFarland EW, Mortara A. 1992. Three-dimensional NMR microscopy: Improving SNR with temperature and microcoils. Magn Reson Imaging 10:279.

Moran PR. 1982. A flow velocity zeugmatographic interlace for NMR imaging in humans. Magn Reson Imaging 1:197.

Mulkern RV, Wong STS, Winalski C, Jolesz FA. 1990. Contrast manipulation and artifact assessment of 2D and 3D RARE sequences. Magn Reson Imaging 8:557.

Peck TL, Magin RL, Lauterbur PC. 1990. Microdomain magnetic resonance imaging. Proc Soc Magn Reson Med 1:207.

Putz B, Barsky D, Schulten K. 1991. Edge enhancement by diffusion: Microscopic magnetic resonance imaging of an ultrathin glass capillary. Chem Phys 183:391.

Rudin M. 1987. MR microscopy on rats in vivo at 4.7 T using surface coils. Magn Reson Med 5:443.

Schoeniger JS, Aiken NR, Blackband SJ. 1991. NMR microscopy of single neurons. Proc Soc Magn Reson Med 2:880.

Smith BR, Johnson GA, Groman EV, Linney E. 1993. Contrast enhancement of normal and abnormal mouse embryo vasculature. Proc Soc Magn Reson Med 1:303.

Suits BH, Wilken DE. 1989. Improving magnetic field gradient coils for NMR imaging. J Phys E: Sci Instrum 22:565.

Ugurbil K, Garwood M, Bendall R. 1987. Amplitude- and frequency-modulated pulses to achieve 90° plane rotation with inhomogeneous B_1 fields. J Magn Reson 72:177.

Wood ML, Henkelman RM. 1985. NMR image artifacts from periodic motion. Med Phys 12:143.

Xiang Q-S, Henkelman RM. 1991. Motion artifact reduction with three-point ghost phase cancellation. J Magn Reson Imaging 1:633.

Zhong J, Gore JC. 1991. Studies of restricted diffusion in heterogeneous media containing variations in susceptibility. Magn Reson Med 19:276.

Zhou X. 1992. Nuclear magnetic resonance microscopy: New theoretical and technical developments. Ph.D. dissertation, University of Illinois at Urbana-Champaign.

Zhou X, Cofer GP, Mills GI, Johnson GA. 1992. An inductively coupled probe for MR microscopy at 7 T. Proc Soc Magn Reson Med. 1:971.

Zhou X, Cofer GP, Suddarth SA, Johnson GA. 1993. High-field MR microscopy using fast spin-echoes. Magn Reson Med 31:60.

Zhou X, Lauterbur PC. 1992. NMR microscopy using projection reconstruction. In B Blümich, W Kuhn (eds), Magnetic Resonance Microscopy, pp 1–27. Weinheim, Germany, VCH.

Zhou X, Liang Z-P, Cofer GP, et al. 1993. An FSE pulse sequence with circular sampling for MR microscopy. Proc Soc Magn Reson Med 1:297.

Zhou X, Maronpot RR, Mills GI, et al. 1994. Studies on bromobenzene-induced hepatotoxicity using in vivo MR microscopy. Magn Reson Med 31:619.

Further Information

A detailed description of the physics of NMR and MRI can be found in *Principles of Magnetic Resonance*, by C. S. Slichter (3rd edition, Springer-Verlag, 1989), in *NMR Imaging in Biology and Medicine*, by P. Morris (Clarendon Press, 1986), and in *Principles of Magnetic Resonance Microscopy*, by P. T. Callaghan (Oxford Press, 1991). The latter two books also contain detailed discussions on instrumentation, data acquisition, and image reconstruction for conventional and microscopic magnetic resonance imaging.

Magnetic Resonance Microscopy, edited by Blümich and Kuhn (VCH, 1992), is particularly helpful to understand various aspects of MR microscopy, both methodology and applications. Each chapter of the book covers a specific topic and is written by experts in the field.

Proceedings of the Society of Magnetic Resonance (formerly Society of Magnetic Resonance in Medicine, Berkeley, California), published annually, documents the most recent developments in the field of MR microscopy. *Magnetic Resonance in Medicine, Journal of Magnetic Resonance Imaging,* and *Magnetic Resonance Imaging,* all monthly journals, contain original research articles and are good sources for up-to-date developments.

69

Positron-Emission Tomography (PET)

Thomas F. Budinger
University of California
at Berkeley

Henry F. VanBrocklin
University of California
at Berkeley

69.1 Radiopharmaceuticals

Thomas F. Budinger and Henry F. VanBrocklin

Since the discovery of artificial radioactivity a half century ago, radiotracers, radionuclides, and radionuclide compounds have played a vital role in biology and medicine. Common to all is radionuclide (radioactive isotope) production. This section describes the basic ideas involved in radionuclide production and gives examples of the applications of radionuclides. The field of radiopharmaceutical chemistry has fallen into subspecialties of positron-emission tomography (PET) chemistry and general radiopharmaceutical chemistry, including specialists in technetium chemistry, taking advantage of the imaging attributes of technetium-99m.

The two general methods of radionuclide production are neutron addition (activation) from neutron reactors to make neutron-rich radionuclides which decay to give off electrons and gamma rays and charged-particle accelerators (linacs and cyclotrons) which usually produce neutron-deficient isotopes that decay by electron capture and emission of x-rays, gamma rays, and positrons. The production of artificial radionuclides is governed by the number of neutrons or charged particles hitting an appropriate target per time, the cross section for the particular reaction, the number of atoms in the target, and the half-life of the artificial radionuclide:

$$A(t) = \frac{N\sigma\phi}{3.7 \times 10^{10}} \left(1 - e^{\frac{0.693t}{T_{1/2}}}\right) \qquad (69.1)$$

where $A(t)$ is the produced activity in number of atoms per second, N is the number of target nuclei, σ is the cross section (probability that the neutron or charged particles will interact with the nucleus to form the artificial radioisotope) for the reaction, ϕ is the flux of charged particles, and $T_{1/2}$ is the half-life of the product. Note that N is the target mass divided by the atomic weight and

0-8493-8346-3/95/$0.00+$.50
© 1995 by CRC Press, Inc.

multiplied by Avogadro's number (6.024×10^{23}) and σ is measured in cm^2. The usual flux is about 10^{14} neutrons per second or, for charged particles, 10 to 100 μA, which is equivalent to 6.25×10^{13} to 6.25×10^{14} charged particles per second.

Nuclear Reactor–Produced Radionuclides

Thermal neutrons of the order of 10^{14} neutrons/s/cm^2 are produced in a nuclear reactor usually during a controlled nuclear fission of uranium, though thorium or plutonium are also used. High specific activity neutron-rich radionuclides are produced usually through the (n, γ), (n, p), or (n, α) reactions (Fig. 69.1a). The product nuclides usually decay by β^- followed by γ. Most of the reactor-produced radionuclides are produced by the (n, γ) reaction. The final step in the production of a radionuclide consists of the separation of product nuclide from the target container by chemical or physical means.

An alternative method for producing isotopes from a reactor is to separate the fission fragments from the spent fuel rods. This is the leading source of ^{99}Mo for medical applications. The following two methods of ^{99}Mo production are examples of carrier-added and no-carrier-added radionuclide synthesis, respectively. In Fig. 69.1a, the ^{99}Mo is produced from ^{98}Mo. Only a small fraction of the ^{98}Mo nuclei will be converted to ^{99}Mo. Therefore, at the end of neutron bombardment, there is a mixture of both isotopes. These are inseparable by conventional chemical separation techniques, and both isotopes would participate equally well in chemical reactions. The ^{99}Mo from fission of ^{238}U would not contain any other isotopes of Mo and is considered carrier-free. Thus radioisotopes produced by any means having the same atomic number as the target material would be considered carrier-added. Medical tracer techniques obviate the need for carrier-free isotopes.

Accelerator-Produced Radionuclides

Cyclotrons and linear accelerators (linacs) are sources of beams of protons, deuterons, or helium ions that bombard targets to produce neutron-deficient (proton-rich) radionuclides (Fig. 69.1b). The neutron-deficient radionuclides produced through these reactions are shown in Table 69.1. These product nuclides (usually carrier-free) decay either by electron capture or by positron emission tomography or both, followed by γ emission. In Table 69.2, most of the useful charged-particle reactions are listed.

The heat produced by the beam current on the target material can interfere with isotope production and requires efficient heat-removal strategies using extremely stable heat-conducting tar-

(a) **(b)**

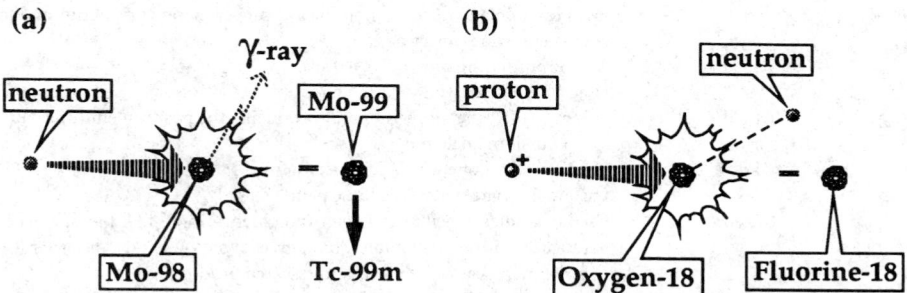

FIGURE 69.1 (a) High specific activity neutron-excess radionuclides are produced usually through the (n, γ), (n, p), or (n, α) reactions. The product nuclides usually decay by $\beta-$ followed by γ. Most of the reactor produced radionuclides are produced by the (n, γ) reaction. (b) Cyclotrons and linear accelerators (linacs) are sources of beams of protons, deuterons, or helium ions which bombard targets to produce neutron-deficient radionuclides.

TABLE 69.1   Radionuclides Used in Biomedicine

Radionuclide	Half-Life	Application(s)
Arsenic-74*	17.9 d	A positron emitting chemical analog of phosphorus
Barium-128*	2.4 d	Parent in the generator system for producing the positron emitting ^{128}Cs, a potassium analog
Beryllium-7*	53.37 d	Berylliosis studies
Bromine-77	57 h	Radioimmunotherapy
Bromine-82	35.3 h	Used in metabolic studies and studies of estrogen receptor content
*Carbon-11**	20.3 min	*Positron emitter for metabolism imaging*
Cobalt-57*	270 d	Calibration of imaging instruments
Copper-62	9.8 min	Heart perfusion
Copper-64	12.8 h	Used as a clinical diagnostic agent for cancer and metabolic disorders
Copper-67	58.5 h	Radioimmunotherapy
Chromium-51	27.8 d	Used to assess red blood cell survival
Fluorine-18	109.7 min	*Positron emitter used in glucose analogs uptake and neuroreceptor imaging*
Gallium-68	68 min	Required in calibrating PET tomographs. Potential antibody label
Germanium-68*	287 d	Parent in the generator system for producing the positron emitting ^{68}Ga
Indium-111*	2.8 d	Radioimmunotherapy
Iodine-122	3.76 min	*Positron emitter for blood flow studies*
Iodine-123*	13.3 h	SPECT brain imaging agent
Iodine-124*	4.2 d	Radioimmunotherapy, *positron emitter*
Iodine-125	60.2 d	Used as a potential cancer therapeutic agent
Iodine-131	8.1 d	Used to diagnose and treat thyroid disorders including cancer
*Iron-52**	8.2 h	*Used as an iron tracer, positron emitter for bone marrow imaging*
Magnesium-28*	21.2 h	Magnesium tracer which decays to 2.3 in aluminum-28
Magnese-52m	5.6 d	Flow tracer for heart muscle
Mercury-195m*	40 h	Parent in the generator system for producing ^{195m}Au, which is used in cardiac blood pool studies
Molybdenum-99	67 h	Used to produce technetium-99m, the most commonly used radioisotope in clinical nuclear medicine
*Nitrogen-13**	9.9 min	*Positron emitter used as ^{13}NH for heart perfusion studies*
Osmium-191	15 d	Decays to iridium-191 used for cardiac studies
*Oxygen-15**	123 s	*Positron emitter used for blood flow studies as $H_2^{15}O$*
Palladium-103	17 d	Used in the treatment of prostate cancer
Phosphorus-32	14.3 d	Used in cancer treatment, cell metabolism and kinetics, molecular biology, genetics research, biochemistry, microbiology, enzymology, and as a starter to make many basic chemicals and research products
Rhenium-188	17 h	Used for treatment of medullary thyroid carcinoma and alleviation of pain in bone metastases
*Rubidium-82**	1.2 min	*Positron emitter used for heart perfusion studies*
Ruthenium-97*	2.9 d	Hepatobiliary function, tumor and inflammation localization
Samarium-145	340 d	Treatment of ocular cancer
Samarium-153	46.8 h	Used to radiolabel various molecules as cancer therapeutic agents and to alleviate bone cancer pain
Scandium-47	3.4 d	Radioimmunotherapy
Scandium-47*	3.4 d	Used in the therapy of cancer
Strontium-82*	64.0 d	Parent in the generator system for producing the positron emitting ^{82}Rb, a potassium analogue
Strontium-85	64 d	Used to study bone formation metabolism
Strontium-89	52 d	Used to alleviate metastatic bone pain
Sulfur-35	87.9 d	Used in studies of cell metabolism and kinetics, molecular biology, genetics research, biochemistry, microbiology, enzymology, and as a starter to make many basic chemicals and research products
Technetium-99m	6 h	The most widely used radiopharmaceutical in nuclear medicine and produced from molybdenum-99
Thalium-201*	74 h	Cardiac imaging agent
Tin-117m	14.0 d	Palliative treatment of bone cancer pain
Tritium (hydrogen-3)	12.3 yr	Used to make tritiated water which is used as a starter for thousands of different research products and basic chemicals; used for life science and drug metabolism studies to ensure the safety of potential new drugs

(continued)

TABLE 69.1　Radionuclides Used in Biomedicine *(continued)*

Radionuclide	Half-Life	Application(s)
Tungsten-178*	21.5 d	Parent in generator system for producing ^{178}Ta, short lived scanning agent
Tungsten-188	69 d	Decays to rhenium-188 for treatment of cancer and rheumatoid arthritis
Vanadium-48*	16.0 d	Nutrition and environmental studies
Xenon-122*	20 h	Parent in the generator system for producing the positron emitting ^{122}I
Xenon-127*	36.4 d	Used in lung ventilation studies
Xenon-133	5.3 d	Used in lung ventilation and perfusion studies
Yttrium-88*	106.6 d	Radioimmunotherapy
Yttrium-90	64 h	Used to radiolabel various molecules as cancer therapeutic agents
Zinc-62*	9.13 h	Parent in the generator system for producing the positron emitting ^{62}Cu
Zirconium-89*	78.4 h	Radioimmunotherapy, positron emitter

*Produced by accelerated charged particles. Others are produced by neutron reactors.

get materials such as metal foils, electroplated metals, metal powders, metal oxides, and salts melted on duralmin plate. All the modern targets use circulating cold deionized water and/or chilled helium gas to aid in cooling the target body and window foils. Cyclotrons used in medical studies have ^{11}C, ^{13}N, ^{15}O, and ^{18}F production capabilities that deliver the product nuclides on demand through computer-executed commands. The radionuclide is remotely transferred into a lead-shielded hot cell for processing. The resulting radionuclides are manipulated using microscale radiochemical techniques: small-scale synthetic methodology, ion-exchange chromatography, solvent extraction, electrochemical synthesis, distillation, simple filtration, paper chromatography, and isotopic carrier precipitation. Various relevant radiochemical techniques have been published in standard texts.

Generator-Produced Radionuclides

If the reactor, cyclotron, or natural product radionuclide of long half-life decays to a daughter with nuclear characteristics appropriate for medical application, the system is called a *medical radionuclide generator*. There are several advantages afforded by generator-produced isotopes. These generators represent a convenient source of short-lived medical isotopes without the need for an on-site reactor or particle accelerator. Generators provide delivery of the radionuclide on demand at a site remote from the production facility. They are a source of both gamma- and positron-emitting isotopes.

The most common medical radionuclide generator is the ^{99}Mo $\rightarrow$ ^{99m}Tc system, the source of ^{99m}Tc, a gamma-emitting isotope currently used in 70% of the clinical nuclear medicine studies. The ^{99}Mo has a 67-hour half-life, giving this generator a useful life of about a week. Another common generator is the ^{68}Ge $\rightarrow$ ^{68}Ga system. Germanium (half-life is 287 days) is accelerator-produced in high-energy accelerators (e.g., BLIP, LAMPF, TRIUMF) through the alpha-particle bombardment of ^{66}Zn. The ^{68}Ge decays to ^{68}Ga, a positron emitter, which has a 68-minute half-life. Gallium generators can last for several months.

The generator operation is fairly straightforward. In general, the parent isotope is bound to a solid chemical matrix (e.g., alumina column, anionic resin, Donux resin). As the parent decays, the daughter nuclide grows in. The column is then flushed ("milked") with a suitable solution (e.g., saline, hydrochloric acid) that elutes the daughter and leaves the remaining parent absorbed on the column. The eluent may be injected directly or processed into a radiopharmaceutical.

Radiopharmaceuticals

^{99m}Tc is removed from the generator in the form of TcO_4^- (pertechnetate). This species can be injected directly for imag-

TABLE 69.2　Important Reactions for Cyclotron-Produced Radioisotopes

1. *p, n*	7. *p, pn*
2. *p, 2n*	8. *p, 2p*
3. *d, n*	9. *d, p*
4. *d, 2n*	10. *d,* ^{4}He
5. *p,* ^{4}He	11. *p, d*
6. *p,* ^{4}He*n*	12. ^{4}He, *n*
	13. ^{3}He, *p*

ing or incorporated into a variety of useful radiopharmaceuticals. The labeling of ^{99m}Tc usually involves reduction complexation/chelation. ^{99m}Tc-Sestamibi (Fig. 69.2) is a radiopharmaceutical used to evaluate myocardial perfusion or in the diagnosis of cancer. There are several reduction methods employed, including Sn(II) reduction in NaHCO$_3$ at pH of 8 and other reduction and complexation reactions such as S$_2$O$_3$ + HCl, FeCl$_3$ + ascorbic acid, LiBH$_4$, Zn + HCl, HCl, Fe(II), Sn(II)F$_2$, Sn(II) citrate, and Sn(II) tartrate reduction and complexation, electrolytic reduction, and in vivo labeling of red cells following Sn(II) pyrophosphate or Sn(II) DTPA administration. ^{131}I, ^{125}I, and ^{123}I labeling requires special reagents or conditions such as chloramine-T, widely used for protein labeling at 7.5 pH; peroxidase + H$_2$O$_2$, widely used for radioassay tracers; isotopic exchange for imaging tracers; excitation labeling as in ^{123}Xe → ^{123}I diazotization plus iodination for primary amines; conjugation labeling with Bolton Hunter agent (*N*-succinimidyl 3-[4-hydroxy 5-(^{131,125,123}I)iodophenyl] propionate); hydroboration plus iodination; electrophilic destannylation; microdiffusion with fresh iodine vapor; and other methods. Radiopharmaceuticals in common use for brain perfusion studies are *N*-isopropyl-*p*-[^{123}I] iodoamphetamine and ^{99m}Tc-labeled hexamethylpropyleneamine.

Sestamibi

^{99m}TcO$_4^-$ + [(CH$_3$)$_2$C(OMe)CH$_2$NC]$_4$CuBF$_4$

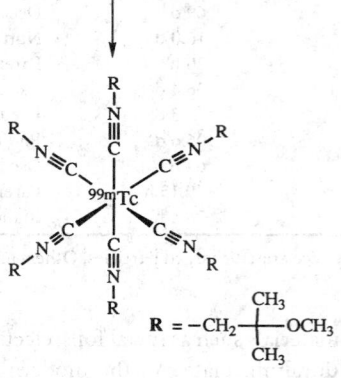

R = —CH$_2$—C(CH$_3$)$_2$—OCH$_3$

FIGURE 69.2 ^{99m}Tc-Sestamibi is a radiopharmaceutical used to evaluate myocardial perfusion or in the diagnosis of cancer using both computed tomography and scintigraphy techniques.

PET Radionuclides

For ^{11}C, ^{13}N, ^{15}O, and ^{18}F, the modes of production of short-lived positron emitters can dictate the chemical form of the product, as shown in Table 69.3. On-line chemistry is used to make various PET agents and precursors. For example, ^{11}C cyanide, an important precursor for synthesis of other labeled compounds, is produced in the cyclotron target by first bombarding N$_2$ + 5% H$_2$ gas target with 20-MeV protons. The product is carbon-labeled methane, ^{11}CH$_4$, which when combined with ammonia and passed over a platinum wool catalyst at 1000°C becomes ^{11}CN$^-$, which is subsequently trapped in NaOH.

Molecular oxygen is produced by bombarding a gas target of ^{14}N$_2$ + 2% O$_2$ with deuterons (6 to 8 MeV). A number of products (e.g., ^{15}O$_2$, C^{15}O$_2$, N^{15}O$_2$, ^{15}O$_3$, and H$_2$^{15}O) are trapped by soda lime followed by charcoal to give ^{15}O$_2$ as the product. However, if an activated charcoal trap at 900°C is used before the soda lime trap, the ^{15}O$_2$ will be converted to C^{15}O. The specific strategies for other on-line PET agents is given in Rayudu [1990].

Fluorine-18 (^{18}F) is a very versatile positron emitting isotope. With a 2-hour half-life and two forms (F$^+$ and F$^-$), one can develop several synthetic methods for incorporating ^{18}F into medically useful compounds [Kilbourn, 1990]. Additionally, fluorine forms strong bonds with carbon and is roughly the same size as a hydrogen atom, imparting metabolic and chemical stability of the molecules without drastically altering biologic activity.

TABLE 69.3 Major Positron-Emitting Radionuclides Produced by Accelerated Protons

Radionuclide	Half-Life	Reaction
Carbon-11	20 min	^{12}C (*p, pn*) ^{11}C
		^{14}N (*p, α*) ^{11}C
Nitrogen-13	10 min	^{16}O (*p, α*) ^{13}N
		^{13}C (*p, n*) ^{13}N
Oxygen-15	2 min	^{15}N (*p, n*) ^{15}O
		^{14}N (*d, n*) ^{15}O
Fluorine-18	110 min	^{18}O (*p, n*) ^{18}F
		^{20}Ne (*d, α*) ^{18}F

Note: A(x, y)B: A is target, x is the bombarding particle, y is the radiation product, and B is the isotope produced.

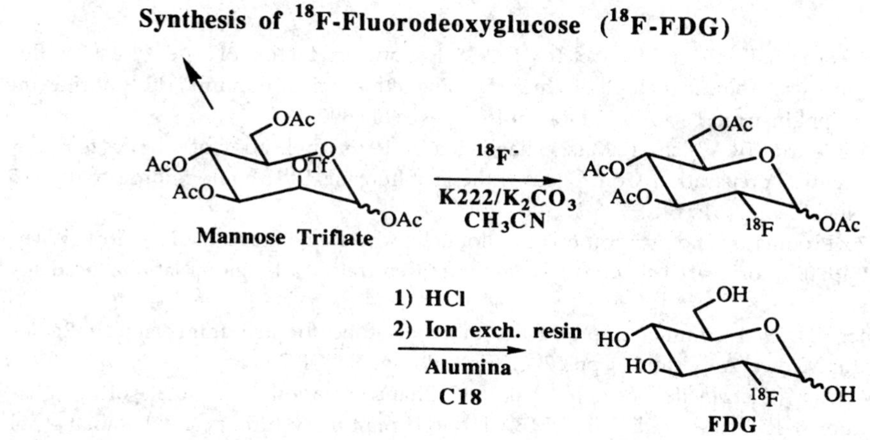

Synthesis of ^{18}F-Fluorodeoxyglucose (^{18}F-FDG)

FIGURE 69.3 Schematic for the chemical production of deoxyglucose labelled with fluorine-18. Here K222 refers to Kryptofix and C18 denotes a reverse-phase high-pressure liquid chromatography column.

The most commonly produced ^{18}F radiopharmaceutical is 2-deoxy-2-[^{18}F]fluoroglucose (FDG). This radiotracer mimics part of the glucose metabolic pathway and has shown both hypo- and hypermetabolic abnormalities in cardiology, oncology, and neurology. The synthetic pathway for the production of FDG is shown in Fig. 69.3.

The production of positron radiopharmaceuticals requires the rapid incorporation of the isotope into the desired molecule. Chemical techniques and synthetic strategies have been developed to facilitate these reactions. Many of these synthetic manipulations require hands-on operations by a highly trained chemist. Additionally, since positrons give off 2- to 511-keV gamma rays upon annihilation, proximity to the source can increase one's personal dose. The demand for the routine production of positron radiopharmaceuticals such as FDG has led to the development of remote synthetic devices. These devices can be human-controlled (i.e., flipping switches to open air-actuated valves), computer-controlled, or robotic. A sophisticated computer-controlled chemistry synthesis unit has been assembled for the fully automated production of ^{18}FDG [Padgett, 1989]. A computer-controlled robot has been programmed to produce 6α-[^{18}F]fluoroestradiol for breast cancer imaging [Brodack, 1986; Mathias, 1987]. Both these types of units increase the availability and reduce the cost of short-lived radiopharmaceutical production through greater reliability and reduced need for a highly trained staff. Additionally, these automated devices reduce personnel radiation exposure. These and other devices are being designed with greater versatility in mind to allow a variety of radiopharmaceuticals to be produced just by changing the programming and the required reagents.

These PET radionuclides have been incorporated into a wide variety of medically useful radiopharmaceuticals through a number of synthetic techniques. The development of PET scanner technology has added a new dimension to synthetic chemistry by challenging radiochemists to devise labeling and purification strategies that proceed on the order of minutes rather than hours or days as in conventional synthetic chemistry. To meet this challenge, radiochemists are developing new target systems to improve isotope production and sophisticated synthetic units to streamline routine production of commonly desired radiotracers as well as preparing short-lived radiopharmaceuticals for many applications.

Acknowledgment

This work was supported in part by the Director, Office of Energy Research, Office of Health and Environmental Research, Medical Applications and Biophysical Research Division of the U.S. Department of Energy, under contract No. DE-AC03-SF00098, and in part by NIH Grant HL25840.

References

Brodack JW, Dence CS, Kilbourn MR, Welch MJ. 1988. Robotic production of 2-deoxy-2-[18F]fluoro-D-glucose: A routine method of synthesis using tetrabutylammonium [18F]fluoride. Int J Radiat Appl Instrum Part A: Appl Radiat Isotopes 39(7):699.

Brodack JW, Kilbourn MR, Welch MJ, Katzenellenbogen JA. 1986. Application of robotics to radiopharmaceutical preparation: Controlled synthesis of fluorine-18 16 alpha-fluoroestradiol-17 beta. J Nucl Med 27(5):714.

Hupf HB. 1976. Production and purification of radionuclides. In Radiopharmacy. New York, Wiley.

Kilbourn MR. 1990. Fluorine-18 Labeling of Radiopharmaceuticals. Washington, National Academy Press.

Lamb J, Kramer HH. 1983. Commercial production of radioisotopes for nuclear medicine. In Radiotracers for Medical Applications, pp 17–62. Boca Raton, Fla, CRC Press.

Mathias CJ, Welch MJ, Katzenellenbogen JA, et al. 1987. Characterization of the uptake of 16 alpha-([18F]fluoro)-17 beta-estradiol in DMBA-induced mammary tumors. Int J Radiat Appl Instrum Part B: Nucl Med Biol 14(1):15.

Padgett HC, Schmidt DG, Luxen A, et al. 1989. Computer-controlled radiochemical synthesis: A chemistry process control unit for the automated production of radiochemicals. Int J Radiat Appl Instrum Part A: Appl Radiat Isotopes 40(5):433.

Rayudu GV. 1990. Production of radionuclides for medicine. Semin Nucl Med 20(2):100.

Sorenson JA, Phelps ME. 1987. Physics in Nuclear Medicine. New York, Grune & Stratton.

Steigman J, Eckerman WC. 1992. The Chemistry of Technetium in Medicine. Washington, National Academy Press.

Stocklin G. 1992. Tracers for metabolic imaging of brain and heart: Radiochemistry and radiopharmacology. Eur J Nucl Med 19(7):527.

69.2 Instrumentation

Thomas F. Budinger

Background

The history of positron-emission tomography (PET) can be traced to the early 1950s, when workers in Boston first realized the medical imaging possibilities of a particular class of radioactive substances. It was recognized then that the high-energy photons produced by annihilation of the positron from positron-emitting isotopes could be used to describe, in three dimensions, the physiologic distribution of "tagged" chemical compounds. After two decades of moderate technological developments by a few research centers, widespread interest and broadly based research activity began in earnest following the development of sophisticated reconstruction algorithms and improvements in detector technology. By the mid-1980s, PET had become a tool for medical diagnosis and for dynamic studies of human metabolism.

Today, because of its million-fold sensitivity advantage over magnetic resonance imaging (MRI) in tracer studies and its chemical specificity, PET is used to study neuroreceptors in the brain and other body tissues. In contrast, MRI has exquisite resolution for anatomic (Fig. 69.4) and flow studies as well as unique attributes of evaluating chemical composition of tissue but in the millimolar range rather than the nanomolar range of much of the receptor proteins in the body. Clinical studies include tumors of the brain, breast, lungs, lower gastrointestinal tract, and other sites. Additional clinical uses include Alzheimer's disease, Parkinson's disease, epilepsy, and coronary artery disease affecting heart muscle metabolism and flow. Its use has added immeasurably to our current understanding of flow, oxygen utilization, and the metabolic changes that accompany disease and that change during brain stimulation and cognitive activation.

MRI

PET

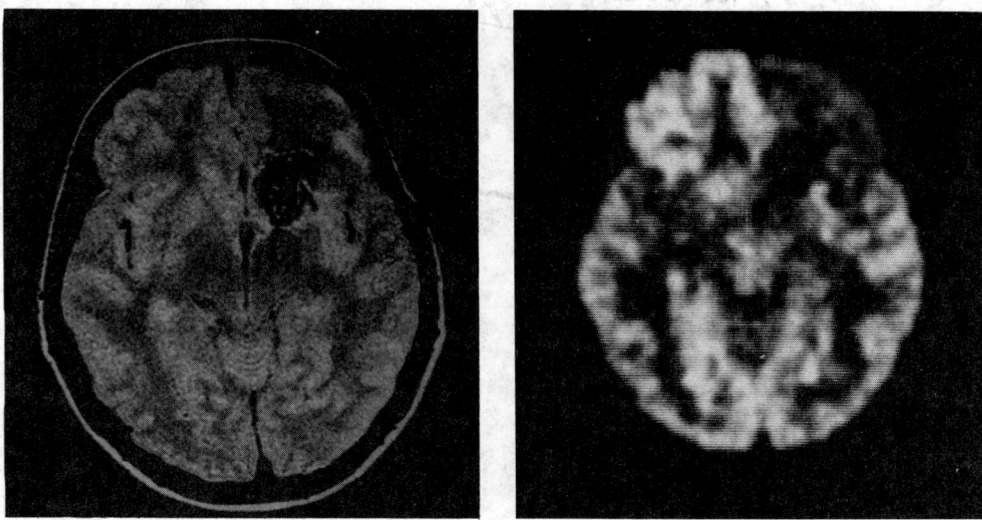

FIGURE 69.4 The MRI image shows the arteriovenous malformation (AVM) as an area of signal loss due to blood flow. The PET image shows the AVM as a region devoid of glucose metabolism and also shows decreased metabolism in the adjacent frontal cortex. This is a metabolic effect of the AVM on the brain and may explain some of the patient's symptoms.

PET Theory

PET imaging begins with the injection of a metabolically active tracer—a biologic molecule that carries with it a positron-emitting isotope (e.g., ^{11}C, ^{13}N, ^{15}O, or ^{18}F). Over a few minutes, the isotope accumulates in an area of the body for which the molecule has an affinity. As an example, glucose labeled with ^{11}C, or a glucose analogue labeled with ^{18}F, accumulates in the brain or tumors, where glucose is used as the primary source of energy. The radioactive nuclei then decay by positron emission. In positron (positive electron) emission, a nuclear proton changes into a positive electron and a neutron. The atom maintains its atomic mass but decreases its atomic number by 1. The ejected positron combines with an electron almost instantaneously, and these two particles undergo the process of annihilation. The energy associated with the masses of the positron and electron particles is 1.022 MeV in accordance with the energy E to mass m equivalence $E = mc^2$, where c is the velocity of light. This energy is divided equally between two photons that fly away from one another at a 180-degree angle. Each photon has an energy of 511 keV. These high-energy gamma rays emerge from the body in opposite directions, to be detected by an array of detectors that surround the patient (Fig. 69.5). When two photons are recorded simultaneously by a pair of detectors, the annihilation event that gave rise to them must have occurred somewhere along the line connecting the detectors. Of course, if one of the photons is scattered, then the line of coincidence will be incorrect. After 100,000 or more annihilation events are detected, the distribution of the positron-emitting tracer is calculated by tomographic reconstruction procedures. PET reconstructs a two-dimensional (2D) image from the one-dimensional projections seen at different angles. Three-dimensional (3D) reconstructions also can be done using 2D projections from multiple angles.

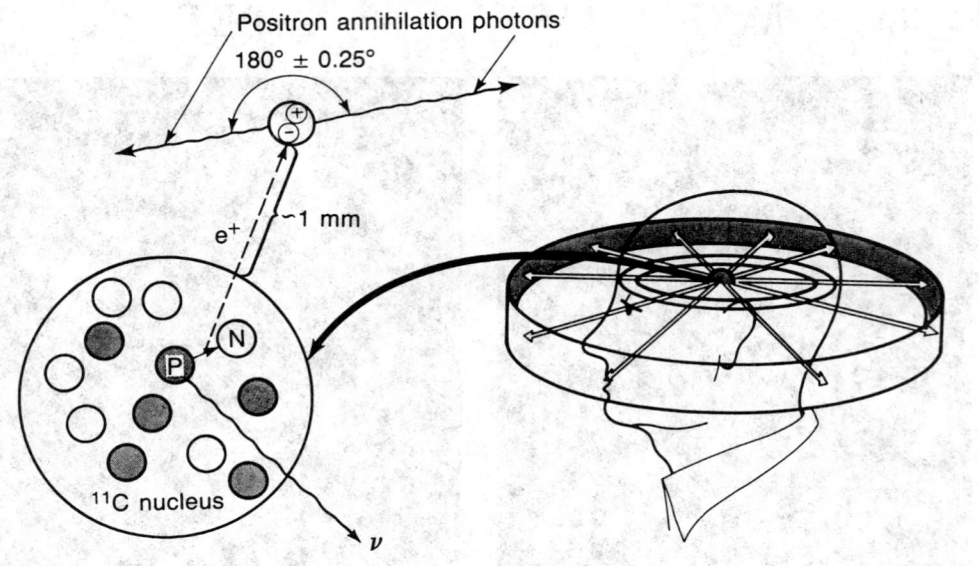

FIGURE 69.5   The physical basis of positron-emission tomography. Positrons emitted by "tagged" metabolically active molecules annihilate nearby electrons and give rise to a pair of high-energy photons. The photons fly off in nearly opposite directions and thus serve to pinpoint their source. The biologic activity of the tagged molecule can be used to investigate a number of physiologic functions, both normal and pathologic.

PET Detectors

Efficient detection of the annihilation photons from positron emitters is usually provided by the combination of a crystal, which converts the high-energy photons to visible-light photons, and a photomultiplier tube that produces an amplified electric current pulse proportional to the amount of light photons interacting with the photocathode. The fact that imaging system sensitivity is proportional to the square of the detector efficiency leads to a very important requirement that the detector be nearly 100% efficient. Thus other detector systems such as plastic scintillators or gas-filled wire chambers, with typical individual efficiencies of 20% or less, would result in a coincident efficiency of only 4% or less.

Most modern PET cameras are multilayered with 15 to 47 levels or transaxial layers to be reconstructed (Fig. 69.6). The lead shields prevent activity from the patient from causing spurious counts in the tomograph ring, while the tungsten septa reject some of the events in which one (or both) of the 511-keV photons suffer a Compton scatter in the patient. The sensitivity of this design is improved by collection of data from cross-planes (Fig. 69.6). The arrangement of scintillators and phototubes is shown in Fig. 69.7.

The "individually coupled" design is capable of very high resolution, and because the design is very parallel (all the photomultiplier tubes and scintillator crystals operate independently), it is capable of very high data throughput. The disadvantages of this type of design are the requirement for many expensive photomultiplier tubes and, additionally, that connecting round photomultiplier tubes to rectangular scintillation crystals leads to problems of packing rectangular crystals and circular phototubes of sufficiently small diameter to form a solid ring.

The contemporary method of packing many scintillators for 511 keV around the patient is to use what is called a *block detector design*. A block detector couples several photomultiplier tubes to a bank of scintillator crystals and uses a coding scheme to determine the crystal of interaction. In the two-

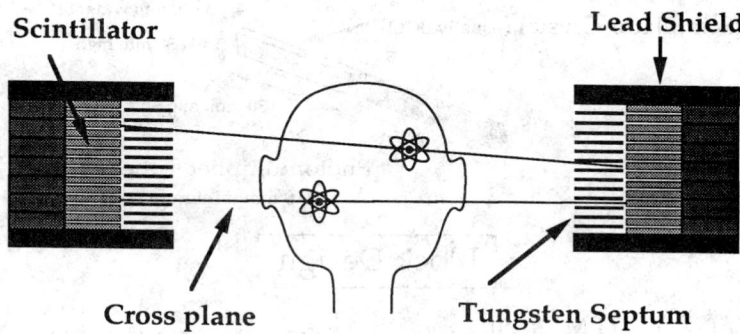

Multi - Layer Detector

Scintillator

Lead Shield

Cross plane

Tungsten Septum

FIGURE 69.6 Most modern PET cameras are multilayered with 15 to 47 levels or transaxial layers to be reconstructed. The lead shields prevent activity from the patient from causing spurious counts in the tomograph ring, while the tungsten septa reject some of the events in which one (or both) of the 511-keV photons suffer a Compton scatter in the patient. The sensitivity of this design is improved by collection of data from cross-planes.

layer block (Fig. 69.7), five photomultiplier tubes are coupled to eight scintillator crystals. Whenever one of the outside four photomultiplier tubes fires, a 511-keV photon has interacted in one of the two crystals attached to that photomultiplier tube, and the center photomultiplier tube is then used to determine whether it was the inner or outer crystal. This is known as a *digital* coding scheme, since each photomultiplier tube is either "hit" or "not hit" and the crystal of interaction is determined by a "digital" mapping of the hit pattern. Block detector designs are much less expensive and practical to form into a multilayer camera. However, errors in the decoding scheme reduce the spatial resolution, and since the entire block is "dead" whenever one of its member crystals is struck by a photon, the dead time is worse than with individual coupling. The electronics necessary to decode the output of the block are straightforward but more complex than that needed for the individually coupled design.

Most block detector coding schemes use an *analog* coding scheme, where the ratio of light output is used to determine the crystal of interaction. In the example above, 4 photomultiplier tubes are coupled to a block of BGO that has been partially sawed through to form 64 "individual" crystals. The depth of the cuts are critical; that is, deep cuts tend to focus the scintillation light onto the face of a single photomultiplier tube, while shallow cuts tend to spread the light over all four photomultiplier tubes. This type of coding scheme is more difficult to implement than digital coding, since analog light ratios place more stringent requirements on the photomultiplier tube linearity and uniformity as well as scintillator crystal uniformity. However, most commercial PET cameras use an analog coding scheme because it is much less expensive due to the lower number of photomultiplier tubes required.

Physical Factors Affecting Resolution

The factors that affect the spatial resolution of PET tomographs are shown in Fig. 69.8. The size of the detector is critical in determining the system's geometric resolution. If the block design is used, there is a degradation in this geometric resolution by 2.2 mm for BGO. The degradation is probably due to the limited light output of BGO and the ratio of crystals (cuts) per phototube.

The angle between the paths of the annihilation photons can deviate from 180 degrees as a result of some residual kinetic motion (Fermi motion) at the time of annihilation. The effect on resolu-

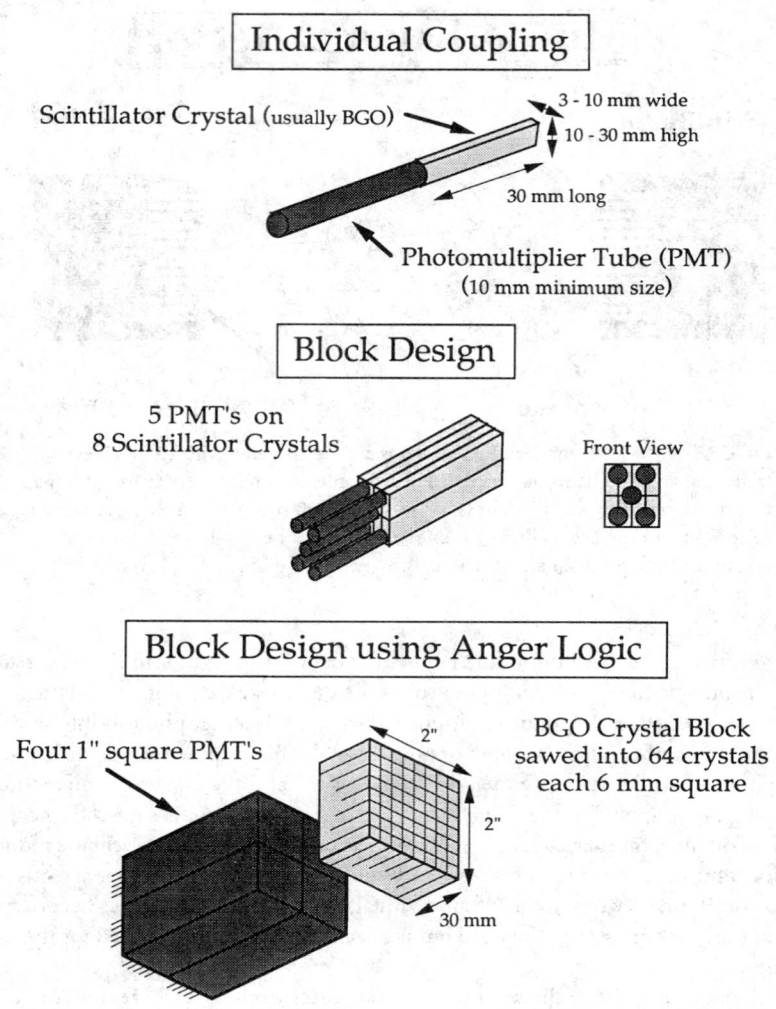

FIGURE 69.7   The arrangement of scintillators and phototubes is shown. The "individually coupled" design is capable of very high resolution, and because the design is very parallel (all the photomultiplier tubes and scintillator crystals operate independently), it is capable of very high data throughput. A block detector couples several photomultiplier tubes to a bank of scintillator crystals and uses a coding scheme to determine the crystal of interaction. In the two-layer block, five photomultiplier tubes are coupled to eight scintillator crystals.

tion of this deviation increases as the detector ring diameter increases so that eventually this factor can have a significant effect.

The distance the positron travels after being emitted from the nucleus and before annihilation causes a deterioration in spatial resolution. This distance depends on the particular nuclide. For example, the range of blurring for ^{18}F, the isotope used for many of the current PET studies, is quite small compared with that of other isotopes. Combining values for these factors for the PET-600 tomograph, we can estimate a detector-pair spatial resolution of 2.0 mm and a reconstructed image resolution of 2.6 mm. The measured resolution of this system is 2.6 mm, but most commercially

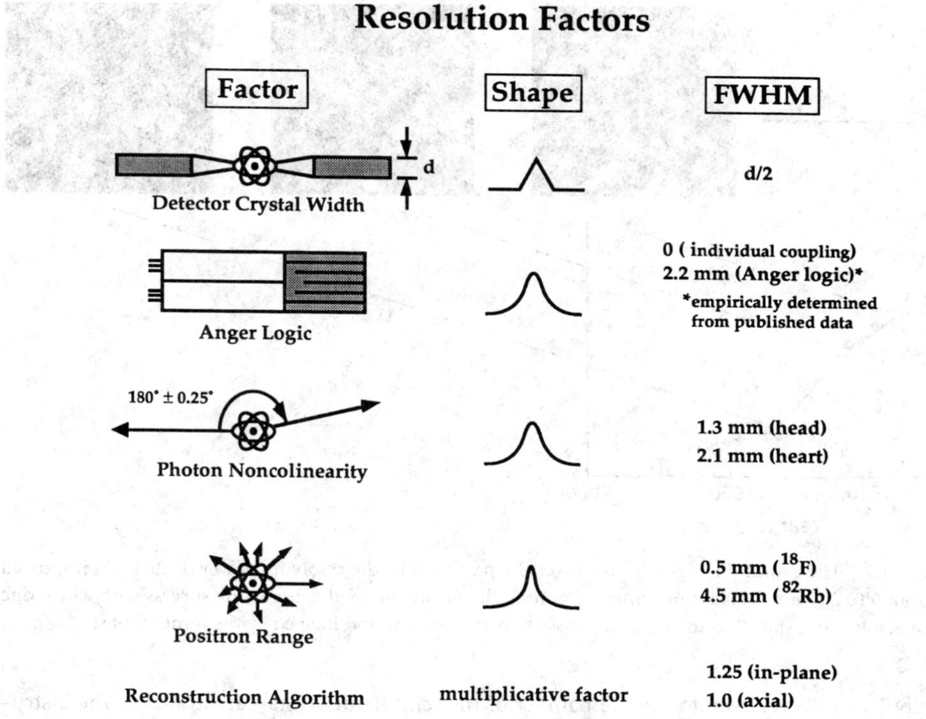

Resolution Factors

Factor	Shape	FWHM
Detector Crystal Width		d/2
Anger Logic		0 (individual coupling) 2.2 mm (Anger logic)* *empirically determined from published data
Photon Noncolinearity		1.3 mm (head) 2.1 mm (heart)
Positron Range		0.5 mm (^{18}F) 4.5 mm (^{82}Rb)
Reconstruction Algorithm	multiplicative factor	1.25 (in-plane) 1.0 (axial)

FIGURE 69.8 Factors contributing to the resolution of the PET tomograph. The contribution most accessible to further reduction is the size of the detector crystals.

available tomographs use a block detector design (Fig. 69.7), and the resolution of these systems is about 5 mm. The evolution of resolution improvement is shown in Fig. 69.9.

The resolution evolutions discussed above pertain to results for the center or axis of the tomograph. The resolution at the edge of the object (e.g., patient) will be less by a significant amount due to two factors. First, the path of the photon from an "off-center" annihilation event typically traverses more than one detector crystal, as shown in Fig. 69.10. This results in an elongation of the resolution spread function along the radius of the transaxial plane. The loss of resolution is dependent on the crystal density and the diameter of the tomograph detector ring. For a 60-cm diameter system, the resolution can deteriorate by a factor of 2 from the axis to 10 cm.

The coincidence circuitry must be able to determine coincident events with 10- to 20-ns resolution for each crystal-crystal combination (i.e., chord). The timing requirement is set jointly by the time of flight across the detector ring (4 ns) and the crystal-to-crystal resolving time (typically 3 ns). The most stringent requirement, however, is the vast number of chords in which coincidences must be determined (over 1.5 million in a 24-layer camera with septa in place and 18 million with the septa removed).

It is obviously impractical to have an individual coincidence circuit for each chord, so tomograph builders use parallel organization to solve this problem. A typical method is to use a high-speed clock (typically 200 MHz) to mark the arrival time of each 511-keV photon and a digital coincidence processor to search for coincident pairs of detected photons based on this time marker. This search can be done extremely quickly by having multiple sorters working in parallel.

The maximum event rate is also quite important, especially in septaless systems. The maximum rate in a single detector crystal is limited by the dead time due to the scintillator fluorescent lifetime

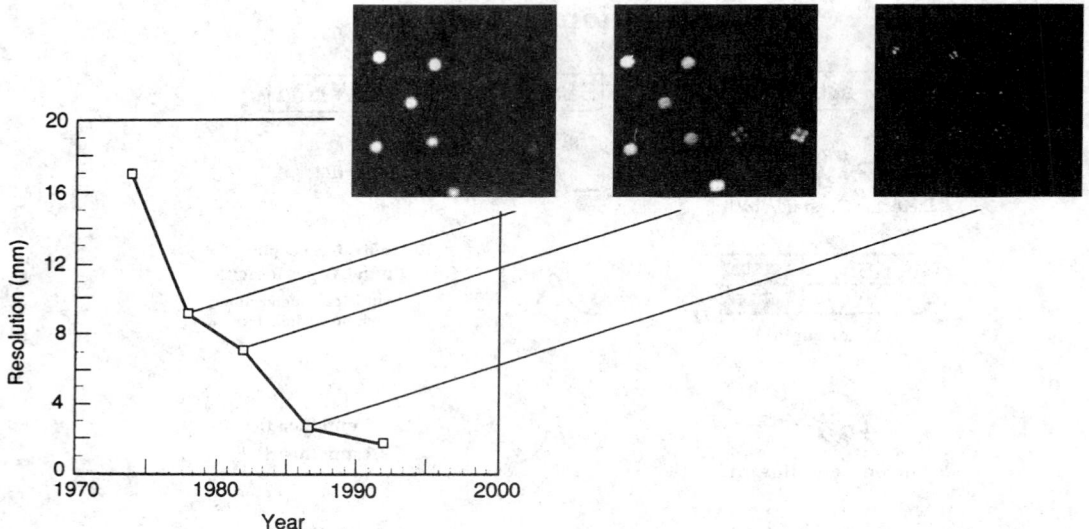

FIGURE 69.9 The evolution of resolution. Over the past decade, the resolving power of PET has improved from about 9 to 2.6 mm. This improvement is graphically illustrated by the increasing success with which one is able to resolve "hot spots" of an artificial sample that are detected and imaged by the tomographs.

(typically 1 μs per event), but as the remainder of the scintillator crystals are available, the instrument has much higher event rates (e.g., number of crystals × 1 μs). Combining crystals together to form contiguous blocks reduces the maximum event rate because the fluorescent lifetime applies to the entire block and a fraction of the tomograph is dead after each event.

Random Coincidences

If two annihilation events occur within the time resolution of the tomograph (e.g., 10 ns), then random coincident "events" add erroneous background activity to the tomograph and are significant at high event rates. These can be corrected for on a chord-by-chord basis. The noncoincidence event rate of each crystal pair is measured by observing the rate of events beyond the coincident timing window. The random rate for the particular chord R_{ij} corresponding to a crystal pair is

$$R_{ij} = r_i \times r_j \times 2\tau \qquad R_{ij} = R_{ij} \tag{69.2}$$

where r_i and r_j are the event rates of crystal i and crystal j, and τ is the coincidence window width. As the activity in the subject increases, the event rate in each detector increases. Thus the random event rate will increase as the square of the activity.

Tomographic Reconstruction

Before reconstruction, each projection ray or chord receives three corrections: crystal efficiency, attenuation, and random efficiency. The efficiency for each chord is computed by dividing the observed count rate for that chord by the average count rate for chords with a similar geometry (i.e., length). This is typically done daily using a transmission source without the patient or object in place. Once the patient is in position in the camera, a transmission scan is taken, and the attenuation factor for each chord is computed by dividing its transmission count rate by its efficiency count rate. The patient is then injected with the isotope, and an emission scan is taken, during which time

Radial Elongation

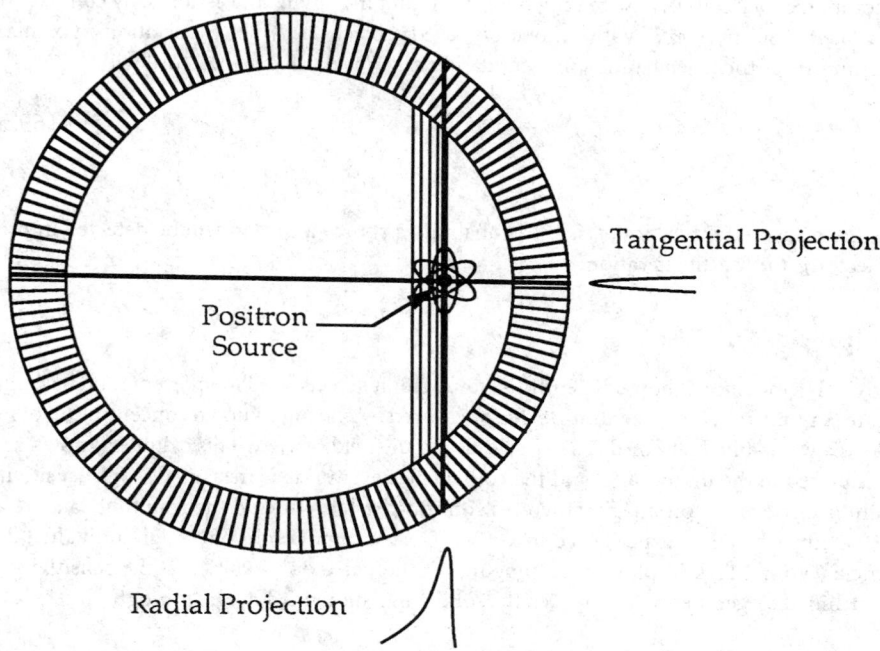

FIGURE 69.10 Resolution astigmatism in detecting off-center events. Because annihilation photons can penetrate crystals to different depths, the resolution is not equal in all directions, particularly at the edge of the imaging field. This problem of astigmatism will be taken into account in future PET instrumentation.

the random count rate is also measured. For each chord, the random event rate is subtracted from the emission rate, and the difference is divided by the attenuation factor and the chord efficiency. (The detector efficiency is divided twice because two separate detection's measurements are made—transmission and emission). The resulting value is reconstructed, usually with the filtered back-projection algorithm. This is the same algorithm used in x-ray computed tomography (CT) and in projection MRI. The corrected projection data are formatted onto parallel- or fan-beam data sets for each angle. These are modified by a high-pass filter and backprojected.

The process of PET reconstruction is linear and shown by operators successively operating on the projections P:

$$A = \sum_{\theta} BPF^{-1} RF(P) \qquad (69.3)$$

where A is the image, F is the Fourier transform, R is the ramp-shaped high-pass filter, F^{-1} is the inverse Fourier transform, BP is the backprojection operation, and ϵ denotes the superposition operation.

The alternative class of reconstruction algorithms involves iterative solutions to the classic inverse problem:

$$P = FA \qquad (69.4)$$

where P is the projection matrix, A is the matrix of true data being sought, and F is the projection operation. The inverse is

$$A = F^{-1}P$$

which is computed by iteratively estimating the data A' and modifying the estimate by comparison of the calculated projection set P' with the true observed projections P. The expectation-maximization algorithm solves the inverse problem by updating each pixel value a_i in accord with

$$a_1^{k+1} = \sum_j p_j \frac{a_i^k f_{ij}}{\sum_i a_1^k f_{ij}} \tag{69.5}$$

where P is the measured projection, f_{ij} is the probability a source at pixel i will be detected in projection detector j, and k is the iteration.

Sensitivity

The sensitivity is a measure of how efficiently the tomograph detects coincident events and has units of count rate per unit activity concentration. It is measured by placing a known concentration of radionuclide in a water-filled 20-cm-diameter cylinder in the field of view. This cylinder, known as a *phantom*, is placed in the tomograph, and the coincidence event rate is measured. High sensitivity is important because emission imaging involves counting each event, and the resulting data are as much as 1000 times less than experienced in x-ray CT. Most tomographs have high individual detection efficiency for 511-keV photons impinging on the detector ($>90\%$), so the sensitivity is mostly determined by geometric factors, i.e., the solid angle subtended by the tomograph:

$$S = \frac{A\varepsilon^2\gamma \times 3.7 \times 10^4}{4\pi r^2} \text{ (events/s)/(mCi/cc)} \tag{69.6}$$

where: r = radius of tomograph
A = area of detector material seen by each point in the object ($2\pi r \times$ axial aperture)
ε = efficiency of scintillator
γ = attenuation factor

For a single layer, the sensitivity of a tomograph of 90 cm diameter (2-cm axial crystals) will be 15,000 events/s/μCi/ml for a disk of activity 20 cm in diameter and 1 cm thick. For a 20-cm-diameter cylinder, the sensitivity will be the same for a single layer with shields or septa that limit the off-slice activity from entering the collimators. However, modern multislice instruments use septa that allow activity from adjacent planes to be detected, thus increasing the solid angle and therefore the sensitivity. This increase comes at some cost due to increase in scatter. The improvement in sensitivity is by a factor of 7, but after correction for the noise, the improvement is 4. The noise equivalent sensitivity S_{NE} is given by

$$S_{NE} = \frac{(\text{true events})^2}{\text{true} \times \text{scatter} \times \text{random}} \tag{69.7}$$

Statistical Properties of PET

The ability to map quantitatively the spatial distribution of a positron-emitting isotope depends on adequate spatial resolution to avoid blurring. In addition, sufficient data must be acquired to allow a statistically reliable estimation of the tracer concentration. The amount of available data depends on the biomedical accumulation, the imaging system sensitivity, and the dose of injected radioactivity. The propagation of errors due to the reconstruction process results in an increase in the noise over that expected for an independent signal (e.g., $\sqrt{\text{signal}}$) by a factor proportional to the square root of the number of resolution elements (true pixels) across the image. The formula that deals with the general case of emission reconstruction (PET or SPECT) is

$$\% \text{ uncertainty} = \frac{1.2 \times 100 \, (\text{total no. of events})^{3/4}}{(\text{total no. of events})^{1/2}} \tag{69.8}$$

The statistical requirements are closely related to the spatial resolution, as shown in Fig. 69.11.

For a given accuracy or a signal-to-noise ratio for a uniform distribution, the ratio of the number of events needed in a high-resolution system to that needed in a low-resolution system is proportional to the 3/2 power of the ratio of the number of effective resolution elements in the two systems. Equation (69.8) and Fig. 69.11 should be used not with the total pixels in the image but with the effective resolution cells. The number of effective resolution cells is the sum of the occupied resolution elements weighted by the activity within each element. Suppose, however, that the activity

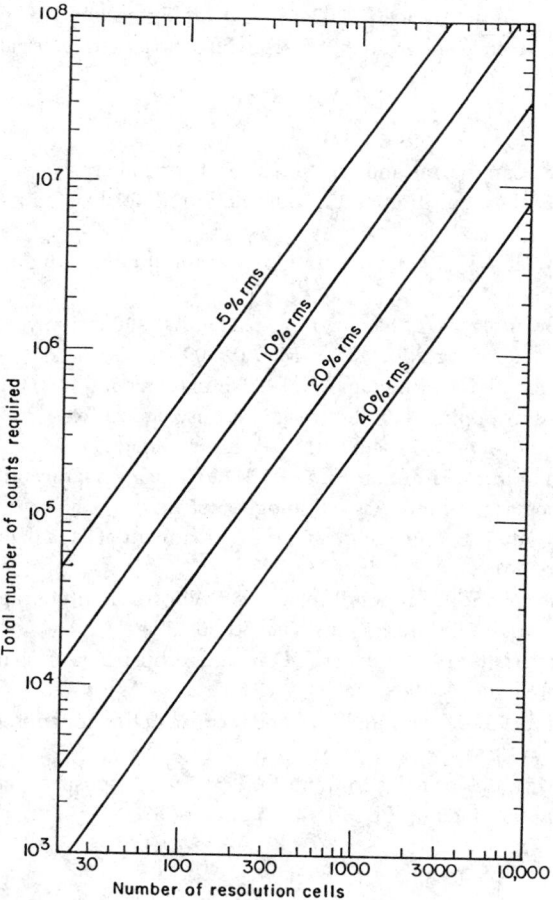

FIGURE 69.11 Statistical requirements and spatial resolution. The general relationship between the detected number of events and the number of resolution elements in an image is graphed for various levels of precision. These are relations for planes of constant thickness.

is mainly in a few resolution cells (e.g., 100 events per cell) and the remainder of the 10,000 cells have a background of 1 event per cell. The curves of Fig. 69.11 would suggest unacceptable statistics; however, in this case, the effective number of resolution cells is below 100. The relevant equation for this situation is

$$\% \text{ uncertainty} = \frac{1.2 \times 100 \text{ (no. of resolution cells)}^{3/4}}{\text{(avg no. of events per resolution cell in target)}^{3/4}} \quad (69.9)$$

The better resolution gives improved results without the requirement for a drastic increase in the number of detected events is that the improved resolution increases contrast. (It is well known that the number of events needed to detect an object is inversely related to the square of the contrast.)

Acknowledgments

This work was supported in part by the Director, Office of Energy Research, Office of Health and Environmental Research, Medical Applications and Biophysical Research Division of the U.S. Department of Energy under contract No. DE-AC03-SF00098 and in part by NIH Grant HL25840. I wish to thank Drs. Stephen Derenzo and William Moses, who contributed material to this presentation.

References

1. Anger HO. 1963. Gamma-ray and positron scintillator camera. Nucleonics 21:56.
2. Bailey DL. 1992. 3D acquisition and reconstruction in positron emission tomography. Ann Nucl Med 6:123.
3. Brownell GL, Sweet WH. 1953. Localization of brain tumors with positron emitters. Nucleonics 11:40.
4. Budinger TF, Greenberg WL, Derenzo SE, et al. 1978. Quantitative potentials of dynamic emission computed tomography. J Nucl Med 19:309.
5. Budinger TF, Gullberg GT, Huesman RH. 1979. Emission computed tomography. In GT Herman (ed), Topics in Applied Physics: Image Reconstruction from Projections: Implementation and Applications, pp 147–246. Berlin, Springer-Verlag.
6. Cherry SR, Dahlbom M, Hoffman EJ. 1991. 3D PET using a conventional multislice tomograph without septa. J Comput Assist Tomogr 15:655.
7. Daube-Witherspoon ME, Muehllehner G. 1987. Treatment of axial data in three-dimensional PET. J Nucl Med 28:1717.
8. Derenzo SE, Huesman RH, Cahoon JL, et al. 1988. A positron tomograph with 600 BGO crystals and 2.6 mm resolution. IEEE Trans Nucl Sci 35:659.
9. Kinahan PE, Rogers JG. 1989. Analytic 3D image reconstruction using all detected events. IEEE Trans Nucl Sci 36:964–968.
10. Shepp LA, Vardi Y. 1982. Maximum likelihood reconstruction for emission tomography. IEEE Trans Med Imaging 1:113.
11. Ter-Pogossian MM, Phelps ME, Hoffman EJ, et al. 1975. A positron-emission transaxial tomograph for nuclear imaging (PETT). Radiology 114:89.

70

Electrical Impedance Tomography

. C. Barber
iversity of Sheffield

70.1 The Electrical Impedance of Tissue

The specific conductance (conductivity) of human tissues varies from 15.4 mS/cm for cerebrospinal fluid to 0.06 mS/cm for bone. The difference in the value of conductivity is large between different tissues (Table 70.1). Cross-sectional images of the distribution of conductivity, or alternatively specific resistance (resistivity), should show good contrast. The aim of electrical impedance tomography (EIT) is to produce such images. It has been shown [Kohn and Vogelius, 1984a, 1984b; Sylvester and Uhlmann, 1986] that for reasonable isotropic distributions of conductivity it is possible in principle to reconstruct conductivity images from electrical measurements made on the surface of an object. Electrical impedance tomography (EIT) is the technique of producing these images. Another early name for this technique was applied potential tomography (APT). This is no longer in common use. In fact, human tissue is not simply conductive. There is evidence that many tissues also demonstrate a capacitive component of current flow [Cole and Cole, 1941], and therefore, it is appropriate to speak of the specific admittance (admittivity) or specific impedance (impedivity) of tissue rather than the conductivity; hence the use of the word *impedance* in electrical impedance tomography.

70.2 Conduction in Human Tissues

Tissue consists of cells with conducting contents surrounded by insulating membranes embedded in a conducting medium. Inside and outside the cell wall is conducting fluid. At low frequencies of applied current, the current cannot pass through the membranes, and conduction is through the extracellular space. At high frequencies, current can flow through the membranes, which act as capacitors. A simple model of bulk tissue impedance based on this structure, which has been proposed by Cole and Cole [1941], is shown in Fig. 70.1.

Clearly, this model as it stands is too simple, since an actual tissue sample would be better represented as a large network of interconnected modules of this form. However, it has been shown that this model fits experimental data if the values of the components are made a power function of the applied frequency ω. The shape of the real and imaginary parts of the admittance of this modified circuit as a function of frequency are given in Fig. 70.2, using some typical values data from human tissues.

Making measurements of the real and imaginary components of tissue impedivity over a range of frequencies will allow the components in this model to be extracted. Since it is known that tissue structure alters in disease and that R, S, C are dependent on structure, it should be possible to use such measurements to distinguish different types of tissue and different disease conditions. It is worth noting that although maximum accuracy in the deter-

TABLE 70.1 Values of Specific Conductance for Human Tissues

Tissue	Conductivity, mS/cm
Cerebrospinal fluid	15.4
Blood	6.7
Liver	2.8
Skeletal muscle	8.0 (longitudinal)
	0.6 (transverse)
Cardiac muscle	6.3 (longitudinal)
	2.3 (transverse)
Neural tissue	1.7
Gray matter	3.5
White matter	1.5
Lung	1.0 (expiration)
	0.4 (inspiration)
Fat	0.36
Bone	0.06

mination of the model components can be obtained if both real and imaginary components are available, in principle, knowledge of the real component alone should enable the values to be determined, provided an adequate range of frequencies is used. This can have practical consequences for data collection, since accurate measurement of the capacitive component can prove difficult.

Although on a microscopic scale tissue is almost certainly electrically isotropic, on a macroscopic scale this is not so for some tissues because of their anisotropic physical structure. Muscle tissue is a prime example (see Table 70.1), where the bulk conductivity along the direction of the fibers is significantly higher than across the fibers. Although unique solutions for conductivity are possible for isotropic conductors, it can be shown that for anisotropic conductors unique solutions for conductivity do not exist. There are sets of different anisotropic conductivity distributions that give the same surface voltage distributions and which therefore cannot be distinguished by these measurements. It is not yet clear how limiting anisotropy is to electrical impedance tomography. Clearly, if sufficient data could be obtained to resolve down to the microscopic level (this is not possible practically), then tissue becomes isotropic. Moreover, the tissue distribution of conductivity, including anisotropy, often can be modeled as a network of conductors, and it is known that a unique solution will always exist for such a network. In practice, use of some prior knowledge about the anisotropy of tissue may remove the ambiguities of conductivity distribution associated with anisotropy. The degree to which anisotropy might inhibit useful image reconstruction is still an open question.

70.3 Determination of the Impedance Distribution

The distribution of electrical potential within an isotropic conducting object through which a low-frequency current is flowing is given by

$$\nabla\phi(\sigma\nabla\phi) = 0 \tag{70.1}$$

where φ is the potential distribution within the object and σ is the distribution of conductivity (generally admittivity) within the object. If the conductivity is uniform, this reduces to Laplace's equation. Strictly speaking, this equation is only correct for direct current, but for the frequencies of alternating current used in EIT (up to 1 MHz) and the sizes of objects being imaged, it can be assumed that this equation continues to describe the instantaneous distribution of potential within the con-

ducting object. If this equation is solved for a
given conductivity distribution and current distribution through the surface of the object, the
potential distribution developed on the surface
of the object may be determined. The distribution of potential will depend on several things.
It will depend on the pattern of current applied
and the shape of the object. It also will depend
on the internal conductivity of the object, and it
is this that needs to be determined. In theory, the
current may be applied in a continuous and
nonuniform pattern at every point across the

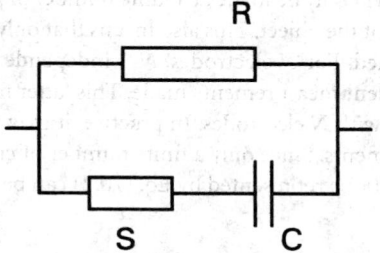

FIGURE 70.1   The Cole-Cole model of tissue impedance.

surface. In practice, current is applied to an object through electrodes attached to the surface of the
object. Theoretically, potential may be measured at every point on the surface of the object. Again,
voltage on the surface of the object is measured in practice using electrodes (possibly different from
those used to apply current) attached to the surface of the object. There will be a relationship, the
forward solution, between an applied current pattern j_i, the conductivity distribution σ, and the surface potential distribution ϕ_i which can be formally represented as

$$\phi_i = R(j_i, \sigma) \tag{70.2}$$

If σ and j_i are known, ϕ_i can be computed. For one current pattern j_i, knowledge of ϕ_i is not in general sufficient to uniquely determine σ. However, by applying a complete set of independent current patterns, it becomes possible to obtain sufficient information to determine σ, at least in the
isotropic case. This is the **inverse solution**. In practice, measurements of surface potential or volt-

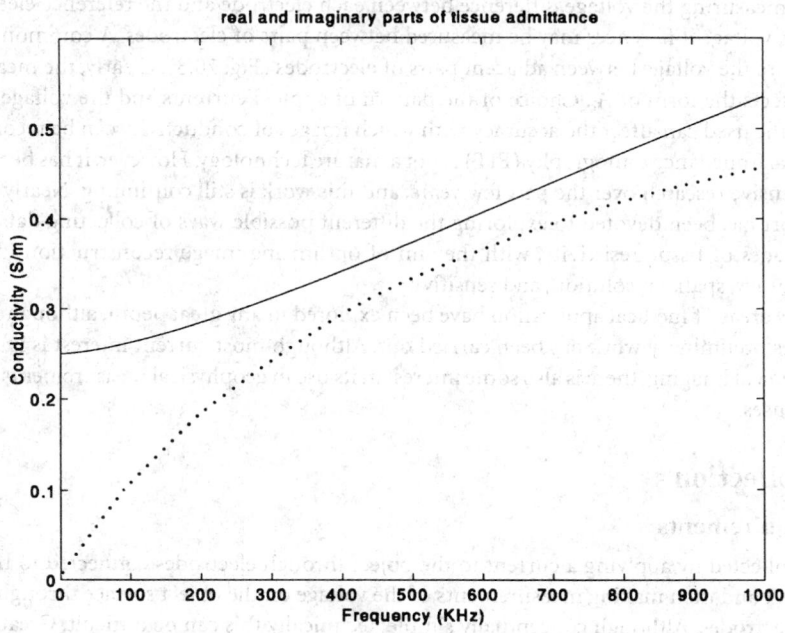

FIGURE 70.2   Theoretical real (−) and imaginary (· · ·)components of the specific admittance of a typical tissue sample as a function of frequency based on the Cole-Cole
model of tissue admittance.

age will only be made at a finite number of positions, corresponding to electrodes placed on the surface of the object. This also means that only a finite number of independent current patterns can be applied. For N electrodes, $N-1$ independent current patterns can be defined and $N(N-1)/2$ independent measurements made. This latter number determines the limit of image resolution achievable with N electrodes. In practice, it may not be possible to collect all possible independent measurements. Since only a finite number of current patterns and measurements is available, the set of equations represented by Eq. (70.2) can be rewritten as

$$\mathbf{v} = A_c \mathbf{c} \qquad\qquad (70.3)$$

where $\mathbf{v}$ is now a concatenated vector of *all* voltage values for *all* current patterns, $\mathbf{c}$ is a vector of conductivity values, representing the conductivity distribution divided into uniform image pixels, and A_c a matrix representing the transformation of this conductivity vector into the voltage vector. Since A_c depends on the conductivity distribution, this equation is nonlinear. Although formally the preceding equation can be solved for $\mathbf{c}$ by inverting A_c, the nonlinear nature of this equation means that this cannot be done in a single step. An iterative procedure will therefore be needed to obtain $\mathbf{c}$.

Examination of the physics of current flow shows that current tends to take the easiest path possible in its passage through the object. If the conductivity at some point is changed, the current path redistributes in such a way that the effects of this change are minimized. The practical effect of this is that it is possible to have fairly large changes in conductivity within the object which only produce relatively small changes in voltage at the surface of the object. The converse of this is that when reconstructing the conductivity distribution, small errors on the measured voltage data, both random and systematic, can translate into large errors in the estimate of the conductivity distribution. This effect forms, and will continue to form, a limit to the quality of reconstructed conductivity images in terms of resolution, accuracy, and sensitivity.

Any measurement of voltage must always be referred to a reference point. Usually this is one of the electrodes, which is given the nominal value of 0 V. The voltage on all other electrodes is determined by measuring the voltage difference between each electrode and the reference electrode. Alternatively, voltage differences may be measured between pairs of electrodes. A common approach is to measure the voltage between adjacent pairs of electrodes (Fig. 70.3). Clearly, the measurement scheme affects the form of A_c. Choice of the pattern of applied currents and the voltage measurement scheme used can affect the accuracy with which images of conductivity can be reconstructed.

Electrical impedance tomography (EIT) is not a mature technology. However, it has been the subject of intensive research over the past few years, and this work is still continuing. Nearly all the research effort has been devoted to exploring the different possible ways of collecting data and producing images of tissue resistivity, with the aim of optimizing image reconstruction in terms of image accuracy, spatial resolution, and sensitivity.

Very few areas of medical application have been explored in any great depth, although in a number of cases preliminary work has been carried out. Although most current interest is in the use of EIT for medical imaging, there is also some interest in its use in geophysical measurements and some industrial uses.

Data Collection

Basic Requirements

Data are collected by applying a current to the object through electrodes connected to the surface of the object and then making measurements of the voltage on the object surface through the same or other electrodes. Although conceptually simple, technically this can be difficult. Great attention must be paid to the reduction of noise and the elimination of any voltage offsets on the measurements. The currents applied are alternating currents usually in the range 10 kHz to 1 MHz. Since tissue has a complex impedance, the voltage signals will contain in-phase and out-of-phase compo-

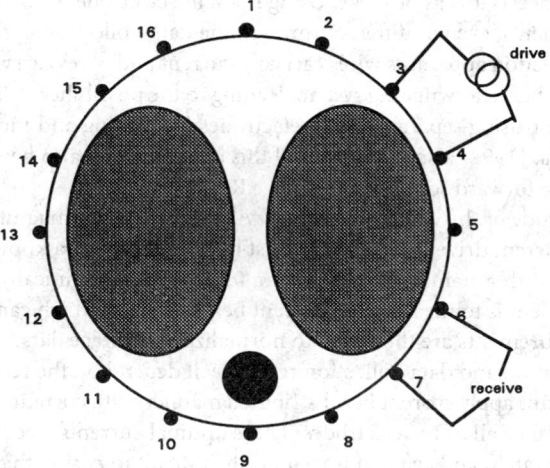

FIGURE 70.3 Idealized electrode positions around a conducting object with typical drive and measurement electrode pairs indicated.

nents. In principle, both of these can be measured. In practice, measurement of the out-of-phase (the capacitive) component is significantly more difficult because of the presence of unwanted (stray) capacitances between various parts of the voltage measurement system, including the leads from the data-collection apparatus to the electrodes. These stray capacitances can lead to appreciable leakage currents, especially at the higher frequencies, which translate into systematic errors on the voltage measurements. The signal measured on an electrode, or between a pair of electrodes, oscillates at the same frequency as the applied current. The magnitude of this signal (usually separated into real and imaginary components) is determined, typically by demodulation and integration. The frequency of the demodulated signal is much less than the frequency of the applied signal, and the effects of stray capacitances on this signal are generally negligible. This realization has led some workers to propose that the signal demodulation and detection system be mounted as close to the electrodes as possible, ideally at the electrode site itself, and some systems have been developed that use this approach, although none with sufficient miniaturization of the electronics to be practical in a clinical setting. This solution is not in itself free of problems, but this approach is likely to be of increasing importance if the frequency range of applied currents is to be extended beyond 1 MHz, necessary if the admittance curve (see Fig. 70.2) is to be adequately sampled.

Various data-collection schemes have been proposed. Most data are collected from a two-dimensional (2D) configuration of electrodes, either from 2D objects or around the border of a plane normal to the principal axis of a cylindrical (in the general sense) object where that plane intersects the object surface. The simplest data-collection protocol is to apply a current between a pair of electrodes (often an adjacent pair) and measure the voltage difference between other adjacent pairs (see Fig. 70.3). Although in principle voltage could be measured on electrodes though which current is simultaneously flowing, the presence of an electrode impedance, generally unknown, between the electrode and the body surface means that the voltage measured is not actually that on the body surface. Various means have been suggested for either measuring the electrode impedance in some way or including it as an unknown in the image-reconstruction process. However, in many systems, measurements from electrodes through which current is flowing are simply ignored. Electrode impedance is generally not considered to be a problem when making voltage measurements on electrodes through which current is not flowing, provided a voltmeter with sufficiently high input impedance is used, although, since the input impedance is always finite, every attempt should be made to keep the electrode impedance as low as possible. Using the same electrode for driving current and making voltage measurements, even at different times in the data-collection cycle, means that at some point in the data-collection apparatus wires carrying current and wires carrying voltage signals will be brought close together in a switching system, leading to the possibility of leakage currents. There is a good argument for using separate sets of electrodes for driving and measuring to reduce this problem. Paulson et al. [1992] also has proposed this approach and also have noted that it can aid in the modeling of the forward solution (see Image Reconstruction).

Clearly, the magnitude of the voltage measured will depend on the magnitude of the current applied. If a constant-current driver is used, this must be able to deliver a known current to a variety of input impedances with a stability of better than 0.1%. This is technically demanding. The best approach to this problem is to measure the current being applied, which can easily be done to this accuracy. These measurements are then used to normalize the voltage data.

The current application and data-collection regime will depend on the reconstruction algorithm used. Several EIT systems apply current in a distributed manner, with currents of various magnitudes being applied to several or all of the electrodes. These optimal currents (see Image Reconstruction) must be specified accurately, and again, it is technically difficult to ensure that the correct current is applied at each electrode. Although there are significant theoretical advantages to using distributed current patterns, the increased technical problems associated with this approach, and the higher noise levels associated with the increase in electronic complexity, may outweigh these advantages.

Although most EIT at present is 2D in the sense given above, it is intrinsically a three-dimensional (3D) imaging procedure, since current cannot be constrained to flow in a plane through a 3D object. 3D data collection does not pose any further problems apart from increased complexity due to the need for more electrodes. Whereas most data-collection systems to date have been based on 16 or 32 electrodes, 3D systems will require four times or more electrodes distributed over the surface of the object if adequate resolution is to be maintained. Technically, this will require 'belts" or "vests" of electrodes that can be rapidly applied [McAdams et al., 1994]. Some of these are already available, and the application of an adequate number of electrodes should not prove insuperable provided electrode-mounted electronics are not required.

Performance of Existing Systems

Several research groups have produced EIT systems for laboratory use [Gisser et al., 1988; Smith, 1990; Griffiths et al., 1992; Jossinet and Trillaud, 1992; Riu et al., 1992]. Two systems have been developed in Sheffield, and Table 70.2 gives some of the performance characteristics of these two systems as typical examples of practical systems. The performance of these systems is typical of current nonoptimal current systems.

The major difference between the two systems is that the Mark II operates in real time at 25 frames per second and is a parallel data-collection system, whereas the Mark I has a serial data-collection system and, although it can collect data at 10 frames per second, cannot reconstruct images at this rate. The parallel data-collection system of the Mark II and other improvements result in a much lower noise level than the Mark I system.

The signal-to-noise ratios (SNRs) given apply to the measurements of voltage profiles. These will determine the ultimate noise levels in the image, but the actual image noise will depend on the re-

TABLE 70.2 Performance of the Sheffield Mark I and Mark II Systems

	Mark I	Mark II
Operating frequency	50	20
Frame rate (frames per second)	10	25
Reconstruction time (s)	2	0.04
Spatial resolution	18.6 (mean)	14.8 (mean)
(% of diameter)	(10.5–23)	(10.9–18)
Signal to noise ratio (dB)	51	68

construction algorithm used. A mean SNR of 60 dB in the profiles will give about 0.1% mean noise in the image, with higher noise toward the center of the image than at the edge. Noise is also related to the rate at which data are collected, so an improvement in noise levels can be expected if data are averaged.

Spatial resolution and noise are the two most important constraints on possible clinical applications. Spatial resolution has to be carefully defined. The figures given are full width at half maximum (FWHM) for a small insulating cylindrical object and are presented as a percentage of the diameter of the field of view. Again, these values will depend to some extent on the reconstruction algorithm used.

Improvements to Be Expected

It is reasonable to ask if the constraints on performance given in Table 70.2 are likely to be relaxed and to ask if other significant improvements in performance can be expected in the near future. Several research workers are working on the development of wide-band or multifrequency data-collection systems [Griffiths et al., 1992; Jossinet and Trillaud, 1992; Kozlowska et al., 1992; Record et al., 1992; Brown et al, 1994]. There is good reason to expect that such systems will enable more information on the electrical properties of tissue to be obtained than is presently possible. For example it should be possible to derive information on the ratio of extracellular to intracellular spaces in the tissue and information on cell membrane integrity.

Spatial resolution is limited by the number of independent measurements that can be made from a given number of electrodes. It follows that if the number of electrodes used is increased, then the spatial resolution might be improved. If the number of electrodes is doubled, then the number of independent measurements will quadruple and the spatial resolution could be improved by a factor of 2. However, increasing the number of electrodes also reduces the SNR, and resolution is also limited by 3D spread of current, so the improvement in resolution will be less than a factor of 2.

Image Reconstruction

Basics of Reconstruction

Although several different approaches to image reconstruction have been tried [Wexler et al., 1985; Barber and Brown, 1986; Isaacson, 1986; Yorkey, 1986; Kim and Woo, 1987; Breckon, 1990], the most accurate approaches are based broadly on the following algorithm. For a given set of current patterns, a forward transform is set up for determining the voltages $\mathbf{v}$ produced from the conductivity distribution $\mathbf{c}$ (Eq. 70.3). A_c is dependent on $\mathbf{c}$, so it is necessary to assume an initial starting conductivity distribution $\mathbf{c_0}$. This is usually taken to be uniform. Using A_c, the expected voltages $\mathbf{v_0}$ are calculated and compared with the actual measured voltages $\mathbf{v_m}$. Unless $\mathbf{c_0}$ is correct (which it will not be initially), $\mathbf{v_0}$ and $\mathbf{v_m}$ will differ. It can be shown that an improved estimate of $\mathbf{c}$ is given by

$$\Delta\mathbf{c} = (S_c^t S_c)^{-1} S_c^t (\mathbf{v_0} - \mathbf{v_m}) \tag{70.4}$$

$$\mathbf{c_1} = \mathbf{c_0} + \Delta\mathbf{c} \tag{70.5}$$

where S_c is the differential of A_c with respect to $\mathbf{c}$, that is,

$$S_c = \frac{dA_c}{d\mathbf{c}} \tag{70.6}$$

and S_c^t is the transpose of S_c. The improved value of $\mathbf{c}$ is then used in the next iteration to compute and improved estimate of $\mathbf{v_m}$, i.e., $\mathbf{v_1}$. This iterative process is continued until some appropriate endpoint is reached. Although convergence is not guaranteed, in practice, convergence to the correct $\mathbf{c}$

in the absence of noise can be expected, provided a good starting value is chosen. Uniform conductivity seems to be a reasonable choice. In the presence of noise on the measurements, iteration is stopped when the difference between $\mathbf{v}$ and $\mathbf{v}_m$ is within the margin of error set by the known noise on the data.

There are some practical difficulties associated with this approach. One is that large changes in $\mathbf{c}$ may only produce small changes in $\mathbf{v}$, and this will be reflected in the structure of S_c, making $S_c^t S_c$ very difficult to invert reliably. Various methods of regularization have been used, with varying degrees of success, to achieve stable inversion of this matrix. The evidence is that this problem is not insoluble. A more difficult practical problem is that for convergence to be possible the computed voltages $\mathbf{v}$ must be equal to the measured voltages $\mathbf{v}_m$ when the correct conductivity values are used in the forward calculation. Although in a few idealized cases analytical solutions of the forward problem are possible, in general, numerical solutions must be used. Techniques such as the finite-element method (FEM) have been developed to solve problems of this type numerically. However, the accuracy of these methods has to be carefully examined [Paulson et al., 1992] and, while they are adequate for many applications, may not be adequate for the EIT reconstruction problem, especially in the case of 3D objects. Accuracies of rather better than 1% appear to be required if image artifacts are to be avoided. Consider a situation in which the actual distortion of conductivity is uniform. Then the initial $\mathbf{v}$ should be equal to the $\mathbf{v}_m$ to an accuracy less than the magnitude of the noise. If this is not the case, then the algorithm will alter the conductivity distribution from uniform, which will clearly result in error. While the required accuracies have been approached under ideal conditions, there is only a limited amount of evidence at present to suggest that they can be achieved with data taken from human subjects.

Optimal Current Patterns

So far little has been said about the form of the current patterns applied to the object except that a set of independent patterns is needed. The simplest current patterns to use are those given by passing current into the object through one electrode and extracting current through a second electrode (a bipolar pattern). This pattern has the virtue of simplicity and ease of application. However, other current patterns are possible. Current can be passed simultaneously through many electrodes, with different amounts passing through each electrode. Indeed, an infinite number of patterns are possible, the only limiting condition being that the magnitude of the current flowing into the conducting object equals the magnitude of the current flowing out of the object. Isaacson [1986] has shown that for any conducting object there is a set of optimal current patterns and has provided an algorithm to compute them even if the conductivity distribution is initially unknown. Isaacson showed that by using optimal patterns, significant improvements in the SNR could be obtained compared with simpler two-electrode current patterns. However, the additional computation and hardware required to use optimal current patterns compared with fixed, nonoptimal patterns is considerable.

Use of suboptimal patterns close to optimum also will produce significant gains. In general, the optimal patterns are very different from the patterns produced in the simple two-electrode case. The optimal patterns are often cosine-like patterns of current amplitude distributed around the object boundary rather than being localized at a pair of points, as in the two-electrode case. Since the currents are passed simultaneously through many electrodes, it is tempting to try and use the same electrodes for voltage measurements. This produces two problems. As noted above, measurement of voltage on an electrode through which an electric current is passing is compromised by the presence of electrode resistance, which causes a generally unknown voltage drop across the electrode, whereas voltage can be accurately measured on an electrode through which current is not flowing using a voltmeter of high input impedance. In addition, it has proved difficult to model current flow around an electrode through which current is flowing with sufficient accuracy to allow the reliable calculation of voltage on that electrode, which is needed for accurate reconstruction. It seems that separate electrodes should be used for voltage measurements with distributed current systems.

Theoretically, distributed (near-) optimal current systems have some advantages. As each of the optimal current patterns is applied, it is possible to determine if the voltage patterns produced contain any useful information or if they are simply noise. Since the patterns can be generated and applied in order of decreasing significance, it is possible to terminate application of further current patterns when no further information can be obtained. A consequence of this is that SNRs can be maximized for a given total data-collection time. With bipolar current patterns this option is not available. All patterns must be applied. Provided the SNR in the data is sufficiently good and only a limited number of electrodes are used, this may not be too important, and the extra effort involved in generating the optimal or near-optimal patterns may not be justified. However, as the number of electrodes is increased, the use of optimal patterns becomes more significant. It also has been suggested that the distributed nature of the optimal patterns makes the forward problem less sensitive to modeling errors. Although there is currently no firm evidence for this, this seems a reasonable assertion.

Three-Dimensional Imaging

Most published work so far on image reconstruction has concentrated on solving the 2D problem. However, real medical objects, i.e., patients, are three-dimensional. Theoretically, as the dimensionality of the object increases, reconstruction should become more robust against systematic error. However, unlike 3D x-ray images, which can be constructed from a set of independent 2D images, EIT data from 3D objects cannot be so decomposed, and strictly speaking, it is necessary to reconstruct a full 3D image from data collected over the whole surface of the object. Although the principles of reconstruction are no different from the 2D case, practically this looks quite formidable, principally because of the need to solve the forward problem in three dimensions. Some preliminary work has been presented on 3D imaging [Goble and Isaacson, 1990].

Single-Step Reconstruction

The complete reconstruction problem is nonlinear and requires iteration. However, each step in the iterative process is linear. Images reconstructed using only the first step of iteration effectively treat image formation as a linear process, an assumption approximately justified for small changes in conductivity from uniform. In this case the functions A_c and S_c often can be precomputed with reasonable accuracy because they usually are computed for the case of uniform conductivity. Although the solution cannot be correct, since the nonlinearity is not taken into account, it may be useful, and first-step linear approximations have gained some popularity. Cheney et al. [1990] have published some results from a first-step process using optimal currents. Most, if not all, of the clinical images produced to date have used a single-step reconstruction algorithm [Barber and Brown, 1986, 1990; Barber and Seagar, 1987]. Although this algorithm uses very nonoptimal current patterns, this has not so far been a limitation because of the high quality of data collected and the limited number of electrodes used (16). With larger numbers of electrodes, this conclusion may need to be revised.

Differential Imaging

Ideally, the aim of EIT is to reconstruct images of the absolute distribution of conductivity (or admittivity). These images are known as absolute (or static) images. However, this requires that the forward problem can be solved to an high degree of accuracy, and this can be difficult. The magnitude of the voltage signal measured on an electrode or between electrodes will depend on the body shape, the electrode shape and position, and the internal conductivity distribution. The signal magnitude is in fact dominated by the first two effects rather than by conductivity. However if a *change* in conductivity occurs within the object, then it can often be assumed that the *change* in surface voltage is dominated by this conductivity change. In differential (or dynamic) imaging, the aim is to image changes in conductivity rather than absolute values. If the voltage difference between a pair of (usually adjacent) electrodes before a conductivity change occurs is $\mathbf{g}_1$ and the value after change occurs is $\mathbf{g}_2$, then a normalized data value is defined as

$$\Delta \mathbf{g}_n = \frac{\mathbf{g}_1 - \mathbf{g}_2}{\mathbf{g}_1} = \frac{\Delta \mathbf{g}}{\mathbf{g}_1} \tag{70.7}$$

Most of the effects of body shape and electrode configuration cancel out in this definition. The normalized data are strongly dependent on the conductivity changes.

The sensitivity matrix must be redefined to include normalization. It is easily shown that the relationship between unnormalized changes in voltage gradients and changes in conductivity is given by a relationship of the form

$$\Delta \mathbf{g} = S_c \Delta \mathbf{c} \tag{70.8}$$

where S_c is a sensitivity matrix of the form of Eq. (70.6). This is converted into a relationship between normalized changes in voltage gradients and conductivity by multiplying both sides by a diagonal matrix G^{-1}, where the diagonal elements of G are the elements of $\mathbf{g}_1$. Equation (70.8) becomes

$$\Delta \mathbf{g}_n = G^{-1} S_c \Delta \mathbf{c}_n = F_c \Delta \mathbf{c}_n \tag{70.9}$$

S_c is sensitive to body shape and electrode configuration, as is G. The combination of these matrices, F_c, is much less sensitive to these effects, and it has proved possible to precompute a general F_c and use it to reconstruct differential images from data taken from human subjects.

The differential algorithm has been used fairly extensively in a variety of exploratory clinical applications. The disadvantages of this algorithm are that it can only image changes in conductivity, which must either be natural or induced, and it is only a single-step reconstruction and so lacks quantitative accuracy. Since a general F_c is used, images produced using this algorithm are distorted relative to the true shape of the object in ways that are not readily correctable, although these distortions appear to be largely "rubber sheet" rather than inconsistency artifacts, at least for 16-electrode systems. Despite these limitations, by analyzing sequences of such images it has proved possible to quantify these temporal changes in a useful way. Figure 70.4 shows a typical differential image. This represents the changes in the conductivity of the lungs between expiration and inspiration.

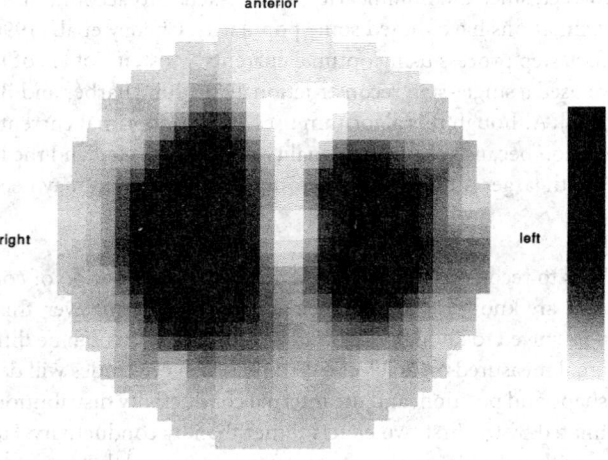

FIGURE 70.4   A differential conductivity image representing the changes in conductivity in going from maximum inspiration (breathing in) to maximum expiration (breathing out). Increasing blackness represents increasing conductivity.

Multifrequency Measurements

Differential algorithms can only image changes in conductivity. Absolute distributions of conductivity cannot be produced using these methods. In addition, any gross movement of the electrodes, either because they have to be removed and replaced or even because of significant patient movement, make the use of this technique difficult for long-term measurements of changes. As an alternative to changes in time, differential algorithms can image changes in conductivity with frequency. Brown et al. [1994] have shown that if measurements are made over a range of frequencies and differential images produced using data from the lowest frequency and the other frequencies in turn, these images can be used to compute parametric images representing the distribution of combinations of the circuit values in Fig. 70.1. For example, images representing the ratio of S to R, a measure of the ratio of intracellular to extracellular volume, can be produced, as well as images of $f_r = 1/2\pi(RC + SC)$, the tissue characteristic frequency. Although not images of the absolute distribution of conductivity, they are images of absolute tissue properties. Since these properties are related to tissue structure, they should produce images with useful contrast. Data sufficient to reconstruct an image can be collected in a time short enough to preclude significant patient movement, which means these images should be robust against movement artifacts. Changes of these parameters with time can still be observed.

70.4 Areas of Clinical Application

There is no doubt that the clinical strengths of EIT relate to its ability to be considered as a functional imaging modality that carries no hazard and can therefore be used for monitoring purposes. The best spatial resolution that might become available will still be much worse than anatomic imaging methods such as magnetic resonance imaging and x-ray computed tomography. However, EIT is able to image small changes in tissue conductivity such as those associated with blood perfusion, lung ventilation, and fluid shifts. Clinical applications seek to take advantage of the ability of EIT to follow rapid changes in physiologic function.

There are several areas in clinical medicine where electrical impedance tomography might provide advantages over existing techniques. These have been reviewed previously [Brown et al., 1985; Dawids, 1987; Holder and Brown, 1990].

Possible Biomedical Applications

Gastrointestinal System

A priori, it seems likely that EIT could be applied usefully to measurement of motor activity in the gut. Electrodes can be applied with ease around the abdomen, and there are no large bony structures likely to seriously violate the assumption of constant initial conductivity. During motor activity, such as gastric emptying or peristalsis, there are relatively large movements of the conducting fluids within the bowel. The quantity of interest is the timing of activity, e.g., the rate at which the stomach empties, and the absolute impedance change and its exact location in space are of secondary importance. The principal limitations of EIT of poor spatial resolution and amplitude measurement are largely circumvented in this application [Avill et al., 1987].

Respiratory System

Lung pathology can be imaged by conventional radiography, x-ray computed tomography, or magnetic resonance imaging, but there are clinical situations where it would be desirable to have a portable means of imaging regional lung ventilation which could, if necessary, generate repeated images over time. Validation studies have shown that overall ventilation can be measured with good accuracy [Harris et al., 1988].

EIT Imaging of Changes in Blood Volume

The conductivity of blood is about 6.7 mS/cm, which is approximately three times that of most intrathoracic tissues. It therefore seems possible that EIT images related to blood flow could be accomplished. The imaged quantity will be the change in conductivity due to replacement of tissue by blood (or vice versa) as a result of the pulsatile flow through the thorax. This may be relatively large in the cardiac ventricles but will be smaller in the peripheral lung fields.

The most interesting possibility is that of detecting pulmonary embolus (PE). If a blood clot is present in the lung, the lung beyond the clot will not be perfused, and under favorable circumstances, this may be visualized using a gated blood volume image of the lung. In combination with a ventilation image, which should show normal ventilation in this region, pulmonary embolism could be diagnosed. Some data [Leathard et al., 1994] indicate that PE can be visualized in human subjects. Although more sensitive methods already exist for detecting PE, the noninvasiveness and bedside availability of EIT mean that treatment of the patient could be monitored over the period following the occurrence of the embolism, an important aim, since the use of anticoagulants, the principal treatment for PE, needs to be minimized in postoperative patients, a common class of patients presenting with this complication.

70.5 Summary and Future Developments

EIT is still an emerging technology. In its development, several novel and difficult measurement and image-reconstruction problems have had to be addressed. Most of these have been satisfactorily solved. The next generation of EIT imaging systems will be multifrequency, with some capable of 3D imaging. These should be capable of greater quantitative accuracy and be less prone to image artifact and are likely to find a practical role in clinical diagnosis. Although there are still many technical problems to be answered and many clinical applications to be addressed, the technology may be close to coming of age.

Defining Terms

Absolute imaging: Imaging the actual distribution of conductivity.

Admittivity: The specific admittance of an electrically conducting material. For simple biomedical materials such as saline with no reactive component of resistance, this is the same as conductivity.

Anisotropic conductor: A material in which the conductivity is dependent on the direction in which it is measured through the material.

Applied current pattern: In EIT, the electric current is applied to the surface of the conducting object via electrodes placed on the surface of the object. The spatial distribution of current flow through the surface of the object is the applied current pattern.

APT: Applied potential tomography. This is an early name for electrical impedance tomography, now no longer in common used.

Bipolar current pattern: A current pattern applied between a single pair of electrodes.

Conductivity: The specific conductance of an electrically conducting material. The inverse of resistivity.

Differential imaging: An EIT imaging technique that specifically images changes in conductivity.

Distributed current: A current pattern applied through more than two electrodes.

Dynamic imaging: The same as differential imaging.

EIT: Electrical impedance tomography.

Forward transform or problem or solution: The operation, real or computational, that maps or transforms the conductivity distribution to surface voltages.

Impedivity: The specific impedance of an electrically conducting material. The inverse of admittivity. For simple biomedical materials such as saline with no reactive component of resistance, this is the same as resistivity.

Inverse transform or problem or solution: The computational operation that maps voltage measurements on the surface of the object to the conductivity distribution.

Optimal current: One of a set of current patterns computed for a particular conductivity distribution that produce data with maximum possible SNR.

Pixel: The conductivity distribution is usually represented as a set of connected piecewise uniform patches. Each of these patches is a pixel. The pixel may take any shape, but square or triangular shapes are most common.

Resistivity: The specific electrical resistance of an electrical conducting material. The inverse of conductivity.

Static imaging: The same as absolute imaging.

References

Avill RF, Mangnall RF, Bird NC, et al. 1987. Applied potential tomography: A new non-invasive technique for measuring gastric emptying. Gastroenterology 92:1019.

Barber DC, Brown BH. 1986. Recent developments in applied potential tomography. In S Bacharach (ed), Information Processing in Medical Imaging, pp 106–121. Dordrecht, Martinus Nijhoff.

Barber DC, Brown BH. 1990. Progress in electrical impedance tomography. In D Colton, R Ewing, W Rundell (eds), Inverse Problems in Partial Differential Equations, pp 149–162. New York, SIAM.

Barber DC, Seagar AD. 1987. Fast reconstruction of resistive images. Clin Phys Physiol Meas 8(A):47.

Breckon WR. 1990. Image Reconstruction in Electrical Impedance Tomography. PhD thesis, School of Computing and Mathematical Sciences, Oxford Polytechnic, Oxford, U.K.

Brown BH, Barber DC, Seagar AD. 1985. Applied potential tomography: possible clinical applications. Clin Phys Physiol Meas 6:109.

Brown BH, Barber DC, Wang W, et al. 1994. Multifrequency imaging and modelling of respiratory related electrical impedance changes. Physiol Meas 15:A1.

Cheney MD, Isaacson D, Newell J, et al. 1990. Noser: An algorithm for solving the inverse conductivity problem. Int J Imag Sys Tech 2:60.

Cole KS, Cole RH. 1941. Dispersion and absorption in dielectrics: I. Alternating current characteristics. J Chem Phys 9:341.

Dawids SG. 1987. Evaluation of applied potential tomography: A clinician's view. Clin Phys Physiol Meas 8(A):175.

Gisser D, Isaacson D, Newell JC. 1988. Theory and performance of an adaptive current tomography system. Clin Phys Physiol Meas 9(A):35.

Goble J, Isaacson D. 1990. Fast reconstruction algorithms for three-dimensional electrical tomography. In IEEE EMBS Proceedings of the 12th Annual International Conference, Philadelphia, pp 285–286.

Griffiths H, Leung HTL, Williams RJ. 1992. Imaging the complex impedance of the thorax. Clin Phys Physiol Meas 13(A):77.

Harris ND, Sugget AJ, Barber DC, Brown BH. 1988. Applied potential tomography: A new technique for monitoring pulmonary function. Clin Phys Physiol Meas 9(A):79.

Holder DS, Brown BH. 1990. Biomedical applications of EIT: A critical review. In D Holder (ed), Clinical and Physiological Applications of Electrical Impedance Tomography, pp 6–41. London, UCL Press.

Isaacson D. 1986. Distinguishability of conductivities by electric current computed tomography. IEEE Trans Med Imaging 5:91.

Jossinet J, Trillaud C. 1992. Imaging the complex impedance in electrical impedance tomography. Clin Phys Physiol Meas 13(A):47.

Kim H, Woo HW. 1987. A prototype system and reconstruction algorithms for electrical impedance technique in medical imaging. Clin Phys Physiol Meas 8(A):63.

Kohn RV, Vogelius M. 1984a. Determining the conductivity by boundary measurement. Comm Pure Appl Math 37:289.

Kohn RV, Vogelius M. 1984b. Identification of an unknown conductivity by means of the boundary. SIAM-AMS Proc 14:113.

Kozlowska K, Rigaud B, Martinez E, et al. 1992. Technical and experimental problems encountered in impedance spectroscopy in the α and β dispersion regions. Clin Phys Physiol Meas 13(A):57.

Leathard AD, Brown BH, Campbell J, et al. 1994. A comparison of ventilatory and cardiac related changes in EIT images of normal human lungs and of lungs with pulmonary embolism. Physiol Meas 15:A137.

McAdams ET, McLaughlin JA, Anderson JMcC. 1994. Multielectrode systems for electrical impedance tomography. Physiol Meas 15:A101.

Paulson K, Breckon W, Pidcock M. 1992. A hybrid phantom for electrical impedance tomography. Clin Phys Physiol Meas 13(A):155.

Record PM, Gadd R, Vinther F. 1992. Multifrequency electrical impedance tomography. Clin Phys Physiol Meas 13(A):67.

Riu PJ, Rosell J, Lozano A, Pallas-Areny RA. 1992. Broadband system for multi-frequency static imaging in electrical impedance tomography. Clin Phys Physiol Meas 13(A):61.

Smith RWM. 1990. Design of a Real-Time Impedance Imaging System for Medical Applications. Ph.D. thesis, University of Sheffield, U.K.

Sylvester J, Uhlmann G. 1986. A uniqueness theorem for an inverse boundary value problem in electrical prospection. Comm Pure Appl Math 39:91.

Wexler A, Fry B, Neuman MR. 1985. Impedance-computed tomography: Algorithm and system. Appl Optics 24:3985.

Yorkey TJ. 1986 Comparing Reconstruction Algorithms for Electrical Impedance Imaging. Ph.D. thesis, University of Wisconsin, Madison, Wisc.

Further Information

All the following conferences were funded by the European commission under the biomedical engineering program. The first two were directly funded as exploratory workshops, the remainder as part of a Concerted Action on Electrical Impedance Tomography. Electrical Impedance Tomography—Applied Potential Tomography. 1987. Proceedings of a conference held in Sheffield, U.K., 1986. Published in Clin Phys Physiol Meas 8:Suppl.A. Electrical Impedance Tomography—Applied Potential Tomography. 1988. Proceedings of a conference held in Lyon, France, November 1987. Published in Clin Phys Physiol Meas 9:Suppl.A. Electrical Impedance Tomography. 1991. Proceedings of a conference held in Copenhagen, Denmark, July 1990. Published by Medical Physics, University of Sheffield, U.K. Electrical Impedance Tomography. 1992. Proceedings of a conference held in York, U.K., July 1991. Published in Clin Phys Physiol Meas 13:Suppl.A. Clinical and Physiologic Applications of Electrical Impedance Tomography. 1993. Proceedings of a conference held at the Royal Society, London, U.K. April 1992. Ed. D.S. Holder, UCL Press, London. Electrical Impedance Tomography. 1994. Proceedings of a conference held in Barcelona, Spain, 1993. Published in Clin Phys Physiol Meas 15:Suppl.A.

71

Medical Applications of Virtual Reality Technology

Walter J. Greenleaf
Greenleaf Medical Systems

Virtual reality (VR) is an emerging technology that radically alters how individuals interact with computers. It consists of a computer-generated *three-dimensional (3D) environment* and interface tools that allow users to do three things:

1. *Immerse* themselves in the environment
2. *Navigate* within the environment
3. *Interact* with objects in the environment

The experience of entering this computer-generated world is compelling. By donning clothing mounted with sensors that communicate movement and location to a computer and by wearing a helmet allowing the user to "see" via a sophisticated graphics system, the user "breaks through" the computer screen and enters a 3D world. Inside virtual reality, one can walk through a virtual house, drive a virtual car, or run a marathon in a park still under design. Recent advances in computer processor speed and graphics make it possible to create very realistic environments. The practical applications are far-reaching. Today, using virtual reality, architects design office buildings, NASA controls robots at remote locations, and physicians plan and practice difficult operations.

Virtual reality is quickly finding wide acceptance in the medical community as researchers and clinicians alike become aware of its potential benefits. Several pioneer research groups have already demonstrated improved clinical performance using VR imaging, planning, and control techniques.

0-8493-8346-3/95/$0.00+$.50
© 1995 by CRC Press, Inc.

71.1 Overview of Virtual Reality Technology

The term *virtual reality* describes a set of techniques that enables users to interact with computer data naturally and intuitively from a first-person perspective.

From a system perspective, virtual reality technology can be segmented as shown in Fig. 71.1.

The computer-generated environment, or virtual world *content,* consists of a *3D graphic model,* typically implemented as a spatially organized, object-oriented database, where each object in the database represents an object in the virtual world.

A separate *modeling program* is used to create the individual objects for the virtual world. For greater realism, *texture maps* are used to create visual surface detail.

The database is manipulated using a real-time *dynamics generator* that allows objects to be moved within the world according to natural laws such as gravity, inertia, or flexibility. These laws are specified for each particular experience by *application-specific programming.*

The dynamics generator also tracks the position and orientation of the user's head and hand using *input peripherals* such as a *head tracker* and *DataGlove.*

Powerful *renderers* are applied to produce 3D images and 3D spatialized sound in real time.

The common method of working with a computer (using a mouse/keyboard/monitor paradigm) is an inefficient means for immersion in virtual worlds. Therefore, one long-term challenge for virtual reality developers has been to replace the conventional computer interface with one that is more natural and intuitive and that will allow the computer to carry a greater proportion of the interface burden (rather than the user). Not surprisingly, this need for improved immersion into computer-generated artificial environments has spawned the development of a new generation of computer interface hardware. To date, three new computer-interface mechanisms have evolved: instrumented clothing, the head-mounted display (HMD), and 3D sound systems.

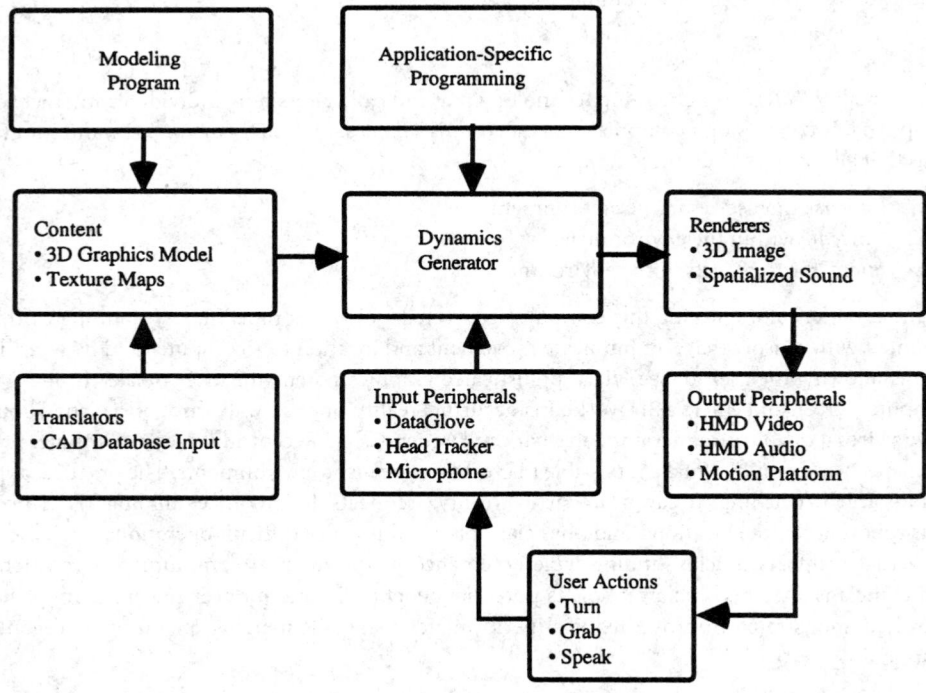

FIGURE 71.1   A complete VR system.

Instrumented Clothing

The DataGlove and DataSuit collect data *dynamically* in 3D space and thereby provide dramatic new methods for the measurement of human motion. The clothing is instrumented with sensors that track the full range of motion of the person wearing the glove or suit as he or she bends, moves, grasps, or waves.

The DataGlove (Fig. 71.2) is a thin Lycra glove with bend sensors running along its dorsal surface. When the joints of the hand bend, the sensors bend, and the angular movement is recorded by the sensors. These recordings are digitized and forwarded to the computer, which calculates the angle at which each joint is bent. On screen, an image of the hand moves in real time, shadowing the movements of the hand in the DataGlove and immediately replicating even the most subtle actions.

The DataSuit is a customized body suit fitted with the same sophisticated bend sensors found in the DataGlove. While the DataGlove is currently in production as both a VR interface and a data-collection instrument, the DataSuit is available only as a custom device.

As noted, DataGlove and DataSuit are utilized as general-purpose computer interface devices for virtual reality. There are several potential applications of this new technology for clinical and therapeutic medicine.

Head-Mounted Display (HMD)

The best-known tool for data output in virtual reality is a *head-mounted display* (HMD). It supports first-person immersion by generating a wide field of view image for each eye, often in true 3D.

Most lower-cost HMDs ($6000 range) use LCD displays; others use small CRTs. The more expensive HMDs ($60,000 and up) use optical fibers to pipe the images from non-head-mounted displays. A HMD requires a position tracker in addition to the helmet. Alternatively, the binocular display can be mounted on an armature for support and tracking (a Boom display) [Bolas, 1994].

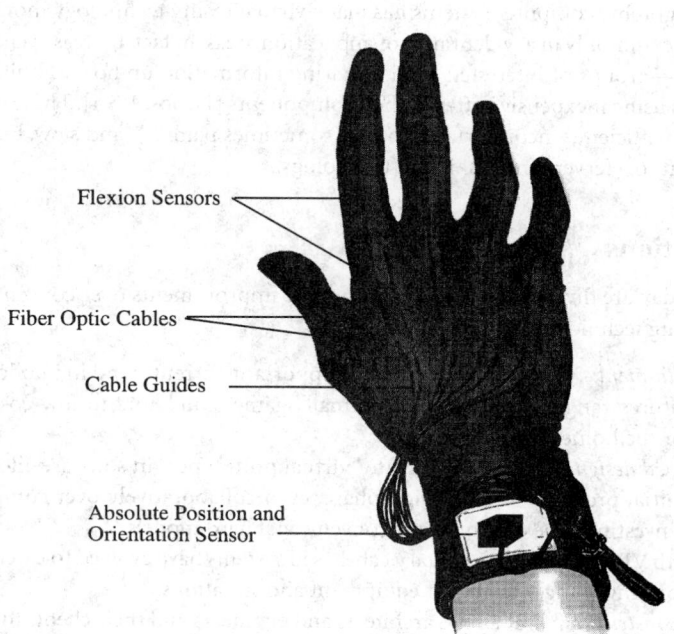

Flexion Sensors

Fiber Optic Cables

Cable Guides

Absolute Position and
Orientation Sensor

FIGURE 71.2 The DataGlove, a VR control device.

3D Spatialized Sound

The impression of immersion within a virtual environment is greatly enhanced by inclusion of 3D spatialized sound [Durlach et al., 1993]. Stereo-pan effects alone are inadequate because they tend to sound as if originating inside the head. Research into 3D audio has shown the importance of modeling the head and pinea and using this model as part of the 3D sound generation. A head-related transfer function (HRTF) can be used to generate the proper acoustics. A number of problems remain, such as the "cone of confusion," wherein sounds behind the head are perceived to be in front of the head.

Other VR Interface Technology

The sense of balance and motion can be generated in a VR system by a motion platform. These have been used in flight simulators to provide motion cues that the mind integrates with other cues to perceive motion.

Haptics is the generation of touch and force feedback information. Most systems to date have focused on force feedback and kinesthetic senses, although some prototype systems exist that generate tactile stimulation. Many of the haptic systems thus far are exoskeletons used for position sensing as well as providing resistance to movement or active force application.

Some preliminary work has been done on generating the sense of temperature in VR. Small electrical heat pumps have been developed that can produce sensations of heat and cold as part of the simulated environment.

71.2 VR Application Examples

Virtual reality has been researched for years in government laboratories and universities, but because of the enormous computing power demands and associated high costs, applications have been slow to migrate from the research world to other areas. Recent improvements in the price/performance ratio of graphic computer systems has made virtual reality technology more affordable and thus used more commonly in a wider range of application areas. In fact, there is even a strong "garage VR" movement—groups of interested parties sharing information on how to build extremely low cost VR systems using inexpensive off-the-shelf components [Jacobs, 1994]. These home-made systems are often inefficient, uncomfortable to use (sometimes painful), and slow, but they exist as a strong testament to a fervent interest in VR technology.

VR Applications

Applications today are diverse and represent dramatic improvements over conventional visualization and planning techniques:

Public entertainment: VR is arguably the most important current trend in public entertainment, with ventures ranging from "shopping mall" game simulators to low-cost virtual reality games for the home.

Computer-aided design: Using VR to create "virtual prototypes" in software allows engineers to test potential products in the design phase, even collaboratively over computer networks, without investing time or money for conventional hard models.

Military: With VR, the military's solitary cab-based systems have evolved to extensive networked simulations involving a variety of equipment and situations.

Architecture/construction: VR allows architects and engineers and their clients to "walk through" structural blueprints. Designs may be seen more clearly by clients who often have difficulty comprehending them even with conventional cardboard models. Atlanta, Georgia credits its

VR model for winning it the site of the 1996 Olympics, while San Diego is using a VR model of a planned convention center addition to compete for the next GOP convention.

Financial visualization: By allowing navigation through an abstract "world" of data, VR helps users to rapidly visualize large amounts of complex financial market data and thus supports faster decision making.

VR is commonly associated with exotic "fully immersive applications" because of the overdramatized media coverage on helmets, body suits, entertainment simulators, and the like. Equally important are the "window into world" applications, where the user or operator is allowed to interact effectively with "virtual" data, either locally or remotely.

71.3 Current Status of Virtual Reality Technology

The commercial market for VR, while taking advantage of advances in VR technology at large, is nonetheless contending with the lack of integrated systems and the lack of reliable equipment suppliers. Typically, researchers buy peripherals and software from separate companies and configure their own systems. Companies that can offer integrated systems for commercial applications are expected to fill this gap over the next few years.

At the same time, the nature of the commercial VR medical market is expected to change as the prices of today's expensive, high-performance graphics systems decrease dramatically. High-resolution display systems also will drop in cost significantly as the VR display business can piggyback on HDTV projection and home entertainment technologies.

Technical advances have been seen in networking applications, improved visual photorealism, decreased tracker latency through predictive algorithms, and variable-resolution image generators. Improved database access methods are underway.

Important hardware advances include eye gear that provides an increased field of view, wireless communications, reductions in bulk and weight, and improved tracking systems.

71.4 Overview of Medical Applications of Virtual Reality Technology

VR is being pursued in the medical community, with the first wave of development efforts having evolved seven key categories:

- Surgical training and surgical planning
- Medical education, modeling, and nonsurgical training
- Anatomically keyed displays with real-time data fusion
- VR-facilitated rehabilitation and motion/ergonomic analysis
- Disability solutions
- Telesurgery and telemedicine
- VR-facilitated patient evaluation and behavioral intervention

The potential of virtual reality in education and information dissemination in general makes it possible to predict that there will be few areas of medicine that will not take advantage of this improved computer interface. However, the latent potential of VR lies in its capacity to be used to manipulate and combine heterogeneous data sets from many sources. This feature is most significant and likely to transform the traditional applications environment in the near future.

Surgical Training and Surgical Planning

Various projects are underway to utilize VR and imaging technology to plan, simulate, and customize invasive (as well as minimally invasive) surgical procedures. See Holler and Breitwieser

[1994], Hon [1994], Johnson [1994], Kuhnapfel [1994], Loftin et al. [1994], Preminger [1994], Schraft et al. [1994], Szabo et al. [1994], and Tendick et al. [1993] for examples. Ranging from advanced imaging technologies for endoscopic surgery to routine hip replacements, these new developments will have a tremendous impact on improving surgical morbidity and mortality. According to Merril [1993, 1994], studies show that doctors are more likely to make errors performing their first few to several dozen diagnostic and therapeutic surgical procedures. Merril claims that operative risk could be substantially reduced by the development of a simulator that allows transference of skills from the simulation to the actual point of patient contact. Overall, with surgical modeling, we should see a much higher degree of precision, reliability, and safety, in addition to cost efficiency.

Several virtual reality–based systems currently under development allow real-time tracking of surgical instrumentation and simultaneous display and manipulation of 3D anatomy corresponding to the simulated procedure [Hon, 1994; McGovern and McGovern, 1994]. With this design surgeons can practice procedures and experience the possible complications and variations in anatomy encountered during surgery. Necessary software tools have been developed to enable the creation of "virtual tissues" which reflect the physical characteristics of physiologic tissues. This technology operates in real time using 3D graphics on a high-speed computer platform.

Virtual Environment for Eye Surgery Simulation

Ophthalmic surgery training in an interactive virtual environment is a new approach that will augment conventional procedures calling for practice on cadavers or animals, progressing through to performing the procedure on a patient under the supervision of an experienced surgeon.

The eye simulation project of the Georgia Institute of Technology and the Medical College of Georgia Department of Ophthalmology is a starting point to demonstrate its potential [Peifer, 1994]. The basic system components required to support this type of training include: (1) the operating station, (2) computer models of anatomy and surgical instruments, (3) a tactile feedback system, (4) a position-tracking system for the surgical instruments, and (5) software that controls interaction and updates the visual and tactile feedback.

The operating station is the physical interface between the surgeon and the virtual operating environment. In practice, ophthalmic surgeons operate on an eye by looking through a stereomicroscope while holding the surgical instruments on a wrist rest that surrounds the patient's head. The operating station for the simulation also includes a stereo operating scope and a wrist rest, but instead of looking directly into the eye, the surgeon interacts with a virtual eye using a virtual surgical instrument controlled by a hand-held, 3D position-tracking stylus that continuously reports position and orientation to the computer.

The simulation also enables the surgeon to change instruments, record and play back training sessions, reset the models, and peel away the outer layers of the eye to reveal interior anatomic components. In addition, the surgeon can rotate the model, change transparency, zoom, and adjust stereo viewing parameters. There are four customized surgical instruments with which the surgeon can "request" a particular kind of action. Both visual and tactile feedback are provided to the user during all the actions.

The simulation environment will become a testbed for designing and evaluating new procedures and instruments. For medical residents, the exploration of basic anatomy and the ability to practice hand-eye coordination in the virtual environment will advance not only their basic training but also provide them unusual anatomy or rare surgical complications as routine presentations. With patient-specific models of anatomy, a surgeon will be able to rehearse the procedure before actually operating on the patient. Selection of the optimal instrument, approach angle, and depth of incision can be predetermined through experimentation on the simulator, and eventually, this technology may be extended to assist the surgeon in performing the surgery itself.

Virtual Reality Surgical Planning and Training System

One example of a virtual reality surgical planning and training system is the computer-based workstation being developed by Ciné-Med of Woodbury, Connecticut [McGovern and McGovern, 1994].

The goal is to develop a realistic, interactive training workstation that helps surgeons make a more seamless transition from surgical simulation to the actual surgical event.

Development has focused on television-controlled endosurgical procedures because of the intensive training required for endosurgery, the adaptability of endosurgery to high-quality imaging, and the fact that tactile response and force feedback issues are not as critical as in a fully immersive, incisional surgical simulation. Surgeons can gain clinical expertise by training on this highly realistic and functional surgical simulator.

Ciné-Med's computer environment includes lifelike virtual organs that react much like their real counterparts and sophisticated details such as the actual surgical instruments that provide system input/output (I/O). To further enhance training, the simulator allows the instructor to adapt clinical instruction to advance the technical expertise of learners. Surgical anomalies and emergency situations can be replicated to allow practicing surgeons to experiment and gain technical expertise on a wide range of surgical problems using the computer model before using an animal model. Since the steps of the procedure can be repeated and replayed at a later time, the learning environment surpasses other skills-training modalities.

The current prototype simulates the environment of laparoscopic cholecystectomy for use as a surgical training device. Development began with the creation of an accurate anatomic landscape, including the liver, the gallbladder, and related structures. Appropriate surgical instruments are used for the system I/O and inserted into a fiberglass replica of a human torso. Four surgical incisional ports are assigned for three scissors grip instruments and camera zoom control. The instruments, retrofitted with switching devices, read and relay the opening and closing of the tips, with position trackers located within the simulator.

The virtual surgical instruments are graphically generated on a display monitor, where they interact with fully textural, anatomically correct, 3D virtual organs. The organs are created as independent objects and conform to object-oriented programming.

To replicate physical properties, each virtual organ must be assigned appropriate values to dictate its reaction when it comes into contact with a virtual surgical instrument. Since rules of free and occupied space programming dictate that only one object can occupy any given space at a time, the physical property values are established to dictate which object occupies which space. Collision algorithms are established to define when the virtual organ is touched by a virtual surgical instrument. Additionally, with the creation of spontaneous objects resulting from the dissection of a virtual organ, each new object is calculated to have independent physical properties using artificial intelligence (AI) subroutines. Collision algorithms drive the programmed creation of spontaneous objects.

To reproduce the patient's physiologic reactions during the surgical procedure, the system employs an expert system. This software subsystem generates patient reactions and probable outcomes derived from surgical stimuli, e.g., bleeding control, heart rate failure, and, in the extreme, a death outcome. The acceptable value ranges of these factors are programmed to be constantly updated by the expert system while important data are displayed on the monitor.

3D graphic representation of a patient's anatomy is the challenge for accurate surgical planning. Technological progress has been seen in the visualization of bone, brain, and soft tissue. Heretofore, 3D modeling of soft tissue has been difficult and often inaccurate owing to the intricacies of the internal organ, its vasculature, its ducts, volume, and connective tissues.

As an extension of the above-described surgical simulator, a functional surgical planning device using VR technology is under development which will enable surgeons to operate on an actual patient, in virtual reality, prior to the actual operation. With the advent of technological advances in anatomic imaging, the parallel development of a surgical planning device incorporating real-time interaction with computer graphics that mimic a patient's anatomy is possible. Identification of anatomic structures to be modeled constitutes the initial phase for development of the surgical planning device. A spiral CT scanning device records multiple slices of the anatomy during a single breath inhalation by the patient. Pin-registered layers of the anatomy are thus provided for the computer to read.

Individual anatomic structures are defined at the scan level according to gray scale. Once the anatomic structures are identified and labeled, the scans are stacked and connected. The result is a volumetric polygonal model of the patient's actual anatomy. A polygon reduction program is initiated to create a wire frame that can be successfully texture mapped and interacted with real time. As each slice of the CT scan is stacked and linked together, the result is a fully volumetric, graphic representation of the human anatomy. Since the model, at this point, is unmanageable by the graphics workstation because of the volume polygons, a polygon reduction program is initiated to eliminate excessive polygons.

Key to the planning device is development of a user-friendly software program that will allow the radiologist to define anatomic structures, incorporate them into graphic representations, and assign physiologic parameters to the anatomy. Surgeons will then be able to diagnose, plan, and prescribe appropriate therapy to their patients using a trial run of a computerized simulation.

Medical Education, Modeling, and Nonsurgical Training

Researchers at the University of California, San Diego, are exploring the value of hybridizing elements of virtual reality (VR), multimedia (MM), and communications technologies into a unified educational paradigm [Hoffman, 1994]. The goal is to develop powerful tools that extend the flexibility and effectiveness of medical teaching and promote lifelong learning. To this end, they have undertaken a multiyear initiative named the VR-MM Synthesis Project. Based on instructional design and user need (rather than technology per se), they have planned a linked three computer array representing the data communications gateway, the electronic medical record system, and the simulation environment. This system supports medical students, surgical residents, and clinical faculty running applications ranging from full surgical simulation to basic anatomic exploration and review, all via a common interface. The plan also supports integration of learning and telecommunications resources (such as interactive MM libraries, on-line textbooks, databases of medical literature, decision support systems, electronic mail, and access to electronic medical records).

Anatomically Keyed Displays with Real-Time Data Fusion

An anatomically keyed display with real-time data fusion is currently in use at NYU Medical Center's Department of Neurosurgery. The system allows both preoperative planning and real-time tumor visualization [Kelly, 1994; Kall et al., 1994]. The technology offers a technique for surgeons to plan and simulate the surgical procedure beforehand in order to reach deep-seated or centrally located brain tumors. The imaging method (volumetric stereotaxis) gathers, stores, and reformats imaging-derived 3D volumetric information that defines an intracranial lesion (tumor) with respect to the surgical field.

Computer-generated information is displayed intraoperatively on computer monitors in the operating room and on a "heads up" display mounted on the operating microscope. These images provide surgeons with a CT (computed tomography) and MRI (magnetic resonance imaging) defined map of the surgical field area scaled to actual size and location. This guides the surgeon in finding and defining the boundaries of brain tumors. The computer-generated images are indexed to the surgical field by means of a robotics-controlled stereotactic frame that positions the patient's tumor within a defined targeting area.

Simulated systems using VR models are being advocated for high-risk techniques, such as the alignment of radiation sources to treat cancerous tumors.

Virtual Reality–Facilitated Rehabilitation

Virtual reality offers the possibility to better shape a rehabilitative program to an individual patient. Greenleaf et al. have theorized that the rehabilitation process can be enhanced through the use of virtual reality technology [Greenleaf, 1994]. The group is currently developing a VR-based rehabilitation workstation that will be used to (1) decompose rehabilitation into small, incremental *functional* steps to facilitate the rehabilitation process and (2) make the rehabilitation process more realistic and less boring and thus enhance motivation and recovery of function (Fig. 71.3).

DataGlove and DataSuit technologies were originally developed as control devices for virtual reality. They are being improved on and applied to the field of functional evaluation of movement in a variety of ways. One system, for example, proposes a glove device coupled with force feedback systems to rehabilitate a damaged hand or to diagnose a range of hand problems [Burdea et al., 1992]. Another system under development incorporates tactile feedback to a glove system to produce feeling in the fingers when virtual objects are "touched" [Burdea et al., 1992]. In order to facilitate accurate goniometric assessment, improvements to the resolution of the standard DataGlove have been developed [Greenleaf, 1992]. The improved DataGlove allows highly accurate measurement of dynamic range of motion of the fingers and wrist and is in use at research centers such as Johns Hopkins and Loma Linda University to measure and analyze functional movements.

Adjacent to rehabilitation evaluation systems are systems utilizing the same measurement technology to provide ergonomic evaluation and injury prevention. Workplace ergonomics has already received a boost from new VR technologies that enable customized workstations tailored to individual requirements [Greenleaf, 1994]. In another area, surgical room ergonomics for medical personnel and patients is projected to reduce the hostile and complicated interface among patients, health care providers, and surgical spaces [Kaplan, 1994].

Motion analysis software (MAS) can assess and analyze upper extremity function from dynamic measurement data acquired by the improved DataGlove. This technology not only provides highly objective measurement but also ensures more accurate methods for collecting data and performing quantitative analyses for physicians, therapists, and ergonomics specialists involved in job-site eval-

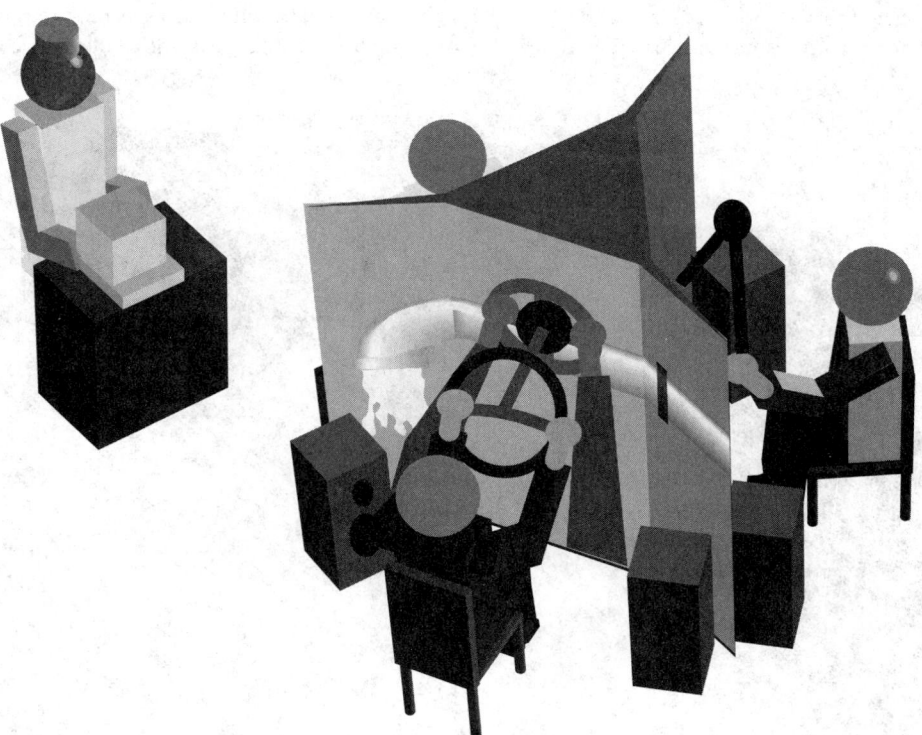

FIGURE 71.3 VR-based rehabilitation workstation.

uation and design. The DataGlove/MAS technology is contributing to a greater understanding of upper extremity biomechanics and kinesiology. Basic DataGlove technology coupled with VR media will offer numerous opportunities for the rehabilitation sector of the medical market, not the least of which is the positive implication for enhancing patient recovery by making the process more realistic and participatory (Fig. 71.4).

Disability Solutions

One exciting aspect of virtual reality technology is the inherent ability to enable individuals with physical disabilities to accomplish tasks and have experiences otherwise denied them (Fig. 71.5). The strategies currently employed for disability-related VR research include head-mounted displays, position/orientation sensing, tactile feedback, eye tracking, 3D sound systems, data input devices, image generation, and optics. For physically disabled persons, VR will provide a new link to capabilities and experiences heretofore unattainable, such as

- An individual with cerebral palsy who is confined to a wheelchair can operate a telephone switchboard, play hand ball, and dance [Greenleaf, 1994] within a virtual environment.
- Disabled individuals can be in one location while their "virtual being" is in a totally different location. This opens all manner of possibilities for participating in work, study, or leisure activities anywhere in the world without leaving home.
- Physically disabled individuals could interact with real-world activities through robotic devices they control from within the virtual world.
- Blind persons could practice and plan in advance navigating through or among buildings if the accesses represented in a virtual world were made up of 3D sound images.

VR also will enable persons with disabilities to experience situations and sensations not accessible in a physical world. Learning and working environments can be tailored to specific needs with VR; for example, since the virtual world can be superimposed over the real world, a learner could

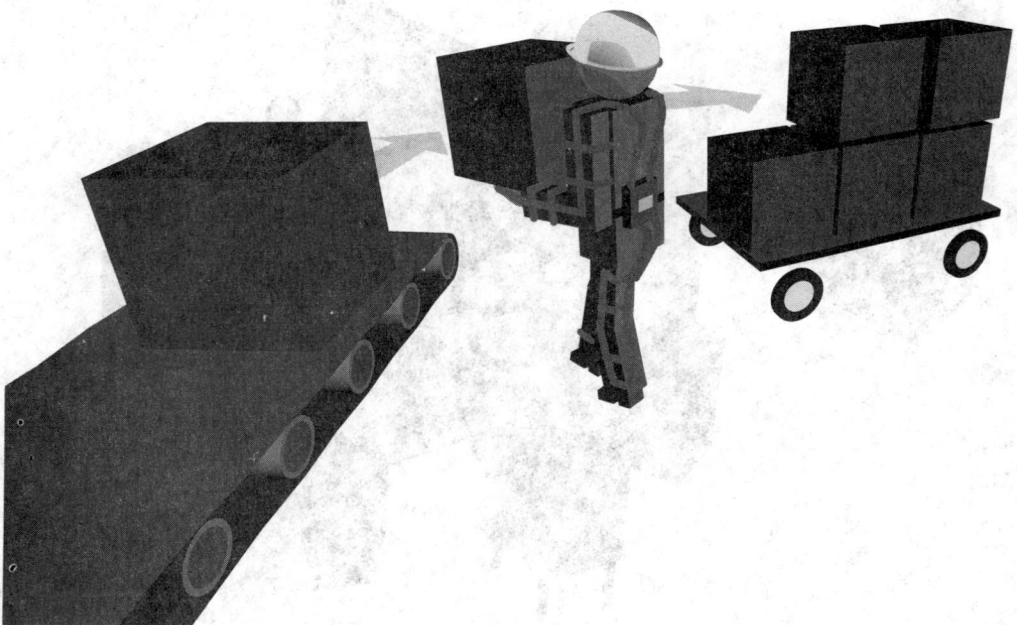

FIGURE 71.4   DataSuit for ergonomic and sports medicine applications.

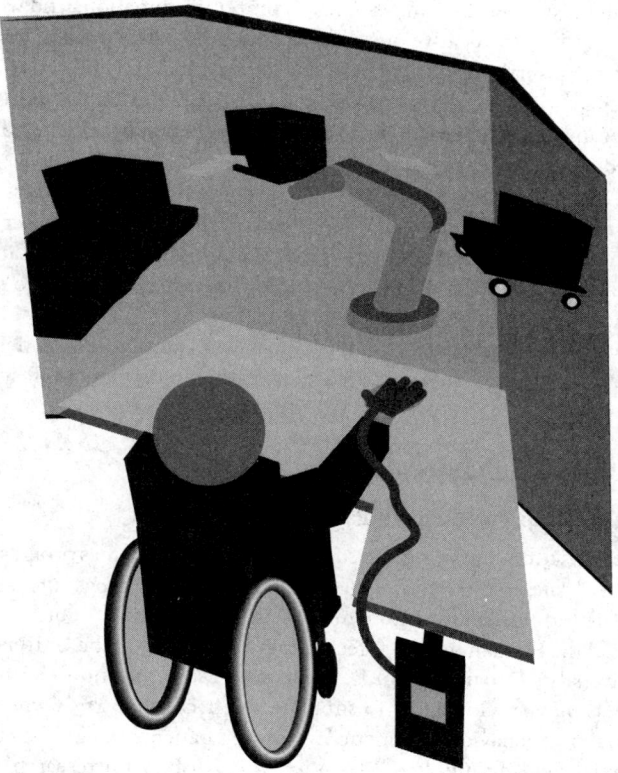

FIGURE 71.5 VR system used as a disability solution.

move progressively from a highly supported mode of performing a task in the virtual world through to performing it unassisted in the real world.

The Wheelchair VR project [Trimble et al., 1992] is a highly specialized architectural software being developed to aid in the design of barrier-free building for persons with disabilities.

Telesurgery and Telemedicine

Telepresence is the "sister field" of virtual reality. Classically defined as the ability to act and interact in an off-site environment by making use of virtual reality technology, telepresence is emerging as an area of development in its own right. Telemedicine (the telepresence of medical experts) is being explored as a way to reduce the cost of medical practice and to bring expertise into remote areas [Burrow, 1994; Rosen, 1994].

Telesurgery is a fertile area for development. On the verge of realization, telesurgery (remote surgery) will help resolve some things that complicate or compromise surgery, among them

- The patient is too ill or injured to be moved for surgery.
- A specialist surgeon is located at some distance from the patient requiring specialized attention.
- Accident victims may have a better chance of survival if immediate, on-the-scene surgery can be performed remotely by an emergency room surgeon at a local hospital.
- Soldiers wounded in battle could undergo surgery on the battlefield by a surgeon located elsewhere.

The surgeon really does operate—on flesh, not a computer animation. And while the distance aspect of remote surgery is a provocative one, telepresence is proving an aid in nonremote surgery as well. It can help surgeons gain dexterity over conventional methods of manipulation. This is expected to be particularly important in laparoscopic surgery. For example, suturing and knot tying will be as easy to see in laparoscopic surgery as it is in open surgery because telepresence enables the surgery to look and fell like open surgery.

As developed at SRI International [Satava, 1992], telepresence not only offers a compelling sense of reality for the surgeon but also allows the surgeon to perform the surgery according to the usual methods and procedures. There is nothing to learn. Hand motions are quick and precise. And the visual field, the instrument motion, and the force feedback can all be scaled to make microsurgery easier than it would be if the surgeon were at the patient's side.

While the current technology has been implemented in prototype, SRI and Telesurgical Corporation, based in Redwood City, California, are collaborating to develop a full system based on this novel concept.

Patient Testing and Behavioral Intervention

Virtual Imaging to Help Parkinson's Patients

For Parkinson disease victims, initiating and sustaining walking becomes progressively difficult. The condition, known as *akinesia,* can be mitigated by treatment with drugs such as L-dopa, a precursor of the natural neural transmitters dopamine, but usually not without unwanted side effects. Now, collaborators at the Human Interface Technology Laboratory at the University of Washington, along with the university's Department of Rehabilitation Medicine and the San Francisco Parkinson's Institute, are using virtual imagery to simulate an effect called *kinesia paradoxa,* or the triggering of normal walking behavior in akinetic Parkinson's patients [Weghorst et al., 1994].

Using a commercial, field-multiplexed, "heads up" video display, the research team has developed an approach that elicits near-normal walking by presenting collimated virtual images of objects and abstract visual cues moving through the patient's visual field at speeds that emulate normal walking. The combination of image collimation and animation speed reinforces the illusion of space-stabilized visual cues at the patient's feet.

This novel, VR-assisted technology also may prove to be therapeutically useful for other movement disorders.

VR and the Treatment of Anxiety, Panic, and Phobia of Heights

Lamson and Meisner [1994] have investigated the diagnostic and treatment possibilities of VR immersion on anxiety, panic, and phobia of heights. By immersing both patients and controls in computer-generated situations, the researchers were able to expose the subjects to anxiety-provoking situations (such as jumping from a height) in a controlled manner. Experimental results indicated a significant subject habituation and desensitization through this approach, and the approach appears clinically useful.

VR Evaluation of Cognitive Deficits

Pugnetti et al. [1994] have explored the potential of enhancing the efficacy of established procedures for the clinical evaluation and management of acquired cognitive impairments in adults. By using a VR-based navigation paradigm, researchers were able to challenge both patients and normal subjects to a complex cognitive activity and simultaneously generate performance data. Behavioral data analysis is then carried out using established scoring criteria.

71.5 Summary

Virtual reality tools and techniques are being rapidly developed in the scientific, engineering, and medical areas. This technology will likely have a direct effect on medical practice. Computer simulation will allow physicians to practice surgical procedures in a virtual environment in which there is no risk to patients and where mistakes can be recognized and rectified immediately by the computer. Procedures can be reviewed from new, insightful perspectives that are not possible in the real world.

Some rather remarkable virtual reality products have progressed beyond prototype, and not surprisingly, some of the technology has already found utility in both clinical medicine and research.

The innovators in medical VR will be called on to refine technical efficiency and increase physical and psychological comfort and capability, while keeping an eye to reducing costs for health care. The mandate is complex, but like VR technology itself, the possibilities are very exciting.

While the possibilities—and the need—for medical VR are immense, approaches and solutions using new VR-based applications require diligent, cooperative efforts among technology developers, medical practitioners, and medical consumers to establish where future requirements and demand will lie.

Further Information

For an excellent treatment of the state of the art of VR and its taxonomy, see the ACM SIGGRAPH publication *Computer Graphics,* vol. 26, no. 3, August 1992. It covers the U.S. Government's National Science Foundation invitational workshop on Interactive Systems Program, March 23–24, 1992, which served to identify and recommend future research directions in the area of virtual environments. A more in-depth exposition of VR taxonomy can be found in the MIT journal *Presence,* vol. 1, no. 2.

Virtual Reality Technology, Grigore Burdea and Philippe Coiffet, New York, Wiley.

HITL (Human Interface Technology Laboratory), University of Washington, FJ-15, Seattle, WA 98195.

UNC Laboratory, University of North Carolina, Chapel Hill, Computer Science Department, Chapel Hill, NC 27599-3175.

CyberEdge Journal. Excellent professional newsletter, Ben Delaney, Editor, 1 Gate Six Road, Suite G, Sausalito, CA 94965.

Presence: Teleoperators and Virtual Environments. Professional Tech Papers and Journal, MIT Press Journals, 55 Hayward St, Cambridge MA 02142

Virtual Reality Report, Meckler Publishing, Sandra Helsel, Editor in Chief, Meckler Corporation, 11 Ferry Lane, Westport CT 06880.

References

Bolas MT. 1994. Human factors in the design of an immersive display. IEEE Comput Graphics Appl 14(1):55.

Burdea G, Zhuang J, Roskos E, et al. 1992. A portable dextrous master with force feedback. Presence 1(1):18.

Burrow M. 1994. A telemedicine testbed for developing and evaluating telerobotic tools for rural health care. In Medicine Meets Virtual Reality II: Interactive Technology and Healthcare: Visionary Applications for Simulation Visualization Robotics, pp 15–18. San Diego, Aligned Management Associates.

Durlach NI, Shinn-Cunningham BG, Held RM. 1993. Supernormal auditory localization: I. General background. Presence 2(2):89.

Greenleaf W. 1992. DataGlove, DataSuit and virtual reality. In Virtual Reality and Persons with Disabilities: Proceedings of the 7th Annual Conference, pp 18–21. Los Angeles, California State University.

Greenleaf WJ. 1995. Rehabilitation, ergonomics, and disability solutions using virtual reality technology. In Morgan K, Satava RM, Sieburg HB, et al. (eds), Interactive Technology and the New Paradigm for Healthcare, IOS Press and Ohmsha.

Hoffman HM. 1994. Virtual reality and the medical curriculum: Integrating extant and emerging technologies. In Medicine Meets Virtual Reality II: Interactive Technology and Healthcare: Visionary Applications for Simulation Visualization Robotics, pp 73–76. San Diego, Aligned Management Associates.

Holler E, Breitwieser H. 1994. Telepresence systems for application in minimally invasive surgery. In Medicine Meets Virtual Reality II: Interactive Technology and Healthcare: Visionary Applications for Simulation Visualization Robotics, pp 77–80. San Diego, Aligned Management Associates.

Hon D. 1994. Ixion's laparoscopic surgical skills simulator. In Medicine Meets Virtual Reality II: Interactive Technology and Healthcare: Visionary Applications for Simulation Visualization Robotics, pp 81–83. San Diego, Aligned Management Associates.

Jacobs L. 1994. Garage Virtual Reality. Indianapolis, Sams Publications.

Johnson AD. 1994. Tactile feedback enhancement to laparoscopic tools (abstract). In Medicine Meets Virtual Reality II: Interactive Technology and Healthcare: Visionary Applications for Simulation Visualization Robotics, p 92. San Diego, Aligned Management Associates.

Kall BA, Kelly PJ, Stiving SO, Goerss SJ. 1994. Integrated multimodality visualization in stereotactic neurologic surgery. In Medicine Meets Virtual Reality II: Interactive Technology and Healthcare: Visionary Applications for Simulation Visualization Robotics, pp 93–94. San Diego, Aligned Management Associates.

Kaplan KL. 1994. Project description: Surgical room of the future. In Medicine Meets Virtual Reality II: Interactive Technology and Healthcare: Visionary Applications for Simulation Visualization Robotics, pp 95–98. San Diego, Aligned Management Associates.

Kelly PJ. 1994. Quantitative virtual reality surgical simulation, minimally invasive stereotactic neurosurgery and frameless stereotactic technologies. In Medicine Meets Virtual Reality II: Interactive Technology and Healthcare: Visionary Applications for Simulation Visualization Robotics, pp 103–108. San Diego, Aligned Management Associates.

Kuhnapfel UG. 1994. Realtime graphical computer simulation for endoscopic surgery. In Medicine Meets Virtual Reality II: Interactive Technology and Healthcare: Visionary Applications for Simulation Visualization Robotics, pp 114–116. San Diego, Aligned Management Associates.

Lamson R, Meisner M., 1994. The effects of virtual reality immersion in the treatment of anxiety, panic, and phobia of heights. In Virtual Reality and Persons with Disabilities: Proceedings of the 2nd Annual International Conference, sponsored by the Center on Disabilities, California State University, Northridge, 18111 Nordhoff Street, DVSS. Northridge, CA.

Loftin RB, Ota D, Saito T, Voss M. 1994. A virtual environment for laparoscopic surgical training. In Medicine Meets Virtual Reality II: Interactive Technology and Healthcare: Visionary Applications for Simulation Visualization Robotics, pp 121–123. San Diego, Aligned Management Associates.

McGovern KT, McGovern LT. 1994. Virtual clinic: A virtual reality surgical simulator. Virtual Reality World 2(2):41.

Merril JR. 1993. Surgery on the cutting edge. Virtual Reality World 1(3–4):34.

Merril JR. 1994. Presentation material: Medicine meets virtual reality II (abstract). In Medicine Meets Virtual Reality II: Interactive Technology and Healthcare: Visionary Applications for Simulation Visualization Robotics, pp 158–159. San Diego, Aligned Management Associates.

Peifer J. 1994. Virtual environment for eye surgery simulation. In Medicine Meets Virtual Reality II: Interactive Technology and Healthcare: Visionary Applications for Simulation Visualization Robotics, pp 166–173. San Diego, Aligned Management Associates.

Preminger GM. 1994. Advanced imaging technologies for endoscopic surgery. In Medicine Meets Virtual Reality II: Interactive Technology and Healthcare: Visionary Applications for Simulation Visualization Robotics, pp 177–178. San Diego, Aligned Management Associates.

Pugnetti L, Mendozzi L, Motta A, et al. 1995. Immersive virtual reality to assist retraining of acquired cognitive deficits. In Morgan K, Satava RM, Sieburg HB, et al. (eds), Interactive Technology and the New Paradigm for Healthcare, IOS Press and Ohmsha.

Rabinowitz WM, Maxwell J, Shao Y, Wei M. 1993. Sound localization cues for a magnified head: Implications from sound diffraction about a rigid sphere. Presence 2(2):125.

Rosen J. 1994. The role of telemedicine and telepresence in reducing health care costs. In Medicine Meets Virtual Reality II: Interactive Technology and Healthcare: Visionary Applications for Simulation Visualization Robotics, pp 187–194. San Diego, Aligned Management Associates.

Satava RM. 1992. Robotics, telepresence and virtual reality: A critical analysis of the future of surgery. Minimally Invasive Therapy 1:357.

Schraft RD, Neugebauer JG, Wapler M. 1994. Virtual reality for improved control in endoscopic surgery. In Medicine Meets Virtual Reality II: Interactive Technology and Healthcare: Visionary Applications for Simulation Visualization Robotics, pp 233–236. San Diego, Aligned Management Associates.

Shimoga KB, Khosla PK, Sclabassi RJ. 1994. Teleneurosurgery: An approach to enhance the dexterity of neurosurgeons. In Medicine Meets Virtual Reality II: Interactive Technology and Healthcare: Visionary Applications for Simulation Visualization Robotics, p 203. San Diego, Aligned Management Associates.

Szabo Z, Hunter JG, Berci G, et al. 1994. Choreographed instrument movements during laparoscopic surgery: Needle driving, knot tying and anastomosis techniques. In Medicine Meets Virtual Reality II: Interactive Technology and Healthcare: Visionary Applications for Simulation Visualization Robotics, pp 216–217. San Diego, Aligned Management Associates.

Tendick F, Jennings RW, Tharp G, Stark L. 1993. Sensing and manipulation problems in endoscopic surgery: Experiment, analysis, and observation. Presence 2(1):66.

Trimble J, Morris T, Crandall R. 1992. Virtual reality. TeamRehab Report 3(8):33.

Wang Y, Sackier J. 1994. Robotically enhanced surgery. In Medicine Meets Virtual Reality II: Interactive Technology and Healthcare: Visionary Applications for Simulation Visualization Robotics, pp 218–220. San Diego, Aligned Management Associates.

Weghorst S, Prothero J, Furness T. 1994. Virtual images in the treatment of Parkinson's disease akinesia. In Medicine Meets Virtual Reality II: Interactive Technology and Healthcare: Visionary Applications for Simulation Visualization Robotics, pp 242–243. San Diego, Aligned Management Associates.

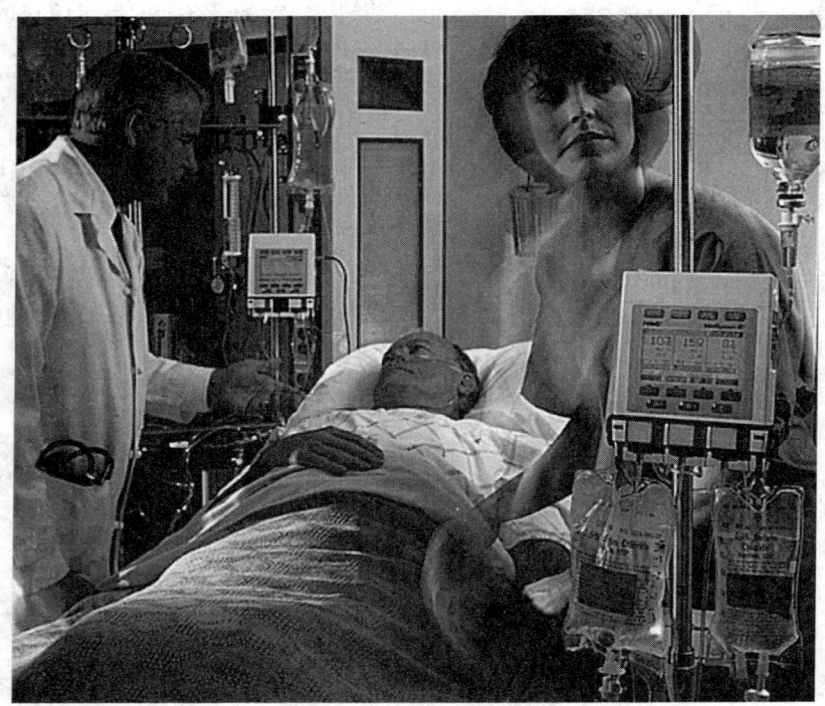

A typical IV infusion system.

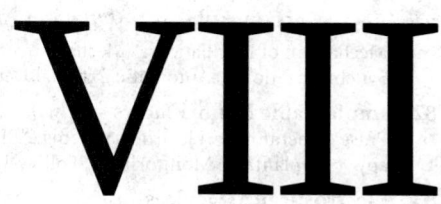

VIII

Medical Instruments and Devices

Wolf W. von Maltzahn
University of Texas at Arlington

N OT TOO LONG AGO, the term *medical instrument* stood for simple hand-held instruments used
by physicians for observing patients, examining organs, making simple measurements, or administering medication. These small instruments, such as stethoscopes, thermometers, tongue depressors,
and a few surgical tools, typically fit into a physician's hand bag. Today's medical instruments are
considerably more complicated and diverse, primarily because they incorporate electronic systems
for sensing, transducing, manipulating, storing, and displaying data or information. Furthermore,
medical specialists today request detailed and accurate measurements of a vast number of physiologic parameters for diagnosing illnesses and prescribe complicated procedures for treating these.
As a result, the number of medical instruments and devices has grown from a few hundred a generation ago to more than 10,000 today, and the complexity of these instruments has grown at the
same pace. The description of all these instruments and devices would fill an entire handbook by
itself; however, due to the limited space assigned to this topic, only a selected number is described.

While medical instruments acquire and process information and data for monitoring patients
and diagnosing illnesses, medical devices use electrical, mechanical, chemical, or radiation energy
for achieving a desired therapeutic purpose, maintaining physiologic functions, or assisting a patient's healing process. To mention only a few functions, medical devices pump blood, remove metabolic waste products, destroy kidney stones, infuse fluids and drugs, stimulate muscles and nerves,
cut tissue, administer anesthesia, alleviate pain, restore function, or warm tissue. Because of their
complexity, medical devices are used mostly in hospitals and medical centers by trained personnel,
but some also can be found in private homes operated by patients themselves or their caregivers.

This section on medical instruments and devices neither replaces a textbook on this subject nor presents the material in a typical textbook manner. The authors assume the reader to be interested in but not knowledgeable of the subject. Therefore, each chapter begins with a short introduction to the subject material, followed by a brief description of current practices and principles, and ends with recent trends and developments. Whenever appropriate, equations, diagrams, and pictures amplify and illustrate the topic, while tables summarize facts and data. The short reference secion at the end of each chapter points toward further resource materials, including books, journal articles, patents, and company brochures.

The chapters in the first half of this section cover the more traditional topics of bioinstrumentation, such as biopotential amplifiers and noninvasive blood pressure, blood flow, and respiration monitors, while those of the second half focus more on recently developed instruments and devices such as pulse oximeters or home-care monitoring devices. Some of this latter material is new or hard to find elsewhere. A few traditional bioinstrumentation topics such as invasive blood pressure measurements, electrocardiography, electromyography, or electroencephalography have been omitted entirely because most textbooks on this subject give excellent introductions and reviews. Transducers, biosensors, and electrodes are covered in other sections of this *Handbook*. Thus this section provides an overview, albeit an incomplete one, of recent developments in the field of medical instruments and devices.

72

Biopotential Amplifiers

Joachim H. Nagel
University of Miami

Biosignals are recorded as potentials, voltages, and electrical field strengths generated by nerves and muscles. The measurements involve voltages at very low levels, typically ranging between 1 μV and 100 mV, with high source impedances and superimposed high-level interference signals and noise. The signals need to be amplified to make them compatible with devices such as displays, recorders, or A/D converters for computerized equipment. Amplifiers adequate to measure these signals have to satisfy very specific requirements. They have to provide amplification selective to the physiologic signal, reject superimposed noise and interference signals, and guarantee protection from damages through voltage and current surges for both patient and electronic equipment. Amplifiers featuring these specifications are known as *biopotential amplifiers*. Basic requirements and features as well as some specialized systems are presented in this chapter.

72.1 Basic Amplifier Requirements

The basic requirements that a biopotential amplifier has to satisfy are:

- The physiologic process to be monitored should not be influenced in any way by the amplifier.
- The measured signal should not be distorted.
- The amplifier should provide the best possible separation of signal and interferences.
- The amplifier has to offer protection of the patient from any hazard of electric shock.
- The amplifier itself has to be protected against damages that might result from high-input voltages as they occur during the application of defibrillators or electrosurgical instrumentation.

A typical configuration for the measurement of biopotentials is shown in Fig. 72.1. Three electrodes, two of them picking up the biologic signal and the third providing the reference potential, connect the subject to the amplifier. The input signal to the amplifier consists of five components: the desired biopotential, undesired biopotentials, a power-line interference signal of 60 Hz and its harmonics, interference signals generated by the tissue/electrode interface, and noise. Proper design of the amplifier provides rejection of a large portion of the signal interferences. The main task of the differential amplifier as shown in Fig. 72.1 is to reject the line frequency interference that is electrostatically or magnetically coupled into the subject. The desired biopotential appears as a voltage between the two input terminals of the differential amplifier and is referred to as the *differential sig-*

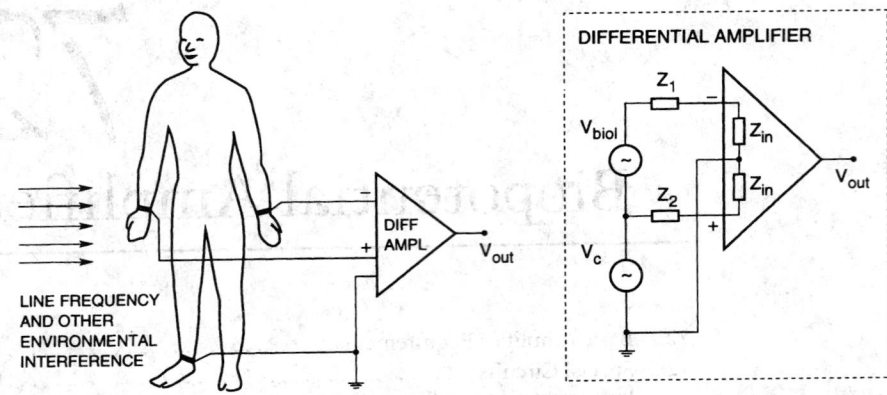

FIGURE 72.1 Typical configuration for the measurement of biopotentials. The biologic signal V_{biol} appears between the two measuring electrodes at the right and left arms of the patient and is fed to the inverting and the noninverting inputs of the differential amplifier. The right leg electrode provides the reference potential for the amplifier with a common node voltage V_c as indicated.

nal. The line frequency interference signal shows only very small differences in amplitude and phase between the two measuring electrodes, causing approximately the same potential at both inputs and thus appears only between the inputs and ground and is called the *common-mode signal*. Strong rejection of the common-mode signal is one of the most important characteristics of a good biopotential amplifier.

The *common-mode rejection ratio* or CMRR of an amplifier is defined as the ratio of the differential mode gain over the common-mode gain. As seen in Fig. 72.1, the rejection of the common-mode signal in a biopotential amplifier is a function of both the amplifier CMRR and the source impedances Z_1 and Z_2. For the ideal biopotential amplifier with $Z_1 = Z_2$ and infinite CMRR of the differential amplifier, the output voltage is the pure biologic signal amplified by the differential mode gain G_D: $V_{out} = G_D \cdot V_{biol}$. With finite CMRR, the common-mode signal is not completely rejected, adding the interference term $G_D \cdot V_c$/CMRR to the output signal. Even in the case of an ideal differential amplifier with infinite CMRR, the common-mode signal will not completely disappear unless the source impedances are equal. The common-mode signal V_c causes currents to flow through Z_1 and Z_2. The related voltage drops show a difference if the source impedances are unequal, thus generating a differential signal at the amplifier input which, of course, is not rejected by the differential amplifier. With amplifier gain G_D and input impedance Z_{in}, the output voltage of the amplifier is:

$$V_{out} = G_D V_{biol} + \frac{G_D V_c}{CMRR} + G_D V_c \left(1 - \frac{Z_{in}}{Z_{in} + Z_1 - Z_2}\right) \qquad (72.1)$$

The output of a real biopotential amplifier will always consist of the desired output component due to a differential biosignal, an undesired component due to incomplete rejection of common-mode interference signals as a function of CMRR, and an undesired component due to source impedance imbalance allowing a small proportion of a common-mode signal to appear as a differential signal to the amplifier. Since source impedance imbalances of 5000 Ω–10,000 Ω, mainly caused by electrodes, are not uncommon, and since sufficient rejection of line frequency interferences requires a minimum CMRR of 100 dB, the input impedance of the amplifier should be at least 10^9 Ω at 60 Hz to prevent source impedance imbalances from deteriorating the overall CMRR of the amplifier. State-of-the-art biopotential amplifiers provide a CMRR of 120–140 dB.

In order to provide optimum signal quality and adequate voltage level for further signal processing, the amplifier has to provide a gain of 100–50,000 and needs to maintain the best possible signal-to-noise ratio. The presence of high-level interference signals not only damages the quality of the physiologic signals but also restricts the design of the biopotential amplifier. Electrode half-cell potentials, for example, limit the gain factor of the first amplifier stage, since their amplitudes can be several orders of magnitude larger than the amplitude of the physiologic signal. To prevent the amplifier from going into saturation, this component has to be eliminated before the required gain can be provided for the physiologic signal.

A typical design of the various stages of a biopotential amplifier is shown in Fig. 72.2. The electrodes that provide the transition between the ionic flow of currents in biologic tissue and the electronic flow of current in the amplifier represent a complex electrochemical system that is described elsewhere in the *Handbook*. The electrodes determine to a large extent the composition of the measured signal. The preamplifier represents the most critical part of the amplifier itself, since the preamplifier sets the stage for the quality of the biosignal. With proper design, the preamplifier can eliminate or at least minimize most of the signals interfering with the measurement of biopotentials.

In addition to electrode potentials and electromagnetic interferences, noise—generated by the amplifier and the connection between biologic source and amplifier—has to be taken into account when designing the preamplifier. The total source resistance R_s, including the resistance of the biologic source and all transition resistances between signal source and amplifier input, causes thermal voltage noise with a root-mean-square (rms) value of

$$E_{rms} = \sqrt{4kTR_sB} \; (Volt) \tag{72.2}$$

where k = Boltzmann constant, T = absolute temperature, R_s = resistance in Ω, and B = bandwidth in Hz.

Additionally, there is the inherent amplifier noise. It consists of two frequency-dependent components: the internal voltage noise source e_n and the voltage drop across the source resistance R_s caused by an internal current noise generator i_n. The total input noise for the amplifier with a bandwidth of $B = f_2 - f_1$ is

$$E_{rms}^2 = \int_{f_1}^{f_2} e_n^2 df + R_s^2 \int_{f_1}^{f_2} i_n^2 df + 4kTR_sB \tag{72.3}$$

High signal-to-noise ratios thus require the use of very low-noise amplifiers and the limitation of banwidth. Current technology offers differential amplifiers with voltage noise of less than 10 nV $\sqrt{Hz}$ and current noise less than 1 pA$\sqrt{Hz}$. Both parameters are frequency dependent and

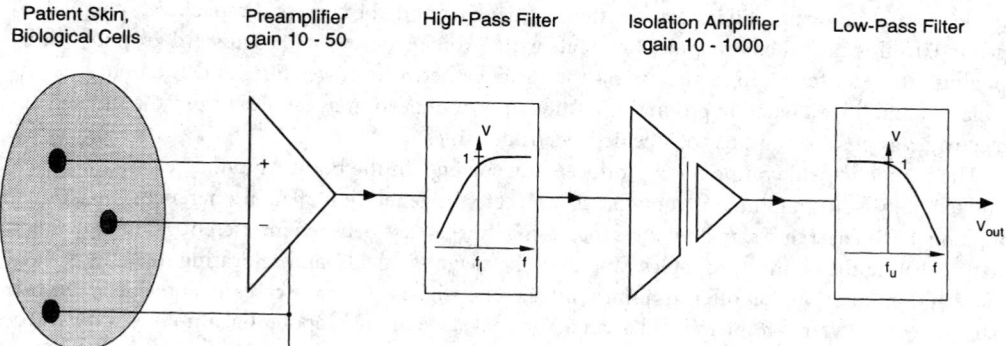

FIGURE 72.2 Schematic design of the main stages of a biopotential amplifier. Three electrodes connect the patient to a preamplifier stage. After removing dc and low-frequency interferences, the signal is connected to an output low-pass filter through an isolation stage which provides electrical safety to the patient, prevents ground loops, and reduces the influence of interference signals.

decrease approximately with the square root of frequency. The exact relationship depends on the technology of the amplifier input stage. Field effect transistor (FET) preamplifiers exhibit about 5 times the voltage noise density compared to bipolar transistors but a current noise density that is about 100 times smaller.

The purpose of the high-pass and low-pass filters in Fig. 72.2 is to eliminate interference signals like electrode half-cell potentials and preamplifier offset potentials and to reduce the noise amplitude by the limitation of the amplifier bandwidth. Since the biosignal should not be distorted or attenuated, higher-order sharp-cutting linear phase filters have to be used. Active Bessel filters are preferred filter types due to their smooth transfer function. Separation of biosignal and interference is in most cases incomplete due to the overlap of their spectra.

The isolation stage serves the galvanic decoupling of the patient from the measuring equipment and provides safety from electrical hazards. This stage also prevents galvanic currents from deteriorating the signal-noise ratio especially by preventing ground loops. Various principles can be used to realize the isolation stage. Analog isolation amplifiers use transformer, optical, or capacitive couplers to transmit the signal through the isolation barrier. Digital isolation amplifiers use a voltage/frequency converter to digitize the signal before it is transmitted easily by optical or inductive couplers to the output frequency/voltage converter. The most important characteristics of an isolation amplifier are low leakage current, isolation impedance, isolation voltage (or mode) rejection (IMR), and maximum safe isolation voltage.

The most critical point in the measurement of biopotentials is the contact between electrodes and biologic tissue. Both the electrode offset potential and the electrode/tissue impedance are subject to changes due to relative movements of electrode and tissue. Thus two interference signals are generated as motion artifacts: the changes of the electrode potential and motion-induced changes of the voltage drop caused by the input current of the preamplifier. These motion artifacts can be minimized by providing high input impedances for the preamplifier, by using electrodes with low half-cell potentials, i.e., nonpolarized electrodes, and by reducing the source impedance by use of electrode gel. Motion artifacts, interferences from external electromagnetic fields, and noise can also be generated in the wires connecting electrodes and amplifier. Reduction of these interferences is achieved by using twisted pair cables, shielded wires, and *input guarding*.

Recording of biopotentials is often done in an environment that is equipped with many electric systems which produce strong electric and magnetic fields. In addition to 60-Hz power line frequency and some strong harmonics, high-frequency electromagnetic fields are encountered. At power line frequency, the electric and magnetic components of the interfering fields can be considered separately. Electric fields are caused by all conductors that are connected to power, even with no flow of current. A current is capacitively coupled into the body where it flows to the ground electrode. If an isolation amplifier is used without patient ground, the current is capacitively coupled to ground. In this case, the body potential floats with a voltage of up to 100 V toward ground. Minimizing interferences requires increasing the distance between power lines and the body, use of isolation amplifiers, separate grounding of the body at a location as far away from the measuring electrodes as possible, and use of shielded electrode cables.

The magnetic field components produce eddy currents in the body. Amplifier, electrode cable, and the body form an induction loop that is subject to the generation of an interference signal. Minimizing this interference signal requires increasing the distance between interference source and patient, twisting the connecting cables, shielding the magnetic fields, and relocating the patient to a place and orientation that offer minimum interference signals. In many cases an additional narrow band-rejection filter is implemented as an additional stage in the biopotential amplifier to provide sufficient suppression of line frequency interferences.

In order to achieve optimum signal quality, the biopotential amplifier has to be adapted to the specific application. Based on the signal parameters, both appropriate bandwidth and gain factor are chosen. Figure 72.3 shows an overview of the most commonly measured biopotentials and specifies the normal ranges for amplitude and bandwidth.

A final requirement for biopotential amplifiers is the need for calibration. Since the amplitude of the biopotential often has to be determined very accurately, there must be provisions to easily determine the gain or the amplitude range referenced to the input of the amplifier. For this purpose, the gain of the amplifier must be well calibrated. In order to prevent difficulties with calibrations, some amplifiers that need to have adjustable gain use a number of fixed gain settings rather than providing a continuous gain control. Some amplifiers have a standard, built-in signal source of known amplitude that can be momentarily connected to the input by the push of a button to check the calibration at the output of the biopotential amplifier.

72.2 Special Circuits

Instrumentation Amplifier

An important stage of all biopotential amplifiers is the input preamplifier, which substantially contributes to the overall quality of the system. The main tasks of the preamplifier are to sense the voltage between two measuring electrodes while rejecting the common mode signal and minimizing the effect of electrode polarization overpotentials. Crucial to the performance of the preamplifier is the input impedance, which should be as high as possible. Such a differential amplifier cannot be realized using a standard single *operational amplifier* (op-amp) design, since this does not provide the necessary high input impedance. The general solution to the problem involves voltage followers, or noninverting amplifiers, to attain high input impedances. A possible realization is shown in Fig. 72.4a. The main disadvantage of this circuit is that it requires high CMRR both in the followers and in the final op-amp. With the input buffers working at unity gain, all the common-mode rejection must be accomplished in the output amplifier, requiring very precise resistor matching. Addition-

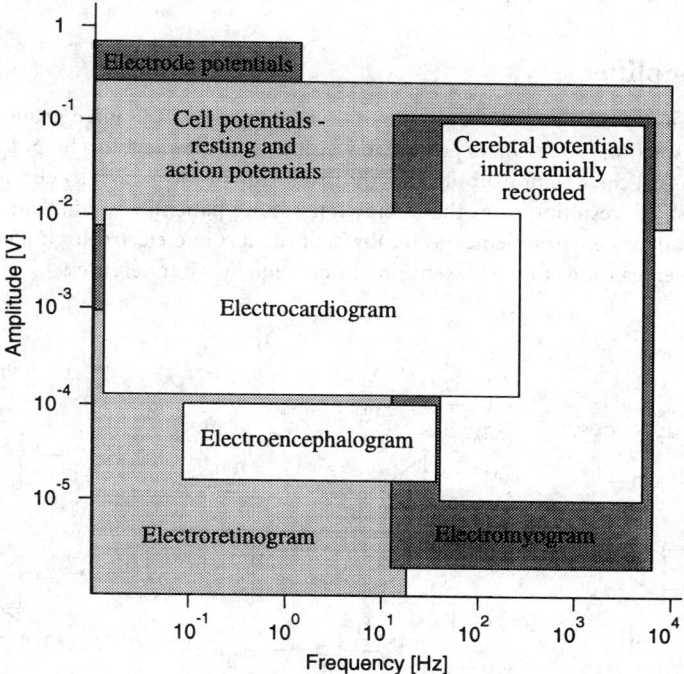

FIGURE 72.3 Amplitudes and spectral ranges of some important biosignals. The various biopotentials completely cover the area from 10^{-6} V to almost 1 V and from dc to 10 kHz.

ally, the noise of the final op-amp is added at a low signal level, decreasing the signal-to-noise ratio unnecessarily. The circuit in Fig. 72.4*b* eliminates this disadvantage. This circuit represents the standard instrumentation amplifier configuration. The two input op-amps provide high differential gain and unity common-mode gain without the requirement of close resistor matching. The differential output from the first stage represents a signal with substantial relative reduction of the common-mode signal and is used to drive a standard differential amplifier which further reduces the common-mode signal. CMRR of the output op-amp as well as resistor matching in its circuit are less critical than in the follower-type instrumentation amplifier. Offset trimming for the whole circuit can be done at one of the input op-amps. Complete instrumentation-amplifier integrated circuits based on this standard instrumentation-amplifier configuration are available from several manufacturers. All components except R_1, which determines the gain of the amplifier, are contained on the integrated circuit chip. Figure 72.4*c* shows another configuration that offers high input impedance with only two op-amps. For good CMRR, however, it requires precise resistor matching.

In applications where dc and very low frequency biopotentials are not to be measured, it would be desirable to block those signal components at the preamplifier inputs by simply adding a capacitor working as a passive high-pass filter. This would eliminate the electrode offset potentials and permit a higher gain factor for the preamplifier. A capacitor between electrodes and amplifier input would, however, result in charging effects from the input bias current. Due to the difficulty of precisely matching capacitors for the two input leads, they would also contribute to an increased source impedance unbalance and thus reduce CMRR. Avoiding the problem of charging effects by adding a resistor between the preamplifier inputs and ground also results in a decrease of CMRR due to the diminished input impedance. Nevertheless, such realizations are used where the specific situation allows. In some applications, a further reduction of the amplifier to a two-electrode amplifier configuration would be convenient, even at the expense of some loss in the CMRR. Figure 72.5 shows a preamplifier design working with two electrodes and providing ac coupling as proposed by Pallás-Areny and Webster [1990].

Isolation Amplifier

Isolation amplifiers can be used to break ground loops, to eliminate source-ground connections, and to provide isolation protection to patient and electronic equipment. In a biopotential amplifier, the main purpose of the isolation amplifier is the protection of the patient by eliminating the hazard of electric shock resulting from the interaction among patient, amplifier, and other electric devices in the patient's environment, specifically defibrillators and electrosurgical equipment. The isolation amplifier also adds to the prevention of line frequency interferences.

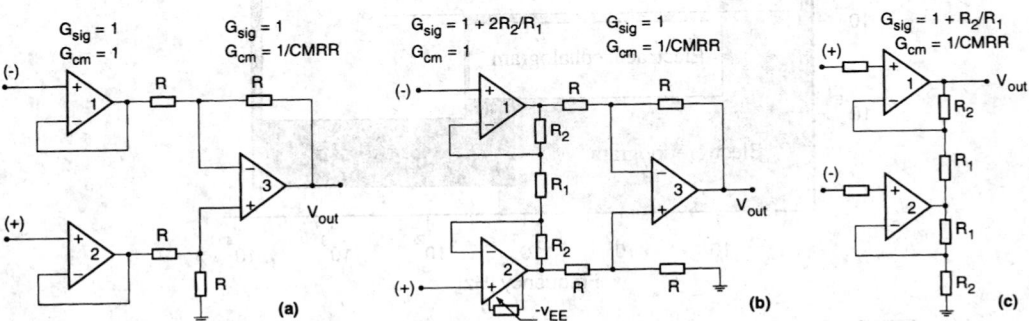

FIGURE 72.4 Circuit drawings for three different realizations of instrumentation amplifiers for biomedical applications. Voltage follower input stage (*a*), improved, amplifying input stage (*b*), and op-amp version (*c*).

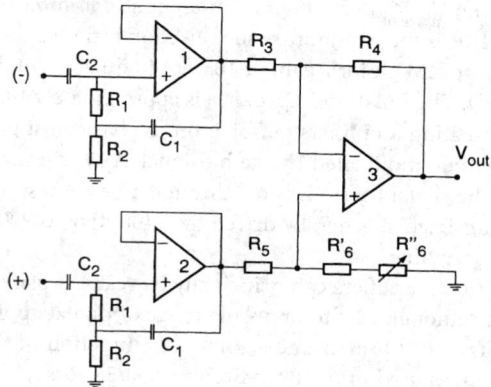

FIGURE 72.5 Composite instrumentation amplifier based on an ac-coupled first stage. The second stage is based on a one op-amp differential amplifier, which can be replaced by an instrumentation amplifier.

Isolation amplifiers are realized in three different technologies: transformer isolation, capacitor isolation, and opto-isolation. An isolation barrier provides a complete galvanic separation of the input side, i.e., patient and preamplifier, from all equipment on the output side. Ideally, there will be no flow of electric current across the barrier. The isolation-mode voltage is the voltage which appears across the isolation barrier, i.e., between the input common and the output common (Fig. 72.6). The amplifier has to withstand the largest expected isolation voltages without damage. Two isolation voltages are specified for commercial isolation amplifiers: the continuous rating and the test voltage. To eliminate the need for lengthy testing, the device is tested at about two times the rated continuous voltage. Thus, for a continuous rating of 2000 V, the device has to be tested at 4000–5000 V for a reasonable period.

Since there is always some leakage across the isolation barrier, the *isolation mode rejection ratio* (IMRR) is not infinite. For a circuit as shown in Fig. 72.6, the output voltage is

$$V_{out} = \frac{G}{R_{G1} + R_{G2} + R_{IN}} \left(V_D + \frac{V_{CM}}{CMRR} \right) + \frac{V_{ISO}}{IMRR} \qquad (72.4)$$

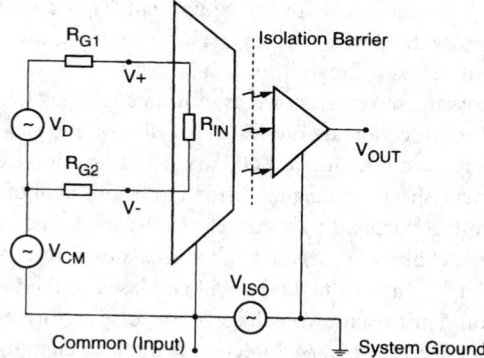

FIGURE 72.6 Equivalent circuit of an isolation amplifier. The differential amplifier on the left transmits the signal through the isolation barrier by a transformer, capacitor, or an opto-coupler.

where G is the amplifier gain; V_D, V_{CM}, and V_{ISO} are differential, common-mode, and isolation voltages, respectively; and CMRR is the common-mode rejection ratio for the amplifier [Burr-Brown Corp., 1994]. Typical values of IMRR for a gain of 10 are 140 dB at dc, and 120 dB at 60 Hz with a source unbalance of 5000 Ω. The isolation impedance is approximately 1.8 pF $\|$ 10^{12} Ω.

Transformer-coupled isolation amplifiers perform on the basis of inductive transmission of a carrier signal that is amplitude modulated by the biosignal. A synchronous demodulator on the output port reconstructs the signal before it is fed through a Bessel response low-pass filter to an output buffer. A power transformer, generally driven by a 400-kHz to 900-kHz square wave, supplies isolated power to the amplifier.

Optically coupled isolation amplifiers can principally be realized using only a single LED and photodiode combination. Although useful for a wide range of digital applications, this design has fundamental limitations as to its linearity and stability as a function of time and temperature. A matched photodiode design, as used in the Burr-Brown 3650/3652 isolation amplifier, overcomes these difficulties [Burr-Brown Corp., 1994]. Operation of the amplifier requires an isolated power supply to drive the input stages. Transformer-coupled low leakage current isolated dc/dc converters are commonly used for this purpose. In some particular applications, especially in cases where the signal is transmitted over a longer distance by fiber optics, such as ECG amplifiers used for gated magnetic resonance imaging, batteries are used to power the amplifier. Fiberoptic coupling in isolation amplifiers is another option that offers the advantage of higher flexibility in the placement of parts on the amplifier board.

Biopotential amplifiers have to provide sufficient protection from electric shock to both user and patient. Electric safety codes and standards specify the minimum safety requirements for the equipment, especially the maximum leakage currents for chassis and patient leads and the power distribution system [AAMI, 1993; Webster, 1992].

Surge Protection

The isolation amplifiers described in the preceding paragraph are used primarily for the protection of the patient from electric shock. Voltage surges between electrodes as they occur during the application of a defibrillator or electrosurgical instrumentation also present a risk to the biopotential amplifier. Biopotential amplifiers should be protected against serious damage to the electronic circuits. This is also part of patient safety, since defective input stages could otherwise apply dangerous current levels to the patient. To achieve this protection, voltage-limiting devices are connected between each measuring electrode and electric ground. Ideally, these devices do not represent a shunt impedance and thus do not lower the input impedance of the preamplifier as long as the input voltage remains in a range considered safe for the equipment. They appear as an open circuit. As soon as the voltage drop across the device reaches a critical value V_b, the impedance of the device changes sharply, and current passes through it to such an extent that the voltage cannot exceed V_b due to the voltage drop across the series resistor R as indicated in Fig. 72.7.

Devices used for amplifier protection are diodes, Zener diodes, and gas-discharge tubes. Parallel silicon diodes limit the voltage to approximately 600 mV. The transition from nonconducting state to conducting state is not very sharp, and signal distortion begins at about 300 mV, which can be within the range of input voltages depending on the electrodes used. The breakdown voltage can be increased by connecting several diodes in series. Higher breakdown voltages are achieved by Zener diodes connected back to back. One of the diodes will be biased in the forward direction and the other in the reverse direction. The breakdown voltage in the forward direction is approximately 600 mV, but the breakdown voltage in the reverse direction is higher, generally in the range of 3–20 V, with a sharper voltage-current characteristic than the diode circuit.

A preferred voltage-limiting device for biopotential amplifiers is the *gas discharge tube.* Due to its extremely high impedance in the nonconducting state, this device appears as an open circuit until it reaches its breakdown voltage. At the breakdown voltage, which ranges from 50–90 V, the tube

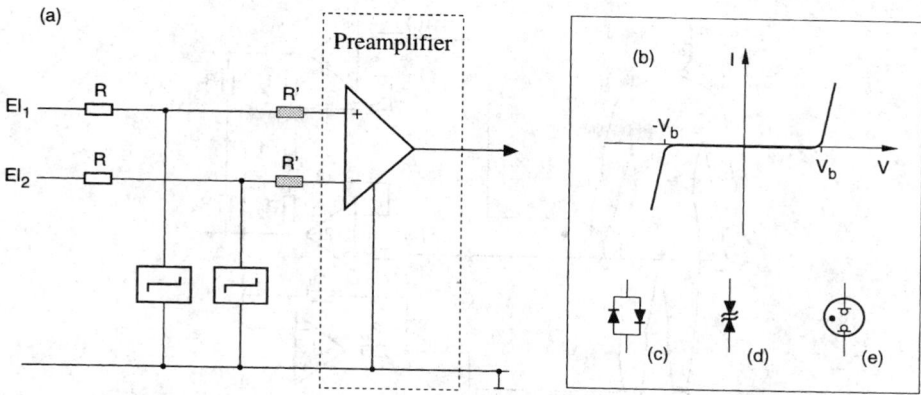

FIGURE 72.7 Protection of the amplifier input against high-voltage transients. The connection diagram for voltage-limiting elements is shown in (*a*) with two optional resistors *R'* at the input. A typical current-voltage characteristic is shown in (*b*). Voltage-limiting elements shown are the antiparallel connection of diodes (*c*), antiparallel connection of Zener diodes (*d*), and gas discharge tubes (*e*).

switches to the conducting state and maintains a voltage that is usually several volts less than the breakdown voltage. Though the voltage maintained by the gas discharge tube is still too high for some amplifiers, it is low enough to allow the input current to be easily limited to a safe value by simple circuit elements such as resistors like the resistors *R'* indicated in Fig. 72.7a. Preferred gas discharge tubes for biomedical applications are miniature neon lamps, which are very inexpensive and have a symmetric characteristic.

Input Guarding

The common-mode input impedance and thus the CMRR of an amplifier can be greatly increased by guarding the input circuit. The common-mode signal can be obtained by two averaging resistors connected between the outputs of the two input op-amps of an instrumentation amplifier as shown in Fig. 72.8. The buffered common-mode signal at the output of op-amp 4 can be used as guard voltage to reduce the effects of cable capacitance and leakage.

In many modern biopotential amplifiers, the reference electrode is not grounded. Instead, it is connected to the output of an amplifier for the common-mode voltage, op-amp 3 in Fig. 72.9, which

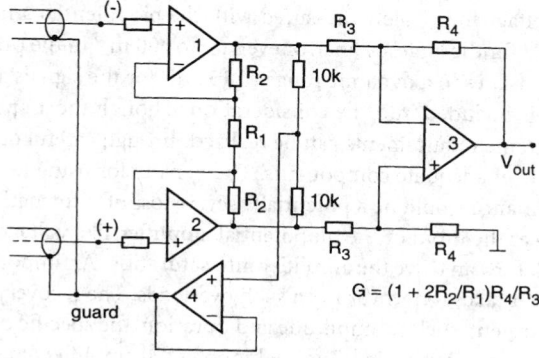

$$G = (1 + 2R_2/R_1)R_4/R_3$$

FIGURE 72.8 Instrumentation amplifier providing input guarding.

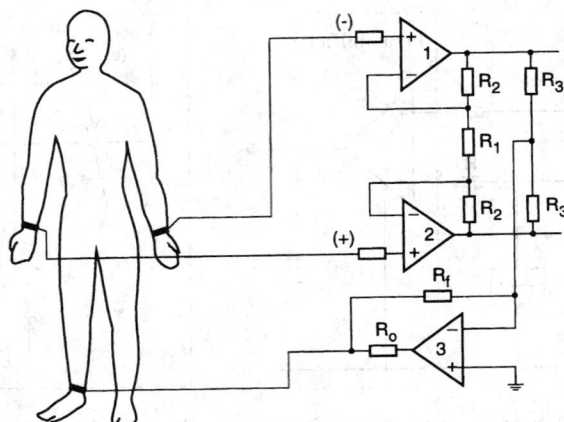

FIGURE 72.9 Driven-right-leg circuit reducing common-mode interference.

works as an inverting amplifier. The inverted common-mode voltage is fed back to the reference electrode. This negative feedback reduces the common-mode voltage to a low value [Webster, 1992]. Electrocardiographs based on this principle are called *driven-right-leg systems*, replacing the right-leg-ground electrode of ordinary electrocardiographs by an actively driven electrode.

Dynamic Range and Recovery

With an increase of either the common-mode or differential input voltage, there will be a point where the amplifier will overload and the output voltage will no longer be representative for the input voltage. Similarly, with a decrease of the input voltage, there will be a point where the noise components of the output voltage cover the output signal to a degree that a measurement of the desired biopotential is no longer possible. The dynamic range of the amplifier, i.e., the range between the smallest and largest possible input signals to be measured, has to cover the whole amplitude range of the physiologic signal of interest. The required dynamic range of biopotential amplifiers can be quite large. In an application such as fetal monitoring, two signals are recorded simultaneously from the electrodes which are quite different in their amplitudes: the fetal ECG and the maternal ECG. Whereas the maternal ECG shows an amplitude of up to 10 mV, the fetal ECG often does not reach more than 1µV. Assuming that the fetal ECG is separated from the composite signal and fed to an analog/digital converter for digital signal processing with a resolution of 10 bit (signed integer), the smallest voltage to be safely measured with the biopotential amplifier is 1/512 µV, or about 2 nV, versus 10 mV for the largest signal, or even up to 300 mV in the presence of an electrode offset potential. This translates to a dynamic range of 134 dB for the signals alone and of 164 dB if the electrode potential is included into the consideration. Though most applications are less demanding, even such extreme requirements can be realized through careful design of the biopotential amplifier and the use of adequate components. The penalty for using less expensive amplifiers with diminished performance would be a potentially severe loss of information.

Transients appearing at the input of the biopotential amplifier, like voltage peaks from a cardiac pacemaker or a defibrillator, can drive the amplifier into saturation. An important characteristic for the amplifier is the time it takes to recover from such overloads. The recovery time depends on the characteristics of the transient, such as amplitude and duration, the specific design of the amplifier, like bandwidth, and the components used. Typical biopotential amplifiers may take several seconds to recover from severe overload. The recovery time can be reduced by disconnecting the amplifier inputs at the discovery of a transient using an electronic switch.

Biopotential amplifiers are crucial components in many medical and biologic measurements and largely determine the quality and information content of the measured signals. The extremely wide range of necessary specifications with regard to bandwidth, sensitivity, dynamic range, gain, CMRR, and patient safety leaves only little room for the application of general purpose biopotential amplifiers, mostly requiring the use of special-purpose amplifiers.

Defining Terms

Common-mode rejection ratio (CMRR): The ratio between the amplitude of a common-mode signal and the amplitude of a differential signal that would produce the same output amplitude or the ratio of the differential gain over the common-mode gain: CMRR $= G_D/G_{CM}$. Expressed in decibels, the common-mode rejection is 20 $\log_{10}$ CMRR. The common-mode rejection is a function of frequency and source-impedance unbalance.

Isolation mode rejection ratio (IMRR): The ratio between the isolation voltage, V_{ISO}, and the amplitude of the isolation signal appearing at the output of the isolation amplifier, or as isolation voltage divided by output voltage V_{out} in the absence of differential and common-mode signal IMRR $= V_{ISO}/V_{out}$.

Operational amplifier (op-amp): A very high gain dc-coupled differential amplifier with single-ended output, high voltage gain, high input impedance, and low output impedance. Due to its high open-loop gain, the characteristics of an op-amp circuit depend only on its feedback network. Therefore, the integrated circuit op-amp is an extremely convenient tool for the realization of linear amplifier circuits [Horowitz & Hill, 1980].

References

AAMI. 1993. AAMI Standards and Recommended Practices, Biomedical Equipment, vol 2, 4th ed, Arlington, Virg.

Burr-Brown Corp. 1994. Burr-Brown Integrated Circuits Data Book, Linear Products, Tucson, Ariz.

Horowitz P, Hill W. 1980. The Art of Electronics, Cambridge Cambridge, University Press.

Hutten H. 1992. Biomedizinische Technik, Berlin, Springer-Verlag.

Pallás-Areny R, Webster JG. 1990. Composite instrumentation amplifier for biopotentials. Ann Biomed Eng 18: 251.

Strong P. 1970. Biophysical Measurements, Beaverton, Ore, Tektronix, Inc.

Webster JG (ed). 1992. Medical Instrumentation, Application and Design, 2d ed, Boston, Houghton Mifflin.

Further Information

Detailed information on the realization of amplifiers for biomedical instrumentation and the availability of commercial products can be found in the references and in the data books and application notes of various manufacturers of integrated circuit amplifiers such as Burr-Brown, Analog Devices, and Precision Monolithics Inc., as well as manufacturers of laboratory equipment such as Gould and Grass.

73

Noninvasive Assessment
of Arterial Blood Pressure
and Mechanics

Gary Drzewiecki
Rutgers University

The beginnings of noninvasive arterial pulse recording can be traced as far back in time as the Renaissance in Poland [Strus, 1555]. At that time the arterial pulse was recognized to possess form. Although instrumentation was simple, early investigators found that changes in the arterial pulse shape and strength could be related to various disease conditions. These altered pulse shapes were associated with the characteristics of various animals. For example, physicians attempted to identify the "snake" or "horse" pulse, each associated with a particular pathology. Today, the instrumentation is more sophisticated, and our knowledge of the physics of the pulse waveform is more detailed, but the method of recording arterial blood pressure remains a fruitful area of research.

In this chapter, the most standard of noninvasive methods for arterial pressure measurements that are employed today will be reviewed, and future trends will be identified. One finds that there are essentially two categories of methods, those that periodically sample the arterial pulse pressure and those that continuously record the pulse waveform. The sampling methods typically provide systolic and diastolic pressure and sometimes mean pressure. These values generally are obtained from different heart beats and over a time span of a half-minute. The continuous recordings methods provide higher resolution of time so that beat-to-beat changes can be monitored in addition to the pulse waveform. Some continuous methods, though, may provide only pulse pressure waveform and timing.

First we will examine some applications for arterial pressure monitoring. The knowledge of systolic and diastolic pressure is particularly important. These values are particularly important not only for evaluating basic cardiovascular function but also to identify the presence of hypertension. High blood pressure is a precursor to many other forms of cardiovascular disease. The monitoring required to study the progression of hypertension, for example, is long term. For this, a conventional noninvasive method that samples blood pressure over the time frame of minutes to months is adequate. The occlusive cuff-based methods of Korotkoff and oscillometry are approaches that fall into this category. These methods have been automated, with recent instruments designed for ambulatory use [Graettinger et al., 1988]. The application of 24- to 48-hour ambulatory monitors have been

0-8493-8346-3/95/$0.00+$.50
© 1995 by CRC Press, Inc.

employed to determine the diurnal variation of a patient's blood pressure. These instruments permit the assessment of the daily mean blood pressure, which may be more valuable in determining the true level of hypertension and the course of treatment. In addition, ambulatory monitoring can alleviate the problem of "white coat hypertension," i.e., the elevation of blood pressure associated with a visit to the physician's office [Pickering et al., 1988].

Short-term hemodynamic information that can be obtained from the noninvasive recording of the arterial pulse waveform is a virtually untapped arena and likely to be the future of blood pressure measurement. Although a great deal of knowledge has been gathered on the physics of the arterial pulse [Noordergraaf, 1978], it has been lacking in application because continuous-pressure waveform monitors have not been available or are deficient in function. A review of methods for continuous pulse monitoring that can potentially fill this gap will be provided.

Some examples of pulse monitoring applications can be found. In the recording time span of less than a minute, the importance of the pressure waveform dominates, as well as beat-to-beat variations in the pulse. This type of monitoring is critical in situations where blood pressure can alter quickly, such as due to trauma or anesthesia. Other applications for acute monitoring have been in aerospace, biofeedback, and lie detection. Moreover, dynamic information becomes available from the pulse, such as the degree of wave reflection [Li, 1986]. Multiple pulse sensors can offer the pulse wave velocity, which is inversely related to arterial compliance. Kelly and coworkers [1989] have shown that elevated systolic pressure can be attributed to pulse waveform changes due to a decrease in arterial compliance and increased wave reflection. Lastly, dynamic information on cardiac control can be obtained from beat-to-beat variation in pulse pressure [Omboni et al., 1993].

Where automatic blood pressure monitoring is available, it has become increasingly popular to provide simultaneous recording of such variables as noninvasive oxygen saturation via pulse oximetry, body temperature, etc. The advances in computer technology improve on this practice, making it a clear trend. While this practice is likely to continue, in the forefront of this approach will be those instruments that provide more than just a mere marriage of technology in a single design. It will be possible to find functional information in addition to just pressure. As an example of this, a method of obtaining the pressure compliance curve of the radial artery using a new type of arterial tonometer will be presented.

73.1 Long-Term Sampling Methods

Vascular Unloading Principle

The vascular unloading principle is fundamental to all occlusive cuff-based methods of determining arterial blood pressure. Vascular unloading is performed by applying an external compression pressure or force to a limb such that the pressure is transmitted to the underlying vessels. It is usually assumed that the external pressure and the pressure (stress) deep within the tissues are in equilibrium. The underlying vessels are then subjected to an altered transmural pressure (internal minus external pressure). It is further assumed [Marey, 1885] that the tension within the wall of the vessel is zero when transmural pressure is zero. Hence, the term *vascular unloading* originated.

Various techniques have been developed that attempt to detect vascular unloading. These techniques generally rely on the fact that once a vessel is unloaded, further external pressure will cause it to collapse. In summary,

$$\text{If } P_a > P_c \rightarrow \text{lumen open}$$

$$\text{or if } P_a < P_c \rightarrow \text{lumen closed}$$

where P_a is the arterial pressure and P_c is the cuff pressure. Most methods that employ the occlusive arm cuff rely on this principle and differ in the means of detecting whether the artery is open or closed. Briefly, some of these techniques are skin flush, palpatory, Korotkoff (auscultatory), oscillometric, and ultrasound [Drzewiecki et al., 1987]. Of these, the methods of Korotkoff and oscillometry currently are in most common use and will be reviewed here.

Occlusive Cuff Mechanics

Before examining specific blood-pressure-measurement methods, it is useful to consider the mechanical properties of the occlusive arm cuff that is so widely employed. The current version of cuff is designed to encircle the upper arm. The cuff consists of a flat rubber bladder with air supply tubing. The bladder is covered by a cloth material with Velcro fasteners at either end for easy placement and removal. While the cuff encircles the entire arm, the internal bladder extends over approximately half the circumference. The bladder is pressurized with air derived from a hand pump, release valve, and manometer combination.

An important property of the cuff is its ability to accurately transmit pressure down to the tissue surrounding the brachial artery. A mechanical analysis [Alexander et al., 1977] revealed that the length of the cuff is required to be a specific fraction of the arm's circumference for pressure equilibrium. A narrow cuff relative to the arm size resulted in the greatest error in pressure transmission and, thus, the greatest error in blood pressure determination. Geddes and Whistler [1978] have examined experimentally the effect of cuff size on blood pressure accuracy for the Korotkoff method. Their results suggest also that a cuff-width-to-arm-circumference ratio of 0.4 be maintained. Cuff manufacturers, therefore, supply a range of cuff sizes appropriate for pediatric use up to large adults.

Another mechanical aspect of the cuff is its pressure response due to either internal air volume change or that of the limb that it encircles. In this sense, the cuff can be thought of as a plethysmograph. The mechanics of the occlusive arm cuff was analyzed by Drzewiecki and coworkers [1993]. The cuff can be examined by considering its pressure-volume characteristics without attention to the details of cuff shape. In an experiment, the cuff properties were isolated from those of the arm by applying the cuff to a rigid cylinder of similar diameter. The pressure-volume curve was then obtained by injecting a known volume of air and noting the pressure. This was performed for a standard bladder cuff (13-cm width) over a typical range of blood pressures.

The cuff pressure-volume data for pressures less than 130 mmHg are nonlinear (Fig. 73.1). For pressures above 130 mmHg, the data asymptotically approach a linear relationship with volume. This implies that the cuff sensitivity to volume change in the arm increases with cuff pressure. In the high range of cuff pressure, the cuff responds with nearly constant sensitivity. This can be seen from the derivative of pressure with respect to volume (Fig. 73.1). Hence, throughout most of the range of blood pressure measurement, the cuff behaves as a nonlinear transducer.

A theory and model of the cuff mechanics has been developed to explain the above cuff experiment [Drzewiecki et al., 1993]. Cuff function consists of two mechanical components. The first is that of the compressibility of air within the cuff and connection tubes. This can be modeled by Boyle's gas law. The second component is that of elastic stretch and shape deformation of the cuff bladder. Since the inside surface of the cuff is constrained by the arm, most of the cuff deformation is due to the outside layer. Cuff shape deformation proceeds until the bladder reaches its final geometry, rendering a nonlinear pressure-volume curve. Then, elastic stretch of the rubber bladder takes over, resulting in a nearly linear function found in the high range of cuff pressures. Solutions for this model are shown to represent the data well in Fig. 73.1 (solid curves) for two cuffs: a standard bladder cuff and the Critikon Dura-cuf. This model is useful in linearizing the cuff for use as a plethysmograph and in understanding oscillometry.

Method of Korotkoff

The auscultatory method or method of Korotkoff was introduced by the Russian army physician N. Korotkoff in 1905. In experiments, Korotkoff discovered that sound was present distal to a partially

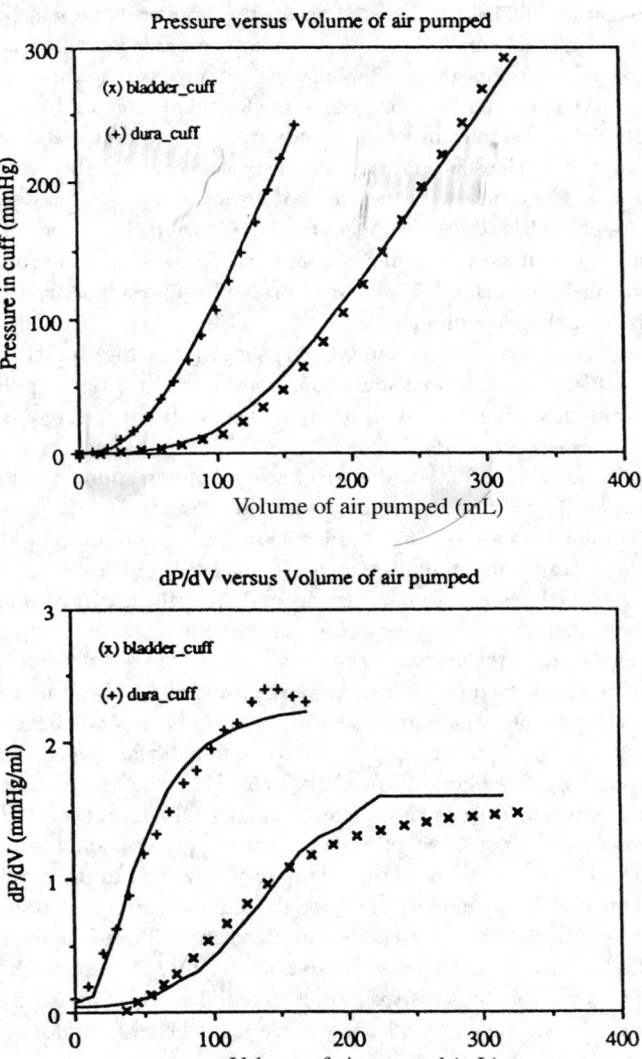

FIGURE 73.1 *Top:* Pressure-volume data obtained from two different occlusive arm cuffs. Inner surface of the cuff in this case to isolate cuff mechanics from that of the arm. *Bottom:* Derivative of the cuff pressure with respect to volume obtained from pressure-volume data of both cuffs. These curves indicate the pressure response of the cuff to volume change and are useful for plethysmography. Solid curves in both figures are the results of the occlusive cuff model.

occluded limb. He realized that this sound was indicative of arterial flow and together with the occlusive cuff could be used to determine blood pressure. The method, as employed today, utilizes a stethoscope placed distal to an arm cuff over the brachial artery at the antecubital fossa. The cuff is inflated to 20–30 mmHg above systolic pressure and then allowed to deflate at a rate of 2–3 mmHg/s. One finds that sound becomes audible coincidently with systolic pressure. These initial "tapping" sounds are referred to as Phase I sound. With falling pressure, the sounds increase in intensity for

Phase II. The maximum intensity is Phase III, where the tapping sound may be followed by a brief murmur due to turbulence. Finally, Phase IV Korotkoff sound is identified as muffled sound and Phase V as the complete disappearance. Phase IV is generally taken to indicate when cuff pressure equals diastolic arterial pressure. The long use of the Korotkoff method has allowed much experimental information. For example, the frequency spectrum of sound, spatial variation along the arm, filtering effects, and timing have been reviewed [Drzewiecki et al., 1989].

It is a long-held misconception that the origin of the Korotkoff sound is due to flow turbulence. Turbulence is thought to be induced by the narrowing of the brachial artery that takes place under an occlusive cuff. There are some arguments against this idea. First, the Korotkoff sound does not sound like turbulence or a murmur. Second, the Korotkoff sound still occurs in low-blood-flow situations. And, last, Doppler ultrasound indicates that peak flow occurs following the time occurrence of Korotkoff sound. A more recent alternative theory suggests that the sound is due to nonlinear distortion of the brachial pulse, such that sound is introduced to the original pulse. This is shown to arise from flow limitation under the cuff in addition to curvilinear pressure-area relationship of the brachial artery [Drzewiecki et al., 1989].

The accuracy of the Korotkoff method is well known. London and London [1967], among others, find that the Korotkoff method routinely underestimates systolic pressure by 5–20 mmHg and overestimates diastolic pressure by 12–20 mmHg. However, certain subject groups, such as hypertensives or the elderly, can compound these errors [Spence et al., 1978]. In addition to this, the arm blood flow can alter the Korotkoff sound intensity and, thus, the accuracy of blood pressure measurement [Rabbany et al., 1993]. Disappearance of Korotkoff sound occurs near Phase III in some subjects and is referred to as the *auscultatory gap*, which can lead to an erroneous indication of diastolic pressure. Errors due to auscultatory gap can be avoided simply by allowing cuff pressure to continue to fall below the gap, where sounds return. A final Phase IV will be present to indicate the true diastolic pressure. This is particularly critical for automatic instruments to take into account. In spite of these errors, the method of Korotkoff is considered an appropriate noninvasive blood pressure reference by which other methods may be evaluated [White et al., 1993].

The conventional site for the Korotkoff method is the upper arm and brachial artery, since it is close to the heart. Thus, the pressures recorded are relatively close to the central arterial or aortic pressures, which are of primary interest. However, the temporal artery has been employed recently [Shenoy et al., 1993]. In this case, a pressure capsule is applied over the temporal artery on the head in place of an occlusive cuff, to provide external pressure. This approach has been shown to be accurate and is applicable to aerospace. Pilots' cerebral vascular pressure often falls in high-acceleration maneuvers, so that temporal artery pressure is a better indicator of this response.

Oscillometry

Oscillometric measurement of blood pressure predates the method of Korotkoff with its introduction by the French physiologist Marey [1885]. In experiments where he placed the arm within a compression chamber, Marey observed that the chamber pressure would fluctuate with the pulse. He also noted that amount of pulsation varied with pressure. Marey believed that the maximum pulsations or the onset of pulsations were associated with equality of blood pressure and chamber pressure. It was not known at that time to what levels of arterial pressure the pulsations correspond. Recently, it has been demonstrated theoretically that the variation in cuff pressure is related to the arterial compliance-pressure curve of the brachial artery [Drzewiecki et al., 1994].

Today, oscillometry is performed using a standard arm cuff. It is only necessary to couple a pressure transducer in line with the cuff tubing to record cuff pressure. Due to the requirement of a pressure sensor, oscillometry is generally not performed manually but is measured with automatic blood pressure instruments. The recorded cuff pressure is then high-pass-filtered above 1 Hz to observe the pulsatile oscillations in cuff pressure (Fig. 73.2). It was determined only recently that the maximum oscillations actually correspond with cuff pressure equal to mean arterial pressure (MAP)

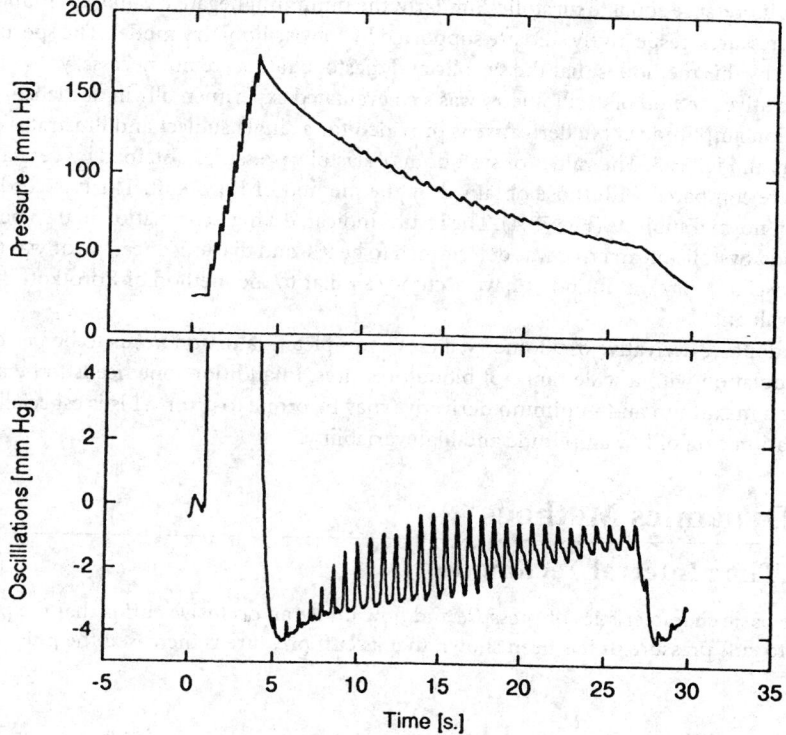

FIGURE 73.2 Sample recording of the cuff pressure during oscillometric blood pressure measurement. Bottom panel shows oscillations in cuff pressure obtained by high-pass filtering above 1/2 Hz.

[Posey et al., 1969; Ramsey, 1979], and the onset of oscillation occurs at a cuff pressure well above systolic pressure, negating Marey's early assumption. It was determined, though, that systolic pressure could be identified when the oscillations, O_s, are a fixed percentage of the maximum oscillations, O_m [Geddes et al., 1983]. In comparisons with the intraarterial pressure recordings, the systolic detection ratio $O_s/O_m = 0.55$. Similarly, the diastolic pressure can be found as a fixed percentage of the maximum oscillations, as $O_d/O_m = 0.85$.

Derivative Oscillometry

Although the above study of the systolic/diastolic detection ratios is not exhaustive, further research can be performed to test their accuracy under different conditions. Most work indicates that the determination of MAP is more accurate than systolic and diastolic levels, since it can be obtained directly from the oscillation amplitude maximum. It is therefore limited by the ability of properly identifying the true maximum from data and experimental error. The systolic and diastolic detection ratio, alternatively, have been determined empirically from a population of subjects. An alternate means was suggested by Link [1987], who employs the oscillation amplitude curve. The derivative of the oscillation amplitude curve with respect to cuff pressure can be applied to Fig. 73.2. When the derivative is plotted against cuff pressure, MAP can be easily identified as the point where the derivative is zero. It can also be seen that the derivative reaches a maximum positive value. This occurs at cuff pressure equal to diastolic. Similarly, the minimum negative value was found to occur at systolic pressures, respectively, and are supported by the oscillometry model. The specific advantage offered by this method is that the systolic and diastolic ratios are not necessary.

The derivative method of oscillometry was also evaluated experimentally in our lab. A sample of the oscillation amplitude curve derivative is provided for a single subject and illustrates derivative oscillometry in Fig. 73.3. The values of systolic and diastolic pressures obtained by derivative oscillometry were compared with those obtained by the method of Korotkoff. Thirty recordings were obtained on normal subjects (Fig. 73.4). The results indicated a high correlation of 0.93 between the two methods. Systolic mean error was determined to be 9% and diastolic mean error was 6%. Thus, derivative oscillometry was found to have accuracy similar to the method of Korotkoff in this preliminary evaluation.

Before adopting derivative oscillometry, a more complete evaluation needs to be performed for subject population with a wide range of blood pressures. In addition, one needs to be aware that identifying a maximum and minimum derivative may be prone to error. This is especially the case with oscillation data of low amplitude and high variability.

73.2 Pulse Dynamics Methods

R-wave Time Interval Technique

One of the basic characteristics of pressure and flow under an occlusive cuff is that the pulse is delayed due to cuff pressure. It has been shown that as cuff pressure is increased the pulse is increas-

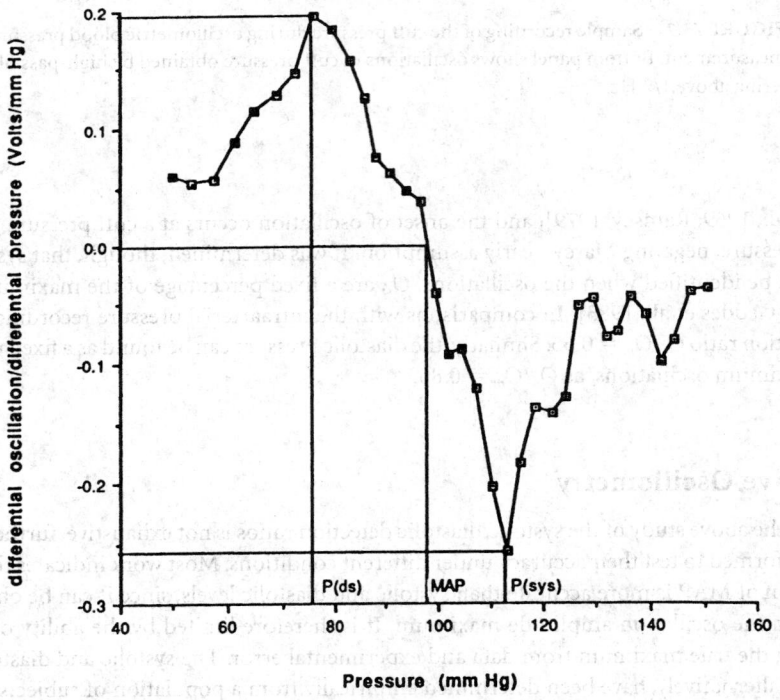

FIGURE 73.3   Method of derivative oscillometry. The derivative of cuff pressure oscillations data with respect to cuff pressure is shown from a single subject. The maximum and minimum values denote diastolic and systolic pressure, respectively. A zero derivative MAP in this plot.

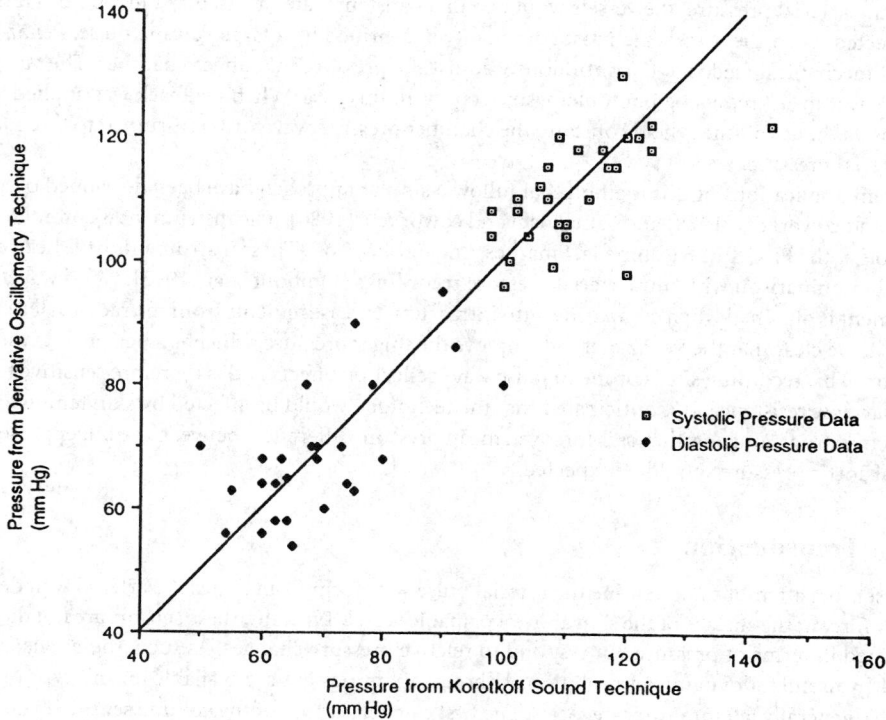

FIGURE 73.4 Experimental evaluation of derivative oscillometry using systolic and diastolic pressure from the method of Korotkoff as reference. The line indicates the result of linear regression to the data.

ingly delayed relative to the cardiac cycle. The *R*-wave of the ECG is often employed as a time reference. Arzbaecher and Novotney [1973] measured the time delay of the Korotkoff sound relative to the *R*-wave. They suggested that the curve obtained by plotting the cuff pressure versus time delay represents the rising portion of the arterial pulse waveform.

A Korotkoff sound model [Drzewiecki et al., 1989] was employed to investigate the cuff delay effect. Time delay of the Korotkoff sound was computed relative to the proximal arterial pulse. Since the arterial pulse waveform was known in this calculation, the pressure-*RK* interval curve can be compared directly. The resemblance to a rising arterial pulse was apparent, but some deviation was noted, particularly in the early portion of the *RK* interval curve. The model indicates that the pulse occurs earlier and with higher derivative than the true pulse waveform. Thus, the model does not completely support this method and indicates it to be, at best, an approximation of the pressure waveform. In particular, the increased derivative that occurs at the foot of the pulse would mislead any study of wave propagation.

Recently, Sharir and coworkers [1993] have performed comparisons of Doppler flow pulse delay and direct arterial pressure recordings. Their results confirm a consistent elevation in pulse compared with intraarterial recording in the early portions of the wave. The average deviation, though, was 10 mmHg. Hence, if waveform accuracy is not important, this method can provide a reasonable measurement of the rising arterial pulse.

Continuous Vascular Unloading

The principle of vascular unloading was discussed relative to occlusive cuff-based measurement of blood pressure. Penaz [1973] reasoned that if the cuff pressure could be continuously altered to equal the arterial pressure, the vessels would be in a constant state of vascular unloading. This can be detected when the vessels are most compliant as identified by a large volume pulse. Penaz employed mechanical feedback to continuously adjust the pressure in a finger chamber. The vascular volume was measured using photoplethysmography, in this case. When feedback was applied such that the vascular volume is held constant, the chamber pressure waveform is assumed to be equal to the arterial pressure.

Recent applications of this method that follow a similar approach have been developed by Wesseling and coworkers [1978] and Yamakoshi and coworkers [1980]. The instrument is commercially available as the FINAPRES (Ohmeda, Finapres, Englewood, Co.). These instruments have been evaluated by comparison with intraarterial pressure recordings [Omboni et al., 1993]. Good waveform agreement is obtained when comparing with intraarterial measurements from the radial artery. But, it should be clear that the Penaz method employs the finger pressure, which is a peripheral vascular location. This recording site is prone to pulse wave reflection effects and is therefore sensitive to the vascular flow resistance. It is anticipated that the technique would be affected by skin temperature, vasoactive drugs, and anesthetics. Moreover, mean pressure differences between the finger pulse and central aortic pressure should be expected.

Pulse Transduction

Pulse sensors attempt to determine the arterial pulse waveform from either the arterial wall deflection or force at the surface of the skin above a palpable vessel. Typically, these sensors are not directly calibrated in terms of pressure but respond to relative pressure changes. As such, these sensors are primarily useful for dynamic information. Although many designs are available for this type of sensor, they generally fall into two categories. The first category is that of the volume sensor (Fig. 73.5). This type of sensor relies on the adjacent tissues surrounding the vessel as a nondeflecting frame of reference. Skin deflections directly above the vessel are then measured relative to a reference frame to represent the arterial pressure. Several different transduction methods may be employed, including capacitive, resistive, inductive, and optical. Ideally, this type of sensor minimally restricts the motion of the skin so that contact force is zero.

The drawback to pulse volume sensing is that the method responds to volume distention and not pressure. Ideally, if the vessel deflects in a linear elastic manner, as a spring, this would not matter. But, the nonlinear and viscoelastic nature of vascular walls results in complex waveform alterations that are difficult to correct in practice. Hence, unless the application is to measure arterial pulse volume, the recordings produced by this class of sensor should not be equated with arterial pressure. The pulse oximeter is used also to provide pulse waveforms in addition to oxygen saturation. This device is a volume sensor and suffers from its inherent problems.

The second category is that of the pressure pulse sensor (Fig. 73.5). This type of sensor depends on part of or all the stress due to arterial pressure to be transmitted through the skin. In this case, force or stress is measured in contact with the skin above the pulse artery. The pressure pulse sen-

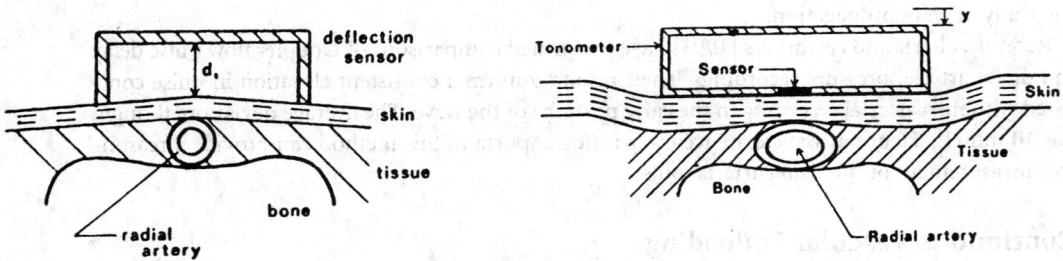

FIGURE 73.5   *Left:* Illustration of volume pulse method. *Right:* Illustration of pressure pulse method and arterial tonometry.

sor requires that surface deflections are zero, as opposed to the volume sensor. Thus, the contact forces are proportionate to arterial pressure at the skin surface. Tonometry, which will be presented later, is a technique by which the contact force can be calibrated.

The differences in pulse waveforms that are provided by the above pulse recording techniques are clear when compared with intraarterial recordings [Van der Hoeven & Beneken, 1970]. In all cases, the pressure pulse method was found to provide superior waveform accuracy, free of the effects of vessel wall nonlinear viscoelasticity. Lastly, it should be noted that various pulse sensors are available commercially that are not designed with particular emphasis on either the volume or pressure pulse concepts. The stiffness of the sensor can then characterize its performance. High stiffness relative to the artery and surrounding tissue is required to best approximate the pressure pulse method.

Motion Artifact Rejection

Arterial pulse recording is typically performed while the subject is stationary and refrains from moving the pulse location. But, it has become of increased interest to record the arterial pressure while the subject is ambulatory. With no subject restraint, pulse recording is quite difficult due to motion artifact. For example, motion of the hand or even a finger can appear in recordings of the radial artery. In addition, the positioning and application force can alter, resulting in another type of artifact. Such motion artifacts are often comparable in magnitude to that of the pulse, making ambulatory recordings impractical. Recently, though, artifact rejection techniques have been applied with good success.

Artifact rejection techniques can eliminate motion artifact from pulse recordings when the motion artifact is common to the entire sensor contact surface. In principle, this is analogous to noise cancellation of common mode signals. Common-mode motion artifact can be found by employing multiple sensors across the pulse artery location. Consider the case of two sensors. One sensor, S_p, is positioned above an artery. It then records pulse and tissue compression force. An adjacent sensor, S_m, is positioned nearby but away from the artery. It records only tissue compression force. If motion artifact affects only the amount of tissue compression, then the compression forces measured by the adjacent sensor can be subtracted from the pulse sensor. Mathematically, this is performed as follows:

$$P = S_p - AS_m - B \qquad (73.1)$$

where the factor A allows sensitivity differences between the two sensors to be corrected. The constant B is determined such that the steady value of contact force is eliminated. This allows the pulse to maintain a constant zero average. In practice, the values of A and B are altered adaptively in real time [Drzewiecki et al., 1992]. Algorithms that continuously monitor the mean squared value of the sensor difference signal attempt to adjust A and B for a minimum average difference. An example of automatic artifact cancellation is provided in Fig. 73.6. Statistical evaluation [Ciaccio et al., 1989] revealed that adaptive cancellation provides the best overall ability to reject motion artifact. More advanced methods may be applied in extension of this concept, but the simplest form of application of Eq. (73.1) is superior to other approaches that were evaluated. Most likely this is because the artifact is unknown and cannot be easily characterized.

Arterial Tonometry

Concept and Application

Whereas the pressure pulse method was shown to possess excellent pulse-recording characteristics, it is deficient in the ability to provide pressure calibration. The method of arterial tonometry [Pressman & Newgard, 1963] was introduced to noninvasively record the pressure in superficial arteries with sufficient bony support, such as the radial artery, and to provide direct pressure calibration.

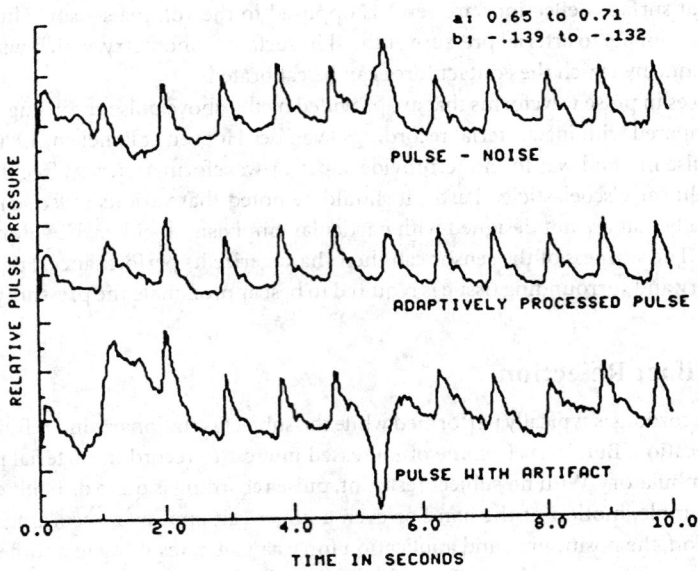

a: 0.65 to 0.71
b: -.139 to -.132

FIGURE 73.6 Sample tonometer records of pulse with motion artifact. Simple subtraction and adaptive cancellation of artifact is applied to the pulse recording. Adaptive processing provides best restoration of the waveform, with simple subtraction offering some improvement.

A tonometer is applied by first centering the sensor area over the vessel. This is accomplished by repositioning the device until the largest pulse is detected. More recent designs employ the use of an array of sensors [Weaver et al., 1978] to accomplish this electronically. Once the vessel is located, the tonometer is depressed toward the vessel. This leads to applanation of the vessel wall (Fig. 73.5). If the vessel is not flattened sufficiently, the tonometer measures a force due to arterial wall tension and bending of the vessel. As depression is continued, the arterial wall is applanated further beneath the sensor area, but not so much as to occlude blood flow. At this position, wall tension is now parallel to the tonometer surface, but arterial pressure is perpendicular to the surface and is the only stress detected by the tonometer sensor. This is termed *contact stress*. Ideally, the sensor does not measure skin shear or frictional stresses. The contact stress is then equal in magnitude to the arterial pressure, and calibration is achieved. The details of arterial tonometer calibration and design were investigated further by Drzewiecki and coworkers [1983, 1987, 1992]. In summary, tonometry requires that the contact stress sensor be flat, stiffer than the vessel and skin system, and small relative to the vessel diameter. Proper calibration can be attained either by monitoring the contact stress distribution or the maximum in measured pulse amplitude.

Recent research in tonometry has focused on miniaturization of semiconductor pressure sensor arrays [Weaver et al., 1978]. Alternatively, electro-optical techniques and fiber optics have been employed by Drzewiecki [1985] and Moubarak and colleagues [1989], allowing extreme size reduction of the contact stress sensor. Commercial technology, though, has been available (Jentow, Colin Electronics, Japan) and evaluated against intraarterial records. Results indicate an average error of −5.6 mmHg for systolic pressure and −2.4 mmHg for diastole. In general, excellent pulse waveform quality was afforded by tonometry [Sato et al., 1993], making it a superior method for noninvasive pulse dynamics applications.

Flexible Diaphragm Tonometer

As an alternative to the high-resolution tonometers under development, a new low-resolution technology is introduced here. The basic advantage becomes one of cost, ease of positioning, and patient comfort, critical for long-term applications. In addition, although most tonometers have employed only the radial artery of the wrist for measurement, this technology is suitable for other superficial vessels and conforms to skin surface irregularities.

The basic principle that will be employed in the flexible tonometer design is that tissue is incompressible in the short term [Bansal et al., 1994]. The tonometer will be made an extension of the tissue by filling it with a similarly incompressible fluid and coupled to the skin by means of a flexible diaphragm. This deviates from previous tonometers that require a rigid and flat surface. Instead, the requirement becomes one of regions of constant volume rather than constant skin deflection. This permits a low-resolution design, thereby relaxing the technology requirements.

The flexible diaphragm tonometer concept is shown in Fig. 73.7 with three volume compartments. These compartments are not physically separated, and fluid can move between them. When the arterial pressure exceeds that in the tonometer, the volume of the artery expands into V_b. Note also, that V_a and V_c must increase to take up this expansion, since water is incompressible. To restore the tonometer to a flat surface, the total volume of the tonometer is increased (Fig. 73.7). In response, the tonometer pressure increases, and the artery flattens. At this point, the volume in each compartment is equal, the tonometer surface is flat, and tonometric calibration is achieved so that the tonometer pressure is equal to arterial pressure. Thus, by maintaining the volume compartments equal, applanation tonometry can be accomplished with a flexible diaphragm rather than a rigid one. In practice, instrumentation continuously adjusts the tonometer volume in order to maintain compartment volume equal as arterial pressure changes.

The flexible diaphragm tonometer was machined from plexiglass for light weight (Fig. 73.8). A rectangular channel was created to contain saline. The front of the tonometer was covered with a sheet of 0.004-in. polyurethane. A water tight seal was obtained using a plexiglass ring and gasket arrangement. Two stainless steel electrodes were placed at each end of the channel. These were used for injecting a current through the length of the tonometer channel. Near the center of the channel, four volume-measuring electrodes were placed at equal spacing. Each pair of electrodes defines a volume compartment, and the voltage across each pair was calibrated in terms of volume using impedance plethysmography. External to the tonometer, a catheter was used to connect the saline channel to an electromechanical volume pump.

Several heart beats of tonometer data were plotted from the volume pulse recordings of the flexible tonometer (Fig. 73.9). Two channels are graphed simultaneously. The pulse volume is shown as a volume deviation from the mean compartment volume. Each record depicts a constant average tonometer pressure and volume. It is apparent that the volume compartments are coupled. In par-

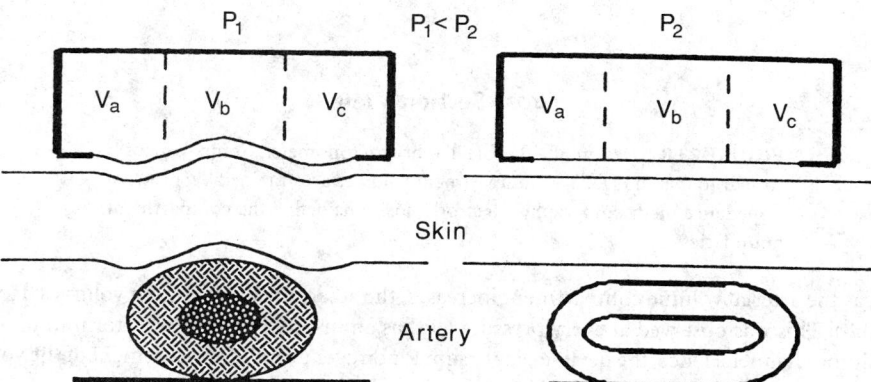

FIGURE 73.7 Concept of flexible diaphragm tonometry. P_1 illustrates inappropriate level of pressure to provide arterial applanation tonometry. P_2 indicates an increase in chamber volume so that the relative compartment volumes, V, are equal. In practice, relative compartment volumes are maintained constant via feedback control, and applanation is continuous. Compartment pressure equals arterial pressure in P_2.

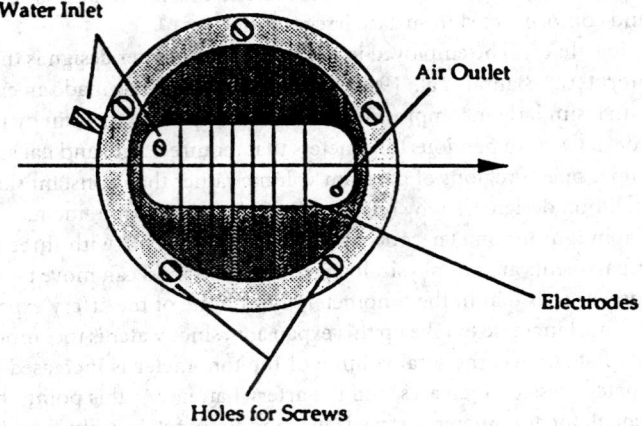

Bottom View

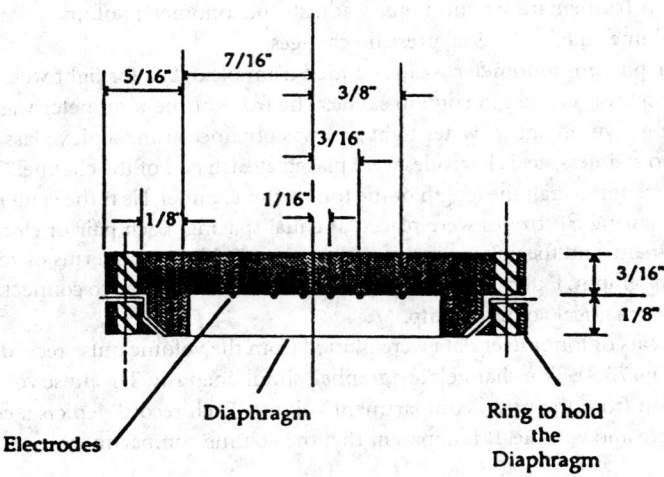

Cross-Section View

FIGURE 73.8 Design of a flexible diaphragm tonometer. Compartment is similar to that in Fig. 73.7. Compartment volumes are obtained by means of impedance plethysmography. Electrode positions define the compartment boundaries.

ticular, as the arterial volume compartment increases, the adjacent compartment volumes decrease (Fig. 73.7). This was observed at every pressure level as an inverted volume waveform in the adjacent volume channel. Hence, the flexible diaphragm tonometer permits measurement of the volume and pressure pulse to be determined at any external applanation pressure.

Arterial Compliance Measurement

The arterial compliance was also obtained using the flexible tonometer. The change in volume was assumed to be the pulse volume. The change in pressure was assumed to be a constant pulse pres-

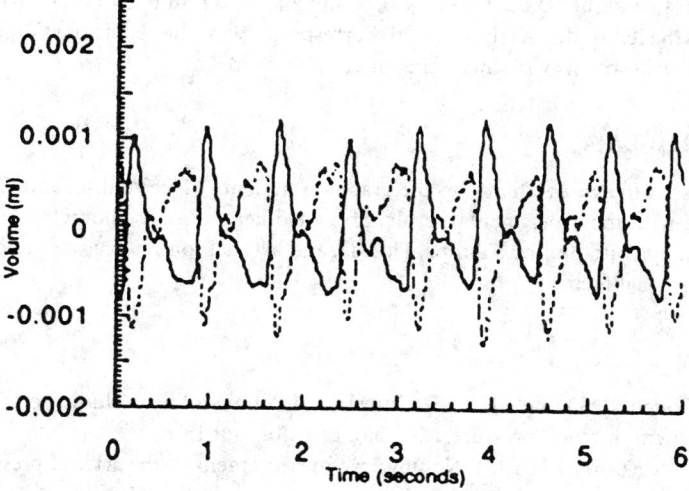

FIGURE 73.9 Sample of radial arterial volume recording from tonometer of Fig. 73.8. Chamber pressure was fixed at 25 mm Hg. Calibrated volume change from mean compartment volume is shown. Solid curve corresponds with V_b of Fig. 73.7, the dashed curve with V_a. Since the volume compartments are fluid-coupled, the side pulse is inverted. This relationship permits lower resolution to be employed as opposed to conventional rigid tonometry.

sure obtained from the systolic minus the diastolic pressure. Then, by definition, the compliance is obtained from the ratio of change in volume to change in pressure. The arterial compliance was found to alter depending on the tonometer pressure (Fig. 73.10). Compliance values were in the range expected for humans. A typical human adult radial artery compliance value is 8.3×10^{-6}

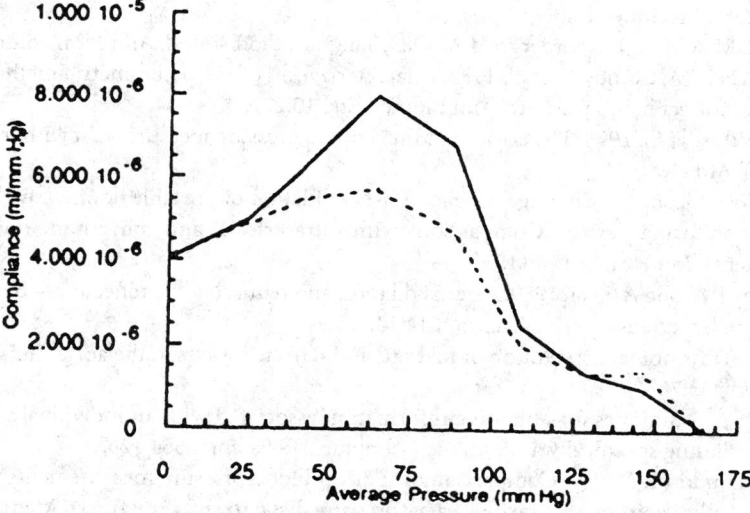

FIGURE 73.10 Arterial compliance obtained noninvasively from the flexible tonometer applied to the radial artery. Pressure is the average tonometer pressure.

mL/mm Hg/cm [Westerhof et al., 1969]. Also, compliance was found to decrease with the tonometer pressure, to the left of the maximum. This corresponds with the classic physiologic observation that the arterial wall stiffens with increasing internal pressure.

Acknowledgments

The author wishes to express thanks to the graduate students Vineet Bansal and Cindy Jacobs for their assistance with the experimental results presented here. Also, oscillometry studies were supported, in part, by Critikon, Inc., Tampa, Florida, and arterial tonometry was supported by IVAC Corp., San Diego, California.

References

Alexander H, Cohen M, Steinfeld L. 1977. Criteria in the choice of an occluding cuff for the indirect measurement of blood pressure. Med Biol Eng Comput 15:2.

Arzbaecher RC, Novotney RL. 1973. Noninvasive measurement of the arterial pressure contour in man. Bibl Cardiol 31:63.

Bansal V, Drzewiecki G, Butterfield R. 1994. Design of a flexible diaphragm tonometer. Thirteenth S Biomed Eng Conf pp 148–151.

Ciaccio EJ, Drzewiecki GM, Karam E. 1989. Algorithm for reduction of mechanical noise in arterial pulse recording with tonometry. Proc 15th Northeast Bioeng Conf pp 161–162.

Drzewiecki GM. 1985. The Origin of the Korotkoff Sound and Arterial Tonometry. Ph.D. thesis. University of Pennsylvania, Philadelphia.

Drzewiecki GM, Butterfield RD, Ciaccio EJ. 1992. Pulse waveform monitor. US Patent 5,154,680.

Drzewiecki G, Hood R, Apple H. 1994. Theory of the oscillometric maximum and the systolic and diastolic detection ratios. Ann Biomed Eng 22:88.

Drzewiecki GM, Karam E, Bansal V, et al. 1993. Mechanics of the occlusive arm cuff and its application as a volume sensor. IEEE Trans Biomed Eng 40:704.

Drzewiecki GM, Melbin J, Noordergraaf A. 1983. Arterial tonometry: Review and analysis. J Biomech 16:141.

Drzewiecki GM, Melbin J, Noordergraaf A. 1987. Noninvasive blood pressure recording and the genesis of Korotkoff sound. In S Chien, R Skalak (eds), Handbook of Bioengineering, pp 8.1–8.36, New York, McGraw-Hill.

Drzewiecki GM, Melbin J, Noordergraaf A. 1989. The Korotkoff sound. Ann Biomed Eng 17:325.

Geddes LA, Voelz M, Combs C, et al. 1983. Characterization of the oscillometric method for measuring indirect blood pressure. Ann Biomed Eng 10:271.

Geddes LA, Whistler SJ. 1978. The error in indirect blood pressure measurement with incorrect size of cuff. Am Heart J 96:4.

Graettinger WF, Lipson JL, Cheung DG, et al. 1988. Validation of portable noninvasive blood pressure monitoring devices: Comparisons with intra-arterial and sphygmomanometer measurements. Am Heart J 116:1155.

Kelly R, Daley J, Avolio A, et al. 1989. Arterial dilation and reduced wave reflection—benefit of Dilevalol in hypertension. Hypertension 14:14.

Li JK-J. 1986. Time domain resolution of forward and reflected waves in the aorta. IEEE Trans Biomed Eng 33:783.

Link WT. 1987. Techniques for obtaining information associated with an individual's blood pressure including specifically a stat mode technique. US Patent 4,664,126.

London SB, London RE. 1967. Comparison of indirect blood pressure measurements (Korotkoff) with simultaneous direct brachial artery pressure distal to cuff. Adv Intern Med 13:127.

Marey EJ. 1885. La Methode Graphique dans les Sciences Experimentales et Principalement en Physiologie et en Medicine. Paris, Masson.

Maurer A, Noordergraaf A. 1976. Korotkoff sound filtering for automated three-phase measurement of blood pressure. Am Heart J 91:584.

Moubarak IF, Drzewiecki GM, Kedem J. 1989. Semi-invasive fiber-optic tonometer. Proc 15th Northeast Bioeng Conf pp 167–168.

Noordergraaf A. 1978. Circulatory System Dynamics, New York, Academic Press.

Omboni S, Parati G, Frattol A, et al. 1993. Spectral and sequence analysis of finger blood pressure variability: Comparison with analysis of intra-arterial recordings. Hypertension 22:26.

Penaz J. 1973. Photoelectric measurement of blood pressure, volume, and flow in the finger. Dig 10th Intl Conf Med Eng 104.

Pickering T, James G, Boddie C, et al. 1988. How common is white coat hypertension? JAMA 259:225.

Posey JA, Geddes LA, Williams H, et al. 1969. The meaning of the point of maximum oscillations in cuff pressure in the indirect measurement of blood pressure: Part 1. Cardiovasc Res Cent Bull 8:15.

Pressman GL, Newgard PM. 1963. A transducer for the continuous external measurement of arterial blood pressure. IEEE Trans Biomed Eng 10:73.

Rabbany SY, Drzewiecki GM, Noordergraaf A. 1993. Peripheral vascular effects on auscultatory blood pressure measurement. J Clin Monitor 9:9.

Ramsey M, III. 1979. Noninvasive blood pressure determination of mean arterial pressure. Med Biol Eng Comp 17:11.

Sato T, Nishinaga M, Kawamoto A, et al. 1993. Accuracy of a continuous blood pressure monitor based on arterial tonometry. Hypertension 21:866.

Sharir T, Marmor A, Ting C-T, et al. 1993. Validation of a method for noninvasive measurement of central arterial pressure. Hypertension 21:74.

Shenoy D, von Maltzahn WW, Buckley JC. 1993. Noninvasive blood pressure measurement on the temporal artery using the auscultatory method. Ann Biomed Eng 21:351.

Spence JD, Sibbald WJ, Cape RD. 1978. Pseuodohypertension in the elderly. Clin Sci Mol Med 55:399s.

Strus J. 1555. Sphygmicae artis jam mille ducentos annos peritae et desideratae. Libri V a Josephi Struthio Posnanience, medico recens conscripti, Basel.

Van der Hoeven, GMA, Beneken JEW. 1970. A reliable transducer for the recording of the arterial pulse wave: Progress report 2. Inst Med Physics. TNO, Utrecht.

Weaver CS, Eckerle JS, Newgard PM, et al. 1978. A study of noninvasive blood pressure measurement technique in noninvasive cardiovascular measurements. Soc Photo-optical Instr Eng 167:89.

Wesseling KH, de Wit B, Snoeck B, et al. 1978. An implementation of the Penaz method for measuring arterial blood pressure in the finger and the first results of an evaluation: Progress Report 6. Inst Med Phys TNO, Utrecht.

Westerhof N, Bosman F, DeVries CJ, et al. 1969. Analog studies of the human systemic arterial tree. J Biomech 2:121.

White WW, Berson AS, Robbins C, et al. 1993. National standard for measurement of resting and ambulatory blood pressures with automated sphygmomanometers. Hypertension 21:504.

Yamakoshi K, Shimazu H, Togawa T. 1980. Indirect measurement of instantaneous arterial blood pressure in the human finger by the vascular unloading technique. IEEE Trans Biomed Eng 27:150.

74

Cardiac Output Measurement

Leslie A. Geddes
Purdue University

Cardiac output is the amount of blood pumped by the right or left ventricle per unit time. It is expressed in liters per minute (L/min) and normalized by division by body surface area in square meters (m²). The resulting quantity is called the cardiac index. Cardiac output is sometimes normalized to body weight, being expressed as mL/min per kilogram. A typical resting value for a wide variety of mammals is 70 mL/min per kg.

With exercise, cardiac output increases. In well-trained athletes, cardiac output can increase five-fold with maximum exercise. During exercise, heart rate increases, venous return increases, and the ejection fraction increases. Parenthetically, physically fit subjects have a low resting heart rate, and the time for the heart rate to return to the resting value after exercise is less than that for subjects who are not physically fit.

There are many direct and indirect (noninvasive) methods of measuring cardiac output. Of equal importance to the number that represents cardiac output is the left-ventricular ejection fraction (stroke volume divided by diastolic volume), which indicates the ability of the left ventricle to pump blood.

74.1 Indicator-Dilution Method

The principle underlying the indicator-dilution method is based on the upstream injection of a detectable indicator and on measuring the downstream concentration-time curve, which is called a *dilution curve*. The essential requirement is that the indicator mixes with all the blood flowing through the central mixing pool. Although the dilution curves in the outlet branches may be slightly different in shape, they all have the same area.

Figure 74.1a illustrates the injection of *m* g of indicator into an idealized flowing stream having the same velocity across the diameter of the tube. Figure 74.1b shows the dilution curve recorded downstream. Because of the flow-velocity profile, the cylinder of indicator and fluid becomes teardrop in shape, as shown in Fig. 74.1c. The resulting dilution curve has a rapid rise and an exponential fall, as shown in Fig. 74.1d. However, the area of the dilution curve is the same as that shown in Fig. 74.1a. Derivation of the flow equation is shown in Fig. 74.1, and the flow is simply the amount of indicator (*m* gm) divided by the area of the dilution curve (gm/mL × s), which provides the flow in mL/s.

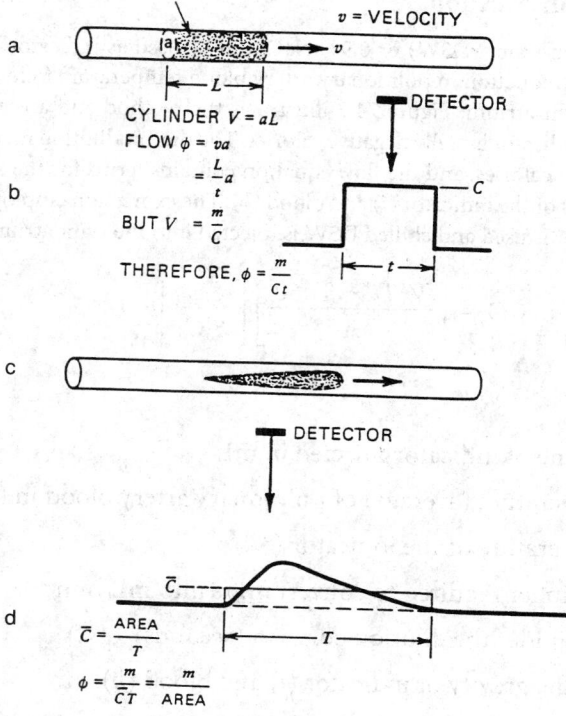

FIGURE 74.1 Genesis of the indicator-dilution curve.

Indicators

Before describing the various indicator-dilution methods, it is useful to recognize that there are two types of indicator, diffusible and nondiffusible. A diffusible indicator will leak out of the capillaries. A nondiffusible indicator is retained in the vascular system for a time that depends on the type of indicator. Whether cardiac output is overestimated with a diffusible indicator depends on the location of the injection and measuring sites. Table 74.1 lists many of the indicators that have been used for measuring cardiac output and the types of detectors used to obtain the dilution curve. It is obvious that the indicator selected must be detectable and not alter the flow being measured. Importantly, the indicator must be nontoxic and sterile.

When a diffusible indicator is injected into the right heart, the dilution curve can be detected in the pulmonary artery, and there is no loss of indicator because there is no capillary bed between these sites; therefore the cardiac output value will be accurate.

TABLE 74.1 Indicators

Material	Detector	Retention Data
Evans blue (TI824)	Photoelectric 640 mu.	50% loss in 5 days
Indocyanine green	Photoelectric 800 mu.	50% loss in 10 minutes
Coomassie blue	Photoelectric 585–600 mu.	50% loss in 15–20 minutes
Saline (5%)	Conductivity cell	Diffusible*
Albumin I^{131}	Radioactive	50% loss in 8 days
NA^{24}, K^{42}, D$_2$O, DHO	Radioactive	Diffusible*
Hot-cold solutions	Thermodetector	Diffusible*

*It is estimated that there is about 15% loss of diffusible indicators during the first pass through the lungs.

Thermal Dilution Method

Chilled 5% dextrose in water (D5W) or 0.9% NaCl can be used as indicators. The dilution curve represents a transient reduction in pulmonary artery blood temperature following injection of the indicator into the right atrium. Figure 74.2 illustrates the method and a typical thermodilution curve. Note that the indicator is really negative calories. The thermodilution method is based on heat exchange measured in calories, and the flow equation contains terms for the specific heat (C) and the specific gravity (S) of the indicator (i) and blood (b). The expression employed when a #7F thermistor-tipped catheter is used and chilled D5W is injected into the right atrium is as follows:

$$CO = \left[\frac{V(T_b - T_i)60}{A} \right] \left[\frac{S_i C_i}{S_b C_b} \right] F$$

where

V = Volume of indicator injected in mL

T_b = Temperature (average) of pulmonary artery blood in (°C)

T_i = Temperature of the indicator (°C)

60 = Multiplier required to convert mL/s into mL/min

A = Area under the dilution curve in (seconds × °C)

S = Specific gravity of indicator (i) and blood (b)

C = Specific heat of indicator (i) and blood (b)

$\left(\dfrac{S_i C_i}{S_b C_b} = 1.08 \text{ for 5\% dextrose and blood of 40\% packed-cell volume} \right)$

F = Empiric factor employed to correct for heat transfer through the injection catheter (for a #7F catheter, F = 0.825 [2]).

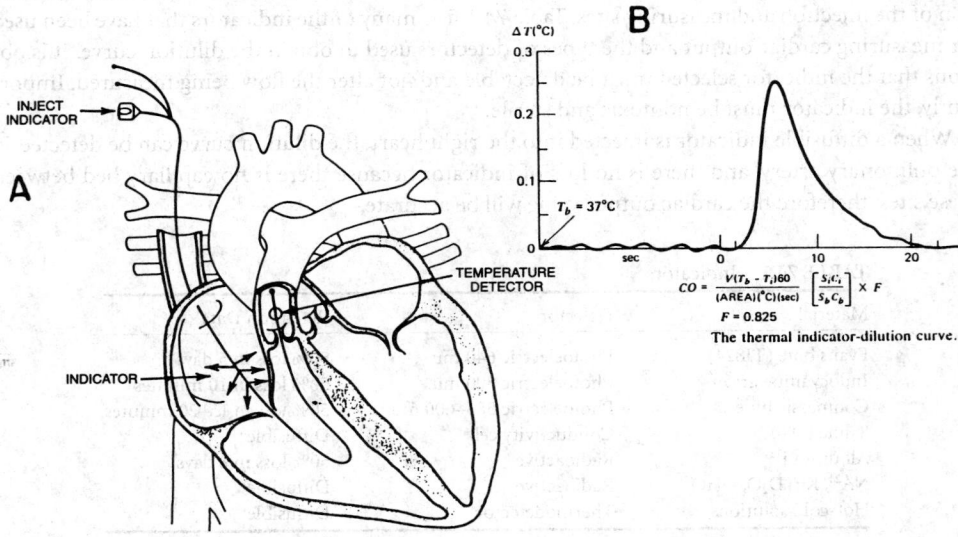

FIGURE 74.2   The thermodilution method (*a*) and a typical dilution curve (*b*).

Entering these factors into the expression gives

$$CO = \frac{V(T_b - T_i)53.46}{A}$$

where

$$CO = \text{cardiac output in mL/min}$$
$$53.46 = 60 \times 1.08 \times 0.825$$

To illustrate how a thermodilution curve is processed, cardiac output is calculated below using the dilution curve shown in Fig. 74.2.

$$V = 5 \text{ mL of 5\% dextrose in water}$$
$$T_b = 37°C$$
$$T_i = 0°C$$
$$A = 1.59°C \text{ s}$$
$$CO = \frac{5(37 - 0)53.46}{1.59} = 6220 \text{mL/min}$$

Although the thermodilution method is *the standard in clinical medicine,* it has a few disadvantages. Because of the heat loss through the catheter wall, several serial 5-mL injections of indicator are needed to obtain a consistent value for cardiac output. If cardiac output is low, i.e., the dilution curve is very broad, it is difficult to obtain an accurate value for cardiac output. There are respiratory-induced variations in PA blood temperature that confound the dilution curve when it is of low amplitude. Although room-temperature D5W can be used, chilled D5W provides a better dilution curve and a more reliable cardiac output value. Furthermore, it should be obvious that if the temperature of the indicator is the same as that of blood, there will be no dilution curve.

Indicator Recirculation

An ideal dilution curve shown in Fig. 74.2 consists of a steep rise and an exponential decrease in indicator concentration. Algorithms that measure the dilution-curve area have no difficulty with such a curve. However, when cardiac output is low, the dilution curve is typically low in amplitude and very broad. Often the descending limb of the curve is obscured by recirculation of indicator or by low-amplitude artifacts. Figure 74.3a is a dilution curve in which the descending limb is obscured by recirculation of indicator. Obviously it is difficult to determine the practical end of the curve, which is often specified as the time when the indicator concentration has fallen to a chosen percentage (e.g., 1%) of the maximum amplitude (C_{max}). Because the descending limb represents a good approximation of a decaying exponential curve (e^{-kt}), fitting the descending limb to an exponential allows reconstruction of the curve without a recirculation error, thereby providing a means for identifying the end for what is called the *first pass of the indicator.*

In Fig. 74.3b, the amplitude of the descending limb of the curve in Fig. 74.3a has been plotted on semilogarithmic paper, and the exponential part represents a straight line. When recirculation appears, the data points deviate from the straight line and therefore can be ignored, and the linear part (representing the exponential) can be extrapolated to the desired percentage of the maximum concentration, say 1% of C_{max}. The data points representing the extrapolated part were replotted on Fig. 74.3a to reveal the dilution curve undistorted by recirculation.

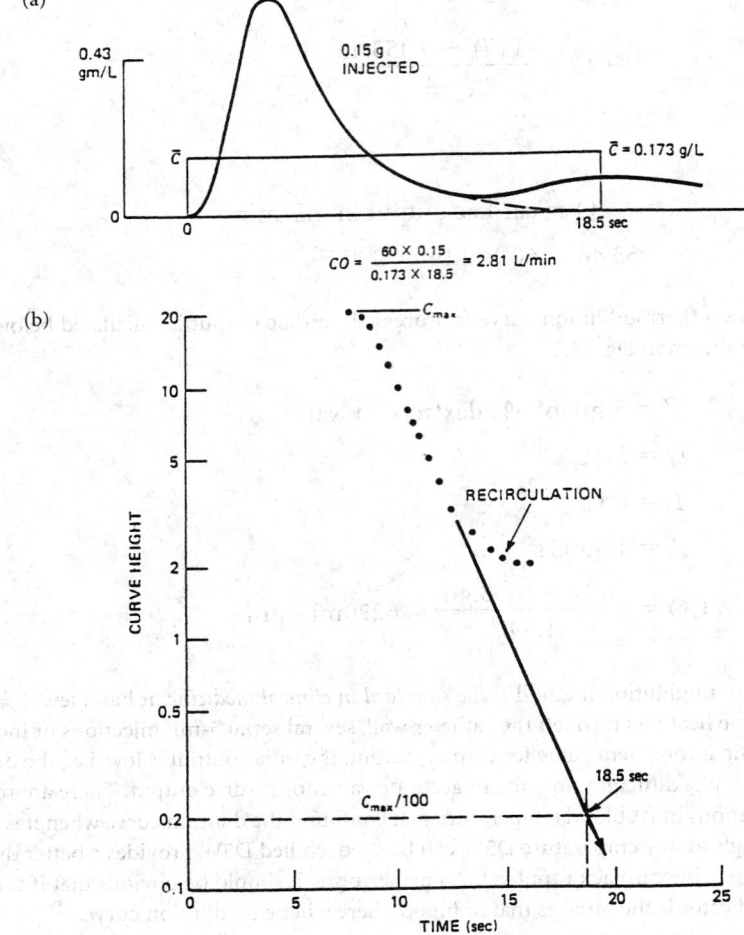

FIGURE 74.3   Dilution curve obscured by recirculation (*a*) and a semilogarithmic plot of the descending limb (*b*).

Commercially available indicator-dilution instruments employ digitization of the dilution curve. Often the data beyond about 30% of C_{max} are ignored, and the exponential is computed on digitally extrapolated data.

74.2 Fick Method

The Fick method *employs oxygen as the indicator* and the increase in oxygen content of venous blood as it passes through the lungs, along with the respiratory oxygen uptake, as the quantities that are needed to determine cardiac output, $CO = O_2$ uptake$/(A - VO_2$ difference). Oxygen uptake (mL/min) is measured at the airway, usually with an oxygen-filled spirometer containing a CO_2 absorber. The $A - VO_2$ difference is determined from the oxygen content (mL/100 mL blood) from any arterial sample and the oxygen content (mL/100 mL) of pulmonary artery blood. The oxygen content of blood used to be difficult to measure. However, the new blood-gas analyzers that measure pH, pO_2, pCO_2, hematocrit, and hemoglobin provide a value for O_2 content by computation using the oxygen-dissociation curve.

There is a slight technicality involved in determining the oxygen uptake because oxygen is consumed at body temperature but measured at room temperature in the spirometer. Consequently, the volume of O_2 consumed per minute displayed by the spirometer must be multiplied by a factor, F. Therefore the Fick equation is

$$CO = \frac{O_2 \text{ uptake/min } (F)}{A - VO_2 \text{ difference}}$$

Figure 74.4 is a spirogram showing tidal volume riding on a sloping baseline that represents the resting expirating level (REL). The slope identifies the oxygen uptake at room temperature. In this subject, the uncorrected oxygen consumption was 400 mL/min at 26°C in the spirometer. With a barometric pressure of 750 mmHg, the conversion factor F to correct this volume to body temperature (37°C) and saturated with water vapor is

$$F = \frac{273 + 37}{273 + T_s} \times \frac{P_b - PH_2O}{P_b - 47}$$

Where T_s is the spirometer temperature, P_b is the barometric pressure, and PH_2O at T_s is obtained from the water-vapor table (Table 74.2).

A sample calculation for the correction factor F is given in Fig. 74.4, which reveals a value for F of 1.069. However, it is easier to use Table 74.3 to obtain the correction factor. For example, for a spirometer temperature of 26°C and a barometric pressure of 750 mmHg, $F = 1.0691$.

Note that the correction factor F in this case is only 6.9%. The error encountered by not including it may be less than the experimental error in making all other measurements.

The example selected shows that the $A - VO_2$ difference is $20 - 15$ mL/100mL blood and that the corrected O_2 uptake is 400×1.069; therefore the cardiac output is:

$$CO = \frac{400 \times 1.069}{(20 - 15)/100} = 8552 \text{mL/min}$$

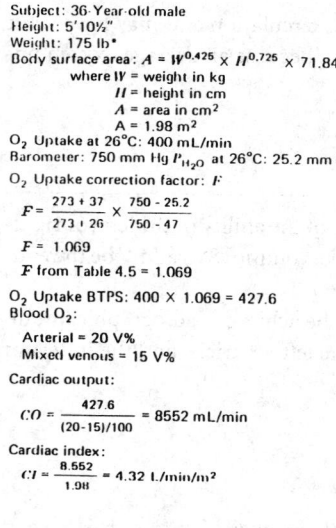

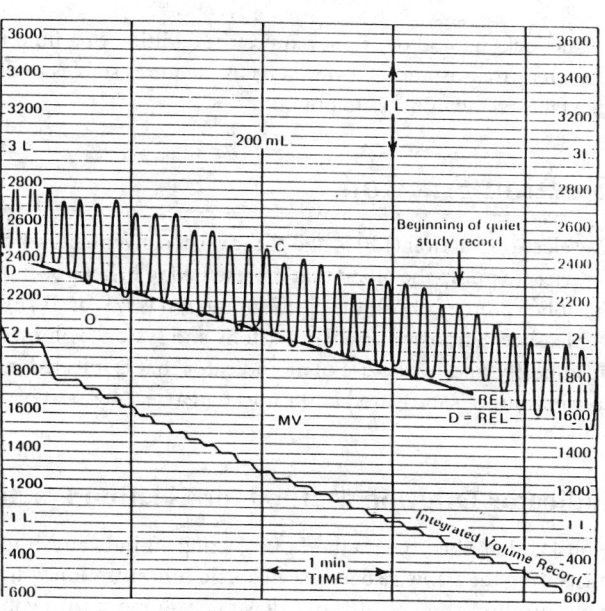

FIGURE 74.4 Measurement of oxygen uptake with a spirometer (*right*) and the method used to correct the measured volume (*left*).

TABLE 74.2 Vapor Pressure of Water

Temp. °C	0.0	0.2	0.4	0.6	0.8
15	12.788	12.953	13.121	13.290	13.461
16	13.634	13.809	13.987	14.166	14.347
17	14.530	14.715	14.903	15.092	15.284
18	15.477	15.673	15.871	16.071	16.272
19	16.477	16.685	16.894	17.105	17.319
20	17.535	17.753	17.974	18.197	18.422
21	18.650	18.880	19.113	19.349	19.587
22	19.827	20.070	20.316	20.565	20.815
23	21.068	21.324	21.583	21.845	22.110
24	22.377	22.648	22.922	23.198	23.476
25	23.756	24.039	24.326	24.617	24.912
26	25.209	25.509	25.812	26.117	26.426
27	26.739	27.055	27.374	27.696	28.021
28	28.349	28.680	29.015	29.354	29.697
29	30.043	30.392	30.745	31.102	31.461
30	31.824	32.191	32.561	32.934	33.312
31	33.695	34.082	34.471	34.864	35.261
32	35.663	36.068	36.477	36.891	37.308
33	37.729	38.155	38.584	39.018	39.457
34	39.898	40.344	40.796	41.251	41.710
35	42.175	42.644	43.117	43.595	44.078
36	44.563	45.054	45.549	46.050	46.556
37	47.067	47.582	48.102	48.627	49.157
38	49.692	50.231	50.774	51.323	51.879
39	52.442	53.009	53.580	54.156	54.737
40	55.324	55.910	56.510	57.110	57.720
41	58.340	58.960	59.580	60.220	60.860

The Fick method does not require the addition of a fluid to the circulation and may have value in such a circumstance. However, its use requires stable conditions, because an average oxygen uptake takes many minutes to obtain.

74.3 Ejection Fraction

The ejection fraction (EF) is one of the most convenient indicators of the ability of the left (or right) ventricle to pump the blood that is presented to it. Let v be the stroke volume (SV) and V be the end-diastolic volume (EDV); the ejection fraction is v/V or SV/EDV.

Measurement of ventricular diastolic and systolic volumes can be achieved radiographically, ultrasonically, and by the use of an indicator that is injected into the left ventricle, and the indicator concentration is measured in the aorta on a beat-by-beat basis.

Indicator-Dilution Method for Ejection Fraction

Holt [1] described the method of injecting an indicator into the left ventricle during diastole and measuring the stepwise decrease in aortic concentration with successive beats (Fig. 74.5). From this concentration-time record, end-diastolic volume, stroke volume, and ejection fraction can be calculated. No assumption need be made about the geometric shape of the ventricle. The following describes the theory of this fundamental method.

TABLE 74.3 Correction Factor F for Standardization of Collected Volume

°C/P_B	640	650	660	670	680	690	700	710	720	730	740	750	760	770	780
15	1.1388	1.1377	1.1367	1.1358	1.1348	1.1339	1.1330	1.1322	1.1314	1.1306	1.1298	1.1290	1.1283	1.1276	1.1269
16	1.1333	1.1323	1.1313	1.1304	1.1295	1.1286	1.1277	1.1269	1.1260	1.1253	1.1245	1.1238	1.1231	1.1224	1.1217
17	1.1277	1.1268	1.1266	1.1249	1.1240	1.1232	1.1224	1.1216	1.1208	1.1200	1.1193	1.1186	1.1179	1.1172	1.1165
18	1.1222	1.1212	1.1203	1.1194	1.1186	1.1178	1.1170	1.1162	1.1154	1.1147	1.1140	1.1133	1.1126	1.1120	1.1113
19	1.1165	1.1156	1.1147	1.1139	1.1131	1.1123	1.1115	1.1107	1.1100	1.1093	1.1086	1.1080	1.1073	1.1067	1.1061
20	1.1108	1.1099	1.1091	1.1083	1.1075	1.1067	1.1060	1.1052	1.1045	1.1039	1.1032	1.1026	1.1019	1.1094	1.1008
21	1.1056	1.1042	1.1034	1.1027	1.1019	1.1011	1.1004	1.0997	1.0990	1.0984	1.0978	1.0971	1.0965	1.0960	1.0954
22	1.0992	1.0984	1.0976	1.0969	1.0962	1.0964	1.0948	1.0941	1.0935	1.0929	1.0923	1.0917	1.0911	1.0905	1.0900
23	1.0932	1.0925	1.0918	1.0911	1.0904	1.0897	1.0891	1.0884	1.0878	1.0872	1.0867	1.0861	1.0856	1.0850	1.0845
24	1.0873	1.0866	1.0859	1.0852	1.0846	1.0839	1.0833	1.0827	1.0822	1.0816	1.0810	1.0805	1.0800	1.0795	1.0790
25	1.0812	1.0806	1.0799	1.0793	1.0787	1.0781	1.0775	1.0769	1.0764	1.0758	1.0753	1.0748	1.0744	1.0739	1.0734
26	1.0751	1.0710	1.0738	1.0732	1.0727	1.0721	1.0716	1.0710	1.0705	1.0700	1.0696	1.0691	1.0686	1.0682	1.0678
27	1.0688	1.0682	1.0677	1.0671	1.0666	1.0661	1.0656	1.0651	1.0640	1.0641	1.0637	1.0633	1.0629	1.0624	1.0621
28	1.0625	1.0619	1.0614	1.0609	1.0604	1.0599	1.0595	1.0591	1.0586	1.0582	1.0578	1.0574	1.0570	1.0566	1.0563
29	1.0560	1.0555	1.0550	1.0546	1.0548	1.0537	1.0533	1.0529	1.0525	1.0521	1.0518	1.0514	1.0519	1.0507	1.0504
30	1.0494	1.0496	1.0486	1.0482	1.0478	1.0474	1.0470	1.0467	1.0463	1.0460	1.0450	1.0453	1.0450	1.0447	1.0444

Source: From Kovach JC, Paulos P, Arabadjis C. 1955. J Thorac Surg **29**:552. $V_s = FV_c$, where V_s is the standardized condition and V_c is the collected condition:

$$V_s = \frac{1 + 37/273}{1 + t°C/273} \times \frac{P_B - PH_2O}{P_B - 47} \quad V_c = FV_c$$

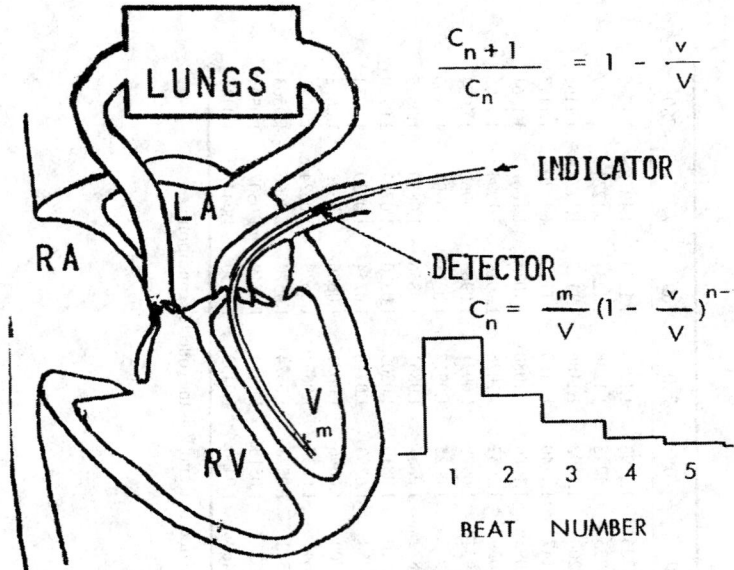

FIGURE 74.5 The saline method of measuring ejection fraction, involving injection of m gm of NaCl into the left ventricle and detecting the aortic concentration (C) on a beat-by-beat basis.

Let V be the end-diastolic ventricular volume, and inject m gm of indicator into this volume during diastole. The concentration (C_1) of indicator in the aorta for the first beat is m/V. By knowing the amount of indicator (m) injected and the calibration for the aortic detector, C_1 is established, and ventricular end-diastolic volume $V = m/C_1$.

After the first beat, the ventricle fills, and the amount of indicator left in the left ventricle is $m - mv/V$. The aortic concentration (C_2) for the second beat is therefore $m - mv/V = m(1 - v/V)$. Therefore the aortic concentration (C_2) for the second beat is

$$C_2 = \frac{m}{V}\left[1 - \frac{v}{V}\right]$$

By continuing the process, it is easily shown that the aortic concentration (C_n) for the nth beat is

$$C_n = \frac{m}{V}\left[1 - \frac{v}{V}\right]^{n-1}$$

Figure 74.6 illustrates the stepwise decrease in aortic concentration for ejection fractions (v/V) of 0.2 and 0.5, i.e., 20% and 50%.

It is possible to determine the ejection fraction from the concentration ratio for two successive beats. For example,

$$C_n = \frac{m}{V}\left[1 - \frac{v}{V}\right]^{n-1}$$

$$C_n + 1 = \frac{m}{V}\left[1 - \frac{v}{V}\right]^{n}$$

$$\frac{C_{n+1}}{C_n} = 1 - \frac{v}{V}$$

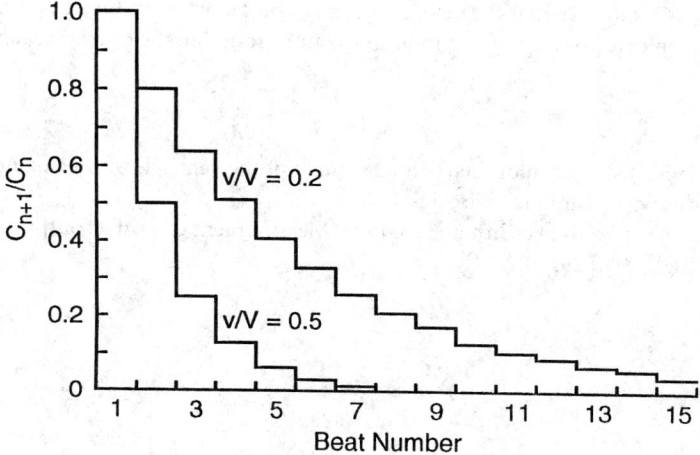

FIGURE 74.6 Stepwise decrease in indicator concentration (C) versus beat number for ejection fractions (v/V) of 0.5 and 0.2.

from which

$$\frac{v}{V} = 1 - \frac{C_{n+1}}{C_n}$$

where v/V is the ejection fraction and C_{n+1}/C_n is the concentration ratio for two successive beats, e.g., C_2/C_1 or C_3/C_2. Figure 74.7 illustrates the relationship between the ejection fraction (v/V) and

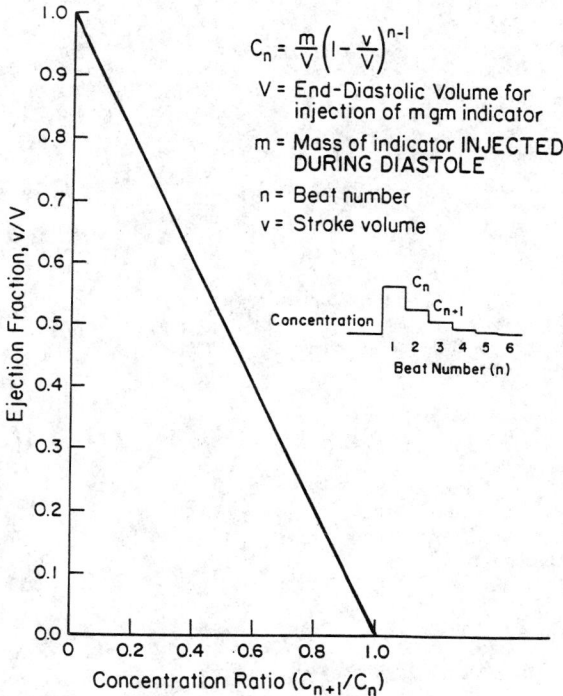

FIGURE 74.7 Ejection fraction (v/V) versus the ratio of concentrations for successive beats (C_{n+1}/C_n).

the ratio of C_{n+1}/C_n. Observe that the detector need not be calibrated as long as there is a linear relationship between detector output and indicator concentration in the operating range.

References

1. Holt JP. 1956. Estimation of the residual volume of the ventricle of the dog heart by two indicator-dilution techniques. Circ Res 4:181.
2. Weissel RD, Berger RL, Hechtman HB. 1975. Measurement of cardiac output by thermodilution. N Engl J Med 292:682.

75

Bioelectric Impedance Measurements

Robert Patterson
University of Minnesota

Bioelectric tissue impedance measurements to determine or infer biologic information has a long history dating back to before the turn of the century. Many of the early physiologists, who studied excitable tissues, made membrane and gross tissue impedance measurements. The start of modern clinical applications of bioelectric impedance (BEI) measurements can be attributed in large part to the reports by Nyboer and associates [1940, 1970]. BEI measurements are commonly used in apnea monitoring, especially for infants, and in the detection of venous thrombus. Many papers report the use of the BEI technique for peripheral blood flow, cardiac stroke volume and output, and body composition. Commercial equipment is available for these later three applications, although the reliability, validity, and accuracy of these applications have been questioned, and therefore, these applications have not received widespread acceptance in the medical community.

BEI measurements can be classified into two types. The first and most common application is in the study of the small pulsatile impedance changes associated with heart and respiratory action. The goal of this application is to give quantitative and qualitative information on the volume changes (plethysmography) in the heart, peripheral arteries, and veins. The second application involves the determination of body characteristics such as total-body fluid volume, intra- and extracellular volume, percent body fat, and cell and tissue viability. In this application, the total impedance is used and in some cases measured as a function of frequency. Applications of BEI to obtain cross-sectional images of the body will not be covered in this chapter.

75.1 Measurement Methods

Most single-frequency BEI measurements are in the range of 50 to 100 kHz (at these frequencies, no significant electric shock hazard exists) using currents from 0.5 to 4 mA RMS. Currents at these levels are usually necessary to obtain a good signal-to-noise ratio when recording the small pulsatile changes that are in the range of 0.1% to 1% of the total impedance. The use of higher frequencies is difficult because stray capacity makes the instrumentation design problem more troublesome.

0-8493-8346-3/95/$0.00+$.50
© 1995 by CRC Press, Inc.

BEI measurements in the 50- to 100-kHz range have typical skin impedance values 2 to 10 times the value of the underlying body tissue of interest. This strongly depends on electrode area. In order to obtain BEI values that can be used to give quantitative biologic information, it is necessary to eliminate the contribution from skin impedance. This is accomplished using the four-electrode impedance measurement method shown in Fig. 75.1, along with other signal-processing blocks used in typical impedance plethysmographs.

Z_{b0} is the internal section of tissue we wish to measure. If we used two electrodes to make the measurement, we would include two skin impedances (i.e., Z_{sk1} and Z_{sk4}) and two internal tissue impedances (i.e., Z_{b1} and Z_{b2}). Since the skin impedance may be 2 to 10 times Z_{b0}, it would be impossible to estimate an accurate value for Z_{b0} without eliminating the skin impedance from the measurement.

A constant current source is used to supply current I_0 to the outside two electrodes 1 and 4. I_0 flows from the constant current source through the skin and body tissue independent of the value of any of this tissue and skin impedances. The voltage V_0 is measured across Z_{b0} with a voltage amplifier using electrodes 2 and 3. Assuming the output impedance of the current source is $\gg Z_{sk1} + Z_{b1} + Z_{b0} + Z_{b2} + Z_{sk4}$ and the input impedance of voltage amplifier is $\gg Z_{sk2} + Z_{b0} + Z_{sk3}$, then

$$Z_{b0} = Z_0 + \Delta Z \qquad Z_0 = \frac{V_0}{I_0} \quad \text{and} \quad \Delta Z = \frac{\Delta V_0}{I_0} \qquad (75.1)$$

where Z_0 is the non-time-varying portion of the impedance, and ΔZ is the impedance change typically associated with the pulsation of blood in the region of measurement.

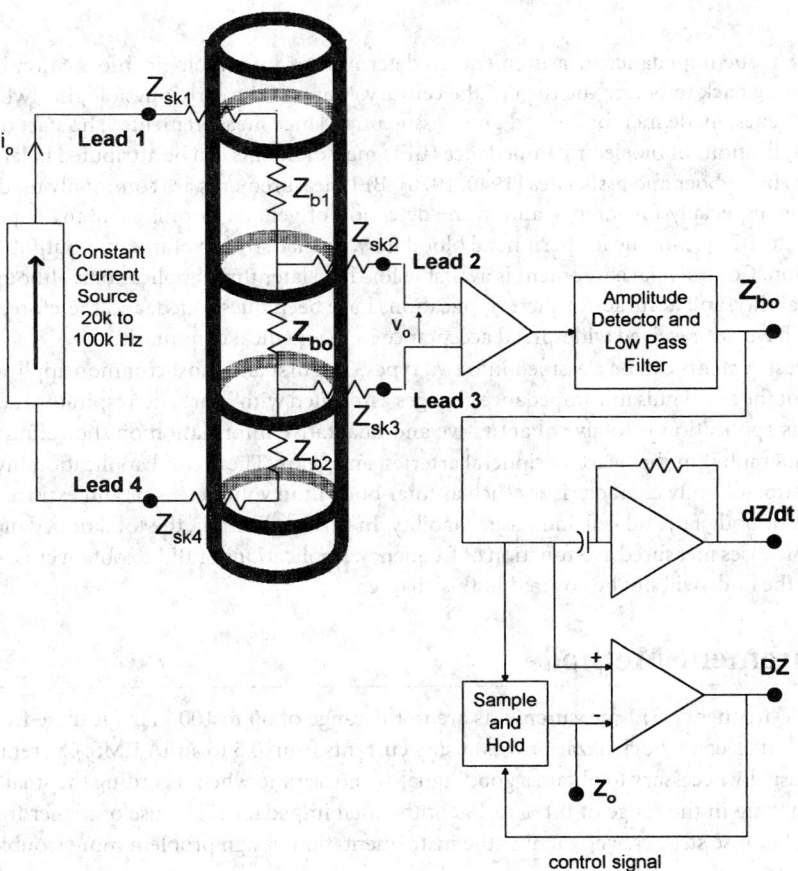

FIGURE 75.1   The four-electrode impedance measurement technique and the associated instrumentation.

The output from the voltage pickup amplifier (see Fig. 75.1) is connected to the amplitude detector and low-pass filter that removes the high-frequency carrier signal, which results in an output voltage proportional to Z_{b0}. Z_{b0} has a large steady part that is proportional to the magnitude of the tissue impedance (Z_0) and a small (0.1% to 1%) part, ΔZ, that represents the change due to respiratory or cardiac activity. In order to obtain a signal representing ΔZ, Z_0 must be removed from Z_{b0} and the signal amplified. This can be accomplished by capacity-coupling or by subtracting a constant that represents Z_0. The latter is usually done because many applications require near dc response. The output of the ΔZ amplifier will be a waveform oscillating around 0 V. The output from the ΔZ amplifier controls the sample and hold circuit. When the ΔZ output exceeds a given value, usually plus or minus a few tenths of an ohm, the sample and hold circuit updates its value of Z_0. The output from the sample and hold circuit is subtracted from Z_{b0} by the ΔZ amplifier. The derivative of Z_{b0} is frequently obtained in instruments intended for cardiac use.

75.2 Modeling and Formula Development

To relate the ΔZ obtained on the thorax or peripheral limbs to the pulsatile blood volume change, the parallel-column model, first described by Nyboer [1970], frequently is used (Fig. 75.2). The model consists of a conducting volume with impedance Z_0 in parallel with a time-varying column with resistivity ρ, length L, and a time-varying cross-sectional area that oscillates from 0 to a finite value. At the time in the cardiac cycle when the pulsatilte volume is at a minimum, all the conducting tissues and fluids are represented by the volume labeled Z_0. This volume can be a heterogeneous mixture of all the non-time-varying tissues such as fat, bone, muscle, etc. in the region under measurement. The only information needed about this volume is its impedance Z_0 and that it is electrically in parallel with the small time-varying column. During the cardiac cycle, the volume change in the right column starts with a zero cross-sectional area and increases in area until its volumes equals the blood volume change. If the impedance of the small time-varying volume is much greater than Z_0, then the following relation holds:

$$\Delta V = \rho \left(L^2/Z_0^2 \right) \Delta Z \tag{75.2}$$

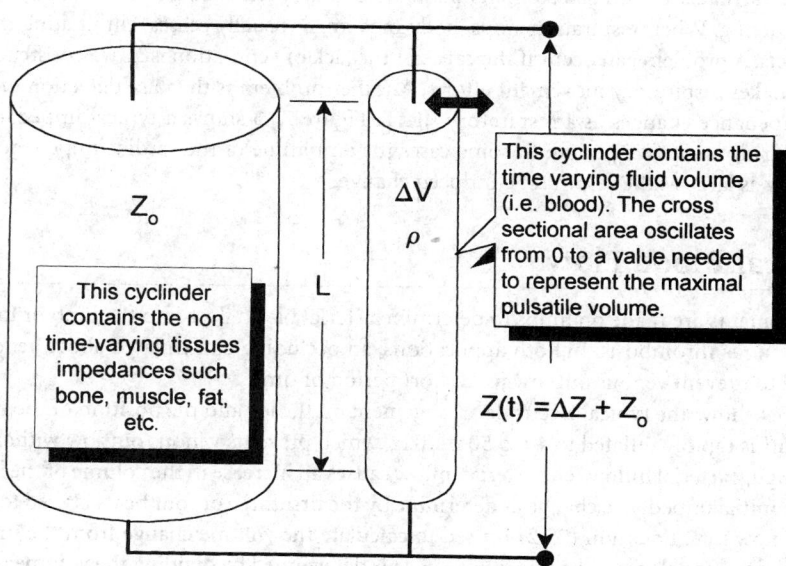

FIGURE 75.2 Parallel-column model.

where ΔV = the pulsatile volume change with resistivity ρ

ρ = the resistivity of the pulsatile volume, in $\Omega \cdot cm$ (typically the resistivity of blood)

L = the length of the cylinder

Z_0 = the impedance measured when the pulsatile volume is at a minimum

ΔZ = the magnitude of the pulsatile impedance change

The resistivity of blood ρ (in $\Omega \cdot cm$) is a function of hematocrit H expressed as a percentage and can be calculated as $\rho = 67.919 \exp(0.0247H)$ [Mohapatra et al., 1977]. The typical value used for blood is 150 $\Omega \cdot cm$.

75.3 Respiration Monitoring and Apnea Detection

If the BEI is measured across the thorax, a small increase in impedance will be observed with inspiration and a decrease with expiration. The most common position of the electrodes is on each side of the thorax along the midaxillary line. The largest signal is generally obtained at the level of the xiphisternal joint, although a more linear signal is obtained higher up near the axilla [Geddes & Baker, 1989]. The typical magnitude of the impedance change is approximately 1 to 2 Ω/liter of lung volume change.

The problems encountered with the quantitative use of BEI for respiration volume are movement artifacts and the change in the response depending on whether diaphragmatic or intercostal muscles are used. For most applications, the most serious problem is body movement and positional change artifacts, which can cause impedance changes significantly larger than the change caused by respiration.

The determination of apnea or whether respiration has stopped [Neuman, 1988] in infants is one of the most widely used application of BEI. Electrodes are typically placed across the midthorax along the midaxillary line. From the same electrodes, the ECG is also obtained. For convenience and due to the lack of space on the thorax of infants, only two electrodes are used. No effort is usually made to quantitate the volume change. Filtering is used to reduce movement artifacts, and automatic gain controls and adaptive threshold detection are used in the breath-detection circuits. Due to movement artifacts, breath detection in infants is not highly reliable when normal respiratory activity is occurring. When respiration stops, body movement usually ceases, eliminating the movement artifacts. A problem can occur if the cause of the lack of ventilation is airway obstruction and the infant makes inspiratory movement efforts. Another problem is the false detection of cardiac-induced impedance changes as a respiratory signal. Figure 75.3 shows a typical impedance measurement during an apneic period. In some cases the amplitude of the cardiac impedance change can be nearly as large as the respiratory-induced change.

75.4 Peripheral Blood Flow

BEI measurements are made on limbs to determine arterial blood flow into the limb or for the detection of venous thrombosis. In both applications, an occluding cuff inflated above venous pressure is used to prevent venous outflow for a short period of time.

Figure 75.4 shows the typical electrode arrangement on the leg and the position of the occluding cuff. The cuff is rapidly inflated to 40 to 50 mmHg, which prevents venous outflow without significantly changing arterial inflow. The arterial inflow causes an increase in the volume of the limb. The slope of the initial impedance change as determine by the first three or four beats is used to measure the arterial flow rate. Equation (75.2) is used to calculate the volume change from the impedance change. The flow (the slope of the line in Fig. 75.4) is determined by dividing the volume change by

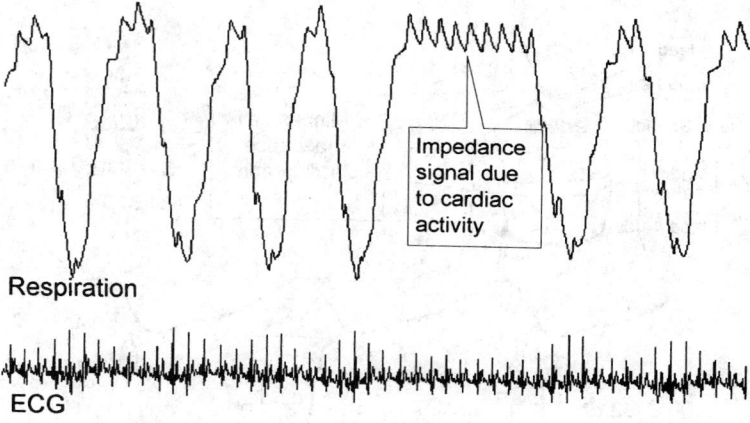

FIGURE 75.3 Example of BEI respiration signal and ECG.

the time over which the impedance change was measured. The volume change that occurs after the impedance change reaches a plateau is a measure of the compliance of the venous system.

After the volume change of the leg has stabilized, the cuff is quickly deflated, which results in an exponential decrease in volume. If a thrombosis exists in the veins, the time constant of the outflow lengthens. The initial slope, the time constant, and the percentage change at 3 seconds after cuff deflation have been used to quantitate the measurement. The percentage change at 3 seconds has been reported to show the best agreement with venograms. The determination of deep venous thrombus frequently is made by combining the maximal volume change with the outflow rate. The agreement with a venogram is 94% for the detection of deep venous thrombus proximal to the knee [Anderson, 1988].

75.5 Cardiac Measurements

The measurements of chest impedance changes due to cardiac activity have been reported since the 1930s. One of the most popular techniques, first reported by Patterson et al. [1964], for quantitative

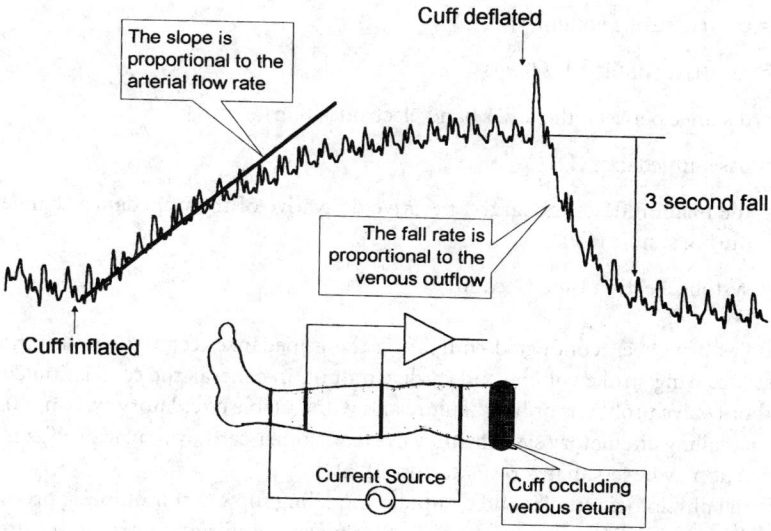

FIGURE 75.4 The measurement of arterial inflow and venous outflow.

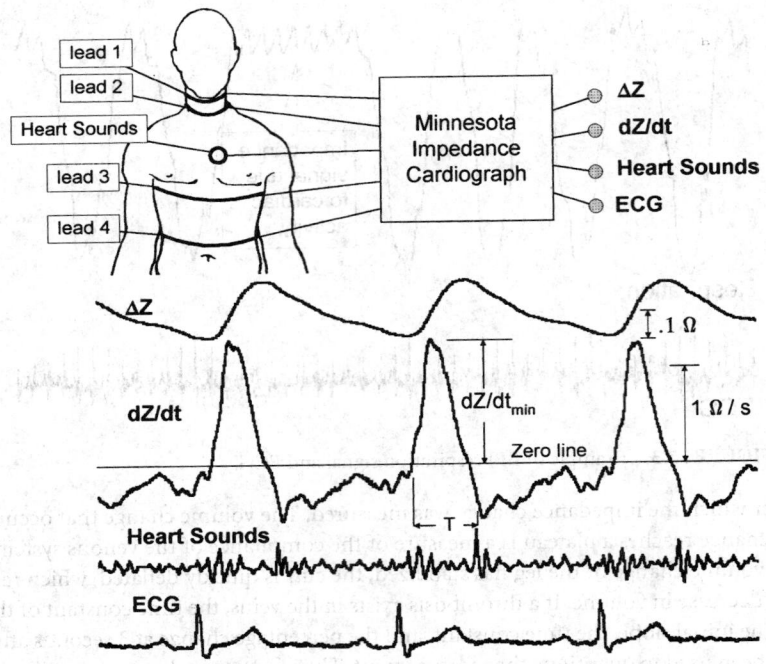

FIGURE 75.5   Impedance cardiographic waveforms.

measurements uses band electrodes around the ends of the thorax, as shown in Fig. 75.5. Each heartbeat causes a pulsatile decrease in impedance of 0.1 to 0.2 Ω (decreasing ΔZ and negative dZ/dt are shown in an upward direction). The empirical formula for stroke volume based on this method follows from Eq. (75.2):

$$\Delta V = \rho (L^2/Z_0^2)\, T\, dZ_{min}/dt \qquad (75.3)$$

where ΔV = cardiac stroke volume (mL)

   ρ = resistivity of blood ($\Omega \cdot$cm)

   L = distance between the inner band electrodes (cm)

   Z_0 = base impedance (Ω)

dZ_{min}/dt = the magnitude of the largest negative derivative of the impedance change occurring during systole (Ω/s)

   T = systolic ejection time (seconds)

   Many studies have been conducted comparing the impedance technique with other standard methods of measuring stroke volume and cardiac output. In general, the correlation coefficient in subjects without valve problems or heart failure and with a stable circulatory system is 0.8 to 0.9. In patients with a failing circulatory system and valvular or other cardiovascular problems, the correlation coefficient may be less than 0.6 [Patterson, 1989a].

   Experimental physiologic studies and computer modeling show that multiple sources contribute to the impedance signal. The anatomic regions that make significant contributions are the aorta, lungs, and atria. Recent studies have reported that the blood resistivity change with flow, pulsatile changes in the neck region, and movement of the heart significantly contribute to the signal [Patterson et al., 1991]. It appears that a number of different sources of the thoracic impedance change combine in a fortuitous manner to allow for a reasonable correlation between BEI-measured stroke volume and other accepted techniques. However, in patients with cardiac problems where the contributions of the different sources may vary, the stroke volume calculated from BEI measurements may have significant error.

75.6 Body Composition

The percentage of body fat has been an important parameter in sports medicine, physical conditioning, weight-loss programs, and predicting optimal body weight. To determine body composition, the body is configured as two parallel cylinders, similar to the model described earlier. One cylinder is represented by fat and the other as fat-free body tissue. Since the resistivity of fat is much larger than that of muscle and other body fluids, the volume determined from the total-body impedance measurement is assumed to represent the fat-free body volume. Studies have been conducted that calculate the fat-free body mass by determining the volume of the fat-free tissue cylinder using both the impedance measured between the right hand and right foot and the subject's height as a measure of cylinder's length [Lukaski et al., 1985]. Knowing the total weight and assuming body density factors, the percentage of body fat can be calculated as the difference between total weight and the weight of the fat-free tissue. Many studies have reported the correlation of the percentage body fat calculated from BEI with other accepted standard techniques to be from approximately 0.88 to 0.98 [Schoeller & Kushner, 1989]. The physical model used for the equation development is a poor approximation to the actual body because it assumes a uniform cross-sectional area for the body between the hand and foot. Patterson [1989b] pointed out the main problem with the technique: The measured impedance depends mostly on the characteristics of the arms and legs and not the trunk. Therefore, determination of body fat with this method often may be inaccurate.

Another BEI technique determines the body composition by measuring impedance over a range of frequencies. Theoretically, this technique can measure the ratio of intra- to extracellular fluid volumes [Kanai et al., 1987]. Quantitative studies evaluating this are currently under way.

75.7 Summary

Electrical impedance instrumentation is relatively low cost, which has encouraged its possible application in many different areas. The impedance measurement is influenced by many different factors, including geometry, tissue conductivity, and blood flow. Because of this complexity, it is difficult to reliably measure an isolated physiologic parameter, which has been the principal factor limiting its use. The applications that are widely used in clinical medicine are apnea monitoring and the detection of venous thrombosis. The other applications described will need more study before becoming reliable and useful measurements.

Defining Terms

Apnea: A suspension of respiration.

Compliance: The volume change divided by the pressure change. The higher the compliance, the more easily the vessel will expand as pressure increases.

Plethysmography: The measurement of the volume change of an organ or body part.

Thrombosis: The formation of a thrombus.

Thrombus: A clot of blood formed within the heart or vessel.

Venogram: An x-ray image of the veins using an injected radiopaque contrast material.

References

Anderson FA Jr. 1988. Impedance plethysmography. In JG Webster (ed), Encyclopedia of Medical Devices and Instrumentation, pp 1632–1643. New York, Wiley.

Geddes LA, Baker LE. 1989. Principles of Applied Biomedical Instrumentation, 3d ed, pp 569–572. New York, Wiley.

Kanai H, Haeno M, Sakamoto K. 1987. Electrical measurement of fluid distribution in human legs and arms. Med Prog Technol 12:159.

Lukaski HC, Johnson PE, Bolonchuk WW, Lykken GI. 1985. Assessment of fat-free mass using bio-electric impedance measurements of the human body. Am J Clin Nutr 41:810.

Mohapatra S. 1981. Non-invasive Cardiovascular Monitoring by Electrical Impedance Technique. London, Pitman Medical.

Mohapatra S. 1988. Impedance cardiography. In JG Webster (ed), Encyclopedia of Medical Devices and Instrumentation, pp 1622–1632. New York, Wiley.

Mohapatra SN, Costeloe KL, Hill DW. 1977. Blood resistivity and its implications for the calculations of cardiac output by the thoracic electrical impedance technique. Intensive Care Med 3:63.

Neuman MR. 1988. Neonatal monitoring. In JG Webster (ed), Encyclopedia of Medical Devices and Instrumentation, pp 2020–2034. New York, Wiley.

Nyboer J, Bango S, Barnett A, Halsey R. 1940. Radiocardiograms. J Clin Invest 19:773.

Nyboer J. 1970. Electrical Impedance Plethysmography, 2d ed. Springfield, Ill, Charles C Thomas.

Patterson RP. 1989a. Fundamentals of impedance cardiography. IEEE Eng Med Biol Magazine 8:35.

Patterson RP. 1989b. Body fluid determinations using multiple impedance measurements. IEEE Eng Med Biol Magazine. 8:16.

Patterson R, Kubicek WG, Kinnen E, et al. 1964. Development of an electrical impedance plethysmography system to monitor cardiac output. In Proceedings of the First Annual Rocky Mountain Bioengineering Symposium, pp 56–71. United States Air Force Academy, Colorado.

Patterson RP, Wang L, Raza SB. 1991. Impedance cardiography using band and regional electrodes in supine, sitting, and during exercise. IEEE Trans Biomed Eng 38:393.

Schoeller DA, Kushner RF. 1989. Determination of body fluids by the impedance technique. IEEE Eng Med Biol Magazine. 8:19.

Further Information

The book by Nyboer entitled *Electrical Impedance Plethysmography* contains useful background information. The *Encyclopedia of Medical Devices and Instrumentation,* edited by J. G. Webster, and *Principles of Applied Biomedical Instrumentation,* by L. A. Geddes and L. E. Baker, give a more in-depth description of many applications and describe some usual measurements.

76

Respiration

Leslie A. Geddes
Purdue University

76.1 Lung Volumes

The amount of air flowing into and out of the lungs with each breath is called the tidal volume (TV). In a typical adult this amounts to about 500 mL during quiet breathing. The respiratory system is capable of moving much more air than the tidal volume. Starting at the *resting expiratory level* (REL in Fig. 76.1), it is possible to inhale a volume amounting to about seven times the tidal volume; this volume is called the *inspiratory capacity* (IC). A measure of the ability to inspire more than the tidal volume is the *inspiratory reserve volume* IRV, which is also shown in Fig. 76.1. Starting from REL, it is possible to forcibly exhale a volume amounting to about twice the tidal volume; this volume is called the *expiratory reserve volume* (ERV). However, even with the most forcible expiration, it is not possible to exhale all the air from the lungs; a *residual volume* (RV) about equal to the expiratory reserve volume remains. The sum of the expiratory reserve volume and the residual volume is designated the *functional residual capacity* (FRC). The volume of air exhaled from a maximum inspiration to a maximum expiration is called the *vital capacity* (VC). The *total lung capacity* (TLC) is the total air within the lungs, i.e., that which can be moved in a vital-capacity maneuver plus the residual volume. All except the residual volume can be determined with a volume-measuring instrument such as a spirometer connected to the airway.

76.2 Pulmonary Function Tests

In addition to the static lung volumes just identified, there are several time-dependent volumes associated with the respiratory act. The *minute volume* (MV) is the volume of air per breath (tidal volume) multiplied by the respiratory rate (R), i.e., MV = (TV) R. It is obvious that the same minute volume can be produced by rapid shallow or slow deep breathing. However, the effectiveness is not the same, because not all the respiratory air participates in gas exchange, there being a dead space volume. Therefore the alveolar ventilation is the important quantity which is defined as the tidal volume (TV) minus the dead space (DS) multiplied by the respiratory rate R, i.e., alveolar ventilation = (TV − DS) R. In a normal adult subject, the dead space amounts to about 150 mL, or 2mL/kg.

Dynamic Tests

Several timed respiratory volumes describe the ability of the respiratory system to move air. Among these are *forced vital capacity* (FVC), *forced expiratory volume* in *t* seconds (FEV$_t$), the *maximum ven-*

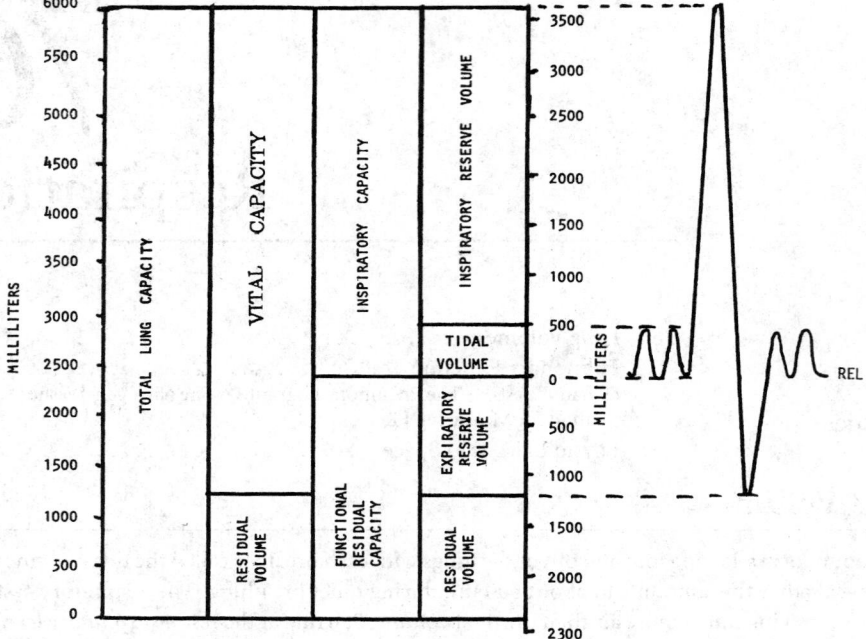

FIGURE 76.1   Lung volumes.

tilatory volume (MVV), which was previously designated the *maximum breathing capacity* (MBC), and the *peak flow* (PF). These quantities are measured with a spirometer without valves and CO_2 absorber or with a pneumotachograph coupled to an integrator.

Forced Vital Capacity

Forced vital capacity (FVC) is shown in Fig. 76.2 and is measured by taking the maximum inspiration and forcing all of the inspired air out as rapidly as possible. Table 76.1 presents normal values for males and females.

Forced Expiratory Volume

Forced expiratory volume in t seconds (FEV_t) is shown in Fig. 76.2, which identifies $FEV_{0.5}$ and $FEV_{1.0}$, and Table 76.1 presents normal values for $FEV_{1.0}$.

Maximum Voluntary Ventilation

Maximum voluntary ventilation (MVV) is the volume of air moved in 1 minute when breathing as deeply and rapidly as possible. The test is performed for 20 s and the volume scaled to a 1-min value; Table 76.1 presents normal values.

Peak Flow

Peak flow (PF) in L/min is the maximum flow velocity attainable during an FEV maneuver and represents the maximum slope of the expired volume-time curve (Fig. 76.2); typical normal values are shown in Table 76.1.

The Water-Sealed Spirometer

The water-sealed spirometer was the traditional device used to measure the volume of air moved in respiration. The Latin word *spirare* means to breathe. The most popular type of spirometer consists

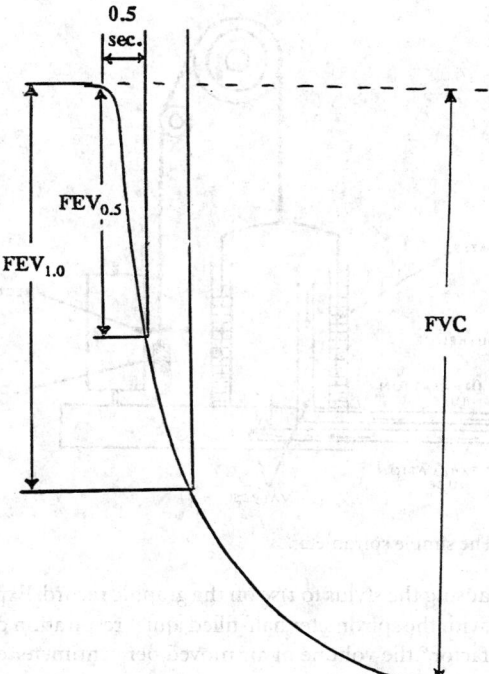

FIGURE 76.2 The measurement of timed forced expiratory volume (FEV_t) and forced vital capacity (FVC).

of a hollow cylinder closed at one end, inverted and suspended in an annular space filled with water to provide an air-tight seal. Figure 76.3 illustrates the method of suspending the counterbalanced cylinder (bell), which is free to move up and down to accommodate the volume of air under it. Movement of the bell, which is proportional to volume, is usually recorded by an inking pen applied to a graphic record which is caused to move with a constant speed. Below the cylinder, in the space that accommodates the volume of air, are inlet and outlet breathing tubes. At the end of one or both of these tubes is a check valve designed to maintain a unidirectional flow of air through the spirometer. Outside the spirometer the two breathing tubes are brought to a Y tube which is connected to a mouthpiece. With a pinch clamp placed on the nose, inspiration diminishes the volume of air under

TABLE 76.1 Dynamic Volumes

Males
  FVC (L) = 0.133H − 0.022A − 3.60 (SEE = 0.58)*
  FEV1 (L) = 0.094H − 0.028A − 1.59 (SEE = 0.52)*
  MVV (L/min) = 3.39H − 1.26A − 21.4 (SEE = 29)*
  PF (L/min) = (10.03 − 0.038A)H†
Females
  FVC (L) = 0.111H − 0.015A − 3.16 (SD = 0.42)‡
  FEV1 (L) = 0.068H − 0.023A − 0.92 (SD = 0.37)‡
  MVV (L/min) = 2.05H − 0.57A − 5.5 (SD = 10.7)‡
  PF (L/min) = (7.44 − 0.0183A)H‡

  H = height in inches, A = age in years, L = liters, L/min = liters per minute,
SEE = standard error of estimate, SD = standard deviation
  *Kory, Callahan, Boren, Syner. 1961. Am J Med 30:243.
  †Leiner, Abramowitz, Small, Stenby, Lewis. 1963. Amer Rev Resp Dis 88:644.
  ‡Lindall, Medina, Grismer. 1967. Amer Rev Resp Dis 95:1061.

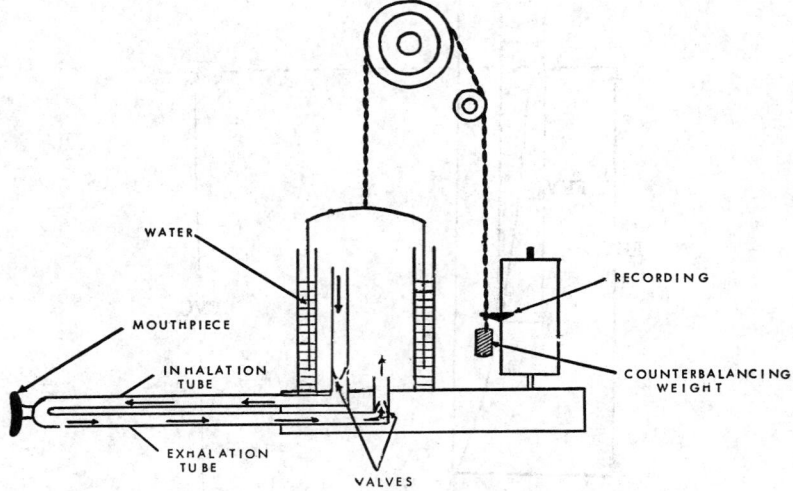

FIGURE 76.3   The simple spirometer.

the bell, which descends, causing the stylus to rise on the graphic record. Expiration produces the reverse effect. Thus, starting with the spirometer half-filled, quiet respiration causes the bell to rise and fall. By knowing the "bell factor," the volume of air moved per centimeter excursion of the bell, the volume change can be quantitated. Although a variety of flowmeters are now used to measure respiratory volumes, the spirometer with a CO_2 absorber is ideally suited to measure oxygen uptake.

Oxygen Uptake

A second and very important use for the water-filled spirometer is measurement of oxygen used per unit of time, designated the *O_2 uptake*. This measurement is accomplished by incorporating a soda-lime, carbon-dioxide absorber into the spirometer as shown in Fig. 76.4a. Soda-lime is a mixture of calcium hydroxide, sodium hydroxide, and silicates of sodium and calcium. The exhaled carbon dioxide combines with the soda-lime and becomes solid carbonates. A small amount of heat is liberated by this reaction.

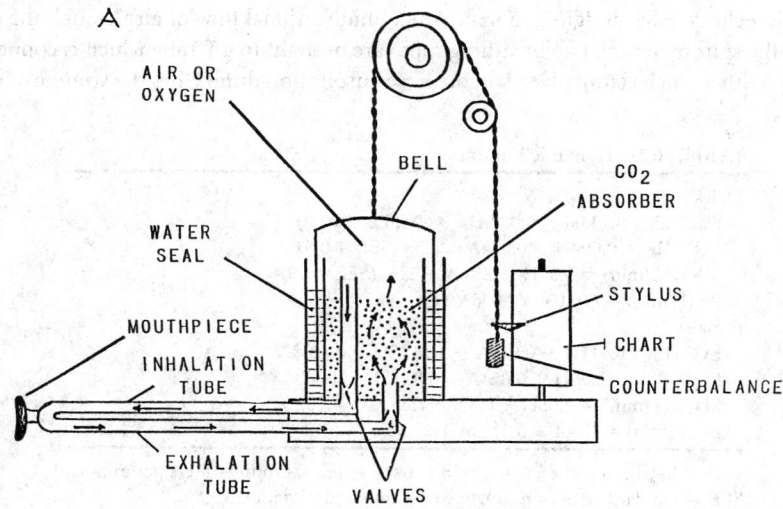

FIGURE 76.4   The spirometer with CO_2 absorber (Fig. 76.5) and a record of oxygen uptake.

Starting with a spirometer filled with oxygen and connected to a subject, respiration causes the bell to move up and down (indicating tidal volume) as shown in Fig 76.5. With continued respiration the baseline of the recording rises, reflecting disappearance of oxygen from under the bell. By measuring the slope of the baseline on the spirogram, the volume of oxygen consumed per minute can be determined. Figure 76.5 presents a typical example along with calculation.

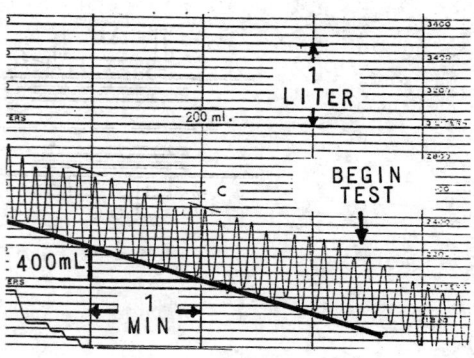

$$V_{BTPS} = V_{MEAS} \times F$$

$$F = \frac{273+37}{273+T} \times \frac{P_B-P_{H_2O}}{P_B - 47}$$

$$V_{MEAS} = 400\text{mL} @ 26^\circ C = T$$
$$(P_B=750 \text{ mmHg})$$

$$F = \frac{273+37}{273+26} \times \frac{750-25.2}{750-47}^*$$

$$= 1.069$$

$$V_{BTPS} = 400 \times 1.069$$
$$= 427.6 \text{ mL}$$

FIGURE 76.5 Oxygen consumption.

The Dry Spirometer

The water-sealed spirometer was the most popular device for measuring the volumes of respiratory gases; however, it is not without its inconveniences. The presence of water causes corrosion of the metal parts. Maintenance is required to keep the device in good working order over prolonged periods. To eliminate these problems, manufacturers have developed dry spirometers. The most common type employs a collapsible rubber or plastic bellows, the expansion of which is recorded during breathing. The earlier rubber models had a decidedly undesirable characteristic which caused their abandonment. When the bellows was in its mid-position, the resistance to breathing was a minimum; when fully collapsed, it imposed a slight negative resistance; and when fully extended it imposed a slight positive resistance to breathing. Newer units with compliant plastic bellows minimize this defect.

The Pneumotachograph

The pneumotachograph is a device which is placed directly in the airway to measure the velocity of air flow. The volume per breath is therefore the integral of the velocity-time record during inspiration or expiration. Planimetric integration of the record, or electronic integration of the velocity-time signal, yields the tidal volume. Although tidal volume is perhaps more easily recorded with the spirometer, the dynamics of respiration are better displayed by the pneumotachograph, which offers less resistance to the air stream and exhibits a much shorter response time—so short in most instruments that cardiac impulses are often clearly identifiable in the velocity-time record.

If a specially designed resistor is placed in a tube in which the respiratory gases flow, a pressure drop will appear across it. Below the point of turbulent flow, the pressure drop is linearly related to air-flow velocity. The resistance may consist of a wire screen or a series of capillary tubes; Fig. 76.6 illustrates both types. Detection and recording of this pressure differential constitutes a pneumotachogram; Fig.76.7 presents a typical air-velocity record, along with the spirogram, which is the integral of the flow signal. The small-amplitude artifacts in the pneumotachogram are cardiac impulses.

For human application, linear flow rates up to 200 L/min should be recordable with fidelity. The resistance to breathing depends upon the flow rate, and it is difficult to establish an upper limit of tolerable resistance. Silverman and Whittenberger [1950] stated that a resistance of 6 mm H_2O is perceptible to human subjects. Many of the high-fidelity pneumotachographs offer 5–10 mm H_2O resistance at 100 and 200 L/min. It would appear that such resistances are acceptable in practice.

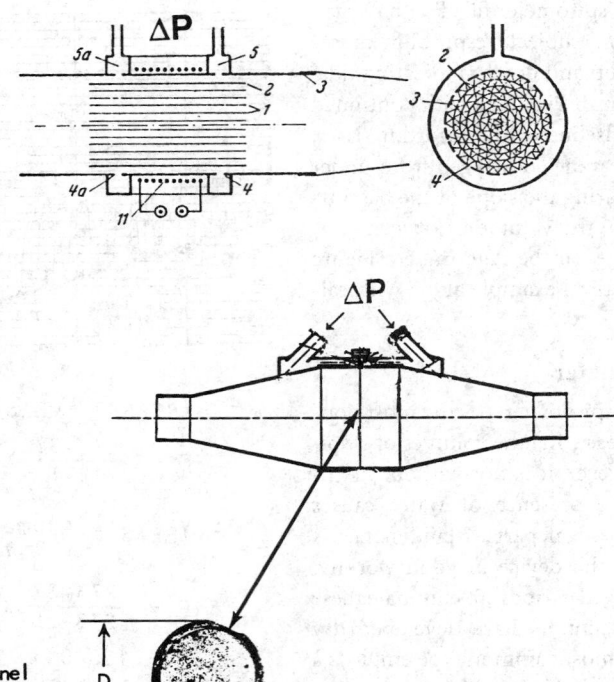

FIGURE 76.6   Pneumotachographs.

Response times of 15–40 ms seem to be currently in use. Fry and coworkers [1957] analyzed the dynamic characteristics of three types of commercially available, differential-pressure pneumotachographs which employed concentric cylinders, screen mesh, and parallel plates for the air resistors. Using a high-quality, differential-pressure transducer with each, they measured total flow resistance ranging from 5–15 cm H_2O. Frequency response curves taken on one model showed fairly uniform response to 40 Hz; the second model showed a slight increase in response at 50 Hz, and the third exhibited a slight drop in response at this frequency.

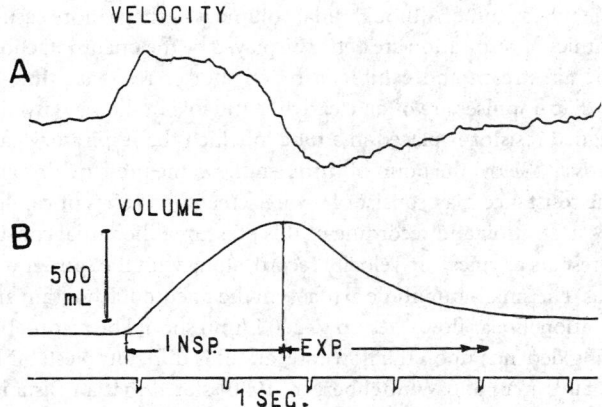

FIGURE 76.7   Velocity (A) and volume changes (B) during normal, quiet breathing; B is the integral of A.

The Nitrogen-Washout Method for Measuring FRC

The *functional residual capacity* (FRC) and the *residual volume* (RV) are the only lung compartments that cannot be measured with a volume-measuring device. Measuring these requires use of the nitrogen analyzer and application of the dilution method.

Because nitrogen does not participate in respiration, it can be called a *diluent.* Inspired and expired air contain about 80% nitrogen. Between breaths, the FRC of the lungs contains the same concentration of nitrogen as in environmental air, i.e., 80%. By causing a subject to inspire from a spirometer filled with 100% oxygen and to exhale into a second collecting spirometer, all the nitrogen in the FRC is replaced by oxygen, i.e., the nitrogen is "washed out" into the second spirometer. Measurement of the concentration of nitrogen in the collecting spirometer, along with a knowledge of its volume, permits calculation of the amount of nitrogen originally in the functional residual capacity and hence allows calculation of the FRC, as now will be shown.

Figure 76.8 illustrates the arrangement of equipment for the nitrogen-washout test. Note that two check valves (I, EX) are on both sides of the subject's breathing tube, and the nitrogen meter is connected to the mouthpiece. Valve V is used to switch the subject from breathing environmental air to the measuring system. The left-hand spirometer contains 100% oxygen, which is inhaled by the subject via valve I. Of course, a nose clip must be applied so that all the respired gases flow through the breathing tube connected to the mouthpiece. It is in this tube that the sampling inlet for the nitrogen analyzer is located. Starting at the resting expiratory level, inhalation of pure oxygen causes the nitrogen analyzer to indicate zero. Expiration closes valve I and opens valve EX. The first expired breath contains nitrogen derived from the FRC (diluted by the oxygen which was inspired); the nitrogen analyzer indicates this percentage. The exhaled gases are collected in the right-hand spirometer. The collecting spirometer and all the interconnecting tubing was first flushed with oxygen to eliminate all nitrogen. This simple procedure eliminates the need for applying corrections and facilitates calculation of the FRC. With continued breathing, the nitrogen analyzer indicates less and less nitrogen because it is being washed out of the FRC and is replaced by oxygen. Figure 76.9 presents a typical record of the diminishing concentration of expired nitrogen throughout the test. In most laboratories, the test is continued until the concentration of nitrogen falls to about 1%. The nitrogen analyzer output permits identification of this concentration. In normal subjects, virtually all the nitrogen can be washed out of the FRC by about 5 minutes.

If the peaks on the nitrogen washout record are joined, a smooth exponential decay curve is obtained in normal subjects. A semilog plot of N_2 versus time provides a straight line. In subjects with trapped air, or poorly ventilated alveoli, the nitrogen-washout curve consists of several exponentials

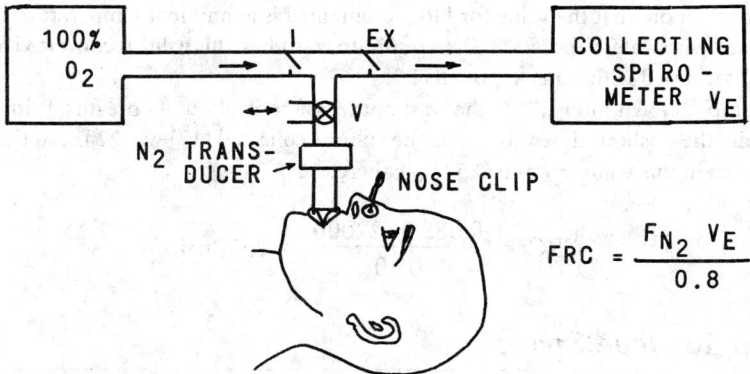

$$FRC = \frac{F_{N_2} \, V_E}{0.8}$$

FIGURE 76.8 Arrangement of equipment for the nitrogen-washout technique. Valve V allows the subject to breathe room air until the test is started. The test is started by operating valve V at the end of a normal breath, i.e. the subject starts breathing 100% O_2 through the inspiratory valve (I) and exhales the N_2 and O_2 mixture into a collecting spirometer via the expiratory valve EX.

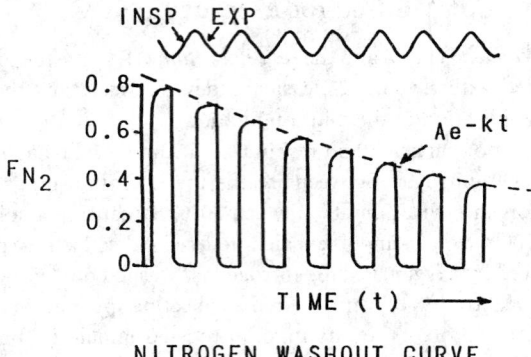

FIGURE 76.9   The nitrogen-washout out curve.

as the multiple poorly ventilated regions give up their nitrogen. In such subjects, the time taken to wash out all the nitrogen usually exceeds 10 min. Thus, the nitrogen concentration-time curve provides useful diagnostic information on ventilation of the alveoli.

If it is assumed that all the collected (washed-out) nitrogen was uniformly distributed within the lungs, it is easy to calculate the FRC. If the environmental air contains 80% nitrogen, then the volume of nitrogen in the functional residual capacity is 0.8 (FRC). Because the volume of expired gas in the collecting spirometer is known, it is merely necessary to determine the concentration of nitrogen in this volume. To do so requires admitting some of this gas to the inlet valve of the nitrogen analyzer. Note that this concentration of nitrogen (F_{N2}) exists in a volume which includes the volume of air expired (V_E) plus the original volume of oxygen in the collecting spirometer (V_0) at the start of the test and the volume of the tubing (V_t) leading from the expiratory collecting valve. It is therefore advisable to start with an empty collecting spirometer ($V_0 = 0$). Usually the tubing volume (V_t) is negligible with respect to the volume of expired gas collected in a typical washout test. In this situation the volume of nitrogen collected is $V_E F_{N2}$, where F_{N2} is the fraction of nitrogen within the collected gas. Thus, 0.80 (FRC) = $F_{N2} (V_E)$. Therefore

$$\text{FRC} = \frac{F_{N2} V_E}{0.80}$$

It is important to note that the value for FRC so obtained is at ambient temperature and pressure and is saturated with water vapor (ATPS). In respiratory studies, this value is converted to body temperature and saturated with water vapor (BTPS).

In the example shown in Fig. 76.9, the washout to 1% took about 44 breaths. With a breathing rate of 12/min, the washout time was 220 s. The volume collected (V_E) was 22 L and the concentration of nitrogen in this volume was 0.085 (F_{N2}); therefore

$$\text{FRC} = \frac{0.085 \times 22000}{0.80} = 2337 \text{mL}$$

76.3 Physiologic Dead Space

The volume of ventilated lung that does not participate in gas exchange is the physiologic dead space (V_d). It is obvious that the physiologic dead space includes anatomic dead space, as well as the volume of any alveoli that are not perfused. In the lung, there are theoretically four types of alveoli, as shown in Fig. 76.10. The normal alveolus (A) is both ventilated and perfused with blood. There are

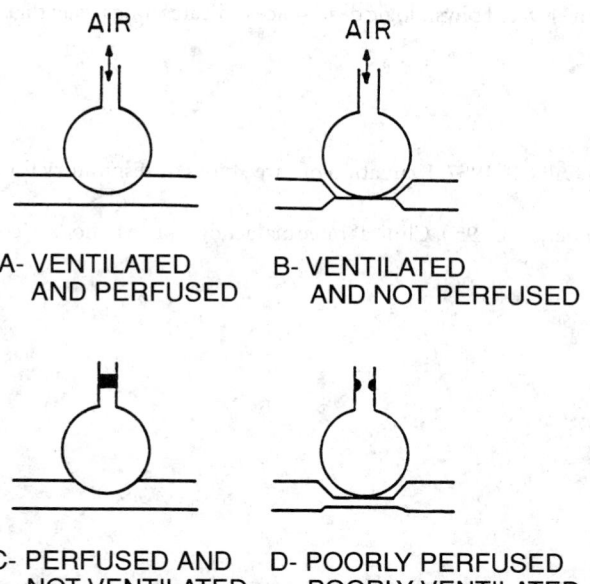

AIR   AIR

A- VENTILATED   B- VENTILATED
AND PERFUSED   AND NOT PERFUSED

C- PERFUSED AND   D- POORLY PERFUSED
NOT VENTILATED   POORLY VENTILATED

FIGURE 76.10   The four types of alveoli.

alveoli that are ventilated but not perfused (B); such alveoli contribute significantly to the physio-logic dead space. There are alveoli that are not ventilated but perfused (C); such alveoli do not pro-vide the exchange of respiratory gases. Finally, there are alveoli that are both poorly ventilated and poorly perfused (D); such alveoli contain high CO_2 and N_2 and low O_2. These alveoli are the last to expel their CO_2 and N_2 in washout tests.

Measurement of physiologic dead space is based on the assumption that there is almost complete equilibrium between alveolar pCO_2 and pulmonary capillary blood. Therefore, the arterial pCO_2 represents mean alveolar pCO_2 over many breaths when an arterial blood sample is drawn for analy-sis of pCO_2. The Bohr equation for physiologic dead space is

$$V_d = \left[\frac{PaCO_2 - pECO_2}{PaCO_2} \right] V_E$$

In this expression, $paCO_2$ is the partial pressure in the arterial blood sample which is withdrawn slowly during the test; $pECO_2$ is the partial pressure of CO_2 in the volume of expired air; V_E is the volume of expired air per breath (tidal volume).

In a typical test, the subject would breathe in room air and exhale into a collapsed (Douglas) bag. The test is continued for 3 min or more, and the number of breaths is counted in that period. An arterial blood sample is withdrawn during the collection period. The pCO_2 in the expired gas is mea-sured, and then the volume of expired gas is measured by causing it to flow into a spirometer of flowmeter by collapsing the collecting bag.

In a typical 3-min test, the collected volume is 33 L, and the pCO_2 in the expired gas is 14.5 mmHg. During the test, the pCO_2 in the arterial blood sample was 40 mmHg. The number of breaths was 60; therefore, the average tidal volume was 33000/60 = 550 mL. The physiologic dead space (V_d) is:

$$V_d = \left[\frac{40 - 14.5}{40} \right] 550 = 350mL$$

It is obvious that an elevated physiologic dead space indicates lung tissue that is not perfused with blood.

References

Fry DI, Hyatt RE, McCall CB. 1957. Evaluation of three types or respiratory flowmeters. Appl Physiol 10:210.

Silverman L, Whittenberger J. 1950. Clinical pneumatachograph. Methods Med Res 2:104.

77

Clinical Laboratory: Separation and Spectral Methods

Richard L. Roa
Baylor University
Medical Center

The purpose of the clinical laboratory is to analyze body fluids and tissues for specific substances of interest and to report the results in a form which is of value to clinicians in the diagnosis and treatment of disease. A large range of tests has been developed to achieve this purpose. Four terms commonly used to describe tests are *accuracy, precision, sensitivity,* and *specificity.* An accurate test, on average, yields true values. Precision is the ability of a test to produce identical results upon repeated trials. Sensitivity is a measure of how small an amount of substance can be measured. Specificity is the degree to which a test measures the substance of interest without being affected by other substances which may be present in greater amounts.

The first step in many laboratory tests is to separate the material of interest from other substances. This may be accomplished through extraction, filtration, and centrifugation. Another step is derivatization, in which the substance of interest is chemically altered through addition of reagents to change it into a substance which is easily measured. For example, one method for measuring glucose is to add o-toluidine which, under proper conditions, forms a green-colored solution with an absorption maximum at 630 nm. Separation and derivatization both improve the specificity required of good tests.

77.1 Separation Methods

Centrifuges are used to separate materials on the basis of their relative densities. The most common use in the laboratory is the separation of cells and platelets from the liquid part of the blood. This requires a relative centrifugal force (RCF) of roughly 1000 *g* (1000 times the force of gravity) for a period of 10 minutes. Relative centrifugal force is a function of the speed of rotation and the distance of the sample from the center of rotation as stated in Eq. (77.1)

$$\text{RCF} = (1.12 \times 10^{-5})\, r\, (\text{rpm})^2 \qquad (77.1)$$

where RCF = relative centrifugal force in *g*, and *r* = radius in cm.

Some mixtures require higher *g*-loads in order to achieve separation in a reasonable period of time. Special rotors contain the sample tubes inside a smooth container, which minimizes air resistance to allow faster rotational speeds. Refrigerated units maintain the samples at a cool temperature throughout long high-speed runs which could lead to sample heating due to air friction on the rotor. Ultracentrifuges operate at speeds on the order of 100,000 rpm and provide relative centrifugal forces of up to 600,000 *g*. These usually require vacuum pumps to remove the air which would otherwise retard the rotation and heat the rotor.

77.2 Chromatographic Separations

Chromatographic separations depend upon the different rates at which various substances moving in a stream (mobile phase) are retarded by a stationary material (stationary phase) as they pass over it. The mobile phase can be a volatilized sample transported by an inert carrier gas such as helium or a liquid transported by an organic solvent such as acetone. Stationary phases are quite diverse depending upon the separation being made, but most are contained within a long, thin tube (column). Liquid stationary phases may be used by coating them onto inert packing materials. When a sample is introduced into a chromatographic column, it is carried through it by the mobile phase. As it passes through the column, the substances which have greater affinity for the stationary phase fall behind those with less affinity. The separated substances may be detected as individual peaks by a suitable detector placed at the end of the chromatographic column.

77.3 Gas Chromatography

The most common instrumental chromatographic method used in the clinical laboratory is the gas-liquid chromatograph. In this system the mobile phase is a gas, and the stationary phase is a liquid coated onto either an inert support material, in the case of a packed column, or the inner walls of a very thin tube, in the case of a capillary column. Capillary columns have the greatest resolving power but cannot handle large sample quantities. The sample is injected into a small heated chamber at the beginning of the column, where it is volatilized if it is not already a gaseous sample. The sample is then carried through the column by an inert carrier gas, typically helium or nitrogen. The column is completely housed within an oven. Many gas chromatographs allow for the oven temperature to be programmed to slowly increase for a set time after the sample injection is made. This produces peaks which are spread more uniformly over time.

Four detection methods commonly used with gas chromatography are thermal conductivity, flame ionization, nitrogen/phosphorous, and mass spectrometry. The thermal conductivity detector takes advantage of variations in thermal conductivity between the carrier gas and the gas being measured. A heated filament immersed in the gas leaving the chromatographic column is part of a Wheatstone bridge circuit. Small variations in the conductivity of the gas cause changes in the resistance of the filament, which are recorded. The flame ionization detector measures the current between two plates with a voltage applied between them. When an organic material appears in the flame, ions which contribute to the current are formed. The NP detector, or nitrogen/phosphorous detector, is a modified flame ionization detector (see Fig. 77.1) which is particularly sensitive to nitrogen- and phosphorous-containing compounds.

Mass spectrometry (MS) provides excellent sensitivity and selectivity. The concept behind these devices is that the volatilized sample molecules are broken into ionized fragments which are then passed through a mass analyzer that separates the fragments according to their mass/charge (m/z) ratios. A mass spectrum, which is a plot of the relative abundance of the various fragments versus m/z, is produced. The mass spectrum is characteristic of the molecule sampled. The mass analyzer most commonly used with gas chromatographs is the quadrupole detector, which consists of four rods that have dc and RF voltages applied to them. The m/z spectrum can be scanned by appropriate changes in the applied voltages. The detector operates in a manner similar to that of a photomultiplier tube except that the collision of the charged particles with the cathode begins the electron cascade, resulting in a measurable electric pulse for each charged particle captured. The MS must operate in a high vacuum, which requires good pumps and a porous barrier between the GC and MS that limits the amount of carrier gas entering the MS.

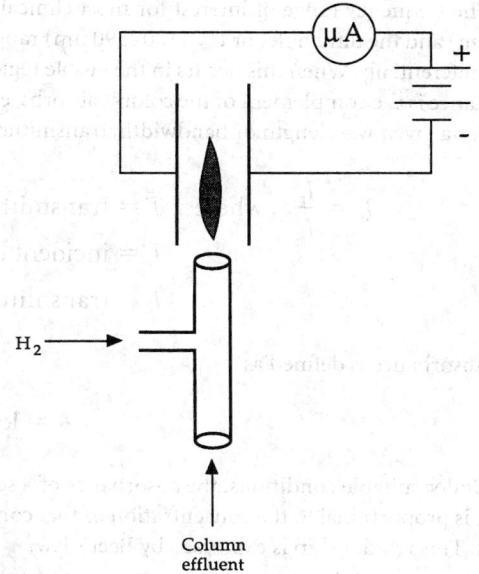

FIGURE 77.1 Flame ionization detector. Organic compounds in the column effluent are ionized in the flame, producing a current proportional to the amount of the compound present.

77.4 High-Performance Liquid Chromatography

In liquid chromatography, the mobile phase is liquid. High-performance liquid chromatography (HPLC) refers to systems which obtain excellent resolution in a reasonable time by forcing the mobile phase at high pressure through a long thin column. The most common pumps used are pistons driven by asymmetrical cams. By using two such pumps in parallel and operating out of phase, pressure fluctuations can be minimized. Typical pressures are 350–1500 psi, though the pressure may be as high as 10,000 psi. Flow rates are in the 1–10 mL/min range.

A common method for placing a sample onto the column is with a loop injector, consisting of a loop of tubing which is filled with the sample. By a rotation of the loop, it is brought in series with the column, and the sample is carried onto the column. A UV/visible spectrophotometer is often used as a detector for this method. A mercury arc lamp with the 254-nm emission isolated is useful for detection of aromatic compounds, while diode array detectors allow a complete spectrum from 190 nm to 600 nm in 10 msec. This provides for detection and identification of compounds as they come off the column. Fluorescent, electrochemical, and mass analyzer detectors are also used.

77.5 Basis for Spectral Methods

Spectral methods rely on the absorption or emission of electromagnetic radiation by the sample of interest. Electromagnetic radiation is often described in terms of frequency or wavelength. Wavelengths are those obtained in a vacuum and may be calculated with the formula

$$\lambda = c/\upsilon \quad \text{where} \quad \lambda = \text{wavelength in meters}$$
$$c = \text{speed of light in vacuum } (3 \times 10^8 \text{ m/s}) \qquad (77.2)$$
$$\upsilon = \text{frequency in Hz}$$

The frequency range of interest for most clinical laboratory work consists of the visible (390–780 nm) and the ultraviolet or UV (180–390 nm) ranges. Many substances absorb different wavelengths preferentially. When this occurs in the visible region, they are colored. In general, the color of a substance is the complement of the color it absorbs, e.g., absorption in the blue produces a yellow color. For a given wavelength or bandwidth, transmittance is defined as

$$T = \frac{I_t}{I_i}$$ where T = transmittance ratio (often expressed as %)

I_i = incident light intensity   (77.3)

I_t = transmitted light intensity

Absorbance is defined as

$$A = \log_{10} 1/T \tag{77.4}$$

Under suitable conditions, the absorbance of a solution with an absorbing compound dissolved in it is proportional to the concentration of that compound as well as the path length of light through it. This relationship is expressed by Beer's law:

$$A = abc$$ where A = absorbance

a = a constant

b = path length   (77.5)

c = concentration

A number of situations may cause deviations from Beer's law, such as high concentration or mixtures of compounds which absorb at the wavelength of interest. From an instrumental standpoint, the primary causes are stray light and excessive spectral bandwidth. Stray light refers to any light reaching the detector other than light from the desired pass-band which has passed through sample. Sources of stray light may include room light leaking into the detection chamber, scatter from the cuvette, and undesired fluorescence.

A typical spectrophotometer consists of a light source, some form of wavelength selection, and a detector for measuring the light transmitted through the samples. There is no single light source that covers the entire visible and UV spectrum. The source most commonly used for the visible part of the spectrum is the tungsten-halogen lamp, which provides continuous radiation over the range of 360 to 950 nm. The deuterium lamp has become the standard for much UV work. It covers the range from 220–360 nm. Instruments which cover the entire UV/visible range use both lamps with a means for switching from one lamp to the other at a wavelength of approximately 360 nm (Fig. 77.2).

Wavelength selection is accomplished with filters, prisms, and diffraction gratings. Specially designed interference filters can provide bandwidths as small as 5 nm. These are useful for instruments which do not need to scan a range of wavelengths. Prisms produce a nonlinear dispersion of wavelengths with the longer wavelengths closer together than the shorter ones. Since the light must pass through the prism material, they must be made of quartz for UV work. Diffraction gratings are surfaces with 1000–3000 grooves/mm cut into them. They may be transmissive or reflective; the reflective ones are more popular since there is no attenuation of light by the material. They produce a linear dispersion. By proper selection of slit widths, pass bands of 0.1 nm are commonly achieved.

The most common detector is the photomultiplier tube, which consists of a photosensitive cathode that emits electrons in proportion to the intensity of light striking it (Fig. 77.3). A series of 10–15 dynodes, each at 50–100 volts greater potential than the preceding one, produce an electron ampli-

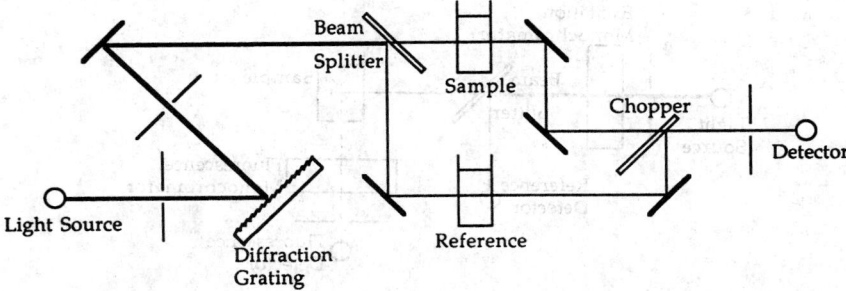

FIGURE 77.2 Dual-beam spectrophotometer. The diffraction grating is rotated to select the desired wavelength. The beam splitter consists of a half-silvered mirror which passes half the light while reflecting the other half. A rotating mirror with cut-out sections (chopper) alternately directs one beam and then the other to the detector.

fication of 4–6 per stage. Overall gains are typically a million or more. Photomultiplier tubes respond quickly and cover the entire spectral range. They require a high voltage supply and can be damaged if exposed to room light while the high voltage is applied.

77.6 Fluorometry

Certain molecules absorb a photon's energy and then emit a photon with less energy (longer wavelength). When the reemission occurs in less than 10^{-8} s, the process is known as *fluorescence*. This physical process provides the means for assays which are 10–100 times as sensitive as those based on absorption measurements. This increase in sensitivity is largely because the light measured is all from the sample of interest. A dim light is easily measured against a black background, while it may be lost if added to an already bright background.

Fluorometers and spectrofluorometers are very similar to photometers and spectrophotometers but with two major differences. Fluorometers and spectrofluorometers use two monochrometers, one for excitation light and one for emitted light. By proper selection of the bandpass regions, all the light used to excite the sample can be blocked from the detector, assuring that the detector sees only fluorescence. The other difference is that the detector is aligned off-axis, commonly at 90°, from the excitation source. At this angle, scatter is minimal, which helps ensure a dark background for the measured fluorescence. Some spectrofluorometers use polarization filters both on the input and output light beams, which allows for fluorescence polarization studies (Fig. 77.4). An intense light source in the visible-to-UV range is desirable. A common source is the xenon or mercury arc lamps, which provide a continuum of radiation over this range.

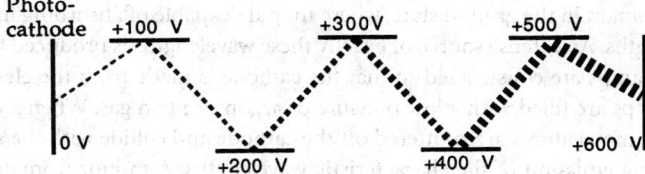

FIGURE 77.3 Photomultiplier tube. Incident photons cause the photocathode to emit electrons which collide with the first dynode which emits additional electrons. Multiple dynodes provide sufficient gain to produce an easily measurable electric pulse from a single photon.

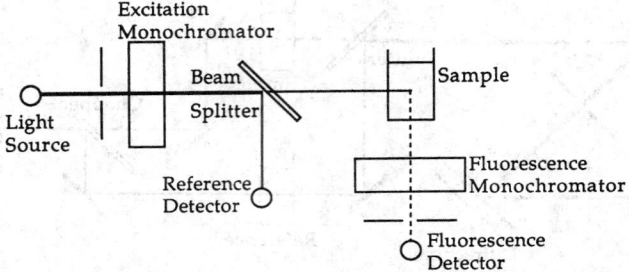

FIGURE 77.4 Spectrofluorometer. Fluorescence methods can be extremely sensitive to the low background interference. Since the detector is off-axis from the incident light and a second monochromator blocks light of wavelengths illuminating the sample, virtually no signal reaches the detector other than the desired fluorescence.

77.7 Flame Photometry

Flame photometry is used to measure sodium, potassium, and lithium in body fluids. When these elements are heated in a flame they emit characteristic wavelengths of light. The major emission lines are 589 nm (yellow) for sodium, 767 nm (violet) for potassium, and 671 nm (red) for lithium. An atomizer introduces a fine mist of the sample into a flame. For routine laboratory use, a propane and compressed air flame is adequate. High-quality interference filters with narrow pass bands are often used to isolate the major emission lines. The narrow band pass is necessary to maximize the signal-to-noise ratio. Since it is impossible to maintain stable aspiration, atomization, and flame characteristics, it is necessary to use an internal standard of known concentration while making measurements of unknowns. In this way the ratio of the unknown sample's emission to the internal standard's emission remains stable even as the total signal fluctuates. An internal standard is usually an element which is found in very low concentration in the sample fluid. By adding a high concentration of this element to the sample, its concentration can be known to a high degree of accuracy. Lithium, potassium, and cesium all may be used as internal standards depending upon the particular assay being conducted.

77.8 Atomic Absorption Spectroscopy

Atomic absorption spectroscopy is based on the fact that just as metal elements have unique emission lines, they have identical absorption lines when in a gaseous or dissociated state. The atomic absorption spectrometer takes advantage of these physical characteristics in a clever manner, producing an instrument with approximately 100 times the sensitivity of a flame photometer for similar elements. The sample is aspirated into a flame, where the majority of the atoms of the element being measured remain in the ground state, where they are capable of absorbing light at their characteristic wavelengths. An intense source of exactly these wavelengths is produced by a hollow cathode lamp. These lamps are constructed so that the cathode is made from the element to be measured, and the lamps are filled with a low pressure of argon or neon gas. When a current is passed through the lamp, metal atoms are sputtered off the cathode and collide with the argon or neon in the tube, producing emission of the characteristic wavelengths. A monochromator and photodetector complete the system.

Light reaching the detector is a combination of that which is emitted by the sample (undesirable) and light from the hollow cathode lamp which was not absorbed by the sample in the flame (desirable). By pulsing the light from the lamp either by directly pulsing the lamp or with a chopper, and

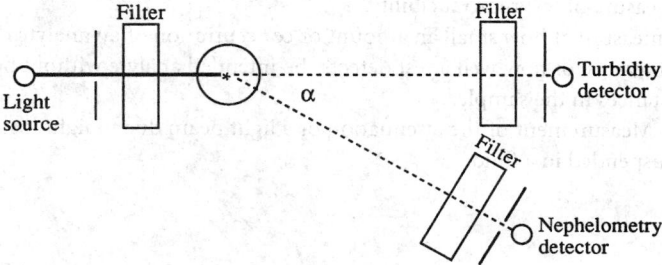

FIGURE 77.5 Nephelometer. Light scattered by large molecules is measured at an angle α away from the axis of incident light. The filters select the wavelength range desired and block undesired fluorescence. When α = 0, the technique is known as turbidimetry.

using a detector which is sensitive to ac signals and insensitive to dc signals, the undesirable emission signal is eliminated. Each element to be measured requires a lamp with that element present in the cathode. Multielement lamps have been developed to minimize the number of lamps required. Atomic absorption spectrophotometers may be either single beam or double beam; the double-beam instruments have greater stability.

There are various flameless methods for atomic absorption spectroscopy in which the burner is replaced with a method for vaporizing the element of interest without a flame. The graphite furnace which heats the sample to 2700° consists of a hollow graphite tube which is heated by passing a large current through it. The sample is placed within the tube, and the light beam is passed through it while the sample is heated.

77.9 Turbidimetry and Nephelometry

Light scattering by particles in solution is directly proportional to both concentration and molecular weight of the particles. For small molecules the scattering is insignificant, but for proteins, immunoglobulins, immune complexes, and other large particles, light scattering can be an effective method for the detection and measurement of particle concentration. For a given wavelength λ of light and particle size d, scattering is described as Raleigh ($d < \lambda/10$), Raleigh-Debye ($d \approx \lambda$), or Mie ($d > 10\lambda$). For particles that are small compared to the wavelength, the scattering is equal in all directions. However, as the particle size becomes larger than the wavelength of light, it becomes preferentially scattered in the forward direction. Light-scattering techniques are widely used to detect the formation of antigen-antibody complexes in immunoassays.

When light scattering is measured by the attenuation of a beam of light through a solution, it is called *turbidimetry*. This is essentially the same as absorption measurements with a photometer except that a large pass-band is acceptable. When maximum sensitivity is required a different method is used—direct measurement of the scattered light with a detector placed at an angle to the central beam. This method is called *nephelometry*. A typical nephelometer will have a light source, filter, sample cuvette, and detector set at an angle to the incident beam (Fig. 77.5).

Defining Terms

Accuracy: The degree to which the average value of repeated measurements approximate the true value being measured.

Fluorescence: Emission of light by an atom or molecule following absorption of a photon of greater energy. Emission normally occurs within 10^{-8} s of absorption.

Nephelometry: Measurement of the amount of light scattered by particles suspended in a fluid.

Precision: A measure of test reproducibility.

Sensitivity: A measure of how small an amount or concentration of an analyte can be detected.

Specificity: A measure of how well a test detects the intended analyte without being "fooled" by other substances in the sample.

Turbidimetry: Measurement of the attenuation of a light beam due to light lost to scattering by particles suspended in a fluid.

References

Burtis CA, Ashwood ER (eds). 1994. Tietz Textbook of Clinical Chemistry, 2d ed, Philadelphia, Saunders.

Hicks MR, Haven MC, Schenken JR, et al. (eds). 1987. Laboratory Instrumentation, 3d ed, Philadelphia: Lippincott.

Kaplan LA, Pesce AJ (eds). 1989. Clinical Chemistry: Theory, Analysis, and Correlation, 2d ed, St. Louis, Mosby.

Tietz NW (ed). 1987. Fundamentals of Clinical Chemistry, 3d ed, Philadelphia, Saunders.

Ward JM, Lehmann CA, Leiken AM. 1994. Clinical Laboratory Instrumentation and Automation: Principles, Applications, and Selection, Philadelphia, Saunders.

78

Clinical Laboratory: Nonspectral Methods and Automation

Richard L. Roa
*Baylor University
Medical Center*

78.1 Particle Counting and Identification

The Coulter principle was the first major advance in automating blood cell counts. The cells to be counted are drawn through a small aperture between two fluid compartments, and the electric impedance between the two compartments is monitored (see Fig. 78.1). As cells pass through the aperture, the impedance increases in proportion to the volume of the cell, allowing large numbers of cells to be counted and sized rapidly. Red cells are counted by pulling diluted blood through the aperture. Since red cells greatly outnumber white cells, the contribution of white cells to the red cell count is usually neglected. White cells are counted by first destroying the red cells and using a more concentrated sample.

Modern cell counters using the Coulter principle often use *hydrodynamic focusing* to improve the performance of the instrument. A sheath fluid is introduced which flows along the outside of a channel with the sample stream inside it. By maintaining laminar flow conditions and narrowing the channel, the sample stream is focused into a very thin column with the cells in single file. This eliminates problems with cells flowing along the side of the aperture or sticking to it and minimizes problems with having more than one cell in the aperture at a time.

Flow cytometry is a method for characterizing, counting, and separating cells which are suspended in a fluid. The basic flow cytometer uses hydrodynamic focusing to produce a very thin stream of fluid containing cells moving in single file through a quartz flow chamber (Fig. 78.2). The cells are characterized on the basis of their scattering and fluorescent properties. This simultaneous measurement of scattering and fluorescence is accomplished with a sophisticated optical system that detects light from the sample both at the wavelength of the excitation source (scattering) as well as at longer wavelengths (fluorescence) at more than one angle. Analysis of these measurements produces parameters related to the cells size, granularity, and natural or tagged fluorescence. High-

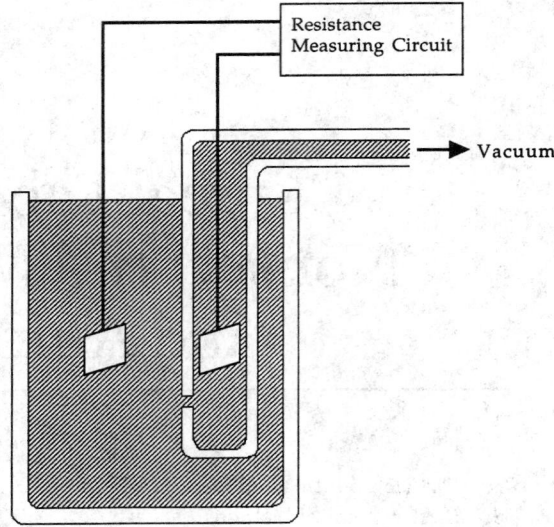

FIGURE 78.1   Coulter method. Blood cells are surrounded by
an insulating membrane, which makes them nonconductive.
The resistance of electrolyte-filled channel will increase slightly
as cells flow through it. This resistance variation yields both the
total number of cells which flow through the channel and the
volume of each cell.

pressure mercury or xenon arc lamps can be used as light sources, but the argon laser (488 nm) is
the preferred source for high-performance instruments.

   One of the more interesting features of this technology is that particular cells may be selected at
rates that allow collection of quantities of particular cell types adequate for further chemical test-

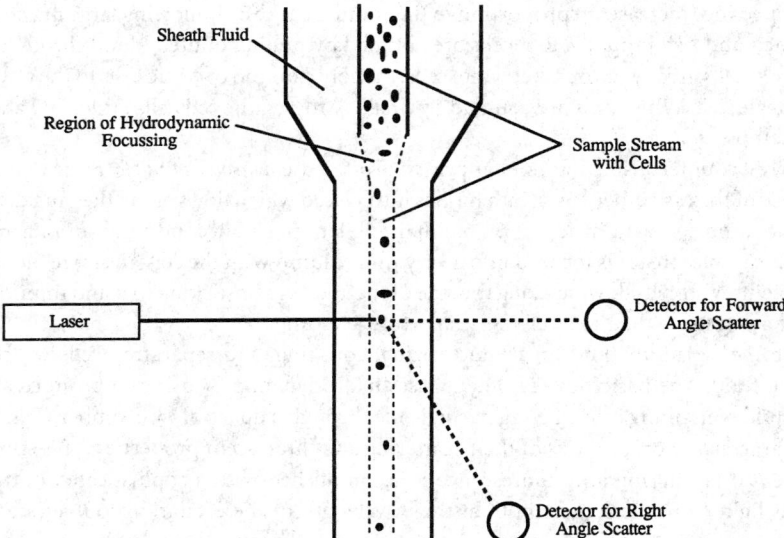

FIGURE 78.2   Flow cytometer. By combining hydrodynamic focusing, state-of-the-art
optics, fluorescent labels, and high-speed computing, large numbers of cells can be characterized and sorted automatically.

ing. This is accomplished by breaking the outgoing stream into a series of tiny droplets using piezo-electric vibration. By charging the stream of droplets and then using deflection plates controlled by the cell analyzer, the cells of interest can be diverted into collection vessels.

The development of monoclonal antibodies coupled with flow cytometry allows for quantitation of T and B cells to assess the status of the immune system as well as characterization of leukemias, lymphomas, and other disorders.

78.2 Electrochemical Methods

Electrochemical methods are increasingly popular in the clinical laboratory, for measurement not only of electrolytes, blood gases, and pH but also of simple compounds such as glucose. *Potentiom-etry* is a method in which a voltage is developed across electrochemical cells as shown in Fig. 78.3. This voltage is measured with little or no current flow.

Ideally, one would like to measure all potentials between the reference solution in the indicator electrode and the test solution. Unfortunately there is no way to do that. Interface potentials develop across any metal-liquid boundary, across liquid junctions, and across the ion-selective membrane. The key to making potentiometric measurements is to ensure that all the potentials are constant and do not vary with the composition of the test solution except for the potential of interest across the ion-selective membrane. By maintaining the solutions within the electrodes constant, the potential between these solutions and the metal electrodes immersed in them is constant. The liquid junction is a structure which severely limits bulk flow of the solution but allows free passage of all ions be-tween the solutions. The reference electrode commonly is filled with saturated KCl, which produces a small, constant liquid-junction potential. Thus, any change in the measured voltage (V) is due to a change in the ion concentration in the test solution for which the membrane is selective.

The potential which develops across an ion-selective membrane is given by the Nernst equation:

$$V = \left(\frac{RT}{zF} \right) \ln \frac{a_2}{a_1} \tag{78.1}$$

where R = gas constant = 8.314 J/K · mol

T = temperature in K

z = ionization number

F = Faraday constant = 9.649×10^4 C/Mol

a_n = activity of ion in solution n

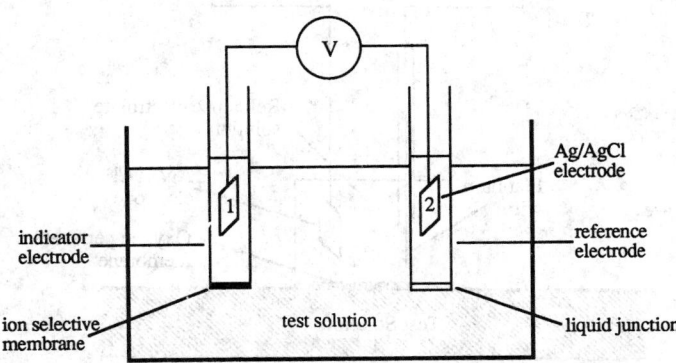

FIGURE 78.3 Electrochemical cell.

When one of the solutions is a reference solution, this equation can be rewritten in a convenient form as

$$V = V_0 + \frac{N}{z} \log_{10} a \qquad (78.2)$$

where V_0 = a constant voltage due to reference solution

$\qquad N$ = Nernst slope $\approx$ 59 mV/decade at room temperature

The actual Nernst slope is usually slightly less than the theoretical value. Thus, the typical pH meter has two calibration controls. One adjusts the offset to account for the value of V_0, and the other adjusts the range to account for both temperature effects and deviations from the theoretical Nernst slope.

78.3 Ion-Specific Electrodes

Ion-selective electrodes use membranes which are permeable only to the ion being measured. To the extent that this can be done, the specificity of the electrode can be very high. One way of overcoming a lack of specificity for certain electrodes is to make multiple simultaneous measurement of several ions which include the most important interfering ones. A simple algorithm can then make corrections for the interfering effects. This technique is used in some commercial electrolyte analyzers. A partial list of the ions that can be measured with ion-selective electrodes includes H^+ (pH), Na^+, K^+, Li^+, Ca^{++}, Cl^-, F^-, NH_4^+, and CO_2.

NH_4^+, and CO_2 both are measured with a modified ion-selective electrode. They use a pH electrode modified with a thin layer of a solution (sodium bicarbonate for CO_2 and ammonium chloride for NH_4^+) whose pH varies depending on the concentration of ammonium ion or CO_2 it is equilibrated with. A thin membrane holds the solution against the pH glass electrode and provides for equilibration with the sample solution. Note that the CO_2 electrode in Fig. 78.4 is a combination

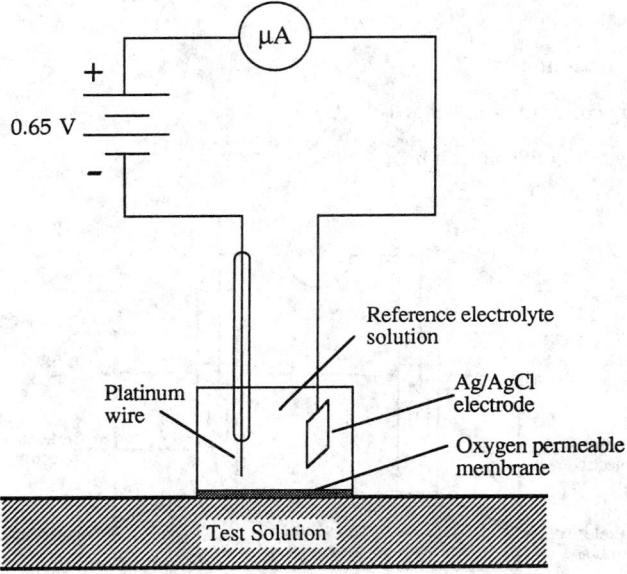

FIGURE 78.4   Clark electrode.

electrode. This means that both the reference and indicating electrodes have been combined into one unit. Most pH electrodes are made as combination electrodes.

The Clark electrode measures pO_2 by measuring the current developed by an electrode with an applied voltage rather than a voltage measurement. This is an example of *amperometry*. In this electrode a voltage of approximately -0.65 V is applied to a platinum electrode relative to a Ag/AgCl electrode in an electrolyte solution. The reaction

$$O_2 + 2H^+ + 2e^- \rightarrow H_2O_2$$

proceeds at a rate proportional to the partial pressure of oxygen in the solution. The electrons involved in this reaction form a current which is proportional to the rate of the reaction and thus to the pO_2 in the solution.

78.4 Radioactive Methods

Isotopes are atoms which have identical atomic number (number of protons) but different atomic mass numbers (protons + neutrons). Since they have the same number of electrons in the neutral atom, they have identical chemical properties. This provides an ideal method for labeling molecules in a way that allows for detection at extremely low concentrations. Labeling with radioactive isotopes is extensively used in radioimmunoassays where the amount of antigen bound to specific antibodies is measured. The details of radioactive decay are complex, but for our purposes there are three types of emission from decaying nuclei: *alpha, beta,* and *gamma radiation*. Alpha particles are made up of two neutrons and two protons (helium nucleus). Alpha emitters are rarely used in the clinical laboratory. Beta emission consists of electrons or positrons emitted from the nucleus. They have a continuous range of energies up to a maximum value characteristic of the isotope. Beta radiation is highly interactive with matter and cannot penetrate very far in most materials. Gamma radiation is a high-energy form of electromagnetic radiation. This type of radiation may be continuous, discrete, or mixed depending on the details of the decay process. It has greater penetrating ability than beta radiation. (See Fig. 78.5.)

The kinetic energy spectrum of emitted radiation is characteristic of the isotope. The energy is commonly measured in electron volts (eV). One electron volt is the energy acquired by an electron

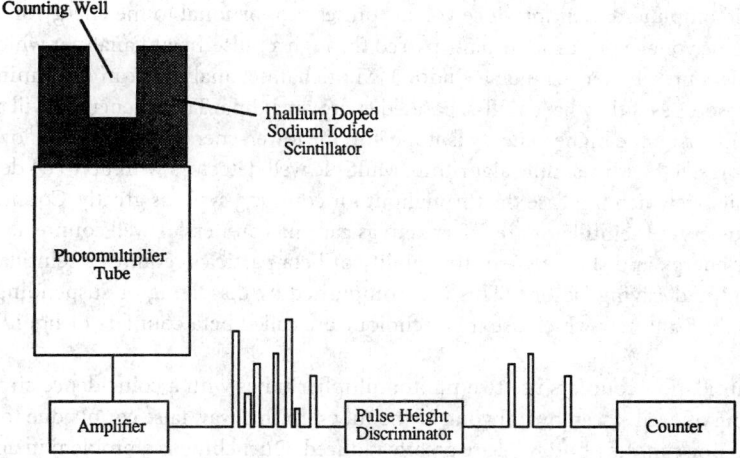

FIGURE 78.5 Gamma counted. The intensity of the light flash produced when a gamma photon interacts with a scintillator is proportional to the energy of the photon. The photomultiplier tube converts these light flashes into electric pulses which can be selected according to size (gamma energy) and counted.

falling through a potential of 1 volt. The isotopes commonly used in the clinical laboratory have energy spectra which range from 18 keV–3.6 MeV.

The activity of a quantity of radioactive isotope is defined as the number of disintegrations per second which occur. The usual units are the curie (Ci), which is defined as 3.7×10^{10} dps, and the becquerel (Bq), defined as 1 dps. Specific activity for a given isotope is defined as activity per unit mass of the isotope.

The rate of decay for a given isotope is characterized by the decay constant λ, which is the proportion of the isotope which decays in unit time. Thus, the rate of loss of radioactive isotope is governed by the equation

$$\frac{dN}{dt} = -\lambda N \tag{78.3}$$

where N is the amount of radioactive isotope present at time t. The solution to this differential equation is:

$$N = N_0 e^{-\lambda t} \tag{78.4}$$

It can easily be shown that the amount of radioactive isotope present will be reduced by half after time

$$t_{1/2} = \frac{0.693}{\lambda} \tag{78.5}$$

This is known as the half-life for the isotope and can vary widely; for example, carbon-14 has a half-life of 5760 years, and iodine-131 has a half-life of 8.1 days.

The most common method for detection of radiation in the clinical laboratory is by scintillation. This is the conversion of radiation energy into photons in the visible or near-UV range. These are detected with photomultiplier tubes.

For gamma radiation, the scintillating crystal is made of sodium iodide doped with about 1% thallium, producing 20 to 30 photons for each electron-volt of energy absorbed. The photomultiplier tube and amplifier circuit produce voltage pulses proportional to the energy of the absorbed radiation. These voltage pulses are usually passed through a pulse-height analyzer which eliminates pulses outside a preset energy range (window). Multichannel analyzers can discriminate between two or more isotopes if they have well-separated energy maxima. There generally will be some spill down of counts from the higher-energy isotope into the lower-energy isotope's window, but this effect can be corrected with a simple algorithm. Multiple well detectors with up to 64 detectors in an array are available which increase the throughput for counting systems greatly. Counters using the sodium iodide crystal scintillator are referred to as gamma counters or well counters.

The lower energy and short penetration ability of beta particles requires a scintillator in direct contact with the decaying isotope. This is accomplished by dissolving or suspending the sample in a liquid fluor. Counters which use this technique are called beta counters or liquid scintillation counters.

Liquid scintillation counters use two photomultiplier tubes with a coincidence circuit that prevents counting of events seen by only one of the tubes. In this way, false counts due to chemiluminescence and noise in the phototube are greatly reduced. Quenching is a problem in all liquid scintillation counters. Quenching is any process which reduces the efficiency of the scintillation counting process, where efficiency is defined as

$$\text{Efficiency} = \text{counts per minute/decays per minute} \tag{78.6}$$

A number of techniques have been developed that automatically correct for quenching effects to produce estimates of true decays per minute from the raw counts. Currently there is a trend away from beta-emitting isotopic labels, but these assays are still used in many laboratories.

78.5 Coagulation Timers

Screening for and diagnosis of coagulation disorders is accomplished by assays that determine how long it takes for blood to clot following initiation of the clotting cascade by various reagents. A variety of instruments has been designed to automate this procedure. In addition to increasing the speed and throughput of such testing, these instruments improve the reproducibility of such tests. All the instruments provide precise introduction of reagents, accurate timing circuits, and temperature control. They differ in the method for detecting clot formation. One of the older methods still in use is to dip a small metal hook into the blood sample repeatedly and lift it a few millimeters above the surface. The electric resistance between the hook and the sample is measured, and when fibrin filaments form, they produce a conductive pathway which is detected as clot formation. Other systems detect the increase in viscosity due to fibrin formation or the scattering due to the large polymerized molecules formed. Absorption and fluorescence spectroscopy can also be used for clot detection.

78.6 Osmometers

The *colligative properties* of a solution are a function of the number of solute particles present regardless of size or identity. Increased solute concentration causes an increase in osmotic pressure and boiling point and a decrease in vapor pressure and freezing point. Measuring these changes provides information on the total solute concentration regardless of type. The most accurate and popular method used in the clinical laboratories is the measurement of freezing point depression. With this method, the sample is supercooled to a few degrees below 0°C while being stirred gently. Freezing is then initiated by vigorous stirring. The heat of fusion quickly brings the solution to a slushy state where an equilibrium exists between ice and liquid, ensuring that the temperature is at the freezing point. This temperature is measured. A solute concentration of 1 osmol/kg water produces a freezing point depression of 1.858°C. The measured temperature depression is easily calibrated in units of milliosmols/kg water.

The vapor pressure depression method has the advantage of smaller sample size. However, it is not as precise as the freezing point method and cannot measure the contribution of volatile solutes such as ethanol. This method is not used as widely as the freezing point depression method in clinical laboratories.

Osmolality of blood is primarily due to electrolytes such as Na^+ and Cl^-. Proteins with molecular weights of 30,000 or more atomic mass units (amu) contribute very little to total osmolality due to their smaller numbers (a single Na^+ ion contributes just as much to osmotic pressure as a large protein molecule). However, the contribution to osmolality made by proteins is of great interest when monitoring conditions leading to pulmonary edema. This value is known as colloid osmotic pressure, or oncotic pressure, and is measured with a membrane permeable to water and all molecules smaller than about 30,000 amu. By placing a reference saline solution on one side and the unknown sample on the other, an osmotic pressure is developed across the membrane. This pressure is measured with a pressure transducer and can be related to the true colloid osmotic pressure through a calibration procedure using known standards.

78.7 Automation

Improvements in technology coupled with increased demand for laboratory tests as well as pressures to reduce costs have led to the rapid development of highly automated laboratory instruments.

Typical automated instruments contain mechanisms for measuring, mixing, and transport of samples and reagents, measurement systems, and one or more microprocessors to control the entire system. In addition to system control, the computer systems store calibration curves, match test results to specimen IDs, and generate reports. Automated instruments are dedicated to complete blood counts, coagulation studies, microbiology assays, and immunochemistry, as well as high-volume instruments used in the clinical chemistry laboratories. The chemistry analyzers tend to fall into one of four classes: continuous flow, centrifugal, pack-based, and dry-slide-based systems. The continuous flow systems pass successive samples and reagents through a single set of tubing, where they are directed to appropriate mixing, dialyzing, and measuring stations. Carry-over from one sample to the next is minimized by the introduction of air bubbles and wash solution between samples.

Centrifugal analyzers use plastic rotors which serve as reservoirs for samples and reagents and also as cuvettes for optical measurements. Spinning the plastic rotor mixes, incubates, and transports the test solution into the cuvette portion of the rotor, where the optical measurements are made while the rotor is spinning.

Pack-based systems are those in which each test uses a special pack with the proper reagents and sample preparation devices built-in. The sample is automatically introduced into as many packs as tests required. The packs are then processed sequentially.

Dry chemistry analyzers use no liquid reagents. The reagents and other sample preparation methods are layered onto a slide. The liquid sample is placed on the slide, and after a period of time the color developed is read by reflectance photometry. Ion-selective electrodes have been incorporated into the same slide format.

There are a number of technological innovations found in many of the automated instruments. One innovation is the use of fiberoptic bundles to channel excitation energy toward the sample as well as transmitted, reflected, or emitted light away from the sample to the detectors. This provides a great deal of flexibility in instrument layout. Multiwavelength analysis using a spinning filter wheel or diode array detectors is commonly found. The computers associated with these instruments allow for innovative improvements in the assays. For instance, when many analytes are being analyzed from one sample, the interference effects of one analyte on the measurement of another can be predicted and corrected before the final report is printed.

78.8 Trends in Laboratory Instrumentation

Predicting the future direction of laboratory instrumentation is difficult, but there seem to be some clear trends. Decentralization of the laboratory functions will continue with more instruments being located in or around ICUs, operating rooms, emergency rooms, and physician offices. More electrochemistry-based tests will be developed. The flame photometer is already being replaced with ion-selective electrode methods. Instruments which analyze whole blood rather than *plasma* or *serum* will reduce the amount of time required for sample preparation and will further encourage testing away from the central laboratory. Dry reagent methods increasingly will replace wet chemistry methods. Radioimmunoassays will continue to decline with the increasing use of methods for performing immunoassays that do not rely upon radioisotopes such as enzyme-linked fluorescent assays.

Defining Terms

Alpha radiation: Particulate radiation consisting of a helium nucleus emitted from a decaying anucleus.

Amperometry: Measurements based on current flow produced in an electrochemical cell by an applied voltage.

Beta radiation: Particulate radiation consisting of an electron or positron emitted from a decaying nucleus.

Colligative properties: Physical properties that depend on the number of molecules present rather than on their individual properties.

Gamma radiation: Electromagnetic radiation emitted from an atom undergoing nuclear decay.

Hydrodynamic focusing: A process in which a fluid stream is first surrounded by a second fluid and then narrowed to a thin stream by a narrowing of the channel.

Isotopes: Atoms with the same number of protons but differing numbers of neutrons.

Plasma: The liquid portion of blood.

Potentiometry: Measurement of the potential produced by electrochemical cells under equilibrium conditions with no current flow.

Scintillation: The conversion of the kinetic energy of a charged particle or photon to a flash of light.

Serum: The liquid portion of blood remaining after clotting has occurred.

References

Burtis CA, Ashwood ER (eds). 1994. Tietz Textbook of Clinical Chemistry, 2d ed, Philadelphia, Saunders Company.

Hicks MR, Haven MC, Schenken JR, et al. (eds). 1987. Laboratory Instrumentation, 3d ed, Philadelphia, Lippincott Company, 1987

Kaplan LA, Pesce AJ (eds). 1989. Clinical Chemistry: Theory, Analysis, and Correlation, 2d ed, St. Louis, Mosby.

Tietz NW (ed). 1987. Fundamentals of Clinical Chemistry, 3d ed, Philadelphia, Saunders.

Ward JM, Lehmann CA, Leiken AM. 1994. Clinical Laboratory Instrumentation and Automation: Principles, Applications, and Selection, Philadelphia, Saunders.

79

Implantable Cardiac Pacemakers

Michael Forde
Medtronic, Inc.

Pat Ridgely
Medtronic, Inc.

The practical use of an implantable device for delivering a controlled, rhythmic electric stimulus to maintain the heartbeat is relatively recent: Cardiac pacemakers have been in clinical use only slightly more than 30 years. Although devices have gotten steadily smaller over this period (from 250 grams in 1960 to 25 grams today), the technological evolution goes far beyond size alone. Early devices provided only single-chamber, asynchronous, *nonprogrammable* pacing coupled with questionable reliability and longevity. Today, advanced electronics afford dual-chamber multi*programmability,* diagnostic functions, rate response, data collection, and exceptional reliability, and lithium-iodine power sources extend longevity to upward of 10 years. Continual advances in a number of clinical, scientific, and engineering disciplines have so expanded the use of pacing that it now provides cost-effective benefits to an estimated 350,000 patients worldwide each year.

The modern pacing system is comprised of three distinct components: pulse generator, lead, and programmer (Fig. 79.1). The pulse generator houses the battery and the circuitry which generates the stimulus and senses electrical activity. The lead is an insulated wire that carries the stimulus from the generator to the heart and relays intrinsic cardiac signals back to the generator. The programmer is a telemetry device used to provide two-way communication between the generator and the clinician. It can alter the therapy delivered by the pacemaker and retrieve diagnostic data that are essential for optimally titrating that therapy. Ultimately, the therapeutic success of the pacing prescription rests on the clinician's choice of an appropriate system, use of sound implant technique, and programming focused on patient outcomes.

This chapter discusses in further detail the components of the modern pacing system and the significant evolution that has occurred since its inception. Our focus is on system design and operations, but we also briefly overview issues critical to successful clinical performance.

79.1 Indications

The decision to implant a permanent pacemaker for bradyarrhythmias usually is based on the major goals of symptom relief (at rest and with physical activity), restoration of functional capacity and

0-8493-8346-3/95/$0.00+$.50
© 1995 by CRC Press, Inc.

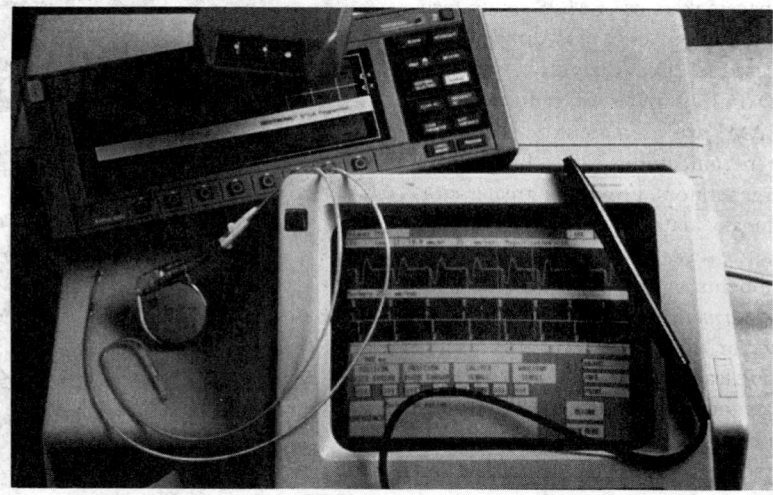

FIGURE 79.1 The pacing systems comprise a programmer, pulse generator, and lead. There are two programmers pictured above; one is portable, and the other is an office-based unit.

quality of life, and reduced mortality. As with other healthcare technologies, appropriate use of pacing is the intent of indications guidelines established by Medicare and other third-party payors.

In 1984 and again in 1991, a joint commission of the American College of Cardiology and the American Heart Association established guidelines for pacemaker implantation [Committee on Pacemaker Implantation, 1991]. In general, pacing is indicated when there is a dramatic slowing of the heart rate or a failure in the connection between the atria and ventricles resulting in decreased cardiac output manifested by such symptoms as syncope, light-headedness, fatigue, and exercise intolerance. Failure of impulse formation and/or conduction is the overriding theme of all pacemaker indications. There are four categories of pacing indications:

1. Heart block (e.g., complete heart block, symptomatic 2° AV block)
2. Sick sinus syndrome (e.g., symptomatic bradycardia, sinus arrest, sinus exit block)
3. Myocardial infarction (e.g., conduction disturbance related to the site of infarction)
4. Hypersensitive carotid sinus syndrome (e.g., recurrent syncope)

Within each of these four categories the ACC/AHA provided criteria for classifying a condition as group I (pacing is considered necessary), group II (pacing may be necessary), or group III (pacing is considered inappropriate).

New indications for cardiac pacing are being evaluated under the jurisdiction of the Food and Drug Administration. For example, *hypertrophic obstructive cardiomyopathy* (HOCM) is one of these new potential indications, with researchers looking at dual-chamber pacing as a means of reducing left ventricular outflow obstruction. Though efforts in these areas are ongoing and expanding, for now they remain unapproved as standard indications for pacing.

79.2 Pulse Generators

The pulse generator contains a power source, output circuit, sensing circuit, and a timing circuit (Fig. 79.2). A telemetry coil is used to send and receive information between the generator and the programmer. *Rate-adaptive* pulse generators include the sensor components along with the circuit to process the information measured by the sensor.

Modern pacemakers use *CMOS circuit* technology. One to 2 kilobytes of read-only memory (ROM) are used to direct the output and sensing circuits; 16–512 bytes of random-access memory (RAM) are used to store diagnostic data. Some manufacturers offer fully RAM-based pulse generators, providing greater storage of diagnostic data and the flexibility for changing feature sets after implantation.

All components of the pulse generator are housed in a *hermetically* sealed titanium case with a connector block that accepts the lead(s). Because pacing leads are available with a variety of different connector sites and configurations, the pulse generator is available with an equal variety of connectors. The outer casing is laser-etched with the manufacturer, name, type (e.g., single- versus dual-chamber), model number,

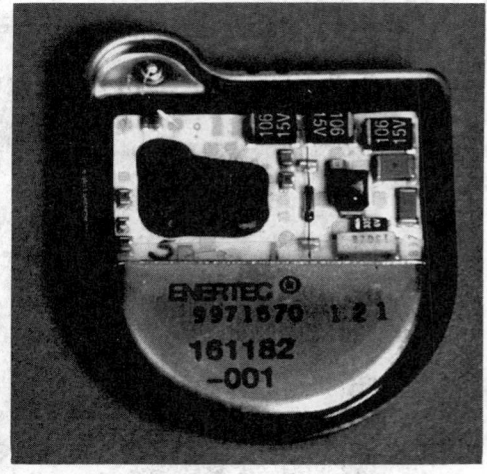

FIGURE 79.2   Internal view of pulse generator.

serial number, and the lead connection diagram for each identification. Once implanted, it may be necessary to use an x-ray to reveal the identity of the generator. Some manufacturers use radiopaque symbols and ID codes for this purpose, whereas others give their generators characteristic shapes.

Sensing Circuit

Pulse generators have two basic functions, pacing and sensing. Sensing refers to the recognition of an appropriate signal by the pulse generator. This signal is the intrinsic cardiac depolarization from the chamber or chambers in which the leads are placed. It is imperative for the sensing circuit to discriminate between these intracardiac signals and unwanted electrical interference such as far-field cardiac events, diastolic potentials, skeletal muscle contraction, and pacing stimuli. An intracardiac electrogram (Fig. 79.3) shows the waveform as seen by the pacemaker; it is typically quite different from the corresponding event as shown on the surface ECG.

Sensing (and pacing) is accomplished with one of two configurations, bipolar and unipolar. In bipolar, the anode and cathode are close together, with the anode at the tip of the lead and the cathode a ring electrode about 2 cm proximal to the tip. In unipolar, the anode and cathode may be 5–10 cm apart. The anode is at the lead tip and the cathode is the pulse generator itself (usually located in the pectoral region).

In general, bipolar and unipolar sensing configurations have equal performance. A drawback of the unipolar approach is the increased possibility of sensing noncardiac signals: The large electrode separation may, for example, sense myopotentials from skeletal muscle movement, leading to inappropriate inhibition of pacing. Many newer pacemakers can be programmed to sense or pace in either configuration.

Once the electrogram enters the sensing circuit, it is scrutinized by a bandpass filter (Fig. 79.4). The frequency of an R-wave is 10 to 30 Hz. The center frequency of most sensing amplifiers is 30 Hz. T-waves are slower, broad signals that are composed of lower frequencies (approximately 5 Hz or less). Far-field signals are also lower-frequency signals, whereas skeletal muscle falls in the range of 10–200 Hz.

At the implant, the voltage amplitude of the *R*-wave (and the *P*-wave, in the case of dual-chamber pacing) is measured to ensure the availability of an adequate signal. *R*-wave amplitudes are typically 5–25 mV, and *P*-wave amplitudes are 2–6 mV. The signals passing through the sense amplifier are compared to an adjustable reference voltage called the *sensitivity*. Any signal below the reference voltage is not sensed, and those above it are sensed. Higher-sensitivity settings (high-reference volt-

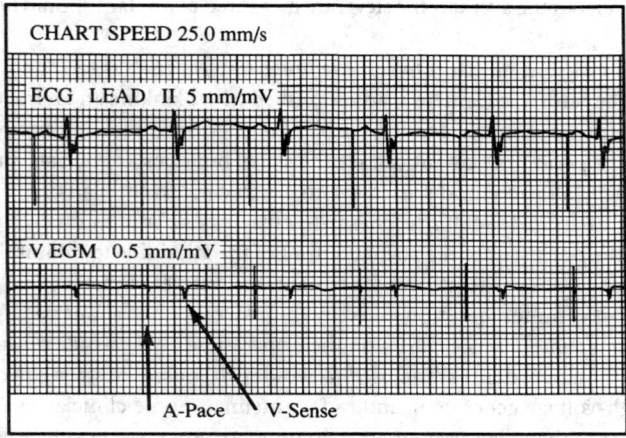

FIGURE 79.3 The surface ECG (ECG LEAD II) represents the sum total of the electrical potentials of all depolarizing tissue. The intracardiac electrogram (V EGM) shows only the potentials measured between the lead electrodes. This allows the evaluation of signals that may be hidden within the surface ECG.

age) may lead to substandard sensing, and a lower reference voltage may result in oversensing. A minimum 2:1 safety margin should be maintained between the sensitivity setting and the amplitude of the intracardiac signal. The circuit is protected from extremely high voltages by a Zener diode.

The slope of the signal is also surveyed by the sensing circuit and is determined by the slew rate (the time rate of change in voltage). A slew rate that is too flat or too steep may be eliminated

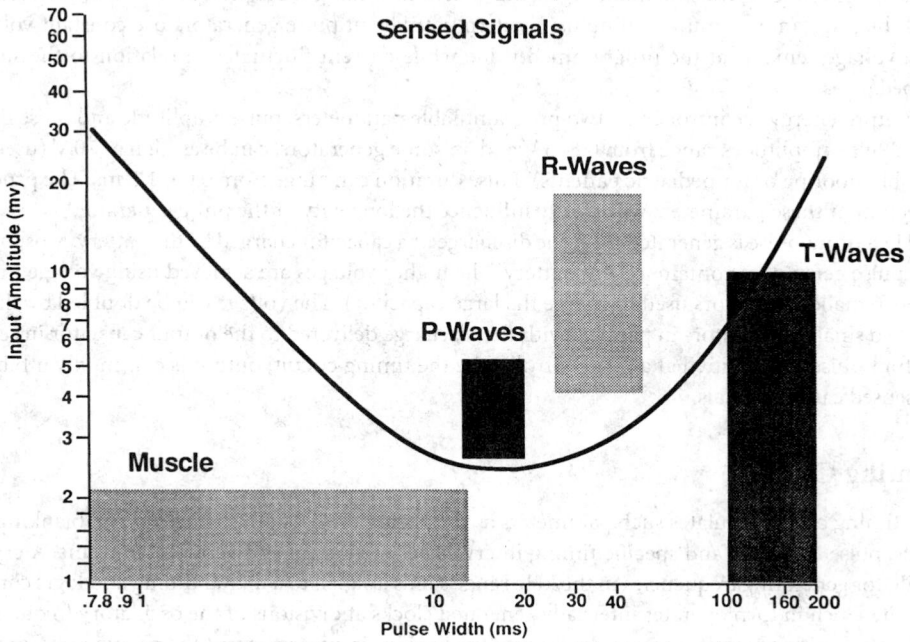

FIGURE 79.4 This is a conceptual depiction of the bandpass filter demonstrating the typical filtering of unwanted signals by discriminating between those with slew rates that are too low and/or too high.

by the bandpass filter. On the average, the slew rate measured at implant should be between 0.75 and 2.50 V/s.

The last line of defense in an effort to remove undesirable signals is to "blind" the circuit at specific times during the cardiac cycle. This is accomplished with blanking and refractory periods. Some of these periods are programmable. During the blanking period the sensing circuit is turned off, and during the refractory period the circuit can see the signal but does not initiate any of the basic timing intervals. Virtually all paced and sensed events begin concurrent blanking and refractory periods, typically ranging from 10–400 ms. These are especially helpful in dual-chamber pacemakers where there exists the potential for the pacing output of the atrial side to inhibit the ventricular pacing output, with dangerous consequences for patients in complete heart block.

Probably the most common question asked by the general public about pacing systems is the effect of electromagnetic interference (EMI) on their operation. EMI outside of the hospital is an infrequent problem, though patients are advised to avoid such sources of strong electromagnetic fields as arc welders, high-voltage generators, and radar antennae. Some clinicians suggest that patients avoid standing near antitheft devices used in retail stores. Airport screening devices are generally safe, though they may detect a pacemaker's metal case. Microwave ovens, ham radio equipment, video games, computers, and office equipment rarely interfere with the operation of modern pacemakers. A number of medical devices and procedures may on occasion do so, however: electrocautery, cardioversion and defibrillation, MRI, lithotripsy, diathermy, TENS units, and radiation therapy.

Pacemakers affected by interference typically respond with temporary loss of output or temporary reversion to asynchronous pacing (pacing at a fixed rate, with no inhibition from intrinsic cardiac events). The usual consequence for the patient is a return of the symptoms that originally led to the pacemaker implant.

Output Circuit

Pacing is the most significant drain on the pulse generator power source. Therefore, current drain must be minimized while maintaining an adequate safety margin between the *stimulation threshold* and the programmed output stimulus. Modern permanent pulse generators use constant voltage. The voltage remains at the programmed value while current fluctuates in relation to the source impedance.

Output energy is controlled by two programmable parameters, pulse amplitude and pulse duration. Pulse amplitudes range from 0.8–5 V and, in some generators, can be high as 10 V (used for troubleshooting or for pediatric patients). Pulse duration can range from 0.05–1.5 ms. The prudent selection of these parameters will greatly influence the longevity of the pulse generator.

The output pulse is generated from the discharge of a capacitor charged by the battery. Most modern pulse generators contain a 2.8 V battery. The higher voltages are achieved using voltage multipliers (smaller capacitors used to charge the large capacitor). The voltage can be doubled by charging two smaller capacitors in parallel, with the discharge delivered to the output capacitor in series. Output pulses are emitted at a rate controlled by the timing circuit; output is commonly inhibited by sensed cardiac signals.

Timing Circuit

The timing circuit regulates such parameters as the pacing cycle length, refractory and blanking periods, pulse duration, and specific timing intervals between atrial and ventricular events. A crystal oscillator generating frequencies in the kHz range sends a signal to a digital timing and logic control circuit, which in turn operates internally generated clocks at divisions of the oscillatory frequency.

A rate-limiting circuit is incorporated into the timing circuit to prevent the pacing rate from exceeding an upper limit should a random component failure occur (an extremely rare event). This is also referred to as "runaway" protection and is typically 180–200 ppm.

Telemetry Circuit

Today's pulse generators are capable of both transmitting information from an RF antenna and receiving information with an RF decoder. This two-way communication occurs between the pulse generator and the programmer at approximately 300 Hz. Real-time telemetry is the term used to describe the ability of the pulse generator to provide information such as pulse amplitude, pulse duration, lead impedance, battery impedance, lead current, charge, and energy. The programmer, in turn, delivers coded messages to the pulse generator to alter any of the programmable features and to retrieve diagnostic data. Coding requirements reduce the likelihood of inappropriate programming alterations by environmental sources of radiofrequency and magnetic fields. It also prevents the improper use of programmers from other manufacturers.

Power Source

Over the years, a number of different battery technologies have been tried, including mercury-zinc, rechargeable silver-modified-mercuric-oxide-zinc, rechargeable nickel-cadmium, radioactive plutonium or promethium, and lithium with a variety of different cathodes. Lithium-cupric-sulfide and mercury-zinc batteries were associated with corrosion and early failure. Mercury-zinc produced hydrogen gas as a by-product of the battery reaction; the venting required made it impossible to hermetically seal the generator. This led to fluid infiltration followed by the risk of sudden failure.

The longevity of very early pulse generators was measured in hours. With the lithium-iodide technology now used, longevity has been reported as high as 15 years. The clinical desire to have a generator that is small and full-featured yet also long-lasting poses a formidable challenge to battery designers. One response by manufacturers has been to offer different models of generators, each offering a different balance between therapy, size, and longevity. Typical *battery capacity* is in the range of 0.8–3.0 amp-hours.

Many factors affect longevity, including pulse amplitude and duration, pacing rate, single- versus dual-chamber pacing, degree to which the patient uses the pacemaker, lead design, and static current drain from the sensing circuits. Improvements in lead design are often overlooked as a factor in improving longevity, but electrodes used in 1960 required a pulse generator output of 675 µJ for effective stimulation, whereas the electrodes of the 1990s need only 3–6 µJ.

Another important factor in battery design lies in the electrolyte that separates the anode and the cathode. The semisolid layer of lithium iodide that is used gradually thickens over the life of the cell, increasing the internal resistance of the battery. The voltage produced by lithium-iodine batteries is inversely related to this resistance and is linear from 2.8 V to approximately 2.4 V, representing about 90% of the usable battery life. It then declines exponentially to 1.8 V as the internal battery resistance increases from 10,000 Ω to 40,000 Ω (Fig. 79.5).

When the battery reaches between 2.0 and 2.4 V (depending on the manufacturer), certain functions of the pulse generator are altered so as to alert the clinician. These alterations are called the elective-replacement indicators (ERI). They vary from one pulse generator to another and include signature decreases in rate, a change to a specific pacing *mode,* pulse duration stretching, and the telemetered battery voltage. When the battery voltage reaches 1.8 V, the pulse generator may operate erratically or cease to function and is said to have reached "end of life." The time period between appearance of the ERI and end-of-life status averages about 3 to 4 months.

79.3 Leads

Implantable pacing leads must be designed not only for consistent performance within the hostile environment of the body but also for easy handling by the implanting physician. Every lead has four major components (Fig. 79.6): the electrode, the conductor, the insulation, and the connector pin(s).

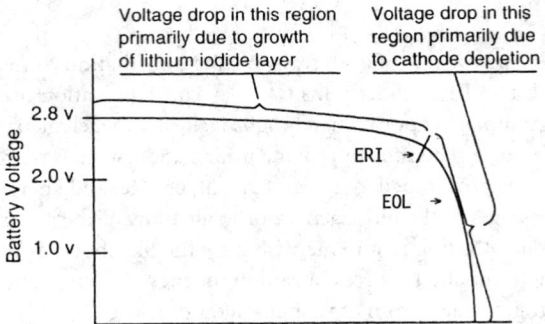

FIGURE 79.5 The initial decline in battery voltage is slow and then more rapid after the battery reaches the ERI voltage. An important aspect of battery design is the predictability of this decline so that timely generator replacement is anticipated.

The electrode is located at the tip of the lead and is in direct contact with the myocardium. Bipolar leads have a tip electrode and a ring electrode (located about 2 cm proximal to the tip); unipolar leads have tip electrodes only. A small-radius electrode provides increased current density resulting in lower stimulation thresholds. The electrode also increases resistance at the electrode-myocardial interface, thus lowering the current drain further and improving battery longevity. The radius of most electrodes is 6–8 mm², though there are clinical trials underway using a "high-impedance" lead with a tip radius as low as 1.5 mm².

Small electrodes, however, historically have been associated with inferior sensing performance. Lead designers were able to achieve both good pacing and good sensing by creating porous-tip electrodes containing thousands of pores in the 20–100 μm range. The pores allow the ingrowth of tissue, resulting in the necessary increase in effective sensing area while maintaining a small pacing area. Some commonly used electrode materials include platinum-iridium, Elgiloy (an alloy of cobalt, iron, chromium, molybdenum, nickel, and manganese), platinum coated with platinized titanium, and vitreous or pyrolytic carbon coating a titanium or graphite core.

Another major breakthrough in lead design is the steroid-eluting electrode. About 1 mg of a corticosteroid (dexamethasone sodium phosphate) is contained in a silicone core that is surrounded by the electrode material (Fig. 79.7). The "leaking" of the steroid into the myocardium occurs slowly over several years and reduces the inflammation that results from the lead placement. It also retards the growth of the fibrous sack that forms around the electrode which separates it from viable myocardium. As a result, the dramatic rise in acute thresholds that is seen with nonsteroid leads over the 8 to 16 weeks postimplant is nearly eliminated. This makes it possible to program a lower pacing output, further extending longevity.

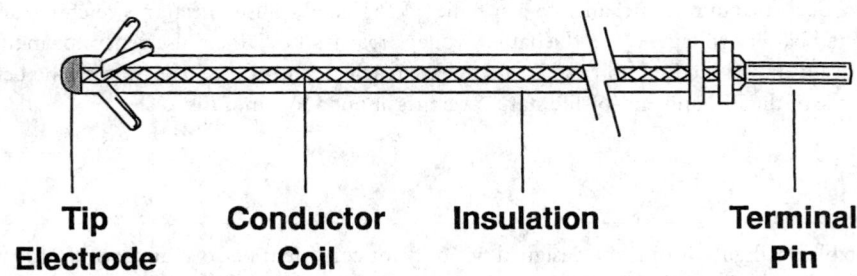

Tip   Conductor   Insulation   Terminal
Electrode   Coil   Pin

FIGURE 79.6 The four major lead components.

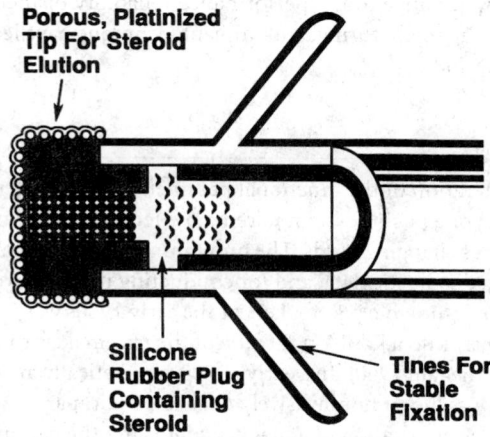

Porous, Platinized Tip For Steroid Elution

Silicone Rubber Plug Containing Steroid

Tines For Stable Fixation

FIGURE 79.7 The steroid elution electrode.

Once a lead has been implanted, it must remain stable (or fixated). The fixation device is either active or passive. The active fixation leads incorporate corkscrew mechanisms, barbs, or hooks to attach themselves to the myocardium. The passive fixation leads are held into place with tines that become entangled into the netlike lining (trabeculae) of the heart. Passive leads generally have better acute pacing and sensing performance but are difficult to remove chronically. Active leads are easier to remove chronically and have the advantage of unlimited placement sites. Some implanters prefer to use active-fixation leads in the atrium and passive-fixation leads in the ventricle.

The conductor carries electric signals to the pulse generator and delivers the pacing pulses to the heart. It must be strong and flexible to withstand the repeated flexing stress placed on it by the beating heart. The early conductors were a single, straight wire that was vulnerable to fracturing. They have evolved into coiled (for increased flexibility) multifilar (to prevent complete failure with partial fractures) conductors. The conductor material is a nickel alloy called MP35N. Because of the need for two conductors, bipolar leads are usually larger in diameter than unipolar leads. Current bipolar leads have a coaxial design that has significantly reduced the diameter of bipolar leads.

Insulation materials (typically silicone and polyurethane) are used to isolate the conductor. Silicone has a longer history and the exclusive advantage of being repairable. Because of low tear strength, however, silicone leads tend to be thicker than polyurethane leads. Another relative disadvantage of silicone is its high coefficient of friction in blood, which makes it difficult for two leads to pass through the same vein. A coating applied to silicone leads during manufacturing has diminished this problem.

A variety of generator-lead connector configurations and adapters are available. Because incompatibility can result in disturbed (or even lost) pacing and sensing, an international standard (IS-1) has been developed in an attempt to minimize incompatibility.

Leads can be implanted epicardially and endocardially. *Epicardial* leads are placed on the outer surface of the heart and require the surgical exposure of a small portion of the heart. They are used when venous occlusion makes it impossible to pass a lead transvenously, when abdominal placement of the pulse generator is needed (as in the case of radiation therapy to the pectoral area), or in children (to allow for growth). *Endocardial* leads are more common and perform better in the long term. These leads are passed through the venous system and into the right side of the heart. The subclavian or cephalic veins in the pectoral region are common entry sites. Positioning is facilitated by a thin, firm wire stylet that passes through the central lumen of the lead, stiffening it. Fluoroscopy is used to visualize lead positioning and to confirm the desired location.

Manufacturers are very sensitive to the performance reliability of their leads. Steady improvements in materials, design, manufacturing, and implant technique have led to reliability well in excess of 99% over 3-year periods.

79.4 Programmers

Noninvasive reversible alteration of the functional parameters of the pacemaker is critical to ongoing clinical management. For a pacing system to remain effective throughout its lifetime, it must be able to adjust to the patient's changing needs. The programmer is the primary clinical tool for changing settings, for retrieving diagnostic data, and for conducting noninvasive tests.

The pacing rate for programmable pacemakers of the early 1960s was adjusted via a Keith needle manipulated percutaneously into a knob on the side of the pacemaker; rotating the needle changed the pacing rate. Through the late 1960s and early 1970s, magnetically attuned reed switches in the pulse generator made it possible to noninvasively change certain parameters such as rate, output, sensitivity, and polarity. The application of a magnet could alter the parameters which were usually limited to only one of two choices. It wasn't until the late 1970s, when radiofrequency energy was incorporated as the transmitter of information, that programmability began to realize its full potential. Radiofrequency transmission is faster, provides bidirectional telemetry, and decreases the possibility of unintended programming from inappropriate sources.

Most manufacturers today are moving away from a dedicated proprietary instrument and toward a PC-based design. The newer designs are generally more flexible, more intuitive to use, and more easily updated when new devices are released. Manufacturers and clinicians alike are becoming more sensitive to the role that time-efficient programming can play in the productivity of pacing clinics, which may provide follow-up for as many as 500–1000 patients a year.

79.5 System Operation

Pacemakers have gotten steadily more powerful over the last three decades, but at the cost of steadily greater complexity. Manufacturers have come to realize the challenge that this poses for busy clinicians and have responded with a variety of interpretive aids (Fig. 79.8).

Much of the apparent complexity of the timing rules that determine pacemaker operation is due to a design goal of mimicking normal cardiac function without interfering with it. One example is the dual-chamber feature that provides sequential stimulation of the atrium before the ventricle.

Another example is rate response, designed for patients who lack the normal ability to increase their heart rate in response to a variety of physical conditions (e.g., exercise). Introduced in the mid-1980s, rate-responsive systems use some sort of sensor to measure the change in a physical variable correlated to heart rate. The sensor output is signal-processed and then used by the output circuit to specify a target pacing rate. The clinician controls the aggressiveness of the rate increase through a variety of parameters (including a choice of transfer function); pacemaker-resident diagnostics provide data helpful in titrating the rate-response therapy.

The most common sensor is the activity sensor, which uses piezoelectric materials to detect vibrations caused by body movement. Systems using a transthoracic-impedance sensor to estimate pulmonary *minute ventilation* are also commercially available. Numerous other sensors (e.g., stroke volume, blood temperature or pH, oxygen saturation, preejection interval, right ventricular pressure) are in various stages of clinical research or have been market released outside the United States. Some of these systems are dual-sensor, combining the best features of each sensor in a single pacing system.

To make it easier to understand the gross-level system operation of modern pacemakers, a five-letter code has been developed by the North American Society of Pacing and Electrophysiology and the British Pacing and Electrophysiology Group [Bernstein et al., 1987]. The first letter indicates the chamber (or chambers) that are paced. The second letter reveals those chambers in which sensing takes place, and the third letter describes how the pacemaker will respond to a sensed event. The

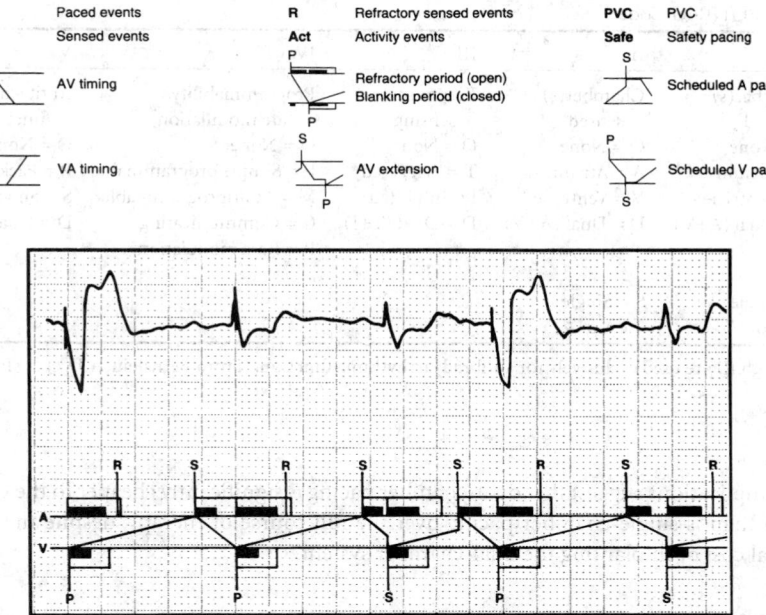

| P | Paced events | | R | Refractory sensed events | | **PVC** | PVC |
| S | Sensed events | | **Act** | Activity events | | **Safe** | Safety pacing |

FIGURE 79.8 The Marker Channel Diagram is just one tool that makes interpretation of the ECG strip faster and more reliable for the clinician. It allows quick checking of the timing operations of the system.

pacemaker will "inhibit" the pacing output when intrinsic activity is sensed or will "trigger" a pacing output based on a specific previously sensed event. For example, in DDD mode:

D: Pacing takes place in the atrium and the ventricle.

D: Sensing takes place in the atrium and the ventricle.

D: Both inhibition and triggering are the response to a sensed event. An atrial output is inhibited with an atrial-sensed event, whereas a ventricular output is inhibited with a ventricular-sensed event; a ventricular pacing output is triggered by an atrial-sensed event (assuming no ventricular event occurs during the A-V interval).

The fourth letter in the code is intended to reflect the degree of programmability of the pacemaker but is typically used to indicate that the device can provide rate response. For example, a DDDR device is one that is programmed to pace and sense in both chambers and is capable of sensor-driven rate variability. The fifth letter is reserved specifically for antitachycardia functions (Table 79.1).

Readers interested in the intriguing details of pacemaker timing operations are referred to the works listed at the end of this chapter.

79.6 Clinical Outcomes and Cost Implications

The demonstrable hemodynamic and symptomatic benefits provided by rate-responsive and dual-chamber pacing have led U.S. physicians to include at least one of these features in over three-fourths of implants in recent years. Also, new prospective data [Andersen et al., 1993] support a hypothesis investigated retrospectively since the mid-1980s: namely, that pacing the atrium in patients with sinus node dysfunction can dramatically reduce the incidence of such life-threatening complications as *congestive heart failure* and stroke associated with chronic *atrial fibrillation*. Preliminary analysis

TABLE 79.1   The NASPE/NPEG Code

Position	I	II	III	IV	V
Category	Chamber(s) paced	Chamber(s) sensed	Response to sensing	Programmability, rate modulation	Antitachyarrhythmia function(s)
	O = None	O = None	O = None	O = None	O = None
	A = Atrium	A = Atrium	T = Triggered	P = Simple programmable	P = Packing
	V = Ventricle	V = Ventricle	I = Inhibited	M = Multiprogrammable	S = Shock
	D = Dual (A+V)	D = Dual (A+V)	D = Dual (T+I)	C = Communicating	D = Dual (P+S)
				R = Rate modulation	
Manufacturers' designation only	S = Single (A or V)	S = Single (A or V)			

Note: Positions I through III are used exclusively for antibradyarrhythmia function. (From Bernstein, A.D. et al., PACE, Vol. 10, July–Aug. 1987.)

of the cost implications suggest that dual-chamber pacing is significantly cheaper to the U.S. health-care system than is single-chamber pacing over the full course of therapy, despite the somewhat higher initial cost of implanting the dual-chamber system.

79.7 Conclusion

Permanent cardiac pacing is the beneficiary of three decades of advances in a variety of key technologies: biomaterials, electrical stimulation, sensing of bioelectrical events, power sources, microelectronics, transducers, signal analysis, and software development. These advances, informed and guided by a wealth of clinical experience acquired during that time, have made pacing a cost-effective cornerstone of cardiac arrhythmia management.

Defining Terms

Atrial fibrillation: An atrial arrhythmia resulting in chaotic current flow within the atria. The effective contraction of the atria is lost, allowing blood to pool and clot, leading to stroke if untreated.

Battery capacity: Given by the voltage and the current delivery. The voltage is a result of the battery chemistry, and current delivery (current × time) is measured in ampere hours and is related to battery size.

CMOS circuit: Abbreviation for complementary metallic oxide semiconductor, which is a form of semiconductor often used in pacemaker technology.

Congestive heart failure: The pathophysiologic state in which an abnormality of cardiac function is responsible for the failure of the heart to pump blood at a rate commensurate with the requirements of the body.

Endocardium: The inner lining of the heart.

Epicardium: The outer lining of the heart.

Hermeticity: The term, as used in the pacemaker industry, refers to a very low rate of helium gas leakage from the sealed pacemaker container. This reduces the chance of fluid intruding into the pacemaker generator and causing damage.

Hypertrophic obstructive cardiomyopathy: A disease of the myocardium characterized by thickening (hypertrophy) of the interventricular septum, resulting in the partial obstruction of blood from the left ventricle.

Minute ventilation: Respiratory rate × tidal volume (the amount of air taken in with each breath) = minute ventilation. This parameter is used as a biologic indicator for rate-adaptive pacing.

Mode: The type of pacemaker response to the patient's intrinsic heartbeat. The three commonly used modes are asynchronous, demand, and triggered.

Programmable: The ability to alter the pacemaker settings noninvasively. A variety of selections exist, each with its own designation.

Rate-adaptive: The ability to change the pacemaker stimulation interval caused by sensing a physiologic function other than the intrinsic atrial rhythm.

Sensitivity: A programmable setting that adjusts the reference voltage to which signals entering the sensing circuit are compared for filtering.

Stimulation threshold: The minimum output energy required to consistently "capture" (cause depolarization) of the heart.

References

Andersen HR, Thuesen L, Bagger JP, et al. 1993. Atrial versus ventricular pacing in sick sinus syndrome: A prospective randomized trial in 225 consecutive patients. Eur Heart J 14(abstr suppl):252.

Bernstein AD, Camm AJ, Fletcher RD, et al. 1987. The NASPE/BPEG generic pacemaker code for antibradyarrhythmia and adaptive-rate pacing and antitachyarrhythmia devices. PACE 10:794.

Committee on Pacemaker Implantation. 1991. Guidelines for implantation of cardiac pacemakers and antiarrhythmic devices. J Am Coll Cardiol 18(1):1.

Further Information

A good basic introduction to pacing from a clinical perspective is the third edition of *A Practical Guide to Cardiac Pacing* by H. Weston Moses, Joel Schneider, Brian Miller, and George Taylor (Little, Brown, 1991).

Cardiac Pacing (Blackwell Scientific, 1992), edited by Kenneth Ellenbogen, is an excellent intermediate treatment of pacing. The treatments of timing cycles and troubleshooting are especially good.

In-depth discussion of a wide range of pacing topics is provided by the third edition of *A Practice of Cardiac Pacing* by Seymour Furman, David Hayes, and David Holmes (Futura, 1993), and by *New Perspectives in Cardiac Pacing 3*, edited by Serge Barold and Jacques Mugica (Futura, 1993).

Detailed treatment of rate-responsive pacing is given in *Rate-Adaptive Cardiac Pacing: Single and Dual Chamber* by Chu-Pak Lau (Futura, 1993) and in *Rate-Adaptive Pacing*, edited by David Benditt (Blackwell Scientific, 1993).

The Foundations of Cardiac Pacing, Part I by Richard Sutton and Ivan Bourgeois (Futura, 1991) contains excellent illustrations of implantation techniques.

Readers seeking a historical perspective may wish to consult "Pacemakers, Pastmakers, and the Paced: An Informal History from A to Z," by Dwight Harken in the July/August 1991 issue of *Biomedical Instrumentation and Technology*.

PACE is the official journal of the North American Society of Pacing and Electrophysiology (NASPE) and of the International Cardiac Pacing and Electrophysiology Society. It is published monthly by Futura Publishing (135 Bedford Road, PO Box 418, Armonk, NY 10504 USA).

80

Implantable Stimulators for Neuromuscular Control

P. Hunter Peckham

Case Western Reserve
University and Veterans
Affairs Medical Center

Brian Smith

Case Western Reserve
University

Implantable neuromuscular stimulators have been developed for many clinical applications, including control of respiration, bowel and bladder, ambulation, and manipulation. Implantable stimulators are used in these applications because they apply electric current to, or near to, the nerves by placement of the electrodes that deliver the current adjacent to the nerve. This is in contrast to surface stimulation systems, in which electrodes are placed on the skin surface and must direct their current through the skin and subcutaneous tissue to achieve neural excitation.

All neuromuscular simulation systems operate on the principle that an electric current can depolarize an electrically excitable nerve. This generates an action potential in the nerve that will propagate across the neuromuscular junction to excite the peripheral actuator, the muscle. These systems have in common a means of generating an electric pulse, a lead wire to route the pulse to the muscle, and an electrode to deliver the pulse to the muscle. Two basic types of implantable neuromuscular stimulators have been developed. They are (1) systems that use percutaneous leads and (2) systems that use totally implantable components.

80.1 Percutaneous Electrode Systems

These systems have the pulse generator located externally and deliver the stimulus through a hardwired link using a small-diameter lead that is passed through the skin. The percutaneous electrode is chronically indwelling and terminates near the motor nerves of interest to affect the excitation of the neural tissue. In this configuration, the conducting electrode is the termination of the lead, formed by removal of the insulation and subsequent modification to ensure stability within the tissue. This modification includes forming barbs or similar locking mechanisms. The percutaneous electrode is implanted using a needle as the trochar for introduction. Withdrawal of the needle results in the electrode remaining in the tissue. A connector at the skin surface allows termination of the electrode lead to the hardwired external stimulator. The neural excitation derived by this tech-

0-8493-8346-3/95/$0.00+$.50
© 1995 by CRC Press, Inc.

nique is similar to that with a surgically implanted stimulation system. The fundamental difference is that the percutaneous interface must be maintained, and the small-diameter wire that is tolerated through the skin can fail. These present clinical limitations to the user. However, this technique has been employed extensively in developing more complex neuromuscular stimulation systems for control of the upper and lower extremities for manipulation and ambulation.

80.2 Implantable Neuromuscular Stimulators

Implantable systems use an encapsulated pulse generator that is surgically implanted and has subcutaneous leads that terminates at electrodes on or near the desired nerves.

Electronic Circuitry

Implantable systems for neuromuscular applications all have used external transmission of a radiofrequency (rf) signal to transmit both power and communication through the skin to the implantable electronics. Thus none of the devices has employed an implantable power source (battery) because the power demands are too great for the anticipated lifetime of the devices, which are generally expected to last on the order of decades. These devices may use from one to twenty or more channels of stimulation, with current levels ranging from less than 1 mA to as high as 20 mA depending on the type of electrode used. The internal power requirements for the device may thus be as high as a few hundred milliwatts.

The form of the implantable neuromuscular stimulation system thus consists of external and implantable components. The external system consists of the external transmitter with an external transmitting coil that is placed over the implanted receiver/stimulator device. This, in turn, is energized by an external controller that is under the command of the operator or patient to perform the desired activation sequence of the implant. The implant receiver/stimulator consists of a coil tuned to resonate with the external coil and electronic circuitry that receives the rf information and decodes it for power and stimulus control information and subsequently generates the stimulus pulses for delivery to the muscles. Depending on the sophistication of the implanted device, it may employ an application-specific integrated circuit (ASIC) and thick-film hybrid circuitry for its implementation. Such circuitry places considerable requirements for hermeticity and protection on the implanted circuit packaging. The output of the implanted circuitry is a train of pulses, which is delivered to the terminal electrode(s). The stimulus may be applied through either monopolar or bipolar electrodes. The *monopolar* electrode is one in which a single active electrode is placed near the excitable nerve and the return pathway is placed remotely, generally at the implantable unit itself. A *bipolar* electrode is one in which both the stimulating poles are placed near the excitable tissue. The pulse waveform used to excite the tissue is generally a biphasic stimulus, in which there is a negative-going component of the pulse (stimulus) followed by a positive-going component (charge recovery). In general, these stimuli are current-regulated ("constant current"), in which the circuitry is designed to be independent of the load impedances of the electrode and tissues over a wide range of impedance. The biphasic stimulus allows for reversal of charge so that no net charge is delivered to the tissue, allowing injection of higher charge levels before degradation of the tissue occurs.

Packaging of Implantable Electronics

The packaging of implantable electronics uses various materials, including polymers (particularly epoxy and silicone rubber), metals (particularly titanium), and ceramics. Epoxy encapsulation was the original choice of designers of implantable neuromuscular stimulators, since other encapsulation techniques had not been well developed. With epoxy encapsulation, the receiving coil is placed around the circuitry to be "potted," and a mold is used to configure the epoxy. The disadvantage of this technique is that moisture ingress ultimately will reach the electronic components, and surface ions will allow electric shorting and degradation of the circuitry and subsequent failure. However, this approach has been used successfully for devices manufactured with discrete electronic components for many years of implantation within the human body.

Metallic packaging generally uses a titanium capsule with hermetic feedthroughs that exit the package and allow passage of the power into and stimulation out from the internal circuitry. The feedthrough assembly utilizes a ceramic insulator to allow one or more wires to exit the package without contact with the package itself. The electronic circuitry is placed in the package and connected internally to the feedthroughs, and the package is welded closed. Assuming integrity of all components, hermeticity with this package is ensured. However, this packaging generally requires that the receiving coil be placed outside the package to avoid significant loss of rf signal or power, thus requiring additional space within the body to accommodate the volume of the entire implant. Generally, an epoxy encapsulant over the metallic receiving antenna provides external electric isolation and stabilizes the entire assembly.

More recently, ceramic packages have been developed that allow hermetic sealing of the electronic circuitry together with enclosure of the receiving coil. This is possible due to the rf transparency of ceramics. The advantage of this approach is that the volume of the implant can be reduced, thus minimizing the biologic response, which is a function of volume.

Leads that exit the device must be sufficiently flexible to move across the joints between the pulse generator and their electrode termination while at the same time sufficiently flexible to last for the decades of intended life of the device. Different configurations of leads have been used, and most include a connector at some point between the implant and the terminal electrode, allowing for replacement of the implanted receiver or leads in the event of failure. The connectors used have been either single-pin in-line connectors located somewhere along the lead length or a multiport/multilead connector at the implant itself. The leads terminate at electrodes placed at or near the effector nerves.

Electrodes

Electrodes used for neuromuscular stimulation generally are called either *nerve* electrodes or *muscle* electrodes. Nerve electrodes generally involve a structure that physically fixes the electrode to the nerve, either a suture technique or a mechanical encircling structure. These electrodes use lower current levels (up to a few milliamps). The muscle electrodes generally use structures that are placed on or within the muscle and adjacent to, but not on, the innervating nerve. These electrodes generally use currents as high as 20 mA and pulse widths as high as 200 μs and are generally less efficient than the nerve cuffs. However, their advantage is that they require less surgical dissection to place, and they are unlikely to damage the nerve because of their remoteness from it.

Surface Stimulation

Surface stimulation has been used extensively in medical rehabilitation for electrical activation of nerve and muscle. These surface stimulation systems typically use conductive electrodes placed at or near the motor point of the muscle to excite the underlying tissue. Surface stimulation generally uses approximately five times the current required for intramuscular stimulation systems. These systems have been used therapeutically to hypertrophy muscle but have not reached practicality for most functional applications. One notable recent exception to this is a surface stimulation–based device for standing and stepping developed by Sigmedics Corporation (Northfield, Ill.) that has recently received FDA approval. In many applications, the inability of surface stimulation to reliably excite the underlying tissue in a repeatable manner requires electrode repositioning. This has limited the clinical applicability. A special issue of *Assistive Technology* (vol. 4, no. 1, 1992) reviews many aspects of surface stimulation.

80.3 Implanted Stimulators in Clinical Use

Implanted stimulators are in clinical use for control of respiration, micturition (urination), and manipulation (grasp and release).

Respiration

Respiratory control systems involve a two-channel implantable stimulator with electrodes applied to the phrenic nerve bilaterally. Most of the devices in clinical use were developed by Avery Laboratories and involve discrete circuitry with epoxy encapsulation of the implant and a lead using a nerve cuff electrode. Approximately 1000 of these devices have been implanted in patients with respiratory disorders such as high-level tetraplegia. Activation of the phrenic nerve results in contraction of each hemidiaphragm in response to electrical stimulation. In order to minimize fatigue to the diaphragms during chronic use, alternation of the diaphragms has been employed, in which one hemidiaphragm will be activated for several hours followed by the second.

Urinary Control Systems

Urinary control systems have been developed for persons with spinal cord injury. The most successful of these devices was developed by Brindley and is manufactured by Finetech, Ltd. (England). The implanted receiver consists of three separate stimulator devices, each with its own coil and circuitry, encapsulated within a single package. The sacral roots (S2, S3, and S4) are placed within a type of encircling electrode, and stimulation of the proper roots will generate contraction of both the bladder and the external sphincter. Cessation of stimulation results in a faster relaxation of the external sphincter than of the bladder wall, which then results in voiding. Repeated trains of pulses applied in this manner will eliminate most urine, with only small residual amounts of urine remaining. Several hundred of these devices have been implanted around the world.

Manipulation

Control of complex functions for movement, such as hand control, requires the use of many channels of stimulation. At Case Western Reserve University, an eight-channel stimulator has been developed for control of grasp and release. This system uses eight channels of stimulation and a titanium-packaged, thick-film hybrid circuit as the pulse generator. This implant is manufactured by BioControl Technologies, Inc. (Indiana, Pa.) and has been implanted in 24 patients in six centers. The implant is controlled by a dual-microprocessor external unit carried by the patient with an input command control signal provided by the user's remaining volitional movement. Activation of the muscles provides two primary grasp patterns and allows the person to achieve functional performance that exceeds his or her capabilities without the use of the implanted system. This neuromuscular prosthesis is presently undergoing clinical trials to achieve regulatory approval. The same implant also has been implanted in the lower extremity musculature to assist incomplete quadriplegics in standing and transfer operations.

80.4 Future Implanted Electric Stimulators

Improvements in the function of implanted stimulators are being developed in two areas. First, more advanced neuroprostheses are anticipated to integrate the control and stimulation functions together. Neuromuscular stimulators are being developed at Case Western Reserve University that have the capability of communicating with implanted sensors, to both power the sensor and telemeter the information derived from the sensor to the external controller, where the processing of information will take place. Communication of stimulation information from the external processor back to the implanted device will then provide the stimulation functions. This type of control is being developed for more advanced neuromuscular applications, in which the command information could be derived from sources such as the position of joints or used in feedback-control loops in a similar way. It also would be applicable to advances in other neuroprostheses in conjunction with sensors that could detect, for example, bladder pressures and be used in a more advanced control system.

Another advancement being pursued by both the A. E. Mann Foundation and the University of Michigan is the development of microinjectable stimulators. The microinjectable stimulator is envisioned to be a small capsule that can be inserted through a small injector into the muscle for activation of nerves. The concept is modular, in which a substantial number of these devices could be implanted within the desired muscles and communicated with via a single external coil that would surround the area within which the microinjectable stimulators were implanted.

Both the bidirectionally communicating single implant and the microinjectable devices are presently reaching a stage of animal testing and may be expected to be undergoing human trials within the next several years. They will provide exciting opportunities for enhancing the function of current neuromuscular stimulation approaches.

References

Durfee WK (ed). 1994. Special issue on practical functional electrical stimulation. *Assistive Technology* 4(1).

Keith MW, Peckham PH, Thrope GB, et al. 1989. Implantable functional neuromuscular stimulation in the tetraplegic hand. J Hand Surg 14A(3):524.

Pourmehdi S, Peckham PH. 1995. Implantable stimulators and control systems. In D Christiansen (ed), IEEE Electronic Engineer's Handbook, 4th ed. New York, McGraw-Hill.

Smith B, Peckham PH, Roscoe DD, Keith MW. 1987. An externally powered, multichannel implantable stimulator for versatile control of paralyzed muscle. IEEE Trans Biomed Eng E-34 (7):499.

Further Information

Information on development of implanted neuroprostheses generally appears in the biomedical engineering literature. The interested reader is referred to the *IEEE Transactions on Biomedical Engineering* and *IEEE Transactions on Rehabilitation Engineering*.

81

External Defibrillators

Willis A. Tacker
Purdue University

Defibrillators are devices used to apply a strong electric shock (often referred to as a *countershock*) to a patient in an effort to convert excessively fast and ineffective heart rhythm disorders to slower rhythms that allow the heart to pump more blood. External defibrillators have been in common use for many decades for emergency treatment of life-threatening cardiac rhythms as well as for elective treatment of less threatening rapid rhythms. Fig. 81.1 shows an external defibrillator.

Cardiac arrest occurs in more than 500,000 people annually in the United States, and more than 70% of the out-of-hospitals are due to cardiac arrhythmia treatable with defibrillators. The most serious arrhythmia treated by a defibrillator is ventricular fibrillation. Without rapid treatment using a defibrillator, ventricular fibrillation causes complete loss of cardiac function and death within minutes. Atrial fibrillation and the more organized rhythms of atrial flutter and ventricular tachycardia can be treated on a less emergent basis. Although they do not cause immediate death, their shortening of the interval between contractions can impair filling of the heart chambers and thus decrease cardiac output. Conventionally, treatment of ventricular fibrillation is called *defibrillation*, whereas treatment of the other tachycardias is called *cardioversion*.

81.1 Mechanism of Fibrillation

Fibrillation is chaotic electric excitation of the myocardium and results in loss of coordinated mechanical contraction characteristic of normal heart beats. Description of mechanisms leading to, and maintaining, fibrillation and other rhythm disorders are reviewed elsewhere [1] and are beyond the scope of this chapter. In summary, however, these rhythm disorders are commonly held to be a result of reentrant excitation pathways within the heart. The underlying abnormality that leads to the mechanism is the combination of conduction block of cardiac excitation plus rapidly recurring depolarization of the membranes of the cardiac cells. This leads to rapid repetitive propagation of a single excitation wave or of multiple excitatory waves throughout the heart. If the waves are multiple, the rhythm may degrade into total loss of synchronization of cardiac fiber contraction. Without synchronized contraction, the chamber affected will not contract, and this is fatal in the case of ventricular fibrillation. The most common cause of these conditions, and therefore of these rhythm disorders, is cardiac ischemia or infarction as a complication of atherosclerosis. Additional

0-8493-8346-3/95/$0.00+$.50
© 1995 by CRC Press, Inc.

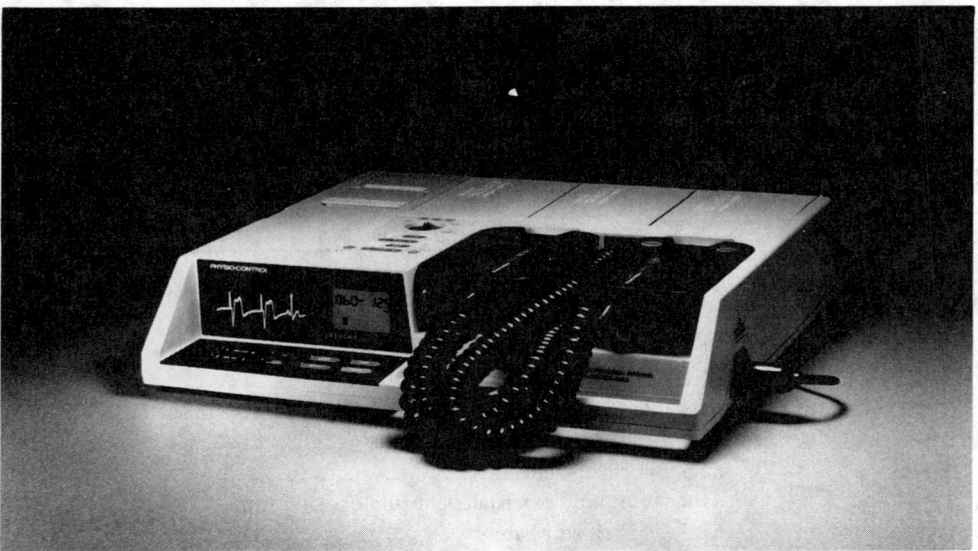

FIGURE 81.1 Photograph of a trans-chest defibrillator (provided by Physio-Control Corporation with permission).

relatively common causes include other cardiac disorders, drug toxicity, electrolyte imbalances in the blood, hypothermia, and electric shocks (especially from alternating current).

81.2 Mechanism of Defibrillation

The corrective measure is to extinguish the rapidly occurring waves of excitation by simultaneously depolarizing most of the cardiac cells with a strong electric shock. The cells then can simultaneously repolarize themselves, and thus they will be back in phase with each other.

Despite years of intensive research, there is still no single theory for the mechanism of defibrillation that explains all the phenomena observed. However, it is generally held that the defibrillating shock must be adequately strong and have adequate duration to affect most of the heart cells. In general, longer duration shocks require less current than shorter duration shocks. This relationship is called the strength-duration relationship and is demonstrated by the curve shown in Fig. 81.2. Shocks of strength and duration above and to the right of the current curve (or above the energy curve) have adequate strength to defibrillate, whereas shocks below and to the left do not. From the exponentially decaying current curve an energy curve can also be determined (also shown in Fig. 81.2), which is high at very short durations due to high current requirements at short durations, but which is also high at longer durations due to additional energy being delivered as the pulse duration is lengthened at nearly constant current. Thus, for most electrical waveforms there is a minimum energy for defibrillation at approximate pulse durations of 3–8 ms. A strength-duration charge curve can also be determined as shown in Fig. 81.2, which demonstrates that the minimum charge for defibrillation occurs at the shortest pulse duration tested. Very-short-duration pulses are not used, however, since the high current and voltage required is damaging to the myocardium. It is also important to note that excessively strong or long shocks may cause immediate refibrillation, thus failing to restore the heart function.

In practice, for a shock applied to electrodes on the skin surface of the patient's chest, durations are on the order of 3–10 milliseconds and have an intensity of a few thousand volts and tens of amperes. The energy delivered to the subject by these shocks is selectable by the operator and is on

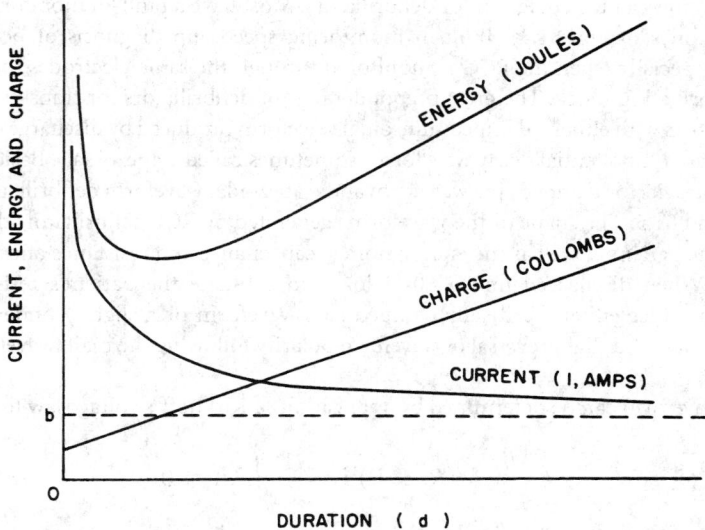

FIGURE 81.2 Strength-duration curves for current, energy, and charge. Adequate current shocks are above and to the right of the current curve. (Modified from Tacker WA, Geddes LA. 1980. *Electrical Defibrillation*, Boca Raton, Fla, CRC Press, with permission.)

the order of 50–360 joules for most defibrillators. The exact shock intensity required at a given duration of electric pulse depends on several variables, including the intrinsic characteristics of the patient (such as the underlying disease problem or presence of certain drugs and the length of time the arrhythmia has been present), the techniques for electrode application, and the particular rhythm disorder being treated (more organized rhythms require less energy than disorganized rhythms).

81.3 Clinical Defibrillators

Defibrillator design has resulted from medical and physiologic research and advances in hardware technology. It is estimated that for each minute that elapses between onset of ventricular fibrillation and the first shock application, survival to leave hospital decreases by about 10%. The importance of rapid response led to development of portable, battery-operated defibrillators and more recently to automatic external defibrillators (AEDs) that enable emergency responders to defibrillate with minimal training.

All clinical defibrillators used today store energy in capacitors. Desirable capacitor specifications include small size, light weight, and capability to sustain several thousands of volts and many charge-discharge cycles. Energy storage capacitors account for at least one pound and usually several pounds of defibrillator weight. Energy stored by the capacitor is calculated from

$$W_S = \frac{1}{2} CE^2 \tag{81.1}$$

where W_S = stored energy in joules, C = capacitance in farads, and E = voltage applied to the capacitor. Delivered energy is expressed as

$$W_d = W_S \times \left(\frac{R}{R_i + R} \right) \tag{81.2}$$

where W_d = delivered energy, W_S = stored energy, R = subject resistance, and R_i = device resistance.

Figure 81.3 shows a block diagram for defibrillators. Most have a built-in monitor and synchronizer (dashed lines in Fig. 81.3). Built-in monitoring speeds up diagnosis of potentially fatal arrhythmias, especially when the ECG is monitored through the same electrodes that are used to apply the defibrillating shock. The great preponderance of defibrillators for trans-chest defibrillation deliver shocks with either a damped sinusoidal waveform produced by discharge of an RCL circuit or a truncated exponential decay waveform (sometimes called trapezoidal). Basic components of exemplary circuits for damped sine waveform and trapezoidal waveform defibrillators are shown in Figs. 81.4 and 81.5. The shape of the waveforms generated by RCL defibrillators depend on the resistance of the patient as well as the energy storage capacitance and resistance and inductance of the inductor. When discharged into a 50-Ω load (to simulate the patient's resistance), these defibrillators produce either a critically damped sine waveform or a slightly underdamped sine waveform (i.e., having a slight reversal of waveform polarity following the main waveform) into the 50-Ω load.

The exact waveform can be determined by application of Kirkhoff's voltage law to the circuit

$$L\frac{di}{dt} + (R_i + R)\,i + \frac{1}{C}\int i\,dt = 0 \tag{81.3}$$

where L = inductance in H, i = instantaneous current in amperes, t = time in seconds, R_i = device resistance, R = subject resistance, and C = capacitance. From this, the second-order differential equation describes the RCL defibrillator.

$$L\frac{d^2i}{dt^2} + (R_i + R)\frac{di}{dt} + \frac{1}{C}\,i = 0 \tag{81.4}$$

Trapezoidal waveform (actually, these are truncated exponential decay waveform) defibrillators are also used clinically. The circuit diagram in Fig. 81.4 is exemplary of one design for producing such a waveform. Delivered energy calculation for this waveform is expressed as

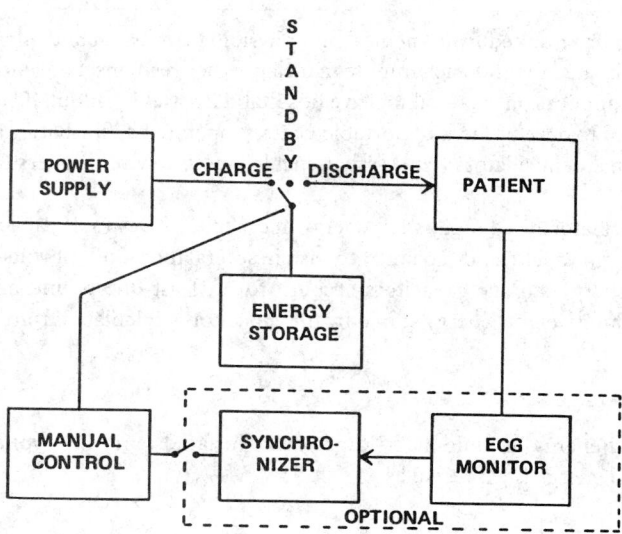

FIGURE 81.3 Block diagram of a typical defibrillator. (From Feinberg B. 1980. *Handbook Series in Clinical Laboratory Science,* vol 2, Boca Raton, Fla, CRC Press, with permission.)

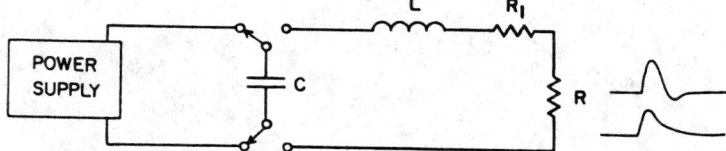

FIGURE 81.4 Resistor-capacitor-inductor defibrillator. The patient is represented by *R*. (Modified from Feinberg B. 1980. *Handbook Series in Clinical Laboratory Science*, vol 2, Boca Raton, Fla, CRC Press, with permission.)

$$W_d = 0.5\, I_i^2 R \left[\frac{d}{\log_e\left(\frac{I_i}{I_f}\right)} \right] \left[1 - \left(\frac{I_f}{I_i}\right)^2 \right] \tag{81.5}$$

where W_d = delivered energy, I_i = initial current in amperes, I_f = final current, R = resistance of the patient, and d = pulse duration in seconds. Both RCL and trapezoidal waveforms defibrillate effectively. Implantable defibrillators now use alternative waveforms such as a biphasic exponential decay waveform, in which the polarity of the electrodes is reversed part way through the shock. Use of the biphasic waveform has reduced the shock intensity required for implantable defibrillators but has not yet been extended to trans-chest use except on an experimental basis.

RCL defibrillators are the most widely available. They store up to about 440 joules and deliver up to about 360 joules into a patient with 50-ohm impedance. Several selectable energy intensities are available, typically from 5–360 J, so that pediatric patients, very small patients, or patients with easily converted arrhythmias can be treated with low-intensity shocks. The pulse duration ranges from 3–6 ms. Because the resistance (*R*) varies between patients (25–150 ohms) and is part of the RCL discharge circuit, the duration and damping of the pulse also varies; increasing patient impedance lengthens and dampens the pulse. Figure 81.6 shows waveforms from RCL defibrillators with critically damped and with underdamped pulses.

81.4 Electrodes

Electrodes for external defibrillation are metal and from 70–100 cm² in surface area. They must be coupled to the skin with an electrically conductive material to achieve low impedance across the electrode-patient interface. There are two types of electrodes: hand-held (to which a conductive liquid or solid gel is applied) and adhesive, for which an adhesive conducting material holds the electrode in place. Hand-held electrodes are reusable and are pressed against the patient's chest by the operator during shock delivery. Adhesive electrodes are disposable and are applied to the chest

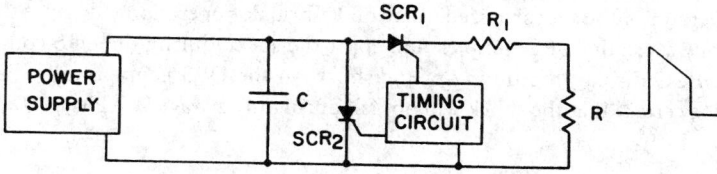

FIGURE 81.5 Trapezoidal wave defibrillator. The patient is represented by *R*. (Modified from Feinberg B. 1980. *Handbook Series in Clinical Laboratory Science*, vol 2, Boca Raton, Fla, CRC Press, with permission.)

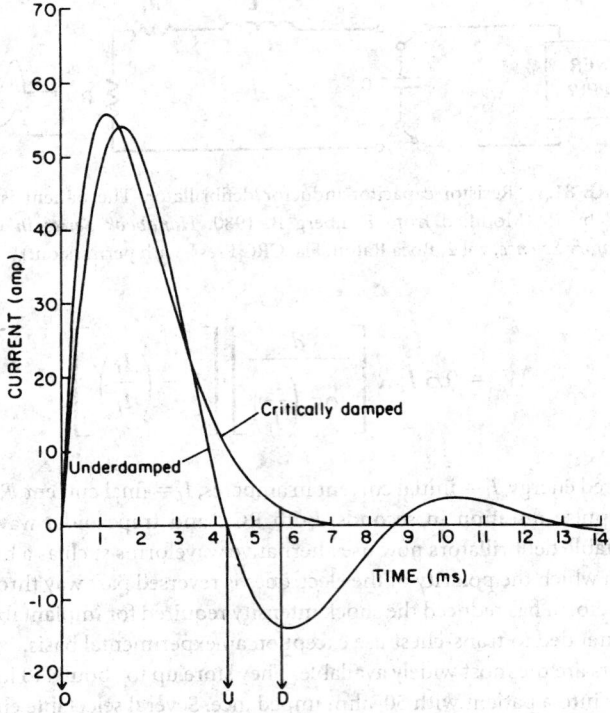

FIGURE 81.6 The damped sine wave. The interval *O–D* represents a duration for the critically and overdamped sine waves. By time *D*, more than 99% of the energy has been delivered. *O–U* is taken as the duration for an underdamped sine wave. (Modified from Tacker WA, Geddes LA. 1980. *Electrical Defibrillation*, Boca Raton, Fla, CRC Press, with permission.)

before the shock delivery and left in place for reuse if subsequent shocks are needed. Electrodes are usually applied with both electrodes on the anterior chest as shown in Fig. 81.7 or in anterior-to-posterior (front-to-back) position, as shown in Fig. 81.8.

81.5 Synchronization

Most defibrillators for trans-chest use have the feature of synchronization, which is an electronic sensing and triggering mechanism for application of the shock during the QRS complex of the ECG. This is required when treating arrhythmias other than ventricular fibrillation, because inadvertent application of a shock during the *T* wave of the ECG often produces ventricular fibrillation. Selection by the operator of the synchronized mode of defibrillator operation will cause the defibrillator to automatically sense the QRS complex and apply the shock during the QRS complex. Furthermore, on the ECG display, the timing of the shock on the QRS is graphically displayed so the operator can be certain that the shock will not fall during the *T* wave (see Fig. 81.9).

81.6 Automatic External Defibrillators

Automatic external defibrillators (AEDs) are defibrillators that automatically or semiautomatically recognize and treat rapid arrhythmias, usually under emergency conditions. Their operation requires less training than operation of manual defibrillators because the operator need not know which ECG

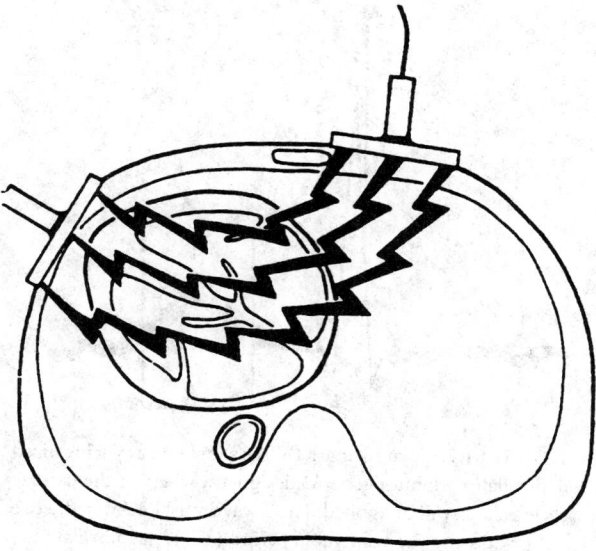

Anterior-Anterior

FIGURE 81.7 Cross-sectional view of the chest showing position for standard anterior wall (precordial) electrode placement. Lines of presumed current flow are shown between the electrodes on the skin surface. (Modified from Tacker WA (ed). 1994. *Defibrillation of the Heart: ICDs, AEDs and Manual*, St. Louis, Mosby-Year Book, with permission.)

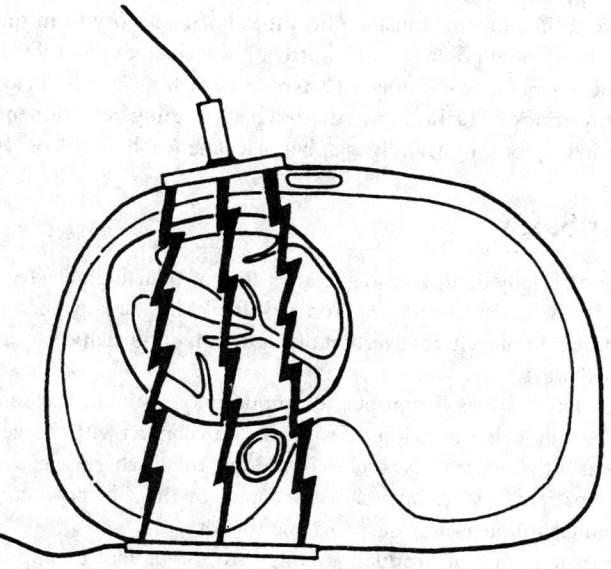

L-Anterior-Posterior

FIGURE 81.8 Cross-sectional view of the chest showing position for front-to-back electrode placement. Lines of presumed current flow are shown between the electrodes on the skin surface. (Modified from Tacker WA (ed). 1994. *Defibrillation of the Heart: ICDs, AEDs and Manual*, St. Louis, Mosby-Year Book, with permission.)

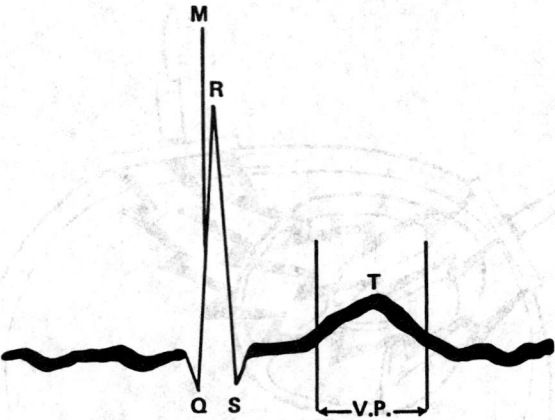

FIGURE 81.9   Timing mark (*M*) as shown on a synchronized defibrillator monitor. The *M* designates when in the cardiac cycle a shock will be applied. The *T* wave must be avoided, since a shock during the vulnerable period (V.P.) may fibrillate the ventricles. This tracing shows atrial fibrillation as identified by the irregular wavy baseline of the ECG. (Modified from Feinberg B. 1980. *Handbook Series in Clinical Laboratory Science*, vol 2, Boca Raton, Fla, CRC Press, with permission.)

waveforms indicate rhythms requiring a shock. The operator applies adhesive electrodes from the AED to the patient and turns on the AED, which monitors the ECG and determines by built-in signal processing whether or not and when to shock the patient. In a completely automatic mode, the AED does not have a manual control as shown in Fig. 81.3 but instead has an automatic control. In semiautomatic mode, the operator must confirm the shock advisory from the AED to deliver the shock. AEDs have substantial potential for improving the changes of survival from cardiac arrest because they enable emergency personnel, who typically reach the patient before paramedics do, to deliver defibrillating shocks. Furthermore, the reduced training requirements make feasible the operation of AEDs in the home by a family member of a patient at high risk of ventricular fibrillation.

81.7 Defibrillator Safety

Defibrillators are potentially dangerous devices because of their high electrical output characteristics. The danger to the patient of unsynchronized shocks has already been presented, as has the synchronization design to prevent inadvertent precipitation of fibrillation by a cardioversion shock applied during the *T* wave.

There are other safety issues. Improper technique may result in accidental shocking of the operator or other personnel in the vicinity, if someone is in contact with the electric discharge pathway. This may occur if the operator is careless in holding the discharge electrodes or if someone is in contact with the patient or with a metal bed occupied by the subject when the shock is applied. Proper training and technique is necessary to avoid this risk.

Another safety issue is that of producing damage to the patient by application of excessively strong or excessively numerous shocks. Although cardiac damage has been reported after high-intensity and repetitive shocks to experimental animals and human patients, it is generally held that significant cardiac damage is unlikely if proper clinical procedures and guidelines are followed.

Failure of a defibrillator to operate correctly may also be considered a safety issue, since inability of a defibrillator to deliver a shock in the absence of a replacement unit means loss of the opportunity to resuscitate the patient. A recent review of defibrillator failures found that operator errors, inadequate defibrillator care and maintenance, and, to a lesser extent, component failure accounted for the majority of defibrillator failures [7].

References

1. Tacker WA Jr (ed). 1994. Defibrillation of the Heart: ICDs, AEDs, and Manual. St. Louis, Mosby-Year Book.
2. Tacker WA Jr, Geddes LA. 1980. Electrical Defibrillation. Boca Raton, Fla, CRC Press.
3. Emergency Cardiac Care Committees, American Heart Association. 1992. Guidelines for cardiopulmonary resuscitation and emergency cardiac care. JAMA 268:2199.
4. American National Standard ANSI/AAMI DF2. 1989 (second edition, revision of ANSI/AAMI DF2-1981). Safety and performance standard: Cardiac defibrillator devices.
5. Canadian National Standard CAN/CSA C22.2 No. 601.2.4-M90. 1990. Medical electrical equipment, part 2: Particular requirements for the safety of cardiac defibrillators and cardiac defibrillator/monitors.
6. International Standard IEC 601-2-4. 1983. Medical electrical equipment, part 2: Particular requirements for the safety of cardiac defibrillators and cardiac defibrillator/monitors.
7. Cummins RO, Chesemore K, White RD, and the Defibrillator Working Group. 1990. Defibrillator failures: Causes of problems and recommendations for improvement. JAMA 264:1019.

Further Information

Detailed presentation of material on defibrillator waveforms, algorithms for ECG analysis, and automatic defibrillation using AED's, electrodes, design, clinical use, effects of drugs on shock strength required to defibrillate, damage due to defibrillator shocks, and use of defibrillators during open-thorax surgical procedures or trans-esophageal defibrillation are beyond the scope of this chapter. Also, the historical aspects of defibrillation are not presented here. For more information, the reader is referred to the publications at the end of this chapter [1–3]. For detailed description of specific defibrillators with comparisons of features, the reader is referred to articles from *Health Devices,* a monthly publication of ECRI, 5200 Butler Pike, Plymouth Meeting, Pa USA. For American, Canadian, and European defibrillator standards, the reader is referred to published standards [3–6] and Charbonnier's discussion of standards [1].

82

Implantable
Defibrillators

Edwin G. Duffin
Medtronic, Inc.

The implantable cardioverter defibrillator (ICD) is a therapeutic device that can detect ventricular tachycardia or fibrillation and automatically deliver high-voltage (750 V) shocks that will restore normal sinus rhythm. Advanced versions also provide low-voltage (5–10 V) pacing stimuli for pain-less termination of ventricular tachycardia and for management of bradyarrhythmias. The proven efficacy of the automatic implantable defibrillator has placed it in the mainstream of therapies for the prevention of sudden arrhythmic cardiac death.

The implantable defibrillator has evolved significantly since first appearing in 1980. The newest devices can be implanted in the patient's pectoral region and use electrodes that can be inserted transvenously, eliminating the traumatic thoracotomy required for placement of the earlier epicar-dial electrode systems. Transvenous systems provide rapid, minimally invasive implants with high assurance of success and greater patient comfort. Advanced arrhythmia detection algorithms offer a high degree of sensitivity with reasonable specificity, and extensive monitoring is provided to document performance and to facilitate appropriate programming of arrhythmia detection and therapy parameters. Generator longevity can now exceed 4 years, and the cost of providing this therapy is declining.

82.1 Pulse Generators

The implantable defibrillator consists of a primary battery, high-voltage capacitor bank, and sensing and control circuitry housed in a hermetically sealed titanium case. Commercially available devices weigh between 197 and 237 grams and range in volume from 113 to 145 cm³. Clinical trials are in progress on devices with volumes ranging from 178 cm³ to 60 cm³ and weights between 275 and 104 grams. Further size reductions will be achieved with the introduction of improved capacitor and integrated circuit technologies and lead systems offering lower pacing and defibrillation thresh-olds. Progress should parallel that made with antibradycardia pacemakers that have evolved from

250-gram, nonprogrammable, VOO units with 600-µJ pacing outputs to 26-gram, multiprogrammable, DDDR units with dual 25-µJ outputs.

Implantable defibrillator circuitry must include an amplifier, to allow detection of the millivolt-range cardiac electrogram signals; noninvasively programmable processing and control functions, to evaluate the sensed cardiac activity and to direct generation and delivery of the therapeutic energy; high-voltage switching capability; dc-dc conversion functions, to step up the low battery voltages; random access memories, to store appropriate patient and device data; and radiofrequency telemetry systems, to allow communication to and from the implanted device. Monolithic integrated circuits on hybridized substrates have made it possible to accomplish these diverse functions in a commercially acceptable and highly reliable form.

Defibrillators must convert battery voltages of approximately 6.5 V to the 600–750 V needed to defibrillate the heart. Since the conversion process cannot directly supply this high voltage at current strengths needed for defibrillation, charge is accumulated in relatively large ($\approx$85–120µF effective capacitance) aluminum electrolytic capacitors that account for 20–30% of the volume of a typical defibrillator. These capacitors must be charged periodically to prevent their dielectric from deteriorating. If this is not done, the capacitors become electrically leaky, yielding excessively long charge times and delay of therapy. Early defibrillators required that the patient return to the clinic periodically to have the capacitors reformed, whereas newer devices do this automatically at preset or programmable times. Improved capacitor technology, perhaps ceramic or thin-film, will eventually offer higher storage densities, greater shape variability for denser component packaging, and freedom from the need to waste battery capacity performing periodic reforming charges. Packaging density has already improved from 0.03 J/cm³ for devices such as the early cardioverter to 0.43 J/cm³ with some investigational ICDs. Capacitors that allow conformal shaping could readily increase this density to more than 0.6 J/cm³.

Power sources used in defibrillators must have sufficient capacity to provide 50–400 full energy charges ($\approx$34 J) and 3 to 5 years of bradycardia pacing and background circuit operation. They must have a very low internal resistance in order to supply the relatively high currents needed to charge the defibrillation capacitors in 5–15 s. This generally requires that the batteries have large surface area electrodes and use chemistries that exhibit higher rates of internal discharge than those seen with the lithium iodide batteries used in pacemakers. The most commonly used defibrillator battery chemistry is lithium silver vanadium oxide.

82.2 Electrode Systems ("Leads")

Early implantable defibrillators utilized patch electrodes (typically a titanium mesh electrode) placed on the surface of the heart, requiring entry through the chest (Fig. 82.1). This procedure is associated with approximately 3–4% perioperative mortality, significant hospitalization time and complications, patient discomfort, and high costs. Although subcostal, subxiphoid, and thoracoscopic techniques can minimize the surgical procedure, the ultimate solution has been development of fully transvenous lead systems with acceptable defibrillation thresholds.

Currently available transvenous leads are constructed much like pacemaker leads, using polyurethane or silicone insulation and platinum-iridium electrode materials. Acceptable thresholds are obtained in 67–95% of patients, with mean defibrillation thresholds ranging from 10.9–18.1J. These lead systems use a combination of two or more electrodes located in the right ventricular apex, the superior vena cava, the coronary sinus, and, sometimes, a subcutaneous patch electrode is placed in the chest region. These leads offer advantages beyond the avoidance of major surgery. They are easier to remove should there be infections or a need for lead system revision. The pacing thresholds of current transvenous defibrillation electrodes are typically 0.96 ± 0.39 V, and the electrogram amplitudes are on the order of 16.4 ± 6.4 mV. The eventual application of steroid-eluting materials in the leads should provide increased pacing efficiency with transvenous lead systems, thereby reducing the current drain associated with pacing and extending pulse generator longevity.

Lead systems are being refined to simplify the implant procedures. One approach is the use of a single catheter having a single right ventricular low-voltage electrode for pacing and detection, and a pair of high-voltage defibrillation electrodes spaced for placement in the right ventricle and in the superior vena cava (Fig. 82.2a). A more recent approach parallels that used for unipolar pacemakers. A single right-ventricular catheter having bipolar pace/sense electrodes and one right ventricular high-voltage electrode is used in conjunction with a defibrillator housing that serves as the second high-voltage electrode (Fig. 82.2b). Mean biphasic pulse defibrillation thresholds with the generator-electrode placed in the patient's left pectoral region are reported to be 9.8 ± 6.6 J ($n = 102$). This approach appears to be practicable only with generators suitable for pectoral placement, but such devices will become increasingly available.

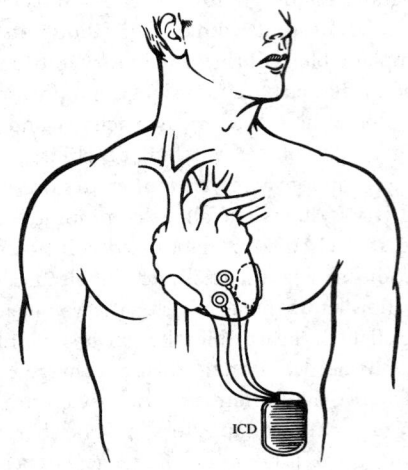

FIGURE 82.1 Epicardial ICD systems typically use two or three large defibrillating patch electrodes placed on the epicardium of the left and right ventricles and a pair of myocardial electrodes for detection and pacing. The generator is usually placed in the abdomen. (Copyright Medtronic, Inc. Used with permission.)

82.3 Arrhythmia Detection

Most defibrillator detection algorithms rely primarily on heart rate to indicate the presence of a treatable rhythm. Additional refinements sometimes include simple morphology assessments, as with the probability density function, and analysis of rhythm stability and rate of change in rate.

The *probability density function* evaluates the percentage of time that the filtered ventricular electrogram spends in a window centered on the baseline. The rate-of-change-in-rate or *onset* evaluation discriminates sinus tachycardia from ventricular tachycardia on the basis of the typically gradual acceleration of sinus rhythms versus the relatively abrupt acceleration of many pathologic tachycardias. The *rate stability* function is designed to bar detection of tachyarrhythmias as long as the variation in ventricular rate exceeds a physician-programmed tolerance, thereby reducing the likelihood of inappropriate therapy delivery in response to atrial fibrillation. This concept appears to be one of the more successful detection algorithm enhancements.

Because these additions to the detection algorithm reduce sensitivity, some defibrillator designs offer a supplementary detection mode that will trigger therapy in response to any elevated ventricular rate of prolonged duration. These *extended-high-rate* algorithms bypass all or portions of the normal detection screening, resulting in low specificity for rhythms with prolonged elevated rates such as exercise-induced sinus tachycardia. Consequently, use of such algorithms generally increases the incidence of inappropriate therapies.

Improvements in arrhythmia detection specificity are desirable, but they must not decrease the excellent sensitivity offered by current algorithms. The anticipated introduction of defibrillators incorporating dual-chamber pacemaker capability will certainly help in this quest, since it will then be possible to use atrial electrograms in the rhythm classification process. It would also be desirable to have a means of evaluating the patient's hemodynamic tolerance of the rhythm, so that the more comfortable pacing sequences could be used as long as the patient was not syncopal yet branch quickly to a definitive shock should the patient begin to lose consciousness.

Although various enhanced detection processes have been proposed, many have not been tested clinically, in some cases because sufficient processing power was not available in implantable

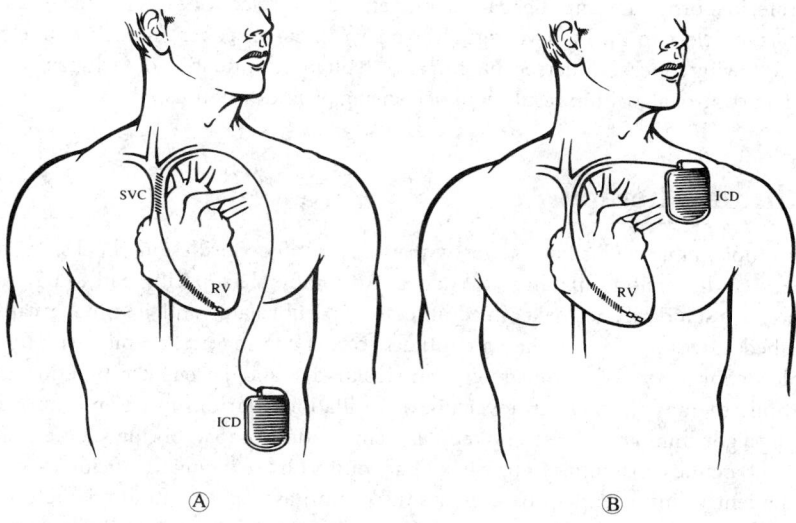

FIGURE 82.2 The latest transvenous fibrillation systems employ a single catheter placed in the right ventricular apex. In panel *a*, a single transvenous catheter provides defibrillation electrodes in the superior vena cava and in the right ventricle. This catheter provides a single pace/sense electrode which is used in conjunction with the right ventricular high-voltage defibrillation electrode for arrhythmia detection and antibradycardia/antitachycardia pacing (a configuration that is sometimes referred to as *integrated bipolar*). With pulse generators small enough to be placed in the pectoral region, defibrillation can be achieved by delivering energy between the generator housing and one high-voltage electrode in the right ventricle (analogous to unipolar pacing) as is shown in panel *b*. This catheter provided bipolar pace/sense electrodes for arrhythmia detection and antibradycardia/antitachycardia pacing. (Copyright Medtronic, Inc. Used with permission.)

systems, and in some cases because sensor technology was not yet ready for chronic implantation. Advances in technology may eventually make some of these very elegant proposals practicable. Examples of proposed detection enhancements include extended analyses of cardiac event timing (PR and RR stability, AV interval variation, temporal distribution of atrial electrogram intervals and of ventricular electrogram intervals, timing differences and/or coherency of multiple ventricular electrograms, ventricular response to a provocative atrial extrastimuli), electrogram waveform analyses (paced depolarization integral, morphology analyses of right ventricular or atrial electrograms), analyses of hemodynamic parameters (right-ventricular pulsatile pressure, mean right atrial and mean right ventricular pressures, wedge coronary sinus pressure, static right ventricular pressure, right atrial pressure, right ventricular stroke volume, mixed venous oxygen saturation and mixed venous blood temperature, left ventricular impedance, intramyocardial pressure gradient, aortic and pulmonary artery flow), and detection of physical motion.

Because defibrillator designs are intentionally biased to overtreat in preference to the life-threatening consequences associated with failure to treat, there is some incidence of inappropriate therapy delivery. Unwarranted therapies are usually triggered by supraventricular tachyarrhythmias, especially atrial fibrillation, or sinus tachycardia associated with rates faster than the ventricular tachycardia detection rate threshold. Additional causes include nonsustained ventricular tachycardias, oversensing of *T* waves, double counting of *R* waves and pacing stimuli from brady pacemakers, and technical faults such as loose lead-generator connections or lead fractures.

Despite the bias for high detection sensitivity, undersensing does occur. It has been shown to result from inappropriate detection algorithm programming, such as an excessively high tachycardia detection rate; inappropriate amplifier gain characteristics; and electrode designs that place the sensing terminals too close to the high-voltage electrodes with a consequent reduction in electrogram amplitude following shocks. Undersensing can also result in the induction of tachycardia should the amplifier gain control algorithm result in undersensing of sinus rhythms.

82.4 Arrhythmia Therapy

Pioneering implantable defibrillators were capable only of defibrillation shocks. Subsequently, synchronized cardioversion capability was added. Antibradycardia pacing had to be provided by implantation of a standard pacemaker in addition to the defibrillator, and, if antitachycardia pacing was prescribed, it was necessary to use an antitachycardia pacemaker. Several currently marketed implantable defibrillators offer integrated ventricular demand pacemaker function and tiered antiarrhythmia therapy (pacing/cardioversion/defibrillation). Various burst and ramp antitachycardia pacing algorithms are offered, and they all seem to offer comparably high success rates. These expanded therapeutic capabilities improve patient comfort by reducing the incidence of shocks in conscious patients, eliminate the problems and discomfort associated with implantation of multiple devices, and contribute to a greater degree of success, since the prescribed regimens can be carefully tailored to specific patient needs. Availability of devices with antitachy pacing capability significantly increases the acceptability of the implantable defibrillator for patients with ventricular tachycardia.

Human clinical trials have shown that biphasic defibrillation waveforms are more effective than monophasic waveforms, and newer devices now incorporate this characteristic. Speculative explanations for biphasic superiority include the large voltage change at the transition from the first to the second phase or hyperpolarization of tissue and reactivation of sodium channels during the initial phase, with resultant tissue conditioning that allows the second phase to more readily excite the myocardium.

Antitachycardia pacing and cardioversion are not uniformly successful. There is some incidence of ventricular arrhythmia acceleration with antitachycardia pacing and cardioversion, and it is also not unusual for cardioversion to induce atrial fibrillation that in turn triggers unwarranted therapies. An ideal therapeutic solution would be one capable of preventing the occurrence of tachycardia altogether. Prevention techniques have been investigated, among them the use of precisely timed subthreshold stimuli, simultaneous stimulation at multiple sites, and pacing with elevated energies at the site of the tachycardia, but none has yet proven practical.

The rudimentary VVI antibradycardia pacing provided by current defibrillators lacks rate responsiveness and atrial pacing capability. Consequently, some defibrillator patients require implantation of a separate dual-chamber pacemaker for hemodynamic support. It is inevitable that future generations of defibrillators will offer dual-chamber pacing capabilities.

Atrial fibrillation, occurring either as a consequence of defibrillator operation or as a natural progression in many defibrillator patients, is a major therapeutic challenge. It is certainly possible to adapt implantable defibrillator technology to treat atrial fibrillation, but the challenge is to do so without causing the patient undue discomfort. Biphasic waveform defibrillation of acutely induced atrial fibrillation has been demonstrated in humans with an 80% success rate at 0.4 J using *epicardial* electrodes. Stand-alone atrial defibrillators are in development, and, if they are successful, it is likely that this capability would be integrated into the mainstream ventricular defibrillators as well. However, most conscious patients find shocks above 0.5 J to be very unpleasant, and it remains to be demonstrated that a clinically acceptable energy level will be efficacious when applied with transvenous electrode systems to spontaneously occurring atrial fibrillation. Moreover, a stand-alone atrial defibrillator either must deliver an atrial shock with complete assurance of appropriate synchronization to ventricular activity or must restrict the therapeutic energy delivery to atrial structures in order to prevent inadvertent induction of a malignant ventricular arrhythmia.

82.5 Implantable Monitoring

Until recently, defibrillator data recording capabilities were quite limited, making it difficult to verify the adequacy of arrhythmia detection and therapy settings. The latest devices record electrograms and diagnostic channel data showing device behavior during multiple tachyarrhythmia episodes. These devices also include counters (number of events detected, success and failure of each programmed therapy, and so on) that present a broad, though less specific, overview of device behavior (Fig. 82.3). Monitoring capability in some of the newest devices appears to be the equivalent of 32 Kbytes of random access memory, allowing electrogram waveform records of approximately 2-min duration, with some opportunity for later expansion by judicious selection of sampling rates and data compression techniques. Electrogram storage has proven useful for documenting false therapy delivery due to atrial fibrillation, lead fractures, and sinus tachycardia, determining the triggers of arrhythmias; documenting rhythm accelerations in response to therapies; and demonstrating appropriate device behavior when treating asymptomatic rhythms.

Electrograms provide useful information by themselves, yet they cannot indicate how the device interpreted cardiac activity. Increasingly, electrogram records are being supplemented with event markers that indicate how the device is responding on a beat-by-beat basis. These records can include measurements of the sensed and paced intervals, indication as to the specific detection zone an event falls in, indication of charge initiation, and other device performance data.

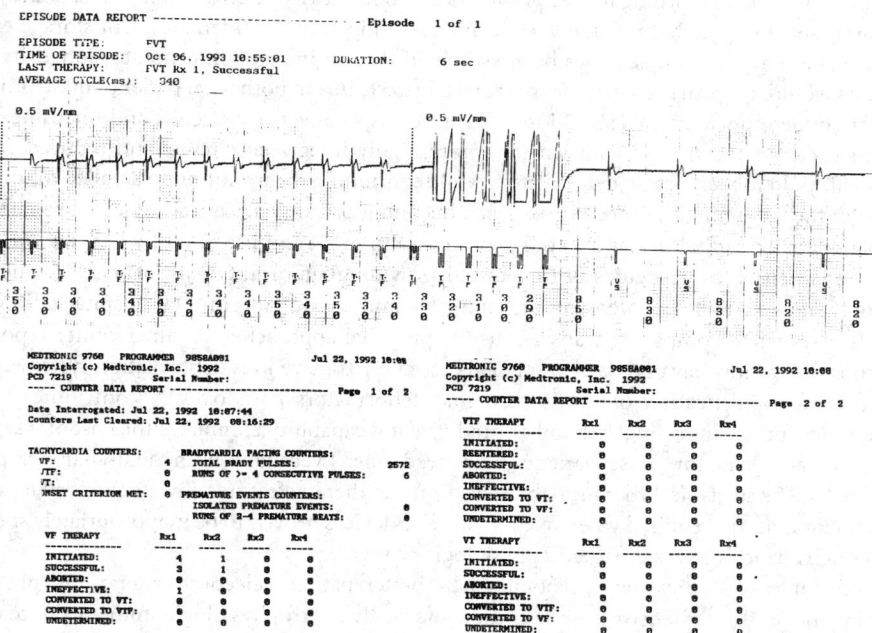

FIGURE 82.3 Typical data recorded by an implantable defibrillator include stored intracardiac electrograms with annotated markers indicating cardiac intervals, paced and sensed events, and device classification of events (TF = fast tachycardia; TP = antitachy pacing stimulus; VS = sensed nontachy ventricular event). In the example, five rapid pacing pulses convert a ventricular tachycardia with a cycle length of 340 ms into sinus rhythm with a cycle length of 830 ms. In the lower portion of the figure is an example of the summary data collected by the ICD, showing detailed counts of the performance of the various therapies (Rx) for ventricular tachycardia (VT), fast ventricular (VTF), and ventricular (VF). (Copyright Medtronic, Inc. Used with permission.)

82.6 Follow-up

Defibrillator patients and their devices require careful follow-up. In one study of 241 ICD patients with epicardial lead systems, 53% of the patients experienced one or more complications during an average exposure of 24 months. These complications included infection requiring device removal in 5%, postoperative respiratory complications in 11%, postoperative bleeding and/or thrombosis in 4%, lead system migration or disruption in 8%, and documented inappropriate therapy delivery, most commonly due to atrial fibrillation, in 22%. A shorter study of eighty patients with transvenous defibrillator systems reported no postoperative pulmonary complications, transient nerve injury (1%), asymptomatic subclavian vein occlusion (2.5%), pericardial effusion (1%), subcutaneous patch pocket hematoma (5%), pulse generator pocket infection (1%), lead fracture (1%), and lead system dislodgement (10%). During a mean follow-up period of 11 months, 7.5% of the patients in this series experienced inappropriate therapy delivery, half for atrial fibrillation and the rest for sinus tachycardia.

Although routine follow-up can be accomplished in the clinic, detection and analysis of transient events depends on the recording capabilities available in the devices or on the use of various external monitoring equipment.

82.7 Economics

The annual cost of ICD therapy is dropping as a consequence of better device longevity and simpler implantation techniques. Early generators that lacked programmability, antibradycardia pacing capability, and event recording had 62% survival at 18 months and 2% at 30 months. Some recent programmable designs that include VVI pacing capability and considerable event storage exhibit 96.8% survival at 48 months. It has been estimated that an increase in generator longevity from 2–5 years would lower the cost per life-year saved by 55% in a hypothetical patient population with a 3-year sudden mortality of 28%. More efficient energy conversion circuits and finer line-width integrated circuit technology with smaller, more highly integrated circuits and reduced current drains will yield longer-lasting defibrillators while continuing the evolution to smaller volumes.

Cost of the implantation procedure is clearly declining as transvenous lead systems become commonplace. Total hospitalization duration, complication rates, and use of costly hospital operating rooms and intensive care facilities all are reduced, providing significant financial benefits. One study reported requiring half the intensive care unit time and a reduction in total hospitalization from 26 to 15 days when comparing transvenous to epicardial approaches. Another center reported a mean hospitalization stay of 6 days for patients receiving transvenous defibrillation systems.

Increasing sophistication of the implantable defibrillators paradoxically contributes to cost efficacy. Incorporation of single-chamber brady pacing capability eliminates the cost of a separate pacemaker and lead for those patients who need one. Eventually even dual-chamber pacing capability will be available. Programmable detection and therapy features obviate the need for device replacement that was required when fixed parameter devices proved to be inappropriately specified or too inflexible to adapt to a patient's physiologic changes.

Significant cost savings may be obtained by better patient selection criteria and processes, obviating the need for extensive hospitalization and costly electrophysiologic studies prior to device implantation in some patient groups. One frequently discussed issue is the prophylactic role that implantable defibrillators will or should play. Unless a means is found to build far less expensive devices that can be placed with minimal time and facilities, the life-saving yield for prophylactic defibrillators will have to be high if they are to be cost-effective. This remains an open issue.

82.8 Conclusion

The implantable defibrillator is now an established and powerful therapeutic tool. The transition to pectoral implants with biphasic waveforms and efficient yet simple transvenous lead systems is simplifying the implant procedure and drastically reducing the number of unpleasant VF inductions required to demonstrate adequate system performance. These advances are making the implantable defibrillator easier to use, less costly, and more acceptable to patients and their physicians.

Acknowledgment

Portions of this text are derived from Duffin EG, Barold SS. 1994. Implantable cardioverter-defibrillators: An overview and future directions, Chapter 28 of I Singer (ed), Implantable Cardioverter-Defibrillator, and are used with permission of Futura Publishing Company, Inc.

References

Josephson M, Wellens H (eds). 1992. Tachycardias: Mechanisms and Management. Mount Kisco, NY, Futura Publishing.

Kappenberger L, Lindemans F (eds). 1992. Practical Aspects of Staged Therapy Defibrillators. Mount Kisco, NY, Futura Publishing.

Singer I (ed). 1994. Implantable Cardioverter-Defibrillator. Mount Kisco, NY, Futura Publishing.

Tacker W (ed). 1994. Defibrillation of the Heart: ICD's, AED's, and Manual. St. Louis, Mosby.

PACE, 14: 865. (Memorial issue on implantable defibrillators honoring Michel Mirowski.)

83

Electrosurgical Devices

Wolf W. von Maltzahn
University of Texas at Arlington

Jeffrey L. Eggleston
Valleylab, Inc.

An electrosurgical unit (ESU) passes high-frequency electric currents through biologic tissues to achieve specific surgical effects such as cutting, coagulation, or desiccation. Although it is not completely understood how electrosurgery works, it has been used since the 1920s to cut tissue effectively while at the same time controlling the amount of bleeding. Cutting is achieved primarily with a continuous sinusoidal waveform, whereas coagulation is achieved primarily with a series of sinusoidal wave packets. The surgeon selects either one of these waveforms or a blend of them to suit the surgical needs. An electrosurgical unit can be operated in two modes, the monopolar mode and the bipolar mode. The most noticeable difference between these two modes is the method in which the electric current enters and leaves the tissue. In the monopolar mode, the current flows from a small active electrode into the surgical site, spreads through the body, and returns to a large dispersive electrode on the skin. The high current density in the vicinity of the active electrode achieves tissue cutting or coagulation, whereas the low current density under the dispersive electrode causes no tissue damage. In the bipolar mode, the current flows only through the tissue held between two forceps electrodes. The monopolar mode is used for both cutting and coagulation. The bipolar mode is used primarily for coagulation.

This chapter begins with the theory of operation for electrosurgical units, outlines various modes of operation, and gives basic design details for electronic circuits and electrodes. It then describes how improper application of electrosurgical units can lead to hazardous situations for both the operator and the patient and how such hazardous situations can be avoided or reduced through proper monitoring methods. Finally, the chapter gives an update on current and future developments and applications.

83.1 Theory of Operation

In principle, electrosurgery is based on the rapid heating of tissue. To better understand the thermodynamic events during electrosurgery, it helps to know the general effects of heat on biologic tissue. Consider a tissue volume that experiences a temperature increase from normal body temperature to 45°C within a few seconds. Although the cells in this tissue volume show neither microscopic nor macroscopic changes, some cytochemical changes do in fact occur. However, these changes are reversible, and the cells return to their normal function when the temperature returns to normal values. Above 45°C, irreversible changes take place that inhibit normal cell functions and lead to cell death. First, between 45°C and 60°C, the proteins in the cell lose their quaternary configuration and solidify into a glutinous substance that resembles the white of a hard-boiled egg. This process, termed *coagulation,* is accompanied by tissue blanching. Further increasing the temperature up to 100°C leads to tissue drying; that is, the aqueous cell contents evaporate. This process is called *desiccation.* If the temperature is increased beyond 100°C, the solid contents of the tissue reduce to carbon, a process referred to as *carbonization.* Tissue damage depends not only on temperature, however, but also on the length of exposure to heat. Thus, the overall temperature-induced tissue damage is an integrative effect between temperature and time that is expressed mathematically by the Arrhenius relationship, where an exponential function of temperature is integrated over time [1].

In the monopolar mode, the active electrode either touches the tissue directly or is held a few millimeters above the tissue. When the electrode is held above the tissue, the electric current bridges the air gap by creating an electric discharge arc. A visible arc forms when the electric field strength exceeds 1 kV/mm in the gap and disappears when the field strength drops below a certain threshold level. In the bipolar mode, two active electrodes touch the tissue.

When the active electrode touches the tissue and the current flows directly from the electrode into the tissue without forming an arc, the rise in tissue temperature follows the bioheat equation

$$T - T_o = \frac{1}{\sigma \rho c} J^2 t \tag{83.1}$$

where T and T_o are the final and initial temperatures (K), σ is the electrical conductivity (S/m), ρ is the tissue density (kg/m^3), c is the specific heat of the tissue (Jkg^{-1}K^{-1}), J is the current density (A/m^2), and t is the duration of heat applications [1]. The bioheat equation is valid for short application times where secondary effects such as heat transfer to surrounding tissues, blood perfusion, and metabolic heat can be neglected. According to Eq. (83.1), the surgeon has primarily three means of controlling the cutting or coagulation effect during electrosurgery: the contact area between active electrode and tissue, the electrical current density, and the activation time. In most commercially available electrosurgical generators, the output variable that can be adjusted is power. This power setting, in conjunction with the output-power-versus-tissue-impedance characteristics of the generator, allow the surgeon some control over current. Table 83.1 lists typical output power and mode settings for various surgical procedures. Table 83.2 lists some typical impedance ranges seen during use of an ESU in surgery. The values are shown as ranges because the impedance increases as the tissue dries out, and at the same time, the output power of the ESU decreases. The surgeon may control current density by selection of the active electrode type and size.

83.2 Monopolar Mode

A continuous sinusoidal waveform cuts tissue with very little hemostasis. This waveform is simply called *cut* or *pure cut.* During each positive and negative swing of the sinusoidal waveform, a new discharge arc forms and disappears at essentially the same tissue location. The electric current concentrates at this tissue location, causing a sudden increase in temperature due to resistive heating. The rapid rise in temperature then vaporizes intracellular fluids, increases cell pressure, and ruptures the cell membrane, thereby parting the tissue. This chain of events is confined to the vicinity of the arc, because from there the electric current spreads to a much larger tissue volume, and the current density is no longer high enough to cause resistive heating damage. Typical output values for ESUs, in cut and other modes, are shown in Table 83.3.

Experimental observations have shown that more hemostasis is achieved when cutting with an interrupted sinusoidal waveform or amplitude modulated continuous waveform. These waveforms

TABLE 83.1   Typical ESU Power Settings for Various Surgical Procedures

Power-Level Range	Procedures
Low power	
< 30 W cut	Neurosurgery
< 30 W coag	Dermatology
	Plastic surgery
	Oral surgery
	Laparoscopic sterilization
	Vasectomy
Medium power	
30 W–150 W cut	General surgery
30 W–70 W coag	Laparotomies
	Head and neck surgery (ENT)
	Major orthopedic surgery
	Major vascular surgery
	Routine thoracic surgery
	Polypectomy
High power	
> 150 W cut	Transurethral resection procedures (TURPs)
> 70 W coag	Thoracotomies
	Ablative cancer surgery
	Mastectomies

Note: Ranges assume the use of a standard blade electrode. Use of a needle electrode, or other small current-concentrating electrode, allows lower settings to be used; users are urged to use the lowest setting that provides the desired clinical results.

are typically called *blend* or *blended cut*. Some ESUs offer a choice of blend waveforms to allow the surgeon to select the degree of hemostasis desired.

When a continuous or interrupted waveform is used in contact with the tissue and the output voltage current density is too low to sustain arcing, desiccation of the tissue will occur. Some ESUs have a distinct mode for this purpose called *desiccation* or *contact coagulation*.

In noncontact coagulation, the duty cycle of an interrupted waveform and the crest factor (ratio of peak voltage to rms voltage) influence the degree of hemostasis. While a continuous waveform reestablishes the arc at essentially the same tissue location concentrating the heat there, an interrupted

TABLE 83.2   Typical Impedance Ranges Seen During Use of an ESU in Surgery

Cut Mode Application	Impedance Range (Ω)
Prostate tissue	400–1700
Oral cavity	1000–2000
Liver tissue	
Muscle tissue	
Gall bladder	1500–2400
Skin tissue	1700–2500
Bowel tissue	2500–3000
Periosteum	
Mesentery	3000–4200
Omentum	
Adipose tissue	3500–4500
Scar tissue	
Adhesions	
Coag Mode Application	
Contact coagulation to stop bleeding	100–1000

TABLE 83.3 Typical Output Characteristics of ESUs

	Output Voltage Range Open Circuit, $V_{peak-peak}$, V	Output Power Range, W	Frequency, kHz	Crest Factor $\left(\dfrac{V_{peak}}{V_{rms}}\right)$	Duty Cycle
Monopolar modes					
Cut	200–5000	1–400	300–1750	1.4–2.1	100%
Blend	1500–5800	1–300	300–1750	2.1–6.0	25–80%
Desiccate	400–6500	1–200	300–800	3.5–6.0	50–100%
Fulgurate/spray	6000–12000	1–200	300–800	6.0–20.0	10–70%
Bipolar mode					
Coagulate/desiccate	400–100	1–70	300–1050	1.6–12.0	25–100%

waveform causes the arc to reestablish itself at different tissue locations. The arc seems to dance from one location to the other raising the temperature of the top tissue layer to coagulation levels. These waveforms are called *fulguration* or *spray*. Since the current inside the tissue spreads very quickly from the point where the arc strikes, the heat concentrates in the top layer, primarily desiccating tissue and causing some carbonization. During surgery, a surgeon can easily choose between cutting, coagulation, or a combination of the two by activating a switch on the grip of the active electrode.

83.3 Bipolar Mode

The bipolar mode concentrates the current flow between the two electrodes, requiring considerably less power for achieving the same coagulation effect than the monopolar mode. For example, consider coagulating a small blood vessel with 3-mm external diameter and 2-mm internal diameter, a tissue resistivity of 360 Ωcm, a contact area of 2×4 mm, and a distance between the forceps tips of 1 mm. The tissue resistance between the forceps is 450 Ω as calculated from $R = \rho L/A$, where ρ is the resistivity, L is the distance between the forceps, and A is the contact area. Assuming a typical current density of 200 mA/cm^2, then a small current of 16 mA, a voltage of 7.2 V, and a power level of 0.12 W suffice to coagulate this small blood vessel. In contrast, during monopolar coagulation, current levels of 200 mA and power levels of 100 W or more are not uncommon to achieve the same surgical effect. The temperature increase in the vessel tissue follows the bioheat equation, Eq. (83.1). If the specific heat of the vessel tissue is 4.2 Jg^{-1}K^{-1} and the tissue density is 1 g/cm^3, then the temperature of the tissue between the forceps increases from 37°C to 57°C in 5.83 s. When the active electrode touches the tissue, less tissue damage occurs during coagulation, because the charring and carbonization that accompanies fulguration is avoided.

83.4 ESU Design

Modern ESUs contain building blocks that are also found in other medical devices, such as microprocessors, power supplies, enclosures, cables, indicators, displays, and alarms. The main building blocks unique to ESUs are control input switches, the high-frequency power amplifier, and the safety monitor. The first two will be discussed briefly here, and the latter will be discussed later.

Control input switches include front panel controls, footswitch controls, and handswitch controls. In order to make operating an ESU more uniform between models and manufacturers, and to reduce the possibility of operator error, the ANSI/AAMI HF 18 standard [5] makes specific recommendations concerning the physical construction and location of these switches and prescribes mechanical and electrical performance standards. For instance, front panel controls need to have their function identified by a permanent label and their output indicated on alphanumeric displays or on graduated scales; the pedals of foot switches need to be labeled and respond to a specified activation force; and if the active electrode handle incorporates two finger switches, their position has to correspond to a specific function. Additional recommendations can be found in reference [5].

Four basic high-frequency power amplifiers are in use currently: the somewhat dated vacuum tube/spark gap configuration, the parallel connection of a bank of bipolar power transistors, the hybrid connection of parallel bipolar power transistors cascaded with metal oxide silicon field effect transistors (MOSFETs), and the bridge connection of MOSFETs. Each has unique properties and represents a stage in the evolution of ESUs.

In a vacuum tube/spark gap device, a tuned-plate, tuned-grid vacuum tube oscillator is used to generate a continuous waveform for use in cutting. This signal is introduced to the patient by an adjustable isolation transformer. To generate a waveform for fulguration, the power supply voltage is elevated by a step-up transformer to about 1600 V rms which then connects to a series of spark gaps. The voltage across the spark gaps is capacitively coupled to the primary of an isolation transformer. The RLC circuit created by this arrangement generates a high crest factor, damped sinusoidal, interrupted waveform. One can adjust the output power and characteristics by changing the turns ratio or tap on the primary and/or secondary side of the isolation transformer, or by changing the spark gap distance.

ESUs that use a parallel bank of bipolar power transistors, the transistors are arranged in a Class A configuration. The bases, collectors, and emitters are all connected in parallel, and the collective base node is driven through a current-limiting resistor. A feedback RC network between the base node and the collector node stabilizes the circuit. The collectors are usually fused individually before the common node connects them to one side of the primary of the step-up transformer. The other side of the primary is connected to the high-voltage power supply. A capacitor and resistor in parallel to the primary create a resonant tank circuit that generates the output waveform at a specific frequency. Additional elements may be switched in and out of the primary parallel RLC circuit to alter the output power and waveform for various electrosurgical modes. Small-value resistors between the emitters and ground improve the current sharing between transistors. This configuration sometimes requires the use of matched sets of high-voltage power transistors.

A similar arrangement exists in amplifiers using parallel bipolar transistors cascaded with a power MOSFET. This arrangement is called a *hybrid cascode amplifier*. In this type of amplifier, the collectors of a group of bipolar transistors are connected, via protection diodes, to one terminal of the primary of the step-up output transformer. The other terminal of the primary is connected to the high-voltage power supply. The emitters of two or three bipolar transistors are connected, via current limiting resistors, to the drain of an enhancement mode MOSFET. The source of the MOSFET is connected to ground, and the gate of the MOSFET is connected to a voltage-snubbing network driven by a fixed amplitude pulse created by a high-speed MOS driver circuit. The bases of the bipolar transistors are connected, via current control RC networks, to a common variable base voltage source. Each collector and base is separately fused. In cut modes, the gate drive pulse is a fixed frequency, and the base voltage is varied according to the power setting. In the coagulation modes, the base voltage is fixed and the width of the pulses driving the MOSFET are varied. This changes the conduction time of the amplifier and controls the amount of energy imparted to the output transformer and its load. In the coagulation modes and in high-power cut modes, the bipolar power transistors are saturated, and the voltage across the bipolar/MOSFET combination is low. This translates to high efficiency and low power dissipation.

The most common high-frequency power amplifier in use is a bridge connection of MOSFETs. In this configuration, the drains of a series of power MOSFETs are connected, via protection diodes, to one terminal of the primary of the step-up output transformer. The drain protection diodes protect the MOSFETs against the negative voltage swings of the transformer primary. The other terminal of the transformer primary is connected to the high-voltage power supply. The sources of the MOSFETs are connected to ground. The gate of each MOSFET has a resistor connected to ground and one to its driver circuitry. The resistor to ground speeds up the discharge of the gate capacitance when the MOSFET is turned on while the gate series resistor eliminates turn-off oscillations. Various combinations of capacitors and/or LC networks can be switched across the primary of the step-up output transformer to obtain different waveforms. In the cut mode, the output power is controlled by varying the high-voltage power supply voltage. In the coagulation mode, the output power is controlled by varying the on time of the gate drive pulse.

83.5 Active Electrodes

The monopolar active electrode is typically a small flat blade with symmetric leading and trailing edges that is embedded at the tip of an insulated handle. The edges of the blade are shaped to easily initiate discharge arcs and to help the surgeon manipulate the incision; the edges cannot mechanically cut tissue. Since the surgeon holds the handle like a pencil, it is often referred to as the "pencil." Many pencils contain in their handle one or more switches to control the electrosurgical waveform, primarily to switch between cutting and coagulation. Other active electrodes include needle electrodes, loop electrodes, and ball electrodes. Needle electrodes are used for coagulating small tissue volumes like in neurosurgery or plastic surgery. Loop electrodes are used to resect nodular structures such as polyps or to excise tissue samples for pathologic analysis. Electrosurgery at the tip of an endoscope or laparoscope requires yet another set of active electrodes and specialized training of the surgeon.

83.6 Dispersive Electrodes

The main purpose of the dispersive electrode is to return the high-frequency current to the electrosurgical unit without causing harm to the patient. This is usually achieved by attaching a large electrode to the patient's skin away from the surgical site. The large electrode area and a small contact impedance reduce the current density to levels where tissue heating is minimal. Since the ability of a dispersive electrode to avoid tissue heating and burns is of primary importance, dispersive electrodes are often characterized by their *heating factor*. The heating factor describes the energy dissipated under the dispersive electrode per Ω of impedance and is equal to I^2t, where I is the rms current and t is the time of exposure. During surgery a typical value for the heating factor is 3 A^2s, but factors of up to 9 A^2s may occur during some procedures [2].

Two types of dispersive electrodes are in common use today, the resistive type and the capacitive type. In disposable form, both electrodes have a similar structure and appearance. A thin, rectangular metallic foil has an insulating layer on the outside, connects to a gel-like material on the inside, and may be surrounded by an adhesive foam. In the resistive type, the gel-like material is made of an adhesive conductive gel, whereas in the capacitive type, the gel is an adhesive dielectric nonconductive gel. The adhesive foam and adhesive gel layer ensure that both electrodes maintain good skin contact to the patient, even if the electrode gets stressed mechanically from pulls on the electrode cable. Both types have specific advantages and disadvantages. Electrode failures and subsequent patient injury can be attributed mostly to improper application, electrode dislodgment, and electrode defects rather than to electrode design.

83.7 ESU Hazards

Improper use of electrosurgery may expose both the patient and the surgical staff to a number of hazards. By far the most frequent hazards are electric shock and undesired burns. Less frequent are undesired neuromuscular stimulation, interference with pacemakers or other devices, electrochemical effects from direct currents, implant heating, and gas explosions [1,3].

Current returns to the ESU through the dispersive electrode. If the contact area of the dispersive electrode is large and the current exposure time short, then the skin temperature under the electrode does not rise above 45°C, which has been shown to be the maximum safe temperature [4]. However, to include a safety margin, the skin temperature should not rise more than 6°C above the normal surface temperature of 29–33°C. The current density at any point under the dispersive electrode has to be significantly below the recognized burn threshold of 100 mA/cm² for 10 seconds.

To avoid electric shock and burns, the American National Standard for Electrosurgical Devices [5] requires that "any electrosurgical generator that provides for a dispersive electrode and that has a rated output power of greater than 50 W shall have at least one patient circuit safety monitor." The most common safety monitors are the contact quality monitor for the dispersive electrode and the patient circuit monitor. A contact quality monitor consists of a circuit to measure the impedance between the two sides of a split dispersive electrode and the skin. A small high-frequency current flows from one section of the dispersive electrode through the skin to the second section of the dispersive electrode. If the impedance between these two sections exceeds a certain threshold, or changes by a certain percentage, an audible alarm sounds, and the ESU output is disabled.

Patient circuit monitors range from simple to complex. The simple ones monitor electrode cable integrity while the complex ones detect any abnormal condition that could result in electrosurgical current flowing in other than normal pathways. Although the output isolation transformer present in most modern ESUs usually provides adequate patient protection, some potentially hazardous conditions may still arise. If a conductor to the dispersive electrode is broken, undesired arcing between the broken conductor ends may occur, causing fire in the operating room and serious patient injury. Abnormal current pathways may also arise from capacitive coupling between cables, the patient, operators, enclosures, beds, or any other conductive surface or from direct connections to other electrodes connected to the patient. The patient circuit monitoring device should be operated from an isolated power source having a maximum voltage of 12 V rms. The most common device is a cable continuity monitor. Unlike the contact quality monitor, this monitor only checks the continuity of the cable between the ESU and the dispersive electrode and sounds an alarm if the resistance in that conductor is greater than 1 kΩ. Another implementation of a patient circuit monitor measures the voltage between the dispersive electrode connection and ground. A third implementation functions similarly to a ground fault circuit interrupter (GFCI) in that the current in the wire to the active electrode and the current in the wire to the dispersive electrode are measured and compared with each other. If the difference between these currents is greater than a preset threshold, the alarm sounds and the ESU is disconnected.

There are other sources of undesired burns. Active electrodes get hot when they are used. After use, the active electrode should be placed in a protective holster, if available, or on a suitable surface to isolate it from the patient and surgical staff. The correct placement of an active electrode will also prevent the patient and/or surgeon from being burned if an inadvertent activation of the ESU occurs (e.g., someone accidentally stepping on a foot pedal). Some surgeons use a practice called *buzzing the hemostat* in which a small bleeding vessel is grasped with a clamp or hemostat and the active electrode touched to the clamp while activating. Because of the high voltages involved and the stray capacitance to ground, the surgeon's glove may be compromised. If the surgical staff cannot be convinced to eliminate the practice of buzzing hemostats, the probability of burns can be reduced by use of a cut waveform instead of a coag (lower voltage), by maximizing contact between the surgeons hand and the clamp, and by not activating until the active electrode is firmly touching the clamp.

Although it is commonly assumed that neuromuscular stimulation ceases or is insignificant at frequencies above 10 kHz, such stimulation has been observed in anesthetized patients undergoing certain electrosurgical procedures. This undesirable side effect of electrosurgery is generally attributed to nonlinear events during the electric arcing between the active electrode and tissue that rectify the high-frequency current and lead to dc or low-frequency current components. These current components can reach magnitudes that stimulate nerve and muscle cells. To minimize the probability of unwanted neuromuscular stimulation, most ESUs incorporate in their output circuit a high-pass filter that suppresses dc and low-frequency current components.

The use of electrosurgery means the presence of electric discharge arcs. This presents a potential fire hazard in an operating room where oxygen and flammable gases may be present. These flammable gases may be introduced by the surgical staff (anesthetics or flammable cleaning solutions) or may be generated within the patient themselves (bowel gases). The use of disposable paper drapes also provides a flammable surface that may be ignited by sparking or by placing a hot active electrode on the drape rather than in a protective holster. Therefore, prevention of fires and explosions depends primarily on the prudence and judgment of the ESU operator.

83.8 Recent Developments

Electrosurgery is being enhanced by the addition of a controlled column of argon gas to the path between the active electrode and the tissue. The flow of argon gas assists in clearing the surgical site of fluid and improves visibility. When used in the coagulation mode, the amount of tissue damage and smoke is reduced, producing a thinner, more flexible eschar. When used with the cut mode, lower power levels may be used.

Many manufacturers have begun to include sophisticated computer-based systems in their ESUs that not only simplify the use of the device but also increase the safety of patient and operator [7]. For instance, in a so-called soft coagulation mode a special circuit continuously monitors the current between the active electrode and the tissue and turns the ESU output only on after the active electrode has contacted the tissue. Furthermore, the ESU output is turned off automatically, once the current has reached a certain threshold level that is typical for coagulated and desiccated tissue. This feature is also used in a bipolar mode termed *autobipolar* to prevent arcing at the beginning of the procedure and to keep the tissue from being heated beyond 70°C. Another feature of some modern devices is the so-called power peak system that delivers a very short power peak at the beginning of electrosurgical cutting to start the cutting arc. Continuous monitoring of current and voltage levels and making automatic adjustments provides for a smooth cutting action from the beginning of the incision to its end. Some manufacturers are developing specific waveforms and instruments designed to achieve a bipolar cutting mode. With the growth and popularity of laparoscopic procedures, additional electrosurgical instruments and waveforms tailored to this surgical specialty should also be expected.

Increased computing power, more sophisticated evaluation of voltage and current waveforms, and the addition of miniaturized sensors will continue to make ESUs more user-friendly and safer.

Defining Terms

Active electrode: Electrode used for achieving desired surgical effect.

Coagulation: Solidification of proteins accompanied by tissue whitening.

Desiccation: Drying of tissue due to the evaporation of intracellular fluids.

Dispersive electrode: Return electrode at which no electrosurgical effect is intended.

Fulguration: Random discharge of sparks between active electrode and tissue surface in order to achieve coagulation and/or desiccation.

Spray: Another term for **fulguration.** Sometimes this waveform has a higher crest factor than that used for fulguration.

References

1. Pearce John A. 1986. Electrosurgery, New York, John Wiley.
2. Gerhard Glen C. 1988. Electrosurgical unit. In JG Webster (ed), Encyclopedia of Medical Devices and Instrumentation, vol 2, pp 1180–1203, New York, John Wiley.
3. Gendron Francis G. 1988. Unexplained Patient Burns: Investigating Iatrogenic Injuries, Brea, Calif, Quest Publishing.
4. Pearce JA, Geddes LA, Van Vleet JF, et al. 1983. Skin burns from electrosurgical current. Med Instrum 17(3):225.

5. American National Standard for Electrosurgical Devices. 1994. HF18, American National Standards Institute.
6. LaCourse JR, Miller WT III, Vogt M, et al. 1985. Effect of high frequency current on nerve and muscle tissue. IEEE Trans Biomed Eng 32:83.
7. Haag R, Cuschieri A. 1993. Recent advances in high-frequency electrosurgery: Development of automated systems. J R Coll Surg Ednb 38:354.

Further Information

American National Standards Institute, 1988. International Standard, Medical Electrical Equipment, Part 1: General Requirements for Safety, IEC 601-1, 2d ed, New York.

American National Standards Institute. 1991. International Standard, Medical Electrical Equipment, Part 2: Particular Requirements for the Safety of High Frequency Surgical Equipment, IEC 601-2-2, 2d ed, New York.

National Fire Protection Association. 1993. Standard for Health Care Facilities, NFPA 99.

84

Mechanical Ventilation

Khosrow Behbehani
*University of Texas at Arlington
and University of Texas
Southwestern Medical Center
at Dallas*

This chapter presents an overview of the structure and function of mechanical ventilators. Mechanical ventilators, which often are also called respirators, are used to artificially ventilate the lungs of patients who are unable to naturally breathe from the atmosphere. In almost 100 years of development, many mechanical ventilators with different designs have been developed [Mushin et al., 1980]. The very early devices used bellows that were manually operated to inflate the lungs. Today's respirators employ an array of sophisticated components such as fast-response servo valves and precision transducers to perform the task of ventilating the lungs. The changes in the design of ventilators have come about as the result of improvements in engineering the ventilator components and the advent of new therapy modes by clinicians. A large variety of ventilators are now available for short-term treatment of acute respiratory problems as well as for long-term therapy for chronic respiratory conditions.

It is reasonable to broadly classify today's ventilators into two groups. The first and indeed the largest group encompasses the intensive care respirators used primarily in hospitals to support patients following certain surgical procedures or to assist patients with acute respiratory disorders. The second group includes less complicated machines that are used primarily at home to treat patients with chronic respiratory disorders.

The level of engineering design and sophistication for the intensive care ventilators is higher than that of the ventilators used for chronic treatment. However, many of the engineering concepts employed in designing intensive care ventilators can also be applied in the simpler chronic care units. Therefore, this chapter focuses on the design of intensive care ventilators; the terms *respirator, mechanical ventilator,* or *ventilator* that will be used from this point on refer to the intensive care unit respirators.

From the beginning, the designers of the mechanical ventilators realized that the main task of a respirator is to ventilate the lungs in a manner as close to natural respiration as possible. Since natural inspiration is a result of negative pressure in the pleural cavity generated by distention of the diaphragm, designers initially developed ventilators that created the same effect. These ventilators are called *negative pressure ventilators.*

84.1 Negative-Pressure Ventilators

The principle of operation of a negative-pressure respirator is shown in Fig. 84.1. In this design, the flow of air to the lungs is created by generating a negative pressure around the patient's thoracic cage. The negative pressure moves the thoracic walls outward, expanding the intrathoracic volume and dropping the pressure inside the lungs. The pressure gradient between the atmosphere and the lungs causes the flow of atmospheric air into the lungs. The inspiratory and expiratory phases of the respiration are controlled by cycling the pressure inside the body chamber between a sub-atmospheric level (inspiration) and the atmospheric level (exhalation). Flow of the breath out the lungs during exhalation is caused by the recoil of thoracic muscles.

Although it may appear that the negative-pressure respirator incorporates the same principles as natural respiration, the engineering implementation of this concept has not been very successful. A major difficulty has been in the design of a chamber for creating negative pressure around the thoracic walls. One approach has been to make the chamber large enough to house the entire body with exception of the head and neck. Using foam rubber around the patient's neck, one can seal the chamber and generate a negative pressure inside the chamber. This design configuration, commonly known as the iron lung, was tried back in 1920s and proved to be deficient in several aspects. The main drawback was that the negative pressure generated inside the chamber was applied to the chest as well as the abdominal wall, thus creating a venous blood pool in the abdomen and reducing cardiac output.

More recent designs have tried to restrict the application of the negative pressure to the chest walls by designing a chamber that goes only around the chest. However, this has not been successful because obtaining a seal around the chest wall (Fig. 84.1) is difficult.

Negative-pressure ventilators also made the patient less accessible for patient care and monitoring. Further, synchronization of the machine cycle with the patient's effort was difficult, and the machines are noisy and bulky [McPherson & Spearman, 1990]. These deficiencies of the negative-pressure ventilators have led to the development of the positive-pressure ventilators.

84.2 Positive-Pressure Ventilators

Positive-pressure ventilators generate the inspiratory flow by applying a positive pressure (greater than the atmospheric pressure) to the airways. Figure 84.2 shows a simplified block diagram of a

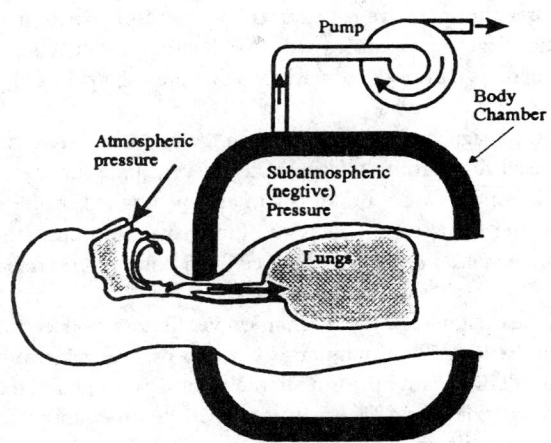

FIGURE 84.1 A simplified illustration of a negative-pressure ventilator.

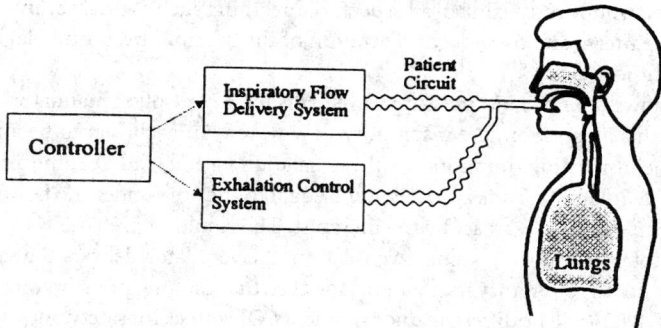

FIGURE 84.2 A simplified diagram of the functional blocks of a positive-pressure ventilator.

positive-pressure ventilator. During inspiration the inspiratory flow delivery system creates a positive pressure in the tubes connected to the patient airway, called *patient circuit,* and the exhalation control system closes a valve at the outlet of the tubing to the atmosphere. When the ventilator switches to exhalation, the inspiratory flow delivery system stops the positive pressure, and the exhalation system opens the valve to allow the patient's exhaled breath to flow to the atmosphere. The use of a positive-pressure gradient in creating the flow allows for treating patients with high lung resistance and low compliance. As a result, positive-pressure ventilators have been very successful in treating a variety of breathing disorders and have become more popular than negative-pressure ventilators.

Positive-pressure ventilators have been employed to treat patients ranging from neonates to adults. Due to anatomic differences between various patient populations, the ventilators and their modes of treating infants are different than those for adults. Nonetheless, their fundamental design principles are similar, and adult ventilators comprise a larger percentage of ventilators manufactured and used in clinics. Therefore, the emphasis here is on the description of adult positive-pressure ventilators. Also, the concepts presented will be illustrated using a microprocessor-based design example, since almost all modern ventilators use microprocessor instrumentation.

84.3 Ventilation Modes

Since the advent of respirators, clinicians have devised a variety of strategies to ventilate the lungs based on patient conditions. For instance, some patients need the respirator to completely take over the task of ventilating their lungs. In this case, the ventilator operates in *mandatory mode* and delivers mandatory breaths. However, some patients are able to initiate a breath and breathe on their own but may need oxygen-enriched air flow or slightly elevated airway pressure. When a ventilator assists a patient who is capable of demanding a breath, the ventilator delivers spontaneous breaths and operates in *spontaneous mode.* In many cases, it is first necessary to treat the patient with mandatory ventilation, and as the patient's condition improves, spontaneous ventilation is introduced; it is used primarily to wean the patient from mandatory breathing.

Mandatory Ventilation

Designers of adult ventilators have employed two rather distinct approaches for delivering mandatory breaths: *volume ventilation* and *pressure ventilation.* Volume ventilation, which presently is more popular, refers to delivering a specified tidal volume to the patient during the inspiratory phase. Pressure ventilation, however, refers to raising and maintaining the airway pressure to a level set by the therapist, during the inspiratory phase of each breath. Regardless of the type, a ventilator operating in mandatory mode must control all aspects of breathing such as tidal volume, respiration rate, inspiratory flow pattern, and oxygen concentration of the breath. This is often labeled as *controlled mandatory ventilation (CMV)*.

Figure 84.3 shows the flow and pressure waveforms for a controlled mandatory volume ventilation (CMV). In this illustration, the inspiratory flow waveform is chosen to be a half-sinewave. In Fig. 84.3a, t_i is the inspiration duration, t_e is the exhalation period, and Q_i is the amplitude of inspiratory flow. The ventilator delivers a tidal volume equal to the area under the flow waveform in Fig. 84.3a at regular intervals $(t_i + t_e)$ set by the therapist. The resulting pressure waveform is shown in Fig. 84.3b. It is noted that during volume ventilation, the ventilator delivers the same volume irrespective of the patient's respiratory mechanics. However, the resulting pressure waveform such as the one shown in Fig. 84.3b will be different among patients. Of course, for safety purposes, the ventilator limits the maximum applied airway pressure according to the therapist's setting.

As can be seen in Fig. 84.3b, the airway pressure at the end of exhalation may not end at atmospheric pressure (zero gauge). The *positive end expiratory pressure* or *PEEP* is sometimes used to keep the alveoli from collapsing during expiration [Norwood, 1990]. In other cases, the expiration pressure is allowed to return to the atmospheric level.

Figure 84.4 shows a plot of the pressure and flow during a mandatory pressure ventilation. In this case, the respirator raises and maintains the airway pressure at the desired level independent of patient airway compliance and resistance. The level of pressure during inspiration, P_i, is set by the therapist. Although the ventilator maintains the same pressure trajectory for patients with different respiratory resistance and compliance, the resulting flow trajectory, shown in Fig. 84.4b, will depend on the respiratory mechanics of each patient.

In the following, the presentation will focus on volume ventilators, since they are more common. Further, in a microprocessor-based ventilator, the mechanism for delivering mandatory volume and pressure ventilation have many similar main components. The primary difference lies in the control algorithms governing the delivery of breaths to the patient.

Spontaneous Ventilation

An important phase in providing respiratory therapy to a recovering pulmonary patient is weaning the patient from the respirator. As the patient recovers and gains the ability to breathe independently,

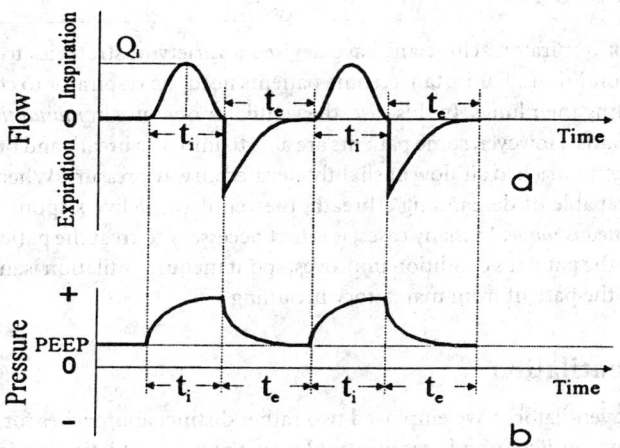

FIGURE 84.3 (a) Inspiratory flow for a controlled mandatory volume ventilation breath. (b) Airway pressure resulting from the breath delivery with a nonzero PEEP.

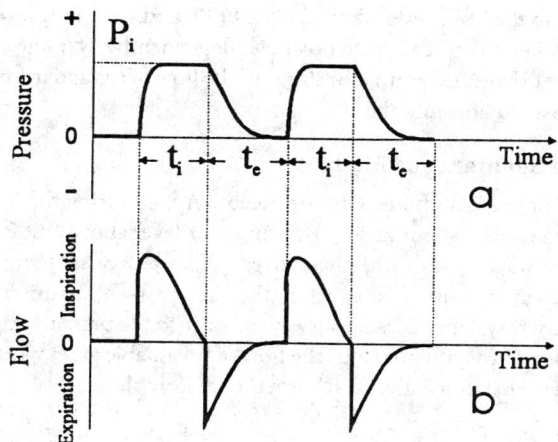

FIGURE 84.4 (*a*) Inspiratory pressure pattern for a controlled mandatory pressure ventilation breath. (*b*) Airway flow pattern resulting from the breath delivery.

the ventilator must allow the patient to initiate a breath and control the breath rate, flow rate, and the tidal volume. Ideally, when a respirator is functioning in the spontaneous mode, it should let the patient take breaths with the same ease as breathing from the atmosphere. This, however, is difficult to achieve, because the respirator has neither an infinite gas supply nor an instantaneous response. In practice, the patient generally has to exert more effort to breathe spontaneously on a respirator than from the atmosphere. However, patient effort is reduced as the ventilator response speed increases [McPherson & Spearman, 1990]. Spontaneous ventilation is often used in conjunction with mandatory ventilation, since the patient may still need breaths that are delivered entirely by the ventilator. Alternatively, when patients can breathe completely on their own but need oxygen-enriched breath or elevated airway pressure, spontaneous ventilation alone may be used.

As in the case of mandatory ventilation, several modes of spontaneous ventilation have been devised by therapists. Two of the most important and popular spontaneous breath delivery modes are described below.

Continuous Positive Airway Pressure (CPAP) in Spontaneous Mode

In this mode, the ventilator maintains a positive pressure at the airway as the patient attempts to inspire. Figure 84.5 illustrates a typical airway pressure waveform during CPAP breath delivery. The therapist sets the sensitivity level lower than PEEP. When the patient attempts to breathe, the pressure drops below the sensitivity level, and the ventilator responds by supplying breathable gases to

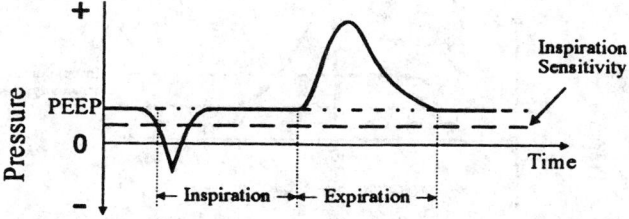

FIGURE 84.5 Airway pressure during a CPAP spontaneous breath delivery.

raise the pressure back to the PEEP level. Typically, the PEEP and sensitivity levels are selected so that the patient will be impelled to exert effort to breathe independently. As in the case of the mandatory mode, when the patient exhales, the ventilator shuts off the flow of gas and opens the exhalation valve to allow the exhaled gases to flow into the atmosphere.

Pressure Support in Spontaneous Mode

This mode is similar to the CPAP mode with the exception that during the inspiration the ventilator attempts to maintain the patient airway pressure at a level above PEEP. Figure 84.6 shows a typical airway pressure waveform during the delivery of a *pressure support* breath. In this mode, when the patient's airway pressure drops below the therapist-set sensitivity line, the ventilator inspiratory breath delivery system raises the airway pressure to the pressure support level (> PEEP) selected by the therapist. The ventilator stops the flow of breathable gases when the patient starts to exhale and controls the exhalation valve to achieve the set PEEP level.

84.4 Breath Delivery Control

Figure 84.7 shows a simplified block diagram for delivering mandatory or spontaneous ventilation. Compressed air and oxygen are normally stored in high-pressure tanks ($\cong$ 1400 kPa) that are attached to the inlets of the ventilator. In some ventilators, an air compressor is used in place of a compressed air tank. Manufacturers of mechanical respirators have designed a variety of blending and metering devices [McPherson & Spearman, 1990]. The primary mission of the device is to enrich the inspiratory air flow with proper level of oxygen and deliver a tidal volume according to the therapist specifications. With the introduction of microprocessors for control of metering devices, electromechanical valves have gained popularity [Puritan-Bennett, 1987]. In Fig. 84.7, the air and oxygen valves are placed in closed feedback loops with the air and oxygen flow sensors. The microprocessor controls each valve to deliver the desired inspiratory air and oxygen flows for mandatory and spontaneous ventilation. During inhalation, the exhalation valve is closed to direct all the delivered flows to the lungs. When exhalation starts, the microprocessor actuates the exhalation valve to achieve the desired PEEP level. The airway pressure sensor, shown on the right side of Fig. 84.7, generates the feedback signal necessary for maintaining the desired PEEP (in both mandatory and spontaneous modes) and pressure support level during spontaneous breath delivery.

Control of Mandatory Breath Inspiratory Flow

In a microprocessor-controlled ventilator (Fig. 84.7), the electronically actuated valves open from a closed position to allow the flow of blended gases to the patient. The control of flow through each valve depends on the therapist's specification for the mandatory breath. That is, the clinician must specify the following parameters for delivery of CMV breaths: (1) respiration rate; (2) flow waveform; (3) tidal volume; (4) oxygen concentration (of the delivered breath); (5) peak flow; and (6)

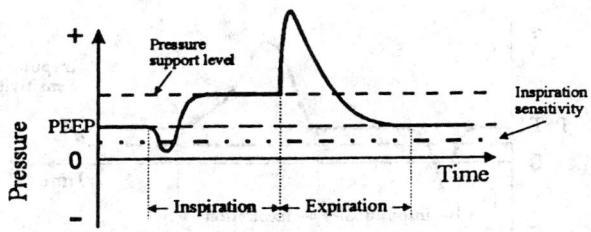

FIGURE 84.6 Airway pressure during a pressure support spontaneous breath delivery.

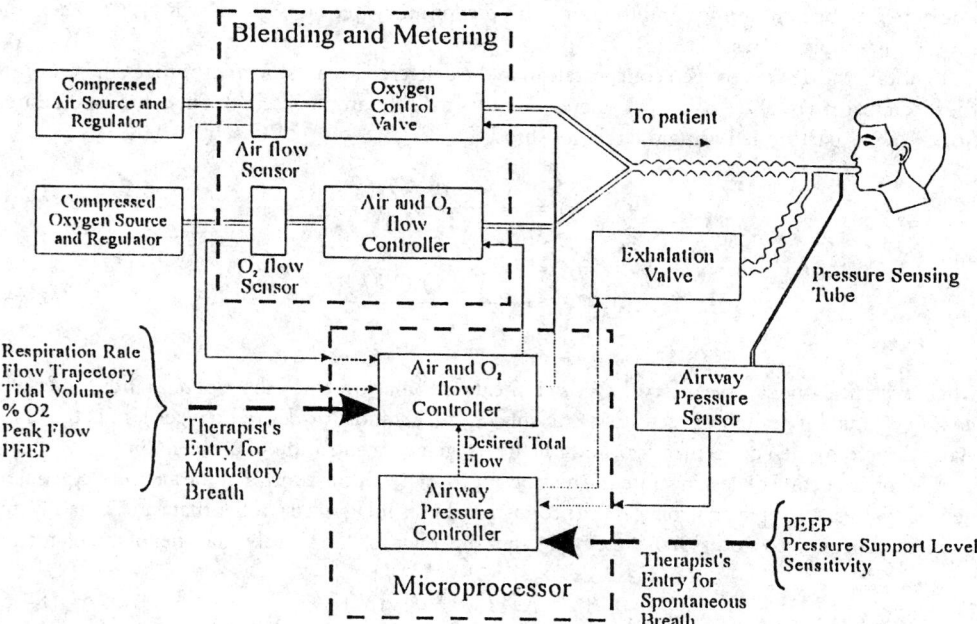

FIGURE 84.7 A simplified block diagram of a control structure for mandatory and spontaneous breath delivery.

PEEP, as shown in the lower left side of Fig. 84.7. It is noted that the PEEP selected by the therapist in the mandatory mode is only used for control of exhalation flow. The microprocessor utilizes the first five of the above parameters to compute the total desired inspiratory flow trajectory. To illustrate this point, consider the delivery of a tidal volume using a half-sinewave as shown in Fig. 84.3. If the therapist selects a tidal volume of $V_t(L)$, a respiration rate of n breaths per minute (bpm), the peak respiratory flow, $Q_i(L/s)$, then the total desired inspiratory flow, $Q_d(t)$, for a single breath can be computed from the following equation:

$$Q_d(t) = \begin{cases} Q_i \sin \dfrac{\pi t}{t_i} & 0 \le t < t_i \\ 0 & t_i < t \le t_e \end{cases} \tag{84.1}$$

where t_i signifies the duration of inspiration and is computed from the relationship

$$t_i = \frac{V_t}{2Q_i} \tag{84.2}$$

The duration of expiration in seconds is obtained from

$$t_e = \frac{60}{n} - t_i \tag{84.3}$$

The ratio of inspiratory period to expiratory period of a mandatory breath often is used for adjusting the respiration rate. This ratio is represented by *I:E (ratio)* and computed as follows. First, the inspiratory and expiratory periods are normalized with respect to t_i. Hence, the normalized inspiratory period becomes unity, and the normalized expiratory period is given by $R = t_e/t_i$. Then, the I:E ratio is simply expressed as 1:R.

To obtain the desired oxygen concentration in the delivered breath, the microprocessor computes the discrete form of $Q_d(t)$ as $Q_d(k)$ where k signifies the kth sample interval. Then, the total desired flow $Q_d(k)$ is partitioned using the relationships

$$Q_{da}(k) = \frac{(1 - m) \, Q_d(k)}{(1 - c)} \tag{84.4}$$

and

$$Q_{dx}(k) = \frac{(m - c) \, Q_d(k)}{(1 - c)} \tag{84.5}$$

where k signifies the sample interval, $Q_{da}(k)$ is the desired air flow (the subscript da stands for desired air), $Q_{dx}(k)$ is the desired oxygen flow (the subscript dx stands for desired oxygen), m is the clinician's desired oxygen concentration, and c is the oxygen concentration of ambient air.

A number of control design strategies may be appropriate for the control of the air and oxygen flow delivery valves. A simple controller is the proportional plus integral controller that can be readily implemented in a microprocessor. For example, the controller for the air valve has the following form:

$$I(k) = K_p E(k) + K_i A(k) \tag{84.6}$$

where $E(k)$ and $A(k)$ are given by

$$E(k) = Q_{da}(k) - Q_{sa}(k) \tag{84.7}$$

$$A(k) = A(k - 1) + E(k) \tag{84.8}$$

where, $I(k)$ is the input (voltage or current) to the air valve at the kth sampling interval, $E(k)$ is the error in the delivered flow, $Q_{da}(k)$ is the desired air flow, $Q_{sa}(k)$ is the sensed or actual air flow (the subscript sa stands for sensed air flow), $A(k)$ is the integral (rectangular integration) part of the controller, and K_p and K_i are the controller proportionality constants. It is noted that the above equations are applicable to the control of either air or oxygen valve. For control of oxygen flow valve, $Q_{dx}(k)$ replaces $Q_{da}(k)$, and $Q_{sx}(k)$ replaces $Q_{sa}(k)$, where $Q_{sx}(k)$ represents the sensed oxygen flow (the subscript sx stands for sensed oxygen flow).

The control structure shown in Fig. 84.7 provides the flexibility of quickly adjusting the percentage of oxygen in the enriched breath gases. That is, the controller can regulate both the total flow and the percentage of oxygen delivered to the patient. Since the internal volume of the flow control valve is usually small ($<$ 50 ml), the desired change in the oxygen concentration of the delivered flow can be achieved within one inspiratory period. In actual clinical applications, rapid change of percentage of oxygen from one breath to another is often desirable, because it reduces the waiting time for the delivery of the desired oxygen concentration. A design similar to the one shown in Fig. 84.7 has been successfully implemented in a microprocessor-based ventilator [Behbehani, 1984] and is deployed in hospitals around the world.

Expiratory Pressure Control in Mandatory Mode

It is often desirable to keep the patient's lungs inflated at the end of expiration at a pressure greater than atmospheric level [Norwood, 1990]. That is, rather than allowing the lungs to deflate during the exhalation, the controller closes the exhalation valve when the airway pressure reaches the PEEP level. When expiration starts, the ventilator terminates flow to the lungs, hence the regulation of the airway pressure is achieved by controlling the flow of patient exhaled gases through the exhalation valve.

In a microprocessor-based ventilator, an electronically actuated valve can be employed that has adequate dynamic response ($\cong$20-ms rise time) to regulate PEEP. For this purpose, the pressure in the patient breath delivery circuit is measured using a pressure transducer (Fig. 84.7). The microprocessor will initially open the exhalation valve completely to minimize resistance to expiratory flow. At the same time, it will sample the pressure transducer's output and starts to close the exhalation valve as the pressure begins to approach the desired PEEP level. Since the patient's exhaled flow is the only source of pressure, if the airway pressure drops below PEEP, it cannot be brought back up until the next inspiratory period. Hence, an overrun (i.e., a drop to below PEEP) in the closed-loop control of PEEP cannot be tolerated.

Spontaneous Breath Delivery Control

The small-diameter ($\cong$ 5 mm) pressure sensing tube, shown on the right side of Fig. 84.7, transmits the pneumatic pressure signal from the patient airway to a pressure transducer placed in the ventilator. The output of the pressure transducer is amplified, filtered, and sampled by the microprocessor. The controller receives the therapist's inputs regarding the spontaneous breath characteristics such as the PEEP, sensitivity, and oxygen concentration, as shown in the lower-right side of Fig. 84.7. The desired airway pressure is computed from the therapist entries of PEEP, pressure support level, and sensitivity. The multiple-loop control structure shown in Fig. 84.7 is used to deliver a CPAP or a pressure support breath. The sensed proximal airway pressure is compared with the desired airway pressure. The airway pressure controller computes the total inspiratory flow level required to raise the airway pressure to the desired level. This flow level serves as the reference input or total desired flow for the flow control loop. Hence, in general, the desired total flow trajectory for the spontaneous breath delivery may be different for each inspiratory cycle. If the operator has specified oxygen concentration greater than 21.6% (the atmospheric air oxygen concentration), the controller will partition the total required flow into the air and oxygen flow rates using Eqs. (84.4) and (84.5). The flow controller then uses the feedback signals from air and oxygen flow sensors and actuates the air and oxygen valves to deliver the desired flows.

For a microprocessor-based ventilator, the control algorithm for regulating the airway pressure can also be a proportional plus integral controller [Behbehani, 1984; Behbehani & Watanabe, 1986]. In this case, the total required flow for maintaining the desired airway pressure $Q_d(k)$ is given by the equation

$$Q_d(k) = C_p E_p(k) + C_i A_p(k) \qquad (84.9)$$

where $E_p(k)$ and $A_p(k)$ are computed using the equations

$$E_p(k) = P_d(k) - P_s(k) \qquad (84.10)$$

$$A_p(k) = A_p(k-1) + E_p(k) \qquad (84.11)$$

In the above equations, $E_p(k)$ is the difference between the desired airway pressure $P_d(k)$ and the sensed airway pressure $P_s(k)$; the parameter $A_p(k)$ represents the integral portion of the controller; C_p and C_i are the proportionality constants; and k represents the sample interval.

If a nonzero PEEP level is specified, the same control strategy as the one described for mandatory breath delivery can be used to achieve the desired PEEP.

84.5 Summary

Today's mechanical ventilators can be broadly classified into negative-pressure and positive-pressure ventilators. Negative-pressure ventilators do not offer the flexibility and convenience that positive-pressure ventilators provide, and hence they have not been very popular in clinical use. Positive-pressure ventilators have been quite successful in treating patients with pulmonary disorders. These ventilators operate in either mandatory or spontaneous mode. When delivering mandatory breaths, the ventilator controls all parameters of the breath such as tidal volume, inspiratory flow waveform, respiration rate, and oxygen content of the breath. Mandatory breaths are normally delivered to the patients that are incapable of breathing on their own. In contrast, spontaneous breath delivery refers to the case where the ventilator responds to the patient's effort to breathe independently. Therefore, the patient can control the volume and the rate of the respiration. The therapist selects the oxygen content and the pressure at which the breath is delivered. Spontaneous breath delivery is typically used for the patients who are on their way to full recovery but are not completely ready to breathe from the atmosphere without mechanical assistance.

Defining Terms

Continuous positive airway pressure (CPAP): A spontaneous ventilation mode in which the ventilator maintains a constant positive pressure, near or below PEEP level, in the patient's airway while patient breathes at will.

Controlled mandatory ventilation: A common term for referring to mandatory ventilation of patients who are not able to initiate or respire on their own.

I:E ratio: The ratio of normalized inspiratory interval to normalized expiratory interval of a mandatory breath. Both intervals are normalized with respect to the inspiratory period. Hence, the normalized inspiratory period is always unity.

Mandatory mode: A mode of mechanically ventilating the lungs where the ventilator controls all breath delivery parameters such as tidal volume, respiration rate, flow waveform, etc.

Patient circuit: A set of tubes connecting the patient airway to the outlet of a respirator.

Positive end expiratory pressure (PEEP): A therapist-selected pressure level for the patient airway at the end of expiration in either mandatory or spontaneous breathing.

Pressure support: A spontaneous breath delivery mode in which the ventilator applies a positive pressure greater than PEEP to the patient's airway during inspiration.

Pressure support level: Refers to the pressure level, above PEEP, that the ventilator maintains during the spontaneous inspiration.

Pressure ventilation: A mandatory mode of ventilation where during the inspiration phase of each breath a constant pressure is applied to the patient's airway independent of the patient's airway resistance and/or compliance.

Spontaneous mode: A ventilation mode in which the patient initiates and breathes from the ventilator supplied gas at will.

Volume ventilation: A mandatory mode of ventilation where the volume of each breath is set by the therapist and the ventilator delivers that volume to the patient independent of patient's airway resistance and/or compliance.

References

Behbehani K. 1984. PLM-implementation of a multiple closed-loop control strategy for a microprocessor-controlled respirator. Proc of AC Conf 574–576.

Behbehani K, Watanabe NT. 1986. A new application of digital computer simulation in the design of a microprocessor-based respirator. Summer Simulation Conf 415–420.

McPherson SP, Spearman CB. 1990. Respiratory Therapy Equipment, 4th ed, St Louis, C.V. Mosby.

Mushin WW, Rendell-Baker L, Thompson PW, et al. 1980. Automatic Ventilation of the Lungs, 3d ed, St. Louis, Blackwell Scientific Publications.

Norwood S. 1990. Physiological principles of conventional mechanical ventilation. In RR Kirby, MJ Banner, JB Downs (eds), Clinical Application of Ventilatory Support, pp 145–172, New York, Churchill Livingstone.

Puritan-Bennett 7200 Ventilator System Series. 1990. Ventilator, options and accessories, Part no 22300A, Carlsbad, Calif.

85

Parenteral Infusion Devices

Gregory I. Voss
IVAC Corporation

Robert D. Butterfield
IVAC Corporation

The circulatory system is the body's primary pathway for both the distribution of oxygen and other nutrients and the removal of carbon dioxide and other waste products. Since the entire blood supply in a healthy adult completely circulates within 60 seconds, substances introduced into the circulatory system are distributed rapidly. Thus intravenous (IV) and intraarterial access routes provide an effective pathway for the delivery of fluid, blood, and medicants to a patient's vital organs. Consequently, about 80% of hospitalized patients receive infusion therapy. Peripheral and central veins are used for the majority of infusions. Umbilical artery delivery (in neonates), enteral delivery of nutrients, and epidural delivery of anesthetics and analgesics comprise smaller patient populations. A variety of devices can be used to provide flow through an intravenous catheter. An intravenous delivery system typically consists of three major components: (1) fluid or drug reservoir, (2) catheter system for transferring the fluid or drug from the reservoir into the vasculature through a venipuncture, and (3) device for regulating and/or generating flow (see Fig. 85.1).

This chapter is separated into five sections. The first describes the clinical needs associated with intravenous drug delivery that determine device performance criteria. The second section reviews the principles of flow through a tube; the third section introduces the underlying electromechanical principles for flow regulation and/or generation and their ability to meet the clinical performance criteria. The fourth section reviews complications associated with intravenous therapy, and the fifth section concludes with a short list of articles providing more detailed information.

85.1 Performance Criteria for Intravenous Infusion Devices

The intravenous pathway provides an excellent route for continuous drug therapy. The ideal delivery system regulates drug concentration in the body to achieve and maintain a desired result. When the drug's effect cannot be monitored directly, it is frequently assumed that a specific blood concentration or infusion rate will achieve the therapeutic objective. Although underinfusion may not provide sufficient therapy, overinfusion can produce even more serious toxic side effects.

The therapeutic range and risks associated with under- and overinfusion are highly drug and patient dependent. Intravenous delivery of fluids and electrolytes often does not require very

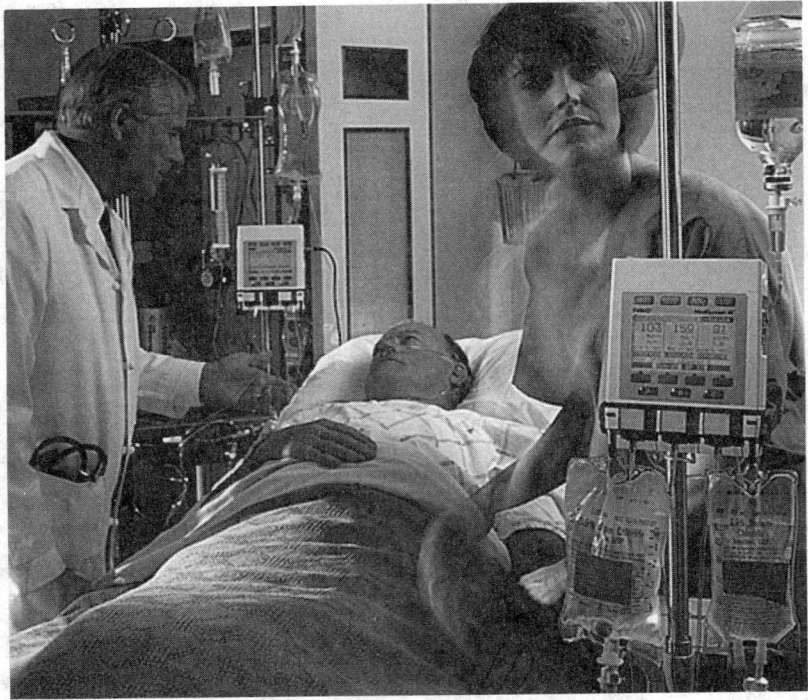

FIGURE 85.1   A typical IV infusion system.

accurate regulation. Low-risk patients can generally tolerate well infusion rate variability of $\pm 30\%$ for fluids. In some situations, however, specifically for fluid-restricted patients, prolonged under- or overinfusion of fluids can compromise the patient's cardiovascular and renal systems.

The infusion of many drugs, especially potent cardioactive agents, requires high accuracy. For example, post-coronary-artery-bypass-graft patients commonly receive sodium nitroprusside to lower arterial blood pressure. Hypertension, associated with underinfusion, subjects the graft sutures to higher stress with an increased risk for internal bleeding. Hypotension associated with overinfusion can compromise the cardiovascular state of the patient. Nitroprusside's potency, short onset delay, and short half-life (30–180 s) provide for very tight control, enabling the clinician to quickly respond to the many events that alter the patient's arterial pressure. The fast response of drugs such as nitroprusside creates a need for short-term flow uniformity as well as long-term accuracy.

The British Department of Health employs *Trumpet curves* in their Health Equipment Information reports to compare flow uniformity of infusion pumps. For a prescribed flow rate, the trumpet curve is the plot of the maximum and minimum measured percentage flow rate error as a function of the accumulation interval (Fig. 85.2). Flow is measured gravimetrically in 30-s blocks for 1 hour. These blocks are summed to produce 120-s, 300-s, and other longer total accumulation intervals. Though the 120-s window may not detect flow variations important in delivery of the fastest acting agents, the trumpet curve provides a helpful means for performance comparison among infusion devices. Additional statistical information such as standard deviations may be derived from the basic trumpet flow measurements.

The short half-life of certain pharmacologic agents and the clotting reaction time of blood during periods of stagnant flow require that fluid flow be maintained without significant interruption. Specifically, concern has been expressed in the literature that the infusion of sodium nitroprusside and other short half-life drugs occur without interruptions exceeding 20 s. Thus, minimization of false alarms and rapid detection of occlusions are important aspects of maintaining a constant

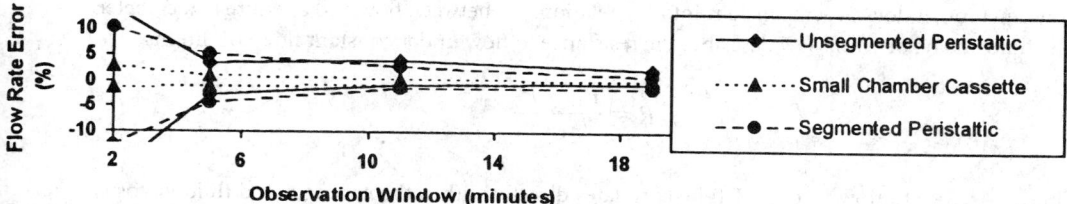

FIGURE 85.2 Trumpet curve for several representative large volume infusion pumps operated a 5 mL/hr. Note that peristaltic pumps were designed for low risk patients.

vascular concentration. Accidental occlusions of the IV line due to improper positioning of stop-cocks or clamps, kinked tubing, and clotted catheters are common.

Occlusions between pump and patient present a secondary complication in maintaining serum drug concentration. Until detected, the pump will infuse, storing fluid in the delivery set. When the occlusion is eliminated, the stored volume is delivered to the patient in a bolus. With concentrated pharmaceutic agents, this bolus can produce a large perturbation in the patient's status.

Occlusions of the pump intake also interrupt delivery. If detection is delayed, inadequate flow can result. During an intake occlusion, in some pump designs removal of the delivery set can produce abrupt aspiration of blood. This event may precipitate clotting and cause injury to the infusion site.

The common practice of delivering multiple drugs through a single venous access port produces an additional challenge to maintaining uniform drug concentration. Although some mixing will occur in the venous access catheter, fluid in the catheter more closely resembles a first-in/first-out digital queue: During delivery, drugs from the various infusion devices mix at the catheter input, an equivalent fluid volume discharges from the outlet. Rate changes and flow nonuniformity cause the mass flow of drugs at the outlet to differ from those at the input. Consider a venous access catheter with a volume of 2 mL and a total flow of 10 mL/hr. Due to the digital queue phenomenon, an incremental change in the intake flow rate of an individual drug will not appear at the output for 12 min. In addition, changing flow rates for one drug will cause short-term marked swings in the delivery rate of drugs using the same access catheter. When the delay becomes significantly larger than the time constant for a drug that is titrated to a measurable patient response, titration becomes extremely difficult leading to large oscillations.

As discussed, the performance requirements for drug delivery vary with multiple factors: drug, fluid restriction, and patient risk. Thus the delivery of potent agents to fluid-restricted patients at risk require the highest performance standards defined by flow rate accuracy, flow rate uniformity, and ability to minimize risk of IV-site complications. These performance requirements need to be appropriately balanced with the device cost and the impact on clinician productivity.

85.2 Flow Through an IV Delivery System

The physical properties associated with the flow of fluids through cylindrical tubes provide the foundation for understanding flow through a catheter into the vasculature. Hagen-Poiseuille's equation for laminar flow of a Newtonian fluid through a rigid tube states

$$Q = \pi \cdot r^4 \cdot \frac{(P_1 - P_2)}{8 \cdot \eta \cdot L}$$

where Q is the flow; P_1 and P_2 are the pressures at the inlet and outlet of the tube, respectively; L and r are the length and internal radius of the tube, respectively; and η is fluid viscosity. Although many drug delivery systems do not strictly meet the flow conditions for precise application of the laminar flow equation, it does provide insight into the relationship between flow and pressure in a catheter. The fluid analog of Ohms law describes the resistance to flow under constant flow conditions

$$R = \frac{P_1 - P_2}{Q}$$

Thus, resistance to flow through a tube correlates directly with catheter length and fluid viscosity and inversely with the fourth power of catheter diameter. For steady flow, the delivery system can be modeled as a series of resistors representing each component, including administration set, access catheter, and circulatory system. When dynamic aspects of the delivery system are considered, a more detailed model including catheter and venous compliance, fluid inertia, and turbulent flow is required. Flow resistance may be defined with units of mmHg/(L/hr), so that 1 fluid ohm = 4.8×10^{-11} Pa s/m^3. Studies determining flow resistance for several catheter components with distilled water for flow rates of 100, 200, and 300 mL/hr appear in Table 85.1.

85.3 Intravenous Infusion Devices

From Hagen-Poiselluie's equation, two general approaches to intravenous infusion become apparent. First, a hydrostatic pressure gradient can be used with adjustment of delivery system resistance controlling flow rate. Complications such as partial obstructions result in reduced flow which may be detected by an automatic flow monitor. Second, a constant displacement flow source can be used. Now complications may be detected by monitoring elevated fluid pressure and/or flow resistance. At the risk of overgeneralization, the relative strengths of each approach will be presented.

Gravity Flow/Resistance Regulation

The simplest means for providing regulated flow employs gravity as the driving force with a roller clamp as a controlled resistance. Placement of the fluid reservoir 60–100 cm above the patient's right atrium provides a hydrostatic pressure gradient P_h equal to 1.34 mmHg per cm of elevation. The modest physiologic mean pressure in the veins, P_v, minimally reduces the net hydrostatic pressure gradient. The equation for flow becomes

$$Q = \frac{P_h - P_v}{R_{mfr} + R_n}$$

where R_{mfr} and R_n are the resistance to flow through the mechanical flow regulator and the remainder of the delivery system, respectively. Replacing the variables with representative values for an infusion of 5% saline solution into a healthy adult at 100 mL/hr yields

$$100 mL/hr = \frac{(68 - 8)\text{mmHg}}{(550 + 50)\dfrac{\text{mmHg}}{(\text{L/hr})}}$$

Gravity flow cannot be used for arterial infusions since the higher vascular pressure exceeds available hydrostatic pressure.

Flow stability in a gravity infusion systems is subject to variations in hydrostatic and venous pressure as well as catheter resistance. However, the most important factor is the change in flow regulator resistance caused by viscoelastic creep of the tubing wall (see Fig. 85.3). Caution must be used in assuming that a preset flow regulator setting will accurately provide a predetermined rate. The clinician typically estimates flow rate by counting the frequency of drops falling through an in-line drip-forming chamber, adjusting the clamp to obtain the desired drop rate. The cross-sectional area of the drip chamber orifice is the major determinant of drop volume. Various manufacturers pro-

TABLE 85.1 Resistance Measurements for Catheter Components Used for Infusion

Component	Length, cm	Flow Resistance, Fluid Ohm, mmHg/(L/hr)
Standard administration set	91–213	4.3–5.3
Extension tube for CVP monitoring	15	15.5
19-gauge epidural catheter	91	290.4–497.1
18-gauge needle	6–9	14.1–17.9
23-gauge needle	2.5–9	165.2–344.0
25-gauge needle	1.5–4.0	525.1–1412.0
Vicra Quick-Cath Catheter 18-gauge	5	12.9
Extension set with 0.22 micron air-eliminating filter		623.0
0.2 micron filter		555.0

Note: Mean values are presented over range of infusions (100, 200, and 300 mL/hr) and sample size ($n = 10$).

vide minidrip sets designed for pediatric (e.g., 60 drops/mL) and regular sets designed for adult (10–20 drops/mL) patients. Tolerances on the drip chamber can cause a 3% error in minidrip sets and a 17% error in regular sets at 125 mL/hr flow rate with 5% dextrose in water. Mean drop size for rapid rates increased by as much as 25% over the size of drops which form slowly. In addition variation in the specific gravity and surface tension of fluids can provide an additional large source of drop size variability.

Some mechanical flow regulating devices incorporate the principle of a Starling resistor. In a Starling device, resistance is proportional to hydrostatic pressure gradient. Thus, the device provides a negative feedback mechanism to reduce flow variation as the available pressure gradient changes with time.

Mechanical flow regulators comprise the largest segment of intravenous infusion systems, providing the simplest means of operation. Patient transport is simple, since these devices require no electric power. Mechanical flow regulators are most useful where the patient is not fluid restricted and the acceptable therapeutic rate range of the drug is relatively wide with minimal risk of serious adverse sequelae. The most common use for these systems is the administration of fluids and electrolytes.

Volumetric Infusion Pumps

Active pumping infusion devices combine electronics with a mechanism to generate flow. These devices have higher performance standards than simple gravity flow regulators. The Association for

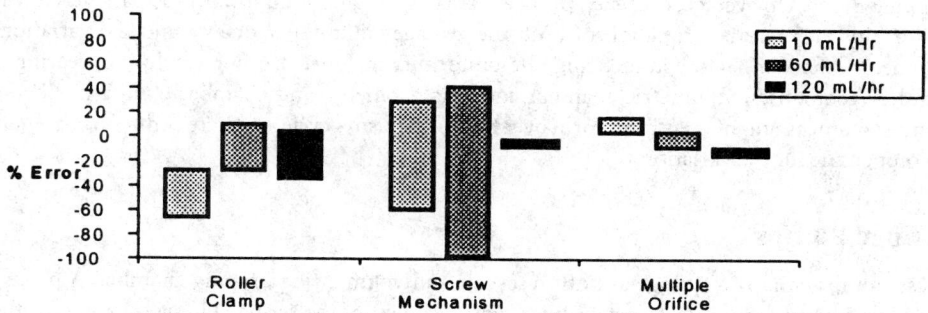

FIGURE 85.3 Drift in flow rate (mean ± standard deviation) over a four-hour period for three mechanical flow regulators at initial flow rates of 10, 60, and 120 mL/hr with distilled water at constant hydrostatic pressure gradient.

the Advancement of Medical Instrumentation (AAMI) recommends that long-term rate accuracy for infusion pumps remain within $\pm 10\%$ of the set rate for general infusion and, for the more demanding applications, that long-term flow remain within $\pm 5\%$. Such requirements typically extend to those agents with narrow therapeutic indices and/or low flow rates, such as the neonatal population or other fluid-restricted patients. The British Department of Health has established three main categories for hospital-based infusion devices: neonatal infusions, high-risk infusions, and low-risk infusions. Infusion control for neonates requires the highest performance standards, because their size severely restricts fluid volume. A fourth category, ambulatory infusion, pertains to pumps worn by patients.

Controllers

These devices automate the process of adjusting the mechanical flow regulator. The most common controllers utilize sensors to count the number of drops passing through the drip chamber to provide flow feedback for automatic rate adjustment. Flow rate accuracy remains limited by the rate and viscosity dependence of drop size. Delivery set motion associated with ambulation and improper angulation of the drip chamber can also hinder accurate rate detection.

An alternative to the drop counter is a volumetric metering chamber. A McGaw Corporation controller delivery set uses a rigid chamber divided by a flexible membrane. Instrument-controlled valves allow fluid to fill one chamber from the fluid reservoir, displacing the membrane driving the fluid from the second chamber toward the patient. When inlet and outlet valves reverse state, the second chamber is filled while the first chamber delivers to the patient. The frequency of state change determines the average flow rate. Volumetric accuracy depends primarily on the dimensional tolerances of the chamber. Although volumetric controllers may provide greater accuracy than drop-counting controllers, their disposables are inherently more complex, and maximum flow is still limited by head height and system resistance.

Beyond improvements in flow rate accuracy, controllers should provide an added level of patient safety by quickly detecting IV-site complications. The IVAC Corporation has developed a series of controllers employing pulsed modulated flow providing for monitoring of flow resistance as well as improved accuracy.

The maximum flow rate achieved by gravimetric based infusion systems can become limited by R_n and by concurrent infusion from other sources through the same catheter. In drop-counting devices, flow rate uniformity suffers at low flow rates from the discrete nature of the drop detector.

In contrast with infusion controllers, pumps generate flow by mechanized displacement of the contents of a volumetric chamber. Typical designs provide high flow rate accuracy and uniformity for a wide rate range (0.1–1000.0 mL/hr) of infusion rates. Rate error correlates directly with effective chamber volume, which, in turn, depends on both instrument and disposable repeatability, precision, and stability under varying load. Stepper or servo-controlled dc motors are typically used to provide the driving force for the fluid. At low flow rates, dc motors usually operate in a discrete stepping mode. On average, each step propels a small quanta of fluid toward the patient. Flow rate uniformity therefore is a function of both the average volume per quanta and the variation in volume. Mechanism factors influencing rate uniformity include: stepping resolution, gearing and activator geometries, volumetric chamber coupling geometry, and chamber elasticity. When the quanta volume is not inherently uniform over the mechanism's cycle, software control has been used to compensate for the variation.

Syringe Pumps

These pumps employ a syringe as both reservoir and volumetric pumping chamber. A precision leadscrew is used to produce constant linear advancement of the syringe plunger. Except for those ambulatory systems that utilize specific microsyringes, pumps generally accept syringes ranging in size from 5–100 mL. Flow rate accuracy and uniformity are determined by both mechanism displacement characteristics and tolerance on the internal syringe diameter. Since syringe mechanisms can generate a specified linear travel with less than 1% error, the manufacturing tolerance on the internal cross-sectional area of the syringe largely determines flow rate accuracy. Although syringes can be manufactured to tighter tolerances, standard plastic syringes provide long-term accuracy of ±5%. Flow rate uniformity, however, can benefit from the ability to select syringe size (see Fig. 85.4). Since many syringes have similar stroke length, diameter variation provides control of volume. Also the linear advancement per step is typically fixed. Therefore selection of a lower-volume syringe provides smaller-volume quanta. This allows tradeoffs among drug concentration, flow rate, and duration of flow per syringe. Slack in the gear train and drive shaft coupling as well as plunger slip cause rate inaccuracies during the initial stages of delivery (see Fig. 85.5a).

Since the syringe volumes are typically much smaller than reservoirs used with other infusion devices, syringe pumps generally deliver drugs in either fluid-restricted environments or for short duration. With high-quality syringes, flow rate uniformity in syringe pumps is generally superior to that accomplished by other infusion pumps. With the drug reservoir enclosed within the device, syringe pumps manage patient transport well, including the operating room environment.

Cassette pumps conceptually mimic the piston type action of the syringe pump but provide an automated means of repeatedly emptying and refilling the cassette. The process of refilling the cassette in single piston devices requires an interruption in flow (see Fig. 85.5b). The length of interruption relative to the drug's half-life determines the impact of the refill period on hemodynamic stability. To eliminate the interruption caused by refill, dual piston devices alternate refill and delivery states, providing nearly continuous output. Others implement cassettes with very small volumes which can refill in less than a second (see Fig. 85.2). Tight control of the internal cross-sectional area of the pumping chamber provides exceptional flow rate accuracy. Manufacturers have recently developed remarkably small cassette pumps that can still generate the full spectrum of infusion rate (0.1–999.0 mL/hr). These systems combine pumping chamber, inlet and outlet valving, pressure sensing, and air detection into a single complex component.

Peristaltic pumps operate on a short segment of the IV tubing. Peristaltic pumps can be separated into two subtypes. Rotary peristaltic mechanisms operate by compressing the pumping segment against the rotor housing with rollers mounted on the housing. With rotation, the rollers push fluid from the container through the tubing toward the patient. At least one of the rollers completely occludes the tubing against the housing at all times precluding free flow from the reservoir to the patient. During a portion of the revolution, two rollers trap fluid in the intervening pumping segment. The captured volume between the rollers determines volumetric accuracy. Linear peristaltic pumps hold the pumping segment in a channel pressed against a rigid backing plate. An array of cam-driven actuators sequentially occlude the segment starting with the section nearest the reservoir forcing fluid toward the patient with a sinusoidal wave action. In a typical design using

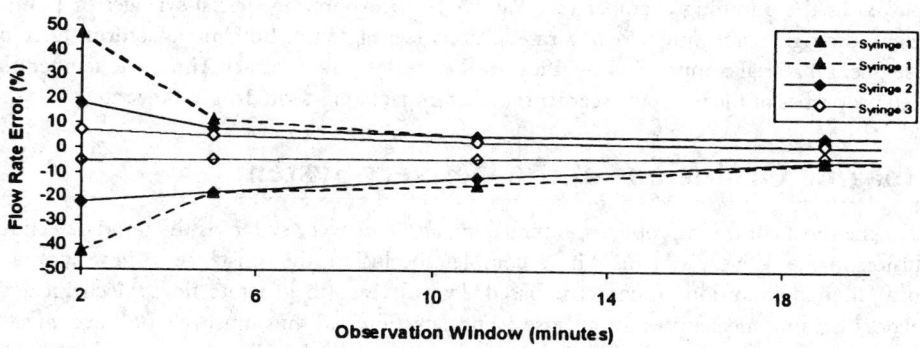

FIGURE 85.4 Effect of syringe type on Trumpet curve of a syringe pump at 1 mL/hr.

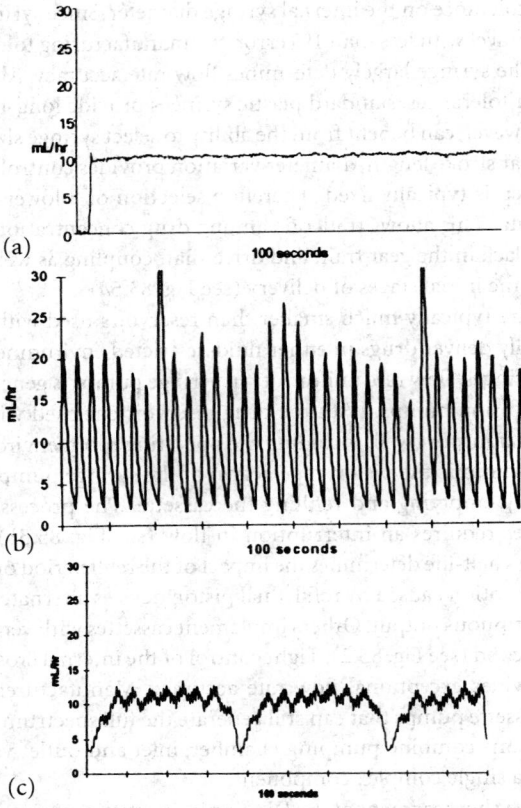

FIGURE 85.5 Continuous flow pattern for a representative, (*a*) syringe, (*b*) cassette, and (*c*) linear peristaltic pump at 10 mL/hr.

uniform motor step intervals, a characteristic flow wave resembling a positively biased sine wave is produced (see Fig. 85.5*c*).

Infusion pumps provide significant advantages over both manual flow regulators and controllers in several categories. Infusion pumps can provide accurate delivery over a wide range of infusion rates (0.1–999.0 mL/hr). Neither elevated system resistance nor distal line pressure limit the maximum the infusion rate. Infusion pumps can support a wider range of applications including arterial infusions, spinal and epidural infusions, and infusions into pulmonary artery or central venous catheters. Flow rate accuracy of infusion pumps is highly dependent on the segment employed as the pumping chamber (see Fig. 85.2). Incorporating special syringes or pumping segments can significantly improve flow rate accuracy (see Fig. 85.6). Both manufacturing tolerances and segment material composition significantly dictate flow rate accuracy. Time- and temperature-related properties of the pumping segment further impact long-term drift in flow rate.

85.4 Managing Occlusions of the Delivery System

One of the most common problems in managing an IV delivery system is the rapid detection of occlusion in the delivery system. With a complete occlusion, the resistance to flow approaches infinity. In this condition, gravimetric-based devices cease to generate flow. Mechanical flow regulators have no mechanism for adverse event detection and thus must rely on the clinician to identify an occlusion as part of routine patient care. Electronic controllers sense the absence of flow and alarm in response to their inability to sustain the desired flow rate.

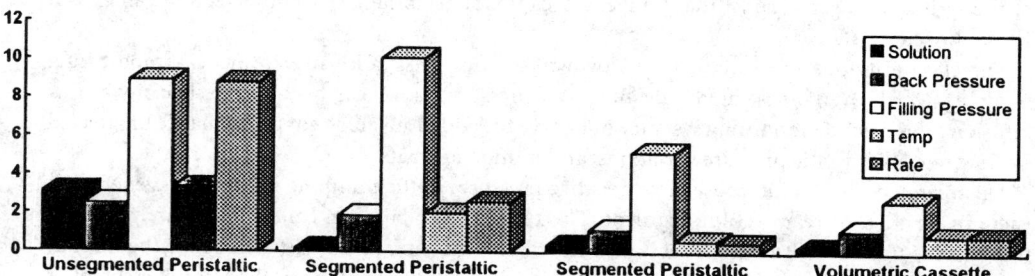

FIGURE 85.6 Impact of 5 variables on flow rate accuracy in 4 different infusion pumps. Variables tested included Solution: Distilled water and 25% dextrose in water; Back Pressure: −100 mmHg and 300 mmHg; Pumping Segment Filling Pressure: −30 inches of water and +30 inches of water; Temperature: 10ºC and 40ºC; and Infusion Rate: 5 mL/hr and 500 mL/hr. Note: First and second peristaltic mechanism qualified for Low Risk patients, while the third peristaltic device qualified for high-risk patients.

The problem of rapidly detecting an occlusion in an infusion pump is more complex. Upstream occlusions that occur between the fluid reservoir and the pumping mechanism impact the system quite differently than downstream occlusions which occur between the pump and the patient. When an occlusion occurs downstream from an infusion pump, the pump continues to propel fluid into the section of tubing between the pump and the occlusion. The time rate of pressure rise in that section increases in direct proportion to flow rate and inversely with tubing compliance (compliance, C, is the volume increase in a closed tube per mmHg pressure applied). The most common approach to detecting downstream occlusion requires a pressure transducer immediately below the pumping mechanism. These devices generate an alarm when either the mean pressure or rate of change in pressure exceeds a threshold. For pressure-limited designs, the time to downstream alarm (TTA) may be estimated as

$$TTA = \frac{P_{alarm} \cdot C_{delivery\text{-}set}}{flow\ rate}$$

Using a representative tubing compliance of 1 μL/mmHg, flow rate of 1 mL/hr, and a fixed alarm threshold set of 500 mmHg, the time to alarm becomes

$$TTA = \frac{500_{mmHg} \cdot 1000^{ml}/_{mmHg}}{1^{mL}/_{hr}} = 30\ min$$

where TTA is the time from occlusion to alarm detection. Pressure-based detection algorithms depend on accuracy and stability of the sensing system. Lowering the threshold on absolute or relative pressure for occlusion alarm reduces the TTA, but at the cost of increasing the likelihood of false alarms. Patient movement, patient-to-pump height variations, and other clinical circumstances can cause wide perturbations in line pressure. To optimize the balance between fast TTA and minimal false alarms, some infusion pumps allow the alarm threshold to be set by the clinician or be automatically shifted upward in response to alarms; other pumps attempt to optimize performance by varying pressure alarm thresholds with flow rate.

A second approach to detection of downstream occlusions uses motor torque as an indirect measure of the load seen by the pumping mechanism. Although this approach eliminates the need for a pressure sensor, it introduces additional sources for error including friction in the gear mechanism or pumping mechanism that requires additional safety margins to protect against false alarms. In syringe pumps, where the coefficient of static friction of the syringe bunge (rubber end of the syringe plunger) against the syringe wall can be substantial, occlusion detection can exceed 1 hr at low flow rates.

Direct, continuous measurement of downstream flow resistance may provide a monitoring modality which overcomes the disadvantages of pressure-based alarm systems, especially at low infusion rates. Such a monitoring system would have the added advantage of performance unaffected by flow rate, hydrostatic pressure variations, and motion artifacts.

Upstream occlusions can cause large negative pressures as the pumping mechanism generates a vacuum on the upstream tubing segment. The tube may collapse and the vacuum may pull air through the tubing walls or form cavitation bubbles. A pressure sensor situated above the mechanism or a pressure sensor below the mechanism synchronized with filling of the pumping chamber can detect the vacuum associated with an upstream occlusion. Optical or ultrasound transducers, situated below the mechanism, can detect air bubbles in the catheter, and air-eliminating filters can remove air, preventing large air emboli from being introduced into the patient.

Some of the most serious complications of IV therapy occur at the venipuncture site; these include extravasation, postinfusion phlebitis (and thrombophlebitis), IV-related infections, ecchymosis, and hematomas. Other problems that do not occur as frequently include speed shock and allergic reactions.

Extravasation (or infiltration) is the inadvertent perfusion of infusate into the interstitial tissue. Reported percentage of patients to whom extravasation has occurred ranges from 10% to over 25%. Tissue damage does not occur frequently, but the consequences can be severe, including skin necrosis requiring significant plastic and reconstructive surgery and amputation of limbs. The frequency of extravasation injury correlates with age, state of consciousness, and venous circulation of the patient as well as the type, location, and placement of the intravenous cannula. Drugs that have high osmolality, vessicant properties, or the ability to induce ischemia correlate with frequency of extravasation injury. Neonatal and pediatric patients who possess limited communication skills, constantly move, and have small veins that are difficult to cannulate require superior vigilance to protect against extravasation.

Since interstitial tissue provides a greater resistance to fluid flow than the venous pathway, infusion devices with accurate and precise pressure monitoring systems have been used to detect small pressure increases due to extravasation. To successfully implement this technique requires diligence by the clinician, since patient movement, flow rate, catheter resistance, and venous pressure variations can obscure the small pressure variations resulting from the extravasation. Others have investigated the ability of a pumping mechanism to withdraw blood as indicative of a patent line. The catheter tip, however, may be partially in and out of the vein such that infiltration occurs yet blood can be withdrawn from the patient. A vein might also may collapse under negative pressure in a patent line without successful blood withdrawal. Techniques currently being investigated which monitor infusion impedance (resistance and compliance) show promise for assisting in the detection of extravasation.

When a catheter tip wedges into the internal lining of the vein wall, it is considered positional. With the fluid path restricted by the vein wall, increases in line resistance may indicate a positional catheter. With patient movement, for example wrist flexation, the catheter may move in and out of the positional state. Since a positional catheter is thought to be more prone toward extravasation than other catheters, early detection of a positional catheter and appropriate adjustment of catheter position may be helpful in reducing the frequency of extravasation.

Postinfusion phlebitis is acute inflammation of a vein used for IV infusion. The chief characteristic is a reddened area or red streak that follows the course of the vein with tenderness, warmth, and edema at the venipuncture site. The vein, which normally is very compliant, also hardens. Phlebitis positively correlates with infusion rate and with the infusion of vesicants.

Fluid overload and speed shock result from the accidental administration of a large fluid volume over a short interval. Speed shock associates more frequently with the delivery of potent medications, rather than fluids. These problems most commonly occur with manually regulated IV systems, which do not provide the safety features of instrumented lines. Many IV sets designed for instrumented operation will free-flow when the set is removed from the instrument without manual clamping. To protect against this possibility, some sets are automatically placed in the occluded state on disengagement. Although an apparent advantage, reliance on such automatic devices may create a false sense of security and lead to manual errors with sets not incorporating these features.

85.5 Summary

Intravenous infusion has become the mode of choice for delivery of a large class of fluids and drugs both in hospital and alternative care settings. Modern infusion devices provide the clinician with a wide array of choices for performing intravenous therapy. Selection of the appropriate device for a specified application requires understanding of drug pharmacology and pharmacokinetics, fluid mechanics, and device design and performance characteristics. Continuing improvements in performance, safety, and cost of these systems will allow even broader utilization of intravenous delivery in a variety of settings.

References

Association for the Advancement of Medical Instrumentation. 1992. Standard for Infusion Devices. Arlington, Virg.

Bohony J. 1993. Nine common intravenous complications and what to do about them. Am J Nursing 10:45.

British Department of Health. 1990. Evaluation of Infusion Pumps and Controllers. HEI Report #198.

Glass PSA, Jacobs JR, Reves JG. 1991. Technology for continuous infusions in anesthesia. Continuous Infusions in Anesthesia. International Anesthesiology Clinics 29(4):39.

MacCara M 1983. Extravasation: A hazard of intravenous therapy. Drug Intelligence Clin Pharm 17:713.

Further Information

Peter Glass provides a strong rationale for intravenous therapy including pharmacokinetic and pharmacodynamic basis for continuous delivery. Clinical complications around intravenous therapy are well summarized by MacCara [1983] and Bohony [1993]. The AAMI Standard for Infusion Devices provides a comprehensive means of evaluating infusion device technology, and the British Department of Health OHEI Report #198 provides a competitive analysis of pumps and controllers.

86

Anesthesia Delivery Systems

A. William Paulsen
West Virginia University

The intent of this chapter is to provide an introductory overview to the technology employed in current anesthesia practice, hopefully impart some insight into a subset of problems that require solutions, and offer a few general considerations that may guide the approach toward possible solutions. Limitations on the length of this work and the enormous size of the topic requires that this chapter rely on other elements within this *Handbook* and other texts cited as general references for many of the details that inquisitive minds desire and deserve.

Today's anesthesia delivery system is composed of six major elements: (1) the primary and secondary sources of gases (O_2, air, N_2O, vacuum, gas scavenging, and possibly CO_2 and helium), (2) the gas blending and vaporization systems, (3) the breathing circuit (including methods for manual and mechanical ventilation), (4) the excess gas scavenging system that minimizes potential pollution of the operating room by anesthetic gases, (5) instruments and equipment to monitor the function of the anesthesia delivery system, and (6) patient monitoring instrumentation and equipment. The traditional anesthesia machine incorporated elements 1, 2, and 3 and, more recently, 4. The evolution to the anesthesia delivery system then included elements 5 and 6. In the text that follows, references to the *anesthesia machine* refer to the basic gas delivery system and breathing circuit, as contrasted with the *anesthesia delivery system,* which includes the basic anesthesia machine and all monitoring instrumentation.

86.1 Gases Used During Anesthesia and Their Sources

Most inhaled anesthetic agents are purchased as liquids and then vaporized in a device within the anesthesia delivery system. However, not all anesthetic agents are inhaled. Many are administered intravenously with the aid of various types of infusion pumps or are infused directly into compartments within the spine. The most common form of anesthesia currently is called a *balanced general anesthetic* and is a combination of inhalation agent plus intravenous analgesic drugs.

Gases needed for the delivery of anesthesia are generally limited to oxygen (O_2), air, nitrous oxide (N_2O), and possibly helium (He) and carbon dioxide (CO_2). Vacuum and gas scavenging lines are also required. There need to be secondary sources of these gases in the event of primary failure or questionable validity. Typically, primary sources are those supplied from a hospital distribution system at 345 kPa (50 psig) through gas columns or wall outlets, with secondary sources hung on the anesthesia delivery system.

Oxygen

Oxygen provides an essential metabolic substrate for all human cells, but it is not without dangerous side effects. Prolonged exposure to high concentrations of oxygen may result in toxic effects within the lung that decrease diffusion of gas into and out of the blood, and the return to breathing air following prolonged exposure to elevated O_2 may result in a debilitating explosive blood vessel growth in infants (retrolentalfibroplasia). Oxygen is usually supplied to the hospital in liquid form (boiling point of $-183°C$) and enters the hospital piping system as a gas. The efficiency of liquid storage is obvious, since 1 liter of liquid becomes 860 liters of gas at standard temperature and pressure. The secondary source of oxygen within an anesthesia delivery system is usually one or more E cylinders filled with gaseous oxygen at a pressure of 15.2 MPa (2200 psig).

Air (78% N_2, 21% O_2, 0.9% Ar, 0.1% Other Gases)

The primary use of air during anesthesia is as a diluent to decrease the inspired oxygen concentration. The typical primary source of medical air (there is an important distinction between air and medical air related to the quality and the requirements for periodic testing) is a special compressor that avoids hydrocarbon-based lubricants for purposes of medical air purity. Dryers are employed to rid the compressed air of water prior to distribution throughout the hospital. Medical facilities with limited need for medical air may use banks of H cylinders of dry medical air. A secondary source of air may be available on the anesthesia machine as an E cylinder containing dry gas at 15.2 MPa.

Nitrous Oxide

Nitrous oxide (N_2O) is a colorless, odorless, and nonirritating gas that does not support human life. Breathing more than 85% N_2O may be fatal. N_2O is not an anesthetic (except under hyperbaric conditions); rather, it is an analgesic and an amnestic. There are many reasons for administering N_2O during the course of an anesthetic, including enhancing the speed of induction and emergence from anesthesia, decreasing the concentration requirements of potent inhalation anesthetics (i.e., halothane, isoflurane, etc.), and as an essential adjunct to narcotic anesthetics. N_2O is supplied to anesthetizing locations from banks of H cylinders that are filled with 90% liquid at a pressure of 5.1 MPa (745 psig). Secondary supplies are available on the anesthesia machine in the form of E cylinders, again containing 90% liquid. Continual exposure to low levels of N_2O in the workplace has been implicated in a number of medical problems, including spontaneous abortion, infertility, birth defects, cancer, liver and kidney disease, and others. Although there is no conclusive evidence to support most of these implications, there is a recognized need to scavenge all waste anesthetic gases and periodically sample N_2O levels in the workplace to maintain the lowest possible levels consistent with reasonable risk to the patient and cost to the institution [Dorsch & Dorsch, 1994].

Carbon Dioxide

Carbon dioxide (CO_2) is colorless and odorless but very irritating to breath in higher concentrations. CO_2 is a by-product of human cellular metabolism and is not a life-sustaining gas. CO_2 influences many physiologic processes either directly or through the action of hydrogen ions by the reaction $CO_2 + H_2O \leftrightarrow H_2CO_3 \leftrightarrow H^+ + HCO_3^-$. Although not very common in the United States today, in the past CO_2 was administered during anesthesia to stimulate respiration that was depressed by anesthetic agents and to cause increased blood flow in otherwise compromised vasculature during some surgical procedures. Like N_2O, CO_2 is supplied as a liquid in H cylinders for distribution in pipeline systems or as a liquid in E cylinders that are located on the anesthesia machine.

Helium

Helium (He) is a colorless, odorless, and nonirritating gas that will not support life. The primary use of helium in anesthesia is to enhance gas flow through small orifices, as in asthma, airway trauma, or tracheal stenosis. Resistance to normal laminar gas flow in a tube can be described in simple terms using the Hagen-Poiseuille relationship:

$$R = \frac{8\eta l}{\pi r^4}$$

where resistance R is proportional to the viscosity η of the gas and the length l of the tube and inversely related to the fourth power of the radius r of the tube. The viscosity of helium is not different from that of other anesthetic gases (Table 86.1) and is therefore of no benefit during routine procedures. However, in the event that ventilation must be performed through abnormally narrow orifices or tubes that create turbulent flow conditions, helium is the preferred carrier gas. Resistance to turbulent flow is proportional to the density rather than viscosity of the gas, and helium is an order of magnitude less dense than other gases. A secondary advantage of helium is that it has a large specific heat relative to other anesthetic gases and therefore can carry the heat from laser surgery out of the airway more effectively than air, oxygen, or nitrous oxide.

86.2 Gas Blending and Vaporization System

The basic anesthesia machine uses primary low-pressure gas sources of 345 kPa (50 psig) available from wall or ceiling column outlets and secondary high-pressure gas sources located on the machine as pictured schematically in Fig. 86.1. Tracing the path of oxygen in the machine demonstrates that oxygen comes from either the low-pressure source or from the 15.2-MPa (2200-psig) high-pressure yokes via cylinder pressure regulators and then branches to service several other functions. First and foremost, the second-stage pressure regulator drops the O_2 pressure to approximately 110 kPa (16 psig) before it enters the needle valve and the rotameter-type flowmeter. From the flowmeter, O_2 mixes with gases from other flowmeters and passes through a calibrated agent vaporizer where specific inhalation anesthetic agents are vaporized and added to the breathing gas mixture. Oxygen is also used to supply a reservoir canister that sounds a reed alarm in the event that the oxygen pressure drops below 172 kPa (25 psig). When the oxygen pressure drops to 172 kPa or lower, then the nitrous oxide pressure sensor shutoff valve closes, and N_2O is prevented from entering its needle valve and flowmeter and is therefore eliminated from the breathing gas mixture. In fact, all machines

TABLE 86.1   Physical Properties of Gases Used During Anesthesia

Gas	Molecular Weight	Density, g/liter	Viscosity, cP	Specific Heat, kJ/kg °C
Oxygen	31.999	1.326	0.0203	0.917
Nitrogen	28.013	1.161	0.0175	1.040
Air	28.975	1.200	0.0181	1.010
Nitrous oxide	44.013	1.836	0.0144	0.839
Carbon dioxide	44.01	1.835	0.0148	0.850
Helium	4.003	0.1657	0.0194	5.190

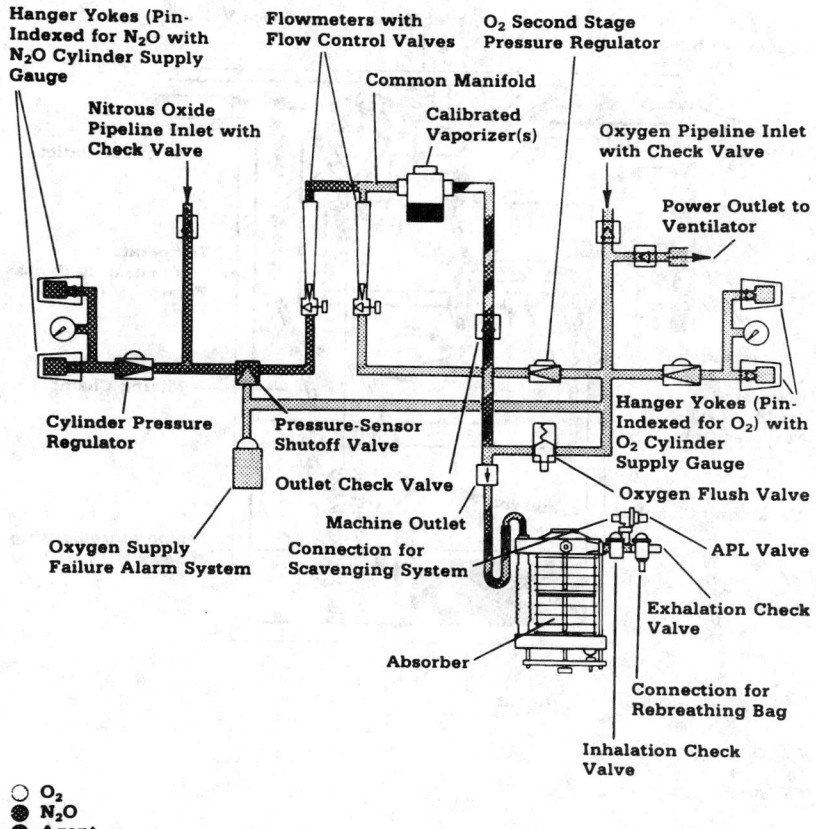

Hanger Yokes (Pin-Indexed for N₂O with N₂O Cylinder Supply Gauge

Nitrous Oxide Pipeline Inlet with Check Valve

Flowmeters with Flow Control Valves

Common Manifold

Calibrated Vaporizer(s)

O₂ Second Stage Pressure Regulator

Oxygen Pipeline Inlet with Check Valve

Power Outlet to Ventilator

Cylinder Pressure Regulator

Pressure-Sensor Shutoff Valve

Outlet Check Valve

Machine Outlet

Connection for Scavenging System

Oxygen Supply Failure Alarm System

Hanger Yokes (Pin-Indexed for O₂) with O₂ Cylinder Supply Gauge

Oxygen Flush Valve

APL Valve

Exhalation Check Valve

Connection for Rebreathing Bag

Inhalation Check Valve

Absorber

○ **O₂**
◉ **N₂O**
● **Agent**

FIGURE 86.1   Schematic diagram of gas piping within a simple two-gas (oxygen and nitrous oxide) anesthesia machine. (Courtesy of Ohmeda of Madison, Wisconsin.)

built in the United States have pressure sensor shutoff valves installed in the lines to every flowmeter except oxygen so that 100% O_2 is the last gas to flow into the breathing circuit following a low-oxygen-pressure failure. The volume of O_2 remaining at 172 kPa may be considerable, and this essentially guarantees that 100% oxygen will fill the breathing circuit before the oxygen is exhausted. Oxygen also may be delivered to the common gas outlet or machine outlet via a momentary normally closed flush valve that typically provides a flow of 65 to 80 liters of O_2 per minute directly into the breathing circuit. New machines are required to have a safety system for limiting the minimum concentration of oxygen that can be delivered to the patient to 25%. The flow paths for nitrous oxide and other gases are much simpler in the sense that after coming from the high-pressure regulator or the low-pressure source, gas is immediately presented to the pressure sensor shutoff valve, from where it travels to its specific needle valve and flowmeter to join the common gas line and enter the breathing circuit.

Currently, all anesthesia machines manufactured in the United States use only calibrated flow through vaporizers, meaning that all the gases from the various flowmeters are mixed in the manifold prior to entering the vaporizer and that any given vaporizer has a calibrated control knob that is specific for the intended agent. Some form of interlock system also must be provided such that only one vaporizer may be activated at any given time. Figure 86.2 schematically illustrates the operation of a purely mechanical vaporizer with temperature compensation. This simple flow-over design permits a fraction of the total gas flow to pass into the vaporizing chamber, where it

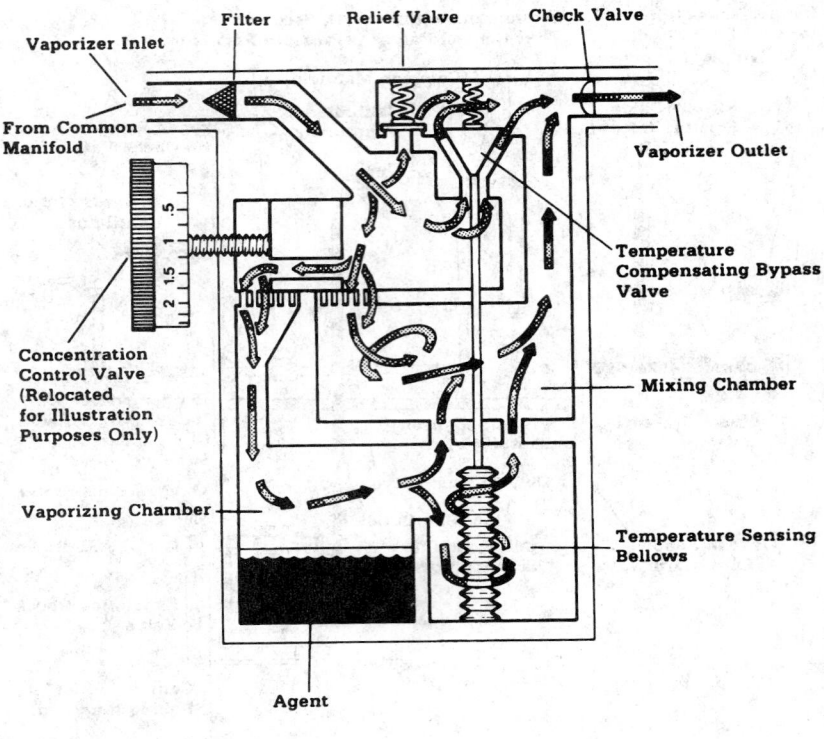

O O₂
⊛ N₂O
● Agent

FIGURE 86.2   Schematic diagram of a calibrated in-line vaporizer that uses the flow-over technique for adding anesthetic vapor to the breathing gas mixture. (Courtesy of Ohmeda of Madison, Wisconsin.)

becomes saturated with vapor before being added back to the total gas flow. Mathematically, this is approximated by

$$F_A = \frac{Q_{VC}P_A}{P_B(Q_{VC} + Q_G) - P_A Q_G}$$

where F_A is the fractional concentration of agent at the outlet of the vaporizer, Q_G is the total flow of gas entering the vaporizer, Q_{VC} is the amount of Q_G that is diverted into the vaporization chamber, P_A is the vapor pressure of the agent (Table 86.2), and P_B is the barometric pressure. From Fig.

TABLE 86.2   Physical Properties of Currently Available Volatile Anesthetic Agents

Agent, Generic Name	Boiling Point (°C) at 760 mmHg	Vapor Pressure (mmHg) at 20°C	Liquid Density, g/mL	MAC*, %
Halothane	50.2	243	1.86	0.75
Enflurane	56.5	175	1.517	1.68
Isoflurane	48.5	238	1.496	1.15
Desflurane	23.5	664	1.45	6.0
Sevoflurane	58.5	160	1.51	2.0

*Minimum alveolar concentration (MAC) is the percentage of the agent required to provide surgical anesthesia to 50% of the population in terms of a cumulative dose-response curve. The lower the MAC, the more potent is the agent.

86.2, the temperature compensator would decrease Q_{VC} as temperature increased. The concentration accuracy over a range of clinically expected gas flows and temperatures is approximately ±15%. Since vaporization is an endothermic process, anesthetic vaporizers must have sufficient thermal mass and conductivity to permit the vaporization process to proceed independent of the rate at which the agent is being used.

86.3 Breathing Circuits

The concept behind an effective breathing circuit is to provide an adequate volume of a controlled concentration of fresh gas to the patient during inspiration and to carry the exhaled gases away from the patient during exhalation. There are several forms of breathing circuits, and these can be classified into two basic types: *open circuits,* meaning no rebreathing of any gases and no CO_2 absorber present, and *closed circuits,* indicating the presence of a CO_2 absorber and some rebreathing of other gases beside CO_2. Figure 86.3 illustrates the Lack modification of a Mapleson open-circuit breathing system. There are no valves and no CO_2 absorber. There is a great potential for the patient to rebreath his or her own exhaled gases unless the fresh gas inflow is two to three times the patient's minute volume. Figure 86.4 illustrates the most popular form of breathing circuit, the circle system, with oxygen monitor, circle pressure gage, volume monitor (spirometer), and airway pressure sensor. The circle is a closed system, or semiclosed when the fresh gas inflow exceeds the patient's requirements. Excess gas evolves into the scavenging device, and some of the exhaled gas is rebreathed after having the CO_2 removed. The inspiratory and expiratory valves in the circle system guarantee that gas flows to the patient from the inspiratory limb and away from the patient through the exhalation limb. In the event of a failure of either or both of these valves, the patient will rebreath exhaled gas that contains CO_2, which is a potentially dangerous situation.

There are two forms of mechanical ventilation used during anesthesia: *volume ventilation,* where the volume of gas delivered to the patient remains constant regardless of pressure that is required, and *pressure ventilation,* where the ventilator provides whatever volume to the patient that is required to produce some desired pressure in the breathing circuit. Volume ventilation is the most popular, since the volume delivered remains constant despite changes in lung compliance. Pressure ventilation is useful when compliance losses in the breathing circuit are high relative to the volume delivered to the lungs.

Humidification is an important adjunct to the breathing circuit because it reduces heat loss and maintains the integrity of the cilia that line the airways and promote the removal of mucus and particulate matter from the lungs. Humidification of dry breathing gases can be accomplished by simple passive heat and moisture exchangers inserted into the breathing circuit at the level of the

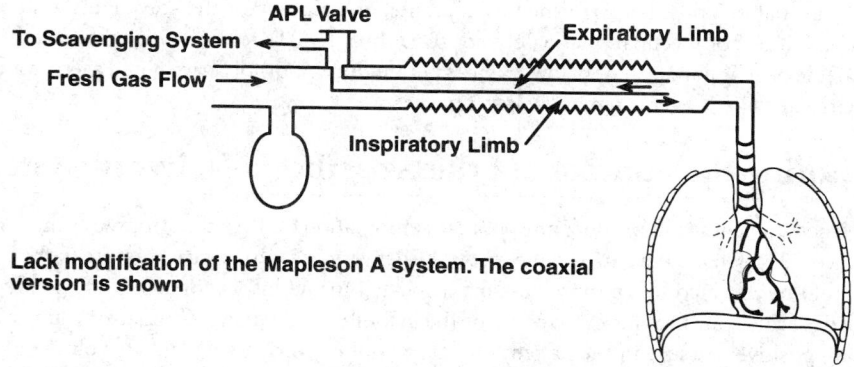

FIGURE 86.3 An example of an open-circuit breathing system that does not use unidirectional flow valves or contain a carbon dioxide absorbent.

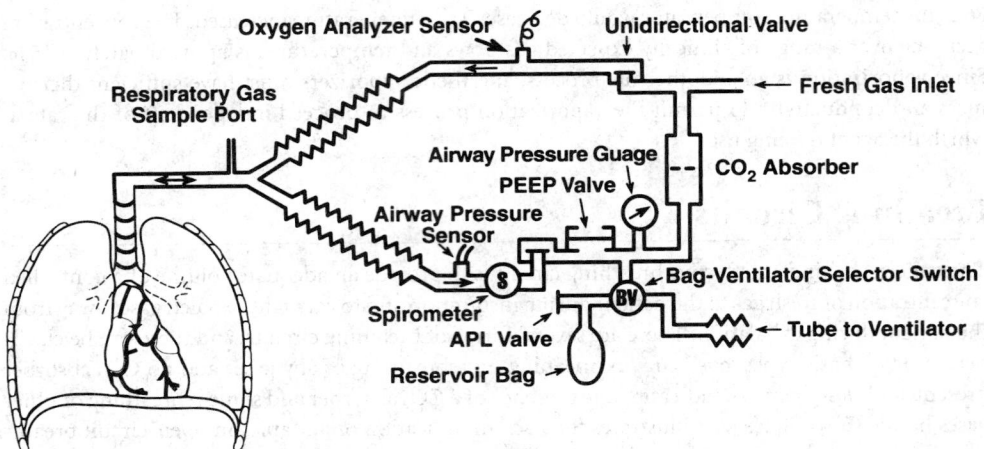

FIGURE 86.4   A diagram of a closed-circuit breathing system with unidirectional valves, inspired oxygen sensor, pressure sensor, and CO_2 absorber.

endotracheal tube connectors or by elegant dual servo electronic humidifiers that heat a reservoir filled with water and also heat a wire in the gas delivery tube to prevent rain-out of the water before it reaches the patient. Electronic safety measures must be included in these active devices due to the potential for burning the patient and the fire hazard.

86.4   Gas Scavenging Systems

The purpose of scavenging exhaled and excess anesthetic agents is to reduce or eliminate the potential hazard to employees who work in the environment where anesthetics are administered, including operating rooms, obstetrical areas, special procedures areas, physicians' offices, dentists' offices, and veterinarians' surgical suites. Typically, more gas is administered to the breathing circuit than is required by the patient, resulting in the need to remove excess gas from the circuit. The scavenging system must be capable of collecting gas from all components of the breathing circuit, including adjustable pressure level valves, ventilators, and sample withdrawal-type gas monitors, without altering characteristics of the circuit, such as pressure or gas flow to the patient. There are two broad types of scavenging systems, as illustrated in Fig. 86.5: the *open interface,* a simple design that requires a large physical space for the reservoir volume, and the *closed interface,* with an expandable reservoir bag, which must include relief valves for handling the cases of no scavenging flow and great excess of scavenging flow.

Trace gas analysis must be performed to guarantee the efficacy of the scavenging system. The National Institutes of Occupational Safety and Health (NIOSH) recommend that trace levels of nitrous oxide be maintained at or below 25 parts per million (ppm) time-weighted average and that halogenated anesthetic agents remain below 2 ppm.

86.5   Monitoring the Function of the Anesthesia Delivery System

The anesthesia machine can produce any possible combination of three catastrophic events, any one of which could be fatal to the patient. The first is the delivery of a hypoxic gas mixture to the patient, which could be detected by an oxygen analyzer located in the inspiratory limb of the breathing circuit. The second catastrophic event could be the inability to adequately ventilate the lungs: by not producing positive pressure in the patient's lungs, by not delivering an adequate volume of gas to the lungs, or by improper breathing circuit connections that permit the patient's lungs to receive only rebreathed gases. Adequacy of ventilation could be monitored by the pressure in the breathing

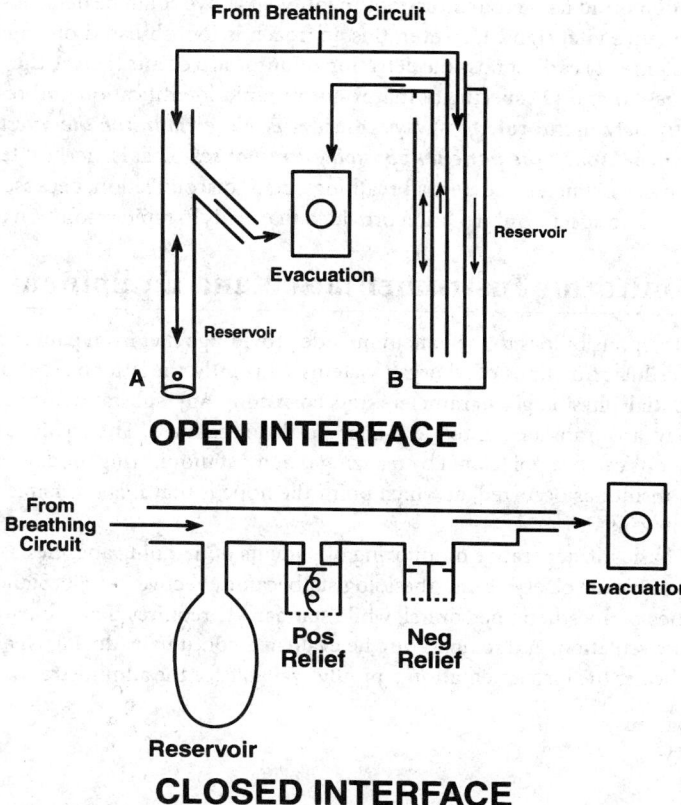

FIGURE 86.5 Examples of open and closed gas scavenger interfaces. The closed interface requires relief valves in the event of scavenging flow failure.

circuit, the volume of gas exhaled from the patient's lungs, and the amount of exhaled carbon dioxide. The third event is the delivery of an overdose of an inhalational anesthetic agent, which could be detected by an agent-specific gas analyzer. The necessary monitoring equipment to guarantee proper function of the anesthesia delivery system is

- *Inspired oxygen concentration monitor* with an absolute low-level alarm of 19%
- *Airway pressure monitor* with alarms for
  1. Low pressure indicative of inadequate breathing volume and possibly a leak
  2. Sustained elevated pressures that could compromise cardiovascular function
  3. High pressures that could cause pulmonary barotrauma
  4. Subatmospheric pressure that could cause collapse of the lungs
- *Exhaled gas volume monitor*
- *Carbon dioxide monitor* (capnography)
- *Inspired and exhaled concentration* of specific anesthetic agents:
  1. Mass spectrometer
  2. Raman spectrometer
  3. Infrared or other optical spectrometer

The mass spectrometer is a very useful, cost-effective device because it alone can provide capnography and inspired and exhaled concentrations of all anesthetic agents plus all breathing gases simultaneously (O_2, N_2, CO_2, N_2O, Ar, He, halothane, enflurane, isoflurane, desflurane, and suprane).

All the catastrophic and dangerous situations mentioned above could be detected through monitoring of the patient's vital signs. However, this approach is foolish based on sound monitoring principles that require (1) earliest possible detection of untoward events (before they result in physiologic derangements) and (2) specificity that result in rapid identification and resolution of the problem. An extremely useful rule to always consider is *Never monitor the anesthesia delivery system performance through the patient's physiologic responses.* That is, never intentionally use a device such as a pulse oximeter to detect a breathing circuit disconnection, because the warning is very late and there is no specific information provided that leads to rapid resolution of the problem.

86.6 Patient Monitoring Instrumentation and Equipment

The anesthetist's responsibilities to the patient include providing relief from pain and preserving all existing normal cellular functions of all organ systems. Currently, the latter obligation is fulfilled by monitoring essential physiologic parameters and correcting any substantial derangements that occur before they are translated into permanent cellular damage. The inadequacy of current monitoring methods can be appreciated by realizing that most monitoring modalities only indicate damage after an insult has occurred, at which point the hope is that it is reversible or that further damage can be prevented.

Standards for basic intraoperative monitoring of patients undergoing anesthesia, developed and adopted by the American Society of Anesthesiologists, became effective in 1990. Standard I concerns the responsibilities of anesthesia personnel, while standard II requires that the patient's oxygenation, ventilation, circulation, and temperature be evaluated continually during all anesthetics. The following list indicates the instrumentation typically available for the administration of anesthetics.

Electrocardiogram
Pulse oximetry
Urine output
Cardiac output
Electroencephalogram (EEG)
Evoked potentials
Noninvasive or invasive blood pressure
Temperature
Nerve stimulators
Mixed venous oxygen saturation
Transesophageal echocardiography (TEE)
Coagulation status
Blood gases and electrolytes (PO_2, PCO_2, pH, BE, Na^+, K^+, Cl^-, Ca^{2+}, and glucose)
Mass spectrometery, Raman spectrometry, or infrared breathing gas analysis

Anesthesia Computer-Aided Record Keeping

Conceptually, every anesthetist desires an automated anesthesia record-keeping system. Anesthesia care can be improved through the feedback provided by correct record keeping, but today's systems have an enormous overhead associated with their use when compared with standard paper record keeping. No doubt that automated anesthesia record keeping reduces the drudgery of routine recording of vital signs, but to enter drugs and drips and their dosages, fluids administered, urine output, blood loss, and other data requires much more time and machine interaction than the current paper system allows. Despite attempts to use every input/output device ever produced by the computer industry from keyboards to bar codes to voice and handwriting recognition, no solution has been found that meets wide acceptance. Tenants of a successful system must include

1. The concept of a user-transparent system, which is ideally defined as no required communication between the computer and the clinician (far beyond the concept of user friendly) and therefore that is intuitively obvious to use even to the most casual users.

2. Recognition of the fact that educational institutions have very different requirements from private-practice institutions.
3. Real-time hard copy of the record produced at the site of anesthetic administration that permits real-time editing and notation.
4. Ability to interface with a great variety of patient and anesthesia delivery system monitors from various suppliers.
5. Ability to interface with a large number of hospital information systems.
6. Inexpensive to purchase and maintain.

Alarms

Vigilance is the key to effective risk management, but maintaining a vigilant state is not easy. The practice of anesthesia has been described as moments of shear terror connected by times of intense boredom. Alarms can play a significant role in redirecting one's attention during the boredom to the most important event regarding patient management, but only if false alarms can be eliminated, alarms can be prioritized, and all alarms concerning anesthetic management can be displayed in a single, clearly visible location.

Ergonomics

The study of ergonomics attempts to improve performance by optimizing the relationship between people and their work environment. *Ergonomics* has been defined as a discipline that investigates and applies information about human requirements, characteristics, abilities, and limitations to the design, development, and testing of equipment, systems, and jobs [Loeb, 1993]. This field of study is only in its infancy, and examples of poor ergonomic design abound in the anesthesia workplace.

Simulation in Anesthesia

Complete patient simulators are hands-on, realistic simulators that interface with physiologic monitoring equipment to simulate patient responses to equipment malfunctions, operator errors, and drug therapies. There are also crisis-management simulators. Complex patient simulators are currently being marketed for training anesthesia personnel. The intended audience for these complex simulators is currently being debated in the sense that training people to respond in a preprogrammed way to a given event is not adequate training.

Reliability

The design of an anesthesia delivery system is unlike the design of most other medical devices because it is a life-support system. As such, its core elements deserve all the considerations of the latest failsafe technologies. Too often in today's quest to apply microprocessor technology to everything, tradeoffs are made among reliability, cost, and engineering elegance. The most widely accepted anesthesia machine designs continue to be based on simple, ultrareliable mechanical systems with a absolute minimum of catastrophic failure modes. The replacement of needle valves and rotameters, for example, with microprocessor-controlled electromechanical valves can only introduce new catastrophic failure modes. However, the inclusion of microprocessors can enhance the safety of anesthesia delivery if they are implemented without adding catastrophic failure modes.

References

Blitt CD (ed). 1990. *Monitoring in Anesthesia and Critical Care Medicine*, 2d ed. New York, Churchill-Livingstone.

Brown BR Jr (ed). 1984. *Future Anesthesia Delivery Systems*. Philadelphia, FA Davis.

Dorsch JA, Dorsch SE. 1994. *Understanding Anesthesia Equipment: Construction, Care and Complications*, 3d ed. Baltimore, Williams & Wilkins.

Ehrenwerth J, Eisenkraft JB. 1993. Anesthesia Equipment: Principles and Applications. St. Louis, Mosby.

Gravenstein JS, Paulus DA. 1987. Clinical Monitoring Practice, 2d ed. Philadelphia, Lippincott.

Lake CL (ed). 1990. Clinical Monitoring. Philadelphia, Saunders.

Loeb R. 1993. Ergonomics of the anesthesia workplace. STA Interface 4(3):18.

Petty C. 1987. The Anesthesia Machine. New York, Churchill-Livingstone.

Saidman LJ, Smith NT (eds). 1993. Monitoring in Anesthesia, 3d ed. Stoneham, Mass, Butterworth-Heinemann.

Schreiber P, Schreiber J. 1987. Anesthesia System Risk Analysis and Risk Reduction. Telford, Pa, North American Drager.

Further Information

An abbreviated list of standards (already published or in progress) related to anesthesia delivery is provided for your information. There are many more standards that apply to anesthesia delivery systems by way of general electrical safety of medical devices, specific requirements for graphical labeling of medical devices, specific requirements for individual forms of monitoring (ECG, blood pressure, heart rate, respiratory rate, pulse oximetry, capnography, etc.), facilities and environmental concerns for anesthetizing locations, and color standards for containers and labels.

American National Standards Institute (New York, New York)

ANSI Z79.8-1979: Minimum performance and safety requirements for components and systems of continuous-flow anesthesia machines.

American Society for Testing and Materials (Philadelphia, Pennsylvania)

ASTM F 1161-88, 1988: Standard specifications for minimum performance and safety requirements for components and systems of anesthesia gas machines, which superseded ANSI Z79.

ASTM F-29 (Committee on Anesthesia and Respiratory Equipment), including specifications for alarm signals in medical equipment used in anesthesia and respiratory care among many other subcommittees.

ASTM E-31 (Committee on computerized systems), standards for computer-based patient records.

Canadian Standards Association (Rexdale, Ontario, Canada)

CSA Q396.1.1-89 and Q396.1.2-89: Quality assurance programs for the development of software used in critical applications.

International Electrotechnical Commission (c/o Health Industries Manufacturers Association, Washington, DC)

IEC 601-2-13, 1989: Medical electrical equipment: Particular requirements for the safety of anesthetic machines.

International Standards Organization

ISO 5356-1, 1980: Anesthetic and respiratory equipment—conical connectors.

ISO 5358, 1980: Continuous flow inhalational anaesthetic apparatus for use with humans.

ISO 5367, 1985: Breathing tubes used with anesthetic apparatus and ventilators.

ISO 7677, 1988: Oxygen analyzers for monitoring patient breathing mixtures—safety requirements.

ISO, 1991 (draft): Anesthesia and respiratory care—visual alarm signals.

ISO 11428 (draft): Ergonomics—visual danger signs.

ISO 7281 (draft proposal): Anesthetic gas scavenging systems.

Military Standard

MIL STD 1629A: Procedures for performing a failure mode, effects and criticality analysis.

National Fire Protection Agency

NFPA-99: Standard for health care facilities, includes requirements for gas piping systems.

87

Biomedical Lasers

Millard M. Judy
Baylor Research Institute

Approximately 20 years ago the *CO₂* laser was introduced into surgical practice as a tool to photothermally ablate, and thus to incise and to debulk, soft tissues. Subsequently, three important factors have led to the expanding biomedical use of laser technology, particularly in surgery. These factors are: (1) the increasing understanding of the wave-length selective interaction and associated effects of *ultraviolet-infrared (UV-IR) radiation* with biologic tissues, including those of acute damage and long-term healing, (2) the rapidly increasing availability of lasers emitting (essentially monochromatically) at those wavelengths that are strongly absorbed by molecular species within tissues, and (3) the availability of both optical fiber and lens technologies as well as of endoscopic technologies for delivery of the laser radiation to the often remote internal treatment site. Fusion of these factors has led to the development of currently available biomedical laser systems.

This chapter briefly reviews the current status of each of these three factors. In doing so, each of the following topics will be briefly discussed:

1. The physics of the interaction and the associated effects (including clinical effects) of UV-IR radiation on biologic tissues
2. The fundamental principles that underlie the operation and construction of all lasers
3. The physical properties of the optical delivery systems used with the different biomedical lasers for delivery of the laser beam to the treatment site
4. The essential physical features of those biomedical lasers currently in routine uses ranging over a number of clinical specialties, and brief descriptions of their use

0-8493-8346-3/95/$0.00+$.50
© 1995 by CRC Press, Inc.

5. The biomedical uses of other lasers used surgically in limited scale or which are currently being researched for applications in surgical and diagnostic procedures and the photosensitized inactivation of cancer tumors

In this review, effort is made in the text and in the last section to provide a number of key references and sources of information for each topic that will enable the reader's more in-depth pursuit.

87.1 Interaction and Effects of UV-IR Laser Radiation on Biologic Tissues

Electromagnetic radiation in the UV-IR spectral range propagates within biologic tissues until it is either scattered or absorbed.

Scattering in Biologic Tissue

Scattering in matter occurs only at the boundaries between regions having different optical refractive indices and is a process in which the energy of the radiation is conserved [Van de Hulst, 1957]. Since biologic tissue is structurally inhomogeneous at the microscopic scale, e.g., both subcellular and cellular dimensions, and at the macroscopic scale, e.g., cellular assembly (tissue) dimensions, and predominantly contains water, proteins, and lipids, all different chemical species, it is generally regarded as a scatterer of UV-IR radiation. The general result of scattering is deviation of the direction of propagation of radiation. The deviation is strongest when wavelength and scatterer are comparable in dimension (Mie scattering) and when wavelength greatly exceeds particle size (Rayleigh scattering) [Van de Hulst, 1957]. This dimensional relationship results in the deeper penetration into biologic tissues of those longer wavelengths which are not absorbed appreciably by pigments in the tissues. This results in the relative transparency of nonpigmented tissues over the visible and near-IR wavelength ranges.

Absorption in Biologic Tissue

Absorption of UV-IR radiation in matter arises from the wavelength-dependent resonant absorption of radiation by molecular electrons of optically absorbing molecular species [Grossweiner, 1989]. Because of the chemical inhomogeneity of biologic tissues, the degree of absorption of incident radiation strongly depends upon its wavelength. The most prevalent or concentrated UV-IR absorbing molecular species in biologic tissues are listed in Table 87.1 along with associated high-absorbance wavelengths. These species include the peptide bonds; the phenylalanine, tyrosine, and tryptophan residues of proteins, all of which absorb in the UV range; oxy- and deoxyhemoglobin of blood which absorb in the visible to near-IR range; melanin, which absorbs throughout the UV to near-IR range, with decreasing absorption occurring with increasing wavelength; and water, which absorbs maximally in the mid-IR range [Hale & Querry, 1973; Miller & Veitch, 1993; White et al., 1968]. Biomedical lasers and their emitted radiation wavelength values also are tabulated also in Table 87.1. The correlation between the wavelengths of clinically useful lasers and wavelength regions of absorption by constituents of biological tissues is evident. Additionally, exogenous light-absorbing chemical species may be intentionally present in tissues. These include:

1. Photosensitizers, such as porphyrins, which upon excitation with UV-visible light initiate photochemical reactions which are cytotoxic to the cells of the tissue, e.g., a cancer which concentrates the photosensitizer relative to surrounding tissues [Spikes, 1989]
2. Dyes such as indocyanine green which when dispersed in a concentrate fibrin protein gel can be used to localize 810 nm *GaAlAs* diode laser radiation and the associated heating to achieve

TABLE 87.1 UV-IR-Radiation-Absorbing Constituent of Biologic Tissues and Biomedical Laser Wavelengths

Constituent	Tissue Type	Optical Absorption Wavelength*, nm	Relative† Strength	Laser Type	Wavelength, nm
Proteins	All				
Peptide bond		<220 (r)	+++++++	ArF	193
Amino acid					
Residues					
Tryptophan		220–290 (r)	+		
Tyrosine		220–290 (r)	+		
Phenylalanine		220–2650 (r)	+		
Pigments					
Oxyhemoglobin	Blood	414 (p)	+++	Ar ion	488–514.5
	vascular	537 (p)	++	Frequency	532
	tissues	575 (p)	++	Doubled	
		970 (p)	+	Nd:YAG	
		(690–1100) (r)		Diode	810
				Nd:YAG	1064
Deoxyhemoglobin	Blood	431 (p)	+++	Dye	400–700
	vascular	554 (p)	++	Nd:YAG	1064
	tissues				
Melanin	Skin	220–1000 (r)	++++	Ruby	693
Water	All	2.1 (p)	+++	Ho:YAG	2100
		3.02 (p)	+++++++	Er:YAG	2940
		>2.94 (r)	++++	CO_2	10,640

*(p): Peak absorption wavelength; (r): wavelength range.
†The number of + signs qualitatively ranks the magnitude of the optical absorbtion.

    localized thermal denaturation and bonding of collagen to effect joining or welding of tissue [Bass et al., 1992; Oz et al., 1989]

  3. Tattoo pigments including graphite (black) and black, blue, green, and red organic dyes [Fitzpatrick, 1994; McGillis et al., 1994].

87.2 Penetration and Effects of UV-IR Laser Radiation into Biologic Tissue

Both scattering and absorption processes affect the variations of the intensity of radiation with propagation into tissues. In the absence of scattering, absorption results in an exponential decrease of radiation intensity described simply by Beers law [Grossweiner, 1989]. With appreciable scattering present, the decrease in incident intensity from the surface is no longer monotonic. A maximum in local internal intensity is found to be present due to efficient back-scattering, which adds to the intensity of the incoming beam as shown, for example, by Miller and Veitch [1993] for visible light penetrating into the skin and by Rastegar and coworkers [1992] for 1.064 μm *Nd:YAG* laser radiation penetrating into the prostate gland. Thus, the relative contributions of absorption and scattering of incident laser radiation will stipulate the depth in a tissue at which the resulting tissue effects will be present. Since the absorbed energy can be released in a number of different ways including thermal vibrations, fluorescence, and resonant electronic energy transfer according to the identity of the absorber, the effects on tissue are in general different. Energy release from both hemoglobin and melanin pigments and from water is by molecular vibrations resulting in a local temperature rise. Sufficient continued energy absorption and release can result in local temperature increases which, as energy input increases, result in protein denaturation (41–65°C), water evaporation and boiling (up to ≈300°C under confining pressure of tissue), thermolysis of proteins, generation of gaseous decomposition products and of carbonaceous residue or char (≥ 300°C). The generation of residual char is minimized by sufficiently rapid energy input to support rapid gasification reactions. The clinical effect of this chain of thermal events is tissue ablation. Much smaller values of energy input result in coagulation of tissues due to protein denaturation.

Energy release from excited exogenous photosensitizing dyes is via formation of free-radical species or energy exchange with itinerant dissolved molecular oxygen [Spikes, 1989]. Subsequent chemical reactions following free-radical formation or formation of an activated or more reactive form of molecular oxygen following energy exchange can be toxic to cells with takeup of the photosensitizer.

Energy release following absorption of *visible (VIS) radiation* by fluorescent molecular species, either endogenous to tissue or exogenous, is predominantly by emission of longer wavelength radiation [Lakowicz, 1983]. Endogenous fluorescent species include tryptophan, tyrosine, phenyl-alanine, flavins, and metal-free porphyrins. Comparison of measured values of the intensity of fluorescence emission from hyperplastic (transformed precancerous) cervical cells to cancerous cervical cells with normal cervical epithelial cells shows a strong potential for diagnostic use in the automated diagnosis and staging of cervical cancer [Mahadevan et al., 1993].

87.3 Effects of Mid-IR Laser Radiation

Because of the very large absorption by water of radiation with wavelength in the IR range $\geq 2.0\ \mu m$, the radiation of *Ho:YAG, Er:YAG,* and CO_2 lasers is absorbed within a very short distance of the tissue surface, and scattering is essentially unimportant. Using published values of the water absorption coefficient [Hale & Querry, 1973] and assuming an 80% water content and that the decrease in intensity is exponential with distance, the depth in the "average" soft tissue at which the intensity has decreased to 10% of the incident value (the optical penetration depth) is estimated to be 619, 13, and 170 micrometers, respectively, for Ho:YAG, Er:YAG, and CO_2 laser radiation. Thus, the absorption of radiation from these laser sources and thermalization of this energy results essentially in the formation of surface heat source. With sufficient energy input, tissue ablation through water boiling and tissue thermolysis occur at the surface. Penetration of heat to underlying tissues is by diffusion alone; thus, the depth of coagulation of tissue below the surface region of ablation is limited by competition between thermal diffusion and the rate of descent of the heated surface impacted by laser radiation during ablation of tissue. Because of this competition, coagulation depths obtained in soft biologic tissues with use of mid-IR laser radiation are typically $\leq 205\text{--}500\ \mu m$, and the ability to achieve sealing of blood vessels leading to hemostatic ("bloodless") surgery is limited [Judy et al., 1992; Schroder et al., 1987].

87.4 Effects of Near-IR Laser Radiation

The 810-nm and 1064-μm radiation, respectively, of the GaAlAs diode laser and Nd:YAG laser penetrate more deeply into biologic tissues than the radiation of longer-wavelength IR lasers. Thus, the resulting thermal effects arise from absorption at greater depth within tissues, and the depths of coagulation and degree of hemostasis achieved with these lasers tend to be greater than with the longer-wavelength IR lasers. For example, the optical penetration depths (10% incident intensity) for 810-nm and 1.024-μm radiation are estimated to be $\simeq 4.6$ and $\simeq 8.6$ mm respectively in canine prostate tissue [Rastegar et al., 1992]. Energy deposition of 3600 J from each laser on to the urethral surface of the canine prostate results in maximum coagulation depths of $\simeq 8$ and 12 mm respectively using diode and Nd:YAG lasers [Motamedi et al., 1993]. Depths of optical penetration and coagulation in porcine liver, a more vascular tissue than prostate gland, of $\simeq 2.8$ and $\simeq 9.6$ mm, respectively, were obtained with a Nd:YAG laser beam, and of 7 and 12 mm respectively with an 810-nm diode laser beam [Rastegar et al., 1992]. The smaller penetration depth obtained with 810-nm diode radiation in liver than in prostate gland reflects the effect of greater vascularity (blood content) on near-IR propagation.

87.5 Effects of Visible-Range Laser Radiation

Blood and vascular tissues very efficiently absorb radiation in the visible wavelength range due to the strong absorption of hemoglobin. This absorption underlies, for example, the use of:

1. The argon ion laser (488–514.5 nm) in the localized heating and thermal coagulation of the vascular choroid layer and adjacent retina, resulting in the anchoring of the retina in treatment of retinal detachment [Katoh & Peyman, 1988]
2. The argon ion laser (488–514.5 nm), frequency-doubled Nd:YAG laser (532 nm), and dye laser radiation (585 nm) in the coagulative treatment of cutaneous vascular lesions such as port wine stains [Mordon et al., 1993]
3. The argon ion (488–514.5 nm) and frequency-doubled Nd:YAG lasers (532 nm) in the ablation of pelvic endometrial lesions which contain brown iron-containing pigments [Keye et al., 1983]

Because of the large absorption by hemoglobin and iron-containing pigments, the incident laser radiation is essentially absorbed at the surface of the blood vessel or lesion, and the resulting thermal effects are essentially local [Miller & Veitch, 1993].

87.6 Effects of UV Laser Radiation

Whereas exposure of tissue to IR and visible-light-range laser energy result in removal of tissue by thermal ablation, exposure to *argon fluoride (ArF)* laser radiation of 193-nm wavelength results predominantly in ablation of tissue initiated by a photochemical process [Garrison & Srinivasan, 1985]. This ablation arises from repulsive forces between like-charged regions of ionized protein molecules that result from ejection of molecular electrons following UV photon absorption [Garrison & Srinivasan, 1985]. Because the ionization and repulsive processes are extremely efficient, little of the incident laser energy escapes as thermal vibrational energy, and the extent of thermal coagulation damage adjacent to the site of incidence is very limited [Garrison & Srinivasan, 1985]. This feature and the ability to tune very finely the fluence emitted by the ArF laser so that micrometer depths of tissue can be removed have led to ongoing clinical trials to investigate the efficiency of the use of the ArF laser to selectively remove tissue from the surface of the human cornea for correction of short-sighted vision to eliminate the need for corrective eyewear [Van Saarloos & Constable, 1993].

87.7 Effects of Continuous and Pulsed IR-Visible Laser Radiation and Associated Temperature Rise

Heating following absorption of IR-visible laser radiation arises from molecular vibration during loss of the excitation energy and initially is manifested locally within the exposed region of tissue. In incidence of the laser energy is maintained for sufficiently long time, the temperature within adjacent regions of biologic tissue increases due to heat diffusion. The mean squared distance $<X^2>$ over which appreciable heat diffusion and temperature rise occur during exposure time t can be described in terms of the thermal diffusion time τ by the equation:

$$<X^2> = \tau t \tag{87.1}$$

where τ is defined as the ratio of the thermal conductivity to the product of the heat capacity and density. For soft biologic tissues τ is approximately 1×10^3 cm^2 s^{-1} [Meijering et al., 1993]. Thus, with continued energy input, the distance over which thermal diffusion and temperature rise occur increases. Conversely, with use of pulsed radiation the distance of heat diffusion can be made very small; for example, with exposure to a 1-μs pulse, the mean thermal diffusion distance is found to be approximately 0.3 μm, or about 3–10% of a biologic cell diameter. If the laser radiation is strongly absorbed and the ablation of tissues is efficient, then little energy diffuses away from the site of incidence, and lateral thermally induced coagulation of tissue can be minimized with pulses of short duration. The effect of limiting lateral thermal damage is desirable in the cutting of cornea [Hibst et al., 1992] and sclera of the eye [Hill et al., 1993], and joint cartilage [Maes & Sherk, 1994], all of which are avascular (or nearly so, with cartilage), and the hemostasis arising from lateral tissue coagulation is not required.

87.8 General Description and Operation of Lasers

Lasers emit a beam of intense electromagnetic radiation that is essentially monochromatic or contains at most a few nearly monochromatic wavelengths and is typically only weakly divergent and easily focused into external optical systems. These attributes of laser radiation depend on the key phenomenon which underlies laser operation, that of light amplification by stimulated emission of radiation, which in turn gives rise to the acronym *LASER*.

In practice, a laser is generally a generator of radiation. The generator is constructed by housing a light-emitting medium within a cavity defined by mirrors which provide feedback of emitted radiation through the medium. With sustained excitation of the ionic or molecular species of the medium to give a large density of excited energy states, the spontaneous and attendant stimulated emission of radiation from these states by photons of identical wavelength (a lossless process), which is amplified by feedback due to photon reflection by the cavity mirrors, leads to the generation of a very large photon density within the cavity. With one cavity mirror being partially transmissive, say 0.1 to 1%, a fraction of the cavity energy is emitted as an intense beam. With suitable selection of a laser medium, cavity geometry, and peak wavelengths of mirror reflection, the beam is also essentially monochromatic and very nearly collimated.

Identity of the lasing molecular species or laser medium fixes the output wavelength of the laser. Laser media range from gases within a tubular cavity, organic dye molecules dissolved in a flowing inert liquid carrier and heat sink, to impurity-doped transparent crystalline rods (solid state lasers) and semiconducting diode junctions [Lengyel, 1971]. The different physical properties of these media in part determine the methods used to excite them into lasing states.

Gas-filled, or gas, lasers are typically excited by dc or rf electric current. The current either ionizes and excites the lasing gas, e.g., argon, to give the electronically excited and lasing Ar+ ion, or ionizes a gaseous species in a mixture also containing the lasing species, e.g., N_2, which by efficient energy transfer excites the lasing molecular vibrational states of the CO_2 molecule.

Dye lasers and so-called solid-state lasers are typically excited by intense light from either another laser or from a flash lamp. The excitation light wavelength range is selected to ensure efficient excitation at the absorption wavelength of the lasing species. Both excitation and output can be continuous, or the use of a pulsed flashlamp or pulsed exciting laser to pump a solid-state or dye laser gives pulsed output with high peak power and short pulse duration of 1 μs to 1 ms. Repeated excitation gives a train of pulses. Additionally, pulses of higher peak power and shorter duration of approximately 10 ns can be obtained from solid lasers by intracavity Q-switching [Lengyel, 1971]. In this method, the density of excited states is transiently greatly increased by impeding the path between the totally reflecting and partially transmitting mirror of the cavity interrupting the stimulated emission process. Upon rapid removal of the impeding device (a beam-interrupting or -deflecting device), stimulated emission of the very large population of excited lasing states leads to emission of an intense laser pulse. The process can give single pulses or can be repeated to give a pulse train with repetition frequencies typically ranging from 1 Hz to 1 kHz.

Gallium aluminum (GaAlAs) lasers are, as are all semiconducting diode lasers, excited by electrical current which creates excited hole-electron pairs in the vicinity of the diode junction. Those carrier pairs are the lasing species which emit spontaneously and with photon stimulation. The beam emerges parallel to the function with the plane of the function forming the cavity and thin-layer surface mirrors providing reflection. Use of continuous or pulsed excitation current results in continuous or pulsed output.

87.9 Biomedical Laser Beam Delivery Systems

Beam delivery systems for biomedical lasers guide the laser beam from the output mirror to the site of action on tissue. Beam powers of up to 100 W are transmitted routinely. All biomedical lasers incorporate a coaxial aiming beam, typically from a HeNe laser (632.8 nm) to illuminate the site of incidence on tissue.

Usually, the systems incorporate two different beam-guiding methods, either (1) a flexible fused silica (SiO_2) optical fiber or light guide, generally available currently for laser beam wavelengths between $\simeq$400 nm and $\simeq$2.1 μm, where SiO_2 is essentially transparent and (2) an articulated arm having beam-guiding mirrors for wavelengths greater than circa 2.1 μm (e.g., CO_2 lasers), for the Er:YAG and for pulsed lasers having peak power outputs capable of causing damage to optical fiber surfaces due to ionization by the intense electric field (e.g., pulsed ruby). The arm comprises straight tubular sections articulated together with high-quality power-handling dielectric mirrors at each articulation junction to guide the beam through each of the sections. Fused silica optical fibers usually are limited to a length of 1–3 m and to wavelengths in the visible-to-low mid-range IR ($<$ 2.1 μm), because longer wavelengths of IR radiation are absorbed by water impurities ($<$ 2.9 μm) and by the SiO_2 lattice itself (wavelengths $>$ 5 μm), as described by Levi [1980].

Since the flexibility, small diameter, and small mechanical inertia of optical fibers allow their use in either flexible or rigid endoscopes and offer significantly less inertia to hand movement, fibers for use at longer IR wavelengths are desired by clinicians. Currently, researchers are evaluating optical fiber materials transparent to longer IR wavelengths. Material systems showing promise are fused Al_2O_3 fibers in short lengths for use with near-3-micrometer radiation of the Er:YAG laser and *Ag halide* fibers in short lengths for use with the CO_2 laser emitting at 10.6 μm [Merberg, 1993]. A flexible hollow Teflon waveguide 1.6 mm in diameter having a thin metal film overlain by a dielectric layer has been reported recently to transmit 10.6 μm CO_2 radiation with attenuation of 1.3 and 1.65 dB/m for straight and bent (5-mm radius, 90-degree bend) sections, respectively [Gannot et al., 1994].

Optical Fiber Transmission Characteristics

Guiding of the emitted laser beam along the optical fiber, typically of uniform circular cross-section, is due to total internal reflection of the radiation at the interface between the wall of the optical fiber core and the cladding material having refractive index n_1 less than that of the core n_2 [Levi, 1980]. Total internal reflection occurs for any angle of incidence θ of the propagating beam with the wall of the fiber core such that $θ > θ_c$ where

$$\sin θ_c = \left(\frac{n_1}{n_2} \right) \tag{87.2}$$

or in terms of the complementary angle $α_c$

$$\cos α_c = \left(\frac{n_1}{n_2} \right) \tag{87.3}$$

For a focused input beam with apical angle $α_m$ incident upon the flat face of the fiber as shown in Fig. 87.1, total internal reflection and beam guidance within the fiber core will occur [Levi, 1980] for

$$NA = \sin (α_m/2) \leq [n_2^2 - n_1^2]^{0.5} \tag{87.4}$$

where *NA* is the numerical aperture of the fiber.

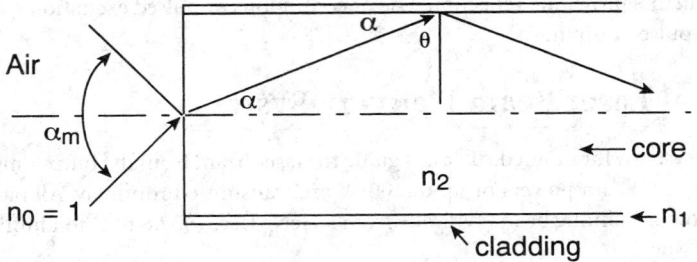

FIGURE 87.1   Critical reflection and propagation within an optical fiber.

This relationship ensures that the critical angle of incidence of the interface is not exceeded and that total internal reflection occurs [Levi, 1980]. Typical values of *NA* for fused SiO_2 fibers with polymer cladding are in the range of 0.36–0.40. The typical value of $\alpha_m = 14$ degrees used to insert the beam of the biomedical laser into the fiber is much smaller than those values ($\simeq$21–23 degrees) corresponding to typical *NA* values. The maximum value of the propagation angle α typically used in biomedical laser systems is $\simeq$4.8 degrees.

Leakage of radiation at the core-cladding interface of the fused SiO_2 fiber is negligible, typically being $\simeq$0.3 dB/m at 400 nm and 0.01 dB/m at 1.064 μm. Bends along the fiber length always decrease the angle of incidence at the core cladding interface. Bends do not give appreciable losses for values of the bending radius sufficiently large that the angle of incidence θ of the propagating beam in the bent core does not become less than θ_c at the core-cladding interface [Levi, 1980]. The relationship given by Levi [1980] between the bending radius r_b, the fiber core radius r_o, the ratio (n_2/n_1) of fiber core to cladding refractive indices, and the propagation angle α in Fig. 87.1 which ensures that the beam does not escape is

$$\frac{n_1}{n_2} > \frac{1 - \rho}{1 + \rho} \cos \alpha \tag{87.5}$$

where $\rho = (r_o/r_b)$. The inequality will hold for all $\alpha \le \alpha_c$ provided that

$$\frac{n_1}{n_2} \le \frac{1 - \rho}{1 + \rho} \tag{87.6}$$

Thus, the critical bending radius r_{bc} is the value of r_b such that Eq. (87.6) is an equality. Use of Eq. (87.6) predicts that bends with radii $\ge$ 12, 18, and 30 mm, respectively, will not result in appreciable beam leakage from fibers having 400-, 600-, and 1000-micron diameter cores, which are typical in biomedical use. Thus, use of fibers in flexible endoscopes usually does not compromise beam guidance.

Because the integrity of the core-cladding interface is critical to beam guiding, the clad fiber is encased typically in a tough but flexible protective fluoropolymer buffer coat.

Mirrored Articulated Arm Characteristics

Typically two or three relatively long tubular sections or arms of 50–80 cm length make up the portion of the articulated arm that extends from the laser output fixturing to the handpiece, endoscope, or operating microscope stage used to position the laser beam onto the tissue proper. Mirrors placed at the articulation of the arms and within the articulated handpiece, laparoscope, or operating microscope stage maintain the centration of the trajectory of the laser beam along the length of the delivery system. Dielectric multilayer mirrors [Levi, 1980] routinely are used in articulated devices. Their low high reflectivity $\ge$ 99.9 + % and power-handling capabilities ensure efficient power transmission down the arm. Mirrors in articulated devices typically are held in kinetically adjustable mounts for rapid stable alignment to maintain beam concentration.

Optics for Beam Shaping on Tissues

Since the rate of heating of tissue, and hence rates of ablation and coagulation, depends directly on energy input per unit volume of tissue, selection of ablation and coagulation rates of various tissues is achieved through control of the energy density (J/cm^2 or $W \cdot s/cm^2$) of the laser beam. This parameter is readily achieved through use of optical elements such as discrete focusing lenses placed in the handpiece or rigid endoscope which control the spot size upon the tissue surface or by affixing a so-called contact tip to the end of an optical fiber. These are conical or spherical in shape with diameter ranging 300–1200 μm and with very short focal lengths. The tip is placed in contact with the tissue and generates a submillimeter-sized focal spot in tissue very near the interface between the tip and tissue. One advantage of using the contact tip over a focused beam is that ablation proceeds with small lateral depth of attendant coagulation [Judy et al., 1993*a*]. This is because the energy of the tightly focused beam causes tissue thermolysis essentially at the tip surface and because the resulting tissue products strongly absorb the beam resulting in energy deposition and ablation essentially at the tip surface. This contrasts with the radiation penetrating deeply into tissue before thermolysis which occurs with a less tightly focused beam from a free lens or fiber. An additional advantage with the use of contact tips in the perception of the surgeon is that the kinesthetics of moving a contact tip along a resisting tissue surface more closely mimics the "touch" encountered in moving a scalpel across the tissue surface.

Recently a class of optical fiber tips has been developed which laterally directs the beam energy from a silica fiber [Judy et al., 1993*b*]. These tips, either a gold reflective micromirror or an angled refractive prism, offer a lateral angle of deviation ranging from 35–105 degrees from the optical fiber axis (undeviated beam direction). The beam reflected from a plane micromirror is unfocused and circular in cross-section, whereas the beam from a concave mirror and refractive devices is typically elliptical in shape, fused with distal diverging rays. Fibers with these terminations are currently finding rapidly expanding, large-scale application in coagulation (with 1.064-μm Nd:YAG laser radiation) of excess tissue lining the urethra in treatment of benign prostatic hypertrophy [Costello et al., 1992]. The capability for lateral beam direction may offer additional utility of these terminated fibers in other clinical specialties.

Features of Routinely Used Biomedical Lasers

Currently four lasers are in routine large-scale clinical biomedical use to ablate, dissect, and to coagulate soft tissue. Two, the carbon dioxide (CO_2) and argon ion (Ar-ion) lasers, are gas-filled lasers. The other two employ solid-state lasing media. One is the Neodymium-yttrium-aluminum-garnet (Nd:YAG) laser, commonly referred to as a solid-state laser, and the other is the gallium-aluminum arsenide (GaAlAs) semiconductor diode laser. Salient features of the operating characteristics and biomedical applications of those lasers are listed in Tables 87.2 to 87.5. The operational descriptions are typical of the lasers currently available commercially and do not represent the product of any single manufacturer.

Other Biomedical Lasers

Some important biomedical lasers have smaller-scale use or currently are being researched for biomedical application. The following four lasers have more limited scales of surgical use:

The Ho:YAG (Holmium:YAG) laser, emitting pulses of 2.1 μm wavelength and up to 4 J in energy, used in soft tissue ablation in arthroscopic (joint) surgery (FDA approved).

TABLE 87.2 Operating Characteristics of Principal Biomedical Lasers

Characteristics	Ar Ion Laser	CO_2 Laser
Cavity medium	Argon gas, 133 Pa	10% CO_2 10% Ne, 80% He; 1330 Pa
Lasing species	Ar+ ion	CO_2 molecule
Excitation	Electric discharge, continuous	Electric discharge, continuous, pulsed
Electric input	208 V_{AC}, 60 A	110 V_{AC}, 15 A
Wall plug efficiency	≃0.06%	≃10%

Characteristics	Nd:YAG Laser	GaAlAs Diode Laser
Cavity medium	Nd-doped YAG	n-p junction, GaAlAS diode
Lasing species	Nd3t in YAG lattice	Hole-electron pairs at diode junction
Excitation	Flashlamp, continuous, pulsed	Electric current, continuous pulsed
Electric input	208/240 V_{AC}, 30 A continuous 110 V_{AC}, 10 A pulsed	110 V_{AC}, 15 A
Wall plug efficiency	≃1%	≃23%

TABLE 87.3 Output Beam Characteristics of Ar-Ion and CO_2 Biomedical Lasers

Output Characteristics	Argon Laser	CO_2 Laser
Output power	2–8 W, continuous	1–100 W, continuous
Wavelength(s)	Multiple lines (454.6–528.7 nm), 488, 514.5 dominant	10.6 μm
Electromagnetic wave propagation mode	TEM_{oo}	TEM_{oo}
Beam guidance, shaping	Fused silica optical fiber with contact tip or flat-ended for beam emission, lensed handpiece. Slit lamp with ocular lens	Flexible articulated arm with mirrors; lensed handpiece or mirrored microscope platen

The Q-switched Ruby (*Cr:Al₂0₃*) laser, emitting pulses of 694-nm wavelength and up to 2 J in energy is used in dermatology to disperse black, blue, and green tattoo pigments and melanin in pigmented lesions (not melanoma) for subsequent removal by phagocytosis by macrophages (FDA approved).

The flashlamp pumped pulsed dye laser emitting 1- to 2-J pulses at either 577- or 585-nm wavelength (near the 537–577 absorption region of blood) is used for treatment of cutaneous vascular lesions and melanin pigmented lesions except melanoma. Use of pulsed radiation helps to localize the thermal damage to within the lesions to obtain low damage of adjacent tissue.

The following lasers are being investigated for clinical uses.

The Er:YAG laser, emitting at 2.94 μm near the major water absorption peak (OH stretch), is currently being investigated for ablation of tooth enamel and dentin [Li et al., 1992].

TABLE 87.4 Output Beam Characteristics of Nd:YAG and GaAlAs Diode Biomedical Lasers

Output Characteristics	Nd:YAG Laser	GaAlAs Diode Laser
Output power	1–100 W continuous at 1.064 millimicron 1–36W continuous at 532 nm (frequency doubled with KTP)	1–25 W continuous
Wavelength(s)	1.064 μm/532 nm	810 nm
Electromagnetic wave propagation modes	Mixed modes	Mixed modes
Beam guidance and shaping	Fused SiO₂ optical fiber with contact tip directing mirrored or refracture tip	Fused SiO₂ optical fiber with contact tip or laterally directing mirrored or refracture tip

TABLE 87.5 Clinical Uses of Principal Biomedical Lasers

Ar-ion laser: Pigmented (vascular) soft-tissue ablation in gynecology; general and oral surgery; otolaryngology; vascular lesion coagulation in dermatology; retinal coagulation in ophthalmology

Nd:YAG laser: Soft-tissue, particularly pigmented vascular tissue, ablation—dissection and bulk tissue removal—in dermatology; gastroenterology; gynecology; general, arthroscopic, neuro-, plastic, and thoracic surgery; urology; posterior capsulotomy (ophthalmology) with pulsed 1.064 millimicron and ocular lens

CO₂ laser: Soft-tissue ablation—dissection and bulk tissue removal in dermatology; gynecology; general, oral, plastic, and neurosurgery; otolaryngology; podiatry; urology

GaAlAs diode laser: Pigmented (vascular) soft-tissue ablation—dissection and bulk removal in gynecology, gastroenterology, general surgery, and urology; FDA approval for otolaryngology and thoracic surgery pending

Dye lasers emitting at 630–690 nm are being investigated for application as light sources for exciting dihematoporphyrin ether or benzoporphyrin derivatives in investigation of the efficacy of these photosensitives in the treatment of esophageal, bronchial, and bladder carcinomas for the FDA approval process.

Defining Terms

Biomedical Laser Radiation Ranges

Infrared (IR) radiation: The portion of the electromagnetic spectrum within the wavelength range 760 nm–1 mm, with the regions 760 nm–1.400 μm and 1.400–10.00 μm, respectively, called the near- and mid-IR regions.

Ultraviolet (UV) radiation: The portion of the electromagnetic spectrum within the wavelength range 100–400 nm.

Visible (VIS) radiation: The portion of the electromagnetic spectrum within the wavelength range 400–760 nm.

Laser Medium Nomenclature

Argon fluoride (ArF): Argon fluoride eximer laser (an eximer is a diatomic molecule which can exist only in an excited state).

Ar ion: Argon ion.

CO₂: Carbon dioxide.

Cr:Al₂0₃: Ruby laser.

Er:YAG: Erbium yttrium aluminum garnet.

GaAlAs: Gallium aluminum laser.

HeNe: Helium neon laser.

Ho:YAG: Holmium yttrium aluminum garnet.

Nd:YAG: Neodymium yttrium aluminum garnet.

Optical Fiber Nomenclature

Ag halide: Silver halide, halide ion, typically bromine (Br) and chlorine (Cl).

Fused silica: Fused SiO₂.

References

Bass LS, Moazami N, Pocsidio J, et al. 1992. Change in type I collagen following laser welding. Lasers Surg Med 12(5):500.

Costello AJ, Johnson DE, Bolton DM. 1992. Nd:YAG laser ablation of the prostate as a treatment for benign prostate hypertrophy. Lasers Surg Med 12(2):121.

Fitzpatrick RE. 1994. Comparison of the Q-switched ruby, Nd:YAG, and alexandrite lasers in tatoo removal. Lasers Surg Med Suppl 6(266):52.

Gannot I, Dror J, Calderon S, et al. 1994. Flexible waveguides for IR laser radiation and surgery applications. Lasers Surg Med 14(2):184.

Garrison BJ, Srinivasan R. 1985. Laser ablation of organic polymers: microscopic models for photo-chemical and thermal processes. J Appl Physiol 58(9):2909.

Grossweiner LI. 1989. Photophysics. In KC Smith (ed), The Science of Photobiology, p 1–47. New York, Plenum.

Hale GM, Querry MR. 1973. Optical constants of water in the 200 nm to 200 μm wavelength region. Appl Optics 12(12):555.

Hibst R, Bende T, Schröder D. 1992. Wet corneal ablation by Er:YAG laser radiation. Lasers Surg Med Suppl 4(236):56.

Hill RA, Le MT, Yashiro H, et al. 1993. Ab-interno erbium (Er:YAG) laser sclerostomy with irido-tomy in dutch cross rabbits. Lasers Surg Med 13(5):559.

Judy MM, Matthews JL, Aronoff BL, et al. 1993a. Soft tissue studies with 805 nm diode laser radia-tion: Thermal effects with contact tips and comparison with effects of 1064 nm Nd:YAG laser radiation. Lasers Surg Med 13(5):528.

Judy MM, Matthews JL, Gardetto WW, et al. 1993b. Side firing laser-fiber technology for minimally invasive transurethral treatment of benign prostate hyperplasia. Proc Soc Photo-Optical Instr Eng (SPIE) 1982:86.

Judy MM, Matthews JL, Goodson JR, et al. 1992. Thermal effects in tissues from simultaneous coax-ial CO_2 and Nd:YAG laser beams. Lasers Surg Med 12(2):222.

Katoh N, Peyman GA. 1988. Effects of laser wavelengths on experimental retinal detachments and retinal vessels. Jpn J Ophthalmol 32(2):196.

Keye WR, Matson GA, Dixon J. 1983. The use of the argon laser in treatment of experimental endometriosis. Fertil Steril 39(1):26.

Lakowicz JR. 1983. Principles of Fluorescence Spectroscopy. New York, Plenum.

Lengyel BA. 1971. Lasers. New York, John Wiley.

Levi L. 1980. Applied Optics, vol 2. New York, John Wiley.

Li ZZ, Code JE, Van de Merve WP. 1992. Er:YAG laser ablation of enamel and dentin of human teeth: determination of ablation rates at various fluences and pulse repetition rates. Lasers Surg Med 12(6):625.

Maes KE, Sherk HH. 1994. Bone and meniscal ablation using the erbium YAG laser. Lasers Surg Med Suppl 6(166):31.

Mahadevan A, Mitchel MF, Silva E, et al. 1993. Study of the fluorescence properties of normal and neoplastic human cervical tissue. Lasers Surg Med 13(6):647.

McGillis ST, Bailin PL, Fitzpatrick RE, et al. 1994. Successful treatments of blue, green, brown and reddish-brown tatoos with the Q-switched alexandrite laser. Laser Surg Med Suppl 6(270):52.

Meijering LJT, VanGermert MJC, Gijsbers GHM, et al. 1993. Limits of radial time constants to approximate thermal response of tissue. Lasers Surg Med 13(6):685.

Merberg GN. 1993. Current status of infrared fiberoptics for medical laser power delivery. Lasers Surg Med 13(5):572.

Miller ID, Veitch AR. 1993. Optical modeling of light distributions in skin tissue following laser irradiation. Lasers Surg Med 13(5):565.

Mordon S, Beacco C, Rotteleur G, et al. 1993. Relation between skin surface temperature and min-imal blanching during argon, Nd:YAG 532, and cw dye 585 laser therapy of port-wine stains. Lasers Surg Med 13(1):124.

Motemedi M, Torres JH, Cammack T, et al. 1993. Thermodynamics of cw laser interaction with pro-static tissue: Effects of simultaneous cooling on lesion size. Lasers Surg Med Suppl 5(314):64.

Oz MC, Chuck RS, Johnson JP, et al. 1989. Indocyanine green dye-enhanced welding with a diode laser. Surg Forum 40(4):316.

Rastegar S, Jacques SC, Motamedi M, et al. 1992. Theoretical analysis of high-power diode laser (810 nm) and Nd:YAG laser (1064 nm) for coagulation of tissue: Predictions for prostate coagulation. Proc Soc Photo-Optical Instr Eng (SPIE) 1646:150.

Schroder T, Brackett K, Joffe S. 1987. An experimental study of effects of electrocautery and various lasers on gastrointestinal tissue. Surgery. 101(6):691.

Spikes JD. 1989. Photosensitization. In KC Smith (ed), The Science of Photobiology, 2d ed, pp 79–110. New York, Plenum.

Van de Hulst HC. 1957. Light Scattering by Small Particles. New York, John Wiley.

Van Saarloos PP, Constable IJ. 1993. Improved eximer laser photorefractive keratectomy system. Lasers Surg Med 13(2):189.

White A, Handler P, Smith EL. 1968. Principles of Biochemistry, 4th ed. New York, McGraw-Hill.

Further Information

Current research on the optical, thermal, and photochemical interactions of radiation and their effect on biologic tissues, are published routinely in the journals: *Lasers in Medicine and Surgery, Lasers in the Life Sciences,* and *Photochemistry Photobiology* and to a lesser extent in *Applied Optics and Optical Engineering.*

Clinical evaluations of biomedical laser applications appear in *Lasers and Medicine and Surgery* and in journals devoted to clinical specialties such as *Journal of General Surgery, Journal of Urology, Journal of Gastroenterological Surgery.*

The annual symposium proceedings of the biomedical section of the Society of Photo-Optical Instrumentation Engineers (SPIE) contain descriptions of new and current research on application of lasers and optics in biomedicine.

The book *Lasers* (a second edition by Bela A. Lengyel), although published in 1971, remains a valuable resource on the fundamental physics of lasers—gas, dye, solid-state, and semiconducting diode. A more recent book, *The Laser Guidebook* by Jeffrey Hecht, published in 1992, emphasizes the technical characteristics of the gas, diode, solid-state, and semiconducting diode lasers.

The *Journal of Applied Physics, Physical Review Letters,* and *Applied Physics Letters* carry descriptions of the newest advances and experimental phenomena in lasers and optics.

The book *Safety with Lasers and Other Optical Sources* by David Sliney and Myron Wolbarsht, published in 1980, remains a very valuable resource on matters of safety in laser use.

Laser safety standards for the United States are given for all laser uses and types in the American National Standard (ANSI) Z136.1-1993, Safe Use of Lasers.

88

Noninvasive Optical Monitoring

Ross Flewelling
Nellcor Incorporated

Optical measures of physiologic status are attractive because they can provide a simple, noninvasive, yet real-time assessment of medical condition. Noninvasive optical monitoring is here taken to mean the use of visible or near-infrared light to directly assess the internal physiologic status of a person without the need of extracting a blood or tissue sample or using a catheter. Liquid water strongly absorbs ultraviolet and infrared radiation, and thus these spectral regions are useful only for analyzing thin surface layers or respiratory gases, neither of which will be the subject of this review. Instead, it is the visible and near-infrared portions of the electromagnetic spectrum that provide a unique "optical window" into the human body, opening new vistas for noninvasive monitoring technologies.

Various molecules in the human body possess distinctive spectral absorption characteristics in the visible or near-infrared spectral regions and therefore make optical monitoring possible. The most strongly absorbing molecules at physiologic concentrations are the hemoglobins, myoglobins, cytochromes, melanins, carotenes, and bilirubin (see Fig. 88.1 for some examples). Perhaps less appreciated are the less distinctive and weakly absorbing yet ubiquitous materials possessing spectral characteristics in the near-infrared: water, fat, proteins, and sugars. Simple optical methods are now available to quantitatively and noninvasively measure some of these compounds directly in intact tissue. The most successful methods to date have used hemoglobins to assess the oxygen content of blood, cytochromes to assess the respiratory status of cells, and possibly near-infrared to assess endogenous concentrations of metabolites, including glucose.

88.1 Oximetry and Pulse Oximetry

Failure to provide adequate oxygen to tissues—*hypoxia*—can in a matter of minutes result in reduced work capacity of muscles, depressed mental activity, and ultimately cell death. It is therefore of considerable interest to reliably and accurately determine the amount of oxygen in blood or tissues. *Oximetry* is the determination of the oxygen content of blood or tissues, normally by optical means. In the clinical laboratory the oxygen content of whole blood can be determined by a benchtop cooximeter or blood gas analyzer. But the need for timely clinical information and the desire to

0-8493-8346-3/95/$0.00+$.50
© 1995 by CRC Press, Inc.

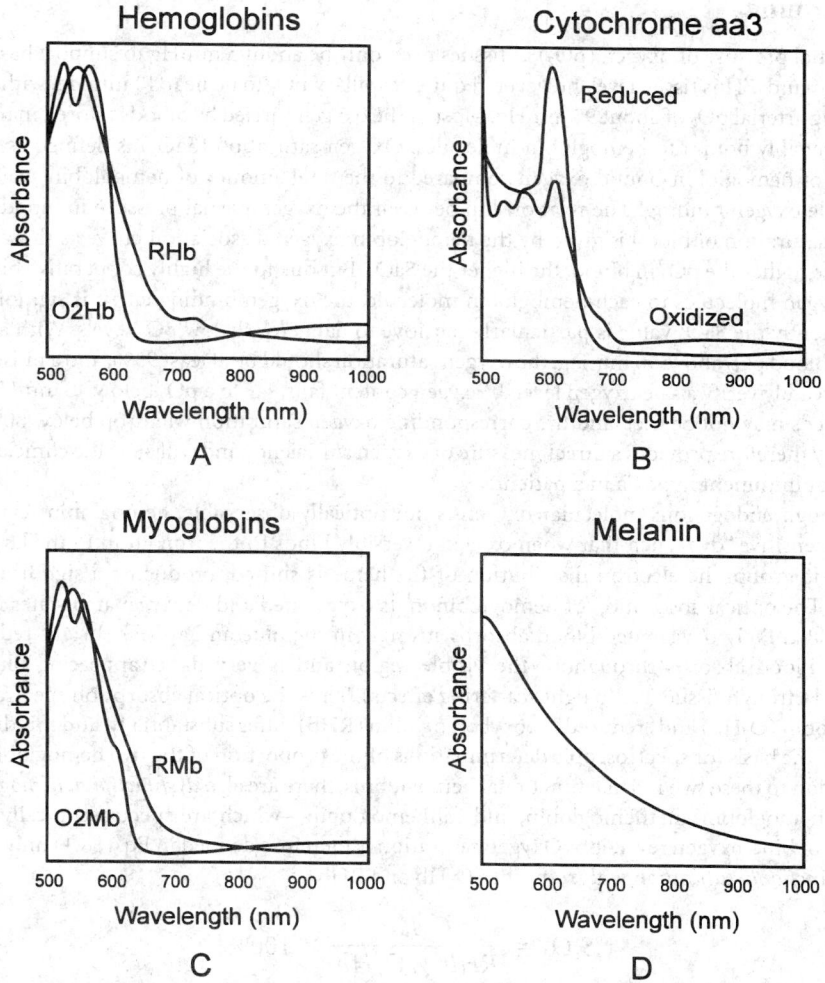

FIGURE 88.1 Absorption spectra of some endogenous biologic materials (*a*) hemoglobins, (*b*) cytochrome *aa3*, (*c*) myoglobins, and (*d*) melanin.

minimize the inconvenience and cost of extracting a blood sample and later analyze it in the lab has led to the search for alternative noninvasive optical methods. Since the 1930s, attempts have been made to use multiple wavelengths of light to arrive at a complete spectral characterization of a tissue. These approaches, although somewhat successful, have remained of limited utility owing to the awkward instrumentation and unreliable results.

It was not until the invention of *pulse oximetry* in the 1970s and its commercial development and application in the 1980s that noninvasive oximetry became practical. Pulse oximetry is an extremely easy-to-use, noninvasive, and accurate measurement of real-time arterial oxygen saturation. Pulse oximetry is now used routinely in clinical practice, has become a standard of care in all U.S. operating rooms, and is increasingly used wherever critical patients are found. The explosive growth of this new technology and its considerable utility led John Severinghaus and Poul Astrup [1986] in an excellent historical review to conclude that pulse oximetry was "arguably the most significant technological advance ever made in monitoring the well-being and safety of patients during anesthesia, recovery and critical care."

Background

The partial pressure of oxygen (pO_2) in tissues need only be about 3 mmHg to support basic metabolic demands. This tissue level, however, requires capillary pO_2 to be near 40 mmHg, with a corresponding arterial pO_2 of about 95 mmHg. Most of the oxygen carried by blood is stored in red blood cells reversibly bound to hemoglobin molecules. Oxygen saturation (SaO_2) is defined as the percentage of hemoglobin-bound oxygen compared to the total amount of hemoglobin available for reversible oxygen binding. The relationship between the oxygen partial pressure in blood and the oxygen saturation of blood is given by the hemoglobin oxygen dissociation curve as shown in Fig. 88.2. The higher the pO_2 in blood, the higher the SaO_2. But due to the highly cooperative binding of four oxygen molecules to each hemoglobin molecule, the oxygen binding curve is sigmoidal, and consequently the SaO_2 value is particularly sensitive to dangerously low pO_2 levels. With a normal arterial blood pO_2 above 90 mmHg, the oxygen saturation should be at least 95%, and a pulse oximeter can readily verify a safe oxygen level. If oxygen content falls, say to a pO_2 below 40 mmHg, metabolic needs may not be met, and the corresponding oxygen saturation will drop below 80%. Pulse oximetry therefore provides a direct measure of oxygen sufficiency and will alert the clinician to any danger of imminent hypoxia in a patient.

Although endogenous molecular oxygen is not optically observable, hemoglobin serves as an oxygen-sensitive "dye" such that when oxygen reversibly binds to the iron atom in the large heme prosthetic group, the electron distribution of the heme is shifted, producing a significant color change. The optical absorption of hemoglobin in its oxygenated and deoxygenated states is shown in Fig. 88.1. Fully oxygenated blood absorbs strongly in the blue and appears bright red; deoxygenated blood absorbs throughout the visible region and is very dark (appearing blue when observed through tissue due to light scattering effects). Thus the optical absorption spectra of oxyhemoglobin (O_2Hb) and "reduced" deoxyhemoglobin (RHb) differ substantially, and this difference provides the basis for spectroscopic determinations of the proportion of the two hemoglobin states. In addition to these two normal functional hemoglobins, there are also *dysfunctional hemoglobins*— carboxyhemoglobin, methemoglobin, and sulfhemoglobin—which are spectroscopically distinct but do not bind oxygen reversibly. Oxygen saturation is therefore defined in Eq. (88.1) only in terms of the *functional saturation* with respect to O_2Hb and RHb:

$$S_aO_2 = \frac{O_2Hb}{RHb + O_2Hb} \times 100\% \qquad (88.1)$$

Cooximeters are bench-top analyzers that accept whole blood samples and utilize four or more wavelengths of monochromatic light, typically between 500 and 650 nm, to spectroscopically determine the various individual hemoglobins in the sample. If a blood sample can be provided, this spectroscopic method is accurate and reliable. Attempts to make an equivalent quantitative analysis noninvasively through intact tissue have been fraught with difficulty. The problem has been to contend with the wide variation in scattering and nonspecific absorption properties of very complex heterogeneous tissue. One of the more successful approaches, marketed by Hewlett-Packard, used eight optical wavelengths transmitted through the pinna of the ear. In this approach a "bloodless" measurement is first obtained by squeezing as much blood as possible from an area of tissue; the arterial blood is then allowed to flow back, and the oxygen saturation is determined by analyzing the change in the spectral absorbance characteristics of the tissue. While this method works fairly well, it is cumbersome, operator dependent, and does not always work well on poorly perfused or highly pigmented subjects.

In the early 1970s, Takuo Aoyagi recognized that most of the interfering nonspecific tissue effects could be eliminated by utilizing only the change in the signal during an arterial pulse. Although an early prototype was built in Japan, it was not until the refinements in implementation and application by Biox (now Ohmeda) and Nellcor Incorporated in the 1980s that the technology became widely adopted as a safety monitor for critical care use.

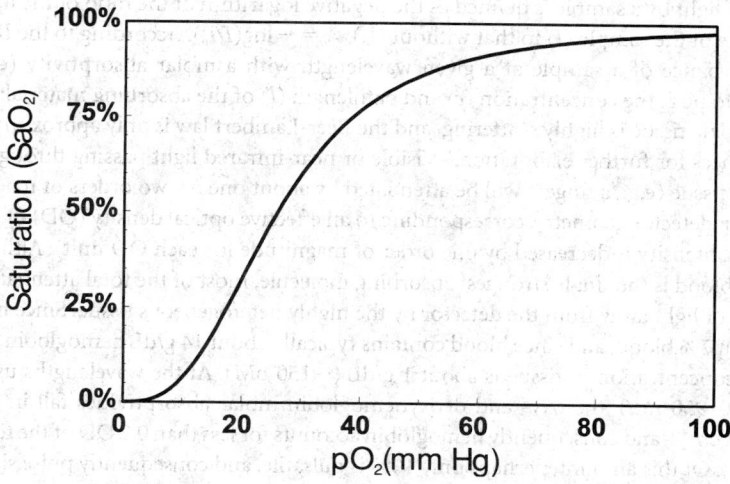

FIGURE 88.2 Hemoglobin oxygen dissociation curve showing the sigmoidal relationship between the partial pressure of oxygen and the oxygen saturation of blood. The curve is given approximately by $\%SaO_2 = 100\%/[1 + P_{50}/pO_2)^n]$, with $n = 2.8$ and $P_{50} = 26$ mm Hg.

Theory

Pulse oximetry is based on the fractional change in light transmission during an arterial pulse at two different wavelengths. In this method the fractional change in the signal is due only to the arterial blood itself, and therefore the complicated nonpulsatile and highly variable optical characteristics of tissue are eliminated. In a typical configuration, light at two different wavelengths illuminating one side of a finger will be detected on the other side, after having traversed the intervening vascular tissues (Fig. 88.3). The transmission of light at each wavelength is a function of the thickness, color, and structure of the skin, tissue, bone, blood, and other material through which the light passes. The

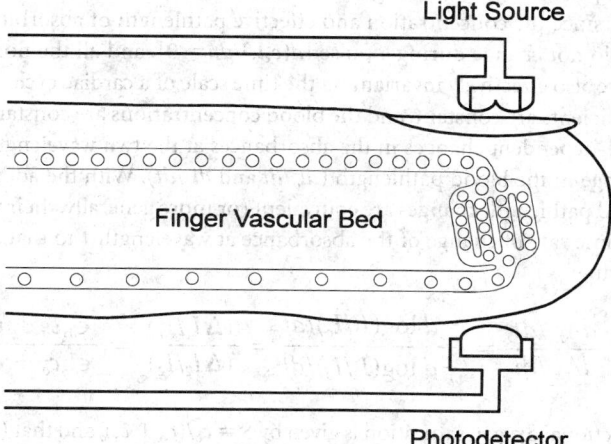

FIGURE 88.3 Typical pulse oximeter sensing configuration on a finger. Light at two different wavelengths is emitted by the source, diffusely scattered through the finger, and detected on the opposite side by a photodetector.

absorbance of light by a sample is defined as the negative logarithm of the ratio of the light intensity in the presence of the sample (I) to that without (I_o): $A = -\log(I/I_o)$. According to the *Beer-Lambert law*, the absorbance of a sample at a given wavelength with a molar absorptivity (ϵ) is directly proportional to both the concentration (c) and pathlength (l) of the absorbing material: $A = \epsilon c l$. (In actuality, biologic tissue is highly scattering, and the Beer-Lambert law is only approximately correct; see the references for further elaboration.) Visible or near-infrared light passing through about one centimeter of tissue (e.g., a finger) will be attenuated by about one or two orders of magnitude for a typical emitter-detector geometry, corresponding to an effective optical density (OD) of 1–2 OD (the detected light intensity is decreased by one order of magnitude for each OD unit). Although hemoglobin in the blood is the single strongest absorbing molecule, most of the total attenuation is due to the scattering of light away from the detector by the highly heterogeneous tissue. Since human tissue contains about 7% blood, and since blood contains typically about 14 g/dL hemoglobin, the effective hemoglobin concentration in tissue is about 1 g/dL ($\sim$150 uM). At the wavelengths used for pulse oximetry (650–950 nm), the oxy- and deoxyhemoglobin molar absorptivities fall in the range of 100–1000 M^{-1}cm^{-1}, and consequently hemoglobin accounts for less than 0.2 OD of the total observed optical density. Of this amount, perhaps only 10% is pulsatile, and consequently pulse signals of only about a few percent are ultimately measured, at times even one-tenth of this.

A mathematical model for pulse oximetry begins by considering light at two wavelengths, λ_1 and λ_2, passing through tissue and being detected at a distant location as in Fig. 88.3. At each wavelength the total light attenuation is described by four different component absorbances: oxyhemoglobin in the blood (concentration c_o, molar absorptivity ϵ_o, and effective pathlength l_o), "reduced" deoxyhemoglobin in the blood (concentration c_r, molar absorptivity ϵ_r, and effective pathlength l_r), specific variable absorbances that are not from the arterial blood (concentration c_x, molar absorptivity ϵ_x, and effective pathlength l_x), and all other non-specific sources of optical attenuation, combined as A_y, which can include light scattering, geometric factors, and characteristics of the emitter and detector elements. The total absorbance at the two wavelengths can then be written:

$$\begin{cases} A_{\lambda_1} = \epsilon_{o_1} c_o l_o + \epsilon_{r_1} c_r l_r + \epsilon_{x_1} c_x l_x + A_{y_1} \\ A_{\lambda_2} = \epsilon_{o_2} c_o l_o + \epsilon_{r_2} c_r l_r + \epsilon_{x_2} c_x l_x + A_{y_2} \end{cases} \qquad (88.2)$$

The blood volume change due to the arterial pulse results in a modulation of the measured absorbances. By taking the time rate of change of the absorbances, the two last terms in each equation are effectively zero, since the concentration and effective pathlength of absorbing material outside the arterial blood do not change during a pulse [$d(c_x l_x)/dt = 0$], and all the nonspecific effects on light attenuation are also effectively invariant on the time scale of a cardiac cycle ($dA_y/dt = 0$). Since the extinction coefficients are constant, and the blood concentrations are constant on the time scale of a pulse, the time-dependent changes in the absorbances at the two wavelengths can be assigned entirely to the change in the blood pathlength (dl_o/dt and dl_r/dt). With the additional assumption that these two blood pathlength changes are equivalent (or more generally, their ratio is a constant), the ratio R of the time rate of change of the absorbance at wavelength *1* to that at wavelength *2* reduces to the following:

$$R = \frac{dA_{\lambda_1}/dt}{dA_{\lambda_2}/dt} = \frac{-d\log(I_1/I_o)/dt}{-d\log(I_2/I_o)/dt} = \frac{(\Delta I_1/I_1)}{(\Delta I_2/I_2)} = \frac{\epsilon_{o_1} c_o + \epsilon_{r_1} c_r}{\epsilon_{o_2} c_o + \epsilon_{r_2} c_r} \qquad (88.3)$$

Observing that functional oxygen saturation is given by $S = c_o/(c_o + c_r)$, and that $(1-S) = c_r/(c_o + c_r)$, the oxygen saturation can then be written in terms of the ratio R as follows:

$$S = \frac{\epsilon_{r1} - \epsilon_{r2} R}{(\epsilon_{r1} - \epsilon_{o1}) - (\epsilon_{r2} - \epsilon_{o2}) R} \qquad (88.4)$$

Equation (88.4) provides the desired relationship between the experimentally determined ratio R and the clinically desired oxygen saturation S. In actual use, commonly available LEDs are used as the light sources, typically a red LED near 660 nm and a near-infrared LED selected in the range 890–950 nm. Such LEDs are not monochromatic light sources, typically with bandwidths between 20 and 50 nm, and therefore standard molar absorptivities for hemoglobin cannot be used directly in Eq. (88.4). Further, the simple model presented above is only approximately true; for example, the two wavelengths do not necessarily have the exact same pathlength changes, and second-order scattering effects have been ignored. Consequently the relationship between S and R is instead determined empirically by fitting the clinical data to a generalized function of the form $S = (a - bR)/(c - dR)$. The final empirical calibration will ultimately depend on the details of an individual sensor design, but these variations can be determined for each sensor and included in unique calibration parameters. A typical empirical calibration for R versus S is shown in Fig. 88.4, together with the curve that standard molar absorptivities would predict.

In this way the measurement of the ratio of the fractional change in signal intensity of the two LEDs is used along with the empirically determined calibration equation to obtain a beat-by-beat measurement of the arterial oxygen saturation in a perfused tissue—continuously, noninvasively, and to an accuracy of a few percent.

Applications and Future Directions

Pulse oximetry is now routinely used in nearly all operating rooms and critical care areas in the United States and increasingly throughout the world. It has become so pervasive and useful that it is now being called the "fifth" vital sign (for an excellent review of practical aspects and clinical applications of the technology see Kelleher [1989]).

The principal advantages of pulse oximetry are that it provides continuous, accurate, and reliable monitoring of arterial oxygen saturation on nearly all patients, utilizing a variety of convenient sensors, reusable as well as disposable. Single-patient-use adhesive sensors can easily be applied to fingers for adults and children and to arms or legs for neonates. Surface reflectance sensors have also

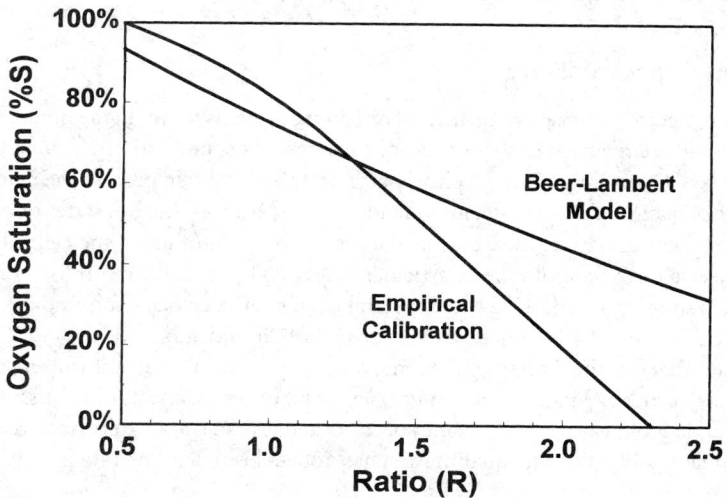

FIGURE 88.4 Relationship between the measured ratio of fractional changes in light intensity at two wavelengths, R, and the oxygen saturation S. Beer-Lambert model is from Eq. (88.4) with $\epsilon_{o_1} = 100$, $\epsilon_{o_2} = 300$, $\epsilon_{r_1} = 800$, and $\epsilon_{r_2} = 200$. Empirical calibration is based on $\%S = 100\% \times (a - bR)/(c - dR)$ with $a = 1000$, $b = 550$, $c = 900$, and $d = 350$, with a linear extrapolation below 70%.

been developed based on the same principles and offer a wider choice for sensor location, though they tend to be less accurate and prone to more types of interference.

Limitations of pulse oximetry include sensitivity to high levels of optical or electric interference, errors due to high concentrations of dysfunctional hemoglobins (methemoglobin or carboxyhemoglobin) or interference from physiologic dyes (such as methylene blue). Other important factors, such as total hemoglobin content, fetal hemoglobin, or sickle cell trait, have little or no effect on the measurement except under extreme conditions. Performance can also be compromised by poor signal quality, as may occur for poorly perfused tissues with weak pulse amplitudes or by motion artifact.

Hardware and software advances continue to provide more sensitive signal detection and filtering capabilities, allowing pulse oximeters to work better on more ambulatory patients. Already some pulse oximeters incorporate ECG synchronization for improved signal processing. A pulse oximeter for use in labor and delivery is currently under active development by several research groups and companies. A likely implementation may include use of a reflectance surface sensor for the fetal head to monitor the adequacy of fetal oxygenation. This application is still in active development, and clinical utility remains to be demonstrated.

88.2 Nonpulsatile Spectroscopy

Background

Nonpulsatile optical spectroscopy has been used for more than half a century for noninvasive medical assessment, such as in the use of multiwavelength tissue analysis for oximetry and skin reflectance measurement for bilirubin assessment in jaundiced neonates. These early applications have found some limited use, but with modest impact. Recent investigations into new nonpulsatile spectroscopy methods for assessment of deep-tissue oxygenation (e.g., cerebral oxygen monitoring), for evaluation of respiratory status at the cellular level, and for the detection of other critical analytes, such as glucose, may yet prove more fruitful. The former applications have led to spectroscopic studies of cytochromes in tissues, and the latter has led to considerable work into new approaches in near-infrared analysis of intact tissues.

Cytochrome Spectroscopy

Cytochromes are electron-transporting, heme-containing proteins found in the inner membranes of mitochondria and are required in the process of oxidative phosphorylation to convert metabolites and oxygen into CO_2 and high-energy phosphates. In this metabolic process the cytochromes are reversibly oxidized and reduced, and consequently the oxidation-reduction states of cytochromes c and aa_3 in particular are direct measures of the respiratory condition of the cell. Changes in the absorption spectra of these molecules, particularly near 600 nm and 830 nm for cytochrome aa_3, accompany this shift. By monitoring these spectral changes, the cytochrome oxidation state in the tissues can be determined (see, for example, Jöbsis [1977] and Jöbsis et al. [1977]). As with all nonpulsatile approaches, the difficulty is to remove the dependence of the measurement on the various nonspecific absorbing materials and highly variable scattering effects of the tissue. To date, instruments designed to measure cytochrome spectral changes can successfully track relative changes in brain oxygenation, but absolute quantitation has not yet been demonstrated.

Near-Infrared Spectroscopy and Glucose Monitoring

Near-infrared (NIR), the spectral region between 780 nm and 3000 nm, is characterized by broad and overlapping spectral peaks produced by the overtones and combinations of infrared vibrational modes. Figure 88.5 shows typical NIR absorption spectra of fat, water, and starch. Exploitation of

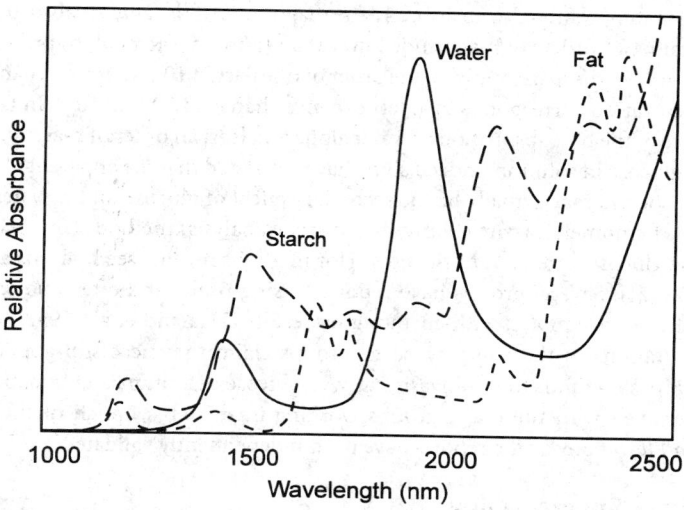

FIGURE 88.5 Typical near-infrared absorption spectra of several biologic materials.

this spectral region for *in vivo* analysis has been hindered by the same complexities of nonpulsatile tissue spectroscopy described above and is further confounded by the very broad and indistinct spectral features characteristic of the NIR. Despite these difficulties, NIR spectroscopy has garnered considerable attention, since it may enable the analysis of common analytes.

Karl Norris and coworkers pioneered the practical application of NIR spectroscopy, using it to evaluate water, fat, and sugar content of agricultural products (see Osborne et al. [1993] and Burns and Cuirczak [1992]). The further development of sophisticated *multivariate analysis* techniques, together with new scattering models (e.g., Kubelka-Munk theory) and high-performance instrumentation, further extended the application of NIR methods. Over the past decade, many research groups and companies have touted the use of NIR techniques for medical monitoring, such as for determining the relative fat, protein, and water content of tissue, and more recently for noninvasive glucose measurement. The body composition analyses are useful but crude and are mainly limited to applications in nutrition and sports medicine. Noninvasive glucose monitoring, however, is of considerable interest.

More than 2 million diabetics in the United States lance their fingers three to six times a day to obtain a drop of blood for chemical glucose determination. The ability of these individuals to control their glucose levels, and the quality of their life generally, would dramatically improve if a simple, noninvasive method for determining blood glucose levels could be developed. Among the noninvasive optical methods proposed for this purpose are optical rotation, NIR analysis, and raman spectroscopy. The first two have received the most attention. Optical rotation methods aim to exploit the small optical rotation of polarized light by glucose. To measure physiologic glucose levels in a 1-cm thick sample to an accuracy of 25 mg/dL would require instrumentation that can reliably detect an optical rotation of at least 1 millidegree. Finding an appropriate in vivo optical path for such measurements has proved most difficult, with most approaches looking to use either the aqueous humor or the anterior chamber of the eye [Coté et al., 1992; Rabinovitch et al., 1982]. Although several groups have developed laboratory analyzers that can measure such a small effect, so far in vivo measurement has not been demonstrated, due both to unwanted scattering and optical activity of biomaterials in the optical path and to the inherent difficulty in developing a practical instrument with the required sensitivity.

NIR methods for noninvasive glucose determination are particularly attractive, although the task is formidable. Glucose has spectral characteristics near 1500 nm and in the 2000–2500 nm band where many other compounds also absorb, and the magnitude of the glucose absorbance in biologic samples is typically two orders of magnitude lower than those of water, fat, or protein. The normal detection limit for NIR spectroscopy is on the order of one part in 10^3, whereas a change of 25 mg/dL in glucose concentration corresponds to an absorbance change of 10^{-4} to 10^{-5}. In fact, the temperature dependence of the NIR absorption of water alone is at least an order of magnitude greater than the signal from glucose in solution. Indeed some have suggested that the apparent glucose signature in complex NIR spectra may actually be the secondary effect of glucose on the water.

Sophisticated chemometric (particularly, multivariate analysis) methods have been employed to try to extract the glucose signal out of the noise (for methods reviews see Martens and Næs [1989] and Haaland [1992]). Several groups have reported using multivariate techniques to quantitate glucose in whole blood samples, with encouraging results [Haaland et al., 1992]. And despite all theoretical disputations to the contrary, some groups claim the successful application of these multivariate analysis methods to noninvasive in vivo glucose determination in patients [Robinson et al., 1992]. Yet even with the many groups working in this area, much of the work remains unpublished, and few if any of the reports have been independently validated.

Time-Resolved Spectroscopy

The fundamental problem in making quantitative optical measurements through intact tissue is dealing with the complex scattering phenomena. This scattering makes it difficult to determine the effective pathlength for the light, and therefore attempts to use the Beer-Lambert law, or even to determine a consistent empirical calibration, continue to be thwarted. Application of new techniques in time-resolved spectroscopy may be able to tackle this problem. Thinking of light as a packet of photons, if a single packet from a light source is sent through tissue, then a distant receiver will detected a photon distribution over time—the photons least scattered arriving first and the photons most scattered arriving later. In principle, the first photons arriving at the detector passed directly through the tissue. For these first photons the distance between the emitter and the detector is fixed and known, and the Beer-Lambert law should apply, permitting determination of an *absolute* concentration for an absorbing component. The difficulty in this is, first, that the measurement time scale must be on the order of the photon transit time (subnanosecond), and second, that the number of photons getting through without scattering will be extremely small, and therefore the detector must be exquisitely sensitive. Although these considerable technical problems have been overcome in the laboratory, their implementation in a practical instrument applied to a real subject remains to be demonstrated. This same approach is also being investigated for noninvasive optical imaging, since the unscattered photons should produce sharp images (see Chance et al., [1988], Chance [1991], and Yoo and Alfano [1989]).

88.3 Conclusions

The remarkable success of pulse oximetry has established noninvasive optical monitoring of vital physiologic functions as a modality of considerable value. Hardware and algorithm advances in pulse oximetry are beginning to broaden its use outside the traditional operating room and critical care areas. Other promising applications of noninvasive optical monitoring are emerging, such as for measuring deep tissue oxygen levels, determining cellular metabolic status, or for quantitative determination of other important physiologic parameters such as blood glucose. Although these latter applications are not yet practical, they may ultimately impact noninvasive clinical monitoring just as dramatically as pulse oximetry.

Defining Terms

Beer-Lambert law: Principle stating that the optical absorbance of a substance is proportional to both the concentration of the substance and the pathlength of the sample.

Cytochromes: Heme-containing proteins found in the membranes of mitochondria and required for oxidative phosphorylation, with characteristic optical absorbance spectra.

Dysfunctional hemoglobins: Those hemoglobin species that cannot reversibly bind oxygen (carboxyhemoglobin, methemoglobin, and sulfhemoglobin).

Functional saturation: The ratio of oxygenated hemoglobin to total nondysfunctional hemoglobins (oxyhemoglobin plus deoxyhemoglobin).

Hypoxia: Inadequate oxygen supply to tissues necessary to maintain metabolic activity.

Multivariate analysis: Empirical models developed to relate multiple spectral intensities from many calibration samples to known analyte concentrations, resulting in an optimal set of calibration parameters.

Oximetry: The determination of blood or tissue oxygen content, generally by optical means.

Pulse oximetry: The determination of functional oxygen saturation of pulsatile arterial blood by ratiometric measurement of tissue optical absorbance changes.

References

Burns DA, Ciurczak EW (eds). 1992. Handbook of Near-Infrared Analysis. New York, Marcel Dekker.

Chance B. 1991. Optical method. Annu Rev Biophys Biophys Chem 20:1.

Chance B, Leigh JS, Miyake H, et al. 1988. Comparison of time-resolved and -unresolved measurements of deoxyhemoglobin in brain. Proc Natl Acad Sci USA 85(14):4971.

Coté GL, Fox MD, Northrop RB. 1992. Noninvasive optical polarimetric glucose sensing using a true phase measurement technique. IEEE Trans Biomed Eng 39(7):752.

Haaland DM. 1992. Multivariate calibration methods applied to the quantitative analysis of infrared spectra. In PC Jurs (ed), Computer-Enhanced Analytical Spectroscopy, vol 3, pp 1–30. New York Plenum.

Haaland DM, Robinson MR, Koepp GW, et al. 1992. Reagentless near-infrared determination of glucose in whole blood using multivariate calibration. Appl Spectros 46(10):1575.

Jöbsis FF. 1977. Noninvasive, infrared monitoring of cerebral and myocardial oxygen sufficiency and circulatory parameters. Science 198(4323):1264.

Jöbsis FF, Keizer JH, LaManna JC, et al. 1977. Reflectance spectrophotometry of cytochrome aa_3 in vivo. J Appl Physiol 43(5):858.

Kelleher JF. 1989. Pulse oximetry. J Clin Monit 5(1):37.

Martens H, Næs T. 1989. Multivariate Calibration. New York, John Wiley.

Osborne BG, Fearn T, Hindle PH. 1993. Practical NIR Spectroscopy with Applications in Food and Beverage Analysis. Essex, England, Longman Scientific & Technical.

Payne JP, Severinghaus JW (eds). 1986. Pulse Oximetry. New York, Springer-Verlag.

Rabinovitch B, March WF, Adams RL. 1982. Noninvasive glucose monitoring of the aqueous humor of the eye: Part I. Measurement of very small optical rotations. Diabetes Care 5(3):254.

Robinson MR, Eaton RP, Haaland DM, et al. 1992. Noninvasive glucose monitoring in diabetic patients: a preliminary evaluation. Clin Chem 38(9):1618.

Severinghaus JW, Astrup PB. 1986. History of blood gas analysis. VI. Oximetry. J Clin Monit 2(4):270.

Severinghaus JW, Honda Y. 1987a. History of blood gas analysis. VII. Pulse oximetry. J Clin Monit 3(2):135.

Severinghaus JW, Honda Y. 1987b. Pulse oximetry. Int Anesthesiol Clin 25(4):205.

Severinghaus JW, Kelleher JF. 1992. Recent developments in pulse oximetry. Anesthesiology 76(6):1018.

Tremper KK, Barker SJ. 1989. Pulse oximetry. Anesthesiology 70(1):98.

Wukitsch MW, Petterson MT, Tobler DR, et al. 1988. Pulse oximetry: Analysis of theory, technology, and practice. J Clin Monit 4(4):290.

Yoo KM, Alfano RR. 1989. Photon localization in a disordered multilayered system. Phys Rev B 39(9):5806.

Further Information

Two collections of papers on pulse oximetry include a book edited by J. P. Payne and J. W. Severinghaus, *Pulse Oximetry* (New York, Springer-Verlag, 1986), and a journal collection—International Anesthesiology Clinics [25(4), 1987]. For technical reviews of pulse oximetry, see J. A. Pologe's 1987 "Pulse Oximetry" [Int Anesthesiol Clin 25(3):137], Kevin K. Tremper and Steven J. Barker's 1989 "Pulse Oximetry" [Anesthesiology 70(1):98], and Michael W. Wukitsch, Michael T. Patterson, David R. Tobler, and coworkers' 1988 "Pulse Oximetry: Analysis of Theory, Technology, and Practice" [J Clin Monit 4(4):290].

For a review of practical and clinical applications of pulse oximetry, see the excellent review by Joseph F. Kelleher [1989] and John Severinghaus and Joseph F. Kelleher [1992]. John Severinghaus and Yoshiyuki Honda have written several excellent histories of pulse oximetry [1987*a*, 1987*b*].

For an overview of applied near-infrared spectroscopy, see Donald A. Burns and Emil W. Ciurczak [1992] and B. G. Osborne, T. Fearn, and P. H. Hindle [1993]. For a good overview of multivariate methods, see Harald Martens and Tormod Næs [1989].

89

Medical Instruments and Devices Used in the Home

Bruce R. Bowman
EdenTec Corporation

Edward Schuck
EdenTec Corporation

89.1 Scope of the Market for Home Medical Devices

The market for medical devices used in the home and alternative sites has increased dramatically in the last 10 years and has reached an overall estimated size of more than $1.6 billion [FIND/SVP, 1992]. In the past, hospitals have been thought of as the only places to treat sick patients. But with the major emphasis on reducing healthcare costs, increasing numbers of sicker patients move from hospitals to their homes. Treating sicker patients outside the hospital places additional challenges on medical device design and patient use. Equipment designed for hospital use can usually rely on trained clinical personnel to support the devices. Outside the hospital, the patient and/or family members must be able to use the equipment, requiring these devices to have a different set of design and safety features. This chapter will identify some of the major market segments using medical devices in the home and discuss important design considerations associated with home use.

Table 89.1 outlines market segments where devices and products are used to treat patients outside the hospital [FIND/SVP, 1992]. The durable medical equipment market is the most established market providing aids for patients to improve access and mobility. These devices are usually not life supporting or sustaining, but in many cases they can make the difference in allowing a patient to be able to function outside a hospital or nursing or skilled facility. Other market segments listed employ generally more sophisticated solutions to clinical problems. These will be discussed by category of use.

The incontinence and ostomy area of products is one of the largest market segments and is growing in direct relationship to our aging society. Whereas sanitary pads and colostomy bags are not very "high-tech," well-designed aids can have a tremendous impact on the comfort and independence of these patients. Other solutions to incontinence are technically more sophisticated, such as use of electric stimulation of the sphincter muscles through an implanted device or a miniature stimulator inserted as an anal or vaginal plug to maintain continence [Wall et al., 1993].

Many forms of equipment are included in the Respiratory segment. These devices include those that maintain life support as well as those that monitor patients' respiratory function. These patients,

TABLE 89.1   Major Market Segments Outside Hospitals

Market Segment	Estimated Equipment Size 1991	Device Examples
Durable medical equipment	$373 M*	Specialty beds, wheelchairs, toilet aids, ambulatory aids
Incontinence and ostomy products	$600 M*	Sanitary pads, electrical stimulators, colostomy bags
Respiratory equipment	$180 M*	Oxygen therapy, portable ventilators, nasal CPAP, monitors, apnea monitors
Drug infusion, drug measurement	$300 M	Infusion pumps, access ports, patient-controlled analgesia (PCA), glucose measurement, implantable pumps
Pain control and functional stimulation	$140 M	Transcutaneous electrical nerve stimulation (TENS), functional electrical nerve stimulation (FES)

Source: FIND/SVP [1992].

with proper medical support, can function outside the hospital at a significant reduction in cost and increased patient comfort [Pierson, 1994]. One area of this segment, infant apnea monitors, provides parents or caregivers the cardio/respiratory status of an at-risk infant so that intervention (CPR etc.) can be initiated if the baby has a life-threatening event. The infant monitor shown in Fig. 89.1 is an example of a patient monitor designed for home use and will be discussed in more detail later in this chapter. Pulse oximetry monitors are also going home with patients. They are used to measure noninvasively the oxygen level of patients receiving supplemental oxygen or ventilator-dependent patients to determine if they are being properly ventilated.

Portable infusion pumps are an integral part of providing antibiotics, pain management, chemotherapy, and parenteral and enteral nutrition. The pump shown in Fig. 89.2 is an example of technology that allows the patient to move about freely while receiving sometimes lengthy drug therapy. Implantable drug pumps are also available for special long-term therapy needs.

Pain control using electric stimulation in place of drug therapy continues to be an increasing market. The delivery of small electric impulses to block pain is continuing to gain medical accep-

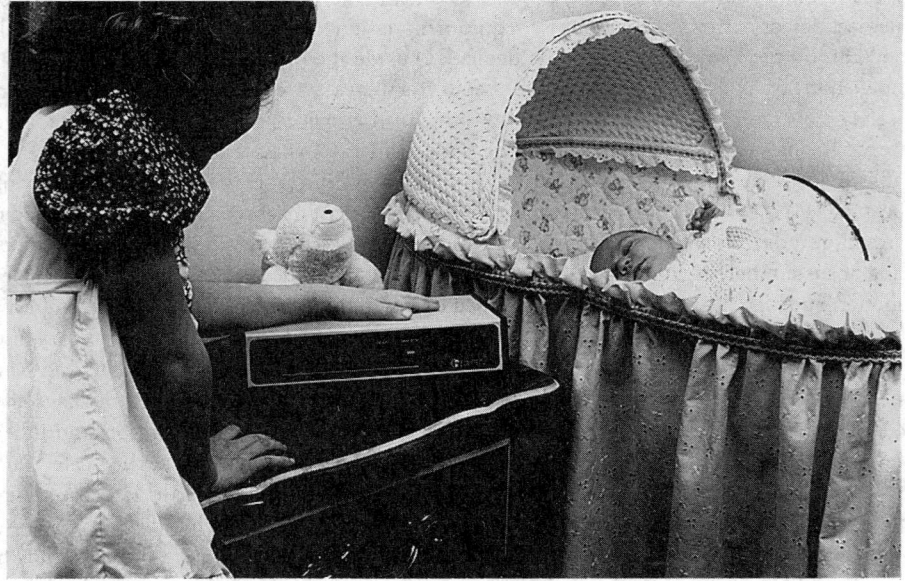

FIGURE 89.1   Infant apnea monitor used in a typical home setting (photo courtesy of EdenTec Corporation).

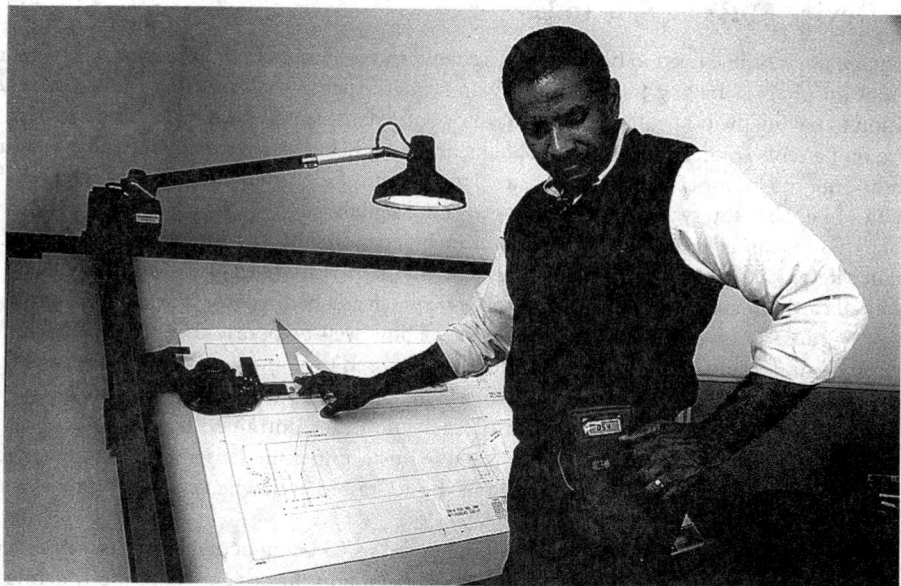

FIGURE 89.2 Portable drug pump used throughout the day (photo courtesy of Pharmacia Deltec Inc.).

tance for treatment outside the hospital setting. A different form of electric stimulation called functional electric stimulation (FES) applies short pulses of electric current to the nerves that control weak or paralyzed muscles. This topic is covered as a separate chapter in this book.

Growth of the homecare business has created problems in overall healthcare costs since a corresponding decrease in hospital utilization has not yet occurred. In the future, however, increased homecare will necessarily result in reassessment and downsizing in the corresponding hospital segment. There will be clear areas of growth and areas of consolidation in the new era of healthcare reform. It would appear, however, that homecare has a bright future of continued growth.

89.2 Unique Challenges to the Design and Implementation of High-Tech Homecare Devices

What are some of the unique requirements of devices that could allow more sophisticated equipment to go home with ordinary people of varied educational levels without compromising their care? Even though each type of clinical problem has different requirements for the equipment that must go home with the patient, certain common qualities must be inherent in most devices used in the home. Three areas to consider when equipment is used outside of the hospital are that the device (1) must provide a positive clinical outcome, (2) must be safe and easy to use, and (3) must be user-friendly enough so that it will be used.

The Device Must Provide a Positive Clinical Outcome

Devices cannot be developed any longer just because new technology becomes available. They must solve the problem for which they were intended and make a significant clinical difference in the outcome or management of the patient while saving money. These realities are being driven by those who reimburse for devices, as well as by the FDA as part of the submission for approval to market a new device.

The Device Must Be Safe to Use

Homecare devices may need to be even *more* reliable and even *safer* than hospital devices. We often think of hospitals as having the best quality and most expensive devices that money can buy. In addition to having the best equipment to monitor patients, hospitals have nurses and aids that keep an eye on patients so that equipment problems may be quickly discovered by the staff. A failure in the home may go unnoticed until it is too late. Thus systems for home use really need extra reliability with automatic backup systems and/or early warning signals.

Safety issues can take on a different significance depending on the intended use of the device. Certain safety issues are important regardless of whether the device is a critical device such as an implanted cardiac pacemaker or a noncritical device such as a bed-wetting alarm. No device should be able to cause harm to the patient regardless of how well or poorly it may be performing its intended clinical duties. Devices must be safe when exposed to all the typical environmental conditions to which the device could be exposed while being operated by the entire range of possible users of varied education and while exposed to siblings and other untrained friends or relatives. For instance, a bed-wetting alarm should not cause skin burns under the sensor if a glass of water spills on the control box. This type of safety issue must be addressed even when it significantly affects the final cost to the consumer.

Other safety issues are not obviously differentiated as to being actual safety issues or simply nuisances or inconveniences to the user. It is very important for the designer to properly define these issues; although some safety features can be included with little or no extra cost, other safety features may be very costly to implement. It may be a nuisance for the patient using a TENS pain control stimulator to have the device inadvertently turned off when its on/off switch is bumped while watching TV. In this case, the patient only experiences a momentary cessation of pain control until the unit is turned back on. But it could mean injuries or death to the same patient driving an automobile who becomes startled when his TENS unit inadvertently turns on and he causes an accident.

Reliability issues can also be mere inconveniences or major safety issues. Medical devices should be free of design and materials defects so that they can perform their intended functions reliably. Once again, reliability does not necessarily need to be expensive and often can be obtained with good design. Critical devices, i.e., devices that could cause death or serious injury if they stopped operating properly, may need to have redundant systems for backup, which likely will increase cost.

The Device Must Be Designed So That It *Will* Be Used

A great deal of money is being spent in healthcare on device for patients that end up not being used. There are numerous reasons for this happening including that the wrong device was prescribed for the patient's problem in the first place; the device works, but it has too many false alarms; the device often fails to operate properly; it is cumbersome to use or difficult to operate or too uncomfortable to wear.

Ease of Use

User-friendliness is one of the most important features in encouraging a device to be used. Technological sophistication may be just as necessary in areas that allow ease of use as in attaining accuracy and reliability in the device. The key is that the technologic sophistication be transparent to the user so that the device does not intimidate the user. Transparent features such as automatic calibration or automatic sensitivity adjustment may help allow successful use of a device that would otherwise be too complicated.

Notions of what makes a device easy to use, however, need to be thoroughly tested with the patient population intended for the device. Caution needs to be taken in defining what "simple" means to different people. A VCR may be simple to the designer because all features can be programmed with one button, but it may not be simple to users if they have to remember that it takes two long pushes and one short to get into the clock-setting program.

Convenience for the user is also extremely important in encouraging use of a device. Applications that require devices to be portable must certainly be light enough to be carried. Size is almost always important for anything that must fit within the average household. Either a device must be able to be left in place in the home or it must be easy to set up, clean, and put away. Equipment design can make the difference between the patient appropriately using the equipment or deciding that it is just too much hassle to bother.

Reliability

Users must also have confidence in the reliability of the device being used and must have confidence that if it is not working properly, the device will tell them that something is wrong. Frequent breakdowns or false alarms will result in frustration and ultimately in reduced compliance. Eventually patients will stop using the device altogether. Most often, reliability can be designed into a product with little or no extra cost in manufacturing, and everything that can be done at no cost to enhance reliability should be done. It is very important, however, to understand what level of additional reliability involving extra cost is necessary for product acceptance. Reliability can always be added by duplicated backup systems, but the market or application may not warrant such an approach. Critical devices which are implanted, such as cardiac pacemakers, have much greater reliability requirements, since they involve not only patient frustration but also safety.

Cost Reimbursement

Devices must be paid for before the patient can realize the opportunity to use new, effective equipment. Devices are usually paid for by one of two means. First, they are covered on an American Medical Association Current Procedural Terminology Code (CPT-code) which covers the medical, surgical, and diagnostic services provided by physicians. The CPT-codes are usually priced out by Medicare to establish a baseline reimbursement level. Private carriers usually establish a similar or different level of reimbursement based on regional or other considerations. Gaining new CPT-codes for new devices can take a great deal of time and effort. The second method is to cover the procedure and device under a capitated fee where the hospital is reimbursed a lump sum for a procedure including the device, hospital, homecare, and physician fees.

Every effort should be made to design devices to be low cost. Device cost is being scrutinized more and more by those who reimburse. It is easy to state, however, that a device needs to be inexpensive. Unfortunately the reality is that healthcare reforms and new regulations by FDA are making medical devices more costly to develop, to obtain regulatory approvals for [FDA, 1993], and to manufacture.

Professional Medical Service Support

The more technically sophisticated a device is, the more crucial that homecare support and education be a part of a program. In fact, in many cases, such support and education are as important as the device itself.

Medical service can be offered by numerous homecare service companies. Typically these companies purchase the equipment instead of the patient, and a monthly fee is charged for use of the equipment along with all the necessary service. The homecare company then must obtain reimbursement from third-party payers. Some of the services offered by the homecare company include training on how to use the equipment, CPR training, transporting the equipment to the home, servicing/repairing equipment, monthly visits, and providing on-call service 24 hours a day. The homecare provider must also be able to provide feedback to the treating physician on progress of the treatment. This feedback may include how well the equipment is working, the patient's medical status, and compliance of the patient.

89.3 Infant Monitor Example

Many infants are being monitored in the home using apnea monitors because they have been identified with breathing problems [Kelly, 1992]. Theses include newborn premature babies who have apnea of prematurity [Henderson-Smart, 1992; NIH, 1987], siblings of babies who have died of sudden infant death syndrome (SIDS) [Hunt, 1992; NIH, 1987], or infants who have had an apparent life-threatening episode (ALTE) related to lack of adequate respiration [Kahn et al. 1992; NIH, 1987]. Rather than keeping infants in the hospital for a problem that they may soon outgrow (1–6 months), doctors often discharge them from the hospital with an infant apnea monitor that measures the duration of breathing pauses and heart rate and sounds an alarm if either parameter crosses limits prescribed by the doctor.

Infant apnea monitors are among the most sophisticated devices used routinely in the home. These devices utilize microprocessor control, sophisticated breath-detection and artifact rejection firmware algorithms, and internal memory that keeps track of use of the device as well as recording occurrence of events and the physiologic waveforms associated with the events. The memory contents can be downloaded directly to computer or sent via modem remotely where a complete 45-day report can be provided to the referring physician (see Fig. 89.3).

Most apnea monitors measure breathing effort through impedance pneumography. A small (100–200 uA) high-frequency (25–100 kHz) constant-current train of pulses is applied across the chest between a pair of electrodes. The voltage needed to drive the current is measured, and thereby the effective impedance between the electrodes can be calculated. Impedance across the chest increases as the chest expands and decreases as the chest contracts with each breath. The impedance change with each breath can be as low as 0.2 ohms on top of an electrode base impedance of 2000 ohms, creating some interesting signal-to-noise challenges. Furthermore, motion artifact and blood volume changes in the heart and chest can cause impedance changes of 0.6 ohms or more that can look just like breathing. Through the same pair of electrodes, heart rate is monitored by picking up the electrocardiogram (ECG) [AAMI, 1988].

Because the impedance technique basically measures motion of the chest, this technique can only be used to monitor central apnea or lack of breathing effort. Another less common apnea in infants called obstructive apnea results when an obstruction of the airway blocks air from flowing in spite of breathing effort. Obstructive apnea can not be monitored using impedance pneumography [Kelly, 1992].

There is a very broad socioeconomic and educational spectrum of parents or caregivers who may be monitoring their infants with an apnea monitor. This places an incredible challenge for the design of the device so that it is easy enough to be used by a variety of caregivers. It also puts special requirements on the homecare service company that must be able to respond to these patients within a matter of minutes, 24 hours a day.

The user-friendly monitor shown in Fig. 89.1 uses a two-button operation, the on/off switch, and a reset switch. The visual alarm indicators are invisible behind a back-lit panel except when an actual alarm occurs. A word describing the alarm then appears. By not showing all nine possible alarm conditions unless an alarm occurs, parent confusion and anxiety is minimized. Numerous safety features are built into the unit, some of which are noticeable but many of which are internal to the operation of the monitor. One useful safety feature is the self-check. When the device is turned on, each alarm LED lights in sequence, and the unit beeps once indicating that the self-check was completed successfully. This gives users the opportunity to confirm that all the alarm visual indicators and the audible indicator are working and provides added confidence for users leaving their baby on the monitor. A dual-level battery alarm gives an early warning that the battery will soon need charging. The weak battery alarm allows users to reset the monitor and continue monitoring their babies for several more hours before depleting the battery to the charge battery level where the monitor must be attached to the ac battery charger/adapter. This allows parents the freedom to leave their homes for a few hours knowing that their child can continue to be monitored.

A multistage alarm reduces the risk of parents sleeping through an alarm. Most parents are sleep-deprived with a new baby. Consequently, it can be easy for parents in a nearby room to sleep through a monitor alarm even when the monitor sounds at 85 dB. A three-stage alarm helps to reduce this risk. After 10 seconds of sounding at 1 beep per second, the alarm switches to 3 beeps per second for

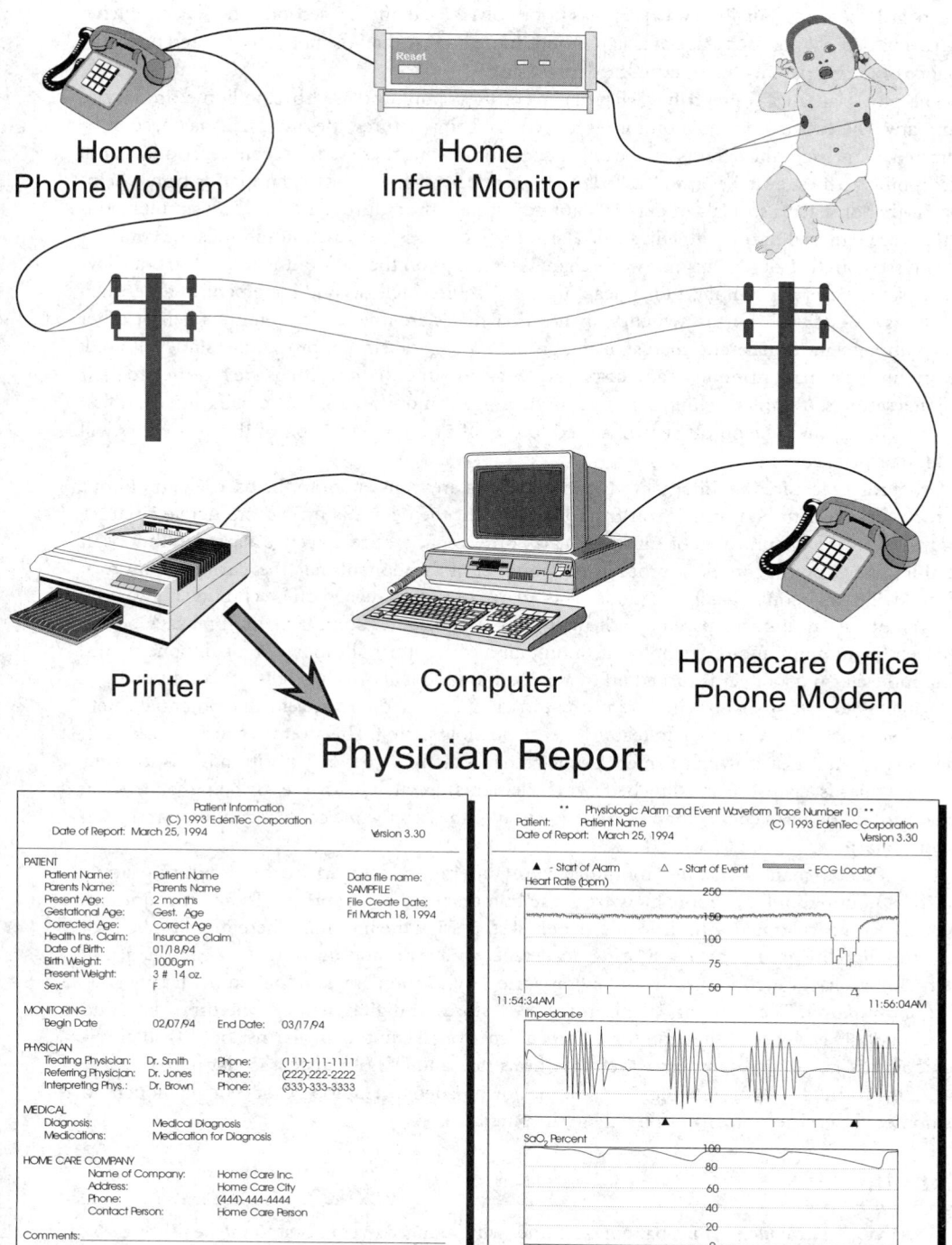

FIGURE 89.3 Infant apnea monitor with memory allows data to be sent by modem to generate physician report (drawing courtesy of EdenTec Corporation).

the next 10 seconds. Finally, if an alarm has not resolved itself after 20 seconds, the alarm switches to 6 beeps per second. Each stage of alarm sounds more intense than the previous one and offers the chance of jolting parents out of even the deepest sleep.

The physician always prescribes what alarm settings should be used by the homecare service company when setting up the monitor. As a newborn baby matures, these settings may need to be adjusted. Sometimes the parents can be relied upon for making these setting changes. To allow both accessibility to these switches as well as to keep them safe from unauthorized tampering from a helping brother or sister, a special tamper-resistant-adjustment procedure is utilized. Two simultaneous actions are required in order to adjust the alarm limit settings. The reset button must be continually pressed on the front of the unit while changing settings on the back of the unit. Heart rate levels are set in beats per minute, and apnea duration is set in single-second increments. Rather than using easy-to-set push-button switches, "pen-set" switches are used which require a pen or other sharp implement to make the change. If the proper switch adjustment procedure is not followed, the monitor alarms continuously and displays a switch alarm until the settings are returned to their original settings. A similar technique is used for turning the monitor Off. The reset button must first be pressed and then the on/off switch turned to the off position. Violation of this procedure will result in a switch alarm.

Other safety features are internal to the monitor and are transparent to the user. The monitor's alarm is designed to be normally on from the moment the device is turned on. Active circuitry controlled by the microprocessor turns the alarm off when there are no active alarm conditions. If anything hangs up the processor or if any of a number of components fail, the alarm will not turn off and will remain on in a fail-safe mode. This "alarm on unless turned off" technique is also used in a remote alarm unit for parents with their baby in a distant room. If a wire breakage occurs between the monitor and the remote alarm unit, or a connector pulls loose, or a component fails, the remote alarm no longer is turned off by the monitor and it alarms in a fail-safe condition.

Switches, connectors, and wires are prone to fail. One way to circumvent this potential safety issue is use of switches with a separate line for each possible setting. The monitor continuously polls every switch line of each switch element to check that "exactly" one switch position is making contact. This guards against misreading bad switch elements, a switch inadvertently being set between two positions, or a bad connector or cable. Violation of the exactly one contact condition results in a switch alarm.

It is difficult to manage an apnea monitoring program in rural areas where the monitoring family may be a hundred miles or more away from the homecare service company. There are numerous ways to become frustrated with the equipment and stop using the monitor. Therefore, simplicity of use and reliability are important. Storing occurrence of alarms and documenting compliance in internal memory in the monitor help the homecare service company and the remote family cope with the situation. The monitor shown in Fig. 89.1 stores in digital memory the time, date, and duration of (1) each use of the monitor; (2) occurrence of all equipment alarms; and (3) all physiologic alarms including respiratory waveforms, heart rate, and ECG for up to a 45-day period. These data in the form of a report (see Fig. 89.3) can be downloaded to a laptop PC or sent via modem to the homecare service company or directly to the physician.

89.4 Conclusions

Devices that can provide positive patient outcomes with reduced overall cost to the healthcare system while being safe, reliable, and user-friendly will succeed based on pending healthcare changes. Future technology in areas of sensors, communications, and memory capabilities should continue to increase the potential effectiveness of homecare management programs by using increasingly sophisticated devices. The challenge for the medical device designer is to provide cost-effective, reliable, and easy-to-use solutions that can be readily adopted by the multidisciplinary aspects of homecare medicine while meeting FDA requirements.

Defining Terms

Apnea: Cessation of breathing. Apnea can be classified as **central, obstructive,** or mixed, which is a combination.

Apnea of prematurity: Apnea in which the incidence and severity increases with decreasing gestational age attributable to immaturity of the respiratory control system. The incidence has increased due to improved survival rates for very-low-birth-weight premature infants.

Apparent life-threatening episode (ALTE):   An episode characterized by a combination of apnea, color change, muscle tone change, choking, or gagging. To the observer it may appear the infant has died.

Capitated fee: A fixed payment for *total* program services versus the more traditional fee for service in which each individual service is charged.

Cardiac pacemaker: A device that electrically stimulates the heart at a certain rate used in absence of normal function of the heart's sino-atrial node.

Central apnea: Apnea secondary to lack of respiratory or diaphragmatic effort.

Chemotherapy: Treatment of disease by chemical agents. Term popularly used when fighting cancer chemically.

Colostomy: The creation of a surgical hole as an alternative opening of the colon.

CPR (cardiopulmonary resuscitation):   Artificially replacing heart and respiration function through rhythmic pressure on the chest.

CPT-code (current procedural terminology code):   A code used to describe specific procedures/tests developed by the AMA.

Electrocardiogram (ECG):   The electric potential recorded across the chest due to depolarization of the heart muscle with each heartbeat.

Enteral nutrition: Chemical nutrition injected intestinally.

Food and Drug Administration (FDA):   Federal agency that oversees and regulates foods, drugs, and medical devices.

Functional electrical stimulation (FES):   Electric stimulation of peripheral nerves or muscles to gain functional, purposeful control over partially or fully paralyzed muscles.

Incontinence: Loss of voluntary control of the bowel or bladder.

Obstructive apnea: Apnea in which effort to breath continues but airflow ceases due to obstruction or collapse of the airway.

Ostomy: Surgical procedure that alters the bladder or bowel to eliminate through an artificial passage.

Parenteral nutrition: Chemical nutrition injected subcutaneously, intramuscularly, intrasternally, or intravenously.

Sphincter: A band of muscle fibers that constricts or closes an orifice.

Sudden infant death syndrome (SIDS):   The sudden death of an infant which is unexplained by history or postmortem exam.

Transcutaneous electrical nerve stimulation (TENS):   Electrical stimulation of sensory nerve fibers resulting in control of pain.

References

AAMI. 1988. Association for the Advancement of Medical Instrumentation Technical Information Report: Apnea Monitoring by Means of Thoracic Impedance Pneumography, Arlington, Virg.

FDA. November 1993. Reviewers Guidance for Premarket Notification Submissions (Draft), Anesthesiology and Respiratory Device Branch. Division of Cardiovascular, Respiratory, and Neurological Devices. Food and Drug Administration. Washington DC.

FIND/SVP. 1992. The Market for Home Care Products, a Market Intelligence Report. New York.

Henderson-Smart, DJ. 1992. Apnea of prematurity. In R Beckerman, R Brouillette, C Hunt (eds), Respiratory Control Disorders in Infants and Children, pp 161–177, Baltimore, Williams and Wilkins.

Hunt, CE. 1992. Sudden infant death syndrome. In R Beckerman, R Brouillette, C Hunt (eds), Respiratory Control Disorders in Infants and Children, pp 190–211, Baltimore, Williams and Wilkins.

Kahn A, Rebuffat E, Franco P, et al. 1992. Apparent life-threatening events and apnea of infancy. In R Beckerman, R Brouillette, C Hunt (eds), Respiratory Control Disorders in Infants and Children, pp 178–189, Baltimore, Williams and Wilkins.

Kelly DH. 1992. Home monitoring. In R Beckerman, R Brouillette, C Hunt (eds), Respiratory Control Disorders in Infants and Children, pp 400–412, Baltimore, Williams and Wilkins.

NIH. 1987. Infantile Apnea and Home Monitoring, Report of NIH Consensus Development Conference, US Department of Health and Human Services, NIH publication 87-2905.

Pierson DJ. 1994. Controversies in home respiratory care: Conference summary. Respir Care 39(4):294.

Wall LL, Norton PA, Dehancey JOL. 1993. Practical Urology, Baltimore, Williams and Wilkins.

Historical Perspectives 3:

Recording of Action Potentials

Leslie A. Geddes
Purdue University

Nerve Action Potential

The quest for the form and nature of the nerve action potential used instruments that we would now call primitive. Yet, in skilled hands, these instruments led directly to discovery of the code used by the nervous system to transmit information. In fact, the code was discovered before the true form of the nerve action potential was known.

Using a slow-speed galvanometer ballistically to measure time [Hoff & Geddes, 1960], Helmholtz [1850, 1851, 1853] measured the velocity of the frog sciatic nerve action potential and determined it to be 30 m/s. This was far below the speed of electricity and caused much controversy among physiologists of the day. Using the rheotome, a slowly responding galvanometer, and an induction coil stimulator [Geddes et al., 1989], Bernstein [1868] reconstructed the action potential of the frog sciatic nerve [Hoff & Geddes, 1957]. The sampling time was 0.3 ms, and the action potential that he obtained is shown in Fig. HP3.1. Not only did Bernstein chart the time course of this 0.5626- to 0.8041-ms action potential, he measured its propagation velocity, obtaining an average of 28.718 m/s, agreeing with the speed obtained by Helmholtz. Thus, with primitive electromechanical instruments, the time course and velocity of the nerve action potential were determined accurately.

When the capillary electrometer appeared in 1876, it was thought that it might be possible to use it to record the nerve action potential. Many attempts were made with variable results because the concept of response time was not fully appreciated. Gotch and Horsley [1888] in the United Kingdom stimulated peripheral nerves in the cat using induction-coil shocks, and with one recording electrode over intact nerve and one in an area of injury, they recorded the action potential. The type of record that they obtained is shown in Fig. HP3.2a. Note that the response (action potential) was in the same direction for the break (b) and make (m) shocks. Recall that the break shock from an induction coil is stronger than the make shock. They knew that the make and break shocks were of opposite polarity and proved it by recording them, as shown in Fig. HP3.2b. After a long discussion about the nerve response being always in the same direction, irrespective of the polarity of the stimulus, they concluded that they had recorded single action potentials in response to single-induction-coil stimuli. They wrote:

> There is thus no doubt that the movement [of the mercury contour] that we obtained and photographed was due to the electromotive change which no doubt that the movement [of the mercury contour] that we obtained and photographed was due to the electromotive change which accompanies the propagation of an excitatory state along the mammalian nerve when thus state is evoked by the application of a single stimulus.

Like Gotch and Horsley [1888], others who attempted recording nerve action potentials with the capillary electrometer were rewarded with a small-amplitude record. When Einthoven's string galvanometer appeared in 1903, it also was used to record nerve action potentials with the same result [Einthoven, 1903]. In 1907 and 1908, De Forest patented the triode (audion), and the vacuum-tube amplifier could be constructed. Therefore, it appeared logical to use a triode amplifier to enlarge nerve action potentials and display them with the string galvanometer and capillary electrometer.

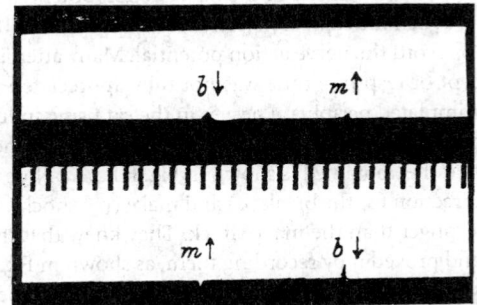

FIGURE HP3.1 Bernstein's reconstruction of the action potential of the frog sciatic nerve. From his experiments, the mean duration was 0.6833 ms. This reconstruction was made with a slow-speed galvanometer and the rheotome. (From Bernstein, 1868.)

The first to put the vacuum-tube amplifier to work in electrophysiology were Forbes and Thacher [1920], who coupled a triode to a string galvanometer and recorded frog nerve and human muscle action potentials. Their paper is essentially a tutorial that describes three ways of coupling the triode to the string galvanometer so that the delicate string would not be damaged. The first method placed the vacuum tube in one arm of a Wheatstone bridge. The string galvanometer was in the detector position, and a resistor constituted the arm adjacent to the triode. The second method employed transformer coupling, and the third method employed capacitor (C) coupling, as shown in Fig. HP3.3a. Of the three methods, the capacitive-coupling method was preferred. Figure HP3.3b is a record obtained by Forbes and Thacher showing the amplified and directly recorded frog sciatic nerve action potential. The timing signal (bottom) is 100 Hz.

Desirous of displaying repetitive nerve action potentials with the string galvanometer, Gasser and Newcomer [1921] employed a two-stage resistance-capacity-coupled amplifier connected to the string galvanometer. They chose the phrenic nerve as the object of their study because of its spontaneous periodic activity in causing the diaphragm to contract tetanically and produce inspiration. The frequency of the phrenic nerve action potentials ranged from 71 to 105 per second, noting that their amplitude appeared to be largest at the peak of inspiration. They also reported a one-to-one correspondence between phrenic nerve and diaphragm action potentials. Their important observations were later to become recognized as the two ways that intensity is signaled in the nervous system.

The addition of amplification to the string galvanometer did not improve its ability to respond to rapidly rising, short-duration action potentials. It required the cathode-ray tube and a multistage amplifier to solve this problem. Gasser and Erlanger [1922] were the first to show the form of the nerve action potential recorded extracellularly using the cathode-ray tube and triode amplifier that they had previously developed for use with the string galvanometer. Not only did they achieve their goal, but they made the fundamental discovery that nerve propagation velocity was proportional to nerve fiber diameter.

FIGURE HP3.2 The first nerve action potentials in response to single stimuli, recorded with the capillary electrometer in response to a break (b) and make (m) induction-coil stimulus (*top*). (*Bottom*) The capillary electrometer record of the break (b) and make (m) stimuli from the induction coil; note that they are of opposite polarity and that of the nerve responses (*top*) are of the same polarity. (From Gotch & Horsley, 1888.)

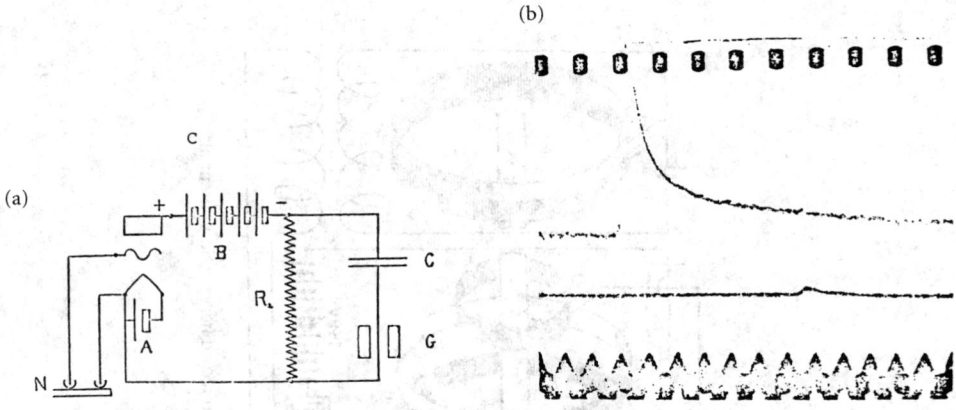

FIGURE HP3.3 Use of the capacitively coupled (*C*) triode to enlarge action potentials from a nerve (*N*) and display them on the string galvanometer (*G*). (*b*) (*upper*) An amplified action potential and (*lower*) the unamplified action potential. At the bottom is a record from a 100-Hz tuning fork [Forbes & Thacher 1920].

Although rapidly responding, the cathode-ray tube is quite insensitive, requiring about 20 to 50 V for a 1-cm deflection of the spot made by the electron beam on the face of the tube. Therefore, considerable amplification was needed to display the millivolt nerve action potentials detected with electrodes on the surface of a nerve trunk. Gasser and Erlanger [1922] built a three-stage amplifier to display nerve action potentials on the cathode-ray tube screen. Figure HP3.4 is the circuit diagram of their equipment. The cathode-ray tube was of the low-voltage (300) type and was provided by J. B. Johnson and E. B. Craft of the Western Electric Company. The tube contained a little argon gas. The fluorescent screen was green with a long persistence (5 to 10 s). The deflection sensitivity was 10 to 20 V/cm.

Before describing the Gasser and Erlanger Nobel prize–winning research, it is of interest to examine how the nerve was stimulated and the action potentials were recorded. Figure HP3-4 shows the nerve (*N*) on the left with the stimulating electrodes (*T*) and the recording electrodes (*E*). The nerve was crushed under the electrode connected to the grid (*G*) of the first vacuum-tube amplifier. Therefore, the nerve action potential appeared under the electrode on the uninjured nerve. Three stages of amplification were used to enlarge the nerve action potential 7000 to 8000 times, which caused the beam of the cathode-ray tube to be deflected vertically.

On the right of Fig. HP3.4 is a rheotome that (1) delivered the stimulus to an induction coil (*PS*) connected to the nerve stimulating electrodes (*T*), (2) started the cathode-ray tube beam moving across the face of the tube to provide a time axis by starting the 1-mF (nowadays μF) capacitor to charge (the voltage on this capacitor was connected to the horizontal deflecting plates in the cathode-ray tube), and (3) later discharged the 1-μF capacitor so that the cycle could be restarted. In this way, the stimulus was delivered to the nerve at the instant when the spot started horizontally across the face of the cathode-ray tube. Typically, 30 stimuli were delivered per second to produce a clear (standing wave) action potential on the cathode-ray tube. Commenting on the action potential recorded from frog sciatic nerve, Gasser and Erlanger [1922] wrote:

> The action current has a gradual ascent, a steep smooth anacrotic limb [rising phase] and a more gradual catacrotic limb [falling phase]. The latter like the former shows a period of great initial acceleration so that the crest is situated near the anacrotic side. In frog nerve and some mammalian nerves there are secondary waves on the catacrotic limb n. Suggestions are made as to the cause of these waves.

Soon an explanation was given for the secondary waves; it came in 1924 when Erlanger and Gasser [1924] published their classic report to be described subsequently.

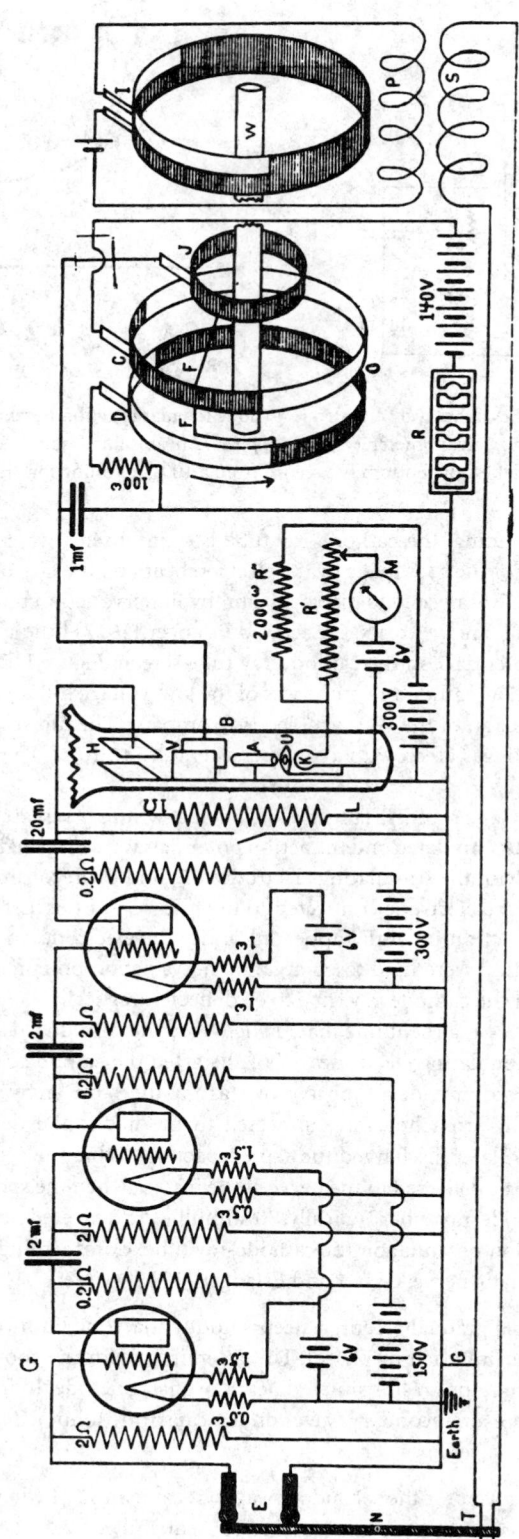

FIGURE HP3.4   Circuit diagram of the three-stage amplifier, cathode-ray tube, and stimulator used by Gasser and Erlanger [1922] to record nerve action potentials.

Having no camera, Gasser and Erlanger either placed tissue paper on the cathode-ray tube face and traced the waveform with a pencil or pressed photographic paper against the face of the tube and obtained a contact print. Figure HP3.5 is such an illustration of the action potential of the bullfrog sciatic nerve.

Erlanger and Gasser knew that their oscilloscope time base was exponential and corrected the oscillograms accordingly. A favorite method employed transilluminating a contact print and tracing the action potential on the back with a pencil to obtain a positive image that was then replotted on semilogarthmic paper. This step was essential because they desired a true temporal display of the compound action potential from a nerve trunk. By varying the distance over which the action potential was propagated, they were able to reveal that the nerve trunk contained groups of fibers that propagated with different velocities. Commenting on their results, they stated:

> Each of the waves of these compound action currents as it progresses along the nerve changes its form just as does the simple action current in the phrenic nerve. It is suggested that these changes are due, in part, at least, to slight differences in the propagation rate in individual, or in many small groups of fibers, whose action currents therefore get slightly out of phase as they progress.

Finally, Erlanger and Gasser [1937] summarized their work in a monograph entitled *Electrical Signs of Nervous Activity*. In it they not only showed how the compound action potential of nerve depends on the velocities of propagation of the different bundles of nerve fibers in a trunk but also provided histograms (fiber maps) of the diameters of different-sized fibers in a nerve trunk. Figure HP3.6 shows the action potentials of the A, B, and C fibers. For this pioneering work Erlanger and Gasser received the Nobel prize in physiology and medicine in 1944.

Meanwhile, in the United Kingdom, Adrian was conducting experiments that showed that a nerve fiber responds in an all-or-none manner and that intensity is signaled in a single nerve fiber by the frequency of action potentials. In addition, he showed that intensity is also signaled by the number of nerve fibers carrying messages. These remarkable discoveries were made with the capillary electrometer, which even then was considered to be a primitive instrument. Adrian [1928] defended his use of the capillary electrometer in the following way:

> The ideal instrument for recording nerve action currents is undoubtedly the cathode-ray oscillograph devised by Erlanger and Gasser, for in this the moving system is a stream of cathode rays, the inertia of which is completely negligible. At present, however, the intensity of the

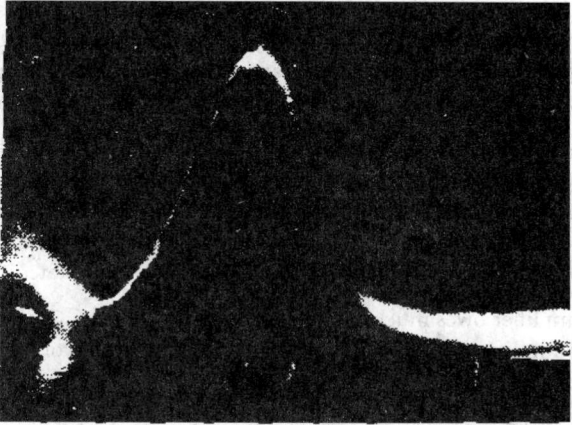

FIGURE HP3.5 Contact print from the cathode-ray tube showing the action potential of the bullfrog sciatic nerve recorded by Erlanger & Gasser [1924].

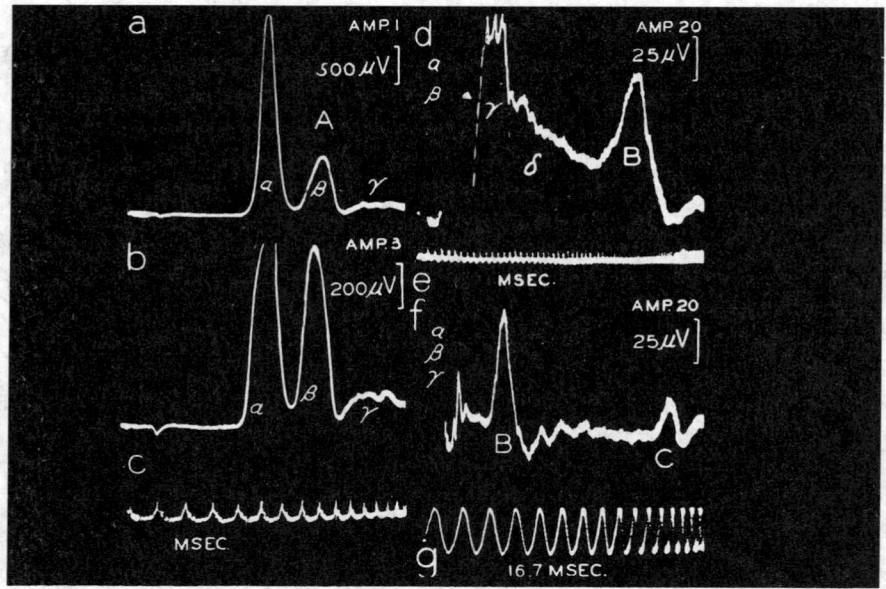

FIGURE HP3.6   Action potential components of the A, B, and C fibers of nerve. (From Erlanger J, Gasser HS. *Electrical Signs of Nervous Activity*. Philadelphia, University of Pennsylvania Press, 1937. With permission.)

illumination from the ray is far too small to allow photographs to be made from a single excursion, and similar excursions must be repeated many times over before the plate or the eye is affected. As a result, the cathode-ray oscillograph can only be used in experiments where the same sequence of action currents can be repeated over and over again, and it is not suitable for recording an irregular series of action currents such as are produced by the activity of the central nervous system. Another instrument in which the inertia factor is extremely small is the capillary electrometer. This has fallen out of favor with the majority of physiologists because its records need analysis and because of its low sensitivity compared with that of the string galvanometer. These objections have now become of little importance. With the advent of reliable valve [vacuum-tube] amplifiers a low sensitivity in the recording instrument is no drawback at all, and the analysis of capillary electrometer records can be made in a few moments by the machine designed by Keith Lucas. As will be seen, the combination of value amplifier and [capillary] electrometer gives us an instrument of such range and precision that it promises access to fields of investigation which are as yet almost unexplored.

In Adrian's first studies [1928] he used the three-valve (vacuum-tube) amplifier shown in Fig. HP3.7 to record action potentials in different nerve fibers. In his next studies with Bronk [Adrian & Bronk, 1928], he used a single-stage amplifier (Fig. HP3.8) that drove a capillary electrometer across which could be connected earphones or another amplifier (*B*) that drove a loudspeaker (*LS*) to enable listening to the nerve action potentials. Adrian stated:

> The three-valve amplifier owes much to the great kindness of Prof. Gasser, who supplied me with details of the amplifier used by him in America, and to the staff of Messers W. G. Pye and Co. of Cambridge, who redesigned an instrument on the same general line and planned the very compact and well shielded lay-out of the apparatus.

Adrian provided details on his capillary electrometer by stating, "The capillary tube at present has a diameter of 0.03 mm at its working part, and a pressure of 140 mmHg is needed to bring the mercury to this point." The working part refers to the sulfuric acid–mercury interface, the contour

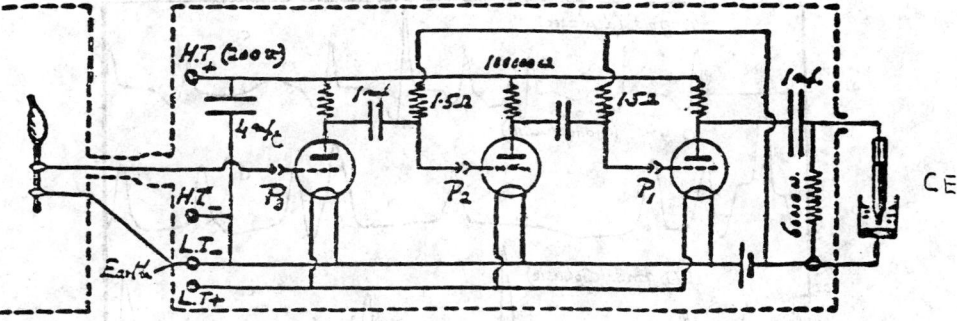

FIGURE HP3.7 The three-stage valve (vacuum-tube) amplifier and capillary electrometer (*CE*) used by Adrian to record action potentials in afferent nerves. The dashed lines represent shielding. (Redrawn from [Adrian, 1926].)

of which changes when current traverses it. Adrian stated that he could detect a voltage as small as 0.01 mV when his electrometer was connected to the three-stage amplifier.

Adrian knew that a photographic recording of the change in contour of the meniscus of the capillary electrometer was not a true representation of the applied voltage; this fact had been pointed out by Burch [1892]. Keith Lucas, a collaborator, devised a mechanical instrument for correcting capillary electrometer records. However, Adrian was less interested in waveform than in the presence or absence of action potentials.

Action Potentials in Afferent Fibers

In the paper that described the three-valve (vacuum-tube) amplifier and capillary electrometer, Adrian [1928] presented numerous examples of the nature of the action potentials in afferent nerve fibers in the frog sciatic nerve when the gastrocnemius muscle was stretched with known weights. He found that the frequency of the action potentials was related to the weight. Fig. HP3.9 shows his corrected capillary electrometer records of this experiment.

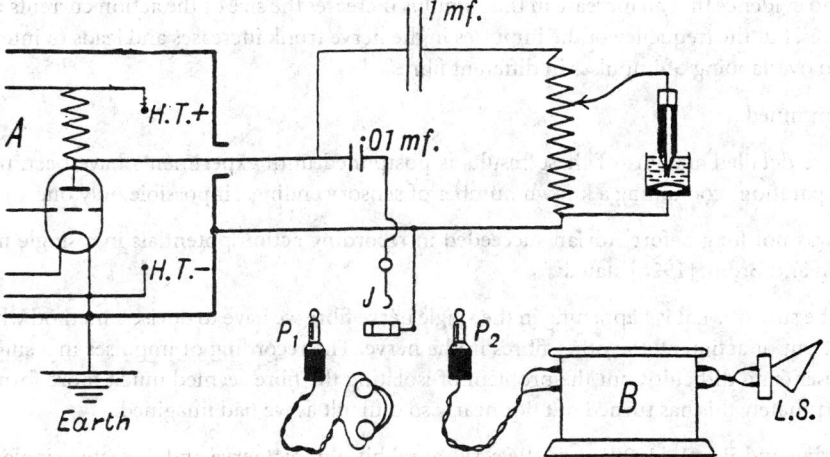

FIGURE HP3.8 Amplifier and capillary electrometer used by Adrian to record nerve action potentials along with headphones, amplifier (*B*), and loudspeaker (*LS*) used to aurally monitor their frequency. (From Adrian & Bronk, 1928.)

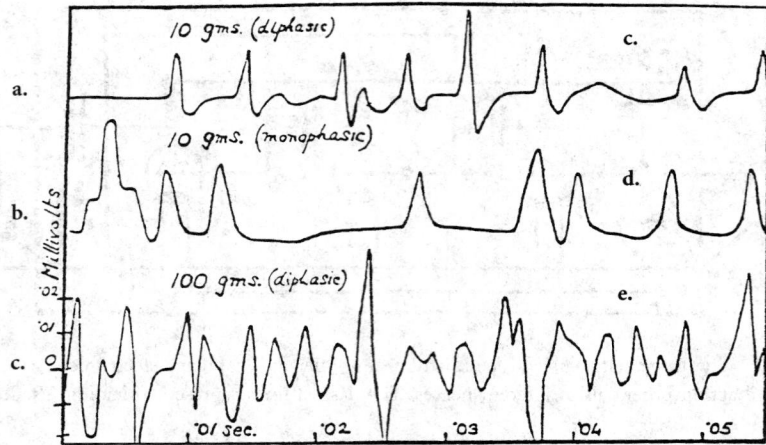

FIGURE HP3.9 Corrected capillary electrometer records of afferent action potentials in a frog sciatic nerve when weights were applied to the gastrocnemius muscle. (*c*) shows the action potentials from 10 g applied for 10 s; (*d*) shows the same weight applied for 24 s; and (*e*) shows the action potentials for 100 g weight applied for 10 s. Note the higher frequency of action potentials with 100-g weight. (From Adrian, 1928.)

After applying strict criteria to test the validity of his results, Adrian then recorded trains of afferent impulses in the saphenous nerve of a decapitated cat when a forcep was used to pinch the skin of the foot. The same result was obtained with a pin prick. He then recorded afferent impulses in the vagus nerve in the spinal and decerebrate cat and in the anesthetized rabbit. He also recorded trains of action potentials in the vagus nerve that were synchronous with the heartbeat and with respiration. Commenting on the latter he wrote: "The striking result is the absence of any sign of renewed discharge of impulses at the moment when the lungs are most deflated."

In the summary to his paper, Adrian stated:

It is probable that many of the oscillations represent action currents in a single nerve fibre, and these same general form and the same general time relations (allowing for temperature differences) in all sensory nerves in which they can be isolated sufficiently for measurement. There is no evidence that an increase in the stimulus increases the size of the action currents in single fibres, but the frequency of the impulses in the nerve trunk increases and leads to interference and overlapping of impulses in different fibres.

He continued:

More detailed analysis of these results is postponed until experiments have been made on preparations containing a known number of sensory endings, if possible only one.

It was not long before Adrian succeeded in recording action potentials in a single nerve fiber. Adrian and Bronk [1928] stated:

To be sure of what is happening in the single nerve fibre we have to devise a method which will put out of action all the other fibres in the nerve. The recording of impulses in a single fibre presents no difficulty, but the problem of isolating the fibre seemed much more formidable. Fortunately this has turned out not nearly so difficult as we had imagined.

Adrian and Bronk [1928] used the cervical rabbit phrenic nerve and dissected single fibers free with a needle and viewed the dissection with a binocular microscope. Teasing out a selected single fiber and sectioning it, electrodes were placed at the distal end. In this way, only afferent information was recorded. The equipment that they used is shown in Fig. HP3.8. Commenting on use of the headphones or a loudspeaker, they stated:

The amplified action currents can be photographed with the capillary electrometer, but until the final stages are reached, it is usually more convenient to lead them to a telephone or loud-speaker and estimate the character of the discharge by the ear instead of the eye.

They continued by showing how aural monitoring aided in the experiment:

When only a few fibres are in action the electrometer excursions may be too small to detect on a screen, but they produce a series of faint clicks in the loudspeaker, and it is thus possible to control the dissection, to expose a plate at the moment when the discharge is at its height, etc., without the inconvenience of wearing telephones.

Adrian and Bronk [1928] investigated the frequency of action potentials in an intact phrenic nerve of the decerebrate cat breathing spontaneously. The single-stage amplifier (Fig. HP3-8) was used. Figure HP3.10a illustrates the phrenic nerve action potentials during spontaneous breathing, and Fig. HP3.10b shows the recordings with the trachea clamped, the breathing becoming labored.

Having shown that the frequency of the action potentials in the phrenic nerve increased with depth of breathing, Adrian and Bronk [1928] set themselves the task of investigating how intrapulmonic pressure was related to the frequency of stimuli applied to the phrenic nerve. Using a rabbit in which the central circulation was occluded above C1, they connected a manometer to the trachea that could be clamped so that the manometer read the negative intrapulmonic pressure when the C4 phrenic nerve root was stimulated. They used a coreless induction coil connected to a rotary switch (rheotome) to enable delivery of stimuli at any desired frequency. By delivering bursts of stimuli of different frequencies, they plotted the negative intrapulmonic pressure as a function of frequency, clearly demonstrating the dependence of the amplitude of inspiration on the frequency of phrenic nerve stimuli.

Adrian published two monographs on his work; one was entitled, *The Mechanism of Nervous Action*, and the other, *The Basis of Sensation*. Interestingly, neither publication contains illustrations obtained with the cathode-ray oscilloscope; however, there are string galvanometer and capillary electrometer recordings. Obviously, Adrian had brought the capillary electrometer to a high degree of perfection, but it is important to remember that Adrian's interest lay in the frequency of the action potentials, not the intimate details of their waveforms.

Perhaps the best summary of Adrian's contributions appear in a single sentence in *The Mechanism of Nervous Action*. The section entitled, "Gradation of Activity," states:

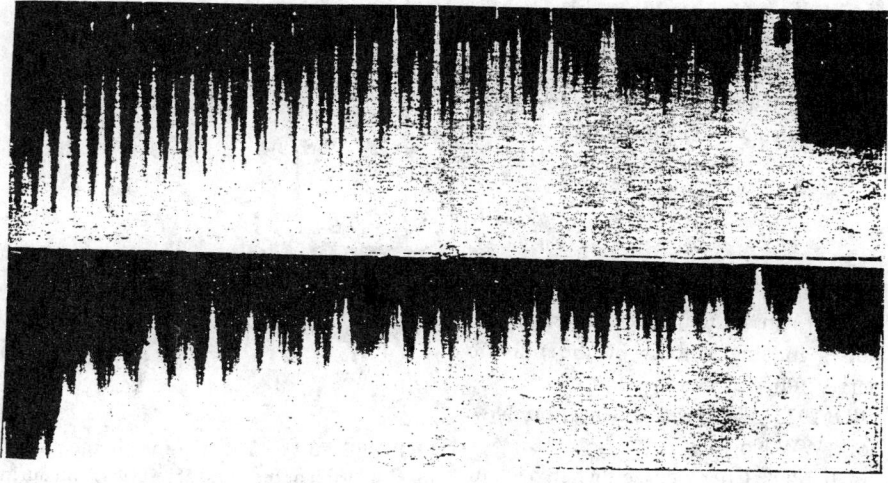

FIGURE HP3.10 Capillary electrometer records from the phrenic nerve of the decerebrate cat breathing spontaneously. (*a*) The airway is open. (*b*) The trachea was clamped. (From Adrian and Bronk, 1928.)

There is certainly no evidence to suggest that the impulses are graded in size, for the fact that sensory messages may produce a small or large effect according to the intensity of the stimulus is naturally explained by the varying number of fibres in action and by the varying frequency of the discharge in each fibre.

In 1932, Adrian shared the Nobel prize in physiology and medicine with Sherrington. The citation read, "For their discoveries regarding the function of the neuron."

Code of the Nervous System

From the impressive research performed by Gasser and Erlanger and by Adrian, the code of the nervous system was discovered. Stated simply, (1) intensity is signaled by the frequency of action potentials in a single axon, the action potentials all being the same, and (2) intensity is also signaled by the number of axons transmitting the information. In modern terms, the nervous system is a communications system that is binary and frequency modulated.

True Form of the Nerve Action Potential

Although the studies by Bernstein, Gasser, Erlanger, and Adrian provided information on the nerve action potential, its true form could not be established until the micropipet electrode was used to measure the transmembrane potential. Hodgkin and Huxley [1939] obtained the true waveform of the nerve action potential and thereby ushered in the modern era of electrophysiology. In a paper published in *Nature* on October 21, 1939, they reported that J. Z. Young [1930] called their attention to the giant axon (500 μm in diameter) of the squid, which was ideal for electrophysiologic studies.

The first micropipet electrode used by Hodgkin and Huxley consisted of a glass tube, 100 μm in diameter, that was slipped into the cut end of the giant axon. The electrode was mounted vertically and filled with seawater, and a silver–silver chloride electrode was inserted. The axon was then dipped into a container of seawater in which a second chlorided silver electrode was placed. The transmembrane potential was found to be −45 mV at 20°C. When the axon was stimulated, the action potential was 90 mV. Figure HP3.11 is a reproduction of this historic record.

The Hodgkin and Huxley experiment clearly demonstrated two important phenomena: (1) there is a measurable resting transmembrane potential, and (2) the action potential is larger than the resting transmembrane potential, the latter indicating that activity represents more than a mere disappearance of the transmembrane potential. The same team later provided the explanation with their classic papers on ion fluxes. Today, the action of many drugs is explained on the basis of ion fluxes.

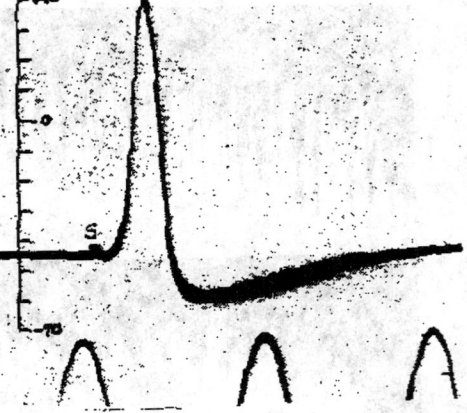

FIGURE HP3.11 The transmembrane potential of the giant axon of the squid at rest (*left*) and during activity. Time marks 2 ms. (From Hodgkin and Huxley, 1939. With permission.)

References

Adrian ED, Bronk DW. 1928. The discharge of impulses in motor nerve fibres: 1. Impulses in single fibres of the phrenic nerve. J Physiol 66:81.

Adrian ED. 1928. The Basis of Sensation. New York, WW Norton.

Bernstein J. 1868. Über den zeitlichen verlauf der negativen Schwankung des nervenstroms. Arch Ges Physiol 1:73–207.

Burch GJ. 1892*a*. On the time relations of the excursions of the capillary electrometer. Phil Trans R Soc (Lond) 83A:81.

Burch GJ. 1892*b*. On a method of determining the value of rapid variations of potential by means of the capillary electrometer communicated by J.B. Sanderson. Proc R Soc (Lond) 48:89.

DeForest L. 1907, 1908. U.S. patent nos. 841,387 (1907) and 879,532 (1908).

Einthoven W. 1903. Ein neues Galvanometer. Ann Phys 12(suppl 4): 1059.

Erlanger J, Gasser HS. 1924. The compound nature of the action current of nerve as disclosed by the cathode ray oscillograph. Am J Physiol 70:624.

Erlanger J, Gasser HS. 1937. Electrical Signs of Nervous Activity. Philadelphia, University of Pennsylvania Press.

Forbes A, Thacher C. 1920. Amplification of action currents with the electron tube in recording with string galvanometer. Am J Physiol 56:409.

Gasser HS, Erlanger J. 1922. A study of the action currents of nerve with the cathode ray oscillograph. Am J Physiol 62:496.

Gasser HS, Newcomer HS. 1921. Physiological action currents in the phrenic nerve. Am J Physiol 57(1):1.

Geddes LA, Foster KS, Senior J, Kahfeld A. 1989. The inductorium: The stimulator associated with discovery. Med Instrum 23(4):308.

Gotch F, Horsley V. 1888. Observations upon the electromotive changes in the mammalian spinal cord following electrical excitation of the cortex cerebri. Proc R Soc (Lond) 45:18.

Helmholtz H. 1850. Note sur la vitesse de propagation de l'agent nerveux dans les nerfs rachidiens. C R Acad Sci 30:204.

Helmholtz H. 1851. Note sur la vitesse de propagation de l'agent nerveux. C R Acad Sci 32:262.

Helmholtz H. 1853. On the methods of measuring very small portions of time and their application to physiological purposes. Phil Mag J Sci 6:313.

Hodgkin AL, Huxley AF. 1939. Action potentials recorded from inside a nerve fiber. Nature 144:710.

Hoff HE, Geddes LA. 1957. The rheotome and its prehistory: A study in the historical interrelation of electrophysiology and electromechanics. Bull Hist Med 31(3):212.

Hoff HE, Geddes LA. 1960. Ballistics and the instrumentation of physiology: The velocity of the projectile and of the nerve impulse. J Hist Med All Sci 15(2):133.

Young JZ. 1930. Structure of nerve fibers and synapses in some invertebrates. Cold Spring Harbor Symp Quant Biol 4:1.

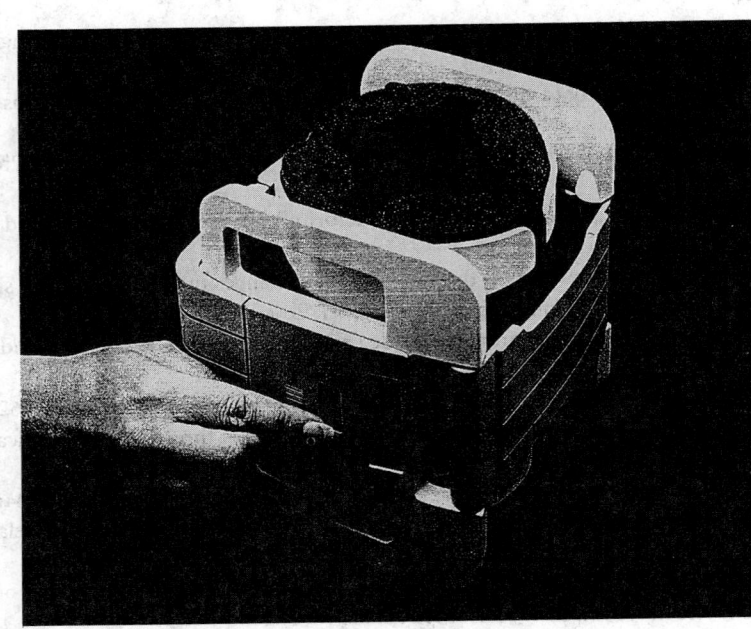

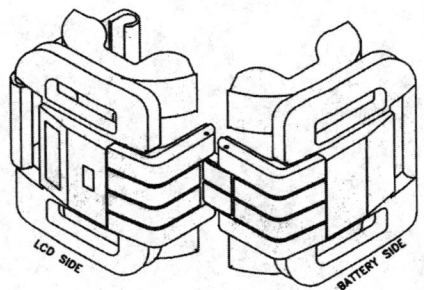

Noninvasive inductive coupling device used to apply low field intensities.

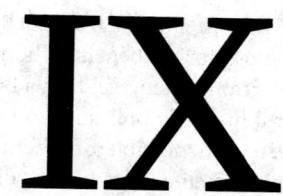

Biologic Effects of Nonionizing Electromagnetic Fields

Charles Polk
University of Rhode Island

T HE PURPOSE OF BIOMEDICAL ENGINEERING is to develop and employ the best available technology for the benefit of human health. Implicitly, the discussion of biologic effects of nonionizing
electromagnetic fields in a biomedical engineering handbook will then be concerned with beneficial medical applications of such fields. However, these applications must be based to as large an
extent as possible on scientific knowledge. This section therefore begins with a description of
experimentally established dielectric properties of biologic materials (Chapter 90). This is followed
by a general discussion of biologic effects—adverse as well as beneficial—of low-frequency magnetic fields (Chapter 91). This chapter is restricted to low-frequency magnetic—rather than electric
and magnetic—fields because the succeeding chapter (Chapter 92), which deals with therapeutic
applications, indicates that time-varying magnetic fields are of greater interest. At the present time,
it is not known whether observed biologic effects of low-frequency magnetic fields (particularly of
those having modest amplitude) are due to the electric fields and currents which they induce in
tissue as a consequence of Faraday's law or are due to an as yet unknown mechanism of direct
magnetic field–tissue interaction.

Since the fundamental equations that characterize field-tissue interaction are very different in
the power to audiofrequency range from those which describe biologic effects at radio and
microwave frequencies, separate chapters are devoted to the different frequency domains. Thus
Chapter 93 is devoted to discussing biologic effects, again not necessarily beneficial, of RF fields,
and Chapter 94 describes methods for their principal medical application, which is the production
of desired hyperthermia.

While Chapters 90 to 93 describe primarily measurements, effects, and applications of relatively
low-intensity fields, Chapter 95 is devoted to the fundamentals of the increasingly important area of
the interaction of short, high-intensity electric field pulses with biologic cells. It is shown that
understanding of "electroporation" is not only important for understanding the nature of electric
injury, but that this phenomenon is becoming a very important tool in biotechnology for transferring genetic material between different cells, as well as being applied for local drug delivery to tissue.

The division of this section along the indicated lines is mandated by the observations that high-
and low-intensity fields have different biologic effects—to consider extremes, electrocution versus
healing of fractured bones—and that different frequencies of electromagnetic energy interact
differently with materials of all types. Of particular importance is the relation between the wavelength λ of electromagnetic waves and the magnitudes L of field-generating and field-absorbing
structures or their distances. Since

$$\lambda = \frac{c}{f} \qquad \text{(IX.1)}$$

where f is the frequency and c is the propagation velocity (3.0×10^8 m/s in free space), it is obvious
that $L \ll \lambda$ at a "low" frequency, even as high as 1 kHz, where $\lambda = 300$ km, when L represents
dimensions that are of interest for interaction with animals, humans, or cell cultures of power transmission lines, motors, or laboratory instruments. When $L \ll \lambda$, all the "quasi-static" approximations discussed in Chap. 91 are applicable, which implies that time retardation effects, i.e., the wave
nature of electromagnetic energy, can essentially be disregarded. At low frequencies, the field amplitude most often decreases as $1/r^2$ or $1/r^3$, where r is the distance from the source, rather than as $1/r$,
as it does in an electromagnetic wave in free space. Furthermore, electric and magnetic fields are
effectively separable at extremely low frequencies (ELF) in the sense that the field from a particular
source in the "near-field region" (i.e., when $L \ll \lambda$) is either "primarily" electric ($E \gg H$) or "primarily" magnetic ($H \gg E$). Here E is the electric and H is the magnetic field intensity. At RFs or
microwaves, on the other hand, one is generally interested in the "far field" or "radiation field" region,
where the ratio between E and H is equal to the "wave impedance" η. It is given in a loss-free medium
by $\eta = \sqrt{\mu/\epsilon}$, where μ and ϵ are, respectively, the magnetic permeability and dielectric permittivity
of the medium in which the wave is propagating. (The magnetic flux density B is given by $B = \mu H$.)

The only precaution that is needed in the application of quasi-statics at ELF is to remember the relation between E and B when the sources involved produce predominantly a magnetic field (such as the application coils in a bone therapy apparatus):

$$\nabla \times \mathbf{E} = -\frac{\partial \mathbf{B}}{\partial t \neq 0} \qquad \text{(IX.2)}$$

Thus in the tissue the curl of the electric field, i.e., the circulation of the electric field per unit area, is not zero, as it is when the applied quasi-static field comes directly from an electric field source. As a consequence, current *distributions* in tissue due to such different sources are likely to be very different even if current *magnitudes* are possibly, in a particular case, identical.

As already mentioned, Chapters 90 to 93 deal primarily (although not exclusively) with low-intensity fields while Chapter 95 describes only high-field-intensity effects. It is of interest here to summarize the known biologic effects of various intensities of dc and low-frequency electric fields (Table IX.1).

The basic laws that give forces (**F**) and torques (**T**) due to electric and magnetic fields are listed on Table IX.2. In this table, q = electric charge, $\mathbf{v}$ = charge velocity, $\mathbf{p}$ = electric dipole moment (magnitude of $\mathbf{p}$ = charge $\times$ separation distance between opposite charges), and $\mathbf{m}$ = magnetic moment (magnitude of $\mathbf{m}$ = magnitude of circulating current $\times$ area enclosed by current; direction of $\mathbf{m}$ is perpendicular to the plane of the circulating current). The derivatives with respect to the distance x are a one-dimensional representation of spatial field gradients. The equations listed on Table IX-2, as well as Maxwell's equations (or the appropriate applicable approximations) and the known laws of classic and/or quantum mechanics, subject to the boundary conditions characteristic for living tissue, must provide a quantitative explanation for the observed biologic effects of electric and magnetic fields. Biologic tissue and cells are obviously extremely complex media; they are not only extremely inhomogeneous and anisotropic, but they are also not in thermodynamic equilibrium (unless dead). Thus the application of physical laws to the explanation of field-tissue interactions becomes a very complex problem, and the physicist and engineer must be careful not to provide "explanations" or to set limits on what should be "possible" or "impossible" based on physical models that are very far from even an approximate representation of biologic conditions.

It is not surprising, therefore, that only relatively gross effects, such as cell damage in electroporation or heating by radiofrequency fields of sufficiently high intensity, are reasonably well (although not completely) understood. Some "nonthermal" microwave effects (Chapter 93) and several low-frequency effects of magnetically induced electric fields of less than 10^{-3} V/m (Table IX.1 and Chapters 91 and 92) or *alternating* magnetic fields of less than about 100 μT are presently not understood. The interested reader may want to consult references given in the following chapters and/or discussions by Adair [1991], Adey [1990], Blanchard and Blackman [1994], Douglass et al. [1993], Kaiser [1993], Kirschvink et al. [1992], Lednev [1991, 1993], Luben [1993], Polk [1992, 1994], Tenforde [1992b], Weaver and Astumian [1990], or additional references listed by these authors. There are numerous, experimentally confirmed in vitro biologic effects at low ELF field intensities. These ef-

TABLE IX.1 Biologic Effects of ELF and Pulsed Electric Fields

	V/m Inside Tissue or Fluid
Electroporation (transient or permanent, depending on amplitude and duration of pulse)	10^5
Cell rotation in insulating fluid	10^4
Nerve/muscle stimulation	
Initiation of firing	10^3
Alteration of firing rate	10
Subtle "long-term" ($t > 10$ min) effects (bone/soft tissue repair, Ca-efflux, transcription)	10^{-3} to 10^{-5}

fects may be beneficial, may be adverse, or may be of no consequence in entire animals or humans. Some epidemiologic data (Chapter 91) suggest the possible existence of adverse health effects. The experimental evidence existing at the present time is insufficient, however, to decide whether any of the more promising physical models that are discussed in the given references can provide an adequate explanation for any of the observed biologic effects.

TABLE IX.2   Forces and Torques on Electric Charges and Electric and Magnetic Dipole Moments

$\mathbf{F} = q\mathbf{E}$	$\mathbf{F} = q\,(v \times \mathbf{B})$
$F = P\,\dfrac{dE}{dx}$	$\mathbf{F} = m\,\dfrac{dB}{dx}$
$\mathbf{T} = \mathbf{p} \times \mathbf{E}$	$\mathbf{T} = \mathbf{m} \times \mathbf{B}$

Two additional observations appear to be appropriate. The first is that the biologic environment is much more complex than the man-made inanimate world, where many different electric and magnetic field effects are used in devices as diverse as large electric motors, Xerox machines, feedback controllers, or television sets. It would therefore be surprising if identical electric or magnetic field "mechanisms" would be responsible for effects of different frequencies or field intensities on different biologic systems (e.g., immune cells versus bone tissue). The second observation concerns the existence and amplitude of the ambient, natural electric and magnetic fields. It is sometimes pointed out—correctly—that humans have been exposed for eons to the natural geomagnetic field of about 500 µT and to the natural dc electric field, which at the earth's surface is about 100 V/m and can be several thousand volts per meter under a thunder cloud. Without conducting contact, *dc electric* fields of this magnitude have indeed not been implicated in any biologic effect, nor have *dc magnetic* fields of about 500 µT, *without the simultaneous presence of an alternating field,* been shown to have significant biologic consequences [Tenforde, 1992a; Frankel and Liburdy, 1995]. Virtually all the reported biologic effects of low-intensity electric and magnetic fields on living organisms, including cells, involve *time variation,* particularly at frequencies below 100 Hz (or microwaves amplitude modulated at these frequencies). The low-frequency effects on animals living outside water appear to be also primarily due to *time-varying magnetic* fields. Clearly, the natural ambient magnetic field of about 500 µT is a *static* field that exhibits diurnal *slow* variations (i.e., with frequency components well below 1 Hz) only of the order of 10^{-3} µT and with "large" variations (taking minutes to hours for one cycle) during magnetic storms occurring a few times each year, rarely as large as 0.5 µT [Matsushita and Campbell, 1967]. The natural background of magnetic fields with "higher" frequencies (10 to 100 Hz) is on the order of 10 pT [Polk, 1982]. Thus the geomagnetic field is clearly a static field that cannot induce an electric field into a stationary object (as a consequence of Faraday's law) anywhere near the magnitude of that induced by a 60-Hz magnitude field even as low as 0.1 µT. Uniform linear motion of an object, such as that of a walking human, in a nearly uniform magnetic field of about 500 µT will produce an induced "Lorentz" electric field proportional to the product of velocity and flux density. However, that field *cannot* produce circulating electric currents as long as the total magnetic flux integrated over the cross-sectional area of the object (animal or human), $\iint \mathbf{B}\, ds$, does not change. Only tumbling motion, such as linear motion by means of somersaults, through the earth's magnetic field could produce induced electric currents comparable in magnitude to those induced by a 1-µT, 60-Hz field. Thus there is no basis for statements, sometimes made, that biologic effects of weak *ELF* magnetic fields are impossible, because animals or humans have been exposed throughout their development to the geomagnetic field.

References

Adair RK. 1991. Constraints on biological effects of weak extremely-low-frequency electromagnetic fields. Phys Rev A 43 (2):1039.

Adey WR. 1981. Tissue interaction with nonionizing electromagnetic fields. Physiol Rev 61:435.

Adey WR. 1990. Electromagnetic fields, cell membrane amplification and cancer promotion. In BW Wilson, RG Stevens, LE Anderson (eds), Extremely Low Frequency Electromagnetic Fields: The Question of Cancer, pp 211–249. Columbus, Ohio, Battelle Press.

Blanchard JP, Blackman CF. 1994. See refs. to Chap. 92.

Douglass JK, Wilkens L, Pantazelou E, Moss F. 1993. Noise enhancement of information transfer in crayfish mechanoreceptors by stochastic resonance. Nature 365:337.

Frankel RB, Liburdy R. 1995. Biological effects of static magnetic fields. In CRC Handbook of Biological Effects of Electromagnetic Fields, 2d ed. Boca Raton, Fla, CRC Press.

Kaiser F. 1993. Explanation of biological effects of low-intensity electric, magnetic and electromagnetic fields by nonlinear dynamics. In 9th Annual Review of Progress in Applied Computational Electromagnetics. Monterey, Calif.

Kirschvink JL, Kobayashi-Kirschvink A, Woodford BJ. 1992. Magnetite biomineralization in the human brain. Proc Natl Acad Sci USA 89(16):7683.

Lednev VV. 1991, 1993. See refs. to Chap. 92.

Liboff AR, McLeod BR. 1988. See refs. to Chap. 92.

Litovitz TA, Montrose CJ, Doinov P, et al. 1994. Superimposing spatially coherent electromagnetic noise inhibits field-induced abnormalities in developing chick embryos. Bioelectromagnetics 15:105.

Luben RA. 1993. See refs. to Chap. 92.

Matsushita S. 1967. Geomagnetic disturbances and storms. In S Matsushita, WM Campbell (eds), Physics of Geomagnetic Phenomena, vol 2, pp 793–821. New York, Academic Press.

Polk C. 1982. Schumann resonances. In H Volland (ed), CRC Handbook of Atmospherics, vol 1, pp 111–178. Boca Raton, Fla, CRC Press.

Polk C. 1992. Dosimetry of extremely-low-frequency magnetic fields. Bioelectromagnetics 13 (S1):209.

Polk C. 1994. Physical/chemical mechanisms and signal-to-noise ratios. In T Tenforde (ed), Proceedings of the 1994 Annual Meeting of the National Council on Radiation Protection. Washington, NCRP.

Tenforde TS. 1992a. Interaction mechanisms and biological effects of static magnetic fields. Automedica 14:271.

Tenforde TS. 1992b. Biological interactions and potential health effects of extremely-low-frequency magnetic fields from power lines and other common sources. Annu Rev Public Health 13:173.

Weaver JC, Astumian RD. 1990. The response of cells to very weak electric fields: The thermal noise limit. Science 347:459.

90

Dielectric Properties of Tissues

Kenneth R. Foster
University of Pennsylvania

The bulk electrical properties of tissues and cell suspensions have been of interest for many reasons for over a century. These properties determine the pathways of current flow through the body. This gives them fundamental importance in studies of biologic effects of electromagnetic fields, in measurements of physiologic parameters using impedance, and in basic and applied studies in electrocardiography, muscle contraction, nerve transmission, and numerous other fields.

I will briefly define the quantities used to characterize the bulk electrical properties of tissues and give some of the background information needed to interpret the data. A more extensive review is presented elsewhere[1]. Other reviews of tissue properties are by Schwan[2], Pethig[3], Grant et al.[4], Schanne and P.-Ceretti[5], and Duck[6]. Other tabulations of tissue properties are by Schwan[2], Geddes and Baker[7], and Stuchly and Stuchly[8]; Schwan[9] has published an extensive review of practical measurement techniques.

90.1 Definitions and Basic Phenomena

The dielectric permittivity $\epsilon\epsilon_0$ and conductivity σ of a material are, respectively, the dipole and current densities induced in response to an applied electric field of unit amplitude.* The significance of these quantities can be illustrated by considering an ideal parallel-plate capacitor, whose plates have surface area A and separation d. The capacitance C and conductance G of the capacitor are then

$$C = \frac{\epsilon\epsilon_0 A}{d}$$

$$G = \frac{\sigma A}{d} \tag{90.1}$$

(This neglects the effects of fringing fields and applies at low frequencies where propagation effects can be neglected.) At radian frequency ω, the admittance Y of the capacitor can be written

---

*In MKS units, the permittivity and conductivity have units of farads per meter and siemens per meter, respectively. For convenience, we write the permittivity as ϵ (the relative permittivity) times ϵ_0, the permittivity of vacuum. $\epsilon_0 = 8.85 \ (10^{-12} \ \text{F/m})$. The resistivity $\rho = 1/\sigma$.

$$Y = (G + j\omega C)$$

$$= (\sigma + j\omega\epsilon\epsilon_0)\frac{A}{d}$$

$$= \sigma^*\frac{A}{d} \tag{90.2}$$

$$= j\omega\epsilon^*\epsilon_0\frac{A}{d}$$

where $\sigma^* = \sigma + j\omega\epsilon\epsilon_0$ is the complex conductivity, and $\epsilon^* = \epsilon - j\sigma/\omega\epsilon_0$ is the complex permittivity.[†] In the usual notation, $\epsilon^* = \epsilon' - j\epsilon''$, where ϵ'' is the loss and tan (ϵ''/ϵ') is the loss tangent. Typically, for soft tissues at low frequencies,

$$\sigma > \omega\epsilon\epsilon_0$$

and the tissue can, for many purposes, be approximated adequately by considering it to be a pure conductor and neglecting the permittivity entirely.

For tissues, both ϵ and σ are strong functions of frequency (Fig. 90.1). This frequency dependence (dispersion) arises from several mechanisms. These mechanisms are discussed, with reference to

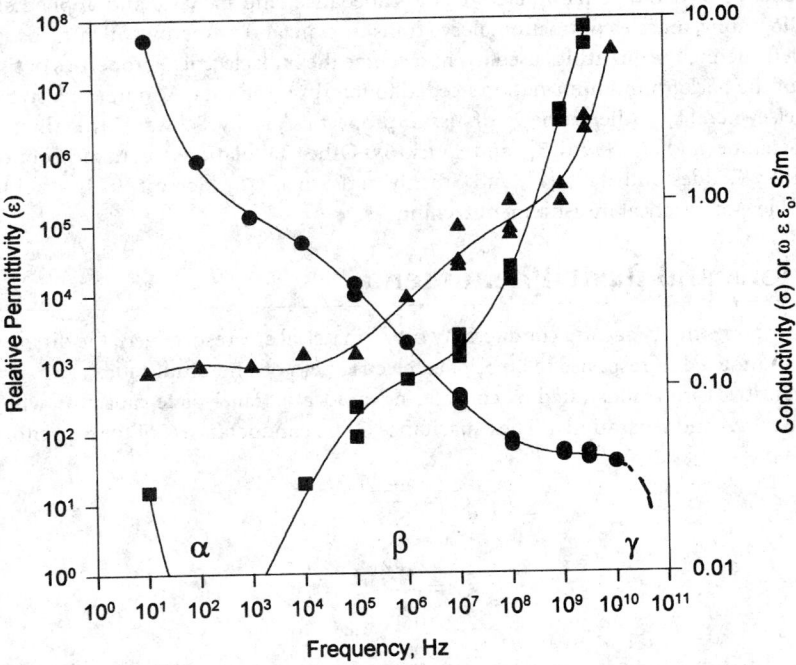

FIGURE 90.1   Data from liver tissue (the composite of several sets of data, from the Table 90.1). (●) Relative permittivity ϵ, (▲) conductivity σ, (■) $\omega\epsilon\epsilon_0$. When $\sigma >> \omega\epsilon\epsilon_0$, the tissue may be regarded for many purposes as a pure conductor. The major dispersion regions (α,β,γ) are indicated on the figure. The lines are regression lines through the data.

[†]The term *dielectric constant* is used, often in the chemical literature, to indicate the relative permittivity of pure liquids at low frequencies, where ϵ is essentially independent of frequency.

simple biophysical models, in Foster and Schwann [1]. For a typical soft tissue, different mechanisms dominate at different frequency ranges:

- At low frequencies (typically below several hundred kilohertz), the conductivity of the tissue is dominated by conduction in the electrolytes in the extracellular space. The bulk conductivity of the tissue is then a sensitive function of the volume fraction of extracellular space and the conductivity of the extracellular medium.
- At low frequencies, the tissue exhibits a dispersion (the alpha dispersion), centered in the low-kilohertz range, due to several physical processes. These include polarization of counterions near charged surfaces in the tissue and possibly the polarization of large membrane-bound structures in the tissue. At frequencies below the alpha dispersion, the relative permittivity of tissue reaches very high values, in the tens of millions.
- At radiofrequencies, the tissue exhibits a dispersion (the beta dispersion), centered in the range 0.1 to 10 MHz, due to the charging of cell membranes through the intracellular and extracellular media. Above the beta dispersion, the cell membranes have negligible impedance, and the current passes through both the extracellular and intracellular media.
- At microwave frequencies (above 1 GHz), the tissue exhibits a dispersion (the gamma dispersion) due to rotational relaxation of tissue water. This dispersion is centered at 20 GHz and is the same as that found in pure liquid water.

In addition to these three major dispersions, other smaller dispersions occur due to rotational relaxation of bound water or tissue proteins, charging of membranes of intracellular organelles, and other effects. These dispersions overlap in frequency and lead to a broad and often featureless dielectric dispersion in tissue.

These dispersions do not affect the permittivity and conductivity in the same way. For a single-time-constant dispersion centered at frequency f_c, the change in permittivity $\Delta\epsilon$ is related to the change in conductivity $\Delta\sigma$:

$$\Delta\sigma = \left|2\pi f_c \Delta\epsilon\epsilon_0\right|$$

Thus the alpha dispersion (at kilohertz frequencies) is associated with a small (usually imperceptible) increase in tissue conductivity but a very large decrease in permittivity. By contrast, the beta dispersion represents a large decrease in the permittivity (from several thousand to less than 100) and a large increase in conductivity (by a factor of 10 or so).

90.2 In Vivo Versus in Vitro Properties

The dielectric properties of the tissues that are summarized in the Table 90.1 pertain, for the most part, to excised tissues. The relation between these properties and the dielectric properties of tissue in vivo is a complicated matter.

At low frequencies (below about 0.1 MHz), electric current largely passes through the extracellular space, and the tissue conductivity is a sensitive function of the extracellular volume fraction. Any changes in the fluid distribution between intracellular and extracellular compartments can lead to a pronounced change in the low-frequency conductivity of the tissue.

For example, substantial (twofold) changes in the conductivity of rat kidney [10] and sheep myocardium [11] have been reported within a few minutes after death of the animal or after experimentally induced ischemia. These changes are almost certainly a result of changes in fluid distribution within the tissue. These changes are likely to be much less pronounced in the permittivity and in the conductivity above about 0.1 MHz.

Most of the data in Table 90.1 were taken from excised tissues within minutes to hours after the death of the animal. This calls for caution in their use.

TABLE 90.1 Dielectric Properties of Selected Tissues

Conductivity (S/m)

Frequency	A — Skeletal Muscle Parallel	B — Skeletal Muscle Perpendicular (Nonoriented)	C — Liver	D — Lung	E — Spleen	F — Kidney	G — Brain White Matter	H — Brain Gray Matter	I — Bone	J — Whole Blood	K — Fat
10 Hz	0.52	0.076	0.12	0.089							0.02–0.07
100 Hz	0.52	0.076	0.13	0.092					0.0126	0.60	
1 kHz	0.52	0.08	0.13	0.096					0.0129	0.68	
10 kHz	0.55	0.085	0.15	0.11	0.62	0.24–0.25	0.12–0.15	0.17	0.0133	0.68	
100 kHz	0.65 0.56–0.59 0.38–0.44	0.40	0.15 0.16	0.15	0.63	0.37–0.39	0.14–0.19	0.21	0.0144	0.55 0.68	0.71
1 MHz	0.83–0.85 0.58–0.63		0.27 0.30						0.0173		
10 MHz	0.86–0.87 0.92–0.96 0.69–0.75 0.95–0.99		0.47 0.46 0.42–0.46 0.72 0.70		0.84 0.55–0.53	0.64–0.68 0.50–0.57	0.21–0.28 0.30 0.29–0.31 0.36–0.48	0.35 0.38 0.45–0.63 0.69	0.0237		1.11 0.02–0.07
100 MHz	0.9 ± 0.08 0.75–0.82 1.38–1.45		0.60–0.71 0.98 1.2	0.80 ± 0.02	1.05 0.53 0.75 ± 0.02 1.2	0.94–1.05 0.73–0.76 0.48–0.51	0.66–0.72 0.52–0.85 0.89–0.94	0.45	0.0574 0.7	1.0	0.7–0.8
1 GHz	1.3 1.5		0.95–1.0 2.0	0.73	1.09–1.13 2.0 2.5 ± 0.03	0.95–0.97 1.0	0.80 0.81–0.82	1.1 0.89–1.17	0.05	1.4–1.6 1.3	0.03–0.09
3 GHz	2.7 ± 0.07 2.8		2.4 2.8		2.7 6.5	2.3 ± 0.05	1.8–2.1 1.5	2.0	0.16	2.5–3.1	0.3–0.4
10 GHz	8.3 7.7 8.8		5.8–6.7 10.0		10.0	4.5–7.4	8	10	0.5–1.7	9.1 10.5	

Relative Permittivity

#	Frequency											
1–3	10 Hz	10^7	10^6	5×10^7	2.5×10^7						1.5×10^5	
4–6	100 Hz	1.1×10^6	3.2×10^5	8.5×10^5	4.5×10^5					3,800		
7–9	1 kHz	2.2×10^5	1.2×10^5	1.3×10^5	8.5×10^4					1,000	5×10^4; 2,900	
10–12	10 kHz	8×10^4	7×10^4	5.5×10^4	2.5×10^4					640	2×10^4; 2,810	
13–15	100 kHz	1.5×10^4; 24,800–27,300; 14,400–15,800	3×10^4	9760; 1.4×10^4		3,260	10,900–12,500	1,960–3,400	3,800	280	4,000; 2,740	
16–18	1 MHz	2,460–2,530; 1,900–2,150		1,970; 1,970		1,450	2,390–2,690	543–827	1,250	87	2,040	
19–21	10 MHz	170–190; 187–204; 162–181		338; 300; 251–265		321; 352–410	431–499; 190–204	163–209; 200; 190–191	352; 380; 237–289	37	200	
22–24	100 MHz	67–72; 68 ± 2; 64–70	35	77; 79; 65–68; 46		83; 71–76; 81 ± 3; 54	89–95; 56–62; 85 ± 1	57–66; 65; 58–64; 40–44	90; 90; 65–80	23	67; 72–74	4.5–7.5
25–27	1 GHz	57–59; 58; 48	35	55; 47–49; 42		50–51; 50; 52 0.6	43; 46	35; 38–39	45; 47–51	8	58–62; 63–67; 63	4.3–7.5; 3–6
28–30	3 GHz	52.5 ± 0.7; 46; 40–42		53		46; 42	47.5 ± 1	35–41; 33	44	7.5	55–56	4–7
31–33	10 GHz	37; 35		42–43; 34–38; 37		38	30–37	25	40	8	50–52; 45	3.5–4.0

(continued)

TABLE 90.1   (*continued*)

			References		
Coordinates	Ref	Tissues	Coordinates	Ref.	Tissues
1 A,B	19	Dog skeletal muscle, 37°C (av of 5 measurements, SD ~ 30%)	33 A,B	23	Dog liver, in situ (av of 20 measurements, SD ~ 25%)
4 A,B			1 C		
7 A,B			4 C		
10 A,B			7 C		
13 A,B			10 C		
15 A,B	20	Nonoriented dog skeletal muscle, 37°C (range of 3 measurements)	1 D	23	Dog lung, inflated, in situ (av of 20 measurements, SD ~ 25%)
18 A,B			4 D		
21 A,B			7 D		
24 A,B			10 D		
14 A,B	20	Nonoriented rat skeletal muscle, 37°C (range of 2 measurements)	7 K	23	Dog fat, in situ
17 A,B			10 K		
20 A,B			19 A,B	24	Cat skeletal muscle, in vivo, 31°C (range of 3 measurements)
13 C	20	Dog liver, 37°C (single specimen)	22 A,B		
16 C			25 A,B		
19 C			20 E	24	Cat spleen, in vivo, 35°C (range of 3 measurements)
22 C			23 E		
14 C	20	Rabbit liver, 37°C (single specimen)	26 E		
17 C			20 F	24	Cat kidney, in vivo, 35°C (range of 3 measurements)
20 C			23 F		
23 C			26 F		
13 E	20	Dog spleen, 37°C (single specimen)	21 G,H	24	Cat brain, in vivo, 33°C (range of 3 measurements)
16 E			24 G,H		
19 E			27 G,H		
22 E			21 C	24	Cat liver, in vivo, 35°C (range of 3 measurements)
13 F	20	Dog kidney, 37°C (range of 2 measurements)	24 C		
16 F			27 C		
19 F			28 C	25	Bovine liver, 37°C
22 F			23 D,J	26	Beef blood
13 G,H	20	Dog brain, white and gray matter, 37°C (range of 2 measurements)	22 K	20	Excised human tissues (deflated lung) 27°C (measurement frequencies 0.2–0.9 GHz)
16 G,H			26 K		
19 G,H			26 D		
22 G,H			27 J		
27 E	21, 22	Dog spleen, 37°C (values at 1,3 GHz interpolated, single specimen)	23 A,B	27	Various cat tissues, in vivo (av ± SD, 55 measurements in 4 animals); value at 10 GHz extrapolated from 8.0 GHz; 1 GHz interpolated
30 E			26 A,B		
33 E			29 A,B		
27 A,B	21, 22	Dog skeletal muscle, 37°C (values at 1,3 GHz interpolated, single specimen)	32 A,B		
30 A,B			24 E		

25 E	17 J		
28 E	20 J		
31 E	13 J	30	Normal human blood, hematocrit 40%, 21°C (50 kHz)
24 F	25 C	16	Various tissues, dog, horse, 38°C (except 25 I, 28 I, 25°C); the
27 F	30 C		measurements were made at 8.6 GHz and extrapolated to
30 F	25 K		10 GHz
33 F	28 K		
26 C	25 J		
29 C	28 J		
32 C	25 I		
4 I	28 I		
7 I	31 A,B,I,K		
10 I	32 J	17	Human (9.4 GHz), 37°C
13 I	20 G,H	31	Dog brain, white and gray matter, 37°C
16 I	23 G,H		
19 I	26 G,H		
22 I	29 G,H		
25 G	32 G,H		
28 G	4 J	29	Sheep blood, 18°C
8 J	7 J		
11 J			
14 J			

21,22 — Dog liver, 37°C (value at 1.3 GHz extrapolated)

28 — Rat femur, 37°C, immersed in Hank's buffered saline, radial direction (single sample)

29 — Mixed brain tissue, mouse, 37°C (value at 3 GHz interpolated)

15 — Rabbit blood, room temperature

Reprinted from Foster and Schwan, 1994.

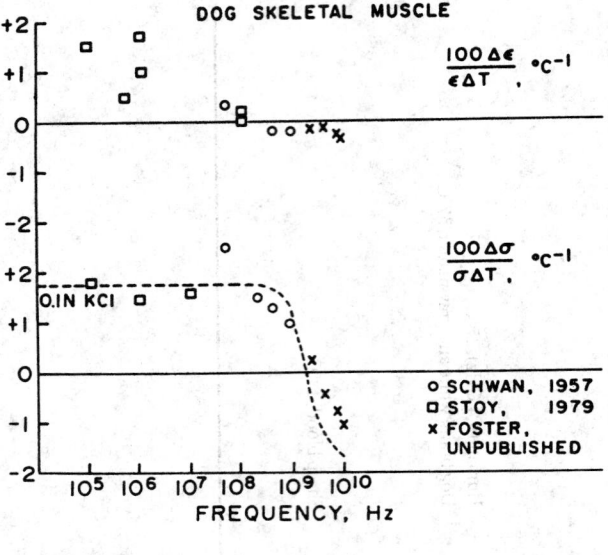

A

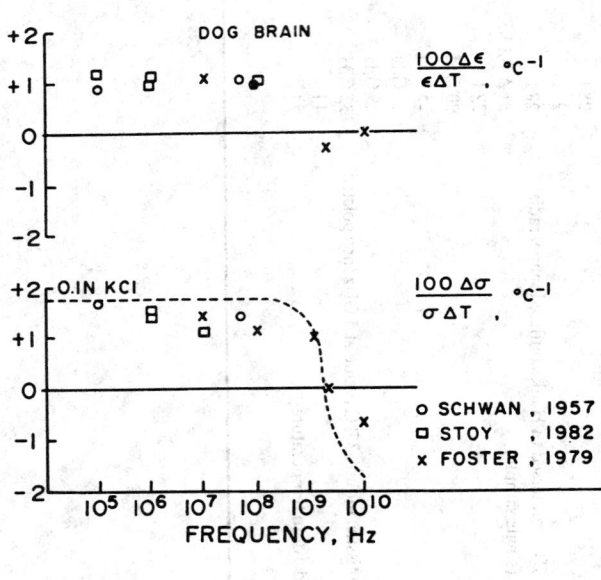

B

FIGURE 90.2 Fractional change with reciprocal temperature of dielectric properties of (*a*) dog muscle and (*b*) brain near 37°C (from Foster and Schwan, ref. 1). In most cases, the temperature coefficients have been calculated from two measurements at 25 to 28 and 37°C.

90.3 Temperature Coefficients

The dielectric properties of tissues change with temperature. Below about 44 to 45°C these changes are generally small and reversible. They can be neglected for many practical purposes. At higher temperatures, irreversible changes occur because of thermally induced tissue damage.

Reversible Changes

The electrical conductivity of tissues at low frequencies (below about 0.1 MHz) reflects the volume fraction of extracellular space and the conductivity of extracellular media; the conductivity above the beta relaxation frequency reflects mostly that of intracellular media. Thus, to a good approximation, the temperature dependence of the conductivity of tissue below about 1 GHz is the same as for typical physiologic electrolytes, +2% per degree Celsius.

Above 1 GHz, the dipolar loss of tissue water (with a temperature coefficient of −2% per degree Celsius below 20 GHz) contributes significantly to the total measured conductivity of a tissue. The combination of dipolar loss and ionic conduction will result in a net temperature coefficient for the conductivity that varies between +2% per degree Celsius (below 1 GHz) and −2% per degree Celsius (above 5 GHz), with a crossover point near 2 GHz.

At all frequencies, the temperature coefficient for the permittivity is smaller but has a more complicated frequency dependence.

Irreversible Changes

Thermally induced damage to tissue will result in irreversible changes in the dielectric properties of tissue. The extent of such changes depends on the tissue type, duration of heating, and other factors. For canine skeleton, such changes occur above 44.5°C[12–14].

Figure 90.2 shows the temperature coefficient, defined in the figure, for the conductivity and permittivity of canine muscle and brain. These data pertain to reversible changes only.

90.4 Dielectric Data: Tabulated

Table 90.1 presents selected permittivity and conductivity data from various tissues. Where available, the table presents up to three values for the tissues, including measurements performed on excised tissues of various species and in vivo. The aim is to present primarily new data; in some cases I have included earlier data. Sources are refs 15 to 31. The large variability in reported properties of these tissues is illustrated in the table. All data pertain to tissues at body temperature (37 to 38°C).

References

1. Foster KR, Schwan HP. 1994. Dielectric properties of tissues. In C Polk, E Postow (eds), Handbook of Biological Effects of Electromagnetic Fields, 2d ed. Boca Raton, Fla, CRC Press.
2. Schwan HP. 1957. Electrical properties of tissue and cell suspensions. In Advances in Biological and Medical Physics, vol 5, p 47. New York, Academic Press.
3. Pethig R. 1979. Dielectric and Electronic Properties of Biological Materials. New York, Wiley.
4. Grant EH, Sheppard RJ, South GP. 1978. Dielectric Behavior of Biological Molecules in Solution. Oxford, Oxford University Press.
5. Schanne OF, P.-Ceretti, ER. 1978. Impedance Measurements in Biological Cells. New York, Wiley.
6. Duck FA. 1990. Physical Properties of Tissue. New York, Academic Press.
7. Geddes LA, Baker LE. 1967. The specific resistance of biological material—A compendium of data for the biomedical engineer and physiologist. Med Biol Eng 5:271.
8. Stuchly MA, Stuchly SS. 1980. Dielectric properties of biological substances—Tabulated. J Microwave Power 15:19.
9. Schwan HP. 1963. Determination of biological impedances. In G Oster et al (eds), Physical Techniques in Biological Research, vol 6, p 323. New York, Academic Press.
10. Löfgren B. 1951. The electrical impedance of a complex tissue and its relation to changes in volume and fluid distribution. Acta Physiol Scand 23(suppl 81):1.

11. Fallert MA, Mirotznik MS, Bogen DK, et al. 1993. Myocardial electrical impedance mapping of ischemic sheep hearts and healing aneurysms. Circulation 87:188.

12. McRae DA, Esrick MA. 1992. The dielectric parameters of excised EMT-6 tumors and their change during hyperthermia. Phys Med Biol 37:2045.

13. McRae DA, Esrick MA. 1993. Changes in electrical impedance of skeletal muscle measured during hyperthermia. Int J Hyperthermia 9:247.

14. Esrick MA, McRae DA. 1994. The effect of hyperthermia-induced tissue conductivity changes on electrical-impedance temperature mapping so physics in medicine and biology. Phys Med Biol 39:133.

15. Fricke H, Curtis HJ. 1935. The electric impedance of hemolyzed suspensions of mammalian erythrocytes. J Gen Physiol 18:821.

16. Herrick JF, Jelatis DG, Lee GM. 1950. Dielectric properties of tissues important in microwave diathermy. Fed Proc Fed Am Soc Exp Biol 9:60 (abstract only; data summarized in ref. 2).

17. England TS, Sharples NA. 1949. Dielectric properties of the human body in the microwave region of the spectrum. Nature 163:487.

18. Schwan HP. 1941. Über die Niederfrequenzleitfahigkeit von Bluten und Blutserum bei verschiedenen Temperaturen. Z Ges Exp Med 109:531.

19. Epstein BR, Foster KR. 1983. Anisotropy in the dielectric properties of skeletal muscle. Med Biol Eng Comput 21:51.

20. Stoy RD, Foster KR, Schwan HP. 1982. Dielectric properties of mammalian tissues from 0.1 to 100 MHz: A summary of recent data. Phys Med Biol 27:501.

21. Schepps JL, Foster KR. 1980. The UHF and microwave dielectric properties of normal and tumor tissues: Variation in dielectric properties with tissue water content. Phys Med Biol 25:1149.

22. Schepps JL. 1980. The measurement and analysis of the dielectric properties of normal and tumor tissues at UHF and microwave frequencies, Ph.D. dissertation, University of Pennsylvania, Philadelphia.

23. Schwan HP, Kay CF. 1957. The conductivity of living tissues. Ann NY Acad Sci 65:1007.

24. Stuchly MA, Athey TW, Stuchly SS, et al. 1981. Dielectric properties of animal tissues in vivo at frequencies 10 MHz–1 GHz. Bioelectromagnetics 2:93.

25. Brady MM, Symonds SA, Stuchly SS. 1981. Dielectric behavior of selected animal tissues in vitro at frequencies from 2 to 4 GHz. IEEE Trans Biomed Eng BME-28:305.

26. Schwan HP, Li K. 1953. Capacity and conductivity of body tissues at ultrahigh frequencies. Proc IRE 41:1735.

27. Kraszewski A, Stuchly MA, Stuchly SS, Smith AM. 1982. In vivo and in vitro dielectric properties of animal tissues at radiofrequencies. Bioelectromagnetics 3:421.

28. Kosterich JD, Foster KR, Pollack SR. 1983. Dielectric permittivity and electrical conductivity of fluid saturated bone. IEEE Trans Biomed Eng BME-30:81.

29. Nightingale NRV, Goodridge VD, Sheppard RJ, Christie JL. 1983. The dielectric properties of cerebellum, cerebrum, and brain stem of mouse brain at radiowave and microwave frequencies. Phys Med Biol 28:897.

30. Pfutzner H. 1984. Dielectric analysis of blood by means of a raster-electrode technique. Med Biol Eng Computing 22:142.

31. Foster KR, Schepps JL, Stoy RD, Schwan HP. 1979. Dielectric properties of brain tissue between 0.01 and 10 GHz. Phys Med Biol 24:1177.

91

Low-Frequency Magnetic Fields: Dosimetry, Cellular, and Animal Effects

Maria A. Stuchly
University of Victoria

Low-frequency magnetic fields are of interest to biomedical engineers for at least two reasons. They have found applications in a few diagnostic procedures, and their therapeutic applications have been growing. The diagnostic applications include the use of strong pulses of magnetic fields for neural stimulation. Another well-established diagnostic use is in magnetic resonance imaging. Therapeutic applications are reviewed in Chapter 92. Information on other applications can be found in a review by Stuchly [1990]. The other reason for the importance of low-frequency magnetic fields is their potential impact on human health. This is an area of considerable research activities and public concern and the subject of this chapter. *Low-frequency magnetic fields,* for the purpose of this review, mostly refer to extremely low frequency (ELF) fields, but the range also encompasses higher frequencies up to a few kilohertz.

The impetus for the inquiry of interactions of ELF magnetic fields with living systems has been provided by epidemiologic reports [e.g., Ahlbom et al., 1993; London et al., 1991; NRPB, 1992; Poole and Trichopoulos, 1991; Savitz et al., 1988; Theriault et al., 1994]. Numerous epidemiologic studies have not provided convincing evidence that ELF, or more specifically the power-line-frequency, magnetic fields are associated with increases in cancer rates. They have shown through some supportive evidence for possible increases in childhood leukemia and brain tumors and some adult leukemias in those exposed occupationally. In an overview that follows, attention is focused on physical interactions of ELF magnetic fields with living systems and reported effects in cellular and animal studies. One general conclusion that can be drawn is that low-frequency magnetic fields at moderate to low levels are biologically active, i.e., interact with various cells or systems of the animal body. What is not known, however, are the biophysical mechanisms responsible for the interactions observed and parameters of the field and biosystem that are essential in eliciting the interactions. Several reviews and reports provide detailed information on the subject [e.g., ORAU, 1992; Tenforde, 1986].

91.1 Physical Interactions: Dosimetry

Basic Principles

ELF magnetic fields interact with conductive bodies such as tissues by inducing electric currents and fields inside them. While, in general, all four of Maxwell's equations have to be satisfied, in the case of ELF fields, certain simplifications apply. As discussed in the preceding chapter, tissues are conductive and nonmagnetic (their bulk magnetic permeability is equal to that of free space). Consideration of the dimensions of the biologic object (e.g., people) in comparison with wavelengths at ELF, the tissue conductivity as compared with the dielectric constant, leads to the following conclusions. Provided that

$$\frac{\sigma}{\omega \epsilon} >> 1 \tag{91.1}$$

and

$$f \mu_0 \sigma L^2 << 1 \tag{91.2}$$

the quasi-static approximation can be applied [Polk 1986, 1990]. This means that the secondary magnetic field induced by the eddy currents produced by the original magnetic field can be neglected. As a result, to determine the induced current and electric field, it suffices to consider Faraday's law and Laplace's equation rather than coupled Maxwell's equations. Faraday's law,

$$\oint_c \overline{E} \cdot d\overline{l} = - \int_s \frac{\partial \overline{B}}{\partial t} \cdot d\overline{s} \tag{91.3}$$

gives the electric field vector $\overline{E}$ over a closed contour c due to the time change of the magnetic flux density vector $\overline{B}$ integrated over the surfaces encompassed by c. Note the scalar products; i.e., only the component of $\overline{B}$ normal to the surface defined by the contour is contributing to the induction of the electric field. For harmonic (sinusoidal) fields and a circular contour in a homogeneous infinite conductor, the magnitude of the electric field is expressed by a simple relationship:

$$E = \pi f B r \tag{91.4}$$

where f is the frequency and r is the radius.

In media that are finite in size and consist of parts having different dielectric properties, the boundary conditions at the interfaces have to be satisfied, and Laplace's equation needs to be solved in the region of interest (subject to the boundary conditions):

$$\nabla^2 V = 0 \tag{91.5}$$

and

$$\overline{E} = -\nabla V \tag{91.6}$$

The induced current density is related to the electric field as:

$$\overline{J} = \sigma \overline{E} \tag{91.7}$$

With an exception of a few simple cases where Eq. (91.4) can be used to determine the induced electric field, more complex analysis, frequently numerical, that considers Eqs. (91.3), (91.5), and (91.6) has to be performed. An example of a valid use of Eq. (91.4) is a conductive solution in a cylindrical dish in a uniform magnetic field parallel to the cylinder axis.

There is no clear indication that the induced electric field and current in tissues, cells, or their parts are responsible for all observed biologic effects. At least some of the effects clearly depend on these parameters [Liburdy, 1995]. Other mechanisms are postulated but not satisfactorily proven to be dependent on the ELF magnetic field itself or its combination with a static magnetic field. Despite this limitation, it appears reasonable to quantify the exposure conditions for in vitro and animal studies in terms of a dosimetric measure that is well based in physics and refers to the biologic system, namely, the induced electric field and current. Evaluations of internal fields and currents are useful in comparing experimental exposures between and within cell preparations and species. Their parameters also can be used in scaling the exposures from one animal to another or to human beings.

People and Animals

Homogeneous spheroids and ellipsoids of sizes and shapes representing humans and rodents have been analyzed [Spiegel, 1977; Hart 1992]. More recently, numerical analysis has been applied to a heterogeneous representation of human beings [Gandhi and Chen, 1992; Xi et al., 1994], and high spatial resolution has been obtained for body parts such as the head [Xi and Stuchly, 1994]. Limited measurements on rats, human, and rodent models have been performed and in general confirm well the results of modeling [Miller, 1991]. Tissue heterogeneity significantly alters the induced fields and currents from those of homogeneous models, as indicated in an insightful analysis [Polk, 1990; Polk and Song, 1990]. Representative data for a heterogeneous human model with cubic cells with a side dimension of 1.3 cm. and homogeneous rodents are given in Table 91.1 to provide some reference for scaling and interspecies comparison. In all cases, the magnetic field orientation is selected to give the maximum values of induced current densities. This means that the magnetic field is directed front to back (and vice versa), translating into a horizontal magnetic field for a person and a vertical field for a rodent. The interspecies scaling values are different from those frequently used which are based on the estimated maximal current paths for various species. For instance, comparing the maximum currents, one gets a ratio of 1:9 for humans versus rats from the modeling results and 1:6 from the weight/volume ratios (maximal current path).

It is worthwhile to note that the induced currents and fields in people exposed to power-line (50- or 60-Hz) magnetic fields in the environment are very weak. Typical levels of magnetic fields at homes are of the order of 0.1 µT and in the proximity of appliances typically less than 1 µT. Therefore, the average induced current density is 0.2 to 2 µA/m², and maximum is 2 to 20 µA/m². In most offices, fields are below 0.2 µT. Use of transportation such as subway trains or Amtrak can result in exposure levels in the range of 0.3 to 10 µT. Some occupational exposures (e.g., work at power substations) are of the order of a few microteslas. The induced current densities from these exposures can be compared with typical endogenous currents associated with action potentials. These current

TABLE 91.1 Induced Currents and Fields from a 60-Hz Uniform Magnetic Field of 1 µT

Subject	Current Density, µA/m²		Electric Field, µV/m	
	Average	Maximum	Average	Maximum
Human, 1.7 m, 70 kg	1.3–1.9*	8 (20)[†]	14–17.7	161 (296)[†]
Rat, 0.3 kg	0.3	1.3	4.4	17.7
Mouse, 0.02 kg	0.12	0.4	1.7	5.7

*The average current density depends on the electrical properties used for the muscle tissue.

[†]Values in parentheses obtained from the analysis with an improved resolution of 0.65 cm instead of 1.3 cm.

Source: Based on Xi et al. [1994] and Xi and Stuchly [1994].

densities are in the brain on the order of 1 mA/m² and higher in the vicinity of the neurons. To obtain similar current densities requires an external magnetic field of about 50 to 100 μT.

Cells and Cell Assemblies

Evaluation of induced current and electric fields is also very important in quantification and interpretation of results of in vitro laboratory studies. This is especially the case when a question is asked if the biologic effect observed is due to the magnetic field or the electric currents and field induced in the test sample by the magnetic field. Also, when results of a study in one laboratory are not corroborated by other data, evaluation of induced fields may prove useful in gaining an insight into hidden differences in apparently identical experiments. For a low density of biologic cells in a conductive medium, the induced current density can be computed based solely on the geometry of the medium contained in the exposure dish and the magnetic field characteristics [Misakian et al., 1993]. Methods of calculation for several dish shapes including an annular ring have been published [McLeod et al., 1983; Misakian and Kaune, 1990; Misakian, 1991; Misakian et al., 1993; Wang et al., 1993]. Some dish configurations and magnetic field orientations facilitate obtaining the same current density in most of the medium volume occupied by cells. However, even at low densities, the presence of biologic cells, because of their low-conductivity membranes, affects the spatial pattern of the induced currents and fields [Polk, 1990]. The effect of cell density becomes much more pronounced at higher densities and when cells form a confluent monolayer [Hart et al., 1993; Stuchly and Xi, 1994].

In a confluent monolayer, the induced currents above the cells depend on the magnetic field characteristics, the dish geometry, and the conductivity of the medium. However, within the monolayer, only very low current densities are induced inside the cells. Their magnitude depends solely on the magnetic flux density, cell diameter, and cytoplasm conductivity. At 60 Hz, 1 μT, and $\sigma = 0.5$ S/m, the maximum current density in a 100-μm-diameter cell is less than 5 nA/m². However, if, for instance, 16 cells are connected by gap junctions forming a ring, numerical modeling indicates a significant increase in the current density. For a realistic gap junction surface area of 0.5% to 5% of the membrane surface area and conductivity of 0.5 S/m, the maximum current density is 12 to 18 times greater than that for a single cell [Stuchly and Xi, 1994]. It can be noted that the estimate from a simplified reasoning considering the radius of the ring gives an increase of only about 3 times. The physical rationale behind the greater increase is that gap junctions occupy only a small fraction of the cross section through which the total current induced in the ring flows. It should be noted that it would require a long ring or other shape of cells connected by gap junctions to produce a significant potential change across the junctions. This discussion merely emphasizes the need for modeling on cellular and subcellular levels. The modeling results referred to here are still for a grossly oversimplified model.

91.2 Biologic Effects

Human Data

Apart from the epidemiologic reports mentioned earlier and clinical reports on therapeutic applications discussed in the next chapter, there are interesting laboratory observations of effects on people of ELF magnetic fields. Even intense magnetic fields are not detected by people in the absence of artifactual cues. Exposure to 20-μT and 9-kV/m 60-Hz fields of healthy male volunteers resulted in statistically significant changes in the heart rate (slowing), components of event-related brain potentials, and errors on a choice reaction-time task. The effects were greatest soon after the field was switched either on or off [Cook et al., 1992]. The fields were not perceived by the subjects. The performance measures such as time estimation, vigilance, digit span, reaction time, and event-related brain potentials were unaffected by the field exposure. Neither were subjective measures such as mood or sleepiness affected. Evidence also has emerged that exposure to 20 μT at night causes suppression of melatonin in individuals who have naturally lower melatonin levels [Graham et al., 1993]. A well-established phenomenon of strong magnetic fields, above 10 mT at frequencies of tens of hertz, is induction of magnetophosphenes, i.e., visual sensations [Tenforde, 1986].

Laboratory Animals

Numerous laboratory investigations of animals, mostly rodents, exposed to magnetic fields have been conducted. More detailed reviews can be found elsewhere [e.g., ORAU, 1992; WHO, 1987; Anderson, 1991]; only a few representative studies are outlined here. Effects of magnetic fields on cancer development have been of primary concern, because of the suggestive indications from epidemiologic studies. Typical animal screening studies that are used in testing carcinogenic potential of various chemicals have been recognized as of very limited value in the case of magnetic fields. The main reason is the difficulty in applying a high "toxic" dose, since what constitutes the dose has not been established. There also exist physiologic and technical limitations on the intensity of magnetic fields that can be applied. From the physiologic point of view, high time-varying magnetic field strengths stimulate excitable cells (muscle, nerve). From the technical point of view, magnetic flux densities of the order of a few milliteslas are the maximum for which artifacts such as excessive vibration, noise, and heating can be avoided at a reasonable cost. With these limitations, even a large number of animals and various exposure conditions used in screening studies may prove to be of little value. The negative outcome of a study with the statistical power of detection of doubling of the number of cancers, which in other screening studies is considered convincing, does not appear to suffice in this case. This is due, in addition to the problems with defining the "dose," to the likelihood that if time-varying magnetic fields affect cancer, it is not through a genotoxic mechanism [McCann et al., 1993] but rather more subtle interaction such as promotion, copromotion, immune system suppression, or others. Furthermore, the expected increases are not large.

Action of time-varying magnetic fields as promoters has been investigated by a few groups. A classic and relatively easy to manipulate model of the mouse skin tumor has been used by investigators in Canada and Sweden [Stuchly et al., 1992; McLean et al., 1992; Rannug et al., 1993a]. Magnetic flux densities were up to 2 mT. No statistically significant effects were found on the tumor development in either of the studies. Mixed results were obtained in a more recent study where intermittent exposures (15 seconds on, 15 seconds off for 19 to 21 hours) were used [Rannug et al., 1994]. Copromoting effects of magnetic fields were investigated in Sencar mice treated with a chemical tumor initiator (DMBA) and promoter (TPA) [Stuchly et al., 1993] and exposed to 2 mT 6 hours per day for 23 weeks. A statistically significant acceleration in the tumor development was observed for animals exposed to magnetic fields, but there was no statistically significant difference at the termination of exposure (neither in the occurrence nor in the cumulative number of tumors). A later attempt to replicate the same finding in the same laboratory was not successful [McLean et al., 1993].

Tumor promotion by magnetic fields also was investigated in the rat liver foci model [Rannug et al., 1993b]. Several exposure levels up to 0.5 mT were used. Prior to exposure, the rats were subjected to partial hepatectomy and treatment with a chemical causing liver cancer. There were no statistically significant differences between the sham- and field-exposed animals in the number of foci, mean focus area, and volume occupied by foci.

Another area of potential health concern is reproductive and teratologic effects. Two comprehensive reviews address this question [Chernoff et al., 1992; Brent et al., 1993]. Most studies of mammalian species have not reported any significant differences in reproduction and development of exposed animals as compared with sham-exposed animals. However, some of the positive findings are provocative and need a follow-up. Perhaps the most interesting is the report by McGiven et al. [1990]. Male offspring of rats exposed to 15-Hz pulsed fields of 0.8 mT and 0.33-ms rise time showed increased accessory sex organ weights and reduced scent-making behavior. Various developmental effects have been reported for avian species. Abnormalities resulting from exposure to low-intensity pulsed magnetic fields were observed in some but not all laboratories, even for an experiment designed to be "identical" in six laboratories [Berman et al., 1990]. Other investigations also reported mixed results [Chernoff et al., 1992; Brent et al., 1993]. There are considerable problems in relating the relevance of these findings to human teratology [Chernoff et al., 1990].

There is evidence indicating that ELF magnetic fields affect nocturnal melatonin production [Anderson, 1991; Reiter and Richardson, 1992].

Overall, studies performed so far have not unambiguously identified any gross detrimental effects at exposures even to relatively high magnetic flux densities on the order of 0.1 to 1 mT. On the other hand, various subtle effects have been observed in some studies, and some of these effects may have implications on human health if the animal data for a specific interaction can be extrapolated to human exposures.

Cellular Systems

Interactions of ELF magnetic fields have been reviewed by Luben [1991], Liburdy [1992], and Tenforde [1993]. A general picture that has been emerging indicates that the fields do not cause genetic damage directly even at relatively high levels [McCann et al., 1993]. The most likely site of interaction is the cell membrane, through the interactions with signal transduction pathways [Luben, 1991]. The possible effects on signal transduction include stimulation or inhibition of receptors or ion channels, alteration of ligand binding, alteration of gene expression, induction of oncogenes, effects in cross-regulation of pathways, and shifts of dose-response curves. Effects of electromagnetic fields resulting from alterations in signal transduction can be synergistic (or antagonistic) with other agents. The calcium ion plays an important role in biosignal transduction. Magnetic fields have been shown in some studies to affect calcium fluxes. A strong magnetic field of 22 mT (induced electric field of 0.1 V/m) affected calcium influx in mitogen-stimulated lympho-cytes. The effect also was correlated with age of the lymphocyte donor. This change did not occur in unstimulated lymphocytes. A study of the dynamics of calcium flux indicated that the magnetic field producing 0.17 V/m in the medium interacted with ligand-mediated channels controlling calcium fluxes but not with the release of calcium from intracellular stores [Liburdy, 1995]. In these studies, dose-response relationships were observed in terms of the induced electric field. Antibody binding to the lymphocyte surface was found to be affected by fields of the same magnitude.

G-protein signal transduction was found to be affected by a magnetic field of 0.1 mT, 60 Hz [Luben, 1991]. Induced electric fields above 0.5 mV/m at 100 Hz were found to affect Na,K-ATPase ion pumps in membranes [Blank, 1992; Liburdy, 1995].

Evidence of various effects on gene expression and protein synthesis at levels of 1 µV/m to 0.1 mV/m was provided by some laboratories. Other laboratories did not corroborate these find-ings. The changes in gene expression can be linked to the ELF field triggering gene transcription by affecting the signal transduction pathways [Liburdy, 1995].

Ornithine decarboxylase (ODC) is an enzyme involved in DNA replication, cell growth, and cell proliferation. Its activity is mediated by cell surface receptor events. ODC activity was affected by magnetic fields producing induced electric fields of 0.01 to 0.1 V/m in three types of normal or transformed cells [Byus et al., 1987]. These findings were corroborated by other laboratories.

91.3 Concluding Remarks

Low-frequency magnetic fields induce electric fields and current in biologic systems. Patterns of these fields and currents are highly nonuniform in cells, tissues, and whole bodies. Very little is known about the actual induced fields on the subcellular, cellular, and even tissue levels and how they may interact with various components of biologic systems. At the same time, laboratory experiments have shown that moderately intense fields can interact with various biologic systems.

These interactions depend on numerous conditions of the exposure and biologic system that are not fully identified. Understanding of underlying biophysical mechanisms of the interactions and quantification of parameters and conditions responsible are important in resolving both the scientific uncertainty and potential public health issue.

References

Ahlbom A, Feychting M, Koskenvue M, et al. 1993. Electromagnetic fields and childhood cancer. Lancet 342:1295.

Anderson LE. 1991. Biological effects of extremely low-frequency electromagnetic fields: In vivo studies. In Plenary Papers: In Vivo Studies, pp 47–89. Workshop, Cincinnati, Ohio. NIOSH publ no 91–111.

Berman E, Chacon L, House D, et al. 1990. Development of chicken embryos in a pulsed magnetic field. Bioelectromagnetics 11:169.

Blank M. 1992. FASEB J 6:2434.

Brent RL, Gordon WE, Bennett WR, Beckman DA. 1993. Reproductive and teratologic effects of electromagnetic fields. Reprod Toxicol Rev 7:535.

Byus CV, Pieper SE, Adey WR., 1987. The effects of low-energy 60-Hz environmental electromagnetic fields upon the growth-related enzyme ornithine decarboxylase. Carcinogenesis 8:1385.

Chernoff N, Rogers JM, Kavet R. 1992. A review of the literature on potential reproductive and developmental toxicity of electric and magnetic fields. Toxicology 74:91.

Cook MR, Graham C, Cohen HD, Gerkovich MM. 1991. A replication study of human exposure to 60-Hz fields: Effect on neurobehavioral measures. Bioelectromagnetics 13:261.

Gandhi OP, Chen J-Y. 1992. Numerical dosimetry at power-line frequencies using anatomically based models. Bioelectromagnetics Suppl 1:43.

Graham C, Cook MR, Cohen HD et al. 1993. EMF suppression of nocturnal melatonin in human volunteers. In Project Abstracts A-31. Savannah, Georgia. Frederick, Md, W/LAssoc Ltd.

Hart FX, Evely K, Finch CD. 1993. Use of a spreadsheet program to calculate the electric field/current density distributions induced in irregularly shaped, inhomogeneous biological structures by low-frequency magnetic fields. Bioelectromagnetics 14:161.

Hart FX. 1992a. Numerical and analytical methods to determine the current density distributions produced in human and rat models by electric and magnetic fields. Bioelectromagnetics Suppl 1:27.

Hart FX. 1992b. Electric fields induced in a rat and human models by 60 Hz magnetic fields: Comparison of calculated and measured values. Bioelectromagnetics 13:313.

Liburdy RP. 1995. Cellular studies and interaction mechanisms of ELF fields. Radio Sci 29:30, in press.

Liburdy RP. 1992. Biological interactions of cellular systems with time-varying magnetic fields. Ann NY Acad Sci 649:74.

London SJ, Thomas DC, Bowman JD, et al. 1991. Exposure to residential electric and magnetic fields and risk of childhood leukemia. Am J Epidemiol 134:923.

Luben RA. 1991. Effects of low-energy electromagnetic fields (pulsed and dc) on membrane signal transduction processes in biological systems. Health Phys 61:15.

McCann J, Dietrich F, Rafferty C, Martin AO. 1993. A critical review of the genotoxic potential of electric and magnetic fields. Mutat Res 297:61.

McGivern RF, Sokol RZ, Adey WR. 1990. Prenatal exposure to a low-frequency electromagnetic field demasculinizes adult scent marking behavior and increases accessory sex organ weights in rats. Teratology 41:1.

McLean J, Lecuyer DW, Davidson C, et al. 1993. Effect of magnetic fields on tumor co-promotion in Sencar mouse skin. BEMS Annual Meeting, June 13–17.

McLean J, Stuchly MA, Mitchel REJ, et al. 1991. Cancer promotion in the mouse skin model by 60 Hz magnetic fields: II. Tumor development and immune response. Bioelectromagnetics 12:273.

McLeod BR, Pilla AA, Sampsel MW. 1983. Electromagnetic fields induced by Helmholtz aiding coils inside saline-filled boundaries. Bioelectromagnetics 4:357.

McLeod KR. 1992. Mecroeklectrode measurements of low frequency electric field effects in cells and tissues. Bioelectromagnetics Suppl 1:161.

Merritt R, Purcell C, Stroink G. 1983. Uniform magnetic fields produced by three, four, and five square coils. Rev Sci Instrum 54:879.

Miller DL. 1991. Miniature-probe measurements of electric fields and currents induced by a 60-Hz magnetic field in rat and human models. Bioelectromagnetics 1:157.

Misakian M. 1991. In-vitro exposure parameters with linearly and circularly polarized ELF magnetic fields. Bioelectromagnetics 12:377.

Misakian M, Kaune WT. 1990. Optimal experimental design for in-vitro studies with ELF magnetic fields. Bioelectromagnetics 11:251.

Misakian M, Kotter FR, Kahler RL. 1978. Miniature ELF electric field probe. Rev Sci Instrum 49:933.

Misakian M, Sheppard AR, Krause D, et al. 1993. Biological, physical, and electrical parameters for in-vitro studies with ELF magnetic and electric fields: a primer. Bioelectromagnetics Suppl 2:1.

NRPB. 1992. Electromagnetic fields and the risk of cancer: Report of an advisory group on non-ionising radiation. National Radiological Protection Board Report 3(1), p. 138.

ORAU. 1992. Health Effects of Low-Frequency Electric and Magnetic Fields. Oak Ridge Associated Universities, Washington, DC.

Polk C. 1986. Introduction. In C Polk, E Postow (eds), Handbook of Biological Effects of Electromagnetic Fields, pp 1–24. Boca Raton, Fla, CRC Press.

Polk C. 1990. Electric fields and surface charges due to ELF magnetic fields. Bioelectromagnetics 11:189.

Polk C. 1992. Dosimetric extrapolations of extremely-low-frequency electric and magnetic fields across biological systems. Bioelectromagnetics Suppl 1:205.

Poole C, Trichopoulos D., 1991. Extremely low-frequency electric and magnetic fields and cancer. Cancer Causes Control 2:267.

Rannug A, Ekstrom T, Hansson Mild K, et al. 1993a. A study on skin tumor formation in mice with 50-Hz magnetic field exposure. Carcinogenesis 14(4):573.

Rannug A, Holmberg B, Hansson Mild K. 1993b. A rat liver foci promotion study with 50-Hz magnetic fields. Environ Res 62:223.

Reiter RJ, Richardson BA. 1992. Magnetic field effects on pineal indoleamine metabolism and possible biological consequences. FASEB J 6:2283.

Savitz DA, Wachtel H, Barnes FA, et al. 1988. Case-control study of childhood cancer and exposure to 60-Hz magnetic fields. Epidemiol 128:21.

Spiegel RJ. 1977. Magnetic coupling to a prolate spheroid model of man. IEEE Trans Power Apparatus Systems PAS-96(1):208.

Stuchly MA. 1990. Applications of time-varying magnetic fields in medicine. Crit Rev Biomed Eng 18:89.

Stuchly MA, McLean JRN, Burnett R, et al. 1992. Modification of tumor promotion in the mouse skin by exposure to an alternating magnetic field. Cancer Lett 65:1.

Stuchly MA, Xi W. 1994. Modeling induced currents in biological cells exposed to low-frequency magnetic fields. Phys Med Biol 39:1319.

Tenforde TS. 1986. Interaction of ELF magnetic fields with living matter. In C Polk, E Postow (eds), Handbook of Biological Effects of Electromagnetic Fields, pp 197–225. Boca Raton, Fla, CRC Press.

Tenforde TS. 1993. Cellular and molecular pathways of extremely low frequency electromagnetic field interactions with living systems. In M Blank (ed), Electricity and Magnetism in Biology and Medicine, pp 1–8. San Francisco, San Francisco Press.

Tenforde TS, Kaune WT. 1987. Interaction of extremely low frequency electric and magnetic fields with humans. Health Phys 53:585.

Theriault G, Goldberg M, Miller AB, et al. 1993 Cancer risk associated with occupational exposure to magnetic fields among electric utility workers in Ontario and Quebec, Canada, and France: 1970–1989. Am J Epidemiol 139(6):550.

Wang W, Litovitz TA, Penafield LM, Meister R. 1992. Determination of the induced ELF electric field distribution in a two layer in vitro system simulating biological cells in nutrient solution. Bioelectromagnetics 14:29.

WHO. 1987. Magnetic Fields: Environmental Health Criteria 69. Geneva, World Health Organization.

Xi W, Stuchly MA. 1994. High spatial resolution analysis of electric currents induced in men by ELF magnetic fields. Appl Comput Electromagnetic Soc J 9:127.

Xi W, Stuchly MA, Gandhi OP. 1994. Induced electric currents in models of men and rodents of 60-Hz magnetic fields. IEEE Trans Biomed Eng 41:1018.

92

Therapeutic Applications of Low-Frequency Sinusoidal and Pulsed Electric and Magnetic Fields

Charles Polk
University of Rhode Island

It has been known for more than 30 years that electric potential differences appear across both living and dead bone subjected to mechanical stress [Fukada and Yasuda, 1957; Bassett and Becker, 1963]. C. A. L. Bassett and R. O. Becker observed that these stress-generated electrical signals decayed very slowly in comparison with similarly initiated signals in piezoelectric crystals and concluded that piezoelectric phenomena "while probably present, were not the sole cause of these potentials." Later analysis and experiments established that the observed signals were primarily due to ion displacement within the porous regions and multiple fluid-filled channels present in all bone [Gross and Williams, 1982].

Having shown that application of a dc electric field to nonexcitable connective tissue cells can produce effects similar to those elicited by mechanical stress, C. A. L. Bassett and his coworkers realized that clinical exploitation of these phenomena would require surgical implantation of electrodes with attendant danger of infection. They proceeded therefore to explore whether non-invasive inductive coupling that gave waveforms similar to those produced endogenously by mechanical stress could lead to beneficial bone development, and they obtained favorable results with pulsed electromagnetic fields on dogs [Bassett et al., 1974]. Signals of this type have generally been identified as PEMF in the orthopedics/electrical stimulation community for the last 20 years and have been applied successfully in a large number of cases for the repair of nonunions [Gossling et al., 1992]. More recently it was found that simultaneous application of dc and sinusoidally time-varying extremely low frequency (ELF) magnetic fields with intensities below 100 µT also could be used for this purpose [Ryaby et al., 1993; Zoltan and Ryaby, 1992].

Although the noninvasive time-varying magnetic field treatment for nonunions (fractures that fail to heal) became—at least in the United States—the most widely used clinical application of subradiofrequency fields, several investigators pursued the application of dc electric fields through implanted electrodes and the application of higher-frequency currents through electrode contacts placed on the skin surface to enhance bone repair [Brighton et al., 1979]. At the same time, laboratory investigations, in vitro and on animals, explored the application of all three modalities—PEMF, implanted dc electrodes, and higher-frequency coupling through skin electrodes—to produce blood vessel regeneration (angiogenesis), soft-tissue healing, nerve repair or regeneration, and regression of tumors. The use of time-varying magnetic fields for the treatment of arthritis also was explored [Trock et al., 1993].

92.1 Bone and Cartilage Repair with PEMF and Other Signals

In the United States, medical devices are approved for clinical use only after it has been shown to the satisfaction of the U.S. Food and Drug Administration (FDA) that they are not only safe but also effective. The devices listed in Table 92.1 are currently (March 1994) approved for one of three applications: the treatment of nonunions (fractures that have failed to heal after standard treatment involving setting and stabilization with casts) and congenital pseudoarthroses [Bassett, 1984] and the promotion of spinal fusion. Although many animal experiments (and possibly a few human trials, especially in Europe) have evaluated the application of electric or magnetic fields for acceleration of fresh fracture healing, for reversal of osteoporosis, and for the treatment of arthritis, no devices are currently approved in the United States for these purposes.

Classified by electrical and mechanical characteristics, the devices in Table 92.1 are either

Noninvasive:

1. Generating time-varying magnetic fields applied by coils to the affected body part (I and PEMF devices A, B, C, and D)
2. Generating time-varying electric fields applied through skin-surface electrodes (capacitively coupled) (E)

Invasive or semi-invasive: dc applied from an implanted battery (F, G) or (semi-invasive) dc applied with percutaneous pins (H).

TABLE 92.1 Electrical Bone Growth Stimulators Approved by the U.S. FDA as of March 1994

Manufacturer	Device	Approved for	Technology	Date	Ref.
Electro-Biology, Inc.	EBI Bone Healing System*	Nonunion, congenital pseudoarthroses, failed fusions	Noninvasive pulsed e.m. field (PEMF)	Nov. 1979	A B
American Medical Electronics, Inc.	Physio-Stim	Nonunions (excluding vertebrae and flat bones)	Noninvasive PEMF	Feb. 1986	C
American Medical Electronics, Inc.	Spinal-Stim	To promote spinal fusion as an adjunct to surgery or as nonoperative treatment when 9 mos. have elapsed since the last surgery	Noninvasive PEMF	Feb. 1990	D
Orthologic Corp.	Orthologic 1000	Nonunion (excluding vertebrae and flat bones)	Noninvasive dc + sinusoidal magnetic fields	March 1994	I
Bioelectron, Inc.	Orthopak BGS System	Nonunions (excluding vertebrae and flat bones)	Noninvasive/capac. coupled	Feb. 1986	E
Electro-Biology, Inc.	Orthogen/Osteogen	Nonunion of long bones	Implantable dc	Jan. 1980	F
Electro-Biology, Inc.	Sp F-4 (2) Implantable BGS†	Spinal fusion adjunct	Implantable dc	April 1987	G
Bioelectron, Inc.	Zimmer direct current bone growth stimulator (DCGBS)	Nonunion fractures	Semi-invasive dc with percutaneous pins	Nov. 1979	H

*Also known as Bi-Osteogen Systems 204.
†Also known as BGS-Osteostim HS 11.

A signal typical for some PEMF (A, C, D) devices is illustrated in Fig. 92.1. Figure 92.1*a* shows the magnetic field versus time, and Fig. 92.1*b* the corresponding electric field induced into a linear, isotropic medium. The waveform shown in Fig. 92.1*b* can be measured by a probe coil having a sufficiently large number of turns. The frequency spectrum of the electric field is shown in Fig. 92.2*a* and *b*. Signals used by the different manufacturers are protected by patents, and FDA approval is for particular signal parameters within specified tolerances on time and amplitude. The pseudoarthrosis signal used by Electrobiology, Inc. (EBI) (B in Table 92.1) consists of single pulses repeated at a rate of 72 pulses per second rather than the pulse bursts illustrated in Figs. 92.1 and 92.2. Each magnetic field pulse increases from 0 to 3.5 mT in 380 µs and then decreases slowly to 0 in approximately 4.5 ms. The signals that are now in use have evolved considerably from those employed in the initial studies, and some have little resemblance to the endogenous electrical signals elicited by mechanical stress.

The PEMF signals employed by the various manufacturers in the United States and Europe can have several different pulse shapes, rise and decay times, pulse widths, pulse repetition rates, and amplitudes. Since it has been shown that all these variables can have a profound effect on the biologic action of a particular signal, it is essential that reports on effectiveness or lack of effectiveness of PEMF give an exact description of the signal that was used. Unfortunately, the medical literature is replete with examples where this information is either incomplete or completely absent. It is particularly important that a PEMF signal not simply be described by its "frequency," when what is meant is the *pulse repetition frequency*. Referring to the legend of Fig. 92.1 and to Fig. 92.2, it is clear that this particular signal should not be identified as a "15-Hz" signal, since it has significant frequency content well into the kilohertz region. Only the spacing between the many different spectral lines is 15 Hz, as is apparent from part *a* of Fig. 92.2.

As a further illustration of the importance of differentiating between simply frequency and pulse repetition frequency, consider the hypothetical signal of Fig. 92.3, which is, however, similar to that of some therapeutic signals. This signal would be correctly described as having a pulse repetition frequency of 20 Hz. However, it should not simply be called a "20-Hz" signal or an "ELF" signal

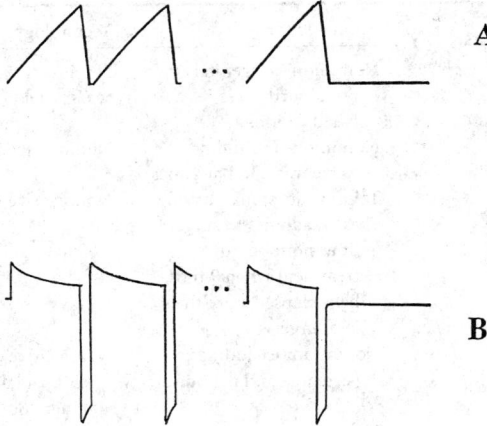

FIGURE 92.1   A typical PEMF signal (signal A of Table 92.1). Signal consists of 15 pulse bursts per second. Each burst is 4.5 ms long and contains 20 magnetic field pulses. In each pulse the magnetic field increases from 0 to approx. 2 mT during 200 µs, decreases to 0 again during 23 µs, and is equal to 0 for 2 µs before the next 225 µs sequence begins. (*a*) Magnetic field versus time. (*b*) Electric field [$\propto/(\partial B/\partial t)$] versus time.

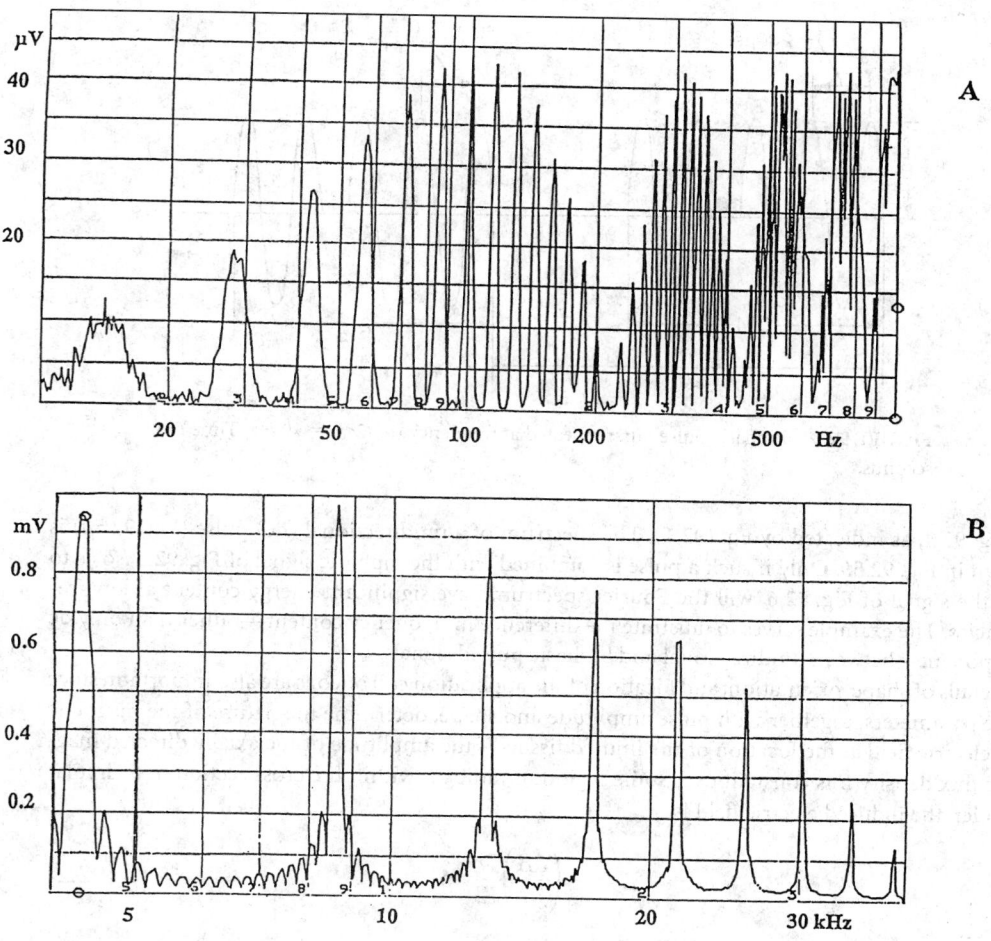

FIGURE 92.2 Electric field spectrum $|E(\omega)|$ of signal in Fig. 92.1 as measured by the output from an air-core coil (self-inductance 0.147 mH, resistance 2.13 Ω, mean radius 1.5 cm). (a) 10 Hz to 1 kHz (frequency resolution: 3 Hz). 100 μV corresponds to 0.6 mT/sHz in a 4.5-ms pulse burst. (b) 1 to 10 kHz (frequency resolution: 10 Hz). 1 mV corresponds to 6 mT/sHz in a 4.5-ms pulse burst.

because very little of its energy is at 20 Hz or even below 1000 Hz. Fourier integral analysis of such a pulse burst [Papoulis, 1962] gives

$$F_1(\omega) = 2\pi \sum_{n=-\infty}^{n=\infty} BT_2\left[\frac{\sin(\omega - \omega_1)T_2}{(\omega - \omega_1)T_2} + \frac{\sin(\omega + \omega_1)T_2}{(\omega + \omega_1)T_2}\right]\delta(\omega - n\omega_0) \quad (92.1)$$

where the delta function $\delta(\omega - n\omega_0)$ indicates discrete spectral lines at multiples of the pulse repetition frequency ($\omega_0/2\pi$), which is 20 Hz in the selected example. The amplitudes of the spectral lines are given by the expression in brackets. The spectral peak for positive frequencies occurs, as illustrated in Fig. 92.4, where $[\sin(\omega - \omega_1)T_2]/(\omega - \omega_1)T_2]$ is equal to 1, which occurs when $\omega = \omega_1$ or at the frequency of the sine wave within each individual burst. In the present example this is $(10^6/200) = 5$ kHz. The duration $2T_2$ of the pulse burst determines the widths of the spectral lobes

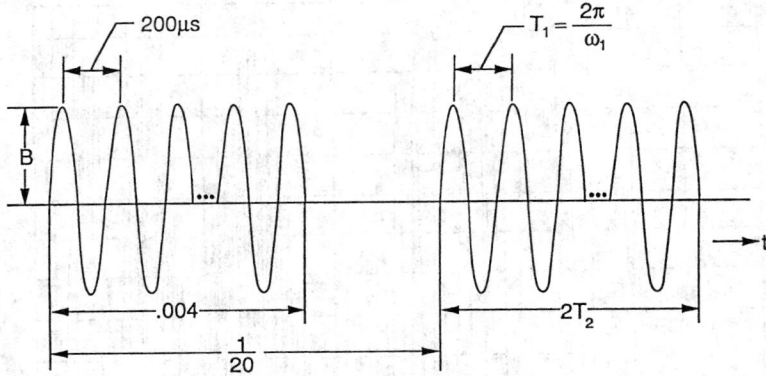

FIGURE 92.3 Biphasic pulse burst repeated at frequency $(\omega_0/2\pi) = 20$ Hz. Time t in seconds.

in Fig. 92.4, as indicated by Eq. (92.1). The spectrum of a unidirectional (dc) pulse (Fig. 92.5*a*) is shown in Fig. 92.5*b*. Only if such a pulse is combined with the biphasic signal of Fig. 92.3, so as to give the signal of Fig. 92.6, will the Fourier spectrum have significant energy content at low frequencies. The example serves to illustrate the difference in frequency content—rather than only dc component—between unidirectional and biphasic pulsed signals.

Details of shape, orientation, and location of the application coil or coils are also important, since these parameters, together with pulse amplitude and shape, determine the nature of the magnetic and electric field at the location of the injured tissue. If the amplitude of the axially directed magnetic flux density B is constant over some region of radius R within the cross section of a circular cylinder, the induced electric field is

$$\mathbf{E} = -\left(\frac{\partial B}{\partial t}\right) \frac{r}{2} \hat{\phi} \tag{92.2}$$

provided the material of the cylinder is electrically homogeneous and isotropic. In Eq. (92.2), $r < R$ is the distance from the center of the cylinder, and $\hat{\phi}$ a unit vector in the circumferential direction. For magnetic fields varying sinusoidally as $B_0 \cos \omega t$, $\mathbf{E} = \omega B_0 (r/2) \sin \omega t \, \hat{\phi}$. Since most biologic objects are neither homogeneous nor isotropic, the actual induced electric fields at various points in the tissue or cells may deviate substantially from the values given by Eq. (92.2) [Polk and Song, 1990; Van Amelsfort, 1990]. Equation (92.2) is useful only for estimating the spatial average value of the induced electric field, which depends in the bone environment, on the point-to-point variation of the electrical properties of muscle, fat, cartilage, periosteum (outer bone membrane), and bone marrow.

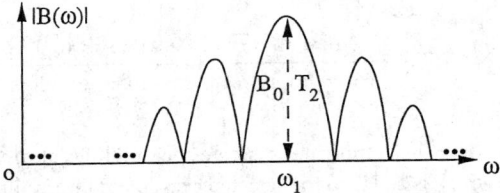

FIGURE 92.4 Spectral envelope of the signal of Fig. 92.3. If a single burst is replaced by bursts repeated at frequency f_0, the continuous spectrum becomes the envelope of spectral lines spaced at intervals f_0.

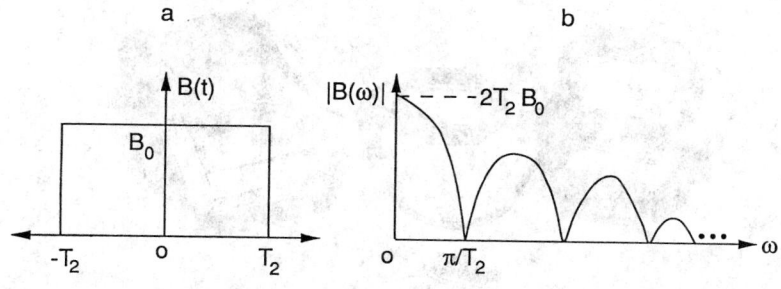

FIGURE 92.5 DC pulse (*a*) and Fourier spectrum (*b*).

Current pulses of the PEMF devices are usually produced by the discharge of capacitor banks controlled by a timing network. The applicator coil cannot be interchanged among different devices because its inductance and resistance are a part of the discharge network. While earlier bone growth stimulators employed Helmholtz coil-pair arrangements, most present devices have single coils which can be custom-shaped for particular limbs. Most commercial units are driven by rechargeable batteries (Fig. 92.7), and control boxes usually include an elapsed-time clock to measure the total time of stimulation of the fracture being treated. A typical treatment time with PEMF devices can be between 2 and 10 hours per day over a period of 6 months and 30 minutes per day with the newer low-field-intensity system (Fig. 92.8, I in Table 92.1).

The so-called capacitively coupled device (E on Table 92.1) generates a continuous sine wave at a frequency of 60 kHz. The total current through the skin contains a not negligible conduction component, since conductive contact is made between the applicator electrodes and the skin that represents a very "leaky" capacitor. Electric fields produced at the tissue level by this device are between 1 and 50 V/m [Pollack and Brighton, 1989]. These levels are very much higher than the average amplitude of the electric fields produced in tissue by PEMF devices and also higher than the instantaneous peak values produced by some of the PEMF systems. It is interesting to note here that in vitro experiments with truly capacitively coupled fields showed enhancement of bone cell proliferation at very much lower amplitude (10^{-5} V/m) when the frequency of the continuous sine wave was 10 Hz rather than 60 kHz [Fitzsimmons et al., 1989].

A typical invasive (implantable) dc device (F, G in Table 92.1) consists of a small (approximately $4 \times 2 \times 0.5$ cm) titanium case and two or four titanium wires. These wires act as the cathode, and the case, which contains the battery that is connected to it, forms the anode. The amplitude of the continuous current is between 5 µA (for some spinal fusion applications) and 20 µA (for nonunion

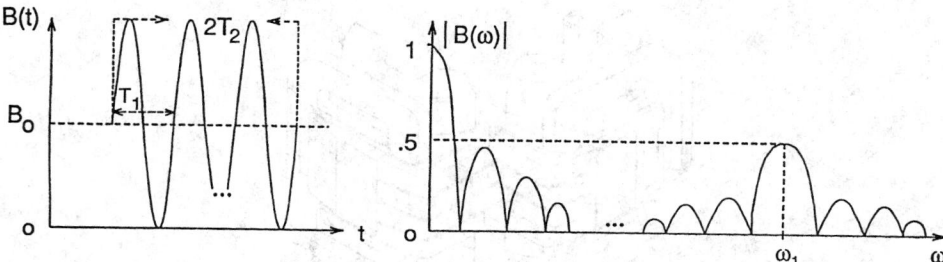

FIGURE 92.6 Unidirectional pulse and spectral envelope. If burst is repeated at frequency f_0, the spectrum consists of discrete spectral lines at f_0 intervals. The illustrated continuous spectrum then becomes the envelope indicating relative amplitudes of the spectral lines.

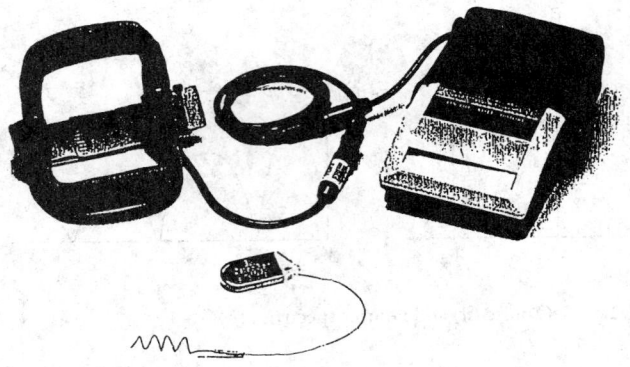

FIGURE 92.7   PEMF applicator and control unit and implantable dc stimulating device (battery with wire electrode) manufactured by Electrobiology, Inc. Systems A and G of Table 92.1. (Photograph courtesy of Electrobiology, Inc.)

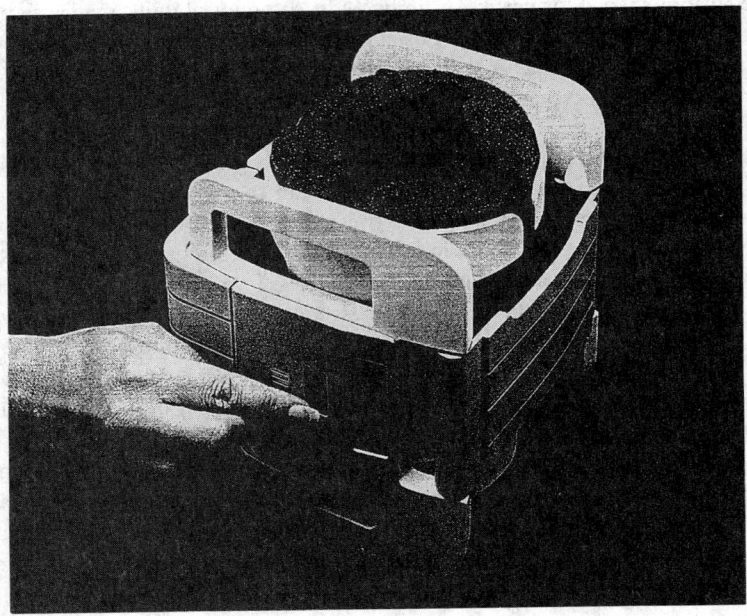

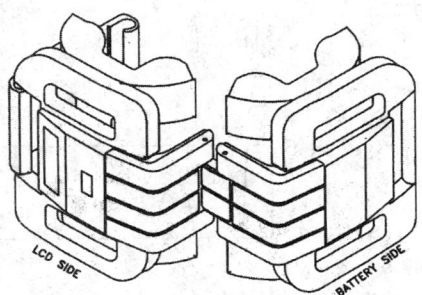

FIGURE 92.8   Applicator of the Orthologic 1000 dc/ac equipment system I of Table 92.1. (Photograph courtesy of Orthologic, Inc.)

of long bones). The cathodes are placed at the location where bone growth is to be enhanced, e.g., at the vertebrae that are surgically fused, while the case is placed in a convenient location some distance from the bone. Treatment details and success rates, in comparison with surgical procedures without use of dc stimulation, are discussed in the medical literature [Nerubay et al., 1986].

Although not used or approved for use in the United States, the German Magnetodyn system [Kraus, 1984] is interesting not only because it employs sinusoidal magnetic fields between 2 and 20 Hz but also because it relies on metallic implants that are used for fixation of the bone to act as the "secondary" of a transformer whose primary is the external applicator. Sometimes an implanted pickup coil (secondary) is connected to fixation bars or to screws (electrically insulated from the bars) on each side of a pseudoarthrotic gap. With this system, peak electric fields of 40 V/m and current densities of 5 A/m^2 have been produced in the gap.

A PEMF signal (similar to B in Table 92.1) also has been used experimentally to arrest osteonecrosis (bone death, possibly due to vascular impairment or toxic agents) of the femoral head. Application for 8 hours per day over 12 months gave substantially better results than the standard surgical (core decompression) treatment [Aaron and Steinberg, 1991].

92.2 Soft-Tissue Repair and Nerve Regeneration

No electric or magnetic system to aid nerve regeneration or soft-tissue repair is approved by the FDA at the present time for nonexperimental therapy. However, considerable animal and in vitro experimentation in this country and abroad suggests the clinical usefulness of electric currents for soft-tissue repair [Canady and Lee, 1991] and possibly also to enhance repair of nerve fibers that have sustained crush or transsection injury [Ito and Bassett, 1983; Siskin et al., 1990]. Since there is a great variety of soft-tissue pathologies that could respond to electric or magnetic fields, the volume of application in this area could in the future become larger than in orthopedics, provided field-tissue and field-cell interactions become better understood and clinical benefits for specific injuries and diseases are established.

Beneficial effects of time-varying electric fields in wound healing are most likely related to promotion of angiogenesis. Wound healing consists of several stages, the first being inflammation, when changes in vascular permeability occur, infiltration of leukocytes and macrophages takes place, and cells migrate, synthesize granulation tissue, collagen, and proteoglycans, and initiate formation of capillaries. This is followed by transitional repair and remodeling phases. Electric currents are probably only important in the first two stages, and the experimental clinical trials performed thus far involve therapy for inflammation [Binder et al., 1984; Ieran et al., 1990].

Very soon after some types of bone injury and pathology were first treated with PEMF, the effects of PEMF on peripheral nerve regeneration became the subject of investigation. Improved neural function that appeared as an unintended "side effect" in the clinical treatment of nonunions lead to a systematic investigation of PEMF effects on neural regeneration in rats [Kort et al., 1980]. Other investigators employed other animal models and also compared PEMF with dc current as agents for neural regeneration. More recent work [Sisken et al., 1990] employed a PEMF signal consisting of 20-ms pulses at a repetition rate of 2 pulses per second with exponential rise and decay times of, respectively, 0.5 and 1 ms. Amplitudes were 0.3 mT for experiments with crush lesions of the sciatic nerve in rats and 0.05 mT for stimulation in vitro of neurite outgrowth in dorsal root ganglia. Estimated values for the induced electric field pulses were 5 mV/m in the animal experiments and 0.7 mV/m in the 60-mm-diameter culture dishes of the in vitro work. Stimulation for 2 hours per day of the in vitro cultures produced approximately 50% enhancement of neurite outgrowth in comparison with controls after 2 days. A report on a very limited (13 subjects) clinical trial [Ellis, 1987] of spinal nerve stimulation in para- and quadriplegics employing pulsed electric current introduced by needle electrodes produced "encouraging results" in terms of increased sensory perception and motor function.

92.3 Mechanisms of Field-Tissue Interaction

It is known that electrokinetic or streaming potentials rather than piezoelectricity make the principal contribution to electric potentials generated by mechanically stressed bone [Gross and Williams, 1982; Lavine and Grodzinsky, 1987]. Thus potential differences appear when mechanical loading displaces fluid that contains "counterions" that normally reside opposite ions fixed to cell or intercellular matrix surfaces. These potentials are likely to play a role in intercellular signaling and in bone as well as cartilage and soft-tissue development. While the original intent of electrical bone therapy was to simply mimic endogenously generated fields, a much wider range of signals was found to be clinically useful. Furthermore, it was found later that some weak ionic currents ($\sim 5 \times 10^{-2}$ A/m^2) appear endogenously without mechanical stress and that extremely weak sinusoidal electric fields can produce profound effects on cells in vitro. For example, transcription (information transfer from DNA to RNA) and translation (formation of new proteins initiated by RNA) have been modified by electric fields estimated at 10^{-5} V/m that were generated inductively by a sinusoidal 60-Hz magnetic field of 5.7 μT [Goodman and Henderson, 1991].

It is likely that the mechanism involved when dc currents are directly applied to injured bone (or other tissue) differs from the transduction sequence that must be acting when low-intensity alternating fields are employed. Even the 5-μA continuous current of the implantable devices (F, G in Table 92.1) when distributed over an (estimated) 5-cm^2 area corresponds to a steady electric field of 1 V/m in bone tissue of 0.01 S/m conductivity. This value is large compared with the average (but not the peak) fields induced in tissue by some PEMF devices [Rubin et al., 1989] or the millivolts per meter ELF sinusoidal fields that affect cartilage and bone development [McLeod and Rubin, 1990]. For example, if one assumes a mean radius of 4 cm for a particular human bone fracture, one obtains from Eq. (92.2) the electric field values between 0.18 and 1.74 V/m shown on Table 92.2.

To clarify the sequence of biologic events that occur when PEMF signals are applied to developing bone, the following in vivo experiment was performed [Aaron, 1989]. Twenty-five milligrams of demineralized rat bone matrix in powdered form was implanted along the thoracic musculature of immature rats. This powder recruits cells from the surrounding tissue leading to formation of cartilage within 6 to 10 days; thereafter, progressive calcification occurs, leading to formation of fibrous particles by days 12 to 14 and formation of a small bone (ossicle). These developments were compared in a large number of paired rats, with equal numbers unexposed and exposed (8 hours per day) to the PEMF signal illustrated on Figs. 92.1 and 92.2 (A in Table 92.1). Estimates of the mean electric fields in the exposed tissues give values equal to about one-fourth those listed on line 1 in Table 92.2. Chemical and histologic analysis of ossicles harvested from animals, sacrificed on every second day, showed that exposure to this PEMF signal at the applied level significantly increased both rate and quantity of cartilage formation and enhanced maturation of the subsequent bone. The experimenters concluded that field exposure either enhanced recruitment or proliferation of cartilage precursor cells, increased differentiation of precursor to cartilage cells, or accelerated maturation of cartilage cells.

Getting closer to fundamental events at the cellular level, both devices A and B (Table 92.1) were used to expose cultured mouse bone cells and mouse skin fibroblasts, as well as explanted mouse

TABLE 92.2   Electric Field (V/m) Induced by Bone Therapy Signals at a Radius of 4 cm into an Electrically Uniform Medium (*B* perpendicular to plane in which radius is defined)

	Positive Peak	Negative Peak	Average of Rectified Signal
PEMF device A (Table 92.1, Figs. 92.1, 92.2, and 92.7)	0.2	1.74	0.024
PEMF device B (Table 92.1)*	0.18	0.015	$(1.4)10^{-4}$
AC-DC device I (Table 92.1, Fig. 92.8)	76.6-Hz sinusoid, peak	$\pm (1.9)10^{-4}$	$(1.2)10^{-4}$

*Signal parameters given on p. 1406 ("pseudoarthrosis" signal).

pineal cells in organ culture [Luben, 1993]. In all three cases, various chemical procedures were employed to examine beta-adrenergic receptors. These are cell surface protein strands that span the cell membrane and emerge from it; they mediate cell response to agents such as epinephrine (adrenaline) and norepinephrine through so-called G-proteins that act essentially as molecular amplifiers at the interior surface of the cell. Other G-proteins are involved in the response to growth factors. The arrangement of the exposure coils and culture plates was such as to give mean electric fields equal to about one-tenth the values shown in Table 92.2. Exposures were of 4 hours duration. Specific types of G-proteins were stimulated by the A signal; others by the B signal. The total number of binding sites on the cells was not affected, but the affinity of the receptors for specific hormones was changed, suggesting a change in receptor conformation. It is interesting to compare this work, which employed peak values on the order of 10^{-2} V/m and time averaged values not greater than $2(10^{-3})$ V/m, with other in vitro experiments showing effects on enzyme activity at the cell surface by ELF sinusoidal fields between $5(10^{-4})$ V/m and 30 V/m [Blank, 1992].

How such weak, low-frequency electric and magnetic fields are translated into biochemical activity is at the present time not known. Field energies are orders of magnitude below levels that would produce thermal effects, and in most cases, potential differences produced across cell membranes also appear to be below thermal equilibrium ("Johnson") noise. References to several possible models of field-to-biochemical process transduction are given in the introduction to Section IX and in Chapter 91. One of the devices (I in Table 92.1) approved by the FDA for the treatment of nonunions is based on either the cyclotron resonance [Liboff and McLeod, 1988] or the parametric resonance model [Lednev, 1991, 1993]. In this device, a dc magnetic field B_0 of 20 μT is used to obtain an ion cyclotron frequency f_c or an integral multiple of it. This frequency is given by

$$f_c = \frac{QB_0}{2\pi m} \tag{92.3}$$

where Q is the charge of the ion and m its mass. The fifth harmonic of f_c for $^{40}Ca^{2+}$ and the third harmonic for $^{24.3}Mg^{2+}$ are equal to 76.6 Hz when $B_0 = 20$ μT. An alternating 76.6-Hz magnetic field of 40 μT is applied through the same coil as the dc field. This parallel field combination has been reported to increase the concentration of the important growth factor IGF-II in a culture medium containing the osteosarcoma cell line TE-85 after 30 minutes of exposure [Fitzsimmons et al., 1993], to affect articular cartilage metabolism [Ryaby et al., 1993a], and to prevent bone loss due to castration in rats [Ryaby et al., 1993b].

Defining Terms

Angiogenesis: Formation of blood vessels.

Biphasic signals (in the context of bone stimulation): An electric or magnetic field signal with both positive and negative components (as opposed to a unidirectional pulse signal).

Capacitively coupled device: An electrical stimulating device (usually for enhancement of bone growth) which employs metallic plates for application of an electric signal to the body part (usually a limb) under treatment. In the 60-kHz device (E) listed in Table 92.1, conductive contact is made with the skin; therefore, current flow consists of both conductive and displacement components.

Cell line: A cell culture derived from a single neoplastic progenitor cell and therefore with homogeneous genetic constitution.

Cyclotron resonance: The condition under which an electrically charged particle continuously gains energy (provided collision damping is not excessive) as it moves in a circular orbit of increasing radius under the simultaneous influence of a dc magnetic field and a circumferential electric field whose frequency is given by Eq. (92.3). This electric field can be generated by an alternating magnetic field whose direction is parallel to that of the dc field.

Extremely low frequency (ELF):   A frequency between 3 and 300 Hz.

Ion cyclotron frequency: The frequency given by Eq. (92.3) for an ion of charge Q (Q is equal to the electronic charge, 1.602×10^{-19} C, or the integral multiple thereof appropriate for the particular ion).

Nonunion: A bone fracture that fails to heal under conventional treatment within the normally expected time.

Parametric resonance: A resonance condition involving Zeeman splitting of a vibrational energy level and consequent changes in the transition probability whose frequency is given by Eq. (92.3). Vibrational levels of an ion within a protein molecule would be at ELF with dc magnetic fields below 100 μT (for details see Lednev, [1991, 1993] and Blanchard and Blackman, [1994]).

Pseudoarthrosis: A false joint formed on the shaft of a long bone. Either congenital or formed at the site of a fracture that failed to fuse.

Pulsed electromagnetic field (PEMF):   A term used frequently in the electrical stimulation literature for a pulsed magnetic field that is capable of inducing an electric field and current as a consequence of Faraday's law. Depending on pulse width and pulse shape, the spectrum of PEMF bone stimulation signals may contain components in the ELF and/or VLF (up to 100 kHz) range.

Spinal fusion: The surgical fusion of two or more vertebral segments in order to eliminate motion between them (sometimes performed to mitigate pain resulting from degenerative bone disease).

References

Aaron RK, Ciombor DM, Grant J. 1989. Stimulation of experimental endochondral ossification by low-energy pulsing electromagnetic fields. J Bone Miner Res 4(2):227.

Aaron RK, Steinberg E. 1991. Electrical stimulation of the femoral head. Semin Arthrop 2–3:214.

Bassett CAL. 1984. Biology of fracture repair, nonunion and pseudoarthrosis. In HR Goosling, SL Pillsbury (eds), Compilations of Fracture Management, pp 1–8. Philadelphia Lippincott.

Bassett CAL, Becker RO. 1963. Generation of electric potentials by bone in response to mechanical stress. Science 137:1063.

Bassett CAL, Pawluck RJ, Pilla AA. 1974. Augmentation of bone repair by inductively coupled electromagnetic fields. Science 184:575.

Binder A, Parr G, Hazelman B, Fitton-Jackson S. 1984. Pulsed electromagnetic field therapy of persistent rotator cuff tendinitis: A double-blind controlled clinical assessment. Lancet 2:695.

Blanchard JP, Blackman CF. 1994. Clarification and application of the ion paramagnetic resonance model for magnetic field interaction with biological systems. Bioelectromagnetics 15:217–238.

Blank M. 1992. Na,K-ATPase function in alternating electric fields. FASEB J 6:2434.

Brighton CT, Friederberg ZB, Black J. 1979. Evaluation of the use of constant direct current in the treatment of nonunion. In CT Brighton, J Blank, SR Pollack (eds), Electrical Properties of Bone and Cartilage, pp 519–545. New York, Grune & Stratton.

Canady DJ, Lee RC. 1991. Scientific basis for clinical applications of electric fields in soft tissue repair. In CT Brighton, SR Pollack (eds), Electromagnetics in Medicine and Biology, pp 275–280. San Francisco, San Francisco Press.

Ellis W. 1987. Pulsed subcutaneous electrical stimulation in spinal cord injury: Preliminary results. Bioelectromagnetics 8:159.

Fitzsimmons RJ, Baylink DJ, Ryaby JT, Magee F. 1993. EMF-stimulated bone-cell proliferation. In M Blank (ed), Electricity and Magnetism in Biology and Medicine, pp 899–901. San Francisco, San Francisco Press.

Fitzsimmons RJ, Farley J, Adey WR, Baylink DJ. 1989. Embryonic bone matrix formation is increased after exposure to a low amplitude capacitively coupled electric field in vitro. Biochim Biophys Acta 882:51.

Fukada E, Yasuda I. 1957. On the piezoelectric effect in bone. J Phys Soc Jpn 12:1158.

Goodman R, Henderson SA. 1991. Transcription and translation in cells exposed to extremely low frequency electromagnetic fields. Bioelectrochem Bioenerget 25:335.

Gossling HR, Bernstein RA, Abbott J. 1992. Treatment of ununited tibial fractures: A comparison of surgery and pulsed electromagnetic fields (PEMF). Orthopaedics 15(6):711.

Gross D, Williams WS. 1982. Streaming potential and the electromechanical response of physiologically moist bone. J Biomech 15:227.

Ieran M, Zaffuto S, Bagnacani M, et al. 1990. Effect of low frequency pulsing electromagnetic fields on skin ulcers of venous origin in humans; A double-blind study. J Orthop Res 8(2):276.

Ito H, Bassett CAL. 1983. Effect of weak, pulsing electromagnetic fields on neural regeneration in the rat. Clin Orthop 181:283.

Kort J, Ito H, Bassett CAL. 1980. Effects of pulsing electromagnetic fields on peripheral nerve regeneration. J Bone Joint Surg Orthop Trans 4:238.

Lavine LS, Grodzinsky AJ. 1987. Electrical stimulation of repair of bone. J Bone Joint Surg 69(4):626.

Lednev VV. 1991. Possible mechanism for the influence of weak magnetic fields on biological systems. Bioelectromagnetics, 12:71.

Lednev VV. 1993. Possible mechanism for the effect of weak magnetic fields on biological systems: Correction of the basic expression and its consequences. In M Blank (ed), Electricity and Magnetism in Biology and Medicine, pp 227–233. San Francisco, San Francisco Press.

Liboff AR, McLeod BR. 1988. Kinetics of channelized membrane ions in magnetic fields. Bioelectromagnetics 9:39.

Luben RA. 1993. Effects of low energy electromagnetic fields on signal transduction by G-protein-linked receptors. In M Blank (ed), Electricity and Magnetism in Biology and Medicine, pp 57–62. San Francisco, San Francisco Press.

McLeod KJ, Rubin CT. 1990. Frequency specific modulation of bone adaptation by induced electric fields. J Theor Biol 145:385.

Nerubay J, Marganit B, Bubis JJ, et al. 1986. Stimulation of bone formation by electrical current on spinal fusion. Spine 11:167.

Papoulis A. 1962. The Fourier Integral and Its Applications. New York, McGraw-Hill.

Polk C, Song JH. 1990. Electric fields induced by low frequency magnetic fields in inhomogeneous biological structures that are surrounded by an electric insulator. Bioelectromagnetics 11:235.

Pollack SR, Brighton CT. 1989. Dosimetry in electrical stimulation. In Bioelectric Repair and Growth Society Transactions, PIX-40.

Rubin CT, McLeod KJ, Lanyon LE. 1989. Prevention of osteoporosis by pulsed electromagnetic fields. J Bone Joint Surg 71A(3):411.

Ryaby JT, Magee FP, Weinstein AM. 1993a. The effect of combined ac/dc magnetic fields on resting articular cartilage metabolism. In M Blank (ed), Electricity and Magnetism in Biology and Medicine, pp 371–374. San Francisco, San Francisco Press.

Ryaby JT, Magee FP, Weinstein AM, et al. 1993b. Prevention of experimental osteopenia by use of combined ac/dc magnetic fields. In M Blank (ed), Electricity and Magnetism in Biology and Medicine, pp 807–810. San Francisco, San Francisco Press.

Siskin BF, Kanje M, Lundborg G, Kurtz W. 1990. Pulsed electromagnetic fields stimulate nerve regeneration in vitro and in vivo. Restor Neurol Neurosci 1:303.

Trock DH, Bollet AJ, Dyer RH, et al. 1993. A double-blind trial of the clinical effect of pulsed electromagnetic fields in osteoarthritis. J Rheumatol 20(3):456.

Van Amelsfort AMJ. 1990. An Analytical Algorithm for Solving Inhomogeneous Electromagnetic Boundary-Value Problems for a Set of Coaxial Circular Cylinders. Eindhoven, The Netherlands, James Clerk Maxwell Foundation.

Zoltan JD, Ryaby YT. 1992. Exogenous signal generators: A review of the electrical stimulation of bone. Int J Orthop Trauma 2:25.

Further Information

Additional information on the application of dc as well as low-frequency and pulsed electric and magnetic fields for bone and soft tissue repair can be found in the following:

Black J. 1987. Electrical Stimulation. New York, Praeger.

Brighton CT, Black J, Pollack S (eds). 1979. Electrical Properties of Bone and Cartilage. New York, Grune & Stratton.

Brighton CT, Pollack SR (eds). 1991. Electromagnetics in Medicine and Biology. San Francisco, San Francisco Press.

Polk C. 1995. Electric and magnetic fields for bone and soft tissue repair. In C Polk, E Postow (eds), CRC Handbook of Biological Effects of Electromagnetic Fields, 2d ed. Boca Raton, Fla, CRC Press.

Transactions of the Bioelectric Repair and Growth Society, vols. I through XIII. Published annually since 1980 by the Bioelectric Repair and Growth Society, P.O. Box 64, Dresher, PA 19025.

93

Biologic Effects of Radiofrequency and Microwave Fields: In Vivo and in Vitro Experimental Results

Edward Elson
Walter Reed Army Institute of Research

Radiofrequency radiation (RFR), defined by the Institute of Electrical and Electronics Engineers (IEEE) as extending from 3 kHz to 300 GHz, is absorbed by biologic systems, which are water-dominated dielectrics richly endowed with electrolytes and intricately packaged polar and nonpolar molecules. At sufficiently high RF intensities, thermal energy is generated that can quickly produce morbidity and, after thermoregulatory mechanisms are overwhelmed, mortality. In recent years, work has focused on possible effects at "nonthermal" levels or under conditions in which physiologic temperature can be maintained by regulatory mechanisms of living systems.

The human perception of microwave heating has been studied [1]. Although the human is the ultimate "test object," the bulk of research has been on animals. This requires an understanding and appreciation of biophysical principles and comparative medicine. Such studies require interspecies "scaling," [2–6] the selection of biomedical parameters that reflect basic physiologic functions, and differentiation of adaptational or compensatory changes from pathologic manifestations. In comparing results of experiments performed in the same or different laboratories, standardization of conditions is important and, unfortunately, all too often not attained.

Even by using approaches where absorbed energy patterns in a test animal are set to approximate as closely as possible the patterns that may exist in humans under certain exposure conditions, the intrinsic physical and physiologic dissimilarities between species further confound the problem of extrapolating between animals and humans. In addition to the obvious external geometric differences, the differences in internal vascular anatomy and mechanisms of heat dissipation in fur-bearing animals compared with humans must be taken into consideration.

Johnson [7] has described factors that affect absorption of electromagnetic energy in animals. This absorption is dependent on the size and geometry of the animal relative to the wavelength and polarization. The wavelength-to-animal size relationship (λ/a, where a is the longest axis dimension of the body and the electric field vector is parallel to the longest axis) is a critical factor in the relative absorption cross section (RAC). The RAC is the ratio of the absorbed power to the power incident on the geometric cross-sectional area of the animal [8]. This produces the immediate result that at a given frequency and power density, the specific absorption rate (SAR) is vastly different in animals depending on size. To produce an identical whole-body average SAR, one must scale from one frequency to another. It is of practical importance to realize that experiments on biologic effects at 2.45 GHz on small animals, such as mice and rats, do not scale to humans at 2.45 GHz but to effects on humans at approximately 100 MHz. In recent years, much modeling and experimental measurement have been done on the variation of localized absorption in animals and humans [9].

93.1 Cellular and Molecular Biology

The mutagenic potential of microwave energy has been evaluated by various techniques, including point mutations in bacterial assays [10], the dominant lethal test in mammalian systems [11], and genetic transmission in *Drosophila* [12], with inconsistent results. Two studies reported effects of RFR on sister chromatid exchange [13,14]. Such changes as were seen appeared to be related to temperature elevations rather than RF exposure. From many studies there is little evidence that exposure to RF radiation induces mutations in bacteria, yeasts, fruit flies, or mammals. One study reported cytogenetic effects at 200 W/m^2 [15], but its finding was contradicted by another study [16] that failed to find any cytogenetic effects at 2 to 5 kW/m^2.

There is a consensus among students of the subject that RF radiation does not initiate carcinogenesis by inflicting direct damage on the genome by any mechanism resembling the effect of ionizing radiation. This is evident from the low photon energies involved. RF radiation as part of a compound stress on intact animals has been studied with conflicting results. Fibroblasts in tissue culture were exposed to benzpyrene and the promoter 12-*o*-tetradecanoylphorbol with and without 2.45-GHz microwaves, SAR 4.4 W/kg. Microwave exposure produced a several-fold increase in transformation frequency [17].

In a study of long-term, low-level microwave exposure of rats, Chou et al. [18] compared 100 rats exposed to 2.45-GHz pulsed microwaves, average SAR 0.15 to 0.4 W/kg, 21 hours per day for 25 months with suitable controls. No adverse effects were found. An increase in malignancies of specific type in exposed animals was found, but a significant increase in malignancies of all types was not found. This was interpreted as minimal evidence of "carcinogenic action."

93.2 Reproduction, Growth, and Development

The effect of microwaves on the testes has been studied extensively [19–21]. Exposure of the scrotal area at high power densities (>500 W/m^2) results in varying degrees of testicular damage, such as edema, necrosis of seminiferous tubules, and atrophy, at 2.45, 3, and 10 GHz.

Lebovitz et al. [22] compared pulse-modulated 1.3-GHz microwaves with conventional heating in rats. Anesthetized animals were sacrificed over the 13-day cycle of maturation of seminiferous epithelium during which test animals were subjected to conventional heating or microwave exposure. At 7.7 W/kg whole-body average SAR for 90 minutes (producing a colonic temperature of 40°C), there was a modest decline in daily sperm production. Exposure for a similar time to 4.2 W/kg (colonic temperature of 38°C) produced no change. Above 7.7 W/kg, all germ cell types were destroyed. Conventional heating in excess of 39°C for 60 minutes produced a significant decrease in daily sperm production. The authors stated that all damage could be explained by heating. Although the general consensus is that damage is thermally mediated, Cleary et al. [23] reported decreases in sperm function in vitro utilizing suspension of mouse sperm exposed to SARs of 50 W/kg or greater but with stringent temperature control.

Effects on embryonic development have been studied. Thermal stress appears to be the primary mechanism by which RF energy absorption exerts a teratogenic action. Chernovetz et al. [24] and others have pointed out evidence that indicates that increases in mortality and resorption are probably related to peak body temperature and its duration regardless of the method by which the temperature elevation is elicited. Rugh and McManaway [25] were able to prevent the increase in incidence of teratogenic activity, which they had previously reported, by lowering the maternal body temperature through controlled use of pentobarbital anesthesia. The most common result from many studies [26] appears to be a reduced or retarded gain of body mass, thermally mediated.

93.3 Effects on the Nervous System

Guy and Chou [27] studied response thresholds in rats for short, high-intensity microwave pulses. Rats were exposed to single 915-MHz RF pulses of 1-μs to 300-ms duration. No reaction occurred until the SAR rose to 28 kJ/kg, which correlated with a temperature rise in the brain of 8°C. Seizures occurred followed by unconsciousness for 4 to 5 minutes. Complete recovery ensued. Postmortem examination revealed some demyelination of neurons 1 day following exposure and focal gliosis 1 month after exposure. More intense exposures could produce a fatal outcome. Brown et al. [28] looked for response thresholds at lower energies, with particular attention to the onset of an involuntary, generalized muscular contraction that did not appear to be injurious.

Studies of low-level chronic effects, mostly dating to the 1960s and 1970s, have yielded inconsistent results. Problems of dosimetric measurement and quantitation of reproducible biologic endpoints have left uncertain whether extended exposure to low-intensity or nonthermal levels of radiofrequency energy produces effects, adverse or not. Electroencephalographic changes have been reported during exposures to RF energy, but inability to standardize dosimetry and reproduce effects from one laboratory to another have left doubt as to the reality of such effects. Much work depended on the insertion of metallic electrodes into the skull. Johnson and Guy [29] pointed out that metallic electrodes perturb the field, produce enhanced absorption of energy in the vicinity of the electrodes, and introduce an artifact in the tissue preparation. Recording artifacts also result from pickup of fields by EEG electrodes during RF exposure. Bawin et al. [30] reported that electromagnetic energy of 147 MHz, amplitude modulated, at brain wave frequencies (8 to 16 Hz), influenced spontaneous and conditioned EEG patterns in the cat at 10 W/m². No effects were seen at other modulation frequencies.

At high field intensities, when death is a result of hyperthermia, pathologic changes are identical to those of hyperthermia. At lower levels of exposure, there are no changes that are specific to RF radiation. From the work of Albert and DeSantis [31], there appears to be a threshold for permanent histologic damage to the brain for exposures lasting several hours per day for up to 3 weeks at between 100 and 250 W/m² at 2.45 GHz CW.

An historically controversial issue has been the effect of radiofrequency radiation on the blood-brain barrier (BBB). This poorly understood functional "barrier" provides resistance to movements of large-molecular-weight, fat-insoluble substances from the blood vessels of the brain into brain tissue, presumably to protect the brain from invasion by various blood-borne pathogens and toxic substances. Early reports asserted that RF radiation reduces the barrier, allowing many substances normally barred from brain tissue to enter. Considerable work was done to verify and characterize this process, which oncologists originally hoped could be exploited to allow the passage of antineoplastic drugs, normally excluded from the brain, to enter and attack brain tumors directly. Much of the work was conflicting, but it does appear that gross hyperthermia (brain tissue elevated to 43°C) compromises the barrier [32]. Such a temperature elevation also produces tissue necrosis and is clinically intolerable. There is even evidence that the level of a drug entering the brain might actually be reduced at "moderate" levels of hyperthermia [32].

A number of studies on isolated nerve preparations have been performed. There is no direct production of a nerve impulse or action potential by CW or PW microwaves, but conduction velocity and amplitude can be changed, mediated by temperature elevations of at least 1°C in the solution. Similar changes can be produced by ambient changes in temperature [33].

93.4 Behavioral Effects

Studies have been conducted on the effects of RFR on performance of trained tasks or operant behavior by rats and rhesus and squirrel monkeys [34,35]. All the studies indicated that the exposure would result in suppressed performance of the trained task and that an energy/dose threshold for achieving the suppression existed. Depending on duration and other parameters of exposure, the threshold power density for affecting trained behavior ranged between 50 and 500 W/m². Lebovitz [36] and Akyel et al. [37] were unable to find any specific effect attributed to pulse power and noted that interference with behavior appeared to be of thermal origin. Raslear et al. [39] and Akyel et al. [38] later found performance deficits at very high-peak, short-pulse powers at low repetition rates, such that no measurable temperature changes occurred in the brains of rats. Peak brain SAR was reported to be 7 MW/kg for 80-ns-wide pulses with an average brain SAR of 0.07 W/kg.

93.5 Effects on the Cardiovascular and Hematopoietic Systems

At nonthermalizing levels of exposure, both bradycardia and tachycardia have been found in different studies of different animals and with inconsistent results in the same animal. The specific conditions of exposure, biologic variability, and other sources of error could account for the findings.

Hyperthermia of RFR or non-RFR origin produces tachycardia and a decrease in total peripheral resistance caused by vasodilation, a heat dissipating response to the thermal burden. Variations from this general principle have been found in unusual circumstances, including the application of localized pulse power to the head, neck, and thoracic region [40].

Changes in the concentrations of circulating blood cells have been observed in a number of animal species exposed to microwave energy. The changes were not consistent within or between species and depended on exposure conditions and thermal changes in tissue. A number of mechanisms have been proposed to explain changes in cellular dynamics, including stimulation of synthesis at thermal levels, recirculation of sequestered cells, and increased hypothalamic-hypophysial-adrenal function following thermal stress. Such changes may be related to changes in immune function noted by a number of investigators [41].

93.6 Auditory and Ocular Effects

Microwave hearing, the perception of a clicking or buzzing in the presence of pulsed microwave energy (but not CW) at low power densities [42], has been attributed to thermoelastic transduction of pulsed microwaves in the head, with detection by the sensory epithelium of the cochlea. The process, familiar to occupationally exposed workers, appears not to be harmful at energies commonly encountered [43].

A threshold for cataract production in the lens of the rabbit eye has been found for 2.45-GHz microwaves at 1.5 kW/m² for 100 minutes. An intraocular temperature elevated to at least 45°C appears to be required [44]. For exposures lower than this there does not appear to be a cumulative effect from microwave exposure, i.e., no pathologic damage following many exposures with time, for which each individual exposure produces no detectable damage.

93.7 Conclusion

Elucidation of the biologic effects of RF exposure requires study of the available literature. Evaluating the research is a difficult task even for scientists specializing in the field. The possible sources of error of the biologic sciences are coupled with the sources of error associated with RF engineering and dosimetry. It is often difficult to make meaningful comparisons between studies. The issue of effects or even hazards at "nonthermal" levels of exposure stimulates continuing debate and research that may affect existing consensus safety standards. Whether existing standards are adequate frequently rests on a determination of whether documented effects constitute actual hazards at energy levels not producing morbidity. The research of the future will continue to affect the issue of safe levels of exposure.

Acknowledgments

I wish to thank Mrs. Doris Michaelson for her support and permission to base this review on Dr. S. Michaelson's monograph that appeared in the *Handbook of Biological Effects of Electromagnetic Fields*, published by CRC Press in 1986. The opinions or assertions contained are private views of the author and are not to be construed as reflecting the official views of the Department of the Army or the Department of Defense.

Defining Terms

Blood-brain barrier: An anatomical and physiologic barrier to the movement of large-molecular-weight, fat-insoluble substances from the blood vessels of the brain into brain tissue.

Bradycardia: An abnormal slowness of the heartbeat, as evidenced by slowing of the pulse rate to 60 or less.

Radiofrequency radiation (RFR): Defined by the Institute of Electrical and Electronics Engineers (IEEE) as that part of the electromagnetic spectrum extending from 3 kHz to 300 GHz.

Relative absorption cross section (RAC): The ratio of the absorbed power to the power incident on the geometrical cross-sectional area of an animal.

Tachycardia: An excessive rapidity in the action of the heart, usually applied to a pulse rate above 100 per minute.

References

1. Biological Effects of Radiofrequency Radiation, EPA-600/8-83-026F, Health Effects Research Laboratory, United States Environmental Protection Agency, Research Triangle Park, NC, 1984, pp 5–76.
2. Durney CH, Johnson CC, Barber PW, et al. 1978. Radiofrequency Radiation Dosimetry Handbook, 2d ed. USAF Report SAM-TR-78-22, Brooks Air Force Base, Texas.
3. Gandhi OP. 1975. Conditions of strongest electromagnetic power deposition in man and animals. IEEE Trans Microwave Theory Technol 23:1021.
4. Gandhi OP. 1980. State of knowledge for electromagnetic absorbed dose in man and animals. Proc IEEE 68:24.
5. Gandhi OP, Hunt EL, D'Andrea JA. 1977. Deposition of electromagnetic energy in animals and in models of man with and without grounding and reflector effects. Radio Sci 12 (6S):39.
6. Guy AW. 1974. Quantitation of induced electromagnetic field patterns and associated biologic effects. In P Czerski et al (eds), Biologic Effects and Health Hazards of Microwave Radiation, p. 203. Warsaw, Polish Medical Publishers.

7. Johnson CC. 1975. Recommendations for specifying EM wave irradiation conditions in bioeffects research. J Microwave Power 10:249.

8. Anne A, Saito M, Salati OM, Schwan HP. 1962. Relative microwave absorption cross sections of biological significance. In MF Peyton (ed), Proceedings of the 4th Annual Tri-Service Conference on the Biological Effects of Microwave Radiating Equipment; Biological Effects of Microwave Radiation, New York, Plenum Press.

9. Gandhi OP. 1990. Electromagnetic energy absorption in humans and animals. In OP Gandhi (ed), Biological Effects and Medical Applications of Electromagnetic Energy, p 175. Englewood Cliffs, New Jersey, Prentice-Hall.

10. Anderstam B, Hamnerius Y, Hussain S, Ehrenberg L. 1983. Studies of possible genetic effects in bacteria of high frequency electromagnetic fields. Hereditas 98:11.

11. Varma MM, Traboulay EA. 1976. Evaluation of dominant lethal test and DNA studies in measuring mutagenicity caused by non-ionizing radiation. In CC Johnson, ML Shore (eds), Biological Effects of Electromagnetic Waves, vol 1, p 386. Publication (FDA) 77-8010, U.S. Department of Health Education, and Welfare, Rockville, Md.

12. Mittler S. 1976. Failure of 2 and 20 meter radio waves to induce genetic damage in Drosophila melanogaster. Environ Res 11:326.

13. Livingston GK, Johnson CC, Dethlefsen LA. 1977. Comparative effects of water bath and microwave-induced hyperthermia on cell survival and sister chromatid exchange in Chinese hamster ovary cells. In Abstracts of the International Symposium on the Biological Effects of Electromagnetic Waves, Airlie, Va, p 106.

14. McRee DI, MacNichols G, Livingston GD. 1981. Incidence of sister chromatid exchange in bone marrow cells of the mouse following microwave exposure. Radiat Res 85:340.

15. Stodolnik-Baranska W. 1974. The effects of microwaves on human lymphocyte cultures. In P Czerski et al (eds), Biologic Effects and Health Hazards of Microwave Radiation, p 189. Warsaw, Polish Medical Publishers.

16. Chen KM, Samuel A, Hoopingavner R. 1974. Chromosomal abberrations of living cells induced by microwave radiation. Environ Lett 6:37.

17. Balcer-Kubiczek EK, Harrison GH. 1985. Evidence for microwave carcinogenesis in vitro. Carcinogenesis 6:859.

18. Chou C-K, Guy AW, Kung LL, et al. 1992. Long-term, low-level microwave irradiation of rats. Bioelectromagnetics 13:469.

19. Ely TS, Goldman D, Hearon JZ, et al. 1964. Heating characteristics of laboratory animals exposed to ten centimeter microwaves. U.S. Naval Medical Research Institute (res. rep. proj. NM 001-056.13.02), Bethesda, Md. IEEE Trans Biomed Eng 11:123.

20. Gorodetskaya SF. 1963. The effect of centimeter radio waves on mouse fertility. Fiziol Zh 9:394.

21. Imig CJ, Thomson JD, Hines HM. 1948. Testicular degeneration as a result of microwave irradiation. Proc Soc Exp Biol 69:382.

22. Lebovitz RM, Johnson L, Samson WK. 1987. Effects of pulse-modulated microwave radiation and conventional heating on sperm production. J Appl Physiol 62:245.

23. Cleary SF, Liu LM, Graham R, East J. 1989. In vitro fertilization of mouse ova by spermatazoa exposed isothermally to radio-frequency radiation. Bioelectromagnetics 10:361.

24. Chernovetz ME, Justesen DR, King NW, Wagner JE. 1975. Teratology, survival, and reversal learning after fetal irradiation of mice by 2450 MHz microwave energy. J Microwave Power 10:391.

25. Rugh R, McManaway M. 1976. Can electromagnetic waves cause congenital anomalies? In International IEEE/AP-S USN/URSI Symposium, Amherst, Mass, p 143.

26. O'Connor ME. 1980. Mammalian teratogenesis and radiofrequency fields. Proc IEEE 68:56.

27. Guy AW, Chou CK. 1982. Effects of high-intensity microwave pulse exposure of rat brain. Radio Sci 17(5S):169.

28. Brown DO, Lu S-T, Elson EC. 1994. Characteristics of microwave evoked body movements in mice. Bioelectromagnetics 15:143.

29. Johnson CC, Guy AW. 1972. Non-ionizing electromagnetic wave effects in biological materials and system. Proc IEEE 60:692.

30. Bawin SM, Adey WR. 1977. Calcium binding in cerebral tissue. In DG Hazzard (ed), Symposium on Biological Effects and Measurement of Radio Frequency/Microwaves. Publication (FDA) 77-8026, U.S. Department of Health, Education and Welfare, Rockville, Md.

31. Albert EN, DeSantis M. 1975. Do microwaves alter nervous system-structure? Ann NY Acad Sci 247:87.

32. Williams WM, Lu S-T, Del Cerro M, et al. 1984. Effects of 2450 MHz microwave energy on the blood-brain barrier: an overview and critique of past and present research. IEEE Trans Microwave Theory Technol 32:808.

33. Chou C-K, Guy AW. 1978. Effects of electromagnetic fields on isolated nerve and muscle preparations. IEEE Trans Microwave Theory Technol 26:141.

34. Gage MI, Guyer WM. 1982. Interaction of ambient temperature and controlled behavior in the rat. Radio Sci 17(5S):179.

35. deLorge JO. 1983. Operant behavior and colonic temperature of Rhesus monkeys, Macaca mulatta, exposed to microwaves at frequencies above and near whole-body resonance. Report no. NAMRL-1289, Naval Aerospace Medical Research Lab., Pensacola, Fla.

36. Lebovitz RM. 1983. Pulse modulated and continuous wave microwave radiation yield equivalent changes in operant behavior of rodents. Physiol Behav 30:391.

37. Akyel Y, Hunt EL, Gambrill C, Vargas C Jr. 1991. Immediate post-exposure effects of high-peak-power microwave pulses on operant behavior of Wistar rats. Bioelectromagnetics 12:183.

38. Akyel Y, Belt M, Raslear TG, Hammer RM. 1993. The effects of high-peak power pulsed microwaves on treadmill performance. In M Blank (ed), Electricity and Magnetism in Biology and Medicine, p 668. San Francisco, San Francisco Press.

39. Raslear TG, Akyel Y, Bates F, et al. 1993. Temporal bisection in rats: The effects of high-peak power pulsed microwave irradiation. Bioelectromagnetics 14:459.

40. Lu S-T, Brown DO, Johnson CE, et al. 1992. Abnormal cardiovascular responses induced by localized high power microwave exposure. IEEE Trans Biomed Eng 39:484.

41. Budd RA, Czerski P. 1985. Modulation of mammalian immunity by electromagnetic radiation. J Microwave Power Electromagnet Energy 20:217.

42. Frey AH. 1962. Human auditory system response to modulated electromagnetic energy. J Appl Physiol 17:689.

43. Lin JC. 1991. Pulsed radiofrequency field effects in biological systems. In JC Lin (ed), Electromagnetic Interaction with Biological Systems, pp 165–177. New York, Plenum Press.

44. Kramar PO, Guy AW, Emergy AF, et al. 1976. Quantitation of microwave radiation effects on the eyes of rabbits and primates at 2450 MHz and 918 MHz. University of Washington, Bioelectromagnetics Research Laboratory Scientific report no. 6, Seattle, Wash.

Further Information

The reader is encouraged to consult the *Handbook of Biological Effects of Electromagnetic Fields*, edited by C. Polk and E. Postow, (CRC Press). *Bioelectromagnetics,* the journal of the Bioelectromagnetics Society and the Society for Physical Regulation in Biology and Medicine, is the leading publication of contemporary research on the biologic effects of electromagnetic radiation.

94

Radiofrequency Hyperthermia in Cancer Therapy

C. K. Chou
City of Hope National
Medical Center

During the last two decades, interest in using hyperthermia in combination with other forms of cancer therapy has significantly increased [Storm, 1983; Anghileri and Robert, 1986; Field and Hand, 1990; Gautherie, 1990; Handl-Zeller, 1992; Gerner and Cetas, 1993]. Currently, hyperthermia is still an experimental treatment in the United States, usually applied only to late-stage patients. However, clinical and experimental results from various countries have indicated a promising future for hyperthermia. Numerous reports have shown the synergistic effects of heat and radiotherapy or heat and chemotherapy [Raaphrost, 1990; Dahl and Mella, 1990]. Hyperthermia has been used in combination with chemotherapy because heating increases membrane permeability and the potency of some drugs. The synergism of radiation and hyperthermia is accomplished by the thermal killing of hypoxic and S-phase (DNA syntheses) cells, which are resistive to radiation alone. Current heating methods include whole-body heating using hot wax, hot air, hot water suits, or infrared radiation and partial-body heating using ultrasound, heated blood, fluid perfusion, radiofrequency fields, or microwaves.

The foremost problem in hyperthermia, however, is the generation and control of heat in tumors. The effective temperature range of hyperthermia is very small: 42 to 45°C. At lower temperatures, the effect is minimal. At temperatures higher than 45°C, normal cells are damaged. Due to this narrow temperature range, the response rate of the tumor is highly dependent on how much of it is heated to a therapeutic level. Tumor temperatures are usually higher than surrounding tissue during hyperthermia treatment because of the difference in tissue blood flow. It is also generally believed that tumors are more sensitive to heat, which is explained by the hypoxic, acidic, and poor nutritional state of tumor cells [Lepock and Kruuv, 1993].

In addition to tissue blood flow and thermal conduction, the final temperature of tumors is also dependent on energy deposition. When electromagnetic (EM) heating methods are used, the energy deposition is a complex function of the frequency, intensity, and polarization of the applied fields, the applicator's size and geometry, as well as the size, depth, geometry, and dielectric property of the tumor [Chou, 1990, 1992]. The material, thickness, and construction of a cooling bolus also influence the amount of energy deposition.

0-8493-8346-3/95/$0.00+$.50

94.1 Methods of EM Heating

The EM energy used in hyperthermia is usually classified by frequency as either microwave energy or radiofrequency (RF) energy. Microwaves occupy the EM frequency band between 300 MHz and 300 GHz. Strictly speaking, RF is between 3 kHz and 300 GHz, but for hyperthermia, it generally refers to frequencies below the microwave range. The most commonly used microwave frequencies in hyperthermia are 433, 915, and 2450 MHz, which are the designated ISM (industrial, scientific, and medical) frequencies in the United States and Europe. Common RF frequencies are 13.56 and 27.12 MHz, which also have been widely used in diathermy. Frequencies higher than 2450 MHz have no practical value due to their limited penetrations. At lower frequencies, field penetration is deeper, but the applicator must be larger and focusing is difficult. Despite these limitations, EM heating methods have been developed for local, regional, and whole-body hyperthermia.

Local Heating

External.   The superficial cooling mechanism of tissue makes deep heating difficult by conductive methods. Two RF methods have been used to provide subcutaneous heating. For the first method, tissues are placed between two capacitor plates and heated by displacement currents. This method is simple, but overheating of the fat, caused by the perpendicular electric field, remains a major problem for obese patients. In planar tissue models, the rate of temperature rise is about 17 times greater in fat than in muscle due to the large differences in their dielectric properties and specific heats [Guy and Chou, 1983; Hand, 1990]. Additionally, blood flow in fat is significantly less than that in muscle. Therefore, the final fat temperature is much higher than the muscle temperature, and a water bolus is necessary to minimize the fat heating.

The second RF method uses solenoidal loops or "pancake" magnetic coils to generate a magnetic field. This field then produces heat in tissue by inducing eddy currents. Since the induced electric fields are parallel to the tissue interface, heating is maximized in muscle rather than in fat. However, the heating pattern is generally toroidal with a null at the center of the coil. Fujita et al. [1993] recently described a paired-aperture-type inductive applicator to produce deep heating in phantom.

In the microwave frequency range, energy is coupled into tissues by waveguides, dipoles, microstrip, or other radiating devices. The shorter wavelengths of microwaves, as compared with RF wavelengths, provide the capability to direct and focus energy into tissues by direct radiation from a small applicator. Many applicators of various sizes operate over a frequency range of 300 to 1000 MHz [Kantor and Witters, 1980; Johnson et al., 1990; Nikawa and Okada, 1991; Lee et al., 1992]. Most of them are dielectrically loaded and have a water bolus for surface cooling. Low-profile, light-weight microstrip applicators, which are easier to use clinically, also have been reported [Samulski et al., 1990; Cerri and Marriani, 1991]. High-permittivity dielectric materials, electric wall boundaries, and magnetic materials have been used to reduce applicator size and weight. For the most part, these applicators are used for treatment of tumors a few centimeters below the skin. Toxicities usually associated with treatment are pain and thermal blistering.

Intracavitary.   Certain tumor sites at hollow visceras or cavities may be treated by intracavitary techniques. The advantages of intracavitary hyperthermia over external hyperthermia include better power deposition due to the proximity of the applicators to the tumors and the reduction of normal tissue exposure. There have been clinical and research studies on hyperthermia and radiation or chemotherapy of the esophagus, rectum, cervix, prostate, and bladder cancers.

Both microwave and RF energies have been used for intracavitary hyperthermia. The main problem, however, is that the tumor temperature is unknown. Most temperatures have been measured on the surface of the applicators, which can be very different from those in the tumor. Furthermore, many investigators have used thermocouples or thermistors to measure temperatures, not knowing the perturbation problem caused by the metallic sensors [Cetas, 1990]. One solution to this problem is to measure tissue temperature in animals and then extrapolate to humans [Chou et al., 1993].

Interstitial.   Methods such as resistive heating, the microwave technique, and ferromagnetic seed implants can be used for interstitial hyperthermia. With resistive heating, tissues can be heated by alternating RF currents conducted through needle electrodes. To prevent excitation of nerve action potentials, an operating frequency greater than 100 kHz should be used. Interstitial techniques for radiation implants as primary or boost treatments have been practiced successfully by radiation oncologists for many years. When hyperthermia was learned to be cytotoxic and synergistic with radiation, it was natural to consider this combination with conventional interstitial radioactive implantation. Other advantages of this technique over external hyperthermia include better control of heat distributions within the tumor and the sparing of normal tissue, especially the overlying skin [Vora et al., 1986].

The microwave technique utilizes small microwave antennas inserted into hollow plastic tubing to produce interstitial heat. In the United States, 915 MHz is a commonly used frequency for this technique. However, satisfactory heating patterns can be produced between 300 and 2450 MHz [Strohbehn et al., 1979; Iskander and Tumeh, 1989]. A small coaxial antenna can irradiate a volume of approximately 60 cc. With a three-node coaxial antenna, the length of the heating pattern can be extended to approximately 10 cm [Lee et al., 1986]. However, since most tumors seen in the clinic are larger than this, a single microwave antenna cannot heat the entire tumor to a therapeutic temperature. It is therefore necessary to use an array of microwave antennas. As in RF resistive hyperthermia, the degree of control of microwave power radiating from these antennas is important in order to achieve homogeneous heating. Since the antennas couple to each other, the spacing, phasing, and insertion depth affect the heating patterns of array applicators [Chan et al., 1989; Zhang et al., 1991].

Interstitial heat also can be produced by using ferromagnetic seed implants. Burton et al. [1971] used thermally self-regulating implants for producing brain lesions. This technique is also applicable for delivering thermal energy to deep-seated tumors. When exposed to RF magnetic fields ($\sim$100 kHz), the implants absorb power and become heated until they reach the Curie point. Here, the implants become nonferromagnetic and no longer produce heat. The surrounding tissues are then heated by thermal conduction. The influence of blood flow and tissue inhomogeneities of the tumor, which may affect the temperature distribution, can be compensated by the self-regulation of the implants. It is therefore possible to maintain a temperature close to the Curie point [Mack et al., 1993]. Another method, exposing magnetic fluid in a tumor to an RF magnetic field (0.3 to 80 MHz), also has been shown to be feasible for inducing selective heating [Jordan et al., 1993].

Regional Heating

Electric Field.   Heating deep-seated tumors is difficult. RF energy can be deposited into the center of the body, but a large region is affected. Differential increases in blood flow in normal and tumor tissues may result in higher temperatures in the tumor than in normal organs. However, this temperature differential cannot be ensured. Strohbehn [1986] used the term "dump and pray" to describe the situation of putting large amounts of EM energy into the region and hoping for satisfactory results. In Japan, the 8-MHz Thermotron system uses a capacitive electric field to heat deep tumors and a water-cooled bolus to minimize the heating of fat tissue [Koga, 1988]. The sizes of two electrodes are adjusted to control the heating patterns in patients.

Most other electric field heating systems generate electric fields parallel to the body surface. These include the annular phased-array systems [Turner, 1984], the CDRH helix system [Ruggera and Kantor, 1984], the coaxial TEM cell [de Leeuw and Legendijk, 1987], the ring electrode [van Rhoon et al., 1988], the segmented cylindrical array [Bach Andersen, 1987], the toroidal inductor [Tiberio et al., 1988], and the loosely coupled TEM system [Harrison, 1989]. The APAS, made by the BSD Company (Salt Lake City, Utah), radiates 16 RF fields in phase toward the patient. A newer heating system using eight dipoles [Turner, 1988] is being evaluated in clinic. These systems, with variations in phase, frequency, amplitude, and orientation of the applied fields, can add more dimensions to the control of heating patterns during treatment. To determine the excitation phases of an array for heating an inhomogeneous medium, the retrofocusing technique was applied [Loane et al., 1986]. A small probe was first inserted into a tumor. A signal was radiated from the probe and received by the array of applicators outside the patient. By the reciprocity theory, conjugate fields were radiated from the applicators and focused at the tumor. The technique was demonstrated experimentally in a water tank. A significant power increase at the desired focus was observed.

In general, superficial heating and hot spots in normal tissues are the limiting factors of treatment effectiveness in the existing systems. Invasive techniques using interstitial hyperthermia have been shown to solve some of the deep-heating problems [Stauffer et al., 1984; Cosset et al., 1985; Vora et al., 1986]. However, no adequate deep EM heating system is available. Scanned ultrasound provides an alternative method [Hynynen, 1990].

Magnetic Field.   Magnetic fields heat tissue by induced eddy currents. The magnetic-loop applicators of the Magnetrode unit (Henry Radio, Los Angeles, Calif.) are self-resonant, noncontact cylindrical coils with built-in impedance-matching circuitry; they operate at 13.56 MHz with a maximum power output of 1000 W. The RF current in the coil creates strong magnetic fields that are parallel to the center axis of the coil where the body or limb of a patient is located. Since the magnitude of the induced eddy current is a function of the radius of the exposed object, there is no energy deposition at the center of the exposed tissue. However, Storm et al. [1983] showed that the heating of tumors deep in the body was possible, as demonstrated in live dogs and humans, with no injury of surface tissue. This was apparently due to the redistribution of the thermal energy by blood flow. Nevertheless, the FDA has forbidden the use of the Magnetrode.

Whole-Body Heating

During the last 20 years, hyperthermia has been used primarily for treating localized tumors. However, tumors that are resistant to conventional therapy tend to be metastatic. For these patients, local and regional hyperthermia can only be palliative. For disseminated disease, whole-body hyperthermia (WBH) in conjunction with chemotherapy and radiation has been studied by many groups [Anhalt et al., 1990; Shen et al., 1991]. Methods of WBH include hot wax, water blankets, water suits, radiant heat, and extracorporeal blood heating. These labor-intensive WBH methods and their morbidity, though, have caused concerns. Except for the extracorporeal blood heating technique, which requires extensive surgical procedures, all other methods depend on conduction of heat from the body surface to the core. Since thermoreceptors are located cutaneously, the heating rate must be slow enough not to trigger pain or cause skin burns.

Volumetric heating using more penetrating methods is a logical alternative. To heat the whole body uniformly with EM energy is impossible. However, it is possible to heat the body regionally so that the blood flow will redistribute the heat to the whole body. In the past, applications of 434- and 468-MHz microwaves have been explored in Europe for WBH, but the results did not produce any significant impact [van der Zee et al., 1990]. Several regional RF systems have been attempted for WBH. The BSD dipole system and the CDRH helix system require that the body be inserted into a tunnel applicator. The BSD system also requires a water bolus in contact with the patient to provide better energy coupling and skin cooling. For hour-long use, the bolus is very heavy and uncomfortable.

The RF electric field system designed by the UCLA group [Harrison, 1989] uses three electrode plates to heat deep-seated tumors in the torso. The patient lies on a table, and the top plate is swung over the abdomen to heat the thoracic region. No water bolus is needed, and there is no contact with the patient. It is very simple to use. After 2 years of extensive phantom and animal studies, it was found to be a very promising system for regional and WBH [Chou et al., 1993].

94.2 Conclusion

There has been much progress in the application of EM energy for clinical hyperthermia. Based on medical demands, many technological advances have been made. As a result, new forms of treatment equipment have been developed, and existing methods have been improved. It is impossible for a single piece of equipment to fulfill all the clinical requirements for patient treatments. Depending on the location and vascularity of the tumor and adjacent tissues and the general physical condition of the patient, the hyperthermia practitioners should have the option of choosing the most appropriate equipment.

Hyperthermia is a complicated technique and should be applied only by individuals well trained in its use. Due to the complexity of EM energy coupling to human tumors, careful heating pattern studies should be performed on all exposure geometries and contingencies prior to treatment to ensure the best treatment conditions for the patient. Since hyperthermia in combination with high-energy radiotherapy cannot be repeated after the tumor receives a maximal dosage of ionizing radiation, the physician must try to reach the critical tumor temperatures in optimal conjunction with radiotherapy. Accurate thermometry is particularly important in all phases of clinical hyperthermia, especially when the patient is anesthetized. The benefit of a good treatment outweighs minor risks. If there is no other choice, it would be more beneficial for the patient to have an effective treatment with a few blisters rather than a safe but ineffective treatment. It is easier to treat the burns than the cancer.

Acknowledgment

This work was supported in part by NCI under Grants CA33572 and CA56116.

References

Anghileri LJ, Robert J (eds). 1986. Hyperthermia in Cancer Treatment. Boca Raton, Fla, CRC Press.

Anhalt D, Hynynen K, Deyoung D, et al. 1990. The CDRH helix: An in-vivo evaluation. Int J Hyperthermia 6:241.

Bach Andersen J. 1987. Electromagnetic power deposition: Inhomogeneous media, applications and phased arrays. In SB Field, C Franconi (eds), Physics and Technology of Hyperthermia, pp 159–188. Amsterdam, Martinus-Nijhoff.

Burton CV, Hill M, Walker AE. 1971. The RF thermal seed: A thermally self-regulating implant for the production of brain lesions. IEEE Trans Biomed Eng 18:104.

Cerri G, Marriani V. 1991. Theoretical and experimental analysis of microstrip spiral antennas. In G Franceschetti, R Pierri (eds), Italian Recent Advances in Applied Electromagnetics, pp 195–210. Napoli, Italy, Liguori.

Cetas TC. 1990. Temperature. In JF Lehmann (ed), Therapeutic Heat and Cold, pp 1–61. Baltimore, Williams & Wilkins.

Chan KW, Chou CK, McDougall JA, Luk KH. 1989. Changes in heating patterns of interstitial microwave antenna arrays at different insertion depths. Int J Hyperthermia 5:499.

Chou CK. 1990. Safety considerations of clinical hypothermia. In SB Field, JW Hand (eds), An Introduction to the Practical Aspects of Clinical Hyperthermia, pp 533–564. London, Taylor & Francis.

Chou CK. 1992. Evaluation of microwave hyperthermia applicators. Bioelectromagnetics 13:581.

Chou CK, McDougall JA, Chan KW, et al. 1993. Intracavitary hyperthermia and radiation of esophageal cancer. In M Blank (ed), Electricity and Magnetism in Biology and Medicine, pp 793–796. San Francisco, San Francisco Press.

Chou CK, McDougall JA, Chan KW, et al. 1993. Whole-body hyperthermia with an RF electric field system. In Proceedings 15th Annual International Conference of the IEEE Engineering in Medicine and Biology Society, part 3, pp 1461–1462.

Cosset JM, Dutreix J, Haie C, et al. 1985. Interstitial thermoradiotherapy: A technical and clinical study of 29 implantations performed at the Institute Gustave-Roussy. Int J Hyperthermia 1:3.

Dahl O, Mella O. 1990. Hyperthermia and chemotherapeutic agents. In SB Field, JW Hand (eds), An Introduction to the Practical Aspects of Clinical Hyperthermia, pp 108–142. London, Taylor & Francis.

de Leeuw AAC, Lagendijk JJW. 1987. Design of a clinical deep-body hyperthermia system based on the "coaxial TEM" applicator. Int J Hyperthermia 3:413.

Field SB, Hand JW (eds). 1990. An Introduction to the Practical Aspects of Clinical Hyperthermia. London Taylor & Francis.

Fujita Y, Kato H, Ishida T. 1993. An RF concentrating method using inductive aperture-type applicator. IEEE Trans Biomed Eng 40:110.

Gautherie M (ed). 1990. Clinical Thermology. Berlin, Springer-Verlag.

Gerner EW, Cetas TC (eds). 1993. Hyperthermic Oncology 1992. Tucson, Arizona Board of Regents.

Guy AW, Chou CK. 1983. Biophysics and technology of electromagnetic hyperthermia. In FK Storm (ed), Hyperthermia in Cancer Therapy, pp 279–304. Boston, GK Hall Medical Publishers.

Hand JW. 1990. Biophysics and technology of electromagnetic hyperthermia. In M Gautherie (ed), Methods of External Hyperthermic Heating, pp 1–59. Berlin, Springer-Verlag.

Handl-Zeller L (ed). 1992. Interstitial Hyperthermia. New York, Springer-Verlag.

Harrison WH. 1989. U.S. patent nos. 4,823,811 and 4,823,813.

Hynynen K. 1990. Biophysics and technology of ultrasound hyperthermia. In M Gautherie (ed), Methods of External Hyperthermic Heating, pp 61–115. Berlin, Springer-Verlag.

Iskander MF, Tumeh AM. 1989. Design optimization of interstitial antennas. IEEE Trans Biomed Eng 36:238.

Johnson RH, Preece AW, Green JL. 1990. Theoretical and experimental comparison of three types of electromagnetic hyperthermia applicator. Phys Med Biol 35:761.

Jordan A, Wust P, Fahling H, et al. 1993. Inductive heating of ferromagnetic particles and magnetic fluids: Physical evaluation of their potential for hyperthermia. Int J Hyperthermia 9:51.

Kantor KG, Witters DM Jr. 1980. A 2450-MHz slab-loaded direct contact applicator with choke. IEEE Trans Microwave Theory Technol 28:1418.

Koga S (ed). 1988. Hyperthermic Oncology in Japan '87. Yonago, Japan, Imai.

Lee DJ, O'Neill MJ, Lam K, et al. 1986. A new design of microwave interstitial applicators for hyperthermia with improved treatment volume Int J Radiat Oncol Biol Phys 12:2003.

Lee ER, Wilsey T, Tarczys-Hornoch P, et al. 1992. Body conformable 915 MHz microstrip array applicators for large surface area hyperthermia. IEEE Trans Biomed Eng 39:470.

Lepock JR, Kruuv J. 1993. Mechanisms of thermal cytoxicity. In EW Gerner, TC Cetas (eds), Hyperthermic Oncology 1992, pp 9–16. Tucson, Arizona Board of Regents.

Loane J, Ling H, Wang BF, Lee SW. 1986. Experimental investigation of a retrofocusing microwave hyperthermia applicator: Conjugate-field matching scheme. IEEE Trans Microwave Theory Technol 34:490.

Mack CF, Stea B, Kittelson JM, et al. 1993. Interstitial thermoradiotherapy with ferromagnetic implants for locally advanced and recurrent neoplasms. Int J Radiat Oncol Biol Phys 27:109.

Nikawa Y, Okada F. 1991. Dielectric loaded lens applicator for microwave hyperthermia. IEEE Trans Microwave Theory Technol 39:1173.

Raaphrost GP. 1990. Fundamental aspects of hyperthermic biology. In SB Field, JW Hand (eds), An Introduction to the Practical Aspects of Clinical Hyperthermia, pp 10–54. London, Taylor & Francis.

Ruggera PS, Kantor G. 1984. Development of a family of RF helical coil applicators which produce transversely uniform axially distributed heating in cylindrical fat-muscle phantoms. IEEE Trans Biomed Eng 31:98.

Samulski TV, Fessenden P, Lee ER, et al. 1990. Spiral microstrip hyperthermia applicators: Technical design and clinical performance. Int J Radiat Oncol Biol Phys 18:233.

Shen RN, Hornback NB, Shidnia H, et al. 1991. Whole body hyperthermia: A potent radioprotector in vivo. Int J Radiat Oncol Biol Phys 20:525.

Stauffer PR, Cetas TC, Fletcher AM, et al. 1984. Observations on the use of ferromagnetic implants for inducing hyperthermia. IEEE Trans Biomed Eng 31:76.

Storm FK (ed). 1983. Hyperthermia in Cancer Therapy. Boston, GK Hall Medical Publishers.

Storm FK, Harrison WH, Elliott RS, Morton DL. 1983. Physical aspects of localized heating by mag-
    netic-loop induction. In FK Storm (ed), Hyperthermia in Cancer Therapy, pp 305–313.
    Boston, GK Hall Medical Publishers.

Strohbehn JW. 1986. Evaluation of hyperthermia equipment. In LJ Anghileri, LJ Robert, J Robert
    (eds), Hyperthermia in Cancer Treatment, pp 179–197. Boca Raton, Fla, CRC Press.

Strohbehn JW, Bowers ED, Walsh JE, Douple EB. 1979. An invasive microwave antenna for locally-
    induced hyperthermia for cancer therapy. J Microwave Power 14:339.

Tiberio CA, Raganella L, Banci G, Franconi C. 1988. The RF toroidal transformer as a heat delivery
    system for regional and focused hyperthermia. IEEE Trans Biomed Eng 35:1077.

Turner PF. 1984. Regional hyperthermia with an annular phased array. IEEE Trans Biomed Eng
    31:106.

Turner PF. 1988. Operational and clinical aspects of the BSD-2000. In Proceedings of Essen
    University and BSD Medical Corporation Symposium, Essen, Germany.

van der Zee J, van Rhoon GC, Faithful NS, van den Berg AP. 1990. Clinical hyperthermic practice:
    Whole-body hyperthermia. In SB Field, JW Hand (eds), An Introduction to the Practical
    Aspects of Clinical Hyperthermia, pp 185–212. London, Taylor & Francis.

van Rhoon GC, Visser AG, van den Berg PM, Reinhold HS. 1988. Evaluation of ring capacitor plats
    for regional deep heating. Int J Hyperthermia 4:133.

Vora N, Shaw S, Forell B, et al. 1986. Primary radiation combined with hyperthermia for advanced
    (stage III–IV) and inflammatory carcinoma of breast. Endocur Hyperthermia Oncol 2:101.

Zhang Y, Joines WT, Oleson JR. 1991. Prediction of heating patterns of a microwave interstitial
    antenna array at various insertion depths. Int J Hyperthermia 7:197.

Further Information

1. *International Journal of Hyperthermia* is published bimonthly by Taylor & Francis, Ltd., 4 John
   Street, London WC1N 2ET, UK. Tel: +44 (0) 71 405 2237; Fax: +44 (0) 71 831 2035.

2. North American Hyperthermia Society, 2021 Spring Road, Suite 600, Oak Brooks, Ill. 60521,
   Tel: (708) 571-2904, Fax: (708) 571-7837.

3. Japanese Society of Hyperthermic Oncology, Contact T. Matsuda, M.D., Division of Radiology, Tokyo Metropolitan Komagome Hospital, 3-18-22, Honko-Magome, Bunkyo-ku, Tokyo,
   Japan.

4. European Society for Hyperthermic Oncology, Contact Clare C. Vernon, M.D., F.R.C.R.,
   Hyperthermia Clinic, Medical Research Council, Cyclotron Unit, Hammersmith Hospital,
   Du Cane Road, London, W12 0HS, Great Britain.

95

Electroporation of Cells and Tissues

James C. Weaver
Massachusetts Institute
of Technology

95.1 Background

Bioelectric phenomena are of great interest and are well established topics in biomedical engineering. Electroporation is of growing interest because of its ability to rapidly and locally deliver molecules across bilayer membrane barriers [1–4]. Although initial applications have used in vitro cellular conditions and have focused almost exclusively on DNA introduction, the use of electroporation with tissue in vivo offers the prospect of "drug delivery" that can be electrically controlled. This is of great potential importance, because medical interventions are increasingly based on molecular rather than physical processes. Electroporation allows reversible or irreversible alteration of the cell membrane, as well as other lipid-based barriers in tissues, such that the barriers to ions and molecules are reduced within microseconds by several orders of magnitude. Simultaneously, the local electric field across the barrier drives molecular transport across the reduced barrier. For short pulses the necessary transient voltage across a single bilayer membrane is about 0.5 to 1 V, which means that electroporation is mild at the molecular level and can result in negligible damage.

95.2 Membrane Barrier Function

A first look at a cell shows that it has an inside and an outside, i.e., intra- and extracellular compartments, and this fundamentally defines the spatial extent of cell and also provides a chemical boundary across which significant chemical concentrations exist. Although there are variable amounts and types of highly specific membrane proteins, the critical barrier-defining element is the thin ($\sim$6 nm) region of low-dielectric-constant ($K_m \approx 2$) lipid. The ability of a thin fluid sheet of low-dielectric-constant material to exclude ions and charged molecules is impressive and can be understood in terms of a Born energy barrier ΔW_{Born} [5]. Briefly, in the case of ion transport, ΔW_{Born} is the change in electrostatic energy associated with electric charge moving from a polarizable liquid medium (here water, dielectric constant $K_w \approx 80$) to a relatively nonpolarizable fluid

0-8493-8346-3/95/$0.00+$.50

lipid region within the membrane (here lipids with dielectric constant $K_m \approx 2$). Formally, W_{Born} is the electrostatic energy needed to assemble a particular configuration of charge and is expressed in terms of the electric field E and the permittivity of the surrounding medium $\epsilon = K\epsilon_0$ (K is the dielectric constant, and $\epsilon_0 = 8.85 \times 10^{-12}$ F/m):

$$W_{Born} \equiv \int_{\substack{\text{all space} \\ \text{except ion}}} \frac{1}{2}\, \epsilon E^2\, dV \tag{95.1}$$

The electrostatic component of the barrier function that excludes ions and molecules from the membrane interior can be understood by considering the change in the Born energy ΔW_{Born} as an ion is moved into the membrane. The maximum value, $\Delta W_{Born,max}$, defines the electrostatic contribution to the barrier and for charged species is the major contribution.

Because W_{Born} increases rapidly as the ion enters the membrane, the magnitude of the membrane barrier can be reasonably estimated by considering the simple problem of moving a charge from water into lipid. The ion exists as a charged sphere of radius r_s and charge $q = ze$ with $z = \pm 1$ and $e = 1.6 \times 10^{-19}$ C. First, the sphere is surrounded by water far from the membrane ($W_{Born,i}$) and is subsequently moved to the center of the membrane ($W_{Born,f}$). The difference in these Born energies is the barrier height. A simple estimate of ΔW_{Born} can be made by recognizing that a small ion diameter, i.e., $2r_s \approx 0.4$ nm, is significantly less than a typical membrane thickness, i.e., $h \approx 3$ to 6 nm (smaller values for artificial planar bilayer membranes, larger for cell membranes). This allows ΔW_{Born} to be estimated by neglecting the finite size of the membrane and replacing the membrane with bulk lipid. This is justified because the greatest contribution to the electric field is in the volume near the ion. Thus,

$$\Delta W_{Born,max} \approx \frac{e^2}{8\pi\epsilon_0 r_s}\left(\frac{1}{K_m} - \frac{1}{K_w}\right) \approx 100 \text{ kT} \tag{95.2}$$

A numerical computation for a thin, low-dielectric-constant region gives $\Delta W_{Born} \approx 65$ kT. A barrier of this magnitude is surmounted at a negligible rate by thermal fluctuations (spontaneous ion movement). Moreover, a transmembrane voltage U_{direct} that is much larger than physiologic values would be needed to provide this energy. This could provide a direct (nonpore) process for forcing an ion across the membrane. Note that molecules that readily partition into the membrane and then cross the membrane by diffusion are not significantly affected by ΔW_{Born}. Instead, their transport is governed by a passive permeability due to the combined effect of dissolution and diffusion. Even large uncharged molecules will not readily cross the membrane, because their combined solubility and effective diffusion constant within the membrane are small.

95.3 Reduction of the Membrane Barrier

Two types of membrane structural "defects" can greatly reduce $\Delta W_{Born,max}$: (1) a mobile aqueous cavity (carrier) and (2) an aqueous perforation (i.e. a pore). Functionally, both structures provide aqueous pathways across the barrier. If they are present, charged molecules can cross the membrane, and indeed biologic systems have evolved specific carriers and channels to regulate ionic and molecular transport. With this as perspective, the rapid and relatively nonspecific reduction in the membrane barrier by transient aqueous hydrophilic pores (Fig. 95.1) can be appreciated. In what follows, the origin of such pores and the constraints they place on membrane electrical behavior and associated molecular transport are presented [5].

At the membrane level, it is believed that structural rearrangements such as those shown in Fig. 95.1 are involved in producing a rapidly changing, heterogeneous population of pores in the

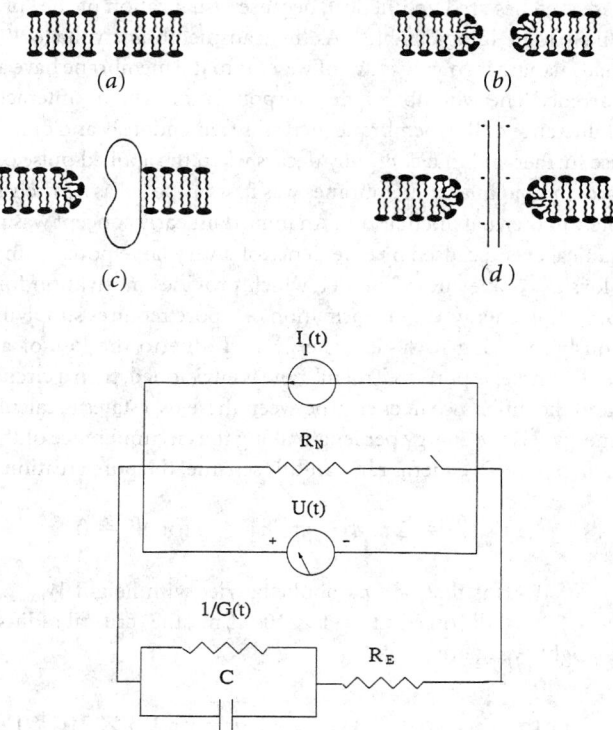

FIGURE 95.1 Illustrations of hypothetical structures of both transient and metastable conformations that may be involved in electroporation and a simple circuit model for a planar bilayer membrane that experiences electroporation. (*Top*) Hypothetical bilayer membrane structures related to electroporation [3]. (*a*) Hydrophobic pore proposed by Chizmadzhev and coworkers. (*b*) Hydrophilic pore proposed by Litster and by Taupin and coworkers; these are usually regarded as the "primary pores" through which ion and molecules pass. (*c*) Composite pore with one or more proteins at the pore's inner edge. (*d*) Composite pore with "foot-in-the-door" charged macromolecule inserted into a hydrophilic core. Although the actual transitions are not known, the transient aqueous pore model assumes that transitions from $A \to B \to C$ or d occur with increasing frequency as ψ is increased. Type d may form by entry of a tethered macromolecule during the time that ψ is significantly elevated and then persist after ψ has decayed to a small value because of pore conduction. These hypothetical structures have not been directly observed but are consistent with a variety of experimental observations and with theoretical models. (Reproduced with permission from Weaver, Cellular Biochem 51:426, 1993). (*Bottom*) Circuit model representing a planar bilayer membrane and the electrical environment with which it interacts during electroporation. The two fixed resistance R_E and R_N represent the external pathway of the bathing electrolyte and of the pulse generator and electrodes, respectively. The membrane capacitance C is essentially constant during electroporation, while the membrane resistance $R(t)$ decreases by orders of magnitude and (for reversible electroporation) then recovers to its original value. (Reproduced with permission from Barnett and Weaver, Bioelectrochem Bioenerg 25:163, 1991.)

membrane [3]. These sketches are hypothetical, because visualization of the "primary pores" [1] of electroporation is likely to be impossible [2]. As the transmembrane voltage $\Psi(t)$ increases, membrane conformational changes involving entry of water into the membrane have a nonlinear increase in frequency of occurrence. The evolution of the pore population is highly interactive; as pores appear and expand, the conductance of the membrane increases tremendously and quickly becomes so large that $\Psi(t)$ cannot rise further and in fact rapidly decays when the applied pulse ceases.

Formation of pores in lipid bilayer membranes was first proposed as a purely spontaneous event, i.e., creation due solely to thermal fluctuations. An important early concept was membrane rupture, a destructive mechanical event, caused by emergence of a very large pore. A simple way of viewing pore creation employs a "cookie cutter" model, which provides motivation for the mathematical form of the pore formation energy $W_p(r)$. Formation of a pore requires supplying an "edge energy" γ while simultaneously receiving in system energy $\pi r^2 \Gamma$ due to the loss of a circular region of membrane. The idea is simple: A pore-free membrane is envisioned, then a circular region is cut out of the membrane, and the difference in energy between these two states is calculated and identified as ΔW_p. The edge energy γ is the energy per length along the circumference of the pore, and Γ is the energy per area of a flat, pore-free membrane. In this scheme, the pore creation energy is

$$\Delta W_p(r) = 2\pi\gamma r - \pi\Gamma r^2 \qquad \text{for } \Psi = 0 \qquad (95.3)$$

The functional form of $W_p(r)$ is that of a parabolic barrier with height $W_{p,\max}$. For typical bilayer membrane values $\gamma \approx 2 \times 10^{-11}$ J/m and $\Gamma \approx 1 \times 10^{-3}$ J/m^2, the "critical radius" at $W_{p,\max}$ and corresponding barrier height $W_{p,\max}$ are

$$r_c = \frac{\gamma}{\Gamma} \approx 20 \text{ nm} \qquad \text{and} \qquad W_{p,\max} = \frac{\pi\gamma^2}{\Gamma} \approx 1.3 \times 10^{-18} \text{ J} \approx 300 \text{ kT} \quad (95.4)$$

Based on structural arguments and interpretation of experiments, the minimum size pore is believed to have $r_{\min} \approx 1$ nm. Significantly, the large size of the barrier suggests that spontaneous rupture of a cell membrane is negligible.

95.4 Basis of Electroporation

The effect of increasing $\Psi(t)$, *viz.* a nonlinear increase in pore formation from negligible basal rates, was first suggested by Chizmadzhev and coworkers [5]. As shown in Fig. 95.1, it was hypothesized that precursor hydrophobic pores occur and that the overall creation and transition to hydrophilic pores are governed by a rate equation with a modified pore barrier function $W_p(r, \Psi)$. A hydrophilic pore (hereafter termed *pore*) is believed to be the primary pore involved in most electroporation phenomena and can be modelled as a "leaky" microscopic capacitor whose parallel resistance for small radii ($r_{\min} \approx 1$ nm) is extremely large $R_p > 10^9$ Ω. As many pores are created and are also increased in size, their combined contribution to the membrane conductance $G(t)$ results in a several order of magnitude drop in membrane resistance. This decrease has been termed *breakdown* in the early literature, even though there is insufficient energy ($\Psi_{\max} \approx 1$ V) for classic dielectric breakdown that involves ionization.

A quantitative model for electroporation of artificial planar bilayer membranes provided the first major insight into the mechanism of electroporation. In this model, in the presence of a transmembrane electric field $E_m = \Psi/h$, the free energy of pore formation is

$$W_p(r, \Psi) = 2\pi\gamma r - \pi\Gamma r^2 - 0.5C_p\Psi^2 r^2 \qquad (95.5)$$

Here Ψ is interpreted as the spatially averaged transmembrane voltage. Later, the local reduction in transmembrane voltage at the site of a conducting pore is included. The change in the pore's specific capacitance is simply $C_p = (\epsilon_w/\epsilon_m - 1)C_0$, where $\epsilon_w = K_w\epsilon_0$ and $\epsilon_m = K_1\epsilon_0$ are the permittivities of the aqueous and lipid interior of the membrane, respectively, and C_0 is the capacitance per area of a pore-free membrane, i.e., $C_0 = \epsilon_m / h$.

The pore creation energy $W_p(r, \Psi)$ is a critically important quantity. When regarded as a barrier, the barrier height $W_{\mathrm{Born,max}}$ and corresponding pore radius r_c both diminish with increasing Ψ. The physical reason for this is that aqueous interior of the pore has a much larger permittivity than the surrounding lipid. As Ψ increases, it becomes progressively more favorable for water to enter the pore; i.e., pore expansion is electrically driven. Qualitatively, this provides a readily visualized explanation of the rupture of planar bilayer membranes. As Ψ increases, $W_{p,\mathrm{max}}$ decreases so that the probability of one or more "supracritical" pores $[r > r(U)_c]$ goes up. But even a single supracritical pore can cause rupture. Once a pore is over the barrier maximum, it can expand until it reaches whatever physical boundary confines the membrane. In the case of experiments with artificial planar bilayer membranes, the membrane is confined to a small but macroscopic aperture (e.g., $r_{\mathrm{aperture}} \approx 10^{-3}$ m). In the case of a cell membrane, it is less clear, but it has been suggested that the cytoskeleton or other cellular structure can play the same role. In either case, expansion of a supracritical pore to a larger boundary is essentially irreversible. This is what is meant by *irreversible breakdown* in the early electroporation literature.

One of the significant successes of the transient aqueous pore model is its quantitative description of rupture, briefly presented here. The extension of Eq. (95.4) to the case $\Psi > 0$ yields

$$r_c(\Psi) = \frac{\gamma}{\Gamma + 0.5 C_p \Psi^2} \quad \text{and} \quad \Delta W_{p,\mathrm{max}}(\Psi) = \frac{\pi \gamma^2}{\Gamma + 0.5 C_p \Psi^2} \quad (95.6)$$

There are two effects. The critical pore radius decreases as Ψ increases, but more significantly, the corresponding pore energy $\Delta W_{p,\mathrm{max}}(\Psi)$ decreases. Physical processes governed by activation energies (barriers) involve Boltzmann factors, and in such cases, including that of pore creation, there is a nonlinear dependence on system parameters such as Ψ. This is the primary source of the nonlinear dependence of pore creation on Ψ. As discussed below, only a moderate increase in Ψ is needed to significantly diminish the stability of a planar membrane and can cause rupture.

Self-consistent electroporation theories predict that pores are located randomly but widely spaced, on average separated by several tens of pore radii. This large separation means that the equipotentials near the membrane have a significant, nonlinear gradient. Thus the current flowing through a pore results in a voltage drop both within the pore and within the electrolyte external to the pore but near the entrance of the pore. This potential drop near a pore's mouth is due to a *spreading resistance* R_s within the bathing electrolyte. A similar localized potential drop is well known to occur for microelectrodes. The spreading resistance associated with a disk electrode, which can be used to approximate the entrance to a pore, is $R_s \approx 1/2\sigma_e r$. The voltage drop associated with R_s is external to the pore and therefore does not contribute to the driving force that tends to expand pores.

For the smallest pores, electrical conduction is suppressed because of Born energy exclusion due to the nearby low-dielectric-constant lipid. That is, ion entry is suppressed due to the energy cost of bringing an ion into a small pore. This leads to a reduction in electrical conductivity within a pore σ_p. Ion movement through a pore slightly larger than the ion itself means that steric hindrance also may be significant. The resistance within a pore is estimated by using a simple cylindrical geometry but a Born energy-reduced conductivity σ_p. This gives $R_p = h/\pi r^2 \sigma_p$, with $\sigma_p < \sigma_e$, where σ_e is the usual, bulk conductivity. The two resistances R_s and R_p are in series, resulting in a voltage divider effect. That is, $\Psi_p \leq \Psi$, and as a result, the electrical expanding force associated with $\partial W_p(r, \Psi)/\partial r$ in pore radius space is diminished. For this reason, pores therefore expand more slowly than expected from using Ψ in Eq. (95.5).

Specifically, the reduced local voltage across an individual pore is

$$\Psi_p = \Psi \left(\frac{R_p}{R_p + R_s} \right) \quad (95.7)$$

Electrical measurements on artificial planar bilayer membranes provide evidence that some small pores remain after Ψ is decreased. In the case of cells, experiments tested the cells' response to the introduction of dyes after electrical pulsing, and these revealed that some cells have a persisting capability to take up these molecules. One hypothesis is that some type of complex pores are created, which may involve a more permanent portion of the cell, e.g., the cytoskeleton or tethered cytoplasmic molecules (see Fig. 95.1). If so, some type of long-lifetime metastable pores may be created. This notion is consistent with experiments involving DNA uptake. DNA is a large, highly charged molecule so that while temporarily occupying a pore, DNA charge groups should have the effect of inhibiting pore closure by coulombic repulsion. This is a "foot-in-the-door" hypothesis (see Fig. 95.1). However, most pores may be destroyed relatively quickly, with pore destruction independent of other pores. This seems reasonable, since pores are predicted to be widely spaced even when the maximum number of pores is transiently present.

A heterogeneous pore size is fundamentally expected, because there are two sources of the energy that contribute to pore formation: (1) thermal fluctuations ("kT energy," stochastic) and (2) an increased transmembrane voltage ("electric field energy," deterministic). The combined contribution is therefore stochastic, and this leads to the expectation that a probabilistic distribution of pore sizes occurs. The flux of pores in pore radius space is described by the equation

$$J_p = -D_p \left(\frac{\partial n}{\partial r} + \frac{n}{kT} \frac{\partial \Delta W_p}{\partial r} \right) \tag{95.8}$$

The diffusion in *pore radius space* is contained in the term with D_p, the diffusion constant of the pores in pore radius space. In keeping with a statistical description, $n = n(r, t)$ is the distribution function of the pores. That is, $n(r, t)$ is a probability density function such that within a radial increment Δr there are $n(r, t)\Delta r$ pores instantaneously present with radii between r and $r + \Delta r$.

This approach leads to the prediction of statistical rupture, with an average membrane lifetime $\bar{\tau}$ given by

$$\bar{\tau} \approx \frac{(kT)^{3/2}}{4\pi c_0 A_m D_p \gamma (\Gamma + 0.5 C_p \Psi^2)^{1/2}} \exp \left[\frac{\pi \gamma^2}{kT(\Gamma + 0.5 C_p \Psi^2)} \right] \tag{95.9}$$

Here A_m is the membrane area, and C_p is the pore concentration (pores per area) within the membrane. Another, simpler approach for estimating $\bar{\tau}$ is based on an absolute rate estimate for critical pore appearance. In this case, the mean lifetime depends on the reciprocal of a Boltzmann factor, in which $W_p(\Psi)$ is an argument. By employing an order-of-magnitude estimate for the prefactor, the mean membrane lifetime against rupture is

$$\bar{\tau} \approx \frac{1}{\nu_0 V_m} \exp \left(+\Delta W_{p,c}/kT \right) \tag{95.10}$$

Here ν_0 is an attempt rate density based on a collision frequency density within the membrane. The order of magnitude of ν_0 was obtained by estimating the volume density of collisions per time in the fluid membrane, and the factor $V_m = h A_m$ is the total volume of the membrane. By choosing a plausible lifetime value (e.g., $\bar{\tau} \approx 1$ s), the value of $\Delta W_{p,c}$, and hence of Ψ_c, can be found. This yields an estimate for the critical voltage for rupture $\Psi_c \approx 0.3$ to 0.4 V. Because of the strong nonlinear behavior of Eqs. (95.9) and (95.10), the choice of lifetime values such as 0.1 or 10 seconds results in only small differences in Ψ_c.

A direct interaction of the membrane and its pore population with its environment also must be considered. Specifically, as shown in Fig. 95.1, there is a current pathway by which bulk electrolyte ions are transported to the membrane in order to charge the membrane capacitance to $\Psi(t)$. During electroporation, the membrane capacitance C changes by less than 2% because only a small fraction of the membrane is occupied by aqueous pores. In contrast, the membrane conductance $G(t) = 1/R(t)$ increases by orders of magnitude. In a typical experiment, a current pulse of amplitude I_i passes through R_N to create a voltage pulse V_0. For a short time ($0 < t < t_{pulse}$) current flows into and/or across the membrane. The membrane can discharge back through the pulse generator, but most of the discharge current passes directly through the membrane, because $G(t)$ approaches $G \approx 10^{-1}$ to $10^{-2} \, \Omega^{-1}$. In the case of a square pulse, the appropriate circuit differential equations are

$$C \frac{d\Psi}{dt} = \begin{cases} \dfrac{I_p R_N}{R_E + R_N} - \Psi \left(G(t) + \dfrac{1}{R_E + R_N} \right) & \text{if } t < t_{pulse} \\ -\dfrac{\Psi}{G(t)} & \text{if } t > t_{pulse} \end{cases} \qquad (95.11)$$

subject to the initial condition $\Psi(0) = 0$ (see Fig. 95.1). These equations are solved numerically in a computer simulation.

Experiments have shown that during rupture $\Psi(t)$ has a much longer discharge time than for reversible electrical breakdown (REB; see below) and that the rupture discharge results in $\Psi(t)$ having a sigmoidal shape. A transient aqueous pore can account for the general aspects of this behavior but does not yet give a completely correct description, since the theoretical result is too fast. The striking phenomenon of REB is observed for both artificial planar bilayer membranes and cell membranes. However, the term *breakdown* is misleading, since REB is actually protective. During REB, the membrane acquires a very large conductance by developing a large pore population, and the resulting highly nonlinear increase in G prevents the membrane from achieving $\Psi(t)$ more than about $\Psi \approx 1.5$ V. Experimentally, for example, if certain types of artificial planar bilayer membranes are challenged by short pulses, a characteristic of REB is observed; there is progressive shortening of the postpulse membrane discharge as larger and larger pulses are used. This is consistent with a progressively smaller membrane resistance $R(t)$ being achieved. Significantly, the transition from irreversible behavior ("rupture") to reversible behavior (REB or incomplete reversible electrical breakdown) can be quantitatively described by the evolution of a dynamic pore population. If the pore population is small (the case of moderate Ψ), then the membrane discharge can be sufficiently slow that one or more pores evolve to rupture the membrane. In contrast, if the pore population is large (large Ψ), then there are so many pores that the membrane discharges before any pores evolve to cause rupture.

Cell membrane destruction appears to be more complicated than rupture of planar membranes. A planar membrane has contact with a meniscus at the edge of the aperture in an experimental apparatus and, for this reason, has a total surface tension (both sides of the membrane) Γ that favors expansion of pores. But there may be no corresponding reservoir of membrane molecules in a cell and almost certainly none in the case of a vesicle (approximately an empty spherical membrane). If the osmotic pressure difference across the cell membrane is zero, the cell membrane has $\Gamma \approx 0$ and therefore is not expected to rupture. However, a portion of a cell membrane that is bounded by the cytoskeleton or other cellular structures may behave like a microscopic planar membrane. If so, one or more portions of a cell membrane may rupture, creating permanent openings and leading to cell death.

95.5 Molecular Transport

From a biomedical engineering viewpoint, tremendously enhanced transport of molecules across the cell membrane (and tissues) is likely to be the most important feature of electroporation. Unlike the electromechanical behavior described in the preceding section, relatively little is yet known quantitatively about the detailed mechanism of electroporative molecular transport. There is, however, evidence that electrophoretic transport through pores is the major contribution for charged molecules. An interesting observation is that charged molecule transport caused by a single exponential pulse can exhibit a plateau, in that net transport is independent of field pulse magnitude for large pulse magnitudes. Initial results from a transient aqueous pore model of electroporation use only an electrophoretic drift contribution through pores, and this predicts a quasi-plateau in net molecular transport. Clearly, however, understanding of molecular transport lags that of the basic electromechanical behavior. As discussed briefly below, this lack of basic understanding has not prevented a number of new applications from being explored.

Most potential applications of electroporation seek controlled molecular transport without significant damage to the cells or tissue. However, assessment of cell viability/death after electroporation is nontrivial. The convenient, short-term viability assays usually assume that membrane openings are themselves evidence for cell death. The fact that electroporation, by definition, causes openings with unknown recovery kinetics means that the usual vital stains and membrane exclusion probes cannot be used without validation. Partly for this reason, cell death by electroporation is not well understood. If the cells of interest can be cultured, then clonal growth is the most stringent test, and this can be carried out relatively rapidly if microcolony (e.g., clones of two to eight cells) formation is assessed.

Chemical stress resulting from nonspecific molecular transport is a likely cause of cell death and could result from electroporation which at the membrane level is either reversible or irreversible. The irreversible case clearly can lead to stress, but in principle, membrane-reversible electroporation that causes large chemical exchange also can create stress. In either case, significant molecular exchange can occur. As already noted, in the case of irreversible electroporation, a portion of the cell membrane may behave much like a microscopic planar membrane and undergo rupture. In the case of reversible electroporation, significant molecular transport between the intra- and extracellular volumes could cause a significant chemical imbalance. It too large, the associated chemical stress (loss of essential compounds, entry of harmful compounds) may kill the cell. If so, the local environment of the cell should be relevant, and the ratio

$$R_{\mathrm{vol}} \equiv \frac{V_{\mathrm{extracellular}}}{V_{\mathrm{intracellular}}} \tag{95.12}$$

should affect the degree of chemical stress and may therefore correlate with cell survival or death. If $R_{\mathrm{vol}} \gg 1$ (typical of in vitro conditions such as cell suspensions and anchorage-dependent cell culture), cell death should be favored, while for the other extreme $R_{\mathrm{vol}} \ll 1$ (typical of in vivo tissue conditions), cell survival should be favored. If this volumetric consideration is correct, then for the same degree of electroporation, significantly less damage may occur in tissue than for cells located in body fluids or under most in vitro conditions.

95.6 In Vitro Applications of Electroporation

Almost all initial applications of electroporation have dealt with the introduction of genetic material into cells under in vitro conditions. In this case, cell survival is not a critical issue, since a typical experiment can begin with a large number of cells and only a few successful clones are needed. The widespread use of electroporation for DNA introduction has involved electroporation of a large number of cell types, including microorganisms with intact cell walls and many mammalian cells. Because of their extremely thick and tough cell walls, plant cells have not been emphasized. However, protoplasts and vesicles (which do not have walls) of many types also have been used. In addition to DNA introduction, imaginative use such as introduction of fluorescent indicators, small particles (including virus), antibodies against specific intracellular targets, and reagents (substrates and cofactors) for in situ enzyme assays have begun to be used. One general application is the in vitro loading of cells with small drug molecules, with the goal of introducing loaded cells into the body for drug delivery purposes.

95.7 In Vivo Tissue Electroporation

Introduction of molecules to desired sites within the body is important to many biomedical interventions. A common problem is overcoming tissue transport barriers, many of which contain lipid bilayer membrane barriers. Recent success in biotechnology has produced new therapeutic molecules, many of which have short biologic lifetimes, and this has motivated a major biomedical engineering effort in "drug delivery." Important engineering goals are the provision of both larger drug delivery rates and greater control over delivery. This has motivated the use of tissue electroporation for enhanced cancer tumor therapy, transdermal drug delivery, and localized gene therapy.

Tissue electroporation for enhanced local chemotherapy of solid cancer tumors is one promising application, with some clinical trials undertaken. In conventional chemotherapy, three sources to treatment resistance are recognized: (1) elevated pressure, (2) large diffusion resistance, and (3) reduced blood perfusion. Tissue electroporation can be expected to significantly reduce this physiologic resistance by creating aqueous pathways across cell membranes. An improvement should result, because electroporation involves creation of new aqueous pathways ("pores") across cell membranes, some of which are large. As a result, the pressure should drop as outflow occurs through these pores. Further, as the pressure decreases, tissue compression should lessen so that diffusion resistance will decrease because of both a "looser tissue" and increased cell membrane permeability. In addition, blood perfusion should increase as the pressure falls and blood vessels and capillaries enlarge. Finally, increased molecular transport across the cell membranes of the tumor tissue should increase intracellular access of anticancer drugs at the cellular level. Most initial studies have utilized an established drug, bleomycin, which ordinarily crosses the membrane poorly but is very potent. Initial animal studies have utilized superficial tumors, which allow tumor growth to be readily measured and convenient placement of electrodes.

There is a nonfundamental dilemma, however, that may prevent electrochemotherapy from being as rapidly used as its potential advantages suggest. All approved drugs are molecules that enter cells by existing pathways (passive and active). Thus, although greatly reduced systemic side effects are expected if local tissue electroporation is used with highly charged drug molecules, such compounds will generally not be approved drugs. Of course, it could be argued that modification of conventional anticancer drugs should be pursued. If, for example, charge groups are purposefully added such that intracellular enzymes can subsequently remove them, then these charged analogues could be locally introduced by electroporation but should not enter cells systemically in other parts of the body. The dilemma is that the charged analogues would presumably have to pass through the full regulatory approval process, and this is extremely expensive.

Gene therapy is being widely pursued as a revolutionary medical intervention. Its potential advantage and initial weakness are the same: In vivo alteration of genes is the aim. Almost all approaches are based on the use of viral vectors for two purposes: (1) delivery to the cell interior and (2) insertion of functioning DNA. However, there are concerns that rare recombinant events could cause the viral vector to become an infectious agent. If the contemplated intervention requires deletion of a cell function, then electroporation may be inappropriate, since achieving treatment of ~100% of the target cells would be difficult. However, if it is sufficient to alter a fraction of the cells (e.g., provision of a cell function such as secretion of a specific protein), then local tissue electroporation may provide a general approach.

A very different type of tissue, the human skin, also may be treatable by electroporation. The main motivation is transdermal drug delivery. Established transdermal methods are limited, in that the skin has such a large barrier that relatively few drugs can be delivered across the skin at therapeutic levels. Generally speaking, passive transdermal drug delivery is limited to small, lipophilic molecules such as scapolamine, nitroglycerine, and nicotine which readily permeate the skin; the much larger number of hydrophilic drugs do not cross the skin in therapeutically useful amounts. Moreover, delivery kinetics are slow, typically with onset times of hours.

The origin of the large barrier function of human skin is the key to understanding this problem. It is generally agreed that the rate-limiting barrier to molecular transport is the stratum corneum (SC). This structure comprises the outermost layer of the skin, is about 10 to 15 μm thick, and is the source of the skin's mechanical and chemical protection capability. The SC can be regarded as a "brick wall" in which the "bricks" are the corneocytes, which are flattened remnants of epidermal cells that are enclosed in an unusual protein-lipid bilayer membrane, the corneocyte envelope. The interior of the corneocytes is occupied with cross-linked keratin, and this region increases several-fold in volume as the skin hydrates. The "mortar" surrounding these "bricks" consists of multi-lamellar lipids, with about five or six bilayers between adjacent corneocytes. It is generally believed that intercellular pathways are responsible for most transdermal transport. This may include pathways between corneocytes within the SC but also may involve the so-called appendages, i.e. the sweat glands and ducts and the hair follicles that penetrate the SC. Creation of aqueous pathways across the lipid bilayers should in principle increase the transport of water-soluble drugs through both translipid and transcorneocyte barriers and also across the layers of cells that line the appendages. Specifically, application of large electric field pulses should lead to aqueous pathway creation in both the corneocyte envelopes and in the multilamellar lipid bilayers. Similarly, smaller electric field pulses should create aqueous pathways across lipid-containing barriers in the appendages. Although only a qualitative argument, the idea that new aqueous pathways should be created by large electric field pulses is supported by the fundamental tendency of lipid-containing barriers to electroporate. Recent experiments support this. Studies using high voltage (50 to 100 V across the skin; this is reasonable because the SC has about 100 bilayer membranes in series) have shown that charged molecules, which ordinarily do not cross the skin at significant rates, can be rapidly transported at rates that could be therapeutic. For this reason, there is considerable interest in pursuing the development of this and other tissue electroporation applications in medicine.

References

1. Chang DC, Chassy BM, Saunders JA, (eds). Sowers AE. 1992. Guide to Electroporation and Electrofusion. New York, Academic Press.
2. Blank M (ed). 1993. Electricity and Magnetism in Biology and Medicine. San Francisco, San Francisco Press.
3. Weaver JC. 1993. Electroporation: A general phenomenon for manipulating cells and tissue. J Cellular Biochem 51:426.
4. Orlowski S, Mir LM. 1993. Cell electropermeabilization: A new tool for biochemical and pharmacological studies. Biochim Biophys Acta 1154:51.
5. Weaver JC, Chizmadzhev Y. 1994. Electroporation. In C Polk, E Postow (eds), CRC Handbook of Biological Effects of Electromagnetic Fields, 2d ed. Boca Raton, Fla, CRC Press.

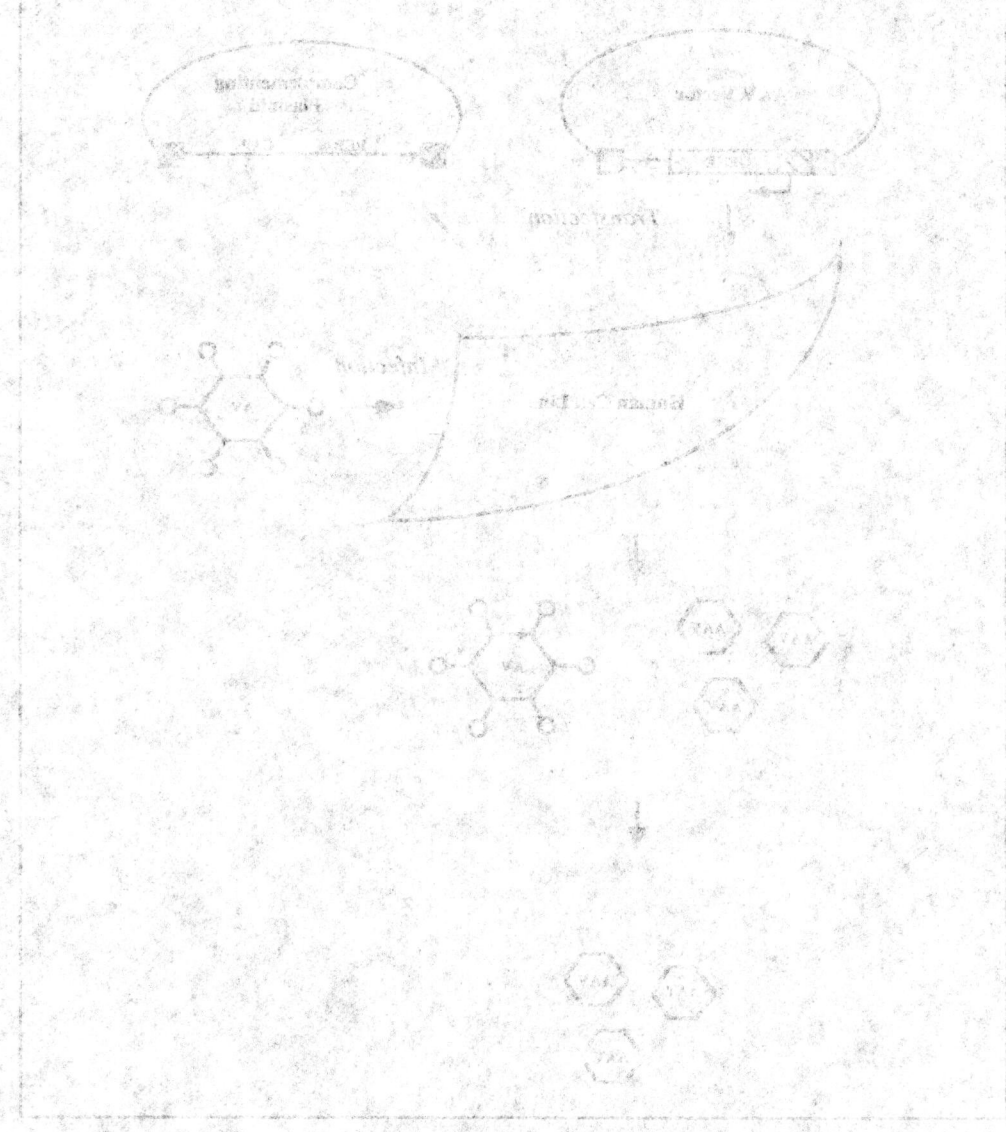

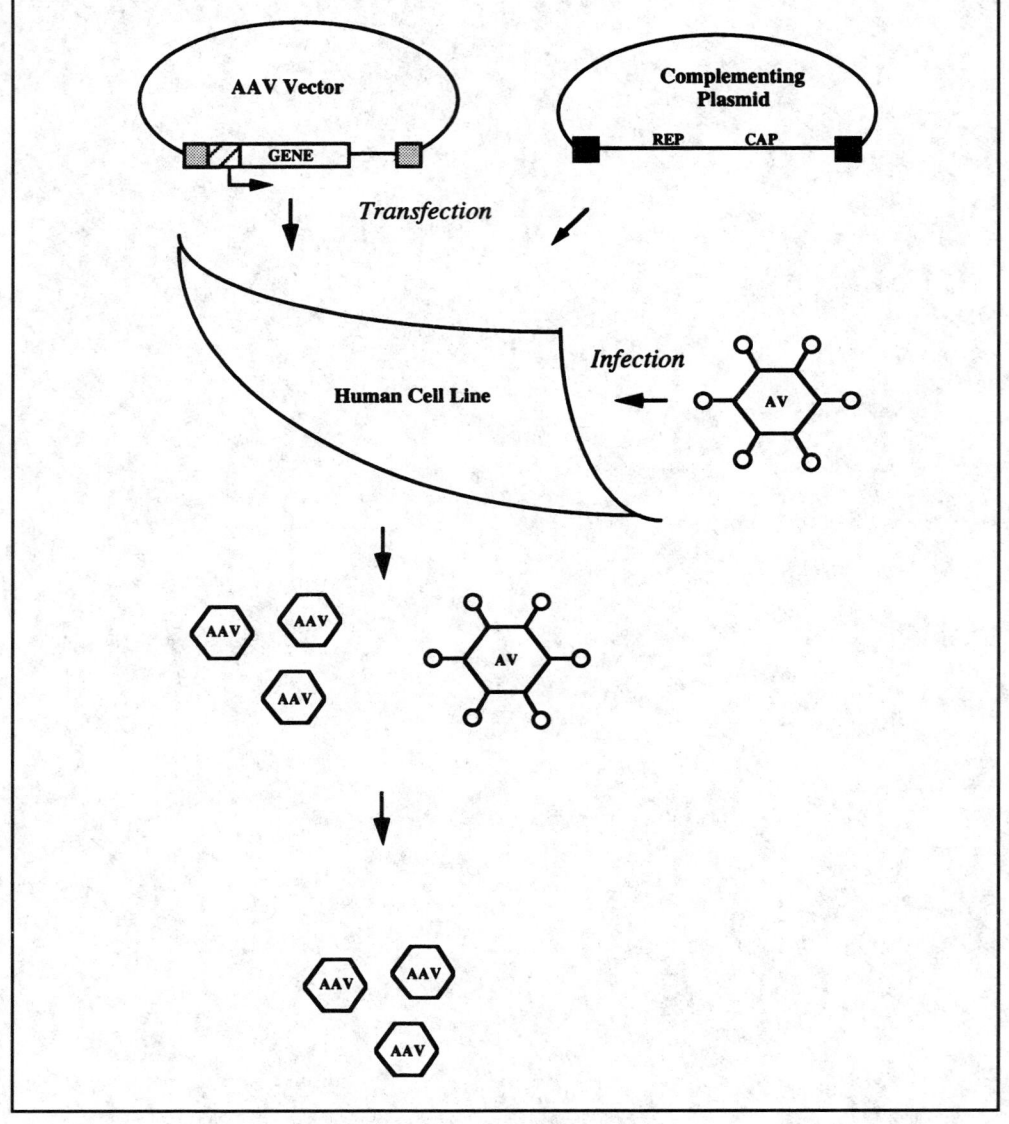

Production of recombinant adeno-associated virus (AAV), which is used in treating cystic fibrosis patients.

X

Biotechnology

Martin L. Yarmush
Rutgers University, Massachusetts General Hospital,
Harvard University Medical School, and the
Shriner Burns Institute

T HE TERM *BIOTECHNOLOGY* HAS UNDERGONE significant change over the past 50 years or so. During the period prior to the eighties, biotechnology referred primarily to the use of microorganisms for large-scale industrial processes such as antibiotic production. Since the 1980s, with the advent of recombinant DNA technology, monoclonal antibody technology, and new technologies for studying and handling cells and tissues, the field of biotechnology has undergone a tremendous resurgence in a wide range of applications pertinent to industry, medicine, and science in general. It is some of these new ideas, concepts, and technologies that will be covered in this section. We have assembled a set of chapters that covers most topics in biotechnology that might interest the practicing biomedical engineer. Absent by design is coverage of agricultural, bioprocess, environmental biotechnology, which is beyond the scope of this *Handbook*.

Chapter 96 deals with our present ability to manipulate genetic material. This new capability, which provides the practitioner with the potential to generate new proteins with improved biochemical and physicochemical properties, has led to the formation of the field of protein engineering. Chapter 97 discusses the field of monoclonal antibody production in terms of its basic technology, diverse applications, and ways that the field of recombinant DNA technology is currently "reshaping" some of the earlier constructs. Chapters 98 and 99 describe applications of nucleic acid chemistry. The burgeoning field of antisense technology is introduced with emphasis on basic techniques and potential applications to AIDS and cancer, and Chapter 99 is dedicated toward identifying the computational, chemical, and machine tools which are being developed and refined for genome analysis. Applied virology is the implied heading for Chapters 100 and 101, in which viral vaccines and viral-mediated gene therapy are the main foci.

Finally, Chapters 102 through 105 focus on important aspects of cell and tissue structure and function as well as fundamental issues and concepts in tissue and organ construction and preservation. These topics share a common approach toward quantitative analysis of cell and tissue behavior in order to develop the principles for cell and tissue growth, function, and preservation. By viewing the world of biomedical biotechnology through our paradigm of proteins and nucleic acids to viruses to cells and tissues, today's biomedical engineer will hopefully be prepared to meet the challenge of participating in the greater field of biotechnology as an educated observer at the very least.

96

Protein Engineering

Alan J. Russell
University of Pittsburgh

Chenzhao Vierheller
University of Pittsburgh

Enzymes have numerous applications in both research and industry. The conformation of proteins must be maintained in order for them to function at optimal activity. Protein stability is dependent on maintaining a balance of forces that include hydrophobic interactions, hydrogen bonding, and electrostatic interactions. Most proteins are denatured, i.e., lose their active conformation, in high-temperature environments (exceptions to this are found among the enzymes from thermophilic microorganisms). Therefore, understanding and maintaining enzyme stability are critical if enzymes are to be widely used in medicine and industry. Protein engineering [1] is used to construct and analyze modified proteins using molecular biologic, genetic engineering, biochemical, and traditional chemical methods (Table 96.1). The generation of proteins with improved activity and stability is now feasible. Recent developments in molecular biology also have enabled a rapid development of the technologies associated with protein engineering (Table 96.2).

96.1 Site-Directed Mutagenesis

Since site-directed mutagenesis was described by Hutchinson et al. [2] in 1978, it has become a powerful tool to study the molecular structure and function of proteins. The purpose of site-directed mutagenesis is to alter a recombinant protein by introducing, replacing, or deleting a specific amino acid. The technique enables a desired modification to be achieved with exquisite precision [3]. Site-directed mutagenesis has been used to change the activity and stability of enzymes, as well as substrate specificity and affinity. Indeed, much of the biologic detergent enzyme sold in the United States (~$200 million per year) is a protein-engineered variant of the native enzyme.

The basic idea behind site-directed mutagenesis is illustrated in Fig. 96.1. The first step of site-directed mutagenesis involves cloning the gene for the protein to be studied into a vector. This non-trivial exercise is discussed elsewhere in this *Handbook*. Next, an oligonucleotide is designed and synthesized. The oligonucleotide will have a centrally located desired mutation (usually a mismatch) that is flanked by sequences of DNA which are complementary to a specific region of interest. Thus the oligonucleotide is designed to bind to a single region of the target gene. The mutation can then be introduced into the gene by hybridizing the oligonucleotide to the single-stranded template. Single-stranded templates of a target gene may be obtained by either cloning the gene to a single-stranded vector, such as bacteriophage M13 [4], or by using phagemids (a chimeric plasmid containing a filamentous bacteriophage replication origin that directs synthesis of single-stranded DNA with a helper bacteriophage) [5]. Alternatively, single-stranded template may be generated by digesting double-stranded DNA with exonuclease III following nicking of the target DNA with DNase or a restriction endonuclease [6].

-8493-8346-3/95/$0.00+$.50
© 1995 by CRC Press, Inc.

TABLE 96.1   Selected Methods for Modification of Proteins

Chemical/biochemical methods	Side chain/amino acid residue modification
	Immobilization
Biologic methods	Site-directed mutagenesis
	Random mutagenesis

The second strand is synthesized with DNA polymerase using the oligonucleotide as a primer, and the DNA can be recircularized with DNA ligase. The vector that carries the newly synthesized DNA (in which one strand is mutated) can be introduced into a bacterial host, where, because DNA duplicates in a semiconservative mode, half the newly synthesized cells containing the DNA will theoretically contain the mutation. In reality, premature DNA polymerization, DNA mismatch repair, and strand displacement synthesis result in much lower yield of mutants. Different strategies have been developed to obtain a higher level of mutation efficiency in order to minimize the screening of mutant. A second mutagenic oligonucleotide containing an active antibiotic resistance gene can be introduced at the same time as the site-directed oligonucleotide. Therefore, the wild-type plasmid will be eliminated in an antibiotic-selective medium [7] (Fig. 96.2). Alternatively, introducing a second mutagenic oligonucleotide can result in the elimination of a unique restriction endonuclease in the mutant strand [8]. Therefore, wild-type plasmid can be linearized with this unique restriction endonuclease, while the circular mutant plasmid can be transformed into bacteria host. Another alternative method is to perform second-strand extension in the presence of 5-methyl-dCTP, resulting in resistance of number of restriction enzymes, including HpaII, MspI, and Sau3A I, in the mutant strand only [9]. The template DNA can then be nicked with these enzymes, followed by digestion with exonuclease III, to increase mutagenesis efficiency.

The recent development of the polymerase chain reaction provides a new approach to site-direct mutagenesis. In 1989, Ho and colleagues [10] developed a method named *overlap extension* (Fig. 96.3), in which four oligonucleotides are used as primers. Two of the primers containing the mutant are complementary to each other. The two other primers are complementary to the opposite strand of the ends of the cloned genes. Polymerase chain reactions are performed three times. The first two polymerase chain reactions are carried out using one end primer and one mutant primer in each reaction. The products contain one double-stranded DNA from one end to the mutation point and the other double-stranded DNA from another end to the mutation point. In other words, the two DNA products are overlapped in the mutated region. The polymerase chain reaction products are purified and used as templates for the third polymerase chain reaction with two end primers. This generates the whole length of DNA with the desired mutation. The advantage of this method is that it can be done quickly with nearly 100% efficiency.

TABLE 96.2   Potentially Useful Modifications to Proteins

Stability	Increased thermostability
	Increased stability at extremes of pH
	Increased stability in organic solvents
	Resistance to oxidative inactivation
	Resistance to proteolysis
Kinetics	Increased maximum velocity
	Altered affinity for substrate
	Altered substrate specificity
	Resistance to substrate/product inhibition
Biology	Altered spectrum of activity
	Altered substrate specificity

Source: Modified from Primrose SB. 1991. In Molecular Biotechnology, 2d ed. New York, Blackwell Scientific.

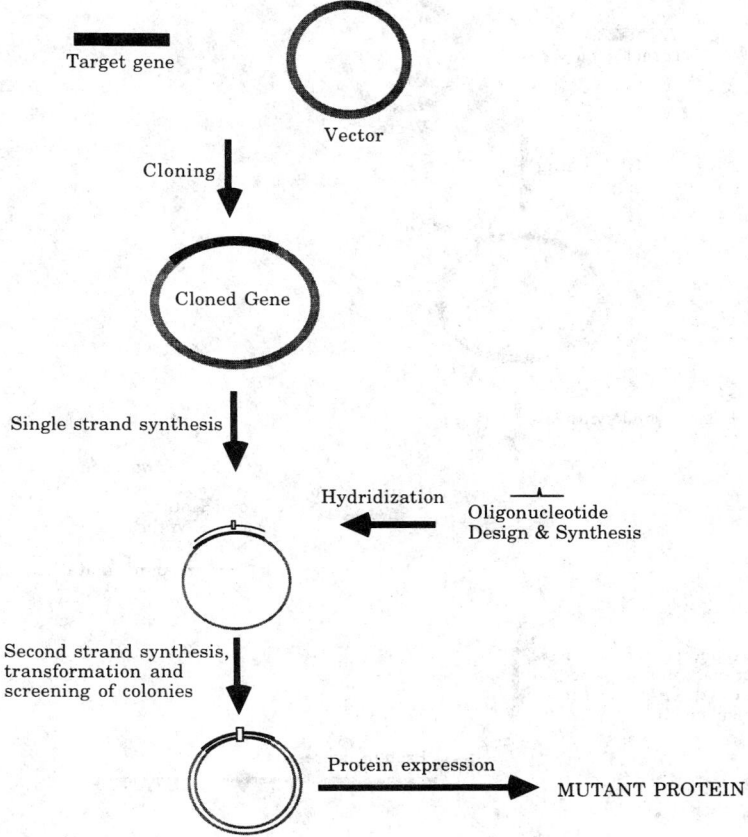

FIGURE 96.1   Overview of site-directed mutagenesis. See text for details.

After screening and selection, a mutation is generally confirmed by DNA sequencing. The mutant then can be subcloned into an expression vector to test the effect of mutation on the activity of the enzyme. Over the last decade, site-directed mutagenesis has become a somewhat trivial technical process, and the most challenging segment of a protein engineering research project is unquestionably the process of determining why a mutant protein has altered properties. The discussion of this particular enterprise lies beyond the scope of this brief review.

96.2 Solvent Engineering

An enzyme-catalyzed reaction can be simplified to its most basic components by considering it as the transfer of a substrate molecule from solvent to the surface of an enzyme molecule. The exchange of substrate-solvent and enzyme-solvent interactions for enzyme-substrate interactions then enables the chemistry of catalysis to take place. *Protein engineering*, as described above, is the process of changing the enzyme in a predictable and precise manner to effect a change on the catalytic process. Since the enzyme is only one side of the balance, however, any changes in the rest of the equation also will alter the catalytic process. Until the late 1980s, for example, substrate specificity could be altered by either protein engineering of the enzyme or by changing the substrate. *Solvent engineering* is now also emerging as a powerful tool in rational control of enzyme activity. Using solvents other than water has successfully led to enzymes with increased thermostability, activity against some substrates, pH dependence, and substrate and enantiospecificity.

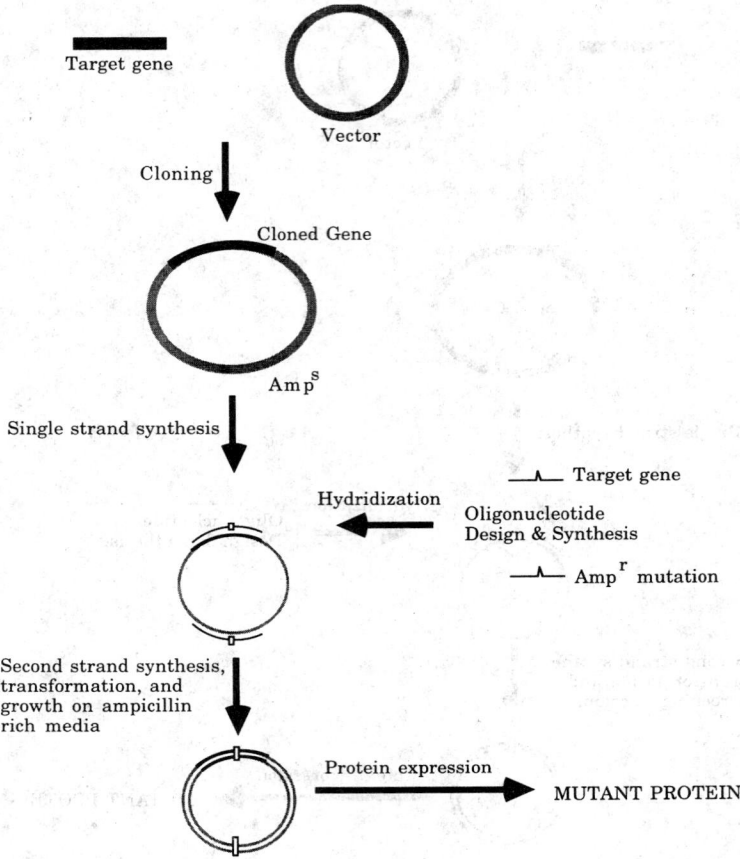

FIGURE 96.2 Selective antibiotic genes as strategy for improvement of site-directed mutagenesis. See text for details.

The simplicity of the solvent-engineering approach is clear. If a protein is not inactivated by a solvent change, then its activity will be dependent on the solvent in which the enzyme and substrate are placed. This strategy has been discussed in detail in recent reviews [11], and we will only summarize the most pertinent information here.

Enzymes that have been freeze-dried and then suspended in anhydrous organic solvents, in which proteins are not soluble, retain their activity and specificity [12]. The enzyme powders retain approximately a monolayer of water per molecule of enzyme during the freeze-drying process. As long as this monolayer of water remains associated with the enzyme in an organic environment, the structure of the enzyme is not disrupted [13], and hence enzyme activity in essentially anhydrous organic solvents can be observed.

The physical properties of a solvent in which an enzyme is placed can influence the level of activity and specificity in a given reaction. For instance, alcohol dehydrogenase can catalyze oxidation-reduction reactions equally well in buffer and heptane, but the level of activity in heptane is sharply dependent on the thermodynamic activity of water in the system. In general, activity can be increased by increasing the hydrophobicity of the solvent used. Interestingly, however, the specificity (both stereo- and substrate) of an enzyme or antibody dispersed in an organic solvent is generally greater in more hydrophilic solvents [14]. Water is involved as a substrate in many of the chemical modification processes that lead to irreversible inactivation of proteins. Not surprisingly, therefore, proteins in anhydrous environments are stable at temperatures exceeding 100°C [15].

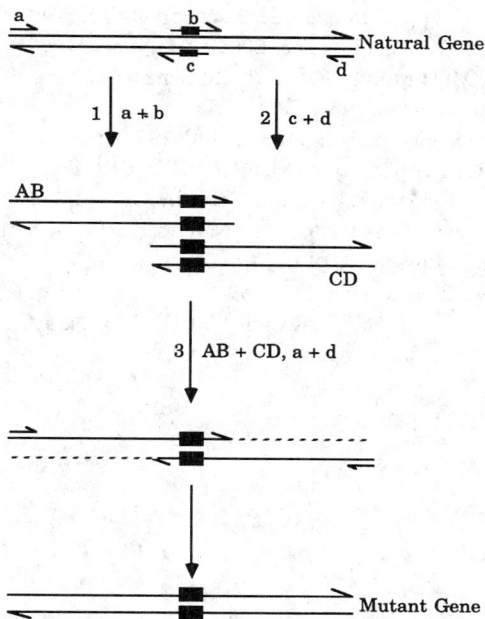

FIGURE 96.3 Site-directed mutagenesis by overlap extension. See text for details.

Considerable attention is now being given to developing the predictability of the solvent-engineering approach. Elucidating the structure-function-environment relationships that govern the activity and specificity of an enzyme is a crucial step for learning how to apply the power of solvent engineering. In recent years, supercritical fluids (materials at temperatures and pressures above their critical point) have been used as a dispersent for enzyme-catalyzed reactions. In addition to being excellent process solvents, the physical properties of supercritical fluids are pressure-dependent. Thus it may be possible to detect which physical properties of a nonaqueous medium have a role in determining a given enzyme function [16].

96.3 Conclusions

The goals of protein and solvent engineering are similar. Ideally, one should be able to predictably alter a given property of an enzyme by either changing the enzyme or its environment. In reality, both approaches are still somewhat unpredictable. Both protein engineering and solvent engineering have been used successfully to alter all the protein properties that appear in Table 96.1. Further research is needed, however, before the results of any given attempt at such biologic engineering can be predicted.

References

1. Alvaro G, Russell AJ. 1991. Methods Enzymol 202:620.
2. Hutchinson C, Phillips S, Edgell M. 1978. J Biol Chem 253:6551.
3. Moody P, Wilkinson A. 1990. Protein Engineering, pp 1–3. IRL Press.
4. Zoller M, Smith M. 1983. Methods Enzymol 100:468.
5. Dente L, Cesareni G, Cortese R. 1983. Nucl Acid Res 11:1645.
6. Rossi J, Zoller M. 1987. In D Oxender, C Fox (eds), Protein Engineering, pp 51–63. New York, Alan R Liss.

7. Promega Protocols and Application Guide, 2d ed, pp 98–105. 1991.
8. Deng W, Nickoloff J. 1992. Anal Biochem 200:81.
9. Vandeyar M, Weiner M, Hutton C, Batt C. 1988. Gene 65:129.
10. Ho N, Hunt H, Horton R, et al. 1989. Gene 77:51.
11. Russell AJ, Chatterjee S, Rapanovich I, Goodwin J. 1992. In A Gomez-Puyon (ed), Biomolecules in Organic Solvents, pp 92–109. Boca Raton, Fla, CRC Press.
12. Zaks A, Klibanov AM. 1985. Proc Natl Acad Sci USA 82:3192.
13. Affleck R, Xu Z-F, Suzawa V, et al. 1992. Proc Natl Acad Sci USA 89:1100.
14. Kamat SV, Beckman EJ, Russell AJ. 1993. J Am Chem Soc 115:8845.
15. Zaks A, Klibanov AM. 1984. Science 224:1249.
16. Kamat S, Iwaskewycz B, Beckman EJ, Russell AJ. 1993. Proc Natl Acad Sci USA 90:2940.

97

Monoclonal Antibodies and Their Engineered Fragments

ikanth Sundaram
tgers University

avid M. Yarmush
tgers University

Antibodies are a class of topographically homologous multidomain glycoproteins produced by the immune system that display a remarkably diverse range of binding specificities. The most important aspects of the immune system are that it is diverse and driven to produce antibodies of the highest possible antigen affinity. The primary repertoire of antibodies consists of about 10^9 different specificities, each of which can be produced by an encounter with the appropriate antigen. This diversity is known to be produced by a series of genetic events each of which can play a role in determining the final function of the antibody molecule. After the initial exposure to the antigen, additional diversity occurs by a process of somatic mutation so that, for any selected antigen, about 10^4 new binding specificities are generated. Thus the immunologic repertoire is the most diverse system of binding proteins in biology. Antibodies also display remarkable binding specificity. For example, it has been shown that antibodies are able to distinguish between *ortho-, meta-,* and *para-* forms of the same haptenic group [Landsteiner, 1945]. This exquisite specificity and diversity make antibodies ideal candidates for diagnostic and therapeutic agents.

Originally, the source of antibodies was antisera, which by their nature are limited in quantity and heterogeneous in quality. Antibodies derived from such sera are termed *conventional antibodies* (*polyclonal antibodies*). Polyclonal antibody production requires methods for the introduction of immunogen into animals, withdrawal of blood for testing the antibody levels, and finally exsanguination for collection of immune sera. These apparently simple technical requirements are complicated by the necessity of choosing a suitable species and immunization protocol that will produce a highly immune animal in a short time. Choice of animal is determined by animal house facilities available, amount of antiserum required (a mouse will afford only 1.0 to 1.5 ml of blood; a goat can provide several liters), and amount of immunogen available (mice will usually respond very well to 50 µg or less of antigen; goats may required several milligrams). Another consideration is the phylogenic relationship between the animal from which the immunogen is derived and that used for antibody production. In most cases, it is advisable to immunize a species phylogenetically unrelated to the immunogen donor, and for highly conserved mammalian proteins, nonmammals (e.g., chickens) should be used for antibody production. The polyclonal antibody elicited by an antigen facilitates the localization, phagocytosis, and complement-mediated lysis of that antigen; thus the usual polyclonal immune response has clear advantages in vivo. Unfortunately, the antibody heterogeneity that increases immune protection in vivo often reduces the efficacy of an antiserum for various in vitro uses. Conventional heterogeneous antisera vary from animal to animal and contain undesirable nonspecific or cross-reacting antibodies. Removal of unwanted specificities from a polyclonal antibody preparation is a time-consuming task, involving repeated adsorption techniques, which often results in the loss of much of the desired antibody and seldom is very effective in reducing the heterogeneity of an antiserum.

After the development of hybridoma technology [Köhler and Milstein, 1975], a potentially unlimited quantity of homogeneous antibodies with precisely defined specificities and affinities (*monoclonal antibodies*) became available, and this resulted in a step change in the utility of antibodies. Monoclonal antibodies (mAbs) have gained increasing importance as reagents in diagnostic and therapeutic medicine, in the identification and determination of antigen molecules, in biocatalysis (catalytic antibodies), and in affinity purification and labeling of antigens and cells.

97.1 Structure and Function of Antibodies

Antibody molecules are essentially required to carry out two principal roles in immune defense. First, they recognize and bind nonself or foreign material (antigen binding). In molecular terms, this generally means binding to structures on the surface of the foreign material (antigenic determinants) that differ from those on the host. Second, they trigger the elimination of foreign material (biologic effector functions). In molecular terms, this involves binding of effector molecules (such as complement) to the antibody-antigen complex to trigger elimination mechanisms such as the complement system and phagocytosis by macrophages and neutrophils, etc.

In humans and other animals, five major immunoglobulin classes have been identified. The five classes include immunoglobulins G (IgG), A (IgA), M (IgM), D (IgD), and E (IgE). With the exception of IgA (dimer) and IgM (pentamer), all other antibody classes are monomeric. The monomeric antibody molecule consists of a basic four-chain structure, as shown in Fig. 97.1. There are two distinct types of chains: the light (L) and the heavy chains (H). The chains are held together by disulfide bonds. The light and heavy chains are held together by interchain disulfides, and the two heavy chains are held together by numerous disulfides in the hinge region of the heavy chain. The light chains have a molecular weight of about 25,000 Da, while the heavy chains have a molecular weight of 50,000 to 77,000 Da depending on the isotype. The L chains can be divided into two subclasses, kappa (κ) and lambda (λ), on the basis of their structures and amino acid sequences. In humans, about 65% of the antibody molecules have κ chains, whereas in rodents, they constitute over 95% of all antibody molecules. The light chain consists of two structural domains: The carboxy-terminal half of the chain is constant except for certain allotypic and isotype variations and is called the C_L (constant: light chain) region, whereas the amino-terminal half of the chain shows much sequence variability and is known as the V_L (variable: light chain) region. The H chains are unique for each immunoglobulin class and are designated by the Greek letter corresponding to the capital letter designation of the immunoglobulin class (α for the H chains of IgA, γ for the H chains of IgG). IgM and IgA have a third chain component, the J chain, which joins the monomeric units. The heavy chain usually consists of four domains: The amino-terminal region (approximately 110 amino acid residues) shows high sequence variability and is called the V_H (variable: heavy chain) region, whereas there are three domains called C_{H1}, C_{H2}, and C_{H3} in the constant part of the chain. The C_{H2} domain is glycosylated, and it has been shown that glycosylation is important in some of the effector functions of antibody molecules. The extent of glycosylation varies with the antibody class and, to some

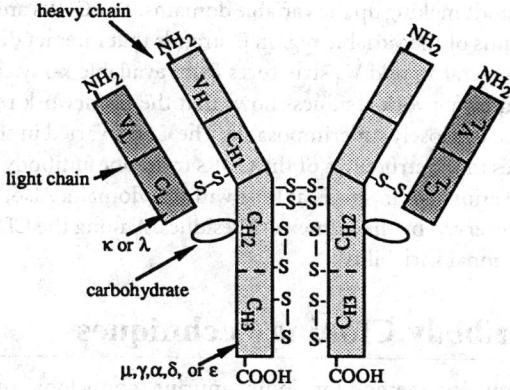

FIGURE 97.1 The structure of a monomeric antibody molecule.

extent, the method of its production. In some antibodies (IgE and IgM), there is an additional domain in the constant part of the heavy chain called the C_{H4} region. The hinge region of the heavy chain (found between the C_{H1} and C_{H2} domains) contains a large number of hydrophilic and proline residues and is responsible for the segmental flexibility of the antibody molecule.

All binding interactions to the antigen occur within the variable domains (V_H and V_L). Each variable domain consists of three regions of relatively greater variability, which have been termed *hypervariable* (HV) or *complementarity-determining regions* (CDR) because they are the regions that determine complementarity to the particular antigen. Each CDR is relatively short, consisting of from 6 to 15 residues. In general, the topography of the six combined CDRs (three from each variable domain) produces a structure that is designed to accommodate the particular antigen. The CDRs on the light chain include residues 24 to 34 (L1), 50 to 56 (L2), and 89 to 97 (L3), whereas those on the heavy chain include residues 31 to 35 (H1), 50 to 65 (H2), and 95 to 102 (H3) in the Kabat numbering system. The regions between the hypervariable regions are called the *framework regions* (FR) because they are more conserved and play an important structural role. The effector functions are, on the other hand, mediated via the two C-terminal constant domains, namely, the C_{H2} and C_{H3}.

Each variable region is composed of several different genetic elements that are separate on the germ line chromosome but rearrange in the B cell to produce a variable-region exon. The light chain is composed of two genetic elements, a variable (V) gene and a joining (J) gene. The V_κ gene generally encodes residues 1 to 95 in a kappa light chain, and the J_κ gene encodes residues 96 to 107, which is the carboxyl end of the variable region. Thus the kappa V gene encodes all the first and second hypervariable regions (L1 and L2) and a major portion of the third hypervariable region (L3). In the human system, there are estimated to be about 100 different V_κ genes and about 5 functional J_κ genes, and the potential diversity is increased by the imprecision of the VJ joining. The heavy-chain variable region is similarly produced by the splicing together of genetic elements that are distant from each other in the germ line. The mature V_H region is produced by the splicing of a variable gene segment (V) to a diversity segment (D) and to a joining (J) segment. There are about 300 V_H genes, about 5 D_H genes, and 9 functional J_H genes [Tizard, 1992]. With respect to the CDRs of the heavy chain, H1 and H2 are encoded by the V_H gene, while the H3 region is formed by the joining of the V, D, and J genes. Additional diversity is generated by recombinational inaccuracies, light- and heavy-chain recombination, and N-region additions.

The three-dimensional structure of several monoclonal antibodies has been determined via x-ray crystallography and has been reviewed extensively [Davies et al., 1990]. Each domain consists of a sandwich of β sheets with a layer of four and three strands making up the constant domains and a layer of four and five strands making up the variable domains. The CDRs are highly solvent exposed and are the loops at the ends of the variable region β strands that interact directly with the antigen. The superimposition of several V_L and V_H structures from available x-ray crystallographic coordinates using the conserved framework residues shows that the framework residues of the antibody variable domains are spatially closely superimposable. The CDRs varied in shape and length, as well as in sequence. Similarities in the structures of the CDRs from one antibody to another suggest that they are held in a fixed relationship in space, at least within a domain. Also, the N and C termini of the CDRs were rigidly conserved by the framework residues. Among the CDRs, L1, L2, H2, and H3 show the most conformational variability.

97.2 Monoclonal Antibody Cloning Techniques

The original, and still dominant, method for cloning murine monoclonal antibodies is through the fusion of antibody-producing spleen B cells and a myeloma line [Köhler and Milstein, 1975]. More recently, "second generation" monoclonal antibodies have been cloned without resorting to hybridoma technology via the expression of combinatorial libraries of antibody genes isolated directly from either immunized or naive murine spleens or human peripheral blood lymphocytes. In addition, display of functional antigen-binding antibody fragments (Fab, sFv, Fv) on the surface of filamentous bacteriophage has further facilitated the screening and isolation of engineered antibody fragments directly from the immunologic repertoire. Repertoire cloning and phage display technology are now readily available in the form of commercial kits [e.g., ImmunoZap and SurfZap Systems from Stratacyte, Recombinant Phage Antibody System (RPAS) from Pharmacia] with complete reagents and protocols.

Hybridoma Technology

In 1975, Kohler and Milstein [1975] showed that mouse myeloma cells could be fused to B lymphocytes from immunized mice resulting in continuously growing, specific monoclonal antibody-secreting somatic cell hybrids, or *hybridoma* cells. In the fused hybridoma, the B cell contributes the capacity to produce specific antibody, and the myeloma cell confers longevity in culture and ability to form tumors in animals.

The number of fusions obtained via hybridoma technology is small, and hence there is a need to select for fused cells. The selection protocol takes advantage of the fact that in normal cells there are two biosynthetic pathways used by cells to produce nucleotides and nucleic acids. The de novo pathway can be blocked using aminopterin, and the salvage pathway requires the presence of functional hypoxanthine guanine phosphoribosyl transferase (HGPRT). Thus, by choosing a myeloma cell line that is deficient in HGPRT as the "fusion partner," Kohler and Milstein devised an appropriate selection protocol. The hybrid cells are selected by using the HAT (hypoxanthine, aminopterin, and thymidine) medium in which only myeloma cells that have fused to spleen cells are able to survive (since unfused myeloma cells are HGPRT−). There is no need to select for unfused spleen cells because these die out in culture.

Briefly, experimental animals (mice or rats) are immunized by injecting them with soluble antigen or cells and an immunoadjuvant. Three or four weeks later, the animals receive a booster injection of the antigen without the adjuvant. Three to five days after this second injection, the spleens of those animals which produce the highest antibody titer to the antigen are excised. The spleen cells are then mixed with an appropriate "fusion partner," which is usually a nonsecreting hybridoma or myeloma cell (e.g., SP2/0 with 8-azaguanine selection) that has lost its ability to produce hypoxanthine guanine phosphoribosyl transferase (HGPRT−). The cell suspension is then briefly exposed to a solution of polyethylene glycol (PEG) to induce fusion by reversibly disrupting the cell membranes, and the hybrid cells are selected for in HAT media. In general, mouse myelomas should yield hybridization frequencies of about 1 to 100 clones per 10^7 lymphocytes. After between 4 days and 3 weeks, hybridoma cells are visible, and culture supernatants are screened for specific antibody secretion by a number of techniques (e.g., radioimmunoassay, ELISA, immunoblotting). Those culture wells which are positive for antibody production are then expanded and subcloned by limiting dilution or in soft agar to ensure that they are derived from a single progenitor cell and to ensure stability of antibody production. Reversion of hybridomas to nonsecreting forms can occur due to loss or rearrangement of chromosomes. The subclones are, in turn, screened for antibody secretion, and selected clones are expanded for antibody production in vitro using culture flasks or bioreactors (yield about 10 to 100 µg/liter) or in vivo as ascites in mice (1 to 10 mg/ml).

The most commonly used protocol is the polyethylene glycol (PEG) fusion technique, which, even under the most efficient conditions, results in the fusion of less than 0.5% of the spleen cells, with only about 1 in 10^5 cells forming viable hybrids. Several methods have been developed to enhance conventional hybrid formation that have led to only incremental improvements in the efficiency of the fusion process (see Neil and Urnovitz [1988] for review). Methods that enhance conventional hybridoma formation include pretreatment of myeloma cells with colcemid and/or in vitro antigen stimulation of the spleen cells prior to fusion, addition of DMSO or phytohemagglutinin (PHA) to PEG during fusion, and addition of insulin, growth factors, human endothelial culture supernatants (HECS), etc. to the growth medium after fusion. In addition, improvements in immunization protocols such as suppression of dominant responses, in vitro or intrasplenic immunization, and antigen targeting also have been developed. Suppression of dominant immune responses is used to permit the expression of antibody-producing cells with specificity for poor immunogens and is achieved using the selective ability of cyclophosphoamide to dampen the immune response to a particular antigen, followed by subsequent immunization with a similar antigen. In in vitro immunization, spleen cells from nonimmunized animals are incubated with small quantities of antigen in a growth medium that has been "conditioned" by the growth of thymocytes. This technique is used most commonly for the production of human hybridomas, where in vivo immunization is not feasible. Intrasplenic immunization involves direct injection of immunogen into the spleen and is typically used when only very small quantities of antigen are available. Other advantages include a shortened immunization time, ability to generate high-affinity monoclonals, and improved diversity in the classes of antibodies generated. Finally, in antigen targeting, the immune response is enhanced by targeting the antigen to specific cells of the immune system, for example, by coupling to anti-class II monoclonal antibodies.

There also have been several advances in fusion techniques such as electrofusion, antigen bridging, and laser fusion. In electrofusion, cells in suspension are aligned using an ac current resulting in cell-cell contact. A brief dc voltage is applied which induces fusion and has resulted in a 30- to 100-fold increase in fusion frequencies in some selected cases. Further improvement in electrofusion yields have been obtained by antigen bridging, wherein avidin is conjugated with the antigen and the myeloma cell membranes are treated with biotin. Spleen cells expressing immunoglobulins of correct specificity bind to the antigen-avidin complex and are in turn bound by the biotinylated cell membranes of the myeloma cells. Finally, laser-induced cell fusion in combination with antigen bridging has been used to eliminate the tedious and time-consuming screening process associated with traditional hybridoma techniques. Here, rather than carry out the fusion process in "bulk," preselected B cells producing antibody of desired specificity and affinity are fused to myeloma cells by irradiating each target cell pair (viewed under a microscope) with laser pulses. Each resulting hybridoma cell is then identified, subcloned, and subsequently expanded.

Despite these improvements, many of the limitations of the hybridoma technique persist. First, it is slow and tedious and labor- and cost-intensive. Second, only a few antibody-producing hybridoma lines are created per fusion, which does not provide for an adequate survey of the immunologic repertoire. Third, as is the case with most mammalian cell lines, the actual antibody production rate is low. Fourth, it is not easy to control the class or subclass of the resulting antibodies, a characteristic that often determines their biologic activity and therefore their usefulness in therapeutic applications. Finally, the production of human monoclonal antibodies by conventional hybridoma techniques has not been very successful due to a lack of suitable human fusion partners, problems related to immunization, difficulty in obtaining human lymphocytes, etc.

Repertoire Cloning Technology

The shortcomings of the hybridoma technology and the potential for improvement of molecular properties of antibody molecules by a screening approach have lead to the expression of the immunologic repertoire in *Escherichia coli.* (repertoire cloning). Two developments were critical to the development of this technology. First, the identification of conserved regions at each end of the nucleotide sequences encoding the variable domains enabled the use of the polymerase chain reaction (PCR) to clone antibody Fv and Fab genes from both spleen genomic DNA and spleen messenger RNA [Orlandi et al., 1989; Sastry et al., 1989]. The amplification of a target sequence via PCR requires two primers, each annealing to one end of the target gene. In the case of immunoglobulin variable-region genes, the J segments are sufficiently conserved to enable the design of universal "downstream" primers. In addition, by comparing the aligned sequences of many variable-region genes, it was found that 5′ ends of the V_H and V_L genes are also relatively conserved so as to enable the design of universal "upstream" primers as well. These primers were then used to establish a repertoire of antibody variable-region genes. Second, the successful expression of functional antigen-binding fragments in bacteria using a periplasmic secretion strategy enabled the direct screening of libraries of cloned antibody genes for antigen binding [Better et al., 1988; Skerra and Pluckthun, 1988].

The first attempt at repertoire cloning resulted in the establishment of diverse libraries of V_H genes from spleen genomic DNA of mice immunized with either lysozyme or keyhole-limpet hemocyanin (KLH). From these libraries, V_H domains were expressed and secreted in *E. coli* [Ward et al., 1989]. Binding activities were detected against both antigens in both libraries; the first library, immunized against lysozyme, yielded 21 clones with lysozyme activity and 2 with KLH activity, while the second library, immunized against KLH, yielded 14 clones with KLH activity and 2 with lysozyme activity. Two V_H domains were characterized with affinities for lysozyme in the 20 nM range. The complete sequences of 48 V_H gene clones were determined and shown to be unique. The problems associated with this single-domain approach are (1) isolated V_H domains suffer from several drawbacks such as lower selectivity and poor solubility and (2) an important source of diversity arising from the combination of the heavy and light chains is lost.

In the so-called combinatorial approach, Huse et al. [1989] used a novel bacteriophage λ vector system (λ-ZAP technology) to express in *E. coli* a combinatorial library of Fab fragments of the murine antibody repertoire. The combinatorial expression library was constructed from spleen mRNA isolated from a mouse immunized with KLH-coupled *p*-nitrophenyl phosphonamidate (NPN) antigen in two steps. In the first step, separate heavy-chain (Fd) and light-chain (κ) libraries were constructed. These two libraries were then combined randomly, resulting in the combinatorial library in which each clone potentially coexpresses a heavy and a light chain. In this case, they obtained 25 million clones in the library, approximately 60% of which coexpressed both chains. One million of these were subsequently screened for antigen binding, resulting in approximately 100 antibody-producing, antigen-binding clones. The light- and heavy-chain libraries, when expressed individually, did not show any binding activity. In addition, the vector systems used also permitted the excision of a phagemid containing the Fab genes; when grown in *E. coli,* these permitted the production of functional Fab fragments in the periplasmic supernatants. While this study did not address the overall diversity of the library, it did establish repertoire cloning as a potential alternative to conventional hybridoma technology.

Repertoire cloning via the λ-ZAP technology (now commercially available as the ImmunoZap kit from Stratacyte) has been used to generate antibodies to influenza virus hemagglutinin (HA) starting with mRNA from an immunized mice [Caton and Kaprowski, 1990]. A total of 10 antigen-binding clones was obtained by screening 125,000 clones from the combinatorial library consisting of 25 million members. Partial sequence analysis of the V_H and V_κ regions of five of the HA-positive recombinants revealed that all the HA-specific antibodies generated by repertoire cloning utilized a V_H region derived from members of a single B-cell clone in conjunction with one of two light-chain variable regions. A majority of the HA-specific antibodies exhibited a common heavy–light-chain combination which was very similar to one previously identified among HA-specific hybridoma monoclonal antibodies. The relative representation of these sequences and the overall diversity of the library also were studied via hybridization studies and sequence analysis of randomly selected clones. It was determined that a single functional V_H sequence was present at a frequency of 1 in 50, while the more commonly occurring light-chain sequence was present at a frequency of 1 in 275. This indicates that the overall diversity of the gene family representation in the library is fairly limited.

The λ-ZAP technology also has been used to produce high-affinity human monoclonal antibodies specific for tetanus toxoid [Mullinax et al., 1990; Persson et al., 1991]. The source of the mRNA in these studies was peripheral blood lymphocytes (PBLs) from human donors previously immunized with tetanus toxoid and boosted with the antigen. Mullinax et al., [1990] estimated that the frequency of positive clones in their library was about 1 in 500, and their affinity constants ranged from 10^6 to 10^9 M (Molar)$^{-1}$. However, the presence of a naturally occurring SacI site (one of the restriction enzymes used to force clone PCR-amplified light-chain genes) in the gene for human C_κ may have resulted in a reduction in the frequency of positive clones. Persson et al. [1991] constructed three different combinatorial libraries using untreated PBLs, antigen-stimulated PBLs (cells cultured in the presence of the antigen), and antigen-panned PBLs (cells that were selected for binding to the antigen). Positive clones were obtained from all three libraries with frequencies if 1 in 6000, 1 in 5000, and 1 in 4000, respectively. Apparent binding constants were estimated to be in the range of 10^7 to 10^9 M^{-1}. Sequence analysis of a limited number of clones isolated from the antigen-stimulated cell library indicated a greater diversity than that described for HA or NPN. For example, of the eight heavy-chain CDR3 sequences examined, only two pairs appeared to be clonally related. The λ-ZAP technology also has been used to rescue a functional human antirhesus D Fab from an EBV-transformed cell line [Burton, 1991].

In principle, repertoire cloning would allow for the rapid and easy identification of monoclonal antibody fragments in a form suitable for genetic manipulation. It also provides for a much better survey of the immunologic repertoire than conventional hybridoma technology. However, repertoire cloning is not without its disadvantages. First, it allows for the production of only antibody fragments. This limitation can be overcome by mounting the repertoire cloned variable domains onto constant domains that possess the desired effector functions and using transfectoma technology to express the intact immunoglobulin genes in a variety of host systems. This has been demonstrated for the case of a human Fab fragment to tetanus toxoid, where the Fab gene fragment obtained via repertoire cloning was linked to an Fc fragment gene and successfully expressed in a CHO cell line [Bender et al., 1993]. The second limitation relates to the use of "immunized" repertoires, which has serious implications in the applicability of this technology for the production of human monoclonal antibodies. The studies reviewed above have all used spleen cells or PBLs from immunized donors. This has resulted in relatively high frequency of positive clones, eliminating the need for extensive screening. Generating monoclonal antibodies from "naive" donors (who have not had any exposure to the antigen) would require the screening of very large libraries. Third, the actual diversity of these libraries is still unclear. The studies reported above show a wide spectrum ranging from very limited (the HA studies) to moderate (NPN) to fairly marked diversity (tetanus toxoid). Finally, the combinatorial approach is disadvantageous in that it destroys the original pairing of the heavy and light chains selected for by immunization. Strategies for overcoming some of these limitations have already been developed and are reviewed below.

Phage Display Technology

A critical aspect of the repertoire cloning approach is the ability to screen large libraries rapidly for clones that possess desired binding properties, e.g., binding affinity or specificity, catalysis, etc. This is especially the case for "naive" human repertoires, wherein the host has not been immunized against the antigen of interest for ethical and/or safety reasons. In order to facilitate screening of large libraries of antibody genes, *phage display* of functional antibody fragments has been developed, which has resulted in an enormous increase in the utility of repertoire cloning technology. In phage display technology, functional antibody fragments (such as the sFv and Fab) are expressed on the surface of filamentous bacteriophages, which facilitates the selection of specific binders (or any other property such as catalysis, etc.) from a large pool of irrelevant antibody fragments. Typically, several hundreds of millions of phage particles (in a small volume of 50 to 100 ml) can be tested for specific binders by allowing them to bind to the antigen of interest immobilized to a solid matrix, washing away the nonbinders, and eluting the binders using a suitable elution protocol.

Phage display of antibody fragments is accomplished by coupling of the antibody fragment to a coat protein of the bacteriophage. Two different coat proteins have been used for this purpose, namely, the major coat protein encoded for by gene VIII and the adsorption protein encoded for by gene III. The system based on gene VIII displays several copies of the antibody fragment (theoretically there are 2000 copies of gene VIII product per phage) and is used for the selection of low-affinity binders. The gene III product is, on the other hand, present at approximately four copies per phage particle and leads to the selection of high-affinity binders. However, since the native gene III product is required for infectivity, at least one copy on the phage has to be a native one.

The feasibility of phage display of active antibody fragments was first demonstrated by McCafferty et al. [1990] when the single-chain Fv fragment (single-chain antibody) of the anti-hen egg white lysozyme (HEL) antibody was cloned into an fd phage vector at the N-terminal region of the gene III protein. This study showed that complete active sFv domains could be displayed on the surface of bacteriophage fd and that rare phage displaying functional sFv (1 in 10^6) can be isolated. Phage that bound HEL were unable to bind to turkey egg white lysozyme, which differs from HEL by only seven residues. Similarly, active Fab fragments also have been displayed on phage surfaces using gene VIII [Kang et al., 1991]. In this method, assembly of the antibody Fab molecules in the periplasm occurs in concert with phage morphogenesis. The Fd chain of the antibody fused to the major coat protein VIII of phage M13 was coexpressed with κ chains, with both chains being delivered to the periplasmic space by the pelB leader sequence. Since the Fd chain is anchored in the membrane, the concomitant secretion of the κ chains results in the assembly of the two chains and hence the display of functional Fab on the membrane surface. Subsequent infection with helper phage resulted in phage particles that had incorporated functional Fab along their entire surface. Functionality of the incorporated Fab was confirmed by antigen-specific precipitation of phage, enzyme-linked immunoassays, and electron microscopy. The production of soluble antibody fragments from selected phages can now be accomplished without subcloning [Hoogenboom et al., 1991]. The switch from surface display to soluble antibody is mediated via the use of an amber stop codon between the antibody gene and phage gene protein. In a *sup*E suppresser strain of *E. coli*, the amber codon is read as Glu and the resulting fusion protein is displayed on the surface of the phage. In nonsuppresser strains, however, the amber codon is read as a stop codon, resulting in the production of soluble antibody.

The combination of repertoire cloning technology and phage display technology was initially used to screen antibody fragments from repertoires produced from immunized animals, namely, the production of Fv fragments specific for the hapten phenyloxazolone using immunized mice [Clackson et al., 1991], human Fab fragments to tetanus toxoid [Barbas et al., 1991], human Fab fragments to gp120 using lymphocytes isolated from HIV-positive individuals [Burton et al., 1991], and human Fab fragments to hepatitis B surface antigen from vaccinated individuals [Zebedee et al., 1992]. These studies established the utility of phage display as a powerful screening system for functional antibody fragments. For example, attempts to generate human Fab fragments against gp120 using the λ-ZAP technology failed to produce any binders. Phage display, on the other handed, resulted in 33 of 40 clones selected via antigen panning possessing clear reactivity with affinity constants of the order of $10^{-8} M^{-1}$. In the case of the tetanus toxoid studies, phage display was used to isolate specific clones from a library that included known tetanus toxoid clones at a frequency of 1 in 170,000.

Bypassing Immunization

The next step was the application of phage display technology to generate antibodies from unimmunized donors (naive repertoires). Marks et al. [1991] constructed two combinatorial libraries starting from peripheral blood lymphocytes of unimmunized human donors, namely, an IgM library using μ-specific PCR primers and an IgG library using γ-specific primers. The libraries were then screened using phage display and sFv fragments specific for nonself antigens such as turkey egg white lysozyme, bovine serum albumin, phenyloxazolone, and bovine thyroglobulin, as well as for self antigens such as human thyroglobulin, human tumor necrosis factor α, cell surface markers, carcinoembryonic antigen, and mucin, and human blood group antigens were isolated [Hoogenboom et al., 1992]. The binders were all isolated from the IgM library (with the exception of six clones for turkey egg white lysozyme isolated from the IgG library), and the affinities of the soluble antibody fragments were low to moderate (2×10^6 to $10^7 M^{-1}$). Both these results are typical of the antibodies produced during a primary response.

The second stage of an immune response in vivo involves affinity maturation, in which the affinities of antibodies of the selected specificities are increased by a process of somatic mutation. Thus one method by which the affinities of antibodies generated from naive repertoires may be increased is by mimicking this process. Random mutagenesis of the clones selected from naive repertoires has been accomplished by error-prone PCR [Gram et al., 1992]. In this study, low-affinity Fab fragments (10^4 to $10^5 M^{-1}$) to progesterone were initially isolated from the library, and their affinities increased 13- to 30-fold via random mutagenesis. An alternative approach to improving the affinities of antibodies obtained from naive repertoires involves the use of chain shuffling [Marks et al., 1992]. This study describes the affinity maturation of a low-affinity antiphenyloxazolone antibody ($3 \times 10^7 M^{-1}$). First, the existing light chain was replaced with a repertoire of in vivo somatically mutated light chains from unimmunized donors resulting in the isolation of a clone with a 20-fold increase in affinity. Next, shuffling of the heavy chain in a similar manner with the exception of retaining the original H3 resulted in a further increase in affinity of about 16-fold. The net increase in affinity (320-fold) resulted in a dissociation constant of 1 nM, which is comparable with the affinities obtained through hybridoma technology.

Other approaches to bypassing human immunization involve the use of semisynthetic and synthetic combinatorial libraries [Barbas et al., 1992] and the immunization of SCID mice that have been populated with human peripheral blood lymphocytes [Duchosal et al., 1992].

97.3 Monoclonal Antibody Expression Systems

Several expression systems are currently available for in vitro production of antibodies such as bacteria, yeast, plants, baculovirus, and mammalian cells. In each of these systems, cloned antibody genes are the starting point for production. These are obtained either by traditional cloning techniques starting with preexisting hybridomas or by the more recent repertoire cloning techniques. Each of the aforementioned systems has its own advantages and drawbacks. For example, bacterial expression systems suffer from the following limitations: They cannot be used for producing intact antibodies, nor can they glycosylate antibodies. Unglycosylated antibodies cannot perform many of the effector functions associated with normal antibody molecules. Proper folding may sometimes be a problem due to difficulty in forming disulfide bonds, and often, the expressed antibody may be toxic to the host cells. On the other hand, bacterial expression has the advantage that it is cheap, can potentially produce large amounts of the desired product, and can be scaled up easily. In addition, for therapeutic products, bacterial sources are to be preferred over mammalian sources due to the potential for the contamination of mammalian cell lines with harmful viruses.

Bacterial Expression

Early attempts to express intact antibody molecules in bacteria were fairly unsuccessful. Expression of intact light and heavy chains in the cytoplasm resulted in the accumulation of the proteins as nonfunctional inclusion bodies. In vitro reassembly was very inefficient [Boss et al., 1984; Cabilly et al., 1984]. These results could be explained on the basis of the fact that the *E. coli* biosynthetic environment does not support protein folding that requires specific disulfide bond formation, post-translational modifications such as glycosylation, and polymeric polypeptide chain assembly.

There has been much more success obtained with antibody fragments. Bacterial expression of IgE "Fc-like" fragments has been reported [Kenten et al., 1984; Ishizaka et al., 1986]. These IgE fragments exhibited some of the biologic properties characteristic of intact IgE molecules. The fragments constituted 18% of the total bacterial protein content but were insoluble and associated with large inclusion bodies. Following reduction and reoxidation, greater than 80% of the chains formed dimers. The fragment binds to the IgE receptor on basophils and mast cells and, when cross-linked, elicits the expected mediator (histamine) release.

Cytoplasmic expression of a Fab fragment directed against muscle-type creatinine kinase, followed by in vitro folding, resulted in renaturation of about 40% of the misfolded protein, with a total active protein yield of 80 μg/ml at 10°C [Buchner and Rudolph, 1991]. Direct cytoplasmic expression of the so-called single-chain antibodies, which are novel recombinant polypeptides composed of an antibody V_L tethered to a V_H by a designed "linker" peptide that links the carboxyl terminus of the V_L to the amino terminus of the V_H or vice versa, was the next important step. Various linkers have been used to join the two variable domains. Bird et al. [1988] used linkers of varying lengths (14 to 18 amino acids) to join the two variable domains. Huston et al. [1988] used a 15 amino acid "universal" linker with the sequence $(GGGGS)_3$. The single-chain protein was found to accumulate in the cell as insoluble inclusion bodies and needed to be refolded in vitro. However, these proteins retained both the affinity and specificity of the native Fabs.

In 1988, two groups reported, for the first time, the expression of functional antibody fragments (Fv and Fab, respectively) in *E. coli* [Better et al., 1988; Skerra and Pluckthun, 1988]. In both cases, the authors attempted to mimic in bacteria the natural assembly and folding pathway of antibody molecules. In eukaryotic cells, the two chains are expressed separately with individual leader sequences that direct their transport to the endoplasmic reticulum (ER), where the signal sequences are removed and correct folding, disulfide formation, and assembly of the two chains occur. By expressing the two chain fragments (V_L and V_H in the case of Fv expression and the Fd and K chains in the case of Fab expression) separately with bacterial signal sequences, these workers were successful in directing the two precursor chains to the periplasmic space, where correct folding, assembly, and disulfide formation occur along with the removal of the signal sequences, resulting in fully functional antibody fragments. Skerra and Pluckthun [1988] report the synthesis of the Fv fragment of MOPC 603 which has an affinity constant identical to that of the intact Ab. Better et al. [1988] report the synthesis of the Fab fragment of an Ig that binds to a ganglioside antigen. While Skerra and Pluckthun obtained a yield of 0.2 mg/liter after a periplasmic wash, Better et al. found that the Fab fragment was secreted into the culture medium with a yield of 2 mg/liter. However, previous attempts to synthesize an active, full-size Ig in *E. coli* by coexpression and secretion mediated by procaryotic signal sequences resulted in poor synthesis and/or secretion of the heavy chain.

Since these early reports, several additional reports have been published (for reviews, see Pluckthun [1992] and Skerra [1993]) which have established the two aforementioned strategies (namely, direct cytoplasmic expression of antibody fragments followed by in vitro refolding and periplasmic expression of functional fragments) as the two standard procedures for the bacterial expression of antibody fragments. Expression of the protein in the periplasmic space has advantages: (1) the expressed protein is recovered in an fully functional form, thereby eliminating the need for in vitro refolding (as is required in the case of cytoplasmically expressed fragments), and (2) it greatly simplifies purification. On the other hand, direct cytoplasmic expression may, in some cases, reduce problems arising from toxicity of the expressed protein and also may increase the total yield of the protein.

Several improvements have been made in the past few years so as to simplify the expression and purification of antibody fragments in bacteria. These include the development of improved vectors with strong promoters for the high-level expression of antibody fragments, the incorporation of many different signal sequences, and the incorporation of cleavable "affinity" handles that simplify purification. Many expression vector systems are now commercially available that enable the rapid cloning, sequencing, and expression of immunoglobulin genes in bacteria within a matter of 2 to 3 weeks.

Expression in Lymphoid and Nonlymphoid Systems (Transfectoma Technology)

Expression of immunoglobulin genes by transfection into eukaryotic cells (*transfectoma technology*) such as myelomas and hybridomas is an alternative approach for producing monoclonal antibodies [Wright et al., 1992; Morrison and Oi, 1989]. Myelomas and hybridomas are known to be capable of high-level expression of endogenous heavy- and light-chain genes and can glycosylate, assemble, and secrete functional antibody molecules and therefore are the most appropriate mammalian cells for immunoglobulin gene transfection. Nonlymphoid expression in CHO and COS cells also has been examined as a potential improvement over expression in lymphoid cells. The biologic properties and effector functions, which are very important considerations for applications involving human therapy and diagnostics, are completely preserved in this mode of expression. However, transfectoma technology still involves working with eukaryotic cell lines with low antibody production rates and poor scale-up characteristics.

Transfectoma technology provides us with the ability to genetically manipulate immunoglobulin genes to produce antibody molecules with novel and/or improved properties. For example, production of "chimeric" and "reshaped" antibodies, wherein the murine variable domains or CDRs are mounted onto a human antibody framework in an attempt to reduce the problem of immunogenicity in administering murine antibodies for in vivo diagnostic and/or therapeutic purposes, would not be possible without the techniques of transfectoma technology. It is also possible to change the isotype of the transfectoma antibodies in order to change their biologic activity. It also has enabled the fusion of antibodies with nonimmunoglobulin proteins such as enzymes or toxins, resulting in novel antibody reagents useful in industrial and medicinal applications.

The most commonly used vectors are the pSV2 vectors that have several essential features. First, they contain a plasmid origin of replication and a marker selectable for procaryotes. This makes it relatively easy to obtain large quantities of DNA and facilitates genetic manipulation. Second, they contain a marker expressible and selectable in eukaryotes. This consists of a eukaryotic transcription unit with an SV40 promoter, splice, and poly A addition site. Into this eukaryotic transcription unit is placed a dominant selectable marker derived from procaryotes (either the *neo* gene or the *gpt* gene).

In order to create the immunoglobulin molecules, the two genes encoding the heavy and light chains must be transfected and both polypeptides must be synthesized and assembled. Several methods have been used to achieve this objective. Both the heavy- and light-chain genes have been inserted into a single vector and then transfected. This approach generates large, cumbersome expression vectors, and further manipulation of the vector is difficult. A second approach is to transfect sequentially the heavy- and light-chain genes. To facilitate this, one gene is inserted into an vector with the *neo* gene, permitting selection with antibiotic G418. The other gene is placed in an expression vector containing the *gpt* gene, which confers mycophenolic acid resistance to the transfected cells. Alternatively, both genes may be introduced simultaneously into lymphoid cells using protoplast fusion.

Heavy- and light-chain genes, when transfected together, produced complete, glycosylated, assembled tetrameric antigen-binding antibody molecules with appropriate disulfide bonds. Under laboratory conditions, these transfected cells yield about 1 to 20 mg/liter of secreted antibody. A persisting problem has been the expression level of the transfected immunoglobulin gene. The expression of transfected heavy-chain genes is frequently seen to approach the level seen in myeloma cells; however, efficient expression of light-chain genes is more difficult to achieve.

Expression in Yeast

Yeast is the simplest eukaryote capable of glycosylation and secretion and has the advantages of rapid growth rate and ease of large-scale fermentation. It also retains the advantage that unlike other mammalian systems, it does not harbor potentially harmful viruses.

Initial attempts to express λ and μ immunoglobulin chains specific for the hapten NP in the yeast *Sacchromyces cerevisiae* under the control of the yeast 3-phosphoglycerate kinase (PGK) promoter resulted in the secretion into culture medium at moderate efficiency (5% to 40%), but secreted antibodies had no antigen-binding activity [Wood et al., 1985]. Subsequent attempts to coexpress heavy and light chains with the yeast invertase signal sequence under the control of the yeast phosphoglycerate kinase (PGK) promoter were more successful, presumably due to differences in the efficiency of different yeast signal sequences in directing the secretion of mammalian proteins from yeast. Culture supernatants contained significant quantities of both light and heavy chains (100 and 50 to 80 mg/liter, respectively) with about 50% to 70% of the heavy chain associated with the light chain. The yeast-derived mouse-human chimeric antibody L6 was indistinguishable from the native antibody in its antigen-binding properties [Horowitz et al., 1988; Better and Horowitz, 1989]. Furthermore, it was superior to the native antibody in mediating antibody-dependent cellular cytotoxicity (ADCC) but was incapable of eliciting complement-dependent cytolysis (CDC). Yeast-derived L6 Fab also was indistinguishable from proteolytically generated Fab as well as recombinant Fab generated from *E. coli*.

Expression in Baculovirus

The baculovirus expression system is potentially a very useful system for the production of large amounts of intact, fully functional antibodies for diagnostic and even therapeutic applications. Foreign genes expressed in insect cell cultures infected with baculovirus can constitute as much as 50% to 75% of the total cellular protein late in viral replication. Immunoglobulin gene expression is achieved by commercially available vectors that place the gene to be expressed under the control of the efficient promoter of the gene encoding the viral polyhedrin protein. The levels of expression seen in this system can be as much as 50- to 100-fold greater per cell than in procaryotes while retaining many of the advantages of an eukaryotic expression system such as glycosylation and extracellular secretion. However, scale-up is not straightforward, since viral infection eventually results in cell death.

There have been at least two reports of antibody secretion in a baculovirus system [Hasemann and Capra, 1990; Putlitz, 1990]. In both cases, the secreted antibody was correctly processed, glycosylated (albeit differently than hybridoma-derived antibody), and assembled into a normal functional heterodimer capable of both antigen binding and complement binding. The secreted antibodies were obtained at a yield of about 5 mg/liter.

Expression in Plants

The development of techniques for plant transformation has led to the expression of a number of foreign genes, including immunoglobulin genes, in transgenic plants [Hiatt and Ma, 1992]. The most commonly used plant cell transformation protocol employs the ability of plasmid Ti of *Agrobacterium tumefaciens* to mediate gene transfer into the plant genome.

The expression of a murine anti-phosphonate ester catalytic antibody in transgenic plants was accomplished by first transforming the heavy-chain and light-chain genes individually into different tobacco plants [Hiatt et al., 1989]. These were then sexually crossed to obtain progeny that expressed both chains simultaneously. It was shown that leader sequences were necessary for the proper expression and assembly of the antibody molecules. The level of antibody expression was determined to be about 3 ng/mg of total protein, and the plant-derived antibody was comparable with ascites-derived antibody with respect to binding as well as catalysis.

97.4 Genetically Engineered Antibodies and Their Fragments

The domain structure of the antibody molecule allows the reshuffling of domains and the construction of functional antibody fragments. A schematic representation of such genetically engineered antibodies and their fragments is shown in Figs. 97.2 and 97.3.

Among intact engineered constructs are chimeric, humanized, and bifunctional antibodies (see Wright et al. [1992] and Sandhu [1992] for reviews). A major issue in the long-term use of murine monoclonal antibodies for clinical applications is the immunogenicity of these molecules or the so-called HAMA response (human antimouse antibody response). Simple chimeric antibodies were constructed by linking murine variable domains to human constant domains in order to reduce immunogenicity of therapeutically administered murine monoclonals. The approach has been validated by several clinical trials that show that chimeric antibodies are much less likely to induce a HAMA response compared with their murine counterparts. In a more sophisticated approach, *CDR grafting* has been used to "humanize" murine monoclonal antibodies for human therapy by transplanting the CDRs of a murine monoclonal antibody of appropriate antigenic specificity onto a human framework. Humanized antibodies are, in some cases, even better than their chimeric counterparts in terms of the HAMA response.

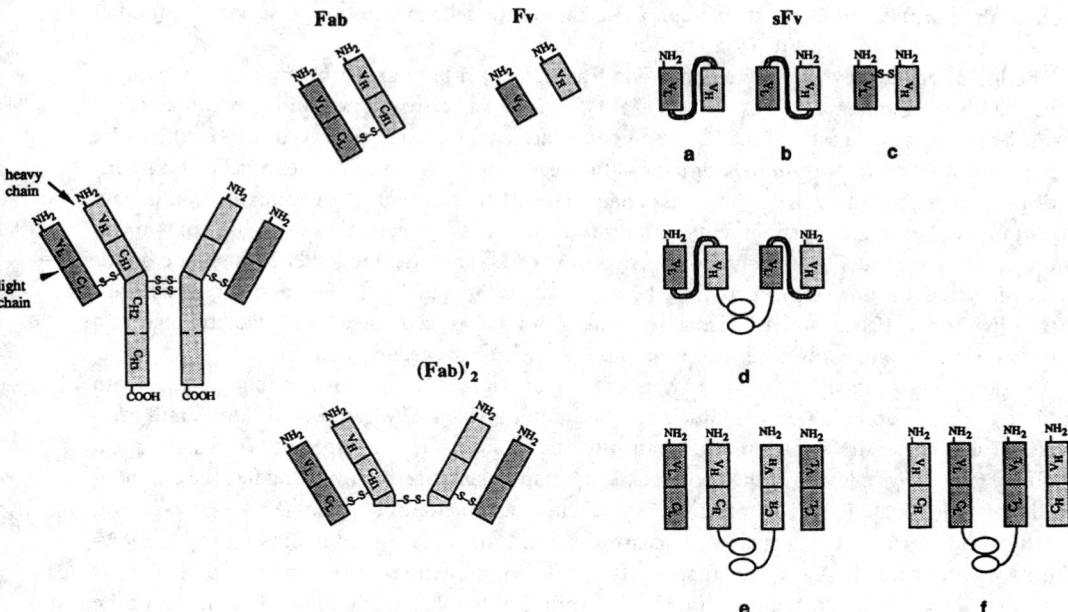

FIGURE 97.2 Schematic of an antibody molecule and its antigen binding fragments. (*a*–*e*) Examples of the fragments expressed in *Escherichia coli*: (*a*) single-chain Fv fragment in which the linking peptide joins the light and heavy Fv segments in the following manner: V_L (carboxyl terminus)–peptide linker–V_H (amino terminus); (*b*) single-chain Fv fragment with the following connection: V_L (amino terminus)–peptide linker–V_H (carboxyl terminus); (*c*) disulfide-linked Fv fragment; (*d*) "miniantibody" comprised of two helix-forming peptides each fused to a single-chain Fv; (*e*) Fab fragments linked by helix-forming peptide fused to heavy chain; (*f*) Fab fragments linked by helix-forming peptide fused to light chain.

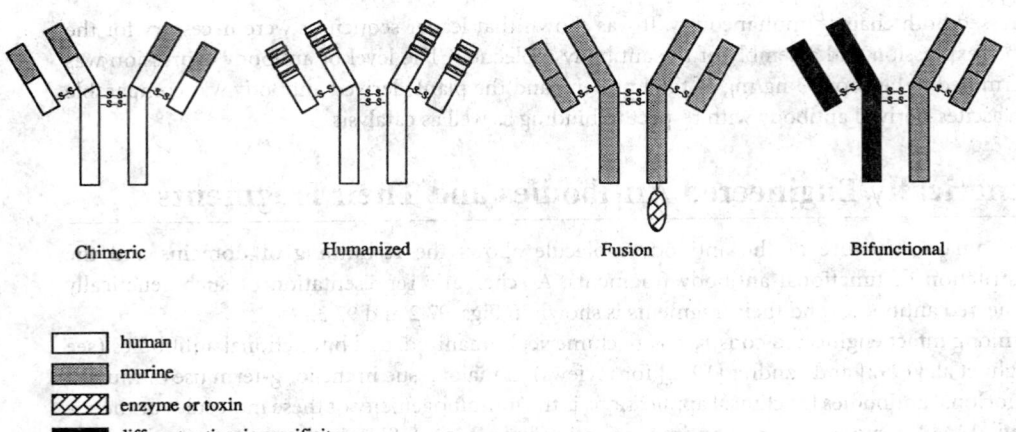

Chimeric   Humanized   Fusion   Bifunctional

☐ human
▨ murine
▧ enzyme or toxin
■ different antigenic specificity

FIGURE 97.3 Schematic of genetically engineered intact monoclonal antibodies prepared with antibody-engineering techniques.

Bifunctional antibodies that contain antigen-specific binding sites with two different specificities have been produced via genetic engineering as well as chemical techniques [Fanger et al., 1992]. The dual specificity of bispecific antibodies can be used to bring together the molecules or cells that mediate the desired effect. For example, a bispecific antibody that binds to target cells such as a tumor cell and to cytotoxic trigger molecules on host killer cells such as T cells has been used to redirect the normal immune system response to the tumor cells in question. Bispecific antibodies also have been used to target toxins to tumor cells.

The list of genetically engineered antibody fragments is a long and growing one [Pluckthun, 1992]. Of these, fragments such as the Fab, F(ab)$'_2$, Fv, and the Fc are not new and were initially produced by proteolytic digestion. The Fab fragment (fragment antigen-binding) consists of the entire light chain and the two N-terminal domains of the heavy chain (V_H and C_{H1}, the so-called Fd chain) and was first generated by digestion with papain. The other fragment that is generated on papain digestion is the Fc fragment (fragment crystallizable), which is a dimeric unit composed of two C_{H2} and C_{H3} domains. The F(ab)$'_2$ fragment consists of two Fab arms held together by disulfide bonds in the hinge region and was first generated by pepsin digestion. Finally, the Fv fragment, which consists of just the two N-terminal variable domains, also was first generated by proteolytic digestion and is now more commonly generated via antibody-engineering techniques.

The other fragments listed in Fig. 97.2 are of genetic origin. These include the sFv (single-chain antibody), the V_H domain (single-domain antibody), multivalent sFvs (miniantibodies), and multivalent Fabs. The multivalent constructs can either be monospecific or bispecific. The single-chain antibody (SCA, sFv) consists of the two variable domain linked together by a long flexible polypeptide linker [Bird et al., 1988; Huston et al., 1988]. The sFv is an attempt to stabilize the Fv fragment, which is known to dissociate at low concentrations into its individual domains due to the low-affinity constant for the V_H-V_L interaction. Two different constructs have been made: the V_L-V_H construct where the linker extends from the C terminus of the V_L domain to the N terminus of the V_H domain, and the V_H-V_L construct, where the linker runs from the C terminus of the V_H domain to the N terminus of the V_L. The linker is usually about 15 amino acids long (the length required to span the distance between the two domains) and has no particular sequence requirements other than to minimize potential interferences in the folding of the individual domains. The so-called universal linker used by many workers in the area is (GGGGS)$_3$. Other strategies to stabilize the Fv fragment include chemical cross-linking of the two domains and disulfide-linked domains [Glockshuber et al., 1990]. Chemical cross-linking via glutaraldehyde has been demonstrated to be effective in stabilizing the Fv fragment in one instance; here, the cross-linking was carried out in the presence of the hapten (phosphorylcholine) to avoid modification of the binding site, an approach that may not be feasible with protein antigens. In the disulfide-linked sFv, Cys residues are introduced at suitable locations in the framework region of the Fv so as to form a natural interdomain disulfide bond. This strategy was shown to be much more effective in stabilizing the Fv fragment against thermal denaturation than either the single-chain antibody approach or chemical cross-linking for the one case where all three approaches were tested [Glockshuber et al., 1990].

The single-domain antibody consists of just the V_H domain and has been shown by some to possess antigen-binding function on its own in the absence of the V_L domain [Ward et al., 1989]. There is some skepticism regarding this approach due to the rather high potential for nonspecific binding (the removal of the V_L domain exposes a very hydrophobic surface), poor solubility, and somewhat compromised selectivity. For example, while the Fv fragment retains its ability to distinguish between related antigenic species, the single-domain antibody does not.

Miniantibodies consist of sFv fragments held together by so-called dimerization handles. sFv fragments are fused via a flexible hinge region to several kinds of amphipathic helices, which then act as dimerization devices [Pack and Pluckthun, 1992]. Alternately, the two sFvs can be fused via a long polypeptide linker, similar to the one linking the individual domains of each Fv but longer to maintain the relative orientation of the two binding sites. Multivalent Fabs use a somewhat similar approach with the dimerization handles comprising of zippers from the transcription factors *jun* and *fos* [Kostelny et al., 1992].

In addition to the constructs described above, a whole new set of genetically engineered fusion proteins with antibodies has been described [Wright at al., 1992]. Antibody fusion proteins are made by replacing a part of the antibody molecule with a fusion partner such as an enzyme or a toxin that confers a novel function to the antibody. In some cases, such as immunotoxins, the variable regions of the antibody are retained in order to retain antigen binding and specificity, while the constant domains are deleted and replaced by a toxin such as ricin or *Pseudomonas* exotoxin. Alternately, the constant regions are retained (thereby retaining the effector functions) and the variable regions replaced with other targeting proteins (such as CD4 for AIDS therapy and IL-2 for cancer therapy).

97.5 Applications of Monoclonal Antibodies and Fragments

The majority of applications for which monoclonal antibodies have been used can be divided into three general categories: (1) purification, (2) diagnostic functions (whether for detecting cancer, analyzing for toxins in food, or monitoring substance abuse by athletes), and (3) therapeutic functions. From the time that monoclonal antibody technology was introduced almost 20 years ago, application methodologies using whole antibody have gradually been transformed into methodologies using antibody fragments such as the Fab_2, Fab', and Fv fragments and even synthetic peptides of a CDR region. Antibody conjugates have come to include bound drugs, toxins, radioisotopes, lymphokines, and enzymes [Pietersz and McKenzie, 1992] and are largely used in the treatment of cancer. Tables 97.1 and 97.2 list some typical examples of monoclonal antibodies and fragments used for diagnostic and therapeutic applications.

Thousands of murine monoclonal antibodies have been made to human carcinomas since the introduction of antibody technology, but very few, if any, of these monoclonal antibodies are entirely specific for malignant cells. In the vast majority of cases, these monoclonal antibodies define tumor-associated differentiation antigens (TADAs), which are either proteins, mucins, proteoglycans, or glycolipids (gangliosides). Examples of TADA proteins are carcinoembryonic antigen (CEA) and α-fetoprotein (AFP), both well-known diagnostic markers. An anti-CEA antibody has been conjugated with the enzyme carboxypeptidase, which, in turn, activates a prodrug at the site of the tumor [Bagshawe, et al., 1992]. This strategy overcomes the inability of monoclonal antibodies conjugated with drugs to deliver a therapeutic dose. Examples of TADA gangliosides are those referred to as GD2 and GD3, for which the respective unmodified monoclonal antibodies have shown to be

TABLE 97.1 Uses of Whole MAb Derived from Hybridoma, Other Cell Fusions, and Genetically Engineered Cell Lines

MAb	Antigen	Ab Source	Actual or Potential Uses
C23	Cytomegalovirus glycoprotein of 130 and 55 kDa	Humab—fusion of human lymphocyte and mouse myeloma (p3 × 63Ag8ul)	Prophylactic agent for viral infection
EV2-7	Cytomegalovirus protein of 82 kDa	Trioma; human × (human × mouse heteromyeloma)	Prophylactic agent for CMV infection
OKT3	CD3 antigen	Murine MAb	Eradication of T lymphocytes involved in graft rejection
Campath 1H	Lymphocyte antigen	"Humanized" chimeric rat/ human MAb; murine CDRs	Prevention of bone marrow and organ rejection
R24	GD2 ganglioside TADA tumor-associated differentiation antigen	Murine MAb	Treatment of melanoma
L72, L55	GD3 ganglioside TADA	Human MAb	Treatment of melanoma
	Digoxin	Murine MAb	Immunodiagnostic for cardiac glycoside digoxin
6H4	*Salmonella* flagella	Murine MAb	Detection of *Salmonella* bacteria in food

effective therapeutics, particularly when intralesionally administered [Irie et al., 1989]. An example of a TADA mucin is the antigens found in colorectal and ovarian carcinoma that react with the antibody 72.3. Chimeric monoclonal antibodies as well as fragments of antibody 72.3 have been constructed and tested [Khazaeli et al., 1991; King et al., 1992].

As mentioned above, monoclonal antibodies defining different TADAs have been used passively (unmodified) and as carriers of, for example, radioisotopes and enzymes. From the results brought forth to date, the passive mode of antibody therapy has produced relatively few remissions in patients, and in those cases where it has shown effects, it is likely that the ability of the antibody to mediate ADCC (antibody-dependent cellular cytotoxicity) and CDC (complement-dependent cytotoxicity) has contributed to the remission. For the case of modified monoclonal antibodies (e.g.,

TABLE 97.2 Immunoconjugates Having Potential for Cancer Therapy

MAb	Conjugate	Antibody Source	Use
A7	Neocarzinostatin	Murine monoclonal (from fusion with murine myeloma P3.X63.Ag8.653)	Eradication of colon cancer
30.6, I-1	*N*-acetylmelphalan	Murine monoclonal	Eradication of colon cancer
	Adriamycin, Mitomycin C	Murine monoclonal	Various cancers
RFB4	RFB4(Fab')-Ricin A (αCD22 (Fab')-Ricin A)	Murine Fab'	B-cell lymphoma
	Anti-CD19-blocked ricin	Murine monoclonal	B-cell lymphoma
	Xomazyme-Mel	Murine monoclonal	Metastatic melanoma
Anti-CEA (carcinoembryonic antigen)	Carboxypeptidase G2	Murine MAb F(ab')$_2$ fragment chemically bound to enzyme	Colon cancer
Recombinant anti-CEA MAb BW431	(DNA coded) human β-glucuronidase	Transfectoma	
B72.3	^{131}I	Murine monoclonal	Ovarian cancer
B72.3	^{131}I	Mouse-human chimeric Ab	Colon cancer
B72.3		Mouse-human chimeric Fab' fragment	Colon cancer
B72.3 (Oncoscint)	Chelated ^{111}In	Murine MAb	Diagnostic imaging agent for colorectal and ovarian cancers

toxin and radioisotope conjugates), success of treatment is varied depending on the type of neoplasm. Antibody conjugate treatment of leukemia and lymphoma results in a relatively greater remission rate than that found in treatments of malignancies having solid tumors (i.e., carcinoma of the ovary, colon, and lung).

The rare case of complete remission for solid tumors is probably due to the inaccessibility of antibody to that tumor. Several barriers impeding access of antibody to cancer cells have been pointed out [Jain, 1988]. A few of these barriers include (1) the high interstitial fluid pressure in tumor nodules, (2) heterogeneous or poor vascularization of tumors, and (3) the long distances extravasated monoclonal antibodies must travel in the interstial mesh of proteoglycans in the tumor. There also exists the possibility that tumor antigen shed from the surface is limiting antibody buildup. In the case of bound toxins or drugs, there is the added concern that organs such as the kidney and liver are quickly processing and eliminating the antibody conjugates. In this respect, immunoconjugates based on antibody fragments (such as the sFv) can be very advantageous. For example, it has been shown that the sFv exhibits rapid diffusion into the extravascular space, increased volume of distribution, enhanced tumor penetration, and improved renal elimination. An assessment of solid tumor therapy with modified antibody has led Riethmüller et al. [1993] to recommend that current cancer therapy be directed toward minimal residual disease, the condition in which micrometastatic cells exist after curatively resecting solid tumors.

With regard to purification, the research literature is replete with examples of immunoaffinity purification of enzymes, receptors, peptides, and small organic molecules. In contrast, commercial applications of immunoaffinity chromatography, even on industrially or clinically relevant molecules, are far less widespread (Table 97.3). Despite its potential utility, immunoadsorption is an expensive process. A significant portion of the high cost is the adsorbent itself, which is related to the cost of materials, preparation, and most important, the antibody. In addition, the binding capacity of the immunoadsorbent declines with repeated use, and a systematic study has shown that significant deactivation can typically take place over 40 to 100 cycles [Antonsen et al., 1991]. A number of factors can contribute to this degradation, including loss of antibody, structural change of the support matrix, nonspecific adsorption of contaminating proteins, incomplete antigen elution, and loss of antibody function. In most cases, this degradation is associated with repeated exposure to harsh elution conditions. Noteworthy commercial applications of immunoaffinity chromatography on useful molecules include the separation of factor VIII used to treat hemophilia A and factor IX, another coagulation factor in the blood-clotting cascade [Tharakan et al., 1992]. The immunoaffinity purification step for factor VIII was one of several additional steps added to the conventional preparation methodology in which plasma cryoprecipitates were heat-treated. The new method contains a virus-inactivation procedure that precedes the immunoaffinity column, followed by an additional chromatographic step (ion exchange). The latter step serves to eliminate the eluting solvent and further reduce virus-inactivating compounds. The often mentioned concern of antibody leakage from the column matrix did not appear to be a problem. Furthermore, with the relatively mild elution conditions used (40% ethylene glycol), one would expect little change in the antibody-binding capacity over many elution cycles.

Typical immunoaffinity matrices contain whole antibody as opposed to antibody fragments. Fragmentation of antibody by enzymatic means contributes additional steps to immunoadsorbent

TABLE 97.3 Clinically or Industrially Relevant Proteins Purified by Immunoaffinity Chromatography

Protein	Use (Actual and Potential)
Factor VIII	Treatment of hemophilia A
Factor IX	Blood coagulant
α-Galactosidase	Improve the food stabilizing properties of guar gum
Alkaline phosphatase	Purify enzyme (a particular glycoform) used as a tumor marker for diagnostic tests
Interferon (recombinant)	Immunotherapeutic
Interleukin 2	Immunotherapeutic

preparation and adds to the overall cost of the separation and is thus avoided. However, fragmentation can lead to a more efficient separation by enabling the orientation of antibody-binding sites on the surface of the immunomatrix [Prisyazhnoy et al., 1988; Yarmush et al., 1992]. Intact antibodies are bound in a random fashion, resulting in a loss of binding capacity upon immobilization. Recombinant antibody fragments could prove to be more useful for immunoaffinity applications due to the potential for production of large quantities of the protein at low cost and improved immobilization characteristics and stability [Spitznagel and Clark, 1993]. In what one could consider the ultimate fragment of a antibody, some investigators have utilized a peptide based on the CDR region of one of the chains (termed *minimal recognition units*) to isolate the antigen. Welling et al. [1990] have synthesized and tested a 13-residue synthetic peptide having a sequence similar to one hypervariable region of an antilysozyme antibody.

Important diagnostic uses of antibody include the monitoring in clinical laboratories of the cardiac glycoside digoxin and the detection of the *Salmonella* bacteria in foods (see Table 97.1). These two examples highlight the fact that despite the exquisite specificity offered by monoclonal antibodies, detection is not failure-proof. Within digoxin immunoassays there are two possible interfering groups: endogenous digoxin-like substances and digoxin metabolites; moreover, several monoclonal antibodies many be necessary to avoid under- or overestimating digoxin concentrations. In the case of bacteria detection in food, at least two antibodies (MOPC 467 myeloma protein and 6H4 antibody) are needed to detect all strains of *Salmonella*.

97.6 Summary

The domain structure of antibodies, both at the protein and genetic levels, facilitates the manipulation of antibody properties via genetic engineering (antibody engineering). Antibody engineering has shown tremendous potential for basic studies and industrial and medical applications. It has been used to explore fundamental questions about the effect of structure on antigen binding and on the biologic effector functions of the antibody molecules. A knowledge of the rules by which the particular sequences of amino acids involved in the binding surface are chosen in response to a particular antigenic determinant would enable the production of antibodies with altered affinities and specificities. Understanding the structures and mechanisms involved in the effector function of antibodies is already starting to result in the production of antibodies with novel biologic effector functions for use as diagnostic and therapeutic reagents. In addition, the production of antibodies via immunoglobulin gene expression has enabled the engineering of novel hybrid, chimeric, and mosaic genes using recombinant DNA techniques and the transfection and expression of these genetically engineered genes in a number of different systems such as bacteria and yeast, plant cells, myeloma or hybridoma cells, and nonlymphoid mammalian cells.

References

Antonsen KP, Colton CK, Yarmush ML. 1991. Elution conditions and degradation mechanisms in long-term immunoadsorbent use. Biotechnol Prog 7:159.

Bagshawe KD, Sharma SK, Springer CJ, et al. 1992. Antibody directed enzyme prodrug therapy (ADEPT). Antibody Immunoconj Radiopharm 54:133.

Barbas CF, Kang AS, Lerner RA, Benkovic SJ. 1991. Assembly of combinatorial antibody libraries on phage surfaces: The gene III site. Proc Natl Acad Sci USA 88:7978.

Barbas CF, Bain JD, Hoekstra DM, Lerner RA. 1992. Semisynthetic combinatorial antibody libraries: achemical solution to the diversity problem. Proc Natl Acad Sci USA 89:4457.

Bender E, Woof JM, Atkin JD, et al. 1993. Recombinant human antibodies: Linkage of an Fab fragment from a combinatorial library to an Fc fragment for expression in mammalian cell culture. Hum Antibod Hybridomas 4:74.

Better M, Chang CP, Robinson RR, Horwitz AH. 1988. Escherichia coli secretion of an active chimeric antibody fragment. Science 240:1041.

Better M, Horowitz AH. 1989. Expression of engineered antibodies and antibody fragments in microorganisms. Methods Enzymol 178:476.

Bird RE, Hardman KD, Jacobson JW, et al. 1988. Single-chain antigen-binding proteins. Science 242:423.

Boss MA, Kenten JH, Wood CR, Emtage JS. 1984. Assembly of functional antibodies from immunoglobulin heavy and light chains synthesized in E. coli. Nucleic Acids Res 12:3791.

Buchner J, Rudolph R. 1991. Renaturation, purification, and characterization of recombinant Fab fragments produced in Escherichia coli. Biotechnology 9:157.

Burton DR. 1991. Human and mouse monoclonal antibodies by repertoire cloning. Trends Biotechnol 9:169.

Burton DR, Barbas CF, Persson MAA, et al. 1991. A large array of human monoclonal antibodies to type 1 human immunodeficiency virus from combinatorial libraries of asymptomatic seropositive individuals. Proc Natl Acad Sci USA 88:10134.

Cabilly S, Riggs AD, Pande H, et al. 1984. Generation of antibody activity from immunoglobulin polypeptide chains produced in Escherichia coli. Proc Natl Acad Sci USA 81:3273.

Caton AJ, Koprowski H. 1990. Influenza virus hemagglutinin-specific antibodies isolated from a combinatorial expression library are closely related to the immune response of the donor. Proc Natl Acad Sci USA 87:6450.

Clackson T, Hoogenboom HR, Griffiths AD, Winter G. 1991. Making antibody fragments using phage display libraries. Nature 352:624.

Davies DR, Padlan EA, Sheriff S. 1990. Antigen-antibody complexes. Annu Rev Biochem 59:439.

Duchosal MA, Eming SA, Fischer P, et al. 1992. Immunization of hu-PBL-SCID mice and the rescue of human monoclonal Fab fragments through combinatorial libraries. Nature 355:258.

Fanger MW, Morganelli PM, Guyre PM. 1992. Bispecific antibodies. Crit Rev Immunol 12:101.

Glockshuber R, Malia M, Pfitzinger I, Pluckthun A. 1990. A comparison of strategies to stabilize immunoglobulin fragments. Biochemistry 29:1362.

Gram H, Lore-Anne M, Barbas CF, et al. 1992. In vitro selection and affinity maturation of antibodies from a naive combinatorial immunoglobulin library. Proc Natl Acad Sci USA 89:3576.

Hassemann CA, Capra JD. 1990. High-level production of a functional immunoglobulin heterodimer in a baculovirus expression system. Proc Natl Acad Sci USA 87:3942.

Hiatt A, Cafferkey R, Bowdish K. 1989. Production of antibodies in transgenic plants. Nature 342:76.

Hiatt A, Ma JK-C. 1992. Monoclonal antibody engineering in plants. FEBS Lett 307:71.

Hoogenboom HR, Griffiths AD, Johnson KS, et al. 1991. Multi-subunit proteins on the surface of filamentous phage: Methodologies for displaying antibody (Fab) heavy and light chains. Nucleic Acids Res 19:4133.

Hoogenboom HR, Marks JD, Griffiths AD, Winter G. 1992. Building antibodies from their genes. Immunol Rev 130:41.

Horowitz AH, Chang PC, Better M, et al. 1988. Secretion of functional antibody and Fab fragment from yeast cells. Proc Natl Acad Sci USA 85:8678.

Huse WD, Sastry L, Iverson SA, et al. 1989. Generation of a large combinatorial library of the immunoglobulin repertoire in phage lambda. Science 246:1275.

Huston JS, Levinson D, Mudgett-Hunter M, et al. 1988. Protein engineering of antibody binding sites: Recovery of specific activity in an anti-digoxin single-chain Fv analogue produced in Escherichia coli. Proc Natl Acad Sci USA 85:5879.

Ishizaka T, Helm B, Hakimi J, et al. 1986. Biological properties of a recombinant human immunoglobulin ε-chain fragment. Proc Natl Acad Sci USA 83:8323.

Jain RK. 1988. Determinants of tumor blood flow: A review. Cancer Res 48:2641.

Kang AS, Barbas CF, Janda KD, et al. 1991. Linkage of recognition and replication functions by assembling combinatorial antibody Fab libraries along phage surfaces. Proc Natl Acad Sci USA 88:4363.

Keneten J, Helm B, Ishizaka T, et al. 1984. Properties of a human immunoglobulin ε-chain fragment synthesized in Escherichia coli. Proc Natl Acad Sci USA 81:2955.

Khazaeli MB, Saleh MN, Liu TP, Meredith RF. 1991. Pharmacokinetics and immune response of 131I-chimeric mouse/human B72.3 (human γ4) monoclonal antibody in humans. Cancer Res 51:5461.

King DJ, Adair JR, Angal S, et al. 1992. Expression, purification, and characterization of a mouse-human chimeric antibody and chimeric Fab′ fragment. Biochem J 281:317.

Kostelny SA, Cole MS, Tso JY. 1992. Formation of bispecific antibody by the use of leucine zippers. J Immunol 148:1547.

Köhler G, Milstein C. 1975. Continuous cultures of fused cells secreting antibody of predefined specificity. Nature 256:495.

Landsteiner K. 1945. The Specificity of Serological Reactions. Cambridge, Mass, Harvard University Press.

Marks JD, Hoogenboom HR, Bonnert TP, et al. 1991. Bypassing immunization: Human antibodies from V-gene libraries displayed on phage. J Mol Biol 222:581.

Marks JD, Griffiths AD, Malmqvist M, et al. 1992. Bypassing immunization: Building high affinity human antibodies by chain shuffling. Biotechnology 10:779.

McCafferty J, Griffiths AD, Winter G, Chriswell DJ. 1990. Phage antibodies: Filamentous phage displaying antibody variable domains. Nature 348:552.

→ Morrison SL, Oi VT. 1989. Genetically engineered antibody molecules. Adv Immunol 41:65.

Mullinax RL, Gross EA, Amberg JR, et al. 1990. Identification of human antibody fragment clones specific for tetanus toxoid in a bacteriophage λ immunoexpression library. Proc Natl Acad Sci USA 87:8095.

Neil GA, Urnovitz HB. 1988. Recent improvements in the production of antibody-secreting hybridoma cells. Trends Biotechnol 6:209.

Orlandi R, Gussow DH, Jones PT, Winter G. 1989. Cloning immunoglobulin variable domains for expression by the polymerase chain reaction. Proc Natl Acad Sci USA 86:3833.

Pack P, Pluckthun P. 1992. Miniantibodies: Use of amphipathic helices to produce functional flexibly linked dimeric Fv fragments with high avidity in Escherichia coli. Biochemistry 31:1579.

Perrson MAA, Caothien RH, Burton DR. 1991. Generation of diverse high-affinity human monoclonal antibodies by repertoire cloning. Proc Natl Acad Sci USA 88:2432.

Pietersz GA, McKenzie IFC. 1992. Antibody conjugates for the treatment of cancer. Immunol Rev 129:57.

Plückthun A. 1992. Mono- and bivalent antibody fragments produced in Escherichia coli: Engineering, folding and antigen-binding. Immunol Rev 130:150.

Prisyazhnoy VS, Fusek M, Alakhov YB. 1988. Synthesis of high-capacity immunoaffinity sorbents with oriented immobilized immunoglobulins or their Fab′ fragments for isolation of proteins J Chromatogr 424:243.

Putlitz JZ, Kubasek WL, Duchene M, et al. 1990. Antibody production in baculovirus-infected insect cells. Biotechnology 8:651.

Riethmüller G, Schneider-Gädicke E, Johnson JP. 1993. Monoclonal antibodies in cancer therapy. Curr Opin Immunol 5:732.

Sandhu JS. 1992. Protein engineering of antibodies. Crit Rev Biotechnol 12:437.

Sastry L, Alting-Mees M, Huse WD, et al. 1989. Cloning of the immunological repertoire in Escherichia coli for generation of monoclonal catalytic antibodies: Construction of a heavy chain variable region-specific cDNA library. Proc Natl Acad Sci USA 86:5728.

Skerra A, Plückthun A. 1988. Assembly of a functional immunoglobulin Fv fragment in Escherichia coli. Science 240:1038.

Skerra A. 1993. Bacterial expression of immunoglobulin fragments. Curr Opin Biotechnol 5:255.

Spitznagel TM, Clark DS. 1993. Surface density and orientation effects on immobilized antibodies and antibody fragments. Biotechnology 11:825.

Tizard IR. 1992. The genetic basis of antigen recognition. In Immunology: An Introduction, 3d ed. Orlando, Fla, Saunders Coolege Publishing.

Ward ES, Gussow D, Griffiths AD, et al. 1989. Binding activities of a repertoire of single immunoglobulin variable domains secreted from Escherichia coli. Nature 341:544.

Wood CR, Boss MA, Kenten JH, et al. 1985. The synthesis and in vivo assembly of functional antibodies in yeast. Nature 314:446.

Welling GW, Guerts T, Van Gorkum J, et al. 1990. Synthetic antibody fragment as ligand in immunoaffinity chromatography. J Chromatogr 512:337.

Wright A, Shin S-U, Morrison SL. 1992. Genetically engineered antibodies: progress and prospects. Crit Rev Immunol 12:125.

Yarmush ML, Lu X, Yarmush D. 1992. Coupling of antibody-binding fragments to solid-phase supports: Site-directed binding of F(ab')2 fragments. J Biochem Biophys Methods 25:285.

Zebedee SL, Barbas CF, Yao-Ling H, et al. 1992. Human combinatorial libraries to hepatitis B surface antigen. Proc Natl Acad Sci USA 89:3175.

98

Antisense Technology

Joseph M. Le Doux
Rutgers University

Jeffrey R. Morgan
Rutgers University, Massachusetts General Hospital, Harvard University Medical School, and the Shriners Burns Institute

Martin L. Yarmush
Rutgers University, Massachusetts General Hospital, Harvard University Medical School, and the Shriners Burns Institute

Antisense molecules can selectively inhibit the expression of one gene among the 100,000 present in a typical human cell. This inhibition is based on simple Watson-Crick base-pairing interactions between nucleic acids and makes possible, in principle, the rational design of therapeutic drugs that can specifically inhibit any gene whose sequence is known. The intervention into disease states at the level of gene expression may potentially make drugs based on antisense techniques significantly more efficient and specific than other standard therapies. Indeed, antisense technology is already an indispensable research tool and may one day be an integral part of future antiviral and anticancer therapies.

Zamecnik and Stephenson [1978] were the first to use antisense DNA to modulate gene expression. They constructed antisense oligodeoxynucleotides (oligos) complementary to the 3′ and 5′ ends of Rous sarcoma virus (RSV) 35 S RNA and added them directly to a culture of chick embryo fibroblasts infected with RSV. Remarkably, viral replication was inhibited, indicating that the cells had somehow internalized the antisense DNA.

Natural antisense inhibition was first observed in bacteria as a means of regulating the replication of plasmid DNA [Tomizawa and Itoh, 1981; Tomizawa et al., 1981]. RNA primers required for the initiation of replication were bound by (i.e., formed duplexes with) antisense RNA. The concentration of these RNA primers, and therefore the initiation of replication, was controlled by the formation of these duplexes. Shortly after this discovery, investigators developed antisense RNA constructs to control gene expression in mammalian cells. Antisense RNA, encoded on expression plasmids that were transfected into mouse cells, successfully blocked expression of target genes [Izant and Weintraub, 1985]. These early successes launched what is now a massive effort into exploring the use of antisense molecules for research and therapeutic purposes.

98.1 Background

Antisense are DNA or RNA molecules whose sequences are complementary to RNA transcribed from the target gene. These molecules block the expression of a gene by interacting with its RNA transcript. Only antisense DNA molecules, which mimic the target gene's antisense strand and thus hybridize to RNA transcribed from the gene, will be discussed in detail in this chapter. These antisense molecules are typically short, single-stranded oligos with a sequence complementary to a sequence within the target RNA transcript. The oligos bind to this sequence via Watson-Crick base pairing [adenosine binds to thymidine (DNA) or uracil (RNA) and guanosine binds to cytidine], form a DNA:RNA duplex, and block the expression of the RNA (Fig. 98.1).

Antisense RNA also can inhibit gene expression. Cells are transfected with a plasmid encoding the antisense RNA, the plasmid is transcribed, and the resulting antisense RNA transcript inhibits gene expression. Unfortunately, difficulties in controlling the expression of the transfected plasmid hinder the effective use of antisense RNA for therapeutic purposes. For a review of antisense RNA, see Green et al. [1986]. Other methods for blocking gene expression are being explored, such as using molecules that competitively bind to regulatory proteins required for their expression (protein traps) or molecules designed to prevent transcription by binding to the target gene and forming a DNA triplex (antigene). Although promising, these approaches are preliminary and are beyond the scope of this chapter.

Many technical issues limit the therapeutic usefulness of current antisense oligos. Our understanding of the mechanism of antisense inhibition must be improved before the development of therapeutically useful antisense molecules is possible. Most oligos currently used are too unstable and lack adequate specificity for use in vivo, and their delivery to cells is often nonspecific and inefficient. The impact of these problems and approaches to solving them will be discussed. In addition, potential applications of antisense techniques to antiviral and anticancer therapies and their evaluation in animal models and clinical trials also will be highlighted.

98.2 Mechanisms of Inhibition

The inhibition of gene expression by antisense molecules occurs by two distinct mechanisms: RNase H degradation of the RNA and steric hindrance of the RNA [Helene and Toulme, 1990]. Some oligos, after hybridizing to the target RNA, activate RNase H, an enzyme normally involved in DNA replication, which specifically recognizes the RNA:DNA duplex and cleaves the RNA portion. The antisense oligo is not degraded and is free to bind to and catalyze the destruction of other target RNA transcripts [Milligan et al., 1993]. Oligos that activate RNase H, therefore, are capable of destroying many RNA transcripts in their lifetime, which suggests that small concentrations of these oligos may be sufficient to significantly inhibit gene expression [Helene and Toulme, 1990].

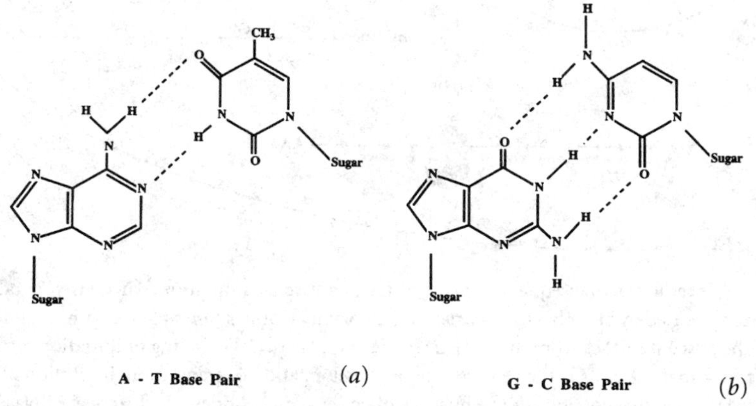

A - T Base Pair   (a)   G - C Base Pair   (b)

FIGURE 98.1 Watson-Crick base-pairing interactions between adenosine and thymidine (A-T) and between guanosine and cytidine (G-C). In DNA, the sugar is 2'-deoxyribose. In RNA, the sugar is ribose.

However, not all oligos activate RNase H enzymes. Some oligos inhibit gene expression by interfering with the RNA's normal lifecycle. In theory, virtually any step in an RNA's lifecycle can be
blocked by an oligo (Fig. 98.2). Newly transcribed RNA must be spliced, polyadenylated, and transported to the cytoplasm before being translated into protein. These oligos (which do not activate
RNase H) block RNA maturation by binding to sites on the RNA important for posttranscriptional
processing [Nagel et al., 1993]. For example, oligos that bind to the splice site may interfere with
spliceosome complex formation and/or splicing of the nascent transcript. Oligos that bind to the
polyadenylation sequence may prevent the addition of a poly A tail. Oligos bound to an RNA may
prevent its proper transport from the nucleus to the cytoplasm, and oligos that bind to the initiation codon region of mRNA may prevent translation and/or the binding of ribosomes. Oligos
designed to block the elongation of translation by binding to coding sequences downstream of the
initiation codon region have rarely succeeded, presumably because ribosomes destabilize and read
through DNA:RNA duplexes [Nagel et al., 1993].

Inhibition by both these mechanisms, RNase H degradation and steric hindrance, was demonstrated in a recent study in which the expression of an intracellular adhesion molecule (ICAM-1)
was blocked using two different oligos [Bennett et al., 1994a]. One oligo, complementary to the 3'
untranslated region of the ICAM-1 mRNA, reduced the number of transcripts, presumably by
RNase H degradation. The second oligo, complementary to the initiation codon of the ICAM-1
mRNA, did not reduce the number of transcripts but did reduce the production of protein, presumably by blocking the initiation of translation.

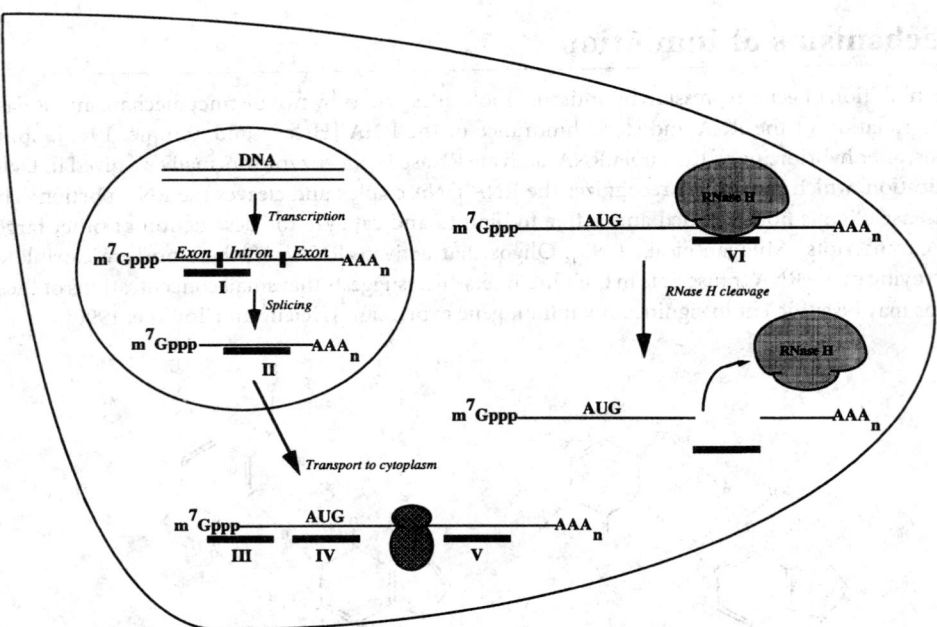

FIGURE 98.2   Several possible sequence-specific sites of antisense inhibition. Antisense oligodeoxynucleotides are represented by black bars. Antisense oligodeoxynucleotides can interfere with (I) splicing, (II)
transport of the nascent mRNA from the nucleus to the cytoplasm, (III) binding of initiation factors, (IV)
assembly of ribosomal subunits at the start codon, or (V) elongation of translation. Inhibition of capping
and polyadenylation is also possible. (VI) Antisense oligodeoxynucleotides which activate RNase H (e.g.,
oligos with phosphodiester and phosphorothioate backbones) also can inhibit gene expression by binding to their target mRNA, catalyzing the RNase H cleavage of the mRNA into segments, which are rapidly
degraded by exonucleases.

The mechanism of inhibition influences the specificity of antisense molecules. Oligos that activate RNase H can inactivate slightly mismatched RNA transcripts by transiently binding to them and catalyzing their cleavage and destruction by RNase H [Woolf et al., 1992]. This nonspecific inactivation of RNA could lead to unwanted toxic side effects. In contrast, oligos that do not activate RNase H and therefore can only inhibit gene expression by steric hindrance are less likely to inactivate slightly mismatched RNA transcripts. These oligos, like the ones that activate RNase H, transiently bind to RNA transcripts. However, they do not catalyze the enzymatic cleavage of the RNA by RNase H, and since transient binding is unlikely to significantly impede translation of the transcript, they are less likely to reduce the expression of slightly mismatched nontargeted RNA transcripts [Herschlag, 1991].

Choosing an effective target site in an mRNA is largely an empirical process. Generally, several candidate oligos are tested for their ability to inhibit gene expression, and the most effective one is used for future studies [Milligan et al., 1993]. The effectiveness of an antisense oligo often depends on the region of the RNA to which it is complementary. RNA molecules are typically folded into complex three-dimensional structures that are formed by self-base pairing and by protein:RNA interactions. If an oligo is complementary to a sequence embedded in the three-dimensional structure, it may not be able to bind to it, and therefore, gene expression will not be inhibited [Lima et al., 1992]. For oligos that block gene expression by steric hindrance and not by RNase H degradation, the number of potential target sites is even more limited because for these oligos the site must not only be accessible for hybridization but also must be a site at which steric hindrance alone is sufficient to interfere with gene expression. Binding sites that are often effective include the 5' cap region and the initiation (AUG) codon region [Goodchild et al., 1988].

98.3 Chemically Modified Oligos

Perhaps the most limiting property of natural oligodeoxynucleotides (PO oligos, oligos with a phosphodiester backbone) is their susceptibility to nuclease degradation (Fig. 98.3). PO oligos are rapidly degraded by 3' to 5' exonucleases and have half-lives as short as 15 minutes [Nagel et al., 1993]. The stability of PO oligos in serum-supplemented culture media is improved by the addition of methylphosphonate diester end groups to their 3' ends, but these modified oligos are still degraded intracellularly [Tidd and Warenius, 1989].

The need for oligos that are stable in vivo prompted the development of chemical derivatives of the phosphodiester backbone (see Fig. 98.3). Phosphorothioate (PS) DNA derivatives have a sulfur atom substituted for a nonbridge oxygen atom in the sugar-phosphate backbone. PS oligos are significantly more stable than PO oligos, with reported intracellular half-lives of greater than 24 hours [Agrawal et al., 1991]. PS oligos have the same negative charge as PO oligos and are equally soluble in aqueous solutions. Like PO oligos, they are believed to be internalized by receptor-

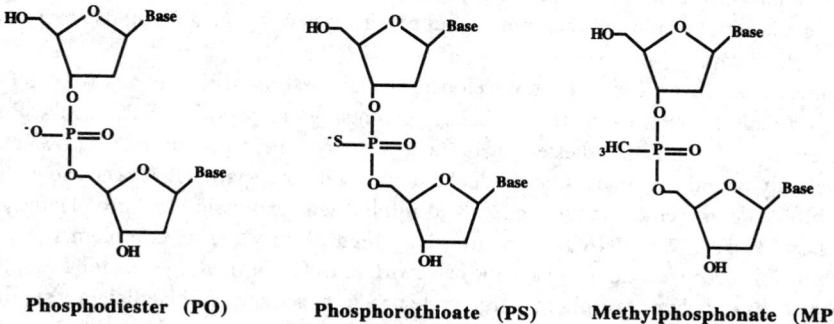

Phosphodiester (PO)   **Phosphorothioate (PS)**   **Methylphosphonate (MP)**

FIGURE 98.3   The structures of the internucleotide backbone of phosphodiester (PO), phosphorothioate (PS), and methylphosphonate (MP) oligodeoxynucleotides.

mediated endocytosis [Loke et al., 1989]. Their affinity for complementary RNA is not as high as that observed with PO oligos. Nevertheless, PS oligos have been shown to efficiently inhibit gene expression [Stein et al., 1988]. One concern with PS oligos (and all chemically modified oligos) is their potential for causing toxic side effects. The metabolic by-products of PS oligos could be incorporated into cellular DNA and cause mutations [Neckers and Whitesell, 1993]. Short-term toxic effects have not been observed, but future studies on the long-term effects are clearly necessary prior to the clinical use of PS oligos.

Another chemical derivative is methylphosphonate (MP) oligos. MP oligos have a methyl group substituted for a nonbridged oxygen atom in the sugar-phosphate backbone. They are resistant to nuclease degradation, neutrally charged, and less soluble in aqueous solutions than PO or PS oligos [Milligan et al., 1993; Nagel et al., 1993]. MP oligos are highly lipophilic and are inefficiently internalized [Nagel et al., 1993]. It was initially thought that MP oligos entered cells by passive diffusion through the plasma membranes, but recent studies suggest that they enter by an active transport process distinct from PO or PS entry mechanisms [Akhtar et al., 1991; Miller, 1991]. The inefficiency of MP oligo internalization may be due in part to their inability to escape lysosomal degradation and gain entry into the cytoplasm. MP oligos, primarily because their methyl groups are sterically unfavorable for oligo:RNA duplex formation, have a lower affinity than PO oligos for their RNA substrates. Nevertheless, MP oligos have been shown to specifically inhibit gene expression [Kibler-Herzog et al., 1991].

A major difference between MP oligos and PO/PS oligos is their mechanism of inhibition [Milligan et al., 1993]. MP oligos, unlike PO and PS oligos, do not activate RNase H enzymatic cleavage of complementary RNA. This may explain why the concentrations typically needed to block gene expression with MP oligos (50 to 100 μM) are significantly higher than those typically required to block gene expression with PS or PO oligos (0.1 to 10 μM).

PS and MP oligos, unlike PO oligos, are chiral molecules, i.e., molecules that are not identical to their mirror image. Current techniques used to synthesize these oligos do not control the orientation of each internucleotide bond, and the resulting oligos are therefore a mixture of $2^{(n-1)}$ diastereomers (where n = the number of bases). It has been demonstrated that not all diastereomers bind their complementary sequences with equal affinity [Lesnikowski et al., 1990]. Two investigators purified a mixture of 9-mer PS oligos (therefore containing 256 diastereomers) by affinity chromatography using a column containing complementary 20-mer PO oligo [Tidd and Warenius, 1988]. They were able to separate the mixture of diastereomers into two groups, high-affinity and low-affinity. Using hybridization experiments, they demonstrated that the high-affinity 9-mers had a significantly higher melting temperature ($T_m \approx 39°C$) than the low-affinity 9-mers ($T_m \approx 31°C$). This demonstrated that there can be significant differences between the affinity of various diastereomers for their intended substrates, and it is likely that their biologic activity also will vary. Mixtures of diastereomers, formed with current synthesis methods, may result in undesirable variability between different oligo stocks [Milligan et al., 1993]. Presently, it is not possible to purify or synthesize large quantities of pure diastereomers, but efforts to develop such methods are in progress [Milligan et al., 1993].

As an alternative, investigators have developed and are testing achiral oligos (e.g., phosphodithioate and peptide nucleic acids). Particularly promising are peptide nucleic acids (PNA) in which the entire ribose-phosphodiester backbone is replaced with a polyamide (Fig. 98.4c). PNA, with a covalently bound terminal lysine residue to prevent self-aggregation, has been shown to preferentially bind to complementary sequences and inhibit gene expression in vitro [Hanvey et al., 1992; Nielsen et al., 1993]. PNA has an unusually high affinity for its complementary target sequence, possibly because it can form a triple helix with RNA (2 PNA:1 RNA) [Egholm et al., 1992]. PNA oligos are especially promising for large-scale use because they can be efficiently synthesized using existing peptide coupling chemistry [Milligan et al., 1993].

Several other chemical modifications to the natural oligodeoxynucleotide structure have been synthesized in an effort to develop oligos with improved stability, affinity, specificity, and cell

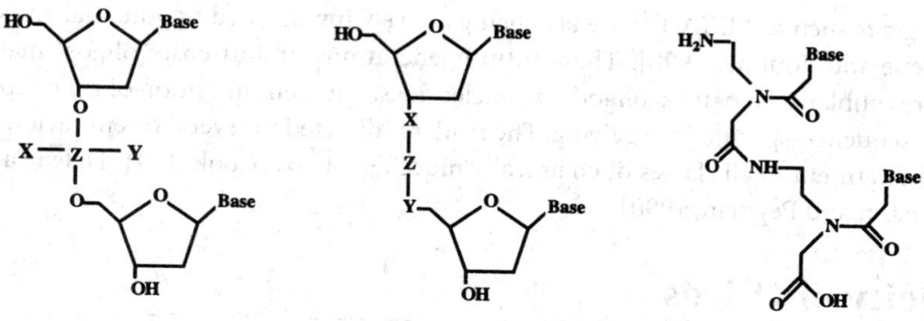

FIGURE 98.4 Backbone analogues of natural phosphodiester backbones. (*a*) Structures in which the phosphorus bridge atom is retained. (*b*) Structures in which the phosphorus bridge atom is replaced. (*c*) Peptide nucleic acids—the entire backbone is replaced with amino acids. See Table 98.1 for legend.

permeability (see Fig. 98.4 and Table 98.1). Modifications to every major component of the oligodeoxynucleotide chain have been explored, including the sugar-phosphate backbone (e.g., sulfur- and carbon-based linkages and peptide nucleic acids), sugars (e.g., α-anomeric and 2'-O-allyl oligos), and bases (e.g., 5-methyl or 5-bromo-2'-deoxycytidine and 7'-deazaguanosine and 7'-deazaadenosine oligos) [Milligan et al., 1993]. Oligonucleotides covalently linked to active groups (e.g., intercalators such as acridine, photoactivated cross-linking agents such as psoralens, and

TABLE 98.1 The Names and Key Characteristics of Several Phosphodiester Oligo Analogues. (Their Chemical Structures can be Determined by Cross-referencing Columns *X*, *Y*, and *Z* with Fig. 98.4.)

	RNase H Activation	Nuclease Resistance	Chiral Center	Affinity	Charge	X (Fig. 98.4)	Y (Fig. 98.4)	Z (Fig. 98.4)
Phosphorus analogues (Fig. 98.3a)								
Phosphodiester (PO)	Yes	No	No	=PO	Negative	O^-	O	P
Phosphorothioate (PS)	Yes	Yes	Yes	<PO	Negative	S^-	O	P
Methylphosphonate (MP)	No	Yes	Yes	<PO	Neutral	CH_3	O	P
Phosphoramidate	No	Yes	Yes	<PO	Neutral	NH-R	O	P
Phosphorodithioate	Yes	Yes	No	<PO	Negative	S^-	S	P
Phosphoethyltriester	No	Yes	Yes	>PO	Neutral	$O-C_2H_5$	O	P
Phosphoroselenoate	Yes	Yes	Yes	<PO	Negative	Se^-	O	P
Nonphosphorus analogues (Fig. 98.3b)								
Formacetal	?	Yes	No	<PO	Neutral	O	O	CH_2
3' Thioformacetal	?	Yes	No	>PO	Neutral	S	O	CH_2
5'-N-Carbamate	?	Yes	No	< or > PO	Neutral	O	NH	C=O
Sulfonate	?	Yes	No	<PO	Neutral	O	CH_2	SO_2
Sulfamate	?	Yes	No	<PO	Neutral	O	NH	SO_2
Sulfoxide	?	Yes	No	<PO	Neutral	CH_2	CH_2	SO
Sulfide	?	Yes	No	<PO	Neutral	CH_2	CH_2	S
α-Analogues	No	Yes	N/A^a	<PO	N/A^a	N/A^b	N/A^b	N/A^b
Peptide nucleic acids								
(Fig. 98.3c)	No	Yes	No	>PO	Positive[c]	N/A^d	N/A^d	N/A^d

? = unknown.

[a]Chirality and charge depends on backbone structure used.

[b]Structure not drawn; The bond between the sugar and base (an *N*-glycosidic bond) of α-analogues have the reverse orientation (α-configuration) from natural (β-configuration) oligonucleotides.

[c]Typically, C terminus is covalently linked to positively charged lysine residue, giving the PNA a positive charge.

[d]See Fig. 98.4c for chemical structure.

X, Y, Z: these columns reference Fig. 98.4; Replace the designated letter in Fig. 98.4 with the molecule indicated in the Table 98.1 to determine the chemical structure of the oligo.

chelating agents such as EDTA-Fe) are also being actively investigated as potential antisense molecules [Helene and Toulme, 1990]. These future generations of antisense "oligos" may bear little structural resemblance to natural oligodeoxynucleotides, but their inhibition of gene expression will still rely on sequence-specific base pairing. The reader is directed to several recent reviews for a comprehensive treatment of all classes of chemically modified oligos [Cook, 1991; Helene and Toulme, 1990; Uhlmann and Peyman, 1990].

98.4 Specificity of Oligos

The ability to block the expression of a single gene without undesired side effects (specificity) is the major advantage of antisense-based strategies. This specificity is primarily determined by the length (i.e., the number of bases) of the oligo. Recent experimental and theoretical data suggest that there is an optimal length at which specific inhibition of gene expression is maximized and nonspecific effects are minimized [Herschlag, 1991; Woolf et al., 1992].

Affinity and specificity limit the minimum effective length of oligos. Oligos that are too short do not inhibit gene expression because they do not bind with sufficient affinity to their substrates. The shortest oligo reported to affect gene expression in mammalian cells was 11 base pairs long (11-mer) [Chang et al., 1991]. In addition, an oligo that is too short is less likely to represent a unique sequence in a given cell's genome and therefore loses specificity. If an oligo is too short, and therefore its sequence is not unique, then it might bind to a complementary sequence in a nontargeted RNA and inhibit its expression. The minimum length a sequence must be before it is statistically likely to be a unique sequence in a pool of mRNAs has been estimated [Woolf et al., 1992]. Since each position in a given sequence can be occupied by any of four nucleotides (A, C, G, or U), the total number of different possible sequences of length N bases is 4^N. Letting R equal the total number of bases in a given mRNA pool and assuming that it is a random and equal mixture of the four nucleotides, then the frequency F of occurrence in that pool of a sequence of length N is given by

$$F = R/4^N \tag{98.1}$$

For a typical human cell, which contains approximately 10^4 unique mRNA species whose average length is 2000 bases, R is approximately equal to 2×10^7. Therefore, for a sequence to be unique ($F < 1$), N must be greater than or equal to 13 bases long [Woolf et al., 1992].

Clearly, there is a minimum length for oligos below which they are either not unique or they cannot bind with high enough affinity to inhibit gene expression. However, oligos cannot be made arbitrarily long because the longer an oligo is the more likely that it will contain internal sequences complementary to nontargeted RNA molecules to which it can hybridize and inactivate. This also has been expressed mathematically [Woolf et al., 1992]. The expected number of complementary sites S of length L for an oligo of length N in an mRNA pool with R bases is given by

$$S = \frac{(N - L + 1) \times R)}{4^L} \tag{98.2}$$

For example, an 18-mer ($N = 18$) has 6 internal 13-mers. Since a 13-mer is expected to occur 0.3 times in an mRNA pool containing 2×10^7 bases, the 18-mer is expected to match 1.8 (i.e., 6×0.3) 13-mers in the mRNA pool. Equation (98.2) also gives this result ($N = 18$, $L = 13$, and $R = 2 \times 10^7$; therefore, $S = 1.8$).

Woolf et al. [1992] have demonstrated that significant degradation of nontargeted mRNAs can occur. They compared the effectiveness of three different 25-mers in suppressing the expression of fibronectin mRNA in xenopus oocytes. Nearly 80% of the fibronectin mRNA was degraded after the oocytes were microinjected with a 25-mer in which all 25 of its bases were complementary to the mRNA. However, when the oocytes were microinjected with 25-mers that had only 17 or 14 complementary bases flanked by random sequences, greater than 30% of the fibronectin mRNA was still degraded. They also showed that a single mismatch in an oligo did not completely eliminate its antisense effect. Over 40% of the target mRNA was degraded when oocytes were treated with a 13-mer with one internal mismatch.

Although these studies were conducted at lower temperatures and therefore under less stringent hybridization conditions than those found in mammalian cells, they clearly showed that complementary oligos flanked by unrelated sequences and even oligos with mismatched sequences can lead to significant degradation of RNA. The possibility of undesired inhibition of partially complementary sequences must be considered when designing and testing any antisense oligo. In summary, an oligo of optimal length is one that is long enough to be unique but which is short enough to minimize side effects due to nonspecific degradation of nontargeted mRNAs.

Chimeric oligos, composed of partly MP and partly PO backbones, can be used to minimize nonspecific effects. Investigators have recently demonstrated that greater than four consecutive PO linkages are required to activate RNase H degradation of a targeted RNA substrate [Giles et al., 1993]. The relative position of this PO sequence in the chimeric oligo:RNA duplex greatly influences its ability to activate RNase H. This property of chimeric oligos could significantly increase their specificity by reducing the nonspecific RNase H cleavage of partially complementary RNAs. Future studies must be conducted to elucidate the biologic effects of partial degradation of nontargeted RNAs and to develop oligos with superior specificity.

98.5 Oligo Delivery

The effectiveness of antisense oligos also can be improved by increasing their uptake by target cells. PS and PO oligos are believed to be internalized by receptor mediated endocytosis [Loke et al., 1989]. MP oligos appear to be internalized by an active transport process such as fluid phase or adsorptive endocytosis [Stein and Cheng, 1993]. In most cases, the concentrations required to achieve a biologic effect are currently too large to be of any therapeutic value.

Four major methods that enhance the delivery of oligos to cells are being investigated: (1) chemical modification of the oligo to increase its hydrophobicity, (2) conjugation of the oligo to a polycation, (3) conjugation of the oligo to a ligand, and (4) encapsulation of the oligo in a liposome.

The hydrophobicity of an oligo can be increased by conjugation with cholesterol derivatives (chol-oligo). The increased hydrophobicity of chol-oligos reportedly improves their ability to permeate cell membranes, and they are therefore more readily internalized by cells than are nonconjugated oligos. Ryte et al. [1992] synthesized chol-oligos with cholesterol residues at the 5′ end and demonstrated improved uptake by cells. Krieg et al. [1993] showed that chol-oligos with cholesterol at the 5′ end could be bound by low-density lipoprotein (LDL) and that this markedly increased the association of the oligo with the cell membrane and its internalization in vitro. It is thought that free chol-oligo was in equilibrium with bound LDL–chol-oligo and that the oligo was internalized by both receptor-mediated endocytosis of the LDL particle and by direct partitioning of the hydrophobic chol derivative into the plasma membrane of the cell. LDL–chol-oligos were 8-fold more effective than PO oligo controls.

Oligos conjugated with polycations such as poly-L-lysine (PLL) have improved cellular uptake. These conjugates are constructed by coupling the 3′ end of the oligo to the epsilon amino groups of the lysine residues [Leonetti et al., 1993]. Oligo-PLL conjugates complementary to the translation initiation site of the *tat* gene (a key HIV regulatory protein) protected cells from HIV-1 infection with concentrations 100-fold lower than nonconjugated oligos [Degols et al., 1992]. Low concentrations of oligo-PLL conjugates (100 nM), in which the 15-base-long oligo was complementary to the initiation region of the virus' N protein mRNA, also inhibited vesicular stomatitis virus (VSV) infection [Leonetti et al., 1993].

Internalization of oligos also has been improved by conjugation to ligands. One such ligand, transferrin, is internalized by receptor-mediated endocytosis. Mammallian cells acquire iron carried by transferrin. Oligo-PLL complexes have been conjugated to transferrin to take advantage of this pathway. For example, an 18-mer complementary to *c-myb* mRNA (an oncogene that is responsible for the hyperproliferation of some leukemia cells) was complexed with a transferrin-PLL conjugate and rapidly internalized by human leukemia (HL-60) cells [Citro et al., 1992]. The expression of *c-myb* was greatly reduced and the uncontrolled proliferation of these cells inhibited. Because an oligo-PLL conjugate (without transferrin) was not tested, it is not clear whether the improved antisense effects were due to the PLL moiety, the transferrin moiety, or a combination thereof.

Oligo-ligand conjugates also have been used to target oligos to specific cells. Hepatocytes of the liver express receptors for asialoglycoprotein. These receptors bind and internalize serum glycoproteins that have had sialic acid residues removed from their carbohydrate chains and have exposed galactose residues at their termini. Using the asialoglycoprotein receptor, hepatocytes rapidly internalize abnormal glycoproteins by receptor-mediated endocytosis and destroy them in their lysosomes. Oligos complexed to asialoglycoprotein, containing terminal galactose residues, are rapidly internalized by hepatocytes. Wu et al. [1992] targeted HepG2 cells, a cell line derived from a human hepatocarcinoma, with an asialoglycoprotein-PLL conjugate complexed to a 21-mer complementary to the polyadenylation signal for human hepatitis B virus (HBV). Expression of virus-related surface antigens was 80% lower than that observed with noncomplexed oligo controls.

Other oligo-ligand conjugates have been tested. Boado and Pardridge [1992] coupled biotin to a 21-mer and complexed this with avidin, a 70-kDa cationic protein that binds biotin with high affinity. These complexes were internalized by absorptive endocytosis, and the oligo was protected from serum exonuclease degradation. Cellular uptake and oligo stability was improved, but no biologic antisense effects were reported.

Another promising means to deliver oligos is lipofection. Oligos are mixed with cationic lipids that condense around the negatively charged polynucleotide backbone forming a lipid vesicle (liposome). The positively charged lipids reduce the electrostatic repulsion between the negatively charged oligo and the similarly charged cell surface. Bennett et al. [1994a] prepared such liposomes using DOTMA [*N*-{1-(2,3-dioleyloxy)propyl)}-*N*,*N*,*N*-trimethylammonium chloride] as the cationic lipid and an oligo complementary to the translation initiation codon of human intracellular adhesion molecule 1 (ICAM-1). These liposomes increased the potency of the antisense oligo by more than 1000-fold over noncomplexed oligos.

Efforts are underway to use antibodies to target the delivery of liposomes (containing oligos) to specific cell types. Protein A, which binds to many immunoglobulin G antibodies, is covalently bound to the liposome to form an liposome–oligo–protein A complex. An antibody specific for the target cell's surface is bound to the protein A, and these complexes are incubated with the target cells. Leonetti et al. [1990] synthesized such a complex which contained a 15-mer complementary to the 5′ end of mRNA encoding the N protein of VSV. The antibody used was specific for the mouse major histocompatibility complex–encoded H-2K molecule. The complexes were administered to mouse L929 cells infected with the virus and inhibited viral replication by more than 95%. Unconjugated liposomes, and liposomes conjugated to antibodies specific for a nonexpressed antigen, had no effect.

98.6 Potential Applications of Antisense Oligos

Human Immunodeficiency Virus

One of the many potential therapeutic applications of antisense technology is the treatment of infectious viral diseases (Table 98.2). The use of antisense oligos as an antiviral agent is particularly promising because viral nucleic acid sequences are unique to the infected cell and are not found in normal healthy cells. The goal of antiviral therapy is to block the expression of key viral proteins that are vital to the lifecycle of the virus. This has been achieved in vitro with several viruses, including HIV, HSV, influenza, and human papillomavirus [Milligan et al., 1993]. The work with HIV is representative of other viruses and will be highlighted here.

TABLE 98.2 A Representative Sample of in Vitro Studies Using Antisense Oligodeoxynucleotides. (Only Studies Which Focused on Developing Antisense Oligos for Therapeutic Applications are Included. Potential Applications of Antisense Technology Include the Treatment of Cancer, Infectious Diseases, and Heart Disease.)

Target Disease	Target Gene	Oligo Characteristics			Cell Type	Reference
		Type	No. of Bases	μM		
Cancer						
Autocrine cancer cells	IL-2	PO	15	5–10	Helper T	Harel-Bellan et al., 1988, J Exp Med 168:2309
Autocrine cancer cells	IL-4	PO	15	5–10	Helper T	Harel-Bellan et al., 1988, J Exp Med 168:2309
Acute myelogenous leukemia	N-ras	PO	18	40–80 μg/ml	T lymphocyte depleted mononuclear cells and progenitors (AT-MNC CD-34+)	Skorski et al., 1992, J Exp Med 175:743
Human malignant keratinocytes	Retinoic acid receptor α	PO	15	20–40	Human malignant keratinocytes (SCC-25)	Cope et al., 1989, PNAS USA 86:5590
Leukemia	c-myc	PO	15	4–10	Human promyelocytic leukemia (HL-60)	Wickstrom et al., 1988, PNAS USA 85:1028
Malignant glioblastoma	bFGF	PS	15	5–20	Human malignant glioblastoma (U87-MG)	Murphy et al., 1992, Mol Endocrinol 6:877
Malignant glioma (immune suppression of TIL's due to TGF-β_2 expression)	TGF-β_2	PS	14	1–5	Peripheral blood mononuclear cells	Jachimczak et al., 1993, J Neurosurg 78:944
Metastatic tumor cells	MHC-1	PO	21	5–30 μmol/ml	Melanoma (B16F$_1$)	Kanbe et al., 1992, Anticancer Drug Des 7:341
Myeloma	IL-6	PO	15	10–100	Human myeloma (U266)	Schwab et al., 1991, Blood 77:587
Infectious diseases						
Influenza type A	3' end of all 8 viral RNAs	PO*	7	50	MDCK	Zerial et al., 1987, Nucleic Acids Res 15:9909
Human immunodeficiency virus	rev	PS	27	25	H9	Matsukura et al., 1989, PNAS USA 86:4244
Human immunodeficiency virus	Nonspecific	PS	dc-28+	1	Human T cells (ATH8)	Matsukura et al., 1987, PNAS USA 84:7706
Herpes simplex virus	UL13	PS	21	4	HeLa	Hoke et al., 1991, Nucleic Acids Res 19:5743
Herpes simplex virus	IE4	MP	12	500	Vero	Kulka et al., 1993, Antiviral Res 20:115
Herpes simplex virus	Nonspecific	PS	dc-28+	1	HeLa	Gao et al., 1990, J Biol Chem 265:20172
Human papillomavirus (genital warts)	E6 and E7	PS	20	5–7	HeLa and CaSki	Storey et al., 1991, Nucleic Acids Res 15:4109
Human papillomavirus (genital warts)	E2	PS	20	5	C127 mouse	Cowsert et al., 1993, Antimicrob Agents Chemother 37:171
Other disorders						
Restenosis	Proliferating cell nuclear antigen (PCNA)	PO	18	10–100	Vascular smooth muscle cells (rats)	Speir et al., 1992, Circulation 86:538

PO = phosphodiester backbone.
PS = phosphorothioate backbone.
MP = methylphosphonate backbone.
* this phosphodiester oligo was covalently linked to an acridine derivative.
+ 28-mer homodeoxycytidine.

Retroviruses, and HIV in particular, have high rates of mutation and genetic recombination. The effectiveness of many anti-HIV drugs has been severely reduced because drug-resistant viral strains often arise after prolonged drug treatment. This is especially relevant to strategies that use an anti-sense approach that relies on specific nucleotide sequences for their effectiveness. One strategy to inhibit HIV replication is to target conserved sequences in key regulatory proteins such as *tat* and *rev*. Part of the *rev* sequence is highly conserved, and all known 16 isolates of HIV differ by at most one base pair in this conserved region [Stein and Cheng, 1993].

The importance of targeting a highly conserved region as is found in *rev* and the profound impact of the rapid mutation rate of HIV on drug effectiveness were demonstrated by Lisziewicz et al. [1992]. They blocked HIV-1 replication with several 28-mers targeted to different regions of the virus' RNA, including the conserved region in *rev*. Initially, all the oligos inhibited viral replication. However, after 25 days, mutant viruses developed that were resistant to oligo treatment. Only those oligos directed at the highly conserved *rev* regions continued to inhibit HIV replication.

Viruses also can be inhibited by PS oligos in a non-sequence-specific manner; i.e., they inhibit gene expression even though their sequences are not complementary to any viral sequences. These unexpected nonspecific effects are due primarily to the polyanionic nature of these oligos. For example, 28-mer phosphorothioate oligodeoxycytidines (S-dc-28) interfere with viral adsorption to the cell surface, block viral polymerases, or interfere with the release of internalized viruses from endosomes into the cytoplasm of the host cells [Stein and Cheng, 1993]. An S-dc-28 oligo inhibited the de novo synthesis of DNA and syncytia formation in cells infected with HIV [Matsukura et al., 1987; Stein et al., 1991]. An 8-mer PS oligo (TTGGGGTT) also inhibited HIV infection by a non-sequence-specific mechanism. These 8-mer PS oligos form tetramers that bind to the V3 loop of the envelope protein (gp120) of HIV and prevent infection by blocking the ability of the V3 loop to bind to CD-4, its cell surface receptor [Matsukura et al., 1987].

The high rate of mutation of HIV makes the development of an effective antisense therapy particularly difficult. As previously discussed, this mutation rate gives rise to resistant strains of the virus that escape the inhibitory effects of most antiviral drugs. It is likely that resistant strains also will develop in response to treatment with nonspecific oligos, such as S-dc-28. The most promising oligo candidates for HIV are directed against [Lisziewicz et al., 1992] conserved sequences such as *rev* which are essential for HIV replication. A second concern in treating HIV and other viruses is that viral replication can restart after antisense treatment is stopped [Stein and Cheng, 1993]. Can oligos be continuously administered to prevent viral replication without toxic side effects? These issues and others common to all antisense-based therapies (oligo stability, specificity, affinity, and delivery) must be addressed prior to the successful implementation of antisense-based HIV therapies.

Cancer

In principle, antisense technology can be used against cancer, but the target is more challenging. Oncogenes are typically genes that play a vital regulatory role in the growth of a cell, the mutation or inappropriate expression of which can result in the overzealous growth of the cell and the development of cancer. In the case of mutation, it is often difficult to distinguish an oncogene from its normal counterpart because they may differ by as little as one base. Thus attempts to inhibit oncogene expression might block the expression of the normal gene in noncancerous cells and cause cytotoxic effects. Despite these challenges, steady progress has been made in the development of effective antisense oligos that have inhibited many types of oncogenes, including transcription factors such as *c-myc* and *c-myb* as well as growth factors and their receptors such as *c-ras, neu/erbB2*, and *bFGF* [Carter and Lemoine, 1993; Nagel et al., 1993].

Recent studies targeting *ras* oncogenes are encouraging and are representative of progress against other classes of oncogenes. Chang et al. [1991] targeted the *ras p21* gene with an antisense oligo. The mutated gene had a point mutation and therefore differed from the wild-type gene by a single base. They mixed cultures of two identical cell lines with the exception that one cell line expressed the mutant *ras* gene and the other expressed the normal gene. The mixed culture was exposed to oligos for the mutant gene. Only the expression of the mutated genes was inhibited, suggesting that it is possible to selectively inhibit an oncogene that differs by as little as a single base from the normal gene.

Recent successes in inhibiting oncogene expression in vitro are encouraging, but many problems remain to be solved before antisense oligos are therapeutically useful for cancer patients. For example, finding a suitable oncogene to target is difficult. Even if a genetic defect is common to all cells of a given cancer, there is no guarantee that inhibition of that oncogene will halt cancer cell proliferation [Carter and Lemoine, 1993]. Even if cell growth is inhibited, tumor growth may restart after antisense treatment is stopped. Oligos are needed that induce cancer cell terminal differentiation or death [Carter and Lemoine, 1993]. In order to avoid inhibiting normal gene expression (and the accompanying toxic side effects), oligos that specifically target cancer cells are required. Even if appropriate antisense oligos are developed, they will still be ineffective against solid tumors unless they can reach the interior of the tumor at biologically effective concentrations.

98.7 In Vivo Pharmacology

The first in vivo antisense studies were designed to test the biodistribution and toxicity of antisense oligos. These studies demonstrated that oligos are rapidly excreted from the body. PS oligos were retained longer than MP or PO oligos. One study injected 30 mg/kg of a 20-mer PS oligo complementary to the HIV *tat* splice acceptor site either intravenously or intraperitoneally into mice [Agrawal et al., 1991]. The authors noted that PS oligos were retained significantly longer than a chimeric 20-mer that contained 15 phosphodiester bonds and only 4 phosphorothioate bonds. Only 30% of the PS oligo was excreted in the urine after 24 hours, whereas 75% of the chimeric oligo was excreted after only 12 hours. A similar study demonstrated that over 70% of an MP oligo was excreted within 1 hour after administration to rats as opposed to a PS oligo that was retained in the body with a half-life of 20 to 40 hours [Iversen, 1991].

These studies suggest that antisense oligos may need to be administered repeatedly to maintain a therapeutic effect for chronic disorders. A recent study demonstrated that antisense oligos could be repeatedly or continuously injected without toxic effects [Iversen, 1991]. A 27-mer PS oligo complementary to HIV *rev* was injected daily for 12 days or continuously infused with subcutaneous osmotic pumps for 4 weeks into rats. The liver, kidneys, and lungs achieved maximum levels of oligo after 6 to 9 days. Body and organ weights were not effected by the treatment, and no other signs of toxicity were noted. It is not known if the immune system will respond to repeated injections of oligo.

The targeted delivery of oligos has been proposed as a way to improve the effectiveness of systemically administered antisense oligos. Targeted delivery could maximize oligo concentration in the desired cells and minimize any nonspecific side effects. The ability to target oligos to a specific organ has been demonstrated recently. As previously discussed, a soluble DNA carrier system has been developed in which the DNA is bound to a poly-L-lysine:asialoglycoprotein complex, and this complex is recognized by receptors for asialoglycoprotein on liver hepatocytes [Wu et al., 1989]. This system was used to target a 67-mer PO oligo (complementary to the 5′ end of rat serum albumin mRNA) to the liver [Lu et al., 1994]. Following tail vein injection into rats, the complex rapidly and preferentially accumulated in the liver, but the efficiency of this targeting method was limited by the rapid dissociation of the oligo from the poly-L-lysine:asialoglycoprotein complex (30% dissociated within 7 minutes).

98.8 Animal Models

The effectiveness of antisense oligos at inhibiting gene expression in vivo has been demonstrated in several animal models. Immunodeficient mice bearing a human myeloid leukemia cell line were continuously infused with 100 μg/day of a 24-mer PS oligo complementary to *c-myb* mRNA

[Ratajczak et al., 1992]. Mice that received the antisense oligo survived up to 8.5 times longer than control mice that received either sense oligos, scrambled oligos, or no treatment. The treated animals also had a significantly lower tumor burden in the ovaries and brain.

Antisense oligos also have inhibited the growth of solid tumors in vivo. Immunodeficient mice bearing a fibrosarcoma or melanoma were injected subcutaneously twice weekly with 1.4 mg of PS oligos complementary to the 5′ end of the p65 subunit of the NF-κB transcription factor mRNA (NF-κB activates a wide variety of genes and is believed to be important in cell adhesion and tumor cell metastasis) [Higgins et al., 1993]. Greater than 70% of antisense-treated mice exhibited a marked reduction in their tumor size. Administration of control oligos complementary to GAPDH and *jun-D* had no effect on tumor size.

The capability of antisense oligos to inhibit viral replication in vivo also has been studied. Fourteen 1-day-old ducklings were infected with duck hepatitis B virus (DHBV), which is closely related to hepatitis B virus, a major cause of chronic liver disease and cancer [Offensperger et al., 1993]. Two weeks later, the ducks were injected daily, for 10 consecutive days, with 20 µg/g of body weight of an 18-mer PS oligo complementary to the start site of the pre-S region of the DHBV genome. The antisense oligos blocked viral gene expression and eliminated the appearance of viral antigens in the serum and liver of all treated ducks. No toxic effects due to the oligos were noted. Unfortunately, residual amounts of DNA precursors of viral transcripts were detected in the nuclei of liver cells, which resulted in a slow restart of viral replication after antisense treatment was stopped. Further studies are needed to determine if prolonged treatment with antisense will eliminate this residual viral DNA.

Antisense oligos also have been evaluated in the treatment of restenosis, a narrowing of an artery following corrective surgery. A major cause of restenosis is the mitogen-induced proliferation of vascular smooth muscle cells (SMC). Several studies have tested the ability of antisense oligos to inhibit genes whose expression is important in SMC proliferation, including *c-myc, c-myb, cdc2,* and *cdk2* [Abe et al., 1994; Bennett et al., 1994b; Simons et al., 1992]. In one study, the left common carotid artery of male rats was injured by balloon catheter dilatation [Bennett et al., 1994b]. Then 200 µg of 15-mer PS oligos complementary to the 5′ end of *c-myc* mRNA was applied in a pluronic gel to 9 rats immediately after the injury. The arteries were examined 14 days later. The formation of a thick intimal layer (neointima) in the areas where the gel was applied was significantly reduced in all the antisense-treated rats when compared with control rats treated with sense oligo or gel alone. Maximum *c-myc* expression was reduced by 75% in the antisense-treated rats. These studies indicate that *c-myc* expression can be suppressed in vivo by antisense oligos and that inhibiting this gene may be an effective treatment for restenosis. More studies are needed to determine if the suppression of restenosis is maintained long term and what effect these antisense oligos are having on the vascular smooth muscle cells.

98.9 Clinical Trials

Despite the many obstacles that still impede the use of antisense oligos in vivo, the first clinical trial of an antisense drug has been approved by the Food and Drug Administration [Reynolds, 1992]. This study is designed to aid in the treatment of chronic myelogenous leukemia. Other clinical trials have since been approved and are in progress [Stein and Cheng, 1993]. In one trial, 5 patients with relapsed or refractory acute myeloid leukemia or myelodysplastic syndrome were continuously infused with a PS oligo complementary to p53 mRNA for 10 days at 0.05 mg/kg/h [Bayever et al., 1993]. No major toxicity was noted. Between 9% and 18% of the oligo was excreted intact in the patients' urine. In future phases of the trial, higher doses will be used to test toxicity and clinical effectiveness.

98.10 Summary

Antisense deoxyribonucleotides have the potential to selectively inhibit the expression of any gene whose sequence is known. Realizing this potential is extremely difficult because of problems with oligo stability, specificity, affinity, and delivery. Natural deoxyribonucleotides contain a phosphodiester backbone that is highly susceptible to degradation and inactivation. Chemically modified oligos (PS and PO oligos) have been synthesized that are more stable. However, these modified oligos are sometimes not very soluble, and often, prohibitively high concentrations are required to inhibit gene expression. PS oligos are typically more effective than MP oligos but are still required in concentrations too large for therapeutic use. Another issue for chemically modified oligos is their large-scale production and purification. Alternative chemistries are needed that are more biologically active and more amenable to large-scale production. Another challenge to the development of therapeutically useful antisense oligos is drug delivery. Targeted delivery of antisense oligos is needed to minimize toxic side effects and maximize oligo concentration in target cells. Attempts to improve delivery include chemical modification of the oligos to increase their cellular permeability, the conjugation of oligos to specific ligands to utilize more efficient receptor mediated internalization pathways, and the use of antibody-conjugated liposomes to deliver oligos to specific cells.

The potential applications of antisense oligos to the treatment of disease are vast. Antisense-based therapies are under development for the treatment of infectious diseases such as HIV, herpes simplex virus, influenza, hepatitis, and human papillomavirus, as well as the treatment of complex genetic disorders such as cancer. Animal models are being developed to study the in vivo effects of antisense oligos, and these studies are needed to determine if (1) antisense oligos can be delivered to target cells at high enough concentrations to be effective, (2) repeated treatment with oligos is toxic or elicits an immune response, and (3) antisense oligos directed against a single gene can be effective against complex genetic diseases such as cancer. Improvements to our understanding of the mechanisms of antisense inhibition, the pharmacology of antisense oligos in vivo, and the development of chemically modified oligos with high affinity, specificity, and stability are needed to realize the clinical potential of antisense-based strategies for the treatment of a wide variety of diseases.

Defining Terms

Antisense: Any DNA or RNA molecule whose sequence is complementary to the sense strand of RNA transcribed from a target gene.

Chiral: A molecule whose configuration is not identical with its mirror image.

Complementary: A nucleic acid sequence is complementary to another if it is able to form a perfectly hydrogen-bonded duplex with it, according to the Watson-Crick rules of base pairing (A opposite U or T, G opposite C).

Diastereomer: Optically active isomers that are not enantiomorphs (mirror images).

Exonuclease: An enzyme that catalyzes the release of one nucleotide at a time, serially, from one end of a polynucleotide.

In vitro: In an artificial environment, referring to a process or reaction occurring therein, as in a test tube or culture dish.

In vivo: In the living body, referring to a process or reaction occurring therein.

Lipofection: Delivery of therapeutic drugs (antisense oligos) to cells using cationic liposomes.

Lipophilic: Capable of being dissolved in lipids (organic molecules that are the major structural elements of biomembranes).

Liposome: A spherical particle of lipid substance suspended in an aqueous medium.

Plasmid: A small, circular extrachromosomal DNA molecule capable of independent replication in a host cell.

Receptor-mediated endocytosis: The selective uptake of extracellular proteins, oligonucleotides, and small particles, usually into clathrin-coated pits, following their binding to cell surface receptor proteins.

Restenosis: A narrowing of an artery or heart valve following corrective surgery on it.

RNase H: An enzyme that specifically recognizes RNA:DNA duplexes and cleaves the RNA portion, leaving the DNA portion intact.

Spliceosome: A cluster of small ribonucleoprotein particles (which are assemblies of small nuclear RNA and proteins) found in eukaryotes, which form on pre-mRNA and carry out its splicing reaction.

References

Abe J, Zhou W, Taguchi J, et al. 1994. Suppression of neointimal smooth muscle cell accumulation in vivo by antisense cdc2 and cdk2 oligonucleotides in rat carotid artery. Biochem Biophys Res Commun 198(1):16.

Agrawal S, Temsamani J, Tang JY. 1991. Pharmacokinetics, biodistribution, and stability of oligodeoxynucleotide phosphorothioates in mice. Proc Natl Acad Sci USA 88:7595.

Akhtar S, Basu S, Wickstrom E, Juliano RL. 1991. Interactions of antisense DNA oligonucleotide analogues with phospholipid membranes (liposomes). Nucleic Acids Res 19(20):5551.

Bayever E, Iversen PL, Bishop MR, et al. 1993. Systemic administration of a phosphorothioate oligonucleotide with a sequence complementary to p53 for acute myelogenous leukemia and myelodysplastic syndrome: Initial results of a phase I trial. Antisense Res Dev 3(4):383.

Bennett CF, Condon TP, Grimm S, et al. 1994a. Inhibition of endothelial cell adhesion molecule expression with antisense oligonucleotides. J Immunol 152:3530.

Bennett MR, Anglin S, McEwan JR, et al. 1994b. Inhibition of vascular smooth muscle cell proliferation in vitro and in vivo by c-myc antisense oligodeoxynucleotides. J Clin Invest 93:820.

Boado RJ, Pardridge WM. 1992. Complete protection of antisense oligonucleotides against serum nuclease degradation by an avidin-biotin system. Bioconjug Chem 3(6):519.

Carter G, Lemoine NR. 1993. Antisense technology for cancer therapy: Does it make sense? Br J Cancer 67:869.

Chang EH, Miller PS, Cushman C, et al. 1991. Antisense inhibition of ras p21 expression that is sensitive to a point mutation. Biochemistry 30:8283.

Citro G, Perrotti D, Cucco C, et al. 1992. Inhibition of leukaemia cell proliferation by receptor-mediated uptake of c-myb antisense oligodeoxynucleotides. Proc Natl Acad Sci USA 89:7031.

Cook PD. 1991. Medicinal chemistry of antisense oligonucleotides—Future opportunities. Anticancer Drug Des 6:585.

Degols G, Leonetti JP, Benkirane M, et al. 1992. Poly(L-lysine)-conjugated oligonucleotides promote sequence-specific inhibition of acute HIV-1 infection. Antisense Res Dev 2(4):293.

Egholm M, Nielsen PE, Buchardt O, Berg RH. 1992. Recognition of guanine and adenine in DNA by cytosine and thymine containing peptide nucleic acids (PNA) J Am Chem Soc 114:9677.

Giles RV, Spiller DG, Tidd DM. 1993. Chimeric oligodeoxynucleotide analogues: Enhanced cell uptake of structures which direct ribonuclease H with high specificity. Anticancer Drug Des 8(1):33.

Goodchild J, Carroll E III, Greenberg JR. 1988. Inhibition of rabbit beta-globin synthesis by complementary oligonucleotides: Identification of mRNA sites sensitive to inhibition. Arch Biochem Biophys 263:401.

Green PJ, Pines O, Inouye M. 1986. The role of antisense RNA in gene regulation. Annu Rev Biochem 55:569.

Hanvey JC, Peffer NJ, Bisi JE, et al. 1992. Antisense and antigene properties of peptide nucleic acids. Science 258:1481.

Helene C, Toulme JJ. 1990. Specific regulation of gene expression by antisense, sense and antigene nucleic acids. Biochim Biophys Acta 1049:99.

Herschlag D. 1991. Implications of ribozyme kinetics for targeting the cleavage of specific RNA molecules in vivo: More isn't always better. Proc Natl Acad Sci USA 88:6921.

Higgins KA, Perez JR, Coleman TA, et al. 1993. Antisense inhibition of the p65 subunit of NF-kB blocks tumorigenicity and causes tumor regression. Proc Natl Acad Sci USA 90:9901.

Iversen P. 1991. In vivo studies with phosphorothioate oligonucleotides: Pharmacokinetics pro-
logue. Anticancer Drug Des 6:531.

Izant JG, Weintraub H. 1985. Constitutive and conditional suppression of exogenous and endogenous genes by anti-sense RNA. Science 229:345.

Kibler-Herzog L, Zon G, Uznanski B, et al. 1991. Duplex stabilities of phosphorothioate,
methylphosphonate and RNA analogues of two DNA 14-mers. Nucleic Acids Res 19:2979.

Krieg AM, Tonkinson J, Matson S, et al. 1993. Modification of antisense phosphodiester oligodeoxynucleotides by a 5' cholesteryl moiety increases cellular association and improves efficacy. Proc Natl Acad Sci USA 90:1048.

Leonetti JP, Degols G, Clarenc JP, et al. 1993. Cell delivery and mechanisms of action of antisense
oligonucleotides. Prog Nucleic Acid Res Mol Biol 44:143.

Leonetti JP, Machy P, Degols G, et al. 1990. Antibody-targeted liposomes containing oligodeoxyri-
bonucleotides complementary to viral RNA selectively inhibit viral replication. Proc Natl
Acad Sci USA 87:2448.

Lesnikowski ZJ, Jaworska M, Stec WJ. 1990. Octa(thymidine methanephosphonates) of partially
defined stereochemistry: Synthesis and effect of chirality at phosphorus on binding to
pentadecadeoxyriboadenylic acid. Nucleic Acids Res 18:2109.

Lima WF, Monia BP, Ecker DJ, Freier SM. 1992. Implication of RNA structure on antisense oligonucleotide hybridization kinetics. Biochemistry 31:12055.

Lisziewicz J, Sun D, Klotman M, et al. 1992. Specific inhibition of human immunodeficiency virus
type 1 replication by antisense oligonucleotides: An in vitro model for treatment. Proc Natl
Acad Sci USA 89:11209.

Loke SL, Stein CA, Zhang XH, et al. 1989. Characterization of oligonucleotide transport into living
cells. Proc Natl Acad Sci USA 86:3474.

Lu XM, Fischman AJ, Jyawook SL, et al. 1994. Antisense DNA delivery in vivo: Liver targeting by
receptor-mediated uptake. J Nucl Med 35:269.

Matsukura M, Shinozuka K, Zon G, et al. 1987. Phosphorothioate analogs of oligodeoxynucleotides:
Inhibitors of replication and cytopathic effects of human immunodeficiency virus. Proc Natl
Acad Sci USA 84:7706.

Miller PS. 1991. Oligonucleotide methylphosphonates as antisense reagents. Biotechnology 9:358.

Milligan JF, Matteucci MD, Martin JC. 1993. Current concepts in antisense drug design. J Med Chem
36(14):1923.

Nagel KM, Holstad SG, Isenberg KE. 1993. Oligonucleotide pharmacotherapy: An antigene strategy.
Pharmacotherapy 13(3):177.

Neckers L, Whitesell L. 1993. Antisense technology: Biological utility and practical considerations.
Am J Physiol 265:L1.

Nielsen PE, Egholm M, Berg RH, Buchardt O. 1993. Peptide nucleic acids (PNAs): Potential antisense and anti-gene agents. Anticancer Drug Des 8:53.

Offensperger W-B, Offensperger S, Walter E, et al. 1993. In vivo inhibition of duck hepatitis B virus
replication and gene expression by phosphorothioate modified antisense oligodeoxynucleotides. EMBO J 12(3):1257.

Ratajczak MZ, Kant JA, Luger SM, et al. 1992. In vivo treatment of human leukemia in a scid mouse
model with c-myb antisense oligodeoxynucleotides. Proc Natl Acad Sci USA 89:11823.

Reynolds T. 1992. First antisense drug trials planned in leukemia. J Natl Cancer Inst 84:288.

Ryte AS, Karamyshev VN, Nechaeva MV, et al. 1992. Interaction of cholesterol-conjugated alkylating oligonucleotide derivatives with cellular biopolymers. FEBS Lett 299:124.

Simons M, Edelman ER, DeKeyser J, et al. 1992. Antisense c-myb oligonucleotides inhibit intimal
arterial smooth muscle cell accumulation in vivo. Nature 359:67.

Stein CA, Cheng YC. 1993. Antisense oligonucleotides as therapeutic agents—Is the bullet really
magical? Science 261:1004.

Stein CA, Ranajit P, DeVico AL, et al. 1991. Mode of action of 5′-linked cholesterol phosphorothioate oligodeoxynucleotides in inhibiting synctia formation and infection by HIV-1 and HIV-2 in vitro. Biochemistry 30:2439.

Stein CA, Subasinghe C, Shinozuka K, Cohen JS. 1988. Physicochemical properties of phosphorothioate oligodeoxynucleotides. Nucleic Acids Res 16:3209.

Tidd DM, Hawley P, Warenius HM, Gibson I. 1988. Evaluation of N-ras oncogene antisense, sense and nonsense sequence methylphosphonate oligonucleotide analogues. Anticancer Drug Des 3:117.

Tidd DM, Warenius HM. 1989. Partial protection of oncogene antisense oligodeoxynucleotides against serum nuclease degradation using terminal methylphosphonate groups. Br J Cancer 60:343.

Tomizawa JI, Itoh T. 1981. Plasmid ColE1 incompatibility determined by interaction of RNA I with primer transcript. Proc Natl Acad Sci USA 78:6096.

Tomizawa JI, Itoh T, Selzer G, Som T. 1981. Inhibition of ColE1 RNA primer formation by a plasmid-specified small RNA. Proc Natl Acad Sci USA 78:1421.

Uhlmann E, Peyman A. 1990. Antisense oligonucleotides: A new therapeutic principle. Chem Rev 90:544.

Woolf TM, Melton DA, Jennings CG. 1992. Specificity of antisense oligonucleotides in vivo. Proc Natl Acad Sci USA 89:7305.

Wu CH, Wilson JM, Wu GY. 1989. Targeting genes: Delivery and persistent expression of a foreign gene driven by mammalian regulatory elements in vivo. J Biol Chem 264:16985.

Wu GY, Wu CH. 1992. Specific inhibition of hepatitis B viral gene expression in vitro by targeted antisense oligonucleotides. J Biol Chem 267(18):12436.

Zamecnik PC, Stephenson ML. 1978. Inhibition of Rous sarcoma virus replication and cell transformation by a specific oligodeoxynucleotide. Proc Natl Acad Sci USA 75:280.

Further Information

The book *Antisense Nucleic Acids and Proteins: Fundamentals and Applications,* edited by Joseph N. M. Mol and Alexander R. van der Krol, is a collection of reviews in the use of antisense nucleic acids to modulate or downregulate gene expression. The book *Antisense RNA and DNA,* edited by James A. H. Murray, explores the use of antisense and catalytic nucleic acids for regulating gene expression.

The journal *Antisense Research and Development,* published by Mary Ann Liebert, Inc., presents original research on antisense technology. For subscription information, contact Antisense Research and Development, Mary Ann Liebert, Inc., 1651 Third Avenue, New York, NY 10128, (212) 289-2300, Fax (212) 289-4697. The biweekly journal *Nucleic Acids Research* publishes papers on physical, chemical, and biologic aspects of nucleic acids, their constituents, and proteins with which they interact. For subscription information, contact IRL Press at Oxford University Press, Inc., 2001 Evans Road, Cary, NC 27513.

99

Tools for
Genome Analysis

Robert Kaiser
University of Washington

The development of sophisticated and powerful recombinant techniques for manipulating and analyzing genetic material has led to the emergence of a new biologic discipline, often termed *molecular biology.* The tools of molecular biology have enabled scientists to begin to understand many of the fundamental processes of life, generally through the identification, isolation, and structural and functional analysis of individual or, at best, limited numbers of genes. Biology is now at a point where it is feasible to begin a more ambitious endeavor—the complete genetic analysis of entire genomes. Genome analysis aims not only to identify and molecularly characterize all the genes that orchestrate the development of an organism but also to understand the complex and interactive regulatory mechanisms of these genes, their organization in the genome, and the role of genetic variation in disease, adaptability, and individuality. Additionally, the study of homologous genetic regions across species can provide important insight into their evolutionary history.

As can be seen in Table 99.1, the genome of even a small organism consists of a very large amount of information. Thus the analysis of a complete genome is not simply a matter of using conventional techniques that work well with individual genes (comprised of perhaps 1000 to 10,000 base pairs) a sufficient (very large) number of times to cover the genome. Such a brute-force approach would be too slow and too expensive, and conventional data-handling techniques would be inadequate for the task of cataloging, storing, retrieving, and analyzing such a large amount of information. The amount of manual labor and scientific expertise required would be prohibitive. New technology is needed to provide high-throughput, low-cost automation and reduced reliance on expert intervention at intermediate levels in the processes required for large-scale genetic analysis. Novel computational tools are required to deal with the large volumes of genetic information produced. Individual tools must be integrated smoothly to produce an analytical system in which samples are tracked through the entire analytical process, intermediate decisions and branch points are few, a stable, reliable and routine protocol or set of protocols is employed, and the resulting information is presented to the biologic scientist in a useful and meaningful format. It is important to realize that the development of these tools requires the interdisciplinary efforts of biologists, chemists, physicists, engineers, mathematicians, and computer scientists.

Genome analysis is a complex and extended series of interrelated processes. The basic processes involved are diagrammed in Fig. 99.1. At each stage, new biologic, chemical, physical (mechanical, optical), and computational tools have been developed within the last 10 years that have begun to

TABLE 99.1   DNA Content of Various Genomes in Monomer Units (Base Pairs)

Organism	Type	Size
Phage T4	Bacteriophage (virus)	160,000
Escherichia coli	Bacterium	4,000,000
Saccharomyces	Yeast	14,000,000
Arabidopsis thaliana	Plant	100,000,000
Caenorhabditis elegans	Nematode	100,000,000
Drosophila melanogaster	Insect (fruit fly)	165,000,000
Mouse	Mammal	3,000,000,000
Human	Mammal	3,500,000,000

Source: Adapted from [1] and [2].

enable large-scale (megabase) genetic analysis. These developments have largely been spurred by the goals of the Human Genome Project, a worldwide effort to decipher the entirety of human genetics. However, biologists are still a significant ways away from having a true genome analysis capability [3], and as such, new technologies are still emerging.

This chapter cannot hope to describe in depth the entire suite of tools currently in use in genome analysis. Instead, it will attempt to present the basic principles involved and to highlight some of the recent enabling technological developments that are likely to remain in use in genome analysis for the foreseeable future. Some fundamental knowledge of biology is assumed; in this regard, an

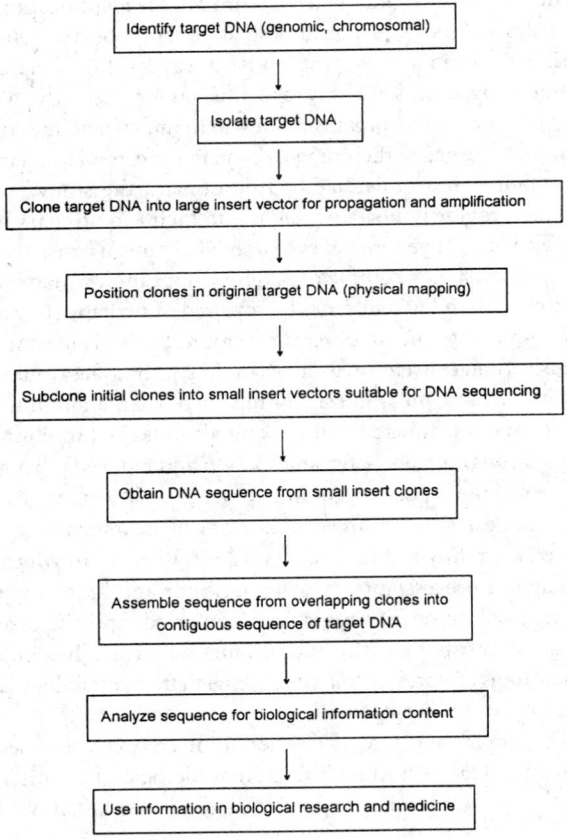

FIGURE 99.1   Basic steps in genome analysis.

excellent beginning text for individuals with a minimal background in molecular biology is that by Watson et al. [1].

99.1 General Principles

The fundamental blueprint for any cell or organism is encoded in its genetic material, its deoxyribonucleic acid (DNA). DNA is a linear polymer derived from a four-letter biochemical alphabet— A, C, G, and T. These four letters are often referred to as *nucleotides* or *bases*. The linear order of bases in a segment of DNA is termed its *DNA sequence* and determines its function. A gene is a segment of DNA whose sequence directly determines its translated protein product. Other DNA sequences are recognized by the cellular machinery as start and stop sites for protein synthesis, regulate the temporal or spatial expression of genes, or play a role in the organization of higher-order DNA structures such as chromosomes. Thus a thorough understanding of the DNA sequence of a cell or organism is fundamental to an understanding of its biology.

Recombinant DNA technology affords biologists the capability to manipulate and analyze DNA sequences. Many of the techniques employed take advantage of a basic property of DNA, the molecular complementarity of the two strands of the double helix. This complementarity arises from the specific hydrogen-bonding interactions between pairs of DNA bases, A with T and C with G. Paired double strands of DNA can be denatured, or rendered into the component single strands, by any process that disrupts these hydrogens bonds—high temperature, chaotropic agents, or pH extremes. Complementary single strands also can be renatured into the duplex structure by reversing the disruptive element; this process is sometimes referred to as *hybridization* or *annealing*, particularly when one of the strands has been supplied from some exogenous source.

Molecular biology makes extensive use of the DNA-modifying enzymes employed by cells during replication, translation, repair, and protection from foreign DNA. A list of commonly used enzymes, their functions, and some of the experimental techniques in which they are utilized is provided in Table 99.2.

99.2 Enabling Technologies

The following are broadly applicable tools that have been developed in the context of molecular biology and are commonly used in genome analysis.

Cloning.   Cloning is a recombinant procedure that has two main purposes: First, it allows one to select a single DNA fragment from a complex mixture, and second, it provides a means to store, manipulate, propagate, and produce large numbers of identical molecules having this single ancestor. A cloning vector is a DNA fragment derived from a microorganism, such as a bacteriophage or yeast, into which a foreign DNA fragment may be inserted to produce a chimeric DNA species. The vector contains all the genetic information necessary to allow for the replication of the chimera in an appropriate host organism. A variety of cloning vectors have been developed which allow for the insertion and stable propagation of foreign DNA segments of various sizes; these are indicated in Table 99.3.

TABLE 99.2   Enzymes Commonly Used in Genome Analysis

Enzyme	Function	Common Use
Restriction endonuclease	Cleave double-stranded DNA at specific sites	Mapping, cloning
DNA polymerase	Synthesize complementary DNA strand	DNA sequencing, amplification
Polynucleotide kinase	Adds phosphate to 5′ end of single-stranded DNA	Radiolabeling, cloning
Terminal transferase	Adds nucleotides to the 3′ end of single-stranded DNA	Labeling
Reverse transcriptase	Makes DNA copy from RNA	RNA sequencing, cDNA cloning
DNA ligase	Covalently joins two DNA fragments	Cloning

TABLE 99.3   Common Cloning Vectors

Vector	Approximate Insert Size Range (Base Pairs)
Bacteriophage M13	100–5000
Plasmid	100–10,000
Bacteriophage lambda	10,000–15,000
Cosmid	25,000–50,000
Yeast artificial chromosome (YAC)	100,000–1,000,000

Electrophoresis.   Electrophoresis is a process whereby nucleic acids are separated by size in a sieving matrix under the influence of an electric field. In free solution, DNA, being highly negatively charged by virtue of its phosphodiester backbone, migrates rapidly toward the positive pole of an electric field. If the DNA is forced instead to travel through a molecularly porous substance, such as a gel, the smaller (shorter) fragments of DNA will travel through the pores more rapidly than the larger (longer) fragments, thus effecting separation. Agarose, a highly purified derivative of agar, is commonly used to separate relatively large fragments of DNA (100 to 50,000 base pairs) with modest resolution (50 to 100 base pairs), while cross-linked polyacrylamide is used to separate smaller fragments (10 to 1,000 base pairs) with single base-pair resolution. Fragment sizes are generally estimated by comparison with standards run in another lane of the same gel. Electrophoresis is used extensively as both an analytical and a preparative tool in molecular biology.

Enzymatic DNA Sequencing.   In the late 1970s, Sanger and coworkers [4] reported a procedure employing DNA polymerase to obtain DNA sequence information from unknown cloned fragments. While significant improvements and modifications have been made since that time, the basic technique remains the same: DNA polymerase is used to synthesize a complementary copy of an unknown single-stranded DNA (the template) in the presence of the four DNA monomers (deoxynucleotide triphosphates, or dNTPs). DNA polymerase requires a double-stranded starting point, so a single-stranded DNA (the primer) is hybridized at a unique site on the template (usually in the vector), and it is at this point that DNA synthesis is initiated. Key to the sequencing process is the use of a modified monomer, a dideoxynucleotide triphosphate (ddNTP), in each reaction. The ddNTP lacks the 3′-hydroxyl functionality (it has been replaced by a hydrogen) necessary for phosphodiester bond formation, and its incorporation thus blocks further elongation of the growing chain by polymerase. Four reactions are carried out, each containing all four dNTPs and one of the four ddNTPs. By using the proper ratios of dNTPs to ddNTP, each reaction generates a nested set of fragments, each fragment beginning at exactly the same point (the primer) and terminating with a particular ddNTP at each base complementary to that ddNTP in the template sequence. The products of the reactions are then separated by electrophoresis in four lanes of a polyacrylamide slab gel. Since conventional sequencing procedures utilize radiolabeling (incorporation of a small amount of ^{32}P- or ^{35}S-labeled dNTP by the polymerase), visualization of the gel is achieved by exposing it to film. The sequence can be obtained from the resulting autoradiogram, which appears as a series of bands (often termed a *ladder*) in each of the four lanes. Each band is composed of fragments of a single size, the shortest fragments being at the bottom of the gel and the longest at the top. Adjacent bands represent a single base pair difference, so the sequence is determined by reading up the ladders in the four lanes and noting which lane contains the band with the next largest sized fragments. The enzymatic sequencing process is diagrammed in Fig. 99.2. It should be noted that although other methods exist, the enzymatic sequencing technique is currently the most commonly used DNA sequencing procedure due to its simplicity and reliability.

Polymerase Chain Reaction (PCR).   PCR [5] is an in vitro procedure for amplifying particular DNA sequences up to 10^8-fold that is utilized in an ever-increasing variety of ways in genome analysis. The sequence to be amplified is defined by a pair of single-stranded primers designed to

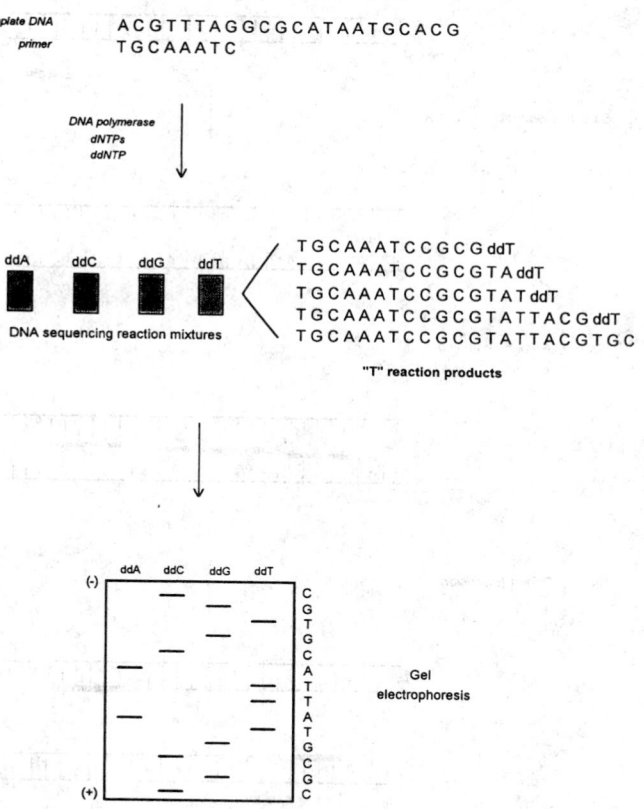

template DNA ACGTTTAGGCGCATAATGCACG
primer TGCAAATC

DNA polymerase
dNTPs
ddNTP

ddA ddC ddG ddT

DNA sequencing reaction mixtures

TGCAAATCCGCG ddT
TGCAAATCCGCGTA ddT
TGCAAATCCGCGTAT ddT
TGCAAATCCGCGTATTACG ddT
TGCAAATCCGCGTATTACGTGC

"T" reaction products

ddA ddC ddG ddT

(-)

Gel
electrophoresis

(+)

FIGURE 99.2 Enzymatic DNA sequencing. A synthetic oligonucleotide primer is hybridized to its complementary site on the template DNA. DNA polymerase and dNTPs are then used to synthesize a complementary copy of the unknown portion of the template in the presence of a chain-terminating ddNTP (see text). A nested set of fragments beginning with the primer sequence and ending at every ddNTP position is produced in each reactions (the ddTTP reaction products are shown). Four reactions are carried out, one for each ddNTP. The products of each reaction are then separated by gel electrophoresis in individual lanes, and the resulting ladders are visualized. The DNA sequence is obtained by reading up the set of four ladders, one base at a time, from smallest to largest fragment.

hybridize to unique sites flanking the target sequence on opposite strands. DNA polymerase in the presence of the four dNTPS is used to synthesize a complementary DNA copy across the target sequence starting at the two primer sites. The amplification procedure is performed by repeating the following cycle 25 to 50 times (see Fig. 99.3). First, the double-stranded target DNA is denatured at high temperature (94 to 96°C). Second, the mixture is cooled, allowing the primers to anneal to their complementary sites on the target single strands. Third, the temperature is adjusted for optimal DNA polymerase activity, initiating synthesis. Since the primers are complementary to the newly synthesized strands as well as the original target, each cycle of denaturation/annealing/synthesis effectively doubles the amount of target sequence present in the reaction, resulting in a 2^n amplification (n = number of cycles). The initial implementation of PCR utilized a polymerase that was unstable at the high temperatures required for denaturation, thus requiring manual addition of polymerase prior to the synthesis step of every cycle. An important technological development was the isolation of DNA polymerase from a thermophilic bacterium, *Thermus aquaticus (Taq)*, which

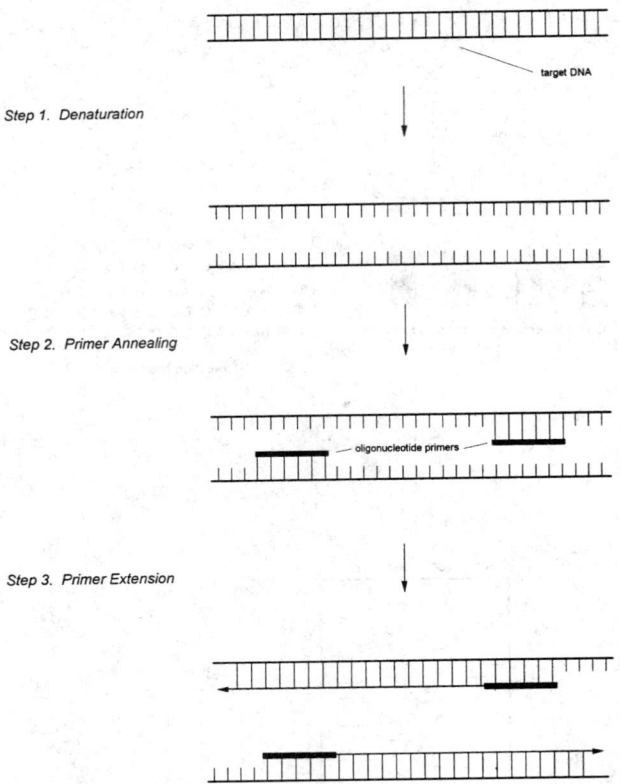

Step 1. Denaturation

Step 2. Primer Annealing

oligonucleotide primers

Step 3. Primer Extension

FIGURE 99.3 The first cycle in the polymerase chain reaction. In step 1, the double-stranded target DNA is thermally denatured to produce single-stranded species. A pair of synthetic primers, flanking the specific region of interest, are annealed to the single strands to form initiation sites for DNA synthesis by polymerase (step 2). Finally, complementary copies of each target single strand are synthesized by polymerase in the presence of dNTPs, thus doubling the amount of target DNA initially present (step 3). Repetition of this cycle effectively doubles the target population, affording one million-fold or greater amplification of the initial target sequence.

can withstand the high denaturation temperatures [6]. Additionally, the high optimal synthesis temperature (70 to 72°C) of *Taq* polymerase improves the specificity of the amplification process by reducing spurious priming from annealing of the primers to nonspecific secondary sites in the target.

While PCR can be performed successfully manually, it is a tedious process, and numerous thermal cycling instruments have become commercially available. Modern thermal cyclers are programmable and capable of processing many samples at once, using either small plastic tubes or microtiter plates, and are characterized by accurate and consistent temperature control at all sample positions, rapid temperature ramping, and minimal temperature over/undershoot. Temperature control is provided by a variety of means (Peltier elements, forced air, water) using metal blocks or water or air baths. Speed, precise temperature control, and high sample throughput are the watchwords of current thermal cycler design.

PCR technology is commonly used to provide sufficient material for cloning from genomic DNA sources, to identify and characterize particular DNA sequences in an unknown mixture, to rapidly produce templates for DNA sequencing from very small amounts of target DNA, and in cycle sequencing, a modification of the enzymatic sequencing procedure that utilizes *Taq* polymerase and thermal cycling to amplify the products of the sequencing reactions.

Chemical Synthesis of Oligodeoxynucleotides.   The widespread use of techniques based on DNA polymerase, such as enzymatic DNA sequencing and the PCR, as well as of numerous other techniques utilizing short, defined-sequence, single-stranded DNAs in genome analysis, is largely due to the ease with which small oligodeoxynucleotides can be obtained. The chemical synthesis of oligonucleotides has become a routine feature of both individual biology laboratories and core facilities. The most widely used chemistry for assembling short (<100 base pair) oligonucleotides is the phosphoramidite approach [7], which has developed over the past 15 years or so. This approach is characterized by rapid, high-yield reactions and stable reagents. Like modern peptide synthesis chemistry, the approach relies on the tethering of the growing DNA chain to a solid support (classically glass or silica beads, more recently cross-linked polystyrene) and is cyclic in nature. At the end of the assembly, the desired oligonucleotide is chemically cleaved from the support, generally in a form that is sufficiently pure for its immediate use in a number of applications. The solid phase provides two significant advantages: It allows for the use of large reagent excesses, driving the reactions to near completion in accord with the laws of mass action while reducing the removal of these excesses following the reactions to a simple matter of thorough washing, and it enables the reactions to be performed in simple, flow-through cartridges, making the entire synthesis procedure easily automatable. Indeed, a number of chemical DNA synthesis instruments ("gene machines") are commercially available, capable of synthesizing one to several oligonucleotides at once. Desired sequences are programmed through a keyboard or touchpad, reagents are installed, and DNA is obtained a few hours later. Improvements in both chemistry and instrument design have been aimed at increasing synthesis throughput (reduced cycle times, increased number of simultaneous sequence assemblies), decreasing scale (most applications in genome analysis require subnanomole quantities of any particular oligonucleotide), and concomitant with these two, reducing cost per oligonucleotide.

99.3 Tools for Genome Analysis

Physical Mapping.   In the analysis of genomes, it is often useful to begin with a less complex mixture than an entire genomic DNA sample. Individual chromosomes can be obtained in high purity using a technology known as *chromosome sorting* [8], a form of flow cytometry. A suspension of chromosomes stained with fluorescent dye is flowed past a laser beam. As a chromosome enters the beam, appropriate optics detect the scattered and emitted light. Past the beam, the stream is acoustically broken into small droplets. The optical signals are used to electronically trigger the collection of droplets containing chromosomes by electrostatically charging these droplets and deflecting them into a collection medium using a strong electric field. Chromosomes can be differentiated by staining the suspension with two different dyes that bind in differing amounts to the various chromosomes and looking at the ratio of the emission intensity of each dye as it passes the laser/detector. Current commercial chromosome sorting instrumentation is relatively slow, requiring several days to collect sufficient material for subsequent analysis.

As mentioned previously, whole genomes or even chromosomes cannot yet be analyzed as intact entities. As such, fractionation of large nucleic acids into smaller fragments is necessary to obtain the physical material on which to perform genetic analysis. Fractionation can be achieved using a variety of techniques: limited or complete digestion by restriction enzymes, sonication, or physical shearing through a small orifice. These fragments are then cloned into an appropriate vector, the choice of which depends on the size range of fragments involved (see Table 99.3). The composite set of clones derived from a large nucleic acid is termed a *library*. In general, it is necessary to produce several libraries in different cloning vectors containing different-sized inserts. This is necessary because the mapping of clones is facilitated by larger inserts, while the sequencing of clones requires shorter inserts.

The library-generating process yields a very large number of clones having an almost random distribution of insert endpoints in the original fragment. It would be very costly to analyze all clones in a library, and unnecessary as well. Instead, a subset of overlapping clones is selected whose inserts span the entire starting fragment. These clones must be arrayed in the linear order in which they are found in the starting fragment; the process for doing this is called *physical mapping*. The conventional method for physically mapping clones uses restriction enzymes to cleave each clone at enzyme-specific sites, separating the products of the digestion by electrophoresis, and comparing the resulting patterns of restriction fragment sizes for different clones to find similarities. Clones exhibiting a number of the same-sized fragments likely possess the same subsequence and thus overlap. Clearly, the longer the inserts contained in the library, the faster a large genetic region can be covered by this process, since fewer clones are required to span the distance. Physical mapping also provides landmarks, the enzyme cleavage sites in the sequence, that can be used to provide reference points for the mapping of genes and other functional sequences. Mapping by restriction enzyme digestion is simple and reliable to perform; however, manual map assembly from the digest data is laborious, and significant effort is currently being expended in the development of robust and accurate map assembly software.

Normal agarose gel electrophoresis can effectively separate DNA fragments less than 10,000 base pairs and fragments between 10,000 and 50,000 base pairs less effectively under special conditions. However, the development of very large insert cloning vectors, such as the yeast artificial chromosome [9], necessitated the separation of fragments significantly larger than 10,000 base pairs to allow for use in physical mapping. In order to address this issue, a technology called *pulsed-field gel electrophoresis* (PFGE) was developed. Unlike conventional electrophoresis, in which the electric field remains essentially constant, homogeneous, and unidirectional during a separation, PFGE utilizes an electric field that periodically changes its orientation. The principle of PFGE is thought to be as follows: When DNA molecules are placed in an electric field, the molecules elongate in the direction of the field and then begin to migrate through the gel pores. When the field is removed, the molecules relax to a more random coiled state and stop moving. Reapplication of the field in another orientation causes the DNA to change its conformation in order to align in that direction prior to migration. The time required for this conformational change to occur has been found to be very dependent on the size of the molecules, with larger molecules reorienting more slowly than small ones. Thus longer DNAs move more slowly under the influence of the constantly switching electric field than shorter ones, and size-based separation occurs. PFGE separations of molecules as large as 10 million base pairs have been demonstrated. Numerous instruments for PFGE have been constructed, differing largely in the strategy employed to provide electric field switching [10].

Physical maps based on restriction sites are of limited long-term utility, since they require the provision of physical material from the specific library from which the map was derived in order to be utilized experimentally. A more robust landmarking approach based on the PCR has been developed recently [11], termed *sequence-tagged site* (STS) *content mapping*. An STS is a short, unique sequence in a genome that can be amplified by the PCR. Clones in a library are screened for the presence of a particular STS using PCR; if the STS is indeed unique in the genome, then clones possessing that STS are reliably expected to overlap. Physical mapping is thus reduced to choosing and synthesizing pairs of PCR primers that define unique sequences in the genome. Additionally, since STSs are defined by pairs of primer sequences, they can be stored in a database and are thus universally accessible.

DNA Sequencing.   Early in the development of tools for large-scale DNA analysis, it was recognized that one of the most costly and time-consuming processes was the accumulation of DNA sequence information. Two factors, the use of radioisotopic labels and the manual reading and recording of DNA sequence films, made it impossible to consider genome-scale (10^6 to 10^9 base pairs) sequence analysis using the conventional techniques. To address this, several groups embarked on the development of automated DNA sequencing instruments [12–14]. Today, automated DNA sequencing is one of the most highly advanced of the technologies for genome analysis, largely due to the extensive effort expended in instrument design, biochemical optimization, and software development.

Key to the development of these instruments was the demonstration that fluorescence could be employed in the place of autoradiography for detection of fragments in DNA sequencing gels and that the use of fluorescent labels enabled the acquisition of DNA sequence data in an automated fashion in real time. Two approaches have been demonstrated: the "single-color, four-lane" approach and the "four-color, single-lane" approach. The former simply replaces the radioisotopic label used in conventional enzymatic sequencing with a fluorescent label, and the sequence is determined by the order of fluorescent bands in the four lanes of the gel. The latter utilizes a different-colored label for each of the four sequencing reactions (thus A might be "blue," C, "green," G, "yellow," and T, "red"). The four base-specific reactions are performed separately and upon completion are combined and electrophoresed in a single lane of the gel, and the DNA sequence is determined from the temporal pattern of fluorescent colors passing the detector. For a fixed number of gel lanes (current commercial automated DNA sequencers have 24 to 36), the four-color approach provides greater sample throughput than the single-color approach. Instruments employing the four-color technology are more widely used for genome analysis at present, and as such, this strategy will be discussed more fully.

In order to utilize fluorescence as a detection strategy for DNA sequencing, a chemistry had to be developed for the specific incorporation of fluorophores into the nested set of fragments produced in the enzymatic sequencing reactions. The flexibility of chemical DNA synthesis provided a solution to this problem. A chemistry was developed for the incorporation of an aliphatic primary amine in the last cycle of primer synthesis (i.e., at the 5' terminus) using standard DNA synthesis protocols [15,16]. This amine was then conjugated with any of several of readily available amine-reactive fluorochromes that had been developed previously for the labeling of proteins to produce the desired labeled sequencing primers. The purified dye-primer was demonstrated to perform well in DNA sequencing, exhibiting both efficient extension by the polymerase and the necessary single-base resolution in the electrophoretic separation [12]. A set of four spectrally discriminable, amine-reactive fluorophores has been developed [16] for DNA sequencing.

While dye-primers are relatively easy to obtain by this method, they are costly to prepare in small quantities and require sophisticated chromatographic instrumentation to obtain products pure enough for sequencing use. Thus they are generally prepared in large amounts and employed as vector-specific "universal" primers, as in situations in which a very large number of inserts cloned in a given vector need to be sequenced [17]. For occasions where small amounts of sample-specific primers are needed, as in the sequencing of products from the PCR, a simpler and more economical alternative is the use of dideoxynucleotides covalently coupled to fluorescent dyes (so-called dye-terminators), since these reagents allow the use of conventional unlabeled primers [18].

Special instrumentation (Fig. 99.4) has been developed for the fluorescence-based detection of nucleic acids in DNA sequencing gels. An argon ion laser is used to excite the fluorescent labels in order to provide sufficient excitation energy at the appropriate wavelength for high-sensitivity detection. The laser beam is mechanically scanned across the width of the gel near its bottom in order to interrogate all lanes. As the labeled DNA fragments undergoing electrophoresis move through the laser beam, their emission is collected by focusing optics onto a photomultiplier tube located on the scanning stage. Between the photomultiplier tube and the gel is a rotating four-color filter wheel. The emitted light from the gel is collected through each of the four filters in the wheel in turn, generating a continuous four-point spectrum of the detected radiation. The color of the emission of the passing bands is determined from the characteristic four-point spectrum of each fluorophore, and the identified color is then translated into DNA sequence using the associated dye/base pairings. Sequence acquisition and data analysis are handled completely by computer; the system is sufficiently sophisticated that the operator can load the samples on the gel, activate the electrophoresis and the data acquisition, and return the next day for the analyzed data. The current commercial implementation of this technology produces about 450 to 500 bases per lane of analyzed DNA sequence information at an error rate of a few percent in a 12- to 14-hour period.

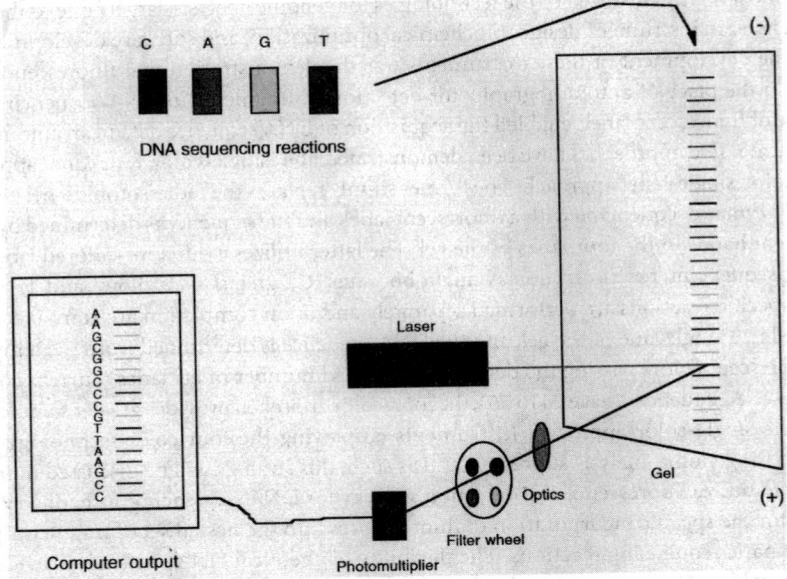

FIGURE 99.4 Schematic illustration of automated fluorescence-based DNA sequencing using the "four-color, single-lane" approach. The products of each of the four
enzymatic sequencing reactions are "color-coded" with a different fluorescent dye, either
through the use of dye-labeled primers or dye-terminators. The four reaction mixtures
are then combined and the mixture separated by gel electrophoresis. The beam of an
argon ion laser is mechanically scanned across the width of the gel near its bottom to
excite the labeled fragments to fluorescence. The emitted light is collected through a
four-color filter wheel onto a photomultiplier tube. The color of each fluorescing band
is determined automatically by a computer from the characteristic four-point spectrum
of each dye, and the order of colors passing the detector is subsequently translated into
DNA sequence information.

The rate of data production of current DNA sequencers is still too low to provide true genome-
scale analytical capabilities, although projects in the few hundred kilobase pair range have been
accomplished. Improvements such as the use of gel-filled capillaries [19] or ultrathin slab gels
(thicknesses on the order of 50 to 100 μm as opposed to the conventional 200 to 400 μm) [20,21]
are currently being explored. The improved heat dissipation in these thin-gel systems allows for the
use of increased electric field strengths during electrophoresis, with a concomitant reduction in run
time of fivefold or so.

The greatly increased throughput of the automated instruments over manual techniques has
resulted in the generation of a new bottleneck in the DNA sequencing process that will only be exacerbated by higher-throughput systems: the preparation of sufficient sequencing reaction products
for analysis. This encompasses two preparative processes, the preparation of sequencing templates
and the performance of sequencing reactions. Automation of the latter process has been approached
initially through the development of programmable pipetting robots that operate in the 96-well
microtiter plate format commonly used for immunoassays, since a 96-well plate will accommodate
sequencing reactions for 24 templates. *Sequencing robots* of this sort have become important tools
for large-scale sequencing projects. Template preparation has proven more difficult to automate. No
reliable system for selecting clones, infecting and culturing bacteria, and isolating DNA has been
produced, although several attempts are in progress. It is clear that unlike in the case of the sequencing robots, where instrumentation has mimicked manual manipulations with programmable

mechanics, successful automation of template preparation will require a rethinking of current techniques with an eye toward process automation. Furthermore, in order to obtain true genome-scale automation, the entire sequencing procedure from template preparation through data acquisition will need to be reengineered to minimize, if not eliminate, operator intervention using the principles of systems integration, process management, and feedback control.

Genetic Mapping. Simply stated, genetic mapping is concerned with identifying the location of genes on chromosomes. Classically, this is accomplished using a combination of mendelian and molecular genetics called *linkage analysis,* a complete description of which is too complex to be fully described here (but see Watson et al. [1]). However, an interesting approach to physically locating clones (and the genes contained within them) on chromosomes is afforded by a technique termed *fluorescence in situ hybridization* (FISH) [22]. Fluorescently labeled DNA probes derived from cosmid clones can be hybridized to chromosome spreads, and the location of the probe-chromosome hybrid can be observed using fluorescence microscopy. Not only can clones be mapped to particular chromosomes in this way, but positions and distances relative to chromosomal landmarks (such as cytogenetic bands, telomere, or centromere) can be estimated to as little as 50,000 base pairs in some cases, although 1 million base pairs or larger is more usual. The technique is particularly useful when two or more probes of different colors are used to order sequences relative to one another.

Computation. Computation plays a central role in genome analysis at a variety of levels, and significant effort has been expended on the development of software and hardware tools for biologic applications. A large effort has been expended in the development of software that will rapidly assemble a large contiguous DNA sequence from the many smaller sequences obtained from automated instruments. This assembly process is computationally demanding, and only recently have good software tools for this purpose become readily available. Automated sequencers produce 400 to 500 base pairs of sequence per template per run. However, in order to completely determine the linear sequence of a 50,000-base-pair cosmid insert (which can be conceptually represented as a linear array of 100 adjacent 500-base-pair templates), it is necessary to assemble sequence from some 300 to 1000 clones to obtain the redundancy of data needed for a high-accuracy finished sequence, depending on the degree to which the clones can be preselected for sequencing based on a previously determined physical map. Currently, the tools for acquiring and assembling sequence information are significantly better than those for physical mapping; as such, most large-scale projects employ strategies that emphasize sequencing at the expense of mapping [23]. Improved tools for acquiring and assembling mapping data are under development, however, and it remains to be seen what effect they will have on the speed and cost of obtaining finished sequence on a genome scale relative to the current situation.

Many software tools have been developed in the context of the local needs of large-scale projects. These include software for instrument control (data acquisition and signal processing), laboratory information-management systems, and local data-handling schemes. The development of process approaches to the automation of genome analysis will necessitate the continued development of tools of these types.

The final outcome of the analysis of any genome will be a tremendous amount of sequence information that must be accessible to researchers interested in the biology of the organism from which it was derived. Frequently, the finished genomic sequence will be the aggregate result of the efforts of many laboratories. National and international information resources (databases) are currently being established worldwide to address the issues of collecting, storing, correlating, annotating, standardizing, and distributing this information. Significant effort is also being expended to develop tools for the rapid analysis of genome sequence data that will enable biologists to find new genes and other functional genetic regions, compare very large DNA sequences for similarity, and study the role of genetic variation in biology. Eventually, as the robust tools for predicting protein tertiary structure and function from primary amino acid sequence data are developed, genome analysis will extend to the protein domain through the translation of new DNA sequences into their functional protein products.

99.4 Conclusions

Genome analysis is a large-scale endeavor whose goal is the complete understanding of the basic blueprint of life. The scale of even the smallest genomes of biologic interest is too large to be effectively analyzed using the traditional tools of molecular biology and genetics. Over the past 10 years, a suite of biochemical techniques and bioanalytical instrumentation has been developed that has allowed biologists to begin to probe large genetic regions, although true genome-scale technology is still in its infancy. It is anticipated that the next 10 years will see developments in the technology for physical mapping, DNA sequencing, and genetic mapping that will allow for a 10- to 100-fold increase in our ability to analyze genomes, with a concomitant decrease in cost, through the application of process-based principles and assembly-line approaches. The successful realization of a true genome analysis capability will require the close collaborative efforts of individuals from numerous disciplines in both science and engineering.

Acknowledgments

I would like to thank Dr. Leroy Hood, Dr. Maynard Olson, Dr. Barbara Trask, Dr. Tim Hunkapiller, Dr. Deborah Nickerson, and Dr. Lee Rowen for the useful information, both written and verbal, that they provided me during the preparation of this chapter.

References

1. Watson JD, Gilman M, Witkowski J, Zoller M (eds). 1992. Recombinant DNA, 2d ed. New York, Scientific American Books, WH Freeman.
2. Lewin B. 1987. Genes III, 3d ed. New York, Wiley.
3. Olson MV. 1993. The human genome project. Proc Natl Acad Sci USA 90:4338.
4. Sanger F, Nicklen S, Coulson AR. 1977. DNA sequencing with chain-terminating inhibitors. Proc Natl Acad Sci USA 74:5463.
5. Saiki RK, Scharf SJ, Faloona F, et al. 1985. Enzymatic amplification of betaglobin sequences and restriction site analysis for diagnosis of sickle cell anemia. Science 230:1350.
6. Saiki RK, Gelfand DH, Stoffel S, et al. 1988. Primer-directed enzymatic amplification of DNA with a thermostable DNA polymerase. Science 239:487.
7. Gait MJ (ed). 1984. Oligonucleotide Synthesis: A Practical Approach. Oxford, England, IRL Press.
8. Engh Gvd. 1993. New applications of flow cytometry. Curr Opin Biotechnol 4:63.
9. Burke DT, Carle GF, Olson MV. 1987. Cloning of large segments of exogenous DNA into yeast by means of artificial chromosome vectors. Science 236:806.
10. Lai E, Birren BW, Clark SM, Hood L. 1989. Pulsed field gel electrophoresis. Biotechniques 7:34.
11. Olson M, Hood L, Cantor C, Botstein D. 1989. A common language for physical mapping of the human genome. Science 245:1434.
12. Smith LM, Sanders JZ, Kaiser RJ, et al. 1986. Fluorescence detection in automated DNA sequence analysis. Nature 321:674.
13. Prober JM, Trainor GL, Dam RJ, et al. 1987. A system for rapid DNA sequencing with fluorescent chain terminating dideoxynucleotides. Science 238:336.
14. Ansorge W, Sproat B, Stegemann J, et al. 1987. Automated DNA sequencing: Ultrasensitive detection of fluorescent bands during electrophoresis. Nucleic Acids Res 15:4593.

15. Smith LM, Fung S, Hunkapiller MW, et al. 1985. The synthesis of oligonucleotides containing an aliphtic amino group at the 5′ terminus: Synthesis of fluorescent DNA primers for use in DNA sequencing. Nucleic Acids Res 15:2399.

16. Connell C, Fung S, Heiner C, et al. 1987. Bio techniques 5:342.

17. Kaiser R, Hunkapiller T, Heiner C, Hood L. 1993. Specific primer-directed DNA sequence analysis using automated fluorescence detection and labeled primers. Methods Enzymol 218:122.

18. Lee LG, Connell CR, Woo SL, et al. 1992. DNA sequencing with dye-labeled terminators and T7 DNA polymerase: Effect of dyes and dNTPs on incorporation of dye-terminators and probability analysis of termination fragments. Nucleic Acids Res 20:2471.

19. Mathies RA, Huang XC. 1992. Capillary array electrophoresis: an approach to high-speed, high-throughput DNA sequencing. Nature 359:167.

20. Brumley RL Jr, Smith LM. 1991. Rapid DNA sequencing by horizontal ultrathin gel electrophoresis. Nucleic Acids Res 19:4121.

21. Stegemann J, Schwager C, Erfle H, et al. 1991. High speed on-line DNA sequencing on ultrathin slab gels. Nucleic Acids Res 19:675.

22. Trask BJ. 1991. Gene mapping by in situ hybridization. Curr Opin Genet Dev 1:82.

23. Hunkapiller T, Kaiser RJ, Koop BF, Hood L. 1991. Large-scale and automated DNA sequencing. Science 254:59.

100

Vaccine Production

John G. Aunins
Merck Research Laboratories

Ann L. Lee
Merck Research Laboratories

David B. Volkin
Merck Research Laboratories

Vaccines are biologic preparations that elicit immune system responses that protect an animal against pathogenic organisms. The primary component of the vaccine is an antigen, which can be a weakened (attenuated) version of an infectious pathogen or a purified molecule derived from the pathogen. Upon oral administration or injection of a vaccine, the immune system generates humoral (antibody) and cellular (cytotoxic, or killer T cell) responses that destroy the antigen or antigen-infected cells. When properly administered, the immune response to a vaccine has a long-term memory component, which protects the host against future infections. Vaccines often contain adjuvants to enhance immune response, as well as formulation agents to preserve the antigen during storage or upon administration, to provide proper delivery of antigen, and to minimize side reactions.

Table 100.1 presents a simple classification scheme for vaccines according to the type of organism and antigen. *Live, attenuated whole-organism vaccines* have been favored for simplicity of manufacture and for the strong immune response generated when the organism creates a subclinical infection before being overwhelmed. These are useful when the organism can be reliably attenuated in pathogenicity (while maintaining immunogenicity) or when the organism is difficult to cultivate ex vivo in large quantities and hence large amounts of antigen cannot be prepared. Conversely, *subunit antigen vaccines* are used when it is easy to generate large amounts of the antigen or when the whole organism is not reliably attenuated. Since there is no replication in vivo, subunit vaccines rely on administering relatively large amounts of antigen mass and are almost always adjuvanted to try to minimize the antigen needed. Subunit preparations have steadily gained favor, since biologic, engineering, and analytical improvements make them easily manufactured and characterized to a consistent standard. *Passive vaccines* are antibody preparations from human blood serum. These substitute for the patient's humoral response for immune-suppressed persons, for postexposure prophylaxis of disease, and for high infection risk situations where immediate protection is required, such as for travelers or medical personnel. Even more so than subunit vaccines, large amounts of antibodies are required. These vaccines do not provide long-term immune memory.

0-8493-8346-3/95/$0.00+$.50
© 1995 by CRC Press, Inc.

TABLE 100.1   Examples of Vaccines Against Human Pathogens, and Their Classification

Type of Organism	Live, Attenuated Cells/Particles	Killed, Inactivated Cells/Particles	Subcellular/ Particle Vaccines	Passive Immunization
Virus	Measles, mumps, rubella, polio, yellow fever, varicella*, rotavirus*	Polio, hepatitis B, rabies, yellow fever, Japanese encephalitis, influenza, hepatitis A*	*Virus-like particles* Hepatitis B, HIV gp120-vaccinia* *Characterized single/ combined antigens* Influenza HA + NA, herpes simplex gD*	*Immune serum globulin* Rabies, hepatitis B, cytomegalovirus *Monoclonal antibody* Anti-HIV gp120*
Bacterium	Tuberculosis (BCG), typhoid	Pertussis, cholera, plague bacillus	*Toxoids* Tetanus, diphtheria *Characterized single/ combined antigens* Pertussis PT + FHA + LPF + PSA + 69kD, *Pneumococcus* poly-saccharides (23), *Meningococcus* polysaccharides *Polysaccharide-protein conjugates* *Haemophilus* b, *Pneumococcus**	*Immune serum globulin* Tetanus, Nonspecific Ig

*Denotes vaccines in development.

The organism and the nature of the antigen combine to determine the technologies of manufacture for the vaccine. Vaccine production generally involves growing the organism or its antigenic parts (cultivation), treating it to purify and/or detoxify the organism and antigen (downstream processing), and in many cases further combining the antigen with adjuvants to increase its antigenicity and improve storage stability (formulation). These three aspects of production will be discussed, in addition to future trends in vaccine technology. This chapter does not include vaccines for parasitic disease [see Barbet, 1989], such as malaria, since such vaccines are not yet commercially available.

100.1 Antigen Cultivation

Microbial Cultivation

Bacterial Growth

As far as cultivation is concerned, the fundamental principles of cell growth are identical for the various types of bacterial vaccines. Detailed aspects of bacterial growth and metabolism can be found in Ingraham et al. [1983]. In the simplest whole-cell vaccines, obtaining cell mass is the objective of cultivation. Growth is an autocatalytic process where the cell duplicates by fission; growth is described by the differential equation

$$\frac{dX}{dt} = \mu X_v \qquad (100.1)$$

where X is the total mass concentration of cells, X_v is the mass concentration of living, or viable, cells, and μ is the specific growth rate in units of cells per cell time. In this equation, the growth rate of the cell is a function of the cells' physical and chemical environment:

$$\mu = f(\text{temperature, pH, dissolved oxygen, } C_1, C_2, C_3, \ldots, C_n) \qquad (100.2)$$

All bacteria have a narrow range of temperatures permissive to growth; for human pathogens, the optimal temperature is usually 37°C; however, for attenuated strains, the optimal temperature may be purposefully lowered by mutation. At the end of culture, heat in excess of 50°C is sometimes used to kill pathogenic bacteria. Dissolved oxygen concentration is usually critical, since the organism will either require it or be inhibited by it. Cultivation of *Clostridium tetani*, for example, is conducted completely anaerobically.

In Eq. (100.2), C_i is the concentration of nutrient i presented to the cells. Nutrient conditions profoundly affect cell growth rate and the ultimate cell mass concentration achievable. At a minimum, the cells must be presented with a carbon source, a nitrogen source, and various elements in trace quantities. The carbon source, usually a carbohydrate such as glucose, is used for energy metabolism and as a precursor for various anabolites, small chemicals used to build the cell. The nitrogen source, which can be ammonia, or a complex amino acid mix such as a protein hydrolysate, also can be used to produce energy but is mainly present as a precursor for amino acid anabolites for protein production. The elements K, Mg, Ca, Fe, Mn, Mo, Co, Cu, and Zn are cofactors required in trace quantities for enzymatic reactions in the cell. Inorganic phosphorus and sulfur are incorporated into proteins, polysaccharides, and polynucleotides.

Historically, bacterial vaccines have been grown in a batchwise fashion on complex and ill-defined nutrient mixtures, which usually include animal and/or vegetable protein digests. An example is *Bordetella pertussis* cultivation on Wheeler and Cohen medium [World Health Organization, 1977c], which contains corn starch, an acid digest of bovine milk casein, and a dialyzed lysate of brewer's yeast cells. The starch serves as the carbon source. The casein digest provides amino acids as a nitrogen source. The yeast extract provides amino acids and vitamins, as well as some trace elements, nucleotides, and carbohydrates. Such complex media components make it difficult to predict the fermentation performance, since their atomic and molecular compositions are not easily analyzed, and since they may contain hidden inhibitors of cell growth or antigen production. More recently, defined media have been used to better reproduce cell growth and antigen yield. In a defined medium, pure sugars, amino acids, vitamins, and other anabolites are used. When a single nutrient concentration limits cell growth, the growth rate can be described by Monod kinetics

$$\mu = \frac{\mu_{max} C_i}{C_i + K} \tag{100.3}$$

Here, μ_{max} is the maximum specific growth rate, and K is the Monod constant for growth on the nutrient, an empirically determined number. It is seen from this equation that at high nutrient concentrations, the cell grows at maximum rate, as if the substrate were not limiting. At low concentration as the nutrient becomes limiting, the growth rate drops to zero, and the culture ends.

Antigen Production

Cultivation of microbes for subunit vaccines is similar to that of whole-cell vaccines, but here one is concerned with the production of an antigenic protein, polysaccharide, or antigen-encoding polynucleotide as opposed to the whole cell; thus cell growth is not necessarily the main objective. The goal is to maintain the proper environmental and nutritional factors for production of the desired product. Similarly to Eqs. (100.1) and (100.2) above, one can describe antigen production by

$$\frac{dP}{dt} = q_p X_v - k_d P \text{ where } q_p \text{ and} \tag{100.4}$$

$$k_d = f(\text{temperature pH, dissolved O}_2, C_1, \ldots, C_n)$$

where P is the product antigen concentration, q_p is the cell-specific productivity, and k_d is a degradation rate constant. For example, the production of pertussis toxin occurs best at slightly alkaline pH, about 8.0 [Jagicza et al., 1986]. *Corynebacterium diphtheriae* toxin production is affected by the concentration of iron [Relyveld, 1980]. Nutrient effects on degradation can be found for hepatitis B virus vaccine, whose production is actually a microbial cultivation. Here, recombinant DNA inserted into *Saccharomyces cerevisiae* yeast cells produces the hepatitis B surface antigen protein (HBsAg), which spontaneously assembles into virus-like particles (about 100 protein monomers per particle) within the cell. Prolonged starvation of the yeast cells can cause production of cellular proteases that degrade the antigen protein to provide nutrition. Consequently, maximum production of antigen is accomplished by not allowing the yeast culture to attain maximum cell mass but by harvesting the culture prior to nutrient depletion.

Cultivation Technology

Cultivation vessels for bacterial vaccines were initially bottles containing stagnant liquid or agar-gelled medium, where the bacteria grew at the liquid or agar surface. These typically resulted in low concentrations of the bacteria due to the limited penetration depth of diffusion-supplied oxygen and/or due to the limited diffusibility of nutrients through the stagnant liquid or agar. Despite the low mass, growth of the bacteria at the gas-liquid interface can result in cell differentiation (pellicle formation) and improved production of antigen (increased q_p). For the past several decades, however, glass and stainless steel fermentors have been used to increase production scale and productivity. Fermentors mix a liquid culture medium via an impeller, thus achieving quicker growth and higher cell mass concentrations than would be achievable by diffusive supply of nutrients. For aerobic microbe cultivations, fermenters oxygenate the culture by bubbling air directly into the medium. This increases the oxygen supply rate dramatically over diffusion supply. Due to the low solubility of oxygen in water, oxygen must be continuously supplied to avoid limitation of this nutrient.

Virus Cultivation

Virus cultivation is more complex than bacterial cultivation because viruses are, by themselves, nonreplicating. Virus must be grown on a host cell substrate, which can be animal tissue, embryo, or ex vivo cells; the host substrate determines the cultivation technology. In the United States, only Japanese encephalitis virus vaccine is still produced from infected mature animals. Worldwide, many vaccines are produced in chicken embryos, an inexpensive substrate. The remainder of vaccines are produced from ex vivo cultivated animal cells. Some virus-like particle vaccines are made by recombinant DNA techniques in either microbial or animal cells, e.g., hepatitis B virus vaccine, which is made in yeast as mentioned above, or in Chinese hamster ovary cells. An interesting synopsis of the development of rabies vaccine technology from Pasteur's use of animal tissues to modern use of ex vivo cells can be found in Sureau [1987].

In Vivo Virus Cultivation

Virus cultivation in vivo is straightforward, since relatively little control can be exercised on the host tissue. Virus is simply inoculated into the organ, and after incubation, the infected organ is harvested. Influenza virus is the prototypical in vivo vaccine; the virus is inoculated into the allantoic sac of 9- to 11-day-old fertilized chicken eggs. The eggs are incubated at about 33°C for 2 to 3 days, candled for viability and lack of contamination from the inoculation, and then the allantoic fluid is harvested. The process of inoculating, incubating, candling, and harvesting hundreds of thousands of eggs can be highly automated [Metzgar and Newhart, 1977].

Ex Vivo Virus Cultivation

Use of ex vivo cell substrates is the most recent technique in vaccine cultivation. In the case of measles and mumps vaccines, the cell substrate is chicken embryo cells that have been generated by trypsin enzyme treatment that dissociates the embryonic cells. Similarly, some rabies vaccines use cells derived from fetal rhesus monkey kidneys. Since the 1960s, cell lines have been generated that can be characterized, banked, and cryopreserved. Cryopreserved cells have been adopted to ensure reproducibility and freedom from contaminating viruses and microorganisms and to bypass the ethical problem of extensive use of animal tissues. Examples of commonly used cell lines are WI-38 and MRC-5, both human embryonic lung cells, and Vero, an African green monkey kidney cell line.

Ex vivo cells must be cultivated in a bioreactor, in liquid nutrient medium, with aeration. The principles of cell growth are the same as for bacterial cells described above, with some important additions. First, ex vivo animal cells cannot synthesize the range of metabolites and hormones necessary for survival and growth and must be provided with these compounds. Second, virus production is usually fatal to the host cells. Cells also become more fragile during infection, a process that is to an extent decoupled from cell growth. Virus growth and degradation and cell death kinetics can influence the choice of process or bioreactor. Third, all ex vivo cells used for human vaccine manufacture require a surface to adhere to in order to grow and function properly. Finally, animal cells lack the cross-linked, rigid polysaccharide cell wall that gives physical protection to microorganisms. These last three factors combine to necessitate specialized bioreactors.

Cell Growth.   Supplying cells with nutrients and growth factors is accomplished by growing the cells in a complex yet defined medium, which is supplemented with 2% to 10% (v/v) animal blood serum. The complex medium will typically contain glucose and L-glutamine as energy sources, some or all of the 20 predominant L-amino acids, vitamins, nucleotides, salts, and trace elements. For polio virus, productivity is a function of energy source availability [Eagle and Habel, 1956] and may depend on other nutrients. For polio and other viruses, the presence of the divalent cations Ca^{2+} and Mg^{2+} promotes viral attachment and entry into cells and stabilizes the virus particles. Serum provides growth-promoting hormones, lipids and cholesterol, surface attachment-promoting proteins such as fibronectin, and a host of other functions. The serum used is usually of fetal bovine origin, since this source is particularly rich in growth-promoting hormones and contains low levels of antibodies that could neutralize virus. After cell growth, and before infection, the medium is usually changed to serum-free or low-serum medium. This is done both to avoid virus neutralization and to reduce the bovine protein impurities in the harvested virus. These proteins are immunogenic and can be difficult to purify away, especially for live-virus vaccines.

Virus Production Kinetics.   An intriguing aspect of ex vivo virus cultivation is that each process depends on whether the virus remains cell-associated, is secreted, or lyses the host cells and whether the virus is stable in culture. With few exceptions, a cell produces a finite amount of virus before dying, as opposed to producing the virus persistently. This is because the host cell protein and DNA/RNA synthesis organelles are usually commandeered by virus synthesis, and the host cannot produce its own proteins, DNA, or RNA. The goal then becomes to maximize cell concentration, as outlined above for bacterial vaccines, while maintaining the cells in a competent state to produce virus. Since infection is transient and often rapid, cell-specific virus productivity is not constant, and productivity is usually correlated with the cell state at inoculation. Specific productivity can be a function of the cell growth rate, since this determines the available protein and nucleic acid synthetic capacity. Although virus production can be nutrient-limited, good nutrition is usually ensured by the medium exchange at inoculation mentioned above. For viruses that infect cells slowly, nutrition is supplied by exchanging the medium several times, batchwise or by continuous perfusion.

For many viruses, the degradation term in Eq. (100.4) can be significant. This can be due to inherent thermal instability of the virus, oxidation, or proteases released from lysed cells. For an unstable virus, obtaining a synchronized infection can be key to maximizing titers. Here, the multiplicity of infection (MOI), the number of virus inoculated per cell, is an important parameter. An MOI greater than unity results in most cells being infected at once, giving the maximum net virus production rate.

Cultivation Technology.   The fragility of animal cells during infection and the surface attachment requirement create a requirement for special reactors [Prokop and Rosenberg, 1989]. To an extent, reactor choice and productivity are determined by the reactor surface area. Small, simple, and uncontrolled vessels, such as a flat-sided T-flask or Roux bottle, made of polystyrene or glass, can be used for small-scale culture. With these flasks the medium is stagnant, so fragile infected cells are not exposed to fluid motion forces during culture. Like bacterial cultures, productivity can be limited due to the slow diffusion of nutrients and oxygen. To obtain larger surface areas, roller bottles or Cell Factories are used, but like egg embryo culture, robotic automation is required to substantially increase the scale of production. Even larger culture scales ($\geq$50 liters) are accommodated in glass or stainless steel bioreactors, which are actively supplied with oxygen and pH controlled. The growth surface is typically supplied as a fixed bed of plates, spheres, or fibers or, alternately, as a dispersion of about 200-μm spherical particles known as *microcarriers* [Reuveny, 1990]. Microcarrier bioreactors are used for polio and rabies production [Montagnon et al., 1984]. The stirred-tank microcarrier reactors are similar to bacterial fermentors but are operated at much lower stirring speeds and gas sparging rates so as to minimize damage to the fragile cells. Packed-bed reactors are used for hepatitis A virus vaccine production [Aboud et al., 1994]. These types of reactors can give superior performance for highly lytic viruses because they subject the cells to much lower fluid mechanical forces. Design considerations for animal cell reactors may be found in Aunins and Henzler [1993].

100.2 Downstream Processing

Following cultivation, the antigen is recovered, isolated in crude form, further purified, and/or inactivated to give the unformulated product; these steps are referred to collectively as the *downstream process*. The complexity of a downstream process varies greatly depending on whether the antigen is the whole organism, a semipurified subunit, or a highly purified subunit. Although the sequence and combination of steps are unique for each vaccine, there is a general method to purification. The first steps reduce the volume of working material and provide crude separation from contaminants. Later steps typically resolve molecules more powerfully but are limited to relatively clean feed streams. Some manufacturing steps are classic small laboratory techniques, because many vaccine antigens are quite potent, requiring only micrograms of material; historically, manufacturing scale-up has not been a critical issue.

Purification Principles

Recovery

Recovery steps achieve concentration and liberation of the antigen. The first recovery step consists of separating the cells and/or virus from the fermentation broth or culture medium. The objective is to capture and concentrate the cells for cell-associated antigens or to clarify the medium of particulates for extracellular antigens. In the first case, the particle separation simultaneously concentrates the antigen. The two methods used are centrifugation and filtration. Batch volume and feed solids content determine whether centrifugation or filtration is appropriate; guidelines for centrifugation are given by Datar and Rosen [1993] and Atkinson and Mavituna [1991]. Filtration is used increasingly as filter materials science improves to give filters that do not bind antigen. Filtration can either be dead-end or cross-flow. Dead-end filters are usually fibrous depth filters and are used when the particulate load is low and the antigen is extracellular. In cross-flow filtration, the particles are retained by a microporous ($\geq$0.1 μm) or ultrafiltration ($\leq$0.1 μm) membrane. The feed stream is circulated tangential to the membrane surface at high velocity to keep the cells and other particulates from forming a filter cake on the membrane [Hanisch, 1986].

If the desired antigen is subcellular and cell-associated, the next recovery step is likely to be cell lysis. This can be accomplished by high-pressure valve homogenization, bead mills, or chemical lysis with detergent or chaotropic agents, to name only a few techniques. The homogenate or cell lysate may subsequently be clarified, again using either centrifugation or membrane filtration.

Isolation

Isolation is conducted to achieve crude fractionation from contaminants that are unlike the antigen; precipitation and extraction are often used here. These techniques rely on large differences in charge or solubility between antigen and contaminants. Prior to isolation, the recovered process stream may be treated enzymatically with nucleases, proteases, or lipases to remove DNA/RNA, protein, and lipids, the major macromolecular contaminants. Nonionic detergents such as Tween and Triton can serve a similar function to separate components, provided they do not denature the antigen. Subsequent purification steps must be designed to remove the enzyme(s) or detergent, however.

Ammonium sulfate salt precipitation is a classic method used to concentrate and partially purify various proteins, e.g., diphtheria and tetanus toxins. Alcohol precipitation is effective for separating polysaccharides from proteins. Cohn cold alcohol precipitation is a classic technique used to fractionate blood serum for antibody isolation. Both techniques concentrate antigen for further treatment.

Liquid-liquid extraction, either aqueous-organic or aqueous-aqueous, is another isolation technique suitable for vaccine purification. In a two-phase aqueous polymer system, the separation is based on the selective partitioning of the product from an aqueous liquid phase containing, e.g., polyethylene glycol (PEG), into a second, immiscible aqueous liquid phase that contains another polymer, e.g., dextran, or containing a salt [see Kelley and Hatton, 1992].

Final Purification

Further purification of the vaccine product is to remove contaminants that have properties closely resembling the antigen. These sophisticated techniques resolve molecules with small differences in charge, hydrophobicity, density, or size.

Density-gradient centrifugation, although not readily scalable, is a popular technique for final purification of viruses [Polson, 1993]. Either rate-zonal centrifugation, where the separation is based on differences in sedimentation rate, or isopycnic equilibrium centrifugation, where the separation is based solely on density differences, is used. Further details on these techniques can be found in Dobrota and Hinton [1992].

Finally, different types of chromatography are employed to manufacture highly pure vaccines; principles can be found in Janson and Ryden [1989]. Ion-exchange chromatography (IEC) is based on differences in overall charge and distribution of charge on the components. Hydrophobic-interaction chromatography (HIC) exploits differences in hydrophobicity. Affinity chromatography is based on specific stereochemical interactions common only to the antigen and the ligand. Size-exclusion chromatography (SEC) separates on the basis of size and shape. Often, multiple chromatographic steps are used, since the separation mechanisms are complementary. IEC and HIC can sometimes be used early in the process to gain substantial purification; SEC is typically used as a final polishing step. This technique, along with ultrafiltration, may be used to exchange buffers for formulation at the end of purification.

Inactivation

For nonattenuated whole organisms or for toxin antigens, the preparation must be inactivated to eliminate pathogenicity. This is accomplished by heat pasteurization, by cross-linking using formaldehyde or glutaraldehyde, or by alkylating using agents such as β-propiolactone. The agent is chosen for effectiveness without destruction of antigenicity. For whole organisms, the inactivation abolishes infectivity. For antigens such as the diphtheria and tetanus toxins, formaldehyde treatment removes the toxicity of the antigen itself as well as killing the organism. These detoxified antigens are known as *toxoids*.

The placement of inactivation in the process depends largely on safety issues. For pathogen cultures, inactivation traditionally has been immediately after cultivation to eliminate danger to manufacturing personnel. For inactivation with cross-linking agents, however, the step may be placed later in the process in order to minimize interference by contaminants that either foil inactivation of the organism or cause carryover of antigen-contaminant cross-linked entities that could cause safety problems, i.e., side-reactions in patients.

Purification Examples

Examples of purification processes are presented below, illustrating how the individual techniques are combined to create purification processes.

Bacterial Vaccines

Salmonella typhi Ty21, a vaccine for typhoid fever, and BCG (bacille Calmette-Guérin, a strain of *Mycobacterium bovis*) vaccine against *Myobacterium tuberculosis,* are the only vaccines licensed for human use based on live, attenuated bacteria. Downstream processing consists of collecting the cells by continuous-flow centrifugation or using cross-flow membrane filtration. For *M. bovis* that are grown in a liquid submerged fermenter culture, Tween 20 is added to keep the cells from aggregating, and the cultures are collected as above. Tween 20, however, has been found to decrease virulence. In contrast, if the BCG is grown in stagnant bottles as a surface pellicle, the downstream process consists of collecting the pellicle sheet, which is a moist cake, and then homogenizing the cake using a ball mill. Milling time is critical, since prolonged milling kills the cells and too little milling leaves clumps of bacteria in suspension.

Most current whooping cough vaccines are inactivated whole *B. pertussis.* The cells are harvested by centrifugation and then resuspended in buffer, which is the supernate in some cases. This is done because some of the filamentous hemagglutinin (FHA) and pertussis toxin (PT) antigens are released into the supernate. The cell concentrate is inactivated by mild heat and stored with thimerosal and/or formaldehyde. The inactivation process serves the dual purpose of killing the cells and inactivating the toxins.

C. diphtheria vaccine is typical of a crude protein toxoid vaccine. Here the 58 kDa toxin is the antigen, and it is converted to a toxoid with formaldehyde and crudely purified. The cells are first separated from the toxin by centrifugation. Sometimes the pathogen culture is inactivated with formaldehyde before centrifugation. The supernate is treated with formaldehyde to 0.75%, and it is stored for 4 to 6 weeks at 37°C to allow complete detoxification [Pappenheimer, 1984]. The toxoid is then concentrated by ultrafiltration and fractionated from contaminants by ammonium sulfate precipitation. During detoxification of crude material, reactions with formaldehyde lead to a variety of products. The toxin is internally cross-linked and also cross-linked to other toxins, beef peptones from the medium, and other medium proteins. Because detoxification creates a population of molecules containing antigen, the purity of this product is only about 60% to 70%.

Due to the cross-linking of impurities, improved processes have been developed to purify toxins before formaldehyde treatment. Purification by ammonium sulfate fractionation, followed by ion-exchange and/or size-exclusion chromatography, is capable of yielding diphtheria or tetanus toxins with purities ranging from 85% to 95%. The purified toxin is then treated with formaldehyde or glutaraldehyde [Relyveld and Ben-Efraim, 1983] to form the toxoid. Likewise, whole-cell pertussis vaccine is being replaced by subunit vaccines. Here, the pertussis toxin (PT) and the filamentous hemagglutinin (FHA) are purified from the supernate. These two antigens are isolated by ammonium sulfate precipitation, followed by sucrose density-gradient centrifugation to remove impurities such as endotoxin. The FHA and PT are then detoxified with formaldehyde [Sato et al., 1984].

Bacterial components other than proteins also have been developed for use as subunit vaccines. One class of bacterial vaccines is based on capsular polysaccharides. Polysaccharides from *Meningococcus, Pneumococcus,* and *Haemophilus influenzae* type b are used for vaccines against these organisms. After separating the cells, the polysaccharides are typically purified using a series of alcohol precipitations. As described below, these polysaccharides are not antigenic in infants. As a consequence, the polysaccharides are chemically cross-linked, or conjugated, to a highly purified antigenic protein carrier. After conjugation, there are purification steps to remove unreacted polysaccharide, protein, and small-molecular-weight cross-linking reagents. Several manufacturers have introduced pediatric conjugate vaccines against *H. influenzae* type b (Hib-conjugate).

Viral Vaccines

Live viral vaccines have limited downstream processes. For secreted viruses such as measles, mumps, and rubella, cell debris is simply removed by filtration and the supernate frozen. In many cases it is necessary to process quickly and at refrigerated temperatures, since live virus can be unstable [Cryz and Gluck, 1990].

For cell-associated virus such as herpesviruses, e.g., varicella zoster (chickenpox virus), the cells are washed with a physiologic saline buffer to remove medium contaminants and are harvested. This can be done by placing them into a stabilizer formulation (see below) and then mechanically scraping the cells from the growth surface. Alternately, the cells can be harvested from the growth surface chemically or enzymatically. For the latter, the cells are centrifuged and resuspended in stabilizer medium. The virus is then liberated by disrupting the cells, usually by sonication, and the virus-containing supernate is clarified by dead-end filtration and frozen.

Early inactivated influenza virus vaccines contained relatively crude virus. The allantoic fluid was harvested, followed by formaldehyde inactivation of the whole virus, and adsorption to aluminum phosphate (see below), which may have provided some purification as well. The early vaccines, however, were associated with reactogenicity. For some current processes, the virus is purified by rate-zonal centrifugation, which effectively eliminates the contaminants from the allantoic fluid. The virus is then inactivated with formaldehyde or β-propiolactone, which preserves the antigenicity of both the hemagglutinin (HA) and neuraminidase (NA) antigens. Undesirable side reactions have been even further reduced with the introduction of *split vaccines,* where the virus particle is disrupted by an organic solvent or detergent and then inactivated. By further purifying the split vaccine using a method such as zonal centrifugation to separate the other virion components from the HA and NA antigens, an even more highly purified HA + NA vaccine is available. These antigens are considered to elicit protective antibodies against influenza [Tyrrell, 1976].

Recently, an extensive purification process was developed for hepatitis A vaccine, yielding a >90% pure product [Aboud et al., 1994]. The intracellular virus is released from the cells by Triton detergent lysis, followed by nuclease enzyme treatment for removal of RNA and DNA. The virus is concentrated and detergent removed by ion-exchange chromatography. PEG precipitation and chloroform solvent extraction purify away most of the cellular proteins, and final purification and polishing are achieved by ion-exchange and size-exclusion chromatography. The virus particle is then inactivated with formaldehyde. In this case, inactivation comes last for two reasons. First, the virus is attenuated, so there is no risk to process personnel. Second, placing the inactivation after the size-exclusion step ensures that there are no contaminants or virus aggregates that may cause incomplete inactivation.

The first hepatitis B virus vaccines were derived from human plasma [Hilleman, 1993]. The virus is a 22-nm-diameter particle, much larger than most biologic molecules. Isolation was achieved by ammonium sulfate or PEG precipitation, followed by rate zonal centrifugation and isopycnic banding to take advantage of the large particle size. The preparation was then treated with pepsin protease, urea, and formaldehyde or heat. The latter steps ensure inactivation of possible contaminant viruses from the blood serum. More recently, recombinant DNA–derived hepatitis B vaccines are expressed as an intracellular noninfectious particle in yeast and use a completely different purification process. Here, the emphasis is to remove the yeast host contaminants, particularly high levels of nucleic acids and polysaccharides. Details on the various manufacturing processes have been described by Sitrin et al. [1993].

Antibody Preparations

Antibody preparation starts from the plasma pool prepared by removing the cellular components of blood. Cold ethanol is added in increments to precipitate fractions of the blood proteins, and the precipitate containing IgG antibodies is collected. This is further redissolved and purified by ultrafiltration, which also exchanges the buffer to the stabilizer formulation. Sometimes ion-exchange chromatography is used for further purification. Although the plasma is screened for viral contamination prior to pooling, all three purification techniques remove some virus.

100.3 Formulation and Delivery

Successful vaccination requires both the development of a stable dosage form for in vitro storage and the proper delivery and presentation of the antigen to elicit a vigorous immune response in vivo. This is done by adjuvanting the vaccine and/or by formulating the adjuvanted antigen. An adjuvant is defined as an agent that enhances the immune response against an antigen. A formulation con-tains an antigen in a delivery vehicle designed to preserve the (adjuvenated) antigen and to deliver it to a specific target organ or over a desired time period. Despite adjuvanting and formulation efforts, most current vaccines require multiple doses to create immune memory.

Live Organisms

Live viruses and bacteria die relatively quickly in liquid solution (without an optimal environment) and are therefore usually stored in the frozen state. Preserving the infectivity of frozen live-organism vaccines is typically accomplished by lyophilization or freeze-drying. The freeze-drying process involves freezing the organism in the presence of stabilizers, followed by sublimation of both bulk water (primary drying) and more tightly bound water (secondary drying). The dehydra-tion process reduces the conformational flexibility of the macromolecules, providing protec-tion against thermal denaturation. Stabilizers also provide conformational stability and protect against other inactivating mechanisms such as amino acid deamidation, oxidation, and light-catalyzed reaction.

Final water content of the freeze-dried product is the most important parameter for the drying process. Although low water content enhances storage stability, overdrying inactivates biologic molecules, since removal of tightly bound water disrupts antigen conformation. Influenza virus suspensions have been shown to more stable at 1.7% (w/w) water than either 0.4% to 1% or 2.1% to 3.2% [Greiff and Rightsel, 1968]. Other lyophilization parameters that must be optimized per-tain to heat and mass transfer, including (1) the rate of freezing and sublimation, (2) vial location in the freeze-drier, and (3) the type of vial and stopper used to cap the vial. Rates of freezing and drying affect phase transitions and compositions, changing the viable organism yield on lyophiliza-tion and the degradation rate of the remaining viable organisms on storage.

Stabilizers are identified by trial-and-error screening and by examining the mechanisms of inactivation. They can be classified into four categories depending on their purpose: specific, non-specific, competitive, and pharmaceutical. *Specific stabilizers* are ligands that naturally bind biologic macromolecules. For example, enzyme antigens are often stabilized by their natural substrates or closely related compounds. Antigen stabilizers for the liquid state also stabilize during freezing. *Nonspecific stabilizers* such as sugars, amino acids, and neutral salts stabilize proteins and virus struc-tures via a variety of mechanisms. Sugars and polyols act as bound water substitutes, preserving conformational integrity without possessing the chemical reactivity of water. Buffer salts preserve optimal pH. *Competitive inhibitors* outcompete the organism or antigen for inactivating conditions, such as gas-liquid interfaces, oxygen, or trace-metal ions [Volkin and Klibanov, 1989]. Finally, *pharmaceutical stabilizers* may be added to preserve pharmaceutical elegance, i.e., to prevent collapse of the lyophilized powder during the drying cycle, which creates difficult redissolution. Large-molecular-weight polymers such as carbohydrates (dextrans or starch) or proteins such as albumin or gelatin are used for this purpose. For example, a buffered sorbitol-gelatin medium has been used successfully to preserve the infectivity of measles virus vaccine during lyophilized storage for several years at 2 to 8°C [Hilleman, 1989]. An example of live bacterium formulation to preserve activity on administration is typhoid fever vaccine, administered orally. *S. typhi* bacteria are lyophilized to a powder to preserve viability on the shelf, and the powder is encapsulated in gelatin to preserve bacterial viability when passing through the low-pH stomach. The gelatin capsule dissolves in the intestine to deliver the live bacteria.

Oral polio vaccine is an exception to the general rule of lyophilization, since polio virus is inherently quite stable relative to other viruses. It is formulated as a frozen liquid and can be used for a limited time after thawing [Melnick, 1984]. In the presence of specific stabilizers such as $MgCl_2$, extended 4°C stability can be obtained.

Subunit Antigens

Inactivated and/or purified viral and bacterial antigens inherently offer enhanced stability because whole-organism infectivity does not need to be preserved. However, these antigens are not as immunogenic as live organisms and thus are administered with an adjuvant. They are usually formulated as an aqueous liquid suspension or solution, although they can be lyophilized under the same principles as above. The major adjuvant recognized as safe for human use is alum. *Alum* is a general term referring to various hydrated aluminum salts; a discussion of the different alums can be found in Shirodkar et al. [1990]. Vaccines can be formulated with alum adjuvants by two distinct methods: adsorption to preformed aluminum precipitates or precipitation of aluminum salts in the presence of the antigen, thus adsorbing and entrapping the antigen. Alum's adjuvant activity is classically believed to be a "depot" effect, slowly delivering antigen over time in vivo. In addition, alum particles are believed to be phagocytized by macrophages.

Alum properties vary depending on the salt used. Adjuvants labeled aluminum hydroxide are actually aluminum oxyhydroxide, AlO(OH). This material is crystalline, has a fibrous morphology, and has a positive surface charge at neutral pH. In contrast, aluminum phosphate adjuvants are networks of platelike particles of amorphous aluminum hydroxyphosphate and possess a negative surface charge at neutral pH. Finally, alum coprecipitate vaccines are prepared by mixing an acidic alum solution of $KAl(SO_4)_2 \cdot 12H_2O$ with an antigen solution buffered at neutral pH, sometimes actively pH-controlled with base. At neutral pH, the aluminum forms a precipitate, entrapping and adsorbing the antigen. The composition and physical properties of this alum vary with processing conditions and the buffer anions. In general, an amorphous aluminum hydroxy(buffer anion)sulfate material is formed.

Process parameters must be optimized for each antigen to ensure proper adsorption and storage stability. First, since antigen adsorption isotherms are a function of the antigen's isoelectric point and the type of alum used [Seeber et al., 1991], the proper alum and adsorption pH must be chosen. Second, the buffer ions in solution can affect the physical properties of alum over time, resulting in changes in solution pH and antigen adsorption. Finally, heat sterilization of alum solutions and precipitates prior to antigen adsorption can alter their properties. Alum is used to adjuvant virtually all the existing inactivated or formaldehyde-treated vaccines, as well as purified subunit vaccines such as HBsAg and Hib-conjugate vaccines. The exception is for some bacterial polysaccharide vaccines and for new vaccines under development (see below).

An interesting vaccine development challenge was encountered with Hib-conjugate pediatric vaccines, which consist of purified capsular polysaccharides. Although purified, unadjuvanted polysaccharide is used in adults, it is not sufficiently immunogenic in children under age 2, the population at greatest risk [Ellis, 1992; Howard, 1992]. Chemical conjugation, or cross-linking, of the PRP polysaccharide to an antigenic protein adjuvant elicits T-helper cell activation, resulting in higher antibody production. Variations in conjugation chemistry and protein carriers have been developed; example proteins are the diphtheria toxoid (CRM 197), tetanus toxoid, and the outer membrane protein complex of *N. meningitidis* [Ellis, 1992; Howard, 1992]. The conjugated polysaccharide is sometimes adsorbed to alum for further adjuvant action.

100.4 Future Trends

The reader will have noted that many production aspects for existing vaccines are quite archaic. This is so because most vaccines were developed before the biotechnology revolution, which is creating a generation of highly purified and better-characterized subunit vaccines. As such, for older vaccines "the process defines the product," and process improvements cannot readily be incorporated into these poorly characterized vaccines without extensive new clinical trials. With improved scientific capabilities, we can understand the effects of process changes on the physicochemical properties of new vaccines and on their behavior in vivo.

Vaccine Cultivation

Future cultivation methods will resemble existing methods of microbial and virus culture. Ill-defined medium components and cells will be replaced to enhance reproducibility in production. For bacterial and ex vivo cultivated virus, analytical advances will make monitoring the environment and nutritional status of the culture more ubiquitous. However, the major changes will be in novel product types—single-molecule subunit antigens, virus-like particles, monoclonal antibodies, and gene-therapy vaccines, each of which will incorporate novel processes.

Newer subunit vaccine antigens will be cultivated via recombinant DNA in microbial or animal cells. Several virus-like particle vaccines are under development using recombinant baculovirus (nuclear polyhedrosis virus) to infect insect cells (spodoptera frugipeeda or trichoplusia ni). Like the hepatitis B vaccine, the viral antigens spontaneously assemble into a noninfectious capsid within the cell. Although the metabolic pathways of insect cells differ from vertebrates, cultivation principles are similar. Insect cells do not require surface attachment and are grown much like bacteria. However, they also lack a cell wall and are larger and hence more fragile than vertebrate cells.

Passive antibody vaccines have been prepared up to now from human blood serum. Consequently, there has been no need for cultivation methods beyond vaccination and conventional harvest of antibody-containing blood from donors. Due to safety concerns over using human blood, passive vaccines will likely be monoclonal antibodies or cocktails thereof prepared in vitro by the cultivation of hybridoma or myeloma cell lines. This approach is under investigation for anti-HIV-1 antibodies [Emini et al., 1992]. Cultivation of these cell lines involves the same principles of animal cell cultivation as described above, with the exception that hybridomas can be less fastidious in nutritional requirements, and they do not require surface attachment for growth. These features will allow for defined serum-free media and simpler cultivation vessels and procedures.

For the gene-therapy approach, the patient actually produces the antigen. A DNA polynucleotide encoding protein antigen(s) is injected intramuscularly into the patient. The muscle absorbs the DNA and produces the antigen, thereby eliciting an immune response [Ulmer et al., 1993]. For cultivation, production of the DNA plasmid is the objective, which can be done efficiently by bacteria such as *Escherichia coli*. Such vaccines are not sufficiently far along in development to generalize the factors that influence their production; however, it is expected that producer cells and process conditions that favor high cell mass, DNA replication, and DNA stability will be important. A potential beauty of this vaccination approach is that for cultivation, purification, and formulation, many vaccines can conceivably be made by identical processes, since the plasmids are inactive within the bacterium and possess roughly the same nucleotide composition.

Downstream Processing

Future vaccines will be more highly purified in order to minimize side effects, and future improvements will be to assist this goal. The use of chemically defined culture media will impact favorably on downstream processing by providing a cleaner feedstock. Advances in filtration membranes and in chromatographic support binding capacity and throughput will improve ease of purification.

Affinity purification methods that rely on specific "lock and key" interactions between a chromatographic support and the antigen will see greater use as well. Techniques amenable to larger scales will be more important to meet increased market demands and to reduce manufacturing costs. HPLC and other analytical techniques will provide greater process monitoring and control throughout purification.

As seen during the evolution of diphtheria and tetanus toxoid vaccines, the trend will be to purify toxins prior to inactivation to reduce their cross-linking with other impurities. New inactivating agents such as hydrogen peroxide and ethyl dimethylaminopropyl carbodiimide have been investigated for pertussis toxin, which do not have problems of cross-linking or reversion of the toxoid to toxin status.

Molecular biology is likely to have an even greater impact on purification. Molecular cloning of proteins allows the addition of amino acid sequences that can facilitate purification, e.g., polyhistidine or polyalanine tails for metal ion, or ion-exchange chromatography. Recent efforts also have employed genetic manipulation to inactivate toxins, eliminating the need for the chemical treatment step.

Vaccine Adjuvants and Formulation

Many new subunit antigens lack the inherent immunogenicity found in the natural organism, thereby creating the need for better adjuvants. Concomitantly, the practical problem of enhancing worldwide immunization coverage has stimulated development of single-shot vaccine formulations in which booster doses are unnecessary. Thus future vaccine delivery systems will aim at reducing the number of doses via controlled antigen release and will increase vaccine efficacy by improving the mechanism of antigen presentation (i.e., controlled release of antigen over time or directing of antigen to specific antigen-presenting cells). Major efforts are also being made to combine antigens into single-shot vaccines to improve immunization rates for infants, who currently receive up to 15 injections during the first 2 years of life. Coadministration of antigens presents unique challenges to formulation as well.

Recent advances in the understanding of in vivo antigen presentation to the immune system has generated considerable interest in developing novel vaccine adjuvants. The efficacy of an adjuvant is judged by its ability to stimulate specific antibody production and killer cell proliferation. Developments in biology now allow analysis of activity by the particular immune cells that are responsible for these processes. Examples of adjuvants currently under development include saponin detergents, muramyl dipeptides, and lipopolysaccharides (endotoxin), including lipid A derivatives. As well, cytokine growth factors that stimulate immune cells directly are under investigation.

Emulsion and liposome delivery vehicles are also being examined to enhance the presentation of antigen and adjuvant to the immune system [Edelman, 1992; Allison and Byars, 1992]. Controlled-release delivery systems are also being developed that encapsulate antigen inside a polymer-based solid microsphere. The size of the particles typically varies between 1 and 300 µm depending on the manufacturing process. Microspheres are prepared by first dissolving the biodegradable polymer in an organic solvent. The adjuvanted antigen, in aqueous solution or lyophilized powder form, is then emulsified into the solvent-polymer continuous phase. Microspheres are then formed by either solvent evaporation, phase separation, or spray-drying, resulting in entrapment of antigen [Morris et al., 1994]. The most frequently employed biodegradable controlled-released delivery systems use FDA-approved poly(lactide-co-glycolide) copolymers (PLGA), which hydrolyze in vivo to nontoxic lactic and glycolic acid monomers. Degradation rate can be optimized by varying the microsphere size and the monomer ratio. Antigen stability during encapsulation and during in vivo release from the microspheres remains a challenge. Other challenges to manufacturing include encapsulation process reproducibility, minimizing antigen exposure to denaturing organic solvents, and ensuring sterility. Methods are being developed to address these issues, including the addition of stabilizers for processing purposes only. It should be noted that microsphere technology may permit vaccines to be targeted to specific cells; they can potentially be delivered orally or nasally to produce a mucosal immune response.

Other potential delivery technologies include liposomes and alginate polysaccharide and poly-(dicarboxylatophenoxy)phosphazene polymers. The latter two form aqueous hydrogels in the presence of divalent cations [Khan et al., 1994]. Antigens can thus be entrapped under aqueous conditions with minimal processing by simply mixing antigen and soluble aqueous polymer and dripping the mixture into a solution of $CaCl_2$. The particles erode by Ca^{2+} loss, mechanical and chemical degradation, and macrophage attack. For alginate polymers, monomer composition also determines the polymer's immunogenicity, and thus the material can serve as both adjuvant and release vehicle.

For combination vaccines, storage and administration compatibility of the different antigens must be demonstrated. Live-organism vaccines are probably not compatible with purified antigens, since the former usually require lyophilization and the latter are liquid formulas. Within a class of vaccines, formulation is challenging. Whereas it is relatively straightforward to adjuvant and formulate a single antigen, combining antigens is more difficult because each has its own unique alum species, pH, buffer ion, and preservative optimum. Nevertheless, several combination vaccines have reached the market, and others are undergoing clinical trials.

100.5 Conclusions

Although vaccinology and manufacturing methods have come a considerable distance over the past 40 years, much more development will occur. There will be challenges for biotechnologists to arrive at safer, more effective vaccines for an ever-increasing number of antigen targets. If government interference and legal liability questions do not hamper innovation, vaccines will remain one of the most cost-effective and logical biomedical technologies of the next century, as disease is prevented rather than treated.

Challenges are also posed in bringing existing vaccines to technologically undeveloped nations, where they are needed most. This problem is almost exclusively dominated by the cost of vaccine manufacture and the reliability of distribution. Hence it is fertile ground for engineering improvements in vaccine production.

Defining Terms

Adjuvant: A chemical or biologic substance that enhances immune response against an antigen. Used here as a verb, the action of combining an antigen and an adjuvant.

Antigen: A macromolecule or assembly of macromolecules from a pathogenic organism that the immune system recognizes as foreign.

Attenuation: The process of mutating an organism so that it no longer causes disease.

Immunogen: A molecule or assembly of molecules with the ability to invoke an immune system response.

Pathogen: A disease-causing organism, either a virus, mycobacterium, or bacterium.

References

Aboud RA, Aunins JG, Buckland BC, et al. 1994. Hepatitis A Virus Vaccine. International patent application, publication number WO 94/03589, Feb. 17, 1994.

Allison AC, Byars NE. 1992. Immunological adjuvants and their mode of action. In RW Ellis (ed), Vaccines: New Approaches to Immunological Problems, p 431. Reading, Mass, Butterworth-Heinemann.

Atkinson B, Mavituna F. 1991. Biochemical Engineering and Biotechnology Handbook, 2d ed. London, Macmillan.

Aunins JG, Henzler H-J. 1993. Aeration in cell culture bioreactors. In H-J Rehm et al (eds), Biotechnology, 2d ed., vol 3, p 219. Weinheim, Germany, VCH Verlag.

Bachmayer H. 1976. Split and subunit vaccines. In P. Selby (ed), Influenza Virus, Vaccines, and Strategy, p 149. New York, Academic Press.

Barbet AF. 1989. Vaccines for parasitic infections. Adv Vet Sci Comp Med 33:345.

Cryz SJ, Reinhard G. 1990. Large-scale production of attenuated bacterial and viral vaccines. In GC Woodrow, MM Levine (eds), New Generation Vaccines, p 921. New York, Marcel Dekker.

Datar RV, Rosen C-G. 1993. Cell and cell debris removal: Centrifugation and crossflow filtration. In H-J Rehm et al (eds), Biotechnology, 2d ed, vol 3, p 469. Weinheim, Germany, VCH Verlag.

Dobrota M, Hinton R. 1992. Conditions for density gradient separations. In D Rickwood (ed), Preparative Centrifugation: A Practical Approach, p 77. New York, Oxford U Press.

Eagle H, Habel K. 1956. The nutritional requirements for the propagation of poliomyelitis virus by the HeLa cell. J Exp Med 104:271.

Edelman R. 1992. An update on vaccine adjuvants in clinical trial. AIDS Res Hum Retrovir 8(8):1409.

Ellis RW. 1992. Vaccine development: Progression from target antigen to product. In JE Ciardi et al (eds), Genetically Engineered Vaccines, p 263. New York, Plenum Press.

Emini EA, Schleif WA, Nunberg JH, et al. 1992. Prevention of HIV-1 infection in chimpanzees by gp120 V3 domain-specific monoclonal antibodies. Nature 355:728.

Greiff D, Rightsel WA. 1968. Stability of suspensions of influenza virus dried to different contents of residual moisture by sublimation in vacuo. Appl Microbiol 16(6):835.

Hanisch W. 1986. Cell harvesting. In WC McGregor (ed), Membrane Separations in Biotechnology, p 66. New York, Marcel Dekker.

Hewlett EL, Cherry JD. 1990. New and improved vaccines against pertussis. In GC Woodrow, MM Levine (eds), New Generation Vaccines, p 231. New York, Marcel Dekker.

Hilleman MR. 1989. Improving the heat stability of vaccines: Problems, needs and approaches. Rev Infect Dis 11(suppl 3):S613.

Hilleman MR. 1993. Plasma-derived hepatitus B vaccine: A breakthrough in preventive medicine. In R Ellis (ed), Hepatitis B Vaccines in Clinical Practice, p 17. New York, Marcel Dekker.

Howard AJ. 1992. Haemophilus influenzae type-b vaccines. Br J Hosp Med 48(1):44.

Ingraham JL, Maaløe O, Neidhardt FC. 1983. Growth of the Bacterial Cell. Sunderland, Mass, Sinauer.

Jagicza A, Balla P, Lendvai N, et al. 1986. Additional information for the continuous cultivation of Bordetella pertussis for the vaccine production in bioreactor. Ann Immunol Hung 26:89.

Janson J-C, Ryden L (eds). 1989. Protein Purification Principles, High Resolution Methods, and Applications. Weinheim, Germany, VCH Verlag.

Kelley BD, Hatton TA. 1993. Protein purification by liquid-liquid extraction. In H-J Rehm et al (eds), Biotechnology, 2d ed, vol 3, p 594. Weinheim, Germany, VCH Verlag.

Khan MZI, Opdebeeck JP, Tucker IG. 1994. Immunopotentiation and delivery systems for antigens for single-step immunization: Recent trends and progress. Pharmacol Res 11(1):2.

Melnick JL. 1984. Live attenuated oral poliovirus vaccine. Rev Infect Dis 6(suppl 2):S323.

Metzgar DP, Newhart RH. 1977. U.S. patent no. 4,057,626, Nov. 78, 1977.

Montagnon B, Vincent-Falquet JC, Fanget B. 1984. Thousand litre scale microcarrier culture of vero cells for killed polio virus vaccine: Promising results. Dev Biol Stand 55:37.

Morris W, Steinhoff MC, Russell PK. 1994. Potential of polymer microencapsulation technology for vaccine innovation. Vaccine 12(1):5.

Pappenheimer AM. 1984. Diphtheria. In R Germanier (ed), Bacterial Vaccines, p 1. New York, Academic Press.

Polson A. 1993. Virus Separation and Preparation. New York, Marcel Dekker.

Prokop A, Rosenberg MZ. 1989. Bioreactor for mammalian cell culture. In A Fiechter (ed), Advances in Biochemical Engineering, vol 39: Vertebrate Cell Culture II and Enzyme Technology, p 29. Berlin, Springer-Verlag.

Rappuoli R. 1990. New and improved vaccines against diphtheria and tetanus. In GC Woodrow, MM Levine (eds), New Generation Vaccines, p 251. New York, Marcel Dekker.

Relyveld EH. 1980. Current developments in production and testing of tetanus and diphtheria vaccines. In A Mizrahi et al (eds), Progress in Clinical and Biological Research, vol 47: New Developments with Human and Veterinary Vaccines, p 51. New York, Alan R Liss.

Relyveld EH, Ben-Efraim S. 1983. Preparation of vaccines by the action of glutaraldehyde on toxins, bacteria, viruses, allergens and cells. In SP Colowic, NO Kaplan (eds), Methods in Enzymology, vol 93, p 24. New York, Academic Press.

Reuveny S. 1990. Microcarrier culture systems. In AS Lubiniecki (ed), In Large-Scale Mammalian Cell Culture Technology, p 271. New York, Marcel Dekker.

Sato Y, Kimura M, Fukumi H. 1984. Development of a pertussis component vaccine in Japan. Lancet 1(8369):122.

Seeber SJ, White JL, Hem SL. 1991. Predicting the adsorption of proteins by aluminum-containing adjuvants. Vaccine 9:201.

Shirodkar S, Hutchinson RL, Perry DL, et al. 1990. Aluminum compounds used as adjuvants in vaccines. Pharmacol Res 7(12):1282.

Sitrin RD, Wampler DE, Ellis R. 1993. Survey of licensed hepatitis B vaccines and their product processes. In R Ellis (ed), Hepatitus B Vaccines in Clinical Practice, p 83. New York, Marcel Dekker.

Sureau P. 1987. Rabies vaccine production in animal cell cultures. In A Fiechter (ed), Advances in Biochemical Engineering and Biotechnology, vol 34, p 111. Berlin, Springer-Verlag.

Tyrrell DAJ. 1976. Inactivated whole virus vaccine. In P Selby (ed), Influenza, Virus, Vaccines and Strategy, p 137. New York, Academic Press.

Ulmer JB, Donnelly JJ, Parker SE, et al. 1993. Heterologous protection against influenza by injection of DNA encoding a viral protein. Science 259(5102):1745.

Volkin DB, Klibanov AM. 1989. Minimizing protein inactivation. In TE Creighton (ed), Protein Function: A Practical Approach, pp 1–12. Oxford, IRL Press.

Further Information

A detailed description of all the aspects of traditional bacterial vaccine manufacture may be found in the World Health Organization technical report series for the production of whole-cell pertussis, diphtheria, and tetanus toxoid vaccines:

World Health Organization. 1997a. BLG/UNDP/77.1 Rev. 1. Manual for the Production and Control of Vaccines: Diphtheria Toxoid.

World Health Organization. 1997b. BLG/UNDP/77.2 Rev. 1. Manual for the Production and Control of Vaccines: Tetanus Toxoid.

World Health Organization. 1997c. BLG/UNDP/77.3 Rev. 1. Manual for the Production and Control of Vaccines: Pertussis Vaccine.

A description of all the aspects of cell culture and viral vaccine manufacture may be found in Spier RE, Griffiths JB. 1985. Animal Cell Biotechnology, vols 1 to 3. London, Academic Press.

For a review of virology and virus characteristics, the reader is referred to Fields BN, Knipe DM (eds). 1990. Virology, 2d ed, vols 1 and 2. New York, Raven Press.

101

Gene Therapy

Joseph M. Le Doux
Rutgers University

Jeffrey R. Morgan
Rutgers University, Massachusetts General Hospital, Harvard University Medical School, and the Shriners Burns Institute

Martin L. Yarmush
Rutgers University, Massachusetts General Hospital, Harvard University Medical School, and the Shriners Burns Institute

Gene therapy is a revolutionary approach to the treatment of disease. In its broadest sense, *gene therapy* is the introduction of nucleic acids into cells for a therapeutic effect. Generally, the nucleic acid is double-stranded DNA that encodes a therapeutic protein. However, it also can be antisense RNA or DNA that binds to and inhibits the expression of complementary sequences in the afflicted cell. In either case, the ultimate goal is to commandeer cellular machinery to execute genetic instructions that result in some desired effect such as producing an enzyme that is missing due to a defective gene.

The first clinically applicable systems for efficiently delivering genes into mammalian cells were developed in the early 1980s. They were constructed from genetically engineered retroviruses which, as part of their lifecycles, stably integrate their genomes into their host cell's genetic material. Using recombinant DNA technology perfected in the mid-1970s, investigators harnessed this viral machinery to introduce therapeutic genes into eukaryotic cells. Since that time, an explosion of research has led to improved recombinant retroviruses as well as alternative methods for introducing genes into cells.

The potential applications of gene therapy are vast (Table 101.1). There are over 4000 known human genetic diseases, and virtually every human disease is profoundly influenced by genetic factors [Anderson, 1992]. Gene therapy could someday become a vital element in the treatment of hundreds of diseases, some of which today have no viable treatment. Gene therapy has already been used to treat patients with ADA (adenosine deaminase) deficiency, a genetic defect that causes severe combined immune deficiency (SCID) and death at an early age [Anderson, 1992]. In this first therapeutic human gene therapy protocol, a young child's lymphocytes were isolated and transduced (insertion of a foreign gene into the genome of a cell) by recombinant retroviruses encoding a functional ADA gene. These transduced cells were expanded in culture and then reinfused back to the patient. This procedure resulted in improved amounts of cellular ADA and response to certain immunologic tests for the first time. These protocols were conducted after an exhaustive peer-review process that laid the groundwork for future gene therapy protocols.

TABLE 101.1   Target Diseases for Gene Therapy

Target Disease	Target Tissues	Corrective Gene	Gene Delivery Systems Used
Inherited			
ADA deficiency	Hematopoietic cells	ADA	RV, RM
Alpha-1 antitrypsin deficiency	Fibroblasts	Alpha-1 antitrypsin	RV
	Hepatocytes		RV
	Lung epithelia cells		AV
	Peritoneal mesothelial cells		AV
Alzheimer's Disease	Nervous system	Nerve growth factor	RV, AV, HSV
Cystic fibrosis	Lung epithelial cells	CFTR	AV, AAV, RM, L
Diabetes	Fibroblasts	Human insulin	RV
	Hepatocytes		L
Duchenne muscular dystrophy	Muscle cells	Dystrophin	AV, DI
Familial hypercholesterolemia	Hepatocytes	LDL receptor	RV, AV, RM
Gaucher disease	Hematopoietic cells	Glucocerebrosidase	RV
	Fibroblasts		RV
Growth hormone deficiency	Endothelial cells	Human growth hormone	RV
	Fibroblasts		TR
	Keratinocytes		RV
	Muscle cells		RV
Hemoglobinopathies	Hematopoietic cells	α or β-globin	RV, AAV
Hemophilia	Fibroblasts	Factor VIII, IX	RV, DI, L
	Keratinocytes		RV
	Hepatocytes		RV, AV, RM, L
	Muscle cells		RV
Leukocyte adhesion deficiency	Hematopoietic cells	CD-18	RV
Parkinson's disease	Nervous system	Tyrosine hydroxylase	RV, AV, HSV
Phenylketonuria	Hepatocytes	Phenylalanine hydroxylase	RV
Purine nucleoside phosphorylase deficiency	Fibroblasts	Purine nucleoside phosphorylase	RV
Urea cycle disorders	Hepatocytes	Ornithine transcarbamylase or arginosuccinate synthetase	AV
Acquired			
Cancer	Acute lymphoblastic leukemia	p53	RV
	Brain tumors	HSV thymidine kinase	RV
	Carcinoma	γ-interferon	TR
	Melanoma	Tumor necrosis factor	RV
	Retinoblastoma	Retinoblastoma gene	RV
Infectious diseases	HIV	Dominant negative Rev	RV
		TAR decoy	RV
		RRE decoy	TR
		Diptheria toxin A	RV
		(Used reporter gene)	DI
Cardiomyopathy	Muscle cells		DI
Emphysema	Lung epithelial cells	Alpha-1 antitrypsin	AV
Local thrombosis	Endothelial cells	Anti-clotting factors	RV
Vaccines	Muscle cells	Various	DI

AAV = recombinant adeno-associated viruses
AV = recombinant adenoviruses
DI = direct injection
HSV = recombinant herpes simplex virus
L = lipofection
RM = receptor mediated
RV = recombinant retroviruses
TR = transfection

Successful treatment of other genetic diseases such as cystic fibrosis, familial hypercholesterolemia, and hemophilia B is likely to be achieved in the future [Levine and Friedmann, 1993; Roemer and Friedmann, 1992]. Other viable targets for gene therapy include more prevalent disorders that show a complex genetic dependence (i.e., cancer and heart disease) as well as infectious diseases [i.e., human immunodeficiency virus (HIV) and human T-cell leukemia virus (HTLV)] [Anderson, 1992].

101.1 Background

Most current gene therapy protocols conduct gene transfer ex vivo [Mulligan, 1993]. Target cells or tissue are removed from the patient, grown in culture, transduced (typically with recombinant retroviruses), and then reinfused or retransplanted into the patient [Ledley, 1993]. Ex vivo gene therapy is limited to those tissues which can be removed, cultured in vitro, and returned to the patient. It cannot be applied to many important target tissues and organs such as the lungs, brain, and heart. An alternative approach is to transduce target tissues in vivo. Unfortunately, it is difficult to achieve long-term gene expression in vivo, and often, nontargeted cells are transduced [Mulligan, 1993]. Gene delivery systems that specifically target diseased cells are needed.

Gene delivery systems can be classified as either viral or nonviral. Viruses are natural vehicles for gene delivery and were the first obvious choice [Friedmann, 1992]. Recombinant viruses have had the sequences required for their self-replication removed and replaced with the foreign DNA sequences. The viral proteins necessary for efficient cell entry and gene delivery are supplied by packaging cell lines. Viruses, in general, efficiently transduce cells and in some cases (retroviruses and adeno-associated viruses) permanently integrate the transgene into the host cell's genome. Retroviruses, adenoviruses, and adeno-associated viruses are the most commonly used viral gene delivery systems (Table 101.2).

Effective nonviral gene transfer systems have been developed which deliver genes to target cells without the inherent disadvantages of viral-based systems such as antigenicity, potential for recombination with wild-type viruses, and possible cellular damage due to persistent or repeated exposure to the viral vectors [Felgner and Rhodes, 1991]. These synthetic systems are also easier to manufacture on a large scale because they typically use plasmid constructs that can be grown with existing fermentation technology [Felgner and Rhodes, 1991]. In addition, tedious measurements of viral titers and tests for replication-competent virus are avoided [Felgner and Rhodes, 1991]. Direct plasmid injection, lipofection, and receptor-mediated delivery vectors are the most promising nonviral systems. There are many other nonviral transfection techniques that are too inefficient (i.e., coprecipitation of DNA with calcium phosphate [Chen and Okayama, 1987], DNA complexed with

TABLE 101.2   Physical Characteristics of Recombinant Virions

Characteristic	Units	Recombinant Retroviruses	Recombinant Adenoviruses	Recombinant AAV
Genome type		ss RNA (2 per virion)	ds DNA	ss DNA
Genome size	Bases	8300	36000	4700
Genome MW	Daltons	3×10^6	$20\text{--}25 \times 10^6$	$1.2\text{--}1.8 \times 10^6$
Particle diameter	nm	90–147	65–80	20–24
Particle mass	Grams	3.6×10^{-16}	2.9×10^{-16}	1.0×10^{-17}
Composition				
DNA/RNA	%	2	13	26
Protein	%	62	87	74
Lipid	%	36	0	0
Density	g/cm³ CsCl	1.15–1.16	1.33–1.35	1.39–1.42
Enveloped?	Yes/no	Yes	No	No
Shape		Spherical	Icosahedral	Icosahedral
Surface projections	Yes/no	Yes	Yes	No
Number		~60–200	12	
Length	nm	5	25–30	
Max diameter	nm	8	4	
Virus titer	pfu/ml	$10^6\text{--}10^7$	$10^{10}\text{--}10^{12}$	$10^5\text{--}10^7$
Integration?		Yes, random	No, episomal	Yes, chromosome 19

DEAE-dextran [Pagano et al., 1967], electroporation [Neumann et al., 1982]) or laborious (i.e., microinjection of DNA [Capecchi, 1980]) for clinical use.

Only those gene delivery systems (viral and nonviral) with potential for clinical application will be discussed in this chapter. Technical problems with each of these technologies (Table 101.3) will be described and specific examples of their applications highlighted.

101.2 Recombinant Retroviruses

Most currently approved clinical gene therapy trials utilize recombinant retroviruses for gene delivery. Retroviruses are the preferred gene transfer system because they accurately integrate a

TABLE 101.3 Advantages and Disadvantages of Gene Transfer Methods

Advantages	Disadvantages
Recombinant retroviruses	
1. Transduces many cell types	1. Limited gene size (8 kb)
2. Stably integrates into host cell genome	2. Transduces only dividing cells
3. High efficiency of *ex-vivo* transduction	3. Low virus titers
4. Biology well understood	4. Inefficient *in-vivo* infection
	5. Difficult to purify or concentrate
Recombinant adenoviruses	
1. Infects nondividing cells	1. Limited gene size (7 kb)
2. High virus titers	2. Gene remains episomal (transient expression)
3. Readily purified and concentrated	3. Complicated vector design
4. High efficiency of *in-vivo* transduction	4. May recombine with natural adenoviruses
5. Biology well understood	5. Immune reaction to vector encoded viral proteins
Recombinant adeno-associated viruses	
1. Infects nondividing cells (DNA may not integrate into nondividing cells)	1. Limited gene size (4.7 kb)
2. Integrates into a specific site on chromosome 19	2. Low virus titers
3. Resistant to detergents, solvents and heat	3. Infection efficiency is often low
4. Readily purified and concentrated	4. Producer cell line requires wild type adenovirus as helper
	5. Integration mechanism results in tandem repeats of the transgene
Direct Injection	
1. Simple technique	1. Gene remains episomal (transient expression)
2. Can be used to vaccinate	2. Very low transduction efficiency
3. Contains no viral sequences	3. Can only transduce skeletal and cardiac muscle
4. Unlimited gene size	
Liposomes	
1. Simple to prepare	1. Gene remains episomal (transient expression)
2. Long-term stability	2. Cannot target specific cell types (may transduce cells nonspecifically)
3. Can transduce any cell type	3. Less efficient transduction than viral based methods
4. Contains no viral sequences	
Receptor mediated	
1. Can target specific cell types	1. Gene remains episomal (transient expression)
2. No limit to gene size	2. Inefficient transduction
3. Contains no viral sequences	3. Unstable; can be degraded in serum and intracellularly in lysosomes
Future challenges for all gene delivery methods	
Challenges	Motivation
1. Tightly regulate expression of the delivered gene	1. Tight regulation needed for many target diseases such as thalessemia and growth hormone deficiency
2. Minimize or eliminate the immune response to the therapeutic protein and delivery system antigens such as viral proteins, liposome lipids etc.	2. An immune response against the therapeutic protein and/or the delivery vehicle may destroy genetically altered cells and/or reduce effectiveness of subsequent treatments

single copy of the therapeutic gene into the target cell's genome [Anderson, 1992]. The molecular biology of these viruses is well understood so that manipulation of their genomes is relatively straightforward.

Retroviral particles contain two copies of identical RNA genomes that are wrapped in a protein coat and further encapsidated by a lipid-bilayer membrane. The virus attaches to specific cell surface receptors via surface proteins that protrude from the viral membrane. The particle is then internalized and its genome is released into the cytoplasm, reverse transcribed from RNA to DNA, transported into the nucleus, and then integrated into the cell's genome. The integrated viral genome has LTRs (long terminal repeats) at both ends that encode the regulatory sequences that drive the expression of the viral genome [Weiss et al., 1982].

Retroviruses used for gene transfer are derived from wild-type murine retroviruses. The recombinant viral particles are structurally identical to the wild-type virus but carry a genetically engineered genome (retroviral vector) that encodes the therapeutic gene of interest. These recombinant viruses are incapable of self-replication but can infect and insert their genomes into a target cell's genome [Morgan and Anderson, 1993].

Recombinant retroviruses, like all other recombinant viruses, are produced by a two-part system composed of a packaging cell line and a recombinant vector (Fig. 101.1) [Anderson, 1992; Levine and Friedmann, 1993]. The packaging cell line expresses all the structural viral genes (*gag, pol,* and *env*) necessary for the formation of an infectious virion. *Gag* encodes the capsid proteins and is necessary for encapsidation of the vector. *Pol* encodes the enzymatic activities of the virus, including reverse transcriptase. *Env* encodes the surface proteins that are necessary for attachment to the target cell's receptors.

The retroviral vector is essentially the wild-type genome with all the viral genes removed. This vector encodes the transgene(s) and the regulatory sequences necessary for their expression as well as a special packaging sequence (Ψ) that is required for encapsidation of the genome into an infectious viral particle [Morgan and Anderson, 1993]. The retroviral vector is transfected into the packaging cell line. The structural proteins expressed by the packaging cell line recognize the packaging sequence on RNAs transcribed from the transfected vector and encapsidate them into an infectious virion, which is subsequently exocytosed by the cell and released into the culture medium. This medium containing infectious recombinant viruses is harvested and used to transduce target cells.

Many different retroviral vector designs have been used (Fig. 101.2). A commonly used vector encodes two genes, one expressed from the LTR and the other from an internal promoter (Fig. 101.2c) [Miller, 1992b]. Often, one gene expresses a therapeutic protein and the other a selectable marker that makes transduced cells resistant to selective media or a drug. This allows the researcher to establish a culture composed solely of transduced cells by growing them under the selective conditions. Several configurations are possible, but the optimal vector design is often dictated by the transgene(s) being expressed and the cell type to be transduced. Vector configuration is crucial for maximizing viral titer and transgene expression [Roemer and Friedmann, 1992].

Recombinant retroviruses are being used for several approved clinical protocols. Examples include the correction of genetic disease (ADA deficiency), treatment of brain cancer (herpes simplex thymidine kinase gene into tumor cells in the brain, making them sensitive to the antibiotic ganciclovir), and treatment of HIV (transduction of cells with a transdominant negative form of *rev*) [Nabel, 1993].

There are several technical problems that hamper the use of recombinant retroviruses. Retroviruses cannot infect quiescent cells because integration requires passage of the target cells through mitosis [Roe et al., 1993]. This is a significant disadvantage because it limits the type of cells and tissues that can be transduced by recombinant retroviruses. Nondividing or fully differentiated cells such as hepatocytes and neurons cannot be transduced unless they are stimulated to divide. Another drawback of retroviral vectors is that they can only accommodate genes that are less than 8 kilobases long [Roemer and Friedmann, 1992]. Larger genes are not efficiently packaged into infectious viral particles.

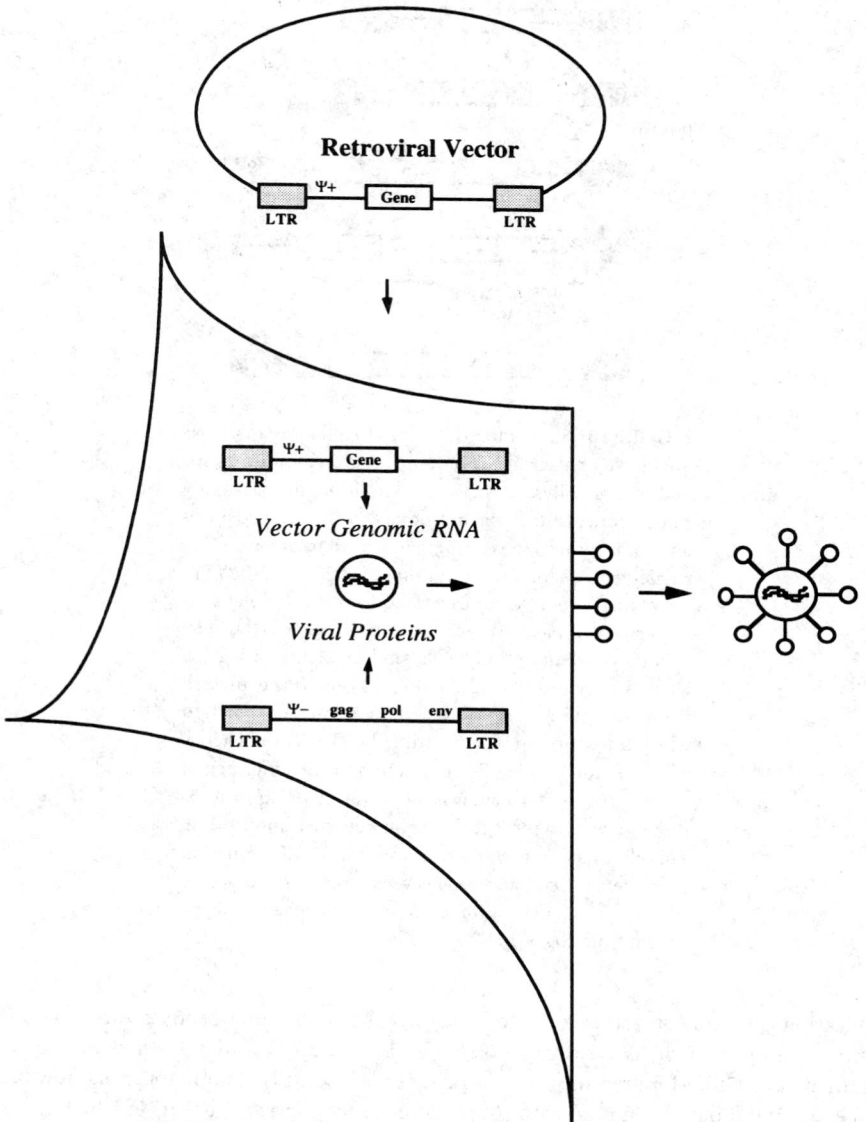

FIGURE 101.1 Packaging cell line for retrovirus. A simple retroviral vector composed of 2 LTR regions which flank sequences encoding the packaging sequence (Ψ) and a therapeutic gene. A packaging cell line is transfected with this vector. The packaging cell line expresses the three structural proteins necessary for formation of a virus particle (*gag, pol*, and *env*). These proteins recognize the packaging sequence on the vector and form an infectious virion around it. Infectious virions bud from the cell surface into the culture medium. The virus-laden culture medium is filtered to remove cell debris and then either immediately used to transduce target cells or the virions are purified and/or concentrated and frozen for later use.

Producer cell lines typically produce virus in relatively low titers (10^5 to 10^7 infectious particles per milliliter) [Paul et al., 1993]. For many in vivo applications, higher titers are required for an adequate therapeutic benefit. The viral titer is a function of several factors, including the producer cell line, the type of transgene, and the vector construction.

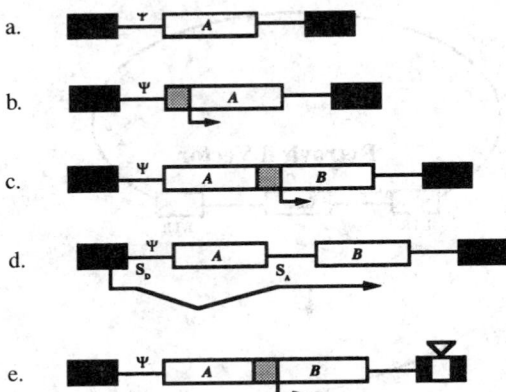

FIGURE 101.2 Standard retroviral vector designs. LTRs are shown as black boxes. S_D and S_A represent splice donor and acceptor sites, respectively. Ψ indicates the packaging signal sequence. Internal promoters are the stippled boxes and transcription start sites are indicated by arrows. (*a*) A single-gene vector. Transcription is driven from the LTR. (*b*) A single-gene vector expressed from an internal promoter. (*c*) A typical two-gene vector. One gene is the therapeutic gene, and the other is a selectable marker gene. Gene *A* is driven from the LTR, and gene *B* is expressed from the internal promoter. (*d*) A two-gene vector in which transcription is driven from the LTR. The efficiency of expression of gene *B* is a function of the efficiency of splicing. (*e*) A self-inactivating vector. A deletion in 3′ LTR is copied to the 5′ LTR during reverse transcription. This eliminates any transcription from the LTR. Internal promoters are still active. This vector reduces the chance of insertional activation of a proto-oncogene downstream from the 3′ LTR.

Purification and concentration of retroviruses without loss of infectivity are very difficult. Standard techniques such as centrifugation, column filtration, and ultrafiltration have failed [McGrath et al., 1978]. More recently, hollow fiber [Paul et al., 1993] and tangential flow filtration [Kotani et al., 1994] have been used with some success. A chimeric retrovirus in which the normal envelope proteins were replaced by VSV (vesicular stomatitis virus) envelope proteins was readily concentrated by centrifugation, but its utility is limited because the cell line that produces it is viable for only a short time due to the toxicity of the VSV envelope proteins [Burns et al., 1993]. Future work on more gentle concentration procedures and improved designs of chimeric retroviruses that can be easily concentrated may lead to significantly higher viral titers.

Stability and level of expression also have been cited as significant drawbacks for retrovirally transduced cells. Although long-term expression has been documented in some systems such as bone marrow, fibroblasts, hepatocytes, and muscle cells, there also have been reports of transient expression in retrovirally transduced cells [Roemer and Friedmann, 1992]. This unstable expression has been attributed to several causes, including methylation of the DNA and in some cases rearrangement or loss of the proviral sequences [Roemer and Friedmann, 1992]. Another major cause of transient expression, common to all gene transfer techniques, is the rejection of transduced cells by the immune system. If the patient does not normally make the therapeutic protein, or if the therapeutic protein contains an epitope not present on the patient's mutated protein, then an immune response may be mounted against the transduced cells. It is possible that successful long-term expression of transduced cells may only occur in patients who already produce a small amount of the therapeutic protein [Verma, 1990].

The use of recombinant retroviruses has raised some safety concerns. These concerns have been thoroughly documented and have centered on two areas [Roemer and Friedmann, 1992; Temin, 1990]. The early retroviral packaging cell lines occasionally produced replication-competent virus by homologous recombination between the retroviral vector and the packaging cell line's retroviral sequences. Recent advances in the construction of these cell lines have made the production of replication-competent viruses essentially impossible [Danos and Mulligan, 1988]. The other main safety concern was the possibility that the retrovirus, due to its integration into the host cell's genome, would activate a proto-oncogene and cause a neoplastic cell to become cancerous. The probability of insertion adjacent to a proto-oncogene is very low, however, and several mutations are required for a cell to become cancerous. Consequently, the risk of cellular transformation by retroviral vectors is extremely low and is typically outweighed by the potential therapeutic benefits to the patient [Temin, 1990].

Although recombinant retroviruses are the most commonly used gene transfer system, there are clearly several technical issues that need to be addressed to improve their reliability and range of applicability. Perhaps the most important of these is the need for increased viral titers. This could be obtained by optimizing production procedures and viral vectors and by developing chimeric viruses with improved stability. Attempts to genetically engineer recombinant retroviruses that can infect nondividing cells are also underway [Deminie and Emerman, 1993]; success in this area would vastly increase the potential target tissue and diseases to which retroviral-based vectors could be applied.

101.3 Recombinant Adenoviruses

Adenoviruses provide a useful alternative to retroviral gene transfer vectors. Their primary advantage is their ability to infect nondividing cells [Mulligan, 1993]. This makes the in vivo transduction of tissues composed of fully differentiated or slowly dividing cells such as the liver and lung possible. Adenoviruses can be grown to very high titers (10^{10} infectious particles per milliliter) and can be concentrated another 100-fold without significant loss of infectivity [Roemer and Friedmann, 1992].

Adenoviruses are large (36-kilobase double-stranded DNA genome), nonenveloped, icosahedral viruses from which protrude several long protein fibers. These fibers bind to specific cell-surface receptors prior to the viruses' internalization into cellular endosomes by clathrin-coated pits. Adenoviruses escape these vesicles by an acidic pH–activated endosomolytic activity and are transported to the nucleus, which they enter via pores in its membrane [Greber et al., 1993].

The wild-type adenovirus genome consists primarily of five early genes (E1 to E5), each of which is expressed from its own promoters [Horwitz, 1990]. There are also five late genes (L1 to L5) that are expressed from the major late promoter (MLP). Recombinant adenoviral vectors are based on a mutant adenovirus in which the E1 region (and in some cases the E3 region) is deleted. The E1 region is required for replication on normal cells. However, E1-minus mutants can be grown on a specialized packaging cell line (293 cells) that expresses the E1 gene products and therefore provides the necessary functions for virus production [Levine and Friedmann, 1993].

Recombinant adenovirus is generated using homologous recombination between the gene of interest (which is inserted into a plasmid vector so that it is flanked by adenovirus sequences) and the genome of an E1-minus mutant (Fig. 101.3). This plasmid is transfected into 293 cells which are actively replicating the E1-minus mutant. The virus stock is screened for the rare recombinants in which the gene of interest has correctly recombined with the E1-minus mutant. These recombinant virions are purified and grown to high titer on 293 cells [Morgan et al., 1994].

Several clinical protocols have been approved recently that utilize recombinant adenoviruses to transfer a corrected copy of the CFTR (cystic fibrosis transmembrane conductance regulator) gene into the nasal epithelium and lungs of cystic fibrosis patients [Boucher and Knowles, 1993; Welsh,

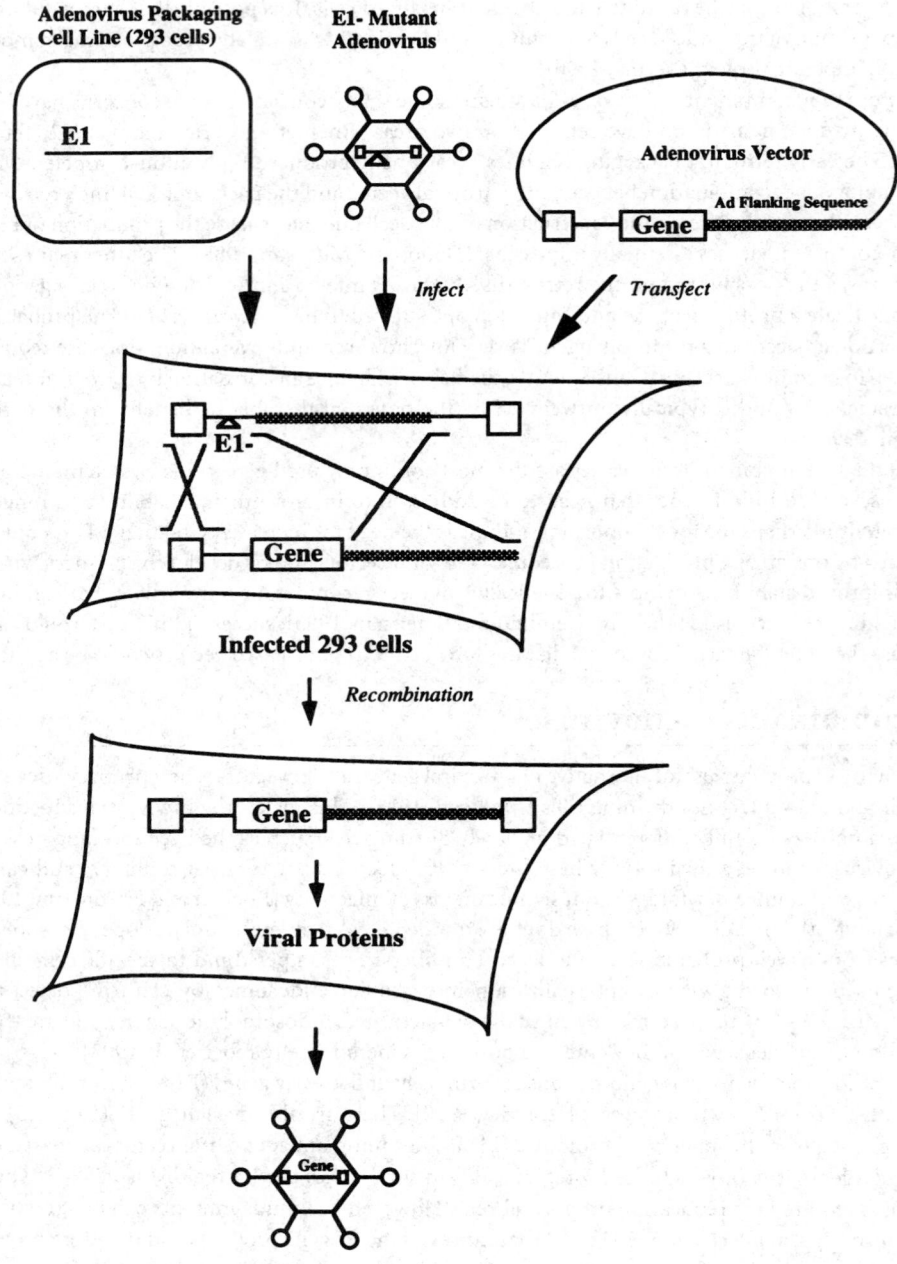

FIGURE 101.3 Isolation of recombinant adenovirus. A packaging cell line (293 cells) which expresses the E1 gene is infected with an E1-minus mutant adenovirus. The adenovirus is derived from a plasmid encoding the wild-type adenovirus genome. The E1 region of the adenovirus genome is replaced with the therapeutic gene, and the resultant plasmid (the adenovirus vector) is transfected into the 293 cell line which is infected by the mutant adenovirus. Since the therapeutic gene is flanked by adenoviral sequences, the mutant adenovirus genome and the adenovirus vector will occasionally undergo homologous recombination and form an infectious recombinant adenovirus whose genome encodes the therapeutic gene. These rare recombinants are isolated then grown on another 293 cell line.

1993; Wilmott and Whitsett, 1993]. Recombinant adenoviruses were chosen for this application because they have a natural tropism for the lung and they can be concentrated to the high titers required to achieve a therapeutic effect [Mastrangeli et al., 1993].

Significant technical issues limit the usefulness of adenoviral-based vectors. Adenoviruses can only support the packaging of therapeutic genes that are smaller than 7 kilobases [Miller, 1992a]. In addition, the genome of adenoviruses does not integrate into the host cells' genetic material but instead remains episomal [Miller, 1992a]. This often results in transient gene expression due to loss of the vector DNA from the transduced cells over time. It is likely that repeated treatments of the patient will be required for continuous relief of chronic disorders. Unfortunately, repeat treatments may provoke an immune response to the viral proteins that could significantly reduce their effectiveness. Recombinant adenoviruses also tend to induce a mild, transient, and dose-dependent inflammatory response that also may limit their usefulness for gene therapy. In addition, the current generation of adenoviral vectors express low levels of viral proteins that may be cytotoxic or can stimulate an immune response that may destroy the genetically modified cells [Levine and Friedmann, 1993; Roemer and Friedmann, 1992]. A recent study demonstrated that hepatocytes transduced by recombinant adenoviruses were eliminated by a cellular immune response that was stimulated by low-level expression of viral proteins [Yang et al., 1994]. The endosomolytic activity of the virus as well as repeated exposure to the virus also may damage cells [Roemer and Friedmann, 1992]. These concerns are tempered somewhat by the good safety record of the military, which has vaccinated thousands of its personnel with inactivated adenovirus [Top, 1975]. Continued work is clearly necessary to address these technical issues and to develop a recombinant adenovirus with no toxicity and long-term gene expression.

101.4 Recombinant Adeno-Associated Viruses

Another viral-based gene transfer system with potential application to gene therapy is the adeno-associated virus (AAV). This virus can transduce a wide range of tissues, but its main advantage is that it stably integrates into a specific position on chromosome 19, which reduces the probability of inadvertent activation of a proto-oncogene [Levine and Friedmann, 1993].

AAV are small nonenveloped viruses that are not known to cause any human disease [Levine and Friedmann, 1993]. AAV vectors are of particular interest for treating cystic fibrosis patients. Recent in vivo transduction of rabbit airway epithelium with an AAV-CFTR vector demonstrated stable expression of the CFTR gene for several months and indicates that AAV-based vectors may be useful for human gene therapy [Flotte et al., 1993].

Several technical problems with AAV vectors must be addressed prior to their use in patients. AAV vectors can package only small transgenes (up to 4.7 kilobases), and production of the recombinant vector is frequently contaminated with wild-type adenovirus, which must be separated or inactivated (Fig. 101.4) [Levine and Friedmann, 1993]. The integration mechanism of AAV vectors is not as precise as retroviral vectors and generally results in tandem repeats of the transgene being inserted into the host chromosome [Mulligan, 1993]. The impact of these tandem repeats and the overall mechanism of AAV vector integration should be deduced prior to its approval for use in human gene therapy clinical trials.

101.5 Direct Injection of Naked DNA

Direct injection of plasmid DNA is the simplest and most direct technique for transducing cells in vivo. A plasmid encoding the therapeutic gene is injected intramuscularly, and the DNA is internalized by cells proximal to the injection site [Wolff et al., 1990]. Gene expression after direct injection has been demonstrated in skeletal muscle cells of rodents and nonhuman primates [Levine and Friedmann, 1993].

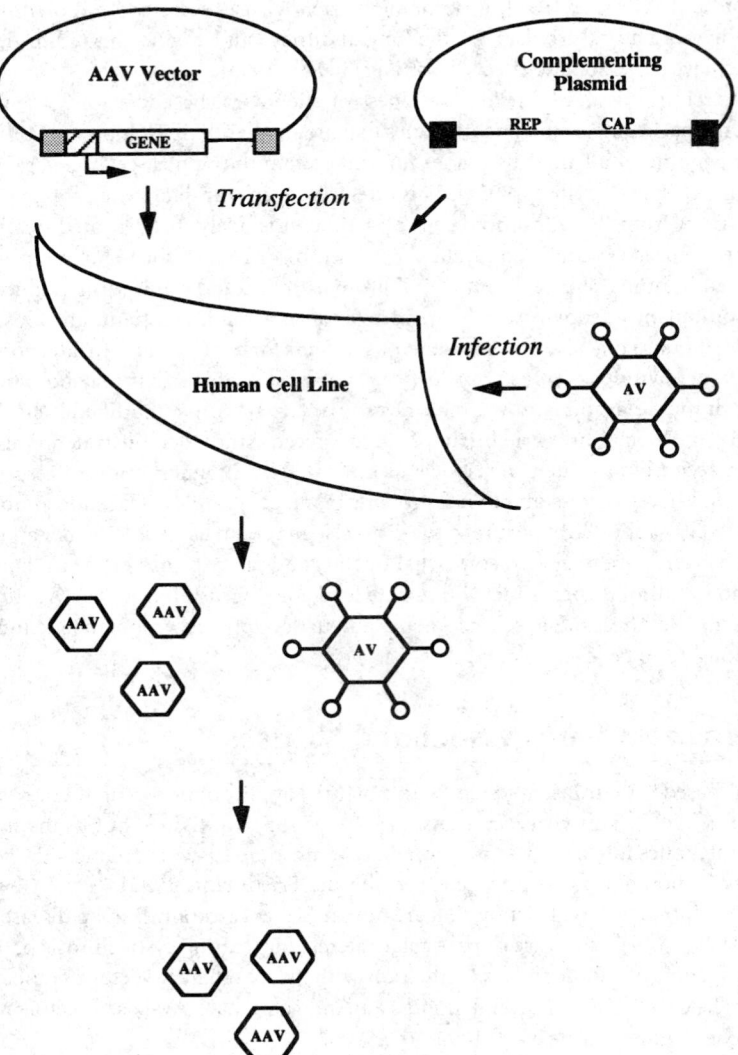

FIGURE 101.4 Production of recombinant AAV. Human cells are transfected with a plasmid encoding the therapeutic gene which is driven from a heterologous pro-moter (*cross-hatched box*) and flanked with AAV terminal repeats (*stippled boxes*). The cells are also transfected with a complementing plasmid encoding the AAV *rep* and *cap* genes, which cannot be packaged because they are not flanked by AAV ter-minal repeats. The *rep* and *cap* genes, whose products are required for particle for-mation, are flanked by adenovirus 5 terminal fragments (*black boxes*) which enhance their expression. The transfected cells are infected with wild-type adenovirus which supplies helper functions required for amplification of the AAV vector. The virus stock contains both AAV recombinant virus and adenovirus. The adenovirus is either separated by density gradient centrifugation or heat inactivated.

This technique could be useful for the treatment of genetic diseases of the muscle such as muscular dystrophy, as demonstrated by recent experiments that transduced 1% of mouse myofibers with plasmids encoding a functional dystrophin gene [Acsadi et al., 1991a]. Direct injec-tion also could be used to vaccinate patients, as demonstrated by a novel method in which rats were immunized by direct injection of a plasmid encoding an antigen. Vaccination by direct injection of nucleic acids could be financially beneficial because it could eliminate the need for the expensive production and purification of recombinant proteins [Geissler et al., 1994].

However, direct injection is extremely inefficient. One study reported as little as 60 to 100 myocardial cells being transduced per injection [Acsadi et al., 1991b]. Improved efficiency has been noted when plasmids are injected into regenerating muscle cells [Wells, 1993] or when coinjected with recombinant adenoviruses [Yoshimura et al., 1993]. Application of direct injection appears to be limited to skeletal and cardiac muscle cells, and the mechanism of internalization is not known. Improved gene transfer frequencies and the longevity of gene expression, as well as susceptibility of human cells to genetic modification by direct injection, must still be demonstrated.

101.6 Liposome-Mediated Gene Delivery

Liposome-mediated gene delivery (lipofection) is more efficient than direct injection and can deliver DNA to virtually any cell type. Liposomes require no viral sequences and appear to be relatively nontoxic [Nabel et al., 1993; Zhu et al., 1993]. Cationic liposomes are prepared by sonicating an aqueous suspension of cationic lipids (e.g., DOTMA) and neutral lipids (e.g., DOPE) (Fig. 101.5). The unilamellar liposomes (roughly 100 nm in diameter) are mixed with the plasmid DNA, whose negatively charged backbone forms a noncovalent complex with the positively charged cationic lipids [Felgner and Ringold, 1989]. The positively charged liposome masks the electrostatic repulsion between the negatively charged cell surface and the similarly charged DNA.

Lipofection has already been used in clinical trials. The first human gene therapy protocol utilizing lipofection was recently completed in which malignant nodules of patients with stage IV melanoma and negative for HLA-B7 (a foreign major histocompatability complex protein) were injected with liposomes carrying plasmid DNA encoding HLA-B7 [Nabel et al., 1993]. The expression of HLA-B7 in tumor cells was expected to stimulate an immune response against the modified and unmodified tumor cells. The treatment transduced 1% to 10% of tumor cells near the site of injection and resulted in regression of injected nodules in at least one patient [Nabel et al., 1993]. More studies are needed to determine the mechanism of the antitumor response and ways to improve it.

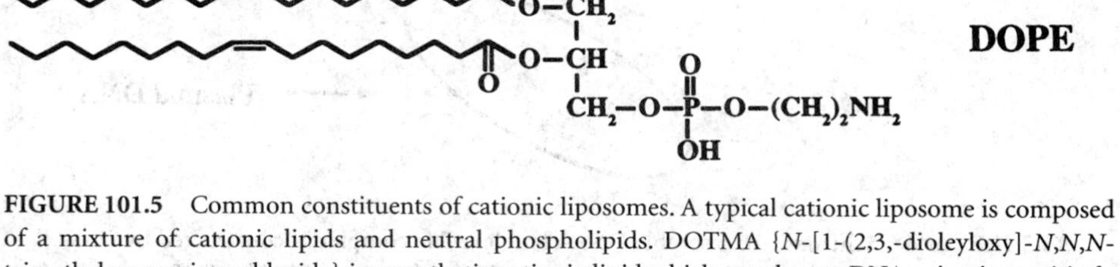

FIGURE 101.5 Common constituents of cationic liposomes. A typical cationic liposome is composed of a mixture of cationic lipids and neutral phospholipids. DOTMA {*N*-[1-(2,3,-dioleyloxy]-*N,N,N*-trimethylammonium chloride} is a synthetic cationic lipid which attaches to DNA using its positively charged head group. DOPE {1,2-Di[(*cis*)-9-octadecenoyl]-sn-glycero-3-phosphoethanolamine} is a neutral phospholipid which enhances the activity of these cationic liposomes. The resultant DNA-liposome complex is positively charged and reduces or eliminates the repulsive electrostatic forces between the negatively charged DNA and the negatively charged cell surface.

Another potential application of lipofection is the treatment of lung disorders, such as cystic fibrosis, with aerosolized liposome vectors. Aerosol delivery is advantageous because it is noninvasive and can deliver genes to cells that are otherwise difficult to access. The feasibility of the technique was demonstrated by delivery of the chloramphenicol acetyltransferase (CAT) reporter gene to mouse lungs in vivo which resulted in its expression for 3 weeks [Stribling et al., 1992].

The major drawback of lipofection is the inability to target specific cell types. Use of lipofection in vivo typically results in nonspecific genetic modification, which is not desirable for many applications. Lipofection also results in only transient expression of the transgene; repeated treatments would therefore be necessary to maintain any therapeutic effect [Morgan et al., 1993].

101.7 Receptor-Mediated Gene Delivery

Methods that rely on receptor-mediated endocytosis are promising alternatives to lipofection. These vectors are constructed by conjugating the DNA to a ligand that can only be internalized by cells expressing receptors for that ligand (Fig. 101.6). These soluble DNA complexes have several advantages. They can target specific cells by using a ligand that can only be internalized by that specific cell type [Levine and Friedmann, 1993]. There are essentially no size limitations to the transgene because the DNA is not packaged inside a virus particle [Felgner, 1993]. It is potentially safer than viral-based systems because it does not carry any active viral gene elements. The design is easily modified to target a particular cell type as long as a ligand is available that is internalized specifically and exclusively by that cell type.

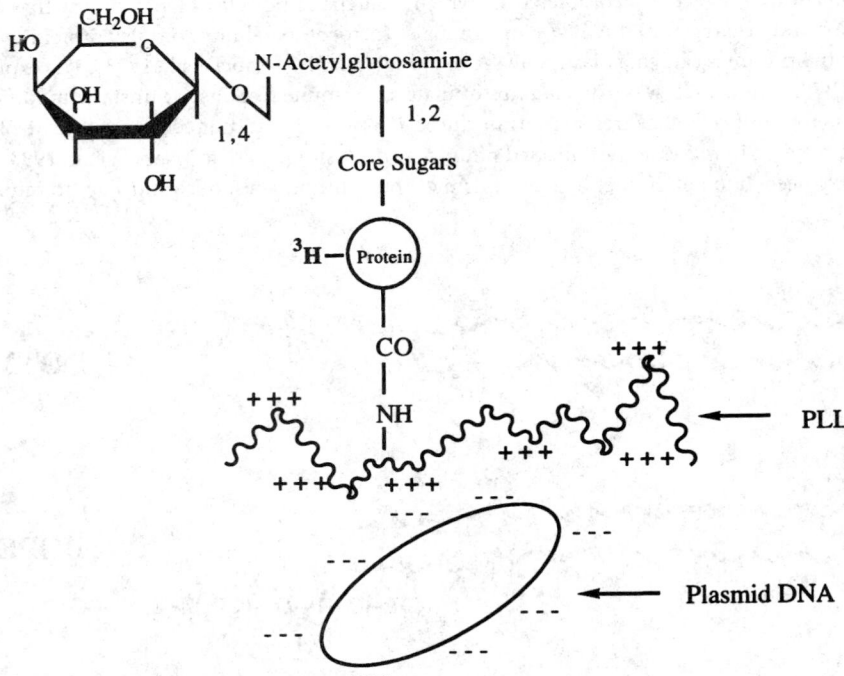

FIGURE 101.6 Schematic of a soluble DNA-complex. The complex is constructed by covalently linking an enzymatically desialyated orosomucoid [asialo-orosomucoid (ASOR)] to poly-L-lysine (PLL), a polycation. The protein–poly-L-lysine conjugate is mixed with the DNA to form a noncovalent complex between the negatively charged groups of the phosphodiester backbone of the DNA and the positively charged groups of the poly-L-lysine. A typical complex has the following molar ratios: 50 ASOR:25 PLL (MW = 3800 Da): 1 plasmid.

One such gene transfer system was devised by Wu et al. [1991] in which asialoglycoprotein (a glycoprotein with exposed galactose residues) was covalently linked by disulfide bonds to poly-L-lysine. The negatively charged DNA molecules were added and bound to the positively charged poly-L-lysine via strong electrostatic interactions.

This system has not yet reached clinical trials, but some encouraging results have been obtained in animal models. Efficient localization to the liver after intravenous injection into rats was demonstrated when over 80% of the injected radiolabeled vector localized to their livers [Wu et al., 1988]. Watanabe rabbits, which have high levels of cholesterol in their blood due to a defective LDL (low-density lipoprotein) receptor, were injected with a soluble DNA complex that encoded the wild-type LDL receptor. The disorder was partially and transiently corrected. The cholesterol levels of the rabbits dropped a maximum of 25% to 30% after treatment and remained below preinjection levels for up to 6 days [Wilson et al., 1992].

The efficiency of a similar conjugate, which used transferrin as the ligand instead of asialoglycoprotein, was improved by coupling it to inactivated adenovirus. The adenovirus was coupled to the poly-L-lysine moiety of the conjugate by an antibody bridge. The adenovirus capsid proteins catalyzed the release of the vesicle-bound virus and the targeting vehicle to which it is bound and reduced the amount of DNA degraded by lysosomal enzymes. This improved conjugate was used to transfer the luciferase reporter gene under the transcriptional control of the cytomegalovirus (CMV) promoter into the airway epithelium of cotton rats. Transient gene expression was detected for up to 1 week [Gao et al., 1993].

These conjugated genes are still too inefficient to achieve useful therapeutic results. The genes remain episomal, and expression is transient. Further improvements in efficiency and the incorporation of an integration mechanism resulting in long-term gene expression would greatly enhance the utility of these vectors [Gao et al., 1993].

101.8 Clinical Applications

Gene therapy is applicable not only to single-gene disorders such as those discussed earlier but also to complex genetic disorders such as cancer and even to infectious diseases such as HIV. The major approaches for treating these complex disorders are outlined in Table 101.4 [Anderson, 1994a, 1994b]. A recently approved protocol targeting cancer is briefly reviewed below to illustrate one such approach.

This protocol, submitted by Raffel and Culver [1993], takes advantage of a fundamental characteristic of all known retroviruses (with the exception of HIV): the inability to infect nondividing cells. This characteristic, usually considered a "disadvantage" of recombinant retroviruses, is exploited to specifically target dividing tumor cells in the brain. A packaging cell line, producing a recombinant retrovirus encoding the herpes simplex thymidine kinase (HS-tk) gene, is injected into human brain tumors. These retroviruses transduce only dividing cells (tumor cells), and expression of the HS-tk gene sensitizes transduced cells to an antibiotic, ganciclovir. After the brain cells are sufficiently transduced, ganciclovir is administered to the patient, and eradication of the tumor cells is expected. The protocol is based on previous experiments with brain tumors in rats in which transduction of only 10% to 50% of the tumor cells was required to completely eradicate the tumor and which resulted in little to no toxicity to surrounding normal tissue [Culver et al., 1992]. This protocol was approved September 3, 1993, and clinical trials are currently in progress [Raffel and Culver, 1993].

101.9 Conclusions

Future applications of gene therapy are practically limitless and are restricted only by the imagination and ingenuity of today's scientists. However, current gene therapy methodologies are severely limited by complex technical problems. Critical issues such as cell targeting and the integrity, regu-

TABLE 101.4 Major Approaches for Gene Therapy

Type of Disorder	Gene Therapy Approaches
Single-gene disorders e.g., cystic fibrosis	1. Gene augmentation: introduction of a functional copy of the gene into the nucleus or target cell's genome
Cancer	1. Tumor vaccine: insertion of gene for cytokine into tumor cells or the in-situ injection of a gene encoding a foreign antigen into a tumor mass to stimulate the immune system to recognize and destroy tumor cells
	2. Suicide genes: insertion of a suicide gene which either kills the transduced cell outright or makes it susceptible to a drug which is administered after transduction. [e.g., HS-tk (herpes simplex thymidine kinase) gene makes transduced cells susceptible to ganciclovir, an antibiotic].
	3. Multiple drug resistance: delivery of a gene (typically to bone marrow cells) which confers increased resistance to drugs used for chemotherapy. This permits use of drug doses which would otherwise be toxic.
	4. Tumor suppressor genes: deliver a functional copy of a tumor suppressor gene (e.g., p53) to cells that are defective for that gene; transduce tumor cells (harboring activated oncogenes) with gene encoding the antisense to an oncogene; the antisense binds to and inactivates the oncogene
HIV	1. Extracellular: transduce cells with a gene encoding an HIV antigen to stimulate the immune system; transduce cells with a gene encoding a secretable protein which interferes with the normal lifecycle of HIV (sCD4-IgG)
	2. Intracellular *Kill infected cells:* insert cytotoxic genes which are expressed only when HIV regulatory proteins are present *Interfere with HIV lifecycle:* insert genes which express antisense sequences to inactivate regulatory proteins vital for HIV lifecycle (*tat* and *rev*); insert genes which express dominant negative mutants of HIV regulatory proteins (*tat* and *rev*) which compete with normal regulatory sequences for DNA binding sites; deliver genes which express TAR or RRE sequences and sequester HIV regulatory proteins (act as decoys); deliver genes that express highly specific ribozymes to cleave HIV transcripts; transduce cells with genes that express single chain antibodies specific for critical HIV proteins (e.g., gp-120). These antibodies are engineered to stay associated with the endoplasmic reticulum thus preventing the HIV proteins from participating in the formation of infectious HIV virions.

lation, and stability of transferred genes must be addressed. Vector toxicity and immunogenicity must be reduced, and the frequency and efficiency of transduction must be improved. Techniques to mass produce, purify, concentrate, and store genetic vectors must be developed before gene therapy can become a standard therapeutic option. These challenges are imposing but can be solved if scientists and engineers combine their talents and skills to address the many and varied technical issues of gene therapy. The potential reward of solving these problems is a medical revolution in which once incurable and debilitating genetic diseases, cancers, and infectious diseases are cured or controlled by the tools of gene therapy.

Defining Terms

Chimeric retrovirus: A recombinant retrovirus whose structural proteins are derived from two or more different viruses.

Ex vivo: Outside the living body, referring to a process or reaction occurring therein.

In vitro: In an artificial environment, referring to a process or reaction occurring therein, as in a test tube or culture dish.

In vivo: In the living body, referring to a process or reaction occurring therein.

Lipofection: Delivery of genetic material to cells using cationic liposomes.

Liposome: A spherical particle of lipid substance suspended in an aqueous medium.

Packaging cell line: Cells that express all the structural proteins required to form an infectious viral particle.

Plasmid: A small, circular extrachromosomal DNA molecule capable of independent replication in a host cell, typically a bacterial cell.

Recombinant: A virus or vector that has DNA sequences not originally (naturally) present in its DNA.

Retrovirus: A virus that possesses RNA-dependent DNA polymerase (reverse transcriptase) which reverse transcribes the virus's RNA genome into DNA and then integrates that DNA into the host cell's genome.

Transduce: To effect transfer and integration of genetic material to a cell by infection with a recombinant retrovirus.

Vector: A plasmid or viral DNA molecule into which a DNA sequence (typically encoding a therapeutic protein) is inserted.

References

Acsadi G, Dickson G, Love DR, et al. 1991a. Human dystrophin expression in mdx mice after intramuscular injection of DNA constructs. Nature 352:815.

Acsadi G, Jiao S, Jani A, et al. 1991b. Direct gene transfer and expression into rat heart in vivo. New Biol 3:71.

Anderson WF. 1992. Human gene therapy. Science 256:808.

Anderson WF. 1994a. Gene therapy for AIDS. Hum Gene Ther 5:149.

Anderson WF. 1994b. Gene therapy for cancer. Hum Gene Ther 5:1.

Boucher RC, Knowles MR. 1993. Gene therapy for cystic fibrosis using E1 deleted adenovirus: A phase I trial in the nasal cavity. In Human Gene Transfer Protocol 9303-042. Office of Recombinant DNA Activity, NIH, 31/4B11, Bethesda, Md.

Burns JC, Friedmann T, Driever W, et al. 1993. Vesicular stomatitis virus G glycoprotein pseudotyped retroviral vectors: Concentration to very high titer and efficient gene transfer into mammalian and nonmammalian cells. Proc Natl Acad Sci USA 90:8033.

Capecchi M. 1980. High efficiency transformation by direct microinjection of DNA into cultured mammalian cells. Cell 22:479.

Chen C, Okayama H. 1987. High-efficiency transformation of mammalian cells by plasmid DNA. Mol Cell Biol 7(8):2745.

Culver KW, Ram Z, Wallbridge S, et al. 1992. In vivo gene transfer with retroviral vector-producer cells for treatment of experimental brain tumors. Science 256:1550.

Danos O, Mulligan RC. 1988. Safe and efficient generation of recombinant retroviruses with amphotropic and ecotropic host ranges. Proc Natl Acad Sci USA 85:6460.

Deminie CA, Emerman M. 1993. Incorporation of human immunodeficiency virus type 1 gag proteins into murine leukemia virus virions. J Virol 67(11):6499.

Felgner PL. 1993. Genes in a bottle. Lab Invest 68(1):1.

Felgner PL, Rhodes G. 1991. Gene therapeutics. Nature 349:351.

Felgner PL, Ringold GM. 1989. Cationic liposome-mediated transfection. Nature 337:387.

Flotte TR, Afione SA, Conrad C, et al. 1993. Stable in vivo expression of the cystic fibrosis transmembrane conductance regulator with an adeno-associated virus vector. Proc Natl Acad Sci USA 90:10613.

Friedmann T. 1992. A brief history of gene therapy. Nature Genet 2:93.

Gao L, Wagner E, Cotten M, et al. 1993. Direct in-vivo gene transfer to airway epithelium employing adenovirus-polylysine-DNA complexes. Hum Gene Ther 4:17.

Geissler EK, Wang J, Fechner JHJ, et al. 1994. Immunity to MHC class I antigen after direct DNA transfer into skeletal muscle. J Immunol 152(2):413.

Greber UF, Willetts M, Webster P, Helenius A. 1993. Stepwise dismantling of adenovirus 2 during entry into cells. Cell 75:477.

Horwitz MS. 1990. Adenoviridae and their replication. In BN Fields et al (eds), Fields Virology, 2d ed, pp 1679–1721. New York, Raven Press.

Kotani H, Newton PB III, Zhang S, et al. 1994. Improved methods of retroviral vector transduction and production for gene therapy. Hum Gene Ther 5:19.

Ledley FD. 1993. Hepatic gene therapy: Present and future. Hepatology 18:1263.

Levine F, Friedmann T. 1993. Gene therapy. Am J Dis Child 147:1167.

Mastrangeli A, Danel C, Rosenfeld MA, et al. 1993. Diversity of airway epithelial cell targets for in vivo recombinant adenovirus-mediated gene transfer. J Clin Invest 91:225.

McGrath M, Witte O, Pincus T, Weissman IL. 1978. Retrovirus purification: Method that conserves envelope glycoprotein and maximizes infectivity. J Virol 25(3):923.

Miller AD. 1992a. Human gene therapy comes of age. Nature 357:455.

Miller AD. 1992b. Retroviral vectors. Curr Top Microbiol Immunol 158:1.

Morgan JR, Tompkins RG, Yarmush ML. 1993. Advances in recombinant retroviruses for gene delivery. Adv Drug Delivery Rev 12:143.

Morgan JR, Tompkins RG, Yarmush ML. 1994. Genetic engineering and therapeutics. In RS Greco (ed), Implantation Biology: The Host Responses and Biomedical Devices, pp 387–400. Boca Raton, Fla, CRC Press.

Morgan RA, Anderson WF. 1993. Human gene therapy. Annu Rev Biochem 62:191.

Mulligan RC. 1993. The basic science of gene therapy. Science 260:926.

Nabel GJ. 1993. A molecular genetic intervention for AIDS: Effects of a transdominant negative form of rev. In Human Gene Transfer Protocol 9306-049. Office of Recombinant DNA Activity, NIH, 31/4B11, Bethesda, Md.

Nabel GJ, Nabel EG, Yang Z-Y, et al. 1993. Direct gene transfer with DNA-liposome complexes in melanoma: Expression, biologic activity, and lack of toxicity in humans. Proc Natl Acad Sci USA 90:11307.

Neumann E, Schaefer-Ridder M, Wang Y, Hofschneider PH. 1982. Gene transfer into mouse lyoma cells by electroporation in high electric fields. EMBO J 1:841.

Pagano J, McCutchan JH, Vaheri A. 1967. Factors influencing the enhancement of the infectivity of poliovirus ribonucleic acid by diethylaminoethyl-dextran. J Virol 1:891.

Paul RW, Morris D, Hess BW, et al. 1993. Increased viral titer through concentration of viral harvests from retroviral packaging lines. Hum Gene Ther 4:609.

Raffel C, Culver K. 1993. Gene therapy for the treatment of recurrent pediatric malignant astrocytomas with in vivo tumor transduction with the herpes simplex thymidine kinase gene. In Human Gene Transfer Protocol 9306-050. Office of Recombinant DNA Activity, NIH, 31/4B11, Bethesda, Md.

Roe T, Reynolds TC, Yu G, Brown PO. 1993. Integration of murine leukemia virus DNA depends on mitosis. EMBO J 12(5):2099.

Roemer K, Friedmann T. 1992. Concepts and strategies for human gene therapy. Eur J Biochem 208:211.

Stribling R, Brunette E, Liggitt D, et al. 1992. Aerosol gene delivery in vivo. Proc Natl Acad Sci USA 89:11277.

Temin HM. 1990. Safety considerations in somatic gene therapy of human disease with retrovirus vectors. Hum Gene Ther 1:111.

Top FHJ. 1975. Control of adenovirus acute respiratory disease in US Army trainees. Yale J Biol Med 48:185.

Verma IM. 1990. Gene therapy. Sci Am 263(5):68.

Weiss R, Teich N, Varmus H, Coffin J. 1982. Molecular Biology of Tumor Viruses. Cold Spring Harbor, NY, Cold Spring Harbor Laboratory.

Wells DJ. 1993. Improved gene transfer by direct plasmid injection associated with regeneration in mouse skeletal muscle. FEBS Lett 332(1,2):179.

Welsh MJ. 1993. Adenovirus-mediated gene transfer of CFTR to the nasal epithelium and maxillary sinus of patients with cystic fibrosis. In Human Gene Transfer Protocol 9312-067. Office of Recombinant DNA Activity, NIH, 31/4B11, Bethesda, Md.

Wilmott RW, Whitsett J. 1993. A phase I study of gene therapy of cystic fibrosis utilizing a replication deficient recombinant adenovirus vector to deliver the human cystic fibrosis transmembrane conductance regulator cDNA to the airways. In Human Gene Transfer Protocol 9303-041. Office of Recombinant DNA Activity, NIH, 31/4B11, Bethesda, Md.

Wilson JM, Grossman M, Wu CH, et al. 1992. Hepatocyte-directed gene transfer in vivo leads to transient improvement of hypercholesterolemia in LDL receptor-deficient rabbits. J Biol Chem 267:963.

Wolff JA, Malone RW, Williams P, et al. 1990. Direct gene transfer into mouse muscle in vivo. Science 247:1465.

Wu GY, Wu CH. 1988. Receptor-mediated gene delivery and expression in vivo. J Biol Chem 263:14621.

Wu GY, Wu CH. 1991. Delivery systems for gene therapy. Biotherapy 3:87.

Yang Y, Nunes FA, Berencsi K, et al. 1994. Cellular immunity to viral antigens limits E1-deleted adenoviruses for gene therapy. Proc Natl Acad Sci USA 91:4407.

Yoshimura K, Rosenfeld MA, Seth P, Crystal RG. 1993. Adenovirus-mediated augmentation of cell transfection with unmodified plasmid vectors. J Biol Chem 268(4):2300.

Zhu N, Liggitt D, Liu Y, Debs R. 1993. Systemic gene expression after intravenous DNA delivery into adult mice. Science 261:209.

Further Information

A comprehensive work on retroviruses is presented in *RNA Tumor Viruses*, edited by Robin Weiss, Natalie Teich, Harold Varmus, and John Coffin. The book *Gene Transfer and Gene Therapy: Proceedings of an E.I. du Pont de Nemours–UCLA Symposium Held at Tamarron, Colorado, February 6–12, 1988*, edited by Arthur L. Beaudet, Richard Mulligan, and Inder M. Verma, presents several articles on early gene therapy technology.

The monthly journal *Human Gene Therapy* publishes papers on original investigations into the transfer and expression of genes in mammals including humans. Technological advances as well as ethical and legal papers relating to gene therapy of humans are included. For subscription information, contact Human Gene Therapy, Mary Ann Liebert, Inc., 1651 Third Avenue, New York, NY 10128, (212) 289-2300, Fax (212) 289-4697. The bimonthly journal *Gene Therapy* focuses on all aspects of gene therapy and its application to human disease, including animal experiments performed as part of a therapeutic development program. It also contains commissioned news and views section and review articles. For subscription information, contact Gene Therapy, Subscription Department, 65 Bleeker St., 12th Floor, New York, NY 10012. Fax (212) 477-8020.

102

Cell Engineering

Douglas A.
Lauffenburger
*Massachusetts Institute
of Technology*

Cell engineering can be defined either academically, as "application of the principles and methods of engineering to the problems of cell and molecular biology of both a basic and applied nature" [Nerem, 1991], or functionally, as "manipulation of cell function by molecular approaches" [Lauffenburger and Aebischer, 1993]. However defined, there is no question that cell engineering is becoming a central area of biomedical engineering. Applications to health care technology include design of molecular therapies for wound healing, cancer, and inflammatory disease, development of biomaterials and devices for tissue regeneration and reconstruction, introduction of gene therapies to remedy a variety of disorders, and utilization of mammalian cell culture technology for production of therapeutic proteins.

Cell engineering has its roots in revolutions that have occurred in the field of molecular cell biology over the past few decades (see Darnell et al. [1986, Chap. 1] for an excellent historical summary). Key advances upon which this field was built include electron microscopy in the 1940s, permitting intracellular structural features to be seen; the identification of DNA as the biochemical basis of genetics, also in the 1940s; the elucidation of the structure and function of DNA in the 1950s; the discovery of gene regulation in the 1960s; and progress in areas such as molecular genetics, light microscopy, and protein biochemistry in the 1970s, 1980s, and 1990s. Combining the powerful set of information and techniques from molecular cell biology with the analytical and synthetic approaches of engineering for purposeful exploitation and manipulation of cell function has given rise to the wide range of applications listed above. Engineering contributions include elucidation of kinetic, transport, and mechanical effects; identification and measurement of system parameters; and production of novel materials and devices required for control of cell and tissue functions by molecular mechanisms. All these aspects of engineering are essential to development of reliable technological systems requiring reproducible performance of cells and tissues.

The central paradigm of cell engineering is employment of an engineering perspective of understanding system function in terms of underlying component properties, with the cells and tissues being the system and the molecular mechanisms being the components. Thus cell and tissue functions must be quantified and related to molecular properties that serve as the key design parameters. This paradigm is made especially powerful by the capability derived from molecular cell biology to alter molecular properties intentionally, permitting rational system design based on the identified parameters.

102.1 Basic Principles

The fundamental aspects of cell engineering are twofold: (1) quantitative understanding of cell function in molecular terms and (2) ability to manipulate cell function through molecular mecha-

0-8493-8346-3/95/$0.00+$.50
© 1995 by CRC Press, Inc.

nisms, whether by pharmacologic or genetic intervention or by introduction of materials or devices. Elucidation of basic technical principles that will stand a relatively long-term test of time is difficult because the field of molecular cell biology continues to experience incredibly rapid and unpredictable advances. However, an attempt can be made to at least outline central principles along the two fundamental lines cited above. First, one can consider the basic categories of cell function that may be encountered in cell engineering applications. These include proliferation, adhesion, migration, uptake and secretion, and differentiation. Second, one can consider basic categories of regulation of these functions. Two major loci of regulation are gene expression and structural/enzymatic protein activity; these processes act over relatively long-term (hours) and short-term (seconds to minutes) time spans, respectively. Thus a cell can change the identities and quantities of the molecular components it makes as well as their functional productivity. A third locus of regulation, which essentially encompasses the other, is receptor-mediated signaling. Molecular ligands interacting with cell receptors generate intracellular chemical and mechanical signals that govern both gene expression and protein activity and thus essentially control cell function.

At the present time, bioengineering efforts to manipulate cell behavior in health care technologies are primarily centered on development of materials, devices, and molecular or cellular therapies based on receptor-ligand interactions. These interactions are amenable to engineering approaches when relevant biochemical and biophysical properties of receptors and their ligands are identified [Lauffenburger and Linderman, 1993]. Examples of such efforts and the basic principles known at the present time to be involved are described below in three categories of current major activity: cell proliferation, cell adhesion, and cell migration.

102.2 Cell Proliferation

Proliferation of mammalian tissue and blood cells is regulated by signaling of growth factor receptors following ligand binding. In some cases, the resulting regulation is that of an on/off switch, in which the fraction of cells in a population that are stimulated to move into a proliferative state is related to the level of receptor occupancy; an example of this is the control of blood cell proliferation in the bone marrow [Kelley et al., 1993]. In other cases, the rate of progression through the cell cycle, governed by the rate of movement into the DNA synthesis phase, is related to the level of receptor occupancy. For two examples at least, epidermal growth factor stimulation of fibroblast proliferation [Knauer et al., 1984] and interleukin 2 stimulation of T-lymphocyte proliferation [Robb, 1982], DNA synthesis rate is linearly proportional to the number of growth factor-receptor complexes, perhaps with a minimum threshold level.

In engineering terms, two key principles emerge from this relationship. One is that the details of the biochemical signal transduction cascade are reflected in the coefficient relating DNA synthesis to the number of complexes, which represents an intrinsic mitogenic sensitivity. Thus, for a specified number of complexes, the cell proliferation rate can be altered by modifying aspects of the signal transduction cascade. The second principle is that mechanisms governing the number, and perhaps location, of growth factor-receptor complexes can influence cell proliferation with just as great an effect as signal transduction mechanisms. At the present time, it is more straightforward for cell engineering purposes to manipulate cell proliferation rates by controlling the number of signaling complexes using a variety of methods. Attempts to quantitatively analyze and manipulate components of receptor signal transduction cascades are also beginning [Mahama and Linderman, 1994; Renner et al., 1994].

Engineering methods helpful for providing desired growth factor concentrations include design of controlled-release devices [Powell et al., 1990] and biomaterials [Cima, 1994]. Endogenous alteration of ligand concentration and receptor number can be accomplished using gene transfer methods to introduce DNA that can increase ligand production or receptor expression or antisense therapy to introduce RNA that can decrease ligand production or reduce receptor expression. Levels of growth factor-receptor binding can be tuned by rational design of ligands; these might be antagonists that block binding of the normal growth factor and hence decrease complex levels or super-agonist growth factor mimics that provide for increased levels of complex formation over that of the normal growth factor. Rates or extents of receptor and ligand trafficking processes can be altered by modification of the receptor, ligand, or accessory components. Such alterations can affect the number of signaling complexes by increasing or decreasing the amount of receptor down-regulation, ligand depletion, or compartmentation of complexes from the cell surface to intracellular locations.

Regulation of fibroblast proliferation by epidermal growth factor (EGF) offers an instructive example of some of these approaches. Under normal circumstances, fibroblasts internalize EGF-receptor complexes efficiently via ligand-induced endocytosis, leading to substantial down-regulation of the EGF-receptor and depletion of EGF from the extracellular medium. The latter phenomenon helps account for the requirement for periodic replenishment of serum in cell culture; although growth factors present in serum could in principle operate as catalysts generating mitogenic signals through receptor binding, they generally behave as pseudonutrients because of endocytic internalization and subsequent degradation. Use of a controlled-release device for EGF delivery thus improved wound-healing responses compared with topical administration by helping compensate for growth factor depletion due to cell degradation as well as proteolysis in the tissue and loss into the bloodstream [Buckley et al., 1985]. Transfecting the gene for EGF into fibroblasts can allow them to become a self-stimulating autocrine system not requiring exogenous supplementation [Will et al., 1995]. Altering EGF/EGF-receptor trafficking can be similarly useful. Fibroblasts possessing variant EGF receptors for which ligand-induced endocytic internalization is abrogated exhibit dramatically increased proliferation rates at low EGF concentrations, primarily due to a diminished depletion of EGF from the medium [Reddy et al., 1994]. Increasing the proportion of ligands or receptors sorted in the endosome to recycling instead of degradation also reduces ligand depletion and receptor down-regulation, thus increasing the number of growth factor-receptor complexes. An instance of this is the difference in response of cells to transforming growth factor alpha compared with EGF [French et al., 1994]; the receptor-binding affinity of TGFα is diminished at endosomal pH, permitting most of the TGFα-receptor complexes to dissociate with consequently increased receptor recycling, in contrast to EGF, which remains predominantly bound to the receptor in the endosome, leading to receptor degradation. TGFα has been found to be a more potent wound-healing agent, likely due to this alteration in trafficking [Schultz et al., 1987]. Hence ligands can be designed to optimize trafficking processes for most effective use in wound-healing, cell culture, and tissue engineering applications.

Proliferation of many tissue cell types is additionally regulated by attachment to extracellular matrices via interactions between adhesion receptors and their ligands. The quantitative dependence of proliferation on adhesion receptor-ligand interactions is not understood nearly as well as that for growth factors, though a relationship between the extent of cell spreading and DNA synthesis has been elucidated [Ingber et al., 1987] and has been applied in qualitative fashion for engineering purposes [Singhvi et al., 1994]. It is likely that a quantitative dependence of proliferation on adhesion receptor-ligand binding, or a related quantity, analogous to that found for growth factors will soon be developed and exploited in similar fashion by design of attachment substrata with appropriate composition of attachment factors. Properties of the cell environment affecting molecular transport [Yarmush et al., 1992] and mechanical stresses [Buschmann et al., 1992] are also important in controlling cell proliferation responses.

102.3 Cell Adhesion

Attachment of mammalian tissue and blood cells to other cells, extracellular matrices, and biomaterials is controlled by members of the various families of adhesion receptors, including the integrins, selectins, cadherins, and immunoglobulins. Interaction of these receptors with their ligands—which are typically accessed in an insoluble context instead of free in solution—is responsible for both physical attachment and chemical signaling events. (For clarity of discussion, the term *receptor* will refer to the molecules on "free" cells, while the term *ligand* will refer to the complementary molecules present on a more structured substratum, even if that substratum is a cell layer such as blood vessel endothelium.) It is essential to note at the outset that biologic adhesion is a dissipative phenomenon, one which in general is nonreversible; the energy of adhesion is typically less than the energy of deadhesion. Thus cell adhesion cannot be analyzed solely in terms of a colloidal adhesion framework. Cell spreading following adhesion to a substratum is an active process requiring expenditure of energy for membrane protrusion and intracellular (cytoskeletal) motile force generation rather than being a purely passive, thermodynamic phenomenon. Similarly, migration of cells over two-dimensional and through three-dimensional environments requires involvement of adhesion receptors not only for physical transmission of motile force via traction to the substratum but also perhaps for active signaling leading to generation of the cytoskeletal motile force.

An engineering approach can be applied to design of cells, ligands, and ligand-bearing biomaterials to optimize attachment and subsequent signaling. For instance, material bearing synthetic peptides to which only a specific, desired cell type will adhere can be developed; an example is the immobilization of a unique amino acid sequence on a vascular-graft polymer to promote attachment and spreading of endothelial cells but not fibroblasts, smooth muscle cells, or platelets [Hubbell et al., 1991]. Moreover, the substratum density of a particular adhesive ligand required for proper cell spreading and leading to desired behavior can be quantitatively determined [Massia and Hubbell, 1991]. Design of substratum matrices with appropriate ligands for attachment, spreading, and proliferation in wound-healing and tissue-regeneration applications can be based on such information. These matrices also must possess suitable biodegradation properties along with appropriate mechanical properties for coordination with forces generated by the cells themselves as well as external loads [Cima et al., 1991b, Tranquillo et al., 1992].

Analyses of cell-substratum adhesion phenomena have elucidated key design parameters of receptor-ligand interactions as well as cell and substratum mechanics. An important principle is that the strength of adhesion is proportional to the receptor-ligand equilibrium binding affinity in a logarithmic manner [Kuo and Lauffenburger, 1993], so to alter adhesion strength by an order of magnitude requires a change in binding affinity by a factor of roughly 10^3. Cells possess the capability to accomplish this via covalent modification of proteins, leading to changes in effective affinity (i.e., avidity) either through direct effects on receptor-ligand binding or through indirect effects in which the state of receptor aggregation is modified. Aggregation of adhesion receptors into organized structures termed *focal contacts* leads to dramatic increases in adhesion strength because distractive forces are distributed over many receptor-ligand bonds together, as demonstrated experimentally [Lotz et al., 1989] and explained theoretically [Ward and Hammer, 1993]. Hence biochemical processes can lead to changes in biophysical properties. The fact that physical forces can affect distribution of receptor-ligand bonds and probably other protein-protein interactions suggests that biophysical processes can similarly alter cellular biochemistry [Ingber, 1993].

Cells are able to regulate the mode of detachment from a substratum, with a variety of alternative sites at which the linkage can be disrupted. Between the intracellular cytoskeleton and the extracellular matrix are generally a number of intermolecular connections involving the adhesion receptor. The receptor can be simply associated with membrane lipids or can be anchored by linkages to one or more types of intracellular components, some of which are also linked to actin filaments. Thus cell-substratum detachment may take place by simple ligand-receptor dissociation or extraction of the intact ligand-receptor bond from the membrane or extraction of the bond along with some intracellularly linked components. Biochemical regulation by the cell itself, likely involving covalent modification of the receptor and associated components, may serve as a means to control the mode of detachment when that is an important issue for engineering purposes. It is likely that the different superfamilies of adhesion receptors possess distinct characteristics of their micromechanical and biochemical regulation properties leading to different responses to imposed stresses generated either intracellularly or extracellularly.

A different situation involving cell adhesion is that of cell capture by a surface from a flowing fluid. Instances of this include homing of white blood cells to appropriate tissues in the inflammatory and immune responses and metastatic spread of tumor cells, both by adhesion to microvascular endothelial cells, as well as isolation of particular cell subpopulations by differential cell adhesiveness to ligand-coated materials to facilitate cell-specific therapies. In such cases, it may be desired to express appropriate attachment ligands at required densities on either the target cells or capturing surfaces or to use soluble receptor-binding competitors to block attachment in the circulation. This is a complicated problem involving application of quantitative engineering analysis of receptor-ligand binding kinetics as well as cell and molecular mechanics. Indeed, properties of adhesion receptors crucial to facilitating attachment from flowing fluid are still uncertain; they appear to include the bond-formation rate constant but also bond mechanical parameters such as strength (i.e., ability to resist dissociation or distraction from the cell membrane) and compliance (i.e., ability to transfer stress into bond-dissociating energy).

Cell-substratum attachment during encounter in fluid flow conditions can be considered under equilibrium control if the strength or affinity of bonds is the controlling parameter, whereas it is under kinetic control when the rate of bond formation is controlling [Hammer and Lauffenburger, 1987]. Most physiologic situations of cell capture from the flowing bloodstream by blood vessel endothelium appear to be under kinetic control. That is, the crucial factor is the rate at which the first receptor-ligand bond can be formed; apparently the bond strength is sufficiently great to hold the cell at the vessel wall despite the distracting force due to fluid flow. Rolling of neutrophils along the endothelium is mediated by members of the selectin family, slowing the cells down for more stable adhesion and extravasation mediated by members of the integrin family. It is not yet clear what special property of the selectins accounts for their ability to yield rolling behavior; one candidate is a combination of both fast association and dissociation rate constants [Lawrence and Springer, 1991], whereas another is a low compliance permitting the dissociation rate constant to be relatively unaffected by stress [Hammer and Apte, 1992]. It will be important to determine what the key properties are for proper design of capture-enhancing or -inhibiting materials or regimens.

102.4 Cell Migration

Movement of cells across or through two- and three-dimensional substrata, respectively, is governed by receptor-ligand interactions in two distinct ways. First, active migration arising from intracellular motile forces requires that these forces can be effectively transmitted to the substratum as differential traction. Adhesion receptors, mainly of the integrin superfamily, are involved in this process. Integrin interactions with their extracellular matrix ligands can influence the linear cell translocation speed. Second, the intracellular motile forces must be stimulated under the specific conditions for which movement is desired. Often, the ligands that stimulate cytoskeletally generated motile forces can do so in a spatially dependent fashion; i.e., cells can be induced to extend membrane lamellipodia preferentially in the direction of higher ligand concentrations, leading to net movement up a ligand concentration gradient. These ligands are termed *chemotactic attractants;* many such attractants can additionally modulate movement speed and are thus also termed *chemokinetic agents.* Chemotactic and chemokinetic ligands include some growth factors as well as other factors seemingly more dedicated to effects on migration.

Two different types of intracellular motile forces are involved, one that generates membrane lamellipod extension and one that generates cell body contraction; it is the latter force that must be transmitted to the substratum as traction in order for locomotion to proceed. Indeed, it must be transmitted in a spatially asymmetrical manner so that attachments formed at the cell front can remain adhered, while attachments at the cell rear are disrupted. Since the contraction force is likely to be isotropic in nature, this asymmetry must arise at the site of the force-transmission linkage. Migration speed of a particular cell type on a given ligand-coated surface thus depends on (1) generation of intracellular motile forces leading to lamellipod extension and to subsequent cell body contraction, stimulated by chemokinetic and/or chemotactic ligand binding to corresponding receptors or by adhesion receptor binding to appropriate soluble or substratum-bound ligands, (2) an appropriate balance between intracellular contractile force and overall level of cell-substratum traction, and (3) a significant front versus rear difference in cell-substratum traction. Speed should be roughly proportional to the first and last quantities but dependent on the middle quantity in biphasic fashion—maximal at an intermediate level of motile force-to-traction-force ratio [DiMilla et al., 1991].

Since many adhesion ligands stimulate intracellular motile force generation, an important parameter for design purposes is thus the effective density at which they are present on the substratum. Migration should be maximized at an intermediate density at which the cell contraction force is roughly in balance with the cell-substratum adhesiveness, consistent with observations for both two-dimensional [DiMilla et al., 1993] and three-dimensional [Parkhurst and Saltzman, 1992] movement environments. Since adhesive force is related to the ligand-receptor binding affinity, use of ligands with different affinities provides a means for migration under conditions of different ligand densities. Recalling also that the degree of receptor organization into aggregates can dramatically increase cell-substratum adhesiveness, use of ligands yielding different degrees of receptor aggregation can similarly influence migration speed. Engineering attempts to development useful substrata for cell migration, e.g., for wound-healing scaffolding or tissue-regeneration biomaterials also need to consider possible effects of microarchitecture, i.e., the physical geometry of three-dimensional matrices through which the cells may crawl and ligands or nutrients may diffuse [Cima and Langer, 1993].

Addition of soluble receptor-binding ligand competitors into the extracellular medium is another approach to affecting cell migration speed by means of altered cell-substratum adhesiveness. As the concentration of a competitor is increased, adhesiveness should decrease. However, since migration speed varies with adhesiveness in biphasic manner, the result of adding the competitor can be either a decrease or an increase in motility, depending on whether the adhesiveness in the absence of the competitor is below or above optimal [Wu et al., 1994]. For example, the rate of blood capillary formation, which is related to the speed of microvessel endothelial cell migration, can be either diminished or enhanced by addition of soluble integrin-binding competitors [Nicosia and Bonnano, 1991; Gamble et al., 1993].

Finally, migration speed may be altered genetically, e.g., by changing the expression level of an adhesion receptor [Schreiner et al., 1989]. An increase in the number of receptors may lead to either an increase or a decrease in motility, depending on whether the change in adhesiveness is helpful or detrimental. At the same time, signaling for motile force generation, if it occurs through the same receptor, will provide an accompanying positive influence. Receptors may be altered in their ligand-binding or cytoskeleton-coupling capabilities as well, providing alternative approaches for affecting force transmission.

Attempts to manipulate the direction of cell migration fall into three categories: soluble chemotactic ligands, immobilized haptotactic ligands, and contact guidance. *Haptotaxis* is commonly referred to as directed migration on a density gradient of an immobilized ligand, regardless of whether it is due to differential adhesiveness or to spatially dependent membrane extension. If the latter effect is causative, the phenomenon should be more precisely termed *chemotaxis* but merely with an immobilized ligand; the classic definition of haptotaxis requires an adhesion effect. Examples in which efforts have been made to manipulate the direction of cell migration including homing of cytotoxic lymphocytes to tumor sites, neovascularization of healing wound tissue, and neuron outgrowth.

Contact guidance can be produced using either patterned substrata, in which pathways for cell migration are delineated by boundaries of adhesiveness [Kleinfeld et al., 1988], or by alignment of matrix fibers for directional orientation of cell movement [Dickinson et al., 1994]. A useful technology for generation of ligand concentration gradients is controlled release of chemotactic ligands from polymer matrices [Edelman et al., 1991]. Gradients required for effective cell guidance have been found to be approximately a few percent in concentration across a cell length, and they must persist for many multiples of the cell mean path length; this is the product of the persistence time (i.e., the mean time between significant direction changes) and the linear speed. Analysis has predicted that the affinity of a chemotactic ligand or, more precisely, the dissociation rate constant may be a key parameter in governing the sensitivity of a cell to a chemotactic ligand concentration gradient [Tranquillo et al., 1988]. Data on directional responses of neutrophil leukocytes to gradients of interleukin 8 show that these cells respond more sensitively to variants of IL-8 possessing lower binding affinities [Clark-Lewis et al., 1991]. Although this finding is consistent with theory, involvement of multiple forms of the IL-8 receptor with possibly varying signaling capabilities also must be considered as an alternative cause. Work with platelet-derived growth factor as a chemotactic attractant has elucidated features of the PDGF receptor involved in sensing ligand gradients, permitting approaches for pharmacologic or genetic manipulation of chemotactic receptors to modify directional migration responses [Kundra et al., 1994].

References

Buckley A, Davidson JM, Kamerath CD, et al. 1985. Sustained release of epidermal growth factor accelerates wound repair. Proc Natl Acad Sci USA 82:7340.

Buschmann MD, Gluzband YA, Grodzinsky AJ, et al. 1992. Chondrocytes in agarose culture synthesize a mechanically functional extracellular matrix. J Orthop Res 10:745.

Cima LG. 1994. Polymer substratas for controlled biological interactions. J Coll Biochem 56:155.

Cima LG, Vacanti JP, Vacanti C, et al. 1991. Tissue engineering by cell transplantation using degradable polymer substrates. ASME Trans J Biomec Eng 113:143.

Cima LG, Langer R. 1993. Engineering human tissue. Chem Eng Progr June:46.

Clark-Lewis I, Schumacher C, Baggiolini M, Moser B. 1991. Structure-activity relationships of IL-8 determined using chemically synthesized analogs. J Biol Chem 266:23128.

Darnell J, Lodish H, Baltimore D. 1986. Molecular Cell Biology. New York, Scientific American Books.

Dickinson RB, Guido S, Tranquillo RT. 1994. Correlation of biased cell migration and cell orientation for fibroblasts exhibiting contact guidance in oriented collagen gels. Ann Biomed Eng 22:342.

DiMilla PA, Barbee K, Lauffenburger DA. 1991. Mathematical model for the effects of adhesion and mechanics on cell migration speed. Biophys J 60:15.

DiMilla PA, Stone JA, Quinn JA, et al. 1993. An optimal adhesiveness exists for human smooth muscle cell migration on type-IV collagen and fibronectin. J Cell Biol 122:729.

Edelman ER, Mathiowitz E, Langer R, Klagsbrun M. 1991. Controlled and modulated release of basic fibroblast growth factor. Biomaterials 12:619.

French AR, Sudlow GP, Wiley HS, Lauffenburger DA. 1994. Postendocytic trafficking of EGF-receptor complexes is mediated through saturable and specific endosomal interactions. J Biol Chem 269:15749.

Gamble JR, Mathias LJ, Meyer G, et al. 1993. Regulation of in vitro capillary tube formation by anti-integrin antibodies. J Cell Biol 121:931.

Hammer DA, Apte SA. 1992. Simulation of cell rolling and adhesion on surfaces in shear flow: General results and analysis of selectin-mediated neutrophil adhesion. Biophys J 63:35.

Hammer DA, Lauffenburger DA. 1987. A dynamical model for receptor-mediated cell adhesion to surfaces. Biophys J 52:475.

Hubbell JA, Massia SP, Desai NP, Drumheller PD. 1991. Endothelial cell-selective materials for tissue engineering in the vascular graft via a new receptor. Biotechnology 9:568.

Ingber DE. 1993. The riddle of morphogenesis: a question of solution chemistry or molecular cell engineering? Cell 75:1249.

Ingber DE, Madri JA, Folkman J. 1987. Endothelial growth factors and extracellular matrix regulate DNA synthesis through modulation of cell and nuclear expansion. In Vitro Cell Dev Biol 23:387.

Kelly JJ, Koury MJ, Bondurant MC, et al. 1993. Survival or death of individual proerythroblasts results from differing erythropoietin sensitivities: A mechanism for controlled rate of erythrocyte production. Blood 82:2340.

Kleinfeld D, Kahler KH, Hockberger PE. 1988. Controlled outgrowth of dissociated neurons on patterned substrates. J Neurosci 8:4098.

Knauer DJ, Wiley HS, Cunningham DD. 1984. Relationship between epidermal growth factor receptor occupancy and mitogenic response: Quantitative analysis using a steady-state model system. J Biol Chem 259:5623.

Kundra V, Escobedo JA, Kazlauskas A, et al. 1994. Regulation of chemotaxis by the PDGF-receptor β. Nature 367:474.

Kuo SC, Lauffenburger DA. 1993. Relationship between receptor/ligand binding affinity and adhesion strength. Biophys J 65:2191.

Lauffenburger DA, Aebischer P. 1993. Cell and tissue engineering: overview. In Research Opportunities in Biomolecular Engineering: The Interface Between Chemical Engineering and Biology. US Dept of Health and Human Services Administrative Document, pp 109–113.

Lauffenburger DA, Lindermann JJ. 1993. Receptors: Models for Binding, Trafficking, and Signaling. New York, Oxford University Press.

Lotz MM, Burdsal CA, Erickson HP, McClay DR. 1989. Cell adhesion to fibronectin and tenascin: Quantitative measurements of initial binding and subsequent strengthening response. J Cell Biol 109:1795.

Mahama P, Linderman JJ. 1994. Monte Carlo study on the dynamics of G-protein activation. Biophys J 67:1345.

Massia SP, Hubbell JA 1991. An RGD spacing of 440 nm is sufficient for integrin $\alpha_v\beta_3$-mediated fibroblast spreading and 140 nm for focal contact and stress fiber formation. J Cell Biol 114:1089.

Nerem RM. 1991. Cellular engineering. Ann Biomed Eng 19:529.

Nicosia RF, Bonanno E. 1991. Inhibition of angiogenesis in vitro by RGD-containing synthetic peptide. Am J Pathol 138:829.

Parkhurst M, Saltzman WM. 1992. Quantification of human neutrophil motility in three-dimensional collagen gels: Effect of collagen concentration. Biophys J 61:306.

Powell EM, Sobarzo MR, Saltzman WM. 1990. Controlled release of nerve growth factor from a polymeric implant. Brain Res 515:309.

Reddy CC, Wells A, Lauffenburger DA. 1994. Proliferative response of fibroblasts expressing internalization-deficient EGF receptors is altered via differential EGF depletion effects. Biotech Progr 10:377.

Renner WA, Hatzimanikatis V, Eppenberger HM, Bailey JE. 1994. Recombinant cyclin E overexpression enables proliferation of CHO K1 cells in serum- and protein-free medium. Preprint from Institute for Biotechnology, ETH-Hoenggerberg, Zurich, Switzerland.

Robb RJ. 1982. Human T-cell growth factor: Purification, biochemical characterization, and interaction with a cellular receptor. Immunobiology 161:21.

Schreiner CL, Bauer JS, Danilov YN, et al. 1989. Isolation and characterization of chinese hamster ovary cell variants deficient in the expression of fibronectin receptor. J Cell Biol 109:3157.

Schultz GS, White M, Mitchell R, et al. 1987. Epithelial wound healing enhanced by TGFα and VGF. Science 235:350.

Singhvi R, Kumar A, Lopez GP, et al. 1994. Engineering cell shape and function. Science 264:696.

Tranquillo RT, Lauffenburger DA, Zigmond SH. 1988. A stochastic model for leukocyte random motility and chemotaxis based on receptor binding fluctuations. J Cell Biol 106:303.

Tranquillo RT, Durrani MA, Moon AG. 1992. Tissue engineering science: Consequences of cell traction force. Cytotechnology 10:225.

Ward MD, Hammer DA. 1993. A theoretical analysis for the effect of focal contact formation on cell-substrate attachment strength. Biophys J 64:936.

Will BH, Lauffenburger DA, Wiley NS. 1995. Studies on engineered autocrine systems: Requirements for ligand release from cells producing an artificial growth factor. Tissue Engineering 1:81.

Wu P, Hoying JB, Williams SK, et al. 1994. Integrin-binding peptide in solution inhibits or enhances endothelial cell migration, predictably from cell adhesion. Ann Biomed Eng (in press).

Yarmush ML, Toner M, Dunn JCY, et al. 1992. Hepatic tissue engineering: Development of critical technologies. Ann NY Acad Sci 21:472.

103

Metabolic Engineering

Craig Zupke
Massachusetts General Hospital
and the Shriners Burns Institute

Metabolic engineering can be defined as the modification of cellular metabolism to achieve a specific goal. Metabolic engineering can be applied to both prokaryotic and eukaryotic cells, although applications to prokaryotic organisms are much more common. The goals of metabolic engineering include improved production of chemicals endogenous to the host cell, alterations of the substrate required for growth and product synthesis, synthesis of new products foreign to the host cell, and addition of new detoxification activities. As metabolic engineering has evolved, some general principles and techniques have emerged. In particular, developments in genetic engineering enable highly specific modification of cellular biochemical pathways. However, the complexity of biologic systems and their control severely limits the ability to implement a rational program of metabolic engineering. Early attempts at metabolic engineering were based on a simplistic analysis of cellular biochemistry and did not live up to expectations [Stephanopoulos and Sinskey, 1993]. An important realization is that metabolism must be considered as a network of interrelated biochemical reactions. The concept of a single rate-limiting step usually does not apply—instead, the control of a metabolic pathway is frequently distributed over several steps. The choice of specific modifications to achieve a desired goal is difficult because of this distributed nature of control. These issues are especially relevant in medical applications of metabolic engineering, where there is the added complication of interacting organ systems.

　　The field of metabolic engineering is still young, and advancements are continuing, especially in the analysis of metabolic networks and their control. Recent advances include techniques for the experimental determination of kinetic or control parameters necessary to apply established mathematical formalisms to metabolic networks. Coupled with computer optimization and simulation, these techniques should lead to a greater success rate for the directed modification of cellular metabolism. In addition, the knowledge and experience gained from engineering cellular metabolism can be applied to individual organs or to the whole body to help guide the development and evaluation of new drugs and therapies.

8493-8346-3/95/$0.00+$.50
© 1995 by CRC Press, Inc.

103.1 Basic Principles

Metabolic engineering is inherently multidisciplinary, combining knowledge and techniques from cellular and molecular biology, biochemistry, chemical engineering, mathematics, and computer science. The basic cycle of metabolic engineering is summarized in the flowsheet in Fig. 103.1. The first step in the process is to define the problem or goal to which metabolic engineering will be applied. The next step is to analyze the relevant biochemistry to determine the specific modifications that will be attempted. Recombinant DNA techniques are then used to implement the modifications, and the analysis of their impact completes one pass through the metabolic engineering cycle. This process is continued in an iterative fashion until the desired result is achieved. In the discussion that follows, each step of the cycle will be addressed individually.

103.2 Problem Definition

As mentioned above, the typical goals of metabolic engineering include improving the production of endogenous chemicals, altering the organism substrate requirements, synthesizing new products, and adding new detoxification activities. There are a variety of ways that these goals can be achieved through genetic engineering and mutation and selection. Through genetic engineering, heterologous enzymes can be added to a cell, either singly or in groups. The addition of new enzymatic activities can be used to meet any of the metabolic engineering goals. Mutation and selection can be used to affect the regulation of particular enzymes and thus are most useful for altering metabolite flow.

Addition of New Activities

The distinction between product formation, substrate utilization, and detoxification is simply a matter of emphasizing different aspects of a metabolic pathway. In product formation, the end of a metabolic pathway is the focal point. In substrate utilization and detoxification, it is the input to the pathway that is important. With detoxification, there is the additional requirement that the toxin is converted to less harmful compounds, but what they are is not important. In the discussion that follows, the addition of new activity for the synthesis of new products will be emphasized. However, since they all involve adding new activity to a metabolic pathway, the same techniques used for the synthesis of new products also can be used to alter substrate requirements or add new detoxification activity.

There are several possible strategies for the synthesis of new products. The choice of strategy depends on the biochemistry present in the host organism and the specific product to be synthesized. In many instances, pathway completion can be used, which only involves the addition of a few enzymes that catalyze the steps missing from the existing metabolic pathway. Entire biochemical pathways also can be transferred to a heterologous host. The motivation for this type of transfer is that the host organism may be more robust, have a more desirable substrate requirement, or have inherently higher productivities than the organism that naturally possesses the biochemical pathway of interest. The transfer of multistep pathways to heterologous hosts has been used frequently for the production of antibiotics because of the clustering of the genes in-

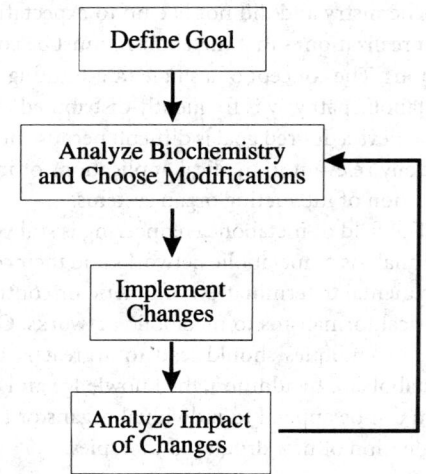

FIGURE 103.1   The metabolic engineering cycle.

volved [Malpartida, 1990]. When the genes are clustered, they can be cloned and inserted into the host organism as a single unit.

The procedures described above involve the transfer of a known metabolic activity from one organism to another. It is also possible to create completely new products, because many enzymes can function with multiple substrates. If an enzyme is introduced into a cell and is thus presented with a metabolite similar to its normal substrate but which was not present in the donor cell, a completely new reaction may be catalyzed. Similarly, if a foreign enzymatic activity produces an intermediate foreign to the host cell, that intermediate may undergo further reactions by endogenous enzymes and produce a novel product. This phenomenon has been used to synthesize novel antibiotics in recombinant *Streptomyces* [McAlpine, 1987; Epp, 1989] and to engineer an *Escherichia coli* for the degradation of trichlorethylene [Winter, 1989]. Of course, the production of new products also may be an undesirable side effect of the introduction of a heterologous enzyme and could interfere with the production of the desired product. The complexity of enzyme activities makes the prediction of negative side effects extremely difficult.

Improving Existing Metabolism

Although a cell or organism may possess a particular metabolic pathway, the flow of material through that pathway (metabolic flux) may be suboptimal. Both recombinant DNA techniques and classic mutation-selection techniques can help to redirect metabolic fluxes. The principal ways to redirect metabolic fluxes are by increasing or decreasing the activity of specific enzymes and by changing their regulation. The choice of which enzymes and how to alter them can be very complicated because of the distributed nature of metabolic control. However, some basic concepts can be illustrated by the analysis of an idealized metabolic network for threonine synthesis, as shown in Fig. 103.2. Aspartate is the biosynthetic precursor for threonine, as well as for lysine, methionine, and isoleucine. If our goal is to maximize the production of threonine, then we may want to decrease the activity of the enzymes that catalyze the production of the other amino acids derived from aspartate. This would result in less of the carbon flow from aspartate being drawn off by the unwanted amino acids, and thus a larger flux to threonine might be achieved. An alternative way of increasing the flux to threonine is to amplify the activity of the enzymes along the pathway from aspartate to threonine. Finally, accumulation of the desired product, threonine, will lead to the reduction of flux from aspartate to ASA and from ASA to homoserine because of feedback inhibi-

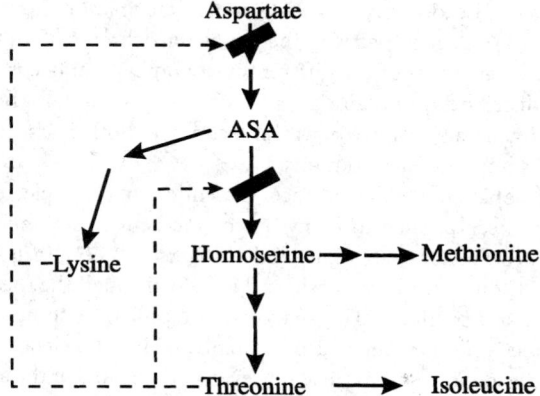

FIGURE 103.2   A simple metabolic network for threonine synthesis. The solid arrows represent enzyme catalyzed biochemical reactions. The dotted arrows indicate allosteric inhibition (ASA=aspartate semialdehyde).

tion. This would result in a reduction in threonine synthesis as well. If the feedback inhibition were removed, threonine could then accumulate without affecting its rate of synthesis. In practice, multiple modifications would probably be required to achieve the desired goal.

103.3 Analysis of Metabolic Networks

Metabolic Flux Analysis

The measurement or estimation of metabolic fluxes is useful for the evaluation of metabolic networks and their control. Direct measurement of intracellular fluxes is possible with in vivo nuclear magnetic resonance (NMR) spectroscopy. However, the inherent insensitivity of NMR limits its applicability. A more general strategy combines material balances with carefully chosen measurements to indirectly estimate metabolic fluxes. In isotopic tracer methods, a material balance is performed on the labeled isotope, and the measured isotope distribution is used to estimate the fluxes of interest. Alternatively, a total mass or carbon balance can be combined with extensive measurements of the rates of change of extracellular metabolite concentrations to calculate intracellular fluxes. Used individually or together, these methods can provide a great deal of information about the state of a biochemical system.

In isotope tracer methods, the cells to be studied are provided with a substrate specifically labeled with a detectable isotope (usually ^{14}C or ^{13}C). The incorporation of label into cellular material and by-products is governed by the fluxes through the biochemical pathways. The quantity and distribution of label are measured and combined with knowledge of the biochemistry to determine the intracellular fluxes. The choices of substrate labeling patterns, as well as which by-products to measure, are guided by careful analysis of the assumed biochemical network. These experiments are usually performed at isotopic steady state so that the flow of isotope into each atom of a metabolite equals the flux out. For the nth atom of the kth metabolite, the flux balance is [Blum, 1982]:

$$\sum_i V_{i,k} S_i(m) = S_k(n) \sum_o V_{o,k} \tag{103.1}$$

where $S_i(m)$ is the specific activity of the mth atom of the ith metabolite that contributes to the labeling of the nth atom of the kth metabolite, $S_k(n)$, and $V_{i,k}$ and $V_{o,k}$ are the input and output fluxes of the kth metabolite, respectively. The system of equations represented by Eq. (103.1) can be solved for the fluxes ($V_{i,k}, V_{o,k}$) from measurements of the specific activities. A similar analysis can be applied to the isotope isomers, or isotopomers, yielding more information from a single experiment. Isotopomer analysis is not just concerned with the average enrichment of individual atoms. Instead, it involves quantifying the amounts of the different isotopomers that occur at a specific metabolic state. The isotopomer distribution contains more information than that obtained from positional enrichments, making it generally a more powerful technique. Both mass spectrometry and NMR can be used to analyze isotopomer distributions.

Flux estimation based only on material balances is identical, in principle, to flux estimation using isotopic tracers and has been applied to many biochemical processes, including lysine synthesis [Vallino, 1989] and rat heart metabolism [Safer and Williamson, 1973]. Instead of following the fate of specific atoms (i.e., ^{13}C or ^{14}C), all are considered equally through the measurement of the rates of change of substrates and products. The analysis is simplified in some ways because only the stoichiometry of the biochemical reactions is important, and no knowledge of the chemical mechanisms is needed. Some resolving power is lost, however, with the loss of the ability to determine the source of individual reactions. The analysis is usually formulated as a matrix equation:

$$\mathbf{r} = \mathbf{Ax} \tag{103.2}$$

where $\mathbf{r}$ is a vector of metabolite rates of change, $\mathbf{A}$ is the matrix of stoichiometric coefficients for the biochemical network, and $\mathbf{x}$ is a vector of the metabolic fluxes. If the rates of change of the metabolites are measured, then Eq. (103.2) can be solved for the flux vector **x** by the method of least squares:

$$\mathbf{x} = (\mathbf{A}^T\mathbf{A})^{-1}\mathbf{A}^T\mathbf{r} \tag{103.3}$$

Typically, extracellular metabolites are measured, while intracellular metabolites are assumed to be at pseudo-steady state and their rates of change are taken to be zero.

Metabolic Control Analysis

A *biochemical network* is a system of enzyme-catalyzed reactions that are interconnected through shared metabolites. At steady state, the fluxes through each pathway will be a function of the individual enzyme kinetic properties, as well as the network architecture. The activity of a particular enzyme will affect the concentration of its reactants and products and thus will influence the flux through pathways upstream and downstream. Metabolic control analysis (MCA) grew from the work originally presented by Kacser and Burns [1973] and Heinrich and Rapoport [1977]. MCA provides a framework for analyzing and quantifying the distributed control that enzymes exert in biochemical networks.

In the discussion of that follows, a metabolic network consists of enzymes e, metabolites X, substrates S, and products P. For simplicity, we assume that the reaction rate v_i is proportional to the enzyme concentration e_i. If this is not true, then some modifications of the analysis are required [Liao and Delgado, 1993]. The concentrations of the products and substrates are fixed, but the metabolite concentrations are free to change in order to achieve a steady-state flux J. An example of a simple, unbranched network is

$$S \rightarrow X_1 \rightarrow X_2 \rightarrow X_3 \rightarrow P$$
$$e_1 \quad e_2 \quad e_3 \quad e_4$$

MCA is essentially a sensitivity analysis that determines how perturbations in a particular parameter (usually enzyme concentration) affect a variable (such as steady-state flux). The measures of the sensitivities are control coefficients defined as follows:

$$C_{e_i}^J \equiv \frac{e_i}{J}\frac{\partial J}{\partial e_i} = \frac{\partial \ln |J|}{\partial \ln e_i} \tag{103.4}$$

The flux control coefficient $C_{e_i}^J$ is a measure of how the flux J changes in response to small perturbations in the concentration or activity of enzyme i. The magnitude of the control coefficient is a measure of how important a particular enzyme is in the determination of the steady-state flux. The summation theorem relates the individual flux control coefficients:

$$\sum_i C_{e_i}^J = 1 \tag{103.5}$$

A large value for $C_{e_i}^J$ indicates that an increase in the activity of enzyme $i(e_i)$ should result in a large change in the metabolic flux. Thus enzymes with large flux control coefficients may be good targets for metabolic engineering. Usually, there are several enzymes in a network with comparably large C values, indicating that there is no single rate-limiting enzyme.

The challenge in analyzing a metabolic network is determination of the flux control coefficients. It is possible to determine them directly by "enzyme titration" combined with the measurement of the new steady-state flux. For in vivo systems, this would require alteration of enzyme expression through an inducible promoter and is not very practical for a moderately sized network. A more common method of altering enzyme activities involves titration with a specific inhibitor. However, this technique can be complicated by nonspecific effects of the added inhibitor and unknown inhibitor kinetics [Liao and Delgado, 1993].

    Although the control coefficients are properties of the network, they can be related to individual enzyme kinetics through elasticity coefficients. If a metabolite concentration X is altered, there will be an effect on the reaction rates in which X is involved. The elasticity coefficient $\epsilon_X^{v_i}$ is a measure of the effect changes in X have on v_i, the rate of reaction catalyzed by enzyme e_i:

$$\epsilon_X^{v_i} \equiv \frac{X}{v_i}\frac{\partial v_i}{\partial X} = \frac{\partial \ln v_i}{\partial \ln X} \tag{103.6}$$

The flux control connectivity theorem relates the flux control coefficients to the elasticity coefficients:

$$\sum_i C_{e_i}^J \epsilon_{X_k}^{v_i} = 0 \qquad \text{for all } k \tag{103.7}$$

In principle, if the enzyme kinetics and steady-state metabolite concentrations are known, then it is possible to calculate the elasticities and through Eq. (103.7) determine the flux control coefficients.

Flux Control Coefficients from Transient Metabolite Concentrations

Recent efforts to address the difficulty of determining MCA parameters include the use of transient measurements of metabolite concentrations to give good estimates of the flux control coefficients [Delgado and Liao, 1992]. The key assumption in the dynamic approach is that the reaction rates are reasonably linear around the steady state. When this is true and a transient condition is induced (by changing substrate or enzyme concentration), the transient fluxes $v_i(t)$ are constrained by the following equation:

$$\sum_{i=1}^{r} C_{e_i}^J v_i(t) = J \tag{103.8}$$

where r equals the number of reactions in the network. Measurements of transient metabolite concentration allow the determination of regression coefficients α_i from the following equation:

$$\sum_{i=1}^{n} \alpha_i [X_i(t) - X_i(0)] = 0 \tag{103.9}$$

where n equals the number of metabolites measured. The flux control coefficients are then determined from

$$[C_{e_1}^J \quad C_{e_2}^J \quad \cdots \quad C_{e_r}^J] = J[\alpha_1 \quad \alpha_2 \quad \cdots \quad \alpha_n]\mathbf{A} \tag{103.10}$$

where $\mathbf{A}$ is the matrix of stoichiometric coefficients. Using this method requires the measurements of transient metabolite concentrations, which are used to calculate the α_i values, and the accumulation or depletion of external metabolites to determine the steady-state flux J. The measurement of transient metabolite concentrations can be difficult but is possible with in vivo NMR or from cell extracts taken at different time points.

"Top Down" MCA

The traditional approach of MCA can be considered to be "bottom up," since all the individual enzyme flux control coefficients are determined in order to describe the control structure of a large network. The "top down" approach makes extensive use of lumping of reactions together to determine group flux control coefficients [Brown, 1990]. These can give some information about the overall control of a metabolic network without its complete characterization.

Consider a simple, multireaction pathway:

$$S \rightarrow \rightarrow \rightarrow X \rightarrow \rightarrow \rightarrow P$$

$$\text{produces } X \qquad \text{consumes } X$$

$$J_1 \qquad\qquad\qquad J_2$$

The reactions of a metabolic network are divided into two groups, those which produce a particular metabolite X and those which consume it. By manipulating the concentration of X and measuring the resulting fluxes J_1 and J_2, "group" or "overall" elasticities $*\epsilon$ of the X producers and X consumers can be determined. Application of the connectivity theorem (Eq. 103.7) then permits the calculation of the group control coefficient for both groups of reactions. Each pathway can subsequently be divided into smaller groups centered around different metabolites, and the process repeated. The advantage of the top-down approach is that useful information about the control architecture of a metabolic network can be obtained more quickly. This approach is particularly appropriate for highly complex systems such as organ or whole-body metabolism.

Large Deviations

One of the limitations of MCA is that it only applies when the perturbations from the steady state are small. Experimentally, it is much easier to induce large changes in enzyme or metabolite concentrations, and in terms of metabolic engineering, the desired perturbations are also likely to be large. Small and Kacser [1993a, 1993b] have developed an analysis based on large deviations and related it to MCA.

In this discussion, e_i^0 is the original concentration of enzyme i, $e_i^r = re_i^0$, where r is noninfinitesimal. Thus e_i^r represents a large perturbation to the system. J^0 is the flux at the original steady state, and J^r is the flux after the large perturbation. A deviation index D is used to characterize the change from the original steady state:

$$D_{e_i}^{J^r} = \left(\frac{\Delta J}{\Delta e_i}\right)\frac{e_i^r}{J^r} \tag{103.11}$$

where $\Delta J = J^r - J^0$ and $\Delta e_i = e_i^r - e_i^0$. By assuming that each individual enzymatic reaction rate is a linear function of the participating metabolites, it can be shown that the deviation index and control coefficients are equivalent:

$$D_{e_i^r}^{J^r} = C_{e_i^0}^{J^0} \tag{103.12}$$

Similarly, an alternate deviation index $*D$ can be defined as

$$*D_{e_i}^{J^r} = \left(\frac{\Delta J}{\Delta e_i}\right)\frac{e_i^0}{J^0} \tag{103.13}$$

and it is equivalent to the control coefficient at the new steady state:

$$D_{e_i^r}^{J^r} = C_{e_i^r}^{J^r} \tag{103.14}$$

Thus, with a single large perturbation, the control coefficients at the original and new steady states can be estimated. This analysis has been extended to branched pathways, but relationships between the deviation indices and the flux control coefficients are more complicated and depend on the magnitude of the deviation (r). If the subscript a designates one branch and b another, the following relationship holds:

$$D_{e_a^r}^{J_b^r} = C_{e_a^0}^{J_b^0} \frac{1}{1 - \left(C_{e_a^0}^{J_a^0} - C_{e_a^0}^{J_b^0} \right) \frac{r-1}{r}} \qquad (103.15)$$

Metabolic control analysis, especially with the recent innovations for determining flux control coefficients, is a powerful tool for the analysis of metabolic networks. It can describe the control architecture of a biochemical reaction network and identify which steps are the most promising targets for efforts at metabolic engineering.

Pathway Synthesis

The diversity of biochemical reactions found in nature is quite extensive, with many enzymes being unique to a particular organism. Through metabolic engineering, it is possible to construct a metabolic network that performs a specific substrate-to-product transformation not found in nature. When exploring the possibility of synthesizing new biochemical pathways, there are several key issues that must be addressed. Given a database of possible enzymatic activities and a choice of substrate and product, one must first generate a complete set of possible biochemical reactions that can perform the desired conversion. Once they are generated, the set of possible biochemical pathways must be checked for thermodynamic feasibility and evaluated in terms of yields, cofactor requirements, and other constraints that might be present. In addition, the impact of an engineered metabolic pathway on the growth and maintenance of the host cell is also important to evaluate.

The problem of synthesizing a complete set of possible biochemical pathways subject to constraints on allowable substrates, intermediates, and by-products has been solved [Mavrovouniotis, 1990]. A computer algorithm allows the efficient determination of a complete and correct set of biochemical pathways that connect a substrate to a product. In addition, a complementary computer algorithm evaluates metabolic pathways for thermodynamic feasibility [Mavrovouniotis, 1993]. The key concept in the thermodynamic analysis is that evaluation of the feasibility of biologic reactions requires the specification of the concentrations of the products and reactants. The standard free-energy change ΔG^0 is not sufficient because physiologic conditions are significantly different from standard conditions. Both local and distributed thermodynamic bottlenecks can be determined by incorporating knowledge of the metabolite concentration ranges. This thermodynamic analysis of a biochemical pathway can pinpoint specific reactions or groups of reactions that should be modified or bypassed in order to better favor product formation.

The addition of new biochemical pathways or the modification of existing pathways is likely to affect the rest of the cellular metabolism. The new or altered pathways may compete with other reactions for intermediates or cofactors. To precisely predict the impact of a manipulation of a metabolic network is virtually impossible, since it would require a perfect model of all enzyme kinetics and of the control of gene expression. However, with relatively simple linear optimization techniques, it is possible to predict some of the behavior of a metabolic network. The procedure involves the solution of Eq. (103.2) for the metabolic fluxes for networks that have more unknowns $\mathbf{x}$ than knowns $\mathbf{r}$. An underdetermined system of linear equations can be solved uniquely using linear optimization techniques if a "cellular objective function" is postulated. Examples of objective functions used in the literature include minimizing ATP or NADH production [Savinell, 1992] and maximizing growth or product formation [Varma, 1993]. Examination of the fluxes gotten from the linear optimization can indicate potential effects of a proposed metabolic change. For example, the maximum growth rate of *E. coli* was found to decrease in a piecewise linear fashion as leucine production increased [Varma, 1993]. In principle, linear optimization also could be applied to whole-body metabolism to evaluate the effects of metabolically active drug or genetic therapies.

3.4 Implementing Changes

The techniques available to implement specific changes in both eukaryotic and prokaryotic cells are quite powerful. Through classic mutation-selection and modern genetic engineering, it is possible to amplify or attenuate existing enzyme activity, add completely new activities, and modify the regulation of existing pathways. A detailed description of all the genetic engineering techniques available is beyond the scope of this discussion, and only a general overview will be presented.

Mutation-Selection

Mutation and selection constitute a method of manipulating the phenotype of a cell. Cells are exposed to a mutagenic environment and then placed in a selective medium in which only those cells which have a desired mutation can grow. Alternatively, cells can be screened by placing them in a medium in which it is possible to visibly detect those colonies which possess the desired phenotype. Although it is a random process, careful design of selection or screening media can result in alterations in specific enzymes. For example, growth in a medium that contains an allosteric inhibitor may be the result of the loss of the allosteric inhibition. By altering metabolite concentrations or adding substrate analogues, it is possible to select for increased or decreased activity or for changes in regulation. The major drawback of mutation and selection for metabolic engineering is the lack of specificity. There may be multiple ways that a particular phenotype can be generated, so there is no guarantee that the enzyme that was targeted was affected at all.

Recombinant DNA

Recombinant DNA techniques are very flexible and powerful tools for implementing specific metabolic changes. The cloning of genes encoding a specific enzyme is relatively routine, and the subsequent insertion and expression are also straightforward for many host cells. With the choice of a very active promoter, the activity of a cloned enzyme can be greatly amplified. In addition, insertion of a heterologous activity into a host cell can serve to alter the regulation of a metabolic pathway, assuming the foreign enzyme has different kinetics than the original. Enzyme activity also can be attenuated by antisense sequences that produce mRNA complementary to the endogenous mRNA and thus form double-stranded RNA complexes that cannot be translated. Finally, heterologous recombination can be used to completely remove a particular gene from the host genome.

03.5 Analysis of Changes

The techniques used to analyze the biochemistry at the beginning of the metabolic engineering cycle are also applicable for assessing the effects of any attempted changes. The effect of the specific change can be evaluated, as well as its impact on the activity of the whole metabolic network. It is quite possible for a desired change to be made successfully at the enzyme level but not have the desired effect on the metabolic network. If a change was partially successful, then the resulting cells can be put through another iteration of metabolic engineering in order to make further improvements. If, on the other hand, a particular change was not successful, then any information which that failure gives about the regulation and control of the metabolic network can be used to make another attempt at implementing the desired change.

03.6 Summary

Metabolic engineering is an evolving discipline that tries to take advantage of the advances which have been made in the genetic manipulation of cells. Through genetic engineering we have the capability of making profound changes in the metabolic activity of both prokaryotic or eukaryotic cells. However, the complexity of the regulation of biochemical networks makes the choice of modifications difficult. Recent advances in the analysis of metabolic networks via MCA or other techniques have provided some of the tools needed to implement a rational metabolic engineering program. Finally, metabolic engineering is best viewed as an iterative process, where attempted modifications are evaluated and the successful cell lines improved further.

Defining Terms

Flux: The flow of mass through a biochemical pathway. Frequently expressed in terms of moles of metabolite or carbon per unit time.

Heterologous enzyme: An enzyme from a foreign cell that has been expressed in a host cell. Frequently used to provide activity normally not present or to alter the control structure of a metabolic network.

Host: The cell that has had foreign DNA inserted into it.

Isotopomers: Isomers of a metabolite that contain different patterns of isotopes (for metabolic studies, the carbon isotopes ^{12}C, ^{13}C, and ^{14}C are the most commonly analyzed).

Metabolic engineering: The modification of cellular metabolism to achieve a specific goal. Usually performed with recombinant DNA techniques.

Metabolic network: A system of biochemical reactions that interact through shared substrates and allosteric effectors.

Pathway completion: The addition of a small number of heterologous enzymes to complete a biochemical pathway.

References

Blum JJ, Stein RB. 1982. On the analysis of metabolic networks. In RF Goldberger, KR Yamamoto (eds), Biological Regulation and Development, pp 99–125. New York, Plenum Press.

Brown GC, Hafner RP, Brand MD. 1990. A "top-down" approach to the determination of control coefficients in metabolic control theory. Eur J Biochem 188:321.

Delgado J, Liao JC. 1992. Determination of flux control coefficients from transient metabolite concentrations. Biochem J 282:919.

Epp JK, Huber MLB, Turner JR, et al. 1989. Production of a hybrid macrolide antibiotic in Streptomyces ambofaciens and Streptomyces lividans by introduction of a cloned carbomycin biosynthetic gene from Streptomyces thermotolerans. Gene 85:293.

Heinrich R, Rapoport TA. 1974. Linear steady-state treatment of enzymatic chains: General properties, control, and effector strength. Eur J Biochem 42:89.

Kascer H, Burns JA. 1973. Control of [enzyme] flux. Symp Soc Exp Biol 27:65.

Liao JC, Delgado J. 1993. Advances in metabolic control analysis. Biotechnol Prog 9:221.

Malpartida F, Niemi J, Navarrete R, Hopwood DA. 1990. Cloning and expression in a heterologous host of the complete set of genes for biosynthesis of the Streptomyces coelicolor antibiotic undercylprodigiosin. Gene 93:91.

Mavrovouniotis ML, Stephanopoulos G, Stephanopoulos G. 1990. Computer-aided sysnthesis of biochemical pathways. Biotechnol Bioeng 36:1119.

Mavrovouniotis ML. 1993. Identification of localized and distributed bottlenecks in metabolic pathways. In Proceedings of the International Conference on Intelligent Systems for Molecular Biology, Washington.

McAlpine JB, Tuan JS, Brown DP, et al. 1987. New antibiotics from genetically engineered Actinomycetes: I. 2-Norerythromycins, isolation and structural determination. J Antibiot 40:1115.

Safer B, Williamson JR. 1973. Mitochondrial-cytosolic interactions in perfused rat heart. J Biol Chem 248:2570.

Savinell JM, Palsson BO. 1992. Network analysis of intermediary metabolism using linear optimization: I. Development of mathematical formalism. J Theor Biol 154:421.

Small JR, Kacser H. 1993a. Responses of metabolic systems to large changes in enzyme activities and effectors: I. The linear treatment of unbranched chains. Eur J Biochem 213:613.

Small JR, Kacser H. 1993b. Responses of metabolic systems to large changes in enzyme activities and effectors: II. The linear treatment of branched pathways and metabolite concentrations. Assessment of the general non-linear case. Eur J Biochem 213:625.

Stephanopoulos G, Sinskey AJ. 1993. Metabolic engineering—Methodologies and future prospects. TIBTECH 11:392.

Vallino JJ, Stephanopoulos G. 1989. Flux determination in cellular bioreaction networks: Applications to lysine fermentations. In SK Sikdar et al (eds), Frontiers in Bioprocessing, pp 205–219. Boca Raton, Fla, CRC Press.

Varma A, Boesch BW, Palsson BO. 1993. Biochemical production capabilities of Escherichia coli. Biotechnol Bioeng 42:59.

Winter RB, Yen K-M, Ensley BD. 1989. Efficient degradation of trichloroethylene by recombinant Escherishia coli. Biotechnology 7:282.

Further Information

An extensive review of recent applications of metabolic engineering can be found in Cameron DD, Tong IT. 1993. Cellular and metabolic engineering: An overview. *Appl Biochem Biotechnol* 38:105. A pioneering discussion of the emerging field of metabolic engineering can be found in Bailey JE. 1991. Toward a science of metabolic engineering. *Science* 252:1668. A good source of information about recombinant DNA techniques is Gliman M, Watson JD, Witkowski J, et al. 1992. *Recombinant DNA,* 2d ed. San Francisco, WH Freeman.

104

Tissue Engineering

François Berthiaume
Massachusetts General Hospital, Harvard University Medical School, and the Shriners Burns Institute

Martin L. Yarmush
Rutgers University, Massachusetts General Hospital, Harvard University Medical School, and the Shriners Burns Institute

Tissue engineering can be defined as the application of scientific principles to the design, construction, modification, growth, and maintenance of living tissues. Tissue engineering can be divided into two broad categories: (1) in vitro construction of bioartificial tissues from cells isolated by enzymatic dissociation of donor tissue and (2) in vivo alteration of cell growth and function. The first category of applications includes bioartificial tissues (i.e., tissues that are composed of natural and synthetic substances) to be used as an alternative to organ transplantation. Besides their potential clinical use, reconstructed organs also may be used as tools to study complex tissue functions and morphogenesis in vitro. For tissue engineering in vivo, the objective is to alter the growth and function of cells in situ, an example being the use of implanted polymeric tubes to promote the growth and reconnection of damaged nerves. Some representative examples of applications of tissue engineering currently being pursued are listed in Table 104.1.

Conceptually, bioartificial tissues involve three-dimensional structures with cell masses that are orders of magnitude greater than those used in traditional two-dimensional cell culture techniques. In addition, bioartificial organ technology often involves highly differentiated somatic and parenchymal cells isolated from normal tissues. This chapter will provide an overview on tissue reconstruction in vitro with particular emphasis on the techniques used to control cell function and organization and to scale up bioartificial tissues. Other equally important issues in tissue engineering, such as cell isolation and biomaterial fabrication, will not be presented here. A chapter on cell preservation is presented next (chap. 105).

104.1 Basic Principles and Considerations

Cell Type and Source

In tissue engineering, differentiated cells offer some advantages over tumor cell lines: (1) tumor cells often do not express the full spectrum of functions at the same level as the somatic cell lines they originated from, (2) tumor cell growth can be very rapid and uncontrollable, which can cause design

0-8493-8346-3/95/$0.00+$.50
© 1995 by CRC Press, Inc.

TABLE 104.1 Representative Applications of Tissue Engineering

Application	Examples
Implantable device	Endothelialized vascular grafts
	Bone and cartilage implants
	Bioartificial skin
	Bioartificial pancreatic islets
	Neurotransmitter-secreting cells
Extracorporeal device	Bioartificial liver
Cell production	Hematopoiesis in vitro
In situ tissue growth and repair	Nerve regeneration
	Artificial skin

problems (e.g., clogging of microchannels), and (3) there is a potential risk of seeding tumor cells in the patient. Notwithstanding these limitations, appropriate selection of procedures can be used to derive tumor cell lines that are easily propagated, are contact-inhibited, and maintain most of the parent somatic cell features.

Certain human cell types can be propagated easily using standard culture techniques, such as human keratinocytes [Parenteau et al., 1991]. Conversely, other cell types, such as adult hepatocytes or pancreatic islet cells, do not replicate to any appreciable extent in vitro. Because there is currently a shortage of human organs, animal sources are also considered. Success in using xenogeneic cells will depend largely on our ability to control the immunologic response of the host to these cells as well as the proteins they produce. Genetic engineering offers the possibility of creating new cells (i.e., cells that perform a new function) that are easy to grow (e.g., fibroblasts); however, care must be taken to verify that these cells also exhibit the necessary control mechanisms for responding appropriately to the host's metabolic changes.

Control of Cell Function by the Extracellular Matrix

Since the vast majority of mammalian cells are anchorage-dependent, they must attach and spread on a substrate to proliferate and function normally. Cell adhesion is generally mediated by certain extracellular matrix proteins such as fibronectin, vitronectin, laminin, and collagen, as well as various glycosaminoglycans. Adsorption of these proteins to surfaces and the conformation of the adsorbed proteins appear to be important factors influencing cell attachment and growth on synthetic substrates [Grinnell and Feld, 1981]. Small sequences of the cell binding region of these proteins (RGDS in fibronectin and vitronectin, YIGSR in laminin) also can be covalently attached to surfaces to promote cell-substrate adhesion [Massia and Hubbel, 1990].

In general, seeding density is important for normal cell function, especially if cell-cell communications must be established, either by direct cell-cell contacts or via the secretion of trophic factors by the cells. Efficient cell seeding will mainly depend on (1) the affinity of certain cell surface proteins for extracellular matrix components, (2) the density of cell-substrate binding sites on the material surface, and (3) the presence or absence of certain nutritional factors. While the first two factors can be controlled independently of the number of cells placed on the surface, the last issue can be problematic because attempts at seeding large numbers of cells can significantly deplete nutrients, with the result that fewer cells than expected will attach. This point is discussed below in the section on metabolic requirements of cells.

After seeding, the cells spread on the surface and reach a stable shape. The final morphology of the cells depends on three factors: (1) adherence of the substrate for the cells, which is a function of the affinity and number of the adhesion sites, (2) rigidity of the substrate (i.e., ability to resist cell-generated tractional forces), and (3) cell-cell adherence. The effect of substrate adherence and compliance on cell shape and function has been studied on hepatocytes. Increased adherence by increasing the amount of fibronectin adsorbed on a surface leads to increased cell spreading, increased DNA synthesis, and reduced expression of liver-specific functions [Mooney et al., 1992]. Conversely, reduced adherence or the use of a compliant substrate where little spreading is observed helps maintain liver-specific function but reduces DNA synthesis [Lindblad et al., 1991]. The quantitative difference between cell-substrate and cell-cell adhesion strength on a rigid substrate is also a potential factor that may dramatically affect the organization of cells on the substrate. A thermodynamic view of the problem suggests that the overall system (consisting of the cells and the extracellular support) ultimately reaches an equilibrium state when the surface free energy is minimized [Martz et al., 1974]. According to this hypothesis, the existence of large cell-substrate adhesion forces relative to cell-cell adhesion forces may be a sufficient condition to prevent cell-cell overlapping. In contrast, the opposite situation would lead to cell clumping or multilayered growth on the substrate. This prediction is in agreement with the observation of cellular aggregate formation when hepatocytes are plated on a nonadherent surface as opposed to a highly adherent surface such as type I collagen [Koide et al., 1990].

One of the most striking features of endothelial and epithelial cells (as opposed to connective tissue cells such as fibroblasts) is the organization of the membrane, which exhibits distinct basal and apical domains, where different proteins and receptors are found. Most epithelial cells can be cultured on a single surface of plastic or extracellular matrix materials, which allows the basal surface to be in contact with the substrate and the apical surface to be exposed to the liquid medium. Changing the extracellular matrix configuration can induce these cells to adopt different morphologies. For example, capillary endothelial cells grown on a single collagen gel reorganize into branching capillary-like structures when overlaid with a second layer of collagen [Montesano et al., 1983]. Unlike most epithelial cells, which exhibit only two distinct membrane domains (one apical and one basal), hepatocytes possess two basolateral surfaces separated by a belt of apical membrane. To express and maintain this particular phenotype, these cells have been cultured between two layers of extracellular matrix, thereby creating a "sandwich" configuration that closely mimics the in vivo geometry. Examples of the effect of the extracellular matrix on cell shape and function are summarized in Table 104.2.

Control of Tissue Organization

New ways to control cell distribution and shape on surfaces are being developed. These methods provide finer control of cell distribution and creation of microstructures (e.g., microchannels) at the a scale that rivals that of natural organs.

The current approach to control cell distribution at size scales down to cell size (10 μm) involves micropatterning techniques. A micropatterning technique based on the utilization of photoreactive

TABLE 104.2 Effect of Extracellular Matrix (ECM) on Cell Shape and Function

ECM Characteristic			Hepatocytes*	
Surface Chemistry	Geometry	Cell shape[†]	Liver-Specific Function	Capillary Endothelial Cell Shape[‡]
1 ng/cm² fibronectin on polystyrene	Single surface	Round (1.2)	+	
1000 ng/cm² fibronectin on polystyrene	Single surface	Spread, flat (5)	−	
0.1% w/v collagen gel	Single surface	Spread, flat (3.5)	−	Cobblestone, flat
	Sandwich	Cuboidal, flat (1.5)	+	Capillary network
Heat denatured collagen	Single surface	Round, cell aggregates	+	
Basement membrane extract	Single surface	Round, cell aggregates	+	Capillary network

*Data from Mooney et al. [1992], Lindblad et al. [1990], and Ezzell [1993].
[†]The number in parentheses indicates the projected surface area relative to that of isolated hepatocytes (~1200 μm²).
[‡]Data from Montesano et al. [1983] and Madri and Williams [1983].

cross-linking of hydrophobic or hydrophilic compounds to a polymeric surface has been described recently. Cells attach and grow along the less hydrophilic micropatterned domains. Micropatterned surfaces produced with this technique have been used to produce two-dimensional neuronal networks with neuroblastoma cells [Matsuda et al., 1992]. Small micropatterned adherent squares of different sizes have been used to control the extent of spreading of hepatocytes [Bhatia et al., 1994; Singhvi et al., 1994].

The control of cell orientation may be important when nonisotropic connective tissues are desired. For example, cells can be mixed with a chilled solution of collagen in physiologic buffer followed by exposure to 37°C to induce the gellation of the collagen. The result is a loose gel comprised of small collagen fibrils where cells and fluid are entrapped. Fibroblasts embedded in a collagen gel cause the contraction of the gel [Bell et al., 1979]. The contraction process can be controlled to a certain extent by mechanically restricting the motion along certain directions; this also induces a preferential alignment of the collagen fibers as well as the cells within it. A mathematical description of the effect of cell tractional forces on the deformation of collagen-cell lattices and the resulting alignment of the collagen fibers has been presented by Tranquillo et al. [1994]. Other strategies to align cells have been reported: (1) alignment of fibroblasts in collagen gels where collagen fibrils were aligned by a magnetic field during gellation [Guido and Tranquillo, 1993], (2) repetitive stretching of endothelial cells cultured on an extensible surface [Banes, 1993], and flow-induced alignment of endothelial cells [Girard et al., 1993].

Heterotypic cell systems or "coculture" systems have been used for the production of skin grafts, in long-term cultures of hepatocytes, and in long-term cultures of mixed bone marrow cells. These systems take advantage of the trophic factors (for the most part unknown) secreted by "feeder" cells. Greater use of different cell types in coculture will enable engineered cell systems to closely mimic in vivo organization, with potential benefits including increased cell function and viability and greater range of functions expressed by the bioartificial tissue. The organization of multicellular three-dimensional structures may not be obvious. Provided that the adherence of homotypic and heterotypic interactions is known, a thermodynamic analysis similar to that used to describe the morphology of a pure cell culture on a surface can be used to predict how cells will organize in these systems [Wiseman et al., 1972]. The process of cell-cell sorting in multicellular systems may be altered by changing the composition of the medium or altering the expression of proteins mediating cell-cell adhesion via genetic engineering [Kuhlenschmidt et al., 1982; Nose et al., 1988].

Metabolic Requirements of Cells

Oxygen is very often the limiting nutrient in reconstructed tissues. The oxygen requirements vary largely with cell type. Among cells commonly used in bioartificial systems, hepatocytes and pancreatic islet cells are particularly sensitive to the availability of oxygen. Oxygen is required for efficient cell attachment and spreading to planar surfaces as well as microcarriers [Foy et al., 1993; Rotem et al., 1994].

Based on a simple mathematical model, we can estimate the critical distance at which the oxygen concentration at the cell surface becomes limiting (this concentration is arbitrarily set equal to K_m) if an unstirred aqueous layer is placed between the gas phase (air) and a confluent monolayer of cells [Yarmush et al., 1992]. In the case of a confluent monolayer of hepatocytes (2×10^5 cells/cm^2), this distance is 0.95 mm. Thus, in a first approximation, a successful bioartificial liver system containing hepatocytes will have to keep the diffusional distance between the oxygen-carrying medium and the cells to below 1 mm (assuming a confluent cell monolayer on the surface).

Figure 104.1 can be used to estimate the maximum half-thickness of a cell mass surrounded by a membrane or external diffusion barrier before the nutrient concentration in the center falls below the Michaelis-Menten constant for nutrient uptake, a sign of nutrient limitation at the cellular level. Oxygen uptake rate parameters for different cell types are given by Fleischaker and Sinskey [1981]. Values for hepatocytes and pancreatic islets can be found in Yarmush et al. [1992], Rotem et al.

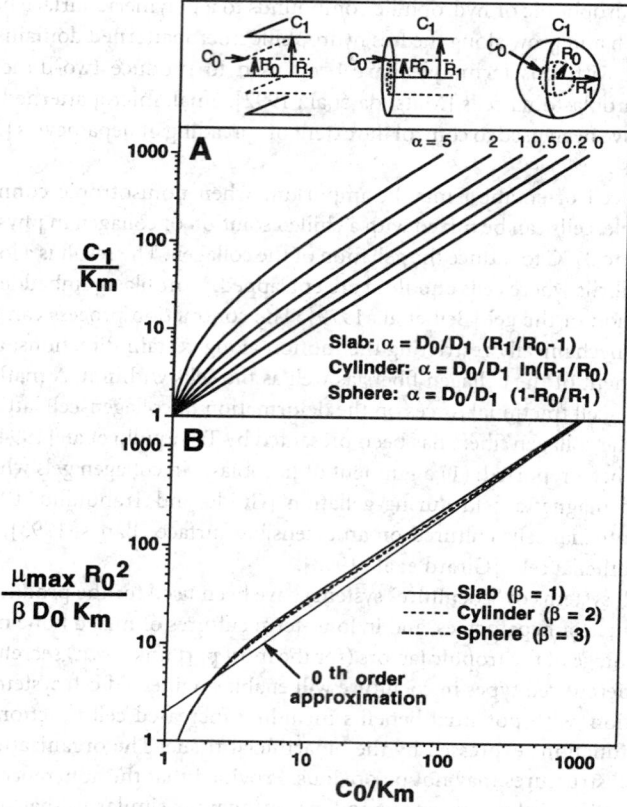

FIGURE 104.1 Correlation to predict the maximum half-thickness R of a cell mass surrounded by a shell of thickness $R_1 - R_0$ without nutrient limitation, assuming that diffusion is the only transport mechanism involved. (*a*) The nutrient concentration at the surface of the cell mass normalized to the Michaelis-Menten constant for the nutrient uptake by the cells (C_0/K_m) is obtained from the normalized bulk nutrient concentration (C_1/K_m) and the aspect ratio of the system (R_1/R_0). D_0 and D_1 are the diffusivities for the nutrient within the cell mass and the external diffusion barrier, respectively. The partition coefficient between the cell mass and the surrounding shell is assumed to be equal to 1. (*b*) The half-thickness R for which $C/K_m = 1$ in the center ($R = 0$) is obtained from the value of the y axis corresponding to C_0/K_m, knowing, in addition to the parameters listed above, the maximum nutrient uptake rate by the cells (μ_{max}). If K_m is unknown, a zero-order approximation may be used, in which case K_m is set arbitrarily so that C_1/K_m falls in the linear portion of the curve in (*a*). In (*b*), R_0 is obtained using the line labeled "0th order approximation" and corresponds to the half-thickness R for which $C = 0$ at the center ($R = 0$).

[1992], and Dionne et al. [1989]. For illustrative purposes, we will use cylindrical hepatocyte aggregates as an example. We assumed the following: no external diffusion barrier (R_1/R_0) = 1; medium saturated with air at 37°C at the aggregate surface (160 mmHg = 190 mmol/cm³); diffusivity of oxygen in aggregates (D_0) similar to that in water (2×10^{-5} cm²/s); a packed cell mass (given a cell diameter of approximately 20 μm, this corresponds to 1.25×10^8 cells/cm³). The oxygen uptake parameters for hepatocytes were $\mu_{max} = 0.4$ nmol/10^6 cells/s (thus 50 nmol/cm³/s for the preceding cell concentration) and $K_m = 0.5$ mmHg (e.g., 0.6 nmol/cm^3). We obtain $C_1/K_m = C_0/K_m = 320$, $(\mu_{max}R^2)/(D_0K_m) = 724$, 1370, and 2010 for the slab, cylindrical, and spherical geometries, respectively, and thus the corresponding maximum half-thicknesses obtained are $R = 132$, 181, and 220 μm, respectively. We now consider the case where there is a 100-μm-thick membrane around a cylindrical cell aggregate assuming that the diffusivity of oxygen in the membrane (D_1) is the same as in the cell mass. An aspect ratio (α) must be assumed, and the values of C_0/K_m, $(\mu_{max}R^2)/(D_0K_m)$, and R_0 are calculated. R_1 is then obtained from the assumed aspect ratio. Calculations must be performed with several aspect ratios until the difference $R_1 - R_0$ equates the membrane thickness. Here, we found that $\alpha = 0.6$ generates $C_0/K_m = 141$, $(\mu_{max}R^2)/(D_0K_m) = 622$, and $R_0 = 122$ μm. For a cylinder, $\alpha = D_0/D_1 \ln(R_1/R_0)$, and thus in this case $R_1 = 222$ μm. Thus the maximum half-thickness of the cell mass is 122 μm, as compared with 181 μm in the absence of the membrane. These estimates can be used as first guidelines to design a bioartificial liver, and they clearly suggest that the thickness of the cell mass must be limited to a few hundred microns to prevent the formation of an anoxic core.

4.2 Reconstruction of Connective Tissues

The most simple method to create connective tissue in vitro is to incorporate connective tissue cells within a loose network of extracellular matrix components. A dermal equivalent has been produced by embedding fibroblasts in collagen gels [Bell et al., 1979]. When fibroblasts (2.5×10^4/ml) were seeded in collagen, the collagen lattice contracted 30- to 50-fold after 4 days of culture. The result is a dense cell-collagen matrix that can be used to support a cultured epidermis. Another example is the production of a bioartificial vascular media by seeding smooth muscle cells in collagen tubes [Weinberg and Bell, 1986]. In the latter case, orientation of the cells along the circumference of the tube may be necessary in order to eventually obtain a tissue with contractile properties similar to that exhibited by native blood vessels.

When reconstructing connective tissue, it may be advantageous to use a relatively low seeding density with the expectation that cell replication together with the migration of blood vessels from the host's surrounding tissue would occur after implantation. This approach may not be appropriate for tissues that grow slowly and that are subjected to high stresses after implantation. This is the case of bioartificial cartilage, which would be best implanted once its mechanical properties are similar to those of the authentic tissue. Chondrocytes seeded at high density (10^7 cells/cm^3) in agarose gels and in serum-free medium retain their phenotype and remain viable for up to 6 months [Bruckner et al., 1989]. In this system, the deposition of type II collagen and highly charged proteoglycans can be observed over a period of 43 days [Buschmann et al., 1992]. The cartilage obtained in the latter studies had a stiffness of approximately one-third that of the cartilage explants used to isolate the cells. It should be recognized that in these experiments the cell density was considerably lower than that found in the native cartilage explants (7.5×10^7 cells/cm^3). Higher chondrocyte seeding density in the initial gel could potentially yield a material with mechanical properties closer to that of native cartilage.

Meshes made of slowly biodegradable polymers may be particularly suitable for dense connective tissue synthesis, such as bone and cartilage. Loose meshes made of lactic and glycolic acid copolymer seeded with calf chondrocytes (5×10^7/ml) have been shown to harbor the production of cartilage in vitro [Freed et al., 1993]. In the same studies, meshes seeded with cells were implanted in nude mice and recovered at different times following implantation. Implants excised at the 7-week time point consisted almost entirely of cartilage-like tissue with an overall shape similar to that of the original synthetic matrix. Histochemical analysis of the specimens revealed the presence of type II collagen and sulfated glycosaminoglycans at week 7 and later.

Angiogenesis may be necessary if there is cell growth in the reconstructed tissue after implantation. Because open matrices are used mainly to reconstruct these tissues, the host's capillaries can migrate into the implant. The presence of angiogenic factors (e.g., heparin-binding growth factor 1) may be used to improve the kinetics of implant vascularization [Thompson et al., 1989].

104.3 Reconstruction of Epithelial or Endothelial Surfaces

Cells Embedded in Extracellular Matrix Materials

A simple way to maintain certain epithelial cells in a three-dimensional matrix is to seed them in gels or meshes in a similar manner as connective tissues are constructed. For example, hepatocytes can be maintained in the same mesh-type matrices made of biodegradable materials used to create bioartificial cartilage [Cima et al., 1991]. In this configuration, hepatocytes have a tendency to aggregate; such aggregates (sometimes called *organoids*) are known to contain cells that have maintained their phenotypic stability [Koide et al., 1990]. However, this process may be somewhat limited unless the aggregate size can be controlled to prevent the formation of large aggregates with anoxic cores. Also, this method may not be used to produce continuous epithelial cell sheets.

Culture on a Single Surface

Bioartificial vascular grafts have been produced by seeding endothelial cells on the luminal surface of small-diameter (6 mm or less) synthetic vascular grafts. These prostheses have given poor results because of inflammatory responses at the anastomotic sites and the poor retention of the seeded endothelium under in vivo conditions. A more intrinsically biocompatible approach to vascular graft production is to reproduce more closely the organization of actual blood vessels. For instance, a bioartificial media has been produced by embedding vascular smooth muscle cells in a collagen gel annulus and the intima reestablished by seeding endothelial cells on the inside surface of the gel [Weinberg and Bell, 1986].

A dermal equivalent consisting of fibroblasts embedded in collagen has been used to support a stratified layer of human keratinocytes [Parenteau et al., 1991]. Exposure to air induces the terminal differentiation of the keratinocytes near the air-liquid interface, which is characterized by the formation of tight cell-cell contacts and cornified envelopes. The resulting bioartificial skin has a morphologic and biochemical organization very similar to that of real skin, including a stratum corneum that exhibits a high resistance to chemical damage. This type of bioartificial skin has been tested successfully in animals, but acceptance of allogeneic skin grafts remains problematic in humans, which means that the production of grafts requires that both fibroblasts and keratinocytes be obtained from the patient and propagated in vitro.

Culture in a Sandwich Configuration

This culture technique has been used successfully to maintain hepatocyte polarity and function in vitro. Hepatocytes are first plated on a single gel of collagen, and then a top layer of type I collagen is placed on the cells after 1 day in culture. The resulting extracellular geometry closely mimics that found in vivo and maintains a wide spectrum of liver-specific functions, including protein secretion (e.g., albumin, transferrin, and fibrinogen) and detoxification (e.g., cytochrome P450–dependent pathways), for up to 6 to 8 weeks [Dunn et al., 1991].

104.4 Bioreactor Design in Tissue Engineering

A *bioreactor* is a system containing a large number of cells that transform an input of reactants into an output of products. Bioreactors have been designed primarily for use as bioartificial liver or pancreas and more recently for the production of blood cells from hematopoietic tissue. These systems require the maintenance of the function of a large number of cells in a small volume. For example, a hypothetical bioartificial liver device possessing 10% of the detoxification and protein-synthesis capacity of the normal human liver (a rough estimate of the minimum processing and secretory capacities that can meet a human body's demands) would contain a total of 10^{10} adult hepatocytes. Thus, to keep the total bioreactor volume within reasonable limits (1 liter or less), 10^7 cells per milliliter or more are required. For comparison, the normal human liver contains approximately 10^8 hepatocytes per milliliter. Two main types of bioreactor designs have been considered in tissue engineering: (1) hollow-fiber systems and (2) microcarrier systems.

Hollow-Fiber Systems

Hollow-fiber systems consist of a shell traversed by a large number of small-diameter tubes. The cells may be placed within the fibers in the intracapillary space or on the shell side in the extracapillary space. The compartment that does not contain the cells is generally perfused with culture medium or the patient's plasma or blood. The fiber walls may provide the attaching surface for the cells and/or act as barrier against the immune system of the host. Some of these systems are essentially designed to be implanted as vascular shunts but also may be perfused with the patient's blood or plasma extracorporeally.

For the selection of fiber dimensions, spacing, and reactor length, the reader is referred to previously published experimental and theoretical studies [Chresand et al., 1988; Piret and Cooney, 1991]. If the pressure gradient across the fiber length is sufficiently high and relatively permeable fibers are used, the pressure difference between the inlet and outlet induces convective flow (called *Starling flow*) across the fiber wall and through the shell compartment [Kelsey et al., 1990; Pillarella and Zydney, 1990]. The maintenance of Starling flow in implanted hollow-fiber devices is contingent on the prevention of a gradual decrease in fiber permeability due to protein deposition over time on the fiber walls, which may be difficult to achieve with fluids containing high levels of proteins such as plasma.

There are several reports in the literature describing the use of hollow-fiber systems in the development of a bioartificial pancreas [Colton and Avgoustiniatos, 1991; Ramírez et al., 1992]. Most designs place the islets on the shell side while perfusing the fibers with the animal's plasma or blood. Recent studies using implantable devices connected to the vascular system of the patient have given some encouraging results [Sullivan et al., 1991], but it appears that none of the pancreatic islet devices tested to date has shown long-term function in a reproducible manner. It is interesting to note that none of the studies involving pancreatic islets encapsulated in hollow-fiber systems has recognized that oxygen transport can be severely compromised within the isolated islets alone, resulting in a substantial reduction in the insulin secretion capacity of the islets in response to glucose changes [Dionne et al., 1993].

It may be advantageous to place cells in the lumina of small fibers because the diffusional distance between the shell (where the nutrient supply would be) and the cells is essentially equal to the fiber diameter, which is easier to control than the interfiber distance. In one configuration, cells have been suspended in a collagen solution and injected into the lumen of fibers where the collagen is allowed to gel. Contraction of the collagen lattice by the cells creates a void in the intraluminal space [Scholz and Hu, 1991]. Such a configuration has been described for the construction of a bioartificial liver using adult hepatocytes [Nyberg et al., 1993]. It has been further proposed that the lumen be perfused with culture medium containing the appropriate hormones for cell maintenance, while the patient's plasma would flow on the shell side.

Microcarrier-Based Systems

Microcarriers are small beads (usually less than 500 μm in diameter) with surfaces treated to support cell attachment. The surface area available per microcarrier can be increased by using porous microcarriers, where cells can migrate and proliferate within the porous matrix as well as on the microcarrier surface. Porous ceramic beads have been used to support a rat cell line transfected with the human proinsulin gene [Park and Stephanopoulos, 1993]; under certain conditions, intraparticle flow significantly enhances mass transport (especially that of oxygen) to the cells in the beads [Stephanopoulos and Tsiveriotis, 1989].

Maintaining a constant number of microcarriers while increasing the number of cells increases the surface coverage of the microcarriers as long as the concentration of nutrients (especially oxygen) is not limiting. With the adult rat hepatocyte–Cytodex 3 microcarrier system, we observed that sufficient supply of oxygen to the hepatocytes is required for the efficient attachment (approximately 90%) of cells to microcarriers. A simple oxygen diffusion-reaction model indicated that a cell surface oxygen partial pressure greater than 0.1 mmHg was needed [Foy et al., 1993].

Two bioreactor configurations using microcarriers may find potential use in tissue engineering: (1) packed or fluidized bed and (2) microcarriers incorporated in hollow-fiber cartridges. A packed bed of microcarriers consists of a column filled with microcarriers with porous plates at the inlet and outlet of the column to allow perfusion while preventing microcarrier entrainment by the flow. Total flow rate is mainly dependent on cell number and the nutrient uptake rate of the cells. Reactor volume is proportional to the microcarrier diameter. From this point of view, it is therefore advantageous to reduce the microcarrier size as much as possible. However, packed beds with small beads may be potentially more prone to clogging, and the cells may have tendency to accumulate in the channels between the microcarrier surfaces. The aspect ratio of the bed (height/diameter) is adjusted so that the magnitude of fluid mechanical forces (proportional to the aspect ratio) within the bed is below damaging levels. Given a fixed flow rate and microcarrier diameter, decreasing column diameter increases fluid velocity and therefore increases the shear stress at the surface of the microcarriers and cells, with potential mechanical damage to cells. On the other hand, low aspect ratios may be difficult to perfuse evenly. Fluidized beds differ from packed beds in that the perfusing fluid motion maintains the microcarriers in suspension [Runstadler and Cerneck, 1988].

Packed-bed systems have been used to support high densities (5×10^8 cells/ml) of anchorage-dependent cell lines seeded on microporous microcarriers (589 to 850 μm in diameter) [Park and Stephanopoulos, 1993]. In addition, packed beads (1.5 mm diameter) have been used to entrap aggregates of hepatocytes. This system was shown to maintain a relatively stable level of albumin secretion (a liver-specific product) for up to 3 weeks [Li et al., 1993].

Microcarriers also have been used as a way to provide an attachment surface for anchorage-dependent cells introduced in the shell side of hollow-fiber devices, as in the case of a hollow fiber bioartificial liver device [Demetriou et al., 1986]. A flat-bed device, which is in principle similar to a hollow-fiber system (cells are separated from the circulating medium by a membrane), for the maintenance of cultured human bone marrow at high densities on porous microcarriers has been recently described [Palsson et al., 1993].

References

Banes AJ. 1993. Mechanical strain and the mammalian cell. In JA Frangos (ed), Physical Forces and the Mammalian Cell, pp 81–123. San Diego, Academic Press.

Bell E, Ivarsson B, Merill C. 1979. Production of a tissue-like structure by contraction of collagen lattices by human fibroblasts of different proliferative potential in vitro. Proc Natl Acad Sci USA 76:1274.

Bhatia SN, Toner M, Tompkins RG, Yarmush ML. 1994. Selective adhesion of hepatocytes on patterned surfaces in vitro. Ann NY Acad Sci 745:187.

Bruckner P, Hoerler I, Mendler M, et al. 1989. Induction and prevention of chondrocyte hypertrophy in culture. J Cell Biol 109:2537.

Buschmann MD, Gluzband YA, Grodzinsky AJ, et al. 1992. Chondrocytes in agarose culture synthesize a mechanically functional extracellular matrix. J Orthop Res 10:745.

Chresand TJ, Gillies RJ, Dale BE. 1988. Optimum fiber spacing in a hollow fiber bioreactor. Biotechnol Bioeng 32:983.

Cima LG, Vacanti JP, Vacanti C, et al. 1991. Tissue engineering by cell transplantation using degradable polymer substrates. J Biomech Eng 113:143.

Colton CK, Avgoustiniatos ES. 1991. Bioengineering in development of the hybrid artificial pancreas. J Biomech Eng 113:152.

Demetriou A, Chowdhury NR, Michalski S, et al. 1986. New method of hepatocyte transplantation and extracorporeal liver support. Ann Surg 204:259.

Dionne KE, Colton CK, Yarmush ML. 1993. Effect of hypoxia on insulin secretion by isolated rat and canine islets of Langherans. Diabetes 42:12.

Dunn JCY, Tompkins RG, Yarmush ML. 1991. Long-term in vitro function of adult hepatocytes in a collagen sandwich configuration. Biotechnol Prog 7:237.

Ezzell RM, Toner M, Hendricks K, et al. 1993. Effect of collagen gel configuration on the cytoskeleton in cultured rat hepatocytes. Exp Cell Res 208:442.

Fleischaker RJ Jr, Sinskey AJ. 1981. Oxygen demand and supply in culture. Eur J Appl Microbiol Biotechnol 12:193.

Foy BD, Lee J, Morgan J, et al. 1993. Optimization of hepatocyte attachment to microcarriers: Importance of oxygen. Biotechnol Bioeng 42:579.

Freed LE, Marquis JC, Nohria A, et al. 1993. Neocartilage formation in vitro and in vivo using cells cultured on synthetic biodegradable polymers. J Biomed Mater Res 27:11.

Girard PR, Helmlinger G, Nerem RM. 1993. Shear stress effects on the morphology and cytomatrix of cultured vascular endothelial cells. In JA Frangos (ed), Physical Forces and the Mammalian Cell, pp 193–222. San Diego, Academic Press.

Grinnell F, Feld MK. 1981. Adsorption characteristics of plasma fibronectin in relationship to biological activity. J Biomed Mater Res 15:363.

Guido S, Tranquillo RT. 1993. A methodology for the systematic and quantitative study of cell contact guidance in oriented collagen gels. J Cell Sci 105:317.

Kelsey LJ, Pillarella MR, Zydney AL. 1990. Theoretical analysis of convective flow profiles in a hollow-fiber membrane bioreactor. Chem Eng Sci 45:3211.

Koide N, Sakaguchi K, Koide Y, et al. 1990. Formation of multicellular spheroids composed of adult rat hepatocytes in dishes with positively charged surfaces and under other nonadherent environments. Exp Cell Res 186:227.

Kuhlenschmidt MS, Schmell E, Slife CF, et al. 1982. Studies on the intercellular adhesion of rat and chicken hepatocytes: Conditions affecting cell-cell specificity. J Biol Chem 257:3157.

Li AP, Barker G, Beck D, et al. 1993. Culturing of primary hepatocytes as entrapped aggregates in a packed bed bioreactor: A potential bioartificial liver. In Vitro Cell Dev Biol 29A:249.

Lindblad WJ, Schuetz EG, Redford KS, Guzelian PS. 1991. Hepatocellular phenotype in vitro is influenced by biphysical features of the collagenous substratum. Hepatology 13:282.

Madri JA, Williams SK. 1983. Capillary endothelial cell cultures: Phenotypic modulation by matrix components. J Cell Biol 97:153.

Martz E, Phillips HM, Steinberg MS. 1974. Contact inhibition of overlapping and differential cell adhesion: A sufficient model for the control of certain cell culture morphologies. J Cell Sci 16:401.

Massia SP, Hubbell JA. 1990. Covalently attached GRGD on polymer surfaces promotes biospecific adhesion of mammalian cells. Ann NY Acad Sci 589:261.

Matsuda T, Sugawara T, Inoue K. 1992. Two-dimensional cell manipulation technology: An artificial neural circuit based on surface microphotoprocessing. ASAIO J 38:M243.

Montesano R, Orci L, Vassalli P. 1983. In vitro rapid organization of endothelial cells into capillary-like networks is promoted by collagen matrices. J Cell Biol 97:1648.

Mooney D, Hansen L, Vacanti J, et al. 1992. Switching from differentiation to growth in hepatocytes: Control by extracellular matrix. J Cell Physiol 151:497.

Nose A, Nagafuchi A, Takeichi M. 1988. Expressed recombinant cadherins mediate cell sorting in model systems. Cell 54:993.

Nyberg SL, Shatford RA, Peshwa MV, et al. 1993. Evaluation of a hepatocyte-entrapment hollow fiber bioreactor: A potential bioartificial liver. Biotechnol Bioeng 41:194.

Palsson BO, Paek S-H, Schwartz RM, et al. 1993. Expansion of human bone marrow progenitor cells in a high cell density continuous perfusion system. Bio/Technology 11:368.

Parenteau NL, Nolte CM, Bilbo P, et al. 1991. Epidermis generated in vitro: Practical considerations and applications. J Cell Biochem 45:245.

Park S, Stephanopoulos G. 1993. Packed bed bioreactor with porous ceramic beads for animal cell culture. Biotechnol Bioeng 41:25.

Pillarella MR, Zydney AL. 1990. Theoretical analysis of the effect of convective flow on solute transport and insulin release in a hollow fiber bioartificial pancreas. J Biomech Eng 112:220.

Piret JM, Cooney CL. 1991. Model of oxygen transport limitations in hollow fiber bioreactors. Biotechnol Bioeng 37:80.

Ramírez CA, López M, Stephens CL. 1992. In vitro perfusion of hybrid artificial pancreas devices at low flow rates. ASAIO J 38:M443.

Rotem A, Toner M, Bhatia S, et al. 1994. Oxygen is a factor determining in vitro tissue assembly: Effects on attachment and spreading of hepatocytes. Biotechnol Bioeng 43:654.

Runstadler PW, Cerneck SR. 1988. Large-scale fluidized-bed, immobilized cultivation of animal cells at high densities. In Animal Cell Biotechnology, pp 306–320. London, Academic Press.

Scholz M, Hu W-S. 1991. A two-compartment cell entrapment bioreactor with three different holding times for cells, high and low molecular weight compounds. Cytotechnology 4:127.

Singhvi R, Kumar A, Lopez GP, et al. 1994. Engineering cell shape and function. Science 264:696.

Stephanopoulos GN, Tsiveriotis K. 1989. The effect of intraparticle convection on nutrient transport in porous biological pellets. Chem Eng Sci 44:2031.

Sullivan SJ, Maki T, Borland KM, et al. 1991. Biohybrid artificial pancreas: Long-term implantation studies in diabetic, pancreatomized dogs. Science 252:718.

Thompson JA, Haudenschild CC, Anderson KD, et al. 1989. Heparin-binding growth factor 1 induces the formation of organoid neovascular structures in vivo. Proc Natl Acad Sci USA 86:7928.

Tranquillo RT, Durrani MA, Moon AG. 1992. Tissue engineering science: Consequences of cell traction force. Cytotechnology 10:225.

Weinberg CB, Bell E. 1986. A blood vessel model constructed from collagen and cultured vascular cells. Science 230:669.

Wiseman LL, Steinberg MS, Phillips HM. 1972. Experimental modulation of intercellular cohesiveness: Reversal of tissue assembly patterns. Dev Biol 28:498.

Yarmush ML, Toner M, Dunn JCY, et al. 1992. Hepatic tissue engineering: Development of critical technologies. Ann NY Acad Sci 21:472.

Further Information

Books, reviews, and special issues of scientific and engineering journals on tissue engineering that may be of interest to the reader are listed below.

Special issue on tissue engineering. 1994. Biotechnol Bioeng, vol 43, nos 7 and 8.

Bell E (ed). 1993. Tissue Engineering: Current Perspectives. Boston, Birkhauser.

Berthiaume F, Toner M, Tompkins RG, Yarmush ML. 1993. Tissue engineering. In Implantation Biology: The Response of the Host. Boca Raton, Fla, CRC Press.

Special issue on tissue engineering. 1992. Cytotechnology, vol 10, no 3.

Special issue on tissue engineering. 1991. J Biomech Eng, vol 113, no 2.

Special issue on tissue engineering. 1991. J Cell Biochem, vol 45, nos 4–5.

Skalak R, Fox CF (eds). 1988. Tissue Engineering. UCLA symposia on molecular and cellular biology, new series, vol 107. New York, Alan R Liss.

105

Preservation Techniques for Biomaterials

Robin Coger
Massachusetts General Hospital, Harvard University Medical School, and the Shriners Burns Institute

Mehmet Toner
Massachusetts General Hospital, Harvard University Medical School, and the Shriners Burns Institute

Biomaterials—i.e., proteins, cells, tissues, and organs—are used daily to preserve life. Uses such as blood transfusions, artificial insemination, burn repair, transplantation, and pharmaceuticals rely on their availability. Natural materials, however, are labile and often deteriorate over time. To counter this effect, preservation procedures for retarding deterioration rates have been developed. Furthermore, since each biomaterial is characterized by unique compositional and physical complexities, a variety of storage techniques exists.

Table 105.1 lists examples of biomaterials that have been preserved successfully using various procedures. The list, although abbreviated, illustrates the wide range of cells, tissues, organs, and macromolecule structures that have been stored successfully and demonstrates how, in some cases (e.g., red blood cells), multiple preservation techniques may be appropriate. In the discussion that follows, four biomaterial storage procedures—nonfreezing, freeze-thaw, freeze-drying (lyophilization), and vitrification—are summarized. Nonfreezing techniques enable biomaterial storage by retarding metabolic processes and chemical reactions during cooling from physiologic to nonfreezing temperatures. With freeze-thaw techniques, the biomaterial is stored at low temperatures (usually less than $-70°C$) in crystalline form and then thawed for actual use. Lyophilized biomaterials are first frozen, then dehydrated by sublimation for storage at ambient temperature, and finally reconstituted for use. With vitrification, the biomaterial is cooled to subzero temperature in such a way that it is transformed to an amorphous solid for storage and then rewarmed for use. Each procedure—i.e., its applications and risks—will be described in more detail below. This discussion is not a comprehensive review but a general overview of the principles governing each of these four common biomaterial storage techniques.

105.1 Phase Behavior

As mentioned previously, biomaterials in their naturally occurring forms tend to deteriorate over time. Hence to achieve safe long-term storage, it is generally necessary to alter the physicochemical state of the biomaterial. One approach is to promote the transformation of the original substance

TABLE 105.1   Some Examples of Biomaterials Stored
Using Various Storage Techniques

Nonfreezing	Liver
	Kidney
	Heart valves
	Protein solutions
Freeze-thaw	Red blood cells
	Cartilage
	Bone marrow
	Skin
Lyophilization (freeze-dry)	Red blood cells
	Platelets
	Penicillin
	Collagen
	Liposomes
Vitrification	Embryos
	Islets of Langerhans
	Corneal tissue
	Drosophila melanogaster

to a form that can be stored safely and then, when needed, restored to its original state. These types of transformations can best be represented using phase diagrams.

Figure 105.1 illustrates a temperature versus concentration phase diagram, where concentration corresponds to the quantity of a hypothetical solute additive present in the solution. The diagram is particularly useful for describing phase transformations in which a thermodynamic phase of reduced energy nucleates within a parent phase. Crystallization is one example of this type of phase transformation and is a two-step process of nucleation of the new phase and its subsequent growth. If the formation of the new phase is catalyzed from the surface of foreign particles or a substrate, the growth process is triggered by heterogenous nucleation (T_{HET}). If, however, the new phase develops from the clustering of individual water molecules, growth of the new phase occurs from homogeneous nucleation (T_{HOM}) [Hobbs, 1974]. The latter type of nucleation requires higher activation energies than heterogeneous nucleation and thus occurs at lower temperatures. Figure 105.1 also illustrates the relative positions of the melting (T_M) and the glass-transition (T_G) temperature

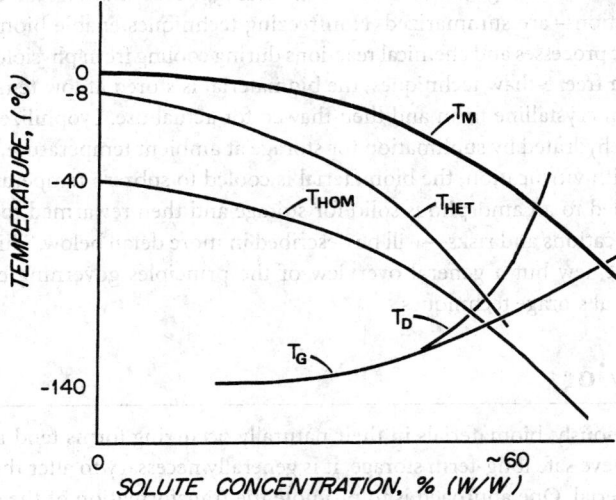

FIGURE 105.1 Phase diagram for a hypothetical solute additive.
[Adapted from Fahy et al., 1984]

curves. The melting-temperature curve shows the melting-point depression of a crystalline sample relative to solute concentration. The glass-transition curve signifies the temperatures for which a supercooled solution becomes glassy during cooling. The final curve in Fig. 105.1 (T_D) demonstrates the devitrification temperature profile and illustrates the conditions for which a substance may experience crystallization damage during warming. For glasslike solids, damage is incurred as the glass transforms to a crystalline form at T_D, while for previously crystalline or partially vitrified solids, recrystallization (the coalescence of small crystals during warming) produces damage. The described elements of the phase diagram are relevant because all the biomaterial storage techniques described in this chapter involve either a phase transformation or its avoidance. Furthermore, if a phase transformation is improperly controlled, the effects can be detrimental to the biomaterial. Four techniques relevant to biomaterial storage are now described.

105.2 Nonfreezing Storage: Hypothermic

Given the high cost of organ transplantation, longer preservation times are urgently needed to make the procedure cost-effective [Evans, 1993] and expand the geographic area over which organs can be harvested and transplanted. Presently, hypothermic storage is the clinically employed organ preservation technique.

There are essentially two techniques for hypothermic preservation of organs for subsequent transplantation. The first is static cold storage by ice immersion at ~4°C—to reduce metabolism as much as possible without the formation of deleterious ice crystals [Belzer and Southard, 1988]. The second procedure is continuous cold machine perfusion at ~10°C to provide diminished metabolism and to remove deleterious end products [Southard and Belzer, 1988]. The perfusate used for static cold storage mimics the intracellular ionic composition of the organ and has impermeant solutes added to prevent cell swelling. However, for perfusion preservation techniques in general, modified plasma or solutions of plasma-like composition usually have been preferred. This is presumably due to the slightly higher temperatures used in perfusion techniques that permit some degree of metabolism to occur during storage.

In most practical instances, simple cold storage is the preservation mode of choice, since the storage time is only slightly increased by using continuous perfusion. Furthermore, the development of the University of Wisconsin (UW) solution has dramatically extended the preservation times. In the case of human liver, for example, the storage time increased from less than 10 to about 30 hours in human liver, thus alleviating the need for continuous-perfusion storage. As a result of extensive studies, it seems that lactobionate is an essential component of the UW solution, which is believed to act as an effective osmotic agent while suppressing cell swelling in metabolically depressed cells and tissues [Southard and Belzer, 1993].

Another nonfreezing technique that can be used to retard the chemical reaction rates of a biomaterial is undercooled storage. During undercooled storage, the biomaterial is exposed to subzero temperatures in the absence of deleterious ice crystal formation. Such a method may be particularly applicable to the medium-term (months) storage of proteins. Small droplets of aqueous-based solutions are dispersed in an inert oil phase, and the final preparation is then put into test tubes for freezer storage at $T \geq -20°C$. By keeping the quantity of aqueous droplets much greater than the number of heterogeneous nucleation sites in the bulk solution, one can effectively deter heterogeneous nucleation during storage. When needed, the dispersions are removed from the freezer and warmed to room temperature and reconstituted [Franks, 1988].

Unfortunately, a chief problem in using the undercooled storage technique in biochemical applications lies in the scale-up of the procedure to the larger volumes needed for clinical and commercial applications. Furthermore, methods for "efficiently" separating the innocuous oil from the biomaterial are a problem that must be solved if the previously stored protein solutions are to be used in therapeutic applications. Apparently, it is also difficult to conduct all steps of the undercool procedure under sterile conditions [Franks, 1988].

105.3 Freeze-Thaw Technology

Freeze-thaw technology is the most commonly used method for storing cells and tissues; hence it is an important cryopreservation methodology. When a transplantation emergency arises, the preserved biomaterial can be thawed and used to save lives. In addition, the development of cell and tissue transplantation procedures also benefits the growing field of tissue engineering—where frozen biomaterials are utilized in organ replacement devices (e.g., bioartificial liver) [Borel-Rinkes et al., 1992; Karlsson et al., 1993]. Even the simple cell, however, is thermophysically complex. Consequently, the design of feasible cryopreservation protocols must incorporate knowledge from biology, engineering, and medicine to be successful.

In 1949, Polge and coworkers made an important contribution to biomaterial preservation research. In work with sperm, they were the first to report the protective effects of additives or cryoprotectant agents (CPAs), i.e., glycerol, on biomaterials at low temperatures. The mechanisms by which CPAs protect cells from freeze injury are of fundamental importance but are, unfortunately, poorly understood. There are four major protective actions of these compounds. First, CPAs act to stabilize the proteins of biomaterials under low-temperature conditions. Experimental evidence indicates that for cells, this effect results from the interaction of sugars with the polar head groups of phospholipids [McGann, 1978]. Recent thermodynamic analyses demonstrate that the preferential exclusion of CPAs from the protein hydration shell, at low temperatures, results in stabilization [Arakawa et al., 1990]. Second, CPAs lower the electrolyte concentration of the suspending medium of the cell at a given temperature by altering the phase relationship during cooling. Third, CPAs reduce the temperature at which cells undergo lethal intracellular ice formation. Fourth, CPAs promote the formation of the vitreous, rather than crystalline, phases inside the cell during cooling and help prevent intracellular ice formation (see Fig. 105.1) [Karlsson et al., 1994].

Unfortunately, the addition and removal of CPAs from the biomaterial introduce a separate set of problems. In the case of penetrating additives (i.e., dimethyl sulfoxide and glycerol), the permeability of the cell membrane is typically several orders of magnitude less than the permeability of the membrane to water [McGrath, 1988]. During the prefreeze addition of these compounds, the biomaterial recognizes the CPA as another extracellular solute. Hence the cell responds by initiating the rapid transport of water across the cell membrane and into the extracellular medium. Meanwhile, if the CPA is permeable, it gradually diffuses into the cell, thus contributing to the state of chemical nonequilibrium experienced by the cell. These transport processes continue (usually for minutes) until equilibrium is regained, at which time the volume of the biomaterial returns to normal. If the initial concentration of CPA is too large, the cell volume variations may be so severe that the biomaterial experiences osmotic stress damage. The reverse process, of cell swelling and the subsequent return to normal volume, is observed during the removal of CPAs. Osmotic injury from the addition or removal of penetrating compounds can be minimized by incrementally increasing or decreasing, respectively, their concentration.

Unfortunately, the benefits of using stepwise CPA addition and removal in reducing osmotic damage is counterbalanced by the increased risk of toxic damage to the biomaterial from longer exposure times [Fahy, 1986]. Also, in some cases, a single-step CPA removal process has been shown to be effective [Friedler et al., 1988]. The balance between these considerations can be optimized if both the permeability of the biomaterial to CPAs and the effects of the CPA on the biomaterial are known. Methodologies for measuring these critical parameters are discussed in McGrath [1988].

In the case of impermeable CPAs (i.e., polyvinylpyrrolidone, hydroxyethyl starch), the potentially injurious effects of exosmosis are also experienced. However, because impermeable CPAs remain in the extracellular medium, they are relatively easier to remove from the biomaterial than permeable additives. Their major disadvantage is believed to be their inability to afford direct protection to intracellular structures during freezing.

Figure 105.2 illustrates extrema observed when cooling biologic substances to subzero temperatures. To minimize cryoinjury, a suitable CPA is added to the biomaterial before the actual freeze-

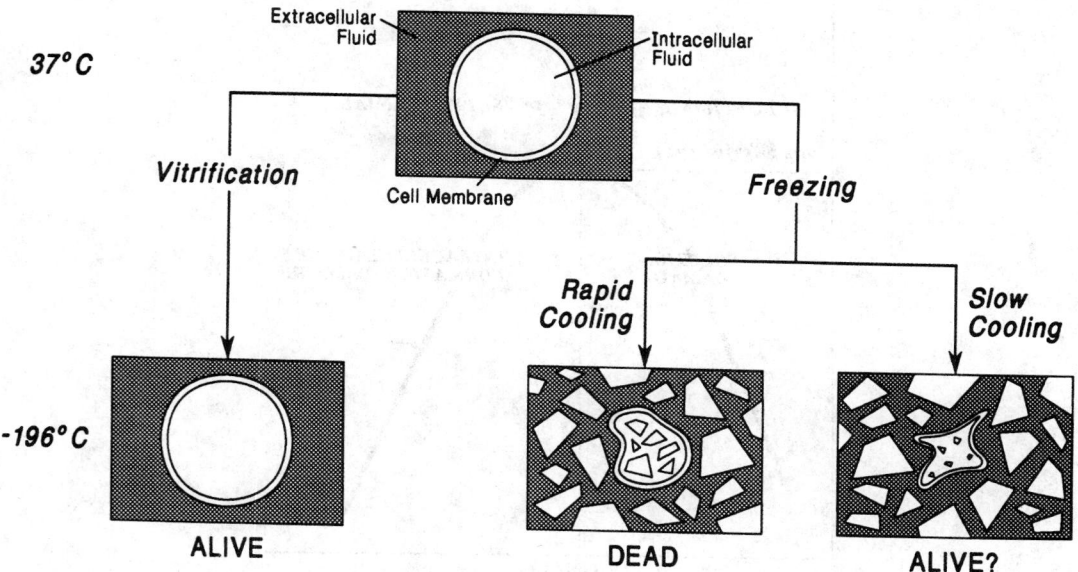

FIGURE 105.2 Schematic of the physiochemical processes experienced by cells during cryopreservation.

thaw protocol is begun. Cooling then proceeds at a controlled rate. As the material is cooled along the freezing path (Fig. 105.2), ice formation initiates first in the extracellular medium. This phase transformation is initiated either by external seeding or by heterogeneous nucleation from the walls of the container and is crucial because it corresponds to the initial temperature at which physico-chemical changes occur within the biomaterial during cooling. The formation of extracellular ice results in a chemical potential gradient across the cell membrane that can be balanced by exosmo-sis of the intracellular water. If the freezing process occurs at slow cooling rates, the intracellular fluid has sufficient time to leave the cell. However, if excessive exosmosis occurs, the result is excessive cell dehydration and shrinkage and subsequent cell death from the high concentration of solutes remaining within the cell after water diffusion. If the freezing rate is rapid, however, water entrapped in the cell becomes supercooled. Then, at some subzero temperature, thermodynamic equilibrium is achieved through intracellular ice formation. Unfortunately, intracellular ice formation is usually associated with irreversible cell damage. Although the exact damage mechanism is not known, mechanical effects and high electrolyte concentrations caused by the crystal formation are believed to be major modes of cell damage [Mazur, 1984].

Figure 105.3 schematically illustrates the relationship between cell survival and cooling rate during a freeze-thaw protocol. As shown, cell damage at suboptimal cooling rates is predominantly caused by "solution" effects (e.g., exposure to high electrolyte concentrations, decreased unfrozen fractions, excessive dehydration), until a range of peak survival is obtained at the optimal cooling rate. Experimental evidence suggests that the optimal cooling rate for maximum cellular survival is the fastest rate that will not result in intracellular ice formation. Beyond this peak, cells are exposed to supraoptimal cooling conditions, in which damage from intracellular ice formation dominates.

Theoretical models have been developed to describe both the kinetics of water loss and the prob-ability of intracellular ice formation [Mazur, 1984; Pitt, 1992; Muldrew and McGann, 1993]. The value of these models in designing effective freezing protocols for biomaterial preservation also has been demonstrated [e.g., Karlsson et al., 1993].

Once a cell or tissue sample has been frozen successfully, it can then be stored in liquid nitrogen in a −70°C freezer until needed. This step is usually not very crucial, since, as long as the freezer temperature is kept stable, storage does not cause cell damage.

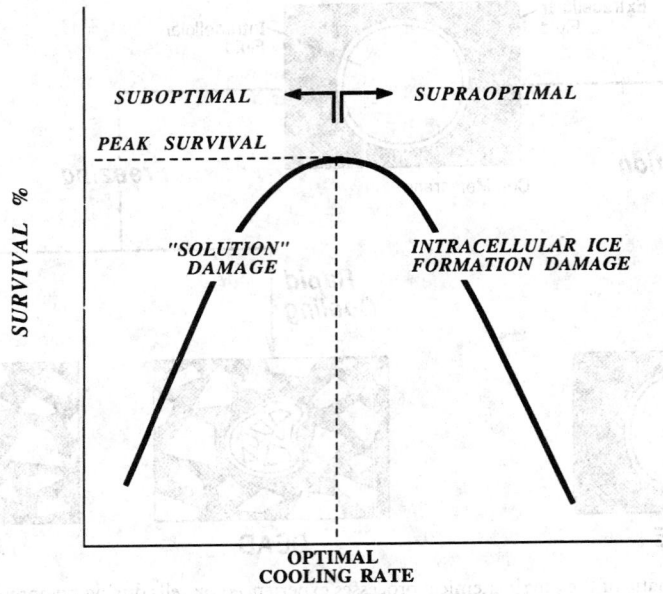

FIGURE 105.3 A diagram illustrating the relationship between cell survival and cooling rate during a freeze-thaw protocol.

   The next challenge in freeze-thaw technology is to thaw the biomaterial using a warming protocol that minimizes the risk of recrystallization, or devitrification if applicable, and promotes high survival. The optimal thawing rate correlates directly with the rate at which the sample was cooled before storage. If the material was frozen slowly at a suboptimal rate (Fig. 105.3), a wide range of thawing rates usually can be utilized with negligible effects on survival. If the biomaterial experienced slightly supraoptimal cooling rates (Fig. 105.3), rapid thawing is almost exclusively required to avoid recrystallization of small intracellular ice crystals formed during the initial cooling step. The rapid thawing of volumes of appreciable size is particularly difficult because the thermal mass of the specimen dictates the warming rate that can be achieved.

105.4 Freeze-Drying

Freeze-drying, or lyophilization, is a dehydration storage technique that is advantageous because it produces a final product that can be stored at suprazero temperatures and reconstituted with the addition of an appropriate solvent. The procedure is commonly applied to protein products (e.g., collagen, penicillin) and less frequently applied to cells (e.g., platelets, red blood cells) [Doebbler et al., 1966; Goodrich and Sowemimo-Coker, 1993]. Freeze-drying techniques also have been applied to liposomes—vesicles utilized in drug delivery systems that can trap water-soluble substances within their lumina. Lyophilization is a dual stage process that consists of rapidly cooling the liquid material to its solid form and subsequent drying (or removing) of the solidified solvent. The intricacies of the procedures employed directly influence the shelf life of the final dehydrated product. The drying stage of the process utilizes vacuum sublimation (transformation of a solid phase directly to the vapor phase) and may itself consist of multiple steps. The complexities of the drying procedure are determined by the continuity of the ice phase throughout the frozen specimen [MacKenzie, 1976]. Franks [1982] explains that the quality of the final lyophilized product partially depends on the freezing protocol experienced by the original sample, the size and distribution of the resultant ice crystals, the degree of heterogeneity, the presence or absence of amorphous regions, and the conditions imposed on the sample during drying. As one might expect, these factors can produce differentiations between the desired goals of the freeze-drying process and the actual final product.

The effects of the freezing protocol and the size and distribution of the resultant crystals are important for the reasons discussed previously. It should be mentioned that in the case of protein lyophilization, carbohydrates are often added for protection, while for cells, glycerol is a common lyoprotectant. The next two factors—the degree of heterogeneity and presence of amorphous regions—directly relate to the drying procedure. For simple cases in which large areas of ice (e.g., continuous channels) have formed in the sample, ice is removed by direct sublimation. However, for the more complex configurations commonly encountered with biomaterials, sublimation alone is inadequate because the ice crystal formation is discontinuous and amorphous regions are present. The amorphous regions correspond to pockets of water bound by freeze-concentrated solutes and biomaterial components (e.g., cell membranes). Water bound in this way serves to satisfy the hydration shell requirements of the specimen [Steinbrecht and Müller, 1987], hence contributing to the stabilization of the biomaterial. It is now recognized that the formation of amorphous regions is necessary for the successful lyophilization of biomaterials [Crowe et al., 1993a; Levine and Slade, 1992]. Since material destabilization is one source of damage during freeze-drying, this is an important area of lyophilization research.

Regardless of the complexity of the frozen matrix, biomaterial injury can occur during drying. Factors such as the effective drying temperature and the rate of drying are important in determining the degree of damage incurred. The drying step entails the removal of first the free water and then the bound water. However, the complete removal of this bound water during freeze-drying can be injurious to biomaterials and can promote protein denaturation and possibly aggregation into insoluble precipitates. Denaturation is the disruption of the folded structure of a protein and is affected by variables such as pH, surface interactions, and thermal and chemical changes [Darby and Creighton, 1993]. It is unfavorable because the final lyophilized product may no longer resemble the original biomaterial once denaturation occurs. Hence the avoidance of protein denaturation is crucial to effective biomaterial lyophilization. Investigations with liposomes and proteins reveal that the survival of biomaterials in the dry state is linked to the stabilizing influence of disaccharides (such as sucrose and trehalose) present in the system [Crowe et al, 1993b]. However, to minimize denaturation during freeze-drying protocols, lyoprotectants and CPAs should be used [Cleland et al., 1993]. It should be mentioned that the removal of these additives can be problematic in the large-scale industrial use of freeze-drying techniques.

Once a biomaterial has been lyophilized successfully, it is stored for future use. For the special case of protein storage—an area that is of particular interest to the pharmaceutical industry—the stability of the drug or protein must be guaranteed throughout a reasonable shelf life (the time period, measured in years, for which the drug maintains its original physical and functional properties). Two means of biomaterial destabilization during storage are the occurrence of oxidative and chemical reactions after lyophilization. Oxidation effects can be reduced by the exclusion of oxygen from containers of the dried materials and the use of antioxidants. The chemical reactions can be inhibited through the maintenance of low residual moisture levels [Cleland et al., 1993].

The final step, in the use of freeze-drying techniques for biomaterial storage, is the reconstitution of the lyophilized product. If pure water is used as the rehydration solvent, concentration gradients and osmotic imbalances can result in severe injury. To counter these effects, biomaterials are commonly rehydrated using isotonic solutions or media. The effects of using additives in the reconstituting solvent of biomaterials has recently been addressed. Apparently sugars are also effective in reducing damage during this rehydration step [Crowe et al., 1993b].

105.5 Vitrification

The hazards of ice crystal formation are significantly reduced by rapidly cooling the biomaterial to low temperatures at sufficient rates to produce an amorphous solid. This alternative, depicted in

Fig. 105.2, was originally proposed in the 1930s and is called *vitrification* [Luyet, 1937; Goetz and Goetz, 1938]. Vitrification is the kinetic process by which a liquid solidifies into a glass. It requires the rapid cooling of the liquid to the glass-transition temperature T_G and is most easily achieved in high-viscosity liquids [Doremus, 1973]. The molecular configuration of the supercooled liquid $(T \geq T_G)$ is the same as that of the glass $(T \leq T_G)$. Hence rapid cooling is necessary to prevent the supercooled liquid molecules from reorganizing into a regular (e.g., lattice) configuration. Vitrification is a second-order phase transition. Hence, by definition, the specific volumes of both phases (near T_G) are identical, although the thermodynamic property values (i.e., heat capacity, coefficient of thermal expansion) are not [Kauzmann, 1948]. The difficulty in successfully vitrifying a material lies in reaching its glass transition temperature T_G prior to crystal formation. Hence reducing the distance between T_M and T_G by increasing the solute concentration (Fig. 105.1) increases the probability that a given liquid will form a glass. Two alternative ways to achieve glassy state are (1) to cool biomaterials at ultrarapid rates such that T_G is reached before nucleation can proceed and (2) to increase the pressure of the system such that the intersection of T_{HOM} and T_G (Fig. 105.1) occurs at lower CPA concentrations [Fahy et al., 1984; Kanno and Angell, 1977]. Since glass formation circumvents the deleterious effects of freeze injury during cooling, it is becoming an increasingly important biomaterial storage technique.

We have already mentioned the roles of viscosity and rapid cooling in vitrification. The more viscous a liquid, the slower it can be cooled to achieve its vitrified form. Fairly large cryoprotectant concentrations are necessary to obtain the vitrified form of aqueous solutions by slow cooling, and the requirement increases with specimen volume. This is undesirable, since high concentrations of CPAs are toxic to biomaterials. Hence, in practical applications of vitrification technology, a balance between the thermodynamic conditions necessary to achieve vitrification and the physicochemical conditions suitable for survival is crucial.

The most common difficulty encountered in attempts to vitrify biologic materials is their susceptibility to ice crystal formation. As mentioned previously, the larger the sample volume, the higher the CPA concentration necessary to reduce the probability of crystallization [Coger et al., 1990]. *Drosophila melanogaster* cells, corneal tissue, and pancreatic islets of Langerhans are three examples of biomaterials that have been vitrified successfully [Steponkus et al, 1990; Bourne, 1986; Jutte et al., 1987]. Of these, only *D. melanogaster* has not been preserved previously by the freeze-thaw technique. In fact, the freeze-thaw technique remains the chief method of cell storage. For many cell and tissue types, the appropriate combination of effective temperature, cryoprotectant concentration, and cooling and warming rate conditions necessary for their vitrification have yet to be determined. For long-term organ storage, the freeze-thaw technique is not an alternative, because the mechanical stress and toxic damage that the organ would incur during freezing would be lethal [Bernard et al., 1988; Fahy et al., 1984]. Organ vitrification attempts, although unsuccessful, have demonstrated that the CPA toxicity limitation is especially evident in organ preservation such that toxic death prevention is an unavoidable challenge in organ vitrification [Fahy, 1986]. With respect to cooling rate, the relatively large volumes of organs require the use of slow cooling protocols to ensure a uniform thermal history throughout the total volume. Organs therefore require high-pressure, high-cryoprotectant concentrations and slow cooling conditions to achieve the vitreous state.

Once a biomaterial has been vitrified successfully, it must be stored at temperatures below T_G (Fig. 105.1) to encourage stability. When restoring the sample to physiologic conditions, special care must be taken to avoid crystallization during the warming protocol. Crystallization under these circumstances, termed *devitrification*, is possible (or even probable) since at temperatures greater than T_G, the crystalline phase is more stable than the amorphous solid. If such a transformation occurs, cryoinjury is unavoidable. The probability of devitrification is significantly reduced by warming the biomaterial at rates equivalent to those imposed during the original cooling [Fahy, 1988; MacFarlane et al., 1992]. The use of vitrification as a biomaterial storage technique is an ongoing and important area of cryopreservation research. Presently, it is the only apparent solution for the long-term storage of organs.

105.6 Summary

Biomaterial storage is an exciting research area whose advances are of value to a variety of fields, including medicine, biologic research, and drug design. However, the compositional and physical complexities of the various biosubstances (e.g., proteins, cells, tissues, and organs) require the development of specialized preservation procedures. In the present discussion, four storage techniques—nonfreezing, freeze-thaw, lyophilization, and vitrification—and their relevance to specific biomaterial examples have been reviewed. Although there have been definite advances, important challenges still remain for future investigations.

Defining Terms

Cryopreservation: Techniques utilized to store cells, tissues, and organs under subzero conditions for future use in clinical applications.

Cryoprotectant: Chemical additive used to protect biomaterials during cooling to low temperatures by reducing freezing injury.

Devitrification: Crystallization of an amorphous substance during warming.

Freeze-drying: Dehydration of a sample by vacuum sublimation.

Lyoprotectant: Expedients added to lyophilization formulations to protect the biomaterial from the damaging effects of the process.

Recrystallization: The coalescence of small ice crystals during warming.

Shelf life: Length of time in which the stability of the components of a biomaterial (e.g., pharmaceutical drugs) is guaranteed during storage.

Vitrification: Solidification process in which an amorphous (glasslike) solid, devoid of crystals, is formed.

References

Arakawa T, Carpenter JF, Kita YA, Crowe JH. 1990. The basis for toxicity of certain cryoprotectants: A hypothesis. Cryobiology 27:401.

Belzer FO, Southard JH. 1988. Principles of solid-organ preservation by cold storage. Transplantation 45:673.

Bernard A, McGrath JJ, Fuller BJ, et al. 1988. Osmotic response of oocytes using a microscope diffusion chamber: A preliminary study comparing murine and human ova. Cryobiology 25:495.

Borel-Rinkes IHM, Toner M, Tompkins RG, Yarmush ML. 1993. Long-term functional recovery of hepatocytes after cryopreservation in a three-dimensional culture configuration. Cell Transplant 1:281.

Bourne WM. 1986. Clinical and experimental aspects of corneal cryopreservation. Cryobiology 23:88.

Cleland JL, Powell MF, Shire SJ. 1993. The development of stable protein formulations: A close look at protein aggregation, deamidation, and oxidation. In S Bruck (ed), Crit Rev Ther Drug Carrier Syst 10:307.

Coger R, Rubinsky B, Pegg DE. 1990. Dependence of probability of vitrification on time and volume. Cryo-Letters 11:359.

Crowe JH, Crowe LM, Carpenter JF. 1993a. Preserving dry biomaterials: The water replacement hypothesis, part 1. Biopharm 6:28.

Crowe JH, Crowe LM, Carpenter JF. 1993b. Preserving dry biomaterials: The water replacement hypothesis, part 2. Biopharm 6:40..

Darby NJ, Creighton TE. 1993. Protein Structure. Oxford, Oxford University Press.

Doebbler FG, Rowe AW, Rinfret AP. 1966. Freezing of mammalian blood and its constituents. In HT Meryman (ed), Cryobiology, pp 407–450. London, Academic Press.

Doremus RH. 1973. Glass Science. New York, Wiley.

Evans RW. 1993. A cost-outcome analysis of retransplantation the need for accountability. Transplant Rev 7:163.

Fahy GM. 1988. Vitrification. In JJ McGrath, KR Diller (eds), Low Temperature Biotechnology, vols 10 and 98, pp 113–146. New York, ASME.

Fahy GM. 1986. The relevance of cryoprotectant "toxicity" to cryobiology. Cryobiology 23:1.

Fahy GM, MacFarlane DR, Angell CA, Meryman HT. 1984. Vitrification as an approach to cryopreservation. Cryobiology 21:407.

Franks F. 1988. Storage in the undercooled state. In JJ McGrath, KR Diller (eds), Low Temperature Biotechnology, vols 10 and 98, pp 107–112. New York, ASME.

Franks F. 1982. The properties of aqueous solutions at subzero temperatures. In F Franks (ed), Water: A Comprehensive Treatise, vol 7, pp 215–338. New York, Plenum Press.

Friedler S, Giudice L, Lamb E. 1988. Cryopreservation of embryos and ova. Fertil Steril 49:743.

Goetz A, Goetz SS. 1938. Vitrification and crystallization of organic cells at low temperatures. J Appl Physiol 9:718.

Goodrich RP, Sowemimo-Coker SO. 1993. Freeze drying of red blood cells. In PL Steponkus (ed), Advances in Low-Temperature Biology, vol 2, pp 53–99. London, JAI Press.

Hobbs PV. 1974. Ice Physics. Oxford, Oxford University Press.

Jutte NHPM, Heyse P, Jansen HG, et al. 1987. Vitrification of human islets of langerhans. Cryobiology 24:403.

Kanno H, Angell CA. 1977. Homogenous nucleation and glass formation in aqueous alkali halide solutions at high pressure. J Phys Chem 81(26):2639.

Karlsson JOM, Cravalho EG, Borel-Rinkes IHM, et al. 1993. Nucleation and growth of ice crystals inside cultured hepatocytes during freezing in the presence of dimethyl sulfoxide. Biophys J 65:2524.

Karlsson JOM, Cravalho EG, Toner M. 1994. A model of diffusion-limited ice growth inside biological cells during freezing. J Appl Physiol 75:4442.

Kauzmann W. 1948. The nature of the glassy state and the behavior of liquids at low temperatures. Chem Rev 43:219.

Levine H, Slade L. 1992. Another view of trehalose for drying and stabilizing biological materials. Biopharm 5:36.

Luyet B. 1937. The vitrification of organic colloids and of protoplasm. Biodynamica 1:1.

MacFarlane DR, Forsyth M, Barton CA. 1992. Vitrification and devitrification in cryopreservation. In PL Steponkus (ed), Advances in Low Temperature Biology, vol 1, pp 221–278. London, JAI Press.

MacKenzie AP. 1976. Principles of freeze-drying. Transplant Proc 8(suppl 1):181.

Mazur P. 1984. Freezing of living cells: Mechanisms and implications. Am J Physiol 143:C125.

McGann LE. 1978. Differing actions of penetrating and nonpenetrating cryoprotective agents. Cryobiology 15:382.

McGrath JJ. 1988. Membrane transport properties. In JJ McGrath, KR Diller (eds), Low Temperature Biotechnology, vols 10 and 98, pp 273–330. New York, ASME.

Muldrew K, McGann LE. 1994. The osmotic rupture hypothesis of intracellular freezing injury. Biophys J 66:532.

Pitt RE. 1992. Thermodynamics and intracellular ice formation. In PL Steponkus (ed), Advances in Low-Temperature Biology, vol 1, pp 63–99. London, JAI Press.

Polge C, Smith AU, Parkes AS. 1949. Revival of spermatozoa after vitrification and dehydration at low temperatures. Nature 164:666.

Rall WP, Mazur P, McGrath JJ. 1983. Depression of the ice-nucleation temperature of rapidly cooled mouse embryos by glycerol and dimethyl sulfoxide. Biophys J 41:1.

Southard JH, Belzer FO. 1993. The University of Wisconsin organ preservation solution: components, comparisons, and modifications. Transplant Rev 7:176.

Southard JH, Belzer FO. 1988. Kidney preservation by perfusion. In GJ Cerilli (ed), Organ Transplantation and Replacement, pp 296–311. Philadelphia, Lippincott.

Steponkus PL, Myers SP, Lynch DV, et al. 1990. Cryopreservation of Drosophila melanogaster embryos. Nature 345:170.

Steinbrecht RA, Muller M. 1987. Freeze substitution and freeze-drying. In RA Steinbrecht, K Zierold (eds), Cryotechniques in Biological Electon Microscopy, pp 149–172. Berlin, Springer-Verlag.

Further Information

In addition to the review works cited throughout the text, the following publications also may be of interest.

For more detailed information concerning lyophilization, as applied specifically to proteins, see *The development of stable protein formulations: A close look at protein aggregation, deamidation, and oxidation,* by Cleland et al., an especially helpful article (1993. *Crit. Rev. Ther. Drug Carrier Syst* 10:307).

A good introduction to the fields of cryobiology and cryopreservation is presented in *The Clinical Applications of Cryobiology,* by B. J. Fuller and B. W. W. Grout (CRC Press, Boca Raton, Fla., 1991). For review work relevant to vitrification and organ preservation, *The Biophysics of Organ Cryopreservation,* edited by D. E. Pegg and A. M. Karow Jr. (Plenum Press, New York, 1987) should be consulted.

For additional information on the physicochemical processes encountered during cooling of biomaterials, refer to Korber's 1988 review (*Q. Rev. Biophys.* 21:229). For an overview of bioheat transfer processes, refer to Diller's review in *Bioengineering Heat Transfer* 22:157, 1992. For additional information on the fundamental principles of intracellular ice formation, consult the 1993 review by Toner (pp. 1–51 in *Advances in Low Termperature Biology,* edited by P. L. Steponkus, vol. 2, JAI Press, London).

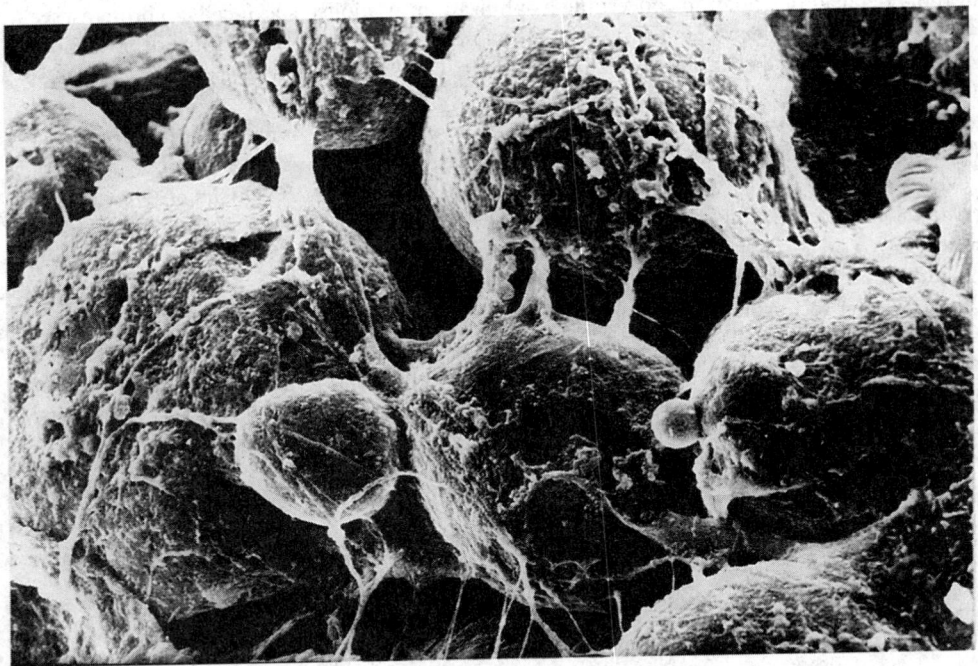

Scanning electron micrographs of bone marrow cultures on a nylon screen template showing myeloid cells of a hematopoietic colony.

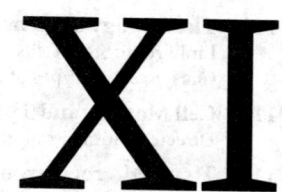

Tissue Engineering

Bernhard Ø. Palsson
University of Michigan

Jeffrey A. Hubbell
California Institute of Technology

T ISSUE ENGINEERING IS A NEW field that is rapidly growing in both scope and importance within biomedical engineering. It represents a marriage of the rapid developments in cellular and molecular biology on the one hand and materials, chemical, and mechanical engineering on the other. The ability to manipulate and reconstitute tissue function has tremendous clinical implications and is likely to play a major role in cell and gene therapies during the next few years in addition to expanding the tissue supply for transplantation therapies.

Tissue function is complex and involves an intricate interplay of biologic and physicochemical rate processes. A major difficulty with selecting topics for this section was to define its scope. After careful consideration we focused on three goals: first, to cover some of the generic engineering issues; second, to cover generic cell biologic issues; and third, to review the status of tissue engineering of specific organs.

In the first category we have two common engineering themes of material properties and development and the analysis of physical rate processes. The role of materials is treated in terms of two length scales—the molecular and the cellular size scales. On the smaller size scale, Chapter 106 deals with engineering the biomolecular properties of a surface, and Chapter 107 deals with protein adsorption onto surfaces to which cells will be exposed. Chapters 108 and 109 deal with the engineering of scaffolds and templates on which cells are grown for transplantation purposes. The effects of physical rate processes are treated in Chapters 110 and 111. Both fluid mechanical forces and mass transfer rates influence important attributes of tissue function and relate to the physical constraints under which tissues operate. The issues associated with materials and the physical rate process represent important engineering challenges that need to be met to further the development of tissue engineering.

In the second category we have common cell biologic themes: stem cell biology, cell motion, the tissue microenvironment, and the role of stroma in tissue function. Its is now believed that many tissues contain stem cells from which the tissue is generated. Chapter 112 describes the basic concepts of stem cell biology. Cell motion is an important process in tissue function and tissue development. Basic concepts of cell motility are covered in Chapter 113, and the manipulation of this process is likely to become an essential part of tissue engineering. It is well established that the cellular microenvironment in vivo is critical to tissue function. This complex set of tissues is treated in Chapter 114. The specific interaction between cells performing a tissue-specific function and the accessory cells (or stroma) found in tissues has proved to be a key to reconstituting tissue function ex vivo. The important role of the stroma in tissue engineering is described in Chapter 115. The understanding and mastery of these cell biologic issues are essential for the future tissue engineer.

Chapters in the third and last category describe progress with the engineering of specific tissues. Six tissues where much progress has been made were selected: bone marrow, liver, the nervous system, skeletal muscle, cartilage, and kidney. These chapters provide a concise review of the accomplishments to date and the likely clinical implications of these developments.

By focusing on these three categories we hope that the reader will acquire a good understanding of the engineering and cell biological fundamentals of tissue engineering and of the progress that has been made to date and will develop ideas for further development of this emerging and important field.

106

Surface Immobilization of Adhesion Ligands for Investigations of Cell-Substrate Interactions

Paul D. Drumheller
Gore Hybrid Technologies, Inc.

Jeffrey A. Hubbell
California Institute of Technology

The interaction between cells and surfaces plays a major biologic role in cellular behavior. Cell membrane receptors responsible for adhesion may influence cell physiology in numerous ways. Examples of these interactions are the rolling and activation of leukocytes on vascular endothelium, the spatial differentiation of embryonic basement membranes in development, the extension of neurites on adhesion proteins, the proliferation of cells induced by mitogenic factors, and the spreading and recruitment of platelets onto the vascular subendothelium. These and other cell-surface interactions influence or control many aspects of cell physiology, such as adhesion, spreading, activation, recruitment, migration, proliferation, and differentiation.

There is great interest in understanding cell-surface interactions. This understanding is paramount to the development of pharmaceutical compounds to enhance or inhibit cell-substrate interactions, such as agents to enhance cell adhesion for tissue regeneration or biomaterials integration or to reduce cell adhesion in metastasis or fibrosis. In the emerging area of tissue engineering, the adhesion of cells to a culture support is essential for many products such as biohybrid dermal dressings, synthetic articular cartilage, and hepatocyte scaffolds. Investigations of cell-surface interactions are central to many areas of biomedicine and bioengineering, including tissue engineering, biomaterials design, immunology, oncology, haematology, and developmental biology.

To examine the interactions of cells with substrates and how they may influence cell behavior, simplified models that simulate basement membranes, cell surfaces, or extracellular matrices have been developed. These models involve the immobilization of biologically active ligands of natural and synthetic origin onto various substrates to produce chemically defined bioactive surfaces. Ligands that have been immobilized include cell-membrane receptor fragments, antibodies, adhesion peptides, enzymes, adhesive carbohydrates, lectins, membrane lipids, and glycosaminoglycan matrix components. Functionalized two-dimensional surfaces are important tools to elucidate the molecular mechanisms of cell-mediated bioadhesion.

Techniques for preparing these ligand-functionalized two-dimensional substrates for investigation of cell adhesion are similar to methods for labeling ligands, preparing immunomatrices, or immobilizing enzymes. This brief tutorial review will focus primarily on schemes for immobilizing bioactive ligands specifically for purposes of investigating cell-surface interactions. Topics that will be addressed include: (1) general considerations of bioconjugation; (2) examples of surface bioconjugation; (3) preparation of surfaces for ligand immobilization; (4) examples of ligand-containing copolymers; (5) techniques for characterizing these surfaces; and (6) examples of applications of surface immobilized ligands in cell-substrate investigations.

106.1 General Considerations

Numerous reviews are available that describe the chemistry of ligand conjugation and immobilization, and the reader is encouraged to consult them for more detailed descriptions [1–12]. When immobilizing ligands for the preparation of cell-adhesive substrates, several factors must be considered to retain maximum bioactivity. Ligand surface immobilization may proceed in low yields due to sterically inaccessible reactive sites on the ligand molecule; the immobilized ligand may not have optimum cell-receptor interactions due to physical constraints imposed by the surface or by the active site being buried; or the immobilized ligand may be partially denatured upon immobilization. The inclusion of spacer arms on the surface may help relieve these limitations [13]. If the ligand has a directionality, then the cell adhesive response may vary depending upon the orientation of the immobilized ligand [14,15] or upon the length of the spacer arm [16].

Ligands have been physicochemically absorbed onto polymeric substrates to investigate cell-surface interactions. The advantage of covalently immobilizing a ligand is that a chemical bond is present to prevent desorption. The general chemical scheme for grafting a ligand onto a surface is shown in Fig. 106.1. Activation usually is a necessary step to produce highly reactive species to enable surface immobilization under mild conditions. Typically the surface is activated, since the chemical steps are somewhat simpler than for ligand activation, but each strategy may have its own advantages and limitations.

The activation of ligands may require suitable protective schemes to prevent homopolymerization or cross-linking if these competing reactions are not desired. Ligands may also be activated at more than one site, some of which may remain unconsumed after coupling is complete and have biological activity. In contrast, the activation of surfaces usually does not require protective schemes; nonetheless, activated surfaces may contain unconsumed sites after immobilization that may require deactivation so as not to influence cell-mediated adhesive responses.

Because most ligands immobilized for cell-surface studies are biologic in origin, water is often the only choice of solvent as the coupling medium. Water is nucleophilic, and hydrolysis can be a competing reaction during activation and coupling, especially at higher pH (>9–10). To reduce hydrolysis, surfaces are commonly activated in nonaqueous solvents; ligands are then coupled using concentrated aqueous solutions (> 1 mg/ml) for extended periods (> 12 hr). Some ligands are soluble in polar solvents such as dimethylsulfoxide (DMSO), dimethylformamide (DMF), acetone, dioxane, or ethanol, or their aqueous cosolvents, and these combinations may be used to reduce hydrolysis during coupling.

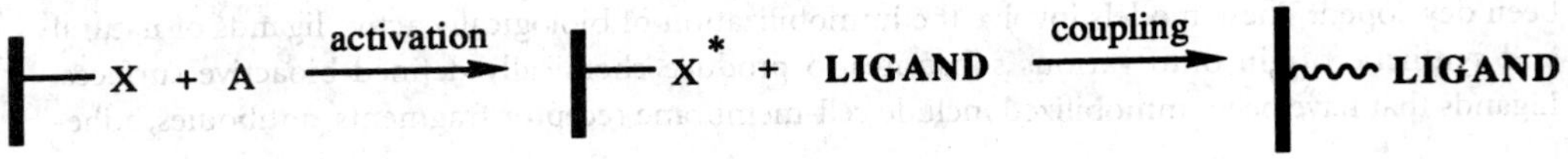

$$\vdash\!\!- X + A \xrightarrow{\text{activation}} \vdash\!\!- X^* + \text{LIGAND} \xrightarrow{\text{coupling}} \vdash\!\!\sim\!\!\text{LIGAND}$$

FIGURE 106.1 General chemical scheme for grafting a ligand onto a surface.

106.2 Surface Bioconjugation

The typical chemical groups involved in immobilizing ligands for cell-surface studies are hydroxyls, amines, carboxylic acids, and thiols. Other groups, such as amides, disulfides, phenols, guanidines, thioethers, indoles, and imidazoles, have also been modified, but these will not be described.

Hydroxyls and carboxylic acids are commonly activated to produce more reactive agents for ligand acylation. Elimination is a possible competing reaction for secondary and aryl alcohols. Primary amines, present on many biologic ligands from N-amino acid termini and lysine, are good nucleophiles when unprotonated ($pK_a \sim 9$); moderately basic pH (8–10) ensures their reactivity. Thiols, present on cysteine ($pK_a \sim 8.5$), are stronger nucleophiles than amines, and as such they can be selectively coupled in the presence of amines at lower pH (5–7). Sulfhydryl groups often exist as their disulfide form and may be reduced to free thiols using mild agents such as dithiothreitol.

The following paragraphs review activation schemes for particular chemical groups present on the surface, giving brief coupling schemes. Due to the advantages of surface versus ligand activation, only general methods involving surface activation will be discussed.

Immobilization to Surface Alcohols

A hydroxyl-bearing surface may be activated with numerous reagents to produce more reactive species for substitution, the most common example being the cyanogen bromide activation of cellulose and agarose derivatives [2–5, 11, 17]. Due to problems with high volatility of the cyanogen bromide, sensitivity of the activated species to hydrolysis, competing reactions during activation and coupling, and the desire to use culture substrates other than polysaccharides, other activation schemes have been developed for more defined activation and coupling. These schemes have been used to modify functionalized glasses and polymers for cell-mediated adhesion studies.

Alcohols react with sulfonyl halides [18–25] carbonyldiimidazole [26, 27], succinimidyl chloroformate [28], epoxides [29, 30] isocyanates [31–33] and heterocyclic [34, 35] and alkyl halides [21]. Activation of surface alcohols with these agents can be performed in organic solvents such as acetonitrile, methylene chloride, acetone, benzene, dioxane, diethyl ether, toluene, or DMF.

Reactive Esters

Alcohols can be activated to reactive sulfonic ester leaving groups by reaction with sulfonyl halides [18–25] (Fig. 106.2) such as p-toluenesulfonyl chloride (tosyl chloride), trifluoroethanesulfonyl chloride (tresyl chloride), methanesulfonyl chloride (mesyl chloride), or fluorobenzenesulfonyl chloride (fosyl chloride). The resulting sulfonic esters are readily displaced in mild aqueous conditions with amines or thiols to produce amino- or thioether-bound ligands. Aryl alcohols should not be activated in this manner, since the sulfonate group may irreversibly transfer to the aromatic nucleus [36]. Sulfonic esters differ in their ease of nucleophilic substitution and resistance to hydrolysis, tosyl esters being low in coupling potential [23] and fosyl esters being high in hydrolysis resistance [24]. Activation can be performed in many organic solvents that are properly dry: Trace water and other species such as ammonia will react. DMSO should not be used as a solvent, as it will react with sulfonyl halides. A tert-amino base such as pyridine, dimethylaminopryidine, triethylamine, diisopropylethyl amine, or ethylmorpholine can be added in equimolar amounts to serve as a nucleophilic catalyst and to combine with the liberated HCl. It has been suggested that hydroxyls

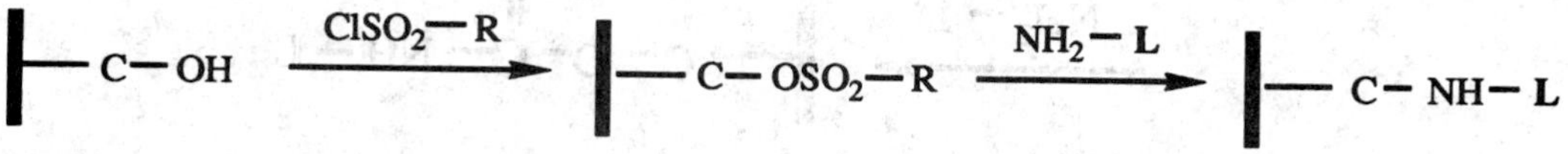

$$\mathord{\mid}\!\!-\!\text{C}\!-\!\text{OH} \xrightarrow{\text{ClSO}_2\!-\!\text{R}} \mathord{\mid}\!\!-\!\text{C}\!-\!\text{OSO}_2\!-\!\text{R} \xrightarrow{\text{NH}_2\!-\!\text{L}} \mathord{\mid}\!\!-\!\text{C}\!-\!\text{NH}\!-\!\text{L}$$

FIGURE 106.2 Alcohols can be activated with sulfonyl halides, which are readily displaced with amine- (shown) or thiol-containing (not shown) ligands.

be converted to alkoxides prior to sulfonic ester activation in the presence of ethers as they may be sensitive to the HCl generated during activation [25].

An alcohol-containing surface is typically incubated with the sulfonyl halide for 0.5–6.0 hr. Any precipitated salts can be rinsed away with 1 mM HCl. The ligand is coupled to the surface for 12–24 hr in borate or carbonate buffer (pH 9–10) at a concentration of 1 mg/ml. Coupling can proceed at more mild pH (~7) with more concentrated solutions (>10 mg ligand/ml) or with thiol-bearing ligands. Excess sulfonic esters can be displaced with aqueous solutions (10–50 mM, pH = 8–9) of tris(hydroxymethyl)aminomethane, aminoethanol, glycine, or mercaptoethanol, or by hydrolysis.

Other Acylating Agents

Surface hydroxyls may be activated to groups other than sulfonic esters. Alcohols react readily with carbonyldiimidazole [26, 27] (Fig. 106.3) and succinimidyl chloroformate [28] (Fig. 106.4) to produce reactive imidazole-N-carboxylates and succinimidyl carbonates, respectively. These species acylate amines to urethane linkages. Activation typically proceeds in organic solvent for 2–6 hr. Dimethylaminopyridine catalyzes formation of the succinimidyl carbonate. Amine-bearing ligands (>10 mg/ml) are coupled to the surface in borate or phosphate buffer (pH 8–9) for 12–24 hr, or 4°C, 2–3 days. Thiol-bearing groups may also be immobilized onto these activated groups; however the thiocarbamate linkage can be sensitive to hydrolysis and may not be generally applicable to preparing well-defined substrates for long-term biologic investigations.

Bifunctional Bridges

In lieu of alcohol conversion to activated reactive groups, the hydroxyl may be added to homo- or heterobifunctional bridges, wherein alcoholysis consumes one terminus to produce newly functionalized surfaces (Figure 106.5). Epoxide bridges can be added to surface-bound alcohols in aqueous base (to reduce hydrolysis or polymerization of the epoxide, 10–100 mM NaOH) or in organic solvent, 12 hr. Isocyanate bridges are added to surface alcohols in organic solvents with organotin catalysts (such as dibutyltin dilaurate), 12 hr. Halo alkylation of surface-bound alcohols or alkoxides proceeds in organic solvents, 2–3 days, or with heat (~80°C), 12 hr. The unconsumed free group (isocyanate, epoxide, or alkyl halide) is substituted with amine- or thiol-bearing ligands in buffered aqueous conditions, pH 8–10, 1–10 mg/ml, 12–24 hr. Hydroxyl-bearing ligands, such as carbohydrates, can be coupled in aqueous DMSO, dioxane, or DMF, 12–24 hr, 60–80°C. Hydroxyl coupling

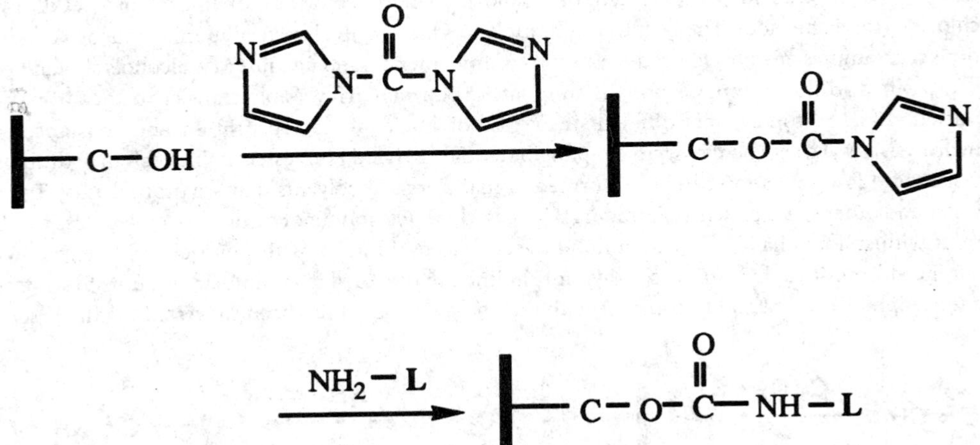

FIGURE 106.3 Alcohols react readily with carbonyldiimidazole to produce reactive imidazole-N-carboxylates for coupling to amine-containing ligands.

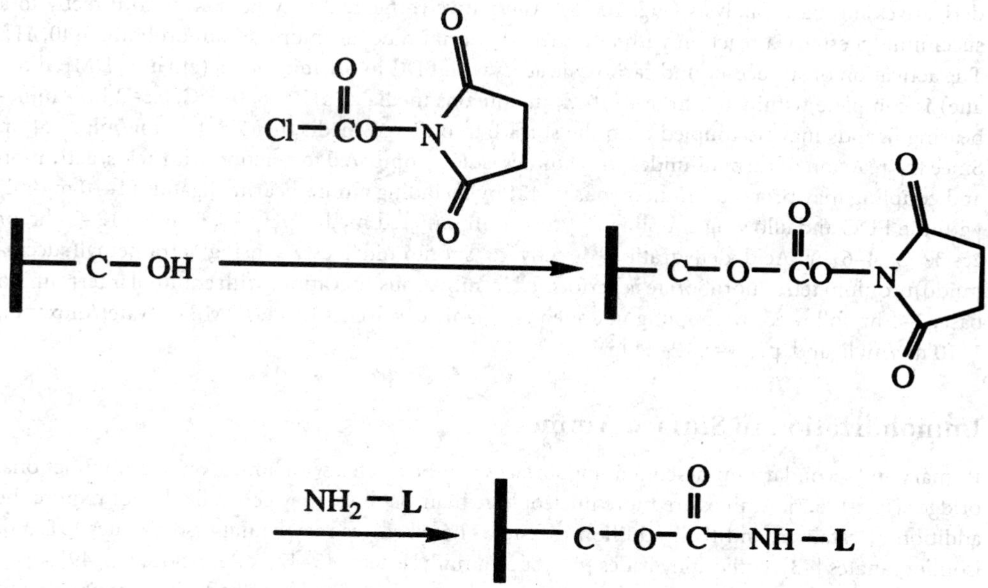

FIGURE 106.4 Alcohols react readily with succinimidyl chloroformate to produce a succinimidyl carbonate for coupling to amine-containing ligands.

may also be performed in aqueous base (10–100 mM NaOH) for ligands that are resistant to ester- or amide hydrolysis, such as mono- or polysaccharides.

Heterocyclic aryl halides, such as cyanuric chloride [34, 35], react with free hydroxyl groups in polar solvents containing sodium carbonate, 40–50°C, 30 min. Amine-bearing ligands are immobilized to the surface in borate buffer, pH 9, 1–10 mg/ml, 5–10°C, 12–24 hr.

Immobilization to Surface Carboxylic Acids

Acids may be converted to activated leaving groups by reaction with carbodiimides [36]. The generated O-acylureas react with amines to produce amide linkages and can react with alcohols to produce ester linkages with acid or base catalysts. An undesirable competing reaction is urea rearrangement to nonreactive N-acylurea; this effect may be accelerated in aprotic polar solvents such as DMF but is reduced at low temperatures (0–10°C) or by the addition of agents such as hydroxybenztriazole to convert the O-acylurea to benztriazole derivatives. Acids may also be activated with carbonyldiimidizole to produce easily amino- and alcoholyzed imidazolide intermediates; however, imidazolides are highly susceptible to hydrolysis and necessitate anhydrous conditions for activation and coupling [37].

Water-soluble carbodiimides such as ethyl(dimethylaminopropyl)-carbodiimide (EDC) can be used in either aqueous or organic media for the immobilization of ligands to produce bioactive substrates [20, 38, 39]. To reduce hydrolysis of the O-acylurea, conversion to more resistant succinimidyl esters can be performed using EDC and N-hydroxysuccinimide or its water-soluble sulfonate

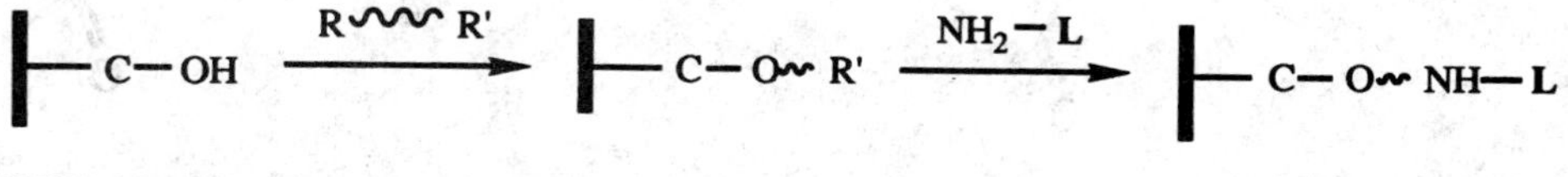

FIGURE 106.5 Bifunctional coupling agents may be used, e.g., to couple an amine-containing ligand to a hydroxyl-containing surface via a spacer.

derivative, and base catalysts (Fig. 106.6). Alternatively, the acid may be converted directly to a succinimidyl ester via reaction with tetramethyl(succinimido)uronium tetrafluoroborate [40, 41]. The activation of surface-bound carboxylic acids with EDC in organic media (ethanol, DMF, dioxane) is complete within 1–2 hr at 0–10°C; in aqueous media at pH 4–6, 0–5°C, 0.5–2 hr. Amine-bearing ligands may be coupled onto the surface in buffered media, pH 7.5–9, 1 mg/ml, 2–24 hr. Since the reaction of carbodiimides with amines is slow compared to reaction with acids, activation and coupling may proceed simultaneously [42] by including amine-bearing ligands (1–10 mg/ml) with the EDC and allowing coupling to proceed in buffered media, pH 5–7, 0–10°C, 12–24 hr, or 25–30°C, 4–6 hr. Acid dehydration directly to succinimidyl esters using tetramethyl(succinimido)uronium tetrafluoroborate is performed in anhydrous conditions with equimolar tert-amino base, 2–4 hr, followed by coupling in aqueous organic cosolvents (water/DMF or water/dioxane), 1–10 mg/ml ligand, pH 8–9, 12–24 hr.

Immobilization to Surface Amines

Primary and secondary amine-containing surfaces may be reacted with homo- or heterobifunctional bridges (Fig. 106.7). Amines are more nucleophilic than alcohols, they generally do not require the addition of catalysts, and their addition is faster. These bridges may contain isocyanates [31, 33], isothiocyanates [43], cyclic anhydrides [44], succinimidyl esters [45–47], or epoxides [48, 49].

Isocyanates add to amines with good efficiency but are susceptible to hydrolysis; epoxides and cyclic anhydrides are somewhat less reactive yet are still sensitive to hydrolysis. Hydrolysis-resistant diisothiocyanates have been used for many years to label ligands with reporter molecules; however, the thiourea linkage may be hydrolytically labile (especially at lower pH) and may be unsuitable for investigations of cell-surface interactions. Succinimidyl esters, although not as resistant to hydrolysis as isothiocyanates, have very good reactivity to amines and form stable amide linkages. Hydrolysis of all these reagents is accelerated at higher pH ($\geq$9–10).

Coupling to surface-bound amines is performed in organic conditions (DMF, DMSO, acetone) for 1–3 hr. Coupling of amine-bearing ligands onto immobilized bridges is performed in buffered media, pH 8–10.5, 2–12 hr, 1–10 mg/ml. Excess reagent can be displaced with buffered solutions of tris(hydroxymethyl)aminomethane, aminoethanol, glycine, or mercaptoethanol, or hydrolysis.

Bifunctional aldehydes, such as glutaraldehyde and formaldehyde, have been used classically as crosslinkers for purposes of immunohistochemistry and ultrastructural investigations. They have been used also to couple ligands onto amine-bearing substrates [50–52]. Hydrolysis of aldehydes is usually not a concern, since the hydrolysis product, alkyl hydrate, is reversible back to the carbonyl. Amines add to aldehydes to produce imine linkages over a wide range of pH (6–10). These Schiff bases are potentially hydrolytically labile; reductive amination can be performed with mild reducing agents such as sodium cyanoborohydride, pH 8–9, without substantial losses in ligand bioactivity [53]. Acetalization of polyhydric alcohols may commence in the presence of Lewis acid cata-

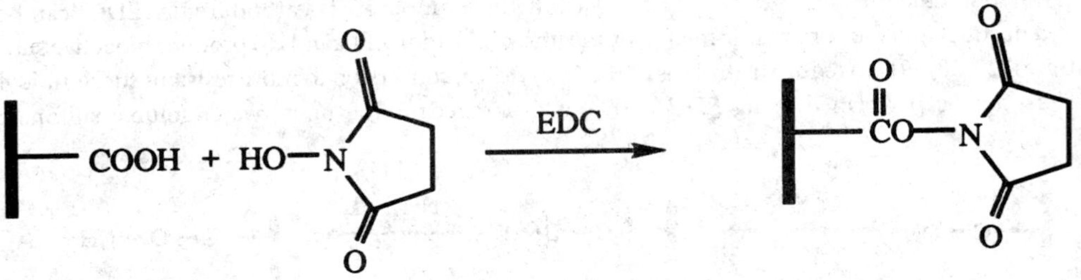

FIGURE 106.6 Carboxylated surfaces can be activated to succimydil esters to subsequently couple amine-containing ligands.

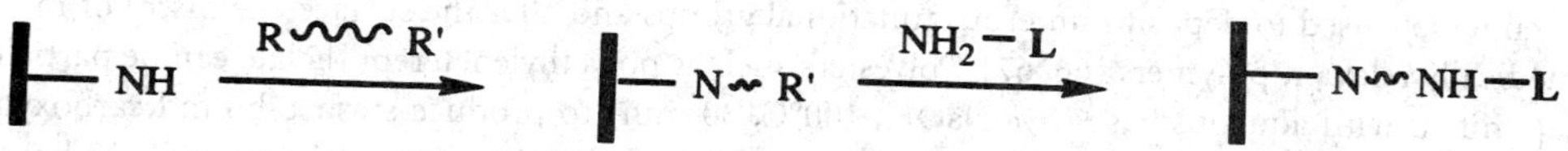

FIGURE 106.7 Primary and secondary amine-containing surfaces may be reacted with homo- or heterobifunctional bridges.

lysts followed by dehydrating the hemiacetal linkage an acetal [54, 55]. The dehydration conditions (air-drying followed by 70–90°C, 2 hr) may damage many biologic ligands.

Alkyl halide-bearing surfaces can be coupled to amine-bearing ligands [49, 56, 57]; their reaction is slower, but they are resistant to hydrolysis. Ligands can be immobilized in buffered medium (pH 9–10), 12–24 hr, 1–10 mg/ml, or in organic medium. Heat may be used to increase yields (60–80°C).

Immobilization to Surface Thiols

Thiols are more nucleophilic than amines or alcohols and may be selectively coupled in their presence at more neutral pH. Thiols can be reacted with reagents that are not reactive toward amines, such as homo- or heterobifunctional maleimide bridges [32, 58–60]. Surface-bound thiols react with maleimides in acetone, methanol, DMF, etc., for 1–2 hr, to produce a thioether linkage (Fig. 106.8). Thiol-bearing ligands can be immobilized to surface maleimides by incubating in mild buffered media, pH 5–7, 12–24 hr, 1–10 mg/ml. More basic pH should be avoided as hydrolysis of the maleimide to nonreactive maleamic acid may occur.

Photoimmobilization

Surfaces can be modified using photoactivated heterobifunctional bridges in one of three schemes: (1) the bridge may be immobilized onto a functionalized surface, followed by photocoupling of the ligand onto the photoactivated group [58, 61]; (2) the reagent may be photocoupled onto the surface, followed by immobilization onto the free terminus [58, 62]; or (3) the ligand may be coupled to the reagent, followed by photoimmobilization to the surface [63, 64]. The photoactivatible group may be light-sensitive azides, benzophenones, diazinines, or acrylates; polymerization initiator-transfer agent-terminators [65] and plasma-deposited free radicals [64] have also been used. Photoactivation produces highly reactive radical intermediates that immobilize onto the surface via a nonspecific insertion of the radical into a carbon-carbon bond. Photolabile reagents may be coupled to amine- or thiol-bearing ligands using succinimidyl esters or maleimides. One utility of photoimmobilization is the ability to produce patterns of ligands on the surface by lithography.

106.3 Surface Preparation

Polymeric materials can be functionalized using plasma deposition or wet chemical methods to produce surfaces containing reactive groups for ligand bioconjugation. Plasma polymerization has

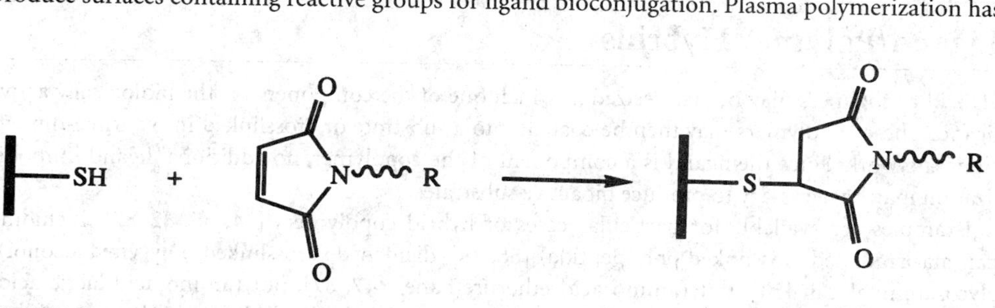

FIGURE 106.8 Thiol-containing surfaces may be coupled to malcimide activated species, either heterobifunctional linkers or ligands.

been widely used to deposit numerous functional groups and alter the surface chemistry of many medically relevant polymers [66, 67]. Polyesters such as polyethyleneterephthalate can be partially saponified with aqueous base (5% NaOH, 100°C, 30 min) to produce surface-bound carboxylic acids [39], partially aminolyzed with diamines such as ethylenediamine (50% aqueous, 12 hr) to produce surface-bound amines [68] or electrophilically substituted with formaldehyde (20% in 1 M acetic acid) to produce surface-bound alcohols [19].

Polyurethanes can be carboxylated via a bimolecular nucleophilic substitution [69]. Carbamate anions are prepared by abstraction of hydrogen from the urethane nitrogen at low temperatures to prevent chain cleavage ($-5°C$), followed by coupling of cyclic lactones such as β-propiolactone. Ligands are then immobilized onto the grafted carboxylic acids.

Polytetrafluoroethylene can be functionalized with a number of reactive groups using wet chemical or photochemical methods. Fluoropolymers are reduced with concentrated benzion dianion solutions to form carbonaceous surface layers which can then be halogenated, hydroxylated, carboxylated, or aminated [70]. Photochemical modification of fluoropolymers is possible by incubating the polymer in solutions of alkoxides or thiolate anions and exposing to UV light [71]. The patterning of surfaces is possible using this technique in conjunction with photolithography.

Glasses and oxidized polymers can be functionalized with bifunctional silanating reagents to generate surfaces containing alkyl halides, epoxides, amines, thiols, or carboxylic acids [19, 49, 59, 72]. The substrate must be thoroughly clean and free of any contaminating agents. Glass is soaked in strong acid or base for 30–60 min. Polymers are cleaned with plasma etching or with strong oxidizers such as chromic acid. Clean substrates are immersed in silane solutions (5–10% in acetone, toluene, or ethanol/water 95%/5%) for 1 hr and cured 50–100 °C, 2–4 hr, or at 25°C, 24 hr, for oxidation-sensitive silanes such as mercaptosilanes. Prepared surfaces stored under Ar are stable for several weeks.

Metals such as gold can be functionalized via the chemisorption of self-assembled monolayers of alkanethiols [73–75]. Gold substrates, prepared by evaporating gold on chromium-primed silicon substrates, are immersed in organic solutions of alkanethiol (1–10 mM) for 5–60 min. The monolayer is adsorbed via a gold-sulfur bond; competitive displacement of the alkanethiol may occur [75], and it is unclear if these surfaces are applicable for use in reducing media. Similar substrates can be prepared from the chemisorption of carboxylic acids onto alumina [76]. Prepared substrates stored under Ar are stable for several months.

Amine-bearing surfaces have been produced by the adsorption of biologically inert proteins such as albumin. Cells do not have adhesion receptors for albumin, and for this reason albumin has been used to passivate surfaces against cell adhesion. Bioactive ligands can be amino-immobilized onto the albumin-coated surfaces [45, 46, 48].

Functional polymers and copolymers containing alcohols, amines, alkyl halides, carboxylic acids, or other groups, can be synthesized, coated onto a surface, and used as the substrate for immobilization of bioactive ligands [77, 78]. Examples include poly(vinyl alcohol) [31, 33], chloromethyl polystyrene [56], aminopolystyrene [79, 80], poly(acrylic acid) [20, 38], polyallylamine [80], poly(maleic acid anhydride) [12], poly(carbodiimide) [81], and poly(succinimide) [82].

106.4 Ligand/Polymer Hybrids

Hybrid copolymers may be synthesized in which one of the components is the biologically active ligand. These copolymers may then be coated onto a substrate or crosslinked into a three-dimensional network. Since the ligand is a component of the copolymer, no additional ligand immobilization may be necessary to produce bioactive substrates.

Examples are available for particular cases of hybrid copolymers [54, 55, 82–87], including gamma-irradiated crosslinked poly(peptide) [86, 88], dialdehyde crosslinked poly(vinyl alcohol)-glycosaminoglycan [54], poly(amino acid-etherurethane) [47, 87], poly(amino acid-lactic acid) [89], poly(amino acid-carbonate) [90], poly(peptide-styrene) [84], and linear [83] or crosslinked [82] poly(glycoside-acrylamide).

106.5 Determining Ligand Surface Densities

The concentration of ligands immobilized upon a surface can be measured using radiolabeling, photochrome labeling, surface analysis, or gravimetry. Since most materials can support the nonspecific adsorption of bioactive ligands, especially proteins, controls must be utilized to differentiate between covalent immobilization and physicochemical adsorption occurring during coupling. For example, ligands immobilized onto unactivated versus activated substrates give relative differences between nonspecific adsorption and specific bioconjugation.

The surface immobilization of radiolabeled ligands with markers such as ^3H, ^{35}S, or ^{125}I, can be followed to give information on the kinetics of coupling, the coupling capacity of the substrate, and the surface density of ligands. Densities on the order of pmol-fmol/cm^2 are detectable using radiolabeled molecules.

The coupling capacity and density of immobilized acids, amines, and thiols can be evaluated using colorimetric procedures. Substrates can be incubated in solutions of Ellman's reagent [91, 92]; the absorbances of the reaction products give the surface density. Antigens which have been immobilized can be exposed to photochrome-labeled antibodies and surface concentrations calculated using standard enzyme immunosorbent assays [49, 93].

Verification of ligand immobilization may be performed using a number of surface analysis techniques. Mass spectroscopy, x-ray photoelectron spectroscopy, and dynamic contact angle analysis can give information on the chemical composition of the substrate's outmost layers. Changes in composition are indicative of modification. Ellipsometry can be used to gauge the thickness of overlapping surface layers; increases imply the presence of additional layers. Highly sensitive gravimetric balances, such as quartz crystal microbalances, can detect *in situ* changes in the mass of immobilized ligand in the nanogram range [65].

106.6 Applications of Immobilized Ligands

Extracellular matrix proteins such as fibronectin, laminin, vitronectin and collagen, or adhesion molecules such as ICAM-1, VCAM-1, PCAM-1, and sialyl Lewis X, interact with cell surface receptors and mediate cell adhesion. The tripeptide adhesion sequence Arg-Gly-Asp (RGD) is a ubiquitous signal present in many cell adhesion proteins. It interacts with the integrin family of cell surface adhesion receptors, and comprises the best studied ligand-receptor pair [94–96]. In lieu of immobilizing complex multifunctional proteins for purposes of cell adhesion studies, synthetic RGD sequences have instead been immobilized onto many substrates as simplified models to understand various molecular aspects of cell adhesion phenomena. The following paragraphs cite examples of RGD-grafted substrates that have been used in biomedicine and bioengineering.

The density of RGD necessary to mediate cell adhesion has been determined in a number of fashions. RGD-containing peptides and protein fragments have been physicochemically adsorbed onto tissue culture substrates [97, 98] or covalently bound to albumin-coated substrates [45, 46] to titrate the dependency of cell adhesion function upon RGD surface densities. To remove potential complications due to desorption of ligands or albumin, RGD has been covalently bound onto functionalized substrates. Immobilization also restricts the number of conformations the peptide may assume, helping to ensure that all the peptide is accessible to the cells. RGD has been immobilized onto silanated glasses by its amino [19, 99] and carboxyl [15] termini. The effects of RGD density on cell adhesion, spreading, and cytoskeletal organization was examined [99] using this well-defined system. Other peptides have been immobilized in identical fashion to determine if they influence cell physiology [100].

RGD peptides have been immobilized onto highly cell-resistant materials to ensure that the peptide is the only cell adhesion signal responsible for cell adhesion to diminish signals borne of nonspecifically adsorbed serum proteins. Hydrogels of polyacrylamide [101], poly(vinyl alcohol) [31] and poly(ethylene glycol) [85] and nonhydrogel networks of polyacrylate/poly(ethylene glycol)

[102] have been grafted with RGD; these background materials were highly resistant to the adhesion of cells even in the presence of serum proteins, demonstrating that the RGD sequence was solely responsible for mediating cell adhesion.

RGD-containing peptides have been immobilized onto medically relevant polymers in an effort to enhance their biocompatibilities by containing an adhered layer of viable cells. RGD-grafted surfaces can be more efficient in supporting the number and strength of cell adhesion by the peptide facilitating cell adhesion additionally to adsorbed adhesion proteins from the biological milieu. RGD has been conjugated onto surfaces by means of photoimmobilization [103] and plasma glow discharge [64]. In an effort to promote cell adhesion onto biodegradable implants, RGD peptides have been covalently grafted onto poly(amino acid-lactic acid) copolymers [89]. In this manner, cells adherent on the degradable material can eventually obtain a completely natural environment. Self-assembled monolayers of biologic ligands have been immobilized onto gold substrates by adsorbing functionalized thiol-containing bridges followed by covalent grafting of the ligand [93] or by adsorbing alkanethiol-containing ligands [104]. It has been suggested [105] that RGD-containing peptides could be immobilized onto gold substrates in these manners to engineer highly defined surfaces for cell culture systems.

These examples only partially illustrate the utility of ligand-grafted substrates for bioengineering and biomedicine. These substrates offer simplified models of basement membranes to elucidate mechanisms and requirements of cell adhesion. They have applications in biomedicine as biocompatible, cell-adhesive biomaterials for tissue engineering or for clinical implantation.

References

1. Brinkley M. 1992. A brief survey of methods for preparing protein conjugate with dyes, haptens, and cross-linking reagents. Bioconjugate Chem 3:2.
2. Means GE, Feeney RE. 1990. Chemical modification of proteins: History and applications. Bioconjugate Chem 1:2.
3. Wong SS. 1991. Chemistry of Protein Conjugation and Cross-Linking, Boca Raton, Fla, CRC Press.
4. Pharmacia Inc. 1988. Affinity chromatography principles and methods, Tech Bull, Uppsala, Sweden.
5. Trevan MD. 1980. Immobilized Enzymes: An Introduction and Applications in Biotechnology, New York, Wiley.
6. Wimalasena RL, Wilson GS. 1991. Factors affecting the specific activity of immobilized antibodies and their biologically active fragments. J Chromatogr 572:85.
7. Matson RS, Little MC. 1988. Strategy for the immobilization of monoclonal antibodies on solid-phase supports. J Chromatogr 458:67.
8. Wingard LB Jr, Katchalski-Katzir E, Goldstein L. 1976. Applied Biochemistry and Bioengineering: Immobilized Enzyme Principles, vol 1, New York, Academic.
9. Smalla K, Turkova J, Coupek J, et al. 1988. Influence on the covalent immobilization of proteins to modified copolymers of 2-hydroxyethyl methacrylate with ethylene dimethacrylate. Biotech Appl Biochem 10:21.
10. Schneider C, Newmanm RA, Sutherland DR, et al. 1982. A one-step purification of membrane proteins using a high efficiency immunomatrix. J Biol Chem 257:10766.
11. Scouten W. 1987. A survey of enzyme coupling techniques. Methods Enzymol 135:30.
12. Maeda H, Seymour LW, Miyamoto Y. Conjugates of anticancer agents and polymers: advantages of macromolecular therapeutics in vivo. Bioconjugate Chem 3:351.
13. Nojiri C, Okano T, Park KD, et al. 1988. Suppression mechanisms for thrombus formation on heparin-immobilized segmented polyurethane-ureas. Trans. ASAIO, 34:386.
14. Fassina G. 1992. Oriented immobilization of peptide ligands on solid supports. J Chromatogr 591:99.

15. Hubbell JA, Massia SP, Drumheller PD. 1992. Surface-grafted cell-binding peptides in tissue engineering of the vascular graft. Ann NY Acad Sci 665:253.

16. Beer JH, Coller BS. (1989). Immobilized Arg-Gly-Asp (RGD) peptides of varying lengths as structural probes of the platelet glycoprotein IIb/IIIa receptor. Blood 79:117.

17. Axen R, Porath J, Ernback S, Chemical coupling of peptides and proteins to polysaccharides by means of cyanogen halides, Nature 214:1302.

18. Delgado C, Patel JN, Francis GE, et al. 1990. Coupling of poly(ethylene glycol) to albumin under very mild conditions by activation with tresyl chloride: Characterization of the conjugate by partitioning in aqueous two-phase systems. Biotech Appl Biochem 12:119.

19. Massia SP, Hubbell JA. 1991. Human endothelial cell interactions with surface-coupled adhesion peptides on a nonadhesive glass substrate and two polymeric biomaterials J Biomed Mater Res 25:223.

20. Nakajima K, Hirano Y, Iida T, et al. 1990. Adsorption of plasma proteins on Arg-Gly-Asp-Ser peptide-immobilized poly(vinyl alcohol) and ethylene-acrylic acid copolymer films. Polym J 22:985.

21. Testoff MA, Rudolph AS. 1992. Modification of dry 1,2-dipalmitoylphosatidylcholine phase behavior with synthetic membrane-bound stabilizing carbohydrates. Bioconjugate Chem 3:203.

22. Fontanel M-L, Bazin H, Teoule R. 1993. End attachment of phenololigonucleotide conjugates to diazotized cellulose. Bioconjugate Chem 4:380.

23. Nilsson K, Mosbach K. 1984. Immobilization of ligands with organic sulfonyl chlorides. Methods Enzymol 104:56.

24. Chang Y-A, Gee A, Smith A, et al. Activating hydroxyl groups of polymeric carriers using 4-fluorobenzenesulfonyl chloride. Bioconjugate Chem 3:200.

25. Harris JM, Struck EC, Case MG, 1984. Synthesis and characterization of poly(ethylene glycol) derivatives. J Polym Sci Polym Chem Edn 22:341.

26. Sawhney AS, Hubbell JA. 1992. Poly(ethylene oxide)-graft-poly(L-lysine) copolymers to enhance the biocompatibility of poly(L-lysine)-alginate microcapsule membranes. Biomaterials 13:863.

27. Hearn MTW. 1987. 1,1′-Carbonyldiimidazole-mediated immobilization of enzymes and affinity ligands. Methods Enzymol 135:102.

28. Miron T, Wilchek M. 1993. A simplified method for the preparation of succinimidyl carbonate polyethylene glycol for coupling to proteins. Bioconjugate Chem 4:568.

29. Uy R, Wold F. 1977. 1,4-Butanediol diglycidyl ether coupling of carbohydrates to sepharose: affinity adsorbents for lectins and glycosidases. Anal Biochem 81:98.

30. Sundberg L, Porath J. 1974. Preparation of adsorbents for biospecific affinity chromatography: I. Attachment of group-containing ligands to insoluble polymers by means of bifunctional oxiranes. J Chromatogr 90:87.

31. Kondoh A, Makino K, Matsuda T. 1993. Two-dimensional artificial extracellular matrix: bioadhesive peptide-immobilized surface design. J Appl Polym Sci 47:1983.

32. Annunziato ME, Patel US, Ranade M, et al. 1993. p-Maleimidophenyl isocyanate: A novel heterobifunctional linker for hydroxyl to thiol coupling. Bioconjugate Chem 4:212.

33. Kobayashi H, Ikada Y. 1991. Covalent immobilization of proteins onto the surface of poly(vinyl alcohol) hydrogel. Biomaterials 12:747.

34. Shafer SG, Harris JM. 1986. Preparation of cyanuric-chloride activated poly(ethylene glycol). J Polym Sci Polym Chem Edn 24:375.

35. Kay G, Cook EM. 1967. Coupling of enzymes to cellulose using chloro-s-triazine. Nature (London) 216:514.

36. Bodanszky M. 1988. Peptide Chemistry, Berlin, Springer-Verlag.

37. Staab HA. 1962. Syntheses using heterocyclic amides (azolides). Angew Chem Internat Edn 7:351.

38. Hirano Y, Okuno M, Hayashi T, et al. 1993. Cell-attachment activities of surface immobilized oligopeptides RGD, RGDS, RGDT, and YIGSR toward five cell lines. J Biomater Sci Polym Edn 4:235.

39. Ozaki CK, Phaneuf MD, Hong SL, et al. 1993. Glycoconjugate mediated endothelial cell adhesion to Dacron polyester film. J Vasc Surg 18:486.

40. Barnwarth W, Schmidt D, Stallard RL, et al. 1988. Bathophenanthroline-ruthenium(II) complexes as non-radioactive labels for oligonucleotides which can be measured by time-resolved fluorescence techniques. Helv Chim Acta 71:2085.

41. Drumheller PD, Elbert DL, Hubbell JA. 1994. Multifunctional poly(ethylene glycol) semi-interpenetrating polymer networks as highly selective adhesive substrates for bioadhesive peptide grafting. Biotech Bioeng 43:772.

42. Liu SQ, Ito Y, Imanishi Y. 1993. Cell growth on immobilized cell growth factor: 9. Covalent immobilization of insulin, transferrin, and collagen to enhance growth of bovine endothelial cells. J Biomed Mater Res 27:909.

43. Wachter E, Machleidt W, Hofner H, Otto J. 1973. Aminopropyl glass and its p-phenylene diisothiocyanate derivative, a new support in solid-phase Edman degradation of peptides and proteins. FEBS Lett 35:97.

44. Maisano F, Gozzini L, de Haen C. 1992. Coupling of DTPA to proteins: A critical analysis of the cyclic dianhydride method in the case of insulin modification. Bioconjugate Chem 3:212.

45. Streeter HB, Rees DA. 1987. Fibroblast adhesion to RGDS shows novel features compared with fibronectin. J Cell Biol 105:507.

46. Singer II, Kawka DW, Scott S, et al. 1987. The fibronectin cell attachment Arg-Gly-Asp-Ser promotes focal contact formation during early fibroblast attachment and spreading. J Cell Biol 104:573.

47. Nathan A, Bolikal D, Vyavahare N, et al. 1992. Hydrogels based on water-soluble poly(ether urethanes) derived from L-lysine and poly(ethylene glycol). Macromolecules 25:4476.

48. Elling L, Kula M-R. 1991. Immunoaffinity partitioning: Synthesis and use of polyethylene glycol-oxirane for coupling to bovine serum albumin and monoclonal antibodies. Biotech Appl Biochem 13:354.

49. Pope NM, Kulcinski DL, Hardwick A, et al. 1993. New applications of silane coupling agents for covalently binding antibodies to glass and cellulose solid supports. Bioconjugate Chem 4:166.

50. Werb Z, Tremble PM, Behrendtsen O, et al. 1989. Signal transduction through the fibronectin receptor induces collagenase and stromelysin gene expression. J Cell Biol 109:877.

51. Yamagata M, Suzuki S, Akiyama SK, et al. 1989. Regulation of cell-substrate adhesion by proteoglycans immobilized on extracellular substrates. J Biol Chem 264:8012.

52. Robinson PJ, Dunnill P, Lilly MD. 1971. Porous glass as a solid support for immobilization or affinity chromatography of enzymes. Biochim Biophys Acta 242:659.

53. Harris JM, Dust JM, McGill RA, et al. 1991. New polyethylene glycols for biomedical applications. ACS Symp Ser 467:418.

54. Cholakis CH, Zingg W, Sefton MV. 1989. Effect of heparin-PVA hydrogel on platelets in a chronic arterio-venous shunt. J Biomed Mater Res 23:417.

55. Cholakis CH, Sefton MV. 1984. Chemical characterization of an immobilized heparin: heparin-PVA. In SW Shalaby, AS Hoffman, BD Ratner, et al (eds), Polymers as Biomaterials, New York, Plenum.

56. Gutsche AT, Parsons-Wingerter P, Chand D, et al. 1994. N-Acetylglucosamine and adenosine derivatized surfaces for cell culture: 3T3 fibroblast and chicken hepatocyte response. Biotech Bioeng 43:801.

57. Jagendorf AT, Patchornik A, Sela M. 1963. Use of antibody bound to modified cellulose as an immunospecific adsorbent of antigen. Biochim Biophys Acta 78:516.

58. Collioud A, Clemence J-F, Sanger M, et al. 1993. Oriented and covalent immobilization of target molecules to solid supports: Synthesis and application of a light-activatible and thiol-reactive cross-linking reagent. Bioconjugate Chem 4:528.

59. Bhatia SK, Shriver-Lake LC, Prior KJ, et al. Use of thiol-terminal silanes and heterobifunctional crosslinkers for immobilization of antibodies on silica surfaces. Anal Biochem 178:408.

60. Moeschler HJ, Vaughan M. 1983. Affinity chromatography of brain cyclic nucleotide phosphodiesterase using 3-(2-pyridyldithio)proprionyl-substituted calmodulin linked to thiol-Sepharose. Biochemistry 22:826.

61. Tseng Y-C, Park K. 1992. Synthesis of photoreactive poly(ethylene glycol) and its application to the prevention of surface-induced platelet activation. J Biomed Mater Res 26:373.

62. Yan M, Cai SX, Wybourne MN, et al. 1993. Photochemical functionalization of polymer surfaces and the production of biomolecule-carrying micrometer-scale structures by deep-UV lithography using 4-substituted perfluorophenyl azides. J Am Chem Soc 115:814.

63. Guire PE. 1993. Biocompatible device with covalently bonded biocompatible agent, U.S. Patent 5,263,992.

64. Ito Y, Suzuki K, Imanishi Y. 1994. Surface biolization by grafting polymerizable bioactive chemicals. ACS Symp Ser 540:66.

65. Nakayama Y, Matsuda T, Irie M. 1993. A novel surface photo-graft polymerization method for fabricated devices. ASAIO J 39:M542.

66. Ratner BD, Chilkoti A, Lopez GP. 1990. Plasma deposition and treatment for biomaterial applications. In R d'Agostino (ed), Plasma Deposition, Treatment, and Etching of Polymers, p 463, New York, Academic Press.

67. Ratner BD. 1992. Plasma deposition for biomedical applications: a brief review. J Biomater Sci Polym Edn 4:3.

68. Desai NP, Hubbell JA. 1991. Biological responses to polyethylene oxide modified polyethylene terephthalate surfaces. J Biomed Mater Res 25:829.

69. Lin H-B, Zhao Z-C, Garcia-Echeverria C, et al. 1992. Synthesis of a novel polyurethane co-polymer containing covalently attached RGD peptide. J Biomater Sci Polymer Edn 3:217.

70. Costello CA, McCarthy TJ. 1987. Surface-selective introduction of specific functionalities onto poly(tetrafluoroethylene). Macromolecules 20:2819.

71. Allmer K, Feiring AE. 1991. Photochemical modification of a fluoropolymer surface. Macromolecules 24:5487.

72. Ferguson GS, Chaudhury MK, Biebuyck HA, et al. 1993. Monolayers on disordered substrates: self-assembly of alkyltrichlorosilanes on surface-modified polyethylene and poly(dimethylsiloxane). Macromolecules, 26:5870.

73. Plant AL. 1993. Self-assembled phospholipid/alkanethiol biomimetic bilayers on gold. Langmuir 9:2764.

74. Prime KL, Whitesides GM. 1993. Adsorption of proteins onto surfaces containing end-attached oligo(ethylene oxide): A model system using self-assembled monolayers. J Am Chem Soc 115:10714.

75. Biebuyck HA, Whitesides GM. 1993. Interchange between monolayers on gold formed from unsymmetrical disulfides and solutions of thiols: evidence for sulfur-sulfur bond cleavage by gold metal. Langmuir 9:1766.

76. Laibinis PE, Hickman JJ, Wrightson MS, et al. 1989. Orthogonal self-assembled monolayers: Alkanethiols on gold and alkane carboxylic acids on alumina. Science 245:845.

77. Veronese FM, Visco C, Massarotto S, et al. 1987. New acrylic polymers for surface modification of enzymes of therapeutic interest and for enzyme immobilization. Ann NY Acad Sci 501:444.

78. Scouten WH. 1987. A survey of enzyme coupling techniques. Methods Enzymol 135:30.

79. Mech C, Jeschkeit H, Schellenberger A. 1976. Investigation of the covalent bond structure of peptide-matrix systems by Edman degradation of support-fixed peptides. Eur J Biochem 66:133.

80. Iio K, Minoura N, Aiba S, et al. 1994. Cell growth on poly(vinyl alcohol) hydrogel membranes containing biguanido groups. J Biomed Mater Res 28:459.

81. Weinshenker NM, Shen C-M. 1972. Polymeric reagents: I. Synthesis of an insoluble polymeric carbodiimide. Tetrahedron Lett 32:3281.

82. Schnaar RL, Brandley BK, Needham LK, et al. 1989. Adhesion of eukaryotic cells to immobilized carbohydrates. Methods Enzymol 179:542.

83. Sparks MA, Williams KW, Whitesides GM. 1993. Neuraminidase-resistant hemagglutination inhibitors: acrylamide copolymers containing a C-glycoside of N-acetylneuramic acid. J Med Chem 36:778.

84. Ozeki E, Matsuda T. 1990. Development of an artificial extracellular matrix. Solution castable polymers with cell recognizable peptidyl side chains. ASAIO Trans 36:M294.

85. Drumheller PD. 1994. Polymer Networks of Poly(Ethylene Glycol) as Biospecific Cell Adhesive Substrates, PhD dissertation, University of Texas at Austin.

86. Nicol A, Gowda DC, Parker TM, et al. 1993. Elastomeric polytetrapeptide matrices: Hydrophobicity dependence of cell attachment from adhesive $(GGIP)_n$ to nonadhesive $(GGAP)_n$ even in serum. J Biomed Mater Res 27:801.

87. Kohn J, Gean KF, Nathan A, et al. 1993. New drug conjugates: attachment of small molecules to poly(PEG-Lys). Polym Mater Sci Eng 69:515.

88. Nicol A, Gowda DC, Urry DW. 1992. Cell adhesion and growth on synthetic elastomeric matrices containing ARG-GLY-ASP-SER. J Biomed Mater Res 26:393.

89. Barrera DA, Zylstra E, Lansbury PT, et al. 1993. Synthesis and RGD peptide modification of a new biodegradable copolymer: Poly(lactic acid-colysine). J Am Chem Soc 115:11010.

90. Pulapura S, Kohn J. 1992. Tyrosine-derived polycarbonate: Backbone-modified "pseudo"-poly(amino acids) designed for biomedical applications. Biopolymers 32:411.

91. Ngo TT. Coupling capacity of solid-phase carboxyl groups. Determination by a colorimetric procedure. Appl Biochem Biotech 13:207.

92. Ngo TT. 1986. Colorimetric determination of reactive amino groups of a solid support using Traut's and Ellman's reagents. Appl Biochem Biotech 13:213.

93. Duan C, Meyerhoff ME. 1994. Separation-free sandwich enzyme immunoassays using microporous gold electrodes and self-assembled monolayer/immobilized capture antibodies. Anal Chem 66:1369.

94. Albeda SM, Buck CA. 1990. Integrins and other cell adhesion molecules. FASEB J 4:2868.

95. Ruoslahti E. 1991. Integrins. J Clin Invest 87:1.

96. Humphries MJ. 1990. The molecular basis and specificity of integrin-ligand interactions. J Cell Sci 97:585.

97. Underwood PA, Bennett FA. 1989. A comparison of the biological activities of the cell-adhesive proteins vitronectin and fibronectin. J Cell Sci 93:641.

98. Yamada KM, Kennedy DW. 1985. Amino acid sequence specificities of an adhesive recognition signal. J Cell Biochem 28:99.

99. Massia SP, Hubbell JA. 1991. An RGD spacing of 44 nm is sufficient for integrin $\alpha_v\beta_3$-mediated fibroblast spreading and 140 nm for focal contact and stress fiber formation. J Cell Biol 114:1089.

100. Hubbell JA, Massia SP, Desai NP, et al. 1992. Endothelial cell-selective materials for tissue engineering in the vascular graft via a new receptor. Bio/Technology 9:568.

101. Brandley BK, Schnaar RL. 1989. Tumor cell haptotaxis on covalently immobilized linear and exponential gradients of a cell adhesion peptide. Dev Biol 135:74.

102. Drumheller PD, Elbert DL, Hubbell JA. 1994. Multifunctional poly(ethylene glycol) semi-interpenetrating polymer networks as highly selective adhesive substrates for bioadhesive peptide grafting. Biotech Bioeng 43:772.

103. Clapper DL, Daws KM, Guire PE. 1994. Photoimmobilized ECM peptides promote cell attachment and growth on biomaterials. Trans Soc Biomater 17:345.

104. Spinke J, Liley M, Guder H-J, et al. 1993. Molecular recognition at self-assembled monolayers: The construction of multicomponent multilayers. Langmuir 9:1821.

105. Singhvi R, Kumar A, Lopez GP, et al. 1994. Engineering cell shape and function. Science 264:696.

107

Biomaterials: Protein-Surface Interactions

Joseph A. Chinn
CarboMedics, Inc.

A common assumption in biomaterials research is that cellular interactions with natural artificial surfaces are mediated through adsorbed proteins. Such diverse processes as thrombosis and hemostasis, hard and soft tissue healing, infection, and inflammation are each affected by protein adsorption to surfaces in vivo. Many in vitro diagnostic analyses and genetic engineering processes also involve protein adsorption.

Successful application of biomedical devices requires that cell-protein-surface interactions be addressed. For example, some cardiovascular device applications require chronic anticoagulation therapy, whereas orthopedic applications exploit surface properties to encourage bone healing. Protein-mediated device mineralization and degradation can significantly impair device performance. An understanding of basic principles of protein adsorption is essential for both engineering professionals involved in design and manufacture of medical products and services and medical professionals involved in clinical and diagnostic application of those products and services.

The adsorption of fibrinogen has been extensively studied, because of its role in thrombosis and hemostasis, as has adsorption of albumin, because it is thought to inhibit the adhesion of blood platelets [Young et al., 1982]. However, the importance of the state of an adsorbed protein in mediating cellular interactions is now becoming evident. Molecularly sensitive indirect measurement techniques, e.g., circular dichroism (CD), differential scanning calorimetry (DSC), enzyme-linked immunosorbent assay (ELISA), Fourier transform infrared spectroscopy/attenuated total reflectance (FTIR/ATR), radio-immunoassay (RIA), or total internal reflection fluorescence (TIRF), must be used to characterize the conformation and organization of adsorbed proteins. (The amount of protein adsorbed to a substrate is best measured directly using radiolabeled proteins. The thickness of an adsorbed protein film can be calculated from ellipsometry measurements.) Highly specific monoclonal (MAb) (against specific protein epitopes) [Shiba et al., 1991] and polyclonal (PAb) [Lindon et al., 1986] antibodies provide direct probes of adsorbed protein conformation and organization. Thus, cellular response can be compared not only with the amounts of proteins adsorbed but also with the organization of the proteins.

Whereas previous studies confirmed roles for adsorbed proteins in subsequent cell-surface interactions, much current research aims to better understand cell-protein-surface interactions on a molecular level. Recently, peptide sequences contained within the cell-binding domains of adhesive proteins have been identified and characterized, synthesized, and demonstrated to bind cellular receptors [Yamada, 1991] called integrins [Ruoslahti, 1991]. Current and potential applications range from selective or enhanced in vitro cell culture to selective in vivo cellular responses such as endothelialization in the absence of inflammation, infection, or thrombosis [Hubbell et al., 1991].

107.1 Fundamentals of Protein Adsorption

Detailed and comprehensive reviews of protein adsorption have been published [Andrade, 1985; Andrade & Hlady, 1986; Horbett, 1982; Norde & Lyklema, 1991]. Thorough understanding of key basic principles will prove helpful in critically evaluating reports in literature. Particularly important concepts are protein structure and heterogeneity that dramatically affect thermodynamics and kinetics of adsorption, reversibility of adsorption, and the dynamics of multicomponent adsorption.

A protein is a complex molecule comprised of amino acid copolymer (polyamide) chains that interact with each other to give the molecule a three-dimensional structure. Each amino acid in the polymer contributes to the chemical and physical properties of the protein. Protein structure and function are relevant to protein adsorption and have been described on four different scales or order [Andrade & Hlady, 1986]. Primary structure refers to the order and number of the amino acids in a copolymer chain. The 20 amino acid building blocks that are polymerized to make proteins are called residues. Of these, 8 have nonpolar side chains, 7 have neutral polar side chains, and 5 have charged polar side chains [Stryer, 1988]. Secondary structure results from hydrogen bonding associated with the amide linkages in the polymer chain backbone to form structures such as the α-helix and β-pleated sheet. Tertiary structure results from associations within chains, including hydrogen bonding, ionic and hydrophobic interactions, salt bridges, and disulfide bonds. Quaternary structure results from associations between chains. It is often this structure that dictates how a protein interacts with surfaces and cells. Many blood proteins contain polar, nonpolar, and charged residues. In polar media such as buffered saline or blood plasma, hydrophilic residues tend to self-associate (often at the outer, water-contacting surface of the protein), as do hydrophobic residues (often "inside" the protein). This results in distinct domains (Fig. 107.1) that dictate higher-order protein structure.

When a single, static protein solution is contacted with a substrate, the rate of adsorption depends upon transport of the protein to and from the bulk to the surface. Andrade and Hlady [1986] identify four primary transport mechanisms, diffusion, thermal convection, flow convection, and coupled convection-diffusion. In isothermal, parallel laminar flow or static systems, protein transport to the interface occurs exclusively by diffusion. In turbulent or stirred systems, each of the four transport modes can be significant.

When adsorption is reaction limited, the net rate of adsorption can sometimes be described by the classic Langmuir theory of gas adsorption [Smith, 1981]

$$r_A = k_A \cdot C_b \cdot (1 - \Theta) - k_D \cdot \Theta \qquad (107.1)$$

where r_A is the net adsorption rate, k_A is the adsorption rate constant, C_b is the bulk concentration of the protein in solution, Θ is fractional surface coverage, and k_D is the desorption rate constant. At equilibrium, the net rate of adsorption, r_A, is zero, and Θ can be calculated from Eq. (107.1) as the Langmuir adsorption isotherm

$$\Theta = \frac{K \cdot C_b}{1 + K \cdot C_b} \qquad (107.2)$$

where $K = k_A/k_D$. This model assumes reversible monolayer adsorption, no conformational changes upon adsorption, and no interactions between adsorbed molecules. It is most applicable to dilute solutions and nonhydrophobic substrates. When adsorption is diffusion limited, the initial rate of adsorption is equivalent to the rate of diffusion, described mathematically [Andrade & Hlady, 1986] as

$$r_A = r_{\mathscr{D}} = 2 \cdot C_b \cdot \sqrt{\frac{\mathscr{D}}{\pi t}} \qquad (107.3)$$

where $\mathscr{D}$ is the diffusivity of the protein, and t is time.

Protein adsorption to hydrophobic substrates differs from that to hydrophilic substrates. The primary driving force for adsorption to hydrophilic substrates is often enthalpic, whereas that to hydrophobic substrates is entropic [Norde, 1986]. Water near a hydrophobic surface tends to hydrogen bond to neighboring water molecules, resulting in a highly ordered water structure [Andrade & Hlady, 1986]. Disruption of this structure (dehydration) by adsorption of a protein to the surface increases the entropy of the system and is therefore thermodynamically favored, whereas desorption is disfavored. As a result, adsorption to hydrophilic substrates is generally reversible, whereas that to hydrophobic substrates is not. Denaturation of the adsorbed protein by hydrophobic-hydrophobic interactions with the substrate can also contribute to irreversible adsorption [Feng & Andrade, 1994].

The amount of a specific protein adsorbed to a substrate can be measured directly if the protein is radiolabeled. Gamma-emitting isotopes are preferred because their signal is directly proportional to the amount of protein present. Radioisotopes of iodine (^{125}I, [129]I, and ^{131}I) are commonly used because iodine readily attaches to tyrosine residues [Macfarlane, 1958]. An ^{125}I monochloride radiolabeling technique has been published [Horbett, 1986]. If neither the ^{125}I-protein nor the unlabeled protein preferentially adsorbs to the substrate at the expense of the other, then the amount of that protein adsorbed to a substrate from multicomponent media such as plasma can be measured by adding a small amount of ^{125}I-protein to the adsorption medium. (^{125}I-fibrinogen generally behaves like its unlabeled

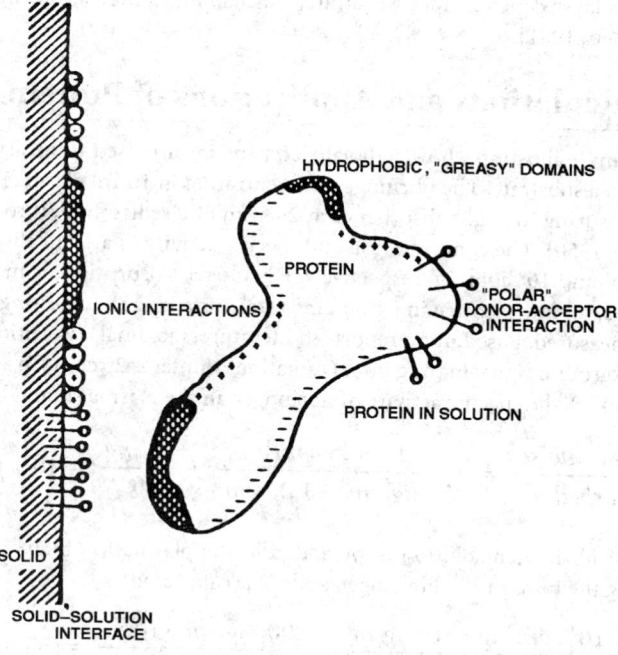

FIGURE 107.1 Schematic view of protein interacting with a well characterized surface. The protein has a number of surface domains with hydrophobic, charged, and polar character. The solid surface has a similar domainlike character (Andrade & Hlady, 1986.)

analog.) Substrates are incubated with the medium, then the radioactivity originating from the ^{125}I-protein adsorbed to the samples is measured. The total amount of the protein adsorbed (both unlabeled and ^{125}I-protein) is calculated by dividing the measured radioactivity by the specific activity of the protein in the medium. (Specific activity is determined by dividing the gamma activity in a measured aliquot of the adsorption medium by the total amount of the protein in the aliquot.)

Indirect methods are also used to study proteins adsorbed to a substrate. ELISA and RIA analytical techniques exploit specific antibody-antigen interactions as follows. Antibodies against specific epitopes of an adsorbed protein are either conjugated to an enzyme (ELISA) or radiolabeled (RIA). Substrates are incubated with the medium, then with a solution containing the antibody or antibody conjugate. In the case of ELISA, the substrates are subsequently incubated with substrate solution. As the substrate is converted to product, the color of the solution changes proportional to the amount of antiprotein bound and is measured spectrophotometrically. However, extensive calibration is required to quantify results. In the case of RIA, the radioactivity originating from the ^{125}I-antiprotein (bound to the protein adsorbed to the substrate) is measured. The amount of antiprotein bound can be calculated from the retained radioactivity. With both methods, the relative amount of the adsorbed protein to which the antiprotein has bound, rather than the total amount of protein adsorbed, is measured. Antiprotein binding is a function of not only the amount of protein adsorbed but also the particular antibody used, total protein surface loading, and protein residence time. Thus, although antibody techniques provide direct probes of adsorbed protein conformation and organization, measurements are not necessarily reflective of the absolute amounts of protein adsorbed. Other indirect methods used to study adsorbed proteins include ellipsometry, electron microscopy, high-performance liquid chromatography (HPLC), and staining techniques.

Although single component adsorption is easily described, multicomponent adsorption is not. Upon contact with blood, a biomaterial is rapidly covered by an adsorbed protein layer that drives subsequent cellular reactions [Horbett 1982; Horbett & Brash, 1987; Young et al., 1982]. The composition of this layer depends upon substrate, plasma bulk composition, and adsorption time [Brash, 1981; Horbett, 1981].

107.2 Example Calculations and Applications of Protein Adsorption

The following example illustrates how radiolabeled proteins are used to measure the amount of protein adsorbed to a substrate. The fibrinogen concentration in 10-ml plasma is determined to be 5.00 mg/ml by measuring the light absorbance at 280 nm of a redissolved, thrombin-induced clot [Ratnoff & Menzie, 1950]. The concentration and specific activity of a 10-μl aliquot of ^{125}I-fibrinogen are 1.00 mg/ml and 10^9 cpm/μg, respectively. Fibrinogen adsorption from dilute plasma to a series of polymer samples, each having 1.00 cm^2 total surface area (counting both sides of the sample), is to be measured. Based upon reports in literature, maximal adsorption of 250 ng/cm^2 is expected. The background signal in the gamma radiation counter is 25 cpm. To achieve a maximum signal/noise ratio of 10, the specific activity of fibrinogen in the plasma should be

$$\frac{(signal/noise) \cdot noise}{mass\ adsorbed} = \frac{10 \cdot 25\ cpm}{250\ ng/cm^2 \cdot 1.00\ cm^2} \cdot \frac{10^3\ ng}{\mu g} = 10^3\ cpm/\mu g \quad (107.4)$$

The volume of ^{125}I-fibrinogen solution to be added to the plasma to obtain 10^3 cpm/μg specific activity (neglecting the mass of ^{125}I-fibrinogen added) is calculated as

$$\frac{10^3\ cpm/\mu g \cdot 10^3\ \mu g/mg \cdot 5.00\ mg/ml \cdot 10\ ml}{10^9\ cpm/mg \cdot 1.00\ mg/ml \cdot ml/10^3\ \mu l} = 50\ \mu l \quad (107.5)$$

Addition of 50 μl ^{125}I-fibrinogen solution should increase the total fibrinogen concentration in the plasma by only a small fraction

$$\frac{50 \ \mu l \cdot ml/10^3 \ \mu l \cdot 1.00 \ mg/ml}{10 \ ml \cdot 5.00 \ mg/ml} = 10^{-3} \qquad (107.6)$$

To determine the amount of protein adsorbed to the substrate, the radioactivity of samples incubated with plasma is measured and compared with the specific activity of the protein in the plasma. In this example, if the amount of radioactivity retained by a sample is measured to be 137 cpm, then the mass of fibrinogen adsorbed is calculated as,

$$\frac{(137 \ cpm/sample - 25 \ cpm \ background) \cdot 10^3 \ ng/\mu g}{10^3 \ cpm/\mu g \ fibrinogen \cdot 1.00 \ cm^2/sample} = 112 \ ng/cm^2 \quad (107.7)$$

To verify that neither labeled nor unlabeled fibrinogen preferentially adsorbs to the substrates, the specific activity of fibrinogen in a small aliquot of the plasma dilution from which adsorption was maximum should be increased 10 times and adsorption from that dilution again measured. Changes in calculated adsorption values should be attributable only to the variability in the data and differences in the signal-to-noise ratio, not the ratio of labeled to unlabeled fibrinogen in the plasma. Similarly, to verify that adsorption of free ^{125}I in the buffer is not significant, adsorption from dilute plasma to which 0.01M unlabeled free iodide is added should be measured.

Adsorption of proteins to polymeric substrates is measured because adsorbed proteins influence cellular processes. Adsorbed albumin is proposed to favor biocompatibility, whereas adsorbed fibrinogen is proposed to discourage biocompatibility because of its role in mediating initial adhesion of blood platelets [Young et al., 1982]. This simplified view inadequately describes biocompatibility in vivo for several reasons. First, the relationships between processes involved in thrombosis, hemostasis, inflammation, and healing (e.g., adhesions of platelets, fibroblasts, white blood cells, endothelial cells) and long-term biocompatibility remains mostly unknown. For example, Sakariassen and coworkers [1979] proposed that exclusively adsorbed von Willebrand factor (vWF) mediates platelet adhesion to vascular subendothelial structures, yet although some people that lack serum vWF in their blood exhibit symptoms of hemophilia, others remain asymptomatic. Second, biologic processes that do not require fibrinogen-mediated cell adhesion (e.g., contact activation [Kaplan, 1978], complement activation [Chenowith, 1988]) are also related to material biocompatibility. Third, biologic factors and serum proteins other than fibrinogen and albumin (e.g., vWF, fibronectin, vitronectin, laminin) significantly affect cellular processes. Fourth, the reactivity of adsorbed proteins depends upon their organization upon the substrate.

Studies of fibrinogen adsorption in vitro illustrate the dynamic nature of protein adsorption from plasma. Vroman and Adams [1969] reported that oxidized silicon and anodized tantalum incubated 2s with plasma bind fibrinogen antiserum, whereas the same materials incubated 25s with plasma do not. Ellipsometry measurements indicated that the observed decrease in antibody binding was not due to loss of protein. Brash and ten Hove [1984] and Horbett [1984] reported that maximal equilibrium fibrinogen adsorption to different materials occurred from intermediate dilutions of plasma. The adsorption maximum is sometimes called a Vroman peak, which describes the shape of the adsorption versus log (plasma concentration) curve referred to as an adsorption isotherm. Both the location and the magnitude of the peak depend upon the surface chemistry of the substrate. (For this reason, it is wise to fully characterize any substrate prior to measuring protein adsorption. Electron spectroscopy for chemical analysis, ESCA [Ratner & McElroy, 1986], and secondary ion mass spectroscopy, SIMS, are often appropriate.) Wojciechowski and colleagues [1986] reported that at short contact times, adsorption was greatest from undiluted plasma. As contact time increased, the plasma concentration at which adsorption was greatest decreased. Because Vroman pioneered much of this work, these phenomena are collectively referred to as the Vroman effect. This principle is most applicable to hydrophilic substrates and is commonly used in biocompatibility studies to vary the composition of the protein layer adsorbed from plasma in a controlled manner.

The unusual observed adsorption behavior occurs because fibrinogen adsorption is driven initially by mass action, i.e., a gradient between surface and bulk concentration. However, as coverage of the surface increases, bulk proteins must compete for surface-binding sites. The composition of the adsorbed layer continues to change as proteins of higher surface activity displace adsorbed proteins of lower surface activity [Horbett, 1984]. Vroman and coworkers [1980] called this process *conversion of the fibrinogen layer* and proposed that fibrinogen adsorbed at early time is at later time displaced by other plasma proteins, possibly high-molecular-weight kininogen (HMWK). A Vroman effect has been reported for other protein-surface systems as well [Horbett & Schway, 1988].

Slack and Horbett [1989] postulated the existence of two distinct types of adsorbed fibrinogen molecules, displaceable and nondisplaceable. Protein adsorption from plasma was modeled as competitive adsorption from a binary solution of fibrinogen and a hypothetical protein H (representing all other plasma components). In this model, protein H adsorbs to unoccupied surface sites in a nondisplaceable state, and fibrinogen molecules first adsorb to unoccupied surface sites in a displaceable state, then are displaced by protein H or spread to become resistant to displacement. The latter process is referred to as *fibrinogen transition*. Neglecting desorption and mass transfer limitations, rate equations for surface coverage by protein H, displaceable fibrinogen, and nondisplaceable fibrinogen were solved simultaneously for a surface initially free of adsorbate. The analytical solution is given by Eq. (107.8) and Eq. (107.9).

$$\Theta_1(t) = \beta(e^{r_1 \cdot t} - e^{r_2 \cdot t}) \tag{107.8}$$

$$\Theta_2(t) = \left(\frac{\beta \cdot k_2}{r_1 \cdot r_2}\right) \cdot [r_1(1 - e^{r_2 \cdot t}) - r_2(1 - e^{r_1 \cdot t})] \tag{107.9}$$

where Θ_1, Θ_2, and Θ_3 are fractional coverages by displaceable fibrinogen, nondisplaceable fibrinogen, and the hypothetical protein, respectively, k_1 is the fibrinogen adsorption rate constant, k_2 is the fibrinogen transition rate constant, k_3 is the hypothetical protein adsorption rate constant, k_4 is the fibrinogen displacement rate constant, C_F is the bulk concentration of fibrinogen, and C_H is the bulk concentration of the hypothetical protein in solution, and β, r_1, and r_2 are constants related to rate constants and bulk concentrations. (See Slack and Horbett [1989] for definitions.) This model predicts maximal fibrinogen coverage at intermediate adsorption time (Fig. 107.2), consistent with reported experimental results. Surface exclusion and molecular mobility arguments have also been proposed to explain the Vroman effect [Willems et al., 1991].

The biologic activity of an adsorbed protein differs from that of the same protein in solution, as illustrated by the observation that fibrinogen in solution does not bind platelets (unless the platelets are first stimulated with adenosine diphosphate, ADP) [Bennett & Vilaire, 1979], whereas platelets do adhere to adsorbed fibrinogen [Young et al., 1982]. Proteins at interfaces can undergo both covalent (e.g., conversion of fibrinogen to fibrin) and noncovalent (e.g., change in conformation, decrease in receptor accessibility) organizational changes. It is these changes that define the state of an adsorbed protein, whose importance in mediating cellular interactions is becoming more evident.

Changes in protein conformation upon adsorption have been inferred from different indirect measurements. Soderquist and Walton [1980] proposed conformational changes in bovine serum albumin (BSA) and fibrinogen upon adsorption to polyaminoacids (after long adsorption times) based upon changes in CD spectra. Similarly Castillo and coworkers [1984] inferred substrate, adsorption time, and residence-time-dependent conformational changes in human serum albumin (HSA) adsorbed to different hydrogels based upon changes in FTIR/ATR and CD spectra. Specific conformational changes, i.e., decreased α-helix and increased random coil and β-pleated sheet content upon adsorption were proposed. Similarly, Norde and colleagues [1986] reported lower α-helix content in HSA first adsorbed to, then desorbed from different substrates compared with native HSA. Castillo and coworkers [1985] also reported that lysozyme became increasingly denatured

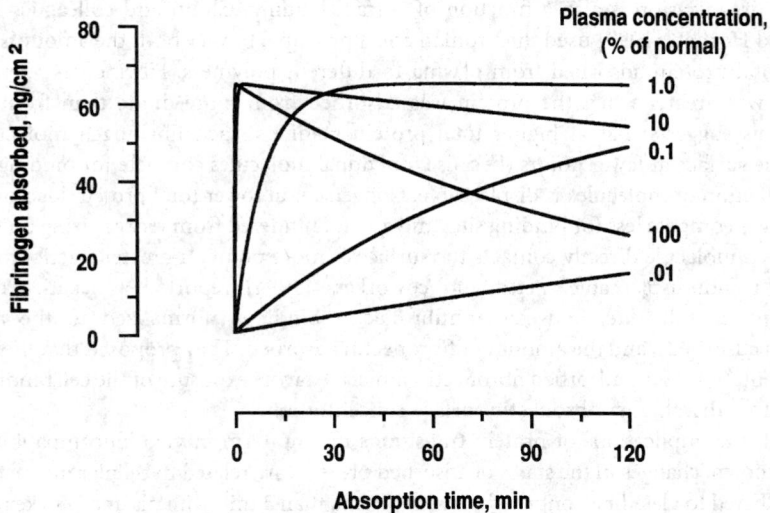

FIGURE 107.2   Time course of fibrinogen adsorption to a polymeric substrate as predicted by the model proposed by Slack and Horbett [1989].

with increased adsorption time and residence time and that denatured lysozyme adsorbed irreversibly to contact lens materials. De Baillou and colleagues [1984] proposed conformational change in fibrinogen upon adsorption to glass based upon DSC measurements. Denaturation of adsorbed proteins is reflected as a phase transition in the DSC thermogram. Based upon similar measurements, Feng and Andrade [1994] proposed that low-temperature isotropic (LTI) carbon significantly denatures adsorbed proteins through hydrophobic interactions. Rainbow and coworkers [1987] proposed conformational change in albumin upon adsorption to quartz, based upon changes in fluorescence lifetimes calculated from TIRF measurements.

Whereas indirect methods provide evidence for changes in protein organization upon adsorption, antibodies against specific protein epitopes provide direct evidence. Antibody-binding measurements reflect the availability of different protein epitopes. Epitopes available in solution might not remain so upon adsorption of the protein. For example, binding of receptor-induced binding site (RIBS) antifibrinogens bind to adsorbed but not free fibrinogen molecules [Zamarron et al., 1990]. Further, if the adsorbed protein reorganizes, changes conformation, or completely denatures upon the surface, epitope availability may change as well. Because an MAb binds to a single protein epitope, and a PAb binds to multiple epitopes of the protein, MAbs rather than PAbs should be more sensitive to such changes. Epitope availability is also a function of protein loading upon the surface. Epitopes available at low surface loadings may become unavailable due to stearic hinderance by proteins adsorbed to neighboring surface sites.

Horbett and Lew [1994] used the Vroman effect principle to maximize the amount of fibrinogen adsorbed from plasma to different polymers, then measured binding of different MAbs against different epitopes of fibrinogen. Binding was reported substrate dependent and, with some MAbs, changed with protein residence time. Thus, different fibrinogen epitopes become more or less available as the adsorbed molecule reorganizes upon the surface. Although this method cannot distinguish between changes in protein conformation (higher-order structure) and changes in surface orientation (e.g., rotation, stearic effects), several authors reported that with increased adsorption time or residence time adsorbed proteins became less readily displaced by plasma or surfactant-eluting agents [Bohnert & Horbett, 1986; Chinn et al., 1992; Rapoza & Horbett, 1990; Slack & Horbett, 1992]. These results suggest that postadsorptive transitions in adsorbed proteins are primarily structural.

Protein organization is also a function of surface loading. Chinn and colleagues [1992] and Rapoza and Horbett [1990] used the Vroman effect principle to vary both the amounts of fibrinogen and total protein adsorbed from plasma to different polymers. Fibrinogen retention by all substrates was greater when the protein was adsorbed from more-dilute than from less-dilute plasma. This suggests that at higher total protein loadings, each fibrinogen molecule directly contacts the surface at fewer points (because individual molecules compete for binding sites), and a greater fraction of molecules is displaceable. Conversely, at lower total protein loadings, individual molecules compete less for binding sites and are not hindered from reorganizing on the surface. Because each molecule directly contacts the surface at more points, a greater fraction of adsorbed molecules is nondisplaceable. Pettit and coworkers [1994] reported a negative correlation, independent of substrate, between antifibronectin binding (normalized to the amount of fibronectin adsorbed), and the amount of fibronectin adsorbed. They proposed that the conformation or orientation of the adsorbed fibronectin molecule favors exposure of the cell binding domain at lower rather than higher fibronectin surface concentrations.

Although the implications of protein transitions in long-term in vivo biocompatibility remain largely unknown, changes in the states of adsorbed proteins are related to cellular interactions. More platelets adhered to glass first contacted 5 s with plasma than 3 min with plasma [Zucker & Vroman, 1969]. Platelet adhesion in vitro to polymers upon which the Vroman effect principle was used to vary the composition of adsorbed protein layer was reported related not to total fibrinogen binding but to antifibrinogen binding [Lindon et al., 1986; Shiba et al., 1991], as well as the fraction of adsorbed protein that can be eluted by surfactant such as sodium dodecyl sulfate (SDS) [Chinn et al., 1991].

It is readily apparent that the organization and not the amount of adsorbed fibrinogen is relevant to its biological activity. However, decreased displaceability (increased retention) of adsorbed fibrinogen with residence time might reflect how tenaciously the fibrinogen molecule is bound to the substrate rather than decreased availability of platelet binding domains. Other studies suggest relationships between protein-binding tenacity and cellular interactions. [Gaebel & Feuerstein, 1991; Goodman et al., 1990].

107.3 Summary, Conclusions, and Directions

Clearly, adsorbed proteins affect biocompatibility in ways that are not entirely understood. Fibrinogen has been extensively studied because blood platelets involved in thrombosis and hemostasis have a receptor for this protein [Phillips et al., 1988]. Adsorbed fibrinogen is often proposed to discourage biocompatibility, but this view does not consider that adsorbed proteins exist in different states, depending upon adsorption condition, residence time, and substrate. Evidence suggests that fibrinogen adsorbed from blood to substrates upon which the protein readily denatures (e.g., LTI carbon [Feng & Andrade, 1994]) may in fact promote biocompatibility. Because it is the organization and not the amount of an adsorbed protein that determines its biological activity, what happens to proteins after they adsorb to the substrate must be determined to properly evaluate the biocompatibility of a material. Further, a material might be made blood compatible if protein organization can be controlled such that the cell-binding epitopes become unavailable for cell binding [Horbett et al., 1994]. Much current research aims to understand the relationship between the states of adsorbed proteins and cell-protein-surface interactions.

Fundamental to better understanding of material biocompatibility is understanding the importance of protein and surface structure and heterogeneity in determining the organization of proteins at the solid-liquid interface, the dynamics of multicomponent adsorption from complex media (e.g., the Vroman effect), and the significance of postadsorptive events and subsequent cellular interactions. MAbs against specific protein epitopes provide direct evidence of changes in the states of adsorbed proteins, and indirect methods provide corroborative evidence. Molecular imaging techniques such as atomic (AFM), lateral force (LFM), and scanning tunneling (STM [Hansma & Tersoff, 1987]) microscopies, might someday be used to better define the states of adsorbed proteins, but adaptation of these methods to aqueous systems has been mostly unsuccessful.

Identification and characterization of the cell-binding domains of adhesive proteins has led to better understanding of cell adhesion at the molecular level. Pierschbacher and colleagues [1981] used monoclonal antibodies and proteolytic fragments of fibronectin to identify the location of the cell attachment site of the molecule. Subsequently, residue sequences within the cell-binding domains of other adhesive proteins were identified as summarized by Yamada [1991]. The RGD sequence first isolated from fibronectin was later found present within vitronectin, osteopontin, collagens, thrombospondin, fibrinogen, and vWF [Ruoslahti & Pierschbacher, 1987]. (See Stryer [1988] for key to amino acid residue abbreviations.) Different adhesive peptides exhibit cell line dependent biological activity in vitro, but relatively few in vivo studies of adhesive peptides have been reported.

Haverstick and coworkers [1985] reported that addition of RGDS containing peptides to protein-free platelet suspension inhibited thrombin-induced platelet aggregation as well as platelet adhesion in vitro to fibronectin, fibrinogen, and vWF coated polystyrene. These results suggest that binding of the peptide to the platelet renders the platelet's receptor for the proteins unavailable for further binding. Similarly, Hanson and colleagues [1988] used MAbs against the platelet glycoprotein IIb/IIIa (fibrinogen binding) complex to prevent thrombus formation upon Dacron vascular grafts placed within a chronic baboon AV shunt. Controlled release of either MAbs or adhesive peptides at the site of medical device implant might allow localized control of thrombosis. Locally administered adhesive peptides might also be used to selectively control cancerous cells, as Ruoslahti [1992] used RGD containing peptides to inhibit tumor invasion in vitro and dissemination in vivo.

Alternatively, adhesive peptides can be used to promote cell proliferation. Hubbell and coworkers [1991] reported that immobilization of different adhesive peptides resulted in selective cell response in vitro. Whereas the immobilized RGD and YIGSR peptides both enhanced spreading of human foreskin fibroblasts, human vascular smooth muscle cells, and human vascular endothelial cells, immobilization of REDV enhanced spreading of only endothelial cells. If this concept can be applied in vivo, then endothelialization in the absence of inflammation, infection, or thrombosis might be achieved.

Defining Terms

Conformation: Higher-order protein structure that describes the spatial relationship between the amino acid chains that comprise a protein.

Epitopes: Particular regions of a protein to which an antibody or cell can bind.

Hemostasis: Mechanism by which damaged blood vessels are repaired without compromising normal blood flow.

Integrins: Cellular transmembrane proteins that act as receptors for adhesive extracellular matrix proteins such as fibronectin. The tripeptide RGD is the sequence recognized by many integrins.

Organization: The manner in which a protein resides upon a surface, in particular, the existence, arrangement, and availability of different protein epitopes.

Plasma concentration: Not the concentration of total protein in the plasma but rather the volume fraction of plasma in the adsorption medium when protein adsorption from different dilutions of plasma is measured.

Postadsorptive transitions: Changes in protein conformation and organization that occur when adsorbed proteins reside upon a surface.

Radiolabel: A radioactive isotope incorporated within or attached to a protein such that the amount of the protein within a sample can be measured.

Residue: The amino acids that comprise a peptide or protein.

Specific activity: The amount of radioactivity detected per unit mass of the protein.

State: The reactive state of an adsorbed protein as determined by its conformation and organization.

Thrombosis: Formation of plug comprising blood platelets and fibrin that stops blood flow through damaged blood vessels. Embolized thrombus refers to a plug which has detached from the wound site and entered the circulation.

Vroman effect: Collective term describing (1) maximal adsorption of a specific protein from multicomponent medium at early time, (2) maximal equilibrium adsorption from intermediate dilution, and (3) decrease with increased adsorption time in the plasma concentration at which adsorption is maximum.

Vroman peak: The adsorption maximum in the adsorption versus log (plasma concentration) curve when protein adsorption from different dilutions of plasma is measured.

References

Andrade JD. 1985. Principles of protein adsorption. In JD Andrade (ed), Surface and Interfacial Aspects of Biomedical Polymers, vol 2, Protein Adsorption, pp 1–80, New York, Plenum.

Andrade JD, Hlady V. 1986. Protein adsorption and materials biocompatibility: A tutorial review and suggested hypotheses. In Advances in Polymer Science 79. Biopolymers/Non-Exclusion HPLC, pp 1–63, Berlin, Springer-Verlag.

Bennett JS, Vilaire G. 1979. Exposure of platelet fibrinogen receptors by ADP and epinephrine. J Clin Invest 81:149.

Bohnert JL, Horbett TA. 1986. Changes in adsorbed fibrinogen and albumin interactions with polymers indicated by decreases in detergent elutability. J Colloid Interface Sci 25:267.

Brash JL. 1981. Proteins interactions with artificial surfaces, In EW Salzman (ed), Interactions of the Blood with Natural and Artificial Surfaces, pp 37–60, New York, Marcel Dekker.

Brash JL ten Hove P. 1984. Effect of plasma dilution on adsorption of fibrinogen to solid surfaces. Thromb Haemostas 51:326.

Castillo EJ, Koenig JL, Anderson JM, et al. 1984. Characterization of protein adsorption on soft contact lenses: I. Conformational changes of adsorbed human serum albumin. Biomaterials 5:319.

Castillo EJ, Koenig JL, Anderson JM, et al. 1985. Characterization of protein adsorption on soft contact lenses: II. Reversible and irreversible interactions between lysozyme and soft contact lens surfaces. Biomaterials 6:338.

Chenowith DE. 1988. Complement activation produced by biomaterials. Artif. Organs 12:502.

Chinn JA, Posso SE, Horbett TA, et al. 1991. Postabsorptive transitions in fibrinogen adsorbed to Biomer: Changes in baboon platelet adhesion, antibody binding, and sodium dodecyl sulfate elutability. J Biomed Mater Res 25:535.

Chinn JA, Posso SE, Horbett TA, et al. 1992. Postadsorptive transitions in fibrinogen adsorbed to polyurethanes: Changes in antibody binding and sodium dodecyl sulfate elutability. J Biomed Mater Res 26:757.

De Baillou N, Dejardin P, Schmitt A, et al. 1984. Fibrinogen dimensions at an interface: Variations with bulk concentration, temperature, and pH. J Colloid Interface Sci 100:167.

Feng L, Andrade JD. 1994. Protein adsorption on low temperature isotropic carbon: I. Protein conformational change probed by differential scanning calorimetry. J Biomed Mater Res 28:735.

Gaebel K, Feuerstein IA. 1991. Platelets process adsorbed protein: A morphological study. Biomaterials 12:597.

Goodman SL, Lai QJ, Park K, et al. 1990. Fibrinogen receptor movement on the ventral surface of platelets. In Proceedings of the XII International Congress for Electron Microscopy, pp 22, San Francisco, San Francisco Press.

Hansma PK, Tersoff J. 1987. Scanning tunneling microscopy. J Appl Phys 28:735.

Hanson SR, Pareti FI, Ruggeri ZM, et al. 1988. Effects of monoclonal antibodies against the platelet glycoprotein complex on thrombosis and hemostasis in the baboon. J Clin Invest 81:149.

Haverstick DM, Cowan JF, Yamada KM, et al. 1985. Inhibition of platelet adhesion to fibronectin, fibrinogen, and von Willebrand factor substrates by a synthetic tetrapeptide derived from the cell-binding domain of fibronectin. Blood 66:946.

Horbett TA. 1981. Adsorption of proteins from plasma to a series of hydrophilic-hydrophobic copolymers: 2. Compositional analysis with the prelabeled protein technique. J Biomed Mater Res 15:673.

Horbett TA. 1982. Protein adsorption on biomaterials. In SL Cooper, NL Peppas (eds), Biomaterials: Interfacial Phenomena and Applications, ACS Advances in Chemistry Series, vol 199, pp 233–244, Washington, DC, American Chemical Society.

Horbett TA. 1984. Mass action effects on competitive adsorption of fibrinogen from hemoglobin solutions and from plasma. Thromb Haemostas 51:174.

Horbett TA. 1986. Techniques for protein adsorption studies. In DF Williams (ed), Techniques of biocompatibility testing, pp 183–214, Boca Raton, Fla, CRC Press.

Horbett TA, Brash JL. 1987. Proteins at interfaces: Current issues and future prospects. In TA Horbett, JL Brash (eds), Proteins at Interfaces: Physicochemical and Biochemical Studies, ACS Symposium Series, vol 343, pp 1–33, Washington, DC, American Chemical Society.

Horbett TA, Grunkemeier JM, Lew KR. 1994. Fibrinogen orientation of a surface coated with a GPIIb/IIIa peptide detected with monoclonal antibodies. Trans Soc Biomaterials 17:335.

Horbett TA, Lew KR. In press. Residence time effects on monoclonal antibody binding to adsorbed fibrinogen. J Biomater Sci Polym Ed.

Horbett TA, Schway MS. 1988. Correlations between mouse 3T3 cell spreading and serum fibronectin adsorption on glass and hydroxyethylmethacrylate-ethylmethacrylate copolymers. J Biomed Mater Res 22:763.

Hubbell JA, Massia SP, Desai NP, et al. 1991. Selective endothelial cell binding surfaces for vascular grafts. Bio/Technology 9:568.

Kaplan AP. 1978. Initiation of the intrinsic coagulation and fibrinolytic pathway of man: The role of surfaces, Hageman factor, prekallikrein, high molecular weight kininogen, and factor XI. Prog Hemostas Thromb 4:127.

Lindon JN, McManama G, Kushner L, et al. 1986. Does the conformation of adsorbed fibrinogen dictate platelet interactions with artificial surfaces? Blood 68:355–362.

Macfarlane AS. 1958. Efficient trace-labelling of proteins with Iodine-131 monochloride. Nature 182:52.

Norde W, MacRitchie F, Nowicka G, et al. 1986. Protein adsorption at solid-liquid interfaces: reversibility and conformation aspects. J Colloid Interface Sci 112:447.

Norde W. 1986. Adsorption of proteins from solution at the solid liquid interface. Adv Colloid Interface Sci 25:267.

Norde W, Lyklema J. 1991. Why proteins prefer interfaces. J. Biomater Sci Polym Ed 2:183.

Pettit DK, Hoffman AS, Horbett TA. 1994. Correlation between corneal epithelial cell outgrowth and monoclonal antibody binding to the cell domain of fibronectin. J Biomed Mater Res 28:685.

Pierschbacher MD, Hayman EG, Ruoslahti E. 1981. Location of the cell attachment site in fibronectin with monoclonal antibodies and proteolytic fragments of the molecule. Cell 26:259.

Rainbow MR, Atherton S, Eberhart RE. 1987. Fluorescence lifetime measurements using total internal reflection fluorimetry: Evidence for a conformational change in albumin adsorbed to quartz. J Biomed Mater Res 21:539.

Rapoza RJ, Horbett TA. 1990. Changes in the SDS elutability of fibrinogen adsorbed from plasma to polymers. J Biomater Sci Polym Ed 1:99.

Ratner BD, McElroy BJ. 1986. Electron spectroscopy for chemical analysis: Applications in the biomedical sciences. In RM Gendreau (ed), Spectroscopy in the Biomedical Sciences, pp 107–140, Boca Raton, Fla, CRC Press.

Ratnoff OD, Menzie C. 1950. A new method for the determination of fibrinogen in small samples of plasma. J Lab Clin Med 37:316.

Ruoslahti E. 1991. Integrins. J Clin Invest 87:1.

Ruoslahti E. 1992. The Walter Herbert Lecture. Control of cell motility and tumour invasion by extracellular matrix interactions. Br J Cancer 66:239.

Ruoslahti E, Pierschbacher MD. 1987. New perspectives in cell adhesion: RGD and integrins. Science 238:497.

Sakariassen KS, Bolhuis PA, Sixma JJ. 1979. Human blood platelet adhesion of artery subendothelium is mediated by factor VIII-von Willebrand factor bound to the subendothelium. Nature 279:636.

Shiba E, Lindon JN, Kushner L, et al. 1991. Antibody-detectable changes in fibrinogen adsorption affecting platelet activation on polymer surfaces. Am J Physiol 260:C965.

Slack SM, Horbett TA. 1989. Changes in strength of fibrinogen attachment to solid surfaces: An explanation of the influence of chemistry on the Vroman effect. J Colloid Interface Sci 133:148.

Slack SM, Horbett TA. 1992. Changes in fibrinogen adsorbed to segmented polyurethanes and hydroxyethylmethacrylate-ethylmethacrylate copolymers. J Biomed Mater Res 26:1633.

Smith JM. 1981. Chemical Engineering Kinetics, 3d ed, New York, McGraw-Hill.

Stryer L. 1988. Biochemistry, 3d ed, San Francisco, W H Freeman.

Vroman L, Adams AL. 1969. Identification of rapid changes at plasma solid interfaces. J Biomed Mater Res 3:43.

Vroman L, Adams AL, Fischer GC, et al. 1980. Interaction of high molecular weight kininogen, Factor XII, and fibrinogen in plasma at interfaces. Blood 55:156.

Willems GM, Hermens WT, Hemker HC. 1991. Surface exclusion and molecular mobility may explain Vroman effects in protein adsorption. J Biomater Sci Polym Ed 2:217.

Wojciechowski P, ten Hove P, Brash J. 1986. Phenomenology and mechanism of the transient adsorption of fibrinogen from plasma (Vroman effect). J Colloid Interface Sci 111:455.

Yamada KM. 1991. Adhesive recognition sequences. J Biol Chem 20:12809.

Young BR, Lambrecht LK, Cooper SL, et al. 1982. Plasma proteins: their role in initiating platelet and fibrin deposition on biomaterials. In SL Cooper, NL Peppas (eds), Biomaterials: Interfacial Phenomena and Applications, ACS Advances in Chemistry Series, vol 199, pp 317–350, Washington, DC, American Chemical Society.

Zamarron C, Ginsberg MH, Plow EF. 1990. Monoclonal antibodies specific for a conformationally altered state of fibrinogen. Thromb Haemostas 64:41.

Zucker MB, Vroman L. 1969. Platelet adhesion induced by fibrinogen adsorbed to glass. Proc Soc Exp Biol Med 131:318.

Further Information

The American Society for Artificial and Internal Organs (ASAIO) publishes original articles in the *ASAIO Journal* through J.B. Lippincott Company (12107 Insurance Way, Suite 114, Hagerstown, MD 21740), and meeting transactions in *Trans. Am. Soc. Artif. Intern. Organs*.

The Society for Biomaterials (SFB) publishes original articles in *J Biomed Mater Res* through John Wiley and Sons, Inc. (605 Third Ave., New York, NY 10158) and meeting transactions in *Trans. Soc. Biomaterials*.

Various industrial sponsors support an annual symposium entitled, "Cardiovascular Science and Technology," that is well attended by leading research groups.

Comprehensive references summarizing applications of protein adsorption and biocompatibility include: *Biomaterials: Interfacial Phenomena and Applications, ACS Advances in Chemistry Series*, vol. 199, edited by S.L. Cooper and N.L. Peppas and published by the American Chemical Society, Washington, D.C., in 1982; *Proteins at Interfaces: Physicochemical and Biochemical Studies, ACS Symposium Series*, vol. 343, edited by T.A. Horbett and J.L. Brash and published by the American Chemical Society, Washington, D.C., in 1987; and "Cardiovascular biomaterials and biocompatibility," *Cardiovasc Path* 2(3) Suppl., 1993.

J Colloid Interface Sci often contains articles related to protein-surface interactions, and *Nature* and *Science* (AAAS) often contain excellent review articles and very current developments.

108

Engineering Biomaterials for Tissue Engineering: The 10–100 Micron Size Scale

David J. Mooney
Massachusetts Institute of Technology

Robert S. Langer
Massachusetts Institute of Technology

A significant challenge in tissue engineering is to take a biomaterial and process it into a useful form for a specific application. All devices for tissue engineering transplant cells and/or induce the ingrowth of desirable cell types from the host organism. The device must provide sufficient mechanical support to maintain a space for tissue to form or serve as a barrier to undesirable interactions. Also, the device can be designed to provide these functions for a defined period before biodegradation occurs or on a permanent basis.

Generally speaking, devices can be broken down into two types. Immunoprotective devices contain semipermeable membranes that prevent elements of the host immune system (e.g., IgG antibodies and lymphocytes) from entering the device. In contrast, open devices have large pores (>10 μm) and allow free transport of molecules and cells between the host tissue and transplanted cells. These latter devices are utilized to engineer a tissue that is completely integrated with the host tissue. Both types of devices can range in size from microns to centimeters or beyond, although the larger sizes are usually repetitions on the structure found at the scale of hundreds of microns.

A fundamental question in designing a device is whether to use synthetic or natural materials. Synthetic materials (e.g., organic polymers) can be easily processed into various structures and can be produced cheaply and reproducibly; it also is possible to tightly control various properties such as the mechanical strength, hydrophobicity, and degradation rate of synthetic materials. Whereas natural materials (e.g., collagen) sometimes exhibit a limited range of physical properties and can be difficult to isolate and process, they do have specific biologic activity. In addition, these molecules generally do not elicit unfavorable host tissue responses, a condition which is typically taken to indicate that a material is biocompatible. Some synthetic polymers, in contrast, can elicit a long-term inflammatory response from the host tissue [Bostman, 1991].

A significant challenge in fabricating devices is either to develop processing techniques for natural biomaterials that allow reproducible fabrication on a large-scale basis [Cavallaro et al., 1994] or to develop materials that combine the advantages of synthetic materials with the biologic activity of natural biomaterials [Barrera et al., 1993; Massia & Hubbell, 1991]. Computer-aided-design–computer-aided-manufacturing (CAD-CAM) technology may possibly be employed in the future to custom-fit devices with complex structures to patients.

108.1 Fundamentals

The interaction of the host tissue with the device and transplanted cells can be controlled by both the geometry of the device and the internal structure. The number of inflammatory cells and cellular enzyme activity around implanted polymeric devices has been found to depend on the geometry of the device [Matlaga et al., 1976], with device geometries that contain sharp angles provoking the greatest response. The surface geometry, or microstructure, of implanted polymer devices also has been found to affect the types and activities of acute inflammatory cells recruited to the device as well as the formation of a fibrous capsule [Taylor & Gibbons, 1983].

The pore structure of a device dictates the interaction of the device and transplanted cells with the host tissue. The pore structure is determined by the size, size distribution, and continuity of the individual pores within the device. Porous materials are typically defined as microporous (pore diameter $d < 2\,nm$), mesoporous ($2\,nm < d < 50\,nm$), or macroporous ($d > 50\,nm$) [Schaeffer, 1994]. Only small molecules (e.g., gases) are capable of penetrating microporous materials. Mesoporous materials allow transport of larger molecules, such as small proteins, but transport of large proteins and cells is prevented. Macroporous materials allow free transport of large molecules, and, if the pores are large enough ($d > 10^4\,nm$), cells are capable of migrating through the pores of the device. The proper design of a device can allow desirable signals (e.g., a rise in serum sugar concentration) to be passed to transplanted cells while excluding molecular or cellular signals which would promote rejections of transplanted cells (e.g., IgG protein).

Fibrovascular tissue will invade a device if the pores are larger than approximately 10 μm, and the rate of invasion will increase with the pore size and total porosity of a device [Mikos et al., 1993c; Weslowski et al., 1961; White et al., 1981]. The degree of fibrosis and calcification of early fabric leaflet valves has been correlated to their porosity [Braunwald et al., 1965], as has the nonthrombogenicity of arterial prosthesis [DeBakey et al., 1964] and the rigidity of tooth implants and orthopedic prosthesis [Hamner et al., 1972; Hulbert et al., 1972].

It is important to realize that many materials do not have a unimodal pore size distribution or a continuous pore structure, and the ability of molecules or cells to be transported through such a device will often be limited by bottlenecks in the pore structure. In addition, the pore structure of a device may change over time in a biologic environment. For example, absorption of water into polymers of the lactic/glycolic acid family results in the formation first of micropores, and eventually of macropores as the polymer itself degrades [Cohen et al., 1991]. The porosity and pore-size distribution of a device can be determined utilizing a variety of techniques [Smith et al., 1994].

Specific properties (e.g., mechanical strength, degradability, hydrophobicity, biocompatibility) of a device are also often desirable. These properties can be controlled both by the biomaterial itself and by the processing technique utilized to fabricate the device. An advantage of fabricating devices from synthetic polymers is the variety of processing techniques available for these materials. Fibers, hollow fibers, and porous sponges can be readily formed from synthetic polymers. Natural biomaterials must be isolated from plant, animal, or human tissue and are typically expensive and suffer from large batch-to-batch variations. Although the wide range of processing techniques available for synthetic polymers is not available for these materials, cells specifically interact with certain types of natural biomaterials, such as extracellular matrix (ECM) molecules [Hynes, 1987]. The known ability of ECM molecules to mediate cell function in vitro and in vivo may allow precise control over the biologic response to devices fabricated from ECM molecules.

108.2 Applications

The applications of tissue engineering are very diverse, encompassing virtually every type of tissue in the human body. However, the devices utilized in these areas can be divided into two broad types.

The first type, immunoprotective devices, utilizes a semipermeable membrane to limit communication between cells in the device and the host. The small pores in these devices ($d < 10$ nm) allow low-molecular-weight proteins and molecules to be transported between the implant and the host tissue, but they prevent large proteins (e.g., immunoglobulins) and host cells (e.g., lymphocytes) of the immune system from entering the device and mediating rejection of the transplanted cells. In contrast, open structures with large pores are typically utilized ($d > 10$ μm) if one desires that the new tissue be structurally integrated with the host tissue. Applications that utilize both types of devices are described below.

Immunoprotective Devices

Devices that protect transplanted cells from the immune system of the host can be broken down into two types, microencapsulation and macroencapsulation systems [Emerich et al., 1992]. Individual cells or small clusters of cells are surrounded by a semipermeable membrane and delivered as a suspension in microencapsulation systems (Fig. 108.1a). Macroencapsulation systems utilize hollow semipermeable membranes to deliver multiple cells or cell clumps (Fig. 108.1b). The small size, thin wall, and spherical shape of microcapsules all optimize diffusional transport to and from the microencapsulated cells. Macroencapsulation devices typically have greater mechanical integrity than microencapsule devices, and they can be easily retrieved after implantation. However, the structure of these devices is not optimal for diffusional transport. Nonbiodegradable materials are the preferred choice for fabricating both types of devices, as the barrier function is typically required over the lifetime of the implant.

A significant effort has been made to cure diabetes by transplanting microencapsulated pancreatic islet cells. Transplantation of nonimmunoprotected islets has led to short-term benefits [Lim & Sun, 1980], but the cells were ultimately rejected. To prevent this, islets have been immobilized in alginate (a naturally occurring polymer derived from seaweed) microbeads coated with a layer of poly(L-lysine) and a layer of polyethyleneimine [Lim & Sun, 1980]. Alginate is ionically crosslinked in the presence of calcium, and the permeability of alginate/poly(L-lysine) microbeads is determined by the formation of ionic or hydrogen bonds between the polyanion alginate and the polycation poly(L-lysine). This processing technique allows cells to be immobilized without exposure to organic solvents or high temperatures. The outer layer of polyethyleneimine was subsequently replaced by a layer of alginate to prevent the formation of fibrous capsules around the implanted microcapsules [O'Shea et al., 1984]. Smaller microbeads (250–400 μm) have been generated with an electrostatic pulse generator [Lum et al., 1992] to improve the in vivo survival and the response time of encapsulated cells [Chicheportiche & Reach, 1988]. These devices have been shown to be effective in a variety of animal models [Lim & Sun, 1980; Lum et al., 1992], and clinical trials of microencapsulated islets in diabetic patients are in progress [Soon-Shiong et al., 1994]. Synthetic analogs to alginate have also been developed [Cohen et al., 1990].

The superior mechanical stability of macroencapsulation devices, along with the possibility of retrieving the entire device, makes these types of devices especially attractive when the transplanted cells have limited lifetimes and/or when one needs to ensure that the transplanted cells are not migrating out of the device. Macroencapsulation devices have been utilized to transplant a variety of cell types, including pancreatic cells [Lacy et al., 1991], NGF-secreting cells [Winn et al., 1994], dopamine-secreting cells [Emerich et al., 1992], and Chromaffin cells [Sagen et al., 1993]. The nominal molecular mass cutoff of the devices was 50 kD, allowing immunoprotection without interfering with transport of therapeutic agents from the encapsulated cells. To prevent cell aggregation, and subsequent large-scale cell death due to nutrient limitations, macroencapsulated islets have been immobilized in alginate [Lacy et al., 1991].

Devices with Open Structures

Devices with large, interconnected pores ($d > 10$ μm) are utilized in applications where one wishes the transplanted cells to interact directly with host tissue and form a structurally integrated tissue.

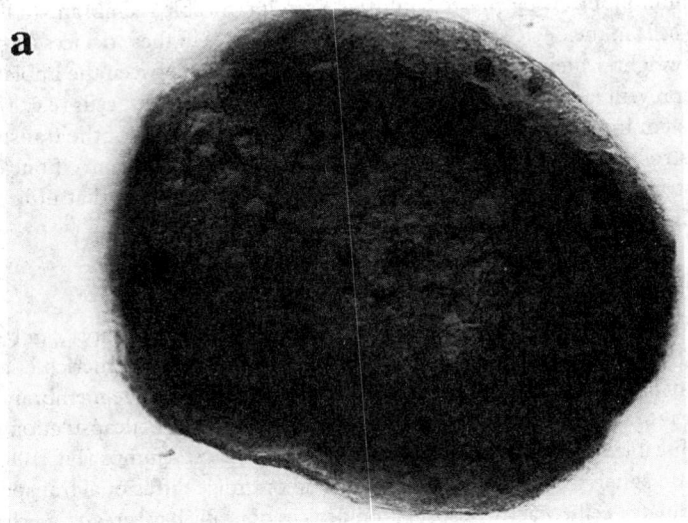

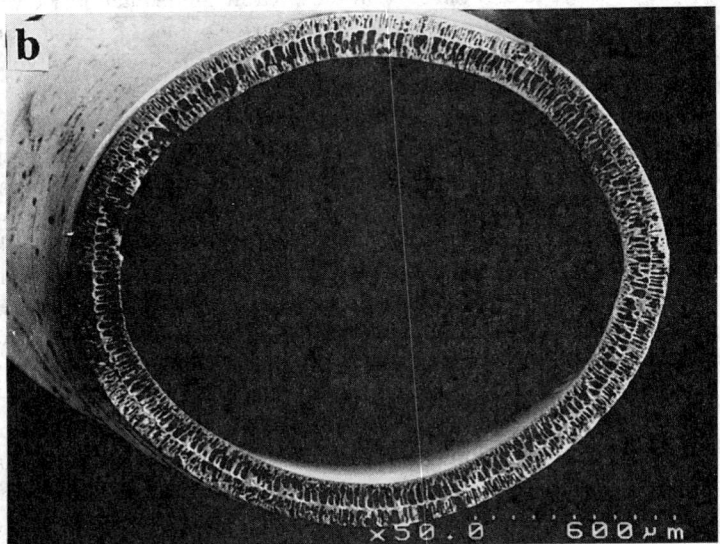

FIGURE 108.1 Examples of microencapsulated cells and a device used for macroencapsulation of cells. (*a*) Phase contrast photomicrograph of hybridoma cells encapsulated in a calcium crosslinked polyphosphazene gel [Cohen et al., 1993]. Original magnification was 100×. Used with permission of Editions de Sante. (*b*) A SEM photomicrograph of a poly(acrylonitrile-co-vinyl chloride) hollow fiber formed by phase inversion using a dry-jet wet-spinning technique [Schoichet et al., 1994]. Used with permission of John Wiley and Sons, Inc.

The open structure of these devices provides little barrier to diffusional transport and often promotes the ingrowth of blood vessels from the host tissue. Degradable materials are often utilized in these applications, since once tissue structure is formed the device is not needed.

These types of devices typically fall into two categories. The first type is fabrics, either woven or nonwoven, of small-diameter (approximately 10–40 μm) fibers (Fig. 108.2*a*). High porosity (>95%) and large average pore size can be easily obtained with this type of material, and these materials can

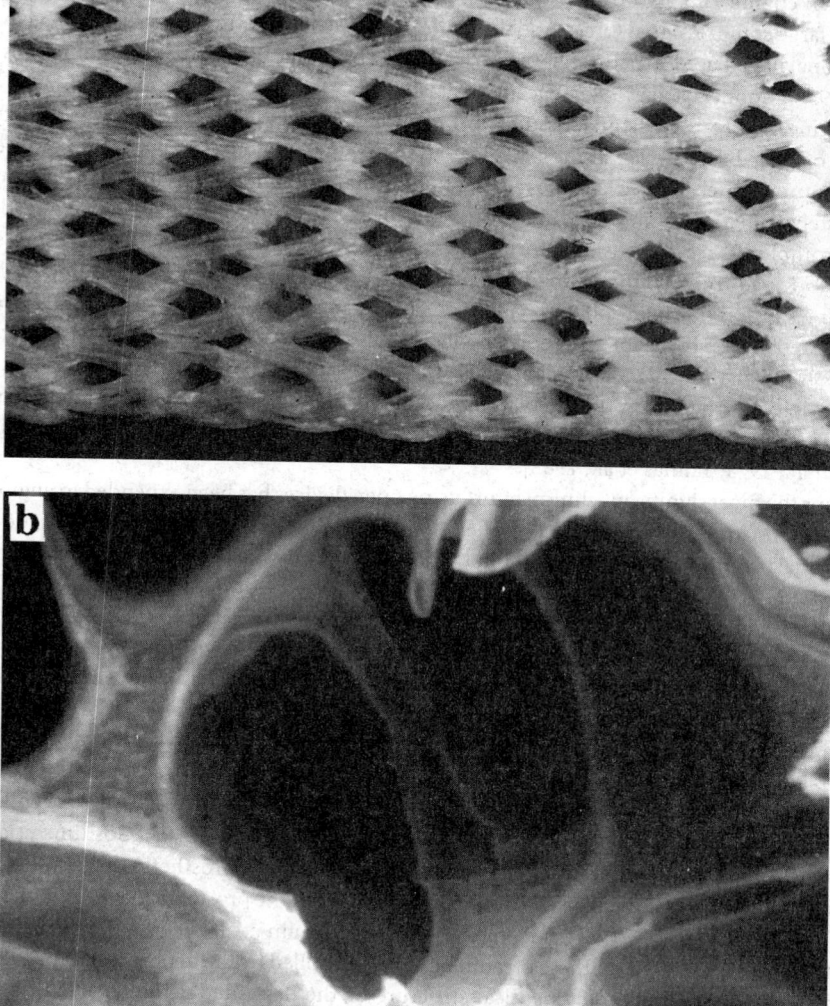

FIGURE 108.2 Examples of a fiber-based fabric and a porous sponge utilized for tissue engineering. (*a*) A photomicrograph of type I collagen fibers knitted into a fabric. Fiber diameters can be as small as 25 μm, and devices constructed from these fibers can be utilized for a variety of tissue engineering applications [Cavallaro et al., 1994]. Used with permission of John Wiley and Sons, Inc. (*b*) A SEM photomicrograph of a formaldehyde-crosslinked polyvinyl alcohol sponge. These devices have been utilized for a variety of applications, including hepatocyte transplantation [Uyama et al., 1993].

be readily shaped into different geometries. Fibers can be formed from synthetic, crystalline polymers such as polyglycolic acid by melt extrusion [Frazza & Schmitt, 1971]. Fibers and fabrics also can be formed from natural materials such as type I collagen, a type of ECM molecule, by extrusion of soluble collagen into a bath where gelling occurs followed by dehydration of the fiber [Cavallaro et al., 1994]. The tensile strength of fibers is dependent on the extent of collagen crosslinking, which can be controlled by the processing technique [Wang et al., 1994]. Processed collagen fibers can be subsequently spooled and knitted to form fabrics [Cavallaro et al., 1994]. These devices are often ideal when engineering two-dimensional tissues. However, these fabrics typically are incapable of resisting large compressional forces, and three-dimensional devices are often crushed in vivo. Three-dimensional fiber-based structures have been stabilized by physically bonding adjacent fibers [Mikos et al., 1993a; Mooney et al., 1994a; Vacanti et al., 1992].

To engineer three-dimensional tissues, porous sponge devices (Fig. 108.2b) are utilized typically in place of fiber-based devices. These devices are better capable of resisting larger compressional forces (approximately 10^4 Pa) [Mikos et al., 1993a] than are unbonded fiber-based devices (approximately 10^2 Pa) [Mooney et al., 1994a] due to the continuous solid phase and can be designed to have complex, three-dimensional forms [Mikos et al., 1993b; White et al., 1972]. Porous sponges can be fabricated from synthetic polymers utilizing a variety of techniques, including performing the polymerization of a hydrophobic polymer in an aqueous solution [Chirila et al., 1993], exploiting phase separation behavior of dissolved polymers in specific solvents [Lo et al., 1994], and combining solvent casting with particulate leaching [Mikos et al., 1993b; Mikos et al., 1994]. Porous sponges can be formed from type I collagen and other ECM molecules by chemically crosslinking gels or assembling the collagen in nonnatural polymeric structures [Bell et al., 1981; Chvapil, 1979; Stenzel et al., 1974; Yannas et al., 1982].

Perhaps the most significant clinical effort using open devices has been expended to engineer skin tissue to treat burn victims. Both natural [Bell et al., 1981; Yannas et al., 1982] and synthetic degradable materials [Hansbrough et al., 1992] in the form of porous sponges or fiber-based fabrics have been utilized to transplant various cellular elements of skin. One device fabricated from ECM molecules has also been combined with an outer coat of silicone elastomer to prevent dehydration of the wound site [Yannas et al., 1982]. The various approaches have shown efficacy in animal models, and tissue-engineered skin has progressed to clinical trials [Burke et al., 1981; Compton et al., 1989; Heimbach et al., 1988; Stern et al., 1990].

Another area with great clinical potential is the engineering of bone and cartilage tissue. Various ceramics and biodegradable synthetic polymers have been utilized to fabricate devices for these purposes. Porous calcium phosphate devices loaded with mesenchymal stem cells have been shown to promote bone formation when implanted into soft tissue sites of animals [Goshima et al., 1991; Haynesworth et al., 1992]. Ceramics also have been coated onto prosthetic devices (e.g., hip replacements) to promote bone ingrowth and bonding between the prosthetic device and the host tissue (Furlong & Osborn, 1991). The degradation rate [de Bruijn et al., 1994] and mechanical properties [Yoshinari et al., 1994] of these ceramics can be controlled by the deposition technique, which determines the crystallinity and chemical structure of the deposited ceramic. The brittleness of ceramic materials limits them in certain applications, and to bypass this problem composite ceramic/polymer devices have been developed [Stupp et al., 1993]. Fiber-based fabrics of biodegradable polymers have also been utilized to transplant cells derived from periosteal tissue and form new bone tissue [Vacanti et al., 1993]. To engineer cartilage tissue with specific structures such as an ear or nasal septum, devices have been fabricated from a nonwoven mesh of biodegradable synthetic polymers molded to the size and shape of the desired tissue. These devices, after seeding with chondrocytes and implantation, have been shown to induce the formation of new cartilage tissue with the same structure as the polymer device utilized as the template [Puelacher et al., 1993; Vacanti et al., 1991, 1992]. After tissue development is complete, the device itself degrades to leave a completely natural tissue.

Liver tissue [Uyama et al., 1993], ligaments [Cavallaro et al., 1994], and neural tissue [Guenard et al., 1992; Madison et al., 1985] also have been engineered with open devices. Tubular tissues, including blood vessels [Weinberg & Bell, 1986], intestine [Mooney et al., 1994b; Organ et al., 1993], and urothelial structures [Atala et al., 1992] have been engineered utilizing open devices fabricated into a tubular structure.

108.3 Conclusions

A variety of issues must be addressed to design and fabricate a device for tissue engineering. Do the transplanted cells need immunoprotection, or should they structurally integrate with the host tissue? If immunoprotection is desired, will a micro- or macroencapsulation device be preferred? If a structurally integrated new tissue is desired, will a fiber-based device or a porous sponge be more suitable? The specific roles that the device will play in a given application and the material itself will dictate the design of the device and the fabrication technique.

Defining Terms

Biocompatible: A material which does not elicit an unfavorable response from the host but instead performs with an appropriate host response in a specific application [Williams, 1987].

Biodegradation: The breakdown of a material mediated by a biologic system [Williams et al., 1992]. Biodegradation can occur by simple hydrolysis or via enzyme- or cell-mediated breakdown.

Extracellular matrix (ECM) molecules: Various substances present in the extracellular space of tissues that serve to mediate cell adhesion and organization.

Immunoprotective: Serving to protect from interacting with the immune system of the host tissue, including cellular elements (e.g., lymphocytes) and proteins (e.g., IgG).

Open devices: Devices with large ($d > 10$ μm) interconnected pores which allow unhindered transport of molecules and cells within the device and between the device and the surrounding tissue.

References

Barrera DA, Zylstra E, Lansbury PT, et al. 1993. Synthesis and RGD peptide modification of a new biodegradable copolymer: poly(lactic acid-co lysine). J Am Chem Soc 115:11010.

Bell E, Ehrlich HP, Buttle DJ, Nakatsuji T. 1981. Living tissue formed in vitro and accepted as skin-equivalent tissue of full thickness. Science 211:1052.

Bostman OM. 1991. Absorbable implants for the fixation of fractures. J Bone Joint Surg 73-A(1):148.

Braunwald NS, Reis RL, Pierce GE. 1965. Relation of pore size to tissue ingrowth in prosthetic heart valves: an experimental study. Surgery 57:741.

Burke JF, Yannas IV, Quinby WC, et al. 1981. Successful use of a physiological acceptable artificial skin in the treatment of extensive burn injury. Ann Surg 194:413.

Cavallaro JF, Kemp PD, Kraus KH. 1994. Collagen fabrics as biomaterials. Biotech Bioeng 43:781.

Chicheportiche D, Reach G. 1988. In vitro kinetics of insulin release by microencapsulated rat islets: effect of the size of the microcapsules. Diabetologia 31:54.

Chirila TV, Constable IJ, Crawford GJ, et al. 1993. Poly(2-hydroxyethyl methacrylate) sponges as implant materials: in vivo and in vitro evaluation of cellular invasion. Biomaterials 14(1):26.

Chvapil M. 1979. Industrial uses for collagen. In DAD Parry, LK Creamer (eds), Fibrous proteins:scientific, industrial, and medical aspects, London, L.K. Academic Press.

Cohen S, Allcock HR, Langer R. 1993. Cell and enzyme immobilization in ionotropic synthetic hydrogels. In AA Hincal, HS Kas (eds), Recent advances in pharmaceutical and industrial biotechnology, Editions de Sante, Paris.

Cohen S, Bano MC, Visscher KB, et al. 1990. Ionically cross-linkable phosphazene: a novel polymer for microencapsulation. J Am Chem Soc 112:7832.

Cohen S, Yoshioka T, Lucarelli M, et al. 1991. Controlled delivery systems for proteins based on poly(lactic/glycolic acid) microspheres. Pharm Res 8(6):713.

Compton C, Gill JM, Bradford DA. 1989. Skin regenerated from cultured epithelial autografts on full-thickness wounds from 6 days to 5 years after grafting: A light, electron microscopic, and immunohistochemical study. Lab Invest 60:600.

DeBakey ME, Jordan GL, Abbot JP, et al. 1964. The fate of dacron vascular grafts. Arch Surg 89:757.

De Bruijn JD, Bovell YP, van Blitterswijk CA. 1994. Structural arrangements at the interface between plasma sprayed calcium phosphates and bone. Biomaterials 15(7):543.

Emerich DF, Winn SR, Christenson L, et al. 1992. A novel approach to neural transplantation in Parkinson's disease: Use of polymer-encapsulated cell therapy. Neurosci Biobeh Rev 16:437.

Frazza EJ, Schmitt EE. 1971. A new absorbable suture. J Biomed Mater Res Symp 1:43.

Furlong RJ, Osborn JF. 1991. Fixation of hip prostheses by hydroxylapatite ceramic coatings. J Bone Jt Surg 73-B(5):741.

Goshima J, Goldberg VM, Caplan AI. 1991. The origin of bone formed in composite grafts of porous calcium phosphate ceramic loaded with marrow cells. Clin Orthop Rel Res 191:274.

Guenard V, Kleitman N, Morissey, TK, Bunge RP, and Aebischer P. 1992. Syngeneic schwann cells derived from adult nerves seeded in semipermeable guidance channels enhance peripheral nerve regeneration. J Neurosci 12:3310–3320.

Hamner JE, Reed OM, Greulich RC. 1972. Ceramic root implantation in baboons. J Biomed Mater Res Symp 6:1.

Hansbrough JF, Cooper ML, Cohen R, et al. 1992. Evaluation of a biodegradable matrix containing cultured human fibroblasts as a dermal replacement beneath meshed skin grafts on athymic mice. Surgery 111(4):438.

Haynesworth SE, Goshima J, Goldberg VM, et al. 1992. Characterization of cells with osteogenic potential from human marrow. Bone 13:81.

Heimbach D, Luterman A, Burke J, et al. 1988. Artificial dermis for major burns. Ann Surg 208(3):313.

Hulbert SF, Morrison SJ, Klawitter JJ. 1972. Tissue reaction to three ceramics of porous and non-porous structures. J Biomed Mater Res 6:347.

Hynes RO. 1987. Integrins: A family of cell surface receptors. Cell 48:549.

Lacy PE, Hegre OD, Gerasimidi-Vazeou A, et al. 1991. Maintenance of normoglycemia in diabetic mice by subcutaneous xenografts of encapsulated islets. Science 254:1782.

Lim F, Sun AM. 1980. Microencapsulated islets as bioartificial endocrine pancreas. Science 210:908.

Lo H, Kadiyala S, Guggino SE, et al. 1994. Biodegradable foams for cell transplantation. In R Murphy, A. Mikos (eds), Biomaterials for drug and cell delivery, Materials Research Society Proceedings, vol 331.

Lum Z, Krestow M, Tai IT, et al. 1992. Xenografts of rat islets into diabetic mice. Transplantation 53(6):1180.

Madison R, Da Silva CR, Dikkes P, et al. 1985. Increased rate of peripheral nerve regeneration using bioresorbable nerve guides and a laminin-containing gel. Exp Neurol 88:767.

Massia SP, Hubbell JA. 1991. An RGD spacing of 440 nm is sufficient for integrin $\alpha_v\beta_3$-mediated fibroblast spreading and 140 nm for focal contact and stress fiber formation. J Cell Biol 115(5):1089.

Matlaga BF, Yasenchak LP, Salthouse TN. 1976. Tissue response to implanted polymers: the significance of sample shape. J Biomed Mater Res 10:391.

Mikos AG, Bao Y, Cima LG, et al. 1993a. Preparation of poly(glycolic acid) bonded fiber structures for cell attachment and transplantation. J Biomed Mater Res 27:183.

Mikos AG, Sarakinos G, Leite SM, et al. 1993b. Laminated three-dimensional biodegradable foams for use in tissue engineering. Biomaterials 14(5):323.

Mikos AG, Sarakinos G, Lyman MD, et al. 1993c. Prevascularization of porous biodegradable polymers. Biotech Bioeng 42:716.

Mikos AG, Thorsen AJ, Czerwonka LA, et al. 1994. Preparation and characterization of poly(L-lactic) foams. Polymer 35(5):1068.

Mooney DJ, Mazzoni CL, Organ GM, et al. 1994*a*. Stabilizing fiber-based cell delivery devices by physically bonding adjacent fibers. In R Murphy, A Mikos (eds), Biomaterials for Drug and Cell Delivery, Materials Research Society Proceedings, Pittsburgh, Pennsylvania, vol 331, 47–52.

Mooney DJ, Organ G, Vacanti JP. 1994*b*. Design and fabrication of biodegradable polymer devices to engineer tubular tissues. Cell Trans 3(2)203.

Organ GM, Mooney DJ, Hansen LK, et al. 1993. Enterocyte transplantation using cell-polymer devices causes intestinal epithelial-lined tube formation. Transplan Proc 25:998.

O'Shea GM, Goosen MFA, Sun AM. 1984. Prolonged survival of transplanted islets of Langerhans encapsulated in a biocompatible membrane. Biochim Biophys Acta 804:133.

Puelacher WC, Vacanti JP, Kim WS, et al. 1993. Fabrication of nasal implants using human shape specific polymer scaffolds seeded with chondrocytes. Surgical Forum 44:678–680.

Sagen J, Wang H, Tresco PA, et al. 1993. Transplants of immunologically isolated xenogeneic chromaffin cells provide a long-term source of pain-reducing neuroactive substances. J Neuroscience 13(6):2415.

Schaeffer DW. 1994. Engineered porous materials. MRS Bulletin April 1994:14.

Schoichet MS, Winn SR, Athavale S, et al. 1994. Poly(ethylene oxide)-grafted thermoplastic membranes for use as cellular hybrid bio-artificial organs in the central nervous system. Biotech Bioeng 43:563.

Smith DM, Hua D, Earl WL. 1994. Characterization of porous solids. MRS Bulletin April 1994:44.

Soon-Shiong P, Sandford PA, Heintz R, et al. 1994. First human clinical trial of immunoprotected islet allografts in alginate capsules. Society for Biomaterials Annual Meeting, Boston, Mass, abstract 356.

Stenzel KH, Miyata T, Rubin AL. 1974. Collagen as a biomaterial. Ann Rev Biophys Bioeng 3:231.

Stern R, McPherson M, Longaker MT. 1990. Histologic study of artificial skin used in the treatment of full-thickness thermal injury. J Burn Care Rehab 11:7.

Stupp SI, Hanson JA, Eurell JA, et al. 1993. Organoapatites: Materials for artificial bone: III. Biological testing. J Biomed Mater Res 27(3):301.

Taylor SR, Gibbons DF. 1983. Effect of surface texture on the soft tissue response to polymer implants. J Biomed Mat Res 17:205.

Uyama S, Takeda T, Vacanti JP. 1993. Delivery of whole liver equivalent hepatic mass using polymer devices and hepatotrophic stimulation. Transplantation 55(4):932.

Vacanti CA, Cima LG, Ratkowski D, et al. 1992. Tissue engineered growth of new cartilage in the shape of a human ear using synthetic polymers seeded with chondrocytes. In LG Cima, ES Ron (eds), Tissue Inducing Biomaterials, pp 367–374, Materials Research Society Proceedings, Pittsburgh, Pennsylvania, vol 252.

Vacanti CA, Kim W, Upton J, et al. 1993. Tissue engineered growth of bone and cartilage. Transplan Proc 25(1):1019.

Vacanti CA, Langer R, Schloo B, et al. 1991. Synthetic polymers seeded with chondrocytes provide a template for new cartilage formation. Plast Reconstr Surg 88(5):753.

Wang MC, Pins GD, Silver FH. 1994. Collagen fibers with improved strength for the repair of soft tissue injuries. Biomaterials 15:507.

Weinberg CB, Bell E. 1986. A blood vessel model constructed from collagen and cultured vascular cells. Science 231:397.

Weslowski SA, Fries CC, Karlson KE, et al. 1961. Porosity: Primary determinant of ultimate fate of synthetic vascular grafts. Surgery 50(1):91.

White RA, Hirose FM, Sproat RW, et al. 1981. Histopathologic observations after short-term implantation of two porous elastomers in dogs. Biomaterials 2:171.

White RA, Weber JN, White EW. 1972. Replamineform: A new process for preparing porous ceramic, metal, and polymer prosthetic materials. Science 176:922.

Williams DF. 1987. Definitions in Biomedicals. Progress in Biomedical Engineering, vol 4, New York, Elsevier.

Williams DF, Black J, Doherty PJ. 1992. Second consensus conference on definitions in biomaterials. In PJ Doherty, RL Williams, DF Williams, et al. (eds), Advances in Biomaterials vol 10, Biomaterials-Tissue Interactions pp 525–533, New York, Elsevier.

Winn SR, Hammang JP, Emerich DF, et al. 1994. Polymer-encapsulated cells genetically modified to secrete human nerve growth factor promote the survival of axotomized septal cholinergic neurons. Proc Natl Acad Sci. 91:2324–2328.

Yannas IV, Burke JF, Orgill DP, et al. 1982. Wound tissue can utilize a polymeric template to synthesize a functional extension of skin. Science 215:174.

Yoshinari M, Ohtsuka Y, Derand T. 1994. Thin hydroxyapatite coating produced by the ion beam dynamic mixing method. Biomaterials 15:529.

Further Information

The Society for Biomaterials, American Society for Artificial Internal Organs, Cell Transplantation Society, and Materials Research Society all sponsor regular meetings and/or sponsor journals on topics relevant to this topic. The following *Materials Research Society Symposium Proceedings* contain a collection of relevant articles: volume 252, *Tissue Inducing Biomaterials* (1992); volume 331, *Biomaterials for Drug and Cell Delivery* (1994). Another good source of relevant material is *Tissue Engineering*, edited by R Skalak and CF Fox, New York, Alan Riss (1988).

109

Regeneration Templates

Ioannis V. Yannas
*Massachusetts Institute
of Technology*

109.1 The Problem of the Missing Organ

Drugs typically replace or correct a missing function at the molecular scale; by contrast, regeneration templates replace the missing function at the scale of tissue or organ. An organ may be lost to injury or may fail in disease: The usual response of the organism is repair, which amounts to contraction and synthesis of scar tissue. Tissues and organs in the adult mammal typically do not regenerate. There are exceptions, such as epithelial tissues of the skin, gastrointestinal tract, genitals, and the cornea, all of which regenerate spontaneously; the liver also shows ability to synthesize substantial organ mass, though without recovery of the original organ shape. There are reports that bone and the elastic ligaments regenerate. These exceptions underscore the fact that the loss of an organ by the adult mammal almost invariably is an irreversible process, since the resulting scar tissue largely or totally lacks the structure and function of the missing organ. The most obvious examples involve losses due to injury, such as the loss of a large area of skin following a burn accident or the loss of substantial nerve mass following an automobile accident. However, irreversible loss of function can also occur following disease, although over a lengthy time: Examples are the inability of a heart valve to prevent leakage during diastole as a result of valve tissue response to an inflammatory process (rheumatic fever), and the inability of liver tissue to synthesize enzymes due to its progressive replacement by fibrotic tissue (cirrhosis).

Five approaches have been used to solve the problem of the missing organ. In autografting, a mass of similar or identical tissue from the patient (autograft) is surgically removed and used to treat the area of loss. The approach can be considered to be spectacularly successful until one considers the long-term cost incurred by the patient. An example is the use of sheet autograft to treat extensive areas of full-thickness skin loss; although the patient incorporates the autograft fully with excellent recovery of function, the "donor" site used to harvest the autograft remains scarred. When the autograft is not available, as is common in cases of burns extending over more than 30% of body surface area, the autograft is meshed in order to make it extensible enough to cover the large wound areas. However, the meshed autograft provides cover only where the graft tissue provides direct cover; where there is no cover, scar forms, and the result is one of low cosmetic value. Similar problems of donor site unavailability and scarring must be dealt with in heart bypass surgery, another widespread example of autografting. In transplantation, the donor tissue is typically harvested from a cadaver, and the recipient has to cope with the problems of rejection and the risk of transmission of viruses from this allograft. Another approach has been based on efforts to synthesize tissues in vitro using autologous cells from the patient; this approach has yielded so far a cultured epidermis (a tissue which regenerates spontaneously provided there is a dermal substrate underneath) about 2–3 weeks after the time when the patient was injured. In vitro synthesis of the dermis, a tissue which does not regenerate, has not been accomplished so far. Perhaps the most successful approach from the commercial standpoint has been the one in which engineered biomaterials are used; these materials are typically required by their designers to remain intact themselves without interfering with the patient's physiologic functions during the entire lifetime; overwhelmingly, this requirement is observed in its breach. A fifth approach is based on the discovery that an analog of the extracellular matrix (ECM) induces partial regeneration of the dermis, rather than of scar, in full-thickness skin wounds in adult mammals (human, guinea pig, pig) where it is well known that no regeneration occurs spontaneously. This fifth approach of solving the problem of organ loss, in situ regeneration, will be described in this chapter.

Efforts to induce regeneration have been successful with only a handful of ECM analogs. Evidence of regeneration is sought after the ECM analog has been implanted in situ, i.e., at the lesion marking the site of the missing organ. When morphogenesis is clearly evident, based on tests of recovery both of the original tissue structure and function, the matrix which has induced these physiologic or nearly physiologic tissues is named a regeneration template. In the absence of evidence of such morphogenetic activity of the cell-free matrix, the latter is not referred to as a regeneration template.

109.2 Design Principles for Regeneration Templates

Several parameters have been incorporated in the design of organ regeneration templates. Briefly, these parameters account for the performance of the implant during the early or acute stage following implantation (physicochemical parameters) as well as for the long-term or chronic stage following implantation (biologic parameters).

Immediately upon making contact with the wound bed, the implant must achieve physicochemical nanoadhesion (i.e., adhesion at a scale of 1 nm) between itself and the lesion. Without contact of this type it is not possible to establish and maintain transport of molecules and cells between implant and host tissue. The presence of adequate adhesion can be studied by measurements of the force necessary to peel the implant from the wound bed immediately after grafting.

Empirical evidence has supported a requirement for an implant which is capable of isomorphous tissue replacement, i.e., the synthesis of new tissue at a rate which is of same order as the rate of degradation of the matrix.

$$\frac{t_b}{t_h} = O(1) \tag{109.1}$$

In Eq. (109.1), t_b denotes a characteristic time constant for biodegradation of the implant *at that tissue site,* and t_h denotes a time constant for healing, the latter occurring by synthesis of new tissue inside the implant.

A third requirement refers to the *critical cell path length* l_c, beyond which migration of a cell into the implant deprives it of an essential nutrient, assumed to be transported from the host tissue by diffusion alone. The emphasis is on the characteristic diffusion path for the nutrient during the early stages of wound healing, before significant angiogenesis occurs several days later. Calculation of the critical cell path can be done by use of the *cell lifeline number, S,* a dimensionless number expressing the relative importance of a chemical reaction, which leads to consumption of an essential nutrient by the cell, and of diffusion of the nutrient which alone makes the latter accessible to the cell. This number is defined as

$$S = \frac{rl^2}{Dc_o} \tag{109.2}$$

where r is the rate of consumption of the nutrient by the cell in mole/cm³/s, l is the diffusion length, D is the diffusivity of the nutrient in the medium of the implant, and c_o is the nutrient concentration at or near the surface of the wound bed, in mole/cm³. When $S = O(1)$ the value of l is the critical path length l_c along which cells can migrate, away from host tissue, without requirement of nutrient in excess of that supplied by diffusion. Eq. (109.2) can, therefore, be used to define the maximum implant thickness beyond which cells require the presence of capillaries.

The chemical composition of the implant which has induced regeneration was designed on the basis of studies of wound-healing kinetics. In most mammals, full-thickness skin wounds close partly by contraction of the wounds edges and partly by synthesis of scar tissue. Clearly, skin regeneration over the entire area of skin loss cannot occur unless the wound edges are kept apart and, in addition, the healing processes in the wound bed are modified drastically enough to yield a physiologic dermis rather than scar. Although several synthetic polymers, such as porous (poly)dimethyl siloxane, delay contraction to a small but significant extent, they do not degrade and therefore violate isomorphous tissue replacement, Eq. (109.1). Synthetic biodegradable polymers, such as (poly)lactic acid, can be modified, e.g., by copolymerization with glycolic acid, to yield polymers which satisfy Eq. (109.1); however, evidence is lacking that these synthetic polymers delay contraction and prevent synthesis of scar. By contrast, there is considerable evidence that a certain analog of the extracellular matrix (ECM analogs) not only delays contraction significantly but also leads to synthesis of partly physiologic skin. Systematic use of the delay in contraction as an essay has been made to identify the structural features of the skin regeneration template (SRT), as shown schematically in Fig. 109.1.

Summarized in Fig. 109.1 are three modes of wound-healing behavior, each elicited by an ECM analog of different design. Mode O of healing is described by a very short time for onset of contraction, followed by contraction and definitive closure of the wound with formation of a thin linear scar. Mode I is characterized by a significant delay in onset of contraction, following which contraction proceeds and eventually leads to a linear scar. Mode II is characterized by a significant delay in onset of contraction (somewhat smaller than in mode I), followed by contraction and then by reversal of contraction, with expansion of the original wound perimeter at a rate which exceeds significantly the growth rate of the entire animal. Mode II healing leads to synthesis of a partly physiologic dermis and a physiologic epidermis within the perimeter of the expanded wound bed. Mode O healing occurs when an ECM analog which lacks specificity is used to graft the wound. Mode O is also observed when the wound bed remains ungrafted. Mode I healing occurs when an ECM analog of highly specific structure (the SRT) is grafted on the wound bed. Mode II healing occurs when the SRT, previously identified as the ECM analog which leads to mode I healing, is seeded with autologous epidermal cells before being grafted. Although contraction is a convenient screening method for identification of structural features of ECM analogs which induce skin regeneration, a different procedure has been used to identify the features of an implant that induces regeneration of the peripheral nerve. The structural features of the nerve regeneration template (NRT) were identified using an essay focused on the long-term return of function of the nerve following treatment with candidate ECM analogs.

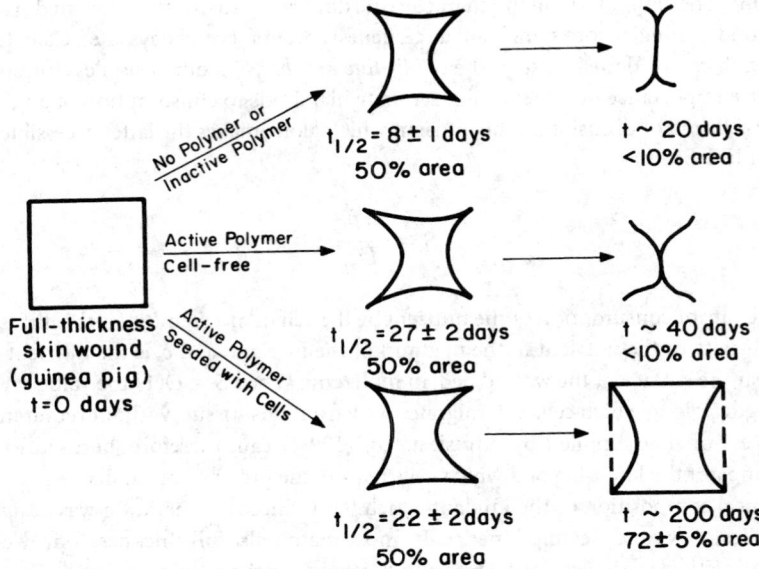

FIGURE 109.1   The kinetics of contraction of full-thickness guinea pig skin wounds can be used to separate collagen-*graft*-glycosaminoglycan copolymers into three classes, as shown. The wound half-life, $t_{1/2}$, is the number of days necessary to reduce the original wound area to 50%. (Courtesy of Massachusetts Institute of Technology.)

Of several ECM analogs that have been prepared, the most commonly studied is a graft copolymer of type I collagen and chondroitin 6-sulfate. The structure of the latter glycosaminoglycan (GAG) is illustrated below in terms of the repeat unit of the disaccharide, an alternating copolymer of D-glucuronic acid and of an O-sulfate derivative of N-acetyl D-galactosamine:

sodium chondroitin 6-sulfate

The principle of isomorphous replacement, Eq. (109.1), cannot be satisfied unless the *biodegradation time constant* of the network, t_b, can be adjusted to an optimal level, about equal to the rate of synthesis of new tissue at that site. Reduction of the biodegradation rate of collagen can be achieved either by grafting GAG chains onto collagen chains or by crosslinking collagen chains to each other. The chemical grafting of GAG chains on polypeptide chains proceeds by previously coprecipitating the two polymers under conditions of acidic pH, followed by covalent crosslinking of the freeze-dried precipitate. A particularly useful procedure for crosslinking collagen chains to GAG, or collagen chains to each other, is a self-crosslinking reaction, requiring no use of crosslinking agent. This condensation reaction principally involves carboxylic groups from glutamyl/aspartyl residues on polypeptide chain P_1 and ϵ-amino groups of lysyl residues on an adjacent chain P_2 to yield covalently bonded collagen chains; as well as condensation of amine groups of collagen with carboxylic groups of glucuronic acid residues on GAG chains to yield *graft*-copolymers of collagen and GAG:

$$P_1\text{-COOH} + P_2\text{-NH}_2 \rightarrow P_2\text{-NHCO-}P_1 + H_2O \qquad (109.3a)$$

$$\text{GAG-COOH} + P_2\text{-NH}_2 \rightarrow P_2\text{-NHCO-GAG} + H_2O \qquad (109.3b)$$

In each case above the reaction proceeds to the right, with formation of a three-dimensional crosslinked network when the moisture content of the protein, or protein-GAG coprecipitate, drops below about 1 wt%. As illustrated by Eq. (109.3), removal of water, the volatile product of the condensation, is favored by conditions which drive the reaction towards the right, with formation of a crosslinked network. Thus, the reaction proceeds to the right when both high temperature and vacuum are used. Another crosslinking reaction, used extensively in preparing implants that have been employed in clinical studies as well as in animal studies, involves use of glutaraldehyde. Dehydration crosslinking, which amounts to self-crosslinking as described above, obviously does not lend toxicity to these implants. Glutaraldehyde, on the other hand, is a toxic substance, and devices treated with it require thorough rinsing before use until free glutaraldehyde cannot be detected in the rinse water. Network properties of crosslinked collagen-GAG copolymers can be analyzed structurally by studying the swelling behavior of small specimens. The method is based on the theory of Flory and Rehner, who showed that the volume fraction of a swollen polymer v_2 depends on the average molecular weight between crosslinks, M_c, through the following relationship:

$$\ln(1 - v_2) + v_2 + \chi v_2 - (\rho V_1/M_c)(v_2^{1/3} - v_2/2) = 0 \qquad (109.4)$$

In Eq. (109.4), V_1 is the molar volume of the solvent, ρ is the density of the dry polymer, and χ is a constant characteristic of a specific polymer-solvent pair at a particular temperature.

Although the chemical identity of collagen-GAG copolymers is a necessary element of their biologic activity, it is not a sufficient one. In addition to chemical composition and the crosslink density, biologic activity also depends strongly on the *pore architecture* of these ECM analogs. Pores are incorporated first by freezing a very dilute suspension of the collagen-GAG coprecipitate and then by inducing sublimation of the ice crystals by exposing to vacuum at low temperatures. The resulting pore structure is, therefore, a negative replica of the network of ice crystals (dendrites). It follows that control of the conditions of ice crystal nucleation and growth can lead to a large variety of pore structures. In practice, the average pore diameter decreases with decreasing temperature of freezing while the orientation of pore channel axes also depends on the magnitude of the heat flux vector during freezing. The dependence of pore channel orientation on heat transfer parameters is illustrated by considering the dimensionless Mikic number Mi, a ratio of the characteristic freezing time of the aqueous medium of the collagen-GAG suspension, t_f, to the characteristic time for entry, t_e, of a container filled with the suspension which is lowered at constant velocity into a well-stirred cooling bath:

$$Mi = \frac{t_f}{t_e} = \frac{\rho_w h_{fg} r V}{10 k_j \Delta T} \qquad (109.5)$$

In Eq. (109.5), ρ_w is the density of the suspension, h_{fg} is the heat of fusion of the suspension, r is an arbitrary length scale, V is the velocity with which the container is lowered into the bath, k_j is the thermal conductivity of the jacket, and ΔT is the difference between freezing temperature and bath temperature. The shape of the isotherms near the freezing front is highly dependent on the value of Mi. The dominant heat flux vector is normal to these isotherms, i.e., ice dendtites grow along this vector. It has been observed that, for $Mi < 1$ (slow cooling), the isotherms, are shallow, flat-shaped parabolae, and the ice dendrites exhibit high axial orientation. For $Mi > 1$ (rapid cooling), the isotherms are steep parabolae, and ice dendrites are oriented along the radial direction.

The structure of the porous matrix is defined by quantities such as the volume fraction, specific surface, mean pore size, and orientation of pores in the matrix. Determination of these properties is based on principles of stereology, the discipline which relates the quantitative statistical properties of three-dimensional structures to those of their two-dimensional sections or projections. In reverse, stereologic procedures allow reconstruction of certain aspects of three-dimensional objects from a quantitative analysis of planar images. A plane which goes through the two-phase structure of pores and collagen-GAG fibers may be sampled by random points, by a regular pattern of points, by a near-total sampling using a very dense array of points, or by arranging the sampling points to form a continuous line. The volume fraction of pores, V_V, is equal to the fraction of total test points which fall inside pore regions, P_P, also equal to the total area fraction of pores, A_A, and, finally, equal to the line fraction of pores, L_L, for a linear point array in the limit of infinitely close point spacing

$$V_V = P_P = A_A = L_L \tag{109.6}$$

Whether cells of a particular type should be part of a regeneration template depends on predictions derived from models of developmental biology as well as empirical findings obtained with well-defined wound-healing models. During morphogenesis of a large variety of organs, an interaction between epithelial and mesenchymal cells, mediated by the basal lamina which is interleaved between the two types of cells, is both necessary and sufficient for development of local physiologic structures involving two types of tissue in juxtaposition. In particular, skin morphogenesis in a full-thickness wound model requires the presence of this interaction between the two cell types and the basal lamina over a critical period. In skin wound–healing experiments with adult mammals, wound healing proceeds with formation of scar, rather than physiologic skin, if the wound bed contains epithelial cells and mesenchymal cells (fibroblasts) but no ECM structure which could act temporarily as a basal lamina. If, by contrast, an analog of the basal lamina is present, wound healing proceeds with nearly physiologic morphogenesis of skin. Furthermore, no epidermis is formed unless epithelial cells become involved in wound healing early during wound healing and continue being involved until they have achieved confluence. It is also known that no dermis forms if fibroblasts are not available early during wound healing. These observations suggest the requirement for a SRT which is an analog of the basal lamina and is designed to encourage the migration and interaction of both epithelial cells and fibroblasts within its volume.

Nerve regeneration following injury essentially amounts to elongation of a single nerve cell across a gap resulting from the injury. During nerve development many nerve cells are elongated by processes which eventually become axons. Interaction of elongating processes with basal lamina are credited as being essential in the formation of nerves during development, and it will be assumed here that such interactions are essential in regeneration following adult injury as well. It is also known that Schwann cells, which derive from neural crest cells during development, are essential contributors to regeneration following injury to the adult peripheral nerve. These considerations suggest a nerve regeneration template which is structured as an analog of the basal lamina, interacting with the elongating axons in the presence of Schwann cells.

109.3 Design Optimization for Skin Regeneration Template (SRT)

The major events accompanying skin wound healing can be summarized as contraction and scar synthesis. Conventional wisdom prescribes the need for a treatment that accelerates wound healing. A large number of devices that claim to speed up various aspects of the healing process has been described in the literature . The need to achieve healing within as short a time as possible is certainly well founded, especially in the clinical setting where the risk to patient's life as well as the morbidity increase with extension of time to heal. However, the discovery of partial skin regeneration by use of the skin regeneration template has introduced the option of a drastically improved healing result for the patient in exchange for a slightly extended hospital stay.

The SRT was optimized in studies with animals in which it was observed that skin regeneration did not occur unless the test ECM analog effectively delayed, rather than accelerated, wound contraction. The length of delay in onset of contraction eventually was used as a quantitative basis for preliminary optimization of the structural features of the SRT. Optimization studies are currently continuing on the basis of a new criterion, namely, the fidelity of regeneration achieved.

Systematic use of the criterion of contraction inhibition has been made to select the biodegradation rate and the average pore diameter of SRT. The kinetics of contraction of full-thickness skin wounds in the guinea pig have been studied for each of the three modes of healing schematically presented in Fig. 109.1. The results, presented in Fig. 109.2, show that mode O healing is characterized by early onset of contraction, whereas mode I and mode II healing show a significant delay in onset of contraction. A measure of the delay is the wound half-life $t_{1/2}$, the time required for the wound area to decrease to 50% of the original value. Use of this index of contraction rate has been made in Figs. 109.3 and 109.4, which present data on the variation of wound half-life with average pore diameter and degradation rate for a type I collagen-chondroitin 6-sulfate copolymer. In Fig. 109.2, mode I kinetics are observed using a cell-free copolymer with average pore diameter and biodegradation rate that correspond to the regions of Figs. 109.3 and 109.4 in which the values of half-life are maximal; these regions characterize the structure of SRT which possesses maximal activity. Maximum delay in wound half-life up to 27 ± 3 days is seen to have occurred when the average pore diameter has ranged from values as low as 20 ± 4 μm to an upper limit of 125 ± 35 μm. In addition, significant delay in wound healing has been observed when the degradation rate has become less than 115 ± 25 enzyme units. The latter index of degradation has been based on the in vitro degradation rate of the copolymer in a standardized solution of bacterial collagenase.

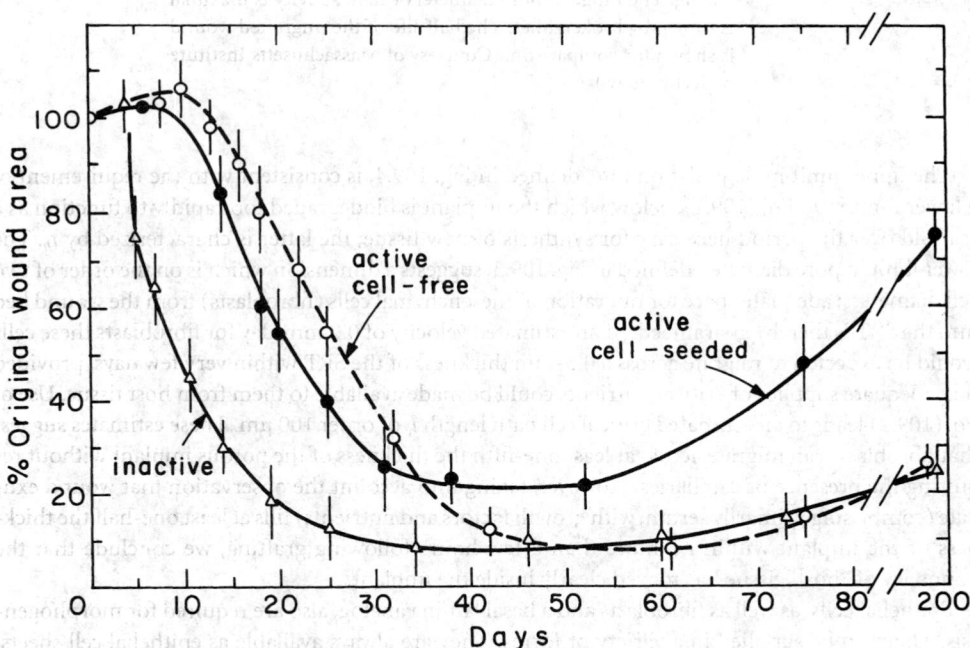

FIGURE 109.2 The kinetics of guinea pig skin wound contraction following grafting with three classes of ECM analogs. Inactive ECM analogs delay the onset of contraction only marginally over the ungrafted wound, whereas active cell-free ECM analogs delay the onset of contraction significantly. When seeded with epithelial cells, not only does an active ECM analog delay the onset of contraction significantly, but it also induces formation of a confluent epidermis and then arrests and reverses the direction of movement of wound edges, leading to expansion of the wound perimeter and to synthesis of partly physiologic skin. (Courtesy of Massachusetts Institute of Technology.)

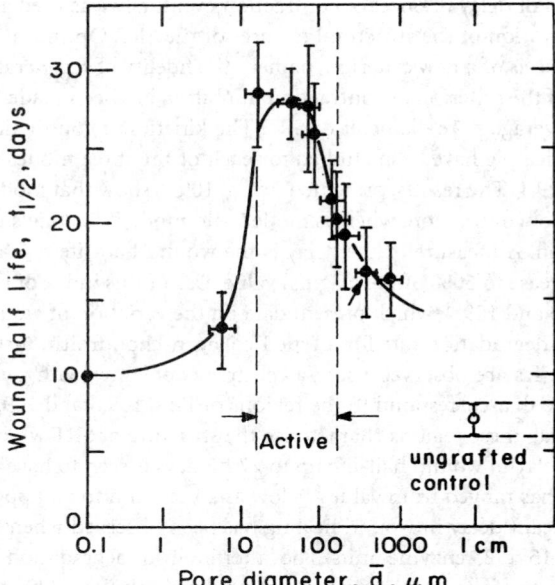

FIGURE 109.3 The half-life of wounds, $t_{1/2}$, grafted with ECM analogs varies with the average pore diameter of the analog. The range of pore diameters where activity is maximal is shown by broken lines. The half-life of the ungrafted wound is shown for comparison. (Courtesy of Massachusetts Institute of Technology.)

The upper limit in degradation rate, defined in Fig. 109.4, is consistent with the requirement of a lower limit in t_b, Eq. (109.1), below which the implant is biodegraded too rapidly to function as a scaffold over the period necessary for synthesis of new tissue; the latter is characterized by t_h. The lower limit in pore diameter, defined in Fig. 109.3, suggests a dimension which is on the order of two cell diameters; adequate space for migration of mesenchymal cells (fibroblasts) from the wound bed into the SRT is thereby guaranteed. At an estimated velocity of 0.2 mm/day for fibroblasts these cells would be expected to migrate across a 0.5-mm thickness of the SRT within very few days, provided that adequate supplies of critical nutrients could be made available to them from host tissue. Use of Eq. (109.2) leads to an estimated critical cell path length l_c of order 100 μm. These estimates suggest that fibroblasts can migrate across at least one-fifth the thickness of the porous implant without requiring the presence of capillaries. However, taking into account the observation that wound exudate (comprising primarily serum, with growth factors and nutrients) fills at least one-half the thickness of the implant within no more than a few hours following grafting, we conclude that the boundary of "host" tissue has moved clearly inside the implant.

Epithelial cells, as well as fibroblasts and a basal lamina analog, also are required for morphogenesis. They can be supplied in a variety of forms. They are always available as epithelial cell sheets, migrating from the wound edges toward the center of the wound bed. However, when the area of skin loss is several centimeters, as with a severely burned patient, these cell sheets, migrating with speeds of about 0.5 mm/day from opposite edges, would not be expected to cover one-half the characteristic wound dimension in less than the time constant t_h for synthesis of new tissue. In the absence of epithelial cells, therefore, at the center of the wound bed, Eq. (109.1) would be violated. To overcome this limitation, which is imposed by the scale of the wound, it has been necessary to resort to a variety of procedures. In the first, uncultured autologous epidermal cells, extracted from a

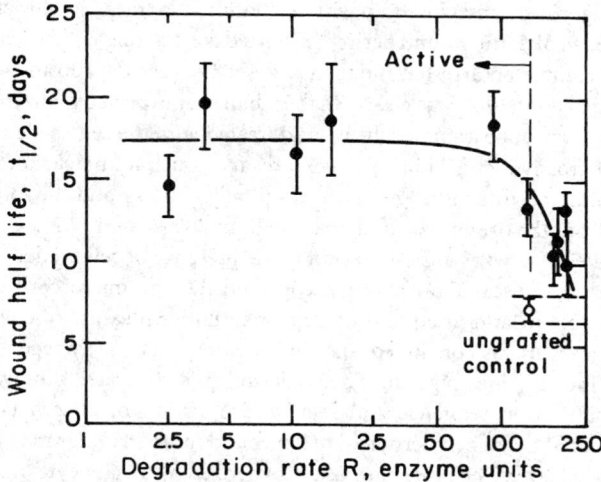

FIGURE 109.4 Variation of wound half-life with degradation rate *R* of the ECM analog used as graft for a full-thickness guinea pig skin wound. *R* varies inversely as the biodegradation time constant, tf. The region of maximal activity is indicated by the broken line. The half-life of the ungrafted wound is shown for comparison. (Courtesy of Massachusetts Institute of Technology.)

skin biopsy by controlled enzymatic degradation, have been seeded into ECM analogs by centrifugation into the porours matrix prior to grafting of the latter on the wound bed. Tested with animals, the procedure leads to formation of a confluent epidermis by about 2 weeks, provided that at least 5×10^4 epithelial cells per cm^2 of SRT area have been seeded. In another procedure, a very thin epidermal layer has been surgically removed from an intact area of the patient and has been grafted on the dermal layer which has been synthesized about 2 weeks after grafting with the SRT. The latter procedure has been tested clinically with reproducible success. A third procedure, studied with animals, has made use of cultured epithelia, prepared by a 2- to 3-week period of culture of autologous cells in vitro and grafted on the newly synthesized dermal bed. Approximately equivalent fidelity of skin regeneration has been obtained by each of these procedures for supplying epithelial cells to the SRT in the treatment of skin wounds of very large area.

109.4 In Situ Synthesis of Skin with SRT

The skin regeneration template SRT induces regeneration of skin to a high degree of fidelity. Fidelity of regeneration has been defined in terms of the degree of recovery of structural and functional features which are present in the intact organ.

The first test of fidelity of skin regeneration following use of the SRT was a study of treatment of full-thickness skin loss in guineas pigs. In this study the lesion was produced by surgery on healthy animals. The characteristic dimension of the wound was about 3 cm, and the desired period for cover by a confluent epidermis was 2 weeks. Covering a wound of such a scale within the prescribed time would have been out of reach of epithelial cells migrating from the wound edges. Accordingly, autologous epithelial cells were extracted from a skin biopsy and seeded into the SRT under conditions of carefully controlled centrifugation.

A clear and unmistakable difference between healing in the presence and absence of SRT was provided by observing the gross anatomy of the wound (Fig. 109.2). In the absence of the SRT, the wound contracted vigorously and closed up with formation of a linear scar by about day 30. In the presence of a cell-seeded SRT, the wound perimeter started contracting with a delay of about 10 days, and contraction was completely arrested and then reversed between days 30 and 40. The wound then continued to expand at a rate that was clearly higher than that expected from the rate of growth of the animal. The long-term appearance of the wound treated with the cell-seeded SRT was that of an organ that appeared grossly identical in color, texture, and touch to intact skin outside the wound perimeter. However, the newly synthesized skin was totally hairless, and the total area of new skin was smaller in area from the original wound area by about 30% (Fig. 109.2).

Morphologic studies of newly synthesized skin in the presence of cell-seeded SRT included comparison with intact skin and scar. Optical microscopy and electron microscopy were supplemented by laser light scattering, the latter used to provide a quantitative measure of collagen fiber orientation in the dermal layer. It was concluded that, in most respects, partly regenerated skin was remarkably similar to intact guinea pig skin. The epidermis in regenerated skin was often hyperplastic; however, the maturation sequence and relative proportion of all cell layers were normal. Keratohyaline granules of the neoepidermis were larger and more irregular in contour than those of the normal granular cell layer. The new skin was characterized by melanocytes and Langerhans cells, as well as a well-formed pattern of rete ridges and interdigitations with dermal papillae, all of which appear in normal skin. Newly synthesized skin was distinctly different morphologically from scar. Scar showed characteristic thinning (atrophy) of the epidermis, with absence of rete ridges and of associated dermal papillae. Elastic fibers in regenerated skin formed a delicate particulate structure, in contrast with scar, where elastic fibers were thin and fragmented. The dermal layer in regenerated skin comprised collagen fibers which were not oriented in the plane of the epidermis, as well as fibroblasts which were not elongated; in scar, collagen fibers were highly oriented in the plane and fibroblasts were elongated. Both normal and regenerated skin comprised unmyelinated nerve fibers within dermal papillae, closely approximated to the epidermis; scar had few, if any, nerves. There were no hair follicles or other skin appendages either in regenerated skin or in scar.

Laser light–scattering measurements of the orientation of collagen fibers in tissue sections of the dermal layer were based on use of the Hermans orientation function

$$f = 2 \langle \cos^2\alpha \rangle - 1 \tag{109.7}$$

In Eq. (109.7), α is the angle between an individual fiber and the mean axis of the fibers, and $\langle \cos^2\alpha \rangle$ is the square cosine of α averaged over all the fibers in the sample. For a random arrangement of fibers, $\langle \cos^2\alpha \rangle$ equals 1/2, while for a perfectly aligned arrangement it is equal to 1. Accordingly, S varies from 0 (truly random) to 1 (perfect alignment). Measurements obtained by use of this procedure showed that S took the values 0.20 ± 0.11, 0.48 ± 0.05 and 0.75 ± 0.10 for normal dermis, regenerated dermis, and scar dermis, respectively. These results provided objective evidence that regenerated dermis had a morphology of collagen fibers that was clearly not scar (n = 7; p <0.001), and was intermediate between that of scar and normal dermis.

Functional studies of regenerated skin showed that the moisture permeability of intact skin and regenerated skin had values of 4.5 ± 0.8 and 4.7 ± 1.9 g/cm/h, insignificantly different from each other (n = 4; p <0.8). Mechanical behavior studies showed a positive curvature for the tensile stress-strain curve of regenerated skin as well as of normal skin. However, the tensile strength of regenerated skin was 14 ± 4 MPa, significantly lower than the strength of intact skin, 31 ± 4 MPa (n = 4; p <0.01).

The second test of fidelity of skin regeneration was a study of treatment of 106 massively burned humans with the cell-free SRT. The characteristic dimension of the wound in this study was of order 15 cm, and the desired period for cover by a confluent epidermis was 2 weeks. The scale of the wound necessitated the introduction of epithelial cells, and this was accomplished by grafting the newly synthesized dermal layer, 2 weeks after grafting with SRT, with a very thin epidermal layer (epidermal autograft), which was removed from an intact area of the patient. The results of the histologic study of the patient population showed that physiologic dermis, rather than scar, had been synthesized in sites that had been treated with SRT and had later been covered with an epidermal graft.

109.5 Advantages and Disadvantages of Clinical Treatment of Skin Loss with SRT

When skin is the missing organ, the patient faces threats to life posed by severe dehydration and infection. These threats can be eliminated permanently only if the area of missing skin is covered with a device that controls moisture flux within physiologic limits and presents an effective barrier to airborne bacteria. Both of these functions can be returned over a period of about 2–4 weeks by use of temporary dressings. The latter include the allograft (skin from a cadaver) and a very large variety of membranes based on synthetic or natural polymers. None of these dressings solves the problem of missing skin over the lifetime of the patient: The allograft does not support synthesis of physiologic skin and must be removed to avoid rejection, and the devices based on the vast majority of engineered membranes do not make effective biologic contact with the patient's tissues, and all lead to synthesis of scar.

Three devices have been tested extensively for their ability to provide long-term physiologic cover to patients with massive skin loss: the patient's own skin (autograft), the skin regeneration template (SRT), and cultured epithelia (CE). All three of these treatments have been studied extensively with massively burned patients. Of these, the autograft and SRT are effective even when the loss of skin extends through the full thickness of the dermis (e.g., third-degree burns), whereas CE is effective when the loss of skin is through part of its thickness only.

The basis for these differences among the three treatments lies in the intrinsic response of skin to injury. Skin comprises three layers: the epidermis, a 100-μm thick cellular layer; the dermis, a 1- to 5-mm layer of connective tissue with very few cells; and the subcutis, a 2- to 4-mm layer of primarily adipose tissue. In the adult mammal, an epidermis lost through injury regenerates spontaneously provided that a dermal substrate is present underneath. When the dermis is lost, whether through part thickness or full thickness, none of the injured mass regenerates; instead, a nonphysiologic tissue, scar, forms. Scar is epithelialized and can, therefore, control moisture flux within physiologic limits as well as provide a barrier to bacterial invasion. However, scar does not have the mechanical strength of physiologic skin. Also, scar synthesis frequently proceeds well beyond what is necessary to cover the wound, and the result of such proliferation is hypertrophic scarring, a cosmetically inferior integument which, when extending over a large area or over hands or face, reduces significantly the mobility of the patient's joints as well as the patient's cosmetic appearance. Autograft can, if used without meshing, provide an excellent permanent cover; if, however, as commonly practiced, autograft is meshed before grafting in order to extend the wound area that becomes covered, the result is new integument which comprises part physiologic skin and part scar and provides the patient with a solution of much lower quality than unmeshed (sheet) autograft. The clinical use of skin regeneration template has led to a new integument comprising a dermal layer, which has been synthesized by the patient, and an epidermal layer, which has been harvested as a very thin epidermal autograft and has been placed on top of the newly synthesized dermis.

The chief advantages of SRT over the meshed autograft are the shorter time that it takes to heal the donor site, from which the epidermal graft was harvested, and a superior cosmetic result at the site of the wound. The main disadvantage in the clinical use of SRT is the subjection of the patient to two surgical treatments rather than one (first graft SRT, then graft the epidermal layer after about 2 weeks). The clinical advantages of CE are the ability to grow a very large area, about 10,000 times as large as the area of the skin biopsy, thereby providing cover over the entire injured skin area of the patient. The disadvantages of cultured epithelia are the lengthy period required to culture the epidermis from the patient's biopsy and the inability of the CE to form a mechanically competent bond with the wound bed.

109.6 Modifications of SRT: Use of a Living Dermal Equivalent

The design concept of a skin regeneration template outlined above has been adopted and modified. One modification involves the replacement of the collagen-GAG matrix with a biodegradable mesh consisting of either (poly) glycolic acid (PGA) or polyglactin-910 (PGL) fibers. The latter is used as a matrix for the in vitro culture of human fibroblasts isolated from neonatal skin. Fibroblasts synthesize extracellular matrix inside the synthetic polymeric mesh, and this "living dermal equivalent" has been cryopreserved for a specified period prior to use.

The living dermal equivalent has been used to graft full-thickness skin wounds in athymic mice. Following grafting of wounds, these PGA/PGL fibroblast grafts were covered with meshed allograft. The latter is human cadaver skin that was meshed in this study to expand it and achieve coverage of maximum possible wound area. This composite graft became vascularized and that, additionally, epithelial cells from the cadaver graft had migrated to the matrix underneath. After a period of about 100 days following grafting, the reported result was an epithelialized layer covering a densely cellular substratum that resembled dermis. A variant of this design, in which the meshed allograft is not used, has been reported; epidermal cells are cultured with the fibroblast mesh before grafting. Studies of these designs are in progress.

109.7 The Bilayered Skin-Equivalent Graft

In one widely reported development, in vitro cell culture procedures have been used to synthesize a bilayered tissue which has been reported to be a useful model of human skin. Briefly, fibroblasts from humans or from rats have been placed inside a collagen gel. Under these conditions, fibroblasts exert contractile forces, trapping the cells inside the contracted collagen lattice. Human epithelial cells, which have been plated onto this contracted dermal equivalent, have been observed to attach to the collagen substrate, multiply, and spread to form a continuous sheet. Differentiation of this sheet has led to formation of specialized epidermal structures, such as a multilayered cell structure with desmosomes, tonofilaments, and keratohyalin granules. Further differentiation events have included the formation of a basement membrane (basal lamina) in vitro when a rat epidermis was formed on top of a dermal equivalent produced from rat fibroblasts.

Grafts prepared from the bilayered skin equivalent have been grafted on animals. When grafted on animals, these structures have been reported to become well vascularized with a network of capillaries within 7 to 9 days. It has been reported that the best grafts have blocked wound contraction, but no systematic data have been presented which could be used to compare the in vivo performance of these skin equivalents with grafts based on SRT (see above). Gross observations of the area grafted with skin equivalents have shown pink hairless areas which were not hypertrophically scarred. A systematic comparison between scar and the tissue synthesized in sites that have been grafted with skin equivalents has not yet been made.

109.8 Design Optimization of Nerve Regeneration Template (NRT)

The design principles for regeneration templates presented above have been used to design implants for regeneration of peripheral nerves. The medical problem typically involves the loss of innervation in arms and legs, leading to loss of motor and sensory function (paralysis). The nerves involved are peripheral, and the design problem becomes the regeneration of injured peripheral nerves, with recovery of function.

A widely used animal model for peripheral nerve injury is a surgically generated gap in the sciatic nerve of the rat. Interruption of nerve function in this case is localized primarily in the region of plantar muscles of the foot involved. This relatively well defined area of loss of function can then be studied neurologically in relative isolation from other neurologic events. Furthermore, the rate of recovery of function can be studied by electrophysiologic methods, a procedure which provides continuous data over the entire period of healing. In the peripheral nerve the healing period extends to about 10 weeks, clearly longer than healing in skin, which occurs largely within a period of only 3 weeks.

When the sciatic nerve is cut and a gap forms between the two nerve ends, the distal part of the nerve is isolated from its cell body in the spinal cord. Communication between the central nervous system and the leg is no longer possible. The lack of muscle innervation leads to inactivity, which in turn leads to muscle atrophy. At the site of injury there is degeneration of the myelin sheath of axons, dissociation of Schwann cells and formation of scar. It has been hypothesized that the formation of scar impedes, more than any other single cause, the elongation of axons across the gap. Axonal elongation through a gap of substantial length becomes, therefore, a parameter of prime importance in the design of a nerve regeneration template (NRT).

Intubation of severed nerve ends is a widely used procedure for isolating axons from the tissue environment of the peripheral nerve. The lumen of the tube serves to isolate the process of nerve regeneration from wound-healing events involving connective tissues outside the nerve; the tube walls, for example, prevent proliferation of scar tissue inside the tube and the subsequent obstruction of the regenerating nerve. Silicone tubes are the most widely used method of intubation. These tubes are both nonbiodegradable and nonpermeable to large molecules. In this isolated environment it is possible to study the substrate preferences of elongating axons by incorporating well-defined ECM analogs and studying the kinetics of functional recovery continuously with electrophysiologic procedures for about 40 weeks following implantation. As in studies of dermal regeneration described above, the ECM analogs which were used in the study of substrate preferences of axons were graft copolymers of type I collagen and chondroitin 6-sulfate. Controls used included the autograft, empty silicone tubes, as well as tubes filled with saline. In these studies it was necessary to work with a gap dimension large enough to preclude spontaneous regeneration, i.e., regeneration in the absence of an ECM analog. It was observed that a gap length of 10 mm was occasionally innervated spontaneously in the rat, whereas no instances of spontaneous regeneration were observed with a 15-mm gap length. Gap lengths of 10 and 15 mm were used in these studies with rats.

Three structural parameters of ECM analogs were varied systematically. The degradation rate had a significant effect on the fidelity of regeneration, and an abbreviated optimization procedure led to an ECM analog which degraded much faster than the SRT. In combination with Eq. (109.1), this empirical finding suggests that a healing nerve wound contains a much smaller concentration of the degrading enzyme, collagenase; this suggestion is qualitatively consistent with observations of collagenolyitc activity in injured nerves. The average pore diameter also was found to have a significant effect on fidelity of regeneration, and the optimization procedure led to a value of 5 μm, significantly smaller than the average pore diameter in the SRT. Finally, use of Eq. (109.5) led to procedures of preparing ECM analogs, the pore channels of which were either highly aligned along the tube axis, randomly oriented, or radially oriented. ECM analogs with axially aligned pore channels were found to be superior to analogs with other types of alignment.

These results have led to a design for an NRT consisting of a specified degradation rate, average pore diameter, and pore channel alignment as shown in Table 109.1. Studies of NRT with humans have not been conducted, in anticipation of replacement of the nondegradable silicone tube (which necessitates a secondary operation to remove the tube) with a collagen tube. This replacement is in progress.

Nerves regenerated with use of NRT have led to recovery of signal conduction velocity of about 90% of physiologic value. Neurologic studies of regenerated nerves are in progress. Optimization of design parameters for the SRT and the NRT has led to results compared in Table 109.1.

Studies of Nerve Regeneration Using Degradable Tubes

Porous collagen tubes without matrix content have been extensively studied as guides for peripheral nerve regeneration in rodents and nonhuman primates. The walls of these collagen tubes had

TABLE 109.1 Design Parameters for Two Regeneration Templates

Design Parameter of ECM Analog	SRT	NRT
Degradation rate, enzyme units	<120	>150
Average pore diameter, μm	20–125	5
Pore channel orientation	random	axial

an average pore diameter which was considered sufficiently large for transport of molecules as large as bovine serum albumen (MW = 68 kDa). A 4-mm gap in the sciatic nerve of the rat was the standard injury studied. Other injury models that were studied included the 4-mm gap and the 15-mm gap in the adult monkey.

The use of an empty tube did not allow for any degree of optimization of tube parameters to be achieved in this study. Nevertheless, the long-term results showed almost complete recovery of motor and sensory responses, at rates that approximated the recovery obtained following use of the nerve autograft, currently the best conventional treatment in cases of massive loss of nerve mass. The success obtained suggests that collagen tubes can be used instead of autografts, the harvesting of which subject the patient to nerve-losing surgery. Studies of collagen tubes are in progress.

109.9 In Situ Synthesis of Meniscus Using a Meniscus Regeneration Template (MRT)

The meniscus of the knee performs a variety of functions which amount to joint stabilization and lubrication, as well as shock absorption. Its structure is that of fibrocartilage, consisting primarily of type I collagen fibers populated with meniscal fibrochondrocytes. The architecture of collagen fibers is complex. In this tissue, which has a shape reminiscent of one-half a doughnut, the collagen fibers are arranged in a circumferential pattern which is additionally reinforced by radially placed fibers. The meniscus can be torn during use, an event which causes pain and disfunction. Currently, the accepted treatments are partial or complete excision of torn tissue. The result of such treatment is often unsatisfactory, since the treated meniscus has an altered shape which is incompatible with normal joint motion and stability. The long-term consequence of such incompatibility is joint degeneration, eventually leading to osteoarthritis.

An effort to induce regeneration of the surgically removed meniscus was based on the use of a type I collagen-chondroitin 6-sulfate copolymer. The precise structural parameters of this matrix have not been reported, so it is not possible to discuss the results of this study in terms of possible similarities and differences with SRT and NRT. The study focused on the canine knee joint, since the latter is particularly sensitive to biomechanical alterations; in this model, joint instabilities rapidly lead to osteoarthritic changes, which can be detected experimentally. Spontaneous regeneration of the canine meniscus following excision is partial and leads to a biomechanically inadequate tissue which does not protect the joint from osteoarthritic changes. The latter condition provides the essential negative control for the study. In this study knee joints were subjected to 80% removal (resection) of the medial meniscus, and the lesion was treated either by an autograft or by an ECM analog or was not treated at all. Evaluation of joint function was performed by studying joint stability, gait, and treadmill performance and was extended up to 27 months. No evidence was presented to show that the structure of the ECM analog was optimized to deliver maximal regeneration.

The results of this study showed that two-thirds of the joints implanted with the ECM analog, two-thirds of the joints which were autografted, and only 25% of the joints which were resected without further treatment showed regeneration of meniscal tissue. These results were interpreted to suggest that the ECM analog, or meniscus regeneration template (MRT), supported significant meniscal regeneration and provided enough biomechanical stability to minimize degenerative osteoarthritis in the canine knee joint.

Defining Terms

Autograft: The patient's own tissue or organ, harvested from an intact area.

Cell lifeline number, S: A dimensionless number that expresses the relative magnitudes of chemical reaction and diffusion. This number, defined as S in Eq. (109.2), can be used to compute the maximum path length l_c over which a cell can migrate in a scaffold while depending on diffusion alone for transport of critical nutrients that it consumes. When the critical length is exceeded, the cell requires transport of nutrients by angiogenesis in order to survive.

Cultured epithelia: A mature, keratinizing epidermis synthesized in vitro by culturing epithelial cells removed from the patient by biopsy. A relatively small skin biopsy (1 cm²) can be treated to yield an area larger by about 10,000 in 2–3 weeks and can then be grafted on patients.

Dermal equivalent: A term which has been loosely used in the literature to describe a device that replaces, usually temporarily, the functions of the dermis following injury.

Dermis: A 1–5 mm layer of connective tissue populated with quiescent fibroblasts which lies underneath the epidermis. It is separated from the former by a very thin basement membrane. The dermis of adult mammals does not regenerate spontaneously following injury.

ECM analog: A model of extracellular matrix, consisting of a highly porous graft copolymer of collagen and a glycosaminoglycan.

Epidermis: The cellular outer layer of skin, about 0.1 mm thick, which protects against moisture loss and against infection. An epidermal graft, e.g., cultured epithelium or a thin graft removed surgically, requires a dermal substrate for adherence onto the wound bed. The epidermis regenerates spontaneously following injury, provided there is a dermal substrate underneath.

Isomorphous tissue replacement: A term used to describe the synthesis of new, physiologic tissue within a regeneration template at a rate of the same order as the degradation rate of the template. This relation, described by Eq. (109.1), is the defining equation for a biodegradable scaffold which couples with, or interacts in this unique manner with, the inflammatory response of the wound bed.

Meniscus regeneration template (MRT):   A graft copolymer of type I collagen and an unspecified glycosaminoglycan, average pore diameter unspecified, which has induced partial regeneration of the knee meniscus in dogs following 80% excision of the meniscal tissue.

Mikic number, *Mi*:   Ratio of the characteristic freezing time of the aqueous medium of the collagen-GAG suspension, t_f, to the characteristic time for entry, t_e, of a container filled with the suspension which is lowered at constant velocity into a well-stirred cooling bath. *Mi*, defined by Eq. (109.5), can be used to design implants which have high alignment of pore channels along a particular axis, or no preferred alignment.

Morphogenesis: The shaping of an organ during embryologic development or during wound healing, according to transcription of genetic information and local environmental conditions.

Nerve regeneration template (NRT):   A graft copolymer of type I collagen and chondroitin 6-sulfate, average pore diameter 5 mm, degrading in vivo to an extent of about 50% in 6 weeks, which has induced partial regeneration of the sciatic nerve of the rat across a 15-mm gap.

Regeneration: The synthesis of new, physiologic tissue at the site of a tissue (one cell type) or organ (more than one cell type) which either has been lost due to injury or has failed due to a chronic condition.

Regeneration template: A biodegradable device which, when attached to a missing organ, induces its regeneration.

Scar: The end result of a repair process in skin and other organs. Scar is morphologically different from skin, in addition to being mechanically less extensible and weaker than skin. The skin regeneration template induces synthesis of nearly physiologic skin rather than scar. Scar is also formed at the site of severe nerve injury.

Self-crosslinking: A procedure for reducing the biodegradation rate of collagen, in which collagen chains are covalently bonded to each other by a condensation reaction which is driven by drastic dehydration of the protein. This reaction, illustrated by Eqs. (109.3*a*) and (109.3*b*), is also used to graft glycosaminoglycan chains to collagen chains without use of an extraneous crosslinking agent.

Skin regeneration template (SRT): A graft copolymer of type I collagen and chondroitin 6-sulfate, average pore diameter 20–125 μm, degrading in vivo to an extent of about 50% in 2 weeks, which induces partial regeneration of the dermis in wounds from which the dermis has been fully excised. When seeded with keratinocytes prior to grafting, this analog of extracellular matrix has induced simultaneous synthesis both of a dermis and an epidermis.

Stereology: The discipline which relates the quantitative statistical properties of three-dimensional structures to those of their two-dimensional sections or projections. In reverse, stereologic procedures allow reconstruction of certain aspects of three-dimensional objects from a quantitative analysis of planar images. Its rules are used to determine features of the pore structure of ECM analogs.

References

Chang AS, Yannas IV. 1992. Peripheral nerve regeneration. In B Smith, G Adelman (eds), Neuroscience Year (Supplement 2 to the Encyclopedia of Neuroscience), pp 125–126, Boston, Birkhäuser.

Hansbrough JF, Boyce ST, Cooper ML, et al. 1989. Burn wound closure with autologous keratinocytes and fibroblasts attached to a collagen-glycosaminoglyacn substrate. JAMA 262:2125.

Hull BE, Sher SS, Rosen S, et al. 1983. Structural integration of skin equivalents grafted to Lewis and Sprague-Dawley rats. J Invest Derm 81:429.

Madison RD, Archibald SJ, Krarup C. 1992. Peripheral nerve injury. In IK Cohen, RF Diegelmann, WJ Lindblad (eds), Wound Healing, pp 450–487, Philadelphia, Saunders.

Stone KR, Rodkey WK, Webber RJ, et al. 1990. Collagen based prostheses for meniscal regeneration. Clin Orth 252:129.

Yannas IV. 1982. Wound tissue can utilize a polymeric template to synthesize a functional extension of skin. Science 215:174.

Yannas IV. 1989. Skin: regeneration templates. In Encyclopedia of Polymer Science and Engineering, vol 15, pp 317–334, New York, Wiley.

Yannas IV, Burke JF. 1980. Design of an artificial skin: I. Basic design principles. J Biomed Mater Res 14:65.

Yannas IV, Lee E, Orgill DP, et al. 1989. Synthesis and characterization of a model extracellular matrix that induces partial regeneration of adult mammalian skin. Proc Natl Acad Sci USA 86:933.

Further Information

Boykin JV Jr, Molnar JA. 1992. Burn scar and skin equivalents. In IK Cohen, RF Diegelmann, WJ Lindblad, (eds), Wound Healing, pp 523–540, Philadelphia, Saunders.

Burke JF, Yannas IV, Quinby WC Jr, et al. 1981. Successful use of a physiologically acceptable artificial skin in the treatment of extensive burn injury. Ann Surg 194:413.

Hansbrough JF, Cooper ML, Cohen R. 1992. Evaluation of a biodegradable matrix containing cultured human fibroblasts as a dermal replacement beneath meshed skin grafts on athymic mice. Surg 111:438.

Hansbrough JF, Morgan JL, Greenleaf GE, et al. 1993. Composite grafts of human keratinocytes grown on a polyglactin mesh-cultured fibroblast dermal substitute function as a bilayer skin replacement in full-thickness wounds on athymic mice. J Burn Care Rehab 14:485.

Heimbach D, Luterman A, Burke J, et al. 1988. Artificial dermis for major burns. Ann Surg 208:313.

Rodkey WG, Stone KR, Steadman JR. 1992. Prosthetic meniscal replacement. In GAM Finerman, FR Noyes (eds), Biology and Biomechanics of the Traumatized Synovial Joint: The Knee as a Model pp 221–231, Amer Acad Orth Surg, Chicago, IL.

Yannas IV. 1988. Regeneration of skin and nerves by use of collagen templates. In ME Nimni (ed), Collagen, vol 3, pp 87–115, Boca Raton, CRC Press.

Yannas IV. 1990. Biologically active analogues of the extracellular matrix: Artificial skin and nerve. Angew Chemie Int Ed Engl 29:20.

Yannas IV, Burke JF, Gordon PL, et al. 1977. Multilayer membrane useful as synthetic skin. US Patent 4,060,081.

Yannas IV, Burke JF, Orgill DP, et al. 1982. Regeneration of skin following closure of deep wounds with a biodegradable template. Trans Soc Biomat 5:1.

Yannas IV, Burke JF, Warpehoski M, et al. 1981. Prompt, long-term functional replacement of skin. Trans Am Soc Artif Intern Organs 27:19.

110

Fluid Shear Stress Effects on Cellular Function

Charles W. Patrick, Jr.
Rice University

Rangarajan Sampath
Rice University

Larry V. McIntire
Rice University

Cells of the vascular system are constantly exposed to mechanical (hemodynamic) forces due to the flow of blood. The forces generated in the vasculature include the frictional force or a fluid shear stress caused by blood flowing tangentially across the endothelium, a tensile stress caused by circumferential vessel wall deformations, and a net normal stress caused by a hydrodynamic pressure differential across the vessel wall. We will restrict our discussion to examining fluid shear stress modulation of vascular cell function. The endothelium is a biologically active monolayer of cells providing an interface between the flowing blood and tissues of the body. It can synthesize and secrete a myriad of vasoconstrictors, vasodilators, growth factors, fibrinolytic factors, cytokines, adhesion molecules, matrix proteins, and mitogens that modulate many physiologic processes, including wound healing, hemostasis, vascular remodeling, vascular tone, and immune and inflammatory responses. In addition to humoral stimuli, it is now well accepted that endothelial cell synthesis and secretion of bioactive molecules can be regulated by the hemodynamic forces generated by the local blood flow. These forces have been hypothesized to regulate neovascularization and the structure of the blood vessel [Hudlicka, 1984]. Clinical findings further show that arterial walls undergo an endothelium-dependent adaptive response to changes in blood flow, with blood vessels in high flow regions tending to enlarge and vessels in the low flow region having reduced lumen diameter, thereby maintaining a nearly constant shear stress at the vessel wall [Zarins et al., 1987]. In addition to playing an active role in the normal vascular biology, hemodynamic forces have also been implicated in the pathogenesis of a variety of vascular diseases. Atheroslerotic lesion-prone regions, characterized by the incorporation of Evans blue dye, enhanced accumulation of albumin, fibrinogen, and LDL, increased recruitment of monocytes, and increased endothelial turnover rates exhibit polygonal endothelial cell morphology typically seen in a low-shear environment, as opposed to nonlesion regions that have elongated endothelial cells characteristic of high-shear regions [Nerem, 1993].

0-8493-8346-3/95/$0.00+$.50
© 1995 by CRC Press, Inc.

In vivo studies of the distribution of atherosclerosis and the degree of intimal thickening have shown preferential plaque localization in low-shear regions. Atherosclerotic lesions were not seen in random locations but were instead found to be localized to regions of arterial branching and sharp curvature, where complex flow patterns develop, as shown in Fig. 110.1 [Asakura & Karino, 1990; Friedman et al., 1981; Gibson et al., 1993; Glagov et al., 1988; Ku et al., 1985; Levesque et al., 1989; Zarins et al., 1983]. Morphologically, intact endothelium over plaque surfaces showed variation in shape and size and loss of normal orientation, characteristic of low-shear conditions [Davies et al., 1988]. Flow in the vascular system is by and large laminar, but extremely complex time dependent flow patterns can develop in localized regions of complex geometry. Zarins and coworkers [1983] have shown that in the human carotid bifurcation, regions of moderate-to-high shear stress where flow remains unidirectional and axially aligned, were relatively free of intimal thickening, whereas extensive plaque localization was seen in the regions where low shear stress, fluid separation from the wall, and complex flow patterns were predominant. Asakura and Karino [1990] presented a technique for flow visualization by using transparent arteries where they directly correlated flow patterns to regions of plaque formation in human coronary arteries. They observed that the flow divider at the bifurcation point, a region of high shear stress, was relatively devoid of plaque deposition, whereas the outer wall, a region of low shear stress, showed extensive plaque formation. Similar patterns were also seen in curved vessels, where the inner wall or the hip region of the curve, a region of low shear and flow separation, exhibited plaque formation. In addition to the direct shear-stress-mediated effects, the regions of complex flow patterns and recirculation also tend to increase the residence time of circulating blood cells in susceptible regions, whereas the blood cells are rapidly cleared away from regions of high wall shear and unidirectional flow [Glagov et al., 1988]. This increased transit time could influence plaque deposition by favoring margination of monocytes and platelets, release of vasoactive agents, or altered permeability at the intercellular junctions to extracellular lipid particles and possible concentration of procoagulant materials [Nollert et al., 1991].

The endothelium forming the interface between blood and the surrounding tissues is believed to act as a sensor of the local hemodynamic environment in mediating both the normal response and

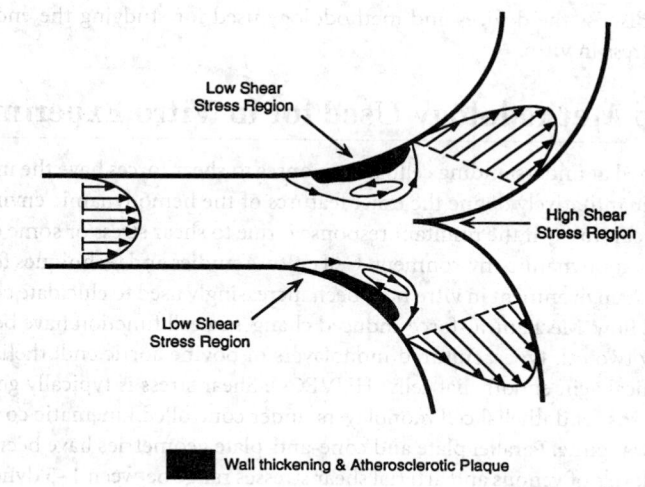

FIGURE 110.1 Atherosclerotic plaques develop in regions of arteries where the flow rate (and resultant wall shear stress) is relatively low, which is often downstream from a vessel bifurcation, where there can be flow separation from the outer walls and regions of recirculation. These regions of low shear stress are pathologically prone to vessel wall thickening and thrombosis.

the pattern of vascular diseases. In vivo studies have shown changes in the actin microfilament localization in a shear-dependent manner. Actin stress fibres have been observed to be aligned with the direction of flow in high-shear regions, whereas they were mostly present in dense peripheral bands in the low-shear regions [Kim et al., 1989]. Langille and Adamson [1981] showed that the cells in large arteries, away from branches, were aligned parallel to the long axes of the artery in rabbit and mouse. Similar results were shown in coronary arteries of patients undergoing cardiac transplantation [Davies et al., 1988]. Near the branch points of large arteries, however, cells aligned along the flow streamlines. In smaller blood vessels, where secondary flow patterns did not develop, the cell alignment followed the geometry of the blood vessel. In fact, endothelial cell morphology and orientation at the branch may be a natural marker of the detailed features of blood flow [Nerem et al., 1981].

Another cell type that is likely to be affected by hemodynamic forces is the vascular smooth muscle cell (SMC) present in the media. In the early stages of lesion development, SMCs proliferate and migrate into the intima [Ross, 1993; Schwartz et al., 1993]. Since the endothelium is intact in all but the final stages of atherosclerosis, SMCs are unlikely to be directly affected by shear stress. Most of the direct force they experience come from the cyclical stretch forces experienced by the vessel itself due to pressure pulses [Grande et al., 1989]. Shear forces acting on the endothelium, however, can release compounds such as endothelin, nitric oxide, and platelet-derived growth factors that act as SMC mitogens and can modulate SMC tone. Ono and colleagues [1991] showed that homogenate of shear-stressed endothelial cells contained increased amounts of collagen and stimulated SMC migration in vitro, compared to endothelial cells grown under static condition. The local shear environment could thus act directly or indirectly on the cells of the vascular wall in mediating a physiologic response.

This chapter presents what is currently known regarding how the mechanical agonist of shear stress modulates endothelial cell function in the context of vascular physiology and pathophysiology. In discussing this topic we have adopted an outside-in approach. That is, we first discuss how shear stress affects endothelial cell-blood cell interactions, then progress to how shear stress affects the endothelial cell cytoskeleton, signal transduction, and protein secretion, and finally end with how shear stress modulates endothelial cell gene expression. We close with gene therapy and tissue engineering considerations related to how endothelial cells respond to shear stress. Before proceeding, however, we discuss the devices and methodology used for studying the endothelial cell responses to shear stress in vitro.

110.1 Devices and Methodology Used for in Vitro Experiments

In vivo studies aimed at understanding cellular responses to shear forces have the inherent problem that they cannot quantitatively define the exact features of the hemodynamic environment. Moreover, it is very difficult to say if the resultant response is due to shear stress or some other feature associated with the hemodynamic environment. Cell culture studies and techniques for exposing cells to a controlled shear environment in vitro have been increasingly used to elucidate cellular responses to shear stress and flow. Mechanical-force-induced changes in cell function have been measured in vitro using mainly two cell types, cultured monolayers of bovine aortic endothelial cells (BAECs) and human umbilical vein endothelial cells (HUVECs). Shear stress is typically generated in vitro by flowing fluid across endothelial cell monolayers under controlled kinematic conditions, usually in the laminar flow regime. Parallel plate and cone-and-plate geometries have been the most common. Physiologic levels of venous and arterial shear stresses range between 1–5 dynes/cm^2 and 6–40 dynes/cm^2, respectively.

The use of the parallel plate flow chamber allows one to have a controlled and well-defined flow environment based on the chamber geometry (fixed) and the flow rate through the chamber (variable). In addition, individual cells can be visualized in real time using video microscopy. Assuming parallel plate geometry and Newtonian fluid behavior, the wall shear stress on the cell monolayer in the flow chamber is calculated as

$$\tau_w = \frac{6Q\mu}{(bh^2)} \qquad (110.1)$$

where Q is the volumetric flow rate, μ is the viscosity of the flowing fluid, h is the channel height, b is the channel width, and τ_w is the wall shear stress. The flow chambers are designed such that the entrance length is very small compared to the effective length of the chamber [Frangos et al., 1985]. Therefore, entry effects can be neglected, and the flow is fully developed and parabolic over nearly the entire length of the flow chamber. Flow chambers usually consist of a machined block, a gasket whose thickness determines in part the channel depth, and a glass coverslip to which is attached a monolayer of endothelial cells (Fig. 110.2a). The individual components are held together either by a vacuum, or by evenly torqued screws, thereby ensuring a uniform channel depth. The flow chamber can have a myriad of entry ports, bubble ports, and exit ports. For short-term experiments, media are drawn through the chamber over the monolayer of cells using a syringe pump. For long-term experiments, the chamber is placed in a flow loop. In a flow loop (Fig. 110.2b), cells grown to confluence on glass slides can be exposed to a well-defined shear stress by recirculation of culture medium driven by gravity [Frangos et al., 1985]. Culture medium from the lower reservoir is pumped to the upper reservoir at a constant flow rate such that there is an overflow of excess medium back into the lower reservoir. This overflow serves two purposes: (1) It maintains a constant hydrostatic head between the two reservoirs, and (2) it prevents entry of air bubbles into the primary flow section upstream of the flow chamber that could be detrimental to the cells. The pH of the medium is maintained at physiologic levels by gassing with a humidified mixture of 95% air and 5% CO_2. The rate of flow in the line supplying the chamber is determined solely by gravity and can be altered by changing the vertical separation between the two reservoirs. A sample port in the bottom reservoir allows periodic sampling of the flowing medium for a time-dependent assay.

As mentioned above, cone-and-plate geometries can also be utilized. A schematic of a typical cone-and-plate viscometer is shown in Fig. 110.2c. Shear stress is produced in the fluid contained between the rotating cone and the stationary plate. Cells grown on coverslips can be placed in the shear field (up to 12 at a time). For relatively small cone angles and low rates of rotation, the shear stress throughout the system is independent of position. The cone angle compensates for radial effects seen in plate-and-plate rheometers. The wall shear stress (τ_w) on the cell monolayer in the cone-and-plate viscometer is calculated as

$$\tau_w = \frac{3\,T}{2\pi R^3} \qquad (110.2)$$

where T is the applied torque and R is the cone radius. The flow becomes turbulent, however, at the plate's edge and at high rotational speeds. Modifications from the basic design have allowed use of an optical system with the rheometer, enabling direct microscopic examination and real-time analysis of the cultured cells during exposure to shear stress [Dewey et al., 1981; Schnittler et al., 1993]. For a more complete description of in vitro device design and applications, refer to the text edited by Frangos [Tran-son-Tay, 1993].

110.2 Shear Stress-Mediated Cell-Endothelium Interactions

Cell-cell and cell-substrate interactions in the vascular system are of importance in a number of physiologic and pathologic situations. Lymphocytes, platelets, or tumor cells in circulation may arrest at a particular site as a result of interaction with the endothelium or the subendothelial matrix. While the margination of leukocyte/lymphocyte to the vessel wall may be a normal physiologic response to injury or inflammation, adhesion of blood platelets to the subendothelium and subsequent platelet aggregation could result in a partial or complete occlusion of the blood vessel lead-

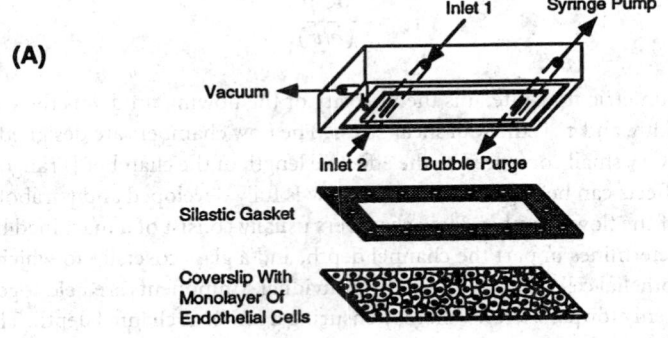

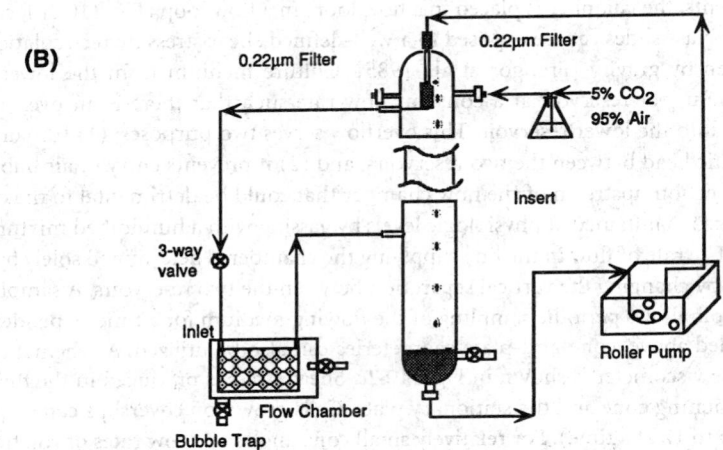

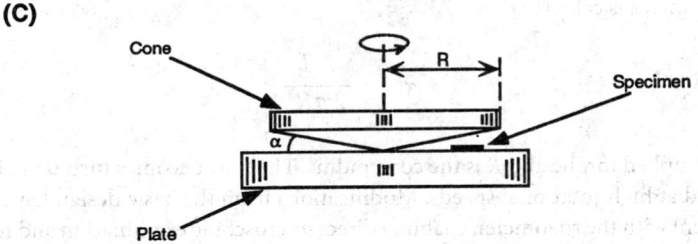

FIGURE 110.2 Devices used for in vitro study of shear stress effects on vascular endothelial cells. (*a*) Parallel plate flow chamber, (*b*) flow loop, (*c*) cone-and-plate viscometer.

ing to thrombosis or stroke. In addition, the adhesion of tumor cells to the endothelium is often the initial step in the development of secondary metastases. The adhesion of leukocytes, platelets, and tumor cells is not only mediated by adhesion molecules on the endothelium but also mediated by the hemodynamic force environment present in the vasculature. In fact, the specific molecular mechanisms employed for adhesion often vary with the local wall shear stress [Alevriadou et al., 1993; Lawrence et al., 1990].

Targeting of circulating leukocytes to particular regions of the body is an aspect of immune system function that is currently of great research interest. This targeting process consists of adhesion of a specific subpopulation of circulating leukocytes to a specific area of vascular endothelium via cell surface adhesion receptors. The large number of receptors involved and the differential regulation of their expression on particular cell subpopulations make this process very versatile but also quite complicated. An extremely important additional complication arises from the fact that these interactions occur within the flowing bloodstream. Study of these various types of adhesive interactions requires accurate recreation of the flow conditions experienced by leukocytes and endothelial cells. Lawrence and coworkers examined neutrophil adhesion to cytokine-stimulated endothelial cells under well-defined postcapillary venular flow conditions in vitro [Lawrence et al., 1987, Lawrence, et al, 1990; Lawrence & Springer, 1991]. They also demonstrated that under flow conditions neutrophil adhesion to cytokine-stimulated endothelial cells is mediated almost exclusively by CD18-independent mechanisms but that subsequent neutrophil migration is CD18-dependent [Lawrence & Springer, 1991; Smith et al., 1991]. The initial flow studies were followed by many further studies both in vitro [Abbassi et al., 1991, 1993; Anderson et al., 1991; Hakkert et al., 1991; Jones et al., 1993; Kishimoto et al., 1991] and in vivo [Ley et al., 1991; Perry & Granger, 1991; von Andrian et al., 1991; Watson et al., 1991] which clearly distinguish separate mechanisms for initial adhesion/rolling and firm adhesion/leukocyte migration. Research has further shown that in a variety of systems, selectin/carbohydrate interactions are primarily responsible for initial adhesion and rolling, and firm adhesion and leukocyte migration are mediated primarily by integrin/peptide interactions. Methodology discussed for studying receptor specificity of adhesion for leukocytes under flow can also be utilized for studying red cell–endothelial cell interactions [Barabino et al., 1987; Wick et al., 1987, 1993].

The interaction of tumor cells with endothelial cells is an important step in tumor metastasis. To adhere to the vessel wall, tumor cells that come into contact with the microvasculature must resist the tractive force of shear stress that tends to detach them from the vessel wall [Weiss, 1992]. Hence, studies of the mechanisms involved in the process of tumor metastasis must take into account the physical forces acting on the tumor cells. Bastida and coworkers [1989] have demonstrated that tumor cell adhesion depends not only on tumor cell characteristics and endothelial cell adhesion molecule expression but on shear stress in the interaction of circulating tumor cells with the endothelium. The influence of shear stress on tumor cell adhesion suggests that attachment of tumor cells to vascular structures occurs in areas of high shear stress, such as the microvasculature [Bastida et al., 1989]. This is supported by earlier pathologic observations that indicate preferential attachment of tumor cells on the lung and liver capillary system [Warren, 1973]. Some tumor cell types roll and subsequently adhere on endothelial cells using selectin-mediated mechanisms similar to leukocytes, whereas others adhere without rolling using integrin-mediated receptors on endothelial cells [Bastida et al., 1989; Giavazzi et al., 1993; Kojima et al., 1992; Menter et al., 1992; Patton et al., 1993; Pili et al., 1993]. It has been postulated that some tumor cell types undergo a stabilization process prior to firm adhesion that is mediated by transglutaminase crosslinking [Menter et al., 1992; Patton et al., 1993]. Recently, Pili and colleagues [1993] demonstrated that tumor cell contact with endothelial cells increases Ca^{2+} release from endothelial cell intracellular stores, which may have a fundamental role in enhancing cell-cell adhesion. The factors and molecular mechanisms underlying tumor cell and endothelial cell interactions remain largely undefined and are certain to be further explored in the future.

The endothelium provides a natural nonthrombogenic barrier between circulating platelets and the endothelial basement membrane. However, there are pathologic instances in which the endothelium integrity is compromised, exposing a thrombogenic surface. Arterial thrombosis is the leading cause of death in the United States. Among the most likely possibilities for the initiation of arterial platelet thrombi are: (1) adhesion of blood platelets onto the subendothelium of injured arteries and arterioles or on ruptured atherosclerotic plaque surfaces, containing collagen and other matrix proteins, with subsequent platelet aggregation, or (2) shear-induced aggregation of platelets in areas of the arterial circulation partially constricted by atherosclerosis or vasospasm. Various experimental models have been developed to investigate the molecular mechanisms of platelet attachment to surfaces (adhesion) and platelet cohesion to each other (aggregation) under shear stress conditions. Whole-blood perfusion studies using annular or parallel-plate perfusion chambers simulate the first proposed mechanism of arterial thrombus formation in vivo, that may occur as a result of adhesion on an injured, exposed subendothelial or atherosclerotic plaque surface [Hubbel & McIntire, 1986; Weiss et al., 1978, 1986]. Platelets arriving subsequently could, under the right conditions, adhere to each other, forming aggregates large enough to partially or completely occlude the blood vessel. In vitro studies have shown an increase in thrombus growth with local shear rate, an event that is believed to be the result of enhanced arrival and cohesion of platelets near the surface at higher wall shear stresses [Turitto et al., 1987]. Video microscopy provides information on the morphologic characteristics of thrombi and enables the reconstruction of three-dimensional models of thrombi formed on surfaces coated with biomaterials or endothelial cell basement membrane proteins. Macroscopic analysis of thrombi can provide information on platelet mass transport and reaction kinetics with the surface, and microscopic analysis allows dynamic real-time study of cell-surface and intercellular interactions. Such a technology enables the study of key proteins involved in mural thrombus formation, such as vWF [Alevriadou et al., 1993; Folie & McIntire, 1989]. In addition, tests of antithrombotic agents and investigation of the thrombogenicity of various purified components of the vessel wall or polymeric biomaterials can be performed.

110.3 Shear Stress Effects on Cell Morphology and Cytoskeletal Rearrangement

In addition to mediating cell–endothelial cell interactions, shear stress can act directly on the endothelium. It has been demonstrated for almost a decade that hemodynamic forces can modulate endothelial cell morphology and structure [Barbee et al., 1994; Coan et al., 1993; Eskin et al., 1984; Franke et al., 1984; Girard & Nerem, 1991, 1993; Ives et al., 1986; Langille et al., 1991; Levesque et al., 1989; Wechezak et al., 1985]. Conceivably, the cytoskeletal reorganization that occurs in endothelial cells several hours after exposure to flow may, in conjunction with shape change, transduce mechanical signals to cytosolic and nuclear signals (mechanotransduction), thereby playing a role in gene expression and signal transduction [Ingber, 1993; Resnick et al., 1993; Watson, 1991]. In fact, investigators have shown specific gene expression related to cytoskeletal changes [Botteri et al., 1990; Breathnach et al., 1987; Ferrua et al., 1990; Werb et al., 1986]. F-actin has been implicated as the principal transmission element in the cytoskeleton and appears to be required for signal transduction [Watson, 1991]. Actin filaments are anchored in the plasma membrane at several sites, including focal adhesions on the basal membrane, intercellular adhesion proteins, integral membrane proteins at the apical surface, and the nuclear membrane [Davies & Tripathi, 1993]. Substantiating this, Barbee and coworkers [1994] have recently shown, utilizing atomic force microscopy, that F-actin fiber stress bundles are formed in the presence of fluid flow and the fibers are coupled to the apical membrane. Moreover, endothelial cell shape change and realignment with flow can be inhibited by drugs that interfere with microfilament turnover [Davies & Tripathi, 1993]. Although all evidence leads one to believe that the endothelial cell cytoskeleton can respond to flow and that F-actin is involved, the exact mechanism involved remains to be elucidated.

110.4 Shear Stress Effects on Signal Transduction and Mass Transfer

Shear stress and resultant convective mass transfer are known to affect many important cytosolic second messengers in endothelial cells. For instance, shear stress is known to cause ATP-mediated increases in calcium ions (Ca^{2+}) [Ando et al., 1988; Dull & Davies, 1991; Mo et al., 1991; Nollert & McIntire, 1992]. Changes in flow influence the endothelial boundary layer concentration of ATP by altering the convective transport of exogenous ATP, thereby altering ATP's interaction with both the

P_{2y}-purinoreceptor and ecto-ATPase. At low levels of shear stress, degradation of ATP by ecto-ATPase exceeds the rate of diffusion, and the steady state concentration of ATP remains low. In contrast, at high levels of shear stress, convection enhances the delivery of ATP from upstream to the P_{2y}-purinoreceptor, and diffusion exceeds the rate of degradation by the ecto-ATPase [Mo et al., 1991]. Whether physiologic levels of shear stress can directly increase intracellular calcium remains unclear. Preceding the calcium increases are increases in inositol-1,4,5 trisphosphate (IP_3) [Bhagyalakshmi et al., 1992; Bhagyalakshmi & Frangos, 1989b; Nollert et al., 1990; Prasad et al., 1993], which binds to specific sites on the endoplasmic reticulum and causes release of Ca^{2+} from intracellular stores, and diacylglycerol (DAG) [Bhagyalakshmi & Frangos, 1989a]. Elevated levels of both DAG and Ca^{2+} can activate several protein kinases, including protein kinase C (PKC). Changes in Ca^{2+}, IP_3, and DAG are evidence that fluid shear stress activates the PKC pathway. In fact, the PKC pathway has been demonstrated to be activated by shear stress [Bhagyalakshmi & Frangos, 1989b; Hsieh et al., 1992, 1993; Kuchan & Frangos, 1993; Milner et al., 1992]. In addition to the PKC pathway, pathways involving cyclic adenosine monophosphate (cAMP) and cyclic guanosine monophosphate (cGMP) may also be modulated by shear stress, as evidenced by increases in cAMP [Bhagyalakshmi & Frangos, 1989b] and cGMP [Kuchan & Frangos, 1993; Ohno et al., 1993] with shear stress. Moreover, it has been shown recently that shear stress causes acidification of cytoslic pH [Ziegelstein et al., 1992]. Intracellular acidification of vascular endothelial cells releases Ca^{2+} into the cytosol [Ziegelstein et al., 1993]. This Ca^{2+} mobilization may be linked to endothelial synthesis and release of vasodilatory substances during the pathological condition of acidosis.

10.5 Shear Stress Effects on Endothelial Cell Metabolite Secretion

The application of shear stress in vitro is accompanied by alterations in protein synthesis that are detectable within several hours after initiation of the mechanical agonist. Shear stress may regulate the expression of fibrinolytic proteins by endothelial cells; tPA is an antithrombotic glycoprotein and serine protease that is released from endothelial cells. Once released, it rapidly converts plasminogen to plasmin which, in turn, dissolves fibrin clots. Diamond and coworkers [1989] have shown that venous levels of shear stress do not affect tPA secretion, whereas arterial levels increase the secretion rate of tPA. Arterial flows lead to a profibrinolytic state that would be beneficial in maintaining a clot-free artery. In contrast to tPA, neither venous nor arterial levels of shear stress cause significant changes in plasminogen activator inhibitor-1 (PAI-1) secretion rates [Diamond et al., 1989; Kuchan & Frangos, 1993]. Increased proliferation of smooth muscle cells is one of the early events of arteriosclerosis. The secretion rate of endothelin-1 (ET-1), a potent smooth muscle cell mitogen, has been shown to increase in response to venous levels of shear stress and decrease in response to arterial levels of shear stress [Kuchan & Frangos, 1993; Milner et al., 1992; Nollert et al., 1991; Sharefkin et al., 1991; Yoshizumi et al., 1989]. Both the in vitro tPA and ET-1 results are consistent with in vivo observations that atherosclerotic plaque development occurs in low shear stress regions as opposed to high shear stress regions. The low shear stress regions usually occur downstream from vessel branches. In these regions we would expect low secretion of tPA and high secretion of ET-1, leading to locally increased smooth muscle cell proliferation (intimal thickening of the vessel) and periodic problems with clot formation (thrombosis). Both of these observations are observed pathologically and are important processes in atherogenesis [McIntire, 1994].

Important metabolites in the arachidonic acid cascade via the cyclooxygenase pathway; prostacylin (PGI_2) and prostaglandin (PGF_{2a}) are also known to increase their secretion rates in response to arterial levels of shear stress [Frangos et al., 1985; Grabowski et al., 1985; Nollert et al., 1989]. In addition, endothelial cells have been shown to increase their production of fibronectin (FN) in response to shear stress [Gupte & Frangos, 1990]. Endothelial cells may respond to shear stress by secreting FN in order to increase their attachment to the extracellular matrix, thereby resisting the applied fluid shear stress. Endothelial cells have been shown to modulate their receptor expression of intercellular adhesion molecule-1 (ICAM-1), vascular cell adhesion molecule-1 (VCAM-1), and monocyte chemotactic peptide-1 (MCP-1) in response to shear stress [Sampath et al., 1995; Shyy et al., 1994]. The adaptive expression of these adhesion molecules in response to hemodynamic shear stresses may aid in modulating specific adhesion localities for neutrophils, leukocytes, and monocytes.

110.6 Shear Stress Effects on Gene Regulation

In many cases, the alterations in protein sythesis observed with shear stress are preceded by modulation of protein gene expression. The molecular mechanisms by which mechanical agonists alter the gene expression of proteins are under current investigation. Diamond and colleagues [1990] and Nollert and colleagues [1992] have demonstrated that arterial levels of shear stress upregulate the transcription of tPA mRNA, concomitant with tPA protein secretion. The gene expressions of ET-1 and PDGF, both of which are potent smooth muscle cell mitogens and vasoconstrictors, are also known to be modulated by hemodynamic forces. For instance, arterial levels of shear stress cause ET-1 mRNA to be downregulated [Malek et al., 1993; Malek & Izumo, 1992; Sharefkin et al., 1991]. ET-1 mRNA downregulation is sensitive to the magnitude of the shear stress in a dose-dependent fashion, reaching a saturation at 15 dynes/cm². Conversely, Yoshizumi and coworkers [1989] have shown that venous levels of shear stress cause a transient increase in ET-1 mRNA, peaking at 4 hours and returning to basal levels by 12–24 hours. However, they had previously reported downregulation of ET-1 mRNA expression [Yanagisawa et al., 1988]. PDGF is expressed as a dimer composed of PDGF-A and PDGF-B subunits. There are conflicting reports as to how arterial shear stresses affect PDGF-B mRNA expression. Malek and colleagues [1993] have shown that arterial levels of shear stress applied to BAECs cause a significant decrease in PDGF-B mRNA expression over a 9-hr period. In contrast, Mitsumata and coworkers [1993] and Resnick and coworkers [1993] have shown increases in BAEC mRNA expression of PDGF-B when arterial shear stresses were applied. The discrepancy in the results may be attributed to differences in BAEC cell line origins or differences in the passage number of cells used. In support of the latter two investigators, Hsieh and colleagues [1992] have reported upregulation of PDGF-B mRNA in HUVECs in the presence of arterial shear stress. As with the B chain of PDGF, there are conflicting reports as to the affect of arterial shear stress on PDGF-A. Mitsumata and coworkers [1993] have reported no change in PDGF-A mRNA expression, whereas Hsieh and coworkers [1991, 1992] have reported a shear-dependent increase in the mRNA expression from 0–6 dynes/cm² which then plateaus from 6–51 dynes/cm². Endothelial cell expression of ET-1 and PDGF may be important in blood vessel remodeling. In blood vessels exposed to increased flow, the chronic vasculature response is an increase in vessel diameter [Langille & O'Donnell, 1986]. Hence, it is tempting to postulate that hemodynamic-force-modulated alterations in ET-1 and PDGF mRNA expression may account for much of this adaptive change.

The gene expression of various adhesion molecules involved in leukocyte recruitment during inflammation and disease has also been investigated. ICAM-1 mRNA has been shown to be transiently upregulated in the presence of venous or arterial shear stresses [Nagel et al., 1994; Sampath et al., 1995]. Its time-dependent response peaked at 1–3 hr following exposure to shear, before declining below basal levels with prolonged exposure of 6–24 hr. In contrast, VCAM-1 mRNA level was downregulated almost immediately upon onset of flow and was found to drop significantly below basal levels within 6 hr of initiation of flow at all magnitudes of shear stresses. E-selectin mRNA expression appeared to be generally less responsive to shear stress, especially at the lower magnitudes. After an initial downward trend 1 hr following exposure to shear stress (2 dynes/cm²), E-selectin mRNA remained at stable levels for up to 6 hr [Sampath et al., 1995]. Recent evidence shows that the expression of MCP-1, a monocyte-specific chemoattractant expressed on endothelial cells, also follows a similar biphasic response with shear stress like ICAM-1 [Shyy et al., 1994]. In addition to adhesion molecules, the gene expression of several growth factors has been investigated. The mRNA expression of heparin-binding epidermal growth factor like growth factor (HB-EGF), a smooth muscle-cell mitogen, transiently increases in the presence of minimal arterial shear stress [Morita et al.,

1993]. Transforming growth factor-β1 (TGF-β1) mRNA has been reported to be upregulated in the presence of arterial shear stresses within 2 hr and remain elevated for 12 hr [Ohno et al., 1992]. In addition, Malek and coworkers [1993] have shown that basic fibroblast growth factor (bFGF) mRNA is upregulated in BAECs in the presence of arterial shear stresses. In HUVECs, however, no significant changes in bFGF message were observed [Diamond et al., 1990]. This difference is probably due to differences in cell source (human versus bovine).

Proto-oncogenes code for binding proteins that either enhance or repress transcription and, therefore, are ideal candidates to act as gene regulators [Cooper, 1990]. Komuro and colleagues [1990, 1991] were the first to demonstrate that mechanical loading causes upregulation of c-*fos* expression. Recently, Hsieh and coworkers [1993] investigated the role of arterial shear stress on the mRNA levels of nuclear proto-oncogenes c-*fos*, c-*jun*, and c-*myc*. Gene expression of c-*fos* was transiently upregulated, peaking at 0.5 hr and returning to basal levels within an hour. In contrast, both c-*jun* and c-*myc* mRNA were upregulated to sustainable levels within an hour. The transcribed protein products of c-*fos*, c-*jun*, and c-*myc* may act as nuclear-signaling molecules for mechanically induced gene modulation [Nollert et al., 1992; Ranjan & Diamond, 1993].

110.7 Mechanisms of Shear Stress-Induced Gene Regulation

Although no unified scheme to explain mechanical signal transduction and modulation of gene expression is yet possible, many studies provide insight in an attempt to elucidate which second messengers are involved in gene regulation mediated by hemodynamic forces. There is substantial evidence that the PKC pathway may be involved in the gene regulation. A model of the PKC transduction pathway is shown in Fig. 110.3. Mitsumata and colleagues [1993] have shown that PDGF mRNA modulation by shear stress could be partially attributed to a PKC pathway. Hsieh and coworkers [1992] have shown that shear-induced PDGF gene expression in HUVECs is mainly mediated by PKC activation and requires Ca^{2+} and the involvement of G proteins. In addition, they demonstrated that cAMP and cGMP dependent protein kinases are not involved in PDGF gene expression. Morita and colleagues [1993] have shown that shear-induced HB-EGF mRNA expression is mediated through a PKC pathway and that Ca^{2+} may be involved in the pathway [Morita et al., 1993]. PKC was also found to be an important mediator in flow-induced c-*fos* expression, with the additional involvement of G proteins, phospholipase C (PLC), and Ca^{2+} [Hsieh et al., 1993]. Moreover, Levin and coworkers [1988] have shown that tPA gene expression is enhanced by PKC activation and Iba and coworkers [1992] have shown that cAMP is not involved in tPA gene expression . As depicted in Fig. 110.3, the PKC pathway may be involved in activating DNA-binding proteins via phosphorylation.

In addition to second messengers, it has been proposed that cytoskeletal reorganization may play a role in regulating gene expression [Ingber, 1993; Resnick et al., 1993]. Morita and colleagues [1993] have shown that shear stress-induced ET-1 gene expression is mediated by the disruption of the actin cytoskeleton and that microtubule integrity is also involved. Gene expression of other bioactive molecules may also be regulated by actin disruption. The actual molecular mechanisms involved in cytoskeletal-mediated gene expression remain unclear. However, the cytoskeleton may activate membrane ion channels and nuclear pores.

In addition to second messengers and the cytoskeletal architecture, it has been postulated by Nollert and others [1992] that transcriptional factors that bind to the DNA may play an active role mediating the signal transduction between the cytosol and nucleus (Fig. 110.4) It is known that nuclear translocation of transcriptional factors and DNA-binding activity of the factors can be mediated by phosphorylation [Bohmann, 1990; Hunter & Karin, 1992]. Many of the transcription factors are protein products of proto-oncogenes. It has previously been stated that shear stress increases expression of c-*fos* and c-*jun*. The gene products of c-*fos* and c-*jun* form protein dimers that bind to transcriptional sites on DNA promoters and act as either transcriptional activators or repressors.

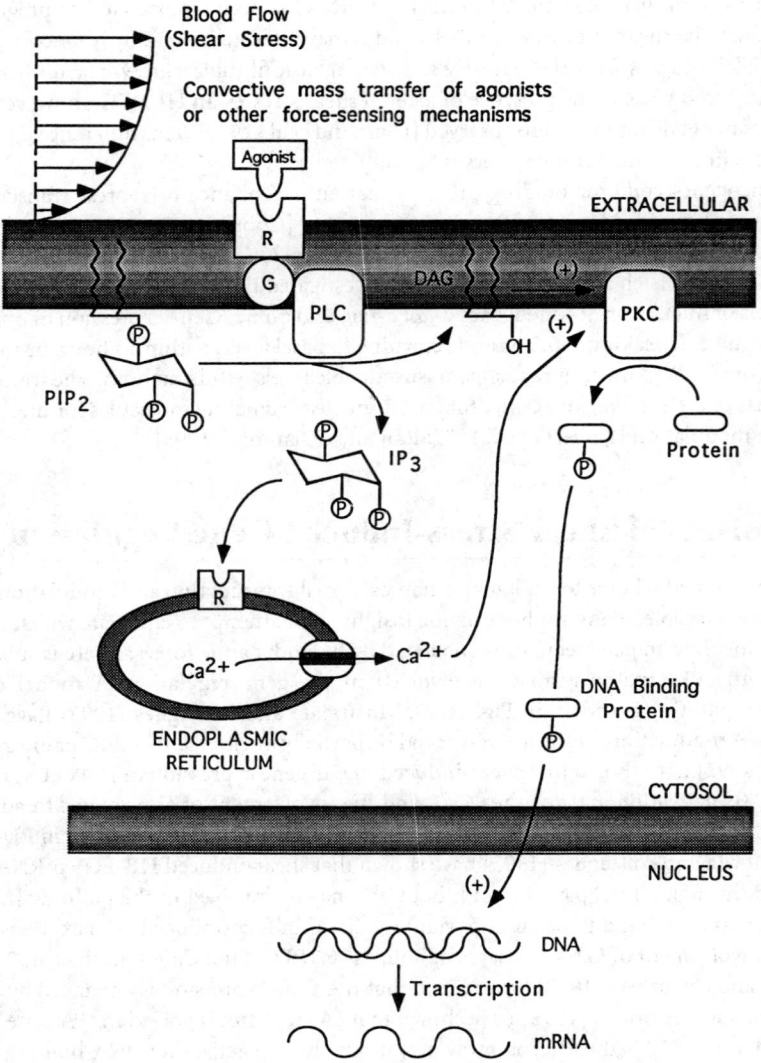

FIGURE 110.3   Model for shear stress induced protein kinase C (PKC) activation leading to modulation of gene expression. Mechanical agonists enhance membrane phosphoinositide turnover via phospholipase C (PLC), producing inositol-1,4,5 trisphosphate (IP_3), and diacylglycerol (DAG). DAG can then activate PKC. IP_3 may also activate PKC via Ca^{2+} release. PKC phosphorylates DNA-binding proteins, thereby making them active. The nuclear binding proteins then alter mRNA transcription. R = receptor, G = G protein, PIP_2 = phosphatidylinositol 4,5-bisphosphate, (+) = activation.

Two of the transcriptional sites to which the *fos* and *jun* family dimers bind are the TRE (tumor promoting agent response element) and CRE (cAMP response element). These have consensus sequences of TGACTCA and TGACGTCA, respectively. It is known that the promoter regions of tPA, PAI-1, ET, and TGF-β1 possess sequences of homology to the CRE and TRE [Nollert et al., 1992]. In addition to mediating known transcription factor binding in perhaps novel ways, mechanical perturbations may initiate molecular signaling through specific stress- or strain-sensitive promoters that can activate gene expression. In fact, Resnick and colleagues [1993] have described a cis-acting shear stress response element (SSRE) in the PDGF-B promoter, and this sequence is also found in the promoters of tPA, ICAM-1, TGF-β1, c-*fos*, and c-*jun* but not in VCAM-1 or E-Selectin pro-

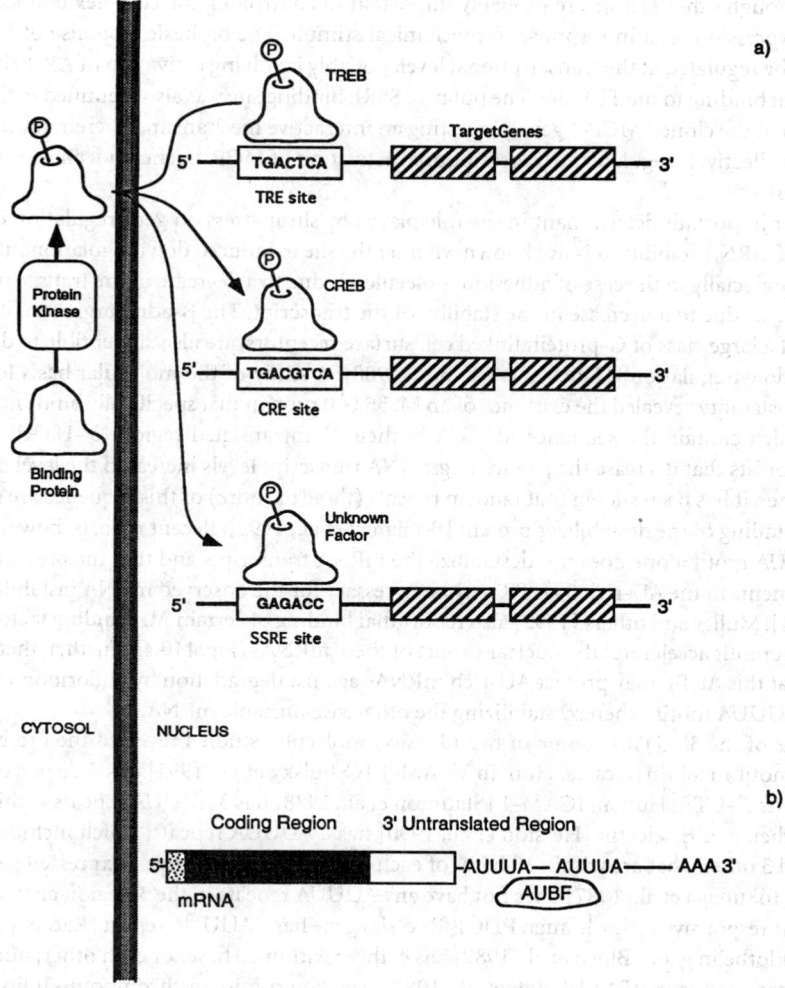

FIGURE 110.4 Gene expression regulated by transcription/translation factors and mechanically sensitive promoters. (*a*) Phosphorylation of transcription factors allows their translocation to the nucleus and subsequent DNA binding. The transcription factors can activate or inhibit transcription. TRE = tumor promoting agent response element, TREB = tumor promoting agent response element binding protein, CRE = cAMP response element, CREB = cAMP response element binding protein, SSRE = shear sensitive response element. (*b*) The AU-binding factor binds the AUUUA motif located in the 3′ untranslated regions of some mature mRNA and could play an important role in mediating stability and/or transport of these mRNAs; AUBF = AU-binding factor.

moters. A core-binding sequence of GAGACC was identified that binds to transcriptional factors found in BAEC nuclear extracts. The identity of transcriptional factors that bind this sequence remains unknown. In addition, Malek and coworkers [1993] have shown that shear-stress mediated ET-1 mRNA expression is not dependent on either the PKC or cAMP pathways, but rather shear stress regulates the transcription of the ET-1 gene via an upstream cis element in its promoter. It remains to be seen if ET-1 is shown to have this same response element as that proposed by Resnick and colleagues. As mentioned previously, Mitsumata and coworkers [1993] found that PDGF mRNA modulation was not solely dependent on a PKC pathway. The PKC independent mechanism may very well involve the cis-acting shear stress response element that Resnick and colleagues described, though other factors are probably important in controlling the complex temporal pattern of gene expression seen in response to mechanical stimuli. The biphasic response of MCP-1 was shown to be regulated at the transcriptional level, possibly involving activation of AP-1 sites and the subsequent binding to the TRE site. The putative SSRE binding site was also identified in the 5' flanking region of the cloned MCP-1 gene suggesting an interactive mechanism, wherein these cis-acting elements collectively regulate the transcriptional activation of MCP-1 gene under shear stress [Shyy et al., 1994].

Another important determinant in the role played by shear stress on gene regulation could be at the level of mRNA stability. It is not known whether the shear-induced downregulation that has been reported, especially in the case of adhesion molecules, is due to a decrease in the transcriptional rate of the gene or due to a decrease in the stability of the transcript. The β-adrenergic receptors, which are part of a large class of G-protein linked cell surface receptors, are also susceptible to desensitization and downregulation [Hadcock & Malbon, 1988]. A study of the molecular basis for agonist-induced instability revealed the existence of an M_r 35,000 protein that specifically binds mRNA transcripts which contain the sequence AUUUA in their 3' untranslated region (3'-UTR) [Port et al. 1992]. Agonists that decrease the β-adrenergic RNA transcript levels increased the level of this protein. Further, it has been shown that tandem repeats (three or more) of this sequence are needed for efficient binding of the destabilizer protein [Bohjanen et al., 1992]. Recent reports, however, suggest that AUUUA motif alone does not destabilize the mRNA transcripts and that the presence of additional elements in the AU-rich 3'-UTR may be necessary for the observed mRNA instability [Peppel et al., 1991]. Muller and others [1992] also report that binding of certain AU-binding factors (AUBF) to AUUUA motif accelerates the nuclear export of these mRNAs (Fig. 110.4). Further, their study indicates that this AUBF may protect AU-rich mRNAs against degradation by endoribonuclease V, by binding AUUUA motifs, thereby stabilizing the otherwise unstable mRNA.

Analysis of the 3'-UTR of some of the adhesion molecules studied revealed the presence of the AUUUA motif in all three cases. Human VCAM-1 [Cybulsky et al., 1991] has 6 dispersed AUUUA repeats in its 3'-UTR. Human ICAM-1 [Staunton et al., 1988] has 3 AUUUA repeats within 10 bases of each other, and E-selectin [Hession et al., 1990] has 8 AUUUA repeats, which include 1 tandem repeat and 3 others that are within 10 bases of each other. The constitutively expressed gene human GAPDH [Tokunaga et al., 1987] does not have any AUUUA repeats in the 3' region analyzed. Of the other shear responsive genes, human PDGF-B (c-sis) gene has 1 AUUUA repeat [Ratner et al., 1985]; human endothelin gene [Bloch et al., 1989] has 4, three within 10 bases of each other; human tissue plasminogen activator (tPA) [Reddy et al., 1987] has 2; and human thrombomodulin [Jackman et al., 1987] has 9 AUUUA boxes, including 1 tandem repeat. The steady state levels of the tPA and PDGF have been shown to be increased, and those of the adhesion molecules and endothelin have been shown to be decreased by arterial shear stress [Diamond et al., 1990; Hsieh et al., 1992; Sampath et al., 1995], suggesting a possible mechanism of shear-induced destabilization of adhesion molecule mRNA. However, the observed changes can be at the transcriptional level, with the AUUUA motifs playing a role only in the transport of these mRNAs to the cytoplasm. As shown by Muller and colleagues [1992], transport of low-abundance mRNAs like cytokine mRNAs, whose cellular concentrations are one-hundredth or less of that of the high abundance mRNAs, are the ones that are prone to modulation by transport-stimulatory proteins such as AUBF. This can explain the presence of AUUUA boxes in the 3'-UTR of adhesion molecules and other modulators of vascular tone and not in that of the constitutively expressed GAPDH, which is an essential enzyme in the metabolic pathway and is expressed in high copy numbers. A more detailed study using transcription run-on assays is needed to address these specific issues.

110.8 Gene Therapy and Tissue Engineering in Vascular Biology

Endothelial cells, located adjacent to the flowing blood stream, are ideally located for use as vehicles for gene therapy, since natural or recombinant proteins of therapeutic value can be expressed directly into the blood to manage cardiovascular diseases or inhibit vascular pathology. One could drive gene expression only in regions of vasculature where desired by using novel cis-acting stress- or strain-sensitive promoter elements or stress-activated transcription factors. For instance, endothelial cells in regions of low shear stress could be modified to express tPA so as to inhibit atherosclerotic plaque formation. An appropriate vector driven by the ET-1 promoter (active at low stress but downregulated at high stress) attached to the tPA gene would be a first logical construct in this application. Likewise, endothelial cells could be modified to increase proliferation rates in order to endothelialize vascular grafts or other vascular prosthesis, thereby inhibiting thrombosis. In addition, endothelial cells could be modified to decrease expression of smooth muscle cell mitogens (ET-1, PDGF) to prevent intimal thickening and restenosis. The endothelial cells could even be modified so as to secrete components that would inactivate toxic substances in the blood stream. Work has already begun to develop techniques to express foreign proteins in vivo [Nabel et al., 1989; Wilson et al., 1989; Zwiebel et al., 1989]. Vical and Gen Vec are currently examining ways to express growth factors in coronary arteries to stimulate angiogenesis following balloon angioplasty [Glaser, 1994]. In addition, Tularik Inc is modifying endothelial cells to over express low density lipoprotein (LDL) receptors to remove cholesterol from the blood stream so as to prevent atherosclerotic plaque formation. The application of gene therapy to cardiovascular diseases is in its infancy and will continue to grow as we learn more about the mechanisms governing endothelial cell gene expression. Since endothelial cells lie in a mechanically active environment, predicting local secretion rates of gene products from transfected endothelial cells will require a knowledge of how these mechanical signals modulate gene expression for each target gene and promoter [McIntire, 1994].

In addition to gene therapy applications, there are tissue engineering applications that can be realized once one gains a fundamental understanding of the function-structure relationship intrinsic to vacular biology. This includes understanding how hemodynamic forces modulate endothelial cell function and morphology. Of primary concern is the development of an artificial blood vessel for use in the bypass and replacement of diseased or occluded arteries [Jones, 1982; Nerem, 1991; Weinberg & Bell, 1986]. This is particularly important in the case of small-diameter vascular grafts (such as coronary bypass grafts), which are highly prone to reocclusion. The synthetic blood vessels must provide the structural support required in its mechanically active environment as well as provide endothelial-like functions, such as generating a nonthrombogenic surface.

110.9 Conclusions

This chapter has demonstrated the intricate interweaving of fluid mechanics and convective mass transfer with cell metabolism and the molecular mechanisms of cell adhesion that occur continuously in the vascular system. Our understanding of these mechanisms and how they are modulated by shear stress is really in the initial stages—but this knowledge is vital to our understanding of thrombosis, atherosclerosis, inflammation, and many other aspects of vascular physiology and pathophysiology. Knowledge of the fundamental cellular and molecular mechanisms involved in adhesion and mechanical force modulation of metabolism under conditions that mimic those seen in vivo is essential for real progress to be made in vascular biology and more generally in tissue engineering.

Defining Terms

CRE: *cAMP response element*; its consensus sequence TGACGTCA is found on genes responsive to cAMP agonists such as forskolin.

Gene regulation: Transcriptional and posttranscriptional control of expression of genes in eukaryotes where regulatory proteins bind specific DNA sequences to turn a gene either on (positive control) or off (negative control).

Gene therapy: The modification or replacement of a defective or malfunctioning gene with one that functions adequately and properly, for instance, addition of gene regulatory elements such as specific stress- or strain-sensitive response elements to specifically drive gene expression only in regions of interest in the vasculature so as to control proliferation, fibrinolytic capacity, etc.

Shear: Shear refers to the relative parallel motion between adjacent fluid (blood) planes during flow. The difference in the velocity between adjacent layers of blood at various distances from the vessel wall determines the local shear rate, expressed in cm/s/cm, or s^{-1}.

Shear stress: Fluid shear stress, expressed in dynes/cm^2, is a measure of the force required to produce a certain rate of flow of a viscous liquid and is proportional to the product of shear rate and blood viscosity. Physiologic levels of venous and arterial shear stresses range between 1–5 dynes/cm^2 and 6–40 dynes/cm^2, respectively.

SSRE: Shear stress response element; its consensus GAGACC has been recently identified in genes responsive to shear stress.

Transcription factor: A protein that binds to a cis-regulatory element in the promoter region of a DNA and thereby directly or indirectly affects the initiation of its transcription to an RNA.

TRE: Tumor promoting agent response element; its consensus sequence TGACTCA is commonly located in genes sensitive to phorbol ester stimulation.

References

Abbassi O, Kishimoto TK, McIntire LV, et al. 1993. E-selectin supports neutrophil rolling in vitro under conditions of flow. J Clin Invest 92:2719.

Abbassi OA, Lane CL, Krater S, et al. 1991. Canine neutrophil margination mediated by lectin adhesion molecule-1 in vitro. J Immunol 147:2107.

Alevriadou BR, Moake JL, Turner NA, et al. 1993. Real-time analysis of shear-dependent thrombus formation and its blockade by inhibitors of von Willebrand factor binding to platelets. Blood 81:1263.

Anderson DC, Abbassi OA, McIntire LV, et al. 1991. Diminished LECAM-1 on neonatal neutrophils underlies their impaired CD18-independent adhesion to endothelial cells in vitro. J Immunol 146:3372.

Ando J, Komatsuda T, Kamiya A. 1988. Cytoplasmic calcium response to fluid shear stress in cultured vascular endothelial cells. In Vitro Cell Devel 24:871.

Asakura T, Karino T. 1990. Flow patterns and spatial distribution of atherosclerotic lesions in human coronary arteries. Circ Res 66:1045.

Barabino GA, McIntire LV, Eskin SG, et al. 1987. Endothelial cell interactions with sickle cell, sickle trait, mechanically injured, and normal erythrocytes under controlled flow. Blood 70:152.

Barbee KA, Davies PF, Lal R. 1994. Shear stress-induced reorganization of the surface topography of living endothelial cells imaged by atomic force microscopy. Circ Res 74:163.

Bastida E, Almirall L, Bertomeu MC, et al. 1989. Influence of shear stress on tumor-cell adhesion to endothelial-cell extracellular matrix and its modulation by fibronectin. Int J Cancer 43:1174.

Bhagyalakshmi A, Berthiaume F, Reich KM, et al. 1992. Fluid shear stress stimulates membrane phospholipid metabolism in cultured human endothelial cells. J Vasc Res 29:443.

Bhagyalakshmi A, Frangos JA. 1989a. Mechanism of shear-induced prostacyclin production in endothelial cells. Biochem Biophys Res Comm 158:31.

Bhagyalakshmi A, Frangos JA. 1989b. Membrane phospholipid metabolism in sheared endothelial cells. Proc 2nd Int Symp Biofluid Mechanics and Biorheology, Munich, Germany 240.

Bloch KD, Friedrich SP, Lee ME, et al. 1989. Structural organization and chromosomal assignment of the gene encoding endothelin. J Biol Chem 264:10851.

Bohjanen PR, Petryniak B, June CH, et al. 1992. AU RNA-binding factors differ in their binding specificities and affinities. J Biol Chem 267:6302.

Bohmann D. 1990. Transcription factor phosphorylation: A link between signal transduction and the regulation of gene expression. Cancer Cells 2:337.

Botteri FM, Ballmer-Hofer K, Rajput B, et al. 1990. Disruption of cytoskeletal structures results in the induction of the urokinase-type plasminogen activator gene expression. J Biol Chem 265:13327.

Breathnach R, Matrisian LM, Gesnel MC, et al. 1987. Sequences coding part of oncogene-induced transin are highly conserved in a related rat gene. Nucleic Acids Res 15:1139.

Coan DE, Wechezak AR, Viggers RF, et al. 1993. Effect of shear stress upon localization of the Golgi apparatus and microtubule organizing center in isolated cultured endothelial cells. J Cell Sci 104:1145.

Cooper GM. 1990. Oncogenes, Boston, Jones and Bartlett.

Cybulsky MI, Fries JW, Williams AJ, et al. 1991. Gene structure, chromosomal location, and basis for alternative mRNA splicing of the human VCAM-1 gene. Proc Natl Acad Sci USA 88:7859.

Davies MJ, Woolf N, Rowles PM, et al. 1988. Morphology of the endothelium over atherosclerotic plaques in human coronary arteries. Br Heart J 60:459.

Davies PF, Tripathi SC. 1993. Mechanical stress mechanisms and the cell: An endothelial paradigm. Circ Res 72:239.

Dewey CF Jr, Bussolari SR, Gimbrone MA Jr, et al. 1981. The dynamic response of vascular endothelial cells to fluid shear stress. J Biomech Eng 103:177.

Diamond SL, Eskin SG, McIntire LV. 1989. Fluid flow stimulates tissue plasminogen activator secretion by cultured human endothelial cells. Science 243:1483.

Diamond SL, Sharefkin JB, Dieffenbach C, et al. 1990. Tissue plasminogen activator messenger RNA levels increase in cultured human endothelial cells exposed to laminar shear stress. J Cell Physiol 143:364.

Dull RO, Davies PF. 1991. Flow modulation of agonist (ATP)-response (Ca^{++}) coupling in vascular endothelial cells. Am J Physiol 261:H149.

Eskin SG, Ives CL, McIntire LV, et al. 1984. Response of cultured endothelial cells to steady flow. Microvasc Res 28:87.

Ferrua B, Manie S, Doglio A, et al. 1990. Stimulation of human interleukin-1 production and specific mRNA expression by microtubule-disrupting drugs. Cell Immunol 131:391.

Folie BJ, McIntire LV. 1989. Mathematical analysis of mural thrombogenesis. Biophys J 56:1121.

Frangos JA, Eskin SG, McIntire LV, et al. 1985. Flow effects on prostacyclin production by cultured human endothelial cells. Science 227:1477.

Franke RP, Grafe M, Schnittler H. 1984. Induction of human vascular endothelial stress fibres by shear stress. Nature 307:648.

Giavazzi R, Foppolo M, Dossi R, et al. 1993. Rolling and adhesion of human tumor cells on vascular endothelium under physiological flow conditions. J Clin Invest 92:3038.

Girard PR, Nerem RM. 1991. Fluid shear stress alters endothelial cell structure through the regulation of focal contact-associated proteins. Adv Bioeng 20:425.

Girard PR, Nerem RM. 1993. Endothelial cell signaling and cytoskeletal changes in response to shear stress. Front Med Biol Eng 5:31.

Glagov S, Zarins CK, Giddens DP, et al. 1988. Hemodynamics and atherosclerosis. Arch Pathol Lab Med 112:1018.

Glaser V. 1994. Targeted injectable vectors remain the ultimate goal in gene therapy. Genetic Eng News 14:8.

Grabowski EF, Jaffe EA, Weksler BB. 1985. Prostacyclin production by cultured endothelial cell monolayers exposed to step increases in shear stress. J Lab Clin Med 105:36.

Grande JP, Glagov S, Bates SR, et al. 1989. Effect of normolipemic and hyperlipemic serum on biosynthesis response to cyclic stretching of aortic smooth muscle cells. Arteriosclerosis 9:446.

Gupte A, Frangos JA. 1990. Effects of flow on the synthesis and release of fibronectin by endothelial cells. In Vitro Cell Devel Biol 26:57.

Hadcock JR, Malbon CC. 1988. Down-regulation of beta-adrenergic receptors: Agonist-induced reduction in receptor mRNA levels. Biochemistry 85:5021.

Hakkert BC, Kuijipers TW, Leeuwenberg JFM, et al. 1991. Neutrophil and monocyte adherence to and migration across monolayers of cytokine-activated endothelial cells: the contribution of CD18, ELAM-1, and VLA-4. Blood 78:2721.

Hession C, Osborn L, Goff D, et al. 1990. Endothelial leukocyte adhesion molecule-1: Direct expression cloning and functional interactions. Proc Natl Acad Sci USA 87:1673.

Hsieh HJ, Li NQ, Frangos JA. 1991. Shear stress increases endothelial platelet-derived growth factor mRNA levels. Am J Physiol H642.

Hsieh H, Li NQ, Frangos JA. 1992. Shear-induced platelet-derived growth factor gene expression in human endothelial cells is mediated by protein kinase C. J Cell Physiol 150:552.

Hsieh H, Li NQ, Frangos JA. 1993. Pulsatile and steady flow induces c-*fos* expression in human endothelial cells. J Cell Physiol 154:143.

Hubbel JA, McIntire LV. 1986. Technique for visualization and analysis of mural thrombogenesis. Rev Sci Instrum 57:892.

Hudlicka O. 1984. Growth of vessels—historical review. In F Hammerson, O Hudlicka (eds), Progress in Applied Microcirculation Angiogenesis, vol 4, 1–8, Basel, Karger.

Hunter T, Karin M. 1992. The regulation of transcription by phosphorylation. Cell 70:375.

Iba T, Mills I, Sumpio BE. 1992. Intracellular cyclic AMP levels in endothelial cells subjected to cyclic strain in vitro. J Surgical Res 52:625.

Ingber D. 1993. Integrins as mechanochemical transducers. Curr Opin Cell Biol 3:841.

Ives CL, Eskin SG, McIntire LV. 1986. Mechanical effects on endothelial cell morphology: In vitro assessment. In Vitro Cell Dev Biol 22:500.

Jackman RW, Beeler DL, Fritze L, et al. 1987. Human thrombomodulin gene is intron depleted: Nucleic acid sequences of the cDNA and gene predict protein structure and suggest sites of regulatory control. Proc Natl Acad Sci USA 84:6425.

Jones DA, Abbassi OA, McIntire LV, et al. 1993. P-selectin mediates neutrophil rolling on histamine-stimulated endothelial cells. Biophys J 65:1560.

Jones PA. 1982. Construction of an artificial blood vessel wall from cultured endothelial and smooth muscle cells. J Cell Biol 74:1882.

Kim DW, Gotlieb AI, Langille BL. 1989. In vivo modulation of endothelial F-actin microfilaments by experimental alterations in shear stress. Arteriosclerosis 9:439.

Kishimoto TK, Warnock RA, Jutila MA, et al. 1991. Antibodies against human neutrophil LECAM-1 and endothelial cell ELAM-1 inhibit a common CD18-independent adhesion pathway in vitro. Blood 78:805.

Kojima N, Shiota M, Sadahira Y, Handa K, Hakomori S. 1992. Cell adhesion in a dynamic flow system as compared to static system. J Biol Chem 267:17264–17270.

Komuro I, Kaida T, Shibazaki Y, et al. 1990. Stretching cardiac myocytes stimulates protooncogene expression. J Biol Chem 265:3595.

Komuro I, Katoh Y, Kaida T, et al. 1991. Mechanical loading stimulates cell hypertrophy and specific gene expression in cultured rat cardiac myocytes. J Biol Chem 266:1265.

Kuchan MJ, Frangos JA. 1993. Shear stress regulates endothelin-1 release via protein kinase C and cGMP in cultured endothelial cells. Am J Physiol 264:H150.

Langille BL, Adamson SL. 1981. Relationship between blood flow direction and endothelial cell orientation at arterial branch sites in rabbit and mice. Circ Res 48:481.

Langille BL, Graham JJ, Kim D, et al. 1991. Dynamics of shear-induced redistribution of F-actin in endothelial cells in vivo. Arterioscler Thromb 11:1814.

Langille BL, O'Donnell F. 1986. Reductions in arterial diameter produced by chronic diseases in blood flow are endothelium-dependent. Science 231:405.

Lawrence MB, McIntire LV, Eskin SG. 1987. Effect of flow on polymorphonuclear leukocyte/endothelial cell adhesion. Blood 70:1284.

Lawrence MB, Smith CW, Eskin SG, et al. 1990. Effect of venous shear stress on CD18-mediated neutrophil adhesion to cultured endothelium. Blood 75:227.

Lawrence MB, Springer TA. 1991. Leukocytes roll on a selectin at physiologic flow rates: distinction from and prerequisite for adhesion through integrins. Cell 65:859.

Levesque MJ, Sprague EA, Schwartz CJ, et al. 1989. The influence of shear stress on cultured vascular endothelial cells: The stress response of an anchorage-dependent mammalian cell. Biotech Prog 5:1.

Levin EG, Santell L. 1988. Stimulation and desensitization of tissue plasminogen activator release from human endothelial cells. J Biol Chem 263:9360.

Ley K, Gaehtgens P, Fennie C, et al. 1991. Lectin-like adhesion molecule 1 mediates leukocyte rolling in mesenteric venules in vivo. Blood 77:2553.

Malek AM, Gibbons GH, Dzau VJ, et al. 1993a. Fluid shear stress differentially modulates expression of genes encoding basic fibroblast growth factor and platelet-derived growth factor B chain in vascular endothelium. J Clin Invest 92:2013.

Malek AM, Greene AL, Izumo S. 1993b. Regulation of endothelin 1 gene by fluid shear stress is transcriptionally mediated and independent of protein kinase C and cAMP. Proc Natl Acad Sci 90:5999.

Malek A, Izumo S. 1992. Physiological fluid shear stress causes downregulation of endothelin-1 mRNA in bovine aortic endothelium. Am J Physiol 263:C389.

McIntire LV. 1994. Bioengineering and vascular biology. Ann Biomed Eng 22:2.

Menter DG, Patton JT, Updike TV, et al. 1992. Transglutaminase stabilizes melanoma adhesion under laminar flow. Cell Biophys 18:123.

Milner P, Bodin P, Loesch A, et al. 1992. Increased shear stress leads to differential release of endothelin and ATP from isolated endothelial cells from 4- and 12-month-old male rabbit aorta. J Vasc Res 29:420.

Mitsumata M, Fishel RS, Nerem RM, et al. 1993. Fluid shear stress stimulates platelet-derived growth factor expression in endothelial cells. Am J Physiol 265:H3.

Mo M, Eskin SG, Schilling WP. 1991. Flow-induced changes in Ca^{2+} signaling of vascular endothelial cells: Effect of shear stress and ATP. Am J Physiol 260:H1698.

Morita T, Yoshizumi M, Kurihara H, et al. 1993. Shear stress increases heparin-binding epidermal growth factor-like growth factor mRNA levels in human vascular endothelial cells. Biochem Biophys Res Comm 197:256.

Muller WEG, Slor H, Pfeifer K, et al. 1992. Association of AUUUA-binding Protein with A + U-rich mRNA during nucleo-cytoplasmic Transport. J Mol Biol 226:721.

Nabel EG, Plautz G, Boyce FM, et al. 1989. Recombinant gene expression in vivo within endothelial cells of the arterial wall. Science 244:1342.

Nagel T, Resnick N, Atkinson W, et al. 1994. Shear stress selectively upregulates intercellular adhesion molecule-1 expression in cultured vascular endothelial cells. J Clin Invest 94:885.

Nerem RM. 1991. Cellular engineering. Ann Biomed Eng 19:529.

Nerem RM. 1993. Hemodynamics and the vascular endothelium. J Biomech Eng 115:510.

Nerem RM, Levesque MJ, Cornhill JF. 1981. Vascular endothelial morphology as an indicator of the pattern of blood flow. J Biomech Eng 103:172.

Nollert MU, Diamond SL, McIntire LV. 1991. Hydrodynamic shear stress and mass transport modulation of endothelial cell metabolism. Biotech Bioeng 38:588.

Nollert MU, Eskin SG, McIntire LV. 1990. Shear stress increases inositol trisphosphate levels in human endothelial cells. Biochem Biophys Res Comm 170:281.

Nollert MU, Hall ER, Eskin SG, et al. 1989. The effect of shear stress on the uptake and metabolism of arachidonic acid by human endothelial cells. Biochim Biophys Acta 1005:72.

Nollert MU, McIntire LV. 1992. Convective mass transfer effects on the intracellular calcium response of endothelial cells. J Biomech Eng 114:321.

Nollert MU, Panaro NJ, McIntire LV. 1992. Regulation of genetic expression in shear stress stimulated endothelial cells. Ann NY Acad Sci 665:94.

Ohno M, Gibbons GH, Dzau VJ, et al. 1993. Shear stress elevates endothelial cGMP. Role of potassium channel and G protein coupling. Circulation 88:193.

Ohno M, Lopez F, Gibbons GH, et al. 1992. Shear stress induced TGFβ1 gene expression and generation of active TGFβ1 is mediated via a K^+ channel. Circulation 86:I-87.

Ono O, Ando J, Kamiya A, et al. 1991. Flow effects on cultured vascular endothelial and smooth muscle cell functions. Cell Struct Funct 16:365.

Patton JT, Menter DG, Benson DM, et al. 1993. Computerized analysis of tumor cells flowing in a parallel plate chamber to determine their adhesion stabilization lag time. Cell Motility and the Cytoskeleton 26:88.

Peppel K, Vinci JM, Baglioni C. 1991. The AU-rich sequences in the 3' untranslated region mediate the increased turnover of interferon mRNA induced by glucocorticoids. J Exp Med 173:349.

Perry MA, Granger DN. 1991. Role of CD11/CD18 in shear rate-dependent leukocyte-endothelial cell interactions in cat mesenteric venules. J Clin Invest 87:1798.

Pili R, Corda S, Passaniti A, et al. 1993. Endothelial cell Ca^{2+} increases upon tumor cell contact and modulates cell-cell adhesion. J Clin Invest 92:3017.

Port JD, Huang LY, Malbon CC. 1992. β-adrenergic agonists that down-regulate receptor mRNA up-regulate a M, 35,000 protein(s) that selectively binds to β-adrenergic receptor mRNAs. J Biol Chem 267:24103.

Prasad AR, Logan SA, Nerem RM, et al. 1993. Flow-related responses of intracellular inositol phosphate levels in cultured aortic endothelial cells. Circ Res 72:827.

Ranjan V, Diamond SL. 1993. Fluid shear stress induces synthesis and nuclear localization of c-fos in cultured human endothelial cells. Biochem Biophys Res Comm 196:79.

Ratner L, Josephs SF, Jarrett R, et al. 1985. Nucleotide sequence of transforming human c-sis cDNA clones with homology to platelet derived growth factor. Nucl Acids Res 13:5007.

Reddy VB, Garramone AJ, Sasak H, et al. 1987. Expression of human uterine tissue-type plasminogen activator using BPV vectors. DNA 6:461.

Resnick N, Collins T, Atkinson W, et al. 1993. Platelet-derived frowth factor B chain promoter contains a cis-acting fluid shear-stress-responsive-element. Proc Natl Acad Sci 90:4591.

Ross R. 1993. The pathogenesis of atherosclerosis: a perspective for the 1990s. Nature 362:801.

Sampath R, Kukielka GL, Smith CW, et al. 1995. Shear stress mediated changes in the expression of leukocyte adhesion receptors on human umbilical vein endothelial cells in vitro. Ann Biomed Eng.

Schnittler HJ, Franke RP, Akbay U, et al. 1993. Improved in vitro rheological system for studying the effect of fluid shear stress on cultured cells. Am J Physiol 265:C289.

Schwartz CJ, Valente AJ, Sprague EA. 1993. A modern view of atherogenesis. Am J Cardiol 71:9B.

Sharefkin JB, Diamond SL, Eskin SG, et al. 1991. Fluid flow decreases preproendothelin mRNA levels and suppresses endothelin-1 peptide release in cultured human endothelial cells. J Vasc Surg 14:1.

Shyy YJ, Hsieh HJ, Usami S, et al. 1994. Fluid shear stress induces a biphasic response of human monocyte chemotactic protein 1 gene expression in vascular endothelium. Proc Natl Acad Sci (USA) 91:4678.

Smith CW, Kishimoto TK, Abbassi OA, et al. 1991. Chemotactic factors regulate LECAM-1 dependent neutrophil adhesion to cytokine-stimulated endothelial cells in vitro. J Clin Invest 87:609.

Staunton DE, Marlin SD, Stratowa C, et al. 1988. Primary structure of ICAM-1 demonstrates interaction between members of the immunoglobulin and integrin supergene families. Cell 52:925.

Tokunaga K, Nakamura Y, Sakata K, et al. 1987. Enhanced expression of a glycearldehyde-3-phosphate dehydrogenase. Cancer Res 47:5616.

Tran-son-Tay R. 1993. Techniques for studying the effects of physical forces on mammalian cells and measuring cell mechanical properties. In JA Frangos (ed), Physical Forces and the Mammalian Cell, p 1, New York, Academic Press.

Turitto VT, Weiss HJ, Baumgartner HR, et al. 1987. Cells and aggregates at surfaces. In EF Leonord, VT Turitto, L Vroman (eds), Blood in Contact with Natural and Artificial Surfaces, vol 516, pp 453–467, New York, Annals of the New York Academy of Sciences.

Von Andrian UH, Chambers JD, McEvoy LM, et al. 1991. Two-step model of leukocyte-endothelial cell interaction in inflammation. Proc Natl Acad Sci 88:7538.

Warren BA. 1973. Evidence of the blood-borne tumor embolus adherent to vessel wall. J Med 6:150.

Watson PA. 1991. Function follows form: Generation of intracellular signals by cell deformation. FASEB J 5:2013.

Watson SR, Fennie C, Lasky LA. 1991. Neutrophil influx into an inflammatory site inhibited by a soluble homing receptor-IgG chimaera. Nature 349:164.

Wechezak AR, Viggers RF, Sauvage LR. 1985. Fibronectin and F-actin redistribution in cultured endothelial cells exposed to shear stress. Lab Invest 53:639.

Weinberg CB, Bell E. 1986. A blood vessel model constructed from collagen and cultured vascular cells. Science 231:397.

Weiss HJ, Turitto VT, Baumgartner HR. 1978. Effect of shear rate on platelet interaction with subendothelium in citrated and native blood. J Lab Clin Med 92:750.

Weiss HJ, Turitto VT, Baumgartner HR. 1986. Platelet adhesion and thrombus formation on subendothelium in platelets deficient in GP IIb-IIIa, Ib, and storage granules. Blood 67:905.

Weiss L. 1992. Biomechanical interactions of cancer cells with the microvasculature during hematogenous metastasis. Cancer Metastasis Rev 11:227.

Werb Z, Hembry RM, Murphy G, et al. 1986. Commitment to expression of metalloendopeptidases, collagenase, and stromelysin: Relationship of inducing events to changes in cytoskeletal architecture. J Cell Biol 102:697.

Wick TM, Moake JL, Udden MM, et al. 1987. ULvWF multimers increase adhesion of sickle erythrocytes to human endothelial cells under controlled flow. J Clin Invest 80:905.

Wick TM, Moake JL, Udden MM, et al. 1993. ULvWF multimers preferentially promote young sickle and non-sickle erythrocyte adhesion to endothelial cells. Am J Hematol 42:284.

Wilson JM, Birinyi LK, Salomon RN, et al. 1989. Implantation of vascular grafts lined with genetically modified endothelial cells. Science 244:1344.

Yanagisawa M, Kurihara H, Kimura S, et al. 1988. A novel potent vasoconstrictor peptide produced by vascular endothelial cells. Nature 332:411.

Yoshizumi M, Kurihara H, Sugiyama T, et al. 1989. Hemodynamic shear stress stimulates endothelin production by cultured endothelial cells. Biochem Biophys Res Commun 161:859.

Zarins C, Zatina MA, Giddens DP. 1987. Shear stress regulation of artery lumen diameter in experimental atherogenesis. J Vasc Surg 5:413.

Zarins CK, Giddens DP, Bharadvaj BK, et al. 1983. Carotid bifurcation atherosclerosis. Circ Res 53:502.

Ziegelstein RC, Cheng L, Blank PS, et al. 1993. Modulation of calcium homeostasis in cultured rat aortic endothelial cells by intracellular acidification. Am J Physiol 265:H1424.

Ziegelstein RC, Cheng L, Capogrossi MC. 1992. Flow-dependent cytosolic acidification of vascular endothelial cells. Science 258:656.

Zwiebel JA, Freeman SM, Kantoff PW, et al. 1989. High-level recombinant gene expression in rabbit endothelial cells transduced by retroviral vectors. Science 243:220.

111

The Roles of Mass Transfer in Tissue Function

Edwin N. Lightfoot
University of Wisconsin

Mass transfer lies at the heart of physiology and to a large extent determines the anatomy of living organisms. Limitations on the speed of mass transport, particularly of dissolved oxygen, is a major constraint at size scales from the whole bodies of higher animals down to the microscopic functional units comprising the major organs, e.g., the lobules of the liver, nephrons of the kidney, or Krogh cylinders of the brain. At the intracellular level mass transfer can be too fast, and elaborate barriers such as selectively permeable cell membranes have evolved to slow mass transport and to segregate the large numbers of simultaneous reactions required for functioning of even the simplest organisms.

The purposes of this chapter are to describe a few of the many roles of mass transfer in living systems and to show how they relate to the form and functioning of organisms. It is hoped that this discussion will be helpful both in metabolic engineering and in devising artificial organs and cell culture devices.

To accomplish these purposes it will be necessary to describe selected mass transport fundamentals and then to provide examples illustrating characteristic behavior. However, it will first be necessary to provide a structural overview of these systems and to show how the almost infinite variety of organisms relate to each other. We therefore begin with a specialized overview of comparative physiology.

111.1 Topology and Transport Characteristics of Living Organisms (Schmidt-Nielsen 1983)

If one includes viruses, the size scales of living systems range from nanometers to meters: a linear ratio of 10^9 and a mass ratio of over 10^{27}, which is greater than Avogadro's number! Moreover, as indicated in Fig. 111.1, the higher animals are organized into spatial hierarchies of discrete struc-

0-8493-8346-3/95/$0.00+$.50
© 1995 by CRC Press, Inc.

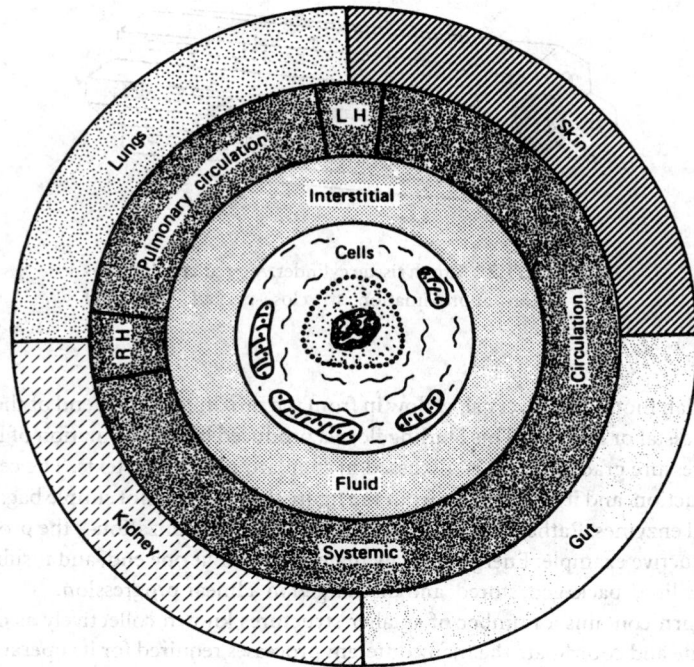

FIGURE 111.1   Diffusional topology of the mammalian body. Convective transport takes place in the blood and interstitial fluid, tangentially in the diagram, and between the four "external" organs and the environment. Diffusional transport is primarily at the cellular level, radially in the two inner rings in this diagram. Inspired by Dr. Peter Abbrecht, University of Michigan. Reprinted with permission from Lightfoot (1974). Copyright 1974 by John Wiley and Sons, Inc.

tures which span this whole size range (see Table 111.1). At the largest scales animals may be considered as organ networks connected by major blood vessels, with each organ carrying out its own set of specialized tasks. Several of these organs, notably the liver and kidney, are described in some detail elsewhere in this volume.

Organs are in turn composed essentially of large numbers of microcirculatory functional units organized in parallel and perfused by capillaries or other microscopic ducts which supply oxygen and other nutrients, carry away waste products, and interchange information with other structures through hormones and other chemical messengers. The Krogh tissue cylinder of Fig. 111.2 is representative and corresponds approximately to the functional units of the brain (see, however, Popel [1989]). It is typical in connecting with the rest of the body through the smallest of blood vessels, in this case capillaries.

The microcirculatory units are in turn comprised of cells which, as suggested in Fig. 111.3, are themselves complex structures comparable in organization to modern chemical plants. Shown schematically in the figure is a pancreatic beta cell which produces, stores, and excretes insulin, a hormone needed in the control of blood glucose levels. Cells connect with each other and the capillaries through a combination of diffusion, primarily the result of

TABLE 111.1   The Spatial Hierarchy in Mammals, Characteristic Lengths

Entity	Length Scale, m
Whole body	10^{-1}–10^{0}
Organs	10^{-2}–10^{-1}
Microcirculatory units	10^{-4}
Cells	10^{-5} (eukaryiots)
	10^{-6} (prokaryiots)
Intracellular organelles	10^{-6}
Molecular complexes	10^{-8}

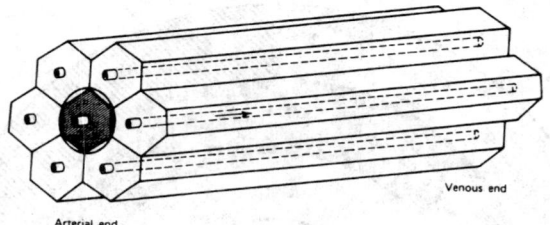

FIGURE 111.2 Krogh tissue cylinder. A circular cylinder is used as an approximation to close-packed hexagonal elements.

random Brownian motion, and very slow flow in from the proximal or inlet end of the capillary and back out at the distal or exit end. This Starling flow is produced by a combination of hydrodynamic and osmotic pressure gradients and is discussed in standard physiology texts. The cells are the seat of metabolic reaction, and it may be seen from the figure that they are not simple bags of well mixed metabolites and enzymes. Rather there is an elaborate internal organization—the production of insulin is an instructive example: Energy and raw materials enter at one end, and insulin is produced on an "assembly line," packaged, stored, and discharged in a linear progression.

The cell in turn contains a number of smaller structures known collectively as organelles that serve to segregate and coordinate the many different processes required for its operation and maintenance. Prominent in the diagram are the mitochondria, which use various carbon sources and oxygen to form high-energy phosphate bonds as in ATP. These are used as energy sources in the

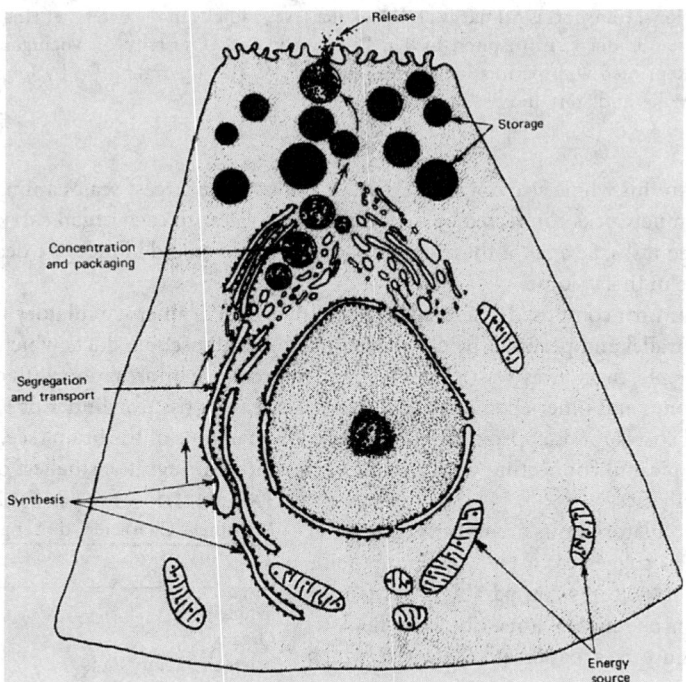

FIGURE 111.3 Structure and organization of a representative eukaryotic cell. Schematic cross-section of a pancreatic beta cell. Reprinted with permission from Lightfoot (1974). Copyright 1974 by John Wiley and Sons.

biochemical networks needed for energy transduction and chemical synthesis. Also shown are the cell nucleus where DNA is stored, ribosomes in which RNA is used to produce individual proteins, and the endoplasmic reticulum which holds ribosomes and channels the proteins produced by them to Golgi apparatus (not shown) for packaging. Organization and structure of the cells is described in standard works on histology.

At the smallest level of organization to be discussed here are enzyme clusters and substructures of the cell membranes used for selective transport across the cell boundary. Enzyme complexes are of particular interest here, but the complex processes by which chemical messengers enter and function in cells are also important (see Lauffenberger & Linderman [1993]).

Underlying all these structures are complex biochemical reaction networks which are largely shared by all species. In addition, all are composed of the same basic elements, primarily proteins, carbohydrates, and lipids. As a result there are a great deal of interspecies similarities [Schmidt-Nielsen, 1983], which we shall find very helpful.

This elaborate organization just described is dictated to a very large extent by mass transfer considerations and in particular by the effect of characteristic time and distance scales on the effectiveness of different mass transport mechanisms. At the larger size scales, only flow or convection is fast enough to transport oxygen and major nutrients, and convective transport is a major function of the larger blood vessels. Diffusive transport begins to take precedence at the level of microcirculatory units; at the cellular level and below, diffusion may even be too fast. Therefore, a variety of specialized intracellular structures, typically selectively permeable membranes, have evolved to maintain spatial segregation against the randomizing forces of diffusion.

111.2 Fundamentals: The Bases of a Quantitative Description

Underneath the bewildering complexity of living organisms are some very simple underlying principles which make a unified description of mass transport feasible. Of greatest utility are observed similarities across the enormous range of system sizes and common magnitudes of key thermodynamic, reaction, and transport parameters. Some simplifying features must still be accepted as justified by repeated observation, and others can be understood from the first principles of molecular kinetic theory. Here we summarize some of the most useful facts and approximations in preparation for the examples of the next section.

Macroscopic Regularity: Allometric Correlations and Physicochemical Data

Impressive macroscopic interspecies similarities have been known about for over 60 years [Schmidt-Nielsen, 1984], and they are often expressed in the form of allometric correlations

$$P = aM^b \tag{111.1}$$

where P is any property, M is average species mass, and a and b are constants specific to the property. A very large number of allometric relations are now available [Adolph, 1949; Calder, 1984; Schmidt-Nielsen, 1984], and those of most interest to us deal with metabolic rate, for example specific oxygen consumption. It is, for example, now widely agreed that total *basal* rates of oxygen consumption for whole animals is given to a good approximation by

$$R_{O_2,\text{tot}} \approx 3.5M^{3/4} \tag{111.2}$$

where $R_{O_2,\text{tot}}$ is oxygen consumption rate in ml O_2 (STP)/hr, and M is body mass in g. Moreover, under basal conditions fat is the primary fuel, and heat generation is about 4.7 Kcal per milliliter of oxygen (STP) consumed.

Equation (111.2) correctly states that small animals have higher specific metabolic rates than large ones, but this is in part because a higher proportion of their body mass is made up of highly active organs such as kidneys and liver. Specific metabolic activity of these organs is much less sensitive to body mass, and for the important case of brain tissue it is invariant at about

$$R_{O_2} \text{ (brain)} \quad 3.72 \times 10^{-5} \text{ mmols } O_2/cm^3 \cdot s \qquad (111.3)$$

for all species. For the liver and kidneys, specific metabolic activity is somewhat lower and falls off slowly with an increase in animal size, but this may be due to an increasing proportion of supporting tissue such as blood vessels and connective tissue. Accurate data valid under physiologic conditions are difficult to find, and to a first approximation specific metabolic activity of parenchymal cells, those actually engaged in the primary activity of the organ, may be close to that of brain for both liver and kidneys. Oxygen consumption may be even higher in specialized preparations such as Chinese hamster ovary hybridoma cells, but reports in the literature vary widely.

The sizes of both microcirculatory units and cells are also very insensitive to animal size. Capillaries are typically about 3–4 µm in radius and about 50–60 µm apart. Typical mammalian cells are about 10–50 µm in diameter, and organelles such as mitochondria are about the size of prokaryotic cells, about 1 µm in diameter. Approximate characteristics of a cerebral tissue cylinder are given in Table 111.2.

The oxygen-carrying capacity of blood, the ionic makeup of body fluids, and the solubility of gases and oxygen diffusivities in body fluids are also largely invariant across species, and some representative data are provided in Tables 111.3, 111.4, and 111.5.

Allometric correlations of this type are essentially empirical and cannot be predicted from any fundamental physical principles. Moreover, most measurements, except solubility and diffusivity data, are of doubtful accuracy.

Time Constants: The Key to Quantitative Modeling

The first step in a priori descriptions is to establish orders of magnitudes of key parameters, and the most important of these for our purposes are time constants, which are estimates of the time required for a given transient process to be "effectively complete." Time constant or order of magnitude analysis is useful because dynamic response times are insensitive to geometric detail and boundary conditions at the order of magnitude level. For example, if a compromise must be made between two processes, the optimum solution very frequently occurs when the ratio of the respective time constants is of the order of unity, i.e., greater than 1/10 and less than 10. Time constants are, however, essentially heuristic quantities and can only be understood on the basis of experience [Lightfoot & Lightfoot, in press]. Here we shall consider diffusion times as our primary example and then go on to flow and chemical reaction.

TABLE 111.2   Characteristic Cerebral Tissue Cylinder

Item	Magnitude
Outer radius	30 µm
Capillary radius	3 µm
Length	180 µm
Blood velocity	400 µm/s
Arterial oxygen tension	0.125 atm
Arterial oxygen concentration (total)	8.6 mM
Arterial oxygen concentration (dissolved O_2)	0.12
Venous oxygen tension	0.053 atm
Venous oxygen concentration (total)	5.87 mM
Venous oxygen concentration (dissolved O_2)	0.05
Tissue oxygen diffusivity	1.5 E-5 cm^2/s (estd.)
Oxygen respiration rate (zero order)	0.0372 mmols O_2/liter-s

TABLE 111.3 Oxygen Solubilities

Solvent	Temperature, °C	O_2 Pressure, atm	Concentration, mM/atm
Water	25		1.26
	30		1.16
	35		1.09
	40		1.03
Plasma	37		1.19
Red cell interior (dissolved O_2 only)	37		1.18
Extracellular tissue (estd.)	37		1.1
Oxygen gas	37		39.3
Alveolar air	37	0.136	
Air (0.21 atm of oxygen)	37	0.21	

Once characteristic system time scales have been established, one can restrict attention to individual processes with response times of the same order: Those an order of magnitude faster can be treated as instantaneous and those ten times longer can be assumed not to happen at all. Both fast and slow terms in the dynamic equations defining the system, for example, the diffusion equation of transport phenomena [Bird et al., 1960], can then be eliminated. Such simplification often provides valuable insights as well simplifying integration. Quantitative descriptions are particularly valuable at the microcirculatory level, for example in diagnostic procedures, and they have been well studied [Bassingthwaighte & Goresky,]. Here we shall stay with relatively simple examples to illustrate selected characteristics of tissue mass transfer, and we begin with diffusion. We then briefly introduce time constants characterizing flow, chemical reaction, and boundary conditions.

Brownian Motion and Concentration Diffusion

The basis of most species selective transport is the relatively slow observable motion of molecules or particles resulting from intermolecular collisions with the surrounding fluid [Lightfoot & Lightfoot, in press]. Such *Brownian motion* does not take any predictable direction, but the particles under observation do tend to move farther from their starting point with increasing time. This motion is best described as the probability of finding any reference particle a distance r from its initial position. For an unbounded quiescent fluid this is [Einstein, 1905]

$$P(r) = \frac{\exp\left[\dfrac{-r^2}{4D_{PF}t}\right]}{8\,(\pi D_{PF}t)^{3/2}} \tag{111.4}$$

This equation defines the *Brownian particle diffusivity* D_{PF} of a particle relative to a surrounding fluid. Here P is a spherically symmetrical normalized probability density defined such that

$$4\pi \int_0^\infty P(r)r^2dr = 1$$

TABLE 111.4 Effective Oxygen Diffusivities

Solvent	Temperature, °C	Pressure	Diffusivity, cm^2/s
Water	25		2.1 E-5
Water	37		3.0 E-5
Blood plasma	37		2.0 E-5
Normal blood	37		1.4 E-5
Red cell interior	37		0.95 E-5
Air	25	1 atm	0.20

TABLE 111.5   Intracellular Diffusion Coefficients

Compound	MW	Radius, Å	Diffusivity in Water cm²/s × 10⁷	Intracell Diffusivity; cm²/s × 10⁷	Diffusivity Ratio
Sorbitol	170	2.5	94	50	1.9
Methylene blue	320	3.7	40	15	2.6
Sucrose	324	4.4	52	20	2.6
Eosin	648	6.0	40	8	5.0
Dextran	3600	12.0	18	3.5	5.0
Inulin	5500	13.0	15	3.0	5.0
Dextran	10,000	23.3	9.2	2.5	3.7
Dextran	24,000	35.5	6.3	1.5	4.2
Actin	43,000	23.2	5.3	0.03	167
Bovine serum albumin	68,000	36.0	6.9	0.10	71

where r is distance (in spherical coordinates) from the initial position, and t is time. The mean net distance traveled from the initial point in unbounded quiescent three-dimensional space is easily determined from the above distribution, as

$$\text{(point)} \quad r_m^2 = \int_0^\infty r^2 P(4\pi r^2)dr = 6D_{PF}t \tag{111.5}$$

The corresponding results from lines and planes through the initial position are

$$\text{(line)} \quad r_m^2 = 4D_{PF}t$$

$$\text{(plane)} \quad x_m^2 = 2D_{PF}t$$

These results provide useful insight in suggesting *characteristic diffusion times t* as the time required for "most" of a transient diffusion process to be complete. Some commonly accepted values are shown in Table 111.6. The numbers in the last column are the fractional changes in solute inventory for a sudden change in surface concentration on a particle initially at a different uniform concentration. For the hollow cylinder the outer surface of radius R_T is assumed impermeable to diffusion, and the inner surface of radius R_C is permeable. The length L is assumed large compared to either radius. Fractional completion for this shape depends in a complex way on the radius ratio, but the diffusion time given is a good approximation.

For large numbers of the reference particles or molecules, species P, nonuniformly distributed in a moving fluid F, the above approach of following undirected Brownian motion of individual molecules becomes too cumbersome to use. We must therefore average behavior over large numbers of molecules to obtain a *continuum approximation* known as Fick's law [Bird et al., 1960], which describes the relative motion of solute and solvent and may be written in the form

TABLE 111.6   Characteristic Diffusional Response Times

Shape	T_{dif}	L	Fractional Completion
Sphere	$L^2/6D_{PF}$	Radius	>0.99
Cylinder	$L^2/4D_{PF}$	Radius	>0.99
Slab	$L^2/2D_{PF}$	Half-thickness	>0.93
Hollow cylinder	$(L^2/2D_{PF})\ln(R_T/R_c)$	Outer radius, R_T.	

$$(v_p - v_F) \cdot \left[\frac{x_P x_F}{D_{PF}} \right] = -\nabla xp \tag{111.6}$$

Here

v_p = observable velocity of species P

x_P = mole fraction of species P, as before

D_{PF} = binary mutual mass diffusivity of solute P relative to solvent fluid F

For situations of interest in this chapter, the Fick's law diffusivity may be considered equal to the Brownian diffusivity just introduced, and it will be written as D_{PF} henceforth. This equation is valid for binary solutions of liquids, gases, and homogeneous solids not acted on by any other diffusional forces than those of mole fraction gradients, and some typical magnitudes for biologic situations are shown in Tables 111.4 and 111.5. For dilute solutions, the hydrodynamic theory of diffusion [Bird et al., 1960] provides useful insight in the form of the Stokes-Einstein equation

$$\frac{D_{PF}\mu}{T} = C = \text{a constant} \tag{111.7}$$

where

$$C = \begin{cases} \dfrac{K}{6\pi} R_P \text{ for } R_P >> R_F \\[2ex] \dfrac{K}{4\pi} R_P \text{ for } R_P \approx R_F \end{cases}$$

Here μ is solvent viscosity, and R_P and R_F are effective spherical solute and solvent radii. Hydrodynamic diffusion theory has been extended to diffusion of isolated solute diffusing through small fluid-filled pores [Deen, 1987]. This work is useful for characterizing transport in microporous membranes.

More Complex Situations

Most biologic transport processes occur in multicomponent solutions, and other sources of species selective transport may occur in addition to the Brownian motion introduced above. A more complete diffusional formulation is needed for such situations, and the most satisfactory is a generalization of the *Maxwell-Stefan* equations described in standard references [Hirschfelder et al., 1954; Lightfoot & Lightfoot, in press; Taylor & Krishna, 1993]. However, for lack of data it is usually necessary to neglect multicomponent diffusional interactions and to assume dilute solutions with constant species activity coefficients. For these purposes transport of both molecules and particles is adequately described by the simplified Maxwell-Stefan equation in Table 111.7. In spite of its somewhat formidable appearance, the equation simply states the relative velocity of a particle or molecule P through a fluid F is proportional to the sum of "driving forces" acting on it.

Flow, Chemical Reaction, and Boundary Conditions.

We now introduce additional time constants in order to characterize the interactions of diffusion with flow and chemical reaction and to show that dynamic boundary conditions can have an important bearing on system behavior.

We begin with flow where mean solute residence time, T_m, forms a convenient time scale. For flow through a cylindrical duct of length L with constant volumetric average velocity $<v>$, we may write

$$T_m = \frac{L}{<v>} \tag{111.8}$$

TABLE 111.7　Particle-Molecular Analogs Dilute Binary Diffusion in a Quiescent Continuum

Particles

$$(v_P - v_F) = -D_{PF} \left\{ \nabla \ln n_p + \frac{1}{\kappa T} \left[V_P(1 - \rho_p^0/\rho)(\nabla p)_\infty - \mathbf{F}_{em} + (\rho_p^0 + \tfrac{1}{2}\rho_f)V_P \frac{dv_P}{dt} \right. \right.$$
$$\left. \left. - 6(\pi\mu\rho_F^0)^{1/2}R_P^2 I + \text{thermal diffusion}\right] \right\}$$

where

$$I = \int_0^t [v_p'(\tau)/(t - \tau)^{1/2}]d\tau$$

Molecules (interdiffusion of species P and F)

$$(v_P - v_F) = -D_{PF}\{\nabla \ln x_P + (1/RT)[V_P(1 - \rho_P^0/\rho)\nabla_p - \mathbf{F}_{em}]\}$$

Both:

$$D_{PF} = \frac{\kappa T}{6\pi\mu R_P}$$

Here:

κ = the Boltzmann constant, or molecular gas constant
n_p = number concentration of particles
R_p = particle or molecular radius
V_P = particle volume or partial molal volume of species P
$\mathbf{F}_{em}$ = total electromagnetic force per particle
$\mathbf{F}_{em}$ = molar electromagnetic force on species P
ρ = density of fluid phase
ρ_p^0 = density of particle or reciprocal of partial specific volume of species P in solution
v' = instantaneous acceleration of particle P
The subscript ∞ refers to conditions near the particle but outside its hydrodynamic boundary layer.

More generally, for constant volumetric flow at a rate Q through a system of volume V with a single inlet and outlet and no significant diffusion across either, T_m is equal to V/Q.

For chemical reaction we choose as our system a reactive solid open to diffusion over at least part of its surface where concentration of a solute i under consideration is maintained at a uniform value c_{i0}, and where the average volumetric rate of consumption of that solute is $<R_i>$. We then define a reaction time constant as

$$T_{rxn} = \frac{c_{i0}}{<R_i>} \tag{111.9}$$

Note that both c_{i0} and $<R_i>$ are measurable, at least in principle [Damköhler, 1937; Weisz, 1973].

Finally we consider as an illustrative situation decay of solute concentration c_i in the inlet stream to a flow system according to the expression

$$c_i(t, \text{inlet}) = c_i(0, \text{inlet})\, e^{-t/T_{BC}} \tag{111.10}$$

where t is time and T_{BC} is a constant.

We now have enough response times for the examples we have selected below, and we turn to illustrating their utility.

111.3 Characteristic Behavior: Selected Examples

We now consider some representative simple processes illustrating the mass transfer behavior of living tissues, and we start with diffusion alone. We then go on to successively more complex examples and finish with a speculation concerning enzyme function.

Alveolar Transients

At the ends of the branching channels comprising the flow channels of the lung are the alveoli, irregular sacs of air surrounded by blood-filled capillaries and with effective diameters of about 75–300 micrometers. The blood residence time is of the order of a second, and it is desired to determine whether gas-phase mass transfer resistance is appreciable.

To answer this question we take the worst possible scenario: flat-plate geometry with a half-thickness of 150 micrometers or 0.0105 cm. From Table 111.4 we find the oxygen diffusivity to be about 0.2 cm²/s. It then follows that the time required for the bulk of gas in an alveolus is

$$T_{\text{dif}} \approx \frac{(0.015)^2}{0.4} \text{ s} = 0.56 \text{ ms}$$

This is extremely fast, with respect to both the 1 s residence time assumed for alveolar blood and the one-twelfth of a minute between breaths: Gas-phase mass transfer resistance is indeed negligible. This is the normal situation for absorption of a sparingly soluble gas like oxygen into aqueius solutions, and a similar situation would normally occur during bubble oxygenation in cell culture vessels.

Mass Transfer Between Blood and Tissue

We next attempt to identify those blood vessels which are capable of transferring appreciable amounts of dissolved solute between the flowing blood and surrounding tissue. To be effective we assume that the mean residence time of the blood should at least equal the radial diffusion time:

$$\frac{L}{<v>} \geq \frac{R^2}{4D_{PF}} = \frac{D^2}{16D_{PF}}$$

or

$$\frac{LD_{PF}}{D^2} <v> \geq \frac{1}{16} = 0.0625$$

where D is vessel diameter. If we now examine the data for a 13-kg dog in Table 111.8, we see that the great majority of vessels are much too short and that only the three smallest classes—arterioles, capillaries, and venules—are at all capable of transferring appreciable mass. These, especially the capillaries, are quite effective; they have long been classified as the microcirculation on the basis of being invisible to the unaided eye. This simple order of magnitude analysis provides a functional definition and a guide to the design of hollow fiber cell culture vessels.

TABLE 111.8 Mass Transfer Effectiveness of Blood Vessels (13-kg Dog, #39)

Vessel	Radius, cm	Length, cm	$<v>$, cm/s	$LD^2/D_{PF}<v>$
Aorta	0.5	10	50	0.00003
Larger arteries	0.15	20	13.4	0.00003
Secondary arteries	0.05	10	8	0.005
Terminal arteries	0.03	1.0	6.0	0.002
Arterioles	0.001	0.2	.032	6.25
Capillaries	0.0004	0.1	0.07	89.4
Venules	0.0015	0.2	0.07	12.7
Terminal veins	0.075	1.0	1.3	0.0014
Secondary veins	0.12	10	1.48	0.0047
Larger veins	0.3	20	3.6	0.0006
Venae cavae	0.625	40	33.4	0.00003

A more refined analysis [Lightfoot, 1974] based on the parameter magnitudes of Table 111.2 shows that lateral diffusional resistance of capillaries is in fact rather small, even for highly active organs like the brain. Oxygenation of tissue has been the subject of much detailed analysis (see, for example, Popel [1989]), but this literature has been long on sophistication and short on reliable histologic data.

Analyses of convection and diffusion in parallel [Lightfoot & Lightfoot, in press] are also of interest, but these processes are much more complicated because of convective dispersion. It can, however, be shown by careful numeric analysis that the behavior of the lung shows a sharp transition between convective ducts and those which can be assumed well-mixed by axial diffusion [Hobbs & Lightfoot, 1974]. This has long been known to pulmonary physiologists who normally model the adult human lung as a plug-flow channel ("dead space") of about 500 ml leading to a well-mixed volume of about 6000 ml.

Intercapillary Spacing in the Microcirculation

It has been shown [Damköhler, 1937; Weisz, 1973] that optimized commercial catalysts normally exhibit ratios of diffusion to reaction times, as defined in Table 111.6 in the relatively narrow range

$$\frac{1}{3} < \frac{T_{\text{dif}}}{T_{\text{rxn}}} < 1$$

Moreover, Weisz has shown that this ratio holds for many biologic systems as well so that enzyme activities can often be inferred from their size, shape, and function.

Here we compare this expectation for cerebral tissue cylinders using the data of Tables 111.2 and 111.6. Throughout the tissue cylinder

$$T_{\text{dif}} = \frac{9 \cdot 10^{-6}\,\text{cm}^2}{3 \cdot 10^{-5}\,\text{cm}^2/\text{s}} \cdot \ln(10) = 0.69\,\text{s}$$

For venous conditions, which are the more severe,

$$T_{\text{rxn}} = \frac{0.0372}{0.0584}\,\text{s} = 0.64\,\text{s}$$

and

$$\frac{T_{\text{dif}}}{T_{\text{rxn}}} \approx 1\ \text{(venous)}$$

For arterial conditions, T_{rxn} is about 1.54 s and

$$\frac{T_{\text{dif}}}{T_{\text{rxn}}} \approx 0.5\ \text{(arterial)}$$

These numbers are reasonable considering the uncertainty in the data and the approximation used for diffusion time. The brain, for example, is far from homogeneous. More elaborate calculations suggest somewhat more conservative design. However, these figures are correct in suggesting that the brain is "designed" for oxygen transport and that the safety factor is small. The body's control mechanisms will shut down other vital organs such as the gut, liver, and kidneys when blood cardiac output or oxygen supply drops to keep the brain as well supplied as possible.

Intraparticle Dispersion

We now ask approximately how long it will take a protein that is initially concentrated in a very small region to disperse throughout the interior of a cell, and to do this we shall assume the cell to be a sphere with a 25-micrometer radius. We begin by noting that the cell interior or cytoplasm is a concentrated solution of polymeric species and that the diffusivity of large molecules is considerably slowed relative to water. We therefore assume a diffusivity of 10^{-8} cm^2/s as suggested by the last entry. In Table 111.5, we note that this situation corresponds closely to the Brownian motion introduced above.

Then if the protein is originally at the center of the sphere, the dispersion time is

$$T_{\text{disp}} \approx T_{\text{dif}} \equiv \frac{(6.25 \cdot 10^{-3})^2}{6 \cdot 10^{-8}} \text{ s} \approx 100 \text{ s}$$

If the protein is initially near the cell periphery, the diffusion will take about 4 times as long, or about 400 s.

It is important to have accurate intracellular diffusion coefficients for this type of calculation, since the corresponding numbers for aqueous solution would have been about $1\frac{1}{2}$ s and $5\frac{1}{2}$ s, respectively! This example is therefore merely illustrative and not accurate for any particular intracellular protein.

Diffusion Controlled Reaction

We now wish to calculate the rate at which a very dilute protein solution in the above cell is adsorbed on a spherical adsorbent particle of radius 5 nanometers if the adsorption is diffusion controlled. That is, we assume that the free protein concentration immediately adjacent to the adsorbent surface is always effectively zero because of the speed and strength of the adsorption reaction.

Now, it is a characteristic of diffusion to a sphere that only the region within a few diameters of the surface offers any effective resistance to transport [Carslaw & Jaeger, 1959]. (More complex problems are dealt with by Özisik [1993]. A simple example of microelectrode operation in Lightfoot [1974, p. 205] is also instructive and very simple.) This is the situation here, since the ratio of adsorbent to cell is only about $2 \cdot 10^{-4}$. The rate at which protein is adsorbed on the sphere surface per unit area is then

$$N_P = \frac{D_{PF}c_{P\infty}}{R_{\text{ads}}} \left(1 + \frac{1}{\sqrt{\pi \tau}}\right)$$

where $c_{P\infty}$ is the protein concentration far from the sphere, and it may be assumed to be uniform, since we are about to see that it adjusts rapidly on the time scale of the adsorption process. The radius of the adsorbent is R_{ads}, and the dimensionless time τ is defined by

$$\tau \equiv \frac{tD_{PF}}{R_{\text{ads}}^2} = \frac{t}{2.5 \cdot 10^{-5} \text{ s}}$$

The transient term in this expression clearly decays very rapidly, and it can be neglected for all practical purposes.

We are therefore ready to calculate the rate of change of protein concentration in the cytoplasm, and to do this we write a macroscopic mass balance of the form

$$-V_{\text{cell}} \frac{dc_{P\infty}}{dt} = A_{\text{ads}}N_P$$

where V_{cell} is the volume of the cell, and A_{ads} is the surface area of the adsorbent. Putting the above expression for N_P into this equation gives

$$-\frac{4}{3}\,\pi R_{cell}{}^3\,\frac{dc_{P\infty}}{dt} = 4\pi R_{ads}{}^2 \cdot \frac{D_{PF}c_{P\infty}}{R_{ads}}$$

or

$$\frac{c_{P\infty}(t)}{c_{P\infty}(0)} = e^{-3D_{PF}R_{ads}t/R_{cell}{}^3}$$

Half the protein will have been adsorbed when the argument of this exponential is minus 0.693 so that the half adsorption time is

$$t_{1/2} = \left(\frac{0.693}{3}\right)\left[\frac{125 \cdot 10^{-9}}{10^{-8} \cdot 5 \cdot 10^{-7}}\right]\,s \approx 6 \cdot 10^6\,s$$

This is clearly a long time compared to the dispersion time of the last example, and the assumed time scale separation of adsorption and dispersion processes is amply justified.

If the protein concentration is now interpreted as the probability of finding a given protein in any position, this example describes the probability of a protein promoter having reached a 25 micrometer DNA site in order to start a genetic reaction. Moreover, the half-time above is the average time such a search will take, and it can be seen that it is *very slow!* It is for this reason that DNA evolved a general binding affinity for promoter molecules and an ability for the adsorbed protein to undergo one-dimensional diffusion along the DNA chain—to increase the effective size of the binding site. We have thus used order of magnitude analysis to simplify an otherwise difficult diffusion problem that has been much discussed in the literature [Berg & von Hipple, 1985].

The Energy Cost of Immobility

Many of the constituents of cells, from small metabolites to organelles, are free to move through the cytoplasm and yet must be limited in their spatial distribution. Many such entities are transported by mechanochemical enzymes which have become known as nanomotors and which depend upon consumption of metabolic energy for their action. Here we attempt to estimate the energy cost of using such processes to maintain spatial segregation, and we do this without detailed knowledge of the mechanisms used.

The basis of our analysis [Okamoto & Lightfoot, 1992] is the Maxwell-Stefan equation of Table 111.7 and more particularly the fact that migration velocities are related to the motive forces of Brownian motion and any mechanically transmitted force through the same diffusivity. Moreover, we shall use the diffusivity of Table 111.7, obtained from hydrodynamic diffusion theory and valid for molecules much larger than water; we shall see that this will suffice.

The heart of our argument is that the mechanical force applied by the nanomotor must produce a migration equal and opposite to that resulting from the dispersive force of Brownian motion:

$$(v_P - v_F)_{tot} = (v_P - v_F)_{dif} + (v_P - v_F)_{mech} = 0$$

$$(v_P - v_F)_{dif} = D_{PF}\,\nabla \ln n_P$$

$$(v_P - v_F)_{mech} = \frac{D_{PF}F}{\kappa T}$$

TABLE 111.9 Energetics of Forced Diffusion

| Particle | Radius, Å | Dilute Solution | | Cytoplasm | |
		Rel. Diff.	$\hat{P}/\Delta G$	Rel. Diff.	Estimated $\hat{P}/\Delta G$
Small metabolite	3	1	7×10^6	1	7×10^6
Globular protein	30	1	7×10^2	0.01	7
Typical organelle	10^4	1	6×10^{-8}	10^4	6×10^{-12}

Now the power required for transporting a particle back against diffusional motion is the product of the mechanical force and mechanical migration velocity

$$P_P = F \cdot (V_P - V_F)_{mech} = \kappa T D_{PF} \, \nabla \ln n_P^2$$

and the power per unit mass for a particle of mass

$$m_P = \frac{4}{3} \pi R_P^3 \rho_P$$

is

$$\frac{P_P}{m_P} = \frac{(\kappa T)^2 \, \nabla \ln n_P^2}{8 \pi \mu_{eff} \rho_P R_P^4} \equiv \hat{P}$$

where μ_{eff} is the effective viscosity of the cytoplasm, ρ_P is particle density, and R_P is effective particle radius. This very strong effect of particle radius suggests that nanomotors will be most effective for larger particles, and calculations of Okamoto and Lightfoot [1992] bear out this suggestion.

If the center of mass of the particle is to be held for the most part within one micrometer of the desired position and the free energy transduction of the cell as a whole corresponds to that of brain tissue, the cost of mechanical motion is negligible for organelles, prohibitive for small metabolites and problematic for proteins, as shown in Table 111.9. Here relative diffusion is the ratio relative to pure water. The quantity $\hat{P}/\Delta G$ is the ratio of power consumption to mean cellular energy transduction.

These numbers are so striking that the conclusions for organelles and small metabolites are not questionable, and it is important to note that no very difficult calculations were required to reach them. It was only necessary to understand the significance of the diffusion equation in Table 111.7. The ability to make useful generalizations with little effort is one of the peculiar strengths of transport phenomena, and we will stop our detailed discussion here.

It remains to note that estimating the cost of organelle transport accurately requires additional information, and some such is available [Okamoto & Lightfoot, 1992]. It is impossible for the cell to transport the large number of small metabolites, and a number of alternate means of segregation have developed. Among them are permselective membranes and compact enzyme clusters, making it difficult for intermediate metabolites to escape into the general cytoplasmic pool. These topics must be discussed elsewhere.

Defining Terms

Allometry: A special form of similarity in which the property of interest scales across species with some constant power of organism mass.

Alveolus: A pulmonary air sac at the distal end of an airway.

Arterioles: The smallest subdivision of the arterial tree proximal to the capillaries.

ATP: Abbreviation for adenosine triphosphate, a source of chemical energy for a wide variety of energy-demanding metabolic reactions.

Capillaries: The smallest class of blood vessel, between an arteriole and venule, whose walls consist of a single layer of cells.

Cell: The smallest unit of living matter capable of independent functioning, composed of protoplasm and surrounded by a semipermeable plasma membrane.

Convection: Mass transport resulting directly from fluid flow.

Cytoplasm: The protoplasm or substance of a cell surrounding the nucleus, carrying structures within which most of the life processes of the cell take place.

Distal: At the downstream end of a flow system.

Microcirculation: The three smallest types of blood vessels—arterioles, capillaries, and venioles.

Mitochondrion: Compartmentalized double-membrane self-reproducing organelle responsible for generating useable energy by formation of ATP. In the average cell there are several hundred mitochondria each about 1.5 micrometers in length.

Organelle: A specialized cytoplasmic structure of a cell performing a specific function.

Parenchyma: The characteristic tissue of an organ or a gland, as distinguished from connective tissue.

Proximal: At the upstream end of a flow system.

Venules: The smallest vessels of the venous tree, distal to the capillaries.

References

Adolph EF. 1949. Quantitative relations in the physiological constitutions of mammals, Science 109: 579.

Bassingthwaighte JB, Goresky CA. Modeling in the Analysis of Solute and Water Exchange in the Microvasculature, Chapter 13, Handbook of Physiology—The Cardiovascular System IV.

Berg OG, von Hippel PH. 1985. Diffusion controlled macromolecular interactions. Ann Rev Biophys Biophys Chem 14:131.

Bird RB, Stewart WE, Lightfoot EN. 1960. Transport Phenomena, New York, Wiley.

Calder WA III. 1984. Size, Function and Life History, Cambridge, Mass, Harvard University Press.

Carslaw HS, Jaeger JC. 1959. Conduction of Heat in Solids, 2d ed, Oxford.

Damköhler G. 1937. Einfluss von Diffusion, Strömung und Wärmetransport auf die Ausbeute bei chemische-technische Reaktionen, Der Chemieingenieur, Bd. 3, p 359.

Deen WM. 1987. Hindered Transport of Large Molecules in Liquid-filled Pores, A I Ch E J, 33 (9): 1409.

Einstein A. 1905. Annalen der Physik 17:549.

Hirschfelder JO, Curtiss CF, Bird RB. 1954. Molecular Theories of Gases and Liquids, New York, Wiley.

Hobbs SH, Lightfoot EN. 1979. A Monte-Carlo simulation of convective dispersion in the large airways. Resp Physiol 37:273.

Lauffenberger DA, Linderman JJ. 1993. Receptors, Oxford, .

Lightfoot EN. 1974. Transport Phenomena and Living Systems, New York, Wiley-Interscience.

Lightfoot EN, Lightfoot EJ. In press. Mass transfer. In Kirk-Othmer Encyclopedia of Chemical Technology, 4th ed, New York, Wiley.

Okamoto GH, Lightfoot EN. 1992. Energy cost of intracellular organization. Ind Eng Chem Res 31 (3):732.

Özisik MN. 1993. Heat Conduction, 2d ed, New York, Wiley.

Popel AS. 1989. Theory of oxygen transport to tissue. Clin Rev Biomed Eng 17 (3):257.

Schmidt-Nielsen Knut. 1983. Animal Physiology: Adaptation and Environment, 3d ed, Cambridge,

Schmidt-Nielsen Knut. 1984. Scaling: Why Is Animal Size So Important?, Cambridge,

Taylor R, Krishna R. 1993. Multicomponent Mass Transfer, New York, Wiley.

Weisz PB. 1973. Diffusion and chemical transformation—an interdisciplinary excursion. Science, 179:433.

112

The Biology of Stem Cells

Craig T. Jordan
Somatix Therapy Corp.

Gary Van Zant
University of Kentucky Medical Center

Life for most eukaryotes, and certainly all mammals, begins as a single totipotent stem cell, the zygote. This cell contains the same complement of genes—no more and no less—as does every adult cell that will make up the organism once development is complete. Nonetheless, this cell has the unique characteristic of being able to implement every possible program of gene expression and is thus totipotent. How is this possible? It is now known that the selective activation and repression of genes distinguishes cells with different developmental potentials. Unraveling this complex series of genetic changes accompanying the progressive restriction of developmental potential during ontogeny is the realm of modern developmental biology. In contrast to the zygote, which has unlimited developmental potential, an intestinal epithelial cell or a granulocyte, for example, is a highly developed cell type that is said to be differentiated. These cells are fixed with respect to their developmental potential and thus no longer possess the ability to contribute to other tissue types. Indeed, intestinal epithelial cells and granulocytes are incapable of undergoing further division and are said to be terminally differentiated. These mature cells have therefore undergone a process whereby they each have acquired a unique and complex repertoire of functions. These functions are usually associated with the cellular morphologic features and/or enzymatic profiles required to implement a specific developmental or functional program. We will come back to the tissue dynamics of these two cell types in a later section of this chapter.

Between the extremes of developmental potency represented by the zygote and terminally differentiated cells, there is obviously a tremendous number of cell divisions (roughly 2^{44}) and an accompanying restriction of this potential in zygotic progeny. The human body, for example, is composed of greater than 10^{13} cells—all ultimately derived from one, the zygote. Where during the developmental sequence does restriction occur? Is it gradual or quantal? These questions are fundamental to an understanding of developmental biology in general and stem cell biology in particular.

112.1 Embryonic Stem Cells

Let us consider first the ultimate human stem cell, the zygote, in more detail. As cellular growth begins, the early embryonic cells start to make a series of irreversible decisions to differentiate along various developmental pathways. This process is referred to as developmental commitment. Importantly, such decisions do not occur immediately; rather, the zygote divides several times and proceeds to the early blastocyst stage of development while maintaining totipotency in all its daughter cells. This is evident most commonly in the phenomenon of identical twins, where two distinct yet genetically matched embryos arise from the same zygote. The ability of early embryonic cells to maintain totipotency has been utilized by developmental biologists as a means to experimentally manipulate these embryonic stem cells, or ES cells, as they are commonly known. In 1981, two scientists at Cambridge, Evans and Kaufman, were able to isolate ES cells from a blastocyst-stage mouse embryo and demonstrate that such cells could be cloned and grown for many generations in vitro [Kaufman et al., 1983]. Remarkably, under the appropriate culture conditions, such cells remained completely totipotent. That is to say, upon reimplantation into another embryo, the stem cells could grow and contribute to the formation of an adult mouse. Importantly, the ES cells retained the developmental potential to differentiate into all the possible adult phenotypes, thereby proving their totipotency.

Thus, in culture, the ES cells were said to self-renew without any subsequent loss of developmental potential. Upon reintroduction into the appropriate environment, the ES cells were able to differentiate into any of the various mature cell types. This basic decision of whether to self-renew or differentiate is a common theme found in stem cells of many developmental systems. Generally self-renewal and differentiation go hand in hand, i.e., the two events are usually inseparable. The important findings of Evans and Kaufman demonstrated that self-renewal and differentiation could be uncoupled and that an extended self-renewal phase of growth was attainable for mammalian embryonic cells.

The advent of ES cell technology has had an enormous impact on the field of mammalian molecular genetics. The ability to culture ES cells was quickly combined with molecular techniques which allow for the alteration of cellular DNA. For example, if an investigator were interested in the function of a gene, he or she might elect to mutate the gene in ES cells so that it was no longer functional. The genetically altered ES cells would then be used to generate a line of mice which carry the so-called gene knockout [Koller & Smithies, 1992; Robertson, 1991]. By examining the consequences of such a mutation, clues to the normal function of a gene may be deduced. Techniques such as these have been widely used over the past 10 years and continue to develop as even more powerful means of studying basic cellular function become available.

112.2 Control of Stem Cell Development

The concepts of self-renewal and differentiation are central to the description of a stem cell; indeed, the potential to manifest these two developmental options is the only rigorous criterion used in defining what constitutes a true stem cell. Consequently, in studying stem cells, one of the most important questions to consider is how the critical choice whether to self-renew or differentiate is made. As seen in the case of ES cells, the environment of the stem cell or extrinsic signals determine the outcome of the self-renewal decision. In other words, such cells are not intrinsically committed to a particular developmental fate; rather, their environment mediates the differentiation decision. Surprisingly, for ES cells this decision is dictated by a single essential protein, or growth factor, known as Leukemia inhibitory factor (LIF) [Hilton & Gough, 1991; Smith et al., 1992]. In the presence of sufficient concentrations of LIF, ES cells will self-renew indefinitely in culture. Although ES cells eventually lose their totipotency in vitro, this is thought to be due to technical limitations of ex vivo culture rather than developmental decisions by the cells themselves.

Interestingly, the default decision for ES cells appears to be differentiation, i.e., unless the cells are prevented from maturing by the presence of LIF, they will quickly lose their totipotent phenotype. Upon beginning the differentiation process, ES cells can be steered along a variety of developmental pathways simply by providing the appropriate extrinsic signal, usually in the form of a growth factor.

Unfortunately, the control of other types of stem cells has proven more difficult to elucidate. In particular, the control of blood-forming, or hematopoietic, stem cells has been extensively studied, but as yet the developmental control of these cells is poorly understood.

112.3 Adult Stem Cells

As the mammalian embryo develops, various organ systems are formed, and tissue-specific functions are elaborated. For the majority of mature tissues, the cells are terminally differentiated and will continue to function for extended periods of time. However, some tissues operate in a much more dynamic fashion, wherein cells are continuously dying and being replenished. These tissues require a population of stem cells in order to maintain a steady flow of fresh cells as older cells turn over. Although there are several examples of such tissue types, perhaps the best characterized are the hematopoietic system and the intestinal epithelia. These two cell types have population parameters that call for their continuous and rapid production: Both cell types occur in very large numbers (approximately 10^{11} to 10^{12} for the human hematopoietic system) and have relatively short life spans that can often be measured in days or sometimes even hours [Koller & Palsson, 1993]. These two tissues in adults are therefore distinct (along with skin epithelium) in that they require tissue-specific stem cells in order to satisfy the inherent population dynamics of the system.

Stem cells of this nature represent a population arrested at an intermediate level of developmental potency that permits them to perform the two classic stem cell functions: They are able to replenish and maintain their own numbers through cell divisions that produce daughter cells of equivalent potency, that is, self-renew. And, they have the capacity, depending on need, to differentiate and give rise to some, if not all, of the various mature cell types of that tissue. Stem cells of the small intestine, to the best of our knowledge, give rise to at least four highly specialized lineages found in the epithelium: Paneth, goblet, enteroendocrine, and enterocytes; these stem cells are therefore pluripotent (i.e., they have the potential to give rise to many different, but not all, lineages) [Potten & Loeffler, 1990]. Similarly, pluripotent stem cells of the hematopoietic system give rise to an even wider variety of mature cells, including at least eight types of blood cells: the various lymphocytes, natural killer cells, megakaryocytes, erythroid cells, monocytes, and three types of granulocytes [Metcalf & Moore, 1971].

Proof of the existence of gut and hematopoietic stem cells came from studies of the effects of ionizing radiation on animals. This research, in the 1940s and 1950s, was spurred by concern over military and peaceful uses of atomic energy. It became recognized that the organ/tissue systems most susceptible to radiation damage were those that normally had a high turnover rate and were replenished by stem cell populations, i.e., the gut lining and the hematopoietic system. In particular, the latter was found to be the radiation dose-limiting system in the body. It was subsequently discovered that mice could be rescued from imminent death from radiation "poisoning" by the transfusion of bone marrow cells following exposure [Barnes et al., 1959]. Initially it was not clear whether the survival factor was humoral or cellular, but mounting evidence pointed to a cell-mediated effect, and, as the dose of bone marrow cells was titrated to determine the number required for survival, it was found that low numbers of cells resulted in the development of macroscopic nodules on the spleens of irradiated mice.* These nodules were composed of cells of some but not all lineages of blood formation—lymphopoiesis was notably missing [Till & McCulloch, 1961]. Low-level radiation was then used to induce unique chromosomal aberrations in bone marrow cells prior to transplantation into lethally irradiated recipients. In this way, unique, microscopically identifiable translocations would be passed on to all progeny of an altered cell. It was found that the spleen

---

*Injected bone-marrow-derived stem cells lodge and develop in several types of hematopoietic tissue, including spleen. Apparently, the splenic microenvironment can at least transiently support stem cell growth and development.

nodules were, in fact, colonies of hematopoietic cells, all possessing an identical chromosomal marker [Becker et al., 1963]. This observation strongly suggested that the nodule was a clonal population, derived from a single stem cell. Since several lineages were represented in the spleen colony, the stem cell responsible was pluripotent. Moreover, single spleen colonies could be isolated and injected into secondary irradiated recipients and give rise to additional spleen colonies. This suggested that the cell giving rise to a spleen colony was capable of some degree of self-renewal as well as multilineage differentiation [Till et al., 1964]. The cells which give rise to spleen colonies were termed CFU-S for colony-forming unit—spleen and have been studied extensively in the characterization of pluripotent hematopoietic stem cells.

More recent studies employing a similar strategy have used retroviruses to mark stem cells. The site of viral integration in an infected host cell genome is random and is passed with high fidelity to all progeny, thus by molecular means stem cell clones may be identified. Such an approach allows for the analysis not only of spleen colonies but of all anatomically dispersed lymphohematopoietic sites, including bone marrow, spleen, thymus, lymph nodes, and mature blood cells in the circulation [Dick et al, 1985; Keller et al., 1985; Lemischka et al., 1986]. These analyses unequivocally showed that the same stem cell may give rise to all lineages, including lymphocytes. Repetitive blood cell sampling and analysis gave a temporal picture of the usage and fate of the stem cell population. In the first few weeks and months after transplant of nonlimiting numbers of stem cells, polyclonal hematopoiesis was the rule; however, after approximately 4–6 months, the number of stem cell clones was reduced. In fact, in some cases, a single stem cell clone was responsible for all hematopoiesis for over a year—about half the mouse's lifetime [Jordan & Lemischka, 1990]. These data were interpreted to mean that many stem cell clones were initially active in the irradiated recipient mice, but over time a subset of stem cells grew to dominate the hematopoietic profile. This implies either that not all the stem cells were equivalent in their developmental potential or that the stem cells were not all seeded in equivalent microenvironments and therefore manifest differing developmental potentials. Both these possibilities have been supported by a variety of subsequent experiments; however, the details of this observation remain cloudy.

One piece of evidence suggesting intrinsic differences at the stem cell level comes from studies of allophenic mice [Mintz, 1971]. These artificially generated strains of laboratory mice are created by aggregating the early embryos of two distinguishable mouse strains. As mentioned previously, early embryonic cells are totipotent; thus, upon combining such cells from two strains, a chimeric mouse will arise in which both cell sources contribute to all tissues, including the stem cell population. Patterns of stem cell contribution in allophenic mice show that one strain can cycle more rapidly and thus contribute to mature blood cells early in life, whereas the other slower-growing strain will arise to dominate at later times. Importantly, upon reimplantation of allophenic bone marrow into a secondary irradiated recipient, the two phases of stem cell activity are recapitulated. Thus, the stem cells which had become completely quiescent in the primary animal were reactivated initially, only to be followed by a later phase of activity from the second strain [Van Zant, 1992]. These data suggest that intrinsic differences at the stem cell level rather than the local microenvironment can mediate differences in stem cell activity.

Unlike most organ systems, mature cells of the lymphohematopoietic system are dispersed either in the circulation or in scattered anatomic sites such as the thymus, lymph nodes, spleen, and, in the case of macrophages, in virtually all tissues of the body. The site of production of most of the mature cells, the bone marrow, is a complex tissue consisting of stromal elements, stem and progenitor cells, maturing cells of multiple lineages, and capillaries and sinusoids of the circulatory system into which mature cells are released. Spatial relationships between these different components are not well understood because of their apparently diffuse organization and because of the paucity of some of the critical elements, most notably the stem cells and early progenitors.

In contrast, the small intestinal epithelium has a much more straightforward organization that has expedited the understanding of some of the critical issues having to do with stem cell differentiation. Numerous fingerlike projections of the epithelium, called *villi*, extend into the intestinal lumen to effectively increase the surface area available for absorption. Each villus is covered with approximately 3500 epithelial cells, of which about 1400 are replaced on a daily basis [Potten & Loeffler, 1990]. Surrounding each villus are 6–10 crypts from which new epithelial cells are produced. They subsequently migrate to villi, and as senescent cells are shed from the villus tip, a steady progression of epithelial cells proceed unidirectionally to replace them. Crypts consist of only about 250 cells, including what is now estimated to be 16 stem cells. Since there are about 16 cells in the circumference of the crypt, stem cells occupy one circumferential ring of the crypt interior. This ring has been identified as the fourth from the bottom, directly above the Paneth cells. In addition, the fifth circumferential ring is occupied by direct progeny of stem cell which retain pluripotency and, in emergencies, may function as stem cells. Given the detailed quantitative information available regarding stem cell numbers and epithelial cell turnover rates, the number of stem cell doublings occurring during a human life span of 70 years has been estimated to be about 5000. Whether this demonstrates that tissue-specific stem cells are immortal is the topic of the following section.

112.4 Aging of Stem Cells

Given the zygote's enormous developmental potential and that ES cells represent cells of apparently equivalent potency that can be propagated as cell lines, it is reasonable to ask whether aging occurs at the cellular level. Put another way, can normal cells, other than ES cells, truly self-replicate without differentiation or senescence? Or do ES cells represent unique examples of cells capable of apparently indefinite self-renewal without differentiation? One of the definitions of hematopoietic stem cells, alluded to above, is that they self-replicate. Without self-renewal, it might be argued, a stem cell population may be exhausted in a time-frame less than a lifetime of normal hematopoiesis or in far less time in the event of unusually high hematopoietic demands associated with disease or trauma. If, for example, hematopoietic stem cells can be propagated in vitro without differentiation, it could have a tremendous impact on a number of clinically important procedures including bone marrow transplantation and gene therapy.

In classic experiments studying fibroblast growth in vitro, Hayflick [1965] observed that there were a finite number of divisions (about 50) that a cell was capable of before reaching senescence. It has been thought that totipotent and pluripotent stem cells may be exempt from this constraint. An analysis above of intestinal epithelial stem cells suggested that in a lifetime they undergo several thousand replications, apparently without any loss in developmental potential. However, several lines of evidence call into question the immortality of hematopoietic stem cells and point to at least a limited self-renewal capacity. For example, studies in which marrow was serially transplanted from primary recipients to secondary hosts, and so on, the number of effective passages is only about four to five [Siminovitch et al., 1964]. After the first transplant, normal numbers of relatively late progenitors are produced, but the number of repopulating stem cells is either diminished or the cells' developmental potential attenuated, or both, resulting in a requirement for successively larger numbers of transplanted cells to achieve engraftment. Another interpretation of these results is that the transplantation procedure itself is responsible for the declining repopulating ability of marrow, rather than an intrinsic change in the self-renewal capacity of the stem cells. According to this argument, the repetitive dissociation of stem cells from their normal microenvironmental niches in the marrow, and the required reestablishment of those contacts during seeding and serial engraftment, irreversibly alter their self-renewal capacity [Harrison et al., 1978]. A mechanistic possibility for this scenario is that differentiation is favored when stem cells are not in contact with their stromal microenvironment. In this context, exposure to growth factors has an overwhelming differentiating influence on stem cells in suspension that is normally tempered by stromal associations.

Recently, an intriguing series of findings has emerged which may at least partially explain cellular aging. At the end of chromosomes there is a specialized region of DNA known as a telomere. This segment of DNA is comprised of hundreds of short six-nucleotide repeats of the sequence

TTAGGG. It has been found that the length of telomeres varies over the life of a cell. Younger cells have longer telomeres, and as replication occurs the telomeres can be seen to shorten. It is thought that via the normal DNA replication process, the last 50–200 nucleotides of the chromosome fail to be synthesized, and thus telomeres are subject to loss with every cell division (reviewed in Blackburn [1992] and Greider [1991]). Consequently, telomeric shortening may act as a type of molecular clock. Once a cell has undergone a certain number of divisions, i.e., aged to a particular extent, it becomes susceptible to chromosome destabilization and subsequent cell death. Importantly, the rate at which telomeric sequence is lost may not be constant. Rather, some cells have the ability to regenerate their telomeres via an enzymatic activity known as telomerase. By controlling the loss of telomeric sequence, certain cell types may be able to extend their ability to replicate. Perhaps primitive tissue such as ES cells, when cultured with LIF, are able to express high levels of telomerase and thereby maintain their chromosomes indefinitely. Similarly, perhaps early hematopoietic stem cells express telomerase, and, as differentiation occurs, the telomerase activity is downregulated. Although intriguing, these hypotheses are very preliminary, and much more basic research will be required to elucidate the mechanisms of stem cell replication and aging.

In contrast to normal mechanisms of preserving replicative ability, a type of aberrant self-renewal is observed in the phenomenon of malignant transformation, or cancer. Some hematopoietic cancers are thought to originate with a defect at an early stem or progenitor cell level (e.g., chronic myelogenous leukemia). In this type of disease, normal differentiation is blocked, and a consequent buildup of immature, nonfunctional hematopoietic cells is observed. Malignant or neoplastic growth comes as a consequence of genetic damage or alteration. Such events range from single nucleotide changes to gross chromosomal deletions and translocations. Mechanistically, there appear to be two general types of mutation which cause cancer. One, activation of so-called oncogenes, is a dominant event and only needs to occur in one of a cell's two copies of the gene. Second, inactivation of tumor-suppressor genes removes the normal cellular control of growth and results in unchecked replication. These two categories of genetic alteration are analogous to stepping on a car's accelerator versus releasing the brake; both allow movement forward. Importantly, malignancy often comes as the result of a multistep process, whereby a series of genetic alterations occur. This process has been shown to involve different combinations of genes for different diseases [Vogelstein & Kinzler, 1993].

112.5 Other Types of Stem Cells

Other tissues may also have stem cell populations contributing to the replacement of effete mature cells. For example, in the liver only a very small fraction (2.5–5×10^{-5}) of hepatocytes is dividing at any given time, resulting in a complete turnover time of about 1 year [Sell, 1994]. This compares with the complete turnover of intestinal epithelia or granulocytes in a period of a few days. Nonetheless, growing evidence, some of which remains controversial, suggests that hepatic stem cells play a role in this tissue turnover. A moderate loss of liver tissue due to mild or moderate insult is probably replaced by the division of mature hepatocytes. However, a severe loss of hepatic tissue is thought to require the enlistment of the putative stem cell population, morphologically identified as oval cells.

Similarly, Noble's group in London has identified cells in the rat optic nerve that have the requisite functions of stem cells [Wren et al., 1992]. These cells, called *oligodendrocyte-type 2 astrocyte (O-2A) progenitors,* are capable of long-term self-renewal in vitro and give rise to oligodendrocytes through asymmetric divisions resulting in one new progenitor and one cell committed to differentiation. Conversion in vitro of O-2A progenitors into rapidly dividing and differentiating cells has been shown to be regulated extrinsically by platelet-derived growth factor (PDGF) and the basic form of fibroblast growth factor (bFGF) [Wolswijk & Noble, 1992]. Since these two growth factors are known to be produced in vivo after brain injury, a mechanism is suggested for generation of the large numbers of new oligodendrocytes required subsequent to trauma and demyelination.

112.6 Summary

- The zygote is the paradigm of a totipotent stem cell.
- ES cells derived from early embryos can be propagated indefinitely and maintain totipotency when cultured in the presence of LIF. Experimental control of differentiation and self-renewal in adult stem cells is being extensively investigated.
- Stem cells are defined by two characteristic traits: (1) Stem cells can self-renew, and (2) they can produce large numbers of differentiated progeny. Stem cells possess the intrinsic ability to manifest either trait; however, extrinsic factors mediate their developmental fate.
- Tissue-specific stem cells are pluripotent but not totipotent.
- Intestinal, epithelial, and hematopoietic tissues are classical self-renewing systems of the adult. In addition, recent studies have indicated the presence of stem cells in several other tissues (e.g., liver, nervous system).
- Although stem cells clearly have an extensive replication potential, it is not clear whether they are truly immortal. Stem cells may possess the ability to circumvent normal cellular processes that determine aging at the cellular level.
- Mutations at the DNA level can alter normal cellular control of stem cell replication and differentiation. This type of event can lead to aberrant development and subsequent malignancy.

Defining Terms

Commitment: The biologic process whereby a cell decides which of several possible developmental pathways to follow.

Differentiation: Expression of cell- or tissue-specific genes which results in the functional repertoire of a distinct cell type.

ES cells: Mouse stem cells originating from early embryonic tissue, capable of developing into any of the adult cell types.

Gene knockout: Deletion or alteration of a cellular gene using genetic engineering technology (generally performed on ES cells).

Hematopoietic: Blood forming.

Ontogeny: The process of development, generally referring to development from the zygote to adult stages.

Pluripotent: Capable of differentiation into multiple cell types.

Self-renew: Term describing cellular replication wherein no developmental commitment or differentiation takes place.

Terminally differentiated: The final stage of development in which all cell-specific features have been attained and cell division is no longer possible.

Totipotent: Capable of differentiation into all possible cell types.

References

Barnes DWH, Ford CE, Gray SM, et al. 1959. Progress in Nuclear Energy, series VI: Spontaneous and Induced Changes in Cell Populations in Heavily Irradiated Mice, London, Pergamon Press.

Becker AJ, McCulloch EA, Till JE. 1963. Cytological demonstration of the clonal nature of spleen colonies derived from transplanted mouse marrow cells. Nature 197:452.

Blackburn EH. 1992. Telomerases. Annu Rev Biochem 61:113.

Dick JE, Magli MC, Huszar D, et al. 1985. Introduction of a selectable gene into primitive stem cells capable of long-term reconstitution of the hemopoietic system of W/W^v mice. Cell 42:71.

Evans MJ, Kaufman MH. 1981. Establishment in culture of pluripotent cells from mouse embryos. Nature 292:154.

Greider CW. 1991. Telomeres. Curr Opin Cell Biol 3(3):444.

Harrison DE, Astle CM, Delaittre JA. 1978. Loss of proliferative capacity in immumohemopoietic stem cells caused by serial transplantation rather than aging. J Exp Med 147:1526.

Hayflick L. 1965. The limited in vitro lifetime of human diploid cell strains. Exp Cell Res 37:614.

Hilton DJ, Gough NM. 1991. Leukemia inhibitory factor: A biological perspective. J Cell Biochem 46(1):21.

Jordan CT, Lemischka IR. 1990. Clonal and systemic analysis of long-term hematopoiesis in the mouse. Genes Dev 4:220.

Kaufman MH, Robertson EJ, Handyside AH, et al. 1983. Establishment of pluripotential cell lines from haploid mouse embryos. J Embryol Exp Morphol 73:249.

Keller G, Paige C, Gilboa E, et al. 1985. Expression of a foreign gene in myeloid and lymphoid cells derived from multipotent hematpoietic precursors. Nature 318:149.

Koller BH, Smithies O. 1992. Altering genes in animals by gene targeting. Annu Rev Immunol 10:705.

Koller MR, Palsson BØ. 1993. Tissue engineering: Reconstitution of human hematopoiesis ex vivo. Biotechnol Bioeng 42:909.

Lemischka IR, Raulet DH, Mulligan RC. 1986. Developmental potential and dynamic behavior of hematopoietic stem cells. Cell 45:917.

Metcalf D, Moore MAS. 1971. Haemopoietic Cells, Amsterdam, Elsevier/North-Holland.

Mintz B. 1971. Methods in Mammalian Embryology, San Francisco, WH Freeman.

Potten CS, Loeffler M. 1990. Stem cells: Attributes, cycles, spirals, pitfalls and uncertainties. Lessons for and from the crypt. Develop 110:1001.

Robertson EJ. 1991. Using embryonic stem cells to introduce mutations into the mouse germ line. Biol Reprod 44(2):238.

Sell S. 1994. Liver stem cells. Mod Pathol 7(1):105.

Siminovitch L, Till JE, McCulloch EA. 1964. Decline in colony-forming ability of marrow cells subjected to serial transplantation into irradiated mice. J Cell Comp Physiol 64:23.

Smith AG, Nichols J, Robertson M, et al. 1992. Differentiation inhibiting activity (DIA/LIF) and mouse development. Dev Biol 151 (2):339.

Till JE, McCulloch EA. 1961. A direct measurement of the radiation sensitivity of normal mouse bone marrow cells. Radiat Res 14:213.

Till JE, McCulloch EA, Siminovitch L. 1964. A stochastic model of stem cell proliferation based on the growth of spleen colony-forming cells. Proc Natl Acad Sci 51:29.

Van Zant G, Scott-Micus K, Thompson BP, et al. 1992. Stem cell quiescence/activation is reversible by serial transplantation and is independent of stromal cell genotype in mouse aggregation chimeras. Exp Hematol 20:470.

Vogelstein B, Kinzler KW. 1993. The multistep nature of cancer. Trends Genet 9(4):138.

Wolswijk G, Noble M. 1992. Cooperation between PDGF and FGF converts slowly dividing O-2A adult progenitors cells to rapidly dividing cells with characteristics of O-2A perinatal progenitor cells. J Cell Biol 118(4):889.

Wren D, Wolswijk G, Noble M. 1992. In vitro analysis of the origin and maintenance of O-2A adult progenitor cells. J Cell Biol 116(10):167.

113

Cell Motility
and Tissue Architecture

Graham A. Dunn
King's College London

The characteristic architecture of a tissue results from an interplay of many cellular processes. In addition to the secretion of extracellular matrix, we may distinguish between processes related to the cell cycle—cell growth, division, differentiation, and death—and processes related to cell motility—cell translocation, directed motile responses, associated movements, and remodeling of the extracellular matrix. These processes are controlled and directed by cell-cell interactions, by cell-matrix interactions, and by cellular interactions with the fluid phase of the tissue. It is known that all three types of interactions can control both the speed and direction of cell translocation. This control results in the directed motile responses, which are the main subject of this chapter. Learning how to manipulate these motile responses experimentally will eventually become an essential aspect of tissue engineering.

Probably the greatest challenge to tissue engineering lies in understanding the complex dynamic systems that arise as a result of feedback loops in these motile interactions. Not only is cell translocation controlled by the fluid phase, by the matrix, and by other cells of the tissue, but cell motility can profoundly influence the fluid phase, remodel the matrix, and influence the position of other cells by active cell-cell responses or by associated movements. It is often forgotten that, especially in "undifferentiated" types of tissue cells such as fibroblasts, the function of the cell's motile apparatus is not only to haul the cell through the extracellular matrix of the tissue spaces but also to remodel this matrix and to change the positions of other cells mechanically by exerting tension on cell-matrix and cell-cell adhesions. These complex dynamic systems lie at the heart of pattern formation in the tissue, and indeed in the developing embryo, and understanding them will require not only a knowledge of the motile responses but also an understanding of the mechanism of cell motility itself.

In the study of cell motility, a great deal is now known about the relative dispositions of specific molecules that are thought to contribute to the motile process, and the dynamics of their interactions are beginning to be unraveled, yet there appears to have been comparatively little progress toward a satisfactory explanation of how a cell moves. There are some molecular biologists who still believe that it is just a question of time before the current molecular genetic thrust will alone come

0-8493-8346-3/95/$0.00+$.50

up with the answers. But there is a rapidly growing climate of opinion, already prevalent among physicists and engineers, that nonlinear dynamic processes such as cell motility have emergent properties that can never be completely understood solely from a knowledge of their molecular basis. Cell locomotion, like muscle contraction, is essentially a mechanical process, and a satisfactory explanation of how it works will inevitably require a study of its mechanical properties. Unlike muscle, the cellular motile apparatus is a continuously self-organizing system, and we also need to know the overall dynamics of its capacity for reorganization. These outstanding areas of ignorance are essentially problems in engineering. There is a nice analogy for this conceptual gap between the molecular and engineering aspects of biologic pattern formation in Harrison's new book on the kinetic theory of living pattern [Harrison, 1993]: ". . . one cannot supplant one end of a bridge by building the other. They are planted in different ground, and neither will ever occupy the place of the other. But ultimately, one has a bridge when they meet in the middle." This chapter is intended to encourage the building of that bridge.

113.1 Directed Motile Responses in Vivo

Cellular Interactions with the Fluid Phase

Cellular responses to the fluid phase of tissue spaces are thought to be mediated largely by specific diffusible molecules in the fluid phase. By far the most important directed response is chemotaxis: the unidirectional migration of cells in a concentration gradient of some chemoattractant or chemorepellent substance. Its study dates back to long before the advent of tissue culture, since it is a widespread response among the free-living unicellular organisms. The most widely studied system in vertebrates is the chemotaxis of neutrophil leukocytes in gradients of small peptides. In the case of tissue cells, it has long been conjectured, usually on the basis of surprisingly little evidence, that the direction of certain cell migrations also might be determined by chemotaxis, and it is recently becoming clear that chemotaxis can in fact occur in several vertebrate tissue cells in culture, particularly in gradients of growth factors and related substances. Yet whether it does occur naturally, and under what circumstances, is still an area of dispute. The concentration gradients themselves are usually speculated to arise by molecular diffusion from localized sources, although a nonuniform distribution of sinks could equally explain them, and they are only likely to arise naturally in conditions of very low convective flow. Besides controlling the migration of isolated cells, there is some evidence that gradients of chemoattractants also may control the direction of extension of organized groups of cells, such as blood capillary sprouts, and of cellular processes, such as nerve axons. Although the mechanisms of these responses may be closely allied to those of chemotaxis, they should more properly be classed as chemotropism, since the effect is to direct the extension of a process rather than the translocation of an isolated cell. The *influence on tissue architecture* of chemotaxis and chemotropism is possibly to determine the relative positions of different cell types and to determine the patterns of angiogenesis and innervation—though this is still largely conjectural. Chemotaxis is potentially a powerful pattern generator if the responding cells can modify and/or produce the gradient field.

Apart from chemotaxis, there also exists the possibility of mechanically mediated cellular responses to flow conditions in the fluid phase. The principal situation in vivo where this is likely to be important is in the blood vessels, and the mechanical effects of flow on the endothelial cells that line the vessel walls has been investigated.

Cellular Interactions with the Acellular Solid Phase

In a tissue, the acellular solid phase is the extracellular matrix, which is usually a fibrillar meshwork, though it may take the laminar form of a basement membrane. One directed response to the fibrillar extracellular matrix is the guidance of cell migrations, during embryonic development, for example, along oriented matrix fibrils. The discovery of this response followed soon after the dawn of tissue culture and is generally attributed to Paul Weiss, who named it contact guidance in the 1930s, though Loeb and Fleisher had already observed in 1917 that cells tend to follow the "path of least resistance" along oriented matrix fibrils (see [Dunn, 1982]). In culture, contact guidance constrains cell locomotion to be predominantly bidirectional, along the alignment axis of the matrix, whereas many embryonic migrations are predominantly unidirectional. This raises the question of whether contact guidance alone can account for these directed migrations in vivo or whether other responses are involved. The *influence on tissue architecture* of contact guidance is less conjectural than that of chemotaxis, since matrix alignment is more easily observed than chemical gradients, and the cells themselves are often coaligned with the matrix. Directed motion can be inferred since, in culture, this orientation of the cell shape on aligned surfaces is strongly correlated with an orientation of locomotion. In conjunction with cellular remodeling of the matrix, contact guidance becomes a potentially powerful generator of pattern. Since the cells, by exerting tension, can align the matrix, and the matrix alignment can guide the cells, a mutual interaction can arise whereby cells are guided into regions of higher cell density. Harris and colleagues [1984] have shown that such a feedback loop can result in the spontaneous generation of a regular array of cell clusters from a randomly distributed field of cells and matrix. The pattern of feather formation in birds' skin, for example, might arise by just such a mechanism.

Several other types of directed response may be mediated by the properties of the solid phase of the cell's environment. One is chemoaffinity, which Sperry [1963] proposed could account for the specific connections of the nervous system by guiding nerve fibers along tracks marked out by specific molecules adsorbed to the surface of substratum. A similar response has been proposed to account for the directional migration of primordial germs cells.

Cellular Interactions with Other Cells

Neighboring cells in the tissue environment may be considered as part of the solid phase. Thus it has been reported that when cells are used as a substratum for locomotion by other cells, directed responses such as contact guidance or chemoaffinity may occur, and these responses may persist even if the cells used as a substratum are killed by light fixation. However, the reason that cell-cell interactions are dealt with separately here is that cells show a directed response on colliding with other living cells that they do not show on colliding with cells that have been lightly fixed. Contact inhibition of locomotion, discovered by Abercrombie and Heaysman [1954], is a response whereby a normal tissue cell, on collision with another, is halted and eventually redirected in its locomotion. The effect of the response is to prevent cells from using other cells as a substratum, and a distinguishing feature of the response to living cells is a temporary local paralysis of the cell's active leading edge at the site of contact, which does not generally occur with a chemoaffinity type of response. The *influence on tissue architecture* of contact inhibition is probably profound but not easily determined. It is possibly the main response by which cells are kept more or less in place within a tissue, rather than milling around, and failure of contact inhibition is thought to be responsible for the infiltration of a normal tissue by invasive malignant cells. Contact inhibition can cause cell locomotion to be directed away from centers of population and thus gives rise to the radial pattern of cell orientation that is commonly observed in the outgrowths from explant cultures. A major question is whether this motile response is related, mechanistically, to the so-called contact inhibition of growth, which is also known to fail in malignant cells but which is probably mediated by diffusion of some signal rather than by cell-cell contact.

113.2 Engineering Directed Motile Responses in Vitro

The investigation of the directed motile responses, using tissue culture, can reveal many aspects of the mechanisms that control and direct cell motility in vivo and also give a valuable insight into the mechanism of cell motility. In fact, most of what we know about these responses in vivo is deduced from experiments in culture. On the other hand, many of the responses discovered in culture may never occur naturally, and yet their study is equally important because it may yield further clues to the mechanism of cell motility and result in valuable techniques for tissue engineering. However, responses to properties of the culture environment, such as electric or magnetic fields, that are not yet known to have any counterparts in vivo will not be dealt with here.

A general experimental approach to engineering motile responses is first to try to reproduce in culture some response that appears to occur in vivo. The main reason is that the cell behavior can be observed in vitro, whereas this is possible in vivo only in very few instances. Another important reason is that once achieved in vitro, the response may be "dissected," by progressively simplifying the culture environment, until we isolate one or more well-defined properties that can each elicit a response. To be successful, this approach not only requires the design of culture environments that each isolate some specific environmental property and simultaneously allow the resulting cell behavior to be observed but also requires methods for adequately quantifying this resulting behavior.

When designing an artificial environment, it is important to consider its information content. Obviously, a uniform field of some scalar quantity is isotropic and cannot, therefore, elicit a directed motile response. A nondirected motile response, such as a change in speed caused by a change in some scalar property, is generally called a kinesis. Anisotropic uniform fields may be vector fields or higher-order tensor fields. In a uniform vector field, such as a linear concentration gradient, a cell may be able to distinguish opposite directions in the field and exhibit a unidirectional response, generally known as a taxis. Or cell movement perpendicular to the vector may predominate, which is sometimes known as a diataxis. In the case of a uniform field of some symmetric second-order tensor, such as strain or surface curvature, there is simply no information to distinguish opposite directions in the field, and yet orthogonal axes may be distinguished. This can give rise to a bidirectional response or, in three-dimensional fields, also to a response where translocation along one axis is suppressed. There is no generally agreed on name to cover all such possible responses, but the term guidance will be used here. Some examples of culture environments with specific physicochemical properties are given below.

Environments with Specific Properties of the Fluid Phase

A Linear Concentration Gradient

The most common method of reproducing the chemotaxis response in vitro is to use a Boyden chamber in which a gradient of some specific chemical is formed by diffusion across a membrane filter. The resulting directed cell translocation is inferred from the relative number of cells that migrate through the pores of the filter from its upper to its lower surface. While this system is very useful for screening for potential chemoattractants, its usefulness for investigating the mechanism of the motile response is strictly limited, since it does not fulfill our two main criteria for an in vitro system. In the Boyden chamber, the properties of the environment are not well defined (since the gradient within the narrow, often tortuous pores of the filter is unpredictable), and the cell response cannot be observed directly. The Zigmond chamber was introduced to overcome these difficulties, by allowing the cell behavior to be observed directly, but the gradient is very unstable and cannot be maintained reliably for longer than an hour or two. Zicha and colleagues [1991] have recently developed a direct viewing chemotactic chamber with much greater stability and better optical properties. The chamber is constructed from glass and has an annular bridge separating concentric wells (Fig. 113.1). When covered by a coverslip carrying the cells, a gap of precisely 20 μm is formed between coverslip and bridge in which the gradient develops. The blind central well confers the greater stability, which allows chemotactic gradients to be maintained for many hours and thus permits the chemotactic responses of slowly moving tissue cells and malignant cells to be studied for the first time. Weber Scientific International, Ltd., manufactures this as the Dunn chamber.

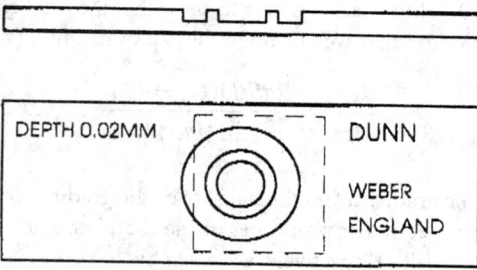

FIGURE 113.1   The Dunn Chemotaxis chamber.

In use, both wells of the chamber are initially filled with control medium. The coverslip carrying the cells is then inverted over the wells, firmly seated, and sealed with wax in a slightly offset position (shown by the dashed lines) to allow access to the outer well. The outer well is then emptied using a syringe, refilled with medium containing the substance under test at known concentration, and the narrow opening is sealed with wax.

Assuming that diffusion is the only mechanism of mass transport in the 20-μm gap between coverslip and bridge, whereas convection currents keep the bulk contents of the two wells stirred, then the concentration in the 20-μm gap as a function of distance r from the center of the inner well is given by

$$C(r) = \frac{C_i \ln(b/r) + C_o \ln(r/a)}{\ln(b/a)} \tag{113.1}$$

where C_i and C_o are the concentrations in the inner and outer wells, respectively, and a and b are the inner and outer radii of the bridge. Because the bridge is annular, the gradient is slightly convex, but the deviation from linearity is very small.

Figure 113.2 shows the formation of the gradient during the first hour for a molecule with diffusion coefficient $D = 13.3 \times 10^{-5}$ mm²/s, such as a small globular protein of molecular weight 17 kD, and chamber dimensions $a = 2.8$ mm, $b = 3.9$ mm. The equations describing gradient formation

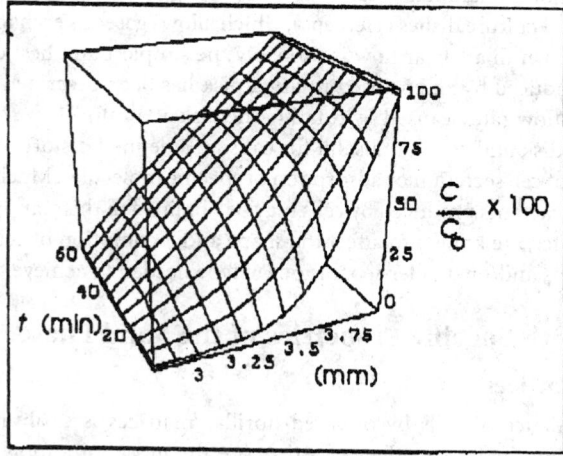

FIGURE 113.2   Formation of the gradient in the Dunn chemotaxis chamber (see text).

are given in Zicha et al. [1991], but it suffices here to show that the gradient is almost linear after 30 minutes. The flux from outer to inner well through the gap of height h (= 20 μm) is given by

$$\frac{dQ}{dt} = \frac{2\pi h D (C_o - C_i)}{\ln(b/a)} \tag{113.2}$$

This flux tends to destroy the gradient, and the half-life of the gradient is equal to $(\ln 2)/kD$, where k is a constant describing the geometric properties of the chamber. For a chamber with volumes v_o and v_i of the outer and inner wells, respectively, k is given by

$$k = \frac{2\pi h(v_i + v_o)}{\ln(b/a)v_i v_o} \tag{113.3}$$

Thus, for our small protein, a chamber with v_o = 30 μl, v_i = 14 μl, and other dimensions as before gives a gradient with a half-life of 33.6 hours. This is ample time to study the chemotaxis of slowly moving tissue cells, with typical speeds of around 1 μm per minute, as well as permitting the study of long-term chemotaxis in the more rapidly moving leukocytes with typical speeds of around 10 μm per minute.

From the point of view of information content, a linear concentration gradient may be viewed as a nonuniform scalar field of concentration or as a uniform vector field of concentration gradient. Thus, if the cell can distinguish between absolute values of concentration, as well as being able to detect the gradient, then the chemotaxis response may be complicated by a superimposed **chemokinesis** response. A stable linear concentration gradient is a great advantage when trying to unravel such complex responses. Other sources of complexity are the possibilities that cells can modify the gradient by acting as significant sinks, can relay chemotactic signals by releasing pulses of chemoattractant, or can even generate chemotactic signals in response to nonchemotactic chemical stimulation. These possibilities offer endless opportunities for chaotic behavior and pattern generation.

A Gradient of Shear Flow

The flow conditions in the fluid phase of the environment can have at least two possible effects on cell motility. First, by affecting mass transport, they can change the distribution of molecules, and second, they can cause a mechanical shear stress to be exerted on the cells. Figure 113.3 shows a culture chamber designed by Dunn and Ireland [1985] that allows the behavior of cells to be observed under conditions of laminar shear flow. If necessary, the cells may be grown on the special membrane in Petriperm culture dishes (Heraeus), which allows gaseous exchange into the medium beneath the glass disk. Laminar shear flow is probably the simplest and best defined flow regime, and the shear flow produced by an enclosed rotating disk has been described in detail [Daily and Nece, 1960]. Very low flow rates, caused by rotating the disk at around 1 rpm with a separation of about 1 mm between disk and cells, are useful for causing a defined distortion to diffusion gradients arising as a result of cell secretion or adsorption of specific molecules. Much information about, for example, chemoattractants produced by cells may be obtained in this way. Higher shear stresses, around 100 times greater, are known to affect the shape and locomotion of cells mechanically, and higher rotational speeds and/or smaller separations will be needed to achieve these.

Environments with Specific Properties of the Solid Phase

Aligned Fibrillar Matrices

The bidirectional guidance of cells by oriented fibrillar matrices is easily replicated in culture models. Plasma clots and hydrated collagen lattices are the most commonly used subtrates, and alignment may be achieved by shear flow, mechanical stress, or strong magnetic fields during the gelling process. The magnitude and direction of orientation may be monitored, after suitable calibration, by measuring the birefringence in a polarizing microscope equipped with a Brace-Köhler

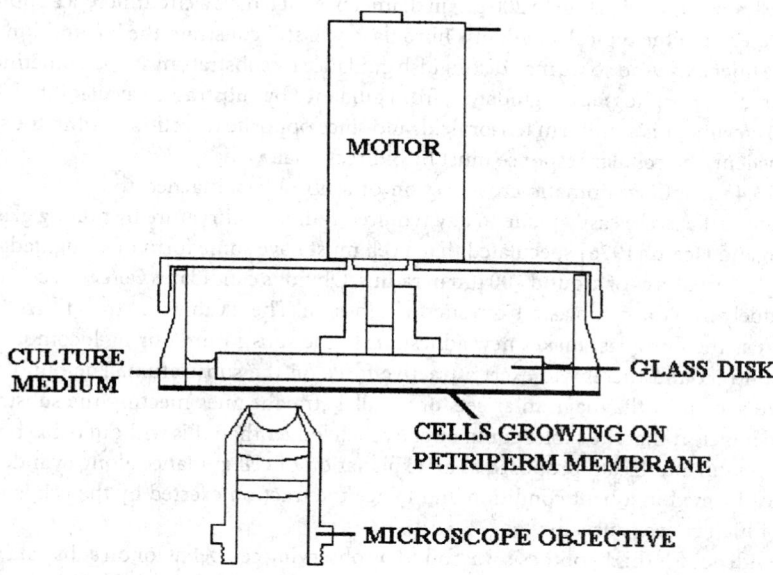

FIGURE 113.3   A culture chamber for laminar shear flow.

compensator. These methods of alignment result in environments that are approximately described as uniform tensor fields, since mechanical strain is a familiar second-order tensor, and they generally give rise to bidirectional motile responses. In three dimensions, the strain tensor that results from applying tension along one axis can be described as a prolate ellipsoid, whereas applying compression along one axis results in an oblate ellipsoid. Thus we might distinguish between prolate guidance, in which bidirectional locomotion predominates along a single axis, and oblate guidance, in which locomotion is relatively suppressed along one of the three axes. But unidirectional information can be imposed on an oriented fibrillar matrix. Boocock [1989] achieved a unidirectional cellular response, called desmotaxis, by allowing the matrix fibrils to form attachments to the underlying solid substratum before aligning them using shear flow. This results in an asymmetrical linkage of the fibrils, and similar matrix configurations may well occur in vivo.

Fibrillar environments in culture are probably good models for the type of cell guidance that occurs in vivo, but they are so complex that it is difficult to determine which anisotropic physicochemical properties elicit the cellular response. Among the possibilities are morphologic properties (the anisotropic shape or texture of the matrix), chemical properties (an oriented pattern of adhesiveness or specific chemical affinity), and mechanical properties (an anisotropic viscoelasticity of the matrix). One approach to discovering which properties are dominant in determining the response is to try to modify each in turn while leaving the others unaffected. This is difficult, though some progress has been made. Another approach is to design simpler environments with better defined properties, as described in the sections that follow.

Specific Shapes and Textures

Ross Harrison, the inventor of tissue culture, placed spiders' webs in some cultures and reported in 1912 that "The behavior of cells . . . shows not only that the surface of a solid is a necessary condition but also that when the latter has a specific linear arrangement, as in the spider web, it has an action in influencing the direction of movement." It is hardly surprising to us today that a cell attached to a very fine fiber, in a fluid medium, is constrained to move bidirectionally. Nevertheless, such stereotropism or guidance by substratum availability is a guidance response and may have relevance to the problem of guidance by aligned fibrillar matrices. Moreover, in the hands of Paul Weiss, the guidance of cells on single cylindrical glass fibers was shown to have a more subtle aspect, and it is now known that fibers up to 200 μm in diameter, which have a circumference approximately 10 times greater than the typical length of a fibroblast, will still constrain the locomotion to be parallel with the fiber axis. And so we may distinguish guidance by substratum shape, sometimes known as topographic or morphographic guidance, from guidance by substratum availability. The surface curvature of a cylinder is a uniform tensor field, and since opposite directions within the surface are always equivalent, the cellular response must be bidirectional.

Figure 113.4a is a diagrammatic cross section of a fibroblast attached to a convex cylindrical surface. These surfaces are easily made to any required radius of curvature by pulling glass rod in a flame. Dunn and Heath [1976] speculated that a cell must have some form of straightedge in order to detect slight curvatures of around 100 μm in radius. Obvious candidates were the actin cables that extend obliquely into the cytoplasm from sites of adhesion. These cables or stress fibers are continually formed as the fibroblast makes new adhesions to the substratum during locomotion and are known to contract and thereby to exert a tractive force on the substratum. The bundles of actin filaments are shown in the diagram as sets of parallel straight lines meeting the substratum at a tangent, and it is clear that the cables could not be much longer than this without being bent around the cylinder. Dunn and Heath proposed as an explanation of cell guidance along cylinders that the cables do not formed in a bent condition and hence the traction exerted by the cell is reduced in directions of high convex curvature.

Further evidence for this hypothesis was found by observing cell behavior on substrata with other shapes. On concave cylindrical surfaces, made by drawing glass tubing in a flame, the cells are not guided along the cylindrical axis but tend to become bipolar in shape and oriented perpendicular to the axis [Dunn, 1982]. This is to be expected, since, as shown in Fig. 113.4b, concave surfaces do not restrict the formation of unbent cables but allow the cells to spread up the walls, which lifts the body of the cell clear of the substratum and thus prevents spreading along the cylinder axis. On substrata made with a sharp change in inclination like the pitched roof of a house, the hypothesis predicts that locomotion across the ridge is inhibited when the angle of inclination is greater than the angle at which the actin cables normally meet a plane substratum, as in Fig. 113.4c. These substrata are more difficult to make than cylinders and require precision optical techniques for grinding and polishing a sharp and accurate ridge angle. Fibroblasts behaved as predicted on these substrata, the limiting angle being about 4 degrees, and high-voltage electron microscopy revealed that actin cables terminate precisely at the ridge on substrata with inclinations greater than this.

Substrata with fine parallel grooves have long been known to be very effective for eliciting morphographic guidance and are interesting because they can be a well-defined mimicry of some of the shape properties of an aligned fibrillar matrix while being mechanically rigid. Effective substrata can easily be made by simply scratching a glass surface with a very fine abrasive, but such substrata are not well defined, and their lack of uniformity may give rise to variations in macro-properties, such as wettability, that cannot be ruled out as causing the guidance. Early attempts to make better-defined substrata used ruling engines such as those used to make diffraction gratings, but Dunn and Brown [1986] introduced electron beam lithography followed by ion milling to make grooves of rectangular cross section down to about 1 μm in width. Clark and colleagues [Clark et al., 1991] have now achieved rectangular grooves with spacings as low as 260 nm using the interference of two wavefronts, obtained by splitting an argon laser beam, to produce a pattern of parallel fringes on a quartz slide coated with photoresist. Groove depths a small as 100 nm can elicit a guidance response from certain cell types, and the main reason for pursuing this line of enquiry is now to discover the molecular mechanism responsible for this exquisite sensitivity.

Figure 113.4c shows a diagrammatic cross section of a fibroblast on a substratum consisting of a parallel array of rectangular grooves. One question that has been debated is whether the cells generally sink into the grooves, as shown here, or bridge across them. In the latter case, the wall and floor of the grooves are not an available substratum, and the cellular response might be a form of guidance by substratum availability. Ohara and Buck [1979] have suggested that this might occur, since the focal adhesions of fibroblasts are generally elongated in the direction of cell movement,

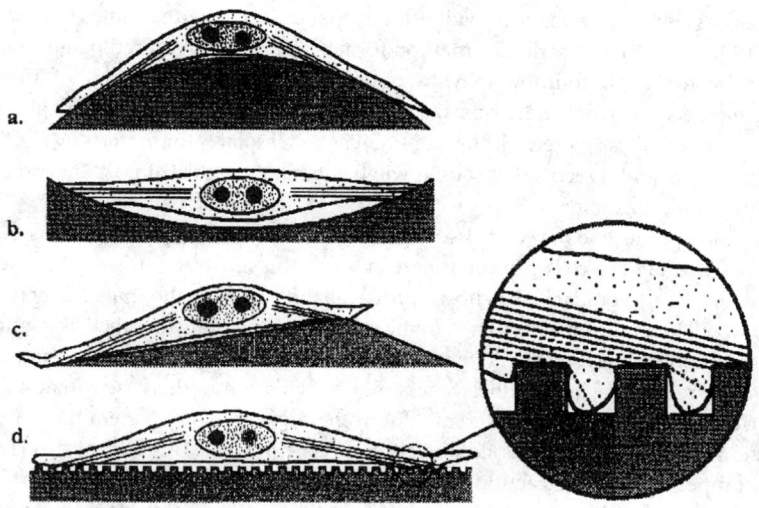

FIGURE 113.4 Diagrammatic cross-sections of fibroblasts on subtrata of various shapes.

and if they are forced to become oriented by being confined to the narrow spaces between grooves, this may force the locomotion into the same orientation. On the other hand, if the cells do generally sink into the grooves, then the Dunn and Heath hypothesis also could account for guidance even by very fine grooves, since individual actin filaments in the bundles, shown as dashed lines in the inset to the figure, would become bent and possibly disrupted if the cell made any attempt to pull on them other than in a direction parallel with the grooves. It is still therefore an unresolved issue whether different mechanisms operate in the cases of cylinders and grooves or whether a common mechanism is responsible for all cases of guidance by the shape of the substratum. Other groove profiles, particularly asymmetrical ones such as sawtooth profiles, will be needed for testing these and other rival hypotheses, and an intriguing possibility is that a unidirectional cell response might be achieved on microfabricated substrata with two orthogonal arrays of parallel sawtooth grooves, as shown in Fig. 113.5.

Specific Patterns of Adhesiveness

The equivalent in culture of the chemoaffinity response is **guidance by differential adhesiveness,** in which cell locomotion is confined to regions of higher adhesiveness patterned on the substrate. As with grooved surfaces, adhesive tracks that guide cells effectively are easily made by a variety of methods, including physically streaking nonadhesive viscous materials on an adhesive substratum or scratching through a nonadhesive film overlying an adhesive substratum. Again, however, these easily made surfaces are not well defined, and in particular, their anisotropic adhesiveness tends to be contaminated by anisotropic surface texture and sometimes by anisotropic mechanical properties. Carter [1965] was probably the first to describe a method of printing a well-defined pattern of adhesiveness onto a substratum; he used the vacuum evaporation of palladium, through a

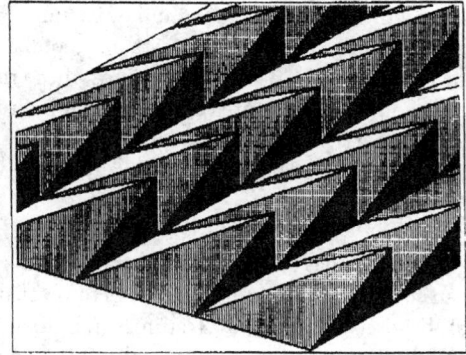

FIGURE 113.5 A proposed microfabricated substratum with two orthogonal arrays of parallel saw tooth grooves.

mask, onto a glass substratum made nonadhesive by first coating it with cellulose acetate. Clark and colleagues [1992] have now described a method for fabricating any required pattern of differential adhesiveness by using photolithography to obtain a hydrophobic pattern of methyl groups covalently coupled to a hydrophilic quartz substratum. The most recent developments in their laboratories are to use these patterns of hydrophobicity as templates for patterning specific proteins onto the substratum, and it seems that soon it will be possible to make almost any required pattern in any combination of proteins.

The explanation of the guidance of cells along tracks of higher adhesiveness appears to be obvious. In extreme cases, when the cells cannot adhere at all to the substrate outside the track, then the response is equivalent to guidance by substratum availability, and if the track happens to be sufficiently narrow, cell locomotion is restricted to the two directions along the track. But guidance along tracks of higher adhesiveness may still be very pronounced even when the cells also can adhere to and move on the regions of lower adhesiveness. The explanation in this case is that on encountering boundaries between regions of different adhesiveness, cells will cross them far more frequently in the direction from lower to higher adhesiveness. It is generally assumed that this results from a tug-of-war competition, since traction can be applied more effectively by the parts of the cell overlapping the region of higher adhesiveness. It is not known, however, how the traction fails in those parts of the cell which lose the competition, whether by breakage or slipping of the adhesions or by a relative failure of the contractile apparatus. Another possibility is simply that the cell spreads more easily over the more highly adhesive regions.

One reason for studying guidance by differential adhesiveness is to discover whether it can account for guidance by oriented extracellular matrices. An array of very narrow, parallel stripes of alternately high and low adhesiveness mimics the linear arrangement of substratum availability in an aligned matrix. Dunn [1982] found that if the repeat spacing is so small that a cell can span several stripes, there is no detectable cell orientation or directed locomotion even though an isolated adhesive stripe can strongly guide cells. Clark and colleagues [1992] confirmed this observation with one cell type (BHK) but found that cells of another type (MDCK) could become aligned even when spanning several stripes but would become progressively less elongated as the repeat spacing decreased. It is not yet clear, therefore, whether the linear arrangement of substratum availability in an aligned matrix might contribute to the guidance response in some cell types. It is clear from the work of Clark and colleagues, however, that the adhesive stripes become less effective in eliciting guidance as their repeat spacing decreases, whereas the opposite is true for grooved surfaces. Thus it seems unlikely that substratum availability is the mechanism of guidance by grooved surfaces and, conversely, unlikely that adhesive stripes guide cells by influencing the orientation of the focal adhesions as suggested for grooved surfaces by Ohara and Buck [1979].

Binary patterns of adhesiveness were not the only ones studied by Carter [1965]. His technique of shadowing metallic palladium by vacuum evaporation onto cellulose acetate also could produce a graded adhesiveness. By placing a rod of 0.5 mm diameter on the substratum before shadowing, he found that the penumbral regions of the rod's shadow acted as steep gradients of adhesiveness that would cause cultured cells to move unidirectionally in the direction of increasing adhesiveness. This is therefore a taxis as distinct from a guidance response, and he named it haptotaxis. It is still not clear whether haptotaxis plays any role in vivo.

Specific Mechanical Properties

As yet, there has been no demonstration that anisotropic mechanical properties of the substratum can elicit directed motile responses. However, it is known that isotropic mechanical properties, such as the viscosity of the substratum, can influence cell locomotion [Harris, 1982], and it appears that changing the mechanical properties of aligned matrices can reduce cell guidance [Dunn, 1982; Haston et al., 1983], although it is probable that other properties are altered at the same time. Moreover, the phenomenon of desmotaxis suggests that it is the asymmetrical mechanical linkage of the fibrils that biases the locomotion. Guidance by anisotropic mechanical properties therefore remains a distinct possibility, but further progress is hampered by the difficulty of fabricating well-defined substrata. An ideal substratum would be a flat, featureless, and chemically uniform surface with anisotropic viscoelastic properties, and it is possible that liquid crystal surfaces will provide the answer.

Environments with Specific Arrangements of Neighboring Cells

Although contact inhibition of locomotion is of primary importance in determining patterns that develop in populations of cells, it is not easy to control the effects of contact inhibition in culture. If the cells are seeded on the substratum at nonuniform density, the response will generally cause cell locomotion to be biased in the direction of decreasing cell density. This can give a unidirectional bias if superimposed on a guidance response, and it has been conjectured that certain cell migrations in vivo are biased in this way. Cellular contact responses also can lead to the mutual orientation of confluent neighboring cells, and this can lead to wide regions of cooriented cells arising spontaneously in uniformly seeded cultures.

A typical culture arrangement for studying contact inhibition is to seed two dense populations of cells, often primary explants of tissue, about 1 mm apart on the substratum [Abercrombie and Heaysman, 1976]. Homologous contact inhibition causes the cells to migrate radially from these foci, usually as confluent sheets, until the two populations collide. With noninvasive cells, their locomotion is much reduced after the populations have met, and there is little intermixing at the population boundary. If one of the two populations is of an invasive type, however, failure of heterologous contact inhibition will cause it to infiltrate the other population, and their invasiveness can be measured by the depth of interpenetration.

Defining Terms

Associated movements: Occur when cells passively change position as a result of external forces, generated by cell motility elsewhere, that are transmitted either through the extracellular matrix or through cell-cell contacts.

Cell motility: A blanket term that covers all aspects of movement actively generated by a cell. It includes changes in cell shape, cell contraction, protrusion and retraction of processes, intracellular motility, and cell translocation.

Cell translocation, cell locomotion, or cell migration: All describe active changes in position of a cell in relation to its substratum. The translocation of tissue cells always requires a solid or semisolid substratum. In seeking a more rigorous definition, *position* must first be defined for both the cell and its substratum. This is not always easy, since both may change continually in shape.

Chemoaffinity: The directional translocation of cells or extension of cellular protrusions along narrow tracks of specific molecules adsorbed to the substratum.

Chemokinesis: A *kinesis* (q.v.) in which the stimulating scalar property is the concentration of some chemical.

Chemotaxis: The directional translocation of cells in a concentration gradient of some chemoattractant or chemorepellent substance.

Chemotropism: The directional extension of a cellular protrusion or multicellular process in a concentration gradient of some chemoattractant or chemorepellent substance.

Contact guidance: The directional translocation of cells in response to some anisotropic property of the substratum.

Contact inhibition of locomotion: Occurs when a cell collides with another and is halted and/or redirected so that it does not use the other cell as a substratum.

Desmotaxis: Describes a unidirectional bias of cell translocation in a fibrillar matrix that is allowed to attach to a solid support and then oriented by shear flow.

Diataxis: A *taxis* (q.v.) in which translocation perpendicular to the field vector predominates. This leads to a bidirectional bias in two dimensions.

Directed motile responses: The responses of cells to specific properties of their environment that can control the direction of cell translocation or, in the case of nerve growth, for example, can control the direction of extension of a cellular protrusion.

Guidance: Used here to indicate a directed response to some high-order tensor-like property of the environment in which opposite directions are equivalent. Translocation is biased bidirectionally in two dimensions.

Guidance by differential adhesiveness: A form of *guidance by substratum availability* (q.v.) in which cell locomotion is wholly or largely confined to narrow tracks of higher adhesiveness on the substratum. The response may be absent or much reduced if the cell spans several parallel tracks.

Guidance by substratum availability: Occurs when the translocation of a cell is confined to an isolated narrow track either because no alternative substratum exists or because the cell is unable to adhere to it.

Guidance by substratum shape, topographic guidance, or morphographic guidance: All refer to the guidance of cells by the shape or texture of the substratum. It is not known whether all types of morphographic guidance are due to a common mechanism.

Haptotaxis: The tendency of cells to translocate unidirectionally up a steep gradient of increasing adhesiveness of the substratum.

Heterologous contact inhibition: The *contact inhibition of locomotion* (q.v.) that may occur when a cell collides with another of different type. Contact inhibition is called nonreciprocal when the responses of the two participating cells are different. A cell type that is invasive with respect to another will generally fail to show contact inhibition in heterologous collisions.

Homologous contact inhibition: The *contact inhibition of locomotion* (q.v.) that may occur when a cell collides with another of the same type. It is not always appreciated that invasive cell types can show a high level of homologous contact inhibition.

Kinesis: The dependence of some parameter of locomotion, usually speed or rate of turning, on some scalar property of the environment. In an adaptive kinesis, the response is influenced by the rate of change of the scalar property, and if the environment is stable but spatially nonuniform, this can lead to behavior indistinguishable from a *taxis* (q.v.). Current nomenclature is inadequate to deal with such situations [Dunn, 1990].

Oblate guidance: A form of guidance in three dimensions in which translocation is suppressed along a single axis.

Prolate guidance: A form of guidance in three dimensions in which translocation along a single axis predominates.

Stereotropism: A form of *guidance by substratum availability* (q.v.) in which the only solid support available for locomotion consists of isolated narrow fibers.

Taxis: A directed response to some vectorlike property of the environment. Translocation is usually biased unidirectionally, either along the field vector or opposite to it, except in the case of *diataxis* (q.v.).

References

Abercrombie M, Heaysman JEM. 1954. Observations on the social behaviour of cells in tissue culture. Exp Cell Res 6:293.

Boocock CA. 1989. Unidirectional displacement of cells in fibrillar matrices. Development 107:881.

Carter SB. 1965. Principles of cell motility: The direction of cell movement and cancer invasion. Nature 208:1183.

Clark P, Connolly P, Curtis ASG, et al. 1991. Cell guidance by ultrafine topography in vitro. J Cell Sci 99:73.

Clark P, Connolly P, Moores GR. 1992. Cell guidance by micropatterned adhesiveness in vitro. J Cell Sci 103:287.

Daily JW, Nece RE. 1960. Chamber dimension effects on induced flow and frictional resistance of enclosed rotating disks. Trans Am Soc Mech Engrs D82:217.

Dunn GA. 1982. Contact guidance of cultured tissue cells: A survey of potentially relevant properties of the substratum. In R Bellairs, A Curtis, G Dunn (eds), Cell Behaviour: A Tribute to Michael Abercrombie, pp 247–280. Cambridge, Cambridge University Press.

Dunn GA. 1990. Conceptual problems with kinesis and taxis. In JP Armitage, JM Lackie (eds), Biology of the Chemotactic Response, pp 1–13. Society for General Microbiology Symposium, 46. Cambridge, Cambridge University Press.

Dunn GA, Brown AF. 1986. Alignment of fibroblasts on grooved surfaces described by a simple geometric transformation. J Cell Sci 83:313.

Dunn GA, Heath JP. 1976. A new hypothesis of contact guidance in tissue cells. Exp Cell Res 101:1.

Dunn GA, Ireland GW. 1984. New evidence that growth in 3T3 cell cultures is a diffusion-limited process. Nature 312:63.

Harris AK. 1982. Traction and its relation to contraction in tissue cell locomotion. In R Bellairs, A Curtis, G Dunn (eds), Cell Behaviour: A Tribute to Michael Abercrombie, pp 109–134. Cambridge, Cambridge University Press.

Harris AK, Stopak D, Warner P. 1984. Generation of spatially periodic patterns by a mechanical instability: A mechanical alternative to the Turing model. J Emb Exp Morph 80:1.

Harrison LG. 1993. Kinetic Theory of Living Pattern, Cambridge, Cambridge University Press.

Haston WS, Shields JM, Wilkinson PC. 1983. The orientation of fibroblasts and neutrophils on elastic substrata. Exp Cell Res 146:117.

Ohara PT, Buck RC. 1979. Contact guidance in vitro: A light, transmission and scanning electron microscopic study. Exp Cell Res 121:235.

Sperry RW. 1963. Chemoaffinity in the orderly growth of nerve fiber patterns and connections. Proc Natl Acad Sci USA 50:703.

Zicha D, Dunn GA, Brown AF. 1991. A new direct-viewing chemotaxis chamber. J Cell Sci 99:769.

114

Tissue Microenvironments

Michael W. Long
University of Michigan

Tissue development is regulated by a complex set of events in which cells of the developing organ interact with each other, with general and specific growth factors, and with the surrounding extracellular matrix (ECM) [Long, 1992]. These interactions are important for a variety of reasons such as localizing cells within the microenvironment, directing cellular migration, and initiating growth-factor-mediated developmental programs. It should be realized, however, that simple interactions such as those between cells and growth factor are not the sole means by which developing cells are regulated. Further complexity occurs via interactions of cells and growth factors with extracellular matrix or via other interactions which generate specific developmental responses.

Developing tissue cells interact with a wide variety of regulators during their ontogeny. Each of these interactions is mediated by defined, specific receptor-ligand interactions necessary to stimulate both the cell proliferation and/or motility. For example, both chemical and/or extracellular matrix gradients exist which signal the cell to move along "tracks" of molecules into a defined tissue area. As well, high concentrations of the attractant, or other signals, next serve to "localize" the cell, thus stopping its nonrandom walk. These signals which stop and/or regionalize cells in appropriate microenvironments are seemingly complex. For example, in the hematopoietic system, complexes of cytokines and extracellular matrix molecules serve to localize progenitor cells [Long et al., 1992], and similar mechanisms of cell/matrix/cytokine interactions undoubtedly exist in other developing systems. Thus, the regulation of cell development, which ultimately leads to tissue formation, is a complex process in which a number of elements work in cohort to bring about coordinated organogenesis: stromal and parenchymal cells, growth factors and extracellular matrix. Each of these is a key component of a localized and highly organized microenvironmental regulatory system.

Cellular interactions can be divided into three classes: cell-cell, cell-extracellular matrix, and cell-growth factor, each of which is functionally significant for both mature and developing cells. For example, in a number of instances blood cells interact with each other and/or with cells in other tissues. Immunologic cell-cell interactions occur when lymphocytes interact with antigen-presenting cells, whereas neutrophil or lymphocyte egress from the vasculature exemplifies blood cell–endothelial cell recognition. Interactions between cells and the extracellular matrix (the complex protinaceous substance surrounding cells) also play an important role. During embryogenesis matrix molecules are involved both in cell migration and in stimulating cell function. Matrix components are also important in the growth and development of precursor cells; they also serve either as cytoadhesion molecules for these cells or to compartmentalize growth factors within specific microenvironmental locales. For certain tissues such as bone marrow, a large amount of information exists concerning the various components of the nature of the microenvironment. For others such as bone, much remains to be learned of the functional microenvironment components. Many experimental designs have examined simple interactions (e.g., cell-cell, cell-matrix). However, the situation in vivo is undoubtedly much more complex. For example, growth factors are often bound to matrix molecules which, in turn, are expressed on the surface of underlying stromal cells. Thus, very complex interactions occur (e.g., accessory cell–stromal cell–growth factor–progenitor cell–matrix, see Fig. 114.1), and these can be further complicated by a developmental requirement for multiple growth factors.

The multiplicity of tissue-cell interactions requires highly specialized cell surface structures (i.e., receptors) to both mediate cell adhesion and transmit intracellular signals from other cells, growth factors, and/or the ECM. Basically, two types of receptor structures exist. Most cell surface receptors are proteins which consist of an extracellular ligand-binding domain, a hydrophobic membrane-spanning region, and a cytoplasmic region which usually functions in signal transduction. The amino acid sequence of these receptors often defines various families of receptors (e.g., immunoglobulin and integrin gene superfamilies). However, some receptors are not linked to the cell surface by protein, as certain receptors contain phosphotidylinositol-based membrane linkages. This type of receptor is usually associated with signal transduction events mediated by phospholipase C activation [Springer, 1990]. Other cell surface molecules important in receptor-ligand interactions are surface proteins which function as a coreceptors. Coreceptors function with a well-defined receptor, usually to amplify stimulus-response coupling.

The goal of this chapter is to examine the common features of each component of the microenvironment (cellular elements, soluble growth factors, and extracellular matrix). As each tissue or organ undergoes its own unique and complex developmental program, this review cannot cover these elements for all organs and tissue types. Rather, two types of microenvironments (blood and bone) will be compared in order to illustrate commonalities and distinctions.

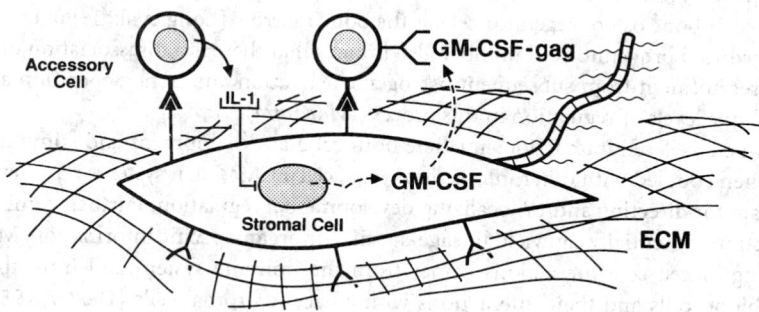

FIGURE 114.1   Hematopoietic cellular interactions. This figure illustrates the varying complexities of putative hematopoietic cell interactions. A conjectural complex is shown in which accessory cell–stromal cell, hematopoietic cell–stromal cell, and stromal cell–PG–growth factor complexes localize developmental signals. ECM = extracellular matrix, gag = glycosaminoglycan side chain bound to proteoglycan (PG) core protein (indicated by cross-hatched curved molecule); IL-1 = interleukin-1; GM-CSF = granulocyte-macrophage colony-stimulating factor. Modified from Long [1992] and reprinted with permission.

114.1 Cellular Elements

Cells develop in a distinct hierarchical fashion. During the ontogeny of any organ, cells migrate to the appropriate region for the nascent tissue to form and there undergo a phase of rapid proliferation and differentiation. In tissues which retain their proliferative capacity (bone marrow, liver, skin, the gastrointestinal lining, and bone), the complex hierarchy of proliferation cells is retained throughout life. This is best illustrated in the blood-forming (hematopoiesis) system. Blood cells are constantly produced, such that approximately 70-times an adult human's body weight of blood cells is produced throughout the human life span. This implies the existence of a very primitive cell type that retains the capacity for self-renewal. This cell is called a *stem cell,* and it is the cell responsible of the engraphment of hematopoiesis in recipients of bone marrow transplantation. Besides a high proliferative potential, the stem cell also is characterized by its multipotentiality in that it can generate progeny (referred to as *progenitor cells*) which are committed to each of the eight blood cell lineages. As hematopoietic cells proliferate, they progressively lose their proliferative capacity and become increasingly restricted in lineage potential. As a result, the more primitive progenitor cells in each lineage produce higher colony numbers, and the earliest cells detectable in vitro produce progeny of 2–3 lineages (there is no in vitro assay for transplantable stem cells). Similar stem cell hierarchies exist for skin and other regenerating tissues, but fewer data exist concerning their hierarchical nature.

The regulation of bone cell development is induced during bone morphogenesis by an accumulation of extracellular and intracellular signals [Urist et al., 1983a]. Like other systems, extracellular signals are known to be transferred from both cytokines and extracellular matrix molecules [Urist et al., 1983a] to responding cell surface receptors, resulting in eventual bone formation. The formation of bone occurs by two mechanisms. Direct development of bone from mesenchymal cells (referred to as *intramembranous ossification,* as observed in skull formation) occurs when mesenchymal cells directly differentiate into bone tissue. The second type of bone formation (the endochondral bone formation of skeletal bone) occurs via an intervening cartilage model. Thus, the familiar cell hierarchy exists in the development and growth of long bones, beginning with the proliferation of mesenchymal stem cells, their differentiation into osteogenic progenitor cells, and then into osteoblasts. The osteoblasts eventually calcify their surrounding cartilage and/or bone matrix to form bone. Interestingly, the number of osteoprogenitor cells in adult bone seems too small to replace all the large mass of bone normally remodeled in the process of aging of the skeleton [Urist et al., 1983a]. Observations from this laboratory confirm this concept by showing that one (unexpected) source of bone osteoprogenitor cells is the bone marrow [Long et al., 1990; Long & Mann, 1993]. This reduced progenitor cell number also implies that there is a disassociation of bone progenitor cell recruitment from subsequent osteogenic activation and bone deposition and further suggests multiple levels of regulation in this process (*vide infra*).

As mentioned, cell-cell interactions mediate both cellular development and stimulus-response coupling. When coupled with other interactions (e.g., cell-ECM), such systems represent a powerful mechanism for directing and/or localizing developmental regulation. Further, combinations of these interactions potentially can yield lineage-specific or organ-specific information. Much of our understanding of cell-cell interactions comes from the immune system and from the study of developing blood cells and their interactions with adjacent stromal cells [Dexter, 1982; Gallatin et al., 1986; Springer, 1990]. For example, the isolation and cloning of immune cell ligands and receptors resulted in the classification of gene families which mediate cell-cell interactions within the immune and hematopoietic system, and similar systems undoubtedly play a role in the development of many tissues.

There are three families of molecules which mediate cell-cell interactions (Table 114.1). The immunoglobulin superfamily is expressed predominantly on cells mediating immune and inflammatory responses (and is discussed only briefly here). The integrin family is a large group of highly versatile proteins which is involved in cell-cell and cell-matrix attachment. Finally, the selectin family

TABLE 114.1   Cell Adhesion Molecule Superfamilies

Immunoglobulin superfamily of adhesion receptors

LFA 2 (CD2)	T-cell receptor (CD3)
LFA 3 (CD58)	CD4 (TCR coreceptor)
ICAM 1 (CD54)	CD8 (TCR coreceptor)
ICAM 2	MHC class I
VCAM-1	MHC class II

Integrins
β₁ integrins (VLA proteins)
   P150,95 (CD11$_c$/CD18)
   VLA 1–3, 6
   VLA 4 (LPAM 1, CD49d/CD29)
   Fibronectin receptor (VLA 5, CD-/CD29)
   LPAM 2
β₂ Integrins
   LFA 1 (CD11$_a$/CD18)
   Mac 1 or Mo1 (CD11$_b$/CD18)
β₃ Integrins
   Vitronectin receptor
   Platelet gp-IIb/IIIa
Selectin/LEC-CAMS
   Mel 14 (LE-CAM-1, LHR, LAM-1, Leu 8, Ly 22, gp90 MEL)
   ELAM-1 (LE-CAM-2)
   GMP 140 (LE-CAM-3, PADGEM, CD62)

Source: Originally adapted from Springer [1990] and Brand-ley and coworkers [1990] and reprinted from Long [1992] with permission.

is comprised of molecules which are involved in lymphocyte, platelet, and leukocyte interactions with endothelial cells. Interestingly, this class of cell surface molecules utilizes specific glycoconjugates (encoded by glycoslytransferase genes) as their ligands on endothelial cell surfaces.

Immunoglobulin Gene Superfamily

These molecules function in both antigen recognition and cell-cell communication. The immunoglobulin superfamily (Table 114.2) is defined by a 90–100 base pair immunoglobulinlike domain found within a dimer of two antiparallel β strands [Sheetz et al., 1989; Williams & Barclay, 1988]; for a review, see Springer [1990]. Two members of this family, the T-cell receptor and immunoglobulin, function in antigen recognition. The T-cell receptor recognizes antigenic peptides in the context of two other molecules on the surface of antigen-presenting cells: major histocompatibility (MHC) class I and class II molecules [Bierer et al., 1989; Sheetz et al., 1989; Springer, 1990]. Whereas the binding of T-cell receptor to MHC/antigenic peptide complexes seems sufficient for cell-cell adhesion, cellular activation also requires the binding of either of two coreceptors, CD8 or CD4. Neither coreceptor can directly bind the MHC complex, but, rather, each seems to interact with the T-cell receptors to synergistically amplify intercellular signalling [Shaw et al., 1986; Spits et al., 1986; Springer, 1990].

Integrin Gene Superfamily

Integrin family members are involved in interactions between cells and extracellular matrix proteins [Giancotti & Ruoslahti, 1990]. Cell attachment to these molecules occurs rapidly (within minutes) and is a result of increased avidity rather than increased expression (see Lawrence and Springer [1991] and references therein). The binding sequence within the ligand for most, but not all, inte-

TABLE 114.2   Cell Surface Molecules Mediating Cell-Cell Interactions

Cell receptor	Receptor: cell expression	Ligand, co-, or counter-receptor	Ligand co- or counter-receptor cell expression	References
Ig superfamily				
MHC I	Macroph, T cell	CD8, TCR	T cells	Springer, 1990
MHC II	Macroph, T cell	CD4, TCR	T cells	Springer, 1990
ICAM-1	Endo, neut. HPC, B cells, T cells, macroph*	LFA-1	Mono, T and B cells	Springer, 1990
ICAM-2	Endo	LFA-1	Mono, T and B cells	Springer, 1990
LFA-2	T cells	LFA-3	T cells, eryth	Springer, 1990
Integrins				
Mac1	Macroph, neut	Fibrinogen, C3bi	Endo, plts	Springer, 1990
LFA-1	Macroph, neut	(See above)	(See above)	
VCAM	Endo	VLA4	Lymphocytes, monocytes, B cells	Brandley et al., 1990 Miyamake, 1990
gp150,95	Macro, neut.	(See above)	(See above)	
FN-R	Eryth lineage	Fibronectin	N.A.	see Table 114.3
IIb/IIIa	Plts, mk	Fibrinogen, TSP, VN, vWF	Endo	Springer, 1990
Selectins				
LEC-CAM-1 (Mel 14)	Endo	Addressins, neg. charged oligosaccrides	Lymphocytes	Brandley et al., 1990
ELAM-1 (LE-CAM-2)	Endo	sialyl-Lewis X[†]	Endo[‡] Neut, tumor cells	Lowe et al., 1990
LEC-CAM-3 (GMP-140)	Plt gran Weible-Palade bodies, endo	Lewis X (CD15)	Endo Neut	Brandley et al., 1990

*Source: Modified from Long [1992] and reprinted with permission. Macroph = macrophage; Mono = Monocyte; Endo = endothelial cell; Eryth = erythroid cells; Plts = Platelets; Neut = neutrophil; Mk = megakarocyte.
[†]Constituatively expressed by few cells, upregulated by TNF- and IL-1.
[‡]Sialylated, fucosylated lactosaminoglycans. Modified from Long [1992] and reprinted with permission.

grins is the tripeptide sequence arganine-glycine-asparagine (RGD) [Ruoslahti & Pierschbacher, 1987]. Structurally, integrins consist of two membrane-spanning alpha and beta chains. The alpha subunits contain three to four tandem repeats of a divalent-ion-binding motif and require magnesium or calcium to function. The alpha chains are (usually) distinct and bind with common or related β subunits to yield functional receptors [Giancotti & Ruoslahti, 1990]. The β subunits of integrins have functional significance, and integrins can be subclassified based on the presence of a given beta chain. Thus, integrins containing $\beta1$ and $\beta3$ chains are involved predominantly in cell-extracellular matrix interactions, whereas molecules containing the $\beta2$ subunits function in leukocyte-leukocyte adhesion (Tables 114.1 and 114.2). The cytoplasmic domain of many integrin receptors interacts with the cytoskeleton. For example, several integrins are known to localize near focal cell contacts where actin bundles terminate [Giancotti & Ruoslahti, 1990; Springer, 1990]. As a result, changes in receptor binding offer an important mechanism for linking cell adhesion to cytoskeletal organization.

Selectins

The selectin family of cell-adhesion receptors contain a single N-terminus, calcium-dependent, lectin-binding domain, an EGF receptor (EFGR) domain, and a region of cysteine-rich tandem repeats (from two to seven) which are homologous to complement-binding proteins [Bevilacqua et al., 1989; Springer, 1990; Stoolman, 1989]. Selectins (e.g., MEL14, gp90MEL, ELAM-1, and GMP140/PADGEM, Table 114-2) are expressed on neutrophils and lymphocytes. They recognize specific glycoconjugate ligands on endothelial and other cell surfaces. Early studies demonstrated that fucose or mannose could block lymphocyte attachment to lymph node endothelial cells [Brandley et al., 1990]. Therefore, the observation that the selectin contain a lectin-binding domain [Bevilacqua et al., 1989] led to the identification of the ligands for two members of this family; for review see Brandley and coworkers [1990]. Lowe and coworkers first demonstrated that alpha (1,3/1,4) fucosyltransferase cDNA converted nonmyeloid COS or CHO cells to selectin (sialyl-Lewis X) positive cells which bound to both HL60 cells and neutrophils in an ELAM-1-dependent manner [Lowe et al., 1990]. Conversely, Goelz and coworkers screened an expression library using a monoclonal antibody which inhibited ELAM-mediated attachment which yielded a novel alpha (1,3) fucosyltransferase whose expression conferred ELAM binding activity on target cells [Goelz et al., 1990].

Unlike mature neutrophils and lymphocytes, information on cell-cell interactions among hematopoietic progenitor cells is less well developed (see Table 114.3). Data concerning the cytoadhesive capacities of hematopoietic progenitor cells deal with the interaction of these cells with underlying, preestablished stromal cell layers [Dexter, 1982]. Gordon and colleagues documented that primitive hematopoietic human blast-colony forming cells (Bl-CFC) adhere to preformed stromal cell layers [Gordon et al., 1985, 1990b] and showed that the stromal cell ligand is not one of the known cell adhesion molecules [Gordon et al., 1987a]. Other investigators have shown that hematopoietic (CD34-selected) marrow cell populations attach to stromal cell layers and that the attached cells are enriched for granulocyte/macrophage progenitor cells [Liesveld et al., 1989]. Highly enriched murine spleen colony-forming cells (CFC-S) attach to stromal cell layers, proliferate, and differentiate into hematopoietic cells [Spooncer et al., 1985]. Interestingly, underlying bone marrow stromal cells can be substituted for by NIH 3T3 cells [Roberts et al., 1987], suggesting that these adherent cells supply the necessary attachment ligand for CFU-S attachment [Roberts et al., 1987; Yamazaki et al., 1989].

114.2 Soluble Growth Factors

Soluble specific growth factors are an obligate requirement for the proliferation and differentiation of developing cells. These growth factors differ in effects from the endocrine hormones such as anabolic steroids or growth hormone. Whereas the endocrine hormones affect general cell function and are required and/or important to tissue formation, their predominant role is one of homeostasis. Growth *factors*, however, specifically drive the developmental programs of differentiating cells. Whether these function in a permissive or an inductive capacity has been the subject of considerable past controversy, particularly with respect to blood cell development. However, the large amount of data demonstrating linkages between receptor-ligand interaction and gene activation argues persuasively for an inductive/direct action on gene expression and, hence, cell proliferation and differentiation.

TABLE 114.3 Hematopoietic Cell–Stromal Cell Interactions (Unknown Receptor-Ligand)

Cell Phenotype	Stromal Cell	References
B cells	Fibroblasts	Ryan et al., 1990; Witte et al., 1987
Pre-B cell	Heter stroma	Palacios et al., 1989
BFC-E	Fibroblasts	Tsai et al., 1986; Tsai et al., 1987
CFC-S	Fibroblasts (NIH 3T3)	Roberts et al., 1987
CFC-S, Bl-CFC	Heter stroma*	Gordon et al., 1985, 1990a, 1990b
CFC-GM	Heter stroma	Tsai et al., 1987; Campbell et al., 1985
CFC-Mk	Heter stroma	Tsai et al., 1987; Campbell et al., 1985

*Methylprednisolone stimulated stromal cells, unstimulated fail to bind—see Gordon and coworkers [1985]. Heter = heterologous; BFC-E = burst forming cell-erythroid; CFC = colony = forming cell; S = spleen; Bl = blast; GM = granulocyte/macrophage; Mk = megakaryocyte. From Long [1992], reprinted with permission.

Again, a large body of knowledge concerning growth factors comes from the field of hematopoiesis (blood cell development). Hematopoietic cell proliferation and differentiation is regulated by numerous growth factors; for reviews see Metcalf [1989] and Arai and colleagues [1990]. Within the last decade, approximately 29 stimulatory cytokines (13 interleukins, M-CSF, erythropoietin, G-CFS, GM-CSF, c-kit ligand, gamma-interferon, and thrombopoietin) have been molecularly cloned and examined for their function in hematopoiesis. Clearly, this literature is beyond the scope of this review. However, the recent genetic cloning of eight receptors for these cytokines has led to the observation that a number of these receptors have amino acid homologies [Arai et al., 1990], showing that they are members of one or more gene families (Table 114.4). Hematopoietic growth factor receptors structurally contain a large extracellular domain, a transmembrane region, and a sequence-specific cytoplasmic domain [Arai et al., 1990]. The extracellular domains of interleukin-1, interleukin-6, and gamma-interferon are homologous with the immunoglobulin gene superfamily, and weak but significant amino-acid homologies exist among the interleukin-2 (beta chain), IL-6, IL-3, IL-4, erythropoietin, and GM-CSF receptors [Arai et al., 1990].

Like other developing tissues, bone responds to bone-specific and other soluble growth factors. TGF-β is a member of a family of polypeptide growth regulators which affects cell growth and differentiation during developmental processes such as embryogenesis and tissue repair [Sporn & Roberts, 1985]. TGF-β strongly inhibits proliferation of normal and tumor-derived epithelial cells and blocks adipogenesis, myogenesis, and hematopoiesis [Sporn & Roberts, 1985]. However, in bone, TGF-β is a positive regulator. TGF-β is localized in active centers of bone differentiation (cartilage canals and osteocytes) [Massague, 1987], and TGF-β is found in high quantity in bone, suggesting that bone contains the greatest total amount of TGF-β [Gehron Robey et al., 1987; Massague, 1987]. During bone formation, TGF-β promotes chrondrogenesis [Massague, 1987]—an effect presumably related to its ability to stimulate the deposition of extracellular matrix (ECM) components [Ignotz & Massague, 1986]. Besides stimulating cartilage formation, TGF-β is synthesized and secreted in bone cell cultures and stimulates the growth of subconfluent layers of fetal bovine bone cells, thus showing it to be an autocrine regulator of bone cell development [Sporn & Roberts, 1985].

In addition to TGF-β, other growth factors or cytokines are implicated in bone development. Urist and coworkers have been able to isolate various regulatory proteins which function in both in vivo and in vitro models [Urist et al., 1983b]. Bone morphogenic protein (BMP), originally an extract of demineralized human bone matrix, has now been cloned [Wozney et al., 1988] and, when implanted in vivo, results in a sequence of events leading to functional bone formation [Muthukumaran & Reddi, 1985; Wozney et al., 1988]. The implanting of BMP is followed by mesenchymal cell migration to the area of the implant, differentiation into bone progenitor cells, deposition of new bone, and subsequent bone remodeling to allow the establishment of bone marrow [Muthukumaran & Reddi, 1985]. A number of additional growth factors which regulate bone development

TABLE 114.4   Hematopoietic Growth Factor Receptor Families

Receptors with homology to the immunoglobulin gene family
    Interleukin-1 receptor
    Interleukin-6 receptor
    Gamma-interferon receptor
Hematopoietic growth factor receptor family
    Interleukin-2 receptor (β-chain)
    Interleukin-3 receptor
    Interleukin-4 receptor
    Interleukin-6 receptor
    Erythropoietin receptor
    G/M-CSF receptor

Source: Modified from Long [1992]. Reprinted with permission.

exists. In particular, bone-derived growth factors (BDGF) stimulate bone cells to proliferate in serum-free media [Hanamura et al., 1980; Linkhart et al., 1986]. However, these factors seem to function at a different level from BMP [Urist et al., 1983a].

114.3 Extracellular Matrix

The extracellular matrix (ECM) varies in its tissue composition throughout the body and consists of various molecules such as laminin, collagens, proteoglycans, and other glycoproteins [Wicha et al., 1982]. Gospodarowicz and coworkers demonstrated that ECM components greatly affect corneal endothelial cell proliferation in vitro [Gospodarowicz et al., 1980; Gospodarowicz & Ill, 1980]. Studies by Reh and coworkers indicate that the ECM protein laminin is involved in inductive interactions which give rise to retinal-pigmented epithelium [Reh & Gretton, 1987]. Likewise, differentiation of mammary epithelial cells is profoundly influenced by ECM components; mammary cell growth in vivo and in vitro requires type IV collagen [Wicha et al., 1982]. A number of investigations elucidated a role for ECM and its components in hematopoietic cell function. These studies have identified the function of both previously known and newly identified ECM components in hematopoietic cell cytoadhesion (Table 114.5).

As mentioned, soluble factors, stromal cells, and extracellular matrix (the natural substrate surrounding cells in vivo) are critical elements of the hematopoietic microenvironment. Work by Wolf and Trenton on the hematopoietic microenvironment in vivo provided the first evidence that (still unknown) components of the microenvironment are responsible for the granulocytic predominance of bone marrow hematopoiesis and the erythrocytic predominance of spleen [Wolf & Trentin, 1968]. Dexter and coworkers observed that the in vitro development of adherent cell populations is essential for the continued proliferation and differentiation of blood cells in long-term bone marrow cell cultures [Dexter & Lajtha, 1974; Dexter et al., 1976]. These stromal cells elaborate specific ECM components such as laminin, fibronectin, and various collagens and proteoglycans, and the presence of these ECM proteins coincided with the onset of hematopoietic cell proliferation [Zuckerman & Wicha, 1983]. The actual roles for extracellular matrix versus stromal cells in supporting cell development remains somewhat obscure, as it often is difficult to disassociate stromal cell effects from those of the ECM, since stromal cells are universally observed to be enmeshed in the surrounding extracellular matrix.

TABLE 114.5   Proteins and Glycoproteins Mediating Hematopoietic Cell–Extracellular Matrix Interactions

Matrix Component	Cell Surface Receptor	Cellular Expression	References
Fibronectin	FnR	Erythroid; BFC-E; B cells; Lymphoid cells; HL60 cells	Patel, 1984, 1986, 1987; Patel et al., 1985; Ryan et al., 1990; Tsai et al., 1987) Van de Water et al., 1988
	IIb/IIIa	Platelets and megakaryocytes	Giancotti et al., 1987
Thrombospondin	TSP-R	Monocytes and platelets	Silverstein and Nachman, 1987; Leung, 1984
		Human CFC,	Long and Dixit, 1990
		CFC-GEMM	Long and Dixit, 1990
Hyaluronic acid	CD44	T and B cells	Aruffo et al., 1990; Dorshkind, 1989; Horst et al., 1990; Miyake et al., 1990
		Neutrophils Tumor cells	
Hemonectin	Unk	CFC-GM, BFC-E Immat. neutr. BFU-E	Campbell et al., 1985, 1987, 1990
Proteoglycans:			
Heparan sulfate	Unk	Bl-CFC	Gordon, 1988; Gordon et al., 1988
Unfract ECM	Unk	Bl-CFC, bm Stroma	Gordon et al., 1988; Campbell et al., 1985

R = receptor; BFC-E and erythroid progenitor cell = the burst-forming cell-erythrocyte; HL60 = a promyelocytic leukemia cell line; CFC = colony = forming cell; GEMM = granulocyte erythrocyte macrophage megakarocyte; GM = granulocyte/macrophage; unk = unknown; Bl = blast cell; bm = bone marrow. Modified and reprinted from Long [1992] with permission.

Bone extracellular matrix contains both collagenous and noncollagenous proteins. A number of noncollagenous matrix proteins, isolated from demineralized bone, are involved in bone formation. Osteonectin is a 32 kDa protein which, binding to calcium, hydroxypatite, and collagen, is felt to initiate nucleation during the mineral phase of bone deposition [Termine et al., 1981]. In vivo analysis of osteonectin message reveals its presence in a variety of developing tissues [Holland et al., 1987; Nomura et al., 1988]. However, osteonectin is present in its highest levels in bones of the axial skeleton, skull, and the blood platelet (megakaryocyte) [Nomura et al., 1988]. Bone gla protein (BGP, osteocalcin) is a vitamin-K-dependent, 5700 Da calcium-binding bone protein which is specific for bone and may regulate $Ca^2 +$ deposition [Price et al., 1976, 1981; Termine et al., 1981]. Other bone proteins seem to function as cytoadhesion molecules [Oldberg et al., 1986; Somerman et al., 1987] or have unresolved functions [Reddi, 1981]. Moreover, bone ECM also contains a number of the more common mesenchymal growth factors such as PDGF, basic, and acidic fibroblast growth factor [Canalis, 1985; Hauschka et al., 1986; Linkhart et al., 1986; Urist et al., 1983a]. These activities are capable of stimulating the proliferation of mesenchymal target cells (BALB/c 3T3 fibroblasts, capillary endothelial cells, and rat fetal osteoblasts). As well, bone-specific proliferating activities such as the BMP exist in bone ECM. Although these general and specific growth factors undoubtedly play a role in bone formation, little is understood concerning the direct inductive/permissive capacity of bone-ECM or bone proteins themselves on human bone cells or their progenitors. Nor is the role of bone matrix in presenting growth factors understood—such "matricrine" (factor-ECM) interactions may be of fundamental importance in bone cell development.

When bone precursor cells are cultured on certain noncollagenous proteins, they show an increase in proliferation and bone protein expression (MWL, unpublished observation). Moreover, we have shown, using the hematopoietic system as a model, that subpopulations of primitive progenitor cells require both a mitogenic cytokine and a specific extracellular matrix (ECM) molecule in order to proliferate [Long et al., 1992]. Indeed, without this obligate matrix-cytokine ("matricrine") signal, the most primitive of blood precursor cells fail to develop in vitro [Long et al., 1992]. Although poorly understood, a similar requirement exists for human bone precursor cells, and complete evaluation of osteogenic development (or that of other tissues) thus requires additional studies of ECM molecules. For example, we have demonstrated the importance of three bone ECM proteins in human bone cell growth: osteonectin, osteocalcin, and type I collagen [Long et al., 1990; Long et al., 1994]. Additional bone proteins such as bone sialoprotein and osteopontin are no doubt important to bone structure and function, but their role is unknown [Nomura et al., 1988; Oldberg et al., 1986].

The above observations on the general and specific effects of ECM on cell development have identified certain matrix components which seem to appear as a recurrent theme in tissue development. These are proteoglycans, thrombospondin, fibronectin, and the collagens.

Proteoglycans and Glycosaminoglycans

Studies on the role of proteoglycans in blood cell development indicate that both hematopoietic cells [Minguell & Tavassoli, 1989] (albeit as demonstrated by cell lines) and marrow stromal cells [Gallagher et al., 1983; Kirby & Bentley, 1987; Spooncer et al., 1983; Wight et al., 1986] produce various proteoglycans. Proteoglycans (PG) are polyanionic macromolecules located both on the stromal cell surface and within the extracellular matrix. They consist of a core protein containing a number of covalently linked glycosaminoglycan (GAG) side chains, as well as one or more O- or N-linked oligosaccharides. The GAGs consist of nonbranching chains of repeating N-acetylglucosamine or N-acetylglactosamine disaccharide units. With the exception of hyaluronic acid, all glycosaminoglycans are sulfated. Interesting, many extracellular matrix molecules (fibronectin, laminin, and collagen) contain glycosaminoglycan-binding sites, suggesting that complex interactions occur within the matrix itself.

Proteoglycans play a role in both cell proliferation and differentiation. Murine stromal cells produce hyaluronic acid, heparan sulfate, and chondroitin sulfate [Gallagher et al., 1983], and in vitro studies show PG to be differentially distributed between stromal cell surfaces and the media, with heparan sulfate being the primary cell-surface molecule and chondroitin sulfate the major molecular species in the aqueous phase [Spooncer et al., 1983]. In contrast to murine cultures, the human hematopoietic stromal cells in vitro contain small amounts of heparan sulfate and large amounts of dermatin and chondroitin sulfate, which seem to be equally distributed between the aqueous phase and extracellular matrix [Wight et al., 1986]. The stimulation of proteoglycan/GAG synthesis is associated with an increased hematopoietic cell proliferation, as demonstrated by an increase in the percentage of cells in S-phase [Spooncer et al., 1983]. Given the general diversity of proteoglycans, it is reasonable to expect that they may encode both lineage-specific and organ-specific information. For example, organ-specific PGs stimulate differentiation, as marrow-derived ECM directly stimulates differentiation of a human progranulocytic cells (HL60), whereas matrix derived from skin fibroblasts lacks this inductive capacity [Luikart et al., 1987]. Moreover, organ-specific effects are seen in studies of human blood precursor cell adhesion to marrow-derived heparan sulfate but not to heparan sulfates isolated from bovine kidney [Gordon et al., 1988].

Interestingly, cell-surface-associated PGs are involved in the compartmentalization or localization of growth factors within the microenvironment. Thus, the proliferation of hematopoietic cells in the presence of hematopoietic stroma is associated with a glycosaminoglycan-bound growth factor (GM-CSF) [Gordon et al., 1987b], and determination of the precise GAG molecules involved in this process (i.e., heparan sulfate) has showed that heparan sulfate side chains bind two blood cell growth factors: GM-CSF and interleukin-3 [Roberts et al., 1988]. These data imply that ECM components and growth factors combine to yield lineage-specific information and indicate that, when PG- or GAG-bound, growth factor is presented to the progenitor cells in a biologically active form.

Thrombospondin (TSP)

Thrombospondin is a large, trimeric disulfide-linked glycoprotein (molecular weight 450,000, subunit molecular weight 180,000) having a domainlike structure [Frazier, 1987]. Its protease-resistant domains are involved in mediating various TSP functions such as cell binding and binding of other extracellular matrix proteins [Frazier, 1987]. Thrombospondin is synthesized and secreted into extracellular matrix by most cells; for review see Lawler [1986] and Frazier [1987]. Matrix-bound TSP is necessary for cell adhesion [Varani et al., 1986], cell growth [Majack et al., 1986], and carcinoma invasiveness [Riser et al., 1988] and is differentially expressed during murine embryogenesis [O'Shea & Dixit, 1988].

Work from our laboratories shows that thrombospondin functions within the hematopoietic microenvironment as a cytoadhesion protein for a subpopulation of human hematopoietic progenitor cells [Long et al., 1992; Long & Dixit, 1990]. Interestingly, immunocytochemical and metabolic labeling studies show that hematopoietic cells (both normal marrow cells and leukemic cell lines) synthesize TSP, deposit it within the ECM, and are attached to it. The attachment of human progenitor cells to thrombospondin is not mediated by its integrin-binding RGD sequence because this region of the TSP molecule is cryptic, residing within the globular carboxy-terminus of the molecule. Thus, excess concentrations of a tetrapeptide containing the RGD sequence did not inhibit attachment of human progenitor cells [Long & Dixit, 1990], and similar observations exist in other cell systems [Asch et al., 1987; Roberts et al., 1987; Varani et al., 1988]. Other studies from this author's laboratories show that bone marrow ECM also plays a major role in hematopoiesis in that complex ECM extracts greatly augment LTBMC cell proliferation [Campbell et al., 1985] and that marrow-derived ECM contains specific cytoadhesion molecules [Campbell et al., 1987, 1990; Long et al., 1990, 1992; Long & Dixit, 1990].

Fibronectin

Fibronectin is a ubiquitous extracellular matrix molecule that is known to be involved in the attachment of paryenchymal cells to stromal cells [Bentley & Tralka, 1983; Zuckerman & Wicha,

1983]. As with TSP, hematopoietic cells synthesize, deposit, and bind to fibronectin [Zuckerman & Wicha, 1983]. Extensive work by Patel and coworkers shows that erythroid progenitor cells attach to fibronectin in a developmentally regulated manner [Patel et al., 1985; Patel & Lodish, 1984, 1986, 1987]. In addition to cells of the erythroid lineage, fibronectin is capable of binding lymphoid precursor cells and other cell phenotypes [Bernardi et al., 1987; Giancotti et al., 1986]. Structurally, cells adhere to two distinct regions of the fibronectin molecule, one of which contains the RGD sequence; the other is within the carboxy terminal region and contains a high-affinity binding site for heparan [Bernardi et al., 1987].

Collagen

The role of various collagens in blood cell development remains uncertain. In vitro marrow cells produce types I, III, IV, and V collagen [Bentley, 1982; Bentley & Foidart, 1981; Castro-Malaspina et al., 1980; Zuckerman and Wicha, 1983], suggesting a role for these extracellular matrix components in the maintenance of hematopoiesis. Consistent with this, inhibition of collagen synthesis with 6-hydroxyprolene blocks or reduces hematopoiesis in vitro [Zuckerman et al., 1985]. Type I collagen is the major protein of bone, comprising approximately 90 percent of its protein.

114.4 Considerations for ex Vivo Tissue Generation

The microenvironmental complexities discussed above suggest that the ex vivo generation of human (replacement) tissue (e.g., marrow, liver) will be a difficult process. However, many of the needed tissues (liver, marrow, bone, and kidney) have a degree of regenerative or hyperplastic capacity which allows their in vitro cultivation. Thus, in vivo growth of many of these tissue types is routinely performed, albeit at varying degrees of success. The best example of this is bone marrow. If unfractionated human bone marrow is established in culture, the stromal and hematopoietic cells attempt to recapitulate in vivo hematopoiesis. Both soluble factors and ECM proteins are produced [Dexter & Spooncer, 1987; Long & Dixit, 1990; Zuckerman & Wicha, 1983], and relatively long-term hematopoiesis occurs. However, if long-term bone marrow cultures are examined closely, they turn out to not faithfully reproduce the in vivo microenvironment [Dexter & Spooncer, 1987; Spooncer et al., 1985; Schofield & Dexter, 1985]. Over a period of 8–12 weeks (for human cultures) or 3–6 months (for murine cultures), cell proliferation ceases, and the stromal/hematopoietic cells die. Moreover, the pluripotentiality of these cultures is rapidly lost. In vivo, bone marrow produces a wide variety of cells (erythroid, megakaryocyte/platelet, four types of myeloid cells, and B-lymphocytes). Human long-term marrow cultures produce granulocytes and megakaryocytes for 1–3 weeks, and erythropoiesis is only seen if exogenous growth factors are added. Thereafter, the cultures produce granulocytes and macrophages. These data show that current culture conditions are inadequate and further suggest that other factors such as rate of fluid exchange (perfusion) or that the three-dimensional structure of these cultures is limiting.

Recent work by Emerson, Palsson, and colleagues demonstrated the effectiveness of altered medium exchange rates in the expansion of blood cells in vitro [Caldwell et al., 1991; Schwartz et al., 1991*a*, 1991*b*]. These studies showed that a daily 50% medium exchange affected stromal cell metabolism and stimulated a transient increase in growth factor production [Caldwell et al., 1991]. As well, these cultures underwent a 10-fold expansion of cell numbers [Schwartz et al., 1991*b*]. While impressive, these cultures nonetheless decayed after 10–12 weeks. Recently, this group utilized continuous-perfusion bioreactors to achieve a longer ex vivo expansion and showed a 10–20-fold expansion of specific progenitor cell types [Koller et al., 1993]. These studies demonstrate that bioreactor technology allows significant expansion of cells, presumably via better mimicry of in vivo conditions.

Another aspect of tissue formation is the physical structure of the developing organ. Tissues exist as three-dimensional structures. Thus, the usual growth in tissue culture flasks is far removed from the in vivo setting. Essentially, cells grown in vitro proliferate at a liquid/substratum interface. As a result, primary tissue cells grow until they reach confluence and then cease proliferating, a process known as *contact inhibition*. This, in turn, severely limits the degree of total cellularity of the system. For example, long-term marrow cultures (which do not undergo as precise a contact inhibition as do cells from solid tissues) reach a density of $1-2 \times 10^6$ per milliliter. This is three orders of magnitude *less* than the average bone marrow density in vivo. A number of technologies have been applied to this three-dimensional growth problem (e.g., hollow fibers). However, the growth of cells on or in a nonphysiologic matrix is less than optimal in terms of replacement tissue, since such implants trigger a type of immune reaction (foreign body reaction) or are thrombogenic.

Recently, another type of bioreactor has been used to increase the ex vivo expansion of cells. Rotating wall vessels are designed to result in constant, low-shear suspension of tissue cells during their development. These bioreactors thus simulate a microgravity environment. The studies of Goodwin and associates document a remarkable augmentation of mesenchymal cell proliferation in low-shear bioreactors. Their data show that mesenchymal cell types show an average three- to six-fold increase in cell density in these bioreactors, reaching a cellularity of approximately 10^7 cells/mL [Goodwin et al., 1993a, 1993b]. Importantly, this increase in cell density was associated with a 75% reduction in glucose utilization as well as an approximate 85% reduction in the enzymatic markers of anabolic cellular metabolism (SGOT and LDH) [Goodwin et al., 1993a]. Importantly, further work by Goodwin and colleagues shows that the growth of mesenchymal cells (kidney and chondrocyte) under low-shear conditions leads to the formation of tissuelike cell aggregates which is enhanced by growing these cells on collagen-coated microcarriers [Duke et al., 1993; Goodwin et al., 1993a].

The physical requirements for optimal bone precursor cell (i.e., osteoprogenitor cells and pre-osteoblasts) proliferation both in vivo and ex vivo are poorly understood. In vivo, bone formation most often occurs within an intervening cartilage model (i.e., a three-dimensional framework referred to as endochondral ossification). This well-understood bone histogenesis is one of embryonic and postnatal chondrogenesis, which accounts for the shape of bone and the subsequent modification and calcification of bone cell ECM by osteoblasts. Recent work in this laboratory has examined the physical requirements for bone cell growth. When grown in suspension cultures (liquid/substratum interface), bone precursor cells develop distinct, clonal foci. These cells, however, express low amounts of bone-related proteins, and they rapidly expand as "sheets" of proliferating cells. As these are nontransformed (i.e., primary) cells, they grow until they reach confluence and then undergo contact inhibition and cease proliferating. We reasoned that growing these cells in a three-dimensional gel might augment their development. It is known from other systems that progenitor cell growth and development in many tissues requires the presence of at least one mitogenic growth factor, and that progenitor cell growth in a three-dimensional matrix results in the clonal formation of cell colonies by restricting the outgrowth of differentiated progeny [Metcalf, 1989]. Thus, bone precursor cells were overlayered with chemically defined, serum-free media containing a biopolymer, thus providing the cells with a three-dimensional scaffold in which to proliferate. In sharp contrast to bone precursor cell growth at a planar liquid/substratum interface, cells grown in a three-dimensional polymer gel show a marked increase in proliferative capacity and an increased per-cell production of the bone-specific proteins (MWL, unpublished observations).

114.5 Conclusions and Perspectives

As elegantly demonstrated by the composite data above, the molecular basis and function of the various components of tissue microenvironments are becoming well understood. However, much remains to be learned regarding the role of these and other, as yet unidentified, molecules in tissue development. One of the intriguing questions to be asked is how each interacting molecule contributes to defining the molecular basis of a given microenvironment—for example, the distinct differences in hematopoiesis as it exists in the marrow versus the spleen (i.e., a predominance of granulopoiesis and erythropoiesis, respectively) [Wolf & Trentin, 1968]. Another rapidly advancing area is the dissection of the molecular basis of cell trafficking into tissues. Again, the immune system offers a paradigm for the assessment of this process. Thus, interaction of the lymphocyte receptors with specific glycoconjugates or vascular addressins [Goldstein et al., 1989; Idzerda et al., 1989; Lasky et al., 1989] suggests that similar recognition systems are involved in other tissues, particularly the bone marrow. Another interesting observation is that hematopoietic progenitor cells synthesize and bind to their own cytoadhesion molecules, independent of the matrix molecules contributed by the stromal cells. For example, developing cells in vitro synthesize and attach to fibronectin, thrombospondin, and hemonectin, suggesting that these molecules function solely in an autochthonous manner to localize or perhaps stimulate development. Such a phenomenon may be a generalized process, as we have noted similar patterns of ECM expression/attachment in osteopoietic cell cultures. Coupled with data from the bioreactor studies, this suggests that, under appropriate biologic/physical conditions tissue cells may spontaneously reestablish their structure. Finally, the elucidation of the various requirements for optimal progenitor cell growth (cell interactions, specific growth factors and matrix components, and/or accessory cells which supply them) should allow the improvement of ex vivo culture systems to yield an environment in which tissue reconstitution is possible. Such a system would have obvious significance in organ-replacement therapy.

References

Arai K, Lee F, Miyajima A, et al. 1990. Cytokines: Coordinators of immune and inflammatory responses. Annu Rev Biochem 59:783.

Aruffo A, Staminkovic I, Melnik M, et al. 1990. CD44 is the principal cell surface receptor for hyaluronate. Cell 61:1303.

Asch AS, Barnwell J, Silverstein RL, et al. 1987. Isolation of the thrombospondin membrane receptor. J Clin Invest 79:1054.

Bentley SA. 1982. Collagen synthesis by bone marrow stromal cells: a quantitative study. Br J Haematol 50:491.

Bentley SA, Foidart JM. 1981. Some properties of marrow derived adherent cells in tissue culture. Blood 56:1006.

Bentley SA, Tralka TS. 1983. Fibronectin-mediated attachment of hematopoietic cells to stromal elements in continuous bone marrow cultures. Exp Hematol 11:129.

Bernardi P, Patel VP, Lodish HF. 1987. Lymphoid precursor cells adhere to two different sites on fibronectin. J Cell Biol 105:489.

Bevilacqua MP, Stengelin S, Gimbrone MA, et al. 1989. Endothelial leukocyte adhesion molecule 1: An inducible receptor for neutrophils related to complement regulatory proteins and lectins. Science 243:1160.

Bierer BE, Sleckman BP, Ratnofsky SE, et al. 1989. The biologic roles of CD2, CD4, and CD8 in T-cell activation. Annu Rev Immunol 7:579.

Brandley BK, Swiedler SJ, Robbins PW. 1990. Charbohydrate ligands of the LEC cell adhesion molecules. Cell 63:861.

Caldwell J, Palsson BO, Locey B, et al. 1991. Culture perfusion schedules influence the metabolic activity and granulocyte-macrophage colony-stimulating factor production rates of human bone marrow stromal cells. J Cell Physiol 147:344.

Campbell A, Sullenberger B, Bahou W, et al. 1990. Hemonectin: A novel hematopoietic adhesion molecule. Prog Clin Biol Res 352:97.

Campbell A, Wicha MS, Long MW. 1985. Extracellular matrix promotes the growth and differentiation of murine hematopoietic cells in vitro. J Clin Invest 75:2085.

Campbell AD, Long MW, Wicha MS. 1987. Haemonectin, a bone marrow adhesion protein specific for cells of granulocyte lineage. Nature 329:744.

Campbell AD, Long MW, Wicha MS. 1990. Developmental regulation of granulocytic cell binding to hemonectin. Blood 76:1758.

Canalis E. 1985. Effect of growth factors on bone cell replication and differentiation. Clin Orth Rel Res 193:246.

Castro-Malaspina H, Gay RE, Resnick G, et al. 1980. Characterization of human bone marrow fibroblast colony-forming cells and their progeny. Blood 56:289.

Coulombel L, Vuillet MH, Tchernia G. 1988. Lineage- and stage-specific adhesion of human hematopoietic progenitor cells to extracellular matrices from marrow fibroblasts. Blood 71:329.

Dexter TM. 1982. Stromal cell associated haemopoiesis. J Cell Physiol 1:87.

Dexter TM, Allen TD, Lajtha LG. 1976. Conditions controlling the proliferation of haemopoietic stem cells in vitro. J Cell Physiol 91:335.

Dexter TM, Lajtha LG. 1974. Proliferation of haemopoietic stem cells in vitro. Br J Haematol 28:525.

Dexter TM, Spooncer E. 1987. Growth and differentiation in the hemopoietic system. Annu Rev Cell Biol 3:423.

Dorshkind K. 1989. Hemopoietic stem cells and B-lymphocyte differentiation. Immunol Today 10:399.

Duke PJ, Daane EL, Montufar-Solis D. 1993. Studies of chondrogenesis in rotating systems. J Cell Biochem 51:274.

Frazier WA. 1987. Thrombospondin: A modular adhesive glycoprotein of platelets and nucleated cells. J Cell Biol 105:625.

Gallagher JT, Spooncer E, Dexter TM. 1983. Role of the cellular matrix in haemopoiesis: I. Synthesis of glycosaminoglycans by mouse bone marrow cell cultures. J Cell Sci 63:155.

Gallatin M, St John TP, Siegleman M, et al. 1986. Lymphocyte homing receptors. Cell 44:673.

Gehron Robey P, Young MF, Flanders KC, et al. 1987. Osteoblasts synthesize and respond to transforming growth factor-type beta (TGF-beta) in vitro. J Cell Biol 105:457.

Giancotti FG, Comoglio PM, Tarone G. 1986. Fibronectin-plasma membrane interaction in the adhesion of hemopoietic cells. J Cell Biol 103:429.

Giancotti FG, Languino LR, Zanetti A, et al. 1987. Platelets express a membrane protein complex immunologically related to the fibroblast fibronectin receptor and distinct from GPIIb/IIIa. Blood 69:1535.

Giancotti FG, Ruoslahti E. 1990. Elevated levels of the alpha 5 beta 1 fibronectin receptor suppress the transformed phenotype of Chinese hamster ovary cells. Cell 60:849.

Goelz SE, Hession C, Goff D, et al. 1990. ELFT: A gene that directs the expression of an ELAM-1 ligand. Cell 63:1349.

Goldstein LA, Zhou DF, Picker LJ, et al. 1989. A human lymphocyte homing receptor, the hermes antigen, is related to cartilage proteoglycan core and link proteins. Cell 56:1063.

Goodwin TJ, Prewett TI, Wolf DA, et al. 1993a. Reduced shear stress: A major component in the ability of mammalian tissues to form three-dimensional assemblies inn simulated microgravity. J Cell Biochem 51:301.

Goodwin TJ, Schroeder WF, Wolf DA, et al. 1993b. Rotating vessel coculture of small intestine as a prelude to tissue modeling: Aspects of simulated microgravity. Proc Soc Exp Biol Med 202:181.

Gordon MY. 1988. The origin of stromal cells in patients treated by bone marrow transplantation. Bone Marrow Transplant 3:247.

Gordon MY, Bearpark AD, Clarke D, et al. 1990a. Haemopoietic stem cell subpopulations in mouse and man: discrimination by differential adherence and marrow repopulation ability. Bone Marrow Transplant 5:6.

Gordon MY, Clarke D, Atkinson J, et al. 1990b. Hemopoietic progenitor cell binding to the stromal microenvironment in vitro. Exp Hematol 18:837.

Gordon MY, Dowding CR, Riley GP, et al. 1987a. Characterisation of stroma-dependent blast colony-forming cells in human marrow. J Cell Physiol 130:150.

Gordon MY, Hibbin JA, Dowding C, et al. 1985. Separation of human blast progenitors from granulocytic, erythroid, megakaryocytic, and mixed colony-forming cells by "panning" on cultured marrow-derived stromal layers. Exp Hematol 13:937.

Gordon MY, Riley GP, Clarke D. 1988. Heparan sulfate is necessary for adhesive interactions between human early hemopoietic progenitor cells and the extracellular matrix of the marrow microenvironment. Leukemia 2:804.

Gordon MY, Riley GP, Watt SM, et al. 1987b. Compartmentalization of a haematopoietic growth factor (GM-CSF) by glycosaminoglycans in the bone marrow microenvironment. Nature 326:403.

Gospodarowicz D, Delagado D, Vlodavsky I. 1980. Permissive effect of the extracellular matrix on cell proliferation in vitro. Proc Natl Acad Sci USA 77:4094.

Gospodarowicz D, Ill C. 1980. Extracellular matrix and control of proliferation of vascular endothelial cells. J Clin Invest 65:1351.

Hanamura H, Higuchi Y, Nakagawa M, et al. 1980. Solubilization and purification of bone morphogenetic protein (BMP) from dunn osteosarcoma. Clin Orth Rel Res 153:232.

Hauschka PV, Mavrakos AE, Iafrati MD, et al. 1986. Growth factors in bone matrix. Isolation of multiple types by affinity chromatography on heparinsepharose. J Biol Chem 261:12665.

Holland PWH, Harmper SJ, McVey JH, et al. 1987. In vivo expression of mRNA for the Ca++-binding protein SPARC (osteonectin) revealed by in situ hybridization. J Cell Biol 105:473.

Horst E, Meijer CJML, Radaszkiewicz T, Ossekoppele GP, VanKrieken JHJM, and Pals ST. 1990. Adhesion molecules in the prognosis of diffuse large-cell lymphoma: expression of a lymphocyte homing receptor (CD44), LFA-1 (CD11a/18), and ICAM-1 (CD54). Leukemia 4, 595–599.

Idzerda RL, Carter WG, Nottenburg C, et al. 1989. Isolation and DNA sequence of a cDNA clone encoding a lymphocyte adhesion receptor for high endothelium. Proc Natl Acad Sci USA 86:4659.

Ignotz RA, Massague J. 1986. Transforming growth factor-beta stimulates the expression of fibronectin and collagen and their incorporation into the extracellular matrix. J Biol Chem 261:4337.

Kirby SL, Bentley SA. 1987. Proteoglycan synthesis in two murine bone marrow stromal cell lines. Blood 70:1777.

Koller MR, Emerson SG, Palsson BO. 1993. Large-scale expansion of human stem and progenitor cells from bone marrow mononuclear cells in continuous perfusion cultures. Blood 82:378.

Lasky LA, Singer MS, Yednock TA, et al. 1989. Cloning of a lymphocyte homing receptor reveals a lectin domain. Cell 56:1045.

Lawler J. 1986. The structural and functional properties of thrombosponidn. Blood 67, 1197–1209.

Lawrence MB, Springer TA. 1991. Leukocytes roll on a selectin at physiologic shear flow rates: Distinction from and prerequisite for adhesion through integrins. Cell 65:859.

Leung LLK. 1984. Role of thrombospondin in platelet aggregation. J Clin Invest 74:1764.

Liesveld JL, Abboud CN, Duerst RE, et al. 1989. Characterization of human marrow stromal cells: Role in progenitor cell binding and granulopoiesis. Blood 73:1794.

Linkhart TA, Jennings JC, Mohan S, et al. 1986. Characterization of mitogenic activities extracted from bovine bone matrix. Bone 7:479.

Long, MW. 1992. Blood cell cytoadhesion molecules. Exp Hematol 20:288.

Long MW, Ashcraft A, Mann KG. 1994. Regulation of human bone marrow-derived osteoprogenitor cells by osteogenic growth factors. Submitted.

Long MW, Briddell R, Walter AW, et al. 1992. Human hematopoietic stem cell adherence to cytokines and matrix molecules. J Clin Invest 90:251.

Long MW, Dixit VM. 1990. Thrombospondin functions as a cytoadhesion molecule for human hematopoietic progenitor cells. Blood 75:2311.

Long MW, Mann KG. 1993. Bone marrow as a source of osteoprogenitor cells. In MW Long, MS Wicha (eds), The Hematopoietic Microenvironment, pp 110–123, Baltimore, Johns Hopkins University.

Long MW, Williams JL, Mann KG. 1990. Expression of bone-related proteins in the human hematopoietic microenvironment. J Clin Invest 86:1387.

Lowe JB, Stoolman LM, Nair RP, et al. 1990. ELAM-1-dependent cell adhesion to vascular endothelium determined by a transfected human fucosyl transferase cDNA. Cell 63:475.

Luikart SD, Sackrison JL, Maniglia CA. 1987. Bone marrow matrix modulation of HL-60 phenotype. Blood 70:1119.

Majack RA, Cook SC, Bornstein P. 1986. Control of smooth muscle cell growth by components of the extracellular matrix: Autocrine role for thrombospondin. Proc Natl Acad Sci USA 83:9050.

Massague J. 1987. The TGF-beta family of growth and differentiation factors. Cell 49:437.

Metcalf D. 1989. The molecular control of cell division, differentiation commitment and maturation in haematopoietic cells. Nature 339:27.

Minguell JJ, Tavassoli M. 1989. Proteoglycan synthesis by hematopoietic progenitor cells. Blood 73:1821.

Miyake K, Medina KL, Hayashi S, et al. 1990. Monoclonal antibodies to Pgp-1/CD44 block lymphohemopoiesis in long-term bone marrow cultures. J Exp Med 171:477.

Miyake K, Weissman IL, Greenberger JS, et al. 1991. Evidence for a role of the integrin VLA-4 in Lympho-hematopoiesis. J Exp Med 173:599.

Miyamake K, Medina K, Ishihara K, et al. 1991. A VCAM-like adhesion molecule on murine bone marrow stromal cells mediates binding of lymphocyte precursors in culture. J Cell Biol 114:557.

Muthukumaran N, Reddi AH. 1985. Bone matrix-induced local bone induction. Clin Orth Rel Res 200:159.

Nomura S, Wills AJ, Edwards DR, et al. 1988. Developmental expression of 2ar (osteopontin) and SPARC (osteonectin) RNA as revealed by in situ hybridization. J Cell Biol 106:441.

O'Shea KS, Dixit VM. 1988. Unique distribution of the extracellular matrix component thrombospondin in the developing mouse embryo. J Cell Biol 107:2737.

Oldberg A, Franzen A, Heinegard D. 1986. Cloning and sequence analysis of rat bone sialoprotein (osteopontin) cDNA reveals an Arg-Gly-Asp cell-binding sequence. Proc Natl Acad Sci USA 83:8819.

Palacios R, Stuber S, Rolink A. 1989. The epigenetic influences of bone marrow and fetal liver stroma cells on the developmental potential of pre-B lymphocyte clones. Eur J Immunol 19:347.

Patel VP, Ciechanover A, Platt O, et al. 1985. Mammalian reticulocytes lose adhesion to fibronectin during maturation to erythrocytes. Proc Natl Acad Sci USA 82:440.

Patel VP, Lodish HF. 1984. Loss of adhesion of murine erythroleukemia cells to fibronectin during erythroid differentiation. Science 224:996.

Patel VP, Lodish HF. 1986. The fibronectin receptor on mammalian erythroid precursor cells: Characterization and developmental regulation. J Cell Biol 102:449.

Patel VP, Lodish HF. 1987. A fibronectin matrix is required for differentiation of murine erythroleukemia cells into reticulocytes. J Cell Biol 105:3105.

Ploemacher RE, Brons NHC. 1988. Isolation of hemopoietic stem cell subsets from murine bone marrow: II. Evidence for an early precursor of day-12 CFU-S and cells associated with radioprotective ability. Exp Hematol 16:27.

Price PA, Otsuka AS, Poser JW, et al. 1976. Characterization of a gamma-carboxyglutamic acid-containing protein from bone. Proc Natl Acad Sci USA 73:1447.

Price PA, Lothringer JW, Baukol SA, et al. 1981. Developmental appearance of the vitamin K-dependent protein of bone during calcification. Analysis of mineralizing tissues in human, calf, and rat. J Biol Chem 256:3781.

Reddi AH. 1981. Cell biology and biochemistry of endochondral bone development. Coll Res 1:209.

Reh TA, Gretton H. 1987. Retinal pigmented epithelial cells induced to transdifferentiate to neurons by laminin. Nature 330:68.

Riser BL, Varani J, Carey TE, et al. 1988. Thrombospondin binding and thrombospondin synthesis by human squamous carcinoma and melanoma cells: relationship to biological activity. Exp Cell Res 174:319.

Roberts DD, Sherwood JA, Ginsburg V. 1987*a*. Platelet thrombospondin mediates attachment and spreading of human melanoma cells. J Cell Biol 104:131.

Roberts RA, Spooncer E, Parkinson EK, et al. 1987*b* . Metabolically inactive 3T3 cells can substitute for marrow stromal cells to promote the proliferation and development of multipotent haemopoietic stem cells. J Cell Physiol 132:203.

Roberts R, Gallagher J, Spooncer E, et al. 1988. Heparan sulphate bound growth factors: A mechanism for stromal cell mediated haemopoiesis. Nature 332:376.

Ruoslahti E, Pierschbacher MD. 1987. New perspectives in cell adhesion: RGD and integrins. Science 238:491.

Ryan DH, Nuccie BL, Abboud CN, et al. 1990. Maturation-dependent adhesion of human B cell precursors to the bone marrow microenvironment. J Immunol 145:477.

Schofield R, Dexter TM. 1985. Studies on the self-renewal ability of CFU-S which have been serially transferred in long-term culture or in vivo. Leuk Res 9:305.

Schwartz RM, Emerson SG, Clarke MF, et al. 1991*a*. In vitro myelopoiesis stimulated by rapid medium exchange and supplementation with hematopoietic growth factors. Blood 78:3155.

Schwartz RM, Palsson BO, Emerson SG. 1991*b*. Rapid medium perfusion rate significantly increases the productivity and longevity of human bone marrow cultures. Proc Natl Acad Sci USA 88:6760.

Shaw S, Luce GE, Quinones R, et al. 1986. Two antigen-independent adhesion pathways used by human cytotoxic T-cell clones. Nature 323:262.

Sheetz MP, Turney S, Qian H, et al. 1989. Nanometre-level analysis demonstrates that lipid flow does not drive membrane glycoprotein movements. Nature 340:284.

Silverstein RL, Nachman RL. 1987. Thrombospondin binds to monocytes-marophages and mediates platelet-monocyte adhesion. J Clin Invest 79:867.

Somerman MJ, Prince CW, Sauk JJ, et al. 1987. Mechanism of fibroblast attachment to bone extracellular matrix: Role of a 44kilodalton bone phosphoprotein. J Bone Miner Res 2:259.

Spits H, van Schooten W, Keizer H, et al. 1986. Alloantigen recognition is preceded by nonspecific adhesion of cytotoxic T cells and target cells. Science 232:403.

Spooncer E, Gallagher JT, Krizsa F, et al. 1983. Regulation of haemopoiesis in long-term bone marrow cultures: IV. Glycosaminoglycan synthesis and the stimulation of haemopoiesis by beta-D-xylosides. J Cell Biol 96:510.

Spooncer E, Lord BI, Dexter TM. 1985. Defective ability to self-renew in vitro of highly purified primitive haematopoietic cells. Nature 316:62.

Sporn MB, Roberts AB. 1985. Autocrine growth factors and cancer. Nature 313:745.

Springer TA. 1990. Adhesion receptors of the immune system. Nature 346:425.

Stoolman LM. 1989. Adhesion molecules controlling lymphocyte migration. Cell 56:907.

Termine JD, Kleinman HK, Whitson SW, et al. 1981. Osteonectin, a bone-specific protein linking mineral to collagen. Cell 26:99.

Tsai S, Sieff CA, Nathan DG. 1986. Stromal cell-associated erythropoiesis. Blood 67:1418.

Tsai S, Patel V, Beaumont E, et al. 1987. Differential binding of erythroid and myeloid progenitors to fibroblasts and fibronectin. Blood 69:1587.

Urist MR, DeLange RJ, Finerman GAM. 1983*a*. Bone cell differentiation and growth factors. Science 220:680.

Urist MR, Sato K, Brownell AG, et al. 1983*b*. Human bone morphogenic protein (hBMP). Proc Soc Exp Biol Med 173:194.

Van de Water L, Aronson D, Braman V. 1988. Alteration of fibronectin receptors (integrins) in phorbol ester-treated human promonocytic leukemia cells. Cancer Res 48:5730.

Varani J, Dixit VM, Fligiel SEG, et al. 1986. Thrombospondin-induced attachment and spreading of human squamous carcinoma cells. Exp Cell Res 156:1.

Varani J, Nickloff BJ, Risner BL, et al. 1988. Thrombospondin-induced adhesion of human kertinocytes. J Clin Invest 81:1537.

Wicha MS, Lowrie G, Kohn E, et al. 1982. Extracellular matrix promotes mammary epithelial growth and differentiation in vitro. Proc Natl Acad Sci USA 79:3213.

Wight TN, Kinsella MG, Keating A, et al. 1986. Proteoglycans in human long-term bone marrow cultures: Biochemical and ultrastructural analyses. Blood 67:1333.

Williams AF, Barclay AN. 1988. The immunoglobulin superfamily—domains for cell surface recognition. Annu Rev Immunol 6:381.

Witte PL, Robinson M, Henley A, et al. 1987. Relationships between B-lineage lymphocytes and stromal cells in long-term bone marrow cultures. Eur J Immunol 17:1473.

Wolf NS, Trentin JJ. 1968. Hemopoietic colony studies: V. Effect of hemopoietic organ stroma on differentiation of pluripotent stem cells. J Exp Med 127:205.

Wozney JM, Rosen V, Celeste AJ, et al. 1988. Novel regulators of bone formation: Molecular clones and activities. Science 242:1528.

Yamazaki K, Roberts RA, Spooncer E, et al. 1989. Cellular interactions between 3T3 cells and interleukin-3-dependent multipotent haemopoietic cells: A model system for stromal-cell-mediated haemopoiesis. J Cell Physiol 139:301.

Zuckerman KS, Rhodes RK, Goodrum DD, et al. 1985. Inhibition of collagen deposition in the extracellular matrix prevents the establishment of a stroma supportive of hematopoiesis in long-term murine bone marrow cultures. J Clin Invest 75:970.

Zuckerman KS, Wicha MS. 1983. Extracellular matrix production by the adherent cells of long-term murine bone marrow cultures. Blood 61:540.

115

The Importance of Stromal Cells

Brian A. Naughton
Advanced Tissue Sciences, Inc.

All tissue is composed of *parenchymal* (from Greek, *that poured in beside*) and *stromal* (Greek, *framework* or *foundation*) cells. Parenchyma are the functional cells of a tissue (e.g., for liver, hepatic parenchymal cells or hepatocytes; for bone marrow, hematopoietic cells), whereas stroma comprises primarily connective tissue elements which, together with their products, form the structural framework of tissue. Parenchymal cells can be derivatives of any of the three germ layers, and during development they usually grow into areas populated by stromal cells or their progenitors. Under the strictest definition, stromal cells are derivatives of mesenchyme and include fibroblasts, osteogenic cells, myofibroblasts, and fat cells which appear to arise from a common stem/progenitor cell [Friedenstein et al., 1970; Owen, 1988] (Fig. 115.1). Some investigators apply the term *stromal cell* to all the nonparenchymal cells that contribute to the microenvironment of a tissue and include endothelial cells and macrophages (histiocytes) in this classification as well [Strobel et al., 1986]. However, the ontogeny of both endothelial cells and macrophages is distinct from that of mesenchymal tissue-derived cells [Wilson, 1983]. In this chapter, the more expansive definition of stroma will be used. A partial listing of tissue cells that may influence the function of organ parenchyma is in Table 115.1. For the sake of brevity, migrating cells of bone marrow origin will not be discussed in the text (e.g., mast cells, B lymphocytes, natural killer cells), although these cells can influence parenchyma either directly or via cytokine-mediated modulation of stromal cell function.

Stromal and parenchymal cell components are integrated to form a multifunctional tissue in vivo. This chapter will focus on the contribution of stromal cells to the microenvironment and their use in culture to support parenchymal function.

115.1 Tissue Composition and Stromal Cells

Some similarities in the spatial organization of cells of different tissues are apparent. Epithelial cells are a protective and regulatory barrier not just for skin but for all surfaces exposed to blood or to the external environment (e.g., respiratory tract, tubular digestive tract). These cells rest atop a

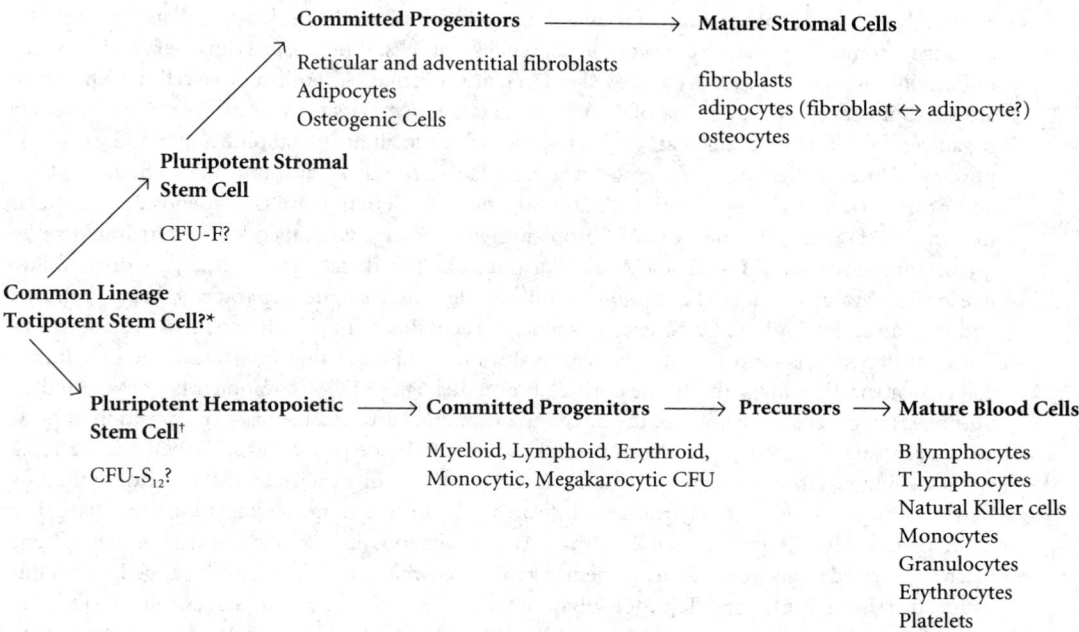

FIGURE 115.1 Hypothetical relationship between the ontogeny of stromal and parenchymal (hematopoietic) cells of the bone marrow. Note that stromal cell is defined in this chart as only those cells that are derivatives of mesenchyme. Hematopoietic stem and progenitor cells express CD 34. This epitope also is expressed by stromal cell precursors (CFU-F) [Simmons & Torok-Storb, 1991] and adherent stromal cells develop from cell populations selected for the CD 34 antigen. In addition, fetal marrow elements with CD 34+, CD 38−, HLA-DR-phenotypes were reported to develop not only the hematopoietic microenvironment but also the hematopoietic cells themselves [Huang & Terstappen, 1992].

* Indicates the possibility that, at least in the fetus, there may be a common stem cell for bone marrow stromal and hematopoietic elements.

† There are several schools of thought relating to single or multiple stem cell pools for the lymphoid versus the other lineages.

TABLE 115.1 Cells That Contribute to the Tissue Microenvironment

Stromal cells: derivates of a common precursor cell
  Mesenchyme
  Fibroblasts
  Myofibroblasts
  Osteogenic/chondrogenic cells
  Adipocytes
Stromal-associated cells: histogenically distinct from stromal cells, permanent residents of a tissue
  Endothelial cells
  Macrophages
Transient cells: cells that migrate into a tissue for host defense either prior to or following an inflammatory stimulus
  B lymphocytes/plasma cells
  Cytotoxic T cells and natural killer (NK) cells
  Granulocytes
Parenchymal cells: cells that occupy most of the tissue volume, express functions that are definitive for the tissue, and interact with all other cell types to facilitate the expression of differentiated function

selectively permeable basement membrane. The composition of the underlying tissue varies, but it contains a connective tissue framework for parenchymal cells. If the tissue is an artery or a vein, the underlying connective tissue is composed of circularly arranged smooth-muscle cells which in turn are surrounded by an adventitia of loose connective tissue. Tissues within organs are generally organized into functional units around capillaries which facilitate metabolite and blood gas transport by virtue of their lack of a smooth muscle layer (*tunica media*) and the thinness of their adventitial covering. Connective tissue cells of the tissue underlying capillaries deposit extracellular matrix (ECM) which is a mixture of fibrous proteins (collagens) embedded in a hydrated gel of glycosaminoglycans (GAGs). The GAGs, as distinguished by their sugar residues, are divided into five groups: hyaluronic acid, the chondiotin sulfates, dermatan sulfate, heparan and heparin sulfate, and keratan sulfate. All the GAGs except hyaluronic acid link with proteins to form proteoglycans. These proteoglycans bind to long-chained hyaluronic acid cores that interweave the crosslinked collagen fibers that form the framework of the tissue. These ECM components are secreted by fibroblasts or other stromal cells of the microenvironment. However, the basic composition of ECM as well as its density of deposition can vary from tissue to tissue [Lin & Bissell, 1993]. Figure 115.2 is a scanning electron micrograph (SEM) depiction of the intricacies of the ECM deposited by human bone marrow–derived stromal cells growing on a three-dimensional culture template. The ECM forms a sievelike arrangement for diffusion in an aqueous environment, and a number of bone marrow–derived migratory cells are present also. Parenchymal cells in tissue are arranged within this connective tissue framework. The most ubiquitous of these cells are macrophages (histiocytes), but normal tissue interstitium may also contain varying amounts of B lymphocyte/plasma cells, T cells, and natural killer cells. The numbers of these cells are enhanced during inflammatory episodes when neutrophils or other granulocytes and/or mononuclear leukocytes infiltrate the tissue. Although tissue function in toto is measured by parenchymal cell output (e.g., for liver, protein synthesis, metabolism; for bone marrow, blood cell production), this is influenced by and in some instances (e.g., bone marrow hematopoiesis) orchestrated by the stromal cell microenvironment.

Regulation of parenchymal cell function or proliferation by stromal cells is manifested in several ways including the synthesis of the proper ECM proteins for cell seeding/attachment, the modulation of gene expression in parenchymal cells by events triggered by cytoskeleton-mediated transduction [Ben-Ze'ev et al., 1988], the deposition of the proper ECM proteins to sequester growth and regulatory factors for use by developing parenchyma [Roberts et al., 1988], deposition of ECM of the right density to permit diffusion of nutrients, metabolites, and oxygen (and egress of CO_2 and waste) to the extent necessary to maintain the functional state of the tissue, by forming the appropriate barriers to minimize cell migration or intrusion, and by synthesizing and/or presenting cytokines that regulate parenchymal cell function, either constitutively or following induction by other humoral agents.

Creating cultures that contain the multiplicity of cell types found in vivo presents a daunting task for several reasons: (1) Culture media that are rich in nutrients select the most actively mitotic cells at the expense of more mitotically quiescent cells. (2) Cell phenotypic expression and function is related to its location in tissue to some extent. It is difficult, especially using a flat culture template, to create a microenvironment that is permissive or inductive for the formation of tissuelike structures. (3) Localized microenvironmental niches regulate different parenchymal cell functions or, in the case of bone marrow, hematopoietic cell differentiation. These milieu are difficult to reproduce in culture, since all cells are exposed to essentially the same media components. However, a major goal of tissue culture is to permit normal cell-cell associations and the reestablishment of tissue polarity so that parenchymal cell function is optimized. The question of three-dimensionality will be addressed later in this chapter. A brief survey of the various types of stromal elements follows:

Fibroblasts

Fibroblasts are responsible for the synthesis of many GAGs and for the deposition and organization of collagens. Although present in most tissues, fibroblasts exhibit specialization with respect to the

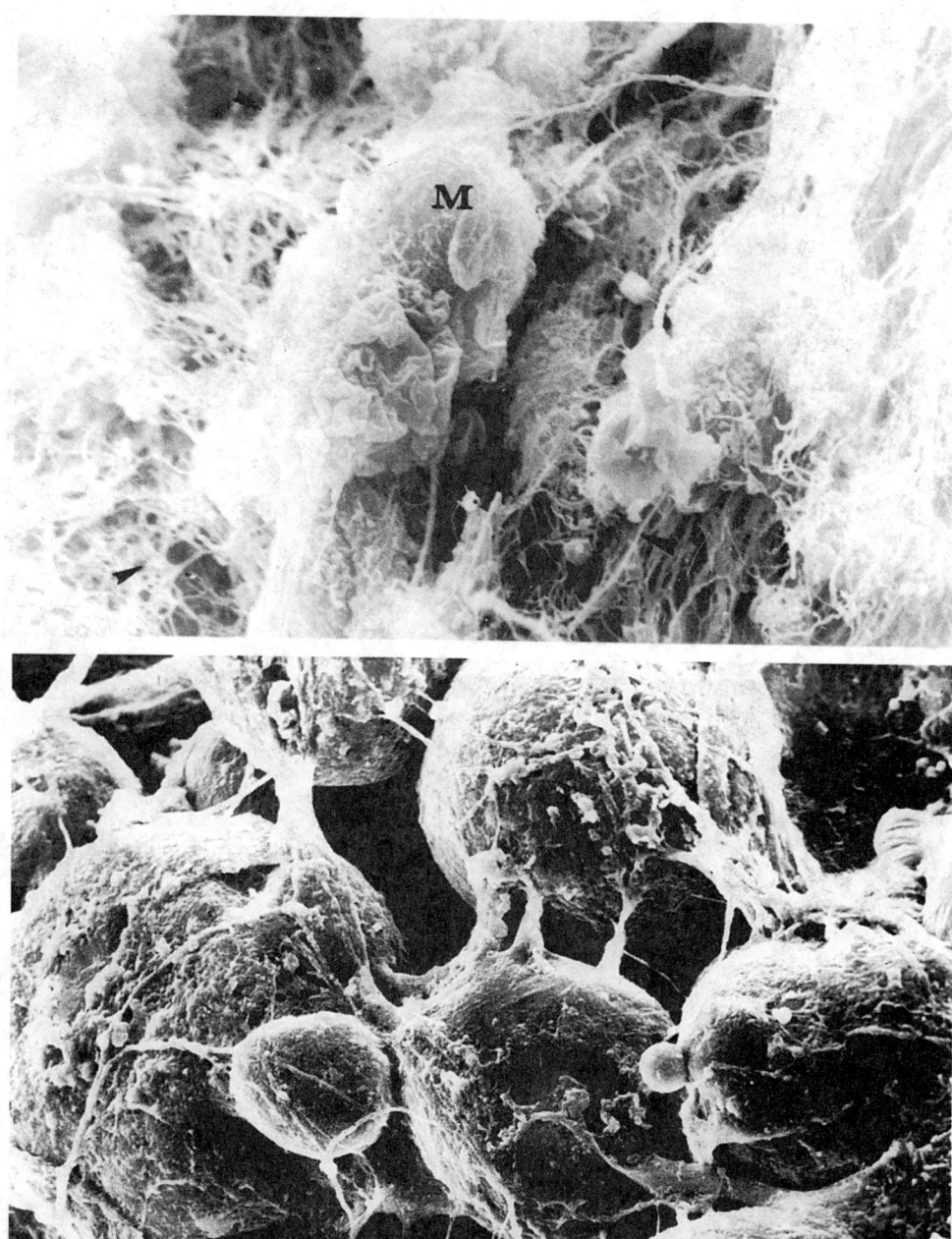

FIGURE 115.2 Scanning electron micrographs of bone marrow cultures on nylon screen templates. (*a*) Photograph depicting a portion of a macrophage (M) associated with the numerous, delicate, interweaving strands of ECM (arrows) that are deposited between the openings of the nylon screen of a bone marrow stromal cell culture. (*b*) Myeloid cells of a hematopoietic colony growing in a coculture of human stromal cells and hematopoietic cells. Note the pattern of attachment of individual cells to matrix and the large open area between the cells for nutrient access. (*c*) The photograph depicts the intimate association of cells of a myeloid or mixed myeloid/monocytic colony (arrow) with enveloping fibroblastic cells (F) in a bone marrow coculture. A filament of the nylon (n) screen is also present in the field. (*d*) An erythroid colony (E) in a human bone marrow coculture on nylon screen. Note that the more mature erythroid cells are on the periphery of the colony and that it is in close apposition to a macrophage (M). A nylon filament is also present (n).

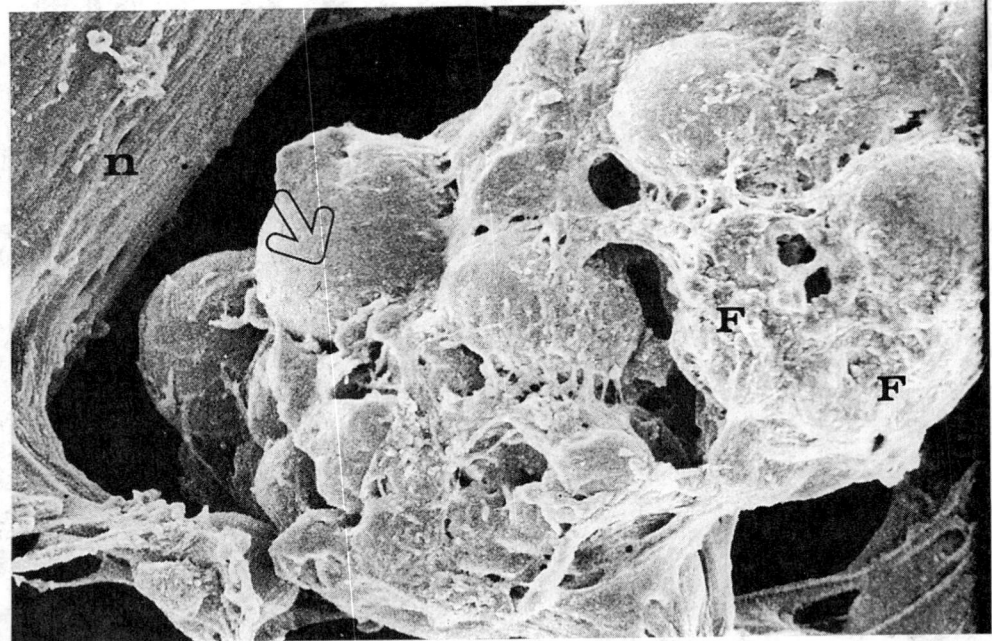

(c)

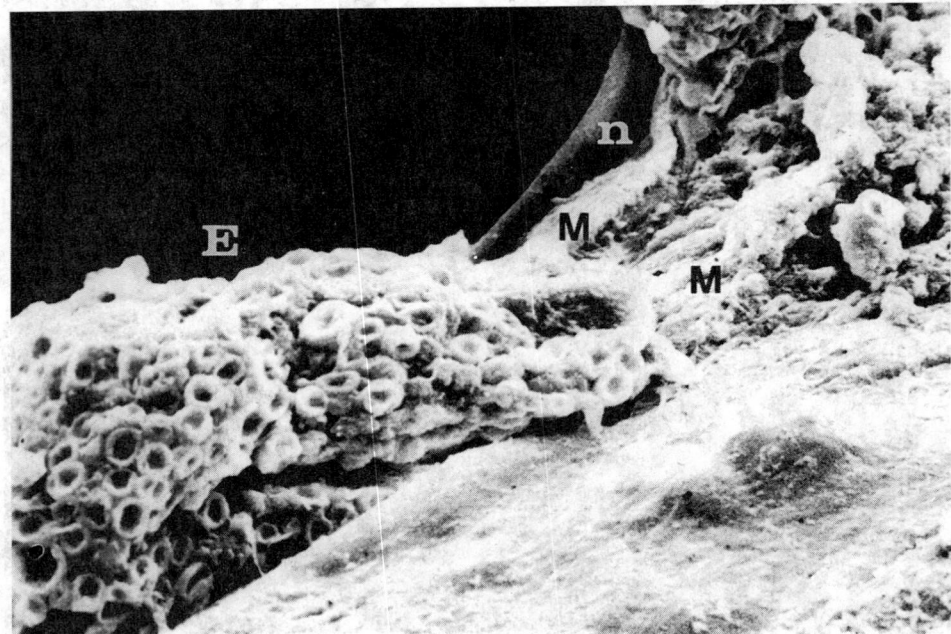

(d)

FIGURE 115.2 *(continued)*

type of ECM that they secrete. For example, liver tissue contains type I and type IV collagen, whereas type II collagen is found in cartilaginous tissues. Bone marrow contains types I, III, IV, and V collagen [Zuckerman, 1984]. Heterogeneity of collagen deposition as well as GAG composition exists not only between different tissues but in developmentally different stages of the same tissue [Thonar & Kuettner, 1987]. Fibroblast activity can be modulated by circulating or locally diffusible factors including IL-1 [Yang et al., 1988]. For example, the most prevalent GAGs in long-term bone marrow cultures are chondroitin sulfate (54%), hyaluronic acid (40%) and heparan sulfate (6%) [Wight et al., 1986]. Treatment of bone marrow stromal cell cultures with the steroid methylprednisolone reduces the concentration of hyaluronic acid and heparan sulfate relative to other proteins [Siczkowski et al., 1993]. In addition, a steroid, hydrocortisone, was found to be a necessary ingredient if the horse serum used to condition medium was to support hematopoiesis in long-term bone marrow cultures [Greenberger et al., 1979]. We found that it was also necessary to supplement medium with hydrocortisone or other corticosteroids to maintain the function of cocultures of liver-derived stromal cells and parenchymal hepatocytes for long-terms [Naughton et al., 1994]. The function of this steroid is clearly to modulate the stromal microenvironment.

Fibroblastic cells in tissue are heterogeneous with respect to support function. Early morphometric studies of bone marrow associated granulopoiesis with alkaline-phosphatase-positive fibroblastic cells [Weston & Bainton, 1979] and erythropoiesis with acid-phosphatase-positive macrophages [Dexter et al., 1981]. The development of highly specific monoclonal antibodies in the intervening years made possible a much more detailed analysis of bone marrow and other stromal cells. When a single cell suspension of bone marrow is inoculated into flasks containing liquid medium, stromal cells can be separated from hematologic cells by virtue of their adherence. However, the numbers of these cells are generally small compared with the hematopoietic marrow elements.

In addition to matrix deposition, fibroblasts synthesize the cytokines of the fibroblast growth factor (FGF) family, a variety of interleukins, and GM-CSF, as well as other regulatory cytokines (Table 115.2). Induction of fibroblast cytokine synthesis by interleukin-1 (IL-1) [Tjota et al., 1992] or other moieties enhances the ability of stromal cells to support hematopoiesis *in vitro*.

Endothelial Cells

For nonglandular tissues such as bone marrow, the endothelial cells are vascular lining cells and can be distinguished by the expression of or the message for von Willebrand factor and surface major histocompatibility complex-II (MHC-II) antigens. As cells of the vascular *tunica intima,* they, along with the basement membrane, form a selective barrier to regulate the transport of substances to and from the blood supply. In addition, their expression of integrins following stimulation with IL-1 or other mediators regulates the attachment of immunocompetent cells during acute (neutrophils) or chronic (T lymphocytes, monocytes) inflammation. Endothelial cells also regulate other vascular functions. They synthesize the vasodilatory effector nitric oxide after induction with acetylcholine [Furchgott & Zawadzki, 1980] and secrete regulatory peptides, the endothelins, which counteract this effect [Yanagisawa et al., 1988]. Specialized vascular endothelia are present in bone marrow, where they permit the egress of mature leukocytes from the marrow into the sinusoids, and in the liver, where the surfaces of the cells lining sinusoids are fenestrated to facilitate transport. In a more general context, endothelial cells also produce collagen IV for basement membranes and secrete several cytokines including IL-1, fibronectin, M-CSF, and GM-CSF and release platelet-activating factor (Table 115.2). Vascular endothelia are nonthrombogenic and contribute to angiogenesis by mitotically responding to locally secreted factors such as bFGF and aFGF. These endothelia possess LDL receptors and degrade this lipoprotein at substantially higher rates than other types of cells. These cells also have receptors for Fc, transferrin, mannose, galactose, and Apo-E, as well as for scavenger receptors [Van Eyken & Desmet, 1993]. Endothelia tend to assemble into tubular structures in culture, but their contribution to parenchymal cell growth in vitro is contingent on the generation of the proper tissue polarity.

In addition to vascular endothelial cells, some organs possess nonvascular endothelial cells such as the bile duct lining cells of the liver. These cells possess antigenic profiles and secretory potentials that are similar to vascular endothelia.

Adipocytes, Fat-Storing Cells

These cells are represented in varying concentrations in different tissues. They are related to fibroblasts (Fig. 115.2), and transformation of fibroblasts to adipocytes in vitro can be induced by

TABLE 115.2   Stromal Cell Phenotypes and Secretory Profiles

Phenotypes*	Cytokine/Protein Secretion
MHC I (all)	IL-1 (mφ, E, F, A)
MHC II (E, mφ)	M-CSF (mφ, E, F)
CD 10 (neural endopeptidase)[†]	G-CSF (mφ, F)
CD 29 (β$_2$ integrin) (all)	GM-CSF (mφ, E)
CD 34 (CFU-F)	LIF (mφ, F)
CD 36 (IA 7) (mφ)	GM-colony enhancing factor (mφ)
CD 44 (H-CAM)†	TGFβ (mφ, F)
CD 49b (α$_2$ chain of VLA-2)[†]	TNFα (mφ, F)
CD 49d (α$_4$ chain of VLA-4)[†]	PAF (E)
CD 49e (α$_5$ chain of VLA-5)[†]	BPA (mφ, E)
CD 51 (vitronectin receptor)[†]	IFNα (mφ, F, E)
CD 54 (ICAM-1) (all)	IFNγ (F)
CD 58 (LFA-3) (all)	IL-6 (mφ)
CD 61 (GP 111a)	c-kit ligand (mφ, F)
VCAM-1 (E)	acidic and basic FGF (F)
α SM actin (F)	angiotensinogen (A)
vimentin (F)	lipoprotein lipase (A)
decorin (Mes)	adipocyte P2 (A)
fibronectin (F, mφ)	MIP-1α (mφ)
laminin (E)	Complement proteins C1–C5 (mφ)
collagen I (F)	Factor B, properdin (mφ)
collagen III (F)	transcobalamin II (mφ)
collagen IV (E)	transferrin (mφ)
von Willebrand factor (E)	arachidonic acid metabolites (mφ, E)
adipsin (A)	(IL-3, IL-7, IL-9, IL-11, neuroleukin)[†]

*Phenotypic expression of stroma in bone marrow cultures. Parentheses indicate localization according to cell type (mφ = macrophage, F = fibroblast, E = endothelial cell, A = adipocyte, Mes = mesenchyme). Many of these phenotypes were identified in the original work of Cicuttini et al. [1992] and Moreau et al. [1993].

†Indicates the presence of mRNA and/or protein expression in bone marrow cultures but not localized to a particular cell type.

Abbreviations: BPA = erythroid burst promoting activity, CD = cluster determinant, MHC = major histocompatibility complex, M = monocyte, G = granulocyte, CSF = colony stimulating factor, CFU-F = colony forming unit-fibroblast, MIP = macrophage inflammatory protein, IL = interleukin, IFN = interferon, TGF = transforming growth factor, TNF = tumor necrosis factor, PAF = platelet activating factor, FGF = fibroblast growth factor, Factor B and properdin = proteins of the alternate complement pathway.

supplementation of the medium with hydrocortisone or other steroids [Brockbank & van Peer, 1983; Greenberger, 1979] which induce the expression of lipoproteinlipase and glycerolphosphate dehydrogenase as well as an increase in insulin receptors [Gimble et al., 1989]. Like fibroblasts, marrow adipocytes are heterogeneous and display different characteristics related to their distribution in red or yellow marrow [Lichtman, 1984]. These characteristics include insulin independence but glucocorticoid dependence in vitro, positive staining with perfomic acid-Schiff, and higher concentrations of neutral fats and unsaturated fatty acids in triglycerides. In bone marrow in vivo, there appears to be an inverse relationship between adipogenesis and erythropoiesis: phenylhydrazine-induced anemia causes a rapid conversion of yellow marrow (containing adipocytes) to red marrow due to compensatory erythroid heperplasia [Maniatis et al., 1971]. However, the role of the adipocyte in supporting hematopoiesis in culture is controversial. Although Dexter and coworkers [1977] associated declining myelopoiesis in long-term murine bone marrow cultures with the gradual disappearance of adipocytes from the stromal layer, these cells may not be necessary to support hematopoiesis in human bone marrow cultures [Touw & Lowenberg, 1983]. In this regard, IL-11 suppressed adipogenesis but stimulated human CD34+ HL-DR+ progenitor cells cocultured with human bone marrow stroma and enhanced the numbers of myeloid progenitor cells [Keller et al., 1993]. Hematopoiesis in vivo requires the proper ECM for cell attachment and differentiation as well as regulation by cytokines elaborated by stromal cells [Metcalf, 1993]. Although there is considerable redundancy in the synthesis of regulatory factors by different stromal cell populations, no single cell population has been identified that can provide an entire hematopoietic microenvironment. The use of cell lines to provide hematopoietic support will be discussed later in this chapter.

In the liver, purified fat-storing cells are capable of broad-scale synthetic activity that includes collagens I, III, IV, fibronectin, heparan sulfate, chondroitin sulfate, and dermatan sulfate [DeLeeuw et al., 1984]. Adipocytes also synthesize colony-stimulating factors and other regulatory cytokines (Table 115.2). In addition to the above characteristics, adipocytes are desmin positive and therefore are phenotypically related to myogenic cells or myofibroblasts. The function of adipocytes may vary depending on their location. Adipocytes in the bone marrow are in close apposition to the sinusoidal endothelial cells and in the liver are found in the space of Disse under the endothelial cells. Hepatic fat-storing cells are finely integrated into several contiguous parenchymal cells and contain fat droplets that are qualitatively different than those found in hepatic parechymal cells in that they contain high levels of retinols. Liver adipocytes are responsible for the metabolism and storage of vitamin A [DeLeeuw et al., 1984], provide some of the raw materials for the synthesis of biologic membranes and also contribute to local energy metabolism needs. Adipocytes of other tissues also act as a type of "progenitor" cell that can be converted to different phenotypes (e.g., osteoblasts or chondroblasts) under the appropriate conditions and are capable of stimulating osteogenesis via their secretion of cytokines [Benayahu et al., 1993].

Macrophages

Macrophages are derivatives of peripheral blood monocytes and are, therefore, bone-marrow–derived. They seed and remain on the surfaces of sinusoidal vessels in organs such as the liver and the spleen or migrate into the interstitial spaces of virtually all tissues. Macrophages are quintessential immunocompetent cells and are central components of many defense strategies, including randomized microbial phagocytosis and killing; antibody-dependent cellular cytotoxicity (ADCC), where they are directed against microbial or other cells that are opsonized with antibody; nonrandomized (specific) phagocytosis mediated by the association of immunoglobulins with a multiplicity of F_c receptors on their surfaces; the presentation of processed antigen to lymphocytes; secretion of and reaction to chemotaxins; and an enzymatic profile enabling them to move freely through tissue. The secretory capacity of macrophages is prodigious. In addition to plasma components such as complement proteins C1 through C5, they synthesize the ferric iron– and vitamin B_{12}–building proteins, transferrin and transcobalamin II, as well as a host of locally acting bioreactive metabolites of arachidonic acid. Macrophage secretory activity appears to influence two simultaneous events in vivo, inflammation and tissue repair. One monokine, IL-1, enhances the adhesion of neutrophils to vascular endothelial cells and activates B and T lymphocytes and other macrophages while stimulating the formation of acute phase proteins inducing collagen, ECM, and cytokine synthesis by fibroblasts and other stromal cells. IL-1, as well as a host of other humoral regulatory factors, originate in macrophages, including TNFα, IFNα, GM-CSF, and MIP-1α (Table 115.2). The ability of macrophages to secrete regulatory cytokines makes them an important contributor to the tissue microenvironment.

Macrophages have been intrinsically associated with erythropoiesis in the bone marrow [Bessis & Breton-Gorius, 1959] and [Naughton et al., 1979]. As such, these "nurse cells" destroy defective erythroblasts and the fetal and regenerating liver, and provide recycled iron stores for hemoglobin synthesis by developing red cells. They also synthesize and/or store erythropoietin.

115.2 Stromal Cells as "Feeder Layers" for Parenchymal Cell Culture

Irradiated stromal feeder layers were first used by Puck and Marcus [1955] to support the attachment and proliferation of HeLa cells in culture. Direct contact with feeder layers of cells also permits the growth of glioma cells and epithelial cells derived from breast tissue and colon [Freshney et al., 1982]. Enhanced attachment of parenchymal cells and production of factors to regulate growth and differentiation are two important benefits of coculturing parenchymal and stromal cells.

Bone Marrow

Bone marrow was the first tissue to be systematically investigated in regard to the influence of ECM and stromal cells on the production of blood cells. By the mid 1970s, the influence of microenvironmental conditions [Trentin, 1970; Wolf & Trentin, 1968] and ECM deposition [McCuskey et al., 1972; Schrock et al., 1973] upon hematapoiesis was well established in the hematology literature. Dexter and coworkers [1977] were the first to apply the feeder-layer–based coculture technology to hematopoietic cells by inoculating mouse bone marrow cells onto preestablished, irradiated feeder layers of marrow-derived stromal (adherent) cells. These cultures remained hematopoietically active for several months. By comparison, bone marrow cells cultured in the absence of feeder layers or supplementary cytokines terminally differentiated within the first two weeks in culture; stromal cells were the only survivors [Brandt et al., 1990; Chang & Anderson, 1971]. If the cultures are not supplemented with exogenous growth factors, then myeloid cells, monocytic cells, and nucleated erythroblasts are present for the first 7–10 days of culture. This trilineage pattern is narrowed over successive weeks in culture so that from about 2–4 weeks myeloid and monocytic cells are produced, and, if cultured for longer terms, the products of the culture are almost entirely monocytic. However, the nature of hematopoietic support can be modulated by changing the environmental conditions. In this regard, cocultures established under identical conditions as the above produce B lymphocytes if the steroid supplementation of the medium is removed and the ambient temperature is increased [Whitlock & Witte, 1982]. Static bone marrow coculture systems are generally categorized as declining because of this and the finding that the hematopoietic progenitor cell concentrations decrease as a function of time in culture. However, this trend can be offset by coculturing bone marrow in bioreactors that provide constant media exchange and optimize oxygen delivery [Palsson et al., 1993] or by supplementing the cocultures with cocktails of the various growth factors elaborated by stromal cells [Keller et al., 1993].

Connective tissue feeder layers had originally been hypothesized to act by conditioning medium with soluble factors that stimulated growth and by providing a substratum for the selective attachment of certain types of cells [Puck & Marcus, 1955]. These are functions that have since been proven for bone marrow and other tissue culture systems. The stromal population of bone marrow (Table 115.1) is heterogeneous for lineage support and perhaps also for stem cell renewal. This is accomplished in part by the creation of niches by select stromal cell populations in vivo. Foci of erythropoiesis in bone marrow, and in bone marrow cultures, are generally associated with acid-phosphatase-positive macrophages [Dexter et al., 1981] (Fig. 115.2c). In contrast, granulocytic cells are associated with alkaline phosphatase positive reticular fibroblasts (Fig. 115.2d) [Weston & Bainton, 1979].

It is very difficult to recreate the marrow microenvironment in vitro. One reason is that the marrow stromal cell populations proliferate at different rates; if expanded vigorously using nutrient-rich medium, the culture selects for fibroblastic cells at the expense of the more slowly dividing types of stroma. We established rat bone marrow cocultures using stromal cells that were passaged for 6 months, and these cultures produced lower numbers of progenitor cells (CFU-C) in the adherent zone as compared to cocultures established with stroma that was only passed three to four times (Fig. 115.3). Cells released from cultures using the older stroma were almost entirely monocytic,

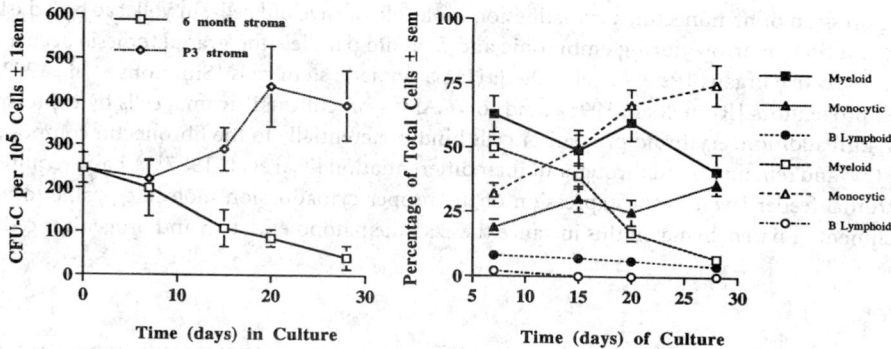

FIGURE 115.3 *Left.* Mean CFU-C progenitor concentration of the adherent zone of a three-dimensional coculture of rat bone hematopoietic cells and rat bone marrow stroma. Stock cultures to generate the stromal cells for the cocultures were seeded onto the three-dimensional template either after passage (P3) or following expansion in monolayer culture for 6 months. Stroma at early passage is substantially more supportive of CFU-C progenitor cells that "old" stroma that is primarily fibroblastic in nature. Vertical lines through the means = ±1 standard error of the mean (sem). *Right.* Analysis of the cellular content of the nonadherent zone of rat bone marrow hematopoietic cell:stromal cell cocultures on three-dimensional templates by flow cytometry. Cocultures were established either with P3 stroma (closed figures) or stroma that was grown in monolayer culture for 6 months (open figures). The mean percentages of cells recognized by the phenotyping antibodies MOM/3F12/F2 (myeloid), ED-1 (monocytic), and OX-33 (B lymphoid) (Serotec, UK) are depicted. Vertical lines through the means = ±1 sem. Whereas low passage stroma generates myeloid, B lymphoid, and monocytic cells in cocultures and releases them into the nonadherent zone, 6-month-old stroma supports mainly the production of macrophages.

even at earlier terms of culture. In a related experiment, we suspended nylon screen cocultures of passage 3–4 stroma and bone marrow hematopoietic cells in flasks containing confluent, 6-month-old stromal cell monolayers and found that these monolayer cells inhibited hematopoiesis in the coculture [Naughton et al., 1989].

We use early passage stroma for our cocultures in order to retain a representation of all the stromal cell types. If hematopoietic cells from cocultures are removed after about a month in vitro and reinoculated onto a new template containing passage 3–4 stromal cells and cultured for an additional month, the progenitor cell concentrations of the adherent zones are considerably higher than in cocultures where no transfer took place [Naughton et al., 1994]. This experiment indicated that continued access to "fresh" stroma enhances hematopoiesis. The maintenance of mixed populations of stromal cells are desirable for a number of reasons. The same cytokine may be synthesized by different stromal cells, but its mode of action is usually synergistic with other cytokines for the differentiation of a specific blood cell lineage(s). Differentiation may not occur in the absence one of these cytokines, although some degree of redundancy in cytokine expression is intrinsic to the stromal system [Metcalf, 1993]. The fibroblastic cells that "grow out" of later passage human and rodent bone marrow stroma share some phenotypic properties with muscle cells (αSM actin+, CD34-, STRO-1-). These cells (endothelial cells and macrophages are absent or present in negligible quantities) supported hematopoietic progenitors for up to 7 weeks of culture but not longer [Moreau et al., 1993], indicating that other types of cells are necessary for long-term hematopoiesis in vitro.

Cytoadhesive molecule expression and its modulation is also an important consideration for the engineering of bone marrow and other tissues. In the case of bone marrow, this regulates "homing" or seeding, restricting cells in specific areas within tissues both to expose them to regulatory factors and to the release of cells from the supportive stroma upon maturation. For example, the sequential expression of hemonectin, a cytoadhesion molecule of myeloid cells, in yolk sac blood islands, liver, and bone marrow during embryonic and fetal life parallels the granulopoiesis occurring in these respective organs [Peters et al., 1990]. Hematopoietic stem cells [Simmons et al., 1992] and B-cell progenitors [Ryan et al., 1991] bind to VCAM-1 on cultured stromal cells by expression of VLA-4. In addition, erythroid progenitor cells bind preferentially to the fibronectin component of the ECM and remain bound throughout their differentiation [Tsai et al., 1987]. A basic requirement of stromal feeder layers is the expression of the proper cytoadhesion molecule profile to permit attachment of parenchyma; in this instance these are hematopoietic stem and progenitor cells.

Liver

Liver is an hematopoietic organ during fetal life, and it contains many of the same stromal cell populations found in bone marrow (Table 115.3). Research trends in liver cell and bone marrow culture have followed a somewhat parallel course. Both tissues are difficult to maintain in vitro; the parenchymal cell numbers either declined (hematopoietic progenitors) or lost function and dedifferentiated (hepatocytes) over time in culture. When mixed suspensions of hepatic cells are inoculated into liquid medium, approximately 20% of the total cells attach. The nonadherent population remains viable for about 72 hours. The adherent cells, although they proliferate for only 24–48 hours after inoculation, can survive for substantially longer periods. However, many of these adherent parenchymal cells undergo drastic phenotypic alterations, especially if the medium is conditioned with serum. These changes include a flattening and spreading on plastic surfaces as well as a propensity to undergo nuclear division in the absence of concomitant cytoplasmic division. The appearance of these bizarre, multinucleated, giant cells herald the loss of liver-specific functions such as

TABLE 115.3   Cells Contributing to the Hepatic Microenvironment

Cell Type	Size, μm	Relative Percent of Total Cells	Characteristics
Stroma			
Kupffer cells	12–16	8	MHC-1+, MHC-II+, Fcr, C3r, mannose and D-acetylglucosamine receptors, acid phosphatase+, density = 1.076 gm/ml,* 1.036gm/ml†
Vascular endothelia	11–12	9	MHC-I+, MHC-II+, vWF+, F$_c$r, TFr, mannose, apo-E, and scavenger receptors, density = 1.06–1.08 gm/ml,* 1.036 gm/ml†
Biliary endothelia	10–12	5	MHC-I+, positive for cytokeratins 7,8,18,19, β2 microglobulin+, positive for VLA-2,3,6 integrins, agglutinate with UEA, WGA, SBA, PNA, density = 1.075–1.1 gm/ml,* 1.0363 gm/ml†
Fat-storing cells	14–18	3	MHC-I+, desmin+, retinol+, ECM expression, collagen I, IV, and laminin expression, density = 1.075–1.1 gm/ml*
Fibroblasts	11–14	7	MHC-I+, ECM expression, collagen I, IV expression, density = 1.025 gm/ml,* 1.063 gm/ml†
Pit cells	11–15	1–2 (variable)	MHC-I+, asialo-GM+, CD8+, CD-5-
Parenchymal cells			
Mononuclear (type I)	17–22	35	MHC-I-, MHC-II-, blood group antigen-, density = 1.10–1.14 gm/ml,* 1.067 gm/ml†
Binuclear (type II)	20–27	27	MHC-I±, MHC-II-, blood group antigen-, density = 1.10–1.14 gm/ml,* 1.071 gm/ml†
Acidophilic (type III)	25–32	5	MHC-I±, MHC-II-, blood group antigen-, density = 1.038 gm/ml†

Abbreviations: ECM = extracellular matrix, MHC = major histocompatability complex, PNA = peanut agglutinin, SBA = soybean agglutinin, WGA = wheat germ agglutinin, UEA = Ulex europaeus agglutinin.

albumin synthesis and the metabolism of organic chemicals by cytochrome P450 enzymes. The percentage of hepatocytes attaching to the flask, the maintenance of rounded parenchymal cell phenotype, and the expression of specialized hepatic function in vitro can be enhanced by precoating the flasks with ECM components such as type I collagen [Michalopoulos & Pitot, 1975], fibronectin [Deschenes et al., 1980], homogenized liver tissue matrix [Reid et al., 1980], laminin, and type IV collagen [Bissell et al., 1987]. Hepatocyte survival and functional expression also improved when hepatocytes were cocultured with liver-derived [Fry & Bridges, 1980] and murine 3T3 [Kuri-Harcuch & Mendoza-Figueroa, 1989] fibroblasts as well as a preestablished layer of adherent liver epithelial cells [Guguen-Guillouzo et al., 1983]. As with bone marrow culture on feeder layers, cells derived from the liver itself usually provide the best support in culture. However, we have found that hepatic parenchyma will express a differentiated function in vitro if supported by bone marrow stroma. Conversely, liver-derived stromal cells support hematopoiesis in culture, but this microenvironment favors erythropoisis (unpublished observations).

In contrast to the role of bone marrow stroma on hematopoiesis, the influence of hepatic stromal cells on the function and/or growth of parenchymal hepatocytes has not been exhaustively investigated. However, several studies indicate that Kupffer cells, fat-storing cells, and perhaps other stroma influence parenchymal cell cytochrome P450 enzyme expression [Peterson & Renton, 1984] and act in tandem with parenchymal cells to metabolize lipopolysaccharide [Treon et al., 1979]. In addition, adipocytes and hepatic fibroblasts synthesize collagen type I and the proteoglycans heparan sulfate, dermatan sulfate, and chondroitin sulfate as well as hyaluronic acid, which is unsulfated in the liver and occurs as a simple GAG. Stromal cells as well as parenchyma deposit fibronectin. Liver adipocytes, like their relatives in bone marrow, express phenotypes (vimentin+, actin+, tubulin+) linking them histogenically to fibroblasts and myogenic cells [DeLeeuw et al., 1984]. Fat-storing cells as well as vascular endothelia apparently synthesize the type IV collagen found in the space of Disse, and fibrin originating from parenchymal cell fibrinogen synthesis is a significant part of liver matrix, at least in culture. As with the hematopoietic cells in bone marrow cultures, hepatic parenchymal cell gene expression is modulated by attachment to ECM and influenced by factors released by stromal cells. For example, parenchymal cells attaching to laminin-coated surfaces express the differentiation-associated substance α-fetoprotein, whereas the synthesis of albumin synthesis is favored when parenchymal cells bind to type IV collagen [Michalopoulous & Pitot, 1975]. Hepatocytes bind to fibronectin using the $\alpha_5\beta$, integrin heterodimer and AGp110, a nonintegrin glycoprotein. Cytoadhesion molecule expression by hepatic cells and cells of other tissues changes with and perhaps controls development [Stamatoglou & Hughes, 1994]. Just as differential hemonectin expression occurred during the development of the hematopoietic system [Peters et al., 1990], a differential expression of liver proteins occurs during ontogeny. Although fibronectin and its receptor are strongly expressed in liver throughout life, AGp110 appears later in development and may guide the development of parenchyma into a polarized tissue. It will probably be necessary to incorporate the various stromal support cells found in liver into hepatocyte cultures.

Tumor Cells

Fibroblasts and other stromal cells derived from malignant tissue have been demonstrated to stimulate the growth of tumor cells in vitro using coculture techniques [Degrassi et al., 1993; Horgan et al., 1987]. Breast cancer cell growth in culture can be stimulated by fibroblast-conditioned medium and apparently does not require direct cell contact [Horgan et al., 1987; van Roozendaal et al., 1992]. In contrast, the primary culture of murine plasmacytomas depends upon the presence of a stromal cell feeder layer. In a manner similar to bone marrow culture, where steroids altered the ECM composition and consequently the hematopoietic support function of stroma, anti-inflammatory drugs alter the microenvironment and prevent plasmacytoma growth in vivo and in vitro [Degrassi et al., 1993].

115.3 Support of Cultured Cells Using Cell Lines

The precise roles of the various cellular constituents of the tissue microenvironment have not been fully defined. One approach to understanding these mechanisms is to develop stromal cell lines with homogeneous and well-defined characteristics and then ascertain the ability of these cells to support parenchyma in coculture. A brief survey of some of these lines is found in Table 115.4. Stromal cell lines derived from bone marrow are usually either fibroblastic (F) or a mixture of fibroblastic and adipocytic cells which contain a subpopulation of fibroblastic cells that can be induced to undergo lipogenesis with dexamethasone or hydrocortisone (A) (reviewed by Gimble, [1990]). In general, fibroblastic lines support myelopoiesis and monocytopoiesis and stroma with both fibroblastic and adipocytic cells supports myelopoiesis as well as B lymphopoiesis. The MBA-14 cell line, which consists of stroma bearing fibroblastic as well as monocytic phenotypes, stimulated the formation of CFU-C (bipotential myeloid/monocytic) progenitors in coculture. Different cell lines that were transformed using the large T oncogene of simian virus 40 (U2) were used as feeder layers for bone marrow hematopoietic cells. Cocultures established using bone-marrow-derived stroma exhibited considerably better maintenance of the primitive stem cell CFU-S$_{12}$ in culture than similarly transfected skin, lung, or kidney tissue cells [Rios & Williams, 1990]. Although feeder layers share a number of characteristics (cytokine production, ECM deposition), it is probably best to derive your feeder cells from the tissue that you wish to coculture rather than use xenogeneic feeder cells or cells derived from a completely dissimilar tissue. In this respect, we found that total cell output and progenitor cell concentrations were substantially higher in rat bone marrow cocultures supported with rat bone marrow stroma as compared to those established using immortalized human skin fibroblasts or fetal lung cell lines [Naughton & Naughton, 1989].

115.4 Stereotypic (Three-Dimensional) Culture Versus Monolayer Culture

Tissue is a three-dimensional arrangement of various types of cells that are organized into a functional unit. These cells also are polarized with respect to their position within tissue and the microenvironment, and therefore the metabolic activity and requirements of the tissue are not uniform throughout. Three-dimensional culture was first performed successfully by Leighton [1951] using cellulose sponge as a template. Collagen gel frameworks [Douglas, 1980] also have been and are currently being employed to culture tissues such as skin, breast epithelium, and liver. In addition, tumor tissue cocultured with stroma in collagen gels respond to drugs in a manner similar to that observed in vivo [Rheinwald & Beckett, 1981].

We developed three-dimensional coculture templates using nylon filtration screens and felts made of polyester or bioresorbable polyglycolic acid polymers [Naughton et al., 1987, 1994]. Rodent or human bone marrow cocultures retained multilineage hematopoietic expression in these stereotypic cultures, a phenomenon that is possible in plastic flask or suspension cultures only if the medium is supplemented with cocktails of cytokines [Peters et al., 1993]. Cocultures of rat hepatic parenchymal and stromal cells on three-dimensional templates also displayed a number of liver-specific functions for at least 48 days in culture, including the active synthesis of albumin, fibrinogen, and other proteins and the expression of dioxin-inducible cytochrome P450 enzyme activity for up to 2 months in culture [Naughton et al., 1994]. Furthermore, hepatic parenchyma in these stereotypic cocultures proliferated in association with stromal elements and the ECM they deposited until all "open" areas within the template were utilized. Our method is different from others because we use stromal cells derived from the tissue we wish to culture to populate the three-dimensional template. These cells secrete tissue-specific ECM and other matrix components that are indigenous to the normal microenvironment of the tissue. Parenchymal cells associate freely within the template after their inoculation and bind to other cells and/or matrix based upon their natural cytoadhesion molecule profiles. We do not add exogenous proteins.

TABLE 115.4 Some Representative Stromal Cell Lines Used to Support Hematopoietic Cells or Hepatocytes

Cell line	Species	Phenotype*	Support Capability
Bone marrow			
AC-4	Mouse	A	Myeloid, monocytic, B lymphoid
ALC	Mouse	A	Myeloid, monocytic, B lymphoid
GM 1380	Human	F	Short-term myelo- + monopoiesis
GY-30	Mouse	A	Myeloid, monocytic, B lymphoid myelopoiesis
K-1	Mouse	A	
MBA-14	Mouse	F/M	Enhances CFU-C numbers myelopoiesis
MS-1	Mouse	F	
U2	Mouse	F†	Maintenance of CFU-S$_{12}$ myelopoiesis
3T3	Mouse	F	
10 T1/2	Mouse	F	Stimulates CFU-GEMM, -GM
10 T1/2 clone D	Mouse	A	Stimulates CFU-GM only
266 AD	Mouse	A	Myeloid, monocytic, B lymphoid
Liver			
3T3	Mouse	F	Enhanced lipid metabolism, extends period of cytochrome P450 activity‡
Detroit 550	Human	F	Prolonged cytochrome P450 and NADPH-cytochrome C reductase activity‡

Source: Adapted from Anklesaria et al. [1987] and Gimble [1990].

*Major phenotype of the cell line (F = fibroblastic, M = monocytic, A = capable of supporting adipocyte phenotypes).

†A bone marrow–derived cell line that was transformed with the large T oncogene of simian virus 40.

‡Support functions are compared to liquid cultures of rat hepatocytes without stroma.

Abbreviations: CFU = colony-forming unit; G = granulocyte; M = macrophage; S = spleen; GEMM = granulocyte, erythrocyte, megakaryocyte, monocyte; NADPH = nicotinamide adenine dinucleotide phosphate.

Three-dimensional scaffolds such as nylon screen or polyester felt provide large surface areas for cell attachment and growth. Although mass transfer limitations of diffusion dictate the maximum thickness (density) of a tissue culture, suspended three-dimensional cultures have the advantage of being completely surrounded by medium. This arrangement effectively doubles the maximum tissue thickness that is possible with a plastic flask-based culture. These stereotypic cultures also appear to form tissuelike structure in vitro and, when implanted after coculture on bioresorbable polymer templates, in vivo.

Defining Terms

When hematopoietic cells are inoculated into semisolid or liquid medium containing the appropriate growth factors, some of the cells are clonal and will form colonies after approximately 2 weeks in culture. These colonies arise from hematopoietic progenitor cells and are called **colony-forming units** or **CFU.** These colonies can consist of granulocytic cells (**G**), monocytic cells (**M**), a mixture of these two cell types (**GM**), or erythroid cells (**E**). Less mature progenitor cells have a greater potential for lineage expression. For example, a **CFU-GEMM** contains granulocytic, erythroid, megakaryocytic, and monocytic cells and is therefore the least mature progenitor of this group.

The text also mentions **CFU-S.** Whereas the other assays quantify colony formation in vitro, this is an in vivo assay. Briefly, irradiated mice are infused with hematopoietic cells. Some of these cells will colonize the spleen and will produce blood cells that "rescue" the animal. As with the in vitro assays, colonies that arise later in culture originate from less mature cells. The **CFU-S$_{12}$** therefore is a more primitive hematopoietic cell than the **CFU-S$_9$.**

References

Anklesaria P, Kase K, Glowacki J, et al. 1987. Engraftment of a clonal bone marrow stromal cell line *in vivo* stimulates hematopoietic recovery from total body irradiation. Proc Natl Acad Sci USA 84:7681.

Benayahu D, Zipori D, Wientroub S. 1993. Marrow adipocytes regulate growth and differentiation of osteoblasts. Biochem Biophys Res Comm 197:1245.

Ben-Ze'ev A, Robinson GS, Bucher NLR, et al. 1988. Cell-cell and cell-matrix interactions differentially regulate the expression of hepatic and cytoskeletal genes in primary cultures of rat hepatocytes. Proc Nat Acad Sci (USA) 85:2161.

Bessis M, Breton-Gorius J. 1959. Nouvelles observations sur l'ilot erythroblastique et la rhopheocytose de la ferritin. Rev Hematol 14:165.

Bissell DM, Arenson DM, Maher JJ, et al. 1987. Support of cultured hepatocytes by a laminin-rich gel: Evidence for a functionally significant subendothelial matrix in normal rat liver. J Clin Invest 790:801.

Brandt J, Srour EF, Van Besien K, et al. 1990. Cytokine-dependent long term culture of highly enriched precursors of hematopoietic progenitor cells from human bone marrow. J Clin Invest 86:932.

Brockbank KGM, van Peer CMJ. 1983. Colony stimulating activity production by hemopoietic organ fibroblastoid cells in vitro. Acta Haematol 69:369.

Chang VT, Anderson RN. 1971. Cultivation of mouse bone marrow cells: I. Growth of granulocytes. J Reticuloendoth Soc 9:568.

Cicuttini FM, Martin M, Ashman L, et al. 1992. Support of human cord blood progenitor cells on human stromal cell lines transformed by SV_{40} large T antigen under the influence of an inducible (metallothionein) promoter. Blood 80:102.

Degrassi A, Hilbert DM, Rudikoff S, et al. 1993. In vitro culture of primary plasmacytomas requires stromal cell feeder layers. Proc Nat Acad Sci (USA) 90:2060.

DeLeeuw AM, McCarthy SP, Geerts A, et al. 1984. Purified rat liver fat-storing cells in culture divide and contain collagen. Hepatology 4:392.

Dexter TM, Allen TD, Lajtha LG. 1977. Conditions controlling the proliferation of haematopoietic stem cells in vitro. J Cell Physiol 91:335.

Dexter TM, Testa NG, Allen TD, et al. 1981. Molecular and cell biologic aspects of erythropoiesis in long-term bone marrow cultures. Blood 58:699.

Douglas WHJ, Moorman GW, Teel RW. 1980. Visualization of cellular aggregates cultured on a three-dimensional collagen sponge matrix. In Vitro 16:306.

Freshney RI, Hart E, Russell JM. 1982. Isolation and purification of cell cultures from human tumours. In E Reid, GMW Cook, DJ Moore (eds), Cancer Cell Organelles. Methodological Surveys: Biochemistry, pp 97–110, Chichester, England, Horwood Press.

Friedenstein AJ, Chailakhyan RK, Gerasimov UV. 1970. Bone marrow osteogenic stem cells: In vitro cultivation and transplantation in diffusion chambers. Cell Tiss Kinet 20:263.

Furchgott RF, Zawadzki JV. 1980. The obligatory role of endothelial cells in the relaxation of arterial smooth muscle by acetylcholine. Nature 286:373.

Gallagher JT, Spooncer E, Dexter TM. 1983. Role of extracellular matrix in haemopoiesis: I. Synthesis of glycosaminoglycans by mouse bone marrow cultures. J Cell Sci 63:155.

Gimble JM. 1990. The function of adipocytes in the bone marrow stroma. New Biol 2:304.

Gimble JM, Dorheim MA, Cheng Q, et al. 1989. Response of bone marrow stromal cells to adipogenetic antagonists. Mol Cell Biol 9:4587.

Greenberger JS. 1979. Corticosteroid-dependent differentiation of human marrow preadipocytes in vitro. In Vitro 15:823.

Guguen-Guilluozo C, Clement B, Baffet G, et al. 1983. Maintenance and reversibility of active albumin secretion by adult rat hepatocytes co-cultured with another cell type. Exp Cell Res 143:47.

Horgan K, Jones DL, Marsel RE. 1987. Mitogenicity of human fibroblasts *in vivo* for human breast cancer cells. Brit J Surg 74:227.

Huang S, Terstappen LWMM. 1992. Formation of haematopoietic microenvironment and haematopoietic stem cells from single human bone marrow cells. Nature 360:745.

Keller D, Ou XX, Srour EF, et al. 1993. Interleukin-II inhibits adipogenesis and stimulates myelopoiesis in human long-term marrow cultures. Blood 82:1428.

Kuri-Harcuch W, Mendoza-Figueroa T. 1989. Cultivation of adult rat hepatocytes on 3T3 cells: Expression of various liver differentiated functions. Differentiation 41:148.

Leighton J. 1951. A sponge matrix method for tissue culture: Formation of organized aggregates of cells in vitro. J Natl Cancer Inst 12:545.

Lichtman MA. 1984. The relationship of stromal cells to hemopoietic cells in marrow. In DG Wright, JS Greenberger (eds), Long-term Bone Marrow Culture, pp 3–30, New York, A.R. Liss.

Lin CQ, Bissell MJ. 1993. Multi-faceted regulation of cell differentiation by extracellular matrix. FASEB J 7:737.

Maniatis A, Tavassoli M, Crosby WH. 1971. Factors affecting the conversion of yellow to red marrow. Blood 37:581.

McCuskey RS, Meineke HA, Townsend SF. 1972. Studies of the hemopoietic microenvironment: I. Changes in the microvascular system and stroma during erythropoietic regeneration and suppression in the speens of CF_1 mice. Blood 5:697.

Metcalf D. 1993. Hematopoietic growth factors. Redundancy or subtlety? Blood 82:3515.

Michalopoulos G, Pitot HC. 1975. Primary culture of parenchymal liver cells on collagen membranes. Exp Cell Res 94:70.

Moreau I, Duvert V, Caux C, et al. 1993. Myofibroblastic stromal cells isolated from human bone marrow induce the proliferation of both early myeloid and B-lymphoid cells. Blood 82:2396.

Naughton BA, Kolks GA, Arce JM, et al. 1979. The regenerating liver: A site of erythropoiesis in the adult long-evans rat. Amer J Anat 156:159.

Naughton BA, Naughton GK. 1989. Hematopoiesis on nylon mesh templates. Ann NY Acad Sci 554:125.

Naughton BA, San Roman J, Sibanda B, et al. 1994. Stereotypic culture systems for liver and bone marrow: Evidence for the development of functional tissue in vitro and following implantation in vivo. Biotech Bioeng 43:810.

Owen ME. 1988. Marrow stromal stem cells. J Cell Sci 10:63.

Palsson BO, Paek S-H, Schwartz RM, et al. 1993. Expansion of human bone marrow progenitor cells in a high cell density continuous perfusion system. Biotechnology 11:368.

Peters C, O'Shea KS, Campbell AD, et al. 1990. Fetal expression of hemonectin: An extracellular matrix hematopoietic cytoadhesion molecule. Blood 75:357.

Peterson TC, Renton KW. 1984. Depression of cytochrome P-450-dependent drug biotransofrmation in hepatocytes after the activation of the reticuloendothelial system by dextran sulfate. J Pharmacol Exp Ther 229:229.

Puck TT, Marcus PI. 1955. A rapid method for viable cell titration and clone production with HeLa cells in tissue culture: The use of X-irradiated cells to supply conditioning factors. Proc Natl Acad Sci (USA) 41:432.

Reid LM, Gaitmaitan Z, Arias I, et al. 1980. Long-term cultures of normal rat hepatocytes on liver biomatrix. Ann NY Acad Sci 349:70.

Rios M, Williams DA. 1990. Systematic analysis of the ability of stromal cell lines derived from different murine adult tissues to support maintenance of hematopoietic stem cells in vitro. J Cell Physiol 145:434.

Roberts R, Gallagher J, Spooncer E, et al. 1988. Heparan sulfate bound growth factors: A mechanism for stromal cell-mediated haemopoiesis. Nature 332:376.

Ryan DH, Nuccie BL, Abboud CN, et al. 1991. Vascular cell adhesion molecule-1 and the integrin VLA-4 mediate adhesion of human B cell precursors to cultured bone marrow adherent cells. J Clin Invest 88:995.

Schrock LM, Judd JT, Meineke HA, et al. 1973. Differences in concentration of acid mucopolysaccharides between spleens of normal and polycythemic CF1 mice. Proc Soc Exp Biol Med 144:593.

Siczkowski M, Amos AS, Gordon MY. 1993. Hyaluronic acid regulates the function and distribution of sulfated glycosaminoglycans in bone marrow stromal cultures. Exp Hematol 21:126.

Simmons PJ, Masinovsky B, Longenecker BM, et al. 1992. Vascular cell adhesion molecule-1 expressed by bone marrow stromal cells mediates the binding of hematopoietic progenitor cells. Blood 80:388.

Simmons PJ, Torok-Storb B. 1991. CD 34 expression by stromal precursors in normal human adult bone marrow. Blood 78:2848.

Strobel E-S, Gay RE, Greenberg PL. 1986. Characterization of the in vitro stromal microenvironment of human bone marrow. Int J Cell Cloning 4:341.

Stamatoglou SC, Hughes RC. 1994. Cell adhesion molecules in liver function and pattern formation. FASEB J 8:420.

Thonar EJ-MA, Kuettner KE, 1987. Biochemical basis of age-related changes in proteoglycans. In: TN Wight, RP Mecham (eds), Biology of Proteoglycans, pp 211–246, New York, Academic Press.

Tjota A, Rossi TM, Naughton BA. 1992. Stromal cells derived from spleen or bone marrow support the proliferation of rat natural killer cells in long-term culture. Proc Soc Exp Biol Med 200:431.

Touw I, Lowenberg B. 1983. No stimulative effect of adipocytes on hematopoiesis in long-term human bone marrow cultures. Blood 61:770.

Trentin JJ. 1970. Influence of hematopoietic organ stroma (Hematopoietic inductive microenvironment) on stem cell differentiation. In AS Gordon (ed), Regulation of Hematopoiesis, New York, Appleton-Century-Crofts.

Treon SP, Thomas P, Baron J. 1979. Lipopolysaccharide (LPS) processing by Kupffer cells releases a modified LPS with increased hepatocyte binding and decreased tumor necrosis-α stimulatory capacity. Proc Soc Exp Biol Med 202:153.

Tsai S, Patel V, Beaumont E, et al. 1987. Differential binding to erythroid and myeloid progenitors to fibroblasts and fibronectin. Blood 69:1587.

Van Eyken P, Desmet VJ. 1993. Bile duct cells. In AV LeBouton (ed), Molecular and Cell Biology of the Liver, pp 475–524, Boca Raton, Fla, CRC Press.

Van Roozendaal CEP, van Ooijen B, Klijn JGM, et al. 1992. Stromal influences on breast cancer cell growth. Brit J Cancer 65:77.

Weston H, Bainton DF. 1979. Association of alkaline phosphatase positive reticulum cells in bone marrow with granulocytic precursors. J Exp Med 150:919.

Whitlock CA, Witte ON. 1982. Long term culture of B lymphocytes and their precursors from murine bone marrow. Proc Nat Acad Sci (USA) 77:4756.

Wight TN, Kinsella MG, Keating A, et al. 1986. Proteoglycans in human long-term bone marrow cultures: Biochemical and ultrastructural analysis. Blood 67:1333.

Wilson D. 1983. The origin of the endothelium in the developing marginal vein of the chick wing-bud. Cell Differ 13:63.

Wolf NS, Trentin JJ. 1968. Hematopoietic colony studies: V. Effects of hemopoietic organ stroma on differentiation of pluripotent stem cells. J Exp Med 127:205.

Yanagisawa M, Jurihara HJ, Kimura S, et al. 1988. A novel potent vasoconstrictor peptide produced by vascular endothelial cells. Nature 332:411.

Yang Y-C, Tsai S, Wong GG, et al. 1988. Interleukin-1 regulation of hematopoietic growth factor production by human stromal fibroblasts. J Cell Physiol 134:292.

Zuckerman KS. 1984. Composition and function of the extracellular matrix in the stroma of long-term bone marrow cell cultures. In DG Wright, JS Greenberger (eds), Long-term Bone Marrow Culture, pp 157–170, New York, A.R. Liss.

Zuckerman KS, Rhodes RK, Goodrum DD, et al. 1985. Inhibition of collagen depostion in the extracellular matrix prevents the establishment of stroma supportive of hematopoiesis in long term murine bone marrow cultures. J Clin Invest 75:970.

Further Information

There are a number of different methodologies for isolating cells including gradient density centrifugation, sedimentation at unit gravity, lectin agglutination, and reaction with specific antibodies followed by immunoselection via panning or immunomagnetic microspheres. These methods are described and illustrated well in volumes 1–5 of *Cell Separation: Methods and Selected Applications,* New York, Academic Press, 1987. For additional details concerning the relevance of ECM deposition to the development and functional expression of various types of tissue cells, the reader is referred to the serial reviews of this subject that appeared in *The FASEB Journal* from volume 7, number 9 (1993) to volume 8, number 4 (1994). Information about the various cell types of the liver, their interaction with matrix components, and their mechanisms of gene expression can be found in *Molecular and Cell Biology of the Liver,* Boca Raton, Florida, CRC Press (1993). Similarly, for more details concerning bone marrow cells and the mechanisms of hematopoiesis, consult *The Human Bone Marrow,* volume 1, Boca Raton, Florida, CRC Press (1992).

116

Tissue Engineering
of Bone Marrow

Manfred R. Koller
Aastrom Biosciences Inc.

Bernhard Ø. Palsson
University of Michigan

The human body consumes a staggering 400 billion mature blood cells every day, and this number increases dramatically under conditions of stress such as infection or bleeding. A complex scheme of multilineage proliferation and differentiation, termed *hematopoiesis* (Greek for blood forming), has evolved to meet this demand. This regulated production of mature blood cells from immature stem cells, which occurs mainly in the bone marrow (BM) of adult mammals, has been the focus of considerable research effort. Ex vivo models of human hematopoiesis now exist that have significant scientific value and promise to have an impact on clinical practice in the near future. This endeavor is spread across many fields, including cell biology, molecular biology, bioengineering, and medicine.

This chapter introduces the reader to the fundamental concepts of hematopoiesis, the clinical applications which drive much of the effort to reconstitute hematopoiesis ex vivo, and the progress made to date toward achieving this goal.

116.1 Biology of Hematopoiesis

The Hematopoietic System: Function and Organization

There are eight major types of mature blood cells which are found in the circulation (see Fig. 116.1). The blood cell population is divided into two major groups: the myeloid and lymphoid. The myeloid lineage includes erythrocytes (red blood cells), monocytes, the granulocytes (neutrophils, eosinophils, and basophils), and platelets (derived from noncirculating megakaryocytes). Thymus-derived (T) lymphocytes and BM-derived (B) lymphocytes constitute the lymphoid lineage. Most

0-8493-8346-3/95/$0.00+$.50
© 1995 by CRC Press, Inc.

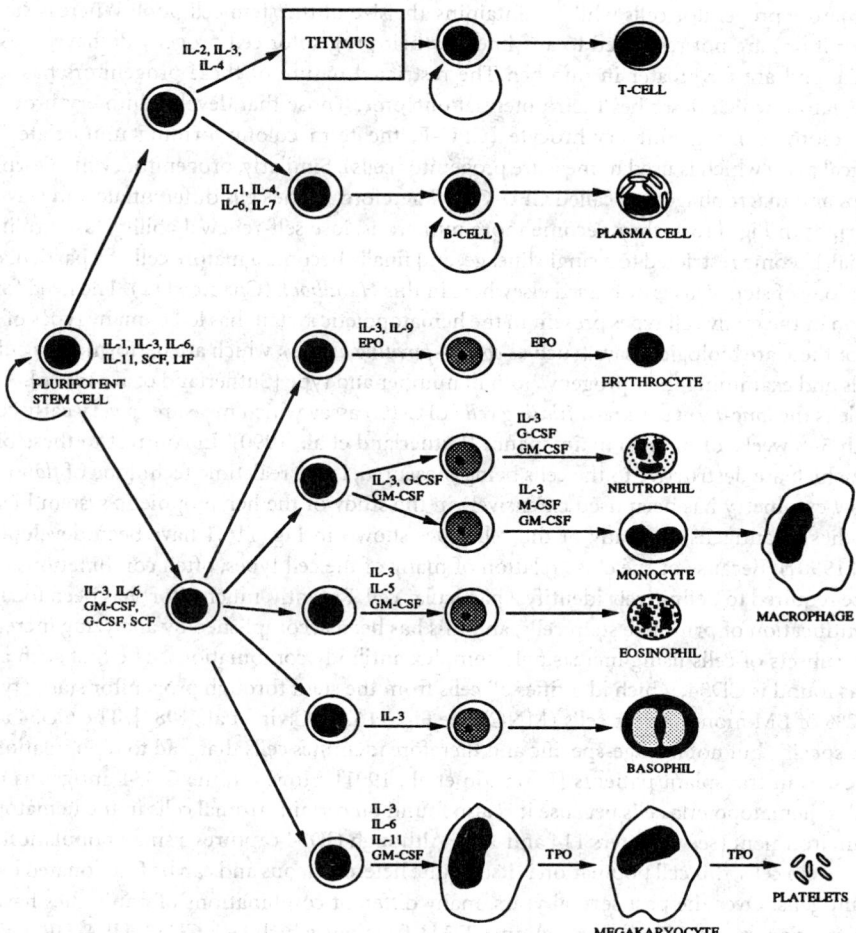

FIGURE 116.1 The hematopoietic system hierarchy. Dividing pluripotent stem cells may undergo self-renewal to form daughter stem cells without loss of potential or may experience a concomitant differentiation to form daughter cells with more restricted potential. Continuous proliferation and differentiation along each lineage results in the production of many mature cells. This process is under the control of many growth factors (GFs) (see Table 116.1). The site of action of some of the better-studied GFs are shown. The mechanisms that determine which lineage a cell will develop into are not understood, although many models have been proposed.

mature blood cells exhibit a limited lifespan in vivo. Although some lymphocytes are thought to survive for many years, it has been shown that erythrocytes and neutrophils have lifespans of 120 days and 8 hours, respectively [Cronkite, 1988]. As a result, hematopoiesis is a highly prolific process which occurs throughout our lives to fulfill this demand.

Mature cells are continuously produced from *progenitor cells,* which in turn are produced from earlier cells which originate from *stem cells.* There are many levels in this hierarchical system, which is usually diagrammed as shown in Fig. 116.1. At the left are the very primitive stem cells, the majority of which are in a nonproliferative state (G_o) [Lajtha, 1979]. These cells are very rare (1 in 100,000 BM cells) but collectively have enough proliferative capacity to last several lifetimes [Boggs et al., 1982; Spangrude et al., 1988]. Through some unknown mechanism, at any given time a small number of these cells are actively proliferating, differentiating, and self-renewing, thereby producing more mature progenitor cells while maintaining the size of the stem cell pool. Whereas stem cells (by definition) are not restricted to any lineage, their progenitor cell progeny do have a restricted potential and are far greater in number. The restricted nature of these progenitors has led to a nomenclature which describes their potential outcome. Those that develop into erythrocytes are called colony-forming unit–erythrocyte (CFU-E, the term colony-forming unit relates to the biological assay which is used to measure progenitor cells). Similarly, progenitors which form granulocytes and macrophages are called CFU-GM. Therefore, as the cells differentiate and travel from left to right in Fig. 116.1, they become more numerous, lose self-renewal ability, lose proliferative potential, become restricted to a single lineage, and finally become a mature cell of a particular type. The biology of stem cells is discussed elsewhere in this *Handbook* (Chapter 112). The need for identification of the many cell types present in the hematopoietic system has led to many types of assays. Many of these are biologic assays (such as *colony-forming assays*), which are performed by culturing the cells and examining their progeny, both in number and type [Sutherland et al., 1991a]. Another example is the *long-term culture-initiating cell* (LTC-IC) assay which measures a very early cell type through 5–8 weeks of in vitro maintenance [Sutherland et al., 1990]. In contrast to these biologic assays, which are destructive to the cells being measured, is the real-time technique of *flow cytometry*. Flow cytometry has been used extensively in the study of the hematopoietic system hierarchy. Antibodies to antigens on many of the cell types shown in Fig. 116.1 have been developed (see [Civin, 1990]). Because of the close relation of many of the cell types, often combinations of antigens are required to definitively identify a particular cell. Recently, much effort has been focused on the identification of primitive stem cells, and this has been accomplished by analyzing increasingly smaller subsets of cells using increasingly complex antibody combinations. The first such antigen that was found is CD34, which identifies all cells from the stem through progenitor stage (typically about 2% of BM mononuclear cells (MNC), see Fig. 116.2) [Civin et al., 1984]. The CD34 antigen is stage-specific but not lineage-specific and therefore identifies cells that lead to repopulation of all cell lineages in transplant patients [Berenson et al., 1991]. However, the CD34 antigen is not restricted to hematopoietic cells because it is also found on certain stromal cells in the hematopoietic microenvironment (see Chapters 114 and 115). Although CD34 captures a small population which contains stem cells, this cell population is itself quite heterogeneous and can be fractionated by many other antigens. Over the past several years, many different combinations of antibodies have been used to fractionate the CD34$^+$ population. CD34$^+$ fractions which lack CD33, HLA-DR, CD38, or CD71 appear to be enriched in stem cells [Civin & Gore, 1993]. Conversely, CD34$^+$ populations which coexpress Thy-1 or *c-kit* appear to contain the primitive cells [Civin & Gore, 1993]. These studies have revealed the extreme rarity of stem cells within the heterogeneous BM population (see Fig. 116.2). Of the *mononuclear cell* (MNC) subset ($\sim$40% of whole BM), only $\sim$2% are CD34$^+$, and of those, only $\sim$5% may be CD38$^+$. Furthermore, this extremely rare population is still heterogeneous with respect to stem cell content. Consequently, stem cells as single cells have not yet been identified.

Molecular Control of Hematopoiesis: The Hematopoietic Growth Factors

A large number of hematopoietic growth factors (GFs) regulate both the production and functional activity of hematopoietic cells. The earliest to be discovered were the colony-stimulating factors (CSFs, because of their activity in the colony-forming assay), which include interleukin-3 (IL-3), granulocyte-macrophage (GM)-CSF, granulocyte (G)-CSF, and monocyte (M)-CSF. These GFs, along with erythropoietin, have been relatively well characterized because of their obvious effects on mature cell production and/or activation. The target cells of some of the better-studied GFs are shown in Fig. 116.1. Subsequent intensive research continues to add to the growing list of GFs that affect hematopoietic cell proliferation, differentiation, and function (Table 116.1). However, new GFs have been more difficult to find and characterize because their effects are more subtle, often

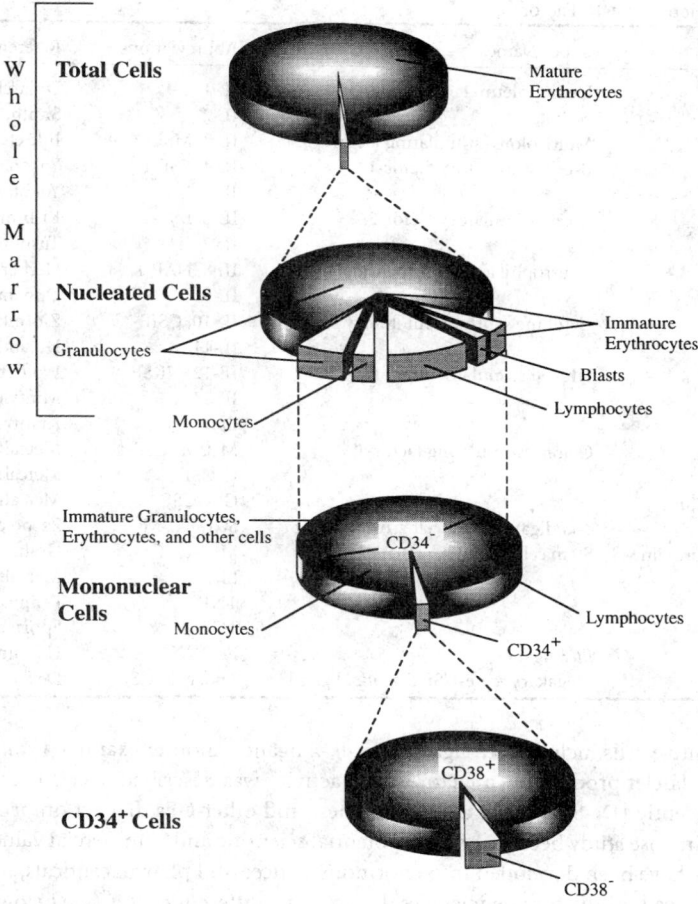

FIGURE 116.2 Relative frequency of the different cell subsets within the BM population. A BM aspirate typically contains 99% mature erythroid cells (mostly from blood contamination), and therefore usually only the nucleated cell fraction is studied. Simple density gradient centrifugation techniques, which remove most of the mature erythrocytes and granulocytes, yield what is known as the mononuclear cell (MNC) fraction (about 40% of the nucleated cells). CD34$^+$ cells, about 2% of MNC, can be isolated by a variety of methods to capture the primitive cells, although the population is quite heterogeneous. The most primitive cells are found in subsets of CD34$^+$ cells (e.g., CD38$^-$), which identify about 5% of the CD34$^+$ population. These rare subsets can be obtained by flow cytometry but are still somewhat heterogeneous with respect to stem cell content. Consequently, although methods are available to fractionate BM to a great extent, individual stem cells have not yet been identified. This diagram conveys the heterogeneous nature of different BM populations as well as the incredible rarity of the primitive cell subset, which is known to contain the stem cells.

providing a synergistic effect which potentiates other known GFs. In addition, there appears to be a significant amount of redundancy and pleotropy in this GF network, which makes the discovery of new GFs difficult [Metcalf, 1993]. In fact, more recent discoveries have focused on potential receptor molecules on the target cell surface, which then have been used to isolate the appropriate ligand GF. Examples of such recently discovered GFs which exhibit synergistic interactions with other GFs

TABLE 116.1 Hematopoietic Growth Factors

Growth Factor Name	Other Names	Abbreviations	Reference
Interleukin-1	Hemopoietin-1	IL-1	Dinarello et al., 1981
Interleukin-2		IL-2	Smith, 1988
Interleukin-3	Multicolony-stimulating factor	IL-3, Multi-CSF	Ihle et al., 1981
Interleukin-4	B-cell-stimulatory factor-1	IL-4, BSF-1	Yokota et al., 1988
Interleukin-5		IL-5	Yokota et al., 1988
Interleukin-6	B-cell-stimulatory factor-2	IL-6, BSF-2	Kishimoto, 1989
Interleukin-7		IL-7	Tushinski et al., 1991
Interleukin-8	Neutrophil activating peptide-1	IL-8, NAP-1	Herbert and Baker, 1993
Interleukin-9		IL-9	Donahue et al., 1990
Interleukin-10	Cytokine synthesis inhibitory factor	IL-10, CSIF	Zlotnik and Moore, 1991
Interleukin-11		IL-11	Du and Williams, 1994
Interleukin-12	NK cell stimulatory factor	IL-12, NKSF	Wolf et al., 1991
Interleukin-13		IL-13	Minty et al., 1993
Erythropoietin		Epo	Krantz, 1991
Monocyte-CSF	Colony-stimulating factor-1	M-CSF, CSF-1	Metcalf, 1985
Granulocyte-CSF		G-CSF	Metcalf, 1985
Granulocyte-macrophage-CSF		GM-CSF	Metcalf, 1985
Stem cell factor	c-*kit* ligand, Mast cell growth factor	SCF, KL, MGF	Zsebo et al., 1990
Macrophage inflammatory protein	Stem cell inhibitor	MIP-1, SCI	Graham et al., 1990
Leukemia inhibitory factor		LIF	Metcalf, 1991
Tumor necrosis factor		TNF	Pennica et al., 1984
Transforming growth factor		TGF	Sporn and Roberts, 1989
flk-2 ligand	*flt*-3 ligand	FL	Hannum et al., 1994
Thrombopoietin	Megakaryocyte-CSF, C = *mpl* ligand	Tpo, MK-CSF	De Sauvage et al., 1994

to act on primitive cells include *c-kit* ligand and *flk-2* ligand. Another example is *thrombopoietin*, a stimulator of platelet production, a factor whose activity was described over 30 years ago but was cloned only recently [De Sauvage et al., 1994]. These and other GFs that act on primitive cells are the subject of intense study because of their potential scientific and commercial value. Already, several of the GFs have been developed into enormously successful pharmaceuticals, used in patients who have blood cell production deficiencies due to many different causes (see below).

The Bone Marrow Microenvironment

Hematopoiesis occurs in the BM cavity in the presence of many accessory and support cells (or *stromal cells*). In addition, like all other cells in vivo, hematopoietic cells have considerable interaction with the extracellular matrix (ECM). These are the chief elements of what is known as the BM microenvironment. Further details on the function of stroma and the microenvironment, and their importance in tissue engineering, are found in Chapters 114 and 115.

Bone Marrow Stromal Cells

Due to the physiology of marrow, hematopoietic cells have a close structural and functional relationship with stromal cells. Marrow stroma includes fibroblasts, macrophages, endothelial cells, and adipocytes. The ratio of these different cell types varies at different places in the marrow and as the cells are cultured in vitro. The term stromal layer therefore refers to an undefined mixture of different adherent cell types which grow out from a culture of BM cells. In vitro, stem cells placed on a stromal cell layer will attach to and often migrate underneath the stromal layer [Yamakazi et al., 1989]. Under the stromal layer, some of the stem cells will proliferate, and the resulting progeny will be packed together, trapped under the stroma, forming a characteristic morphologic feature known as a cobblestone area (see below). It is widely believed that primitive cells must be in contact with stromal cells to maintain their primitive state. However, much of the effect of stromal cells has been attributed to the secretion of GFs. Consequently, there have been reports of successful hematopoietic cell growth with the addition of numerous soluble GFs in the absence of stroma

[Bodine et al. 1989; Brandt et al., 1990, 1992; Haylock et al. 1992; Koller et al. 1992a; Verfaillie, 1992]. However, this issue is quite controversial, and stromal cells are still likely to be valuable because they synthesize membrane-bound GFs [Toksoz et al., 1992], ECM components [Long, 1992], and probably some as yet undiscovered cytokines. In addition, stromal cells can modulate the GF environment in a way that would be very difficult to duplicate by simply adding soluble GFs [Koller et al., 1995]. This modulation may be responsible for the observations that stroma can be both stimulatory and inhibitory [Zipori, 1989].

The Extracellular Matrix

The ECM of BM consists of collagens, laminin, fibronectin [Zuckerman & Wicha, 1983], vitronectin [Coulombel et al., 1988], hemonectin [Campbell et al., 1987], and thrombospondin [Long & Dixit, 1990]. The heterogeneity of this system is further complicated by the presence of various proteoglycans, which are themselves complex molecules with numerous glycosaminoglycan chains linked to a protein core [Minguell & Tavassoli, 1989; Spooncer et al., 1983; Wight et al., 1986]. These glycosaminoglycans include chondroitin, heparan, dermatan, and keratan sulfates and hyaluronic acid. The ECM is secreted by stromal cells of the BM (particularly endothelial cells and fibroblasts) and provides support and cohesion for the marrow structure.

There is a growing body of evidence indicating that ECM is important for the regulation of hematopoiesis. Studies have shown that different glycosaminoglycans bind and present different GFs to hematopoietic cells in an active form [Gordon et al., 1987; Roberts et al., 1988]. This demonstrates that ECM can sequester and compartmentalize certain GFs in local areas and present them to hematopoietic cells, creating a number of different hematopoietically inductive microenvironments. Another important ECM function is to provide anchorage for immature hematopoietic cells. Erythroid precursors have receptors which allow them to attach to fibronectin. As cells mature through the BFU-E to the reticulocyte stage, adherence to fibronectin is gradually lost, and the cells are free to enter the circulation [Patel et al., 1985]. It has also been shown that binding to fibronectin renders these erythroid precursors more responsive to the effects of Epo [Weinstein et al., 1989]. Another adhesion protein termed hemonectin has been shown to selectively bind immature cells of the granulocyte lineage in an analogous fashion [Campbell et al., 1987]. This progenitor binding by ECM has led to the general concept of stem cell homing. When BM cells are injected into the circulation of an animal, a sufficient number are able to home to the marrow and reconstitute hematopoiesis [Tavassoli & Hardy, 1990]. It is therefore likely that homing molecules are present on the surface of the primitive cells. Studies suggest that lectins and CD44 on progenitor cells may interact with ECM and stromal elements of the marrow to mediate cellular homing [Aizawa & Tavassoli, 1987; Kansas et al., 1990; Lewinsohn et al. 1990; Tavassoli and Hardy, 1990]. These concepts have recently been reviewed in detail [Long, 1992].

116.2 Applications of Reconstituted ex Vivo Hematopoiesis

The hematopoietic system, as described above, has many complex and interacting features. The reconstitution of functional hematopoiesis, which has long been desired, must address these features to achieve a truly representative ex vivo system. A functioning ex vivo human hematopoietic system would be a valuable analytic model to study the basic biology of hematopoiesis. The clinical applications of functional ex vivo models of human hematopoiesis are numerous and are just beginning to be realized. Most of these applications revolve around cancer therapies and, more recently, gene therapy. The large-scale production of mature cells for transplantation represents an important goal that may be realized in the more distant future.

Bone Marrow Transplantation

In 1980, when *bone marrow transplantation* (BMT) was still an experimental procedure, fewer than 200 BMTs were performed worldwide [Gratwohl, 1991]. Over the past decade, BMT has become an established therapy for many diseases. In 1990, over 10,000 BMTs were performed, primarily in the United States and Western Europe, for more than a dozen different clinical indications [Bortin et al. 1992; Gratwohl, 1991]. The number of BMTs performed annually is increasing at a rate of 20–30% per year and is expected to continue to rise in the foreseeable future.

BMT is required as a treatment in a number of clinical settings because the highly prolific cells of the hematopoietic system are sensitive to many of the agents used to treat cancer patients. Chemotherapy and radiation therapy usually target rapidly cycling cells, so hematopoietic cells are ablated along with the cancer cells. Consequently, patients undergoing these therapies experience neutropenia (low neutrophil numbers), thrombocytopenia (low platelet numbers), and anemia (low red blood cell numbers), rendering them susceptible to infections and bleeding. A BMT dramatically shortens the period of neutropenia and thrombocytopenia, but the patient may require repeated transfusions. The period during which the patient is neutropenic represents the greatest risk associated with BMT. In addition, some patients do not achieve *engraftment* (when cell numbers rise to safe levels). As a result, much effort is focused on reducing the severity and duration of the blood cell nadir period following chemotherapy and radiation therapy.

There are several sources of hematopoietic cells for transplantation. BMT may be performed with patient marrow (autologous) that has been removed and cryopreserved prior to administration of chemotherapy or with donor marrow (allogeneic). The numbers of autologous and allogeneic transplants performed are roughly equal, and there are advantages and disadvantages with both techniques.

Autologous Bone Marrow Transplantation

Autologous BMTs have been used in the treatment of a variety of diseases including acute lymphoblastic leukemia (ALL), acute myelogenous leukemia (AML), chronic myelogenous leukemia (CML), various lymphomas, breast cancer, neuroblastoma, and multiple myeloma [Gale et al., 1991]. Currently, autologous BM transplantation is hampered by the long hospital stay that is required until engraftment is achieved and the possibility of reintroducing tumor cells along with the cryopreserved marrow. Long periods of neutropenia, anemia, and thrombocytopenia require parenteral antibiotic administration and repeated blood component transfusions.

Autologous transplantation could also be used in gene therapy procedures. The basic concept underlying gene therapy of the hematopoietic system is the insertion of a therapeutic gene into the hematopoietic stem cell, so that a stable transfection is obtained. Engineered retroviruses are the gene carriers currently used. However, mitosis of primitive cells is required for integration of foreign DNA [Bodine et al., 1989]. A culture system which contains dividing stem cells is therefore critical for the enablement of retroviral-based gene therapy of the hematopoietic system. This requirement holds true whether or not the target stem cell population has been purified prior to the transfection step. To date, only very limited success has been achieved with retroviral transfection of human BM cells, whereas murine cells are routinely transfected. A comprehensive and accessible accounting of the status of gene therapy has been presented elsewhere [Larrick & Burck, 1991].

Allogeneic Bone Marrow Transplantation

In patients with certain hematologic malignancies, or with genetic defects in the hematopoietic population, allogeneic transplants are currently favored when suitable matched donors are available. With these leukemias, such as CML, it is likely that the patient's marrow is diseased and would not be suitable for autotransplant. A major obstacle in allogeneic transplantation, however, is the high incidence of *graft-versus-host disease* (GVHD).

Alternative Sources of Hematopoietic Cells for Transplantation

Although hematopoiesis occurs mainly in the BM of adult mammals, during embryonic development, pluripotent stem cells first arise in the yolk sac, are later found in the fetal liver, and at the time of delivery are found in high concentrations in umbilical cord blood. In adults, stem cells are found in peripheral blood only at very low concentrations, but the concentration increases dramatically after stem cell mobilization. Mobilization of stem cells into peripheral blood is a phenomenon that occurs in response to chemotherapy or GF administration. Therefore, hematopoietic stem cells can be collected from cord blood [Gluckman et al., 1989; Wagner et al., 1992] or from mobilized peripheral blood [Schneider et al., 1992] as well as from BM. Disadvantages of cord blood are the limited number of cells that can be obtained from one individual and the question of whether this amount is sufficient to repopulate an adult patient. Mobilized peripheral blood results in more rapid patient engraftment than BM, but the number of stem cells mobilized varies widely in different patients, and multiple multihour apheresis sessions are required to obtain enough cells for transplant. Currently, these procedures are less popular than BMT, but the use of mobilized peripheral blood stem cells is growing rapidly.

Tissue Engineering and Improved Transplantation Procedures

BMT would be greatly facilitated by reliable systems and procedures for ex vivo stem cell maintenance, expansion, and manipulation. For example, the harvest procedure, which collects 1–2 liters of marrow, is currently a painful and involved operating room procedure. The complications and discomfort of marrow donation are not trivial and can affect donors for a month or more [Stroncek et al., 1993]. Through cell expansion techniques, a small marrow specimen taken under local anesthesia in an outpatient setting could be expanded into the large number of cells required for transplant, thereby eliminating the large harvest procedure. Engraftment may be accelerated by increasing the numbers of progenitors and immature cells available for infusion. In addition, it may be possible to cryopreserve expanded cells to be infused at multiple time points, thereby allowing multiple cycles of chemotherapy (schedule intensification). Finally, the use of expanded cells may allow increasing doses of chemotherapy (dose intensification), facilitating tumor reduction while ameliorating myeloablative side effects.

The expansion of alternative hematopoietic cell sources would also facilitate transplant procedures. For example, multiple rounds of apheresis, each requiring ~4 hours, are required to collect enough mobilized peripheral blood cells for transplant. Expansion of a small amount of mobilized peripheral blood may reduce the number of aphereses required or eliminate them altogether by allowing the collection of enough cells from a volume of blood that has not been apheresed. With cord blood, there is a limit on the number of cells that can be collected from a single donor, and it is currently thought that this number is inadequate for an adult transplant. Consequently, cord blood transplants to date have been performed on children. Expansion of cord blood cells may therefore enable adult transplants from the limited number of cord blood cells available for collection.

Large-Scale Production of Mature Blood Cells

Beyond the ability to produce stem and progenitor cells for transplantation purposes lies the promise to produce large quantities of mature blood cells. Large-scale hematopoietic cultures could potentially provide several types of clinically important mature blood cells. These include red blood cells, platelets, and granulocytes. About 12 million units of red blood cells are transfused in the United States every year, the majority of them during elective surgery and the rest in acute situations. About 4 million units of platelets are transfused every year into patients who have difficulty exhibiting normal blood clotting. Mature granulocytes, which constitute a relatively low-usage market of only a few thousand units administered each year, are involved in combating infections. This need arises in situations when a patient's immune system has been compromised and requires assistance in combating opportunistic infections, such as during chemotherapy and the healing of burn wounds.

All in all, the market for these blood cells totals about $1–1.5 billion in the United States annually, with a worldwide market that is about three to four times larger. The ability to produce blood cells on demand ex vivo would alleviate several problems with the current blood cell supply. The first of these problems is the availability and stability of the blood cell supply. The availability of donors has traditionally been a problem, and, coupled with the short shelf-life of blood cells, the current supply is unstable and cannot meet major changes in demand. The second problem is the usual blood-type compatibility problem resulting in shortages of certain types at various times. The third problem is the safety of the blood supply. This last issue has received much attention recently due to the contamination of donated blood with the human immunodeficiency virus (HIV). However, the three forms of hepatitis currently pose an even more serious viral contamination threat to the blood supply.

Unlike ex vivo expansion of stem and progenitor cells for transplantation, the large-scale production of fully mature blood cells for routine clinical use is less developed and represents a more distant goal. The large market would require systems of immense size, unless major improvements in culture productivity are attained. For example, the recent discovery of thrombopoietin [De Sauvage et al., 1994] may make the large-scale production of platelets feasible. At present, there are ongoing attempts in several laboratories to produce large numbers of neutrophils from CD34-selected cell populations. Thus, large-scale production of mature cells may soon become technically feasible, although the economic considerations are still unknown.

116.3 The History of Hematopoietic Cell Culture Development

As outlined above, there are many compelling scientific and clinical reasons for undertaking the development of efficient ex vivo hematopoietic systems. Such achievement requires the use of in vivo mimicry, sophisticated cell culture technology, and the development of clinically acceptable cell cultivation devices. The foundations for these developments lie in the BM cell culture methods which have been developed over the past 20 years. The history of BM culture will therefore be described briefly, as it provides the backdrop for tissue engineering of the hematopoietic system. More complete reviews have been published previously [Dexter et al., 1984; Eaves et al., 1991; Greenberger, 1984].

The Murine System

In the mid 1970s, Dexter and coworkers were successful in developing a culture system in which murine hematopoiesis could be maintained for several months [Dexter et al., 1977]. The key feature of this system was the establishment of a BM-derived stromal layer during the first three weeks of culture which was then recharged with fresh BM cells. One to 2 weeks after the cultures were recharged, active sites of hematopoiesis appeared. These sites are often described as cobblestone regions, which are the result of primitive cell proliferation (and accumulation) underneath the stromal layer. Traditionally, the cultures are fed by replacement of one-half of the medium either once or twice weekly. In these so-called Dexter cultures, myelopoiesis proceeds to the exclusion of lymphopoiesis. The selection of a proper lot of serum for long-term BM cultures (LTBMCs) was found to be very important. In fact, when using select lots of serum, one-step LTBMCs were successfully performed without the recharging step at week 3 [Dexter et al., 1984]. It is thought that good serum allows rapid development of stroma before the primitive cells are depleted, and once the stroma is developed, the culture is maintained from the remaining original primitive cells without need for recharging. The importance of stroma has often been demonstrated in these Dexter cultures, because the culture outcome was often correlated with stromal development.

The Human System

The adaptation of one-step LTBMC for human cells was first reported in 1980 [Gartner & Kaplan, 1980]. A mixture of fetal bovine serum and horse serum was found to be required for human

LTBMC, and a number of other medium additives such as sodium pyruvate, amino acids, vitamins, and antioxidants were found to be beneficial [Gartner & Kaplan, 1980; Greenberg et al., 1981; Meagher et al., 1988]. Otherwise, the culture protocol has remained essentially the same as that used for murine culture. Unfortunately, human LTBMCs have never attained the productivity or longevity which is observed in cultures of other species [Dexter et al., 1984; Greenberger et al., 1986]. The exponentially decreasing numbers of total and progenitor cells with time in human LTBMC [Eastment & Ruscetti, 1984; Eaves et al., 1991] renders the cultures unsuitable for cell expansion and indicates that primitive stem cells are lost over time. The discovery of hematopoietic GFs was an important development in human hematopoietic cell culture, because addition of GFs to human LTBMC greatly enhanced cell output. However, GFs did not prolong the longevity of the cultures, indicating that primitive cell maintenance was not improved [Coutinho et al., 1990; Lemoli et al., 1992]. Furthermore, although the total number of progenitors obtained was increased by GFs, it was still usually less than the number used to initiate the culture. Therefore, a net expansion in progenitor cell numbers was not obtained. The increased cell densities that were stimulated by GF addition were not well supported by the relatively static culture conditions.

The disappointing results from human LTBMCs led to the development of other culture strategies. The development of an increasing number of recombinant GFs was soon joined by the discovery of the CD34 antigen (see above). As protocols for the selection of CD34$^+$ cells became available, it was thought that the low cell numbers generated by enrichment could be expanded in GF-supplemented cultures without the impediment of numerous mature cells in the system. Because the enrichment procedure results in a cell population depleted of stromal cells, CD34$^+$ cell cultures are often called suspension cultures, due to the lack of an adherent stromal layer. A number of groups have reported experiments in which CD34$^+$ cells were incubated with high doses of up to seven recombinant GFs in suspension culture [Brandt et al., 1992; Haylock et al. 1992]. Although 500–1000-fold cell expansion numbers are often obtained, the magnitude of CFU-GM expansion is usually less than 10-fold, suggesting that differentiation, accompanied by depletion of primitive cells, is occurring in these systems. In fact, when LTC-IC have been measured, the numbers obtained after static culture of enriched cells have always been significantly below the input value [Sutherland et al., 1991b, 1993; Verfaillie, 1992]. A further consideration in CD34$^+$ cell culture is the loss of cells during the enrichment procedure. It is not uncommon to experience 70–80% loss of progenitors with most CD34$^+$ cell purification protocols [Traycoff et al., 1994], and this can be very significant when trying to maximize the final cell number obtained (such as in clinical applications, see below). Nevertheless, cultures of purified CD34$^+$ cells, and especially the smaller subsets (e.g., CD33$^-$, CD38$^-$), have yielded valuable information on the biology of hematopoietic stem cells.

An alternative approach has also been taken to improve human hematopoietic cell culture. Most of these advances have come from the realization that the traditional culture protocols are highly nonphysiologic and that these deficiencies can be corrected by in vivo mimicry. Therefore, these techniques do not involve cell purification or high-dose cytokine stimulation. Because these cultures attain fairly high densities, it was thought that the tradition of changing one-half of the culture medium either once or twice weekly was inadequate. When Dexter-type cultures were performed with more frequent medium exchanges, progenitor cell production was supported for at least 20 weeks [Schwartz et al., 1991b]. This increase in culture longevity indicates that primitive cells were maintained for a longer period, and this was accompanied by an increase in progenitor cell yield. Although the precise mechanisms of increased medium exchange are unknown, the increased feeding rate enhances stromal cell secretion of GFs [Caldwell et al., 1991].

As previously noted, recombinant GFs can significantly improve culture productivity, but GF-stimulated cell proliferation exacerbates the problems of nutrient depletion because cell proliferation and the consumption of metabolites increases many-fold. Therefore, increased feeding protocols also benefit GF-stimulated cultures. Cultures supplemented with IL-3/GM-CSF/Epo and fed with 50% daily medium exchanges were found to result in significant cell and progenitor expansion while maintaining culture longevity [Schwartz et al., 1991a].

Tissue Engineering Challenges

Although a daily feeding schedule significantly enhanced the productivity and longevity of hematopoietic cultures, the labor required to feed each culture daily is a daunting task. In addition, the cultures are subjected to physical disruption and large discontinuous daily changes in culture conditions and may be exposed to contamination at each daily feeding. These complications frustrate the optimization of the culture environment for production of hematopoietic cells and limit the clinical usefulness of the cultures. A perfusion system, if properly designed and constructed, would eliminate many of the problems currently associated with these cultures.

Two reports have described the cultivation of murine BM in continuous perfusion systems [Koller et al., 1992*b*; Wang & Wu, 1992]. More recent reports have shown that human hematopoietic cells can be successfully cultivated in continuous perfusion bioreactors [Koller et al., 1993*a*; Palsson et al., 1993*b*]. Slow medium flow rates without recirculation and internal oxygenation have given the best results to date and yielded cell densities in excess of 3 million cells per square centimeter, which was accompanied by significant progenitor and primitive cell expansion [Oh et al., 1994; Palsson et al., 1993*b*]. These systems have also been amenable to scale-up, first by a factor of 10 [Koller et al., 1993*b*] and then by a further factor of 7.5 [Armstrong et al., 1993]. The perfusion bioreactors also support the development and maintenance of accessory cell populations, resulting in significant endogenous GF production in a controlled manner, which likely contributes to culture success [Koller et al., 1995].

116.4 Challenges for Scale-Up

To gauge the scale-up challenges, one first needs to state the requirements for clinically useful systems. The need to accommodate stroma that supports active hematopoiesis represents perhaps the most important consideration for the selection of a bioreactor system.

Bioreactors and Stroma

If stroma is required, the choices are limited to systems that can support the growth of adherent cells. This requirement may be eliminated in future systems if the precise GF requirements become known and if the microenvironment that the stroma provides is not needed for hematopoietic stem and progenitor cell expansion.

Currently, there are at least three culture systems that may be used for adherent cell growth. Fluidized bed bioreactors with macroporous bead carriers provide one option. Undoubtedly, significant effort will be required to develop the suitable bead chemistry and geometry, since the currently available systems are designed for homogeneous cell cultures. Beads for hematopoietic culture probably should allow for the formation of functional colonies comprised of a mixed cell population within each bead. Since it is likely that tolerance for inhomogenieties in the nutritional environment is lower for primary cultures than for continuous cell lines, beads of relatively small diameters will probably be required. Cell sampling from fluidized beds would be relatively easy, but final cell harvesting may require stressful procedures, such as prolonged treatment with collagenase and/or trypsin.

Flatbed bioreactors are a second type of system which can support stromal development. Such units can be readily designed to carry the required cell number, and, further, they can allow for direct microscopic observation of the cell culture. Flatbed bioreactors provide perhaps the most straightforward scale-up and automation of LTBMC. However, the large area required may prove to be an obstacle in routine clinical use unless the cell surface density is improved. Some recent reports indicate the feasibility of this approach [Koller et al., 1993*a*, 1993*b*; Palsson et al., 1993*b*].

Finally, membrane-based systems, such as hollow fiber units, could be used to carry out hematopoietic cell cultures of moderate size. Special design of the hollow fiber bed geometry with respect to axial length and radial fiberspacing should eliminate all undesirable spatial gradients. Such units have been made already and have proved effective for their use for in vivo NMR analysis of metabolic behavior of homogeneous cell cultures [Mancuso et al., 1990]. However, hematopoietic cell observation and harvesting may prove to be troublesome with this approach, as one report has suggested [Sardonini & Wu, 1993].

It is possible that the function of accessory cells may be obtained by the use of spheroids without classical adherent cell growth. This approach to the growth of liver cells in culture has meet with some success (see Chapter 117). In fact, there have been reports of functional heterogeneous cell aggregates within BM aspirates [Blazsek et al., 1990; Funk et al., 1994]. If successfully developed, suspension cultures containing these aggregates could be carried out in a variety of devices, including the rotating wall vessels that have been developed by NASA [Schwarz et al., 1992].

Alternatives

The precise arrangement of future large-scale systems will be significantly influenced by continuing advances in the understanding of the molecular and microenvironmental regulation of the hematopoietic process. Currently, the proximity of a supporting stromal layer is believed to be important. It is thought to function through the provision of both soluble and membrane-bound GFs and by providing a suitable microenvironment. The characterization of the microenvironment is uncertain at present, but its chemistry and local geometry are both thought to play a role. If the proximity of stroma is found to be unimportant, one could possibly design culture systems in which the stroma and BM cells are separated [Verfaillie, 1992], resulting in the ability to control each function separately. Finally, if the GF requirements can be defined and artificially supplied, and the stromal microenvironment is found to be unimportant, large-scale hematopoietic suspension cultures would become possible.

Production of Mature Cells

Culture systems for generic allogeneic BMT, or for the large-scale production of mature cells, will pose more serious scale-up challenges. The number of cells required for these applications, in particular the latter, may be significantly higher than that for autologous BMT. Of the three alternatives discussed above, the fluidized bed system is the most readily scalable. The flatbed systems can be scaled by a simple stacking approach, whereas hollow fiber units are known for their shortcomings with respect to large-scale use.

116.5 Recapitulation

Rapid advances in our understanding of hematopoietic cell biology and the molecular control of hematopoietic cell replication, differentiation, and apoptosis are providing some of the basic information that is needed to reconstitute human hematopoiesis ex vivo. Compelling clinical applications provide a significant impetus for developing systems that produce clinically useful cell populations in clinically meaningful numbers. Use of in vivo mimicry and the bioreactor technologies that were developed in the 1980s are leading to the development of perfusion-based bioreactor systems that will meet some of the clinical needs. Further tissue engineering of human hematopoiesis is likely to continue to grow in scope and sophistication and lead to definition of basic structure-function relationships and the enablement of many needed clinical procedures.

Defining Terms

Colony-forming assay: Assay carried out in semisolid medium under GF stimulation. Progenitor cells divide, and progeny are held in place so that a microscopically identifiable colony results after 2 weeks.

Differentiation: The irreversible progression of a cell or cell population to a more mature state.

Engraftment: The attainment of a safe number of circulating mature blood cells after a BMT.

Flow cytometry: Technique for cell analysis using fluorescently conjugated monoclonal antibodies which identify certain cell types. More sophisticated instruments are capable of sorting cells into different populations as they are analyzed.

Graft-versus-host disease: The immunologic response of transplanted cells against the tissue of their new host. This response is often a severe consequence of allogeneic BMT and can lead to death (acute GVHD) or long-term disability (chronic GVHD).

Hematopoiesis: The regulated production of mature blood cells through a scheme of multilineage proliferation and differentiation.

Lineage: Refers to cells at all stages of differentiation leading to a particular mature cell type, i.e., one branch on the lineage diagram shown in Fig. 116.1.

Long-term culture-initiating cell: Cell that is measured by a 7–12-week in vitro assay. LTC-IC are thought to be very primitive, and the population contains stem cells. However, the population is heterogeneous, so not every LTC-IC is a stem cell.

Microenvironment: Refers to the environment surrounding a given cell in vivo.

Mononuclear cell: Refers to the cell population obtained after density centrifugation of whole BM. This population excludes cells without a nucleus (erythrocytes) and polymorphonuclear cells (granulocytes).

Progenitor cells: Cells that are intermediate in the development pathway, more mature than stem cells but not yet mature cells. This is the cell type measured in the colony-forming assay.

Self-renewal: Generation of a daughter cell with identical characteristics as the original cell. Most often used to refer to stem cell division, which results in the formation of new stem cells.

Stem cells: Cells with unlimited proliferative and lineage potential.

Stromal cells: Heterogeneous mixture of support or accessory cells of the BM. Also refers to the adherent layer which forms in BM cultures.

References

Aizawa S, Tavassoli M. 1987. In vitro homing of hemopoietic stem cells is mediated by a recognition system with galactosyl and mannosyl specificities. Proc Natl Acad Sci 84:4485.

Armstrong RD, Koller MR, Paul LA, et al. 1993. Clinical scale production of stem and hematopoietic cells ex vivo. Blood 82:296a.

Berenson RJ, Bensinger WI, Hill RS, et al. 1991. Engraftment after infusion of CD34+ marrow cells in patients with breast cancer or neuroblastoma. Blood 77:1717.

Blazsek I, Misset J-L, Benavides M, et al. 1990. Hematon, a multicellular functional unit in normal human bone marrow: Structural organization, hemopoietic activity, and its relationship to myelodysplasia and myeloid leukemias. Exp Hematol 18:259.

Bodine DM, Karlsson S, Nienhuis AW. 1989. Combination of interleukins 3 and 6 preserves stem cell function in culture and enhances retrovirus-mediated gene transfer into hematopoietic stem cells. Proc Natl Acad Sci 86:8897.

Boggs DR, Boggs SS, Saxe DF, et al. 1982. Hematopoietic stem cells with high proliferative potential. J Clin Invest 70:242.

Bortin MM, Horowitz MM, Rimm AA. 1992. Progress report from the international BM transplant registry. Bone Marrow Transplant 10:113.

Brandt, JE, Briddell, RA, Srour, EF, Leemhuis, TB, and Hoffman, R. 1992. Role of c-*kit* ligand in the expansion of human hematopoietic progenitor cells. Blood 79:634–641.

Brandt JE, Srour EF, Van Besien K, et al. 1990. Cytokine-dependent long-term culture of highly enriched precursors of hematopoietic progenitor cells from human bone marrow. J Clin Invest 86:932.

Caldwell J, Palsson BØ, Locey B, et al. 1991. Culture perfusion schedules influence the metabolic activity and granulocyte-macrophage colony-stimulating factor production rates of human bone marrow stromal cells. J Cell Physiol 147:344.

Campbell AD, Long MW, Wicha MS. 1987. Haemonectin, a bone marrow adhesion protein specific for cells of granulocyte lineage. Nature 329:744.

Civin CI. 1990. Human monomyeloid cell membrane antigens. Exp Hematol 18:461.

Civin CI, Gore SD. 1993. Antigenic analysis of hematopoesis: A review. J Hematotherapy 2:137.

Civin CI, Strauss LC, Brovall C, et al. 1984. Antigenic analysis of hematopoiesis: III. A hematopoietic progenitor cell surface antigen defined by a monoclonal antibody raised against KG-Ia cells. J Immunol 133:157.

Coulombel L, Vuillet MH, Leroy C, et al. 1988. Lineage- and stage-specific adhesion of human hematopoietic progenitor cells to extracellular matrices from marrow fibroblasts. Blood 71:329.

Coutinho LH, Will A, Radford J, et al. 1990. Effects of recombinant human granulocyte colony-stimulating factor (CSF), human granulocyte macrophage-CSF, and gibbon interleukin-3 on hematopoiesis in human long-term bone marrow culture. Blood 75:2118.

Cronkite EP. 1988. Analytical review of structure and regulation of hemopoiesis. Blood Cells 14:313.

De Sauvage FJ, Hass PE, Spencer SD, et al. 1994. Stimulation of megakaryocytopoiesis and thrombopoiesis by the c-Mpl ligand. Nature 369:533.

Dexter TM, Allen TD, Lajtha LG. 1977. Conditions controlling the proliferation of haemopoietic stem cells in vitro. J Cell Physiol 91:335.

Dexter TM, Spooncer E, Simmons P, et al. 1984. Long-term marrow culture: An overview of techniques and experience. In DG Wright, JS Greenberger (eds), Long-Term Bone Marrow Culture, pp 57–96 New York, Alan R. Liss.

Dinarello CA, Rosenwasser LJ, Wolff SM. 1981. Demonstration of a circulating suppressor factor of thymocyte proliferation during endotoxin fever in humans. J Immunol 127:2517.

Donahue RE, Yang Y-C, Clark SC. 1990. Human P40 T-cell growth factor (interleukin 9) supports erythroid colony formation. Blood 75:2271.

Du XX, Williams DA. 1994. Interleukin-11: A multifunctional growth factor derived from the hematopoietic microenvironment. Blood 83:2023.

Eastment CE, Ruscetti FW. 1984. Evaluation of hematopoiesis in long-term bone marrow culture: Comparison of species differences. In DG Wright, JS Greenberger (eds), Long-Term Bone Marrow Culture, pp 97–118, New York, Alan R. Liss.

Eaves CJ, Cashman JD, Eaves AC. 1991. Methodology of long-term culture of human hemopoietic cells. J Tiss Cult Meth 13:55.

Funk PE, Kincade PW, Witte PL. 1994. Native associations of early hematopoietic stem cells and stromal cells isolated in bone marrow cell aggregates. Blood 83:361.

Gale RP, Armitage JO, Dicke KA. 1991. Autotransplants: Now and in the future. Bone Marrow Transplant 7:153.

Gartner S, Kaplan HS. 1980. Long-term culture of human bone marrow cells. Proc Natl Acad Sci 77:4756.

Gluckman E, Broxmeyer HE, Auerbach AD, et al. 1989. Hematopoietic reconstitution in a patient with Fanconi's anemia by means of umbilical-cord blood from an HLA-identical sibling. NE J Med 321:1174.

Gordon MY, Riley GP, Watt SM, et al. 1987. Compartmentalization of a haematopoietic growth factor (GM-CSF) by glycosaminoglycans in the bone marrow microenvironment. Nature 326:403.

Graham GJ, Wright EG, Hewick R, et al. 1990. Identification and characterization of an inhibitor of haemopoietic stem cell proliferation. Nature 344:442.

Gratwohl A. 1991. Bone marrow transplantation activity in Europe 1990. Bone Marrow Transplant 8:197.

Greenberg HM, Newburger PE, Parker LM, et al. 1981. Human granulocytes generated in continuous bone marrow culture are physiologically normal. Blood 58:724.

Greenberger JS. 1984. Long-term hematopoietic cultures. In DW Golde (ed), Hematopoiesis, pp 203–242, New York, Churchill Livingstone.

Greenberger JS, Fitzgerald TJ, Rothstein L, et al. 1986. Long-term culture of human granulocytes and granulocyte progenitor cells. In Transfusion Medicine: Recent Technological Advances, pp 159–185, New York, Alan R. Liss.

Hannum C, Culpepper J, Campbell D, et al. 1994. Ligand for FLT3/FLK2 receptor tyrosine kinase regulates the growth of haematopoietic stem cells and is encoded by variant RNAs. Nature 368:643.

Haylock DN, To LB, Dowse TL, et al. 1992. Ex vivo expansion and maturation of peripheral blood CD34$^+$ cells into the myeloid lineage. Blood 80:1405.

Herbert CA, Baker JB. 1993. Interleukin-8: A review. Cancer Invest 11:743.

Hoffman R, Benz EJ Jr, Shattil SJ, et al. 1991. Hematology: Basic Principles and Practice, New York, Churchill Livingstone.

Ihle JN, Pepersack L, Rebar L. 1981. Regulation of T cell differentiation: In vitro induction of 20 alpha-hydroxysteroid dehydrogenase in splenic lymphocytes is mediated by a unique lymphokine. J Immunol 126:2184.

Kansas GS, Muirhead MJ, Dailey MO. 1990. Expression of the CD11/CD18, leukocyte adhesion molecule 1, and CD44 adhesion molecules during normal myeloid and erythroid differentiation in humans. Blood 76:2483.

Kishimoto T. 1989. The biology of interleukin-6. Blood 74:1.

Koller MR, Bender JG, Miller WM, et al. 1993a. Expansion of human hematopoietic progenitors in a perfusion bioreactor system with IL-3, IL-6, and stem cell factor. Biotechnology 11:358.

Koller MR, Bender JG, Papoutsakis ET, et al. 1992a. Effects of synergistic cytokine combinations, low oxygen, and irradiated stroma on the expansion of human cord blood progenitors. Blood 80:403.

Koller MR, Bender JG, Papoutsakis ET, et al. 1992b. Beneficial effects of reduced oxygen tension and perfusion in long-term hematopoietic cultures. Ann NY Acad Sci 665:105.

Koller MR, Emerson SG, Palsson BØ. 1993b. Large-scale expansion of human stem and progenitor cells from bone marrow mononuclear cells in continuous perfusion culture. Blood 82:378.

Koller MR, Bradley MS, Palsson BØ. 1995. Growth factor consumption and production in perfusion cultures of human bone marrow correlates with specific cell production. Experimental Hematology, in press.

Krantz SB. 1991. Erythropoietin. Blood 77:419.

Lajtha LG. 1979. Stem cell concepts. Differentiation 14:23.

Larrick JW, Burck KL. 1991. Gene Therapy: Application of Molecular Biology, New York, Elsevier.

Lemoli RM, Tafuri A, Strife A, et al. 1992. Proliferation of human hematopoietic progenitors in long-term bone marrow cultures in gaspermeable plastic bags is enhanced by colony-stimulating factors. Exp Hematol 20:569.

Lewinsohn DM, Nagler A, Ginzton N, et al. 1990. Hematopoietic progenitor cell expression of the H-CAM (CD44) homing-associated adhesion molecule. Blood 75:589.

Long MW. 1992. Blood cell cytoadhesion molecules. Exp Hematol 20:288.

Long MW, Dixit VM. 1990. Thrombospondin functions as a cytoadhesion molecule for human hematopoietic progenitor cells. Blood 75:2311.

Mancuso A, Fernandez EJ, Blanch HW, et al. 1990. A nuclear magnetic resonance technique for determining hybridoma cell concentration in hollow fiber bioreactors. Biotechnology 8:1282.

Meagher RC, Salvado AJ, Wright DG. 1988. An analysis of the multilineage production of human hematopoietic progenitors in long-term bone marrow culture: Evidence that reactive oxygen intermediates derived from mature phagocytic cells have a role in limiting progenitor cell self-renewal. Blood 72:273.

Metcalf D. 1985. The granulocyte-macrophage colony-stimulating factors. Science 229:16.

Metcalf D. 1991. The leukemia inhibitory factor (LIF). Int J Cell Cloning 9:95.

Metcalf D. 1993. Hematopoietic regulators: Redundancy or subtlety? Blood 82:3515.

Minguell JJ, Tavassoli M. 1989. Proteoglycan synthesis by hematopoietic progenitor cells. Blood 73:1821.

Minty A, Chalon P, Derocq JM, et al. 1993. Interleukin-13 is a new human lymphokine regulating inflammatory and immune responses. Nature 362:248.

Palsson BØ, Oh DJ, and Koller MR. 1995. Replating of bioreactor expanded human bone marrow results in extended growth of primitive and mature cells. Cytotechnology, in press.

Oh DJ, Koller MR, Palsson BØ. 1993. Extended growth of stem and progenitor cells from adult human bone marrow in sequential bioreactor cultures. Blood 82:17a.

Oh DJ, Koller MR, Palsson BØ. 1994. Frequent harvesting from perfused bone marrow cultures results in increased overall cell and progenitor expansion. Biotechnology & Bioengineering 44:609.

Palsson BØ, Bradley MS, Koller MR. 1993a. Growth factor consumption and production in ex vivo perfusion cultures of human bone marrow. Blood 82:373.

Palsson BØ, Paek S-H, Schwartz RM, et al. 1993b. Expansion of human bone marrow progenitor cells in a high cell density continuous perfusion system. Biotechnology 11:368.

Patel VP, Ciechanover A, Platt O, et al. 1985. Mammalian reticulocytes lose adhesion to fibronectin during maturation to erythrocytes. Proc Natl Acad Sci 82:440.

Pennica D, Nedwin GE, Hayflick JS, et al. 1984. Human tumour necrosis factor: Precursor structure, expression and homology to lymphotoxin. Nature 312:724.

Roberts R, Gallagher J, Spooncer E, et al. 1988. Heparan sulphate bound growth factors: A mechanism for stromal cell mediated haemopoiesis. Nature 332:376.

Sardonini CA, Wu Y-J. 1993. Expansion and differentiation of human hematopoietic cells from static cultures through small scale bioreactors. Biotechnol Prog

Schneider JG, Crown J, Shapiro F, et al. 1992. Ex vivo cytokine expansion of CD34-positive hematopoietic progenitors in bone marrow, placental cord blood, and cyclophosphamide and G-CSF mobilized peripheral blood. Blood 80:268a.

Schwartz RM, Emerson SG, Clarke MF, et al. 1991a. In vitro myelopoiesis stimulated by rapid medium exchange and supplementation with hematopoietic growth factors. Blood 78:3155.

Schwartz RM, Palsson BØ, Emerson SG. 1991b. Rapid medium perfusion rate significantly increases the productivity and longevity of human bone marrow cultures. Proc Natl Acad Sci 88:6760.

Schwarz RP, Goodwin TJ, Wolf DA. 1992. Cell culture for three-dimensional modeling in rotating-wall vessels: An application of simulated microgravity. J Tiss Cult Meth 14:51.

Smith KA. 1988. Interleukin-2: Inception, impact, and implications. Science 240:1169.

Spangrude GJ, Heimfeld S, Weissman IL. 1988. Purification and characterization of mouse hematopoietic stem cells. Science 241:58.

Spooncer E, Gallagher JT, Krizsa F, et al. 1983. Regulation of haemopoiesis in long-term bone marrow cultures: IV. Glycosaminoglycan synthesis and the stimulation of haemopoiesis by β-D-xylosides. J Cell Biol 96:510.

Sporn MB, Roberts AB. 1989. Transforming growth factor-β: Multiple actions and potential clinical applications. JAMA 262:938.

Stroncek DF, Holland PV, Bartch G, et al. 1993. Experiences of the first 493 unrelated marrow donors in the national marrow donor program. Blood 81:1940.

Sutherland HJ, Eaves AC, Eaves CJ. 1991a. Quantitative assays for human hemopoietic progenitor cells. In AP Gee (ed), Bone Marrow Processing and Purging, pp 155–167, Boca Raton, Fla, CRC Press.

Sutherland HJ, Eaves CJ, Lansdorp PM, et al. 1991b. Differential regulation of primitive human hematopoietic stem cells in long-term cultures maintained on genetically engineered murine stromal cells. Blood 78:666.

Sutherland HJ, Hogge DE, Cook D, et al. 1993. Alternative mechanisms with and without steel factor support primitive human hematopoiesis. Blood 81:1465.

Sutherland HJ, Lansdorp PM, Henkelman DH, et al. 1990. Functional characterization of individual human hematopoietic stem cells cultured at limiting dilution on supportive marrow stromal layers. Proc Natl Acad Sci 87:3584.

Tavassoli M, Hardy CL. 1990. Molecular basis of homing of intravenously transplanted stem cells to the marrow. Blood 76:1059.

Toksoz D, Zsebo KM, Smith KA, et al., 1992. Support of human hematopoiesis in long-term bone marrow cultures by murine stromal cells selectively expressing the membrane-bound and secreted forms of the human homolog of the steel gene product, stem cell factor. Proc Natl Acad Sci 89:7350.

Traycoff CM, Abboud MR, Laver J, et al. 1994. Evaluation of the in vitro behavior of phenotypically defined populations of umbilical cord blood hematopoietic progenitor cells. Exp Hematol 22:215.

Tushinski RJ, McAlister IB, Williams DE, et al. 1991. The effects of interleukin 7 (IL-7) on human bone marrow in vitro. Exp Hematol 19:749.

Verfaillie CM. 1992. Direct contact between human primitive hematopoietic progenitors and bone marrow stroma is not required for long-term in vitro hematopoiesis. Blood 79:2821.

Wagner JE, Broxmeyer HE, Byrd RL, et al. 1992. Transplantation of umbilical cord blood after myeloablative therapy: Analysis of engraftment. Blood 79:1874.

Wang T-Y, Wu JHD. 1992. A continuous perfusion bioreactor for long-term bone marrow culture. Ann NY Acad Sci 665:274.

Weinstein R, Riordan MA, Wenc K, et al. 1989. Dual role of fibronectin in hematopoietic differentiation. Blood 73:111.

Wight TN, Kinsella MG, Keating A, et al. 1986. Proteoglycans in human long-term bone marrow cultures: Biochemical and ultrastructural analyses. Blood 67:1333.

Wolf SF, Temple PA, Kobayashi M, et al. 1991. Cloning of cDNA for natural killer cell stimulatory factor, a heterodimeric cytokine with multiple biologic effects on T and natural killer cells. J Immunol 146:3074.

Yamakazi K, Roberts RA, Spooncer E, et al. 1989. Cellular interactions between 3T3 cells and interleukin-3-dependent multipotent haemopoietic cells: A model system for stromal-cell-mediated haemopoiesis. J Cell Physiol 139:301.

Yokota T, Arai N, de Vries JE, et al. 1988. Molecular biology of interleukin-4 and interleukin-5 genes and biology of their products that stimulate B cells, T cells and hemopoietic cells. Immunol Rev 102:137.

Zipori D. 1989. Stromal cells from the bone marrow: Evidence for a restrictive role in regulation of hemopoiesis. Eur J Haematol 42:225.

Zlotnik A, Moore KW. 1991. Interleukin 10. Cytokine 3:366.

Zsebo KM, Wypych J, McNiece IK, et al. 1990. Identification, purification, and biological characterization of hematopoietic stem cell factor from buffalo rat liver-conditioned medium. Cell 63:195.

Zuckerman KS, Wicha MS. 1983. Extracellular matrix production by the adherent cells of long-term murine bone marrow cultures. Blood 61:540.

Further Information

The American Society of Hematology (ASH) is the premier organization dealing with both the experimental and clinical aspects of hematopoiesis. The society journal, *BLOOD,* is published twice per month, and can be obtained through ASH, 1200 19th Street NW, Suite 300, Washington, DC 20036 (phone: 202-857-1118). The International Society of Experimental Hematology (ISEH) publishes *Experimental Hematology* monthly. Two recent textbooks [Hoffman et al., 1991; Sutherland et al., 1991a] contain a wealth of information on all aspects of experimental and clinical hematopoiesis.

117

Tissue Engineering of the Liver

Tae Ho Kim
*Harvard University and Boston
Children's Hospital*

Joseph P. Vacanti
*Harvard University and Boston
Children's Hospital*

Liver transplantation has been established as a curative treatment for end-stage adult and pediatric liver disease [Starzl et al., 1989], and over recent years, many innovative advances have been made in transplantation surgery. Unfortunately, a fundamental problem of liver transplantation has been severe donor shortage, and no clinical therapeutic bridge exists to abate the progression of liver failure (see Table 117.1). As the demand for liver transplantation surgery increases, still fewer than 3500 donors are available annually for the approximately 25,000 patients who die from chronic liver disease [National Vital Statistic System, 1991, 1992]. Currently, cadaveric and living-related donors are the only available sources. Xenograft [Starzl et al., 1993] and split liver transplantation [Merion & Campbell, 1991] are under experimental and clinical evaluation. The research effort to engineer a functional liver tissue has been vigorous, since tissue engineering of the liver offers, in theory, an efficient use of limited organ availability.

Whereas other experimental hepatic support systems such as extracorporeal bioreactors and hemoperfusion devices [Yarmush et al., 1992] attempt to temporarily support the metabolic functions of the liver, transplantation of hepatocyte systems is a possible temporary or permanent alternative therapy to liver transplantation for treatment of liver failure. An experimental model system of hepatocellular transplantation should provide optimal cell survival, proliferation, and maintenance of sufficient functional hepatocyte mass to replace liver function. Direct hepatocellular injection or infusion into various organs or tissues and a complex hepatocyte delivery system utilizing polymer matrices have been two major areas of research interest. Just as the liver is one of the most sophisticated organs in the human body, the science of hepatocyte or liver tissue construction has proved to be equally complex.

117.1 Background

The causes of end-stage liver disease are many, including alcoholic or viral cirrhosis, biliary atresia, inborn errors of metabolism, and sclerosing cholangitis. With chronic and progressive liver injury, hepatic necrosis occurs followed by fatty infiltration and inflammation. Scar tissue and nodular regeneration replace the normal liver architecture and increase the microcirculatory resistance, which results in portal hypertension; the liver is further atrophied as important factors in the portal

blood which regulate liver growth and maintenance are shunted away from the liver. Currently, end-stage liver disease must be present to
be considered for orthotopic liver transplantation therapy, but a significant difference exists
between alcohol- or viral-induced liver injury
and congenital liver diseases such as isolated
gene defects and biliary atresia. With alcohol- or
viral-induced chronic hepatic injury, the degree
of liver injury is unknown until metabolic functions are severely impaired and signs of progressive irreversible hepatic failure including portal
hypertension, coagulopathy, progressive jaundice, and hepatic encephalopathy have devel-

TABLE 117.1 UNOS Liver Transplantation Data
Summary from 1989 to 1993 in the United States:
Total Number of Liver Transplant Candidates and
Deaths Reported per Year While on Transplant
Waiting List.

Year	No. of Patients	No. of Deaths Reported
1989	3096	39
1990	4008	45
1991	4866	67
1992	5785	104
1993	7040	141

Source: United Network for Organ Sharing and the
Organ Procurement and Transplantation Network. Data
as of January 12, 1994.

oped. In congenital liver diseases, normal hepatic metabolic functions exist until dangerous toxins
build up and destroy the liver parenchyma. Hepatocellular transplantation could potentially *prevent*
hepatic injury and preserve host hepatic function for congenital inborn errors of liver metabolism.

As liver transplantation emerged as an important therapeutic modality, research activity intensi-
fied to improve or understand many areas of liver transplantation such as immunological tolerance,
preservation techniques, and the mechanism of healing after acute and chronic liver injury. Liver
growth and regulation, in particular, have been better understood: For example, after partial
hepatectomy, several *mitogens*—epidermal growth factor, alpha fibroblastic growth factor, hepatocyte growth factor, and transforming growth factor-alpha—are produced early after injury to stimulate liver regeneration. Comitogens—including insulin, glucagon, estrogen, norepinephrine, and
vasopressin—also aid with liver regeneration [Michalopoulos, 1993]. These stimulation factors help
govern the intricate regulatory process of liver growth and regeneration, but much about what
controls these factors is still unknown. In vitro and in vivo experiments with mitogens such as hepatocyte growth factor, epidermal growth factor, and insulin have yielded only moderate improvement
in hepatic proliferation.

The importance of hepatocyte proliferation and hepatic regeneration becomes evident when one
considers the difficulty in delivering large numbers of hepatocytes in hepatocyte replacement
systems. The potential advantage of hepatocyte cellular transplantation is to take a small number of
hepatocytes and proliferate these cells, in vitro or in vivo, to create functional liver equivalents for
replacement therapy. Without hepatocyte regeneration, delivery of a very large number of hepatocytes is required. Asonuma and coworkers [1992] have determined that approximately 12% of the
liver by heterotopic liver transplantation can significantly correct hyperbilirubinemia in the Gunn
rat, which is deficient in uridine diphosphate glucuronyl transferase. Although long-term efficacy
remains unclear, 10–12% of the liver is an approximate critical hepatocellular mass thought necessary to replace the metabolic functions of the liver. The inability to mimic normal liver growth and
regeneration in *in vitro* and *in vivo* systems has been one significant obstacle for hepatocyte tissue
construction thus far.

117.2 Hepatocyte Transplantation Systems

Hepatocyte transplant systems offer the possibilities of creating many functional liver equivalents,
storing hepatocytes by cryopreservation for later application [Yarmush et al., 1992], and using
autologous cells for gene therapy [Jauregui & Gann, 1991]. The two systems discussed below differ
in the amount of hepatocytes delivered, use of implantation devices, and implantation sites and techniques. Yet, in both systems, one significant roadblock in proving the efficacy of hepatocyte transplantation has been in the lack of a definitive, reproducible isolated liver defect model. Previous
studies using syngeneic rat models such as the jaundice Gunn rat, the analbuminemic Nagase rat, or

acute and chronic liver injury rat models have attributed significant correction of their respective deficit from hepatocyte transplantation. However, either inconsistencies or variations of animal strains and lack of consistent reproducible results have made accurate scientific interpretations and conclusions difficult. For instance, a study assessing hepatocyte delivery with microcarrier beads reported significant decrease in bilirubin in the hyperbilirubinemic Gunn rat and elevation of albumin in the Nagase analbuminemic rat after intraperitoneal implantation [Demetriou et al., 1986]; other studies have not demonstrated significant hepatocyte survival with intraperitoneal injection of hepatocytes with or without microcarriers; histology showed predominant cell necrosis and granuloma formation after 3 days [Henne-Bruns et al., 1991]. In *allogeneic* models, the possibility of immunological rejection further complicates the evaluation of the hepatocyte transplant system. Clearly, determining the efficacy of hepatocyte transplantation in liver metabolic-deficient models requires significant chemical results, and histologic correlation without confounding variables.

Hepatocellular Injection Model

Hepatocytes require an extracellular matrix for growth and differentiation, and the concept of utilizing existing **stromal** tissue as a vascular extracellular matrix is inviting. Isolated hepatocytes have been injected directly into the spleen or liver or into the portal or splenic vein. Several studies have reported significant but temporary correction of acute and metabolic liver defects in rat models as a result of intrahepatic, intraportal [Matas et al., 1976], or intrasplenic injections [Vroemen et al., 1985]. However, elucidating the efficacy of hepatocellular injection transplantation has been difficult for three significant reasons: (1) Differentiation of donor transplanted hepatocytes from host liver parenchyma has not been well established in an animal liver defect model, (2) how much hepatocyte mass needed to inject for partial or total liver function replacement has not been determined [Onodera et al., 1992], and (3) establishing a definitive animal liver defect model to prove efficacy of hepatocyte injection has been difficult.

Transgenic animal strains have been developed and offer a reproducible model in differentiating host from transplanted hepatocytes. Using transgenic mouse lines, donor hepatocytes injected into the spleen were histologically shown to migrate to the host liver, survive, and maintain function [Ponder et al., 1991]. Recently, a transgenic liver model in a mouse was used to evaluate the replicative potential of adult mouse hepatocytes. Normal adult mouse hepatocytes from two established transgenic lines were injected into the spleen of an Alb-uPA transgenic mouse that had an endogenous defect in hepatic growth potential and function (see Fig. 117.1). The adult mouse hepatocytes were shown to translocate to the liver and undergo up to 12 cell doublings; however, function of the transplanted hepatocytes was not fully reported [Rhim et al., 1994]. Rhim's study suggests that a hepatocyte has the potential to replicate many-fold so long as the structural and chemical milieu is optimal for survival and regeneration. If a small number of transplanted hepatocytes survive and proliferate many-fold in the native liver, sufficient hepatocyte mass to replace liver function would be accomplished, ameliorating the need to deliver a large quantity of donor hepatocytes.

Although many questions about hepatocyte injection therapy remain, the transgenic liver model has been used to test the safety and efficacy of ex vivo gene therapy for metabolic liver diseases. The Watanabe heritable hyperlipidemic rabbit, a strain deficient in low density lipoproteins (LDL) receptors, has been used to evaluate the possible application of gene therapy by hepatocyte injection. *Autologous* hepatocytes were obtained from a liver segment, genetically modified *ex vivo*, and infused into the inferior mesenteric vein through a catheter placed intraoperatively without postoperative sequelae to the rabbit. Decreased levels of LDL have been reported out to 6 months [Wilson et al., 1992]. Larger animal models have shown engraftment of the genetically altered hepatocytes for as long as 1.5 years. The first clinical application of hepatocellular injection has been performed on a patient diagnosed with homozygous familial hypercholesterolemia. The patient has had decreased levels of cholesterol and has maintained expression of the transfected gene after 18 months [Grossman et al., 1994]. This is an important step forward as we await long-term results.

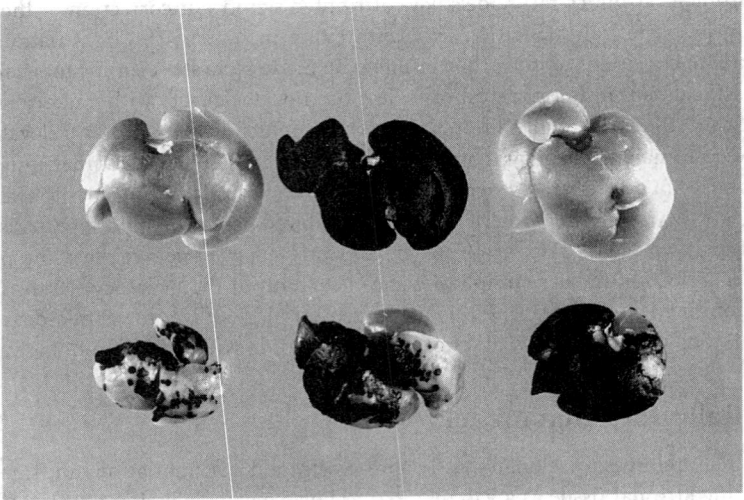

FIGURE 117.1   Control and transgenic liver specimens: a nontransgenic (normal mouse) control with normal liver color (top, left); a *transgenic (MT-lacZ)* liver with normal function which is stained in blue and served as a positive control (top, center); a *nontransgenic* control transplanted with *transgenic MIT-lacZ* hepatocytes (top, right); and three livers with a different *transgene Alb-uPA* transplanted with *transgenic (MT-lacZ)* hepatocytes. A deficiency in hepatic growth potential and function is induced by the *Alb-uPA transgene,* resulting in a chronic stimulus for liver growth. The liver with *Alb-uPA transgene* has the same color as the *nontransgenic* control liver but is partially replaced by the blue-stained *transgenic (MT-lacZ)* normal functioning hepatocytes, showing the regenerative response of normal hepatocytes in a mouse liver with a chronic stimulus for liver growth. (Rhim, Sandgren, and Brinster, University of Pennsylvania, reprinted with permission from American Association for the Advancement of Science.)

Hepatocyte Transplantation on Polymer Matrices

Since the practical application of implanting few hepatocytes to proliferate and replace function is not yet possible, hepatocyte tissue construction, using polymer as a scaffold, relies on transplanting a large number of hepatocytes to allow survival of enough hepatocyte mass to replace function. The large surface area of the polymer accommodates hepatocyte attachment in large numbers so that many cells may survive initially by diffusion of oxygen and other vital nutrients (see Fig. 117.2). The polymer scaffold is constructed with a high porosity to allow vascular ingrowth, and vascularization of surviving cells then can provide permanent nutritional access [Cima et al., 1991]. The cell-polymer system has been used in several other tissue-engineering applications such as cartilage, bone, intestine, and urologic tissue construction [Langer & Vacanti, 1993]. Hepatocytes adhere to the polymer matrix for growth and differentiation as well as locate into the interstices of the polymer. The polymer-hepatocyte interface can be manipulated with surface proteins such as laminin, fibronectin, and growth factors to improve adherence, viability, function, or growth [Mooney et al., 1992]. Hepatocyte proliferation by attaching mitogenic factors like hepatocyte growth factor, epidermal growth factor, or transforming growth factor-alpha is under current investigation.

Synthetic polymer matrices, both degradable and nondegradable, have been evaluated for hepatocyte-polymer construction. As degradable polymers were being studied and evaluated for tissue engineering, a nondegradable polymer, polyvinyl alcohol (PVA), was used for *in vitro* and *in vivo* systems. The polyvinyl alcohol sponge offered one significant advantage: a uniform, noncollapsable

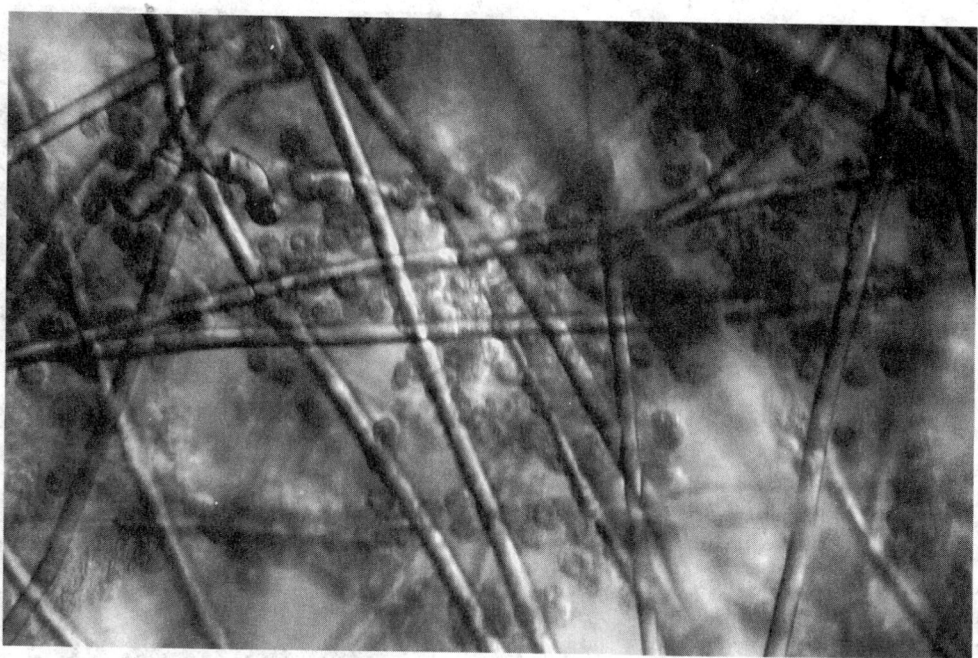

FIGURE 117.2   Hepatocytes are seen adhering to polyglycolic acid polymer in culture (Mooney, unpublished data).

structure which allowed quantification of hepatocyte engraftment [Uyama et al., 1993]. *In vitro* and *in vivo* studies have demonstrated hepatocyte survival on the polyvinyl alcohol scaffold. However, the polyvinyl alcohol sponge will not degrade and could act as a nidus for infection and chronic inflammation. A degradable polymer conceptually serves as a better implantable scaffold for hepatocyte-polymer transplantation, since the polymer dissolves to leave only tissue. Polyglycolic acid (PGA), polylactic acid (PLA), and copolymer hybrids have been employed in several animal models of liver insufficiency (see Fig. 117.3). Histologic analyses have shown similar survival of hepatocytes when compared to studies with polyvinyl alcohol.

The experimental design for the hepatocyte-polymer model has been standardized as follows: (1) an end-to-side portacaval shunt is performed to provide hepatotrophic stimulation to the graft, (2) hepatocytes are isolated and seeded onto degradable polyglycolic acid polymer, (3) the hepatocyte-polymer construct is implanted into the abdominal cavity on vascular beds of small intestinal mesentery and omentum, (4) pertinent chemical studies are obtained and analyzed at periodic intervals, and (5) histologic analysis of the specimens is performed at progressive time points. Early studies have shown that a large percentage of hepatocytes perish from hypoxia within 6–24 hours after implantation. To improve hepatocyte survival, implantation of hepatocytes onto large vascular surface areas for engraftment and exposing the hepatocytes to hepatotrophic factors were two important maneuvers. The small intestinal mesentery and omentum have offered large vascular surface areas. Hepatocyte survival has been reported at other sites such as the peritoneum [Demetriou et al., 1991], renal capsule [Ricordi et al., 1989], lung [Sandbichler et al., 1992], and pancreas [Vroemen et al., 1988], but these sites do not provide enough vascular surface area to allow survival of a large number of hepatocytes.

The concept of hepatotrophic factors originated when atrophy and liver insufficiency was observed with heterotopic liver transplantation. Later studies have confirmed that important factors regulating liver growth and maintenance existed in the portal blood [Jaffe et al., 1991]. Thus, when a portacaval shunt to redirect hepatotrophic factors from the host liver to the hepatocyte-polymer construct was performed, survival of heterotopically transplanted hepatocytes significantly improved [Uyama et al., 1993]; consequently, portacaval shunts were instituted in all experimental models. Studies thus far have shown survival of functional hepatocytes over 6 months in rat and dog models (unpublished data); replacement of liver function has been of shorter duration.

A study using the Dalmatian dog model of hyperuricosuria typifies the current status of the hepatocyte-polymer system. The hepatocyte membrane of the Dalmatian dog has a defect in the uptake of uric acid, which results in hyperuricemia and hyperuricosuria [Giesecke & Tiemeyer, 1984]. The study has shown a significant but temporary correction of the liver uric acid metabolic defect after implantation of normal beagle hepatocytes, which has normal uric acid metabolism, on degradable polyglycolic acid polymer [Takeda et al., 1994]. Cyclosporine was administered for immunosuppression. The results of the Dalmatian dog study suggest that (1) successful engraftment of the hepatocyte-polymer construct occurred, (2) maintenance of functional hepatocytes under current conditions was temporary, and (3) loss of critical hepatocyte mass to replace the liver uric acid metabolism defect occurred at 5–6 weeks after hepatocyte-polymer transplantation. The temporary effect could be attributed to suboptimal immunosuppression, suboptimal regulation of growth factors and hormones involved with hepatic growth, regeneration, and maintenance, or both.

Coculture of hepatocytes with pancreatic islet cells also has been under investigation to aid in hepatocyte survival, growth, and maintenance. Trophic factors from islet cells have been shown to improve hepatocyte survival [Ricordi et al., 1988], and cotransplantation of hepatocytes with islet cells on a polymer matrix has been shown to improve hepatocyte survival as well [Kaufmann et al., 1994]. Coculture with other cell types such as the biliary epithelial cell also may improve hepatocyte survival. Other studies with biliary epithelial cells have shown

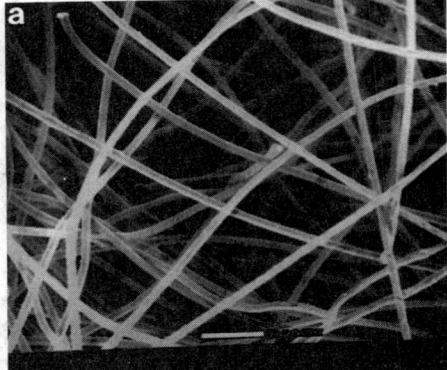
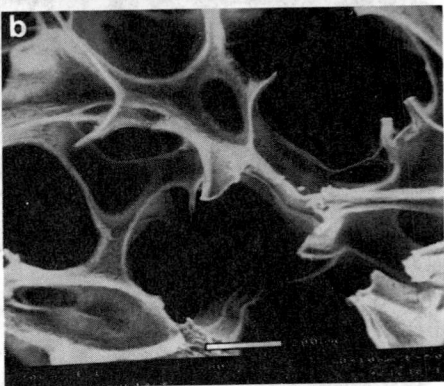
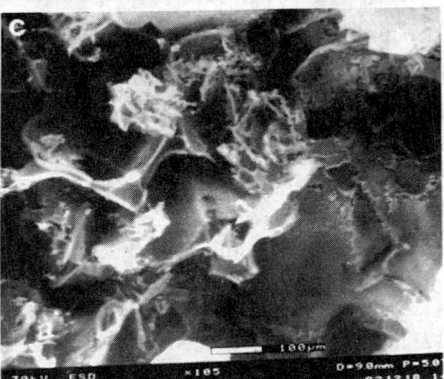

FIGURE 117.3 Scanning electron microscopic photographs of polyglycolic acid (top), polyvinyl alcohol (middle), and polylactic acid (bottom) demonstrate the high porosity of these polymers (Mooney, reprinted with permission from W.B. Saunders Company).

ductular formation in in vitro and in vivo models [Sirica et al., 1990], and vestiges of ductular formation in hepatocyte-polymer tissue have been histologically observed [Hansen & Vacanti, 1992]. A distinct advantage of the cell-polymer engineered construct is that one can manipulate the polymer to direct function. Thus far, diseases involving the biliary system, primarily biliary atresia, are not amenable to hepatocyte transplantation. An attempt to develop a biliary drainage system with biliary epithelial cells, hepatocytes, and polymer has been initiated. In the future, the potential construction of a branching polymer network could serve as the structural cues for the development of an interconnecting ductular system.

Ex vivo gene therapy with the hepatocyte-polymer system is also an exciting potential application as demonstrated by the recent clinical trial with hepatocyte injection therapy. Genetically altered hepatocytes transplanted on polymer constructs have been studied with encouraging results [Fontaine et al., 1993].

117.3 Conclusion

Studies in hepatocyte transplantation through tissue engineering methods have made important advances in recent years. The research in the hepatocellular injection and the research in the hepatocyte-polymer construct models have complemented each other in understanding the difficulties as well as the possibilities of liver replacement therapy. In order to make further advances with hepatocyte replacement systems, the process of liver development, growth, and maintenance need to be better understood. Currently, the amount of hepatocyte engraftment, proliferation, and the duration of hepatocyte survival remain undetermined in both systems. The amount of functional hepatocyte engraftment necessary may vary for different hepatic diseases. For instance, isolated gene defects of the liver may require a small number of functional transplanted hepatocytes to replace function, whereas end-stage liver disease may require a large amount of hepatocyte engraftment.

Current hepatic replacement models have both advantages and disadvantages. For hepatocellular injection, the application of ex vivo gene therapy for an isolated gene defect of liver metabolism is promising. However, the small amount of hepatocyte delivery and significant potential complications for patients with portal hypertension may preclude application of the hepatocellular injection method for end-stage liver disease. A significant amount of intrapulmonary shunting of hepatocytes was observed in rats with portal hypertension after intrasplenic injection of hepatocytes, which resulted in increased portal pressures, pulmonary hypertension, pulmonary infarction, and reduced pulmonary compliance [Gupta et al., 1993]. With the hepatocyte-polymer system, delivery of a large number of hepatocytes is possible. In patients with portal hypertension, portal blood-containing hepatotrophic factors are shunted away from the liver, obviating the need for a portacaval shunt. Thus, patients with end-stage liver disease and portal hypertension may need only transplantation of the hepatocyte-polymer construct. However, an end-to-side portacaval shunt operation is needed in congenital liver diseases with normal portal pressures to deliver hepatotrophic factors to the heterotopically placed hepatocytes. In the future, each hepatocyte transplant system could have specific and different clinical applications. More important, both offer the hope of increasing therapeutic options for patients requiring liver replacement therapy. Approximately 260,000 patients out of 634,000 patients hospitalized for liver diseases have liver diseases which could have been considered for hepatic transplantation. The total acute care nonfederal hospital costs for liver diseases in 1992, which does not include equally substantial outpatient costs, exceeded $9.2 billion [HCIA Inc., 1992].

Defining Terms

Allogeneic: Pertaining to different genetic compositions within the same species.

Cadaveric: Related to a dead body. In transplantation, *cadaveric* is related to a person who has been declared brain dead; organs should be removed prior to cardiac arrest to prevent injury to the organs.

Heterotopic: Related to a region or place where an organ or tissue is not present in normal conditions.

Mitogens: Substances that stimulate mitosis or growth.

Orthotopic: Related to a region or place where an organ or tissue is present in normal conditions.

Portacaval shunt: A surgical procedure to partially or completely anastomose the portal vein to the inferior vena cava to divert portal blood flow from the liver to the systemic circulation.

Stroma: The structure or framework of an organ or gland usually composed of connective tissue.

Transgenic: Referred to introduction of a foreign gene into a recipient which can be used to identify genetic elements and examine gene expression.

Xenograft: A graft transferred from one animal species to another species.

References

Asonuma K, Gilbert JC, Stein JE, et al. 1992. Quantitation of transplanted hepatic mass necessary to cure the Gunn rat model of hyperbilirubinemia. J Ped Surg 27(3):298.

Asonuma K, Vacanti JP. 1992. Cell transplantation as replacement therapy for the future. Pediatr Transplantation 4(2):249.

Cima L, Vacanti JP, Vacanti C, et al. 1991. Tissue engineering by cell transplantation using degradable polymer substrates. J Biomech Eng 113:143.

Demetriou AA, Felcher A, Moscioni AD. 1991. Hepatocyte transplantation. A potential treatment for liver disease. Dig Dis Sci 12(9):1320.

Demetriou AA, Whiting JF, Feldman D, et al. 1986. Replacement of liver function in rats by transplantation of microcarrier-attached hepatocytes. Science 233:1190.

Fontaine MJ, Hansen LK, Thompson S, et al. 1993. Transplantation of genetically altered hepatocytes using cell-polymer constructs leads to sustained human growth hormone secretion in vivo. Transplant Proc 25(1):1002–4.

Giesecke D, Tiemeyer W. 1984. Defect of uric acid in Dalmatian dog liver. Experientia 40:1415.

Grossman M, Roper SE, Kozarsky K, et al. 1994. Successful ex vivo gene therapy directed to liver in a patient with familial hypercholesterolemia. Nature Genetics 6:335.

Gupta S, Yerneni PR, Vemuru RP, et al. 1993. Studies on the safety of intrasplenic hepatocyte transplantation: relevance to ex vivo gene therapy and liver repopulation in acute hepatic failure. Hum Gene Ther 4(3):249.

Hansen LK, Vacanti JP. 1992. Hepatocyte transplantation using artificial biodegradable polymers. 1992. In MA Hoffman (ed), Current Controversies in Biliary Atresia. The Medical Intelligence Unit Series pp 96–106, (CRC Press), Austin, Tex, R.G. Landes.

HCIA Inc. 1992. Survey of costs in non-Federal, acute care hospitals in the United States prepared for the American Liver Foundation, Baltimore.

Henne-Bruns D, Kruger U, Sumpelman D, et al. 1991. Intraperitoneal hepatocyte transplantation: morphological results. Virchows Arch A, Path Anat Histopathol 419(1):45.

Jaffe V, Darby H, Bishop A, et al. 1991. The growth of liver cells in the pancreas after intrasplenic implantation: the effects of portal perfusion. Int J Exp Pathol 72(3):289.

Jauregui HO, Gann KL. 1991. Mammalian hepatocytes as a foundation for treatment in human liver failure [Review]. J Cell Biochem 45(4):359.

Kaufmann P-M, Sano K, Uyama S, et al. 1994. Heterotopic hepatocyte transplantation using three dimensional polymers. Evaluation of the stimulatory effects by portacaval shunt or islet cell co-transplantation. Second International Congress of the Cell Transplant Society, Minneapolis, Minnesota.

Langer R, Vacanti J. 1993. Tissue Engineering. Science 260:920.

Matas AJ, Sutherland DER, Steffes MW, et al. 1976. Hepatocellular transplantation for metabolic deficiencies: decrease of plasma bilirubin in Gunn rats. Science 192:892.

Merion RM, Campbell DA Jr. 1991. Split liver transplantation: One plus one doesn't always equal two. Hepatology 14(3):572.

Michalopoulos G. 1993. HGF and liver regeneration. Gasterologica Japonica 28(suppl 4):36.

Mooney DJ, Hansen LK, Vacanti JP, et al. 1992. Switching from differentiation to growth in hepatocytes: Control by extracellular matrix. J Cell Physiol 151:497.

National Vital Statistic System. 1991, 1992. Data derived from National Center for Health Statistics.

Onodera K, Ebata H, Sawa M, et al. 1992. Comparative effects of hepatocellular transplantation in the spleen, portal vein, or peritoneal cavity in congenitally ascorbic acid biosynthetic enzyme-deficient rats. Transplant Proc 24(6):3006.

Ponder KP, Gupta S, Leland F, et al. 1991. Mouse hepatocytes migrate to liver parenchyma and function indefinitely after intrasplenic transplantation. Proc Natl Acad Sci USA 88(4):1217.

Rhim JA, Sandgren EP, Degen JL, et al. 1994. Replacement of diseased mouse liver by hepatic cell transplantation. Science 263:1149.

Ricordi C, Lacy PE, Callery MP, et al. 1989. Trophic factors from pancreatic islets in combined hepatocyte-islet allografts enhance hepatocellular survival. Surgery 105:218.

Sandbichler P, Then P, Vogel W, et al. 1992. Hepatocellular transplantation into the lung for temporary support of acute liver failure in the rat. Gastroenterology 102(2):605.

Sirica AE, Mathis GA, Sano N, et al. 1990. Isolation, culture, and transplantation of intrahepatic biliary epithelial cells and oval cells. Pathobiology 58:44.

Starzl TE, Demetris AJ, Van Thiel D. 1989. Chronic liver failure: Orthotopic liver transplantation. N Eng J Med 321:1014.

Starzl TE, Fung J, Tzakis A, et al. 1993. Baboon-to-human liver transplantation. Lancet 341(8837):65.

Takeda T, Kim TH, Lee SK, et al. 1994. Hepatocyte transplantation in biodegradable polymer scaffolds using the dalmation dog model of hyperuricosuria. Fifteenth Congress of the Transplantation Society, Kyoto Japan. Submitted.

Uyama S, Takeda T, Vacanti JP. 1993. Delivery of whole liver equivalent hepatic mass using polymer devices and heterotrophic stimulation. Transplantation 55(4):932.

Uyama S, Takeda T, Vacanti JP. In press. Hepatocyte transplantation equivalent to whole liver mass using cell-polymer devices. Polymer Preprints.

Vacanti JP, Morse MA, Saltzman WM, et al. 1988. Selective cell transplantation using bioabsorbable artificial polymers as matrices. J Ped Surg 23(1):3.

Vroemen JPAM, Blanckaert N, Buurman WA, et al. 1985. Treatment of enzyme deficiency by hepatocyte transplantation in rats. J Surg Res 39:267.

Vroemen JPAM, Buurman WA, van der Linden CJ, et al. 1988. Transplantation of isolated hepatocytes into the pancreas. Eur Surg Res 20:1.

Wilson JM, Grossman M, Raper SE, et al. 1992. Ex vivo gene therapy of familial hypercholesterolemia. Human Gene Ther 3(2):179.

Yarmush ML, Toner M, Dunn JCY, et al. 1992. Hepatic tissue engineering: Development of critical technologies. Ann NY Acad Sci 665:238.

118

Tissue Engineering in the Nervous System

Ravi Bellamkonda
*Lausanne University
Medical School*

Patrick Aebischer
*Lausanne University
Medical School*

Tissue engineering in the nervous system facilitates the controlled application and/or organization of neural cells to perform appropriate diagnostic, palliative, or therapeutic tasks. As the word *tissue* implies, tissue engineering in general involves cellular components and their organization. Any cell, given its broad genetic program, expresses a particular phenotype in a manner that is dependent on its environment. The extracellular environment consists of cells, humoral factors, and the extracellular matrix. Research in genetic engineering and the intense focus on growth factors and extracellular matrix biology have made it possible to manipulate both the cell's genetic program and its phenotypic expression.

In the nervous system, degeneration or injury to neurons or glia and/or an aberrant extracellular environment can cause a wide variety of ailments. Diseases such as Parkinson's may require the replacement of diminished levels of a particular neurochemical, e.g., dopamine. Other pathologies such as injured nerves or reconnection of severed neural pathways may require regeneration of nervous tissue.

Tissue engineering efforts in the nervous system have currently been addressing the following goals:

1. Functional replacement of a missing neuroactive component
2. Rescue or regeneration of damaged neural tissue
3. Human-machine interfaces: neural coupling elements

118.1 Delivery of Neuroactive Molecules to the Nervous System

Deficiency of specific neuroactive molecules has been implicated in several neurologic disorders. These factors may be neurotransmitters, neurotrophic agents, or enzymes. For example, part of the basal ganglia circuitry that plays a role in motor control consists of striatal neurons receiving dopaminergic input from the mesencephalic substantia nigra neurons. It has been shown that a lesioned nigrostriatal dopaminergic pathway is responsible for Parkinson's disease [Ehringer & Hornykiewicz, 1960]. In chronic cancer patients, the delivery of antinociceptive neurotransmitters such as enkephalins, endorphins, catecholamines, neuropeptide Y, neurotensin, and somatostatin to the cerebrospinal fluid may improve the treatment of severe pain [Akil et al., 1984; Joseph et al., in press]. Neurotrophic factors may play a role in the treatment of several neurodegenerative disorders. For example, local delivery of nerve growth factor (NGF) [Hefti et al., 1984; Williams et al., 1986] and/or brain-derived growth factor (BDNF) may be useful in the treatment of Alzheimer's disease [Anderson et al., 1990; Knüsel et al., 1991]. BDNF [Hyman et al., 1991; Knüsel et al., 1991] and glial cell line–derived nerve growth factor (GDNF) may be beneficial in Parkinson's disease [Lin et al., 1993]. Other neurotrophins such as ciliary neurotrophic factor (CNTF) [Oppenheim et al., 1991; Sendtner et al., 1990], BDNF [Yan et al., 1992], neurotrophin-3 (NT-3), neurotrophin-4 (NT-4/5) [Hughes et al., 1993] and GDNF [Zurn et al., 1994] also could have an impact on amyotrophic lateral sclerosis (ALS) or Lou Gehrig's disease.

Therefore, augmentation or replacement of any of the above-mentioned factors in the nervous system would be a viable therapeutic strategy for the treatment of the pathologies listed above. There are several issues that ought to be considered in engineering a system to deliver these factors. The stability of the factors, the dosage required, the solubility, the target tissue, and possible side effects all are factors that influence the choice of the delivery mode. Pumps, slow-release polymer systems, and cells from various sources that secrete the compound of interest are the main modes by which these factors can be delivered. Table 118.1 lists all the means employed to deliver dopamine to alleviate the symptoms of Parkinson's disease.

TABLE 118.1 Engineering Solutions for Parkinson's Disease

Mode of Delivery	Rodents	Monkey	Human	Reference
Infusion	Rat striatum			Hargraves et al., 1987
		Cerebroventricular		De Yebenes et al., 1988
			Systemic	Hardie et al., 1984
Polymer slow release	Rat striatum (EVA rods)			Winn et al., 1989
	Rat subcutaneous (EVA rods)			Sabel et al., 1990
	Rat striatum (Si pellet)			Becker et al., 1990
	Rat striatum (liposomes)			During et al., 1992
Cell transplantation				
Fetal				
Substantia nigra	Rat striatum			Björklund et al., 1980; Freund et al., 1985
Ventral mesencephalon	Rat striatum			Bolam et al., 1987
Human DA neurons			Putamen	Lindvall et al., 1990
Autologuous primary				
Genetically altered skin fibroblasts	Rat striatum			Chen et al., 1991
Genetically altered skin fibroblasts with myoblasts	Rat striatum			Jiao et al., 1993
Encapsulated xenogeneic tissue				
Bovine adrenal chromaffin cells	Striatum (microcapsules)			Aebischer et al., 1991
PC12 cells	Rat striatum (microcapsules)			Winn et al., 1991
	Rat striatum (macrocapsule)			Aebischer et al., 1988
		Striatum (macrocapsule)		Aebischer et al., 1994
Mouse mesencephalon	Rat parietal cortex (macrocapsule)			Aebischer et al., 1988

Pumps

Pumps are used to deliver opiates epidurally to relieve severe pain [Ahlgren et al., 1987]. Pumps also have been used to deliver neurotrophic factors such as NGF intraventricularly as a prelude or supplement to transplantation of chromaffin cells for Parkinson's disease [Olson et al., 1991] or as a potential therapy for Alzheimer's disease [Olson et al., 1992]. Pumps also have been used to experimentally deliver dopamine or dopamine receptor agonists in Parkinson's disease models [De Yebenes et al., 1988; Hargraves et al., 1987]. While pumps have been employed successfully in these instances, they may need to be refilled every 4 weeks, and this may be a limitation. Other potential drawbacks include susceptibility to "dumping" of neuroactive substance due to presence of a large reservoir of neuroactive element, infections, and diffusion limitations. Also, some factors such as dopamine and ciliary neurotrophic factor (CNTF) are very unstable chemically and have short half-life periods, rendering their delivery by such devices difficult. Some of these problems may be eliminated by well-designed slow-release polymer systems.

Slow-Release Polymer Systems

Slow-release polymer systems essentially trap the molecule of interest in a polymer matrix and release it slowly by diffusion over a period of time. Proper design of the shape and composition of the polymer matrix may achieve stabilization of the bioactive molecule and facilitate a steady, sustained release over a period of time. For instance, it has been shown that the dopamine precursor L-dopa may be effective in alleviating some motor symptoms of Parkinson's disease [Birkmayer, 1969], fluctuations in the plasma levels of L-dopa due to traditional, periodic oral administration and difficulties in converting L-dopa to dopamine may cause the clinical response to fluctuate as well [Albani et al., 1986; Hardie et al., 1984; Muenter et al., 1977; Shoulson et al., 1975]. It has been demonstrated that a slow-release ethylene vinyl acetate polymer system loaded with L-dopa can sustain elevated plasma levels of L-dopa for at least 225 days when implanted subcutaneously in rats [Sabel et al., 1990]. Dopamine can only be released directly in the CNS, since it does not pass the blood-brain barrier. It has been demonstrated that experimental parkinsonism in rats can be alleviated by intrastriatal implantation of dopamine-releasing ethylene vinyl acetate rods [Winn et al., 1989]. Silicone elastomer as well as resorbable polyester pellets loaded with dopamine also have been implanted intrastriatally and shown to induce a behavioral recovery in parkinsonian rats [Becker et al., 1990; McRae et al., 1991].

Slow-release systems also may be employed to deliver trophic factors to the brain either to avoid side affects that may come about due to systemic administration or to overcome the blood-brain barrier, getting the factor delivered to the brain directly [During et al., 1992; Hoffman et al., 1990]. Therefore, polymeric systems with the molecule of interest trapped inside may be able to achieve many of the goals of an ideal delivery system, including targeted local delivery and zero-order continuous release [Langer, 1981; Langer et al., 1976]. However, some of the disadvantages of this system are the finite amounts of loaded neuroactive molecules and difficulties in shutting off release or adjusting rate of release once the polymer is implanted. Also, for long-term release in humans, the device size may become a limiting factor. Some of these limitations may be overcome by the transplantation of cells that release neuroactive factors to the target site.

Cell Transplantation

Advances in molecular biology and gene transfer techniques have given rise to a rich array of cellular sources, which have been engineered to secrete a wide range of neurologic compounds. These include cells that release neurotransmitters, neurotrophic factors, and enzymes. Transplantation of these cells leads to functional replacement or augmentation of the original source of these compounds in the host. They can deliver neuroactive molecules as long as they survive, provided they maintain their phenotype and/or transgene expression, in the case of gene therapy. Some of the disadvantages of the slow-release systems, such as the presence of a large reservoir for long-term release or reloading of an exhausted reservoir, can thus be overcome. Some of the tissues transplanted so far may be classified in the following manner.

Transplantation of Autologous Primary Cells

This technique involves the procurement of primary cells from the host, expanding them if necessary to generate requisite amounts of tissue, engineering them if so required by using gene transfer techniques, and then transplanting them back into the "donor" at the appropriate site. For instance, autologous Schwann cells have been isolated and transplanted experimentally into the brain and have been shown to enhance retinal nerve regeneration, presumably by the release of factors that influence regeneration [Morrissey et al., 1991]. Schwann cells also express various neurologically relevant molecules [Bunge & Bunge, 1983; Muir et al., 1989]. Autologous Schwann cells also can work as nerve bridges to help reconstruction of rat sciatic nerve after axotomy [Guénard et al., 1992]. Primary skin fibroblasts also have been genetically engineered to secrete L-dopa and transplanted successfully into the autologous host's striatum in an experimental model of Parkinson's disease in rats [Chen et al., 1991]. The same group also has reported that nerve growth factor, tyrosine hydroxylase, glutamic acid decarboxylase, and choline acetyltransferase genes may be introduced successfully and expressed in primary fibroblasts [Gage et al., 1991]. More recently, muscle cells have been engineered to express tyrosine hydroxylase and transplanted successfully in a rat model of Parkinson's disease [Jiao et al., 1993].

Thus nonneural cells such as a fibroblast or muscle cells may be selected, in part, for the ease with which they can be engineered genetically and made neurologically relevant. It is therefore possible to engineer cells to suit particular pathologies as a step toward being able to engineer biomimetic tissues and then place them in appropriate locations and contexts in vivo. However, it may not always be technically possible to procure sufficient amounts of autologous tissue. Other sources of tissues have therefore been explored, and these include fetal tissue, used usually in conjunction with immunosuppression.

Fetal Tissue Transplantation

One of the important advantages of fetal tissue is its ability to survive and integrate into the host adult brain. Transplantation of fetal neural tissue allografts might be useful in treating Parkinson's disease [Lindvall et al., 1990]. While promising results have been reported using neural fetal tissue [Björklund, 1991; Björklund et al., 1980], availability of donor tissue and potential ethical issues involved with the technique may be potential shortcomings. One promising strategy to obtain allogeneic fetal tissue in large quantities is to isolate neural stem cells and have them proliferate in vitro. It has been demonstrated recently that CNS progenitor cells may be selected using epidermal growth factor (EGF). The cells thus selected have been shown to proliferate in vitro under appropriate culture conditions. With time and appropriate culture conditions, they differentiate into mature CNS neurons and glia [Reynolds et al., 1992; Vescovi et al., 1993]. When optimized, this technique could be useful to select and expand fetal neurons of interest in vitro and then transplant them. Transplantation of xenogeneic fetal tissue with immunosuppression using cyclosporin A is another alternative to using fetal tissue [Wictorin et al., 1992], and this approach might yield more abundant amounts of tissue for transplantation and overcome some of the possible ethical dilemmas in using human fetal tissue. However, immunosuppression may not be sufficient to prevent long-term rejection and may have other undesirable side-effects.

Transplantation of Encapsulated Xenogeneic Tissue

Polymeric encapsulation of xenogeneic cells might be a viable strategy to transplant cells across species in the absence of systemic immunosuppression [Aebischer et al., 1988; Tresco et al., 1992]. Typically, the capsules have pores large enough for nutrients to reach the transplanted tissue and let the neuroactive factors out, but the pores are too small to let the molecules and the cells of the immune system reach the transplanted tissue (Fig. 118.1). At the same time, this strategy retains all the advantages of using cells as controlled, local manufacturers of the neuroactive molecules. The use of encapsulation also eliminates the restriction of having to use postmitotic tissue for transplantation to avoid tumor formation. The physical restriction of the polymeric capsule prevents

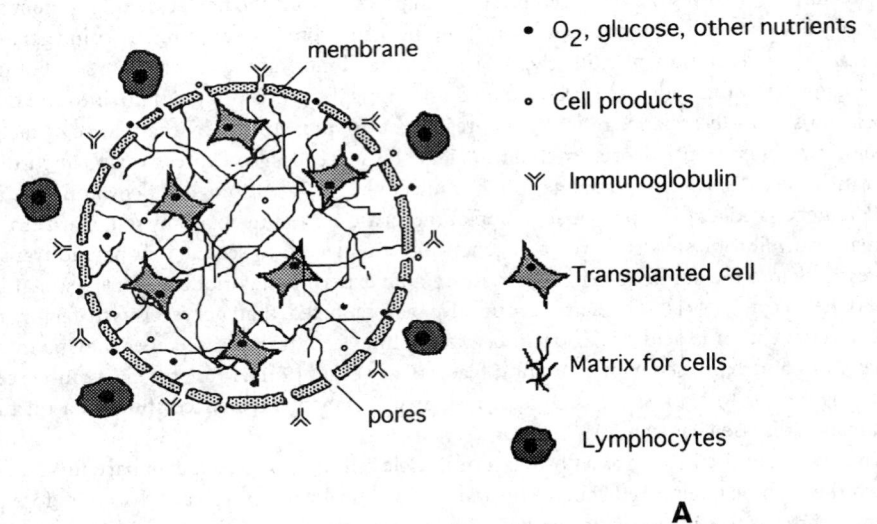

- O_2, glucose, other nutrients
- Cell products
- Immunoglobulin
- Transplanted cell
- Matrix for cells
- Lymphocytes

A

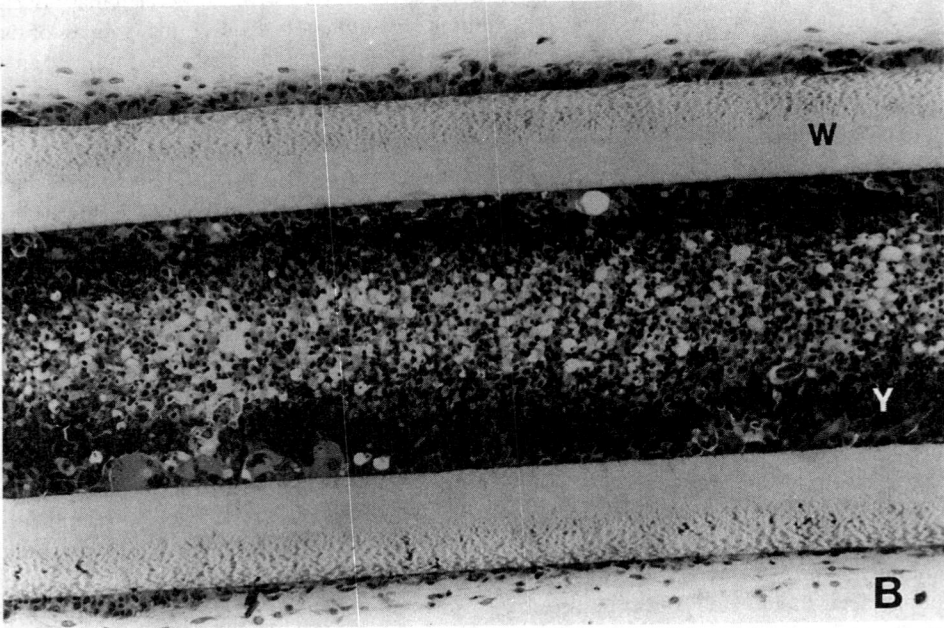

B

FIGURE 118.1 (*a*) Schematic illustration of the concept of immunoisolation involved in the transplantation of xenogeneic tissue encapsulated in semipermeable polymer membranes. (*b*) Light micrograph of a longitudinal section showing baby hamster kidney cells encapsulated in a polyacrylonitrile-vinylchloride membrane and transplanted in an axotomized rat pup after 2 weeks in vivo. *W* denotes the capsule's polymeric wall, and *Y* shows the cells.

escape of the encapsulated tissue. Should the capsule break, the transplanted cells are rejected and eliminated by the host immune system. However, no integration of the transplanted tissue into the host is possible with this technique.

Some of the tissue engineering issues involved in optimizing the encapsulation technique are (1) the type and configuration of the encapsulating membrane, (2) the various cells to be used for encapsulation, and the (3) matrix in which the cells are immobilized.

Type and Configuration of the Encapsulating Membrane. One important factor determining the size of the device is oxygen diffusion and availability to the encapsulated cells. This consideration influences the device design and encourages situations where the distances between the oxygen source, usually a capillary, and the inner core of transplanted tissue are kept as minimal as possible. The size and configuration of the device also influence the kinetics of release of the neuroactive molecules, the "response time" being slower in larger capsules with thicker membrane walls.

The capsule membrane may be a water-soluble system stabilized by ionic or hydrogen bonds formed between two weak polyelectrolytes—typically an acidic polysaccharide, such as alginic acid or modified cellulose, and a cationic polyaminoacid, such as polylysine or polyornithine [Goosen et al., 1985; Lim & Sun, 1980; Winn et al., 1991]. Gelation of the charged polyelectrolytes is caused by ionic cross-linking in the presence of di- or multivalent counterions. However, the stability and mechanical strength of these systems are questionable in the physiologic ionic environments. The major advantage of using these systems is that they obviate the need of organic solvent use in the making of the capsules and might be less cytotoxic in the manufacturing process.

The capsule membrane also may be a thermoplastic, yielding a more mechanically and chemically stable membrane. This technique involves loading of cells of interest in a preformed hollow fiber and then sealing the ends either by heat or with an appropriate glue. The hollow fibers are typically fabricated by a dry jet wet-spinning technique involving a phase-inversion process [Aebischer et al., 1991]. The use of thermoplastic membranes allows the manipulation of membrane structure, porosity, thickness, and permeability by appropriate variation of polymer solution flow rates, viscosity of the polymer solution, the nonsolvent used etc.

Long-term cross-species transplants of dopaminergic xenogeneic tissues and functional efficacy in the brain have been reported [Aebischer et al., 1991, 1994] using the preceding system. PC12 cells, a catecholaminergic cell line derived from a rat pheochromocytoma, ameliorated experimental Parkinson's disease when encapsulated within thermoplastic PAN/PVC capsules and implanted in the striatum of adult guinea pigs [Aebischer et al., 1991].

The Choice of Cells and Tissues for Encapsulation. Three main types of cells can be used for encapsulation. Cells may be postmitotic, cell lines that differentiate under specific conditions, or slow-dividing cells. The latter two types of cells lend themselves to genetic manipulation.

Postmitotic Cells. Primary xenogeneic tissue may be encapsulated and transplanted across species. For instance, chromaffin cells release various antinociceptive substances such as enkephalins, catecholamines, and somatostatin. Allografts of adrenal chromaffin cells have been shown to alleviate pain when transplanted in the subarachnoid space in rodent models and terminal cancer patients [Sagen et al., 1993]. Transplantation of encapsulated xenogeneic chromaffin cells may provide a long-term source of pain-reducing neuroactive substances [Sagen et al., 1993]. In our laboratory, clinical trials are currently underway using the transplantation of encapsulated bovine chromaffin tissue into human cerebrospinal fluid as a strategy to alleviate chronic pain in terminal cancer patients. [Aebischer et al., 1994]. This may circumvent the problem of the limited availability of human adrenal tissue in grafting procedures of chromaffin tissue.

Cell Lines that Differentiate under Specific Conditions. Postmitotic cells are attractive for transplantation applications because the possibility of tumor formation, loss of phenotypic expression, is potentially lower. Also, when encapsulated, there is less debris accumulation inside the capsule due to turnover of dividing cells. However, the disadvantage is that the amount of postmitotic tissue is usually too limited in quantity for general clinical applications. Therefore, the use of cells that are mitotic and then are rendered postmitotic under specific conditions is attractive for transplantation applications.

Under appropriate culture conditions, primary myoblasts undergo cell division for at least 50 passages. Fusion into resting myoblasts can be obtained by controlling the culture conditions. Alternatively, a transformed myoblast cell line C_2C_{12} derived from a C_2H mouse thigh differentiates and forms myotubes when cultured under low serum conditions [Yaffe & Saxel, 1977]. Therefore, these cells could be genetically altered, expanded in vitro, and then made postmitotic by varying the culture conditions. They can then be transplanted with the attendent advantages of using postmitotic tissue. Since myoblasts can be altered genetically, they have the potential to be a rich source for augmentation of tissue function via cell transplantation.

Slow-Dividing Cells.   Slow-dividing cells that reach a steady state in a capsule either due to contact inhibition or due to the encapsulation matrix are an attractive source of cells for transplantation. Potentially, their division can result in a self-renewing supply of cells inside the capsule. Dividing cells are also easier to transfect reliably with retroviral methods and therefore lend themselves to genetic manipulation. It is therefore possible to envisage the transplantation of various genetically engineered cells for the treatment of several neurologic disorders. This technique allows access to an ever-expanding source of xenogeneic tissues that have been engineered to produce the required factor of interest. For instance, Horellou and Mallet [1989] have retrovirally transferred the human TH cDNA into mouse anterior pituitary AtT-20 cell line, potentially resulting in a plentiful supply of dopamine-secreting cells that can then be encapsulated and transplanted into the striatum.

Another promising area for the use of such techniques is in the treatment of some neurodegenerative disorders where a lack of neurotrophic factors is believed to be part of the pathophysiology. Neurotrophic factors are soluble proteins that are required for the survival of neurons. These factors often exert a trophic effect; i.e., they have the capability of attracting growing axons. The "target" hypothesis describes the dependence of connected neurons on a trophic factor that is retrogradely transported along the axons after release from the target neurons. In the absence of the trophic factors, the neurons shrink and die, presumably to avoid potential misconnections. Experimentally, fibroblast lines have been used in CNS transplantation studies because of their convenience for gene transfer techniques [Gage et al., 1991]. The transplantation of encapsulated genetically engineered fibroblasts to produce NGF has been shown to prevent lesion-induced loss of septal ChaT expression following a fimbria-fornix lesion [Hoffman et al., 1993]. The fimbria-fornix lesion is characterized by deficits in learning and memory resembling those of Alzheimer's disease.

Matrices for Encapsulation.   The physical, chemical, and biologic properties of the matrix in which the cells have been immobilized may play an important role in determining the transplanted cell's state and function. Broadly, matrices can be classified into the following types: cross-linked polyelectrolytes, collagen in solution or as porous beads, naturally occurring extracellular matrix derivatives such as Matrigel, fibrin clots, and biosynthetic hydrogels with appropriate biologic cues bound to them to elicit a specific response from the cells of interest. The matrix has several functions: It can prevent the formation of large cell aggregates that lead to the development of central necrosis as a consequence of insufficient oxygen and nutrient access; it may allow anchorage-dependent cells to attach and spread on the matrix substrate; and it may induce differentiation of a cell line and therefore slow down or stop its division rate.

Negatively charged polyelectrolytes such as alginate have been used successfully for the immobilization of adrenal chromaffin cells [Aebischer et al., 1991]. Positively charged substrates, such as those provided by the amine groups of chitosan, allow attachment and spreading of fibroblasts [Zielinski et al., in press]. Biologically derived Matrigel induces differentiation of various cell lines such as Chinese hamster ovary (CHO) cells, astrocyte lines, or fibroblast lines (unpublished observations). Spongy collagen matrices, as well as fibrin matrices, seem to possess similar qualities. Our laboratory is currently evaluating the use of biosynthetic hydrogel matrices with biologically relevant peptides covalently bound to the polymer backbone. It is hypothesized that these matrices may elicit a specific designed response from the encapsulated cells.

118.2 Tissue Reconstruction: Nerve Regeneration

Most of the techniques described above were attempts at identifying the missing molecules of various neuropathologies, finding an appropriate source for those molecules and, if necessary, designing a cellular source via genetic engineering, and ultimately, choosing an optimal mode of delivery of the molecules, be it chemical or cellular. This approach, however, falls short of replacing the physical neuroanatomic synaptic circuits in the brain, which, in turn, may play an important role in the physiologic feedback regulation mechanisms of the system. Attempts to duplicate in vivo predisease neuronal structure have been made. For instance, the bridging of the nigrostriatal pathway, which when disrupted may cause Parkinson's disease, and the septohippocampal pathway, which may serve as a model for Alzheimer's disease, has attracted some attention. Wictorin and colleagues [1992] have reported long-distance directed axonal growth from human dopaminergic mesencephalic neuroblasts implanted along the nigrostriatal pathway in 6-hydroxydopamine–lesioned rats. In this section we shall examine the use of synthetic guidance channels and extracellular matrix cues to guide axons to their appropriate targets. Thus a combination of all these techniques may render the complete physical and synaptic reconstruction of a degenerated pathway feasible.

The promotion of nerve regeneration is an important candidate task for tissue reconstruction in the nervous system. Synthetic nerve guidance channels (NGCs) have been used to study the underlying mechanisms of mammalian peripheral nerve regeneration after nerve injury and enhance the regeneration process. Guidance channels may simplify end-to-end repair and may be useful in repairing long nerve gaps. The guidance channel reduces tension at the suture line, protects the regenerating nerve from infiltrating scar tissue, and directs the sprouting axons toward their distal targets. The properties of the guidance channel can be modified to optimize the regeneration process. Nerve guidance channels also may be used to create a controlled environment in the regenerating site. In the peripheral nervous system, NGCs can influence the extent of nerve gap that can be bridged and the quality of regeneration. The channel properties, the matrix filling the NGC, the cells seeded within the channel lumen, and polymer-induced welding of axons all can be strategies used to optimize and enhance nerve regeneration and effect nervous tissue reconstruction (see Fig. 118.2 for a schematic). Table 118.2 lists some of the kinds of nerve guidance channels used so far.

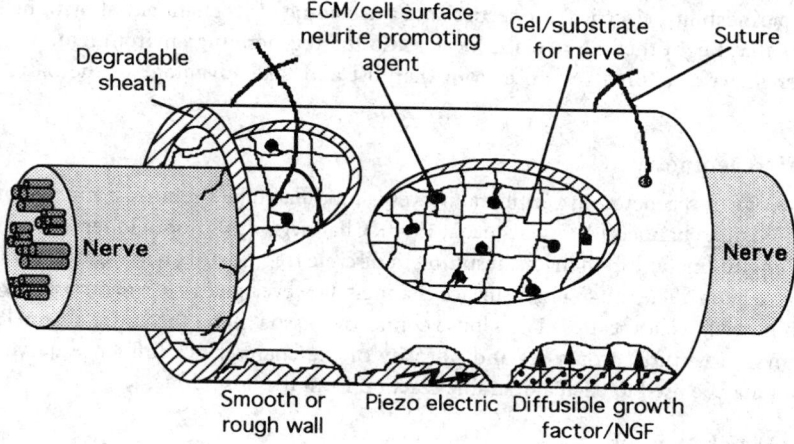

FIGURE 118.2   Schematic illustration of a nerve guidance channel and some of the possible strategies for influencing nerve regeneration.

TABLE 118.2   Nerve Guidance Channels

I. The Channel Wall	
1. *Passive polymeric channels*	
Silicone elastomer	Lundborg et al., 1982
Polyvinyl chloride	Scaravalli, 1984
Polyethylene	Madison et al., 1988
2. *Permeable polymer channels*	
Acrylonitrile vinylchloride	
copolymer	Uzman and Villegas, 1983
Collagen	Archibald et al., 1991
Expanded polytetrafluoroethylene	Young et al., 1984
3. *Resorbable polymer channels*	
Polyglycolic acid	Molander et al., 1989
Poly-L-lactic acid	Nyilas et al., 1983
Collagen	Archibald et al., 1991
4. *Electrically charged polymer channels*	
Silicone channels with electrode cuffs	Kerns and Freeman, 1986; Kerns et al., 1991
Polyvinylidenefluoride (piezoelectric)	Aebischer et al., 1987
Polytetrofluoroethylene (electret)	Valentini et al., 1989
5. *Polymer channels releasing trophic factors*	
Ethylene vinylacetate copolymer	Aebischer et al., 1989
II. Intrachannel, luminal matrices	
1. Fibrin matrix	Williams et al., 1987
2. Collagen-glycosaminoglycan template	Yannas et al., 1985
3. Matrigel	Valentini et al., 1987
III. Cell seeded lumens for trophic support	
1. Schwann cell–seeded lumens (PNS)	Guénard et al., 1992
2. Schwann cell–seeded lumens (CNS)	Guénard et al., 1993; Kromer and Cornbrooks, 1985, 1987; Smith and Stevenson, 1988

The Active Use of Channel Properties

In the past, biocompatability of a biomaterial was evaluated by the degree of its passivity or lack of "reaction" when implanted into the body. However, the recognition that the response of the host tissue is related to the mechanical, chemical, and structural properties of the implanted biomaterial has lead to the design of materials that promote a beneficial response from the host. In the context of a synthetic nerve guidance channel, this may translate to manipulation of its microstructural properties, permeability, electrical properties, and the loading of its channel wall with neuroactive components that might then be released locally into the regenerating environment. The strategy here is to engineer a tailored response from the host and take advantage of the natural repair processes.

Surface Microgeometry

The morphology of regenerating peripheral nerves is modulated by the surface microgeometry of polymeric guidance channels [Aebischer et al., 1990]. Channels with smooth inner walls give rise to organized, longitudinal fibrin matrices, resulting in discrete free-floating nerve cables with numerous myelinated axons. The rough inner surface channels, however, give rise to an unorganized fibrin matrix with nerve fascicles scattered in a loose connective tissue filling the entire channel's lumen. Thus the physical textural properties and porosity of the channel can influence nervous tissue behavior and may be used to elicit a desirable reaction from the host tissue.

Molecular Weight Cutoff

The molecular weight cutoff of the NGCs influences peripheral nerve regeneration in rodent models [Aebischer et al., 1989]. The molecular weight cutoff may influence nerve regeneration possibly by controlling the exchange of molecules between the channel lumen and the external wound-healing environment. This may be important because the external environment consists of humoral factors that can play a role in augmenting regenerative processes in the absence of a distal stump.

Electrical Properties

In vivo regeneration following transection injury in the peripheral nervous system has been reported to be enhanced by galvanotropic currents produced in silicone channels fitted with electrode cuffs [Kerns & Freeman, 1986; Kerns et al., 1991]. Polytetrafluoroethylene (PTFE) "electret" tubes show more myelinated axons compared with uncharged tubes in peripheral nerves [Valentini et al., 1989]. Dynamically active piezoelectric polymer channels also have been shown to enhance nerve regeneration in the sciatic nerves of adult mice and rats [Aebischer et al., 1987; Fine et al., 1991].

Release of Bioactive Factors from the Channel Wall

Polymer guidance channels can be loaded with various factors to study and enhance nerve regeneration. Basic fibroblast growth factor released from an ethylene–vinyl acetate copolymer guidance channel facilitates peripheral nerve regeneration across long nerve gaps after a rat sciatic nerve lesion [Aebischer et al., 1989]. The possible influence of interleukin-1 (IL-1) on nerve regeneration also was studied by the release of IL-1 receptor antagonist (IL-1ra) from the wall of an EVA copolymer channel [Guénard et al., 1991]. It is conceivable that the release of appropriate neurotrophic factors from the channel wall may enhance specifically subsets of axons, e.g., ciliary neurotrophic factor on motor neurons and nerve growth factor on sensory neurons.

Resorbable Channel Wall

Bioresorbable nerve guidance channels are attractive because once regeneration is completed, the channel disappears without further surgical intervention. Mice sciatic nerves have been bridged with poly-L-lactic acid channels [Nyilas et al., 1983] and polyester guidance channels [Henry et al., 1985]. Rabbit tibial nerves also have been bridged with guidance channels fabricated from polyglycolic acid [Molander et al., 1989]. Resorbable guidance channels need to retain their mechanical integrity over 4 to 12 weeks. At the same time, their degradation products should not interfere with the regenerative processes of the nerve. These issues remain the challenging aspects in the development of bioresorbable nerve guidance channels for extensive use in animals and humans.

Intraluminal Matrices for Optimal Organization of Regeneration Microenvironment

The physical support structure of the regenerating environment may play an important role in determining the extent of regeneration. An oriented fibrin matrix placed in the lumen of silicone guidance channels accelerates the early phases of peripheral nerve regeneration [Williams et al., 1987].

Silicone channels filled with a collagen-glycosaminoglycan template bridged a 15-mm nerve gap in rats, whereas no regeneration was observed in unfilled tubes [Yannas et al., 1985]. However, even matrices known to promote neuritic sprouting in vitro may impede peripheral nerve regeneration in semipermeable guidance channels if the optimal physical conditions are not ensured [Madison et al., 1988; Valentini et al., 1987]. Therefore, the structural, chemical, and biologic aspects of the matrix design may all play a role in determining the fate of the regenerating nerve. The importance of the effect of the physical environment on regeneration, mediated by its influence on fibroblast and Schwann cell behavior, has been demonstrated in several studies and has been reviewed by Schwartz [1987] and Fawcett & Keynes [1990]. Thus the choice of a hydrogel with physical, chemical, and biologic cues conducive to nerve regeneration may enhance nerve regeneration. This strategy is currently being explored [Bellamkonda et al., in press]. Neurite-promoting oligopeptides from the basement membrane protein laminin (LN) were covalently coupled to agarose hydrogels. Agarose gels derivatized with LN oligopeptides specifically enhance neurite extension from cells that have receptors to the LN peptides in vitro [Bellamkonda et al., in press]. Preliminary results show that the presence of an agarose gel carrying the LN peptide CDPGYIGSR inside the lumen of a synthetic guidance channel enhances the regeneration of transected peripheral nerves (Fig. 118.3) in rats. Thus it is feasible to tailor the intraluminal matrices with more potent neurite-promoting molecules such as the cell adhesion molecules (CAMs) L1, N-CAM, or tenascin and "engineer" a desired response from the regenerating neural elements.

Cell-Seeded Lumens for Trophic Support

Cells secreting various growth factors may play an important role in organizing the regeneration environment, e.g., Schwann cells in the peripheral and central nervous system. It has been reported that regenerating axons do not elongate through acellular nerve grafts if Schwann cell migration was impeded [Hall et al., 1986]. Syngeneic Schwann cells derived from adult nerves and seeded in semi-permeable guidance channels enhance peripheral nerve regeneration [Guénard et al., 1992]. Schwann cells in the preceding study orient themselves along the axis of the guidance channel, besides secreting various neurotrophic factors. Schwann cells could play a role in organizing the fibrin cable formed during the initial phases of nerve regeneration. Schwann cells may be effective in inducing regeneration in the CNS, too [Kromer & Cornbrook, 1985, 1987; Smith & Stevenson, 1988]. The use of tailored intraluminal matrices and presenting exogeneic Schwann cells to the regeneration environment in a controlled matter are strategies aimed at engineering the desired tissue response by creating the optimal substrate, trophic, and cellular environments around the regenerating nerves.

CNS glial cells have a secretory capacity that can modulate neuronal function. Astrocytes release proteins that enhance neuronal survival and induce neuronal growth and differentiation. When a silicone channel was seeded with astrocytes of different ages, ranging from P9 to P69 (postnatal), it was observed that while P9 astrocytes did not interfere with peripheral nerve regeneration, adult astrocytes downregulate axonal growth [Kalderon, 1988]. However, the presence of Schwann cells

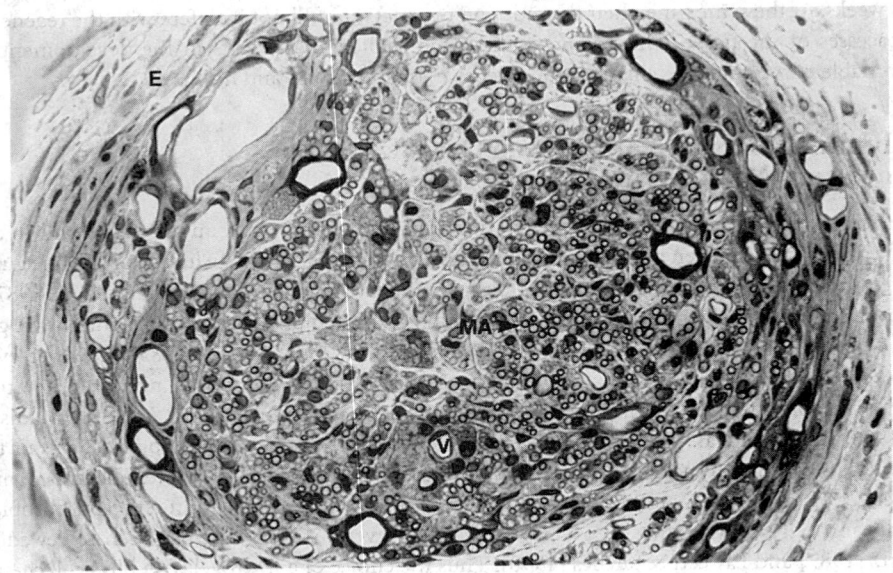

FIGURE 118.3   Light micrograph of a cross-sectional cut of a sural nerve regenerating through a polymer guidance channel 4 weeks after transection. The nerve guidance channel had been filled with a CDPGYIGSR derivatized agarose gel. *E* is the epineurium; *V* shows neovascularization; and *MA* is myelinated axon.

reverses the inhibition of PNS regeneration due to adult astrocytes [Guénard et al., 1994]. Thus the cellular environment in the site of injury may play an important role in determining the extent of regeneration. Knowledge of these factors also may be employed in designing optimal environments for nerve regeneration.

Polyethyleneglycol-Induced Axon Fusion

Rapid morphologic fusion of severed myelinated axons may be achieved by the application of poly-ethylene glycol (PEG) to the closely apposed ends of invertebrate-myelinated axons [Krause & Bittner, 1990]. Selection of appropriate PEG concentration and molecular mass, tight apposition, and careful alignment of the cut ends of the nerve may facilitate the direct fusion of axons. However, this technique is only applicable when the two ends of the severed nerve are closely apposed to each other, before the onset of wallerian degeneration.

CNS Nerve Regeneration

Most of the preceding studies have been conducted in the peripheral nervous system (PNS). In the CNS, however, endogenous components express poor support for axonal elongation. Significant regeneration may, however, occur with supporting substrates. Entubulation with a semipermeable acrylic copolymer tube allows bridging of a transected rabbit optic nerve with a cable containing myelinated axons [Aebischer et al., 1988]. Cholinergic nerve regeneration into basal lamina tubes containing Schwann cells has been reported in a transected septohippocampal model in rats [Kromer & Cornbrooks, 1985].

Thus the appropriate combination of physical guidance, matrices, and growth factors can create the right environmental cues and may be effective in inducing regeneration in the CNS. Therefore, both in the PNS and CNS, manipulation of the natural regenerative capacities of the host either by guidance factors or stimulation by electrical or trophic factors or structural components of the regenerating microenvironment can significantly enhance regeneration and help the reconstruction of severed or damaged neural tissue.

118.3 In Vitro Neural Circuits and Biosensors

The electrochemical and chemoelectrical transduction properties of neuronal cells can form the basis of a cell-based biosensing unit. The unique information-processing capabilities of neuronal cells through synaptic modulation may form the basis of designing simple neuronal circuits in vitro. Both the preceding applications necessitate controlled neuronal cell attachment, tightly coupled to the substrate, and a sensitive substrate to monitor changes in the cell's electrical activity.

The use of bioactive material systems tailored to control neuronal cell attachment on the surface and still amenable to the incorporation of electrical sensing elements like an field effect transistor (FET) could be one feasible design. Therefore, composite material systems, which might incorporate covalently patterned bioactive peptides on their surface to control cell attachment and neurite extension, may be a step toward the fulfillment of the preceding goal. Oligopeptides derived from larger extracellular proteins like laminin have been shown to mediate specific cell attachment via cell surface receptors [Graf et al., 1987; Iwamoto et al., 1987; Kleinman et al., 1988]. Cell culture on poly-meric membranes modified with the preceding bioactive peptidic components may give rise to a system where neuronal cell attachment and neuritic process outgrowth may be controlled. This control may help in designing microelectronic leads to complete the cell-electronic junction. Preliminary recordings from a FET-based neuron-silicon junction using leech Retzius cells [Fromherz et al., 1991] have been reported. Though there are many problems, such as attaining optimal coupling, this could form the basis of a "neural chip." A neural chip could potentially link neurons to external electronics for applications in neuronal cell–based biosensors, neural circuits, and limb prosthesis. Polymer surface modification and intelligent use of extracellular matrix components through selective binding could help attain this goal.

Studies in our laboratory have been trying to understand the underlying mechanisms involving protein adsorption onto polymeric substrates and their role in influencing and controlling nerve cell attachment [Ranieri et al., 1993]. Controlled neuronal cell attachment within a tolerance range of 20 μm may be achieved either nonspecifically via monoamine surfaces or specifically via oligopeptides derived from ECM proteins like laminin and fibronectin (Fig. 118.4), mediated by integrin cell surface receptors [Ranieri et al., in press]. Molecular control of neuronal cell attachment

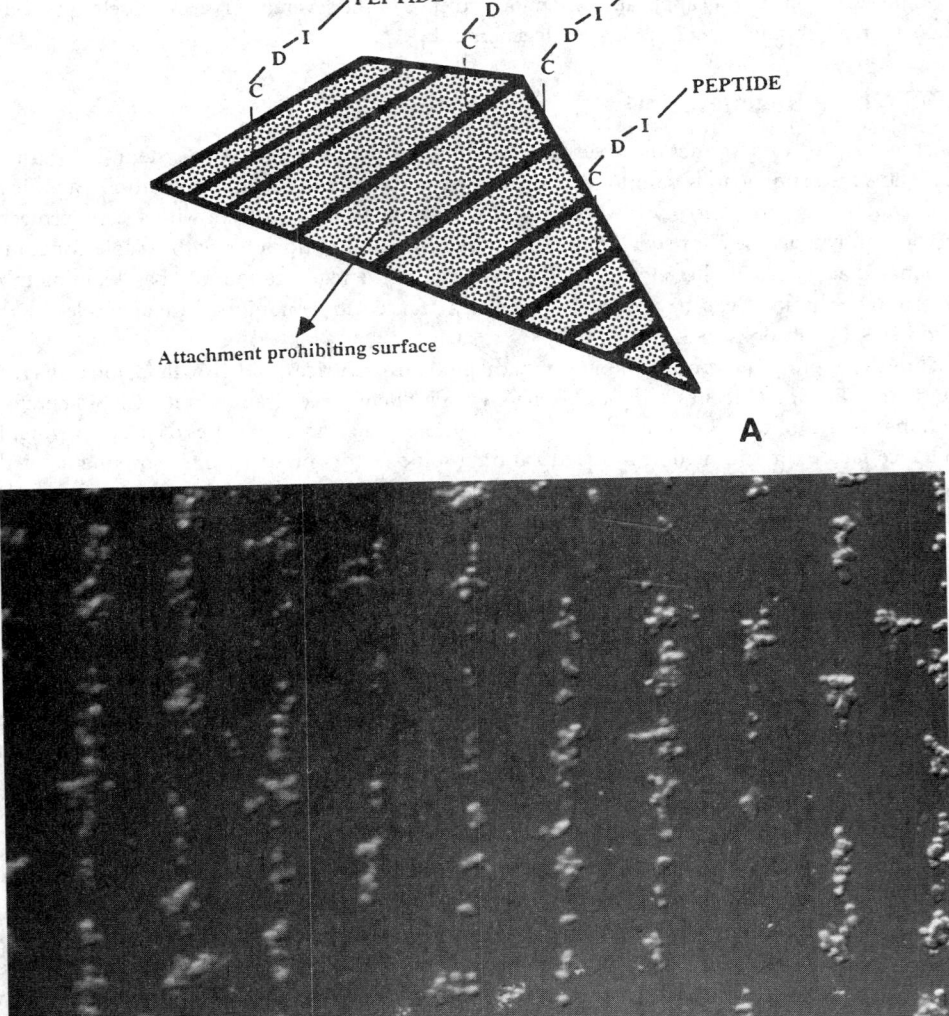

FIGURE 118.4 (*a*) Schematic of fluorinated ethylene propylene membrane modified in a "striped" fashion with bioactive oligopeptides using carbonyldiimidazole homobifunctional linking agent. (*b*) Light micrograph of Ng108-15 cells "striping" on FEP membrane surfaces selectively modified with CDP-GYIGSR oligopeptide.

and interfacing neuronal cells with electrodes may find applications in the design and fabrication of high-sensitivity neuron-based biosensors with applications in detection of low level neuro-transmitters.

Studies are also currently in progress involving polymeric hydrogels and controlling neuronal cell behavior in a three-dimensional (3D) tissue culture environs as a step toward building 3D neuronal tissues [Bellamkonda et al., in press]. The choice of an appropriate hydrogel chemistry and struc-ture, combined with the possibility of the gel serving as a carrier for ECM proteins or their peptidic analogues, can enable one to enhance regeneration when seeded in a nerve guidance channel. Also, the use of appropriate hydrogel chemistries in combination with the chemical modification of the polymer backbone by laser-directed photochemistry may be feasible in controlling the direction and differentiation of neuronal cells in three dimensions. Covalent binding of bioactive components like the laminin oligopeptides to the hydrogel backbone gives a specific character to the gel so that it elicits specific responses from anchorage-dependent neuronal cells [Bellamkonda et al., in press] (Fig. 118.5). Such a system could be useful in organizing nerves in 3D either for bridging different regions of the brain with nerve cables or for the 3D organization of nerves for optimal coupling with external electronics in the design of artificial limb prosthesis. In either case, development of such systems presents an interesting challenge for tissue engineering.

118.4 Conclusion

Advances in gene transfer techniques and molecular and cell biology offer potent tools in the functional replacement of various tissues of the nervous system. Each of these cells' functions can be optimized with the design and selection of its optimal extracellular environment. Substrates that support neuronal differentiation in two and three dimensions may play an important role in taking advantage of the advances in molecular and cell biology. Thus research aimed at tailoring extracel-

3-D Neuronal cell culture in bioactive hydrogels

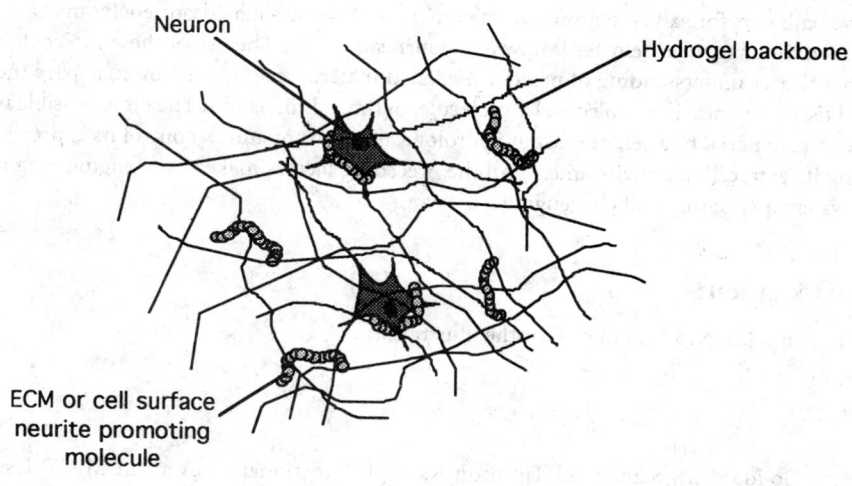

A

FIGURE 118.5 (*a*) Schematic of hydrogel derivatized with bioactive peptides with an anchorage-dependent neuron suspended in 3D. (*b*) Light micrograph of a E14 chick superior cervical ganglion suspended in 3D and extending neurites in an agarose gel derivatized with the laminin oligopeptide CDPGYIGSR.

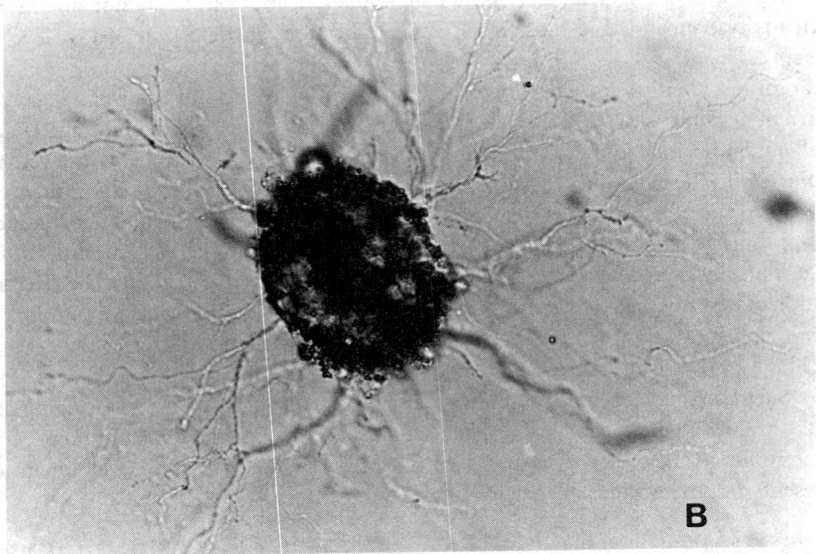

FIGURE 118.5   *(continued)*

lular matrices with the appropriate physical, chemical, and biologic cues may be important in optimizing the function of transplanted cells, inducing nerve regeneration, or in the construction of neuronal tissues in two and three dimensions in a controlled fashion. Controlled design and fabrication of polymer hydrogels and polymer scaffolds on a scale that is relevant for single cells also may be important. This would presumably control the degree and the molecular location of permissive, attractive, and repulsive regions of the substrate and in turn control cellular and tissue response both in vitro and in vivo.

Biologic molecules like laminin, collagen, fibronectin, and tenascin may provide attractive and permissive pathways for axons to grow. On the other hand, some sulfated proteoglycans have been shown to inhibit or repulse neurites [Snow & Letourneau, 1992]. The use of these molecules coupled with a clearer understanding of protein-mediated material-cell interaction may pave the way for neural tissue engineering, molecule by molecule, in three dimensions. Thus it is possible to tailor the genetic material of a cell to make it neurologically relevant and to control its expression by optimizing its extracellular environment. All the preceding factors make tissue engineering in the nervous system an exciting and challenging endeavor.

Acknowledgments

We wish to thank Mr. Nicolas Bouche for the illustrations.

References

Aebischer P, Goddard M, Signore A, Timpson R. 1994. Functional recovery in MPTP lesioned primates transplanted with polymer encapsulated PC12 cells. Exp Neurol 26:1.

Aebischer P, Buchser E, Joseph JN. 1994. Transplantation in humans of encapsulated xenogeneic cells without immunosuppression. Transplantation 58:1275.

Aebischer P, Guénard V, Brace S. 1989a. Peripheral nerve regeneration through blind-ended semipermeable guidance channels: effect of the molecular weight cutoff. J Neurosci 9:3590.

Aebischer P, Guénard V, Valentini RF. 1990. The morphology of regenerating peripheral nerves is modulated by the surface microgeometry of polymeric guidance channels. Brain Res 531:211.

Aebischer P, Salessiotis AN, Winn SR. 1989b. Basic fibroblast growth factor released from synthetic guidance channels facilitates peripheral nerve regeneration across long nerve gaps. J Neurosci Res 23:282.

Aebischer P, Tresco PA, Winn SR, et al. 1991a. Long-term cross-species brain transplantation of a polymer-encapsulated dopamine-secreting cell line. Exp Neurol 111:269.

Aebischer P, Tresco PA, Sagen J, Winn SR. 1991b. Transplantation of microencapsulated bovine chromaffin cells reduces lesion-induced rotational asymmetry in rats. Brain Res 560:43.

Aebischer P, Wahlberg L, Tresco PA, Winn SR. 1991c. Macroencapsulation of dopamine secreting cells by coextrusion with an organic polymer solution. Biomaterials 12:50.

Aebischer P, Winn SR, Galletti PM. 1988a. Transplantation of neural tissue in polymer capsules. Brain Res 448:364.

Aebischer P, Valentini RF, Dario P, et al. 1987. Piezoelectric guidance channels enhance regeneration in the mouse sciatic nerve after axotomy. Brain Res 436:165.

Aebischer P, Valentini RF, Winn SR, Galletti PM. 1988b. The use of a semipermeable tube as a guidance channel for a transected rabbit optic nerve. Brain Res 78:599.

Ahlgren FI, Ahlgren MB. 1987. Epidural administration of opiates by a new device. Pain 31:353.

Akil H, Watson SJ, Young E, et al. 1984. Endogenous opioids: biology and function. Annu Rev Neurosci 7:223.

Albani C, Asper R, Hacisalihzade SS, Baumgartner F. 1986. Individual levodopa therapy in Parkinson's disease. In Advances in Neurology: Parkinson's Disease, pp 497–501. New York, Raven Press.

Anderson RF, Alterman AL, Barde YA, Lindsay RM. 1990. Brain-derived neurotrophic factor increases survival and differentiation of septal cholinergic neurons in culture. Neuron 5:297.

Archibald SJ, Krarup C, Shefner J, et al. 1991. A collagen-based nerve guide conduit for peripheral nerve repair: an electrophysiological study of nerve regeneration in rodents and nonhuman primates. J Comp Neurol 306:685.

Becker JB, Robinson TE, Barton P, et al. 1990. Sustained behavioral recovery from unilateral nigrostriatal damage produced by the controlled release of dopamine from a silicone polymer pellet placed into the denervated striatum. Brain Res 508:60.

Bellamkonda R, Ranieri JP, Aebischer P. Laminin oligopeptide derivatized agarose gels allow three-dimensional neurite outgrowth in vitro. J Neurosci Res. In press.

Bellamkonda R, Ranieri JP, Bouche N, Aebischer P. In press. A hydrogel-based three-dimensional matrix for neural cells. J Biomed Nat Res. In press.

Birkmayer W. 1969. Experimentalle ergebnisse uber die kombinationsbehandlung des Parkinson-syndroms mit 1-dopa und einem decarboxylasehemmer. Wiener Klin Wochenschr 81:677.

Björklund A. 1991. Neural transplantation—An experimental tool with clinical possibilities. TINS 14:319.

Björklund A, Dunnett SB, Stenevi U, et al. 1980. Reinnervation of the denervated striatum by substantia nigra transplants: Functional consequences as revealed by pharmacological and sensorimotor testing. Brain Res 199:307.

Bolam JP, Freund TF, Björklund A, et al. 1987. Synaptic input and local output of dopaminergic neurons in grafts that functionally reinnervate the host neostriatum. Exp Brain Res 68:131.

Bunge RP, Bunge MB. 1983. Interrelationship between Schwann cell function and extracellular matrix production. TINS 6:499.

Chen LS, Ray J, Fisher LJ, et al. 1991. Cellular replacement therapy for neurologic disorders: potential of genetically engineered cells. J Cell Biochem 45:252.

De Yebenes JG, Fahn S, Jackson-Lewis V, et al. 1988. Continuous intracerebroventricular infusion of dopamine and dopamine agonists through a totally implanted drug delivery system in animal models of Parkinson's disease. J Neural Transplant 27:141.

During MJ, Freese A, Deutch AY, et al. 1992. Biochemical and behavioral recovery in a rodent model of Parkinson's disease following stereotactic implantation of dopamine-containing liposomes. Exp Neurol 115:193.

Ehringer H, Hornykiewicz O. 1960. Vetreilung von Noradrenalin und Dopamin (3-Hydroxytyramin) im Gehirn des menschen und ihr Verhalten bei Erkrankungen des extrapyramidalen systems. Klin Ther Wochenschr 38:1236.

Fawcett JW, Keynes RJ. 1990. Peripheral nerve regeneration. Annu Rev Neurosci 13:43.

Fine EG, Valentini RF, Bellamkonda R, Aebischer P. 1991. Improved nerve regeneration through piezoelectric vinylidenefluoride-trifluoroethylene copolymer guidance channels. Biomaterials 12:775.

Fromherz P, Offenhausser A, Vetter T, Weis J. 1991. A neuron-silicon junction: A Retzius cell of the leech on an insulated-gate field-effect transistor. Science 252:1290.

Gage FH, Kawaja MD, Fisher LJ. 1991. Genetically modified cells: Applications for intracerebral grafting. TINS 14:328.

Goosen MFA, Shea GM, Gharapetian HM, et al. 1985. Optimization of microencapsulation parameters: semipermeable microcapsules as a bioartificial pancreas. Biotech Bioeng 27:146.

Graf J, Ogle RC, Robey FA, et al. 1987. A pentapeptide from the laminin B1 chain mediates cell adhesion and binds the 67,000 laminin receptor. Biochemistry 26:6896.

Guénard V, Aebischer P, Bunge R. 1994. The astrocyte inhibition of peripheral nerve regeneration is reversed by Schwann cells. Exp Neurol 126:44.

Guénard V, Dinarello CA, Weston PJ, Aebischer P. 1991. Peripheral nerve regeneration is impeded by interleukin 1 receptor antagonist released from a polymeric guidance channel. J Neurosci Res 29:396.

Guénard V, Kleitman N, Morrissey TK, et al. 1992. Syngeneic Schwann cells derived from adult nerves seeded in semipermeable guidance channels enhance peripheral nerve regeneration. J Neurosci 2:3310.

Guénard V, Xu XM, Bunge MB. 1993. The use of Schwann cell transplantation to foster central nervous system repair. Semin Neurosci 5:401.

Hall SM. 1986. The effect of inhibiting Schwann cell mitosis on the re-innervation of acellular autografts in the peripheral nervous system of the mouse. Neuropathol Appl Neurobiol 12:27.

Hardie RJ, Lees AJ, Stern GM. 1984. On-off fluctuations in Parkinson's disease: A clinical and neuropharmacological study. Brain 107:487.

Hargraves R, Freed WJ. 1987. Chronic intrastriatal dopamine infusions in rats with unilateral lesions of the substantia nigra. Life Sci 40:959.

Hefti F, Dravid A, Hartikka J. 1984. Chronic intraventricular injections of nerve growth factor elevate hippocampal choline acetyltransferase activity in adult rats with partial septo-hippocampal lesions. Brain Res 293:305.

Henry EW, Chiu TH, Nyilas E, et al. 1985. Nerve regeneration through biodegradable polyester tubes. Exp Neurol 90:652.

Hoffman D, Breakefield XO, Short MP, Aebischer P. 1993. Transplantation of a polymer-encapsulated cell line genetically engineered to release NGF. Exp Neurol 122:100.

Hoffman D, Wahlberg L, Aebischer P. 1990. NGF released from a polymer matrix prevents loss of ChaT expression in basal forebrain neurons following a fimbria-fornix lesion. Exp Neurol 110:39.

Horellou P, Guibert B, Leviel V, Mallet J. 1989. Retroviral transfer of a human tyrosine hydroxylase cDNA in various cell lines: Regulated release of dopamine in mouse anterior pituitary AtT-20 cells. Proc Natl Acad Sci USA 86:7233.

Hughes RA, Sendtner M, Thoenen H. 1993. Members of several gene families influence survival of rat motoneurons in vitro and in vivo. J Neurosci Res 36:663.

Hyman C, Hofer M, Barde YA, et al. 1991. BDNF is a neurotrophic factor for dopaminergic neurons of the substantia nigra. Nature 350:230.

Iwamoto Y, Robey FA, Graf J, et al. 1987. YIGSR, a synthetic laminin pentapeptide, inhibits experimental metastasis formation. Science 238:1132.

Jiao S, Gurevich V, Wolff JA. 1993. Long-term correction of rat model of Parkinson's disease by gene therapy. Nature 362:450.

Joseph JM, Goddard MB, Mills J, et al. 1994. Transplantation of encapsulated bovine chromaffin cells in the sheep subarachnoid space: a preclinical study for the treatment of cancer pain. Cell Transplant 3:355.

Kalderon N. 1988. Differentiating astroglia in nervous tissue histogenesis regeneration: studies in a model system of regenerating peripheral nerve. J Neurosci Res 21:501.

Kerns JM, Fakhouri AJ, Weinrib HP, Freeman JA. 1991. Electrical stimulation of nerve regeneration in the rat: The early effects evaluated by a vibrating probe and electron microscopy. J Neurosci 40:93.

Kerns JM, Freeman JA. 1986. DC electrical fields promote regeneration in the rat sciatic nerve after axotomy. Soc Neurosci Abstr 12:13.

Kleinman H, Ogle RC, Cannon FB, et al. 1988. Laminin receptors for neurite formation. Proc Natl Acad Sci USA 85:1282.

Knüsel B, Winslow JW, Rosenthal A, et al. 1991. Promotion of central cholinergic and dopaminergic neuron differentiation by brain derived neurotrophic factor but not neurotrophin-3. Proc Natl Acad Sci USA 88:961.

Krause TL, Bittner GD. 1990. Rapid morphological fusion of severed myelinated axons by polyethylene glycol. Proc Natl Acad Sci USA 87:1471.

Kromer LF, Cornbrooks CJ. 1985. Transplants of Schwann cell culture cultures promote axonal regeneration in adult mammalian brain. Proc Natl Acad Sci USA 82:6330.

Kromer LF, Cornbrooks CJ. 1987. Identification of trophic factors and transplanted cellular environments that promote CNS axonal regeneration. Ann NY Acad Sci 495:207.

Langer R. 1981. Polymers for sustained release of macromolecules: Their use in a single-step method for immunization. In JJ Langone, J Van Vunakis (eds), Methods of Enzymology pp 57–75. San Diego, Academic Press.

Langer R, Folkman J. 1976. Polymers for sustained release of proteins and other macromolecules. Nature 263:797.

Lim F, Sun AM. 1980. Microencapsulated islets as bioartificial endocrine pancreas. Science 210:908.

Lin HL-F, Doherty DH, Lile JD, et al. 1993. GDNF: A glial derived neurotrophic factor for midbrain dopaminergic neurons. Science 260:1130.

Lindvall O. 1991. Prospects of transplantation in human neurodegenerative diseases. TINS 14:376.

Lindvall O, Brundin P, Widner H, et al. 1990. Grafts of fetal dopamine neurons survive and improve motor function in Parkinson's disease. Science 247:574.

Lundborg G, Dahlin LB, Danielsen N, et al. 1982. Nerve regeneration in silicone chambers: Influence of gap length and of distal stump components. Exp Neurol 76:361.

Madison RD, Da Silva CF, Dikkes P. 1988. Entubulation repair with protein additives increases the maximum nerve gap distance successfully bridged with tubular prosthesis. Brain Res 447:325.

McRae A, Hjorth S, Mason DW, et al. 1991. Microencapsulated dopamine (DA)–induced restitution of function in 6-OHDA denervated rat striatum in vivo: Comparison between two microsphere excipients. J Neural Transplant Plast 2:165.

Molander H, Olsson Y, Engkvist O, et al. 1989. Regeneration of peripheral nerve through a polygalactin tube. Muscle Nerve 5:54.

Morrissey TK, Kleitman N, Bunge RP. 1991. Isolation and functional characterization of Schwann cells derived from adult nerve. J Neurosci 11:2433.

Muenter MD, Sharpless NS, Tyce SM, Darley FL. 1977. Patterns of dystonia (I-D-I) and (D-I-D) in response to 1-dopa therapy for Parkinson's disease. Mayo Clin Proc 52:163.

Muir D, Gennrich C, Varon S, Manthorpe M. 1989. Rat sciatic nerve Schwann cell microcultures: Responses to mitogens and production of trophic and neurite-promoting factors. Neurochem Res 14:1003.

Nyilas E, Chiu TH, Sidman RL, et al. 1983. Peripheral nerve repair with bioresorbable prosthesis. Trans Am Soc Artif Intern Organs 29:307.

Olson L, Backlund EO, Ebendal T, et al. 1991. Intraputaminal infusion of nerve growth factor to support adrenal medullary autografts in Parkinson's disease: One year follow-up of first clinical trial. Arch Neurol 48:373.

Olson L, Nordberg A, Von-Holst H, et al. 1992. Nerve growth factor affects ^{11}C-nicotine binding, blood flow, EEG, and verbal episodic memory in an Alzheimer patient (case report). J Neural Transm Park Dis Dement Sect 4:79.

Oppenheim RW, Prevette D, Yin QW, et al. 1991. Control of embryonic motoneuron survival in vivo by ciliary neurotrophic factor. Science 251:1616.

Ranieri JP, Bellamkonda R, Bekos E, et al. 1994. Spatial control of neural cell attachment via patterned laminin oligopeptide chemistries. Int J Dev Neurosci 12: 725.

Ranieri JP, Bellamkonda R, Jacob J, et al. 1993. Selective neuronal cell attachment to a covalently patterned monoamine on fluorinated ethylene propylene films. J Biomed Mater Res 27:917.

Reynolds BA, Tetzlaff W, Weiss S. 1992. A multipotent EGF-responsive striatal embryonic progenitor cell produces neurons and astrocytes. J Neurosci 12:4565.

Sabel BA, Dominiak P, Hauser W, et al. 1990. Levodopa delivery from controlled release polymer matrix: Delivery of more than 600 days in vitro and 225 days elevated plasma levels after subcutaneous implantation in rats. J Pharmacol Exp Ther 255:914.

Sagen J, Pappas GD, Winnie AP. 1993a. Alleviation of pain in cancer patients by adrenal medullary transplants in the spinal subarachnoid space. Cell Transplant 2:259.

Sagen J, Wang H, Tresco PA, Aebischer P. 1993b. Transplants of immunologically isolated xenogeneic chromaffin cells provide a long-term source of pain-reducing neuroactive substances. J Neurosci 13:2415.

Scaravalli F. 1984. Regeneration of perineurium across a surgically induced gap in a nerve encased in a plastic tube. J Anat 139:411.

Schwartz M. 1987. Molecular and cellular aspects of nerve regeneration. CRC Crit Rev Biochem 22:89.

Sendtner M, Kreutzberg GW, Thoenen H. 1990. Ciliary neurotrophic factor prevents the degeneration of motor neurons after axotomy. Nature 345:440.

Shoulson I, Claubiger GA, Chase TN. 1975. On-off response. Neurology 25:144.

Smith GV, Stevenson JA. 1988. Peripheral nerve grafts lacking viable Schwann cells fail to support central nervous system axonal regeneration. Exp Brain Res 69:299.

Snow DM, Letourneau PC. 1992. Neurite outgrowth on a step gradient of chondroitin sulfate proteoglycan (CS-PG). J Neurobiol 23:322.

Tresco PA, Winn SR, Aebischer P. 1992. Polymer encapsulated neurotransmitter secreting cells: Potential treatment for Parkinson's disease. ASAIO J 38:17.

Uzman BG, Villegas GM. 1983. Mouse sciatic nerve regeneration through semipermeable tubes: A quantitative model. J Neurosci Res 9:325.

Valentini RF, Aebischer P, Winn SR, Galletti PM. 1987. Collagen- and laminin-containing gels impede peripheral nerve regeneration through semipermeable nerve guidance channels. Exp Neurol 98:350.

Valentini RF, Sabatini AM, Dario P, Aebischer P. 1989. Polymer electret guidance channels enhance peripheral nerve regeneration in mice. Brain Res 48:300.

Vescovi AL, Reynolds BA, Fraser DD, Weiss S. 1993. bFGF regulates the proliferative fate of unipotent (neuronal) and bipotent (neuronal/astroglial) EGF-generated CNS progenitor cells. Neuron 11:951.

Wictorin K, Brundin P, Sauer H, et al. 1992. Long distance directed axonal growth from human dopaminergic mesencephalic neuroblasts implanted along the nigrostriatal pathway in 6-hydroxydopamine lesioned rats. J Comp Neurol 323:475.

Williams LR, Danielsen N, Muller H, Varon S. 1987. Exogenous matrix precursors promote functional nerve regeneration across a 15-mm gap within a silicone chamber in the rat. J Comp Neurol 264:284.

Williams LR, Varon S, Peterson GM, et al. 1986. Continuous infusion of nerve growth factor prevents basal forebrain neuronal death after fimbria-fornix transection. Proc Natl Acad Sci USA 83:9231.

Winn SR, Tresco PA, Zielinski B, et al. 1991. Behavioral recovery following intrastriatal implantation of microencapsulated PC12 cells. Exp Neurol 113:322.

Winn SR, Wahlberg L, Tresco PA, Aebischer P. 1989. An encapsulated dopamine-releasing polymer alleviates experimental parkinsonism in rats. Exp Neurol 105:244.

Yaffe D, Saxel O. 1977. Serial passaging and differentiation of myogenic cells isolated from dystrophic mouse muscle. Nature 270:725.

Yan Q, Elliott J, Snider WD. 1992. Brain-derived neurotrophic factor rescues spinal motor neurons from axotomy-induced cell death. Nature 360:753.

Yannas EV, Orgill DP, Silver J, et al. 1985. Polymeric template facilitates regeneration of sciatic nerve across 15 mm gap. Trans Soc Biomater 11:146.

Young BL, Begovac P, Stuart D, Glasgow GE. 1984. An effective sleeving technique for nerve repair. J Neurosci Methods 10:51.

Zielinski B, Aebischer P. 1994. Encapsulation of mammalian cells in chitosan-based microcapsules: effect of cell anchorage dependence. Biomaterials.

Zurn AD, Baetge EE, Hammang JP, et al. 1994. Glial cell line-derived neurotrophic factor (GDNF): A new neurotrophic factor for motoneurones. Neuroreport 6:113.

119

Tissue Engineering
of Skeletal Muscle

Susan V. Brooks
University of Michigan

Neil M. Cole
University of Michigan

John A. Faulkner
University of Michigan

Contractions of skeletal muscles generate the stability and power for all movement. Consequently, any impairment in skeletal muscle function results in at least some degree of instability or immobility. Muscle function can be impaired as a result of injury, disease, or old age. The goal of tissue engineering is to restore the structural and functional properties of muscles to permit the greatest recovery of normal movement. Impaired movement at all ages, but particularly in the elderly, increases the risk of severe injury, reduces participation in the activities of daily living, and impacts on the quality of life.

Contraction is defined as the activation of muscle fibers with a tendency of the fibers to shorten. Contraction occurs when an increase in the cytosolic calcium concentration triggers a series of molecular events that includes the binding of calcium to the muscle regulatory proteins, the formation of strong interactions between the myosin cross-bridges and the actin filaments, and the generation of the cross-bridge driving stroke. In vivo, muscles perform three types of contractions depending on the interaction between the magnitude of the force developed by the muscle and the external load placed on the muscle. When the force developed by the muscle is greater than the load on the muscle, the fibers shorten during the contraction. When the force developed by the muscle is equal to the load, or if the load is immovable, the overall length of the muscle remains the same. If the force developed by the muscle is less than the load placed on the muscle, the muscle is stretched during the contraction. The types of contractions are termed *miometric, isometric,* and *pliometric,* respectively. Most normal body movements require varying proportions of each type of contraction.

119.1 Skeletal Muscle Structure

Each of the some 660 skeletal muscles in the human body is composed of hundreds to hundreds of thousands of single muscle fibers (Fig. 119.1). The plasma membrane of a muscle fiber is termed the *sarcolemma.* Contractile, structural, metabolic, regulatory, and cytosolic proteins, as well as many myonuclei and other cytosolic organelles are contained within the sarcolemma of each fiber

0-8493-8346-3/95/$0.00+$.50
© 1995 by CRC Press, Inc.

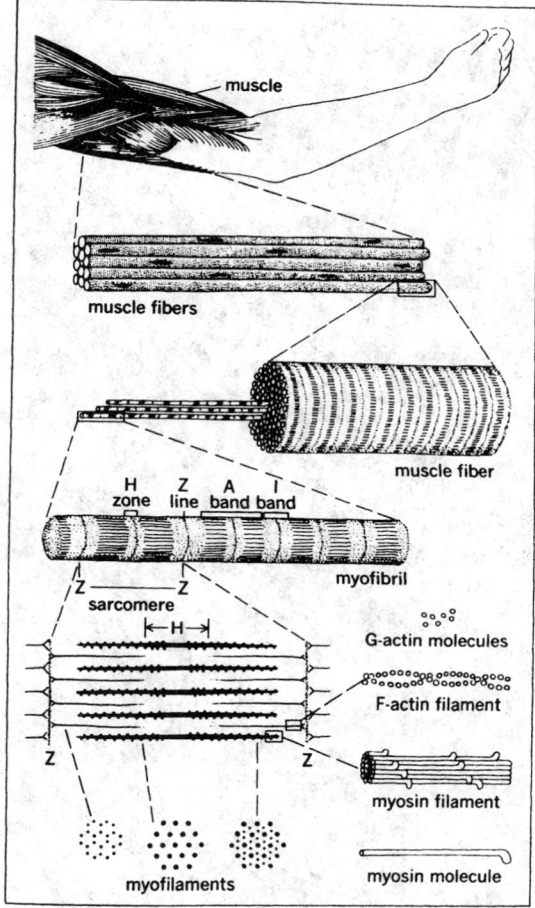

FIGURE 119.1   Levels of anatomical organization within a skeletal muscle. *Source:* Bloom W, Fawcett DW. 1968. A Textbook of Histology, 9th ed., Philadelphia, Saunders. With permission.

(Fig. 119.2). The contractile proteins myosin and actin are incorporated into thick and thin myofilaments, respectively, which are arrayed in longitudinally repeated banding patterns termed *sarcomeres* (Fig. 119.1). Sarcomeres in series form myofibrils, and many parallel myofibrils exist within each fiber. The number of myofibrils arranged in parallel determines the cross-sectional area (CSA) of single fibers and, consequently, the force-generating capability of the fiber. During a contraction, the change in the length of a sarcomere occurs as thick and thin filaments slide past each other, but the overall length of each actin and myosin filament does not change. An additional membrane, referred to as the *basement membrane* or the *basal lamina,* surrounds the sarcolemma of each fiber (Fig. 119.2).

In mammals, the number of fibers in a given muscle is determined at birth and changes little throughout the life span except in cases of injury or disease. In contrast, the number of myofibrils can change dramatically, increasing with normal growth or hypertrophy induced by strength training and decreasing with atrophy associated with immobilization, inactivity, injury, disease, or old age. A single muscle fiber is innervated by a single branch of a motor nerve. A motor unit is composed of a single motor nerve, its branches, and the muscle fibers innervated by the branches.

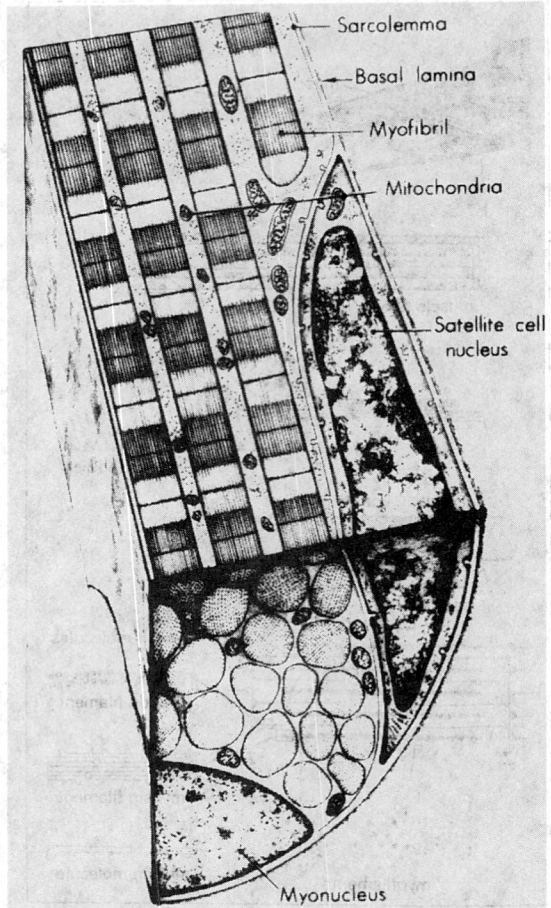

FIGURE 119.2 Drawing of a muscle fiber-satellite cell complex. Note that the satellite cell is located between the muscle fiber sarcolemma and the basal lamina. *Source:* Carlson BM, Faulkner JA. 1983. Med Sci Sports Exer 15:187. With permission.

The motor unit is the smallest group of fibers within a muscle that can be activated volitionally. Activation of a motor unit occurs when action potentials emanating from the motor cortex depolarize the cell bodies of motor nerves. The depolarization generates an action potential in the motor nerve that is transmitted to each muscle fiber in the motor unit, and each of the fibers contracts more or less simultaneously. Motor units range from small slow units to large fast units dependent on the CSA of the motor nerve.

119.2 Skeletal Muscle Function

Skeletal muscles may contract singly or in groups, working synergistically. On either side of limbs, muscles contract against one another or antagonistically. The force or power developed during a contraction depends on the frequency of stimulation of the motor units, the total number of motor units, and the size of the motor units recruited. The frequency of stimulation, particularly for the generation of power, is normally on the shoulder of the frequency-power relationship. Consequently, the total number of motor units recruited is the major determinant of the force or power developed.

Motor units are classified into three general categories based on their functional properties [Burke et al., 1973]. Slow (S) units have the smallest single muscle fiber CSAs, the fewest muscle fibers per motor unit, and the lowest velocity of shortening. The cell bodies of the S units are the most easily depolarized to threshold [Henneman et al., 1965]. Consequently, S units are the most frequently recruited during tasks that require low force or power but highly precise movements. Fast-fatigable (FF) units are composed of the largest fibers, have the most fibers per unit, and have the highest velocities of shortening. The FF units are the last to be recruited and are recruited for high-force and power movements. The fast-fatigue-resistant (FR) units are intermediate in terms of the CSAs of their fibers, the number of fibers per motor unit, the velocity of shortening, and the frequency of recruitment. The force normalized per unit CSA is ~280 kN/m^2 for each type of fiber, but the maximum normalized power (W/kg) developed by FF units is as much as four-fold greater than that of the S units due to a four-fold higher velocity of shortening for FF units. Motor units may also be identified by histochemical techniques as Type I (S), IIA (FR), and IIB (FF). Classifications based on histochemical and functional characteristics are usually in good agreement with one another, but differences do exist, particularly following experimental interventions. Consequently, in a given experiment, the validity of this interpretation should be verified.

119.3 Injury and Repair of Skeletal Muscle

Injury to skeletal muscles may occur as a result of disease, such as dystrophy; exposure to myotoxic agents, such as Marcaine or lidocaine; sharp or blunt trauma, such as punctures or contusions; ischemia, such as that which occurs with transplantation; exposure to excessively hot or cold temperatures; and contractions of the muscles. Pliometric contractions are much more likely to injure muscle fibers than are isometric or miometric contractions [McCully & Faulkner, 1985]. Regardless of the factors responsible, the manner in which the injuries are manifested appears to be the same, varying only in severity. In addition, the processes of fiber repair and regeneration appear to follow a common pathway regardless of the nature of the injurious event [Carlson & Faulkner, 1983].

Injury of Skeletal Muscle

The injury may involve either some of or all the fibers within a muscle [McCully & Faulkner, 1985]. In an individual fiber, focal injuries, localized to a few sarcomeres in series or in parallel (Fig. 119.3), as well as more widespread injuries, spreading across the entire cross-section of the fiber, are observed using electron microscopic techniques [Newham et al., 1983b]. Although the data are highly variable, many injuries also give rise to increases in serum levels of muscle enzymes, particularly creatine kinase, leading to the conclusion that sarcolemmal integrity is impaired [McNeil & Khakee, 1992; Newham et al., 1983a]. This conclusion is further supported by an influx of circulating proteins, such as serum albumin [McNeil & Khakee, 1992], and of calcium [Jones et al., 1984]. An increase in intracellular calcium concentration may activate a variety of proteolytic enzymes leading to further degradation of sarcoplasmic proteins.

In cases when the damage involves a large proportion of the sarcomeres within a fiber, the fiber becomes necrotic. If blood flow is impaired, fibers remain as a necrotic mass of noncontractile tissue [Carlson & Faulkner, 1983]. In contrast, in the presence of an adequate blood supply, the injured fibers are infiltrated by monocytes and macrophages [McCully & Faulkner, 1985]. The phagocytic cells remove the disrupted myofilaments, other cytosolic structures, and the damaged sarcolemma (Fig. 119.4). The most severe injuries result in the complete degeneration of the muscle fiber, leaving only the empty basal lamina. The basal lamina appears to be highly resistant to any type of injury and generally remains intact [Carlson & Faulkner, 1983].

An additional indirect measure of injury is the subjective report by human beings of delayed-onset muscle soreness, common following intense or novel exercise [Newham et al., 1983a]. Because of the focal nature of the morphological damage, the variability of serum enzyme levels and the subjectivity of reports of soreness, the most quantitative and reproducible measure of the totality of a

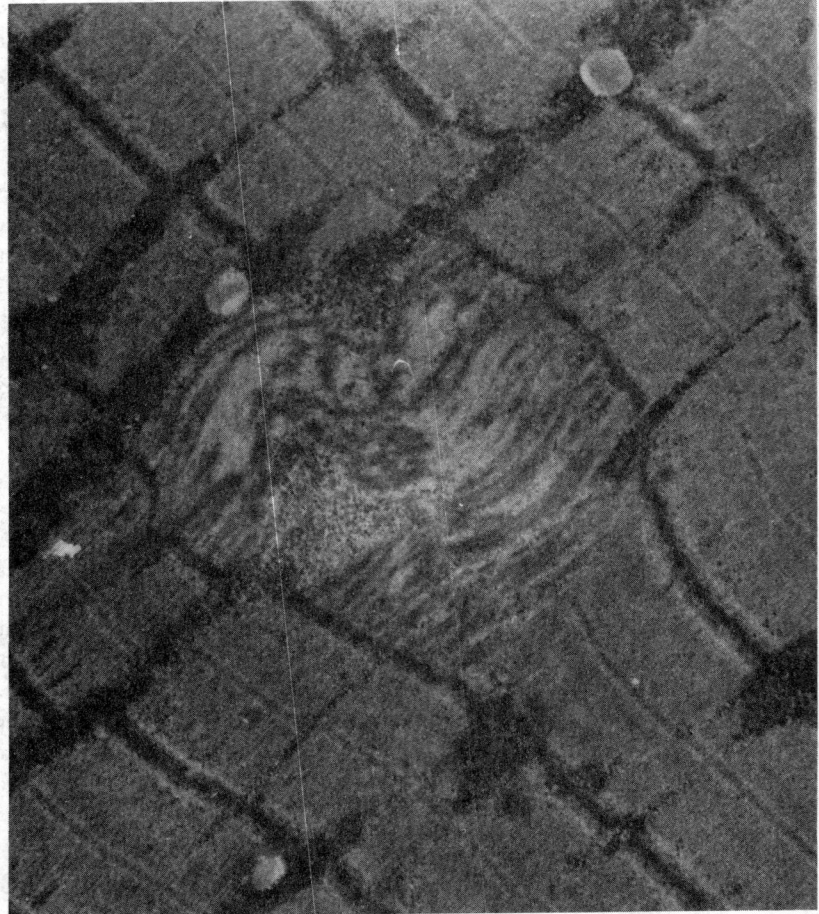

FIGURE 119.3   Focal area of disruption immediately after pliometric contractions affecting two adjacent myofibrils. The myofilaments are disorganized, and there is displacement of the Z-lines. Original magnification ×19,000. *Source:* Newham DJ, McPhail G, Mills KR, et al. 1983. J Neurol Sci 61:109. With permission.

muscle injury is the decrease in the ability of the muscle to develop force [McCully & Faulkner, 1985; Newham et al., 1983*a*, 1983*b*].

Repair of Injured Skeletal Muscles

Under circumstances when the injury involves only minor disruptions of the thick or thin filaments of single sarcomeres, the damaged molecules are likely replaced by newly synthesized molecules available in the cytoplasmic pool [Russell et al., 1992]. In addition, contraction-induced disruptions of the sarcolemma are often transient and repair spontaneously, allowing survival of the fiber [McNeil & Khakee, 1992]. Following more severe injuries, complete regeneration of the entire muscle fiber will occur.

Satellite Cell Activation

A key element in the initiation of muscle fiber regeneration following a wide variety of injuries is the activation of satellite cells [Carlson & Faulkner, 1983]. Satellite cells are quiescent myogenic stem

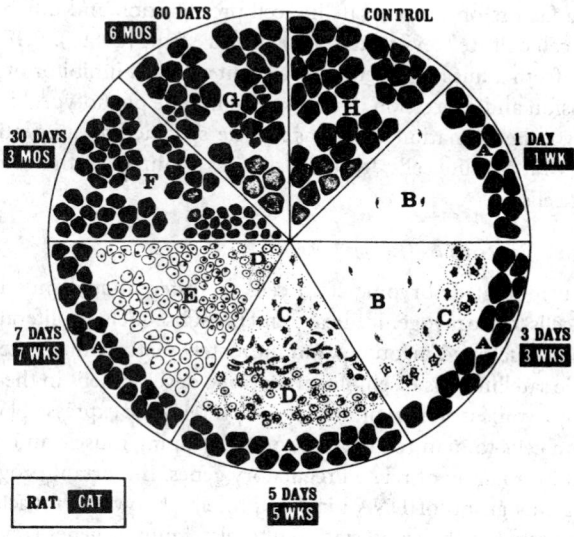

FIGURE 119.4 Schematic representation of the cellular responses during the processes of degeneration and regeneration following transplantation of extensor digitorum longus muscles in rats and cats. The diagram is divided into segments that represent the histological appearance of the muscle cross-section at various times after transplantation. The times given in days refer to rat muscles and those given in weeks refer to the larger cat muscles. The letters indicate groups of muscle fibers with similar histological appearances. (*a*): surviving fibers, (*b*): fibers in a state of ischemic necrosis, (*c*): fibers invaded by phagocytic cells, (*d*): myoblasts and early myotubes, (*e*): early myofibers, (*f*): immature regenerating fibers, (*g*): mature regenerated fibers, (*h*): normal control muscle fibers [Carlson & Faulkner, 1983]. *Source:* Mauro A. 1979. Muscle Regeneration, pp 493–507, New York, Raven Press. With permission.

cells located between the basal lamina and the sarcolemma (Fig. 119.2). Upon activation, satellite cells divide mitotically to give rise to myoblasts. The myoblasts can then fuse with existing muscle fibers, acting as a source of new myonuclei. This is the process by which a muscle fiber increases the total number of myonuclei in fibers that are increasing in size [Moss & Leblond, 1971] and may be necessary to repair local injuries. Alternatively, the myoblasts can fuse with each other to form multinucleated myotubes inside the remaining basal lamina of the degenerated fibers [Carlson & Faulkner, 1983]. The myotubes then begin to produce muscle specific proteins and ultimately differentiate completely into adult fast- or slow-muscle fibers [Carlson & Faulkner, 1983].

The factors that activate muscle satellite cells following injury are not well understood. Following a closed contusion injury, mitotic activation of satellite cells has been observed within the first day after the injury and is correlated in time with the appearance of phagocytes and newly formed capillaries [Hurme & Kalimo, 1992]. Similarly, DNA synthesis by the satellite cells is observed within the first day following crush injuries [Bischoff, 1986] and exercise-induced injuries [Darr & Schultz, 1987] in rats. These observations have led to speculations that satellite cells are activated by factors either synthesized and secreted by the macrophages [Hurme & Kalimo, 1992] or endogenous to the injured tissue itself [Bischoff, 1986]. Candidates for these factors include fibroblast growth factor (FGF), the insulinlike growth factors (IGFs), and transforming growth factor beta (TGF-β).

The effects of these factors on muscle satellite cell proliferation and differentiation have been studied extensively in cell culture (reviewed in Florini and Magri [1989]). FGF is a powerful mitogen for myogenic cells from adult rat skeletal muscle, but a potent inhibitor of terminal differentiation, i.e., myoblast fusion and expression of the skeletal muscle phenotype. Similarly, the presence of TGF-β prevents myotube formation as well as muscle-specific protein synthesis by rat embryo myoblasts and by adult rat satellite cells. In contrast, IGFs stimulate both proliferation and differentiation of myogenic cells.

Myogenic Regulatory Factors

The conversion of pluripotent embryonic stem cells to differentiated muscle cells involves the commitment of these cells to the myogenic lineage and the subsequent proliferation, differentiation, and fusion to form multinucleated myotubes and ultimately mature muscle cells. New muscle cell formation from muscle satellite cells resembles embryonic development in the sense that in regenerating muscle cells embryonic isoforms of the muscle proteins are expressed [Whalen et al., 1985]. The conversion of stem cells to mature fibers in both developing muscle and regenerating muscle appears to be directed by a family of related regulatory genes. Important progress has been made recently in identifying this group of DNA-binding proteins known as muscle regulatory factors (MRFs) that interact to regulate the transcription of skeletal muscle genes (reviewed in Weintraub and coworkers [1991]).

The existence of myogenic regulatory genes was first demonstrated directly when a cDNA, referred to as MyoD1, was isolated and shown to induce muscle-specific genes when transfected in fibroblasts. Subsequently, three other related genes were identified, including myogenin, MRF4 (also called herculin or Myf-6), and Myf-5 [Weintraub et al., 1991]. Since each of these factors has the ability to independently convert fibroblasts to stable myogenic cells, the original conclusion was that the functions of these MRFs were largely redundant. Currently, the totality of the evidence supports each MRF playing a separate and distinct role in myogenesis.

The patterns of expression of these regulatory factors have been studied in cell cultures of various embryonic myoblasts and satellite cells derived from muscles of newborn and adult animals, as well as in fetal, postnatal, and adult limb muscles [Hinterberger et al., 1991; Smith et al., 1993, 1994]. The four MRFs appear to be expressed in vitro with similar sequential patterns for late embryonic, fetal, and newborn myogenic cells, as well as in adult rat satellite cells. MyoD1 is clearly the first member of this family to be expressed in these myogenic cell types [Smith et al., 1993, 1994]. MyoD1 appears to be followed by myogenin and Myf-5 in embryonic and fetal myogenic cells, whereas myogenin lags Myf-5 by ~24 hours in satellite cell cultures [Smith et al., 1993, 1994]. The muscle regulatory factor MRF4 accumulates slowly, and its expression is maintained in the adult muscle, whereas expression of MyoD1, myogenin, and Myf-5 declines to low levels in adult muscle fibers [Hinterberger et al., 1991]. In addition to the characterization of MRF expression in vitro, investigators have recently turned to studies of the expression of MRFs in satellite cells and reexpression in mature muscle myonuclei in vivo.

In spite of the extensive study of this family of proteins, their specific roles in normal myogenesis during development or regeneration are not well defined. The family of MRFs is likely to also be regulated by as yet unidentified factors [Russell et al., 1992a]. The complex interactions between growth factors and MRFs that provide both positive and negative control of satellite cell proliferation, myotube formation, and muscle cell differentiation are topics of current research [Florini et al., 1991; Hardy et al., 1993].

119.4 Reconstructive Surgery of Whole Skeletal Muscles

When an injury or impairment is so severe that the total replacement of the muscle is required, a whole donor muscle must be transposed or transplanted into the recipient site [Faulkner et al., 1994]. One of the most versatile muscles for transpositions is the latissimus dorsi (LTD) muscle. LTD transfers have been used to restore elbow flexion, replace the pectoralis major in breast reconstruction [Moelleken et al., 1989], and function as a heart assist pump [Carpentier & Chachques, 1985]. Thompson [1974] popularized the use of small free standard grafts to treat patients with partial facial paralysis. The transplantation of large skeletal muscles in dogs with immediate restoration of blood flow through the anastomosis of the artery and vein provided an operative technique with numerous applications [Tamai et al., 1970]. Coupled with cross-face nerve grafts, large skeletal muscles are transplanted with microneurovascular repair to correct deficits in the face [Harii et al., 1976] and adapted for reconstructive operations to treat impairments in function of the limbs, anal and urinary sphincters, and even the heart [Freilinger & Deutinger, 1992].

Transposition and transplantation of muscles invariably results in structural and functional deficits [Guelinckx et al., 1992]. The deficits are of the greatest magnitude during the first month and then a gradual recovery results in the stabilization of structural and functional variables between 90–120 days [Guelinckx et al., 1992]. In stabilized vascularized grafts ranging from 1–3 grams in rats to 90 grams in dogs, the major deficits are a ∼30% decrease in muscle mass and in most grafts a ∼40% decrease in maximum force [Faulkner et al., 1994a]. The decrease in power is more complex, since it depends on both the average shortening force and the velocity of shortening. As a consequence, the deficit in maximum power may be either greater or less than the deficit in maximum force [Kadhiresan et al., 1993]. Tenotomy and repair are major factors responsible for the deficits [Guelinckx et al., 1988]. When a muscle is transplanted to act synergistically with other muscles, the action of the synergistic muscles may contribute to the deficits observed [Miller et al., 1994]. Although the data are limited, skeletal muscle grafts appear to respond to training stimuli in a manner not different from that of control muscles [Faulkner et al., 1994a]. The training stimuli include traditional methods of endurance and strength training [Faulkner et al., 1994b], as well as chronic electrical stimulation [Pette & Vrbova, 1992]. In spite of the deficits, transposed and transplanted muscles develop sufficient force and power to function effectively to maintain posture and patent sphincters and to move limbs or drive assist devices in parallel or in series with the heart [Faulkner et al., 1994a].

119.5 Myoblast Transfer and Gene Therapy

Myoblast transfer and gene therapy are highly pursued forms of tissue engineering aimed at delivering viable genetic constructs to diseased cells. Myoblast transfer is a cell-mediated technique designed to treat inherited myopathies by intramuscular injection of myoblasts containing a normal functional genome. The ultimate goal is to correct for a defective or missing gene in the myopathic tissue through the fusion of normal myoblasts with growing or regenerating diseased cells. Gene therapy presents a more complex and flexible approach, whereby genetically engineered DNA constructs are delivered to a host cell to specifically direct production of a desired protein. By reengineering the coding sequence of both the gene and its regulatory regions, the function, quantity of expression, and the protein itself can be altered. For many years cells have been genetically altered to induce the production of a variety of useful proteins, such as human growth hormone and interferon. Theoretically, by manipulating the genetic "blueprint" of a cell in a specific and rational manner, one can explore the role and importance of proteins naturally synthesized within the cell. Furthermore, spontaneous mutations that eliminate or alter the expression of cellular proteins necessary for normal cell function may be corrected through genetic engineering. The implications of myoblast and gene therapy hold great promise for skeletal muscle research and those afflicted with inherited myopathies such as Duchenne and Becker muscular dystrophy (DMD and BMD).

As a focus in skeletal muscle tissue engineering, DMD is the most common severe childhood degenerative disease of skeletal muscle affecting approximately 1 in 3500 males. Patients affected by DMD first exhibit clinical manifestations of muscle weakness at 3–6 years of age. A progressive wasting of viable muscle tissue leaves those afflicted severely weakened and wheelchair-bound by 10–12 years of age. Premature death occurs primarily due to respiratory failure usually in the second or third decade of life [Emery, 1988]. In BMD, an allelic form of DMD, the myopathy is less severe, ranging from very mild to very debilitating phenotypic expressions. An X-linked genetic deficiency in the coding of the large, 427 kDalton protein dystrophin has been implicated as the primary cause of both DMD and BMD. The genetic defect leads to the absence or marked deficiency in the expression or functional stability of dystrophin [Hoffman et al., 1988]. Dystrophin is associated with the sarcolemmal membrane and is believed to have a structural function, but its specific role is unknown [Bonilla et al., 1988; Tidball & Law, 1991].

Animal models have played an important role in the study of dystrophic muscle diseases. The discovery of the X-linked murine muscular dystrophy in the *mdx* mouse [Bulfield et al., 1984] has placed the mouse model at the forefront in studies leading toward the elucidation of the biochemical and mechanical processes involved in the progressive wasting of dystrophic muscle tissue. The *mdx* mouse has a homologous genetic defect to human DMD. A nonsense mutation in the gene leads to the complete absence of the protein dystrophin in muscle and brain tissues of the mouse [Hoffman et al., 1987; Sicinski et al., 1989]. Unlike DMD patients, the *mdx* mouse displays a minimal pathology in limb skeletal muscle [Dangain & Vrbova, 1984]. Nonetheless, a number of phenotypic abnormalities have been documented in the mouse. The *mdx* mouse exhibits elevated levels of serum creatine kinase, massive degeneration and regeneration of skeletal muscle fibers between 2–4 weeks of age with the persistence of centrally located nuclei and muscle necrosis in many fibers, progressive wasting of the diaphragm muscle, absence of the dystrophin associated proteins, and depressed levels of skeletal muscle specific force [Cox et al., 1993; Dangain & Vrbova, 1984; Ohlendieck & Campbell, 1991].

The *mdx* mouse provides an accurate model of dystrophin deficiency to explore the processes of the dystrophic disease and test proposed therapies or cures. The focus of treatment of myopathies such as DMD and BMD is to replace the missing or defective protein dystrophin. Two potential approaches of treatment of the myopathy are myoblast transfer and gene therapy.

Myoblast Transfer Therapy

The concept of myoblast transfer is based on the role satellite cells play in muscle fiber growth and repair [Carlson & Faulkner, 1983]. As a therapy for DMD, the idea is to obtain satellite cells from a healthy compatible donor, containing a completely functional dystrophin gene, have the cells multiply in culture, and then inject them into the muscles of the patient. The objective is for the implanted precursors to fuse with growing or regenerating muscle fibers to form a mosaic fiber in which the cytoplasm will contain normal myoblast nuclei capable of producing a functional form of dystrophin.

Experiments involving *mdx* mice and DMD patients have had varying success. Implantation of healthy myoblasts into muscles of *mdx* mice led to the production of the protein dystrophin in considerable quantities [Morgan et al., 1990; Partridge et al., 1989]. The successful transfer and fusion of donor myoblasts were greatly enhanced by X-ray irradiation of *mdx* muscles prior to myoblast injection to prevent the proliferation of myoblasts endogenous to the host and encourage the growth of donor myoblasts [Morgan et al., 1990]. In contrast to these studies with mice, delivery of myoblasts to DMD patients has shown very limited success characterized by very low levels of fusion efficiency and immune rejection [Gussoni et al., 1992; Morgan, 1994]. Unfortunately, the use of X-ray irradiation in an attempt to enhance transfer efficiency is not applicable to DMD boys due to substantial health risks. Furthermore, it may be necessary to apply methods of immunosuppression to circumvent immune rejection, which carries risks of its own. Much more work is needed to assess the viability of myoblast transfer as a treatment of DMD.

Gene Therapy

The aim of gene therapy is to transfer a functional dystrophin gene directly into skeletal muscle tissue. The challenge behind gene therapy is not only obtaining a functional genetic construct of the dystrophin gene and regulatory region but the effective delivery of the gene to the cell's genetic machinery. There exist several methods to effectively transfer genetic material into a muscle cell, such as direct injection and the use of retroviral and adenoviral vectors. Each of these strategies possess the potential for treating myopathies such as DMD, but they present highly technical difficulties that to date remain unresolved.

Transgenic Mice

To explore the feasibility of gene therapy for DMD, Cox and colleagues [1993] examined the introduction of an exogenous dystrophin gene into the germ line of *mdx* mice to produce transgenic animals. The transgenic mice were created by microinjection of a full-length murine dystrophin complementary DNA (cDNA) vector controlled by regulatory regions of the mouse muscle creatine kinase gene, for tissue specific expression, into the pronuclei of fertilized mouse embryos. The transgenic *mdx* mice were found to express an overabundance of dystrophin in skeletal muscles throughout the animal, nearly 50 times the level of endogenous dystrophin found in muscles from control C57BL/10 mice. Nevertheless, the transgenic procedure prevented the morphological, immunohistological, and functional symptoms of the murine muscular dystrophy. Although transgenic technology does not provide an appropriate means for treating humans, these results demonstrate the efficacy of gene therapy to correct pathologic genetic defects such as DMD. Furthermore, since it is presently impossible to regulate how and where the recombinant DNA becomes integrated into a chromosome, and subsequently the extent of gene expression, it is important that overexpression of dystrophin have no deleterious side effects.

Direct Intramuscular Injection

The straightforward gene delivery method of direct injection of large quantities of human dystrophin plasmid DNA into skeletal and heart muscles has been proposed as a treatment for DMD and BMD. The idea is that dystrophic cells will incorporate the genetic constructs, whereby the genes will use the cell's internal machinery to produce the protein dystrophin. When naked plasmid RNA and DNA constructs were injected into rodent skeletal muscles, genetic expression was observed for many weeks and even months later [Lin et al., 1990; Ono et al., 1994; Wolff et al., 1990]. Acsadi and coworkers [1991] demonstrated that a 12-kilobase full-length human dystrophin cDNA gene and a 6.3-kilobase Beckerlike gene can be made to express in cultured cells and in vivo. Direct intramuscular injection of these plasmids into *mdx* mice led to the expression of human dystrophin in approximately 1% of the muscle fibers. These results demonstrate that direct injection of DNA shows potential for gene delivery and may be beneficial as a therapeutic treatment of DMD. Nevertheless, the method must be improved upon to create a much larger number of transfected myofibers for this method to prove clinically effective. Furthermore, it is not known whether human muscle cells will incorporate and express the genetic material as will cells of rodents. The advantages of direct injection of DNA as a gene delivery system are its simplicity, and it presents no chance of viral infection or the potential of cancer development that can occur with viral vectors [Morgan, 1994].

Retrovirus-Mediated Gene Transfer

The use of retroviral and adenoviral vectors represent the two primary means of viral-mediated gene transfer strategies. Retroviruses reverse the normal process by which DNA is transcribed into RNA. A single-stranded viral RNA genome enters into a host cell, and a double helix comprised of two DNA copies of the viral RNA is created by the enzyme reverse transcriptase. Catalyzed by a viral enzyme, the DNA copy then integrates into a host cell chromosome where transcription, via the host cell RNA polymerase, produces large quantities of viral RNA molecules identical to the infecting genome [Alberts et al., 1989]. Eventually, new viruses emerge and bud from the plasma membrane ready to infect other cells. Consequently, retroviral vectors used for gene therapy are, by design, rendered replication defective. Once they infect the cell and integrate into the genome, they cannot make functional retroviruses to infect other cells. After the infective process is completed, cells are permanently altered with the presence of the viral DNA that causes the synthesis of proteins not originally endogenous to the host cell. A primary obstacle to the efficiency of a retroviral gene delivery system is its dependence on host cell division. The cell must be mitotically active for the virus to be incorporated into the host cell genetic machinery [Morgan, 1994]. This presents a problem for DMD treatment, since differentiated skeletal muscle is in a permanent postmitotic state. Nonetheless, skeletal muscle fibers regenerating from injury depend on the fusion of myoblasts. Since degeneration and regeneration of muscle cells is a continuous ongoing process in DMD patients, viral transfection of myoblasts may be an effective route for gene delivery to skeletal muscle.

For treatment of DMD and BMD, the obvious goal would be to deliver a viable dystrophin construct to the skeletal and cardiac muscles of the patient. Unfortunately, retroviruses are limited to the delivery of small genes, up to approximately 7 kilobases, precluding the delivery of a full-length dystrophin construct of 12–14 kilobases [Dunckley et al., 1993; Morgan, 1994]. Therefore, studies of the functional viability of truncated forms of dystrophin are presently being pursued. A viable reduced size 6.3-kilobase dystrophin construct has received a great deal of attention since its discovery in a BMD patient expressing a very mild phenotype. The 6.3-kilobase size is the result of a large in-frame deletion corresponding to the absence of over 40% of the central domain of the dystrophin protein.

Retroviral infection of cultured *mdx* myoblasts in vitro with the Becker dystrophin minigene has successfully led to the production of a truncated dystrophin protein product observed at the sarcolemma of the cultured myotubes [Dunckley et al., 1992]. Single injection of a retrovirus containing the dystrophin minigene into the quadriceps or anterior tibalis muscle of the *mdx* mouse led to the sarcolemmal expression of dystrophin in an average of 6% of the myofibers [Dunckley et al., 1993]. Restoration of the 43-kDalton dystrophin-associated glycoprotein was observed, and expression of the recombinant dystrophin was found in muscle tissues for up to 9 months following treatment. Transduction of the minigene was significantly enhanced when muscles were pretreated with an intramuscular injection of the myotoxic agent bupivacaine to experimentally induce muscle regeneration. These findings established that retroviral-mediated transfer of dystrophin into activated myoblasts within the host is a feasible route for delivery of a viable dystrophin gene into muscle tissues in vivo.

Adenovirus-Mediated Gene Transfer

Adenoviruses are large stable DNA-containing viruses that have the ability to infect human cells. Use of adenoviral vectors has an advantage over retroviral vectors, since they are capable of infecting nondividing or slowly proliferating cells. After intravenous administration of a recombinant adenovirus into mice, reporter gene expression was observed in skeletal and cardiac muscles for at least 12 months [Stratford-Perricaudet et al., 1992]. The potential for using adenoviral vectors containing the Beckerlike dystrophin minigene as a treatment for DMD and BMD is presently under investigation using the *mdx* mouse as a patient model. Initial studies with 5–9-day-old *mdx* mice have demonstrated that after a single intramuscular injection of the Beckerlike 6.3-kilobase cDNA driven by the Rous Sarcoma Virus promoter, up to 50% of the muscle fibers were found to contain dystrophin [Ragot et al., 1993]. Furthermore, 6 months after a single injection, expression of the minigene was still observed in the treated muscle. The truncated dystrophin gene product was correctly localized on the sarcolemmal membrane and was observed to protect myofibers from the degeneration process characteristic of *mdx* muscles [Vincent et al., 1993].

Adenoviral vectors have the potential to be used for systemic delivery of exogenous DNA. Through the use of tissue-specific promoters it may be possible to target specific tissues such as skeletal muscle for transfection via intravenous injection. Further investigations are necessary before adenoviral vectors can be applied to treat DMD patients. The efficiency and long-term corrective ability of adenovirus-mediated gene therapy need to be explored in a variety of animal models and at various stages of development. Furthermore, there are possible risks associated with adenoviral vector treatments that need to be considered. The potential exists for inhibition of host cell protein synthesis, the development of cancer, or even an immune response targeted against infected cells

[Morgan, 1994]. Also, an immune response against the adenovirus itself would likely prevent attempts at subsequent treatments because the virus would be quickly cleared from the bloodstream preventing the infection of targeted tissues.

Acknowledgments

The research from our laboratory and the preparation of this chapter was supported by a grant from the United States Public Health Service, National Institute on Aging, AG-06157 (JAF) and a Multidisciplinary Training Program on Aging, AG-00114 (SVB and NMC).

References

Acsadi G, Dickson G, Love DR, et al. 1991. Human dystrophin expression in mdx mice after intramuscular injection of DNA constructs. Nature 352:815.

Alberts B, Bray D, Lewis J, et al. 1989. Molecular Biology of the Cell, 2d ed, p 254, New York, Garland Publishing.

Bischoff R. 1986. A satellite cell mitogen from crushed adult muscle. Dev Biol 115:140.

Bonilla E, Samitt CE, Miranda AF, et al. 1988. Duchenne muscular dystrophy: Deficiency of dystrophin at the muscle cell surface. Cell 54:447.

Bulfield G, Siller WG, Wight PAL, et al. 1984. X chromosome-linked muscular dystrophy (mdx) in the mouse. Proc Natl Acad Sci USA 81:1189.

Burke RE, Levin DN, Tsairis P, et al. 1973. Physiological types and histochemical profiles in motor units of the cat gastrocnemius muscle. J Physiol (Lond) 234:723.

Carlson BM, Faulkner JA. 1983. The regeneration of skeletal muscle fibers following injury: A review. Med Sci Sports Exer 15:187.

Carpentier A, Chachques JC. 1985. Myocardial substitution with a stimulated skeletal muscle: first successful clinical case. Lancet 1(8440):1267.

Cox GA, Cole NM, Matsumura K, et al. 1993. Overexpression of dystrophin in transgenic mdx mice eliminates dystrophic symptoms without toxicity. Nature 364:725.

Dangain J, Vrbova G. 1984. Muscle development in mdx mutant mice. Muscle Nerve 7:700.

Darr KC, Schultz E. 1987. Exercise-induced satellite cell activation in growing and mature skeletal muscle. J Appl Physiol 63:1816.

Dunckley MG, Love DR, Davies KE, et al. 1992. Retroviral-mediated transfer of a dystrophin minigene into mdx mouse myoblasts in vitro. FEBS Lett 296:128.

Dunckley MG, Wells DJ, Walsh FS, et al. 1993. Direct retroviral-mediated transfer of a dystrophin minigene into mdx mouse muscle in vivo. Hum Mol Genet 2:717.

Emery AEH. 1988. Duchenne Muscular Dystrophy, 2d ed, New York, Oxford University Press.

Faulkner JA, Carlson BM, Kadhiresan VA. 1994. Whole muscle transplantation: Mechanisms responsible for functional deficits. Biotech Bioeng 43:757.

Faulkner JA, Green HJ, White TP. 1994. Response and adaptation of skeletal muscle to changes in physical activity. In C Bouchard, RJ Shephard, T Stephens (eds), Physical Activity Fitness and Health, pp 343–357, Champaign, Ill, Human Kinetics Publishers.

Florini JR, Ewton DZ, Roof SL. 1991. Insulin-like growth factor-1 stimulates terminal myogenic differentiation by induction of myogenic gene expression. Mol Endocrinol 5:718.

Florini JR, Magri KA. 1989. Effects of growth factors on myogenic differentiation. Am J Physiol 256 (Cell Physiol 25):C701.

Freilinger G, Deutinger M. 1992. Third Vienna Muscle Symposium, Vienna, Blackwell-MZV.

Guelinckx PJ, Carlson BM, Faulkner JA. 1992. Morphologic characteristics of muscles grafted in rabbits with neurovascular repair. J Recon Microsurg 8:481.

Guelinckx PJ, Faulkner JA, Essig DA. 1988. Neurovascular-anastomosed muscle grafts in rabbits: Functional deficits result from tendon repair. Muscle Nerve 11:745.

Gussoni E, Pavlath GK, Lancot AM, et al. 1992. Normal dystrophin transcrips detected in Duchenne muscular dystrophy patients after myoblast transplantation. Nature 356:435.

Hardy S, Kong Y, Konieczny SF. 1993. Fibroblast growth factor inhibits MRF4 activity independently of the phosphorylation status of a conserved threonine residue within the DNA-binding domain. Mol Cell Biol 13:5943.

Harii K, Ohmori K, Torii S. 1976. Free gracilis muscle transplantation with microneurovascular anastomoses for the treatment of facial paralysis. Plast Recon Surg 57:133.

Henneman E, Somjen G, Carpenter D. 1965. Functional significance of cell size in spinal motor neurons. J Neurophysiol 28:560.

Hinterberger TJ, Sassoon DA, Rhodes SJ, et al. 1991. Expression of the muscle regulatory factor MRF4 during somite and skeletal myofiber development. Dev Biol 147:144.

Hoffman EP, Brown RH Jr, Kunkel LM. 1987. Dystrophin: The protein product of the Duchenne muscular dystrophy locus. Cell 51:919.

Hoffman EP, Fischbeck RH, Brown RH, et al. 1988. Characterization of dystrophin in muscle-biopsy specimens from patients with Duchenne's or Becker's muscular dystrophy. N Eng J Med 318:1363.

Hurme T, Kalimo H. 1992. Activation of myogenic precursor cells after muscle injury. Med Sci Sports Exer 24:197.

Jones DA, Jackson MJ, McPhail G, et al. 1984. Experimental mouse muscle damage: The importance of external calcium. Clin Sci 66:317.

Kadhiresan VA, Guelinckx PJ, Faulkner JA. 1993. Tenotomy and repair of latissimus dorsi muscles in rats: implications for transposed muscle grafts. J Appl Physiol 75:1294.

Lin H, Parmacek MS, Morle G, et al. 1990. Expression of recombinant genes in myocardium in vivo after direct injection of DNA. Circulation 82:2217.

McCully KK, Faulkner JA. 1985. Injury to skeletal muscle fibers of mice following lengthening contractions. J Appl Physiol 59:119.

McNeil PL, Khakee R. 1992. Disruptions of muscle fiber plasma membranes. Role in exercise-induced damage. Am J Path 140:1097.

Miller SW, Hassett CA, White TP, et al. 1994. Recovery of medial gastrocnemius muscle grafts in rats: Implications for the plantarflexor group. J Appl Physiol (accepted.)

Moelleken BRW, Mathes SA, Chang N. 1989. Latissimus dorsi muscle-musculocutaneous flap in chest-wall reconstruction. Surg Clin North Am 69(5):977.

Morgan JE. 1994. Cell and gene therapy in Duchenne muscular dystrophy. Hum Gene Ther 5:165.

Morgan JE, Hoffman EP, Partridge TA. 1990. Normal myogenic cells from newborn mice restore normal histology to degenerating muscles of the mdx mouse. J Cell Biol 111:2437.

Moss FP, Leblond CP. 1971. Satellite cells as the source of nuclei in muscles of growing rats. Anat Rec 170:421.

Newham DJ, McPhail G, Jones DA, et al. 1983a. Large delayed plasma creatine kinase changes after stepping exercise. Muscle Nerve 6:380.

Newham DJ, McPhail G, Mills KR, et al. 1983b. Ultrastructural changes after concentric and eccentric contractions of human muscle. J Neurol Sci 61:109.

Ohlendieck K, Campbell KP. 1991. Dystrophin-associated proteins are greatly reduced in skeletal muscle from mdx mice. J Cell Biol 115:1685.

Ono T, Ono K, Mizukawa K, et al. 1994. Limited diffusability of gene products directed by a single nucleus in the cytoplasm of multinucleated myofibres. FEBS Lett 337:18.

Partridge TA, Morgan JE, Coulton GR, et al. 1989. Conversion of mdx myofibers from dystrophin-negative to -positive by injection of normal myoblasts. Nature 337:176.

Pette D, Vrbova G. 1992. Adaptation of mammalian skeletal muscle fibers to chronic electrical stimulation. Rev Physiol Biochem Pharmcol 120:115.

Ragot T, Vincent N, Chafey P, et al. 1993. Efficient adenovirus-mediated transfer of a human minidystrophin gene to skeletal muscle of mdx mice. Nature 361:647.

Russell B, Dix DJ, Haller DL, et al. 1992. Repair of injured skeletal muscle: A molecular approach. Med Sci Sports Exer 24:189.

Russell B, Wenderoth MP, Goldspink PH. 1992. Remodeling of myofibrils: Subcellular distribution of myosin heavy chain mRNA and protein. Am J Physiol 262 (Regulatory Integrative Comp Physiol 31):R339.

Sicinski P, Geng Y, Ryder-Cook AS, et al. 1989. The molecular basis of muscular dystrophy in the *mdx* mouse: A point mutation. Science 244:1578.

Smith CK II, Janney MJ, Allen RE. 1994. Temporal expression of myogenic regulatory genes during activation, proliferation, and differentiation of rat skeletal muscle satellite cells. J Cell Physiol 159:379.

Smith TH, Block NE, Rhodes SJ, et al. 1993. A unique pattern of expression of the four muscle regulatory factor proteins distinguishes somitic from embryonic, fetal and newborn mouse myogenic cells. Development 117:1125.

Stratford-Perricaudet LD, Makeh I, Perricaudet M, et al. 1992. Widespread long-term gene transfer to mouse skeletal muscles and heart. J Clin Invest 90:626.

Tamai S, Komatsu S, Sakamoto H, 1970. Free-muscle transplants in dogs with microsurgical neuro-vascular anastomoses. Plast Recon Surg 46:219.

Thompson N. 1974. A review of autogenous skeletal muscle grafts and their clinical applications. Clin Plast Surg 1:349.

Tidball JG, Law DJ. 1991. Dystrophin is required for normal thin filament-membrane associations at myotendinous junctions. Am J Pathol 138:17.

Vincent N, Ragot T, Gilgenkrantz H, et al. 1993. Long-term correction of mouse dystrophic degeneration by adenovirus-mediated transfer of a minidystrophin gene. Nature Genetics 5:130.

Weintraub H, Davis R, Tapscott S, et al. 1991. The *myoD* gene family: nodal point during specification of the muscle cell lineage. Science 251:761.

Whalen RG, Butler-Browne GS, Bugaisky LB, et al. 1985. Myosin isozyme transitions in developing and regenerating rat muscle. Adv Exp Med Biol 182:249.

Wolff JA, Malone RW, Williams P, et al. 1990. Direct gene transfer into mouse muscle in vivo. Science 247:1465.

Lisa E. Freed
*Massachusetts Institute
of Technology and Harvard
University*

**Gordana Vunjak-
Novakovic**
*Massachusetts Institute
of Technology*

Cartilage has only a small capacity for self-repair due to the avascular nature of the tissue [Buck-walter et al., 1990; Campbell, 1969]. Reconstructive plastic and orthopedic surgeries are done on a daily basis in order to treat the many patients with defective cartilage due to arthritis, congenital abnormalities, or trauma. Current therapies include cartilage transplantation and the implantation of artificial prosthetic devices. However, transplants are limited by the availability of donor tissue and technical difficulties related to graft sizing and fixation [Zukor et al., 1990], and prostheses are complicated by loosening and toxicity due to adhesive breakdown at the host-device interface [McKee, 1982; Peterson et al., 1988]. The clinical need for improved methods for cartilage repair or replacement has motivated research aimed at creating tissue-engineered cartilage that could bene-fit an estimated 1 million patients per year [Langer & Vacanti, 1993]. *Tissue engineering* has been defined as "the use of living cells, together with extracellular components, either natural or synthetic, in the development of implantable parts or devices for the restoration or replacement of function" [Nerem, 1991]. This chapter reviews the current state of the art of in vivo cartilage repair based on implanted cartilage cells (chondrocytes) and/or biomaterials (Table 120.1), and focuses on tissue engineering of cartilage for in vivo use based on the in vitro cultivation of chondrocytes on synthetic biodegradable polymer scaffolds [Freed et al., 1993a, 1993b, 1994a, 1994b, 1994c, 1994d; Freed & Vunjak-Novakovic, 1994a, 1994b].

120.1 Literature Review

Table 120.1 chronologically lists a large number of studies showing that implantation of chondro-cytes and/or biomaterials promotes in vivo cartilage formation (chondrogenesis). Several key parameters varied greatly from study to study: (1) the model system (rabbits, dogs, and roosters for articular cartilage and meniscal repairs; nude mice for subcutaneous chondrogenesis), (2) the age of animals (host, donor) and the cell source (articular, epiphyseal or costal cartilage obtained from the various species), (3) the surgical techniques used to create cartilage defects and implant the cells and/or biomaterial, (4) the defect size and the healing time in vivo (6 weeks to 1 year), and (5) the

0-8493-8346-3/95/$0.00+$.50
© 1995 by CRC Press, Inc.

methods used to assess cartilage repair or chondrogenesis, e.g., qualitative or quantitative histology, biochemical analyses of cartilage tissue components, and biomechanical tests.

Isolated chondrocytes were first shown to enhance articular cartilage repair by Chesterman and Smith [1968] and Bently and Greer [1971]. Periosteal flaps have been successfully used to immobilize the cells at the site of the defect [Grande et al., 1989]; in this case both the cellular and periosteal components of the implant are chondrogenic [O'Driscoll & Salter, 1984; Upton et al., 1981]. Fibrin-based glues have also been used for chondrocyte delivery [Itay et al., 1987], but have cytotoxic side effects [Messner, 1993; Nevo et al., 1992]. *Chondrocytes cultured in vitro* on demineralized bone have been used to repair cartilage defects in rabbits [Green, 1977], and chondrocytes cultured in vitro on Vicryl surgical sutures have been used to create subcutaneous neocartilage in nude mice [Vacanti et al., 1991].

A variety of *biomaterials,* naturally occurring and synthetic, degradable or nondegradable, also promoted articular cartilage repair in the absence of cultured cells (Table 120.1). Naturally occurring biodegradable materials included collagen sponges and gels [Speer et al., 1979; Wakitani et al., 1989], collagen and glycosaminoglycan (GAG) composites [Stone et al., 1992], and hyaluronic acid (HA) [Nevo et al., 1992; Robinson et al., 1990]. Naturally occurring nonbiodegradable materials included agarose [Buschmann et al., 1992]. Synthetic biodegradable materials included polyesters, e.g., polylactic acid [Von Schroeder et al., 1991], polyglycolic acid [Freed et al., 1993a,c 1994a], Vicryl [Vacanti et al., 1991] and Dacron [Messner & Gillquist, 1993a], and some polyurethanes [DeGroot et al., 1990; Elema et al., 1990; Klompmaker et al., 1992]. Synthetic nonbiodegradable materials included polyvinylalcohol (Ivalon) [Speer et al., 1979], carbon fibers [Minns et al., 1982, 1989], and Teflon [Messner 1994; Messner & Gillquist, 1993a, 1993b].

In the majority of studies listed in Table 120.1, the repair tissue was found to be of variable morphological quality, ranging from fibrous to hyaline cartilage with biomechanical properties that were subnormal and tended to deteriorate over time. These findings can be attributed to insufficient regeneration of cartilaginous matrix in conjunction with in vivo loading of the nascent repair tissue. The use of in-vitro-grown tissue constructs with histologic, biochemical, and mechanical properties that match the requirements of the given implant site could presumably further improve cartilage repair. Our approach to cartilage tissue engineering is therefore based on the in vitro cultivation of chondrocytes on specifically designed polymer scaffolds to obtain custom-designed cartilaginous implants for in vivo use (Freed et al., 1993a, 1993b, 1994a, 1994b, 1994c, 1994d; Freed & Vunjak-Novakovic, 1995a, 1995b Vunjak-Novakovic et al., 1995).

120.2 Cartilage Tissue Engineering Based on Cell-Polymer Constructs

Model System

Tissue constructs with clinically useful dimensions and structures and compositions resembling natural cartilage can be grown in vitro using the cell-polymer model system (Fig. 120.1). The biodegradable polyglycolic acid (PGA) scaffold provides a three-dimensional (3D) structure for cell attachment and defines the shape and size of the engineered tissue. Under appropriate in vitro culture conditions, the chondrocytes proliferate within the scaffold and secrete cartilaginous extracellular matrix (ECM) consisting of GAG and collagen. Scaffold degradation in parallel with tissue regeneration provides long-term construct biocompatibility.

One advantage of this approach is that the scaffold can be designed to meet specific tissue engineering criteria. Ideally, the material should: (1) be reproducibly processible into a highly porous 3D structure that permits a spatially uniform cell distribution and minimizes diffusional constraints during in vitro cultivation, (2) stimulate cell proliferation and ECM secretion without inflammatory or toxic side effects, and (3) biodegrade at a controlled rate. Other potential advantages include: (1) the use of either autografted or allografted chondrocytes, (2) the immunoprotection offered by

TABLE 120.1 Literature Review

Study	Model System: Animal, site*	Chondrocyte†	Biomaterial‡ (Biodegradable: yes or no)	Other Material	Time In vitro	Time In vivo	Repair Tissue (Assessment)§	References
1	Rabbit, articular	Articular	—	—	—	6 wks	Fibrocartilage (H)	Chesterman & Smith, 1968
2,3	Rabbit, articular	Articular, epiphyseal	—	—	—	8 wks–1 yr	Fibrocartilage (H,B)	Bently et al., 1971, 1989
4	Rabbit, articular	Articular	Demin. bone	—	10 days	10 days	Hyaline cartilage (H,B)	Green, 1977
5	Rabbit, articular	—	Collagen (y), PVA (n)	—	—	11 mos	Fibrocartilage (H)	Speer, 1979
6	Rabbit, articular	—	—	Perichondrium	—	1 yr	Fibrocartilage (H)	Upton et al., 1981
7,8	Rabbit, articular	—	Carbon (n)	—	—	6 mos	Fibrocartilage (H,M)	Minns et al., 1982, 1989
9,10	Rabbit, articular	—	—	Periosteum	—	1 mo	Hyaline cartilage (H,B)	O'Driscoll et al., 1984, 1986
11	Nude mouse, subcutaneous	Costal	—	—	Serial passage	1 mo	Cartilage nodule (H,B)	Takigawa et al., 1987
12	Rooster, articular	Epiphyseal	—	Fibrin glue	Several days	6 mos	Hyaline cartilage (H,B)	Itay et al., 1987
13	Rabbit, articular	Articular	Collagen gel (y)	—	—	6 mos	Hyaline cartilage (H,B)	Wakitani et al., 1989
14	Rabbit, articular	Articular	—	Periosteum	2 wks	6 wks	Hyaline cartilage (H,B)	Grande et al., 1989
15,16	Dog, meniscal	—	PU/PLLA (y)	—	—	8 mos	Fibrocartilage (H)	De Groot et al., 1990; Elema et al., 1990
17	Rabbit, articular	—	PU/PLLA (y)	—	—	1 yr	Fibro-hyaline cartilage (H,B)	Klompmaker et al., 1992
	Dog, articular	—	PU/PLLA (y)	—	—	6 mos	Fibrocartilage (H,B)	
18,19	Chicken, articular	Epiphyseal	Hyaluronate gel (y), Demin. bone	—	—	6 mos	Hyaline cartilage (H,B)	Robinson et al., 1990; Nevo et al., 1992
20	Rabbit, articular	—	PMMA, pHEMA(n)	Periosteum	—	2 mos	Hyaline cartilage (H,B,M)	Mow et al., 1991
21	Rabbit, articular	—	PLLA (y)	Periosteum	—	3 mos	Hyaline cartilage (H,B,M)	Von Schroeder et al., 1991

	Species, site†	Chondrocytes†	Biomaterial‡	Supplement			Repair tissue§	Reference
22,23	Nude mouse, subcutaneous	Articular	PLGA (y)	—	0–10 days	3–9 mos	Cartilage nodule (H)	Vacanti et al, 1991; Cima et al, 1991
24	Bovine, *in vitro*	Articular	Agarose (n)	—	10 wks	—	Hyaline matrix (H,B,M)	Buschmann et al, 1992
25	Dog, meniscal	—	Collagen/GAG (y)	—	—	1 yr	Fibrocartilage (H,B)	Stone et al, 1992
26	Rabbit, articular	—	PE (y), PTFE (n), PTFE/PU (n)	Fibrin glue	—	3 mos	Fibrocartilage (H,M)	Messner and Gillquist, 1993a
27	Rabbit, articular	—	PE (y), Hydroxylapatite	Periosteum	—	1 yr	Fibro-hyaline cartilage (H,M)	Messner, 1993
28	Rabbit, meniscus	—	PU/PE (n) PU/PTFE (n)	—	—	3 mos	Fibrocartilage (H,M)	Messner and Gillquist, 1993b
29	Rabbit, meniscal	—	PTFE (n)	Periosteum	—	3 mos	Graft failure (H,M)	Messner, 1994
30	Nude mouse, subcutaneous	Articular, costal	PGA, PLLA (y)	—	2–3 wks	6 mos	Cartilage nodule (H,B)	Freed et al, 1993a
31	Equine, *in vitro*	Articular	Collagen (y)	—	3 wks	—	Fibro-hyaline matrix (H,B)	Nixon et al, 1993
32	Rabbit, articular	Articular	PGA (y)	—	3–4 wks	6 mos	Fibro-hyaline cartilage (H)	Freed et al, 1994a
33	Bovine, *in vitro*	Articular	PGA (y)	—	3 days–8 wks	—	Fibro-hyaline matrix (H,B)	Freed et al, 1993b, 1994b, 1994c, 1994d; Freed & Vunjak-Novakovic, 1995a, 1995b

*Site of implant: articular—joint surface in knee joint; meniscal—meniscus in knee joint; *in vitro*—cells cultured but not implanted.

†Chondrocytes: articular—cells from joint surfaces; costal—cells from cartilaginous rib; epiphyseal—cells from developing epiphysis.

‡Biomaterial: demin. bone = demineralized bone, PE = polyester (Dacron), pHEMA = polyhydroxy-ethylmethacrylate, PGA = polyglycolic acid (Dexon), PLGA = polyglycolic-co-lactic acid (Vicryl), PLLA = poly-L-lactic acid, PMMA = polymethylmethacrylate, PTFE = polytetrafluoroethylene (Teflon), PU = polyurethane, PVA = polyvinyl alcohol (Ivalon).

§Assessment of repair tissue: B = biochemical, H = histological, M = mechanical

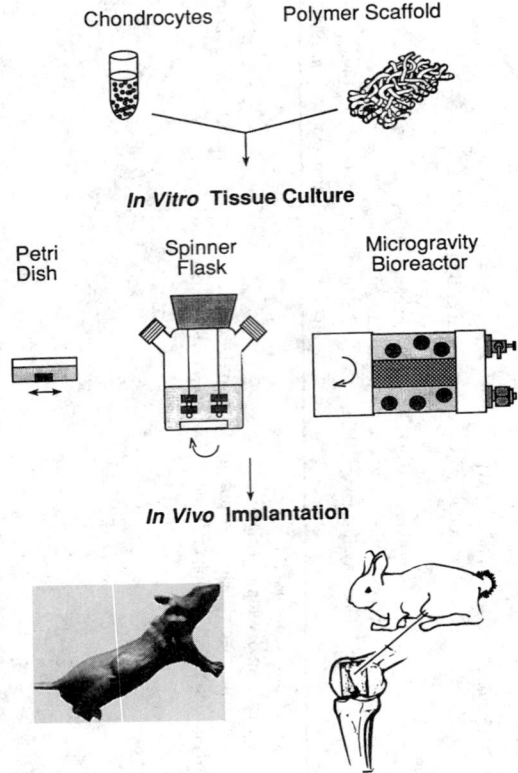

FIGURE 120.1 Model system: Chondrocytes isolated from a harvested cartilage sample are seeded on a synthetic, biodegradable polymer scaffold, and cultured in vitro in petri dishes, spinner flasks, or microgravity bioreactors prior to in vivo implantation, e.g., to form subcutaneous neocartilage or to repair damaged articular cartilage.

sequestration of cell surface antigens by ECM generated during in vitro cultivation [Langer & Gross, 1974], (3) the ability to control in vitro culture conditions, (4) the ability of in-vitro-grown cartilage constructs to continuously remodel and thus completely integrate with the host tissue following in vivo implantation, and (5) the extension of the same methodologies to other cell types to engineer a variety of clinically useful tissues.

Experimental Methods

Scaffolds

Fibrous polyglycolic acid (PGA) mesh was produced commercially at Albany International (Mansfield, MA). PGA was extruded into 13-μm diameter fibers, processed to form a nonwoven mesh with a porosity of 97%, punched into discs (e.g., 10 mm in diameter × 2–5 mm thick), and sterilized with ethylene oxide (see discussion of scaffold design later in the chapter).

Chondrocytes

Animal cartilage was obtained from the articular surfaces of 2 to 4-week-old bovine calves or 2 to 8-month-old rabbits; human cartilage was obtained following repair of a congenital rib defect in an 11-year-old male [Freed et al., 1993a, 1994a]. Chondrocytes were isolated by digestion with type II collagenase [Freed et al., 1993a]. When the amount of donor tissue was limited, primary chondrocytes were serially passaged up to four times in monolayer cultures prior to seeding on polymer scaffolds (Freed et al., 1994a).

In Vitro Studies. The *static petri dish* culture system is described in detail in Freed and coworkers [1993a]. Dry PGA scaffolds (10 mm diameter × 2 mm thick discs) were seeded with freshly isolated cells (5×10^6 cells in 100–300 μl of medium) by capillary action. Constructs were cultured statically for 6 h in a 37°C humidified 5% CO_2 incubator; 1.5 cm³ of medium was then added after which the medium was replaced every 2–3 days.

The *mixed petri dish* culture system is described in detail in Freed and coworkers [1994b, 1994c]. In contrast to the static petri dish culture, PGA scaffolds (10 mm diameter × 2 mm thick discs) were prewetted for 12 h in culture medium prior to seeding (5×10^6 cells and 4 cm³ medium per well). During both the cell seeding and tissue culture, the dishes were placed on an orbital shaker (85 rpm) in a 37°C/5% CO_2 incubator.

The *spinner flask* culture system is described in detail in Freed and Vunjak-Novakovic [1995] and Vunjak-Novakovic and coworkers [1995]. Conventional spinner flasks obtained from Bellco were 5.5 cm in diameter and contained a nonsuspended 4-cm long magnetic stir bar (Fig. 120.1). Prewetted PGA scaffolds (10 mm diameter × 5 mm thick discs) were threaded onto 4-in long needles, and 4 needles each with 2 scaffolds apiece were fixed to the stopper in the mouth of the flask. To seed polymer scaffolds, medium (110 cm³) and chondrocytes (5×10^5 cells/cm³) were added, and the flasks were stirred for 3 days at a speed of 50 rpm in a 37°C/5% CO_2 incubator. Constructs were then cultivated under mixed culture conditions (i.e., in flasks mixed at 50–100 rpm) or statically. Medium was completely replaced every other day.

The *microgravity bioreactor* culture system is described in detail by Schwarz and colleagues (1992) and by Freed and Vunjak-Novakovic (1995a). The NASA-developed slow-turning lateral vessel (STLV) consists of a 5.75-cm diameter outer cylinder and a concentric gas exchange membrane (Fig. 120.1). Prewetted PGA scaffolds, medium (110 cm³), and chondrocytes (5×10^5 cells/cm³) were added such that all air was displaced. The vessel was attached to a custom-designed base, placed in a 37°C/5% CO_2 incubator, and rotated around its central axis at a speed of 15–20 rpm; gas exchange was established across the membrane using a positive pressure air pump. The medium was completely replaced every other day.

In Vivo Studies. The athymic (nude) *mouse model system* was adapted from Vacanti and coworkers [1991] as described by Freed and coworkers [1993a]. Cell-polymer constructs based on bovine or human chondrocytes were cultivated in static petri dishes for 2–3 weeks in vitro and then implanted subcutaneously in nude mice as follows. Mice (Swiss CD1 nu/nu males weighing 22–25 g) were anesthetized, and subcutaneous pouches (2 cm × 2 cm) were created on the left and right sides using sterile technique. Constructs were implanted into one pouch, and scaffolds without cultured cells were inserted into the opposite pouch. Explants were removed after in vivo intervals of 1–6 months.

The *rabbit model system* was adapted from Grande and coworkers (1989) as described by Freed and coworkers (1994a). Cell-polymer constructs based on allograft chondrocytes were cultivated in static petri dishes for 3–4 weeks in vitro and then implanted intra-articularly in New Zealand white rabbits as follows. Rabbits (8-month-old males weighing approximately 4.5 kg) were anesthetized, and medial parapatellar arthrotomies were performed. A pointed 3-mm diameter drill was used to create bilateral full thickness defects in the femoropatellar grooves; an attempt was made to extend these defects just through the subchondral plate without violating the subchondral bone (i.e., 1–2 mm deep). A 4-mm diameter × 1–2 mm thick disc was punched out of a cell-polymer construct using a surgical trephine and press-fit into the defect on one side. A 4-diameter × 2-mm thick polymer scaffold without cells was press-fit into the defect on the opposite side. Knee joints were not immobilized postoperatively. Explants were removed after in vivo intervals of 1–6 months.

Analytical Techniques

Histologic samples were fixed in neutral buffered formalin, embedded in parrafin, and cross-sectioned (8-μm thick). Sections were stained for cells (with hematoxylin and eosin, H&E), GAG (with safranin-O), cross-linked collagen (with trichrome), and types I and II collagen with poly-clonal goat-anti-bovine antibodies (Southern Biotechnology, Birmingham, AL) and a labeled strep-tavidin biotin alkaline phosphatase staining kit (DAKO, Carpinteria, CA) [Freed et al., 1993a; Freed & Vunjak-Novakovic, 1994a].

Biochemical analyses were done following papain digestion of lyophilized samples. Cell number was assessed from the amount of DNA measured using Hoechst 33258 dye [Kim et al., 1988]. Sulfated GAG content was determined by dimethylmethylene blue dye binding [Farndale et al., 1986]. Total collagen content was determined from hydroxyproline content by acid hydrolysis and reaction with p-dimethylaminobenzaldehyde and chloramine-T [Woessner et al., 1961].

Scaffold Design

Synthetic, biodegradable scaffolds were custom-designed, reproducibly made on a commercial scale, and studied with respect to biocompatibility, structure, and biodegradation rate [Freed et al., 1994c]. Polyglycolic acid (PGA) was selected because it meets all the criteria listed above for a tissue-engineering scaffold and is approved for clinical use by the Food and Drug Administration (FDA) [Frazza & Schmitt, 1971]. PGA fibers were extruded and processed to form a highly porous, mechanically stabilized mesh (Fig. 120.2).

The PGA had an initial weight average molecular weight (M_W) of about 70 kD and a number average molecular weight (M_n) of 25 kD $(M_w/M_n = 2.75)$, as measured by gel permeation chromatography. A multifilament yarn with a tenacity of 4–5 grams per denier was formed by polymer extrusion, stretching and relaxation at elevated temperatures. The yarn was crimped, cut, carded into a lofty web, and formed as a nonwoven mesh using barbed needles to entangle the fibers and lock them together. Heat setting increased the dimensional stability of the mesh and smoothed the top and bottom surfaces. A multihole die was used to punch the mesh into 1-cm diameter × 2–5-mm thick discs; 3000 discs were produced in a single run. Fiber diameter was 13 μm, scaffold porosity was 97%, and scaffolds had sufficient structural integrity to maintain their dimensions when seeded with isolated chondrocytes and cultured in vitro at 37°C.

The degradation rate of PGA scaffolds was measured without cultured cells in 37°C buffer containing 10% serum [Freed et al., 1994c]. The scaffold mass passed through a flat maximum over the first week due to hydration and nonspecific protein adsorption and then decreased according to first-order kinetics in two stages. Between weeks 1–4, the PGA degraded relatively quickly and the crystallinity of the remaining polymer increased; both the mass and crystallinity changed more slowly thereafter. These findings are consistent with previous reports that the amorphous polymer regions degrade more rapidly than the crystalline regions [Zhang et al., 1993].

Chondrocytes (bovine, rabbit, human; articular, costal) attached to the PGA fibers as multiple layers of cells that retained their spherical morphology (Fig. 120.3a and 120.3b). GAG secretion was highest for cells located near the polymer (Fig. 120.3c), which is consistent with the general hypothesis that a cell expresses its differentiated phenotype in vitro when cultured on a substrate that maintains the cell's in vivo configuration [Watt, 1986]. Cardiac myocytes also attached to PGA scaffolds and formed tissue constructs 10 mm in diameter × 2-mm thick that contracted spontaneously and synchronously [Freed and Vunjak-Novakovic, 1995b]. The PGA scaffold thus appears to be an excellent cell culture substrate for a variety of tissue engineering applications.

In Vivo Feasibility Studies

In-vitro-grown constructs based on xenograft chondrocytes (bovine articular or costal; human costal) and polymer scaffolds were implanted subcutaneously in nude mice [Freed et al., 1993a].

Processing: **Chemistry:**

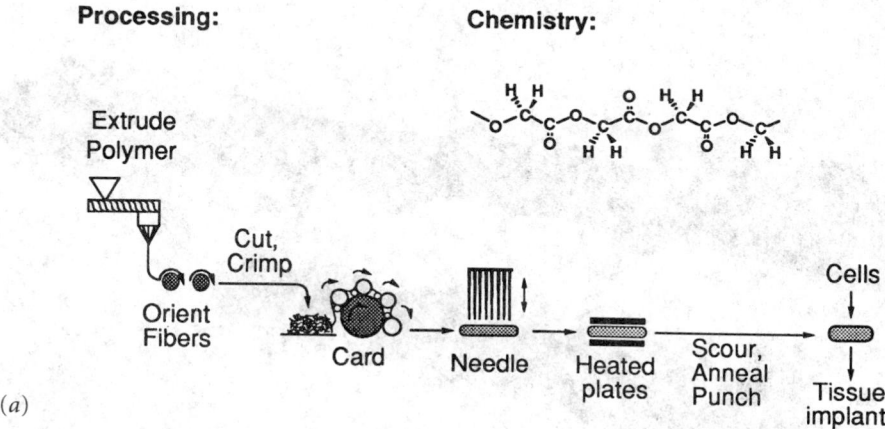

(a)

Scanning Electron Micrograph:

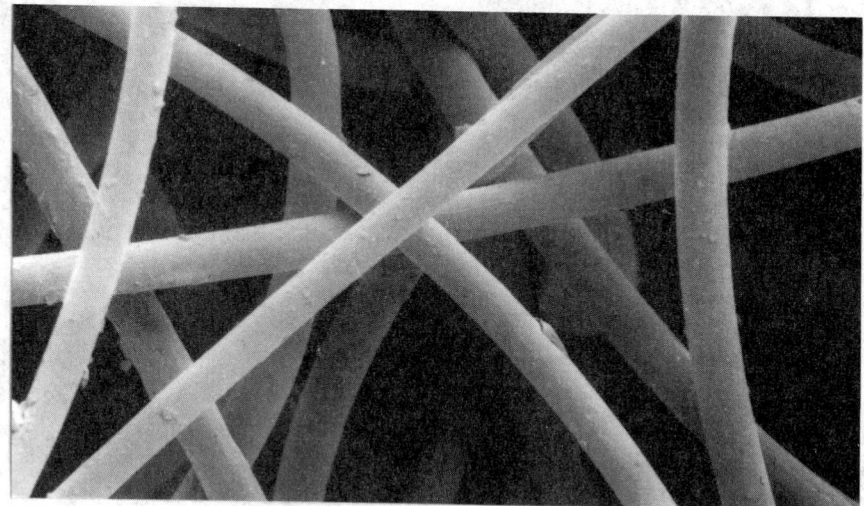

(b)

FIGURE 120.2 Polymer scaffold: (*a*) chemical structure, large-scale processing technology; (*b*) appearance.

Subcutaneous neocartilage formed that retained the shape of the polymer scaffold and contained GAG and collagen types I and II in amounts that increased over time. In a separate study, in-vitro-grown constructs based on allograft chondrocytes were implanted intra-articularly in rabbits [Freed et al., 1994a]. At the time of implantation, the total amount of GAG and collagen in the allograft was one-third that in the host cartilage. Full-thickness, 3 mm-diameter defects were repaired with fibro-hyaline cartilage with varying degrees of success; representative good results at 1 and 6 months are shown in Fig. 120.4.

Chondrocytes dedifferentiated by serial passage in monolayer culture regain their potential to regenerate cartilage tissue when transferred to a 3D culture environment [Benya & Shaffer, 1982; Takigawa et al., 1987]. Three-dimensional cell-PGA constructs based on chondrocytes that had been serially passaged three times had similar cellularities and higher amounts of GAG and collagen as constructs based on primary chondrocytes [Freed et al., 1994a]. Chondrogenesis also depends on

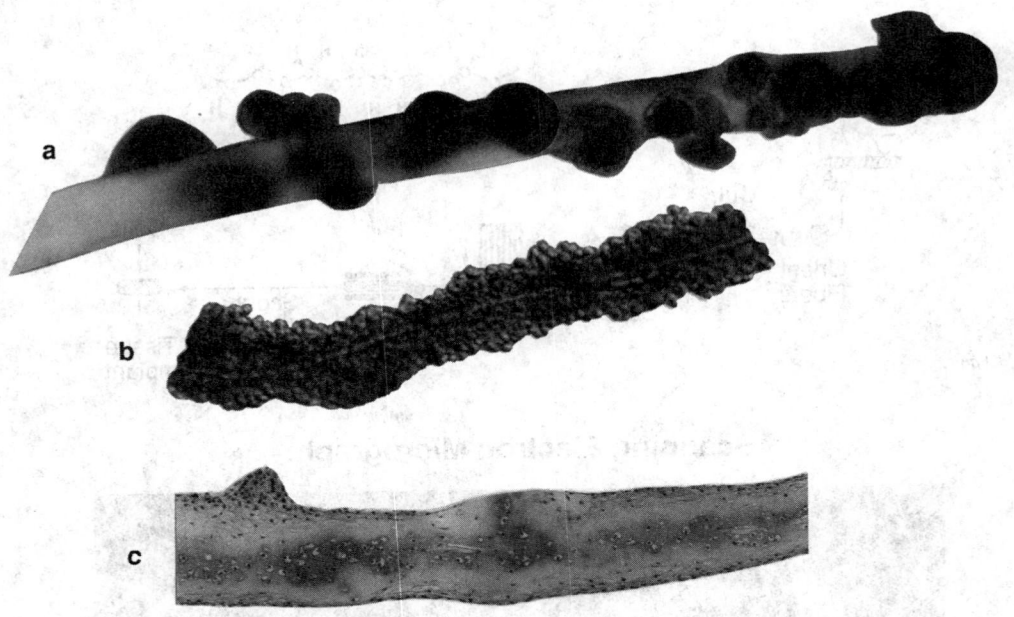

FIGURE 120.3 Chondrocyte attachment and differentiated morphology on PGA fibers: (*a*), (*b*) 3 days after cell seeding—note the spherical morphology and multiple cell layers (*a*) (H&E stain, (*b*) Hoffman modulation contrast); (*c*) after 6 weeks of cultivation—note a higher concentration of GAG around the PGA remnants (safranin-O stain).

the age of the cartilage donor; chondrocytes from immature donors are in general metabolically more active [Nevo et al., 1992]. One-month cell-PGA constructs based on chondrocytes obtained from 1–2-week-old bovine calves contained significantly more GAG and collagen than constructs based on chondrocytes obtained from 2–8-month-old rabbits and cultured under identical conditions [Freed et al., 1994a, 1994b].

Implantation of PGA scaffolds both with and without cultured chondrocytes promoted the repair of articular cartilage defects in rabbits [Freed et al., 1994a]. In the absence of cultured cells, the PGA scaffold presumably guided host cells into the defect and provided a favorable environment for chondrogenesis. Six-month cartilage repair was qualitatively judged to be better after implantation of cell-polymer allografts than PGA scaffolds alone with respect to surface smoothness, columnar alignment of chondrocytes, uniformity of GAG distribution, reconstitution of the subchondral plate, and bonding of the repair tissue to the underlying bone. A minor inflammatory response characterized by moderate numbers of lymphocytes localized in the bone marrow spaces underlying the defect was observed following implantation of scaffolds with and without cultured cells at 1 month and had completely resolved at 6 months [Freed et al., 1994a]. The lack of any specific immune response to the allograft chondrocytes was attributed to sequestration of cell surface antigens by ECM generated during the in vitro culture period that preceded in vivo implantation [Langer & Gross, 1974].

These initial pilot studies demonstrated: (1) the feasibility of using in-vitro-grown cell-polymer constructs to form subcutaneous neocartilage or repair articular cartilage defects, and (2) the continuation of the chondrogenesis process in vivo.

Joint resurfacing
(1-month explant)

Repair tissue
(6-month explant)

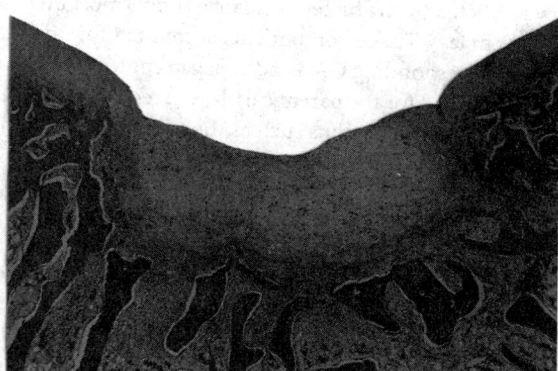
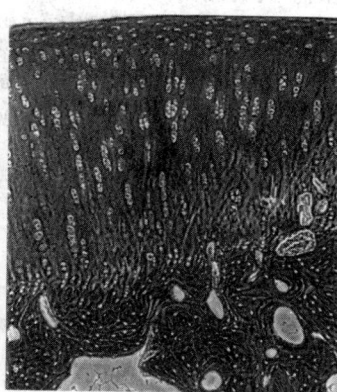

FIGURE 120.4 Joint resurfacing with cell-polymer allografts: (*a*) 1-month explant stained with H&E, original magnification ×40; (*b*) 6-month explant stained with trichrome, original magnification ×200.

In Vitro Chondrogenesis

During natural cartilage formation, chondrocytes proliferate and secrete collagen and proteoglycan (PG) that represent 50–79% and 14–35%, respectively, of the tissue dry weight (dw) [Buckwalter et al., 1990; Mow et al., 1992]. Collagen provides a fibrillar framework which gives the tissue its form, and mechanically traps and/or binds other matrix components. The major collagens in fibro- and hyaline cartilage are type I and type II, respectively [Zanetti & Solursh, 1989]. PG consists of GAG and HA and interacts with collagen and tissue fluid to give cartilage its compressive stiffness [Mow et al., 1992]. The outermost 10% of the tissue consists of flattened cells and thin collagen fibers oriented parallel to the surface; the deeper zone has round cells arranged in columns oriented perpendicular to the surface, a higher GAG content, and thicker collagen fibers [Buckwalter et al., 1990]. In vitro chondrogenesis in the cell-polymer model system (Fig. 120.1) should ideally resemble natural in vivo chondrogenesis. The isolated chondrocytes must first attach to polymer surfaces throughout the PGA scaffold, and then regenerate a cartilaginous ECM in parallel with scaffold degradation. This requires a high chondrocyte density [Tacchetti et al., 1992] in conjunction with several biochemical and biomechanical factors [Mow et al., 1991].

Petri Dish Cultures

Under static cell-seeding conditions, gravity caused the cells to settle to the base of the scaffold. Except for very thin (≤1mm) scaffolds, constructs appeared bilaminar, and consisted mainly of undifferentiated cells and small areas of cartilaginous tissue; subsequent cultivation of statically seeded constructs under mixed conditions could not compensate for an initially nonuniform cell distribution [Freed et al., 1994*b*]. Mixing was found to improve the uniformity of cell seeding throughout the polymer scaffold and the rates of cell proliferation and ECM regeneration. Cell-polymer constructs seeded and grown in mixed petri dishes consisted of mature chondrocytes, cartilaginous ECM, and remnant polymer and maintained the dimensions of the original scaffold. Histologic assessment of 8-week constructs showed the presence of GAG (with safranin-O), collagen types I and II (immunohistochemically), and a 200–300 μm thick outer capsule consisting of multiple layers of flat cells and collagen (Fig. 120.5*a*) [Freed et al., 1994*c*].

The kinetics of tissue regeneration in cell-polymer constructs is shown in Fig. 120.5*b*. The amounts of cells, GAG, and collagen increased over time (filled squares), and the amount of PGA decreased to about 30% of the initial polymer mass after 8 weeks of in vitro culture (open squares) [Freed et al., 1994*c*]. The total construct dw predicted by the material balance (uppermost line) accounted for 100% of the measured dw (filled circles). Tissue components accounted for approximately 50% of the dw of 8-week constructs; the corresponding GAG and collagen contents per gram wet weight (ww) were 33% and 19% of those measured for the parent cartilage [Freed et al., 1994*c*]. These findings imply that well-defined in vitro culture conditions such as those provided by tissue culture bioreactors are required to cultivate clinically sized cartilage constructs.

Bioreactor Cultures

Tissue culture bioreactors offer a number of potential advantages over static or mixed petri dishes: (1) uniform and efficient mixing coupled with increased mass transfer rates, (2) regulation of shear stress within the vessel, (3) maintenance of pH, gas partial pressures (pO_2, pCO_2) and nutrient levels (e.g., glucose), and (4) process control strategies which can match the changing needs of a growing tissue over the entire duration of its cultivation.

Cell-polymer constructs were seeded in mixed flasks and then cultivated under either static or mixed conditions for 8 weeks (Fig. 120.1). In static cultures, the constructs had a relatively uniform distribution of round cells, GAG, and collagen and only one or two layers of spherical cells at the surface (Fig. 120.6*a*). In contrast, mixing induced the formation of a capsule consisting of flat, elongated cells and collagen surrounding a central area that resembled a construct grown statically (Fig. 120.6*b*).Mixing significantly improved the biochemical compositions of cartilage constructs (Figs. 120.7b, 120.7c). Constructs grown for 8 weeks in mixed cultures were 30% thicker, more regular in shape, and contained 70% more cells, 60% more GAG, and 125% more collagen than constructs

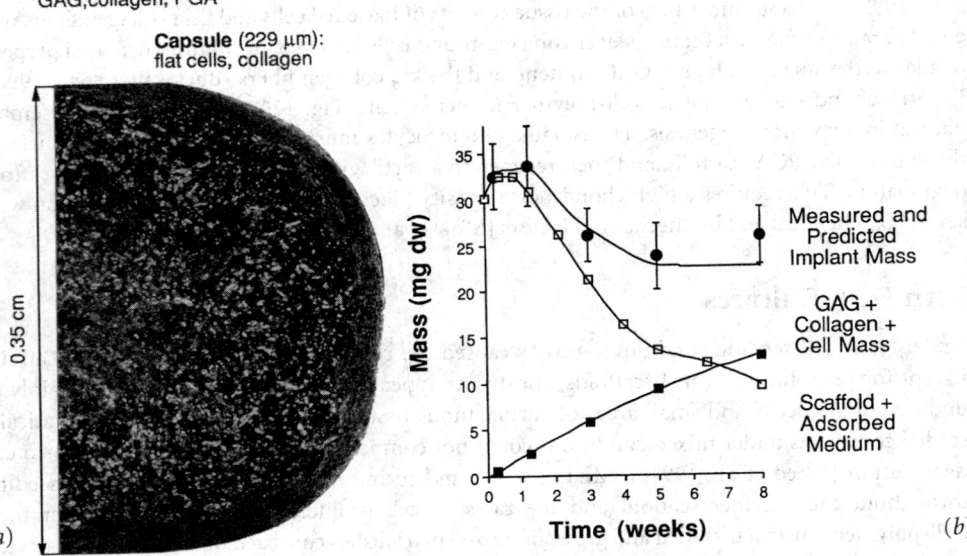

FIGURE 120.5   Cell-polymer constructs grown in mixed petri dishes: (*a*) 8-week construct consisting of cells, GAG, collagen, and PGA remnants surrounded by a collagenous capsule (dark field microscopy of full cross-section); (*b*) tissue regeneration kinetics: (1) accumulation of tissue components (filled squares), (2) degradation of scaffold (open squares), and (3) measured construct dry weights (filled circles) compared to those accounted for by the sum of (1) and (2) above (uppermost line).

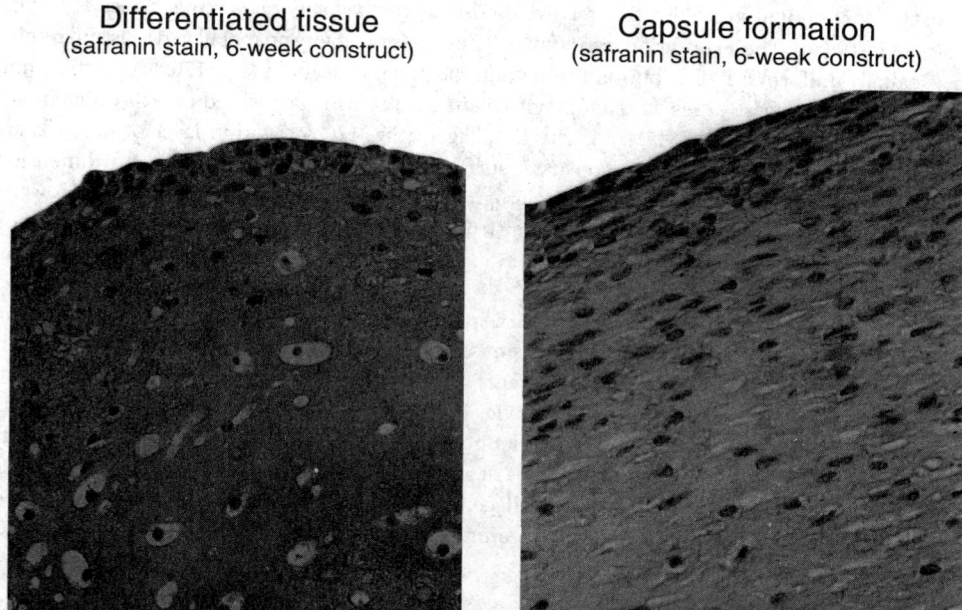

Differentiated tissue
(safranin stain, 6-week construct)

Capsule formation
(safranin stain, 6-week construct)

(*a*)   (*b*)

FIGURE 120.6   Histologic appearance of 8-week cell-polymer constructs grown in: (*a*) a static flask; (*b*) a flask mixed at 100 rpm (GAG stained with safranin-O).

grown statically [Vunjak-Novakovic et al., 1995]. The observed effects of mixing can be attributed both to increased mass transfer rates of chemical species and direct effects of hydrodynamic forces on cell shape and function.

Cell-polymer constructs were seeded and cultivated under well-defined fluid-dynamic conditions using bioreactors developed at the National Aeronautics and Space Administration (NASA) (Fig. 120.1) [Schwarz et al., 1992]. Rotation of the vessel around its central axis maintained the construct

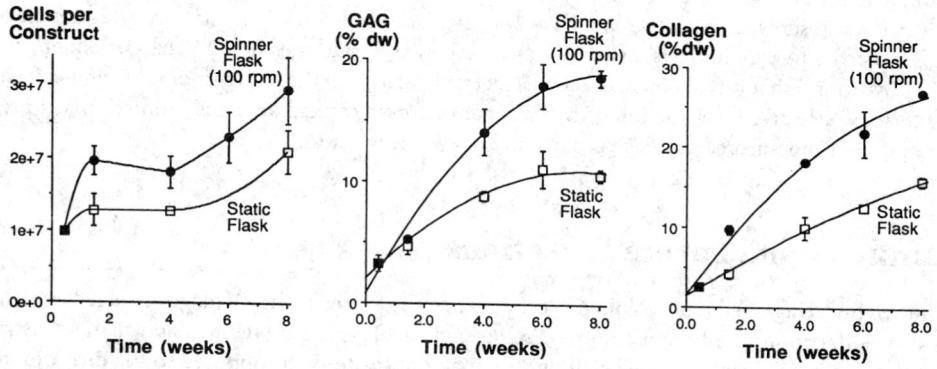

FIGURE 120.7   Biochemical composition of cell-polymer constructs: (*a*) cells (per construct); (*b*), (*c*) GAG or collagen content (as percent of construct dry weight). Constructs grown for 0–8 weeks statically are compared to those grown in spinner flasks mixed at 100 rpm (open and closed symbols, respectively).

in a state of continual free-fall with a relative fluid-construct velocity of 2–3cm/s [Freed & Vunjak-Novakovic, 1995a]. These conditions randomized the effects of gravity on inoculated cells and resulted in a spatially uniform cell distribution throughout the polymer scaffold (Fig. 120.8a). Cartilaginous tissue regenerated over 1 week of microgravity tissue culture which consisted of well-differentiated chondrocytes, GAG (Fig. 120.8b) and type II collagen (Fig. 120.8c). A thin layer of flat cells and type I collagen was present at the construct surface (Fig. 120.8d). The weights and dimensions were comparable for constructs grown in microgravity vessels and control spinner flasks. However, microgravity conditions resulted in 1-week constructs with 39% fewer cells (Fig. 120.9a), 37% more GAG per g dw (Fig. 120.9b), and similar amounts of collagen (Fig. 120.9c) [Freed & Vunjak-Novakovic, 1995a].

Two basic criteria have to be met to achieve a spatially uniform, high yield during cell seeding of polymer scaffolds in vitro: a uniform suspension of isolated cells and relative velocity between the cells and the polymer fibers. These requirements can be met using either spinner flasks or micro-gravity bioreactors [Freed & Vunjak-Novakovic, 1995a, 1995b]. Mixing was observed to increase chondrocyte growth rates both on microcarrier beads and in cell-polymer constructs [Freed et al., 1993b, 1994d, Vunjak-Novakovic et al., 1995]. In addition, constructs grown in mixed vessels were larger and contained more cells, GAG, and collagen than constructs grown statically. These findings indicate that tissue culture bioreactors are required for the in vitro cultivation of clinically sized cartilage constructs and that mixing decreases the time required for the in vitro cultivation of constructs with given properties.

Previous studies have shown that: (1) exogenous forces determine cellular production and 3D assembly of tissue ECM in vivo [Koch, 1917; Thompson, 1977], (2) environmental stresses stimu-late cell spreading and proliferation [Ingber & Folkman, 1989] and the formation of protective, cytoskeletal "stress fibers" [Franke et al., 1984], (3) cells cultured in laminar flow chambers flatten and elongate in the direction of fluid flow [Levesque et al., 1985], and (4) extracellular tension or-ganizes extracellular collagen into the form of a peripheral capsule [Harris et al., 1981]. It is likely that the capsule observed at the surfaces of constructs grown under mixed conditions represents the response of the growing tissue to hydrodynamic forces in the in vitro culture environment.

Continuous passive motion (CPM) enhances chondrogenesis in experimental animals [O'Driscoll & Salter, 1984] and cartilage healing in humans [Salter, 1990] due to improve cellular nutrition and stimulation of differentiated cellular function. Note that in natural cartilage, applied pressures are thought to generate microcirculatory currents which facilitate transport of oxygen and nutrients to the cells through tissue macro- and micropores [Poole et al., 1987], since the cells lie 1–3 mm from a nutrient artery [Shapiro et al., 1991]. The synthesis of cartilage ECM (GAG, colla-gen) was increased 20–40% when explanted cartilage tissue was subjected to dynamic compression at frequencies of 0.01–1 Hz but not when explants were compressed statically [Sah et al., 1989]. Another study showed that GAG synthesis was increased by 25% when chondrocyte monolayers were subjected to dynamic hydrostatic pressure cycles at frequencies of 0.25 Hz [Parkkinen et al., 1993]. We found that mixing increased construct cellularity and the contents of GAG and collagen; whether the selective introduction of hydrodynamic forces can enhance the biomechanical prop-erties of tissue engineered cartilage is currently under investigation.

120.3 Summary and Future Directions

Tissue engineering offers a new biologically based therapy for repairing cartilage damaged by arthri-tis, congenital abnormalities, or trauma. Engineered cartilage is here defined as a tissue construct grown in vitro, e.g., using isolated cells and biomaterial scaffolds, as opposed to the direct in vivo implantation of either the isolated chondrocytes or the biomaterial scaffold (Table 120.1). At this time, cartilaginous constructs with clinically useful dimensions can be successfully grown in vitro using chondrocytes, synthetic biodegradable polymer scaffolds and mixed culture vessels [Freed & Vunjak-Novakovic, 1994a, 1994b; Freed et al., 1994b, 1994c]. These constructs consist of viable

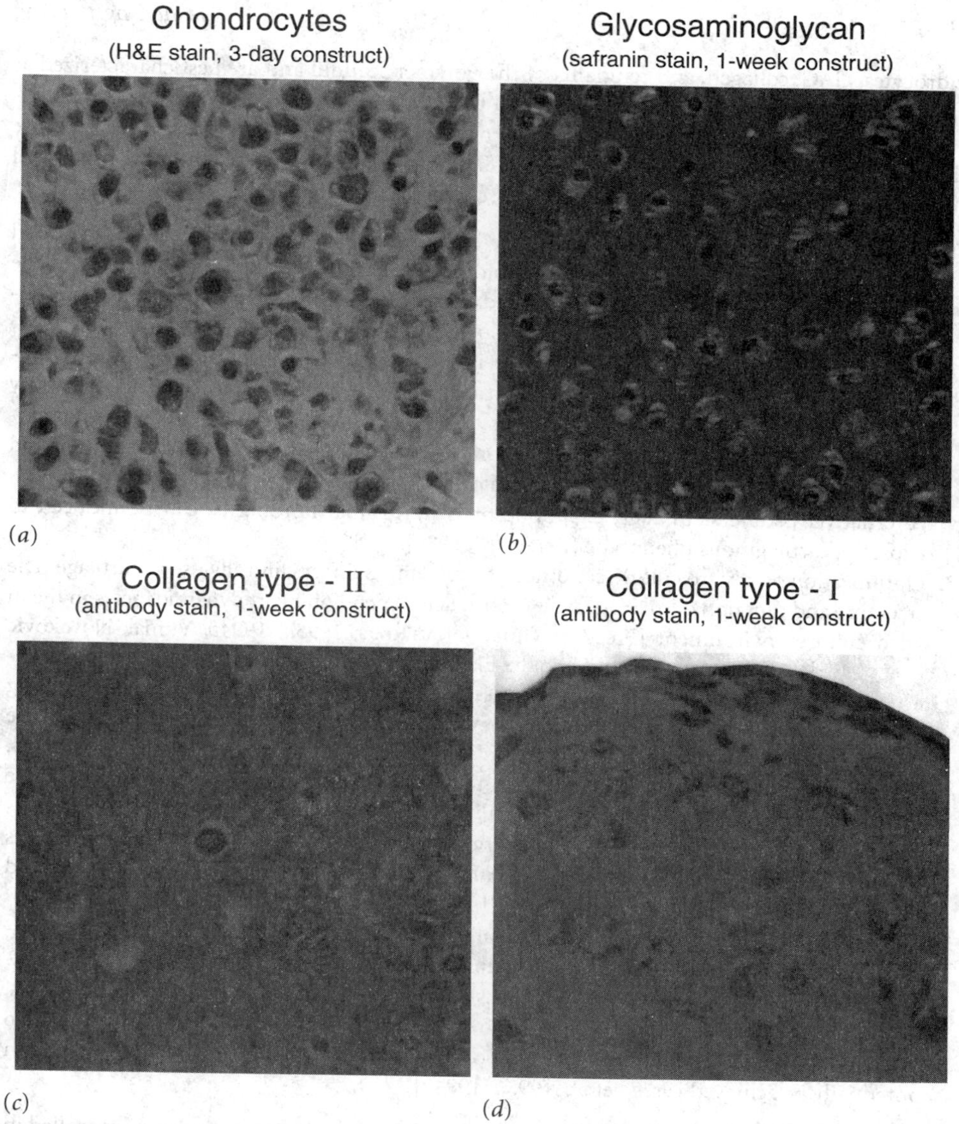

Chondrocytes
(H&E stain, 3-day construct)

Glycosaminoglycan
(safranin stain, 1-week construct)

(a)

(b)

Collagen type - II
(antibody stain, 1-week construct)

Collagen type - I
(antibody stain, 1-week construct)

(c)

(d)

FIGURE 120.8 Histologic appearance of constructs grown in NASA microgravity bioreactors: (a) 3-day construct (cells stained with H&E); (b) 1-week construct (GAG stained with safranin-O); (c), (d) 1-week constructs (type-II or type-I-collagen–stained immunochemically, respectively).

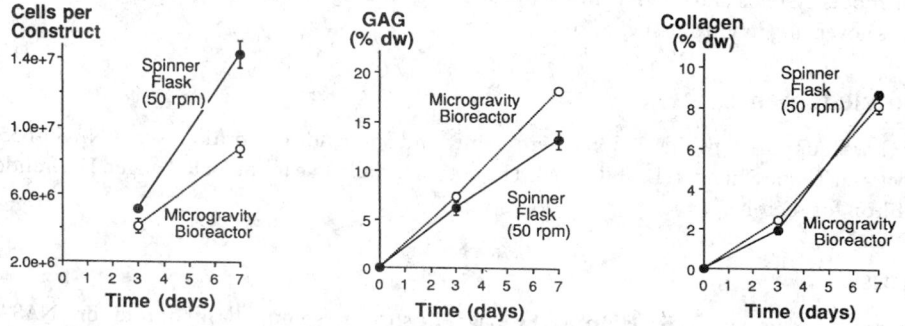

FIGURE 120.9 Biochemical composition of cell-polymer constructs: (a) cells (per construct); (b), (c) GAG or collagen content (%dw). Constructs grown for 0–7 days in microgravity bioreactors are compared to those grown in spinner flasks mixed at 50 rpm (open and closed symbols, respectively).

chondrocytes, GAG, collagen, and remnants of the polymer scaffold and are best characterized as fibro-hyaline cartilage. However, several basic and practical problems still need to be resolved before tissue-engineered cartilage becomes a tool of orthopedic and reconstructive surgeons. Future work should focus on fundamental studies of the factors regulating the 3D assembly of functional cartilage tissue, both in vitro and in vivo. Current research needs include:

1. Establishment of design criteria for tissue-engineered cartilage constructs. The required dimensions, structure, composition, and biomechanical properties of the construct at the time of implantation will necessarily depend on the specific clinical application (e.g., articular cartilage repair, meniscal replacement, cartilage for reconstructive surgery).

2. Development of reliable methods to source, isolate, amplify, and cryopreserve human chondrocytes. Chondrocytes can be isolated from autogenous cartilage harvested by needle biopsy and amplified in the presence of growth factors. If a larger cell mass is needed, allograft cartilage from cadavers can be harvested. Embryonal cells have a higher mitotic potential and are immunoprivileged as compared to chondrocytes from older donors [Nevo et al., 1992]. Alternatively, some stem cells, e.g., bone marrow stromal fibroblasts, can be induced to express a cartilaginous phenotype [Beresford, 1989].

3. Optimization of in vitro culture conditions to custom-engineer clinically useful cartilage. The structure and function of cartilage tissue constructs depend on hydrodynamic forces in the in vitro culture environment [Freed & Vunjak-Novakovic, 1995a, 1994b, Vunjak-Novakovic et al., 1995]. We are currently studying the histologic, biochemical, and biomechanical properties of constructs grown in bioreactor vessels with defined fluid flow fields (e.g., rotating bioreactors, perfused chambers). An attempt will be made to quantify the forces acting on the constructs and to define algorithms for optimizing bioreactor design and operating conditions.

4. Matching the strength of the graft with the biomechanical requirements in vivo. The mechanical properties of tissue-engineered cartilage, like natural cartilage, depend on its composition and structure (e.g., distribution of cells and ECM, molecular interactions between GAG and type II collagen in articular cartilage) which in turn depend on scaffold design and in vitro culture conditions.

5. Further in vivo studies to define construct properties required for successful in vivo integration (e.g., biochemical composition, mechanical strength, outer capsule presence and thickness) and to develop methods of fixing constructs to large defects to resurface entire joints. Continued chondrogenesis of in-vitro-grown cell-polymer constructs following in vivo implantation indicates that full integration of the graft with the surrounding host tissue can potentially be achieved [Freed et al., 1993a, 1994a].

Tissue engineering based on isolated chondrocytes and degradable scaffolds under controlled in vitro culture conditions represents a relatively straightforward procedure to custom-design cartilage constructs. The same approaches and methodologies could potentially be extended to other cell-polymer model systems and should enhance our understanding of the biological and engineering principles governing in vitro tissue morphogenesis.

Acknowledgments

This work was supported by the National Aeronautics and Space Administration (grant NAG9-655) and Advanced Tissue Sciences (La Jolla, CA). The authors would like to thank R. Langer, D. Grande, and R. Biron for their help.

Defining Terms

Bioreactors: Tissue culture vessels mixed by magnetic stirring (spinner flask) or rotation (NASA-developed microgravity bioreactor).

Chondrocytes: Cartilage cells.

Chondrogenesis: The process of cartilage formation.

Extracellular matrix (ECM):   The biochemical components present in the extracellular space of a tissue, e.g., collagen and glycosoaminoglycan (GAG) in cartilage.

Polymer scaffold: A synthetic material designed for cell cultivation, characterized by its specific chemical composition (e.g., polyglycolic acid, PGA) and 3D structure (e.g., fibrous mesh).

Tissue construct: The tissue engineered in vitro by cultivating isolated cells on polymer scaffolds.

References

Bently G. 1989. Grafts and implants for cartilage repair and replacement. Crit Rev Biocompat 5: 245.

Bently G, Greer RB. 1971. Homotransplantation of isolated epiphyseal and articular cartilage chondrocytes into joint surfaces of rabbits. Nature 230:385.

Benya PD, Shaffer JD. 1982. Dedifferentiated chondrocytes reexpress the differentiated collagen phenotype when cultured in agarose gels. Cell 30:215.

Beresford JN. 1989. Osteogenic stem cells and the stromal system of bone and marrow. Clin Orthop 240:270.

Buckwalter JA, Rosenberg LC, Hunziker EB. 1990. Articular cartilage: Composition, structure, response to injury, and methods of facilitating repair. In JW Ewing (ed), Articular Cartilage and Knee Function: Basic Science and Arthroscopy, Ch 2, pp 19–55, New York, Raven Press.

Buschmann MD, Gluzband YA, Grodzinsky AJ, et al. 1992. Chondrocytes in agarose culture synthesize a mechanically functional extracellular matrix. J Orthop Res 10:745.

Campbell CJ. 1969. The healing of cartilage defects. Clin Orthop Rel Res 64:45.

Chesterman PJ, Smith AU. 1968. Homotransplantation of articular cartilage and isolated chondrocytes: an experimental study in rabbits. J Bone Joint Surg 50B:184.

Cima LG, Vacanti JP, Vacanti C, et al. 1991. Tissue engineering by cell transplantation using degradable polymer substrates. J Biomech Eng 113:143.

De Groot JH, Nijenhuis AJ, Bruin P, et al. 1990. Use of porous biodegradable polymer implants in meniscus reconstruction: 1) Preparation of porous biodegradable polyurethanes for the reconstruction of meniscus lesions. Colloid Polym Sci 268:1073.

Elema H, de Groot JH, Nijenhuis AJ et al. 1990. Use of porous biodegradable polymer implants in meniscus reconstruction: 2) Biological evaluation of porous biodegradable polymer implants in menisci. Colloid Polym Sci 268:1082.

Farndale RW, Buttle DJ, Barrett AJ. 1986. Improved quantitation and discrimination of sulphated glycosaminoglycans by the use of dimethylmethylene blue. Biochim Biophys Acta 883:173.

Franke RP, Grafe M, Schnittler H, et al. 1984. Induction of human vascular endothelial stress fibres by fluid shear stress. Nature 307:648.

Frazza EJ, Schmitt EE. 1971. A new absorbable suture. J Biomed Mater Res Symp 1:43.

Freed LE, Grande DA, Emmanual J, et al. 1994a. Joint resurfacing using allograft chondrocytes and synthetic biodegradable polymer scaffolds. J Biomed Mater Res 28:891.

Freed LE, Marquis JC, Nohria A, et al. 1993a. Neocartilage formation in vitro and in vivo using cells cultured on synthetic biodegradable polymers. J Biomed Mat Res 27:11.

Freed LE, Marquis JC, Vunjak-Novakovic G, et al. 1994b. Composition of cell-polymer cartilage implants. Biotech Bioeng 43:605.

Freed LE, Vunjak-Novakovic G. 1995a. Cultivation of cell-polymer constructs in simulated microgravity. Biotech Bioeng 46:306–313.

Freed LE, Vunjak-Novakovic G. 1995b. Microgravity tissue engineering. In Vitro Cell Dev Biol (in press).

Freed LE, Vunjak-Novakovic G, Biron RJ, et al. 1994c. Biodegradable scaffolds for tissue engineering. Biotechnology 12:689–693.

Freed LE, Vunjak-Novakovic G, Langer R. 1993b. Cultivation of cell-polymer cartilage implants in bioreactors. J Cell Biochem 51:257.

Freed LE, Vunjak-Novakovic G, Marquis JC, et al. 1994*d*. Kinetics of chondrocyte growth in cell-polymer implants. Biotech Bioeng 43:597.

Glowacki J, Trepman E, Folkman J. 1983. Cell shape and phenotypic expression in chondrocytes. Proc Soc Exp Biol Med 172:93.

Goodwin TJ, Jessup JM, Wolf DA. 1992: Morphological differentiation of colon carcinoma cell lines HT-29 & HT-29KM in rotating-wall vessels. In Vitro Cell Dev Biol 28A:47.

Grande DA, Pitman MI, Peterson L, et al. 1989. The repair of experimentally produced defects in rabbit articular cartilage by autologous chondrocyte transplantation. J Orthop Res 7:208.

Green WT. 1977. Articular cartilage repair: behavior of rabbit chondrocytes during tissue culture and subsequent allografting. Clin Orthop Rel Res 124:237.

Gristina AG. 1987. Biomaterial-centered infection: Microbial adhesion versus tissue integration. Science 237:1588.

Harris GK, Stopak D, Wild P. 1981. Fibroblast traction as a mechanism for collagen morphogenesis. Nature 290:249.

Ingber DE, Folkman J. 1989. Tension and compression as basic determinants of cell form and function: utilization of a cellular tensegrity mechanism. In W Stein, F Bronner (eds), Cell Shape: Determinants, Regulation and Regulatory Role, pp 1–32, Orlando, Fla, Academic Press.

Itay S, Abramovici A, Nevo Z. 1987. Use of cultured embryonal chick epiphyseal chondrocytes as grafts for defects in chick articular cartilage. Clin Orth Rel Res 220:284.

Kim YJ, Sah RL, Doong JYH, et al. 1988. Fluorometric assay of DNA in cartilage explants using Hoechst 33258. Anal Biochem 174:168.

Klompmaker J, Jansen HWB, Veth RPH, et al. 1992. Porous polymer implants for repair of full-thickness defects of articular cartilage: and experimental study in rabbit and dog. Biomaterials 13:625.

Koch, J. 1917. The laws of bone architecture. Am J Anat 21:177–298.

Langer F, Gross AE. 1974. Immunogenicity of allograft articular cartilage. J Bone Joint Surg 56A:297.

Langer R, Vacanti JP. 1993. Tissue engineering. Science 260:920.

Levesque MJ, Nerem RM. 1985. The elongation and orientation of cultured endothelial cells in response to shear stress. J Biomech Eng 107:341.

McKee GK. 1982. Total hip replacement—past, present and future. Biomaterials 3:130.

Messner K. 1993. Hydroxylapatite supported Dacron plugs for repair of isolated full-thickness osteochondral defects of the rabbit femoral condyle: mechanical and histological evaluations from 6–48 weeks. J Biomed Mater Res 27:1527.

Messner K, Gillquist J. 1993*a*. Synthetic implants for the repair of osteochondral defects of the medial femoral condyle: A biomechanical and histological evaluation in the rabbit knee. Biomaterials 14:513.

Messner K, Gillquist J. 1993*b*. Prosthetic replacement of the rabbit medial meniscus. J Biomed Mater Res 27:1165.

Messner K. 1994. Meniscal substitution with a Teflon-periosteal composite graft: a rabbit experiment. Biomaterials. 15:223–230.

Minns RJ, Muckle DS. 1989. Mechanical and histological response of carbon fibre pads implanted in the rabbit patella. Biomaterials 10:273.

Minns RJ, Muckle DS, Donkin JE. 1982. The repair of osteochondral defects in osteoarthritic rabbit knees by the use of carbon fibre. Biomaterials 3:81.

Mow VC, Ratcliffe A, Poole AR. 1992. Cartilage and diarthrodial joints as paradigms for hierarchical materials and structures. Biomaterials 13:67.

Mow VC, Ratcliffe A, Rosenwasser MP, et al. 1991. Experimental studies on the repair of large osteochondral defects at a high weight bearing area of the knee joint: a tissue engineering study. Trans ASME 113:198.

Nerem RM. 1991. Cellular engineering. Ann Biomed Eng 19:529.

Nevo Z, Robinson D, Halperin N. 1992. The use of grafts composed of cultured cells for repair and regeneration of cartilage and bone. In BK Hall (ed), Bone: Fracture Repair and Regeneration, pp 123–152, Boca Raton, Fla, CRC Press.

Nixon AJ, Sams AE, Lust G, et al. 1993. Temporal matrix synthesis and histologic features of a chondrocyte-laden porous collagen cartilage analogue. Amer J Vet Res 54:349.

O'Driscoll SW, Kelley FW, Salter RB. 1986. The chondrogenic potential of free autogenous periosteal grafts for biological resurfacing of major full-thickness defects in joint surfaces under the influence of continuous passive motion. J Bone Joint Surg 68A:1017.

O'Driscoll SW, Salter RB. 1984. The induction of neochondrogenesis in free intra-articular periosteal autografts under the influence of continuous passive motion: an experimental study in the rabbit. J Bone Joint Surg 66A:1248.

Parkkinen JJ, Ikonen J, Lammi MJ, et al. 1993. Effects of cyclic hydrostatic pressure on proteoglycan synthesis in cultured chondrocytes and articular cartilage explants. Arch Biochem Biophys 300:458.

Peterson CD, Hillberry BM, Heck DA. 1988. Component wear of total knee prostheses using Ti-6A1-4V, titanium nitride coated Ti-6Al–4V, and cobalt-chromium-molybdenum femoral components. J Biomed Mater Res 22:887.

Poole CA, Flint MH, Beaumont BW. 1987. Chondrons in cartilage: ultrastructural analysis of the pericellular microenvironment in adult human articular cartilages. J Orthop Res 5:509.

Robinson D, Halperin N, Nevo Z. 1990. Regenerating hyaline cartilage in articular defects of old chickens using implants of embryonal chick chondrocytes embedded in a new natural delivery substance. Calcif Tiss Int 46:246.

Sah RL, Kim YJ, Doong JY, et al. 1989. Biosynthetic response of cartilage explants to dynamic compression. J Orthop Res 7:619.

Salter RB. 1990. The biological concept of continuous passive motion of synovial joints: The first 18 years of basic research and its clinical application. In JW Ewing (ed), Articular Cartilage and Knee Function: Basic Science and Arthroscopy, pp 335–352, New York, Raven Press.

Schwarz RP, Goodwin TJ, Wolf DA. 1992. Cell culture for three-dimensional modeling in rotating-wall vessels: An application of simulated microgravity. J Tiss Cult Meth 14:51.

Shapiro IM, Tokuoka T, Silverton SF. 1991. Energy metabolism in cartilage. In BK Hall, SA Newman (eds), Cartilage: Molecular Aspects, pp 97–130, Boca Raton, Fla, CRC Press.

Speer DP, Chvapil M, Volz RG, et al. 1979. Enhancement of healing in osteochondral defects by collagen sponge implants. Clin Orthop Rel Res 144:326.

Stone KR, Rodkey WG, Webber R, et al. 1992. Meniscal regeneration with copolymeric collagen scaffolds. Amer J Sports Med 20:104.

Tacchetti C, Tavella S, Dozin B, et al. 1992. Cell condensation in chondrogenic differentiation. Exper Cell Res 200:26.

Takigawa M, Shirai E, Fukuo K, et al. 1987. Chondrocytes dedifferentiated by serial monolayer culture form cartilage nodules in nude mice. Bone Miner 2:449.

Thompson DW. 1977. On Growth and Form, pp 221–267, New York, Cambridge University Press.

Upton J, Sohn SA, Glowacki J. 1981. Neocartilage derived from transplanted perichondrium: What is it? Plast Reconst Surg 68:166.

Vacanti C, Langer R, Schloo B, et al. 1991. Synthetic biodegradable polymers seeded with chondrocytes provide a template for new cartilage formation *in vivo*. Plast Reconstr Surg 88:753.

Von Schroeder HP, Kwan M, Amiel D, et al. 1991. The use of polylactic acid matrix and periosteal grafts for the reconstruction of rabbit knee articular defects. J Biomed Mater Res 25:329.

Vunjak-Novakovic G, Freed LE, Biron RJ, et al.,1995. Effects of mixing on tissue engineered cartilage. J AICHE (submitted).

Wakitani S, Kimura T, Hirooka A, et al. 1989. Repair of rabbit articular surfaces with allograft chondrocytes embedded in collagen gel. J Bone Joint Surg 71B:74.

Watt F. 1986. The extracellular matrix and cell shape. Trends Biochem Sci 11:482.

Woessner JF. 1961. The determination of hydroxyproline in tissue and protein samples containing small proportions of this amino acid. Arch Biochem Biophys 93:440.

Zanetti NC, Solursh M. 1989. Effect of cell shape on cartilage differentiation. In WD Stein, F Bronner (eds), Cell Shape, Determinants, Regulation and Regulatory Role, pp 291–327, San Diego, Academic Press.

Zhang X, Goosen MFA, Wyss UP, et al. 1993. Biodegradable polymers for orthopedic applications. J Macromol Sci Rev Macromol Chem Phys C33:81.

Zukor DJ, Oakeshott RD, Brooks PJ, McAuley, et al. 1990. Fresh, small fragment osteochondral allografts for posttraumatic defects of the knee. In JW Ewing (ed), Articular Cartilage and Knee Joint Function: Basic Science and Arthroscopy, New York, Raven Press.

Further Information

Ewing JW. 1990. Articular Cartilage and Knee Joint Function: Basic Science and Arthroscopy, New York, Raven Press.

Hall BK. 1992. Bone: Fracture Repair and Regeneration, Boca Raton, Fla, CRC Press.

Hall BK, Newman SA. 1991. Cartilage: Molecular Aspects, Boca Raton, Fla, CRC Press.

Maroudas A, Kuettner K. 1990. Methods in Cartilage Research, London, Academic Press.

Mow VC, Ratcliffe A, Poole AR. 1992. Cartilage and diarthrodial joints as paradigms for hierarchical materials and structures. Biomaterials 13:67.

Skalak R, Fox CF. 1988. Tissue Engineering, New York, Alan Liss.

Van den Berg WB, van der Kraan PM, van Lent PL. 1993. Joint Destruction in Arthritis and Osteoarthritis. Agents Actions Suppl 39.

121

Tissue Engineering of the Kidney

H. David Humes
University of Michigan

Tissue engineering is one of the most intriguing and exciting areas in biotechnology due to its requirements for state-of-the-art techniques from both biologic and engineering disciplines. This field is on the threshold of the development of an array of products and devices comprised of cell components, biologic compounds, and synthetic materials to replace physiologic function of diseased tissues and organs.

Successful tissue and organ constructs depend on a thorough understanding and creative application of molecular, cellular, and organ biology and the principles of chemical, mechanical, and material engineering to produce appropriate structure-function relationships to restore, maintain, or improve tissue or organ function. This approach depends on the most advanced scientific methodologies, including stem cell culture, gene transfer, growth factors, and biomaterial technologies.

The kidney was the first solid organ whose function was approximated by a machine and a synthetic device. In fact, renal substitution therapy with hemodialysis or chronic ambulatory peritoneal dialysis (CAPD) has been the only successful long-term ex vivo organ substitution therapy to date [1]. The kidney was also the first organ to be successfully transplanted from a donor individual to an autologous recipient patient. However, the lack of widespread availability of suitable transplantable organs has kept kidney transplantation from becoming a practical solution to most cases of chronic renal failure.

Although long-term chronic renal replacement therapy with either hemodialysis or CAPD has dramatically changed the prognosis of renal failure, it is not complete replacement therapy, since it only provides filtration function (usually on an intermittent basis) and does not replace the homeostatic, regulatory, metabolic, and endocrine functions of the kidney. Because of the nonphysiologic manner in which dialysis performs or does not perform the most critical renal functions, patients with ESRD on dialysis continue to have major medical, social, and economic problems [2]. Accordingly, dialysis should be considered as renal substitution rather than renal replacement therapy.

Tissue engineering of a biohybrid kidney comprised of both biologic and synthetic components will most likely have substantial benefits for the patient by increasing life expectancy, increasing mobility and flexibility, increasing quality of life with large savings in time, less risk of infection, and reduced costs. This approach could also be considered a cure rather than a treatment for patients.

121.1 Fundamentals of Kidney Function

The kidneys are solid organs located behind the peritoneum in the posterior abdomen and are critical to body homeostasis because of their excretory, regulatory, metabolic, and endocrinologic functions. The excretory function is initiated by filtration of blood at the glomerulus, which is an enlargement of the proximal end of the tubule incorporating a vascular tuft. The structure of the glomerulus is designed to provide efficient ultrafiltration of blood to remove toxic waste from the circulation yet retain important circulating components, such as albumin. The regulatory function of the kidney, especially with regard to fluid and electrolyte homeostasis, is provided by the tubular segments attached to the glomerulus.

The ultrafiltrate emanating from the glomerulus courses along the kidney tubule, which resorbs fluid and solutes to finely regulate their excretion in various amounts in the final urine. The kidney tubules are segmented, with each segment possessing differing transport characteristics for processing the glomerular ultrafiltrate efficiently and effectively to regulate urine formation. The segments of the tubule begin with the proximal convoluted and straight tubules, where most salt and water are resorbed. This segment leads into the thin and thick segments of Henle's loop, which are critical to

the countercurrent system for urinary concentration and dilution of water. The distal tubule is next and is important for potassium excretion. The final segment is the collecting duct, which provides the final regulation of sodium, hydrogen, and water excretion. The functional unit of the kidney is therefore composed of the filtering unit (the glomerulus) and the regulatory unit (the tubule). Together they form the basic component of the kidney, the nephron. In addition to these excretory and regulatory functions, the kidney is an important endocrine organ. Erythropoietin, active forms of vitamin D, renin, angiotensin, prostaglandins, leukotrienes, and kallikrein-kinins are some of the endocrinologic compounds produced by the kidney.

In order to achieve its homeostatic function for salt and water balance in the individual, the kidney has a complex architectural pattern (Fig. 121.1). This complex organization is most evident in the exquisitely regulated structure-function interrelationships between the renal tubules and vascular structures to coordinate the countercurrent multiplication and exchange processes to control water balance with urinary concentration and dilution [3]. This complex structure is the result of a long evolutionary process in which animals adapted to many changing environmental conditions. Although well suited for maintaining volume homeostasis, the mammalian kidney is an inefficient organ for solute and water excretion. In humans, approximately

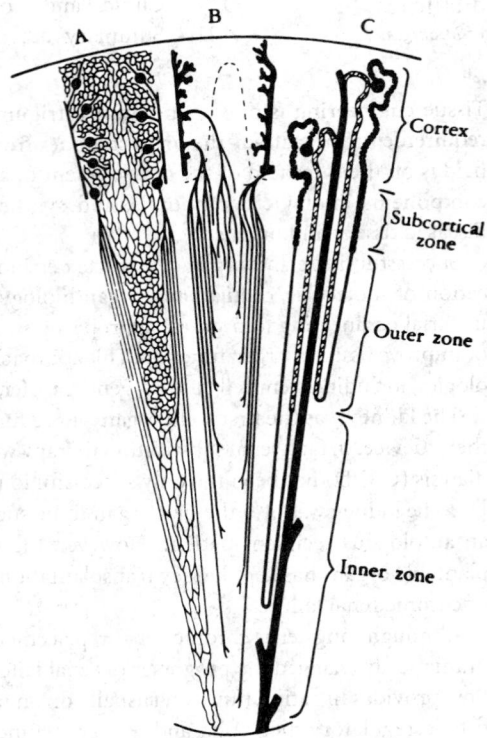

FIGURE 121.1 Representation of the complex morphologic architecture of a section of a mammalian kidney in which these components are schematized separately: (*a*) arterial and capillary blood vessels; (*b*) venous drainage; (*c*) two nephrons with their glomeruli and tubule segments. (*Source:* From [3] with permission.)

180 liters of fluid are filtered into the tubules daily, but approximately 178 liters must be reabsorbed into the systemic circulation. Because of the importance of maintaining volume homeostasis in an individual to prevent volume depletion, shock, and death, multiple redundant physiologic systems exist within the body to maintain volume homeostasis. No such redundancy, however, exists to replace renal excretory function of soluble metabolic toxic byproducts of metabolic activity. Accordingly, chronic renal disease becomes a clinical disorder due to loss of renal excretory function and buildup within the body of metabolic toxins which require elimination by the kidneys. Because of the efficiency inherent in the kidneys as an excretory organ, life can be sustained with only 5–10% of normal renal excretory function. With the recognition that the complexity of renal architectural organization is driven by homeostatic rather than excretory function and that renal excretory function is the key physiologic process which must be maintained or replaced to treat clinical renal failure, the approach to a tissue engineering construct becomes easier to entertain, especially since only a fraction of normal renal excretory function is required to maintain life.

For elimination of solutes and water from the body, the kidney utilizes simple fundamental physical principles which govern fluid movement (Fig. 121.2). The kidney's goal in excretory function is to transfer solutes and water from the systemic circulation into tubule conduits in order to eliminate toxic byproducts from the body in a volume of only several liters. Solute and fluid removal from the systemic circulation is the major task of the renal filtering apparatus, the glomerulus. The force responsible for this filtration process is the hydraulic pressure generated within the systemic circulation due to myocardial contraction and blood vessel contractile tone. Most of the filtered fluid and solutes must be selectively reabsorbed by the renal tubule as the initial filtrate courses along the renal tubule. This reabsorptive process depends upon osmotic forces generated by active solute transport by the renal epithelial cell and the colloid oncotic pressure within the peritubular capillary (Fig. 121.2). The approach of a tissue-engineering construct for renal replacement is to mimic these natural physical forces to duplicate filtration and reabsorption processes to attain adequate excretory function lost in renal disorders.

Glomerular Ultrafiltration

The process of urine formation begins within the capillary bed of the glomerulus [4]. The glomerular capillary wall has evolved into a structure with the property to separate as much as one-third of the plasma entering the glomerulus into a solution of a nearly ideal ultrafiltrate. This high rate of ultrafiltration across the glomerular capillary is a result of hydraulic pressure generated by the pumping action of the heart and the vascular tone of the preglomerular and postglomerular vessels as well as the high hydraulic permeability of the glomerular capillary walls. This hydraulic pressure and hydraulic permeability of the glomerular capillary bed is at least two times and two orders of magnitude higher, respectively, than most other capillary networks within the body [5]. Despite this high rate of water and solute flux across the glomerular capillary wall, this same structure retards the filtration of important circulating macromolecules, especially albumin, so that all but the lower-molecular-weight plasma proteins are restricted in their passage across this filtration barrier.

A variety of experimental studies and model systems have been employed to characterize the sieving properties of the glomerulus. Hydrodynamic models of solute transport through pores have been successfully used to describe the size selective barrier function of this capillary network to macromolecules [6]. This pore model, in its simplest form, assumes the capillary wall to contain cylindrical pores of identical size and that macromolecules are spherical particles. Based upon the steric hindrances that macromolecules encounter in the passage through small pores, whether by diffusion or by convection (bulk flow of fluid), definition of the glomerular capillary barrier can be defined by solving hydrodynamic equations governing the movement of a spherical particle through a fluid-filled cylindrical pore (Fig. 121.3). This modeling characterizes the glomerular capillary barrier as a membrane with uniform pores of 50Å radius [7]. This pore size predicts that molecules with radii smaller than 14Å appear in the filtrate in the same concentration as in plasma water. Since

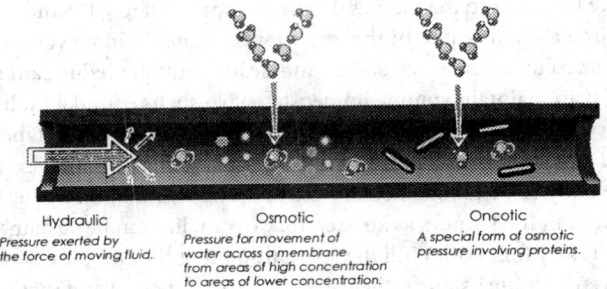

Hydraulic
Pressure exerted by the force of moving fluid.

Osmotic
Pressure for movement of water across a membrane from areas of high concentration to areas of lower concentration.

Oncotic
A special form of osmotic pressure involving proteins.

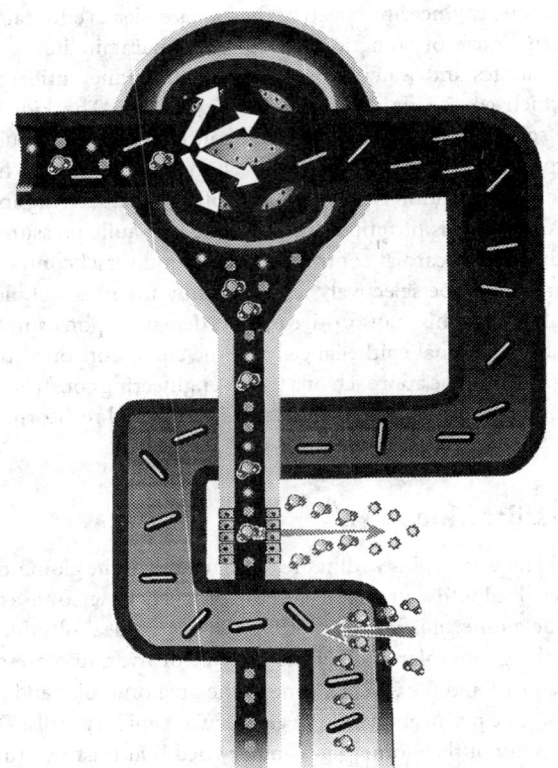

FIGURE 121.2 Physical forces which govern fluid transfer within the kidney.

there is no restriction to filtration, fractional clearance of this size molecule is equal to one. The filtration of molecules of increasing size decreases progressively, so that the fractional clearance of macromolecules the size of serum albumin (36Å) is low.

The glomerular barrier, however, does not restrict molecular transfer across the capillary wall only on the basis of size (Fig. 121.4). This realization is based upon the observation that the filtration of the circulating protein, albumin, is restricted to a much greater extent than would be predicted from size alone. The realization that albumin is a polyanion at physiologic pH suggests that molecular charge, in addition to molecular size, is another important determination of filtration of macro-molecules [8]. The greater restriction to the filtration of circulating polyanions, including albumin, is due to the electrostatic hindrance by fixed negatively charged components of the glomerular

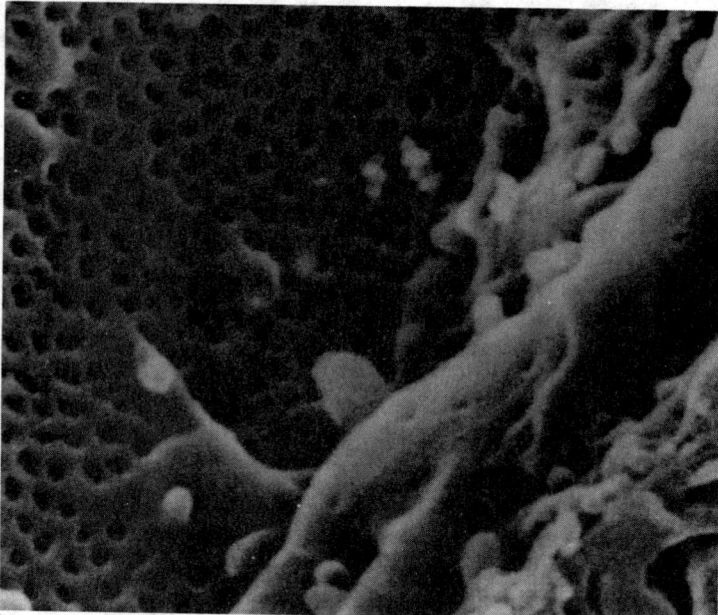

FIGURE 121.3 Scanning electron micrograph of the glomerular capillary wall demonstrating the fenestrae (pores) of the endothelium within the glomerulus (mag ×50,400). Reprinted with permission from Schrier RW, Gottschalk CW. 1988. Diseases of the Kidney, p 12, Boston, Little, Brown.

capillary barrier. These fixed negative charges, as might be expected, simultaneously enhance the filtration of circulating polycations.

Thus, the formation of glomerular ultrafiltrate, the initial step in urine formation, depends upon the pressure and flows within the glomerular capillary bed and the intrinsic permselectivity of the glomerular capillary wall. The permselective barrier excludes circulating macromolecules from

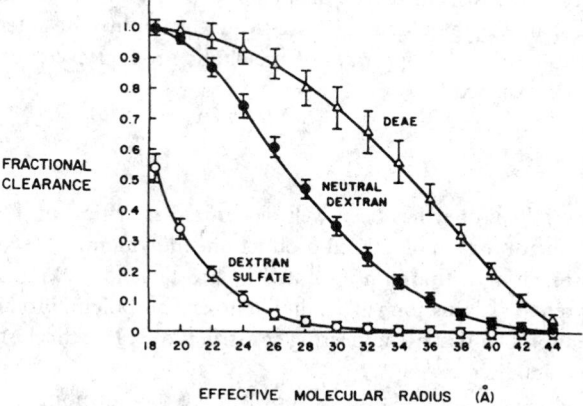

FIGURE 121.4 Fractional clearances of negatively charged (sulfate) dextrans, neutral dextrans, and positively charged (DEAE) dextrans of varying molecular size. These data demonstrate that the glomerular capillary wall behaves as both a size-selective and charge-selective barrier [8].

filtration based upon size as well as net molecular charge, so that for any given size, negatively charged macromolecules are restricted from filtration to a greater extent than neutral molecules.

Tubule Reabsorption

Norman human kidneys form approximately 100 ml of filtrate every minute. Since daily urinary volume is roughly 2 L more than 98% of the glomerular ultrafiltrate must be reabsorbed by the renal tubule. The bulk of the reabsorption, 50–65%, occurs along the proximal tubule. Similar to glomerular filtration, fluid movement across the renal proximal tubule cell is governed by physical forces. Unlike the fluid transfer across the glomerular capillary wall, however, tubular fluid flux is principally driven by osmotic and oncotic pressures rather than hydraulic pressure (Fig. 121.2). Renal proximal tubule fluid reabsorption is based upon active Na^+ transport, requiring the energy-dependent $Na^+K^+ATPase$ located along the basolateral membrane of the renal tubule cell to promote a small degree of luminal hypotonicity [9]. This small degree of osmotic difference (2–3 mOsm/kg H_2O) across the renal tubule is sufficient to drive isotonic fluid reabsorption due to the very high diffusive water permeability of the renal tubule cell membrane. Once across the renal proximal tubule cell, the transported fluid is taken up by the peritubular capillary bed due to the favorable oncotic pressure gradient. This high oncotic pressure within the peritubular capillary is the result of the high rate of protein-free filtrate formed in the proximate glomerular capillary bed [10]. As can be appreciated, the kidney has evolved two separate capillary networks to control bulk fluid flow from various fluid compartments of the body. The glomerular capillary network has evolved an efficient structure to function as a highly efficient filter to allow water and small solutes, such as urea and sodium, to cross the glomerular capillary wall while retaining necessary macro-molecules, such as albumin. This fluid transfer is driven by high hydraulic pressures within the glomerular capillary network generated by the high blood flow rates to the kidney and a finely regulated vascular system. The permselectivity of the filter is governed by an effective pore size to discriminate macromolecular sieving based upon both size and net molecular charge. The high postglomerular vascular resistance and the protein-free glomerular filtrate results, respectively, in low hydraulic pressure and high oncotic pressure within the peritubular capillary system which follows directly in series from the glomerular capillary network. The balance of physical forces within the peritubular capillaries, therefore, greatly favors the uptake of fluid back into the systemic circulation. The addition of a renal epithelial monolayer with high rates of active Na^+ transport and high hydraulic permeability assists further in the high rate of salt and water reabsorption along the proximal tubule. Thus, an elegant system has evolved in the nephron to filter and reabsorb large amounts of fluid in bulk to attain high rates of metabolic product excretion while maintaining regulatory salt and water balance.

Endocrine

As an endocrine organ, the kidney has been well recognized as critical in the production of ery-thropoietin, a growth factor for red blood cell production, and vitamin D, a compound important in calcium metabolism, along with, but not limited to, prostaglandins, kinins, and renin. For the purposes of this chapter, this discussion will be limited to erythropoietin production as an example of a potential formulation of a tissue-engineering construct to replace this lost endocrine function in chronic end-stage renal disease.

More than 40 years ago erythropoietin was shown to be the hormone that regulates erythro-poiesis, or red blood cell production, in the bone marrow [11]. In adults, erythropoietin is produced primarily (greater than 90%) by specialized interstitial cells in the kidney [12]. Although the liver also synthesizes erythropoietin, the quantity is not adequate (less than 10%) to maintain adequate red cell production in the body [13]. The production of erythropoietin by the kidney is regulated by a classic endocrinologic feedback loop system. As blood flows through the kidney, the erythropoietin-producing cells are in an ideal location to sense oxygen delivery to tissues by red cells in the bloodstream, since they are located adjacent to peritubular capillaries in the renal interstitium.

As demonstrated in Fig. 121.5, erythropoietin production is inversely related to oxygen delivery to the renal interstitial cells. With hypoxemia or decline in red blood cell mass, a decline in oxygen delivery occurs to these specialized cells, and increased erythropoietin production develops. Upon return to normal oxygen delivery with normoxia and red blood cell mass, the enhanced production of erythropoietin is suppressed, closing the classic feedback loop. Of importance, the regulation of erythropoietin in the kidney cells depends upon transcriptional control, not upon secretory control, as seen with insulin [14]. The precise molecular mechanism of the oxygen sensor for tissue oxygen availability has not been delineated but appears to depend on a heme protein.

Once erythropoietin is released, it circulates in the bloodstream to the bone marrow, where it signals the marrow to produce red blood cells. In this regard, all blood cells, both white and red cells, originate from a subset of bone marrow cells, called *multipotent stem cells*. These stem cells develop during embryonic development and are maintained through adulthood via self-regulation. Under appropriate stimulation, stem cells proliferate and produce committed, more highly differentiated progenitor cells which are then destined to a specific differentiated line of blood cells, including neutrophils, lymphocytes, platelets, and red cells. Specifically, erythropoietin binds to receptors on the outer membrane of committed erythroid progenitor cells, stimulating the terminal steps in erythroid differentiation. Nearly 200 years ago, it was first recognized that anemia is a complication of chronic renal failure. Ordinarily an exponential increase in serum erythropoietin levels are observed when the hemoglobin level in patients declines below 10 gm/dl. In the clinical state of renal disease, however, the normal increase in erythropoietin in response to anemia is impaired [14]. Although the oxygen delivery (or hemoglobin) to erythropoietin feedback loop is still intact, the response is dramatically diminished. In patients with end-stage renal disease (ESRD), the hematocrit levels are directly correlated to circulating erythropoietin levels. In fact, ESRD patients with bilateral nephrectomies have the lowest hematocrits and lowest rates of erythropoiesis, demon-

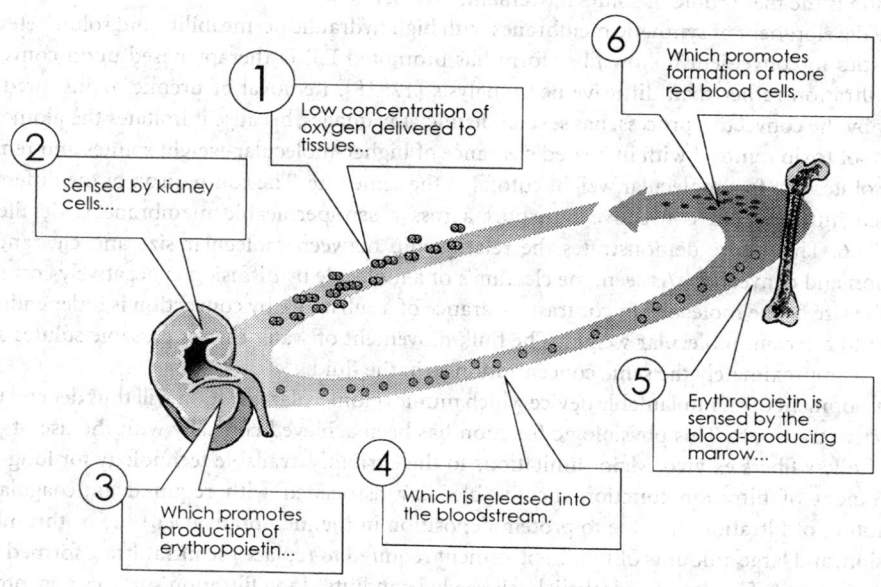

FIGURE 121.5 Endocrinologic feedback loop which regulates erythropoietin production by the kidney.

strating that even the small amount of erythropoietin produced by the end-stage kidney is important. Thus, the loss of renal function due to chronic disease results in an endocrine deficiency of a hormone normally produced by the kidney and results in a clinical problem that complicates the loss of renal excretory function.

121.2 Tissue-Engineering Formulation Based upon Fundamentals

In designing an implantable bioartificial kidney for renal replacement function, essential functions of kidney tissue must be utilized to direct the design of the tissue-engineering project. The critical elements of renal function must be replaced, including the excretory, regulatory (reabsorptive), and endocrinologic functions. The functioning excretory unit of the kidney, as detailed previously, is composed of the filtering unit, the glomerulus, and the regulatory or reabsorptive unit, the tubule. Therefore, a bioartificial kidney requires two main units, the glomerulus and the tubule, to replace renal excretory function.

Bioartificial Glomerulus: The Filter

The potential for a bioartificial glomerulus has been achieved with the use of polysulphone fibers ex vivo with maintenance of ultrafiltration in humans for several weeks with a single device [15, 16]. The availability of hollow fibers with high hydraulic permeability has been an important advancement in biomaterials for replacement function of glomerular ultrafiltration. Conventional hemodialyses for ESRD have used membranes in which solute removal is driven by a concentration gradient of the solute across the membranes and is, therefore, predominantly a diffusive process. Another type of solute transfer also occurs across the dialysis membrane via a process of ultrafiltration of water and solutes across the membrane. This convective transport is independent of the concentration gradient and depends predominantly on the hydraulic pressure gradient across the membrane. Both diffusive and convective processes occur during traditional hemodialysis, but diffusion is the main route of solute movement.

The development of synthetic membranes with high hydraulic permeability and solute retention properties in convenient hollow fiber form has promoted ESRD therapy based upon convective hemofiltration rather than diffusive hemodialysis [17, 18]. Removal of uremic toxins, predominantly by the convective process, has several distinct advantages, because it imitates the glomerular process of toxin removal with increased clearance of higher-molecular-weight solutes and removal of all solutes (up to a molecular weight cutoff) at the same rate. The comparison of the differences between diffusive and convective transport across a semipermeable membrane is detailed in Fig. 121.6. This figure demonstrates the relationship between molecular size and clearance by diffusion and convection. As seen, the clearance of a molecule by diffusion is negatively correlated with the size of the molecule. In contrast, clearance of a substance by convection is independent of size up to a certain molecular weight. The bulk movement of water carries passable solutes along with it in approximately the same concentration as in the fluid.

Development of an implantable device which mimics glomerular filtration will thus depend upon convective transport. This physiologic function has been achieved clinically with the use of polymeric hollow fibers ex vivo. Major limitations to the currently available technology for long-term replacement of filtration function include bleeding associated with required anticoagulation, diminution of filtration rate due to protein deposition in the membrane over time or thrombotic occlusion, and large amounts of fluid replacement required to replace the ultrafiltrate formed from the filtering unit. The use of endothelial-cell-seeded conduits along filtration surfaces may provide improved long-term hemocompatibility and hemofiltration in vivo [19, 20, 21], as schematized in Fig. 121.7.

In this regard, endothelial cell seeding of small-caliber vascular prosthesis has been shown experimentally to reduce long-term platelet deposition, thrombus formation, and loss of graft

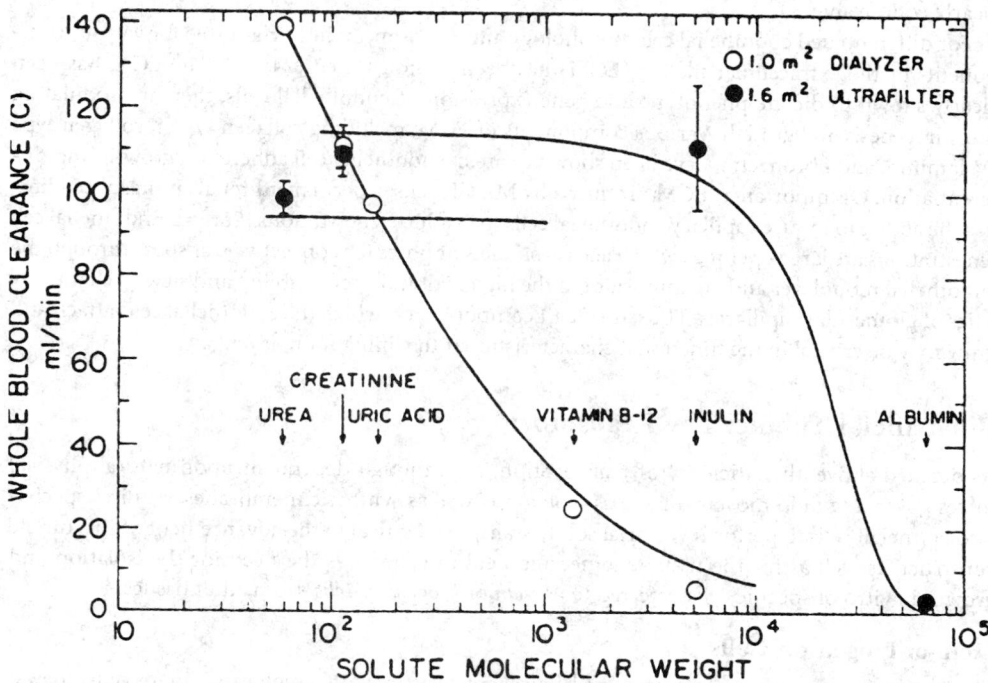

FIGURE 121.6 Relationship between solute molecular size and clearance by diffusion (open circles) and convection (closed circles). Left curve shows solute clearance for a 1.0 m² dialyzer with no ultrafiltration where solute clearance is by diffusion. Right curve shows clearance for a 1.6 m² ultrafilter where solute clearance is by convection. Smaller molecules are better cleared by diffusion; larger molecules by convection. Normal kidneys clear solutes in a pattern similar to convective transport. (Figure adapted from [18].)

patency [21]. Recent results in humans have demonstrated success in autologous endothelial cell seeding in small caliber grafts after growth of these cells along the graft lumen ex vivo to achieve a confluent monolayer prior to implantation. Long-term persistent endothelialization and patency of the implanted graft has been reported [19]. A potential rate-limiting step in endothelial-cell-lined hollow fibers of small caliber is thrombotic occlusion, which limits the functional patency of this filtration unit. In this regard, gene transfer into seeded endothelial cells for constitutive expression of anticoagulant factors can be envisioned to minimize clot formation in these small-caliber hollow fibers. Since gene transfer for in vivo protein production has been clearly achieved with endothelial

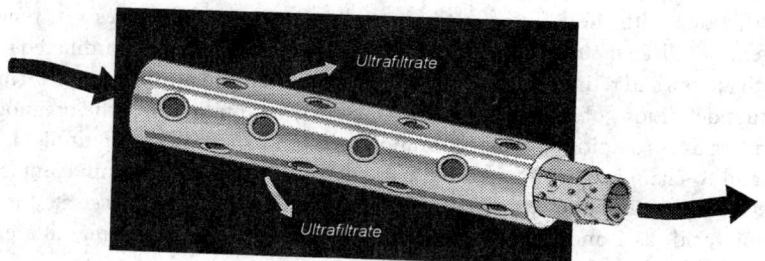

FIGURE 121.7 Conceptual schematization of bioartificial glomerulus.

cells [22, 23], gene transfer into endothelial cells for the production of an anticoagulant protein is clearly conceivable.

For differentiated endothelial cell morphology and function, an important role for various components of the extracellular matrix (ECM) has been demonstrated [24, 25]. The ECM has been clearly shown to dictate phenotype and gene expression of endothelial cells, thereby modulating morphogenesis and growth. Various components of ECM, including collagen type I, collagen type IV, laminin, and fibronectin, have been shown to affect endothelial cell adherence, growth, and differentiation. Of importance, ECM produced by MDCK cells, a permanent renal epithelial cell line, has the ability to induce capillary endothelial cells to produce fenestrations [25, 26]. Endothelial cell fenestrations are large openings which act as channels or pores for convective transport through the endothelial monolayer and are important in the high hydraulic permeability and sieving characteristics of glomerular capillaries. Thus, the ECM component on which the endothelial cells attach and grow may be critical in the functional characteristics of the lining monolayer.

Bioartificial Tubule: The Reabsorber

As detailed above, the efficiency of reabsorption, even though dependent upon natural physical forces governing fluid movement across biologic as well as synthetic membranes, requires specialized epithelial cells to perform vectorial solute transport. Critical to the advancement of this tubule construct, as well as for the tissue-engineering field in general, is the need for the isolation and growth in vitro of specific cells, referred to as *stem* or *progenitor cells,* from adult tissues.

Stem or Progenitor Cells

These cells are those that possess stem-cell-like characteristics with a high capacity for self-renewal and the ability to differentiate under defined conditions into specialized cells to develop correct structure and functional components of a physiologic organ system [27, 28, 29]. Stem cells have been extensively studied in three adult mammalian tissues: the hematopoietic system, the epidermis, and the intestinal epithelium. Recent work has also suggested that stem cells may also reside in the adult nervous system [30]. Little insight into possible renal tubule stem cells had been developed until recent data demonstrating methodology to isolate and grow renal proximal tubule stem or progenitor cells from adult mammalian kidneys [31, 32]. This series of studies was promoted by the clinical and experimental observations suggesting that renal proximal tubule progenitor cells must exist, because they have the ability to regenerate after severe nephrotoxic or ischemic injury to form a fully functional and differentiated epithelium [33, 34]. Whether proximal tubule progenitor cells are pluripotent, possessing the ability to differentiate into cells of other segments (such as loop of Henle, distal convoluted tubule) as in embryonic kidney development, is presently unclear; the clinical state of acute tubular necrosis certainly supports the idea that proximal tubule progenitor cells have the ability to replicate and differentiate into proximal tubule cells with functionally and morphologically differentiated phenotypes.

In this regard, recent data have demonstrated, using renal proximal tubule cells in primary culture, that the growth factors transforming growth factor-β1 (TGF-β1) and epidermal growth factor (EGF), along with the retinoid, retinoic acid, promoted tubulogenesis in renal proximal tubule progenitor cells in tissue culture [31]. These observations defined a coordinated interplay between growth factors and retinoids to induce pattern formation and morphogenesis. This finding is one of the first definitions of inductive factors which may be important in the organogenesis of a mammalian organ. In addition, using immunofluorescence microscopy, retinoic acid induced laminin A- and B$_1$-chain production in these cells and purified soluble laminin completely substituted for retinoic acid in kidney tubulogenesis. These results clearly demonstrate the manner in which retinoic acid, as a morphogen, can promote pattern formation and differentiation by regulating the production of an extracellular matrix molecule.

Further work has demonstrated, in fact, that a population of cells resides in the adult mammalian kidney which have retained the capacity to proliferate and morphogenically differentiate into tubule structures in vitro [32]. These experiments have identified non-serum-containing growth conditions, which select for proximal tubule cells with a high capacity for self-renewal and an ability to differentiate phenotypically, collectively and individually, into proximal tubule structures in collagen gels. Regarding the high capacity for self-renewal, genetic marking of the cells with a recombinant retrovirus containing the *lacZ* gene and dilution analysis demonstrated that in vitro tubulogenesis often arose from clonal expansion of a single genetically tagged progenitor cell. These results suggest that a population of proximal tubule cells exist within the adult kidney in a relatively dormant, slowly replicative state, but with a rapid potential to proliferate, differentiate, and pattern-form to regenerate the lining proximal tubule epithelium of the kidney following severe ischemic or toxic injury.

Bioartificial Tubule Formulation

The bioartificial renal tubule is now clearly feasible when conceived as a combination of living cells supported on polymeric substrata [35]. A bioartificial tubule uses epithelial progenitor cells cultured on water and solute-permeable membranes seeded with various biomatrix materials so that expression of differentiated vectorial transport and metabolic and endocrine function is attained (Figs. 121.8, 121.9, 121.10). With appropriate membranes and biomatrices, immunoprotection of cultured progenitor cells can be achieved concurrent with long-term functional performance as long as conditions support tubule cell viability [35, 36]. The technical feasibility of an implantable epithelial cell system derived from cells grown as confluent monolayers along the luminal surface of polymeric hollow fibers has been achieved [35]. These previously constructed devices, however, have used permanent renal cell lines which do not have differentiated transport function. The ability to purify and grow renal proximal tubule progenitor cells with the ability to differentiate morphogenically may provide a capability for replacement renal tubule function.

A bioartificial proximal tubule satisfies a major requirement of reabsorbing a large volume of filtrate to maintain salt and water balance within the body. The need for additional tubule equivalents to replace another nephronal segment function, such as the loop of Henle, to perform more refined homeostatic elements of the kidney, including urine concentration or dilution, may not be necessary. Patients with moderate renal insufficiency lose the ability to finely regulate salt and water homeostasis—because they are unable to concentrate or dilute, yet are able to maintain reasonable

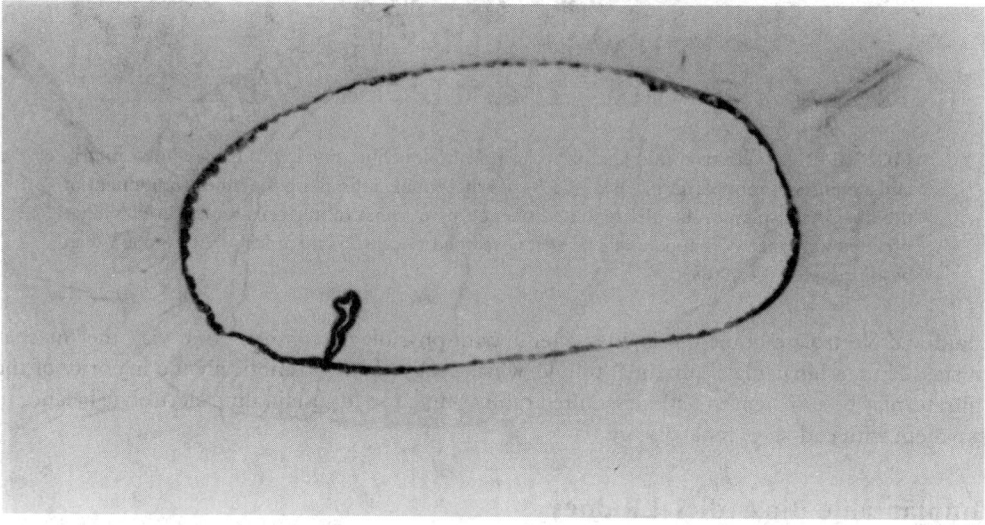

FIGURE 121.8 Light micrograph of an H&E section (100×) of hollow fiber lined with collagen type IV and confluent monolayer of human renal tubule epithelial cells along the inner component of the fiber. In this fixation process, the hollow fiber is clear with the outer contour of the hollow fiber identified by the irregular line (disregard artifact in lower left quadrant).

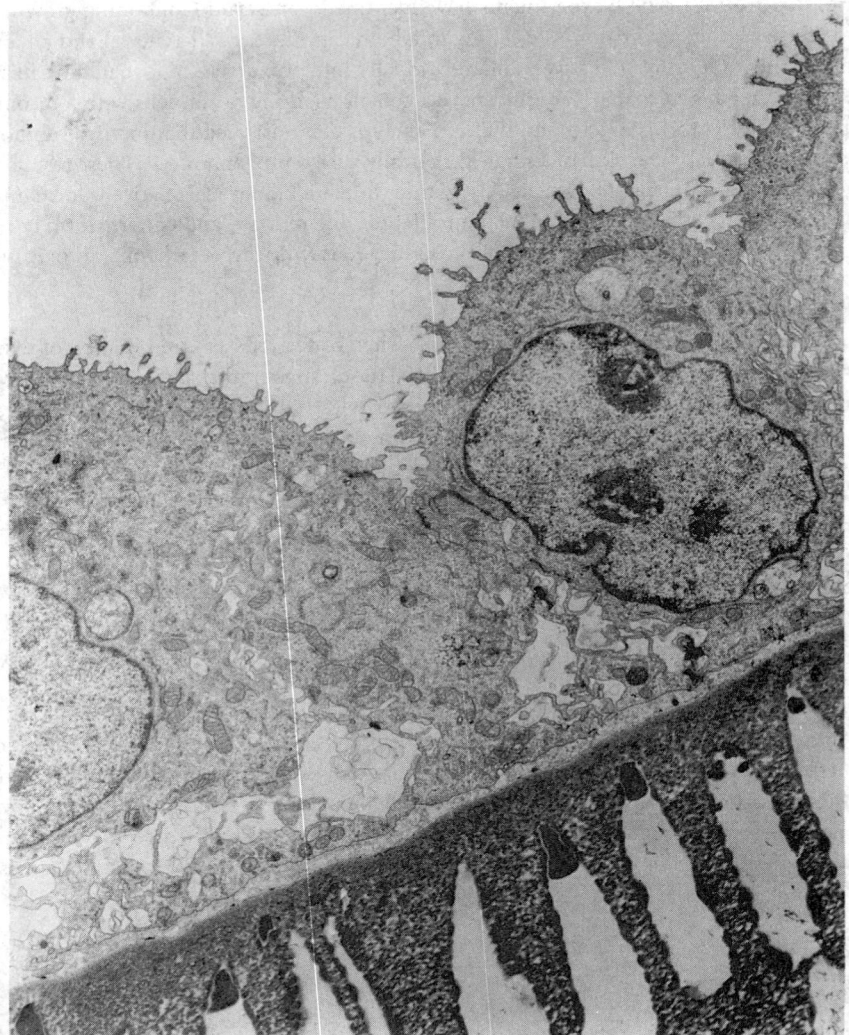

FIGURE 121.9 Electron micrograph of a single hollow fiber lined with extracellular matrix and a confluent monolayer (see Fig. 121.8) of renal tubule cells along the inner component of the fiber. As displayed, the differentiated phenotype of renal tubule cells on the hollow fiber prelined with matrix is apparent. The well developed microvilli and apical tight junctions can be appreciated (14,000×).

fluid and electrolyte homeostasis due to redundant physiologic compensation via other mechanisms. Thus, a bioartificial proximal tubule, which reabsorbs iso-osmotically the majority of the filtrate, may be sufficient to replace required tubular function to sustain fluid electrolyte balance in a patient with end-stage renal disease.

Implantable Bioartificial Kidney

The development of a bioartificial filtration device and a bioartificial tubule processing unit would lead to the possibility of an implantable bioartificial kidney, consisting of the filtration device followed in series by the tubule unit (Fig. 121.11). The filtrate formed by this device will flow directly

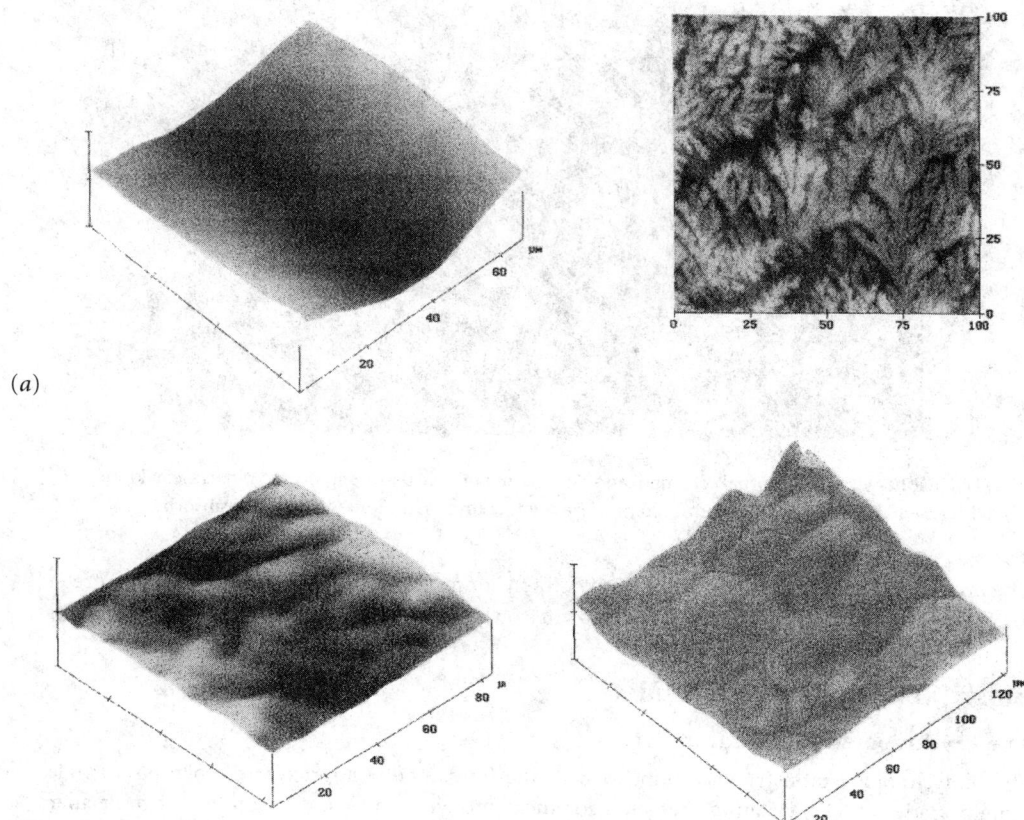

(a)

(b)

FIGURE 121.10 (a) Atomic force microscopy (AFM) images (100 μm by 100 μm) of polysulphone hollow fiber cut longitudinally and opened in buffered saline solution (left) and hollow fibers with adherent synthetic extracellular matrix material, ProNectin F, along the inner surface (right). Notice the reorganization of the ProNectin into fernlike islands. (b) Atomic force microscopy (AFM) images (100 μm by 100 μm) of human umbilical-vein endothelial cells (HUVEC) (left) and renal proximal tubule cells (right) grown for 7–10 days on a polysulphone hollow fiber with preadhered ProNectin F. Notice the cobblestone appearance of the confluent monolayer of both types of cells. Microvilli are clearly seen along the apical luminal border of the tubule cells. (AFM images performed by J. P. Anderson from the College of Engineering, University of Michigan.)

into the tubule unit. The tubule unit should maintain viability, because metabolic substrates and low-molecular-weight growth factors are delivered to the tubule cells from the ultrafiltration unit. Furthermore, immunoprotection of the cells grown within the hollow fiber is achievable due to the impenetrance of immunologically competent cells through the hollow fiber. Rejection of transplanted cells will, therefore, not occur. This arrangement thereby allows the filtrate to enter the internal compartments of the hollow fiber network, which are lined with confluent monolayers of renal tubule cells for regulated transport function.

This device could be used either extracorporeally or implanted within a patient. In this regard, the specific implant site for a bioartificial kidney will depend upon the final configuration of both the bioartificial filtration and tubule device. As presently conceived, the endothelial-lined bioartificial filtration hollow fibers can be placed into an arteriovenous circuit using the common iliac artery and vein, similar to the surgical connection for a renal transplant. The filtrate is connected in series to a bioartificial proximal tubule, which is embedded into the peritoneal membrane, so that reabsorbate will be transported into the peritoneal cavity and reabsorbed into the systemic circulation.

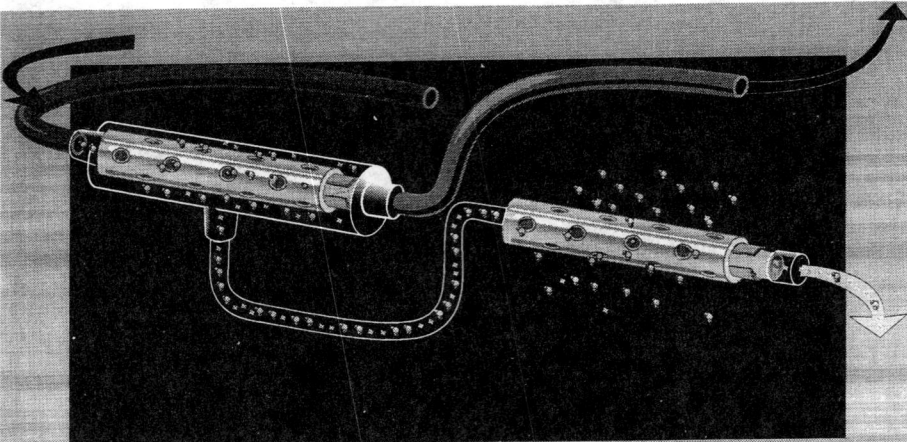

FIGURE 121.11   Conceptual schematization of an implantable tissue engineered bioartificial kidney with an endothelial-cell-lined hemofilter in series with a proximal tubule-cell-lined reabsorber.

The processed filtrate exiting the tubule unit is then connected via tubing to the proximate ureter for drainage and urine excretion via the recipient's own urinary collecting system.

Bioartificial Endocrine Gland

The Erythropoietin Generator

The biotechnology industry was founded with the fundamental approach of isolating a single protein made by cells, isolating the genes for these proteins, and using recombinant molecular biologic techniques to introduce these genes into prokaryotic or eukaryotic expression systems to produce large quantities of the gene product. Human growth hormone, human insulin, and human erythropoietin are key examples of the implementation and success of this strategy. Such successes, however, have been less common than anticipated, since the use of a single protein for identifiable useful purposes has been difficult for several reasons. First, complex interactions and networks of multiple proteins, as opposed to a single protein, are needed to promote a therapeutic effect. Second, targeted delivery to the site of disease is difficult to attain. And finally, adequate dosage without toxic effects may not be achievable.

Cell therapy may be the next successful strategy in biotechnology to overcome these prior difficulties [37]. Because specialized cells are programmed to carry out specific biologic tasks, cell therapy may deliver several key proteins in a coordinated cascade to promote a biologic or physiologic process, such as wound healing. Targeted delivery of a specific deficient protein, hormone, or neurotransmitter may be achieved with site-specific implantation of cells which can produce this deficient compound after being encapsulated in special polymeric membranes. The membranes allow cell nutrients into the encapsulated space to maintain cell viability and allow cellular metabolic wastes to exit along with the desired protein, hormone, or neurotransmitter while shielding the cells from the host's destructive immune response. This strategy is being employed, for example, to deliver dopamine produced by bovine adrenal cells to the substantia nigra where a deficiency of this neurotransmitter at this site leads to Parkinson's Disease [37].

Regulated and homeostatic drug dosing may also be achieved with cell therapy. For hormonal therapy, such as insulin for diabetes mellitus, appropriate insulin levels within the body are only crudely attained with once-a-day or twice-a-day dosing. Any hormone-producing cell has a highly evolved biologic sensing system to monitor the ambient environment and respond with graded production and release of the hormone to regulate the sensed level of the moiety which is regulated.

The circulating level of a protein or a hormone may be regulated at several levels: at the gene level by transcriptional mechanisms, at the protein level by translational processes, or at the secretory level by cellular processes. The complexity of regulation increases several-fold, as control progresses from transcriptional to translational to excretory processes. Accordingly, a more refined differentiated cell phenotype is required to maintain a regulated secretory process compared to a transcriptional process. The lack of success of encapsulation of insulin-producing cells is due to the fact that the cells are unable to maintain a viable, highly differentiated state to sense ambient glucose levels and release preformed insulin in a regulated, differentiated secretory pathway. In contrast, since erythropoietin production is regulated by transcriptional mechanisms, the ability to identify and perhaps grow cells from adult mammalian kidneys with the ability to regulate erythropoietin production in response to oxygen delivery may allow the design of an implantable cell therapy device to sense circulating oxygen levels and regulate erythropoietin production based upon a biologic sensing mechanism.

121.3 Clinical and Economic Implications

Although long-term chronic renal replacement therapy with either hemodialysis or CAPD has dramatically changed the prognosis of renal failure, it is not complete replacement therapy, since it only provides filtration function (usually in an intermittent basis) and does not replace the excretory, regulatory, and endocrine functions of the kidney. Because of the nonphysiologic manner in which dialysis performs or does not perform the most critical renal functions, patients with ESRD on dialysis continue to have major medical, social, and economic problems. Renal transplant addresses some of these issues, but immunologic barriers and organ shortages keep this approach from being ideal for a large number of ESRD patients.

Although dialysis or transplantation therapies can prolong the life of a patient with ESRD disease, it is still a serious medical condition, with ESRD patients having only one-fifth the life expectancy of a normal age-matched control group. ESRD patients also experience significantly greater morbidity. Patients with ESRD have five times the hospitalization rate, nearly twice the disability rate, and five times the unemployment rate of age-matched non-ESRD individuals [2]. Accordingly, this new technology based upon the proposed bioengineering prototypes would most likely have substantial benefits to the patient by increasing life expectancy, increasing mobility and flexibility, increasing quality of life with large savings in time, less risk of infection, and reduced costs.

Besides the personal costs to the patient and family, care of chronic kidney failure is monetarily expensive on a per-capita basis in comparison to most forms of medical care [1, 2]. The 1989 estimated Medicare payment (federal only) per ESRD patient during the entire year averaged $30,900. The patient and private insurance obligations were an additional $6900 per patient. The total cost of a patient per year with end-stage renal disease, therefore, is approximately $40,000. In 1988 the expected life span after beginning dialysis for an ESRD patient was approximately 4 years; therefore, the total costs per patient of ESRD during his or her lifetime was approximately $160,000 in 1988.

The total cost in 1989 of direct medical payments for ESRD, by both public and private payors, was $6 billion per year. These estimates do not include a number of indirect cost items, since they do not include patient travel costs, outpatient drugs, and lost labor production. The current number of patients receiving chronic dialytic therapy in the United States is over 200,000 with a current growth rate of new patients with ESRD in the United States receiving chronic dialytic therapy at 8–9%. The 1995 estimated total annual cost of treatment is approximately $10 billion for the treatment of patients with end-stage renal disease in the United States. It is conceivable that in the not-too-distant future this tissue-engineering technology could supplant current treatments for ESRD. Although it is difficult to estimate the value of a technology, a purely economic evaluation suggests a major objective cost savings of this technology.

With regard to erythropoietin therapy, the development of an injectable form of recombinant human erythropoietin has brought tremendous benefit to the patient on dialysis with end-stage renal disease [38]. The dependency on blood transfusions in this patient population was decreased; enhanced exercise capacity was achieved in patients; major improvements in patient symptoms and sense of well-being were demonstrated with this agent. Regression of left ventricular hypertrophy and enhanced cognitive brain function were also commonly observed. As with any new biotechnologic therapy, substantial cost can be attributed to this new treatment program. On average, human recombinant erythropoietin costs $5300 per dialysis patient per year [38]. The exact incremental cost for the treatment of ESRD patients, however, is difficult to quantitate, since this treatment has decreased the requirements of blood transfusions in these patients and limited the cardiac symptoms of these patients.

The overall cost of erythropoietin in the treatment of anemia of chronic renal failure in 1992 was approximately $500 million. The high cost of this agent is due to the continuing need to administer the recombinant protein. Once a patient with chronic anemia due to erythropoietin deficiency is begun on replacement therapy, the need for this agent in the treatment of anemia is required for the rest of the patient's lifetime with repeated administration on a three-times-a-week basis with careful monitoring and dose adjustment to maintain adequate hematocrit and hemoglobin levels. A new, more efficacious and cost-effective therapeutic strategy can be entertained with the use of cell therapy as a drug delivery vehicle as detailed in the previous section. Regulated homeostatic drug dosing will optimize drug dosing and eliminate the need and cost of repeated drug administration.

121.4 Summary

Three technologies will most likely dominate medical therapeutics in the next century. One is "cell therapy"—the implantation of living cells to produce a natural substance in short supply from the patient's own cells due to injury and destruction from various clinical disorders. Erythropoietin cell therapy is an example of this approach to replace a critical hormone deficiency in end-stage renal disease. A second therapy is tissue engineering, wherein cells are cultured to replace masses of cells that normally function in a coordinated manner. Growing a functional glomerular filter and tubule reabsorber from a combination of cells, biomaterials and synthetic polymers to replace renal excretory and regulatory functions is an example of this formulation. Finally, a third technology that will dominate future therapeutics is gene therapy, in which genes are transferred into living cells either to deliver a gene product to a cell in which it is missing or to produce a foreign gene product by a cell to promote a new function. The use of genes which encode for anticoagulant proteins as a means to deliver in a targeted and local fashion an anticoagulant to maintain hemocompatibility of a tissue engineered hemofilter is an example of the application of this third technology.

The kidney was the first organ whose function was substituted by an artificial device. The kidney was also the first organ to be successfully transplanted. The ability to replace renal function with these revolutionary technologies in the past was due to the fact that renal excretory function is based upon natural physical forces which govern solute and fluid movement from the body compartment to the external environment. The need for coordinated mechanical or electrical activities for renal substitution was not required. Accordingly, the kidney may well be the first organ to be available as a tissue-engineered implantable device as a fully functional replacement part for the human body.

References

1. Iglehart JK. 1993. The American Health Care System: The End Stage Renal Disease Program. N Engl J Med 328:366.
2. Excerpts from United States Renal Data System 1991 Annual Data Report. Prevalence and cost of ESRD therapy. Am J Kidney Diseases 18(5)(supp)2:21.
3. Kriz W, Lever AF. 1969. Renal countercurrent mechanisms: Structure and function. Am Heart J 78:101.

4. Brenner BM, Humes HD. 1977. Mechanisms of glomerular ultra-filtration. N Engl J Med 297:148.

5. Landis EM, Pappenheimer JR. Exchange of substances through the capillary walls. In WF Hamilton, P Dow (eds), Handbook of Physiology: Circulation, sec 2, vol 2, p 961, Washington DC, American Physiological Society.

6. Anderson JL, Quinn JA. 1974. Restricted transport in small pores. A model for steric exclusion and hindered particle motion. Biophys J 14:130.

7. Chang RLS, Robertson CR, Deen WM, et al. 1975. Permselectivity of the glomerular capillary wall to macromolecules: I. Theoretical considerations. Biophys J 15:861.

8. Brenner BM, Hostetter TH, Humes HD. 1978. Molecular basis of proteinuria of glomerular origin. N Engl J Med 298:826.

9. Andreoli TE, Schafer JA. 1978. Volume absorption in the pars recta: III. Luminal hypotonicity as a driving force for isotonic volume absorption. Am J Physiol 234(4):F349.

10. Knox FG, Mertz JI, Burnett JC, et al. 1983. Role of hydrostatic and oncotic pressures in renal sodium reabsorption. Circ Res 52:491.

11. Jacobson LO, Goldwasser E, Fried W, et al. 1957. Role of kidney in erythropoiesis. Nature. 179:633.

12. Maxwell PH, Osmond MK, Pugh CW, et al. 1993. Identification of the renal erythropoietin-producing cells using transgenic mice. Kidney Int 44:1149.

13. Fried W. 1972. The liver as a source of extrarenal erythropoietin production. Blood 40:671.

14. Jelkmann W. 1992. Erythropoietin: Structure, control of production, and function. Physiolog Rev 72(2):449.

15. Golper TA. 1986. Continuous arteriorvenous hemofiltration in acute renal failure. Am J Kidney Dis 6:373.

16. Kramer P, Wigger W, Rieger J, et al. 1977. Arterior-venous haemofiltration: A new and simple method for treatment of overhydrated patients resistant to diuretics. Klin Wochenschr 55:1121.

17. Colton CK, Henderson LW, Ford CA, et al. 1975. Kinetics of hemodiafiltration. In vitro transport characteristics of a hollow-fiber blood ultrafilter. J Lab Clin Med 85:355.

18. Henderson LW, Colton CK, Ford CA. 1975. Kinetics of hemodiafiltration: II. Clinical characterization of a new blood cleansing modality. J Lab Clin Med 85:372.

19. Kadletz M, Magometschnigg H, Minar E, et al. 1992. Implantation of in vitro endothelialized polytetrafluoroethylene grafts in human beings. J Thorac Cardiovasc Surg 104:736.

20. Schnider PA, Hanson SR, Price TM, et al. 1988. Durability of confluent endothelial cell monolayers of small-caliber vascular prostheses in vitro. Surgery 103:456.

21. Shepard AD, Eldrup-Jorgensen J, Keough EM, et al. 1986. Endothelial cell seeding of small-caliber synthetic grafts in the baboon. Surgery 99:318.

22. Zweibel JA, Freeman SM, Kantoff PW, et al. 1989. High-level recombinant gene expression in rabbit endothelial cells transduced by retroviral vectors. Science 243:220.

23. Wilson JM, Birinyi LK, Salomon RN, et al. 1989. Implantation of vascular grafts lined with genetically modified endothelial cells. Science 244:1344.

24. Carey DJ. 1991. Control of growth and differentiation of vascular cells by extracellular matrix proteins. Annu Rev Physiol 53:161.

25. Carley WW, Milici AJ, Madri JA. 1988. Extracellular matrix specificity for the differentiation of capillary endothelial cells. Exp Cell Res 178:426.

26. Milici AJ, Furie MB, Carley WW. 1985. The formation of fenestrations and channels by capillary endothelium in vitro. Proc Natl Acad Sci 82:6181.

27. Garlick JA, Katz AB, Fenjves ES, et al. 1991. Retrovirus-mediated transduction of cultured epidermal keratinocytes. J Invest Dermatol 97:824.

28. Hall PA, Watt FM. 1989. Stem cells: The generation and maintenance of cellular diversity. Development 106:619.

29. Potten CS, Lieffler M. 1990. Stem cells; lessons for and from the crypt. Development 110:1001.

30. Reynolds BA, Weiss S. 1992. Generation of neurons and astrocytes from isolated cells of the adult mammalian central nervous system. Science 255:1707.

31. Humes HD, Cieslinski DA. 1992. Interaction between growth factors and retinoic acid in the induction of kidney tubulogenesis. Exp Cell Res 201:8.

32. Humes HD, Krauss JC, Cieslinski DA, et al. Tubulogenesis from isolated single cells of adult mammalian kidney: Clonal analysis with a recombinant retrovirus (submitted).

33. Coimbra T, Cieslinski DA, Humes HD. 1990. Exogenous epidermal growth factor enhances renal repair in mercuric chloride-induced acute renal failure. Am J Physiol 259:F483.

34. Humes HD, Cieslinski DA, Coimbra T, et al. 1989. Epidermal growth factor enhances renal tubule cell regeneration and repair and accelerates the recovery of renal function in postischemic acute renal failure. J Clin Invest 84:1757.

35. Ip TK, Aebischer P. 1989. Renal epithelial-cell-controlled solute transport across permeable membranes as the foundation for a bioartificial kidney. Artif Organs 13:58.

36. Aebischer P, Wahlberg L, Tresco PA, et al. 1991. Macroencapsulation of dopamine-secreting cells by coextrusion with an organic polymer solution. Biomaterials 12:50.

37. Tai IT, Sun AM. 1993. Microencapsulation of recombinant cells: A new delivery system for gene therapy. FASEB J 7:1061.

38. Aebischer P, Tresco PA, Winn SR, et al. Long-term cross-species brain transplantation of a polymer-encapsulated dopamine-secreting cell line. Exp Neurol 111:269.

39. Nissenson AR (ed). 1993. Proceedings from ESRD patient management: Strategies for meeting the clinical and economic challenges. Am J Kidney Dis 22(2):Supplement 1.

Photograph of Carp...ttee...w...ws...um...dith...the

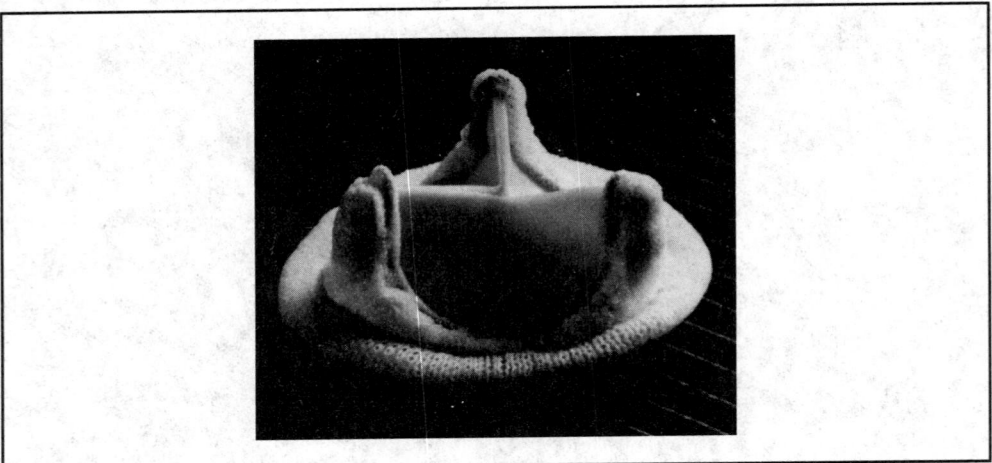

Photograph of Carpentier-Edwards pericardial valve.

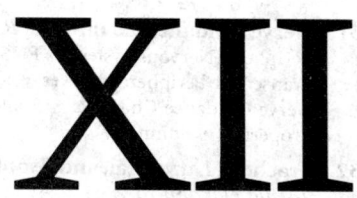

XII

Prostheses and Artificial Organs

Pierre M. Galletti
Brown University

XII.1 Substitutive Medicine

Over the past 50 years, humanity has progressively discovered that an engineered device or the transplantation of organs, tissues, or cells can substitute for most, and perhaps all, organs and body functions. The devices are human-made, whereas the living replacement parts can be obtained from the
patient, a relative, a human cadaver, or a live animal or can be prospectively developed through
genetic engineering. The concept that a disease state may be addressed not only by returning the
malfunctioning organ to health using chemical agents or physical means but also by replacing
the missing function with a natural or an artificial counterpart has brought about a revolution in
therapeutics. Currently in the United States alone, 2 to 3 million patients a year are treated with a
human-designed spare part (assist device, prosthesis, or implant), with the result that over
20 million people enjoy a longer or better quality of life thanks to artificial organs. In comparison,
a shortage of donor organs limits the number of transplantation procedures to about 20,000 a year,
and the total population of transplant survivors is on the order of 200,000.

The fundamental tenet of substitutive medicine is that beyond a certain stage of failure, it is more
effective to remove and replace a malfunctioning organ than to seek in vain to cure it. This ambitious proposition is not easy to accept. It goes against the grain of holistic views of the integrity of
the person. It seems at odds with the main stream of twentieth-century scientific medicine, which
strives to elucidate pathophysiologic mechanisms at the cellular and molecular level and then to correct them through a specific biochemical key. The technology of organ replacement rivals that of
space travel in complexity and fanfare and strikes the popular imagination by its daring, its
triumphs, and its excesses. Although the artificial organ approach does not reach the fundamental
objective of medicine, which is to understand and correct the disease process, it is considerably more
effective than drug therapy or corrective surgery in the treatment of many conditions, e.g., cardiac
valve disease, heart block, malignant arrhythmia, arterial obstruction, cataract.

A priori, functional disabilities due to the destruction or wear of body parts can be addressed in
two ways: the implantation of prosthetic devices or the transplantation of natural organs. For a
natural organ transplants, we typically borrow a spare part from a living being or from an equally
generous donor who before death volunteered to help those suffering from terminal organ failure.
Transplanted organs benefit from refinements acquired over thousands of years of evolution. They
are overdesigned, which means they will provide sufficient functional support even though the

donated part may not be in perfect condition at the time of transfer to another person. They have the same shape and the same attachment needs as the body part they replace, which means that surgical techniques are straightforward. The critical problem is the shortage of donors, and therefore only a small minority of patients currently benefit from this approach.

Artificial organs have different limitations. Seen on the scale of human evolution, they are still primitive devices, tested for 40 years at most. Yet they have transformed the prognosis of many heretofore fatal diseases, which are now allowed to evolve past what used to be their natural termination point. In order to design artificial organs, inventive engineers, physiologists, and surgeons think in terms of functional results, not anatomical structures. As a result, artificial organs have but a distant similarity to natural ones. They are mostly made of synthetic materials (often called biomaterials) which do not exist in nature. They use different mechanical, electrical, or chemical processes to achieve the same functional objectives as natural organs. They adapt but imperfectly to the changing demands of human activity. They cannot easily accommodate body growth and therefore are more beneficial to adults than to children. Most critically, artificial organs, as is the case for all machines, have a limited service expectancy because of friction, wear, or decay of construction materials in the warm, humid, and corrosive environment of the human body. Such considerations limit their use to patients whose life expectancy matches the expected service life of the replacement part or to clinical situations where repeated implantations are technically feasible. In spite of these obstacles, the astonishing reality is that millions of people are currently alive thanks to cardiac pacemakers, cardiac valves, artificial kidneys or hydrocephalus drainage systems, all of which address life-threatening conditions. An even larger number of people enjoy the benefits of hip and knee prostheses, vascular grafts, intraocular lenses, and dental implants, which correct dysfunction, pain, inconvenience, or merely appearance. In short, the clinical demonstration of the central dogma of substitutive medicine over the span of two generations can be viewed demographically as the first step in an evolutionary jump which humans cannot yet fully appreciate.

Hybrid artificial organs, or bioartificial organs, are more recent systems which include living elements (organelles, cells, or tissues) as part of a device made of synthetic materials. They integrate the technology of natural organ transplantation and the refinements which living structures have gained through millions of years of evolution with the purposeful design approach of engineering science and the promises of newly developed synthetic materials. Table XII.1 provides a current snapshot in the continuing evolution of substitutive medicine.

Depending upon medical needs and anticipated duration of use, artificial organs can be located outside of the body yet attached to it (paracorporeal prostheses or assist devices) or implanted inside the body in an appropriate location (internal artificial organs or implants). The application of artificial organs may be temporary, i.e., a bridge procedure to sustain life or a specific biologic activity while waiting for either recovery of natural function (e.g., the heart-lung machine), or permanent organ replacement (e.g., left ventricular assist devices). It can be intermittent and repeated at intervals over extended periods of time when there is no biologic necessity for continuous replacement of the missing body functions (e.g., artificial kidney). It can pretend to be permanent, at least within the limits of a finite life span.

Up to 1950, organ replacement technology was relatively crude and unimaginative. Wooden legs, corrective glasses and dental prostheses formed the bulk of artificial organs. Blood transfusion was the only accepted form of transplantation of living tissue. Suddenly, within a decade, the artificial kidney, the heart-lung machine, the cardiac pacemaker, the arterial graft, the prosthetic cardiac valve, and the artificial hip joint provided the first sophisticated examples of engineering in medicine. More recently, the membrane lung, the implantable lens, finger and tendon prostheses, total knee replacements, and soft-tissue implants for maxillo-facial, ear, or mammary reconstruction have reached the stage of broad clinical application. Ventricular assist devices and the total artificial heart have been extensively tested in animals and validated for clinical evaluation. Artificial skin is increasingly used in the treatment of ulcers and burns. Soft- and hard-tissue substitutes function effectively for several years. Sexual and sensory prostheses offer promises for the replacement of complex human functions. Interfacing of devices with the peripheral and central nervous systems appears as promising today as cardiovascular devices were 30 years ago. Perhaps the brightest future

TABLE XII.1 Evolution of Organ Replacement Technology: A 1995 perspective

Current Status	Artificial Organs	Transplantation
Broadly accepted clinically	Heart-lung machine	Blood transfusion
	Large-joint prostheses	Corneal transplants
	Bone fixation systems	Banked bone
	Cardiac pacemakers	Bone marrow
	Implantable defibrillators	Kidney—living related donor
	Large vascular grafts	Kidney—cadaveric donor
	Prosthetic cardiac valves	Heart
	Intra-aortic balloon pump	Liver
	Intraocular lenses	
	Middle ear ossicle chain	
	Hydrocephalus shunts	
	Dental implants	
	Skin and tissue expanders	
	Maintenance hemodialysis	
	Chronic ambulatory peritoneal dialysis	
Accepted with reservations	Breast implants	Whole pancreas
	Sexual prostheses	Single and double lung
	Small joint prostheses	Combined heart-lung
	ECMO in children	
Limited clinical application	ECMO in adults	Cardiomyoplasty
	Ventricular assist devices	Pancreatic islets
	Cochlear prostheses	Liver lobe or segment
	Artificial tendons	Small intestine
	Artificial skin	
	Artificial limbs	
Experimental stage	Artificial pancreas	Bioartificial pancreas
	Artificial blood	Bioartificial liver
	Intravenous oxygenation	CNS implants of secreting tissue
	Artificial esophagus	Gene therapy products
	Total artificial heart	
	Nerve guidance channels	
Conceptual stage	Artificial eye	Striated muscle implants
	Neurostimulator	Smooth muscle implants
	Blood pressure regulator	Cardiac muscle implants
	Implantable lung	Functional brain implants
	Artificial trachea	Bioartificial kidney
	Artificial gut	
	Artificial fallopian tube	

belongs to "information prostheses" which bring to the human body signals which the organism can no longer generate by itself (e.g., pacemaker functions), signals which need to be modulated differently to correct a disease state (e.g., electronic blood pressure regulators) or signals which cannot be perceived by the nervous system through its usual channels of information gathering (e.g., artificial eye or artificial ear).

XII.2 Biomaterials

The materials of the first generation of artificial organs—those which are widely available at the moment—are for the most part standard commodity plastics and metals developed for industrial purposes. Engineers have long recognized the limitations of construction materials in the design and performance of machines. However, a new awareness arose when they started interacting with surgeons and biologic scientists in the emerging field of medical devices. In many cases the intrinsic and well established physical properties of synthetic materials, such as mechanical strength, hardness, flexibility, or permeability to fluids and gases were not as immediately limiting as the detrimental effects deriving from the material's contact with living tissues. As a result, fewer than 20 chemical compounds among the 1.5 million candidates have been successfully incorporated into clinical devices. Yet some functional implants require material properties which exceed the limits of current polymer, ceramic, or metal alloy technology. This is an indirect tribute to the power of evolution, as well as a challenge to scientists to emulate natural materials with synthetic compounds, blends, or composites.

The progressive recognition of the dominant role of phenomena starting at the tissue-material interface has led to two generalizations:

1. All materials in contact with body fluids or living tissues undergo almost instantaneous and then continuing surface deposition of body components which alter their original properties.
2. All body fluids and tissues in contact with foreign material undergo a dynamic sequence of biologic reactions which evolve over weeks or months, and these reactions may remain active for as long as the contact persists and perhaps even beyond.

The recognition of biologic interactions between synthetic materials and body tissues has been translated into the twin operational concepts of biomaterials and compatibility.

Biomaterials is a term used to qualify materials which can be placed in intimate contact with living structures without harmful effects. Compatibility characterizes a set of material specifications and constraints which address the various aspects of material-tissue interactions. More specifically, hemocompatibility defines the ability of a biomaterial to stay in contact with blood for a clinically relevant period of time without causing alterations of the formed elements and plasma constituents of the blood or substantially altering the composition of the material itself. The term biocompatibility is often used to highlight the absence of untoward interactions with tissues other than blood (e.g., hard or soft tissues).

It is worth observing that hemocompatibility and biocompatibility are virtues demonstrated not by the presence of definable favorable properties but rather by the absence of adverse effects on blood or other tissues. Although these terms imply positive characteristics of the material, the presumption of compatibility is actually based on the accumulation of negative evidence over longer and longer periods of time, using an increasingly complex battery of tests, which must eventually be confirmed under the conditions of clinical use.

The clinical success of materials incorporated into actual devices is altogether remarkable, considering how limited is our understanding of the physical and biologic mechanisms underlying tissue-material interactions. Indeed the most substantial conclusion one can draw from a review of records of literally millions of implants is how few major accidents have been reported and how remarkably uncommon and benign have been the side effects of implanting substantial amounts of synthetic substances into the human body. Artificial organs are by no means perfect. Their performance must be appreciated within the same limits that the inexorable processes of disease and aging impose on natural organs.

XII.3 Outlook for Organ Replacement

Now emerging is a second generation of implantable materials through the confluence of biomaterial science and cell biology (Fig. XII.1). Cell culture technology, taking advantage of biotechnology products and progressing to tridimensional tissue engineering on preformed matrices, now provides building blocks which incorporate the peptide or glycoprotein sequences responsible for cell-to-cell interactions. This combination leads to a new class of biohybrid devices which includes

1. Cellular transplants for continuing secretion of bioactive substances (e.g., transplants of insulin-producing xenograft tissue protected against immune rejection by permselective envelopes)
2. Composites of synthetic materials with living cells (often called organoids) to accelerate implant integration within the body (e.g., endothelial cell-lined polymer conduits designed for vascular grafts)
3. Replacement parts in which natural tissue regeneration is activated by the presence of supportive cells (e.g., Schwann cell-seeded nerve guidance channels)
4. Vehicles for gene therapy in which continued gene expression is enhanced by a synthetic polymer substrate with appropriate mechanical, chemical, or drug release properties (e.g., epicardial transplants of genetically modified skeletal or cardiac muscle grown on a distensible polymer matrix)

In many respects, the new wave of organ replacement systems exemplifies the synergy of the two original currents in substitutive medicine: prostheses and transplants. It expands the feasibility of

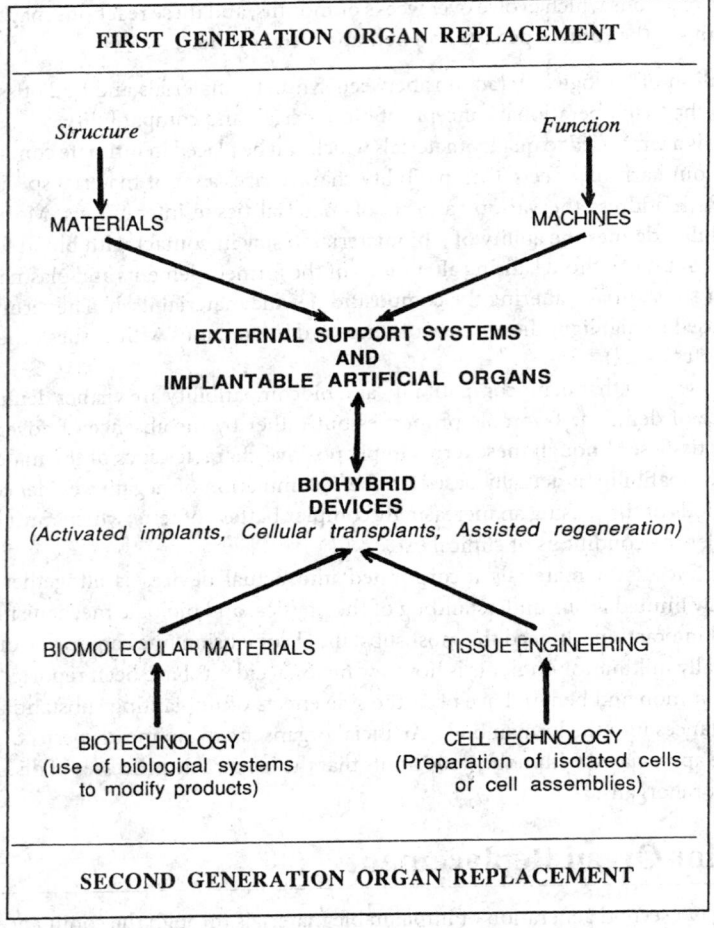

FIGURE XII.1 Schematic description of the advances in engineering, biologic, and medical technology which led to the first generation of artificial organs (read from the top) and the newer developments in body replacement parts (read from the bottom).

cell and tissue transplantation beyond the boundaries of autografts and related donor allografts, opening the way to xenogeneic and genetically engineered replacement parts. It also confronts the "foreign body" limitations of human-made synthetic implants by adding the molecular and cellular elements that favor permanent biointegration.

XII.4 Design Considerations

Natural organ transplants, if ideally preserved, should be able to fulfill all functions of the original body part except for those mediated by the nervous system, since a transplanted organ is by definition a denervated structure. In actuality, transplants always present some degree of ischemic damage caused by interruption of the blood supply during transfer from donor to recipient. This may be reflected by a temporarily impaired function in the postoperative period or by permanent necrosis of the most delicate components of the transplant, resulting in some degree of functional limitation. In the long run, transplanted organs may also exhibit functional alterations because of cell or tissue damage associated with an underlying systemic disease. They may be damaged by the immunosuppression protocol, which at the current stage is needed for all organ replacements except for autografts, identical-twin homografts, and some types of fetal tissue transplants. The second-order limitations of transplanted organs are usually ignored, and the assumption is made that all original functions are restored in the recipient.

Artificial organs, however, can only replace those bodily functions which have been incorporated into their design because these functions were scientifically described and known to be important. Therefore, in the design of an artificial organ, the first task is to establish the specifications for the device, i.e., to describe in quantitative terms the function or functions which must be fulfilled by a human-made construct and the physical constraints that apply because the device must interface with the human body. Each human organ fulfills multiple functions of unequal importance in terms of survival. Consequently, it is critical to distinguish the essential functions which must be incorporated into an effective spare part from those which can be neglected.

Defining specifications and constraints is the first step in the conceptualization of an artificial organ. Only when this is done can one think realistically about design alternatives, the limitations of available materials, and the clinical constraints which will apply, of which the key ones are connections to the body and duration of expected service.

Once all these considerations have been integrated (modelling is often useful at that stage), the next step is typically the construction of a prototype. Ideally the device should achieve everything it was expected to do, but usually it exhibits some level of performance and durability which falls short of design specifications, either because of some misjudgment in terms of required function or because of some unanticipated problem arising at the interface between the device and the body.

The following step of development may be called *optimization*, if the specifications were well defined from the outset, or *reevaluation*, if they were not. More commonly it is the reconciliation of competing and at times contradictory design criteria which leads to a second prototype.

At this point, new experiments are needed to establish the reliability and effectiveness of the device in animal models of the target disease (if such exist) or at least in animals in which the natural organ can be removed or bypassed. This is the stage of *validation* of the device, which is first conducted in acute experiments and must later be extended to periods of observation approximating the duration of intended use in humans. These criteria, however, cannot always be met for long-term implants, since the life expectancy of most animals is shorter than that of humans. By this point, the diverse vantage points of the theoretician, the manufacturer, the performance evaluator, and the clinical user have been articulated for some specific devices and generalized in terms of quality control for classes of devices.

The final stage of design, for many artificial organs, is *individualization*, i.e., the ability to fit the needs of diverse individuals. Humans come in a wide range of body sizes. In some cases, the prostheses must fit very strict dimensional criteria, which implies that they must be fabricated over an extended range of sizes (e.g., cardiac valves). In other cases, there is enough reserve of function in the device that one pediatric model and one adult size model may suffice (e.g., blood oxygenator for cardiac surgery).

XII.5 Evaluation Process

The evaluation of an artificial organ typically is done in six phases:

1. In vitro bench testing
2. Ex vivo appraisal
3. In vivo studies with healthy experimental animals
4. In vivo studies with animal models of disease
5. Controlled clinical trials
6. General clinical use

In Vitro Bench Testing

In vitro bench testing of a completed prototype has three major purposes:

1. To observe the mode of operation of the device and assess its performance under tightly controlled circumstances
2. To define performance in quantitative terms over a wide range of environmental or input conditions
3. To assess the device's reliability and durability in a manner which can be extrapolated to the intended clinical use

For all of its value, there are limitations to in vitro testing of devices. Devices are made to work while in contact with body fluids or body tissues. This complex environment modifies materials in ways which are not always predictable. To duplicate this effect as closely as possible, a laboratory bench system can be made to match the body's environment in terms of temperature and humidity. Operating pressures and external forces can also be imitated but not perfectly reproduced (e.g., the complex pulsatile nature of cardiovascular events). Other fluid dynamic conditions such as viscosity, wall shear stress, and compliance of device-surrounding structures call for sophisticated laboratory systems and can only be approximated. The chemical environment is the most difficult to reproduce in view of the complexity of body fluids and tissue structures. Some in vitro testing systems make use of body fluids such as plasma or blood. This in turn brings in additional intricacies because these fluids are not stable outside of the body without preservatives and must be kept sterile if the experiment is to last more than a few hours.

Accelerated testing is a standard component in the evaluation of machines. It is critical for permanent implants with moving parts which are subject to the repeated action of external forces. Fatigue testing provides important information on progressive wear or catastrophic failure of device components. For example, the human heart beats about 40 million times per year. Manufacturers and regulatory agencies conduct testing of prosthetic cardiac valves over at least 400 million cycles. With a testing apparatus functioning at 1200 cycles per minute, this evaluation can be compressed by a factor of about 15, i.e., to about a year.

Ex Vivo Appraisal

Because of the difficulty of keeping blood in its physiologic state in a container, the evaluation of some blood processing or blood contacting devices is performed by connecting them through the skin to an artery or vein or both if the blood must be returned to the cardiovascular system to avoid excessive hemorrhage. Such experiments retain the advantage of keeping the device under direct observation while allowing longer experiments than are feasible in vitro, particularly if the animal does not require general anesthesia. It is also possible in some cases to evaluate several devices in parallel or sequentially under quite realistic conditions and therefore to conduct comparative experiments under reasonably standardized conditions.

In Vivo Evaluation with Healthy Experimental Animals

There comes a stage in the development of most devices where they must be assessed in their target location in a living body. The matching of device size and shape with available experimental sites in the appropriate animal species is a necessary condition. Such experiments typically last weeks, months, or years and provide information about body-device and tissue-material interactions either through noninvasive measurement techniques or through device retrieval at the end of the observation period. Rodents, felines, and dogs raised for research purposes are usually too small for the evaluation of human-sized devices. Farm animals such as sheep, goats, pigs, and calves are commonly used. Here again the limited life expectancy of experimental animals prevents studies for periods of service as long as can be expected with permanent implants in man.

In Vivo Evaluation with Animal Models of Disease

A first approximation of the effectiveness of a device in replacing a physiologic function can be obtained after removing the target organ in a normal animal. However, when the organ failure is only the cardinal sign of a complex systemic disease, the interactions between the device and the persisting manifestations of the disease cannot be evaluated in a healthy subject. Animal models of human disease occur spontaneously in some species and in other cases can be obtained by chemical, physical, or surgical intervention. Where such models of disease exist in animals which can be fitted with a device, useful information is obtained which helps to refine the final prototypes.

Controlled Clinical Trials

Although some devices can be evaluated with little risk in normal volunteers who derive no health benefit from the experiment, our culture frowns on this approach and legal considerations discourage it. Once reliability and effectiveness have been established through animal experiments and the device appears to meet a recognized clinical need, a study protocol is typically submitted to an appropriate ethics committee or institutional review board and, upon their approval, a series of clinical trials is undertaken. The first step often concentrates on the demonstration of safety of the device with a careful watch for side effects or complications. If the device passes this first hurdle, a controlled clinical trial will be carried out with patients to evaluate effectiveness as well as safety on a scale which allows statistical comparison with a control form of treatment. This protocol may extend from a few months to several years depending upon the expected benefits of the device and the natural history of the disease.

General Clinical Use

Once a device is deemed successful by a panel of experts, it may be approved by regulatory agencies for commercial distribution. Increasingly a third stage of clinical evaluation appears necessary, namely postmarket surveillance, i.e., a system of clinical outcomes analysis under conditions of general availability of the device to a wide range of doctors and patients.

Postmarket surveillance is a new concept which is not yet uniformly codified. It may take the form of a data collection and analysis network, a patient registry to allow continuing follow-up and statistical analysis, a device-tracking system aimed at early identification of unforeseen types of failure, or ancillary controls such as inspection of facilities and review of patient histories in institutions where devices are used. Protocols of surveillance on a large scale are difficult and costly to implement, and their cost-effectiveness is therefore open to question. They are also impaired by the shortage of broadly available and minimally invasive diagnostic methods for assessing the integrity or function of a device prior to catastrophic failure. Worthwhile postmarket surveillance requires a constructive collaboration between patients, doctors, device manufacturers, government regulatory agencies, and study groups assessing health care policy issues in the public and private sectors.

Acknowledgments

The chapters that follow are derived to a substantial extent from lecture notes used in graduate courses at Brown University, the Massachusetts Institute of Technology, and the Georgia Institute of Technology. Colleagues at other institutions have also contributed chapters in their own area of specialization. The authors are also indebted to successive generations of students of biomedical engineering who through a fresh, unencumbered look at the challenges of organ replacement have demonstrated their curiosity, their creativity, and their analytical skills.

Defining Terms

Artificial organs: Human-made devices designed to replace, duplicate, or augment, functionally or cosmetically, a missing, diseased, or otherwise incompetent part of the body, either temporarily or permanently, and which requires that a nonbiologic material interface with living tissue.

Assist device: An apparatus used to support or partially replace the function of a failing organ.

Bioartificial organ: Device combining living elements (organelles, cells, or tissues) with synthetic materials in a therapeutic system.

Biocompatibility: The ability of a material to perform with an appropriate host tissue response when incorporated for a specific application in a device, prosthesis, or implant.

Biomaterial: Any material or substance (other than a drug) or combination of materials, synthetic or natural in origin, which can be used as a whole or as a part of a system which treats, augments, or replaces any tissue, organ, or function of the body.

Compatibility: A material property which encompasses a set of specifications and constraints relative to material-tissue interactions.

Device: Defined by Congress as ". . . an instrument, apparatus, implement, machine, contrivance, implant, in vitro reagent, or other similar or related article, including any component, part, or accessory, which is . . . intended for use in the diagnosis of disease or other conditions, or in the cure, mitigation, treatment, or prevention of disease, in man or other animals, . . . and which does not achieve any of its principal intended purposes through chemical action within or on the body of man or other animals and which is not dependent upon being metabolized for the achievement of any of its principal intended purposes."

Hemocompatibility: The ability of a biomaterial to stay in contact with blood for a clinically relevant period of time without causing alterations of the blood constituents.

Hybrid artificial organs: Synonym of *bioartificial organs,* stressing the combination of cell transplantation and artificial organ technology.

Implant: Any biomaterial or device which is actually embedded within the tissues of a living organism.

Organs: Differentiated structures or parts of a body adapted for the performance of a specific operation or function.

Organoid: An organlike aggregate of living cells and synthetic polymer scaffolds or envelopes, designed to provide replacement or support function.

Organ transplant: An isolated body part obtained from the patient, a living relative, a compatible cadaveric donor, or an animal and inserted in a recipient to replace a missing function.

Prosthesis: An artificial device to replace a missing part of the body.

Substitutive medicine: A form of medicine which relies on the replacement of failing organs or body parts by natural or human-made counterparts.

Tissue-material interface: The locus of contact and interactions between a biomaterial, implant, or device and the tissue or tissues immediately adjacent.

References

Cauwels JM. 1986. The Body Shop: Bionic Revolutions in Medicine, St. Louis, Mosby.

Galletti PM. 1991. Organ replacement: A dream come true. In R Johnsson-Hegyeli, AM Marmont du Haut Champ (eds), Discovering New Worlds in Medicine, pp 262–277, Milan, Farmitalia Carlo Erba.

Galletti PM. 1992. Bioartificial organs. Artif Organs 16(1):55.

Galletti PM. 1993. Organ replacement by man-made devices. J Cardiothor Vasc Anesth 7:624.

Harker LA, Ratner BD, Didisheim P. 1993. Cardiovascular biomaterials and biocompatibility. A guide to the study of blood-tissue-material interactions. Cardiovasc Pathol 2 (3)(suppl):IS-2245.

Helmus MN. 1992. Designing critical medical devices without failure. Spectrum, Diagnostics, Medical Equipment Supplies Ophthalmics, pp 37-1–37-17, Decision Resources, Inc.

Richardson PD. 1976. Oxygenator testing and evaluation: Meeting ground of theory, manufacture and clinical concerns. In WM Zapol, J Qvist (eds), Artificial Lungs for Acute Respiratory Failure. Theory and Practice. pp 87–102, New York, Academic Press.

Further Information

The articles and books listed above provide different overviews in the field of organ replacement. Historically most contributions to the field of artificial organs were described or chronicled in the 40 annual volumes of the *Transactions of the American Society of Artificial Internal Organs* (1955 to present). The principal journals in the field of artificial organs are *Artificial Organs* (currently published by Blackwell Scientific Publications, Inc.), the *ASAIO Journal* (published by J. B. Lippincott Company), and the *International Journal of Artificial Organs* (published by Wichtig Editore s.r.l. Milano, Italy). Publications of the Japanese Society for Artificial Organs (typically in Japanese with English abstracts, *Artificial Organs Today,* for example) contain substantial information.

122

Artificial Heart and Circulatory Assist Devices

Gerson Rosenberg
Pennsylvania State University

In 1812, LeGallois (LeGallois, 1813) postulated the use of mechanical circulatory support. In 1934, DeBakey proposed a continuous flow blood transfusion instrument using a simple roller pump (DeBakey, 1934). In 1961, Dennis et al, performed left heart bypass by inserting cannulae into the left atrium and returning blood through the femoral artery (Dennis, 1979). In 1961, Kolff and Moulopoulos developed the first intra-aortic balloon pump (Moulopoulos et al., 1962). In 1963, Liota performed the first clinical implantation of a pulsatile left ventricular assist device (Liota et al., 1963). In 1969, Dr. Denton Cooley performed the first total artificial heart implantation in a human (Cooley et al., 1969). Since 1969, air driven artificial hearts and ventricular assist devices have been utilized in over 200 and 600 patients, respectively. The primary use of these devices has been as a bridge to transplant. Recently, electrically powered ventricular assist devices have been utilized in humans as a bridge to transplant. These electrically powered systems utilize implanted blood pumps and energy converters with percutaneous drive cables and vent tubes.

Completely implanted heart assist systems requiring no percutaneous leads have been implanted in calves with survivals over eight months. The electric motor–driven total artificial hearts being developed by several groups in the United States are completely implanted systems employing transcutaneous energy transmission and telemetry [Rosenberg, 1991. Appendix C, *The Artificial Heart, Prototypes, Policies, and Patients*]. One total artificial heart design has functioned in a calf for over five months[Snyder, 1993].

There has been steady progress in the development of artificial heart and circulatory assist devices. Animal survivals have been increasing, and patient morbidity and mortality with the devices has been decreasing. It does not appear that new technologies or materials will be required for the first successful clinical application of long-term devices. There is no doubt that further advances in energy systems, materials, and electronics will provide for smaller and more reliable devices, but for the present, sound engineering design using available materials and methods appears to be adequate to provide devices satisfactory for initial clinical trials.

122.1 Engineering Design

A definition for design is given by Pahl and Beitz (1977): "Designing is the intellectual attempt to meet certain demands in the best possible way. It is an engineering activity that impinges on nearly every sphere of human life, relies on the discoveries and laws of science, and creates the conditions for applying these laws to the manufacture of useful products." Designing is a creative activity that calls for sound grounding in mathematics, physics, chemistry, mechanics, thermodynamics, hydrodynamics, electrical engineering, production engineering, materials technology, and design theory together with practical knowledge and experience in specialist fields. Initiative, resolution, economic insight, tenacity, optimism, sociability, and teamwork are all qualities that will assist the designer. Engineering design has been broken into many steps or phases by various authors. In general, though, each of these definitions include some common tasks. No matter what device is being designed, be it a complicated device such as a totally implantable artificial heart or a simpler device, such as a new fastener, sound engineering design principles utilizing a methodical approach will help ensure satisfactory outcome of the design process. The engineering design process can be broken down into at least four separate stages.

1. *Define the problem—clarification of the task.* At first, it may appear that defining the problem or clarifying the task to be accomplished is an easy matter. In general, this is not the case. Great care should be taken in defining the problem, being very specific about the requirements and specifications of the system to be designed. Very often, a complex system can be reduced to the solution of one core problem. An excellent way to begin defining the problem or clarifying the task to be accomplished is to begin by writing a careful design specification or design requirement. This is a document that lists all the requirements for the device. Further, this design requirement may elucidate one or two specific problems which, when solved, will yield a satisfactory design.

2. *Conceptual design—plan treatment.* After the problem has been defined, the designer must plan the treatment of the problem and begin conceptual design. In this phase possible solutions to the problem at hand are examined. Various methods of determining possible solutions include brainstorming, focus groups, Delphi method. This is the phase of the design process where a thorough review of the literature and examination of similar problems is valuable. In this phase of design each of the proposed solutions to the problem should be examined in terms of a hazard analysis or failure modes and effects analysis to determine which solution appears the most feasible. Economic considerations should also be examined in this phase.

3. *Detailed design—Execute the plan.* In this phase of engineering design, a detailed design is formulated. Perhaps two designs may be evaluated in the initial detailed design phase. As the detailed design or designs near completion, they must be examined with reference to the design specifications. Here, each of the proposed designs may be evaluated with regard to its ability to perform. Such aspects as system performance, reliability, manufacturability, cost, and user acceptance are all issues which must be considered before a final design is chosen.

4. *Learn and generalize.* Finally, after the design is complete, the designer should be able to learn and generalize from the design. This educational process will include manufacturing of prototypes and testing. General concepts and principles may be gleaned from the design process that can be applied to further designs.

The remainder of this chapter will deal with the application of this engineering design method to the design of artificial heart and circulatory assist devices.

122.2 Engineering Design of Artificial Heart and Circulatory Assist Devices

Define the Problem—Clarification of the Task

In the broadest sense, this step can best be accomplished by writing the detailed design requirement or specification for the device. In defining the problem, it is often easiest to begin with the most obvious and imperative requirements and proceed to the subtler and less demanding. A general statement of the problem for a total artificial heart or assist device is "to develop a device (perhaps totally implantable) that when implanted in the human will provide a longer and better quality of life than conventional pharmacologic or transplant therapy." The devices considered will be assumed to be permanent implantable devices, not necessarily totally implantable; they may utilize percutaneous wires or tubes. In general, it will be assumed that they will be intended for long-term use (one year or longer) but may also be utilized for short-term applications.

Fit of the System

One must first decide who the device is intended for. Will it be used in men and women, and of what size? No matter how good the device is, it must first "fit" the patient. For our example, let us assume the device will be used in men and women in the size range of 70–100 kg. The device must then fit in these patients and cause minimal or no pathologic conditions. When considering the fit of the implanted device, one must consider the volume and mass of the device, as well as any critical dimension such as the length, width, or height and the location of any tubes, conduits, or connectors. Careful consideration must be given to the physical attributes of the system such as whether the system should be hard, soft, rough, or smooth and the actual shape of the system in terms of sharp corners or edges that may damage tissue or organs. The design specification must give the maximum length, height, and width of the device, these dimensions being dictated by the patient's anatomy. The designer must not be limited by existing anatomy; the opportunity to surgically alter the anatomy should be considered. Nontraditional locations for devices should be considered.

The device should not reject heat in such a way that surfaces in contact with tissue or blood are subjected to a temperature rise 5°C above core temperature on a chronic basis. The use of heat spreaders or fins, along with insulation, may be required. Heat transfer analysis may be helpful.

The effect of device movement and vibration should be considered in the design specification. The acceptable sound levels at various frequencies must be specified. Acceptable levels of magnetic and electrical fields should be specified. A device should meet existing standards for electromagnetic interference and susceptibility.

The use of any percutaneous tubes will require the choice of an exit site. This site must not be in a location of constant or excessive movement or tissue breakdown will be experienced at the interface.

Pump Performance

Pump performance must be specified in terms of cardiac output range. In a 70-kg person, a normal resting cardiac output is approximately 70 ml/min/kg or 5 l/min. Choosing a maximum cardiac output of approximately 8 l/min will allow the patient the ability to perform light exercise. The cardiac output performance must be obtained at physiologic pressures, that is, the device, be it a heart assist or total artificial heart device, must be able to pump a cardiac output ranging up to 8 l/min with physiologic inlet and outlet pressures (central venous pressure ~5 mmHg mean, left atrial pressure ~7 mmHg mean, pulmonary artery pressure ~15 mmHg mean, aortic pressure ~100 mmHg mean).

Control of the device is critical and must be included in the design specification. For an assist pump, it may be as simple as stating that the pump will pump all the blood delivered to it by the native heart while operating under physiologic inlet and outlet pressures. Or, the design specification may include specific requirements for synchronization of the device with the natural heart. For the total artificial heart, the device must always maintain balance between the left and right pumps. It must not let left atrial pressure rise above a value that will cause pulmonary congestion (approximately 20 mmHg). The device must respond to the patient's cardiac output requirements. The device must either passively or through an active controller vary its cardiac output upon patient demand.

Biocompatibility

Biocompatibility has already been alluded to in the design requirements by saying that the device must not cause excessive damage to the biologic system. Specifically, the device must be minimally thrombogenic and minimally hemolytic. It should have a minimal effect on the immune system. It should not promote infection, calcification, or tissue necrosis. Meeting these design requirements will require careful design of the pumping chamber and controller and careful selection of materials.

Reliability

The design specification must assign a target reliability for the device. For total artificial hearts and circulatory assist devices, the NIH has proposed a reliability of 80% with an 80% confidence for a 2-year device life. This is the value that the NIH feels is a reliability goal to be achieved before devices can begin initial clinical trials, but the final design reliability may be much more stringent, perhaps 90% reliable with 95% confidence for a 5-year life. The design specification must state which components of the system could be changed if necessary. The design specification must deal with any service that the device may require. For instance, the overall design life of the device may be 5 years, but battery replacement at 2-year intervals may be allowed. The reliability issue is very complex and involves moral, ethical, legal, and scientific issues. A clear goal must be stated and is necessary before the detailed design can begin.

Quality of Life

The design specification must address the quality of life for the patient. The designers must specify what is a satisfactory quality of life. Again, this is not an easy task. Quantitative measures of the quality of life are difficult to achieve. One person's interpretation of a satisfactory quality of life may not be the same as another's. It must always be kept in mind that the quality of life for these patients without treatment would generally be considered unsatisfactory by the general public. The prognosis for patients before receiving artificial hearts and circulatory assist devices is very poor. The quality of life must thus be considered in relation to the patient's quality of life without the device without ignoring the quality of life of individuals unaffected by cardiac disease [Rosenberg, 1991].

The design specification must state the weight of any external power supplies. The designer must consider how much weight an older patient will be able to carry. How long should this patient be able to be free-roaming and untethered? How often will the energy source require a "recharge"? What sound level will be acceptable? These are all issues that must be addressed by the designer.

All the foregoing must be considered and included in the definition of the problem and clarification of the task. Each of these issues should be clearly described in the design specification or requirement. In many instances there are no right and wrong answers to these questions.

Conceptual Design—Plan Treatment

In the conceptual design phase, the designer must plan the treatment of the problem and consider various designs that meet the design specification. In the design specification, it must be stated whether the blood pump is to be pulsatile or nonpulsatile. If there is no requirement in the design specification, then in the conceptual design phase, the designer may consider various nonpulsatile and pulsatile flow devices. Nonpulsatile devices include centrifugal pumps, axial flow pumps, shear flow pumps, and peristaltic pumps. Pulsatile pumps have traditionally been sac- or diaphragm-type devices. At the present time there is no definitive work describing the absolute requirement for pulsatility in the cardiovascular system; thus, both types of devices can be considered for assist and total artificial hearts.

In the conceptual design phase, the designer should consider other nontraditional solutions to the problem such as devices that employ micro machines or magneto-hydrodynamics. Careful consideration must be given for the source of energy. Sources that have been considered include electrical energy stored in batteries or derived from piezoelectric crystals, fuel cells, and thermal energy created either thermonuclearly or through thermal storage. The performance of each of these energy sources must be considered in the conceptual design phase. Public considerations and cost for a thermonuclear source, at the present time, have essentially eliminated this as an implantable energy source. Thermal storage has been shown to be a feasible energy source, and adequate insulation has been developed and demonstrated to be reliable for short periods of time [Unger, 1989].

Steady flow devices that employ seals within the blood stream deserve very careful consideration of the seal area. These seals have been prone to failure, causing embolization. Active magnetic levitation has been proposed for component suspension and may be considered as a possible design. A device that utilizes a rotating member such as a rotating electric motor that would drive an impeller or mechanical mechanism will create forces on the tissue when the patient moves due to gyroscopic or coriolis accelerations. These forces must be considered.

Pump performance, in terms of purely hydraulic considerations, can be achieved with any of the pumping systems described. Control of these devices may be more difficult. Designs that include implanted sensors such as pressure or flow sensors must deal with drift of these signals. Very often, signal-to-noise ratios are poor in devices that must operate continuously for several years. Designs that employ few or no sensors are preferable.

Systems such as sac-type blood pumps have been described as having intrinsic automatic control. That is, these devices can run in a fill limited mode, and, as more blood is returned to the pump, it will increase its stroke volume. Intrinsic control is desirable, but, unfortunately, this generally provides for only a limited control range. Nearly all devices currently being developed employ some form of automatic electronic control system. These automatic control systems are utilized on both total artificial hearts and assist devices. In some designs system parameters such as blood pump fill time, electric current, voltage, or speed are utilized to infer the state of the circulatory system. These types of systems appear to demonstrate good long-term stability and eliminate the potential for device malfunction associated with transducer drift.

Consideration of pump performance and the interaction with the biologic system is important in the conceptual design phase. Two pump designs may be capable of pumping the same in a hydrodynamic sense in terms of pressures and flows, but one pump may have much higher shear stresses than the other and thus be more hemolytic. One device may have much more mechanical vibration or movement compromising surrounding tissue.

The subject of biocompatibility for circulatory assist and artificial hearts is a very complex one. No matter what type device is designed, its interaction with the environment is paramount. Blood-contacting materials must not cause thrombosis and should have a minimal effect on formed elements in the blood. In terms of tissue biocompatibility, the device should not have sharp corners or areas where pressure necrosis can occur. Both smooth and rough exterior surfaces of devices have been investigated. It appears that devices in contact with the pleura tend to form a thinner encapsulation when they are rough surfaced. Compliance chambers form much thinner capsules when they have a rough surface. In other areas, it is not entirely clear if a rough surface is advantageous. Tissue ingrowth into a rough surface makes removal of the device difficult.

The selection of materials in the design of these devices is limited. The designer's job would be made much easier if there were several completely biocompatible materials available. If the designer only had a perfectly nonthrombogenic material that had outstanding fatigue properties, the design of these devices would be greatly simplified! Unfortunately, at the present time the designer is limited to existing materials. Traditionally, metals that have been employed in blood pumps include various stainless steels, cobalt, cobalt chromium alloys, and titanium. Each of these materials has adequate performance when in contact with tissue and blood under certain circumstances. Ceramic materials such as pyrolytic carbon, alumina, and zirconia have been used in contact with both tissue and blood with varying degrees of success. The range of polymeric materials that have been utilized for these devices is much greater. These materials include various polyurethanes, silicone rubber, Kel-F, Teflon, Delrin, butyl rubber, Hexsyn rubber, polysulfone, polycarbonate, and others [Williams, 1981]. The designer must carefully consider all the properties of these materials when employing them. The designer must look at the strength, durability, hardness, wear resistance, modulus of elasticity, surface energy, surface finish, and biocompatibility before choosing any of these materials.

The interaction between the biologic system and these materials is complex and may be strongly influenced by fluid mechanics if in contact with blood. The designer should carefully consider surface modification of any of these materials. Surface modification can be performed, including ion implantation or grafting of various substances to the surface to promote improved compatibility. Manufacturing and fabrication processes have a profound effect on the properties of these materials and must be carefully analyzed and controlled.

T e designer must give a great deal of consideration to the fluid mechanics involved. It is well known that excessive shear stresses can promote hemolysis and activation of the clotting system, as well as damage to the other formed elements in the blood. Not only the actual design of the blood pump, but the operation of the blood pump can affect phenomena such as cavitation, which can be hemolytic and destructive to system components. Thrombosis is greatly affected by blood flow. Regions of stagnation, recirculation, and low wall shear stress should be avoided. The magnitude of "low" shear stress is reported in the literature with wide range [Folie & McIntire, 1989; Hashimoto et al., 1985; Hubbell & McIntire, 1986].

Many of the analytical tools available today in terms of computational fluid dynamics and finite element analysis are just beginning to be useful in the design of these devices. Most of these systems have complex flow (unsteady, turbulent, non-Newtonian with moving boundaries) and geometries and are not easily modeled.

Once a reliability goal has been established, the designer must ensure that this goal is met. The natural heart beats approximately 40 million times a year. This means that an artificial heart or assist device with a 5-year life may undergo as many as 200,000,000 cycles. The environment in which this device is to operate is extremely hostile. Blood and extracellular fluids are quite corrosive and can promote galvanic or crevice corrosion in most metallic materials. Devices that employ polymeric materials must deal with diffusion of mass across these materials. Water, oxygen, nitrogen, carbon dioxide, and so on may all diffuse across these polymeric materials. If temperature fluctuations occur or differences exist, liquid water may form due to condensation. With carbon dioxide present, a weak acid can be formed. Many polymeric materials are degraded in the biologic environment. A careful review of the literature is imperative. The use of any "new" materials must be based upon careful testing. The designer must be aware of the difficulty in providing a sealed system. The designer may need to utilize hermetic connectors and cables which can tolerate the moist environment. All these affect the reliability of the device.

External components of the system which may include battery packs or monitoring and perhaps control functions have reliability requirements that differ from the implanted components. System components which are redundant may not require the same level of reliability as do nonredundant implanted components. Externally placed components have the advantage of being amenable to preventative maintenance or replacement. Systems that utilize transcutaneous energy transmission through inductive coupling may have advantages over systems that utilize a percutaneous wire. Although the percutaneous wire can function for long periods of time, perhaps up to 1 year, localized infection is almost always present. This infection can affect the patient's quality of life and be a source of systemic infection.

In the conceptual design phase, one must carefully weigh quality of life issues when evaluating solutions to the problem. Careful consideration needs to be given to the traditional quality of life issues such as the patient's emotional, social, and physical well-being, as well as to the details of day-to-day use of the device. What are the frequency and sound level requirements for patient prompts or alarms, and are certain kinds of alarms useful at all? For visible information for the patient, from what angles can this information be viewed, how bright does the display need to be, should it be in different languages, or should universal symbols be used? A great deal of thought must be given to all aspects of device use, from charging of the batteries to dealing with unexpected events. All these issues must be resolved in the conceptual design phase so that the detailed design phase will be successful.

Detailed Design—Execute the Plan

This is the phase of engineering design where the designer and other members of the team must begin to do what is generally considered the designer's more traditional role, i.e., calculations and drawings. This phase of design may require some initial prototyping and testing before the detailed design can be complete. Akutsu and Koyanagi [1993] provide several results of various groups' detailed designs for artificial hearts and circulatory assist devices.

Learn and Generalize

Substantial research and development of artificial hearts and circulatory assist devices has been ongoing for almost 30 years. During this period there have been literally thousands of publications related to this research, not only descriptions of device designs, but experimental results, detailed descriptions of fluid dynamic phenomena, hemolysis, thrombosis, investigation of materials selection and processing, consideration of control issues, and so on. The artificial organs and biomaterials literature has numerous references to materials utilized in these devices. A thorough review of the literature is required to glean the general principles that can be applied to the design of these devices. Many of these principles or generalities apply only to specific designs. In some design circulatory assist devices, a smooth surface will function satisfactorily, whereas a rough surface may cause thrombosis or an uncontrolled growth of neointima. Yet, in other design devices, a textured or rough surface will have performance superior to that of an extremely smooth surface. Wide ranges of sheer stresses are quoted in the literature that can be hemolytic. Although considerable research has been performed examining the fluid mechanics of the artificial hearts and circulatory assist devices, there is really no current measure of what is considered a "good" blood flow within these devices. We know that the design must avoid regions of stasis, but how close to stasis one can come, or for how long, without thrombosis is unknown.

It is up to the designer to review current literature and determine what fundamental principles are applicable to his or her design. Then, when the design is complete, the designer can learn and generalize specific principles related to her or his device. Hopefully, general principles that can apply to other devices will be elucidated.

122.3 Conclusions

The design of artificial hearts and circulatory assist devices is a very complex process involving many engineering disciplines along with medicine and other life science areas. Social issues must enter into the design process. The design of such devices requires sound engineering design principles and an interdisciplinary design team dedicated to the development and ultimate clinical application of these devices.

References

Akutsu T, Koyanagi H. 1993. Heart Replacement. Artificial Heart 4, Tokyo, Springer-Verlag.

Cooley DA, Liota D, Hallman GL, et al. 1969. Orthotopic cardiac prosthesis for 2-stage cardiac replacement. Am J Card 24:723.

DeBakey ME. 1934. A simple continuous flow blood transfusion instrument. New Orleans Med Surg J 87:386.

Dennis C. 1979. Historical background. In F Unger (ed), Assisted Circulation, pp 1–2, New York, Springer-Verlag.

Folie BJ, McIntire LV. 1989. Mathematical analysis of mural thrombogenesis, concentration profiles of platelet-activating agents and effects of viscous shear flow. Biophys J 56:1121.

Hashimoto S, Maeda H, Sasada T. 1985. Effect of shear rate on clot growth at foreign surfaces. Artif Organs 9:345.

Hubbell JA, McIntire LV. 1986. Visualization and analysis of mural thrombogenesis on collagen, polyurethane and nylon. Biomaterials 7:354.

LeGallois CJJ. 1813. Experience on the Principles of Life, Philadelphia, Thomas. (Translation of CJJ LeGallois. 1812. Experiences sur les Principles de Vie. Paris, France.)

Liota D, Hall CW, Walter SH, et al. 1963. Prolonged assisted circulation during and after cardiac and aortic surgery. Prolonged partial left ventricular bypass by means of an intra-corporeal circulation. Am J Card 12:399.

Moulopoulos D, Topaz SR, Kolff WJ. 1962. Extracorporeal assistance to the circulation at intra-aortic balloon pumping. Trans Am Soc Artif Intern Organs 8:86.

Pahl G, Beitz W. 1977. Engineering Design, Berlin, Heidelberg, Springer-Verlag. (First English edition published 1984 by The Design Council, London.)

Rosenberg G. 1991. Technological opportunities and barriers in the development of mechanical circulatory support systems (Appendix C). In Institute of Medicine, The Artificial Heart, Prototypes, Policies, and Patients, National Academy Press.

Snyder AJ, Rosenberg G, Weiss WJ, et al. 1993. *In vivo* testing of a completely implanted total artificial heart system. ASAIO J 39(3):M415.

Unger Felix. 1989. Assisted Circulation 3, Berlin, Heidelberg, Springer-Verlag.

Williams DF. 1981. Biocompatibility of Clinical Implant Materials, Boca Raton, Fla, CRC Press.

Cardiac Valve Prostheses

Ajit P. Yoganathan
Georgia Institute of Technology

The first clinical use of a cardiac valvular prosthesis took place in 1952, when Dr. Charles Hufnagel implanted the first artificial caged ball valve for aortic insufficiency. The Plexiglas cage contained a ball occluder and was inserted into the descending aorta without the need for cardiopulmonary bypass. It did not cure the underlying disease, but it did relieve regurgitation from the lower two-thirds of the body.

The first implant of a replacement valve in the anatomic position took place in 1960, with the advent of cardiopulmonary bypass. Since then, the achievements in valve design and the success of artificial heart valves as replacements have been remarkable [Roberts, 1976]. More than 50 different cardiac valves have been introduced over the past 35 years. Unfortunately, after many years of experience and success, problems associated with heart valve prostheses have not been eliminated. The most serious problems and complications [Bodnar, Frater, 1991; Butchart, Bodnar, 1992; Giddens et al. 1993; Roberts, 1976] are:

- Thrombosis and thromboembolism
- Anticoagulant-related hemorrhage
- Tissue overgrowth
- Infection
- Paravalvular leaks due to healing defects, and
- Valve failure due to material fatigue or chemical change.

New valve designs continue to be developed. Yet to understand the future of valve replacements, it is important to understand their history.

0-8493-8346-3/95/$0.00+$.50

123.1 A Brief History of Heart Valve Prostheses

This section on replacement valves highlights a relatively small number of the many various forms which have been made. However, those that have been included are either the most commonly used today or those which have made notable contributions to the advancement of replacement heart valves [Brewer, 1969; Yoganathan et al., 1992].

Mechanical Valves

The use of the caged-ball valve in the descending aorta became obsolete with the development in 1960 of what today is referred to as the *Starr-Edwards ball-and-cage valve*. Similar in concept to the original Hufnagel valve, it was designed to be inserted in place of the excised diseased natural valve. This form of intracardiac valve replacement was used in the mitral position and for aortic and multiple replacements. Since 1962 the Starr-Edwards valve has undergone many modifications to improve its performance in terms of reduced hemolysis and thromboembolic complications. However, the changes have involved materials and techniques of construction and have not altered the overall concept of the valve design in any way (Fig. 123.1a).

Other manufacturers have produced variations of the ball and cage valve, notably the Smeloff-Cutter valve and the Magovern prosthesis. In the case of the former, the ball is slightly smaller than the orifice. A subcage on the proximal side of the valve retains the ball in the closed position with its equator in the plane of the sewing ring. A small clearance around the ball ensures easy passage of the ball into the orifice. This clearance also gave rise to a mild regurgitation which was felt, but not proven, to be beneficial in preventing thrombus formation. The Magovern valve is a standard ball-and-cage format which incorporates two rows of interlocking mechanical teeth around the orifice ring. These teeth are used for inserting the valve and are activated by removing a special valve holder once the valve has been correctly located in the prepared tissue annulus. The potential hazard of dislocation from a calcified annulus due to imperfect placement was soon observed. This valve is no longer in use.

Due to the high-profile design characteristics of the ball valves, especially in the mitral position, low-profile caged disc valves were developed in the mid-1960s. Examples of the caged disc designs are the Kay-Shiley and Beall prostheses, which were introduced in 1965 and 1967, respectively

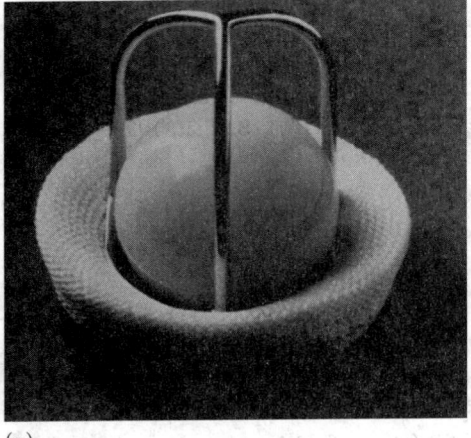
(a)

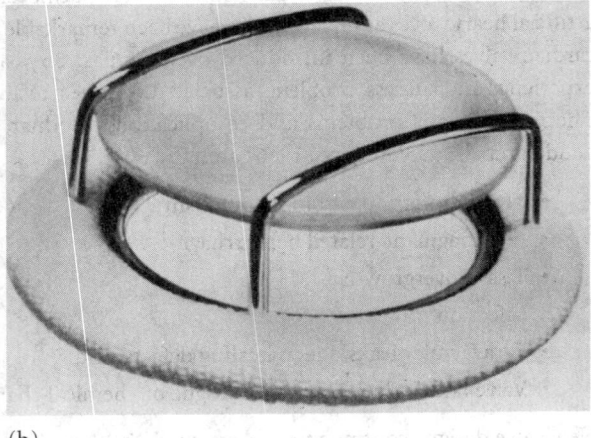
(b)

FIGURE 123.1   (*a*) Photograph of Starr-Edwards ball and cage valve; (*b*) photograph of Kay-Shiley disc valve; (*c*) photograph of Bjork-Shiley tilting disc valve; (*d*) photograph of Medtronic-Hall tilting disc valve; (*e*) photograph of St. Jude bileaflet valve; (*f*) photograph of CarboMedics bileaflet valve; (*g*) photograph of Parallel bileaflet valve.

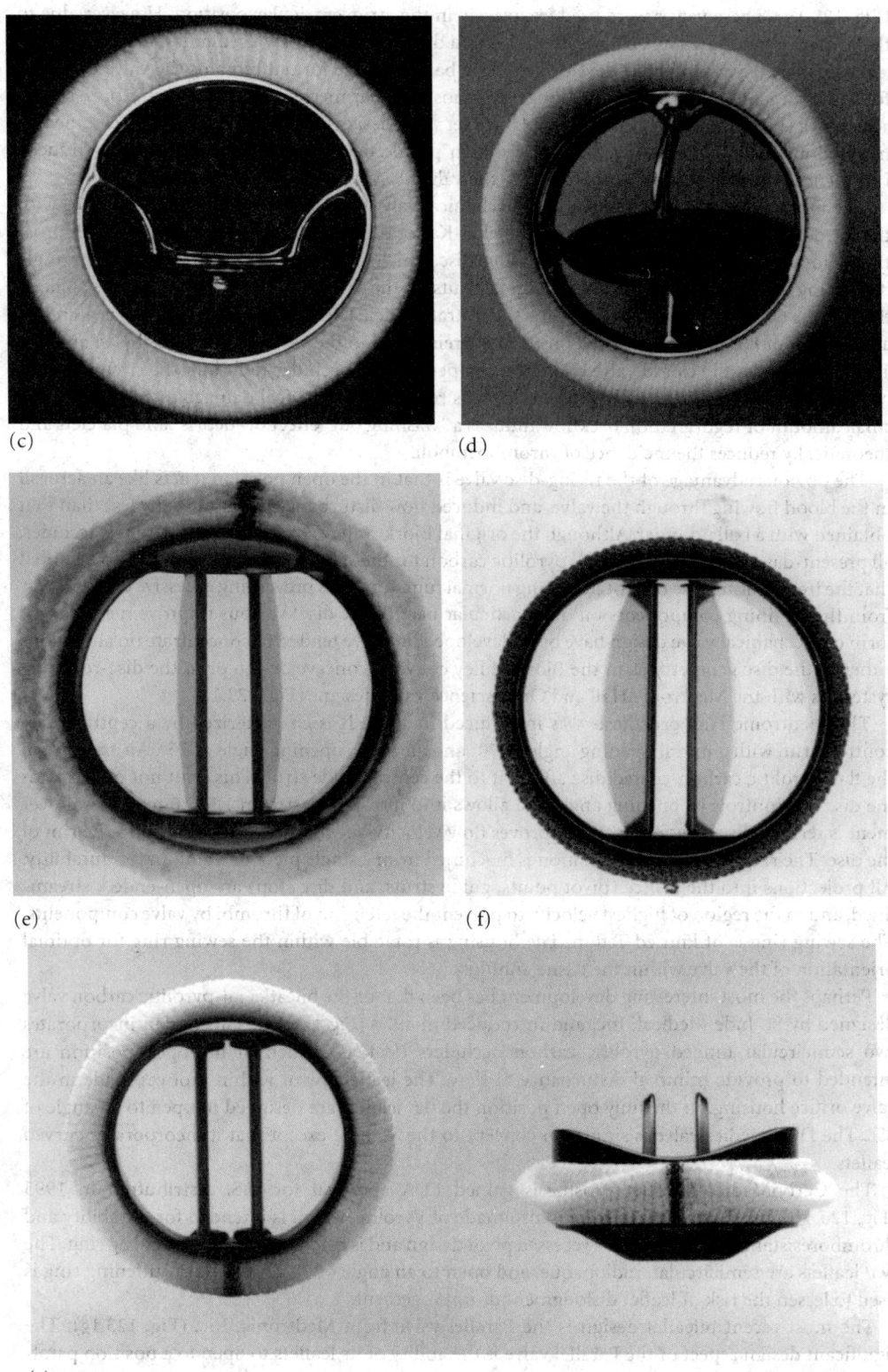

FIGURE 123.1   *(continued)*

(Fig. 123.1*b*). These valves were used exclusively in the atrioventricular position. However, due to their inferior hemodynamic characteristics, caged disc valves are rarely used today.

Even after 35 years of valve development, the ball-and-cage format remains the valve of choice for some surgeons. However, it is no longer the most popular mechanical valve, having been superseded, to a large extent, by tilting-disc and bileaflet valve designs. These valve designs overcome two major drawbacks of the ball valve, namely, high profile heights and excessive occluder-induced turbulence in the flow through and distal to the valve.

The most significant developments in mechanical valve design occurred in 1969 and 1970 with the introduction of the Bjork-Shiley and Lillehei-Kaster tilting-disc valves (Fig. 123.1*c*). Both prostheses involve the concept of a free-floating disc which in the open position tilts to an angle depending on the design of the disc-retaining struts. In the original Bjork-Shiley valve, the angle of the tilt was 60° for the aortic and 50° for the mitral model. The Lillehei-Kaster valve has a greater angle of tilt of 80° but in the closed position is preinclined to the valve orifice plane by an angle of 18°. In both cases the closed valve configuration permits the occluder to fit into the circumference of the inflow ring with virtually no overlap, thus reducing mechanical damage to erythrocytes. A small amount of regurgitation backflow induces a "washing out" effect of "debris" and platelets and theoretically reduces the incidence of thromboemboli.

The obvious advantage of the tilting-disc valve is that in the open position it acts like an aerofoil in the blood flowing through the valve, and induced flow disturbance is substantially less than that obtained with a ball occluder. Although the original Bjork-Shiley valve employed a Delrin occluder, all present-day tilting-disc valves use pyrolitic carbon for these components. It should also be noted that the free-floating disc can rotate during normal function, thus preventing excessive contact wear from the retaining components on one particular part of the disc. Various improvements to this form of mechanical valve design have been developed but have tended to concentrate on alterations either to the disc geometry as in the Bjork-Shiley convexo-concave design or to the disc-retaining system as with the Medtronic Hall and Omniscience valve designs (Fig. 123.1*d*).

The Medtronic Hall prosthesis was introduced in 1977. It is characterized by a central, disc-control strut, with a mitral opening angle of 70° and an aortic opening angle of 75°. An aperture in the flat, pyrolitic carbon-coated disc affixes it to the central guide strut. This strut not only retains the disc but controls its opening angle and allows it to move downstream 1.5–2.0 mm; this movement is termed disc *translation* and improves flow velocity between the orifice ring and the rim of the disc. The ring and strut combination is machined from a single piece of titanium for durability. All projections into the orifice (pivot points, guide struts, and disc stop) are open-ended, streamlined, and in the region of highest velocity to prevent the retention of thrombi by valve components. The sewing ring is of knitted Teflon. The housing is rotatable within the sewing ring for optimal orientation of the valve within the tissue annulus.

Perhaps the most interesting development has been that of the bileaflet all-pyrolitic carbon valve designed by St. Jude Medical, Inc. and introduced in 1978 (Fig 123.1*e*). This design incorporates two semicircular hinged pyrolitic carbon occluders (leaflets) which in the open position are intended to provide minimal disturbance to flow. The leaflets pivot within grooves made in the valve orifice housing. In the fully open position the flat leaflets are designed to open to an angle of 85°. The Duromedics valve is similar in concept to the St. Jude except that it incorporates curved leaflets.

The CarboMedics bileaflet prosthesis gained FDA approval for U.S. distribution in 1993 (Fig. 123.1*f*). The CarboMedics valve is also made of Pyrolite, which is intended for durability and thromboresistance. The valve has a recessed pivot design and is rotatable within the sewing ring. The two leaflets are semicircular, radiopaque, and open to an angle of 78°. A titanium stiffening ring is used to lessen the risk of leaflet dislodgment or impingement.

The most recent bileaflet design is the Parallel valve from Medtronic, Inc. (Fig. 123.1*g*). The significant design aspect of the Parallel valve is the ability of its leaflets to open to a position parallel to flow. This is intended to reduce the amount of turbulence that is created in the blood and therefore should improve hemodynamics and reduce thromboembolic complications. European clinical implants began in the Spring of 1994.

The most popular valve design in use today is the bileaflet. Approximately 75% of the valves implanted today are bileaflet prostheses.

Tissue Valves

Two major disadvantages with the use of mechanical valves is the need for life-long anticoagulation therapy and the accompanying problems of bleeding [Butchart & Bodnar, 1992]. Furthermore, the hemodynamic function of even the best designed valves differs significantly from that of the natural healthy heart valve. An obvious step in the development of heart valve substitutes was the use of naturally occurring heart valves. This was the basis of the approach to the use of antibiotic or cryo-treated human aortic valves (homografts: from another member of the same species) removed from cadavers for implantation in place of a patient's own diseased valve.

The first of these homograft procedures was performed by Ross in 1962, and the overall results so far have been satisfactory. This is, perhaps, not surprising since the homograft replacement valve is optimum both from the point of view of structure and function. In the open position these valves provide unobstructed central orifice flow and have the ability to respond to deformations induced by the surrounding anatomical structure. As a result, such substitutes are less damaging to the blood when compared with the rigid mechanical valve. The main problem with these cadaveric allografts, as far as may be ascertained, is that they are no longer living tissue and therefore lack that unique quality of cellular regeneration typical of normal living systems. This makes them more vulnerable to long-term damage. Furthermore, they are only available in very limited quantities.

An alternative approach is to transplant the patient's own pulmonary valve into the aortic position. This operation was also the first carried out by Ross in 1967, and his study of 176 patients followed up over 13 years showed that such transplants continued to be viable in their new position with no apparent degeneration [Wain et al., 1980]. This transplantation technique is, however, limited in that it can only be applied to one site.

The next stage in development of tissue valve substitutes was the use of autologous fascia lata (a wide layer of membrane that encases the thigh muscles) either as free or frame-mounted leaflets. The former approach for aortic valve replacement was reported by Senning in 1966, and details of a frame-mounted technique were published by Ionescu and Ross in 1966 [Ionescu, 1969] The approach combined the more natural leaflet format with a readily available living autologous tissue. Although early results seemed encouraging, Senning expressed his own doubt on the valve of this approach in 1971, and by 1978 fascia lata was no longer used in either of the above, or any other, form of valve replacement. The failure of this technique was due to the inadequate strength of this tissue when subjected to long-term cyclic stressing in the heart.

In parallel with the work on fascia lata valves, alternative forms of tissue leaflet valves were being developed. In these designs, however, more emphasis was placed on optimum performance characteristics than on the use of living tissue. In all cases the configuration involved a three-leaflet format which was maintained by the use of a suitably designed mounting frame. It was realized that naturally occurring animal tissues, if used in an untreated form, would be rejected by the host. Consequently, a method of chemical treatment had to be found which prevented this antigenic response but did not degrade the mechanical strength of the tissue.

Formaldehyde has been used by histologists for many years to arrest autolysis and "fix" tissue in the state in which it is removed. It had been used to preserve biologic tissues in cardiac surgery but, unfortunately, was found to produce shrinkage and increase the stiffness of the resulting material. For these reasons, formaldehyde was not considered ideal as a method of tissue treatment.

Glutaraldehyde is another histologic fixative which has been used especially for preserving fine detail for electron microscopy. It is also used as a tanning agent by the leather industry. In addition to arresting autolysis, glutaraldehyde produces a more flexible material due to increased collagen crosslinking. Glutaraldehyde has the additional ability of reducing the antigenicity of xenograft tissue to a level at which it can be implanted into the heart without significant immunologic reaction.

In 1969, Kaiser and coworkers described a valve substitute using an explanted glutaraldehyde-treated porcine aortic valve which was mounted on to a rigid support frame. Following modification in which the rigid frame was replaced by a frame having a rigid base ring with flexible posts, this valve became commercially available as the Hancock Porcine Xenograft in 1970 (Fig. 123.2a). It remains one of the two most popular valve substitutes of this type, the other being the Carpentier-Edwards Bioprosthesis introduced commercially by Edwards Laboratories in 1976. This latter valve uses a totally flexible support frame.

In 1977 production began of the Hancock Modified Orifice (M.O.) valve, a refinement of the Hancock Standard valve. The Hancock M.O. is of a composite nature—the right coronary leaflet containing the muscle shelf is replaced by a noncoronary leaflet of the correct size from another porcine valve. This high-pressure fixed valve is mounted into a Dacron-covered polypropylene stent. The Hancock II and Carpentier-Edwards supra-annular porcine bioprostheses are second-generation bioprosthetic valve designs which were introduced in the early 1980s. The porcine tissue is initially fixed at 1.5 mmHg and then at high pressure. This fixation method is designed to ensure good tissue geometry. Both valves are treated with antimineralization treatments. Neither valve has been FDA approved for clinical use in the United States.

In porcine prostheses, the use of the intact biologically formed valve makes it unnecessary to manufacture individual valve cusps. Although this has the obvious advantage of reduced complexity of construction, it does require a facility for harvesting an adequate quantity of valves so that an appropriate range of valve sizes of suitable quality can be made available. This latter problem did not occur in the production of the three-leaflet calf pericardium valve developed by Ionescu and colleagues; the construction of this valve involved the molding of fresh tissue to a tricuspid configuration around a support frame. As the tissue is held in this position, it is treated with a glutaraldehyde solution. The valve, marketed in 1976 as the Ionescu-Shiley Pericardial Xenograft, was discontinued in the mid-1980s due to structural failure problems. Early clinical results obtained with tissue valves indicated their superiority to mechanical valves with respect to a lower incidence of thromboembolic complications [Bodnar & Yacoub 1991]. For this reason the use of tissue valves increased significantly during the late 1970s.

The Carpentier-Edwards pericardial valve consists of three pieces of pericardium mounted completely within the Elgiloy wire stent to reduce potential abrasion between the Dacron-covered

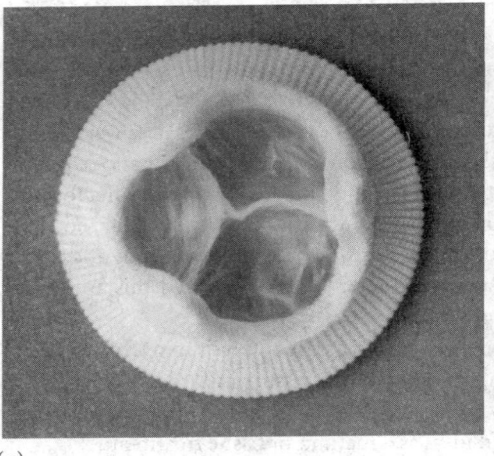   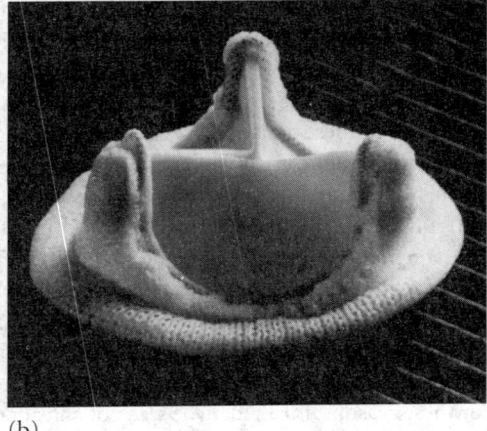

(a)   (b)

FIGURE 123.2   (*a*) Photograph of Hancock porcine valve; (*b*) photograph of Carpentier-Edwards pericardial valve.

frame and the leaflets. The pericardium is retained inside the stent by a Mylar button rather than by holding sutures. Its clinical implantation began in July 1980, and it is currently approved for clinical use in the United States (Fig. 123.2*b*).

Clinical experiences with different tissue valve designs have increasingly indicated time-dependent (5- to 7-year) structural changes such as calcification and leaflet wear, leading to valve failure and subsequent replacement [Ferrans et al., 1980; Oyer et al., 1979; Bodnar, Yacoub, 1986]. The problem of valve leaflet calcification is more prevalent in children and young adults. Therefore, tissue valves are rarely used in children and young adults at the present time. Such problems have not been eliminated by the glutaraldehyde tanning methods so far employed, and it is not easy to see how these drawbacks are to be overcome, unless either living autologous tissue is used or the original structure of the collagen and elastin are chemically enhanced. On the latter point there is, as yet, much room for further work. For instance, the fixing of calf pericardium under tension during the molding of the valve cusps will inevitably produce "locked-in" stresses during fixation, thus changing the mechanical properties of the tissue.

123.2 Current Types of Prostheses

At present, over 175,000 prosthetic valves are implanted each year throughout the world. Currently, the four most commonly used basic types of prostheses are:

1. Caged ball
2. Tilting disc
3. Bileaflet
4. Bioprostheses (tissue valves)

Valve manufacturers continue to develop new designs of mechanical and tissue valves. The ideal heart valve prosthesis does not yet exist and may never be realized. However, the characteristics of the "perfect" prostheses should be noted. The ideal heart valve should:

- Be fully sterile at the time of implantation and be nontoxic
- Be surgically convenient to insert at or near the normal location of the heart
- Conform to the heart structure rather than the heart structure conforming to the valve (i.e., the size and shape of the prosthesis should not interfere with cardiac function)
- Show a minimum resistance to flow so as to prevent a significant pressure drop across the valve
- Have a minimal reverse flow necessary for valve closure, so as to keep the incompetence of the valve at a low level
- Show long resistance to mechanical and structural wear
- Be long-lasting (25 years) and maintain its normal functional performance (i.e., must not deteriorate over time)
- Cause minimal trauma to blood elements and the endothelial tissue of the cardiovascular structure surrounding the valve
- Show a low probability for thromboembolic complications without the use of anticoagulants
- Be sufficiently quiet so as not to disturb the patient
- Be radiographically visible
- Have an acceptable cost

123.3 Tissue Versus Mechanical

Tissue prostheses gained widespread use during the mid-1970s. The major advantage of tissue valves compared to mechanical valves is that tissue valves have a lower incidence of thromboembolic complications [Butchart & Bodnar, 1992]. Therefore, most patients receiving tissue valves do not have to take anticoagulants long-term. The major disadvantages to tissue valves are large pressure drops compared to some mechanical valves (particularly in the smaller valve sizes), jetlike flow through the valve leaflets, material fatigue and/or wear of valve leaflets, and calcification of valve leaflets, especially in children and young adults. Valve deterioration, however, usually takes place slowly with tissue valves, and patients can be monitored by echocardiography and other noninvasive techniques.

The clear advantage of mechanical valves is their long-term durability. Current mechanical valves are manufactured from a variety of materials, such as pyrolitic carbon and titanium. Structural failure of mechanical valves is rare, but, when it occurs, is usually *catastrophic* [Giddens et al., 1993]. One major disadvantage of the use of mechanical valves is the need for continuous, life-long anticoagulation therapy to minimize the risk of thrombosis and thromboembolic complications. Unfortunately, the anticoagulation therapy may lead to bleeding problems; therefore, careful control of anticoagulation medication is essential for the patient's well-being and quality of life. Another concern is the hemodynamic performance of the prosthesis. The hemodynamic function of even the best designs of mechanical valves differs significantly from that of normal heart valves.

123.4 Engineering Concerns and Hemodynamic Assessment of Prosthetic Heart Valves

In terms of considerations related to heart valve design, the basic engineering concerns are

- Hydrodynamics/hemodynamics
- Durability (structural mechanics and materials)
- Biologic response to the prosthetic implant

The ideal heart valve design from the hemodynamic point of view should [Giddens et al., 1993]

- Produce minimal pressure gradient
- Yield relatively small regurgitation
- Minimize production of turbulence
- Not induce regions of high shear stress
- Contain no stagnation or separation regions in its flow field, especially adjacent to the valve superstructure

No valve design as yet, other than normal native valves, satisfies all these criteria.

Pressure Gradient

The heart works to maintain adequate blood flow through a prosthetic valve; a well-designed valve will not significantly impede that blood flow and will therefore have as small a pressure gradient as possible across the valve.

Because of the larger separation region inherent in flow over bluff bodies, configurations such as the caged disc and caged ball have notably large pressure gradients. Porcine bioprostheses have relatively acceptable pressure gradients for larger diameter valves because they more closely mimic natural valve geometry and motion, but the smaller sizes (<23 mm) generally have higher pressure gradients than their mechanical valve counterparts, as shown in Fig. 123.3 [Yoganathan et al., 1984]. Tilting disc and bileaflet valve designs present a relatively streamlined configuration to the flow, and, although separation regions may exist in these designs, the pressure gradients are typically smaller than for the bluff shapes. The clinical importance of pressure gradients in predicting long-term performance is not clear. The fact that these gradients are a manifestation of energy losses resulting from viscous-related phenomena makes it intuitive that minimizing pressure gradients across an artificial valve is highly desirable in order to reduce the workload of the pump (i.e., left ventricle).

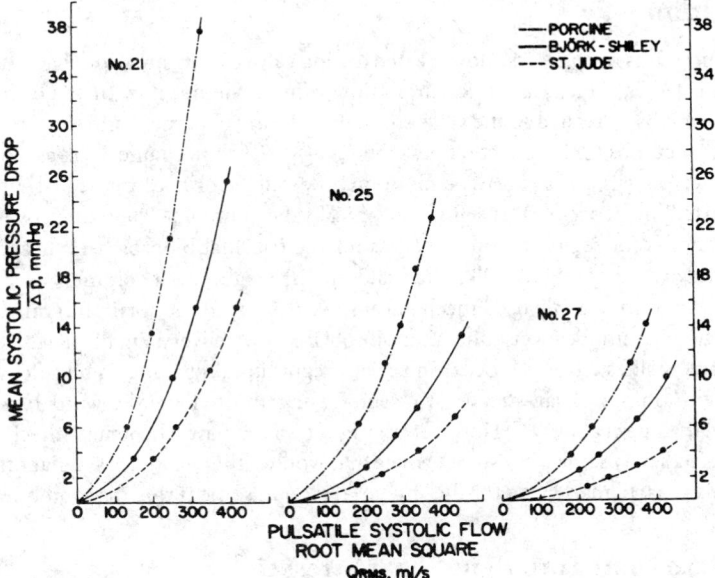

FIGURE 123.3 Examples of in vitro pulsatile flow pressure gradients across tilting disc (Bjork-Shiley convexo-concave), bileaflet (St. Jude Medical), and porcine aortic valves of three different sizes (27, 25, and 21 mm).

Effective Orifice Area (EOA)

The EOA is an index of how well a valve design utilizes its primary or internal stent orifice area. In other words, it is related to the degree to which the prosthesis itself obstructs the flow of blood. A larger EOA corresponds to a smaller pressure drop and therefore a smaller energy loss. It is desirable to have as large an EOA as possible. EOA is calculated from in vitro pressure drop measurements for a particular valve using the following formula [Yoganathan et al., 1984]:

$$EOA(cm^2) = \frac{Q_{rms}}{51.6\sqrt{\Delta \bar{p}}}$$

Q_{rms} is the root mean square systolic/diastolic flow rate (cm³/s), $\Delta\bar{p}$ is the mean systolic/diastolic pressure drop (mmHg).

Table 123.1 lists EOAs obtained in vitro, for different size mechanical and tissue valve designs in clinical use today. These results illustrate the fact that, size for size, the newer mechanical valve designs have better pressure gradient characteristics than porcine bioprostheses in current clinical use.

TABLE 123.1 Effective Orifice Areas of Different Prosthetic Aortic Valve Designs

Valve Sewing Ring Diam, mm	Medtronic-Hall Tilting Disc, cm²	St. Jude Bileaflet, cm²	Carbomedics Bileaflet, cm²	Hancock I Porcine, cm²	Hancock MO Porcine, cm²	Carpentier-Edwards Pericardial, cm²	Starr-Edwards 1260 Ball, cm²
19/20	1.74	1.21	1.12	1.01	1.22	1.56	1.04
21	1.74	1.81	1.66	1.31	1.43	1.88	1.23
23	2.26	2.24	2.28	1.73	1.94	2.25	1.45
25	3.07	3.23	3.14	1.93	2.16	3.25	1.59
27	3.64	4.05	3.75	2.14	–	3.70	1.75

Regurgitation

Regurgitation results from reverse flow created during valve closure and from backward leakage once closure is effected (see Fig. 123.4). Regurgitation reduces the net flow through the valve. Closing regurgitation is closely related to the valve shape and closing dynamics, and the percentage of stroke volume that succumbs to this effect ranges from 2.0–7.5% for mechanical valves. For tissue valves it is typically less: 0.1–1.5%. Leakage depends upon how well the orifices are "sealed" upon closure, and it has a reported incidence of 0–10% in mechanical valves and 0.2–3% in bioprosthetic valves. The overall tendency is for regurgitation to be less for the trileaflet bioprosthetic heart valves than for mechanical valve designs. Figure 123.5 illustrates in vitro regurgitant volumes (closing and leakage) measured on three commonly used mechanical valve designs in the aortic and mitral positions.

Regurgitation has implications other than simply for flow delivery. On the negative side, back flow through a narrow slit, such as can occur in leakage regurgitation through a bileaflet valve, can create relatively high laminar shear stresses, thus increasing the tendency toward blood cell damage [Baldwin, 1990; Cape et al., 1993]. However, regurgitation can have a beneficial effect in that the back-flow over surfaces may serve to wash out zones that would otherwise have stagnant flow throughout the cycle. This is particularly true for the "hinge" region in some tilting disc and bileaflet designs.

Flow Patterns and Turbulent Shear Stresses

Thrombosis and embolism, tissue overgrowth, hemolysis, and damage to endothelium adjacent to the valve are directly related to the velocity and turbulence fields created by various valve designs and have been addressed in detail during the past decade by investigators studying cardiovascular fluid mechanics [Chandran et al., 1983, 1984; Woo & Yoganathan 1985, 1986; Yoganathan et al., 1986a, 1986b; Yoganathan et al., 1988].

It has been established that shear stresses in the order of 1500–4000 dynes/cm^2 can cause lethal damage to red cells [Nevaril et al., 1969]. However, in the presence of foreign surfaces, red cells can be destroyed by shear stresses on the order of 10–100 dynes/cm^2 [Mohandas et al., 1974]. It has also been observed that sublethal damage to red cells can occur at turbulent shear stress levels of 500 dynes/cm^2 [Sutera & Merjhardi, 1975]. Platelets appear to be more sensitive to shear and can be damaged by shear stress on the order of 100–500 dynes/cm^2 [Ramstack et al., 1979; Wurzinger et al., 1983]. Evidence that platelet activation, aggregation, and thrombosis is induced by fluid shear forces has been predominantly generated by viscometric studies performed under well-defined fluid mechanical conditions. In viscometers, the extent and reversibility of shear-induced platelet aggregation are a function of both the magnitude and duration of the applied shear stress. For example, at 150 dynes/cm^2, platelet aggregation is not observed until shear is applied for 300 s. But, as the

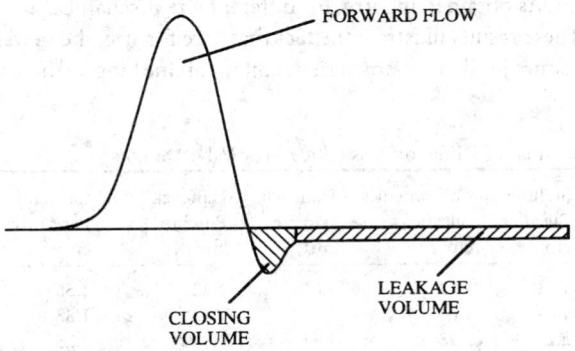

FIGURE 123.4   Flow cycle divided into forward flow, closing volume, and leakage volume.

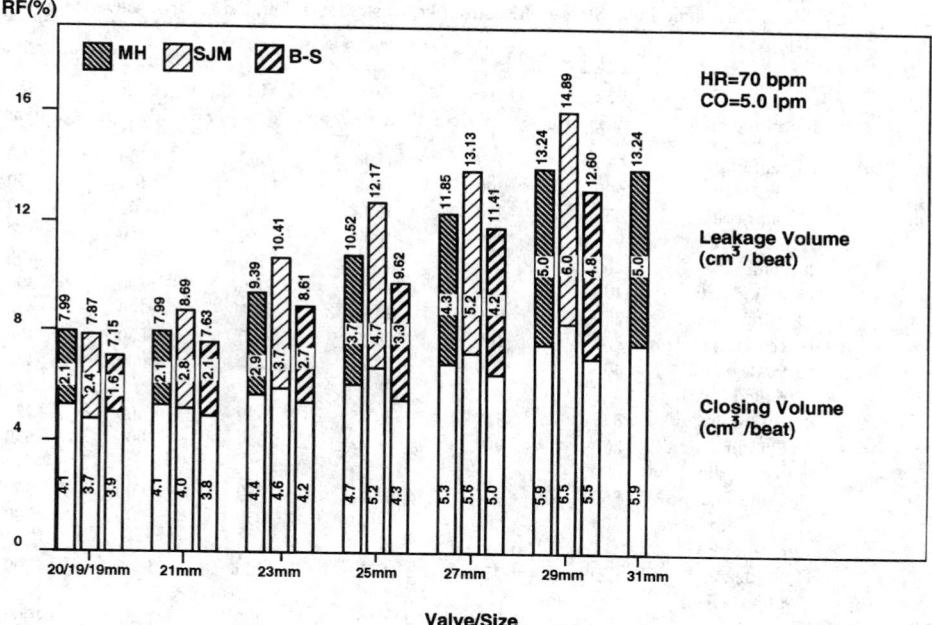

FIGURE 123.5 Examples of in vitro regurgitant volumes (closing and leakage) with three mechanical valve designs (MH—Medtronic-Hall; SJM—St. Jude Medical; B—Bjork-Shiley mono-strut).

intensity of the applied shear stress increases, platelet activation and aggregation occur more rapidly. For example, at a shear stress of 600 dynes/cm^2, platelet aggregation occurs within 30 s, and at 6500 dynes/cm^2, platelet activation occurs in fewer than 5 ms. As the magnitude of the applied shear increases, formed platelet aggregates tend not to separate when the shear forces are discontinued. Furthermore, platelet damage increases linearly with time of exposure to constant shear stress, indicating that shear-induced platelet damage is cumulative [Anderson & Hellums, 1978; Brown et al., 1977; Colantuoni et al., 1977].

Although the exact mechanism of turbulent stress damage to the cell is not precisely known, there is no disagreement that cell damage can be created by high turbulent stresses; minimizing these is conducive to better valve performance from the standpoints of thrombus formation, thromboembolic complications, and hemolysis and from energy loss considerations.

To illustrate the abnormal flow fields and elevated levels of turbulent shear stresses created by prosthetic valves, in vitro measurements conducted on 27-mm aortic valve designs in current clinical use in the United States (i.e., FDA approved) are presented below.

The figures of the in vitro flow field studies are presented as schematic diagrams and represent velocity and turbulence profiles obtained at peak systole, at a cardiac output of 6.0 l/min and a heart rate of 70 beats/min. All downstream distances are measured from the valve sewing ring. Tables 123.2 and 123.3 list the maximum and cross sectionally averaged mean turbulent shear stresses measured downstream of the valves at different times during systole and diastole.

Starr-Edwards Caged-Ball Valve (Model 1260)

The flow emerging from the valve formed a circumferential jet that separated from the ball, hit the wall of the flow chamber, and then flowed along the wall. The flow had very high velocities in the annular region. The maximum velocity, measured 12 mm downstream of the valve, was 220 cm/s at peak systole. The peak systolic velocity, measured 30 mm downstream of the valve, was 180 cm/s, as shown in Fig. 123.6. High-velocity gradients were observed at the edges of the jet. The maximum

TABLE 123.2   Peak and Mean Turbulent Shear Stresses Measured Downstream of Different Aortic Valve Designs

Valve	Location, mm	Acceleration Phase		Peak Systole		Deceleration Phase	
		Peak, dynes/cm²	Mean, dynes/cm²	Peak, dynes/cm²	Mean, dynes/cm²	Peak, dynes/cm²	Mean, dynes/cm²
Starr-Edwards (1260)	26, centerline	750	450	1800	1000	1400	700
	30, centerline	600	200	1850	1100	1300	750
Medtronic Hall	7, major orifice	450	250	1200	450	600	300
	7, minor orifice	950	400	1000	350	850	450
	13, centerline	1200	600	1000	550	800	400
	13, major orifice	400	320	1500	370	700	300
	13, minor orifice	1250	550	1450	700	700	450
	16, centerline	300	100	2000	1000	850	450
	15, 90 degree rotated (Fig.)	300	170	1450	700	900	450
St. Jude	8, centerline	820	450	1150	500	600	320
	8, 6.25 mm lateral to centerline	1600	1050	2000	1000	1000	650
	13, centerline	950	470	1500	750	1400	900
	13, 6.25 mm lateral to centerline	1400	800	2000	1050	1000	700
	11, 90-degree rotated (Fig.)	950	550	1700	1200	1000	700
Carpentier Edwards (2625 Porcine)	10, centerline	900	400	2750	1200	1750	1000
	15, centerline	1400	700	4500	2000	1700	900
Hancock MO (250 Porcine)	10, centerline	1000	400	2900	1100	1150	550
	15, centerline	1750	950	2450	1900	2100	1400
Carpentier Edwards (Pericardial)	17, centerline	500	100	850	200	1000	350
	33, centerline	850	200	1130	450	900	370

velocity gradient (1700 cm s⁻¹/cm) was observed in the annular region adjacent to the surface of the ball during peak systole. A large-velocity defect was observed in the central part of the flow chamber as a wake developed distal to the ball. A region of low velocity reverse flow was observed at peak systole and during the deceleration phase, with a diameter of about 8 mm immediately distal to the apex of the cage. The maximum reverse velocity measured was −25 cm/s; it occurred at peak systole 30 mm downstream of the valve (Fig. 123.6). The intensity of the reverse flow during the deceleration phase was not as high as that observed at peak systole. No reverse flow was observed during the acceleration phase. However, the velocity in the central part of the flow channel was low.

High turbulent shear stresses were observed at the edges of the jet. The maximum turbulent shear stress measured was 1850 dynes/cm², which occurred at the location of the highest-velocity gradient (Fig. 123.6). The intensity of turbulence during peak systole did not decay very rapidly downstream of the valve. Elevated turbulent shear stresses occurred during most of systole. Turbulent shear stresses as high as 3500 dynes/cm² were estimated in the annular region between the flow channel wall and the ball.

Medtronic Hall Tilting Disc Valve

High-velocity jetlike flows were observed from both the major and minor orifice outflow regions. The orientation of the jets with respect to the axial direction changed as the valve opened and closed. The major orifice jet was larger than the minor orifice jet and had a slightly higher velocity. The peak velocities measured 7 mm downstream of the valve were 210 cm/s and 200 cm/s in the major and the minor orifice regions, respectively (Fig. 123.7). A region of reverse flow was observed adjacent to the wall in the minor orifice region at peak systole, which extended 2 mm from the wall with a maximum reverse velocity of −25 cm/s. The size of this region increased during the deceleration phase to 8 mm from the wall. A small region of flow separation was observed adjacent to the wall in

TABLE 123.3 Peak and Mean Turbulent Shear Stresses Measured Downstream of Different Mitral Valve Designs

Valve	Location, mm	Acceleration Phase		Peak Diastole		Deceleration Phase	
		Peak, dynes/cm^2	Mean, dynes/cm^2	Peak, dynes/cm^2	Mean, dynes/cm^2	Peak, dynes/cm^2	Mean, dynes/cm^2
Beall	11, centerline	500	150	1950	450	800	250
	11, 10 mm above centerline	360	150	1300	400	425	150
	17, centerline	375	125	700	225	400	175
Bjork-Shiley (cc)	8, 13 mm above centerline	320	70	235	60	240	60
	8, 10 mm below centerline	40	18	30	17	25	19
	12, centerline	100	40	330	75	150	55
	15, 90-degree rotated	310	85	375	100	280	60
	18, centerline	90	60	300	110	225	80
	18, 13 mm above centerline	155	80	350	240	210	140
	18, 10 mm below centerline	60	25	210	70	70	25
Medtronic Hall	8, centerline	300	170	1800	400	650	180
	8, 12 mm above line center	850	300	1150	450	500	200
	8, 9 mm below centerline	900	230	1200	350	225	130
	14, 90-degree rotated	620	230	1200	320	670	230
	18, centerline	340	100	500	230	300	150
	18, 12 mm above centerline	600	230	2600	900	950	500
	18, 9 mm below centerline	280	130	670	280	360	180
St. Jude	10, centerline	170	95	250	95	175	85
	10, 10 mm above centerline	310	120	440	150	185	100
	12, 90-degree rotated	725	270	770	300	670	250
	19, centerline	130	80	335	130	165	90
	19, 10 mm above centerline	115	50	575	170	250	110

the major orifice region as illustrated by Fig. 123.7. In the minor orifice region, a profound velocity defect was observed 7 and 11 mm distal to the minor orifice strut (Fig. 123.7). Furthermore, the region adjacent to the wall immediately downstream from the minor orifice was stagnant during the acceleration and deceleration phases and had very low velocities (<15 cm/s) during peak systole.

In the major orifice region, high turbulent shear stresses were confined to narrow regions at the edges of the major orifice jet (Fig. 123.7). The peak turbulent shear stresses measured at peak systole were 1200 and 1500 dynes/cm^2, 7 and 13 mm downstream of the valve, respectively. During the acceleration and deceleration phases the turbulent shear stresses were relatively low. High turbulent shear stresses were more dispersed in the minor than those in the major orifice region as shown by Fig. 123.7. The turbulent shear stress profiles across the major and minor orifices 15 mm downstream of the valve (Fig. 123.7) showed a maximum turbulent shear stress of 1450 dynes/cm^2 at the lower edge of the minor orifice jet.

St. Jude Medical Bileaflet Valve

The St. Jude Medical valve has two semicircular leaflets which divide the area available for forward flow into three regions: two lateral orifices and a central orifice. The major part of the forward flow

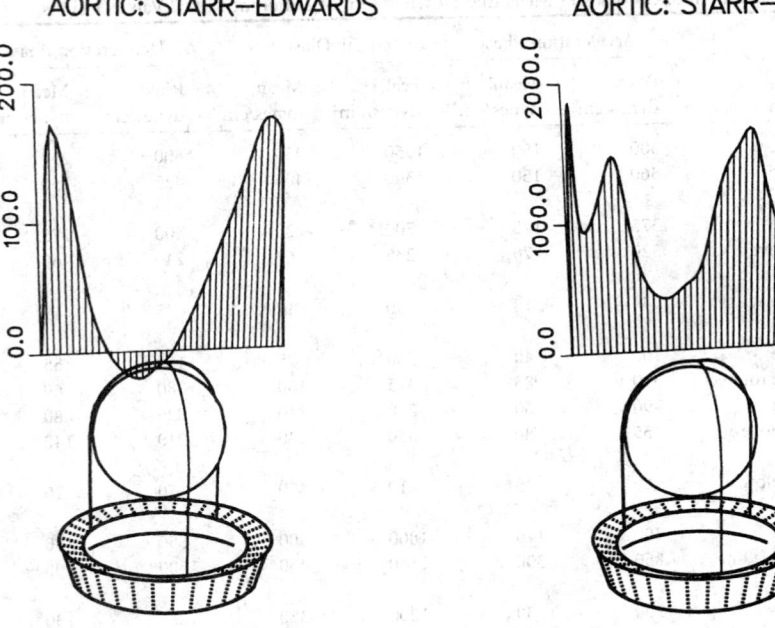

NUMBERS ARE VELOCITIES IN CM/S   NUMBERS ARE TURBULENT SHEAR STRESSES IN DYNES/CM²
(a)   (b)

FIGURE 123.6 (*a*) Velocity profile 30 mm downstream on the centerline for the Starr-Edwards ball valve, at peak systole; (*b*) turbulent shear stress profile 30 mm downstream on the centerline for the Starr-Edwards ball valve, at peak systole.

emerged from the two lateral orifices. The measurements along the centerline plane 8 mm downstream of the valve showed at peak systole a maximum velocity of 220 cm/s and 200 cm/s for the lateral and central orifice jets, respectively. The velocity of the jets remained about the same as the flow traveled from 8 to 13 mm downstream (Fig. 123.8). The velocity profiles showed two defects which corresponded to the location of the two leaflets. The velocity measurements indicated that the flow was more evenly distributed across the flow chamber during the deceleration than during the acceleration phase. Regions of flow separation were observed around the jets adjacent to the flow channel wall as the flow separated from the orifice ring. The measurements across the central orifice illustrated in Fig. 123.8 show that the maximum velocity in the central orifice was 220 cm/s. Small regions of low-velocity reverse flow were observed adjacent to the pivot/hinge mechanism of the valve (Fig. 123.8). More flow emerged from the central orifice during the deceleration phase than during the acceleration phase.

High turbulent shear stresses occurred at locations of high-velocity gradients and at locations immediately distal to the valve leaflets (Fig. 123.8). The flow along the centerline plane became more disturbed as the flow traveled from 8 to 13 mm downstream of the valve. The peak turbulent shear stresses measured along the centerline plane at peak systole were 1150 and 1500 dynes/cm² at 8 and 13 mm downstream of the valve, respectively. The profiles across the central orifice showed that the flow was very disturbed in this region. The maximum turbulent shear stress measured in the central orifice as shown in Fig. 123.8 (1700 dynes/cm²) occurred peak systole. Since these high turbulent shear stresses across the central orifice were measured 11 mm downstream, it is probable that even higher turbulent shear stresses occurred closer to the valve.

Carpentier-Edwards Porcine Valve (Model 2625)

The velocity profiles taken 10 mm downstream of the valve, along the centerline plane, showed that the peak velocity of the jetlike flow emerging from the valve was as high as 220 cm/s at peak systole

AORTIC: MEDTRONIC—HALL

AORTIC: MEDTRONIC—HALL

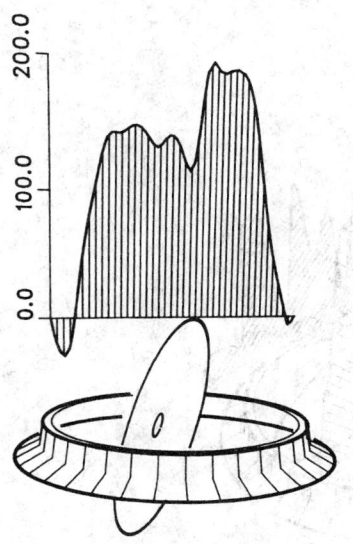

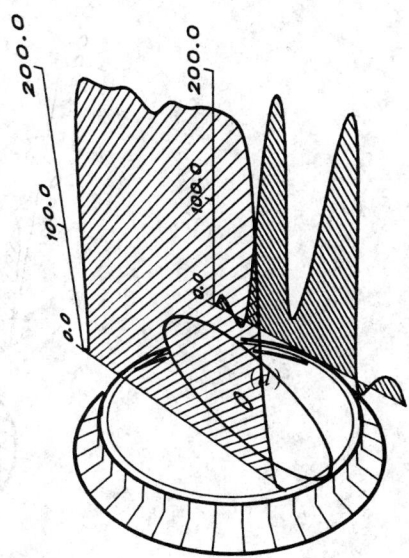

(a) NUMBERS ARE VELOCITIES IN CM/S (b) NUMBERS ARE VELOCITIES IN CM/S

AORTIC: MEDTRONIC—HALL

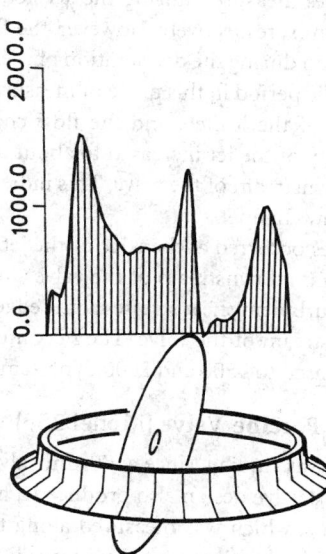

(c) NUMBERS ARE TURBULENT SHEAR STRESSES IN DYNES/CM²

FIGURE 123.7 (*a*) Velocity profile 15 mm downstream on the centerline across the major and minor orifices of the Medtronic-Hall tilting disc valve (major orifice to the right), at peak systole; (*b*) velocity profiles 13 mm downstream in the major and minor orifices of the Medtronic-Hall tilting disc valve, at peak systole; (*c*) turbulent shear stress profile 15 mm downstream on the centerline across the major and minor orifices of the Medtronic-Hall tilting disc valve (major orifice to the right), at peak systole; (*d*) turbulent shear stress profiles 13 mm downstream in the major and minor orifices of the Medtronic-Hall tilting disc valve, at peak systole.

AORTIC: MEDTRONIC—HALL

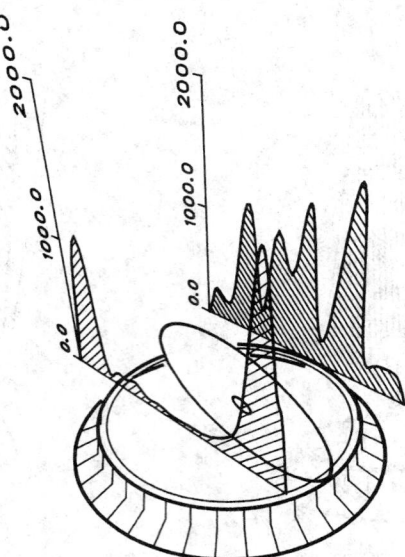

(d)   NUMBERS ARE TURBULENT SHEAR STRESSES IN DYNES/CM²

FIGURE 123.7   *(continued)*

(Fig. 123.9). The peak velocities measured during the acceleration and deceleration phases were about the same, 175 and 170 cm/s, respectively. However, the flow was much more evenly distributed during the acceleration than during the deceleration phase. No regions of flow separation were observed throughout the systolic period in this plane of measurement. However, the annular region between the outflow surfaces of the leaflets and the flow chamber wall was relatively stagnant throughout systole. The velocity of the jet increased to about 370 cm/s at peak systole, as the flow traveled from 10 to 15 mm downstream of the valve. This indicated that the flow tended to accelerate toward the center of the flow channel.

High turbulent shear stresses occurred at the edge of the jet (Fig. 123.9). The maximum turbulent shear stress measured 10 mm downstream of the valve along the centerline plane at peak systole was 2750 dynes/cm². The turbulent shear stresses at the edge of the jet increased as the flow traveled from 10 to 15 mm downstream of the valve. The maximum and mean turbulent shear stress measured at peak systole increased to 4500 and 2000 dynes/cm², respectively (Table 123.2).

Hancock Modified Orifice Porcine Valve (Model 250)

In this design, a 25-mm valve was studied, since a 27-mm valve is not manufactured. The velocity measurements showed that this valve design also produced a high-velocity jetlike flow field with a maximum velocity of 330 cm/s, which was measured along the centerline plane, 10 mm downstream. The jet, however, started to dissipate very rapidly as it flowed downstream. The maximum velocity measured 15 mm downstream of the valve was 180 cm/s, as shown in Fig. 123.10. A velocity defect was observed 15 mm downstream in the central part of the flow channel peak systole and during the deceleration phase but was not observed along the centerline plane 10 mm downstream of the valve. Once again, the annular region between the outflow surfaces of the leaflets and the flow chamber wall was relatively stagnant during systole.

Turbulent shear stress measurements showed that the high turbulent shear stresses measured 10 mm downstream of the valve were confined to a narrow region at the edge of the jet, with a peak

AORTIC: ST. JUDE

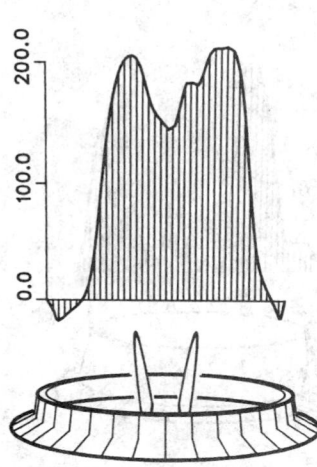

(a)   NUMBERS ARE VELOCITIES IN CM/S

AORTIC: ST. JUDE

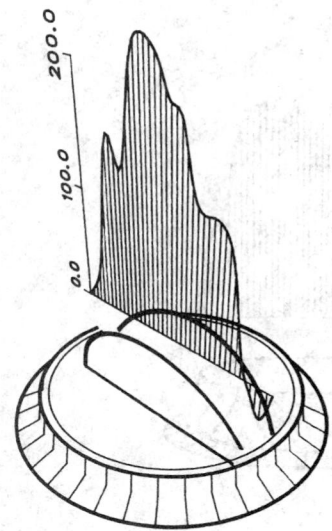

(b)   NUMBERS ARE VELOCITIES IN CM/S

AORTIC: ST. JUDE

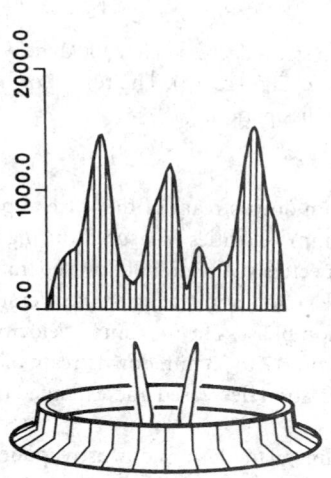

(c)

NUMBERS ARE TURBULENT SHEAR STRESSES IN DYNES/CM²   (d)

AORTIC: ST. JUDE

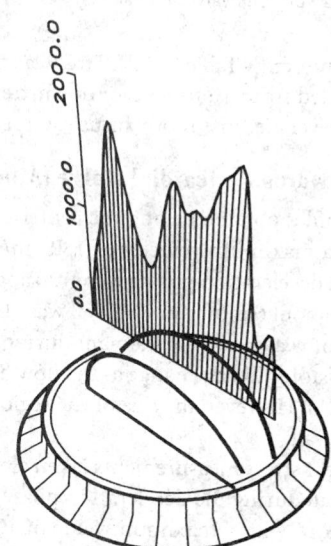

NUMBERS ARE TURBULENT SHEAR STRESSES IN DYNES/CM²

FIGURE 123.8   (*a*) Velocity profile 13 mm downstream on the centerline for the St. Jude Medical bileaflet valve, at peak systole; (*b*) velocity profile 13 mm downstream across the central orifice for the St. Jude Medical bileaflet valve, at peak systole; (*c*) turbulent shear stress profile 13 mm downstream of the centerline orifice for the St. Jude Medical bileaflet valve, at peak systole; (*d*) turbulent shear stress profile 13 mm downstream across the central orifice for the St. Jude Medical bileaflet valve, at peak systole.

AORTIC: C–E 2625 PORCINE

AORTIC: C–E PORCINE (2625)

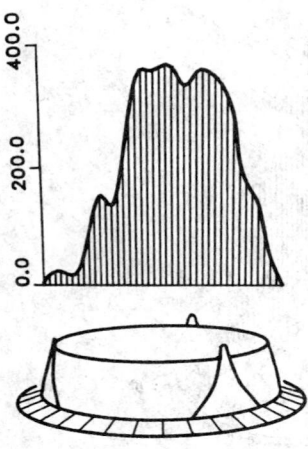

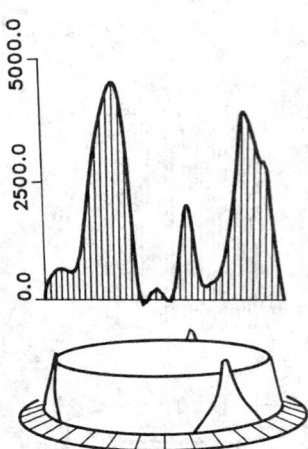

NUMBERS ARE VELOCITIES IN CM/S

(a)

NUMBERS ARE TURBULENT SHEAR STRESSES IN DYNES/CM²

(b)

FIGURE 123.9 (*a*) Velocity profile 15 mm downstream on the centerline for the Carpentier-Edwards 2625 porcine valve, at peak systole; (*b*) turbulent shear stress profile 15 mm downstream on the centerline for the Carpentier-Edwards 2625 porcine valve, at peak systole.

value of 2900 dynes/cm² (Table 123.2). This peak turbulent shear stress decreased to 2400 dynes/cm² as the flow traveled from 10 to 15 mm downstream of the valve (Fig. 123.10). The region of high turbulence, however, became more diffuse as a result of energy dissipation.

Carpentier-Edwards Pericardial Valve (Model 2900)

The velocity profiles obtained along the centerline plane 17 mm downstream of the valve at peak systole showed a maximum velocity of 180 cm/s. The maximum velocities measured during the acceleration and deceleration phases were 120 and 80 cm/s, respectively. A region of flow separation which extended about 6 mm from the wall was observed at peak systole and during the deceleration phase. This region was relatively stagnant during the acceleration phase. The maximum velocity of the jet at peak systole did not change as the flow field traveled from 17 to 33 mm downstream of the valve (Fig. 123.11). However, the size of the region of flow separation decreased and extended only 1 mm from the wall.

Turbulent shear stress measurements taken along the centerline plane 17 mm downstream of the valve showed that, during the deceleration phase, elevated turbulent shear stresses were spread out over a wide region (with a maximum value of 100 dynes/cm²). At peak systole, the high turbulent shear stresses were confined to a narrow region, with a maximum value of 850 dynes/cm² (Fig. 123.11). The intensity of turbulence at peak systole increased as the flow traveled from 17 to 33 mm downstream of the valve (Table 123.2).

123.5 Implications for Thrombus Deposition

In the vicinity of mechanical aortic heart valves, where peak shear stresses can easily exceed 1500 dynes/cm² and mean shear stresses are frequently in the range of 200–600 dynes/cm² (Table 123.2),

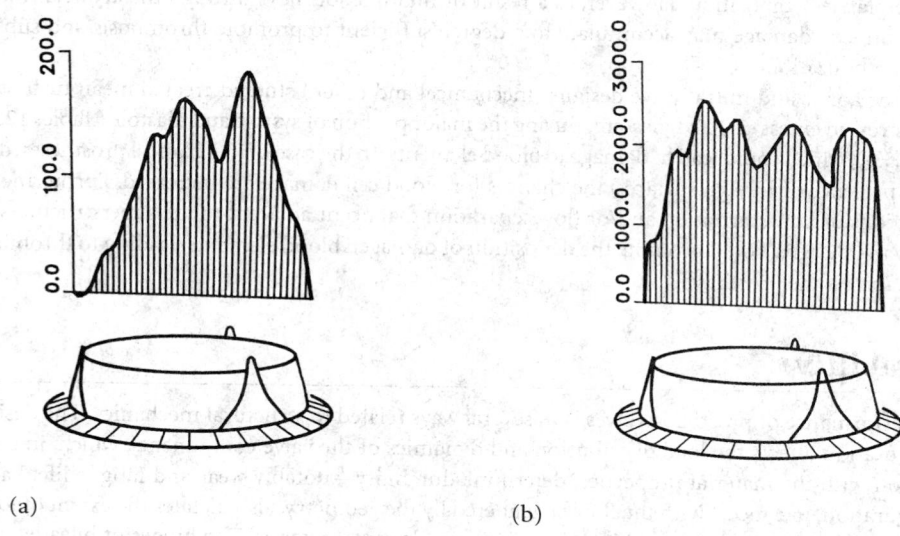

FIGURE 123.10 (*a*) Velocity profile 15 mm downstream on the center for the Hancock modified orifice porcine valve, at peak systole; (*b*) turbulent shear stress profile 15 mm downstream on the centerline for the Hancock modified orifice porcine valve, at peak systole.

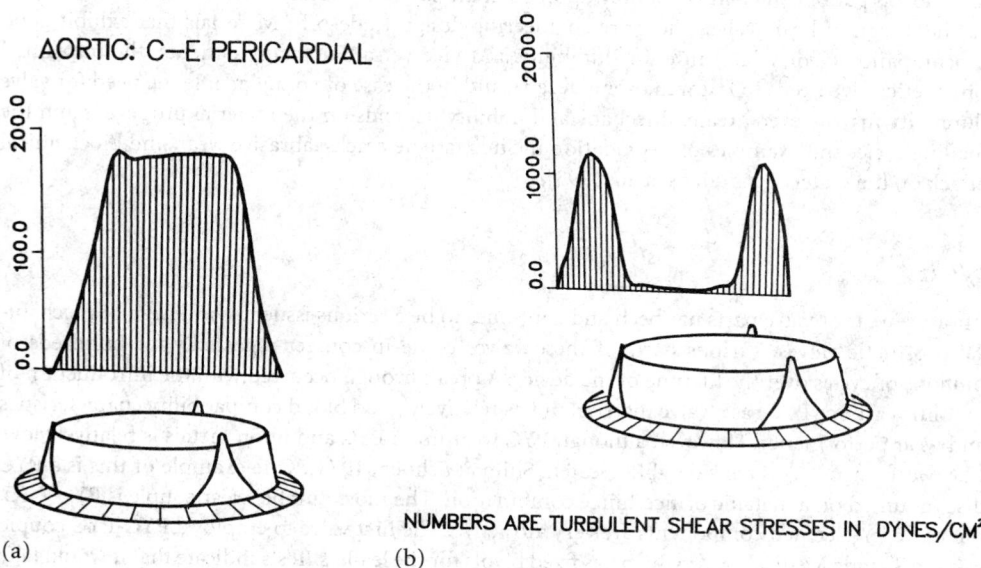

FIGURE 123.11 (*a*) Velocity profile 17 mm downstream on the centerline for the Carpentier-Edwards pericardial valve, at peak systole; (*b*) turbulent shear stress profile 17 mm downstream on the centerline for the Carpentier-Edwards pericardial valve, at peak systole.

platelet activation and aggregation can readily occur. Data indicating that shear-induced platelet damage is cumulative are particularly relevant to heart valves. During an individual excursion through the replacement valve, the combination of shear magnitude and exposure time may not induce platelet aggregation. However, as a result of multiple journeys through the artificial valve, shear-induced damage may accumulate to a degree sufficient to promote thrombosis and subsequent embolization.

All the aortic and mitral valve designs (mechanical and tissue) studied created mean turbulent shear stress in excess of 200 dynes/cm^2 during the major portion of systole and diastole (Tables 123.2 and 123.3), which could lead to damage to blood elements. In the case of mechanical prostheses, due to the presence of foreign surfaces, the chances for blood cell damage are increased. Furthermore, the regions of flow stagnation and/or flow separation that occur adjacent to the superstructures of these valve designs, could promote the deposition of damaged blood elements, leading to thrombus formation on the prosthesis.

123.6 Durability

The performance of prosthetic valves is in several ways related to structural mechanics. The design configuration affects the load distribution and dynamics of the valve components, which, in conjunction with the material properties, determine durability—notably wear and fatigue life. Valve configuration, in concert with the flow engendered by the geometry, also dictates the extent of low-wear (e.g., flow separation) and high-shear (e.g., gap leakage) regions. The hinges of bileaflet and tilting disc valves are vulnerable—their design can produce sites of stagnant flow, which may cause localized thrombosis, which may in turn restrict occluder motion. In addition, as discussed earlier, the rigid circular orifice ring is an unnatural configuration for a heart valve, since the elliptically shaped natural valve annulus changes in size and shape during the cardiac cycle.

The choice of valve materials is closely related to structural factors, since the fatigue and wear performance of a valve depend not only on its configuration and loading but on the material properties as well. In addition, the issue of biocompatibility is crucial to prosthetic valve design— and biocompatibility depends not only upon the material itself but also on its in vivo environment. In the design of heart valves there are engineering design trade-offs: Materials that exhibit good biocompatibility may have inferior durability and vice versa. For many patients, the implanted prosthetic valve needs to last well over a decade, and in the case of young people the need for valve durability may be even greater. Mechanical durability depends on the material properties and the loading cycle, and examples of degradation include fatigue cracks, abrasive wear, and biochemical attack on the material [Giddens et al., 1993].

Wear

Abrasive wear of valve parts has been and continues to be a serious issue in the design of mechanical prosthetic valves. Various parts of these valves come in contact repeatedly for hundreds of millions of cycles over the lifetime of the device. A breakthrough occurred with the introduction of pyrolitic carbon (PYC) as a valve material: It has relatively good blood compatibility characteristics and wear performance. However, although PYC wear upon PYC and upon metals is relatively low, PYC wear by metals is considerably greater [Shim & Schoen, 1974]. One example of this is a PYC disc mounted on a metallic orifice/hinge combination. The most durable wear couple is PYC-PYC, therefore PYC-coated components are very attractive. The first valve to employ a PYC-PYC couple was the St. Jude Medical valve, which has fixed pivots for the leaflets. Tests indicate that it would take 200 years to wear halfway through the PYC coating on a leaflet pivot [Gombrich et al., 1979]. By creating designs that allow wear surfaces to be distributed rather than focal (i.e., the Omnicarbon valve, which has a PYC-coated disc that is free to rotate), it is possible to reduce wear even further.

Thus, materials technology continues to progress and in fact has reached the point where wear need not negatively impact the performance of prosthetic mechanical valves.

Fatigue

Metals are prone to fatigue failure. Their polycrystalline nature contains structural characteristics that may produce dislocations under mechanical loading. These dislocations can migrate when subjected to repeated loading cycles and can accumulate at intercrystalline boundaries, and the end result is tiny cracks. These tiny cracks are sites of stress concentration, and the fissures can worsen until fracture occurs. The Haynes 25 Stellite Bjork-Shiley valve, which used a chromium-cobalt alloy, experienced the most severe fatigue problem for a mechanical valve [Lindblom et al., 1986]. Previous investigations suggested that fatigue was not a problem for PYC; however, recent data contradict this, suggesting that cyclic fatigue-crack growth occurs in graphite/pyrolitic carbon composite material [Ritchie et al., 1990]. This work suggests a fatigue threshold that is as low as 50% of the fracture toughness, and those authors view cyclic fatigue as an essential consideration in the design and life prediction of heart valves constructed from PYC. The FDA now requires detailed characterization of PYC materials used in different valve designs (December 1993 FDA heart valve guidelines).

Mineralization

The major cause of both porcine aortic and pericardial bioprosthetic valve failure is calcification, which stiffens and frequently causes cuspal tears [Levy et al., 1991]. Calcific deposits occur most commonly at the commissures and basal attachments. Calcification is most extensive deep in (intrinsic to) the cusps in the spongiosa layer. Ultrastructurally, calcific deposits are associated with cuspal connective tissue cells and collagen. Degenerative cuspal calcific deposits are composed of calcium phosphates that are chemically and structurally related to physiologic bone mineral (hydroxyapatite). The flexing bladders in cardiac assist devices, flexing polymeric heart valves, and vascular grafts have also been found to be vulnerable to calcific deposits. In such cases, calcification is usually related to inflammatory cells adjacent to the blood-contacting surface, rather than to the implanted material itself.

The mechanisms of calcification, and the methods of preventing calcification are active areas of current research [Webb et al., 1991]. The most common methods of studying calcification involves valve tissue implanted either subcutaneously in 3-week-old weanling rats or valves implanted as mitral replacements in young sheep or calves. Results of both types of studies show that bioprosthetic tissue calcifies in a fashion similar to clinical implants but at a greatly accelerated rate. The subcutaneous implantation mode is a well-accepted, technically convenient, economical, and quantifiable model for investigating mineralization issues. It is also very useful for determining the potential of new antimineralization treatments.

Host, implant, and biomechanical factors impact the calcification of tissue valves. Patients who are young or have renal failure are vulnerable to valve mineralization, but immunologic factors seem to be unimportant. Pretreatment of valve tissue with an aldehyde crosslinking agent has been found to cause calcification in rat subcutaneous implants; nonpreserved cusps do not mineralize. Calcification of bioprosthetic valves is greatest at the cuspal commissures and bases, where leaflet flexion is the greatest and deformations are maximal. Most data suggest that the basic mechanisms of tissue valve mineralization result from aldehyde pretreatment, which changes the tissue microstructure.

In both clinical and experimental bioprosthetic tissue, the earliest mineral deposits are observed to be localized to transplanted connective tissue cells. The collagen fibers are involved later. Mineralization of the connective tissue cells of bioprosthetic tissue is thought to result from glutaraldehyde-induced cellular "revitalization" and the resulting disruption of cellular calcium regulation. Normal animal cells have a low intracellular free calcium concentration (approximately 10^{-7} M), whereas extracellular free calcium is much higher (approximately 10^{-3} M), yielding a 10,000-fold gradient across the plasma membrane. In healthy cells, cellular calcium is maintained in low concentration by energy-requiring metabolic mechanisms. In addition, organellar and plasma membranes and cell nuclei, the observed sites of early nucleation of bioprosthetic tissue mineralization, contain considerable phosphorus, mainly in the form of phospholipids. In cells modified by aldehyde crosslinking, passive calcium entry occurs unimpeded, but the mechanisms for calcium removal are dysfunctional. This calcium influx reacts with the preexisting phosphorus and contributes to the mineralization [Schoen et al., 1986]. A very recent article discusses the approaches to preventing heart valve mineralization [Schoen, 1993].

123.7 Current Trends in Valve Design

The long-term clinical durability of bioprosthetic valves is the major impediment to their use. Before long-term durability data became available, improvement of hemodynamic performance was the focus of development. The clinical introduction of the bovine pericardial valve solved the hemodynamic problem, and such valves exhibit hemodynamics equal to or better than some mechanical prostheses.

The long-term durability of porcine and bovine bioprostheses can be improved through innovative stent designs that minimize stress concentrations and through improved processing fixation techniques that yield more pliable tissue. The most recent tissue valve design is the stentless bioprosthesis, used for aortic valve replacement. These aortic root bioprostheses are similar in concept to homografts. Absence of the stent is thought to improve hemodynamics, as there is less obstruction in the orifice. The absence of the stent is also thought to improve durability of the tissue, as there is less mechanical wear. Currently, three designs of stentless aortic valves (Medtronic's Freestyle, Baxter's Prima, and St. Jude's Toronto Non-Stented) are undergoing clinical evaluation in the United States and Europe. New antimineralization treatments are also being developed with the goal of increasing the durability of the tissue.

If the above-mentioned design challenges are met, so that bioprostheses can be produced that are durable and thromboresistant, and anticoagulant therapy is not required, there most likely will be another swing toward increased bioprosthesis use.

123.8 Conclusion

Direct comparison of the "total" performance of artificial heart valves is difficult, if not impossible. The precise definition of criteria used to benchmark valve performance varies from study to study. To study long-term performance, large numbers of patients and lengthy observation periods are required. During these periods there may be an evolution in valve materials, or design, and in the medical treatment of patients with prosthetic heart valves. The age of the patient at implant and the underlying valvular heart disease are extremely important factors in valve choice and longevity as well. A valve design suited for the aortic position may be inappropriate for the mitral position. Consequently, it is not possible to categorize a particular valve as *the best*. All valves currently in use, mechanical and bioprosthetic, produce relatively large turbulent stresses (that can cause lethal and or sublethal damage to red cells and platelets) and greater pressure gradients and regurgitant volumes than normal heart valves.

There are three promising directions for further advances in heart valves (and therefore three challenges for engineers designing new heart valves):

- Improved thromboresistance with new and better artificial materials
- Improved durability of new tissue valves, through the use of nonstented tissue valves, new anticalcification treatments, and better fixation treatments
- Improved hemodynamic characteristics, especially reduction or elimination of low shear stress regions near valve and vessel surfaces and of high turbulent shear stresses along the edges of jets produced by valve outflow and/or leakage of flow

Whereas the artificial valves certainly have room for further improvement, the superior prognosis for the patient with a replacement heart valve is dramatic and convincing.

Acknowledgments

The technical writing assistance of Ms. Julie Cerlson made the writing of this chapter an enjoyable experience.

References

Anderson GH, Hellums JD. 1978. Platelet lysis and aggregation in shear fields. Blood Cells 4:499.

Baldwin, T. 1990. An investigation of the mean fluid velocity and Reynolds stress fields within an artificial heart ventricle. Ph.D. thesis, Penn State University, PA.

Bodnar E, Frater R. 1991. Replacement Cardiac Valves, New York, Pergamon Press.

Bodnar E, Yacoub M. 1986. Biologic & Bioprosthetic Valves, New York, York Medical Books.

Brewer LA III. 1969. Prosthetic Heart Valves, Springfield, Ill, Charles C Thomas.

Brown CH III, Lemuth RF, Hellums JD, et al. 1977. Response of human platelets to shear stress. Trans ASAIO 21:35.

Butchart EG, Bodnar E. 1992. Thrombosis, Embolism and Bleeding, ICR Publishers.

Cape EG, Nanda NC, Yoganathan AP. 1993. Quantification of regurgitant flow through bileaflet heart valve prostheses: theoretical and in vitro studies. Ultrasound Med Biol 19(6):461.

Chandran KG, Cabell GN, Khalighi B, et al. 1983. Laser anemometry measurements of pulsatile flow past aortic valve prostheses. J Biomech 16:865.

Chandran KG, Cabell GN, Khalighi B, et al. 1984. Pulsatile flow past aortic valve bioprosthesis in a model human aorta. J Biomech 17:609.

Colantuoni G, Hellums JD, Moake JL, et al. 1977. The response of human platelets to shear stress at short exposure times. Trans ASAIO 23:626.

Ferrans VJ, Boyce SW, Billingham ME, et al. 1980. Calcific deposits in porcine bioprostheses: Structure and pathogenesis. Am J Cardiol 46:721.

Giddens DP, Yoganathan AP, Schoen FJ. 1993. Prosthetic cardiac valves. Cardiovasc Pathol 2(3)(suppl.):167S.

Gombrich PP, Villafana MA, Palmquist WE. 1979. From concept to clinical—the St. Jude Medical bileaflet pyrolytic carbon cardiac valve. Presented at Association for the Advancement of Medical Instrumentation, 14th Annual Meeting, Las Vegas, Nev.

Ionescu MF, Ross DN. 1969. Heart valve replacement with autologous fascia lata. Lancet. 2:335.

Lefrak EA, Starr A. 1979. Cardiac Valve Prostheses, New York, Appleton-Century-Crofts.

Levy RJ, Schoen FJ, Anderson HC, et al. 1991. Cardiovascular implant calcification: a survey and update. Biomaterials 12:707.

Lindblom D, Bjork VO, Semb KH. 1986. Mechanical failure of the Bjork-Shiley valve. J Thorac Cardiovasc Surg 92:894.

Mohandas H, Hochmuth RM, Spaeth EE. 1974. Adhesion of red cells to foreign surfaces in the presence of flow. J Biomed Mater Res 8:119.

Nevaril C, Hellums J, Alfrey C Jr, et al. 1969. Physical effects in red blood cell trauma. J Am Inst Chem Engr 15:707.

Oyer PE, Stinson EB, Reitz BA, et al. 1979. Long term evaluation of the porcine xenograft bioprosthesis. J Thorac Cardiovasc Surg 78:343.

Ramstack JM, Zuckerman L, Mockros, LF. 1979. Shear induced activation of platelets. J Biomech 12:113.

Ritchie RO, Dauskart RH, Yu W. 1990. Cyclic fatigue-crack propagation, stress-corrosion, and fracture-toughness in pyrolytic carbon-coated graphite for prosthetic heart valve applications. J Biomed Mater Res 24:189.

Roberts WC. 1976. Choosing a substitute cardiac valve; type, size, surgeon. Am J Cardiol 38:633.

Schoen FJ, Libby P, Diddersheim P. 1993. Future directions and therapeutic approaches. Cardiovasc. Pathol. 2(3) (Suppl.):2095.

Schoen FJ, Tsao JW, Levy RJ. 1986. Calcification of bovine pericardium used in cardiac valve bioprostheses: implications for the mechanisms of bioprosthetic tissue mineralization. Am J Pathol 123:134.

Shim HS, Schoen FJ. 1974. The wear resistance of pure and silicon alloyed isotropic carbons. Biomater Med Dev Artif Organs 2:103.

Sutera SP, Merjhardi MH. 1975. Deformation and fragmentation of human red cells in turbulent shear flow. Biophys J 15:1.

Wain EH, Greco R, Ignegen A, et al. 1980. Int J Artif Organs 3:169.

Webb CL, Schoen FJ, Alfrey AC, et al. 1991. Inhibition of mineralization of glutaraldehyde-pretreated bovine pericardium by A1Cl$_3$ and other metallic salts in rat subdermal model studies. Am J Pathol 38:971.

Woo Y-R, Yoganathan AP. 1985. In vitro pulsatile flow velocity and turbulent shear stress measurements in the vicinity of mechanical aortic l heart valve prostheses. Life Support Syst 3:283.

Woo Y-R, Yoganathan AP. 1986. In vitro pulsatile flow velocity and shear stress measurements in the vicinity of mechanical mitral heart valve prostheses. J Biomech 19:39.

Wurzinger LJ, Opitz R, Blasberg P, et al. 1983. The role of hydrodynamic factors in platelet activation and thrombotic events. In G Schettler (ed), The Effects of Shear Stress of Short Duration, Fluid Dynamics as a Localizing Factor for Atherosclerosis, pp 91–102, Berlin, Springer.

Yoganathan AP, Chaux A, Gray R, et al. 1984. Bileaflet, tilting disc and porcine aortic valve substitutes: in vitro hydrodynamic characteristics. JACC. 3(2):313.

Yoganathan AP, Reul H, Black MM. 1992. Heart valve replacements: Problems and developments. In GW Hastings (ed), Cardiovascular Biomaterials, London, Springer-Verlag.

Yoganathan AP, Sung H-W, Woo Y-R, et al. 1988. In vitro velocity and turbulence measurements in the vicinity of three new mechanical aortic heart valve prostheses. J Thorac Cardiovasc Surg 95:929.

Yoganathan AP, Woo Y-R, Sung H-W, et al. 1986a. In vitro haemodynamic characteristics of tissue bioprostheses in the aortic position. J Thorac Cardiovasc Surg 92:198.

Yoganathan AP, Woo Y-R, Sung H-W. 1986b. Turbulent shear stress measurements in the vicinity of aortic heart valve prostheses. J Biomech 19:433.

124

Vascular Grafts

David N. Ku
Georgia Institute of Technology

Robert C. Allen
Emory University

The use of natural or synthetic replacement parts in vascular repair and vascular reconstruction is extensive, with a vascular graft market of approximately $200 million worldwide. A multitude of biologic grafts and synthetic prostheses are available, each with distinct qualities and potential applications [Rutherford, 1989; Veith et al., 1994]. The ideal vascular graft would (1) be biocompatible, (2) be nonthrombogenic, (3) have long-term potency (4) be durable yet compliant, (5) be infection resistant, and (6) be technically facile. There is currently no ideal conduit available, but, overall, the autogenous saphenous vein is preferred for small-vessel reconstruction, and synthetic prostheses are best suited for large-vessel replacement. Large-diameter (>10 mm) vascular grafts are predominantly used for aortic/iliac artery reconstruction with Dacron (80%) and PTFE (20%) being the standard construction materials. Synthetic grafts function well in these high-flow, low-resistance circuits with high long-term patencies. Small-caliber (<10 mm) vascular grafts are used for a variety of indications including lower-extremity bypass procedures, coronary artery bypass grafting (CABG), hemodialysis access, and extra-anatomic bypasses. Saphenous vein is the conduit of choice for lower-extremity revascularization and CABG procedures and shows superior patency rates compared to synthetic grafts. Internal mammary artery (IMA) grafts are used extensively for CABG with better long-term patency than saphenous vein grafts. Synthetic prostheses are used for hemodialysis access and extra-anatomic bypass grafting, especially PTFE due to its durability and resistance to external pressure. Bovine carotid heterografts are also used for hemodialysis access with fair success, but their value is questionable because of aneurysmal changes over time due to graft degeneration.

124.1 History of Vascular Grafts

Vascular surgery was first defined as a field with the initial publication of Alexis Carrel's work in 1902. Goyanes performed the first arterial graft in 1906 by using the popliteal vein *in situ* to replace an excised popliteal artery aneurysm. Lexer, in 1907, performed the first free autogenous vein graft by replacing an axillary artery defect with a segment of greater saphenous vein from the same patient. It was not until 1949, however, that Kunlin performed the first successful femoropopliteal bypass with reversed saphenous vein. The Korean War was the true advent of reconstructive surgery for arterial injuries as initiated by Shumacker and reported by Hughes and Bowers in 1952. The first report of a synthetic graft also appeared in 1952 when Voorhees described his initial work in dogs using tubes

0-8493-8346-3/95/$0.00+$.50
© 1995 by CRC Press, Inc.

of Vinyon-N cloth to bridge arterial defects. In the late 1950s and 1960s DeBakey firmly established the clinical usefulness of Dacron grafts; Dacron arterial prostheses became commercially available in 1957. Microporous expanded polytetrafluoroethylene (ePTFE) grafts, introduced in the 1970s, were the next generation of successful synthetic grafts but bear no clear superiority to Dacron grafts.

124.2 Synthetic Grafts

Synthetic prostheses are the preferred conduit for large-vessel reconstruction and the primary alternative to saphenous vein in small-vessel repair. Thankfully, the saphenous vein is of adequate quality and length in 70–75% of patients requiring small-vessel grafting. The two major choices available for prosthetic reconstruction are Dacron (polyethylene terephthalate) and PTFE (polytetrafluoroethylene). The tensile strength of these grafts remains unchanged even after years of implantation, whereas Nylon (Polyamide), Ivalon, and Orlon lose significant tensile strength over a period of months.

Dacron grafts are constructed from multifilamentous yarn and fabricated by weaving or knitting [Rutherford, 1989; Sawyer, 1987]. Woven fabric is interlaced in an over-and-under pattern resulting in a nonporous graft with no stretch. Knitted fabrics have looped threads forming a continuous interconnecting chain with variable stretch and porosity. Knitted velour is a variant in which the loops of yarn extend upward at right angles to the fabric surface resulting in a velvety texture. The velour finish may be created on the internal, the external, or both surfaces to enhance preclotting and tissue incorporation. Porous knitted Dacron prostheses may be made impervious by impregnation or coating with albumin/collagen to obviate preclotting and minimize blood loss while maintaining the superior handling characteristics of knitted Dacron grafts. Dacron prostheses are often crimped to impart elasticity, maintain shape during bending, and facilitate vascular anastomosis formation. The use of external support for vascular grafts is an alternative to crimping which uses externally attached polyprophylene rings to avoid kinking with angulation and to create dimensional stability. Woven Dacron grafts possess poor handling characteristics and poor compliance and elicit a poor healing response and, therefore, are used predominantly in the repair of the thoracic aorta, ruptured abdominal aortic aneurysms, and patients with coagulation defects. Knitted Dacron prostheses are used in the remainder of cases involving the abdominal aorta, iliac, femoral, and popliteal vessels, and in extra-anatomic repair/bypass. Dacron grafts are not advocated in small-vessel reconstruction, such as the below-knee popliteal or tibial, because of poor patency rates. An active infective process or contaminated field contraindicate the use of Dacron prostheses. Vascular grafts are named after the vessel they replace or the arterial segments they connect.

Expanded Teflon (ePTFE) is a synthetic polymer of carbon and fluorine produced by mechanical stretching [Rutherford, 1989; Sawyer, 1987]. The result is a series of solid nodes of ePTFE with interconnecting small fibrils. The pore size is variable and averages 30 microns. The chief advantages of ePTFE in comparison to knitted Dacron include impermeability to blood, resistance to aneurysmal formation, and ease of declotting; ePTFE is used clinically mainly for femoropopliteal bypasses, hemodialysis angioaccess, and extra-anatomic reconstructions. The addition of an external support coil can be used to enhance graft stability against external pressures and to prevent kinking at points of angulation.

The primary area of failure in prosthetic grafting with Dacron and PTFE is the patency of small-caliber grafts, which remains poor. The inherent thrombogenicity of these prosthetic grafts in conjunction with neointimal hyperplasia, which is limited to the anastomotic areas, are the prime factors. The seeding of prosthetic grafts with endothelial cells and subsequent proliferation of these cells into a confluent monolayer along the graft has been suggested as an attractive solution to this problem for a number of years. The technology and techniques devoted to develop this solution to small-caliber graft patency have been impressive, but the results have been variable and certainly not the panacea envisioned by early investigators. The clinical utility of endothelial cell seeding onto prosthetic grafts remains to be defined.

TABLE 124.1   Patency Data for Representative Vascular Grafts

Graft	Conduit	5-Year Patency, percent
Aortobifemoral	Dacron	90
Aortobifemoral	ePTFE	90
Femorofemoral	Dacron	80
Femorofemoral	ePTFE	80
Femoropopliteal	Saphenous vein	70
Femoropopliteal	Dacron	50
Femoropopliteal	ePTFE	40
Dialysis access	ePTFE	60 (3 years)
Dialysis access	Bovine heterograft	25 (3 years)

124.3 Regional Patency

Patency data for any vascular graft depend on multiple factors including the conduit and vessel size. Large-diameter vessels have a high rate of patency, and therefore, synthetic grafts are the conduit of choice and display high short- and long-term patencies. Saphenous vein is the primary graft for small-caliber vessel reconstruction with good patency rates, and prosthetic grafts demonstrate acceptable short-term patencies but poor long-term results. Extra-anatomic bypasses utilize synthetic conduits with external support to reduce kinking. Dacron versus PTFE graft trials have shown no significant difference in patency rates [Rutherford, 1989]. Hemodialysis access grafts are constructed primarily of PTFE with a minority of bovine carotid heterografts still present. PTFE is preferred due to resistance to infection, decreased pseudoaneurysm formation, and improved patency rates. Patency data for representative vascular grafts is summarized in Table 124.1 by anatomical location and conduit [Imparato et al., 1972; Rutherford, 1989; Veith et al., 1994].

Vascular grafts have a finite life span which is usually reported in the form of a life-table of graft patency. The patency rate falls to about 50% in 4 years after implantation for the most common PTFE femoral-popliteal grafts. Graft failures are typically caused by: (1) thrombosis in the early postoperative period of 1 month, (2) tissue ingrowth or neointimal hyperplasia at the anastomoses after several years, and (3) graft infections. Thrombosis in the early postoperative period is usually caused by a technical error at time of implantation and is readily fixed. The longer-term growth of tissue at the anastomoses is more insidious. Late failure of these grafts as a result of neointimal hyperplasia is a major problem confronting the vascular surgeon. Increasing the longevity of these grafts would greatly benefit the patient and have an important economic impact, nationally.

124.4 Thrombosis

When an artificial vascular graft is first exposed to blood, a clot will typically form at the surface. The clot is formed initially of platelet aggregates, and then the coagulation cascade is activated to lay down fibrin and thrombin. The tissue which forms this inner lining of the graft is often called pseudointimal hyperplasia. Pseudointimal hyperplasia is devoid of cellular ingrowth and is composed mainly of fibrin, platelet debris, and trapped red blood cells [Greisler, 1991]. The blood clots immediately on contact and will occlude the vessel if the blood is stagnant or very sluggish. Platelet activity is generally most intense during the first 24 hours and subsides to a very low level after 1 week.

Various artificial surfaces are more or less thrombogenic. Many approaches have been developed in an attempt to make the grafts less thrombogenic [Greisler, 1991]. Typically, the surface characteristics have been modified to prevent adherence or activation of platelets. The surfaces have been modified by seeding with endothelial cells and other exotic treatments such as photopolymerization, plasma-gas coatings, and antisense genetics. Although many of these theories have promise, few have been shown to yield long-term improvements over the existing materials of Dacron and PTFE.

124.5 Neointimal Hyperplasia

Tissue ingrowth onto the artificial surface of a PTFE graft occurs at the anastomoses and is called *neointimal hyperplasia*. Initially, platelets and thrombin/fibrin cover the entire graft surface within the first 24 hours. After this initial phase, smooth-muscle cells migrate from the native artery into the graft, variously referred to as pannus ingrowth, neointimal hyperplasia, and fibromuscular hyperplasia. The pannus advances from the edge of the graft at a rate of approximately 0.1 mm per week but does not cover the entire surface in humans. Typically, the maximum extent of ingrowth in humans is 1–2 cm. In the first few hours, a thrombotic stage of platelet, fibrin, and red blood cell accumulation occurs (stage I). Days 3–4 consist of cellular recruitment in which the thrombus is coated with an endothelial layer (stage II). Cell proliferation of actin-positive cells which resorb and replace the residual thrombus are the major events in stage III, at approximately 7–9 days. This description leads to a conclusion that thrombosis and cell proliferation are the two controll-ing events affecting graft patency. However, this process is one of normal healing which creates no significant stenosis in most cases. Recent findings indicate that a fourth stage should be added in which the tissue grows in volume primarily by synthesis and deposition of large amounts of extracellular substance over the following months, as shown in Fig. 124.1. This stage IV leads to a hemodynamically significant stenosis.

The ingrowth has been characterized by Glagov as having two different forms: intimal fibromuscular hypertrophy (IFMH) and intimal hyperplasia (IH) [Glagov et al., 1991]. The first form of IFMH is basically a normal healing process which consistently takes place on all grafts and does not become highly stenotic. Initial healing is well organized with smooth-muscle cells organized in lamellae and little extracellular proteins or mucopolysaccharide material. A second form of abnormal healing creates stenotic and occlusive thickening, called *intimal hyperplasia* (IH). Intimal hyperplasia is characterized by a chaotic appearance of randomly oriented cells embedded in a field of extracellular matrix material. The histologic appearance is one of hyperplasia or tumorlike behavior. Little is known on the exact stimulant which causes healing to proceed by IFMH or IH, although Glagov speculates that hemodynamic shear stress may play a role. The events in graft neointimal hyperplasia appear to be similar to that of restenotic hyperplasia.

Although the underlying etiology of neointimal hyperplasia has not been fully elucidated, a large number of theories have been proposed to explain this process. The theories generally fall into several broad categories: platelet deposition with local release of PDGF, other growth factor stimulation of SMC proliferation (e.g., TGF-β, FGF), monocyte recruitment, complement activation, leukocyte deposition, chronic inflammation, and mechanical stimuli such as stress and shear abnormalities [Greisler, 1991].

Many studies have focused on preventing graft intimal thickening by attacking either thrombosis or cell proliferation. Cell culture studies clearly demonstrate that certain pharmacologic agents can profoundly affect the platelet adhesiveness and cell proliferation. However, the effectiveness of these agents in vivo is variable, depending on which animal species is used. A large number of human restenosis trials using a wide variety of antithrombotic agents, steroids, lipid-lowering therapies, and ACE inhibitors have largely been negative. Arteriovenous fistula graft studies in baboons suggest that modifying graft surfaces and infusing antithrombotic agents have little effect on the rate of obstruction of the prostheses.

Compliance mismatch, medial tension, and hemodynamic shear stress are additional putative agents which have been hypothesized to be important in arterial adaptation and neointimal hyperplasia. Arteries tend to adapt in size to maintain a specific wall shear stress under conditions of increased blood flow. Wall shear stress appears to play a major role in the pathogenesis of atherosclerosis and in arterially transplanted autogenous veins, and elevations in shear stress inhibits SMC proliferation and neointimal thickening in porous PTFE grafts in baboons.

We have recently characterized the quantitative relationship between the amount of shear stress and the associated neointimal thickness, shown graphically in Fig. 124.2.

This relationship can be written as the mathematical relationship

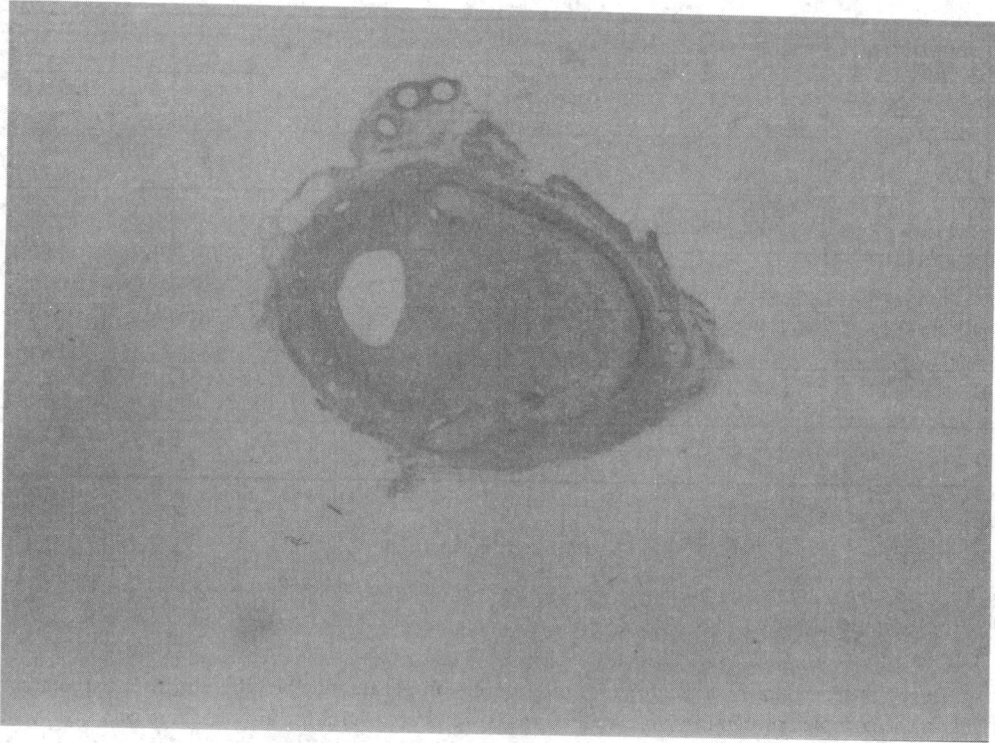

FIGURE 124.1 High-power sections of the anastomotic neointimal hyperplasia in a PTFE graft. This endothelium-lined layer is formed of highly disorganized spindle-shaped cells surrounded by a large amount of extracellular matrix material.

$$\text{Intimal thickness} = A \times \frac{1}{\text{wall shear rate}} + C \qquad (124.1)$$

where C is a constant which would depend on the implantation age of the graft. This relationship appears to be dominant over proximal or distal positioning or absolute flow rate. This inverse, non-linear relationship between neointimal thickening and wall shear stress shown in Fig. 124.2 is strikingly similar to that seen for early atherosclerotic intimal thickening in arteries [e.g., Ku & Zhu, 1993]. Thus, neointimal hyperplasia appears to respond to low shear stress in the same consistent, stereotypic way as do other vascular cells in vivo. Since wall shear is primarily determined by the graft diameter, selection of an optimal-size graft for typical flow rates may increase the long-term patency of prosthetic grafts [Binns et al., 1989]. These results apply to in vivo PTFE grafts composed of the pore-size and material configuration used most commonly in clinical vascular surgery today.

Surprisingly, the pseudointima of thrombus material consistently shows the same thickening as the anastomotic neointima, even though there are no nucleated cells in the pseudointima [Binns et al., 1989]. The advancing front exhibits an unusual shape in which the endothelial cells grow over the existing thrombus at the lumen, but the smooth-muscle cells stay at the graft surface underneath the thrombus. Thus, the two cell types do not touch each other at the advancing edge of the pannus. The distances between the two types of cells suggest that direct cellular communication is not present at the advancing edge.

Although there is clearly a large body of knowledge on intimal hyperplasia, the more general question of what biologic material is actually causing occlusions is not clear. The in vitro cell culture studies are elegant in their ability to probe the molecular regulators of synthesis and proliferation.

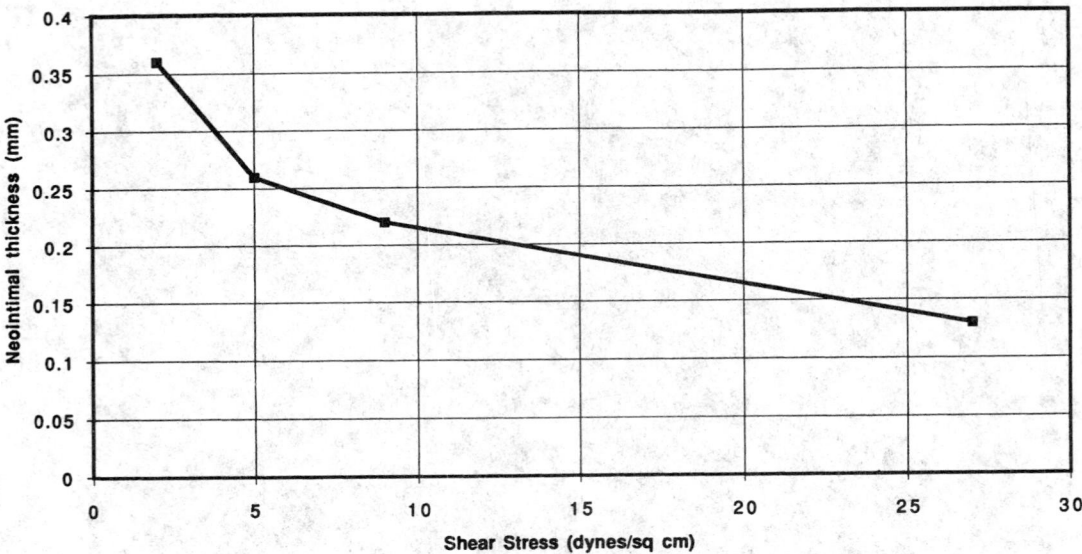

FIGURE 124.2 Graph of neointimal thickness versus mean shear stress for PTFE tapered grafts in a canine model of intimal hyperplasia.

However, the response of cells grown as monolayers on plastic may be different from tissue growing in the complex milieu in vivo. Small animal studies are useful for initial testing of a wide variety of potential therapeutic agents. Unfortunately, many agents which are successful in rats and rabbits turn out to be unsuccessful in large animals or humans. Large animals such as dogs, pigs, and baboons appear to develop lesions similar to humans and respond to therapies in a similar manner. The major drawback, however, is that the lesions typically take approximately one year to develop into advanced stenoses which mimic the clinical human problem. An accurate large-animal model of high-grade neointimal hyperplastic lesions is needed in order to generate a comprehensive characterization of lesion development in vivo.

The cellular mechanism by which shear stress influences the development of neointimal hyperplasia is not well understood. The pannus ingrowth is likely to be composed predominantly of smooth-muscle cells. However, the fluid-wall shear stress interface is primarily experienced by the endothelial cell. One mechanism for neointimal thickening may be that the endothelial cells sense the local wall shear and regulate the amount of underlying smooth muscle cell growth. Clearly, endothelial cells can change their physiologic behavior and morphologic appearance in response to wall shear stress [Nerem, 1992]. Shear-sensitive endothelial cells mechanoreceptors have been postulated as regulators of the adaptation process seen in arteries in response to increased shear stress. Such receptors, however, have not been identified. An "endothelial-derived relaxation factor" and an "endothelial-derived constriction factor" appear to play an important role in the acute response of the arterial wall to alterations in shear stress. A separate humoral factor acting on the media in response to alterations in shear stress has been suggested. The fact that most of these mediators are endothelium-derived or endothelium-dependent may explain the localization of neointimal hyperplasia in PTFE grafts to the juxta-anastomotic region. In contrast to native vessels, the commonly used human prosthetic grafts are rarely, if ever, fully lined with endothelium except for a short distance adjacent to the anastomosis.

The morphology of endothelial cells grown in low shear or static conditions are random in orientation without a preferred direction. As the intimal thickening progresses, one would expect the deeper layers to be more insulated from the shear effects of hemodynamics and to experience a more static environment. PTFE grafts are essentially nondistensible under physiologic pressure conditions. Thus, the perigraft cells would be expected to experience the least amount of stress from pressure pulses and circumferential stretch as well.

Recently, there has been greater recognition of the importance of extracellular matrix (ECM) in vascular lesions [Bell, 1992]. In general, we have observed that the deepest layers of cells in the perigraft region exhibited the most disorganization and extracellular matrix material. The appearance of the intimal hyperplasia in this region strongly suggests that growth of neointima in this region from the production of extracellular matrix is the dominant mechanism by which intimal hyperplasia becomes occlusive. ECM is dominant in advanced lesions, often to the virtual exclusion of cellular elements. The ECM is also directly responsible for a variety of tissue signals which can augment or reduce cellular proliferation and protein production. The ECM can act directly or act as a repository for other growth factors. Several investigators are attempting to recreate the detailed architecture of ECM in order to develop future biologic substrates for arteries.

Low compliance of PTFE grafts is associated with higher rates of intimal hyperplasia. Rodbard [1970] has hypothesized that the normal adaptive response of cells to static conditions is the production of large amounts of ECM. It is possible that the lack of stretch in the PTFE graft removes any mechanical stimulus to the smooth-muscle cells in this layer and transforms the cells into a synthetic mode with production of large amounts of ECM. The highly synthetic mode of these cells and the hypocellularity in this region would suggest that the major culprit of late graft occlusion is synthesis instead of proliferation. Studies of the response of endothelial cells to very low levels of wall shear stress and the response of underlying smooth muscle cells to endothelial cell products should provide important information on the cellular and molecular mechanisms producing the transformation of thin, organized healing into occlusive growth.

124.6 Graft Infections

Vascular graft infections are catastrophic and challenging problems that threaten life and limb. The incidence of synthetic graft infection is approximately 2% and has remained stable despite advances in aseptic surgical technique, vascular graft production, and immunology. Prosthetic grafts are involved in infections four times as often as autogenous vein. The infection rates for PTFE and Dacron prostheses are about the same. The mechanism of infectious complications may involve direct inoculation during surgery or hematogenous seeding, but most occur due to contamination at the time of surgery. Contact of the prosthesis with the skin of the patient is felt to be a key event. The highest incidence anatomically occurs in the inguinal areas due to perineal proximity, lymphatic disruption, and poor wound healing. Antibiotic prophylaxis, both systemically and locally, decreases the incidence of graft infection. The bonding of antibiotics to the prosthesis has been attempted in various forms to prevent prosthetic graft infection but to date is not clinically available. *Staphylococcus epidermidis* is the most common organism involved in graft infections, with Staphylococcus aureus also a prevalent organism. Early graft infections commonly are superficial infections (inguinal) with virulent organisms such as *Staphylococcus aureus* or *Pseudomonas aeruginosa*. Late graft infections usually involve contamination of an abdominal graft with less virulent species such as *Staphylococcus epidermidis*. The reported mortality rates vary with the anatomic location of the graft and the aggressiveness of the infecting organism. These may range from 5–10% for femoropopliteal grafts to 50–75% for aortobifemoral grafts. The associated amputation rate varies from 25–75%.

Vascular grafts are important tools in the clinical treatment of end-stage arteriosclerosis. Large-diameter grafts made of artificial material have high success and longevity. For small-diameter grafts, autogenous venous grafts are superior in longevity and patency than artificial grafts. The main problems for artificial vascular grafts are early thrombosis, late neointimal hyperplasia, and iatrogenic infection. Some active areas of research include the prevention of flowing blood thrombosis on surfaces, control of the pathogenic process causing neointimal hyperplasia occlusions, and facilitation of the immunogenic response to bacterial infection of a graft.

Defining Terms

Extra-anatomic bypass: Vascular graft used to bypass a blocked artery where the graft is placed in a different location than the original artery. One example is an axillo-femoral graft which brings blood from the arm to the leg through a tube placed under the skin along the side of the person.

Hemodialysis access: Arterial-venous connection surgically placed to provide a large amount of blood flow for hemodialysis. These are often loops of ePTFE placed in the arm.

Neointimal hyperplasia: Fibroblast and smooth-muscle cell growth covering a vascular graft on the inside surface.

Pannus: Neointimal hyperplasia tissue ingrowth at the anastomoses.

Pseudointimal hyperplasia: Fibrin/thrombin deposition on the inside surface of an arterial vascular graft. This accumulation of material is acellular.

Stenosis: Tissue ingrowth into vessel causing a narrow lumen and reduction of blood flow.

Vascular graft: Tube replacement of an artery or vein segment.

Vascular reconstruction: Reconstruction of an artery or vein after trauma, surgery, or blockage of blood flow from disease.

References

Bell E. 1992. Tissue Engineering, Current Perspectives, Boston, Birkhouser.

Binns RL, Ku DN, Stewart MT, et al. 1989. Optimal graft diameter: Effect of wall shear stress on vascular healing. J Vasc Surg 10:326.

Glagov S, Giddens DP, Bassiouny H, et al. 1991. Hemodynamic effects and tissue reactions at grafts to vein anastomosis for vascular access. In BG Sommer, ML Henry (eds), Vascular Access for Hemodynamics—II, pp 3–20, Precept Press.

Greisler HP. 1991. New Biologic and Synthetic Vascular Prosthesis, Austin, Tex, RG Landes.

Imparato AM, Bracco A, Kim GE, et al. 1972. Intimal and neointimal fibrous proliferation causing failure of arterial reconstructions. Surgery 72:1007.

Ku DN, Zhu C. 1993. The mechanical environment of the artery. In B Sumpio (ed), Hemodynamic Forces and Vascular Cell Biology, pp 1–23, Austin, Tex, RG Landes.

Nerem RM. 1992. Vascular fluid mechanics, the arterial wall, and atherosclerosis. J Biomech Eng 114:274.

Rodbard S. 1970. Negative feedback mechanisms in the architecture and function of the connective and cardiovascular tissues. Perspect Biol Med 13:507.

Rutherford RB. 1989. Vascular Surgery, pp 404–486, Philadelphia, Saunders.

Sawyer PN. 1987. Modern Vascular Grafts, New York, McGraw-Hill.

Veith FJ, Hobson RW, Williams RA, et al. 1994. Vascular Surgery, pp 523–535, New York, McGraw-Hill.

Further Information

Greisler HP. 1991. New Biologic and Synthetic Vascular Prosthesis, Austin, Tex, RG Landes.

Ku DN, Salam TA, Chen C. 1994. The development of intimal hyperplasia in response to hemodynamic shear stress. Second World Congress of Biomechanics, 31b, Amsterdam.

Veith FJ, Hobson RW, Williams RA, et al. 1994. Vascular Surgery, pp 523–535, New York, McGraw-Hill.

125

Artificial Lungs
and Blood-Gas
Exchange Devices

Pierre M. Galletti
Brown University

Clark K. Colton
Massachusetts Institute of Technology

The natural lung is the organ in which blood exchanges oxygen and carbon dioxide with the body environment. In turn, blood brings oxygen to all body tissues, so as to oxidize the nutrients needed to sustain life. The end products of the chemical reactions that take place in tissues (globally referred to as metabolism) include carbon dioxide, water, and heat, which must all be eliminated. In mammals, oxygen is obtained from the air we breathe through diffusion at the level of the pulmonary alveoli and then carried to the tissues by the hemoglobin in the red blood cells. The carbon dioxide produced by living cells is picked up by the circulating blood and brought to the pulmonary capillaries from where it diffuses into the alveoli and is conveyed out by ventilation through the airways. These processes can be slowed down to a fraction of resting levels by hypothermia or accelerated up to 20-fold when the demand for fuel increases, as for instance with hyperthermia, fever, and muscular exercise.

Only a fraction of the oxygen in the air is actually transferred from the pulmonary alveoli to the pulmonary capillary blood, only a fraction of the oxygen carried by arterial blood is actually extracted by the tissues, and only a fraction of the oxygen present in tissues is actually replenished in a single blood pass. Similarly, only a fraction of the CO$_2$ present in tissues is conveyed to the circulating blood, only a fraction of the mixed venous blood CO$_2$ content is actually discharged in the alveoli, and only a fraction of the CO$_2$ in the alveolar gas is eliminated into each breath. Delicately poised physiologic mechanisms, further balanced by chemical buffer systems, maintain the gas exchange system in equilibrium.

The challenge of replacing the function of the natural lungs by an exchange device allowing continuous blood flow and continuous blood arterialization was first outlined by physiologists at the end of the 19th century but could not be met reliably until the 1950s. The large transfer areas needed for blood-gas exchange in an artificial lung were initially obtained by continuous foaming and defoaming in a circulating blood pool or by spreading a thin film of blood in an oxygen atmosphere. Because the direct blood-gas interface was found to be damaging to blood as well as difficult to stabilize over extended periods, membrane-mediated processes were introduced and are now almost universally preferred.

125.1 Gas Exchange Systems

Artificial lungs are often called blood oxygenators because oxygen transfer has traditionally been seen as the most important function being replaced and, in most situations, has proved more limiting than CO_2 transfer. The change in blood color between inlet and outlet also encourages the term *oxygenator*, considering that changes in blood CO_2 content are not visible to the eye and are more difficult to measure than oxygen transfer.

As is the case for most artificial organs, artificial lungs may be called upon to *replace* entirely the pulmonary gas exchange function (when the natural organ is totally disabled or, while still sound, must be taken out of commission for a limited time to allow a surgical intervention) or to *assist* the deficient gas transfer capacity of the natural organ, either temporarily, with the hope that the healing process will eventually repair the diseased organ, or permanently, when irreversible lung damage leaves the patient permanently disabled.

Since most artificial lungs cannot be placed in the anatomical location of the natural lung, venous blood must be diverted from its normal path through the central veins, right heart, and pulmonary vascular bed and rerouted, via catheters and tubes, through an extracorporeal circuit which includes the artificial lung before being returned, by means of a pump, to the arterial system.

The procedure in which the pulmonary circulation is temporarily interrupted for surgical purposes and gas exchange is provided by an artificial lung is often referred to as extracorporeal circulation (ECC) because, for convenience sake in the operating room, the gas exchange device as well as the pumps which circulate the blood are located outside the body.

The vision of coupling extracorporeal blood pumping with extracorporeal gas exchange at a level of performance sufficient to permit unhurried surgical interventions in adult patients originated with Gibbon [1939] whose initial laboratory models relied on rotating cylinders to spread blood in a continuously renewed thin film, in the tradition of 19th-century physiologists. Gibbon's clinical model [1954], built with technical support from IBM, was a stationary film oxygenator, a bulky device in which venous blood was evenly smeared over a stack of vertical wire screen meshes in an oxygen atmosphere, flowing gently downward to accumulate in a reservoir from where blood could be returned to a systemic artery. The main problems with that design, besides its cumbersome dimensions, were to avoid blood streaming and to maintain a constant blood-gas exchange area. Other investigators tried to increase the flexibility of the system by replacing the stationary film support with rotating screens or rotating discs partly immersed in a pool of blood. This allowed some control of gas transfer performance by changing the rational speed, but minimizing the blood content of the device dictated a tight fit between the discs and the horizontal glass cylinder surrounding them. Foaming and hemolysis were encountered at high disc spinning velocity, and these designs were eventually abandoned.

The very first strategy of physiologists for exchanging oxygen and carbon dioxide in venous blood had been to bubble pure oxygen through a stationary blood pool. To turn this batch process into a continuous operation for total body perfusion, blood was collected through cannulae from the central veins by a syphon or a pump, driven upward in a vertical chimney, mixed with a stream of oxygen gas bubbles, and finally passed through filters and defoaming sponges so as to collect bubble-free arterialized blood, which could then be used to perfuse the arterial tree. The efficiency of bubble oxygenators is extremely high because the smaller the bubbles, the larger the blood-oxygen exchange area developed by a steady current of gas. In the limiting case, it is even possible to saturate venous blood by introducing no more oxygen into the blood than is consumed by the tissues. This process, however, does not remove any carbon dioxide. Since the partial pressure of CO_2 in the excess gas vented from a bubble oxygenator cannot exceed the CO_2 partial pressure in arterialized blood (and in actuality is much lower), it follows that the carbon dioxide transfer rate of bubble oxygenators is a direct function of the volume inflow rate of oxygen, which must exceed oxygen uptake severalfold to transfer both O_2 and CO_2. Thus, the operating conditions for a bubble oxygenator are dictated to a major extent by the requirements for adequate CO_2 removal.

Three major advances propelled bubble oxygenators ahead of film oxygenators in the pioneer decades of cardiac surgery. The first was the identification of silicone-based defoaming compounds which could be smeared on top of the bubble chimney and proved much more effective in coalescing the blood foam than previously used chemicals. The second was the quantitative process analysis by Clark [1950] and Gollan [1956] which showed that, since small bubbles favor oxygen transfer and large bubbles are needed for CO_2 removal, an optimum size could be found in between, or alternatively a mix of small and large bubbles should be used. The third and practically decisive advance was made simultaneously by Rygg [1956] and DeWall [1957], who replaced the assembly of glass, steel, and ceramic parts of early bubble oxygenators with inexpensive plastic components and thereby paved the way for the industrial manufacturing of disposable bubble oxygenators. As a result, reusable stationary film and disc oxygenators, which required careful cleaning and sterilization, slowly disappeared, and disposable bubble oxygenators dominated the field of extracorporeal gas exchange from 1960 to the early 1980s. The oxygenator and pumps designed during the pioneer phase of extracorporeal circulation are described in a book by Galletti and Brecher [1962].

In the 1970s, the bubble oxygenator was integrated with a heat exchanger (usually a stainless steel coil) and placed within a clean plastic container that also served as a venous reservoir with a capacity of several liters of blood. The level of blood-air interface allowed direct observation of changes of blood volume in the extracorporeal circuit. This simple design feature gave the equipment operator (who eventually became known as the perfusionist) plenty of time in which to react to a sudden blood loss and make compensating changes in operation.

Yet a number of problems occurred with bubble oxygenators because of their large blood-gas interface. If the blood foam did not coalesce completely, gaseous microemboli could be carried into the arterialized bloodstream. Plasma proteins were denatured at the gas interface, leading to blood trauma associated with platelet activation and aggregation, complement activation, and hemolysis. These problems could be ameliorated by placement of a gas-permeable membrane between the blood and gas phases. The idea of using membranes permeable to respiratory gases in order to separate the blood phase from the gas phase in an artificial lung, and consequently avoid the risk of foaming or the formation of thick blood rivulets inherent in bubble or film oxygenators, was stimulated after World War II by the growing availability of commercially produced thin plastic films for the packaging industry. The two major challenges for membrane oxygenators were, and indeed remain, that no synthetic membrane could be fabricated as thin as the pulmonary alveolar wall, and no manifolding and blood distribution system could match the fluid dynamic efficiency of the pulmonary circulation, where a single feed vessel—the pulmonary artery—branches over a short distance and with minimal resistance to flow into millions of tiny gas exchange capillaries the size of an erythrocyte. Membrane oxygenators have progressively captured the largest share of the market for clinical gas exchange devices not only because their operation is less traumatic for blood but also because the blood content of the gas exchange unit is fixed, thereby limiting volume fluctuations to calibrated reservoirs and minimizing the risk of major shifts in intracorporeal blood volume during total body perfusion.

The interposition of a membrane between flowing gas and flowing blood reduces the gas transfer efficiency of the system as a consequence of the additional mass transfer resistances associated with the membrane itself and the geometry of the blood layer. The permeability of various polymeric materials to oxygen and carbon dioxide is summarized in Table 125.1. The very first plastic films used, such as thin sheets of polyethylene and polytetrafluoroethylene (PTFE), showed such a low diffusional permeability that 5–10 m^2 were needed to meet even the minimal oxygen needs of an anesthetized hypothermic adult [Clowes et al., 1956]. The advent of silicone elastomer films (either as solid sheets or cast over a textile support mesh) in the 1960s established the technical feasibility of membrane oxygenators [Bramson et al., 1965; Galletti et al., 1966; Peirce et al., 1967]. Silicone rubber is about 140 times more permeable to oxygen and 230 times more permeable to CO_2

TABLE 125.1 O_2 and CO_2 Permeability of Various Materials

Chemical Composition	Common Name	O_2 Permeability $\dfrac{cm^3(STP)\cdot mil}{min\cdot m^2\cdot atm}$	$\dfrac{CO_2 \text{ Permeability}}{O^2 \text{ Permeability}}$
Air		5×10^7	0.8
Polydimethylsiloxane	Silicone rubber	1100	5
Water		150	18
Polystyrene		55	5
Polyisoprene	Natural rubber	50	6
Polybutadiene		40	7
Regenerated cellulose	Cellophane	25	18
Polyethylene		12	5
Polytetrafluoroethylene	Teflon	8	3
Polyamide	Nylon	0.1	4
Polyvinylidene chloride	Saran	0.01	6

Permeability is the product of the diffusion coefficient D and the Bunsen solubility coefficient α. The gas flux J [cm^3 (STP)/min·m²] across a membrane of thickness h with a partial pressure difference Δr is given by $J = P\Delta r/h$.

than is PTFE for equivalent thickness. Even though silicone rubber and related elastomers cannot be cast as thin as PTFE, their permeability is so high that they became the standard material for early membrane oxygenator prototypes.

Extensive research was carried out in the 1960s and 1970s to develop improved membrane oxygenator designs with more efficient oxygen transport across the blood boundary layer. These designs are discussed later in this chapter. The clinical motivation was to provide continuous full or partial replacement of pulmonary gas exchanges for periods of weeks to patients with advanced respiratory failure, with the hope that in the interval the natural lung would recover. Since extensive blood trauma limited the use of bubble oxygenators beyond 12–24 hours, membrane oxygenators became the key to this application. In the mid-1970s, an NIH-sponsored clinical study [Zapol, 1975] demonstrated that with the protocols used lung function was not regained after 1–3 weeks of extracorporeal circulatory with a membrane oxygenator. The major intended application of membrane oxygenators having vanished, and the high cost of silicone rubber making these devices much more expensive than bubble oxygenators, research and development almost came to a halt, leaving bubble oxygenators in control of the remaining field of use, namely cardiopulmonary bypass.

Two technical advances have over the following two decades reversed this trend: (1) the discovery that hydrophobic microporous membranes, through which gas can freely diffuse, have a high enough surface tension to prevent plasma filtration at the moderate pressures prevailing in the blood phase of an artificial lung; (2) the large-scale fabrication of defect-free hollow fibers of microporous polypropylene, which can be assembled in bundles, potted and manifolded at each extremity to form an artificial capillary bed of parallel blood pathways immersed in a cylindrical hard shell through which oxygen circulates.

Microporous hollow fiber membrane oxygenators now dominate the market. The most common embodiment of the hollow fiber membrane oxygenator features gas flow through the lumen of the fibers and blood flow in the interstices between fibers. This arrangement not only utilizes the larger outer surface area of the capillary tubes as gas transfer interface, instead of the luminal surface, it also promotes blood mixing in a manner which enhances oxygen transport, as will become apparent below.

125.2 Cardiopulmonary Bypass

Cardiopulmonary bypass (CPB), also called heart-lung bypass, allows the temporary replacement of the gas exchange function of the lungs and the blood-pumping function of the heart. As a result blood no longer flows through the heart and lungs, which then presents the surgeon with a bloodless operative field.

The terms pump-oxygenator and heart-lung machine graphically describe the equipment used. Cardiopulmonary bypass is the procedure. Open-heart surgery strictly speaking refers to interventions inside the heart cavities, which once provided the most frequent demand for cardiopulmonary bypass technology. By extension, the term is also applied to surgical procedures which take place primarily on the external aspects of the heart, such as creating new routes for blood to reach the distal coronary arteries from the aorta, e.g., coronary artery bypass grafting (CABG) or, popularly, *bypass surgery*. In these operations the cardiac cavities are temporarily vented (i.e., open to atmospheric pressure) to avoid the build-up of pressure which could damage the cardiac muscle.

As usually employed for cardiac surgery, the heart-lung machine is part of a total, venoarterial cardiopulmonary bypass circuit, meaning that all the venous blood returning to the right heart cavities is collected in the extracorporeal circuit and circulated through the gas exchange device, from where it is pumped back into the arterial tree, thereby "bypassing" the heart cavities and the pulmonary circulation. On the blood side, this procedure usually involves hemodilution, some degree of hypothermia, nonpulsatile arterial perfusion at a flow rate near the resting cardiac output, and continuous recirculation of blood in an extracorporeal circuit in series with the systemic circulation of the patient. On the gas side, oxygen or an oxygen-enriched gas mixture (with or without a low concentration of CO_2) flows from a moderately pressurized source in a continuous, nonrecycling manner and is vented to the room atmosphere.

CPB hinges on twin postulates: that blood circulation can be sustained by mechanical pumps while the heart is arrested and that venous blood can be artificially arterialized in an extracorporeal gas exchange device while blood flow is excluded from the lungs. Each of these claims was established separately through animal experimentation over the course of over 100 years (see Galletti and Brecher [1962]). Then surgeons and engineers combined the advances made by physiologists and pharmacologists and turned them, in the 1950s, into the basic tool of cardiac surgery. A recent update on the evolution of artificial membrane lungs for CPB surgery has been provided by Galletti [1993]. It is estimated that each year about 650,000 disposable membrane lungs are used in the operating room worldwide, with each gas exchange unit selling for a price in the range of $250–400, i.e., a market close to $2 billion.

Typical operating conditions for total cardiopulmonary bypass in an adult are summarized in Fig. 125.1 and Table 125.2. Most notable are the large differences in driving forces for O_2 and CO_2. An approximate comparison can be made using the inlet conditions. Thus, under normothermia and with pure oxygen fed to the gas phase, the initial driving force is approximately $45 - 0 = 45$ mmHg for CO_2 and $760 - 47 = 713$ mmHg for O_2 yielding a ratio of CO_2 to O_2 driving forces of about 0.06. The ratio of CO_2 to O_2 permeability for silicone rubber is roughly 5 (Table 125.2), and the corresponding flux ratio is 0.35, less than half that of the metabolically determined respiratory quotient. Under these conditions, CO_2 is the limiting gas, and the device should be sized on the basis of CO_2 transport rather than O_2 transport requirements. This is why silicone rubber membranes have been replaced by microporous polypropylene membrane, where the solubility of CO_2 in the membrane material, and consequently its permeability, is no longer the limiting factor. Indeed, with some modern membrane oxygenators, gas flow through the device may have to be controlled to avoid an excessive loss of CO_2.

125.3 Artificial Lung Versus Natural Lung

In the *natural lungs*, the factors underlying exchange across the alveolo-capillary barrier and transport by the blood can be grouped into four classes:

1. The ventilation of the lungs (the volume flow rate of gas) and the composition of the gas mixture to which mixed venous (pulmonary artery) blood will be exposed

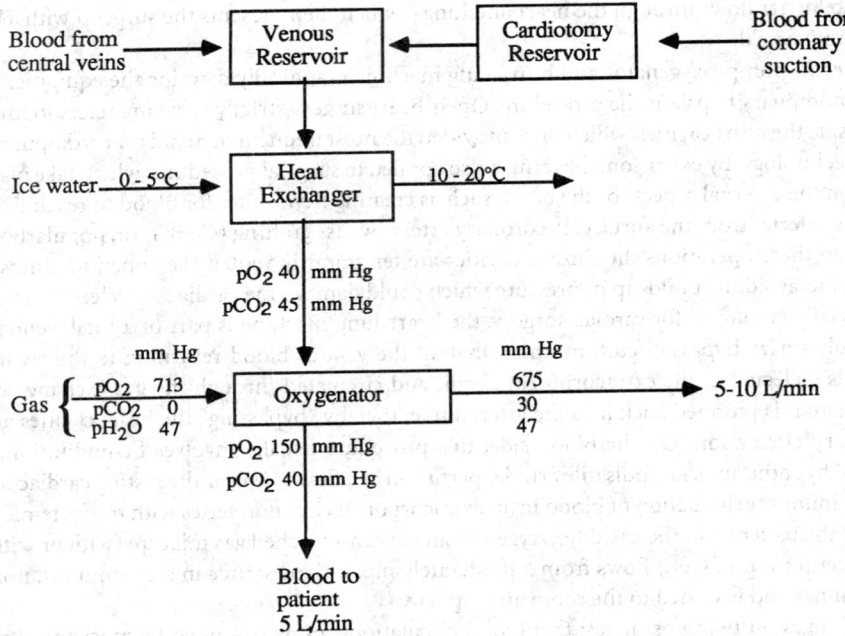

FIGURE 125.1 Scheme of standard operating conditions during cardiopulmonary bypass.

2. The permeability of the materials which separate the gas phase from the blood phase in the pulmonary alveoli
3. The pattern of pressure and flow through the airways and through the pulmonary vascular bed and the distribution of inspired air and circulating blood among the various zones of the exchange system
4. The gas carrying capacity of the blood as regards oxygen and carbon dioxide (and secondarily nitrogen and anesthetic gases)

In an *artificial lung*, replacing the gas transfer function of the natural organ implies that blood circulation can be sustained by mechanical pumps for extended periods of time to achieve a continuous, rather than a batch process, and that venous blood can be arterialized in that device by exposure to a gas mixture of appropriate composition. The external gas supply to an artificial lung does not pose particular problems, since pressurized gas mixtures are readily available. Similarly the components of blood which provide its gas-carrying capacity are well identified and can be adapted to the task at hand. In clinical practice, it is important to minimize the amount of donor blood needed to fill the extracorporeal circuit, or priming volume. Therefore a heart-lung machine is

TABLE 125.2   Typical Operating Parameters for Cardiopulmonary Bypass in an Adult

Oxygen transfer requirement	250 mL/min	
CO_2 elimination requirement	200 mL/min	
Respiratory gas exchange ratio (respiratory quotient)	0.8	
Blood flow rate	5 L/min	
Gas flow rate	5–10 L/min	
Gas partial pressures (in mmHg)		
Blood in	$pO_2 = 40$	$pCO_2 = 45$
Blood out	$pO_2 = 100$–300	$pCO_2 = 30$–40
Gas in (humidified)	$pO_2 = 250$–713	$pCO_2 = 0$–20
Gas out	$pO_2 = 150$–675	$pCO_2 = 10$–30

generally filled with an electrolyte or plasma expander solution (with or without donor blood), resulting in hemodilution upon mixing of the contents of the extracorporeal and intracorporeal blood circuits. The critical aspects for the operation of an artificial lung are blood distribution to the exchanger, diffusion resistances in the blood mass transfer boundary layer, and stability of the gas exchange process.

Artificial lungs are expected to perform within acceptable limits of safety and effectiveness. The most common clinical situation in which an artificial lung is needed is typically of short duration, with resting or basal metabolism in anesthetized patients. Table 125.3 compares the structures and operating conditions of the natural lung and standard hollow fiber artificial membrane lungs with internal blood flow.

An artificial lung designed to replace the gas exchange function of the natural organ during cardiac surgery must meet specifications which are far less demanding than the range of capability of the mammalian lung would suggest. Nonetheless, these specifications must embrace a range of performance to cover all metabolic situations which a patient undergoing cardiopulmonary bypass might present. These conditions range in terms of metabolic rate from the slightly depressed resting me-

TABLE 125.3 Comparison of Natural and Artificial Membrane Lung

Natural Lung	Hollow Fiber Oxygenator
Performance	
Must meet demand at rest and during exercise, fever, etc.	Must meet demand at rest and under anesthesia
Constant temperature process around 37° C	Can be coupled with heat exchanger to lower body temperature
O_2 and CO_2 transfer are matched to achieve the respiratory quotient imposed by foodstuff metabolism (around 0.8)	O_2 and CO_2 transfer are largely independent of each other and must be controlled by the operator
Continuous over a lifetime	Usually limited to few hours
Exchange surface area	
Wide transfer area (~ 70 m^2)	Limited transfer area (1–3 m^2)
Highly permeable alveolar-capillary membrane	Diffusion barriers in synthetic membrane and blood oxygenation boundary layer
Short diffusion distances (1–2 μm)	Relatively thick membranes (50–100 μm)
Hydrophilic membrane	Hydrophobic polymers
No hemocompatibility problems	Hemocompatibility problems
Self-cleaning membrane	Protein build-up on membrane
Gas side	
To-and-fro ventilation	Steady cross flow gas supply
Operates with air	Operates with oxygen-rich mixture
Membrane structure sensitive to high oxygen partial pressure	Membrane insensitive to high oxygen partial pressure
Pressure below that in blood phase to avoid capillary collapse	Pressure below that on blood side to avoid bubble formation
Operates under water vapor saturation conditions	Can be clogged by water vapor condensation
Ventilation linked to perfusion by built-in control mechanisms	Ventilation dissociated from perfusion, with risks of hyper- or hypoventilation
Can be used for gaseous anesthesia	Can be used for gaseous anesthesia
Blood side	
Short capillaries (0.5–1 mm)	Long blood path (10–15 cm)
Narrow diameter (3–7 μm)	Thick blood film (150–250 μm)
Short exposure time (0.7 s)	Long exposure time (5–15 s)
Low resistance to blood flow	Moderate to high resistance to blood flow
Sophisticated branching	Crude manifolding of entry and exit ports
Minimal priming volume	Moderate to large priming volume
Capillary recruitment capability	Fixed geometry of blood path
No recirculation	Possibility of recirculation
Limited venous admixture	Risk of uneven perfusion of parallel beds
No on-site blood mixing	Possibility of blood stirring and mixing
Operates with normal hemoglobin concentration	Hemodilution is common
Does not require anticoagulation	Requires anticoagulation

tabolism characteristic of an anesthetized patient, lightly clad in a cool operating room, to moderate (25–28° C) and occasionally deep (below 20° C) hypothermia. Hyperthermia and high blood flow are occasionally encountered in patients with septic shock. In terms of body mass, patients range from the 2–5-lb newborn with congenital cardiac malformations to the 250-lb obese, diabetic elderly patient suffering from coronary artery disease and scheduled for aortocoronary bypass surgery.

Whereas it is appropriate to match in advance the size and therefore the transfer capability of the gas exchange unit in the heart-lung machine to the size of the patient (largely out of concern for the volume of fluid needed to fill or "prime" the extracorporeal circuit), each gas exchange unit, once in use, must be capable of covering the patient's requirement under any circumstances. This is the responsibility of the perfusionist, who controls the system in the light of what is happening to the patient in the operative field. In fact, the perfusionist substitutes his or her own judgment for the natural feedback mechanisms which normally control ventilation and circulation to the natural lungs. The following analysis indicates how these requirements can be met in the light of the gas transport properties of blood and the characteristics of diffusional and convective transport in membrane lung devices.

125.4 Oxygen Transport

The starting point for analysis of O_2 transport is the conservation of mass relation, which is derived from a material balance in a differential element within the flowing blood. By way of example, the relation commonly employed for oxygen transport of blood flowing in a tube is

$$V\left(\frac{\partial[O_2]}{\partial x} + \frac{\partial[HbO_2]}{\partial x}\right) = DO_2 \frac{1}{r}\frac{\partial}{\partial r}\left(r\frac{\partial[O_2]}{\partial x}\right) \qquad (125.1)$$

where x is the axial coordinate, r is the radial coordinate, V is the velocity in the axial direction, DO_2 is the effective diffusion coefficient of O_2 in flowing blood, $[O_2]$ is the concentration of physically dissolved O_2, and $[HbO_2]$ is the concentration of O_2 bound to hemoglobin. The terms on the left side of Eq. (125.1) represent convection in the axial direction of O_2 in its two forms, dissolved in aqueous solution and bound to hemoglobin. The right-side term represents the diffusion of dissolved O_2 in the radial direction.

By making the usual assumption that the concentration of dissolved O_2 is linearly proportional to the O_2 partial pressure p, $[O_2] = \alpha p$, where α is the Bunsen solubility coefficient, and by using the definition of oxyhemoglobin saturation: $[HbO_2] = C_T S$ where C_T is the oxygen-carrying capacity of hemoglobin (per unit volume of blood) and S is its fractional saturation, Eq. (125.1) can be rewritten in a modified form

$$V\frac{\partial p}{\partial x}\left(1 + \frac{C_T}{a}\frac{\partial S}{\partial p}\right) = DO_2 \frac{1}{r}\frac{\partial}{\partial r}\left(r\frac{\partial p}{\partial x}\right) \qquad (125.2)$$

which shows that the convective contribution is proportional to the slope of the saturation curve. Equation (125.2) must be solved subject to the appropriate initial and boundary conditions, which for a tube are

$$x = 0, \quad p = p_i \qquad (125.3)$$

$$r = 0, \quad \frac{\partial p}{\partial r} = 0 \qquad (125.4)$$

$$r = R, \quad \alpha DO_2 \frac{\partial p}{\partial r} = P_m\left(p_o - p\right) \qquad (125.5)$$

where p_i and p_o are the oxygen partial pressures in the inlet blood and in the gas, respectively, and P_m is the membrane permeability for O_2 diffusion, defined so as to include the membrane thickness. These conditions represent, in order, a uniform inlet concentration, symmetry about the tube axis, and the requirement that the O_2 diffusion flux at the blood-membrane interface be equal to the O_2 diffusion flux through the membrane.

Implicit in the derivation of Eq. (125.2) are two important assumptions. The first is that, on a macroscopic scale, blood can be treated as a homogeneous continuum, even though as a suspension of red blood cells in plasma, blood is microscopically heterogeneous. This simplification is acceptable as long as the volume element in which oxygen transport occurs is large compared to the size of a single red cell but small compared to the size of the overall diffusion path. This seems reasonable when applied to transport in membrane lungs, where the blood diffusion path thickness is usually equivalent to 20–30 red cell diameters or more.

The second important assumption is that the rate of reaction between O_2 and hemoglobin is sufficiently fast, when compared to the rate of diffusion of O_2 within the red cell, that the reaction can be considered at equilibrium, with the concentration of hemoglobin-bound O_2 in the red blood cells directly related to the concentration of dissolved O_2 in plasma via the oxyhemoglobin dissociation curve (ODC). Implicit in the use of this relationship is the assumption that the O_2 diffusion resistance of the red cell membrane is insignificant.

The human ODC for normal physiologic conditions is shifted to the right by increased temperature or decreased pH because of decreased hemoglobin affinity for O_2. The ODC is shifted to the right by an increase in the concentration of various organic phosphates, especially 2,3-diphosphoglycerate (DPG).

Under typical venous physiologic conditions (37°C, boundary O_2 partial pressures of 40 and 95 mmHg), the reaction between hemoglobin and oxygen reaches equilibrium during the time of contact between the blood and the gas phase. The ratio of the effective permeability of blood to that of plasma in a model system is 0.87 at a hematocrit of 45%; without any facilitation within the red cell, the ratio would be 0.75. Using the most reliable data for the O_2 solubility and diffusion coefficient in plasma leads to an estimate of 1.7×10^{-5} cm^2/s for the effective diffusion coefficient of O_2 in normal whole blood.

We can now return to the analysis of convective transport of oxygen in a membrane lung, specifically the solution of Eq. (125.2) or its equivalent for other geometrics, on the assumption of equilibrium for the hemoglobin oxygenation reaction in such devices. The various theoretical analyses that have been carried out differ primarily in the means by which the saturation curve is handled. The most common approach is to retain its intrinsic nonlinearity and to approximate it by a suitable analytical expression. The resulting nonlinear partial differential equation does not permit analytical solution, and it is therefore necessary to resort to numerical solution with a finite difference scheme on a digital computer. This approach yields numerical values for p and S as a function of x and r. To relate theoretical prediction with experimental measurement, one must calculate the velocity-weighted bulk average values of p and S [Colton, 1976]. The average O_2 partial pressure, p, and oxyhemoglobin saturation, S, that would be measured if the blood issuing from the tube were physically mixed are then calculated from

$$\frac{1}{\int_0^R Vr\, dr} \left[\alpha \int_0^R Vpr\, dr + C_T \int_0^R VSr\, dr \right] = \alpha\bar{p} + C_T\bar{S} \qquad (125.6)$$

Numerical solutions provide accurate predictions. However they apply only to specific operating conditions and cannot be generalized for design purposes. Two methods have been used to simplify the ODC and provide approximate yet useful analytical solutions.

The first is known as the advancing front theory [Marx et al., 1960; Thews, 1957]. The oxyhemoglobin saturation curve is approximated as a step function between the saturation values corresponding to the O_2 partial pressure and that of the gas phase or the blood-membrane interface. The blood is treated as two regions of uniform oxyhemoglobin saturation separated by a front that moves rapidly inward. Outside the front, blood is saturated at a value corresponding to the blood-gas or blood-membrane interface, and the rest of the blood is relatively unsaturated. Oxygen diffuses through the saturated blood to the interface, where it reacts with unsaturated hemoglobin. The advancing front approximation reasonably represents the calculated saturation profiles and has proved useful in developing analytical design expressions for membrane lungs in terms of satura-tion changes effected. However, it can be in error by a very wide margin for the prediction of O_2 partial pressure changes. A modification of advancing front theory, involving approximation of the ODC by several straight line segments, retains the ability to provide an analytical solution and gives better accuracy than the conventional step function approximation of the ODC.

The second type of simplification is to approximate the ODC by a straight line drawn between the inlet and boundary O_2 partial pressures, which makes $\partial S/\partial p$, the slope of the saturation curve, constant and renders Eq. (125.2) linear. Use can then be made of existing solutions for analogous convective heat and mass transfer problems without chemical reaction.

For typical operating conditions in the clinic, the initial and boundary O_2 partial pressures lie on the upper portion of the ODC, and the advancing front solution provides an overestimation of the rate of O_2 transport, whereas the constant slope solution provides an underestimate. Conversely, on the lower portion of the ODC at very low O_2 partial pressures, the advancing front estimate of O_2 transport rate is too low and constant slope too high. The constant slope approximation is most ac-curate over the steep portion of the saturation curve, where it is nearly linear. Since the O_2 transport rate per unit membrane surface area is much more sensitive to blood inlet O_2 partial pressure than would be expected solely from the change in the overall driving force, comparative testing of mem-brane lungs must be carried out with identical inlet blood O_2 partial pressure and oxyhemoglobin saturation.

Theoretical prediction of membrane lung performance is useful for design purposes and for providing a guide to the effect of permissive design variables. However, theoretical prediction cannot substitute for experimental data under closely controlled conditions where control of pH, temper-ature, and CO_2 partial pressure in fresh blood allow the definition of the appropriate ODC.

125.5 CO_2 Transport

The CO_2 dissociation curve for normal human blood is far more linear in its normal operating range than the ODC. The fractional volume of CO_2 that is removed in the process of arterialization of venous blood is also considerably less than the corresponding fractional loss of oxygen (about 10 percent of blood CO_2 content, versus 25 percent for oxygen). As is the case for oxygen, the total CO_2 concentration is far larger than that of gas physically dissolved in the aqueous component of blood. Plasma accounts for about two-thirds of all the CO_2 carried in blood, whereas typically about 98% of O_2 is carried in the red cells.

The main vehicles for CO_2 transport in blood are bicarbonate, the primary carrier in both plasma and red cells, and carbamino hemoglobin, where CO_2 is combined with the amino groups of hemoglobin (Fig. 125.2a). Arrows on Fig. 125.2b indicate the direction and relative rate of each re-action whereby CO_2 is removed in a membrane lung. Carbonate and hydrogen ions form bicar-bonate, which decomposes to CO_2 or combines with another hydrogen ion to form carbonic acid; the latter is dehydrated to liberate CO_2. Since the reactions that form CO_2 in plasma are very slow, biocarbonate is the predominant species. Biocarbonate can diffuse into the red cell, albeit slowly, in exchange for chloride, leading to the same chain of reactions. In the red cell, however, dehydration of carbonic acids is catalyzed by the enzyme carbonic anhydrase. This reaction liberates CO_2, which, in turn, diffuses out of the red cell into the plasma and then across the blood-membrane interface. Decomposition of carbamino hemoglobin is a significant additional source of CO_2. Carbamate compounds that arise from combination of CO_2 with plasma proteins have a much smaller effect

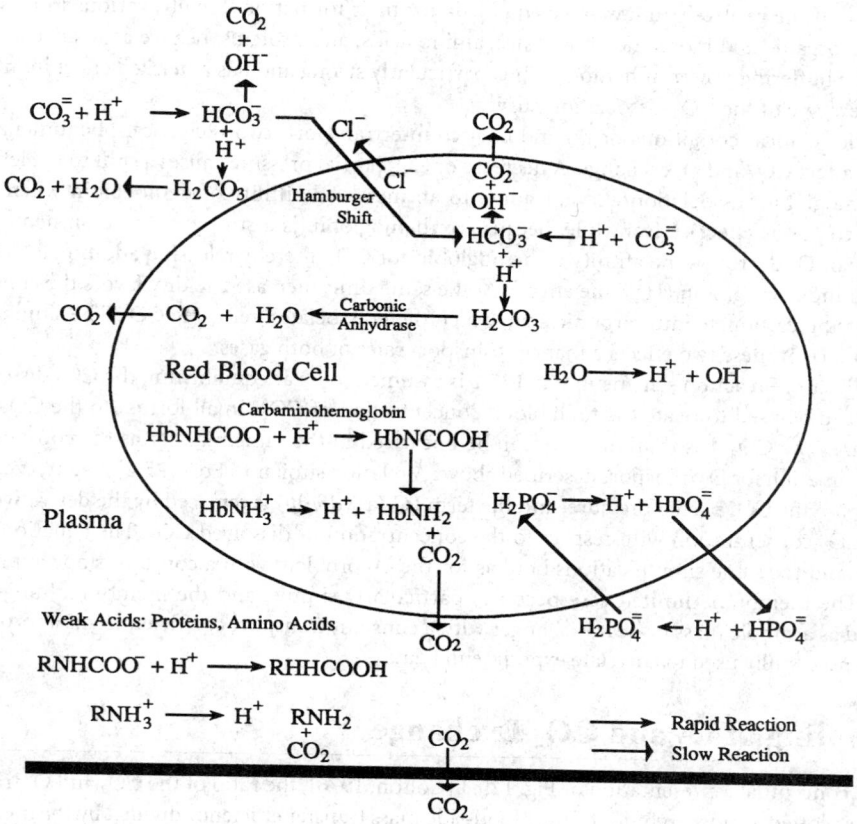

FIGURE 125.2a Schematic representation of CO_2 transfer from red blood cell to plasma and into alveolar gas, emphasizing the various buffer systems involved.

CO_2 transport form		Mixed venous blood		Arterial blood		Veno-arterial difference	
		mM/L	%	mM/L	%	mM/L	%
Bicarbonate	plasma	14.41	61.8	13.42	62.4	.99	55.0
	RBC	5.92	25.4	5.88	27.3	.04	2.2
Dissolved CO_2	plasma	.76	3.3	.66	3.1	.10	5.6
	RBC	.51	2.2	.44	2.0	.07	3.9
Carbamino CO_2	plasma	-	-	-	-	-	-
	RBC	1.70	7.3	1.10	5.1	.60	33.3
Total in whole blood		23.30	100%	21.50	100%	1.80	100%

FIGURE 125.2b. Blood CO_2 content. CO_2 transport forms in mixed venous and arterial blood, and as components of the veno-arterial CO_2 difference. Observe that the red blood cells (RBC) bicarbonate content, although it represents a large fraction of CO_2 transport, does not contribute significantly to the arteriovenous difference in CO_2 content. Conversely, hemoglobin-bound CO_2, though less abundant than bicarbonate in red blood cells, constitutes a larger fraction of the veno-arterial difference.

because of the relatively unfavorable equilibria for their formation. Finally, various ionic species, such as organic and inorganic phosphates, amino acids, and proteins, behave as weak acids at pH 7.4. The buffering power of hemoglobin is particularly strong and has a marked effect in influencing the shape of the CO_2 dissociation curve.

Under clinical conditions of O_2 and CO_2 countertransport, two reciprocal phenomena occur which affect CO_2 and O_2 exchange. A decrease of CO_2 partial pressure causes a shift to the left of the oxyhemoglobin dissociation curve, leading to an increased affinity of hemoglobin when CO_2 is removed (Bohr effect). Meanwhile, because oxyhemoglobin is a stronger acid than hemoglobin, uptake of O_2 decreases the affinity of hemoglobin for CO_2, thereby releasing additional CO_2 from carbamino hemoglobin (Haldane effect). At the same time, increased acidity favors the conversion of more biocarbonate into carbonic acid, which then dissociates, releasing CO_2. The simultaneous occurrence of these two effects enhances transport rates of both gases.

If the entire reaction scheme in Fig. 125.2 is assumed to be at equilibrium, the CO_2 dissociation curve can be used to relate the total blood concentration of CO_2 (in all forms) to the CO_2 partial pressure. The CO_2 dissociation curve can be linearized in the same manner as the constant slope approximation for O_2 transport described above. A relation similar to Eq. (125.2) results, except that p refers to the CO_2 partial pressure, and the term $(C_T/a)\,(\partial S/\partial p)$ is replaced by the derivative of the total CO_2 concentration with respect to the concentration of dissolved CO_2. The equation is now linear, and the same simplifications hold as for the O_2 problem with a constant slope approximation. The membrane-limited case becomes particularly simple, and the membrane lung can be treated as a simple mass or heat exchanger with a constant transport coefficient. This approach has been successfully used to correlate experimental data.

125.6 Coupling of O_2 and CO_2 Exchange

In the conceptual representation of Fig. 125.3 [Colton, 1976], the ratio of the CO_2 and O_2 transport rates is plotted against an index of the blood-side mass transfer efficiency divided by the membrane permeability on a logarithmic scale. With a constant slope approximation for both O_2 and CO_2 transport, a unique curve is obtained for a specific membrane lung design if the abscissa is taken to be the ratio of the blood-side log-mean average CO_2 mass transfer coefficient divided by the CO_2 membrane permeability, and the curve is parameterized by unique values of three dimensionless quantities: (1) the ratio of the membrane permeabilities for O_2 and CO2, (2) the ratio of the average blood-side mass transfer coefficients for O_2 and CO_2, and (3) the ratio of the log-mean average

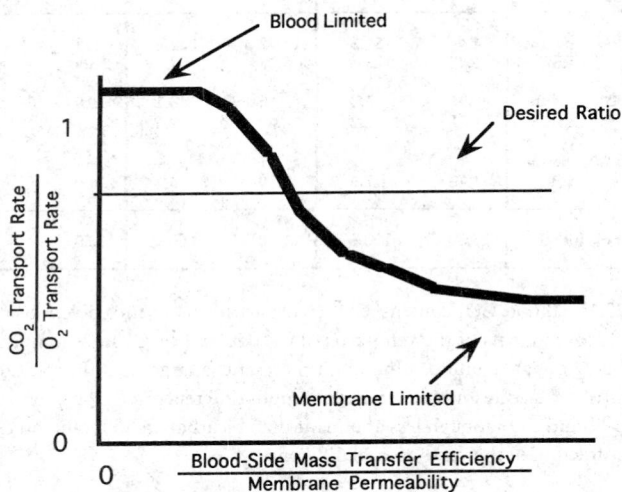

FIGURE 125.3 Relative CO_2 and O_2 transport in a membrane lung.

O_2 and CO_2 partial pressure driving force. The asymptotic limits plotted are very approximate characteristic values of a capillary or flat plate (sandwich) gas exchange device in which the limiting factor is either the blood mass transfer boundary layer or the membrane itself.

When transport of both O_2 and CO_2 is blood phase–limited—that is, there is a relatively low blood-side mass transfer coefficient or high membrane permeability—the CO_2 transport rate is higher than the O_2 rate, and it is necessary to add CO_2 to the inlet gas or to decrease gas flow rate to prevent excessive CO_2 removal. At the other extreme, if gas transport is membrane limited, the ratio of CO_2 to O_2 transport is always lower than the physiological value (0.8), because no existing gas-permeable membrane has a sufficiently high CO_2/O_2 permeability ratio to overcome the unfavorable driving force ratio of the O_2 and CO_2 partial pressures (14:1) under the actual operating conditions of a membrane lung. Under either limiting condition, it is necessary to design the membrane lung on the basis of the gas that limits transport, O_2 for blood-limited conditions and CO_2 for membrane-limited conditions.

A priori, it seems undesirable to operate under blood-limited conditions because full advantage is not taken of the membrane permeability. Therefore, an increase in the blood-side mass transfer efficiency is valuable, but only to the point where the ratio of CO_2 to O_2 transport rates is equal to the respiratory quotient. Beyond that point, further improvements in design will not reduce the size of the device required unless membrane permeability to CO_2 is increased, thereby moving the operating point on the curve to the left and justifying the use of a more efficient exchange device. For example, conventional solid silicone rubber membranes cannot take advantage of high-efficiency designs because gas transport is membrane limited and has to be designed on the basis of CO_2 transport rate. To make effective use of the most effective devices, it is necessary to employ microporous membranes or ultrathin membranes on microporous substrates where the CO_2 permeability is no longer a limiting factor.

125.7 Shear-Induced Transport Augmentation and Devices for Improved Gas Transport

There is evidence that flow-dependent properties of blood can substantially influence the transport of O_2 and CO_2. The presence of velocity gradient in a stream can enhance mass transfer through blood either by shear-induced collision diffusion wherein interactions between red blood cells produce net lateral displacements and associated motions in the surrounding phase or by rotation of individual cells, which gives rise to local mechanical stirring of the adjacent fluid. Both mechanisms can lead to transport augmentation of species present in the dispersed or continuous phases. Only the first mechanism can cause dispersive migration of the particles themselves, and available evidence suggests that it is the dominant factor [Cha & Bessinger, 1994]. The shear-induced diffusion coefficient of particles in suspension increases linearly with the shear rate and can be orders-of-magnitude larger than the Brownian motion diffusivity. The effect of lateral cell movement in oxygen transport in capillary tubes depends on both the shear rate and the slope of the ODC, with a maximum at the steepest portion of the curve, i.e., below the operating range of a clinical oxygenator. The extent to which such phenomena occur in blood under the clinical operating conditions of membrane lungs in cardiopulmonary bypass has not been investigated, but the effect on oxygen transport is thought to be significant.

The earliest oxygenator configurations featuring rubber membranes made the blood flow in simple enclosed geometries, such as a flat plate or hollow fiber, that were inherently inefficient from a mass transfer standpoint. It was soon recognized that the gas transport rate was limited almost entirely by transport within the blood oxygenation boundary layer. There followed extensive efforts in the 1960s and early 1970s to investigate new approaches for improving gas transfer in membrane oxygenators, as summarized in Table 125.4. These approaches relied on one or more mechanisms: (1) increasing shear rate or producing turbulence; (2) keeping the oxygenation boundary layer very thin by using an appropriate contacting geometry or pulsatile blood flow; and (3) making use of

TABLE 125.4   Approaches for Improving Mass Transport in Membrane Oxygenators

Passive designs	Active designs
Obstacles in blood path	Oscillating toroidal chamber
Membrane undulations from external supports	Enclosed rotating disc
Membrane texturing or embossing	Pulsed flow vortex shedding
Helical flow systems	Couette flow
External blood flow over hollow fibers	Annulus, inner cylinder rotating axial flow, tangential flow

Mixed designs
Helical flow systems with controlled blood flow pulsation

secondary flow, which incorporates significant velocity components normal to the membrane surface. All these approaches are demonstrably effective under laboratory conditions, but few have achieved successful commercialization because of the constraints imposed by the geometry of available membrane materials (flat sheets and capillary tubes) and the clinical demand for simple, reliable, and inexpensive devices.

In Table 125.4, *passive designs* for inducing secondary flows are those for which no energy source is needed except that required for steady blood flow. A common technique has been to place obstacles, for example screens, in the blood path to induce secondary fluid movements and/or flow separation on a small scale and thereby increase blood mixing in flat plate devices. A similar result has been obtained by creating undulations in a flat membrane with grooved or multiple point supports or by using textured membranes to direct blood flow through the exchanger.

Active signs are those in which there is energy input to achieve high shear rates or create secondary flows. Highly efficient oxygenator prototypes have been described, and at least two, the enclosed rotating disc and a pulsed-flow vortex shedding device, have been commercialized, but neither has achieved widespread clinical acceptance, in part because of the complexity or cumbersomeness of their operating mechanisms in an operating room setting.

Another widely investigated approach has been to use flow geometries that naturally induce secondary flow, for example helical coils, where, superimposed on the primary flow, is a swirling motion in each half of the tube. The secondary flow trajectory which results from centrifugal effects takes particles from the periphery and carries them into the core, back to the periphery, back to the core in a continuously repeated fashion. Such secondary motion, by continuously sweeping oxygenated blood away from the membrane and replacing it with venous blood from the central core of the channel, can be extremely effective in increasing gas transport rates to the point where the dominant resistance to diffusion lies in the membrane. However, the practical difficulty of constructing such complex devices which are also disposable has thus far prevented industrial development.

When the potential market for continuous extracorporeal membrane oxygenation collapsed, so did the intensive research and development effort in developing new devices. However, three developments, two technical and one marketing-related, over the next decade eventually led to dominance of membrane oxygenators for cardiopulmonary bypass.

The first major technical advance was the fabrication of hydrophobic microporous capillary hollow fiber membranes at prices considerably lower than for silicone rubber membranes. The driving force for the initial development of these materials was their potential in another technology, membrane plasmapheresis for the separation of plasma from the cellular components of blood. Hollow fibers for that application had nominal pore sizes, around 0.5 μm, which were too large for membrane oxygenation because plasma could seep through the fiber wall under pressure leading to a catastrophic decrease in membrane permeability (Table 125.1). In the early 1980s, microporous polypropylene hollow fibers with a nominal pore size around 0.1 μm became available and proved satisfactory for membrane oxygenation. In addition to reduced trauma and competitive pricing with bubble oxygenators, membrane lungs could be employed with a reduced, fixed blood-priming volume, thereby minimizing transfusion and hemodilution problems. Surprisingly, this advantage

TABLE 125.5 Comparison of Membrane Oxygenator Performance (Blood flow rate = gas flow rate = 5 l/min; AAMI conditions)

Model	Membrane Form	Blood Path Configuration	O_2 Flux, $cm^3(STP)/min \cdot m^2$	CO_2/O_2 Flux Ratio
Silicone Rubber				
Sci Med SM35	Sheet	Spiral coil embedded fabric	90	0.6
Microporous polypropylene				
Cobe CMI	Sheet	Flat plate	130	1.4
Shiley M-2000	Sheet	Blood screens	120	1.0
Bentley Bos CM-40	Hollow fiber	Internal flow	70	0.7
Terumo Capiox II 43	Hollow fiber	Internal flow	60	0.9
Bard William Harvey 4000	Hollow fiber	External cross flow	140	0.9
Johnson & Johnson Maxima	Hollow fiber	External cross flow	150	0.9
Sarns	Hollow fiber	External cross flow	150	1.0
Bentley Univox	Hollow fiber	External cross flow	160	1.0

was initially viewed as a drawback by perfusionists who were used to having a large venous blood reservoir with a visible gas-blood interface.

The key marketing development of the mid-1980s was to make a membrane oxygenator by attaching it, along with a heat exchanger, to a clear plastic venous reservoir with a visible gas-blood interface. This astute move was the breakthrough which put membrane oxygenators into the operating room. Their clear advantage in minimizing blood trauma and postoperative complications was so overwhelming that within a year membrane oxygenators captured the dominant market share. Shortly thereafter, bubble oxygenators were virtually eliminated from the U.S. marketplace.

The most recent technical development has been the inversion of the usual internal flow arrangement so that, now, gas flows through the lumen of the hollow fibers while blood is pumped over the external surface of the capillary membrane. This arrangement is most effective when the blood flow is at right angles to the hollow fiber. In that configuration the flowing blood successively encounters different fibers, and a new oxygenation boundary layer forms on each fiber. Because the boundary layer is thinnest where it begins (in this case, at the front of each fiber), and the mass transfer rate is correspondingly highest, the transport of oxygen averaged over the periphery of each fiber is much higher than with the conventional internal (luminal) flow of blood. Thus the transport of oxygen averaged over the periphery of each fiber is much higher than with the conventional internal (luminal) flow of blood. The performance of various membrane oxygenators is compared in Table 125.5. The data clearly demonstrate the superior performance attainable with microporous hollow fibers operated with external crossflow of blood.

The state of the art is now fairly advanced for membrane blood oxygenators, but there is still room for improvement. Further increases in flux would further reduce cost and minimize priming volume and blood consumption. Now that membrane oxygenators are fully entrenched, it is more likely that the reduced priming volume and improved control of a closed system can be realized. Lastly, the residual gas-blood interface that still exists at the microporous membrane surface could be eliminated by coating with a very thin skin in an asymmetric or composite structure.

Defining Terms

Advancing front theory: A type of exchanger theory addressing the limitation of oxygen transport in a blood film through a fully saturated boundary layer leading to a front where the hemoglobin in flowing blood reacts with the dissolved oxygen.

Arterialization: A gas exchange process whereby oxygen and carbon dioxide concentrations in venous blood are changed to levels characteristic of arterial blood.

Artificial lung: A device which allows for continuous exchange of oxygen and carbon dioxide between circulating blood and a controlled gas atmosphere.

Blood oxygenator: Synonymous with artificial lung, with the accent placed on oxygen transport, which is the most critical aspect of natural lung replacement, since the body oxygen reserves are very limited. Depending upon the physical process used for blood-gas transfer, artificial lungs are classified as bubble oxygenators, stationary or rotating film oxygenators, and membrane oxygenators.

Boundary layer: The film of blood adjacent to a permeable membrane, which, by reason of local fluid dynamics, is not renewed at the same rate as blood in the core of the flow path, thereby creating an additional diffusion barrier between the blood and the gas phase.

Bubble oxygenator: Blood-gas transfer device in which a large exchange surface is obtained by the dispersion of oxygen bubbles in a venous blood stream, followed by coalescence of the foam and venting of excess gas (cocurrent blood and gas flow) or by spreading of venous blood over a continuously renewed column of foam generated by bubbling oxygen at the bottom of a reservoir (countercurrent blood and gas flow).

Bypass: Derivation or rerouting of blood around an organ or body part, to diminish its blood supply, to abolish local circulation for the duration of a surgical intervention, or to increase blood flow permanently beyond an obstruction. The qualifier used with the word *bypass* designates the organ so isolated (e.g., *left ventricular* bypass, *coronary artery* bypass).

Cardiopulmonary bypass (CPB):   A procedure whereby blood is prevented from circulating through the heart cavities and the lungs. Cardiopulmonary bypass (also known as *heart-lung bypass*) can be *partial* if no obstacle is placed on venous return to the right heart cavities and consequently some of the blood continues to flow through the pulmonary circulation. In that case the arterial system is fed in part by left ventricular output and in part by the arterialized blood perfusion from the heart-lung machine. The balance between the internal and extracorporeal blood circuits depends on the setting of the pumps and the relative resistance to flow in the two venous drainage pathways. During *total* cardiopulmonary bypass, the cardiac muscle must receive arterial blood from the extracorporeal circuit (intermittently or continuously) to prevent hypoxic myocardial damage. Since coronary venous blood drains into the cardiac cavities, this blood must be drained to the outside to prevent an intracavitary pressure increase which could be damaging to the heart.

Catheter: A long hollow cylinder designed to be introduced in a body canal to infuse or withdraw materials into or out of the body.

Coronary artery bypass graft (CABG):   The construction of new blood conduits between the aorta (or other major arteries) and segments of coronary arteries beyond lesions which partially or totally obstruct the lumen of those vessels, for the purpose of providing an increased blood supply to regions of the myocardium made ischemic by those lesions.

Extracorporeal circulation: Artificial maintenance of blood circulation by means of pumps located outside of the body, with blood fed through catheters advanced in an appropriate blood vessel and returning the blood to another blood vessel.

Film oxygenator: Blood-gas transfer device in which a large exchange surface is obtained by spreading venous blood in a thin film over a stationary or moving physical support in an oxygen-rich atmosphere.

Heart-lung bypass: Synonymous with *cardiopulmonary bypass.*

Heart-lung machine: A mechanical system capable of pumping venous blood around the heart and the lungs and arterializing it in an appropriate gas exchange unit.

Hemodilution: Temporary reduction in blood erythrocyte concentration (and consequently hemoglobin content, hematocrit, oxygen-carrying capacity, and viscosity) resulting from mixing with the erythrocyte-free or erythrocyte-poor content of the liquid used to prime an extracorporeal circuit.

Hemolysis: The destruction of red blood cells with liberation of hemoglobin in surrounding plasma, caused by mechanical damage of the erythrocyte membrane, osmotic imbalance between intracorpuscular and extracorpuscular ion concentration, or uncontrolled freezing-thawing cycles.

Hollow fiber: A capillary tube of polymeric material produced by spinning a melted or dissolved polymer through an annular orifice.

Membrane: A solid or liquid phase which acts as a barrier to prevent coalescence of neighboring compartments while allowing restricted or regulated passage of one or more molecular species.

Membrane lung or **Membrane oxygenator:** Blood-gas transfer device in which the blood compartment is shielded from the gas phase by a porous or solid, hydrophobic polymer membrane permeable to gases but not to liquids (in particular, blood plasma).

Metabolism: The sum of the chemical reactions occurring within a living body including build up (anabolism) and break down (catabolism) of chemical substances.

Open heart surgery: Interventions taking place inside the cardiac cavities, such as for the replacement or reconstruction of cardiac valves, or the closure of abnormal communications between cardiac chambers, and which for reasons of convenience and safety, require the interruption of blood flow through the heart. By extension this term is often used for cardiac interventions under total cardiopulmonary bypass, which address structures on the outside surface of the heart (such as coronary arteries) when drainage of the cardiac cavities through a vent is needed to avoid accumulation of coronary venous blood.

Oxygenation boundary layer: Stationary or slowly moving blood layer adjacent to a gas-permeable membrane, which progressively develops along the blood path and, once enriched with oxygen diffusing through the membrane, effectively becomes a barrier to oxygen transport perpendicular to the direction of flow.

Perfusion: A technique for keeping an organ or body part alive, though severed from its normal blood circulation, by introducing blood under pressure into the appropriate feeder artery.

Perfusionist: The operator of the heart-lung machine during cardiac surgery or respiratory assist procedures.

Priming volume: The volume of liquid (blood, plasma, synthetic plasma expanders, or electrolyte solutions) needed to fill all components of an extracorporeal circuit (oxygenator, heat exchanger, blood pumps, filter, tubing, and catheters) so as to avoid exsanguination once the intracorporeal and extracorporeal circulation systems are joined.

Pump-oxygenator: Equipment used to circulate blood through an extracorporeal circuit by means of mechanical blood pumps and to arterialize mixed venous blood by means of a gas exchange device. In most embodiments, the pump-oxygenator also serves to control blood temperature by means of a heat exchanger, typically incorporated in the gas exchange device. Synonymous with *heart-lung machine.*

Respiratory quotient: The ratio of carbon dioxide produced by tissues or eliminated by the lungs to oxygen consumed by tissues or taken in through the lungs.

Secondary flow: Any type of fluid motion, steady or periodic, in which the fluid is moving in a direction different from that of the primary flow. Secondary flow systems may be continuous in distribution, occupying the entire flow path, or comprise local elements that produce periodic remixing of the fluid.

Total body perfusion: Maintenance of blood circulation through the arterial and venous system by means of a positive displacement pump introducing blood into an artery under pressure and collecting it from a vein for continuous recirculation.

References

Bartlett RH, Drinker PA, Galletti PM (eds). 1971. Mechanical Devices for Cardiopulmonary Assistance, Basel, Karger.

Bramson ML, Osborn JJ, Main FB, et al. 1965. A new disposable membrane oxygenator with integral heat exchange. J Thorac Cardiovasc Surg 50: 391.

Cha W, Beissinger RL. In press. Augmented mass transport of macromolecules in sheared suspension to surfaces: Part B (Borine serum interface). J Colloid Interfac Sci.

Clark LC Jr, Gollan F, Gupta V. 1950. The oxygenation of blood by gas dispersion. Science 111:85.

Clowes GHA Jr, Hopkins AL, Neville WE. 1956. An artificial lung dependent upon diffusion of oxygen and carbon dioxide through plastic membranes. J Thor Surg 32:630.

Colton CK. 1976. Fundamentals of gas transport in blood. In WM Zapol, J Qvist (eds), Artificial Lungs for Acute Respiratory Failure. Theory and Practice, pp. 3–41, New York, Academic Press.

Colton CK, Drake RF. 1971. Effect of boundary conditions on oxygen transport to flowing blood in a tube. Chem Eng Prog Symp 67(114):88.

Curtis RM, Eberhart RC. 1974. Normalization of oxygen transfer data in membrane oxygenators. Trans Am Soc Artif Intern Organs 20:210.

Dawids SG, Engell HC (eds). 1976. Physiological and Clinical Aspects of Oxygenator Design, Amsterdam, Elsevier.

DeWall RA, Lillelei CW, Vareo RL, et al. 1957. The helix reservoir pump-oxygenator. Surg Gyn Obstet 104:699.

Dorson WJ Jr, Voorhees ME, 1974. Limiting models for the transfer of CO_2 and O_2 in membrane oxygenators. Trans Am Soc Artif Intern Organs 20: 219.

Dorson WJ Jr, Voorhees ME. 1976. Analysis of oxygen and carbon dioxide transfer in membrane lungs. In WM Zapol, J Qvist (eds), Artificial Lungs for Acute Respiratory Failure. Theory and Practice, pp 43–68, New York, Academic Press.

Galletti PM. 1993. Cardiopulmonary bypass: A historical perspective. Artif Organs 17:675.

Galletti PM, Brecher GA. 1962. Heart-Lung Bypass, Principles and Techniques of Extracorporeal Circulation, New York, Grune & Stratton.

Galletti PM, Richardson PD, Snider MT, et al. 1972. A standardized method for defining the overall gas transfer performance of artificial lungs. Trans Am Soc Artif Internal Organs 18:359.

Galletti PM, Snider MT, Silbert-Aidan D. 1966. Gas permeability of plastic membrane for artificial lungs. Med Res Eng 20.

Gibbon JH Jr. 1939. An oxygenator with a large surface-volume ratio. J Lab Clin Med 24:1192.

Gibbon JH Jr. 1954. Application of a mechanical heart and lung apparatus to cardiac surgery. Minnesota Med 37:71.

Gollan, F. 1956. Oxygenation of circulating blood by dispersion, coalesence and surface tension separation. J Appl Physiol 8:571.

Hagl S, Klovekorn WP, Mayr N, et al. (eds). 1984. Thirty Years of Extracorporeal Circulation, Munich, Deutches Herzzentrum

Harris GW, Tompkins FC, de Filippi RP. 1970. Development of capillary membrane blood oxygenators. In D Hershey (ed), Blood Oxygenation, pp 333–354, New York, Plenum.

Marx TI, Snyder WE, St John AD, et al. 1960. Diffusion of oxygen into a film of whole blood. J Appl Physiol 15:1123.

Mockros LF, Gaylor JDS. 1975. Artificial lung design: Tubular membrane units. Med Biol Eng 13:171.

Peirce EC II. 1967. The membrane lung, its excuse, present status, and promise. J Mt Sinai Hosp 34:437.

Richardson PD. 1971. Effects of secondary flows in augmenting gas transfer in blood. Analytical considerations. In RH Bartlett, PA Drinker, PM Galletti (eds), Mechanical Devices for Cardiopulmonary Assistance, pp 2–16, Basel, Karger.

Richardson PD. 1976. Oxygenator testing and evaluation: Meeting ground of theory, manufacture and clinical concerns. In WM Zapol, J Qvist, (eds), Artificial Lungs for Acute Respiratory Failure. Theory and Practice, pp 87–102, New York, Academic Press.

Richardson PD, Galletti PM. 1976. Correlation of effects of blood flow rate, viscosity, and design features on artificial lung performance. In SG Davids, HC Engell (eds), Physiological and Clinical Aspects of Oxygenator Design, pp 29–44, Amsterdam, Elsevier.

Rygg IH, Kyvsgaard E. 1956. A disposable polyethylene oxygenator system applied in a heart-lung machine. Acta Chir Seond 112:433.

Snider MT, Richardson PD, Friedman LI, et al. 1974. Carbon dioxide transfer rate in artificial lungs. J Appl Physiol 36:233.

Spaan JAE, Oomens JMM. 1976. Scaling rules for flat plate and hollow fiber membrane oxygenators. In SG Dawids, HC Engell (eds), Physiological and Clinical Aspects of Oxygenator Design, pp 13–28, Amsterdam, Elsevier.

Thews G. 1957. Verfahren zur Berechnung des O_2-Diffusionskoeffizienten aus Messungen der Sauerstoffdiffusion in Haemoglobin und Myoglobin Loesungen. Pfluegers Arch 2:138.

Villarroel F, Lanham CE, Bischoff KB, et al. 1970. A mathematical model for the prediction of oxygen, carbon dioxide, and pH profiles with augmented diffusion in capillary blood oxygenators. In D Hershey (ed), Blood Oxygenation, pp 321–333, New York, Plenum.

Zapol WM. 1975. Membrane lung perfusion for acute respiratory failure. Surg Clin N Am 55:603.

Zapol WM, Qvist J (ed). 1976. Artificial Lungs for Acute Respiratory Failure. Theory and Practice, New York, Academic Press.

Further Information

Over the years, a number of books and monographs have reviewed the scientific and technical literature on gas exchange devices and their application. These include J.G. Allen, ed., *Extracorporeal Circulation,* Thomas, Springfield, 1958; P.M. Galletti and G.A. Brecher, *Heart-Lung Bypass, Principles and Techniques of Extracorporeal Circulation,* Grune and Stratton, New York, 1962; D. Hershey, ed., *Blood Oxygenation,* Plenum, New York, 1970; R.H. Bartlett, P.A. Drinker, and P.M. Galletti, eds., *Mechanical Devices for Cardiopulmonary Assistance,* Karger, Basel, 1971; W.M. Zapol and J. Qvist, eds., *Artificial Lungs for Acute Respiratory Failure. Theory and Practice.* Academic Press, New York, 1976; G.G. Dawids and H.G. Engell, *Physiological and Clinical Aspects of Oxygenator Design,* Elsevier, Amsterdam, 1976; S. Hagl, W.P. Klövekorn, N. Mayr, and F. Sebening, *Thirty Years of Extracorporeal Circulation,* Deutsches Herzzentrum, Munich, 1984; P.A. Casthely and D. Bregman, *Cardiopulmonary Bypass: Physiology, Related Complications and Pharmacology,* Futura, Mount Kisco, N.Y., 1991.

Topical advances in artificial lungs are typically published in the *Transactions of the American Society for Artificial Internal Organs* or in journals such as the *ASAIO Journal,* the *International Journal of Artificial Organs, Artificial Organs,* the *Japanese Journal of Artificial Organs,* and the *Journal of Thoracic and Cardiovascular Surgery,* as well as the *Proceedings of the American Institute for Chemical Engineering* and, occasionally, *Chemical Engineering Symposium Series.*

126

Artificial Kidney

Pierre M. Galletti
Brown University

Clark K. Colton
Massachusetts Institute of Technology

Michael J. Lysaght
CytoTherapeutics, Inc

126.1 Structure and Function of the Kidney

The key separation functions of the kidney are:

1. To eliminate the water-soluble nitrogenous end-products of protein metabolism
2. To maintain electrolyte balance in body fluids and get rid of the excess electrolytes
3. To contribute to obligatory water loss and discharge excess water in the urine
4. To maintain acid-base balance in body fluids and tissues

To fulfill these functions, the kidney processes blood—or more accurately, plasma water—which in turn exchanges water and solutes with the extravascular water compartments: extracellular, intracellular, and transcellular. The solute concentrations in body fluids vary from site to site, yet all compartments are maintained remarkably constant in volume and composition despite internal and external stresses. The global outcome of normal renal function is a net removal of water, electrolyte, and soluble waste products from the blood stream. The kidney provides the major regulatory mechanisms for the control of volume, osmolality, and electrolyte and nonelectrolyte composition as well pH of the body fluids and tissues.

Renal function is provided by paired, fist-sized organs, the kidneys, located behind the peritoneum against the posterior abdominal wall on both sides of the aorta. Each kidney is made up of over a million parallel mass transfer units which receive their common blood supply from the renal arteries, return the processed blood to the systemic circulation through the renal veins, and collect the waste fluids and solutes through the calyx of each kidney into the ureter and from there into the

0-8493-8346-3/95/$0.00+$.50
© 1995 by CRC Press, Inc.

urinary bladder. These functional units are called *nephrons* and can be viewed as a sequential arrangement of mass transfer devices (glomerulus, proximal tubule, and distal tubule) for two fluid streams: blood and urine.

Kidney function is served by two major mechanisms: *ultrafiltration*, which results in the separation of large amounts of extracellular fluid through plasma filtration in the glomeruli, and a combination of passive and active *tubular transport* of electrolytes and other solutes, together with the water in which they are dissolved, in the complex system provided in the rest of the nephron.

Glomerular Filtration

The volume of blood flowing into the natural kidneys far exceeds the amount needed to meet their requirements for oxygen and nutrients: The primary role of the kidneys is chemical processing. As blood flows through the glomerular capillaries, about one-fifth of the plasma water is forced through permeable membranes to enter the proximal portion of the renal tubule and form the primary urine, which henceforth becomes the second fluid phase of the renal mass exchanger. The concentrated blood remaining in the vascular system is collected in the efferent arterioles and goes on to perfuse the tubules via the peritubular capillaries of the "vasa recta" system, where it recovers some of the lost water and eventually coalesces with the other blood drainage channels to form the renal vein. The plasma water removed from the blood in the glomerulus is termed the *glomerular filtrate*, and the process of removal is called *glomerular filtration*. Glomerular filtrate normally contains no blood cells and very little protein. Glomerular filtration is a passive process driven by the differences in hydrostatic and oncotic pressures across the glomerular membrane. Solutes which are sufficiently small and not bound to larger molecules pass quite freely through the glomerular membrane. All major ions, glucose, amino acids, urea, and creatinine appear in the glomerular filtrate at nearly the same concentrations as prevail in plasma.

The normal glomerular filtration rate (GFR) averages 120 ml/min. This value masks wide physiologic fluctuations (e.g., up to 30% decrease during the night, and a marked increase in the postprandial period). Although the kidneys produce about 170 liters of glomerular filtrate per day, only 1–2 liters of urine is formed. A minimum volume of about 400 ml/day is needed to excrete the metabolic wastes produced under normal conditions (often called *obligatory water loss*).

Tubular Function

In the tubule, both solute and water transport take place. Some materials are transported from the lumen across the tubular epithelium into the interstitial fluid surrounding the tubule and thence into the blood of the peritubular capillaries. This process is called *reabsorption* and results in the return of initially filtered solutes to the blood stream. Other substances are transported from the peritubular blood to the interstitial fluid across the tubular epithelium and into the lumen. This process is called *secretion* and leads to elimination of those substances to a greater extent than would be possible solely through glomerular filtration. The return of filtered molecules from the kidney tubule to the blood is accompanied by the passive reabsorption of water through osmotic mechanisms.

The *proximal tubule* reabsorbs about two-thirds of the water and salt in the original glomerular filtrate. The epithelial cells extrude $Na+$ (and with it $Cl-$) from the glomerular filtrate into the interstitial fluid. Water follows passively and in proportionate amounts because of the osmotic pressure gradient (the proximal tubular membrane is freely permeable to water). In the loop of Henle, the glomerular filtrate, now reduced to one-third of its original volume, and still isoosmotic with blood, is processed to remove another 20% of its water content. The active element is the ascending limb of the loop of Henle, where cells pump out $Na+$, $K+$, and $Cl-$ from the filtrate and move the $Na+$ and $Cl-$ to the interstitial fluid. Because the ascending limb is not permeable to water, tubular fluid becomes increasingly more dilute along the ascending loop. The blood vessels around the loop do not carry back all the extruded salt to the general circulation, and therefore the $Na+$

concentration builds up down the descending limb of the loop of Henle, reaching a concentration 4–5 times higher than isoosmolar. As a result, the Na+ concentration in tubular fluid increases as its volume is decreased by passive transport into interstitial fluid and from there into the blood.

Countercurrent multiplication refers to the fact that the more Na+ the ascending limb extrudes, the higher the concentration in the interstitial fluid, the more water removed from the descending limb by osmosis, and the higher the Na+ concentration presented to the ascending limb around the bend of the loop. Overall, the countercurrent multiplier traps salt in the medullary part of the nephron because it recirculates it locally. *Countercurrent exchange* refers to the interaction of the descending and ascending branches of the circulatory loops (vasa recta) with the loop of Henle which flows in the opposite direction. Substances which pass from the tubule into the blood accumulate in high concentrations in the medullary tissue fluid. Na+ and urea diffuse into the blood as it descends along the loop but then diffuse out of the ascending vessels and back into the descending vessels where the concentration is lower. Solutes are therefore recirculated and trapped (short-circuited) in the medulla, but water diffuses out of the descending vessel and into the ascending vessel to be transported out.

The distal tubule of the kidney, located in the cortex, is the site of fine adjustments of renal excretion. Here again the primary motor is the Na+/K+ pump in the baso-lateral membrane, which creates a Na+ concentration gradient. The walls of the collecting duct, which traverses through a progressively hypertonic renal medulla tissue, are permeable to water but not to Na+ and Cl−. As a result, water is drawn out and transported by capillaries to the general circulation. The osmotic gradient created by the countercurrent multiplier system provides the force for water reabsorption from the collecting duct. However, the permeability of the cell membrane in the collecting duct is modulated by the concentration of antidiuretic hormone (ADH). A decrease in ADH impairs the reabsorption of water and leads to the elimination of a larger volume of more dilute urine.

The terms *reabsorption* and *secretion* denote direction of transport rather than a difference in physiologic mechanism. In fact, a number of factors may impact on the net transport of any one particular solute. For example, endogenous creatinine (an end product of protein metabolism) is removed from plasma water through glomerular filtration in direct proportion to its concentration in plasma. Since it is neither synthesized nor destroyed anywhere in the kidney, and it is neither reabsorbed nor secreted in the tubule, its eventual elimination in the urine directly reflects glomerular filtration. Therefore, creatinine clearance can be used to measure glomerular filtration rate. However, glucose, which initially passes in the glomerular filtrate at the same concentration as in plasma, is completely reabsorbed from the tubular urine into peritubular capillaries as long as its plasma concentration does not exceed a threshold value somewhat above the level prevailing in normal subjects. As a result, there should be no glucose in the urine. When the threshold is exceeded, the amount of glucose excreted in the urine increases proportionately, producing glycosuria.

Several weak organic acids such as uric acid and oxalic acid, and some related but not naturally occuring substances such as p-aminohippuric acid (PAH), barbiturates, penicillates, and some x-ray contrast media, have the special property of being secreted in the proximal tubule. For example, PAH concentration in glomerular filtrate is the same as in plasma water. So avid is the tubular transport system for PAH that tubular cells remove essentially all the PAH from the blood perfusing them. Therefore, the removal of PAH is almost complete, and the rate of appearance of PAH in the urine mirrors the rate of presentation of PAH to the renal glomeruli, that is to say, renal plasma flow. Therefore, PAH clearance can be used, in association with the hematocrit, to estimate the rate of renal blood flow.

Urea appears in the glomerular filtrate at the same concentration as in plasma. However, one-third of urea diffuses back into the blood in the proximal tubule. In the distal nephron, urea (as an electrically neutral molecule without specific transport system) follows the fate of water (*solvent drag*). If large amounts of water are reabsorbed in the distal tubule and the collecting duct, then an additional third of the urea can be reabsorbed. However, if water diuresis is large, then correspondingly more urea is excreted.

126.2 Kidney Disease

The origin of kidney disease may be infectious, genetic, traumatic, vascular, immunologic, metabolic, or degenerative [Brenner & Rector, 1986]. The response of the kidneys to a pathologic agent may be rapid or slow, reversible or permanent, local or extensive. Under most circumstances, an abnormal body fluid composition is more likely to arise from the unavailability or excess of a raw material than from some intrinsic disturbance of renal function. This is why many clinical problems are corrected by fluid or electrolyte therapy and secondarily by dietary measures and pharmacologic agents which act on the kidney itself. Only as a treatment of last resort, where kidney disease progresses to renal failure, do clinicians use extracorporeal body fluid processing techniques that come under the generic concept of *dialysis*. These invasive procedures are intended to reestablish the body's fluid and electrolyte homeostasis and to eliminate toxic waste products. Processing can address the blood (e.g., *hemodialysis*) or a proxy fluid introduced in body cavities (e.g., *peritoneal dialysis*).

Even in healthy subjects, the GFR falls steadily from age 40 onward. Beyond age 80, it is only half of its adult value of 120 ml/min. However this physiologic deterioration is not extensive enough to cause symptoms. Since nature has provided kidneys with an abundance of overcapacity, patients do not become identifiably sick until close to 90% of original function has been lost. When kidneys keep deteriorating and functional loss exceeds 95%, survival is no longer possible without some form of replacement therapy.

Supplementation (as distinct from replacement) of renal function by artificial means is occasionally used in case of poisoning. Toxic substances are often excreted into the urine by glomerular filtration and active tubular secretion, but the body load at times exceeds the kidneys' clearing capacity. There are no methods known to accelerate the active transport of poisons into urine. Similarly, enhancement of passive glomerular filtration is not a practical means to facilitate elimination of toxic chemicals. Processing of blood in an extracorporeal circuit may be life-saving when the amount of poison in the blood is large compared to the total body burden and binding of the compound to plasma proteins is not extensive. In such cases (e.g., methanol, ethylene glycol, or salicylates poisoning) extracorporeal processing of blood for removing the toxic element from the body is indicated. If the poison is distributed in the entire extracellular space or tightly bound to plasma proteins, dialytic removal is unlikely to affect the clinical outcome because it can only eliminate a small fraction of the toxic solute.

Unfortunately in some situations either the glomerular or the tubular function of the kidneys, or both, fails and cannot be salvaged by drug and diet therapy. Failure can be temporary, self-limiting, and potentially reversible, in which case only temporary substitution for renal function will be needed. Failure can also be the expression of progressive, intractable structural damage, in which case permanent replacement of renal function will eventually be needed for survival. However, the urgency of external intervention in end-stage renal disease (ESRD) is never as acute as is the case for the replacement of cardiac or respiratory function: The signs of renal dysfunction (water retention, electrolyte shifts, accumulation of metabolic end products normally eliminated by the kidneys) develop over days, weeks, or even months and are not immediately life threatening. Even in the end stage, renal failure can be addressed by intermittent rather than continuous treatment.

126.3 Renal Failure

There are two types of renal failure: acute (days or weeks) and chronic (months or years). *Acute renal failure* is typically associated with ischemia (reduction in blood flow), acute glomerulonephritis, tubular necrosis, or poisoning with "nephrotoxins" (e.g., heavy metals, some aminoglycosides, and excessive loads of free hemoglobin). *Chronic renal failure* is usually caused by chronic glomerulonephritis (of infectious or immune origin), pyelonephritis (ascending infection of the urinary tract), hypertension (leading to nephrosclerosis), or vascular disease (most commonly secondary to diabetes).

Renal insufficiency elicits the clinical picture of *uremia*. Although the word *uremia* means that there is too much urea in the blood, urea level in itself is not the cause of the problem. Uremia, often expressed in the United States as blood urea nitrogen concentration or BUN (which is actually half the urea concentration), serves as an indicator of the severity of renal disease. Urea is a metabolic end product in the catabolism of proteins that is hardly toxic even in high concentration. However, it mirrors the impaired renal elimination and the resulting accumulation in body fluids of other toxic substances, some of which have been identified (e.g. phenols, guanidine, diverse polypeptides); others remain unknown and are therefore referred to as *uremic toxins* or, for reasons to be discussed later, *middle molecules*. The attenuation of uremic symptoms by protein restriction in the diet and by various dialytic procedures underscores the combined roles of retention, removal, and metabolism in the constellation of signs of uremia. Toxicity may result from the synergism of an entire spectrum of accumulated molecules [Vanholder & Ringoir, 1992]. It may also reflect the imbalance that results from a specific removal through mechanisms which eliminate physiologic compounds together with potential toxins.

Not until the GFR (as estimated by its proxy, creatinine clearance) falls much below a third of normal do the first signs of renal insufficiency become manifest. At that point the plasma or extracellular concentration of substances eliminated exclusively through the glomeruli, such as creatinine or urea, increase measurably, and the possibility of progressive renal failure must be considered. In such cases, over a period of months to years, the kidneys lose their ability to excrete waste materials, to achieve osmoregulation, and to maintain water and electrolyte balance. The signs of ESRD become recognizable as creatinine clearance approaches 15 ml/min, eventually leading to uremic coma as water and solute retention depress the cognitive functions of the central nervous system. Empirically, it appears that the lowest level of creatinine clearance that is compatible with life is on the order of 8 ml/min, or 11.5 liters per day, or 80 liters per week. (These numbers have a bearing on the definition of adequate dialysis in ERSD patients, because they represent the time-averaged clearance which must be achieved by much more effective but intermittent blood processing). Human life cannot be sustained for more than 7–10 days in the total absence of kidney function. Clinical experience also shows that even a minimum of *residual renal clearance* (K_R) below the level necessary for survival can be an important factor of well-being in dialyzed patients, perhaps because the natural kidney, however sick, remains capable of eliminating middle molecular weight substances, whereas the artificial kidney is mostly effective in eliminating water and small molecules.

The incidence of ESRD (*incidence* is defined as the number of new patients entering treatment during a given year) has increased dramatically in the past 25 years in the United States and elsewhere. Whereas in the 1960s it was estimated at 700–1000 new cases a year in the United States (nearly three-quarters of them between the ages of 25 and 54), the number of new patients reached 16,000 per year at the end of the 1970s (still with the majority of cases under age 54) and 40,000 at the end of the 1980s, with the largest contingent between 65 and 74 years old. Serious kidney disease now strikes between 1 in 5000 and 1 in 10,000 people per year in our progressively aging population. The fastest rate of growth is in the age group over 75, and the incidence of ESRD shows no signs of abating.

The prevalence of ESRD (*prevalence* is defined as the total number of patients present in the population at a specific time) has grown apace: In the United States, about 1000 people were kept alive by dialysis in 1969; 58,253 in 1979; 163,017 in 1989; close to 200,000 now. This is the result of a combination of factors which include longer survival of patients on hemodialysis and absolute growth of an elderly population suffering from an increasing incidence of diseases leading to ESRD such as diabetes. Worldwide, over 500,000 people are being kept alive by various modalities of "artificial kidney" treatment: about a third in the United States, a third in Europe, and a third in Japan and Pacific Rim countries. Another 500,000 or so have benefitted from dialytic treatment in the past but have since died or received transplants [Lysaght & Baurmeister, 1993]. Close to 85% of current patients are treated by maintenance hemodialysis, and 15% are on peritoneal dialysis. These numbers do not include about 100,000 people with a functional renal transplant, most of whom required hemodialysis support while waiting for a donor organ, and who may need it again, if only for a limited period, in case of graft rejection.

The mortality of ESRD patients in the United States has inched upward from 12%–16% percent per year in the 1970s and 1980s and has risen abruptly in recent years to levels in the order of 20%–25%. This has led to extensive controversy as to the origin of this deterioration, which has not been observed to the same extent in other regions with a similarly large population of ESRD patients, such as Western Europe and Japan, and may reflect for the United States insufficient dialysis as well as the burden of an increasingly older population.

126.4 Treatment of Renal Failure

Profound uremia, whether caused by an acute episode of renal failure or by the chronic progressive deterioration of renal function, used to be a fatal condition until the middle of the twentieth century. The concept of clearing the blood of toxic substances while removing excess water by a membrane exchange process was first suggested by the experiments of Abel, Rowntree, and Turner at the Johns Hopkins Medical School. Back in 1913, these investigators demonstrated the feasibility of blood dialysis to balance plasma solute concentrations with those imposed by an appropriately formulated washing solution. However, their observation was not followed by clinical application, perhaps because experiments were limited by the difficulty of fabricating suitable exchange membranes, and blood anticoagulation was then extremely precarious. Collodion, a nitrocellulose film precipitated from an alcohol, ether, or acetone solution was the sole synthetic permeable membrane material available until the advent of cellophane in the 1930s. The unreliability of anticoagulants before the discovery of heparin also made continuous blood processing a hazardous process even in laboratory animals.

In 1944, Kolff in the Netherlands developed an artificial kidney of sufficient yet marginal capacity to treat acute renal failure in man. This device consisted of a long segment of cellophane sausage tubing coiled around a drum rotating in a thermostabilized bath filled with a hypertonic, buffered electrolyte solution, called the *dialysate*. Blood was allowed to flow from a vein into the coiled cellophane tube. Water and solute exchange occurred through the membrane with a warm dialysate pool, which had to be renewed every few hours because of the risk of bacterial growth. The cleared blood was returned to the circulatory system by means of a pump. After World War II, a somewhat similar system was developed independently by Alwall in Sweden. Because of the technical difficulty of providing repeated access to the patient's circulation, and the overall cumbersomeness of the extracorporeal clearing process, hemodialysis was limited to patients suffering from acute, and hopefully reversible, renal failure, with the hope that their kidneys would eventually recover. To simplify the equipment, Inouye and Engelberg [1953] devised a coiled cellophane tube arrangement that was stationary and disposable, and shortly thereafter Kolff and Watschinger (by then at the Cleveland Clinic) reported a variant of this design, the Twin Coil, that became the standard for clinical practice for a number of years.

Repeated treatment, as needed for chronic renal failure, was not possible until late 1959, when Scribner and Quinton introduced techniques for chronic access to the blood stream which, combined with improvements in the design and use of hemodialysis equipment, allowed the advent of chronic intermittent hemodialysis for long-term maintenance of ESRD patients. This was also the time when Kiil first reported results with a flat plate dialyzer design in which blood was made to flow between two sheets of cellophane supported by solid mats with grooves for the circulation of dialysate. This design—which had been pioneered by Skeggs and Leonard, McNeill, and Bluemle and Leonard—not only needed less blood volume to operate then the coiled tube devices, it also had the advantage of requiring a relatively low head of pressure to circulate the blood and the dialysate. This meant that the two fluids could circulate without high pressure differences across the membrane. Therefore, in contrast to coil dialyzers, where a long blood path necessitated a high blood pressure at the entrance of the exchanger, flat plate dialyzers could transfer metabolites through the membrane by diffusion alone, without coupling it with the obligatory water flux deriving from high transmembrane pressure. When ultrafiltration was needed, it could be achieved by circulating the dialysate at subatmospheric pressures.

Device development was also encouraged by the growing number of home dialysis patients. By 1965, the first home dialysate preparation and control units were produced industrially. Home dialysis programs based on the twin coil or flat plate dialyzers were soon underway. At that time the cost of home treatment was substantially lower than hospital care, and in the United States, Social Security was not yet underwriting the cost of treatment of ESRD.

In 1965 also, Bluemle and coworkers analyzed means to pack the maximum membrane area in the minimum volume, so as to reduce the bulkiness of the exchange device and diminish the blood loss associated with large dialyzers and long tubing. They concluded that a tightly packed bundle of parallel capillaries would best fit this design goal. Indeed by 1967, Lipps and colleagues reported the initial clinical experience with hollow fiber dialyzers, which have since become the mainstay of hemodialysis technology.

In parallel developments, Henderson and coworkers [1967] proposed an alternative solution to the problem of limited mass transfer achievable by diffusion alone with hemodialysis equipment. They projected that a purely convective transport (ultrafiltration) through membranes more permeable to water than the original cellulose would increase the effective clearance of metabolites larger than urea. The lost extracellular volume was to be replaced by infusing large volumes of fresh saline into the blood at the inlet or the outlet of the dialyzer to replace the lost water and electrolytes. The process was called *hemodiafiltration* or, sometimes, *diafiltration*. (The procedure in which solutes and water are removed by convective transport alone, using large pore membranes and without substantial replacement of the fluid, is now known as *hemofiltration* and is used primarily in patients presenting with massive fluid retention.)

As is intuitively apparent, the effectiveness of hemodialysis with a given device is related to the duration of the procedure. In the pioneer years, dubbed "the age of innocence" by Colton [1987], patients were treated for as many as 30 hours a week. Economics and patient convenience promoted the development of more efficient transfer devices. Nowadays, intermittent maintenance dialysis can be offered with 10 hours (or even less) of treatment divided in 3 sessions per week. Conversely, nephrologists have developed (mostly for use in the intensive care unit) the procedure known as *continuous arterio-venous hemodialysis* (with its variant continuous arterio-venous hemofiltration) in which blood pressure from an artery (aided or not by a pump) drives blood through the exchange device and back into a vein. Continuous operation compensates for the relatively low blood flow and achieves stable solute concentrations, as opposed to the seesaw pattern that prevails with periodic treatment.

The concept of using a biologic membrane and its blood capillary network to exchange water and solutes with a washing solution underlies the procedure known as *peritoneal dialysis,* which relies on the transfer capacity of the membranelike tissue lining the abdominal cavity and the organs it contains. In 1976, Popovich and Moncrief described continuous ambulatory peritoneal dialysis (CAPD), a procedure in which lavage of the peritoneal cavity is conducted as a continuous form of mass transfer through introduction, equilibration, and drainage of dialyzate on a repetitive basis 4–6 times a day. In CAPD, a sterile solution containing electrolytes and dextrose is fed by gravity into the peritoneal cavity through a permanently installed transcutaneous catheter. After equilibriation with capillary blood over several hours, this dialyzate is drained by gravity into the original container and the process is repeated with a fresh solution. During the dwell periods, toxins and other solutes are exchanged by diffusional processes. Water transfer is induced by the osmotic pressure difference due to the high dextrose concentration in the treatment fluid. This procedure is analyzed in detail in Chapter 127.

Plasmapheresis, i.e., the extraction of plasma from blood by separative procedures (see Chapter 128), has been used in the treatment of renal disease [Samtleben & Gurland, 1989]. However, the cost of providing fresh plasma to replace the discarded material renders plasmapheresis impractical for frequent, repeated procedures, and plasmapheresis is used mainly for other clinical indications.

Most hemodialysis is performed in free-standing treatment centers, although it may also be provided in a hospital or performed by the patient at home. The hemodialysis circuit consists of two fluid pathways. The blood circuitry is entirely disposable, though many centers reuse some or all circuit components in order to reduce costs. It comprises a 16-gauge needle for access to the circulation (usually through an arteriovenous fistula created in the patient's forearm), lengths of plasticized polyvinyl chloride tubing (including a special segment adapted to fit into a peristaltic blood pump), the hemodialyzer itself, a bubble trap and an open mesh screen filter, various ports for sampling or pressure measurements at the blood outlet, and a return cannula. Components of the blood side circuit are supplied in sterile and nonpyrogenic condition. The dialysate side is essentially a machine capable of (1) proportioning out glucose and electrolyte concentrates with water to provide a dialysate of appropriate composition; (2) sucking dialysate past a restrictor valve and through the hemodialyzer at subatmospheric pressure; and (3) monitoring temperature, pressures, and flow rates. During treatment the patient's blood is anticoagulated with heparin. Typical blood flow rates are 200–350 ml/min; dialysate flow rates are usually set at 500 ml/min. Simple techniques have been developed to prime the blood side with sterile saline prior to use and to return to the patient nearly all the blood contained in the extracorporeal circuit after treatment. Whereas most mass transport occurs by diffusion, circuits are operated with a pressure on the blood side, which may be 100–500 mmHg higher than on the dialysate side. This provides an opportunity to remove 2–4 liters of fluid along with solutes. Higher rates of fluid removal are technically possible but physiologically unacceptable. Hemodialyzers must be designed with high enough hydraulic permeabilities to provide adequate fluid removal at low transmembrane pressure but not so high that excessive water removal will occur in the upper pressure range.

Although other geometries are still employed, the current preferred format is a "hollow fiber" hemodialyzer about 25 cm in length and 5 cm in diameter, resembling the design of a shell and tube heat exchanger. Blood enters at the inlet manifold, is distributed to a parallel bundle of capillary tubes (potted together with polyurethane), and exits at a collection manifold. Dialysate flows countercurrent in an external chamber. The shell is typically made of an acrylate or polycarbonate resin. Devices typically contain 6000–10,000 capillaries, each with an inner diameter of 200–250 microns and a dry wall thickness as low as 10 microns. The total membrane surface area in commercial dialyzers varies from 0.5 to 1.5 m², and units can be mass-produced at a relatively low cost (selling price around $10–$15, not including tubing and other disposable accessories). Several reference texts (see For Further Information) provide concise and comprehensive coverage of all aspects of hemodialysis.

126.5 Renal Transplantation

The uremic syndrome resembles complex forms of systemic poisoning and is characterized by multiple symptoms and side effects. Survival requires that the toxins be removed, and the resulting quality of life depends on the quantity of toxins which are actually eliminated. Ideally, one would like to clean blood and body fluids to the same extent as is achieved by normal renal function. This is only possible at the present time with an organ transplant.

The feasibility of renal transplantation as a therapeutic modality for ESRD was first demonstrated in 1954 by Murray and coworkers in Boston, and Hamburger and coworkers in Paris, in homozygous twins. Soon the discovery of the first immunosuppressive drugs led to the extension of transplantation practice to kidneys of live, related donors. Kidney donation is thought to be innocuous since removal of one kidney does not lead to renal failure. The remaining kidney is capable of hypertrophy, meaning that the glomeruli produce more filtrate, and the tubules become capable of increased reabsorption and secretion. A recent Canadian study indicates that the risk of ESRD is not higher among living kidney donors than in the general population, meaning that a single kidney has enough functional capacity for a lifetime. Nonetheless, cadaver donors now constitute the main organ source for the close to 10,000 renal transplants performed in the United States every year. Even though under ideal circumstances each cadaver donor allows two kidney transplants, the scarcity of donors is the major limitation to this form of treatment of ESRD. Most patients aspire to renal transplant because of the better quality of life it provides and the freedom from the time constraints of repeated procedures. However, the incidence of ESRD is such that only one patient in five can be kept alive by transplantation. Dialysis treatment remains a clinical necessity while waiting for a transplant, as a safety net in case of organ rejection, and for the many patients for whom transplantation is either contraindicated or simply not available.

126.6 Mass Transfer in Dialysis

In artificial kidneys, the removal of water and solutes from the blood stream is achieved by

1. Solute diffusion in response to concentration gradients
2. Water ultrafiltration and solute convection in response to hydrostatic and osmotic pressure gradients
3. Water migration in response to osmotic gradients

In most cases, these processes occur simultaneously and in the same exchange device, rather than sequentially as they do in the natural kidney with the cascade of glomerular filtration, tubular reabsorption, and final adjustments in the collecting tubule.

Mechanistically, the removal of water and solutes from blood is achieved by passive transport across thin, leaky, synthetic polymer sheets or tubes similar to those used in the chemical process call dialysis. Functionally, an artificial kidney (also called *hemodialyzer*, or *dialyzer* or *filter* for short) is a device in which water and solutes are transported from one moving fluid stream to another. One fluid stream is blood; the other is dialysate: a human-made solution of electrolytes, buffers, and nutrients. The solute concentrations as well as the hydrostatic and osmotic pressures of the dialysate are adjusted to achieve transport in the desired direction (e.g., to remove urea and potassium ions while adding glucose or bicarbonate to the bloodstream).

Efficiency of mass transfer is governed by two and only two independent parameters. One, which derives from mass conservation requirements, is the ratio of the flow rates of blood and dialysate. The other is the rate constant for solute transport between the two fluid streams. This rate constant depends upon the overall surface area of membrane available for exchange, its leakiness or *permeability*, and such design characteristics as fluid channel geometry, local flow velocities, and boundary layer control, all of which affect the thickness of stationary fluid films, or diffusion barriers, on either side of the membrane.

126.7 Clearance

The overall mass transfer efficiency of a hemodialyzer is defined by the fractional depletion of a given solute in the blood as it passes through the unit. Complete removal of a solute from blood during a single pass defines the dialyzer clearance for that solute as equal to dialyzer blood flow. In other terms, dialyzer blood flow asymptotically limits the clearance of any substance in any device, however efficient.

Under conditions of steady-state dialysis, the mass conservation requirement is expressed as

$$N = Q_B (C_{Bi} - C_{Bo}) = Q_D (C_{Do} - C_{Di}) \qquad (126.1)$$

where N is the overall solute transfer rate between blood and dialysate, Q_B and Q_D are blood flow and dialysate flow rates respectively, and C_{Bi}, C_{Bo}, C_{Di}, and C_{Do} are the solution concentrations C in blood, B, or dialysate, D, at the inlet, i, or the outlet, o of the machine.

Equation (126.1) about mass conservation leads to the first and oldest criterion for dialyzer effectiveness, namely clearance K, modeled after the concept of renal clearance. Dialyzer clearance is defined as the mass transfer rate N divided by the concentration gradient prevailing at the inlet of the artificial kidney.

$$K = \frac{N}{C_{Bi} - C_{Di}} \qquad (126.2)$$

Since mass transfer rate also means the amount of solute removed from the blood per unit of time, which in turn is equal to the amount of solute accepted in the dialysate per unit of time, there are two expressions for dialysance

$$K_B = \frac{Q_B \, (C_{Bi} - C_{Bo})}{C_{Bi} - C_{Di}} \qquad (126.3)$$

$$= K_D = \frac{Q_D \, (C_{Do} - C_{Di})}{(C_{Bi} - C_{Di})} \qquad (126.4)$$

which afford two methods for measuring it. Any discrepancy must remain within the error of measurements, which under the conditions of clinical hemodialysis easily approaches $\pm$ 10%. As in the natural kidney, the clearance of any solute is defined by the flow rate of blood which is completely freed of that solute while passing through the exchange device. The dimensions of clearance are those of flow (a *virtual* flow, one may say), which can vary only between zero and blood flow (or dialysate flow, whichever is smaller), much in the way the renal clearance of a substance can only vary between zero and effective renal plasma flow.

Since dialyzer clearance is a function of blood flow, a natural way to express the efficiency of a particular exchange device consists of "normalizing" clearance with respect to blood flow as a dimensionless ratio

$$\frac{K}{Q_B} = \frac{C_{Bi} - C_{Bo}}{C_{Bi} - C_{Di}} \qquad (126.5)$$

or

$$\frac{K}{Q_B} = \frac{C_{Do} - C_{Di}}{C_{Bi} - C_{Di}} \text{ (extraction fraction)} \qquad (126.6)$$

K/Q_B can vary only between zero and one and represents the highest attainable solute depletion in the blood which is actually achieved in a particular device for a particular solute under a particular set of circumstances.

Another generalization of the dialysance concept may be useful in the case where the direction of blood flow relative to the direction of dialysate flow is either parallel, random, or undetermined, as occurs with the majority of clinical hemodialyzers. Under such circumstances, the best performance which can be achieved is expressed by the equality of solute concentration in outgoing blood and outgoing dialysate ($C_{Bo} = C_{Do} = C_e$ or equilibrium concentration). This limit defines, after algebraic rearrangement of Eqs. (126.3) and (126.4), the maximal achievable clearance at any combination of blood and dialysate flow rates without reference to solute concentrations.

$$K_{max} = \frac{Q_B \times Q_D}{Q_B + Q_D} \qquad (126.7)$$

Since blood and dialysate flows can usually be measured with a reasonable degree of accuracy, the concept of K_{max} provides a practical point of reference against which the effectiveness of an actual dialyzer can be estimated.

126.8 Filtration

So far we implicitly assumed that differences in concentration across the membrane provide the sole driving force for solute transfer. In clinical hemodialysis, however, the blood phase is usually subject to a higher hydrostatic pressure than the dialysate phase. As a result, water is removed from the plasma by ultrafiltration, dragging with it some of the solutes into the dialysate. Ultrafiltration capability is a necessary consequence of the transmural pressure required to keep the blood path open with flat sheet or wide tubular membranes. It is also clinically useful to remove the water accumulated in the patient's body in the interval of dialysis. Ultrafiltration can be enhanced by increasing the resistance to blood flow at the dialyzer outlet, and thereby raising blood compartment pressure, by subjecting the dialysate to a negative pressure or by utilizing membranes more permeable to water than the common cellophanes.

Whenever water is removed from the plasma by ultrafiltration, solutes are simultaneously removed in a concentration equal to or lower than that present in the plasma. For small, rapidly diffusible molecules such as urea, glucose, and the common electrolytes, the rate of solute removal almost keeps pace with that of water, and ultrafiltrate concentration is the same as that in plasma. With compounds characterized by a larger molecular size, the rate of solute removal lags behind that of water. Indeed with some of the largest molecules of biological interest, ultrafiltration leads to an actual increase in plasma concentration during passage through the artificial kidney.

Defining *ultrafiltration* as the difference between blood flow entering the dialyzer and blood flow leaving the dialyzer

$$F = Q_{Bi} - Q_{Bo}$$

one can rewrite the mass conservation requirement as

$$Q_{Bi}C_{Bi} \text{ (Amount of solute in the incoming blood)}$$
$$= Q_{Bo}C_{Bo} \text{ (amount of solute in the outgoing blood)}$$
$$+ K_B(C_{Bi} - C_{Di}) \text{ (amount cleared in the dialyzer)}$$

The clearance equations can then be rewritten as

$$K_B = \frac{Q_{Bi}\left(C_{Bi} - \dfrac{Q_{Bo}}{Q_{Bi}}C_{Bo}\right)}{C_{Bi} - C_{Di}} \quad (126.8)$$

$$K_D = \frac{Q_{Di}\left(\dfrac{Q_{Do}}{Q_{Di}}C_{Do} - C_{Di}\right)}{C_{Bi} - C_{Di}} \quad (126.9)$$

The clearance is now defined as the amount of solute removed from the blood phase per unit of time, *regardless of the nature of the driving force,* divided by the concentration difference between incoming blood and incoming dialysate.

When $C_{Di} = 0$

$$K_B = Q_{Bi} - Q_{Bo}\left(\frac{Q_{Bo}}{Q_{Bi}}\right) \quad (126.10)$$

$$K_D = \frac{Q_{Do} \, C_{Do}}{C_{Bi}} \qquad (126.11)$$

When $C_{Di} = 0$ and $C_{Bo} = C_{Bi}$

$$K_B = F \qquad (126.12)$$

The practical value of these equations is somewhat limited, since their application requires a high degree of accuracy in the measurement of flows and solute concentrations. The special case where there is no solute in the incoming dialysate ($C_{Di} = 0$) is important for in vitro testing of artificial kidneys.

126.9 Permeability

The definition of clearance is purely operational. Based upon considerations of conservation of mass, it is focused primarily on the blood stream from which a solute must be removed, thus, in final analysis, on the patient herself or himself. Clearance describes the artificial kidney as part of the circulatory system and of the fluid compartments which must be cleared of a given solute. To relate the performance of a hemodialyzer to its design characteristics, clearance is of limited value.

To introduce into the picture the surface area of membrane and the continuously variable (but predictable) concentration difference between blood and dialysate within the artificial kidney, one must define the rate constant of solute transfer, or *permeability* P_Σ.

$$P_\Sigma = \frac{N}{A \times \overline{\Delta C}} \qquad (126.13)$$

where N is the overall solute transport rate between blood dialysate, A is the membrane area, and $\overline{\Delta C}$ is the average solute concentration difference between the two moving fluids.

Permeability is defined by Eq. (126.13) as the amount of solute transferred per unit area and per unit of time, under the influence of a unit of concentration driving force. The proper average concentration, $\overline{\Delta C}$, driving force is the logarithmic mean of the concentration differences prevailing at the inlet and at the outlet

$$\overline{\Delta C} = \frac{\Delta C_i - \Delta C_o}{\ln \dfrac{\Delta C_i}{\Delta C_o}} \qquad (126.14)$$

The boundary conditions on the concentration driving force (ΔC_i and ΔC_o) are uniquely determined by the geometry of the dialyzer. The three most common cases to consider are: (1) cocurrent flow of blood and dialysate; (2) laminar blood flow, with completely mixed dialysate flow; and (3) countercurrent blood and dialysate flow. The boundary conditions on concentration driving force follow.

Cocurrent flow is

$$C_{Bi} - C_{Di} \quad \text{and} \quad C_{Bo} - C_{Do}$$

Mixed dialysate flow is

$$C_{Bi} - C_{Do} \quad \text{and} \quad C_{DBo} - C_{Do}$$

Countercurrent flow is

$$C_{Bi} - C_{Do} \quad \text{and} \quad C_{Bo} - C_{Di}$$

Thus permeability can be expressed as in the following equations. Cocurrent flow is

$$P_\Sigma = \frac{N \dfrac{\ln\left(C_{Bi} - C_{Di}\right)}{C_{Bo} - C_{Do}}}{A\left(C_{Bi} - C_{Di}\right) - \left(C_{Bo} - C_{Do}\right)} \tag{126.15}$$

Mixed dialysate flow is

$$P_\Sigma = \frac{N \dfrac{\ln\left(C_{Bi} - C_{Do}\right)}{C_{Bo} - C_{Do}}}{A\left(C_{Bi} - C_{Do}\right) - \left(C_{Bo} - C_{Do}\right)} \tag{126.16}$$

Countercurrent flow is

$$P_\Sigma = \frac{N \dfrac{\ln\left(C_{Bi} - C_{Do}\right)}{C_{Bo} - C_{Di}}}{A\left(C_{Bi} - C_{Do}\right) - \left(C_{Bo} - C_{Di}\right)} \tag{126.17}$$

By simultaneous solution of Eqs. (126.3), (126.4), and (126.12), and use of the formal definition of the logarithmic mean concentration driving force (126.14), the clearance ratio (K/Q_B) can be expressed as a function of two dimensionless parameters (Z and R), neither of which involves solute concentration terms [Leonard & Bluemle, 1959; Michaels, 1966]. Cocurrent flow is

$$\frac{K}{Q_B} = \frac{1}{1 + Z}\left[1 - \exp(-R(1 + Z))\right] \tag{126.18}$$

Mixed dialysate flow is

$$\frac{K}{Q_B} = \frac{1 - \exp(-R)}{1 + Z\left[1 - \exp(-R)\right]} \tag{126.19}$$

Countercurrent flow is

$$\frac{K}{Q_B} = \frac{1 - \exp\left[R(1 - Z)\right]}{Z - \exp\left[R(1 - Z)\right]} \tag{126.20}$$

where $Z = Q_B/Q_D$ and $R = P_\Sigma A/Q_B$

Michaels has expressed graphically Eqs. (126.18–126.20) as plots of clearance ratio (K/Q_B) versus flow ratio (Q_B/Q_D) with various solute transport ratios ($P_\Sigma, A/Q_B$) as parameters. These plots give an appreciation of the relative importance of the variables affecting dialyzer efficiency and permit one to recognize readily the factors which limit mass transfer under a particular set of conditions.

For the computation of actual permeability coefficients, from pooled data obtained at varying solute concentrations, Eqs. (126.15–126.17) can be rearranged, using definitions of N, C_{Bo}, and C_{Do} from Eqs. (126.2–126.4). Cocurrent flow is

$$P_\Sigma = \frac{Q_B Q_{D;}}{A(Q_B + Q_D)} \ln \frac{1}{1 - K/Q_B - K/Q_D} \tag{126.21}$$

Mixed dialysate flow is

$$P_\Sigma = \frac{Q_B}{A} \ln \frac{1 - K/Q_D}{1 - K/Q_B - K/Q_D} \tag{126.22}$$

Countercurrent flow is

$$P_\Sigma = \frac{Q_B Q_D}{A(Q_D - Q_B)} \ln \frac{1 - K/Q_D}{1 - K/Q_B} \qquad (126.23)$$

As remarked by Leonard and Bluemle [1959], when, and only when, Q_D is much greater than Q_B, the above equations (126.18–126.23) reduce to Renkin's [1956] formula.

$$P_\Sigma = \frac{Q_B}{A} \ln \frac{1}{1 - K/Q_B} \qquad (126.24)$$

or

$$\frac{K}{Q_B} = 1 - \exp\left(\frac{P_\Sigma A}{Q_B}\right) \qquad (126.25)$$

Historically, Eq. (126.25) played an important role in pointing out to designers that the clearance ratio (K/Q_B) can be improved equally well by an increase in exchange area (A) or in permeability (P). However, caution is required in applying the equation to some of the efficient modern dialyzers. First, the assumption that dialysate flow is "infinitely" large with respect to blood flow is seldom verified. Furthermore, the functions relating permeability to dialysance, Eqs. (126.21–126.24), or to the individual solute concentrations and flows, Eqs. (126.15–126.17), have an exponential form. When the overall permeability approaches that of the membrane alone, when the outgoing solute concentrations approach the equilibrium conditions, or when clearance approaches blood flow, one deals with the steep part of that exponential function. Any slight error in the experimental measurements will lead to a disproportionately larger error in calculated permeability.

126.10 Overall Transport

In a dialyzer, separation occurs because small molecules diffuse more rapidly than larger ones and because the degree to which membranes restrict solute transport usually increases with permeant size (permselectivity). Fick's equation states that solute will move from a region of greater concentration to a region of lower concentration in a rate proportional to the difference in concentration on opposite sides of the membrane

$$\phi = -D \frac{\partial c}{\partial x} \qquad (126.26)$$

where ϕ = unit solute flux in g/cm²-s; D = diffusion coefficient cm²/s; c = concentration in g/cm³; and x = distance in cm. The minus sign accounts for the convention that flux is considered positive in the direction of decreasing concentration. Diffusion coefficient decreases roughly in proportion to the square root of molecular weight.

Ignoring boundary layer effects for the moment, and assuming that diffusion within the membrane is analogous to that in free solution, Eq. (126.26) can be integrated across a homogenous membrane of thickness d to yield

$$\phi = \frac{S D_m \Delta c}{d} \qquad (126.27)$$

where S represents the dimensionless solute partition coefficient, i.e., the ratio of solute concentration in external solution to that at the membrane surface, and D_m represents solute diffusion within the membrane and is assumed to be independent of solute concentration in the membrane. If two or more solutes are dialysing at the same time, the degree of separation or enrichment will be proportional to the ratio of their permeabilities. The closer the permeability of a membrane is to that of an equivalent thickness of free solution, the more rapid will be the resultant dialytic transport. Equation (126.27) is often further simplified to this expression for flux per unit of membrane area

$$\phi = P_\Sigma \, \overline{\Delta C} \tag{126.28}$$

where thickness is incorporated into an overall membrane mass transfer coefficient with units of cm/s, and $\overline{\Delta C}$ is the logarithmic mean concentration.

Chemical engineers provided a firm foundation for describing the overall performance of hemodialyzers by recognizing the importance of understanding and describing mass transfer in each of the three phases of a hemodialyzer (blood, membrane, dialysate), the individual mass transfer resistances of which sum to the overall mass transfer resistance of the device [Colton, 1987]. Solutions adjacent to the membranes are rarely well mixed, and the resistance to transport resides not just in the membrane but also in the fluid regions termed *boundary layers,* on both the dialysate and blood side. Moreover, some dialyzers are designed to direct flow parallel to the surface of the membrane rather than expose it to a well-mixed bath. Boundary layer effects typically account for 25–75% of the overall resistance to solute transfer [Lysaght & Baurmeister, 1993]. In many exchanger designs, boundary layer effects can be minimized by rapid convective flow targeted to the surface of the membrane where fluid pathways are thin, flow near the membrane is laminar, and boundary layer resistance decreases with increasing wall shear rates. When geometry permits higher Reynolds numbers, flow becomes turbulent, and fluid resistance varies with net tangential velocity. Geometric obstacles (e.g., properly spaced obstacles) or fluid mechanical modulation (e.g., superimposed pulsation) are often-used tactics to minimize boundary layer effects, but all result in higher energy utilization. Quantitatively, the membrane resistance becomes part of an overall mass transfer parameter P_Σ which for conceptual purposes can be broken down into three independent and reciprocally additive components for the triple laminate: blood boundary layer (subscript B), membrane (subscript M), and dialysate boundary layer (subscript D), such that

$$\frac{1}{P_\Sigma} = \frac{1}{P_B} + \frac{1}{P_M} + \frac{1}{P_D} \tag{126.29}$$

or reciprocally

$$R_\Sigma = R_B + R_M + R_D \tag{126.30}$$

where P_Σ is the device-averaged mass transfer coefficient (or permeability) in cm/s and R_Σ is the device-averaged resistance in s/cm. P_B can be estimated for many revelant conditions of geometry and flow using mass transport analysis based upon wall Sherwood numbers [Colton et al., 1971]. P_M is best obtained by measurements employing special test fixtures in which boundary layer resistances are negligible or known [Klein et al., 1977]. P_D is more problematic and is usually obtained by extrapolations based upon Wilson plots [Leonard & Bluemle, 1960]. Boundary layer theory, as well as technique for correlation, estimation, and prediction of the constituent mass transfer coefficients, is reviewed in detail by Colton and coworkers [1971] and Klein and coworkers [1977]. Overall solute transport is obtained from local flux by mass balance and integration; for the most common case of countercurrent flow

$$\Phi = (C_{Bi} - C_{Di}) \, \frac{Q_B}{A} \, \frac{\exp\left[\dfrac{P_\Sigma A}{Q_B} \left(1 - \dfrac{Q_B}{Q_D} \right) \right] - 1}{\exp\left[\dfrac{P_\Sigma A}{Q_B} \left(1 - \dfrac{Q_B}{Q_D} \right) \right] - \dfrac{Q_B}{Q_D}} \tag{126.31}$$

where C_{Bi} and C_{Di} represent inlet concentrations in the blood and dialysate streams in g/cm³, A represents membrane surface area in cm², Q_B and Q_D are blood and dialysate flow rates in cm³/min, and Φ and P_Σ are as defined in Eqs. (126.28) and (126.29). Derivations of this relationship and similar expressions for cocurrent or crossflow geometries can be found in reviews by Colton and Lowrie [1981] and Gotch and colleagues [1972].

As pointed out by Lysaght and Baurmeister [1993], hemodialysis is a highly constrained process. Molecular diffusion is slow, and the driving forces are set by the body itself, decreasing in the course of purification and not amenable to extrinsic augmentation. The permeant toxic species are not to be recovered, and their concentrations are necessarily more dilute in the dialysate than in the incoming blood. The slow and gentle nature of dialysis has a special appeal for biologic applications, particularly when partial purification of the feed stream, rather than recovery of a product, is intended.

126.11 Membranes

Hemodialysis membranes vary in chemical composition, transport properties, and, as we will see later, biocompatibility. Hemodialysis membranes are fabricated from three classes of materials: regenerated cellulose, modified cellulose, and synthetics [Lysaght & Baurmeister, 1993]. Regenerated cellulose is most commonly prepared by the cuproamonium process and are macroscopically homogenous. These extremely hydrophillic structures sorb water, bind it tightly, and form a true hydrogel. Solute diffusion occurs through highly water-swollen amorphous regions in which the cellulose polymer chains are in constant random motion and would actually dissolve if they were not tied down by the presence of crystalline regions. Their principle advantage is low unit cost, complemented by the strength of the highly crystalline cellulose, which allows polymer films to be made very thin. These membranes provide effective small-solute transport in relatively small exchange devices. The drawbacks of regenerated cellulose are their limited capacity to transport middle molecules and the presence of labile nucleophilic groups which trigger complement activation and transient leukopenia during the first hour of exposure to blood. The advantages appear to outweigh the disadvantages, since over 70% of all hemodialyzers are still prepared from cellulosics, the most common of which is supplied by Akso Faser AG under the trade name Cuprophan.

A variety of other hydrophilic polymers account for 20% of total hemodialyzer production, including derivatized cellulose, such as cellulose acetate, diacetate, triacetate, and synthetic materials such as polycarbonate (PC), ethylenevinylalcohol (EVAL), and polyacrylonitrile-sodium methallyl sulfonate copolymer (PAN-SO₃), which can all be fabricated into homogenous films.

At the opposite end of the spectrum are membranes prepared from synthetic engineered thermoplastics, such as polysulfones, polyamides, and polyacylonitrile-polyvinylchloride copolymers. These hydrophobic materials, which account for about 10% of the hemodialyzer market, form asymmetric and anisotropic membranes with solid structures and open void spaces (unlike the highly mobile polymeric structure of regenerated cellulose). These membranes are characterized by a skin on one surface, typically a fraction of a micron thick, which contains very fine pores and constitutes the discriminating barrier determining the hydraulic permeability and solute retention properties of the membrane. The bulk of the membrane is composed of a spongy region, with interstices that cover a wide size range and with a structure ranging from open to closed cell foam. The primary purpose of the spongy region is to provide mechanical strength; the diffusive permeability of the membrane is usually determined by the properties of this matrix. As the convective and diffusive transport properties of these membranes are, to a large extent, associated independently with the properties of the skin and spongy matrix, respectively, it is possible to vary independently the convective and diffusive transport properties with these asymmetric structures. There is often a second skin on the other surface, usually much more open than the primary barrier. These materials are usually less activating to the complement cascade than are cellulosic membranes. The materials are also less restrictive to the transport of middle and large molecules. Drawbacks are increased cost and such high hydraulic permeability as to require special control mechanisms to avoid excess fluid loss and to raise concerns over the biologic quality of dialysate fluid because of the possibility of back filtration carrying pyrogenic substances to the blood stream.

The discovery of asymmetric membrane structures launched the modern era of membrane technology by motivating research on new membrane separation processes. Asymmetric membranes proved useful in ultrafiltration, and a variety of hydrophobic materials have been used including polysulfone (PS), polyacrylonitrile (PAN), its copolymer with polyvinylchloride (PVC), polyamide (PA), and polymethyl methacrylate (PMMA). PMMA does not form an obvious skin surface and should perhaps be placed in a class of its own.

126.12 Hemofiltration

Although low rates of ultrafiltration have been used routinely for water removal since the beginning of hemodialysis, the availability of membranes with very high hydraulic permeabilities led to radically new approaches to renal substitutive therapy. Such membranes allowed uniformly high clearance rates of solutes up to moderate molecular weights (several thousands) by the use of predominantly convective transport, thereby mimicking the separation capabilities of the natural kidney glomeruli. Progress in the development of this pressure-driven technique, which has come to be known as *hemofiltration*, has been reviewed by Henderson [1982], Lysaght [1986], and Ofsthum et al. [1986].

In ultrafiltration, the solute flux J_S (the rate of solute transport per unit membrane surface area) is equal to the product of the ultrafiltrate flux J_F (the ultrafiltrate flow rate per unit membrane surface area) and the solute concentration in the filtrate, c_F. In turn c_F is related to the retentate concentration c_R in the bulk solution above the membrane by the observed rejection coefficient R:

$$J_S = J_F c_F = J_F (1 - R) c_R \qquad (126.32)$$

Thus, knowledge of the ultrafiltrate flux and observed rejection coefficient permits prediction of the rate of solute removal.

With increasing transmembrane pressure difference, the ultrafiltrate flux increases and then levels off to a pressure-independent value. This behavior arises from the phenomenon of *concentration polarization* [Colton 1987]. Macromolecules (e.g., proteins) that are too large to pass through the membrane build up in concentration in a region near the membrane surface. At steady state, the rate at which these rejected macromolecules are convected by the flow of fluid towards the membrane surface must be balanced by the rate of convective diffusion away from the surface. Estimation of the ultrafiltrate flux reduces largely to the problem of estimating the rate of back transport of macromolecules away from the membrane surface

$$J_F = k \ln \frac{c_{pw}}{c_{pb}} \qquad (126.33)$$

where k is the mass transfer coefficient for back transport of the rejected species, and c_{pw} and c_{pb} are the plasma concentrations of rejected species at the membrane surface and in the bulk plasma, respectively. Attainment of an asymptotic, pressure-independent flux is consistent with the concentration at the wall c_{pw} reaching a constant value. As with diffusive membrane permeability, solute rejection coefficients must be measured experimentally, since the available theoretical models and details of membrane structure are inadequate for prediction.

In hemofiltration the magnitude of the maximum clearance is determined by the blood and ultrafiltrate flow rates and whether the substitution fluid is added before or after filtration. Solutes with molecular weights up to several thousand are cleared at essentially the same rate in hemofiltration, whereas there is a monotonic decrease with increasing molecular weight in hemodialysis. If a comparison is made with devices of equal membrane surface area, it is generally found that hemodialysis provides superior clearance for low-molecular-weight solutes such as urea. The superiority of hemofiltration becomes apparent at molecular weights of several hundred.

Hemodialysis and hemofiltration represent two extremes with membranes having relatively low and relatively high hydraulic permeabilities, respectively. As a variety of new membranes became available with hydraulic permeabilities greater than that of regenerated cellulose, various groups began to examine new treatment modalities in which hemodialysis was combined with controlled rates of ultrafiltration which were higher than those employed in conventional hemodialysis but smaller than those used in hemofiltration [Funck-Brenato et al., 1972; Lowrie et al., 1978; Ota et al., 1975]. The advantage of such an approach is that it retains the high clearance capabilities of hemodialysis for low-molecular-weight solutes while adding enhanced clearance rates for the high-molecular-weight solutes characteristic of hemofiltration. A variety of systems is now commercially available and in clinical use, mainly in Europe and Japan. The proliferation of mixed-mode therapies has led to a panopoly of acronyms: hemodialysis (HD), hemofiltration (HF), high-flux dialysis (HFD), hemodiafiltration (HDF), biofiltration (BF), continuous arteriovenous hemofiltration (CAVH), continuous arteriovenous hemodialysis (CAVHD), slow continuous ultrafiltration (SCUF), simultaneous dialysis and ultrafiltration (SDUF), and so on.

Rigorous description of simultaneous diffusion and convection in artificial kidneys has not yet been carried out. Available analyses span a wide range of complexity and involve, to varying degrees, simplifying assumptions. Their predictions have not been systematically compared with experimental data. In view of the growing interest in various "high-flux" membranes and their application for enhanced solute removal rates and/or shortened treatment times, further refinement may be helpful.

126.13 Pharmacokinetics

Whereas the above analysis is founded on understanding the solute-removal capabilities of hemodialyzers, clinical application must also consider the limitations imposed by the transport of solute between body fluid compartments. The earliest physiologic models were produced by chemical engineers [Bell et al., 1965; Dedrick & Bischoff, 1968] using techniques which had been developed to describe the flow of material in complex chemical processes and were applied to the distribution of drugs and metabolites in biologic systems. This approach has progressively found its way into the management of uremia by hemodialysis [e.g., Farrell, 1983; Gotch & Sargent, 1983; Lowrie et al., 1976; Sargent et al., 1978].

Pharmacokinetics summarizes the relationships between solute generation, solute removal, and concentration in the patient's blood stream. It is most readily applied to urea as a surrogate for other uremic toxins in the quantitation of therapy and in attempts to define its adequacy. In the simplest case, the patient is assumed to have no residual renal function and to produce no urea during the relatively short periods of dialysis. Urea is generated in the body from the breakdown of dietary protein, which empirically has been found to approximate

$$G = 0.11\,I - 0.12 \tag{126.34}$$

where G is the urea generation rate and I the protein intake (both in mg/min). If reliable measurements of I are not available, one assumes an intake of 1 gram of protein per kg of body weight per day.

Urea accumulates in a single pool equivalent to the patient's total body water and is removed uniformly from that pool during hemodialysis. Mass balance yields the following differential equation:

$$\frac{d(cV)}{dt} = G - Kc \tag{126.35}$$

where c is the blood urea concentration (equal to total body water urea concentration) in mg/ml; V is the urea distribution volume in the patient in ml; G is the urea generation rate in mg/min; t is the time from onset of hemodialysis in minutes; and K is the urea clearance in ml/min. V can be measured by tritiated water dilution studies but is usually 58% of body weight. Generation is calculated from actual measurement or estimate of the patient's protein intake (each gram of protein consumed produces about 250 mg of urea). Therefore, a 70-kg patient, consuming a typical 1.0 g of protein per kilogram of body weight per day, would produce 28 g of urea distributed over a fluid volume of 40.6 L. In the absence of any clearance, urea concentration would increase by 70 mg/100ml every 24 hours. The reduction of urea concentration during hemodialysis is readily obtained from Eq. (126.32) by neglecting intradialytic generation and changes in volume:

$$c^t = c^i \exp\left(\frac{Kt}{V}\right) \tag{126.36}$$

where c^i and c^t represent the urea concentrations in the blood at the beginning and during the course of treatment. A 3-1/2-hour treatment of a 70-kg patient ($V = 40.6$L) with a urea clearance of 200 ml/min would lead to a 64% reduction in urea concentration or a value of 0.36 for the c^t/c^i ratio. (This parameter almost always falls between 0.30 and 0.45.)

The increase in urea concentration between hemodialysis treatments is obtained from Eq. (126.33), again assuming a constant V:

$$c^t = c^f + \frac{G}{V}t \tag{126.37}$$

where c^f is the urea concentration in the patient's blood at the end of the hemodialysis and c^t the concentration at time t during the intradialytic interval. Urea concentration typically increases by about 50–100 mg/100ml/24 hours. Even a small residual renal clearance will prove numerically significant. Therefore in oliguric patients who still exhibit a minimum of kidney function, one should use the slightly more complex equations given by Sargent and Gotch [1989] or Farrell [1988].

The exponential decay constant in Eq. (126.33), Kt/v, expresses the net normalized quantity of hemodialysis therapy received by a uremic patient. It is calculated simply by multiplying the urea clearance of the dialyzer (in ml/min) by the duration of hemodialysis (in min) and dividing by the distribution volume (in ml) which in the absence of a better estimate is taken as $0.58 \times$ body weight. Gotch and Sargent [1983] first recognized that this parameter provides an index of the adequacy of hemodialysis. Based upon a retrospective analysis of various therapy formats, they suggested a value of 1.0 or greater as representing an adequate amount of hemodialysis for most patients. Although not immune to criticism, this approach has found widespread clinical acceptance and represents the current prescriptive norm in hemodialysis therapy.

126.14 Adequacy of Dialysis

As outlined in Table 126.1, the uremic syndrome under dialysis is more complex than observed in ESRD before the institution of treatment. The pathology observed not only is related to insufficient removal of toxic solutes but also comprises some unavoidable adverse effects of extracorporeal blood processing, including the interactions of blood with foreign materials [Colton et al., 1994]. The attenuation of uremic syndrome symptoms by protein restriction in the patient's diet and by various dialytic procedures underscores the combined roles of retention, removal, and metabolism in the constellation of signs of the disease. Toxicity may result from the synergism of the entire spectrum of accumulated molecules, which is surprisingly large (see Table 126.2 and Vanholder and Ringoir [1992]). The uremic syndrome resembles complex forms of systemic poisoning and is characterized by multiple symptoms and side effects. Survival requires that the toxins be removed, and

TABLE 126.1   Uremic Syndrome under Dialysis

Adverse effects of uremia can be attributed to:

1. Retention of solutes normally degraded or excreted by the kidneys.
2. Overhydration associated with inadequate balance between fluid intake and water removal.
3. Absence of factors normally synthesized by the kidneys.
4. Pathophysiologic response to the decline in renal function on the part of other organ systems.
5. Pathologic response of the organism to repeated exposure to damaging procedures and foreign materials.

survival quality depends on the quantity of toxins that are actually eliminated. Ideally, one would like to clean blood and body fluids to the same extent as is achieved by normal renal function. This is possible with an organ transplant that works without interruption but is only asymptotically approached with intermittent dialysis.

There is a compelling need for objective definition of the adequacy of ESRD treatment: How much removal in how much time is necessary for each individual? The answer is indirect and approximate. Some define adequacy of dialysis by clinical assessment of patient well-being. More sophisticated procedures, such as electromyography, electroencephalography, and neuropsychologic

TABLE 126.2   Uremic Solutes with Potential Toxicity

Urea	Middle molecules
Guanidines	Ammonia
Methylguanidine	Alkaloids
Guanidine	Trace metals (e.g., bromine)
β-guanidinipropionic acid	Uric acid
Guanidinosuccinic acid	Cyclic AMP
Gamma-guanidinobutyric acid	Amino acids
Taurocyanine	Myoinositol
Creatinine	Mannitol
Creatine	Oxalate
Arginic acid	Glucuronate
Homoarginine	Glycols
N-a-acetylarginine	Lysozyme
Phenols	Hormones
O-cresol	Parathormone
P-cresol	Natriuretic factor
Benzylalcohol	Glucagon
Phenol	Growth hormone
Tyrosine	Gastrin
Phenolic acids	Prolactin
P-hydroxyphenylacetic acid	Catecholamines
β-(m hydroxyphenyl)-	Xanthine
hydracrylic acid	Hypoxanthine
Hippurates	Furanpropionic acid
p-(OH)hippuric acid	Amines
o-(OH)hippuric acid	Putrescine
Hippuric acid	Spermine
Benzoates	Spermidine
Polypeptides	Dimethylamine
β_2-microglobulin	Polyamines
Indoles	Endorphins
Indol-3-acetic acid	Pseudouridine
Indoxyl sulfate	Potassium
5-hydroxyindol acetic acid	Phosphorus
Indo-3-acrylic acid	Calcium
5-hydroxytryptophol	Sodium
N-acetyltryptophan	Water
Tryptophan	Cyanides

tests, may refine the clinician's perception of inadequate dialysis. Yet inadequate therapy can remain unrecognized when therapeutic decisions are based exclusively on clinical parameters. The inverse is also true, and follow-up of dialysis adequacy should never be restricted to static markers of toxicity or dynamic biochemical parameters such as clearance, kinetic modeling, and the like.

Most patients undergoing dialysis do not work or function as healthy people do, and often their physical activity and employment status does not go beyond the level of taking care of themselves. In many centers, the best patients in a hemodialysis program are selectively removed for transplantation. Hospitalization rate is an approximate index of dialysis inadequacy. About 25 percent of all hospitalizations are due to vascular access problems. Comparison among centers may be difficult, however, because of differences in local conditions for hospital admission. Vanholder and Ringoir [1992] have attempted to relate the adequacy of dialysis to the relevant solute concentrations in blood and distinguish among between solute-related factors, patient-related factors, and dialysis-related factors (Table 126.3). Their analysis constitutes a useful point of departure for adjusting the quantity of dialysis to the specific needs of an individual patient, which is a complex problem, since it requires not only an appreciation of what the removal process can do, but also of the generation rate of metabolic end products (related to nutrition, physical activity, fever, etc.) and the dietary load of water and electrolytes. Dialysis patients are partially rehabilitated, but their condition rarely compares to that of recipients of a successful renal transplant.

126.15 Outlook

The treatment of chronic renal failure by artificial kidney dialysis represents one of the most common, and certainly the most expensive, component of substitutive medicine. From an industrial viewpoint, 500,000 patients each "consuming" perhaps 100 heamodialysis filters per year (allowing for some reuse from the 150 units per year that would be needed for 3 times per week treatment) means a production of 50 million filters. With each unit selling for an approximate price of 15 dollars, the world market is on the order of $750 million. From a public health viewpoint, if one is to take the U.S. figure of $30,000 for the world average annual cost of a single dialysis patient, the aggregate economic impact of the medical application of hemodialysis approaches $15 billion a year (of which less than 10 percent is spent on the purchase of technology; health care personnel costs are the most expensive component of the treatment).

TABLE 126.3   Factors Influencing Solute Concentration in Dialyzed Patients

Solute-related factors	Patient-related factors
Compartmental distribution	Body weight
Intracellular concentration	Distribution volume
Resistance of cell membrane	Intake and generation of solutes metabolic precursors
Protein binding	Residual renal function
Electrostatic charge	Quality of vascular access
Steric configuration	Absorption from the intestine
Molecular weight	Hematocrit
Dialysis-related factors	Blood viscosity
Dialysis duration	Absorption of solutes on the membrane, on other parts of the circuit
Interdialytic intervals	Ultrafiltration rate
Blood flow	Intradialytic changes in efficiacy
Mean blood flow	Changes with indirect effect on solute-related factors
Blood flow pattern	Blood pH
Concentration gradients	Heparinization
Dialysate flow	Free fatty acid concentration
Dialyzer surface	
Dialyzer volume	
Dialyzer membrane resistance	
Dialyzer pore size	

Yet "maintenance dialysis on the whole is non-physiological and can be justified only because of the finiteness of its alternative" [Burton, 1976]. Dialytic removal remains nonspecific, with toxic as well as useful compounds eliminated indiscriminately. A better definition of disturbed metabolic pathways will be necessary to formulate treatment hypotheses and design adapted equipment. Sensors for on-line monitoring of appropriate markers may also help to evaluate the modeling of clearance processes. The confusing interference of interactions between the patient and the foreign materials in the dialysis circuit may be reduced as more compatible materials become available. A better clinical condition of the ESRD patient remains the ultimate goal of dialysis therapy because at the moment it seems unlikely that either preventative measures or organ transplantation will reduce the number of patients whose lives depend on the artificial kidney.

Defining Terms

Arteriovenous fistula: A permanent communication between an artery and an adjacent vein, created surgically, leading to the formation of a dialated vein segment which can be punctured transcutaneously with large bore needles so as to allow connecting the circulatory system with an extracorporeal blood processing unit.

Artificial kidney: A blood purification device based on the removal of toxic substances through semipermeable membranes washed out by an acceptor solution which can safely be discarded.

Blood urea nitrogen (BUN): The concentration of urea in blood, expressed as the nitrogen content of the urea (BUN is actually 0.47 times, or approximately half, the urea concentration).

Boundary layer: The region of fluid adjacent to a permeable membrane, across which virtually all (99%) of the concentration change within the fluid occurs.

Catheter: A tube used to infuse a fluid in or out of the vascular system or a body cavity.

Clearance: A measure of the rate of mass removal expressed as the volume of blood which per unit of time is totally cleared of a substance through processing in a natural or artificial kidney. Clearance has the dimensions of a flow rate and can be defined only in relation to a specific solute. Clearance can also be viewed as the minimal volume flow rate of blood which would have to be presented to a processing device to provide the amount actually recovered in the urine or the dialysate if extraction of that material from blood were complete. Clearance is measured as the mass transfer rate of a substance divided by the blood concentration of that substance.

Continuous ambulatory peritoneal dialysis: A modality of peritoneal dialysis in which uninterrupted—although not evenly effective—treatment is provided by 4–6 daily cycles of filling and emptying the peritoneal cavity with a prepared dialysate solution. Solute removal relies on diffusive equalization with molecular species present in capillary blood. Water removal relies on the use of hyperosmotic dialysate.

Continuous arteriovenous hemodialysis: A dialytic procedure in which blood, propelled either by arterial pressure or by a pump, flows continuously at a low flow rate through a dialyzer, from where it returns to a vein, providing for uninterrupted solute and fluid removal and nearly constant equilibration of body fluids with the dialysate solution.

Dialysate: A buffered electrolyte solution, usually containing glucose at or above physiologic concentration, circulated through the water compartment of a hemodialyzer to control diffusional transport of small molecules across the membranes and achieve the blood concentrations desired.

Dialysis: A membrane separation process in which one or more dissolved molecular species diffuse across a selective barrier in response to a difference in concentration.

Dwell time: The duration of exposure of a solution used to draw waste products and excessive water out of the blood during peritoneal dialysis.

ESRD: End-stage renal disease.

Glomerular filtration rate: The volume of plasma water, or primary urine, filtered in the glomerulus per unit of time. Measured, for instance, by creatinine clearance, it expresses the level of remaining renal function in end-stage renal disease.

Hemodiafiltration: Removal of water and solutes by a combination of diffusive and convective transport (paired filtration-dialysis) across a dialysis membrane to achieve effective transport of small and middle molecules. To compensate for the water loss, a large volume of saline or balanced electrolyte solution must be infused in the blood circuit to prevent hemoconcentration.

Hemodialysis: A modality of extracorporeal blood purification in which blood is continuously circulated in contact with a permeable membrane, while a large volume of balanced electrolyte solution circulates on the other side of the membrane. Diffusion of dissolved substances from one stream to the other removes molecules that are in excess in the blood and replaces those for which there is a deficiency. Increased removal can be achieved by increasing the duration of the procedure, the overall membrane area, or the membrane permeability.

Hemofiltration: Removal of water and solutes by convective transport, controlled by a large hydrostatic pressure difference between blood and a liquid compartment across a large-pore, high-water-flux membrane.

Membrane: A thin film of natural or synthetic polymer which allows the passage of dissolved molecules and solvents in response to a concentration or pressure difference (diffusion or filtration) across the polymer.

Middle molecules: Molecules of intermediate molecular weight (roughly of 1000 to 30,000 daltons) which are presumed to be responsible for the toxic manifestations of end-stage renal disease and therefore should be eliminated by substitutive therapy.

Peritoneal dialysis: A process in which metabolic waste products, toxic substances, and excess body water are removed through a membranelike tissue that lines the internal abdominal wall and the organs in the abdominal cavity.

Permeability: The ability of a membrane to allow the passage of certain molecules while maintaining a physical separation between two adjacent phases.

Permselectivity: The property of a membrane whereby a differential rate of molecular transport between two phases is achieved based on characteristics such as molecular weight, molecular size, degree of hydration, affinity for membrane material, and electric charge. The most common feature leading to permselectivity is membrane pore size.

Residual renal clearance: The small level of renal function (measured as creatinine clearance by the diseased kidneys) remaining in some patients in end-stage renal disease, particularly in the early years of dialytic treatment.

Ultrafiltration: The process whereby plasma water flows through a membrane in response to a hydrostatic pressure gradient, dragging with it solute molecules at concentrations equal or lower to that prevailing in plasma.

Uremia: A condition in which the urea concentration in blood is chronically elevated, reflecting an inability to remove from the body the end products of protein metabolism.

Uremic toxins: Partly unidentified and presumably toxic substances appearing in the blood of patients in end-stage renal failure, which can be eliminated to a variable extent by chemical processing of body fluids.

References

Abel JJ, Rowntree LG, Turner BB. 1913. On the removal of diffusible substances from the circulating blood by means of dialysis. Trans Assoc Am Physicians 28:50.

Babb AL, Maurer CJ, Fry DL, et al. 1968. The determination of membrane permeabilities and solute diffusivities with applications to hemodialysis. Chem Eng Prog Symp Ser 63:59.

Brunner H, Mann H. 1985. What remains of the "middle molecule" hypothesis today? Contr Nephrol 44:14.

Burton BJ. 1976. Overview of end stage renal disease. J Dialysis 1:1.

Chenoweth DE. 1984. Complement activation during hemodialysis: clinical observations, proposed mechanisms and theoretical implications. Artif Organs 8:281.

Colton CK. 1987a. Analysis of membrane processes for blood purification. Blood Purification 2:202.

Colton CK. 1987b. Technical foundations of renal prostheses. In HG Gurland (ed), Uremia Therapy, pp 187–217, Berlin, Heidelberg. Springer Verlag.

Colton CK, Smith KA, Merril EW, et al. 1971. Permeability studies with cellulosic membranes. J Biomed Mat Res 5:459.

Colton CK, Ward RA, Shaldon S. 1994. Scientific basis for assessment of biocompatibility in extracorporeal blood treatment. J Nephol Dial Transplant 9 (suppl 2):11.

Dedrick RA, Bischoff KB. 1968. Pharmacokinetics in applications of the artificial kidney. Chem Eng Prog Ser 64:32.

Gotch FA, Autian J, Colton CK, et al. 1972. The Evaluation of Hemodialyzers, Washington, DC, Department of Health, Education and Welfare Publ. No. NIH-72-103.

Gotch FA, Sargent JA, Keen ML, et al. 1974. Individualized, quantified dialysis therapy of uremia. Proc Clin Dial Transplant Forum 4:27.

Jaffrin MY, Butruille Y, Granger A, et al. 1978. Factors governing hemofiltration (HF) in a parallel plate exchanger with highly permeable membranes. Trans Am Soc Artif Intern Organs 24:448.

Jaffrin MY, Gupta BB, Malbraneq JM. 1981. A one-dimensional model of simultaneous hemodialysis and ultrafiltration with highly permeable membranes. J Biomech Eng 103:261.

Kedem O, Katchalsky A. 1958. Thermodynamic analysis of the permeability of biological membranes to nonelectrolytes. Biochim Biophys Acta 27:229.

Kiil F. 1960. Development of a parallel flow artificial kidney in plastics. Acta Chir Scand [Suppl] 253:143.

Klein E, Holland FF, Donnaud A, et al. 1977. Diffusive and hydraulic permeabilities of commercially available cellulosic hemodialysis films and hollow fibers. J Membr Sci. 2:349–364.

Leonard EF, Bluemle LW. 1960. The permeability concept as applied to dialysis. Trans Am Soc Artif Intern Organs 6:33.

Lysaght MJ, Colton CK, Ford CA, et al. 1978. Mass transfer in clinical blood ultrafiltration devices—a review. In TH Frost (ed), Technical Aspects of Renal Dialysis, pp 81–95, London, Pittman Medical.

Michaels AS. 1966. Operating parameters and performance criteria for hemodialyzers and other membrane separation devices. Trans Am Soc Artif Intern Organs 12:387.

Quinton W, Dillard D, Scribner BH. 1960. Cannulation of blood vessels for prolonged hemodialysis. Trans Am Soc Artif Intern Organs 6:104.

Renkin EM. 1956. The relationship between dialysance, membrane area, permeability, and blood flow in the artificial kidney. Trans Am Soc Artif Intern Organs 2:102.

Sargent JA, Gotch FA, Borah M, et al. 1978. Urea kinetics: A guide to nutritional management of renal failure. Am J Clin Nutr 31:1692.

Solomon BA, Castino F, Lysaght MJ, et al. 1978. Continuous flow membrane filtration of plasma from whole blood. Trans Am Soc Artif Intern Organs 24:21.

Vanholder R, Hsu C, Ringoir S. 1993. Biochemical definition of the uremic syndrome and possible therapeutic implications. Artif Organs 17:234.

Vanholder R, Ringoir S. 1992. Adequacy of dialysis, a critical analysis. Kidney Int 42:540.

Vanholder RC, De Smet RV, Ringoir SM. 1992. Validity of urea and other "uremic markers" for dialysis quantification. Clin Chem 38:1429.

Wilson EE. 1915. A basis for rational design of heat transfer apparatus. Trans Am Soc Mech Eng 37:47.

Further Information

An extensive review of renal pathophysiology is to be found in: B.M. Brenner and F.C. Rector, eds., *The Kidney*, 3d ed., Saunders Publishing Co., Philadelphia, 1986. Two volumes addressing the clinical aspects of dialysis are A.R. Nissanson, R. Fine, and D. Gentile, *Clinical Dialysis*, Appleton Lange Century Crofts, Norwalk, 1984; and H.J. Gurland, ed., *Uremia Therapy*, Springer Verlag, Berlin, 1987. The principles of designs and functions of dialysis therapy are outlined in P.C. Farrel, *Dialysis Kinetics, ASAIO Primers in Artificial Organs*, vol. 4, J.B. Lippincott, Philadelphia, 1988; and J.F. Maher, *Replacement of Renal Function by Dialysis*, 3d ed., Klumer, Boston, 1989. Recent reviews of specific aspects in the operation of artificial kidneys are C.K. Colton, "Analysis of Membrane Processes for Blood Purification," *Blood Purification* 5: 202–251, 1987; C. K. Colton and E. G. Lowrie, "Hemodialysis: Physical Principles and Technical Considerations," in B. M. Brenner and F. C. Rector, Jr., eds., *The Kidney*, 2d ed., vol. 2, Saunders, Philadelphia; and C.K. Colton, R.A. Ward, and S. Shaldon, "Scientific Basis for Assessment of Biocompatibility in Extracorporeal Blood Treatment," *Nephrology, Dialysis, Transplantation*, 9 (Suppl. 2):11, 1994.

Ongoing contributions to the field of artificial kidney therapy are often found in biomaterials journals (e.g., the *Journal of Biomaterials Research*) and in artificial organ publications (e.g., the *Transactions of the American Society for Artificial Organs*, the *ASAIO Journal*, the *International Journal of Artificial Organs* and *Artificial Organs*). Clinical contributions can be found in *Kidney International, Nephron,* and *Blood Purification*.

127

Peritoneal Dialysis Equipment

Michael J. Lysaght
CytoTherapeutics, Inc.

John Moran
Baxter Healthcare Corporation

Irreversible end-stage kidney disease occurs with an annual frequency of about 1 in 5000 to 10,000 in the general population, and this rate is increasing. Until the 1960s, such disease was universally fatal. In the last four decades, various interventions have been developed and implemented for preserving life after loss of all or most of a patient's own kidney function. Continuous ambulatory peritoneal dialysis (CAPD), the newest and most rapidly growing of renal replacement therapies, is one such process in which metabolic waste products, electrolytes, and water are removed through the peritoneum, an intricate membranelike tissue that lines the abdominal cavity and covers the liver, intestine, and other internal organs. This review begins with a brief summary of the development of CAPD and its role in the treatment of contemporary renal failure. The therapy format and its capacity for solute removal are then described in detail. Bioengineering studies of peritoneal transport, in which the peritoneum is described in terms analogous to the mass transfer properties of a planar membrane separating well-mixed pools of blood and dialysate, are then reviewed. The transport properties of the equivalent peritoneal membrane are summarized and compared to those of hemodialysis membranes. Models to describe and predict fluid and solute removal rates are examined. Finally, current developments and emerging trends are summarized.

The early history of peritoneal dialysis, as reviewed by Boen [1985], is contemporaneous with that of hemodialysis (HD). Small-animal experiments were reported in the 1920s and 1930s in the United States and Germany. Earliest clinical trials in acute reversible cases of kidney failure began in the late 1930s in the form of a continuous "lavage" in which dialysate was continuously infused and withdrawn from dual trochar access sites. Acute treatments were continued through the 1940s, and about 100 case reports appeared in the literature by 1950; sequential inflow, dwell, and withdrawal was increasingly favored over continuous flow. Chronic therapy was introduced in the early 1960s, followed shortly by indwelling peritoneal catheters. From 1960 onward, peritoneal dialysis clearly lagged behind HD, as the latter became more streamlined, efficient, and cost-effective. Although endorsed by a small group of enthusiasts and proponents, peritoneal dialysis had evolved into a specialized or niche therapy. This changed dramatically in 1976 when Popovich, a biomedical engineer, and Moncrief, a clinical nephrologist, announced the development of a new form of peritoneal dialysis in which ambulatory patients were continuously treated by two liters of dialysis dwelling in the peritoneal cavity and exchanged four times daily [Popovich et al., 1976]. Two years later Baxter began to offer CAPD fluid in flexible plastic containers, along with necessary ancillary equipment and supplies. The rapid subsequent growth of the process is tabulated in Fig. 127.1. At this writing, approximately 90,000 patients are treated by CAPD (versus 490,000 by HD and 130,000 with kidney transplants). A more recent development is the introduction of automated peritoneal dialysis (APD), in which all fluid exchanges are performed by a simple pump console, usually while the patient sleeps. About one peritoneal dialysis patient in six now receives some form of APD; this approach is discussed more fully in a later section on emerging developments.

Both CAPD and HD have advantages and disadvantages, and neither therapy is likely to prove better for all the patients all the time. The principal attraction of CAPD is that it frees the patient from the pervasive life-style invasions associated with thrice weekly in-center HD. CAPD is particularly popular with patients living in rural areas distant from a hemodialysis treatment center. The continuous nature of CAPD eliminates fluctuations in the concentrations of uremic metabolites and avoids the sawtooth pattern of hemodialysis peak toxin concentrations. Fluid and dietary constraints are less restrictive for patients on CAPD than those on HD. A major complication of CAPD is peritonitis. The rate of peritonitis was initially around 2 episodes per patient year; this has fallen to fewer than 0.5 episodes per patient year due to advances in administration set design and use. The morbidity of peritonitis has also decreased with increased experience in its treatment. In most cases, detected early and treated promptly, peritonitis can be managed without requiring hospitalization. Peritonitis caused by certain organisms including Staphylococcus aureus, Pseudomonas, and fungi remains a clinical problem. Other drawbacks of CAPD include the daily transperitoneal administration of 100–150 g of glucose providing ~600 calories, and the tedium of the exchanges. APD and new solution formulations are being developed to address both issues. Little doubt now exists that risk-adjusted survival and morbidity for patients treated by CAPD is equivalent to that for patients

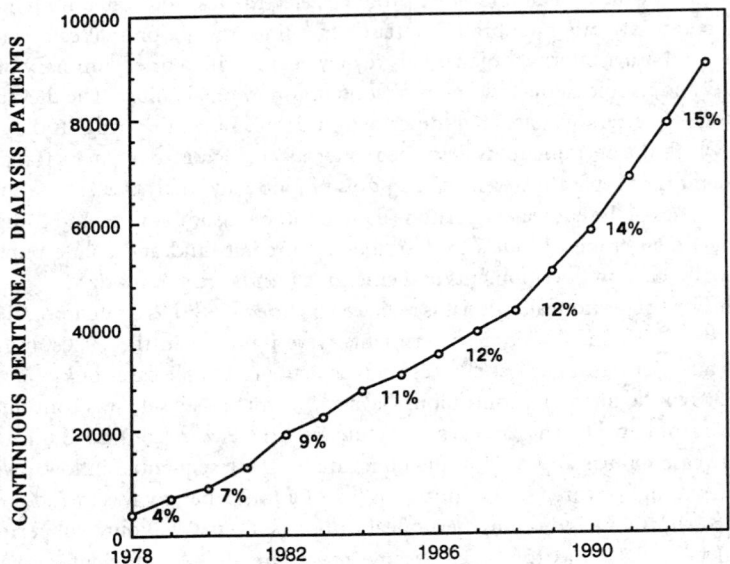

FIGURE 127.1 The growth of peritoneal dialysis. Line and points refer to the total estimated worldwide peritoneal dialysis population; the numbers adjacent to the points are PD patients as a percent of total dialysis population. At the end of 1993, 14,000 of the 90,000 peritoneal dialysis patients utilized some version of APD; the remainder were treated with CAPD. Data compiled taken from various patient registries and industrial sources.

treated with HD. On balance, the therapy seems well suited to many patients, and it continues to grow more rapidly than alternative treatment modalities.

127.1 Therapy Format

The process of CAPD is technically simple. Approximately 2 L of a sterile, nonpyrogenic, and hypertonic solution of glucose and electrolyte are instilled via gravity flow into the peritoneal cavity through an indwelling catheter 4 times per day. A single exchange is illustrated in Fig. 127.2. Intraperitoneal fluid partially equilibrates with solutes in the plasma, and plasma water is ultrafiltered due to osmotic gradients. After 4–5 hours, except at night where the exchange is lengthened to 9–11 hours to accommodate sleep, the peritoneal fluid is drained and the process repeated. Patients perform the exchanges themselves in 20–30 minutes, at home or in the work environment after a training cycle which lasts only 1–2 weeks. In APD, 10–15 L are automatically exchanged overnight; 2 L remain in the peritoneal cavity during the day for a "long dwell" exchange.

As will be discussed in more detail below, the drained fluid contains solute at concentrations around 90–100% of plasma for urea, 65–70% for creatinine, and 15–25% for inulin and β_2 microglobulin. Net fluid removal ranges up to 1000 ml per exchange. CAPD generally removes the same quantity of toxins and fluid as HD (a little thought will show that this is a requirement of steady state, provided that generation is unaltered between the two treatment formats); however, CAPD requires a higher plasma concentration as the driving force for this removal. Steady-state concentrations during CAPD are typically close to the peak, i.e., pretreatment, concentrations of small solutes during HD but much lower than the corresponding peaks for larger species.

Access to the peritoneum is usually via a double-cuff Tenckhoff catheter, essentially a 50–100-cm length of silicone tubing with side holes at the internal end, a dacron mesh flange at the skin line, and connector fittings at the end of the exposed end. Several variations have evolved, but little hard evidence supports the selection of one design format over another [Dratwa et al., 1986]. Most are implanted in a routine surgical procedure requiring about 1 hour and are allowed to heal for 1–2 weeks prior to routine clinical use. Sterile and nonpyrogenic fluid is supplied in 2-L containers fabricated from dioctyl phthalate plasticized polyvinyl chloride. The formulation is essentially potassium-free lactated Ringers to which has been added from 15–42.5 g/L of glucose (dextrose monohydrate). The solution is buffered to a pH of 5.1–5.5, since the glucose would caramelize during autoclaving at higher pH levels. Several different exchange protocols are in use. In the original design, the patient simply rolls up the empty bag after instillation and then drains into the same bag following exchange. The bag filled with drain fluid is disconnected and a fresh bag is reconnected. Patients are trained to use aseptic technique to perform the connect and disconnect. Many ingenious aids were developed to assist in minimizing breaches of sterility including enclosed ultraviolet-sterilized chambers and heat splicers. More recent approaches, known as the "O" set and "Y" set or more generically as "flush before fill" disconnect, invoke more complex tubing sets to allow the administration set to be flushed (often with antiseptic) prior to instillation of dialysate and generally

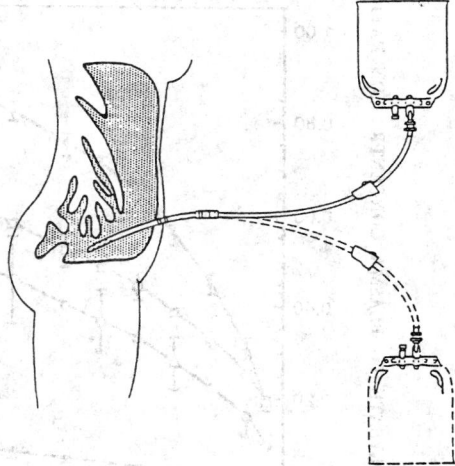

FIGURE 127.2 Illustration of the three steps involved in a single CAPD exchange: fluid infusion, dwell, and drain. Some administration sets require the bag to stay connected during dwell (it is rolled and fits in a girdle around the waist); others allow it to be disconnected. Drain and infusion take about 10 minutes each; three daytime dwells are 4–6 hours each; the overnight dwell lasts 8–10 hours.

permit the patient to disconnect the empty bag during the dwell phase. Initial reports of the success of these protocols in reducing peritonitis were regarded with skepticism, but definite improvement over earlier systems has now been documented in well-designed and carefully controlled clinical trials [Churchill et al., 1989].

127.2 Fluid and Solute Removal

The rate at which solutes are removed during peritoneal dialysis depends primarily upon the rate of equilibration between blood and instilled peritoneal fluid. This is usually quantified as the ratio of dialysate to plasma concentration as a function of dwell time, often in graphs called simply "D over P" (dialysate over plasma) curves. A typical plot of dialysate-to-plasma ratio for solutes of various molecular weight is given in Fig. 127.3. Smaller species equilibrate more rapidly than do larger ones, because diffusion coefficient varies in inverse proportion to the square root of a solute's molecular weight. Dialysate equilibration rates vary considerably from patient to patient; error bars on the plot represent standard error of the mean for duplicate determinations with five patients.

The rate of mass removal during dialysis, ϕ, is simply the volume of fluid, V_D, removed from the peritoneal cavity at the end of a dwell period lasting time t, multiplied by the concentration C_D of the solute in the removed fluid

$$\phi = V_D C_D \qquad (127.1)$$

The whole blood clearance, Cl, is the rate of mass removal divided by the solute concentration in blood C_B

$$Cl = \frac{\phi}{t\,C_B} = \frac{V_D C_D}{t\,C_B} \qquad (127.2)$$

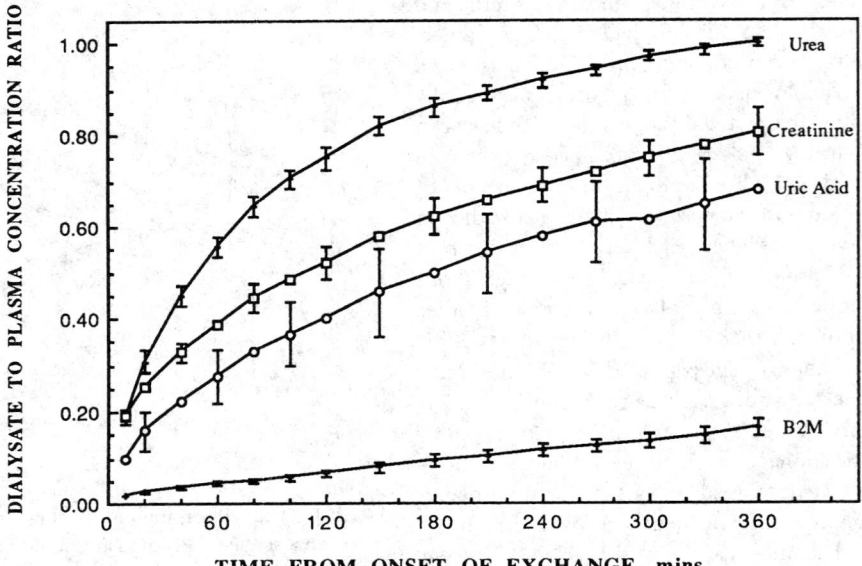

FIGURE 127.3 Ratio of plasma to dialysate concentration for urea (60 daltons), creatinine (113 daltons), uric acid (158 daltons), and β_2 microglobulin (~12,000 daltons). Data were obtained by withdrawing and analyzing a sample of dialysate at each time point and comparing it to plasma concentration. Each point is the average of two determinations on five patients. Error bars are standard error of the mean [Lysaght, 1989].

In Eqs. (127.1) and (127.2), time conventionally is reported in minutes, volume in milliliters, and concentration in any consistent units. Equations (127.1) and (127.2) are based on mass balances; they are thus general and unaffected by the complexity of underlying phenomena such as bidirectional selective connective transport and lymphatic uptake. Equation (127.2) requires that solute concentration in the denominator be reported as whole blood concentration, rather than as plasma concentration, which is often reported clinically. With many small solutes (urea, creatinine, and uric acid), only small error is introduced by considering blood and plasma concentration as interchangeable. With larger solutes, especially those excluded from the red blood cell, care must be taken to correct for differences in plasma and blood concentrations.

Since urea is nearly completely equilibrated during CAPD, i.e., $c_D/c_B = \sim1.0$, urea clearance is commonly equated with total drainage volume. Four 2-L exchanges and 2 L of ultrafiltration would thus result in a continuous urea clearance of 10 L/day or ~7 ml/min. The situation is more complex with APD, which involves several (4–6) short exchanges at partial equilibrium and one very long exchange. In any case, no meaningful direct or *a priori* comparison of clearance with hemodialysis is possible because one therapy is intermittent and the other continuous.

The volume of fluid in the peritoneal cavity increases during an exchange but at a decreasing rate. The driving force for fluid transfer from the blood to the peritoneal cavity is the osmotic pressure of the glucose in the infused dialysate. Typical CAPD solutions contain $\sim1.5\%$, $\sim2.5\%$, or $\sim4.25\%$ by weight of glucose monohydrate, leading to an initial maximum osmotic force (across an ideally semipermeable membrane) of approximately 1000–5000 mmHg. In the first few minutes of an exchange, the rate of ultrafiltration may be as high as 10–30 ml/min. The driving force rapidly dissipates as glucose diffuses from the peritoneal cavity into the bloodstream. After the first hour, rates of 1.0–2.0 ml/min are common. Throughout the exchange, the peritoneal lymphatics are draining fluid from the peritoneal cavity at a rate of 0.5–2.0 ml/min. Fluid balance is thus the difference between removal by a time-dependent rate of ultrafiltration and return via a more constant lymphatic drainage. Net fluid removal is very easily determined in the clinical setting simply by comparing the weight of fluid drained to that instilled. Instantaneous rates of ultrafiltration may be estimated in study protocols by a serious of tedious mass balances around high-molecular-weight radiolabeled markers added to the dialysate fluid. The results of a typical study are plotted in Figs. 127.4 and 127.5 showing both the instantaneous rate of ultrafiltration and the net intraperitoneal volume as a function of time. On average, these patients removed 500 ml of fluid in a single 6-hour exchange or roughly 2 L/day, which permits far more liberal fluid intake than is possible with patients on HD. But here again patient variation is high. Commercial CAPD fluid is available in a variety of solute concentrations; physicians base their prescription for a particular patient on his or her fluid intake and residual urine volume.

3 The Peritoneal Membrane: Physiology and Transport Properties

In contrast to synthetic membranes employed during HD, the peritoneum is not a simple selective barrier between two phases. As implied by its Latin root (*peritonere* = to stretch tightly around), the primary physiologic function of the peritoneum is to line the walls of the abdominal cavity and encapsulate its internal organs (stomach, liver, spleen, pancreas, and parts of the intestine). Most CAPD literature, including this review, uses the terms *peritoneum* and *peritoneal membrane* interchangeably and conveniently extends both expressions to include underlying and connective tissue. Overall adult peritoneal surface is approximately 1.75 ± 0.5 m^2, which generally is considered equal on an individual basis to skin surface area. The peritoneum is not physically homogeneous. The visceral portion ($\sim80\%$) covering the internal organs differs somewhat from the parietal portion overlaying the abdominal walls, which in turn is different from the folded or pleated mesentery connecting the two.

The physiology of the peritoneum, its normal ultrastructure, and variations induced by CAPD have been increasingly elucidated over the past decade. Morphologically, the peritoneum is a smooth, tough, somewhat translucent sheath. Its thickness ranges from under 200 to over 1000

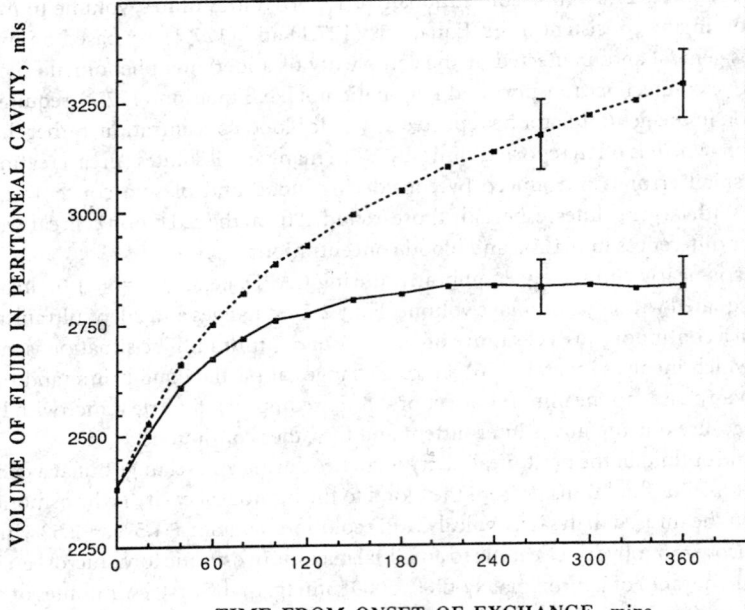

FIGURE 127.4 Volume of fluid in the peritoneal cavity versus time during an exchange with ~2.5% glucose dialysis fluid. Solid line is actual volume. Dotted line represents estimate of the volume in the absence of lymphatic flow. Results represent an average of duplicate determinations on five patients. Volume was estimated by dilution of radiolabeled tracers (too large to diffuse across the peritoneal membrane) added to dialysate prior to instillation; lymphatic flow was calculated from a mass balance on net recovered marker. Each point is the average of two determinations on five patients. Error bars are standard error of the mean [Lysaght, 1989].

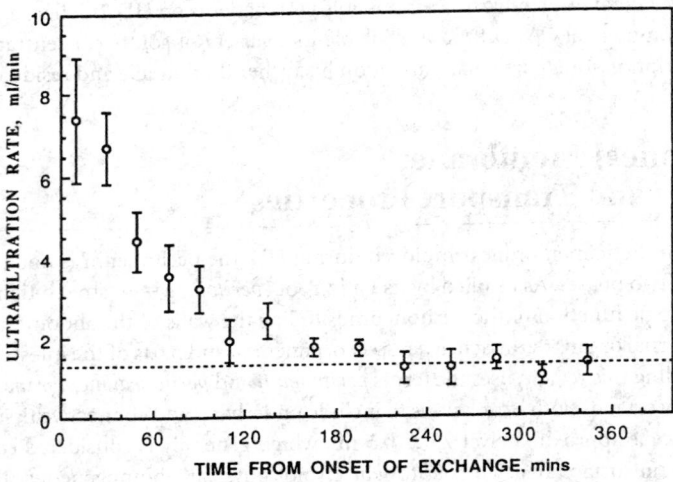

FIGURE 127.5 Comparisons of rates of ultrafiltration of fluid into the peritoneal cavity (open circles) and lymphatic drainage of fluid from the peritoneal cavity back to the patient (dotted line). Same study and methods as in Fig. 127.4.

microns. The topmost layer, which presents to the dialysate during CAPD, is formed from a single layer of mesothelial cells, densely covered by microvilli (hairlike projections), although the latter tend to disappear gradually during the first few weeks of CAPD. Immediately underneath is the interstitium, a thick sheath of dense mucopolysaccharide hydrogel interlaced with collagenous fibers, microfibrillar structures, fibroblasts, adipocytes, and granular material. Most important for CAPD, the interstitium is perfused with a network of capillaries through which blood flows from the mesenteric arteries and the vasculature of the abdominal wall to the portal and systemic venous circulations. Blood-flow rate has been estimated to be in the range of 30–60 ml/min, but this is not well established. The interstitial layer is a hydrogel; its water content, and thus its transport properties, will vary in response to the osmolarity of the peritoneal dialysate.

Peritoneal mass transfer characteristics are most commonly obtained by back-calculating basic membrane properties from results in standard or modified peritoneal dialysis. Three membrane parameters will be described: Lp, the hydraulic permeability; R, the rejection coefficient; and K_oA, the mass transfer coefficient ($=$ area $A \times$ diffusive permeability K_o). The formal definitions of these parameters are given in Eqs. (127.3) through (127.5), with R and K_oA defined for the limiting conditions of pure convection and pure diffusion.

$$Lp = \frac{\text{Filtration rate}}{\text{Area} \cdot \text{pressure driving force}} = \frac{J_F}{A(\Delta P - \Sigma \sigma_i \pi_i)} \qquad (127.3)$$

$$R = 1 - \frac{\text{Concentration in bulk filtrate}}{\text{Concentration in bulk retentate}} = \left[\frac{C_B - C_D}{C_B} \right]_{\phi d = 0} \qquad (127.4)$$

$$K_oA = \frac{\text{Solute transport}}{\text{Concentration driven force}} = \left[\frac{\phi_d}{C_B - C_D} \right]_{J_F R = 0} \qquad (127.5)$$

where $J_F =$ filtration rate, $A =$ area, $\sigma =$ Staverman reflection coefficient, $\pi =$ osmotic pressure, and other terms are as defined previously.

At the onset of a CAPD exchange using 4.25% dextrose, the ultrafiltration rate is 10–30 ml/min. Relative to a perfectly semipermeable membrane, the glucose osmotic pressure of the solution is 4400 mmHg. Overall membrane hydraulic permeability is the quotient of these terms and is thus of the order of 0.2 ml/hr-mmHg, in the units commonly employed for HD membranes. This estimate needs to be corrected for the osmotic back-pressure, which is primarily due to urea in the blood (conc $\sim$ 1.3 g/L) as well as the fact that the membrane is only partially semipermeable. The best results are not obtained from a single point measurement but either from curve fitting to the ultrafiltration profile during the entire course of dialysis or from data taken at different osmotic gradients. A review [Lysaght & Farrell, 1989] of reports from several different investigators suggests an average value of $\sim$ 2 ml/hr-mmHg or, roughly, 2 gal/ft^2/day (GSFD) at 100 PSI. This is higher than desalination membranes, just slightly lower than conventional regenerated cellulose hemodialysis membranes, and much lower than anisotropic ultrafiltration membranes.

Rejection coefficients, R, numerically equal to unity minus sieving coefficient are obtained either from kinetic modeling as described below or experimentally by infusing a hypertonic solution into the peritoneum with a permeant concentration equal to that in the plasma. After a suitable period of ultrafiltration, the ratio of solute to water flux is calculated from the dilution of the recovered solution. Both methods are approximate and results from different investigators may vary substantially. Reported values are observed average rejection coefficients. These are often described as the Staverman rejection coefficient, σ, which is somewhat overreaching, since filtration velocity is not recorded and differences between bulk and wall concentrations are not known. Representative values, from a review of the literature [Lysaght & Farrell, 1989], are summarized in Table 127.1. Thus the membrane appears quite tight, possibly rejecting about 10–20% of urea and other small molecules, about 50% of intermediate-molecular-weight species, and over 99% of plasma proteins.

TABLE 127.1 Equivalent Transport Coefficients for the Peritoneal Membrane

Permeant Species, MW	Rejection Coefficient, dimensionless	K_oA, cm³/min
Urea, 60	0.26 ± 0.08	21 ± 4
Creatinine, 113	0.35 ± 0.07	10 ± 2
Uric acid, 158	0.37	10
B-12, 1355		5
Inulin, 5200	0.5 ± 0.2	4 ± 1.5
$\beta_2$microglobulin, 12,000		0.8 ± 0.4
Albumin, 69,000	0.99	

Note: *SD* not given if $n < 3$. Equivalent ultrafiltration coefficient is ~2.0 ml/min-m²-mmHg. Data taken from a review by Lysaght and Farrell [1989].

The diffusive permeability of the membrane is obtained by back calculation from measurements of blood and dialysate concentration versus time during an exchange, as will be further elaborated below. Values are given as the product of membrane permeability and estimated peritoneal area (K_oA), and the results of various investigators have been reasonably consistent. Critical values from a review of the literature are summarized in Table 127.1. A K_oA value of about 20 ml/min for urea is around one order of magnitude less than comparable values for contemporary hollow-fiber hemodialyzers. If the area of the peritoneum is taken as 1.75 m², then urea transfers through the peritoneum analogously to urea diffusing through a stagnant film of water roughly a centimeter thick. Alternatively, given a peritoneal thickness range of 200–2000 microns, the diffusion of urea inside the membrane is about 20% of what would be found in a film of stagnant water of the same thickness.

It should once more be noted that the physiologic peritoneum is a complex and heterogeneous barrier, and its transport properties would be expected to vary over different regions of its terrain. For example, studies in animal models have suggested that transport during peritoneal dialysis is little affected when large segments of the visceral membrane are surgically excised. It is also repeated for emphasis that the terms Lp, R, and K_oA do not describe this membrane itself but rather a hypothetical barrier that is functionally and operationally equivalent and thus capable of producing the same mass transfer characteristics in response to the same driving forces.

127.4 Transport Modeling

Several investigators have developed mathematic models to describe, correlate, and predict relationships among the time-course of solute removal, fluid transfer, treatment variables, and physiologic properties [Lysaght & Farrell, 1989; Vonesh et al., 1991; Waniewski et al., 1991]. Virtually all kinetic studies start with the model illustrated in Fig. 127.6. The patient is considered to be a well-mixed compartment with a distribution volume V_B set equal to some fraction of total body weight. (For example, urea distributes over total body water, which is ~ 0.58 times body weight.) Dialysate occupies a second, much smaller compartment, $V_D = 2$–3 L, which is also considered well-mixed but which changes in size during the course of exchange. These two compartments are separated by a planar membrane capable of supporting bidirectional transport and characterized by the terms Lp, R, and K_oA previously defined by Eqs. (127.3)–(127.5). Fluid drains from the peritoneum to the blood at a rate of Q_L. From this point forward, the complexity and appropriate utility of the models depend upon the investigators' choices of simplifying assumptions. The simplest model, proposed by Henderson and Nolph [1969], considers ultrafiltration rate and lymphatic flow to be negligible and treats all parameters except dialysate concentration as constant with time. The basic differential equation describing this model is

$$\frac{d(V_D C_D)}{dt} = V_D \frac{dC_D}{dt} = K_0 A (C_B - C_D) \qquad (127.6)$$

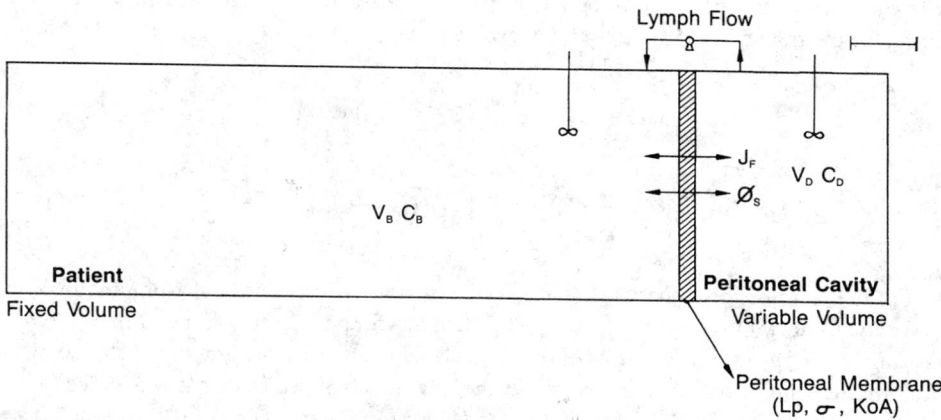

FIGURE 127.6 Single pool model for peritoneal dialysis. Solute diffuses across a planar selective membrane from a large well-mixed plasma space at constant volume and concentration to a smaller well-mixed space in which concentration and volume both increase with time. Fluid and solute are selectively ultrafiltered across the peritoneal membrane from plasma to dialysate; they are also nonselectively transported by the lymphatics from the dialysate to the body compartment.

Equation 127.6 may be readily solved, either to obtain K_oA from a knowledge of concentration versus time data Eq. (127.7), or to predict dialysate concentration from a knowledge of mass transfer coefficient, blood concentration, and initial dialysate concentration Eq. (127.8) where:

$$K_0A = \frac{V_D}{t} \ln\left(\frac{C_B - C_D^0}{C_B - C_D^t}\right) \tag{127.7}$$

$$C_D^t = C_B - (C_B - C_D^0)e^{\frac{-K_0At}{V_D}} \tag{127.8}$$

In these equations, the superscript t represents the value at time t, and the superscript 0 designates the value at $t = 0$. This model provides a very easy way of measuring K_oA if it is applied during the isovolemic interval that often occurs $\sim$30–90 min after the beginning of an exchange.

Several years later, investigators at the University of New South Wales [Garred et al., 1983] proposed a slightly more complex model that included ultrafiltration, subject to the assumptions that: (1) blood concentration was constant, (2) the membrane was nonselective ($R = O$), and (3) lymphatic involvement could be ignored. The appropriate differential equation is now:

$$\frac{d(V_D C_D)}{dt} = K_0A(C_B - C_D) + C_B\frac{dV_D}{dt} \tag{127.9}$$

This equation can be solved in two ways. Over either relatively short time intervals or small differences in dialysate volume, an average volume V_D is obtained as the mean of initial and final volumes. In that case K_oA is given by

$$K_0A = \frac{\overline{V}_D}{t} \ln\left[\frac{V_D^o(\overline{C}_B - C_D^0)}{V_D^t(\overline{C}_B - C_D^t)}\right] \tag{127.10}$$

where variables overlined with a solid diachrin are treated as constant during the integration of Eq. (127.9). The similarity of Eqs. (127.9) and (127.10) to Eqs. (127.7) and (127.8) should be noted.

Where a series of data points for blood and dialysate concentrations are available at various times during the treatment, Eq. (127.10) may be rewritten as

$$C_D^t = \overline{C}_B - \frac{V_D^o}{V_D^t}(\overline{C}_B - C_D^o)\, e^{\left(\frac{-K_oAt}{V_D}\right)} \tag{127.11}$$

$$\ln[V_D^t(\overline{C}_B - C_D^t)] = \ln[V_D^o(\overline{C}_B - C_D^o)] - \frac{K_oAt}{V_D} \tag{127.12}$$

Data in the form of this equation may be readily regressed to obtain K_oA from a knowledge of V_D, C_B, and C_D at various times in an exchange. The values for peritoneal volume V_D may be obtained experimentally from tracer dilution studies, calculated from an algorithm, in which case it varies with time, or simply averaged between initial and final values, in which case it is assumed constant. Equations (127.11) and (127.12) are recommended for routine modeling of patient kinetics.

Several investigators, reviewed by Lysaght and Farrell [1989], have produced far more elaborate models which incorporate lymphatic drainage, deviations from ideal semipermeability of the peritoneal membrane, time-dependent ultrafiltration rates, and coupling between bidirectional diffusive and connective transport. Although potent in the hands of their developers, none of the numerical models has been widely adopted, and the current trend is toward simpler approaches. In comparative studies [Lysaght, 1989; Waniewski et al., 1991], only small differences were found between the numeric values of transport parameters calculated from simple analytic models [Eqs. (127.6)–(127.12)] and those we obtained by far more complex numerical methods. In peritoneal dialysis, solute is being exchanged through an inefficient membrane between a large body compartment through an inefficient membrane and a second compartment only 5% as large, and treatment times have been chosen so that the smaller compartment will reach saturation. These physical circumstances, and the very forgiving nature of exponential asymptotes, perhaps explain why simple analytic solutions perform nearly as well as their more complex numeric counterparts.

127.5 Emerging Developments

Modified therapy formats and new formulations for exchange solutions constantly are being proposed and evaluated. APD is the most successful of the new formats; at the end of 1993, about one in six peritoneal dialysis patients received some variant of automated overnight treatment. APD is carried out by a small console (Fig. 127.7) which automatically instills and drains dialysate at 1.5–3-hour intervals while the patient sleeps, typically over 8–10 hours each night. The peritoneum is left full during the day. Since the short exchanges do not permit complete equilibration even for urea, the process is somewhat wasteful of dialysate. However, reference to Fig. 127.3 will readily demonstrate that small-solute removal is most efficient in the early portion of an exchange; for example, two 2-hour exchanges will provide 75% more urea clearance than one 4-hour exchange. As currently prescribed, APD requires 84–105 L per week of dialysate (versus 56 for CAPD) and increases total small-solute clearance per 24 hours by up to 50% over that achieved by CAPD. The number of patients on APD is increasing by half every year, a phenomenon driven by two main factors. The first relates to quality of life; APD is far-and-away the least invasive of the maintenance dialysis protocols. The patient performs one connection at night and one disconnection in the morning and is thereby freed from the tedium and inconvenience of daily exchanges or the need to spend a significant portion of 3 days per week at an HD treatment facility. In addition, small-solute clearance is higher than in other continuous peritoneal therapies, which helps address increasing concern about the adequacy of the standard four 2-L CAPD exchanges per day, especially with large

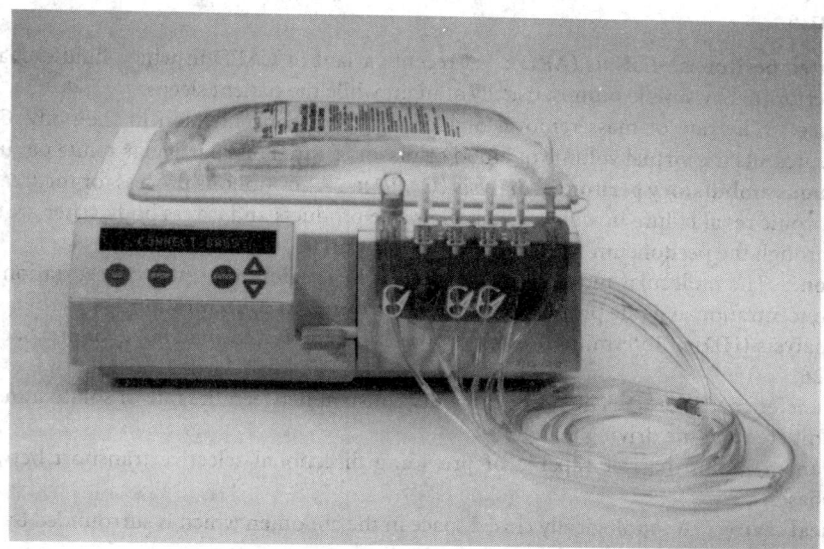

FIGURE 127.7 Contemporary equipment module for APD (Home Choice, Renal division, Baxter Healthcare) which automatically controls and monitors the delivery of 10–15 L of dialysate from 5-L bags via a multipronged disposable administration set. The console incorporates a diaphragm pump used to emulate gravity, and a derivative of the ideal gas law measures fluid volume, eliminating the need for scales. Setup and operation are designed to be straightforward and convenient.

muscular patients and those with no residual renal function. A group of patients who may benefit from APD are those who have rapid transport of glucose across the peritoneal membrane; because of the consequent loss of the osmotic gradient, they have difficulty achieving adequate ultrafiltration. The short dwell times of APD circumvent this problem. The counterbalancing disadvantage of APD is increased expense associated with the larger fluid consumption and the fluid cyclers.

Virtually all solution development comprises attempts to replace glucose with an alternative osmotic agent, preferably one which diffuses more slowly and thus provides a more stable osmotic gradient and one which obviates the obligatory load of about 600 calories of sugar. However glucose is cheap and safe, and it will be difficult to find a satisfactory alternative. A competing osmotic agent must be safe to administer in amounts of tens of grams per day over years to patients who have little or no ability to clear accumulated material via the kidney—but an osmotic agent which is readily metabolizable provides no caloric "advantage" over glucose. A glucose polymer, termed polyglucose, has been recently introduced in England [Mistry & Gokal, 1993]. This disperse oligodextrin has a weight-averaged MW of 18,700 daltons and number-averaged molecular weight of 7300 daltons. At a concentration of 7.5% (i.e., 30 g per 2-L exchange), it provides more stable ultrafiltration during long dwell exchanges; however, administration is limited to one exchange per day because of the accumulation of maltose and higher MW polysaccharides; an alternative approach, recently introduced in Europe and in clinical trails in the United States, is a solution in which glucose is replaced with 1.1% amino acids, enriched for essential amino acids [Jones et al., 1992]. This solution also improves nitrogen balance, a significant feature, since dialysate patients are frequently malnourished. Concern about excessive nitrogen intake, however, limits its use to one or two exchanges per day, and the amino acid solution is necessarily more expensive than glucose.

Defining Terms

Automated peritoneal dialysis (APD):   A recent variant of CAPD in which fluid exchanges are performed by simple pumps, usually at night while the patient sleeps.

Clearance: The rate of mass removal divided by solute concentration in the body. Clearance represents the virtual volume of blood or plasma cleared of a particular solute per unit time.

Continuous ambulatory peritoneal dialysis (CAPD):   A continuous process for the treatment of chronic renal failure in which metabolic waste products and excess body water are removed through the peritoneum with four exchanges of up to 3 L every 24 hours.

Diffusion: The molecular movement of matter from a region of greater concentration to lesser concentration at a rate proportional to the difference in concentration.

Hemodialysis (HD):   Intermittent extracorporeal therapy for chronic renal failure. See Chapter 126.

Mass transfer coefficient: The proportionality constant between the rate of solute transport per unit area and the driving force.

Membrane: A thin barrier capable of providing directional selective transport between two phases.

Peritoneal cavity: A topologically closed space in the abdomen which is surrounded by the peritoneum.

Peritoneum: An intricate, vascularized, membranelike tissue that lines the internal abdominal walls and covers the liver, intestine, and other internal organs. Used interchangeably with the expression *peritoneal membrane*.

References

Boen ST. History of peritoneal dialysis. 1985. In KD Nolph (ed), Peritoneal Dialysis, pp 1–22, The Hague, Martinus Nijhoff.

Churchill DN, Taylor DW, Vas SI, et al. 1989. Peritonitis in continuous ambulatory peritoneal dialysis (CAPD): A multi-centre randomized clinical trial comparing the Y connector disinfectant system to standard systems. Perit Dial Int 19:159.

Dratwa M, Collart F, Smet L. 1986. CAPD peritonitis and different connecting devices: A statistical comparison. In JF Maher, JF Winchester (eds), Frontiers in Peritoneal Dialysis, pp 190–197, New York, Field Rich.

Garred LJ, Canaud B, Farrell PC. 1983. A simple kinetic model for assessing peritoneal mass transfer in chronic ambulatory peritoneal dialysis. ASAIO J 6:131.

Henderson LW, Nolph KD. 1969. Altered permeability of the peritoneal membrane after using hypertonic peritoneal dialysis fluid. J Clin Invest 48: 992.

Jones MR, Martis L, Algrim CE, et al. 1992. Amino acid solutions for CAPD: Rationale and clinical experience. Miner Electrolyte Metab 18:309.

Lysaght MJ. 1989. The Kinetics of Continuous Peritoneal Dialysis. PhD thesis, Center for Biomedical Engineering, University of New South Wales.

Lysaght MJ, Farrell PC. 1989. Membrane phenomena and mass transfer kinetics in peritoneal dialysis. J Mem Sci 44:5.

Mistry CD, Gokal R. 1993. Single daily overnight (12-h dwell) use of 7.5% glucose polymer (Mw 18700; Mn 7300) + 0.35% glucose solution: A 3-month study. Nephrol Dial Transplant 8:443.

Popovich RP, Moncrief JW, Decherd JF, et al. 1976. The definition of a novel portable/wearable equilibrium peritoneal technique. Abst Am Soc Artif Intern Organs 5:64.

Vonesh EF, Lysaght MJ, Moran J, et al. 1991. Kinetic modeling as a prescription aid in peritoneal dialysis. Blood Purif 9:246.

Waniewski J, Werynski A, Heimburger O, et al. 1991. A comparative analysis of mass transport models in peritoneal dialysis. ASAIO Trans 37:65.

Further Information

The literature on continuous peritoneal dialysis is abundant. Among several reference texts the most venerable and popular is *Peritoneal Dialysis* edited by K. Nolph and published by Kluwer; this is regularly updated. Also recommended is *Continuous Ambulatory Peritoneal Dialysis* edited by R Gokal and published by Churchill Livingston. The journal *Peritoneal Dialysis International* (published by MultiMed; Toronto) is published quarterly and is devoted exclusively to CAPD. The continuing education department of the University of Missouri-Columbia organizes a large annual conference on peritoneal dialysis with plenary lectures and submitted papers. The International Society of Peritoneal Dialysis holds its conference biannually and usually publishes proceedings. Peritoneal dialysis is also discussed in the meeting and journals of the other major artificial organ societies (American Society of Artificial Internal Organs; European Dialysis and Transplant Association; Japanese Society of Artificial Organs) and the American and International Societies of Nephrology. *Blood Purification* (published by Karger; Basel) attracts many outstanding papers dealing with engineering and transport issues in peritoneal dialysis. For the insatiable, Medline now contains over 10,000 citations to CAPD and peritoneal dialysis.

128

Therapeutic Apheresis and Blood Fractionation

Andrew L. Zydney
University of Colorado at Boulder

Apheresis is the process in which a specific component of blood (either plasma, a plasma component, white cells, platelets, or red cells) is separated and removed with the remainder of the blood returned to the patient (often in combination with some type of replacement fluid). Donor apheresis is used for the collection of specific blood cells or plasma components from blood donors, resulting in a much more effective use of limited blood-based resources. Donor apheresis developed during World War II as a means for increasing the supply of critically needed plasma, and clinical trials in 1944 demonstrated that it was possible to safely collect donations of a unit of plasma (approximately 300 ml) on a weekly basis if the cellular components of blood were returned to the donor. Therapeutic apheresis is used for the treatment of a variety of diseases and disorders characterized by the presence of abnormal proteins or blood cells in the circulation which are believed to be involved in the progression of that particular condition. Therapeutic apheresis thus has its roots in the ancient practice of bloodletting, which was used extensively well into the 19th century to remove "bad humors" from the patient's body, thereby restoring the proper balance between the "blood, yellow bile, black bile, and phlegm."

The term *plasmapheresis* was first used by Abel, Rowntree, and Turner in 1914 in their discussion of a treatment for toxemia involving the repeated removal of a large quantity of plasma, with the cellular components of blood returned to the patient along with a replacement fluid [Kambic & Nosé, 1993]. The first successful therapeutic applications of plasmapheresis were reported in the late 1950s in the management of macroglobulinemia (a disorder characterized by a large increase in blood viscosity due to the accumulation of high-molecular-weight globulins in the blood) and in the treatment of multiple myeloma (a malignant tumor of the bone marrow characterized by the production of excessive amounts of immunoglobulins).

By 1990, there were well over 50 diseases treated by therapeutic apheresis [Sawada et al., 1990] with varying degrees of success. Plasmapheresis is used in the treatment of: (1) protein-related diseases involving excessive levels of specific proteins (e.g., macroglobulins in Waldenstrom's syndrome and lipoproteins in familial hypercholesterolemia) or excessive amounts of protein-bound substances (e.g., toxins in hepatic failure and thyroid hormone in thyrotoxicosis), (2) antibody-related or *autoimmune diseases* (e.g., glomerulonephritis and myasthenia gravis), and (3) immune-complex-related diseases (e.g., rheumatoid arthritis and systemic lupus erythematosus).

Cytapheresis involves the selective removal of one (or more) of the cellular components of blood, and it has been used in the treatment of certain leukemias (for the removal of leukocytes) and in the treatment of polycythemia. Table 128.1 provides a more complete listing of some of the diseases and blood components that are removed during therapeutic apheresis. This list is not intended to be exhaustive, and there is still considerable debate over the actual clinical benefit of apheresis for a number of these diseases.

The required separation of blood into its basic components (red cells, white cells, platelets, and plasma) can be accomplished using centrifugation or membrane filtration; the more specific removal of one (or more) components from the separated plasma generally involves a second membrane filtration or use of an appropriate sorbent. The discussion that follows focuses primarily on the technical aspects of the different separation processes currently in use. Additional information on the clinical aspects of therapeutic apheresis is available in the references listed at the end of this chapter.

128.1 Plasmapheresis

The therapeutic application of plasmapheresis can take one of two forms: plasma exchange or plasma perfusion. In *plasma exchange* therapy, a relatively large volume of plasma, containing the toxic or immunogenic species, is separated from the cellular components of blood and replaced with an equivalent volume of a replacement fluid (either fresh frozen plasma obtained from donated blood or an appropriate plasma substitute). In *plasma perfusion,* the separated plasma is treated by an adsorptive column or second membrane filtration to remove a specific component (or components) from the plasma. This treated plasma is then returned to the patient along with the blood cells, thereby eliminating the need for exogenous replacement fluids. The different techniques that can be used for plasma perfusion are discussed subsequently.

The reduction in the concentration (C_i) of any plasma component during the course of a plasmapheresis treatment can be described using a single compartment pharmacokinetic model as

$$V_p \frac{dC_i}{dt} = -\alpha_i Q_p C_i + G_i \qquad (128.1)$$

where V_p is the volume of the patient's plasma (which is assumed to remain constant over the course of the therapy through the use of a replacement fluid or through the return of the bulk of the plasma after a plasma perfusion), Q_p is the volumetric rate of plasma collection, G_i is the rate of component generation, and α_i is a measure of the effectiveness of the removal process. In membrane plasmapheresis, α_i is equal to the observed membrane sieving coefficient, which is defined as the ratio of the solute concentration in the filtrate collected through the membrane to that in the plasma entering the device; α_i is thus equal to 1 for a small protein that can pass unhindered through the membrane but can be less than 1 for large proteins and immune complexes. In plasma perfusion systems, α_i is equal to the fraction of the particular component removed from the collected plasma by the secondary (selective) processing step. The generation rate is typically negligible over the relatively short periods (fewer than 3 hours) involved in the actual plasmapheresis; thus the component concentration at the end of a single treatment is given as

$$\frac{C_i}{C_{io}} = \exp\left(-\frac{\alpha_i Q_p t}{V_p}\right) = \exp\left(-\frac{\alpha_i V_{exc}}{V_p}\right) \qquad (128.2)$$

where $V_{exc} = Q_p t$ is the actual volume of plasma removed (or exchanged) during the process. Plasma exchange thus reduces the concentration of a given component by 63% after an exchange of one plasma volume (for $\alpha_i = 1$) and by 86% after two plasma volumes. This simple single compartment model has been verified for a large number of plasma components, although immuno-

TABLE 128.1   Disease States Treated by Therapeutic Apheresis

Disease	Components Removed
Hematologic	
Hemophilia	AntiFactor VIII Ab
Idiopathic Thrombocytopenia Purpura	Antiplatelet Ab, immune complexes
Thrombotic Thrombocytopenia Purpura	Antiplatelet Ab, immune complexes
AIDS, HIV	Antilymphocyte Ab, immune complexes
Autoimmune Hemolytic Anemia	Anti-red cell Ab, red cells
Rh Incompatibility	Anti-Rh Ab
Cryoglobulinemia	Cryoglobulins
Hyperviscosity Syndrome	Macroglobulins, immunoglobulin M
Waldenstrom's Syndrome	Immunoglobulin M
Paraproteinemia	Paraproteins
Sickle Cell Anemia	Red blood cells
Thrombocythemia	Platelets
Collagen/rheumatologic	
Systemic Lupus Erythematosus	Anti-DNA Ab, immune complexes
Progressive Systemic Sclerosis	Antinonhistone nuclear Ab
CREST Syndrome	Anticentromere Ab
Sjorgen Syndrome	Antimitochondrial Ab
Rheumatoid Arthritis	Rheumatoid factor, cryoglobulins, immunoglobulins
Periarteritis Nodosa	Cryoglobulins, immune complexes
Raynaud's Disease	Cryoglobulins, macroglobulins
Scleroderma	Immune complexes
Mixed Connective Tissue Diseases	Immunoglobulins
Neurologic	
Myasthenia Gravis	Antiacetylcholine receptor Ab, cryoglobulins
Multiple Sclerosis	Antimyelin Ab
Guillain-Barre Syndrome	Antimyelin Ab
Polyneuropathy	Cryoglobulins, macroglobulins
Polyradiculoneuropathy	Antibodies
Lambert-Eaton Syndrome	Antibodies
Hepatic	
Chronic Active Hepatitis	Antimitochondrial Ab
Hepatic Failure	Protein-bound toxins
Primary Biliary Cirrhosis	Protein-bound toxins, antimitochondrial Ab
Renal	
Goodpasture's Syndrome	Antiglomerular basement membrane Ab
Glomerulonephritis	Immune complexes
Lupus Nephritis	Immune complexes
Transplant Rejection	Immune complexes, anti-HLA Ab
Malignant diseases	
Cancer	Tumor-specific Ab, immune complexes
Multiple Myeloma	Immunoglobulins
Leukemia	Leukocytes
Miscellaneous	
Addison's Disease	Antiadrenal Ab
Autoimmune Thyroiditis	Antimicrosomal Ab
Chronic Ulcerative Colitis	Anticolonic epithelial cell Ab
Diabetes Mellitus	Antiinsulin receptor Ab
Hashimoto's Disease	Antithyroglobulin Ab
Insulin Autoimmune Syndrome	Antiinsulin Ab
Pemphigus	Antiepidermal cell membrane Ab
Ulcerative Colitis	Anticolonic lipopolysaccharide Ab
Asthma	Immunoglobulin E
Hypercholesterolemia	Cholesterol, lipoproteins
Hyperlipidemia	Low- and very low density lipoproteins
Thyrotoxicosis	Thyroid hormone

globulin G actually appears to have about 50% extravascular distribution with the re-equilibration between these compartments occurring within 24–48 hr following the plasmapheresis.

There is still considerable variability in the frequency and intensity of the plasmapheresis used in different therapeutic applications, and this is due in large part to uncertainties regarding the metabolism, pharmacokinetics, and pathogenicity of the different components that are removed during therapeutic apheresis. The typical plasma exchange therapy currently involves the removal of 2–3 L of plasma (approximately one plasma volume) at a frequency of 2–4 times per week, with the therapy continued for several weeks. There have also been a number of studies of the long-term treatment of several diseases via plasmapheresis, with the therapy performed on a periodic basis (ranging from once per week to once every few months) over as much as 5 years (e.g., for the removal of cholesterol and lipoproteins in the treatment of severe cases of hypercholesterolemia).

Centrifugal Devices

Initially, all plasmapheresis was performed using batch centrifuges. This involved the manual removal of approximately one unit (500 ml) of blood at a time, with the blood separated in a centrifuge so that the target components could be removed. The remaining blood was then returned to the patient before drawing another unit and repeating the entire process. This was enormously time-consuming and labor-intensive, requiring as much as 5 hours for the collection of only a single liter of plasma. Batch centrifugation is still the dominant method for off-line blood fractionation in most blood-banking applications, but almost all therapeutic plasmapheresis is performed using on-line (continuous) devices.

The first continuous flow centrifuge was developed in the late 1960s by IBM in conjunction with the National Cancer Institute, and this basic design was subsequently commercialized by the American Instrument Co. (now a division of Travenol) as the Aminco Celltrifuge [Nosé et al., 1983]. A schematic diagram showing the general configuration of this, and most other, continuous flow centrifuges is shown in Fig. 128.1. The blood is input at the bottom of the rotating device and passes through a chamber in which the actual separation into plasma, white cells/platelets, and red cells occurs. Three separate exit ports are located at different radial positions to remove the separated components continuously from the top of the chamber using individual roller pumps. The position of the buffy coat layer (which consists of the white cells and platelets) is controlled by adjusting the centrifugal speed and the relative plasma and red cell flow rates to obtain the desired separation. Probably the most difficult engineering problem in the development of the continuous flow centrifuge was the design of the rotating seals through which the whole blood and separated components must pass without damage. The seal design in the original NCI/IBM device used saline lubrication to prevent intrusion of the cells between the contacting surfaces.

In order to obtain effective cell separation in the continuous flow centrifuge, the residence time in the separation chamber must be sufficiently large to allow the red cells to migrate to the outer region of the device. The degree of separation can thus be characterized by the packing factor

$$P = \frac{G\, V_{sed}\, t}{h} \tag{128.3}$$

where G is the g-force associated with the centrifugation, V_{sed} is the sedimentation velocity at 1 g, t is the residence time in the separation chamber, and h is the width of the separation chamber (i.e., the distance over which the sedimentation occurs). The packing factor thus provides a measure of the radial migration compared to the width of the centrifuge chamber, with adequate cell separation obtained when $P > 1$. The residence time in the separation chamber is inversely related to the blood flow rate (Q_B) as

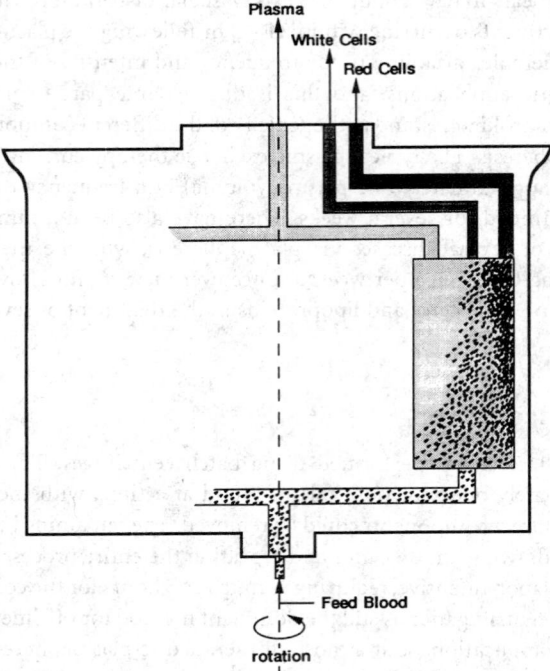

FIGURE 128.1 Schematic diagram of a generic continuous flow centrifuge for fractionation of blood into red cells, white cells/platelets, and plasma.

$$t = \frac{AL}{Q_B} \tag{128.4}$$

where L and A are the length and cross-sectional area of the chamber, respectively.

Rotational speeds in most continuous flow centrifuges are maintained around 1500 rpm (about 100 g) to obtain a relatively clean separation between the red cells and buffy coat, to avoid the formation of a very highly packed (and therefore highly viscous) region of cells at the outer edge of the chamber, and to minimize excessive heating around the rotating seals [Rock, 1983]. The width of the separation chamber must be large enough to permit effective removal of the different blood components from the top of the device, while minimizing the overall extracorporeal blood volume. For example, a packing factor of 10 requires a residence time of about 20 s for a device operated at 100 g with a 0.1-cm-wide separation chamber. The blood flow rate for this device would need to be maintained below about 120 ml/min for a chamber volume of 40 ml. Most of the currently available devices operate at $Q_B \approx 50$ ml/min and can thus collect a liter of plasma in about 30–40 minutes.

More recent models for the continuous flow centrifuge have modified the actual geometry of the separation chamber to enhance the cell separation and reduce the overall cost of the device [Sawada et al., 1990]. Examples include tapering the centrifuge bowl to improve flow patterns and optimizing the geometry of the collection region to obtain purer products. The IBM 2997 (commercialized by Cobe Laboratories) uses a disposable semirigid plastic rectangular channel for the separation chamber, which eliminates some of the difficulties involved in both sterilizing and setting up the device. Fenwal Laboratories developed the CS-3000 Cell Separator (now sold by Baxter Healthcare), which uses a continuous J-shaped multichannel tubing connected directly to the rotating element. This eliminates the need for a rotating seal, thereby minimizing the possibility of leaks. The tubing in this device actually rotates around the centrifuge bowl during operation, using a "jump rope" principle to prevent twisting of the flow lines during centrifugation.

In addition to the continuous flow centrifuge, Haemonetics has developed a series of intermittent flow centrifuges [Rock, 1983]. Blood flows into the bottom of a separation chamber similar to that shown in Fig. 128.1, but the red cells simply accumulate in this chamber while the plasma is drawn to the center of the rotating bowl and removed through an outlet port at the top of the device. When the process is complete, the pump action reverses, and the red cells are forced out of the bowl and reinfused into the patient (along with any replacement fluid). The entire process is then automatically repeated to obtain the desired level of plasma (or white cell) removal. This device was originally developed for the collection of leukocytes and platelets, but it is now used extensively for large-scale plasmapheresis as well. Maximum blood flow rates are typically about 70–80 ml/min, and the bowl rotates at about 5000 rpm. The device as a whole is more easily transported than most of the continuous flow centrifuges, but it requires almost 50% more time for the collection of an equivalent plasma volume due to the intermittent nature of the process. In addition, the total extracorporeal volume is quite high (about 500 ml compared to only 250 ml for most of the newer continuous flow devices) due to the larger chamber required for the red cell accumulation [Sawada et al., 1990].

All these centrifugal devices have the ability to carry out effective plasma exchange, although the rate of plasma collection tends to be somewhat slower than that for the membrane devices discussed in the next section. These devices can also be used for the collection of specific cell fractions, providing a degree of flexibility that is absent in the membrane systems. The primary disadvantage of the centrifugal units is the presence of a significant number of platelets in the collected plasma (typically about 10^5 platelets per μl). Not only can this lead to considerable platelet depletion during repeated applications of plasma exchange, it can also interfere with many of the secondary processing steps employed in plasma perfusion.

Membrane Plasmapheresis

The general concept of blood filtration using porous membranes is quite old, and membranes with pores suitably sized to retain the cellular components of blood and pass the plasma proteins have been available since the late 1940s. Early attempts at this type of blood filtration were largely unsuccessful due to severe problems with membrane plugging (often referred to as *fouling*) and red cell lysis. Blatt and coworkers at Amicon recognized that these problems could be overcome using a cross-flow configuration [Solomon et al., 1978] in which the blood flow was parallel to the membrane and thus perpendicular to the plasma (filtrate) flow as shown schematically in Fig. 128.2. This geometry minimizes the accumulation of retained cells at the membrane surface, leading to much higher filtration rates and much less cell damage than could be obtained in conventional dead-end filtration devices [Solomon et al., 1978]. This led to the development of a large number of membrane devices using either flat sheet or hollow-fiber membranes made from a variety of polymers including polypropylene (Travenol Laboratories, Gambro, Fresenius), cellulose diacetate (Asahi Medical), polyvinyl alcohol (Kuraray), polymethylmethacrylate (Toray), and polyvinyl chloride (Cobe Laboratories).

These membrane devices all produce essentially cell-free plasma with minimal protein retention using membranes with pore sizes of 0.2–0.6 μm. In addition, these devices must be operated under conditions that cause minimal red cell lysis, while maintaining a sufficiently high plasma filtrate flux to reduce the cost of the microporous membranes. Typical experimental data for a parallel plate membrane device are shown in Fig. 128.3 [Zydney & Colton, 1987]. The results are plotted as a function of the mean transmembrane pressure drop (ΔP_{TM}) at several values of the wall shear rate (γ_w), where γ_w is directly proportional to the inlet blood flow rate (Q_B). The filtrate flux initially increases with increasing ΔP_{TM}, reaching a maximum pressure independent value which increases with increasing shear rate. The flux under all conditions is substantially smaller than that obtained when filtering pure (cell-free) saline under identical conditions (dashed line in Fig. 128.3). No measurable

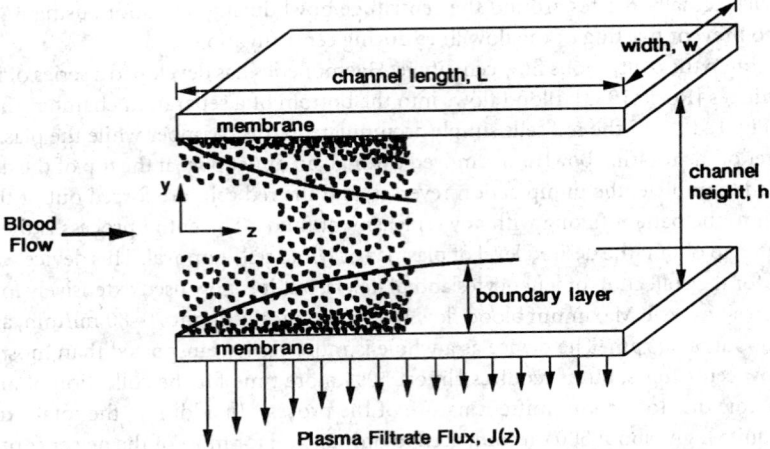

FIGURE 128.2   Schematic diagram of a parallel plate device for cross-flow membrane plasmapheresis.

hemolysis was observed at low ΔP_{TM}, even when the flux was in the pressure-independent regime. Hemolysis does become significant at higher pressures, with the extent of hemolysis decreasing with increasing γ_w and with decreasing membrane pore size [Solomon et al., 1978]. The dashed diagonal line indicates the pressure at which the filtrate hemoglobin concentration exceeds 20 mg/dl.

The pressure-independent flux at high ΔP_{TM} generally has been attributed to the formation of a concentration polarization boundary layer consisting of a high concentration of the formed elements in blood, mainly the red blood cells, which are retained by the microporous membrane (Fig. 128.2). This dynamic layer of cells provides an additional hydraulic resistance to flow, causing the flux to be substantially smaller than that obtained during filtration of a cell-free solution. At steady-state, this boundary layer is in dynamic equilibrium, with the rate of convection of formed elements toward the membrane balanced by the rate of mass transport back into the bulk suspen-

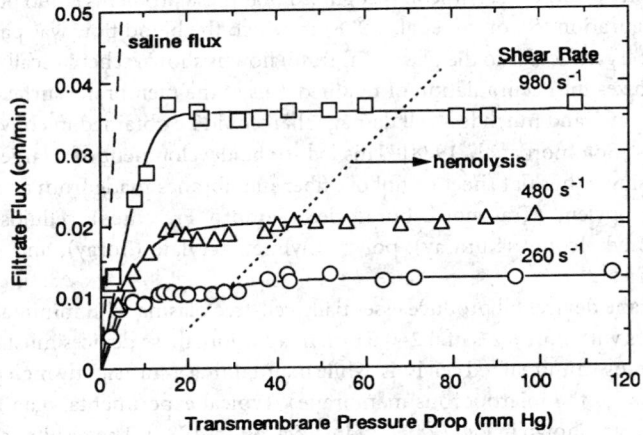

FIGURE 128.3   Experimental data for the filtrate flux as a function of the applied transmembrane pressure drop in a parallel plate membrane plasmapheresis device. Red cell hemolysis, defined as a filtrate hemoglobin concentration exceeding 20 mg/dl, occurs to the right of the dashed line. Data have been adapted from Zydney and Colton [1987].

sion. There has been some debate in the literature over the actual mechanism of cell transport in these devices, and the different models that have been developed for the plasma flux during membrane plasmapheresis are discussed elsewhere [Zydney & Colton, 1986].

Zydney and Colton [1982] proposed that cell transport occurs by a shear-induced diffusion mechanism in which cell-cell interactions and collisions give rise to random cell motion during the shear flow of a concentrated suspension. This random motion can be characterized by a shear-induced diffusion coefficient, which was evaluated from independent experimental measurements as

$$D = a^2 \gamma f(C) \tag{128.5}$$

where γ is the local shear rate (velocity gradient), a is the cell radius (approximately 4.2 μm for the red blood cells), and C is the local red cell concentration. The function $f(C)$, which reflects the detailed concentration dependence of the shear-induced diffusion coefficient, is approximately equal to 0.03 for red cell suspensions over a broad range of cell concentrations.

The local filtrate flux can be evaluated using a stagnant film analysis in which the steady-state mass balance is integrated over the thickness of the concentration boundary layer yielding [Zydney & Colton, 1986]

$$J(z) = k_m \ln \frac{C_w}{C_b} \tag{128.6}$$

where z is the axial distance measured from the device inlet, and C_w and C_b are the concentrations of formed elements at the membrane surface and in the bulk suspension, respectively. The bulk mass transfer coefficient (k_m) can be evaluated using the Leveque approximation for laminar flow in either a parallel plate or hollow fiber device

$$k_m = 0.516 \left(\frac{D^2 \gamma_w}{z} \right)^{1/3} = 0.047 \left(\frac{a^4}{z} \right)^{1/3} \gamma_w \tag{128.7}$$

where the second expression has been developed using the shear-induced diffusion coefficient given by Eq. (128.5) with $f(C) = 0.03$. The wall shear rate is directly proportional to the blood flow rate with

$$\gamma_w = \frac{4Q_B}{N\pi R^3} \tag{128.8}$$

for a hollow-fiber device with N fibers of inner radius R and

$$\gamma_w = \frac{6Q_B}{wh^2} \tag{128.9}$$

for a parallel plate device with channel height h and total membrane width w.

At high pressures, C_w approaches its maximum value which is determined by the maximum packing density of the cells (about 95% under conditions typical of clinical plasmapheresis). The plasma flux under these conditions becomes independent of the transmembrane pressure drop, with this pressure-independent flux varying linearly with the wall shear rate and decreasing with increasing bulk cell concentration as described by Eqs. (128.6) and (128.7). A much more detailed numeric model for the flux [Zydney & Colton, 1987], which accounts for the concentration and shear rate dependence of both the blood viscosity and shear-induced cell diffusion coefficient as well as the compressibility of the blood cell layer that accumulates at the membrane, has confirmed the general behavior predicted by Eqs. (128.6) and (128.7).

The volumetric filtrate (plasma) flow rate (Q_p) in a hollow-fiber membrane filter can be evaluated by integrating Eqs. (128.6)–(128.8) along the length of the device accounting for the decrease in the blood flow rate (and thus γ_w) due to the plasma removal [Zydney & Colton, 1986]. The resulting expression for the fractional plasma yield is

$$\frac{Q_p}{Q_B} = 1 - \exp\left[-0.62 \left(\frac{a^2 L}{R^3}\right)^{2/3} \ln \frac{C_w}{C_b}\right] \tag{128.10}$$

An analogous expression can be evaluated for a parallel plate device with the channel height h replacing R and the coefficient 0.62 becoming 0.84. Even though the development leading to Eq. (128.10) neglects the detailed variations in the bulk cell concentration and velocity profiles along the fiber length, the final expression has been shown to be in good agreement with experimental data for the plasma flow rate in actual clinical devices [Zydney & Colton, 1986]. Equation (128.10) predicts that the volumetric plasma flow rate is independent of the number of hollow fibers (or the membrane width for a parallel plate membrane device), a result which is consistent with a number of independent experimental investigations.

According to Eq. (128.10), the plasma flow rate increases significantly with decreasing fiber radius. There are, however, a number of constraints on the smallest fiber radius that can actually be employed in these hollow-fiber membrane devices. For example, blood clotting and fiber blockage can become unacceptable in very narrow bore fibers. The blood flow in such narrow fibers also causes a very high bulk shear stress, which potentially can lead to unacceptable levels of blood cell damage (particularly for white cells and platelets). Finally, the hollow-fiber device must be operated under conditions which avoid hemolysis.

Zydney and Colton [1982] developed a model for red cell lysis during membrane plasmapheresis in which the red cells are assumed to rupture following their deformation into the porous structure of the membranes. A given red cell is assumed to lyse if it remains in a pore for a sufficient time for the strain induced in the red cell membrane to exceed the critical strain for cell lysis. Since the red cell can be dislodged from the pore by collisions with other cells moving in the vicinity of the membrane or by the fluid shear stress, the residence time in the pore will be inversely related to the wall shear rate.

The tension (σ) in the red cell membrane caused by the deformation in the pore is evaluated using Laplace's law [Zydney & Colton, 1987]

$$\sigma = \frac{\Delta P_{TM} R_p}{2} \tag{128.11}$$

where R_p is the pore radius. Hemolysis is assumed to occur at a critical value of the strain in the red cell membrane (S); thus the time required for lysis is given implicitly by

$$S = \sigma\, g(t) = \sigma\, \{0.0010 + 0.0012\, [1 - \exp(-8t)] + 4.5 \times 10^{-6}\, t\} \tag{128.12}$$

The function $g(t)$ represents the temporal dependence of the lytic phenomenon and has been evaluated from independent experimental measurements [Zydney & Colton, 1982]. Cell lysis occurs when $S \geq 0.03$ in Eq. (128.12) where σ is given in dyne/cm and t is in sec. This simple model has been shown to be in good agreement with experimental data for red cell lysis during cross-flow membrane plasmapheresis [Zydney & Colton, 1987].

This physical model for red cell lysis implies that hemolysis can be avoided by operating at sufficiently high shear rates to reduce the residence time in the membrane pores. However, operation at high shear rates also causes the inlet transmembrane pressure drop to increase due to the large axial pressure drop associated with the blood flow along the length of the device [Zydney & Colton, 1982]:

$$\Delta P_{TM}(0) = \Delta P_{TM}(L) + 2\mu\gamma_w \frac{L}{R} \qquad (128.13)$$

where $\Delta P_{TM}(0)$ and $\Delta P_{TM}(L)$ are the inlet and exit transmembrane pressure drops, respectively, and μ is the average blood viscosity. $\Delta P_{TM}(L)$ is typically maintained at a small positive value (about 20 mmHg) to ensure that there is a positive transmembrane pressure drop along the entire length of the device. Since the increase in $\Delta P_{TM}(0)$ with increasing γ_w has a greater effect on hemolysis than the reduction in the residence time for the red cells in the membrane pores, there is also an upper bound on the shear rate for the safe operation of any given clinical device.

The predicted safe operating regime for a clinical membrane plasmapheresis device can be determined using Eq. (128.11), with the maximum transmembrane pressure drop occurring at the device inlet, Eq. (128.13). The results are shown schematically in Fig. 128.4. Hemolysis occurs at very low shear rates due to the long residence time in the membrane pores, whereas lysis at high shear rates is due to the large value of the inlet transmembrane pressure drop associated with the axial flow. Note that there is a critical fiber length [at fixed values of the fiber radius and $\Delta P_{TM}(L)$] above which there is no longer any safe operating condition.

To avoid some of the constraints associated with the design of both parallel plate and hollow-fiber membrane devices, Hemasciences has developed a rotating membrane filter for use in both donor and therapeutic plasmapheresis. A nylon membrane is placed on an inner cylinder and rotated at about 3600 rpm inside a concentric outer cylindrical chamber using a magnetic coupling device. The rotating membrane causes a very high shear rate (on the order of 10,000 s^{-1}) in the narrow gap between the cylinders. However, these high shear rates do not result in a large axial pressure drop, as found in the parallel plate and hollow-fiber devices, due to the decoupling of the axial blood flow and the shear rate in this system (the shear is now due almost entirely to the membrane rotation). The fluid flow in this rotating cylinder system also leads to the development of fluid instabilities known as Taylor vortices, and these vortices dramatically increase the rate of cell mass transport away from the membrane and back into the bulk suspension. This leads to a dramatic increase in the plasma filtrate flux and a dramatic reduction in the required membrane area. The Autopheresis-C (the rotating filter currently sold by Baxter Healthcare) uses only 70 cm^2 of membrane, which is more than an order of magnitude less than that required in competitive hollow-fiber and parallel plate devices.

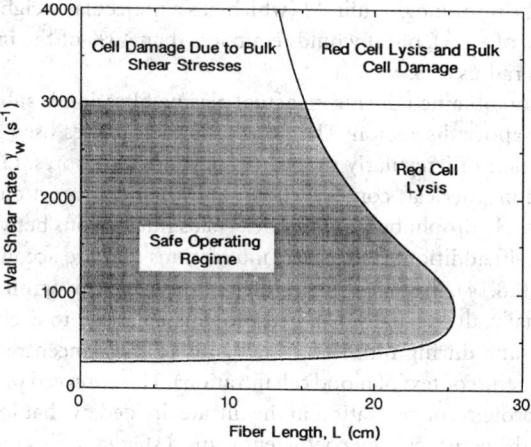

FIGURE 128.4 Schematic representation of the safe operating regime for a clinical membrane plasmapheresis device.

128.2 Plasma Perfusion

In repeated applications of plasma exchange, it is necessary to use replacement fluids that contain proteins to avoid the risks associated with protein depletion. One approach to minimizing the cost of these protein-containing replacement fluids (either albumin solutions, fresh frozen plasma, or plasma protein fraction) is to use a saline or dextran solution during the initial stages of the process and to then switch to a protein-containing replacement fluid toward the end of the treatment. Alternatively, a number of techniques have been developed to selectively remove specific toxic or immunogenic components from the plasma, with this treated plasma returned to the patient along with the cellular components of blood. This effectively eliminates the need for any expensive protein-containing replacement fluids.

Plasma perfusion (also known as on-line plasma treatment) is typically performed using either membrane or sorbent-based systems. Membrane filtration separates proteins on the basis of size and is thus used to selectively remove the larger molecular weight proteins from albumin and the smaller plasma solutes (salts, sugars, amino acids, and so on). A variety of membranes has been employed for this type of plasma fractionation, including cellulose acetate (Terumo), cellulose diacetate (Asahi Medical and Teijin), ethylene vinyl alcohol (Kuraray), and polymethylmethacrylate (Toray). These membranes are generally hydrophilic to minimize the extent of irreversible protein adsorption, with pore sizes ranging from 100–600 Å depending on the specific objectives of the membrane fractionation.

The selectivity that can be obtained with this type of plasma filtration can be examined using available theoretical expressions for the actual sieving coefficient (S_a) for a spherical solute in a uniform cylindrical pore:

$$S_a = (1 - \lambda)^2 [2 - (1 - \lambda)^2] \exp(-0.711 \lambda^2) \qquad (128.14)$$

where λ is the ratio of the solute to pore radius. Equation (128.14) is actually an approximate expression which has been shown to be in good agreement with more rigorous theoretical analyses. This expression for the actual sieving coefficient, where S_a is defined as the ratio of the protein concentration in the filtrate to that at the upstream surface of the membrane, is valid at high values of the plasma filtrate flux, since it implicitly assumes that the diffusive contribution to protein transport is negligible. To avoid excessive albumin loss, it is desirable to have $S_a > 0.8$, which can be achieved using a membrane with an effective pore size greater than about 160 Å (albumin has a molecular weight of 69,000 and a Stokes-Einstein radius of 36 Å). This membrane would be able to retain about 80% of the immunoglobulin M (which has a molecular weight of about 900,000 and a Stokes-Einstein radius of 98 Å), but it would retain less than 40% of the immunoglobulin G (with MW = 155,000 and a radius of 55 Å).

The protein retention obtained during an actual plasma filtration is substantially more complex than indicated by the above discussion. The polymeric membranes used in these devices actually have a broad distribution of irregularly shaped (noncylindrical) pores. Likewise, the proteins can have very different (nonspherical) conformations, and their transport characteristics also can be affected by electrostatic, hydrophobic, and van der Waals interactions between the proteins and the polymeric membrane, in addition to the steric interactions that are accounted for in the development leading to Eq. (128.14). Protein-protein interactions can also significantly alter the observed protein retention. Finally, the partially retained proteins will tend to accumulate at the upstream surface of the membrane during filtration (analogous to the concentration polarization effects described previously in the context of blood cell filtration). The observed protein-sieving coefficient, which is equal to the protein concentration in the filtrate divided by that in the bulk plasma, can be evaluated in terms of the actual sieving coefficient using a stagnant film model as

$$S_o = \frac{S_a}{(1 - S_a)\exp(-J/k_m) + S_a} \qquad (128.15)$$

where J is the average filtrate flux and k_m is the bulk mass transfer coefficient, which is a function of the detailed flow characteristics and geometry of the particular membrane device. This concentration polarization phenomenon will tend to increase the transmission of both small- and large-molecular-weight proteins. This effect can, however, be used to enhance the overall selectivity through the use of relatively small pore membranes which retain a high percentage of the larger immunoglobulins but still have a reasonable albumin flux due to the increase in the albumin concentration at the membrane surface and the corresponding increase in the observed sieving coefficient.

This type of secondary plasma filtration, which is generally referred to in the literature as *cascade filtration,* is primarily effective at removing large immune complexes (molecular weight of approximately 700,000) and immunoglobulin M (MW of 900,000) from smaller proteins such as albumin. Several studies have, however, found a higher degree of albumin–immunoglobulin G separation than would be expected based on purely steric considerations [Eq. (128.14)]. This enhanced selectivity is probably due to some type of long-range (e.g., electrostatic) interaction between the proteins and the membrane in combination with the concentration polarization phenomenon discussed previously.

A number of different techniques have also been developed to enhance the selectivity of these plasma filtration devices. For example, Malchesky and coworkers at the Cleveland Clinic [Malchesky et al., 1980] developed the process of *cryofiltration* in which the temperature of the plasma is lowered to about 10 °C prior to filtration. A number of diseases are known to be associated with the presence of large amounts of cryo- (cold) precipitable substances in the plasma, including a number of autoimmune diseases such as systemic lupus erythematosus and rheumatoid arthritis. Lowering the plasma temperature causes the aggregation and/or gelation of these cryoproteins, making it much easier for these components to be removed by membrane filtration. About 10 g of cryogel can be removed in a single cryofiltration, along with significant amounts of the larger-molecular-weight immune complexes and IgM. The actual extent of protein removal during cryofiltration depends on the specific composition of the plasma and thus on the nature as well as the severity of the particular disease state [Sawada et al., 1990]. There is thus considerable uncertainty over the actual components that are removed during cryofiltration under different clinical and/or experimental conditions. The cryogel layer that accumulates on the surface of the membrane also affects the retention of other plasma proteins, which potentially could lead to unacceptable losses even of small proteins such as albumin.

It is also possible to alter the selectivity of the secondary membrane filtration by heating the plasma up to or even above physiologic temperatures. This type of *thermofiltration* has been shown to increase the retention of low- (LDL) and very low (VLDL) density lipoproteins, and this technique has been used for the on-line removal of these plasma proteins in the treatment of hypercholesterolemia. LDL removal can also be enhanced by addition of a heparin/acetate buffer to the plasma, which causes precipitation of LDL and fibrinogen with the heparin [Sawada et al., 1990]. These protein precipitates then can be removed relatively easily from the plasma by membrane filtration. The excess heparin is subsequently removed from the solution by adsorption, with the acetate and excess fluid removed using bicarbonate dialysis.

An attractive alternative to secondary membrane filtration for the selective removal of plasma components is the use of sorbent columns such as: (1) activated charcoal or anion exchange resins for the removal of exogenous toxins, bile acids, and bilirubin; (2) dextran sulfate cellulose for the selective removal of cholesterol, LDL, and VLDL; (3) immobilized protein A for the removal of immunoglobulins (particularly IgG) and immune complexes; and (4) specific immobilized ligands like DNA (for the removal of anti-DNA Ab), tryptophan (for the removal of antiacetylcholine receptor antibodies), and insulin (for the removal of anti-insulin antibodies). These sorbents provide a much more selective separation than is possible with any of the membrane processes; they thus have the potential to significantly reduce the side effects associated with the depletion of needed plasma components. The sorbent columns generally are used in combination with membrane plasmapheresis, since the platelets that are present in the plasma collected from available centrifugal devices can clog the columns and interfere with the subsequent protein separation.

The development of effective sorbent technology for on-line plasma treatment has been hindered by the uncertainties regarding the actual nature of the plasma components that must be removed for the clinical efficacy of therapeutic apheresis in the treatment of different disease states. In addition, the use of biologic materials in these sorbent systems (e.g., protein A or immobilized DNA) presents particular challenges, since these materials may be strongly immunogenic if they desorb from the column and enter the circulation.

128.3 Cytapheresis

Cytapheresis is used to selectively remove one (or more) of the cellular components of blood, with the other components (including the plasma) returned to the patient. For example, leukocyte (white cell) removal has been used in the treatment of leukemia, autoimmune diseases with a suspected cellular immune mechanism (e.g., rheumatoid arthritis and myasthenia gravis), and renal allograft rejection. Erythrocyte (red cell) removal has been used to treat sickle cell anemia, severe autoimmune hemolytic anemia, and severe parasitemia. Plateletapheresis has been used to treat patients with thrombocythemia.

Most cytapheresis is performed using either continuous or intermittent flow centrifuges, with appropriate software and/or hardware modifications used to enhance the collection of the specific cell fraction. It is also possible to remove leukocytes from whole blood by depth filtration, which takes advantage of the strong adherence of leukocytes to a variety of polymeric materials (e.g., acrylic, cellulose acetate, polyester, or nylon fibers). Leukocyte adhesion to these fibers is strongly related to the configuration and the diameter of the fibers, with the most effective cell removal obtained with ultrafine fibers less than 3 μm in diameter. Available leukocyte filters (Sepacell, Cellsorba, and Cytofrac from Asahi Medical Co.) have packing densities of about 0.1–0.15 g fiber/cm³ and operate at blood flow rates of 20–50 ml/min, making it possible to process about 2 L of blood in 1.5 hr.

Leukocyte filtration is used most extensively in blood-banking applications to remove leukocytes from the blood prior to transfusion, thereby reducing the likelihood of antigenic reactions induced by donor leukocytes and minimizing the possible transmission of white-cell-associated viral diseases such as cytomegalovirus. The adsorbed leukocytes can also be eluted from these filters by appropriate choice of buffer solution and pH, making it possible to use this technique for the collection of leukocytes from donated blood for use in the subsequent treatment of leukopenic recipients. Depth filtration has also been considered for on-line leukocyte removal from the extracorporeal circuit of patients undergoing cardiopulmonary bypass as a means to reduce the likelihood of postoperative myocardial or pulmonary reperfusion injury which can be caused by activated leukocytes.

A new therapeutic technique that involves on-line cytapheresis is the use of extracorporeal photochemotherapy, which is also known in the literature as *photopheresis*. Photopheresis can be used to treat a variety of disorders caused by aberrant T-lymphocytes [Edelson, 1989], and it has been examined most extensively in the treatment of advanced cutaneous T-cell lymphoma. In this case, the therapy involves the use of photoactivated 8-methoxypsoralen, which blocks DNA replication causing the eventual destruction of the immunoactive T-cells. The psoralen compound is taken orally prior to the phototherapy. Blood is drawn from a vein and separated by centrifugation. The white cells and plasma are collected, diluted with a saline solution, and then pumped through a thin plastic chamber in which the cells are irradiated with a high-intensity UV light that activates the psoralen. The treated white cells are then recombined with the red cells and returned to the patient. Since the photoactivated psoralen has a half-life of only several microseconds, all its activity is lost prior to reinfusion of the cells, thereby minimizing possible side effects on other organs. The removal of the red cells (which have a very high absorptivity to UV light) makes it possible to use a much lower energy UV light, thereby minimizing the possible damage to normal white cells and platelets.

Photopheresis has also been used in the treatment of scleroderma, systemic lupus erythematosus, and pemphigus vulgaris. The exact mechanism for the suppression effect induced by the phototherapy in these diseases is uncertain, although the T-cell destruction seem to be highly specific for the immunoactive T-cells [Edelson, 1989]. The response is much more involved than simple direct photoinactivation of the white cells; instead, the return of the photo-treated cells to the circulation appears to elicit an immunologic response against the entire immunoactive T-cell line [Edelson, 1989]. This allows for an effective "vaccination" against a particular T-cell activity without the need for isolating or even identifying the particular cells that are responsible for that activity [Edelson, 1989].

Phototherapy has also been used for virus inactivation, particularly in blood-banking applications prior to transfusion. This can be done using high-intensity UV light alone or in combination with specific photoactive chemicals to enhance the virus inactivation. For example, hematoporphyrin derivatives have been shown to selectively destroy hepatitis and herpes viruses in contaminated blood. This technique shows a high degree of specificity toward this type of enveloped virus, which is apparently due to the affinity of the photoactive molecules for the lipids and glycolipids that form an integral part of the viral envelope.

Another interesting therapeutic application involving cytapheresis is the ex vivo activation of immunologically active white cells (lymphokine-activated killer cells, tumor-infiltrating lymphocytes, or activated killer macrophages) for the treatment of cancer. The detailed protocols for this therapy are still being developed, and there is considerable disagreement regarding its actual clinical efficacy. A pool of activated cells is generated in vivo by several days of treatment with interleukin-2. These cells are then collected from the blood by centrifugal cytapheresis and further purified using density gradient centrifugation. The activated cells are cultured for several days in a growth media containing additional interleukin-2. These ex-vivo-activated cells are then returned to the patient, where they have been shown to lyse existing tumor cells and cause regression of several different metastatic cancers.

128.4 Summary

Apheresis is unique in terms of the range of diseases and metabolic disorders which have been successfully treated by this therapeutic modality. This broad range of application is possible because apheresis directly alters the body's immunologic system through the removal or alteration of specific immunologically active cells and/or proteins.

Although there are a number of adverse reactions that can develop during apheresis (e.g., fluid imbalance, pyrogenic reactions, depletion of important coagulation factors, and thrombocypenia), the therapy is generally well tolerated even by patients with severely compromised immune systems. This has, in at least some instances, led to the somewhat indiscriminate use of therapeutic apheresis for the treatment of diseases in which there was little physiologic rationale for the application of this therapy. This was particularly true in the 1980s, where dramatic advances in the available technology for both membrane and centrifugal blood fractionation allowed for the relatively easy use of apheresis in the clinical milieu. In some ways, apheresis in the 1980s was a medical treatment that was still looking for a disease. Although apheresis is still evolving as a therapeutic modality, it is now a fairly well-established procedure for the treatment of a significant number of diseases (most of which are relatively rare) in which the removal of specific plasma proteins or cellular components can have a beneficial effect on the progression of that particular disease. Furthermore, continued advances in the equipment and procedures used for blood fractionation and component removal have, as discussed in this chapter, provided a safe and effective technology for the delivery of this therapy.

The recent advances in sorbent-based systems for the removal of specific immunologically active proteins and in the development of techniques for the activation or inactivation of specific cellular components of the immune system has led Applied ImmuneSciences to develop an integrated package of apheresis technologies that they describe as an "artificial lymph node." Although this description may be somewhat overstated given the current state of the available technology, it does reflect the enormous potential of therapeutic apheresis for the alteration and even control of the body's immunologic response through: (1) the direct removal of specific antibodies or immune complexes (using membrane plasmapheresis with appropriate immunosorbent columns), (2) the inactivation or removal of specific lymphocytes (using centrifugal cytapheresis in combination with appropriate extracorporeal phototherapy or chemotherapy), and/or (3) the activation of a disease-specific immunologic response (using cytapheresis and ex vivo cell culture with appropriate lymphokines and cell stimuli). New advances in our understanding of the immune system and in our ability to selectively manipulate and control the immunologic response should thus have a major impact on therapeutic apheresis and the future development of this important medical technology.

Defining Terms

Autoimmune diseases: A group of diseases in which pathological antibodies are produced that attack the body's own tissue. Examples include glomerulonephritis (characterized by the inflammation of the capillary loops in the glomeruli of the kidney) and myasthenia gravis (characterized by an inflammation of the nerve/muscle junctions).

Cascade filtration: The combination of plasmapheresis with a second on-line membrane filtration of the collected plasma to selectively remove specific toxic or immunogenic components from blood based primarily on their size.

Cytapheresis: A type of therapeutic apheresis involving the specific removal of red blood cells, white cells (also referred to as *leukapheresis*), or platelets (also referred to as *plateletapheresis*).

Donor apheresis: The collection of a specific component of blood (either plasma or one of the cellular fractions), with the return of the remaining blood components to the donor. Donor apheresis is used to significantly increase the amount of plasma (or a particular cell type) that can be donated for subsequent use in blood banking and/or plasma fractionation.

Immune complexes: Antigen-antibody complexes that can be deposited in tissue. In rheumatoid arthritis this deposition occurs primarily in the joints, leading to severe inflammation and tissue damage.

Photopheresis: The extracorporeal treatment of diseases characterized by aberrant T-cell populations using visible or ultraviolet light therapy, possibly in combination with specific photoactive chemicals.

Plasma exchange: The therapeutic process in which a large volume of plasma (typically 3 L) is removed and replaced by an equivalent volume of a replacement fluid (typically fresh frozen plasma, a plasma substitute, or an albumin-containing saline solution).

Plasma perfusion: The therapeutic process in which a patient's plasma is first isolated from the cellular elements in the blood and then subsequently treated to remove specific plasma components. This secondary treatment usually involves a sorbent column designed to selectively remove a specific plasma component or a membrane filtration designed to remove a broad class of plasma proteins.

Plasmapheresis: The process in which plasma is separated from the cellular components of blood using either centrifugal or membrane-based devices. Plasmapheresis can be employed in donor applications for the collection of source plasma for subsequent processing into serum fractions or in therapeutic applications for the treatment of a variety of disorders involving the presence of abnormal circulating components in the plasma.

Therapeutic apheresis: A process involving the separation and removal of a specific component of the blood (either plasma, a plasma component, or one of the cellular fractions) for the treatment of a metabolic disorder or disease state.

References

Edelson RL. 1989. Photopheresis: A new therapeutic concept. Yale J Biol Med 62:565.

Kambic HE, Nosé Y. 1993. Plasmapheresis: Historical perspective, therapeutic applications, and new frontiers. Artif Organs 17(10):850.

Malchesky PS, Asanuma Y, Zawicki I, et al. 1980. On-line separation of macromolecules by membrane filtration with cryogelation. Artif Organs 400:205.

Nosé' Y, Kambic HE, Matsubara S. 1983. Introduction to therapeutic apheresis. In Y Nosé', PS Malchesky, JW Smith, et al. (eds), Plasmapheresis: Therapeutic Applications and New Techniques, pp 1–22, New York, Raven Press.

Rock G. 1983. Centrifugal apheresis techniques. In Y Nosé', PS Malchesky, JW Smith, et al. (eds), Plasmapheresis: Therapeutic Applications and New Techniques, pp 75–80, New York, Raven Press.

Sawada K, Malchesky P, Nosé' Y. 1990. Available removal systems: State of the art. In UE Nydegger (ed), Therapeutic Hemapheresis in the 1990s, pp 51–113, New York, Karger.

Solomon BA, Castino F, Lysaght MJ, et al. 1978. Continuous flow membrane filtration of plasma from whole blood. Trans Am Soc Artif Intern Organs 24:21.

Zydney AL, Colton CK. 1982. Continuous flow membrane plasmapheresis: Theoretical models for flux and hemolysis prediction. Trans Am Soc Artif Intern Organs 28:408.

Zydney AL, Colton CK. 1986. A concentration polarization model for filtrate flux in cross-flow microfiltration of particulate suspensions. Chem Eng Commun 47:1.

Zydney AL, Colton CK. 1987. Fundamental studies and design analyses of cross-flow membrane plasmapheresis. In JD Andrade, JJ Brophy, DE Detmer (eds), Artificial Organs, pp 343–358, VCH Publishers.

Further Information

Several of the books listed above provide very effective overviews of both the technical and clinical aspects of therapeutic apheresis. In addition, the Office of Technology Assessment has published *Health Technology Case Study 23: The Safety, Efficacy, and Cost Effectiveness of Therapeutic Apheresis,* which has an excellent discussion of the early clinical development of apheresis. Several journals also provide more detailed discussions of current work in apheresis, including *Artificial Organs* and the *Journal of Clinical Apheresis*. The abstracts and proceedings from the meetings of the International Congress of the World Apheresis Association and the Japanese Society for Apheresis also provide useful sources for current research on both the technology and clinical applications of therapeutic apheresis.

129

Liver Support Systems

Pierre M. Galletti
Brown University

Hugo O. Jauregui
Rhode Island Hospital

129.1 Morphology of the Liver

The liver is a complex organ that operates both in series and in parallel with the gastrointestinal tract. After entering the portal system, the products of digestion come in contact with the liver parenchymal cells, or hepatocytes, which remove most of the carbohydrates, amino acids, and fats from the feeder circulation, therefore preventing excessive increases throughout the body after a meal. In the liver, these products are then stored, modified, and slowly released to better advantage of the whole organism.

The liver can be considered a complex large-scale biochemical reactor, since it occupies a central position in the *metabolism*, i.e., the sum of the physical and chemical processes by which living matter is produced, maintained, and destroyed, and whereby energy is made available for the functioning of liver cells as well as tissues from all other organs.

The adult human liver (weighing 1500 g) receives its extensive blood supply (on the order of 1 L/min or 20% of cardiac output) from two sources: the portal vein (over two-thirds) and the hepatic artery (about one-third). Blood from the liver drains through the hepatic veins into the inferior vena cava. Macroscopically, the liver is divided into 4 or 5 lobes with individual blood supply and bile drainage channels. Some of these lobes can be surgically separated, although not without difficulty.

Microscopically, human hepatocytes ($250–500 \times 10^9$ in each liver) are arranged in plates (Fig. 129.1) that are radially distributed around the central (drainage) vein [Jones & Spring-Mills, 1977] and form somewhat hexagonal structures, or liver lobules, which are much more clearly demarcated in porcine livers. Present in the periphery of these lobules are the so-called *portal triads*, in the ratio of three triads for each central vein. In each portal triad, there are tributaries of the portal vein, branches of the hepatic artery, and collector ducts for the bile (Fig. 129.1). Blood enters the liver lobule at the periphery from terminal branches of the portal vein and the hepatic arteries and is distributed into capillaries which separate the hepatocyte plates. These capillaries, called sinusoids, characteristically have walls lined by layers of endothelial cells that are not continuous but are perforated by small holes (fenestrae). Other cells are present in the sinusoid wall, e.g., phagocytic

0-8493-8346-3/95/$0.00+$.50
© 1995 by CRC Press, Inc.

Branches of:

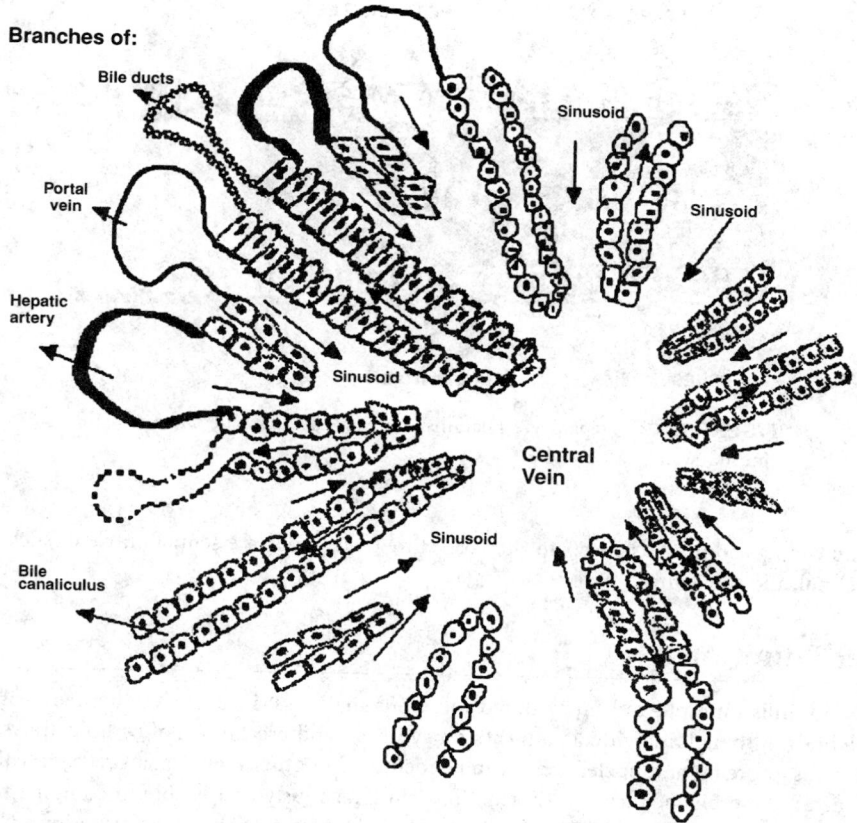

FIGURE 129.1 The liver lobule.

Kuppfer cells, fat-storing Ito cells, and probably a few yet undefined mesenchymal cells. It is important to emphasize that blood-borne products (with the exception of blood cells) have free access to the perisinusoidal space, called the space of Disse, which can be visualized by electron microscopy as a gap separating the sinusoidal wall from the hepatocyte plasma membrane (Fig. 129.2). In this space, modern immunomicroscopic studies have identified three types of collagens: Type IV (the most abundant), Type I, and Type III. Fibronectin and glycosaminoglycans are also found there, but laminin is only present in the early stages of liver development not in adult mammalian livers [Martinez-Hernandez, 1984].

The hepatocytes themselves are large (each side about 25 microns), multifaceted, polarized cells with an apical surface which constitutes the wall of the bile canaliculus (the channel for bile excretion) and basolateral surfaces which lie in close proximity to the blood supply. Hepatocytes constitute 80–90% of the liver cell mass. Kuppfer cells (about 2%) belong to the reticulo-endothelial system, a widespread class of cells which specialize in the removal of particulate bodies, old blood cells, and infectious agents from the blood stream.

The cytoplasm of hepatocytes contains an abundance of smooth and rough endoplasmic reticulum, ribosomes, lysosomes, and mitochondria. These organelles are involved in complex biochemical processes: fat and lipid metabolism, synthesis of lipoproteins and cholesterol, protein metabolism, and synthesis of complex proteins, e.g., serum albumin, transferrin, and clotting factors from amino acid building blocks. The major aspects of detoxification take place in the cisternae of the smooth endoplasmic reticulum, which are the site of complex oxidoreductase enzymes known collectively as the cytochrome P-450 system. In terms of excretion, hepatocytes produce bile, which contains bile

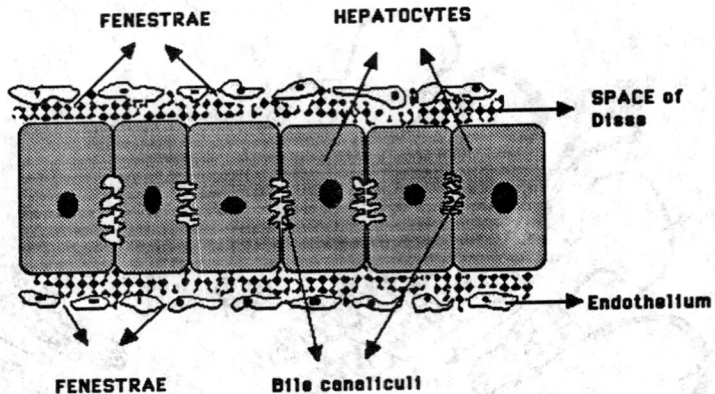

FIGURE 129.2 Hepatocyte relationships with the space of Disse and the sinusoid wall.

salts and conjugated products. Hepatocytes also store large pools of essential nutrients such as folic acid, retinol, and cobalamin.

129.2 Liver Functions

The liver fulfills multiple and finely tuned functions that are critical for the homeostasis of the human body. Although individual pathways for synthesis and breakdown of carbohydrates, lipids, amino acids, proteins, and nucleic acids can be identified in other mammalian cells, only the liver performs all these biochemical transformations simultaneously and is able to combine them to accomplish its vital biologic task. The liver is also the principal site of biotransformation, activation or inactivation of drugs and synthetic chemicals. Therefore, this organ displays a unique biologic complexity. When it fails, functional replacement presents one of the most difficult challenges in substitutive medicine.

Under normal physiologic requirements, the liver modifies the composition and concentration of the incoming nutrients for its own usage and for the benefit of other tissues. Among the major liver functions, the detoxification of foreign toxic substances (*xenobiotics*), the regulation of essential nutrients, and the secretion of transport proteins and critical plasma components of the blood co-agulation system are probably the main elements to evaluate in a successful organ replacement [Jau-regui, 1991]. The liver also synthesizes several other critical proteins, excretes bile, and stores excess products for later usage, functions that can temporarily be dispensed with but must eventually be provided.

The principal functions of the liver are listed in Table 129.1. The challenge of liver support in case of organ failure is apparent from the complexity of functions served by liver cells and from our still imperfect ability to rank these functions in terms of urgency of replacement.

129.3 Hepatic Failure

More than any other organ, the liver has the property of regeneration after tissue damage. Removal or destruction of a large mass of hepatic parenchyma stimulates controlled growth to replace the missing tissue. This can be induced experimentally, e.g., two thirds of a rat liver can be excised with no ill effects and will be replaced within 6 to 8 days. The same phenomenon can be observed in humans and is a factor in the attempted healing process characteristic of the condition called liver *cirrhosis*. Recent attempts at liver transplantation using a liver lobe from a living donor rely on the

TABLE 129.1   Liver Functions

Carbohydrate metabolism: Glyconeogenesis and glycogenolysis
Fat and lipid metabolism: Synthesis of lipoproteins and cholesterol
Synthesis of plasma proteins, for example:
    Albumin
    Globulins
    Fibrinogen
    Coagulation factors
    Transferrin
    α-fetoprotein
Conjugation of bile acids; conversion of heme to bilirubin and biliverdin
Detoxification: Transformation of metabolites, toxins, and hormones into water-soluble compounds
    (e.g., cytochrome P-450 oxidation, glucuronyl transferase conjugation)
Biotransformation and detoxification of drugs
Metabolism and storage of vitamins
Storage of essential nutrients
Regeneration

same expectation of recovery of lost liver mass. Liver regeneration is illustrated by the myth of Prometheus, a giant who survived in spite of continuous partial hepatectomy through the good offices of a vulture (a surgical procedure inflicted on him as punishment for having stolen the secret of fire from the gods and passing it on to humanity).

Hepatic failure may be acute or chronic according to the time span it takes for the condition to develop. Mechanisms and toxic by-products perpetuating these two conditions are not necessarily the same. Acute *fulminant hepatic failure* (FHF) is the result of massive necrosis of hepatocytes induced over a period of days or weeks by toxic substances or viral infection. It is characterized by jaundice and mental confusion which progresses rapidly to stupor or coma. The latter condition, *hepatic encephalopathy* (HE), is currently thought to be associated with diminished hepatic catabolism. Metabolites have been identified which impair synaptic contacts and inhibit neuromuscular and mental functions (Table 129.2). Although brain impairment is the rule in this condition, there is no anatomic damage to any of the brain structures, and therefore, the whole process is potentially reversible. The mortality rate of FHF is high (70–90%), and death is quite rapid (a week or two). Liver transplantation is currently the only effective form of treatment for FHF. Transplantation procedures carried out in life-threatening circumstances are much more risky than interventions in relatively better compensated patients. The earlier the transplantation procedure takes place, the greater is the chance for patient survival. However, 10–30% of FHF patients will regenerate their liver under proper medical management without any surgical intervention. Hence, liver transplantation presents the dilemma of choosing between an early intervention, which might be unnecessary in some cases, or proceeding to a late procedure, with a statistically higher mortality [Jauregui et al., 1994].

Chronic hepatic failure, the more common and progressive form of the disease, is often associated with morphologic liver changes known as cirrhosis in which fibrotic tissue gradually replaces liver

TABLE 129.2   Metabolic Products with Potential Effects in Acute Liver Failure

Substance	Mode of action
Ammonia	Neurotoxic interaction with other neurotransmitters
	Contributes to brain edema
Benzodiazepinelike substances	Neural inhibition
GABA	Neural inhibition
Mercaptans	Inhibition of Na-K ATPase
Octopamine	Acts as a false neurotransmitter

tissue as the result of long-standing toxic exposure (e.g., alcoholism) or secondary to viral hepatitis. More than 30,000 people died of liver failure in the United States in 1990.

In chronic hepatic failure, damaged hepatocytes are unable to detoxify toxic nitrogenous products that are absorbed by intestinal capillaries and carried to the liver by the portal system. Ammonia probably plays the major role in the deterioration of the patient's mental status, leading eventually to "hepatic coma." An imbalance of conventional amino acids (some abnormally high, some low) may also be involved in the pathogenesis of the central nervous system manifestations of hepatic failure, the most dramatic of which is cerebral edema. Impaired blood coagulation (due to decreased serum albumin and clotting factors), hemorrhage in the gastro-intestinal system (increased resistance to blood flow through the liver leads to portal hypertension, ascites formation, and bleeding from esophageal varices), and hepatic encephalopathy with glial cell damage in the brain are the standard landmarks of chronic hepatic failure. In fact, HE in chronic liver failure is often precipitated by episodes of bleeding and infection, and progression to deep coma is an ominous sign of impending death.

Intensive management of chronic liver failure includes fluid and hemodynamic support, correction of electrolyte and acid-base abnormalities, respiratory assistance, and treatment of cerebral edema if present. Aggressive therapy can diminish the depth of the coma and improve the clinical signs, but the outcome remains grim. Eventually, 60–90% of the patients require transplantation. About 2500 liver transplants are performed every year in the United States, with a survival rate ranging from 68–92%. The most serious limitation to liver transplantation (besides associated interrelated diseases) remains donor scarcity. Even if segmented transplants and transplants from living related donors become acceptable practices, it is unlikely that the supply of organs will ever meet the demand. Further, the problem of keeping alive a patient with terminal hepatic failure, either chronic or acute, while waiting for an adequately matched transplant is much more difficult than the parallel problem in end-stage renal disease, where dialysis is a standardized and effective support modality.

An appreciation of the modalities of presentation of the two types of hepatic coma encountered in liver failure is needed for a definition of the requirements for the proper use of liver assist devices. In the case of FHF, the hepatologist wants an extracorporeal device that will circulate a large volume of blood through a detoxifying system [Jauregui & Muller, 1992] allowing either the regeneration of the patient's damaged liver (and the avoidance of a costly and risky liver transplantation procedure) or the metabolic support needed for keeping the patient alive while identifying a cadaveric donor organ. In the first option, the extracorporeal liver assist device functions as an organ substitute for the time it takes the liver to regenerate and recover its function; in the second, it serves as a temporary bridge to transplantation.

In the case of chronic liver failure today, spontaneous recovery appears impossible. The damaged liver needs to be replaced by a donor organ, although not with the urgency of FHF. The extracorporeal liver assist device (LAD) is used as a bridge while waiting for the availability of a transplant. It follows that the two different types of liver failure may require different bioengineering designs.

129.4 Liver Support Systems

The concept of artificial liver support is predicated on the therapeutic benefit of removing toxic substances accumulating in the circulation of liver failure patients. These metabolites reflect the lack of detoxification by damaged hepatocytes, the lack of clearance of bacterial products from the gut by impaired Kupffer cells, and possibly the release of necrotic products from damaged cells which inhibit liver regeneration. Systemic endotoxemia as well as massive liver injury give rise to an inflammatory reaction with activation of monocytes and macrophages and release of cytokines which may be causally involved in the pathogenesis of multiorgan failure commonly encountered in liver failure.

Technologies for temporary liver support focus on the detoxifying function, since this appears to be the most urgent problem in liver failure. The procedures and devices which have been considered for this purpose include the following.

Hemodialysis

Hemodialysis with conventional cellulosic membranes (cut-off point around 2000 daltons) or more permeable polysulfone or polyacrylonitrile [de Groot et al., 1984] (cut-off 1500–5000 daltons) helps to restore electrolyte and acid-base balance and may decrease the blood ammonia levels but cannot remove large molecules and plasma protein-bound toxins. Improvement of the patient's clinical condition (e.g., amelioration of consciousness and cerebral edema) is temporary. The treatment appears to have no lasting value and no demonstrated effect on patient survival. In addition, hemodialysis may produce a respiratory distress syndrome caused by a complement-mediated polymorphonuclear cell aggregation in the pulmonary circulatory bed. Because some of the clinical benefit seems related to the removal of toxic molecules, more aggressive approaches focused on detoxification have been attempted.

Hemofiltration

Hemofiltration with high cut-off point membranes (around 50,000 daltons with some polyacrylonitrile-polyvinyl chloride copolymers, modified celluloses, or polysulfones) clears natural or abnormal compounds within limits imposed by convective transport across the exchange membrane. These procedures again have a temporary favorable effect on hepatic encephalopathy (perhaps because of the correction of toxic levels of certain amino acids) with reversal of coma, but they do not clearly improve survival rates.

Hemoperfusion

Hemoperfusion, i.e., extracorporeal circulation of blood over nonspecific sorbents (e.g., activated charcoal) [Chang, 1975] or more complex biochemical reactors which allow the chemical processing of specific biologic products, such as ammonia, have not yet met clinical success in spite of encouraging experimental results, except in the case of hepatic necrosis induced by poisonous mushrooms such as Amanita phalloides. Anion exchange resins and affinity columns similar to those used in separative chromatography may help in removing protein-bound substances (e.g., bilirubin) which would not pass through hemodialysis or hemofiltration membranes, but nonspecific sorbents may also deplete the plasma of biologically important substances. Further, these techniques are complicated by problems of hemocompatibility, related in part to the entrainment of dust ("fines") associated with the sorbent material itself and in part to platelet activation in patients with an already compromised coagulation status. To minimize this problem, direct blood or plasma contact with the sorbent material can be avoided by polymer coating of the sorbent particles using either albumin, cellulose nitrate, or similar thin films, but hemocompatability remains a concern. Here again, there is anecdotal evidence of clinical improvement of hepatic failure with hemoperfusion, with some reports claiming a higher survival rate in hepatic encephalopathy, but these reports have not been supported by well-controlled studies. As is the case for hemodialysis and hemofiltration, the possible beneficial effect of hemoperfusion should be evaluated in the context of the clinical variability in the course of FHF.

Lipophilic Membrane Systems

Because lipophilic toxins dominate in fulminant hepatic failure, it is conceivable to eliminate such compounds with a hydrophobic (e.g., polysulfone) membrane featuring large voids filled with a nontoxic oil [Brunner & Tegtimeier, 1984]. After diffusion, the toxins can be made water-soluble through reaction with a NaOH-based acceptor solution, thereby preventing their return to the blood stream. A standard, high-flux dialyzer in series with the lipophilic membrane device allows the removal of hydrophilic solutes. Such a system has proved effective in removing toxins such as phenol and p-cresol as well as fatty acids without inducing detrimental side effects of its own.

Immobilized Enzyme Reactors

To address the problem of specificity in detoxification, enzymes such as urease, tyrosinase, L-asparaginase, glutaminase, and UDP-glucuronyl transferase have been attached to hollow fibers or circulated in the closed dialysate compartment of an artificial kidney or still incorporated into microcapsules or "artificial cells" exposed to blood. There is considerable in vitro evidence for the effectiveness of this approach, and some indication of therapeutic value from in vivo animal experiments [Brunner et al., 1979]. However, no clinical report has documented the superiority of enzyme reactors over the various modalities of dialysis. Again there are clinical observations of clearing of the mental state of patients in hepatic coma, but no statistically demonstrated effect on survival. It is unclear whether the lack of success is due to the inability of specific enzymes to remove all offending toxins or is evidence of the need for more than detoxification for effective treatment.

Parabiotic Dialysis

Also referred to as *cross-dialysis*, parabolic dialysis is a variant of hemodialysis in which the dialysate compartment of a solute exchange device is perfused continuously with blood from a living donor. Because of membrane separation of the two blood streams, the procedure can be carried out even if the two subjects belong to different blood groups or different animal species. However, the risk of the procedure to a human donor (control of blood volume, transfer of toxic substances, mixing of blood streams in case of dialyzer leak) and the difficulty of introducing a live animal donor into the hospital environment have relegated this approach to the class of therapeutic curiosities.

Exchange Transfusion

Exchange transfusion, i.e., the quasi-total replacement of the blood volume of a patient in liver failure by alternating transfusion and bleeding, is occasionally used in severe hyperbilirubinemia of the newborn, which used to carry an ominous prognosis because of its association with cerebral edema. The rationale is that exchange transfusion will reduce the level of toxins and replenish the deficient factors in the blood stream while the underlying condition is corrected by natural processes or drugs [Trey et al., 1966]. With the advent of blood component therapy, specific plasma components can also be administered to treat identified deficiencies. Mortality rates of patients treated with exchange blood transfusion have been reported as greater than those observed with conventional therapies.

Plasmapheresis

Plasmapheresis, i.e., the combination of withdrawal of blood, centrifugation, or membrane processing to separate and discard the patient's plasma, and return of autologous cells diluted with donor plasma, was practiced initially as a batch process. Techniques now exist for a continuous exchange process, in which plasma and cells are separated by physical means outside of the body (membrane separation or centrifugation), and the patient's plasma replaced by banked plasma (up to 5000 ml per day) [Lepore et al., 1972]. There is evidence from controlled clinical trials for the effectiveness of this form of therapy, but the mortality rate remains high in patients with hepatic failure, whether from insufficient treatment or the risks of the procedure. It appears, however, that plasma exchange can be beneficial in the preoperative period prior to liver transplantation so as to correct severe coagulopathy. Plasmapheresis is used in conjunction with the placement of a hepatocyte-seeded extracorporeal hollow-fiber device to treat acute and chronic liver failure [Rozga et al., 1993].

Combined Therapy

Endotoxins and cytokines can be removed by hemoperfusion over activated charcoal and adsorbent resins, but it may be more effective to process plasma than whole blood. This has led to the concept of combining plasmapheresis with continuous plasma treatment for removal of substances such as tumor necrosis factor (TNF), interleukin-6 (IL-6), and bile acids by a resin column, and then ultrafiltration or dialysis for fluid removal, since patients with liver failure often develop secondary renal failure.

129.5 Global Replacement of Liver Function

Because of the complexity and interplay of the various functions of the liver, more success can be expected from global approaches, which allow many or all hepatic functions to be resumed. These include the following.

Cross-circulation

Cross-circulation of the patient in hepatic coma with a compatible, healthy donor is one approach. This procedure is more than a prolonged exchange transfusion since it allows the donor's liver to substitute for the patient's failing organ and to process chemicals from the patient's blood stream as long as the procedure lasts [Burnell, 1973]. It had been attempted in isolated cases, but reports of effectiveness are entirely anecdotal, and the procedure has not been accepted clinically because of ambiguous results and the perceived risk for the donor.

Hemoperfusion over Liver Tissue Slices

The incorporation of active hepatocytes in a hemoperfusion circuit was suggested by the laboratory practice of biochemists who, since Warburg, have investigated metabolic pathways in tissue slices. For liver replacement, this technology has been pioneered primarily in Japan as a substitute for organ transplantation, which is culturally frowned upon in that country, in spite of a major incidence of severe liver disease. The procedure may improve biochemical markers of liver failure but has no demonstrated clinical value [Koshino et al., 1975].

Ex Vivo Perfusion

Ex vivo perfusion uses an isolated animal liver (pig or baboon) connected to the patient's cardiovascular system [Saunders et al., 1968]. This is a cleaner and more acceptable form of treatment than cross-circulation or hemoperfusion over tissue pieces. Nevertheless, it is limited by the need for thorough washing of the animal's blood from the excised liver, the requirement for a virus-free donor organ source, the limited survival capacity of the excised, perfused organ, which must be replaced at intervals of approximately 24 hours, and the cost of the procedure. Success has recently been reported in isolated clinical trials [Chari, 1994].

Heterotopic Hepatocyte Transplantation

This procedure may someday offer an alternative to whole organ transplantation, especially in cases of chronic liver failure, if a sufficient number of cells can be grafted. Freshly isolated hepatocytes have damaged cell surfaces and must be cultured to regain their integrity and display the surface receptors needed for attachment or binding of xenobiotics or endogenous toxic products [McMillan et al., 1988]. At the clinical level, this procedure could rely in part on banking frozen hepatocytes from livers which are not usable for whole organ transplants but constitute a reliable source of cells [Bumgardner et al., 1988]. The procedure does not require removal of the recipient's liver and provides the following advantages: (1) minimal surgery, (2) repeatability as needed, and (3) interim strategy to whole organ transplant. There is no agreement as to the best anatomic site for hepatocyte transplantation, the type of matrix needed for cell attachment and differentiation, and the number of cells needed. It has been reported that hepatocyte culture supernatants were as effective as transplanted hepatocytes in treating rats with chemically induced liver failure [LaPlante-O'Neill et al., 1982]. The tridimensional reconstruction of high-density, functional liver tissue will be the greatest challenge in view of the cell mass required. Structural organization and differentiated functions may be achieved by using an asialoglycoprotein model polymer as the synthetic substrate for a primary culture of hepatocytes to develop functional modules for implantation in humans [Akaike et al., 1989].

Whole Organ in Situ Transplantation

This is currently the procedure of choice, most particularly in children. Although progress in clinical and surgical skills certainly accounts in large part for the growing success rate of this procedure over the past 20 years, it is worth noting that the introduction of extracorporeal circulation techniques in the surgical protocol to support the donor organ while waiting for completion of the anastomosis has paralleled the steepest increase in success rate of liver transplantation in the past few years. Whereas most liver transplants rely on the availability of cadaver organs, the recent advent of segmented transplants allows consideration of living related donors and possibly the sharing of a donor organ among two or more recipients.

129.6 Hybrid Replacement Procedures

The complexity of hepatic functions, coupled with the shortage of human donor organs, has encouraged the development of procedures and devices which rely on xenogeneic living elements attached to synthetic structures and separated from the most host by a permselective membrane to replace temporarily, and perhaps someday permanently, the failing organ.

The *incorporation of liver microsomes* in microcapsules, hydrogels, or polymer sheets, with or without additional enzymes or pharmacologic agents, goes one step beyond the immobilized enzyme reactor inasmuch as it calls on cell components endowed with a variety of enzymatic properties to process blood or other body fluids. The feasibility of this technique has been demonstrated in vitro [Denti et al., 1976] but has not been investigated extensively in animal experiments.

Cellular hybrid devices—the incorporation of functional cells in a device immersed in body fluids or connected to the vascular system (extracorporeally or somewhere inside the body of the recipient)—are a promising application of the concept of bioartificial organs. However, the problems faced by the "hepatocyte bioreactor" are formidable:

1. The mass of functional cells required is much larger than in the case of secretory or endocrine organs, since a normal liver weighs about 1.5 kg and since as much as 10–30% of that mass (i.e., several billion cells) may be required for life-sustaining replacement of function. Taking into account the need for supporting structures, the shear size of the device will be an obstacle to implantation.

2. The liver features a double feeder circulation (portal and hepatic) and a complex secretory-excretory system which utilizes both blood and bile to dispose of its waste products. How to duplicate such a complex manifolding in an artificial organ and whether it is worth the resulting complexity are questions not yet resolved.

3. With membrane separation of recipient and donor cells, the size of some natural macromolecules to be exchanged (e.g., low-density lipoproteins) precludes the use of standard diffusion membranes. Allowing relatively free solute exchange between the compartments in a device without endangering the immune sequestration of the donor tissue remains a challenge for membrane technology. However, the low immunogenicity of hepatocytes (which lack type I HLA antigens) allows the consideration of relatively open membranes for the construction of extracorporeal reactors.

At the moment, most of the extracorporeal liver assist devices (ELAD) utilize xenogeneic mammalian hepatocytes seeded on solid, isotropic hollow fibers. Membrane selectivity limits the rate of diffusion of liposoluble toxins which are bound to plasma proteins for transport. Hence manipulation of membrane transport properties and concentrations of acceptor proteins can affect the clearance of polar materials.

Also, most devices focus on replacing the detoxification function of the natural liver and avoid the more complex "cascade" dialysis circuitry which could either (1) allow to return the macromolecules synthesized by hepatocytes to the blood stream (or another body fluid compartment) through a high cut-off point membrane or (2) provide an excretory path to clear toxic products manufactured by the hepatocytes, on the model of the bile excretory system. Nonetheless, such circuitry might be valuable to prolong the life of the seeded cells, since the combination of bile salts and bile acids has a damaging detergent effect on the lipid components of the hepatocyte membrane.

The development of bioreactors including cells capable of performing liver functions, and therefore capable of providing temporary liver support, finds applications in the treatment of acute, reversible liver failure or as a bridge for liver transplantation. Designs for a bioartificial liver can be classified according to (1) the type of cells selected to replace the hepatic functions or (2) the geometry and chemical nature of the polymer structure used to organize the hepatocytes.

Source of Functional Cells

Two main methods of hepatocyte isolation (mechanical and enzymatic) can be used, separately or in combination. Mechanical methods (tissue dissociation) have largely failed in terms of long-term cell viability, although this is not always recognized by investigators developing liver assist systems. Collagenase perfusion [Seglen, 1976] is today the method of choice, yet there is evidence that hepatocytes lose some of their oligosaccharide-lectin binding capacity in the process and do not recover their glycocalyx until after a day or two in culture. Collagenase is thought to loosen the cell junctions and secondarily to digest the connective tissue around the hepatocytes. Chemical methods using citrate, EDTA, and similar substances weaken cell junctions by depleting calcium ions without altering the cell membranes and presumably result in better preservation of natural enzymatic functions. Although the yield of chemical methods is lower than that of enzymatic dissociation methods, it may be of interest once a reliable technology for separating viable from nonviable cells on a large scale is perfected.

A priori, an effective bioartificial liver would require either all the multifunctional characteristics of normal hepatocytes in vivo or only the specific functional activity that happens to be missing in the patient. Unfortunately, in most cases, clinical signs do not allow us to distinguish between these two extremes, justifying a preference for highly differentiated cells.

Differentiation and proliferation are usually at opposite ends of a biologic continuum in most cell types (Fig. 129.3) [Jauregui, 1991]. Hence, there is a difficulty of obtaining large numbers of multifunctional hepatocytes. Several options are available:

1. The simplest approach is to use *adult mammalian liver cells* isolated in sufficient number from large animals. Porcine hepatocytes are preferred for clinical applications because of the availability of virus-free donors. Large-scale isolation of porcine hepatocytes is becoming a routine procedure, and Demetriou has been able to treat several patients with such a system. The expectation is that hepatocytes in suspension or attached to synthetic microcarriers will remain metabolically active even though separated from neighboring cells and normal

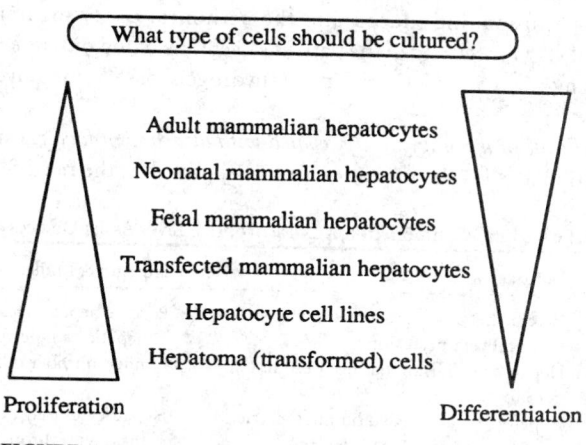

What type of cells should be cultured?

Adult mammalian hepatocytes
Neonatal mammalian hepatocytes
Fetal mammalian hepatocytes
Transfected mammalian hepatocytes
Hepatocyte cell lines
Hepatoma (transformed) cells

Proliferation   Differentiation

FIGURE 129.3 Cellular choices based on proliferation and differentiation.

supportive structures. This approach, which appeared almost beyond practicality a few years ago, seems now less formidable because of expanded knowledge of the molecular factors which favor both hepatocyte attachment to polymeric substrates and functional differentiation. The potential contribution of Kupffer cells to a bioartificial liver has not yet been extensively investigated.

2. The use of *liver tumor cells*—preferably nonmalignant hepatoma—has been pioneered by Wolf and Munkelt [1975] because such cells can proliferate indefinitely and therefore require a minimal seeding dose. They are also less anchor-dependent than normal cells. The drawbacks are the loss of specialized hepatic functions often encountered in tumor cell lines, and the theoretical risk of escape of tumor cells in the recipient.

3. A modified, functionally differentiated, *human hepatoblastoma cell line* capable of growing to high densities, yet strongly contact-inhibited by containment with membranes, has been patented and used in animals and man by Sussman and colleagues [1992]. Evidence for metabolic effectiveness has been reported, and clinical trials are now in progress. The uncertainty associated with the use of a human tumor cell line remains a source of concern.

4. Potentially *replicating hepatocytes,* such as those obtained from embryonic liver, neonatal animals, or recently hepatectomized adults, have been proposed as a means to obtain a stem cell population with enhanced proliferation capacity. Neonatal hepatocyte-based bioartificial devices have been built on that principle [Hager et al., 1983] and have shown to produce albumin, to metabolize urea, to deaminate cytidine, and to detoxify drugs such as a diazepam. The reliance on "juvenile" cells has become less important with the identification of molecular mechanisms for growth control mitogens such as EGF, TGFa, hepatopoietin B, HSS (hepatic stimulatory substance) and HGF (hepatocyte growth factor), co-mitogenic factors such as norepinephrine and growth inhibitors such as TGFβ, and interleukin-1β.

5. *Transfected or transgenic hepatocytes* may provide the ultimate solution to the cell supply problem. However, they are usually selected for the monoclonal expression of a single function and therefore may not be suitable except when a single cause of hepatic failure has been identified. Alternatively, a combination of different transfected hepatocytes may be considered.

Table 129.3 illustrates the choices made by three different groups of investigators for clinical liver assist devices.

Supporting Structures

Microencapsulation in a nutrient liquid or a polymer gel surrounded by a conformal membrane provides a suspension of metabolically active units which can either be placed in a container for extracorporeal hemoperfusion, introduced into the peritoneal cavity for implantation, or even infused into the portal vein for settling in the patient's liver. The blood or tissue reaction to multiple implants and the long-term in vivo stability of hydrogels based on polyelectrolytes remain unresolved problems.

A flat sheet of membrane or a spongy matrix coated with attachment factors can be used to anchor a suspension of functional cells. The limitation of this approach is the need for vascularization of

TABLE 129.3   Present Choice of the Cellular Component for Extracorporeal Liver Assist Devices

Sussman & Kelly (1993)	Neuzil et al.	Jauregui & Muller (1992)
Hepatoblastoma-derived cell line	Porcine hepatocytes separated via portal vein perfusion	Porcine hepatocytes separated via hepatic vein perfusion
Cells divide indefinitely	Hepatocyte division has not been tested (5 to 8)	Limited number of hepatocyte doublings
Cells are cultured in the device	Hepatocytes are seeded on microcarriers and introduced in the device immediately before clinical use	Hepatocytes may be seeded or cultured in the device through a proprietary technology

the implant, since the cells are metabolically active and therefore are quite avid of oxygen and nutrients.

Microcarrier-attached hepatocytes are attractive because the technology of suspension cultures is amenable to the proliferation of a large number of cells. The bulk of the carrier beads probably limits this approach to extracorporeal circuits similar to those used for hemoperfusion [Rozga et al., 1993].

Hollow-fiber ELADs are constructed by filling the interstices within a bundle of parallel hollow fibers with live cells, using the lumen of the tubes to provide metabolic support and an excretion channel, typically by circulating blood from an extracorporeal circuit. Alternatively, a hybrid organ can be built by filling the lumen of the hollow fibers with functional cells and implanting the bundle in the body cavity to allow exchanges with the surrounding fluid. One could combine such a device with an oxygenation system, e.g., by filling the peritoneal cavity with a high-oxygen-capacity fluid such as a fluorocarbon and a gas exchange system for that fluid analogous to the intravenous oxygenator (IVOX).

129.7 Outlook

Medical trials with extracorporeal hollow-fiber systems are already in progress, although there are some unanswered questions in the proper design of a hepatocyte-seeded ELAD. A review of Table 129.4 will indicate that there is no consensus for implementing cellular choices in the construction of such systems.

Some researchers believe that the culture of hepatocytes on a synthetic matrix prior to chemical application is a complicated proposition that impairs the practical application of this technology. An alternative could be the isolation, freezing, and shipping of porcine hepatocytes to the medical centers treating patients with acute and chronic liver failure (usually transplantation centers). This approach may offer a direct and economically sound solution. Unfortunately, many FHF patients require emergency liver support and are managed in secondary care medical institutions which have neither a transplantation program nor a tissue culture facility for the seeding of hollow-fiber devices. Part of the argument for the porcine hepatocyte isolation, shipment, seeding, and immediate use in a bioartificial liver system relies on the earlier concept that primary mammalian hepatocytes do not grow in vitro or are very difficult to maintain in hollow-fiber devices. In fact, rodent hepatocytes have shown excellent detoxification activities when cultured on perfused hollow fiber cultures. Rabbit hepatocytes also survive in hollow-fiber bioreactors which have proved successful in treating one of the most representative animal models of human FHF.

The technology for manufacturing ELADs may also need further attention. For instance, the efficiency of hollow fibers in maintaining hybridoma cultures and producing specific proteins is known to be inferior to that of cellular bioreactors based on microcarrier technology. The surface of hollow fibers has been optimized for blood compatibility but not for hepatocyte attachment, and therefore new materials or structures may have to be developed.

At the conceptual level, primary hepatocytes may need to be cultured either in combination with other cells that will provide parabiotic support or on substrates that imitate the composition of the extracellular matrix found in situ in the space of Disse. Our own experience [Naik et al., 1990] and

TABLE 129.4 Consideration in the Choice of the Cellular Component of Extracorporeal Liver Assist Devices

Advantages	Disadvantages
Hepatoblastoma cell lines are easy to culture and are free of other cell contaminants	Hepatoblastoma cell lines are tumorigenic
Tumor cell lines are not anchorage dependent	Tumor cell lines may not respond to physiologic regulation
Porcine or primary hepatocytes respond to physiologic stimulation	Porcine hepatocytes have limited proliferation ability
Porcine hepatocytes express P450 (detoxification activity)	Porcine hepatocytes show limited life span

that of others [Singhvi et al., 1994] raise some questions about the role of substrates in maintaining long-term hepatocyte viability in vitro. In fact, most of them operate in a rather indiscriminate fashion by providing an anchor for hepatocytes. Collagen, types I, III, IV, and fibronectin contribute to cytoplasmic spreading which in the long term does not favor maintenance of the phenotypic expression of hepatocytes. Polymer compositions expressing surface sugar residues responsible for hepatocyte attachment through the asialoglycoprotein receptor (a plasma membrane complex present mainly in the bile canalicular area which internalizes plasma asialoglycoprotein) appear able to maintain hepatocytes in culture with extended functional activities [Akaike et al., 1989]. Other investigators have shown the value of extracellular glycoproteins and glycosaminoglycans rich in laminin (e.g., Matrigel) [Caron & Bissell, 1989]. Hepatocytes immobilized on these substrates do not spread but maintain their tridimensional morphology, as well as their functional activity. Suchobservations suggest that long-term expression of hepatocyte-specific functions depend on maintaining the in situ cell shape and their spacial interrelations [Koide et al., 1990]. Future ELAD designs should provide not only ideal polymer substrates for cell attachment but also a spacial configuration that will maintain the tridimensional structure of hepatic tissue.

Experience with artificial organs shows that the development of these devices tends to underestimate the effort and the technical advances needed to pass from a "proof of principle" prototype for animal evaluation to fabrication of a clinically acceptable system for human use. Full-scale design, cell procurement, cell survival, and device storage are all major bottlenecks on the way to a clinical product. One of the gray areas remains in the molecular weight cut-off of the hollow fiber wall. Which substances are responsible for the development of FHF and must therefore be cleared? Are they protein-bound, middle-molecular-, or low-molecular-size compounds? In the absence of clear answers to these questions, the designer of separation membranes is in an ambiguous position; some investigators use low molecular cut-off membranes to guarantee immunoseparation of the xenograft, whereas others prefer high-molecular cut-off to enhance functionality. The use of microporous membranes in human subjects has not led, as of yet, to any hypersensitivity reactions in spite of potential passage of immunoglobulins.

A reliable way to restore consciousness in animal models of FHF is to cross-circulate the blood with a normal animal. To the extent that ELADs may function in patients as in these animal models, they may prove successful only in relieving the symptoms of the disorder without increasing the survival rate. For instance, when 147 patients with advanced stage of HE were treated with charcoal hemoperfusion over a 10-year period, all showed symptomatic improvement, but the survival rate of 32% was the same as in five control groups. Therefore, enthusiasm generated by preliminary human trials with hollow-fiber devices should be tempered with a cautious approach. Without reliable control studies, we will remain in the position defined by Benhamou and coworkers [1972], "The best future one can wish for a sufferer from severe acute hepatic failure is to undergo a new treatment and have his case published—Be published or perish!"

Defining Terms

Bioartificial liver: A liver assist or liver replacement device incorporating living cells in physical or chemical processes normally performed by liver tissue.

Catabolism: The aspect of metabolism in which substances in living tissues are transformed into waste products or solutes of simpler chemical composition. (The opposite process is called *anabolism*.)

Cirrhosis: A degenerative process in the liver marked by excess formation of connective tissue, destruction of functional cells, and, often, contraction of the organ.

Conjugated: The joining of two compounds to produce another compound, such as the combination of a toxic product with some substance in the body to form a detoxified product, which is then eliminated.

ELAD: Extracorporeal liver assist device.

Homeostasis: A tendency to stability in the normal body states (internal environment) of the organism. This is achieved by a system of control mechanisms activated by negative feedback, e.g., a high level of carbon dioxide in extracellular fluid triggers increased pulmonary ventilation, which in turn causes a decrease in carbon dioxide concentration.

Mesenchymal cells: The meshwork of embryonic connective tissue in the mesoderm from which are formed the connective tissues of the body and the blood vessels and lymphatic vessels.

Metabolism: The sum of all the physical and chemical processes by which living organized substance is produced and maintained (anabolism) and the transformation by which energy is made available for the uses of the organism (*catabolism*).

Parenchymal cells: The essential elements of an organ.

Phagocytic: Pertaining to or produced by any cells that ingest microorganisms or other cells and foreign particles.

Portal triad: These are microscopic areas of collagen type I–III fibroblasts as well as other connective tissue elements. These triads have a branch of the portal vein, a branch of the hepatic artery, and intermediate caliber bile ducts.

Xenobiotic: A chemical foreign to the biologic system.

References

Akaike T, Kobayashi A, Kobayashi K, et al. 1989. Separation of parenchymal liver cells using a lactose-substituted styrene polymer substratum. J Bioact Compat Polym 4:51.

Benhamou JP, Rueff B, Sicot C. 1972. Severe hepatic failure: a critical study of current therapy. In F Orlandi, AM Jezequel (eds), Liver and Drugs, New York, Academic Press.

Brunner G, Holloway CJ, Lösgen H. 1979. The application of immobilized enzymes in an artificial liver support system. Artif Organs 3:27.

Brunner G, Tegtimeier F. 1984. Enzymatic detoxification using lipophilic hollow fiber membranes. Artif Organs 8:161.

Bumgardner GL, Fasola C, Sutherland DER. 1988. Prospects for hepatocyte transplantation. Hepatology 8:1158.

Burnell JM, Runge C, Saunders FC, et al. 1973. Acute hepatic failure treated by cross circulation. Arch Intern Med 132:493.

Caron JM, Bissel DM. 1989. Extracellular matrix induces albumin gene expression in cultured rat hepatocytes. Hepatology 10:636.

Chang TMS. 1975. Experience with the treatment of acute liver failure patients by haemoperfusion over biocompatible microencapsulated (coated) charcoal. In R Williams, IM Murray-Lyon (eds), Artificial Liver Support, Tunbridge Wells, England, Pitman Medical.

Chari RS, Collins BH, Magee JC, et al. 1994. Brief Report: Treatment of hepatic failure with ex vivo pig-liver perfusion followed by liver transplantation. N Engl J Med 331:234.

De Groot GH, Schalm SW, Schicht I, et al. 1984. Large-pore hemodialytic procedures in pigs with ischemic hepatic necrosis; a randomized study. Hepatogastroenterology 31:254.

Denti E, Freston JW, Marchisi M, et al. 1976. Toward a bioartificial drug metabolizing system: gel immobilized liver cell microsomes. Trans Am Soc Artif Intern Organs 22:693.

Hager JC, Carman R, Porter LE, et al. 1983. Neonatal hepatocyte culture on artificial capillaries: A model for drug metabolism and the artificial liver. ASAIO J 6:26–35.

Jauregui HO. 1991. Treatment of hepatic insufficiency based on cellular therapies. Int J Artif Organs 14:407.

Jauregui HO, Muller TE. 1992. Long-term cultures of adult mammalian hepatocytes in hollow fibers as the cellular component of extracorporeal (hybrid) liver assist devices. Artif Organs 16(2):209.

Jauregui HO, Naik S, Santangini H, et al. 1994. Primary cultures of rat hepatocytes in hollow fiber chambers. In Vitro Cell Dev Biol 30A:23.

Jones AL, Spring-Mills E. 1977. The liver and gallbladder. In Weiss, RO Greep, (eds), Histology, 4th ed, New York, McGraw-Hill.

Koide N, Sakaguchi K, Koide Y, et al. 1990. Formation of multicellular spheroids composed of adult rat hepatocytes in dishes with positively charged surfaces and under other nonadherent environments. Exper Cell Res 186:227.

Koshino I, Castino F, Yoshida K, et al. 1975. A biological extracorporeal metabolic device for hepatic support. Trans Amer Soc Artif Intern Organs 21:492.

LaPlante-O'Neill P, Baumgartner D, Lewis WI, et al. 1982. Cell-free supernatant from hepatocyte cultures improves survival of rats with chemically induced acute liver failure. J Surg Res 32:347.

Lepore MJ, Stutman LJ, Bonnano CA, et al. 1972. Plasmapheresis with plasma exchange in hepatic coma. II. Fulminant viral hepatitis as a systemic disease. Arch Intern Med 129:900.

Martinez-Hernandez A. 1984. The hepatic extracellular matrix: I. Electron immunohistochemical studies in normal rat liver. Lab Invest 51:57.

McMillan PN, Hevey KA, Hixson DC, et al. 1988. Hepatocyte cell surface polarity as demonstrated by lectin binding to isolate and cultured hepatocytes. J Histochem Cytochem 36:1561.

Naik S, Santangini H, Jauregui HO. 1990. Culture of adult rabbit hepatocytes in perfused hollow membranes. In Vitro Cell Dev Biol 26:107

Neuzil DF, Rozga J, Moscioni AD, Ro MS, Hakim R, Arnaout WS, Demetriou AA. 1993. Use of a novel bioartificial liver in a patient with acute liver insufficiency Surgery 113:340.

Rozga J, Williams F, Ro M-S, et al. 1993. Development of a bioartificial liver: Properties and function of a hollow-fiber module inoculated with liver cells. Hepatology 17:258.

Saunders SJ, Bosman SCW, Terblanche J, et al. 1968. Acute hepatic coma treated by cross circulation with a baboon and by repeated exchange transfusions. Lancet 2:585.

Seglen PO. 1976. Preparation of isolated rat liver cells. Meth Cell Biol 13:29.

Singhvi R, Kumar A, Lopez GP, et al. 1994. Engineering cell shape and function. Science 264:696.

Sussman NL, Chong MG, Koussayer T, et al. 1992. Reversal of fulminant hepatic failure using an extracorporeal liver assist device. Hepatology 16:60

Sussman NL, Kelly JH. 1993. Extracorporeal liver assist in the treatment of fulminant hepatic failure. Blood Purif 11:170.

Trey C, Burns DG, Saunders SJ. 1966. Treatment of hepatic coma by exchange blood transfusion. N Eng J Med 274:473.

Wolf CFW, Munkelt BE. 1975. Bilirubin conjugation by an artificial liver composed of cultured cells and synthetic capillaries. Trans Amer Soc Artif Internal Organs 21:16.

Further Information

Two books of particular interest in hepatic encephalopathy are *Hepatic Encephalopathy: Pathophysiology and Treatment* edited by Roger F. Butterworth and Gilles Pomier Layrargues, published by The Humana Press (1989), and *Hepatology: A Textbook of Liver Disease* edited by David Zakim and Thomas D. Boyer, published by W. B. Saunders Company (1990).

Articles pertaining to extracorporeal liver assist devices appear periodically in the following journals: *ASAIO Journal,* the official journal for the American Society for Artificial Internal Organs (for subscription information, write to J.B. Lippincott, P.O. Box 1600, Hagerstown, MD 21741-9932); *Artificial Organs,* official journal of the International Society for Artificial Organs (for subscription information, write to Blackwell Scientific Publications, Inc., 328 Main Street, Cambridge, MA 02142); and *Cell Transplantation,* official journal of the Cell Transplantation Society (for subscription information, write to Elsevier Science, P.O. Box 64245, Baltimore, MD 21264-4245).

130
Artificial Pancreas

Pierre M. Galletti
Brown University

Clark K. Colton
Massachusetts Institute of Technology

Michel Jaffrin
Université de Technologie de Compiègne

Gerard Reach
Hôpital Hotel-Dieu Paris

130.1 Structure and Function of the Pancreas

The pancreas is a slender, soft, lobulated gland (ca. 75 g in the adult human), located transversally in the upper abdomen in the space framed by the three portions of the duodenum and the spleen. Most of the pancreas is an *exocrine* gland which secretes proteolytic and lipolytic enzymes, conveying more than 1 L per day of digestive juices to the gastrointestinal tract. This liquid originates in cell clusters called *acini* and is collected by a system of microscopic ducts, which coalesce in a channel (the canal of Wirsung) which courses horizontally through the length of the organ and opens into the duodenum next to, or together with, the main hepatic duct (choledocous). Interspersed throughout the exocrine tissue are about 1 million separate, highly vascularized and individually innervated cell clusters known as islets of Langerhans, which together constitute the *endocrine* pancreas (1–2% of the total pancreatic mass). Blood is supplied to the islets by the pancreatic artery and drained into the portal vein. Therefore the entire output of pancreatic hormones is first delivered to the liver.

Human islets average 150 µm in diameter, each cluster including several endocrine cell types. Alpha cells (about 15% of the islet mass) are typically located at the periphery of the cluster. They are the source of glucagon, a fuel-mobilizing (catabolic) hormone which induces the liver to release into the circulation energy-rich solutes such as glucose and aceto-acetic and β-hydroxybutyric acids. Beta cells, which occupy the central portion of the islet, comprise about 80% of its mass. They secrete insulin, a fuel-storing (anabolic) hormone that promotes sequestration of carbohydrate, protein, and fat in storage depots in the liver, muscle, and adipose tissue. Delta cells, interposed between alpha and beta cells, produce somatostatin, one role of which seems to be to slow down the secretion of insulin and digestive juices, thereby prolonging the absorption of food. The PP cells secrete a "pancreatic polypeptide" of yet unknown significance. Other cells have the potential to produce gastrin, a hormone that stimulates the production of gastric juice.

0-8493-8346-3/95/$0.00+$.50
© 1995 by CRC Press, Inc.

130.2 Endocrine Pancreas and Insulin Secretion

The term *artificial pancreas* is used exclusively for systems aimed at replacing the endocrine function of that organ. Although the total loss of exocrine function (following removal of the gland for polycystic disease, tumor, or trauma) can be quite debilitating, no device has yet been designed to replace the digestive component of the pancreas. Since insulin deficiency is the life-threatening consequence of the loss of endocrine function, the artificial pancreas focuses almost exclusively on insulin supply systems, even though some of the approaches used, such as islet transplantation, of necessity include an undefined element of delivery of other hormones.

Insulin is the most critical hormone produced by the pancreas because, in contradistinction to glucagon, it acts alone in producing its effects, and survival is not possible in its absence. Endogenous insulin secretion is greatest immediately after eating and is lowest in the interval between meals. Coordination of insulin secretion with fluctuating demands for energy production results from beta-cell stimulation by metabolites, other hormones, and neural signals. The beta cells monitor circulating solutes (in humans, primarily blood glucose) and release insulin in proportion to needs, with the result that in normal individuals, blood glucose levels fluctuate within quite narrow limits. The response time of pancreatic islets to an increase in blood glucose is remarkably fast: 10 to 20 sec for the initial burst of insulin release (primarily from intracellular stores), which is then followed, in a diphasic manner, by a gradual increase in secretion of newly synthesized hormone up to the level appropriate to the intensity and duration of the stimulus. Under fasting condition the pancreas secretes about 40 µg (1 unit) of insulin per hour to achieve a concentration of insulin of 2–4 µg/ml (50 to 100 µU/ml) in portal blood and of 0.5 µg/ml (12 µU/ml) in the peripheral circulation.

130.3 Diabetes

Insulin deficiency leads to a disease called *diabetes mellitus,* which is the most common endocrine disease in advanced societies, affecting as many as 3–5% of the population in the United States, with an even higher incidence in specific ethnic groups.

Diabetes is a chronic systemic disease resulting from a disruption of fuel metabolism either because the body does not produce enough insulin or because the available insulin is not effective. In either case, the result is an accumulation of glucose in the blood or *hyperglycemia*, and, once the renal tubular threshold for glucose is exceeded, a spillover of glucose into the urine or "glycosuria." Hyperglycemia is thought to be the main determinant of microvascular alterations which affect several organs (renal glomerulus, retina, myocardium). It is considered as an important factor in large-blood-vessel pathology (aorta and peripheral arteries, such as carotid and lower limb vessels) often observed in diabetes. Neuropathies of the autonomic, peripheral, and central nervous systems are also common in diabetics, although the pathogenic mechanism is not known.

When blood glucose levels are abnormally high, an increasing fraction of the hemoglobin in the red blood cells tends to conjugate with glucose forming a compound identifiable by chromatography and called HbA_{1C}. This reaction serves as a tool in diabetes management and control. The fraction of hemoglobin that is normally glycosylated (relative to total Hb) is between 6% and 9%. If elevated, HbA_{1C} reflects the time-averaged level of hyperglycemia over the lifetime of the red blood cells (3–4 months). It can be interpreted as an index of the severity of diabetes or the quality of control by dietary measures and insulin therapy.

There are two main forms of diabetes: *Type I,* juvenile onset diabetes (typically diagnosed before age 30), or insulin-dependent diabetes; and *type II,* maturity onset diabetes (typically observed after age 40), or non-insulin-dependent diabetes.

Type I appears abruptly (in a matter of days or weeks) in children and young people, although there is evidence that the islet destruction pattern may start much earlier but remain undiagnosed until close to 90% of the islets have been rendered ineffective. Type I represents only 10% of all cases of diabetes, yet it still affects close to 1 million patients in the United States alone. Endogenous insulin is almost totally absent, and an exogenous supply is therefore required immediately to avoid life-threatening metabolic accidents (ketoacidosis) as well as the more insidious degenerative processes which affect the cardiovascular system, the kidneys, the peripheral nervous system and the retina. For some unknown reason, 15% of juvenile diabetics never develop complications. Because the cellular and molecular mechanisms of hyperglycemic damage appear experimentally to be reversible by tight control of glucose levels, and the progress of vascular complications is said to be proportional to the square of the blood glucose concentration, early and rigorous control of insulin administration is believed to be essential to minimize the long term consequences of the disease.

In contrast, type II diabetes, which affects close to 90% of all patients, develops slowly and can often be controlled by diet alone or by a combination of weight loss and/or oral hypoglycemic drugs. Endogenous insulin is often present in normal and sometimes exaggerated amounts, reflecting an inability of cells to make use of available insulin rather than a true hormonal deficiency. Only 20–30% of type II diabetics benefit from insulin therapy. Keto-acidosis is rare, and the major problems are those associated with vascular wall lesions and arterial obstruction. Adult onset diabetics develop the same vascular, renal, ocular, and neural complications as type I diabetics, suggesting that even if the origin of the disease is not identical, its later evolution is fundamentally the same as in juvenile diabetics (Table 130.1).

Diabetes is the leading cause of blindness in the United States. It is also responsible for the largest fraction of the population of patients with end-stage renal disease who are being kept alive by maintenance dialysis. It is one of the most frequent causes of myocardial infarction and stroke, and the most common factor in arterial occlusion and gangrene of the lower extremities leading to limb amputation. With the diabetic population increasing by about 5% per year, diabetes has become one of the major contributors to health expenditures in advanced societies.

It is currently thought that destruction of the pancreatic islets in juvenile diabetes is the result of an autoimmune process, occurring in genetically predisposed individuals, perhaps in relation to an intercurrent infectious disease. This has led to clinical attempts to salvage the remaining intact islets at the earliest recognizable stage of the disease using standard immunosuppressive drugs such as cyclosporin A. The effectiveness of this approach has not been demonstrated.

Diabetologists have also recognized that, at the onset of juvenile diabetes, hyperglycemia exerts a deleterious effect on the function of the still surviving islets, and that in the short term, intensive exogenous insulin therapy may actually lead to an apparent cure of the disease. However, this phenomenon, occasionally referred to as the *honeymoon period* of insulin treatment is transitory. After a period of weeks to months, diabetes reappears, and an exogenous source of insulin administration becomes necessary for survival. The need for insulin to protect borderline functioning islets against hyperglycemic damage has also been recognized in the early stage of islet transplantation.

130.4 Insulin

Insulin is the mainstay for the treatment of diabetes type I and, to a lesser extent, type II. Since it is the key substance produced by beta cells, it is important to define its chemical nature and its mode of action.

Insulin is a 51 amino acid peptide with a molecular weight of about 5800 daltons, made up of two chains (A and B) connected by disulfide bridges. Insulin is formed in the beta cell as a cleavage product of a larger peptide, proinsulin, and is stored there as crystals in tiny intracellular vesicles until released into the blood. The other cleavage product, the "connecting" or C-peptide, though biologically inactive, passes into the blood stream together with insulin, and therefore its concentration reflects, in a patient receiving exogenous insulin, the amount of insulin secreted by the pancreas itself, if any.

Active extracts of islet tissue, obtained from animals following ligation of the pancreatic duct to avoid autolysis, were first prepared by Banting and Best in 1922. Insulin was crystallized by Abel in 1926. In 1960, Sanger established the sequence of amino acids that make up the molecule and shortly thereafter the hormone was synthesized.

The exact composition of insulin varies slightly among animal species. The presence of disulfide bonds between the A and the B chain is critical. Loss of the C-terminal alanine of the B chain by carboxypeptidase hydrolysis results in no loss of biologic activity. The octapeptide residue that remains after splitting off the last eight amino acids of the B chain has a biologic activity amounting to about 15% of the original insulin molecule. About one-half of the insulin disappears in its passage through the liver. Only a small fraction normally goes to peripheral tissues. Plasma halflife is on the order of 40 min, most of the degradation occurring in the liver and kidneys. No biologically active insulin is eliminated in the urine.

Since insulin is a polypeptide, it cannot be taken orally because it would be digested and inactivated in the gastrointestinal tract. In an emergency, insulin can be administered intravenously, but standard treatment relies on subcutaneous administration. This port of entry differs from physiologic secretion of insulin in two major ways: The adsorption is slow and does not mimic the rapid rise and decline of secretion in response to food ingestion, and the insulin diffuses into the systemic veins rather than into the portal circulation.

TABLE 130.1 Pathogenesis of Diabetes

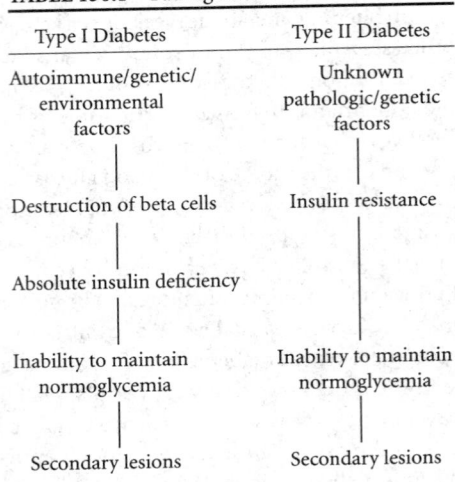

Type I Diabetes	Type II Diabetes
Autoimmune/genetic/ environmental factors	Unknown pathologic/genetic factors
Destruction of beta cells	Insulin resistance
Absolute insulin deficiency	
Inability to maintain normoglycemia	Inability to maintain normoglycemia
Secondary lesions	Secondary lesions

130.5 Insulin Therapy

Preparations of insulin are classified according to their species of origin and their duration of action. Human insulin (synthesized by recombinant DNA techniques) and porcine insulin (which is obtained by chemical extraction from slaughterhouse-retrieved organs and differs from human insulin by only one amino-acid at the carboxyl-terminus of the B chain) are in principle preferable to bovine insulin (which differs from the human form by three amino acid residues). In practice, all three are equipotent, and all three can, in a minority of patients, stimulate an immune response and cause hypersensitivity reactions. Because of insulin's relatively short duration of action, formulations delaying the absorption of subcutaneously injected hormone and hence prolonging its effectiveness have greatly facilitated the treatment of diabetes. The mode of administration of insulin influences its plasma concentration and bioavailability. The usual treatment schemes rely on the use of one or more types of insulin (Table 130.2).

Pharmacologists classify the available insulin formulations according to their latency and duration of action as fast acting, intermediate-acting, and slow acting using a terminology of *regular, semilente, lente,* and *ultralente* (Table 130.3). Crystalline insulin is prepared by precipitating the polypeptide in the presence of zinc in a suitable buffer solution. Insulin complexed with a strongly basic protein, protamine, and stabilized with zinc is relatively insoluble at physiological pH and is therefore released only slowly from the site of injection. However, one must keep in mind that onset and duration of action may be quite variable from one patient to another.

Whereas insulin was hailed as a life-saving drug in the years following its discovery (which it was, as evidenced by the much reduced incidence of hyperglycemic coma and the much longer life

TABLE 130.2 Types of Insulin

Fast acting	Multiple injections (basal and preprandial)
Intermediate	Two injections (morning and evening)
Slow acting	One injection (to prevent hyperglycemia at night)

TABLE 130.3   Properties of Insulin Preparations

Type	Appearance	Added Protein	Zinc Content mg/100 U	Time of Action (h) Onset	Peak	Duration
Rapid						
Crystalline (regular)	Clear	None	0.01–0.04	0.3–0.7	2–4	5–8
Insulin-zinc suspension (semilente)	Cloudy	None	0.2–0.25	0.5–1.0	2–8	12–16
Intermediate						
NPH (Isophane insulin suspension)	Cloudy	Protamine	0.016–0.04	1–2	6–12	18–24
Lente (insulin zinc suspension)	Cloudy	None	0.2–0.25	1–2	6–12	18–24
Slow						
Ultralente (extended insulin zinc suspension)	Cloudy	None	0.2–0.25	4–6	16–18	20–36
PZI (Protamine zinc insulin suspension)	Cloudy	Protamine	0.2–0.25	4–6	14–20	24–36

Source: Modified from Table 71-1 in *The Pharmacological Basis of Therapeutics*, 3rd ed., Goodman and Gillman.

expectancy of juvenile diabetics, as compared to the period before 1930), it has not turned out to be quite the universal panacea it was expected to be. Some of the problems that have surfaced relate to the limitations associated with the mode of administration of the drug. Other problems are thought to derive from our inability to mimic the finely tuned feedback system which normally maintains the blood glucose levels within very narrow limits (Table 130.4).

130.6 Therapeutic Options in Diabetes

Experimental studies of blood glucose regulation and empirical observations in diabetic patients have revealed three major characteristics of blood glucose regulation by the pancreas:

1. The natural system operates as a closed-loop regulatory mechanism within narrow limits.
2. Portal administration is more effective than systemic administration because insulin reaches the liver first.
3. Pulsatile administration of insulin is more effective than continuous administration.

There are several stages in the evolution of diabetes where a medical intervention might be helpful (Table 130.5). Many interventions have been attempted with various degrees of success. Since diabetes expresses a disturbance of a biologic feedback mechanism between blood glucose levels and insulin secretion, there might be possibilities to influence the biologic regulation process through its natural sensing or amplifying mechanisms. However, no practical solution has yet emerged from this approach. As a result the accent has been placed primarily on pharmacologic forms of treatment (diverse insulin formulations and routes of administration), engineered delivery systems (extracorporeal or implanted pumps), and substitution by natural insulin production sources (organ, islet,

TABLE 130.4   Problems with Insulin Treatment

Problem	Answers
Poor compliance with multiple injections	Better syringes and needles
	Subcutaneous ports
	Intravenous ports
	Insulin pens
Inadequate pharmacokinetics of insulin preparations	Enhance immediate effect
	Prolong duration of effect
Hyperinsulinemia	Release insulin in portal circulation
Lack of feedback control	Servo-controlled administration
	Natural control by transplant
	Bioartificial pancreas

TABLE 130.5   Potential Approaches to Diabetes Treatment

Prevent destruction of beta cells
Prevent beta cell exhaustion
Increase insulin output
Amplify glucose signal
Overcome insulin resistance
Replace beta cells by:
    Insulin administration
    Electromechanical delivery system
    Whole organ transplantation
    Islet transplantation
    Biohybrid device

or individual beta cell transplantation, with or without genetic manipulation and with or without membrane immunoprotection). An overview of the recently investigated approaches is given in Table 130.6.

130.7 Insulin Administration Systems

Syringes and Pens

Insulin traditionally has been administered subcutaneously by means of a syringe and needle, from a vial containing insulin at a concentration of 40 units per ml.

TABLE 130.6   Biologic and Engineered Insulin Delivery Systems

Insulin Administration Systems	
Standard insulin	Routes of administration (subcutaneous, intravenous, intraperitoneal, nasal spray)
Insulin release systems	Injection systems (syringes, pens)
	Passive release from depot forms
	Bioresponsive insulin depot
	Implanted, permeable reservoirs
	Programmed release systems
Insulin delivery pumps	
Open loop	Osmotic pumps
	Piston and syringe pumps
	Peristaltic (roller) pumps
	Bellow frame pumps
	Pressurized reservoir pumps
Closed loop	Glucose sensors
	Electromechanical, servo-controlled delivery systems

Insulin Synthesis Systems	
Pancreas transplantation	Simultaneous with kidney transplant
	After kidney transplant
	Before kidney transplant
Islet transplantation	Autologous tissue
	Allogeneic tissue
	Xenogeneic tissue
Encapsulated islets or beta cell transplants	Microencapsulated cells
	Macroencapsulated cells
Genetically engineered cell transplants	Unprotected gene therapy
	Protected gene therapy

When insulin was first proposed to treat diabetic patients in 1922, glass syringes were used. The burden linked to repeated sterilization disappeared when disposable syringes became available in the early 1970s. Yet patients still had to perform the boring and, for some, difficult task of refilling the syringe from a vial. From a pragmatic viewpoint the development of pens in which insulin is stored in a cartridge represented a major advance in diabetes management. In France, for instance, a recent survey indicates that more than half of the patients use a pen for daily therapy. A needle is screwed on the cartridge and should ideally be replaced before each injection. Cartridges containing either 1.5 or 3 ml of 100 U/ml regular or intermediate insulin are available. Unfortunately, long-acting insulin cannot be used in pens because it crystallizes at high concentrations. Attempts are being made toward developing soluble, slow-acting analogs of insulin to overcome this problem.

A common insulin regimen consists of injecting regular insulin before each meal with a pen and long-acting insulin at bedtime with a syringe. Typically half of the daily dosage is provided in the form of regular insulin. Since patients often need 50 units of insulin per day, a pen cartridge of 150 units of regular insulin must be replaced every 6 days or so. The setting of the appropriate dose is easy. However, most pens cannot deliver more than 36 units of insulin at a time, which in some patients may place a limit on their use. In those countries where insulin comes in vials of 40 U/ml for use with syringes, patients must be aware that insulin from cartridges is 2.5 times more concentrated than standard vial insulin. The major advantage of insulin pens is that they do not require refilling and therefore can be used discretely. Pens are particularly well accepted by teenagers.

Reservoirs, Depots, and Sprays

Attempts have been made to develop distensible, implantable reservoirs or bags made of silicone elastomers, fitted with a small delivery catheter, and refillable transcutaneously. In the preferred embodiment, insulin drains at a constant rate into the peritoneal cavity. Assuming uptake by the capillary beds in the serosal membranes which line the gastrointestinal tract, insulin reaches first the portal valve and hence the liver, which enhances its effectiveness. This is an attractive concept but not without serious handicaps. The implanted reservoir may elicit an untoward tissue reaction or become a site of infection. The delivery catheter may be plugged by insulin crystals if a high insulin concentration is used, or the catheter may be obstructed by biologic deposits at the tip. The system only provides a baseline insulin delivery and needs to be supplemented by preprandial injections. Its overall capacity constitutes a potential risk should the reservoir accidentally rupture and flood the organism with an overdose of insulin.

Insulin depots, in the form of bioerodible polymer structures in which insulin—amorphous or in crystalline form—is entrapped and slowly released as hydrolytic decay of the carrier polymer progressively liberates it, present some of the same problems as reservoirs. In addition, the initial burst which often precedes zero-order release can prove unpredictable and dangerous. No reliable long-term delivery system has yet been developed on that principle.

New routes of introduction of insulin are being investigated, in particular, transmucosal adsorption. Nasal sprays of specially formulated insulin may become a practical modality of insulin therapy if means are found to control reliably the dose administered.

Insulin Pumps

Externally carried portable pumps, based on the motorized syringe or miniature roller pump designs, were evaluated in the 1970s with the anticipation that they could be both preprogrammed for baseline delivery and overridden for bolus injections at the time of meals without the need for repeated needle punctures. In actual practice, this system did not find wide acceptance on the part of patients, because it was just too cumbersome and socially unacceptable.

The first *implantable* insulin pump was evaluated clinically in 1980. Unlike heparin delivery or cancer chemotherapy, insulin administration requires programmable pumps with adjustable flow rates. Implantable pumps provide better comfort for the patient than portable pumps, since the former are relatively unobtrusive and involve no danger of infection at the skin catheter junction. They also permit intraperitoneal insulin delivery, which is more efficient than subcutaneous administration. However, these pumps operate without feedback control, since implantable glucose sensors are not yet available, and the patient must program the pump according to his/her needs.

The vapor pressure driven *Infusaid* pump relies on a remarkably astute mechanism for an implantable device. A rigid box is separated in two compartments by a metal bellow with a flat diaphragm and an accordion-pleated seal (bellow frame). One compartment is accessible from the outside through a subcutaneously buried filling port and contains a concentrated insulin solution. The other compartment (the bellows itself) is filled with a liquid freon which vaporizes at 37° C with a constant pressure of 0.6 bar. With no other source of energy but body heat (which is continuously replenished by metabolism and blood circulation), the freon slowly evaporates, and the pressure developed displaces the diaphragm and forces insulin at a constant flow rate through a narrow delivery catheter. The freon energy is restored each time the insulin reservoir is refilled, since the pressure needed to move the bellow liquifies the freon vapor within a smaller compartment.

The housing is a disc-shaped titanium box. The insulin reservoir contains 15 to 25 ml of insulin stabilized with polygenol at a concentration of either 100 or 400 U/ml, providing an autonomy of 1 to 3 months. The self-sealing septum on the filling port can be punctured through the skin up to 500 times. The pump is implanted under general or local anesthesia between skin and muscle in the lateral abdominal area. The tip of the catheter can be located subcutaneously or intraperitoneally.

The original device provided a constant flow of insulin which still needed to be supplemented by the patient at meal time. The most recent model (*Infusaid* 1000) weighs 272 g, contains 22 ml of insulin, and has a diameter of 9 cm and a height of 2.2 cm. It is designed for 100 U/ml insulin and is equipped with a side port which allows flushing of the catheter when needed. To dissipate the pressure generated by freon evaporation before it reaches the catheter, the insulin must cross a 0.22 μm bacteriologic filter and pass through a steel capillary 3 cm long and 50 μm in diameter. Basal flow rate can be adjusted from 0.001–0.5 ml/h, and a bolus can be superposed by releasing a precise amount of insulin stored in a pressurized accumulator through the opening of a valve leading to the catheter. These control features require an additional source of energy in the form of lithium thionile batteries with a service life of about 3 years. Control is achieved with a handheld electronic module or programs connected to the pump by telemetry.

The current *Minimed* pump (INIP 2001) has a dry weight of 162 g and a diameter of 8.1 cm and contains 14 ml of insulin at a concentration of 400 U/ml, allowing up to 3 months' autonomy between refills. This pump relies on a reservoir from which insulin can be delivered in a pulsatile form by a piston mechanism under the control of solenoid-driven valves. The basal rate can be adjusted 0.13–30 U/h (0.0003 to 0.07 ml/h), and boluses from 1 to 32 U over intervals 1–60 min can be programmed. The reservoir is permanently under negative pressure to facilitate filling.

The Siemens *Infusor* (1D3 model) replaced an earlier type based on a peristaltic miniature roller pump (discontinued in 1987). It is somewhat similar in design and dimensions to the Minimed pumps, but it has now been withdrawn from the market.

The Medtronic *Synchromed* pump, which was originally designed for drug therapy and relied on a roller pump controlled by an external programmer, was evaluated for insulin therapy but is seldom used for that purpose because it lacks the required flexibility.

Between 1989 and 1992, 292 insulin pumps were implanted in 259 patients in France, where most of the clinical experience has been collected (205 Minimed, 47 Infusaid, and 7 Siemens). The treatment had to be permanently discontinued in 14 patients (10 because of poor tissue tolerance, 3 due to catheter obstruction, and 1 due to pump failure). The pump was replaced in 33 patients, with 28 cases of component failure: battery, microelectronic control, flow rate decline due to insulin precipitation in Infusaid pumps, insulin reflux in Minimed pumps, perceived risk of leak from septum. The overall frequency of technical problems was 0.10 per patient-year. There were 46 surgical interventions without pump replacement because of catheter obstructions, and 24 related to poor tissue tolerance at the site of implantation. Glucose regulation was satisfactory in all cases, and the mean blood glucose concentration dropped appreciably after 6 and 18 months of treatment. A major gain with the intraperitoneal delivery was the reduction in the incidence of severe hypoglycemia associated with improved metabolic control. For the sake of comparison, other methods used for intensive insulin therapy showed a threefold increase in the frequency of serious hypoglycemic episodes.

Servo-Controlled Insulin Delivery Systems

Sensor-actuator couples which allow insulin delivery in the amount needed to maintain a nearly constant blood glucose level are sometimes designated as the *artificial beta cell* because of the analogy between the components of the electromechanical system and the biologic mechanisms involved in sensing, controlling, and delivering insulin from the pancreas (Table 130.7).

From a technology viewpoint, the key aspects are the glucose sensor, the control systems applicable to a biologic situation where both hyperglycemia and hypoglycemia must be prevented, and the practicality of the overall system.

Glucose Sensors

A glucose sensor provides a continuous reading of glucose concentration. The device consists of a detection part, which determines for the specificity of the glucose measurement, and a transducing element, which transforms the chemical or physical signals associated with glucose recognition into an electric signal. The most advanced technology is based on enzymatic and amperometric detection of glucose. Glucose is recognized by a specific enzyme, usually glucose oxidase, layered on the anode of an electrode, generating hydrogen peroxide which is then oxidized and detected by the current generated in the presence of a fixed potential between the anode and the cathode. Alternatively, a chemical mediator may serve as a shuttle between the enzyme and the electrode to avoid the need for a potential difference at which other substances, such as ascorbate or acetaminophen, may be oxidized and generate an interfering current. Other approaches such as the direct electrocatalytic oxidation of glucose on the surface of the electrode or the detection of glucose by a combination with a lectin have not reached the stage of clinical evaluation.

Ideally, a blood glucose sensor would be permanently installed in the bloodstream. Because of the difficulty of building a hemocompatible device and the inconvenience of a permanent blood access, several investigators have turned to the subcutaneous site for glucose sensing. Indeed, glucose concentration in the interstitial fluid is very close to that of blood and reflects quite directly changes associated with meals or physical activity as observed in diabetic patients. Two types of subcutaneous glucose sensors have been developed. Those with electrodes at the tip of a needle may be shielded from their environment by the inflammatory reaction in tissues contacting the electrode membrane and occasionally cause pain or discomfort. Nonetheless, reliable measurements have been obtained for up to 10 days, whereupon the sensor needed to be changed. Sensing can also be based on microdialysis through an implanted, permeable hollow fiber, providing fluid which is then circulated to a glucose electrode. This system has not yet been miniaturized and industrialized.

TABLE 130.7 Component Mechanisms of Insulin Delivery Systems

	Natural β cell	Artificial β cell
Sensor of glucose level	Intracellular glycolysis	Polarographic or optoelectronic sensor
Energy source	Mitochondria	Implantable battery
Logic	Nucleus	Minicomputer chip
Insulin reserve	Insulin granules	Insulin solution reservoir
Delivery system	Cell membrane	Insulin pump
Set point	Normally 80–120 mg %	Adaptable
Fail-safe	Glucagon and hunger	Glucose infusion

In either case, the concept is to develop an external monitor such as a wrist watch, which could receive its analyte from the implanted catheter and/or sensor and trigger a warning when glucose concentration is abnormally high or low. Such a monitor could eventually be incorporated in a closed-loop insulin delivery system, but this objective is not yet realizable.

Noninvasive technology has been suggested to monitor blood glucose, e.g., by near-infrared spectroscopy or optical rotation applied to transparent fluid media of the eye. No reliable technology has yet emerged.

The Artificial Beta Cell

The standard equipment for feedback-controlled insulin administration is the artificial beta cell, also referred to in the literature as the extracorporeal artificial pancreas. It consists of a system for continuous blood sampling, a blood glucose sensor, and minicomputer which, through preestablished algorithms, drives an insulin infusion pump and a glucose infusion pump according to the needs of the patient. Accessories provide a minute-by-minute recording of blood glucose levels, insulin delivery, and glucose delivery.

In the first clinically oriented artificial beta cell (Miles Laboratories' *Bioslator*), the glucose sensor was located in a flow-through chamber where blood from a patient's vein was sucked continuously, at the rate of 2 ml/h, through a double-lumen catheter. The double lumen allowed the infusion of a minute dose of heparin at the tip of the catheter to prevent thrombosis in the glucose analyzer circuit. Glucose diffused through a semipermeable membrane covering the electrode and was oxidized by the enzyme. The hydrogen peroxide generated by this reaction crossed a second membrane, the role of which was to screen off substances such as urate and ascorbate. The resulting electric current was fed to a computer which controlled the flow rate of the insulin pump when the readings were in the hyperglycemic range and administered a glucose solution in case of hypoglycemia.

Three forms of oversight of blood glucose levels and insulin needs can be achieved with the artificial beta cell:

Blood glucose monitoring is the technique employed to investigate the time course of blood glucose levels in a particular physiologic situation without any feedback control from the artificial beta cell, that is, without insulin administration to correct the fluctuations of blood glucose levels.

Blood glucose control is the standard feedback mode of application of the artificial beta cell, which entails an arbitrary choice of the level of blood glucose desired and provides a recording of the rate of administration and the cumulative dose of intravenous insulin needed to achieve a constant blood glucose level.

Blood glucose clamp involves intravenous insulin administration at a constant rate to obtain a stable, high blood insulin level. The desired value of blood glucose level is arbitrarily selected (typically in the normal range), and the feedback-control capability of the artificial beta cell is used to measure the amount of exogenous glucose needed to "clamp" blood glucose at the desired level in the presence of a slight excess of insulin. With this technique, a decrease in the rate of glucose administration signals a decrease in insulin biologic activity.

The artificial beta cell is primarily a clinical research tool, applicable also for therapy in high-risk conditions such as pregnancy in poorly controlled diabetic mothers or cardiac surgery in brittle diabetics [Galletti et al., 1985], where hypothermia and a massive outpouring of adrenergic agents alter the response to insulin [Kuntschen et al., 1986]. The primary drawbacks of current servo-controlled insulin delivery systems are the instability of the glucose sensor (in terms of both risk of thrombosis and the need for intermittent recalibration), the complexity of the system (up to four pumps can be needed for continuous blood sampling, heparinization, insulin administration, and glucose administration), and the risks involved. The dose of intravenous insulin required for rapid correction of hyperglycemia may cause an overshoot, which in turn calls for rapid administration of glucose. Such fluctuations may also influence potassium uptake by cells and in extreme conditions lead to changes in potassium levels which must be recognized and corrected [Kuntschen et al., 1983]. Finally, the general cumbersomeness of the extracorporeal system, to which the patient must be tethered by sampling and infusion lines, limits its applicability. Modeling of blood glucose control by insulin has allowed the development of algorithms that are remarkably efficient in providing metabolic feedback in most clinical situation. The physiologic limits of closed-loop systems have been lucidly analyzed by Sorensen and coworkers [1982] and Kraegen [1983].

130.8 Insulin Production Systems

The exacting requirement placed on insulin dosage and timing of administration in diabetic patients, as well as the many years of safe and reliable treatments expected from the insulin delivery technology, have pointed to the advantages of implantable systems in which insulin would be synthesized as needed and made available to the organism on demand.

As already outlined in Table 130.6, four avenues have been considered and undergone chemical evaluation: whole organ transplantation, human islet and xenogeneic islet transplantation, immunoisolation of normal or tumoral insulin-secreting tissue, and transplantation of cells genetically engineered to replace the functions of the beta cells.

Pancreas Transplantation

Human allograft transplantation, first attempted over 20 years ago, has been slow in reaching clinical acceptance because of the difficulty of identifying healthy cadaver organs (the pancreas is also a digestive gland which undergoes autolysis soon after death) and the need to deal with the gland exocrine secretion, which serves no useful purpose in diabetes but nonetheless must be disposed of. After many ingenious attempts to plug the secretory channels with room-temperature vulcanizing biopolymers, a preferred surgical technique has been developed whereby the pancreas is implanted in the iliac fossa, its arterial supply and venous drainage vessels anastomosed to the iliac artery and vein, and the Wirsung canal implanted in the urinary bladder. Surprisingly, the bladder mucosa is not substantially damaged by pancreatic enzymes, and the exocrine secretion dries up after a while.

The success rate of pancreatic transplantation is now approaching that of heart and liver transplantation. Since it is mostly offered to immunosuppressed uremic diabetic patients who previously received or concurrently receive a kidney transplant, preventative therapy against organ rejection does not constitute an additional risk. The main limitation remains the supply of donor organs, which in the United States will probably not exceed 2000 per year, that is to say, very far from meeting the incidence of new cases of juvenile diabetes [Robertson & Sutherland, 1992]. Therefore, human organ transplantation is not a solution to the public health problems of diabetes and ensuing complications.

Human Islet Transplantation

Interest in the transplantation of islets of Langerhans, isolated from exocrine, vascular, and connective tissue by enzymatic digestion and cell separation techniques, has received a boost following the clinical demonstration that it can lead to insulin independence in type I diabetic patients [Scharp et al., 1990]. However, this "proof of principle" has not been followed by widespread application. Not only is the overall supply of cadaveric organs grossly insufficient in relation to the need (by as much as two orders of magnitude), but the islet separation techniques are complex and incompletely standardized. Therefore, it is difficult to justify at this point cutting into the limited supply of human pancreata for whole organ transplantation, the more so that whole organ replacement has become increasingly successful. Autologous islet transplantation can be successfully performed in relatively uncommon cases of pancreatic and polycystic disease, where the risk of spilling pancreatic juice in the peritoneal cavity necessitates the removal of the entire organ. Allogeneic islet transplantation under the cover of pharmacologic immunosuppression is useful inasmuch as it provides a benchmark against which to evaluate islet transplantation from animal sources and the benefits of membrane immunoisolation.

Xenogeneic Islet Transplantation

The term bioartificial pancreas refers to any insulin-production–glycemia-regulation system combining living pancreatic beta cells or equivalents with a synthetic polymer membrane of gel to protect the transplant against immune rejection. A wide variety of device designs, cell sources and processing techniques, implant location, and biomaterial formulation and characterization have been investigated (Table 130.8). Common to all is the belief that if transplantation of insulin-producing tissue is to serve the largest number of insulin-dependent diabetic patients possible, xenogeneic tissue sources will have to be identified. In that context, protection by a semipermeable membrane may be the most effective way to dispense with drug immunosuppression therapy [Lysaght et al., 1994]. However, a number of issues must be addressed and resolved before the bioartificial pancreas becomes a clinically acceptable treatment modality [Colton, 1994].

Tissue Procurement

In the evolution of type I diabetes, the oral glucose tolerance test does not become abnormal until about 70% of the islets are destroyed. Therefore, roughly 250,000 human islets, or about 3500 islets per kilogram of body weight, should suffice to normalize blood glucose levels. In reality, clinical observations of transplanted patients indicate a need for a considerably larger number (3500–6000 islets/kg, and perhaps more). This suggests that many processed islets are either nonviable or not functional because they have been damaged during the isolation procedure or by the hyperglycemic environment of the transplanted patient [Eizirik et al., 1992].

TABLE 130.8   Membrane-Encapsulated Cell Transplants

Technology	Microencapsulation	
	Macroencapsulation	
	Coextrusion	
Location	Vascular release	Intravascular
		Perivascular
	Portal release	Intraperitoneal
		Intrahepatic
		Intrasplenic
	Systemic release	Subcutaneous
		Intramuscular
Cell source	Human islets or beta cells } fetal or adult	
	Animal islets or beta cells	
	Functionally active tumor tissue	
	Immortalized cell lines	
	Genetically engineered cell lines	
Cell processing	Isolation and purification	
	Culture and banking	
	Cryopreservation	
	Implant manufacturing	
Membrane characterization	Envelope mechanical stability	
	Envelope chemical stability	
	Diffusion and filtration kinetics	
	Immunoprotection	
	Bioacceptance	

To procure such large numbers of islets an animal source must be identified. Porcine islets are favored because of the size of the animal, the availability of virus-free herds, and the low antigenicity of porcine insulin. Pig islet separation procedures are not yet fully standardized, and there are still considerable variations in terms of yield, viability, and insulin secretory function. Quality control and sterility control present serious challenges to industrialization.

Alternative tissue sources are therefore being investigated. *Insulinomas* provided the first long-term demonstration of the concept of encapsulated endocrine tissue transplant [Altman et al., 1984]. Genetically engineered cell lines which can sense glucose concentration and regulate it with-in the physiologic range have been reported, but so far none has matched the secretory ability of normal pancreatic tissue or isolated islets. This approach remains nonetheless attractive for large-scale device production, even though no timetable can be formulated for successful development.

Device Design

Immunoisolation of allogeneic or xenogeneic islets can be achieved by two main classes of technology: microencapsulation and macroencapsulation. *Microencapsulation* refers to the formation of a spherical gel around each islet, cell cluster, or tissue fragment. Calcium alginate, usually surrounded with a polyanion such as poly-L-lysine to prevent biodegradation, and at times overcoated with an alginate layer to improve the biocompatibility, has been the most common approach, although other polymers may be substituted. Suspension of microcapsules are typically introduced in the peritoneal cavity to deliver insulin to the portal circulation.

Technical advances have permitted the fabrication of increasingly smaller microcapsules (order of 150–200 µm) which do not clump, degrade, or elicit too violent a tissue reaction. Control of diabetes has been achieved in mice, rats, dogs, and, on a pilot basis, in humans [Soon-Siong et al., 1994]. An obstacle to human application has been the difficulty, if not the impossibility, of retrieving the very large number of miniature implants, many of which adhere to tissue. There is also a concern for the antigenic burden that may arise upon polymer degradation and liberation of islet tissue, whether living or necrotic.

Macroencapsulation refers to the reliance on larger, prefabricated envelopes in which a slurry of islets or cell clusters is slowly introduced and sealed prior to implantation. The device configuration can be tubular or planar. The implantation site can be perivascular, intravascular, intraperitoneal, subcutaneous, or intravascular.

Intravascular Devices

In the most successful intravascular device (which might be more accurately designated as *perivascular*), a semipermeable membrane is formed into a wide-bore tube connected between artery and vein or between the severed ends of an artery as if it were a vascular graft. The islets are contained in a gel matrix within a compartment surrounding the tube through which blood circulates. In other embodiments, the islets are contained in semipermeable parallel hollow fibers or coiled capillaries attached to the external wall of a macroporous vascular prosthesis. In all cases, a rising glucose concentration in the blood stream leads to glucose diffusion into the islet compartment, which stimulates insulin production, raises its concentration in the gel matrix, and promotes diffusion into the blood stream.

In an earlier type of perivascular device, blood is forced to circulate through the lumina of a tight bundle of hollow fibers, and the islet suspension is placed in the extracapillary space between fibers and circumscribed by a rigid shell, as was the case in the design which established the effectiveness of immunoprotected islets [Chick et al., 1987]. A truly intravascular device design has been proposed in which the islets are contained within the lumina of a bundle of hollow fibers which are plugged at both ends and placed surgically in the blood stream of a large vein or artery, in a mode reminiscent of the intravenous oxygenator (IVOX). Hemocompatibility has been the major challenge with that approach.

There have also been attempts to develop extracorporeal devices with a semipermeable tubular membrane connected transcutaneously, through flexible catheters, to an artery or vein. The islets are seeded in the narrow "extravascular" space separating the membrane from the device external wall and can therefore be inspected and, in case of need, replaced. This concept has evolved progressively to wider-bore (3–6 mm ID), spirally coiled tubes in a disc-shaped plastic housing. Such devices have remained patent for several months in dogs in the absence of anticoagulation and have shown the ability to correct hyperglycemia in spontaneous or experimentally induced diabetes.

In order to accelerate glucose and insulin transport across synthetic membranes and shorten the reactive time lag of immuno-protected islets, Reach and Jaffrin [1984] have proposed to take advantage of a Starling-type ultrafiltration cycle made possible, in blood-perfused devices, by the arteriovenous pressure difference between device inlet and outlet. An outward-directed ultrafiltration flux in the first half of the blood conduit is balanced by a reverse readsorption flux in the second half, since the islet compartment is fluid-filled, rigid, and incompressible. An acceleration of the response time to fluctuations in blood glucose levels has been demonstrated both by modeling and experimentally. This system may also enhance the transport of oxygen and nutrients and improve the metabolic support of transplanted tissue.

The primary obstacle to clinical acceptance of the intravascular bioartificial pancreas is the risk of thrombosis (including obstruction and embolism) of a device expected to function for several years. The smaller the diameter of the blood channel, and the greater the surface of polymeric material exposed to blood, the more likely are thrombotic complications. These devices also share with vascular grafts the risk of a small but definite incidence of infection of the implant and the potential sacrifice of a major blood vessel. Therefore, their clinical application is likely to remain quite limited.

Intratissular Devices

Tubular membranes with diameters on the order of 0.5–2 mm have also been evaluated as islet containers for subcutaneous, intramuscular, or intracavitary implantation: The islets are contained inside the membrane envelope at a low-volume fraction in a gel matrix. A problem is that small-diameter tubes require too much length to be practical. Larger-diameter tubes are mechanically fragile and often display a core of necrotic tissue because diffusion distances are too long for adequate oxygen and nutrient transport to the islets. Both systems are subject to often unpredictable foreign body reactions and the development of scar tissue which further impairs metabolic support of the transplanted tissue. However materials that elicit a minimal tissue reaction have been identified [Galletti, 1992], and further device design and evaluation is proceeding at a brisk pace [Scharp et al., 1994].

Some microporous materials display the property of inducing neovascularization at the tissue-material interface and in some cases within the voids of a macroporous polymer. This phenomenon is thought to enhance mass transport for nutrient and secretory products by bringing capillaries in closer proximity to immuno-separated cells. Pore size, geometry, and interconnections are critical factors in vascularization [Colton, 1994]. Some encapsulated cell types also stimulate vascularization beyond the level observed with empty devices. Chambers made by laminating a 5-μm porosity expanded polytetrafluoroethylene (Gore PTFE) on a 0.45-μm Biopore (Millipore) membrane have shown the most favorable results [Brauker et al., 1992]. The laminated, vascularized membrane structure has been fabricated in a sandwichlike structure that can be accessed through a port to inject an islet suspension once the empty device has been fully integrated in the soft tissues of the host. This organoid can nonetheless be separated from adjacent tissues, exteriorized and retrieved.

Polymers for Immunoisolation

The polymeric materials used in bioartificial endocrine devices serve two major purposes: (1) As a scaffold and an extracellular matrix, they favor the attachment and differentiation of functional cells or cell clusters and keep them separate from one another, which in some cases has proven critical; (2) as permselective envelopes they provide immunoisolation of the transplant from the host, while inducing a surrounding tissue reaction which will maximize the diffusional exchange of solutes between the transplant and its environment. A number of materials can be used for these purposes (Table 130.9).

The matrix materials typically are gels made of natural or synthetic polyelectrolytes, with quite specific requirements in terms of viscosity, porosity, and electric charge. In some cases specific attachment or growth factors may be added.

For immunoisolation, the most commonly used envelopes are prepared from polyacrylonitrile-polyvinyl chloride copolymers. These membranes display the anisotropic structure typical of most ultrafiltration membranes, in which a thin retentive skin is supported on a spongy matrix [Colton, 1994]. The shape and dimensions of the interconnecting voids and the microarchitecture of the inner and outer surfaces of the membrane are often critical characteristics for specific cell types and implant locations.

Protection from Immune Rejection

The central concept of immunoisolation is the placement of a semipermeable barrier between the host and transplanted tissue. It has been tacitly assumed that membranes with a nominal 50,000–100,000-daltons cutoff would provide adequate protection, because they would prevent the passage of cells from the host immune system and impair the diffusion of proteins involved in the humoral component of immune rejection.

This belief has been largely supported by empirical observations of membrane-encapsulated graft survival, with occasional failures rationalized as membrane defects.

However, the cut-off point of synthetic semipermeable membranes is not as sharp as one may believe, and there is often a small number of pores which theoretically at least allow the transport of much larger molecules than suggested by the nominal cut-off definition. Therefore, complex issues of rate of transport, threshold concentration of critical proteins, adsorption and denaturation in contact with polymeric materials, and interactions between proteins involved in immune reactions in an environment where their relative concentrations may be far from normal may all impact in immunoprotection. The possibility of antigen release from living or necrotic cells in the sequestered environment must also be considered. The cellular and luminal mechanisms of immunoseparation by semipermeable membranes and the duration of the protection they afford against both immune rejection of the graft and sensitizations of the host call for considerably more study.

TABLE 130.9   Polymer Technology for Cell Transplantation

Component	Function	Polymer
Scaffold	Synthetic or semisynthetic extracellular matrix	Collagen
		Gelatin
		Alginate
		Agarose
	Physical separation of cells or cell aggregates	Chitosan
		Hyaluronan
Envelope		
Microencapsulation	Stabilization of cell suspension and immunoseparation	Alginate
		Poly-L-lysine
Macroencapsulation	Physical immunoseparation	Polyacrylonitrile
		Polyvinyl copolymers
		Polysulfones
		Modified celluloses
	Transport-promoting tissue-material interface	PTFE-Biopore laminate

130.9 Outlook

Replacement of the endocrine functions of the pancreas presents a special challenge in substitutive medicine. The major disease under consideration, diabetes, is quite common, but a reasonably effective therapy already exists with standard insulin administration. The disease is not immediately life-threatening, and therefore optimization of treatment is predicated on the potential for reducing the long-term complications of diabetes. Therefore, complete clinical validation will require decades of observations, not merely short-term demonstration of effectiveness in controlling blood glucose levels.

Standard insulin treatment is also relatively inexpensive. Competitive therapeutic technologies will therefore be subject to a demanding cost-benefit analysis before they are widely recognized. Finally, the patient self-image will be a major factor in the acceptance of new diagnostic or treatment modalities. Already some demonstrably useful devices, such as subcutaneous glucose sensors, portable insulin pumps, and the extracorporeal artificial beta cell, have failed in the marketplace for reasons of excessive complexity, incompatibility with all activities of daily life, physicians' skepticism, or cost. Newer technologies involving the implantation of animal tissue or genetically engineered cells will bring about a new set of concerns, whether justified or imaginary. There is perhaps no application of the artificial organ concept where human factors are so closely intertwined with the potential of science and technology as is already the case with the artificial pancreas.

Defining Terms

Anabolism: The aspect of metabolism in which relatively simple building blocks are transformed into more complex substances for the purpose of storage or enhanced physiologic action.

Artificial beta cell: A system for the control of blood glucose levels based on servo-controlled administration of exogenous insulin based on continuous glucose level monitoring.

Artificial pancreas: A device or system designed to replace the natural organ. By convention, this term designates substitutes for the endocrine function of the pancreas and specifically glucose homeostasis through the secretion of insulin.

Autolysis: Destruction of the components of a tissue, following cell death, mediated by enzymes normally present in that tissue.

Bioartificial pancreas: A device or implant containing insulin-producing, glycemia-regulating cells in combination with polymeric structures for mechanical support and/or immune protection.

Catabolism: The aspect of metabolism in which substances in living tissues are transformed into waste products or solutes of simpler chemical composition.

Endogenous: Originating in body tissues.

Exogenous: Introduced in the body from external sources.

Extracorporeal artificial pancreas: An apparatus including a glucose sensor, a minicomputer with appropriate algorithms, an insulin infusion pump, and a glucose infusion pump, the output of which are controlled so as to maintain a constant blood glucose level. (Synonymous with *artificial beta cell.*)

Hyperglycemia: Abnormally high blood glucose level (in humans, above 140 mg/100 ml).

Hypoglycemia: Abnormally low blood glucose level (in humans, below 50 mg/100 ml).

Immunoisolation: Separation of transplanted tissue from its host by a membrane or film which prevents immune rejection of the transplant by forming a barrier against the passage of immunologically active solutes and cells.

Insulinoma: A generally benign tumor of the pancreas, originating in the beta cells and functionally characterized by a secretion of insulin and the occurrence of hypoglycemic coma. Insulinoma cells are thought to have lost the feedback function and blood-glucose-regulating capacity of normal cells, or to regulate blood glucose around an abnormally low set point.

Ketoacidosis: A form of metabolic acidosis encountered in diabetes mellitus, in which fat is used as a fuel instead of glucose (because of the lack of insulin), leading to high concentration of metabolites such as acetoacetic acid, β hydroxybutyzic acid, and, occasionally, acetone in the blood and intestinal fluids.

Organoid: A device—typically an implant—in which cell attachment and growth in the scaffold provided by a synthetic polymer sponge or mesh leads to a structure resembling that of a natural organ including, in many cases, revascularization.

References

Altman JJ, Houlbert D, Callard P, et al. 1986. Long-term plasma glucose normalization in experimental diabetic rats using microencapsulated implants of benign human insulinomas. Diabetes 35:625.

Altman JJ, Houlbert D, Chollier A, et al. 1984. Encapsulated human islet transplantation in diabetic rats. Trans Am Soc Artif Intern Organs 30:382.

Brauker JH, Martinson LA, Young S, et al. 1992. Neovascularization at a membrane-tissue interface is dependent on microarchitecture. Abstracts, Fourth World Biomaterials Congress, Berlin FRG: 685.

Chick WL, Like AA, Lauris V, et al. 1975. A hybrid artificial pancreas. Trans Am Soc Artif Intern Organs 21:8.

Chick WL, Perna JJ, Lauris V, et al. 1977. Artificial pancreas using living beta cells: effects on glucose homeostasis in diabetic rats. Science 197:780.

Colton CK. 1992. The engineering of xenogeneic islet transplantation by immunoisolation. Diab Nutr Metab 5:145.

Colton CK. 1994. Engineering issues in islet immunoisolation. In R Lanza, W Chick (eds), Pancreatic Islet Transplanation, vol III: Immunoisolation of Pancreatic Islets, RG Landes.

Colton CK, Avgoustiniatos ES. 1991. Bioengineering in development of the hybrid artificial pancreas. J Biomech Eng 113:152.

Dionne KE, Colton CK, Yarmush ML. 1993. Effect of hypoxia on insulin secretion by isolated rat and canine islets of Langerhans. Diabetes 42:12.

Eizirik DL, Korbutt GS, Hellerstrom C. 1992. Prolonged exposure of human pancreatic islets to high glucose concentrations in vitro impairs the β-cell function. J Clin Invest 90:1263.

Galletti PM. 1992. Bioartificial organs. Artif Organs 16(1):55.

Galletti PM, Altman JJ. 1984. Extracorporeal treatment of diabetes in man. Trans Am Soc Artif Intern Organs 30:675.

Galletti PM, Kuntschen FR, Hahn C. 1985. Experimental and clinical studies with servo-controlled glucose and insulin administration during cardiopulmonary bypass. Mt Sinai J Med 52:500.

Jaffrin MY, Reach G, Notelet D. 1988. Analysis of ultrafiltration and mass transfer in a bioartificial pancreas. ASME J Biomech Eng 110:1.

Kraegen EW. 1983. Closed loop systems: Physiological and practical considerations. In P Brunetti, KGMM Alberti, AM Albisser, et al. (eds), Artificial Systems for Insulin Delivery, New York, Raven Press.

Kuntschen FR, Galletti PM, Hahn C. 1986. Glucose-insulin interactions during cardiopulmonary bypass. Hypothermia versus normothermia. J Thorac Cardiovasc Surg 91:45.

Kuntschen FR, Taillens C, Hahn C, et al. 1983. Technical aspects of Biostator operation during coronary artery bypass surgery under moderate hypothermia. In Artificial Systems for Insulin Delivery, pp 555–559, New York, Raven Press.

Lanza RP, Butler DH, Borland KM, et al. 1991. Xenotransplantation of canine, bovine and porcine islets in diabetic rats without immunosuppression. PNAS 88:11100.

Lanza RP, Sullivan SJ, Chick WL. 1992. Islet transplantation with immunoisolation. Diabetes 41:1503.

Lysaght MJ, Frydel B, Winn S, et al. 1994. Recent progress in immunoisolated cell therapy. J Cell Biochem 56:1.

Mikos AG, Papadaki MG, Kouvroukogiou S, et al. 1994. Mini-review: Islet transplantation to create a bioartificial pancreas. Biotechnol Bioeng 43:673.

Pfeiffer EF, Thum CI, Clemens AH. 1974. The artificial beta cell. A continuous control of blood sugar by external regulation of insulin infusion (glucose controlled insulin infusion system). Horm Metab Res 6:339.

Reach G, Jaffrin MY, Desjeux J-F. 1984. A U-shaped bioartificial pancreas with rapid glucose-insulin kinetics. In vitro evaluation and kinetic modelling. Diabetes 33:752.

Ricordi C. (ed). 1992. Pancreatic Islet Transplantation, Austin, Tex, RG Landes.

Robertson RP, Sutherland DE. 1992. Pancreas transplantation as therapy for diabetes mellitus. Annu Rev Med 43:395.

Scharp DW, Lacy PE, Santiago JV, et al. 1990. Insulin independence after islet transplantation into a Type I diabetes patient. Diabetes 39:515.

Scharp DW, Swanson CJ, Olack BJ, et al. 1994. Protection of encapsulated human islets implanted without immunosuppression in patients with Type I and II diabetes and in nondiabetic controls. Diabetes (accepted for publication in September 1994 issue).

Soon-Siong P, Heintz RE, Merideth N, et al. 1994. Insulin independenence in a type 1 diabetic patient after encapsulated islet transplantation. Lancet 343:950.

Sorensen JT, Colton CK, Hillman RS, et al. 1982. Use of a physiologic pharmacokinetic model of glucose homeostasis for assessment of performance requirements for improved insulin therapies. Diabetes Care 5:148.

Sullivan SJ, Maki T, Borland KM, et al. 1991. Biohybrid artificial pancreas: Long-term implantation studies in diabetic, pancreatectomized dogs. Science 252:718.

Further Information

A useful earlier review of insulin delivery systems is to be found in: *Artificial Systems for Insulin Delivery,* edited by P. Brunetti, K.G.M.M. Alberti, A.M. Albisser, K.D. Hepp, and M. Massi Benedetti, Serono Symposia Publications from Raven Press, New York, 1983. An upcoming review, focused primarily on islet transplantation, will be found in *Pancreatic Islet Transplantation,* vol. III: *Immunoisolation of Pancreatic Islets,* edited by R.P. Lanza and W.L. Chick, R.G. Landes Company, Austin, Texas, 1994. A volume entitled *Implantation Biology: The Host Response and Biomedical Devices,* edited by R.S. Greco, from CRC Press, 1994, provides a background in the multiple aspects of tissue response to biomaterials and implants.

Individual contributions to the science and technology of pancreas replacement are likely to be found in the following journals: *Artificial Organs,* the ASAIO Journal, *International Journal of Artificial Organs,* the *Journal of Cell Transplantation,* and *Transplantation.* Reports on clinically promising devices are often published in *Diabetes* and *Lancet.*

131

Nerve Guidance Channels

Robert F. Valentini
Brown University

In adult mammals, including humans, the peripheral nervous system (PNS) is capable of regeneration following injury. The PNS consists of neural structures located outside the central nervous system (CNS), which is comprised of the brain and spinal cord. Unfortunately, CNS injuries rarely show a return of function, although recent studies suggest a limited capacity for recovery under optimal conditions. Neural regeneration is complicated by the fact that neurons, unlike other cell types, are not capable of proliferating. In successful regeneration, sprouting axons from the proximal nerve stump traverse the injury site, enter the distal nerve stump, and make new connections with target organs. Current surgical techniques allow surgeons to realign nerve ends precisely when the lesion does not require excision of a large nerve segment. Nerve realignment increases the probability that extending axons will encounter an appropriate distal neural pathway, yet the incidence of recovery in the PNS is highly variable, and the return of function is never complete. Surgical advances in the area of nerve repair seem to have reached an impasse, and biologic rather than technical factors now limit the quality of regeneration and functional recovery. The use of synthetic nerve guidance channels facilitates the study of nerve regeneration in experimental studies and shows promise in improving the repair of injured human nerves. Advances in the synthesis of biocompatible polymers have provided scientists with a variety of new biomaterials which may serve as nerve guidance channels, although the material of choice for clinical application has not yet been identified.

The purpose of this chapter is to review the biologic aspects of PNS regeneration (CNS regeneration will be discussed in a subsequent chapter) and the influence of nerve guidance channels on the regeneration process. The biologic mechanisms and the guidance channel characteristics regulating regeneration will be emphasized, since the rational design of guidance systems hinges on the integration of engineering (polymer chemistry, materials science, and so on) and biologic (cellular and molecular events) principles.

-8493-8346-3/95/$0.00+$.50
© 1995 by CRC Press, Inc.

131.1 Peripheral Nervous System

Peripheral nerve trunks are responsible for the innervation of the skin and skeletal muscles and contain electrically conductive fibers termed *axons,* whose cell bodies reside in or near the spinal cord (Fig. 131.1). Nerve cells are unique in that their cellular processes may extend for up to one meter or longer (e.g., for axons innervating the skin of the foot). Three types of neuronal fibers can be found in peripheral nerves: (1) motor fibers, whose axons originate in the anterior horn of the spinal cord and terminate in the neuromuscular endings of skeletal muscle; (2) sensory fibers, which are the peripheral projections of dorsal root ganglion neurons and terminate at the periphery either freely or in a variety of specialized receptors; and (3) sympathetic fibers, which are the postganglionic processes of neurons innervating blood vessels or glandular structures of the skin. These three fiber types usually travel within the same nerve trunk, and a single nerve can contain thousands of axons All axons are wrapped by support cells named *Schwann cells.* Larger axons are surrounded by a multilamellar sheath of myelin, a phospholipid-containing substance which serves as an insulator and enhances nerve conduction. An individual Schwann cell may ensheath several unmyelinated axons but only one myelinated axon, within its cytoplasm. Schwann cells are delineated by a fine basal lamina and are in turn surrounded by a complex structure made of collagen fibrils interspersed with fibroblasts and small capillaries, forming a tissue termed the *endoneurium.* A layer of flattened cells with associated basement membrane and collagen constitute the *perineurium,* which envelops all endoneurial constituents. The presence of tight junctions between the perineurial cells creates a diffusion barrier for the endoneurium and thus functions as a blood-nerve barrier. The perineurium and its endoneurial contents constitute a *fascicle,* which is the basic structural unit of a peripheral nerve. Most peripheral nerves contain several fascicles, each containing numerous myelinated and unmyelinated axons. Since the fascicular tracts branch frequently and follow a tortuous pathway, the cross-sectional fascicular pattern changes significantly along a nerve trunk. Outside the perineurium is the *epineurium,* a protective, structural connective tissue sheath

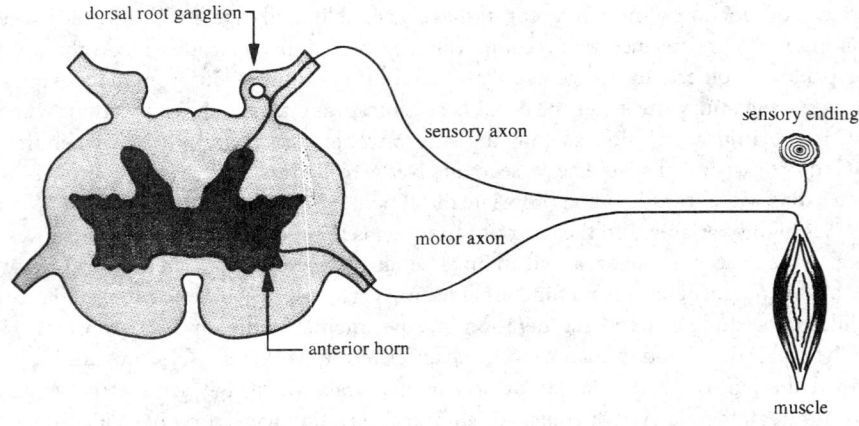

FIGURE 131.1 Spinal cord in cross-section. Relationship between motor and sensory cell bodies and their axons. Motor neurons (black) are located in the anterior horn of the gray matter within the spinal cord. Sensory neurons (white) are located in dorsal root ganglia just outside the spinal cord. Axons exit via dorsal (sensory) and ventral (motor) spinal roots and converge to form peripheral nerves, which connect to target structures (sensory endings and muscles). Note that the distance between axons and their corresponding cell bodies can be quite long.

made of several layers of flattened fibroblastic cells interspersed with collagen, blood vessels, and adipocytes (fat cells). Peripheral nerves are well vascularized, and their blood supply is derived either from capillaries located within the epineurium and endoneurium (i.e., vasa nervosum) or from peripheral vessels which penetrate into the nerve from surrounding arteries and veins.

131.2 PNS Response to Injury

Nerves subjected to mechanical, thermal, chemical, or ischemic insults exhibit a typical combination of degenerative and regenerative responses. The most severe form of injury results from complete transection of the nerve, which interrupts communication between the nerve cell body and its target, disrupts the interrelations between neurons and their support cells, destroys the local blood-nerve barrier, and triggers a variety of cellular and humoral events. Injuries close to the nerve cell body are more detrimental than injuries occurring more peripherally.

The cell bodies and axons of motor and sensory nerves react in a characteristic fashion to transection injury. The central cell body (which is located within or just outside the spinal cord) and its nucleus swell. Neurotransmitter (e.g., the chemicals which control neuronal signaling) production is diminished drastically, and carbohydrate metabolism is shifted to the pentose-phosphate cycle. These changes indicate a metabolic shift toward production of the substrates necessary for reconstituting the cell membrane and other structural components. For example, the synthesis of the protein tubulin, which is the monomeric element of the microtubule, the structure responsible for axoplasmic transport, is increased dramatically. Following injury, tubulin and other substrates produced in the cell soma are transported, via slow and fast axoplasmic transport, to the distal nerve fiber.

Immediately after injury, the tip of the proximal stump (i.e., the nerve segment closest to the spinal cord) swells to two or three times its original diameter, and the severed axons retract. After several days, the proximal axons begin to sprout vigorously and growth cones emerge. Growth cones are axoplasmic extrusions of the cut axons which flatten and spread when they encounter a solid, adhesive surface. They elicit numerous extensions (fillipodia) which extend outward in all directions until the first sprout reaches an appropriate target (i.e., Schwann cell basal lamina). The lead sprout is usually the only one to survive, and the others quickly die back.

In the distal nerve stump, the process of Wallerian degeneration begins within 1 to 2 hours after transection. The isolated axons and their myelin sheaths are degraded and phagocytized by Schwann cells and macrophages, leading to a complete dissociation of neurotubules and neurofilaments. This degradation process is accompanied by a proliferation of Schwann cells which retain the structure of the endoneurial tube by organizing themselves into ordered columns termed *bands of Bunger*. While the Schwann cells multiply, the other components of the distal nerve stump atrophy or are degraded, resulting in a reduction in the diameter of the overall structure. Severe retrograde degeneration can lead to cell atrophy and, eventually, cell death. Peripheral nerve transection also leads to marked atrophy of the corresponding target muscle fibers.

131.3 PNS Regeneration

In successful regeneration, axons sprouting from the proximal stump bridge the injury gap and encounter an appropriate Schwann cell column (band of Bunger). In humans, axons elongate at an average rate of 1 mm per day. The bridging axons are immediately engulfed in Schwann cell cytoplasm, and some of them become myelinated. Induction of myelogenesis by the Schwann cell is thought to depend on axonal contact. Some of the axons reaching the distal stump traverse the length of the nerve to form functional synapses, but changes in the pattern of muscular and sensory reinnervation invariably occur. The misrouting of growing fibers occurs primarily at the site of injury, since once they reach the distal stump their paths do not deviate further. The original Schwann cell basal lamina in the distal stump persists and may aid in the migration of axons and proliferating Schwann cells. Axons which fail to reach an appropriate end organ or fail to make a functional synapse eventually undergo Wallerian degeneration. Abnormal regeneration may lead to the formation of a *neuroma*, a dense, irregular tangle of axons which can cause painful sensations. Some nerve injuries result from clean transections of the nerve which leave the fascicular pattern intact. More often, a segment of nerve is destroyed (e.g., during high-energy trauma or avulsion injuries in which tissue is torn), thus creating a nerve deficit. The resulting nerve gap is the separation between the proximal and distal stumps of a damaged nerve that is due to elastic retraction of the nerve stumps and tissue loss. The longer the nerve gap, the less likely regeneration will occur.

131.4 Surgical Repair of Transected Peripheral Nerves

In the absence of surgical reconnection, recovery of function following a transection or gap injury to a nerve is negligible, since (1) the cell bodies die due to severe retrograde effects, (2) the separation between nerve ends precludes sprouting axons from finding the distal stump, (3) connective tissue ingrowth at the injury site acts as a physical barrier to neurite elongation, and (4) the proximal and distal fascicular patterns differ so much that extending axons cannot find an appropriate distal pathway.

Efforts to repair damaged peripheral nerves by surgical techniques date back many years, although histologic evidence of regeneration was not reported by Ramon y Cajal until the first part of this century. Early attempts to reconnect severed peripheral nerves utilized a crude assortment of materials, and anatomic repair rarely led to an appreciable return of function. In the 1950s, the concept of end-to-end repair was refined by surgeons who directly reattached individual nerve fascicles or groups of fascicles. Further refinements occurred during the 1960s with the introduction of the surgical microscope and the availability of finer suture materials and instrumentation. Microsurgical nerve repair led to a significant improvement in the return of motor and sensory function in patients to the point that success rates of up to 70% can currently be achieved. In microsurgical nerve repair the ends of severed nerves are apposed and realigned by placing several strands of very fine suture material through the epineurial connective tissue without entering the underlying nerve fascicles. Nerve-grafting procedures are performed when nerve retraction or tissue loss prevents direct end-to-end repair. Nerve grafts are also employed when nerve stump reapproximation would create tension along the suture line, a situation which is known to hinder the regeneration process. In grafting surgery, an autologous nerve graft from the patient, such as the sural nerve (whose removal results in little functional deficit), is interposed between the ends of the damaged nerve.

131.5 Repair with Nerve Guidance Channels

In repair procedures using nerve guidance channels, the mobilized ends of a severed nerve are introduced in the lumen of a tube and anchored in place with sutures (Fig. 131.2). Tubulation repair provides: (1) a direct, unbroken path between nerve stumps; (2) prevention of scar tissue invasion into the regenerating environment; (3) directional guidance for elongating neurites and migrating cells; (4) proximal-distal stump communication without suture-line tension in cases of extensive nerve deficit; (5) minimal number of epineurial stay sutures, which are known to stimulate connective tissue proliferation; and (6) preservation, within the guidance channel lumen, of endogenous trophic or growth factors released by the traumatized nerve ends. Guidance channels are also useful from an experimental perspective: (1) The gap distance between the nerve stumps can be precisely controlled; (2) the fluid and tissue entering the channel can be evaluated; (3) the properties of the channel can be varied; and (4) the channel can be filled with various drugs, gels, and the like. Nerves with various dimensions from several mammalian species, including mice, rats, rabbits, hamsters, and nonhuman primates have been tested. The regenerated tissue in the guidance channel is evaluated morphologically to quantify the outcome of regeneration. Parameters analyzed

Creation of Nerve Deficit

Placement of Guidance Channel

Controlled Nerve Gap

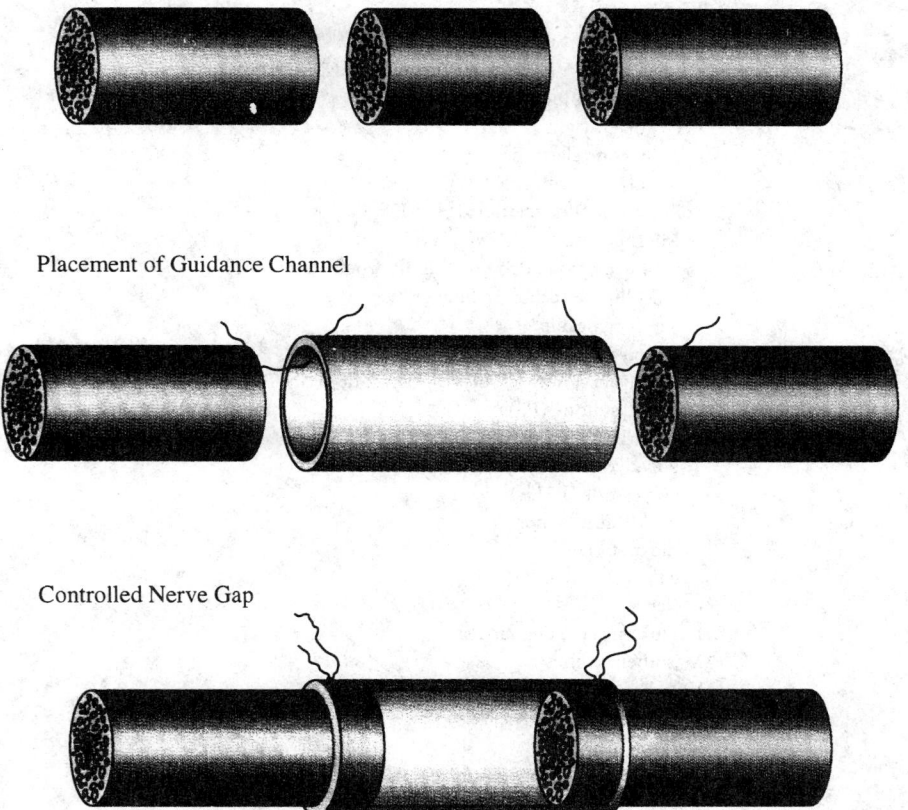

gap

FIGURE 131.2 Tube to repair nerve. Surgical placement of nerve guidance channel.

include the cross-sectional area of the regenerated nerve cable, the number of myelinated and unmyelinated axons, and the relative percentages of cellular constituents (i.e., epineurium, endoneurium, blood vessels, and so on). Electrophysiologic and functional evaluation can also be performed in studies conducted for long periods (e.g., several weeks or more).

The frequent occurrence of nerve injuries during the world wars of this century stimulated surgeons to seek simpler, more effective means of repairing damaged nerves. A variety of biologic and synthetic materials shaped into cylinders were investigated (Table 131.1). Bone, collagen membranes, arteries, and veins (either fresh or freeze-dried to reduce antigenicity) were used from the late 1800s through the 1950s to repair nerves. These materials did not enhance the rate of nerve regeneration when compared to regular suturing techniques, so clinical applications were infrequent. Magnesium, rubber, and gelatin tubes were evaluated during World War I, and cylinders of parchment paper and tantalum were used during World War II. The poor results achieved with these materials can be attributed to poor biocompatibility, since the channels elicited an intense tissue response which limited the ability of growing axons to reach the distal nerve stump. Following World War II, polymeric materials with more stable mechanical and chemical properties became available. Millipore (cellulose acetate) and Silastic (silicone elastomer) tubing received the greatest attention. Millipore, a filter material with a maximum pore size of 0.45 μm, showed early favorable results. In

TABLE 131.1   Materials Used for Nerve Guidance Channels

Synthetic materials
  Nonresorbable
    Nonporous
      Ethylene-Vinyl Acetate Copolymer (EVA)
      Polytetrafluoroethylene (PTFE)
      Polyethylene (PE)
      Silicone elastomers (SE)
      Polyvinyl chloride (PVC)
      Polyvinylidene fluoride (PVDF)
    Microporous
      Gortex, expanded polytetrafluoroethylene (ePTFE)
      Millipore (cellulose filter)
    Semipermeable
      Polyacrylonitrile (PAN)
      Polyacrylonitrile/Polyvinyl chloride (PAN/PVC)
      Polysulfone (PS)
  Bioresorbable
    Polyglycolide (PGA)
    Polylactide (PLLA)
    PGA/PLLA blends
Biologic materials
  Artery
  Collagen
  Hyaluronic acid derivatives
  Mesothelial tubes
  Vein
Metals
  Stainless steel
  Tantalum

human trials, however, Millipore induced calcification and eventually fragmented several months after implantation so that its use was discontinued. Silastic tubing, a biologically inert polymer with rubberlike properties, was first tested in the 1960s. Thin-walled Silastic channels were reported to support regeneration over large gaps in several mammalian species. Thick-walled tubing was associated with nerve necrosis and neuroma production. The material showed no long-term degradation nor did it elicit a sustained inflammatory reaction. As a result, thin-walled Silastic tubing has been used, on a very limited basis, in the clinical repair of severed nerves.

131.6 Recent Studies with Nerve Guidance Channels

The availability of a variety of new biomaterials has led to a resurgence of tubulation studies designed to elucidate the mechanisms of nerve regeneration. The spatial-temporal progress of nerve regeneration across a 10-mm rat sciatic nerve gap repaired with a silicone elastomer tube has been analyzed in detail (Fig. 131.3). During the first hours following repair, the tube fills with a clear, protein-containing fluid exuded by the cut blood vessels in the nerve ends. The fluid contains the clot-forming protein, fibrin, as well as factors known to support nerve survival and outgrowth. By the end of the first week, the lumen is filled with a longitudinally oriented fibrin matrix which coalesces and undergoes syneresis to form a continuous bridge between the nerve ends. The fibrin matrix is soon invaded by cellular elements migrating from the proximal and distal nerve stumps, including fibroblasts (which first organize along the periphery of the fibrin matrix), Schwann cells, macrophages, and endothelial cells (which form capillaries). At 2 weeks, axons advancing from the proximal stump are engulfed in the cytoplasm of Schwann cells. After 4 weeks some axons have

Filling of Tube by Blood Derived Fluid and Proteins (day 1)

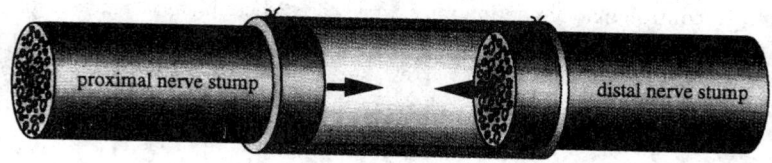

Formation and Coalescence of Fibrin Cable (days 2-6)

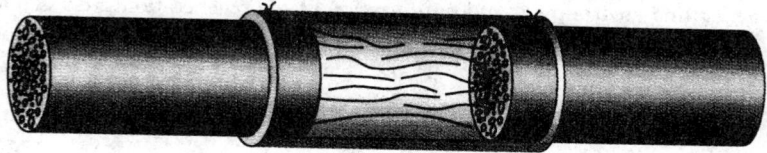

Invasion of Cable by Schwann Cells, Fibroblasts, and Endothelial Cells (days 7-14)

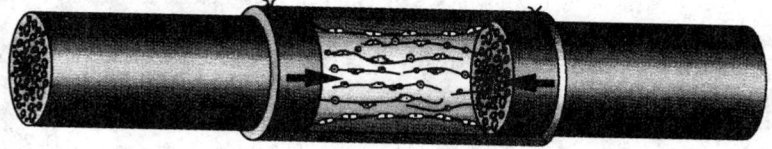

Axonal Elongation and Myelination (days 15-28)

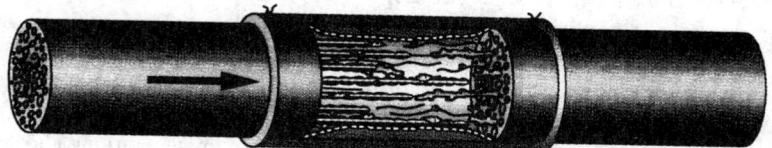

FIGURE 131.3　Regeneration process. Nerve regeneration through a guidance channel.

reached the distal nerve stump, and many have become myelinated. The number of axons reaching the distal stump is related to the distance the regenerating nerve has to traverse and the length of original nerve resected. Silicone guidance channels do not support regeneration if the nerve gap is greater than 10 mm and if the distal nerve stump is left out of the guidance channel. The morphology and structure of the regenerated nerve is far from normal. The size and number of axons and the thickness of myelin sheaths are less than normal. Electromyographic evaluation of nerves regenerated through silicone tubes reveals that axons can make functional synapses with distal targets, although nerve conduction velocities and signal amplitudes are slower than normal, even after many months. Attempts to improve the success rate and quality of nerve regeneration have led to the use of other tubular biomaterials as guidance channels (Table 131.1). Biodurable materials such as acrylic copolymers, polyethylene, and porous stainless steel and bioresorbable materials including polyglycolides, polylactides, and other polyesters have been investigated. There is some concern that biodurable materials may cause long-term complications via compression injury to nerves or soft tissues. Biodegradable materials offer the advantage of disappearing once regeneration is complete, but success thus far has been limited by swelling, increased scar tissue induction, and difficulty in controlling degradation rates. In all cases, these materials have displayed variable degrees of success in bridging transected nerves, and the newly formed nerves are morphologically quite different from normal peripheral nerves. The general spatial-temporal progress of nerve regeneration, however, resembles that described for the silicone channel model.

131.7 Enhancing Regeneration by Optimizing Nerve Guidance Channel Properties

Manipulating the physical, chemical, and electrical properties of guidance channels allows control over the regenerating environment and optimization of the regeneration process. The following features of synthetic nerve guidance channels have been studied: (1) transmural permeability, (2) surface texture or microgeometry, (3) electric charges, (4) release of soluble factors, (5) inclusion of insoluble factors, and (6) seeding with neuronal support cells.

Transmural Permeability

The synthetic nerve guidance channel controls the regeneration process by influencing the cellular and metabolic aspects of the regenerating environment. Since transected nerves lose the integrity of their blood-nerve barrier (which controls oxygen and carbon dioxide tensions, pH, and the concentrations of nutrients and essential proteins), the guidance channel's transmural mass transfer characteristics modulate solute exchange between the regenerating tissue and the surrounding fluids. Nerves regenerated through permselective tubes display more normal morphologic characteristics than nerves regenerated in impermeable silicone elastomer (SE) and polyethylene (PE) or freely permeable expanded polytetrafluoroethylene (ePTFE) tubes. Nerves found in semipermeable tubes feature more myelinated axons and less connective tissue. Nerve cables regenerated in semipermeable or impermeable tubes are both round-shaped and free from attachment to the inner wall of the guidance channel. Nerves regenerated in highly porous, open structures do not form a distinct cable but contain connective tissue and dispersed neural elements. The range of permselectivity is very important, and optimal regeneration is observed with a molecular weight (MW) cut-off of 50,000–100,000 daltons (D). Permselective PAN/PVC channels with an MW cut-off of 50,000 D support regeneration even in the absence of a distal nerve stump.

These observations suggest that controlled solute exchange between the internal regenerative and external wound-healing environments is essential in controlling regeneration. The availability of oxygen and other nutrients may minimize connective tissue formation in permeable PAN/PVC and PS tubes. Decreased oxygen levels and waste buildup may increase connective tissue formation in SE and PE tubes. Regeneration may also be modulated by excitatory and inhibitory factors released by the wound-healing environment. Semipermeable channels may sequester locally generated growth factors while preventing the inward flux of molecules inhibitory to regeneration.

Surface Texture or Microgeometry

The microgeometry of the luminal surface of the guidance channel plays an important role in regulating tissue outgrowth. Expanded microfibrillar polytetrafluoroethylene (ePTFE) tubes exhibiting different internodal distances (1, 5, and 10 μm) were compared to smooth-walled, impermeable PTFE tubes. Larger internodal distances result in greater surface irregularity and increased transmural porosity. Rough-walled tubes contained isolated fascicles of nerves dispersed within a loose connective tissue stroma. The greater the surface roughness, the greater the spread of fascicles. In contrast, smooth-walled, impermeable PTFE tubes contained a discrete nerve cable delineated by an epineurium and located within the center of the guidance channel. Similar results were observed with semipermeable PAN/PVC tubes with the same chemistry and MW cut-off but with either smooth or rough surfaces. Nerves regenerated in tubes containing alternating sections of smooth and rough inner walls showed similar morphologies with an immediate change from single-cable to numerous fascicle morphology at the interface of the smooth and rough segments.

These studies suggest that the microgeometry of the guidance channel lumen also modulates the nerve regeneration process. Wall structure changes may alter the protein and cellular constituents of the regenerating tissue bridge. For example, the orientation of the fibrin matrix is altered in the presence of a rough inner wall. Instead of forming a single, longitudinally oriented bridge connecting the nerve ends, the fibrin molecules remain dispersed throughout the lumen. As a result, cells migrating in from the nerve stumps loosely fill the entire lumen rather than form a dense central structure.

Electric Charge Characteristics

Applied electric fields and direct dc stimulation are known to influence nerve regeneration in vitro and in vivo. Certain dielectric polymers may be used to study the effect of electric activity on nerve regeneration in vivo and in vitro. These materials are advantageous in that they provide electric charges without the need for an external power supply, can be localized anatomically, are biocompatible, and can be formed into a variety of shapes including tubes and sheets.

Electrets are a broad class of dielectric polymers which can be fabricated to display surface charges because of their unique molecular structure. True electrets, such as polytetrafluoroethylene (PTFE), can be modified to exhibit a static surface charge due to the presence of stable, monopolar charges located in the bulk of the polymer. The sign of the charge depends on the poling conditions. Positive, negative, or combined charge patterns can be achieved. The magnitude of surface charge density is related to the number and stability of the monopolar charges. Charge stability is related to the temperature at which poling occurs. Crystalline piezoelectric materials such as polyvinylidene fluoride (PVDF) display transient surface charges related to dynamic spatial reorientation of molecular dipoles located in the polymer bulk. The amplitude of charge generation depends on the degree of physical deformation (i.e., dipole displacement) of the polymer structure. The sign of the charge is dependent on the direction of deformation, and the materials show no net charge at rest.

Negatively and positively poled PVDF and PTFE tubes have been implanted as nerve guidance channels. Poled PVDF and PTFE channels contain significantly more myelinated axons than unpoled, but otherwise identical, channels. In general, positively poled channels contained larger neural cables with more myelinated axons than negatively poled tubes. It is not clear how static or transient charge generation affects the regeneration process. The enhancement of regeneration may be due to electrical influences on protein synthesis, membrane receptor mobility, growth cone motility, cell migration, and other factors.

Release of Soluble Factors

The release of soluble agents, including growth factors and other bioactive substances from synthetic guidance channels, may improve the degree and specificity of neural outgrowth. Using single or multiple injections of growth factors has disadvantages including early burst release, poor control over local drug levels, and degradation in biologic environments. Guidance channels can be prefilled with drugs or growth factors, but the aforementioned limitations persist. Advantages of using a local, controlled delivery system are that the rate and amount of factor release can be controlled and that the delivery can be maintained for long periods (several weeks). Channels composed of an ethylene-vinyl acetate (EVA) copolymer have been fabricated and designed to release incorporated macromolecules in a predictable manner. The amount of drug loaded, its molecular weight, and geometry of the drug-releasing structure affect the drug release kinetics. It is also possible to restrict drug release to the luminal side of the guidance channel by coating its outer wall with a film of pure polymer.

Growth or neuronotrophic factors that ensure the survival and general growth of neurons are produced by support cells (e.g., Schwann cells) or by target organs (e.g., muscle fibers). Some factors support neuronal survival, others support nerve outgrowth, and some do both. Numerous growth factors have been identified, purified, and synthesized through recombinant technologies (Table 131.2). In vivo, growth factors are found in solution in the serum or extracellular fluid or bound to extracellular matrix (ECM) molecules. Nerve guidance channels fabricated from EVA and designed to slowly release basic fibroblast growth factor (bFGF) or nerve growth factor (NGF) support regeneration over a 15-mm gap in a rat model. Control EVA tubes supported regeneration over a maximum gap of only 10 mm withnoregenerationin 15-mm gaps. The concurrent release of growth factors which preferentially control the survival and outgrowth of motor and sensory neurons may further enhance regeneration, since the majority of peripheral nerves contain both populations. For example, NGF and b-FGF control sensory neuronal survival and outgrowth, whereas brain-derived growth factor (BDGF) and ciliary neuronotrophic factor (CNTF) control motor neuronal survival and outgrowth. Growth factors released by guidance channels may also allow regeneration over large nerve deficits, an important consideration in nerve injuries with severe tissue loss. The local release of other pharmacologic agents (e.g., anti-inflammatory drugs) may also be useful in enhancing nerve growth.

Inclusion of Insoluble Factors

Several neural molecules found on cell membranes and in the extracellular matrix are potent modulators of neural attachment and outgrowth (Table 131.3). Proteins responsible for eliciting and stimulating axon elongation are termed *neurite promoting factors*. The glycoprotein laminin, an ECM component present in the basal lamina of Schwann cells, has been reported to promote nerve elongation in vitro and in vivo. Other ECM products, including the glycoprotein fibronectin and the proteoglycan heparan sulphate, also have been reported to promote nerve extension in vitro. Some subtypes of the ubiquitous protein collagen also support neural attachment. Filling guidance channels with gels of laminin and collagen has been shown to improve and accelerate nerve repair. The addition of longitudinally oriented fibrin gels to SE tubes has also been shown to accelerate regeneration. Collagen, laminin, and glycosaminoglycans (another ECM component) introduced in the guidance channel lumen support some degree of regeneration over a 15–20-mm gap in adult rats. The concentration of ECM gel is important, as thicker gels impede regeneration in semipermeable tubes.

The activity of these large, insoluble ECM molecules (up to 10^6 D MW) can be mimicked by short sequences only 3–10 amino acids long (e.g., RGD, YIGSR) (Table 131.3). The availability of small, soluble, bioactive agents allows more precise control over the chemistry, conformation, and binding of neuron-specific substances. Additionally, their stability and linear structure facilitate their use instead of labile (and more expensive) proteins which require three-dimensional structure for

TABLE 131.2   Growth Factors Involved in Peripheral Nerve Regeneration

Growth Factor	Possible function
NGF—nerve growth factor	Neuronal survival, axon-Schwann cell interaction
BDNF—brain-derived neurotrophic factor	Neuronal survival
CNTF—ciliary neuronotrophic factor	Neuronal survival
NT-3—neuronotrophin 3	Neuronal survival
NT-4—neuronotrophin 4	Neuronal survival
IGF-1—insulinlike growth factor-1	Axonal growth, Schwann cell migration
IGF-2—Insulinlike growth factor-2	Motoneurite sprouting, muscle reinnervation
PDGF—platelet-derived growth factor	Cell proliferation, neuronal survival
aFGF—acidic fibroblast growth factor	Neurite regeneration, cell proliferation
bFGF—basic fibroblast growth factor	Neurite regeneration, neovascularisation

TABLE 131.3 Neuronal Attachment and Neurite-Promoting Factors

Factor	Minimal Peptide Sequence
Collagen	RGD
Fibronectin	RGD
Laminin	RGD, SIKVAV, YIGSR
Neural cell adhesion molecule (N-CAM)	Unknown
N-cadherin	Unknown

activity. Two- and three-dimensional substrates containing peptide mimics have been shown to promote neural attachment and regeneration in vitro and in vivo.

Seeding Neuronal Support Cells

Adding neural support cells to the lumen of guidance channels is another strategy being used to improve regeneration or to make regeneration possible over otherwise irreparable gaps. For example, Schwann cells cultured in the lumen of semipermeable guidance channels have been shown to improve nerve repair in adult rodents. Cells harvested from inbred rats were first cultured in PAN/PVC tubes using various ECM gels as stabilizers. The Schwann cells and gel formed a cable at the center of the tube after several days in culture. Once implanted, the cells were in direct contact with the nerve stumps. A dose-dependent relationship between the density of seeded cells and the extent of regeneration was noted. Another approach toward nerve repair involves the use of Schwann cells, fibroblasts, and the like which are genetically engineered to secrete growth factors. The use of support cells which release neuronotrophic and neurite-promoting molecules may enable regeneration over large gaps. There is increasing evidence that PNS elements, especially Schwann cells, are capable of supporting CNS regeneration as well. For example, Schwann-cell-seeded semipermeable channels support regeneration at the level of the dorsal and ventral spinal cord roots and the optic nerve, which are CNS structures.

131.8 Summary

The permeability, textural, and electrical properties of nerve guidance channels can be optimized to impact favorably on regeneration. The release of growth factors, addition of growth substrates, and inclusion of neural support cells and genetically engineered cells also enhance regeneration through guidance channels. Current limitations in PNS repair, especially the problem of repairing long gaps, and in CNS repair, where brain and spinal cord trauma rarely result in appreciable functional return, may benefit from advances in engineering and biology. The ideal guidance system has not been identified but will most likely be a composite device that contains novel synthetic or bioderived materials and that incorporates genetically engineered cells and new products from biotechnology.

References

Aebischer P, Salessiotis AN, Winn SR. 1989. Basic fibroblast growth factor released from synthetic guidance channels facilitates peripheral nerve regeneration across nerve gaps. J Neurosci Res 23:282.

Dyck PJ, Thomas PK. 1993. Peripheral Neuropathy, 3d ed, vol 1, Philadelphia, London, WB Saunders.

Guenard V, Kleitman N, Morrissey TK, et al. 1992. Syngeneic Schwann cells derived from adult nerves seeded in semi permeable guidance channels enhance peripheral nerve regeneration. J Neurosci 12:3310–3320.

LeBeau JM, Ellisman MH, Powell HC. 1988. Ultrastructural and morphometric analysis of long-term peripheral nerve regeneration through silicone tubes. J Neurocytol 17:161.

Longo FM, Hayman EG, Davis GE, et al. 1984. Neurite-promoting factors and extracellular matrix components accumulating in vivo within nerve regeneration chambers. Exp Neurol 81:756.

Lundborg G. 1987. Nerve regeneration and repair: A review. Acta Orthop Scand 58:145.

Lundborg G, Dahlin LB, Danielsen N, et al. 1982. Nerve regeneration in silicone chambers: Influence of gap length and of distal stump components. Exp Neurol 76:361.

Lundborg G, Longo FM, Varon S. 1982. Nerve regeneration model and trophic factors in vivo. Brain Res 232:157.

Raivich G, Kreutzberg GW. 1993. Peripheral nerve regeneration: role of growth factors and their receptors. Int J Dev Neurosci 11(3): 311.

Sunderland S. 1991. Nerve Injuries and Their Repair, Edinburgh, London, Churchill Livingstone.

Valentini RF, Aebischer P. 1991. The role of materials in designing nerve guidance channels and chronic neural interfaces. In P Dario, G Sandini, P Aebischer (eds), Robots and Biological Systems: Towards a New Bionics?, pp 625–636, Berlin, Germany, Springer-Verlag.

Valentini RF, Aebischer P, Winn SR, et al. 1987. Collagen- and laminin-containing gels impede peripheral nerve regeneration through semi-permeable nerve guidance channels. Exp Neurol 98:350.

Valentini RF, Sabatini AM, Dario P, et al. 1989. Polymer electret guidance channels enhance peripheral nerve regeneration in mice. Brain Res 480:300.

Weiss P. 1944. The technology of nerve regeneration: A review. Sutureless tubulation and related methods of nerve repair. J Neurosurg 1:400.

Williams LR, Longo FM, Powell HC, et al. 1983. Spatial-temporal progress of peripheral nerve regeneration within a silicone chamber: Parameters for a bioassay. J Comp Neurol 218:460.

132

Tracheal, Laryngeal, and Esophageal Replacement Devices

Tatsuo Nakamura
Kyoto University

Yasuhiko Shimizu
Kyoto University

As the ability to reconstruct parts of the body has increased, so has the potential for complications associated with the replacement devices used to do so. Some of the most significant complications associated with replacement devices, such as vascular prostheses, cardiac valves, and artificial joints, are caused by infections at the implantation site. It is well known that the presence of a foreign material impairs host defenses and that prolonged infections cannot be cured unless the foreign material is removed from the site of infection. As the trachea, larynx, and esophagus are located at sites facing the "external environment," these prostheses are exposed to a high risk of infections and severe complications. The development of an artificial trachea, esophagus, and larynx is way behind that of artificial vascular grafts even though they are all tubular organs. In this chapter, we review conventional prostheses and their problems and limitations and discuss the current state of developments in this field.

132.1 Tracheal Replacement Devices

End-to-end anastomosis has been one of the standard operations for tracheal reconstruction. However, in patients in whom a large length of trachea has to be resected, this procedure is often difficult (the resectable limit is now considered to be approximately 6 cm). In such patients, alternative methods are required to reconstruct the airway. Such reconstructive methods can be classified into the following three categories: (1) reconstruction with autologous tissue, (2) reconstruction with nonautologous trachea (that is, transplantation), and (3) reconstruction with artificial material. The only one of these operative techniques which achieves good clinical results in the long term is the first (reconstruction with autologous tissue), particularly cervical tracheal reconstruction using an autologous skin flap conduit.

Designs of Artificial Tracheae

The artificial tracheae developed previously were designed according to one of two concepts. One is that the implanted prosthesis alone replaces the resected area of trachea, and the inner surface of the reconstructed trachea is not endothelialized. The other is that the implanted prosthesis is incorporated by the host tissue and its inner surface is endothelialized. These two types of prosthesis are called *nonporous* and *mesh types*, respectively, which reflects the materials from which they are made.

Nonporous Tube–Type Artificial Tracheae

The study of nonporous tube–type trachea has a long history, and many materials have been tried repeatedly for artificial tracheae. However, the results have been unsatisfactory, and now only one prosthesis of this type remains on the market, the *Neville artificial trachea,* which comprises a silicone tube with two suture rings attached to each of its ends (Fig. 132.1). Neville used this trachea in 62 patients, from 1970 to 1988, some of whom survived for a long time [1]. However, late complications, such as migration of the artificial trachea and granular tissue formation at the anastomosis, were inevitable in many cases and occurred within several months and even as late as 2 years after implantation. Therefore, the Neville prosthesis is not used for patients with benign tracheal disease, because clinically, even if a large portion of the trachea up to the bifurcation has to be resected, the airway can be reconstructed easily by tracheotomy using a skin flap with sternal resection. For the alleviation of tracheal stenosis, *silicone T-tubes* (Fig. 132.2) are widely indicated. The major advantage of such nonporous tubular prostheses is that airway patency can be ensured. Therefore, for patients for whom end-to-end anastomosis is impossible, nonporous prostheses may be used as a last resort to avoid threatened suffocation (asphyxiation).

Tracheal replacement using the Neville artificial trachea requires the following operative procedure:

1. *Right-sided posterolateral skin incision and 4th or 5th intercostal thoracotomy.* Up to the stage of tracheal resection, the operative procedure is similar to that for standard tracheal resection. However, because the tension at the anastomosis is not as high as that with an end-to-end anastomosis, neither hilar nor laryngeal release is often necessary.

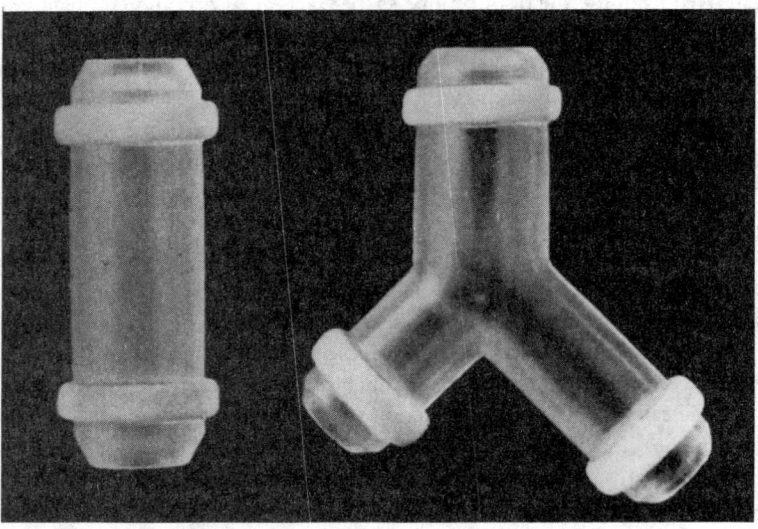

FIGURE 132.1 Neville artificial trachea constructed with a nonporous silicone tube with Dacron suture rings.

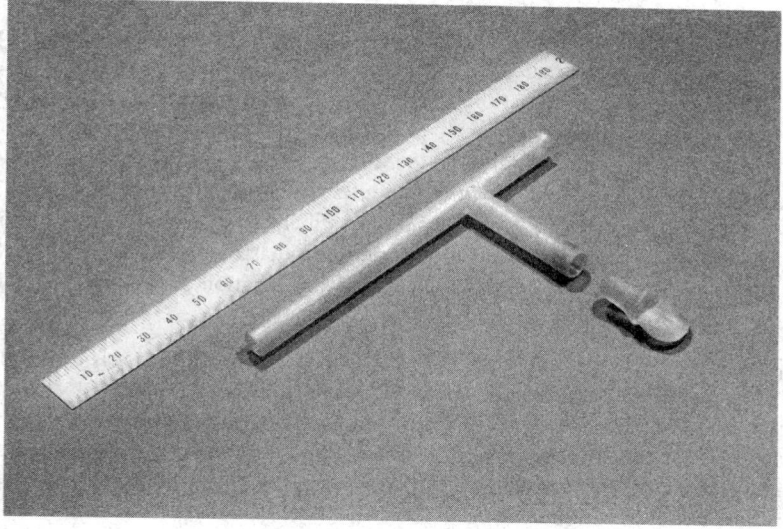

FIGURE 132.2   Silicone T-Tube.

2. *Reconstruction with an artificial trachea.* After resection of the tracheal lesion, the oral intubation tube is drawn back, and the trachea is reintubated via the operative field (Fig. 132.3). In patients who require resection that reaches to near the bifurcation, the second intubation tube should be placed in the left main bronchus. An artificial trachea with a diameter similar to that of the tracheal end is used. Any small differences in their diameters can be compensated

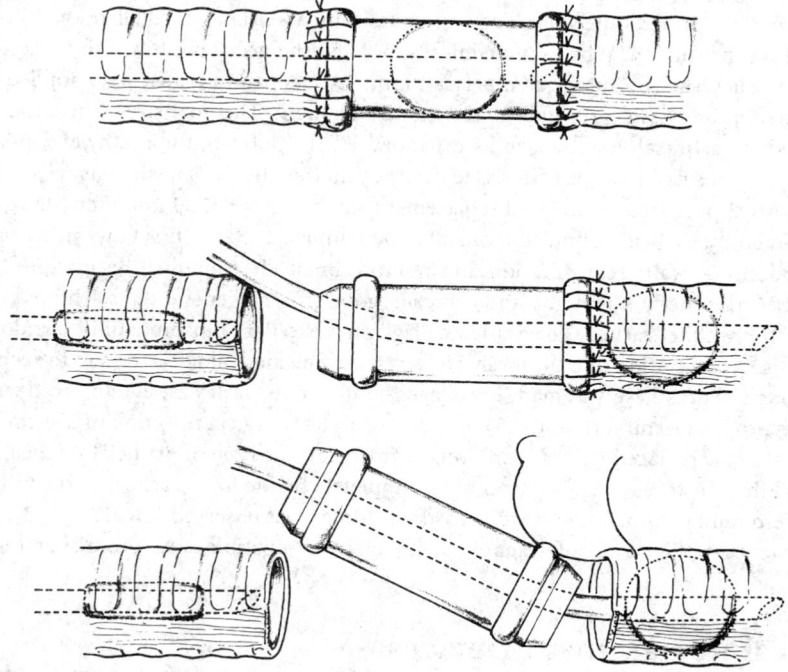

FIGURE 132.3   Operation proceeding of tracheal reconstruction using an artificial trachea.

for by suturing. Anastomosis is carried out using 4-0 absorbable sutures, 2 mm apart, with interrupted suturing. The tracheal sutures are attached to the tracheal cartilage. On completion of the anastomosis on one side, the oral intubation tube is readvanced, and the other side is anastomosed under oral ventilation. After anastomosis, an air leakage test at a pressure of 30 cmH_2O is carried out. In order to avoid rupture of the great vessels near the implanted artificial trachea, they should not be allowed to touch each other. In cases at risk of this occurring, wrapping of the artificial trachea with the greater omentum is also recommended.

3. *Postoperative care.* Frequent postoperative broncofiberscopic checks should be performed to ensure sputum does not come into contact with the anastomosis sites. The recurrent laryngeal nerves on both sides are often injured during the operation, so the movement of the vocal cords should be checked at extubation.

The major reason for the poor results with the Neville tracheal prosthesis during long-term follow-up is considered to be the structure of the prosthesis, that is, the nonelasticity of the tube and suture rings. A variety of improvements to this prosthesis have been tried, especially at the areas of interface with the host tissue by suture reinforcement with mesh skirts, increasing the flexibility of the tube, and application of hydroxyapatite to the suture rings. However, the problems at the anastomosis have not been conquered yet.

In an attempt to overcome the problems described above, a new mesh-type artificial trachea has been designed that is intended to be incorporated into the host tissue so that eventually there is no foreign-body–external-environment interface.

Mesh-Type Artificial Tracheae

Porous artificial tracheae are called *mesh-type* because the prosthetic trunk is made of mesh. In the 1950s, several trials of tracheal reconstruction using metallic meshes made of tantalum and stainless steel were conducted. In the 1960s, heavy Marlex mesh was used clinically for tracheal reconstruction, and good short-term results were reported. However, long-term observations showed that this mesh caused rupture of the adjacent great vessels, which was fatal, so it fell gradually out of use for tracheal reconstruction. When used clinically, because the heavy mesh was rough and not airtight, other tissues, such as autografted pericardium, fascia, or dura mater, were applied to seal it until the surrounding tissue grew into it and made it air-tight. The pore size of materials conventionally used for artificial vessels, such as expanded PTFE (polytetrafluoroethylene, pore size of $15 \sim 30$ μm), is so small that the host tissue cannot penetrate the mesh, which is rejected eventually. The optimal pore size for tracheal replacement mesh is $200 \sim 300$ μm. Fine Marlex mesh is made of polypropylene with a pore size of $200 \sim 300$ μm (Fig. 132.4). It is now widely used clinically for abdominal wall reconstruction and reinforcement after inguinal herniation. Collagen-grafted fine Marlex mesh is air-tight, and clinically, good tissue regeneration is achieved when it is used to patch-graft the trachea. The grafted collagen has excellent biocompatibility and promotes connective tissue infiltration into the mesh. However, the fine mesh alone is too soft to keep the tube open, so a tracheal prosthesis was made of collagen-grafted fine Marlex mesh reinforced with a continuous polypropylene spiral (Fig. 132.5). In dogs, complete surgical resection of a 4-cm length of trachea, which was replaced with a 5-cm long segment of this type of artificial trachea, was performed, and the prostheses were incorporated completely by the host tracheae and confluent formation of respiratory epithelium on each prosthetic lumen was observed (Fig. 132.6) [2]. These results indicate that this artificial trachea is highly biocompatible and promising for clinical application.

132.2 Laryngeal Replacement Devices

Total laryngectomy is one of the standard operations for laryngeal carcinomas. As radiation therapy and surgery have progressed, the prognosis associated with laryngeal carcinoma has improved. The

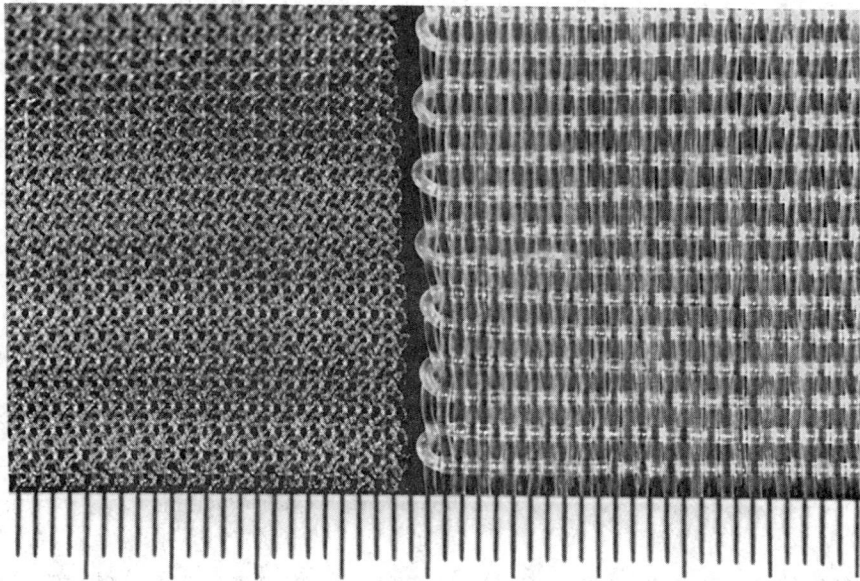

FIGURE 132.4 Marlex Mesh, fine (left) and heavy (right) (division of the scale: mm).

curability of total laryngeal carcinoma is now almost 70%, and therefore many patients survive for a long time after surgery. Individuals who have undergone laryngectomy are called *laryngectomees* or *laryngectomized patients*, and for them, laryngeal reconstruction is of the utmost importance. However, because the larynx is situated just beneath the oral cavity, where the danger of infection is high, successful reconstruction with foreign materials is very difficult. As yet, no total replacement device for the larynx has been developed, and laryngeal transplantation, although apparently feasible, is still at the animal experiment stage.

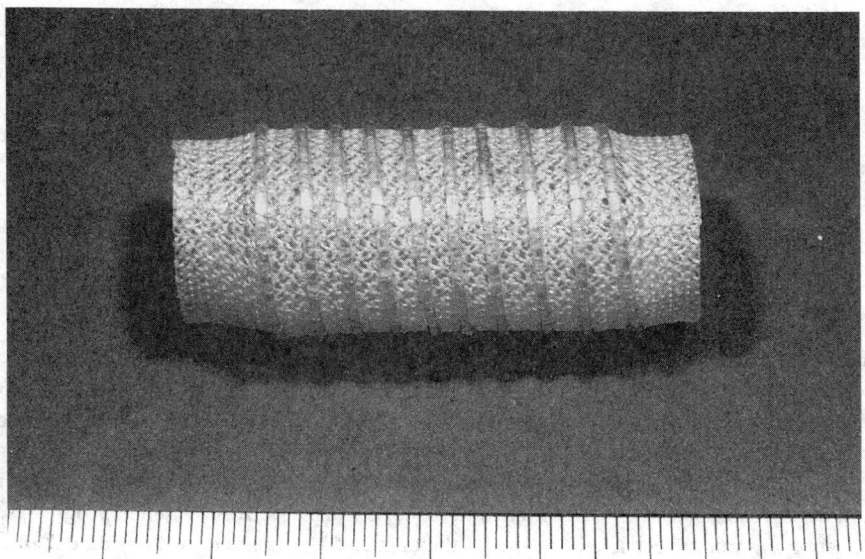

FIGURE 132.5 New artificial trachea made from collagen-conjugated fine Marlex mesh.

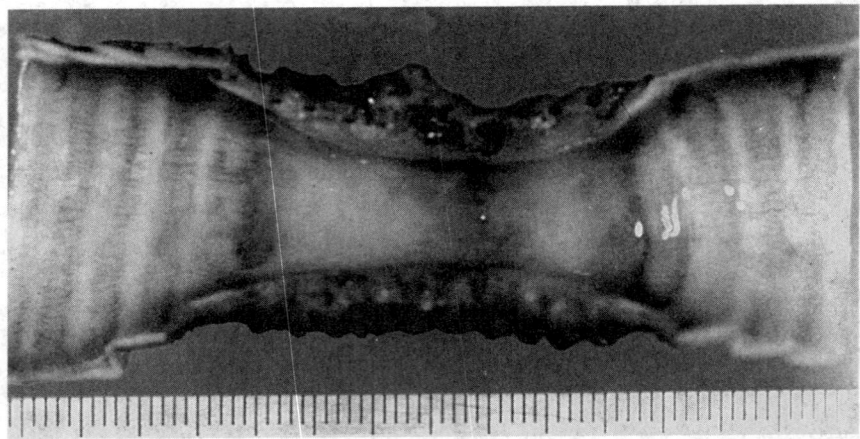

FIGURE 132.6   Macroscopic inner view of the reconstructed trachea 6 months after operation. Inner surface is covered with smooth and lustrous soft regenerated tissue.

The larynx has three major functions: (1) phonation, (2) respiration, and (3) protection of the lower airway during swallowing. Of these, phonation is considered to be the most important. The conventional so-called *artificial larynx* can only substitute phonation. A variety of methods have been developed to recover phonation after total laryngectomy, which is called *vocal rehabilitation*. Methods for vocal rehabilitation are classified as (1) esophageal speech, (2) artificial larynx, and (3) surgical laryngoplasty. Two-thirds of laryngectomees learn esophageal speech as their means of communication. For the rest, an artificial larynx and surgical laryngoplasty are indicated. The typical devices are the *pneumatic* and *electrical larynx*, which are driven by the expiratory force and electric energy, respectively. Tracheo-esophageal (T-E) fistula with voice prosthesis is the most popular method in surgical laryngoplasty. Figure 132.7 illustrates the mechanical structures of typical artificial larynxes.

Pneumatic Larynxes

The first pneumatic mechanical device was developed by Tapia in 1883. Several variations of pneumatic larynxes are now used. In Fig. 132.8, the pneumatic device uses expired air from the tracheo stoma to vibrate a rubber band or reed to produce a low frequency sound, which is transmitted to the mouth via a tube. Pneumatic transoral larynxes produce excellent natural speech, which is better than that with other artificial larynxes, but their disadvantages are that they are conspicuous and that regular cleaning and mopping of saliva leakage is necessary.

Electrical Artificial Larynxes

The *transcervical electrolarynx* is an electric, handheld vibrator that is placed on the neck to produce sound (Fig. 132.9). The frequency used is $100 \sim 200$ Hz. The vibrations of the electrolarynx are conducted to the neck tissue and create a low-frequency sound in the hypopharynx. This is the most popular artificial larynx. The *transoral artificial laryngeal device* is a handheld electric device that produces a low-pitched sound which is transmitted to the back of the mouth by a connecting tube placed in the patient's mouth. As microelectronic science progresses, great hopes of applying microelectric techniques to the artificial larynx are now entertained, and some devices have been designed, although implantable laryngeal prostheses have not achieved widespread use.

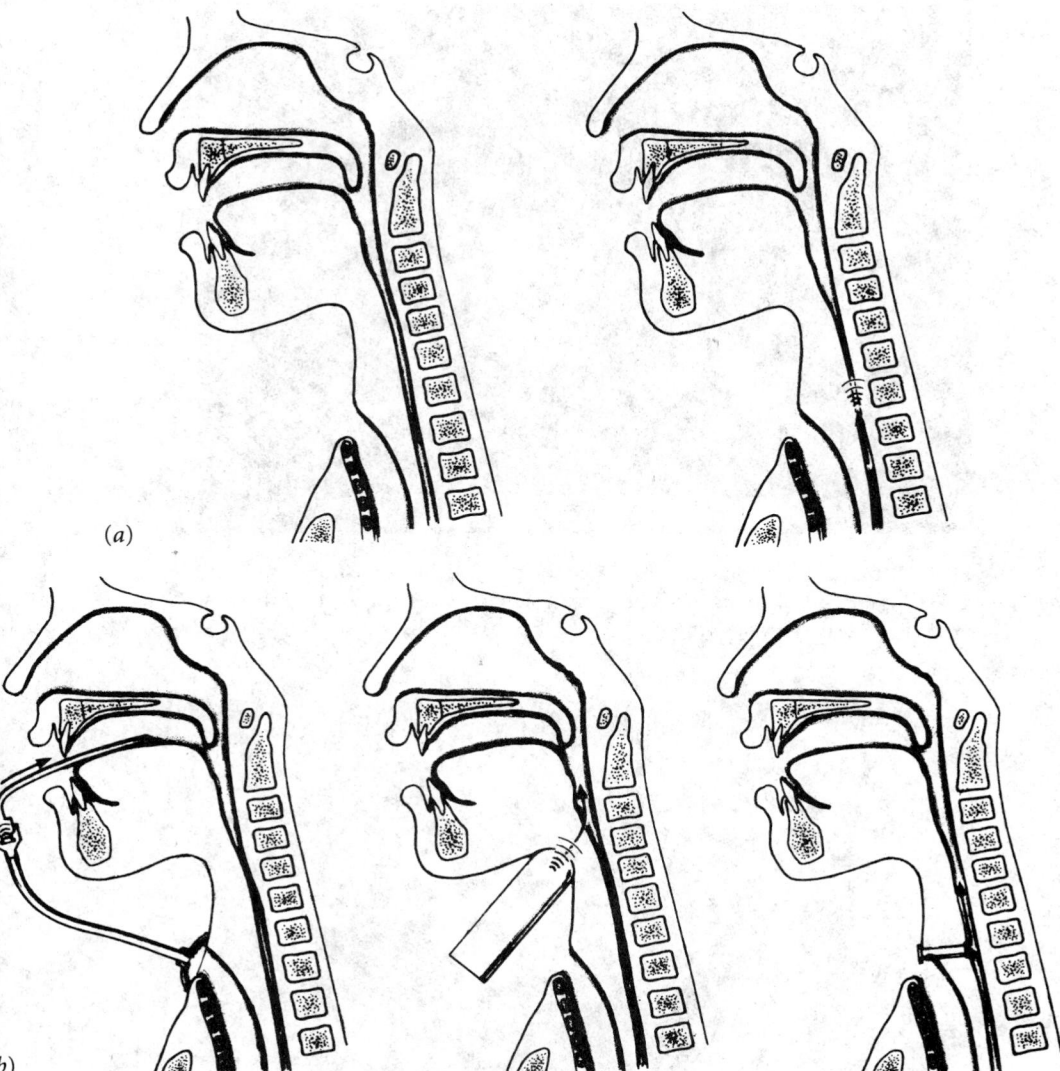

FIGURE 132.7 (*a*) Sagital views of the laryngectomee (left) and esophageal speech (right). Air flow from the esophagus makes the sound. (*b*) Pneumatic larynx (reed type) (left); electrical artificial larynx (transcervical type), (center); voice prosthesis (T-E shut) of Blom-& Singer method, right.

Voice Prostheses

As well as the artificial larynxes described above, tracheo-esophageal (T-E) fistula prostheses are now widely used for vocal rehabilitation, and excellent speech and voice results have been achieved. In 1980, Singer and Blom developed and introduced the first simple method, which is called Blom and Singer's voice prosthesis. The principle of the tracheo-esophageal fistula technique is to shunt expired pulmonary air through a voice prosthesis device into the esophagus to excite the mucosal tissue to vibrate. A fistula is made by puncturing the posterior wall of the trachea 5 mm below the upper margin of the tracheal stoma, and when a patient speaks, he/she manually occludes the stoma to control the expiratory flow through the fistula to the oral cavity. The voice prosthesis has a one-way value to prevent saliva leakage (Fig. 132.10).

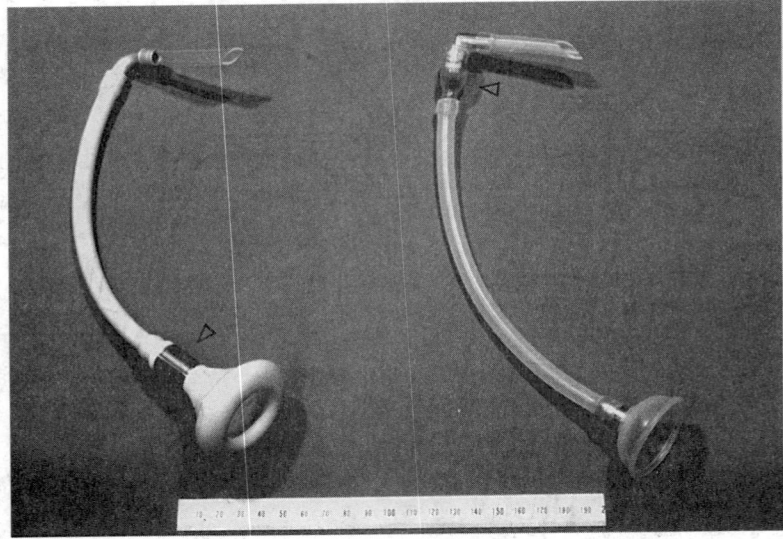

FIGURE 132.8 Pneumatic larynxes: Myna (left) (Nagashima Medical Instrument Tokyo, Japan) and Okumura Artificial larynx (Okumura, Osaka, Japan) (right). Arrow marks indicate the portions of reed and rubber band, respectively.

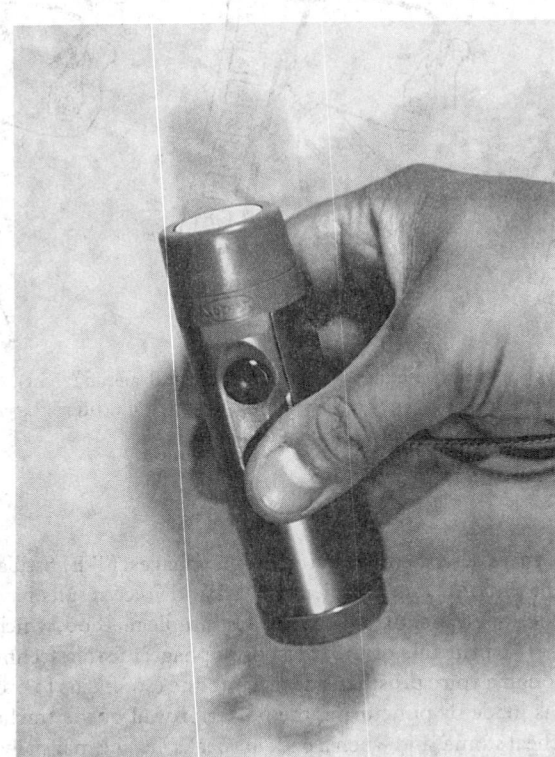

FIGURE 132.9 Electric artificial larynx (transcervical type): Servox (Dr Kuhn & Co. GmBH, Köln, Germany).

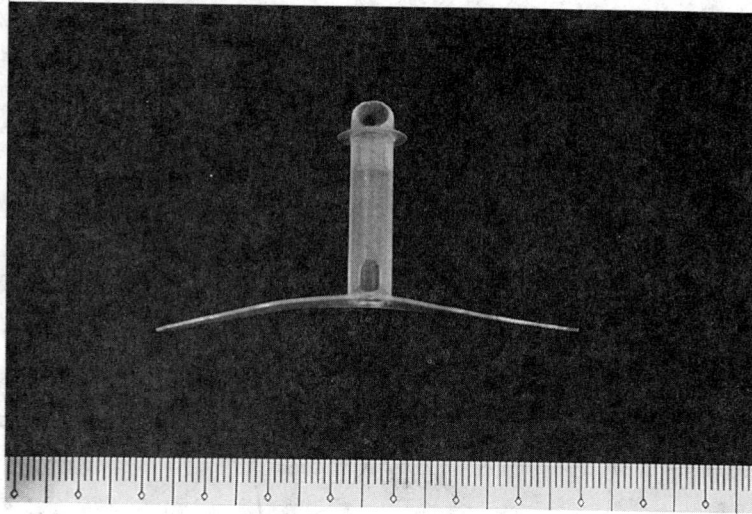

FIGURE 132.10 Voice prosthesis (Bivona, Indiana, USA). This valved tube is inserted into a surgically placed tracheo-esophageal fistula for voice restoration following laryngectomy.

132.3 Artificial Esophagi (Esophageal Prostheses)

In patients with esophageal cancer, the esophagus is resected and reconstructed using a piece of pediculated alimentary tract, such as the gastric conduit, colon, or ileum. However, in some cases, it is impossible to use autologous alimentary tract, for example, in patients who have undergone gastrectomy. In such cases, an artificial esophagus is indicated. However, with the exception of extracorporeal-type esophagi and intraesophageal stent tubes, the esophageal replacement devices developed have remained far from useful in clinical reconstructive practice. The main reason is anastomosis dehiscence, which often leads to fatal infections, as well as prosthetic dislodgement, migration, and narrowing at a late stage.

The conventional artificial esophagi now used in the clinic can be broadly classified into two types: extracorporeal and intraesophageal stents. *Extracorporeal artificial esophagi* are used as bypasses from cervical esophageal to gastric fistulae (Fig. 132.11). They are used during the first stage of two-stage esophageal reconstruction. They are made of latex rubber or silicone, but since the development of IVH method, their use is now extremely rare.

Intraesophageal stent types of artificial esophagus are made from a rubber or plastic tube, which is inserted in the stenotic part of the esophagus (Fig. 132.12). They are used only for unresectable esophageal carcinoma, i.e., they are not indicated for resectable cases. Therefore, conventional artificial esophagi are only palliative devices for use as stop-gap measures.

Development of New Artificial Esophagi

In contrast to the palliative artificial esophagi, the ideal artificial esophagus would replace the resected part of the esophagus by itself. The artificial esophagi of this type are classified according to the materials from which they are made, namely natural substances, artificial materials, and their composites (hybrids).

Artificial Esophagi Made of Natural Substances

The first report of an artificial esophagus made of a natural substance was the skin conduit developed by Bircher in 1907. Subsequently, esophageal reconstruction using a variety of natural

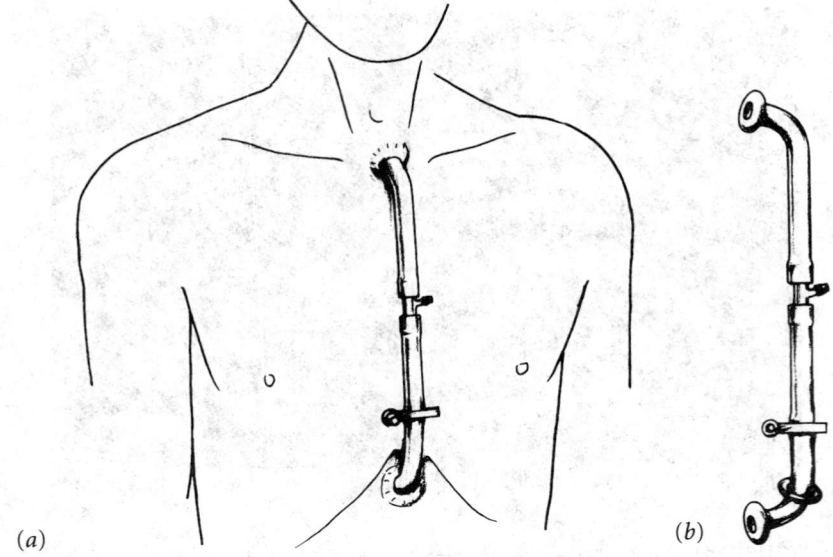

(a)   *(b)*

FIGURE 132.11   Extracorporeal artificial esophagus (Tokyo University type).

substances—muscle fasciae, isolated jejunum; autologous aorta; aortic homograft, autologous esophagus; connective tissue conduit; trachea; and freeze-dried dura mater homograft—has been reported. However, none of these has overcome the problems of stenosis, which necessitates continuous bougieing, and other complications at the anastomosis sites.

Artificial Esophagi Made of Artificial Materials

The first trial of an esophagus made of an artificial material was carried out by Neuhof, who, in 1922, used a rubber tube to reconstruct the cervical esophagus. Subsequently, several artificial materials have been tried repeatedly, such as polyethylene, Dacron, stainless steel mesh, tantalum mesh, dimethylpolysiloxane, polyvinylformal sponge, Teflon, nylon, silicone rubber, collagen-silicone, Dacron-silastic, acrylresin, and expanded PTFE tubes, but all the trials ended in failure. These materials were foreign bodies, after all, and the host tissues continuously rejected them, which caused anastomotic dehiscence followed by infections. Even rare cases, whose artificial esophagi escaped early rejection, did not avoid the late complications, such as prosthetic migration and esophageal stenosis.

Hybrid Artificial Esophagi

Cultured cells are now widely used for hybrid artificial organs, especially for metabolic organs, such as the liver and pancreas. A hybrid artificial esophagus comprising a latissimus dorsi muscle tube, the inner surface of which is epithelialized by human cultured esophageal epithelial cells, is being studied by the Keio University group [3]. Human esophageal epithelial cells cultured on collagen gel for 10 days were transplanted onto the surfaces of the lattisimus dorsi muscles of athymic mice, and new epithelial cells were observed, which indicates it may be possible to develop an artificial esophagus incorporating cultured epithelial cells.

New Concepts in Artificial Esophageal Design

The previous studies on artificial esophagi are a history of how to prevent the host tissue from recognizing the artificial esophagus as a foreign body, and all the trials, without exception, resulted in failure. Currently, an artificial esophagus made according to a completely new design concept is

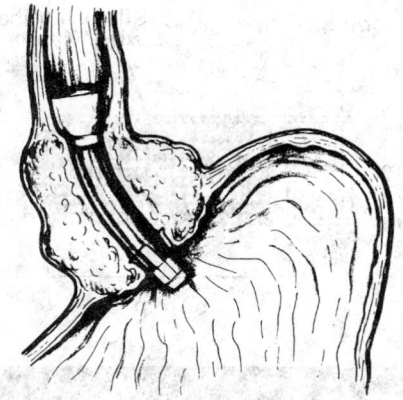

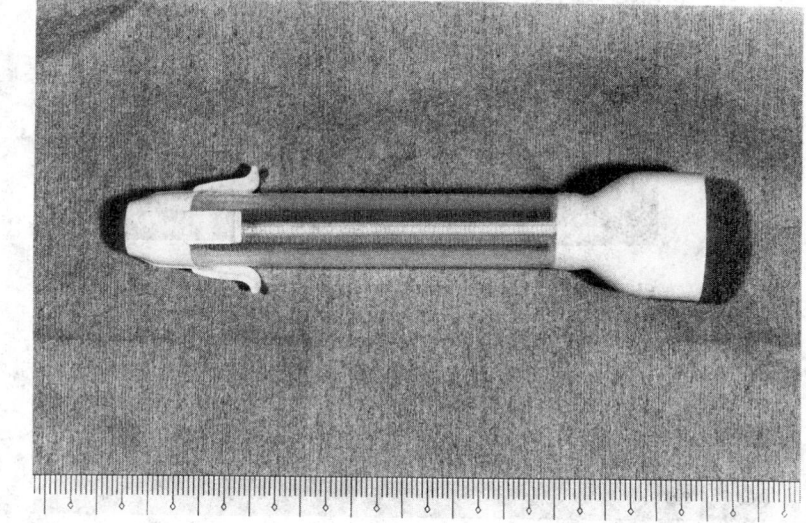

(a)

FIGURE 132.12 Intraesophageal type of artificial esophagus. (Sumitomo Bakelite Co., Ltd., Tokyo, Japan).

undergoing trials. The outer collagen sponge layer of the prosthesis is intended to be replaced with host tissue over a period of time, and its inner tube acts as a palliative (temporary) stent until the outer layer has been replaced by host tissue. This type of artificial esophagus comprises an inner silicone tube and an outer tube of collagen sponge (Fig. 132.13), which is nonantigenic and has excellent biocompatibility, as well as promoting tissue regeneration in the form of an extracellular matrix. In dogs implanted with a 5-cm length of this artificial esophagus, esophageal regeneration was accomplished in 3 weeks, and all the early complications at the anastomosis were overcome. However, in dogs from which the inner stents were removed as soon as mucosal regeneration was accomplished, stenosis developed rapidly, and the regenerated esophagus began to constrict. Such stenosis and constriction could not be overcome, even when autologous buccal mucosal cells were seeded onto the collagen sponge. Accordingly, on the basis of the hypothesis that stenosis and constriction depend on the maturity of the regenerated submucosal tissue, stent removal was postponed for at least 1 week after mucosal epithelialization of the artificial esophagus was complete. Late stenotic complications did not occur, and regeneration of muscle tissue and esophageal glands was observed (Fig. 132.14) [4]. The regenerated esophagus showed adequate physiologic function and

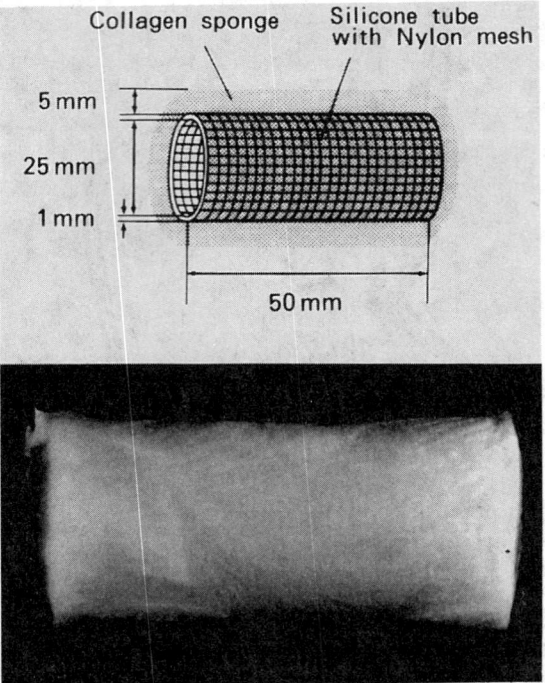

FIGURE 132.13   An artificial esophagus made of collagen sponge which is intended to be replaced with host tissue.

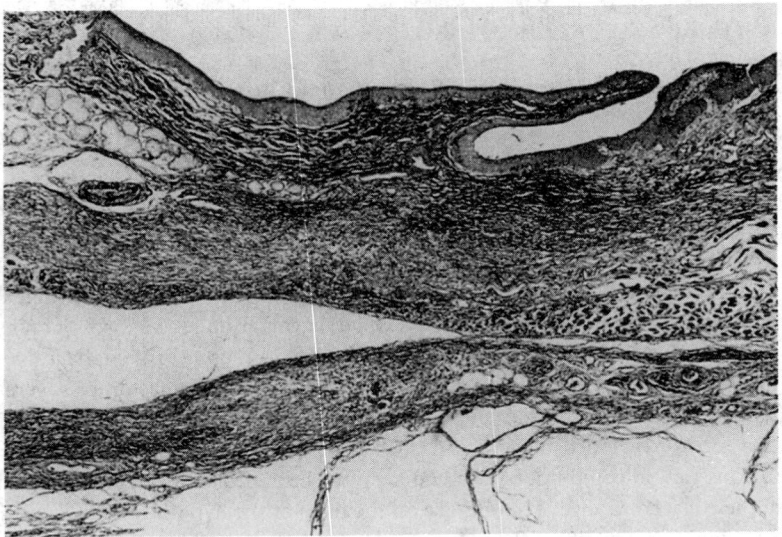

FIGURE 132.14   Pathologic finding of a regenerated esophageal tissue in a dog using the artificial esophagus (Fig. 132.13). Continuous epithelial layer and the muscle and esophageal gland were regenerated at the interposed area.

pathologically satisfactory results. The limit to the length of the esophagus that can be resected successfully was reported to be 9 cm, and the longest successful artificial esophagus developed hitherto was 5 cm. In order to achieve more widespread use, artificial esophagi which can be used for longer reconstructions are needed. Although still at the stage of animal experiments, the long-term observations indicate that typical difficulties, such as anastomotic leakage, ablation, and dislocation of the prosthesis, have been overcome, which suggests this type of prosthesis will have a promising future in clinical practice.

Defining Terms

Collagen: A main supportive protein of connective tissue, bone, skin, and cartilage. One-third of protein of vertebrate animal consists of collagen.

End-to-end anastomosis: An operative union after resecting the lesion, each end to be joined in a plane vertical to the ultimate flow through the structures.

Expanded PTFE (polytetrafluoroethylene): PTFE is polymer made from tetrafluoroethylene $(CF_2 = CF_2)$, with the structure of $-CF_2-CF_2-$. It provides excellent stability chemically and thermally. Teflon is the trade mark of PTFE of Du Pont Co. Expanded PTFE has a microporous structure which has elastisity and antithrombogenisity in the body and is medically applied for vascular grafts or surgical seats.

Extracellular matrix (ECM): The substances which are produced by connective tissue cells. The two major components of the extracellular matrix are collagen and proteoglycans. There are a number of other macromolecules which provide important functions such as tissue growth, regeneration, or aging.

Heavy Marlex mesh and fine Marlex mesh: Surgical mesh is used for reconstruction of the defect that results from massive resection. Most popular surgical meshes are Marlex meshes. Heavy mesh is made of high-density polyethylene and has been used for reconstruction of chest wall. Fine mesh is made of polypropylene and is now widely used for abdominal wall reconstruction or reinforcement of inguinal herniation operation.

Hilar release and laryngeal release: The pulmonis hilus is the depression of the mediastinal surface of the lung where the blood vessels and the bronchus enter. The hilus is fixed by the pulmonary ligament to downward. In order to reduce the tension at the tracheal anastomoses, the pulmonary ligament is released surgically. This method is called *hilar release*. At the resection and reconstruct of upper trachea, the larynx can be also released from its upper muscular attachment. This method is called *laryngeal release* and up to 5 cm of tracheal mobilization may be achieved.

Hydroxyapatite: An inorganic compound, $Ca_{10}(PO_4)_6(OH)_2$, found in the matrix of bone and the teeth which gives rigidity to these structures. The biocompatibility of hydroxyapatite has attracted special interest.

IVH (intravenous hyperalimentation): An alimentation method for patients who cannot eat. A catheter is placed in the great vessel, through which high concentration alimentation is given continuously.

Silicone T-tube: A self-retaining tube in the shape of a *T* which is made of silicone. Tracheal T-tube is used popularly for tracheal stenotic disease and serves both as a tracheal stent and tracheotomy tube. One side branchi of T-tube projects from the tracheotomy orifice.

References

1. Neville WE, Bolanowski PJP, Kotia GG. 1990. Clinical experience with the silicone tracheal prosthesis. J Thorac Cardiovasc Surg 99:604.
2. Okumura N, Nakamura T, Takimoto Y, et al. 1993. A new tracheal prosthesis made from collagen grafted mesh. ASAIO J 39:M475.

3. Sato M, Ando N, Ozawa S, et al. 1993. A hybrid artificial esophagus using cultured human esophageal cells. ASAIO J 39:M554.
4. Takimoto Y, Okumura N, Nakamura T, et al. 1993. Long-term follow up of the experimental replacement of the esophagus with a collagen-silicone composite tube. ASAIO J 39:M736.

Further Information

Proceedings of the American Society of Artificial Internal Organs Conference are published annually by the American Society of Artificial Internal Organs (ASAIO). These proceedings include the latest developments in the field of reconstructive devices each year. The monthly journal *Journal of Thoracic and Cardiovascular Surgery* reports advances in tracheal and esophageal prosthetic instruments. An additional reference is H.F. Mahieu, ``Voice and speech rehabilitation following laryngectomy, Groningen,'' the Netherlands, Rijksuniversiteit Groningen, 1988.

133

Artificial Blood

Marcos Intaglietta
*University of California
at San Diego*

Robert M. Winslow
*University of California
at San Diego*

Blood is a key therapeutic component in the treatment of injury, and its availability is a critical factor that limits effective recovery of victims of severe blood losses. The need for an artificial substitute to blood has been present since the roles of the heart, the blood vessel, and blood were established in the 17th century. An artificially made material provides the possibility of introducing features not available in the natural product, such as freedom from transmission of infectious diseases, elimination of the need for cross-matching, universal compatibility, long-term stability at ambient conditions, and reduced cost.

Central to the need for an artificial blood substitute is the fact that transfusion of red blood cells is associated with risks, mainly the hemolytic transfusion reaction and infection of the recipient with agents transmitted by donor blood. The magnitude and nature of this risk is variable and controversial, being generally accepted to be of the order of 1% (1 adverse outcome per 100 units transfused) for minor reactions, to a probability of 0.001% of undergoing a fatal hemolytic reaction. Current risks of becoming infected with hepatitis B virus is in the range of 0.002%, and non-A non-B hepatitis is 0.03%. Current probability of becoming infected with the human immunodeficiency virus from transfused blood is 1 adverse reaction per 225,000 units of blood transfused.

133.1 Modern History of Blood Transfusion and Blood Substitutes

Physiologic saline as a blood substitute was introduced around 1875. The substances that are responsible for the incompatibility reactions and hemolysis of blood were discovered in 1900, which led to blood typing. The finding that sodium citrate and glucose prevented coagulation of blood was the final step in the introduction and relatively safe use of blood transfusion. World War II caused the development of the blood banking system, and the American Red Cross begun establishing blood banks in 1947.

Early experiments with saline solutions showed that addition of potassium and calcium ions significantly improved the effectiveness of this fluid in maintaining the viability of tissue. Presently lactate is added to this composite solution, which is gradually converted into sodium bicarbonate, which prevents alkalosis. This constitutes "lactate-Ringers," which is the most widely used solution for intravenous delivery.

Gum-saline gained popularity as a plasma expander after World War I. The oncotic material is galactoso-gluconic acid with molecular weight 1500. This material was used to treat hemorrhagic shock and had a half-life in the circulation of approximately 30 h.

Blood plasma (the fluid in which red blood cells are suspended) and serum, the same fluid from which coagulation factors and platelets have been removed, were recognized early on to be superior to crystalloid solutions in maintaining tissue viability, and this effect was correctly attributed to the oncotic pressure produced by the large molecules in solution, mainly albumin whose molecular weight is 69 kDA. In 1947, it was shown that bovine plasma could be used if globulins were removed.

Dextrans are high-molecular-weight polysaccharides consisting of linked glucose molecules which are produced in the range of molecular weights ranging from 4–250 kDA [Hint, 1968]. Clinically used molecules have molecular weights 40, 60, and 70 kDA. They have proven to be quite safe as colloidal substitute for albumin, and their use has promoted the development of *hemodilution* both as a means of reestablishing blood volume with a noncellular blood substitute and as a therapeutic procedure in ischemia. Dextrans have a long half-life in the circulation and are completely metabolized into CO_2 and H_2O. In Europe they were regarded as the colloid of choice for volume replacement and shock treatment until recently, being gradually replaced by hydroxyethyl starch, a chemically modified material with molecular weight from 40–450 kDA depending on the type and formulation.

Gelatins with molecular weight in the range of 30–35 kDA were in use in the United States until 1978, when they were declared unsafe and withdrawn by the FDA.

Perfluorocarbons were introduced in the 1960s. These materials are fluorinated polymers, similar to Teflon, which bind reversibly with oxygen. They are water insoluble but can be introduced in water in the form of an emulsion. A drawback is that perfluorocarbon's binding to oxygen is linearly related to pO_2, and therefore in order to carry sufficient oxygen the lungs must be exposed to high oxygen atmospheres.

Hemoglobin was considered early on as a potential oxygen-carrying blood substitute because of the high oxygen-carrying capacity. The introduction of *stroma-free hemoglobin* eliminated many of the toxic effects noted with the use of these solutions. An early problem due to the dissociation of native hemoglobin into dimers and their rapid secretion by the kidney is now resolved through crosslinking, polymerization, and binding with dextran and polyethylene glycol. Recombinant DNA techniques are also being studied to produce molecules with the desired properties.

Ultimately it is likely that the universal blood substitute of choice will be an encapsulated material which allows for introduction of the oxygen carrier at relatively high concentrations, while reducing its oncotic and biologic activity, in the same way that red blood cells are constructed. This is becoming possible through the advances of liposome technology.

133.2 Blood Components and Characteristics

The primary function of blood is tissue oxygen supply and extraction of carbon dioxide. It collects food from the gastrointestinal tact, eliminates metabolites through the kidneys, neutralizes foreign biologic agents, and dissipates heat generated by the metabolic processes.

Whole blood is a "fluid" tissue composed of cellular and molecular elements suspended in water. Red cells are the predominant cellular component of blood and occupy on the order of 40–50% of the blood volume (5×10^6 cells/mm³). This fraction is termed the *hematocrit*. For every 1000 red blood cells there is 1 white cell, in conditions of normal health. The major function of red cells is to transport oxygen, which is accomplished through the reversible binding with the contained hemoglobin. Each 100 ml of blood contain approximately 15 g of hemoglobin, which, when saturated with oxygen, binds 20 ml of O_2 (760 mmHg, 37°C). Blood O_2 transport is determined by the O_2-binding properties of hemoglobin and the transport properties of blood and the circulation. Red cells have a density of 1.08 g/ml and average life in circulation of 120 days. Red cells are in osmotic equilibrium with the sodium chloride dissolved in plasma at a concentration of 0.85–0.90% by weight. The thickness of the red cell membrane is 60–200 Å. The red cell membrane is impermeable to cations but permeable to anions, which move through porelike structures estimated to be of the order of 7 Å diameter.

Red cells behave like polyanions when in suspension. The are very flexible and present a bidiscoidal shape. These two factors determine that they can undergo large deformations without altering their surface area.

Plasma is about 90% water by weight, where most of the solid content is plasma protein (7%), inorganic materials (1%), and the reminder different organic substances. Free ions cause an osmotic pressure of approximately 8 atmospheres, equivalent to a NaCl solution of 0.9% by weight (physiologic saline). The wall of the exchange vessels is freely permeable to water and ions, and therefore the significant osmotic pressure is that due to the larger molecules, namely albumin, which produces an oncotic pressure on the order of 25 mmHg.

The concentration of inorganic substances in serum is given in Table 133.1. The concentrations are given in milliequivalents per liter. To obtain the concentration mg/100 ml, multiply by the molecular weight and divide by 10. The number in milliequivalents is directly related to the osmotic effects exerted by the amount if material is equal to 1 mole.

Plasma contains a variety of proteins, which are the prime determinants in producing the oncotic pressure needed to maintain water in the circulatory compartment. Albumin and globulins with molecular weights of 69 kDA and 90–160 kDA, respectively, provide the largest contribution. The ratio albumin/globulin, A/G, by weight ranges from 1.5:1 to 2.0/1.

Viscosity

The viscosity of blood is a complex issue from both theoretical and experimental considerations. The basic studies on the viscosity of suspensions were made by Einstein, who determined that the viscosity of a suspension η_s is related to the viscosity of the suspending medium η_0 by the equation

$$\eta_s = \eta_o(1 + 2.5c)$$

where c is the volumetric concentration of the particles (hematocrit, in the case of blood). This expression is valid for concentration up to 1%. A formula that predicts the viscosity of the suspension up to approximately 40% concentration is

$$\eta_s = \frac{\eta_o}{1 - 2.5c} = \eta_o(1 + 2.5c + 6.25\,c^2 + \cdots)$$

TABLE 133.1 Concentrations of Inorganic Substances in Serum

	Cations				Anions			
	Na^+	K^+	Ca^{++}	Other	Cl^-	HCO_3^-	Phos.	Other
mEq/L	140	4	5	6	103	29	2	21
Range	±5	±0.5	±1.0	±5	±0.5		±1.0	
mg/100 ml	330	16	10	365	64		34	
Total		155 mEq/L					155 mEq/L	

The viscosity of blood is approximately described by this equation because the particles are non-spherical and flexible, and the concentration is high. The viscosity of blood is shear dependent, where the relationship between shear stress τ and shear rate γ is relatively well fitted by Casson's equation

$$\tau^{1/2} = K\gamma^{1/2} + \tau_o^{1/2}$$

where K is the "Casson viscosity" and τ_o is the yield stress. This equation has been found to be accurate in the range of shear rates of 1–100,000 s^{-1}. The nonlinear behavior of Casson's equation is due to the yield stress; however, in normal circumstances this parameter is small (0.1 dyne/cm^2).

In physiologic conditions the principal determinant of blood viscosity is hematocrit [Lipowsky et al., 1980]. There is a linear relationship between hematocrit and the logarithm of viscosity, which is relatively independent of shear rate in the range of 40–200 s^{-1}. The relationship between hematocrit, vascular resistance, and blood flow velocity is nonlinear because the reduced hematocrit changes the distribution of pressure losses in the circulation in a nonlinear manner. As a result of the decreased systemic viscosity, a greater portion of the systemic pressure is delivered to the capillary bed, thus improving perfusion. Some of this pressure is transmitted to the end point, the right atrium, which improves cardiac filling thus improving cardiac output and blood flow velocity, which further decreases blood viscosity.

Oxygen Transport

Red blood cells contain hemoglobin approximately in the amount of 35% by volume. This molecule is a globular protein of 68.4 kDA. It is composed of 4 subunits with molecular weight 16.1 kDA, each containing an iron compound or heme. In humans several hemoglobins occur normally, but their differences are limited to the amino acid sequence.

The relationship between the fractional saturation of hemoglobin with oxygen relative to the oxygen that is dissolved in the plasma surrounding the red blood cells is the *oxygen equilibration curve*. An important point is that the value P_{50} is the pO_2 at which the molecule is half-saturated. If oxygen affinity increases, P_{50} is reduced, and the curve shifts to the left, and vice versa. The principal factors responsible for these shifts are pH, the concentration of 2,3-diphosphocerate (2,3-DPG), CO_2, and temperature.

As a consequence of the sigmoidal shape of the oxygen/hemoglobin equilibration curve, a significant amount of oxygen can be unloaded into the microcirculation where pO_2 is low. Myoglobin, which also binds oxygen reversibly, has such a high affinity for oxygen that it will not release it in the tissue. The iron atom that is part of the hemoglobin molecule is a ferrous ion (Fe^{++}), which can be converted to a ferric ion (F^{+++}) by the process of oxidation. This resulting oxidized hemoglobin is called *methemoglobin*. This material does not bind reversibly to oxygen and is not useful as an oxygen carrier. Normally about 3% of the body's hemoglobin is converted into methemoglobin per day. This process is a source of oxygen free radicals, and the red blood cells are protected from their effects by the presence of comparatively large amounts of methemoglobin reductase.

Blood Products

In blood transfusion therapy, red cells are separated from donated blood, and after determining compatibility they are infused into a patient. Platelets and white cells are separated and transfused to treat bleeding disorders and infections. Coagulation proteins such as the antihemophilic factor are isolated from plasma by fractionation procedures and administered in purified forms. Albumin and gamma globulins are separated from blood and are used clinically. Whole blood or packed red blood cells are the only products currently available to improve or restore oxygen transport in patients. Red blood cells can be stored as blood up to 42 days with appropriate refrigeration and can be stored frozen up to 25 years. However, when frozen and thawed for infusion, they must be used within 24 hours.

133.3 Blood Substitutes and Hemodilution

In general it is possible to survive very low hematocrits, corresponding to losses of the red blood cell mass on the order of 70%; however, our ability to compensate for comparatively smaller losses of blood volume is limited. A 30% deficit in blood volume can lead to irreversible shock if not rapidly corrected.

Maintenance of normovolemia is the objective of most forms of blood substitution or replacement, leading to the dilution of the original blood constituents. This hemodilution produces systemic and microvascular phenomena that underlie all forms of blood replacement and provides a physiologic reference for comparison for blood substitutes. The fluids available to accomplish volume restitution can be broadly classified as crystalloid solutions, colloidal solutions, and oxygen-carrying solutions. For non-oxygen-carrying volume replacement, the variables that can be manipulated in the selection of transport properties for the fluid with which to implement substitution or restitution are oncotic pressure, viscosity, and the oxygen-carrying capacity of the mixture of original blood and substitute.

The end point of any alteration of the transport properties of blood is whether tissue metabolism is sustained, i.e., whether the tissue is adequately oxygenated, a phenomenon that takes place in the microvasculature. Therefore hemodilution must be analyzed not only in terms of systemic effects but also in terms of how these, coupled with the altered composition of blood, influence the transport properties of the microcirculation.

Hematocrit and Blood Viscosity

Blood viscosity is primarily determined by the hematocrit in the larger vessels, whereas it is a weaker function of the systemic hematocrit in the microcirculation. At a given shear rate blood viscosity is approximately proportional to the hematocrit squared and inversely proportional to shear rate according to the relationship

$$\eta = a_s + b_s H^2$$

while microvascular blood viscosity can be empirically described by a relation of the form

$$\eta = a_m + b_m H$$

where η is the blood viscosity in centipoise and a_i's and the b_i's are parameters that depend on shear rate and vessel size [Dintenfass, 1971; Quemada, 1971]. In the microcirculation, blood viscosity is relatively insensitive to shear rate. These relationships show that when hematocrit is reduced, systemic viscous pressure losses decrease much more rapidly than those in the microvasculature, although in the microcirculatory the A-V pressure drop is not very much affected. The net result is that if arterial pressure remains constant, hemodilution produces a significant pressure redistribution in the circulation [Mirhashemi et al., 1987b].

An important systemic pressure effect produced by the lowered hematocrit and blood viscosity occurs in the venous return where central venous pressure is increased, which improves cardiac performance and increases cardiac output. This effect translates into an increased blood flow velocity and shear rate and therefore lowers blood viscosity in the systemic circulation [Richardson & Guyton, 1959].

Hemodilution and Oxygen Transport

The decrease in hematocrit lowers the intrinsic oxygen-carrying capacity of blood, but this effect is compensated by the increased blood flow velocity due to the lowered blood viscosity, which increases the rate at which the oxygen-carrying red blood cells are delivered to the microcirculation.

As a consequence of hemodilution, both systemic and capillary oxygen-carrying capacities improve up to hematocrit 33% and are at the normal value at arterial hematocrits on the order of 27%. The maximum improvement in oxygen-carrying capacity is small and at most on the order of 10%. The effect is not sufficient to explain the improvement of tissue oxygenation attributed to hemodilution [Messmer et al., 1972].

The architecture of the microcirculation determines additional effects that support the maintenance of capillary oxygen delivery capacity. The principal barrier for the exit of oxygen from the blood vessels is the resistance to diffusion through the tissue, characterized by the diffusion constant which is fairly uniform and of the same order as that of oxygen through water. This is valid for most soft tissues, including the blood vessel wall. As a consequence, oxygen leaks out continuously from the blood column to the extent that upon arrival to the microcirculation virtually half of the oxygen gathered in the lung has been lost [Duling & Berne, 1973; Mirhashemi et al., 1987*b*].

Oxygen mass balance of a vessel segment into which blood with oxygen-carrying capacity *C* flows with an average velocity *v* shows that the blood pO$_2$ will fall as a function of the distance *x* travelled along the blood vessel according to the expression:

$$P_{\text{blood}} = K_1 e^{-\frac{K_2 D x}{C v}}$$

where K_1 and K_2 are constants and *D* is the diffusion constant for oxygen in the tissue. This equation shows the critical role played by the velocity of blood in lowering the diffusional oxygen losses. However, since the increased velocity is usually due to decreased intrinsic oxygen-carrying capacity of blood, the improved oxygen delivery will manifest itself only when the product *Cv* is higher than normal. Furthermore, any decrease in the intrinsic blood oxygen-carrying capacity not accompanied by increased flow velocities augments diffusional oxygen loss.

The fact that venules are juxtaposed to arterioles in a counter-current configuration provides an additional mechanism for oxygen shunting; thus increased blood flow velocity diminishes transit time and therefore leakage and shunting from the distributing arterioles and collecting venules. This mechanism allows more oxygen to reach the capillaries, improving the utilization of the available oxygen, and is responsible for the observation that venular blood pO$_2$ increases as blood emerges from the microcirculation.

At the capillary level, where red blood cells become discrete oxygen sources, flow velocity also impacts on the extent by which oxygen can diffuse out of the capillary and penetrate the surrounding tissue; thus high velocities provide significant oxygenation, and low velocities oxygenate a larger tissue radius at the beginning of the capillary [Tsai & Intaglietta, 1989].

Hemodilution and Leukocytes

The distribution of leukocytes in the cross-section of the microvascular lumen is a flow-dependent phenomenon, whereby as the velocity of the flow increases, the leukocrit is highest in the blood-cell-rich core of arterioles and venules. This situation changes as velocity decreases, causing the leukocytes to migrate toward the vessel wall; therefore, with decreasing flow rate the possibility for endothelium-leukocyte interaction is enhanced [Goldsmith & Spain, 1984].

The attachment of leukocytes to the microvascular vessel wall, a sign of inflammation potentially leading to vessel wall damage, is the resultant of a balance between the adhesive forces generated at their activated surface and the shear stress imparted by the flowing blood. An increased shear stress proportionally lowers the number of adhering cells, which may be one of the factors responsible for the decrease in leukocyte adhesion noted when dextran-based hemodilution is used prophylactically prior to an ischemic injury.

The replacement of blood with a volume expander lowers the number of leukocytes. Conversely, most forms of artificial blood replacement cause some level of endothelial/leukocyte activation, and therefore the quantity of potentially harmful leukocytes that become adhered to the microvascular wall is the result of a balance between the hydrodynamic effects due to changes in flow velocity and blood viscosity, the level of activation, and the rate of delivery of activated cells [Menger et al., 1989].

Hemodilution and Functional Capillary Density

Tissue oxygenation is also dependent on a normal and spatially uniform distribution system for oxygen delivery. Although a significant fraction of oxygen is delivered directly by the larger vessels as evidenced by the decrease in pO_2 of blood as it nears the microcirculation, the mechanism that ensures that oxygen is delivered to every tissue microdomain is capillary blood flow.

It is generally assumed that capillaries are inert endothelium-lined tunnels [Fung et al., 1966], which unless adversely affected by thrombosis remain essentially open to the passage of plasma and blood-formed elements. Internal capillary diameter may vary significantly due to changes of volume of the endothelium and the state of hydration of the tissue; however, the capillary diameter must be greater than 2.8 μm to allow passage of red blood cells [Secomb et al., 1987].

When all the factors that determine tissue oxygenation are taken into account, the parameter m_{Oxygen} that characterizes the rate of oxygen delivery to the tissue from a microscopic basis is defined to be

$$m_{Oxygen} = QC_{Oxygen} \, FCD$$

where Q is the capillary flow, C_{Oxygen} is the local oxygen content of circulating mixture of blood and substitute, and FCD is the functional capillary density, i.e., the number of capillaries per unit volume of tissue in which there is through-flow [Vetterlein & Schmidt, 1980].

133.4 Crystalloid Solutions as Volume Expanders

Ringer's Lactate

One of the most widely used fluids for volume replacement are crystalloid solutions, particularly Ringer's lactate, which must be administered in volumes that are as much as 3 times the blood loss to be perfected, since the dilution of plasma proteins lowers the plasma oncotic pressure, causing an imbalance of the fluid exchange favoring microvascular fluid extravasation and edema. The advantage of crystalloid solutions is that large volumes can be given over short periods with low danger of increasing pulmonary wedge pressure. Excess volumes are rapidly cleared from the circulation by diuresis, which in many instances is a beneficial side effect in the treatment of trauma.

The rapid clearance of crystalloid solutions from the intravascular compartment is at the expense of the expansion of the tissue compartment and edema. This effect is significantly reduced when colloidal solutions are used. Peripheral edema has been speculated to impair oxygen delivery, the healing of wounds, and the resistance to infection, but these effects have not been proved. A more important effect is the development of pulmonary edema, or adult respiratory distress syndrome (ARDS); however, the relationship between the use of large volumes of salt solutions and ARDS is not firm.

Blood volume replacement with Ringer's lactate is accompanied by all the effects of hemodilution related to lowered blood viscosity. Consequently this form of artificial blood improves oxygen delivery at moderate level of blood substitution, since the forementioned Cv product is higher than normal at hematocrit 35 ± 5% in humans. The often-encountered massive edema resulting from sustained transfusions needed to maintain circulating volume have led to the supposition that microvascular flow may be impaired by capillary compression from edema; however, at present there is no definitive experimental or clinical proof of this effect.

Hypertonic Fluid Resuscitation

Small volumes of 2400 mOsm saline given in the amount of 10% of the total blood volume loss have been shown to produce a rapid improvement in blood pressure and cardiac output [Velasco et al.,

1980]. The mechanism behind this effect is the plasma expansion consequent to osmotically induced fluid shifts from the cellular to extracellular compartment, the decrease of peripheral vascular resistance due to arteriolar vasodilation, a reflex decrease in venular capacitance that shifts cardiac output to the kidney and visceral organs, increased heart contractility, osmotic diuresis, and improved microvascular perfusion due to endothelial deswelling.

The initial rapid restoration of systemic cardiovascular function is due to the increased osmolarity per se. High concentrations of sodium salt initiate the pulmonary vagal reflex, whereas chloride and nonelectrolytes do not. Hyperosmotic salt solutions cause a rapid (1–3 min) restoration of cardiovascular function, which is only transient, lasting on the order of 1 hour. The addition of an hyperoncotic component to the solution such as 10% dextran 70 kDA significantly prolongs the effect [Kramer et al., 1986].

This form of blood volume replacement would appear to fulfill many of the requirements set forth for an ideal blood substitute, since it is easily storable, has virtually immediate effects, and is artificial and therefore free of potential disease transmission. However, it is being explored only reluctantly because there is little clinical experience with the significance of the rapid fluid shift induced by the hyperosmolarity. Furthermore, its use implicitly requires understanding of the cardiac status of the patient, and the sustained elevation of blood pressure is counterindicated in surgical interventions.

133.5 Colloidal Solutions as Blood Substitutes

Albumin could be used as a plasma expander for emergency volume restitution, but due to cost considerations the synthetic colloids dextran and hydroxyethyl starch are used more frequently. These materials are free of viral contaminations but may cause anaphylactic reaction and have a tendency to alter platelet function thus interfering with hemostasis. It is not well established whether these materials increase bleeding per se or the effect is due to improved perfusion.

The beneficial effect of this form of volume replacement resides in the high oncotic pressure which it generates, maintaining intravascular volume in the amount of about 20 ml of fluid per gram of circulating colloid. In this context dextran 70 kDA and hydroxyethyl starch have the highest retention capacity, being respectively 22 and 17 ml/g, while albumin is 15 ml/g. Furthermore, this form of volume replacement lowers blood viscosity with all the associated positive transport effects described for hemodilution.

133.6 Oxygen-Carrying Artificial Blood

Although all aqueous fluids carry oxygen to the extent that it is dissolved in water, this amount is inconsequential in the overall demand of oxygen supply to the tissue, and therefore when intrinsic oxygen-carrying capacity is a requirement for artificial blood, it becomes necessary to include a component that provides this property. Intrinsic oxygen-carrying capacity is differentiated from "derived" capacity resulting from changes in the carrying capacity of the circulation, as, for instance, those attributable to the changed transport properties of the circulation due to hemodilution.

There presently are two materials that possess the desired oxygen-carrying properties: modified hemoglobins, which bind oxygen chemically and reversibly, and fluorocarbons, which have a high capacity for dissolving oxygen. These compounds present important differences which will ultimately determine in what form of blood substitution and replacement they will be collocated.

Hemoglobin separated from the red cell membrane, i.e., stroma-free hemoglobin, carries oxygen with a high affinity and therefore reduces release to the tissues. These materials have intrinsically higher oxygen-carrying capacity; however, they are based on a biologically active molecule, which to the present requires specialized storage procedures. By contrast, fluorocarbons carry a limited amount of oxygen under normal atmospheric conditions but are biologically inert, can be stored at room temperature, and are excreted as gas through the lung.

Hemoglobin Derivatives

When hemoglobin is diluted relative to the concentration present in red blood cells, the tetrameric molecule tends to spontaneously dissociate into smaller molecular weight dimers and monomers which are rapidly extravasated from the vascular compartment. This phenomenon is prevented by chemically crosslinking the tetrameric form, thus increasing retention in the circulation and reducing exposure of the renal tubules to hemoglobin. When hemoglobin is free in the circulation, it has an oxygen affinity that is too high for tissue oxygenation. As a consequence, strategies for the modification of hemoglobin by chemical means are aimed at prolongation of intravascular retention and reduction of oxygen affinity [Greenburg, 1988].

Hemoglobin can be prevented from dissociating by chemically crosslinking the dimers such as the widely used agent glutaraldehyde. Direct crosslinking with this agent produces a spectrum of different high-molecular-weight hemoglobin derivatives, since glutaraldehyde is nonspecific and reacts with any amino group. A more homogenous product can be obtained by reacting human hemoglobin first with the 2,3-DPG analog PLP, which reduces oxygen affinity, and then polymerizing the compound with glutaraldehyde. This product is called *PLP-polyHB* and has near normal oxygen-carrying capacity and a plasma half-life retention (in rats) of about 40 hours.

Diaspirins are another group of crosslinking agents. The reaction of native hemoglobin with bis(3,5-dibromosalicy)fumarate (DBBF) leads to the linking of the two α chains of the hemoglobin molecule, producing a compound called ααHb that has an oxygen affinity (P_{50}) of 30 mmHg and an intravascular retention time on the order of 15 in rats. Phosphorylated compounds added to purified hemoglobin also change the P_{50} value of the resulting compound and have been studied extensively. An increasing variety of hemoglobin compounds are being developed; however, at this time ααHb is the most widely studied compound, since it was produced in quantity by the U.S. Army Letterman Institute, San Francisco, and made available to different laboratories for investigation.

Genetically Engineered Hemoglobin

Hemoglobin can be produced as a recombinant protein leading to the construction of either the naturally occurring molecule or variants that have different crosslinking and oxygen affinity. It is presently possible to produce both alpha and beta chains of human hemoglobin in bacteria, yeast, and transgenic animals. Although it is in principle possible to produce large amounts of a specific product by these means, there remain problems of purification, elimination of other bacterial products, and endotoxins that may be expressed in parallel.

Human hemoglobin genes have been induced into transgenic mammals, leading to the potential production of large amounts of human hemoglobin. However, the production is not 100% pure, and some of the original animal material is also present, causing an important purification problem. This problem may be compounded by potential immunogenicity of animal hemoglobin and the potential transmission of animals diseases to humans.

133.7 Hemoglobin-Based Artificial Blood

Many hemoglobin-based artificial blood substitutes are being developed which may be classified relative to the technology used and whether the hemoglobin is either of human, animal, or bacterial origin. It is now established that hemoglobin containing red blood cell substitutes deliver oxygen to the issue and maintain tissue function. However, problems of toxicity and efficacy are not yet resolved and are shared by many of the hemoglobin solutions presently available. Renal toxicity is one of the primary problems, since hemoglobin toxicity to the kidney is a classic model for kidney failure. The mechanism of toxicity includes tubular obstruction, renal arterial vasospasm, and direct toxicity to tubular cells. It is not clear whether hemoglobin must be filtered by the kidney to be toxic, and the tolerance of the kidney to different types of hemoglobins and concentrations is not established [Paller, 1988].

There are many reports of anaphylaxis/anaphylactoid reactions to hemoglobin infusion. This may result from heme release from hemoglobin, the presence of endotoxins bound to hemoglobin or preexisting in the circulation, or from oxygen-derived free radicals released after exposure to hemoglobin. Vasoconstriction of coronary, cerebral, and renal vessels has also been attributed to the presence of free hemoglobin in the circulation, a phenomenon that may be due to the intrinsic capacity of hemoglobin to scavenge nitric oxide or metabolic autoregulation.

To the present there have been a number of clinical trials where more than 200 human subjects received hemoglobin solutions. Early studies in the 1960s were made before it was appreciated that hemoglobin solutions need to be rigorously purified. The study of Savitsky and colleagues [1978] using modern materials provides a well-documented report of some of the reactions to the injection of purified stroma-free hemoglobin, including bradycardia, hypertension, and oliguria. There is evidence that hemoglobin is not toxic if filtration in the kidney is prevented.

Toxicity of hemoglobin may be due to special characteristics of the manufacturing procedure, the given molecule, or problems due to purification. It may also be inherent to the presence of large quantities of a molecular species for which the circulation has a very limited tolerance when present in solution. This problem may be circumvented by separating hemoglobin from the circulation by encapsulating this material in a synthetic membrane, in the same way that the red cell membrane encapsulates hemoglobin.

Encapsulation of hemoglobin has been accomplished by introducing the molecule into a liposome. To the present this technology has a variety of problems, which include poor efficiency of hemoglobin incorporation into the liposome; physical instability of liposomes in storage; and chemical instability of the lipid-hemoglobin interface leading to lipid peroxidation and hemoglobin denaturation. These factors translate to decreased oxygen-carrying capacity, increased viscosity of the circulating blood/liposome mixture, and reticuloendothelial blockade. This situation notwithstanding, lipid encapsulation may ultimately provide the artificial blood of choice once a quality hemoglobin becomes consistently available and liposome production can be scaled up to quantities commensurate with demand.

133.8 Fluorocarbons

Fluorocarbons, and in particular perfluorochemicals (PFCs), are materials that exhibit a very high solubility of oxygen and whose oxygen transport capacity is directly proportional to their concentration and pO_2. Although they are virtually insoluble in water, they can be formulated in stable water soluble emulsions that are metabolically inert and dissolve 50% or more of their own volume of oxygen at ambient pressure [Riess, 1991].

PFCs emulsion consists of droplets of fluorochemicals in the range of 0.1–0.2 µm diameter coated by a thin film of egg yolk phospholipids. These products can be heat sterilized and can be stored under ambient conditions ready for use or, when refrigerated, have shelf lives on the order of 1 year. The technology for large-scale production of this compound is well established, and the products are well characterized and commercially available. Their half-life in the circulation is in the range of 4–12 h.

PFCs have high oxygen solubilities. These materials are diluted when they are infused, and the actual change in oxygen-carrying capacity that is introduced for most clinically recommended dosages (of the order of 3 ml/kg b.w.) reflects the change in oxygen carried in solution (rather than that bound chemically) or the change in oxygen-carrying capacity of plasma. As stated earlier, the amount of delivered oxygen in plasma is on the order of 0.3 ml at 100 mmHg; therefore, the actual effects on blood oxygen-carrying capacity is relatively small at normal blood pO_2s.

Although PFCs do not carry much oxygen when the lungs are exposed to atmospheric pO_2, they do not saturate and therefore transport progressively more oxygen as partial pressure is increased, an effect not available with blood and hemoglobin solutions, which become saturated. This effect is further magnified by the fact that in hemodilution the amount of plasma and plasma flow velocity increases, and therefore the rate of delivery of dissolved oxygen, thus magnifying the contribution of PFCs. These factors determine that if a patient breaths pure oxygen, the hematocrit at which the infusion of blood (red cells or hemoglobin solution, also referred to as *hematocrit trigger*) becomes necessary in order to maintain tissue metabolism is significantly lowered.

In terms of side effects, whenever particulate matter is introduced in the vasculature, protein is absorbed unto the particle surface, a process termed *opsonization*. These proteins eventually denature, causing the transient response of the macrophage system leading to the release of material in the arachidonic acid cascade and cytokines. These events may be the cause of some of the side effects consistently seen when PFCs have been used in clinical trails, namely occasional skin flushing, lower back pain, and delayed flulike symptoms including headache and nausea.

133.9 Cardiovascular Stabilization Time and Intravascular Retention

One of the primary uses of blood substitutes is to correct for acute losses of blood. Under the assumption that a safe substitute is available, a further consideration is the time required for the circulatory system to return to normal stable conditions after the blood loss has been corrected, and how long stable conditions are maintained before further interventions are necessary.

Small-volume resuscitation with hiperosmotic/hyperoncotic solutions presents the fastest normalization times, given that mean arterial blood pressure and cardiac output are normalized within 3–5 min of volume restitution. This effect has been analyzed by phenomenological treatment of transport [Mazzoni et al., 1988] and is due to the osmotic equilibration that takes place between intra and extravascular fluid. Since the primary osmotic agent is NaCl, the effect is not sustained and falters within 1 h, at which time additional fluid therapy becomes necessary.

Normalization of the circulation is achieved over approximately 1 h when colloidal solutions are used, which is similar to the effects obtained with blood. By contrast the use of Ringer's lactate may require periods in excess of 2 h. This disparity in reactions is primarily due to the difference in osmotic/oncotic properties of the fluid replacement, which also determine the duration of the effect. Colloids have retention times on the order of hours.

Hemoglobin-based oxygen-carrying substitutes possess in principle the same retention time as dextran and albumin, which is dictated by their molecular weight, provided that the molecule does not split into dimers, which are actively excreted by the kidney. Stable crosslinked hemoglobin in principle would allow for the introduction of all the material present in normal blood into the circulation in the form of a solution, with a potentially lower viscosity than normal blood, while maintaining intrinsic oxygen-carrying capacity of the fluid. This, however, is not possible due to osmotic considerations.

The osmotic pressure π of colloidal solutions is a function of the concentration of colloid c and has the form

$$\pi = k_1 c + k_2 c^2$$

where k_1 and k_2 are constants. As a consequence, whereas a 5–6% by concentration by weight of albumin normally present in blood provides an osmotic effect in the range of 20–25 mmHg, the presence of the hemoglobin contained in the red blood cell in solution would create an effect in the range of 100 mmHg, leading to the disruption of fluid balance. Consequently, unless the hemoglobin molecule is polymerized or contained within an enclosure, the oxygen-carrying capacity of blood cannot be achieved solely by solutions of individual hemoglobin molecules.

Fluorocarbons emulsions have particle size that is too large to yield relevant osmotic properties. They have the oncotic properties of the fluid medium in which they are prepared, which can be designed accordingly.

133.10 Summary and Assessment

If we accept the concept that lethality consequent to blood losses results from hypovolemia and not anemia, it is apparent that there are presently in existence a number of artificial bloods that sustain metabolism even though they carry oxygen only to the extent of its plasma solubility. This is a consequence of the "derived" increase of oxygen-carrying capacity resulting from lowered viscosity. Even in the absence of derived oxygen delivery enhancement, experience in humans that do not accept homologous blood because of religious convictions demonstrates that in appropriate clinical settings the red blood cell loss that can be tolerated is very high and in all probability not attained in most situations.

The positive feature of non-oxygen-carrying artificial blood is the virtual (by comparison) lack of side effects, a feature shared to some extent with fluorocarbons. It is generally accepted that blood losses on the order of 50% can be readily remedied with Ringer's lactate and colloidal solutions. Hypertonic/hyperosmotic solutions, or small-volume resuscitation, provide an additional dimension, voiding the requirement for availability and delivery of large volumes under field conditions. However, this option may not be viable under prevailing efficacy criteria.

An oxygen-carrying volume replacement with a capacity commensurate to blood is a condition sine qua non for extreme blood losses. For lesser blood losses the need for an oxygen-carrying blood substitute is a matter of balance between the level of clinical care required for a patient of intrinsically precarious conditions to which is superposed the effects of diminished vascular oxygen-carrying capacity, versus the benefit of providing a fluid (which may include blood) that has enhanced oxygen-carrying capacity. How this balance is perceived and established is fundamentally a question of the circumstances in which blood (or its artificial substitute) is required. Large-scale emergencies and the absence of or delayed access to primary care medical facilities are deciding factors in selecting an optimal blood substitute and point to the need for artificial blood.

Hemoglobin-based oxygen-carrying artificial blood possesses the intrinsic capacity for oxygen delivery not present in fluorocarbons. However, hemoglobin is an aggressive biologic material that in natural conditions is tolerated only when protected by the red blood cell membrane. It may not be feasible to introduce hemoglobin in large quantities in an organism that is already compromised because of events that have led to a severe blood loss. It is probable that tolerance to hemoglobin equivalent to that given by the red blood cell membrane may be partially accomplished by encapsulation in liposomes or other artificial membranes. Such a development will also require the solution of the problem of opsonization. It may be that the goal of developing artificial blood that is free of side effect may not be fully achievable, and therefore the deployment of this material will ultimately depend on a balance between its life-giving properties and the type and severity of side effects.

Acknowledgment

This work was supported by USPHS Grant HLBI 48018.

Defining Terms

Hemodilution: The replacement of natural blood with a compatible fluid that reduces the concentration of red blood cells.

Liposome: Microscopic phospholipid vesicle used to encapsulate materials for slow release. The use of liposomes to encapsulate hemoglobin is a departure from the conventional use of liposomes, exploiting encapsulation, and requires their modification to ensure sustained entrapment.

Oncotic: Refers to colligative properties due to the presence of macromolecules, for instance oncotic pressure, which is differentiated from osmotic pressure, which is that due to the presence of all molecular species in solution.

Oxygen-carrying capacity: The total amount of oxygen that is being transported by blood or the fluid in the circulation. Differentiated from oxygen delivery capacity, which involves considerations of flow rate.

Stroma-free hemoglobin: Hemoglobin derived from red blood cells where all materials related to cell membrane and other components within the red blood cella have been removed.

References

Dintenfass L. 1971. Blood Microrheology: Viscosity Factors in Blood Flow, Ischemia and Thrombosis, New York, Appleton-Century-Crofts.

Duling BR, RM Berne. 1973. Longitudinal gradients of perivascular oxygen tension. Circ Res 27:669.

Fung YC, Zweifach BW, Intaglietta M. 1966. Elastic environment of the capillary bed. Circ Res 19:441.

Goldsmith HL, Spain S. 1984. Margination of leukocytes in blood flow through small tubes. Microvasc Res 27:204.

Greenburg AG. 1988. An overview of chemical modification of stroma free hemoglobin. Biomater Artif Cells Artif Organs 16:71.

Hint H. 1968. The pharmacology of dextran and physiological background of the clinical use of Rheomacrodex. Acta Anaesthesiol Belg 2:119.

Kramer GC, Perron PR, Lindsey DC, et al. 1986. Small volume resuscitation with hyperosmotic saline dextran solutions. Surgery 100:239.

Lipowsky HH, Usami S, Chien S. 1980. In vivo measurement of apparent viscosity and microvessel hematocrit in the mesentery of the cat. Microvasc Res 19:297.

Lipowsky HH, Firrel JL. 1986. Microvascular hemodynamics during systemic hemodilution and hemoconcentration. Am J Physiol 250:H908.

Mazzoni MC, Borgström P, Arfors K-E, et al. 1988. Dynamic fluid redistribution in hyperosmotic resuscitation of hypovolemic hemorrhage. Am J Physiol 255:H629.

Menger MD, Thierjung C, Hammersen F, et al. 1989. Influence of isovolemic hemodilution with Dextran 60 and HAES on the PMN-endothelium interaction in postischemic skeletal muscle. Eur Surg Res 21:74.

Messmer K, Sunder-Plasman L, Klövekorn WP, et al. 1972. Circulatory significance of hemodilution: Rheological changes and limitations. Adv Microcirc 4:1.

Mirhashemi S, Breit GA, Chávez RH, et al. 1988. Effects of hemodilution on skin microcirculation. Am J Physiol 254:H411.

Mirhashemi S, Ertefai S, Messmer K, et al. 1987a. Model analysis of the enhancement of tissue oxygenation by hemodilution due to increased microvascular flow velocity. Microvasc Res 34:290.

Mirhashemi S, Messmer K, Intaglietta M. 1987b. Tissue perfusion during normovolemic hemodilution investigated by a hydraulic model of the cardiovascular system. Int J Microcirc: Clin Exp 6:123.

Paller MS. 1988. Hemoglobin and myoglobin-induced acute renal failure: Role of iron nephrotoxicity. Am J Physiol 255:F539.

Quemada D. 1978. Rheology of concentrated dispersed systems: III. General features of the proposed non-Newtonian model: Comparison with experimental data. Rheol Acta 17:643.

Richardson TQ, Guyton AC. 1959. Effects of polycythemia and anemia on cardiac output and other circulatory factors. Am J Physiol 197:1167.

Riess IG. 1991. Fluorocarbon based in vivo oxygen transport delivery systems. Vox Sang 61:225.

Savitsky JP, Doczi J, Black J, et al. 1978. A clinical safety trial of stroma free hemoglobin. Clin Pharmacol Ther 23:F539.

Secomb TW, Fleishman GJ, Papenfuss H-D, et al. 1987. Effects of reduced perfusion and hematocrit on flow distribution in capillary networks. Prog Appl Microcirc 12:205.

Tsai AG, Intaglietta M. 1989. Local tissue oxygenation during constant red blood cell flux: A discrete source analysis of velocity and hematocrit changes. Microvasc Res 37:308.

Velasco IT, Lopes OU, Pontieri V, et al. 1980. Hyperosmotic NaCl and severe hemorhaggic shock. Am J Physiol 239:H664.

Vetterlein F, Schmidt G. 1980. Functional capillary density in skeletal muscle during vasodilation unduced by isoprenaline and muscular exercise. Microvasc Res 20:156.

Further Information

Chang TMS (ed). 1993. Blood Substitutes and Oxygen Carriers, New York, Marcel Dekker.

Chang TMS (ed). 1994. Artificial Cells, Blood Substitutes and Immobilization Biotechnology, New York, Marcel Dekker.

Dodd RY. 1992. The risk of transfusion transmitted infection. N Eng J Med 327:419.

Tuma RR, White JV, Messmer K (eds). 1989. The Role of Hemodilution in Optimal Patient Care, Munich, Zuckeschwerdt Verlag GmbH.

Winslow RM. 1992. Hemoglobin-based Red Cell Substitutes, The Johns Hopkins University Press.

134

Artificial Skin and Dermal Equivalents

Ioannis V. Yannas
*Massachusetts Institute
of Technology*

134.1 The Vital Functions of Skin

Skin is a vital organ, in the sense that loss of a substantial fraction of its mass immediately threatens the life of the individual. Such loss can result suddenly, either from fire or from a mechanical accident. Loss of skin can also occur in a chronic manner, as in skin ulcers. Irrespective of the time scale over which skin loss is incurred, the resulting deficit is considered life threatening primarily for two reasons: Skin is a barrier to loss of water and electrolytes from the body, and it is a barrier to infection from airborne organisms. A substantial deficit in the integrity of skin leaves the individual unprotected either from shock, the result of excessive loss of water and electrolyte, or from sepsis, the result of a massive systemic infection. It has been reported that burns alone account for 2,150,000 procedures every year in the United States. Of, these, 150,000 refer to individuals who are hospitalized, and as many as 10,000 die.

Four types of tissue can be distinguished clearly in normal skin. The *epidermis,* outside, is a 0.1-mm-thick sheet, comprising about 10 layers of keratinocytes at levels of maturation which increase from the inside out. The *dermis,* inside, is a 2–5-mm-thick layer of vascularized and innervated connective tissue with very few cells, mostly quiescent fibroblasts. The dermis is a massive tissue, accounting for 15–20% of total body weight. Interleaved between the epidermis and the dermis is the *basement membrane,* an approximately 20–nm-thick multilayered membrane (Fig. 134.1). A fourth layer, the *subcutis,* underneath the dermis and 0.4–4-mm in thickness, comprises primarily fat tissue. In addition to these basic structural elements, skin contains several appendages (*adnexa*), including hair follicles, sweat glands, and sebaceous glands. The latter are mostly embedded in the dermis, although they are ensheathed in layers of epidermal tissue.

The functions of skin are quite diverse, although it can be argued that the single function of skin is to provide a viable interface with the individual's environment. In addition to the specific vital

0-8493-8346-3/95/$0.00+$.50
© 1995 by CRC Press, Inc.

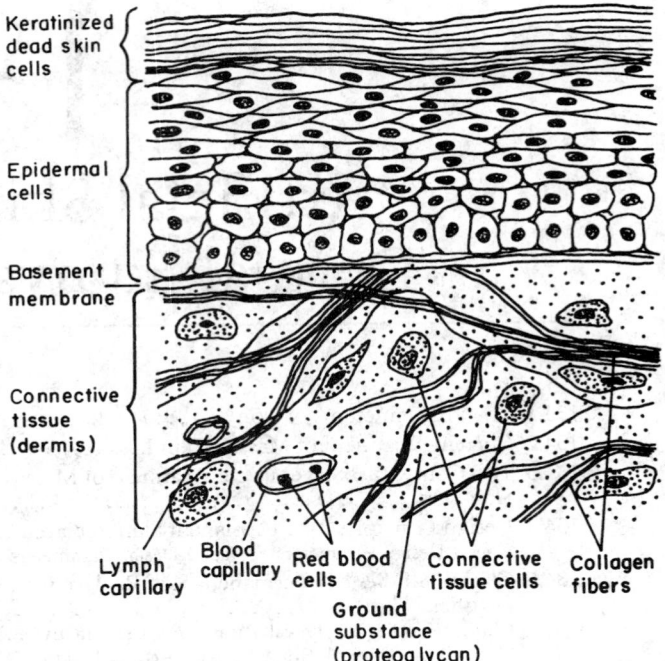

Keratinized
dead skin
cells

Epidermal
cells

Basement
membrane

Connective
tissue
(dermis)

Lymph capillary   Blood capillary   Red blood cells   Connective tissue cells   Collagen fibers

Ground
substance
(proteoglycan)

FIGURE 134.1   Schematic view of skin which highlights the epidermis, the basement membrane interleaved between the epidermis and the dermis, and the dermis underneath. Only a small fraction of the thickness of the dermis is shown. (Redrawn with permission from J. Darnell, J. Lodish, and D. Baltimore, *Molecular Cell Biology,* Scientific American Books, New York, Chapter 5, Fig. 552, 1986.)

functions mentioned above (protection from water and electrolyte loss and from infection), skin also protects from heat and cold, mechanical friction, chemicals, and from UV radiation. Skin is responsible for a substantial part of the thermoregulatory and communication needs of the body, including the transduction of signals from the environment such as touch, pressure, and temperature. Further, skin transmits important emotional signals to the environment, such as paleness or blushing of the face and the emission of scents (pheromones). Far from being a passive membrane that keeps the internal organs in shape, skin is a complex organ.

134.2 Current Treatment of Massive Skin Loss

The treatment of skin loss has traditionally focused on the design of a temporary wound closure. Attempts to cover wounds and severe burns have been reported from historical sources at least as far back as 1500 B.C., and a very large number of temporary wound dressings have been designed. These include membranes or sheets fabricated from natural and synthetic polymers, skin grafts from human cadavers (homografts, or *allografts*), and skin grafts from animals (heterografts, or *xenografts*). Although a satisfactory temporary dressing helps to stem the tide, it does not provide a permanent cover. Polymeric membranes which lack specific biologic activity, such as synthetic polymeric hydrogels, have to be removed after several days due to incidence of infection and lack of formation of physiologic structures. Patients with cadaver allografts and xenografts are frequently immunosuppressed to avoid rejection; however, this is a stop-gap operation which is eventually terminated by removal of the graft after several days. In all cases where temporary dressings have been used, the routine result has been an open wound. Temporary dressings are useful in delaying the time at which a permanent graft, such as an autograft, is necessary and are therefore invaluable aids in the management of the massively injured patient.

The use of an autograft has clearly shown the advantages of a permanent wound cover. This treatment addresses not only the urgent needs of the patient with massive skin loss but also the long-term needs. The result of treatment of a third-degree burn with a split-thickness autograft is an almost fully functional skin which has become incorporated into the patient's body and will remain functional over a lifetime. Autografts usually lack hair follicles and certain adnexa as well. However, the major price paid is the removal of the split thickness graft from an intact area of the patient's body: The remaining dermis eventually becomes epithelialized but not without synthesis of scar over the entire area of trauma (donor site). To alleviate the problem associated with the limited availability of autograft, surgeons have resorted to meshing, a procedure in which the sheet autograft is passed through an apparatus which cuts slits into the sheet autograft, allowing the expansion of the graft by several times and thereby extending greatly the area of use. An inevitable long-term result of use of these meshed autografts is scar synthesis in areas coinciding with the open slits of the meshed graft and a resulting pattern of scar which greatly reduces the value of the resulting new organ (Fig. 134.2). An important aspect of the use of the autograft is the requirement for early excision of dead tissue and the provision, thereby, of a viable wound bed to "take" the autograft.

134.3 Two Conceptual Stages in the Treatment of Massive Skin Loss

Loss of the epidermis alone can result from a relatively mild burn, such as an early exposure to the sun. Controlled loss of epidermis in a laboratory experiment with an animal can result from the repeated use of adhesive tape to peel off the keratinocyte layers. In either case, the long-term outcome is an apparently faithful regeneration of the epidermis by migration of epithelial cells from the wound edge, and from roots of hair follicles, over the underlying basement membrane and

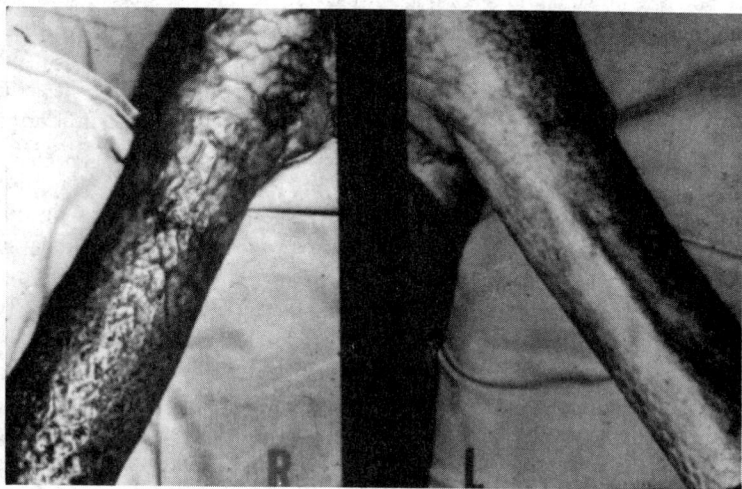

FIGURE 134.2 Comparison between treatment with the meshed autograft (R) and treatment with the artificial skin (L). Autograft is usually meshed before grafting; scar forms in areas coinciding with the open slits of the autograft. The artificial skin treatment consists of grafting the excised wound bed with a skin regeneration template, followed by grafting on about day 14 with a very thin epidermal autograft. (Photo courtesy of J. F. Burke.)

dermis. It has been shown that the epidermis can regenerate spontaneously provided there is a dermal substrate over which epithelial migration and eventual anchoring to the inderlying connective tissue can occur.

Loss of the dermis has quite a different outcome. Once lost, the dermis does not regenerate spontaneously. Instead, the wound closes by contraction of the wound edges toward the center of the skin deficit, and by synthesis of *scar*. Scar is a distinctly different type of connective tissue than is dermis. The depth of skin loss is, therefore, a critical parameter in the design of a treatment for a patient who has a skin deficit. In the treatment of burns, physicians distinguish among a first-degree burn (loss of epidermis alone), a second-degree burn (loss of epidermis and a fraction of the thickness of the dermis), and a third-degree burn (loss of the epidermis and the entire dermis down to muscle tissue). A similar classification, based on depth of loss, is frequently applied to mechanical wounds, such as abrasion. The area of skin which has been destroyed needs also to be specified in order to assess the clinical status of the patient.

A massively injured patient, such as a patient with about 30% body surface area or more destroyed from fire through the full thickness of skin, presents an urgent problem to the clinician, since the open wound is an ongoing threat to survival. A large number of temporary wound coverings have been used to help the patient survive through this period while waiting for availability of autografts which provide permanent cover. If autograft is unavailable over a prolonged period while the patient has survived the severe trauma, contraction and scar synthesis occur over extensive areas. In the long run, the patient therefore has to cope with deep, disfiguring scars or with crippling contractures. Thus, even though the patient has been able to survive the massive trauma and has walked out of the clinic, the permanent loss of skin which has been sustained prevents, in many cases, resumption of an active, normal life.

134.4 Design Principles for a Permanent Skin Replacement

The analysis of the plight of the patient who has suffered extensive skin loss, presented above, leads logically to a wound cover which treats the problem in two stages. Stage 1 is the early phase of the clinical experience, one in which protection against severe fluid loss and against massive infection are defined as the major design objectives. Stage 2 is the ensuing phase, one in which the patient needs protection principally against disfiguring scars and crippling contractures. Even though the conceptual part of the design is separated in two stages for purposes of clarity, the actual treatment is to be delivered continuously, as will be become clear below. The sequential utilization of features inherent in stages 1 and 2 in a single device can be ensured by designing the graft as a bilayer membrane (Fig. 134.3). In this approach, the top layer incorporates the features of a stage 1 device, while the bottom layer delivers the performance expected from a stage 2 device. The top layer is subject to disposal after a period of about 10–15 days, during which time the bottom layer has already induced substantial synthesis of new dermis. Following removal of the top layer, the epidermal cover is provided either by covering with a thin epidermal graft or by modifying the device (cell seeding) so that an epidermis forms spontaneously by about 2 weeks after grafting.

Stage 1 Design Parameters

The overriding design requirement at this stage is based on the observation that air pockets ("dead space") at the graft-wound bed interface readily become sites of bacterial proliferation. Such sites can be prevented from forming if the graft surface wets, in the physicochemical sense, the surface of the wound bed on contact and thereby displaces the air from the graft-tissue interface (Fig. 134.4). It follows that the physicochemical properties of the graft must be designed to ensure that this leading requirement is met, not only when the graft is placed on the wound bed but for several days thereafter, until the function of the graft has moved clearly into its stage 2, in which case the graft–

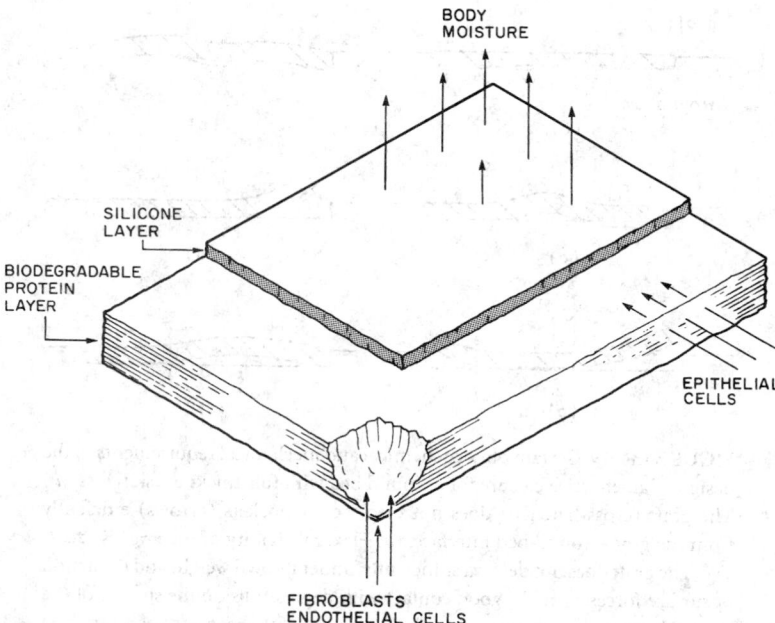

FIGURE 134.3 Schematic of the bilayer membrane which has become known as the artificial skin. The top layer is a silicone film which controls moisture flux through the wound bed to nearly physiologic levels, controls infection of the wound bed by airborne bacteria, and is strong enough to be sutured on the wound bed. The bottom layer is the skin regeneration template, which consists of a graft copolymer of type I collagen and chondroitin 6-sulfate, with critically controlled porosity and degradation rate. About 14 days after grafting, the silicone layer is removed and replaced with a thin epidermal autograft. The bottom layer induces synthesis of a nearly physiologic dermis and eventually is removed completely by biodegradation. (From Yannas IV, Burke JF, Orgill DP, et al. 1982. Science 215: 74.)

wound bed interface has been synthesized de novo and the threat of dead space has been thereby eliminated indefinitely.

First, the flexural rigidity of the graft, i.e., the product of Young's modulus and moment of inertia of a model elastic beam, must be sufficiently low to provide for a flexible graft which drapes intimately over a geometrically nonuniform wound bed surface and thus ensures that the two surfaces will be closely apposed. In practice, these requirements can be met simply by adjusting both the stiffness in tension and the thickness of the graft to appropriately low values. Second, the graft will wet the wound bed if the surface energy of the graft–wound bed interface is lower than that of the air–wound bed surface, so that the graft can adequately displace air pockets from the air–wound bed surface. Although the measurement of a credible value of the surface energy is not a simple matter when the graft is based on certain natural polymers in the form of a hydrated gel, the requirement of adequate adhesion can be met empirically by chemical modification of the surface or by proper use of structural features such as porosity.

Third, the moisture flux through the graft must be maintained within bounds which are set by the following considerations. The upper bound to the moisture flux must be kept below the level where excessive dehydration of the graft occurs, thereby leading to alteration of the surface energy of the graft–wound bed interface and loss of the adhesive bond between graft and wound bed. Further, when the moisture flux exceeds the desired level, the graft is desiccated, and shrinkage stresses develop which pull the graft away from the wound bed. An estimate of the maximum

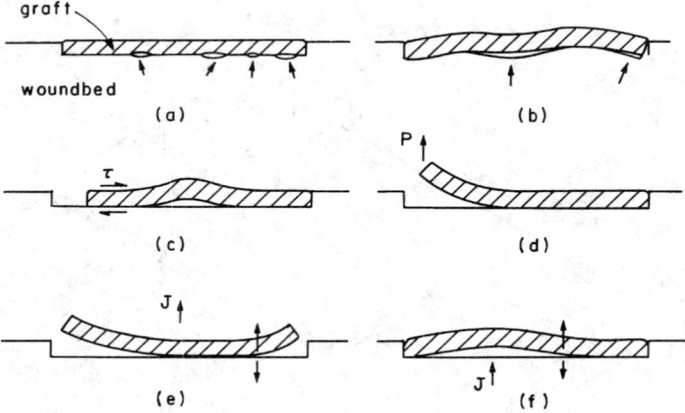

FIGURE 134.4   Certain physicochemical and mechanical requirements in the design of an effective closure for a wound bed with full-thickness skin loss. (*a*) The graft (cross-hatched) does not displace air pockets (arrows) efficiently from the graft–wound bed interface. (*b*) Flexural rigidity of the graft is excessive. The graft does not deform sufficiently, under its own weight and the action of surface forces, to make good contact with depressions on the surface of the wound bed; as a result, air pockets form (arrows). (*c*) Shear stresses τ (arrows) cause buckling of the graft, rupture of the graft–wound bed bond and formation of an air pocket. (*d*) Peeling force P lifts the graft away from the wound bed. (*e*) Excessively high moisture flux rate J through the graft causes dehydration and development of shrinkage stresses at the edges (arrows), which cause lift-off away from the wound bed. (*f*) Very low moisture flux J causes fluid accumulation (edema) at the graft–wound bed interface and peeling off (arrows). (From Yannas IV, Burke JF. 1980. J Biomed Mater Res 14:65.)

normal stress σ_m can be obtained by modeling the desiccating graft in one dimension as a shrinking elastic beam bonded to a rigid surface

$$\sigma_m = 0.45\alpha(V_2 - V_1)E \tag{134.1}$$

In Eq. (134.1), α is the coefficient of expansion of a graft which swells in water, V_1 and V_2 are initial and final values of the volume fraction of moisture in the graft, and E is Young's modulus of the graft averaged over the range V_1 to V_2, the latter range being presumed to be narrow. If, by contrast, the moisture flux through the graft is lower than the desired low bound, water accumulates between the graft and the wound bed, and edema results with accompanying loss of the adhesive bond between the two surfaces.

Stage 2 Design Parameters

The leading design objectives in this stage are two: synthesis of new, physiologic skin and the eventual disposal of the graft.

The lifetime of the graft, expressed as the time constant of biodegradation t_b, was modeled in relation to the time constant for normal healing of a skin incision t_h. The latter is about 25 days. In preliminary studies with animals, it was observed that when matrices were synthesized to degrade at a very rapid rate, amounting to $t_b \ll t_h$, the initially insoluble matrix was reduced early to a liquidlike state, which was incompatible with an effective wound closure. At the other extreme, matrices were synthesized which degraded with exceptional difficulty within 3–4 weeks, compatible with

$t_b \gg t_h$. In these preliminary studies it was observed that a highly intractable matrix, corresponding to the latter condition, led to formation of a dense fibrotic tissue underneath the graft which eventually led to loss of the bond between graft and wound bed. Accordingly, it was hypothesized that a rule of *isomorphous matrix replacement*, equivalent to assuming a graft degradation rate of order of magnitude similar to the synthesis rate for new tissue, and represented by the relation

$$\frac{t_b}{t_h} = O(1) \tag{134.2}$$

would be optimal. Control of t_b is possible by adjustment of the crosslink density of the matrix. Equation (134.2) is the defining equation for a biodegradable scaffold which is coupled with, and therefore interacts with, the inflammatory process in a wound.

Migration of cells into the matrix is necessary for synthesis of new tissue. Such migration can proceed very slowly, defeating Eq. (134.2), when fibroblasts and other cells recruited below the wound surface are required to wait until degradation of a potentially solid-like matrix has progressed sufficiently. An easier pathway to migrating cells can be provided by modifying a solid-like matrix into one which has an abundance of pore channels, where the average pore is at least as large as one cell diameter (about 10 μm) for ready access. Although this rationale is supported by experiment, results with animal studies have shown that not only is there a lower limit to the average pore diameter, but there is also an upper limit (see below).

Migration of cells into the porous graft can proceed only if nutrients are available to these cells. Two general mechanisms are available for transport of nutrients to the migrating cells, namely, diffusion from the wound bed and transport along capillaries which may have sprouted within the matrix (angiogenesis). Since capillaries would not be expected to form for at least a few days, it is necessary to consider whether a purely diffusional mode of transport of nutrients from the wound bed surface into the graft could immediately supply the metabolic needs of the invading cells adequately. The cell has been modled as a reactor which consumes a critical nutrient with a rate r, in units of mole/cm^3/s; the nutrient is transported from the wound bed to the cell by diffusion over a distance l, the nutrient concentration at or near the surface of the wound bed is c_0, in units of mole/cm^3, and the diffusivity of the nutrient is D, in cm^2/s. The appropriate conditions were expressed in terms of a dimensionless number S, the *cell lifeline number*, which expresses the relative importance of reaction rate for consumption of the nutrient by the cell to rate of transport of the nutrient by diffusion alone:

$$S = \frac{rl^2}{Dc_0} \tag{134.3}$$

Eq. (134.3) suggests that when $S = 1$, the critical value of the path length, l_c, corresponds to the maximum distance along which cells can migrate inside the graft without requiring angiogenesis (vascularization) for nutrient transport. The value of l_c defines the maximum thickness of graft that can be populated with cells within a few hours after grafting, before angiogenesis has had time to occur.

These conceptual objectives have been partially met by designing the graft as an analog of *extracellular matrix* (ECM) which possesses morphogenetic activity since it leads to partial regeneration of dermis. The discovery of the specific ECM analog that possesses this activity has been based on the empirical observation that, whereas the vast majority of ECM analogs apparently do not inhibit wound contraction almost at all, one of the analogs does. The activity of this analog, for which the term *regeneration template* has been coined, is conveniently detected as a significant delay in the onset of wound contraction. When seeded with (uncultured) autologous keratinocytes, an active regeneration template is capable of inducing simultaneous synthesis both of a dermis and an epidermis in the guinea pig and in the swine (Yorkshire pig). The regeneration is almost complete; however, hair follicles and other skin adnexa are not formed. The resulting integument performs the two vital functions of skin, i.e., control of infection and moisture loss, while also providing physiologic mechanical protection to the internal organs and, additionally, providing a cosmetic effect almost identical to that of intact skin.

The morphogenetic specificity of the skin regeneration template depends sensitively on retention of certain structural characteristics. The overall structure is that of an insoluble, three-dimensional covalently crosslinked network. The primary structure can be described as that of a *graft*-copolymer of type I collagen and a glycosaminoglycan (GAG) in the approximate ratio 98/2. The GAG can be either chondroitin 6-sulfate or dermatan sulfate; other GAGs appear capable of contributing approximately equal increments to morphogenetic specificity. The collagen fibers lack banding almost completely although the integrity of the triple helical structure is retained through the network. The resistance of the network to collagenase degradation is such that approximately two-thirds of the mass of the network becomes solubilized in vivo within about 2 weeks. The structure of the network is highly porous. The pore volume fraction exceeds 95% while the average pore diameter is maintained in the range 20–125 μm. The regeneration template loses its activity rapidly when these structural features are flawed deliberately in control studies.

The *skin regeneration template,* a porous matrix unseeded with cells, induces synthesis of a new dermis and solves this old surgical problem. Simultaneous synthesis of a new, confluent epidermis occurs by migration of epithelial cell sheets from the wound edges, over the newly synthesized dermal bed. With wounds of relatively small characteristic dimension, e.g., 1 cm, epithelial cells migrating at speeds of about 0.5 mm/day from each wound edge can provide a confluent epidermis within 10 days. In such cases, the unseeded template fulfills all the design specifications set above. However, the wounds incurred by a massively burned patient are typically of characteristic dimension of several centimeters, often more than 20–30 cm. These wounds are large enough to preclude formation of a new epidermis by cell migration alone within a clinically acceptable timeframe, say 2 weeks. Wounds of that magnitude can be treated by seeding the porous collagen-GAG template, before grafting, with at least 5×10^4 keratinocytes per cm^2 wound area. These uncultured, autologous cells are extracted by applying a cell separation procedure, based on controlled trypsinization, to a small epidermal biopsy.

Details of the synthesis of the skin regeneration template, as well as of other templates which regenerate peripheral nerves and the knee meniscus, are presented elsewhere in this *Handbook* (see Chapter 109). The skin regeneration template described in this section was first reported as a *synthetic skin* and as an *artificial skin* by its designers.

134.5 Clinical Studies of a Permanent Skin Replacement (Prototype Artificial Skin)

Clinical Studies

The skin regeneration template has been tested clinically on two occasions. In the first, conducted in the period 1979–1980, one clinical center was involved, and 10 severely burned patients were studied. In the second, conducted during 1986–1987, 11 clinical centers were involved, and 106 severely burned patients were treated in a prospective, randomized manner. In each case the results have been published in some detail. The second study led to a surgical report, a histologic report, and an immunologic report. There is now adequate information available to discuss the advantages and disadvantages of this prototype artificial skin in the treatment of the severely burned patient.

The artificial skin used in clinical studies so far consists of the bilayer device illustrated in Fig. 134.3. The outer layer is a silicone film, about 100 μm in thickness, which fulfills the requirements of stage 1 of the design (see above), and the inner layer is the skin regeneration template. In these clinical studies this device has not been seeded with keratinocytes. Closure of the relatively large wounds by formation of an epidermis has been achieved instead by use of a 100-μm-thin layer of the patient's epidermis (autoepidermal graft). The latter has been excised from an intact area of the patient's skin; the donor site can, however, be harvested repeatedly, since the excised epidermis regenerates spontaneously in a few days over the relatively intact dermal bed. Briefly, the entire procedure consists of preparation of the wound bed prior to grafting by excision of thermally injured tissue (*eschar*), followed by immediate grafting of the unseeded template on the freshly excised wound and ending, 3 weeks later, by replacing the outer, silicone layer of the device with a thin epidermal graft.

The discussion below focuses on the advantages and disadvantages of the (unseeded) artificial skin, as these emerge from clinical observations during the treatment as well as from a limited number of follow-up observations extending over several years after the treatment. The controls used in the clinical studies included meshed autograft, allograft, and xenografts. Comparative analysis of the clinical data will focus on each of the two stages of treatment for the massively burned patient, i.e., the early (acute) stage and the long term stage, the conceptual basis for which has been discussed above.

Clinical Parameters Used in the Evaluation

The clinical parameters during the early stage of treatment (about 3 weeks) include the *take* of the graft, expressed as a percentage of graft area which formed an adhesive bond of sufficient strength with the wound bed and became vascularized. In the case of the artificial skin treatment, two different measures of take are reported, namely, that of the bilayer membrane on the freshly excised wound bed and the take of the epidermal graft applied on the neodermal bed about 3 weeks later. Another parameter is the thickness of dermis that has been excised from the donor site in order to obtain the autograft that is used to close the wound definitively. An additional parameter which characterizes the cost of the donor site to the patient is the time to heal the donor site. The surgeon's overall qualitative evaluation of the treatment (relative to controls) during the early stage is also reported.

The long-term evaluation has extended at least 1 year in approximately one-quarter of the patients. The first long-term parameter is based on the patients' reports of the relative incidence of nonphysiologic sensations, including itching, dryness, scaliness, lack of elasticity (lack of deformability), sweating, sensation, and erythema. The second parameter is based on the physicians' report of the relative presence of hypertrophic scarring in the grafted area. A third parameter is the patient's evaluation of the physiologic feel and appearance of the donor sites. Finally, there is an overall evaluation and preference of the patients for a given grafted site as well as the physicians' evaluation of the same grafted sites.

Short-Term Clinical Evaluation of Artificial Skin

The median percentage take of the artificial skin was 80%, compared with the median take of 95% for all controls. Use of the Wilcoxin Rank Sum Test for the bimodally distributed data led to the conclusion that the take of the artificial skin was lower than that of all controls with a p value of <0.0001. The reported difference reflected primarily the significantly lower take of the artificial skin relative to the meshed autograft. There was no significant difference in take when the artificial skin was compared with allograft (Wilcoxin Rank Sum $p > 0.10$). The take of the epidermal autograft was 86%.

Mean donor site thickness was 0.325 ± 0.045 mm for control sites and only 0.15 ± 0.0625 mm for epidermal grafts which were harvested for placement over the newly synthesized dermis; the difference was found to be significant by t test with a p value of <0.001. The thinner donor sites used in the artificial skin procedures healed, as expected, significantly faster, requiring 10.6 ± 5.8 d compared to 14.3 ± 6.9 d for control sites, with a p value of <0.001 by t test. It is worth noting that donor sites used in the artificial skin procedure were frequently reharvested sites from previous autografting; reharvested donor sites healed more slowly than primary sites.

The subjective evaluation of the operating surgeons at the conclusion of the acute stage of treatment was a response to the question, "Was artificial dermis (artificial skin) advantageous in the management of this particular patient?" Sixty-three percent of the comments were affirmative, whereas in 36% of the responses, the acute (early) results were believed to be no better than by use of routine methods. The physicians who responded positively to the use of artificial skin commented on the ability to use thin donor sites that healed quickly, relative to the thicker donor sites which were harvested in preparation for an autograft. Positive comments also cited the handling characteristics of the artificial skin relative to the allograft as well as the ability to close the wound without fear of rejection while awaiting healing of the donor site. Negative comments included a less-than-adequate drainage of serum and blood through the unperforated silicone sheet, the seemingly poor resistance of the artificial skin to infection, and the need for a second operation.

Long-Term Clinical Evaluation of Artificial Skin

One year after treatment, the allografted and xenografted sites had been long ago covered definitively with autograft; therefore, the experimental sites included, in the long term, either autografts (referred to occasionally as *controls* below) or the test sites, comprising the new integument induced as a result of treatment with the artificial skin (partially regenerated dermis closed with an epidermal graft).

The patients reported that itching was significantly less (Wilcoxin Rank Sum test $p < 0.02$) in the artificial skin site than in control sites. Dryness, scaliness, elasticity (deformability), sweating, sensation, and erythema were similar at both control and artificial skin sites. Hypertrophic scarring was reported to be less in artificial skin in 42% of sites and was reported to be equivalent on test and control sites 57% of the time. No patient reported that the artificial skin sites had more hypertrophic scar than the autografted sites. Even though donor sites that were used during treatment with the artificial skin were harvested repeatedly (recropping), 72% of patients reported that these artificial skin donor sites felt "more normal," 17% felt that there was no difference, and 11% felt that the control donor site was "more normal."

The results of the histologic study on this patient population showed that, in sites where the artificial skin was used, an intact dermis was synthesized as well as definitive closure of a complete epidermal layer with a minimum of scarring. The results of the immunologic study led to the conclusion that, in patients who had been treated with the artificial skin, there was increased antibody activity to bovine skin collagen, bovine skin collagen with chondroitin sulfate, and human collagen; however, it was concluded that these increased levels of antibody were not immunologically significant.

The overall evaluation by the patients showed that 26% preferred the new integument generated by use of the artificial skin whereas 64% found that the sites were equivalent and 10% showed preference for the autografted site. Physicians' overall evaluation showed that 39% preferred the artificial skin site, 45% found the sites to be equivalent, and 16% preferred the autografted site.

Clinical Results

The take of the artificial skin was comparable to all other grafts and was inferior only to the meshed autograft. The latter showed superior take in part because meshing reduces drastically the flexural rigidity of the graft (see above) leading thereby to greater conformity with the wound bed (see Fig. 134.4). The interstices in the meshed autograft also provided an outlet for drainage of serum and blood from the wound, thereby allowing removal of these fluids. By contrast, the continuity of the silicone sheet in the artificial skin accounted for the increased flexural rigidity of the graft and prevented drainage of wound fluids with a resulting increased incidence of fluid accumulation underneath the graft. Fluid accumulation is probably the cause of the reduced take of the artificial skin, since immediate formation of a physicochemical bond between the graft and the wound bed was thereby prevented (see Fig. 134.4). The development of infection underneath the artificial skin, noted by physicians in certain cases, can also be explained as originating in the layer of wound fluid which presumptively collected underneath the artificial skin. This analysis suggests that meshing of the silicone layer of the artificial skin, without affecting the continuity of the collagen-GAG layer, could lead to improved take and probably to reduced incidence of infection.

The healing time for donor sites associated with use of the artificial skin was shorter by about 4 days than for donor sites that were used to harvest autograft. An even shorter healing time for donor sites for artificial skin can be realized by reducing the thickness of the epidermal graft which is required to close the dermal bed. The average epidermal graft thickness reported in this study, 0.15 mm, was significantly higher than thicknesses in the range 0.05–0.07 mm, corresponding to an epidermal graft with adequate continuity but negligible amount of attached dermis. Increasing familiarity of surgeons with the procedure for harvesting these thin epidermal grafts is expected to lead to harvesting of thinner grafts in future studies. The importance of harvesting a thin graft cannot be overestimated, since the healing time of the donor site decreases rapidly with decreasing thickness. It has been reported that the mean healing time for donor sites for the artificial skin reported in this study, about 11 days, is reduced to 4 days provided that a pure epidermal graft, free of dermis, can be harvested.

Not only does the time to heal increase, but the incidence of hypertrophic scarring at a donor site also increases with the thickness of the harvested graft. This observation explains the higher incidence of hypertrophic scarring in donor sites associated with the harvesting of autografts, since the latter were thicker by about 0.175 mm than the epidermal grafts used with the artificial skin. An additional advantage associated with use of a thin epidermal graft is the opportunity to reharvest (recropping) within a few days; this reflects the ability of epithelial tissues to regenerate spontaneously provided there is an underlying dermal bed. When frequent recropping of donor graft is possible, the surface area of a patient that can be grafted within a clinically acceptable period increases rapidly. In the clinical study described here, a patient with deep burns over as much as 85% body surface area was covered with artificial skin grafts for 75 days while the few donor sites remaining were being harvested several times each.

In the long term rarely did a patient or a physician in this clinical study prefer the new skin provided by the autograft to that provided by the artificial skin treatment. This result is clearly related to the use of meshed autografts, a standard procedure in the treatment of massively burned patients. Meshing increases the wound area which can be autografted by between 1.5 and 6 times, thereby alleviating a serious resource problem. However, meshing destroys the dermis as well as the epidermis; although the epidermis regenerates spontaneously and fills in the defects, the dermis does not. The long-term result is a skin site with the meshed pattern permanently embossed on it. The artificial skin is a device that, in principle, is available in unlimited quantity; accordingly, it does not suffer from this problem (Fig. 134.2). The result is a smooth skin surface which was clearly preferred on average by patients and physicians alike.

Summary

The prototype artificial skin leads to a new skin which appears closer to the patient's intact skin than does the meshed autograft. Take of the artificial skin is as good as all comparative materials except for the autograft, which is superior in this respect. Donor sites associated with the artificial skin treatment heal faster, can be recropped much more frequently, and eventually heal to produce sites that look closer to the patient's intact skin than do donor sites harvested for the purpose of autografting. In comparison to the allograft, the artificial skin is easier to use, has the same take, does not get rejected, and is free of the risk of viral infection associated with use of allograft.

134.6 Alternative Approaches: Cultured Epithelia and Skin Equivalents

The use of cultured epithelia has been studied clinically. In this approach autologous epidermal cells are removed by biopsy and are then cultured in vitro for about 3 weeks until a mature keratinizing epidermis has formed; the epidermis is then grafted onto the patient. The epithelial cells spread and cover the dermal substrate, eventually covering the entire wound. Results with this approach have been somewhat encouraging, especially in cases where the skin has not been lost through its full thickness. However, the take has been unsatisfactory when cultured epithelia have been grafted on full-thickness wounds.

In another development, a *skin equivalent* which consists of a collagen gel, previously contracted by fibroblasts cultured therein, has been studied with animals. Clinical studies to date with this device are very limited, and no conclusions can be drawn on its potential in treating the patient with skin loss.

An attempt has been made to correct the erratic cover provided by split-thickness autografts; the latter are normally applied in a meshed form (meshed autograft) and, consequently, fail to cover the entire wound bed with a dermal layer. The attempted improvement consisted in grafting underneath the meshed autograft a living dermal tissue replacement, consisting of a synthetic polymeric mesh (polyglactin-910) which had been cultured in vitro over a period of 2 to 3 weeks with fibroblasts isolated from neonatal foreskin. Seventeen patients with full-thickness burn wounds were included in a preliminary clinical trial. Epithelialization of the interstices of the meshed autograft led to complete wound closure in 14 days both in sites where the dermal living replacement had been grafted underneath the meshed autograft (experimental sites) and in those where it was omitted (control sites). Take of the meshed autograft was slightly reduced when the living dermal tissue replacement was underneath. Basement membrane structures developed both in control and experimental sites. Elastic fibers (elastin) were not observed in neodermal tissue either in control or experimental sites at periods up to one year after grafting. These incompletely reported results do not allow a definitive assessment of the relative value of this treatment over the artificial skin treatment described above.

Allograft is human cadaver skin, which is frequently stored in frozen state in skin bank. It is a temporary cover. If left on the wound longer than about 2 weeks, allograft is rejected by the severely burned patient, even though the latter is in an immunocompromised condition. When rejection is allowed to occur, the wound bed is temporarily ungraftable and is subject to infection. In a modification of this basic use of the allograft, the latter has been used as a dermal equivalent prior to grafting with cultured epithelia. Since the allograft is rejected if allowed to remain on the wound long enough for the epithelia to spread across the wound bed, the allograft has been treated in a variety of media in an effort to eliminate its immunogenicity. The experience with this procedure is limited.

Defining Terms

Adnexa: Accessory parts or appendages of an organ. Adnexa of skin include hair follicles and sweat glands.

Allograft: Human cadaver skin, usually maintained frozen in a skin bank and used to provide a temporary cover for deep wounds. About 2 weeks after grafting, the allograft is removed and replaced with autograft which has become available by that time. Previously referred to as *homograft.*

Artificial skin: A graft consisting of an upper layer of silicone and a lower layer of skin regeneration template. The template is a cell-free, highly porous analog of extracellular matrix.

Autograft: The patient's own skin, harvested from an intact area in the form of a membrane and used to graft an area of severe skin loss.

Basement membrane: An approximately 20-nm-thick multilayered membrane interleaved between the epidermis and the dermis.

Cell lifeline number: A dimensionless number which compares the relative magnitudes of chemical reaction and diffusion. This number, defined as S in Eq. (134.3) above, can be used to compute the maximum path length l_c over which a cell can migrate in a scaffold while depending on diffusion alone for transport of critical nutrients that it consumes. When the critical length is exceeded, the cell requires transport of nutrients by angiogenesis in order to survive.

Cultured epithelia: A mature, keratinizing epidermis synthesized in vitro by culturing epithelial cells removed from the patient by biopsy. A relatively small skin biopsy (1 cm²) can be treated to yield an area larger by about 10,000 in 2–3 weeks and is then grafted on patients with burns.

Dermal equivalent: A term which has been loosely used to describe a device that replaces, usually temporarily, the functions of the dermis following injury.

Dermis: A 2–5-mm-thick layer of connective tissue populated with quiescent fibroblasts which lies underneath the epidermis. It is separated from the former by a very thin basement membrane. The dermis of adult mammals does not regenerate spontaneously following injury.

Donor site: The skin site from which an autograft has been removed with a dermatome.

Epidermis: The cellular outer layer of skin, about 0.1-mm thick, which protects against moisture loss and against infection. An epidermal graft, e.g., cultured epithelium or a thin graft removed surgically, requires a dermal substrate for adherence onto the wound bed. The epidermis regenerates spontaneously following injury, provided there is a dermal substrate underneath.

Eschar: Dead tissue, typically the result of a thermal injury, which covers the underlying, potentially viable tissue.

Extracellular matrix: A largely insoluble, nondiffusible macromolecular network, consisting mostly of glycoproteins and proteoglycans, which, together with cells embedded therein, forms tissues.

Isomorphous matrix replacement: A term used to describe the synthesis of new, physiologic tissue within a skin regeneration template at a rate which is of the same order as the degradation of the templarte. This relation, Eq. (134.2) above, is the defining equation for a biodegradable scaffold which couples with, or interacts with, the inflammatory process of the wound bed.

Living dermal replacement: A synthetic biodegradable polymeric mesh, previously cultured with fibroblasts, which is placed underneath a conventional meshed autograft.

Meshed autograft: A sheet autograft which has been meshed and then expanded by a factor of 1.5–6 to produce grafts with a characteristic meshed pattern.

Regeneration template: A biodegradable scaffold which, when attached to a missing organ, induces its regeneration.

Scar: The result of a repair process in skin and other organs. Scar is morphologically different from skin, in addition to being mechanically less extensible and weaker than skin. The skin regeneration template induces synthesis of nearly physiologic skin rather than scar.

Sheet autograft: A layer of the patient's skin, comprising the epidermis and about one-third of the dermal thickness, which has not been meshed prior to grafting areas of severe skin loss.

Skin: A vital organ which indispensably protects the organism from infection and dehydration while also providing other functions essential to physiologic life, such as assisting in thermoregulation and providing a tactile sensor for the organism.

Skin equivalent: A collagen gel which has been contracted by fibroblasts cultured therein. In combination with keratinocytes, it has been used to cover deep wounds in animals.

Skin regeneration template: A graft copolymer of type I collagen and chondroitin 6-sulfate, average pore diameter 20–125 μm, degrading in vivo to an extent of about 50% in 2 weeks, which induces partial regeneration of the dermis in wounds from which the dermis has been fully excised. When seeded with keratinocytes prior to grafting, this analog of extracellular matrix has induced simultaneous synthesis both of a dermis and an epidermis.

Split-thickness autograft: An autograft which is about one-half or one-third as thick as the full thickness of skin.

Subcutis: A layer of fat tissue underneath the dermis.

Synthetic skin: A term used to describe the artificial skin in the early literature.

Take: The adhesion of a graft on the woundbed. Without adequate take, there is no physicochemical or biologic interaction between graft and wound bed.

Xenograft: Skin graft obtained from a different species; e.g., pig skin grafted on human. Synthetic polymeric membranes are often referred to as *xenografts*. Previously referred to as *heterograft*.

References

Boykin JV Jr, Molnar JA. 1992. Burn scar and skin equivalent. In IK Cohen, RF Diegelmann, WJ Lindblad (eds), Wound Healing, pp 523–540, Philadelphia, Saunders.

Burke JF, Yannas IV, Quinby WC Jr, et al. 1981. Successful use of a physiologically acceptable artificial skin in the treatment of extensive burn injury. Ann Surg 194:413.

Heimbach D, Luterman A, Burke J, et al. 1988. Artificial dermis for major burns. Ann Surg 208:313.

Michaeli D, McPherson M. 1990. Immunologic study of artificial skin used in the treatment of thermal injuries. J Burn Care Rehab 11:21.

Stern R, McPherson M, Longaker MT. 1990. Histologic study of artificial skin used in the treatment of full-thickness thermal injury. J Burn Care Rehab 11:7.

Tompkins RG, Burke JF. 1992. Artificial skin. Surg Rounds 881.

Yannas IV, Burke JF, Orgill DP, et al. 1982. Wound tissue can utilize a polymeric template to synthesize a functional extension of skin. Science 215:174.

Yannas IV, Burke JF. 1980. Design of an artificial skin: I. Basic design principles. J Biomed Mater Res 14:65.

Yannas IV, Burke JF, Gordon PL, et al. 1977. Multilayer membrane useful as synthetic skin, US Patent 4,060,081, Nov. 29, 1977.

Yannas IV, Burke JF, Warpehoski M, et al. 1981. Prompt, long-term functional replacement of skin. Trans Am Soc Artif Intern Organs 27:19.

Further Information

Boyce ST, Hansbrough JF. 1988. Biologic attachment, growth, and differentiation of cultured human keratinocytes on a graftable collagen and chondroitin 6-sulfate substrate. Surgery 103:421.

Eldad A, Burt A, Clarke JA. 1987. Cultured epithelium as a skin substitute. Burns 13:173.

Gallico GG, O'Connor NE, Compton CC, et al. 1984. Permanent coverage of large burn wounds with autologous cultured human epithelium. N Eng J Med 311:448.

Hausbrough JF, Dore C, Hausbrough WB. 1992. Clinical trials of a living dermal tissue replacement placed beneath meshed, split-thickness skin grafts on excised burn wounds. J Burn Care Rehab 13:519.

Langer R, Vacanti JP. 1993. Tissue engineering. Science 260:920.

O'Connor NE, Mulliken JB, Banks-Schlegel S, et al. 1981. Grafting of burns with cultured epithelium prepared from autologous epidermal cells. Lancet 1:75.

Yannas IV, Lee E, Orgill DP, et al. 1989. Synthesis and characterization of a model extracellular matrix that induces partial regeneration of adult mammalian skin. Proc Natl Acad Sci USA 86:933.

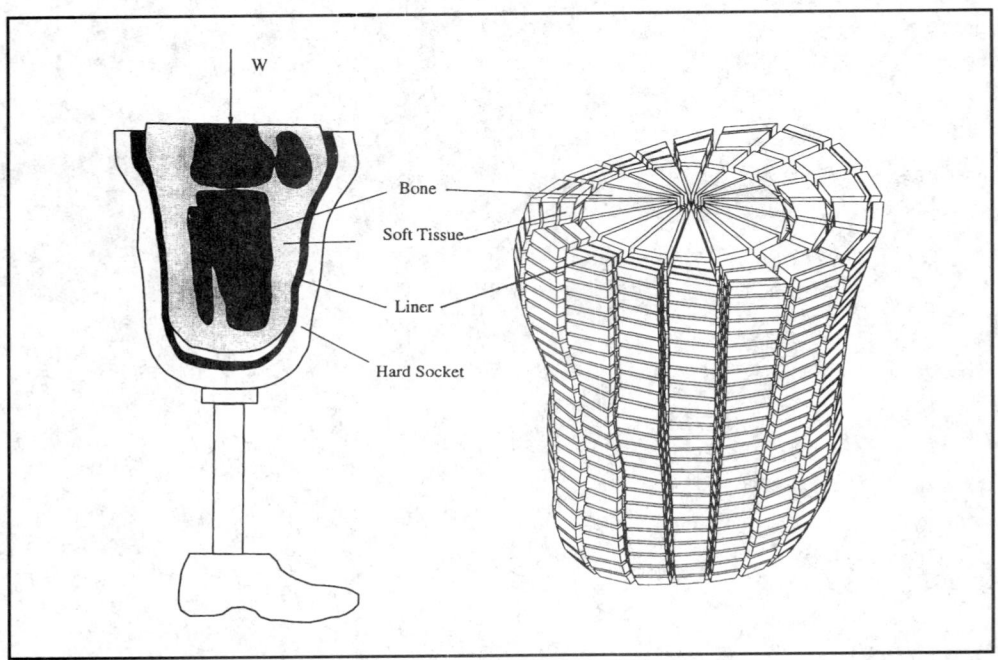

Finite-element analysis employed to determine sensitivity of interface pressures to socket-shape rectification illustrating limb and socket and elements in layers.

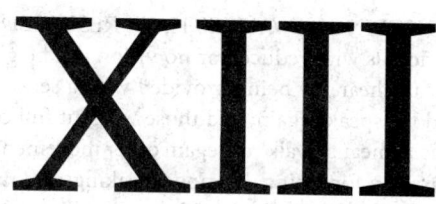

XIII

Rehabilitation Engineering

Charles J. Robinson
University of Pittsburgh and Highland Drive Veterans Affairs Medical Center

ENGINEERING ADVANCES HAVE RESULTED IN enormous strides in the field of rehabilitation. Individuals with reduced or no vision can be given "sight"; those with severe or complete hearing loss can "hear" by being provided with a sense of their surroundings; those unable to talk can be aided to "speak" again; and those without full control of a limb (or with the limb missing) can by artificial means "walk" or regain other movement functions. The present level of available functional restoration for seeing, hearing, speaking, and moving, however, still pales in comparison with the capabilities of individuals without disability. As is readily apparent from the content of many of the chapters in this *Handbook,* the human sensory and motor (movement) systems are marvelously engineered, both within a given system and integrated across systems. The rehabilitation engineer thus faces a daunting task in trying to design augmentative or replacement systems when one or more of these systems are impaired.

Rehabilitation engineering had its origins in the need to provide assistance to individuals who were injured in World War II. *Rehabilitation engineering* can be defined in a number of ways. Perhaps the most encompassing (and the one adopted here) is that proposed by Reswick [1982]: Rehabilitation engineering is the application of science and technology to ameliorate the handicaps of individuals with disabilities. With this definition, any device, technique, or concept used in rehabilitation that has a technological basis falls under the purview of rehabilitation engineering. This contrasts with the much narrower view that is held by some that rehabilitation engineering is only the design and production phase of a broader field called *assistive technology.* Lest one consider this distinction trivial, consider that the U.S. Congress has mandated that rehabilitation engineering and technology services be provided by all states, and an argument has ensued among various groups of practitioners about who can legally provide such services because of the various interpretations of what rehabilitation engineering is.

There is a core body of knowledge that defines each of the traditional engineering disciplines. Biomedical engineering is less precisely defined, but in general, a biomedical engineer must be proficient in a traditional engineering discipline and have a working knowledge of things biologic or medical. The rehabilitation engineer is a biomedical engineer who must not only be technically proficient as an engineer and know biology and medicine but also must integrate artistic, social, financial, psychological, and physiologic considerations to develop or analyze a device, technique, or concept that meets the needs of the population that the engineer is serving. In general, rehabilitation engineers deal with musculoskeletal or sensory disabilities. They often have a strong background in biomechanics. Most work is done in a multidisciplinary team setting [Robinson, 1993a].

Rehabilitation engineering deals with many aspects of rehabilitation, including applied, scientific, clinical, technical, and theoretical. Various topics include, but are not limited to, assistive devices and other aids for those with disability, sensory augmentation and substitution systems, functional electrical stimulation (for motor control and sensory-neural prostheses), orthotics and prosthetics, myoelectric devices and techniques, transducers (including electrodes), signal processing, hardware, software, robotics, systems approaches, technology assessment, postural stability, wheelchair seating systems, gait analysis, biomechanics, biomaterials, control systems (both biologic and external), ergonomics, human performance, and functional assessment [Robinson, 1993b].

In this section of the *Handbook* we focus only on applications of rehabilitation engineering. The concepts of rehabilitation engineering, rehabilitation science, and rehabilitation technology are outlined in Chapter 135. Rehabilitation engineering's traditional strength in the orthopedics area is described in Chapter 136. Chapter 137 discusses the importance of personal mobility and various wheeled modes of transportation (wheelchairs, scooters, cars, vans, and public conveyances). Chapter 138 looks at other nonwheeled ways to enhance mobility and physical performance. Chapter 139 covers techniques available to augment sensory impairments or to provide a substitute way to input sensory information. Conversely, Chapter 140 looks at the output side as it explores augmentative (assistive) communication, control, and computer access. Chapter 141 looks at how one measures the effect of a rehabilitation intervention. Finally, Chapter 142 describes the application of rehabilitation technology in a clinical setting, where engineering principles are applied to the proper selection and design of wheelchairs, seating and postural control systems, and other types of assistive technology.

For the purposes of this *Handbook,* many topics that partially fall under the rubric of rehabilitation engineering are covered elsewhere. These include chapters on electrical stimulation (Chapter 17), hard tissue replacement: long bone repair and joints (Chapters 47.1, 48), biomechanics, analysis of gait (Chapter 27), human factors applications in rehabilitation engineering (Chapter 151), electrical stimulators (Chapter 80), bioactive brain implants (Chapter 118), and tracheal, laryngeal, and esophageal replacement devices (Chapter 132).

Rehabilitation engineering can be described as an engineering systems discipline. Imagine being the design engineer on a project that has an unknown, highly nonlinear plant with coefficients whose variations in time appear to follow no known or solvable model, where time (yours and your client's) and funding are severely limited, and where no known solution has been developed (or if it has, it will need modification for nearly every client so no economy of scale exists). Further, there will be severe impedance mismatches between available appliances and your client's needs. Or the low residual channel capacity of one of your client's senses will require enormous signal compression to get a signal with any appreciable information content through it. Welcome to the world of the rehabilitation engineer!

References

Reswick J. 1982. What is a rehabilitation engineer? In El Pan, et al. (eds), Annual Review of Rehabilitation, vol 2. New York, Springer-Verlag.

Robinson CJ. 1993*a*. Rehabilitation engineering. In RC Dorf (ed), CRC Handbook of Electrical Engineering. Boca Raton, Fla, CRC Press.

Robinson CJ. 1993*b*. Rehabilitation engineering: An editorial. IEEE Trans Rehabil Eng 1(1):1.

135

Rehabilitation Engineering, Science, and Technology

Charles J. Robinson
*University of Pittsburgh
and Highland Drive
Veterans Affairs Medical Center*

Rehabilitation engineering requires a multidisciplinary effort. To put rehabilitation engineering into its proper context, we need to review some of the other disciplines with which rehabilitation engineers must be familiar. Robinson [1993] has reviewed or put forth the following working definitions and discussions:

Rehabilitation is the *(re)integration* of an individual with a disability into society. This can be done either by enhancing existing capabilities or by providing alternative means to perform various functions or to substitute for specific sensations.

Rehabilitation engineering is the "*application* of science and technology to ameliorate the handicaps of individuals with disabilities" [Reswick, 1982]. In actual practice, many individuals who say that they practice rehabilitation engineering are not engineers by training. While this leads to controversies from practitioners with traditional engineering degrees, it also has the de facto benefit of greatly widening the scope of what is encompassed by the term *rehabilitation engineering*.

Rehabilitation medicine is a clinical *practice* that focuses on the physical aspects of functional recovery but that also considers medical, neurologic, and psychologic factors. *Physical therapy, occupational therapy,* and *rehabilitation counseling* are professions in their own right. On the sensory-motor side, other medical and therapeutical specialties practice rehabilitation in vision, audition, and speech.

Rehabilitation technology (or *assistive technology*) narrowly defined is the *selection, design,* or *manufacture* of *augmentative* or *assistive devices* that are appropriate for the individual with a disability. Such devices are selected based on the specific disability, the function to be augmented or restored, the user's wishes, the clinician's preferences, cost, and the environment in which the device will be used.

0-8493-8346-3/95/$0.00+$.50

Rehabilitation science is the *development* of a body of knowledge, gleaned from rigorous basic and clinical research, that describes how a disability alters specific physiologic functions or anatomic structures and that details the underlying principles by which residual function or capacity can be measured and used to restore function of individuals with disabilities.

135.1 Rehabilitation Concepts

Effective rehabilitation engineers must be well versed in all the areas described above because they generally work in a team setting, in collaboration with physical and occupational therapists, orthopedic surgeons, physical medicine specialists, and/or neurologists. Some rehabilitation engineers are interested in certain activities that we do in the course of a normal day that could be summarized as activities of daily living (ADL). These include eating, toileting, combing hair, brushing teeth, reading, etc. Other engineers focus on *mobility* and the limitations to mobility. Mobility can be personal (e.g., within a home or office) or public (automobile, public transportation, accessibility questions in buildings). Mobility also includes the ability to move functionally through the environment. Thus the question of mobility is not limited to that of getting from place to place but also includes such questions as whether one can reach an object in a particular setting or whether a paralyzed urinary bladder can be made functional again. Barriers that limit mobility are also studied. For instance, an ill-fitted wheelchair cushion or support system will most assuredly limit mobility by reducing the time that an individual can spend in a wheelchair before he or she must vacate it to avoid serious and difficult-to-heal pressure sores. Other groups of rehabilitation engineers deal with *sensory disabilities,* such as sight or hearing, or with *communications disorders,* both in the production side (e.g., the nonvocal) and in the comprehension side. For any given client, a rehabilitation engineer might have all these concerns to consider (i.e., ADLs, mobility, sensory, and communication dysfunctions).

A key concept in physical or sensory rehabilitation is that of residual function or residual capacity. Such a concept implies that the function or sense can be quantified, that the performance range of that function or sense is known in a nonimpaired population, and that the use of residual capacity by a disabled individual should be encouraged. These measures of human performance can be made subjectively by clinicians or objectively by some rather clever computerized test devices.

A rehabilitation engineer asks three key questions: Can a diminished function or sense be successfully augmented? Is there a substitute way to return the function or to restore a sense? And is the solution appropriate and cost-effective? These questions give rise to two important rehabilitation concepts: orthotics and prosthetics. An *orthosis* is an appliance that aids an existing function. A *prosthesis* provides a substitute.

An artificial limb is a prosthesis, as is a wheelchair. An ankle brace is an orthosis. So are eyeglasses. In fact, eyeglasses might well be the penultimate rehabilitation device. They are inexpensive, have little social stigma, and are almost completely unobtrusive to the user. They have let many millions of individuals with correctable vision problems lead productive lives. In essence, however, a pair of eyeglasses is an optical device, governed by traditional equations of physical optics. Eyeglasses can be made out of simple glass (from a raw material as abundant as the sands of the earth) or complex plastics such as those which are ultraviolet-sensitive. They can be ground by hand or by sophisticated computer-controlled optical grinders. Thus crude technology can restore functional vision. Increasing the technical content of the eyeglasses (either by material or manufacturing method) in most cases will not increase the amount of function restored, but it might make the glasses cheaper, lighter, and more prone to be used.

135.2 Engineering Concepts in Sensory Rehabilitation

Of the five traditional senses, vision and hearing most define the interactions that permit us to be human. These two senses are the main input channel through which data with high information content can flow. We read; we listen to speech or music; we view art. A loss of one or the other of these senses (or both) can have a devastating impact on the individual affected. Rehabilitation engineers attempt to restore the functions of these senses either through augmentation or via sensory substitution systems. Eyeglasses and hearing aids are examples of augmentative devices that can be used if some residual capacity remains. A major area of rehabilitation engineering research deals with *sensory substitution systems* (see Chapter 139).

The visual system has the capability to detect a single photon of light yet also has a dynamic range that can respond to intensities many orders of magnitude greater. It can work with high-contrast items and with those of almost no contrast and across the visible spectrum of colors. Millions of parallel data channels form the optic nerve that comes from an eye; each channel transmits an asynchronous and quasi-random (in time) stream of binary pulses. While the temporal coding on any one of these channels is not fast (on the order of 200 bits per second or less), the capacity of the human brain to parallel process the entire image is faster than any supercomputer yet built.

If sight is lost, how can it be replaced? A simple pair of eyeglasses will not work, since either the sensor (the retina), the communication channel (the optic nerve and all its relays to the brain), or one or more essential central processors (the occipital part of the cerebral cortex for initial processing, the parietal and other cortical areas for information extraction) has been damaged. For replacement within the system, one must determine where the visual system has failed and whether a stage of the system can be artificially bypassed. If one uses another sensory modality (e.g., touch or hearing) as an alternate input channel, one must determine whether there is sufficient bandwidth in that channel and whether the higher-order processing hierarchy is plastic enough to process information coming via a different route.

While the preceding discussion might seem just philosophical, it is more than that. We normally read printed text with our eyes. We recognize words from their (visual) letter combinations. We comprehend what we read via a mysterious processing in the parietal and temporal parts of the cerebral cortex. Could we perhaps read and comprehend this text or other forms of writing through our fingertips with an appropriate interface? The answer, surprisingly, is yes! And the adaptation actually goes back to one of the earliest applications of coding theory—that of the development of Braille. Braille condenses all text characters to a raised matrix of 2 by 3 dots (2^6 combinations), with certain combinations reserved as indicators for the next character (such as a number indicator) or for special contractions. Trained readers of Braille can read over 250 words per minute of grade 2 Braille (as fast as most sighted readers can read printed text). Thus the Braille code is in essence a rehabilitation engineering concept where an alternate sensory channel is used as a substitute and where a recoding scheme has been employed.

Rehabilitation engineers and their colleagues have designed other ways to read text. To replace the retina as a sensor element, a modern high-resolution, high-sensitivity, fast-imaging sensor (CCD, etc.) is employed to capture a visual image of the text. One method, used by the Kurzweil reading machine, converts the scanned image to text by using optical character-recognition schemes and then outputs the text as speech via text-to-speech algorithms. This machine essentially recites the text, much as a sighted helper might do when reading aloud to a blind individual. The user of the Kurzweil device is thus freed of the absolute need for a helper. Such *independence* is often the goal of rehabilitation.

Another device (the OPTICON) presents the pattern of text scanned by a small hand-held scanner to a matrix of vibrating pins on which the index finger rests [Bliss et al., 1970]. This technique works at the input stage because the fingertip has a high density of vibration detectors, and there is a good match of signal content to the spatial and temporal characteristics of the receiver. While this input mode is completely different from vision or hearing, some users can achieve good reading speeds. This implies that the central processor for text pattern content (i.e., comprehension) does not rely solely on visual neural pathways. A goal of rehabilitation is to find alternate means to perform a task.

Perhaps the most interesting method presents an image of the scanned data directly to the visual cortex via an array of implantable electrodes that are used to electrically activate nearby cortical structures. The visual cortex is laid out in a topographic fashion such that there is an orderly mapping of the signal from different parts of the retina to corresponding parts of the occipital cortex. The goal of stimulation is to mimic the neural activity that would have been evoked had the signal come through normal channels. And such stimulation does produce the sensation of light. Since the "image" stays within the visual system, the rehabilitation solution is said to be *modality-specific*. However, substantial problems remain in the design of the electrode arrays that serve as the interface between the electronics and neurologic tissue in this application, and the surgery required is very invasive.

Deafness is another manifestation of a loss of a communication channel, this time for the sense of hearing. Hearing aids are now commercially available that can adaptively filter out background noise (a predictable signal) while amplifying speech (unpredictable) using autoregressive, moving-average (ARMA) signal processing. Totally deaf individuals use vision as a substitute input channel when communicating via sign language (also a substitute code) and can sign at information rates that match or exceed that of verbal communication.

Deafness is often brought on (or occurs congenitally) by damage to the cochlea. The cochlea normally transduces variations in sound pressure intensity at a given frequency into patterns of neural discharge. This neural code is then carried by the auditory (eighth cranial) nerve to the brainstem, where it is preprocessed and relayed to auditory cortex for initial processing and on to the parietal and other cortical areas for information extraction. Similar to the case for the visual system, the cochlea, auditory nerve, auditory cortex, and all relays in between maintain a topologic map, this time based on tone frequency (tonotopic).

If deafness is solely due to cochlear damage (as is often the case), and if the auditory nerve is still intact, a newly commercialized system called a *cochlear implant* can substitute for the regular transducer array (the cochlea) while still sending the signal through the normal auditory channel (to maintain modality-specificity). A few individuals with cochlear implants have been able to comprehend speech sent over a telephone, but most users simply gain a crude, but needed, sense of their (auditory) environment. This application is discussed in greater detail in the next to the last section of this chapter.

An exciting new development is occurring outside the field of rehabilitation that could have a profound impact on the ability of the deaf to comprehend speech. Electronics companies are beginning to market universal translation aids for travelers, where a phrase spoken in one language is captured, parsed, translated, and restated (either spoken or displayed) in another language. The deaf would simply require that the display be in the language that they use for writing.

135.3 Engineering Concepts in Motor Rehabilitation

Limitations in mobility can severely restrict the quality of life of an individual so affected. A wheelchair is a prime example of a prosthesis that can restore personal mobility to those who cannot walk. Given the proper environment (fairly level floors, roads, etc), modern wheelchairs can be highly efficient. In fact, the fastest times in one of humanity's greatest tests of endurance, the Boston Marathon, are achieved by the wheelchair racers. Although they do gain the advantage of being able to roll, they still must climb the same hills and do so with only one-fifth the muscle power available to an able-bodied marathoner.

While a wheelchair user could certainly go down a set of steps (not recommended), climbing steps in a normal manual or electric wheelchair is a virtual impossibility. Ramps or lifts are engineered to provide accessibility in these cases, or special climbing wheelchairs can be purchased. Wheelchairs also do not work well on surfaces with high rolling resistance or viscous coefficients (e.g., mud, rough terrain, etc.), so alternate mobility aids must be found if access to these areas is to be provided to the physically disabled. Hand-controlled cars, vans, tractors, and even airplanes are now driven by wheelchair users. The design of appropriate control modifications falls to the rehabilitation engineer.

Loss of a limb can greatly impair functional activity. The engineering aspects of artificial limb design increase in complexity as the amount of residual limb decreases, especially if one or more joints are lost. As an example, a person with a midcalf amputation could use a simple wooden stump to extend the leg and could ambulate reasonable well. But such a leg is not cosmetically appealing and completely ignores any substitution for ankle function.

Immediately following World War II, the U.S. government began the first concerted effort to foster better engineering design for artificial limbs. Dynamically lockable knee joints were designed for artificial limbs for above-knee amputees. In the ensuing years, energy-storing artificial ankles have been designed, some with prosthetic feet so realistic that beach thongs could be worn with them. Artificial hands, wrists, and elbows were designed for upper limb amputees. Careful design of the actuating cable system also provided for a sense of hand-grip force so that the user had some feedback and did not need to rely on vision alone for guidance.

Perhaps the most transparent (to the user) artificial arms are the ones that use an electrical activity generated by the muscles remaining in the stump to control the actions of the elbow, wrist, and hand [Stein et al., 1988]. This electrical activity is known as *myoelectricity* and is produced as the muscle contraction spreads through the muscle. Note that these muscles, if intact, would have controlled at least one of these joints (e.g., the biceps and triceps for the elbow). Thus a high level of modality-specificity is maintained, since the functional element is substituted only at the last stage. All the batteries, sensor electrodes, amplifiers, motor actuators, and controllers (generally analog) reside entirely within these myoelectric arms. An individual trained in the use of a myoelectric arm can perform some impressive tasks with this arm. Current engineering research efforts involve the control of simultaneous multijoint movements (rather than the single-joint movement now available) and the provision for sensory feedback from the end effector of the artificial arm to the skin of the stump via electrical means.

135.4 Engineering Concepts in Communication Disorders

Speech is a uniquely human means of interpersonal communication. Problems that affect speech can occur at the initial transducer (the larynx) or at other areas of the vocal tract. They can be of neurologic (due to cortical, brainstem, or peripheral nerve damage), structural, and/or cognitive origin. A person might only be able to make a halting attempt at talking or might not have sufficient control of other motor skills to type or write.

If only the larynx is involved, an externally applied artificial larynx can be used to generate a resonant column of air that can be modulated by other elements in the vocal tract. If other motor skills are intact, typing can be used to generate text, which in turn can be spoken via text-to-speech devices described earlier. And the rate of typing (either whole words or via coding) might be fast enough so that reasonable speech rates could be achieved.

The rehabilitation engineer often becomes involved in the design or specification of *augmentative communication aids* for individuals who do not have good muscle control, either for speech or for limb movement. A whole industry has developed around the design of symbol or letter boards, where the user can point out (often painstakingly) letters, words, or concepts. Some of these boards now have speech output. Linguistics and information theory have been combined in the invention of acceleration techniques intended to speed up the communication process. These include alternative language representation systems based on semantic (iconic), alphanumeric, or other codes and prediction systems, which provide choices based on previously selected letters or words. Goodenough-Trepagnier [1994] edited a good publication dealing with human factors and cognative requirements.

Some individuals can produce speech, but it is dysarthric and very hard to understand. Yet the utterance does contain information. Can this limited information be used to figure out what the individual wanted to say and then voice it by artificial means? Research labs are now employing neural-network theory to determine which pauses in an utterance are due to content (i.e., between a word or sentence) and which are due to unwanted halts in speech production.

135.5 Appropriate Technology

Rehabilitation engineering lies at the interface of a wide variety of technical, biologic, and other concerns. A user might (and often does) put aside a technically sophisticated rehabilitation device in favor of a simpler device that is cheaper and easier to use and maintain. The cosmetic appearance of the device (or *cosmesis*) sometimes becomes the overriding factor in acceptance or rejection of a device. A key design factor often lies in the use of the appropriate technology to accomplish the task adequately given the extent of the resources available to solve the problem and the residual capacity of the client. Adequacy can be verified by determining that increasing the technical content of the solution results in disproportionately diminishing gains or escalating costs. Thus a rehabilitation engineer must be able to distinguish applications where high technology is required from those where such technology results in an incremental gain in cost, durability, acceptance, and other factors. Further, appropriateness very much depends on location. What is appropriate to a client near a major medical center in a highly developed country might not be appropriate to one in a rural setting or in a developing country.

This is not to say that rehabilitation engineers should shun advances in technology. In fact, a fair proportion of rehabilitation engineers work in a research setting where state-of-the-art technology is being applied to the needs of the disabled. However, it is often difficult to transfer complex technology from a laboratory to disabled consumers not directly associated with that laboratory. Such devices are often designed for use only in a structured environment, are difficult to repair properly in the field, and often require a high level of user interaction or sophistication.

Technology transfer in the rehabilitation arena is difficult, due to the limited and fragmented market. Advances in rehabilitation engineering are often piggybacked onto advances in commercial electronics. For instance, the exciting developments in text-to-speech and speech-to-text devices mentioned earlier are being driven by the commercial marketplace and not by the rehabilitation arena. But such developments will be welcomed by rehabilitation engineers no less.

135.6 An Example of Rehabilitation Engineering

In this short chapter it is difficult to convey just how much engineering actually can go into the design of a rehabilitation device. Clearly, mechanical and materials engineering must play an important role in the design of modern orthopedic aids (seating surfaces, artificial limbs or joints, wheelchairs, braces, etc.). However, the influence of electrical and electronics engineering (as opposed to technology) is often more subtle. For instance, there are many rehabilitation applications that use computer technology, but very few of these actually involve applying engineering principles to the rehabilitation problem itself. There are, however, classes of rehabilitation problems where engineering techniques are essential to the development of an appropriate solution. One of these classes involves the use of residual nervous pathways to restore a sense lost by injury, disease, or genetic deficit. A good example of this latter class is the cochlear implant (Fig. 135.1), which was briefly described in a preceding section. At first glance, the design of a cochlear prosthesis to restore hearing appears daunting. The hearing range of a healthy young individual is 20 to 16,000 Hz. The transducing structure, the cochlea, has 3500 inner and 12,000 outer hair cells, each best activated by a specific frequency that causes a localized mechanical resonance in the basilar membrane of the cochlea (see Fig. 135.1a). Deflection of a hair cell causes the cell to fire an all-or-none (i.e., pulsatile) neuronal discharge, whose rate of repetition depends to a first approximation on the amplitude of the stimulus. The outputs of these hair cells have an orderly convergence on the 30,000 to 40,000 fibers that make up the auditory portion of the eighth cranial nerve. These afferent fibers in turn go to brainstem neurons that process and relay the signals on to higher brain centers [Klinke, 1983]. For many causes of deafness, the hair cells are destroyed, but the eighth nerve remains intact. Thus, if one could elicit activity in a specific output fiber by means other than the hair cell motion, perhaps some sense of hearing could be restored.

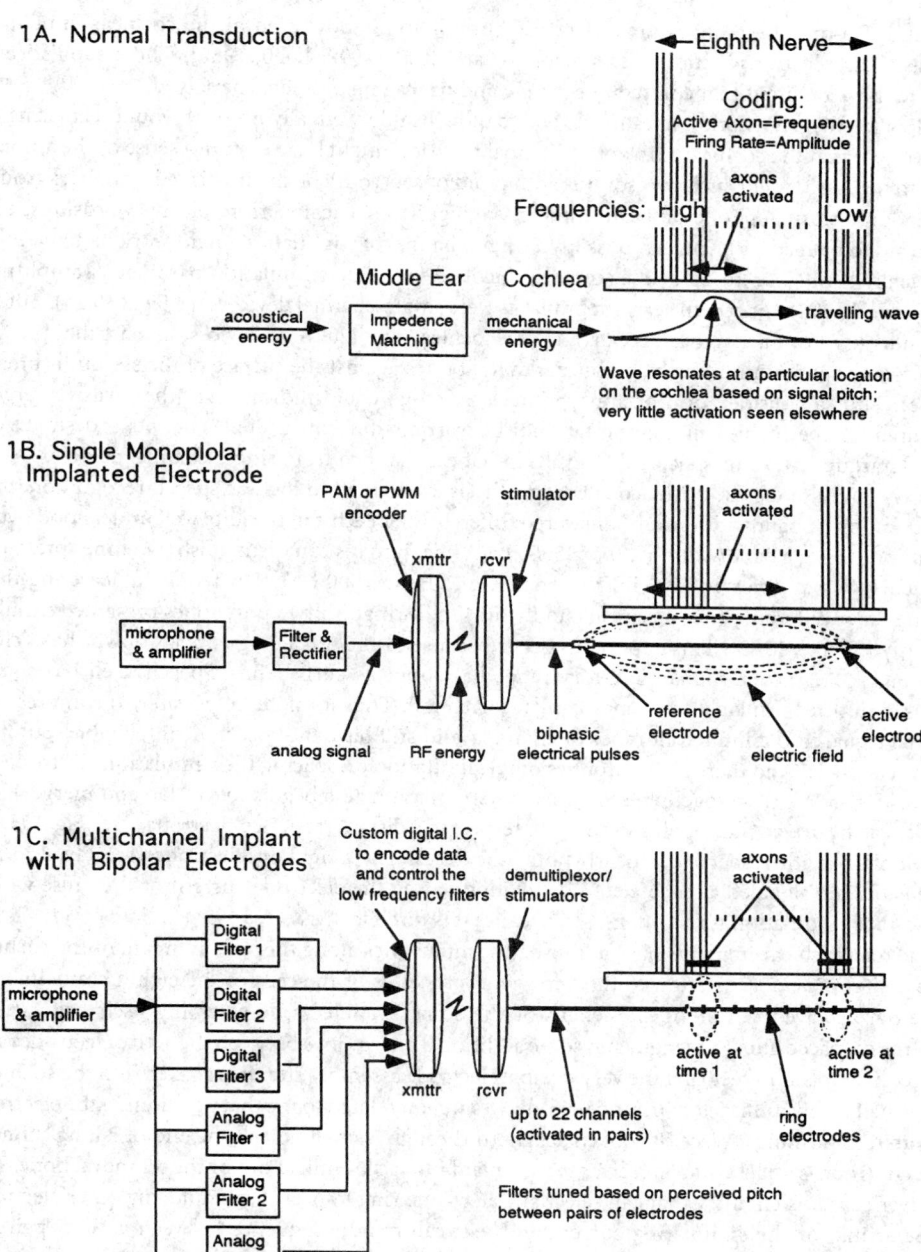

FIGURE 135.1 Mechanisms of normal hearing (1A), and electrical stimulation via a single (1B) or multichannel (1C) cochlear implant. See text for details.

Electrical stimulation can be used to excite axons in a nerve, but the spacing of the hair cells, their size, and convergence are such that its is currently impossible to stimulate just one afferent axon in the eighth nerve. Further, our ability to couple signals into a nerve trunk is also rudimentary and is done by exciting a portion of the nerve bundle from the surface of the nerve. The geometry of the cochlea helps in this regard, since different portions of the nerve are closer to different parts of the cochlea. Despite these limitations, electrical stimulation is now used in the cochlear implant to bypass hair cell transduction mechanisms [Clark et al., 1990; Loeb, 1985]. These sophisticated devices have required that complex electronic and packaging problems be solved.

Now for the engineering questions. What bandwidth do we really need? It would seem sensible to propose that the cochlear implant's principal function might be to restore a sense of the ambient auditory environment such that sounds with rapid onsets could be distinguished from background (e.g., doors closing, phone or alarm ringing, distinguishing fricative from plosive words in speech as an aid to lip reading). For this, possibly a single channel of stimulation might work in many cases, especially if the amplitude of the sound is encoded via some stimulation parameter (amplitude, pulse width, etc.). Indeed, the earliest implants were single-channel devices (see Fig. 135.1*b*). But the stimulus used can activate a large area of the cochlea. And alternate devices do exist that provide single-channel sensation, such as a buzzer that vibrates against the surface of the sternum (breast-bone). Thus a consideration of appropriate technology could indicate that the invasive surgery required for the cochlear implant might not be warranted if only a single channel is desired. As a counterargument, some spectacular results have been claimed from single-channel devices.

If the premise for use of the cochlear prosthesis is enlarged to include speech recognition, then the question of bandwidth will be answered differently. Speech can be quite well understood over a telephone using a bandwidth of 30 to 3500 Hz. While humans can distinguish two tones presented sequentially that differ by 0.3% in frequency (e.g., 3 Hz at 1000 Hz), they require at least one-third of an octave difference (i.e., a critical bandwidth) to distinguish two pure tones presented simultaneously [Klinke, 1983]. This appears to occur because of the way energy travels down the cochlea (see Fig. 135.1*a*). The human auditory range has about 24 such bands. Speech itself has energy focused in three principal frequency bands (formants). Thus it might be possible to compress the speech signal into a limited number of channels and still have the speech be intelligible. But how many channels? And there is a neurophysiologic limitation on spacing the stimulation electrodes. If electrodes are set close together, their effective stimulation area begins to overlap and merge. Electrodes can be driven monopolarly (i.e., with respect to a distant reference electrode—see Fig. 135.1*b*) or bipolarly with respect to a nearby, but not necessarily neighbor, electrode (see Fig. 135.1*c*). Intensities are signaled at each electrode by modulating the electrode current or the pulse width; pulse-rate modulation is not often used because it is not effective.

Current cochlear implants have at most 22 stimulus sites along the scala tympani of the cochlea. Those sites provide excitation to the peripheral processes of the cells of the eighth cranial nerve, which are splayed out along the length of the scala. The electrode assembly itself has 22 ring electrodes spaced along its length and some additional guard rings between the active electrodes and the receiver to aid in securing the very flexible electrode assembly after it is snaked into the cochlea's very small (a few millimeters) round window (a surgeon related to me that positioning the electrode was akin to pushing a piece of cooked spaghetti through a small hole at the end of a long tunnel). The electrode is attached to a receiver that is inlaid into a slot milled out of the temporal bone. The receiver contains circuitry that can select any electrode ring to be a source and any other electrode to be a sink for the stimulating current and that can rapidly sequence between various pairs of electrodes (see Fig. 135.1*c*). The receiver is powered and controlled by a radiofrequency link with an external transmitter, whose alignment is maintained by means of a permanent magnet embedded in the receiver.

A digital signal processor stores information about a specific user and his or her optimal electrode locations for specific frequency bands. The signal frequencies are decomposed into bands by means of analog and digital filters—the voicing frequency and the first and second formant frequencies are filtered digitally, while the frequencies about 2 kHz are filtered with three analog filters. The transmitter receives input from these tunable filters (see Fig. 135.1*c*). However, these filters are assigned to particular electrodes after a very exhaustive testing program that attempts to determine the relative pitch perception produced by each electrode ring or pair. The object is to determine what pair of electrodes best produces the subjective perception of a certain pitch *in the implanted individual* *himself or herself* and then to associate a particular filter with that pair via the controller. Within the limits of threshold and saturation, the amplitude of the stimulus pulse delivered to the pair is determined by the energy in the filter band. The amplitudes are translated into biphasic pulse amplitudes and widths that can be changed dynamically over a wide range as determined by the characteristics of the particular user. The pulse amplitudes can be varied from 15 µA to 1.5 mA; the widths from 200 to 400 µs. Two schemes are used to determine pulse repetition frequency (PRF); the PRF can be set equal to the voicing frequency or it can be fixed at about 250 Hz.

An enormous amount of compression occurs in taking the frequency range necessary for speech comprehension and reducing it to a few discrete channels. At present, the optimal compression algorithm is unknown. But what is amazing is that some totally deaf individuals (albeit a small minority of from 5% to 10% of users) can relearn to comprehend speech exceptionally well without lip reading through the use of these implants. Other individuals find that the implant aids in lip reading. For some, only an awareness of environmental sounds is apparent, and for another group, the implant appears to have had little effect. However, if you could (as I have been able to) finally converse in unaided speech with an individual who had been rendered totally blind and deaf by a traumatic brain injury, you begin to appreciate the power of rehabilitation engineering.

135.7 The Future of Engineering in Rehabilitation

The traditional engineering disciplines permeate many aspects of rehabilitation. Signal processing, control, and information theory, materials design, and computers are all in widespread use from an electrical engineering perspective. Neural networks, microfabrication, fuzzy logic, virtual reality, image processing, and other emerging electrical and computer engineering tools are increasingly being applied. Mechanical engineering principles are used in biomechanical studies, gait and motion analysis, prosthetic fitting, seat cushion and back support design, and the design of artificial joints. Materials and metallurgical engineers provide input on newer biocompatable materials. Chemical engineers are developing implantable sensors. Industrial engineers are increasingly studying rehabilitative ergonomics.

The challenge to rehabilitation engineers is to find advances in *any* field, engineering or otherwise, that will aid their clients who have a disability.

Defining Terms

Activities of daily living (ADL): Personal activities that are done by almost everyone in the course of a normal day, including eating, toileting, combing hair, brushing teeth, reading, etc. ADLs are distinguished from hobbies and from work-related activities (e.g., typing).

Appropriate technology: The technology that will accomplish a task adequately given the resources available. Adequacy can be verified by determining that increasing the technological content of the solution results in diminishing gains or increasing costs.

Disability: Lack of a competent ability to perform a particular function or functions in the manner in which these functions are normally performed due to a physical, medical, or mental incapacity or loss. Compare with *handicap*.

Handicap: A barrier to normal function, a disadvantage to the performance of a task. A person might or might not be handicapped by a disability or even need a disability to be handicapped. And the handicap might be imposed from outside the disability. Indeed, everyone is occasionally handicapped by a step that is too high, but people in wheelchairs are handicapped by steps in general if they need to climb them.

Modality-specific: A task that is specific to a single sense or movement pattern.

Orthosis: A modality-specific appliance that aids the performance of a function or movement by augmenting or assisting the residual capabilities of that function or movement. An orthopedic brace is an orthosis.

Prosthesis: An appliance that substitutes for the loss of a particular function, generally by involving a different modality as an input and/or output channel. An artificial limb, a sensory substitution system, or an augmentative communication aid are prosthetic devices.

Residual function or residual capacity: *Residual function* is a measure of the ability to carry out one or more general tasks using the methods normally used. *Residual capacity* is a measure of the ability to carry out these tasks using any means of performance. These residual measures are generally more subjective than other more quantifiable measures such as residual strength.

References

Much of this material also appeared in Robinson CJ. 1993. Rehabilitation engineering. In RC Dorf (ed), CRC Handbook of Electrical Engineering, chap 107. Boca Raton, Fla, CRC Press.

Bliss JC, Katcher MH, Rogers CH, Shepard RP. 1970. Optical-to-tactile image conversion for the blind. IEEE Trans Man-Machine Syst MMS-11:58.

Clark GM, Tong YC, Patrick JF. 1990. Cochlear Prostheses. Edinburgh, Churchill-Livingstone.

Goodenough-Trepagnier C. 1994. Guest editor of a special issue of Assist Technol 6(1) dealing with mental loads in augmentative communication.

Kaczmarek KA, Webster JG, Bach-y-Rita P, Tompkins WJ. 1991. Electrotactile and vibrotactile displays for sensory substitution. IEEE Trans Biomed Eng 38:1.

Klinke R. 1983. Physiology of the sense of equilibrium, hearing and speech. In RF Schmidt, G Thews (eds), Human Physiology. Berlin, Springer-Verlag.

Loeb GE. 1985. The functional replacement of the ear. Sci Am 252:104.

Reswick J. 1982. What is a rehabilitation engineer? In EL Pan, TE Backer, CL Vash (eds), Annual Review of Rehabilitation, vol 2. New York, Springer-Verlag.

Robinson CJ. 1993. Rehabilitation engineering—An editorial. IEEE Trans Rehabil Eng 1(1):1.

Stein RB, Charles D, James KB. 1988. Providing motor control for the handicapped: A fusion of modern neuroscience, bioengineering, and rehabilitation. In SG Waxman (ed), Advances in Neurology, vol 47: Functional Recovery in Neurological Disease. New York, Raven Press.

Further Information

Readers interested in rehabilitation engineering can contact RESNA, an interdisciplinary association for the advancement of rehabilitation and assistive technologies, 1101 Connecticut Ave., N.W., Suite 700, Washington, DC 20036. RESNA publishes a quarterly journal called *Assistive Technology*. The United States Department of Veterans Affairs puts out a quarterly *Journal of Rehabilitation R&D*. The January issue of each year contains an overview of most of the rehabilitation engineering efforts occurring in the United States and Canada, with over 500 listings. The IEEE Engineering in Medicine and Biology Society has begun publishing the *IEEE Transactions on Rehabilitation Engineering*, a quarterly journal. The reader should contact the IEEE for further details.

136

Orthopedic Prosthetics and Orthotics in Rehabilitation

Marilyn Lord
King's College London

Alan Turner-Smith
King's College London

An *orthopedic prosthesis* is an internal or external device that *replaces* lost parts or functions of the neuroskeletomotor system. In contrast, a *orthopedic orthosis* is a device that *augments* a function of the skeletomotor system by controlling motion or altering the shape of body tissue. For example, an artificial leg or hand is a prosthesis, whereas a calliper (or brace) is an orthosis. This chapter addresses only orthoses and external orthopedic prostheses; internal orthopedic prostheses, such as artificial joints, are a subject on their own.

When a human limb is lost through disease or trauma, the integrity of the body is compromised in so many ways that an engineer may well feel daunted by the design requirements for a prosthetic replacement. Consider the losses from a lower limb amputation. Gone is the structural support for the upper body in standing, along with the complex joint articulations and muscular motor system involved in walking. Lost also is the multimode sensory feedback, from *inter alia* pressure sensors on the sole of the foot, length and force sensors in the muscles, and position sensors in the joints, which closed the control loop around the skeletomotor system. The body also has lost a significant percentage of its weight and is now asymmetrical and unbalanced.

We must first ask if it is desirable to attempt to replace all these losses with like-for-like components. If so, we need to strive to make a bionic limb of similar weight embodying anthropomorphic articulations with equally powerful motors and distributed sensors connected back into the wearer's residual neuromuscular system. Or, is it better to accept the losses and redefine the optimal functioning of the new unit of person-plus-technology? In many cases, it may be concluded that a wheelchair is the optimal solution for lower limb loss. Even if engineering could provide the bionic solution, which it certainly cannot at present despite huge inroads made into aspects of these demands, there remain additional problems inherent to prosthetic replacements to consider. Of these, the unnatural mechanical interface between the external environment and the human body is one of the most difficult. Notably, in place of weight bearing through the structures of the foot that are well adapted for this purpose, load must now be transferred to the skeletal structures via intimate contact between the surface of residual limb and prosthesis; the exact distribution of load becomes critical. To circumvent these problems, an alternative direct transcutaneous fixation to the bone has been attempted in limited experimental trials, but this brings its own problems of materials biocompatability and prevention of infection ingress around the opening through the skin.

Orthotic devices are classified by acronyms that describe the joint which they cross. Thus an AFO is an ankle-foot orthosis, a CO is a cervical orthosis (neck brace or collar), and a TLSO is a thoracolumbosacral orthosis (spinal brace or jacket). The main categories are braces for the cervix (neck), upper limb, trunk, lower limb, and foot. Orthoses are generally simpler devices than prostheses, but because orthoses are constrained by the existing body shape and function, they can present an equally demanding design challenge. Certainly the interaction with body function is more critical, and successful application demands an in-depth appreciation of both residual function and the probable reaction to external interference. External orthotics are often classified as structural or functional, the former implying a static nature to hold an unstable joint and the latter a flexible or articulated system to promote the correct alignment of the joints during dynamic functioning. An alternative orthotic approach utilizes functional electrical stimulation (FES) of the patient's own muscles to generate appropriate forces for joint motion; this is dealt with in Chapter 138.

136.1 Fundamentals

Designers of orthotic and prosthetic devices are aware of the three cardinal considerations—function, structure, and cosmesis.

For requirements of function, we must be very clear about the objectives of treatment. This requires first an understanding of the clinical condition. Functional prescription is now a preferred route for the medical practitioner to specify the requirements, leaving the implementation of this instruction to the prosthetist, orthotist, or rehabilitation technologist. The benefits of this distinction between client specification and final hardware will be obvious to design engineers. Indeed, the influence of design procedures on the supply process is a contribution from engineering that is being appreciated more and more.

The second requirement for function is the knowledge of the biomechanics that underlies both the dysfunction in the patient and the function of proposed device to be coupled to the patient. Kinematics, dynamics, energy considerations, and control all enter into this understanding of function. Structure is the means of carrying the function, and finally both need to be embodied into a design that is cosmetically acceptable. Some of the fundamental issues in these concepts are discussed here.

To function well, the device needs an effective coupling to the human body. To this end, there is often some part that is molded to the contours of the wearer. Achieving a satisfactory mechanical interface of a molded component depends primarily on the shape. The internal dimensions of such components are not made an exact match to the external dimensions of the limb segment, but by a process of *rectification*, the shape is adjusted to relieve areas of skin with low load tolerance. The shapes are also evolved to achieve appropriate load distribution for stability of coupling between prosthetic socket and limb or, in orthotic design, a system of usually three forces that generates a moment to stabilize a collapsing joint (Fig. 136.1). Alignment is a second factor influencing the interface loading. For lower limb prostheses particularly, the alignment of the molded socket to the remainder of the structural components also will be critical in determining the moments and forces transmitted to the interface when the foot is flat on the ground. The same is true for lower limb orthoses, where the net action of the ground reaction forces and consequent moments around the natural joints are highly dependent on the alignment taken up by the combination of orthosis and shoe. Adjustability may be important, particularly for children or progressive medical conditions.

Functional components that enable desirable motions are largely straightforward engineering mechanisms such as hinges or dampers, although the specific design requirements for their dynamic performance may be quite complex because of the biomechanics of the body. An example of the design of knee joints is expanded below. These motions may be driven from external power sources but more often are passive or body-powered mechanisms. In orthoses where relatively small angular motions are needed, these may be provided by material flexibility rather than mechanisms.

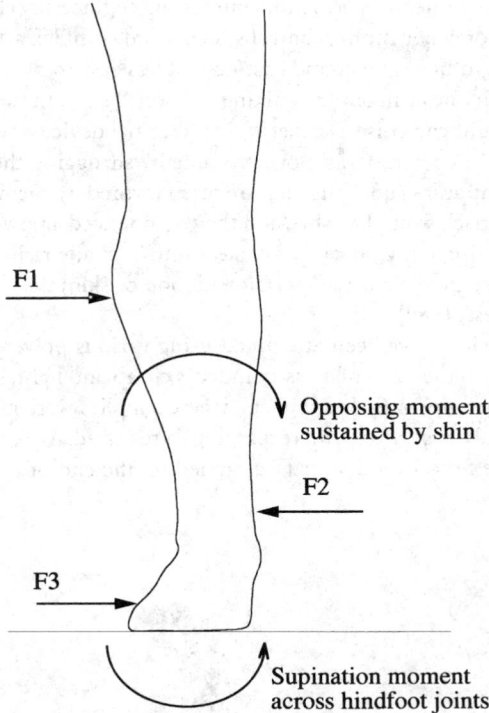

F1

Opposing moment
sustained by shin

F2

F3

Supination moment
across hindfoot joints

FIGURE 136.1 Three-force system required in an orthosis to control a valgus hindfoot due to weakness in the hindfoot supinators.

The structural requirements for lower-limb prosthetics have been laid down at a consensus meeting (1978) based on biomechanical measurement of forces in a gait laboratory, referred to as the *Philadelphia standards* and soon to be incorporated into an ISO standard (ISO 13404,5; ISO 10328). Not only are the load level and life critical, but so is the mode of failure. Sudden failure of an ankle bolt resulting in disengagement of an artificial foot is not only potentially life-threatening to an elderly amputee who falls and breaks a hip but also can be quite traumatic to unsuspecting witnesses of the apparent event of autoamputation. Design and choice of materials should ensure a controlled slow yielding, not brittle fracture. A further consideration is the ability of the complete structure to absorb shock loading, either the repeated small shocks of walking at the heel strike or rather more major shocks during sports activities or falls. This minimizes the shock transmitted through the skin to the skeleton, known to cause both skin lesions and joint degeneration. Finally, the consideration of hygiene must not be overlooked; the user must be able to clean the orthosis or prosthesis adequately without compromising its structure or function.

Added to the two elements of structure and function, the third element of *cosmesis* completes the trilogy. Appearance can be of great psychological importance to the user, and technology has its contribution here, too. As examples, special effects familiar in science fiction films also can be harnessed to provide realistic cosmetic covers for hand or foot prostheses. Borrowing from advanced manufacturing technology, optical shape scanning linked to three-dimensional (3D) computer-aided design, and CNC machining can be pressed into service to generate customized shapes to match a contralateral remaining limb. Up-to-date materials and component design each contribute to minimize the "orthopedic appliance" image of the devices (Fig. 136.2). In providing cosmesis, the views of the user must remain paramount. The wearer will often choose an attractive functional design in preference to a lifelike design that is not felt to be part of his or her body.

Upper limb prostheses are often seen as a more interesting engineering challenge than lower limb, offering the possibilities for active motor/control systems and complex articulations. However, the market is an order of magnitude smaller and cost/benefit less easy to prove—after all, it is possible to function fairly well with one arm, but try walking with one leg. At the simplest end, an arm for a below-elbow amputee might comprise a socket with a terminal device offering a pincer grip (hand or hook) that can be operated through a Bowden cable by shrugging the shoulders. Such body-powered prostheses may appear crude, but they are often favored by the wearer because of a sense of position and force feedback from the cable, and they do not need a power supply. Another, more elegant method of harnessing body power is to take a muscle made redundant by an amputation and tether its tendon through an artificially fashioned loop of skin; the cable can then be hooked through the loop [Childress, 1989].

Externally powered devices have been attempted using various power sources with degrees of success. Pneumatic power in the form of a gas cylinder is cheap and light, but recharging is a problem that exercised the ingenuity of early suppliers; where supplies were not readily available, even schemes to involve the local fire services with recharging were costed. Also, contemplate the prospect of bringing a loaded table fork toward your face carried on the end of a position-controlled arm

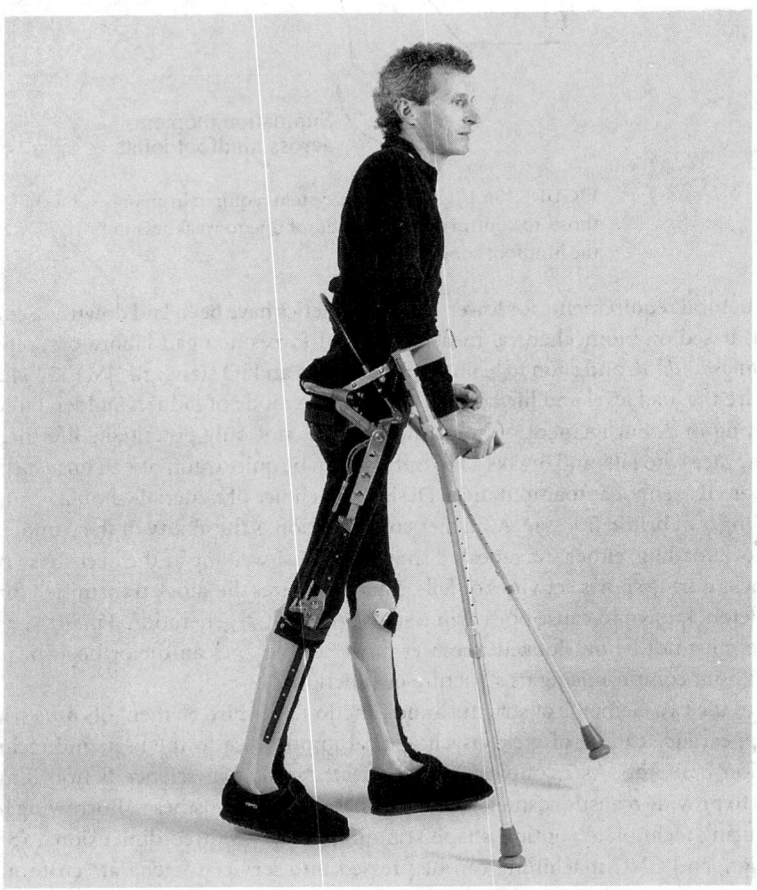

(a)

FIGURE 136.2 The ARGO reciprocating-gait orthosis, normally worn under the clothing, with structural components produced from 3D CAD. (Courtesy of Hugh Steeper, Ltd., U.K.)

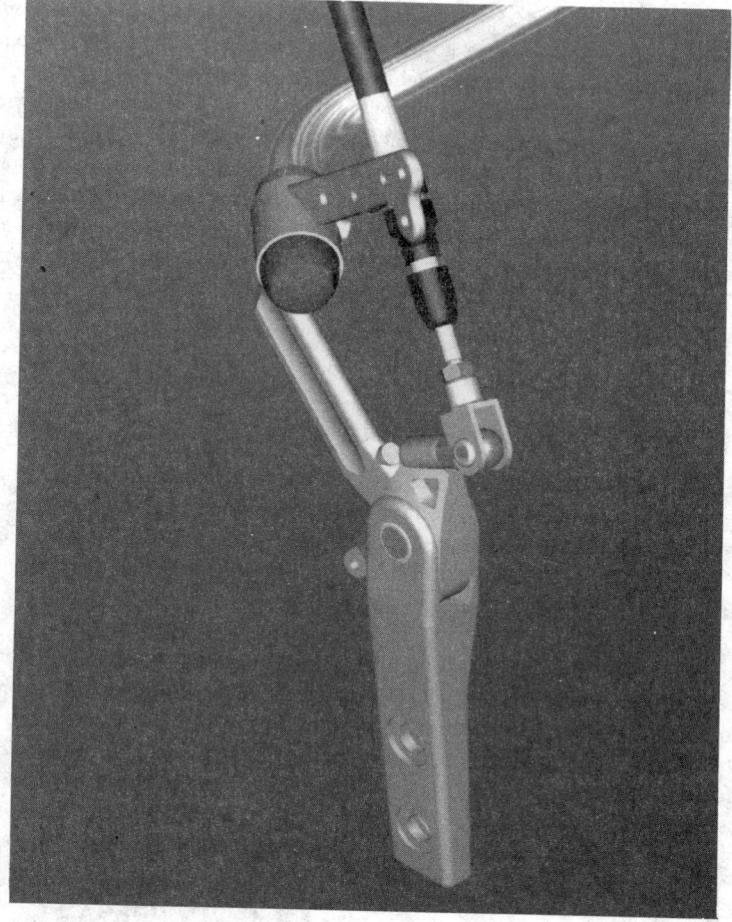

(b)

FIGURE 136.2 *(continued)*

powered with spongy, low-pressure pneumatic actuators, and you will appreciate another aspect of difficulties with this source. Nevertheless, gas-powered grip on a hand can be a good solution. Early skirmishes with stiffer hydraulic servos were largely unsuccessful because of power supply and actuator weight and oil leakage. Electric actuation, heavy and slow at first, has gradually improved to establish its premier position. Input control to these powered devices can be from surface electromyography or by mechanical movement of, for example, the shoulder or an ectromelic limb. Feedback can be presented as skin pressure, movement of a sensor over the skin, or electric stimulation. Control strategies range from position control around a single joint or group of related joints through combined position and force control for hand grip to computer-assisted coordination of entire activities such as feeding.

The physical designs in prosthetic and orthotic devices has changed substantially over the past decade. One could propose that this is solely the introduction of new materials. The sockets of artificial limbs have always been fashioned to suit the individual patient, historically by carving wood, shaping leather, or beating sheet metal. Following the introduction of thermosetting fiber-reinforced plastics hand-shaped over a plaster cast of the limb residuum, substitution of thermoforming plastics that could be automatically vacuum-formed made a leap forward to give light, rapidly made, and cosmetically improved solutions. Polypropylene is the favored material in this application. The same materials permitted the new concept of custom-molded orthoses. Carbon fiber composites substituted for metal have certainly improved the performance of structural components such as limb shanks. But some of the progress owes much to innovative thinking. The flex foot is a fine example, where a traditional anthropomorphic design with imitation ankle joint and metatarsal break is completely abandoned and a functional design adopted to optimize energy storage and return. This is based on two leaf springs made from Kevlar, joined together at the ankle with one splaying down toward the toes to form the forefoot spring and the other rearward to form the heel spring (Fig. 136.3). Apart from the gains for the disabled athletes for whom the foot was designed—and these are so remarkable that there is little point in competing now without this foot—clients across all age groups have benefited from the adaptability to rough ground and shock-absorption capability.

136.2 Applications

Computer-Aided Engineering in Customized Component Design

Computer-aided engineering has found a fertile ground for exploitation in the process of design of customized components to match to body shape. A good example is in sockets for artificial limbs. What prosthetists particularly seek is the ability to produce a well-fitting socket during the course of a single patient consultation. Traditional craft methods of casting the residual limb in plaster of paris, pouring a positive mold, manual rectification, and then socket fabrication over the rectified cast takes too long.

By using advanced technology, residual limb shapes can be captured in a computer, rectified by computer algorithms, and CNC machined to produce the rectified cast in under an hour so that with the addition of vacuum-forming machinery to pull a socket rapidly over the cast, the socket can be ready for trial fitting in one session. There are added advantages too, in that the shape is now stored in digital form in the computer and can be reproduced or adjusted whenever and wherever desired. Although such systems are still in an early stage of introduction, many practicing prosthetists in the United States have now had hands-on experience of this technology, and a major evaluation by the Veterans Administration has been undertaken [Houston et al., 1992].

Initially, much of the engineering development work went into the hardware components, a difficult brief in view of the low cost target for a custom product. Requirements are considerably different from those of standard engineering, e.g., relaxation in the accuracies required (millimeters, not microns); a need to measure limb or trunk parts that are encumbered by the attached body, which may resist being orientated conveniently in a machine and which will certainly distort with the lightest pressure; and a need to reproduce fairly bulky items with strength to be used as a sacrificial mold. Instrumentation for body shape scanning has been developed using methods of silhouettes, Moiré fringes, contact probes measuring contours of plaster casts, and light triangulation. Almost universally the molds are turned by "milling on a spit" [Duncan & Mair, 1983], using an adapted lathe with a milling head to spiral down a large cylindrical plug of a material such as a plaster of

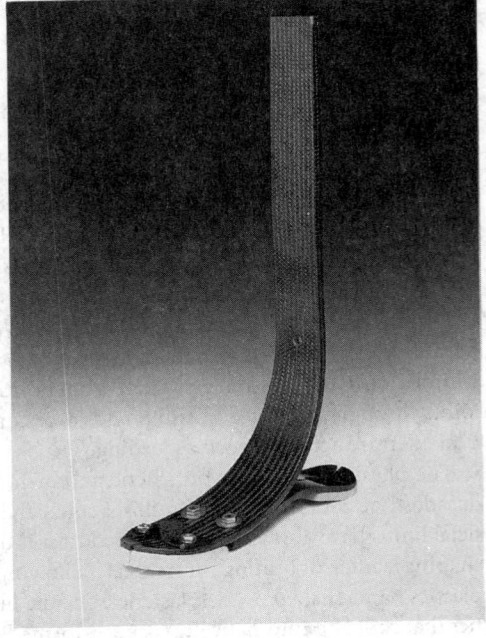

FIGURE 136.3   The Flex Foot.

paris mix. Rehabilitation engineers watch with great interest, some with envy, the developments in rapid prototyping manufacture, which is so successful in reducing the cycle time for one-off developments elsewhere in industry, but alas the costs of techniques such as stereolithography are as yet beyond economic feasibility for our area.

Much emphasis also has been placed on the graphics and algorithms needed to achieve rectification. Opinions vary as to what extent the computer should simply provide a more elegant tool for the prosthetist to exercise his or her traditional skills using 3D modeling and on-screen sculpting as a direct replacement for manual plaster rectification or to what extent the computer system should take over the bulk of the process by an expert systems approach. Systems currently available tend to do a little of each. A series of rectification maps can be held as templates, each storing the appropriate relief or buildup to be applied over a particular anatomic area of the limb. Thus the map might provide for a ridge to be added down the front of the shin of a lower limb model so that the eventual socket will not press against the vulnerable bony prominence of the tibia (Fig. 136.4). Positioning of the discrete regions to match individual anatomy might typically be anchored to one or more anatomic features indicated by the prosthetist. The prosthetist is also able to free-form sculpt a particular region by pulling the surface interactively with reference to graphic representation (Fig. 136.5); this is particularly useful where the patient has some unusual feature not provided for in the templates.

As part of this general development, finite-element analysis has been employed to model the soft tissue distortion occurring during limb loading and to look at the influence of severity of rectification in the resultant distribution of interface stress [e.g., Reynolds & Lord, 1992] (Fig. 136.6). In engineering terms, this modeling is somewhat unusual and decidedly nonlinear. For a start, the tissues are highly deformable but nearly incompressible, which raises problems of a suitable Poisson ratio to apply in the modeling. Values of $n = 0.3$ to $n = 0.49$ have been proposed, based on experimental matching of stress-strain curves from indentation of limb tissue in vivo. In reality, though, compression (defined as a loss of volume) may be noted in a limb segment under localized external pressure due to loss of mass as first the blood is rapidly evacuated and then interstitial fluids are more slowly squeezed out. Also, it is difficult to define the boundaries of the limb segment at the proximal end, still attached to the body, where soft tissues can easily bulge up and out. This makes accurate experimental determination of the stress-strain curves for the tissue matrix difficult. A

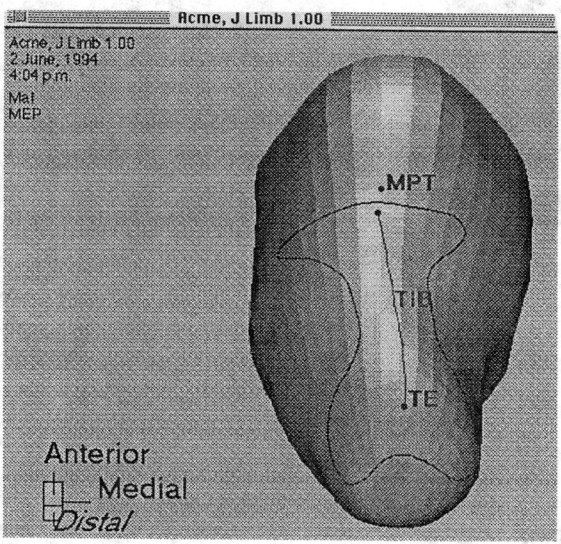

FIGURE 136.4   A rectification require defined over the tibia of lower limb stump using the Shapemaker application for computer-aided socket design.

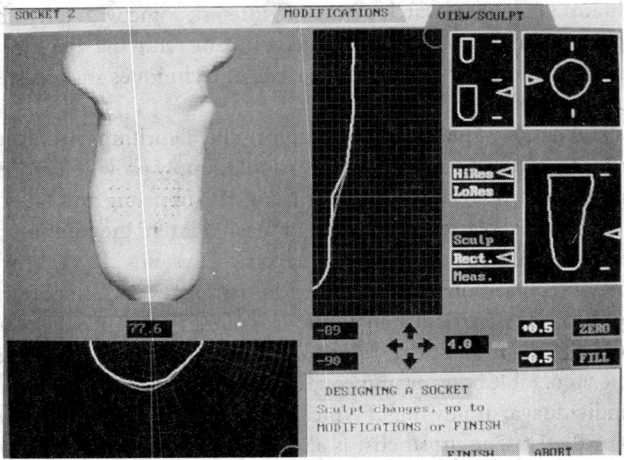

FIGURE 136.5 Adjusting a socket contour with reference to 3D graphics and cross-sectional profiles in the UCL CASD system. (Reproduced from Reynolds and Lord [1992] with permission.)

nonlinear model with interface elements allowing slip to occur between skin and socket at the limit of static friction may need to be considered, since the frictional conditions at the interface will determine the balance between shear and direct stresses in supporting body weight against the sloping sidewalls. Although excessive shear at the skin surface is considered particularly damaging, higher pressures would be required in its complete absence.

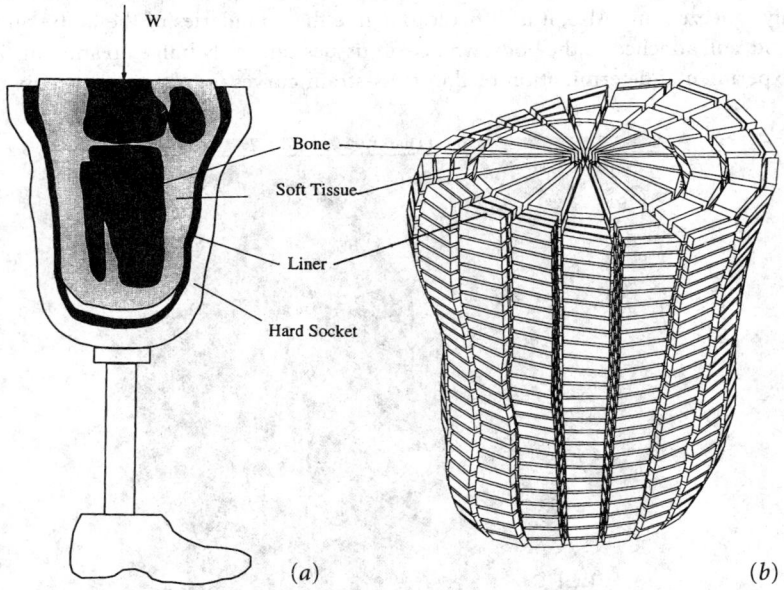

FIGURE 136.6 Finite-element analysis employed to determine the sensitivity of interface pressure to socket shape rectification: (*a*) limb and socket; (*b*) elements in layers representing idealized geometry of bone, soft tissue, and socket liner; (*c*) rectification map of radial differences between the external free shape of the limb and the internal dimensions of socket; and (*d*) FE predictions of direct pressure. (Courtesy of Zhang Ming, King's College London.)

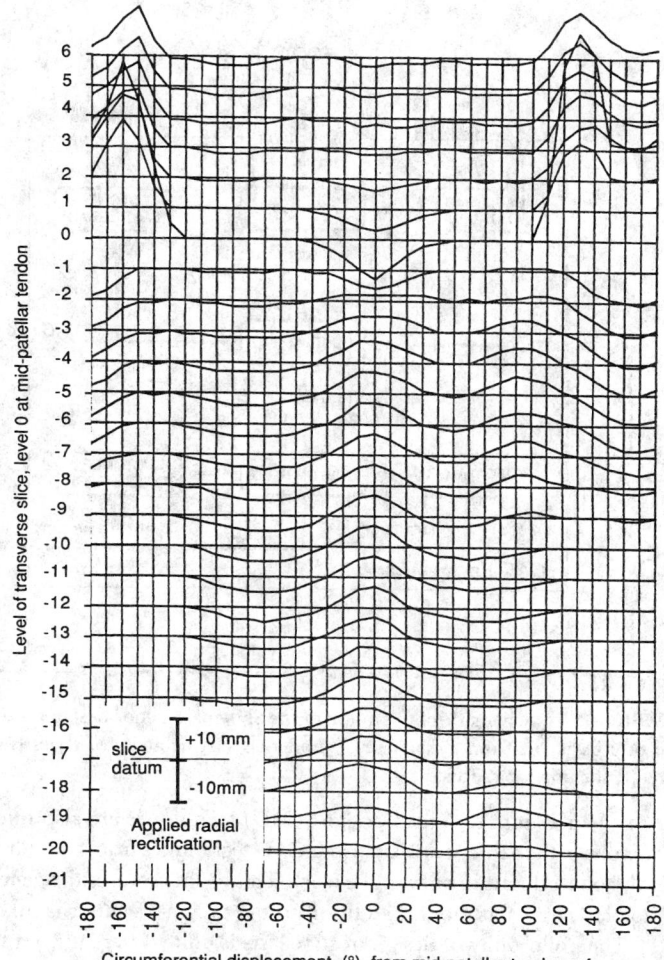

(c) Circumferential displacement (°) from mid-patellar tendon reference

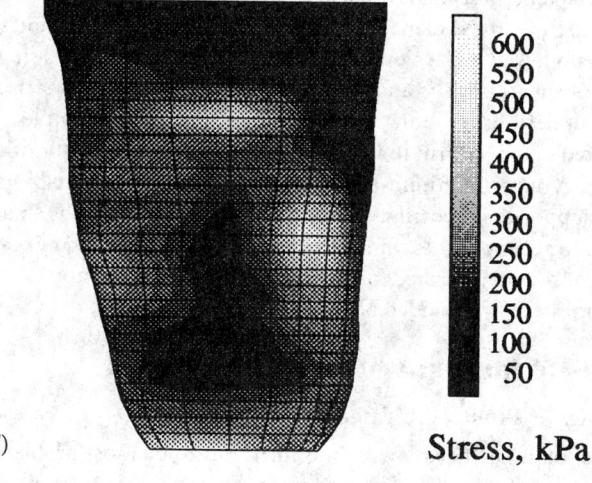

(d)

Stress, kPa

FIGURE 136.6 (continued)

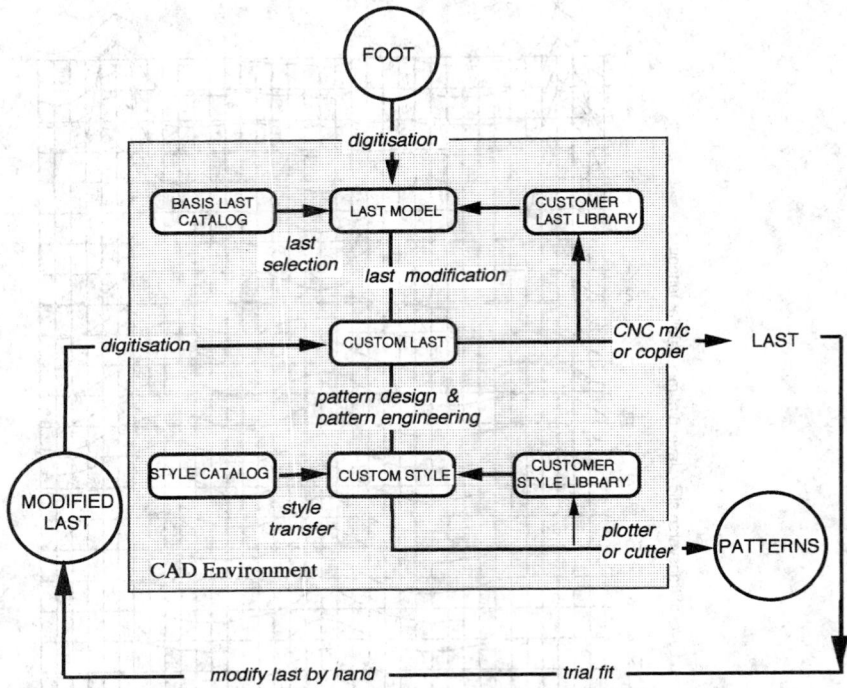

FIGURE 136.7 Schematic of operation of the Shoemaster shoe design system based on selection of a basis last from a database of model lasts. A database of styles is also employed to generate the upper patterns.

In a similar vein, computer-aided design (CAD) techniques are also finding application in the design of bespoke orthopedic footwear, using CAD techniques from the volume fashion trade modified to suit the one-off nature of bespoke work. This again requires the generation of a customized mold, or shoe last, for each foot, in addition to the design of patterns for the shoe uppers [Lord et al., 1991]. The philosophy of design of shoe lasts is quite different from that of sockets, because last shapes have considerable and fundamental differences from foot shapes. In this instance, a library of reference last shapes is held, and a suitable one is selected both to match the client's foot shape and to fulfill the shoemaking needs for the particular style and type of shoe. The schematic of the process followed in development of the Shoemaster system is shown in Fig. 136.7.

Design of shoe inserts is another related application, with systems to capture, manipulate, and reproduce underfoot contours now in commercial use. An example is the Ampfit system, where the foot is placed on a platform to which preshaped arch supports or other wedges or domes may first be attached. A matrix of round-ended cylinders is then forced up by gas pressure through both platform and supports, supporting the foot over most of the area with an even load distribution. The shape is captured from the cylinder locations and fed into a computer, where rectification can be made similar to that described for prosthetic sockets. A benchtop CNC machine then routs the shoe inserts from specially provided blanks while the client waits.

Examples of Innovative Component Design

An Intelligent Prosthetic Knee

The control of an artificial lower limb turns out to be most problematic during the swing phase, during which the foot is lifted off the ground to be guided into contact ahead of the walker. A prosthetic lower limb needs to be significantly lighter than its normal counterpart because the muscular power is not present to control it. Two technological advances have helped. First, carbon fiber construction has reduced the mass of the lower limb, and second, pneumatic or hydraulically controlled damping mechanisms for the knee joint have enabled adjustment of the swing phase to suit an individual's pattern of walking.

Swing-phase control of the knee should operate in three areas:

1. Resistance to flexion at late stance during toe-off controls any tendency to excessive heel rise at early swing.
2. Assistance to extension after midswing ensures that the limb is fully extended and ready for heel strike.
3. Resistance before a terminal impact at the end of the extension swing dampens out the inertial forces to allow a smooth transition from flexed to extended knee position.

In conventional limbs, parameters of these controls are determined by fixed components (springs, bleed valves) that are set to optimum for an individual's normal gait at one particular speed, e.g., the pneumatic controller in Fig. 136.8. If the amputee subsequently walks more slowly, the limb will tend to lead, while if the amputee walks more quickly, the limb will tend to fall behind; the usual compensatory actions are, respectively, an unnatural tilting of the pelvis to delay heel contact or abnormal kicking through of the leg.

In a recent advance, intelligence is built into the swing-phase controller to adjust automatically for cadence variations (Fig. 136.9). A 4-bit microprocessor is used to adjust a needle valve, via a linear stepper motor, according to the duration of the preceding swing phase [Zahedi, in press]. The unit is programmed by the prosthetist to provide optimal damping for the particular amputee's swing phase at slow, normal, and fast walking paces. Thereafter, the appropriate damping is automatically selected for any intermediate speed.

A Hierarchically Controlled Prosthetic Hand

Control of the intact hand is hierarchical. It starts with the owner's intention, and an action plan is formulated based on knowledge of the environment and the object to be manipulated. For gross movements, the numerous articulations rely on "preprogrammed" coordination from the central nervous system. Fine control leans heavily on local feedback from force and position sensors in the joints and tactile information about loading and slip at the skin. In contrast, conventional prostheses depend on the conscious command of all levels of control and so can be slow and tiring to use.

Current technology is able to provide both the computing power and transducers required to recreate some of a normal hand's sophisticated proprioceptive control. A concept of extended physiologic proprioception (EPP) was introduced for control of gross arm movement [Simpson & Kenworthy, 1973] whereby the central nervous system is retrained through residual proprioception to coordinate gross actions applying to the geometry of the new extended limb. This idea can be applied to initiate gross hand movements while delegating fine control to an intelligent controller.

Developments by Chappell and Kyberd [1991] and others provide a fine example of the possibilities. A suitable mechanical configuration is shown in Fig. 136.10. Four 12-V dc electric motors with gearboxes control, respectively, thumb adduction, thumb flexion, forefinger flexion, and flexion of digits 3, 4, and 5. Digits 3, 4, and 5 are linked together by a double-swingletree mechanism that allows all three to be driven together. When one digit touches an object the other two can continue to close until they also touch or reach their limit of travel. The movement of the digits allows one of several basic postures:

- *Three-point chuck:* Precision grip with digits 1, 2, and 3 (thumb set to oppose the midline between digits 2 and 3); digits 4 and 5 give additional support.
- *Two-point grip:* Precision grip with digits 1 and 2 (thumb set to oppose forefinger); digits 3, 4, and 5 fully flexed and not used or fully extended.
- *Fist:* As two-point grip but with thumb fully extended to allow large objects to be grasped.
- *Small fist:* As fist but with thumb flexed and abducted to oppose side of digit 2.

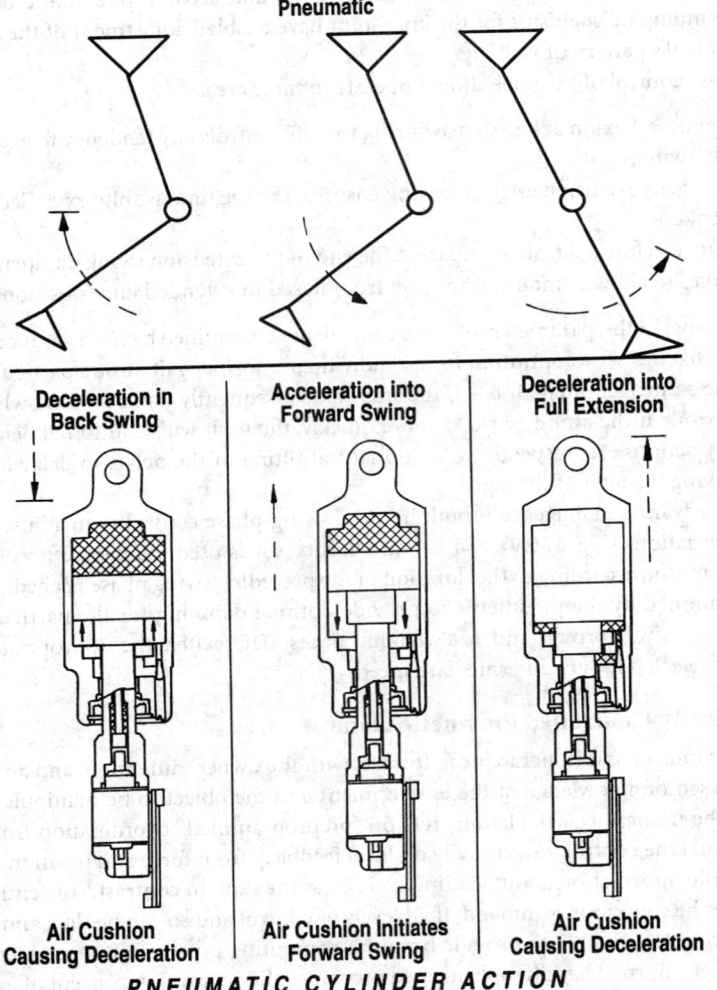

FIGURE 136.8 Pneumatic cylinder action in a swing phase controller. (Reprinted with permission from S. Zahedi, The Results of the Field Trial of the Endolite Intelligent Prosthesis, internal publication, Chas. A. Blatchford & Sons, U.K.)

- *Side, or key:* Digits 2 to 5 half fully flexed with thumb opposing side of second digit.
- *Flat hand:* Digits 2 to 5 fully extended with thumb abducted and flexed, parked beside digit 2.

The controller coordinates the transition between these positions and ensures that trajectories do not tangle. Feedback to the controller is provided by several devices. Potentiometers detect the angles of flexion of the digits; touch sensors detect pressure on the palmer surfaces of the digits; and a combined contact force (Hall effect) and slip sensor (from acoustic frequency output of force sensor) is mounted at the fingertips. The latter detects movement of an object and so controls grip strength appropriate to the task—whether holding a hammer or an egg [Kyberd & Chappell, 1993].

The whole hand may be operated by electromyographic signals from two antagonistic muscles in the supporting forearm stump, picked up at the skin surface. In response to tension in one muscle, the hand opens progressively and then closes to grip with an automatic reflex. The second muscle controls the mode of operation as the hand moves between the states of touch, hold, squeeze, and release.

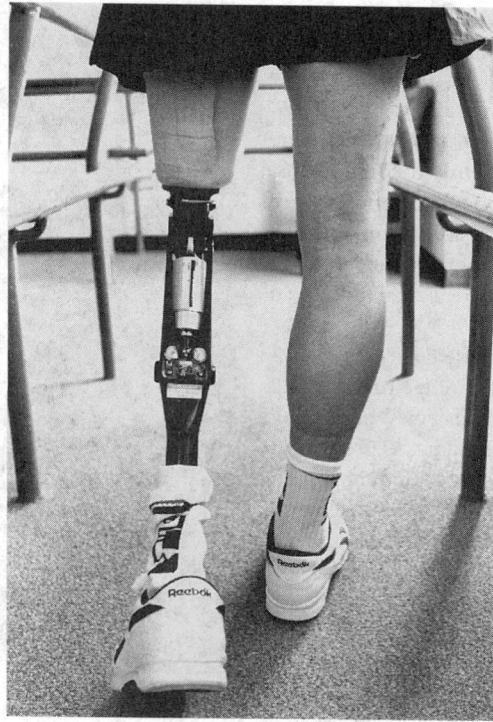

FIGURE 136.9   The Endolite intelligent prosthesis in use, minus its cosmetic covers.

A Self-Aligning Orthotic Knee Joint

Knee orthosis are often supplied to resist knee flexion during standing and gait at an otherwise collapsing joint. The rigid locking mechanisms on these devices are manually released to allow knee flexion during sitting. Fitting is complicated by the difficulty of attaching the orthosis with its joint accurately aligned to that of the knee. The simple diagram in Fig. 136.11 shows how misplacement of a simple hinged orthosis with a notional fixed knee axis would cause the cuffs on the thigh and calf to press into the soft tissues of the limb (known as *pistoning*).

The human knee does not have a fixed axis, though, but is better represented as a polycentric joint. In a sagittal (side) view, it is easy to conceptualize the origin of these kinematics from the anatomy of the cruciate ligaments running crisscross across the joint, which together with the base of the femur and the head of the tibia form a classic four-bar linkage. The polycentric nature of the motion can therefore be mimicked by a similar geometry of linkage on the orthosis.

The problem of alignment still remains, however, and precision location of attachment points is not possible when gripping through soft tissues. In one attempt to overcome this specific problem, the knee mechanism has been designed with not one but two axes (Fig. 136.11). The center of rotation is then free to self-align. This complexity of the joint while still maintaining the ability to fixate the knee and meeting low weight requirements is only achieved by meticulous design in composite materials.

136.3 Summary

The field of prosthetics and orthotics is one where at present traditional craft methods sit alongside the application of high technology. Gradually, advanced technology is creeping into most areas, bringing vast improvements in hardware performance specifications and aesthetics. This is, however, an area where the clinical skills of the prosthetist and orthotist will always be required in specification and fitting and where many of the products have customized components. The successful applications of technology are those which assist the professional to exercise his or her judgment, providing him or her with good tools and means to realize a functional specification.

Since the demand for these devices is thankfully low, their design and manufacture are small scale in terms of volume. This taxes the skills of most engineers, both to design the product at reasonable up-front costs and to manufacture it economically in low volume. For bespoke components, we are moving from a base of craft manufacture through an era when modularization was exploited to allow small-batch production toward the use of CAD. In the latter, the engineering design effort is then embodied in the CAD system, leaving the prosthetist or orthotist to incorporate clinical design for each individual component.

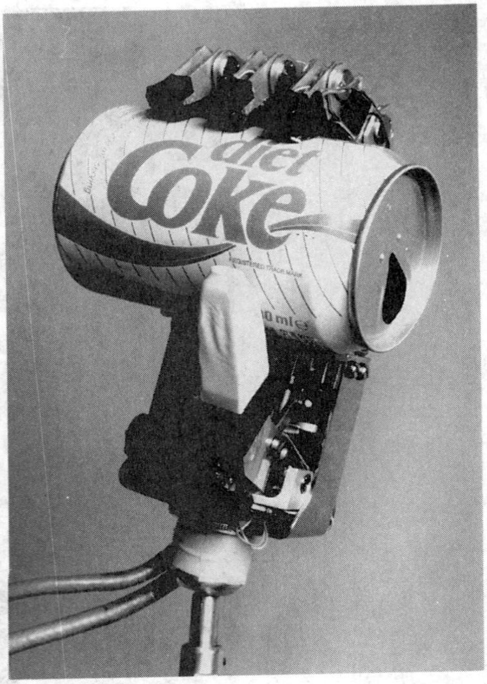

Specific examples of current applications have been described. These can only represent a small part of the design effort that is put into prosthetics and orthotics on a continuing basis, making advances in materials and electronics in particular available.

FIGURE 136.10 The Southampton hand prosthesis with four degrees of freedom in a power grip. An optical/acoustic sensor is mounted on the thumb. (Reprinted from Kyberd and Chappell [1993], Fig. 1.)

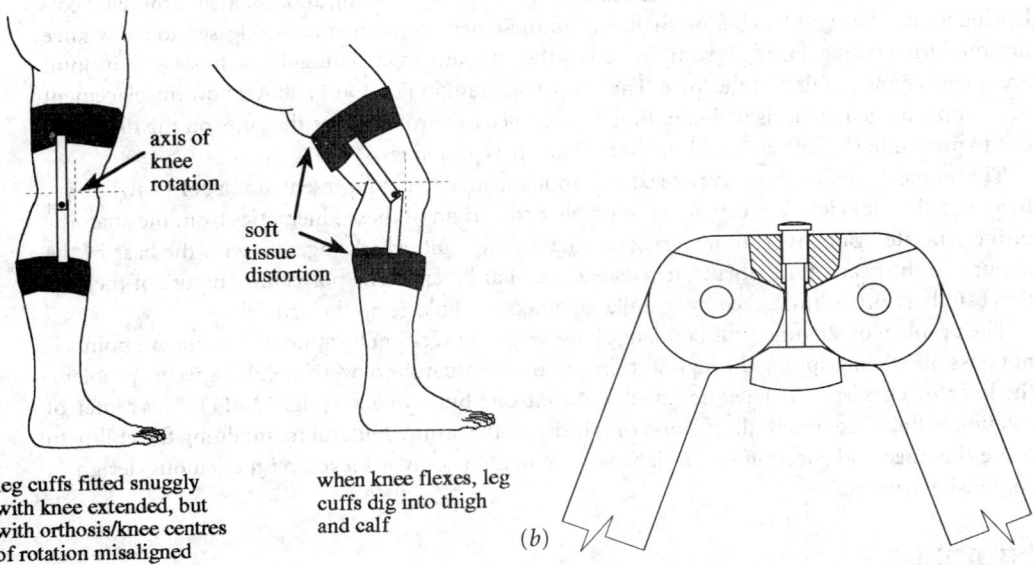

axis of
knee
rotation

soft
tissue
distortion

leg cuffs fitted snuggly
with knee extended, but
with orthosis/knee centres
of rotation misaligned

when knee flexes, leg
cuffs dig into thigh
and calf

(b)

FIGURE 136.11 The problem caused by misplacement of a single-axis orthotic joint (a) is overcome by an orthosis (b) with a self-aligning axis. (The Laser system, courtesy of Hugh Steeper, Ltd., U.K.)

We are also aware that in the space available, it has not been possible to include a discussion of the very innovative work that is being done in intermediate technology for the third world, for which the International Society of Prosthetics and Orthotics (address below) currently has a special working group.

Defining Terms

Biocompatability: Compatibility with living tissue, e.g., in consideration of toxicity, degradability, and mechanical interfacing.

CNC machining: Use of a computer numerically controlled machine.

Cosmesis: Aesthetics of appearance.

Ectromelia: Congenital gross shortening of the long bones of a limb.

Functional prescription: A doctor's prescription for supply of a device written in terms of its function as opposed to embodiment.

Neuroskeletomotor system: The skeletal frame of the body with the muscles, peripheral nerves, and central nervous system of the spine and brain, which together participate in movement and stabilization of the body.

Rectified, rectification: Adjustment of a model of body shape to achieve a desirable load distribution in a custom-molded prosthesis or orthosis.

Soft tissues: Skin, fat, connective tissues, and muscles which, along with the hard tissues of bone, teeth, etc. and the fluids, make up the human body.

Transcutaneous: Passing through the skin.

References

Chappell PH, Kyberd PJ. 1991. Prehensile control of a hand prosthesis by a microcontroller. J Biomed Eng 13:363.

Childress DS. 1989. Control philosophies for limb prostheses. In J Paul, et al. (eds), Progress in Bioengineering, pp 210–215. New York, Adam Hilger.

Duncan JP, Mair SG. 1983. Sculptured Surfaces in Engineering and Medicine. Cambridge, England, Cambridge Univ. Press.

Houston VL, Burgess EM, Childress DS, et al. 1992. Automated fabrication of mobility aids (AFMA): Below-knee CASD/CAM testing and evaluation. J Rehabil Res Dev 29:78.

Kyberd PJ, Chappell PH. 1993. A force sensor for automatic manipulation based on the Hall effect. Meas Sci Technol 4:281.

Lord M, Foulston J, Smith PJ. 1991. Technical evaluation of a CAD system for orthopaedic shoe-upper design. Eng Med Proc Instrum Mech Eng 205:109.

Reynolds DP, Lord M. 1992. Interface load analysis for computer-aided design of below-knee prosthetic sockets. Med Biol Eng Comput 30:419.

Simpson DC, Kenworthy G. 1973. The design of a complete arm prosthesis. Biomed Eng 8:56.

Zahedi S. In press, 1994. Evaluation and biomechanics of the intelligent prosthesis: A two-year study. Orthop Tech.

Further Information

Bowker P, Condie DN, Bader DL, Pratt DJ (eds). Biomechanical Basis of Orthotic Management. Oxford, Butterworth-Heinemann, 1993.

Murdoch G, Donovan RG (eds). 1988. Amputation Surgery and Lower Limb Prosthetics. Boston, Blackwell Scientific Publications.

Nordin M, Frankel V. 1980. Basic Mechanics of the Musculoskeletal System, 2d ed. Philadelphia, Lea & Febiger, 1980.

Smidt GL (ed). 1990. Gait in Rehabilitation. New York, Churchill-Livingstone.

Organizations

International Society of Prosthetics and Orthotics (ISPO), Borgervaenget 5,2100 Copenhagen Ø, Denmark [tel (31) 20 72 60].

Department of Veterans Affairs, VA Rehabilitation Research and Development Service, 103 Gay Street, Baltimore, MD 21202-4051.

Rehabilitation Engineering Society of North America (RESNA), Suite 1540, 1700 North Moore Street, Arlington, VA 22209-1903.

137

Wheeled Mobility: Wheelchairs and Personal Transportation

Rory A. Cooper
*University of Pittsburgh and
Highland Drive Veterans Affairs
Medical Center*

Centuries ago, people with disabilities who survived for an extended period of time were transported on hammocks slung between poles that were carried by others. This was the preferred means of transportation of the upper class and thus carried no stigma. Later, the wheelbarrow was developed and soon became a common mode of transportation for people with disabilities. Because wheelbarrows were used to transport materials, during this period in history, people with disabilities were looked on as outcasts from society. During the renaissance, the French court popularized the first wheelchairs. Wheelchairs were overstuffed arm chairs with wheels placed on them. This enabled movement, with assistance, indoors. Later the wooden wheelchair with wicker matting was developed. This type of chair remained the standard until the 1930s. Franklin D. Roosevelt was not satisfied with the wooden wheelchair and had many common metal kitchen chairs modified with wheels. In the 1930s, a young mining engineer named Everest experienced an accident that left him mobility-impaired. He worked with a fellow engineer, Jennings, to develop steel wheelchairs. Within a few years, they formed a company, Everest and Jennings, to manufacture wheelchairs. Following World War II, medical advances saved the lives of many veterans with spinal cord injuries or lower limb amputations who would have otherwise died. Veterans medical centers issued these veterans steel-framed wheelchairs with 18-inch seat widths. These wheelchairs were designed to provide the veteran some mobility within the hospital and home and not to optimize ergonomic variables. Just as among the ambulatory population, mobility among people with disabilities varies. Mobility is more a functional limitation than a disability-related condition. Powered mobility can have tremendous positive psychosocial effects on an individual. Power wheelchairs provide greater independence to thousands of people with severe mobility impairments.

Power wheelchairs began in the 1940s as standard cross-brace folding manual wheelchairs adapted with automobile starter motors and an automobile battery. The cross-braced wheelchair remained the standard for a number of years. When the rigid power wheelchair frame was developed, space became available under the seat for electronic controls, respirators, communication systems, and reclining devices. By the mid 1970s, wheelchairs had evolved to the point where people had acquired a significant level of mobility.

A personal automobile has a profound affect on a person's mobility and ability to participate in society. A wheelchair is suitable for short distances and for many situations where an unimpaired person would walk. Modifications to vehicles may be as simple as a lever attached to the brake and accelerator pedals or as complex as a complete joystick-controlled fly-by-wire system. Modifications to other components of the vehicle may be required to provide wheelchair access. An automobile may not be appropriate for some people who travel distances too long to be convenient with a wheelchair but not long enough to warrant an adapted automobile. Microcars, enlarged wheelchairs that travel at bicycle speeds, are convenient for many people who wish only to travel to the local grocery store or post office. Microcars are also useful for people who like to travel along bicycle paths or drive short distances off-road.

137.1 Categories of Wheelchairs

There are two basic classes of wheelchairs: manually powered and externally powered. For practical purposes, externally powered wheelchairs are electrically powered wheelchairs. There are approximately 200,000 wheelchairs sold annually within the United States, of which about 20,000 are powered wheelchairs [Cooper, 1991*b*]. Most wheelchairs are purchased by third-party payers (e.g., insurance companies, government agencies). This requires the market to be responsive to wheelchair users' needs, prescriber expertise and experience, third-party payer purchase criteria, and competition from other manufacturers. Despite the complicated interaction between these components and the regulation of products by several government agencies, a number of wheelchairs and options are available.

Depot wheelchairs are intended for institutional use where several people may use the same wheelchair. Generally, these wheelchairs are inappropriate for active people who use wheelchairs for personal mobility. Depot wheelchairs are designed to be inexpensive, to accommodate large variations in body size, to be low maintenance, and often to be attendant-propelled. They are heavy, and their performance is limited. A typical depot wheelchair will have swing-away footrests, removable armrests, a single cross-brace frame, and solid tires.

People who have impairment of an arm and one or both lower extremities may benefit from a *one-arm-drive wheelchair* that uses a linkage connecting the rear wheels. This allows the user to push on the pushrim of one wheel and propel both wheels. To effectively turn the wheelchair, the user must have the ability to disengage the drive mechanism.

Some people have weakness of the upper and lower extremities and can gain maximal benefit from wheelchair propulsion by combining the use of their arms and legs or by using only their legs. The design and selection of a *foot-drive wheelchair* depend greatly on the how the user can take greatest advantage of his or her motor abilities.

Indoor spaces are more limited, and one is often required to get close to furnishings and fixtures to use them properly. Indoor wheelchairs often use rear castors because of the maneuverability of these designs. However, rear-castor designs make the wheelchair less stable in lateral directions. Indoor wheelchairs typically have short wheelbases.

All wheelchairs are not propelled by the person sitting in the wheelchair. In many hospitals and long-term care facilities, wheelchairs are propelled by attendants. Attendant-propelled wheelchair designs must consider the rider and the attendant as users. The rider must be transported safely and comfortably. The attendant must be able to operate and easily maneuver safely and with minimum physical strain.

Active users often prefer highly maneuverable and responsive wheelchairs that fit their physical and psychosocial character. The *ultralight wheelchair* evolved from the desire of wheelchair users to develop functional ergonomic designs for wheelchairs. Ultralight wheelchairs are made of such materials as aluminum, alloy steel, titanium, or composites. The design of ultralight wheelchairs allows a number of features to be customized by the user or be specified for manufacture. The most common features of all are the light weight, the high quality of materials used in their construction, and their functional design. Many people can benefit from ultralight wheelchair designs.

The desire to achieve better performances has lead wheelchair users, inventors, and manufacturers to constantly develop specialized wheelchairs for sports. There is no real typical *sports wheelchair*, since the design depends heavily on the sport. Basketball and tennis wheelchairs are often thought to typify sports wheelchair design. However, racing, field events, and shooting wheelchairs have little in common with the former.

Some wheelchairs are made to change configuration from reclining to sitting and from sitting to standing. Most *stand-up wheelchairs* cannot be driven in the stand-up setting in order to ensure safe and stable operation. Standing gives the user the ability to reach cabinet and counter space otherwise inaccessible. Standing has the additional advantage of providing therapeutic benefits, i.e., hemodynamic improvements and amelioration of osteoporosis.

Stairs and other obstacles persist despite the progress made in universal design. *Stair-climbing wheelchairs* are electrically powered wheelchairs designed to ascend and descend stairs safely under the occupant's control. Stair-climbing wheelchairs are quite complicated and often reconfigure themselves while climbing stairs. The additional power required to climb stairs often reduces the range of the wheelchair when compared with standard power wheelchairs.

137.2 Wheelchair Structure and Component Design

Several factors must be considered when designing a wheelchair frame: What are the intended uses? What are the abilities of the user? What are the resources available? and What are the existing products available? These factors determine if and how the frame will be designed and built. Successful designs of a wheelchairs can only be accomplished with continuous input from and interaction with wheelchair users. The durability, aesthetics, function, ride comfort, and cost of the frame are dependent on the materials for construction, the frame geometry, and fabrication methods. One of the issues that makes wheelchair design more complicated is the fact that many users depend on wheeled mobility everyday, nearly all day.

Materials

Most wheelchairs are made of either aluminum or steel. Some chairs are made of titanium or advanced composite materials, primarily carbon fiber, and in the future, composite frames will probably begin to become more available. All these materials have their strengths and weaknesses.

Commonly, aluminum wheelchairs are tungsten inert gas (TIG) welded (i.e., electrically welded together in a cloud of inert gas). They are sometimes bolted together using lugs. Most aluminum wheelchair frames are constructed of round drawn 6061 aluminum tubing. This is one of the least expensive and most versatile of the heat-treatable aluminum alloys. It has most of the desirable qualities of aluminum. It has good mechanical properties and high corrosion resistance. It can be fabricated using most standard techniques.

Most steel wheelchairs are made of mild steel (1040 or 1060) or chromium-molybdenum alloy (4130 or 4140) seamless tubing commonly called *chro-moly*. Mild steel is very inexpensive and easy to work with. It is wildly available and performs well for many applications. However, it has a low strength-to-weight ratio compared with other materials. Chro-moly is widely used because of its weldability, ease of fabrication, mild hardenability, and high fatigueability. Commonly wheelchairs are made of tubing 0.028 to 0.035 in. in wall thickness, and diameters vary depending on the expected loads from between 0.25 and 1.25 in.

More and more of the high-end wheelchairs are made of titanium. Titanium is a lightweight, strong, nonferrous metal. Titanium wheelchair frames are TIG welded. Titanium is the most exotic of the metals used in production wheelchairs and the most expensive. Titanium requires special tooling and skill to be machined and welded. It has very good mechanical properties and high corrosion resistance. It is resilient to wear and abrasion. Titanium is used because of its availability, appearance, corrosion resistance, very good strength, and light weight. A drawback of titanium, besides cost, is that titanium, once worn or if flawed, may break rapidly (i.e., it has a tendency toward brittle fractures).

Advanced composites have been in use in aerospace and industrial applications for a number of years. These materials include Kevlar, carbon fiber, and polyester-limestone composite. These materials are now making the transition to wheelchair design [MacLeish et al., 1993]. Kevlar is an organic fiber that is yellow in color and soft to the touch. It is extremely strong and tough. It is one of the lightest structural fabrics on today's market. Kevlar is highly resistant to impact, but its compression strength is poor. Carbon fibers are made by changing the molecular structure of Rayon fibers by extreme stretching and heating. Carbon fiber is very stiff (high modulus of elasticity), very strong (high tensile strength), and has very low density (weight for a given volume). Composites come as cloth or yarn. Composite cloth is woven into bidirectional or unidirectional cloth. Unidirectional weaves can add strength along a particular direction. Composites must be bound together by resin or epoxy. Generally, polyester resins or various specialty epoxies (e.g., Safe-T-Poxy) are used. To achieve greatest strength, a minimum amount of epoxy must be used while wetting all the fibers. This is often achieved through a process called *bagging*. To increase the strength and stiffness of structural components, a foam (e.g., styrofoam, urethane, or PVC) core is used. The strengthening occurs because of the separation of the cloth layers (it now becomes more like a tube than a flat sheet). Polyesther-limestone composites have been used widely in industrial high-voltage electrical component enclosures. A blend of polyester and limestone is used to form a mixture that can be molded under pressure and heat to form a stiff and durable finished product. Polyester-limestone composites have high impact strength and hold tolerances well but have substantially lower strength-to-weight ratios than other composites. Their primary advantage is cost; polyester-limestone composite is very inexpensive and readily available. Composite can be molded into elaborate shapes, which opens a multitude of possibilities for wheelchair design.

Frame Design

Presently, all common wheelchair frames center around tubular construction. The tubing can either be welded together or bolted together using lugs [Cooper, 1991*b*]. There are two basic common frame styles: box frame and cantilever frame. The *box frame* is named such because of its rectangular shape and the fact that tubes outline the edges of the box. Box frames can be very strong and very durable. A *cantilever frame* is named so because the front and rear wheels, when viewing the chair from the side, appear to be connected by only one tube; this is similar to having the front wheels attached to a cantilever beam fixed at the rear wheels. Both frame types require cross-bracing to provide adequate strength and stiffness.

The box frame provides great strength and rigidity. If designed and constructed properly, the frame deflects only minimally during normal loading, and most of the suspension is provided by the seat cushion, the wheels, and the wheel mounting hardware. Many manufacturers do not triangulate their box frame designs to allow some flexibility. The cantilever frame is based on a few basic principles: (1) the frame can act as suspension, (2) there are fewer tubes and they are closer to the body, which may makes the chair less conspicuous, and (3) there are fewer parts and fewer welds, which makes the frame easier to construct.

Wheels and Casters

Casters can be as small as 2 in. in diameter or as large as 12 in. in diameter for wheelchairs designed for daily use. Casters are either pneumatic, semipneumatic, or solid (polyurethane). Pneumatic casters offer a smoother ride at the cost of increased maintenance, whereas polyurethane casters are very durable. Semipneumatic tires offer a compromise. Most active users prefer 5-in. polyurethane casters or 8-in. pneumatic casters for daily use. An 8-in. caster offers better ride comfort at the expense of foot clearance. Caster foot clearance is maximized with 2-in. "roller blade" casters often used for court sports (e.g., basketball, tennis, and racquetball). Rear wheels come in three common sizes 22, 24, and 26 in. They come in two styles: spoked and MAG. MAG wheels are typically made of plastic and are die cast. MAG wheels require minimal maintenance and wear well. However, spoked wheels are substantially lighter, more responsive, and generally are preferred by active manual wheelchair users. Rear tires can be two types: pneumatic or puncture-proof. Pneumatic tires can use either a separate tube and tire or a combined tube and tire (sew-up). Commonly, a belted rubber tire with a butyl tube (65 psi) is used. However, those desiring higher performance prefer sew-up tires or Kevlar-belted tires with high-pressure tubes (180 psi). Puncture-proof tires are heavier, provide less suspension, and are less lively than pneumatic tires.

The chair must be designed to optimize the interaction of the wheels with the ground. Four critical performance factors need to be considered: (1) castor flutter, (2) castor float, (3) tracking, and (4) alignment [Cooper, 1991b]. *Castor flutter* is the shimmy (rapid vibration of the front wheels) that may occur on some surfaces above certain speeds. When one of the castors does not touch the floor when on level ground, the wheelchair has castor float. *Castor float* decreases the stability and performance of the wheelchair. Since manual wheelchairs use rear-wheel steering via differential propulsion torque, tracking is the tendency of the wheelchair/rider to maintain its course once control has been relinquished. *Tracking* is important; as the rider propels the handrims periodically (about every second), and if the chair does not track well, it will drift from its course between pushes and force the rider to correct heading. This will waste valuable energy and reduce control over the chair. *Alignment* generally refers to the orientation of the rear wheels with respect to one another. Typically, it is desirable to have the rear wheels parallel to one another without any difference between the distance across the two rear wheels at the front and back. Misalignment on the order of 1/8 in. can cause a noticeable increase in the effort required to propel the wheelchair.

37.3 Ergonomics of Wheelchair Propulsion

The most important area of wheelchair design and prescription is determining the proper interaction between the wheelchair and the user. This can lead to reducing the risk of developing repetitive strain injury while maximizing mobility. Cardiovascular fitness can be improved through exercise, which requires a properly fitted wheelchair.

Kinematics

Kinematic data by themselves do not provide sufficient information for the clinician to implement appropriate rehabilitation intervention strategies or the engineer to incorporate this information into wheelchair design changes. Kinematic data are commonly collected at 60 Hz; this is the maximum frequency of many videotape-based systems. Kinematic data analysis shows that experienced wheelchair users contact the pushrim behind top-dead-center and push to nearly 90 degrees in front of top-dead-center [Asato et al., 1993]. This is significantly longer than non-wheelchair users. Lengthening the stroke permits lowering the propulsion moment and may place less stress on the user's joints.

An important aspect of the evaluation and possible retraining of wheelchair users is to determine the optimal stroke kinetics and kinematics. However, there is typically some degree of variation from one stroke to another. Wheelchair propulsion kinematic data are typically cyclic (i.e., a person repeats or nearly repeats his or her arm motions over several strokes). Each marker of the kinematic model (e.g., shoulder, elbow, wrist, knuckle) of each subject generates an *x* and *y* set of data that are periodic. The frequencies of the *x* and *y* data are dependent on the anthropometry of the individual, the construction of the wheelchair, and the speed of propulsion [Cooper, 1991*a*]. The periodic nature of the kinematic data for wheelchair propulsion can be exploited to develop a characteristic stroke from a set of kinematic data (with the wheelchair's rear hub chosen as the origin) including several strokes.

Kinetics

Recently, the SMART[wheel] was developed to measure the pushrim forces required for evaluating net joint forces and moments to allow the clinician and researcher to study the level of stress experienced by the joint structures during wheelchair propulsion [Asato et al., 1993]. The SMART[wheel] uses a standard wheelchair wheel fitted with three beams 120 degrees apart, each instrumented with two full strain-gauge bridges. The strain-gauge bridges are each interfaced through an instrumentation amplifier to a microcontroller that transmits the data through a mercury slip ring to the serial port of a computer. Kinetics of wheelchair propulsion are affected by speed of propulsion, injury level, user experience, and wheelchair type and fit. Van Der Woude et al. [1989] have reported on an ergometer that detected torque by way of a force transducer located in the wheel center and attached to what is referred to as the *wheel/handrim construction*. The ergometer was adjusted for each subject's anthropometric measurements. Data were sampled at 100 Hz for 7.5-s periods with a digital filter cutoff frequency of 10 Hz. Mean and peak torque increased with mean velocity; a maximum mean peak torque of 31 N·m occurred at 1.27 m/s. Torque curves of inexperienced subjects showed an initial negative deflection and a dip in the rising portion of the curve.

Brauer and Hertig [1981] measured the static torque produced on pushrims that were rigidly restrained by springs and mounted independent of the tires and rims of the wheelchair. The spring system was adjustable for the subject's strength. The wheels were locked in a fixed position. Torque was measured using slide-wire resistors coupled to the differential movements between the pushrim and wheels and recorded using a strip-chart recorder. Subjects were asked to grasp the pushrim at six different test positions (−10, 0, 10, 20, 30, and 40 degrees relative to vertical) and to use maximal effort to turn both wheels forward. Male subjects (combined ambulatory and wheelchair user) produced torques of 27.9 to 46.6 N·m, and female subjects produced torques of 17.1 to 32.1 N·m. Grip location, handedness, grip strength, and how well the test wheelchair fit the anthropometric measurements of the individual affected the torque generated. Problems encountered were slipperiness of the pushrims due to a polished finish and limited contact due to the small diameter of the pushrim tubing (12.7 mm, or 1/2 in.). The use of one wheelchair for all subjects presented the problem of variations due to inappropriate fit for some individuals.

Brubaker et al. [1982] examined the effect of horizontal and vertical seat position (relative to the wheel position) on the generation of static pushrim force. Force was measured using a test platform with a movable seat and strain-gauged beams to which the pushrims were mounted. Pushing and pulling forces were recorded using a strip-chart recorder. Static force was measured for four grip positions (−30, 0, 30, and 60 degrees) with various seat positions. Pushrim force ranged from approximately 500 to 750 N and varied considerably with seat position and rim position.

Net Joint Forces and Moments

Net joint forces and moments acting at the wrist, elbow, and shoulder during wheelchair propulsion provide scientists and clinicians with information related to the level of stress borne by the joint structure. Joint moments and forces are calculated using limb segment and joint models, anthropometric data, kinetic data, and kinematic data. Joint moments data show that forces at each joint vary among subjects in terms of peak forces, where they occur during the propulsion phase, and how quickly they develop. Peak net joint moments occur at different joint angles for different subjects and conditions (e.g., speed, resistance). Convention for joint angles is that 180 degrees at the elbow represents full extension, while at the wrist this is the hand in the neutral position (flexion less than 180 degrees and extension greater than 180 degrees). Joint angles at the shoulder are determined between the arm and the trunk, with zero at the point where the trunk and arm are aligned. Wheelchair users show maximum net shoulder moment between 20 and 40 degrees of extension. Some wheelchair users also show a rapid rise in the elbow extensor moment at the beginning of the stroke with the elbow at about 120 degrees. This moment value begins to decrease between 150 and 170 degrees. At the wrist, the peak moments occur between 190 and 220 degrees. Net joint moment and force models need to take account of hand center of pressure, inaccuracies in anthropometric data, and joint models related to clinical variables.

137.4 Power Wheelchair Electrical Systems

Some people are impaired to an extent that they would have no mobility without a power wheelchair. However, some people may have limited upper body mobility and may have the ability to propel a manual wheelchair for short distances. These people may liken using a power wheelchair to admitting defeat. However, a power wheelchair may provide greater mobility. In such cases, it may be best to suggest a power wheelchair for longer excursions and a manual wheelchair for in-home and recreational use.

User Interface

Power wheelchairs often are used in conjunction with a number of other adaptive devices. For people with severe mobility impairments, power wheelchairs may be used with communication devices, computer access devices, respirators, and reclining seating systems. The integration of the user's multiple needs also must be considered when designing or prescribing a power wheelchair [Schauer et al., 1990].

The joystick is the most common control interface between the user and the wheelchair. Joysticks produce voltage signals proportional to displacement, force, or switch closures. Displacement joysticks are most popular. Displacement joysticks may use either potentiometers, variable inductors (coils), or optical sensors to convert displacement to voltage. Inductive joysticks are most common because they wear well and can be made quite sensitive. Joysticks can be modified to be used for chin, foot, elbow, tongue, or shoulder control. Typically, short-throw joysticks are used for these applications. Force-sensing joysticks use three basic transducers: simple springs and dampeners on a displacement joystick, cantilever beams with strain gauges, and fluid with pressure sensors. Force-sensing joysticks that rely on passive dampers or fluid pressure generally require the user to have range of motion within normal values for displacement joysticks users. Beam-based force-sensing joysticks require negligible motion and hence may be used for people with limited motion abilities.

People who exhibit intention or spastic tremor or with multiple sclerosis may require special control considerations [Riley & Rosen, 1987]. Signal-processing techniques often are required to grant the user greater control over the wheelchair. Typically, signal averaging or a low-pass filter with a cut-off frequency of below 5 Hz is used. The signal processing is typically incorporated into the controller.

Some people lack the fine motor control to effectively use a joystick. An alternative for these people is to use switch control or head-position control. Switch control simply uses either a set of switches or a single switch and a coded input, i.e., Morse code or some other simple switch code. The input of the user is latched by the controller, and the wheelchair performs the task commanded by the user. The user may latch the chair to repeatedly perform a task a specified number of times, e.g., continue straight until commanded to do otherwise. Switch control is quite functional, but it is generally slower than joystick control. Switch inputs can be generated in many ways. Typically, low-pressure switches are used. The input can come from a sip-and-puff mechanism that works off a pressure transducer. A switch contact is detected when the pressure exceeds or drops below a threshold. The pressure sensor may be configured to react to pressure generated by the user blowing into or sipping from an input or by the user simply interrupting the flow in or out of a tube. Sip and puff also may be used as a combination of proportional and switch control. For example, the user can put the control in the "read speed" mode, and then the proportional voltage output from the pressure transducer will be latched as the user-desired speed.

Simple switches of various sizes can be used to control the chair with many parts of the body. Switches may be mounted on the armrests or a lap tray for hand or arm activation, on the footrest(s) for foot activation, or on a headrest for head activation. The motion of the head also can be used for proportional control by using ultrasonic sensors. Ultrasonic sensors can be mounted in an array about the headrest. The signal produced by the ultrasonic sensors is related to the position of the head. Hence motion of the head can be used to create a proportional control signal. Ultrasonic head control and switch control can be combined to give some users greater mastery over their power wheelchair. Switches can be used to select the controller mode, whereas the ultrasonic sensors give a proportional input signal.

A critical consideration when selecting or designing a user interface is that the ability of the user to accurately control the interface is heavily dependent on the stability of the user within the wheelchair. Often custom seating and postural support systems are required for a user interface to be truly effective. The placement of the user interface is also critical to its efficacy as a functional control device.

Integrated Controls

People with severe physical impairments may only be able to effectively manipulate a single input device. Integrated controls are used to facilitate using a single input device (e.g., joystick, head switches, voice recognition system) to control multiple actuators (e.g., power wheelchair, environmental control unit, manipulator). This provides the user with greater control over the environment. The M3S multiple master, multiple slave bus is designed to provide simple, reliable access to a variety of assistive devices. Assistive devices include input devices and actuators, end-effectors. M3S is based on the computer area network (CAN) standard [van Woerden, 1993].

A large number of organizations provide assistive devices that offer the opportunity of functioning in a more independent manner. However, many of these devices and systems are developed without coordination, resulting in incompatible products. Clinicians and users often desire to combine products from various sources to achieve maximal independence. The result is to have several devices with their own input devices and overlapping functions. Integrated controls provide access to various end-effectors with a single input device; M3S provides an electronic communication protocol so that the system operates properly.

M3S is an interface specification with a basic hardware architecture, a bus communication protocol, and a configuration method. The M3S standard incorporates CAN plus two additional lines for greater security (i.e., 7-wire bus, 2 power lines, 2 CAN lines, safety lines, 1 shield, and 1 harness line) [van Woerden, 1993]. The system can be configured to each individual's needs. An M3S system consists of a microcontroller in each device and a control and configuration module (CCM). The CCM ensures proper signal processing, system configuration, and safety monitoring. The CCM is linked to a display (e.g., visual, auditory, tactile) that allows the user to select and operate each end-effector. Any M3S-compatible device can communicate with another M3S-compatible device. M3S is an International Organization of Standards (ISO) open-system communication implementation.

Power System

To implement a motor controller, a servo amplifier is required to convert signal-level power (volts at milliamps) to motor power (volts at amps). Typically, a design requirement for series, shunt, and brushless motor drives is to control torque and speed and hence power. Voltage control often can be used to control speed for both shunt and series motors. Series motors require feedback to achieve accurate control.

Either a linear servo amplifier or a chopper can be used. Linear servo amplifiers are not generally used with power wheelchairs primarily because of their lower efficiency than chopper circuits. A motor can be thought of as a filter to a chopper circuit; in this case, the switching unit can be used as part of a speed and current control loop. The torque ripple and noise associated with phase-control drives can be avoided by the use of high switching frequencies. The response of the speed-control loop is likewise improved with increasing switching frequency.

Motor torque is proportional to the armature current in shunt motors and to the square of the current in series motors. The conduction losses of the motor and servo amplifier are both proportional to current squared. Optimal efficiency is achieved by minimizing the form factor (I_{rms}/I_{mean}). This can be done by increasing the switching frequency to reduce the amplitude of the ripple. A benefit of increased efficiency is increased brush life and gear life and a lower probability of field permanent magnet demagnetization.

Switching or chopper drives are classified as either unidirectional or bidirectional. They are further divided by whether they use dynamic braking. Typically, power wheelchairs use bidirectional drives without dynamic braking. However, scooters may use unidirectional drives. The average voltage delivered to the motor from a switching drive is controlled by varying the duty cycle of the input waveform. There are two common methods of achieving this goal: (1) fixed pulsewidth, variable repetition rate, and (2) pulsewidth modulation (PWM). Power wheelchair servo amplifiers typically employ PWM.

Pulsewidth modulation at a fixed frequency has no minimum on-time restriction. Therefore, current peaking and torque ripple can be minimized. For analysis, a dc motor can be modeled as an RL circuit, resistor, and inductor in series with a voltage source [Powell & Inigo, 1992]. If the motor current is assumed continuous, then the minimum and maximum motor current can be represented by

$$I_{min} = \frac{e^{-(R/L)t_{off}}(1 - e^{-(R/L)t_{on}})}{1 - e^{-(R/L)(t_{on} - t_{off})}} \frac{V_s}{R} - \frac{V_{gen}}{R}$$

$$I_{max} = \frac{1 - e^{-(R/L)t_{on}}}{1 - e^{-(R/L)(t_{on} - t_{off})}} \frac{V_s}{R} - \frac{V_{gen}}{R}$$

(137.1)

Two basic design principals are used when designing switching servo amplifiers: (1) I_{max} should be limited to five times the rated current of the motor to ensure that demagnetization does not occur, and (2) the ripple, $(I_{max} - I_{min})/I_{avg}$, should be minimized to improve the form factor and reduce the conduction loss in the switching devices. To achieve low ripple, either the inductance has to be large or the switching frequency has to be high. Permalloy powder cores can be used to reduce core loss at frequencies above a few kilohertz. However, this comes at the cost of the electrical time constant of the motor, degrading the motor response time. Hence raising the switching frequency is most desirable. A power MOSFET has the ability to switch rapidly without the use of load-shaping components.

There are several motor types that may be suitable for use with power wheelchairs. Most current designs use permanent-magnet dc motors. These motors provide high torque and high starting torque and are simplest to control. Permanent-magnet dc motors can be controlled in what are commonly called either *current mode* or *voltage mode*. These modes developed out of designs based on controlling torque and speed, respectively.

Alternating current (ac) motors can be designed to be highly efficient and can be controlled with modern power circuitry. Because of the development and widespread dissemination of switching dc converters, it is quite feasible to use ac motors with a battery supply. To date, ac motors have been used only in research on power wheelchairs. The output of the motor is controlled by varying the phase or the frequency.

The battery energy storage system is recognized as one of the most significant limiting factors in power wheelchair performance [Kauzlarich et al., 1983]. Battery life and capacity are important. If battery life can be improved, the power wheelchair user will have longer reliable performance from his or her battery. An increase in battery capacity will allow power wheelchair users to travel greater distances with batteries that weigh and measure the same as existing wheelchair batteries. Most important, increases in battery capacity will enable the use of smaller and lighter batteries. Because batteries account for such a large proportion of both the weight and volume of current power wheelchair systems, wheelchair manufacturers must base much of their design around the battery package.

Power wheelchairs typically incorporate 24-V dc energy systems. The energy for the wheelchair is provided by two deep-cycle lead-acid batteries connected in series [Aylor et al., 1992]. Either wet-cell or gel-cell batteries are used. Wet-cell batteries also cost about half as much as gel-cell batteries. Gel cells may be required for transport by commercial air carriers.

Battery technology for wheelchair users remains unchanged despite the call for improvements by power wheelchair users. This may be due in part to the relatively low number of units purchased, about 500,000 per annum, when compared with automotive applications, about 6.6 million per annum by a single manufacturer [Kauzlarich et al., 1983]. Wheelchair batteries are typically rated at 12 V and 30 to 90 A·h capacity at room temperature. A power wheelchair draws about 10 A during use. The range of the power wheelchair is directly proportional to the ampere-hour rating for the operating temperature.

Batteries are grouped by size. Group size is indicated by a standard number. The group size defines the dimensions of the battery (Table 137.1). The ampere-hour rating defines the battery's capacity.

It is important that the appropriate charger be used with each battery set. Many battery chargers automatically reduce the amount of current delivered to the battery as the battery reaches full charge. This helps to prevent damage to the battery from boiling. The rate at which wet- and gel-cell batteries charge is significantly different. Some chargers are capable of operating with both types of batteries. Many require setting the charger for the appropriate battery type. Most wheelchairs batteries connected in series are charged simultaneously with a 24-V battery charger.

Electromagnetic Compatibility

Power wheelchairs have been reported to exhibit unintended movement. Wheelchair manufacturers and the U.S. Food and Drug Administration Center for Devices and Radiological Health (FDA-CDRH) have examined the susceptibility of power wheelchairs and scooters to interference from radio and microwave transmissions [Witters & Ruggera, 1994]. These devices are tested at frequencies ranging from 26 MHz to 1 GHz, which is common for transmissions (e.g., radio, television, microwave, telephones, mobile radios). Power wheelchairs incorporate complex electronics and microcontrollers that can be sensitive to electromagnetic (EM) radiation, electrostatic discharge (ESD), and other energy sources.

Electric-powered wheelchairs may be susceptible to electromagnetic interference (EMI) present in the ambient environment. Some level of EMI immunity is necessary to ensure the safety of power

TABLE 137.1 Standard Power Wheelchair Battery Group Sizes (units in inches)

Group Number	Length	Width	Height
U1	$7^3/_4$	$5^3/_{16}$	$7^5/_{16}$
22NF	$9^7/_{16}$	$5^1/_2$	$8^{15}/_{16}$
24	$10^1/_4$	$6^{13}/_{16}$	$8^7/_8$
27	$12^1/_{16}$	$6^{13}/_{16}$	$8^7/_8$

wheelchair users. *Electromagnetic compatibility* (EMC) is the term used to describe how devices and systems behave in an electromagnetic environment. Because of the complexity of power wheelchairs and scooters and the interaction with an electromagnetic environment, susceptibility to interference cannot be calculated or estimated reliably. A significant number of people attach accessories (e.g., car stereos, computers, communication systems) to their power wheelchairs that share the batteries. This may increase the susceptibility of other system components to EMI. A number of companies make electric-powered devices designed to operate on power wheelchairs to provide postural support, pressure relief, environmental control, and motor vehicle operation. These devices may alter the EMI compatibility of power wheelchairs as provided by the original equipment manufacturer (OEM). Wheelchairs and accessories can be made to function properly within EM environments through testing.

Field strengths have been measured at 20 V/m from a 15-W hand-held cellular telephone and 8 V/m from a 1-W hand-held cellular telephone. The FDA-CDRH has tested power wheelchairs and scooters in a gigahertz transverse electromagnetic (GTEM) cell and in an anechoic chamber with exposure strengths from 3 to 40 V/m [Witters & Ruggera, 1994]. The FDA requires that a warning sticker be placed on each power wheelchair or scooter indicating the risk due to EMI.

Two tests are commonly performed on chairs: brake release and variation in wheel speed. The device(s) used for measuring wheel speed and brake release must not significantly alter the field. The brakes shall not release or the wheels are not to move with a wheel torque equivalent to a 1:6 slope with a 100-kg rider when the wheelchair is exposed to EM radiation. Nonelectrical contact methods (e.g., audio sensing, optical sensing) of measuring brake release or wheelchair movement are preferable. Nominal wheel speed may drift over the length of the test. This drift is primarily due to drop in battery charge over the test interval. Wheel speed must be recorded without EM interference between test intervals. The percentage change in wheel speed during exposure to EM interference shall be referenced to the nominal wheel speed for that test interval. The variation in absolute forward speed, $(v_{emR} + v_{emL})/2$, is to be within 30% of the nominal forward speed, $(v_{nomR} + v_{nomL})/2$. The differential speed between the two wheels should be within 30% of each other, $2 \cdot (v_{emR} - v_{emL})/(v_{nomR} + v_{nomL})$. The test frequency must be held long enough to accommodate the slowest time constant (time required to reach 63% of maximum or minimum) or parameters related to wheelchair driving behavior. Currently, 2 seconds is used by the FDA-CDRH test laboratory.

137.5 Personal Transportation

Special adaptive equipment requirements increase with the degree of impairment and desired degree of independence in areas such as personal care, mobility, leisure, personal transportation, and employment. People are concerned that they receive the proper equipment for them to safely operate their vehicle [Sprigle et al., 1992a, 1992b]. Access and egress equipment have the greatest maintenance requirements. Other devices such as hand controls, steering equipment, securement mechanisms, and interior controls require less maintenance. Most users of adaptive driving equipment are satisfied with the performance of such equipment. Most frequent equipment problems are minor and are repaired by consumers themselves.

Physical functional abilities such as range of motion, manual muscle strength, sensation, grip strength, pinch strength, fine motor dexterity, and hand-eye coordination all may be related to driving potential. Driving characteristics also must be evaluated when determining an individual's potential to safely operate a motor vehicle. Throttle force, brake force, steering force, brake reaction time, and steering reaction time are all factors that influence an individual's driving potential.

Vehicle Selection

It is often a difficult task to find an automobile that meets the specific needs of a particular wheelchair user; no automobile meets the needs of all wheelchair users. Automotive consumers with disabilities are also concerned about ease of entry, stowage space for the wheelchair, and seat positioning. Reduced size, increasingly sloping windshields, lower roofs, and higher sills of new cars make selecting a new vehicle difficult for wheelchair users. The ability to load the wheelchair into a vehicle is essential. Some individuals with sufficient strength and the suitable vehicle are able to stow their wheelchairs inside the vehicle without the use of loading devices. Many people must rely on an external loading device. The selection of the appropriate vehicle should be based on the client's physical abilities and social needs.

An approach some people have used to overcome the problems associated with a smaller car is to use a cartop wheelchair carrying device. These devices lift the wheelchair to the top of the car and fold and stow it. They have been designed to work with four-door sedans, light trucks, and compact automobiles.

There are several critical dimensions to an automobile when determining wheelchair accessibility. The wheelbase of the automobile often is used by automobile manufacturers to determine vehicle size (e.g., full-size, midsize, compact). Typical ranges for passenger vehicles are presented in Table 137.2.

Lift Mechanisms

Many wheelchair users who cannot transfer into a passenger vehicle seat or prefer larger vehicles drive vans equipped with wheelchair lifts. Platform lifts may use a lifting track, a parallelogram lifting linkage, or a rotary lift. Lift devices are either electromechanically powered or electrohydraulically powered. The platform often folds into the side doorway of the van. Crane lifts, also called *swing-out lifts*, have a platform that elevates and folds or rotates into the van. Lifts may either be semiautomatic or automatic. In many cases, semiautomatic lifts require the user to initiate various stages (e.g., unlocking door, door opening, lowering lift) of the lifting process. Automatic lifts are designed to perform all lift functions. They usually have an outside key-operated control box or an interior radio-controlled control box.

Some lifts use electrohydraulic actuators to lift and fold, with valves and gravity used to lower the lift. Crane lifts may swing out from a post on the front or rear of the side door. Interlocking mechanisms are available with some lifts to prevent the lift from being operated while the door is closed. The Society of Automotive Engineers (SAE) has developed guidelines for the testing of wheelchair lift devices for entry and exit from a personal vehicle. The standards are intended to set a acceptable level of reliability and performance for van lifts.

Wheelchair Restraint Mechanisms

Securement systems are used to temporarily attach wheelchairs to vehicles during transport. Many wheelchair users can operate a motor vehicle from their wheelchair but are unable to transfer into a vehicle seat. Automobile safety standards have reduced the number of U.S. automobile accident fatalities despite an increase in the number of vehicles. The crash pulse determines the severity of the collision of the test sled and hence real world. Securement systems are tested with a surrogate wheelchair at 30 mi/h (48 + 2/-0 km/h) with a 20g deceleration [Adams et al., 1992]. Wheelchairs must be safely restrained when experiencing an impact of this magnitude, and no part of the wheelchair shall protrude into the occupant space, where it might cause injury.

Proper use of lap and shoulder belts is critical to protecting passengers in automobiles seats. A similar level of crash protection is required for individuals who remain in their wheelchairs during transportation. Wheelchairs are flexible, higher than a standard automobile seat, and not fixed to the vehicle. The pas-

TABLE 137.2 Typical Ranges of Accessibility Dimensions for Sedans (units in inches)

Wheelbase	93–108
Door height	33–47
Door width	41–47
Headroom	36–39
Max. space behind seat	9–19
Min. space behind seat	4–9
Seat-to-ground distance	18–22
Width of door opening	38–51

senger is restrained using a harness of at least one belt to provide pelvic restraint and two shoulder or torso belts that restrain both shoulders. A head support also may be used to prevent rearward motion of the head during impact or rebound. A three-point restraint is the combination of a lap belt and a shoulder belt (e.g., pelvic torso restraint, lap-sash restraint, lap-shoulder restraint).

The relationship between injury criteria and the mechanics of restraint systems is important to ensure the safety of wheelchair users in motor vehicles. Hip and head deflections are often-used criteria for determining potential injury. The automotive industry has invested considerable research and development effort to protect vehicle passengers. Research is not nearly so extensive for the passenger who remains seated in a wheelchair while traveling. Many wheelchair and occupant restraint systems copy the designs used for standard automobile seats. This type of design may not be appropriate.

Crash tests have shown that for 10g or 20g impacts of 100-ms duration, people may sustain injuries despite being restrained [Adams et al., 1992]. When shoulder belts mounted 60 inches above the floor were used to restrain a 50th percentile male dummy, it was found that the torso was well controlled, and head and chest excursions were limited. When shoulder belts were anchored 36 inches above the floor, they were ineffective in controlling torso movement [Adams & Reger, 1993]. Kinematic results and head injury criteria (HIC) can be used to estimate the extent of injury sustained by a human passenger. An HIC of 1000 or greater indicates a serious or fatal head injury. Generally, an HIC value approaching or exceeding 1000 is indicative of head impact with some portion of the vehicle interior. The open space typically surrounding a wheelchair user in a public bus precludes impact with the bus's interior. High HIC values may occur when the torso is effectively restrained and there is a high degree of neck flexion. If the chin strikes the chest, then there may be an impact great enough to cause head injury.

Hand Controls

Hand controls are available for automatic and manual transmission vehicles. However, hand controls for manual transmission automobiles must be custom-made. There are also portable hand controls and long-term hand controls. Portable hand controls are designed to easily attach to most common automobiles with a minimal number of tools. Hand controls are available for either left- or right-hand control.

Many hand controls are attached to the steering column. Hand controls either clamp to the steering column or are attached to a bracket that is bolted to the steering column or dash, typically where the steering column bolts to the dash. Installation of the hand control should not interfere with driver safety features (e.g., air bags, collapsible steering columns). The pushrods of the hand control clamp directly to either the pedals or the levers connected to them.

Most systems activate the brakes by having the driver push forward on a lever with a hand grip. This allows the driver to push against the back of the seat, creating substantial force, and braces the driver in the event of a collision. The throttle, or gas pedal, is operated in a number of ways. Some systems use a twist knob or motorcycle-type throttle. Other systems actuate the throttle by pulling on the brake throttle lever. Another method is to rotate the throttle-brake lever downward (i.e., pull the lever toward the thigh at a right angle to the brake application to operate the throttle). It is common to have the same vehicle driven by multiple people, which may require the vehicle to be safely operated with hand controls and the OEM foot controls. Care must be taken to ensure that the lever and brackets of the hand controls do not restrict the driving motions of foot-control drivers.

Many people have the motor control necessary to operate a motor vehicle, but they do not have the strength required to operate manual hand controls. Automatic, or *fly-by-wire*, hand controls use external actuators (e.g., air motors, servo mechanisms, hydraulic motors) to reduce the force required to operate various vehicle primary controls. Power steering, power brakes, six-way power seats, and power-adjustable steering columns can be purchased as factory options on many vehicles.

Six-way power seats are used to provide greater postural support and positioning than standard automotive seats. They can be controlled by a few switches to move fore-aft, incline-recline, and superior-inferior. This allows the user to position the seat for easy entry and exit and for optimal driving comfort. Power-adjustable steering columns also make vehicles more accessible. By using a few buttons, the steering column can be tilted upward or downward, allowing positioning for entry/exit into the vehicle and for optimal driving control.

Custom devices are available for people who require more than the OEM options for power assistance. Microprocessor and electronic technology have dramatically changed how motor vehicles are designed. Many functions of an automobile are controlled electronically or with electro-mechanical-electrohydraulic controls. This change in vehicle design has made a wide variety of options available for people who require advanced vehicle controls. Many automobiles use electronic fuel injection. Electronic fuel injection systems convert the position of the accelerator pedal to a serial digital signal that is used by a microcontroller to inject the optimal fuel-air mixture into the automobile at the proper time during the piston stroke. The electronic signal for the accelerator position can be provided by another control device (e.g., joystick, slide bar).

Defining Terms

Alignment: The orientation of the drive wheels with respect to one another. It is desirable to have the all wheels parallel to one another without any difference between the distance across the two sets of wheels.

Castor float: When one of the casters does not touch the floor when on level ground, the wheel-chair has castor float.

Castor flutter: The shimmy (rapid vibration of the caster wheels) that may occur on some surfaces above certain speeds.

Crash pulse: The acceleration time-motion profile that determines the severity of the collision of a test sled and hence real world.

Electromagnetic compatibility (EMC): The term used to describe how devices and systems behave in an electromagnetic environment.

Fly-by-wire: Automotive hand controls that use external actuators (e.g., air motors, servo mechanisms, hydraulic motors) to reduce the force required to operate various vehicle primary controls.

Head injury criteria (HIC): A standard measure used with crash test dummies to estimate the extent of injury sustained by a human passenger.

Kinematics: The study of human motion without regard to the forces that initiate or control the motion.

Kinetics: The study of the forces generated by and acting on the human body.

Multiple master, multiple slave bus (M3S): An interface specification with a basic hardware architecture, a bus communication protocol, and a configuration method.

Tracking: The tendency of the wheelchair/rider to maintain its course once steering control has been relinquished.

References

Adams TC, Reger SI. 1993. Factors affecting wheelchair occupant injury in crash simulation. In Proceedings of the 16th Annual RESNA Conference, Las Vegas, Nev, pp 80–82.

Adams TC, Sauer B, Reger SI. 1992. Kinematics of the wheelchair seated body in crash simulation. In Proceedings of RESNA International '92, Toronto, Ontario, Canada, pp 360–362.

Asato KT, Cooper RA, Robertson RN, Ster JF. 1993. SMART[wheels]: Development and testing of a system for measuring manual wheelchair propulsion dynamics. IEEE Trans Biomed Eng 40(12):1320.

Aylor JH, Thieme A, Johnson BW. 1992. A battery state-of-charge indicator. IEEE Trans Ind Electronics 39(5):398.

Brauer RL, Hertig BA. 1981. Torque generation on wheelchair handrims. In Proceedings of the 1981 Biomechanics Symposium, ASME/ASCE Mechanics Conference, pp 113–116.

Brubaker CE, Ross S, McLaurin CA. 1982. Effect of seat position on handrim force. In Proceedings of the 5th Annual Conference on Rehabilitation Engineering, p 111.

Cooper RA. 1991*a*. System identification of human performance models. IEEE Trans Syst Man Cybernet 21(1):244.

Cooper RA. 1991*b*. High tech wheelchairs gain the competitive edge. IEEE Eng Med Biol Mag 10(4):49.

Kauzlarich JJ, Ulrich V, Bresler M, Bruning T. 1983. Wheelchair batteries: Driving cycles and testing. J Rehabil Res Dev 20(1):31.

MacLeish MS, Cooper RA, Harralson J, Ster JF. 1993. Design of a composite monocoque frame racing wheelchair. J Rehabil Res Dev 30(2):233.

Powell F, Inigo RM. 1992. Microprocessor-based dc brushless motor controller for wheelchair propulsion. In Proceedings of RESNA International '92, Toronto, Canada, pp 313–315.

Riley PO, Rosen MJ. 1987. Evaluating manual control devices for those with tremor disability. J Rehabil Res Dev 24(2):99.

Sprigle SH, Morris BO, Karg PE. 1992*a*. Assessment of transportation technology: Survey of driver evaluators. In Proceedings of RESNA International '92, Toronto, Ontario, Canada, pp 351–353.

Sprigle SH, Morris BO, Karg PE. 1992*b*. Assessment of transportation technology: Survey of equipment vendors. In Proceedings of RESNA International '92, Toronto, Ontario, Canada, pp 354–356.

Schauer J, Kelso DP, Vanderheiden GC. 1990. Development of a serial auxiliary control interface for powered wheelchairs. In Proceedings of RESNA 13th Annual Conference, Washington, DC, pp 191–192.

Van Der Woude LHV, Veeger HEJ, Rozendal RH. 1989. Propulsion technique in handrim wheelchair ambulation. J Med Eng Technol 13(12):136.

van Woerden JA. 1993. M3S, a general purpose interface for the rehabilitation environment. In Proceedings of the European Conference on the Advancement of Rehabilitation Technology ECART 2, 22.1.

Witters DM, Ruggera PS. 1994. Electromagnetic compatibility (EMC) of powered wheelchairs and scooters. In Proceedings of RESNA 17th Annual Conference, Nashville, Tenn, pp 359–360.

Further Information

The quarterly journal *IEEE Transactions on Rehabilitation Engineering* reports on advances in rehabilitation engineering. For subscription information, contact IEEE Service Center, 445 Hoes Lane, P.O. Box 1331, Piscataway, NJ 08855-1331.

The quarterly publication from the U.S. Department of Veterans Affairs *Journal of Rehabilitation Research and Development* publishes articles on recent advances in rehabilitation science and engineering. For subscription information, contact Journal of Rehabilitation Research and Development, Rehabilitation Research and Development Service, US Department of Veterans Affairs, 103 South Gay Street, Baltimore, MD 21202-4051.

RESNA (1700 North Moore Street, Suite 1540, Arlington, VA 22209) and IEEE sponsor several conferences and publish proceedings that address the latest advances in rehabilitation science, engineering, and technology each year.

138

Externally Powered
and Controlled Orthotics
and Prosthetics

Dejan B. Popović
University of Miami and
University of Belgrade

Rehabilitation of physically challenged humans often includes effective use of assistive systems for restoration of motor functions. Some of the features of an effective assistive system are (1) reliability, (2) minimum increase in energy rate and cost with respect to able-bodied subjects performing the same task, (3) minimum disruption of normal activities when employing the assistive system, (4) cosmetics, and (5) practicality. The system should be easy to don and doff and available for daily home use. These requirements and available technology have led to the development of externally powered orthoses and prostheses that interface directly or indirectly with the human neuromuscular system or that are modeled on features possessed by that system. These devices include battery-powered actuators, microprocessor-based controller, and reliable biologic-like sensors.

Hand, arm, and lower extremities assistive systems for amputees and humans with paralysis will be elaborated in this chapter. Two approaches for the restoration of movements in humans with paralysis are described: functional activation of paralyzed muscles called *functional electrical stimulation* (FES) or *functional neuromuscular stimulation* (FNS) and the combined use of FES and a mechanical orthosis. The latter is called a *hybrid assistive system* (HAS). The part dealing with prostheses relates to externally controlled and powered artificial organs, with specific emphasis on so-called *myoelectric controlled* devices.

Available assistive systems meet many of the requirements listed above but still have some drawbacks. The small number of externally powered system users on a daily basis is a significant indicator that these systems are not perfected. Recent neurophysiologic findings on muscle properties and strengthening techniques in addition to improved percutaneous or implantable stimulators may increase the applicability of many assistive systems, mostly in the case of paralyzed limbs. Major limitations in daily use are connected with insufficiently adaptive and robust control methods. The complexity of central nervous system (CNS) control and the interface between voluntary control and external artificial control are still challenging, unanswered questions. Hierarchical control methods, combining symbolic models at the highest level and analytical models at lower levels, give hope for further progress. The controller should allow the user to perform motor tasks while concentrating on his or her normal daily activities.

0-8493-8346-3/95/$0.00+$.50
© 1995 by CRC Press, Inc.

Sensory feedback is essential for effective control of FES systems. In addition to artificial sensors, hopes are directed toward the use of natural sensors and the development of an "intelligent" movement controller.

138.1 FES Systems

Functional electrical stimulation (FES) can help in regaining functional movements in numerous paralyzed humans. FES activates innervated but paralyzed muscles by using an electronic stimulator to deliver trains of pulses to neuromuscular structures. The basic phenomenon of the stimulation is a contraction of muscle due to the controlled delivery of electric charge to neuromuscular structures.

FES systems can restore: (1) goal-oriented (hand and arm) movements and (2) cyclic (walking and standing) movements.

Restoration of Hand Functions

The objective of an upper extremity assistive system must be directed toward establishing independence for the user. Most effort in upper extremity FES has been directed toward the individual with diminished, but preserved, shoulder and elbow functions, with lack of wrist control and grasping ability [Peckham & Keith, 1992].

There have been several designs of FES systems. These systems can be divided based on the source of control signals to trigger or regulate the stimulation pattern: shoulder control [Buckett et al., 1988], voice control [Handa et al., 1992; Nathan & Ohry, 1990], respiratory control [Hoshimiya et al., 1989], joystick control [Peckham & Keith, 1992], and position transducers [Prochazka, 1993; Reberšek & Vodovnik, 1973]. The division can be made based on the method by which patterned electrical stimulation is delivered: one- or two-channel surface electrode systems [Prochazka, 1993; Vodovnik et al., 1981], multichannel surface stimulation system [Nathan & Ohry, 1990], multichannel percutaneous systems with intramuscular electrodes [Buckett et al., 1988; Handa et al., 1992; Hoshimiya et al., 1989], and fully implanted systems with epimysial electrodes [Peckham & Keith, 1992]. Only a few FES grasping systems have been used outside the laboratory.

The first grasping system used to provide prehension and release [Long & Masciarelli, 1963] used a splint with a spring for closure and electrical stimulation of the thumb extensor for release. This attempt was unsuccessful mostly because of the state of the art of technology used but also because of muscle fatigue and erratic contractile response. Rudel et al. [1984], following the work of Vodovnik [Reberšek & Vodovnik, 1973], suggested the use of a simple two-channel stimulation system and a position transducer (sliding potentiometer). The shift of the potentiometer forward from its neutral position causes opening by stimulating the dorsal side of the forearm, and backward causes closing of the hand by stimulating the volar side of the forearm.

The follow-up of initial FES system use was systematically continued in Japan. Japanese groups succeeded in developing the FES Clinic in Sendai, Japan, where many subjects are implanted with up to 30 percutaneous intramuscular electrodes that are used for therapy but not to assist grasping. The Japanese research approach in functional grasping relates to subjects lacking not only hand functions but also elbow control (e.g., C4 complete CNS injuries), and the system uses either voice or suck/puff control and preprogrammed EMG-based stimulation patterns. This preprogrammed EMG-based stimulation is developed by detailed studies of muscle activities with intramuscular electrodes in able-bodied subjects while reaching and grasping [Handa et al., 1989].

The approach taken at Ben Gurion University, Israel [Nathan, 1989], uses a voice-controlled multichannel surface electrode system. As many as 12 bipolar stimulation channels and a splint are used to control elbow, wrist, and hand functions. There is very little practical experience with the system, and the system has to be fine-tuned for the needs of every single user. Surface stimulation most probably does not allow control of the small hand and forearm muscles necessary to provide dexterity while grasping. Daily mounting and fitting of the system are other problems with this approach.

The group at the Institut for Biokibernetik, Karlsruhe, Germany, suggested the use of EMG recordings from the muscle that is stimulated [Holländer et al., 1987]. The aim of this device is to enhance the grasping using weak muscles. Hence, in principle, it could be possible to use retained recordings from the volar side of the forearm to trigger on and off the stimulation of the same muscles. In this case, it is essential to eliminate the stimulation artifact and the evoked potential caused by the stimulus in order to eliminate positive-feedback effects that will generate a tetanic contraction that cannot be turned off using the method presented.

The Case Western Reserve University (CWRU) fully implantable system has a switch to turn the system on and off and select the grasp, and a joystick to proportionally control aperture of the hand for palmar and lateral grasp. These two grasps are synthesized using a preprogrammed synergy. The joystick, mounted on the contralateral shoulder, voluntarily controls the preprogrammed sequence of stimulation. The palmar grasp starts from the extended fingers and thumb (one end position of the joystick), followed by movement of the thumb to opposition and flexing of fingers (other end position of the joystick). The lateral grasp starts from the full extension of fingers and the thumb, followed by flexion of fingers and adduction of the thumb. The system is applicable if the following muscles can be stimulated: extensor pollicis longus, flexor pollicis longus, adductor pollicis, opponens, flexor digitorum profundus and superficialis, and extensor digitorum communis. It is possible to surgically change the grasp permanently [Peckham & Keith, 1992] (pining some joints, tendon transfer, etc.). An important feature of the grasping system is related to daily fitting of the joystick (zeroing the neutral position) and going to hold mode from the movement mode. The hold mode is the regimen where the muscle nerves are stimulated at the level that the same force is maintained, and that level is selected by the user. At this time, the CWRU system uses the joystick with two degrees of freedom or velocity sensor software to switch from active control to hold mode. When the system is in the hold mode, joystick movements do not affect the grasp. The initial CWRU system [Peckham et al., 1980] suggested the use of myoelectric signals obtained from a site, with some regaining voluntary activity. The CWRU implantable system is the only system used for assistance in daily living functions [Peckham & Keith, 1992]. The functional evaluation of the system [Wijman et al., 1990] showed that there is substantial improvement in simple grasping tasks, which is important to a tetraplegic subject, and more than 25 systems are in use around North America.

Prochazka [1993] suggested the use of wrist position to control the stimulation of muscles to enhance this tenodesis grasping, and the device is called a *bionic glove*. A glove with a sensor is used to detect wrist movement, and it contains the contacts for the surface-stimulation electrodes. A microcomputer is built into the battery-operated stimulation unit that detects this movement and controls three channels to stimulate thumb extension and flexion and finger flexors.

Based on EMG recordings from above the lesion [Graupe, 1989], a grasping system with up to three channels of surface stimulation providing similar function to the Prachazka's system was developed [Saxena et al., 1994]. The developer suggested use of myoelectric signals from above-lesion sites (forearm wrist extensors) to trigger the stimulation of thumb and finger flexors. A threshold discrimination of the EMG is done that activates the proper stimulus pattern to be applied to the surface electrodes.

Restoration of Standing and Walking

The application of FES to the restoration of gait was first investigated systematically in Ljubljana, Slovenija [Bajd et al., 1982; Gračanin et al., 1967; Kralj et al., 1980, 1987; Vodovnik et al., 1967; Vodovnik & McLeod, 1965]. Currently, FES for gait rehabilitation is used in a clinical setting in several rehabilitation centers [Andrews et al., 1988; Brindley et al., 1978; Hermens et al., 1986; Jaeger et al., 1989; Kralj & Bajd, 1989; Marsolais & Kobetic, 1983; Mizrahi et al., 1985; Petrofsky & Phillips, 1983; Solomonow et al., 1989; Stein et al., 1990; Thomas et al., 1987; Vossius et al., 1987; Waters, 1985], and there is a growing trend for the design of devices for home use.

Current surface FES systems use various numbers of stimulation channels. The simplest one, from a technical viewpoint, is a single-channel stimulation system. This system is only suitable for stroke patients and a limited group of incomplete spinal cord–injured patients. These individuals can perform limited ambulation with assistance of the upper extremities without an FES system, although this ambulation may be both modified and/or impaired. The FES in these humans is used to activate a single muscle group. The first demonstrated application of this technique was in stroke patients [Gracanin et al., 1967], even though the original patent came from Liberson [1961]. The stimulation is applied to ankle dorsiflexors so that "foot drop" can be eliminated.

A multichannel system with a minimum of four channels of FES is required for ambulation of a patient with a complete motor lesion of the lower extremities and preserved balance and upper body motor control [Kralj & Bajd, 1989]. Appropriate bilateral stimulation of the quadriceps muscles locks the knees during standing. Stimulating the common peroneal nerve on the ipsilateral side while switching off the quadriceps stimulation on that side produces a flexion of leg. This flexion, combined with adequate movement of the upper body and use of the upper extremities for support, allows ground clearance and is considered as the swing phase of the gait cycle. Hand or foot switches can provide the flexion-extension alternation needed for a slow forward or backward progression (Fig. 138.1). Sufficient arm strength must be available to provide balance in parallel bars (clinical application) and with a rolling walker or crutches (daily use of FES). These systems evolved into a commercial product called Parastep-1 (Sigmedics, Chicago, Ill.), which has been approved for home use (Food and Drug Administration approval in April 1994).

Multichannel percutaneous systems for gait restoration, with many channels, were suggested [Brindley, 1979; Marsolais & Kobetic, 1983, 1987]. The main advantage of these systems is the possibility to activate many different muscle groups. A very similar preprogrammed stimulation pattern to the one in an able-bodied human is delivered to ankle, knee, and hip joints, as well as to paraspinal muscles. The experience of the Cleveland research team suggests that 48 channels are

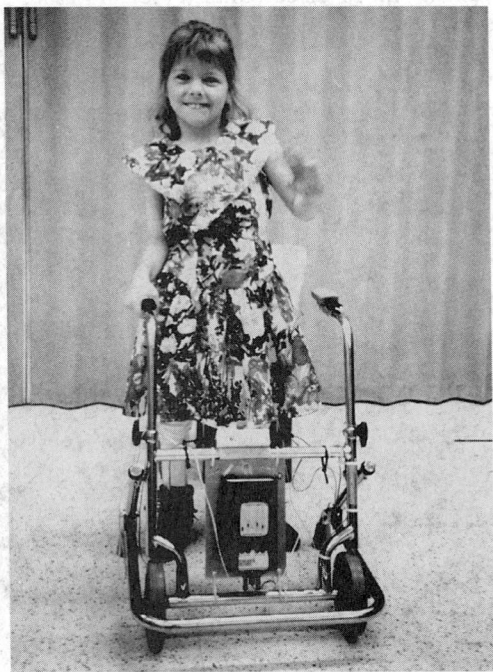

FIGURE 138.1 A paraplegic subject using the four-channel surface stimulation system (Quadstim, Biomech Design, Edmonton, Alberta).

required for a complete SCI walking system to achieve a reasonable walking pattern. Fine-wire intramuscular electrodes are cathodes positioned close to the motor point within selected muscles. Knee extensors (rectus femoris, vastus medialis, vastus lateralis, vastus intermedius), hip flexors (sartorius, tensor fasciae latae, gracilis, iliopsoas), hip extensors (semimembranosus, gluteus maximus), hip abductors (gluteus medius), ankle dorsiflexors (tibialis anterior, peroneus longus), ankle plantar flexors (gastrocnemius lateralis and medialis, plantaris and soleus), and paraspinal muscles are selected for activation. A surface electrode is used as a common anode. Interleaved pulses are delivered with a multichannel, battery-operated, portable stimulator. The hand controller allows the selection of gait activity. These systems have been limited to clinical environments. The application was investigated in complete spinal cord lesions and in stroke patients [Marsolais et al., 1990]. The same strategy and selection criteria for implantation were used for both stroke and SCI patients.

A multichannel totally implanted FES system [Thomas et al., 1983, 1987] was proposed and tested in a few subjects. This system uses a 16-channel implantable stimulator attached to the epineurium electrodes. Femoral and gluteal nerves were stimulated for hip and knee extension. The so-called round-about stimulation was applied, in which four electrodes were located around the nerve and stimulated intermittently. This stimulation method reduces muscle fatigue.

The Cleveland research team started using a fully implantable stimulation system originally developed for upper extremities. Eight channels are used for stimulation of leg muscles in stroke subjects. An eight-channel system was sufficient for stroke patients. An interesting phenomenon of motor control improvement or "short-term carryover" was demonstrated by some stroke patients and not usually demonstrated by SCI patients. *Short-term carryover* refers to changes in neuromuscular activities of impaired structures for a period after the electrical stimulation is discontinued. It is possible to observe improved function for a day or more without the FES device. Repetition of the proper pattern can result in permanent changes in stroke subjects.

The development of stimulation technology is giving new hopes. Two new techniques are specially important: (1) application of remotely controlled wireless microstimulators (Fig. 138.2) [Loeb, personal communication] and (2) the so-called stimulator for all seasons [Strojnik et al., 1990].

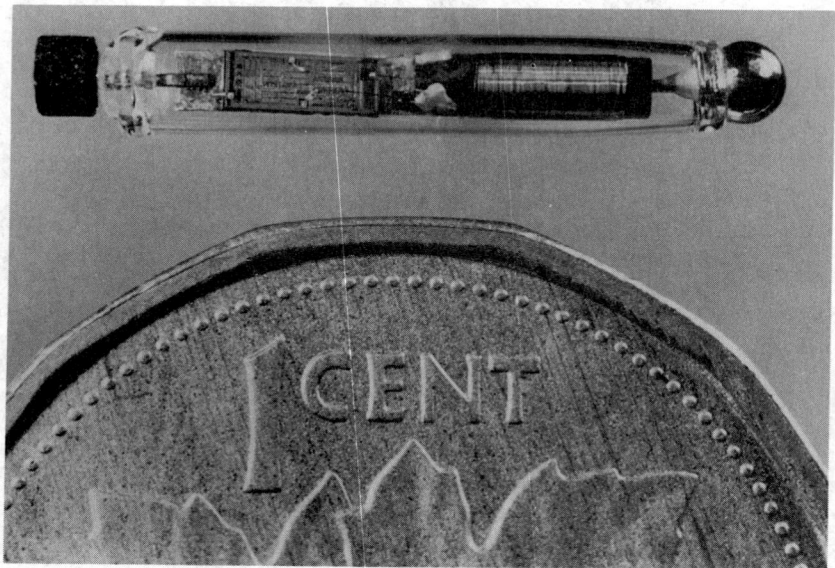

FIGURE 138.2   The microstimulator developed as a part of a NIH contract by Minimed, Sylmar, California.

However, there are some not completely answered questions limiting the effectiveness of FES systems dealing with muscle fatigue, reduced joint torques generated through FES in comparison with CNS-activated torques in healthy subjects, modified reflex activities, spasticity, functional and joint contractures, and osteoporosis and stress fractures. From the engineering point of view, further development of the FES system has to address the following issues: the interface between a FES system and neuromuscular structures in the organism, biocompatibility of the FES system, and overall practicality. The least resolved questions in FES systems deal with interfacing artificial and natural control. A nonconventional method based on symbolic representation of motion in animals and humans, called *artificial reflex control,* was proposed [Tomović, 1984]. The term *symbolic* refers here to representation of motion in the form of discrete events. A *discrete event* is recognized as a specific sensory pattern occurring during a particular motor activity. The current state of the system and a sensory input define the corresponding functional movement to be executed [Tomović, 1984, Tomović et al., 1987]. Different variants of such control systems [Andrews et al., 1987, 1988; Veltink et al., 1990] are currently under development.

In principle, closed-loop systems offer substantial increases in input-output linearity and repeatability, along with a substantial decrease in the sensitivity of the system to parameter variations (internal disturbances) and load changes (external disturbances). Recently, digital closed-loop methods using proportional (P) and proportional plus integral (PI) controllers were studied for both recruitment and fatigue of muscles. The increase in the loop gain in these controllers improved compensation for variation in muscle properties but brought the system closer to instability. The effects of the simultaneous control of interpulse interval and pulse width were investigated, and promising results were obtained [Chizeck, 1992].

The research results indicate that the usual classification of CNS lesions is applicable as a guideline but is not convenient as a selection criterion for FES candidates. FES users and an appropriate FES system must be selected through a functional diagnosis. The term *functional diagnosis* is used to indicate that the functional status after the injury determines the type of treatment. General statements about FES systems indicate that it is suitable for subjects with preserved peripheral neuromuscular structures, moderate spasticity, without joint contractures, and limited osteoporosis. Subjects should be able to control their balance and upper body posture using the upper extremities for assistance (parallel bars, walker, crutches, etc). Subjects with pathologies affecting the heart, lung, or circulation should be treated with extreme care, and often these subjects should not be included in an FES walking program. A satisfactory mental and emotional condition is extremely important, since an FES treatment requires a certain degree of intelligence and understanding of the technical side of the system. High motivation and good cooperation with medical staff are significant aspects of the efficacy of FES. Surface stimulation may be applied only in subjects with limited sensation, because it activates pain receptors. Subjects suitable for FES can be found within groups with head and spinal cord injuries, cerebral paralysis, multiple sclerosis, different types of myelitis, and others.

The final current drawback to FES ambulation is the excessive energy cost of walking. FES walking should be described as a sequence of static states, long stance phase (several seconds), followed by brisk flexion movement and short step, followed by the same movement on the contralateral side. Dynamic walking is a necessary development that will introduce better use of inertial and gravity forces, reduce energy rate and cost, increase the walking distance, and increase the speed of progression, in parallel with decreased fatigue of muscles, because they will not be stimulated for long periods.

A difference in walking performances between able-bodied and paralyzed humans (energy cost, energy rate, amount of the use of upper extremities, and cardiovascular stress measured through pulse rate and blood pressure) is given in Table 138.1.

Hybrid Assistive Systems (HAS)

A specific approach of integration of two assistive systems (FES and an external mechanical orthosis) has been proposed (Fig. 138.3). These systems are called *hybrid assistive systems* (HAS) or

TABLE 138.1   Best Performance with the Use of an Assistive System Compared with the Performance of Able-Bodied Subjects

	Oxygen Rate, ml/kg/min	Oxygen Cost, ml/kg/m	Speed V_{max}, m/min	Heart Rate, beats/min	Blood Pressure, mmHg	Use of Upper Extremities, %
Paralyzed subjects	13.6	0.6	60	~118 (84 rest)	~119/85	28
Able-bodied subjects	12.1	0.15	85	95 (81 rest)	~120/80	0
Control method	Voluntary, hand-switch	Voluntary, sensory driven	Automatic, preprogrammed	Voluntary hand-switch or sensory driven	Voluntary hand-switch or sensory driven	Voluntary, hand-switch or sensory driven
Assistive system used	FES + SFMO FES + RGO	FES + SFMO	FES implant	FES + RGO FES + SFMO	FES + RGO	FES + RGO

Note: The data are collected from Bowker et al., 1992; Nene and Jennings, 1992; Petrofsky & Smith, 1991; Popović et al., 1990; Popović & Schwirtlich, 1993; Solomonow, 1992; Stein et al., 1993; Waters et al., 1989; Waters & Lunsford, 1985. Abbreviations used in the table are RGO = reciprocating gait orthosis; SFMO = self-fitting modular orthosis; FES = functional electrical stimulation. Data for able-bodied subjects are from Waters at el., 1989.

hybrid orthotic systems (HOS) [Popović et al. 1989; Solomonow, 1992]. A few possibilities for HAS design have been suggested combining relatively simple, rigid mechanical structures for passive stabilization of lower limbs during stance phase and FES systems. These systems combine use of a *reciprocating gait orthosis* with multichannel stimulation [Solomonow, 1992], the use of an ankle-foot orthosis or an extended ankle-foot orthosis with a knee cage [Andrews et al., 1987], or the use

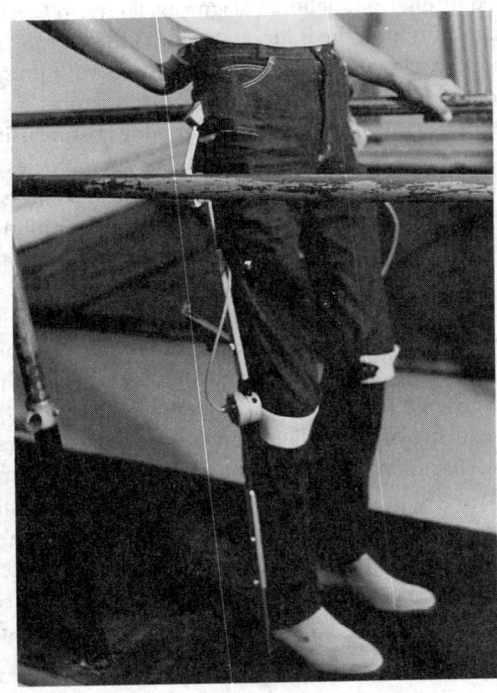

FIGURE 138.3   A paraplegic subject standing with a hybrid assistive system. The particular system incorporates a six-channel surface stimulation system and a self-fitting modular orthosis.

of a self-fitting modular orthosis (SFMO) [Schwirtlich & Popović, 1984]. A few more sophisticated laboratory systems were demonstrated [Andrews et al., 1989; Phillips, 1989]. Each trend in the design of HAS implies different applications as well as specific hardware and control problems. On the basis of accumulated experience, the following features can serve as criteria for a closer description of various HAS designs [Popović et al., 1990]: (1) partial mechanical support, (2) parallel operation of the biologic and mechanical system, and (3) sequential operation of the biologic and the mechanical system. Partial mechanical support refers to the use of braces to assist FES only at specific events within a walking cycle [Andrews et al., 1989].

138.2 Active Prostheses

The role of active prosthesis is to extend the function provided by a "non-externally" powered and controlled artificial organ and hence to improve the overall performance of motor function, ultimately providing a better quality of life.

Active Above-Knee Prostheses

Effective restoration of walking and standing of handicapped humans is an important element to improve the quality of life. Artificial legs of different kinds have been in use for a long time, but in many cases they are inadequate for the needs of amputees, specifically for high above-knee amputations (e.g., hip disarticulation), bilateral amputees, and patients who have demanding biomechanical requirements (e.g., subjects involved in sport).

Modern technology has led to improved designs of below-knee prostheses (BKPs) in recent years. Below-knee amputees perform many normal locomotor activities and participate in many sports requiring running, jumping, and other jerky movements [Inman et al., 1981]. The biggest progress was made using readily available and easy-to-work-with plastic and graphite alloys for building the artificial skeletal portion of the shank and foot [Doane & Holt, 1983]. Below-knee prostheses are light, easy to assemble, and reliable. They provide good support and excellent energy absorption, which prevent impact jerks and allow the push-off phase in the gait cycle. Existing below-knee prostheses, even those without ankle joints, duplicate the behavior of the normal foot-ankle complex during the swing and stance phases of the step cycle.

The same technology has been introduced into the design of above-knee prostheses (AKPs). However, commercially available AKPs suffer from several drawbacks. The requirements for an AKP were stated by Wagner and Catranis [1954]. The prosthesis must support the body weight of the amputee like the normal limb during the stance phase of level walking, on slopes, and on soft or rough terrain. This implies that the prosthesis provides "stability" during weight bearing; i.e., it prevents sudden or uncontrolled flexion of the knee during weight bearing. The second requirement is that the body be supported such that undesirable socket-stump interface pressures and gait abnormalities due to painful socket-stump contact are prevented. The analysis of biomechanical factors that influence the shaping, fitting, and alignment of the socket is a problem in itself. If the fitting has been accomplished, allowing the amputee to manipulate and control the prosthesis in an active and comfortable manner, the socket and stump can be treated as one single body. The third requirement, which is somewhat controversial, is that the prosthesis should duplicate as nearly as possible the kinematics and dynamics of normal gait. The amputee should walk with a normal-looking gait over a useful range of speeds associated with typical activities for normal persons of similar age. The latter requirement has received attention in recent years, and fully integrated systems, so-called self-contained active AKPs, are being incorporated into modern rehabilitation. The self-contained principle implies that the artificial leg contains the energy source, actuator, controller, and sensors.

Devices such as the polycentric knee mechanism [Cappozzo et al., 1980], the polycentric knee mechanism with a hydraulic valve [Radcliffe, 1980], and the AKP with a friction-type brake [Aoyama, 1980] satisfy some of these performance requirements. A logically controlled AKP with a hydraulic valve represents a further bridge between purely passive and fully controllable assistive devices [James et al., 1991; Turajlić & Drakulić, 1978].

Detailed studies of knee joint performance in the stance phase have been done [Flowers & Mann, 1977; Flowers et al., 1978, Mann, 1981; Stein & Flowers, 1980]. From these it is clear that for several gait modes (ramp, stairs), active knee control in the swing phase is desirable. To meet these requirements, self-contained multimode AKPs have been introduced [Koganezawa et al., 1984; Kuzhekin et al., 1984; Popović & Schwirtlich, 1988, Tomović et al., 1982]. The final prototype version of an active self-contained AKP allowing controlled flexion and extension throughout the gait cycle was developed by Kelly James [James et al., 1991], and it will be a product offered by Otto Bock Company, Germany. This leg uses an efficient knee controller with a custom-built hydraulic valve and a single-chip microcontroller with a rule-based control scheme (see Chapter 163).

The advantages of the externally powered and controlled leg (e.g., Belgrade AKP) [Popović et al., 1991] are an increased speed of locomotion, better gait symmetry, and lower energy cost and rate. These accomplishments are due to the fact that the powered leg allows controlled knee bounce after heel contact, limited push-off at the end of the stance phase, and effective flexion and controlled knee extension during the swing phase of gait. The external control allows the amputee to walk almost without any circumduction, which helps gait symmetry considerably. The knee joint of a standard endoskeletal prosthesis is fitted with an actuator having two independent braking units (friction drum–type brake with an azbestum lining to allow control of the knee joint stiffness) and an extension-flexion driver with a ball-screw mechanism. The rechargeable battery power supply is designed for up to 3 hours of continuous level walking. The Motorola 68HC11–based microcontroller has been fitted into the interior of the prosthesis, fulfilling self-containing principles. A hierarchical controller allows for intention recognition (volitional actions of the subject), adaptation to environmental changes and cyclical triggering throughout locomotion, and minimal jerk actuator control (see Chapter 163).

Myoelectric Hand and Arm Prostheses

The popularity of this control strategy comes from the fact that it is "very elegant" one, since control signals going to the prosthesis may come from the myoelectric activity of the muscle that formerly controlled the lost limb [Graupe & Kline, 1975; Jacobsen et al., 1982; Lyman et al., 1974]. Therefore, in some sense, the brain's own signals are used to control the motion of the prosthesis [Sheridan & Mann, 1978]. Although the validity of myoelectric control–based techniques seems reasonable, in practice, the performances are somewhat disappointing. There are a number of reasons for this. In the cases of high-level amputation, the electrical activity of the remaining muscles have only minor correlations with the normal arm movements, and this makes coordinated control of several functions very difficult. A more important problem is that any EMG-controlled prosthesis is inherently open loop (preprogrammed) [Simpson, 1974]. The absence of position proprioception and other related problems of reliability in executing movements [Gibbons et al., 1987] have contributed to the poor success rate of myoelectrically controlled prostheses.

Presently, two systems based on myoelectric control are used with success. The Otto Bock myoelectric hand [Pike, personal communication] uses the technique of detection of the fixed threshold of the integrated rectified surface electromyography. Extension/flexion of the targeted muscle group serves as the on/off control, which causes opening and closing of the hand, respectively. Two sets of electrodes are used to detect this differential signal. The Utah arm [Jacobsen et al., 1982] utilizes the myoelectric signals from two antagonists as the proportional elbow control. These signals are full wave rectified and differentiated to give the command signal. The Utah arm has a wrist rotator, and it can be combined with different grasping systems. Most artificial hands used in everyday activities do not include five-finger dexterity, except in devices that are mechanically preprogrammed.

An interesting approach to overcoming the problems encountered with EMG control has been proposed by Simpson [1974]. The control strategy is termed *extended physiologic proprioception*

(EPP) and uses the positions of intact joints as the controlling input signals to a prosthesis. This strategy is based on a recognition of the facts that intact joints possess inherent position feedback and that most of goal-oriented tasks are highly synergistic [Popović & Popović, 1994]. By establishing a one-to-one relationship between the position of the intact joint and the position in the space of the terminal device (prosthesis), the natural feedback of the intact joint can be "extended" to the prosthesis and thereby provide it with proprioceptive information. Based on this idea, an externally controlled elbow-wrist-hand prosthesis was evaluated [Gibbons et al., 1987]. The shoulder joint position is measured with a potentiometer mounted between the upper arm and trunk. An important feature of the system is that disabled humans can learn how to control the system within minutes using trial-and-error procedure.

Defining Terms

Artificial reflex control: A nonnumeric method for movement control. The artificial reflex is a sensory-driven algorithm based on knowledge representation (production rule-based system).

Externally controlled assistive system: Assistive system for restoration of motor functions with automatic and voluntary control.

Externally powered assistive system: Assistive system for restoration of motor functions which uses external power sources to either stimulate muscles or drive actuators.

Functional electrical stimulation or functional neuromuscular stimulation: Patterned electrical stimulation of neuromuscular structures in an organism dedicated to restore functions lost after paralysis.

Hierarchical control: Multilevel control structure implies that the decision making and implementation are not concentrated in one place. Certain decision activities and implementation processes are delegated to centers distributed to several levels.

Hybrid assistive systems: Combines use of functional electrical stimulation and mechanical bracing.

Myoelectric (EMG) control: Use of voluntary generated myoelectric activity as control signals for an externally controlled and powered assistive system.

Reciprocating gait orthosis: A walking and standing assistive system with a reciprocating mechanism for hip joints that extends the contralateral hip when the ipsilateral hip is flexed.

Self-fitting modular orthosis: A modular, self-fitting mechanical brace with a soft interface between human body and the orthosis.

References

Andrews BJ, Barnett RW, Phillips GF, et al. 1989. Rule-based control of a hybrid FES orthosis for assisting paraplegic locomotion. Automedica 11:175.

Andrews BJ, Baxendale RM, Barnett RW, et al. 1987. A hybrid orthosis for paraplegics incorporating feedback control. In Advances in External Control of Human Extremities IX, pp. 297–331 Belgrade, ETAN.

Andrews BJ, Baxendale RH, Barnett R, et al. 1988. Hybrid FES orthosis incorporating closed loop control and sensory feedback. J Biomed Eng 10:189.

Aoyama F. 1980. Lapoc system leg. In Proceedings of the Rehabilitation Engineering Seminar REIS '80, Tokyo, Japan, pp 59–67.

Bajd T, Kralj A, Turk R. 1982. Standing-up of a healthy subject and a paraplegic patients. J Biomech 15:1.

Bar A, Ishai P, Meretsky P, Koren Y. 1983. Adaptive microcomputer control of an artificial knee in level walking. J Biomed Eng 5:145.

Bowker P, Messenger N, Oglivie C, Rowley DI. 1992. Energetics of paraplegic walking. J Biomed Eng 14:344.

Brindley GS, Polkey CE, Rushton DN. 1978. Electrical splinting of the knee in paraplegia. Paraplegia 16:428.

Buckett JR, Peckham HP, Thrope G, et al. 1988. A flexible, portable system for neuro-muscular stimulation in the paralyzed upper extremities. IEEE Trans Biomed Eng BME-35:897.

Cappozzo A, Leo T, Cortesi S. 1980. A polycentric knee-ankle mechanism for above-knee prostheses. J Biomech 13:231.

Doane NE, Holt LE. 1983. A comparison of the SACH foot and single axis foot in the gait of the unilateral below-knee amputee. Prosthet Orthop Intern 7:33.

Flowers WC, Mann RW. 1977. An electrohydraulic knee-torque controller for a prosthesis simulator. J Biomech Eng 99:3.

Flowers WC, Rowell D, Tanquary A, Cone A. 1978. A microcomputer controlled knee mechanism for A/K prostheses. In Proceedings of the Third CISM-IFToMM International Symposium on Theory and Practice of Robots and Manipulators, Udine, Italy, pp 28–42.

Gibbons DT, O'Riain MD, Philippe-Auguste JS. 1987. An above-elbow prosthesis employing programmed linkages. IEEE Trans Biomed Eng BME-34:251.

Graupe D. 1989. EMG pattern analysis for patient-responsive control of FES in paraplegics for walker-supported walking. IEEE Trans Biomed Eng BME-36:711.

Graupe D, Kline WK. 1975. Functional separation of EMG signals via ARMA identification methods for prosthesis control purposes. IEEE Trans Syst Man Cybernet SMC-5:252.

Gračanin F, Prevec T, Trontelj J. 1967. Evaluation of use of functional electronic peroneal brace in hemiparetic patients. In Advances in External Control of Human Extremities III, pp 198–210. Belgrade, ETAN.

Handa Y, Handa T, Ichie M, et al. 1992. Functional electrical stimulation (FES) systems for restoration of motor function of paralyzed muscles—Versatile systems and a portable system. Frontiers Med Biol Eng 4:241.

Hermens HJ, Mulder AK, Tijhaar WH, et al. 1986. Research on electrical stimulation with surface electrodes. In Proceedings of the 2nd Vienna International Workshop on Functional Electrostimulation, Vienna, pp 321–324.

Holländer HJ, Huber M, Vossius G. 1987. An EMG controlled multichannel stimulator. In D Popović (ed), Advances in External Control of Human Extremities IX, Belgrade, ETAN, pp 291–295.

Hoshimiya N, Naito N, Yajima M, Handa Y. 1989. A multichannel FES system for the restoration of motor functions in high spinal cord injury patients: A respiration-controlled system for multijoint upper extremity. IEEE Trans Biomed Eng BME-36:754.

Inman VT, Ralston JJ, Todd F. 1981. Human Walking. Baltimore, Williams & Wilkins.

Jacobsen SC, Knutti FF, Johnson RT, Sears HH. 1982. Development of the Utah artificial arm. IEEE Trans Biomed Eng BME-29:249.

Jaeger R, Yarkony GY, Smith R. 1989. Standing the spinal cord injured patient by electrical stimulation: Refinement of a protocol for clinical use. IEEE Trans Biomed Eng BME-36:720.

James K, Stein RB, Rolf R, Tepavac D. 1991. Active suspension above-knee prosthesis. In D Goh, A Nathan (eds), Proceedings of the VI International Conference of Biomedical Engineering, pp 317–320.

Keith MW, Peckham PH, Thrope GB, et al. 1988. Functional neuromuscular stimulation for the tetraplegic hand. Clin Orthop 233:25.

Koganezawa E, Fujimoto H, Kato I. 1987. Multifunctional above-knee prosthesis for stairs walking. Prosthet Orthop Intern 11:139.

Kralj A, Bajd T. 1989. Functional Electrical Stimulation, Standing and Walking after Spinal Cord Injury. Boca Raton, Fla, CRC Press.

Kralj A, Bajd T, Turk R. 1980. Electrical stimulation providing functional use of paraplegic patient muscles. Med Prog Technol 7:3.

Kralj A, Bajd T, Turk R, Benko H. 1987. Results of FES application to 71 SCI patients. In Proceedings of RESNA 10th Annual Conference on Rehabilitation Technology, San Jose, pp 645–647.

Kuzhekin AP, Jacobson JS, Konovalov VV. 1984. Subsequent development of motorized above-knee prosthesis. In D Popović (ed), Advances in External Control of Human Extremities VIII, pp 525–530. Belgrade, ETAN.

Lieberson W, Holmquest HJ, Scott D, Dow A. 1961. Functional electrotherapy stimulation of the peroneal nerve synchronized with the swing phase of the gait of hemiplegic patients. Arch Phys Med Rehabil 42:101.

Long C II, Masciarelli CV. 1963. An electrophysiologic splint for the hand. Arch Phys Med Rehabil 44:499.

Lyman JH, Freedy A, Prior R, Solomonow M. 1974. Studies toward a practical computer-aided arm prosthesis system. Bull Prosthet Res 213.

Marsolais EB, Kobetic R. 1983. Functional walking in paralyzed patients by means of electrical stimulation. Clin Orthop 175:30.

Marsolais EB, Kobetic R. 1987. Implantation techniques and experience with percutaneous intramuscular electrode in the lower extremities. J Rehabil Res 23:1.

Marsolais EB, Kobetic R, Jacobs J. 1990. Comparison of FES treatment in the stroke and spinal cord injury patient. In D Popović (ed), Advances in External Control of Human Extremities X, pp 213–218. Belgrade, Nauka.

Mizrahi J, Braun Z, Najenson T, Graupe D. 1985. Quantitative weight bearing and gait evaluation of paraplegics using functional electrical stimulation. Med Biol Eng Comput 23:101.

Nathan RH. 1989. An FNS-based system for generating upper limb function in the C4 quadriplegic. Med Biol Eng Comput 27:549.

Nathan RH, Ohry A. 1990. Upper limb functions regained in quadriplegia: A hybrid computerized neuromuscular stimulation system. Arch Phys Med Rehabil 71:415.

Nene AV, Jennings SJ. 1992. Physiological cost index of paraplegic locomotion using the ORLAU Para Walker. Paraplegia 30:246.

Peckham PH, Keith MW. 1992. Motor prostheses for restoration of upper extremity function. In RB Stein, HP Peckham, DB Popović (eds), Neural Prostheses: Replacing Motor Function after Disease or Disability, pp 162–190. London, Oxford University Press.

Peckham PH, Mortimer JT, Marsolais EB. 1980. Controlled prehension and release in the C5 quadriplegic elicited by functional electrical stimulation of the paralyzed forearm muscles. Ann Biomed Eng 8:369.

Petrofsky JS, Phillips CA. 1983. Computer controlled walking in the paralyzed individual. J Neurol Orthop Surg 4:153.

Petrofsky JS, Smith JB. 1991. Physiologic cost of computer-controlled walking in persons with paraplegia using a reciprocating-gait orthosis. Arch Phys Med Rehabil 72:890.

Phillips CA. 1989. An interactive system of electronic stimulators and gait orthosis for walking in the spinal cord injured. Automedica 11:247.

Popović D, Schwirtlich L. 1988, Belgrade active A/K prosthesis. In J de Vries (ed), Electrophysiological Kinesiology, pp 337–343. Amsterdam, Excerpta Medica.

Popović D, Schwirtlich L, Radosavljević S. 1990. Powered hybrid assistive system. In D Popović (ed), Advances in External Control of Human Extremities X, pp 191–200. Belgrade, Nauka.

Popović D, Tomović R, Schwirtlich L. 1989. Hybrid assistive system—Neuroprosthesis for motion. IEEE Trans Biomed Eng BME-37:729.

Popović M, Popović D. 1994. A new approach to reaching control for tetraplegic subjects. J Electromyogr Kinesiol 4:242–253.

Prochazka A. 1993. Life with the electric glove. Newsletter Alberta Heritage Foundation for Medical Research, April, p 6.

Reberšek S, Vodovnik L. 1973. Proportionally controlled functional electrical stimulation of hand. Arch Phys Med Rehabil 54:378.

Rudel D, Bajd T, Reberšek S, Vodovnik L. 1984. FES assisted manipulation in quadriplegic patients. In D Popović (ed), Advances in External Control of Human Extremities VIII, pp 273–282. Belgrade, Yugoslav Committee for ETAN.

Saxena S, Nikolić S, Popović D. 1994. An EMG controlled FES system for grasping in Tetraplegics. J Rehabil Res Dev 32:17–24.

Sheridan TB, Mann RW. 1978. Design of control devices for people with severe motor impairment. Human Factors 20:321.

Schwirtlich L, Popović D. 1984. Hybrid orthoses for deficient locomotion. In D Popović (ed), Advances in External Control of Human Extremities VIII, pp 23–32. Belgrade, ETAN.

Simpson DC. 1974. The choice of control system for the multimovement prosthesis: Extended physiological proprioception (e.p.p.). In P Herberts (ed), The Control of Upper-Extremity Prostheses and Orthoses. Springfield, Ill, C Thomas.

Solomonow M. 1992. Biomechanics and physiology of a practical powered walking orthosis for paraplegics. In RB Stein, HP Peckham, D Popović, et al. (eds), Neural Prostheses: Replacing Motor Function after Disease or Disability, pp 202–230. London, Oxford University Press.

Solomonow M, Eldred E, Lyman J, Foster J. 1983. Control of muscle contractile force through indirect high-frequency stimulation. Am J Phys 62:71.

Stein RB, Belanger M, Wheeler G, et al. 1993. Assessment of electrical systems for improving locomotion after incomplete spinal cord injury. Arch Phys Med Rehab 74:954.

Stein JL, Flowers WC. 1980. Above-knee prosthesis: A case study of the interdependency of effector and controller design. ASME Winter Annual Meeting, Chicago, Ill, pp 275–277.

Stein RB, Prochazka A, Popović D, et al. 1990. Technology transfer and development for walking using functional electrical stimulation. In D Popović (ed), Advances in External Control of Human Extremities X, pp 161–176. Belgrade, Nauka.

Strojnik P, Whitmoyer D, Schulman J. 1990. An implantable stimulator for all season. In D Popović (ed), Advances in External Control of Human Extremities X, pp 335–344. Belgrade, Nauka.

Thomas H, Benzer H, Bruber H, et al. 1983. First implantation of a 16-channel electric stimulation device in human. Trans Am Soc Artific Intern Organs 12, Toronto, University of Toronto Press.

Thomas H, Frey M, Hole J, et al. 1987. Functional neurostimulation to substitute locomotion in paraplegia patients. In D Andrade (ed), Artificial Organs, pp 515–529. VCH Publishers.

Tomović R. 1984. Control of assistive systems by external reflex arcs. In D Popović (ed), Advances in External Control of Human Extremities IX, pp 7–21. Belgrade, ETAN.

Tomović R, Popović D, Tepavac D. 1987. Adaptive reflex control of assistive systems. In D Popović (ed), Advances in External Control of Human Extremities IX, pp 207–214. Belgrade, ETAN.

Tomović R, Popović D, Turajlić S, McGhee RB. 1982. Bioengineering actuator with nonnumerical control. In Proceedings of the IFAC Conference on Orthotics and Prosthetics, Columbus, Ohio, pp 145–151. New York, Pergamon Press.

Turajlić S, Drakulić B. 1981. Above-knee prosthesis with attitude control. In Advances in External Control of Human Extremities VII, pp. 529–541. Belgrade, ETAN.

Veltink PH, Koopman AFM, Mulder AJ. 1990. Control of cyclical lower leg movements generated by FES. In D Popović (ed), Advances in External Control of Human Extremities X, pp 81–90. Belgrade, Nauka.

Vodovnik L, Bajd T, Kralj A, et al. 1981. Functional electrical stimulation for control of locomotor systems. CRC Crit Rev Bioeng 6:63.

Vodovnik L, Crochetiere WJ, Reswick JB. 1967. Control of a skeletal joint by electrical stimulation of antagonists. Med Biol Eng 5:97.

Vodovnik L, McLeod WD. 1965. Electronic detours of broken nerve paths. Med Electr 20:110.

Vossius G, Mueschen U, Hollander HJ. 1987. Multichannel stimulation of the lower extremities with surface electrodes. In D Popović (ed), Advances in External Control of Human Extremities IX, pp 193–203. Belgrade, ETAN.

Wagner EM, Catranis JG. 1954. New developments in lower-extremity prostheses. In PE Klopsteg, PD Wilson, et al. (eds), Human Limbs and Their Substitutes, New York, McGraw-Hill.

Waters RL, Lunsford BR. 1985. Energy cost of paraplegic locomotion. J Bone Joint Surg 67A:1245.

Waters RL, McNeal DR, Fallon W, Clifford B. 1985. Functional electrical stimulation of the peroneal nerve for hemiplegia. J Bone Joint Surg 67:792.

Waters RL, Yakura JS, Adkins R, Barnes G. 1989. Determinants of gait performance following spinal cord injury. Arch Phys Med Rehabil 70:811.

Wijman AC, Stroh KC, Van Doren CL, et al. 1990. Functional evaluation of quadriplegic patients using a hand neuroprosthesis. Arch Phys Med Rehabil 71:1053.

Further Information

1. Stein RB, Peckham HP, Popović DB. 1992. Neural Prostheses: Replacing Motor Function after Disease or Disability. London, Oxford University Press.

2. Kralj A, Bajd T. 1989. Functional Electrical Simulation: Standing and Walking after Spinal Cord Injury. Boca Raton, Fla, CRC Press.

3. Agnew WV, McCreery DB. 1990. Neural Prostheses: Fundamental Studies. Englewood Cliffs, NJ, Prentice-Hall.

4. Yugoslav Committee for Electronics and Automation, 1964–1987. Advances in External Control of Human Extremities I–IX. Belgrade, Yugoslavia.

5. Popović DB. 1990. Advances in External Control of Human Extremities X. Nauka, Belgrade (available from Demos Publications, New York).

139

Sensory Augmentation and Substitution

Kurt A. Kaczmarek
University of Wisconsin
at Madison

This chapter will consider methods and devices used to present visual, auditory, and tactual (touch) information to persons with sensory deficits. *Sensory augmentation* systems such as eyeglasses and hearing aids enhance the existing capabilities of a functional human sensory system. *Sensory substitution* is the use of one human sense to receive information normally received by another sense. Braille and speech synthesizers are examples of systems that substitute touch and hearing, respectively, for information that is normally visual (printed or displayed text).

The following three sections will provide theory and examples for aiding the visual, auditory, and tactual systems. Because capitalizing on an *existing* sensory capability is usually superior to substitution, each section will consider first augmentation and then substitution, as shown below:

Human Sensory Systems		
Visual	Auditory	Tactual
Visual augmentation	Auditory augmentation	Tactual augmentation
Tactual vision substitution	Visual auditory substitution	Tactual substitution
Auditory vision substitution	Tactual auditory substitution	

139.1 Visual System

With a large number of receptive channels, the human visual system processes information in a parallel fashion. A single glimpse acquires a wealth of information; the field of view for two eyes is 180 degrees horizontally and 120 degrees vertically [Mehr & Shindell, 1990]. The spatial resolution in the central (foveal) part of the visual field is approximately 0.5 to 1.0 minute of arc [Shlaer, 1937], although Vernier acuity, the specialized task of detecting a misalignment of two lines placed end to end, is much finer, approximately 2 seconds of arc [Stigmar, 1970]. Low-contrast presentations substantially reduce visual acuity.

0-8493-8346-3/95/$0.00+$.50
© 1995 by CRC Press, Inc.

The former resolution figure is the basis for the standard method of testing visual acuity, the Snellen chart. Letters are considered to be "readable" if they subtend approximately 5 minutes of arc and have details one-fifth this size. Snellen's 1862 method of reporting visual performance is still used today. The ratio 20/40, for instance, indicates that a test was conducted at 20 ft and that the letters that were recognizable at that distance would subtend 5 minutes of arc at 40 ft (the distance at which a normally sighted, or "20/20," subject could read them). Although the standard testing distance is 20 ft, 10 ft and even 5 ft may be used, under certain conditions, for more severe visual impairments [Fonda, 1981].

Of the approximately 6 to 11.4 million people in the United States who have visual impairments, 90% have some useful vision [NIDRR, 1993]. In the United States, *severe visual impairment* is defined to be 20/70 vision in the better eye with best refractive correction (see below). *Legal blindness* means that the best corrected acuity is 20/200 or that the field of view is very narrow (<20 degrees). People over 65 years of age account for 46% of the legally blind and 68% of the severely visually impaired. For those with some useful vision, a number of useful techniques and devices for visual augmentation can allow performance of many everyday activities.

Visual Augmentation

People with certain eye disorders see better with higher- or lower-than-normal light levels; an illuminance from 100 to 4000 lux may promote comfortable reading [Fonda, 1981]. Ideal illumination is diffuse and directed from the side at a 45-degree angle to prevent glare. The surrounding room is preferably 20% to 50% darker than the object of interest.

Refractive errors cause difficulties in focusing on an object at a given distance from the eye [Mountcastle, 1980]. Myopia (near-sightedness), hyperopia (far-sightedness), astigmatism (focus depth that varies with radial orientation), and presbyopia (loss of ability to adjust focus, manifested as far-sightedness) are the most common vision defects. These normally can be corrected with appropriate eyeglasses or contact lenses and are rarely the cause of a disability.

Magnification is the most useful form of image processing for vision defects that do not respond to refractive correction. The simplest form of image magnification is getting closer; halving the distance to an object doubles its size. Magnifications up to 20 times are possible with minimal loss of field of view. At very close range, eyeglasses or a loupe may be required to maintain focus [Fonda, 1981]. Hand or stand magnifiers held 18 to 40 cm (not critical) from the eye create a virtual image that increases rapidly in size as the object-to-lens distance approaches the focal length of the lens. Lenses are rated in diopters ($D = 1/f$, where f is the focal length of the lens in centimeters). The useful range is approximately 4 to 20 D; more powerful lenses are generally held close to the eye as a loupe, as just mentioned, to enhance field of view. For distance viewing, magnification of 2 to 10 times can be achieved with hand-held telescopes at the expense of a reduced field of view.

Closed-circuit television (CCTV) systems magnify print and small objects up to 60 times, with higher effective magnifications possible by close viewing. Users with vision as poor as 1/400 (20/8000) may be able to read ordinary print with CCTV [Fonda, 1981]. Some recent units are portable and contain black/white image reversal and contrast enhancement features.

Electrical (or, more recently, magnetic) stimulation of the visual cortex produces perceived spots of light called *phosphenes*. Some attempts, summarized in Webster et al. [1985], have been made to map these sensations and display identifiable patterns, but the phosphenes often do not correspond spatially with the specific location on the visual cortex. Although the risk and cost of this technique do not yet justify the minimal "vision" obtained, future use cannot be ruled out.

Tactual Vision Substitution

With sufficient training, people without useful vision can acquire sufficient information via the tactile sense for many activities of daily living, such as walking independently and reading. The traditional long cane, for example, allows navigation by transmitting surface profile, roughness, and elasticity to the hand. Interestingly, these features are *perceived* to originate at the tip of the cane, not at the hand where they are transduced; this is a simple example of *distal attribution* [Loomis, 1992]. Simple electronic aids such as the hand-held Mowat sonar sensor provide a tactile indication of range to the nearest object.

Braille reading material substitutes raised-dot patterns on 2.3-mm centers for visual letters, enabling reading rates up to 30 to 40 words per minute (wpm). Contracted Braille uses symbols for common words and affixes, enabling reading at up to 200 wpm (125 wpm is more typical).

More sophisticated instrumentation also capitalizes on the spatial capabilities of the tactile sense. The Optacon (*op*tical-to-*tac*tile *con*verter) by TeleSensory, Inc. (Mountain View, Calif.) converts the outline of printed letters recorded by a small, hand-held camera to enlarged vibrotactile letter outlines on the user's fingerpad. The camera's field of view is divided into 100 or 144 pixels (depending on the model), and the reflected light intensity at each pixel determines whether a corresponding vibrating pin on the fingertip is active or not. Ordinary printed text can be read at 28 (typical) or 90 (exceptional) wpm.

Spatial orientation and recognition of objects beyond the reach of a hand or long cane are the objective of experimental systems that convert an image from a television-type camera to a matrix of electrotactile or vibrotactile stimulators on the abdomen, forehead, or fingertip. With training, the user can interpret the patterns of tingling or buzzing points to identify simple, high-contrast objects in front of the camera, as well as experience visual phenomena such as looming, perspective, parallax, and distal attribution [Bach-y-Rita, 1972; Collins, 1985].

Access to graphic or spatial information that cannot be converted into text is virtually impossible for blind computer users. Several prototype devices have been built to display computer graphics to the fingers via vibrating or stationary pins. A fingertip-scanned display tablet with embedded electrodes, under development in our laboratory, eliminates all moving parts; ongoing tests will determine if the spatial performance and reliability are adequate.

Auditory Vision Substitution

Electronic speech synthesizers allow access to electronic forms of text storage and manipulation. Until the arrival of graphic user interfaces such as those in the Apple Macintosh and Microsoft Windows computer operating systems, information displayed on computer screens was largely text-based. A number of products appeared that converted the screen information to speech at rates of up to 500 wpm, thereby giving blind computer users rapid access to the information revolution. Fortunately, much of the displayed information in graphic operating systems is not essentially pictorial; the dozen or so common graphic features (e.g., icons, scroll bars, buttons) can be converted to a limited set of words, which can then be spoken. Because of the way information is stored in these systems, however, the screen-to-text conversion process is much more complex, and the use of essentially spatial control features such as the mouse await true spatial display methods [Boyd et al., 1990].

Automated optical character recognition (OCR) combined with speech synthesis grants access to the most common printed materials (letters, office memorandums, bills), which are seldom available in Braille or narrated-tape format. First popularized in the Kurzweil reading machine, this marriage of technologies is combined with a complex set of lexical, phonetic, and syntactic rules to produce understandable speech from a wide variety of, but not all, print styles.

Mobility of blind individuals is complicated, especially in unfamiliar territory, by hazards that cannot be easily sensed with a long cane, such as overhanging tree limbs. A few devices have appeared that convert the output of sonar-like ultrasonic ranging sensors to discriminable audio displays. For example, the Wormald Sonicguide uses interaural intensity differences to indicate the azimuth of an object and frequency to indicate distance [Cook, 1982]; subtle information such as texture can sometimes also be discriminated.

139.2 Auditory System

The human auditory system processes information primarily serially; having at best two receptive channels, spatial information must be built up by integration over time. This later capability, however, is profound. Out of a full orchestra, a seasoned conductor can pinpoint an errant violinist by sound alone.

Human hearing is sensitive to sound frequencies from approximately 16 to 20,000 Hz and is most sensitive at 1000 Hz. At this frequency, a threshold root-mean-square pressure of 20 Pa (200 µbar) can be perceived by normally hearing young adults under laboratory conditions. Sound pressure level (SPL) is measured in decibels relative to this threshold. Some approximate benchmarks for sound intensity are a whisper at 1 m (30 dB), normal conversation at 1 m (60 dB), and a subway train at 6 m (90 dB). Sounds increasing from 100 to 140 dB become uncomfortable and painful, and short exposures to a 160-dB level can cause permanent hearing impairment, while continuous exposure to sound levels over 90 dB can cause slow, cumulative damage [Sataloff et al., 1980].

Because hearing sensitivity falls off drastically at lower frequencies, clinical audiometric testing uses somewhat different scales. With the DIN/ANSI reference threshold of 6.5 dB SPL at 1 kHz, the threshold rises to 24.5 dB at 250 Hz and 45.5 dB at 125 Hz [Sataloff et al., 1980]. Hearing loss is then specified in decibels relative to the reference threshold, rather than the SPL directly, so that a normal audiogram would have a flat threshold curve at approximately 0 dB.

Auditory Augmentation

Loss of speech comprehension, and hence interpersonal communication, bears the greatest effect on daily life and is the main reason people seek medical attention for hearing impairment. Functional impairment begins with 21- to 35-dB loss in average sensitivity, causing difficulty in understanding faint speech [Smeltzer, 1993]. Losses of 36 to 50 dB and 51 to 70 dB cause problems with normal and loud speech. Losses greater than 90 dB are termed *profound* or *extreme* and cannot be remedied with any kind of hearing aid; these individuals require auditory substitution rather than augmentation.

Hearing loss can be caused by conduction defects in the middle ear (tympanic membrane and ossicles) or by sensorineural defects in the inner ear (cochlear transduction mechanisms and auditory nerve). Conduction problems often can be corrected medically or surgically. If not, hearing aids are often of benefit because the hearing threshold is elevated uniformly over all frequencies, causing little distortion of the signal. Sensorineural impairments differentially affect different frequencies and also cause other forms of distortion that cannot be helped by amplification or filtering. The dynamic range is also reduced, because while loud sounds (>100 dB) are often still perceived as loud, slightly softer sounds are lost. Looked at from this perspective, it is easy to understand why the amplification and automatic gain control of conventional hearing aids do not succeed in presenting the 30-dB or so dynamic range of speech to persons with 70+ dB of sensorineural impairment.

Most hearing aids perform three basic functions. (1) Amplification compensates for the reduced sensitivity of the damaged ear. (2) Frequency-domain filtering compensates for hearing loss that is not spectrally uniform. For example, most sensorineural loss disproportionately affects frequencies over 1 kHz or so, so high-frequency preemphasis may be indicated. (3) Automatic gain control (AGC) compresses the amplitude range of desired sounds to the dynamic range of the damaged ear. Typical AGC systems respond to loud transients in 2 to 5 ms (attack time) and reduce their effect in 100 to 300 ms (recovery time).

Sophisticated multiband AGC systems have attempted to normalize the ear's amplitude/frequency response, with the goal of preserving intact the usual intensity relationships among speech elements. However, recent research has shown that only certain speech features are important for intelligibility [Moore, 1990]. The fundamental frequency (due to vocal cord vibration), the first and second formants (the spectral peaks of speech that characterize different vowels), and place of articulation are crucial to speech recognition. In contrast, the overall speech envelope (the contour connecting the individual peaks in the pressure wave) is not very important; articulation information is carried in second-formant and high-frequency spectral information and is not well-represented in the envelope [Van Tasell, 1993]. Therefore, the primary design goal for hearing aids should be to preserve and make audible the individual spectral components of speech (formants and high-frequency consonant information).

The cochlear implant could properly be termed an auditory augmentation device because it utilizes the higher neural centers normally used for audition. Simply stated, the implant replaces the function of the (damaged) inner ear by electrically stimulating the auditory nerve in response to sound collected by an external microphone. Although the auditory percepts produced are extremely distorted and noiselike due to the inadequate coding strategy, many users gain sufficient information to improve their lipreading and speech-production skills. The introductory chapter in this section provides a detailed discussion of this technology.

Visual Auditory Substitution

Lipreading is the most natural form of auditory substitution, requiring no instrumentation and no training on the part of the speaker. However, only about one-third to one-half of the 36 or so phonemes (primary sounds of human speech) can be reliably discriminated by this method. The result is that 30% to 50% of the words used in conversational English look just like, or very similar to, other words (homophenes) [Becker, 1972]. Therefore, word pairs such as buried/married must be discriminated by grammar, syntax, and context.

Lipreading does not provide information on voice fundamental frequency or formants. With an appropriate hearing aid, any residual hearing (less than 90-dB loss) often can supply some of this missing information, improving lipreading accuracy. For the profoundly deaf, technological devices are available to supply some or all of the information. For example, the Upton eyeglasses, an example of a cued-speech device, provide discrete visual signals for certain speech sounds such as fricatives (letters like *f* or *s*, containing primarily high-frequency information) that cannot be readily identified by sight.

Fingerspelling, a transliteration of the English alphabet into hand symbols, can convey everyday words at up to 2 syllables per second, limited by the rate of manual symbol production [Reed et al., 1990]. American Sign Language uses a variety of upper body movements to convey words and concepts rather than just individual letters, at the same effective rate as ordinary speech, 4 to 5 syllables per second.

Closed captioning encodes the full text of spoken words on television shows and transmits the data in a nonvisible part of the video signal (the vertical blanking interval). Since July of 1993, all new television sets sold in the United States with screens larger than 33 cm diagonal have been required to have built-in decoders that can optionally display the encoded text on the screen. Over 1000 hours per week of programming is closed captioned [National Captioning Institute, 1994].

Automatic speech-recognition technology may soon be capable of translating spoken discourse accurately into visually displayed text, at least in quiet environments; this would be a major boon for the profoundly hearing impaired. Presently, such systems must be carefully trained on individual speakers and/or must have a limited vocabulary, e.g., the 10 numeric digits [Ramesh et al., 1992]. Because there is much commercial interest in speech command of computers and vehicle subsystems, this field is advancing rapidly.

Tactual Auditory Substitution

Tadoma is a method of communication used by a few people in the deaf-blind community and is of theoretical importance for the development of tactual auditory substitution devices. While sign language requires training by both sender and receiver, in Tadoma, the sender speaks normally. The trained receiver places his or her hands on the face and neck of the sender to monitor lip and jaw movements, airflow at the lips, and vibration on the neck [Reed et al., 1992]. Experienced users achieve 80% keyword recognition of everyday speech at a rate of 3 syllables per second. Using no instrumentation, this is the highest speech communication rate recorded for any tactual-only communication system.

Alternatively, tactile vocoders perform a frequency analysis of incoming sounds, similarly to the ear's cochlea [Békésy, 1955], and adjust the stimulation intensity of typically 8 to 32 tactile stimulators (vibrotactile or electrotactile) to present a linear spectral display to the user's abdominal or forehead skin. Several investigators [Blamey & Clark, 1985; Boothroyd & Hnath-Chisolm, 1988; Brooks & Frost, 1986; Saunders et al., 1981] have developed laboratory and commercial vocoders. Although vocoder users cannot recognize speech as well as Tadoma users, research has shown that vocoders can provide enough "auditory" feedback to improve the speech clarity of deaf children and to improve auditory discrimination and comprehension in some older patients [Szeto & Riso, 1990] and aid in discrimination of phonemes by lipreading [Hughes, 1989; Rakowski et al., 1989]. An excellent review of earlier vocoders appears in Reed et al. [1982]. The most useful information provided by vocoders appears to be the second-formant frequency (important for distinguishing vowels) and position of the high-frequency plosive and fricative sounds that often delineate syllables [Bernstein et al., 1991].

139.3 Tactual System

Humans receive and combine two types of perceptual information when touching and manipulating objects. *Kinesthetic* information describes the relative positions and movements of body parts as well as muscular effort. Muscle and skin receptors are primarily responsible for kinesthesis; joint receptors serve primarily as protective limit switches [Rabischong, 1981]. *Tactile* information describes spatial pressure patterns on the skin given a fixed body position. Everyday touch perception combines tactile and kinesthetic information; this combination is called *tactual* or *haptic* perception. Loomis and Lederman [1986] provide an excellent review of these perceptual mechanisms.

Geldard [1960] and Sherrick [1973] lamented that as a communication channel, the tactile sense is often considered inferior to sight and hearing. However, the tactile system possesses some of the same spatial and temporal attributes as both of the "primary" senses [Bach-y-Rita, 1972]. With over 10,000 parallel channels (receptors) [Collins & Saunders, 1970], the tactile system is capable of processing a great deal of information if it is properly presented.

The human kinesthetic and tactile senses are very robust and, in the case of tactile, very redundant. This is fortunate, considering their necessity for the simplest of tasks. Control of movement depends on kinesthetic information; tremors and involuntary movements can result from disruption of this feedback control system. Surgically repaired fingers may not have tactile sensation for a long period or at all, depending on the severity of nerve injuries; it is known that insensate digits are rarely used by patients [Tubiana, 1988]. Insensate fingers and toes (due to advanced Hansen's disease or diabetes) are often injured inadvertently, sometimes requiring amputation. Anyone who has had a finger numbed by cold realizes that it can be next to useless, even if the range of motion is normal.

The normal sensitivity to touch varies markedly over the body surface. The threshold forces in dynes for men (women) are lips, 9 (5); fingertips, 62 (25); belly 62 (7); and sole of foot, 343 (79) [Weinstein, 1968]. The fingertip threshold corresponds to a 10-μm indentation Sensitivity to vibration is much higher and is frequency- and area-dependent [Verrillo, 1985]. A 5-cm^2 patch of skin on the palm vibrating at 250 Hz can be felt at 0.16-μm amplitude; smaller areas and lower frequencies require more displacement. The minimal separation for two nonvibrating points to be distinguished is 2 to 3 mm on the fingertips, 17 mm on the forehead, and 30 to 50 mm on many other locations. However, size and localization judgments are considerably better than these standard figures might suggest [Vierck & Jones, 1969].

Tactual Augmentation

Although we do not often think about it, kinesthetic information is reflected to the user in many types of human-controlled tools and machines, and lack of this feedback can make control difficult.

For example, an automobile with power steering always includes some degree of "road feel" to allow the driver to respond reflexively to minor bumps and irregularities without relying on vision. Remote-control robots (telerobots) used underwater or in chemical- or radiation-contaminated environments are slow and cumbersome to operate, partly because most do not provide force feedback to the operator; such feedback enhances task performance [Hannaford & Wood, 1992].

Tactile display of spatial patterns on the skin uses three main types of transducers [Kaczmarek & Bach-y-Rita, 1995; Kaczmarek et al., 1991]. *Static tactile* displays use solenoids, shape-memory alloy actuators, and scanned air or water jets to indent the skin. *Vibrotactile* displays encode stimulation intensity as the amplitude of a vibrating skin displacement (10 to 500 Hz); both solenoids and piezoelectric transducers have been used. *Electrotactile* stimulation uses 1- to 100-mm^2-area surface electrodes and careful waveform control to electrically stimulate the afferent nerves responsible for touch, producing a vibrating or tingling sensation.

Tactile rehabilitation has received minimal attention in the literature or medical community. One research device sensed pressure information normally received by the fingertips and displayed it on the forehead using electrotactile stimulation [Collins & Madey, 1974]. Subjects were able to estimate surface roughness and hardness and detect edges and corners with only one sensor per fingertip. Phillips [1988] reviews prototype tactile feedback systems that use the intact tactile sense to convey hand and foot pressure and elbow angle to users of powered prosthetic limbs, often with the result of more precise control of these devices.

Slightly more attention has been given to tactile augmentation in special environments. Astronauts, for example, wear pressurized gloves that greatly diminish tactile sensation, complicating extravehicular repair and maintenance tasks. Efforts to improve the situation range from mobile tactile pins in the fingertips to electrotactile stimulation on the abdomen of the information gathered from fingertip sensors [Bach-y-Rita et al., 1987].

Tactual Substitution

Because of a paucity of adequate tactual display technology, spatial pressure information from a robot or remote manipulator is usually displayed to the operator visually. A three-dimensional bar graph, for example, could show the two-dimensional pressure pattern on the gripper. While easy to implement, this method suffers from two disadvantages: (1) the visual channel is required to process more information (it is often already heavily burdened), and (2) reaction time is lengthened, because the normal human tactual reflex systems are inhibited. An advantage of visual display is that accurate measurements of force and pressure may be displayed numerically or graphically.

Auditory display of tactual information is largely limited to warning systems, such as excessive force on a machine. Sometimes such feedback is even inadvertent. The engine of a bulldozer will audibly slow down when a heavy load is lifted; by the auditory and vibratory feedback, the operator can literally "feel" the strain.

The ubiquity of such tactual feedback systems suggests that the human-machine interface on many devices could benefit from intentionally placed tactual feedback systems. Of much current interest is the *virtual environment*, a means by which someone can interact with a mathematic model of a place that may or may not physically exist. The user normally controls the environment by hand, head, and body movements; these are sensed by the system, which correspondingly adjusts the information presented on a wide-angle visual display and sometimes also on a spatially localized sound display. The user often describes the experience as "being there," a phenomenon known as *telepresence* [Loomis, 1992]. One can only imagine how much the experience could be enhanced by adding kinesthetic and tactile feedback [Shimoga, 1993], quite literally putting the user in touch with the virtual world.

Defining Terms

Distal attribution: The phenomenon whereby events are normally perceived as occurring external to our sense organs—but also see Loomis' [1992] engaging article on this topic. The environment or transduction mechanism need not be artificial; for example, we visually perceive objects as distant from our eyes.

Electrotactile: Stimulation that evokes tactile (touch) sensations within the skin at the location of the electrode by passing a pulsatile, localized electric current through the skin. Information is delivered by varying the amplitude, frequency, etc. of the stimulation waveform. Also called *electrocutaneous stimulation.*

Illuminance: The density of light falling on a surface, measured in lux. One lux is equivalent to 0.0929 foot-candles, an earlier measure. Illuminance is inversely proportional to the square of the distance from a point light source. A 100-W incandescent lamp provides approximately 1280 lux at a distance of 1 ft (30.5 cm). Brightness is a different measure, depending also on the reflectance of the surrounding area.

Kinesthetic perception: Information about the relative positions of and forces on body parts, possibly including efference copy (internal knowledge of muscular effort).

Sensory augmentation: The use of devices that assist a functional human sense; eyeglasses are one example.

Sensory substitution: The use of one human sense to receive information normally received by another sense. For example, Braille substitutes touch for vision.

Sound pressure level (SPL): The root-mean-square pressure difference from atmospheric pressure (≈ 100 kPa) that characterizes the intensity of sound. The conversion SPL $= 20 \log (P/P_0)$ expresses SPL in decibels, where P_0 is the threshold pressure of approximately 20 Pa at 1 kHz.

Static tactile: Stimulation that is a slow local mechanical deformation of the skin. It varies the deformation amplitude directly rather than the amplitude of vibration. This is "normal touch" for grasping objects, etc.

Tactile perception: Information about spatial pressure patterns on the skin with a fixed kinesthetic position.

Tactual (haptic) perception: The seamless, usually unconscious combination of tactile and kinesthetic information; this is "normal touch."

Vibrotactile: Stimulation that evokes tactile sensations using mechanical vibration of the skin, typically at frequencies of 10 to 500 Hz. Information is delivered by varying the amplitude, frequency, etc. of the vibration.

Virtual environment: A real-time interactive computer model that attempts to display visual, auditory, and tactual information to a human user as if he or she were present at the simulated location. The user controls the environment with head, hand, and body motions. A airplane cockpit simulator is one example.

References

Bach-y-Rita P. 1972. Brain Mechanisms in Sensory Substitution. New York, Academic Press.

Bach-y-Rita P, Webster JG, Tompkins WJ, Crabb T. 1987. Sensory substitution for space gloves and for space robots. In Proceedings of the Workshop on Space Telerobotics, Jet Propulsion Laboratory, Publication 87–13, pp 51–57.

Becker KW. 1972. Speechreading: Principles and Methods. Baltimore, National Educational Press.

Békésy Gv 1955. Human skin perception of traveling waves similar to those of the cochlea. J Acoust Soc Am 27:830.

Bernstein LE, Demorest ME, Coulter DC, O'Connell MP. 1991. Lipreading sentences with vibrotactile vocoders: Performance of normal-hearing and hearing-impaired subjects. J Acoust Soc Am 90:2971.

Blamey PJ, Clark GM. 1985. A wearable multiple-electrode electrotactile speech processor for the profoundly deaf. J Acoust Soc Am 77:1619.

Boothroyd A, Hnath-Chisolm T. 1988. Spatial, tactile presentation of voice fundamental frequency as a supplement to lipreading: Results of extended training with a single subject. J Rehabil Res Dev 25(3):51.

Boyd LH, Boyd WL, Vanderheiden GC. 1990. The Graphical User Interface Crisis: Danger and Opportunity. September, Trace R&D Center, University of Wisconsin-Madison.

Brooks PL, Frost BJ. 1986. The development and evaluation of a tactile vocoder for the profoundly deaf. Can J Public Health 77:108.

Collins CC. 1985. On mobility aids for the blind. In DH Warren, ER Strelow (eds), Electronic Spatial Sensing for the Blind, pp 35–64. Dordrecht, The Netherlands, Matinus Nijhoff.

Collins CC, Madey JMJ. 1974. Tactile sensory replacement. In Proceedings of the San Diego Biomedical Symposium, pp 15–26.

Collins CC, Saunders FA. 1970. Pictorial display by direct electrical stimulation of the skin. J Biomed Syst 1:3.

Cook AM. 1982. Sensory and communication aids. In AM Cook, JG Webster (eds), Therapeutic Medical Devices: Application and Design, pp 152–201. Englewood Cliffs, NJ, Prentice-Hall.

Fonda GE. 1981. Management of Low Vision. New York, Thieme-Stratton.

Geldard FA. 1960. Some neglected possibilities of communication. Science 131:1583.

Hannaford B, Wood L. 1992. Evaluation of performance of a telerobot. NASA Tech Briefs 16(2):item 62.

Hughes BG. 1989. A New Electrotactile System for the Hearing Impaired. National Science Foundation final project report, ISI-8860727, Sevrain-Tech, Inc.

Kaczmarek KA, Bach-y-Rita P. 1995. Tactile displays. In W Barfield, T Furness (eds), Virtual Environments and Advanced Interface Design. New York, Oxford University Press.

Kaczmarek KA, Webster JG, Bach-y-Rita P, Tompkins WJ. 1991. Electrotactile and vibrotactile displays for sensory substitution systems. IEEE Trans Biomed Eng 38:1.

Loomis JM. 1992. Distal attribution and presence. Pres Teleoperators Virtual Environ 1(1):113.

Loomis JM, Lederman SJ. 1986. Tactual perception. In KR Boff et al (eds), Handbook of Perception and Human Performance, vol II: Cognitive Processes and Performance, pp 31.1–31.41. New York, Wiley.

Mehr E, Shindell S. 1990. Advances in low vision and blind rehabilitation. In MG Eisenberg, RC Grzesiak (eds), Advances in Clinical Rehabilitation, vol 3, pp 121–147. New York, Springer.

Moore BCJ. 1990. How much do we gain by gain control in hearing aids? Acta Otolaryngol (Stockh) Suppl. 469:250.

Mountcastle VB (ed). 1980. Medical Physiology. St. Louis, Mosby.

National Captioning Institute, Falls Church, Va, 1994. Personal communication.

NIDRR. 1993. Protocols for choosing low vision devices. U.S. Department of Education. Consensus Statement 1(1–28).

Phillips CA. 1988. Sensory feedback control of upper- and lower-extremity motor prostheses. CRC Crit Rev Biomed Eng 16:105.

Rabischong P. 1981. Physiology of sensation. In R Tubiana (ed), The Hand, pp 441–467. Philadelphia, Saunders.

Rakowski K, Brenner C, Weisenberger JM. 1989. Evaluation of a 32-channel electrotactile vocoder (abstract). J Acoust Soc Am 86(suppl 1):S83.

Ramesh P, Wilpon JG, McGee MA, et al. 1992. Speaker independent recognition of spontaneously spoken connected digits. Speech Commun 11:229.

Reed CM, Delhorne LA, Durlach NI, Fischer SD. 1990. A study of the tactual and visual reception of fingerspelling. J Speech Hear Res 33:786.

Reed CM, Durlach NI, Bradia LD. 1982. Research on tactile communication of speech: A review. AHSA Monogr 20:1.

Reed CM, Rabinowitz WM, Durlach NI, et al. 1992. Analytic study of the Tadoma method: Improving performance through the use of supplementary tactile displays. J Speech Hear Res 35:450.

Sataloff J, Sataloff RT, Vassallo LA. 1980. Hearing Loss, 2d ed. Philadelphia, Lippincott.

Saunders FA, Hill WA, Franklin B. 1981. A wearable tactile sensory aid for profoundly deaf children. J Med Syst 5:265.

Sherrick CE. 1973. Current prospects for cutaneous communication. In Proceedings of the Conference on Cutaneous Communication System Development, pp 106–109.

Shimoga KB. 1993. A survey of perceptual feedback issues in dextrous telemanipulation: II. Finger touch feedback. In IEEE Virtual Reality Annual International Symposium, pp 271–279.

Shlaer S. 1937. The relation between visual acuity and illumination. J Gen Physiol 21:165.

Smeltzer CD. 1993. Primary care screening and evaluation of hearing loss. Nurse Pract 18:50.

Stigmar G. 1970. Observation on vernier and stereo acuity with special reference to their relationship. Acta Ophthalmol 48:979.

Szeto AYJ, Riso RR. 1990. Sensory feedback using electrical stimulation of the tactile sense. In RV Smith, JH Leslie Jr (eds), Rehabilitation Engineering, pp 29–78. Boca Raton, Fla, CRC Press.

Tubiana R. 1988. Fingertip injuries. In R Tubiana (ed), The Hand, pp 1034–1054. Philadelphia, Saunders.

Van Tasell DJ. 1993. Hearing loss, speech, and hearing aids. J Speech Hear Res 36:228.

Verrillo RT. 1985. Psychophysics of vibrotactile stimulation. J Acoust Soc Am 77:225.

Vierck CJ, Jones MB. 1969. Size discrimination on the skin. Science 163:488.

Webster JG, Cook AM, Tompkins WJ, Vanderheiden GC (eds). 1985. Electronic Devices for Rehabilitation. New York, Wiley.

Weinstein S. 1968. Intensive and extensive aspects of tactile sensitivity as a function of body part, sex and laterality. In DR Kenshalo (ed), The Skin Senses, pp 195–218. Springfield, Ill, Charles C Thomas.

Further Information

Presence: Teleoperators and Virtual Environments is a recent quarterly journal focusing on advanced human-machine interface issues. A forthcoming article in *Presence*, "Comparison of human sensory capabilities with technical specifications of virtual environment equipment," by W. Barfield et al. provides detailed summary tables on the visual, auditory, and tactual senses and the technology available to display information to those senses.

The Trace Research and Development Center, Madison, Wisc., publishes a comprehensive resource book on commercially available assistive devices, organizations, etc. for communication, control, and computer access for individuals with physical and sensory impairments.

Electronic Devices for Rehabilitation, edited by J. G. Webster (Wiley, 1985), summarizes the technologic principles of electronic assistive devices for people with physical and sensory impairments.

140

Augmentative Communication/Control/ Computer Access

Barry Romich
Prentke Romich Company

Gregg Vanderheiden
*University of Wisconsin
at Madison*

Perhaps the most limiting of physical disabilities is the inability to express oneself through either speech or writing. Meaningful participation in life is essentially impossible when one is unable to communicate basic information, desires, needs, feelings, and dreams. The potential for education, employment, and independent living is substantially reduced for a person who cannot communicate.

Fortunately, for people who cannot speak or write effectively, there are techniques, therapies, and systems designed to address this situation. The field of augmentative and alternative communication (AAC) is made up of many different professions, including speech-language pathology, regular and special education, occupational and physical therapy, engineering, linguistics, technology, and others. Also, individuals who rely on AAC, as well as their families and friends, contribute to the field.

There are many ways in which augmentative communication can be classified. While there are unaided communication techniques, such as gestures, signs, and eye pointing, this chapter will be limited to a review of technology-aided techniques and related issues.

As with people who rely on AAC, personal achievement and independence can be limited for people who are unable to operate electrical and electronic items in their surroundings. The impact can be particularly acute in the area of computer use and information communication. This chapter also covers these topics.

Engineering has played a significant role in the development of the field of AAC and related assistive technology. Engineering contributions range from relatively independent work to the collaborative development of tools to support the contributions of other professions, such as classical and computational linguistics and speech-language pathology.

Technology-based AAC systems have taken two forms: hardware designed specifically for this application and software that runs on mass-market computer hardware. AAC systems can be considered to have three basic components. These are the user interface, the outputs, and the accel-

0-8493-8346-3/95/$0.00+$.50
© 1995 by CRC Press, Inc.

eration and language access techniques. Generally, a multidisciplinary team would evaluate the current and projected skills and needs of the individual and select a system with characteristics that are a good match.

140.1 User Interface

Most AAC systems have a user interface that is based on the selection of items that will produce the desired output [Vanderheiden & Lloyd, 1986]. Items being selected could be individual letters (as would be used in spelling), could be whole words or phrases, or could be symbols that represent vocabulary.

There are numerous techniques for making selections. Most, however, are based on either direct selection or scanning. *Direct selection* refers to techniques in which the desired item is indicated from a set of choices using a single action. A common example of this would be the use of a computer keyboard. Each key is directly selected. Expanded keyboards could accommodate more gross motor actions, such as using the fist or foot. In some cases, pointing can be enhanced through the use of technology. Sticks are held in the mouth or attached to the head using a headband (Figure 140.1). Light pointers can be used to direct a light beam at a target. Indirect pointing systems might include the common computer mouse, trackball, or joystick. Alternatives to these for people with disabilities are based on head and other movements.

Scanning refers to techniques in which the individual is presented with a time sequence of choices and the individual indicates when the desired choice is presented. A simple linear scanning system might be a clock face–type display with a rotating pointer to indicate a letter, word, or picture. Additional dimensions of scanning can be added to reduce the selection time when the number of possible choices is larger. A common technique involves the arrangement of choices in a matrix of rows and columns. The selection process has two steps. First, rows are scanned, and the user signals when the row containing the desired element is reached. Then the items in the selected row are scanned, and the user signals when the desired item is reached. This is called *row-column scanning* (Figure 140.2). Either by convention or by the grouping of the elements, the order might be reversed. For example, in the United Kingdom, column-row scanning is preferred over row-column scanning. Other scanning techniques also exist, and additional dimensions could be employed.

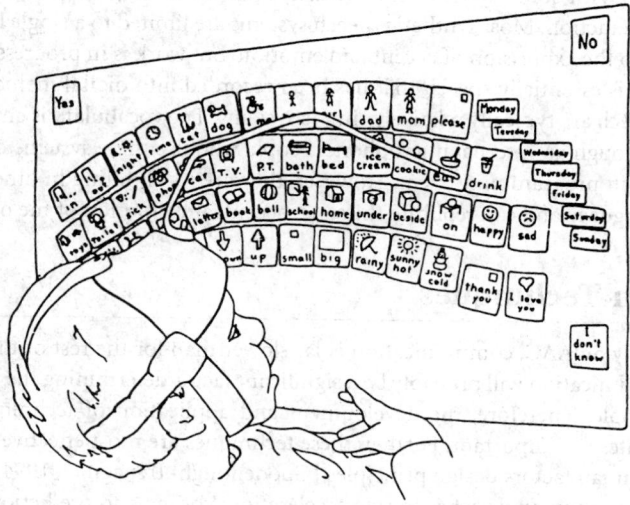

FIGURE 140.1 Direct selection using a headstick. Figure courtesy of Trace Center, Madison, WI.

Both direct selection and scanning can be used to select elements that might not of themselves define an output. In these cases, the output might be defined by a code or sequence of selected elements. A common example is Morse code, in which dots and dashes are directly selected but must be combined to define letters and numbers. Another example, more common to AAC, has an output defined by a sequence of two or more pictures or icons.

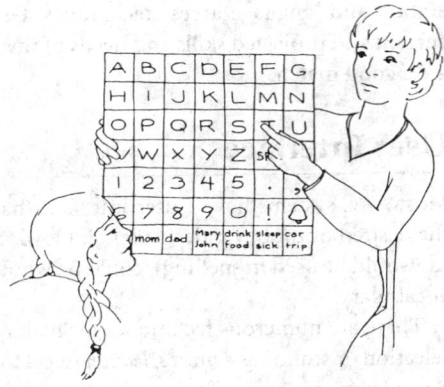

Scanning and, to some degree, direct selection can be faster if the choices are arranged such that those most frequently used are easiest to access. For example, in a row-column scanning spelling system that scans top to bottom and left to right, the most frequently used letters should be grouped toward the upper-left corner.

FIGURE 140.2   Row-column scanning. Figure courtesy of Trace Center, Madison, WI.

Generally, the selection technique of choice would be the one that would result in the fastest communication possible. Consideration of such factors as cognitive load [Cress & French, 1994], changing environment, fatigue, aesthetics, and stability of physical skill would influence the choice of the best selection technique.

140.2 Outputs

AAC system outputs in common use are speech, displays, printers, beeps, data, and other control formats. Outputs are generally directed toward the communication partner but also might be user feedback or for the control of other items.

AAC speech output is normally of two types: synthetic and digitized. *Synthetic speech* usually is generated from text input following a set of rules. Synthetic speech is usually associated with AAC systems that are able to generate text. These systems have unlimited vocabulary, being able to speak anything that can be spelled. Intelligibility has improved over recent years to the point where it is no longer a significant issue. Some offer multiple gender voices, a feature that is valued by many people who rely on AAC. With some systems, it is actually possible to sing songs, again a feature that enhances social interaction. Most synthetic speech systems are limited to a single language. Further limitations relate to the expression of accent and emotion, but work is in progress in this area.

Digitized speech is essentially speech that has been recorded into digital memory. AAC systems using digitized speech are typically relatively simple systems. The vocabulary is entered by speaking into the system through an internal microphone. People who use these systems can say only what someone else said in programming them. However, they are less limiting in other ways. They are independent of language and can replicate the song, accent, and emotion of the original speaker.

140.3 Acceleration Techniques

For people who rely on AAC, communication is far slower than for the rest of the population. Yet the speed of communication will probably be a significant factor determining the personal achievement of these people. Therefore, the development and application of techniques to accelerate communication rates are important. Further, these techniques are most effective when developers pay attention to human factors design principles [Goodenough-Trepagnier, 1994].

There are two common approaches to rate acceleration: coding and prediction. *Coding systems* represent language elements using a number of selections that is typically smaller than that required by spelling or other more traditional approaches. For example, words or sentences might be abbreviated using some principled approach such as vowel elimination or the first letters of salient words. Abbreviation systems can be fast but generally require spelling and reading skills. Also, they develop frequent conflicts with relatively small vocabulary sizes. But even small vocabulary sets can have significant impact on keystrokes required [Vanderheiden & Kelso, 1987]. Demasco [1994] offers additional background and proposes some interesting work in this area.

Morse code actually requires a larger number of selections than the letters being generated. However, the advantage here is that the selection set is very small: dot, dash, and in some implementations a code termination.

Perhaps the most commonly used acceleration technique in AAC is semantic coding [Baker, 1994]. With this system, language is represented using a relatively small set of multimeaning icons. The specific meaning of each icon is a function of the context in which it is used. Semantic coding makes use of a meaningful relationship between the code and the information it represents, does not require spelling and reading skills, yet is powerful even for people with those skills. A virtue of all coding systems, including semantic coding, is that the cognitive process is continuous, resulting in the potential for high speed.

Predictive selection is a technique used with semantic coding and possibly with other coding systems. When this feature is enabled, only those choices which complete a meaningful sequence can be selected. With scanning, for example, the selection process can be significantly faster because the number of possible choices is automatically reduced.

Word prediction systems are available from many sources. Based on previously selected letters and words, the system presents the user with "best guess" choices for completing the word being spelled. The user then chooses one of the predictions or continues spelling, resulting in yet another set of predictions. Prediction systems have consistently demonstrated a reduction in the number of keystrokes but have not consistently shown an increase in the actual rate of communication. Scull and Hill [1988] and Koester and Levine [1994] found no real gain; Newell et al. [1991] found a loss in communication rate with some and a gain with others. Newell et al. [1992] were able to demonstrate an even greater increase in communication rate, even though the technique represented a smaller keystroke saving than Newell et al. [1991]. The appropriateness of a prediction system for a given individual, therefore, would appear to be a function of the importance of reducing keystrokes (fatigue, etc.) and the ability of the particular technique to actually increase the individual's rate of communication.

140.4 Cost-Effectiveness of High- Versus Low-Technology Approaches

Cost is sometimes a factor in the acquisition of communication systems. In many cases, individuals are not provided with technical aids because of the perceived high cost of the aids. However, less expensive aids require the same amount of training time and more frequent assistance from others, thus raising the cost of these aids. In looking at the cost of a communication system, therefore, it is important to examine the costs related to its purchase, training, use (e.g., time for an assistant or interpreter if one is required), and maintenance. For example, when comparing the cost of a manual communication board with that of an electronic conversation and writing aid, it is obvious that the purchase cost for the manual communication board ($50 to $100) is much less than the purchase cost for the advanced electronic aid. However, if the individual is to use the communication system in an educational setting where he or she is required to do homework, written assignments, etc., the manual communication board will require the presence of an assistant, while the electronic aid would not. Also, the electronic aid will provide a more independent and better indication of the user's skills in these areas (written work, etc.). Even when an individual is only watching a person point and reading off the letters, it is amazing how many clues and cues to the correct answer can be gleaned from facial expressions, tone of voice, or variations in the time before the assistant reads out the letter when the user points to a correct letter versus when he or she points to an incorrect letter. As a result, it is important when judging the cost of a communication system to include all the costs, including the need or lack of need for a personal assistant as well as tradeoffs in the benefits of the systems. In the end, individuals who cannot be employed represent the highest cost to our society.

140.5 Intervention and Other Issues

Perhaps the single factor limiting the more widespread use of assistive technology in general and AAC in particular is the lack of awareness of its availability and the impact it can have on the lives of the people who could benefit [Romich, 1993]. This situation exists not only with the general public but even within many of the professions providing services to this population. University programs often are far behind in their integration of this information into professional curricula.

In choosing an AAC system, the overriding factor must be the best interests of the person who will be using the system (Figure 140.3). Since personal achievement will be directly related to the ability to communicate, the choice of a system will have lifelong implications. The process of choosing the most appropriate system is not trivial. As indicated previously, it is best accomplished by a team of skilled professionals. It is worthy of note that the interests of the individual served professionally are not necessarily aligned with those of the AAC professional or the funding agency. There can be a temptation to select a system that is easy to apply or inexpensive to purchase.

Following the selection (and funding) of a system, the next step is the actual intervention program. Early in the history of AAC it became apparent [Rodgers, 1984] that AAC systems are more like tools than appliances. To be effective, there is a need for much more than simply plugging them in and turning them on. The individual who relies on AAC must develop the skills to become a communication craftsperson. In general, as well as specific to AAC, the fastest, most efficient use of a system occurs when the individual operates from knowledge that is in the head, rather than knowledge that must be gathered from the world [Norman, 1980]. The implication for AAC is that an intervention program must include a significant training component to ensure that the needed knowledge is put into the head [Romich, 1994]. Further, a drill component of training develops automaticity [Treviranus, 1994].

Intervention goes well beyond the technical use of the AAC system and includes issues such as language development and communication pragmatics. The intervention program should be under the supervision of professionals with appropriate knowledge and skills.

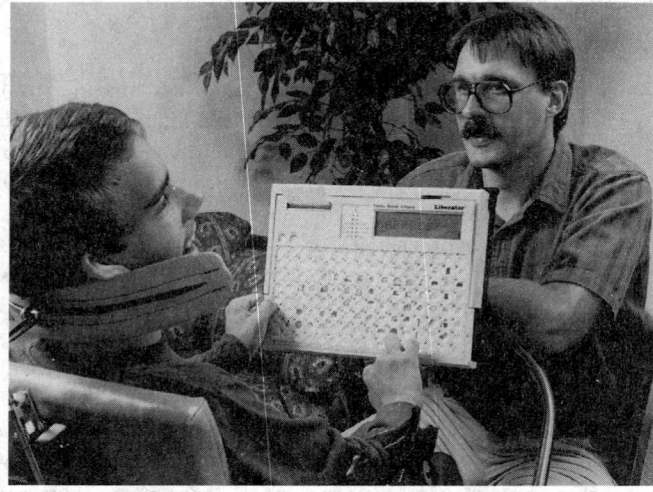

FIGURE 140.3   Individual using an electronic communication system.
Photo courtesy of Prentke Romich Company, Wooster, OH.

Beyond the initial application of the system, there may be an ongoing need for professional services. People who rely on AAC frequently live unstable lives. For people with congenital (from birth) conditions, developmental delays may have occurred that result in educational and training needs that extend well beyond the normal age of public school services. For people with progressive neurologic disorders, such as Lou Gehrig's disease, the physical skill level will change, and accommodation will be needed.

140.6 Environmental Control and Access to Computers and Next-Generation Information Systems

In addition to the communications needs of people who rely on AAC, related needs include environmental control, access to computers, and access to information and transaction systems. These other areas are issues for people with physical and sensory disabilities regardless of communication skills. The *Assistive Technology Sourcebook* [Enders & Hall, 1990] is an excellent resource for these topics.

Environmental control generally refers to the operation of electrical and electronic items in one's surroundings. However, it also can include the operation of items not normally considered electrical that have been automated or powered, such as doors, locks, and drapes. Common functions covered by this area include things such as telephones, entertainment items (TV, VCR, stereo), and lamps. However, one should not rule out other needs for control, such as robotics and mobility [Guerette & Sumi, 1994].

Environmental controls were originally developed for people with polio or high-level spinal cord injury. Typically, early systems were operated using two switches, which could be pressure switches operated by blowing and sucking on a tube. One switch would be used to scan through or otherwise select the item to be controlled, and the other switch would activate it. Today this technique is still useful but has been joined by speech-recognition systems and those which respond to either serial data commands, infrared, or other media.

The computer has continued to become a part of normal life for a growing portion of the population. While the computer can be a powerful tool for people with disabilities, the computer revolution can create additional handicaps for many people. If the computer allows only everyone without a disability to take a step forward, the result is a relative step backward for people with disabilities.

Access to computers is an issue for people with sensory and cognitive as well as motor disabilities. Thus the eventual general need is greater than that for augmentative communication, environmental controls, and many other assistive technologies. Many hardware and software solutions exist that address the computer-access needs of people with disabilities. For people with motor impairments, much of the information presented above relative to input systems and acceleration techniques applies. For people with sensory or cognitive impairments, entirely different approaches are needed. In some cases, features that solve the problems of one population create problems for others. For example, people with cognitive disabilities may be well served by systems that make extensive use of graphics. People with blindness or other visual impairments find this environment particularly adverse.

Related to computers, either directly or indirectly, is the issue of access to information and transaction systems and the "information superhighway." While the individual with a disability can have appropriate adaptive hardware and software on his or her own computer system, there will be increasing needs to interact with systems that are not personal. Thus there is a need to build disability access directly into systems that are intended for the general public [Vanderheiden, 1994]. Comprehensive consideration of this issue means the incorporation of a variety of access techniques from which would be chosen the most appropriate to the individual's needs and capabilities. Further, standardization will be needed to prevent the need to accommodate new systems and techniques.

140.7 Future Developments

It has become apparent that technological development in and of itself will not solve the problems of people with disabilities. However, technology advancements will continue to provide more powerful tools that will allow new and different approaches to be explored. Computational linguistics is one example of where this could be expected.

While computer technology continues to become more powerful, it also becomes less costly. A major cost of assistive technology intervention is the professional time needed for device selection and application. Lower-cost computer systems could stimulate changes in the way training occurs. A related issue is the preparation of assistive technology professionals. Computer technology could be put to better use in helping these people ready themselves for this work.

References

Baker BR. 1994. Semantic compaction: An approach to a formal definition. In Proceedings of the Sixth Annual European Minspeak Conference, Swinstead, Lincs, UK, Prentke Romich Europe.

Cress CJ, French GJ. 1994 The relationship between cognitive load measurements and estimates of computer input control skills. Assist Technol 6.1:54.

Demasco P. 1994. Human factors considerations in the design of language interfaces in AAC. Assist Technol 6.1:10.

Enders A, Hall M (eds). 1990. Assistive Technology Sourcebook. Arlington, Texas RESNA Press.

Goodenough-Trepagnier C. 1994. Design goals for augmentative communication. Assist Technol 6.1:3.

Guerette P, Sumi E. 1994. Integrating control of multiple assistive devices: A retrospective review. Assist Technol 6.1:67.

Horstmann Koester H, Levine SP. 1994. Learning and performance of able-bodied individuals using scanning systems with and without word prediction. Assist Technol 6.1:42.

Norman DA. 1980. The Psychology of Everyday Things. New York, Basic Books.

Newell AF, Arnott JL, Waller A. 1991. On the validity of user-modeling in AAC: Comments on Horstman and Levine. Augment Altern Commun 8:89.

Newell AF, Booth L, Beattie W. 1991. Predictive text entry with PAL and children with learning difficulties. Br J Ed Technol 21.1:23.

Rodgers B. 1984. A future perspective on the holistic use of technology for people with disabilities. Trace Center working paper based on presentation at Discovery '84 Conference, Chicago, Ill.

Romich B. 1993. Assistive technology and AAC: An industry perspective. Assist Technol 5.2:74.

Romich B. 1994. Knowledge in the world vs knowledge in the head: The psychology of AAC systems. Commun Outlook 16(2):19–21.

Scull J, Hill L. 1988. A computerized communication message preparation program that "learns' the user's vocabulary." Augment Altern Commun 4.1:40.

Treviranus J. 1994. Mastering alternative computer access: The role of understanding, trust, and automaticity. Assist Technol 6.1:26.

Vanderheiden GC. 1994a. Building disability access directly into next-generation information and transaction systems. In H Yamada, Y Kambayashi, S Ohta (eds), Computers As Our Better Partners, Proceedings of the IISF/ACM Japan International Symposium, pp 2–6. Singapore: World Scientific.

Vanderheiden GC. 1994b. Use of multiple parallel interface strategies to create a seamless accessible interface for next-generation information systems. In Proceedings of the RESNA Annual Conference, pp 508–510.

Vanderheiden GC, Kelso DP. 1987. Comparative analysis of fixed-vocabulary communication acceleration techniques. In AAC: Augmentative and Alternative Communication, pp 196–206.

Vanderheiden GC, Lloyd LL. 1986. In SW Blackstone (ed), Augmentative Communication: An Introduction. Rockville, Md, American Speech-Language-Hearing Association.

Further Information

There are a number of organizations and publications that relate to AAC, control, and computer access assistive technology.

AAC (Augmentative and Alternative Communication) is the quarterly refereed journal of ISAAC. It is published by Decker Periodicals, Inc., P.O. Box 620, L.C.D. 1, Hamilton, Ontario, L8N 3K7, Canada. Tel: 905-522-7017, Fax: 905-522-7839.

The *American Speech-Language-Hearing Association (ASHA)* is the professional organization of speech-language pathologists. ASHA has a Special Interest Division on augmentative communication. ASHA, 10801 Rockville Pike, Rockville, MD 20852. Tel: 301-897-5700, Fax: 301-571-0457

Augmentative Communication News is published bimonthly by Augmentative Communication, Inc., 1 Surf Way, Suite 215, Monterey, CA 93940. Tel: 408-649-3050, Fax: 408-646-5428.

CAMA (Communication Aid Manufacturers Association) is an organization of manufacturers of AAC systems marketed in North America. CAMA, 518-526 Davis St., Suite 211-212, Evanston, IL 60201. Tel: 800-441-2262, Fax: 708-869-5689.

Communicating Together is published quarterly by Sharing to Learn as a means of sharing the life experiences and communication systems of augmentative communicators with other augmentative communicators, their families, their communities, and those who work with them. Sharing to Learn, PO Box 986, Thornhill, Ontario, L3T 4A5, Canada. Tel: 905-771-1491, Fax: 905-771-7153.

Communication Outlook is an international quarterly addressed to the community of individuals interested in the application of technology to the needs of persons who experience communication handicaps. It is published by the Artificial Language Laboratory, Michigan State University, 405 Computer Center, East Lansing, MI 48824-1042. Tel: 517-353-0870, Fax: 517-353-4766.

Gopher and FTP Servers: A wide variety of disability-related gopher and worldwide web sites can be located by tapping into *trace.waisman.wisc.edu.*

Hear Our Voices is the only international organization governed by people who rely on AAC. Hear Our Voices, 1660 L St NW, Suite 700, Washington, D.C., 20036-5602 Tel: 202-776-0406, Fax: 202-776-0414.

ISAAC is the International Society for Augmentative and Alternative Communication. USSAAC is the United States chapter. Both can be contacted at PO Box 1762 Station R, Toronto, Ontario, M4G 4A3, Canada. Tel: 905-737-9308, Fax: 905-737-0624.

RESNA is an interdisciplinary association for the advancement of rehabilitation and assistive technologies. RESNA has many special-interest groups including those on augmentative and alternative communication and computer applications. RESNA, 1700 North Moore Street, Suite 1540, Arlington, VA 22209-1903, Tel: 703-524-6686, Fax: 703-524-6630.

141

Measurement Tools and Processes in Rehabilitation Engineering

George V. Kondraske
University of Texas at Arlington

In every engineering discipline, measurement facilitates the use of structured procedures and decision-making processes. In rehabilitation engineering, the presence of "a human," the only or major
component of *the system of interest,* has presented a number of unique challenges with regard to measurement. This is especially true with regard to the routine processes of rehabilitation that either do
or could incorporate and rely on measurements. This, in part, is due to the complexity of the human
system's architecture, the variety of ways in which it can be adversely affected by disease or injury, and
the versatility in the way it can be used to accomplish various tasks of interest to an individual.

Measurement supports a wide variety of assistive device design and prescription activities
undertaken within rehabilitation engineering (e.g., Leslie and Smith [1990], Webster et al. [1985],
and other chapters within this section). In addition, rehabilitation engineers contribute to the specification and design of measurement instruments that are used primarily by other service providers
(such as physical and occupational therapists). As measurements of human structure, performance,
and behavior become more rigorous and instruments used have taken advantage of advanced technology, there is also a growing role for rehabilitation engineers to assist these other medical
professionals with the proper application of measurement instruments (e.g., for determining areas
that are most deficient in an individual's performance profile, objectively documenting progress
during rehabilitation, etc.). This is in keeping with the team approach to rehabilitation that has
become popular in clinical settings. In short, the role of measurement in rehabilitation engineering
is dynamic and growing.

0-8493-8346-3/95/$0.00+$.50
© 1995 by CRC Press, Inc.

In this chapter, a top-down overview of measurement tools and processes in rehabilitation engineering is presented. Many of the measurement concepts, processes, and devices of relevance are common to applications outside the rehabilitation engineering context. However, the nature of the human population with which rehabilitation engineers must deal is arguably different in that each individual must be assumed to be unique with respect to at least a subset of his or her performance capacities and/or structural parameters; i.e., population reference data cannot be assumed to be generally applicable. While there are some exceptions, population labels frequently used such as "head-injured" or "spinal cord–injured" represent only a gross classification that should not be taken to imply homogeneity with regard to parameters such as range of motion, strength, movement speed, information processing speed, and other performance capacities. This is merely a direct realization that many different ways exist in which the human system can be adversely affected by disease or injury and recognition of the continuum that exists with regard to the degree of any given effect. The result is that in rehabilitation engineering, compared with standard human factors design tasks aimed at the average healthy population, many measurement values must be acquired directly for the specific client.

Measurement in the present context encompasses actions that focus on (1) the human (e.g., structural aspects and performance capacities of subsystems at different hierarchical levels ranging from specific neuromuscular subsystems to the total person and his or her activities in daily living, including work), (2) assistive devices (e.g., structural aspects and demands placed on the human), (3) tasks (e.g., distances between critical points, masses of objects involved, etc.), and (4) overall systems (e.g., performance achieved by a human-assistive device-task combination, patterns of electrical signals representing the timing of muscle activity while performing a complex maneuver, behavior of an individual before and after being fitted with a new prosthetic device, etc.). Clearly, an exhaustive treatment is beyond the scope of this chapter. Measurements are embedded in every specialized subarea of rehabilitation engineering. However, there are also special roles served by measurement in a broader and more generic sense, as well as principles that are common across the many special applications. Emphasis here is placed on these.

There is no lack of other literature regarding the types of measurement outlined to be of interest here and their use. However, it is diffusely distributed, and gaps exist with regard to how such tools can be integrated to accomplish goals beyond simply the acquisition of numeric data for a given parameter. With rapidly changing developments over the last decade, there is currently no comprehensive source that describes the majority of instruments available, their latest implementations, procedures for their use, evaluation of effectiveness, etc. While topics other than measurement are discussed, Leslie and Smith [1990] produced what is perhaps the single most directly applicable source with respect to rehabilitation engineering specifically, although it too is not comprehensive with regard to measurement, nor does it attempt to be.

141.1 Fundamental Principles

Naturally, the fundamental principles of human physiology manifest themselves in the respective sensory, neuromuscular, information-processing, and life-sustaining systems and impact approaches to measurement. In addition, psychological considerations are vital. Familiarization with this material is essential to measurement in rehabilitation; however, treatment here is far beyond the scope of this chapter. The numerous reference works available may be most readily found by consulting relevant chapters in this *Handbook* and the works that they reference. In this section, key principles that are more specific to measurement and of general applicability are presented.

Structure, Function, Performance, and Behavior

It is necessary to distinguish between structure, function, performance, and behavior and measurements thereof for both human and artificial systems. In addition, hierarchical systems concepts are necessary both to help organize the complexity of the systems involved and to help understand the various needs that exist.

Structural measures include dimensions, masses (of objects, limb segments), moments of inertia, circumferences, contours, compliances, and any other aspects of the physical system. These may be considered hierarchically as being pertinent to the total human (e.g., height, weight, etc.), specific body segments (e.g., forearm, thigh, etc.), or components of basic systems such as tendons, ligaments, and muscles.

Function is the *purpose* of the system of interest (e.g., to move a limb segment, to communicate, to feed and care for oneself). Within the human, there are many single-purpose systems (e.g., those that function to move specific limb segments, process specific types of information, etc.). As one proceeds to higher levels, such as the total human, systems that are increasingly more multifunctional emerge. These can be recognized as higher-level configurations of more basic systems that operate to feed one-self, to conduct personal hygeine, to carry out tasks of a job, etc. This multilevel view of just functions begins to help place into perspective the scope over which measurement can be applied.

In rehabilitation in general, a good deal of what constitutes measurement involves the application of structured subjective observation techniques (see also the next subsection) in the form of a wide range of rating scales [e.g., Fuhrer, 1987; Granger & Greshorn, 1984; Potvin et al., 1985]. These are often termed *functional assessment scales* and are typically aimed at obtaining a global index of an individual's ability to function independently in the world. The global index is typically based on a number of items within a given scale, each of which addresses selected, relatively high-level functions (e.g., personal hygiene, mobility, etc.). The focus of measurement for a given item is often an estimate of the *level* of independence or dependence that the subject exhibits or needs to carry out the respective function. In addition, inventories of functions that an individual is able or not able to carry out (with and without assistance) are often included. The large number of such scales that have been proposed and debated is a consequence of the many possible functions and combinations thereof that exist on which to base a given scale. Functional assessment scales are relatively quick and inexpensive to administer and have a demonstrated role in rehabilitation. However, the nature and levels of measurements obtained are not sufficient for many rehabilitation engineering purposes. This latter class of applications generally begins with a function at the level and of the type used as a constituent component of functional assessment scales, considers the level of performance at which that function is executed more quantitatively, and incorporates one or more lower levels in the hierarchy (i.e., the human subsystems involved in achieving the specific functions of daily life that are of interest and their capacities for performance).

Where functions can be described and inventoried, *performance* measures directly characterize *how well* a physical system of interest executes its intended function. Performance is multidimensional (e.g., strength, range, speed, accuracy, steadiness, endurance, etc.). Of special interest are the concepts of *performance capacity* and *performance capacity measurement*. Performance capacity represents the *limits* of a given system's ability to operate in its corresponding multidimensional performance space. In this chapter, a resource-based model for both human and artificial system performance and measurement of their performance capacities is adopted [e.g., Kondraske, 1990, 1995]. Thus the *maximum* knee flexor strength available (i.e., the resource availability) under a stated set of conditions represents one unique performance capacity of the knee flexor system. In rehabilitation, the terms *impairment, disability,* and *handicap* [World Health Organization, 1980] have been prominently applied and are relevant to the concept of performance. While these terms place an emphasis on what is missing or what a person cannot do and imply not only a measurement but also the incorporation of an assessment or judgment based on one or more observations, the resource-based performance perspective focuses on "what is present" or "what is right" (i.e., performance resource availability). From this perspective, an impairment can be determined to exist if a given performance capacity is found to be less than a specified level (e.g., less than the 5th percentile value of a healthy reference population). A disability exists when performance resource insufficiency exists in a specified task.

While performance relates more to what a system can do (i.e., a challenge or maximal stress is implied), *behavior* measurements are used to characterize what a system does naturally. Thus a given variable such as movement speed can relate to both performance and behavior depending on whether the system (e.g., a human subsystem) was maximally challenged to respond "as fast as possible" (performance) or simply observed in the course of operation (behavior). It is also possible to observe a system that it is behaving at one or more of its performance capacities (e.g., at the maximum speed possible, etc.) (see Table 141.1).

Subjective and Objective Measurement Methods

Subjective measurements are made by humans without the aid of instruments, and objective measurements result from the use of instruments. However, it should be noted that the mere presence of an instrument does not guarantee complete objectivity. For example, the use of a ruler requires a human judgment in reading the scale and thus contains a subjective element. A length-measurement system with an integral data-acquisition system would be more objective. However, it is likely that even this system would involve human intervention in its use, e.g., the alignment of the device and making the decision as to exactly what is to be measured with it by selection of reference points. Measures with more objectivity (less subjectivity) are preferred to minimize questions of bias. However, measurements that are intrinsically more objective are frequently more costly and time-consuming to obtain. Well-reasoned tradeoffs must be made to take advantage of the ability of a human (typically a skilled professional) to quickly "measure" many different items subjectively (and often without recording the results but using them internally to arrive at some decision).

It is important to observe that identification of the variable of interest is not influenced by whether it is measured subjectively or objectively. This concept extends to the choice of instrument used for objective measurements. This is an especially important concept in dealing with human performance and behavior, since variables of interest can be much more abstract than simple lengths and widths (e.g., coordination, postural stability, etc.). In fact, many measurement variables in rehabilitation historically have tended to be treated as if they were inextricably coupled with the measurement method, confounding debate regarding *what should be measured* with *what should be used to measure it* in a given context.

Measurements and Assessments

The basic representation of a measurement itself in terms of the actual units of measure is often referred to as the *raw form*. For measures of performance, the term *raw score* is frequently applied. Generally, some form of *assessment* (i.e., judgment or interpretation) is typically required. Assessments may be applied to (or, viewed from a different perspective, may require) either a single measure or groups of them. Subjective assessments are frequently made that are based on the practitioner's familiarity with values for a given parameter in a particular context. However, due to the large number of parameters and the amount of experience that would be required to gain a sufficient level of familiarity, a more formal and objective realization of the process that takes place in subjective assessments is often employed. This process combines the measured value with objectively determined reference values to obtain new metrics, or scores, that facilitate one or more steps in the assessment process.

For aspects of performance, *percent normal scores* are computed by expressing subject Y's availability of performance resource k [$R_{A_k}(Y)$] as a fraction of the mean availability of that resource in a specified reference population [$R_{A_k}(\text{pop})$]. Ideally, the reference population is selected to match the characteristics of the individual as closely as possible (e.g., age range, gender, handedness, etc.).

$$\text{Percent normal} = \frac{R_{A_k}(Y)}{R_{A_k}(\text{pop})} \times 100 \qquad (141.1)$$

TABLE 141.   The Scope of Measurement in Rehabilitation is Broad

Hierarchical Level	Structure	Function	Performance	Behavior
Global/Composite • Total human • Human with artificial systems	• Height • Weight • Postures • Subjective and instrumented methods	• Multifunction, reconfigurable system • High-level functions: tasks of daily life (work, grooming, recreation, etc.) • Functional assessment scales • Single-number global index • Level of indep. estimates	• No single-number direct measurement is possible • Possible models to integrate lower-level measures • Direct measurement (subjective and instrumented) of selected performance attribute for selected functions	• Subjective self- and family reports • Instrumented ambulatory activity monitors (selected attributes) • See notes under "function"

Complex Body Systems
• Cognitive
• Speech
• Lifting, gait
• Upper extremity
• Cardiovascular/respiratory
• Etc.
	• Dimensions
	• Shape
	• Etc.
	• Instrumented methods
		• Multifunction, reconfigurable systems
		• System-specific functions
			• Function specific subjective rating scales
			  Often based on impairment/ disability concepts
			  Relative metrics
			• Some instrumented performance capacity measures
			  Known also as "functional capacity" (misnomer)
				• Subjective and automated (objective) videotape evaluation
				• Instrumented measures of physical quantities vs time (e.g., angles, forces, motions)
				• Electromyography (e.g., muscle timing patterns, coordination)

Basic Systems
• Visual information processors
• Flexors, extensors
• Visual sensors
• Auditory sensors
• Lungs
• Etc.
	• Dimensions
	• Shape
	• Masses
	• Moments of inertia
	• Instrumented methods
		• Single function
		• System-specific functions
			• Subjective estimates by clinician for diagnostic and routine monitoring purposes
			• Instrumented measures of performance capacities (e.g., strength, extremes/range of motion, speed, accuracy, endurance, etc.)
				• Instrumented systems
				  Measure and log electrophysiologic biomechanical, and other variables vs. time
				  Post-hoc parameterization

Components of basic systems • Muscle • Tendon • Nerve • Etc.	• Mechanical properties • Instrumented methods/imaging	• Generally single-function • Component-specific functions	• Difficult to assess for individual subjects • Infer from measures at "basic system level" • Direct measurement methods with lab samples, research applications	• Difficult to assess for individual subject • Direct measurement methods with lab samples, research applications

Note: Structure, function, performance, and behavior are encompassed at multiple hierarchical levels. Both subjective and objective, instrumented methods of measurement are employed.

Aside from the benefit of placing all measurements on a common scale, a percent normal representation of a performance capacity score can be loosely interpreted as a probability. Consider grip strength as the performance resource. Assume that there is a uniform distribution of demands placed on grip strength across a representative sample of tasks of daily living, with requirements ranging from zero to the value representing mean grip strength availability in the reference population. Further assuming that grip strength was the only performance resource that was in question for subject Y (i.e., all others were available in nonlimiting amounts), the percent normal score would represent the probability that a task involving grip strength, randomly selected from those which average individuals in the reference population could execute (i.e., those for which available grip strength would be adequate), could be successfully executed by subject Y. While the assumptions stated here are unlikely to be perfectly true, this type of interpretation helps place measurements that are most commonly made in the laboratory into daily-life contexts.

In contrast to percent normal metrics, *z-scores* take into account variability within the selected reference population. Subject Y's performance is expressed in terms of the difference between it and the reference population mean, normalized by a value corresponding to one standard deviation unit (σ) of the reference population distribution:

$$z = \frac{R_{A_k}(Y) - R_{A_k}(\text{pop})}{\sigma} \tag{141.2}$$

It is important to note that valid z-scores assume that the parameter in question exhibits a normal distribution in the reference population. Moreover, z-scores are useful in assessing measures of structure, performance, and behavior. With regard to performance (and assuming that measures are based on a resource construct, i.e., a larger numeric value represents better performance), a z-score of zero is produced when the subject's performance equals that of the mean performance in the reference population. Positive z-scores reflect performance that is better than the population mean. In a normal distribution, 68.3% of the samples fall between z-scores of -1.0 and $+1.0$, while 95.4% of the samples fall between z-scores of -2.0 and $+2.0$. Due to variability of a given performance capacity within a healthy population (e.g., some individuals are stronger, faster, more mobile that others), a subject with a raw performance capacity score that produces a percent normal score of 70% could easily produce a z-score of -1.0. Whereas this percent normal score might raise concern regarding the variable of interest, the z-score of -1.0 indicates that a good fraction of healthy individuals exhibit a lower level of performance capacity.

Both percent normal and z-scores require reference population data to compute. The best reference (i.e., most sensitive) is data for that specific individual (e.g., preinjury or predisease onset). In most cases, these data do not exist. However, practices such as preemployment screenings and regular checkups are beginning to provide individualized reference data in some rehabilitation contexts.

In yet another alternative, it is frequently desirable to use values representing demands imposed by tasks $[R_{D_k}(\text{task A})]$ as the reference for assessment of performance capacity measures. Demands on performance resources can be envisioned to vary over the time course of a task. In practice, an estimate of the worst-case value (i.e., highest demand) would be used in assessments that incorporate task demands as reference values. In one form, such assessments can produce binary results. For example, availability can be equal to or exceed demand (resource sufficiency), or it can be less than demand (resource insufficiency). These rule-based assessments are useful in identifying limiting factors, i.e., those performance resources that inhibit a specified type of task from being performed successfully or that prevent achievement of a higher level of performance in a given type of task.

$$\text{If } R_{A_k}(\text{subject Y}) \geq R_{D_k}(\text{task A}), \text{ then} \tag{141.3}$$

$$R_{A_k}(\text{subject Y}) \text{ is sufficient, else}$$

$$R_{A_k}(\text{subject Y}) \text{ is insufficient}$$

These rule-based assessments represent the basic process often applied (sometimes subliminally) by experienced clinicians in making routine decisions, as evidenced by statements such as "not enough strength," "not enough stability," etc. It is natural to extend and build on these strategies for use with objective measures. Extreme care must be employed. It is often possible, for example, for an individual to substitute another performance resource that is not insufficient for one that is. Clinicians take into account many such factors, and objective components should be combined with subjective assessments that provide the required breadth that enhances validity of objective components of a given assessment.

Using the same numeric values employed in rule-based binary assessments, a *performance capacity stress* metric can be computed:

$$\text{Performance capacity stress (\%)} = \frac{R_{D_k}(\text{task A})}{R_{A_k}(\text{subject Y})} \times 100 \qquad (141.4)$$

Binary assessments also can be made using this metric and a threshold of 100%. However, the stress value provides additional information regarding how far (or close) a given performance capacity value is from the sufficiency threshold.

141.2 Measurement Objectives and Approaches

Characterizing the Human System and Its Subsystems

Figure 141.1 illustrates various points at which measurements are made over the course of a disease or injury, as well as some of the purposes for which they are made. The majority of measurements made in rehabilitation are aimed at characterizing the human system.

Measurements of human structure [e.g., Pheasant, 1986] play a critical role in the design and prescription of components such as seating, wheelchairs, workstations, artificial limbs, etc. Just like clothing, these items must "fit" the specific individual. Basic tools such as measuring tapes and rulers are becoming supplemented with three-dimensional digitizers and devices found in computer-aided manufacturing. Measurements of structure (e.g., limb segment lengths, moments of inertia, etc.) are also used with computer models [Vasta & Kondraske, 1995] in the process of analyzing tasks to determine demands in terms of performance capacity variables associated with basic systems such as flexors and extensors.

After nearly 50 years, during which a plethora of mostly disease- and injury-specific functional assessment scales were developed, the *functional independence measure* (FIM) [Hamilton et al., 1987; Keith et al., 1987] is of particular note. It is the partial result of a task-force effort to produce a systematic methodology (Uniform Data System for Medical Rehabilitation) with the specific intent of achieving standardization throughout the clinical service-delivery system. This broad methodology uses subjective judgments exclusively, based on rigorous written guidelines, to categorize demographic, diagnostic, functional, and cost information for patients within rehabilitation settings. Its simplicity to use once learned and its relatively low cost of implementation have helped in gaining a rather widespread utilization for tracking progress of individuals from admission to discharge in rehabilitation programs and evaluating effectiveness of specific therapies within and across institutions.

In contrast, many objective measurement tools of varying degrees of technological sophistication exist [Jones, 1995; Kondraske, 1995; Smith & Leslie, 1990; Potvin et al, 1985; Smith, 1995] (also see Further Information below). A good fraction of these have been designed to accomplish the same purposes as corresponding subjective methods, but with increased resolution, sensitivity, and repeatability. The intent is not always to replace subjective methods completely but to make available alternatives with the advantages noted for situations that demand superior performance in the aspects noted. There are certain measurement needs, however, that cannot be accomplished via subjective means (e.g., measurement of a human's visual information-processing speed, which

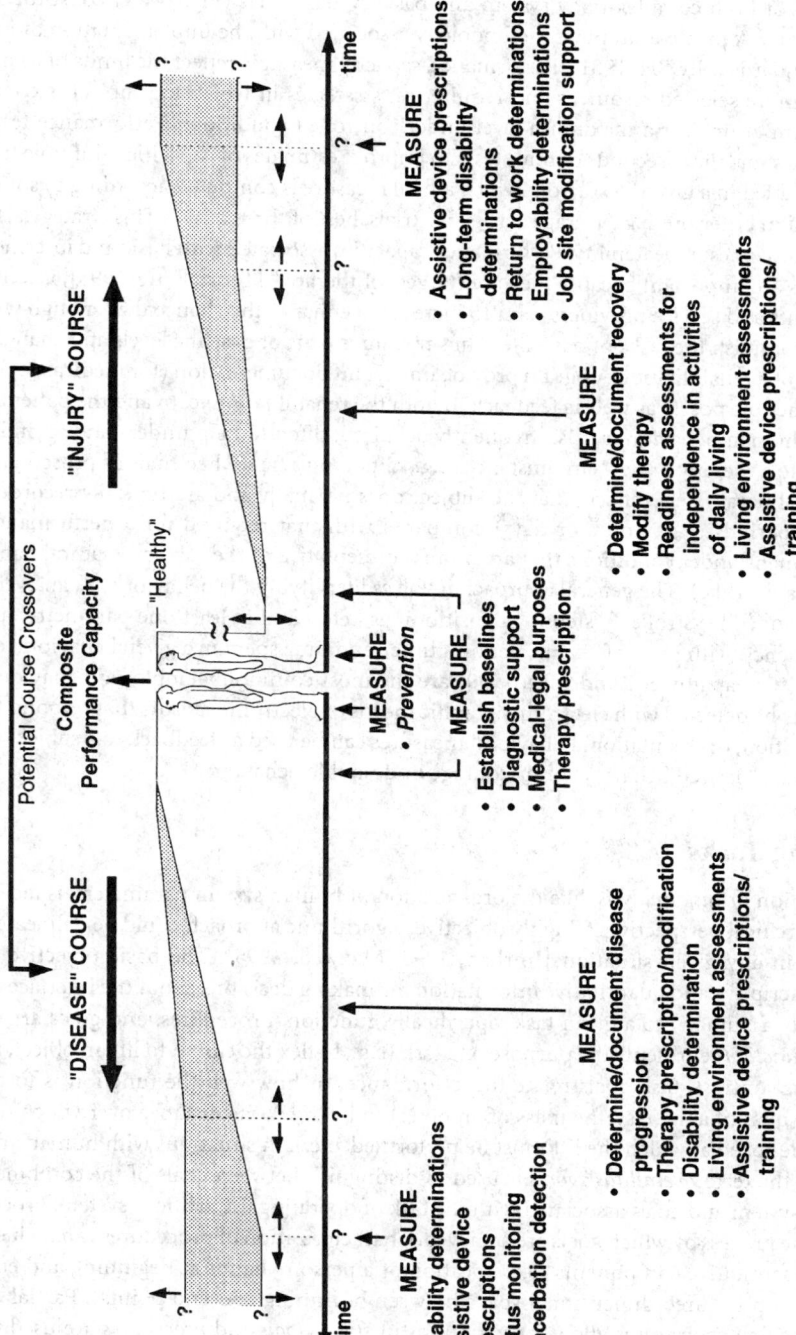

FIGURE 141.1　Measurements of structure, performance, and behavior serve many different purposes at different points over the course of a disease or injury that results in the need for rehabilitation services.

involves the measurement of times of less than 1 second with millisecond resolution). These needs draw on the latest technology in a wide variety of ways, as demonstrated in the cited material.

With regard to instrumented measurements that pertain to a specific individual, performance capacity measures at both complex body system and basic system levels (Fig. 141.1) constitute a major area of activity. A prime example is methodology associated with the implementation of industrial lifting standards [NIOSH, 1981]. Performance-capacity measures reflect the limits of availability of one or more selected resources and require test strategies in which the subject is commanded to perform at or near a maximum level under controlled conditions. Performance tests typically last only a short time (seconds or minutes). To improve estimates of capacities, multiple trials are usually included in a given "test" from which a final measure is computed according to some established reduction criterion (e.g., average across five trials, best of three trials). This strategy also tends to improve test-retest repeatability. Performance capacities associated with basic and intermediate-level systems are important because they are "targets of therapy" [Tourtellotte, 1993], i.e., the entities that patients and service providers want to increase to enhance the chance that enough will be available to accomplish the tasks of daily life. Thus measurements of baseline levels and changes during the course of a rehabilitation program provide important documentation (for medical, legal, insurance, and other purposes) as well as feedback to both the rehabilitation team and the patient.

Parameters of human behavior are also frequently acquired, often to help understand an individual's response to a therapy or new circumstance (e.g., obtaining a new wheelchair or prosethetic device). Behavioral parameters reflect what the subject does normally and are typically recorded over longer time periods (e.g., hours or days) compared with that required for a performance capacity measurement under conditions that are more representative of the subject's natural habitat (i.e., less laboratory-like). The general approach involves identifying the behavior (i.e., an event such as "head flexion," "keystrokes," "steps," "repositionings," etc.) and at least one parametric attribute of it. Frequency, with units of "events per unit time," and time spent in a given behavioral or activity state [e.g., Gonapathy & Kondraske, 1990] are the most commonly employed behavioral metrics. States may be detected with electromyographic means or electronic sensors that respond to force, motion, position, or orientation. Behavioral measures can be used as feedback to a subject as a means to encourage desired behaviors or discourage undesirable behaviors.

Characterizing Tasks

Task characterization or *task analysis,* like the organization of human system parameters, is facilitated with a hierarchical perspective. A highly objective, algorithmic approach could be delineated for task analysis in any given situation [Imrhan, 1995; Maxwell, 1995]. The basic objective is to obtain both descriptive and quantitative information for making decisions about the interface of a system (typically a human) to a given task. Specifically, function, procedures, and goals are of special interest. *Function* represents the purpose of a task (e.g., to flex the elbow, to lift an object, to communicate). In contrast, task goals relate to performance, or how well the function is to be executed, and are quantifiable (e.g., the mass of an object to be lifted, the distance over which the lift must occur, the speed at which the lift must be performed, etc.). In situations with human and artificial systems, the term *overall task goals* is used to distinguish between goals of the combined human-artificial system and goals associated with the task of operating the artificial system. Procedures represent the process by which goals are achieved. Characterization of procedures can include descriptive and quantitative components (e.g., location of a person's hands at beginning and end points of a task, path in three-dimensional space between beginning and end points). Partial or completely unspecified procedures allow for variations in *style. Goals* and *procedures* are used to obtain numeric estimates of task demands in terms of the performance resources associated with the systems anticipated to be used to execute the task. Task demands are time dependent. Worst-case demands, which may occur only at specific instants in time, are of primary interest in task analysis.

Estimates of task demand can be obtained by (1) direct measurement (i.e., of goals and procedures), (2) the use of physics-based models to map direct measurements into parameters that relate more readily to measurable performance capacities of human subsystems, or (3) inference. Examples of direct measurement include key dimensions and mass of objects, three-dimensional spatial locations between "beginning" and "end points" of objects in tasks involving the movement of objects, etc. Instrumentation supporting task analysis is available (e.g., load cells, video and other systems for measuring human position and orientation in real-time during dynamic activities), but it is not often integrated into systems for task analysis per se. Direct measurements of forces based on masses of objects and gravity often must be translated (to torques about a given body joint); this requires the use of static and dynamic models and analysis [e.g., Vasta & Kondraske, 1995; Winter, 1990].

An example of an inferential task-analysis approach that is relatively new is nonlinear causal resource analysis (NCRA) [Kondraske, 1988; Vasta & Kondraske, 1994]. This method was motivated by human performance analysis situations where direct analysis is not possible (e.g., determination of the amount of visual information-processing speed required to drive safely on a highway). Quantitative task demands, in terms of performance variables that characterize the involved subsystems, are inferred from a population data set that includes measures of subsystem performance, resource availabilities (e.g., speed, accuracy, etc.), and overall performance on the task in question. This method is based on the simple observation that the individual with the *least amount* of the given resource (i.e., the lowest performance capacity) who is still able to accomplish a given goal (i.e., achieve a given level of performance in the specified high-level task) provides the key clue. That amount of availability is used to infer the amount of demand imposed by the task.

The ultimate goal to which task characterization contributes is to identify limiting factors or unsafe conditions when a specific subject undertakes the task in question; this goal must not be lost while carrying out the basic objectives of task analysis. While rigorous algorithmic approaches are useful to make evident the true detail of the process, they are generally not performed in this manner in practice at present. Rather, the skill and experience of individuals performing the analysis are used to simplify the process, resulting in a judicious mixture of subjective estimates and objective measurements. For example, some limiting factors (e.g., grip strength) may be immediately identified without measurement of the human or the task requirements because the margin between availability and demand is so great that quick subjective "measurements" followed by an equally quick "assessment" can be used to arrive at the proper conclusion (e.g., "grip strength is a limiting factor in this task").

Characterizing Assistive Devices

Assistive devices can be viewed as artificial systems that either completely or partially bridge a gap between a given human (with his or her unique profile of performance capacities, i.e., available performance resources) and a particular task or class of tasks (e.g., communication, mobility, etc.). It is thus possible to consider the aspects of the device that constitute the user-device interface and those aspects which constitute, more generally, the device-task interface. In general, measurements supporting assessment of the user-device interface can be viewed to consist of (1) those which characterize the human and (2) those which characterize tasks (i.e., "operating" the assistive device). Each of these was described earlier. Measurements that characterize the device-task interface are often carried out in the context of the complete system, i.e., the human–assistive device–task combination (see next subsection).

Characterizing Overall Systems in High-Level-Task Situations

This situation generally applies to a human–artificial system–task combination. Examples include an individual using a communication aid to communicate, an individual using a wheelchair to achieve mobility, etc. Here, concern is aimed at documenting how well the task (e.g., communication, mobility, etc.) is achieved by the composite or overall system. Specific aspects or *dimensions of performance* associated with the relevant function should first be identified. Examples include speed, accuracy, stability, efficiency, etc. The total system is then maximally challenged (tempered by safety considerations) to operate along one or more of these dimensions of performance (usually not more than two dimensions are maximally challenged at the same time). For example, a subject with a communication device may be challenged to generate a single selected symbol "as fast as possible" (stressing speed without concern for accuracy). Speed is measured (e.g., with units of symbols per second) over the course of short trial (so as not to be influenced by fatigue). Then the "total system" may be challenged to generate a subset of specific symbols (chosen at random from the set of those available with a given device) one at a time, "as accurately as possible" (stressing accuracy while minimizing stress on speed capacities). Accuracy is then measured after a representative number of such trials are administered (in terms of "percent correct," for example). To further delineate the speed-accuracy performance envelope, "the system" may be challenged to select symbols at a fixed rate while accuracy is measured. Additional dimensions can be evaluated similarly. For example, endurance (measured in units of time) can be determined by selecting an operating point (e.g., by reference to the speed-accuracy performance envelope) and challenging the total system "to communicate" for "as long as possible" under the selected speed-accuracy condition.

In general, it is more useful if these types of characterizations consider all relevant dimensions with some level of measurements (i.e., subjective or objective) than it would be to apply a high-resolution, objective measurement in a process that considers only one aspect of performance.

141.3 Decision-Making Processes

Measurements that characterize the human, task, assistive device, or combination thereof are themselves only means to an end; the end is typically a decision. As noted previously, decisions are often the result of assessment processes involving one or more measurements. Although not exhaustive, many of the different types of assessments encountered are related to the following questions: (1) Is a particular aspect of performance normal (or impaired)? (2) Is a particular aspect of performance improving, stable, or getting worse? How should therapy be modified? (3) Can a given subject utilize (and benefit from) a particular assistive device? (4) Does a subject possess the required capacities to accomplish a given higher level task (e.g., driving, a particular job after a work-related injury, etc.)?

In Fig. 141.2, several of the basic concepts associated with measurement are used to illustrate how they enter into and facilitate systematic decision-making processes. The upper section shows raw score values as well as statistics for a healthy normal reference population in tabular form (left). It is difficult to reach any decision by simple inspection of just the raw performance capacity values. Tabular data are used to obtain percent normal (middle) and z-score (right) assessments. Both provide a more directly interpretable result regarding subject A's impairments. By examining the "right shoulder flexion extreme of motion" item in the figure, it can be seen that a raw score value corresponding to 51.2% normal yields a very large-magnitude, negative z-score (-10.4). This z-score indicates that virtually no one in the reference population would have a score this low. In contrast, consider similar scores for the "grip strength" item (56.2% normal, z-score $= -1.99$). On the basis of percent normal scores, it would appear that both of these resources are similarly affected, whereas the z-score basis provides a considerably different perspective due to the fact that grip strength is *much more variable* in healthy populations than the extreme angle obtained by a given limb segment about a joint, relatively speaking. As noted, z-scores account for this variability.

The lower section of Fig. 141.2 considers a situation in which the issue is a specific individual (subject A) considered in a specific task. Tabular data now include raw score values (which are the same as in upper section of the figure) and quantitative demands (typically worst case) imposed on the respective performance resources by task X. The lower-middle plot illustrates the process of individually assessing sufficiency of each performance resource in this task context using a rule-based assessment that incorporates the idea of a threshold (i.e., availability must exceed demand for

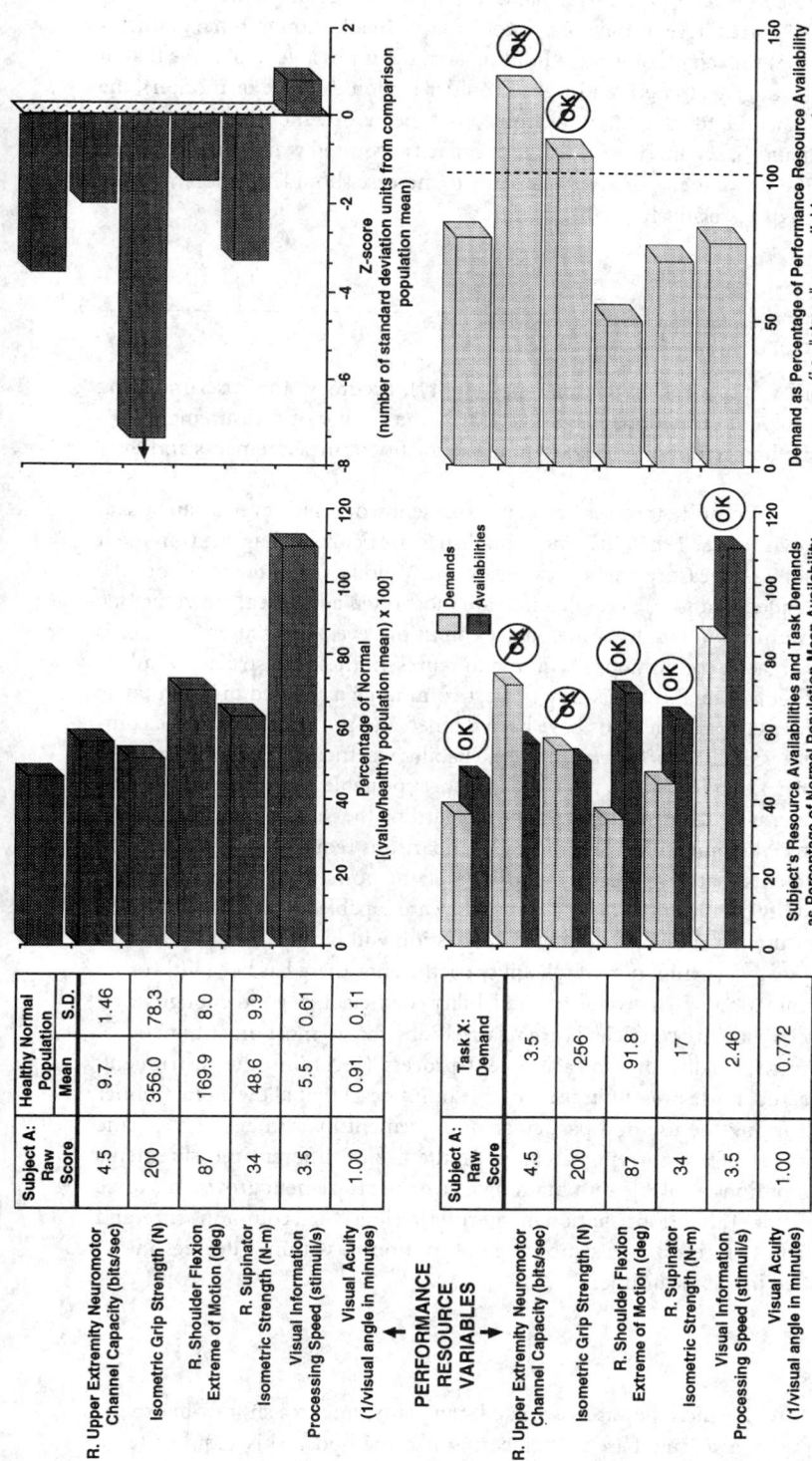

FIGURE 141.2 Examples of different types of assessments that can be performed by combining performance capacity measures and reference values of different types. The upper section shows raw score values as well as statistics for a healthy normal reference population in tabular form (*left*). It is difficult to reach any decision by simple inspection of just the raw performance capacity values. Tabular data are used to obtain a percent normal assessment (*middle*) and a z-score assessment (*right*). Both of these provide a more directly interpretable result regarding subject A's impairments. The lower section shows raw score values (same as in upper section) and quantitative demands (typically worst case) imposed on the respective performance resources by task X. The lower-middle plot illustrates the process of individually assessing sufficiency of each performance resource in this task context using a threshold rule (i.e., availability must exceed demand for sufficiency). The lower-right plot illustrates a similar assessment process after computation of a stress metric for each of the performance capacities. Here, any demand that corresponds to more than a 100% stress level is obviously problematic.

sufficiency). The lower-right plot illustrates an analogous assessment process that is executed after computation of a stress metric for each of the performance capacities. Here, any demand that corresponds to more than a 100% stress level is obviously problematic. In addition to binary conclusions regarding whether a given capacity is or is not a limiting factor, it is possible to observe that of the two limiting resources (e.g., grip strength and right shoulder flexion extreme of motion), the former is more substantial. This might suggest, for example, that the task be modified so as to decrease the grip-strength demand (i.e., gains in performance capacity required would be substantial to achieve sufficiency) and the use of focused exercise therapy to increase shoulder flexion mobility (i.e., gains in mobility required are relatively small).

141.4 Current Limitations

Quality of Measurements

Key issues are measurement validity, reliability (or repeatability), accuracy, and discriminating power. At issue in terms of current limitations is not necessarily the quality of measurements but limitations with regard to methods employed to determine the quality of measurements and their interpretability.

A complete treatment of these complex topics is beyond the present scope. However, it can be said that standards are such [Potvin et al., 1985] that most published works regarding measurement instruments do address quality of measurements to some extent. Validity (i.e., how well does the measurement reflect the intended quantity) and reliability are most often addressed. However, one could easily be left with the impression that these are binary conditions (i.e., a measurement is or is not reliable or valid), when in fact a continuum is required to represent these constructs. Of all attributes that relate to measurement quality, reliability is most commonly expressed in quantitative terms. This is perhaps because statistical methods have been defined and promulgated for the computation of so-called reliability coefficients [Winer, 1971]. Reliability coefficients range from 0.0 to 1.0, and the implication is that 1.0 indicates a perfectly reliable or repeatable measurement process. Current methods are adequate, at best, for making inferences regarding the relative quality of two or more methods of quantifying "the same thing." Even these comparisons require great care. For example, measurement instruments that have greater intrinsic resolving power have a greater opportunity to yield smaller-reliability coefficients simply because they are capable of measuring the true variability (on repeated measurement) of the parameter in question within the system under test. While there has been widespread determination of reliability coefficients, there has been little or no effort directed toward determination of what value of a reliability coefficient is "good enough" for a particular application. In fact, reliability coefficients are relatively abstract to most practitioners.

Methods for determining the quality of a measurement process (including the instrument, procedures, examiner, and actual noise present in the variable of interest) that allow a practitioner to easily reach decisions regarding the use of a particular measurement instrument in a specific application and limitations thereof are currently lacking. As the use of different measurements increases and the number of options available for obtaining a given measurement grows, this topic will undoubtedly receive additional attention. Caution in interpreting literature, common sense, and the use simple concepts such as "I need to measure range of motion to within 2 degrees in my application" are recommended in the meantime.

Standards

Measurements, and concepts with which they are associated, can contribute to a shift from experience-based knowledge acquisition to rule-based, engineering-like methods. This requires (1) a widely accepted conceptual framework (i.e., known to assistive device manufacturers, rehabilitation engineers, and other professionals within the rehabilitation community), (2) a more complete set of measurement tools that are at least standardized with regard to the definition of the quantity measured, (3) special analysis and assessment software (that removes the resistance to the application of more rigorous methods by enhancing the quality of decisions as well as the speed with which they can be reached), and (4) properly trained practitioners. Each is a necessary *but not sufficient* component. Thus balanced progress is required in each of these areas.

Rehabilitation Service Delivery and Rehabilitation Engineering

In a broad sense, it has been argued that all engineers can be considered rehabilitation engineers who merely work at different levels along a comprehensive spectrum of human performance, which itself can represent a common denominator among all humans. Thus an automobile is a mobility aid, a telephone is a communication aid, and so on. Just as in other engineering disciplines, measurement must be recognized not only as an important end in itself (in appropriate instances) but also as an integral component or means within the overall scope of rehabilitation and rehabilitation engineering processes. The service-delivery infrastructure must provide for such means. At present, one should anticipate and be prepared to overcome potential limitations associated with factors such as third-party reimbursement for measurement procedures, recognition of equipment and maintenance costs associated with obtaining engineering-quality measurements, and education of administrative staff and practitioners with regard to the value and proper use of measurements.

Defining Terms

Behavior: A general term that relates to what a human or artificial system does while carrying out its function(s) under given conditions. Often, behavior is characterized by measurement of selected parameters or identification of unique system states over time.

Function: The purpose of a system. Some systems map to a single primary function (e.g., process visual information). Others (e.g., the human arm) map to multiple functions, although at any given time multifunction systems are likely to be executing a single function (e.g., polishing a car). Functions can be described and inventoried, whereas level of performance of a given function can be measured.

Functional assessment: The process of determining, from a relatively global perspective, an individual's ability to carry out tasks in daily life. Also, the result of such a process. Functional assessments typically cover a range of selected activity areas and include (at a minimum) a relatively gross indication (e.g., can or can't do; with or without assistance) of status in each area.

Goal: A desired endpoint (i.e., result) typically characterized by multiple parameters, at least one of which is specified. Examples include specified task goals (e.g., move an object of specified mass from point A to point B in 3 seconds) or estimated task performance (maximum mass, range, speed of movement obtainable given a specified elemental performance resource availability profile), depending on whether a reverse or forward analysis problem is undertaken. Whereas function describes the general process of a task, the goal directly relates to performance and is quantitative.

Limiting resource: A performance resource at any hierarchical level (e.g., vertical lift strength, knee flexor speed) that is available in an amount that is less than the worst-case demand imposed by a task. Thus a given resource can be "limiting" only when considered in the context of a specific task.

Overall task goals: Goals associated with a task to be executed by a human-artificial system combination (to be distinguished from goals associated with the task of operating the artificial system).

Performance: Aspects of a human or artificial system (e.g., strength, speed, accuracy, endurance) that pertain to how well that system executes its function.

Performance capacity: A quantity in finite availability that limits some aspect of a system's ability to execute tasks, or the limit of that aspect itself.

Performance capacity measurement: A general class of measurements, performed at different hierarchical levels, intended to quantify one or more performance capacities.

Procedure: A set of constraints placed on a system in which flexibility exists regarding how a goal (or set of goals) associated with a given function can be achieved. Procedure specification requires specification of initial, intermediate, and/or final states or conditions dictating how the goal is to be accomplished. Such specification can be thought of in terms of removing some degrees of freedom.

Structure: Physical manifestation and attributes of a human or artificial system and the object of one type of measurements at multiple hierarchical levels.

Style: Allowance for variation within a procedure, resulting in the intentional incomplete specification of a procedure or resulting from either intentional or unintentional incomplete specification of procedure.

Task: That which results from (1) the combination of specified functions, goals, and procedures or (2) the specification of function and goals and the observation of procedures utilized to achieve the goals.

References

Fuhrer MJ. 1987. Rehabilitation Outcomes: Analysis and Measurement. Baltimore, Brookes.

Ganapathy G, Kondraske GV. 1990. Microprocessor-based instrumentation for ambulatory behavior monitoring. J Clin Eng 15(6):459.

Granger CV, Greshorn GE. 1984. Functional Assessment in Rehabilitation Medicine. Baltimore, Williams & Wilkins.

Hamilton BB, Granger CV, Sherwin FS, et al. 1987. A uniform national data system for medical rehabilitation. In MJ Fuhrer (ed), Rehabilitation Outcomes: Analysis and Measurement, pp 137–147. Baltimore, Brookes.

Imrhan S. 1995. Task analysis and decomposition: Physical components. In JD Bronzino (ed), Handbook of Biomedical Engineering. Boca Raton, Fla, CRC Press.

Jones RD. 1995. Measurement of neuromotor control performance capacities. In JD Bronzino (ed), Handbook of Biomedical Engineering. Boca Raton, Fla, CRC Press.

Keith RA, Granger CV, Hamilton BB, Sherwin FS. 1987. The functional independence measure: A new tool for rehabilitation. In MG Eisenberg, RC Grzesiak (eds), Advances in Clinical Rehabilitation, vol 1, pp 6–18. New York, Springer-Verlag.

Kondraske GV. 1988. Experimental evaluation of an elemental resource model for human performance. In Proceedings of the Tenth Annual IEEE Engineering in Medicine and Biology Society Conference, New Orleans, pp 1612–13.

Kondraske GV. 1990. Quantitative measurement and assessment of performance. In RV Smith, JH Leslie (eds), Rehabilitation Engineering, pp 101–125. Boca Raton, Fla, CRC Press.

Kondraske GV. 1995. A working model for human system-task interfaces. In JD Bronzino (ed), Handbook of Biomedical Engineering. Boca Raton, Fla, CRC Press.

Kondraske GV, Vasta PJ. 1995. Measurement of information processing performance capacities. In JD Bronzino (ed), Handbook of Biomedical Engineering. Boca Raton, Fla, CRC Press.

Maxwell KJ. 1995. High-level task analysis: Mental components. In JD Bronzino (ed), Handbook of Biomedical Engineering. Boca Raton, Fla, CRC Press.

National Institute of Occupational Safety and Health (NIOSH). 1981. Work Practices Guide for Manual Lifting (DHHS Publication No. 81122). Washington, US Government Printing Office.

Pheasant ST. 1986. Bodyspace: Anthropometry, Ergonomics and Design. Philadelphia, Taylor & Francis.

Potvin AR, Tourtellotte WW, Potvin JH, et al. 1985. The Quantitative Examination of Neurologic Function. Boca Raton, Fla, CRC Press.

Smith RV, Leslie JH. 1990. Rehabilitation Engineering. Boca Raton, Fla, CRC Press.

Smith SS. 1995. Measurement of neuromuscular performance capacities. In JD Bronzino (ed), Handbook of Biomedical Engineering. Boca Raton, Fla, CRC Press.

Tourtellotte WW. 1993. Personal communication.

Vasta PJ, Kondraske GV. 1994. Performance prediction of an upper extremity reciprocal task using non-linear causal resource analysis. In Proceedings of the Sixteenth Annual IEEE Engineering in Medicine and Biology Society Conference, Baltimore.

Vasta PJ, Kondraske GV. 1995. Human performance engineering: Computer based design and analysis tools. In JD Bronzino (ed), Handbook of Biomedical Engineering. Boca Raton, Fla, CRC Press.

Webster JG, Cook AM, Tompkin WJ, Vanderheiden GC. 1985. Electronic Devices for Rehabilitation. New York, Wiley.

Winer BJ. 1971. Statistical Principles in Experimental Design, 2d ed. New York, McGraw-Hill.

Winter DA. 1990. Biomechanics and Motor Control of Human Movement, 2d ed. New York, Wiley.

World Health Organization. 1980. International Classification of Impairments, Disabilities, and Handicaps. Geneva, World Health Organization.

Further Information

The section of this *Handbook* entitled "Human Performance Engineering" contains chapters that address human performance modeling and measurement in considerably more detail.

Manufacturers of instruments used to characterize different aspects of human performance often provide technical literature and bibliographies with conceptual backgrounds, technical specifications, and application examples. A partial list of such sources is included below. (No endorsement of products is implied.)

Baltimore Therapeutic Equipment Co.
7455-L New Ridge Road
Hanover, MD 21076-3105

Chattecx Corporation
P.O. Box 4287
Chattanooga, TN 37405

Cybex
2100 Smithtown Avenue
Ronkonkoma, NY 11779

Human Performance Measurement, Inc.
P.O. Box 1996
Arlington, TX 76004-1996

Lafayette Instrument
3700 Sagamore Parkway North
Lafayette, IN 47903

Loredan Biomedical, Incorporated
P.O. Box 1154
Davis, CA 95617

The National Institute on Disability and Rehabilitation Research (NIDRR), part of the Department of Education, funds a set of Rehabilitation Engineering Research Centers (RERCs) and

Research and Training Centers (RTCs). Each has a particular technical focus; most include measurements and measurements issues. Contact NIDRR for a current listing of these centers.

Measurement devices, issues, and application examples specific to rehabilitation are included in the following journals:

IEEE Transactions on Rehabilitation Engineering
IEEE Service Center
445 Hoes Lane
P.O. Box 1331
Piscataway, NJ 08855-1331

Assistive Technology
RESNA Press
1700 North Moore St.
Suite 1540
Arlington, VA 22209

Rehabilitation Research and Development
Scientific and Technical Publications Section
Rehabilitation Research and Development Service
103 South Gay St., 5th floor
Baltimore, MD 21202-4051

Archives of Physical Medicine and Rehabilitation
Suite 1310
78 East Adams Street
Chicago, IL 60603-6103

American Journal of Occupational Therapy
The American Occupational Therapy Association, Inc.
1383 Piccard Drive
Rockville, MD 20850-4375

Physical Therapy
American Physical Therapy Association
1111 North Fairfax St.
Alexandria, VA 22314

Journal of Occupational Rehabilitation
Subscription Department
Plenum Publishing Corporation
233 Spring St.
New York, NY 10013

Rehab Management
4676 Admiralty Way
Suite 202
Marina Del Rey, CA 90292

142

Rehabilitation Engineering Technologies: Principles of Application

Douglas Hobson
University of Pittsburgh

Elaine Trefler
University of Pittsburgh

Rehabilitation engineering is the branch of *biomedical engineering* that is concerned with the application of science and technology to improve the quality of life of individuals with disabilities. Areas addressed within rehabilitation engineering include wheelchairs and seating systems, access to computers, sensory aids, prosthetics and orthotics, alternative and augmentative communication, home and work-site modifications, and universal design. Because many products of rehabilitation engineering require careful selection to match individual needs and often require custom fitting, rehabilitation engineers have necessarily become involved in service delivery and application as well as research, design, and development. Therefore, as we expand on later, it is not only engineers that practice within the field of rehabilitation engineering.

As suggested above, and as in many other disciplines, there are really two career tracks in the field of rehabilitation engineering. There are those who acquire qualifications and experience to advance the state of knowledge through conducting research, education, and product development, and there are others who are engaged in the application of technology as members of service delivery teams. At one time it was possible for a person to work in both arenas. However, with the explosion of technology and the growth of the field over the past decade, one must now specialize not only within research or service delivery but often within a specific area of technology. Another factor that will differentiate the researcher from the practitioner is that within the next 5 years the practitioner will need to be certified as an assistive technology provider in order to receive payment for his or her services.

One can further differentiate between rehabilitation and assistive technology. *Rehabilitation technology* is a term most often used to refer to technologies associated with the acute-care rehabilitation process. Therapy evaluation and treatment tools, clinical dysfunction measurement and recording instrumentation, and prosthetic and orthotic appliances are such examples. *Assistive technologies* are those devices and services that are used in the daily lives of people in the community to enhance their ability to function independently, examples being specialized seating, wheelchairs, environmental control devices, workstation access technologies, and sensory and communication aids. Recognition and support of assistive technology devices and services are now embedded in all the major disability legislation that has been enacted over the last decade.

The primary focus of this chapter is on the role of the rehabilitation engineering practitioner as he or she carries out the responsibilities demanded by the application of assistive technology.

Before launching into the primary focus of this chapter, let us first set a conceptual framework for the *raison d'etre* for assistive technology and the role of the assistive technology professional.

142.1 The Conceptual Frameworks

The application of assistive technology can be conceptualized as minimizing the handicapping effects of the mismatch between the person and his or her environment. This in reality is what technology does for all of us to varying degrees. For example, if you live in a suburban area that has been designed for access only by car and your car breaks down, you are handicapped. If your house has been designed to be cooled by air conditioning in the "dog days" of summer and you lose a compressor, your comfort is immediately compromised by your incompatibility with your environment. Similarly, if you live in a home that has only access by steps and you have an impairment requiring the use of a wheelchair, you are handicapped because you no longer have abilities that are compatible with your built environment. Because our environments, homes, workplaces, schools, and communities have been designed to be compatible with the abilities of the norm, young children, persons with disabilities, and many elderly people experience the consequences of their mismatch as a matter of course. The long-term utopian solution would be to design environments and their contents so that they can be used by all people of all ages, which is the essence of the universal design concept. However, given that today we do not have very many products and environments that have been universally designed, rehabilitation engineering and assistive technology attempt to minimize the effects of the mismatch by designing, developing, and providing technologies that will allow persons with disabilities to pursue their life goals in a manner similar to any other person. Of course, the rehabilitation engineer cannot accomplish this working in isolation but rather must function as part of a consumer-responsive team that can best deal with the multiplicity of factors that usually impact on the successful application of assistive technology.

Let us now move to another conceptual framework, one that conceptualizes how people actually interact with technology.

The following conceptualization has been adapted from the model proposed by Roger Smith [Smith, 1992]. In Fig. 142.1, Smith suggests that there are three cyclic elements that come into play when humans interact with technology: the human and his or her innate sensory, cognitive, and functional abilities; the human factor's characteristics of the interface between the human and the technology; and the technical characteristics of the technology itself in terms of its output as a result of a specific input by the user. People with disabilities may have varying degrees of dysfunction in their sensory, cognitive, and functional abilities. The interface will have to be selected or adapted to these varying abilities in order to allow the person to effectively interact with the technology. The technology itself will need to possess specific electronic or mechanical capabilities in order to yield the desired outcome. The essence of assistive technology applications is to integrate all three of these elements into a functional outcome that meets the specific needs of a user. This is usually done by selecting commercially available devices and technologies at a cost that can be met by either the individual or his or her third-party payment source. When technologies are not available, then they must be modified from existing devices or designed and fabricated as unique custom solutions. It is

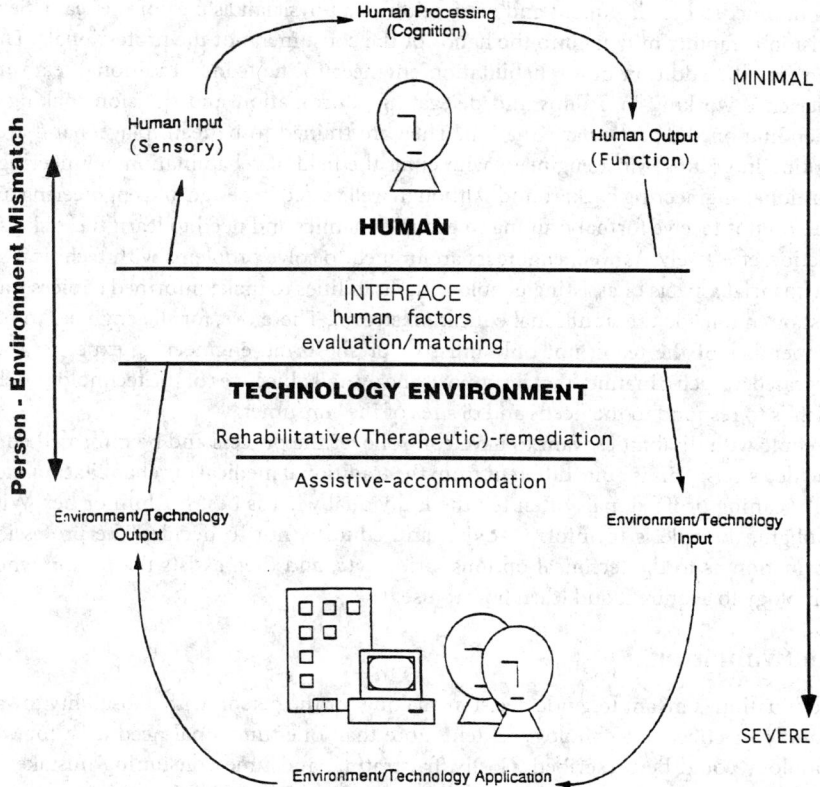

FIGURE 142.1   Conceptual framework of technology and disability. (Modified from Smith [1992].)

particularly in these latter activities that a rehabilitation engineer can make his or her unique contribution to team process.

It should be realized that there are several levels of assistive technology. The first level might be termed *fundamental technology* in contrast to advanced technology. Fundamental technologies, such as walkers, crutches, many wheelchairs, activities of daily living (ADL) equipment, etc., usually do not require the involvement of the rehabilitation engineer in their application. Others on the team can better assess the need, confirm the interface compatibility, and verify that the outcome is appropriate. The rehabilitation engineer is most often involved in the application of advanced technologies, such as powered wheelchairs, computerized workstation designs, etc., that require an understanding of the underlying technological principles in order to achieve the best match with the abilities and needs of the user, especially if custom modifications are required to the original equipment. The rehabilitation engineer is usually the key person if a unique solution is necessary.

Let's now discuss a few fundamental concepts related to the process by which assistive technology is typically provided in various service delivery programs.

142.2 The Provision Process

The Shifting Paradigm

In the traditional rehabilitation model of service delivery, a multidisciplinary team of professionals is already in place. Physicians, therapists, counselors, and social workers meet with the client and, based on the findings of a comprehensive evaluation, plan a course of action. In the field of assistive technology, the rules of the team are being charted anew. First, the decision making often takes place in a nonmedical environment and often without a physician as part of the team. Second, the final decision is rapidly moving into the hands of the consumer, not the professionals. The third major change is the addition of a rehabilitation engineer to the team. Traditional team members have experience working in groups and delegating coordination and decision making to colleagues depending on the particular situation. They are trained to be team players and are comfortable working in groups. Most engineers who enter the field of rehabilitation engineering come with a traditional engineering background. Although well versed in design and engineering principles, they often do not receive formal training in group dynamics and need to learn these skills if they are to function effectively. As well, engineers are trained to solve problems with technical solutions. The psychosocial aspects of assisting people with disabilities to make informed choices must be learned most often outside the traditional education stream. Therefore, for the engineer to be a contributing member of the team, not only must he or she bring engineering expertise, but it must be integrated in such a manner that it supports the overall objectives of the technology delivery process, which is to respond to the needs and desires of the consumer.

People with disabilities want to have control over the process and be informed enough to make good decisions. This is quite different from the traditional medical or rehabilitation model, in which well-meaning professionals often tell the individual what is best for him or her. Within this new paradigm, the role is to inform, advise, and educate, not to decide. The professional provides information as to the technical options, prices, etc. and then assists the person who will use the technology to acquire it and learn how to use it.

The Evaluation

An evaluation is meant to guide decision-making for the person with a disability toward appropriate and cost-effective technology. Often, more than one functional need exist for which assistive technology could be prescribed. Costly, frustrating, and time-consuming mistakes often can be avoided if a thorough evaluation based on a person's total functional needs is performed before any technology is recommended. Following the evaluation, a long-range plan for acquisition and training in the chosen technology can be started.

For example, suppose a person needs a seating system, both a powered and manual wheelchair, an augmentative communication device, a computer workstation, and an environmental control unit (ECU). Where does one begin? Once a person's goals and priorities have been established, the process can be begin. First, a decision would likely be made about the seating system that will provide appropriate support in the selected manual chair. However, the specifications of the seating system should be such that the components also can be interfaced into the powered chair. The controls for the computer and augmentative communication device must be located so that they do not interfere with the vocabulary of the communication device and must in some way be compatible with the controls for the ECU. Only if all functional needs are addressed can the technology be acquired in a logical sequence and in such a manner that all the components will be compatible. The more severely disabled the individual, the more technology he or she will need, and the more essential is the process of setting priorities and ensuring compatibility of technical components.

In summary, as suggested by the conceptual model, the process begins by gaining an understanding of the person's sensory, cognitive, and functional abilities, combined with clarification of his or her desires and needs. These are then filtered through the technology options, both in terms of how the interface will integrate with the abilities of the user and how the technology itself will be integrated to meet the defined needs. This information and the associated pros and cons are conveyed to the user, who then has the means to participate in the ultimate selection decisions.

Service Delivery Models

People with disabilities can access technology through a variety of different service delivery models. A team of professionals might be available in a university setting where faculty not only teach but also deliver technical services to the community. More traditionally, the team of rehabilitation professionals, including a rehabilitation engineer, might be available at a hospital or rehabilitation facility. More recently, technology professionals might be in private practice either individually, as a team, or part of the university, hospital, or rehabilitation facility structure. Another option is the growing number of rehabilitation technology suppliers (RTSs) who offer commercial technology services within the community. They work in conjunction with an evaluation specialist and advise consumers as to the technical options available to meet their needs. They then sell and service the technology and train the consumer in its use. Local chapters of national disability organizations such as United Cerebral Palsy and Easter Seals also may have assistive technology services. In recent years, a growing number of centers for independent living (CILs) have been developed in each state with federal support. Some of these centers have opted to provide assistive technology services, in addition to their information and referral services, which are common to all CILs. And finally, there are volunteers, either in engineering schools or community colleges (student supervised projects) or in industry (high-technology industries often have staff interested in doing community service), such as the Telephone Pioneers. Each model has its pros and cons for the consumer, and only after thoroughly researching the options will the person needing the service make the best choice as to where to go with his or her need in the community. A word of caution. Only if there is timely provision and follow-up available is a service delivery system considered appropriate, even if the cost of the service is less.

A more extensive description of service delivery options may be reviewed in a report that resulted from a RESNA-organized conference on service delivery [ANSI/RESNA, 1987].

142.3 Education and Quality Assurance

Professionals on the assistive technology team have a primary degree in their individual professions. For example, the occupational or physical therapist will have a degree and most often state licensure in occupational or physical therapy. The engineer will have recognized degrees in mechanical, electrical, biomedical, or some other school of engineering. However, in order to practice effectively in the field of assistive technology, almost all will need advanced training. A number of occupational therapy curriculums provide training in assistive technology, but not all. The same is true of several of the others. Consumers and payers of assistive technology need to know that professionals practicing in the field of assistive technology have met a certain level of competency. For this reason, all professionals, including rehabilitation engineers, will soon require credentialing as assistive technology providers. The engineer also will need to be a certified rehabilitation engineer.

RESNA

RESNA, an interdisciplinary association of persons dedicated to the advancement of assistive technology for people with disabilities, is now aggressively working toward a credentialing program that will certify individuals on the assistive technology team. As part of the process, the minimum skills and knowledge base for practitioners is being formulated. Ties with professional organizations are being sought so that preservice programs will include at least some of the knowledge and skills base necessary. Continuing education efforts by RESNA and others also will assist in building the level of expertise of practitioners and consumers. An important, although controversial, component of the credentialing process is the testing that will determine those who can practice in this field with sufficient skills and knowledge to warrant payment for their expertise. At this time, it appears that there will be a first level of qualification that will yield a generalist in assistive technology. Following the base level, individuals can take a second exam to be certified in specific specialty areas, such as seating and wheeled mobility, augmentative and alternative communication, adaptive driving and transportation, computer applications for persons with disabilities, etc. Once in place, this program will go a long way toward the quality assurance that so urgently is needed by consumers, colleagues, and funders.

Payment for technology and the services required for its application is complex and changing rapidly as health care reform evolves. It is beyond the scope of this discussion to detail the very convoluted and individual process required to ensure that people with disabilities receive what they need. However, there are some basic concepts to be kept in mind. Professionals need to be competent. The documentation of need and the justification of selection must be comprehensive. Time for a person to do this must be allocated if there is to be success. Persistence, creativity, education of the payers, and documentation of need seem to be the key issues.

142.4 Specific Impairments and Related Technologies

Current information related to specific technologies is best found in brochures, magazines (*Team Rehab*), exhibit halls of technology-related conferences, and databases such as ABLEDATA, since it is constantly expanding and changing. What follows is only a brief introduction to specific disabilities areas to which assistive technology applications are commonly used.

Mobility

Mobility technologies include wheelchairs, walkers, canes, orthotic devices, FES (functional electrical stimulation), laser canes, and any other assistive device that would assist a person with a mobility disability, be it motor or sensory, to move about in his or her environment. There are very few people who have a working knowledge of all the possible commercial options. Therefore, people usually acquire expertise in certain areas, such as wheelchairs. There are hundreds of varieties of wheelchairs, each offering a different array of characteristics that need to be understood as part of the selection process. Fortunately, there are now several published ways that the practitioner and the consumer can obtain useful information. A classification system has been developed that sets a conceptual framework for understanding the different types of wheelchairs that are produced commercially [Hobson, 1990]. *Paraplegic News* and *Sports and Spokes* annually publish the specifications on most of the manual and powered wheelchairs commonly found in the North American marketplace. These reviews are based on standardized testing that is carried out by manufacturers following the ANSI/RESNA wheelchair standards [ANSI/RESNA, 1990]. Since the testing and measurements are done and reported in a standard way, it is now possible to make accurate comparisons between products, a tremendous recent advancement for the wheelchair specialist and the users they serve [Axelson et al., 1994].

Sitting

Many people cannot use the wheelchairs as they come from the manufacturer. Specialized seating is required to help persons to remain in a comfortable and functional seated posture for activities that enable them to access work and attend educational and recreational activities. Orthotic supports, seating systems in wheelchairs, chairs that promote dynamic posture in the workplace, and chairs for the elderly that fit properly, are safe, and encourage movement all fit into the broad category of sitting technology.

Sensation

People with no sensation are prone to skin injury. Special seating technology can assist in the prevention of tissue breakdown. Specially designed cushions and backs for wheelchairs and mattresses that have pressure-distributing characteristics fall into this category. Technology also has been developed to remind people to relieve pressure at determined intervals or to do it for them mechanically.

Again, a classification system of specialized seating has been developed that provides a conceptual framework for understanding the features of the various technologies and their potential applications. The same reference also discusses the selection process, evaluation tools, biomechanics of supported sitting, and materials properties of weight-relieving materials [Hobson, 1990].

Access (Person-Machine Interface)

In order to use assistive technology, people with disabilities need to be able to operate the technology. With limitations in motor and/or sensory systems, often a specially designed or configured interface system must be assembled. It could be as simple as several switches or a miniaturized keyboard or as complex as an integrated control system that allows a person to drive a wheelchair and operate a computer and a communication device using only one switch.

Communication

Because of motor or sensory limitations, some individuals cannot communicate with spoken or written word. There are communication systems that enable people to communicate using synthesized voice or printed output. Systems for people who are deaf allow them to communicate over the phone or through computer interfaces. Laptop computers with appropriate software can enable persons to communicate faster and with less effort than previously possible. Some basic guidelines for selecting an augmentative communication system, including strategies for securing funding, have been proposed in an overview chapter by James Jones and Winifred Jones [Jones & Jones, 1990].

Transportation

Modified vans and cars enable persons with disabilities to independently drive a vehicle. Wheelchair tie-downs and occupant restraints in personal vehicles and in public transportation vehicles are allowing people to be safely transported to their chosen destination. Fortunately, voluntary performance standards for restraint and tie-down technologies are currently being developed by a task group within the Society for Automotive Engineers (SAE). These standards are due to be completed in 1995. Standards for hand controls have just been revised for another 5 years. Other standards that will be completed by 1995 are van body modifications and wheelchair lifts. These standards provide the rehabilitation engineer with a set of tools that can be used to confirm safety compliance of modified transportation equipment. Currently in process and still requiring several more years of work are transport wheelchair and vehicle power control standards.

Universal-Access Design

Universal-access design is a current issue. The concept is to design environments and their contained products so people with disabilities or who are aging and/or acquire a disability can hopefully use or readily adapt existing built environments or products. Paul Grayson and others have published extensively regarding the need to rethink how we design our living environments [Grayson, 1991]. Vanderheiden and the Denno-lead group of that Honeywell SSD Center have prepared excellent human factor guidelines for product designers. These guidelines provide invaluable information on access characteristics to allow use by the elderly and persons with disabilities [Denno et al., 1992; Vanderheiden & Vanderheiden, 1991].

Activities of Daily Living (ADL)

ADL technology enables a person to live independently as much as possible. Such devices as environmental control units, bathroom aids, dressing assists, automatic door openers, and alarms are all considered aids to daily living. Many are inexpensive and can be purchased through careful selection in stores or through catalogues. Others are quite expensive and must be ordered through vendors who specialize in technology for independent living.

School and Work

Technology that supports people in the workplace or in an educational environment can cover such applications as computer workstations, modified restrooms, and transportation to and from work or school. Students need the ability to take notes and do assignments, and people working have a myriad of special tasks that may need to be analyzed and modified to enable the employee with the disability to be independent and productive. Weisman has printed an extensive overview of rehabilitation engineering in the workplace, which includes a review of different types of workplaces, the process of accommodation, and a dozen or so case examples [Weisman, 1990].

Recreation

A component of living that is often overlooked by the professional community is the desire and, in fact, need of people with disabilities to participate in recreational activities. Many of the adaptive recreational technologies have been developed by persons with disabilities themselves in their effort to participate and be competitive in sports. Competitive wheelchair racing, archery, skiing, bicycles, and technology that enables people to bowl, play pool, and fly their own airplanes are just a few areas in which equipment has been adapted for specific recreational purposes.

Community and Workplace Access

There is probably no other single legislation that is having a more profound impact on the lives of people with disabilities then the Americans with Disabilities Act, signed into law by President Bush in August of 1990. This civil rights legislation mandates that all people with disabilities have access to public facilities and that reasonable accommodations must be made by employers to allow persons with disabilities to access employment opportunities. The impact of this legislation is now sweeping America and leading to monumental changes in the way people view the rights of persons with disabilities.

142.5 Future Developments

The field of rehabilitation engineering, both in research and in service delivery, is at an important crossroad in its young history. Shifting paradigms of services, reduction in research funding, consumerism, credentialing, health care reform, and limited formal educational options all make speculating on what the future may bring rather hazy. Given all this, it is reasonable to say that one group of rehabilitation engineers will continue to advance the state of the art through research, while another group will be in the front lines as members of clinical teams working to ensure that all individuals with disabilities receive devices and services that are most appropriate for their particular needs.

The demarcation between researchers and service providers will become clearer, since the latter will need to be certified in order to get a job. RESNA and its professional specialty group (PSG) on rehabilitation engineering will work out a credentialing process acceptable to other assistive technology providers (ATPs) and the funding agencies. The engineers working in service provision will be certified rehabilitation engineers working as ATPs. They will be recognized as valued members of the clinical team by all members of the rehabilitation community, including third-party payers, who will reimburse them for the rehabilitation engineering services that they provide. They will spend as much or more time working in the community as they will in clinical settings. They will work closely with consumer-managed organizations who will be the gatekeepers of increasing amounts of government-mandated service dollars.

If these predictions come to pass, the need for rehabilitation engineering will continue to grow. As medicine and medical technology continue to improve, more people will survive traumatic injury, disease, and premature birth, and many will acquire functional impairments that impede their involvement in personal, community, educational, vocational, and recreational activities. People continue to live longer lives, thereby increasing the likelihood of acquiring one or more disabling conditions during their lifetime. This presents an immense challenge for the field of rehabilitation engineering. As opportunities grow, more engineers will be attracted to the field. More and more rehabilitation engineering education programs will develop that will support the training of qualified engineers, engineers who are looking for exciting challenges and opportunities to help people live more satisfying and productive lives.

References

ANSI/RESNA. 1990. Wheelchair Standards. RESNA Press, RESNA, 1700 Moore St., Arlington, Va 22209-1903.

Axelson P, Minkel J, Chesney D. 1994. A Guide to Wheelchair Selection: How to Use the ANSI/RESNA Wheelchair Standards to Buy a Wheelchair. Paralyzed Veterans of America (PVA).

Deno JH, et al. 1992. Human Factors Design Guidelines for the Elderly and People with Disabilities. Honeywell, Inc., Minneapolis, Minn 55418 (Brian Isle, MN65-2300).

Hobson DA. 1990. Seating and mobility for the severely disabled. In R Smith, J Leslie (eds), Rehabilitation Engineering, pp 193–252. Boca Raton, Fla, CRC Press.

Jones D, Jones W. 1990. Criteria for selection of an augmentative communication system. In R Smith, J Leslie (eds), Rehabilitation Engineering, pp 181–189. Boca Raton, Fla, CRC Press.

Medhat M, Hobson D. 1992. Standardization of Terminology and Descriptive Methods for Specialized Seating. RESNA Press, RESNA, 1700 Moore St., Arlington, Va 22209-1903.

Smith RO. 1992. Technology and disability. AJOT 1(3):22.

Rehabilitation Technology Service Delivery—A Practical Guide. 1987. RESNA Press, RESNA, 1700 Moore St., Arlington, Va 22209-1903.

Society for Automotive Engineers. 1994. Wheelchair Tie-Down and Occupant Restraint Standard (committee draft). SAE. Warrendale, Pa.

Vanderheiden G, Vanderheiden K. 1991. Accessibility Design Guidelines for the Design of Consumer Products to Increase their Accessibility to People with Disabilities or Who Are Aging. Trace R&D Center, University of Wisconsin, Madison, Wisc.

Weisman G. 1990. Rehabilitation engineering in the workplace. In R Smith, J Leslie (eds), Rehabilitation Engineering, pp 253–297. Boca Raton, Fla, CRC Press.

Further Information

ABLEDATA, 8455 Colesville Rd., Suite 935, Silver Spring, Md. 20910-3319.

Historical Perspectives 4
Electromyography

Leslie A. Geddes
Purdue University

Early Investigations

The study of bioelectricity started with the Galvani-Volta controversy over the presence of electricity in frog muscle [see Geddes and Hoff, 1971]. Galvani likened the sciatic nerve–gastrocnemius muscle to a charged Leyden jar (capacitor) in which the nerve was the inner conductor and the surface of the muscle was the outer conductor. Therefore, Galvani thought that by joining the two with an arc of dissimilar metals, the biologic capacitor was discharged and the muscle twitched. Volta proved conclusively that it was the dissimilar metals in contact with tissue fluid that was the stimulus.

Interestingly, it was found that when the sciatic nerve of a nerve-muscle preparation was laid on the cut end of another frog muscle and the nerve was touched to the intact surface, the muscle of the nerve-muscle preparation twitched. Here was evidence of stimulation without metal conductors; this experiment was performed by Matteucci [1842].

With the first galvanometers, it was shown that current would be indicated when one electrode was placed on the cut end of a frog muscle and the other on the intact surface. This phenomenon became known as the *injury current* or *frog current,* the cut surface being negative to the intact surface.

Whereas the foregoing experiments showed that skeletal muscle possessed electricity, little was known about its relation to contraction. Matteucci [1842] conducted an ingenious experiment in which he placed the nerve of a second nerve-muscle preparation on the intact muscle of a first such preparation and stimulated the nerve of the first using an inductorium. He discovered that both muscles contracted. Here is the first evidence of the electric activity of contracting skeletal muscle.

Matteucci and DuBois-Reymond both found that the injury current disappeared when a muscle was contracted tetanically. This observation led directly to the concept of a resting membrane potential and its disappearance with activity [see Hoff and Geddes, 1957].

That human muscle, as well as frog muscle, produced electric activity was demonstrated by Du Bois-Reymond [1858] in the manner shown in Fig. HP4.1. With electrodes in saline cups connected to a galvanometer, Du Bois-Reymond stated that as soon as the fingers were placed in the cups, the galvanometer needle deflected, and it required some time for a position of equilibrium to be attained. Du Bois-Reymond [1858] stated:

> As soon as this state [equilibrium] is attained, the whole of the muscles of one of the arms must be so braced that an equilibrium may be established between the flexors and the extensors of all the articulations of the limb, pretty much as in a gymnastic school is usually done when one wants to let a person feel the development of one's muscles.
>
> As soon as this is done, the [galvanometer] needle is thrown into movement, its deflection being uniformly in such a sense as to indicate in the braced arm "an inverse current," accord-

0-8493-8346-3/95/$0.00+$.50
© 1995 by CRC Press, Inc.

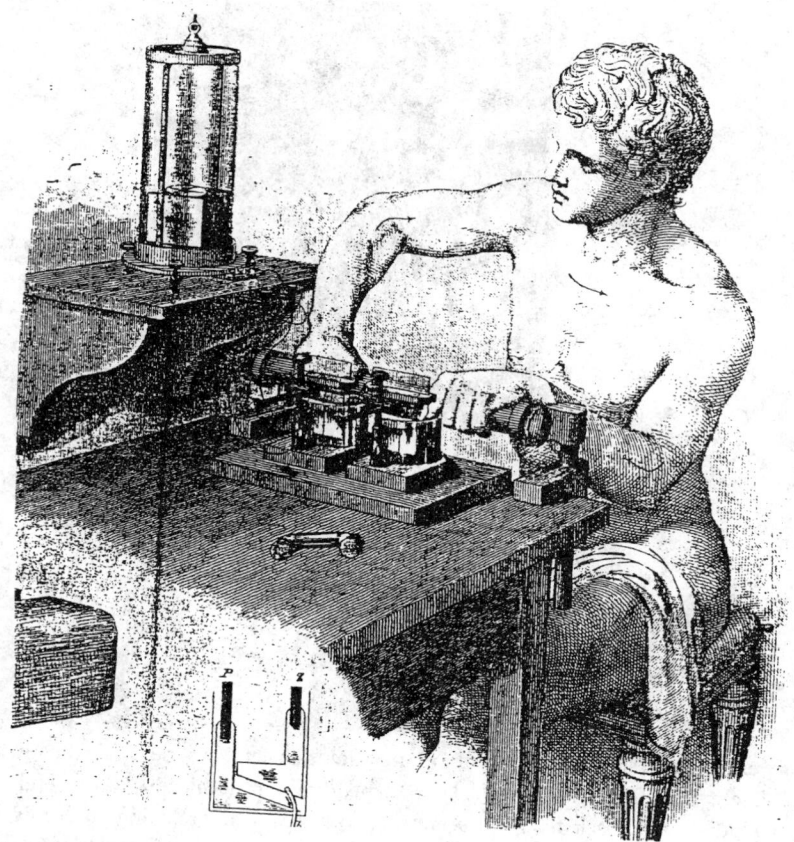

FIGURE HP4.1 The first evidence that contracting skeletal muscle in man produces an electrical signal. (From Du Bois-Reymond [1858].)

ing to Nobili's nomenclature; that is to say, a current passing from the hand to the shoulder. The braced arm then acts the part of the copper in the compound arc of zinc and copper mentioned above. [Du Bois-Reymond was referring to the polarity of a voltaic cell in which zinc and copper are the positive and negative electrodes, respectively.]

The rheotome and slow-speed galvanometer were used to reconstruct the muscle action potential. However, it was desired to know the time course of the electric change associated with a single muscle contraction (twitch), as well as its relationship to the electrical event (action potential). A second item of interest was the so-called latent period, that time between the stimulus and the onset of muscle contraction, which Helmholtz [1853] reported to be 10 ms for frog muscle.

Waller [1887] set himself the task of measuring the latent period and the relationship between the action potential and the force developed by frog gastrocnemius muscle in response to a single stimulus. He found that the onset of the twitch was later than the onset of the action potential, as shown in Fig. HP4.2. However, the true form of the muscle action potential and its relationship to the onset of the twitch had to await the development of the micropipet electrode, the vacuum-tube amplifier, and the cathode-ray oscilloscope. In 1957, Hodgkin and Horowicz [1957] recorded the twitch and action potential of a single muscle fiber of the frog. Figure HP4.3 is a copy of their record. Note that the onset of the action potential precedes the onset of muscle contraction by about 4 ms. We now know that it is the action potential that triggers the release of mechanical energy.

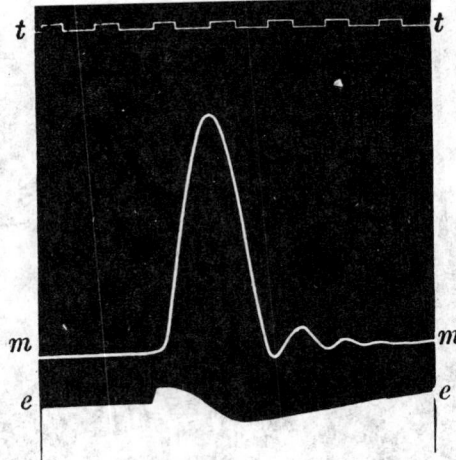

FIGURE HP4.2 Relationship between the twitch (recorded with a myograph, *m*) and the action potential (recorded with a capillary electrometer, *e*) of a frog gastrocnemius muscle. The time marks (*t*) are 1/20 s. (From Waller [1887].)

Clinical Electromyography

It was well known that when a nerve that innervates a skeletal muscle is cut, the muscle is paralyzed immediately; however, days to weeks later (depending on the species), on careful visual examination, the individual muscle fibers are seen to be contracting and relaxing randomly, i.e., fibrillating. The first to bring the facts together regarding normal muscle action potentials and denervation-fibrillation potentials were Denny-Brown and Pennybacker in the United Kingdom [1939]; the date and locale are highly significant. They distinguished between involuntary twitching of innervated muscle and fibrillation of denervated muscle by recording both the electric and mechanical activity of muscles. Two instrumental advances made their study possible: (1) the use of a hypodermic

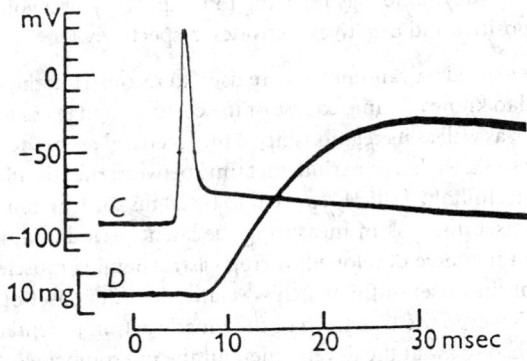

FIGURE HP4.3 The relationship between the muscle action potential and the force of contraction in a single skeletal muscle fiber in the frog. (From Hodgkin and Horowicz [1957].)

needle electrode inserted into the muscle and (2) the use of a rapidly responding, mirror-type photographic recorder, the Matthews [1928] oscillograph.

The cathode-ray tube was not generally available in the United Kingdom when Matthews [1928] constructed his moving-tongue mirror oscillograph. The device consisted of a piece of soft iron mounted on a steel leaf spring, as shown in Fig. HP4.4. A strong electromagnet attracted the soft iron, which bent the steel (leaf-spring) support. Two coils mounted on the pole faces were connected to the output tubes of a five-stage, single-sided, resistance-capacitance coupled amplifier. The amplified potentials altered the current in the electromagnet coils, causing more or less bending of the leaf spring, thereby tilting the mirror mounted on the leaf spring and permitting photographic recording of action potentials.

With the Matthews oscillograph, Denny-Brown and Pennybacker [1939] laid the foundation for clinical electromyography when they reported as follows:

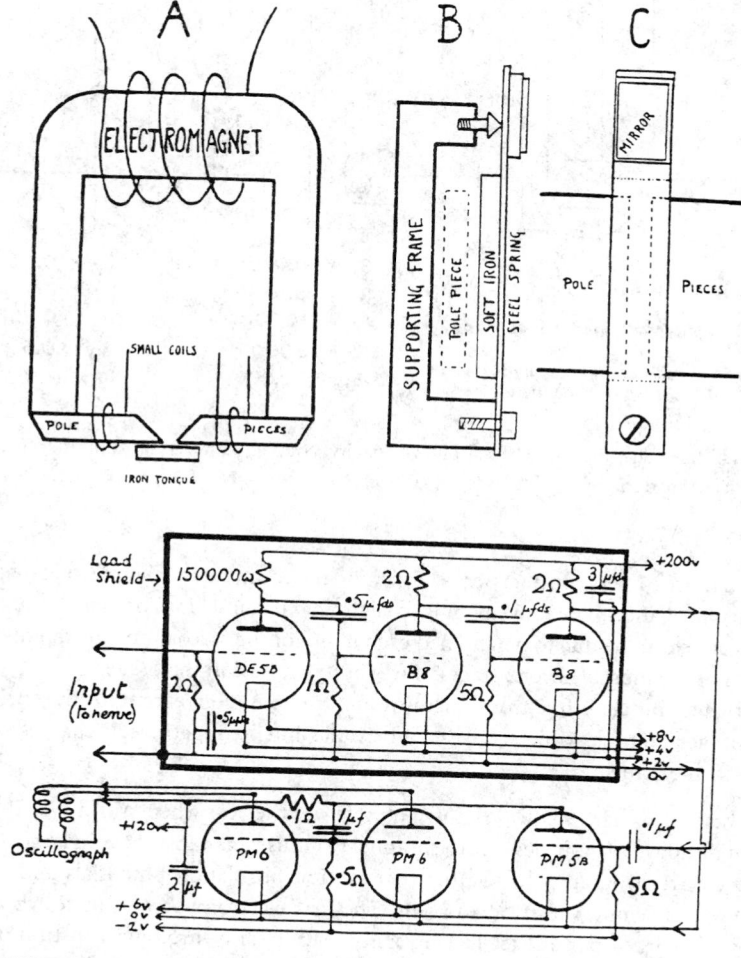

FIGURE HP4.4 The Matthews moving-tongue oscillograph and amplifier used with it. The electromagnetic coil (*A*) provided an attractive force on the tongue (soft iron and steel spring); the signal current applied to the small coils aided or opposed this force and caused the tongue to bend more or less and hence move the mirror which reflected a beam of light on to a recording surface. (From BHC Matthews, 1928, J. Physiol (Lond) 65:225, with permission.)

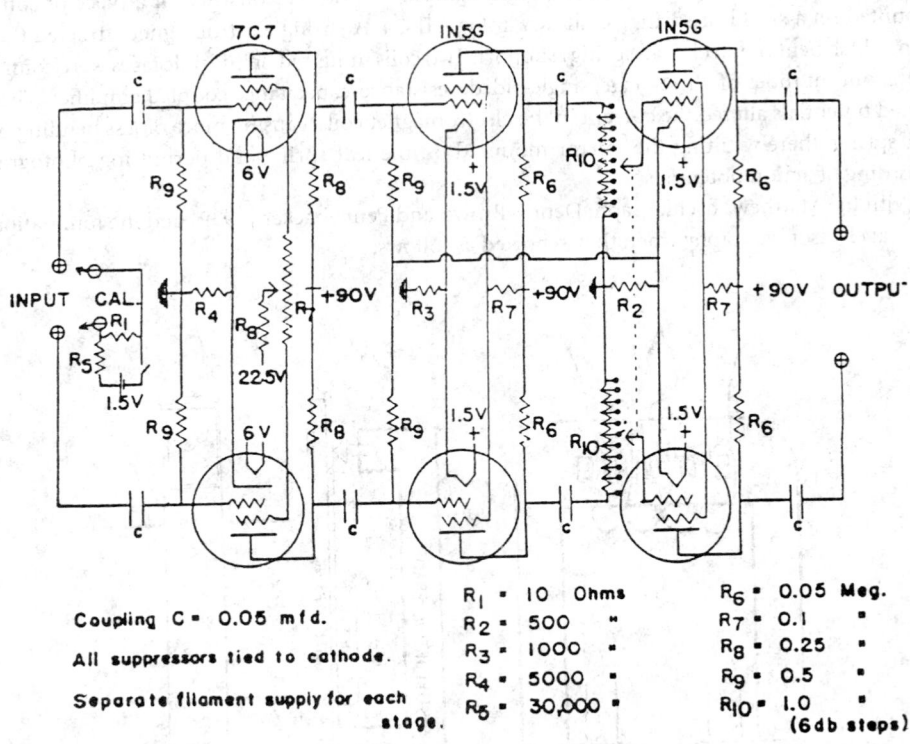

FIGURE HP4.5   The three-stage resistance-capacity coupled differential amplifier used is the RCAMC electromyography. (From Jasper et al. [1945].)

Denervated muscle fibers contract periodically, and the confused medley of small twitches constitutes true fibrillation. The movement is so slight that it can seldom be seen in the clinic. The twitchings appear to be due to heightened excitability of the sarcolemma or rapidly conducting portion of the muscle fibre to traces of free acetylcholine in the tissues.

Reinnervated muscle is free from such involuntary excitation, except for the curious "contracture" of facial muscle, which consists of periodic, intense repetitive discharges which suggest a central mechanism.

Earlier it was stated that 1939 was significant; this was the year when World War II broke out in Europe. Soon motor nerve injuries due to shrapnel wounds began to appear in large numbers, and the need for electromyography to identify denervation fibrillation potentials and their gradual disappearance with reinnervation was urgent. The first electromyograph in North America was developed by Herbert Jasper at McGill University (Montreal Neurological Institute). Starting in 1942, design concepts were developed, and by 1944, prototypes had been built and used clinically. In his report to the Committee on Army Medical Research, Capt. Jasper [1945] stated:

The present equipment has been developed over a period of about 18 months experimentation with different designs of electromyograph for use on hospital wards. Numerous modifications of design have been incorporated in the present model in order to provide simplicity of operation, portability, freedom from electrical interference, and perfection of both the audible and visible analysis of the electrical activity of normal and diseased muscles.

A portable clinical electromyograph has been developed which has proven to be practical in operation on hospital wards to aid in the diagnosis and prognosis of muscles paralyzed by traumatic injuries of their nerve supply. Four complete units have been constructed for use in Special Centers for the treatment of nerve injuries.

The Royal Canadian Army Medical Corps (RCAMC) electromyograph had many unique design features that were incorporated in all later commercially available electromyographs. It consisted of three units, a small battery-operated three-stage differential amplifier (Fig. HP4.5) and an oscilloscope (Fig. HP4.6), both placed on a loudspeaker cabinet on rubber-wheel casters (Fig. HP4.7). Thus simultaneous visual display and aural monitoring of normal motor units and fibrillation potentials was possible.

The preamplifier (Fig. HP4.5) was very carefully constructed, the input tubes being supported by rubber-mounted antimicrophonic sockets. The grid resistors (R9) and plate resistors (R8) were wire wound and carefully matched. A high common-mode rejection ratio was obtained by matching the input tubes and adjustment of the potentiometer (R7) in the screen-grid supply. A common-mode rejection ratio in excess of 10,000 was easily achieved. The overall frequency response extended from 3 to 10,000 Hz.

The cathode-ray oscilloscope (Fig. HP4.6) was of unusual design for that time because the sweep velocity was independent of the number of sweeps per second, a feature to appear much later in

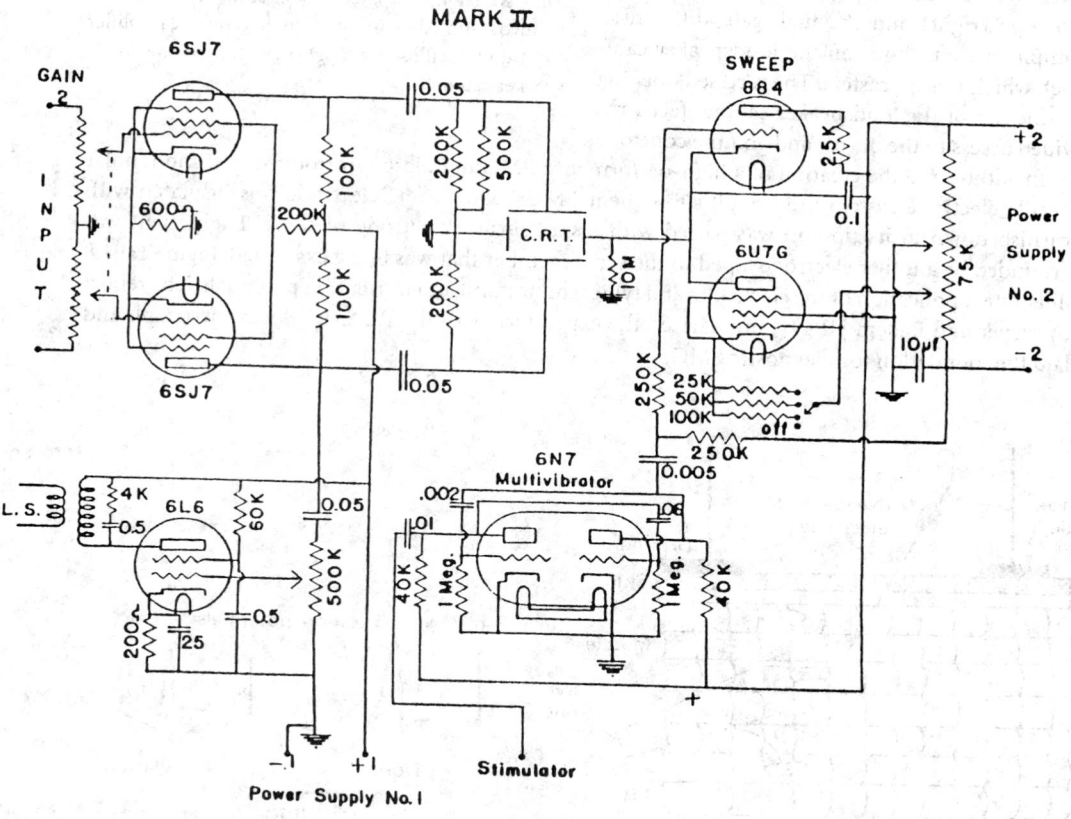

FIGURE HP4.6 The oscilloscope, loudspeaker amplifier, and stimulator unit of the RCAMC electromyograph. (From Jasper et al. [1945].)

oscilloscopes. A linear sweep (time base) was obtained by charging a capacitor (0.1 μF) through a pentode (6U7G) which acted as a constant-current device. The sweep was initiated at a rate of about 7 times per second by the multivibrator (6N7), which also provided an output to enable stimulating a nerve, the stimulus occurring at the beginning of each sweep, thereby permitting nerve conduction–time measurements. The oscilloscope also contained the audio amplifier (6L6). The cathode-ray tube had a short-persistence, blue-white phosphor that produced brilliant blue-white images of remarkable clarity. A camera was used to obtain photographic records of the waveforms, which were optimized by listening to them via the loudspeaker (as advocated by Adrian) as the needle electrode was being inserted and adjusted. Fig. HP4.8 illustrates typical action potentials.

At the end of the war (1945), oscilloscopes became available, and Fig. HP4.7 shows the RCAMC electromyograph with a Cossor oscilloscope (right) and the high-gain differential amplifier (left), both on the loudspeaker cabinet, which was on casters. The recessed opening at the top of the loudspeaker cabinet face provided access to the on-off and volume controls.

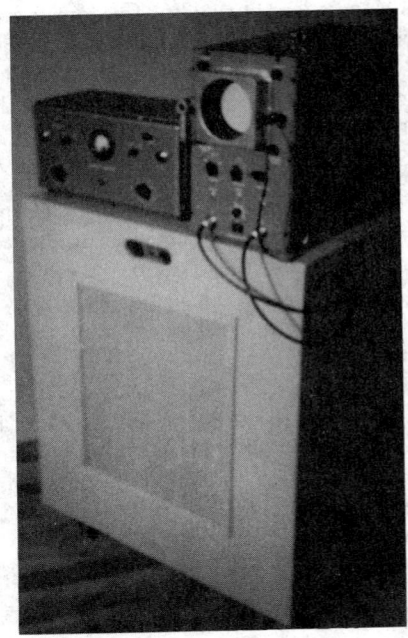

FIGURE HP4.7   A later version of the RCAMC electromyograph showing the high-gain preamplifier (*left*) and oscilloscope (*right*) on top of the loudspeaker cabinet.

In addition to the creation of a high-performance EMG unit, Jasper introduced the monopolar needle electrode system used in all subsequent EMGs. The needle electrode was insulated with varnish down to its tip and was paired with a skin surface electrode of silver. The patient was grounded by another electrode taped to the same member that was being examined. Figure HP4.8 illustrates application of the electrodes and typical motor unit and fibrillation potentials. The report by Jasper and Ballem [1949] summarized the experience with the RCAMC electromyograph and laid the foundation for diagnostic EMG.

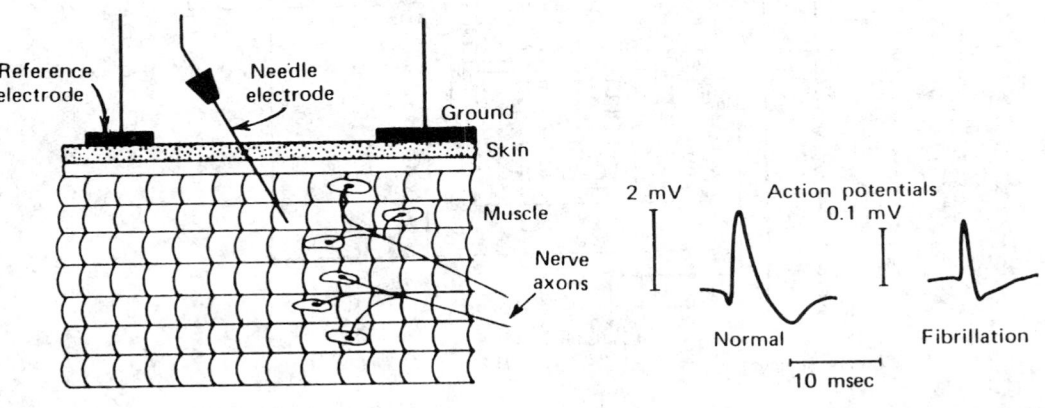

FIGURE HP4.8   Electrode arrangement and action potentials with the RCAMC electromyograph. (Redrawn from Jasper and Ballem [1949].)

World War II ended in 1945, after which electromyographs became available commercially. Their features were essentially the same as those embodied in the RCAMC electromyograph. From the beginning, these units were completely power-line-operated, the author's master's thesis describing the first of these units.

References

Denny-Brown D, Pennybacker JB. 1939. Fibrillation and fasciculation in voluntary muscle. Brain 61:311.

Du Bois-Reymond E. 1858. Untersuchungen uber thierische Elektricitat. Moleschott's Untersuch. Z Natur Mensch 4:1.

Geddes LA, Hoff HE. 1971. The discovery of bioelectricity and current electricity (the Galvani-Volta controversy). IEEE Spect 8(12):38.

Helmholtz H. 1853. On the methods of measuring very small portions of time and their application to physiological purposes. Philos Mag J Sci 6:313.

Hodgkin AL, Horowicz P. 1957. The differential action of hypertonic solutions on the twitch and action potential of a muscle fiber. J Physiol (Lond) 136:17P.

Hoff HE, Geddes LA. 1957. The rheotome and its prehistory: A study in the historical interrelation of electrophysiology and electromechanics. Bull Hist Med 31(3):212.

Jasper HH, Ballem G. 1949. Unipolar electromyograms of normal and denervated human muscle. J Neurophysiol 12:231.

Jasper HH. 1945. The RCAMC electromyograph, Mark II. With the technical assistance of Lt. RH Johnston and LA Geddes. Report submitted to the Associate Committee on Army Medical Research, National Research Council of Canada, 27 April 1945.

Matteucci C. 1842. Deuxieme memoire sur le courant electrique propre de la grenouille et sur celui des animaux a sang chaud. Ann Dhim Phys 3S(6):301.

Matthews BHC. 1928. A new electrical recording system for physiological work. J Physiol (Lond) 65:225.

Waller AD. 1887. A demonstration on man of electromotive changes accompanying the heart's beat. J Physiol (Lond) 8:229.

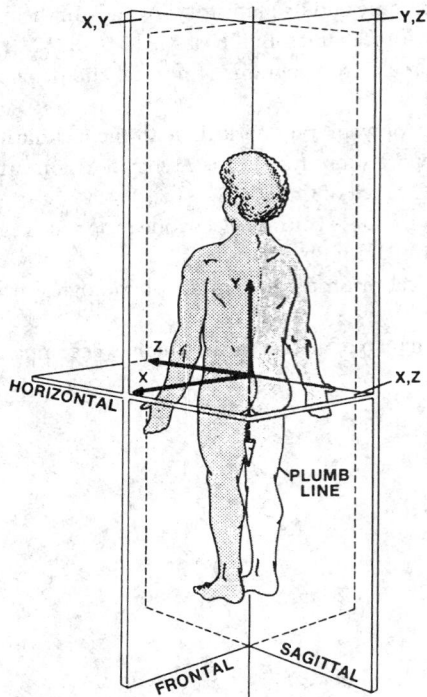

Planes and axes illustrated for human anatomic position.

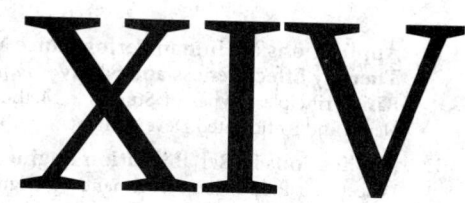

Human Performance Engineering

George V. Kondraske
University of Texas at Arlington

T HE ULTIMATE GOAL OF HUMAN performance engineering is enhancement of the performance and safety of humans in the execution of tasks. The field (in a more formalized sense) was fueled initially by military applications but has become an important component in industrial settings as well. In a biomedical engineering context, the scope of definition applied to the term *human* not only encompasses individuals with capabilities that differ from those of a typical healthy individual in many possible different ways (e.g., individuals who are disabled, injured, unusually endowed, etc.) but also includes those who are "healthy" (e.g., health care professionals). Consequently, one finds a wide range of problems in which human performance engineering and associated methods are employed. Some examples include

- Evaluation of individual's performance capacities for determining the efficacy of new therapeutic interventions or so-called level of disability for worker's compensation and other medical-legal purposes.
- Design of assistive devices and/or work sites in such a way that a person with some deficiency in his or her "performance resource file" will be able to accomplish specified goals.
- Design of operator interfaces for medical instruments that promote efficient, safe, and error-free use.

In basic terms, each of these situations involves one or more of the following: (1) a human, (2) a task or tasks, and (3) the interface of a human and task(s). Human performance engineering emphasizes concepts, methods, and tools that strive toward treatment of each of these areas with the engineering rigor that is routinely applied to artificial systems (e.g., mechanical, electronic, etc.). Importance is thus placed on models (a combination of cause-and-effect and statistical), measurements (of varying degrees of sophistication that are selected to fit needs of a particular circumstance), and various types of analyses. Whereas many specialty areas within biomedical engineering begin with an emphasis on a specific subsystem and then proceed to deal with it at lower levels of detail (sometimes even at the molecular level) to determine how it functions and often why it malfunctions, human performance engineering emphasizes subsystems and their performance capacities (i.e., *how well* a system functions), the integration of these into a whole and their interactions, and their operation in the execution of tasks that are of ultimate concern to humans. These include tasks of daily living, work, and recreation. In recent years, there has been an increased concern with medical communities on issues such as quality of life, treatment outcome measures, and treatment cost-effectiveness. By linking human subsystems into the "whole" and discovering objective quantitative relationships between the human and tasks, human performance engineering can play an important role in addressing these and other related concerns.

Human performance engineering combines knowledge, concepts, and methods from across many disciplines (e.g., biomechanics, neuroscience, psychology, physiology, and many others) which, in their overlapping aspect, all deal with similar problems. Among current difficulties is that these wide-ranging efforts are not linked by a conceptual framework that is commonly employed across contributing disciplines. In fact, few candidate frameworks exist even within the relevant disciplines. One attempt to provide some unification and commonality is presented in Chapter 143 as basis for readers to integrate material in subsequent chapters. In a further attempt to enhance continuity across this section, chapter authors have been requested to consider this perspective and to incorporate basic concepts and terms where applicable.

Chapters 144 through 146 look "toward the human" and focus on measurement of human performance capacities and related issues. Owing to a combination of the complexity of the human system (even when viewed as a collection of rather high-level subsystems) and limited space available, treatment is not comprehensive. For example, measurement of sensory performance capacities (e.g., tactile, visual, auditory) is not included in this first edition. Both systems and tasks can be viewed at various hierarchical levels. Chapters 144 and 145 focus on a rather "low" systems level and discuss basic functional units such as actuator, processor, and memory systems. Chapter 146 moves to a more intermediate level, where speech, postural control, gait, and hand-eye coordination systems could be considered. Measurement of structural parameters, which play important roles in many analyses, also is not allocated the separate chapter it deserves (as a minimum) due to space limitations. Chapters 147 and 148 then shift focus to consider the analysis of different types of tasks in a similar, representative fashion.

Chapters 149 through 153 are included to provide insight into a representative selection of application types. Space constraints, the complexity of human performance, and the great variety of tasks that can be considered limit the level of detail with which such material can reasonably be presented. Work in all application areas will begin to benefit from emerging computer-based tools, which is the theme of Chapter 154. The section concludes with a look to the future (Chapter 155) that summarizes selected current limitations, identifies some specific research and development needs, and speculates regarding the nature of some anticipated developments.

Many have contributed their talents to this exciting field in terms of both research and applications, yet much remains to be done. I am indebted to the authors not only for their contributions and cooperation during the preparation of this section but also for their willingness to accept the burdens of communicating complex subject matter reasonably, selectively, and as accurately as possible within the imposed constraints.

143

A Working Model for Human System–Task Interfaces

George V. Kondraske
University of Texas at Arlington

Humans are complex systems. Our natural interest in ourselves and things that we do has given rise to the study of this complex system at every conceivable level ranging from genetic, through cellular and organ systems, to interactions of the total human with the environment in the conduct of purposeful activities. At each level, there are corresponding practitioners who attempt to discover and rectify or prevent problems at the respective level. Some practitioners are concerned with specific individuals, while others (e.g., biomedical scientists and product designers) address populations as a whole. Problems dealt with span medical and nonmedical contexts, often with interaction between the two. Models play a key role not only in understanding the key issues at each level but also in describing relationships between various levels and providing frameworks that allow practitioners to obtain reasonably predictable results in a systematic and efficient fashion. In this chapter, a working model for human system-task interfaces is presented. Any such model must, of course, not only consider the interface per se but also representations of the human system and tasks. The model presented here, the *elemental resource model* (ERM), represents the most recent effort in a relatively small family of models that attempt to address similar needs.

143.1 Background

The interface between a human and a task of daily living (e.g., work, recreation, or other) represents a level that is quite high in the hierarchy noted above. One way in which to summarize previous efforts directed at this level, across various application contexts, is to recognize two different lines along which study has evolved: (1) *bottom-up* and (2) *top-down*. Taken together, these relative terms imply a focus of interest at a particular level of convergence, which, here, is the human-task interface level. It is emphasized that these terms are used here to characterize the general course of development and not specific approaches applied at a particular instant in time. A broad view is necessary to grapple with the many previous efforts that either are, or could be, construed to be pertinent.

The biomedical community has approached the human-task interface largely along the bottom-up path. This is not surprising given the historical evolution of interest first in anatomy (human structure) and then physiology (function). The introduction of chemistry, giving rise to biochemistry, and the refinement of the microscope provided motivations to include even lower hierarchical levels of inquiry and of a substantially different character. Models in this broad bottom-up category begin with *anatomic components* and include muscles, nerves, tendons (or subcomponents thereof), or subsets of organs (e.g., heart, lungs, vasculature, etc.). They often focus on relationships between components and exhibit a scope that stays within the confines of the human system. Many cause-and-effect models have been developed at these lower levels for specific purposes (e.g., to understand lines of action of muscle forces and their changes during motion about a given joint).

As a natural consequence of linkages that occur between hierarchical levels and our tendency to utilize that which exists, consideration of an issue at any selected level (in this case, the human-task interface level) brings into consideration *all lower levels* and all models that have been put forth with the stated purpose of understanding problems or behaviors at the original level of focus. The amount of detail that is appropriate or required at these original, lower levels results in great complexity when applied to the total human at the human-task interface level. In addition, many lower-level modeling efforts (even those which are quantitative) are aimed primarily at obtaining a basic scientific understanding of human physiology or specific pathologies (i.e., pertaining to *populations* of humans). In such circumstances, highly specialized, invasive, and cumbersome laboratory procedures for obtaining the necessary data to populate models are justified. However, it is difficult and sometimes impossible to obtain data describing *a specific individual* to utilize in analyses when such models are extended to the human-task interface level. Another result of drawing lower-level models (and their approaches) into the human-task interface context is that the results have a specific and singular character (e.g., biomechanical versus neuromuscular control versus psychologic, etc.) [e.g., Card et al., 1986; Delp et al., 1990; Gottlieb et al., 1989; Hemami, 1988; Schoner & Kelso, 1988]. Models that incorporate most or all of the multiple aspects of the human system or frameworks for integrating multiple lower-level modeling approaches have been lacking. Lower-level models that serve meaningful purposes at the original level of focus have provided and will continue to provide insights into specific issues related to human performance at multiple levels of consideration. However, their direct extension to serve general needs at the human-task interface level has inherent problems; a different approach is suggested.

A top-down progression can be observed over the major history in human factors/ergonomic [Gilbreth & Gilbreth, 1917; Taylor, 1911] and vocational assessment [e.g., Botterbusch, 1987] fields (although the former has more recently emphasized a "human-centered" concept with regard to design applications). In contrast to the bottom-up path, in which anatomic components form the initial basis of modeling efforts, the focus along the top-down developmental path begins with consideration of the *task or job* that is to be performed by the total human. The great variety in the full breadth of activities in which humans can be engaged gives rise to one aspect of complexity at this level that pertains to taxonomies for job and task classification [e.g., Fleishman & Quaintance, 1984; Meister, 1989; U.S. Department of Labor, 1992]. Another enigmatic aspect that quickly adds complexity with respect to modeling concerns the appropriate level to be used to dissect the items at the highest level (e.g., jobs) into lower-level components (e.g., tasks and subtasks). In fact, the choice of level is complicated by the fact that no clear definition has evolved for a set of levels from which to choose.

After progressing through various levels at which all model elements represent tasks and are completely outside the confines of the human body, a level is eventually reached where one encounters the human. Attempts to go further have been motivated, for example, by desires to predict performance of a human in a given task (e.g., lifting an object, assembling a product, etc.) from a set of measures that characterizes the human. From the human-task interface, difficulty is encountered with regard to the strategy for approaching a system as complex, multifaceted, and multipurpose as a human [Fleishman & Quaintance, 1984; Wickens, 1984]. In essence, the full scope of options that have emerged from the bottom-up development path is now encountered from the opposite direction. Options range from relatively gross analyses (e.g., estimates of the "fraction" of a task that is physical or mental) to those which are much more detailed and quantitative. The daunting prospect of considering a "comprehensive quantitative model" has led to approaches and models, argued to be "more practical," in which sets of parameters are often selected in a somewhat mysterious fashion based on experience (including previous research) and intuition. The selected parameters are then used to develop predictive models, most of which have been based primarily on statistical methods (i.e., regression models) [Fleishman, 1967; Fleishman & Quaintance, 1984]. Although the basic modeling tools depend only on correlation, it is usually possible to envision a causal link between the independent variables selected (e.g., visual acuity) and the dependent variable to be predicted (e.g., piloting an aircraft). Models (one per task) are then tested in a given population and graded with regard to their prediction ability, the best of which have performed marginally [Kondraske, 1994]. Another characteristic associated with many of the statistically based modeling efforts from the noted communities is the almost exclusive use of healthy, "normal" subjects for model development (i.e., humans with impairments were excluded). Homogeneity is a requirement of such statistical models, leading to the need for one model per task per population (at best). Also, working with a mindset that considers only normal subjects can be observed to skew estimates regarding which of the many parameters that one might choose for incorporation in a model are "most important." The relatively few exceptions that employ cause-and-effect models (e.g., based on physical laws) at some level of fidelity [e.g., Chaffin & Andersonn, 1984] often adopt methods that have emerged from the bottom-up path and are, as noted above, limited in character at the "total human" level (e.g., "biomechanical" in the example cited).

It is critical to note that the issue is *not* that no useful models have emerged from previous efforts but rather that no clear comprehensive strategy has emerged for modeling at the human-task interface level. A fairly recent National Research Council panel on human performance modeling [Baron et al., 1990] considered the fundamental issues discussed here and also underscored needs for models at the human-task interface level. While it was concluded that an all-inclusive model might be desirable (i.e., high fidelity, in the sense that biomechanical, information processing, sensory and perceptual aspects, etc. are represented), such a model was characterized as being highly unlikely to achieve and perhaps ultimately not useful because it would be overly complex for many applications. The basic recommendation made by this panel was to pursue development of more limited scope submodels. The implication is that two or more submodels could be integrated to achieve a broader range of fidelity, with the combination selected to meet the needs of particular situations. The desire to "divide efforts" due to inherent complexity of the problem also surfaces within the histories of the bottom-up and top-down development paths discussed above. While a reasonable concept in theory, one component in the division of effort that has consistently been underrepresented is the part that ties together the so-called submodels. Without a conceptual framework for integration of relatively independent modeling efforts and a set of common modeling constructs, prospects for long-term progress are difficult to envision. This, along with the recognition that enough work had been undertaken in the submodel areas so that key issues and common denominators could be identified, motivated development of the ERM.

The broad objectives of the ERM are most like those of Fleishman and colleagues [Fleishman, 1966, 1972, 1982; Fleishman & Quaintance, 1984], whose efforts in human performance are generally well known in many disciplines. These are the only two efforts known that (1) focus on the total human in a task situation (i.e., directly address the human-task interface level); (2) consider tasks in general, and not only a specific task such as gait, lifting, reading, etc.; (3) incorporate all aspects of the total human system (e.g., sensory, biomechanical, information processing, etc.); and (4) aim at quantitative models. There are also some similarities with regard to the incorporation of the ideas of "abilities" (of humans) and "requirements" (of tasks). The work of Fleishman and colleagues has thus been influential in shaping the ERM either directly or indirectly through its influence of others. However, there are several substantive conceptual differences that have resulted in considerably different end-points. Fleishman's work emerged from "the task" perspective and is rooted in psychology, whereas the ERM emerges from the perspective of "human system architecture" and is rooted in engineering methodology with regard to quantitative aspects of system performance but also incorporates psychology *and* physiology. Both approaches address humans *and* tasks, and both efforts contain aspects identifiable with psychology and engineering, as they ultimately must. These different perspectives, however, may explain in part some of the major differences. Aspects unique to the ERM include (1) its basis on modeling and measurement of *all* aspects of a system's performance using resource constructs, (2) the use of cause-and-effect resource economic principles (i.e., the idea of threshold "costs" for achieving a given level of performance in any given high-level task), (3) the concept of monadology (i.e., the use of a finite set of "elements" to explain a complex phenomenon), and (4) a consistent strategy for identifying performance elements at different hierarchical levels.

The ERM attempts to provide a quantitative and relatively straightforward framework for characterizing the human system, tasks, and the interface of the human to tasks. It depends in large part on, and evolves directly from, a separate body of material referred to collectively as *general systems performance theory* (GSPT). GSPT was developed first and independently, i.e., removed from the human system context. It incorporates resource constructs exclusively for modeling of the abstract idea of *system performance*, including specific rules for measuring performance resource availability and resource economic principles to provide a cause-and-effect analysis of the interface of any system (e.g., humans) to tasks. The concept of a *performance model* is emphasized and distinguished from other model types.

143.2 Basic Principles

The history of the ERM and the context in which it was developed are described elsewhere [Kondraske, 1987a, 1990b, 1994]. It is important to note that the ERM is derived from the combination of GSPT with the philosophy of monadology and their application to the human system. As such, these two constituents are briefly reviewed before presenting and discussing the actual ERM.

General Systems Performance Theory

The concept of performance now pervades all aspects of life, especially decision-making processes that involve both human and artificial systems. Yet it has not been well understood theoretically, and systematic techniques for modeling and its measurement have been lacking. While a considerable body of material applicable to general systems theory exists, the concept of performance has not been incorporated in it, nor has performance been addressed in a general fashion elsewhere. Most of the knowledge that exists regarding performance and its quantitative treatment has evolved within individual application contexts, where generalizations can easily be elusive.

Performance is multifaceted, pertaining to how well a given system executes an intended function and the various factors that contribute to this. It differs from behavior of a system in that "the best of something" is implied. The broad objectives of GSPT are

1. To provide a common conceptual basis for defining and measuring all aspects of the performance of any system.
2. To provide a common conceptual basis for the analysis of any task in a manner that facilitates system-task interface assessments and decision making.
3. To identify cause-and-effect principles, or laws, that explain what occurs when any given system is used to accomplish any given task.

While GSPT was motivated by needs in situations where the human is "the system" of interest and it was first presented in this context [Kondraske, 1987a], application of it has been extended to the context of artificial systems. These experiences range from computer vision and sensor fusion [Yen & Kondraske, 1992] to robotics [Kondraske & Khoury, 1992; Kondraske & Standridge, 1988].

A succint statement of GSPT designed to emphasize key constructs is presented below in a step-like format. The order of steps is intended to suggest how one might approach any system or system-task interface situation to apply GSPT. While somewhat terse and "to-the-point," it is nonetheless an essential prerequisite for a reasonably complete understanding the ERM.

1. Within a domain of interest, select any level of abstraction and identify the system(s) of interest (i.e., the physical structure) and its function (i.e., purpose).

2. Consider "the system" and "the task" separately.

3. Use a resource construct to model the system's *performance*. First, consider the unique intangible qualities that characterize *how well a system executes its function*. Each of these is considered to represent a unique performance resource associated with a specific *dimension of performance* (e.g., speed, accuracy, stability, smoothness, "friendliness," etc.) of that system. Each performance resource is recognized as a *desirable* item (e.g., endurance versus fatigue, accuracy versus error, etc.) "possessed" by the system in a certain quantitative amount. Thus one can consider *quantifying* the amount of given *quality* available. As illustrated, an important consequence of using the resource construct at this stage is that confusion associated with duality of terms is eliminated.

4. Looking toward the system, identify all I dimensions of performance associated with it. In situations where the system does not yet exist (i.e., design contexts), it is helpful to note that dimensions of performance of the system are the same as those of the task.

5a. Keeping the resource construct in mind, define a parameterized metric for each dimension of performance (e.g., speed, accuracy, etc.). If the resource construct is followed, values will be produced with these metrics that are always nonnegative. Furthermore, a larger numeric value will consistently represent *more* of a given resource and therefore *more performance capacity*.

5b. Measure system performance with the system *removed from* the specific intended task. This is a reinforcement of Step 2. The general strategy is to *maximally stress* the system (within limits of comfort and/or safety, when appropriate) to define its *performance envelope*, or more specifically, the envelope that defines *performance resource availability*, $R_{AS}(t)$. Note that $R_{AS}(t)$ is a continuous surface in the system's nonnegative, multidimensional performance space. Also note that unless all dimensions of performance and parameterized metrics associated with each are defined using the resource construct, a performance envelope cannot be guaranteed. Addressing the issue of measurement more specifically, consider resource availability values $R_{A_i}|_{Q_{i,k}}(t)$ for $i = 1$ to I, associated with each of the I dimensions of performance. Here, each $\mathbf{Q}_{i,k}$ represents a unique condition, in terms of a set of values R_i along *other* identified dimensions of performance, under which a specific resource availability (R_{A_i}) is measured; i.e., $\mathbf{Q}_{i,k} = \{R_{1,k}, R_{2,k}, \ldots, R_{p,k}\}$ for all $p \neq i$ ($1 \geq p \geq I$). The subscript k is used to distinguish several possible conditions under which a given resource availability (R_{A_1}, for example) can be measured. These values are measured using a set of "test tasks," each of which is designed to *maximally stress* the system (within limits of comfort and/or safety, when appropriate): (a) along each dimension of performance individually (where $\mathbf{Q}_{i,k} = \mathbf{Q}_{i,0} = \{0,0,\ldots,0\}$) or (b) along selected subsets of dimensions of performance simultaneously (i.e., $\mathbf{Q}_{i,k} = \mathbf{Q}_{i,n}$, where each possible $\mathbf{Q}_{i,n}$ has one or more nonzero elements). The points obtained $[R_{A_i}|_{Q_{i,k}}(t)]$ provide the basis to estimate the performance envelope $R_{AS}(t)$. Note that if only on-axis points are obtained (e.g., maximally stress one specific performance resource availability with minimal or no stress on other performance resources, or the $\mathbf{Q}_{i,0}$ condition), a rectangular or idealized performance envelope is obtained. A more accurate representation, which would be contained within the idealized envelope, can be obtained at the expense of making additional measurements or the use of known mathematic functions based on previous studies that define the shape of envelope in two or more dimensions.

5c. Define estimates of single-number *system figures-of-merit*, or *composite performance capac-ities*, as the mathematical product of all or any selected subset of $R_{A_i}|_{Q_{i,0}}(t)$. If more accuracy is desired and a sufficient number of data points is available from the measurement process described in Step 5b, composite performance capacities can be determined by integration over $R_{AS}(t)$ to determine the volume enclosed by the envelope. The composite performance capacity is a measure of performance at a higher level of abstraction than any individual di-mension of performance at the "system" level, representing the capacity of the system to per-form tasks that place demands on *those performance resources availabilities included in the cal-culation*. Different composite performance capacities can be computed for a given system by selecting different combinations of dimensions of performance. Note that the definition of a composite performance capacity used here preserves dimensionality; e.g., if speed and accu-racy dimensions are included in the calculation, the result has units of speed $\times$ accuracy. (This step is used only when needed, e.g., when two general-purpose systems of the same type are to be compared. However, if decision making that involves the interface of a specific sys-tem to a specific task is the issue at hand, a composite performance capacity is generally of any use only to *rule out* candidates).

6. Assess the "need for detail." This amounts to a determination of the number of hierarchical levels included in the analysis. If the need is to determine if the currently identified "system" can work in the given task or how well it can execute its function, go to Step 7 now. If the need is to determine the *contribution of one or more constituent subsystems* or why a desired level of performance is not achieved at the system level, repeat Steps 1 to 5 for all J functional units (subsystems), or a selected subset thereof based on need, that form the system that was orig-inally identified in Step 1; i.e., go to the next-lowest hierarchical level.

7. At the "system" level, look toward the task(s) of interest. Measure, estimate, or calculate *demands* on system performance resources (e.g., the speed, accuracy, etc. required), $R_{D_i}|_{Q'_{i,k}}(t)$, where the notation here is analogous to that employed in Step 5b. This represents the quanti-tative definition and communication of *goals*, or the set of values P_{HLT} representing level of per-formance P desired in a specific high-level task (*HLT*). Use a worst-case or other less-conservative strategy (with due consideration of the impact of this choice) to summarize variations over time. This will result in a set of M points (R_{D_m}, for $m = 1$ to M) that lie in the multidimensional space defined by the set of I dimensions of performance. Typically, $M \geq I$.

8. Use *resource economic principles* (i.e., require $R_A \geq R_D$ for "success") at the system level *and* at all system-task interfaces at the subsystem level (if included) to evaluate success/failure at each interface. More specifically, for a given system-task interface, all task demand points (i.e., the set of R_{D_m} associated with a given task or subtask) must lie within the performance resource envelope $R_{AS}(t)$ of the corresponding system. This is the key law that governs system-task interfaces. If a two-level model is used (i.e., "system" and "subsystem" levels are incor-porated), map system-level demands to demands on constituent subsystems. That is, functional relationships between P_{HLT} and demands imposed on constituent subsystems [i.e., $R_{D_{ij}}(t, P_{HLT})$] must be determined. The nature of these mappings depends on the type of systems in question (e.g., mechanical, information processing, etc.). The basic process includes application of Step 7 to the subtasks associated with each subsystem. If *resource utilization flexibility* (i.e., redundancy in subsystems of similar types) exists, select the "best" or optimal subsystem configuration (handled in GSPT with the concept of *performance resource substitution*) and *procedure* (i.e., use of performance resources over time) as that which allows *accomplishment of goals* with *minimization of stress* on available performance resources across all subsystems and over the time of task execution. Thus redundancy is addressed in terms of a constrained performance resource optimization problem. Stress on individual performance resources is defined as $0 < R_{D_{ij}}(t, P_{HLT})/R_{A_{ij}}(t) < 1$. It is also useful to define and take note of reserve capacity, i.e., the margin between available and utilized per-formance resources.

The preceding statement is intended to reflect the true complexity that exists in systems, tasks, and their interfaces when viewed primarily from the perspective of performance. This provides a basis for the judicious decision making required to realize "the best" *practical implementation* in a given situation where many engineering tradeoffs must be considered. While a two-level approach is described above, it should be apparent that it can be applied with any number of hierarchical levels by repeating the steps outlined in an iterative fashion starting at a different level each time. A striking feature of GSPT is the *threshold effect* associated with the resource economic principle. This nonlinearity has important implications in quantitative human performance modeling, as well as interesting ramifications in practical applications such as rehabilitation, sports, and education. Note also that no distinction is made as to whether a given performance resource is derived from a human or artificial system; both types of systems, or subcomponents thereof, can be incorporated into models and analyses.

Monadology

Monadology dates back to 384 B.C. [Neel, 1977] and is essentially the idea of "basic elements" vis à vis chemistry, alphabets, genetic building blocks, etc. The concept is thus already well accepted as being vital to the systematic description of human systems from certain perspectives (i.e., chemical, genetic). Success associated with previous application of monadology, whether intentional or unwitting (i.e., discovered to be at play *after* a given taxonomy has emerged), compels its serious a priori consideration for other problems.

Insight into how monadology is applied to human performance modeling is perhaps more readily obtained with reference to a widely known example in which monadology is evident, such as chemistry. Prior to modern chemistry (i.e., prior to the introduction of the periodic table), alchemy existed. The world was viewed as being composed of an infinite variety of unique *substances*. The periodic table captured the notion that this infinite variety of substances could all be defined in terms of a finite set of basic elements. Substances have since been analyzed using the "language" of chemistry and organized into categories of various complexity, i.e., elements, simple compounds, complex compounds, etc. Despite the fact that this transition occurred approximately 200 years ago, compounds remain that have yet to be analyzed. Furthermore, the initial periodic table was incorrect and has undergone revision up to relatively recent times. Analogously, in the alchemy of human performance, the world is viewed as being composed of an infinite variety of unique tasks. A "chemistry" can be envisioned that first starts with the identification of the "basic elements" or, more specifically, *basic elements of performance*. Simple and complex tasks are thus analogous to simple and complex compounds, respectively. The analogy carries over to quantitative aspects of GSPT as well. Consider typical equations of chemical reactions with resources on the left and products (i.e., tasks) on the right. Simple compounds (tasks) are realized by drawing on basic elements in the proper combination and amounts. The amount of "product" (level of performance in a high-level task) obtained depends on availability of the *limiting resource*.

Another informative aspect of this analogy is the issue of how to deal with the treatment of hierarchical level. Clearly, the chemical elements are made up of smaller particles (e.g., protons, neutrons, and electrons). Physicists have identified even smaller, more elusive entities, such as bosons, quarks, etc. Do we need to consider items at this lowest level of abstraction each time a simple compound such as hydrochloric acid is made? Likewise, the term *basic* in basic elements of performance is clearly relative and requires the choice of a particular hierarchical level of abstraction for the identification of systems or basic functional units, a level that is considered to be both natural and useful for the purpose at hand. Just as it is possible but not always necessary or practical to map chemical elements down to the atomic particle level, it is possible to consider mapping a basic element of performance (see below) such as elbow flexor torque production capacity down to the level of muscle fibers, biochemical reactions at neuromuscular junctions, etc.

The Elemental Resource Model

The resource and resource economic constructs used in GSPT specifically to address performance have employed and have become well established in some segments of the human performance field, specifically with regard to attention and information processing [Navon & Gopher, 1979; Wickens, 1984]. However, in these cases, the term *resource* is used mostly conceptually (in contrast to quantitatively), somewhat softly defined, and applied to refer in various instances to systems (e.g., different processing centers), broad functions (e.g., memory versus processing), and sometimes to infer a particular aspect of performance (e.g., attentional resources). In the ERM, through the application of GSPT, these constructs are incorporated universally (i.e., applied to all human subsystems) and specifically to model "performance" at both conceptual and quantitative levels. In addition to the concept of monadology, the insights of others [Shoner & Kelso, 1988; Turvey et al., 1978] were valuable in reinforcing the basic "systems architecture" employed in the ERM and in refining description of more subtle, but important aspects.

As illustrated in Fig. 143.1, the ERM contains multiple hierarchical levels. Specifically, three levels are defined: (1) the basic element level, (2) the generic intermediate level, and (3) the high level. GSPT is to define performance measures at any hierarchical level. This implies that to measure performance, one must isolate the desired system and then stress it maximally along one dimension of performance (or more, if interaction effects are desired) to determine performance resource availability. For example, consider the human "posture stabilizing" system (at the generic intermediate level), which is stressed maximally along a stability dimension. As further illustrated below, the basic element level represents measurable stepping stones in the human system hierarchy between lower-level systems (i.e., ligaments, tendons, nerves, etc.) and higher-level tasks.

A summary representation emphasizing the basic element level of the ERM is depicted in Fig. 143.2. While this figure is intended to be more or less self-explanatory, a brief walk-through is warranted.

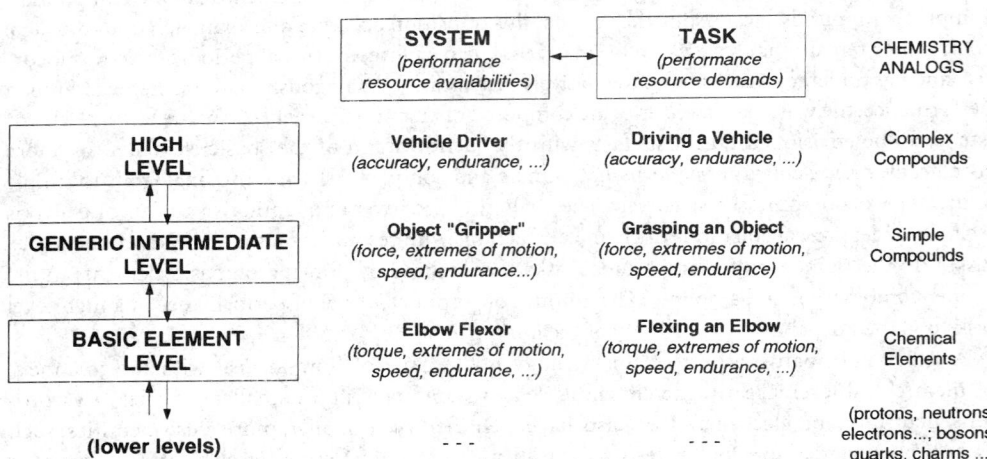

FIGURE 143.1 The elemental resource model contains multiple hierarchical levels. Performance resources (i.e., the basic elements) at the "basic element level" are finite in number, as dictated by the finite set of human subsystems and the finite set of their respective dimensions of performance. At higher levels, new "systems" can be readily created by configuration of systems at the basic element level. Consequently, there are an infinite number of performance resources (i.e., higher-level elements) at these levels. However, rules of general systems performance theory (refer to text) applied at any level in the same way, resulting in the identification of the system, its function, dimensions of performance, performance resource availabilities (system attributes), and performance resource demands (task attributes).

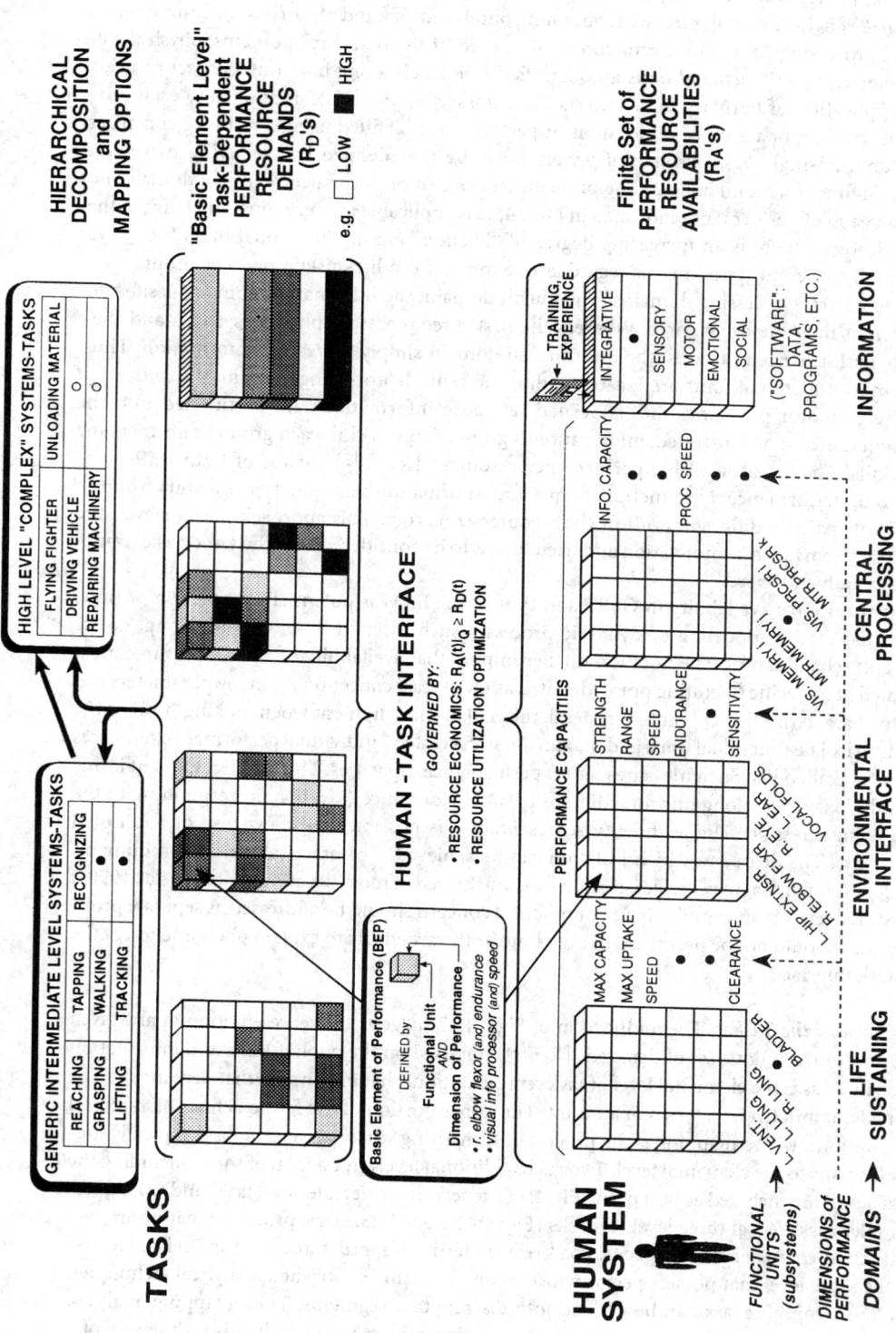

FIGURE 143.2 A summary of the major constructs of the elemental resource model, emphasizing the categorization of performance resources at the basic element level into four life-sustaining, environmental-interface, central-processing, and information domains.

Looking Toward the Human.   The entire human (lower portion of Fig. 143.2) is modeled as a pool of elemental *performance resources* that are grouped into one of four different domains: (1) life-sustaining, (2) environmental interface (containing purely sensory and sensorimotor components), (3) central processing, and (4) information. Within each of the first three domains, physical subsystems referred to as *functional units* are identified (see labels along horizontal aspect of grids) through application of fairly rigorous criteria [Kondraske, 1990b]. GSPT is applied to each functional unit, yielding first a set of dimensions of performance (defined using a resource construct) for each unit. A single *basic element of performance* (BEP) is defined by specifying two items: (1) the basic functional unit and (2) one of its dimensions of performance. Within a domain, not every dimension of performance indicated in Fig. 143.2 is applicable to every functional unit in that domain. However, there is an increasing degree of "likeness" among functional units (i.e., fewer fundamentally different types) in this regard as one moves from life-sustaining to environmental-interface to central-processing domains. The fourth domain, the information domain, is substantially different than the other three. Whereas the first three represent physical systems and their intangible performance resources, the information domain simply represents information. Thus, while memory functional units are located within the central-processing domain, the *contents of memory* (e.g., motor programs and associated reference information) are partitioned into the information domain. As illustrated, information is grouped, but within each group there are many specific skills. The set of available performance resources $[R_{A_{ij}}(t)|_Q]$ consist of both BEPs ($i =$ dimension of performance, $j =$ functional unit) and information sets (e.g., type i within group j). Although intrinsically different, both fit the resource construct. This approach permits even the most abstract items such as motivation and friendliness to be considered with the same basic framework as strength and speed.

Note that resource availability in GSPT and thus in the ERM is potentially a function of time, allowing quantitative modeling of dynamic processes such as child development, aging, disuse atrophy, and rehabilitation. The notation further implies that availability of a given resource must be evaluated at a specific operating point, denoted as **Q**. At least conceptually, many parameters can be used to characterize this **Q** point. In general, the goal of measurement when looking "toward the human" is to isolate functional units and maximally stress (safely) individual performance resources to determine availability. Such measures reflect performance capacities. The simplest **Q** point is one in which there is stress along only one dimension of performance (i.e., that corresponding to the resource being stressed). Higher-fidelity representation is possible at the expense of additional measurements. The degree to which isolation can be achieved is of practical concern in humans. Nonetheless, it is felt that reasonable isolation can be achieved in most situations [Kondraske, 1990a, 1990b]. Moreover, this and similar issues of practical concern should be addressed as separate problems; i.e., they should not be permitted to obfuscate or thwart efforts to explain phenomenon at the human-task interface.

Looking Toward the Task.   The midportion of Fig. 143.2 suggests the representation of any given task in terms of the unique set of demands $[R_D ij(t)]$ imposed on the pool of BEPs and information resources; i.e., this is the elemental level of task representation. Shading implies that demands can be represented quantitatively in terms of amount. The upper portion of the figure defines hierarchical mapping options, where mapping is the process of translating what happens in tasks typically executed by humans to the elemental level. Two such additional levels (for a total of three, including the elemental level) are included as part of the ERM: (1) generic intermediate-level tasks and (2) higher-level complex tasks. At all three levels of tasks (Figs. 143.1 and 143.2) are processes that occur over time and can be characterized by specific goals (e.g., in terms of speed, force, etc.) and related to systems at the same level that possess performance resources. Using established analytical techniques, even the most complex task can be divided into discrete task segments. Then mapping analyses, which take into account task procedures (e.g., a squatting subject with two hands on the side of a box), are applied to each task segment to determine $R_{D_{ij}}(t)$. Once this is found, the worst case or a selected percentile point in the resource demand distribution (over a time period corresponding to a selected task segment) can be used to obtain a single numeric value representation of demand for a given resource *and* the conditions under which the given demand occurs; i.e., the $\mathbf{Q}'$ point (e.g., at what speed and position angle does the worst-case demand on elbow flexor torque occur?). This reduction process requires parameterization algorithms that are similar to those used to process time-series data collected during tests designed to measure performance resource availability.

The Human-Task Interface.　Using GSPT, success in achieving the goals of a given task segment is governed by resource economic principles requiring that $R_{A_{ij}}(t)|_Q \geq R_D ij(t)$ for all i and j (i.e., $R_{A_{11}} \geq R_{D_{11}}$ AND $R_{A_{12}} \geq R_{D_{12}}$ AND $R_{A_{13}} \geq R_{D_{13}}$). In other words, all task demands, when translated to the individual subsystems involved, must fit within the envelopes that define performance resource availability. Adequacy associated with any one resource is a *necessary but not sufficient condition* for success. Concepts and observations in human performance referred to as *compensation* or *redundancy* are explained in terms of *resource utilization flexibility,* which includes the possibility of substituting one performance resource (of the same dimensionality) for another (i.e., *resource substitution*). It has been hypothesized [Kondraske, 1990*b*] that an optimal performance resource utilization is achieved through learning. Furthermore, the optimization rule suggested by GSPT is that the human system is driven to accomplish task goals and use procedures that minimize performance resource stress (i.e., the fraction of available performance resources utilized) over the duration of a given task segment and across all BEPs involved. Minimizing stress is equivalent to maximizing the margin between available and utilized performance resources. Thus optimization is highly dependent on the resource availability profile, and it would be predicted, for instance, that two individuals with different resource availability profiles would not optimally accomplish the same task goals by using identical procedures.

143.3 Application Issues

Implications of the ERM and what it demonstrates regarding intrinsic demands imposed by nature and methods for creatively navigating these demands over both the short and long terms are considered. The ERM offers a number of flexibilities with regard to how it can be applied (e.g., "in whole" or "in part," "conceptually" or "rigorously," with "low tech" or sophisticated "high tech" tools, and to define performance measures or to develop predictive models). While immediate application is possible at a conceptual level of application, it also provides the motivation and potential to consider coordinated, collaborative development of sophisticated tools that allow rigorous and efficient solutions to complex problems by practitioners without extraordinary training.

The ERM provides a basis for obtaining insight into the nature of routine tasks that clinicians and other practitioners are expected to perform; there are both "troublesome" and "promising" insights in this regard. Perhaps the most obvious troublesome aspect is that the ERM makes it painfully evident that *many* BEPs are typically called into play in tasks of daily living, work, and/or recreation and that resource insufficiency associated with *any one* of this subset of BEPs can be the factor that limits performance in the higher-level task. The further implication is that for rigorous application, one must know (via measurement and analyses) the availability and demand associated with each and every one of these unique resources. An additional complexity with which practitioners must cope is the high degree of specificity and complexity of resources in the information domain (i.e., the "software"). There is no simple, rapid way to probe this domain to determine if the information required for a given task is correct; it requires methods analogous to those used to debug software source code.

Aspects that hold promise are associated with (1) the nature of hierarchical systems, (2) the threshold mathematics of resource economics, and (3) the fact that when n resources combine to address a single task, the mathematics of logical combination is employed to arrive at an overall assessment. That is, the individual "$R_A \geq R_D$?" questions result in a set of "OK" or "not OK" results that are combined with logical AND operations to obtain the final "OK" or "not OK" assessment (note that the OR operator is used when resource substitution is possible).

Conceptual, Low-Tech Practical Application

The ERM description alone can be used simply to provide a common conceptual basis for discussing the wide range of concepts, measurements, methods, and processes of relevance in human performance or a particular application area [Frisch, 1993; Mayer & Gatchel, 1988; Syndulko et al., 1988]. It also can be used at this level as a basis for structured assessment [Kondraske, 1988b, 1994, 1995] of individuals in situations, including therapy prescription, assistive device prescription, independent living decision making (e.g., self-feeding, driving, etc.), age or gender discrimination issues in work or recreational tasks, etc. At points in such processes, it is often more important to consider the full scope of different performance resources involved in a task using even a crude level of quantification than it is to consider just a select few in great depth. A "checklist" approach is recommended. The professional uses only his or her judgment and experience to consider both the specific individual and the specific task of interest to make quantitative but relatively gross assessments of resource adequacy using a triage-like categorization process (e.g., with "definitely limiting," "definitely not limiting," or "not sure" categories). This is feasible because of the threshold nature of the system-task interface; in cases where R_A and R_D are widely separated instrumented, high-resolution measurements are not required to determine if a given performance resource is limiting. Any resource(s) so identified as "definitely limiting" becomes an immediate focus of interest. If none is categorized as such, concern moves to those in the "not sure" category, in which case more sensitive measurements may be required. Purely subjective methods of measuring resource availability and/or demands can be augmented with selected, more objective and higher-resolution measurements in "hybrid applications."

Conceptual, Theoretical Application

The ERM can be used to reconsider previous work in human performance. For example, it can be employed to reason why Fleishman [Fleishman & Quaintance, 1984] (as well as others) achieved promising, but limited, success with statistically based predictions of performance in higher-level tasks using regression models with independent variables, which can now be viewed as representing lower-level performance resources (in most cases). Specifically, regression models rely heavily on an assumption that there exists some correlation between dependent and each independent variable, the latter of which typically represent scores from maximal performance tasks and therefore reflect resource availability (using GSPT and ERM logic). Brief reflection results in the realization that correlation is not to be anticipated between the level of performance attainable in a "higher-level task" and *availability* of one of the many performance resources essential to the task (e.g., if 4 cups of flour are needed for a given cake, having 40 cups available will not *alone* result in a larger cake of equal quality—availability of another ingredient may in fact be limiting). Rather, correlation *is* expected between high-level task performance and the amount of resource *utilization*. Unfortunately, as noted above, the independent variables used typically reflect resource availability. The incomplete labeling of performance variables in such studies reflects the general failure to distinguish between utilization and availability. Why not, then, just use measures of resource utilization in such statistical models? Resource availability measures are simple to obtain in the laboratory without requiring that the individual execute *the* high-level task of interest. Resource utilization measures can only be obtained experimentally by requiring the subject to execute the task in question, which is counterproductive with respect to the goal of using a set of laboratory measurements to extrapolate to performance in one or more higher-level task situations. Furthermore, regression models based on linear combination of resource *availability* measures do not reflect the nonlinear threshold effect accounted for with resource economic, GSPT-based performance models. One potential alternative based on GSPT and termed *nonlinear causal resource analysis* has been proposed [Kondraske, 1988a; Vasta & Kondraske, 1994].

Application "in Part"

In this approach, whole domains (i.e., many BEPs) are assessed simultaneously, resulting in an estimate or well-founded assumption that states that "all performance resources in domain X are nonlimiting in task(s) Y." Such assumptions are often well justified. For example, it would be reasonable to assume that a young male with a sports-related knee injury would have only a reduction in performance resource availability in the environmental interface domain. More specifically, it is reasonable to assume that the scope of interest can be confined to a smaller subset of functional units, as in gait or speech. These can then be addressed with rigorous application. Examples of this level and manner of applying the ERM have been or are being developed for head/neck control in the context of assistive communication device prescription [Carr, 1989], workplace design [Kondraske, 1988c], evaluating work sites and individuals with disabilities for employment [Parnianpour & Marras, 1993], gait [Carollo & Kondraske, 1987], measurement of upper extremity motor control [Behbehani et al., 1988], speech production performance [Jafari, 1989; Jafari et al., 1989], and to illustrate changes in performance capacity associated with aging [Kondraske, 1989]. Additionally, in some applications only the generic intermediate level need be considered. For example, one may only need to know how well an individual can walk, lift, etc. While it is sometimes painfully clear just how complex the execution of even a relatively simple task is, it also can be recognized that relatively simple, justifiable, and efficient strategies can be developed to maintain a reasonable degree of utility in a given context.

Rigorous, High-Tech Application

While this path may offer the greatest potential for impact, it also presents the greatest challenge. The ultimate *goal* would be to capture the analytic and modeling capability (as implied by the preceding discussions) for a "total human" (single subject or populations) and "any task" in a desktop computer system (used along with synergistic "peripherals" that adopt the same framework, such as measurement tools [e.g., Kondraske, 1990a]). This suggests a long-term, collaborative effort. However, intermediate tools that provide significant utility are feasible [e.g., Vasta & Kondraske, 1994] and needed [e.g., Allard et al., 1994; Vasta & Kondraske, 1994]. While tools that are useful to practitioners are desirable, they are almost essential for the efficient conduct of in-depth experimental work with the ERM that must accompany the evolution of such tools.

The issue of biologic variability and its influence on numeric analyses can be raised in the context of rigorous numeric application. In this regard, the methods underlying GSPT and the ERM (or any similar cause-and-effect model) are noted to be analogous with those used to design artificial systems. In recent years, conceptual approaches and mathematic tools widely known as *Taguchi methods* [e.g., Bendell et al., 1988] have been shown to be effective for understanding and managing a very similar type of variability that surfaces in the manufacture of artificial systems (e.g., variability associated with performance of components of larger systems and the effect on aspects of performance of the final "product"). Such tools may prove useful in working through engineering problems such as those associated with variability.

143.4 Conclusion

The ERM is a step toward the goal of achieving an application-independent approach to modeling any human-task interface. It provides a systematic and generalizable (across all subsystem types) means of identifying performance measures that characterize human subsystems, as well as a consistent basis for performance measurement definition (and task analysis). It also has served to stimulate focus on a standardized, distinct set of variables that facilitates clear communication of an individual's status among professionals.

After the initial presentation, refinements in both GSPT and the ERM were made. However, the basic approaches, terminology, and constructs used in each have remained quite stable. More recent work has focused on development of various components required for application of the ERM in nontrivial situations. This entails using GSPT and basic ERM concepts to guide a full "fleshing out" of the details of measurement parameterizations and models for different types of human subsystems, definition of standard conventions and notations, and development of computer-based tools. In addition, experimental studies designed to evaluate key constructs of the ERM and to demonstrate the various ways in which it can be applied are being conducted. A good portion of the developmental work is aimed at building a capability to conduct more complex, nontrivial experimental studies. Collaborations with other research groups also have emerged and are being supported to the extent possible. Experiences with it in various contexts and at various levels of application have been productive and encouraging.

The ERM is one, relatively young attempt at organizing and dealing with the complexity of some major aspects of human performance. There is no known alternative that, in a specific sense, attempts to accomplish the same goals as the working model presented here. Is it good enough? For what purposes? Is a completely different approach or merely refinement required? The process of revision is central to the natural course of the history of ideas. Needs for generalizations in human performance persist.

Defining Terms

Basic element of performance (BEP):   A modeling item at the basic element level in the ERM defined by identification of a specific system at this level and one of its dimensions of performance (e.g., functional unit = visual information processor, dimension of performance = speed, BEP = visual information processor speed).

Behavior: A general term that relates to what a human or artificial system does while carrying out its function(s) under given conditions. Often, behavior is characterized by measurement of selected parameters or identification of unique system states over time.

Composite performance capacity: A performance capacity at a higher level of abstraction, formed by combining two or more lower-level performance capacities (e.g., via integration to determine the area or volume within a performance envelope).

Dimension of performance: A unique quality that characterizes how well a system executes its function (e.g., speed, accuracy, torque production); one of axes or the label associated with one of the axes in a multidimensional performance space.

Function: The purpose of a system. Some systems map to a single primary function (e.g., process visual information). Others (e.g., the human arm) map to multiple functions, although at any given time multifunction systems are likely to be executing a single function (e.g., polishing a car). Functions can be described and inventoried, whereas level of performance of a given function can be measured.

Generic intermediate level: One of three major hierarchical levels for systems and tasks identified in the elemental resource model. The generic intermediate level represents new systems (e.g., postural maintenance system, object gripper, object lifter, etc.) formed by the combination of functional units at the basic element level (e.g., flexors, extensors, processors, etc.). The term *generic* is used to imply the high frequency of use of systems at this level in tasks of daily life (i.e., items at the "high level" in the ERM).

Goal: A desired endpoint (i.e., result) typically characterized by multiple parameters, at least one of which is specified. Examples include specified task goals (e.g., move an object of specified mass from point A to point B in 3 seconds) or estimated task performance (maximum mass, range, speed of movement obtainable given a specified elemental performance resource availability profile), depending on whether a reverse or forward analysis problem is undertaken. Whereas function describes the general process of a task, the goal directly relates to performance and is quantitative.

Limiting resource: A performance resource at any hierarchical level (e.g., vertical lift strength, knee flexor speed) that is available in an amount that is less than the worst-case demand imposed by a task. Thus a given resource can only be "limiting" when considered in the context of a specific task.

Performance: Aspects of a human or artifical system (e.g., strength, speed, accuracy, endurance) that pertain to how well that system executes its function.

Performance capacity: A quantity in finite availability that limits some aspect of a system's ability to execute tasks, or the limit of that aspect itself.

Performance envelope: The surface in a multidimensional performance space, formed with a selected subset of a system's dimensions of performance, that defines the limits of a system's performance. Tasks represented by points that fall within this envelope can be performed by the system in question.

Performance resource: A unique quality of a system's performance modeled and quantified using a resource construct.

Performance resource substitution: The term used in GSPT to describe the manner in which intelligent systems, such as humans, utilize redundancy or adapt to unusual circumstances (e.g., injuries) to obtain optimal procedures for executing a task.

Procedure: A set of constraints placed on a system in which flexibility exists regarding how a goal (or set of goals) associated with a given function can be achieved. Procedure specification requires specification of initial, intermediate, and/or final states or conditions dictating how the goal is to be accomplished. Such specification can be thought of in terms of removing some degrees of freedom.

Resource construct: The collective set of attributes that define and uniquely characterize a resource. Usually, the term is applied only to tangible items. A resource is desirable and measurable in terms of amount (from zero to some finite positive value) in such a manner that a larger numeric value indicates a greater amount of the resource.

Resource economic principle: The principle, observable in many contexts, that states that the amount of a given resource that is available (e.g., money) must exceed the demand placed on it (e.g., cost of an item) if a specified task (e.g., purchase of the item) is to be executed.

Resource utilization flexibility: A term used in GSPT to describe situations in which there are more than one possible source of a given performance resource type, i.e., redundant supplies exist.

Structure: Physical manifestation and attributes of a human or artificial system; the object of one type of measurements at multiple hierarchical levels.

Style: Allowance for variation within a procedure, resulting in the intentional incomplete specification of a procedure or resulting from either intentional or unintentional incomplete specification of procedure.

System: A physical structure, at any hierarchical level of abstraction, that executes one or more functions.

Task: That which results from (1) the combination of specified functions, goals, and procedures or (2) the specification of function and goals and the observation of procedures utilized to achieve the goals.

References

Allard P, Stokes IAF, Blanchi JP. 1994. Three-Dimensional Analysis of Human Movement. Champaign, Ill, Human Kinetics.

Baron S, Kruser DS, Huey BM (eds). 1990. Quantitative Modeling of Human Performance in Complex, Dynamic Systems. Washington, National Academy Press.

Behbehani K, Kondraske GV, Richmond JR. 1988. Investigation of upper extremity visuomotor control performance measures. IEEE Trans Biomed Eng 35(7):518.

Bendell A, Disney J, Pridmore WA. 1988. Taguchi Methods: Applications in World Industry. London, IFS Publishing.

Botterbusch KF. 1987. Vocational Assessment and Evaluation Systems: A Comparison. Menomonie, Wisc, Stout Vocational Rehabilitation Institute, University of Wisconsin.

Card SK, Moran TP, Newell A. 1986. The model human processor. In KR Boff, L Kaufman, and JP Thomas (eds), Handbook of Perception and Human Performance, vol II, pp 45.1–45.35. New York, Wiley.

Carollo JJ, Kondraske GV. 1987. The prerequisite resources for walking: Characterization using a task analysis strategy. In J Leinberger (ed), Proceedings of the Ninth Annual IEEE Engineering and Medical Biology Society Conference, p 357.

Carr B. 1989. Head/Neck Control Performance Measurement and Task Interface Model. M.S. thesis, University of Texas at Arlington, Arlington, Texas.

Chaffin DB, Andersson GBJ. 1984. Occupational Biomechanics. New York, Wiley.

Delp SL, Loan JP, Hoy MG, et al. 1990. An interactive graphics-based Model of the lower extremity to study orthopaedic surgical procedures. IEEE Trans Biomed Eng 37(8):757.

Fleishman EA. 1956. Psychomotor selection tests: Research and application in the United States Air Force. Personnel Psychology 9:449.

Fleishman EA. 1966. Human abilities and the acquisition of skill. In EA Bilodeau (ed), Acquisition of Skill, pp 147–167. New York, Academic Press.

Fleishman EA. 1967. Performance assessment based on an empirically derived task taxonomy. Human Factors 9:349.

Fleishman EA. 1972. Structure and measurement of psychomotor abilities. In RN Singer (ed), The Psychomotor Domain: Movement Behavior, pp 78–106. Philadelphia, Lea and Febiger.

Fleishman EA. 1982. Systems for describing human tasks. Am Psychol 37:821.

Fleishman EA, Quaintance MK. 1984. Taxonomies of Human Performance. New York, Academic Press.

Frisch HP. 1993. Man/machine interaction dynamics and performance analysis. In Proceedings of the NATO-Army-NASA Advanced Study Institute on Concurrent Engineering Tools and Technologies for Mechanical System Design. New York: Springer-Verlag.

Gilbreth FB, Gilbreth FM. 1917. Applied Motion Study. New York, Sturgis and Walton.

Gottlieb GL, Corcos DM, Agarwal GC. 1989. Strategies for the control of voluntary movements with one mechanical degree of freedom. Behav Brain Sci 12:189.

Hemami H. 1988. Modeling, control, and simulation of human movement. CRC Crit Rev Bioeng 13(1):1.

Jafari M. 1989. Modeling and Measurement of Human Speech performance Toward Pathology Pattern Recognition. Ph.D. dissertation, University of Texas at Arlington, Arlington, Texas.

Jafari M, Wong KH, Behbehani K, Kondraske GV. 1989. Performance characterization of human pitch control system: An acoustic approach. J Acous Soc Am 85(3):1322.

Kondraske GV. 1987a. Human performance: Science or art? In K Foster (ed), Proceedings of the Thirteenth Northeast Bioengineering Conference, pp 44–47.

Kondraske GV. 1987b. Looking at the study of human performance. SOMA: Eng Human Body (ASME) 2(2):50.

Kondraske GV. 1988a. Experimental evaluation of an elemental resource model for human performance. In G Harris, C Walker (eds), Proceedings of the Tenth Annual IEEE Engineering and Medical Biology Society Conference, pp 1612–1613. New York, IEEE.

Kondraske GV. 1988b. Human performance measurement and task analysis. In A Enders (ed), Technology for Independent Living Sourcebook, 2d ed. Washington, RESNA.

Kondraske GV. 1988c. Workplace design: An elemental resource approach to task analysis and human performance measurements. In Proceedings of the International Conference of the Association of Advanced Rehabilitation Technology, pp 608–611.

Kondraske GV. 1989. Neuromuscular performance: Resource economics and product-based composite indices. In Proceedings of the Eleventh Annual IEEE Engineering and Medical Biology Society Conference, pp 1045–1046. New York, IEEE.

Kondraske GV. 1990*a*. A PC-based performance measurement laboratory system. J Clin Eng 15(66):467.

Kondraske GV. 1990*b*. Quantitative measurement and assessment of performance. In RV Smith, JH Leslie (eds), Rehabilitation Engineering, pp 101–125. Boca Raton, Fla, CRC Press.

Kondraske GV. 1993. The HPI Shorthand Notation System for Human System Parameters. Technical Report 92-001R V1.5. Human Performance Institute, University of Texas at Arlington, Arlington, Texas.

Kondraske GV. 1994. An elemental resource model for the human-task interface. Int J Technol Assess Health Care (in press).

Kondraske GV. 1995. Measurement tools an processes in rehabilitation engineering. In JD Bronzino (ed), Handbook of Biomedical Engineering. Boca Raton, Fla, CRC Press.

Kondraske GV, Beehler PJH. 1994. Applying general systems performance theory and the elemental resource model to gender-related issues in physical education and sport. Women Sport Phys Act J 3(2)1–19.

Kondraske GV, Beehler, PJH, Behbehani K, et al. 1988. Measuring human performance: Concepts, methods, and application examples. SOMA: Eng Human Body 2 (ASME), Jan 6.

Kondraske GV, Khoury GJ. 1992. Telerobotic system performance measurement: Motivation and methods. In Cooperative Intelligent Robotics in Space III, pp 161–172. New York, SPIE.

Kondraske GV, Standridge R. 1988. Robot performance: Conceptual strategies. In Conference of Digest IEEE Midcon/88 Technical Conference, pp 359–362. New York, IEEE.

Mayer TG, Gatchel RJ. 1991. Functional Restoration for Spinal Disorders: The Sports Medicine Approach, pp 66–77. Philadelphia, Lea & Febinger.

Meister D. 1989. Conceptual Aspects of Human Performance. Baltimore, Johns Hopkins University Press.

Navon D, Gopher D. 1979. On the economy of the human processing system. Psych Rev 86:214.

Neel A. 1977. Theories of Psychology: A Handbook. Cambridge, Mass, Schenkman.

Parnianpour M, Marras WS. 1993. Development of clinical protocols based on ergonomics evaluation in response to American Disability Act (1992). In Rehabilitation Engineering Center Proposal to National Institute on Disability and Rehabilitation Research, Ohio State University, Columbus, Ohio.

Schoner G, Kelso JAS. 1988. Dynamic pattern generation in behavioral and neural systems. Science 239:1513.

Syndulko K, Tourtellotte WW, Richter E. 1988. Toward the objective measurement of central processing resources. IEEE Eng Med Biol Soc Magazine 7(1):17.

Taylor FW. 1911. The Principles of Scientific Management. New York, Harper and Brothers.

Turvey MT, Shaw RE, Mace W. 1978. Issues in the theory of action: Degrees of freedom, coordinative structures, and coalitions. In J Requin (ed), Attention and Performance VII. Hillsdale, NJ, Lawrence Earlbaum.

US Department of Labor. 1992. Dictionary of Occupation Titles, 4th ed. Baton Rouge, La, Claitor's Publishing Division.

Vasta PJ, Kondraske GV. 1994. Performance prediction of an upper extremity reciprocal task using non-linear causal resource analysis. In Proceedings of the Sixteenth Annual IEEE Engineering in Medicine and Biology Society Conference. New York, IEEE.

Wickens CD. 1984. Engineering Psychology and Human Performance. Columbus, Ohio, Charles E Merrill.

World Health Organization (WHO). 1980. International classification of impairments, disabilities, and handicaps. WHO Chron 34:376.

Yen SS, Kondraske GV. 1992. Machine shape perception: Object recognition based on need-driven resolution flexibility and convex-hull carving. In Proceedings of the Conference on Intelligent Robots and Computer Vision X: Algorithm Techniques, pp 176–187. New York, SPIE.

Further Information

General discussions of major issues associated with human performance modeling can be found in the following texts:

Fleishman EA, Quaintance MK. 1984. Taxonomies of Human Performance. New York, Academic Press.

Meister D. 1989. Conceptual Aspects of Human Performance. Baltimore, Johns Hopkins University Press.

Neel A. 1977. Theories of Psychology: A Handbook. Cambridge, Mass, Schenkman.

Requin J. 1978. Attention and Performance VII. Hillsdale, NJ, Lawrence Earlbaum.

Wickens CD. 1984. Engineering Psychology and Human Performance. Columbus, Ohio, Charles E Merrill.

More detailed information regarding general systems performance theory, the elemental resource model, and their application is available from the Human Performance Institute, P.O. Box 19180, University of Texas at Arlington, Arlington, TX 76019-0180.

144

Measurement of Neuromuscular Performance Capacities

Susan S. Smith
Southwestern PT

Movements allow us to interact with our environment, express ourselves, and communicate with each other. Life is movement. Movement is constantly occurring at many hierarchical levels, including cellular and subcellular levels. By using the adjective *human* to clarify the term *movement*, we are not only defining the species of interest but also limiting the study to observable performance and its more overt causes. Study of human performance is of interest to a broad range of professionals including rehabilitation engineers, orthopedic surgeons, therapists, biomechanists, kinesiologists, psychologists, and so on. Because of the complexity of human performance and the variety of investigators, the study of human performance is conducted from several theoretical perspectives including (1) anatomic, (2) purpose or character of the movement (such as locomotion), (3) physiologic, (4) biomechanical, (5) psychological, (6) sociocultural, and (7) integrative. The elemental resource model (ERM), presented in Chap. 143, is an integrative model that incorporates aspects of the other models into a singular system accounting for the human, the task, and the human-task interface [Kondraske, 1995].

The purposes of this chapter are to (1) provide reasons for measuring four selected variables of human performance: extremes/range of motion, strength, speed of movement, and endurance; (2) briefly define and discuss these variables; (3) overview selected instruments and methods used to measure these variables; and (4) discuss interpretation of performance for a given neuromuscular subsystem.

144.1 Neuromuscular Functional Units

While the theoretical perspectives listed previously may be useful within specific contexts or within specific disciplines, the broader appreciation of human performance and its control can be gained from the perspective of an integrative model such as the ERM [Kondraske, 1995]. This model organizes performance resources into four different domains. Basic movements, such as elbow flexion, are executed by *neuromuscular functional units* in the environmental interface domain. Intermediate and complex tasks, such as walking and playing the piano, utilize multiple basic functional units. The human performing a movement operates the involved functional units along different dimensions of performance according to the demands of the task. Dimensions of performance are factors such as joint motion, strength, speed of movement, and endurance. Lifting a heavy box off the floor requires, among other things, a specific amount of strength associated with neuromuscular functional units of the back, legs, and arms according to the weight and size of the box. Reaching for a light-weight box from the top shelf of a closet requires specific shoulder ranges of motion according to the height of the shelf.

Whereas four dimensions of performance are considered individually in this chapter, they are *highly interdependent*. For an example, strength availability during a movement is partly dependent on joint angle. Despite interdependence, considering the variables as different dimensions is essential to studying human performance. The components limiting the human's ability to complete a task can only be identified and subsequently enhanced by determining, for example, that the reason the human cannot reach the box off the top shelf is not because of insufficient range of motion of the shoulder but because of insufficient strength of the shoulder musculature required to lift the arm through the range of motion. Isolating the subsystems involved in a task and maximally stressing them along one or more "isolated" dimensions of performance are key concepts in the ERM. *Maximally stressing* the subsystems means that the maximum amount of the resource available is being determined. This differs from determining the amount of the resource that happened to be used while performing a particular task. Often the distinction between obtaining maximal performance from a human and submaximal performance is in the instructions given the subject. For example, in measuring speed, we say "move as fast as you can."

144.2 Purposes for Measuring Selected Neuromuscular Performance Capacities

Range of motion, strength, speed of movement, and/or endurance can be measured for one or more of the following purposes:

1. To determine the amount of the resource available and to compare it to the normal value for that individual. "Normal" is frequently determined by comparisons with the opposite extremity or with normative data when available. This information may be used to develop goals and a program to change the performance.

2. To assist in determining the possible effects of insufficient or imbalanced amounts of the variable on a person's performance of activities of daily living, work, sport, and leisure pursuits. In this case, the amount of the variable is compared with the demands of the task rather than with norms or with the opposite extremity.
3. To assist in diagnosis of medical conditions and the nature of movement dysfunctions.
4. To reassess status in order to determine the effectiveness of a program designed to change the amount of the variable.
5. To motivate persons to comply with treatment or training regimes.
6. To document status and the results of treatment or training and to communicate with other involved persons.
7. To assist in ergonomically designed furniture, equipment, techniques, and environments.
8. To provide information to combine with other measures of human performance to predict functional capabilities.

144.3 Range of Motion and Extremes of Motion

Range of motion (ROM) is the amount of movement that occurs at a joint. *Range* of motion is typically measured by noting the *extremes of motion*. The designated reference or zero position must be specified for measurements of the two extremes of motion. For example, to measure elbow (radiohumeral joint) flexion and extension, the preferred starting position is with the subject supine, sitting, or standing with the arm parallel to the lateral midline of the body with the palm facing forward [Duesterhaus Minor & Duesterhaus Minor, 1985; Moore, 1984]. Measurements are taken with the elbow in the fully flexed position and with the elbow in the fully extended position.

Movement Terminology

Joint movements are described using a coordinate system with the human body in anatomic position. Anatomic position of the body is an erect position, face forward, arms at sides, palms facing forward, and fingers and thumbs in extension. The central coordinate system consists of three cardinal planes and axes with its origin located between the cornua of the sacrum [Panjabi et al., 1974]. Figure 144.1 demonstrates the planes and axes of the central coordinate system. The same coordinate system can parallel the master system at any joint in the body by relocating the origin to any defined point.

The sagittal plane is the *y,z* plane; the frontal (or coronal) plane is the *y,x* plane; the horizontal (or transverse) plane is the *x,z* plane. Movements are described in relation to the origin of the coordinate system. The arrows indicate the positive direction of each axis. An anterior translation is $+z$; a posterior translation is $-z$. Clockwise rotations are $+\theta$, and counterclockwise rotations are $-\theta$.

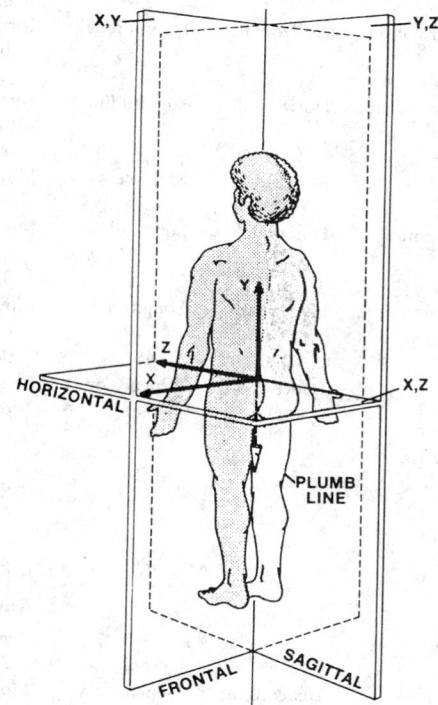

FIGURE 144.1 Planes and axes are illustrated in anatomic position. The central coordinate system with its origin between the cornua of the sacrum is shown. (From White & Panjabi, 1990, with permission.)

Joints are described as having degrees of freedom (dof) of movement. This is the number of independent coordinates in a system that are necessary to accurately specify the position of an object in space. If a motion occurs in one plane and around one axis, the joint is defined as having one dof. Joints with movements in two planes occurring around two different axes have two dof, and so on.

Angular movements refer to motions that cause an increase or decrease in the angle between the articulating bones. Angular movements are flexion, extension, abduction, adduction, and lateral flexion (see Table 144.1). Rotational movements generally occur around a longitudinal (or vertical) axis except for movements of the clavicle and scapula. The rotational movements occurring around the longitudinal axis (internal rotation, external rotation, opposition, horizontal abduction, and horizontal adduction) are described in Table 144.1. Rotation of the scapula is described in terms of the direction of the inferior angle. Movement of the inferior angle of the scapula toward the midline is a medial (or downward) rotation, and movement of the inferior angle away from the midline

TABLE 144.1 Movement Terms, Planes, Axes, and Descriptions of Movements

Movement Term	Plane	Axis	Description of Movement
Flexion	Sagittal	Frontal	Bending of a part such that the anterior surfaces approximate each other. However, flexion of the knee, ankle, foot, and toes refers to movement in the posterior direction.
Extension	Sagittal	Frontal	Opposite of flexion; involves straightening a body part.
Abduction	Frontal	Sagittal	Movement away from the midline of the body or body part; abduction of the wrist is sometimes called *radial deviation*.
Adduction	Frontal	Sagittal	Movement towards the midline of the body or body part; adduction of the wrist is sometimes called *ulnar deviation*.
Lateral flexion	Frontal	Sagittal	Term used to denote lateral movements of the head, neck, and trunk; also called *side bending*.
Internal (medial) rotation	Horizontal	Longitudinal	Turning movement of the anterior surface of a part towards the midline of the body; internal rotation of the forearm is referred to as *pronation*.
External (lateral) rotation	Horizontal	Longitudinal	Turning movement of the anterior surface of a part away from the midline of the body; external rotation of the forearm is referred to as *supination*.
Opposition	Multiple	Multiple	Movement of the tips of the thumb and little finger toward each other.
Horizontal abduction	Horizontal	Longitudinal	Movement of the arm in a posterior direction away from the midline of the body with the shoulder joint in 90° of either flexion or abduction.
Horizontal adduction	Horizontal	Longitudinal	Movement of the arm in an anterior direction toward the midline of the body with the shoulder joint in 90° of either flexion or abduction.
Tilt	Depends on joint	Depends on joint	Term used to describe certain movements of the scapula and pelvis. In the scapula, an anterior tilt occurs when the coracoid process moves in an anterior and downward direction while the inferior angle moves in a posterior and upward direction. A posterior tilt of the scapula is the opposite of an anterior tilt. In the pelvis, an anterior tilt is rotation of the anterior superior iliac spines (ASISs) of the pelvis in an anterior and downward direction; a posterior tilt is movement of the ASISs in a posterior and upward direction. A lateral tilt of the pelvis occurs when the pelvis is not level from side to side, but one ASIS is higher than the other one.
Gliding	Depends on joint	Depends on joint	Movements that occur when one articulating surface slides on the opposite surface.
Elevation	Frontal		A gliding movement of the scapula in an upward direction as in shrugging the shoulders.
Depression	Frontal		Movement of the scapula downward in a direction reverse of elevation.

is lateral (or upward) rotation. In the extremities, the anterior surface of the extremity is used as the reference area. Because the head, neck, trunk, and pelvis rotate about a midsagittal, longitudinal axis, rotation of these parts is designated as right or left. As can be determined from Fig. 144.1, axial rotation of the trunk toward the left can be described mathematically as $+\theta y$.

A communications problem often exists in describing motion using the terms defined in Table 144.1. A body segment can be in a position such as flexion but can be moving toward extension. This confusion is partially remedied by using the form of the word with the suffix *-ion* to indicate a static position and using the suffix *-ing* to denote a movement. Thus an elbow can be in a position of 90 degrees of flex*ion* and also extend*ing*.

Factors Influencing ROM and ROM Measurements

The ROM available at a joint is determined by morphology and the soft tissues surrounding and crossing a joint, including the joint capsule, ligaments, tendons, and muscles. Other factors such as age, gender, swelling, muscle mass development, body fat, passive insufficiency (change in the ROM available at one joint in a two-joint muscle complex caused by the position of the other joint), and time of day (diurnal effect) also affect the amount of motion available. Some persons, because of posture, genetics, body type, or movement habits, normally demonstrate hypermobile or hypomobile joints. Dominance has not been found to significantly affect available ROM. (See discussion in Miller [1985].) The shape of joint surfaces, which are designed to allow movement in particular directions, can become altered by disease, trauma, and posture, thereby increasing or decreasing the ROM. Additionally, the soft tissues crossing a joint can become tight (contracted) or overstretched, altering the ROM.

The type of movement, active or passive, also affects ROM. When measuring active ROM (AROM), the person voluntarily contracts muscles and moves the body part through the available motion. When measuring passive ROM (PROM), the examiner moves the body part through the ROM. PROM is usually slightly greater than AROM due to the extensibility of the tissues crossing and comprising the joint. AROM can be decreased because of restricted joint mobility, muscle weakness, pain, unwillingness to move, or inability to follow instructions. PROM is assessed to determine the integrity of the joint and the extent of structural limitation.

Instrumented Systems Used to Measure ROM

The most common instrument used to measure joint ROM is a goniometer. The universal goniometer, shown in Fig. 144.2a, is most widely used clinically. A number of universal goniometers have been developed for specific applications. Two other types of goniometers are also shown in Fig. 144.2.

Table 144.2 lists and compares several goniometric instruments used to measure ROM. Choice of the instrument used to measure ROM depends on the degree of accuracy required, time available to the examiner, the measurement environment, the body segment being measured, and the equipment available.

Nongoniometric methods of joint measurement are available. Tape measures, radiographs, photography, cinematography, videotape, and various optoelectric movement monitoring systems also can be used to measure or calculate ROM at various joints. These methods are beyond the scope of this chapter.

Key Concepts in Goniometric Measurement

Numerous textbooks [Clarkson & Gilewich, 1989; Duesterhaus Minor & Duesterhaus Minor, 1985; Moore, 1984; Palmer & Epler, 1990] that describe precise procedures for goniometric measurements of each joint are available. Unfortunately, there is a lack of standardization among these references.

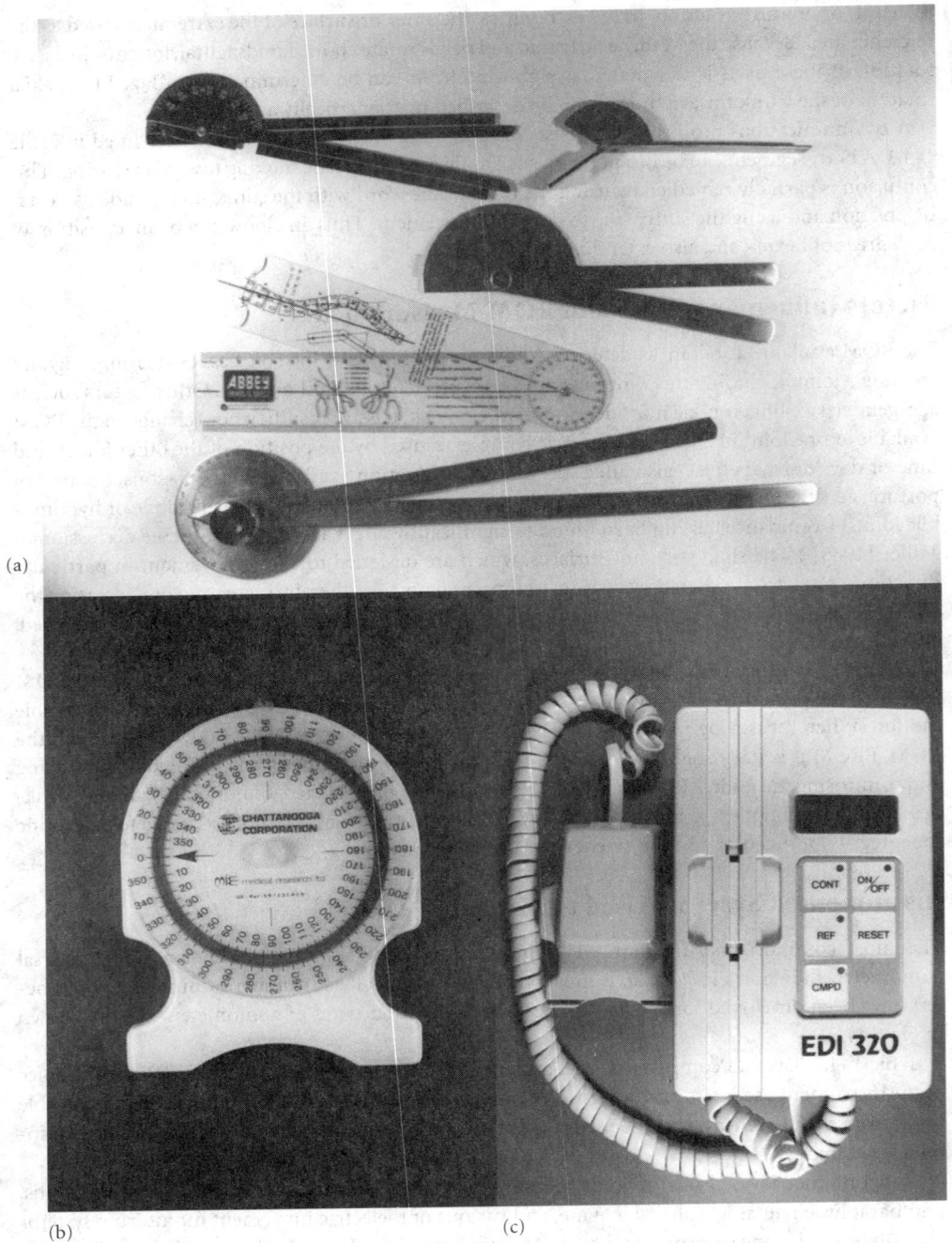

FIGURE 144.2 Three types of goniometric instruments used to measure range of motion are shown: (*a*) typical 180- and 360-degree universal goniometers of various sizes; (*b*) a fluid goniometer, which is activated by the effects of gravity; (*c*) an EDI 320 digital electronic device, which works similarly to a pendulum goniometer.

In general, the anatomic position of zero degrees (*preferred starting position*) is the desired starting position for all ROM measurements except rotation at the hip, shoulder, and forearm. The arms of the goniometer are usually aligned parallel and lateral to the long axis of the moving and the fixed body segments in line with the appropriate landmarks. In the past, some authors contended that

TABLE 144.2 Comparison of Various Goniometers Commonly Used to Measure Joint Range of Motion

Type of Goniometer	Advantages/Uses	Disadvantages/Limitations
Universal goniometer A protractor-like device with one arm considered movable and the other arm stationary; protractor can have a 180- or 360-degree scale and is usually numbered in both directions; available in a range of sizes and styles to accommodate different joints (see Fig. 144.2a).	Inexpensive; portable; familiar devices; size of the joint being measured determines size of the goniometer used; clear plastic goniometers have a line through the center of the arms to make alignment easier and more accurate; finger goniometers can be placed over the dorsal aspect of the joint being measured.	Several goniometers of different sizes may be required, especially if digits are measured; full-circle models may be difficult to align when the subject is recumbent and axis alignment is inhibited by the protractor bumping the surface; the increments on the protractors may vary from 1, 2, or 5 degrees; placement of the arms is a potential source of error.
Fluid (or bubble) goniometer A device with a fluid-filled channel with a 360-degree scale that relies on the effects of gravity (see Fig. 144.2b); dial turns allowing the goniometer to be "zeroed"; some models are strapped on and others must be held against the body part.	Quick and easy to use because it is not usually aligned with bony landmarks; does not have to conform to body segments; useful for measuring neck and spinal movements; using a pair of fluid goniometers permits distinguishing regional spinal motion.	More expensive than universal goniometers; using a pair of goniometers is awkward; useless for motions in the horizontal plane; error can be induced by slipping, skin movement, variations in amount of soft tissue owing to muscle contraction, swelling, or fat, and the examiner's hand pressure changing body segment contour; reliability may be sacrificed from lack of orientation to landmarks and difficulty with consistent realignment [Miller, 1985].
Pendulum goniometer A scaled, inclinometerlike device with a needle or pointer (usually weighted); some models are strapped on, and others must be held against the body part (not shown).	Inexpensive; same advantages as for the fluid goniometer described above.	Some models cannot be "zeroed"; useless for motions in the horizontal plane; same soft tissue error concerns as described above for the fluid goniometer.
"Myrin" OB goniometer A fluid-filled, rotatable container consisting of compass needle that responds to the earth's magnetic field (to measure horizontal motion), a gravity-activated inclination needle (to measure frontal and sagittal motion), and a scale (not shown).	Can be strapped on the body part, allowing the hands free to stabilize and move the body part; not necessary to align the goniometer with the joint axis; permits measurements in all three planes.	Expensive and bulky compared with universal goniometer; not useful for measuring small joints of hand and foot; susceptible to magnetic fields [Clarkson & Gilewich, 1989]; subject to same soft tissue error concerns described above under fluid goniometer.
Arthrodial protractor A large, flat, clear plastic protractor without arms that has a level on the straight edge (not shown).	Does not need to conform to body segments; most useful for measuring joint rotation and axioskeletal motion.	Not useful for measuring smaller joints, especially those with lesser ROMs; usually scaled in large increments only.
EDI 320 Pendulum-type goniometer with digital sensing and electronics; can either perform continuous monitoring or calculate individual ROM from a compound motion function (see Fig. 144.2c.)	Easy to use; provides rapid digital read-out; comes with unique body interfaces for use with different applications; one hand is free to stabilize and move body segments; particularly easy for measuring regional neck and spinal movements.	Expensive compared with most other instruments described; sensing unit must be moved slowly to avoid error messages; not useful for motions in the horizontal plane; subject to the same soft tissue error concerns as described above under fluid goniometer.
Electrogoniometer Arms of a goniometer are attached to a potentiometer and are strapped to the proximal and distal body parts; movement from the device causes resistance in the potentiometer which measures the ROM (not shown).	More useful for dynamic ROM, especially for determining kinematic variables during activities such as gait; provides immediate data; some electrogoniometers permit measurement in one, two, or three dimensions.	Aligning and attaching the device is time-consuming and not amenable to all body segments; device and equipment needed to use it are moderately expensive; essentially laboratory equipment; less accurate for measurement of absolute limb position; device itself is cumbersome and may alter the movement being studied.

placement of the axis of the goniometer should be congruent with the joint axis for accurate measurement [West, 1945; Wiechec & Krusen, 1939]. However, the axis of rotation for joints changes as the body segment moves through its ROM; therefore, a goniometer cannot be placed in a position in line with the joint axis during movement. Robson [1966] described how variations in the placement of the goniometer's axis could affect the accuracy of ROM measurements. Miller [1985] suggested that the axis problem could be handled by ignoring the goniometer's axis and concentrating on the accurate alignment of the arms of the goniometer with the specified landmarks. Potentially, some accuracy may be sacrificed, but the technique is simplified and theoretically more reproducible. The subject's movement is observed for unwanted motions that could result in inaccurate measurement. For example, a subject might attempt to increase forearm supination by laterally flexing the trunk.

Numeric Notation Systems

Three primary systems exist for expressing joint motion in terms of degrees. These are the *0 to 180 system,* the *180 to 0 system,* and the *360 system.* The 0 to 180 system is the most widely accepted system in medical applications and may be the easiest system to interpret. In the 0 to 180 system, the starting position for all movements is considered to be 0 degrees, and movements proceed toward 180 degrees. As the joint motion increases, the numbers on the goniometric scale increase. In the 180 to 0 system, movements toward flexion approach 0 degrees, and movements toward extension approach 180 degrees. Different rules are used for the other planes of motion. The 360 system is similar to the 180 to 0 system. In the 360 system, movements are frequently performed from a starting position of 180 degrees. Movements of extension or adduction that go beyond the neutral position approach 360 degrees. Joint motion can be reported in tables, charts, graphs, or pictures. In the 0 to 180 system, the starting and ending ranges are recorded separately, as 0 to 130 degrees. If a joint cannot be started in the 0-degree position, the actual starting position is recorded such as 10 to 130 degrees.

144.4 Strength

Muscle strength implies the force or torque production capacity of muscles. However, to measure strength, the term must be operationally defined. One definition modified from Clarkson and Gilewich [1989] states that muscular strength is the maximal amount of torque or force that a muscle or muscle groups can voluntarily exert in one maximal effort, when type of muscle contraction, movement velocity, and joint angle(s) are specified.

Strength Testing and Muscle Terminology

Physiologically, skeletal muscle strength is the ability of muscle fibers to generate maximal tension for a brief time interval. A muscle's ability to generate maximal tension and to sustain tension for differing time intervals is dependent on the muscle's cross-sectional area (the larger the cross-sectional area, the greater the strength), geometry (including the muscle fiber arrangement, length, moment arm, and angle of pennation), and physiology. Characteristics of muscle fibers have been classified based on twitch tension and fatigability. Different fiber types have different metabolic traits. Different types of muscle fibers are differentially stressed depending on the intensity and duration of the contraction. Ideally, strength tests should measure the ability of the muscle to develop tension rapidly and to sustain the tension for brief time intervals. In order to truly measure muscle tension, a measurement device must be directly attached to the muscle or tendon. Whereas this direct procedure has been performed [Komi, 1990], it is hardly useful as a routine clinical measure. Indirect measures are used to estimate the strength of muscle groups performing a given function, such as elbow flexion.

Muscles work together in groups and may be classified according to the major role of the group in producing movement. The *prime mover,* or *agonist,* is a muscle or muscle group that makes the major contribution to movement at a joint. The *antagonist* is a muscle or muscle group that has an opposite action to the prime mover(s). The antagonist relaxes as the agonist moves the body part through the ROM. *Synergists* are accessory muscles that contract and work with the agonist to produce the desired movement. Synergists may work by stabilizing proximal joints, preventing unwanted movement, and joining with the prime mover to produce a movement that one muscle group acting alone could not produce.

A number of terms and concepts are important toward understanding the nature and scope of strength capacity testing. Several of these terms' relations to types of contractions are defined below; however, there are no universally accepted definitions for these terms.

Dynamic—the output of muscles moving body segments [Kroemer, 1991].

Isometric—tension develops in a muscle, but the muscle length does not change and no movement occurs.

Static—same as *isometric.*

Isotonic—a muscle develops constant tension against a load or resistance. Kroemer [1991] suggests that the term *isoforce* more aptly describes this condition.

Concentric—a contraction in which a muscle develops internal force that exceeds the external force of resistance, the muscle shortens, and movement is produced [O'Connel & Gowitzke, 1972].

Eccentric—a contraction in which a muscle lengthens while continuing to maintain tension [O'Connel & Gowitzke, 1972].

Isokinetic—a condition where the angular velocity is held constant. Kroemer [1991] prefers the term *isovelocity* to describe this type of muscle exertion.

Isoinertial—a static or dynamic muscle contraction where the external load is held constant [Kroemer, 1983].

Factors Influencing Muscle Strength and Strength Measurement

In addition to the anatomic and physiologic factors affecting strength, other factors must be considered when strength-testing. The ability of a muscle to develop tension depends on the type of muscle contraction. Per unit of muscle, the greatest tension can be generated eccentrically, less can be developed isometrically, and the least can be generated concentrically. These differences in tension-generating capacity are so great that the type of contraction being strength-tested requires specification.

Additionally, strength is partially determined by the ability of the nervous system to cause more motor units to fire synchronously. As one trains, practices an activity, or learns test expectations, strength can increase. Therefore, strength is affected by previous training and testing. This is an important consideration in standardizing testing and in retesting.

A muscle's attachments define the angle of pull of the tendon on the bone and thereby the mechanical leverage at the joint center. Each muscle has a moment arm length, which is the length of a line normal to the muscle passing through the joint center. This moment arm length changes with the joint angle, which changes the muscle's tension output. Optimal tension is developed when a muscle is pulling at a 90-degree angle to the bony segment.

Changes in muscle length alter the force-generating capacity of muscle. This is called the *length-tension relationship. Active* tension decreases when a muscle is either lengthened or shortened relative to its resting length. However, after applying a precontraction stretch, or slightly lengthening a muscle and the series elastic component (connective tissue), prior to a contraction causes a greater amount of *total* tension to be developed [Soderberg, 1992]. Of course, excessive lengthening would reduce the tension-generating capacity.

A number of muscles cross over more than one joint. The length of these muscles may be inadequate to permit complete ROM of all joints involved. When a multijoint muscle simultaneously shortens at all joints it crosses, further effective tension development is prevented. This phenomenon is called *active insufficiency*. For example, when the hamstrings are tested as knee flexors with the hip extended, less tension can be developed than when the hamstrings are tested with the hip flexed. Therefore, when testing the strength of multijoint muscles, the position of all involved joints must be considered.

The *load-velocity relationship* is also important in testing muscle strength. A load-velocity curve can be generated by plotting the velocity of motion of the muscle lever arm against the external load. With concentric muscle contractions, the least tension is developed at the highest velocity of movement, and vice versa. When the external load equals the maximal force that the muscle can exert, the velocity of shortening reaches zero, and the muscle contracts isometrically. When the load is increased further, the muscle lengthens eccentrically. During eccentric contractions, the highest tension can be achieved at the highest velocity of movement [Komi, 1973].

The force generated by a muscle is proportional to the contraction time. The longer the contraction time, the greater is the force development up to the point of maximum tension. Slower contraction leads to greater force production because more time is allowed for the tension produced in contractile elements to be transferred through the noncontractile components to the tendon. This is the *force-time relationship*. Tension in the tendon will reach the maximum tension developed by the contractile tissues only if the active contraction process is of adequate (even up to 300 ms) duration [Sukop & Nelson, 1974].

Subject effort or motivation, gender, age, fatigue, time of day, temperature, occupation, and dominance also can affect force or torque production capacity. Important additional considerations may be changes in muscle function as a result of pain, overstretching, immobilization, trauma, paralytic disorders, neurologic conditions, and muscle transfers.

Grading Systems and Parameters Measured

Clinically, the two most frequently used methods of strength testing are actually noninstrumented tests: the manual muscle test (MMT) and the functional muscle test (see Amundsen [1990] and Palmer and Epler [1990] for more information on functional muscle tests). In each of these cases, interval-scaled grading criteria are operationally defined. However, a distinct advantage of using instruments to measure strength is that quantifiable units can be obtained, usually force or torque. Torque = force × the distance between the point of force application and the axis of rotation,

$$T = Fx \qquad (144.1)$$

An important issue in strength testing is deciding whether to measure force (a linear quantity) or torque (a rotational quantity). If the point of application of a force is closer to the axis of rotation, the muscle being assessed has a mechanical advantage as compared to when the point of contact is more distal. Therefore, when forces are measured, unless the measurement devices are applied at the same anatomic position for each test, force measurements can differ substantially even though actual muscle tension remains the same. If the strength-testing device has an axis of rotation that can be aligned with the anatomic axis of rotation, then torque can be measured directly. When this is not the case, the moment arm can be measured and torque calculated. Force is more typically measured in whole-body exertions, such as lifting. Another issue is whether to measure and record peak or averaged values. However, if strength is defined as maximum torque production capacity, peak values are implied.

In addition to single numeric values, some strength measurement systems display and print force or torque (versus time) curves, angle-torque curves, and graphs. Computerized systems frequently compare the "involved" with the "uninvolved" extremity, calculating *percentage deficits*.

Since strength is considered proportional to body weight (perhaps erroneously; see Delitto [1990]), force and torque measurements are frequently reported as a peak torque to body weight ratio. This is seemingly to facilitate use of normative data where present.

Methods and Instruments Used to Measure Muscle Strength

There are two broad categories of testing force or torque production capacity; one category consists of measuring the capacity of defined, local muscle groups (e.g., elbow flexors), and the second category of tests consists of measuring several muscle groups on a whole-body basis performing a higher-level task (e.g., lifting). The purpose of the test, required level of sensitivity, and expense are primary factors in selecting the method of strength testing. No single method has emerged as being clearly superior or more widely applicable. Like screwdrivers, different types and different sizes are needed depending on job demands.

Many of the instrumented strength-testing techniques, which are becoming more standardized clinically and which are almost exclusively used in engineering applications, are based on the concepts and methods of MMT. Although not used for performance capacity tests, because of the ease, practicality, and speed of manual testing, it is still considered a useful tool, especially diagnostically to localize lesions. Several MMT grading systems prevail. These differ in the actual test positions and premises on which muscle grading is based. For example, the approach promoted by Kendall et al. [1993] tests a specific muscle (e.g., brachioradialis) rather than a motion. The Daniels and Worthingham [1986] method tests motions (e.g., elbow flexion) that involve all the agonists and synergists used to perform the movement. The latter is considered more functional and less time-consuming but less specific. The reader is advised to consult these references directly for more information about MMT methods. Further discussion of noninstrumented tests is beyond the scope of this chapter.

An argument can be made for using isometric testing because the force or torque reflects actual muscle tension as the position of the body part is held constant and the muscle mechanics do not change. Additionally, good stabilization is easier to achieve, and muscle actions can be better isolated. However, some clinicians prefer dynamic tests, perceiving them as more reflective of function. An unfortunate fact is that neither static nor dynamic strength measurements alone can reveal whether strength is adequate for functional activities. However, strength measurements can be used with models and engineering analyses for such assessments.

Selected instrumented methods of measuring force or torque production capacity are listed and compared in Table 144.3. Table 144.3 is by no means comprehensive. More indepth review and comparisons of various methods can be found in Amundsen [1990] and Mayhew and Rothstein [1985]. Figure 144.3 illustrates three common instruments used to measure strength.

Key Concepts in Measuring Strength

Because of the number of factors influencing strength and strength testing (discussed in a previous section), one can become discouraged rather than challenged when faced with the need to measure strength. Optimally, strength testing would be based on the "worst case" functional performance demands required by an individual in his or her daily life. This requires knowing the performance demands of tasks, including the positions required, types of muscle contractions, and so on.

In the absence of such data, current strategy is to choose the instruments and techniques that seem logical based on knowledge of the task, or that have been reported as appropriate and reliable for the population of interest, and to maximally stress the system under a set of representative conditions. An attempt is made to standardize the testing in terms of contraction type, test administration instructions, feedback, warmup, number of trials, time of day, examiner, duration of contraction (usually 4 to 6 seconds), method and location of application of force, testing order, environmental distractions, subject posture and position of testing, degree of stabilization, and rest intervals

TABLE 144.3   Comparison of Various Instrumented Methods Used to Measure Muscle Strength

Instrument/Method	Advantages/Uses	Disadvantages/Limitations
Repetition maximum Amount of weight a subject can lift a given number of times and no more; one determines either a one repetition maximum (1-RM) or a ten repetition maximum (10-RM). A 1-RM is the maximum amount of weight a subject can lift once; a 10-RM is the amount of weight a subject can lift 10 times; a particular protocol to determine RMs is defined [DeLorme & Watkins, 1948]; measures dynamic strength in terms of weight (pounds or kilograms) lifted.	Requires minimal equipment (weights); inexpensive and easy to administer; frequently used informally to assess progress in strength training.	Uses serial testing of adding weights which may invalidate subsequent testing; no control for speed of contraction or positioning; minimal information available on the reliability and validity of this method.
Hand-held dynamometer Device held in the examiner's hand used to test strength; devices use either hydraulics, strain gauges (load-cells), or spring systems (see Fig. 144.3a); used with a "break test" (the examiner exerts a force against the body segment to be tested until the part gives way) or a "make test" (the examiner applies a constant force while the subject exerts a maximum force against it); "make tests" are frequently preferred for use with hand-held dynamometers [Bohannon, 1990; Smidt, 1984]; measures force; unclear whether test measures isometric or eccentric force (this may depend on whether a "make test" or a "break test" is used).	Similar to manual muscle testing (MMT) in test positions and sites for load application; increased objectivity over MMT; portable; easy to administer; relatively inexpensive; commercially available from several suppliers; adaptable for a variety of test sites; provide immediate output; spring and hydraulic systems are non-electrical; load-cell based systems provide more precise digital measurements.	Stabilization of the device and body segment can be difficult; results can be affected by the examiner's strength; limited usefulness with large muscle groups; spring-based systems fatigue over time becoming inaccurate; range and sensitivity of the systems vary; shape of the unit grasped by the examiner and shape of the end-piece vary in comfort, and therefore the force a subject or examiner is willing to exert; more valuable for testing subjects with weakness than for less involved or healthy subjects due to range limits within the device (see discussion in Bohannon [1990]).
Cable tensiometer One end of a cable is attached to an immovable object and the other end is attached to a limb segment; the tensiometer is placed between the sites of fixation; as the cable is pulled, it presses on the tensiometer's riser which is connected to a gauge (see discussion in Mayhew and Rothstein [1985]); measures isometric force.	Mostly used in research settings; evidence presented on reliability when used with normal subjects [Clarke, 1954; Clarke et al., 1952]; relatively inexpensive.	Requires special equipment for testing; testing is time-consuming and some tests require two examiners; unfamiliar to most clinicians; not readily available; less sensitive at low force levels.
Strain gauge Electroconductive material applied to metal rings or rods; a load applied to the ring or bar deforms the metal and a gauge; deformation of the gauge changes the electrical resistance of the gauge causing a voltage variation; this change can be converted and displayed using a strip chart recorder or digital display; measures isometric force.	Mostly used in research settings; increased sensitivity for testing strong and weak muscles.	Strain gauges require frequent calibration and are sensitive to temperature variations; to be accurate the body part must pull or push against the gauge in the same line that the calibration weights were applied; unfamiliar to most clinicians; not commercially available; difficult to interface the device comfortably with the subject.

(continued)

TABLE 144.3　Comparison of Various Instrumented Methods Used to Measure Muscle Strength *(continued)*

Instrument/Method	Advantages/Uses	Disadvantages/Limitations
Isokinetic dynamometer Constant velocity loading device; several models marketed by a number of different companies; most consist of a movable lever arm controlled by an electronic servomotor that can be preset for selected angular velocities usually between 0° and 500° per second; when the subject attempts to accelerate beyond the pre-set machine speed, the machine resists the movement; a load cell measures the torque needed to prevent body part acceleration beyond the selected speed; computers provide digital displays and printouts (see typical device in Fig. 144.3*c*); measures isokinetic-concentric (and in some cases, isokinetic-eccentric) and isometric strength; provides torque (or occasionally force) data; debate exists about whether data are ratio-scaled or not; accounting for the weight of the segment permits ratio-scaling [Winter et al., 1981].	Permits dynamic testing of most major body segments; especially useful for stronger movements; most devices provide good stabilization; measures reciprocal muscle contractions; wide-spread clinical acceptance; also records angular data, work, power, and endurance-related measures; provides a number of different reporting options; also used as exercise devices.	Devices are large and expensive; need calibration with external weights or are "self-calibrating;" signal damping and "windowing" may affect data obtained; angle-specific measurements may not be accurate if a damp is used because torque readings do not relate to the goniometric measurements; joints must be aligned with the mechanical axis of the machine; inferences about muscle function in daily activities from isokinetic test results have not been validated; data obtained between different brands of devices are not interchangeable; adequate stabilization may be difficult to achieve for some movements; may not be usable with especially tall or short persons.
Hand dynamometer Instruments to measure gripping or pinching strength specifically for the hand; usually use a spring scale or strain-gauge system (see typical grip strength testing device in Fig. 144.3*b*); measures isometric force.	Readily available from several suppliers; easy to use; relatively inexpensive; widespread use; some normative data available.	Only useful for the hand; different brands not interchangeable; normative data only useful when reported for the same instrument and when measurements are taken with the same body position and instrument setting; must be recalibrated frequently.

between exertions (usually 30 seconds to 2 minutes) [Chaffin, 1975; Smidt & Rogers, 1982]. In addition, the subject must be observed for muscle group substitutions and "trick" movements.

144.5 Speed of Movement

Speed of movement refers to the rate of movement of the body or body segments. The maximum movement speed that can be achieved represents another unique performance capacity of an iden-tified system that is responsible for producing motion. It is common to hear everyday, work, and sport tasks described in terms of the speed requirements (e.g., repetitions per minute or per hour). For physical tasks, such descriptions translate to translational motion speeds (e.g., as in lifting) as well as rotational motion speeds (i.e., movement about a dof of the joint systems involved). Thus there is important motivation to characterize this capacity.

Speed of Movement Terminology

Speed of movement must be differentiated from *speed of contraction*. Speed of contraction refers to how fast a muscle generates tension. Two body parts may be moving through an arc with the same speed of movement; however, if one has a greater mass, its muscles must develop more tension per unit of time to move the heavier body part at the same speed as the lighter body part.

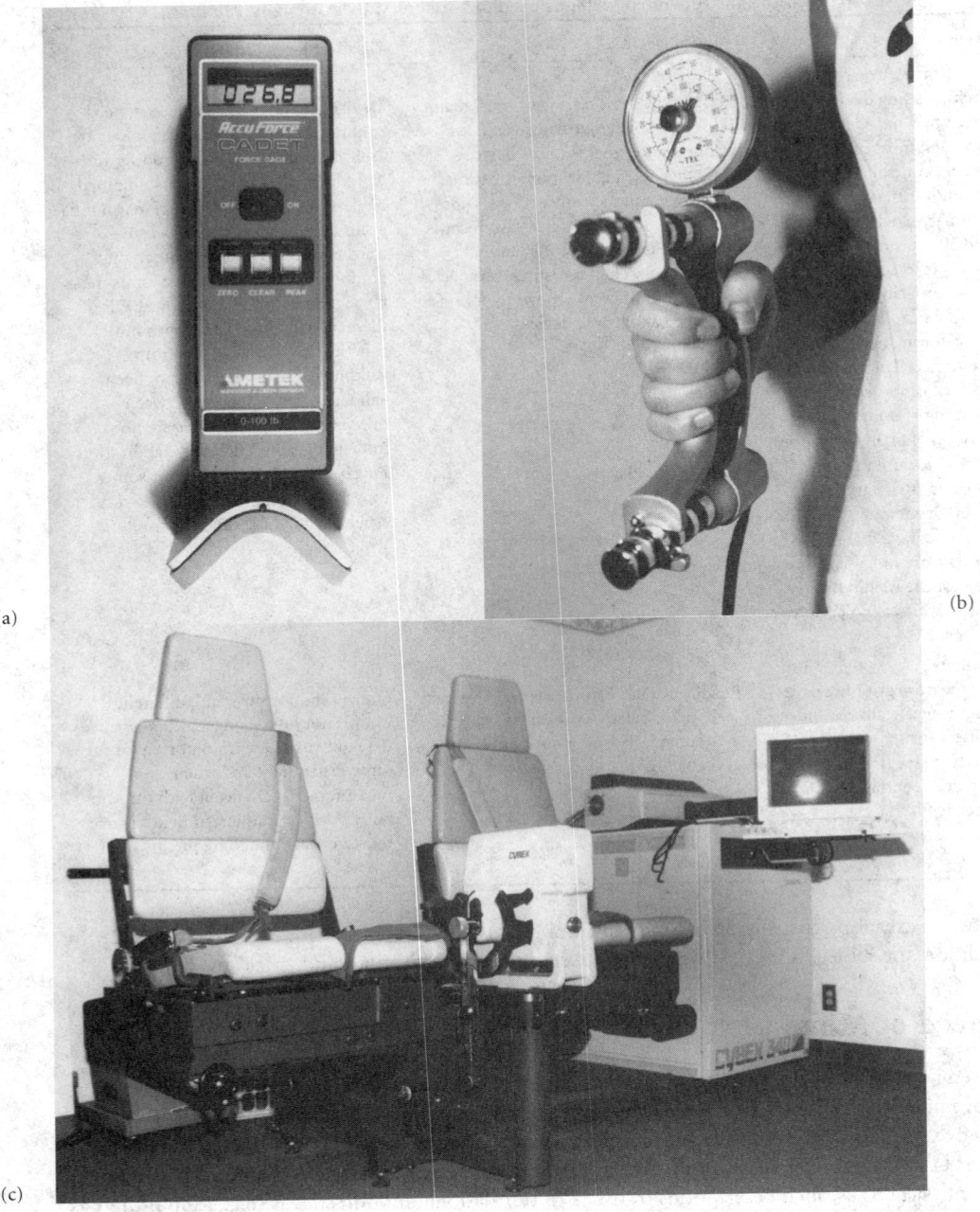

(a)

(b)

(c)

FIGURE 144.3 Three types of instrumented strength testing devices are shown: (*a*) a representative example of a typical hand-held dynamometer; (*b*) an example of an isokinetic strength testing device; (*c*) a hand dynamometer used to measure grip strength.   PAGE 2188

Speed, velocity, and acceleration also can be distinguished. The terms *velocity* and *speed* are often used interchangeably; however, the two quantities are frequently not identical. *Velocity* means the rate of motion *in a particular direction*. *Acceleration* results from a change in velocity. General velocity and acceleration measurements are beyond the intent of this chapter. Reaction speed and response speed are other related variables also not considered.

Factors Influencing Speed of Movement and Speed of Movement Measurements

Muscles with larger moment arms, longer muscle fibers, and less pennation tend to be capable of generating greater speed. Many of the same factors that influence strength, discussed previously, such as muscle length, fatigue, and temperature also affect the muscle's contractile rate. The load-velocity relationship is especially important when testing speed of movement. In addition to these and other physiologic factors, speed can be reduced by factors such as friction, air resistance, gravity, unnecessary movements, and inertia [Jensen & Fisher, 1979].

Parameters Measured

Speed of movement can be measured as a linear quantity or as an angular quantity. Typically, if the whole body is moving linearly in space, as in walking or running, a point such as the center of gravity is picked, and translational motion is measured. Also, when an identified point on a body segment (e.g., the tip of the index finger) is moved in space, translational movement is observed, and motion is measured in translational terms. If the speed of a rotational motion system (e.g., elbow flexors) is being measured, then the angular quantity is determined. Since the focus here is on measuring isolated neuromuscular performance capacities, the angular metric is emphasized. Angular speed of a body segment is obtained by: Angular speed = change in angular position/change in time,

$$\sigma = \frac{\Delta\phi}{\Delta t} \qquad (144.2)$$

Thus speed of movement may be expressed in revolutions, degrees, or radians per unit of time, such as degrees per second (deg/s).

   Another type of speed measure applies to well-defined (over fixed angles or distance) cyclic motions. Here, repetitions per unit time or cycles per unit time measures are sometimes used. However, in almost every one of these situations, it is possible to express speed in degrees per second or meters per second. The latter units are preferred because they allow easier comparison of speeds across a variety of tasks. The only occasion when this is difficult is when translation motion is not in a simple straight line, such as when a person is performing a complex assembly task with multiple subtasks.

   The issue of whether to express speed as maximum, averaged, or instantaneous values also must be decided based on which measure is a more useful indicator of the performance being measured. In addition to numeric reporting of speed data, time-history graphs of speed may be helpful in comparing some types of performance.

Instruments Used to Measure Speed of Movement

When movement time is greater than a few seconds and the distance is known, speed can be measured with a stopwatch or with switch plates, such as the time elapsed in moving between two points or over a specified angle. With rapid angular joint movements, switch plates or electrogoniometers with electronic timing devices are required. Speeds also can be computed from the distance or angle and time data available from cinematography, optoelectric movement monitoring systems, and videotape systems. Some dynamic strength testing devices involve presetting a load and measuring the speed of movement.

   In addition, accelerometers can be used to measure acceleration directly, and speed can be derived through integration. However, piezoelectric models have no steady-state response and may not be useful for slower movements. Single accelerometers are used to measure linear motion. Simple rotatory motions require two accelerometers. Triaxial accelerometers are commercially available that contain three premounted accelerometers perpendicular to each other. Multiple accelerometer outputs require appropriate processing to resolve the vector component corresponding to the desired speed. Accelerometers are most appropriately used to measure acceleration when they are mounted on rigid materials. Accelerometers have the advantage of continuously and directly measuring acceleration in an immediately usable form. They also can be very accurate if well mounted. Because they require soft tissue fixation and cabling or telemetry, they may alter performance, and further error may be induced by relative motion of the device and tissues. The systems are moderately expensive (see discussion of accelerometers in [Robertson & Sprigings, 1987]).

Key Concepts in Speed of Movement Measurement

As discussed, maximum speed is determined when there is little stress on torque production resources. As resistance increases, speed will decrease. Therefore, the load must be considered and specified when testing speed. Because speed-of-movement data are calculated from displacement and temporal data, a key issue is minimizing error that might result from collecting this information. Error can result from inaccurate identification of anatomic landmarks, improper calibration, perspective error, instrument synchronization error, resolution, digitization error, or vibration. The sampling rate of some of measurement systems may become an issue when faster movements are being analyzed. In addition, the dynamic characteristics of signal conditioning systems should be reported.

144.6 Endurance

Endurance is the ability of a system to sustain an activity for a prolonged time (static endurance) or to perform repeatedly (dynamic endurance). Endurance can apply to the body as a whole, a particular body system, or to specific neuromuscular functional units. High levels of endurance imply that a given level of performance can be continued for a long time period.

Endurance Terminology

General endurance of the body as a whole is traditionally considered cardiovascular endurance or aerobic capacity. Cardiovascular endurance most frequently viewed in terms of $\dot{V}O_2$ max. This chapter considers only endurance of neuromuscular systems. Although many central and peripheral anatomic sites and physiologic processes contribute to a loss of endurance, endurance of neuromuscular functional units is also referred to as *muscular endurance.*

Absolute muscle endurance is defined as the amount of time that a neuromuscular system can continue to accomplish a specified task against a constant resistance (load and rate) without relating the resistance to the muscle's strength. Absolute muscle endurance and strength are highly correlated. Conversely, there is an inverse relationship between strength and *relative muscle endurance*. That is, when resistance is adjusted to the person's strength, a weaker person tends to demonstrate more endurance than a stronger person. Furthermore, the same relationships between absolute and relative endurance and strength are correlated by type of contraction; in other words, there is a strong positive correlation between isotonic strength and *absolute* isotonic endurance, and vice versa, for strength and *relative* isotonic endurance. The same types of relationships exist for isometric strength and isometric endurance [Jensen & Fisher, 1979].

Factors Influencing Neuromuscular Endurance and Measurement of Endurance

Specific muscle fiber types, namely, fast-twitch fatigue-resistant fibers (FR), generate intermediate levels of tension and are resistant to short-term fatigue (a duration of about 2 minutes or intermittent stimulation). Slow-twitch fibers (S) generate low levels of tension slowly and are highly resistant to fatigue. Muscle contractions longer than 10 seconds but less than 2 minutes will measure local muscle endurance [Åstrand & Rodahl, 1977]. For durations longer than 2 minutes, the S fibers will be most stressed. A submaximal isometric contraction to the point of voluntary fatigue will primarily stress the FR and S fibers [Thorstensson & Karlsson, 1976]. Repetitive, submaximal, dynamic contractions continued for about 2 to 6 minutes will measure the capacity of FR and S fibers. Strength testing requires short duration and maximal contractions; therefore, to differentiate strength and endurance testing, the duration and intensity of the contractions must be considered.

Because strength affects endurance, all the factors discussed previously that influence strength also influence endurance. In addition to muscle physiology and muscle strength, endurance is dependent on the extensiveness of the muscle's capillary beds, the involved neuromuscular mechanisms, contraction force, load, and the rate at which the activity is performed.

Endurance time, or the time for muscles to reach fatigue, is a function of the contraction force or load [von Rohmert, 1960]. As the load (or torque required) increases, endurance time decreases. Also, as speed increases, particularly with activities involving concentric muscle contractions, endurance decreases.

Parameters Measured

Endurance is *how long* an activity can be performed at the required load and rate level. Thus the basic unit of measure is *time*. Time is the only measure of how long it takes to complete a task. If we focus on a given variable (e.g., strength, speed, or endurance), it is necessary to either control or measure the others. When the focus is endurance, the other factors of force or torque, speed, and joint angle can be described as conditions under which endurance is measured. Because of the interactions of endurance and load, or endurance and time, for example, a number of *endurance-related* measures have evolved. These endurance-related measures have clouded endurance testing.

One endurance-related measure uses either the number of repetitions that can be performed at 20%, 25%, or 50% of maximum peak torque or force. The units used to reflect endurance in this case are number of repetitions at a specified torque or force level. One difficulty with this definition has been described previously, i.e., the issue of relative versus absolute muscle endurance. Rothstein and Rose [1982] demonstrated that elderly subjects with selected muscle fiber type atrophy were able to maintain 50% of their peak torque longer than young subjects. However, if a high force level is required to perform the task, then the younger subject would have more endurance in that particular activity [Rothstein, 1982]. Another difficulty is that this method can be used only for dynamic activities. If isometric activities are involved, then the time an activity can be sustained at a specified force or torque level is measured. Why have different units of endurance? Time could be used in both cases. Furthermore, the issue of absolute versus relative muscle endurance becomes irrelevant if the demands of the task are measured.

Yet another method used to reflect endurance is to calculate an endurance-related work ratio. Many isokinetic testing devices, such as the one shown in Fig. 144.3c, will calculate work (integrate force or torque over displacement). In this case, the total amount of work performed in the first five repetitions is compared with the total amount of work performed in the last five repetitions of a series of repetitions (usually 25 or more). Work degradation *reflects* endurance and is reported as a percentage. An additional limitation of using these endurance ratios is that work cannot be determined in isometric test protocols. Mechanically, there is no movement, and no work is being performed.

Overall, the greatest limitation with most *endurance-related* approaches is that the measures obtained cannot be used to perform task-related assessments. In a workplace assessment, for example, one can determine how long a specific task (defined by the conditions of load, range, and speed) needs to be performed. Endurance-related metrics can be used to reflect changes over time in a subject's available endurance capacity; however, they cannot be compared with the demands of the task. Task demands are measured in time or repetitions (e.g., 10) with a given rate (e.g., 1/0.5 hours) from which total time (e.g., 5 hours) can be calculated. A true endurance measure (versus an endurance-related measure) can serve both purposes. Time reflects changes in endurance as the result of disease, disuse, training, or rehabilitation and also can be linked to task demands.

Methods and Instruments Used to Measure Neuromuscular Endurance

Selection of the method or instrument used to measure endurance depends on the purpose of the measurement and whether endurance or endurance-related measures will be obtained. As in strength testing, endurance tests can involve simple, low-level tasks or whole-body, higher-level activities. The simplest method of measuring endurance is to define a task in terms of performance criteria and then time the performance with a stopwatch. A subject is given a load and a posture and asked to hold it "as long as possible" or to move from one point to another point at a specific rate of movement for "as long as possible."

An example of a static endurance test is the Sorensen test used to measure endurance of the trunk extensors [Biering-Sorensen, 1984]. This test measures how long a person can sustain his or her torso in a suspended prone posture. The individual is not asked to perform a maximal voluntary contraction, but an indirect calculation of load is possible [Smidt & Blanpied, 1987].

An example of a dynamic endurance test is either a standardized or nonstandardized, dynamic isoinertial (see previous description in the section on strength testing) repetition test. In other words, the subject is asked to lift a known load with a specified body part or parts until defined conditions can no longer be met. Conditions such as acceleration, distance, method of performance, or speed may or may not be controlled. The more standardized of these tests, particularly those which involve lifting capacity, are reported, and projections about performance capacity over time are estimated [Snook, 1978]. Ergometers and some of the isokinetic dynamometers discussed previously measure work, and several can calculate endurance-related ratios. These devices could be adapted to measure endurance in time units.

Key Concepts in Measuring Muscle Endurance

Of the four variables of human performance discussed in this chapter, endurance testing is the least developed and standardized. Except for test duration and rest intervals, attention to the same guidelines as described for strength testing is currently recommended.

144.7 Reliability, Validity, and Limitations in Testing

Space does not permit a complete review of these important topics. However, a few key comments are in order. First, it is important to note that reliability and validity are not inherent qualities of instruments but exist in the measurements obtained only within the context in which they are tested. Second, reliability and validity are not either present or absent but are present or absent along a continuum. Third, traditional quantitative measures of reliability might indicate how much reliability a given measurement demonstrates but not how much reliability is actually needed. Fourth, technology has advanced to the extent that it is generally possible to measure physical variables such as time, force, torque, angles, and speed accurately, repeatably, and with high resolution. Lastly, clinical generalizability of human performance capacity measures ultimately results from looking at the body of literature on reliability as a whole and not from single studies.

For these types of variables, results of reliability studies basically report that if the instrumentation is good and if established optimal procedures are carefully followed, then results of repeat testing will usually be in the range of about 5% to 20% of each other. This range of repeatability depends on the particular variable being measured (i.e., repeated endurance measures will differ more than repeated measures of hinge joint ROM) and the magnitude of the given performance capacity (i.e., errors are often in fixed amounts, such as 3 degrees for ROM; thus, 3 out of 180 degrees is smaller percentage-wise than 3 out of 20 degrees). One can usually determine an applicable work-ing value (e.g., 5% or 20%) by careful review of the relevant reliability studies. Much of the differ-ence obtained in test-retest is because of limitations in how well one can reasonably control proce-dures and the actual variability of the parameter being measured, even in the most ideal test subjects. Measurements should be used with these thoughts in mind. If a specific application requires extreme repeatability, then a reliability study should be conducted under conditions that most closely match those in which the need arises. Reliability discussions specific to the some of the focal measures of this chapter are presented in Amundsen [1990], Hellebrandt et al. [1949], Mayhew and Rothstein [1985], and Miller [1985].

Measurements can be reliable but useless without validity. Most validity studies have compared the results of one instrument with those of another instrument or with known quantities. This is the classic type of validity testing, which is an effort to determine whether the measurement reflects the variable being measured. In the absence of a "gold standard," this type of testing is of limited value. In addition to traditional studies of the validity of measurements, the issue of the *validity of the inferences* based on the measurements is becoming increasingly important [Rothstein & Echter-nach, 1993]. That is, can the measurements be used to make inferences about human performance in real-life situations? Unfortunately, measurements that have not demonstrated more than content validity are frequently used as if they were predictive. The validity of the inferences made from human performance data needs to be rigorously addressed.

Specific measurement limitations were briefly addressed in Tables 144.2 and 144.3 and in the written descriptions of various measurement techniques and instruments. Other limitations have more to do with interpreting the data. A general limitation is that performance variables are not fixed human attributes. Another limitation is that population data are limited, and available normative data are, unfortunately, frequently extrapolated to women, older persons, and so on [Chaffin & Andersson, 1991]. Some normative data suggest the amount of resources such as strength, ROM, speed of movement, and endurance *required* for given activities; other data suggest the amount *available*. As previously mentioned, these are two different issues. Performance measurements may yield information about the current status of performance, but testing rarely in-dicates the *cause* or the nature of dysfunction. More definitive diagnostic studies are used to answer these questions. Whereas considerable information exists with regard to measuring performance capacities of human systems, much less energy has been directed to understanding requirements of tasks. The link between functional performance in tasks and laboratory-acquired measurements is a critical question and a major limitation in interpreting test data. The ERM addresses several of these limitations by using a multidimensional, individualized, cause-and-effect model.

144.8 Performance Capacity Space Representations

In both study and practice, performance of neuromuscular systems has been characterized along one or two dimensions of performance at a time. However, human subsystems function within a *multi*dimensional performance space. ROM, strength, movement speed, and endurance capacities are not only interdependent but also may vary uniquely within individuals. Multiple measurements are necessary to characterize a person's performance capacity space, and performance capacity is dependent on the task to be performed. Therefore, both the individual and the task must be considered when selecting measurement tools and procedures [Chaffin & Andersson, 1991].

In many of the disciplines in which human performance is of interest, traditional thinking has often focused on single-number measures of ROM, strength, speed, etc. More recent systems engi-neering approaches [Kondraske, 1995] emphasize consideration of the performance envelope of a given system and suggest ways to integrate single measurement points that define the limits of performance of a given system [Vasta & Kondraske, 1994]. Figure 144.4 illustrates a three-dimensional performance envelope derived from torque, angle, and velocity data for the knee extensor system. The additional dimension of endurance can be represented by displaying this

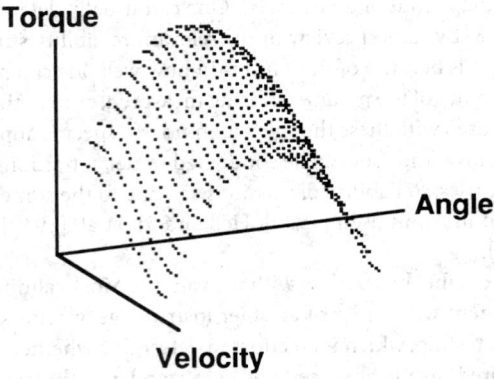

FIGURE 144.4 An example of a torque-angle-velocity performance envelope for the knee extensor system. (From Vasta & Kondraske, 1994, with permission.)

envelope after performing an activity for different lengths of time. A higher-level, composite performance capacity, as is sometimes needed, could be derived by computing the volume enclosed by this envelope. Such representations also facilitate assessment of the given system in a specific task; i.e., a task is defined as a point in this space that will either fall inside or outside the envelope.

144.9 Conclusion

In summary, human movement is so essential that it demands interest and awe from the most casual observers to the most sophisticated scientists. The complexity of performance is truly inspiring. We are challenged to understand it! We want to reduce it to comprehensible units and then enhance it, reproduce it, restore it, and predict it. To do so, we must be able to define and quantify the variables. Hence an array of instruments and methods has emerged to measure various aspects of human performance. To date, measurement of neuromuscular performance capacities along the dimensions of ROM, strength, speed of movement, and endurance represents a giant stride but only the "tip of the iceberg." Progress in developing reliable, accurate, and valid instruments and in understanding the factors influencing the measurements cannot be permitted to discourage us from the larger issues of applying the measurements toward a purpose. Yet single measurements will not suffice; multiple measurements of different aspects of performance will be necessary to fully characterize human movement.

Defining Terms

Endurance: The amount of time a body or body segments can sustain a specified static or repetitive activity.

Extremes of motion: The end ranges of motion at a joint measured in degrees.

Muscle strength: The maximal amount of torque or force production capacity that a muscle or muscle groups can voluntarily exert in one maximal effort, when type of muscle contraction, movement velocity, and joint angle(s) are specified.

Neuromuscular functional units: Systems (i.e., the combination of nerves, muscles, tendons, ligaments, and so on) responsible for producing basic movements.

Range of motion (ROM): The amount of movement that occurs at a joint, typically measured in degrees. ROM is usually measured by noting the extremes of motion.

Speed of movement: The rate of movement of the body or body segments.

References

Amundsen LR. 1990. Muscle Strength Testing: Instrumented and Non-Instrumented Systems. New York, Churchill-Livingstone.

Åstrand P-O, Rodahl K. 1977. Textbook of Work Physiology: Physiological Bases of Exercise, 2d ed. New York, McGraw-Hill.

Biering-Sorensen F. 1984. Physical measurements as risk indicators for low back trouble over a one year period. Spine 9:106.

Bohannon RW. 1990. Muscle strength testing with hand-held dynamometers. In LR Amundsen (ed), Muscle Strength Testing: Instrumented and Non-Instrumented Systems, pp 69–88. New York, Churchill Livingstone.

Chaffin DB. 1975. Ergonomics guide for the assessment of human strength. Am Ind Hyg J 36:505.

Chaffin DB, Andersson GB. 1991. Occupational Biomechanics, 2d ed. New York, Wiley.

Clarke HH. 1954. Comparison of instruments for recording muscle strength. Res Q 25:398.

Clarke HH, Bailey TL, Shay CT. 1952. New objective strength tests of muscle groups by cable-tension methods. Res Q 23:136.

Clarkson HM, Gilewich GB. 1989. Musculoskeletal Assessment: Joint Range of Motion and Manual Muscle Strength. Baltimore, Williams & Wilkins.

Daniels L, Worthingham C. 1986. Muscle Testing: Techniques of Manual Examination, 5th ed. Philadelphia, Saunders.

Delitto A. 1990. Trunk strength testing. In LR Amundsen (ed), Muscle Strength Testing: Instrumented and Non-Instrumented Systems, pp 151–162. New York, Churchill-Livingstone.

DeLorme TL, Watkins AL. 1948. Technics of progressive resistive exercise. Arch Phys Med Rehabil 29:263.

Duesterhaus Minor MA, Duesterhaus Minor S. 1985. Patient Evaluation Methods for the Health Professional. Reston, Va, Reston Publishing Company.

Hellebrandt FA, Duvall EN, Moore ML. 1949. The measurement of joint motion: III. Reliability of goniometry. Phys Ther Rev 29:302.

Jensen CR, Fisher AG. 1979. Scientific Basis of Athletic Conditioning, 2d ed. Philadelphia, Lea & Febiger.

Kendall FP, McCreary EK, Provance PG. 1993. Muscles: Testing and Function, 4th ed. Baltimore, Williams & Wilkins.

Komi PV. 1973. Measurement of the force-velocity relationship in human muscle under concentric and eccentric contractions. In S Cerquiglini, A Venerando, J Wartenweiler (eds), Biomechanics III, pp 224–229. Baltimore, University Park Press.

Komi PV. 1990. Relevance of in vivo force measurements to human biomechanics. J Biomech 23(suppl 1):23.

Kondraske GV. 1995. A working model for human system-task interfaces. In JD Bronzino (ed), Biomedical Engineering Handbook. Boca Raton, Fla, CRC Press.

Kroemer KHE. 1983. An isoinertial technique to assess individual lifting capability. Human Factors 25:493.

Kroemer KHE. 1991. A taxonomy of dynamic muscle exertions. J Hum Muscle Perform 1:1.

Mayhew TP, Rothstein JM. 1985. Measurement of muscle performance with instruments. In JM Rothstein (ed), Measurement in Physical Therapy, pp 57–102. New York, Churchill-Livingstone.

Miller PJ. 1985. Assessment of joint motion. In JM Rothstein (ed), Measurement in Physical Therapy, pp 103–136. New York, Churchill-Livingstone.

Moore ML. 1984. Clinical assessment of joint motion. In JV Basmajian (ed), Therapeutic Exercise, 4th ed., pp 192–224. Baltimore, Williams & Wilkins.

O'Connel AL, Gowitzke B. 1972. Understanding the Scientific Bases of Human Movement. Baltimore, Williams & Wilkins.

Palmer ML, Epler M. 1990. Clinical Assessment Procedures in Physical Therapy. Philadelphia, Lippincott.

Panjabi MM, White AA III, Brand RA. 1974. A note on defining body parts configurations. J Biomech 7:385.

Robertson G, Sprigings E. 1987. Kinematics. In DA Dainty, RW Norman (eds), Standardizing Biomechanical Testing in Sport, pp 9–20. Champaign Ill, Human Kinetics Publishers.

Robson P. 1966. A method to reduce the variable error in joint range measurement. Ann Phys Med 8:262.

Rothstein JM. 1982. Muscle biology: Clinical considerations. Phys Ther 62:1823.

Rothstein JM. Echternach JL. 1993. Primer on Measurement: An Introductory Guide to Measurement Issues. Alexandria, Va, American Physical Therapy Association.

Rothstein JM, Rose SJ. 1982. Muscle mutability: II. Adaptation to drugs, metabolic factors, and aging. Phys Ther 62:1788.

Soderberg GL. 1992. Skeletal muscle function. In DP Currier, RM Nelson (eds), Dynamics of Human Biologic Tissues, pp 74–96, Philadelphia, FA Davis.

Smidt GL. 1984. Muscle Strength Testing: A System Based on Mechanics. Iowa City, SPARK Instruments and Academics.

Smidt GL, Blanpied PR. 1987. Analysis of strength tests and resistive exercises commonly used for low-back disorders. Spine 12:1025.

Smidt GL, Rogers MR. 1982. Factors contributing to the regulation and clinical assessment of muscular strength. Phys Ther 62:1284.

Snook SH. 1978. The design of manual handling tasks. Ergonomics 21:963.

Sukop J, Nelson RC. 1974. Effects of isometric training in the force-time characteristics of muscle contractions. In RC Nelson, CA Morehouse (eds), Biomechanics IV, pp 440–447. Baltimore, University Park Press.

Thorstensson A, Karlsson J. 1976. Fatiguability and fibre composition of human skeletal muscle. Acta Physiol Scand 98:318.

Vasta PJ, Kondraske GV. 1994. A multi-dimensional performance space model for the human knee extensor (technical report 94-001R). University of Texas at Arlington, Human Performance Institute, Arlington, Texas.

von Rohmert W. 1960. Ermittlung von erholungspausen fur statische arbeit des menschen. Int Z Angew Physiol 18:123.

West CC. 1945. Measurement of joint motion. Arch Phys Med 26:414.

White AA III, Panjabi MM. 1990. Clinical Biomechanics of the Spine, 2d ed. Philadelphia, Lippincott.

Wiechec FJ, Krusen FH. 1939. A new method of joint measurement and a review of the literature. Am J Surg 43:659.

Winter DA, Wells RP, Orr GW. 1981. Errors in the use of isokinetic dynamometers. Eur J Appl Physiol 46:397.

Further Information

Journals: Clinical Biomechanics, Journal of Biomechanics, Medicine and Science in Sports and Exercise, Physical Therapy.

Smith SS, Kondraske GV. 1987. Computerized system for quantitative measurement of sensorimotor aspects of human performance. Phys Ther 67:1860.

Task Force on Standards for Measurement in Physical Therapy. 1991. Standards for tests and measurements in physical therapy practice. Phys Ther 71:589.

145

Measurement of Sensory–Motor Control Performance Capacities

Richard D. Jones
Christchurch Hospital

The human nervous system is capable of simultaneous and integrated control of 100 to 150 mechanical degrees of freedom of movement in the body via tensions generated by about 700 muscles. In its widest context, movement is carried out by a sensory-motor system comprising multiple sensors (visual, auditory, proprioceptive), multiple actuators (muscles and skeletal system), and an intermediary processor that can be summarized as a multiple-input multiple-output nonlinear dynamic time-varying control system. This grand control system comprises a large number of interconnected processors and subcontrollers at various sites in the central nervous system, of which the more important are cerebral cortex, thalamus, basal ganglia, cerebellum, and spinal cord. It is capable of responding with remarkable accuracy, speed (when necessary), appropriateness, versatility, and adaptability to a wide spectrum of continuous and discrete stimuli and conditions. Certainly, by contrast, it is orders of magnitude more complex and sophisticated than the most advanced robotic systems currently available—although the latter also have what are often highly desirable attributes, such as precision and repeatability, and a much greater immunity from factors such as fatigue, distraction, and lack of motivation.

This chapter addresses the control function. First, it introduces several important concepts relating to sensory-motor control, accuracy of movement, and performance resources/capacities. Second, it provides an overview of apparatus and methods for the *measurement* and *analysis* of complex sensory-motor performance. The overview focuses on measurement of sensory-motor control performance capacities of the *upper limbs* and by means of *tracking tasks*.

145.1 Basic Principles

Sensory-Motor Control and Accuracy of Movement

From the perspective of Kondraske's [1995] *elemental resource model* of human performance, *sensory-motor control* is the function of the overall sensory-motor control system. This system can be considered as a hierarchy of multiple interconnected sensory-motor controllers sited in the *central processing and skills ("software") domains* (cf. environmental interface domain, comprising sensors and actuators, and life-sustaining domains) of the elemental resource model. These controllers range from low-level elemental-level controllers for control of movement around single joints through intermediate-level controllers needed to generate integrated movements of an entire limb and involving multiple joints and degrees of freedom and high-level controllers and processors to enable coordinated synergistic multilimb movements and the carrying out of *central executive* functions concerned with allocation and switching of resources for execution of multiple tasks simultaneously.

Each of these controllers is considered to possess limited *performance resources* (PRs)—or *performance capacities*—necessary to carry out its control functions. PRs are characterized by *dimensions of performance*, which for controllers are *accuracy of movement* (including steadiness and stability) and *speed of movement*. Accuracy is the most important of these and can be divided into four major classes:

1. *Spatial accuracy.* Required by tasks which are *self-paced* and for which time taken is of secondary or minimal importance and includes tracing (e.g., map-tracking), walking, reaching, and, in fact, most activities of daily living. Limitation in speed PRs should have no influence on this class of accuracy.

2. *Spatial accuracy with time constraints.* Identical to spatial accuracy except that, in addition to accuracy, speed of execution of task is also of importance. Because maximal performance capacities for accuracy and speed of movement cannot, in general, be realized simultaneously, the carrying out of such tasks must necessarily involve speed-accuracy tradeoffs [Fitts, 1954; Fitts & Posner, 1967]. The extent to which accuracy is sacrificed for increased speed of execution, or vice versa, is dependent on the perceived relative importance of accuracy and speed.

3. *Temporal accuracy.* Required by tasks that place minimal demands on positional accuracy and includes single and multifinger tapping and foot tapping.

4. *Spatiotemporal accuracy.* Required by tasks that place considerable demand on attainment of simultaneous spatial and temporal accuracy. This includes *paced* positional tasks such as tracking, driving a vehicle, and playing ball games, sports, and video games. It should be stressed, however, that most of the preceding self-paced tasks also involve a considerable interrelationship between space and time.

Tracking tasks have become well established as being able to provide one of the most accurate and flexible means for laboratory-based measurement of spatiotemporal accuracy and thus of the performance capacity of sensory-motor control or sensory-motor coordination. In addition, they provide an unsurpassed framework for studies of the underlying control mechanisms of motor function [e.g., Lynn et al., 1979; Neilson et al., 1993]. They have achieved this status through their (1) ability to maximally stress the accuracy dimension of performance and hence the corresponding control PR, (2) the continuous nature and wide range of types and characteristics of input target signals they permit, (3) facility for a wide range of one- and two-dimensional (2D) sensors for measuring a subject's motor output, and (4) measure of continuous performance (cf. reaction-time tests).

From this perspective, it will be of little surprise to find that tracking tasks are the primary thrust of this chapter.

The Influence of Lower-Level Performance Resources on Higher-Level Control Performance Resources

By their very nature, tasks that enable one to measure spatiotemporal accuracy are complex or higher-level sensory-motor tasks. These place demands on a large number of lower-level PRs such as visual acuity, dynamic visual perception, range of movement, strength, simple reaction times, acceleration/deceleration, static steadiness, dynamic steadiness, prediction, memory, open-loop movements, concentration span, attention switching (i.e., central executive function or supervisory attentional system for multitask abilities), utilization of preview, and learning.

It is therefore important to ask: If there are so many PRs involved in tracking, can tracking performance provide an accurate estimate of sensory-motor control performance capacities? Or, if differences are seen in tracking performance between subjects, do these necessarily indicate comparable differences in control performance capacities? Yes, they can, but only if the control resource is the *only* resource being maximally stressed during the tracking task. Confirmation that the other PRs are not also being maximally stressed for a particular subject can be ascertained by two means. The first method is by independently measuring the capacity of the other PRs and confirming that these are considerably greater than that determined as necessary for the tracking task in question. For example, if the speed range for a certain reference group on a nontarget speed test is 650 to 1250 mm/s and the highest speed of a tracking target signal is 240 mm/s, then one can be reasonably confident that intragroup differences in performance on the tracking task are unrelated to intragroup differences in speed. Second, where this process is less straightforward or not possible, it may be possible to alter the demands imposed by the task on the PR in question. For example, one could see whether visual acuity was being maximally stressed in a tracking task (and hence be a significant limiting factor to the performance obtained) by increasing or decreasing the eye-screen distance. Similarly, one could look at strength in this context by altering the friction, damping, or inertia of the sensor or at range of movement by altering the gain of the sensor.

The conclusion that a task and a PR are unrelated for a particular group does not, of course, mean that this can necessarily be extrapolated to some other group. For example, strength may be completely uncorrelated with tracking performance in normal males yet be the primary factor responsible for poor tracking performance by the paretic arm of subjects who have suffered a stroke.

The foregoing discussion is based on the concept of an assumption that if a task requires less than the absolute maximum available of a particular PR, then performance on that task will be independent of that PR. Not surprisingly, the situation is unlikely to be this simplistic or clear-cut. If, for example, a tracking task places moderate submaximal demands on several PRs, these PRs will be stressed to varying levels such that the subject may tend to optimize the utilization of those resources [Kondraske, 1995] so as to achieve an acceptable balance between accuracy, speed, stress/effort, and fatigue (physical and cogitive). Thus, although strength available is much greater than strength needed (i.e., resource available $\gg$ resource demand) for both males and females, could the differential in strength be responsible for males performing better on tracking tasks than females [Jones et al., 1986]?

145.2 Measurement of Sensory–Motor Control Performance

Techniques: An Overview

Tracking tasks are the primary methodologic approach outlined in this chapter for measurement of sensory-motor control performance. There are, however, a large number of other approaches, each with its own set of apparatus and methods, which can provide similar or different data on control performance. It is possible to give only a cursory mention of these other techniques in this chapter (see also Further Information).

Hand and foot test boards comprising multiple touch-plate sensors provide measures of accuracy and speed of lateral reaching-tapping abilities [Kondraske et al., 1984, 1988].

Measurement of steadiness and tremor in an upper limb, lower limb, or segment of either, particularly when sustended, can be made using variably sized holes, accelerometers, or force transducers [Potvin et al., 1975]. A dual-axis capacitive transducer developed by Kondraske et al. [1984] provides an improved means of quantifying steadiness and tremor due to it requiring no mechanical connection to subject (i.e., no added inertia) and by providing an output of limb position as opposed to less informative measures of acceleration or force. Interestingly, tests of steadiness can be appropriately considered as a category of tracking tasks in which the target is static. The same is also true for measurement of postural stability using force-balance platforms, whether for standing [Kondraske et al., 1984; Milkowski et al., 1993] or sitting [Riedel et al., 1992] (see also Further Information).

Tracking Tasks: An Overview

A *tracking task* is a laboratory-based test apparatus characterized by a continuous input signal—the target—that a subject must attempt to match as closely as possible by his or her output response by controlling the position of (or force applied to) some sensor. It provides unequaled opportunities for wide-ranging experimental control over sensors, displays, target signals, dimensionality (degrees of freedom), control modes, controlled system dynamics, and sensor-display compatibility, as well as the application of a vast armamentarium of linear and nonlinear techniques for response signal analysis and systems identification. Because of this, the tracking task has proven to be *the* most powerful and versatile tool for assessing, studying, and modeling higher-level functioning of the human "black box" sensory-motor system.

There are three basic categories of tracking tasks, differing primarily in their visual display and in the corresponding control system (Fig. 145.1). The pursuit task displays both the present input and output signals, whereas the compensatory task displays only the difference or error signal between these. The preview task [Jones & Donaldson, 1986; Poulton, 1964; Welford, 1968] (Fig. 145.2) is similar to the pursuit task except that the subject can see in advance where the input signal is going to be and plan accordingly to minimize the resultant error signal. Tracing tasks [Driscoll, 1975;

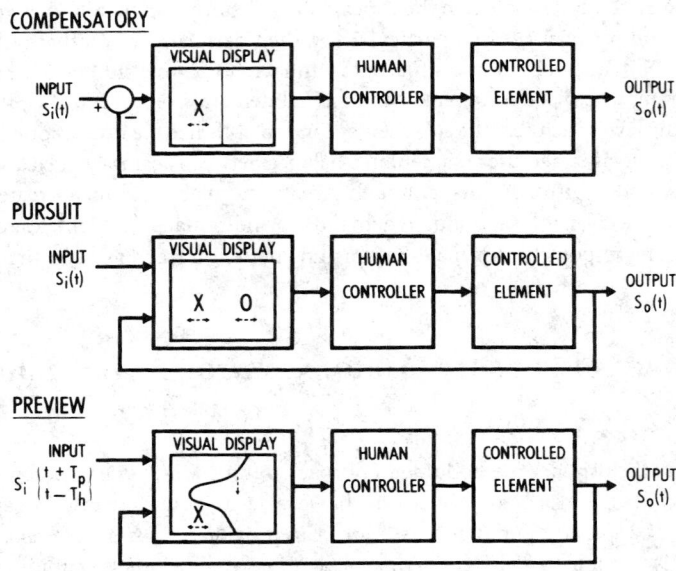

FIGURE 145.1   Modes of tracking (*a*) Compensatory: Subject aims to keep his or her resultant error signal **X** [= input signal − output signal = $s_i(t) - s_o(t)$] on stationary vertical line. (*b*) Pursuit: Subject aims to keep his or her output signal **X**, $s_o(t)$, on the target input signal **O**, $s_i(t)$. (*c*) Preview: Subject aims to keep his or her output signal **X**, $s_o(t)$, on the descending target input signal [$s_i(t+T_p) - s_i(t - T_h)$] (where t = present time, T_p = preview time, T_h = history or postview time).

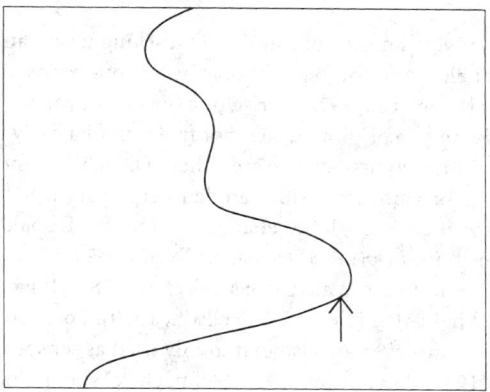

FIGURE 145.2   Visual display for random tracking with a preview of 8.0 s and postview of 1.1 s.

Hocherman & Aharon-Peretz, 1994; Stern et al., 1983] are effectively self-paced 2D preview tracking tasks.

The input-output nature of tracking tasks has made them most suitable for analysis using engineering control theories. This has lead to the common view of pursuit tracking as a task involving continuous negative feedback [Notterman et al., 1982], but there is evidence that tracking viewed as a series of discrete events would be more appropriate [Bösser, 1984]. The inclusion of preview of the input signal greatly complicates characterization of the human controller, and Sheridan [1966] has suggested three models of preview control that employ the notions of constrained preview and nonuniform importance of input. Lynn et al. [1979] and Neilson et al. [1992] also have demonstrated how, by treating the neurologically impaired subject as a black box, control analysis can lead to further information on underlying neurologic control mechanisms.

Despite the widespread utilization and acceptance of tracking tasks as a powerful and versatile means for quantifying and studying sensory-motor control capacities, there is little available on the market in this area. The most obvious exception to this is the photoelectric pursuit rotor that is ubiquitous in the motor behavior laboratories of university psychology departments and has been available since the 1950s [Schmidt, 1982; Siegel, 1985; Welford, 1968]. It is a paced 2D task with a target periodic on each revolution. Although inexpensive, the pursuit rotor is a crude tracking task allowing limited control over target signals and possessing a very gross performance analysis in terms of time on target. Thus nearly all the many and varied tracking tasks that have been used in countless experimental studies around the world have been developed by the users themselves for their specific objectives.

An improvement in this situation appears imminent with the recent arrival on the market of a number of tracking devices from Human Performance Measurement, Inc. (Arlington, Texas). These devices are a natural extension of those developed by Kondraske et al. [1984]. Off-the-shelf availability of computer-based tracking tests, including sensors for both upper and lower limbs, opens up the possibility of a much broader and widespread use of tracking tasks. In particular, one can look forward to a much greater utilization of tracking tasks outside traditional research areas and in more routine assessment applications in clinical, rehabilitative, vocational, sports, and other environments.

Tracking Tasks: Options and Considerations

Whatever the reasons for needing quantification of sensory-motor control capacity via a tracking task, there are a number of options available and factors to be considered in the design and choice of tracking tasks.

Sensors

Sensors for measuring a subject's motor output in 1D tracking tasks can be categorized under (1) movements involving a single degree of freedom such as flexion-extension rotation around a single joint, including the elbow [Lynn et al., 1977], wrist, or a finger, or pronation-supination of the wrist, and (2) movements involving two or more degrees of freedom of a body part (e.g., hand)—i.e., coordinated movement at multiple joints—which are either 1D, such as some form of linear transducer [Baroni et al., 1984; Patrick & Mutlusoy, 1982; van den Berg et al., 1987], or 2D, such as a steering wheel [Buck, 1982; Ferslew et al., 1982; Jones et al., 1993; Jones & Donaldson, 1986], stirring wheel [De Souza et al., 1980], position stick (i.e., 1D joystick) [Neilson & Neilson, 1980; Potvin et al., 1993], joystick [Jones et al., 1993; Kondraske et al., 1984; Miall et al., 1985], finger-controlled rotating knob [Neilson et al., 1993], and light-pen [Neilson & Neilson, 1980]. Force sticks, utilizing strain-gauge transducers mounted on a cantilever, are also commonly used as sensors [Barr et al., 1988; Garvey, 1960; Miller and Freund, 1980; Potvin et al., 1977; Stelmach & Worrington, 1988].

Sensors for 2D tasks must, of course, be capable of moving with and recording two degrees of freedom. Joysticks are commonly used for this and range in size from small, for finger movement [Anderson, 1986] and wrist/forearm movement [Bloxham et al., 1984; Frith et al., 1986], to large floor-mounted joysticks for arm movements primarily involving shoulder and elbow function Anderson, 1986; Behbehani et al., 1988; Dalrymple-Alford et al., 1994; Jones et al., 1993; Jones & Watson, 1993; Kondraske et al., 1984]. Other 2D task sensors include a hand-held stylus for the photoelectric pursuit rotor [Schmidt, 1982; Siegel, 1985], Plexiglas tracing [Driscoll, 1975], and tasks utilizing sonic digitizers [Hocherman & Aharon-Peretz, 1994; Stern et al., 1984]. Abend et al. [1982] and Flash and Hogan [1985] used a two-joint mechanical arm to restrict hand movements to the horizontal plane in the investigation of CNS control of two-joint (shoulder and elbow) movements in trajectory formation. Stern et al. [1983] simply used the subject's finger as the sensor for a tracing task on a vertical Plexiglas "screen"; a video camera behind the screen recorded finger movements. Novel whole-body 2D tracking is also possible by having subjects alter their posture while standing on a dual-axis force platform [Kondraske et al., 1984].

Displays

Early tracking devices used mechanical-based displays such as a rotating smoked drum [Vince, 1948], the ubiquitous pursuit rotor, and a paper-strip preview task [Poulton, 1964; Welford, 1968]. An oscilloscope was, and still is to a much less degree, used in a large number of tracking tasks, initially driven by analog circuitry [Anderson, 1986; Flowers, 1976;] but later by digital/analog (D/A) outputs on digital computers [Cooper et al., 1989; Kondraske et al., 1984; Miall et al., 1985; Sheridan et al., 1987]. Standard raster-based television screens have been used by some workers [Beppu et al., 1984; Potvin et al., 1977]. Nonraster vector graphics displays, such as Digital Equipment's VT11 dynamic graphics unit, proved valuable during the PDP era as a means for generating more complex dynamic stimuli such as squares [Frith et al., 1986; Neilson & Neilson, 1980] and preview [Jones & Donaldson, 1986] (see Fig. 145.2). More recently, raster-based color graphics boards have allowed impressive static displays and simple dynamic tracking displays to be generated on PCs. However, such boards are not, in general, immediately amenable for the generation of flawless dynamic displays involving more complex stimuli, such as required for preview tracking. Jones et al. [1993] have overcome this drawback by the use of specially written high-speed assembly-language routines for driving their display. These generate a display of the target and the subject's response marker by considering the video memory (configured in EGA mode) as four overlapping planes, each switchable (via a mask) and each capable of displaying the background color and a single color from a palette. Two planes are used to display the target, with the remaining two being used to display the subject's pointer. The current target is displayed on one target plane, while the next view of the target, in its new position, is being drawn on the other undisplayed target plane. The role of the two planes is reversed when the computer receives a vertical synchronization interrupt from the graphics controller indicating the completion of a raster. Through a combination of a high update rate of 60.34 Hz (i.e., the vertical interrupt frequency), assembly language, and dual-display buffers, it has been possible to obtain an extremely smooth dynamic color display. Their system for tracking and other quantitative sensory-motor assessments is further enhanced through its facility to generate dynamic color graphics on two high-resolution monitors simultaneously: one for the tracking display and one for use by the assessor for task control and analysis. The two monitors are driven by WinSprint 100 graphic controllers (Artist Graphics, Inc.) in 640 $\times$ 480 VGA and 800 $\times$ 600 EGA modes, respectively.

In contrast to the preceding CRT-based displays, Warabi et al. [1986] used a laser beam spot to indicate a subject's hand position together with a row of LEDs for displaying a step target. Similarly, Gibson et al. [1987] used a galvonometer-controlled laser spot to display smooth and step stimuli on a curved screen together with a white-light spot controlled by subject. Leist et al. [1987] also used a galvonometer-controlled spot but via backprojection to display smooth and step stimuli on a curved screen. Van den Berg et al. [1987] used two rows of 240 LEDs each to display target and response. 2D arrays of LEDs also have been used to indicate step targets in 2D tracking tasks [Abend et al., 1982; Flash & Hogan, 1985].

Target Signals

Tracking targets cover a spectrum from smoothly changing (low-bandwidth) targets, such as sinusoidal and random, through constant-velocity ramp targets to abruptly changing step targets.

Sinusoidal Targets. The periodicity, constancy of task complexity (over cycles), and spectral purity of sine targets make them valuable for measurement of within-run changes in performance (e.g., learning, lapses in concentration) [Jones & Donaldson, 1981], study of the ability to make use of the periodicity to improve tracking performance [Jones & Donaldson, 1989], and study of the human frequency response [Leist et al., 1987]. Several other workers also have incorporated sine targets in their tracking batteries [Ferslew et al., 1982; Jones et al., 1993; Miller & Freund, 1980; Notterman et al., 1982; Potvin et al., 1977].

Bloxham et al. [1984] and Frith et al. [1986] extended the use of sinewaves into the 2D domain by having subjects track a moving circle on the screen.

Random Targets. These are commonly generated via a sum of sines approach in which a number of harmonically or nonharmonically related sinusoids of random phase are superimposed [Baddeley et al., 1986; Barr et al., 1988; Cassell, 1973; Cooper et al., 1989; Frith et al., 1986; Jones et al., 1993; Miall et al., 1985; Neilson & Neilson, 1980; van den Berg et al., 1987]. If harmonically related, this can effectively give a flat spectrum target out to whatever bandwidth is required. Thus, in Jones et al.'s [1993] system, the random signal generation program asks the user for the required signal bandwidth and then calculates the number of equal-amplitude harmonics that must be summed together to give this bandwidth, each harmonic being assigned a randomly selected phase from a uniform phase distribution. Each target comprises 4096 (2^{12}) or more samples, a duration of at least 68 s (4096 samples/60.34 Hz), and a fundamental frequency of 0.0147 Hz (i.e., period of 68 s). By this means, it is possible to have several different pseudorandom target signals that are nonperiodic up to 68-s duration, have flat spectra within a user specified bandwidth, have no components above this bandwidth, and whose spectra can be accurately computed by FFT from any 68-s block of target (or response). Another common approach to the generation of random targets is to digitally filter a sequence of pseudorandom numbers [Kondraske et al., 1984; Lynn et al., 1977; Neilson et al., 1993; Potvin et al., 1977; van den Berg et al., 1987], although this method gives less control over the spectral characteristics of the target. Bösser [1984] summed a number of these filtered sequences in such a way as generate a target having an approximate $1/f$ spectrum. Another smooth pursuit target was generated by linking together short segments of sinewaves with randomly selected frequencies up to some maximum [Gibson et al., 1987] and was thus effectively a hybrid sinusoidal-random target.

Ramp Targets. These have been used in conjunction with sensory gaps of target or response to study predictive tracking and the ability to execute smooth constant-velocity movements in the absence of immediate visual cues in normal subjects [Flowers, 1978*b*] and subjects with cerebellar disorders [Beppu et al., 1987], stroke [Jones et al., 1989], and Parkinson's disease [Cooke et al., 1978; Flowers, 1978*a*].

Step Targets. These have been used in many applications and studies to measure and investigate subjects' abilities to predict, program, and execute ballistic (open-loop) movements. To enable this, spatial and temporal unpredictability have been incorporated into step tasks in various ways:

- *Temporal.* The time of onset of steps has ranged from (1) explicitly predictable, with preview of the stimulus [Day et al., 1984; Jones et al., 1993], to (2) implicitly predictable, with fixed interval between steps [Abend et al., 1982; Cooke et al., 1978; Flowers, 1978*a*; Potvin et al., 1977], to (3) unpredictable, with intervals between steps varied randomly over spans lying somewhere between 1.5 and 7.0 s [Anderson, 1986; Angel et al., 1970; Baroni et al., 1984; Flowers, 1976; Gibson et al., 1987; Jones et al., 1993; Jones & Donaldson, 1986; Jones & Watson, 1993; Kondraske et al., 1984; Sheridan et al., 1987; Warabi et al., 1986].
- *Amplitude.* The amplitude of steps has ranged from (1) explicitly predictable, where the endpoint of the step is shown explicitly before it occurs [Abend et al., 1982; Baroni et al., 1984; Jones et al., 1993; Jones & Watson, 1993; Sheridan et al., 1987], to (2) implicitly predictable, where all steps have the same amplitude [Angel et al., 1970; Potvin et al., 1977; Cooke et al., 1978; Day et al., 1984; Kondraske et al., 1984; Anderson, 1986] or return-to-center steps in variable-amplitude step tasks [Flowers, 1976; Jones et al., 1993; Jones & Donaldson, 1986], to (3) unpredictable, with between two and eight randomly distributed amplitudes [Flowers, 1976; Gibson et al., 1987; Jones et al., 1993; Jones & Donaldson, 1986; Sheridan et al., 1987; Warabi et al., 1986].
- *Direction.* Previous step tasks have had steps whose direction of steps has ranged from (1) all steps explicitly predictable, alternating between right and left [Baroni et al., 1984; Cooke et al., 1978; Flowers, 1976; Kondraske et al., 1984; Potvin et al., 1977], or all in one direction (i.e., a series of discontinuous steps) [Sheridan et al., 1987] or between corners of an invisible square [Anderson, 1986] or having preview [Abend et al., 1982; Jones et al., 1993], to (2) most steps predictable but with occasional "surprises" for studying anticipation [Flowers, 1978*a*], to (3) a combination of unpredictable (outward) and predictable (back-to-center) steps [Angel et al., 1970; Jones et al., 1993; Jones & Donaldson, 1986; Jones & Watson, 1993], and to (4) all steps unpredictable, with multiple endpoints [Gibson et al., 1987; Warabi et al., 1986] or resetting between single steps [Day et al., 1984].

The three elements of unpredictability can be combined in various ways to generate tasks ranging from completely predictable to completely unpredictable (Table 145.1). Several groups have implemented several variations of unpredictability both within and between step tracking tasks to investigate possible loss of ability to use predictability to improve performance in, for example, Parkinson's disease [Day et al., 1984; Flowers, 1978*a*; Jones & Watson, 1993; Sheridan et al., 1987]. In addition to unpredictability, other characteristics can be built into step tasks including explicit target zones [Sheridan et al., 1987] and visual gaps in target [Flowers, 1976; Warabi et al., 1986].

An example of a 1D step-tracking task possessing full spatial and temporal unpredictability is that of Jones and colleagues [Jones et al., 1993; Jones & Donaldson, 1986] (Fig. 145.3*a*). The task comprises 32 abrupt steps alternating between displacement from and return to center screen. In the nonpreview form, spatial unpredictability is present in the outward steps through four randomly distributed amplitude/direction movements (large and small steps requiring 90 and 22.5 degrees on a steering wheel, respectively, and both to right and left of center) with temporal unpredictability achieved via four randomly distributed durations between steps (2.8, 3.4, 4.0, and 4.6 s). This task

TABLE 145.1   Unpredictability in Step Tracking Tasks

| | | Temporal | | | Spatial, Amplitude | | | Spatial, Direction | | | Overall |
		Full	Partial	None	Full	Partial	None	Full	Partial	None	Full
Angel et al. [1970]*	1D	■				■		■		■	
Flowers [1976]*	1D	■			■	■				■	
Potvin et al. [1977]	1D		■			■				■	
Cooke et al. [1978]	1D		■			■				■	
Flowers [1978a]	1D		■			■			■		
Baroni et al. [1984]	1D	■					■			■	
Day et al. [1984]	1D			■		■		■			
Kondraske et al. [1984]	1D	■				■				■	
Warabi et al. [1986]	1D	■			■			■			●
Jones and Donaldson [1986]*	1D	■			■	■		■		■	●
Gibson et al. [1987]	1D	■			■			■			●
Sheridan et al. [1987]*	1D	■			■		■			■	
Jones et al. [1993]*	1D	■		■	■	■		■		■	●
Abend et al. [1982]	2D		■				■			■	
Anderson [1986]	2D	■				■				■	
Jones and Watson [1993]	2D	■					■	■			

*Several authors have several variations of unpredictability within one task or between multiple tasks.

has been used, together with preview random tracking, to demonstrate deficits in sensory-motor control in the asymptomatic arm of subjects who have had a unilateral stroke [Jones et al., 1989].

Jones et al. [1993] also provide an example of a 2D step-tracking task with spatial and temporal unpredictability. In this task, the subject must move a cross from within a central starting square to within one of eight 10 × 10 mm target squares that appear on the screen with temporal and spatial unpredictability (Fig. 145.3b). The centers of the eight surrounding targets are positioned at the vertices and midway along the perimeter of an imaginary 100 × 100 mm square centered on the central square. To initiate the task, the subject places the cross within the perimeter of the central target. After a 2- to 5-s delay, one of the surrounding blue targets turns green, and the subject moves the cross to within the green target square as quickly and as accurately as possible. After a further delay, the central target turns green, indicating onset of the spatially predictive "back-to-center" target. The task, which comprises 10 outward and 10 return targets, was used to show that parkinsonian subjects per-

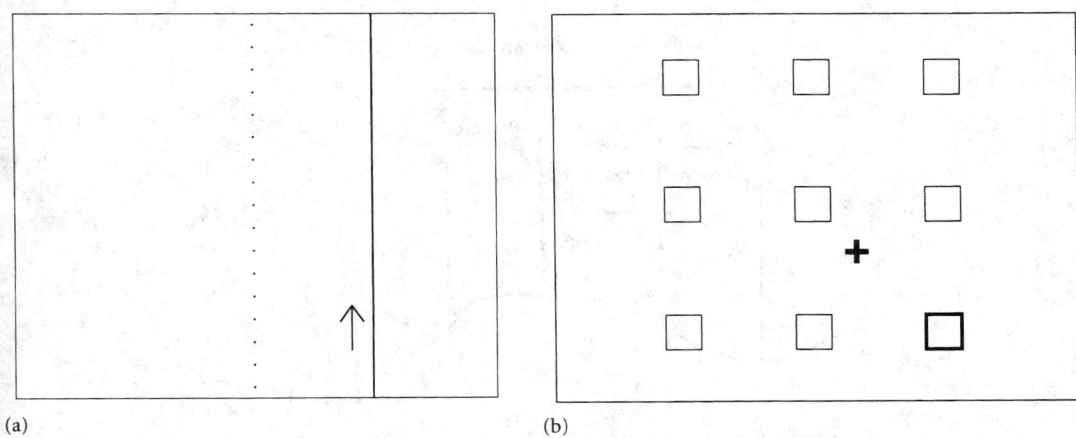

(a)   (b)

FIGURE 145.3   Visual displays for (a) 1D step tracking task and (b) 2D step tracking task (bottom-right square is current target).

form worse than matched controls on all measures of step tracking but are not impaired in their ability to benefit from spatial predictability to improve performance [Jones & Watson, 1993].

Step tasks with explicit target zones, in 1D [Sheridan et al., 1987] or 2D [Jones & Watson, 1993], provide the possibility of altering task difficulty by varying the size of the target. On the basis that subjects need only aim to get their marker somewhere within target zone (see close to center), then, according to Fitt's [1954] ratio rule, the difficulty of the primary movement is proportional to $\log_2 (2A/W)$, where A is the amplitude of the movement and W is the width of the target.

Combination Targets. Jones et al. [1986, 1989, 1993] have combined two quite different modes of tracking within a single task. *Combination* tracking involves alternating between preview random and nonpreview step tracking over 11-s cycles (Fig. 145.4). Thus, while tracking the random target, the preview signal is abruptly and unpredictably replaced by a stationary vertical line at some distance from the random signal, and vice versa. Although the steps occur with a fixed foreperiod (as with the step tasks listed above with implicit temporal predictability) of 7.3 s, subjects are not informed of this, and irrespective, Weber's law [Fitts & Posner, 1967] indicates that the accuracy of prediction of steps with such a long prestimulus warning is very low. Combination tracking allows study of the ability to change *motor set* [Robertson & Flowers, 1990] between quite different modes of tracking and is analogous to having to quickly and appropriately respond to an unexpected obstacle, such as a child running onto the road, while driving a vehicle.

Dimensionality

The number of dimensions of a tracking task usually refers to the number of cartesian coordinates over which the *target* moves, rather than those of the response marker or sensor handle, or the number of degrees of freedom of the target or of the upper limb. Some examples: (1) Most tasks with a 2D joystick sensor or light-pen are 2D, but if the target moves in the vertical direction only [Jones et al., 1993; Kondraske et al., 1984; Miall et al., 1985; Neilson & Neilson, 1980], the task is only considered 1D, irrespective of whether the response marker is confined to vertical movements on the screen or not. (2) If the target trajectory is a circle [Bloxham et al., 1984], the task is 2D despite the target having only one degree of freedom (i.e., radius r is constant). (3) A pursuit rotor is a 2D task because it has a target that moves in two dimensions (whether cartesian or polar) as well as doing so with two degrees of freedom.

Tracking Mode

The two primary modes of tracking—compensatory and pursuit—have been introduced above. The majority of tasks are of the pursuit type, which is appropriate in that it has a more direct parallel

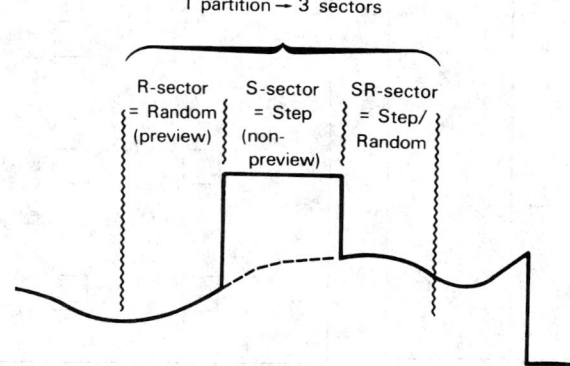

FIGURE 145.4 Section of input waveform in combination tracking in which the target alternates between preview-random and nonpreview-step.

with real-world sensory-motor tasks than the more artificial compensatory task [e.g., Barr et al., 1988; Bösser, 1984; Garvey, 1960; Miller & Freund, 1980; Potvin et al., 1977; Vince, 1948], in which the subject is only shown the instantaneous value of the error signal. The compensatory mode may be preferentially chosen for control theory modeling due to its simpler set of defining equations [Potvin et al., 1977]. The preview task [Jones & Donaldson, 1986; Welford, 1968] is an important variation of pursuit tracking in which a still greater correspondence with everyday tasks is achieved.

Controlled System Dynamics

The majority of tracking tasks have a zero-order controlled system in which the position of the response marker is proportional to the position of the sensor, and the mechanical characteristics of friction, inertial mass, and velocity damping are simply those of the input the device. Van den Berg et al. [1987] eliminated even these by feeding back a force signal from a strain gauge on the tracking handle to the power amplifier of a torque motor connected to their sensor. Conversely, Neilson et al. [1993] artificially introduced mechanical characteristics into the movement of their response marker by having a second-order filter as the controlled system; by an appropriate transfer function [$H(z)$ = $0.4060/(1 - 1.0616z^{-1} + 0.4610z^{-2})$], they were able to introduce inertial lag and underdamping (resonant peak at 2.0 Hz). Miall et al. [1985] introduced an analog delay of 500 ms between their joystick and display so that they could study the effect of delayed visual feedback on performance.

The inclusion of a delay in the controlled system has been extended yet further in *critical tracking,* a rather novel variation of pursuit tracking conceived by Jex [1966] in which there is no external target. Instead, the subject's own instability acts as an input to an increasingly unstable controlled system, $Y(s) = K\lambda/(s - \lambda)$, in which the level of instability, represented by the root λ ($= 1/T$), is steadily increased during the task until a preset error is exceeded. The task has been described as analogous to driving a truck with no brakes down a hill on a winding road [Potvin et al., 1977]. The task has been applied clinically by Potvin et al. [1977] and Kondraske et al. [1984] and shown to be a reliable measure of small changes in neurologic function [Potvin et al., 1977].

Having a torque motor as part of the sensor opens up possibilities for dynamically altering the controlled system characteristics or for adding external force perturbations. The torque motor can be operated as a "torque servo," in which applied torque is independent of position, or a "position servo," in which applied torque is proportional to position error (together with velocity damping if desired) [Thomas et al., 1976]. Despite these possibilities, torque motors do not appear to have been applied in studies of voluntary movements, such as tracking, other than for canceling unwanted controller characteristics [van den Berg et al., 1987]. Instead, they have been used to apply constant-velocity movements [Kondraske et al., 1984] or pulsatile-force [van den Berg et al., 1987], sinusoidal-force [Gottlieb et al., 1984], or random-force [Kearney and Hunter, 1983; van den Berg et al., 1987] perturbations for the measurement/study of neuromuscular reflexes or limb transfer function (i.e., stiffness, viscosity, and inertia).

Sensor-Display Compatibility

It is generally accepted that the level of compatibility between sensor and display in continuous tracking tasks influences the accuracy of performance [Neilson & Neilson, 1980]. The perfectly compatible sensor is the display marker itself [Poulton, 1974], where the subject holds and moves the response marker directly such as with a light pen in tracking [Neilson & Neilson, 1980] or rotary pursuit [Schmidt, 1982; Welford, 1968], handle on a two-joint mechanical arm [Abend et al., 1982], or in self-paced 2D tracing tasks [Driscoll, 1975; Hocherman and Aharon-Peretz, 1994; Stern et al., 1984;]. Similarly, Van den Berg et al. [1987] achieve a high sensor-display compatibility by having the LED arrays for target and response displayed directly above a horizontally moving handle. However, the majority of tracking tasks have sensors that are quite separate from the response marker displayed on an oscilloscope or computer screen. Sensor-display compatibility can be maximized in this case by having the sensor physically close to the display, moving in the same direction as the marker, and with a minimum of controlled system dynamics (e.g., zero-order). In the case of a joystick in a 2D task, for example, direct compatibility (*left-right → left-right*) is easier than inverse compatibility (*left-right → right-left*), which is easier than noncompatibility (*left-right → up-down*). In contrast, fore-aft movements on a joystick appear to possess bidirectional compatibility in that *fore-aft → up-down* seems as inherently natural as *fore-aft → down-up* (i.e., no obvious inverse).

Sensor-display compatibility may not, however, be overly critical to performance. For example, Neilson and Neilson [1980] found no decrement in performance on random tracking of overall error scores, such as mean absolute error, between a light pen and a 1D joystick; nevertheless, the latter did result in a decrease in gain, an increase in phase lag, and an increase in the noncoherent response component.

Response Sampling Rates

Although some workers have manually analyzed tracking data from multichannel analog chart recordings [Beppu et al., 1984; Flowers, 1976] or analog processed results [Potvin et al., 1977], the majority have used computers, sometimes via a magnetic tape intermediary [Day et al., 1984; Miall et al., 1985], to digitize data for automated analyses. Sampling rates used have varied from 10 Hz [Neilson & Neilson, 1980] through 20 Hz [Cooper et al., 1989; Neilson et al., 1993], 28.6 Hz [Jones & Donaldson, 1986; Jones & Watson, 1993], 40 Hz [Frith et al., 1986], 60.3 Hz (= screen's vertical interrupt rate) [Jones et al., 1993], 100 Hz (all 2D tasks) [Abend et al., 1982; Hocherman & Aharon-Peretz, 1994; Stern et al., 1984], and as high as 250 Hz [Day et al., 1984].

For the most part, a relatively low sampling rate is quite satisfactory for analysis of tracking performance as long as the Nyquist criterion is met and there is appropriate analog or digital low-pass filtering to prevent aliasing. Spectral analysis indicates that the fastest of voluntary arm movements have no power above about 8.7 Hz [Jones & Donaldson, 1986]. This is very similar to the maximal voluntary oscillations of the elbow of 4 to 6 Hz [Neilson, 1972; Leist et al., 1987] and to maximum finger tapping rates of 6 to 7 Hz [Muir et al., in press]. The sampling rate can be reduced still further if the primary interest is only in *coherent* performance, whose bandwidth is only on the order of 2 Hz for both kinesthetic stimuli [Neilson, 1972] and visual stimuli [Leist et al., 1987; Neilson et al., 1993]; i.e., performance above 2 Hz must be open-loop and hence learned and preprogrammed [Neilson, 1972]. Thus, from an information theory point of view, there is no need to sample tracking performance beyond, say, 20 Hz. However, a higher rate may well be justified on the grounds of needing better temporal resolution than 50 ms for transient or cross-correlation analysis, unless one is prepared to regenerate the signal between samples by some form of nonlinear interpolation (e.g, sinc, spline, polynomial).

Other Measures

Several researchers have further extended the information that can derived from upper limb tracking performance by comparison with other simultaneously recorded biosignals. The most common of these is the EMG, particularly *integrated* EMG (i.e., full-wave rectification and low-pass filtering of the raw EMG), due to its close parallel to force of contraction [Neilson, 1972] and where the tracking movement is constrained to be around a single joint. The EMG has been used together with step tracking for fractionating reaction times into premotor and motor components [Sheridan et al., 1987] and confirmation of open-loop primary movements [Sheridan et al., 1987; Sittig et al., 1985]. In smooth tracking, correlation/cross-spectral analysis between the EMG and limb position has been used to study limb dynamics [Barr et al., 1988; Neilson, 1972].

In contrast, Cooper et al. [1989] measured the EEG at four sites during 2D random tracking to show that slow changes in the EEG (equivalent to the Bereitschaftspotential preceding self-paced voluntary movement), particularly at the vertex, are correlated with the absolute velocity of the target.

Simultaneous measurement of hand and eye movements has been carried out by Warabi et al. [1986] and Leist et al. [1987] using EOG to measure horizontal eye movements, and by Gibson et al. [1987] using an infrared limbus reflection technique. Interestingly, Leist et al. [1987] found that ocular pursuit and self-paced oscillations were limited to about 1 and 2.2 Hz, respectively, whereas the equivalent values for arm movements are 2 and 4 to 6 Hz, respectively.

Standard Assessment Procedures

Having designed and constructed a tracking task or set of tracking tasks with the characteristics necessary to allow measurement of the sensory-motor control performance capacities under investigation, it is essential that this process be complemented by a well-formulated set of standard assessment procedures. These must include (1) standard physical setup, in which positioning of subject, sensor, and screen are tightly specified and controlled, as well as factors such as screen brightness, room lighting, etc., and (2) standardized instructions. The latter are particularly important in tasks where speed-accuracy tradeoff [Agarwal & Logsdon, 1990; Fitts, 1954; Welford, 1968] is possible. This applies particularly to step tracking in which leaving the tracking strategy completely up to subjects introduces the possibility of misinterpretation of differences in performance on certain measures, such as reaction time, risetime, and mean absolute error. For example, subjects need to know if it is more important to have the initial movement end up close to the target (i.e., emphasis on *accuracy* of primary movement) or to get within the vicinity of the target as soon as possible (i.e., emphasis on *speed* of primary movement); the latter results in greater under/overshooting but also tends to result in lower mean errors. The most common approach taken is to stress the importance of both speed and accuracy with an instruction to subjects of the form: "Follow the target as fast and as accurately as possible."

Test and Experimental Protocols

The design of appropriate test and experimental protocols is also a crucial component of the tracking task design process [Pitrella & Kruger, 1983; Roscoe, 1975]. When comparisons are to be made between different subjects, tasks, and/or conditions, careful consideration needs to be given to the paramount factors of *matching* and *balancing* to minimize the possibility of significant differences being due to some bias or confounding variable other than that under investigation. Matching can be achieved between experimental and control subjects in an intersubject design by having average or one-to-one equivalence on age, gender, education, etc. or through an intrasubject design in which the subject acts as his or her own control in, say, a study of dominant versus nondominant arm performance. Balancing is primarily needed to offset *order effects* due to learning that pervade much of sensory-motor performance [Frith et al., 1986; Jones et al., 1990; Poulton, 1974; Schmidt, 1982; Welford, 1968]. A study by Jones and Donaldson [1989] provides a good example of the application of these principles. Their study, aimed at investigating the effect of Parkinson's disease on predictive motor planning, involved 16 parkinsonian subjects and 16 age- and sex-matched control subjects. These were then divided into 8 subgroups in a three-way randomized crossover design so as to eliminate between- and within-session order effects in the determining the effect of target type, target preview, and medication on tracking performance.

145.3 Analysis of Sensory–Motor Control Performance

Accuracy

Analyses of raw tracking data can provide performance information that is objective and quantitative and which can be divided into two broad classes:

Measures of Global Accuracy of Performance

Measures of *global* (or overall or integrated) sensory-motor control capacities have proven invaluable for

- *Vocational screening* of minimum levels of sensory-motor skills. Tracking tasks, in fact, have their origins in this area during World War II, when they were used to help screen and train aircraft pilots [Poulton, 1974; Welford, 1968].
- *Clinical screening* for sensory-motor deficits (arising from one or more lesions in one or more sites in the sensory-motor system). An excellent example of the application of this in

clinical practice is the provision of objective measures in off-road driving assessment programs [Croft & Jones, 1987; Jones et al., 1983;].

- *Measuring longitudinal changes* in sensory-motor function. There are many examples of subjects being assessed repeatedly on tracking tasks for periods up to 12 or more months. This has been done to quantify recovery following head injury [Jones & Donaldson, 1981] and stroke [De Souza et al., 1980; Jones et al., 1990; Jones & Donaldson, 1981; Lynn et al., 1977] as well as for studies of learning in tracking performance [Frith et al., 1986; Jones et al., 1990; Jones & Donaldson, 1981; Poulton, 1974; Schmidt, 1982]. They also can be used to quantify changes due to medication, such as in Parkinson's disease [Jones & Donaldson, 1989].

Measures of Characteristics of Performance

Measures of global accuracy of tracking performance can detect and quantify the presence of abnormal sensory-motor control performance capacities with considerable sensitivity [Jones et al., 1989; Potvin et al., 1977]. Conversely, they are unable to give any indication of which of the many subsystems or performance resources in the overall sensory-motor system are, or may be, responsible for the abnormal performance. Nor can they provide any particular insight into the underlying neuromuscular control mechanisms of normal or abnormal performance.

Two quite different approaches can be taken to provide information necessary to help identify the sensory-motor subsystems and their properties responsible for the *characteristics* of observed normal and abnormal performance:

- Batteries of neurologic sensory-motor tests. Potvin et al.'s group [Potvin et al., 1985; Potvin & Tourtellotte, 1975;], now led by Kondraske et al. [1984, 1988], have developed what is by far the most comprehensive battery of tests available for quantitative evaluation of neurologic function covering a number of sensory, motor, cognitive, and sensory-motor functions or performance resources. Similarly, Jones et al. [1989, 1993] have developed a battery of *component* function tests, most of which have been specifically designed to isolate and quantify the various performance resources involved in their tracking tasks. There is, therefore, a close resemblance between the component and tracking tests so as to maximize the validity of comparisons made between them. This has been particularly important in the separation and fractionation of the visuoperceptual components involved in tracking [Jones & Donaldson, 1992; Jones & Donaldson, in press].
- Analysis of the characteristics of performance by signal analysis and control systems approaches and techniques.

Measures of Global Accuracy of Performance

The most commonly used measure of global or overall accuracy is the *mean absolute error* (MAE) [Jones & Donaldson, 1986], which indicates the average distance the subject was away from the target irrespective of side; it is also variously called *average absolute error* [Poulton, 1974], *modulus mean error* [Poulton, 1974], *mean rectified error* [Neilson & Neilson, 1980], or simply *tracking error* [Behbehani et al., 1988; Kondraske et al., 1984]. In contrast, the mean error, or constant position error, is of little value because it simply indicates only the extent to which the response is more on one side of the target than the other [Poulton, 1974]. Measures of overall performance that give greater weighting to larger errors include *mean square error* [Neilson et al., 1993], root mean square error [Poulton, 1974], *variance of error* [Neilson & Neilson, 1980], and *standard deviation of error* [Poulton, 1974]. Relative or *normalized error* score equivalents of these can be calculated by expressing the raw error scores as a percentage of the respective scores obtained had the subject simply held the response marker stationary at the mean target position [Day et al., 1984; Neilson & Neilson, 1980; Poulton, 1974]; i.e., no response = 100%.

An issue met in viewing error scores from the perspective of Kondraske's [in press] elemental resource model is the unifying requirement of its associated *general systems performance theory (GSPT)* that all dimensions of performance must be in a form for which a higher numeric value indicates a superior performance. Thus scores that state that a *smaller* score indicates a superior performance, including reaction times, movement times, and all error scores, need to be transformed into *performance scores* [Kondraske, 1988]. For example:

- *Central response speed* = 1/*reaction time*
- *Information processing speed* = 1/(8-*choice reaction time*)
- *Movement speed* = 1/*movement time*
- *Tracking accuracy* = 1/*tracking error*

Since transformation via inversion is nonlinear, the distributions of raw error scores and derived performance will be quite different. This has no effect on ordinal analyses, such as nonparametric statistics, but will have some effect on linear analyses, such as parametric statistics, linear regression/correlation, etc., and may include improvements due to a possible greater normality of the distributions of derived performances. An alternative transformation that would retain a linear relationship with the error scores is

$$Tracking\ accuracy = 100 - relative\ tracking\ error$$

However, while this gives a dimension of performance with the desired "bigger is better" characteristic, it also raises the possibility of negative values, implying an accuracy worse than zero. The author can attest to the fact that some subjects do indeed end up with error scores worse than the "hands off" score. Irrespective of GSPT, there is no doubt that it is beneficial to deal conceptually and analytically with multiple performance measures when *all* measures are consistently defined in terms of "bigger is better."

Time on target is a much cruder measure of tracking performance than all the preceding, but it has been used reasonably widely due to its being the result obtained from the pursuit rotor. The crudeness generally reflects (1) a lack of spatiotemporal sampling during task (i.e., simple integration of time on target only), preventing the possibility of further analysis of any form, and (2) a task's performance *ceiling* due the target having a finite zone within which greater accuracy, relative to centre of zone, is unrewarded. This latter factor can, however, be used to advantage for the case where the investigator wishes to have control over the *difficulty* of a task to gain, for example, similar levels of task difficulty across subjects irrespective of individual ability. This attribute has been used very effectively with 2D random tracking tasks to minimize the confounding effects of major differences in task load between experimental and control subjects in dual-task studies of impairment of central executive function in subjects with Alzheimer's disease [Baddeley et al., 1986] and Parkinson's disease [Dalrymple-Alford et al., 1994].

Measures of Characteristics of Performance

Time Domain (Nonballistic)

There are several run-averaged biases that can indicate the general *form* of errors being made, particularly when the tracking performance is subnormal. Positive *side of target* (%) and *direction of target* (%) biases reflect a greater proportion of errors occurring to the right of target or while the target is moving to the right, respectively [Jones & Donaldson, 1986], which, if substantial, may indicate the presence of some visuoperceptual deficit. Similarly, the *side of screen* bias (assuming mean target position is midscreen) [Jones & Donaldson, 1986] is identical to the mean error or constant position error.

Perhaps the single most important measure of performance, other than mean absolute error, for nontransient targets is that of the average time delay, or *lag*, of a subject's response with respect to the target signal. The lag is most commonly defined as being the shift τ corresponding to the peak of the cross-correlation function, calculated directly in the time domain or indirectly via the inverse of the cross-spectrum in the frequency domain. Although simulation studies indicate that these techniques are at least as accurate and as robust to noise/remnants as the alternatives listed below [Watson, 1994], one needs to be aware of a bias leading to underestimation of the magnitude of the lag (or lead) due to distortion of the standard cross-correlation function but specifically of the peak toward zero shift. The distortion arises as a result of the varying overlap of two truncated signals (i.e., the target and the response) resulting in the multiplication of the cross-correlation function by a triangle (maximum at $\tau = 0$ and zero at $\tau = \pm NT_s$, assuming signals of equal length NT_s). This effect is minimal as long as both signals have a mean value of zero (i.e., zero dc). Temporal resolution is another factor deserving consideration. If desired, greater resolution than that of the sampling period can be obtained by interpolation of the points around the peak of the cross-correlation function by some form of curve fitting (e.g., parabola [Jones et al., 1993]).

An alternative estimate of the lag, which has proven accurate on simulated responses, can be gained from *least-squares time-delay estimation* by finding the time shift between the response and target at which the mean square error is minimized [Fertner & Sjölund, 1986; Jones et al., 1993]. Another approach, *phase-shift time-delay* estimation, calculates lag from the gradient of the straight line providing a best least-squares to the phase points in the cross-spectrum. This technique has, however, proven more sensitive to noncorrelated remnants in the response than the other procedures [Watson, 1994].

Several measures used to help characterize within-run variability in performance include variance of error [Neilson & Neilson, 1980], standard deviation of error [Poulton, 1974], and inconsistency [Jones & Donaldson, 1986].

Time Domain (Ballistic)

Irrespective of any of the preceding nonballistic analyses, evaluation of step tracking performance usually involves separate ballistic or transient analysis of each of the step responses. This generally takes the form of breaking up each response into three phases (Fig. 145.5): (1) reaction time phase, or the time between onset of step stimulus and initiation of movement defined by exit from a visible or invisible reaction zone; (2) primary movement phase, or the open-loop ballistic movement made by most normal subjects aiming to get within the vicinity of the target as quickly as possible, the end of which is defined as the first stationary point; and (3) secondary correction phase, com-

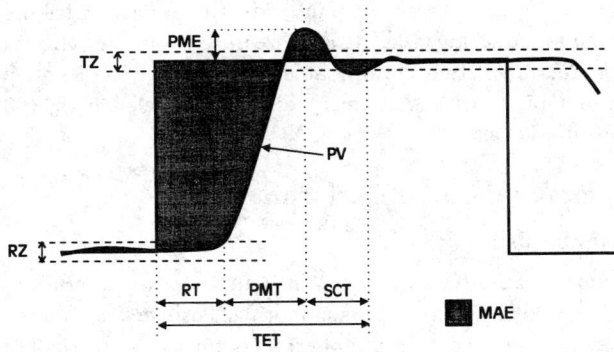

FIGURE 145.5 Transient response analysis. Tolerance zones: RZ = reaction zone; TZ = target zone. Performance parameters: RT = reaction time; PMT = primary movement time; SCT = secondary correction time; TET = target entry time; PV = peak velocity; PME = primary movement error; MAE = mean absolute error over a fixed interval following stimulus.

prising one or more adjustments and the remaining time needed to enter and stay within target zone. The step measures from individual steps can then be grouped into various step categories to allow evaluation of the effect of step size, spatial predictability, arm dominance, etc. on transient performance.

Accuracy of the primary aimed movement also can be characterized in terms of a constant error and a variable error (standard deviation of error), which are considered to be indices of accuracy of central motor programming and motor execution respectively [Guiard et al., 1983].

Phase-plane (velocity-versus-position) plots provide an alternative means for displaying and examining the qualitative characteristics of step tracking responses. In particular, they have proven valuable for rapid detection of gross abnormalities [Potvin et al., 1985]. Behbehani et al. [1988] have introduced a novel quantitative element to phase-plane analysis by deriving an index of coordination: $I_c = V_m^2/A$, where V_m is the maximum velocity during an outward and return step and A is the area within the resultant loop on the phase-plane plot.

Frequency Domain

Cross-correlation and spectral analysis has proven an invaluable tool for quantifying the frequency-dependent characteristics of the human subject. The cross-spectral density function, or cross-spectrum $S_{xy}(f)$, can be obtained from the random target $x(t)$ and random response $y(t)$ by taking the Fourier transform of the cross-correlation function $r_{xy}(\tau)$, i.e., $S_{xy}(f) = F\{r_{xy}(\tau)\}$, or in the frequency domain via $S_{xy}(f) = X(f)Y(f)^*$, or by a nonparametric system identification approach (e.g., "spa.m" in MATLAB). The cross-spectrum provides estimates of the relative amplitude (i.e., gain) and phase lag at each frequency. Gain, phase, and remnant frequency-response curves provide objective measures of pursuit tracking behavior, irrespective of linearity, and are considered a most appropriate quasi-linear tool for obtaining a quantitative assessment of pursuit tracking behavior [Neilson & Neilson, 1980]. From the cross-spectrum one also can derive the *coherence function* that gives the proportion of the response signal linearly related to the target at each frequency: $\gamma_{xy}^2 = |S_{xy}(f)|^2/S_x(f)S_y(f)$. Lynn et al. [1977] emphasize, however, that one must be cognizant of the difficulty representing tracking performance by a quasi-linear time-invariant transfer function, especially if the run is of short duration or if the target waveform is of limited bandwidth, since the results can be so statistically unreliable as to make description by a second- or third-order transfer function quite unrealistic. Van den Berg et al. [1987] chose four parameters to characterize tracking performance: low-frequency performance via the mean gain of transfer function at the three lowest of eight frequencies in target signal, high-frequency performance via the frequency at which the gain has dropped to less than 0.4, mean delay via shift of peak of cross-correlation function, and remnant via power in frequencies introduced by the subject relative to total power. Spectral and coherence analysis has been used to demonstrate that the human bandwidth is about 2 Hz for both kinesthetic tracking [Neilson, 1972] and visual tracking [Neilson et al., 1993], a much greater relative amplitude of second harmonic in the response of cerebellar subjects in sine tracking [Miller & Freund, 1980], a near-constant lag except at low frequencies in normal subjects [Cassell, 1973], adaptation to time-varying signals [Bösser, 1984], and 2D asymmetry in postural steadiness [Milkowski et al., 1993].

Graphic Analysis

Most of the preceding analyses give quantitative estimates of some aspect of performance that is effectively assumed to be constant over time, other than for random fluctuations. This is frequently not the case, especially for more complex sensory-motor tasks such as tracking. Changes in performance over time can be divided into two major classes: class 1, those for which the underlying PRs remain unchanged (these are due to factors such as practice, fatigue, and lapses in concentration), and class II, those for which one or more underlying PRs have changed (these are due to abrupt or gradual alterations at one or more sites in the sensory-motor system and include normal changes, such as due to age, and abnormal changes, due to trauma or pathology).

Studies of class I factors using tracking tasks are complicated most by the intrarun *difficulty* of a task not being constant. Changes in tracking accuracy *during* a run can be viewed via graphs of target, response, and errors [Jones et al., 1993]. The latter is particularly informative for sinusoidal targets for which the mean absolute errors can be calculated over consecutive epochs, corresponding to sine-wave cycles, and plotted both as a histogram form and as a smoothed version of this [Jones & Donaldson, 1986]. Since complexity of task is constant over epochs (cf. random pursuit task), the error graph gives an accurate measure of a subject's time-dependent spatiotemporal accuracy that is not confounded by changes in task difficulty and therefore gives a true indication of changes in performance due to factors such as learning, fatigue, and lapses in concentration. Attempts by the author to derive an instantaneous or short epoch (up to several seconds) function or *index of task difficulty* that would allow equivalent graphs to be generated for random targets were unsuccessful.

By comparison, studies of class II factors using tracking tasks are complicated most by interrun *learning*. Although most learning occurs over the first one or two runs or sessions, tracking performance can continue to improve over extended periods, as evidenced by, for example, significant improvements still being made by normal subjects after nine weekly sessions [Jones & Donaldson, 1981]. Consequently, a major difficulty met in the interpretation of serial measures of performance following acute brain damage is differentiation of neurologic recovery from normal learning. Furthermore, it is not simply a matter of subtracting off the degree of improved performance due to learning seen in normal control subjects. Jones et al. [1990] have developed graphic analysis techniques that provide for the removal of the learning factor, as much as is possible, and which can be applied to generating recovery curves for individual subjects following acute brain damage such as stroke. They demonstrated that, for tracking, percentage improvement in performance (PIP) graphs give more reliable evidence of neurologic recovery than absolute improvement in performance (PIA) graphs due to the former's greater independence from what are often considerably different absolute levels of performance.

Statistical

Parametric statistics (*t* test, ANOVA) are by far the most commonly used in studies of sensory-motor/psychomotor performance, due in large part to their availability and ability to draw out interactions between dependent variables. However, there is also a strong case for the use of non-parametric statistics. For example, the Wilcoxon matched-pairs statistic may be preferable for both between-group and within-subject comparisons due to its greater robustness over its parametric paired *t*-test equivalent, with only minimal loss of power. This is important due to many sensory-motor measures having very nongaussian skewed distributions as well as considerably different variances between normal and patient groups.

Defining Terms

Basic element of performance (BEP): Defined by a *functional unit* and a *dimension of performance,* e.g., right elbow flexor + speed.

Dimension of performance: A basic measure of performance such as speed, range of movement, strength, spatial perception, spatiotemporal accuracy.

Functional unit: A subsystem such as right elbow flexor, left eye, or motor memory.

Performance capacity: The maximal level of performance possible on a particular dimension of performance.

Performance resource (PR): One of a pool of elemental resources from which the entire human is modeled [Kondraske, 1995] and which are available for performing tasks. These resources can be subdivided into life-sustaining, environmental-interface, central-processing, and skills domains and have a parallel with *basic elements of performances.*

Sensor: (In the context of tracking tasks) A device for measuring/transducing a subject's motor output.

Sensory-motor control: The primary (but not only) performance resource responsible for accuracy of movement.

Spatiotemporal accuracy: The class of accuracy most required by tasks that place considerable demand on attainment of simultaneous spatial and temporal accuracy; this refers particularly to *paced* tasks such as tracking, driving, and playing ball games and video games.

Tracking task: A laboratory apparatus and associated procedures that have proven one of the most versatile means for assessing and studying the human "black box" sensory-motor system by providing a continuous record of a subject's response, via some *sensor*, to any one of a large number of continuous and well-controlled stimulus or *target* signals.

References

Abend W, Bizzi E, Morasso P. 1982. Human arm trajectory formation. Brain 105:331.

Agarwal GC, Logsdon JB. 1990. Optimal principles for skilled limb movements and speed accuracy tradeoff. Proc Ann Int Conf IEEE Eng Med Biol Soc 12:2318.

Anderson OT. 1986. A system for quantitative assessment of dyscoordination and tremor. Acta Neurol Scand 73:291.

Angel RW, Alston W, Higgins JR. 1970. Control of movement in Parkinson's disease. Brain 93:1.

Baddeley A, Logie R, Bressi S, et al. 1986. Dementia and working memory. J Exp Psychol 38A:603.

Baroni A, Benvenuti F, Fantini L, et al. 1984. Human ballistic arm abduction movements: Effects of L-dopa treatment in Parkinson's disease. Neurology 34:868.

Barr RE, Hamlin RD, Abraham LD, Greene DE. 1988. Electromyographic evaluation of operator performance in manual control tracking. Proc Ann Int Conf IEEE Eng Med Biol Soc 10:1608.

Behbehani K, Kondraske GV, Richmond JR. 1988. Investigation of upper extremity visuomotor control performance measures. IEEE Trans Biomed Eng 35:518.

Beppu H, Nagaoka M, Tanaka R. 1987. Analysis of cerebellar motor disorders by visually-guided elbow tracking movement: 2. Contributions of the visual cues on slow ramp pursuit. Brain 110:1.

Beppu H, Suda M, Tanaka R. 1984. Analysis of cerebellar motor disorders by visually-guided elbow tracking movement. Brain 107:787.

Bloxham CA, Mindel TA, Frith CD. 1984. Initiation and execution of predictable and unpredictable movements in Parkinson's disease. Brain 107:371.

Bösser T. 1984. Adaptation to time-varying signals and control-theory models of tracking behavior. Psychol Res 46:155.

Buck L. 1982. Location versus distance in determining movement accuracy. J Mot Behav 14:287.

Cassell KJ. 1973. The usefulness of a temporal correlation technique in the assessment of human motor performance on a tracking task. Med Biol Eng 11:755.

Cooke JD, Brown JD, Brooks VB. 1978. Increased dependence on visual information for movement control in patients with Parkinson's disease. Can J Neurol Sci 5:413.

Cooper R, McCallum WC, Cornthwaite SP. 1989. Slow potential changes related to the velocity of target movement in a tracking task. Electroencephalogr Clin Neurophysiol 72:232.

Croft D, Jones RD. 1987. The value of off-road tests in the assessment of driving potential of unlicensed disabled people. Br J Occup Ther 50:357.

Dalrymple-Alford JC, Kalders AS, Jones RD, Watson RW. 1994. A central executive deficit in patients with Parkinson's disease. J Neurol Neurosurg Psychiatry 57:360.

Day BL, Dick JPR, Marsden CD. 1984. Patient's with Parkinson's disease can employ a predictive motor strategy. J Neurol Neurosurg Psychiatry 47:1299.

De Souza LH, Langton Hewer R, Lynn PA, et al. 1980. Assessment of recovery of arm control in hemiplegic stroke patients: 2. Comparison of arm function tests and pursuit tracking in relation to clinical recovery. Int Rehab Med 2:10.

Driscoll MC. 1975. Creative technological aids for the learning-disabled child. Am J Occup Ther 29:102.

Ferslew KE, Manno JE, Manno BR, et al. 1982. Pursuit meter II, a computer-based device for testing pursuit-tracking performance. Percept Mot Skills 54:779–784.

Fertner A, Sjölund SJ. 1986. Comparison of various time delay estimation methods by computer simulation. IEEE Trans Acoust Speech Signal Proc 34:1329.

Fitts PM. 1954. The information capacity of the human motor system in controlling the amplitude of movement. J Exp Psychol 47:381.

Fitts PM, Posner MI. 1967. Human Performance. California, Brooks/Cole.

Flash T, Hogan N. 1985. The coordination of arm movements: An experimentally confirmed mathematical model. J Neurosci 5:1688.

Flowers KA. 1976. Visual "closed-loop" and "open-loop" characteristics of voluntary movement in patients with Parkinsonism and intention tremor. Brain 99:269.

Flowers KA. 1978a. Lack of prediction in the motor behavior of Parkinsonism. Brain 101:35.

Flowers KA. 1978b. The predictive control of behavior: Appropriate and inappropriate actions beyond the input in a tracking task. Ergonomics 21:109.

Frith CD, Bloxham CA, Carpenter KN. 1986. Impairments in the learning and performance of a new manual skill in patients with Parkinson's disease. J Neurol Neurosurg Psychiatry 49:661.

Garvey WD. 1960. A comparison of the effects of training and secondary tasks on tracking behavior. J Appl Psychol 44:370.

Gibson JM, Pimlott R, Kennard C. 1987. Ocular motor and manual tracking in Parkinson's disease and the effect of treatment. Neurology 50:853.

Gottlieb GL, Agarwal GC, Penn R. 1984. Sinusoidal oscillation of the ankle as a means of evaluating the spastic patient. J Neurol Neurosurg Psychiatry 41:32.

Guiard Y, Diaz G, Beaubaton D. 1983. Left-hand advantage in right-handers for spatial constant error: Preliminary evidence in a unimanual ballistic aimed movement. Neuropsychologica 21:111.

Hocherman S, Aharon-Peretz J. 1994. Two-dimensional tracing and tracking in patients with Parkinson's disease. Neurology 44:111.

Jex HR. 1966. A "critical" tracking task for manual control research. IEEE Trans Hum Factors Electronics 7:138.

Jones RD, Donaldson IM. 1981. Measurement of integrated sensory-motor function following brain damage by a preview tracking task. Int Rehab Med 3:71.

Jones RD, Donaldson IM. 1986. Measurement of sensory-motor integrated function in neurological disorders: three computerized tracking tasks. Med Biol Eng Comput 24:536.

Jones RD, Donaldson IM. 1989. Tracking tasks and the study of predictive motor planning in Parkinson's disease. Proc Ann Int Conf IEEE Eng Med Biol Soc 11:1055.

Jones RD, Donaldson IM. 1992. Removal of the visuospatial component from tracking performance and its application to Parkinson's disease. Proc Ann Int Conf IEEE Eng Med Biol Soc 14:1477.

Jones RD, Donaldson IM. Fractionation of visuoperceptual dysfunction in Parkinson's disease. J Neurol Sci (in press).

Jones RD, Donaldson IM, Parkin PJ. 1989. Impairment and recovery of ipsilateral sensory-motor function following unilateral cerebral infarction. Brain 112:113.

Jones RD, Donaldson IM, Parkin PJ, Coppage SA. 1990. Impairment and recovery profiles of sensory-motor function following stroke: single-case graphical analysis techniques. Int Disabil Stud 12:141.

Jones R, Giddens H, Croft D. 1983. Assessment and training of brain-damaged drivers. Am J Occup Ther 37:754.

Jones RD, Sharman NB, Watson RW, Muir SR. 1993. A PC-based battery of tests for quantitative assessment of upper-limb sensory-motor function in brain disorders. Proc Ann Int Conf IEEE Eng Med Biol Soc 15:1414.

Jones RD, Watson RW. 1993. A two-dimensional step tracking task and its application to Parkinson's disease. Proc Ann Int Conf IEEE Eng Med Biol Soc 15:1416.

Jones RD, Williams LRT, Wells JE. 1986. Effects of laterality, sex, and age on computerized sensory-motor tests. J Hum Mot Stud 12:163.

Kearney RE, Hunter IW. 1983. System identification of human triceps surae stretch reflex dynamics. Exp Brain Res 51:117.

Kondraske GV. 1988. Experimental evaluation of an elemental resource model for human performance. Proc Ann Int Conf IEEE Eng Med Biol Soc 10:1612.

Kondraske GV. 1995. An elemental resource model for the human-task interface. Int J Technol Assess Health Care.

Kondraske GV, Behbehani K, Chwialkowski M, et al. 1988. A system for human performance measurement. IEEE Eng Med Biol Mag March:23.

Kondraske GV, Potvin AR, Tourtellotte WW, Syndulko K. 1984. A computer-based system for automated quantitation of neurologic function. IEEE Trans Biomed Eng 31:401.

Leist A, Freund HJ, Cohen B. 1987. Comparative characteristics of predictive eye-hand tracking. Hum Neurobiol 6:19.

Lynn PA, Parker WR, Reed GAL, et al. 1979. New approaches to modelling the disable human operator. Med Biol Eng Comput 17:344.

Lynn PA, Reed GAL, Parker WR, Langton Hewer R. 1977. Some applications of human-operator research to the assessment of disability in stroke. Med Biol Eng 15:184.

Miall RC, Weir DJ, Stein JF. 1985. Visuomotor tracking with delayed visual feedback. Neuroscience 16:511.

Milkowski LM, Prieto TE, Myklebust JB, et al. 1993. Two-dimensional coherence: A measure of asymmetry in postural steadiness. Proc Ann Int Conf IEEE Eng Med Biol Soc 15:1181.

Miller RG, Freund HJ. 1980. Cerebellar dyssynergia in humans: A quantitative analysis. Ann Neurol 8:574.

Muir SR, Jones RD, Andreae JH, et al. Measurement and analysis of single and multiple finger tapping in normal and Parkinsonian subjects. Parkinsonism Related Disorders.

Neilson PD. 1972. Speed of response or bandwidth of voluntary system controlling elbow position in intact man. Med Biol Eng 10:450.

Neilson PD, Neilson MD. 1980. Influence of control-display compatibility on tracking behaviour. Q J Exp Psychol 32:125.

Neilson PD, Neilson MD, O'Dwyer NJ. 1992. Adaptive model theory: Application to disorders of motor control. In JJ Summers (ed), Approaches to the Study of Motor Control and Learning, pp 495–548. New York, Elsevier Science Publishers.

Neilson PD, Neilson MD, O'Dwyer NJ. 1993. What limits high speed tracking performance? Hum Mov Sci 12:85.

Notterman JM, Tufano DR, Hrapsky JS. 1982. Visuo-motor organization: Differences between and within individuals. Percept Mot Skills 54:723.

Patrick J, Mutlusoy F. 1982. The relationship between types of feedback, gain of a display and feedback precision in acquisition of a simple motor task. Q J Exp Psychol 34A:171.

Pitrella FD, Kruger W. 1983. Design and validation of matching tests to form equal groups for tracking experiments. Ergonomics 26:833.

Potvin AR, Albers JW, Stribley RF, et al. 1975. A battery of tests for evaluating steadiness in clinical trials. Med Biol Eng 13:914.

Potvin AR, Doerr JA, Estes JT, Tourtellotte WW. 1977. Portable clinical tracking-task instrument. Med Biol Eng Comput 15:391.

Potvin AR, Tourtellotte WW. 1975. The neurological examination: Advancement in its quantification. Arch Phys Med Rehabil 56:425.

Potvin AR, Tourtellotte WW, Potvin JH, et al. 1985. The Quantitative Examination of Neurologic Function. Boca Raton, Fla, CRC Press.

Poulton EC. 1964. Postview and preview in tracking with complex and simple inputs. Ergonomics 7:257.

Poulton EC. 1974. Tracking Skill and Manual Control. New York, Academic Press.

Riedel SA, Harris GF, Jizzine HA. 1992. An investigation of seated postural stability. IEEE Eng Med Biol Mag 11:42.

Robertson C, Flowers KA. 1990. Motor set in Parkinson's disease. J Neurol Neurosurg Psychiatry 53:583.

Roscoe JT. 1975. Fundamental Research Statistics for the Behavioral Sciences, 2d ed. New York, Holt, Rinehart and Winston.

Schmidt RA. 1982. Motor Control and Learning: A Behavioral Emphasis. Champaigne, Ill, Human Kinetics.

Sheridan MR, Flowers KA, Hurrell J. 1987. Programming and execution of movement in Parkinson's disease. Brain 110:1247.

Sheridan TB. 1966. Three models of preview control. IEEE Trans Hum Factors Electronics 7:91.

Siegel D. 1985. Information processing abilities and performance on two perceptual-motor tasks. Percept Mot Skills 60:459.

Sittig AC, Denier van der Gon JJ, Gielen CC, van Wilk AJ. 1985. The attainment of target position during step-tracking movements despite a shift of initial position. Exp Brain Res 60:407.

Stelmach GE, Worrington CJ. 1988. The preparation and production of isometric force in Parkinson's disease. Neuropsychologica 26:93.

Stern Y, Mayeux R, Rosen J, Ilson J. 1983. Perceptual motor dysfunction in Parkinson's disease: a deficit in sequential and predictive voluntary movement. J Neurol Neurosurg Psychiatry 46:145.

Stern Y, Mayeux R, Rosen J. 1984. Contribution of perceptual motor dysfunction to construction and tracing disturbances in Parkinson's disease. J Neurol Neurosurg Psychiatry 47:983.

Thomas JS, Croft DA, Brooks VB. 1976. A manipulandum for human motor studies. IEEE Trans Biomed Eng 83.

van den Berg R, Mooi B, Denier van der Gon JJ, Gielen CCAM. 1987. Equipment for the quantification of motor performance for clinical purposes. Med Biol Eng Comput 25:311.

Vince MA. 1948. The intermittency of control movements and the psychological refractory period. Br J Psychol 38:149.

Warabi T, Noda H, Yanagisawa N, et al. 1986. Changes in sensorimotor function associated with the degree of bradykinesia of Parkinson's disease. Brain 109:1209.

Watson RW. 1994. Advances in Zero-Based Consistent Deconvolution and Evaluation of Human Sensory-Motor Function. Ph.D. dissertation, University of Canterbury, Christchurch, New Zealand.

Welford AT. 1968. Fundamentals of Skill. London, Methuen.

Further Information

The Quantitative Examination of Neurologic Function, by Potvin et al., [1985], is a two-volume book that provides a superb indepth review of instrumentation and methods for measurement of both normal and abnormal neurologic function.

An excellent overview of control of postural stability is contained in the theme section (edited by G. Harris) of the December 1992 issue of *IEEE Engineering in Medicine and Biology Magazine*.

146

Measurement of Information-Processing Performance Capacities

George V. Kondraske
University of Texas at Arlington

Paul J. Vasta
University of Texas at Arlington

The human brain has been the subject of much scientific research. While a tremendous amount of information exists and considerable progress has been made in unlocking its mysteries, many gaps in understanding exist. However, it is not essential to understand in full detail how a given function of the brain is mediated in order to accept that the function exists or to understand how to maximally isolate it, stress it, and characterize at least selected attributes of its performance quantitatively. In this chapter, a systems view of major functional aspects of the brain is used as a basis for discussing methods employed to measure what can be termed *central processing performance capacities*. Central processing capacities are distinguished from the information that is processed. In humans, the latter can be viewed to represent the contents of memory (e.g., facts, "programs," etc.). Clearly, both the information itself and the characteristics of the systems that process it (i.e., the various capacities discussed below) combine to realize what are commonly observed as skills, whether perceptual, motor, cognitive, or other.

Investigations of how humans process information have been performed within various fields including psychology, cognitive science, and information theory with the primary motivation being to better understand how human information processing works and the factors that influence it. On the basis that it provided a rigorous definition for the measurement of information, it can be argued that Shannon's information theory [Shannon, 1948] has been and continues to be one of the more important developments to influence both the science and engineering associated with human information processing. Several early attempts to apply it to human information processing [Fitts, 1954; Hick, 1952; Hyman, 1953] have stood the test of time and have provided the basis for subsequent efforts of both researchers and practitioners. These works are central to the material presented here. In addition, the work of Wiener [1955] is also noteworthy in that it began the process of viewing human and artificial information processing with a common perspective. Analogies between humans and computers have proven to be very useful up to certain limits.

While there is considerable overlap and frequent interchange, the roles of science and engineering are different. In the present context, the emphasis is on aspects of the latter. It has been necessary to engineer useful measurement tools and processes without complete science to serve a wide variety of purposes that have demanded attention in both clinical and nonclinical contexts. Whether purposeful or accidental, methods of systems engineering have been incorporated and have proven useful in dealing with the complexity of human brain structure and function. While scientific controversies continue to exist, much research has contributed to the now common view of separate (in both function and location) processing subsystems that make up the whole. Various versions of a general distributed, multiprocessor model of human brain function have been popularly sketched [Gazzaniga, 1985; Minsky, 1986; Ornstein, 1986]. For example, it is widely known that the occipital lobe of the brain is responsible for visual information processing, while other areas have been found to correspond to other functions. It is not possible to do justice here to the tremendous scope of work that has been put forth and therefore to the brain itself. Nonetheless, this compartmentalistic or systems approach, which stresses major functional systems that must exist based on overwhelming empirical evidence, has proven to be useful for explaining many normal and pathologic behavioral observations. This approach is essential to the development of meaningful and practical performance measurement strategies such as those described.

146.1 Basic Principles

Many of the past efforts in which performance-related measurements have played a significant role have been directed toward basic research. Furthermore, much of this research has been aimed at uncovering the general operational frameworks of normal human information processing and not the measurement of performance capacities and their use, either alone or in combination with other capacity metrics, to characterize humans of various types (e.g., normal, aged, handicapped, etc.). However, representative models and theories provide direction for, and are themselves shaped by, subsequent measurement efforts. While there are many principles and basic observations that have some relevance, the scope of material presented herein is limited to topics that more specifically support the understanding of human information-processing performance capacity measurement.

Functional Model of Central Information Processing

A simplified, although quite robust, model that is useful within the context of human information processing is illustrated in Fig. 146.1. With this figure, attention is called to systems, their functions, and major interconnectivities. At a functional level that is relatively high within the hierarchy of the human central nervous system, the central processing system can be considered to be composed of two types of subsystems: (1) information processors and (2) memories. As can be seen from the diagram, information from the environment is provided to the information-processing subsystems through human sensor subsystems. These not only include the obvious sensors (e.g., the eyes) that receive input from external sources but also those specifically designed to provide information regarding the internal environment, including proprioception and state of being. The capacity to process information input from multiple sources at a conscious level is finite. Constant overload is prevented by limiting the amount of information simultaneously received; specific sensory information of high priority is controlled by what may be termed an *attention processor*. Information associated with a given sensor system is processed by a corresponding processor. The model further suggests that there are memory subsystems for each sensory modality in bidirectional communications with the associated processor. Thus modality-specific (e.g., visual, auditory, etc.) information may be referenced and processed with new information. As information is received and processed at modality-specific levels, it is combined at a higher level by integrative processors to generate

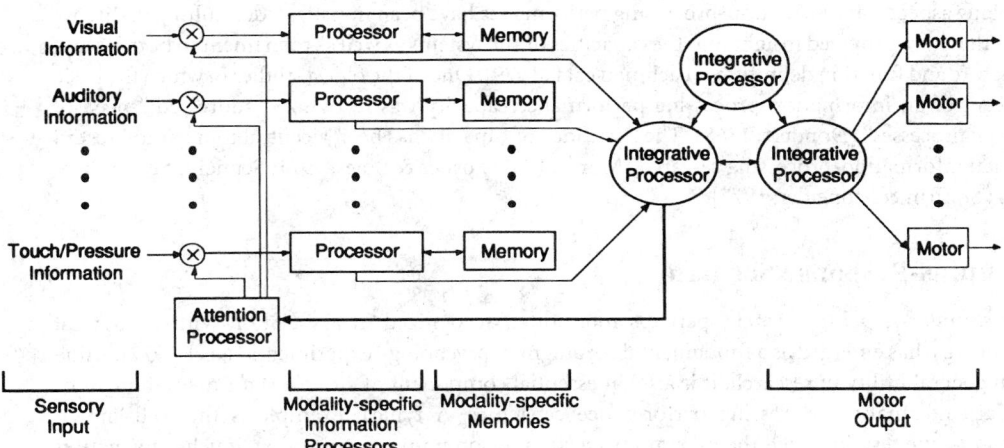

FIGURE 146.1 A functional systems-level block diagram of human information processing that facilitates description of the measurement of subsystem performance capacities.

situation-specific responses. These may be in the form of musculoskeletal, cognitive, or attention-modifying events, as well as any combination of these.

General measurement issues of fidelity, validity, and reliability are natural concerns in measurement of information-processing performance capacities. Special issues emerge that increase the overall complexity of the problem when attempting to measure attributes that reflect *just* the information-processing subsystems. Unlike a computer, where one may remove a memory module, place it in a special test unit, and determine its capacity, the accessibility of the subsystems within the human brain is such that it is impossible to perfectly isolate and directly measure any of the individual components. When measuring characteristics of human information-processing subsystems, it is necessary to address measurement goals that are similar to those applied to analogous artificial systems within the constraint that human sensors and motoric subsystems also must be utilized.

Performance Capacities

In considering the performance of human information-processing systems, the resource-based perspective represented by the elemental resource model [Kondraske, 1995] is adopted here. This model for human performance encompasses all types of human subsystems and is the result of the application of a general theoretical framework for system performance to the human system and its subsystems. A central idea incorporated in this framework, universal to all types of systems, is that of *performance capacity*. This implies a finite availability of some quantity which thereby limits performance. A general two-part approach is used to identify unique performance capacities (e.g., visual information-processor speed): (1) identify the system (e.g., visual information processor) and (2) identify the dimension of performance (e.g., speed). In this framework, system performance capacities are characterized by availability of performance resources along each of the identified dimensions. These *performance resources* are to be distinguished from less rigorously defined general processing resources described by others [e.g., Kahneman, 1973; Wickens, 1984]. However, many of the important basic constructs associated with the idea of "a resource" are employed in a similar fashion in each of these contexts. For processors, key dimensions of performance are speed and accuracy. *Processor speed* and *processor accuracy* capacities are thus identified. For memory systems, key dimensions of performance are storage capacity, speed (e.g., retrieval), and accuracy (e.g., retrieval). Other important attributes of performance capacities are developed in other sections of this chapter.

Many aspects of information-processing performance have been investigated, resulting in discoveries that have provided insight into the capacities of subsystems as well as refinement to both system structure and function definitions [Lachman et al., 1979]. One of the oldest studies in which the basic concept of an information-processing performance capacity was recognized addressed "speed of mental processes" [Donders, 1868]. The basic idea of capacity has been a central topic of interest in human information-processing research [Moray, 1967; Posner & Boies, 1971; Schneider & Shiffrin, 1977; Shiffrin & Schneider, 1977].

Stimulus-Response Scenario

The *stimulus-response scenario,* perhaps most often recognized in association with behavioral psychology, has emerged as a fundamental paradigm in psychology experiments [Neel, 1977]. Aside from general utility in research, it is also an essential component of strategies for measurement of human information-processing performance capacities. A typical example is the well-known reaction-time test, in which the maximum speed (and sometimes accuracy) at which information can be processed is of interest. Here, a subject is presented a stimulus specific to some sensory modality (e.g., visual, auditory, tactile) and is instructed to respond in a prescribed manner (e.g., lift a hand from a switch "as fast as possible" when the identified stimulus occurs). This general approach, which has become so popular and useful in psychology, also can be recognized as one that has been commonly employed in engineering to characterize artificial systems (e.g., amplifiers, motors, etc.). A specific known signal (stimulus) is applied to the system's input, and the corresponding output (response) is observed. Specified, measurable attributes of the output, in combination with the known characteristics of the input, are used to infer various characteristics of the system under test. When the focus of interest is the performance limits of processing systems, these characteristics include processing speed, processing accuracy, memory storage capacity, etc.

In performance capacity tests, an important related component is the *prestimulus set,* or simply the way in which the system is "programmed to respond to the stimulus." This is usually accomplished by one or more components of the instructions given to the subject under test (e.g., respond "as quickly as possible," etc.) just prior to the execution of an actual test.

Measurement of Information (Stimulus Characterization)

Within a given sensory modality, it is easy to understand that different stimuli place different demands or "loads" on information-processing systems. Thus, in order to properly interpret results of performance tests, it is necessary to describe the stimulus. While this remains a topic of ongoing research with inherent controversies, some useful working constructs are available. At issue is not simply a qualitative description, but the *measurement* of stimulus content (or complexity). Shannon's information theory [1948], which teaches how to measure the amount of information associated with a generalized information source, has been the primary tool used in these efforts. Thus a stimulus can be characterized in terms of the amount of information present in it. Simple stimuli (e.g., a light that is "on" or "off") possess less information than complex stimuli (e.g., a computer screen with menus, buttons, etc.). The best successes in attempts to quantitatively characterize stimuli have been achieved for simple, discrete stimuli [Hick, 1952; Hyman, 1953]. From Shannon, the amount of information associated with a given symbol i selected from a source with n such symbols is given by

$$I_i = \log_2 (1/p_i) \tag{146.1}$$

where p_i is the probability of occurrence of symbol i (within a finite symbol set), and the result has the units of "bits." Thus high-probability stimuli contain less information than low-probability stimuli. It is a relatively straightforward matter to control the probabilities associated with symbols that serve as stimuli in test situations. The application of basic information theory to the characterization of stimuli that are more complex (i.e., multiple components, continuous) is challenging both theoretically and practically (e.g., large symbol sets, different sets with different probability distributions that must be controlled, etc.).

If stimuli are not or cannot be characterized robustly in terms of a measure with units of "bits," operationally defined units are frequently used (e.g., "items," "chunks," "stimuli," etc.). In addition, as many stimulus attributes as possible are identified and quantified, and others are simply "described." This at least maximizes the opportunity for obtaining repeatable measurements. However, the additional implication is that the number of "bits per item" or "bits per chunk" is waiting to be delineated and that perhaps a conversion could be substituted at a later time. While this state leaves much to be desired from a rigorous measurement perspective, it is nonetheless quite common in the evolution of measurement for many physical quantities and allows useful work to be conducted.

Speed-Accuracy Tradeoff

Fundamental to all human information-processing systems and tasks is the so-called *speed-accuracy tradeoff*. This basic limitation can be observed in relatively high-level everyday tasks such as reading, writing, typing, listening to a lecture, etc. Psychologists [see Wicklegren, 1977] have studied this tradeoff in many different contexts. Fitts [1966] demonstrated a relationship between measures reflecting actual performance (reaction time and errors) and incentive-based task goals (i.e., were subjects attempting to achieve high speed or high accuracy). As shown in Fig. 146.2, relationships that have been found suggest an upper limit to the combination of speed and accuracy available for information-processing tasks. In this figure, original reaction-time measures have been transformed by simple inversion to obtain true speed measures that also conform to the resource construct used in modeling performance capacities, as described earlier. The result then defines a two-dimensional (e.g., speed-accuracy) performance envelope for information-processing systems. The area within this envelope, given that each dimension represents a resource-based performance capacity, represents a higher-level or composite performance capacity metric (with units of speed × accuracy), analogous in some respects to a gain-bandwidth product or work (force × displacement) metric.

Divided Attention and Time Sharing

An approach sometimes used in a variety of measurement contexts incorporates a *dual-task scenario* that is designed to require use of attention resources in two different simultaneously executed tasks [e.g., Wickens, 1984]. For example, visual tracking (primary task) accuracy *and* speed of response to an embedded visual stimulus (secondary task) can be measured. Details of the potential time-sharing possibilities at play are quite complex [Schneider & Shiffrin, 1977; Shiffrin & Schneider, 1977].

In comparison with single-task performance test situations, in which the attention processor may not be working at capacity, the additional demand is designed to change (compared with a single-task baseline) and sometimes maximizes the stress on attentional resources. Performance on both primary and secondary tasks, compared with levels attained when each task is independently performed, can provide an indirect mea-

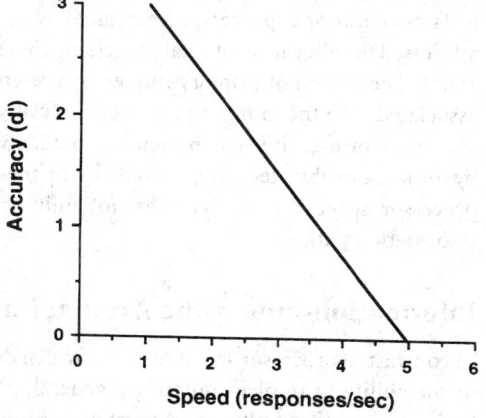

FIGURE 146.2 A typical information-processing performance envelope in two-dimensional speed-accuracy space. Data used were derived from Wicklegren [1977].

sure of capacity associated with attention [Parasuraman & Davies, 1984]. This approach has been useful in determining relative differences in demand imposed by two different primary tasks by comparison of results from respective tests in which a fixed secondary task is used with different primary tasks. Of more direct relevance to the present context, an appropriate secondary task can be used to control in part the conditions under which a given performance capacity (defined in a standard way and measured in association with the primary task) is measured; for example, visual information-processing speed can be measured with no additional attentional load or with several different additional attentional load levels. While it may be possible to rank secondary tasks in terms of the additional load presented, there are no known methods to quantify attentional load in absolute terms.

146.2 General Measurement Paradigms

Despite the complexity of human information processing, a fairly small number of different measurement paradigms have emerged for quantification of the many unique human information-processing performance capacities. This is perhaps in part due to the limited number of system types (e.g., processors and memories). A good portion of the observed complexity can therefore be attributed to the number of different processors and memories, as well as the vastness and diversity of actual information that human's typically possess (i.e., facts, knowledge, skills, etc.). While most of the paradigms described below have been used for decades, it is helpful to recognize that they all conform to the more recently proposed [Kondraske, 1987, 1995] generalized strategy for measuring any aspect of performance for any human subsystem: (1) maximally isolate first the system of interest, (2) maximally isolate the dimension(s) of performance of interest, and (3) maximally stress (tempered by safety considerations when appropriate) the system along the dimension(s) (Table 146.1).

Information-Processing Speed

The paradigm for measuring information-processing speed is commonly referred to as a *reaction-time test* because the elapsed time (i.e., the processing time) between the onset of a given stimulus and the occurrence of a prescribed response is the basic measurable quantity. To obtain a processing-speed measure, the stimulus content in "bits," "chunks," or simply "stimuli" is divided by the processing time to yield measures with units of bits per second, chunks per second, or stimuli per second. Choice of stimulus modality isolates a specific sensory processor, whereas choice of a responder (e.g., index finger, upper extremity motion caused primarily by shoulder flexors, etc.) isolates a motoric processor associated with generation of the response. Much research has addressed the allocation of total processing times to various subsystem components [e.g., Sternberg, 1966]. The system of primary interest as presented here is the sensory processor. Processing times associated with the motoric processor associated with the response are substantially less in normal systems. However, it is recommended that a given processor speed capacity be identified not only by the sensor subsystem stressed but also by the responder (e.g., visual–shoulder flexor information processor speed). This identifies not only the test scenario employed but also the complete information path.

Information-Processing Accuracy and Speed-Accuracy Combinations

In contrast to processor speed capacity, which describes limits on information rate, accuracy relates to the ability to resolve content. In general, paradigms for tests that include accuracy measures typically involve a finite set of symbols with a corresponding set of responses. Various stimulus presentation-response scenarios can be used. For example, a stimulus can be randomly selected from the set with the subject required to identify the stimulus presented. Alternately, a subset of stimuli can be presented and the subject asked to select the response corresponding to the symbol not in

TABLE 146.1 The Combination of the Human Sensor Subsystem (Determined by Stimulus Source) and Responder Isolates Unique Subsystems. Depending on objectives of the test task (as communicated to the subject under test) and metrics obtained, many different unique capacities can be measured.

Capacity Types	Stimulus Type	Responder*	Measurements
Attention	Visual Auditory	Upper extremity Vocal system	Length of time that task can be performed to specification and accuracy (if appropriate for task) when subject is instructed to perform for "as long as possible."
Processor speed	Visual Visual Visual Auditory Auditory Auditory Vibrotactile	Upper extremity Lower extremity — Upper extremity Lower extremity Vocal system Vocal system	Inverse of time required to react to stimulus (i.e. stimuli/second) when subject is instructed to respond "as quickly as possible."
Processor accuracy	Visual Visual Visual Auditory Auditory Auditory Vibrotactile	Upper extremity Lower extremity — Upper extremity Lower extremity Vocal system Vocal system	Subject is asked to perform task (e.g., typically recognition of symbols from set with similar information content across symbols) "as accurately as possible" and without stress on speed of measures of accuracy. The percentage correct (out of a predetermined set size) is often used, although different accuracy measures have been proposed [Green & Swets, 1966; Wicklegren, 1977].
Processor speed-accuracy	Visual Visual Visual Auditory Auditory Auditory Vibrotactile	Upper extremity Lower extremity — Upper extremity Lower extremity Vocal system Vocal system	Basically a combination of test that stress speed and accuracy capacities individually, both speed and accuracy measures are obtained as defined above to get off-axis data points in two-dimensional speed-accuracy space. Both speed and accuracy can be maximally stressed (e.g., by instructing subject to perform "as fast and accurately as possible"), or accuracy can be measured at different speeds by varying time available for responses and stressing accuracy within this constraint.
Memory storage capacity	Visual Visual Visual Auditory Auditory Auditory Vibrotactile	(Same options as above†	Maximum amount of information of type defined by stimulus which subject is able to recall. Stimuli usually consist of sets of symbols of varying complexity in different sets (e.g., spatially distributed lights, alphanumeric characters, words, motions, etc.) but similar amount of information per symbol in a given set. Units of "bits" are ideal but not often possible if number of bits per symbol is unknown. In such cases, units are often reported as "symbols," "chunks," or "items."

*General terms are used in table to illustrate combination options. Very specific definition that controls the motoric functional units involved as precisely as possible should be used for any given capacity test. For example, (1) upper extremity (shoulder flexor vs. elbow flexor vs. digit 2 flexor), (2) vocal system (lingua-dental "ta" vs. labial "pa" response), etc.

†Unless motor memory capacities are being tested, typically chosen to minimize stress on motoric processing and, compared with processor measures, not to isolate unique memory system.

the subset (size of subsets should be small if it is desired to minimize stress on memory capacities). A key element is that, within a poststimulus response window, the subject is forced to select one of the available responses. This allows accuracy of the response to be measured in any of a number of ways ranging from relatively simple to complex [Green & Swets, 1966; Wicklegren, 1977]. The response window is either relatively open-ended, as short as possible, and variable (based on the speed of the subject's response) or fixed at a given length of time. When only accuracy is stressed, subjects are instructed to perform as accurately as possible, and the stress on speed is minimized (e.g., "take your time"). In a second type of speed-accuracy test, subjects are instructed to perform as fast and as accurately as possible, maximally stressing both dimensions, while both accuracy and speed of responses are measured. In a variation of this general paradigm, a fixed response window size is selected to challenge response speed. This provides a known point along the speed dimension of performance. In all three cases, measured response accuracy provides the second coordinate of a point in the two-dimensional speed-accuracy performance space. The combination of different paradigms can be used to determine the speed-accuracy performance envelope (see above).

Memory Capacity

As used here, *memory capacity* refers to the amount of information that can be stored and/or recalled. It is well accepted that separate memory exists for different sensory modalities. Also, short-, medium-, and long-term memory systems have been identified [Crook et al., 1986]. Thus separate capacities can be identified for each. Higher-level capacities also can be identified with processes that utilize memory, such as scanning [Sternberg, 1966]. A comprehensive assessment of memory would require tasks that challenge the various memory systems to determine resources available, singly and along different combinations of their various modalities, most directly relevant to the individual's developmental stage (infant, youth, adolescent, young adult, middle-aged adult, or older adult) and reflecting the diversity and depth of life experiences of that individual. No such comprehensive batteries are available. As noted by Syndulko et al. [1988], "Most typically, a variety of individual tests are utilized that evaluate selected aspects of memory systems under artificial conditions that relate best to college students." This general circumstance is in part due to the lack of generalized performance measurement strategies for memory. Despite such diversity, perhaps the most common variation of the many memory capacity tests involves providing a stimuli of the appropriate modality and requiring complete, accurate recall (i.e., a response) after some specified period of delay. The response window is selected to be relatively long so that processor speed is only minimally stressed. Typically, a test begins with a stimulus that has a low information content (i.e., one that should be within capacity limits of the lowest one expects to encounter). If the response is correct, the information content of the stimuli is increased, and another trial is administered. It is typically assumed that the amount of information added after each successful trial is fairly constant. Examples include adding another light to spatial distributed light pattern, adding another randomly selected digit (0 to 9) to a sequence of such digits, etc. By continuing this process of progressively increasing the amount of stimulus information until an inaccurate response is obtained, the isolated memory capacity is assumed to be maximally stressed. The result is simply the amount of information stored and recalled, in units of bits, chunks, or items.

Attention

Tests for basic attention capacity can be considered to be somewhat analogous to endurance capacity tests for neuromuscular systems. Simply put, the length of time over which a specified information-processing task can be executed provides a measure of attention capacity (or attention span). The test paradigm typically involves presentation at random time intervals of a randomly selected stimulus from a finite predefined symbol set for a relatively short, fixed time (e.g., 1 s). Within a predefined response window (with a maximum duration that is selected so that processing speed resources are minimally stressed), the subject must generate a response corresponding to the stimulus that occurred. Attention is maximally stressed by continuing this process until the subject either (1) makes no response within the allocated response window or (2) produces an incorrect response (i.e., a response associated with a stimulus that was not presented). These criteria thus essentially define the point at which the specified task (i.e., recognize stimuli and respond correctly within a generous allotted time) can no longer be completed. Once again, choice of stimulus modality isolates a specific sensory processor (e.g., visual, auditory, tactile, etc.). Clearly, stimulus complexity is also important. Stress on higher-level cognitive resources can be minimized by choice of simple stimuli (e.g. lights, tones, etc.), although motoric processors associated with response generation are also involved. However, these are minimally stressed, and as long as basic functionality is present, the choice of responder should have little influence on results compared with, for example, the influence occurring during processor speed capacity measurements.

146.3 Measurement Instruments and Procedures

Given the preceding functional systems model for human information processing (see Fig. 146.1) and review of measurement paradigms for information-processing subsystems, a general architecture for instruments capable of measuring information-processing performance capacities can be defined (Fig. 146.3). It is interesting to observe that this architecture parallels the human information-processing system (i.e., compare Fig. 146.1 and Fig. 146.3).

Most such instruments are computer-based, allowing for generation of stimuli with different contents, presentation of stimuli at precisely timed intervals, measurement of processing times (from which processing speeds are derived) with high accuracy (typically, to within 1 ms), and accurate recording of responses and determination of their correctness.

A typical desktop computer system fits the general architecture presented in Fig. 146.3, and as such, it has been widely exploited "as is" physically with appropriate software to conduct information-processing tests. This is adequate for tests that specifically focus on higher-level, complex cognitive processing tasks due to the longer processing times involved. That is, screen refresh times and keyboard response times are smaller fractions of total times measured and contribute less error. However, for measurement of more basic performance capacities and to allow testing of subjects who do not possess normal physical performance capacities, custom test setups are essential. The general design goal for these stimuli generators and response sensors is to minimize the stress on human sensory, motor, and aspects of central processing resources that are not the target of the test. For example, the size of standard keyboard switches imposes demands on positioning accuracy when, for example, visual information-processing accuracy is being tested. According to Fitts' law [Fitts, 1954], the task component involved with hitting the desired response key (i.e., the component that occurs after the visual information processing component) requires longer processing times (associated with the motoric response task) for smaller targets. Thus, to minimize such influences, a relatively large target is suggested. Along the same lines of reasoning, these additional design guidelines are important: (1) key stimulus attributes that are not related to information content should be well above normal minimum human sensing thresholds (e.g., relatively bright lights that do not stress visual sensitivity, large characters or symbols that do not stress visual acuity), and (2) response speeds of stimulus generators and response sensors should be much faster than the fastest human response speed that is anticipated to be measured.

Even the many custom devices reported in the literature (as well as commercially available versions of some) have been devised primarily to support research into fundamental aspects of information processing and are used in studies that typically involve only healthy young college students. While such devices measure the stated or implied capacities well in this population, the often unstated assumption regarding other performance capacities (i.e., that they are available in "normal" amounts) is severely challenged when the subject under test is a member of a population with impairments (e.g., head-injured, multiple sclerosis, Parkinson disease, etc.).

A representative instrument [Kondraske, 1990; Kondraske et. al., 1984] is illustrated in Fig. 146.4. This device incorporates 8 LEDs and 15 high-speed touch sensors ("home," A1–A8, B1–B6) and a

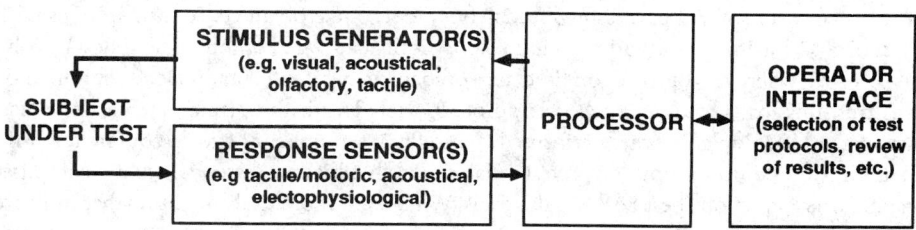

FIGURE 146.3 The general architecture for instruments used to measure human information-processing performance capacities.

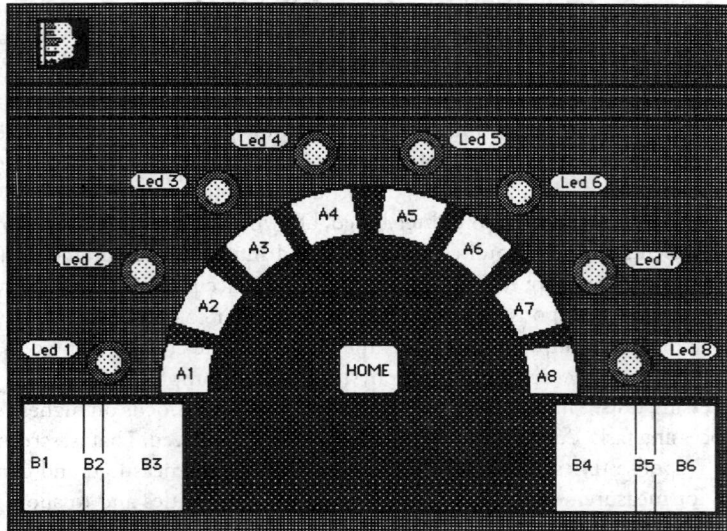

FIGURE 146.4 Major components of a specific microprocessor-based instrument for measurement of a selected subset of information-processing capacities incorporating high-intensity LEDs for visual stimuli and large-contact-area, fast-touch sensors to acquire responses (made by the upper extremity) from the subject under test. (Radius of semicircle is 15 cm.)

dedicated internal microprocessor to measure an array of different performance capacities associated with information processing. Measures at the most basic hierarchical level (visual information-processing speed, visual-spatial memory capacity, visual attention span, etc.) and intermediate level (coordination tasks involving different sets of more basic functional units) are included.

For example, visual–upper extremity information-processing speed is measured in a paradigm whereby the test subject first places his or her hand on the "home" plate. A random time after an audible warning cue, one out of eight LEDs (e.g., LED 4) stimulates the subject to respond "as quickly as possible" by lifting his or her hand off the home plate and touching the sensor (e.g., A4) associated with the lighted LED. Each LED represents a binary (ON or OFF) information source. Since an equiprobable selection scheme is employed, the $\log_2$(number of choices) represents the number of bits of information to be processed when determining which LED is lighted. In this example, the number of choices is eight; prior to the test, the subject was informed that any one of eight LEDs will be selected. Modes reflecting different information loads (1, 2, 4, or 8 choices) are available. Processing speed (in stimuli per second) is obtained as a result from each trial by inverting the total processing time, measured as the time from presentation of the stimulus until the subject's hand is lifted off the home plate. By combining time measures from two or more tests with different information loads, a more direct measure of true processing speed in bits per second is obtained. For example, results from an 8-choice (3-bit load) test and a 1-choice test (0-bit load) are combined as follows: (3 bits—0 bits)/$(t_3 - t_0)$, where t_n is the reaction time measured for an n-bit information load. This method removes transmission and other time delays not associated with the primary visual information-processing task. Multiple trials are performed (typically, 3 × number of choices, but no fewer than 5 trials for any mode) to improve test-retest reliability in the final measures, which are computed by averaging over a fraction (best 80%) of the trials. While even more trials might further improve repeatability of final capacity measures in some subjects, the overall test duration must be considered in light of the desire (from a test design perspective) to minimize stress on attention resources, the availability of which could vary widely over potential test subjects. Careful tradeoffs are necessary.

Visual-spatial memory capacity is measured using the same device. A random sequence of LEDs, beginning with a sequence length of "one," is presented to the subject. The subject responds by contacting (with the preferred hand) the subset of touch sensors (from A1 through A8) corresponding to the LEDs incorporated in a given stimulus presentation in the same order as the LEDs sequence was presented. A correct response causes a new trial to be initiated automatically with the sequence length increased by "one." The maximum length of this sequence (in items) that the subject can repeat without error is used as the measure of visual-spatial memory capacity. The best of two trials is used as a final score. The bright LEDs, relatively large contact area of the touch sensors (5 × 5 cm), and a relatively long poststimulus response window (up to 10 s) ensure that other performance resources are minimally stressed.

A measure of visual attention span is obtained with a task in which random LEDs are lighted for 1 s at random intervals ranging from 4 to 15 s. After each LED is lighted, a response window is entered (3 s maximum) during which the subject is required to indicated that a lighted LED was observed by contacting the corresponding touch sensor. The task continues until either the wrong touch sensor is contacted or no response is received within the defined response window. The time (in seconds) from the beginning of the test until an "end of test" criterion is met is used as the measure of visual attention performance capacity. The simple stimuli ensure that higher-level cognitive resources are minimally stressed. This allows a wide range of populations to be tested, including young children. Some normal subjects can achieve very long attention spans (e.g., hours) with this specific scenario, while some head-injured subjects (for example) produce times less than 60 s.

One example of a more comprehensive, computer-based memory performance test battery is that developed over the past 15 years by Crook and colleagues [1986]. This battery is directed at older adults, evaluates memory in the visual and auditory modalities at each of the three temporal process levels, and utilizes challenges that relate well to the daily activities of the target group. The challenges (i.e., stimulus sets) are computer generated and controlled, administered by means of a color graphics terminal, and in some cases, played for a videodisk player to provide as realistic a stimulus representation as possible outside of using actors in the everyday environment of the subject. The battery takes 60 to 90 minutes to administer and provides a profile of scores across the various measurement domains. Extensive age and gender norms are available to scale the scores in terms of percentiles. Despite its scope, it does not provide, nor was it intended to provide, information about modalities other than visual and auditory (e.g., tactile, kinesthetic, or olfactory). It also does not address long-term memory storage beyond about 45 minutes (consider the test administration complexities in doing so). Nonetheless, it represents one of the most sophisticated memory performance measurement and assessment systems currently available.

146.4 Present Limitations

General methods and associated tools do not exist to quantify the information content of any arbitrary stimulus within a given modality (e.g., visual, auditory, etc.). Success has been achieved only for relatively simple stimuli (e.g., lights which are on or off, at fixed positions spatially, etc.). It can be said, however, that serious attempts to quantify complex stimuli even in one modality appear to be lacking. To the practitioner, this prevents standardization that could occur across many information-processing performance capacity metrics. For example, information-processing speed capacities cannot yet be expressed universally in terms of bits per seconds. Perhaps more significant, this limitation not only impacts looking toward the human and the measurement of intrinsic performance capacities but also the analysis of information-processing tasks in quantitative terms. This, in turn, has limited the way in which information-processing performance capacity measures can be utilized. Whereas one can measure grip strength available in a subject (a neuromuscular capacity) and also the worst-case grip force required to support turning a door knob, it is not yet possible to quantify how much visual information one must process to reach out and find the door knob.

As was also noted, one cannot ideally isolate the systems under test. The required involvement of human sensory and motoric systems also requires the use of ancillary performance tests that establish at least some minimal levels of performance availabilities in these systems (e.g., visual acuity, etc.) in order to lend validity to measures of information-processing performance capacities. New imaging techniques and advanced electroencephalographic and magnetoencephalographic techniques such as brain mapping may offer the basis for new approaches that circumvent in part this limitation. While the cost and practicality of using these techniques routinely are likely to be prohibitive for the foreseeable future, the use of such techniques in research settings to optimize and establish validity of simpler methods can be anticipated.

Moray [1967] was one of many to use the analogy to data and program storage in a digital computer to facilitate understanding of a "limited capacity concept" with regard to human information processing. In the material presented, emphasis has been placed on the components analogous to those within the realm of computer hardware (i.e., processors and memories). These have been dealt with at their most basic operational levels for testing purposes, attempting to intentionally limit stresses on the test subject's acquired "skill" (i.e., stored information itself). It has been implied and is argued that knowledge of these hardware system capacities is in itself quite useful (e.g., it is helpful to know whether your desktop computer's basic information-processing rate is 33 or 60 MHz). However, many tasks that humans perform daily that involve information processing require not only processing and storage capacities but also the use of *unique information* acquired in the past (i.e., training or "programs"). These software components, which like processor and memory performance capacities also represent a necessary but not sufficient resource for completion of the specific task at hand, present even greater challenges to evaluation. If the analogy to computer programs is used (or even musical scores, plans, scripts, etc.), it can be observed that even the smallest "programming error" can lead to a failure of the total system in accomplishing its intended purpose with the intended degree of performance. Checking the integrity of human "programs" can be envisioned to be relatively easy if the desired functionality is in fact found to be present. However, if functionality is not present and diagnostic data points to a "software problem," methods that can be employed to reveal the source of the error in the basic information itself (i.e., the contents of memory) can be expected to be just as tedious as checking the integrity of code written for digital computers.

Defining Terms

Attention: A performance capacity representing the length of time that an information-processing system can carry out a prescribed task when maximally stressed to do so. This is analogous to endurance in neuromuscular subsystems.

Dual-task scenario: A test paradigm characteristic by a primary and secondary task and measurement of subject performance in both.

Memory: One of two major subsystem types of the human information-processing system that performs the function of storage of information for possible later retrieval.

Performance capacity: A quantity in finite availability that limits some aspect of a system's ability to execute tasks, or the limit of that aspect itself.

Prestimulus set: The manner in which a human system is programmed to respond to an ensuing stimulus.

Processor: One of two major subsystem types within the human information-processing system that performs the general function of processing information. Multiple processors at different hierarchical levels can be identified (e.g., those specific to sensory modalities, integrative processors, etc.).

Processor accuracy: The aspect, quality, or dimension of performance of a processor that characterizes the ability to correctly process information.

Processor speed: The aspect, quality, or dimension of performance of an information processor that characterizes the rate at which information is processed.

Speed-accuracy tradeoff: A fundamental limit of human information-processing systems at any level of abstraction that is most likely due to a more basic limit in channel capacity; i.e., channel capacity can be used to achieve more accuracy at the expense of speed or to achieve more speed at the expense of accuracy.

References

Crook T, Salama M, Gobert J. 1986. A computerized test battery for detecting and assessing memory disorders. In Bés et al. (eds), Senile Dementia: Early Detection, pp 79–85. John Libbey Eurotext.

Donders FC. 1868–1869. Over de snelheid van psychische processen. Onderzoekingen gedaan in het Psyiologish Laboratorium der Utrechtsche Hoogescholl. In Attention and Performance II. Translated by WG Koster. Acta Psychol 30:412.

Fitts PM. 1954. The information capacity of the human motor system in controlling the amplitude of movement. J Exp Psychol 47:381.

Fitts PM. 1966. Cognitive aspects of information processing: III. Set for speed versus accuracy. J Exp Psychol 71:849.

Gazzaniga MS. 1985. The Social Brain. New York, Basic Books.

Green DM, Swets JR. 1966. Signal Detection Theory and Psychophysics. New York, Wiley.

Hick W. 1952. On the rate of gain of information. Q J Exp Psychol 4:11.

Hunt E. 1986. Experimental perspectives: Theoretical memory models. In LW Poon (ed), Handbook for Clinical Memory Assessment of Older Adults, pp 43–54. Washington, American Psychological Association.

Hyman R. 1953. Stimulus information as a determinant of reaction time. J Exp Psychol 45:423.

Kahneman D. 1973. Attention and Effort. Englewood Cliffs, NJ, Prentice-Hall.

Kondraske GV. 1987. Human performance: Science or art. In KR Foster (ed), Proceedings of the Thirteenth Northeast Bioengineering Conference, pp 44–47. New York, Institute of Electrical and Electronics Engineers.

Kondraske GV, Potvin AR, Tourtellotte WW, Syndulko K. 1984. A computer-based system for automated quantification of neurologic function. IEEE Trans Biomed Eng 31(5):401.

Kondraske GV. 1990. A PC-based performance measurement laboratory system. J Clin Eng 15(6):467.

Kondraske GV. 1995. A working model for human system-task interfaces. In JD Bronzino (ed), Handbook of Biomedical Engineering. Boca Raton, Fla, CRC Press.

Lachman R, Lachman JL, Butterfield EC. 1979. Cognitive Psychology and Information Processing: An Introduction. Hillsdale, NJ, Lawrence Erlbaum.

Minsky M. 1986. The Society of Mind. New York, Simon & Schuster.

Moray N. 1967. Where is capacity limited? A survey and a model. Acta Psychol 27:84.

Neel A. 1977. Theories of Psychology: A Handbook. Cambridge, Mass, Schenkman Publishing.

Ornstein R. 1986. Multimind. Boston, Hougton Mifflin.

Parasuraman R, Davies DR (eds). 1984. Varieties of Attention. Orlando, Fla, Academic Press.

Posner MI, Boies SJ. 1971. Components of attention. Psychol Rev 78:391.

Sanders MS, McCormick EJ. 1987. Human Factors in Engineering and Design. New York, McGraw-Hill.

Schneider W, Shiffrin RM. 1977. Controlled and automatic human information processing: I. Detection, search, and attention. Psychol Rev 84:1.

Shannon CE. 1948. A mathematical theory of communication. The Bell System Technical Journal 27(3):379.

Shiffrin RM, Schneider W. 1977. Controlled and automatic human information processing: II. Perceptual learning, automatic attending, and a general theory. Psychol Rev 84:127.

Squire LR, Butters N. 1992. Neuropsychology of Memory. New York, Guilford Press.

Sternberg S. 1966. High-speed scanning in human memory. Science 153:652.

Syndulko K, Tourtellotte WW, Richter E. 1988. Toward the objective measurement of central processing resources. IEEE Eng Med Biol Soc Mag 7(1):17.

Wickens CD. 1984. Engineering Psychology and Human Performance. Columbus, Ohio, Charles E Merrill.

Wickelgren WA. 1977. Speed-accuracy tradeoff and information processing dynamics. Acta Psychol 41:67.

Wiener N. 1955. Cybernetics, or Control and Communications in the Animal and the Machine. New York, Wiley.

Further Information

A particularly informative yet concise historical review of the major perspectives in psychology leading up to much of the more recent work involving quantitative measurements of information processing and determination of information processing capacities is provided in *Theories of Psychology: A Handbook,* by A. Neel (Schenkman Publishing, Cambridge, Mass., 1977). Human information processing has long been and continues to be a major topic of interest of the U.S. military. Considerable indepth information and experimental results are available in the form of technical reports, many of which are unclassified. *CSERIAC Gateway,* published by the Crew System Ergonomics Information Analysis Center (CSERIAC), is distributed free of charge and provides timely information on scientific, technical, and engineering knowledge. For subscription information, contact AL/CFH/CSERIAC, Bldg. 248, 2255 H St., Wright-Patterson Air Force Base, Ohio, 45433. Also, the North Atlantic Treaty Organization AGAARD (Advisory Group for Aerospace Research and Development) Aerospace Medical Panel Working Group 12 has worked on standards for a human performance test battery for military environments (much of which addresses information processing) and has defined data exchange formats. Documents can be obtained through the National Technical Information Service (NTIS), 5285 Port Royal Road, Springfield, Va. 22161.

Information regarding the design, construction, and evaluation of instrumentation (including quantitative attributes of stimuli, etc.) is often embedded in journal articles with titles that emphasize the major question of the study (i.e., not the instrumentation). Most appear in the many journals associated with the fields of psychology, neurology, and neuroscience.

147

High-Level
Task Analysis:
Mental Components

Kenneth J. Maxwell
Departure Technology

As advanced information technologies have been increasingly integrated into communications, manufacturing, transportation, power, and medical systems, among others, the predominant requirements of many human-performed tasks have correspondingly shifted from manual to mental (i.e., information-processing) activities. Examples of tasks reflecting this shift include supervisory control of complex systems and operating advanced technology equipment. As a result, data, models, and metrics for describing and understanding mental tasks and the mental capabilities of persons performing them have become very important to engineering decision making. *Task analysis* is a generic term that represents processes and methods for applying task data to improve engineering decisions. This chapter presents a process and associated methods for analyzing the mental components of tasks. It further describes the role of *mental task analysis* along with human performance and machine models (as applicable) in applied decision making and presents a quantitative, performance-based framework for performing a unified human-machine-task analysis. This chapter is not intended as a review. Selected techniques are presented to familiarize the reader with different major approaches that are currently applied to solving real-world engineering problems.

147.1 Fundamentals

The goals of task analysis are to (1) decompose high-level tasks into their constituent, mutually exclusive, lower-level tasks; (2) describe intertask relationships and dependencies; and (3) define each task's goals, procedures, and performance and skill requirements. A major thesis of this chapter is that using task analysis for applied decisions will be improved to the degree that (1) the

0-8493-8346-3/95/$0.00+$.50
© 1995 by CRC Press, Inc.

performance requirements are quantified and (2) they are quantified in a form that is consistent with quantitative models of human performance. A *task* is a goal-directed, procedural activity that is defined with regard to the resources (i.e., capabilities) that performing agents (i.e., humans or machines) must possess to accomplish the goal. *High-level tasks* refer to complex, composite activities that entail performing many simpler but interrelated tasks in meaningful ways. *Mental components* refer to the *perceptual and cognitive* information-processing activities and resources that are necessary or sufficient for accomplishing tasks.

Figure 147.1 depicts the mental task-analysis process in four major steps. Before any data are collected, required data should be defined on the basis of the characteristics of the system and the applied decision. Selection and use of data-collection methods, task models, and task metrics are driven by the system and applied decision.

Figure 147.1 illustrates how task analysis is used with human and machine models as a basis for solving applied problems. Task data by themselves are of limited use in solving applied problems because the task data address only one set of the total system variables that need to be considered. To be applied, task data must be analyzed with human performance and machine performance data (i.e., capacities), as applicable to the applied problem (i.e., *not all problems will involve machines*). This combined human-machine-task system analysis requires that the analysis of each component is accomplished with consistent constructs. Further, the quality and precision of applied decisions

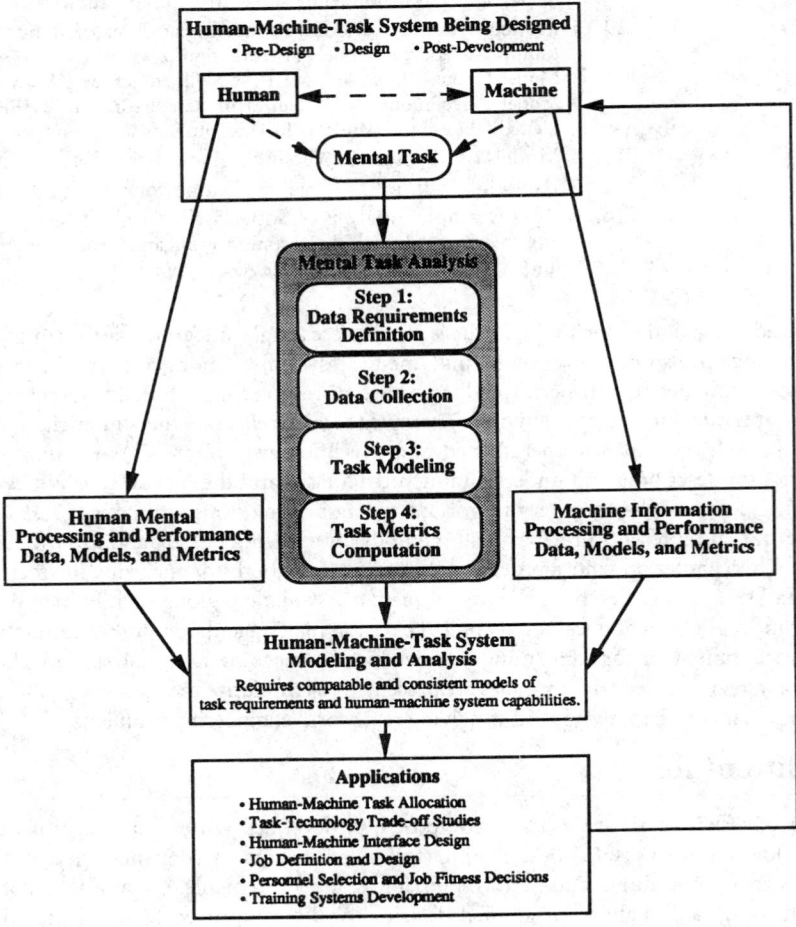

FIGURE 147.1   Mental task analysis is a four-step process that is used in combination with models of human and machine performance, as applicable, to make applied decisions.

are enhanced to the degree that these constructs provide for quantitative treatment. A framework for human-machine-task decision making (described below) combines the use of task decomposition and resource requirement modeling techniques with human performance and machine performance models.

147.2 Mental Task Analysis: Process and Methods

Step 1: Data Requirements Definition

In Step 1, the task data required for the analysis are identified and defined. There are many different dimensions and properties of tasks that can be analyzed. The functional scope of the human-machine-task system being analyzed, the point in the system design process at which the analysis is conducted, and the applied purpose of the analysis all contribute to determining what data are needed. In Fig. 147.1, the functional scope of the real-world, high-level mental task being performed by a human-machine system is represented generically. Identifying the task is necessary to bound the analysis. Task analysis can be applied to existing systems that perform well-defined tasks or to proposed systems for which tasks are in the process of being defined. At different points in the analysis, different decisions are applicable.

When task analysis is used for system design decisions, different types of task data can be collected as the fidelity of system prototypes progresses and operational systems become available. These differences are apparent by examining three points in the system engineering process at which task analysis is of particular utility.

Predesign. After the functional and performance requirements for a system have been established, an analysis of major functions, together with data about technology availability and human performance, can be used to (1) define and allocate tasks, (2) develop procedures to accomplish the tasks, and (3) identify the needed human-machine interfaces. Note that the description of a task depends on the technology assumed. For example, a writing task would be accomplished differently with paper and pencil, a manual typewriter, or a computer with word processing software.

Design Phase. During the design phase, task scenarios, prototypes, and simulations can be used to detail and refine the task procedures, task requirements, allocation decisions, and human-machine interface design.

Postdevelopment. Analyzing well-defined tasks performed by an operational system provides a detailed description of task procedures and resource requirements that can be used to improve task performance and the system design.

The applied purpose of the task analysis has the greatest impact on what type of data are needed. Applications vary greatly and include design and nondesign decisions that may or may not involve machines. Applications include, but are not limited to, those described below.

Human-Machine Task Allocation. Allocation of tasks represents a major systems engineering decision. Task analysis is used to identify task load and performance requirements and contributes to assessing workload. Workload assessment provides a basis for assigning task responsibilities to humans and machines such that performance requirements can be satisfied and workload levels are not excessively low or high. These assessments augment qualitative allocation strategies (e.g., Fitts' lists) in which tasks are assigned on judgments of the relative performance capacities of humans and machines on generic tasks. Allocating tasks requires that the resource demands associated with each lower-level task are assessed and that the human and machine resources available can be matched against these at comparable levels of analysis.

Task-Technology Tradeoffs. Task analyses may be performed for systems that have yet to be developed but for which functional and performance requirements have been defined. In these cases, the analysis will be based on the defined requirements combined with data on human performance capacities and available machine technology. These analyses can be used to assess the workload, technology, and performance tradeoffs expected with different human-machine system configurations.

Human-Machine Interface Design.   Mental task analysis provides not only a basis for allocating task responsibilities to humans and machines but also can be used to define, for example, the spatial aspects of display and control requirements for the interface between humans and machines.

Job Design.   The roles humans satisfy in complex systems and organizations (e.g., manager, operator, maintainer) are generally designed to include many mental tasks. By identifying and describing the mental skills and resources required for task performance, task analysis provides a basis for optimizing job performance in new and existing systems.

Personnel Selection and Job Fitness.   Mental task analysis yields a specification of information-processing resources (e.g., speed, accuracy) required for task performance. This specification can be used in combination with measurements of the available resources individuals possess. Assessing performance resource sufficiency provides a basis for selecting personnel and determining if injured, rehabilitated personnel are sufficiently recovered to safely return to work.

Training Systems Development.   Task analysis identifies and characterizes the skills, knowledge, and mental capabilities that are necessary or sufficient for task performance. More specifically, it can be used to characterize differences in these abilities and in task performance between experts and novices. These differences serve as a basis for designing effective personnel training systems.

These applications reduce to answering the following types of questions:

- What is the best way to structure the task procedures?
- Does a specific individual have the needed mental resources to perform the task?
- What knowledge or skills does an individual need to acquire to perform the task with a given level of technology?
- Can the task be modified to accommodate the special needs of individuals?

If machines are involved:

- What human and machine combinations are most capable of performing the task?
- How should human and machine components interact in performing the task?

To answer these applied questions, the following data must be defined and described:

- The demands imposed on mental capacities by the tasks (e.g., knowledge, required mental actions, speed and accuracy in performing actions).
- The mental capacities of humans in the system (e.g., knowledge, learning, processing speed, processing accuracy).

If machines are involved:

- The information-processing capacities of machine components (e.g., processing speed, algorithms, and data).
- The human-machine interaction demands imposed by the task.
- The human-machine interaction capacities of the humans in the system.
- The human-machine interaction capacities of applicable machines.

Step 2: Data Collection

Once the required task data are defined, they need to be collected. Table 147.1 lists four generic categories of techniques for acquiring data about mental tasks. The categories are not mutually

TABLE 147.1 Task Data-Acquisition Techniques

Technique	Data Collected	Requirements	Application Phase
Knowledge acquisition	Knowledge required to perform tasks	Task performers Interaction instruments, prototypes, and simulations (dependent on techniques used)	All
Protocol analysis	Procedures Strategies Knowledge	Task performers Task scenarios	Design Postdevelopment
Instrumented human-Interface	Overt human action (e.g., keys pressed)	Task performers Applicable hardware and software	Design Postdevelopment
Observation	Overt machine behaviors Overt human behaviors Situation state and state changes	Task performers Prototypes or developed systems Monitoring instruments	Design Postdevelopment

exclusive. For example, all techniques use some form of observation, and instrumented human-interface techniques and protocol analysis are used as knowledge-acquisition techniques. Each generic category is described in more detail below.

Knowledge-Acquisition Techniques. *Knowledge acquisition* refers to the process of eliciting from persons the knowledge they possess. This process was originally applied to elicit knowledge from experts in the development of knowledge-based systems. However, knowledge-acquisition techniques have been used more generally as a means of analyzing the cognitive components of tasks [Lehto et al., 1992]. Knowledge-acquisition methods include those listed below:

- Various interviewing techniques
- Automatic inductive methods that infer and specify knowledge
- Protocol analysis [Ericsson & Simon, 1984]
- Psychological scaling [Cooke & McDonald, 1988]
- Repertory grids from personal construct psychology theory [Boose, 1985]
- Observational techniques [Boy & Nuss, 1988]

Protocol Analysis. *Protocol analysis* refers to various techniques for collecting data in the form of verbal reports. In this methodology, persons generate thinking-aloud protocols of the unobservable (i.e., mental) activities they perform while accomplishing a task [Ericsson & Simon, 1984]. The verbal reports represent behavioral descriptions from which task strategies, requirements, procedures, and problem areas can be derived. Protocols provide data on the sequence in which tasks are performed and thus can be used to identify the strategies used by humans in accomplishing tasks that can be accomplished in multiple ways. There are several issues that need to be considered about the validity of using verbal reports as data and inferring thought processes from them. Ericsson and Simon [1984] address these concerns by demonstrating how verbal protocols are distinct from retrospective responses and classic introspection by trained observers and detailing the methods for collecting and analyzing protocols.

Instrumented Human-Interface Techniques. These techniques are used to passively and unobtrusively collect objective data on task performance and the procedures by instrumenting human-machine interfaces. These techniques are used to record the timing, sequences, and frequencies of explicit actions. For a computer system, examples are keystrokes, button pushes, and mouse movements. In an aircraft, examples are steering and throttle commands, as well as any other actions controlling any onboard systems. By themselves, the data associated with actions can be used to infer workload and to study the frequency of actions, their temporal relationships, and human error. Although these data are objective, they are restricted to overt responses and, by themselves, do not provide a basis for analyzing mental components. Modeling the mental task components involves correlating these action data with data about the situations and system behavior that elicited the actions and the changes in the situations and system state caused by the actions, i.e., knowledge of context is vital.

Observation Techniques. *Observation* is a generic term referring to many techniques that can use a wide range of instruments to monitor situations and the behavior of systems and task performers. Two types of observation are distinguished. In *direct* observation, a human observer is with the task performer as he or she performs the task. In *indirect* observation, a human observer monitors the task performer remotely with audio and visual monitoring systems. Indirect observation can be done as the task is being performed or after the fact by using a recording. Observation techniques may be unobtrusive or invasive, record subjective or objective data, and may be used in controlled testing or real-world environments.

Steps 3 and 4: Data Modeling and Metric Computation

Steps 3 and 4 are the actual analysis steps. In Step 3, the task data are modeled in accordance with a selected modeling method. This task model is employed in Step 4 to compute various task metrics that are useful in solving the applied problem. Table 147.2 lists seven major approaches for analyzing the mental components of tasks. Each has been shown to be useful in applied decision making, and each is described below. For an extended review of techniques, see Linton et al. [1989].

Task-Timeline Analysis. Timeline analysis organizes and relates low-level tasks on the basis of their time of onset, duration, and concurrences in the context of performing a high-level task. Any task taxonomy or decomposition model can be used to define the lower-level tasks that will be mapped to the high-level task timeline. Generally, the task-timeline mapping is constructed by decomposing a high-level task in terms of specific scenarios because different scenarios can have very different task and time requirements.

TABLE 147.2 Analytic Techniques for Modeling Tasks

Technique	Modeled Dimensions/Characteristics	Analysis
Task time-line analysis	Temporal onset, duration, and concurrences	Taskload estimates Task complexity
GOMS, NGOMSL, and keystroke-level analysis	Task and system knowledge required by task performers Overt low-level actions Procedures Temporal relationships	Task complexity Knowledge requirements Performance estimates from production rule simulation
Task-action grammar	Task and system knowledge required by task performers Observable low-level actions Action sequences	Task complexity Task consistency Knowledge requirements
Fleishman and Quaintance's cognitive task taxonomy	Identifies twenty-three cognitive abilities underlying task performance. Tasks are modeled in terms of required abilities.	Cognitive ability requirements Performance requirements
Rasmussen's cognitive task analysis	Generic activities, knowledge states, and dependencies in cognitive task performance	Knowledge requirements Task complexity
Knowledge-representation techniques	Task and system knowledge required by task performers	Knowledge requirements
Elemental resource model	Mental resources needed to perform tasks Resources are defined in terms of function and performance requirements	Functional requirements Performance requirements

This technique is useful for analyzing workload, allocating tasks, and determining human and system performance requirements. When the resource requirements for each lower-level task are mapped to the timeline, the result is a dynamic task-demand profile. Wickens [1984] discusses two limitations of timeline analysis. First, the technique often does not account for time-sharing capabilities in which the performance of multiple tasks can be accomplished efficiently when resource demands are low. Second, the technique is most effective when analyzing forced-pace activities. The more freedom the human has to schedule activities, the harder it is to construct a useful timeline.

GOMS and NGOMSL Analysis. GOMS, an acronym for goals, operators, methods, and selection rules [Card et al., 1983, 1986], is an analytic technique for modeling (1) the knowledge about a task and a machine that a task performer must possess and (2) the operations that a task agent must execute in order to accomplish the task using the machine. It is based on work by Newell and Simon [1972] in human problem solving. The model was extended by Kieras [1988] into NGOMSL (for *natural GOMS language*), which affords a more detailed analysis and specification of tasks. In both GOMS and NGOMSL goals represent what a human is trying to accomplish. Operators are elementary perceptual, cognitive, or motor acts that may be observable or unobservable. Methods are sequences of operations that accomplish a goal. Selection rules are criteria used to select one method to apply when many methods are available.

The NGOMSL analysis uses this model to predict quantitative measures of the complexity of the knowledge required to perform a task with a system. These measures include learning time, amount of transfer, and task execution time. To accomplish this, methods (i.e., procedural knowledge) are represented in the form of production rules. These are IF-THEN rules that describe knowledge in approximately equal-sized units. The number of rules needed to represent a task provides a measure of the complexity of that task. Time predictions are obtained by modeling the production rules in a computer program that simulates the tasks being analyzed.

The keystroke-level task model is an abbreviated application of the GOMS analysis [Card et al., 1983] that models only the overt actions (i.e., the observable operators and methods) taken by the task performer. In this way it does not require the inferences about mental processes required by the full GOMS approach. The model was developed with regard to a computer system and defines six operators: a keystroke or mouse button push, pointing using a mouse, moving the mouse, moving hands between the mouse and keyboard, mental preparation, and system response. Tasks are modeled by identifying the sequence of operators needed to perform the task.

Task-Action Grammar Analysis. Task-action grammar (TAG) [Payne & Green, 1986; Schiele & Green, 1990] is a formalism for modeling the knowledge required to perform simple tasks with a given system. Task knowledge is represented as sequences of simple acts. Similarities in the syntactic representation of simple tasks are used to derive higher-level schemas that apply across tasks possessing a family resemblance. The ability to derive schemas is used to assess the consistency of the tasks performed with a given user interface and has implications for ease of learning and overall usability. In similarity with NGOMSL, the number of grammatical rules and schemas provides a quantitative measure of task and interface complexity.

Rasmussen's Cognitive Task Analysis. Rasmussen [1986] and Rasmussen and Goodstein [1988] define a framework for cognitive task analysis that was derived from an analysis of human-machine interaction in process-control tasks. One element of this framework is a schematic structure for describing cognitive tasks and information requirements. The schematic structure includes a sequence of (1) information-processing activities, (2) states of knowledge resulting from performing the information-processing activities, and (3) conditions (related to the experience of the human performing the task) that allow the processing sequence to be shortened. This structure constitutes a generic processing task model into which specific task data can be mapped. The information processing activities are

- Detecting a need for action
- Observing relevant data
- Identifying the present system state
- Interpreting the present system state
- Evaluating possible consequences of this state with reference to a goal
- Defining a desired target state
- Formulating procedures to achieve the desired state
- Executing the actions required by the procedures

Fleishman and Quaintance's Cognitive Task Taxonomy.   *Task taxonomies* classify tasks on the basis of various characteristics and properties. As such, they can serve a useful purpose in modeling tasks. Tasks of the same taxonomic classification will have similar characteristics and similar requirements. This inference provides a basis for efficiently creating models for analyzed tasks. Fleishman and Quaintance [1984] provide an extensive review of taxonomies of human performance and identify four classifications: (1) behavior descriptions, (2) behavior requirements, (3) ability requirements, and (4) task characteristics. They further detail a taxonomy of human abilities that identifies 23 cognitive factors underlying task performance. These factors were derived from an analysis of empirical performance data collected from a large number of diversified tasks and individuals. The factors constitute a structure for modeling cognitive tasks. That is, these factors can be mapped onto specific tasks and thus specify the cognitive abilities needed to perform the task.

Knowledge-Representation Techniques.   *Knowledge representation* is a generic term that refers to several formalisms for modeling knowledge about tasks, systems, and the physical environment. Major representation schemes include production rules, frames, scripts, and cases. Production rules represent knowledge as a set of condition-consequence (i.e., IF-THEN) associations. Frames, scripts, and cases are different forms of schemas that represent knowledge as stereotypical chunks. Rules and scripts generally represent procedural knowledge, while frames and cases represent declarative knowledge. By formally representing data acquired from knowledge-acquisition techniques, a model of the procedural and declarative knowledge required to perform a task is created.

Elemental Resource Analysis of Tasks.   The *elemental resource model* (ERM) [Kondraske, 1995] defines human performance in terms of the performance and skill resources (capacities) that a human or system *possesses* and which can be brought to bear in performing tasks. Elemental resources are defined at a low-level such that many of them may be required to perform a high-level task. In addition, intermediate-level resources are defined to provide task-analysis targets at a less granular (i.e., higher hierarchical) level. In this model, a *resource* is defined as a paired construct consisting of a functional capability (e.g., visual word recognition) combined with a performance capability (e.g., recognition speed). Thus, even though the functional capability is the same, visual-word-recognition speed and visual-word-recognition accuracy are defined as two distinct resources because they model two distinct dimensions of performance. This model can be applied in task analysis by decomposing the mental components of a task in terms of the resources that a human or system performing them is *required* to possess.

147.3 Models of Human Mental Processing and Performance

The analysis of task data by themselves is of limited use in solving applied problems because task data address only one set of the system variables that need to be considered. For example, a task-timeline analysis provides a model from which a measure of task demand can be computed. However, this analysis does not indicate whether the taskload is acceptable or how it could be optimally distributed among humans and machines. Making these judgments requires consideration of human and machine capabilities. Similarly, using the NGOMSL and TAG models, a measure of task complexity can be computed, indicating that one task or procedure is more complex than another. However, these judgments are based solely on the number of task steps and the amount of information needed to perform each step and do not consider how difficult each step is for a human or machine to perform. Using these task models without incorporating human and machine models forces a general assumption that task difficulty is a linear function of complexity (modeled as more task steps or information requirements). Even with this assumption, the task model by itself provides no indication of the acceptability of the task complexity or expected human or machine performance. Both these judgments require consideration of human and machine processing and performance models.

Because of these issues, task analysis is used in combination with human and machine models to make applied decisions. Using task, human, and machine models in concert requires that the mental components being modeled are described in consistent and compatible terms. Further, the quality and precision of the decision will be enhanced to the degree that the task model describes requirements quantitatively, while the human and machine models describe their capabilities quantitatively.

Five models of human mental processes and performance are listed in Table 147.3 and discussed below. These were selected because they (1) describe concepts that are generally applicable to a wide range of information-processing tasks and (2) are engineering-oriented models for use on applied problems. Connectionist (e.g., neural network) models [Rumelhart & McClelland, 1986; Schneider & Detweiller, 1987] and the optimal control model [Barron & Kleinman, 1969], which represent major but different approaches to modeling human processing, are intentionally not included due to space constraints.

Multiple-Resource Model of Attention and W/INDEX

In psychology, resource models of attention attribute the capability to perform the mental components of tasks to the capacity of applicable and available processing resources, time-sharing skills,

TABLE 147.3 Models of Human Mental Processes and Performance

Model	Description	Modeled Components
Multiple resource model of attention and W/INDEX	Models attention as a collection of separable processing resources. W/INDEX is a computer model of workload that adopts the multiple resource construct and accounts for resource conflict from concurrent processing.	Identifies separable processing resources Time-sharing ability Automatic processing
Model human processor (HMP)	Models human information processing in terms of processing subsystems, memories, and performance parameters.	Performance is modeled by assigning time values to the model's parameters Perceptual, cognitive, motor processing subsystems Long-term and working memories
Keystroke-level performance model	Models the performance (i.e., time) estimated for executing each of six defined actions, from which overall estimated task completion times can be computed.	Performance is modeled by assigning time values to each of six modeled actions.
Skills, rules, and knowledge model	Models human information processing in terms of three levels of behavioral control: skill-based, rule-based, and knowledge-based.	Models the processes and requirements for each level of behavior. Can be used with quantitative models of human performance to estimate task time and errors.
Technique for human error-rate prediction (THERP)	Structured methodology for modeling human error and task completion in terms of probabilities.	Predicts human error and task completion probabilities using a human performance database and expert judgments
Elemental resource model of human and system performance (ERM)	Models human and system performance in terms of basic elements of performance and elemental resources.	Performance is modeled in terms of elemental units that can be combined to provide estimates of high-level task performance and completability.

and automatic processes. Attention is modeled as either a single processing resource or multiple, separable processing resources. In these models, the processing resource or resources afford a capacity to perform information-processing tasks (e.g., perception, cognition, and response selection) but have limited availability. The definition of resources here is different from that used in the ERM, which formally includes a specific performance dimension as part of the definition of a performance resource, which is distinguished from the system itself.

Norman and Bobrow [1975] adopted a single-resource model to examine the theoretical relationships between the application of the resource and performance on single and multiple tasks. For a given task, performance may be limited by insufficient processing resources (resource-limited) or by insufficient data (data-limited). In multitask situations, a human performing the tasks is assumed to be capable of controlling the allocation of a portion of the processing resource to each task. Different allocation strategies result in different relative performance on each task. The relationship between allocation strategies and relative performance is plotted on a graph called the *performance operating characteristic*. Automatic processing (e.g., skill-based) is assumed not to require processing resources.

The multiple-resource model of attention [Navon & Gopher, 1979; Wickens, 1980, 1984] extends and specifies the resource concept by identifying several separate processing resources that are exclusive to a subset of activities. Results of numerous dual-task studies were used to distinguish separable resources. The model identifies different resource structures for verbal and auditory modalities, spatial and verbal codes, manual and vocal responses, and between (1) selection and execution of responses and (2) perceptual and central processing stages.

W/INDEX, for *workload index* [North & Riley, 1989], is a computer model for predicting operator workload that uses the multiple-resource construct and accounts for time-sharing skills. A task-timeline combined with a design model that differentiates different interface channels (e.g., visual or auditory, manual or verbal) is used to compile an interface activity matrix. This matrix specifies, by subjective ratings, the amount of attention the task demands for each channel. A conflict matrix is generated with respect to each design channel that specifies a penalty resulting when the operator must attend simultaneously to multiple channels. The W/INDEX algorithm is then applied to these data, resulting in a workload profile.

The Model Human Processor (MHP)

MHP [Card et al., 1983, 1986] defines three interacting processing subsystems: perceptual, cognitive, and motor. The perceptual and cognitive subsystems include memories. Within each subsystem, processing parameters (e.g., perceptual processor, long-term memory, visual-image memory, and eye movements) and metrics (e.g., capacity, speed, and decay rate) are defined. Using data from numerous empirical studies, the MHP defines typical and range values for 19 parameters. To apply the model, processing parameters are associated with an analysis of the steps involved in accomplishing a task with a given system. Values for each parameter are assigned and summed, providing time estimates for task completion.

Skills, Rules, and Knowledge Model

Rasmussen [1983, 1986] developed a three-level model for describing qualitatively different modes of human information processing. *Skill-based processing* describes sensorimotor performance that is accomplished without conscious control. The behavior exhibited is smooth, automated, and integrated and only moderately based on feedback from the environment. Skill-based processes are generally simple automated behaviors, but they can be combined by higher-level conscious processes into long sequences to fit complex situations. *Rule-based processing* describes performance that is goal-directed and consciously controlled in a feed-forward manner from stored rules that have been developed from experience. Rule-based processing does not use feedback control. *Knowledge-based processing* is the highest level and applies to unfamiliar situations for which rules are available. Performance is goal-controlled and conscious. The goal and plans need to be explicitly developed, and reasoning is accomplished with knowledge (i.e., a mental model) of the system and environment.

This three-level model can be directly related to Rasmussen's framework for cognitive task analysis. Knowledge-based processing requires performing all the activities in the framework. Rule-based processing provides a means to bypass activities by applying rules that have been stored from familiarity. Skill-based processing provides a means to go directly from detection to execution. Thus the processing required is a function of the experience of the task performer and the nature of the task.

Technique for Human Error-Rate Prediction (THERP)

THERP [Swain & Guttmann, 1980] is a widely applied human reliability method [Meister, 1984] used to predict human error rates (i.e., probabilities) and the consequences of human errors. The method relies on conducting a task analysis. Estimates of the likelihood of human errors and the likelihood that errors will be undetected are assigned to tasks from available human performance databases and expert judgments. The consequences of uncorrected errors are estimated from models of the system. An event tree is used to track and assign conditional probabilities of error throughout a sequence of activities.

Elemental Resource Model (ERM) of Human Performance

ERM [Kondraske, 1995] was discussed briefly in the preceding section as a task-analysis technique. That discussion addressed how the ERM uses the same quantitative modeling construct (i.e., elemental performance resources) for task requirements and human capabilities. Major classes of resources include motor, environmental (i.e., sensing), central processing (i.e., perception and cognition), and skills (i.e., knowledge). Central processing and information (skill) resources are of interest in this chapter. When applied to humans or to machines (i.e., agents that perform tasks), the ERM describes the perceptual, cognitive, and knowledge resources available to the agent. If the agent has a deficiency in any of these elemental resources, a task requiring that resource cannot be completed by that agent. In this case, agents with sufficient resources need to be selected, agents with insufficient resources need to be trained, or the task goals or procedures need to be modified to accommodate the resources available to the agents targeted to perform the task.

147.4 Models of Machine Processing Capabilities

Table 147.4 describes models of machine processing and performance. These models vary greatly in scope and detail. They are presented to illustrate that quantitative analysis of performance resources using the ERM extends to machine capabilities. These models are not elaborated further.

147.5 A Human-Machine-Task Analytic Framework

Making applied decisions involves performing a combined human-machine-task analysis of available and required mental capacities. This analysis (1) requires that the mental components of tasks, the mental capabilities of humans, and the information processing capabilities of machines be modeled and analyzed in compatible and consistent terms and (2) is greatly enhanced if the terms are quantitative. From the techniques and models described above for task analysis and human and machine models, a methodology for a unified, quantitative human-machine-task analysis of mental components is described.

The approach first quantifies task requirements by combining techniques that produce detailed task-decomposition analyses of goals, actions, and required procedures (e.g., GOMS, NGOMSL, TAG, keystroke-level task model, or Rasmussen's cognitive framework) with timeline analysis, where

TABLE 147.4   Models of Machine Processes and Capabilities

Machine Model	Description	Components/Parameters
Process models	This refers to a category of models that describe the flow of information and the process performed on information through a system. It is useful for determining the consequences of failures in THERP.	Flow Transformations Dependencies Normal performance
Principles of operation models	In this category machines are modeled in terms of their operating principles. These are also useful for determining the consequences of failures needed to apply THERP.	Physical properties Mathematic formulas Mathematic relationships Logical relationships Normal range of performance
Human interaction models	In this category the characteristics of the machine side of the human-machine interface are modeled.	Physical properties Information content Information display format Performance metrics
Rasmussen's abstraction hierarchy	Developed for modeling process systems. Provides a task-independent description of systems at five levels.	Hierarchy levels that include process, operation, and interaction descriptions
ERM	Models machines in terms of the performance resources they possess. Resource definition is consistent across task, human, and machine domains.	Elemental information-processing performance resources available to the machine.

applicable, and the elementary resource analysis of tasks. The task-decomposition models are used to specify tasks at a level at which the elemental mental resources required to perform the tasks can be specified. The timeline provides a basis for specifying performance requirements. Other performance dimensions also should be used depending on the task.

The next step employs quantitative models of human performance and technology to reach an applied decision that best satisfies the required resources if sufficient resources are available. If sufficient resources are not available, additional performance and skill resources need to be obtained to complete the task, or the task requirements need to be reduced. Quantitative models of human performance include MHP, THERP, and the ERM. Using the MHP, the human processing parameters needed for each task operation are identified. The time values assigned to each parameter are used to compute task time estimates. This approach is limited to estimating performance in terms of time. THERP maps operations to the tasks included in human reliability databases to estimate human error probabilities. The ERM provides a framework for specifying performance and functional capacities at the resource level. It is the only model that (1) incorporates all required dimensions of performance and skills and (2) uses consistent modeling constructs across tasks, humans, and machines.

Using the approach outlined above establishes a basis for making applied decisions objectively. The task-analysis portion of this approach is illustrated by the example below.

147.6 Brief Example: Analysis of Supervisory Control Task

Supervisory control refers to the role a human plays in operating a semiautomatic process or system. Examples include control of large systems such as a nuclear power plant and specific instrumentation such as a robotic or assistive device. Performing supervisory control is a high-level task that predominantly consists of mental components. This task is used to generically illustrate the use of analytic techniques to model a task.

High-Level Goals

Two major modes of operation are distinguished [Wickens, 1984]. In one mode (normal), the system is behaving as expected. The primary role of the human controller is to monitor system activity and modify performance parameters in accordance with planned output goals. In the second mode (fault), the system is faulty. The goal of the human controller, in this case, is to detect and diagnose the fault and intervene to bring the process back into normal performance.

Task Decomposition and Procedures

Sheridan [1987] identifies 10 functions performed by a supervisory controller within these modes of operation. Rasmussen's cognitive task framework, which was developed with regard to process-control tasks, includes 8 functions applicable to the fault mode of operation. Figure 147.2 depicts these 8 generic functions as a top-level breakdown of the supervisory control task in fault mode. For this example, only selected tasks are decomposed to lower levels. At each level, the decomposition is not intended to be complete. Selected tasks at each level are intended to be illustrative and representative of increasingly specific and simple tasks. The arrows within each level provide procedural information. The goals of the lower-level tasks are defined by their titles (e.g., acquire data). Only the situation interpretation task is decomposed. In reference to Rasmussen's human information-processing model, the task is assumed to be knowledge-based. The lower-level tasks represent a hypothesis-testing strategy for knowledge-based diagnosis described by Rasmussen and Goodstein [1988]. However, other models of lower-level tasks could be used. Note that although a Rasmussen model is illustrated, the decomposition could be accomplished with other applicable models (e.g., GOMS).

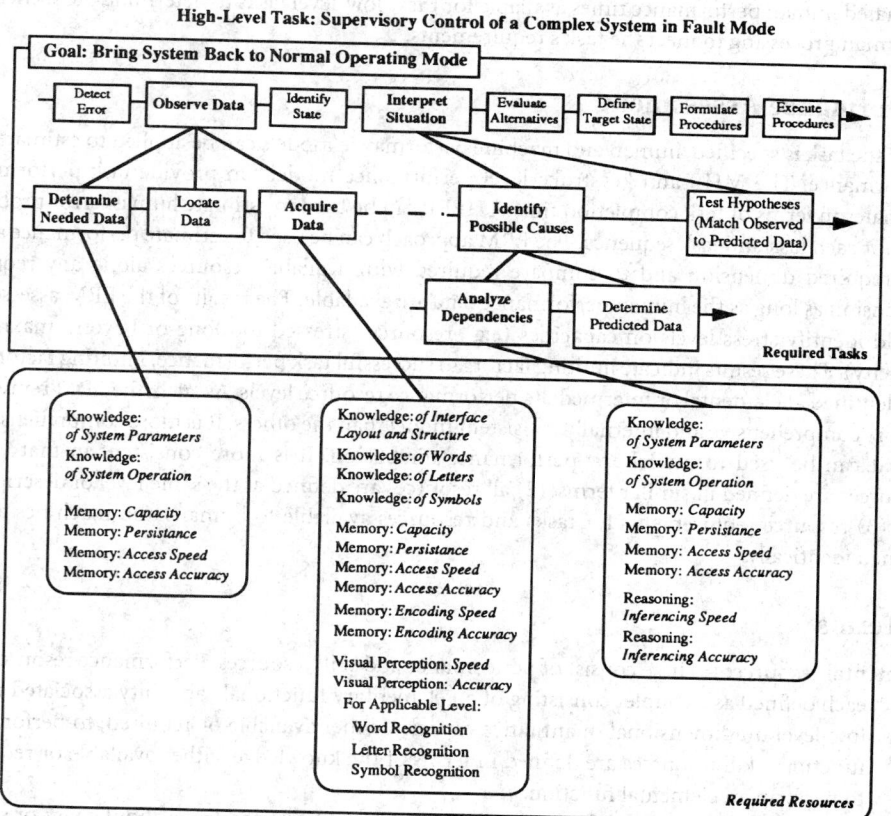

FIGURE 147.2 Selected task decomposition and resource requirements for a high-level supervisory control task.

Required Resources

Of the task-modeling techniques presented above, only Fleishman and Quaintance's cognitive abilities taxonomy and the ERM provide for explicit analysis of required resources. The approach defined by the ERM is illustrated in this example because it defines similar analyses for human and machine performance. As such, it is the only technique that models all three components of a human-machine-task system in the same way. For three of the lowest-level tasks, a set of elemental central processing resources is identified. Humans or machines responsible for performing each task are required to possess these resources to accomplish the task successfully. Four types of elemental mental resources are identified: knowledge, memory, perception, and reasoning. Resources are distinguished by their functional type and the performance dimension they specify. In the example, the performance dimensions are generically identified. In application, values should be assigned to these dimensions to the degree they are available or obtainable. Given time and cost constraints for the analysis, the ability to quantify all resources may not be practical. Task priorities can be used to selectively quantify resources, or the resource model can be used less rigorously as a guide to decision making if specific data are not available [Maxwell, 1995]. Once values are assigned, these required resources can be analyzed in concert with sets of available resources possessed by humans and machines. Available resources will have values that indicate a performance capability.

Although the MHP is a human processing and performance model, it can be adapted for use in a way analogous to the way the ERM is used in task analysis. The MHP would be applied as usual by identifying the processing parameters needed to accomplish each low-level task. However, instead of using the human performance values associated with these parameters, time values *required by the task* would be derived and assigned. These required times could then be compared with the estimated human performance times available for these low-level tasks to determine the sufficiency of human processing to meet the task's requirements.

Performance Assessment

After the task is specified, human and machine performance models can be applied to estimate task performance. The MHP and keystroke-level performance model can provide task performance estimates in terms of task completion time. THERP can be used to estimate human error probabilities for each task and task sequence. The ERM approach can be used to estimate performance along any required dimension and to compare required with available resources along any required dimension as long as the human performance data are available. The results of the ERM assessment would identify stress levels on capacities (e.g., resources stressed too long or beyond maximum capacity). These results indicate limiting factors to successful task performance. Limiting factors can be identified at elemental or intermediate performance resource levels. As such, the ERM represents a more comprehensive and internally consistent model than the others. It is more comprehensive in that it can be used to model any performance dimension. It is more consistent in that (1) all resources are defined in similar terms, (2) all resources are defined at the same level of description, and (3) resource requirements for tasks and resources available to humans and machines are all defined identically.

Defining Terms

Elemental resource: These consist of performance and skill resources. Performance resources are each defined as a couplet consisting of an elementary functional capability associated with a low-level unidimensional quantitative capacity, either available or required, to perform the function. Skill resources are defined in terms of the knowledge, either available or required, to perform an elemental function.

Knowledge acquisition: Any of several techniques for eliciting knowledge about a task or system from a human.

Mental components: The perceptual, cognitive, and knowledge-processing components of a task.

Mental tasks: Tasks that consist predominantly of mental components and, in ERM terms, require mental performance and skill resources to perform.

Protocol analysis: Protocols are verbal reports generated contemporaneously by a person accomplishing a task that describe the unobservable (mental) processes being performed.

Task: A goal-directed, procedural activity that is defined with regard to the resources (i.e., capabilities) that performing agents (i.e., humans or machines) must possess to accomplish the goal.

Task analysis: The process of (1) decomposing high-level tasks into their constituent, mutually exclusive, lower-level tasks; (2) describing intertask relationships and dependencies; and (3) defining each task's goals, procedures, and performance and skill requirements.

Task taxonomy: A classification of tasks in accordance with a defined method, strategy, or set of criteria.

Task timeline: A time-based profile of a high-level task that maps its lower-level tasks by time-of-onset, duration, and concurrences onto a timeline.

References

Bailey RW. 1989. Human Performance Engineering, 2d ed. Englewood Cliffs, NJ, Prentice-Hall.

Barron S, Kleinman DL. 1969. The human as an optimal controller and information processor. IEEE Trans Man-Machine Syst MMS-10:9.

Boose JH. 1985. A knowledge acquisition program for expert systems based on personal construct psychology. Int J Man-Machine Stud 23:495.

Boy G, Nuss N. 1988. Knowledge acquisition by observation: Application to intelligent tutoring systems. In Proceedings of the Second European Knowledge Acquisition Workshop (EKAW-88), pp 11.1–14.

Card SK, Moran TP, Newell A. 1983. The Psychology of Human-Computer Interaction. Hillsdale, NJ, Erlbaum.

Card SK, Moran TP, Newell A. 1986. The model human processor. In KR Boff, L Kaufman, JP Thomas (eds), Handbook of Perception and Human Performance, vol. II, pp 45-1–45-35. New York, Wiley.

Cooke NM, McDonald JE. 1988. The application of psychological scaling techniques to knowledge elicitation for knowledge-based systems. In JH Boose, BR Gaines (eds), Knowledge-Based Systems, vol 1: Knowledge Acquisition for Knowledge-Based Systems, pp 65–82. New York, Academic Press.

Ericsson KA, Simon HA. 1984. Protocol Analysis. Cambridge, Mass, MIT Press.

Fleishman EA, Quaintance MK. 1984. Taxonomies of Human Performance: The Description of Human Tasks. Orlando, Fla, Academic Press.

Kieras DE. 1988. Towards a practical GOMS model methodology for user interface design. In M Helander (ed), Handbook of Human-Computer Interaction, pp 135–157. New York, Elsevier Science Publishers.

Kondraske GV. 1995. A working model of human-system-task interfaces. In JD Bronzino, (ed), The Biomedical Engineering Handbook. Boca Raton, Fla, CRC Press.

Lehto MR, Boose J, Sharit J, Salvendy G. 1992. Knowledge acquisition. In G Salvendy (ed), Handbook of Industrial Engineering, 2d ed. New York, Wiley.

Linton PM, Plamondon BD, Dick AO, et al. 1989. Operator workload for military system acquisition. In GR McMillan et al. (eds), Applications of Human Performance Models to System Design, pp 21–46. New York, Plenum Press.

Maxwell KM. 1995. Human-computer interface design issues. In JD Bronzino (ed), The Biomedical Engineering Handbook pp 2263–2277. Boca Raton, Fla, CRC Press.

Meister D. 1984. Human reliability. In FA Muckler (ed), Human Factors Review, pp 13–54. Santa Monica, Calif, Human Factors and Ergonomics Society.

Navon D, Gopher D, 1979. On the economy of the human processing system. Psychol Rev 86.

Newell A, Simon H. 1972. Human Problem Solving. Englewood Cliffs, NJ, Prentice-Hall.

Norman D, Bobrow D. 1975. On data-limited and resource-limited processing. J Cogn Psychol 7:44.

North RA, Riley VA. 1989. W/INDEX: A predictive model of operator workload. In GR McMillan et al. (eds), Applications of Human Performance Models to System Design, pp 81–90. New York, Plenum Press.

Payne SJ, Green T. 1986. Task-action grammars: A model of mental representation of task languages. Human-Comput Interact 2:93.

Rasmussen J. 1983. Skills, rules, and knowledge: Signals, signs, and symbols and other distinctions in human performance models. IEEE Trans Syst Man Cybernet SMC-13:257.

Rasmussen J. 1986. Information Processing and Human-Machine Interaction. New York, North-Holland.

Rasmussen J, Goodstein LP. 1988. Information technology and work. In M Helander (ed), Handbook of Human-Computer Interaction, pp 175–201. New York, Elsevier Science Publishers.

Rumelhart DE, McClelland JL. 1986. Parallel Distributed Processing, Explorations in the Microstructure of Cognition, vol I: Foundations. Cambridge, Mass, MIT Press.

Schiele F, Green T. 1990. HCI formalisms and cognitive psychology: The case of task-action grammar. In M Harrison, H Thimbleby (eds), Formal Methods in Human-Computer Interaction, pp 9–62. Cambridge, UK, Cambridge University Press.

Schneider W, Detweiller M. 1987. A connectionist/control architecture for working memory. In GH Bower (ed), The Psychology of Learning and Motivation, vol 21, pp 53–119. Orlando, Fla, Academic Press.

Sheridan TB. 1987. Supervisory control. In G Salvendy (ed), Handbook of Human Factors, New York, Wiley.

Swain AD, Guttmann HE. 1980. Handbook of Human Reliability Analysis with Emphasis on Nuclear Power Plant Applications. Report no. NUREG/CR-1278, Nuclear Regulatory Commission, Washington.

Wickens CD. 1980. The structure of attentional resources. In R Nickerson, R Pew (eds), Attention and Performance VIII. Hillsdale, NJ, Erlbaum.

Wickens CD. 1984. Engineering Psychology and Human Performance. Columbus, Ohio, Charles E Merrill.

Further Information

Applications of Human Performance Models to System Design, edited by G.R. McMillan, D. Beevis, E. Salas, M.H. Strub, R. Sutton, and L. Van Breda, includes several chapters that describe task analysis and its relationship to human performance and workload analysis in the context of system design. *Behavioral Analysis and Measurement Methods,* by David Meister, provides a review and practical guide to applying task-analytic methods. The *Handbook of Perception and Human Performance,* Vols. I and II, edited by K. R. Boff, L. Kaufman, and J. P. Thomas, provides a broad range of human factors and ergonomic data related to perceptual and cognitive task performance. The *Handbook of Human Factors,* edited by G. Salvendy, reviews task analytic methods, workload and resource models of mental processing, and human performance models in detail. The *Handbook of Industrial Engineering,* edited by G. Salvendy, reviews task analytic techniques and human performance models in the context of industrial design applications. The journal *Human Factors,* published by the Human Factors and Ergonomics Society, is a source new task analytic techniques and application studies. *Cognitive Psychology and Information Processing,* by R. Lachman, J. L. Lachman, and E. C. Butterfield, presents an extensive discussion of the information-processing approach as applied to research in modern experimental and cognitive psychology.

148

Task Analysis and Decomposition: Physical Components

Sheik N. Imrhan
University of Texas at Arlington

A *task* can be viewed as a sequence of actions performed to accomplish one or more desired objectives. *Task analysis* and *decomposition* involve breaking down a task into identifiable elements or steps and analyzing them to determine the resources (human, equipment, and environmental) necessary for the accomplishment of the task. As indicated in earlier chapters, all human tasks require the interaction of mental and physical resources, but it is often convenient, for analytical purposes, to make a distinction between tasks that require predominantly physical resources of the person performing the tasks and tasks that require predominantly mental resources. These different types of tasks are often analyzed separately. Usually, in physical tasks, the mental requirements are described but are not analyzed as meticulously as the physical requirements. For example, a heavy-lifting task in industry requires musculoskeletal strength and endurance, decision making, and other resources, but the successful completion of such a task is limited by musculoskeletal strength. Decision-making and cognitive resources may be lightly tapped, and so the heavy-lifting task analysis will tend to focus only on those factors which modify the expression of musculoskeletal strength while keeping the other kinds of requirements at a descriptive level. The descriptions and analyses of manual materials handling tasks in Chaffin and Andersson [1991] and Ayoub and Mital [1991] exemplify this kind of focus. The degree with which a resource may be stressed depends on a number factors, among which are the resource availabilities (capacities) of the person performing the task compared with the task demands.

0-8493-8346-3/95/$0.00+$.50
© 1995 by CRC Press, Inc.

This chapter deals with the analysis and decomposition of only the physical aspects of tasks. It is assumed that nonphysical resources are either available in nonlimiting quantities or are not crucial to task accomplishment. While the compartmentalization of task characteristics tends to blur the natural connections among the various human performance resources, it is still the most pragmatic method available for task analysis.

Physical task analysis first achieved scientific respectability in the early part of this century from the work of the industrial engineer Fredrick Winslow Taylor [Taylor, 1911] and, shortly afterward, by Frank and Lillian Gilbreth [Gilbreth & Gilbreth, 1917]. Taylor and the Gilbreths showed how a task can be broken down into a number of identifiable, discrete steps that can be characterized by type of physical motions, energy expenditure, and time required to accomplish the task. By this method, they argued that many task steps, normally taken for granted, may contribute little or nothing to the accomplishment of the task and can therefore be eliminated. As a result of these kinds of analyses, Taylor and the Gilbreths were able to enhance productivity of individual workers on a scale that was considered unrealistic at that time. The basic approach to the highest level of physical task analysis today has evolved from the motion and time studies of Taylor and the Gilbreths (known as *taylorism*), both in the industrial and nonindustrial environments. The exact methods have become more sophisticated and refined, incorporating new technologies and knowledge accumulated about human-task interaction.

From its roots in time and motion studies, task analysis has become a very complex exercise. No longer is a single task considered in isolation, as shoveling was by Taylor and bricklaying by the Gilbreths. Today, different ideas in management and advanced data analytical methods have established the need for cohesion between physical tasks and (1) the more global processes, such as jobs and occupations encompassing them, and (2) the more detailed processes contained within them (the different types of subtasks and basic elements of performance). Campion and Medsker [1992] give examples of the first, and Kondraske [1995] gives examples of the second. This chapter describes physical task analysis, showing the approach for proceeding from higher-level tasks to lower-level ones. Figure 148.1 shows a summary of the overall approach.

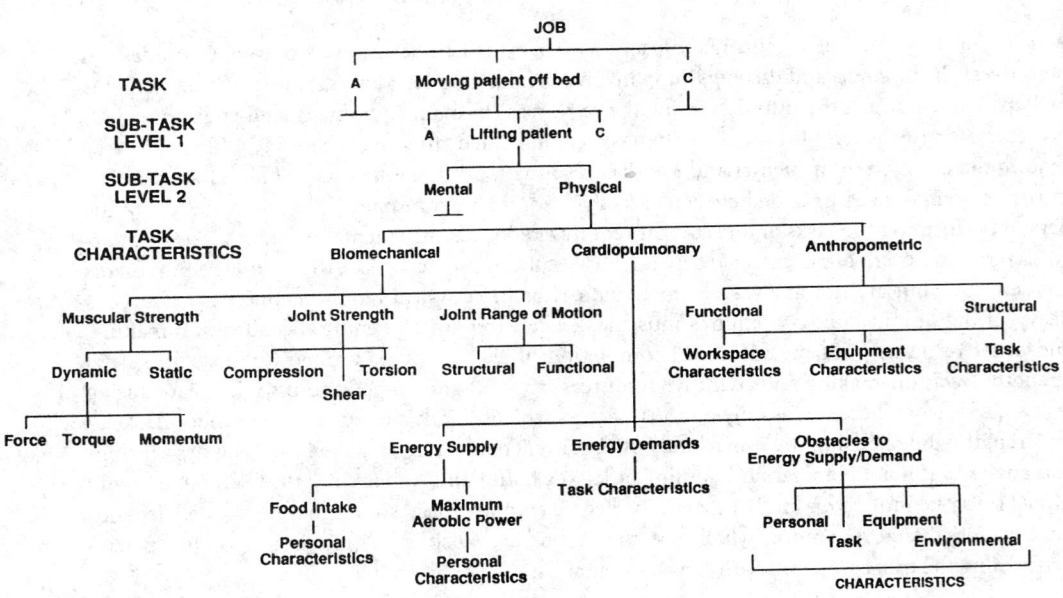

FIGURE 148.1 Diagram showing the concept of a hierarchical task analysis for physical tasks.

148.1 Fundamental Principles

The fundamental principle of physical task analysis is the establishment of the work relationships between the person(s) performing the task and the elements of the task under specified environmental and social conditions. The main driving forces are performance enhancement, protection from injuries and illnesses, and decision making. The order of importance depends on the particular context in which the task analysis is performed. Performance enhancement is a concern in all disciplines that deal with human performance, though the approaches and objectives may differ. In physical rehabilitation, for example, performance enhancement focuses on improving the performance of basic physical functions of the human body, such as handgrip, elbow flexion, etc., that have deteriorated from injury or illness. In athletics, it focuses on improving performance to the highest possible levels, such as the highest jump or the fastest 100-m run. In exercise and fitness, it aims at improving body functions to enhance health and quality of life. Finally, in the discipline of ergonomics, it aims at enhancing task performance as well as the health and safety of people at work.

Speed-Accuracy Principle

Performance enhancement and protection from injuries and illnesses are not necessarily mutually exclusive. In performance enhancement, the aim is to complete a task as accurately and quickly as possible. Both accuracy and speed are important in the work environment, especially in manufacturing, and are influenced by other factors. When lack of accuracy or precision leads to dire consequences, as in air traffic control jobs, then a decision to sacrifice speed is usually made. The basic concept of Fitt's law [1954] is relevant to these situations. It is difficult to find examples of cases where gross inaccuracy is tolerable, but in many cases more speed is required and less accuracy is tolerable, and a different point on the speed-accuracy continuum is selected. In the manufacturing environment, speed translates into productivity and accuracy into quality, and both determine profitability of the production enterprise. Speed and accuracy are rarely attainable at the highest levels simultaneously. In practice, a certain amount of one may be sacrificed for the other. Thus industrial engineers who set these tolerable limits talk of "optimum" speed instead of "fastest" speed and "optimum" quality instead of "perfect" quality. These facts must be borne in mind when analyzing physical tasks. A task analysis indicating that a person can increase his or her speed of performance should not necessarily imply that the task is being done inefficiently, because quality of performance may deteriorate with increased speed. This kind of flawed reasoning can occur when a variable is dealt with in isolation, without regard to its interaction with other variables.

Stress-Strain Concept

In task analysis, it is common practice to distinguish between *stress* and *strain*. However, these terms are sometimes used interchangeably and confusedly. In this chapter, *stress* refers to a condition that may lead to an adverse effect on the body, whereas *strain* refers to the effect of stress on the body. For example, working at a computer job in dim lighting often leads to headaches. The dim lighting is considered the stress, and the headache is the strain. The term *stressor* is also widely used as a synonym for stress. Strain has often been wrongly called stress. These terms must be clearly defined to determine which factors are causative ones (stresses) and which are consequences (strains). Stress is determined by task demands, while strain is determined by the amount of physical resources expended beyond some tolerable level, defined by the person's resource capacities. The stress-strain principle is pivotal to task analysis when one is concerned with errors, cumulative traumas, and injuries in the workplace and is applicable to task situations where task demands are likely to exceed human resource capacities.

Ayoub et al. [1987] developed a quantitative stress-strain index, called the *job severity index* (JSI), from empirical task analysis and epidemiologic data for manual materials handling tasks. This index computes the ratio of "job task physical demands to person physical capacities" from several interacting variables. The application of the JSI is also detailed in Ayoub and Mital [1991]. Also, Kondraske [1995] defines a quantitative measure of stress that can be applied to individual performances resources. In this measure, defined as the "ratio of resource utilization to resource availability," an adverse effect may be noted when the stress level exceeds a threshold, which may be different for different types of performance resources (e.g. strength, range of motion, etc.).

Cumulative Strains

The elimination of motions and other physical actions that do not contribute directly to task performance (tayloristic practice) has led to a concentration of work at specific localities in the body and to consequent overwork at those localities, but this concentration often leads to rapid consumption of the limited resources of the working systems. For example, VDT data entry is a highly repetitive task with very little variation; work is concentrated heavily on the hands (rapid finger motions for operating the keyboard) and in the neck and trunk (prolonged static muscular contraction), and this often leads to cumulative trauma disorders of the hands, wrists, neck, and shoulders. By comparison, traditional typists performed a variety of tasks in addition to using the keyboard—changing paper on the typewriter, filing documents, using the phone, etc.—and this helped to stem the depletion of physiologic resources caused by rapid finger work or sustained static muscular contractions in the neck and shoulders. Also, it is now recognized that some functions of the body that have not been considered "productive" under taylorism are highly stressed and may even be the limiting factors in task performance. In data processing, the muscles of the neck and back maintain prolonged static contractions that often result in muscular strains in the neck and back and limit work time. Traditional task analysis does not always consider this static muscular work as productive, even though it is absolutely necessary for steadying the arms (for keyboard and mouse use) and the head (for viewing the screen and documents). Likewise, work pauses, which have been considered wasteful, are now valued for their recuperative effects on the physical (and mental) working systems of the body. The increasing awareness of the causes of work-related cumulative trauma disorders will continue to influence the interpretation of data derived from task analyses.

148.2 Early Task-Analysis Methods

The history of physical task analysis does not show a trend toward the development of a single generalized model. The direction of physical task analysis has been influenced by taylorism and by specific efforts in the military that were later adapted to the industrial and other nonmilitary environments. A list of influential methods, to which readers are referred, is given below:

1. Time studies of Fredrick Winslow Taylor [Taylor, 1911]
2. Time and motion studies of Frank and Lillian Gilbreth [Gilbreth & Gilbreth, 1917]
3. Job analysis developed by the U.S. Department of Labor in the 1930s [Drury et al., 1987]
4. The U.S. Air Force "method for man-machine task analysis" developed by R. Miller [1953]
5. Singleton's methods [Singleton, 1974]
6. Hierarchical task analysis (HTA) developed by Annette and Duncan [1974]
7. Checklist of worker activities developed by E.J. McCormick and others for the U.S. Office of Naval Research [Drury et al., 1987]
8. Position analysis questionnaire [McCormick et al., 1969]
9. The AET method (*Arbeitswissenschaftliches Erhenbungsverfahen zur Tatigkeitsanalyse*, or ergonomic job analysis) developed by Rohmert and Landau [Drury et al., 1987]

148.3 Methods of Physical Task Analysis

Methods of physical task analysis vary widely. Drury and colleagues [1987] point out that "the variation of task analysis format is the result of different requirements placed on the task analysis." While this is a pragmatic method for short-term results, a more general approach for long-term solutions is needed. Such an approach should aim to proceed from higher- to lower-level tasks, as discussed in other chapters [Kondraske, 1995]. The following general sequence of analysis is recommended:

1. Description of the system within which the tasks reside
2. Identification of jobs (if relevant) within the system
3. Identification of the tasks
4. Identification of subtasks that can stand independently enough to be analyzed as separate entities
5. Determination of the specific starting point of each task
6. Determination of the specific stopping point of each task
7. Characterization of the task as discrete, continuous, or branching [Drury et al., 1987]
8. Determination of task resources (human, equipment, and environmental) required to perform the task (this step is the essence of *task description*)
9. Determination of other support systems (e.g., in work situations, managerial and supervisory help may be needed)
10. Determination of possible areas of person-task conflicts
11. Determination of possible consequences of conflicts, e.g. errors, slowing down of work rate, deterioration of quality of end product, decline in comfort, harm to health, and decline in safety

General Methods for Background Information

Many different techniques for gathering information in physical task analysis have evolved over the years, especially in the industrial and biomedical engineering environments. The quality and quantity of information that the techniques provide are limited by available equipment, and it seems that the quality and quantity of available equipment lag far behind the state of the art in technology. General data-gathering techniques, which are somewhat self-descriptive, include

- Direct observation (predominantly visual)
- Indirect observation (e.g., replay of videotape)
- Document review
- Questionnaire survey
- Personal interview

Specific Techniques

Specialized data-gathering techniques [Chaffin & Andersson, 1991; Niebel, 1993; Winter, 1990] that have evolved into powerful tools in the industrial environment and which can be used for task analysis in other situations include

- Methods analysis—determines the overall relationships among various operations, the workforce, and equipment
- Operations analysis—determines the details of specific operations
- Worker-equipment relationship study—determines the interaction between people and their equipment (cases of person-machine mismatches are determined here)
- Motion study—details the motions made by the various segments of the body while performing the task
- Time study—details the time taken to perform each motion element
- Micromotion study—detailed description of motion using mainly videotapes
- Kinematic analysis—measures or estimates various motion parameters for specified body segments, e.g. displacement, velocity, acceleration. (It involves micromotion studies. The data

are used for subsequent biomechanical analyses, e.g., to determine mechanical strain in the musculoskeletal system [Chaffin & Andersson, 1991])

- Kinetic analysis—measures or estimates forces produced by body segments and other biomechanical parameters (e.g., center of mass, moment of inertia, etc.) and physical parameters of objects (e.g., mass, dimension, etc.) (the data are used for subsequent biomechanical analyses)

Decomposition of Physical Tasks

Physical tasks can be viewed as exchanges of energy within a system consisting of the human, the task, the equipment, and the environment. In task analysis and decomposition, we look at the human on one side and the other system components on the other side and then determine the nature of the exchange. The energy is transmitted by muscular action. Tasks are hierarchical, however, and for systematic decomposition, it is useful to identify the various levels and proceed in a top-down sequence (see Fig. 148.1). The items in the various levels below are self-explanatory, but there is considerable content within each. Detailed descriptions of each is beyond the scope of this chapter, and readers should consult the references [Chaffin & Andersson, 1994; Corlett et al., 1979; Meister, 1985; Niebel, 1993; Singleton, 1974; Winter, 1990] for standard measurement procedures and analyses.

Level I.   Identifying general types of tasks according to levels of energy requirements:

- Tasks requiring great muscular forces
- Tasks requiring medium to low levels of muscular forces

Tasks requiring very low levels of muscular forces are not predominantly physical. Their successful accomplishment is strongly dependent on cognitive resources. The application of strong and weak muscular forces is not necessarily mutually exclusive. Such forces may be exerted simultaneously by different muscular systems or may even alternate within the same system. For example, a typing task may require strong back extensor forces while sitting bent forward (if the workstation is poorly designed) and weak finger flexion forces for activating the keyboard keys, and a weak index finger flexion may be required to activate a trigger on a hand drill while strong handgrip forces stabilize the drill.

Level II.   Identifying the crucial subsystems involved in the generation and transference of forces of varying intensities involved in tasks:

- Musculoskeletal—for great forces
- Cardiopulmonary—for medium to low forces
- General body posture
- Body motion
- Local segmental motion
- Local segmental configuration
- Anthropometry
- Workplace and equipment dimensions

The last three subsystems modify directly the expression of muscular force.

Level III.   Identifying environmental requirements and constraints. Environmental conditions influence performance and functional capacities in humans. They should therefore be measured or estimated in task analyses. Table 148.1 describes common environmental constraints.

Level IV.   Identifying body actions in relation to tasks. These actions can be decomposed into two major types:

TABLE 148.1 Environmental Factors in Task Analysis

Environmental factor	Constraint	Examples of effects
Illumination	Insufficient intensity	Errors
Heat	Excessive heat and humidity	Lowering of physiologic endurance
Cold	Excessive cold	Numbness of hands—inability to grasp handtool properly
Vibration	Excessive amplitude	Loss of grip and control of vibrating tool
Noise	Excessive intensity	Inability to coordinate job with coworkers
Body supporting surface	Slipperiness	Difficulty in balancing body
Space	Insufficient workspace	Inability to position body properly

1. Those which involve body motions. They are used for either changing body positions or moving objects.
2. Those which do not involve body motions. They are used for primarily for balancing and stabilizing the body for performing some task. Body posture is especially important here, especially when great muscular forces must exerted.

These actions are not mutually exclusive during task performance. One part of the body may move, while another part, involved in the task, may be still. For example, the fingers move rapidly when using a keyboard, but the rest of the hand is kept motionless while the fingers are moving. Tables 148.2 through 148.5 depict practical decompositions of these actions as well as those requiring muscular forces.

Level V.   Identifying anthropometric variables. Human anthropometry interacts with workplace and equipment dimensions. Tasks are performed better when the interaction defines a close "match" between human body size and task-related physical dimensions. Therefore, physical task analysis may be inadequate without measurements of the dimensions of people performing the task(s) and the corresponding dimensions of other aspects of the system of which the task is a part. This kind of matching is one of the basic thrusts in the discipline of ergonomics. Grandjean [1988] and Konz [1990] discuss these issues in many types of human-task environments, and Pheasant [1986] gives numerous body dimensions related to task design. Some important examples of human-system dimensions that must be considered during task analysis are shown in Table 148.6.

148.4 Factors Influencing the Conduct of Task Analysis

While task analysis traditionally focuses on what a person does and how he or she does it, other factors must be considered to complete the picture. In general, the characteristics of the task, the equipment used, and environmental conditions must all be accounted for. Human functional

TABLE 148.2 Representative Actions with Motions

Class of Action	Subclass	Purpose of Action	Examples
Whole body		Positioning body	Walking, crawling, running, jumping, climbing
		Transporting object	Lifting, lowering, carrying horizontally, pushing, pulling, rotating
Gross segmental	Arm movement	Applying forces to object	Reaching for object, twisting, turning, lifting, lowering, transporting horizontally, positioning, pressing down, pushing, pulling, rotating
	Leg movement	Applying forces	Rotating (e.g., foot pedal), pushing
	Trunk movement	Generating momentum	Sitting and bending forward, backward, and sideways to retrieve items on a table
Fine segmental	Finger movement	Applying forces	Turning, pushing, pulling, lifting

TABLE 148.3   Representative Actions without Motions

Class of Action	Subclass	Purpose of Action	Examples
Whole body		Balancing body	Standing while preparing meal in kitchen
		Supporting or stabilizing object	Bracing ladder while coworker climbs on it
Segmental	Arm		Holding food item with one hand while cutting it with other hand
	Leg	Supporting body	Forcing foot on ground while sitting in constrained posture

performance cannot be viewed in isolation because the person, the task, the equipment, and the environment form a system in which a change in one factor is likely to affect the way the person reacts to the others. For example, in dim lighting, a VDT operator may read from a document with marked flexion of the neck but with only slight flexion (which is optimal) when reading from the screen. Brighter ambient lighting may prevent sharp flexion when reading from documents but is likely to decrease contrast of characters on the screen. Screen character brightness must therefore be changed to maintain adequate reading performance to prevent sharp flexion of the neck again.

Knowing the Objectives of Task Analysis

Motion, speed, force, environment, and object (equipment) characteristics are common factors for consideration in task analysis. However, the reasons for performing a task are an equally important factor. Tasks that may involve the same equipment and which may seem identical may differ in their execution because of their objectives. Thus a person opening a jar in the battlefield in the midst of enemy fire to retrieve medicines will not perform that task in exactly the same way as a person at home opening a similar jar to retrieve sugar for sweetening coffee. In the former case, speed is more important, and both the type of grasp used and the manual forces exerted are likely to be markedly different from the latter case. Napier [1980] recognized this principle, in relation to gripping tasks,

TABLE 148.4   Representative Actions Requiring Forces, for Different Types of Forces

Class of Action	Subclass	Sub-subclass	Body-Object Contact	Purpose of Action	Examples
Whole body	Whole body	Dynamic	One hand, two hands, or other contact	Generate great forces that must be transmitted over small localized area or large area. The effort produces motion of whole body.	Lift, push, pull
		Static	One hand, two hands, or other contact	Generate great forces that must be transmitted over small localized area or large area. The effort does not produces motion.	Lift, push, pull
Segmental		Static	One hand, two hands, one foot, or two feet	Generate forces (over a wide range of magnitude) that must be transmitted over a relatively small localized area. The effort does not produce motion of the body segment.	Gripping with whole hand, pinching, pressing down, twisting, turning, pushing, pulling, or combinations
		Dynamic	One hand, two hands, one foot, or two feet	Generate great forces that must be transmitted over small localized area or large area. The effort produces motion of the body segment.	Pushing, pulling, pressing down,

TABLE 148.5   Posture While Performing Tasks

Class	Subclass	Purpose	Examples
Whole body	Standing, sitting, kneeling, lying down, other	Optimize body leverage; position body for making proper contact with object; other	Squatting at beginning of a heavy lift to prevent excessive strain in the lower back
Segmental	Arms, legs, trunk, hands, other	Optimize segment leverage; position segment for making proper contact with object	Placing elbow at about right angles while using wrench to prevent excessive shoulder and muscle efforts

when he wrote that the "nature of the intended activity influences the pattern of grip used on an object." These kinds of considerations in task analysis can influence the design of objects and other aids and the nature of education and training programs.

Levels of Effort

The level of required effort when performing similar tasks in different environments is not necessarily the same, and the interpretation of task-analysis data is influenced by these differences. Tasks in the workplace are designed so that human physical effort is minimized, whereas tasks in the competitive athletics environment are designed to tap the limits of human performance resources. There are other differences. An athlete paces himself or herself according to his or her own progress. He or she has greater freedom to stop performing a task should physical efforts become painful or uncomfortable. In the workplace, however, there is often little freedom to stop. Many workers often push themselves to the limits of their endurance in order to maintain (flawed) performance goals set by their employers. This is why cumulative strains are more prevalent in the workplace than in many other environments. These differences in performance levels may influence the way task analyses are performed among the different disciplines and the application of the data derived therefrom.

Criticality of Tasks

An inventory of task elements is necessary for describing the requirements of the task. It can tell us about the person, equipment, and environmental requirements for performing a job, but also we must be able to identify specific elements or factors that can prevent the successful completion of the task or that can lead to accidents and injuries. These critical elements are usually measured in detail or estimated and used for developing quantitative models for predicting success or failure in performance. One such widely researched element is the compression force on the L5/S1 disk in the human spine while performing heavy-lifting tasks [Chaffin & Andersson, 1984]. This force is being used by the National Institute of Occupational Safety and Health as a criterion for determining how safe a lifting activity is. If analysis of task-analysis data indicates that the safety limit (3400 N of compression) is exceeded, then work redesign, based on task-analysis information, must be implemented [National Technical Information Service, 1991; NIOSH, 1981].

TABLE 148.6   Human Anthropometry and System Dimensions

Body Dimensions	System Dimensions
Height, arm length, shoulder width	Workspace—height of shelf, depth of space under work table, circumference of escape hatch
Leg length, knee height	Equipment size—distance from seat reference point to foot pedal of machine, height from floor to dashboard of vehicle
Hand length, grip circumference	Handtool size—trigger length, handle circumference
Crotch height, arm length	Apparel size—leg length of pants, arm length of shirt
Face height, hand width	Personal protective equipment—height of respirator, width of glove

148.5 Measurement of Task Variables

During task analysis, variables must be measured for subsequent data summary and analysis. It is important to know not only what the inventory of task-related variables is but also to what degree the variables are related to or affect overall performance. The measurement of task-related variables allows for quantification of the overall system. For example, the NIOSH lifting equation [National Technical Information Service, 1991] shows how task variables such as the horizontal distance of the load from the body, the initial height of the load, the vertical height of lift, the frequency of lifting, the angular displacement of the load from the saggital plane during lifting, and the type of hand-handle coupling affect the maximal weight of the load that can be lifted safely by most people in a manual materials-handling task. The number of task-related variables measured should be adequate for describing the task and for representing it quantitatively. However, there are often constraints. These include

1. The number of variables that can be identified
2. The number of variables that can be measured at an acceptable level of reliability and accuracy
3. The availability of measurement instruments

Merely summarizing individual measurements seldom yields the desired information. Task performance is essentially a multivariable operation, and variables often must be combined by some quantitative method that can yield models representative of the performance of the task. Sometimes a variable cannot be measured directly but can be estimated from other measured variables. The estimated variable may then be used in a subsequent modeling process. A good example of this is the intraabdominal pressure achieved during heavy lifting. Though it can be predicted by a cumbersome process of swallowing a pressure-sensitive pill, it also can be estimated from the weights of the upper body and load lifted and other variables related to lifting posture. Its estimate can then be used to estimate the compressive force in the L5/S1 disk and the tension in the erector spinae muscles during lifting. Imrhan and Ayoub [1988] also show how estimated velocity and acceleration of elbow flexion and shoulder extension can be used, with other variables, to predict linear pulling strength.

Task-Related Variables

Variables that are usually measured during physical task analysis include

1. Those related to the physical characteristics of task objects or equipment:
   - Weight of load lifted, pushed, carried, etc.
   - Dimensions of load
   - Location of center of mass of load
2. Those related to the nature of the task:
   - The frequency of performance of a cycle of the task
   - The range of heights over which a load must be lifted
   - The speed of performance
   - The level of accuracy of performance
3. Those related to the capacities of various physical resources of the person
   - Muscular strength
   - Joint range of motion
   - Joint motion (velocity and acceleration)
   - Maximal aerobic power
   - Anthropometry
4. Those related to the environment:
   - Temperature
   - Illumination
   - Vibration

5. Those related to workplace design:
   - Amount of space available for the task
   - Geometric and spatial relationships among equipment
   - Furniture dimensions
6. Those related to anthropometry:
   - Length, breadth, depth, or circumference of a body segment
   - Mass and mass distribution of a body segment
   - Range of motion of a skeletal joint

Instruments for Gathering Task-Analysis Data

A great number of instruments are available for measuring variables derived from task analyses. The choice of instruments depends on the type of variables to be measured and the particular circumstances. In general, there should be instruments for recording the sequence of actions during task, e.g., videotape with playback feature, and for measuring kinematic, kinetic, and anthropometic variables [Chaffin & Andersson, 1994; Winter, 1990]. The main kinematic variables include displacement (of a body part), velocity, and acceleration. Kinetic variables include force and torque. Anthropometric variables include body segment length, depth, width, girth, segment center of mass, segment radius of gyration, segment moment of inertia, joint axis of rotation, and joint angle. Some variables are measured directly, e.g., acceleration (with accelerometers), force applied at a point of contact between the body and an object (with load cells), and body lengths (with anthropometers); some may be measured indirectly, e.g., joint angle (from a videotape image) and intraabdominal pressure (using swallowed pressure pill); and others may be estimated by mathematic computations from other measured variables, e.g., compressive force on the lumbosacral (L5/S1) disk in the lower back. Posture targeting, a method for recording and analyzing stressful postures in work sampling [Corlett et al., 1979], is becoming popular.

The measurements of performance capacities associated with human functions should conform to certain criteria. Details can be found in Brand and Crownshield [1981] and Chaffin [1982]. A general set of psychometric criteria is also discussed by Sanders and McCormick [1993]. It includes measurement accuracy, reliability, validity, sensitivity, and freedom from contamination. Meeting these criteria depends not only on the instruments used but also on the methods of analysis and the expertise of the analyst. It is almost impossible to satisfy these criteria perfectly, especially when the task is being performed in its natural environment (as opposed to a laboratory simulation). However, the analyst must always be aware of them and must be pragmatic in measuring task variables. Meister [1985] lists the following practical requirements for measurements: (1) objective, (2) quantitative, (3) unobtrusive, (4) easy to collect, (5) requiring no special data-collection techniques or instrumentation, and (6) of relatively low cost in terms of money and effort by the experimenter. However, these are not necessarily mutually exclusive.

148.6 Uses and Applications of Task Analysis

The uses of task-analysis information depend on the objectives of performing the task, which, in turn, depend on the environment in which the task is performed. Table 148.7 gives different the situations.

148.7 Future Developments

To date, there is no reliable quantitative model that can combine mental and physical resources. A general-purpose task-analysis method that uses active links between the various compartments of human functions would be an ideal method, but our lack of knowledge about the way in which many of these "compartments" communicate precludes the development of such a method. The present approach to compartmentalization seems to be the most pragmatic approach. It offers the analyst

TABLE 148.7   Uses and Applications of Task Analysis

Uses and Applications	Examples of Relevant Situations
Modeling human performance and determining decision-making strategies	A model showing the sequence of the various steps required to perform a task and the type of equipment needed at each step
Predicting human performance	Using a quantitative model to predict whether an elderly person has enough arm strength to lift a pot full of water from a cupboard onto a stove
Redesigning of the existing tasks or designing of new tasks	Eliminating an unnecessary step in the packaging of production items into cartons; designing a different package for a new item based on task analytic data gathered for a related item
Determining whether to use task performance aids	The analysis may show that most elderly persons do not possess enough strength to open many food jars and may, therefore, need a mechanical torqueing aid.
Personnel selection or placement	Matching personnel physical characteristics with task requirements can reveal which persons may be able to perform a task and, hence, be assigned to it.
Determining whether to use aids that enhance health or safety	Task analysis may show that too much dust always gets into the atmosphere when opening packages of a powered material and that workers should wear a respirator.
Determining educational and training procedures	Identification of difficult task steps or the need for using mechanical aids, together with knowledge of workers' skills, may indicate the level of education and training needed.
Allocating humans to machines and machines to humans	Matching people skills and capacities with the resource demands of machines
Determining emergency procedures	Task-analysis information may indicate which steps are likely to result in dangerous situations and, therefore, require contingency plans.

access to paths from a gross task or job to the myriad of basic task elements of performance. Unfortunately, actual systems and subsystems used in practice seem to be loosely defined and inconsistent, often with confusing metrics and terminologies for important variables. Moreover, available task-analysis models deal only with specific classes of application [Drury, 1987]. A general-purpose model is badly needed for handling different mental and physical resources at the same time, dealing with wide ranges in a variable, and bridging the gaps across disciplines. Such a model should help us to perform task analyses and manipulate the resulting data from environments ranging from the workplace, the home (activities of daily living), athletics, exercise and fitness, and rehabilitation. Such a model also can help to eliminate the present trend of performing task analyses that are either too specific to apply to different situations or not specific enough to answer general questions. Fleishman [1982] deals with this issue. At least one recent effort is active [Kondraske, 1995].

There is also a need for better quantification of performance. We need to know not only what kind of shifting in resources a person resorts to when one route to successful task accomplishment is blocked (e.g., insufficient strength for pressing down in a certain sitting posture) but also the quantity and direction of that shift. For example, we need to know not merely that a change in posture can increase manual strength for torqueing but also what the various postures can yield and what quantity of specific mental resources were involved in the change. The models today that answer the quantitative questions are mainly statistical regression ones, and they are limited by the number of variables and the number of levels of each variable that they can deal with.

Defining Terms

Anthropometry: The science that deals with the measure of body size, mass, shape, and inertial properties.

Cumulative trauma: The accumulation of repeated insults to body structures over a period of time (usually months or years) often leading to "cumulative trauma disorders."

Endurance: The maximum time for which a person can perform a task at a certain level under specified conditions without adverse effects on the body.

Fitts' law: The equation, derived by P. Fitts, showing the quantitative relationship between the time for a human (body segment) to move from one specific point to another (the target) as a function of distance of movement and width of the target.

Hierarchical task analysis: The analysis of a task by breaking it down to its basic components, starting from an overall or gross description (e.g., lifting a load manually) and moving down in a series of steps in sequence.

Job analysis: Any of a number of techniques for determining the characteristics of a job and the interactions among workers, equipment, and methods of performing the job.

Job Severity Index: An index indicating the injury potential of a lifting or lowering job. It is computed as the ratio of the physical demands of the job to the physical capacities of the worker.

Local segment: A specific body segment, usually the one in contact with an object required for performing a task or the one most active in the task.

Maximal aerobic power: The maximal rate at which a person's body can consume oxygen while breathing air at sea level.

Motion study: The analysis of a task or job by studying the motions of humans and equipment related to its component activities.

Person-task conflict: The situation in which task demands are beyond a person's capacities and the task is unlikely to be performed according to specifications by that person.

Position analysis questionnaire: A checklist for job analysis, developed by the Office of Naval Research in 1969, requiring the analyst to rate or assess a job from a list of 187 job elements.

Safety limit: The maximum stress (e.g., load to be lifted) that most workers can sustain, under specified job conditions, without adverse effects (injuries or cumulative strains) on their bodies.

Time study: The study of a task by timing its component activities.

Work pause: A short stoppage from work.

References

Ayoub MM, Bethea NJ, Deivanayagam S, et al. 1979. Determination and Modeling of Lifting Capacity. Final report, HEW (NIOSH), grant no. 5R01-OH-00545-02.

Ayoub MM, Mital A. 1991. Manual Materials Handling. London, Taylor and Francis.

Campion MA, Medsker GJ. 1992. Handbook of Industrial Engineering. New York, Wiley.

Chaffin DB, Andersson GD. 1991. Occupational Biomechanics. New York, Wiley.

Corlett EN, Madeley SJ, Manenica I. 1979. Postural targeting: A technique for recording work postures. Ergonomics 22(3):357.

Drury GD, Paramore B, Van Cott HP, et al. 1987. Task analysis. In J Salvendy (ed), Handbook of Human Factors, pp 371–399. New York, Wiley.

Fleishman EA. 1982. Systems for describing human tasks. Am Psychol 37(7):821.

Fitts P. 1954. The information capacity of the human motor system in controlling the amplitude of movement. J Exp Psychol 47:381.

Gilbreth FB, Gilbreth FM. 1917. Applied Motion Study. New York, Sturgis and Walton.

Grandjean E. 1988. Fitting the Task to the Man, 4th ed. New York, Taylor and Francis.

Imrhan SN, Ayoub MM. 1988. Predictive models of upper extremity rotary and linear pull strength. Hum Factors 30(1):83.

Kondraske GV. 1995. A working model for human system task interfaces. In JD Bronzino (ed), Handbook of Biomedical Engineering. Boca Raton, Fla, CRC Press.

Konz S. 1990. Work Design: Industrial Ergonomics. Worthington, Ohio, Publishing Horizon.

Meister D. 1985. Behavioral Analysis and Measurement Methods. New York, Wiley.

Napier JR. 1980. Hands. New York, Pantheon.

National Technical Information Service. 1991. Scientific Support Documentation for the Revised 1991 NIOSH Lifting Equation. PB91-226274, U.S. Department of Commerce, Springfield, Va.

Niebel BW. 1993. Motion and Time Study, 9th ed. Homewood, Ill, Richard D Irwin.

NIOSH. 1981. Work Practices Guide for Manual Lifting. NIOSH technical report no 81-122, US Department of Health and Human Services, National Institute of Occupational Safety and Health, Cincinnati, Ohio.

Pheasant S. 1986. Bodyspace. London, Taylor and Francis.

Singleton. 1974. Man-Machine Systems. London, Penguin.

Taylor FW. 1911. The Principles of Scientific Management. New York, Harper.

Winter DA. 1990. Biomechanics and Motor Control of Human Movement, 2d ed. New York, Wiley.

Further Information

For the design of equipment in human work environments where task analysis is employed, see *Human Factors Design Handbook,* by W. E. Woodson (McGraw-Hill, New York, 1981). For human anthropometric data that are useful to task analysis, see *NASA Reference Publication 1024: Anthropometric Source Book,* vol 1: *Anthropometry for Designers* (Webb Associates, Yellow Springs, Ohio, 1978).

149

Human–Computer Interface Design Issues

Kenneth J. Maxwell
Departure Technology

Purpose of This Chapter

This chapter provides the reader with a structure for addressing human-computer interface (HCI) design issues and making design decisions on the basis of quantitative human performance assessments. HCI design issues are structured in accordance with a dual-component, dual-task HCI architecture and are analyzed using a performance-based usability model. This framework is general and not bound to specific interaction paradigms or limited to assumptions about specific technologies. As such, it is anticipated to serve the needs for making HCI design decisions for any biomedical application. It is beyond the scope of this chapter to identify, categorize, describe, and analyze all HCI design issues. Further, it is not the intent of this chapter to review and compare the specific characteristics of different user-interface systems—there are several commonly used—or to review in detail the voluminous research that has been generated in recent years on HCI design. References for this information are provided in the Further Information section.

HCI Design Challenges

Since the introduction of personal computers approximately 20 years ago, the manner in which humans and computers interact has dramatically changed from computer-centered to user-centered. A major driver of change in HCI design has been a growing understanding of user needs and expectations and of the ways in which humans can use computers in accomplishing applied objectives. This increased user awareness in concert with emerging technology has dramatically expanded the uses and users of computers. This expansion is not simply limited to enabling users to do traditional tasks more effectively and efficiently. New technology can enable work to be done

0-8493-8346-3/95/$0.00+$.50

in ways that were previously impossible and with constructs that previously did not exist. For example, electronic documents can be merged, displayed, and stored in ways that do not have hard-copy analogues. New approaches to computer-based instructional media enable users to discover and experience concepts in ways that traditional multimedia education does not. The use of computer programs as aids for medical, legal, and business decision making has expanded individual's access to expertise.

That computers can be used to accomplish many different tasks and that both experienced and novice users need to use them present a complex challenge for HCI designers. The multitude of user needs creates a diverse set of functional and performance requirements that must be accommodated. Accommodating these diverse requirements is complicated by the advantages of designing user interfaces across applications and platforms using a standard set of generic interface devices and techniques. This approach reduces the need for task-specific devices and software and exploits user experience to reduce training requirements and improve interaction performance. However, it can cause the use of standard devices and techniques to be generalized and applied suboptimally. Another design goal, aimed at accommodating special user groups and individual user differences, pushes designs toward alternative devices and techniques that optimally meet specific requirements.

The emergence of new technologies combined with an awareness among software and hardware developers that users demand intuitive, direct, and easy-to-use interfaces promises to foster continued dramatic change in the near future. Reductions in size and integration of computers in specific instruments and personal devices have increased their portability and applied uses. The integration of digital information technology across information-gathering, communication, and information-delivery devices promises to dramatically change the model of a computer as a single device into a seamless assemblage of devices for assisting in all information-processing tasks. Not surprisingly, the design of human-computer interfaces has become a prominent area of applied research in human factors and ergonomics.

149.1 Fundamentals

User Tasks

When humans and computers interact, two tasks are performed: an interaction task and an application task. The *interaction task* consists of the activities that the user performs to use the computer. These activities include moving a mouse device, typing keyboard inputs, viewing displays, searching for and managing files, managing displays, setting preferences, and executing programs. The *application task* refers to the user's functional objectives. These objectives vary widely and include writing a report, performing a statistical analysis, finding information in a database, controlling a process, making a medical diagnosis, and monitoring/testing the health of a system. The application task is a higher-level task than the interaction task, and consequently, the design issues associated with each task are different. The HCI design process should include a task analysis. Methods for analyzing tasks are presented by Maxwell [1995] and Imrhan [1995] in this *Handbook*.

A Dual-Component, Dual-Task-Level HCI Architecture

HCIs have many components. For the purposes of this chapter, two major types of components are of interest: mental and physical. These components are distinguishable in terms of the performance and skill resources [Kondraske, 1995] that a user needs to perform interaction and application tasks with the computer. Using the mental-interface component requires perceptual-cognitive performance and information (skill) resources. Using the physical-interface component requires sensory-motor performance and skill resources. The relationship of these HCI components with the user are illustrated in Fig. 149.1.

For each HCI component, a design specification associated with each user task is defined. The application task-level design specifies the structure and level of objects, actions, and information

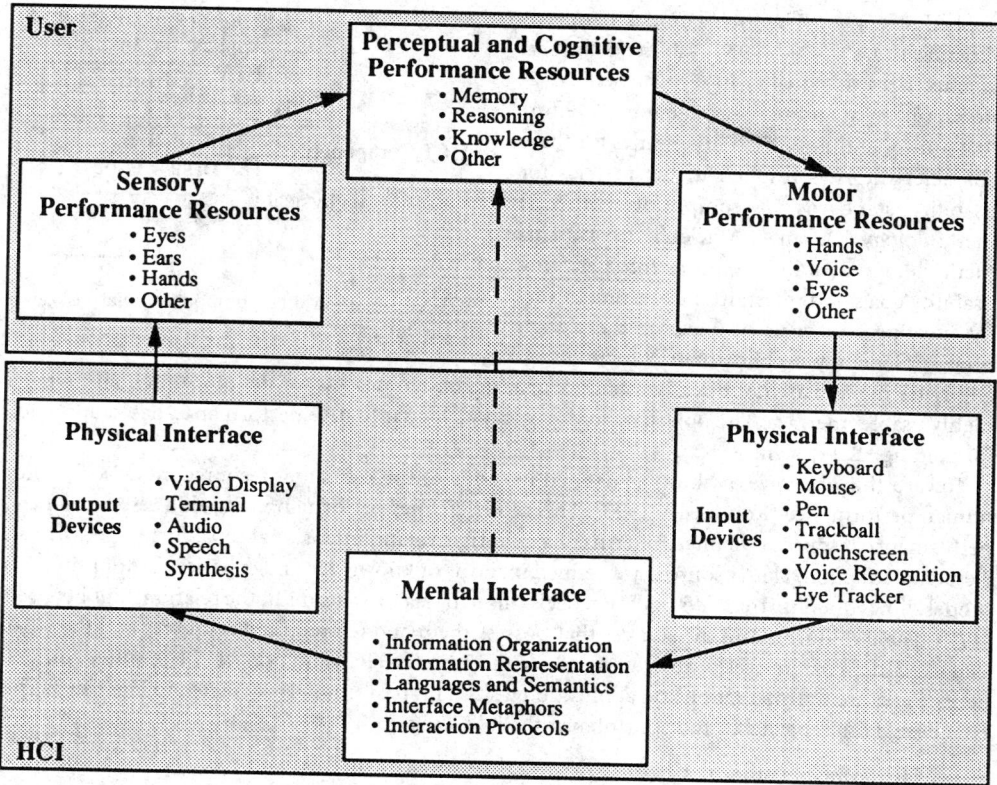

FIGURE 149.1 The mental and physical HCI components fit different user performance resources.

that the user needs, and the procedures, both mental and physical, that a user must take to accomplish applied objectives. The interaction-task-level design specifies the representation and behavior of HCI elements associated with the mental and physical HCI components. This framework, illustrated in Fig. 149.2, reflects the need to enable two user tasks requiring both mental and physical performance and skill resources and is used to structure the analysis of HCI design issues.

Successful HCI design decisions must be made on the basis of (1) knowledge about the user's performance and skill resources, (2) the performance and skill resource requirements of the application task, and (3) the performance capabilities of available HCI technologies. The design of the physical-interface component requires knowledge of the user's sensory-motor performance and skill resources and of the resources required to use various physical HCI devices with regard to the application tasks to be performed. Design of the mental-interface component requires knowledge of the user's perceptual-cognitive performance and skill resources and of the resources required to process information in different organizations and representations with regard to the application tasks to be performed.

149.2 A Quantitative Performance-Based Model of Usability

Achieving a highly usable interface is the HCI designer's primary goal. All HCI design issues are addressed on the basis of their impact on usability. The concept of *usability* is fundamental to the design of any human-system interface and is a major factor affecting the operational performance, availability, maintainability, and reliability of the overall system. Usability is a multidimensional quality that affords the user practical and convenient interaction with the computer for achieving applied objectives. The International Standards Organization's (ISO) [1993] usability definition characterizes this quality in terms of effectiveness, efficiency, and user satisfaction. An effort to define quantitative usability metrics for these characteristics has resulted in the metrics for usability standards in computing (MUSiC) methodology [Bevan & Macleod, 1994]. This methodology uses these metrics for specifying usability goals and intermittently testing to verify meeting the goals as part of the design process. Generally, usability metrics focus on us-

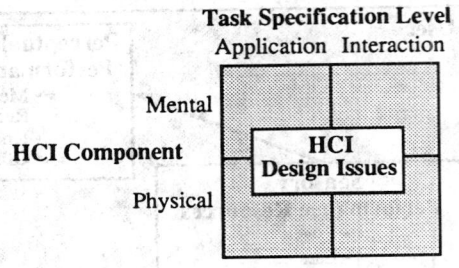

FIGURE 149.2   A dual-component, dual-task-level HCI architecture for design.

ability testing and are not directly useful early in the design process for defining and quantifying a highly usable interface. The objective here is to define a quantitative performance-based approach for guiding HCI design.

Toward this objective, usability is defined in terms of the elemental resource model (ERM) of human performance [Kondraske, 1995]. This model defines performance and skill resources. Each performance resource is defined in terms of a quantitative unidimensional capability to perform an elemental function. Skill resources are defined in terms of knowledge and experience. Adopting this model allows usability tradeoffs in design decisions to be stated in terms of the relationships between (1) available resources and the sources that possess them and (2) required resources and the sinks that expend them. Sources of resources include the user, the HCI, and non-HCI computer components. Sinks are the interaction and application tasks. This basic model is depicted in Fig. 149.3. The HCI designer has partial or full control over the following:

- HCI available resources
- Interaction-task required resources
- Application-task required resources
- Non-HCI computer components available resources

Why Use the ERM?

There are several methods for quantifying various aspects of HCI design. The GOMS (for goals, operators, methods, and selection rules) and keystroke-level models [Card et al., 1983, 1986], when used in combination with human performance models such as the model human processor, provide task performance estimates and knowledge requirements. The NGOMSL (for natural GOMS language) [Kieras, 1988] and TAG (task action grammer) [Payne & Green, 1986; Schiele & Green, 1990] models provide quantitative metrics for interaction task complexity and consistency. However, the ERM is the only model that (1) incorporates all required dimensions of performance and skills, (2) provides a performance-modeling capability at elementary and intermediate levels, and (3) uses

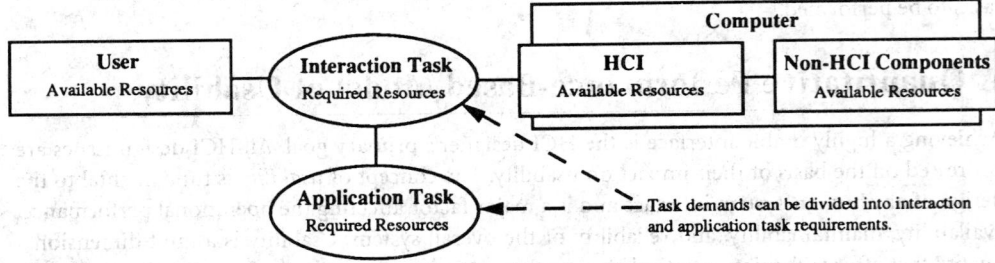

FIGURE 149.3   HCI design goal is to minimize interaction and application task demands.

consistent modeling constructs across tasks, humans, and computers. Also, the ERM can be used in a rigorous way when performance data are obtainable or less rigorously as a set of principles to guide designing for enhanced usability. Finally, the ERM provides a framework for specifying performance and functional capacities that can be used in concert with other models and techniques at various design levels. This is illustrated in the example at the end of this chapter.

Minimal and Optimal Usability

In terms of the ERM, an HCI design is minimally usable when all the user's performance and skill resources needed to accomplish the interaction and application tasks are exhausted in achieving the desired level of application task performance. This means that the user can perform the task using the computer only with maximal effort and expenditure of resources. Note that this definition of usability does not address the design of the HCI specifically. Rather, it addresses the relationship between the performance that can be obtained with a given HCI design and the effort a user needs to expend to achieve it. This means that different users will have different points at which an HCI for a given task will be minimally usable. The concept of optimal usability is more complex. An optimized design will allow users maximal use of their performance and skill resources, allocated at their discretion to the application task, to maximize their performance on the application task. Thus an optimal design minimizes the resources required to perform the interaction task and enhances the utility of the user's resources in performing the application task. This means that the HCI will support the user in performing the portion of the application task allocated to the user. This is accomplished through application-level design issues associated with the organization and level of objects, actions, and information.

Performance-Based Usability Design Decisions

The design strategy for achieving usability follows from an analysis of available and required performance and skill resources and application of HCI design principles that act to reduce resource task demand on users (Fig. 149.4). For example:

- Usability will increase as the resources required of the user to perform the interaction and application tasks decrease.

ERM-Based Approach to Usability Design Decisions

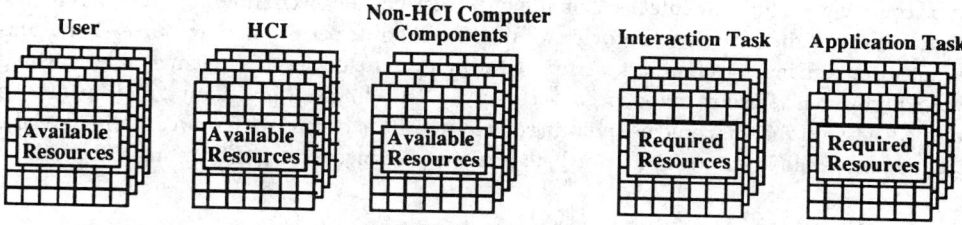

User	HCI	Non-HCI Computer Components	Interaction Task	Application Task
Available Resources	Available Resources	Available Resources	Required Resources	Required Resources

HCI Design Goal:
Use HCI performance resources to minimize performance and skill resource task demands on the user.

HCI Design Approach:
- Apply design principles for reducing the user's performance and skill resource requirements
  - Naturalness and Familiarity of Interaction
  - Simplicity of Interaction
  - Robustness of Design
  - Consistency of Design
  - Accommodate Different User Capabilities
- Apply ERM quantitative analysis techniques

FIGURE 149.4 A quantitative human-performance-based approach to HCI design.

- Usability will increase as the HCI available resources increase (provided the design principles for reducing resource demands are applied).

A detailed discussion regarding performance resources is presented by Kondraske [1995]. Different resource sources and tasks impose different design objectives. One performance-based design objective is to apply HCI resources to minimize the number of performance resources the user needs to perform the interaction task. This approach permits the user to allocate more resources to performing the application task. Achieving this objective includes (1) incorporating appropriate input and display devices to meet the user's sensory-motor resources and (2) use of organizations, representations, and levels of object, actions, and information that fit within the limits of the user's knowledge and perceptual-cognitive resources.

A second performance-based design objective is to apply HCI resources to optimize the resources the user needs to perform the application task. Many of the objects, actions, and information with which the user interacts are application-task-specific. Organization and representation decisions should be based on these task-specific requirements. For example, if the application task involves drawing, the user needs general software and hardware drawing tools and devices. This consideration can be used to illustrate the relationship between application and interaction task-level design issues. A software drawing package can provide different levels of drawing elements (e.g., having a tool to directly draw n-sided polygons versus a line-drawing tool from which a polygon can be drawn segment by segment). Assume that the HCI provides a palette of drawing tools and that it includes primitive and complex tools. The user can draw an n-sided polygon using the line tool or using the polygon tool. Both tools are included in the palette. The issue here is how the decision to develop the polygon tool and include it in the product is made. The decision must be based on the user's application task need to draw polygons. This need is established by an analysis of the application task. The decision to include the polygon tool is an HCI decision at the application-task level. Once this applied need is established, the HCI design needs of how to represent, where to locate, and how to operate the tool are addressed. These design needs are HCI design issues at the interaction-task level.

The decisions at these two task levels can be further used to illustrate interactions in assessing performance-based usability. A decision to include the polygon tool made on the basis of the application-task requirements will increase usability at the application-task level in that the user will need to use fewer sensory-motor resources to create a polygon. However, the inclusion of the polygon tool complicates the interaction-task level in that more items are added to the tool palette and that procedures need to be defined for drawing it. As will be discussed, these complications are addressed by applying HCI design principles that reduce performance and skill resource demands.

Because the ERM defines performance resources at an elemental level, performance-based design can be conducted at the elemental level or at higher intermediate levels. Intermediate levels reduce the granularity of the analysis and provide for use of composite performance resources. For example, analyzing a menu-selection task performed with a mouse device at an elemental level would involve performance resources for speed, accuracy, and steadiness of positioning movements. An intermediate-level analysis could use pointing as a composite performance resource. At this level the selection task would involve two intermediate-level performance resources: pointing and clicking.

Design Principles for Reducing Task Resource Demands

Optimizing usability is accomplished through the application of resource-demand-reducing HCI design principles. As stated earlier, the ERM can be applied rigorously or as a set of guiding principles. Rigorous application requires an analysis of available and required performance and skill resources and performance data associated with each resource. These data are usually not obtainable for all resources. Less rigorous application uses the principles of resource economics, resource stress, and analyses of the performance and skill resources involved in tasks to guide the design toward lower resource demands on the user. Five major design principles that act to reduce task demands on performance and skill resources are described. Each principle can be applied to all HCI architectural design categories.

Naturalness and Familiarity of Interaction.   Usability will be improved to the degree that the interaction is natural and familiar. Naturalness and familiarity reduce training requirements and increase available resources (e.g., available knowledge, sensory-motor performance). For physical components at a task level, this means that the user's sensory and effector modalities are properly matched to the required interactions. For example, keyboards used for typing, keypads for data entry, and mouse, pen, or touch-screen devices for pointing. For physical components at a feature level, this means that (1) user anthropometrics are employed in defining workstation and component configurations and dimensions and (2) that the physical characteristics of controls and displays (e.g., operating force, sensitivity, brightness, intensity, and size of displayed information) are congruous with the users and physical capabilities. For mental components at a task-level, natural interaction means that the HCI models the user's tasks in accordance with the user's knowledge and experience. For mental components at a feature level, natural interaction means that the user's perceptual and cognitive capabilities and limitations are employed in defining HCI features (e.g., icons, names, screen layouts, and the behavior of window controls such as scroll bars). *Direct manipulation* interaction techniques (e.g., drag and drop) are a form of natural interaction in that they create a software mechanism with a physical analogy.

Simplicity of Interaction.   Simplicity applies across a wide variety of design issues and must be incorporated in every architectural category. Applying this principle reduces training requirements, memory demands, perceptual demands, and the cognitive demands for inferencing. For the physical interface component, applying this principle reduces the number of physical steps needed to select and invoke actions and reduces movement precision requirements.

Consistency of Design.   Consistency reduces training requirements and memory requirements and promotes skill development. Consistency applies across a wide variety of design issues and must be incorporated in every architectural category. Examples include object, action, and information organizations, task flows, representations for objects and actions, and procedures. TAG [Payne & Green, 1986; Schiele & Green, 1990] provides a formal technique for analyzing consistency.

Robustness of Design.   *Robustness* refers to the ability of the design to tolerate user error and to span the functional requirements of the user. Error tolerance reduces resources needed to recover from errors and reduces initial accuracy requirements, allowing the user to increase operating speed. Users may commit errors because of a lack of knowledge. In this case, the user may be exploring the system to learn it. These are not errors. But this type of behavior should be expected, and the design should allow the user to do this exploration and to recover from anything he or she may do. Users may commit errors because of a misunderstanding or negative transfer from other systems. Thus a user may infer that a menu item will elicit a given behavior because it does so on another system that he or she has used. Or the user may feel that he or she understands what a given menu item or icon means and be wrong. Users may commit errors through unintentional commands. For example, a user may inadvertently click a wrong button, hit a wrong key, or select a wrong item from a menu. Ensuring adequate functional coverage reduces the functional demands on the user.

User Capabilities Accommodation.   In resource terms, applying this design principle increases the fit between an individual user's available mental and physical resources and those required by the interaction and application tasks. There are two major dimensions on which users vary: experience and capability.

Along the experience dimension users vary between experts and novices on either the interaction or application task. Thus a user could be very experienced with the applied task but not with doing that task on a computer. Similarly, a user may be very used to using computers but not skilled in the applied task. Novice users will (1) need more guidance and feedback, (2) require more structure to the task, (3) rely more on memory-aiding design features (e.g., menus), and (4) benefit more from on-line help facilities than expert users. Expert users (1) will want more flexibility in task control, (2) will want shortcut methods to do high-level actions, (3) will rely more on recall rather than memory aids, and (4) will benefit more from the use of preferences and tailored configurations than novice users [Brown, 1988; Galitz, 1993].

Along the capacity dimension users vary between healthy and impaired. In the ERM, impairments are not defined differently from any other performance or skill differences among users. All differences are defined in terms of the amount of specific performance resources available to an individual. Impaired users will vary greatly in capacity and experience. Only through an analysis of resources demanded by the task and resources available to the user can an adequate design for an impaired user be accomplished successfully.

149.3 Selected HCI Design Issues, Goals, and Resource Requirements

Selected design issues in each architectural category are identified. Design goals for enhancing usability related to each issue are described. These goals are derived by applying the resource-demand-reducing design principles described earlier. The human performance resources associated with each issue are also identified. Thus for each issue the reader is presented with the areas of a human's performance resource profile that need to be assessed to achieve a design that enhances usability. For illustrative purposes, an example design process is presented using issues related to the design of a menu system.

Mental Interface: Application-Task-Level Specification

Design issues in this category are concerned with the organization and level of objects, actions, and information that users need to perform the interaction and applied tasks. Design decisions must consider the perceptual-cognitive performance and skill resources possessed by users. Design goals are to minimize the resources required to accomplish the applied task. Table 149.1 lists selected design issues of this type, along with the design goals and performance and skill resources involved in making design decisions for each issue.

Mental Interface: Interaction-Task-Level Specification

Design issues in this category are concerned with the representation and behavior of HCI elements. Design decisions must consider the perceptual-cognitive performance and skill resources possessed by users. Design goals are to minimize the resources required to accomplish the interaction task. Table 149.2 lists selected design issues of this type, along with the design goals and performance and skill resources involved in making design decisions for each issue.

Physical Interface: Application-Task-Level Specification

Design issues in this category are concerned with (1) the performance and structural characteristics of major physical elements of the workstation and (2) the physical actions required to perform tasks. Design decisions must consider the sensory-motor performance and skill resources possessed by users. Design goals are to minimize the resources required to accomplish the applied task. Table 149.3 lists selected design issues of this type, along with the design goals and performance and skill resources involved in making design decisions for each issue.

TABLE 149.1. Selected Mental-Interface/Application-Task-Level Design Issues

Design Issue	Selected Design Goals (Based on Design Principles)	Selected Performance and Skill Resources Required of the User
Application-task-level interaction structure	Match interaction structure to user's cognitive model of task Minimize the number of steps needed to complete tasks Consistent task syntax Consistent task semantics	User's knowledge of the application task structure
Design of dialogs and query languages	Structure syntax in accordance with natural language Define semantics in accordance with task usage Minimize number of dialogs and queries required Allow for flexible usage Consistency of usage	User's knowledge of the application task structure User's knowledge of application task terminology Dialog or query entry speed Dialog or query entry accuracy
Use of an application-task-level metaphor	Leverage user's prior experience Increase intuitiveness of application-task-level interaction	User's knowledge of the application task structure
Menu structure design	Optimize menu navigation Structure menus in accordance with user's knowledge of task Structure menus in accordance with user's associations among menu set.	User's knowledge of the application task structure

Physical Interface: Interaction-Task-Level Specification

Design issues at the feature level of the physical HCI are concerned with the physical performance parameters associated with using controls and displays. Design decisions must consider the sensory-motor performance and skill resources possessed by users. Design goals are to minimize the resources required to accomplish the interaction task. Table 149.4 lists selected design issues of this type, along with the design goals and performance and skill resources involved in making design decisions for each issue.

TABLE 149.2 Selected Mental-Interface/Interaction-Task-Level Design Issues

Design Issue	Selected Design Goals (Based on Design Principles)	Selected Performance and Skill Resources Required of the User
Interaction-level icon, symbol, and label selection	Select based on strength of association to represented objects and commands Establish consistent usage, i.e., identical icons, symbols, and labels should be used for the same objects and actions.	User's knowledge of computer objects and actions Perceptual accuracy Perceptual speed
Color selection	Consistency with cultural usage	User's existing color associations to application task and HCI objects and actions
Screen and window layout	Consistency of within-screen activity flow with other learned activities (e.g., left to right flow of activity for English speaking users)	Memory speed Memory accuracy Perceptual speed Perceptual accuracy
Number of controls and displays	Optimize Use integrated displays where applicable	Memory speed Memory accuracy Perceptual speed Perceptual accuracy

TABLE 149.3 Selected Physical-Interface/Application-Task-Level Design Issues

Design Issue	Selected Design Goals (Based on Design Principles)	Selected Performance and Skill Resources Required of the User

Input device selection	Account for user familiarity
	Account for naturalness for task (e.g., keyboard for text entry, number pad for data entry, pen, mouse, or touch screen for pointing)
		For manual and ocular controls:
		  Movement speed
		  Movement accuracy
		  Movement steadiness
		  Movement extension

Display selection	The greater the amount of information that has to be displayed simultaneously, the greater the size and resolution requirement. Greater size increases the number of required head and eye movements. Optimize size, resolution, and color needs.	Visual acuity Color sensitivity Visual span angle

Action procedure specification	Minimize the required number of keystrokes, mouse movements, hand movements, head and eye movements
	Use of direct manipulation techniques (e.g., drag and drop interaction, scroll bars, mouse controls for moving and resizing windows)
		For manual and ocular controls:
		  Movement speed
		  Movement accuracy
		  Movement steadiness
		  Movement extension

Use of multiple input and control methods (e.g., keyboard and mouse)	Provide the user with more than one action procedure for doing tasks	For manual and ocular controls:
		  Movement speed
		  Movement accuracy
		  Movement steadiness
		  Movement extension

Brief Example Using Menu System Design

This example identifies the design issues associated with each HCI architectural category and traces the decision process for the design of a menu system. The issues and process are illustrated in Fig. 149.5. The design process begins with the results of an analysis of the application task, the performance and skill resources of the user, and available HCI technology. The analysis of the user will account for user knowledge of the application task, familiarity with computer interfaces, and user performance capabilities. The application-task analysis will provide information about the number of tasks, sequences of required actions to perform tasks, the semantic associations among

TABLE 149.4 Selected Physical-Interface/Interaction-Task-Level Design Issues

Design Issue	Selected Design Goals (Based on Design Principles)	Selected Performance and Skill Resources Required of the User
Keyboard and button devices:		

Size of keys	Greater size will reduce the required accuracy and steadiness of movements
	Smaller size will reduce the required movement length and duration
	Optimize size across these considerations
		For wrist, hand, and fingers:
		  Movement accuracy
		  Movement steadiness
		  Movement speed
		  Movement extension

Force required to press keys	Greater force requires more strength Too little force will not provide adequate feedback to the user. Optimize force across these considerations	Finger strength Proprioceptive feedback sensitivity
Use of audio/visual feedback when key is pressed	User requires feedback to know that the key press has been acknowledged.	Audio/visual acuity Audio/visual sensitivity
Visual display devices:		
Font	Low confusion rate	Visual acuity Visual sensitivity
Brightness	Optimal viewing	

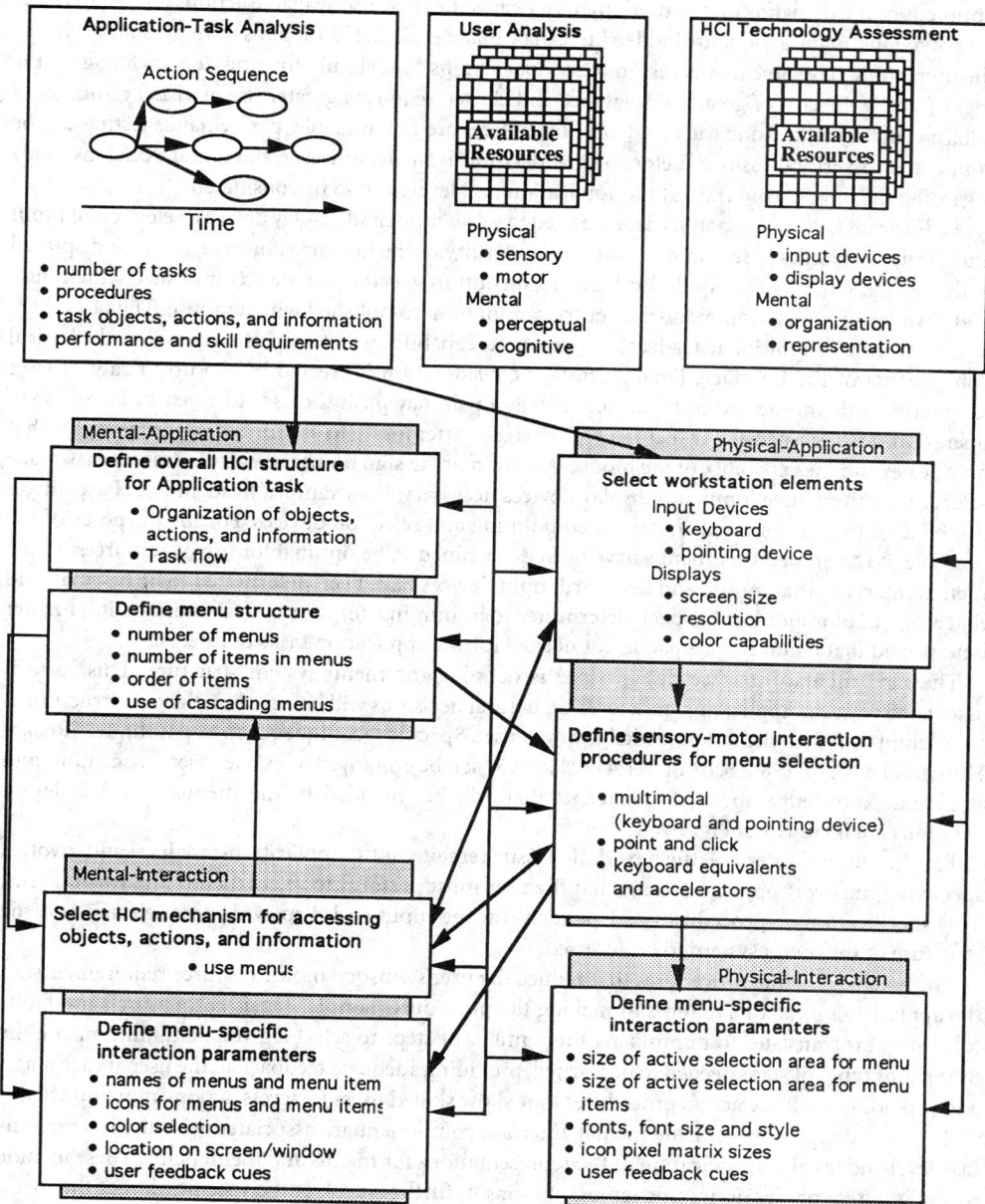

FIGURE 149.5 HCI design decisions for design of a menu system.

tasks and actions, and information to be manipulated. The HCI technology assessment will provide the designer with the set of resources available for application. Data from these analyses are used to make initial mental-interface component and physical-interface component decisions at an application-task level.

The decision to use a menu system to access actions and control the flow of the application task is based on the usability criteria discussed above with regard to performance and skill resources. Specifically, it is based on an assessment of the resources required to perform tasks using menu selection compared with other operating mechanisms. Alternative mechanisms would be command-line input from the user and visually presented buttons for each object and action. Menus and visual buttons both reduce the demands on the user's memory capacities because available actions are listed. In the case of menus, many actions are hidden but can be made explicit. If all actions were constantly visible, the user would have an easier access to individual actions (i.e., eliminating the step of calling up the menu) but at the cost of greater display size and clutter, requiring greater use of visual resources. If data specifically addressing each tradeoff in resources are not available, performance testing can be conducted to verify decisions. Before a final decision is made, however, the initial decisions made regarding the physical interface at the application task level need to be considered.

As illustrated, the task-analysis data are used to select input and display devices. Selection of input and display devices is based on matching the congruity of the information to be input or displayed with the capabilities of the device. Both menu and button selection can be accomplished with mouse and keyboard devices. Command-line entry cannot be accomplished with a mouse. The point here is that there are additional tradeoffs in resource capabilities between the mental and physical components of the interface. Finally, another consideration is created by the user analysis. User familiarity with another pointing device such as a pen may push the user to a pen-based mode of operation. This is especially true if the HCI design is attempting to account for gestural inputs that may be beyond the capability of the mouse. Additionally, design for users with disabilities may make selection of alternative input and display devices necessary. For example, head and ocular controls can be used in place of hand-manipulated pointing and selection devices. For the purposes of the example, it is assumed that menus have been determined to be optimal for use of resources on the mental interface, that mouse and keyboard input devices have been determined to be optimal, and that a 14-in. color monitor has been determined to be minimal for the physical interface. It is further determined that a number keypad is not needed for the application tasks of interest.

The next mental-interface design issue is defining the menu system structure. This issue is associated with the application-task level. Structural decisions will be based on the task structure in an attempt to reflect the task knowledge of the user. Specific techniques such as pathfinder [Roske-Hofstrand & Paap, 1986; Schvaneveldt et al., 1985] can be employed to extract user associations and structural knowledge about the concepts that will be included in the menus. Specific design decisions are included in Fig. 149.5.

For the physical interface, the next design issue remains at the application-task level and involves specifying the overt physical actions that the user must perform to select menus and menu items. This specification of procedures is dependent on the input and display devices selected and the structure of the menu system to be accessed.

The goal is to define procedures that reduce the user's sensory-motor resource requirements. At the application level, this reduces to making the procedures simple, consistent, natural, and fault-tolerant. This translates to minimizing the number of steps to select a given item, minimizing the number of types of steps needed to be learned, providing adequate feedback to the user at each stage, and providing multiple access procedures that allow skilled users to access actions more directly.

The next design issues for the mental-interface component are associated with the interaction-task level and involve specification of the representations for menus and menu items. These include menu and item names or graphic representations. It further involves the specification of the menu box and other menu indications (e.g., an ellipsis for indicating that a dialog box will be opened or an arrow indicating a cascading menu item). The specification of the selection procedures also may impose design considerations at this point. For example, keyboard operation will involve use of a selection cursor that cues the user to the active selection position. The perceptual-cognitive aspects of the design of this cursor will be considered here.

For the physical interface, the next design issues are associated with the interaction-task level. The specified procedures will be used to determine menu-specific, low-level operating parameters for the display and input devices. Menu-specific issues related to menu selection with a multibutton mouse device include the following:

- Size of the active screen selection area of each menu button. Greater size will translate to a reduced demand on pointing (positioning) accuracy resources.

- Size of the active screen selection area for each menu item. Greater size will require less precise pointing.
- Number of items in a selected menu. More items require more access time (or greater processing speed to keep access time fixed), more precise pointing, and create a greater probability of selection errors.
- Use of cascading menus. Selection requires more precise pointing.

Issues related to selection with a keyboard include the following:

- Key binding to selection action. Traditional, familiar, and consistent binding will reduce memory requirements and probability of user error.
- Distinguishability of the displayed selection cursor. Greater distinguishability requires less visual search and detection time.
- Size, sensitivity, required operating force of keyboard device.
- Response lag between keystroke and selection-cursor movement. Greater lag will create greater pointing error and increased pointing time.

Defining Terms

Application task: Refers to the applied objectives the user is employing the computer to accomplish (e.g., writing a report, performing a statistical analysis, finding information in a database, controlling a process, making a medical diagnosis, and monitoring/testing the health of a system).

Direct manipulation: A term coined by Schneiderman [1982, 1983]. Refers to an HCI or style of interaction with the following characteristics:

- Objects are continuously displayed.
- Physical action (e.g., point and click, drag and drop interaction) rather than command line interaction is employed.
- Impact of actions are rapid and directly observable.

Interaction task: Refers to the activities that the user performs to use the computer (e.g., moving a mouse device, typing keyboard inputs, viewing displays, searching for and managing files, managing displays, setting preferences, and executing programs).

Usability: Usability is a multidimensional quality that affords the user practical and convenient interaction with the computer for achieving applied objectives. The concept of usability is fundamental to the design of any human-system interface and is a major factor affecting the operational performance, availability, maintainability, and reliability of the overall system.

User-centered: User-centered design refers to a philosophy of human-machine system design that places the focus of the design process on the needs of the human who uses the system to accomplish a task. The following items characterize a user-centered design approach:

- The system is viewed as a tool that the user employs to accomplish objectives.
- The user is always performing a higher-level task than the system.
- Tasks are allocated away from the user rather than to the user. This is not simply a matter of perspective but rather is fundamental to a human-centered approach. That is, the user is assumed to be performing a high-level task. Lower-level tasks that are better performed by the computer are allocated from the user to the computer. This approach is opposed to one that considers the computer as the high-level task performer and allocates to the user lower-level tasks that the machine cannot do well.
- Tasks allocated to the user are meaningful.
- The user's responsibilities provide job satisfaction and make use of the user's talents and skills.

- Users are involved in all phases of the design process.
- The user's skills and performance capabilities are explicitly considered in and accounted for in design decisions.

References

Bevan N, Macleod M. 1994. Usability measurement in context. Behav Inform Technol 13:132.

Brown CM. 1988. Human-Computer Interface Design Guidelines. Norwood, NJ, Ablex Publishing.

Card SK, Moran TP, Newell A. 1983. The Psychology of Human-Computer Interaction. Hillsdale, NJ, Erlbaum.

Card SK, Moran TP, Newell A. 1986. The model human processor. In KR Boff, L Kaufman, JP Thomas (eds), Handbook of Perception and Human Performance, vol II, pp 45-1–45-35. New York, Wiley.

Galitz WO. 1993. User-Interface Screen Design. Boston, QED Publishing Group.

Imrhan S. 1995. Analysis of high-level tasks: Physical components. In JD Bronzino (ed), The Biomedical Engineering Handbook. Boca Raton, Fla, CRC Press.

ISO. 1993. ISO CD 9241-11, Guidelines for Specifying and Measuring Usability.

Kieras DE. 1988. Towards a practical GOMS model methodology for user interface design. In M Helander (ed), Handbook of Human-Computer Interaction, pp 135–157. New York, Elsevier Science Publishers.

Kondraske GV. 1995. A working model for human-system-task interfaces. In JD Bronzino, (ed), The Biomedical Engineering Handbook, pp 2157–2174. Boca Raton, Fla, CRC Press.

Maxwell KJ. 1995. Analysis of high-level tasks: Mental components. In JD Bronzino (ed), The Biomedical Engineering Handbook, pp 2233–2248. Boca Raton, Fla, CRC Press.

Payne SJ, Green T. 1986. Task-action grammars: A model of mental representation of task languages. Human-Computer Interact 2:93.

Roske-Hofstrand RJ, Paap KR. 1986. Cognitive networks as a guide to menu organization: An application in the automated cockpit. Ergonomics 29:1301.

Schiele F, Green T. 1990. HCI formalisms and cognitive psychology: The case of task-action grammar. In M Harrison, H Thimbleby (eds), Formal Methods in Human-Computer Interaction, pp 9–62. Cambridge, UK, Cambridge University Press.

Schvaneveldt RW, Durso FT, Dearholt DW. 1985. PATHFINDER: Scaling with Network Structures. Report no. MCCS-85-9, Computing Research Laboratory, Las Cruces, NM.

Shneiderman B. 1982. The future of interactive systems and the emergence of direct manipulation. Behav Inform Technol 1:237.

Shneiderman B. 1983. Direct manipulation: A step beyond programming languages. IEEE Comput 16:57.

Further Information

The following publications provide specifications and style guidelines and standards associated with specific user-interface systems.

Apple Computer. 1992. Apple Human Interface Guidelines: The Apple Desktop Interface. Reading, Mass, Addison-Wesley.

IBM. 1989. Systems Application Architecture, Common User Access Advanced Interface Design Guide, SC26-4582-0.

IBM. 1991. Systems Application Architecture, Common User Access Advanced Interface Design Reference, SC26-4582-0.

IBM. 1991. Systems Application Architecture, Common User Access Guide to User Interface Design, SC34-4290-00.

Microsoft Programming Series. 1992. The Windows Interface: An Application Design Guide. Washington, Microsoft Press.

Open Systems Foundation. 1993. OSF/Motif Style Guide. Revision 1.2, Cambridge, Mass.

The following books provide general design standards, guidelines, and methods.

Card SK, Moran TP, Newell A. 1983. The Psychology of Human-Computer Interaction. Hillsdale, NJ, Erlbaum.

Helander M (ed). 1988. Handbook of Human Computer Interaction. New York, Elsevier Science Publishers.

Human Factors and Ergonomics Society (ed). 1988. ANSI Standard HFS 100. American National Standard for Human Factors Engineering of Visual Display Terminal Workstations. Santa Monica, Calif, Human Factors and Ergonomics Society.

ISO. 1993. ISO 9241, Ergonomic Requirements for Office Work and Visual Display Terminals.

ISO. 1993. ISO DIS 9241-10, Dialogue Principles.

ISO. 1993. ISO DIS 9241-14, Menu Dialogues.

Laurel B (ed). 1990. The Art of Human-Computer Interface Design. Reading, Mass, Addison-Wesley.

Mayhew DJ. 1991. Principles and Guidelines in Software User Interface Design. Englewood Cliffs, NJ, Prentice-Hall.

Norman DA, Draper SW (eds). 1986. User Centered System Design, Hillsdale, NJ, Erlbaum.

Peddie J. 1992. Graphical User Interfaces and Graphic Standards. New York, McGraw-Hill.

Shneiderman B. 1987. Designing the User Interface: Strategies for Effective Human-Computer Interaction. Reading, Mass, Addison-Wesley.

Smith SL, Mosier JN. 1986. Guidelines for Designing User Interface Software. Bedford, Mass, MITRE Corporation.

Tognazzini B. 1992. TOG on Interface. Reading, Mass, Addison-Wesley.

The *International Journal of Human-Computer Studies* and *Human Factors* are excellent sources for new research findings on HCI design. The Association for Computing Machinery (ACM) has a *Special Interest Group in Computer-Human Interaction* (SIGCHI). The Human Factors and Ergonomics Society has a technical group on computer systems. Both organizations are an excellent source of information on new research and development through publications, conferences, and professional contacts.

150

Applications of Human Performance Measurements to Clinical Trials to Determine Therapy Effectiveness and Safety

Pamela J. Hoyes
Beehler
University of Texas at Arlington

Karl Syndulko
UCLA School of Medicine

A *clinical trial* is a research study involving human subjects and an intervention (i.e., device, drug, surgical procedure, or other procedure) that is ultimately intended to either enhance the professional capabilities of physicians (i.e., improve the service delivered), improve the quality of life of patients, or contribute to the field of knowledge in those sciences which are traditionally in the medical field setting—e.g., physiology, anatomy, pharmacology, epidemiology, neurology, cognitive psychology, etc. [Levin, 1986]. Clinical trials research is in the business of evaluating therapeutic interventions intended to benefit humans. Its value is directly related to the relevance of the questions "Do our treatments work?" "How well do our treatments work?" and "Are our treatments safe?" For example, drug *A* is designed and anticipated to relieve sinus congestion. Is there a drug interaction when drug *A* is taken with drug *B* and/or moderate levels of alcohol consumption such that while congestion is relieved (i.e., drug *A* is effective), human information processing capacities are reduced (i.e., is drug *A* safe?). And what is the time course of effects with regard to positive and negative (or adverse) effects? Thus it is clear that not only steady-state issues but also dynamic questions are of interest in clinical trials research.

While clinical trials research incorporates many different components, the focus of this chapter is limited to study questions associated with human performance capacity variables and their measurement as they contribute to the determination of therapy effectiveness and safety. Such variables

0-8493-8346-3/95/$0.00+$.50
© 1995 by CRC Press, Inc.

have been incorporated into trials since the use of controlled studies in the medical field began. However, the methodology employed to address human performance variables has been slowly but steadily shifting from mostly subjective to more objective instrumented methods [e.g., Tourtellotte et al., 1965] as both the understanding of the phenomena at play and the demand for improved quality of studies have increased. This chapter begins by briefly examining a classification of typical clinical trials study models, presents a summary of methods employed and key methodologic issues in both the design and conduct of studies (with special emphasis on issues related to the selection of measures and interpretation of results), and ends with a walk-through of a typical example that demonstrates the methods described. Brief discussion of the benefits that can be attributed to the use of objective, instrumented measures of human performance capacities as well as their current limitations in clinical trials research is also presented. While it is emphasized that most methods and issues addressed are applicable to any intervention, the use of human performance variables in pharmaceutial clinical trials has been most prevalent, and special attention has been given here to this application.

150.1 Basic Principles: Types of Studies

Depending on the set of primary and secondary questions to be addressed, considerable variety can exist with respect to the structure of a given trial and the analysis that is performed. Within the focus and scope of this chapter, clinical trials are classified into two categories for discussion: (1) safety-oriented and (2) efficacy-oriented. According to the Food and Drug Administration (FDA) [1977], four phases of research studies are required before a drug can be marketed in the United States. Phase I is known as *clinical pharmacology* and is intended to include the initial introduction of a drug into humans. These studies are safety-oriented; one issue often addressed is determination of the maximum tolerable dose. Phases II and III are known as *clinical investigation* and *clinical trials*, respectively, consisting of controlled and uncontrolled clinical trials research. Phase IV is the *postmarketing of clinical trials* to supplement premarketing data. Both safety and efficacy are addressed in phase II to IV investigations. As specified earlier, not all interventions studied are drugs. However, a similar phased approach is also characteristic of the investigation of therapeutic devices and treatments.

Safety-oriented trials usually involve vital sign measures (e.g., heart rate, blood pressure, respiration rate), clinical laboratory tests (e.g., blood chemistries, urinalysis, ECG), and adverse reaction tests (both mental and physical performance capacities) to evaluate the risk of the intervention. In this chapter we focus on the adverse reaction components, most of which historically have been addressed with subjective reporting methods. In the case of drug interventions, different doses (e.g., small to large) are administered within the trial, and the dose-related effects are examined. Thus the rate at which a drug is metabolized (*pharmacokinetics*), as evidenced by changes in drug concentrations in blood, cerebral spinal fluid, urine, etc., is usually addressed in safety-oriented drug studies, as well as the maximum dosage which subjects can tolerate [Baker et al., 1985; Fleiss, 1986; Jennison & Turnbull, 1993; Tudiver et al., 1992].

Efficacy-oriented trials are usually conducted after initial safety-oriented trials have established that the intervention has met safety criteria, but they will always have safety questions and elements as well. In this type of study, the goal is to objectively determine the therapeutic effect. Whatever the type of intervention, these studies are designed around the bottom-line question "Is the intervention effective?" In many cases (e.g., drugs for neurologic disorders, exercise programs for musculoskeletal injuries, etc.), *effectiveness* implies improvement or retarding the rate of deterioration in one or more aspects of mental and/or physical performance. With regard to disease contexts, it is necessary to distinguish performance changes that merely reflect treatment of systems as opposed to those which reflect the slowing or reversal of the basic disease process. Studies typically include pre- and postintervention measurement points and, whenever feasible, a control group that is administered a placebo intervention [Fleiss, 1986; Tang & Geller, 1993; Weissman, 1991]. The situation is complicated because there are many performance capacities that could be affected. In response to the intervention, some capacities may improve, some may remain unchanged, and some may be adversely affected. Thus efficacy-oriented studies typically include a number of secondary questions that address specificity of effects. When the intervention is a drug, both the pharmaco-kinetics and *pharmacodynamics* are often addressed. Pharmacodynamic studies attempt to relate physiologic and/or metabolic changes in the concentration of the agent over time to corresponding changes in the therapeutic effect. Thus repeated measurement of selected performance capacities are required over relatively short periods of time as part of these protocols.

Clinical trials involving human performance metrics generally use the *randomized clinical trial* (RCT) design. The RCT is a way to compare the efficacy and safety of two or more therapies or regimens. It was originally designed to test new drugs [Hill, 1963]; however, over the last 25 years, it has been applied to the study of vaccinations, surgical interventions, and even social innovations such as multiphasic screening [Levin, 1986]. Levin [1986] describes four key elements of RCTs: (1) the trials are "controlled," i.e., part of the group of subjects receive a therapy that is tested while the other subjects receive either no therapy or another therapy; (2) the significance of its results must be established through statistical analysis; (3) a double-blind experimental design should be used whenever possible; and (4) the therapies being compared should be allocated among the subjects randomly. Levin [1986] further noted that "the RCT is the gold standard for evaluating therapeutic efficacy."

150.2 Methods

Studies are defined and guided by *protocols*, a detailed statement of all procedures and methods to be employed. Figure 150.1 summarizes the major steps in clinical trials in which human perfor-mance variables represent those of primary interest, although the general process is similar for most trials involving human subjects.

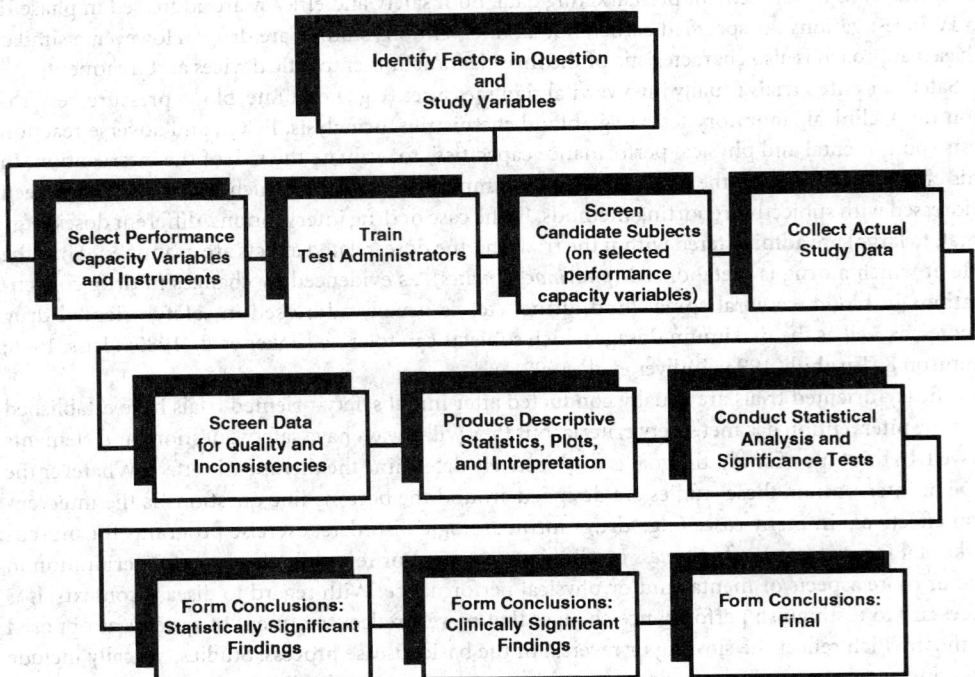

FIGURE 150.1 Summary of major steps in the conduct of a clinical trial involving human performance capacities.

Selecting Study Variables

In many clinical trials, performance measurements must be focused on the specific disease or set of symptoms against which a medication or intervention is directed. The critical element is selection of an outcome assessment that will indicate directly whether the intervention can eliminate key signs or symptoms of the disease, improve function affected by the disease, or even simply delay further disease progression and loss of function. Economic and statistical constraints of such trials often indicate that a minimal set of measures must be used to provide valid, reliable, and sensitive indicators of changes in underlying disease activity related to the treatments. In many instances, there is considerable controversy about what constitutes a valid and reliable assessment of the underlying disease process, or there may be de facto standards adopted by clinicians, pharmaceutical companies, and the FDA as to the choice of outcome assessments. In many diseases, these standards may be physician rating scales of disease severity. Thus objective studies may be required in the case of specific diseases and disorders to delineate the most sensitive set of performance measures for clinical trial evaluations [Mohr & Prouwers, 1991]. Further, it often must be demonstrated to clinicians, drug companies, and the FDA that the objective performance measures selected as outcome assessments actually do provide equal or more sensitive indicators of disease progression (and improvement) than do existing rating scale measures traditionally utilized in clinical trials for that disease. Experience with human performance testing in multiple sclerosis clinical trials, discussed below, illustrates these issues.

While objective measurement of performance capacities has been incorporated into many clinical trials, concepts and tools from human performance engineering can facilitate the selection of variables and shed some light on the issues noted above. In either safety- or efficacy-oriented studies, study variable selection can be characterized as a two-step process: (1) identification of the factors in question (e.g., Table 150.1) and (2) selection of the relevant *performance capacities* to be measured and associated measurement instruments. This link between these two steps often represents a challenge to researchers for a number of reasons. First, duality in terminology must be overcome. Concerns about an intervention are typically initially identified with "negative" terms such as "dizziness" and not in terms of performance capacities such as "postural stability." Human performance models based on systems engineering concepts [e.g., Kondraske, 1995] can be used to facilitate the translation of both formal and lay terms used to identify adverse effects to relevant performance capacities to be measured, as shown in Table 150.1.

In Kondraske's [1995] model, performance capacities are modeled as resources that a given system possesses and draws up to perform tasks. It also provides a basis for delineation of *hierarchical* human systems and their performance capacities as well as a basis to quantitatively explain the interaction of available performance capacities with demands of higher-level tasks (e.g., such as those encountered in daily living). The hierarchical aspect is particularly important in selecting performance capacities to be measured. It is generally good practice to include a combination of carefully selected lower-level and higher-level capacity measures. This combination allows careful tradeoffs between information content (i.e., specificity) and simplicity of the protocol (e.g. number of variables, time for test administration, etc.). Higher-level capacities (characterizing systems responsible for gait, postural stability, complex mental task, etc.) are dependent on the performance capacities of multiple lower-level subsystems. Thus a few higher-level performance capacities can reflect multiple lower-level capacities (e.g., knee flexor strength, visual information processing speed, etc.). However, lower-level capacity measures are typically less variable than higher-level capacities within individuals (i.e., on retest) and within populations. Therefore, small changes in performance can be more readily discriminated statistically if they exist and are attributable primarily to localized lower-level capacities (e.g., see data in Potvin et al. [1985]). Also, more specific information can provide valuable insights into physiologic effects if they are present. By combining both types, broad coverage can be achieved (so that aspects of human performance in which the expectation of an effect is less remain included), as well as a degree of specificity, while keeping the total number of study vari-

TABLE 150.1   Representative Examples of Linking Factors in Question to Specific Measurable Performance Capacities

Factor in Question*	Selected Relevant Performance Capacities[†]
General central nervous system effects (of drug)	Selected activity of daily living execution speed
	Postural stability
	Upper extremity neuromotor channel capacity
	Manual manipulation speed
	Visual–upper extremity information processing speed
	Visual attention span
	Visual-spatial memory capacity
	Visual-numerical memory capacity
Alcohol interaction (of drug)	Selected activity of daily living execution speed
	Postural stability
	Visual information processing speed
	Visual-spatial memory capacity
Dizziness	Postural stability
Drowsiness	Selected activity of daily living execution speed
	Visual attention span
	Visual–upper extremity information processing speed
	Bond-Lader visual analog scale
Slowness of movement, psychomotor retardation	Visual–upper extremity information processing speed
	Upper extremity random reach movement speed
	Index finger (proximal intercarpal phalangeal joint), flexion-extension speed
Mood	Emotional stability (e.g., with Hamilton anxiety scale, Bond-Lader analog scale and other similar tools)
Speed	Reaction time
Coordination	Finger tapping
Tremors, abnormal movements	Limb steadiness
	Postural stability
	Vocal amplitude and pitch steadiness
Joint stiffness or pain	Extremes and range of motion
	Isometric strength (selected joints)
Weakness, strength	Postural stability (one leg, eyes open)
	Isometric grip strength
	Isometric strength (representative set of upper and lower extremity, proximal and distal muscle groups)
Sensation	Vibration sensitivity
	Thermal sensitivity

* Terms used include those often used by pharmaceutical companies to communicate adverse effects to general public.
[†] Lists are illustrative and not exhaustive. More or fewer items can be included depending on time available or willingness to expend for data collection, with commensurate tradeoffs between specificity and protocol simplicity.

ables to a reasonable size. In addition, if an effect is found in both a higher-level capacity and a re-lated lower-level capacity, an internal cross-validation of finding is obtained. Many early studies incorporated variables representing looks across different hierarchical levels but did not distinguish them by level during analysis and interpretation. While such logic begins to remove the guesswork, much work remains to refine variable-selection methodology.

To address the broad, bottom-line questions regarding safety and efficacy, the formation of *composite scores* (i.e., some combination of scores from two or more performance capacity challenges or "tests") is necessary. A resource model and the concept of hierarchical human systems also can be used to develop composite variables for practical use in clinical trials. Component capacities can be selected that are theoretically or empirically most sensitive to the disease or condition under study. The composite variable is then created by calculating a more traditional weighted arithmetic sum [e.g., Potvin et. al., 1985] or product [e.g., Kondraske, 1989] of the component scores. In both cases, the definition of component scores is important (i.e., whether a smaller or larger number represents better performance). Treatments are not approved if only a small subset of individuals is helped. Composite measures provide the only objective means of integrating multidimensional information about an intervention's effects. The primary advantages of the composite variable is the creation of a single, global, succinct measure of the disease, condition, or intervention, which is often essential as the primary outcome assessment for efficacy. The major disadvantage is loss of detailed information about the unique profile of performance changes that each subject or a group as a whole may show. Such tradeoffs are to be expected. Thus both composite and component measures play important but different roles in clinical trials.

It is imperative that the selection of the study measures also consider a test's objectivity (non-biased), reliability (consistency), and validity (measures what it intends to measure) to add to the quality of the measurements. Many complex issues, which are beyond the present scope, are associated with measuring and interpreting the quality of a measurement. (See Baumgartner and Jackson [1993], Hastad and Lacy [1994], and Safrit [1990] for more information.)

Formation of the Subject Pool

Clinical research investigations usually involve a sample group of subjects from a defined population. Selection of the study population so that generalizations from that sample accurately reflect the defined population is a dilemma that must be adequately addressed. If *probability sampling* is chosen, each subject in the defined population theoretically has an equal chance of being included in the sample. The advantage of this kind of sampling is that differences between treatment groups can be detected and the probability that these differences actually exist may be estimated. If *non-probability sampling* is chosen, there is no way to ensure that each subject had an equal chance of being included in the sample. Conclusions of nonprobability sampling therefore have less merit (not as generalizable) than those based on probability sampling.

Studies with healthy subjects are believed to be necessary before exposing sick persons to some interventions because persons with disease or injuries commonly have impaired function of various organs that metabolize drugs and may take medications that can alter the absorption, metabolism, and/or excretion rates of the intervention. Gender issues also should be a concern in clinical trials because of new FDA regulations [Cotton, 1993; Merkatz et al., 1993; Stone, 1993].

All subjects selected as study candidates should be informed of the procedures that will be utilized in the clinical trials investigation by signing an informed consent document, as required by the Department of Health and Human Services *Code of Federal Regulations* [1985] and other federal regulations applicable to research involving human subjects. Using all or a subset of study measurement variables (in addition to medical history and examinations as necessary), a screening procedure is recommended to determine if each subject meets the minimum performance criteria established for subject inclusion. When patients are part of the sample group, this performance screening also can be used to establish that the sample includes the desired balance of subjects with different amounts of "room for improvement" on relevant variables. An added benefit of this screening process is that subjects and test administrators obtain experience with test protocols, equipment, and procedures that will add to the validity of the study.

Unless available from a previous similar study, it is typical for pilot data to be collected to estimate the expected size of outcome effects. With this information, the power of the statistical analysis (i.e., the likelihood that a significant difference will be detected) can be estimated so that sample size can be determined [Cochran & Cox, 1957; Fleiss, 1986; Kepple, 1982]. Another concern is that some of the original subject pool will not complete the study or will have incomplete data. High attrition rates may damage the credibility of the study, and every effort should be made to not lose subjects. DeAngelis [1990] estimates that attrition rates higher than 50% make the interpretation of clinical trial research very difficult. Some researchers believe that no attempt should be made to replace these subjects because even random selection of new subjects will not ensure bias caused by differential participation of all the subjects.

Data Collection

Investigators should seek to minimize sources of variability by careful control of the test conditions and procedures. Proper control can be attained by (1) using rooms that are reasonably soundproof or sound-deadened, well lighted, and of a comfortable temperature; (2) selecting chairs and other accessories carefully (e.g., no wheels for tests in which the subject is seated); (3) testing subjects one at a time without other subjects in the test room; (4) using standardized written instructions for each test to eliminate variability in what is stated; (5) allowing for familiarization with the test instruments and procedures; (6) not commenting about subject performance to avoid biased raising or lowering of expectations; (7) arranging a test order to offset fatigue (mental and physical) or boredom and to include rest periods; and (8) training test administrators and evaluating their training using healthy subjects, especially in multicenter studies, so that consistent results can be obtained.

Data Integrity Screening

Despite all good efforts and features incorporated to ensure high-quality data, opportunities exist for error. It is therefore beneficial to subject data obtained during formal test sessions to quality screenings. This is a step toward forming the official study data set (i.e., the set that will be subjected to statistical and other analyses). Several independent analyses used to screen data, which are typically computer-automated, are described below.

Screening of Baseline Measures Against Inclusionary Criteria.   If human performance study variables with specific performance criteria are used as part of the subject selection process as recommended above, each subject's baseline score can be compared with the score obtained during inclusionary testing. For most variables, baseline scores should not differ from inclusionary testing by more than 20% [Potvin et al., 1985]. Greater deviations point to examiner training, test procedure, or subject compliance problems.

Screening Against Established Norms.   For variables that are not included in inclusionary screenings or in studies where performance variables are not used as part of the subject inclusionary criteria, baseline data can be screened against established reference data (e.g., human performance means and standard deviations). Data are considered acceptable if they fall within an established range (e.g., two standard deviation units of the reference population mean). From the perspective of risk associated with not identifying a data point that could be a potential problem, this is a fairly liberal standard that can still identify problems in data collection and management. Standards that lessen risk can, of course, be employed at the discretion of the investigator, but at the expense of the possible identification of a larger number of data points that require follow-up.

Screening Against Anticipated Effects.   It is more difficult to screen nonbaseline data for quality because of the possible influences of the intervention. However, criteria can be established based on (1) absolute level of variables (both maximums and minimums) and (2) rates and direction of change from one measurement period to the next. Even criteria that allow a rather wide range of data (or changes across repeated measures) can be useful in detecting gross anomalies and is recommended.

   If anomalies are discovered using the screening methods described above, several outcomes are possible: (1) The anomaly can be traced and rectified (e.g., it may be attributable to a human or computer error with backup available); (2) the anomaly may be explainable as a procedural error, but it may not be possible to rectify; and (3) the anomaly may be unexplainable. Data anomalies that are explainable with supporting documentation could justify classification of the given data item as "missing data" or replacement of all data for the corresponding subject in the data set (i.e., the subject could be dropped from the study and replaced with another). There is no justification for eliminating or replacing data anomalies for which a documentable explanation does not exist.

Analysis and Interpretation of Results

Traditional inferential statistical analysis should be performed according to the statistical model and significance levels agreed on by the clinical research team when the study is designed. However, data also should be analyzed and interpreted from a clinical perspective as well.

In experimental research, tests of *statistical significance* are the most commonly used tools for assessing possible associations between independent and dependent variables as well as differences among treatment groups. The purpose of significance (i.e., statistical) tests is to evaluate the research hypothesis at a specific level of probability, or p value. For example, if a p value of 0.05 was chosen, the researcher is asking if the levels of treatment (for example) differ significantly so that these differences are not attributable to a chance occurrence more than 5 times out of 100. By convention, a p value of 0.01 (1%) or 0.05 (5%) is usually selected as the cutoff for statistical significance. Significance tests cannot accept a research hypothesis; all that significance tests can do is reject or fail to reject the research hypothesis [Thomas & Nelson, 1990]. Ultimately, significance tests can determine if treatment groups are different, but not why they are different. Good experimental design, appropriate theorizing, and sound reasoning are used to explain why treatment groups differ.

Exclusive reliance on tests of statistical significance in the present context can mislead the clinical researcher, and interpretation of *clinical significance* is required. The key issue here is the size of the observed effect; p values give little information on the actual magnitude of a finding (i.e., decrement or improvement in performance, etc.). Also, statistical findings are partially a function of sample size. Thus even an effect that is small in size can be detected with tests of statistical significance in a study with a large sample. For example, a mean difference in grip strength of 2 kg may be found in response to drug therapy. This difference is a quite small fraction of the variability in grip strength observed across normal individuals, however. Thus, although statistically significant, such a change would perhaps have a minimal impact on an individual's ability to function in daily activities which make demands on grip strength performance resources. Thus clinical significance addresses cause-and-effect relationships between study variables and performance in activities of daily life or other broad considerations such as the basic disease process. The danger of not defining clinical significance appropriately can be either that a good intervention is not used in practice (e.g., it may be rejected for a safety finding that is statistically significant but small) or that a poor intervention is allowed into practice (e.g., it may result in statistically significant improvements that are small).

Ideally, if empirical data existed that established what amount of a given performance capacity such as visual information processing speed (VIPS) was necessary to perform a task (e.g., driving safely on the highway), then it would be possible to interpret statistically significant findings (e.g., a decrement in VIPS of a known amount) to determine if the change would be of a magnitude that would limit the individual from successfully accomplishing the given task. Unfortunately, while general cause-effect relationships between laboratory-measured capacities and performance in high-level tasks are evident, quantitative models do not yet exist, and completely objective interpretations of clinical significance are not yet possible. As such, the process by which clinical significance is determined is less well developed and structured. More recent concepts introduced by Kondraske [1988a, 1988b, 1989] based on the use of *resource economic* principles (i.e., the idea of a threshold "cost" associated with lower-level variables typically employed in clinical trials for achieving a given level of human performance in any given high-level task) may be helpful in defining objective criteria for clinical significance. This approach directly addresses cause-and-effect relationships between performance capacities and high-level tasks with an approach much like that which an engineer would employ to design a system capable of performing a specified task.

Despite known limitations, interpretation of clinical significance is always incorporated into clinical trials in some fashion. Any change in human performance for a given variable should be first documented to be statistically significant before it is considered to be a candidate for clinical significance (i.e., a statistically significant difference is a necessary but not a sufficient condition for clinical significance). Objective determination of clinical significance can be based in part on previous methods introduced by Potvin et al. [1985] in clinical trials involving neuromotor and central processing performance tests. They advocate the use of an objective criteria whereby a decrease or increase in a human performance capacity (with healthy test subjects, for example) should be greater than 20% to be classified as "clinically significant." Kondraske [1989] uses a similar approach that uses z-scores (i.e., number of standard deviation units from a population mean) as the basis for determining criteria. This accounts for population variability which is different for different performance capacity variables. A recent approach is to assess effect size, a statistical metric that is independent of sample size and which takes into account data variability. This method provides an objective basis for comparison of the magnitude of treatment effects among studies [Cohen, 1988; Ottenbacher & Barrett, 1991].

150.3 Representative Application Examples

Safety-Oriented Example: Drug-Alcohol Interaction

In this section, selected elements of an actual clinical trial are presented to further illustrate methods and issues noted above. To maintain confidentialities, the drug under test is simply denoted as drug A.

Identify Factors in Question.   Upper respiratory infections are among the most frequent infections encountered in clinical practice and affect all segments of the general population. The pharmacologic agent of choice for upper respiratory infections are the antihistamines (reference drug), which possess a wide margin of safety and almost no lethality when taken alone in an overdose attempt. Although quite effective, antihistamines can produce several troublesome side effects (i.e., general CNS impairment, sedation, and drowsiness) and have been incriminated in automobile accidents as well as public transportation disasters. New drugs (e.g., drug A) are being developed to have similar benefits but fewer side effects. From prior animal studies, drug A has been shown to have minimal effects on muscle relaxation and muscular coordination as well as less sedative and alcohol-potentiating effects than those associated with classical antihistamines. Based on drug A's history and concerns, the following factors in question were identified in this clinical trial: general CNS impairment, alcohol interaction, dizziness, drowsiness, mood, and slowness of movement/speed. The purpose of this investigation was to examine the effect of drug A on human performance capacity relative to a reference drug and placebo as well as the drug-alcohol potentiating interaction effects after multiple dose treatment.

Select Performance Capacity Variables and Instruments.   With the factors in question identified, the following performance capacity variables and their testing instruments were selected for the clinical trial: visual information processing speed (VIPS), finger tapping speed (TS), visual arm lateral reach coordination (VALRC), visual spatial memory capacity (VSMC), postural performance (PP), digit symbol substitution task (DSST), and Bond-Lader Visual Analog Scale (BLS). These variables were collectively called the *human performance capacity test battery* (HPCTB) (Table 150.2). Due to space limitations, only one performance capacity variable (VMRS—visual information processing speed, i.e., VIPS) is discussed in this section.

Experimental Design.   The first primary objective of this investigation was to examine after 8 days of oral dosing the relative effects of drug A, reference drug, and placebo on the human performance capacity of healthy male and female adult volunteers (see Table 150.2). This effect was determined by examining the greatest decrease in human performance capacity from day 1 of testing (i.e., baseline at -0.5 hour drug ingestion time) to day 8 of testing at drug ingestion times of 0.0, 1.0, 2.0, 4.0, and 6.0 hours. The second primary objective was to examine after 9 days of oral dosing the relative

TABLE 150.2 Experimental Schedule for Human Performance Capacity Test Battery (HPCTB)

	Drug Ingestion Times (hours)					
Test Day	−0.5	0.0	1.0	2.0	4.0	6.0
1*	HPCTB					
8†		HPCTB	HPCTB	HPCTB	HPCTB	HPCTB
9†,‡		HPCTB	HPCTB	HPCTB	HPCTB	HPCTB

Note: The human performance capacity test battery (HPCTB) was administered in the following order: VIPS, TS, VALRC, VSMC, PP, DSST, and BLS.

* On day 1 of testing only, the −0.5 HPCTB was performed and utilized as the baseline value for test days 8 and 9.

† The peak effect was determined by comparing baseline values (day 1) against the greatest detriment in performance for the eighth and ninth testing days at drug ingestion times of 0.0, 1.0, 2.0, 4.0, and 6.0 hours.

‡ On day 9 of testing, an alcohol drink was served immediately after drug administration and was ingested over a 15-minute period.

effects of drug A, reference drug, and placebo in combination with a single dose of alcohol served immediately after drug administration (male alcohol dose 0.85 g/kg body weight, female alcohol dose 0.75 g/kg body weight) on the human performance capacity of healthy male and female adult volunteers (see Table 150.2). This effect was determined by comparing the greatest decrease in performance on the ninth day of study drug treatment (at drug ingestion times of 0.0, 1.0, 2.0, 4.0, and 6.0 hours) to baseline on day one of testing (−0.5 hour drug ingestion time) for the HPCTB (see Table 150.2). Independent variables were treatment group (1 = drug A, 2 = reference drug, and 3 = placebo) and gender (male/female). The dependent variable was maximum decrease in performance (peak effect) for each human performance capacity study variable and was determined by comparing the baseline value (day 1) against the greatest decrease in performance at drug ingestion times of 0.0, 1.0, 2.0, 4.0, and 6.0 hours for day 8 and day 9 of testing. Inferential statistical analysis of the data was performed using a 3 (treatment group: reference drug, drug A, and placebo) by 5 (hour: 0, 1, 2, 4, and 6) mixed factorial ANOVA with repeated measures on hour for each dependent variable. Statistical tests of significance for all ANOVAs were conducted at the 0.05 level.

Data Screening. For each dependent variable, baseline treatment data were compared against the criteria established for subject inclusion using each subject's performance score from the HPCTB to identify data anomalies. Then the expected increases/decreases in human performance capacity from baseline treatment data were compared against the drug therapy–influenced data to determine if these changes were within "reasonable" limits. Potential anomalies were detected in less than 5% of the data, with most occurring within records for only a few subjects. These cases were investigated, and in consultation with the principal investigator, decisions were made and documented to arrive at the official data set.

Descriptive Statistical Analysis. Figure 150.2 illustrates the visual information processing speed (VIPS) for treatment groups reference drug, drug A, and placebo. On day 1 of testing (baseline), all treatment groups had similar VIPSs, with means between 5.7 and 5.8 stimuli per second. On day 8 of testing and at drug ingestion time of 2 hours, VIPS decreased to 4.9 stimuli per second for drug A, to 5.1 stimuli per second for reference drug, and to 5.65 stimuli per second for the placebo. On day 8, the greatest group impairment of VIPS occurred at drug ingestion time of 4 hours. Drug A appeared to have the greatest impairment of VIPS (4.6 stimuli per second), followed by the reference drug group (4.9 stimuli per second). This decrease in performance was not present with the placebo group (5.61 stimuli per second). By the sixth hour after drug ingestion on day 8, VIPS improved toward baseline for treatment groups reference drug (5.1 stimuli per second) and drug A (5.3 stimuli per second), while the placebo group remained unchanged (5.58 stimuli per second).

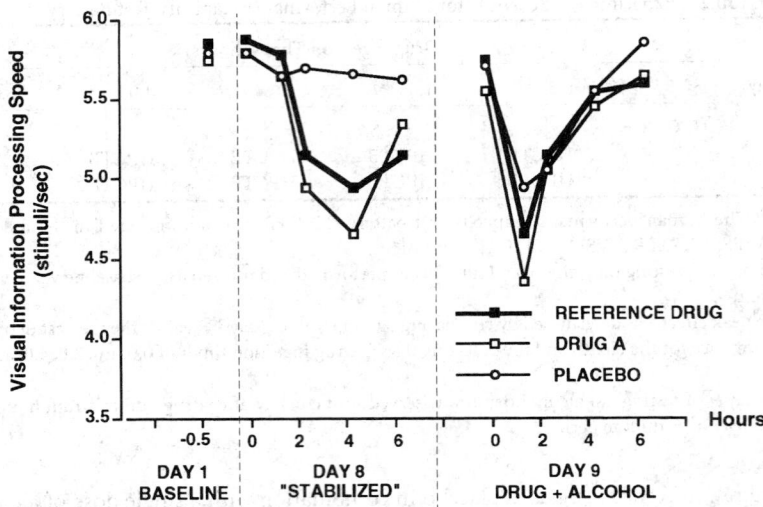

FIGURE 150.2 One performance capacity variable (visual information processing speed) for three treatment groups (drug *A*—the drug under test—reference drug, and placebo) taken from an actual efficacy-oriented study. Note changes from baseline to drug stabilization (day 8) and interaction with alcohol (day 9). See text for further explanation.

On day 9 of testing, all treatment groups received their assigned drug and alcohol. By 1 hour after drug ingestion, all treatment groups' VIPSs were impaired from baseline, with drug *A* showing the greatest impairment (4.3 stimuli per second), followed by reference drug (4.6 stimuli per second) and placebo (4.9 stimuli per second). All treatment groups' VIPSs improved toward baseline values by the second hour after drug ingestion (5.0 to 5.1 stimuli per second) and the fourth hour after drug ingestion (5.4 to 5.5 stimuli per second), respectively. By the sixth hour after drug ingestion, reference drug and drug *A* plateaued between 5.55 and 5.6 stimuli per second, respectively, while the placebo group improved slightly above the baseline value (5.8 stimuli per second). The basic patterns observed (i.e., decrease from baseline, return to baseline, impairment of all groups, including placebo, with alcohol) lend validity to the overall study.

Statistical Analysis and Significance Test Results.   On day 8 of testing, significant differences in VIPS for main effects treatment group and hour were observed. There was a significant interaction, however, between treatment group and hour of drug ingestion. Post hoc analysis demonstrated that treatment groups drug *A* and reference drug were significantly slower in VIPS than the placebo group at drug ingestion times of 2, 4, and 6 hours, but there was no difference in VIPS between treatment groups drug *A* and reference drug. (Simple main effects and simple, simple main effects showed that the placebo group had faster VIPSs than both reference drug and drug *A* treatment groups at drug ingestion times of 2, 4, and 6 hours.)

On day 9 of testing when the drug-alcohol potentiating interaction effect was of primary interest, significant differences in VIPS occurred for main effects treatment group and hour, but there were no interactions between treatment group and hour of drug ingestion. Post hoc analysis demonstrated that treatment groups drug *A* and reference group were significantly slower in VIPS than the placebo group at 1 hour after drug ingestion only, but there was no statistically significant difference in VIPS between treatment groups drug *A* and reference drug at any hour after drug-alcohol ingestion. Also, the drug-alcohol interaction was significant 1 hour after drug-alcohol ingestion for all treatment groups.

Conclusions from Statistically Significant Findings. After 8 days of oral dosing, while a significant difference was found for both drug treatment groups compared with the placebo group, there was no significant difference in VIPS between drug *A* and reference drug treatment groups. The effect was apparent at approximately the same drug ingestion time of 4 hours. It was concluded that drug *A* had the same effect on safety as the reference drug in terms of CNS impairment as measured by VIPS.

After 9 days of oral dosing in combination with alcohol consumption, drug *A* and the reference drug caused a greater decrease in VIPS compared with the placebo group. This effect was most apparent at 1 hour after drug ingestion. The placebo group also decreased its VIPS at 1 hour after drug ingestion at a statistically significant level. It was concluded after 9 days of oral dosing that drug *A* in combination with alcohol produced the same effect as the reference drug in combination with alcohol in terms of CNS impairment as measured by VIPS.

Conclusions from Clinically Significant Findings. Since there was no statistically significant difference between drug *A* and the reference drug on either day 8 or day 9, the only findings requiring an interpretation of clinical significance are the statistically significant findings for both drug *A* and the reference drug relative to the placebo group. On both day 8 and day 9, these findings are clinically significant using either the Potvin et al. [1985] percentage change or Kondraske [1989] *z*-score approach. Using the resource economic model for human performance [Kondraske, 1988a, 1988b, 1989], it can be argued that, for example, during critical events during tasks such as driving, all of an individual's available VIPS resource is drawn on. Clearly, the substantial decrease in VIPS observed can compromise safety during such events.

Efficacy-Oriented Study: Experiences in Neurology

Performance testing in clinical trials in neurology has grown tremendously within the last decade [Mohr & Brouwers, 1991], but within specific disease areas there remains reluctance to accept the replacement of traditional rating-scale evaluations of disease presence and progression by objective performance testing [Syndulko et al., 1993]. The evolution of clinical evaluations in multiple sclerosis clinical trials illustrates this point.

Evaluation of disability change or deterioration in multiple sclerosis (MS) historically has been limited to physician rating scales that attempt to globally summarize some or most of the salient clinical features of the disease. General consensus in the use of rating scales for MS has been achieved in the specification of a minimal record of disability (MRD) for MS that incorporates several physician- and paramedical-administered rating scales for evaluating MS disease status and its effects on the patient's life [International Federation of Multiple Sclerosis Societies, 1984]. However, there has been general dissatisfaction with the use of rating scales in MS clinical trials because of issues of lack of sensitivity to disease change, lack of interrater reliability, and simply the inherent reliance on subjective ratings of signs, symptoms, and unmeasured performance changes [Paty et al., 1992].

As an alternative to MS rating scales, comprehensive, quantitative evaluation of human performance was originally proposed and developed over 25 years ago for use in MS clinical trials [Tourtellotte et al., 1965]. The first application of performance testing in a major MS clinical trial was the multicenter cooperative ACTH study [Rose et al., 1968]. The study proved that human performance testing could be incorporated into a multicenter MS clinical trial and that examiners at multiple centers could be trained to administer the tests in a standardized, repeatable fashion. The results generally supported fairly comparable levels of sensitivity among the outcome measures, including performance testing [Dixon & Kuzma, 1974]. Subsequent analyses showed that a priori composites that provided succinct summary measures of disease change in key functional areas could be formed from the data and that these composite measures were sensitive to treatment effects in relapsing/remitting MS patients [Henderson et al., 1978]. Despite the favorable results of the ACTH study, performance testing did not achieve general acceptance in MS clinical studies. Comprehensive performance testing as conducted in the ACTH trial was considered time-consuming, the instrumentation was not generally available, and despite the use of composites, the number of outcome measures remained too large. In a recent double-blind, placebo-controlled collaborative study in 12 medical centers, the study design included both rating-scale and performance measures as outcome assessments in the largest sample of chronic progressive MS patients studied to date [The Multiple Sclerosis Study Group, 1990]. Analyses of the change in performance composite scores from baseline over the 2-year course of the clinical trial showed that the drug-treated patients worsened significantly less than the placebo-treated patients. In contrast, the EDSS and other clinical rating scores did not show significant treatment effects for the subset of MS patients at the same center [Syndulko et al., 1993]. This indicated that the performance composites were more sensitive than the clinical disability measures to disease progression and treatment effects. A more recent comparative analysis of the full data set also supports the greater sensitivity of composites based on performance testing compared with rating scales to both MS disease progression and to a treatment effect [Syndulko et al., 1994a; Syndulko et al., 1944b]. Although the biomedical community remains divided regarding the best outcome assessment in MS clinical trials, the accumulating evidence favors performance testing over clinical measures.

Another type of efficacy-oriented study of particular note in the context of this chapter involves the combination of pharmacodynamic models with instrumented, objective, and sensitive performance capacity measurements to optimize therapeutic effectiveness by fine-tuning dose prescription for individual subjects. For example, the results from a Parkinson's disease study by Hacisalihzade et al. [1989] suggest that performance capacity measurements, which would play a key role in a strategy to determine pharmacodynamics of a drug for the individual (i.e., not a population), could become a component in the management of some patients receiving long-term drug therapy.

150.4 Future Needs and Anticipated Developments

The field of clinical trials in which human performance variables are of interest has expanded at such a rapid rate in recent years that it has been difficult for researchers to keep up with all the new technologies, instrumentations, and methodologies. The type of evaluation employed has steadily shifted from mostly subjective to more objective, which can be argued to provide improved measurement quality. Increased standardization of human performance measurements has led to greater cost-effectiveness due to computer-based test batteries [Kennedy et al., 1993; Woollacott, 1983]. Thus, even if the quality of measurement were the same with methodologies that used less sophisticated methods, the initial investment would frequently be saved with newer data management techniques. This sentiment has not yet been accepted by all segments of the relevant communities. Also, the speed at which data can now be collected (which is especially important when changes over short time periods are of interest, as in pharmacodynamic studies) has led to greater cost-effectiveness. Furthermore, since instrumented devices are becoming commercially available and more widely used, it is not necessary nor desirable for researchers whose primary interest is the intervention or disease process to "reinvent" measurements (possibly with subtle but significant changes that ultimately inhibit standardization) for use in studies. Also, new measurements that may be different—but not necessarily better—must undergo long and expensive studies prior to their use in clinical trials. Although certain human performance measures are becoming standard in selected situations, more experience is needed before a substantial degree of standardization in human performance measurement is achieved in such situations.

The perfect research strategy in clinical trials involving human performance capacities to determine therapy effectiveness and safety may not be possible due to financial and/or ethical considerations. Thus the challenge of clinical trials research in the future is to maintain scientific integrity while conforming to legal mandates and staying within economic feasibility; i.e., an optimization is almost always necessary. Multidisciplinary research efforts can be useful in these circumstances.

Defining Terms

Clinical significance: An additional level of interpretation of a statistically significant finding that addresses the size of the effect found.

Clinical trial: A research study involving human subjects and an intervention (i.e., device, drug, surgical procedure, or other procedure) that is ultimately intended to either enhance the professional capabilities of physicians, improve the quality of life of patients, or contribute to the field of knowledge in those sciences which are traditionally in the medical field setting.

Composite score: A score derived by combining two of more measured performance capacities.

Efficacy-oriented clinical trial: A study that is conducted to objectively determine an intervention's effectiveness along with any pharmacokinetic or pharmacodynamic interactions.

Nonprobability sampling: A method of sampling whereby no subject in a defined population has an equal chance of being included in the sample.

Performance capacities: Dimensional capabilities or resources (e.g., speed, accuracy, strength, etc.) that a given human subsystem (e.g., visual, central processing, gait production, posture maintenance, etc.) possesses to perform a given task.

Pharmacodynamics: The physiologic and/or metabolic changes in the concentration of a drug over time to corresponding measurable performance capacity changes in the therapeutic effect.

Pharmacokinetics: The rate at which a drug is metabolized, as evidenced by changes in drug concentrations in blood, cerebral spinal fluid, urine, etc.

Probability sampling: A method of sampling whereby each subject in a defined population theoretically has an equal chance of being included in the sample.

Protocol: A detailed statement of all procedures and methods to be employed in a research investigation.

Randomized clinical trial (RCT): A study that uses controlled trials whereby part of the group of subjects receives a therapy that is tested, while the other subjects receive either no therapy or another therapy.

Resource economics: A cause-effect type of relationship between available performance resources (i.e., capacities) and demands of higher-level tasks in which the relevant subsystems are used.

Safety-oriented clinical trial: A study that usually involves vital sign measures (e.g., heart rate, blood pressure, respiration rate), clinical laboratory tests (e.g., blood chemistries, urinalysis, ECG), and adverse reaction tests (both mental and physical performance capacities) to evaluate the risk of an intervention.

Sample: A proportion of the defined population that is studied. When used as a verb (sampling), it refers to the process of subject selection.

Significance (statistical) test: A tool used for assessing possible associations between independent and dependent variables as well as differences among treatment groups.

Statistical significance: An evaluation of the research hypothesis at a specific level of probability so that any differences observed are not attributable to a chance occurrence.

References

Baker SJ, Chrzan GJ, Park CN, Saunders JH. 1985. Validation of human behavioral tests using ethanol as a CNS depressant Model. Neurobehav Toxicol Teratol 7:257.

Baumgartner TA, Jackson AS. 1993. Measurement for Evaluation, 4th ed. Dubuque, Iowa, Wm. C. Brown.

Cochran WG, Cox GM. 1957. Experimental Designs, 2nd ed. New York, Wiley.

Cohen J. 1988. Statistical Power Analysis for the Behavioral Sciences. Hillsdale, NJ, Lawrence Erlbaum Associates.

Cotton P. 1993. FDA lifts ban on women in early drug tests, will require companies to look for gender differences. JAMA 269:2067.

DeAngelis C. 1990. An Introduction to Clinical Research. New York, Oxford University Press.

Department of Health and Human Services. 1985. Code of Federal Regulations of the Department of Health and Human Services, title 45, part 46.

Dixon WJ, Kuzma JW. 1974. Data reduction in large clinical trials. Comm Stat 3:301.

Food and Drug Administration. 1977. General Considerations for the Clinical Evaluation of Drugs. DHEW Publication No. (FDA) 77-3040. Washington.

Fleiss JL. 1986. The Design and Analysis of Clinical Experiments. New York, Wiley.

Hacisalihzade SS, Mansour M, Albani C. 1989. Optimization of symptomatic therapy in Parkinson's disease. IEEE Trans Biomed Eng 36(3):363.

Hastad DN, Lacy AC. 1994. Measurement and Evaluation, 2nd ed. Scottsdale, Ariz, Gorsuch Scarisbrick.

Henderson WG, Tourtellotte WW, Potvin AR, Rose AS. 1978. Methodology for analyzing clinical neurological data: ACTH in multiple sclerosis. Clin Pharmacol Ther 24:146.

Hill AB. 1963. Medical ethics and controlled trials. Br Med J 1:1043.

Horne JA, Gibbons H. 1991. Effects of vigilance performance and sleepiness of alcohol given in the early afternoon (post lunch) vs early evening. Ergonomics 34:67.

International Federation of Multiple Sclerosis Societies. 1984. Symposium on a minimal record of disability for multiple sclerosis. Acta Neurol Scand 70(Suppl):101–217.

Jennison C, Turnbull BW. 1993. Group sequential tests for bivariate response: Interim analyses of clinical trials with both efficacy and safety endpoints. Biometrics 49:741.

Jones B, Kenward MG. 1989. Design and Analysis of Crossover Trials. New York, Chapman and Hall.

Kennedy RS, Turnage JJ, Wilkes RL. 1993. Effects of graded doses of alcohol on nine computerized repeated-measures tests. Ergonomics 36:1195.

Kepple G. 1982. Design and Analysis a Researcher's Handbook, 2nd ed. Englewood Cliffs, NJ, Prentice-Hall.

Kondraske GV. 1988a. Workplace design: An elemental resource approach to task analysis and human performance measurements. International Conference for the Advancement of Rehabilitation Technology, Montreal, Proceedings, pp 608–611.

Kondraske GV. 1988b. Experimental evaluation of an elemental resource model for human performance. Tenth Annual IEEE Engineering in Medicine and Biology Society Conference, New Orleans, Proceedings, pp 1612–1613.

Kondraske GV. 1989. Measurement science concepts and computerized methodology in the assessment of human performance. In T Munsat (ed), Quantification of Neurologic Deficit. Stoneham, Mass, Butterworth.

Kondraske GV. 1995. A working model for human system-task interfaces. In JD Bronzino (ed), Handbook of Biomedical Engineering. Boca Raton, Fla, CRC Press.

Levin RJ. 1986. Ethics and Regulation of Clinical Research, 2nd ed. Baltimore, Urban & Schwarzenberg.

Merkatz RB, Temple R, Sobel S. 1993. Women in clinical trials of new drugs: A change in Food and Drug Administration policy. N Engl J Med 329:292.

Mohr E, Prouwers P. 1991. Handbook of Clinical Trials: The Neurobehavioral Approach. Berwyn, Pa, Swets and Zeitlinger.

Ottenbacher KJ, Barrett KA. 1991. Measures of effect size in the reporting of rehabilitation research. Am J Phys Med Rehabil 70(suppl 1):S131.

Paty DE, Willoughby E, Whitakek J. 1992. Assessing the outcome of experimental therapies in multiple sclerosis. In Treatment of Multiple Sclerosis: Trial Design, Results, and Future Perspectives, pp 47–90. London, Springer-Verlag.

Potvin AR, Tourtellotte WWT, Potvin JH, et al. 1985. Quantitative Examination of Neurologic Function, vols I and II. Boca Raton, Fla, CRC Press.

Rose AS, Kuzma JW, Kurtzke JF, et al. 1968. Cooperative study in the evaluation of therapy in multiple sclerosis: ACTH vs placebo in acute exacerbations. Preliminary report. Neurolology 18:1.

Safrit MJ. 1990. Evaluation in Exercise Science. Englewood Cliffs, NJ, Prentice-Hall.

Salame P. 1991. The effects of alcohol in learning as a function of drinking habits. Ergonomics 34:1231.

Stone R. 1993. FDA to ask for data on gender differences. Science 260:743.

Syndulko K, Ke D, Ellison GW, et al. 1994*a*. Neuroperformance assessment of treatment efficacy and MS disease progression in the Cyclosporine Multicenter Clinical Trial. Brain (submitted).

Syndulko K, Ke D, Ellison GW, et al. 1994*b*. A comparative analysis of assessments for disease progression in multiple sclerosis: I. Signal to noise ratios and relationship among performance measures and rating scales. Brain (submitted).

Syndulko K, Tourtellotte WW, Baumhefner RW, et al. 1993. Neuroperformance evaluation of multiple sclerosis disease progression in a clinical trial. 7:69.

Tang D, Geller NL. 1993. On the design and analysis of randomized clinical trials with multiple endpoints. Biometrics 49:23.

The Multiple Sclerosis Study Group. 1990. Efficacy and toxicity of cyclosporine in chronic progressive multiple sclerosis: A randomized, double-blinded, placebo-controlled clinical trial. Ann Neurol 27:591.

Thomas JR, Nelson JK. 1990. Research Methods in Physical Activity, 2nd ed. Champaign, Il, Human Kinetics Publishers.

Tourtellotte WW, Haerer AF, Simpson JF, et al. 1965. Quantitative clinical neurological testing: I. A study of a battery of tests designed to evaluate in part the neurologic function of patients with multiple sclerosis and its use in a therapeutic trial. Ann NY Acad Sci 122:480.

Tudiver F, Bass MJ, Dunn EV, et al. 1992. Assessing Interventions Traditional and Innovative Methods. London, Sage Publications.

Weissman A. 1991. On the concept "study day zero." Perspect Biol Med 34:579.

Willoughby PD, Whitaker JE. 1992. Assessing the outcome of experimental therapies in multiple sclerosis. In RA Rudick, DE Goodkin (eds), Treatment of Multiple Sclerosis: Trial Design, Results, and Future Perspectives, pp 47–90. London, Springer-Verlag.

Woollacott MH. 1983. Effects of ethanol on postural adjustments in humans. Exp Neurol 80:55.

Further Information

The original monograph, *Experimental and Quasi-Experimental Designs for Research*, by D.T. Campbell and J.C. Stanley (Boston: Houghton Mifflin, 1964), is a classic experimental design text. The book *Statistics in Medicine*, by T. Colton (Boston: Little, Brown, 1982), examines statistical principles in medical research and identifies common perils when drawing conclusions from medical research. The book *Clinical Epidemiology: The Essentials*, R.H. Fletcher, S.W. Fletcher, and E.H. Wagner (2nd ed., Baltimore: Williams & Wilkins, 1982), is a readable text with concise descriptions of various types of studies. *Clinical Trials: Design, Conduct, and Analysis*, by C.L. Meinert (New York: Oxford University Press, 1986), is a comprehensive text covering most details and provides many helpful suggestions about clinical trials research. R.J. Porter and B.S. Schoenberg, *Controlled Clinical Trials in Neurological Disease* (Boston: Kluwer Academic Publishers, 1990), is also a comprehensive text covering clinical trials with a special emphasis on neurologic diseases.

151

Applications in Rehabilitation Engineering

Mark Strauss
*University of Illinois at
Urbana/Champaign*

Jon Gunderson
*University of Illinois at
Urbana/Champaign*

The other chapters in this section have discussed the measurement and expected performance parameters of the human possessing what could be termed *statistically normal functioning*. Disease or trauma can result in acute decrease in performance levels to be regained during the recuperation process, or they could result in permanent diminution or complete loss of functions. Similarly, congenital variation can result in reduced performance of discrete human functions. How does an impairment affect the abilities of that individual? Although the performance level of a discrete test may indicate that this person is in the first percentile for the entire population, how does his or her performance at an integrated task differ from that of the norm?

This chapter discusses the performance of people who have *disabilities*. The reader is cautioned not to assume that the performance level of an individual with a specific disability will be the same for another individual with the same disability, just as not all mobile individuals can successfully compete in a triathalon. Whereas a disability connotes a decrease in performance within an individual, a *handicap* exists when something in the environment prevents a person (with or without a disability) from accomplishing his or her intent. Although a wheelchair user can travel fine on a sidewalk and in a building, if he or she cannot enter the building because of a staircase, then the staircase is the cause of the handicap. Similarly, if the lights in a library are turned off while people are reading, that also will cause a major handicap to people who are sighted but will cause no handicap to someone who is blind. It is just a matter of perspective.

As proposed by Kondraske [1990], the human could be thought of as possessing discrete elements of abilities or performance that have been termed *basic elements of performance* (BEP). It could be assumed that we are all born with the same number and type of BEPs, and that what varies would be the magnitude of each. The statistically average individual would have BEP "scores" that would

0-8493-8346-3/95/$0.00+$.50

be measured to center around the population average, while a person with a disability would have one or more BEP scores either diminished or zero. A person who has had a stroke may have diminished ambulation ability and no ability to speak. In time, with education, therapy, and support, this person will learn to use the still functioning BEPs in order to compensate for lost function. In time, the increased use of these previously underutilized resources may result in an increase in that person's performance levels. Good examples of this are lip reading by people who are deaf and the increased torso musculature of young people with spinal cord injuries who use manual wheelchairs. The field of rehabilitation engineering seeks to maximize the abilities of persons with disabilities so that they can pursue and achieve as many desires as any other person. We all have different desires, often influenced by the stage of life we are in. The child yearns to play and interact on the playground. The young adult may seek to achieve a higher education to enter a career that will allow for independence. The homemaker desires to perform all the necessary tasks at home in order to care for the family. Each person must be considered unique. The combination of his or her disability, tasks he or she wants to accomplish, and the environment he or she must access all combine to present unique challenges. In order to design solutions to overcome handicapping situations, there are two key components. First, the capabilities of the individual must be evaluated to discriminate the areas of high and low performance. Second, the tasks must be analyzed to determine the levels of performance normally required. What is found is that the person possesses elements of performance that are normally used to accomplish some of the tasks and that these tasks require no intervention. What also may be found is that the limb strength or range of motion, sensory acuity, and cognition normally required to accomplish other tasks are not within the repertoire of the performance of the individual. In this latter case, other performance resources can be utilized, sometimes with technology extensions, in order to complete the tasks [Church, 1992].

In the effort to identify the performance resources, many of the same test regimens that have been developed for the average population can be administered to people with disabilities. Examples of these are the common refractory eye examination, range-of-motion evaluations, and standardized cognitive or dexterity tests. These are well documented and widely used, but other performance indicators specific to the disability realm are not as widely available. What follows in this chapter are two examples of how human performance engineering is quantifying the unique resources developed when disability reduces others. The next two sections provide a broad view of how human performance capabilities change and are compensated for in two different populations of people with disabilities. The last section is a case study on employment accommodations for a person with a visual impairment. Space limitations prevents the elaboration of other evaluation techniques or the psychosocial influences on the accommodation process. Some of these very important issues will be addressed in more detail in other chapters.

151.1 Wheelchair Propulsion Performance

There are dozens of wheelchair manufacturers, each producing different model wheelchairs, and many of these chairs have adjustable features. One set of adjustments can vary the rear axle position forward or back and up or down with respect to the user's shoulders. Another adjustment can vary the angle the rear wheels make with respect to the vertical. A big question is what are the optimal adjustments for a particular user? If manual wheelchair propulsion performance could be optimized, then maybe the high incidence of shoulder pain in manual wheelchair users can be avoided or at least reduced. It may be possible to increase the efficiency of the propulsion stroke based on the propulsion characteristics of the individual or to better evaluate these characteristics in order to determine if retraining is necessary. One methodology developed for evaluating propulsion performance uses technology similar to that used in test equipment for the able-bodied population.

The mobile wheelchair *ergometer* allows for three-dimensional resolution of the forces generated by the hand on the handrim of the wheel. Since this can be monitored throughout the entire propulsion cycle, along with information from a system that provides kinematic information about the user, cause-and-effect relationships can be determined. Propulsion performance can be measured in relation to energy output, maximum torque, and the user's position, to name just a few. By using the wheelchair ergometer, the data shown in Fig. 151.1 have been obtained. This figure shows two consecutive propulsion cycles of the left arm. This person is stroking the wheel approximately at once per second. The figure shows the forces of the hand tangential to the hand rim, radially in toward the wheel hub, and directed perpendicular to the plane of the wheel. These curves can be examined for the relative magnitudes between these vectors within a propulsion cycle and between cycles. Even though the two cycles shown in Fig. 151.1 are consecutive, it is observed that they are not the same. Of particular interest is the force applied perpendicular to the plane of the wheel. This force provides no direct propulsive contribution, but for the first cycle the magnitude of this force is 28% of the magnitude of the tangential component. The second cycle shows almost no out-of-plane forces exerted. This would indicate that this person is not performing his or her propulsive activity consistently. What still needs to be determined is which profile is most efficient.

151.2 High-Speed Speech Perception by People with Blindness

The access to computers by people who are blind is frequently accomplished by using a voice output screen access system that takes text information on the computer screen and outputs it through a speech synthesizer for the user to hear [Edwards, 1991]. To increase the rate of interaction with the computer, many people with blindness increase the speech rate of their synthesizer to rates that are more than three times normal conversational rates (typical conversational rates are 150 to 180 words per minute). At high speech rates, the speech generated by the synthesizer sounds unintelligible to the casual untrained listener, but many people with blindness are understanding the information with over 90% accuracy at 350 words per minute (wpm). Figure 151.2 shows the mean of performance of speech intelligibility as speech rate is increased for a group of 24 sighted individuals without any experience with accelerated synthesized speech and for a group of 8 persons with blindness who have used speech synthesis to access computers for at least 2 years prior to the study. The sighted group shows a consistently lower level of performance as speech rate increases. Three of the subjects with blindness demonstrate only a slight decrease in intelligibility as speech rate is increased. The three subjects are understanding the accelerated speech at over twice the level of intelligibility as the

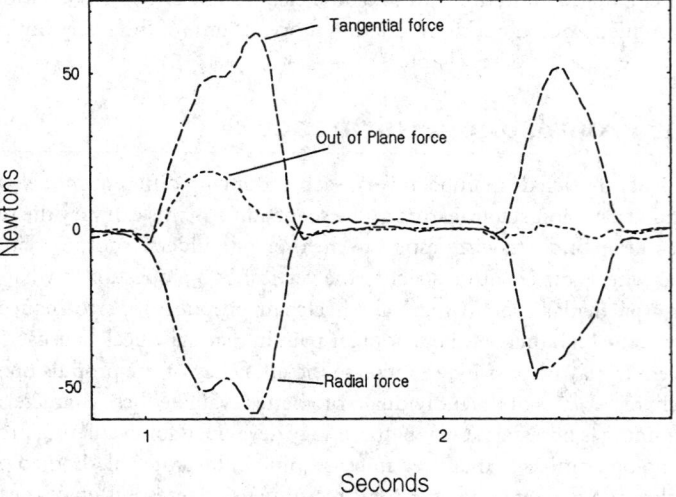

FIGURE 151.1   By using an instrumented wheelchair ergometer, the force profiles of the hand on the handrim during two propulsion cycles are displayed.

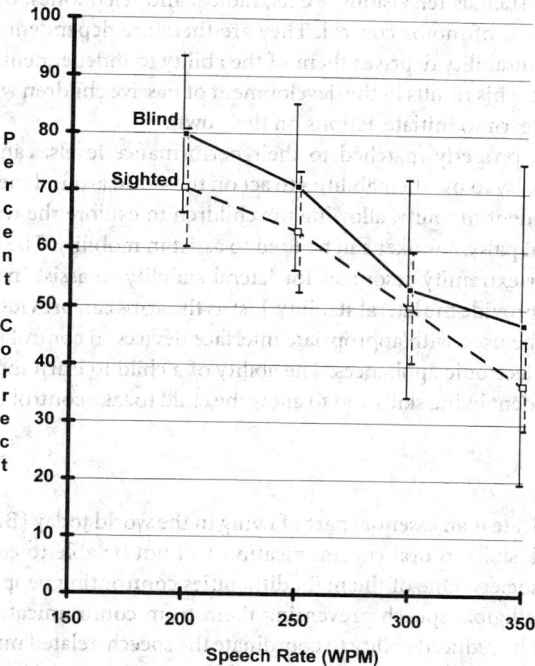

FIGURE 151.2 Mean percentage of words correct versus speech rate by group.

best sighted subjects at the 350-wpm speech rate. Clearly these three people have developed a skill that the average person does not develop. The unique skill can be attributed to the motivation to increase the synthesizer speech rate to improve the rate interaction with the computer and the high level of exposure to synthesized speech the participants receive. People with blindness therefore develop unique resources to help them perform at their highest level when using speech to access computer information.

151.3 Children with Cerebral Palsy

Cerebral palsy is a congenital disability that is the result of oxygen deprivation to the brain during birth which can result in any combination of motor, sensory, and cognitive impairments. The motor characteristics of a person with cerebral palsy can vary from only a slight gait anomaly to severe forms that limit almost all voluntary motion. Many children with cerebral palsy have normal intelligence, but severe physical disabilities can cause developmental delays due to lack of varied age-appropriate experience. Therefore, it is important to integrate children with disabilities into age-appropriate settings as early in life as possible to allow them to develop an awareness that they can affect the world around them. The inclusion needs to provide activities and assistive technology for the children with disabilities to participate and interact with their peers. *Assistive technology* [Church, 1992] is equipment that provides an important bridge between the capabilities of persons with disabilities to interact in their environment [Barrier Free Environments Inc., 1993] and to communicate with peers.

Daily Living

Many activities that most people take for granted in their daily life are impossible for some people with severe forms of cerebral palsy. Children with cerebral palsy may be unable to eat independently, control common items such as televisions, VCRs, radios, and telephones, or independently move themselves due to the loss of motor control. They are therefore dependent on others for most of these daily tasks. Their disability deprives them of the ability to independently explore and manipulate their environment. This results in the development of passive children who respond only when stimulated and do not learn to initiate actions on their own.

Assistive technology, properly matched to their performance levels, can provide a means for children with cerebral palsy to use their abilities to act on the world around them. The use of a wheelchair can offer independent mobility, allowing the children to explore the world on their own. For milder forms of cerebral palsy, a walker can be used to assist in mobility. The walker allows a person to use his or her upper extremity resources for lateral stability to assist in walking, reducing the demands on the legs to provide the lateral stability. Just as the arms can provide assistance in mobility, good head control can be used with appropriate interface devices to control televisions, computers, telephones, and other electronic appliances. The ability of a child to learn independence is essential for developing independent living skills and to allow the child to take control over his or her own life.

Communication

Being able to communicate is an essential part of living in the world today [Bukalmen & Mirendam, 1992]. People who lack skills in oral communication will not be able to easily participate in our information-oriented society. One of the main difficulties confronting people with severe forms of cerebral palsy is unintelligible speech preventing them from communicating their thoughts and needs to other people. The reduced ability to coordinate the speech-related musculature can be overcome by a range of assistive technologies from low-technology pointing boards to high-technology electronic speech output systems. Pointing boards range in simplicity from large cards, with a simple alphabet and a few words printed on it mounted to a wheelchair lap tray, to multipage notebooks with each page containing lists of words and phrases on different topics the user wants to communicate. People with cerebral palsy use their hand- or head-pointing capabilities to spell out words or to directly point to frequently used words or phrases printed on their board. Pointing to complete words or phrases increases the rate of message transfer as long as the time necessary to visually scan the choices and locate the word/phrase is not unduly long.

The pointing techniques can be extended to electronic assistive technology that utilizes speech output. Forming a phrase by pointing to an electronic keyboard with a finger, toe, or the head results in electronic speech production. This is essential when making presentations to groups, talking on the telephone, and in other situations where the listener may not be in a position to see a pointing board or does not understand how to use it. Because cerebral palsy can significantly impede message production, long messages need to be prepared ahead of time or risk loosing the listener's attention while the message is being formed. For example, one person with cerebral palsy uses a high-quality DECTalk speech synthesizer for making group presentations. He prepares his speech ahead of time, utilizing the adjustable voice attributes of the DECTalk to emphasize different points during his presentation. He also programs in a number of potential responses to questions after his main talk. His preparation of materials ahead of time is a skill he needs to develop if he is going to make timely presentations and responses to questions. For people with cerebral palsy, assistive technology can bridge the gap between their physical capabilities and the verbal communication people expect for most conversations.

Literacy

Reading and writing are compromised for people with severe cerebral palsy. Their movement impairments do not allow them to write with their hands or manipulate books for reading. But the cognitive skills of being able to read and write are important resources for people with cerebral palsy to develop. Their physical disabilities will limit their ability to do manual work; therefore, to participate in employment they will need to be in jobs that require primarily cognitive skills. These types of jobs require individuals to effectively read, evaluate, and prepare written materials for other people. For a physically challenged person, a personal computer and readily available assistive technologies will augment limited range-of-motion performance and allow for written communication and access to a plethora of knowledge using CD-ROM technology and worldwide computer networks.

151.4 Independent Living Skills for Stroke Victims

People with brain injuries from a stroke have abrupt changes in their physical, cognitive, and sensory resources. The changes typically result in the loss of capabilities that in some cases can be almost fully restored with speech, physical, and occupational therapies over a period of several months to a year [Wehman & Kreutzer, 1990]. However, in many cases the abilities never fully return, requiring the person to develop new compensatory skills, modify his or her environment, and/or use assistive technology for increasing his or her functional capabilities. Permanent changes in a person's resources can include physical capabilities such as paralysis or weakness, memory loss, hearing and speech disorders, visual and spatial disorders, and cognitive reasoning and personality changes to name a few. The range of possible deficits that can result from head injury varies extensively from person to person and on the location and size of the injury in the brain.

Mobility

One of the key items for living independently is mobility [Hobson, 1990]. Mobility varies from maneuvering in a house to going across town to visit a friend. There are two types of resources required for mobility that can be affected in stroke victims: physical capacity and cognitive processing. Some strokes result in the partial or total loss of muscle control on one side of the body. The loss of innervation results in atrophy of the muscles on the affected side, resulting in asymmetrical physical and proprioception capabilities that adversely affect coordination and posture. Less severe hemiplegia may require only a cane or walker to assist in stability. More severe loss of motor control may require a wheelchair with either a one-hand drive mechanism or motor drive capability. The type of assistive technology for mobility needs to match the level of ability. People who drive an automobile may require additional hand and foot controls to allow them to operate the vehicle with the unaffected areas of their body. The placement of controls within the reach of their unaffected limbs allows them to control the vehicle safely.

Physical capabilities are only one aspect of the mobility problem. Reduction of cognitive resources can cause forgetfulness or disorientation, resulting in the person getting lost. Memory devices such as writing down where the person is going can be used to assist in the short-term memory loss. Confusion requires more mobility retraining to learn new navigation skills. It may require learning to travel during less busy times of the day or to use routes that are less heavily traveled to reduce the distractions that could lead to confusion. Less traveled routes have lower levels of visual and auditory stimulation, which reduces the number of distractions that the user must deal with, increasing the cognitive resources available to concentrate on remembering the route and purpose of the trip. The use of written reminders can be problematic, since the person often forgets to look at them. However, automatic electronic memory aids with voice output can be used to remind the stroke victim of where he or she has to be and at what time. The automatic auditory output does not require the user to remember to look at their notebook to receive the message.

Personal Hygiene/Dressing

For people with reduced physical function due to stroke, the ability to independently perform daily dressing and hygiene activities may require assistance. Simple mechanical reachers can be used to extend the working volume and access items on high shelves. In the bathroom, the addition of grab bars around the toilet and the bathtub can provide stability and support as people sit and stand by allowing them to use the intact performance of their arms and hands in supporting and coordinating movement. A toilet can be raised and a seat put in the bathtub to reduce the distance people need to lift themselves. The adaptations demand fewer physical resources and less coordination. If a wheelchair is used, the environment can be modified to facilitate lateral transfers to beds, toilets, and bathtubs. The use of a lateral transfer technique requires the stroke victim only to have enough strength and coordination to make side-to-side movements, eliminating much of the strength and coordination required for lifting and lowering the body.

Food Preparation and Eating

The ability to use only one hand can make it very difficult to perform basic cooking and eating functions. But loss of the use of one hand can be compensated with the use of simple assistive technologies. Typically, one hand is dominant during cooking and eating, while the other hand has the passive role of holding the food. The dominant hand performs the fine motor skill of cutting, stirring, chopping, and other food-handling operations. Cutting boards can be fitted with small spikes for holding the food, allowing the person to use only one hand to cut. The use of Dycem, a thin sheet that is tacky on both sides, can prevent bowls and plates from moving while mixing or cutting, thus requiring the use of only one hand for these operations. Eating utensils can be purchased with wider grips or straps to reduce the amount of movement or grasp required to use the utensil. There are just a few examples of the wide range of kitchen and eatingware that has been designed specifically for people with physical impairments. They complement existing physical resources in order to reduce the effect of the diminished resources.

Literacy

One potential loss of functional resources associated with strokes is visual processing problems. People will be able to see words but cannot identify them. Their visual processing system may make the words appear unrecognizable. Some people have only half their normal visual field, so they can only see items on their left or right side. The problem is complex because turning the head does not always compensate for the loss of vision on one side to see an entire scene. They have lost the ability to integrate visual information on their left- and right-hand sides, making it difficult to perceive the wholeness of objects, including text and images from books and computer screens. The visual processing problems affect the ability to read, write, and use computers, since people have trouble seeing or integrating the print information. Even though visual processing capabilities are reduced, the auditory system may be intact. If visually presented information is translated to speech form, people can still access the printed material or the information on a computer screen. Optical character-recognition programs for computers can be coupled to a speech synthesizer to provide people access to books and other printed materials. Computer programs to read selected portions of computer screens have been developed to add speech-reading capabilities to computer systems. The concept of redundancy in the display of information is important to allow people with reduction of one sensory resource to compensate with another sensory resource.

151.5 Case Study: Computer Access by People with Blindness

A state agency that employs five people with blindness and two people with severe visual impairments is computerizing its offices around the state. The computers are used for word processing, filling out forms, and accessing a network database on people who use the services of the state agency. All employees of the state agency are required to use the system to reduce secretarial and record-keeping costs. Administrators of the agency are concerned that the employees with visual impairments will not be able to use the computer system because they cannot see the monitors. The employees with visual impairments need to use their nonvisual senses as resources to receive information about what is on the computer screen for writing and access to the computerized management system.

Display Alternatives to the Computer Screen

Information on the computer screen needs to be presented to people with blindness through either a speech synthesizer, tactile imaging device such as a dynamic Braille display (6- to 8-dot patterns used to represent ASCII characters), or a tactile imaging system (images of the object perceived through mechanical or electrical stimulation of the skin). Electronic speech synthesizers convert text on the computer screen to a voice that can be heard by the person with blindness. Dynamic Braille displays provide a means for persons to read character information from the screen with their fingers. Tactile imaging technology is a means for representing pictorial images of text, graphs, pictures, icons, and other graphic information that is difficult to convert to representations in speech or Braille formats. The tactile images that are presented on the skin through mechanical or electrical stimulation are difficult to interpret due to the characteristics and resolution of skin perception. For tactile imaging technology to be usable, people require special training. Even with training, users of the Optacon (a commercial tactile imaging technology) have been measured to have a typical maximum reading rate of only 10 to 12 wpm [Schiff & Foulke, 1982].

The decision of whether to use synthetic speech output, dynamic Braille display, or both is dependent on the type of task the user is trying to complete. From the user's perspective, synthetic speech is less intelligible than human speech, but the intelligibility improves with practice. Most users report that they can acceptably understand the speech after a few weeks of constant use. Experienced computer users with blindness develop unique perceptual resources to understand their speech synthesizers speaking at very fast rates with little loss in understanding (see above). The high rate of speech allows users to increase their abilities to interact with the computer.

Synthesized Speech Displays

Synthesized speech, though very good for many tasks, is not ideal for all tasks. It is difficult to detect spelling mistakes with speech, since the quality of the synthesizer's voices often makes misspelled words sound acceptable. Abbreviations and format information are often difficult to understand. For example, in WordPerfect for MS-DOS, the bottom of the screen has document and cursor status information such as "Doc 1 Pg 1 Ln 1.35″ Pos 2.36″," which the user often hears as a continuous sentence "Doc One Pee Gee One L N one period three five quote Pos two period three six quote." The information would be better spoken as "Document one ⟨pause⟩ Page one ⟨pause⟩ Line one and thirty-five hundredths inch ⟨pause⟩ Position two and thirty-six hundredths inch." The ability of screen review programs (SRP) to make this type of translation requires the user to use less cognitive resources to understand the information presented. This type of translation is currently not available with screen review programs. In this and many other situations, the blind user must devote cognitive resources to the secondary task of making his or her own mental translations of information spoken to what in means in the current computer task, leading to lower performance on the primary task. The result is that useful information may be ignored since it is not readily apparent what the information presented means, or the mental translations are never learned well enough to be used effectively. Speech is most effective when the information is primarily prose text, such as in a word processor or text descriptions in a database program.

Dynamic Braille Displays

Dynamic Braille, the primary alternative to synthetic speech for computer access, is similar to the use of print by sighted persons. Braille allows the blind user to receive more spatial information about screen character relationships and the exact characters presented on the computer screen.

Dynamic Braille displays are usually a single line or dual lines of 20 to 80 Braille cells. Each cell consists of 8 dots that are felt with the user's fingers. The 8 dots are used to represent the 256 ASCII characters used on most computer displays to represent the alphabet, punctuation, and special characters. In general, users of dynamic Braille displays have lower reading rates (50 to 150 wpm) compared with listening to synthetic speech (150 to 600 wpm), but Braille provides greater detail in character formatting. From the user's perspective, dynamic Braille displays can be thought of as a small window of the actual computer screen. The Braille cells are read with the fingers, and therefore, the user has more temporal control over the reading rate of the characters. The user can easily adjust his or her reading rate to the difficulty of the material as it is read, similar to a sighted persons scanning a printed page with his or her eyes. Control over reading rates increases performance by reducing errors and the need to read information more than once. Speech synthesizer technologies do have variable speech rates, but the adjustment is often an off-line process that requires additional time and skill to adjust. Braille also provides detailed character information and relationships. In the preceding example it is easier for people to decode the WordPerfect status line information "Doc 1 Pg 1 Ln 1.35″ Pos 2.36‴" in Braille rather than in speech, since the user can feel the relationships between the characters. Braille is therefore a more natural medium to use where detailed character information is needed, as in programming computers, or where spatial information is important, as in a spreadsheet. A negative aspect of dynamic Braille is that it requires the user to take his or her hands off the keyboard to read the Braille. The user needs to keep moving his or her hands back and forth between the Braille display and the keyboard, which results in slowing down of the interaction between the user and the computer.

Cognitive Resources Required for Screen Review Programs

There are high cognitive demands placed on people with blindness to use computer access systems due to the incomplete translation of the computer screen information to a nonvisual form. The two-dimensional layout of information on the screen is often difficult to translate to an audible form that maintains a sense of the location and meaning of information on the screen. The burden for making these translations is placed on users to take the limited spatial information they receive and then to reconstruct the layout and meaning of items on the computer screen.

In order to use alternative output devices such as speech, Braille, or other nonvisual display technologies, an additional program is needed. The additional program is called a *screen review program*. Screen review programs (SRP) allow the blind user to "view" different areas on a computer screen using speech and/or Braille. SRPs have their own set of keyboard commands to allow the user to control where on the screen information is presented from. SRPs typically have little, if any, knowledge about the application program the user is using, so it places the burden on the user to know where information is on the computer screen. Users issue special SRP commands to "view" the information they want and to keep the reader from presenting information they do not want. The blind user has the difficult task of developing detailed knowledge about what's on a computer screen that he or she has never seen. For novice computer users, the lack of screen layout knowledge is compounded by their lack of familiarity with computer tasks and terminology. The task of learning to use a computer system for a person with blindness is therefore more difficult than for a sighted person. The person with blindness must learn both the commands related to the application program and then another set of different commands for the screen review program to read screen information back in a meaningful way. The user is, in essence, learning to use two programs at the same time and often has little conceptual knowledge of the dual tasks he or she is performing. Some tasks are easier to learn than others, such as reading sentences and words that are on the screen of a word processor. But some other tasks are almost impossible, since spatial formatting information is often lost with synthetic speech (the most common technique for people to interact with computers in the United States), and the resulting speech often sounds like a string of random numbers, letters, and punctuation marks. One example of the translation problem is setting tabs in WordPerfect for MS-DOS where the letters *L, R,* and *C* are used for identifying the tab type. The letters appear below a line of dashes and plus sign characters used to represent a ruler bar for indicating the location of the tab stops. The spatial layout of the characters for the tab stops is important to what the character represents, but the spatial layout information is beyond the capabilities of current speech synthesizer technology to represent the spatial information. Dynamic Braille technologies may help, but only if is a multiline display to view both lines at the same time (very few people have this technology available to them due to the expense). Therefore, the blind computer user must devote more of his or her cognitive resources to understanding, interpreting, and planning of commands to read the computer screen than sighted peers. The diversion of cognitive resources to the screen reading task reduces the resources away from their primary task of what the person is using the computer for originally, such as writing a report, calculating a budget, writing a program, or accessing client information from a database.

The transformation of information from a visual computer display to an alternative nonvisual display places a burden on the blind user's cognitive resources to determine how the nonvisual information he or she receives relates to the visual information on the computer screen and the task the computer is presenting. Sometimes the transformation is straightforward, but in many cases the mental translation is difficult, if not impossible, due to cryptic and sparse information available to the person with blindness resulting from the capabilities of current screen access systems. The transformation results in a higher likely hood of errors, an underutilization of the computer's capabilities, and additional time to complete tasks. An improvement in the design of screen review technologies can increase the capabilities and the level of performance of people with blindness.

Job Accommodation

To accommodate workers in this case study who were blind, the state agency purchased screen review software for use with speech output. The word processor WordPerfect for MS-DOS is used for writing reports and filling out forms. Forms are created using standard WordPerfect documents. Each item on the form is displayed on one line of the document so that the form can be filled out using simple cursor control commands. A special version of the database software was created that placed only one item on each line of the computer screen. A speech cue provides automatic speech prompting to the blind user to indicate which item in the database he or she is on. The use of one item on a line with an autospeak indicator for the screen review program reduces the demands on the blind user to know where information is on the display and eliminates the extra time required to seek out and read information on the computer screen using screen review commands. A dynamic Braille display was not used because none of the tasks required the reading of detailed character information and there was very little spatial information of importance in any of the tasks. Even though some people may have preferred Braille displays, it was felt that the advanced users with blindness could provide better peer support if all the systems were the same.

One important aspect was the extensive training provided to help the employees to develop skill with the screen access technology. The training increased the individual skills and capabilities of each employee to use and apply screen review functions to read the screen and to explore new application programs. Training is critical due to the knowledge needed about screen review commands for them to be used effectively to access the computer screen and achieve a high level of performance in completing the desired task with the computer.

151.6 Conclusion

The passage of the Americans with Disabilities Act of 1990 highlights society's desire for the full inclusion of people with disabilities. For full inclusion to take place, people with disabilities must be provided with the skills and technology they need to participate in the recreational, education, and employment opportunities available to their peers. The role of rehabilitation engineering is to design and develop the assistive technology to bridge the functional capabilities of a person with disabilities to the task he or she wants to complete. In order to meet the challenge, we must be able to quantitatively define the functional capabilities of a person and the task the person is trying to complete. This is why human performance evaluation is critical for the further evolution of a more equitable society.

Defining Terms

Braille: Braille is a reading system for people with blindness. Braille uses 6 to 8 raised dots to represent letters, numbers, and punctuation. Braille is read by using the tips of the fingers to feel the raised dot patterns. There are different grades of Braille. Grade I is a direct character-for-character mapping of printed text to Braille cells. Grades II and III use contractions and codes to compress the number of characters used to represent words and phrases. The contractions increase reading speeds and reduce the physical volume of the Brailled materials.

Cerebral palsy: A condition due to incomplete brain development or trauma during the first few years of life. It results in motor impairments that can show symptoms unilaterally or symmetrically. The physical impairments can include paralysis, weakness, uncontrollable random movements, and/or loss of fine motor control of the extremities, trunk, and head.

Disability: Defined by World Health Organization (WHO) as "any restriction or lack of ability to perform an activity in the manner or within the range considered normal for a human being." Disability refers to a person's physical, sensory, or cognitive capabilities and not to the ability to do a particular task.

Ergonomer: An apparatus for measuring the amount of work done by a human for a particular task.

Handicap: Defined by WHO as "problems in performing highly valued roles." Handicap therefore refers to the ability to do a functional task such as typing a letter on a standard typewriter.

References

Barrier Free Environments Inc. 1993. UFAS Retrofit Guide: Accessibility Modification for Existing Buildings. New York, Van Nostrand Reinhold.

Bukalmen DR, Mirendam P. 1992. Augmentative and Alternative Communication: Management of Severe Communication Disorders in Children and Adults. Baltimore, Paul H Brookes.

Church G. 1992. The Handbook of Assistive Technology. San Diego, Singular Publication Group.

Edwards ADN. 1991. Speech Synthesis: Technology for disabled people. Baltimore, Paul H Brookes.

Kondraske GV. 1990. Quantitative measurement and assessment of function. In RV Smith, JH Leslie (eds), Rehabilitation Engineering, pp 101–126. Boca Raton, Fla, CRC Press.

Hobson DA. 1990. Seating and mobility for the severely disabled. In RV Smith, JH Leslie (eds), Rehabilitation Engineering, pp 193–252. Boca Raton, Fla, CRC Press.

Schiff W, Foulke E (eds). 1982. Tactual Perception: A Sourcebook. New York, Cambridge University Press.

Wehman P, Kreutzer J. 1990. Vocational Rehabilitation: For Persons with Traumatic Brain Injury. Rockville, Md, Aspen Publishers.

Further Information

The *IEEE Transactions on Rehabilitation Engineering* is devoted to engineering research into the design of assistive technology for people with disabilities and is available from IEEE Service Center, 445 Hoes Lane, P.O. Box 1331, Piscataway, NJ 08855-1331. The *Proceedings of RESNA Conferences* is a good source for current issues in the research, design, and application of assistive technology and is available from RESNA PRESS, 1700 North Moore Street, Suite 1540, Arlington, VA 22209. *Assistive Technology* is the official journal of RESNA and publishes articles on both research and clinical practice of applying assistive technology and is available from RESNA Press, 1700 North Moore Street, Suite 1540, Arlington, VA 22209. *Technology and Disability* is a quarterly journal that deals with the application of rehabilitative and assistive technology for persons with disabilities, particularly in the performance of major life functions: education, employment, and recreation; it is available from Journal Fulfillment Department, Andover Medical, 80 Montvale Avenue, Stoneham, MA 02180. *Rehabilitation Research and Development* is a journal supported by the Department of Veterans Affairs and deals with a wide range of engineering design issues of assistive technology primarily for people with physical disabilities; it is available from Scientific and Technical Publications Section, Rehabilitation Research and Development Service, 103 South Gay Street, 5th floor, Baltimore, MD 21202-4051. The National Institute on Disability Rehabilitation Research (NIDRR) is a part of the Department of Education and funds 18 Rehabilitation Engineering Research Centers (RERC) and 40 Research and Training Centers (RTC) around the country. Each research center focuses on different types of research in rehabilitation. Each RERC and RTC also has a clinical and information dissemination component; contact NIDRR for a list of the location and research focus of the current RERCs and RTCs. The Job Accommodation Network is a national information resource on job accommodations for people with disabilities. The Job Accommodation Network is located at P. O. Box 6080, Morgantown, WV, 26506-6080. ABLEDATA is an electronic database (CD-ROM, BBS) of currently available assistive technology for people with disabilities. The database is currently available from Micro International, 8455 Colesville Road, Suite 935, Silver Spring, MD 2010-3319. CO-NET is an electronic database (CD-ROM, Internet) of rehabilitation materials including products, services, and legislation. It is available from the Trace Research and Development Center, 1500 Highland Avenue, Madison, WI, 53705-2280.

152

Applications of Quantitative Assessment of Human Performance in Occupational Medicine

Mohamad Parnianpour
Ohio State University

As early as 1700, Bernardino Ramazzini, one of the founders of occupational medicine, had associated certain physical activities with musculoskeletal disorders (MSD). He postulated that certain violent and irregular motions and unnatural postures of the body impair the internal structure [Snook et al., 1988]. Presently, much effort is directed toward a better understanding of work-related musculoskeletal disorders involving the back, cervical spine, and upper extremities. The World Health Organization (WHO) has defined occupational diseases as those work-related diseases where the relationship to specific causative factors at work has been fully established [WHO, 1985]. Other work-related diseases may have a weaker or unclear association to working conditions. They may be aggravated, accelerated, or exacerbated by workplace factors and lead to impairment of workers' performance. Hence obtaining the occupational history is crucial to proper diagnosis and appropriate treatment of work-related disorders. The occupational physician must consider the conditions of both the workplace and the worker in evaluation of injured workers. Biomechanical and ergonomic evaluators have developed a series of techniques for quantification of the task demands and evaluation of the stresses in the workplace. Functional capacity evaluation also has been advanced to quantify the maximum performance capability of workers. The motto of ergonomics is to avoid the mismatch between the task demand and functional capacity of individuals. A multidisciplinary group of physicians and engineers constitutes the rehabilitation team that will work together to

0-8493-8346-3/95/$0.00+$.50
© 1995 by CRC Press, Inc.

implement the prevention measures. Through proper workplace design, workplace stressors could be minimized. It is expected that one-third of the compensatable low back pain in industry could be prevented by proper ergonomic workplace or task design. In addition to reducing the probability of both the initial and recurring episodes, proper ergonomic design allows earlier return to work of injured workers by keeping the task demands at a lower level. Unfortunately, ergonomists are often asked to redesign the task or the workplace after a high incidence of injuries has already been experienced. The next preventive measure that has been suggested is preplacement of workers based on the medical history, strength, and physical examinations [Snook et al., 1988]. Training and education have been the third prevention strategy in the reduction of musculoskeletal disorders. Some components of these educational packages such as "back schools" and the teaching of "proper body mechanics" have been used in the rehabilitation phase of injured workers as well.

Title I of the Americans with Disability Act [ADA, 1990] prohibits discrimination with regard to any aspect of the employment process. Thus the development of preplacement tests has been impeded by the possibility of discrimination against individuals based on gender, age, or medical condition. The ADA requires physical tests to simulate the "essential functions" of the task. In addition, one must be aware of "reasonable accommodations," such as lifting aids, that may make an otherwise infeasible task possible for a disabled applicant to perform. Healthcare providers who perform physical examinations and provide recommendations for job applicants must consider the rights of disabled applicants. It is extremely crucial to quantify the specific physical requirements of the job to be performed and to examine an applicant's capabilities to perform those specific tasks, taking into account any reasonable accommodations that may be provided. Hence task analysis and functional capacity assessment are truly intertwined.

Work-related disorders of the upper extremities, unlike low back disorders, can better be related to specific anatomic sites such as a tendon or compressed nerve. Examples of the growing number of cumulative trauma disorders of the upper extremities and the neck are carpal tunnel syndrome (CTS), DeQuervain's disease, trigger finger, lateral epicondylitis (tennis elbow), rotator cuff tendinitis, thoracic outlet syndrome, and tension neck syndrome. The prevalence of these disorders is higher among some specific jobs, such as meat cutters, welders, sewer workers, grinders, meat packers, and keyboard operators. Some of the common risk factors leading to pain, impairment, and physical damage in the neck and upper extremities are forceful motion, repetitive motion, vibration, prolonged awkward posture, and mechanical stress [Kroemer et al., 1994].

This chapter is intended to illustrate the application of some principles and practices of human performance engineering, especially quantification of human performance in the field of occupational medicine. I have selected the problem of low back pain to illustrate a series of concepts that are essential to evaluation of both the worker and the workplace, while realizing the importance of the disorders of the neck and upper extremities. By inference and generalization, most of these concepts can be extended to these situations.

152.1 Principles

Assessment of function across various dimensions of performance (i.e., strength, speed, endurance, and coordination) has provided the basis for a rational approach to clinical assessment, rehabilitation strategies, and determination of return-to-work potential for injured employees [Kondraske, 1990]. To understand the complex problem of trunk performance evaluation of low back pain (LBP) patients, the terminology of muscle exertion must first be defined. However, it should be noted that a number of excellent reviews of trunk muscle function have been performed [Andersson, 1991; Beimborn & Morrissey, 1988; Newton & Waddell, 1993; Pope, 1992]. I do not intend to reproduce this extensive literature here, since my motive is to provide a critical analysis that will lead the reader toward an understanding of the future of functional assessment techniques. A more extensive clinical application is presented in Spalski and Parnianpour [1994].

Impairment, Disability, and Handicap

The tremendous human suffering and economic costs of disability present a formidable medical, social, and political challenge in the midst of growing healthcare costs and scarcity of resources. The WHO [1980] distinguished among impairment, disability, and handicap. *Impairment* is any loss or abnormality of psychological, physiologic, or anatomic structure or function—impairment reflects disturbances at the organ level. *Disability* is any restriction or lack of ability (resulting from impairment) to perform an activity in the manner or within the range considered normal for a human being—disability reflects disturbances at the level of person. *Handicap* is a disadvantage for a given individual, resulting from an impairment or a disability, that limits or prevents the fulfillment of a role that is normal (depending on age, sex, and social and cultural factors) for that individual. Since disability is the objectification of an impairment, handicap represents the socialization of an impairment or disability. Despite the immense improvement presented by the International Classification of Impairments, Disabilities, and Handicaps (ICIDH), the classification is limited from an industrial medicine or rehabilitation perspective. The hierarchical organization lacks the specificity required for evaluating the functional state of an individual with respect to task demands.

Kondraske [1990] has suggested an alternative approach using the principles of resource economics. The resource economics paradigm is reflective of the principal goal of ergonomics: fitting the demands of the task to the functional capability of the worker. The Elemental Resource Model (ERM) is based on the application of general performance theory that presents a unified theory for measurement, analysis, and modeling of human performance across all different aspects of performance, across all human subsystems, and at any hierarchical level. This approach uses the same bases to describe both the fundamental dimensions of performance capacity and task demand (available and utilized resources) of each functional unit involved in performance of the high-level tasks. The elegance of the ERM is due to its hierarchical organization, allowing causal models to be generated based on assessment of the task demands and performance capabilities across the same dimensions of performance [Kondraske, 1990].

Muscle Action and Performance Quantification

The details of the complex processes of muscle contraction in terms of the bioelectrical, biochemical, and biophysical interactions are under intense research. Muscle tension is a function of muscle length and its rate of change and can be scaled by the level of neural excitation. These relationships are called the *length-tension* and *velocity-tension relationships*. From a physiologic point of view, the measured force or torque applied at the interface is a function of (1) the individual's motivation (magnitude of the neural drive for excitation and activation processes), (2) environmental conditions (muscle length, rate of change of muscle length, nature of the external load, metabolic conditions, pH level, temperature, and so forth), (3) prior history of activation (fatigue), (4) instructions and descriptions of the tasks given to the subject, (5) the control strategies and motor programs employed to satisfy the demands of the task, and (6) the biophysical state of the muscles and fitness (fiber composition, physiologic cross-sectional area of the muscle, cardiovascular capability). It cannot be overemphasized that these processes are complex and interrelated [Kroemer et al., 1994]. Other factors that may affect the performance of patients are misunderstanding of the degree of effort needed in maximal testing, test anxiety, depression, nociception, fear of pain and reinjury, as well as unconscious and conscious symptom magnification.

The following sections review some methods to quantify performance and lifting capability of isolated trunk muscles during a multilink coordinated manual materials handling task. Relevant factors that influence the static and dynamic strength and endurance measures of trunk muscles will be addressed, and the clinical applications of these assessment techniques will be illustrated.

The central nervous system (CNS) appropriately excites the muscle, and the generated tension is transferred to the skeletal system by the tendon to cause motion, stabilize the joint, and/or resist the effect of external forces on the body. Hence the functional evaluation of muscles cannot be performed without the characterization of the interfaced mechanical environment.

The four fundamental types of muscle exertion or action are isometric, isokinetic, isotonic, and isoinertial. In *isometric* exertion, the muscle length is kept constant, and there is no movement. Although mechanical work is not achieved, physiologic work, i.e., static work, is performed, and energy is consumed. When the internal force exerted by the muscle is greater than the external force offered by the resistance, then concentric, i.e., shortening, muscle action occurs, whereas if the muscle is already activated and the external force exceeds the internal force of the muscle, then eccentric, i.e., lengthening, muscle action occurs. When the muscle moves, either concentrically or eccentrically, dynamic work is performed. If the rate of shortening or lengthening of the muscle is constant, the exertion is called *isokinetic*. When the muscle acts on a constant inertial mass, the exertion is called *isoinertial*. *Isotonic* action occurs when the muscle tension is constant throughout the range of motion.

These definitions are very clear when dealing with isolated muscles during physiologic investigations. However, terminology employed in the literature of strength evaluation is imprecise. The terms are intended to refer to the state of muscles, but they actually refer to the state of the mechanical interface, i.e., the dynamometer. Isotonic exertion, as defined, is not as realizable physiologically because muscular tensions change as its lever arm changes despite the constancy of external loads. Special designs may vary the resistance level in order to account for changes in mechanical efficiency of the muscles. In addition, the rate of muscle length change may not remain constant even when the joint angular velocity is regulated by the dynamometer during isokinetic exertions. During isoinertial action, the net external resistance is not only a function of the mass (inertia) but also a function of the acceleration. The acceleration, however, is a function of the input energy to the mass. Hence, to fully characterize the net external resistance, we need to have both the acceleration and the inertial parameters (mass and moment of inertia) of the load and body parts. Future research should better quantify the inertial effects of the dynamometers, particularly during nonisometric and nonisokinetic exertions.

For any joint or joint complex, muscle performance can be quantified in terms of the basic dimensions of performance: strength, speed, endurance, steadiness, and coordination. Muscle *strength* is the capacity to produce torque or work by voluntary activation of the muscles, whereas muscle endurance is the ability to maintain a predetermined level of motor output—e.g., torque, velocity, range of motion, work, or energy—over a period of time. *Fatigue* is considered to be a process under which the capability of muscles diminish. However, neuromuscular adjustments take place to meet the task demands (i.e., increase in neural excitation) until there is final performance breakdown—endurance time. *Coordination*, in this context, is the temporal and spatial organizations of movement and the recruitment patterns of the muscle synergies.

Despite the proliferation of various technologies for measurement, basic questions such as "What needs to be measured and how can it best be measured?" are still being investigated. However, there is a consensus on the need to measure objectively the performance capability along the following dimensions: range of motion, strength, endurance, coordination, speed, acceleration, etc. Strength is one of the most fundamental dimensions of human performance and has been the focus of many investigations. Despite the general consensus about the abstract definition of strength, there is no direct method for measurement of muscle tension in vivo. Strength has often been measured at the interface of a joint (or joints) with the mechanical environment. A *dynamometer*, which is an external apparatus onto which the body exerts force, is used to measure strength indirectly.

Different modes of strength testing have evolved based on different levels of technologic sophistication. The practical implication of contextual dependencies on the provided mechanical environment of the strength measures must be considered during selection of the appropriate mode of measurement. In this regard, equipment that can measure strength in different modes is more efficient in terms of both initial capital investment, required floor space in the clinics or laboratories, and the amount of time it takes to get the person in and out of the dynamometer.

152.2 Low Back Pain and Trunk Performance

The problem of LBP is selected to present important models that could be used by the entire multidisciplinary rehabilitation team for the measurement, modeling, and analysis of human performance [Kondraske, 1990]. The inability to relate LBP to anatomic findings and the difficulties in quantifying pain have directed much effort toward quantification of spinal performance. The problem is made even more complex by the increasing demand of the healthcare system to quantify the level of impairment of patients reporting back pain without objective findings.

There are three basic impairment evaluation systems, each having their merits and shortcomings: (1) anatomic, based on physical examination findings, (2) diagnostic, based on pathology, and (3) functional, based on performance or work capacity [Luck & Florence, 1988]. The earlier systems were anatomic, based on amputation and ankylosis. Although this approach may be more applicable to the hand, it is very inappropriate for the spine. The diagnostic-based systems suffer from lack of correspondence between the degree of impairment for a given diagnosis and the resulting disability and even more from the lack of a clear diagnosis. A large percentage of symptom-free individuals have anatomic findings detectable by the imaging technologies, while some LBP patients have no structural anomalies.

The function-based systems are more desirable from an occupational medicine perspective for the following reasons: They allow the rehabilitation team to rationally evaluate the prospect for return to light-duty work and the type of "reasonable accommodations" needed (such as assistive devices) that could reduce the task demand below the functional capability of the individual. By focusing on remaining ability and transferable skills rather than the disability or structural impairment of the injured worker, the set of feasible jobs can be identified. These points are extremely important, given the natural history of work disability after a single low back pain episode causing loss of work time: 40% to 50% of workers return to work by 2 weeks, 60% to 80% return by 4 weeks, and 85% to 90% return by 12 weeks. The small portion of disabled workers who become chronic are responsible for the majority of the economic cost of LBP. It is therefore the primary goal of the rehabilitation team to prevent the LBP, which is self-correcting in most cases, no matter what kind of therapy is used, from becoming a chronic disabling predicament. Injured workers should neither be returned to work too early nor too late, since both could complicate the prognosis. The results of functional capacity evaluation and task demand quantification should guide the timing for returning to work. It is clear that psychosocioeconomic factors become increasingly more important than physical factors as the disability progresses into "chronicity syndrome" and play a major role in defining the evolution of a low back disability claim. Future research should further establish the reliability and reproducibility of performance assessment tools to expedite their widespread use [Luck & Florence, 1988; Newton & Waddell, 1993].

Maximal and Submaximal Protocols

Biomechanical strength models of the trunk are usually based on static maximal strength measurement. In real-life work situations, individuals rarely exert lengthy or maximum static effort. In most clinical situations, submaximal protocols are recommended, especially in patients with pain or with cardiovascular problems. Also, submaximal testing is less susceptible to fatigue and injury. The activities of daily living also have a great deal of submaximal efforts at the self-selected pace. Hence it has been argued that testing at the preferred rate may be complementary to the maximal effort protocols. The preferred motion can be solicited by instructing the subject to perform repetitive movement at a pace and through the range of motion which he or she feels is the most comfortable. It has been shown that LBP patients and normal individuals have different resisted preferred flexion/extension motion characteristics. Having the subject perform against resistance is based on the hypothesis that, at higher resistance levels, the separation between the performance levels of patients and normal subjects becomes more evident. It has been shown, for example, that functional impairment of trunk extensors in LBP patients with respect to the normal population is larger at higher velocities during isokinetic trunk extension. However, the proponents of unconstrained testing have argued that separation of these groups can be performed based on the position, velocity, and acceleration profiles of the trunk during self-selected flexion/extension tasks. They have noted that pain and fear of reinjury may become the limiting factors. The sudden surge in acquiring performance measures of LBP patients during the initial rehabilitation process also underscores the validity of this concept.

Static and Dynamic Strength Measurements of Isolated Trunk Muscles

Weakness of the trunk extensor and abdominal muscles in patients with LBP was demonstrated using the cable tensiometer to measure isometric strength. The disadvantage of the cable tensiometer (which records applied force) is that it neglects to measure the lever arm distance from the center of trunk motion. It is also recommended that cable tensiometer be used to determine peak isometric torques rather than the stable average torque exerted over a 3-second period. Dynamometers used for testing dynamic muscle performances contain either hydraulic or servo motor systems to provide constant velocity, e.g., isokinetic devices, or constant resistance, e.g., isoinertial devices. The isokinetic devices can be further categorized into passive and active types. The robotics-based dynamometers can actively apply force on the body and hence allow eccentric muscle performance assessments, while only concentric exertions can be measured by the passive devices. Eccentric muscle action can simulate the lowering phase of a manual materials handling task. Based on sports medicine literature, eccentric action has been implicated for its significant role in the muscle injury mechanism. Using isokinetic dynamometers, the isometric and isokinetic strengths of trunk extensor and abdominal muscles were shown to be weaker in LBP patients compared with healthy individuals. Dedicated trunk testing systems have become the cornerstone of objective functional evaluation and have been incorporated in the rehabilitation programs in many centers.

Two issues of importance for future research are the role of pelvic restraints and the significance of using newly developed triaxial dynamometers as opposed to more traditional uniaxial dynamometers. Studies on healthy volunteers have shown that trunk motions occur in more than one plane—lateral bending accompanies the primary motion of axial rotation. Numerous attempts have been made to measure the segmental range of motion three-dimensionally in the lumbar spine with the purpose of quantifying abnormal coupling and diagnosing instabilities.

The effect of posture on the maximum strength capability can be described based on the length-tension relationship of muscle action. Marras and Mirka [1989] studied the effect of trunk postural asymmetry, flexion angle, and trunk velocity (eccentric, isometric, and concentric) on maximal trunk torque production. It was shown that trunk torque decreased by about 8.5% of the maximum for every 15 degrees of asymmetric trunk angle. At higher trunk flexion angles, extensor strength increased. Complex, significant interaction effects of velocity, asymmetry, and sagittal posture were detected. The ranges of velocity studies were more limited (± 30 degrees per second) than those used customarily in spinal evaluation. Tan et al. [1993] tested 31 healthy males for the effects of standing trunk-flexion positions (0, 15, and 35 degrees) on triaxial torques and did *electromyograms* (EMGs) of 10 trunk muscles during isometric trunk extension at 30%, 50%, 70%, and 100% of maximum voluntary exertions (MVE). Trunk muscle strength was significantly increased at a more flexed position. However, the accessory torques in the transverse and coronal planes were not affected by trunk postures. The recorded lateral bending and rotation accessory torques were less than 5% and 16% of the primary extension torque, respectively. The rectus abdominis muscles were inactive during all the tests. The EMGs of the erector spinae varied linearly with higher values of MVE, while the latissimus dorsi had a nonlinear behavior. The obliques were coactivated only during 100% MVE. The *neuromuscular efficiency ratio* (NMER) was constructed as the ratio of the extension torque over the processed (RMS) EMG of the extensor muscles. It was hoped that NMER could be used in clinical settings where generation of the maximum exertion are not indicated. However, the

NMER proved to have a limited clinical utility because it was significantly affected by both exertion level and posture. The NMER of the extensor muscles increased at more flexed position. Studies that have combined the EMG activities and dynamometric evaluations have the potential of discovering the neuromuscular adaptation during different phases of injury and rehabilitation processes.

Static and Dynamic Trunk Muscle Endurance

The high percentage of type I fibers in the back muscles, in addition to the better vascularization of these muscles groups, contributes to their superior endurance. Physiologic studies indicate that at higher muscle utilization ratios (relative muscle loads), fatigue is detected earlier. Isometric endurance tests have been used to compute the median frequency (MF) of the myoelectrical activities of trunk muscles in both normal and LBP populations. The expected decline of the median frequency with fatigue is parameterized by the intercept (initial MF) and the slope of the fall. It has been shown that trunk range of motion (ROM) and isometric strength suffered from lower specificity and sensitivity than spectral parameters. Trunk muscle endurance does differ between healthy subjects and those reporting LBP. During isometric endurance testing, trunk flexors develop fatigue faster than extensors in symptom-free subjects. The flexor fatigability appeared significantly higher in patients with LBF as compared with controls. Chronicity also influences trunk muscle endurance. Chronic LBP patients showed reduced abdominal as well as back muscle endurance as compared with the healthy controls and lower back muscle endurance as compared with the intermittent LBP group. Individuals with a history of debilitating LBP demonstrated less isometric trunk extensor endurance than either normal individuals or patients with history of lesser LBP.

Soft tissues subjected to repetitive loading, due to their viscoelastic properties, demonstrate creep and load relaxation. The loss of precision, speed, and control of the neuromuscular system induced by fatigue reduces the ability of muscles to protect the weakened passive structure, which may explain many industrial, clinical, and recreational injury mechanisms. These results further indicate the necessity of relating clinical protocols to the job and show how short-duration maximal isometric testing alone cannot provide the complex functional interaction of strength, endurance, control, and coordination.

Parnianpour et al. [1988] studied the effect of isoinertial fatiguing of flexion and extension trunk movements on the movement pattern (angular position and velocity profile) and the motor output (torque) of the trunk. They showed that, with fatigue, there is a reduction of the functional capacity in the main sagittal plane. There is also a loss of motor control enabling a greater range of motion in the transverse and coronal planes while performing the primary sagittal task. Association of sagittal with coronal and transverse movements is considered more likely to induce back injuries; thus the effect of fatigue and reduction of motor control and coordination may be an important risk factor leading to injury-prone working postures. The endurance limit is a more useful predictor of incidence and recurrence of low back disorders than the absolute strength values. Although physiologic criteria used in the *National Institute for Occupational Safety and Health Lifting Guide* [NIOSH, 1981] considered cardiovascular demands of dynamic repetitive lifting tasks, the limits of muscular endurance were not explicitly addressed. Future research should fill this gap, since the maximum strength measures should not guide the design decisions. Maximum level of performance can only be maintained for short periods of time, and muscular fatigue should be avoided to prevent the development of MSD. This caveat should be applied to all dimensions of performance capability [Kondraske, 1990].

A prospective, randomized study among employees in a geriatric hospital showed that exercising during work hours to improve back muscle strength, endurance, and coordination proved cost-effective in preventing back symptoms and absence from work [Gundewall et al., 1993]. Every hour spent by the physiotherapist on the exercise group reduced the work absence by 1.3 days. In this study, both training and testing equipment were very modest. Endurance training is based on exercises with high repetition and low resistance, while strength training requires exercise with high resistance and low repetition.

Lifting Strength Testing

The National Institute for Occupational Safety and Health [NIOSH, 1981] recommended static, i.e., isometric, strength measurement as its standard for lifting tasks. This was based on the evidence that associated LBP with inadequate isometric strength. The incidence of an individual's sustaining an on-the-job back injury increases threefold when the task-lifting requirements approached or exceed the individual's strength capacity. However, lifting strength is not a true measure of trunk function but is a global measure taking into account arm, shoulder, and leg strength as well as the individual's lifting technique and overall fitness. It has been shown that strength tests were more valid and predictive of risk of low back disorders if they simulated the demands of the job. The clinicians must be aided with easy-to-use and validated instruments or questionnaires to gather information about the task demands in order to decide what testing protocol best simulates the applicant's spinal loading conditions.

Static strength measurements have been reported to underestimate significantly the loads on the spine during dynamic lifts. Comparing static and dynamic biomechanical models of the trunk, the predicted spinal loads under static conditions were 33% to 60% less than those under dynamic conditions, depending on the lifting technique. The recruitment patterns of trunk muscles (and thus the internal loading of the spine) are significantly different under isometric and dynamic conditions. General manual materials handling tasks require a coordinated multilink activity that can be simulated using classic psychophysical techniques or the robotics-based lift task simulators. Various lifting tests, including static, dynamic, maximal, and submaximal, are currently available. The experimental results of correlational studies have confirmed the theoretical prediction that strength will be dependent on the measurement technique. Since muscle action requires external resistance, the effect of muscle action will depend on the nature of the resistance. These results refute the implicit assumption that a generic strength test exists that can be used for preplacing workers (pre-employment) and predicting the risk of injury or future occurrence of LBP. The psychometric properties of isokinetic and isoresistive modes of strength testing were recently addressed. The quantification of the surface response of strength as a function of joint angle and velocity was only possible for isokinetic testing, while isoresistive tests yielded a very sparse data set. Figures 152.1 and 152.2 illustrate these points graphically.

The widely conflicting results found in the literature regarding the relationship of an individual's strength to the risk of developing LBP may be due to inappropriate modes of strength measurements, i.e., lack of job specificity. Isometric strength testing of the trunk is still widely used, especially in large-scale industrial or epidemiologic studies, because it has been standardized and studied prospectively in industry. Compared with trunk dynamic strength testing protocols, the trunk isometric strength testing protocols are simpler and less expensive.

One outstanding issue during dynamic testing is the unresolved problem of how the wealth of information can be presented in a succinct and informative fashion. One approach has been to compare the statistical features of the data with the existing normal databases. This is particularly crucial because one does not have the option of comparing the results to the "contralateral asymptomatic joint," as one has with lower or upper extremity joints. Given the large differences between individuals, I recommend comparison be made to job-specific databases. For example, it is more appropriate for the trunk strength of an injured construction worker to be compared with age- and gender-controlled healthy construction workers than with data from healthy college graduate students or office workers. However, given the scarcity of such data, I argue for comparison of performance capacity with job demand based on task analysis. The performance capacity evaluation is once again linked to task demand quantification.

Inverse and Direct Dynamics

A major task of biomechanics has been to estimate the internal loading of musculoskeletal structure and establish the physiologic loading during various daily activities. Kinematic studies deal

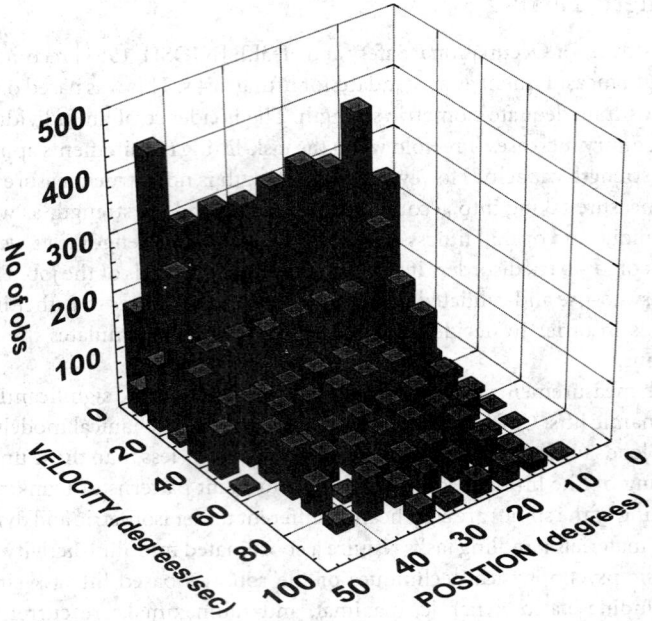

FIGURE 152.1 Bivariate distribution histogram of isokinetic trunk extension for 10 subjects.

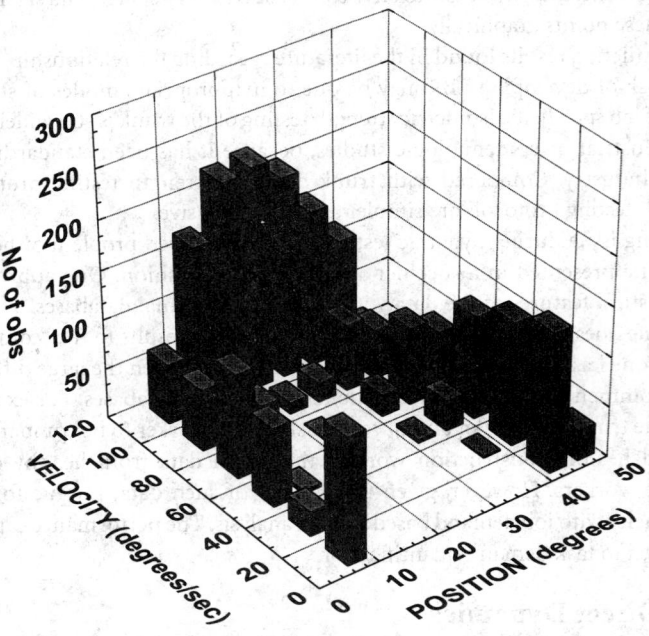

FIGURE 152.2 Bivariate distribution histogram of isotonic trunk extension for 10 subjects.

with joint movement, with no emphasis on the forces involved. However, kinetic studies address the effect of forces that generate such movements. Using sophisticated experimental and theoretical stress/strain analyses, hazardous/failure levels of loads have been determined. The estimated forces and stresses are used to estimate the level of deformation in the tissues. This technique allows one to assess the risk of overexertion injury associated with any physical activity. Given repetitive motions and exertion levels much lower than the ultimate strength of the tissues, an alternative injury mechanism, the cumulative trauma model, has been used to describe much of the musculoskeletal disorders of the upper extremities.

The experimental data on the joint trajectories are differentiated to obtain the angular velocity and acceleration. Appropriate inertial properties of the limb segments are used to compute the net external moments about each joint. This mapping from joint kinematics to net moments is called *inverse dynamics*. *Direct dynamics* refers to studies that simulate the motion based on known actuator torques at each joints. The key issue in these investigations is understanding the control strategies underlying the trajectory planning and performance of purposeful motion. A highly multidisciplinary field has emerged to address these unsolved questions (see Berme and Cappozzo [1990] for a comprehensive treatment of these issues).

It should be pointed out that determination of the external moments about different joints during manual materials-handling tasks is based on the well-established laws of physics (Fig. 152.3). However, the determination of human performance and assessment of functional capacity are based on other disciplines, e.g., psychophysics, that are not as exact or well developed. One can describe easily the job demand, in terms of the required moments about each joint, by analyzing the workers performing the tasks. However, one is unable to predict the ability to perform an arbitrary task based on the incomplete knowledge of functional capacities at the joint levels. A task is easily decomposed to its demands at the joint level; however, one cannot compose (construct) the set of feasible tasks based on one's functional capacity knowledge. The mapping from high-level task demands to the joint-level functional capacity for a given performance trial is unique. However, the mapping from joint-level functional capacity to the high-level task demand is one to many (not unique). The challenge to the human performance research community is to establish this missing link. Much of the integration of ergonomics and functional analysis depends on removal of this obstacle. The question of whether a subject can perform a task based on knowledge of his or her functional capacity at the joint level remains an area of open research. When ergonomists or occupational physicians evaluate the fitness of task demands and worker capability, the following clinical questions will be presented: (1) Which space should be explored for determining normalcy, fit, or equivalence? (2) Should we consider the performance of the multilink system in the joint space or end-effector (cartesian workspace)? These issues have profound effects on both the development of new technologies and the evaluation of trunk or lifting performance.

The enormous degrees of freedom existing in the neuromusculoskeletal system provide the control centers both the kinematic and actuator redundancies. The redundancies provide optimization possibility. Since one can lift an object from point *A* to point *B* with infinite postural possibilities, it can be suggested that certain physical parameters maybe optimized for the learned movements. The possible candidates for objective function to be optimized are movement time, energy, smoothness, muscular activities, etc. This approach, though still in its early stage, may be very important for spine functional assessment. One could compare the given performance with the optimal performance that is predicted by the model. This approach provides specific goals and gives biofeedback with respect to the individual's performance.

Comparison of Task Demands and Performance Capacity

The regression analysis was used to model the dynamic torque, velocity, and power output as a function of resistance level during flexion and extension using the B-200 Isostation [Parnianpour et al., 1990]. Results indicated that the measured torque was not a good discriminator of the tenth, fifti-

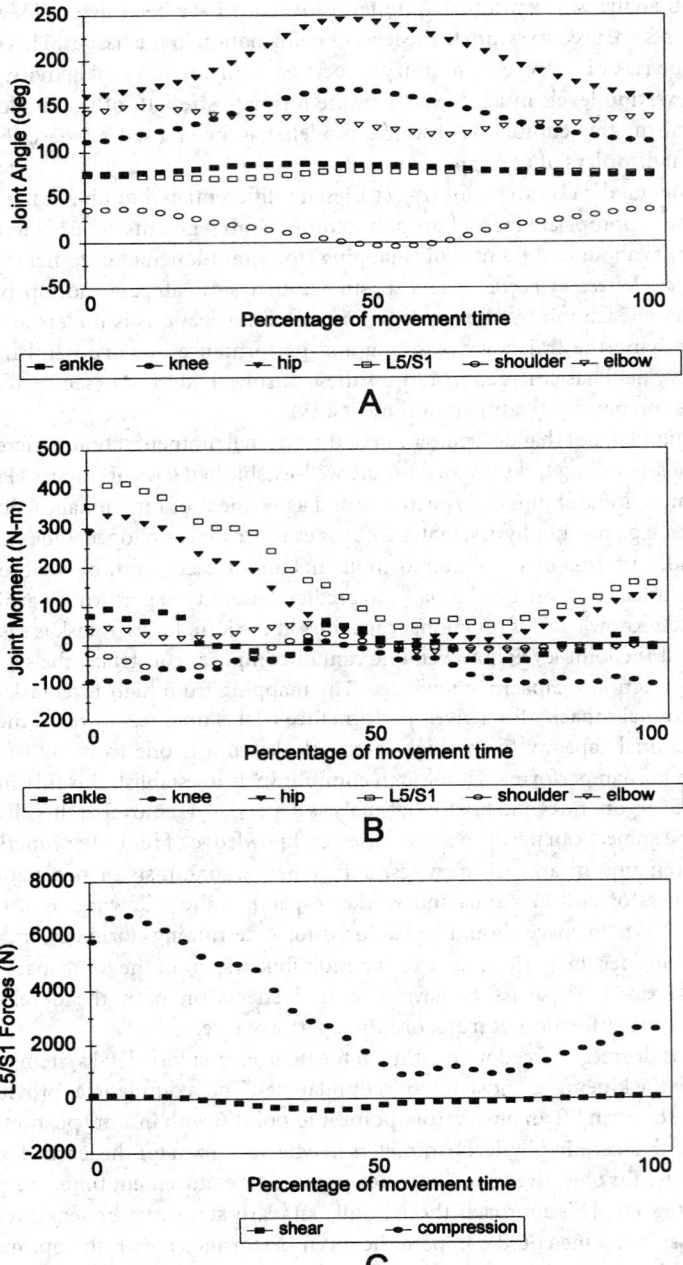

FIGURE 152.3 The dynamic analysis of a sagittal plane symmetrical isokinetic lift (load 21 kg, speed = 51 cm/s, mode = preferred method of lifting): (*a*) joint angle; (*b*) net muscular joint moment; and (*c*) the joint reaction forces at L5/S1.

eth, and ninetieth percentile population. However, velocity and power were shown to effectively discriminate the three populations. Based on these data, it was suggested that during clinical testing, sagittal plane resistance should not be set at higher than about 80 N·m in order to minimize the internal loading of spine while taxing trunk functional capacity. This presentation of data may be useful to the physician or ergonomist in evaluating the functional capacity requirements of workplace manual materials-handling tasks. For example, a manual material-handling task that requires about 80 N·m (61 ft·lb) of trunk extensor strength could be performed by 90% of the population in the normal database if the required average trunk velocity does not exceed 40 degrees per second, while only 50% could perform the task if the velocity requirement exceeds 70 degrees per second. More important, only the top tenth percentile population could perform the task if the velocity requirement approaches 105 degrees per second (Fig. 152.4). A few versions of lumbar motion monitors that can record the triaxial motion in the workplace have been used to provide the trunk movement requirements. The preceding example also illustrates the importance of having the same bases for evaluation of both task and the functional capability of the worker.

152.3 Clinical Applications

Clinical studies have utilized quantitative human performance, i.e., strength and endurance measures, to predict the first incidence or recurrence of LBP and disability outcome and also as a prognosis measure during the rehabilitation process. Training programs to enhance the endurance and strength of workers have been implemented in some industries. More studies on the effectiveness of these programs are needed. It can be hypothesized that these programs complement the stress-management programs to enhance both worker satisfaction and coping strategies with regard to physical and nonphysical stressors at the workplace.

Functional-based impairment evaluation schemes traditionally have used spinal mobility. Given the poor reliability of range of motion (ROM), its large variability among individuals, and the static psychometric nature of ROM, the use of continuous dynamic profiles of motion with the higher-order derivatives has been suggested. Dynamic performances of 281 consecutive patients from the Impairment Evaluation Center at the Mayo Clinic were used. As part of the comprehensive physical and psychological evaluation, 281 consecutive LBP patients underwent isometric and dynamic trunk testing using the B200 Isostation. *Feature extraction* and *cluster analysis* techniques were used to find the main profiles in dynamic patient performances. The middle three cycles of movements were interpolated and averaged into 128 data points; thus the data were normalized with respect to

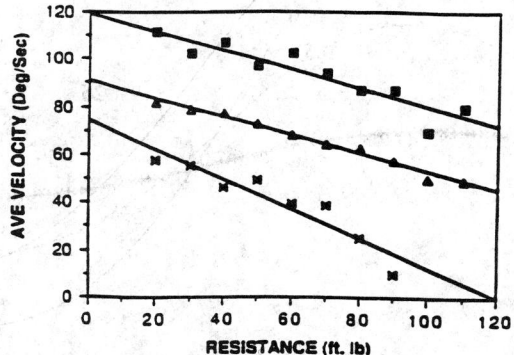

FIGURE 152.4 The average extension velocity measured during maximum trunk extension against a set resistance for 10th (cross), 50th (triangle), and 90th (square) percentile distribution.

cycle time. This allowed for comparison between individuals. Figure 152.5 presents the main profiles of sagittal trunk angular position. The number of patients in each group is also noted on the graph. Patients in the first ($n = 48$) and second ($n = 55$) groups had similar flexion mobility; however, those in the first group had more limited extension mobility. The time to peak sagittal position also varied among the five groups. Forty-seven patients in the fifth group showed extreme impairment in both flexion and extension. The third group (26 patients) showed differential impairments with respect to direction of motion. A marked improvement over the use of ROM has been achieved by preserving information in the continuous profiles. The LBP patients in this study are heterogeneous with respect to their movement profile. Uniform treatment of these patients is questionable, and rehabilitation programs should consider their specific impairments. Future research should incorporate the clinical profiles with these movement profiles to further delineate the heterogeneity of LBP patients. Marras et al. [1993] used similar feature-extraction techniques to characterize the movement profiles of 510 subjects belonging to normal ($n = 339$) and 10 LBP patient groups ($n = 171$). Subjects were asked to perform flexion/extension trunk movement at five levels of asymmetry, while the three-dimensional movement of the spine was monitored by the Lumbar Motion Monitor (an exoskeleton goniometer developed at the Biodynamics Lab of The Ohio State University). Trunk motions were performed against no resistance, and no pelvic stabilization was required. The quadratic discriminant analysis was able to correctly classify over 80% of the subjects. The same technology was used to develop logistic regression models to identify the high-risk jobs in industrial workplaces. Hence principles of human performance can be applied successfully to the worker and the task to avoid the mismatch between performance capability and task demand.

152.4 Conclusions

The outcome of trunk performance is affected by the many neural, mechanical, and environmental factors that must be considered during quantitative assessment. The objective evaluation of the critical dimensions of functional capacity and its comparison with the task demands is crucial to the

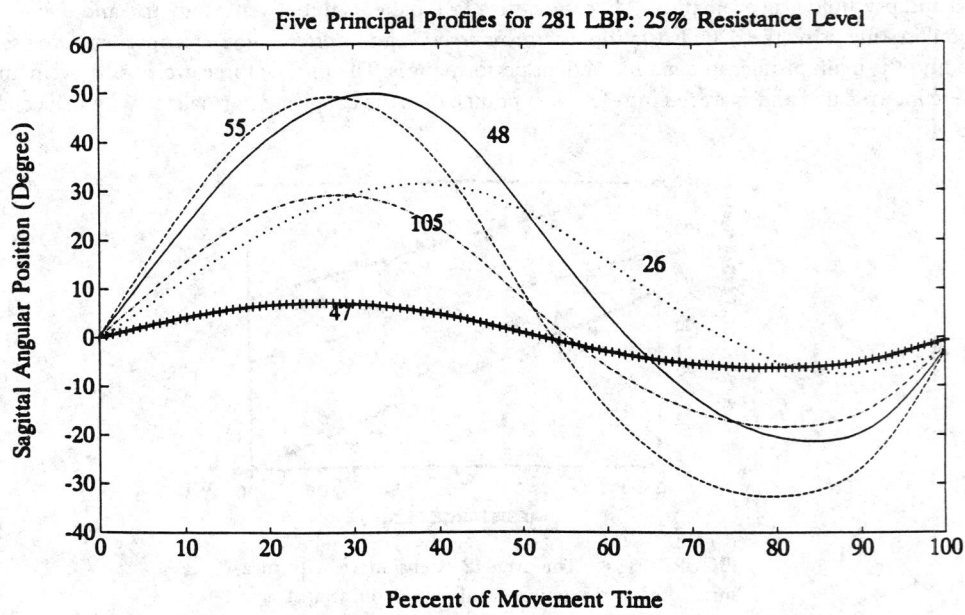

FIGURE 152.5   The five principal profiles of trunk sagittal movement for 281 low back pain patients.

decision-making processes in the different stages of the ergonomic prevention and rehabilitation process. Knowing the tissue tolerance limits from biomechanical studies, task demands from ergonomic analysis, and function capacities from performance evaluation, the rehabilitation team will optimize the changes to the workplace or the task that will maximize the functional reserves (unutilized resources) to reduce the occurrence of fatigue or overexertion. This will enhance worker satisfaction and productivity while reducing the risk of the MSD. Based on ergonomic and motor control literature, the testing protocols that best simulate the loading conditions of the task will yield more valid results and better predictive ability. Ergonomic principles indicate that the ratio of the functional capacity to the task demand (utilization ratio) is critical to the development of muscular fatigue, which may lead to more injurious muscle recruitment patterns and movement profiles due to loss of motor control and coordination. However, large prospective studies are still needed to verify this. The most promising application for these quantitative measures is to be used as a benchmark for the safe return to work of injured workers, given the enormous variations within the normal population. With the advent of technologies to monitor trunk performance in the workplace, one can obtain estimates of the injurious levels of task demands (kinematic and kinetic parameters), which can be used to guide preplacement and rehabilitation strategies. The more functional the clinical tests become, the more clinicians need a complex interpretation scheme. An increasingly complex interpretation scheme opens the possibility of using mathematical modeling with intelligent computer interfaces. The ability to identify subgroups of patients or high-risk individuals based on their functional performance will remain an open area of research to interested biomedical engineers within the multidisciplinary group of experts addressing neuromusculoskeletal occupational disorders.

Defining Terms

Carpal tunnel syndrome (CTS): The result of compression of the median nerve in the carpal tunnel of the wrist.

Cluster analysis: A statistical technique to identify natural groupings in data.

DeQuervain's disease: A special case of tendosynovitis (swelling and irritation of the tendon sheath) which occurs in the abductor and extensor tendons of the thumb, where they share a common sheath.

Electromyogram: Recordings of the electric potentials produced by muscle action.

Feature extraction: A statistical technique to allow efficient representation of variability in the original signals while reducing the dimensions of the data.

Lateral epicondylitis (tennis elbow): Tendons attaching to the epicondyle of the humerus bone become irritated.

Rotator cuff tendinitis: The irritation and swelling of the tendon or the bursae of the shoulder that is caused by continuous muscle or tendon effort to keep the arm elevated.

Tension neck syndrome: An irritation of the levator scapulae and trapezius group of muscles of the neck commonly occurring after repeated or sustained overhead work.

Thoracic outlet syndrome: A disorder resulting from compression of nerves and blood vessels between the clavicle and the first and second ribs at the brachial plexus.

Trigger finger: A special case of tendosynovitis where the tendon becomes nearly locked so that forced movement is not smooth.

Acknowledgments

The author acknowledges the support from OSURF and NIDRR H133E30009. The author would like to thank invaluable comments and contributions of Drs. George V. Kondraske, Margareta Nordin, Victor H. Frankel, Elen Ross, Jackson Tan, Robert Gabriel, Robert R. Crowell, William Marras, Sheldon R. Simon, and Heinz Hoffer and research associates Ali Sheikhzadeh, Jung Yong Kim, Sue Ferguson, Patrick Sparto, and Kinda Khalaf.

References

Andersson GBJ. 1991. Evaluation of muscle function. In JW Frymoyer (ed), The Adult Spine: Principles and Practice, p 241. New York, Raven Press.

Beimborn DS, Morrissey MC. 1988. A review of literature related to trunk muscle performance. Spine 13(6):655.

Berme N, Cappozzo A. 1990. Biomechanics of Human Movement: Applications in Rehabilitation, Sports and Ergonomics. Worthington, Ohio, Bertec Corporation.

Gundewall B, Liljeqvist M, Hansson T. 1993. Primary prevention of back symptoms and absence from work. Spine 18(5):587.

Kondraske GV. 1990. Quantitative measurement and assessment of performance. In RV Smith, JH Leslie (eds), Rehabilitation Engineering. Boca Raton, Fla, CRC Press.

Kroemer KE, Kroemer H, Kroemer-Elbert K. 1994. Ergonomics: How to Design for the Ease and Efficiency. Englewood Cliffs, NJ, Prentice-Hall.

Luck JV, Florence DW. 1988. A brief history and comparative analysis of disability systems and impairment evaluation guides. Office Pract 19:839.

Marras WS, Mirka GA. 1989. Trunk strength during asymmetric trunk motion. Hum Fact 31(6):667.

Marras WS, Parnianpour M, Ferguson SA, et al. 1993. Quantification and classification of low back disorders based on trunk motion. Eur J Med Rehabil 3(6):218.

National Institute for Occupational Safety and Health (NIOSH). 1981. Work practices guide for manual lifting (DHHS Publication No. 81122). Washington, US Government Printing Office.

Newton M, Waddell G. 1993. Trunk strength testing with iso-machines: 1. Review of a decade of scientific evidence. Spine 18(7):801.

Parnianpour M, Nordin M, Kahanovitz N, et al. 1988. The triaxial coupling of torque generation of trunk muscles during isometric exertions and the effect of fatiguing isoinertial movements on the motor output and movement patterns. Spine 13:982.

Parnianpour M, Nordin M, Sheikhzadeh A. 1990. The relationship of torque, velocity and power with constant resistive load during sagittal trunk movement. Spine 15:639.

Pope MH. 1992. A critical evaluation of functional muscle testing. In JN Weinstein (ed), Clinical Efficacy and Outcome in the Diagnosis and Treatment of Low Back Pain, pp 101. New York, Raven Press.

Snook SH, Fine LJ, Silverstein BA. 1988. Musculoskeletal disorders. In BS Levy, DH Wegman (eds), Occupational Health: Recognizing and Preventing Work-Related Disease, pp 345–370. Boston, Little, Brown.

Spalski M, Parnianpour M. 1994. Strength and endurance: Measurement techniques and application. In SW Weisel, JN Weinstein (eds), The Lumbar Spine. Philadelphia. WB Saunders.

Tan JC, Parnianpour M, Nordin M, et al. 1993. Isometric maximal and submaximal trunk exertion at different flexed positions in standing: Triaxial torque output and EMG. Spine 18(16):2480.

World Health Organization. 1980. International Classification of Impairments, Disabilities, and Handicaps. Geneva, WHO.

World Health Organization. 1985. Identification and Control of Work-Related Diseases. Technical report no. 174. Geneva, WHO.

153

Design of Respiratory Protective Masks to Improve Human Performance

Arthur T. Johnson
University of Maryland

Cathryn R. Dooly
University of Maryland

Medical and biologic engineers may find themselves involved with development of many kinds of instruments and apparatuses. They traditionally help to develop medical instrumentation, but there is need for those with the talents, interests, and expertise possessed by medical and biologic engineers to work with other types of equipment, including that for personal protection against environmental contaminants. Material in this chapter illustrates the challenges and approaches used to improve protective equipment. Similar methodologies are found in the development of medical instruments.

Respirator masks are worn to protect wearers against airborne contaminants. As long as filters are effective and seals remain intact, these masks can remove all but 0.1% to 0.01% of the original concentrations of contaminants. If this removal rate is not sufficient, as in the case of some very highly toxic vapors and dusts, masks can be worn that draw their air from tanks instead of the environment. The former type of mask is called *air-purifying*, whereas the second type is called *air-supplied*.

The technology of contaminant removal is largely physical and chemical and can be applied while largely ignoring the fact that a human is the beneficiary of the endeavor. Hence one would likely find that chemists, chemical engineers, and mechanical engineers represent the majority of disciplines contributing to this aspect of respirator design. It is only when considering the untoward effects of respirator wear on the human wearers that the need for biomedical engineers begins to be understood.

Respirator mask design, given an effective filter mechanism, may proceed along many routes. One of these is aesthetic: Design the mask so that it is as pleasing to the eye as possible and has an acceptable appearance from the inside as well as from the outside. There is a strong element of aesthetic content in the design of modern respirator masks. Another possible design criterion would be the alleviation of physiologic stresses incurred while wearing a mask. Experimental studies have shown sometimes higher heart rates, greater heat accumulation, and hypoventilation while wearing

0-8493-8346-3/95/$0.00+$.50
© 1995 by CRC Press, Inc.

masks. Respirator design could be based on minimizing differences in physiologic variables between respirator wearers and those not wearing respirator masks. However, this is a case where physiologists have not clearly identified goals to be attained by designers, and engineers, for their part, have not embraced concepts necessary to interpret physiologic goals in terms related to respirator design.

Mask wearers cannot work as long nor as hard while wearing respirators as they can while not wearing them. Thus it might be seen as a natural respirator design objective to minimize performance decrements associated with mask wear. Choosing performance as a design criterion incorporates economic meaning into a largely objective measure of respirator wear effects. Unlike the aesthetic approach, for which the judgment criteria shift from person to person and from time to time, performance criteria are not subject to interpretation once standardized tests are established; unlike the physiologic approach, there is a clear bottom-line means of assessing design changes, and it does not matter if some physiologic variables increase while others decrease as long as the overall performance of the wearer is improved.

Employers and supervisors can understand performance criteria as well. Performance improvements are associated with increased quality and, especially, with increased profits. Performance decrements cost money, either through poorer quality or through the need to hire more people to complete a job or because of the need for more time to complete the task. And the modern regulatory climate requires that some performance decrements not be tolerated because of unsafe conditions that might result if the wearer could not properly perform the task.

153.1 Exercise Model

An overall model for performance while wearing a respirator mask is given in Fig. 153.1 in schematic form. Like many physiologic systems models, there are a number of relatively simple functional components connected in a complex manner. Mathematical description of each function can be ad-

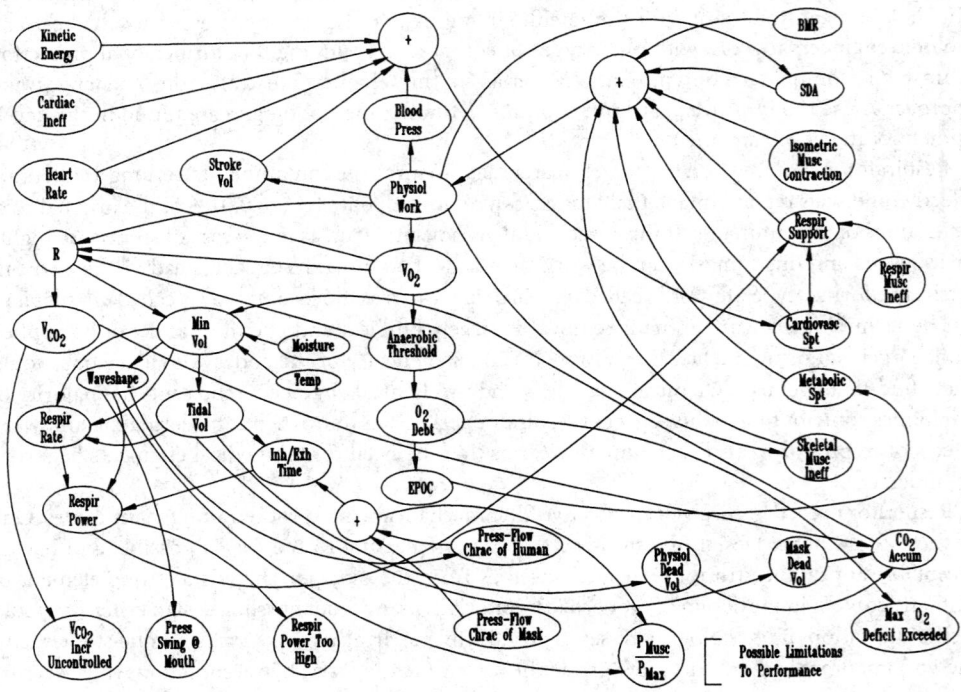

FIGURE 153.1   Schematic overview of the model.

equately given by relatively simple, albeit often nonlinear, equations [Johnson, 1991]. The intricate interconnections connote the complexities in actual physiologic systems.

The model is meant to describe physiologic adjustments to physical activity from rest to heavy exercise. The model includes metabolic measures, cardiovascular measures, and respiratory measures. Thermal measures have not been included as yet but would need to be included for the model to be completely general.

General steps involved with this model are

1. Determine energy costs of muscular work and support functions.
2. Convert total energy costs into oxygen requirements.
3. Obtain respiratory ventilation from oxygen requirements.
4. Obtain carbon dioxide production from oxygen requirements.
5. Account for the metabolic demands of respiration, respiratory flow limitation, and nonaerobic ventilation.
6. Ascertain details of respiration, such as flow rates, respiration rates, wave shapes, and respiratory mechanics.
7. Test various parameters against known or supposed psychophysiologic limits.

There are a number of summation points in Fig. 153.1 designated by a circle including a plus sign. The summation point at the upper right is the place to begin.

To be added at this point are all contributions to *physiologic work*. There are several of these:

1. Skeletal muscle work
2. Basal metabolic processes
3. Additional metabolic support
4. Respiratory and cardiac support in addition to basal support
5. Isometric muscular contraction required to maintain posture
6. The effects of the ingestion of food

Skeletal muscles produce external physical work given as a force (or weight) moved through a distance. Muscles also produce heat as a result of inefficiencies. Both physical work production and heat production place metabolic demands on the body.

Basal metabolic processes require the minimum amounts of energy to sustain life. Included in the *basal metabolic rate* (BMR) are low rates of respiration, blood circulation, chemical activity, central nervous system activity, and kidney activity.

Additional metabolic support is required to meet additional chemical demands during and after active movement. Especially important is the metabolism necessary to produce *excess postexercise oxygen consumption* (EPOC) occurring after exercise above the anaerobic threshold.

Specific dynamic action (SDA) is produced as food is chemically changed and assimilated into the body. SDA effects can be seen many hours after food ingestion but are influenced by physical activity.

Different metabolic demands are placed on lying, sitting, and standing individuals due to posture maintenance. Active muscular contraction is required to sustain bodily position, but this isometric muscular contraction does not result in external physical work because the muscles are used to produce force (muscle tone) but not movement.

Respiration and blood circulation are required to deliver oxygen to and remove carbon dioxide and other metabolic products from active tissues. The energy demands of exercise require blood to flow more rapidly and the quantity of air ventilating the lungs to increase. There is an interaction between respiration and cardiac function because they share space in the chest cavity: Lung inflation squeezes the heart, and heart inflation squeezes the lungs.

Inclusion of respiration and blood circulation as determinants of physiologic work makes this model somewhat iterative, because higher levels of physiologic work require higher rates of respiration and blood circulation. Respiration and circulation, in turn, help to determine physiologic work. Skeletal muscular contraction is the greatest determinant of physiologic work, however.

The summation point at the top, middle of Fig. 153.1, forms energy usage by the heart. Blood pressure, stroke volume, and heart rate are determined by physiologic work. The heart propels the blood, adding a kinetic energy component, and cardiac muscular inefficiency is also included.

The respiratory portion of the model is the most complicated. Respiratory power is determined from air volume flow rate, respiration rate, respiratory mechanics, and respiratory muscular inefficiency. Airflow rate occurs with different wave shapes and different ratios of inhalation time to exhalation time. The respiratory system differs fundamentally from the cardiovascular system because respiratory flow is bidirectional, and power requirements are more complicated as a result.

Pressure-flow characteristics of both the respiratory system and the mask are nonlinear. Resistances of both vary somewhat with flow rate, and since flow rate is calculated from pressure divided by resistance, an implicit solution must be obtained.

Because one determinant of ventilation is the level of carbon dioxide in the blood, and also because mask dead volume affects the level of inhaled carbon dioxide, the model is used to calculate carbon dioxide blood levels. Again, there is a calculation loop here: CO_2 levels determine ventilation, but ventilation helps to determine CO_2 levels through respiratory power.

The *respiratory exchange ratio R* is defined as the ratio of the amount of carbon dioxide produced to the amount of oxygen used. R varies with the metabolic substrate (carbohydrate, fat, or protein) and with the level of exercise. Above the anaerobic threshold, the level of R rises extra rapidly.

Respiratory dead volume and mask dead volume both increase with tidal volume. This should not be surprising, since higher flow rates usually accompany higher tidal volumes and higher flow rates induce turbulence and mixing. Thus air in corners and tube boundaries, where CO_2 can accumulate, is more thoroughly mixed with fresh air at higher flow rates.

Metabolism above the anaerobic threshold is a mixture of aerobic (requiring oxygen) and anaerobic (not requiring oxygen). Anaerobic metabolic products, at least for short-term exercise, must eventually be converted into the same water and carbon dioxide end products that result from aerobic metabolism. The difference between actual oxygen consumption and virtual oxygen consumption (that which would exist if all metabolism were aerobic) is termed the *oxygen deficit*. Repaying the oxygen deficit requires sustained elevated breathing and blood circulation following the cessation of heavy exercise. EPOC is the result.

Many of these metabolic, respiratory, and circulatory processes change levels with exponential time responses. There are also time delays occurring in the system.

Several possible limitations to performance with the mask have been included. Some require checking pressures at the mouth and in the respiratory system. Others require calculation of maximum oxygen deficit, respiratory power, and rate of change of carbon dioxide production.

Human performances with and without a mask are intended to be predicted through the use of this conceptual model. Unfortunately, because of the nature of human physiologic mechanical and control responses, it is not possible to completely separate mask effects from those possessed by the wearer. There is a great deal of possible interaction between the human and the attached apparatus. Therefore, a model such as this, although able to predict exercise responses, still cannot give complete answers required for improved mask designs.

153.2 Performance Rating Tables

The overall physiologic model appearing in Fig. 153.1 will take some time to validate, especially because the limits to exercise performance are not completely understood. Even when they are, the problem of mask design requires more than just prediction of exercise performance. Some tasks involve elements of cognition, dexterity, and motor skills [Fleishman, 1954; Fleishman & Hempel, 1954]; some tasks require quantification of psychological inputs; some tasks may be performed at a pace determined by the worker, whereas other tasks may themselves dictate the rate of work.

As a means to deal with this complexity, the *performance rating table* (PRT) concept was proposed [Johnson et al., 1992*a*].

The PRT quantifies effects of respirator mask factors on the task performance of an individual wearing a mask compared with the no-mask condition. Individual cell entries are thus relative and are scaled by assuming that a cell value of 100 is equivalent to no performance degradation and that a cell value of 0 is equivalent to complete performance degradation. There are very few experimental results upon which to base each cell value. Values were thus estimated from the literature, when possible, and from estimates derived from experiences of the authors and others in the remainder of cases. Therefore, individual cell values may not be entirely correct, but the values that are presently in place, and the PRT method of organizing the data, can be valuable in drawing conclusions regarding mask design and in guiding the conduct of experimental work.

The PRT for temperate environments is given in Table 153.1. The table is organized horizontally by levels of work defined as very light through very heavy (Table 153.2). At the very heavy level, performance time is most likely limited by body biochemistry; for the heavy level, respiratory stress is the most likely limiting factor; for the moderate work rate, thermal burden dominates; and at the light and very light rates of work, long-term factors, such as skin irritation, lack of nourishment, and psychological discomfort, will be the most likely limiting factors.

There are seven mask factors considered in the PRT. Respirators interfere with vision, communications, respiration, heat loss, eating and drinking, compatibility with other equipment, and psychological well-being. The PRT is organized vertically by mask factors (e.g., vision) and contributing mask elements (e.g., acuity and field of view) arranged beneath the mask factors. There are many more possible mask elements that could be included, but efforts were made to reduce the number of elements to a manageable few.

Overall performance rating is obtained from the individual entry values at any particular work rate as the product of all mask element values or as the product of all mask factor values. The rationale for this approach is based on the fact that all mask factor effects are considered to be independent and that the maximum performance, including one factor, cannot be any higher than that determined by the other factors. Performance decrement is the performance rating subtracted from 100.

The PRT is based on several assumptions:

1. The level of technology is the military full-facepiece, air-purifying M-17 mask.
2. Effects are linear.
3. Wearers are normal, healthy, young adults.
4. Work is performed at a constant rate for as long as possible.
5. Masks and hoods are worn before and after work periods.
6. Task variety increases as performance time increases.
7. Temperate environmental conditions prevail.

PRTs for nontemperate environments have been developed as well [Johnson et al., 1992*b*].

How close most performance ratings are to 100 should be noted in this table. Although total performance ratings may be significantly low, individual mask factor ratings are often in the range of 90 to 100. This means that performance because of these particular factors is close to the unencumbered performance. The law of diminishing returns indicates that much more design effort will be needed to remove the last few percents of performance degradation. Thus, although the mask gives an overall low performance rating, most of its individual elements are in the area of diminishing returns. For this reason, the mask and hood must be considered from a total systems viewpoint, and more total effort should be expected to be expended to make marginal gains.

One other implication of the PRT is that it can show that one mask designed for a wide range of tasks and environments, although feasible, does not optimally satisfy any requirement. The result is that all users are unsatisfied to some extent. Producing masks designed for specific uses would solve this problem. Modular mask elements can reduce the logistical burden of this approach, but to expect mask designers to produce masks that perform optimally for all uses in all environments is unrealistic.

TABLE 153.1 Performance Rating Table for Temperate Environments (20°C)*

Mask Factor	Work Rate				
	Very Light	Light	Medium	Heavy	Very Heavy
Vision	93	95	97	99	99
Field size	96	97	98	100	100
Acuity	97	98	99	99	99
Communications	94	95	98	99	100
Attenuation dist.	99	99	99	99	100
Intelligibility	95	97	99	100	100
Direction	100	99	100	100	100
Respiration	100	98	94	80	81
Resistance	100	99	99	84	84
Dead Space	100	99	95	95	96
Thermal factors	100	95	95	100	100
Moisture removal	100	100	100	100	100
Thermal balance	100	95	95	100	100
Personal support	93	94	95	95	95
Drinking/eating	93	94	95	95	95
Medical procedures	100	100	100	100	100
Physical factors	64	69	87	92	97
Physical structure	76	90	98	98	98
Compatibility	85	78	90	95	100
Anthropometry	99	99	99	99	99
Psychological factors	95	95	98	100	100
Total performance rating	49	52	69	69	74
(Total performance degradation)	(51)	(48)	(31)	(31)	(26)

*Values indicate percent performance of an M-17 mask wearer compared with no-mask performance.

The PRT can be an important step toward a computer-aided design procedure that would enable the mask designer to determine the effects of design changes before a prototype is built. Respirator masks traditionally have been designed and prototypes built before they could be tested to ascertain what improvements had been made. This is a very expensive and time-consuming process that could be greatly improved if designs could at least be partially checked by computer while still in the conceptual stage. Respirators consist of many modules, from lenses to valves and filters, and changes in

TABLE 153.2 Essential Features of Work Rates Used in the Performance Rating Table

Work Classification	Physical Work Rate (watts)	Metabolic Rate (watts)	Estimated Performance Time	Example	Description
Very heavy	430	2150	2 min	Sprinting	Very intense work performed for only a short time
Heavy	240	1190	10 min	Running at 4 m/s	Intense work not likely to include much variation of type
Moderate	140	755	50 min	Climbing hills, shoveling fast	Work at high enough level for a long enough time to significantly increase body temperature
Light	10	202	8 hr	Washing clothes, light gymnastics, walking at 0.9 m/s	Significant variation expected in types of tasks performed
Very light	0	105	indefinitely	Reading, answering phone, intermittent typing	A wide variety of performed tasks include many involving information transfer

one of these often affect others. The element of trial and error may not ever be completely eliminated from the design process, but the overall anticipated effect on performance rating could be determined before a prototype is produced. To illustrate the nature of these interactions, two tables are presented.

The translation between PRT mask factors and mask design modules appears in Table 153.3 [Johnson & Grove, 1993]. On the left of Table 153.3 are listed some common mask design modules: lenses, speech, communications, valves, filters, seals, hood, facepiece, drinking, and materials. It is not uncommon that one individual cannot be the most knowledgeable in all these modules, so mask design is accomplished by teams. Entries in the interior of Table 153.3, however, show the interdependence between mask modules and various physiologic effects. Mask seals can affect a full range of mask physiologic factors; lens design affects more than vision. Thus those designers working on modules seemingly far removed from one another must be aware of the effects each has on another and on the overall final product.

In Table 153.4 appear most, if not all, principal interactions between mask factors. Table columns represent primary factors; i.e., the mask factors considered to be those leading to the interaction. Table rows represent secondary factors, or those factors receiving the effects of the interactions. Table entries are not reciprocal; the effect of a change of vision on communication (increased vision allows better close-up communication by allowing mouth and facial expression to be seen better by the person spoken to) is different from the effect of a change in communication on vision (talking leads to lens fogging, thus reducing vision).

153.3 Some Experimental Results

The performance rating table can serve as inspiration for the conduct of experiments. Realizing that PRT cell entries must often be considered as substitutes for more complicated models, experiments can be conducted to determine the dependence of performance ratings on continuums of mask element values. Two illustrations that are presented here are the effects of performance rating on visual acuity for three generic tasks and the effect of performance rating on subject anxiety level when the rate of work can be adjusted.

Visual Acuity

There are many tasks that depend for their satisfactory performance on visual acuity. One class of these tasks involves console monitoring, computer operation, or other uses of video-display terminals. Another of these tasks uses the hands in conjunction with vision, such as, for example, in office filing, on electronic repairs, or in small-scale assembly. Wearing a respiratory protective mask while performing those tasks can impose a burden on the wearer and should cause reduced performance expectations on the part of the supervisor.

The mask used in this investigation was the U.S. Army M-17 full-facepiece respirator mask [Johnson et al., 1994b]. Plastic lenses were clouded by uniformly scratching lens surfaces with fine steel wool to visual acuities of about 20/100, 20/70, 20/50, 20/40, 20/30, and 20/25. Each pair of lenses was applied to a mask, and that pair of lenses remained on that mask throughout the length of the study to ensure that all subjects were tested uniformly with the same pair of lenses. The actual visual acuity represented by each set of lenses was determined by the subjects reading the Snellen eye chart while wearing a mask with clouded lenses. Subjects were allowed up to one incorrect letter identification on a line with the line still representing visual acuity. Four custom-made Snellen charts, differing from the original in order of letter appearance only, were used at various times to circumvent the problem of letter memorization.

These performance tests were chosen because they were easily quantifiable and represented different visual abilities. The saccadics test, representing console monitoring, consisted of a computer program running on an IBM-PC or compatible and displayed on a color monitor. The display screen was divided into a regular matrix of 16×29 squares, and in each square location a letter A or C

TABLE 153.3 Customary Mask Design Modules Affecting Mask Factors

Design Module	Vision	Communication	Respiration	Thermal	Personal Support	Physical	Psychological
					Mask Factor		
Lens design	Field of view Acuity	Size affects close communication	Size can effect flow volume and fogging	Radiated heat transfer thru lens	Allows for subject identification and observation	Size and clamping requirements affect bulk Eye relief affects compatibility	Better field of view and acuity improve psychological reactions
Communications design	Size can cause limits in field of view	Intelligibility distance	Size of communication system can affect dead space	Can add to metabolic burden	Enhances correct medical diagnosis	Size of communication device affects bulk Plug-in compatibility is critical	Better communication improves psychological reactions
Valve design	Size of nosecup valves can affect lens design	Outlet valve openings help communication	Resistances to airflow	Valves can allow for heat transfer	Give mouth access for medical treatment	Size of valving can affect bulk	Improved breathing can reduce psychological burden
Filter design	Size of filter can reduce field of view	Filter can block speech projection	Resistances to airflow	Filter slightly reduces humidity	Provides protection from contaminants	Size of filter affects weight and bulk	Labored breathing causes psychological burden
Seal design	Nosecup sealing can interfere with vision	Nosecup seal can influence communication	Nosecup seal affects dead volume	Warm, humid air can leak into facepiece	None	Can affect weight comfort, and compatibility	Improved seal and comfort can improve psychological reaction
Hood design	Hood can interfere with field of view	Hood material and design affects hearing	Pressurized mode affects breathing	Hood material and design affect convection and conduction	None	Size and material affects bulk	Good flexibility and thermal characteristics improve psychological reaction
Facepiece design	Shape of nose cavity affects vision	Materials and size of nose cavity affects communication	Ducting and dead space affect breathing	Materials and flow patterns affect cooling	Location of drinking system affects ease of operation Eating inhibited	Size and materials affect bulk Size affects compatibility	Improper size affects psychology Clarity can improve feelings
Drinking design	Usually none	Tubes can absorb acoustic power	Can affect dead volume	Improved drinking helps cooling	Flow must be adequate	Size can affect bulk and compatibility	Improved drinking can improve feelings
Materials	Materials affect both physical optics	Materials affect both output power and frequency	Valve and filter materials affect resistance	Materials affect heat transfer	Materials must be impermeable and safe	Materials greatly affect flexibility and bulk	Softer materials help comfort

TABLE 153.4 Principal Interactions Between Respirator Mask Factors

Secondary Factor	Primary Factor						
	Vision	Communication	Respiration	Thermal	Personal Support	Physical	Psychological
Vision	None	Talking leads to fogging and creates lens movement	Respiration helps defog at high flows and can induce fog at low flows	Sweating leads to fogging	Illness may affect vision	Some due to geometry, especially in binocular and lower quadrant	Distraction causes less vision awareness
Communications	Near distance lip clues	Outside noises compete with comprehension	Breathing is picked up in electronic communication devices	Moisture on diaphragm reduces communication ability	Illness can affect hearing, speaking	Geometry affects communications	Distraction causes less communications awareness
Respiration	Increased vision may affect dead space	Communication configuration affects dead space	Breathing can be affected by CO_2 levels	Increased temperature in mask can change respiration	Illness can affect respiration	Geometry and resistances increase physical work	Nervousness causes heavier breathing
Thermal	More vision allows more penetration of radiation in and out	Worse communication means more physical work	Heavier breathing increases physical work. Increased dead space increases moisture accumulation	Increased temperature in mask reduces respiratory heat loss	Easier drinking facilitates sweating. Illness can affect thermoregulation	Increased weight causes increased physical work. Geometry can help moisture accumulation	Nervousness increases heart rate, heat generation, and muscle tension.
Personal support	Vision needed for drinking and medical procedures	Some communications needed for medical support	None	More thermal stress, more drinking	None	Geometry can cause compatibility problem	Psychological state affects drinking and medical condition
Physical	Some interaction in structure and compatibility	Some interaction in structure and compatibility	Respiratory pathways are required	Heat removal affects geometry and materials	Inclusion of drinking affects geometry	Geometry affects compatibility	None
Psychological	More vision causes less psychological problems	More communication causes higher acceptance	Easier breathing causes less stress	Cooler environment causes less stress	Easier to drink and eat causes less stress	Less weight and less fatigue causes more comfort	Psychological problems may generate more stress

would momentarily appear one at a time in random order and location. The seated subject was required to press the keyboard key corresponding to the letter appearing on the screen. Correct response had to be made within 0.67 s, and only the first response was accepted. Once a response was made, another letter was presented; the faster the responses, the larger the number of challenges and the higher the maximum score. The number of correct responses was automatically scored.

The tracking and random hand-eye tests, representing vision and spatial sense tasks, were performed on a 0.8 × 1.3-m wall-mounted board divided into a matrix of 39 × 25 squares that were programmed to light either randomly or in a particular order. When the tracking test was performed, the squares lit one at a time in a serpentine pattern on the board. For the random hand-eye coordination test, the squares were lit in a completely random pattern. Correct scores were obtained by touching the square while it was lit. Touching other squares did not register. Squares were lit for about 0.7 s each. The number of correct responses again was automatically scored.

Performance rating results appear in Fig. 153.2. Percent performance scores suffer when a mask is worn. The difference between the no-mask (control) and unaltered mask condition is nearly zero for the saccadics test, where all information presented to the subjects is immediately in front of them. They could rest their fingers on the two letter choices, so no keyboard searching was necessary. There was about a 5% degradation in performance when an unaltered mask was worn during the tracking test. Although subjects were supposed to keep their eyes fixed on the center of the board, all that could be imposed is that they did not move their heads. Some of the lights were out of the peripheral visual field permitted by the mask lenses, but the effects of this were not too severe, since the sequence of lighted squares always occurred with the next lit square in the vicinity of the preceding one. Thus the serpentine pattern was partially predictable, and subjects made use of this information to overcome some of the effects of the mask.

There was nearly a 13% difference in performance associated with mask wear for the random hand-eye test. Mask peripheral vision limited performance on this test, since some lighted squares

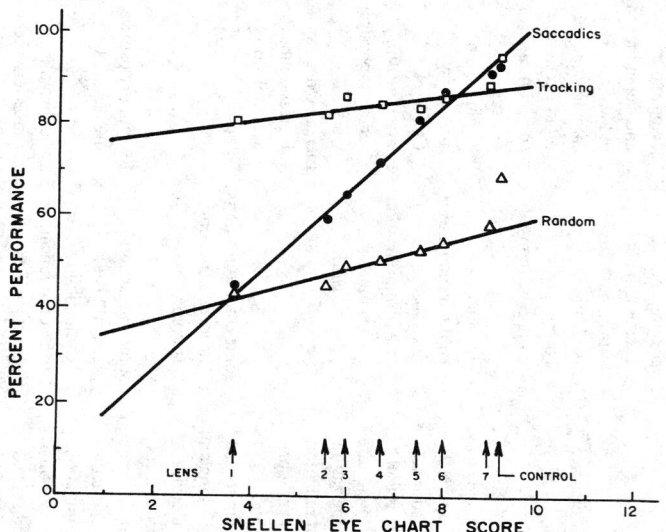

FIGURE 153.2 Percent correct performance while wearing masks with lenses giving seven levels of visual acuity. Mean values of visual acuity, as given by Snellen chart line number, are given for each lens and the control (unmasked). Data shown are means of individual subject data obtained with each lens. Lines are regression lines based on mean data.

were not seen by the subjects, and there was no reliable way they could guess where the next lighted square would be. Performance ratings were determined to be

$$\text{Performance rating} = 12.8 + 9.76S \qquad \text{(saccadics)} \qquad (153.1)$$

$$\text{Performance rating} = 75.2 + 2.21S \qquad \text{(tracking)} \qquad (153.2)$$

$$\text{Performance rating} = 37.4 + 5.64S \qquad \text{(random)} \qquad (153.3)$$

where S = Snellen chart score.

Anxiety Level

The PRT assumes constant rates of work. When the work rate is dictated by the task, the constant-work-rate assumption is valid. For some types of tasks, however, the worker may reduce work rate in response to the increased physiologic burden of the mask. If, in addition, the total amount of work is not fixed, it is not clear that a mask influences performance time, and it is not clear what effect subject anxiety has. A study was designed [Johnson et al., 1994a] to obtain the results when subjects exhibiting varying anxiety levels perform treadmill exercise adjusted to maintain a constant indicator of physiologic stress.

Subjects were administered the Spielberger [Spielberger et al., 1970] State-Trait Anxiety Inventory (STAI), and the results were used to select subjects in order to establish a trait anxiety continuum with scores dispersed as evenly as possible throughout the scoring range of 20 to 80. The range of scores for selected subjects was 23 to 68.

Prior to each exercise session, and after the subject was dressed in the appropriate gear, the STAI was administered in a classroom or office setting with no interruption or time limit. Subjects were then allowed a 4- to 5-minute warmup in which they were given a workload that elicited a heart rate of 80% to 85% of their individual maximum. External workload was manipulated by adjusting treadmill speed and grade throughout exercise sessions to maintain heart rate at the 80% to 85% level.

Performance times for all unmasked subjects appear in Fig. 153.3 and for masked subjects appear in Fig. 153.4. There is a great deal of scatter in the data for both figures for low anxiety scores; above scores of about 30, there are clear downward trends as anxiety scores increase. The lines in both figures were determined by a least-squares procedure while discounting data points below anxiety scores of 30 and excluding data from subjects terminated for excessive core temperature. In addition, data points at anxiety scores of 41, clearly outliners, were not included.

Unmasked subject data yielded the curve

$$\log\,(perf) = 3.131 - 0.01477\,(anx) \qquad (153.4)$$

where *perf* = performance time, minutes
  anx = trait anxiety score, unitless

Masked subject data gave

$$\log\,(perf) = 4.541 - 0.05718\,(anx) \qquad (153.5)$$

Performance rating can be obtained from Eqs. (153.4) and (153.5) by taking the antilog of each and dividing the two. Thus

$$\text{Performance rating} = 409.6e^{-0.04241(anx)} \qquad (153.6)$$

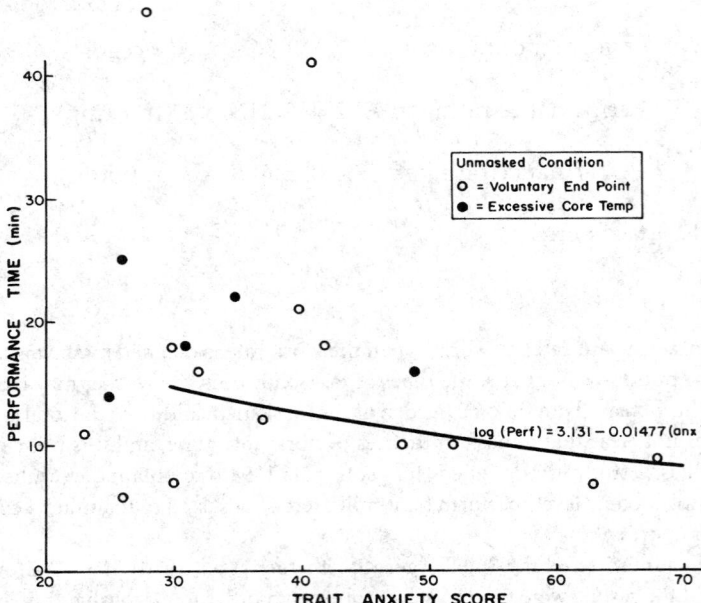

FIGURE 153.3 Performance times of unmasked subjects. The line is the best fit for anxiety scores greater than 30 and with excessive core temperature subject data removed.

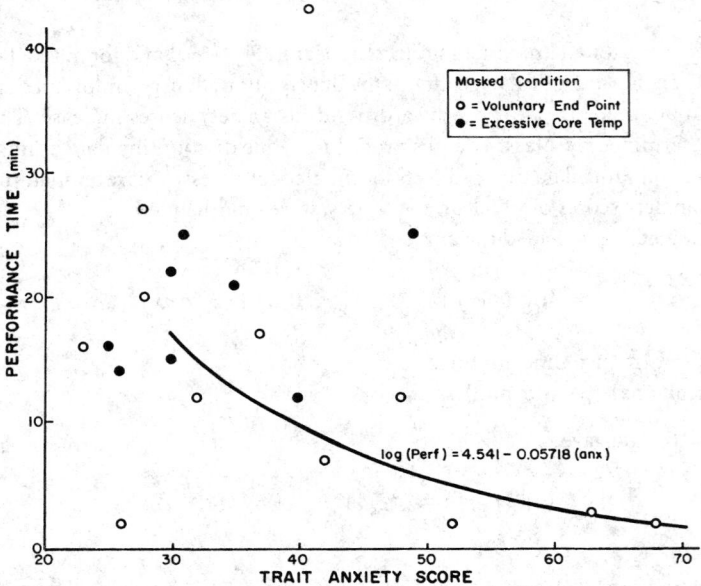

FIGURE 153.4 Performance times of masked subjects. The line is the best fit for anxiety scores greater than 30 and with excessive core temperature subject data removed.

This equation should not be applied below an anxiety score of about 34, where predicted performance rating becomes greater than 100. This equation predicts that masked subjects with anxiety scores of 40 should be able to complete only 75% of the exercise duration that they can tolerate without a mask. At an anxiety score of 70, the predicted performance rating falls to 21%.

153.4 Conclusions

The health of our population depends more on sanitation and nutrition than on care of the infirm. Prevention of disease and trauma can be a very significant contribution made by biomedical engineers to human welfare. Respirator mask design and use are an example of the challenges that are present in the field of occupational health and safety. There is tremendous opportunity to contribute through modeling, experimentation, instrumentation, and design dealing with physiology, environmental medicine, psychology, motor skills, and a broad range of other topics in human performance engineering not normally considered to be the bailiwick of the medical and biologic engineer. There is a need to make the workplace a safer, more hospitable environment for people who must support themselves by being there [Howe, 1992]. The opportunities are limitless, the challenges are exciting, the rewards are heartfelt, and the results can be very worthwhile.

Defining Terms

Anaerobic threshold: The level of exercise at which a significant portion of metabolism occurs without oxygen.

Basal metabolic rate: The amount of heat produced by a completely resting, fasting person in a thermoneutral environment. It includes heat produced by the nervous system, liver, kidneys, heart, and respiratory muscles to sustain life at a very low level.

Dead volume: The volume of air in the respiratory system that does not contribute to air exchange in the lung.

Excess postexercise oxygen consumption: The increase in oxygen consumption following exercise to repay the oxygen deficit incurred during exercise.

Oxygen deficit: The accumulated difference between actual oxygen consumption and the oxygen equivalent of exercise (about 20.9 N · m of work equals 1 liter of oxygen uptake).

Physiologic work: The metabolic demands placed on the body to produce physical or external work. Physiologic work includes energy required to produce external work as well as heat.

Respiratory exchange ratio: The ratio of the rate of carbon dioxide production to the rate of oxygen utilized. At rest, this ratio is determined by the type of food utilized. During exercise, it is an indication of anaerobic metabolism.

Specific dynamic action: Excess heat produced following the ingestion of food during catabolism as food is chemically changed and assimilated into the body.

References

Fleishman EA. 1954. Dimensional analysis of psychomotor abilities. J Exp Psychol 48:437.

Fleishman EA, Hempel WE. 1954. A factor analysis of dexterity tests. Pers Psychol 7:15.

Howe MB. 1992. Safety first, at last. Invention Technol 8(1):54.

Johnson AT. 1976. The energetics of mask wear. Am Ind Hyg Assoc J 35:479.

Johnson AT. 1991. Biomechanics and Exercise Physiology. New York, Wiley.

Johnson AT. 1993. How much work is expended for respiration? Front Med Biol Engr 5:265.

Johnson AT, Dooly CR, Blanchard CA, Brown EY. 1994a. Influence of anxiety level on work performance while wearing a respirator mask. Am Ind Hyg Assoc J (accepted).

Johnson AT, Dooly CR, Brown EY. 1994b. Performance rating with visual acuity while wearing a respirator mask. Am Ind Hyg Assoc J (accepted).

Johnson AT, Grove CM. 1993. Respirator design modules and their interactions. Am Ind Hyg Assoc J 54:749.

Johnson AT, Weiss RA, Grove C. 1992*b*. Respirator performance rating table for mask design. Am Ind Hyg Assoc J 53:193.

Johnson AT, Grove CM, Weiss RA. 1992*a*. Respirator performance rating tables for nontemperate environments. Am Ind Hyg Assoc J 53:548.

Spielberger C, Gorsuch R, Lushene R. 1970. STAI Manual Palo Alto, Calif, Consulting Psychologist Press.

154

Human Performance Engineering: Computer-Based Design and Analysis Tools

Paul J. Vasta
University of Texas at Arlington

George V. Kondraske
University of Texas at Arlington

Computer software applications have been implemented in virtually every aspect of our lives, and the field of human performance has not proven to be an exception. Due to the growing recognition of the role of human performance engineering in many different areas (e.g., clinical medicine, industrial design, etc.) and the resulting increase in requirements of the methods involved, having the "right tool for the job" is becoming of vital importance. Software developers bear the brunt of the responsibility of determining the qualities of a software application that define it as being "the right tool" for the specific job. In contrast, users of this class of tools must determine when their application extends a given tool beyond its intended scope. These abilities require a knowledge base spanning a number of different fundamental concepts and methods encompassing not only the obvious aspects of human performance and computer programing but also many other less obvious issues related to database requirements, parameter standards, systems engineering principles, and software architecture. In addition, foresight about how specific components can best be integrated to fit the needs of a particular use is also necessary.

This chapter addresses selected aspects of computer software tools specifically directed toward human performance design and analysis. The majority of tools currently available emphasize biomechanical models, and as such, this emphasis is reflected here. However, a much broader scope in terms of the body systems incorporated is anticipated, and an effort is made to consider the evolution of more versatile and integrated packages. Selected key functional components of tools are described, and a representative sample of currently emerging state-of-the-art packages is used to illustrate a snapshot not only of the capabilities now available but also of those which are needed and options that exist in terms of the fundamental approach taken to address similar problems.

In general, the development of computer software applications, especially in maturing fields such as human performance engineering, serves multiple purposes. The most apparent is the relative speed and accuracy that can be achieved in computationally intensive tasks (e.g., dynamic analysis) compared with performing the processes by hand. In addition, computers can handle large amounts of data and help keep track of the multitude of parameters associated with the human architecture. This allows otherwise impossible procedures, such as the detailed analysis of a complex *human-task interface*, visualization of a human figure in a *virtual workspace*, or the computation of time-series multibody joint torques, to be realized. Perhaps more important, though, are the indirect benefits provided. For example, relatively complex analytical methods utilized in research facilities can be directly implemented in the field by practitioners, with the need for a complete knowledge only of how to effectively *use* the capability available (which is substantially different from the knowledge required to *create* that ability). Also, because the software environment demands rigor (e.g., coding structure requirements, data handling and storage, etc.), and since the potential scope of end-user needs in terms of functional and parametric components encompassed is broad, decisions are forced and rules must be clearly delineated. These characteristics thus serve as a motivation to develop standards for (or at least decide on the use of) many items, including methods, parameters, parameter definition conventions, and units of measure. Such efforts can expose and correct inadequacies inherent in current standards, while successful software tools (i.e., those which make their way into everyday use) facilitate dissemination of key knowledge and standards to both researchers and practitioners alike.

It can be anticipated that most analysis or decision-making tasks required of practitioners will be made available in computer-based form, including some that are not currently feasible to perform at all except, perhaps, by using intuitive methods that are inconsistently applied and produce results of questionable validity. Given the extent of the possible list of tools within a given package, and considering the substantial overlap of various support functions, classification of packages is difficult. This can already be seen in the relatively modest number of those currently available.

154.1 Selected Fundamentals

It is typical to think of a software capability in terms of a high-level process, e.g., gait analysis, where the end result is of primary interest because the underlying processes are performed "invisibly." Yet these supportive processes, many of which have common mathematic methodologies and modeling approaches, determine the ultimate usability and applicability of the software to a given problem and therefore deserve closer examination. It makes sense to consider these methods generically not only because they are common to several existing packages but also because they will undoubtedly be important in others.

Physics-Based Models and Methods

Physics-based methods are implemented when direct analysis of the system and/or its resources is feasible and required data can be obtained. These methods allow the derivation of unknown parameters from known characteristics of the situation and are based on established physical laws and relationships. With regard to the human system, this approach is exemplified by methods common to biomechanical analysis. For example, the isometric torque that a subject is capable of generating about a given joint degree of freedom at a given angular position is often used to represent musculoskeletal strength. In various task situations, a well-known physics relationship (e.g., $\mathbf{T} = \mathbf{r} \times \mathbf{F}$) can be used to compute a torque requirement (i.e., for that task) from knowledge of the moment arm (e.g., upper extremity length) and end-effector force required (in a given direction). Even simple analyses of the human system often include several joints (e.g., whole body or spine) and many degrees of freedom, greatly adding to the complexity of the analysis. The inclusion of movement adds to the analytical requirements, requiring kinematic or dynamic methods described below. As the analytical complexity (e.g., number of degrees of freedom) of the model increases, the significance of implementing such processes within a computer software application becomes readily apparent.

Physical motion is common to most situations in which the human functions and is therefore fundamental to the analysis of performance. The determination of segment position, orientation, velocity, and acceleration is accomplished through kinematic analysis, which, by definition, is the study of motion without inclusion of the forces that cause motion. Thus the derivation of performance parameters, including range of motion, speed, and accuracy, relies on the defined constructs of kinematics. Depending on the required output, forward (direct) or inverse kinematic analysis may be employed to derive the parameters of interest. This approach is equally appropriate for operations on a single joint system or *linked multibody systems,* such as is typically required for human analysis. For forward kinematic analysis, assuming knowledge of structural parameters (e.g., segment length, joint characteristics), the positions of the end-effector and each joint (i.e., segment endpoints) can be determined in three-dimensional space relative to some global reference frame given the involved joint angles. Alternatively, inverse kinematic analysis provides joint angles (as sets of possible combinations) given the position of the end-effector (or a single solution given the positions of all joints). Both the preceding analyses also can be utilized in analyzing trajectories, resultant forces, velocities, and accelerations in terms of joint angles or segment positions.

Dynamics is an extension of kinematics which relates the forces and torques acting on a body or bodies to their resulting motions. In most task situations, joint torques cannot be directly measured, and it is necessary to derive joint torque from knowledge of motion and structural parameters. By recording joint positions during the task as well as sample intervals, and given the necessary structural characteristics (e.g., mass distribution, inertial moments, etc.) as well as any external forces, joint torques are derived in a similar fashion to joint angle calculations from position data using inverse kinematics. Thus inverse dynamic analysis provides joint torques given motion and force data, while forward dynamic analysis uses joint torques to derive motion. Especially for three-dimensional analyses of multijoint systems, the methods are quite complex and are presently a focal point for computer implementation [Allard et al., 1994]. Even the fastest desktop computers require very noticeable processing times for such tasks.

Physics models used to address biomechanical aspects of human performance are relatively well established and utilized in both research and applied domains. In contrast, concepts and methods directed toward other aspects of human performance, such as information processing (in purely perceptual contexts as well as in neuromotor control contexts), are based on strong science and have been incorporated into one-of-a-kind computer models but, to our knowledge, have not been engineered into any general-purpose computer tools. It can be argued that Shannon's information theory provides the basis for a similar set of "physics-based" cause-and-effect models to support the incorporation of this aspect of human performance into computer-based modeling and analysis tools. Considerable work has gone into the application of information theory to human information processing [e.g., Lachman et al., 1979] within research domains. The definition of neuromotor *channel capacity* [Fitts, 1954] and metrics for the information content of a visual stimulus measured in bits [Hick, 1952; Hyman, 1953] are some examples of the influence of information theory that have become well established. Given the considerable science that now exists, useful computer-based analytical tools that use these ideas as basic modeling constructs are likely to emerge.

Inference-Based Models

Often, direct measurement of a *performance resource* or structural element is not feasible or practical, and estimates must be inferred from models based on representative populations. Inferential-based methods, therefore, utilize derived relationships between parameters to provide an estimation (or prediction) of an unknown quantity based on other available measures. One type of modeling approach in such a situation is through statistical regression. This process uses data measured from a population of subjects with characteristics similar to the subject or population of interest to derive a function that represents a "typical" relationship between the independent (measured) variables and the dependent (desired) variable. Specifically, this is achieved through determination of the function that minimizes the error between the actual and the predicted values across all observations of the independent variable. This process results in an approximation of the desired parameter with a quantified standard error [Remington & Schork, 1985]. Applications of this method require that the dependent variable is distributed normally and with constant variance and, correspondingly, that an estimation of its typical value (for a given population) is desired. Applied to the human system, regression is often implemented to develop *data models,* which are then used to estimate unknown structural parameter values from known parameters, such as the estimation of body segment moments of inertia from stature and weight [McConville et al., 1980]. Regression also has been used to predict task performance from a wide variety of other variables (e.g., height, weight, age, other performance variables, etc.). A specific example is the determination of the maximum acceptable load during lifting tasks as a function of variables such as body weight and arm strength [Jiang & Ayoub, 1987].

A conceptually different and relatively new example of an inferential model, motivated by human performance problems specifically, is Nonlinear Causal Resource Analysis (NCRA) [Kondraske, 1988; Vasta & Kondraske, 1994]. Quantitative task demands, in terms of performance variables that characterize the involved subsystems, are inferred from a population data set that includes measures of subsystem performance resource availabilities (e.g., speed, accuracy, etc.) and overall performance on the task in question. This method is based on the following simple concept. Consider a sample of 100 people, each with a known amount of cash (e.g., a fairly even distribution from $0 to $10,000). Each person is asked to try to purchase a specific computer, the "cost" of which is unknown. In the subgroup that was able to make the purchase (some will not have enough cash), the individual who had the least amount of cash provides the key clue. This "amount of cash availability" provides an estimate of the computer's cost (i.e., the unknown value). Thus, in human performance, demand is inferred from resource availabilities.

Fidelity

An important principle that has not often received the scrutiny it deserves is that of the level of fidelity desired or, perhaps more critically, necessary for a particular application. This includes anything that affects the range of applicability or quality of the results provided in a given application. Fidelity can be characterized in terms of three distinctly different components: (1) model scope, (2) computational quality (e.g., resolution limits, compounding of errors, convergence limits of numerical methods, etc.), and (3) data quality (e.g., noise, intrinsic resolution limits, etc.). Model scope considers the extent to which major systems are incorporated (e.g., neuromuscular, sensory, cognitive, etc.) and, as a separate issue, the extent to which these major subsystems are represented (e.g., peak torque and angle limits versus a three-dimensional torque-angle-speed envelope for neuromuscular systems of rotational joints).

Parameter Conventions

Often, the exact definition of parameters across (and even within) scientific disciplines varies, limiting communication of findings and inhibiting dissemination of knowledge. Careful selection and clear documentation of *parameter conventions* are important principles in producing analytical software that can be understood, accepted, and used.

Within the broad scope of parameters that could possibly be incorporated in analytical and other software tools, there are many parameter convention challenges that arise. Due to the fact that the reported analyses in which various parameters appear have been of restricted scope and largely special purpose, more generalized situations where convention is important have escaped standardization in terms broad enough to support all application needs. As one example, consider the description of relative orientation between two object-attached coordinate systems in three dimensions (in the context of the human system, this specifies joint angle). There are two basic forms of angle-set representations, each derived in terms of the method of rotation of one coordinate system (attached to a moving object) about a specific axis: (1) fixed-angle representation, which involves referencing each rotation of the moving system to some fixed reference frame, and (2) Euler angle representation, indicating that each consecutive rotation of the moving system is referenced to the coordinate axes of its present orientation. Given multiple degrees of freedom, multiple angles result representing the amount of rotation about a specific axis and at a defined position in the order of rotations. The specification of these parameters defines the associated angle-set convention (i.e., fixed or Euler). Utilization of the terms *roll, pitch,* and *yaw* [e.g., Chao, 1980] in communicating this convention, originally used to describe ship and aircraft orientation, also can lead to confusion. This is not only due to the lack of similarity between the defined reference frame of an aircraft and that of a human segment but also due to its altered definition within other disciplines (e.g., fixed-angle representation [Spong & Vidyasagar, 1989]). Thus, depending on the "type" of Euler angle used and the sequence of axes about which the rotations occur, two entirely different orientations are likely to result. This discussion does not even consider the clinical perspective on joint angles, where only angles measured in three orthogonal planes [Panjabi et al., 1974] are considered. Despite the fact that the human architecture has remained constant (unlike many artificial systems), to our knowledge there is no standard convention that defines all angles in a total human link model for three-dimensional motion.

Data Formats

The utilization of data, especially within a software environment, involves both communication and manipulation not only within a single stand-alone application but often across facilities, databases, and platforms. Data formats, in this light, can be considered among the most important of the components fundamental to analytical software. Problematic effects may result from aspects including inconsistent adoption of terminology (e.g., endurance versus fatigue), units of measure specifications, file structures, parameter coding, and database structure. CAD environments in traditional engineering disciplines (e.g., drafting, mechanic design, etc.) have confronted such issues with standardizations such as the .DXF file formats (used for two- and three-dimensional geometric drawings, even accepted by some numeric machining systems) and the Gerber format (used to communicate a printed circuit board specification to board manufacturers). Within the realm of human performance engineering, standards for data formats remain at the forefront of developmental needs. Some weak standards are emerging, such as the relatively consistent use of ASCII text files with either labeled or position-dependent parameters. However, there are currently no known agreed on or de facto standards for positions, labels, units of measure, etc.

154.2 Scope, Functionality, and Performance

As summarized in Fig. 154.1, CAD-like human performance software depends on conceptual issues as well as decisions regarding fidelity, functionality, and implementation. There is also a great deal of interaction among these categories. Topics within each category were derived in part from a review of current packages (e.g., those described below) and an assessment of other issues and needs. These lists are intended to be illustrative and not exhaustive. While *every* major category applies to *any* given software tool, not all topics listed within a category will always be relevant.

Conceptual issues include taxonomies on which a given package is based (e.g., basic approaches to motor control, system performance, task categorizations and analysis, data estimation, etc.),

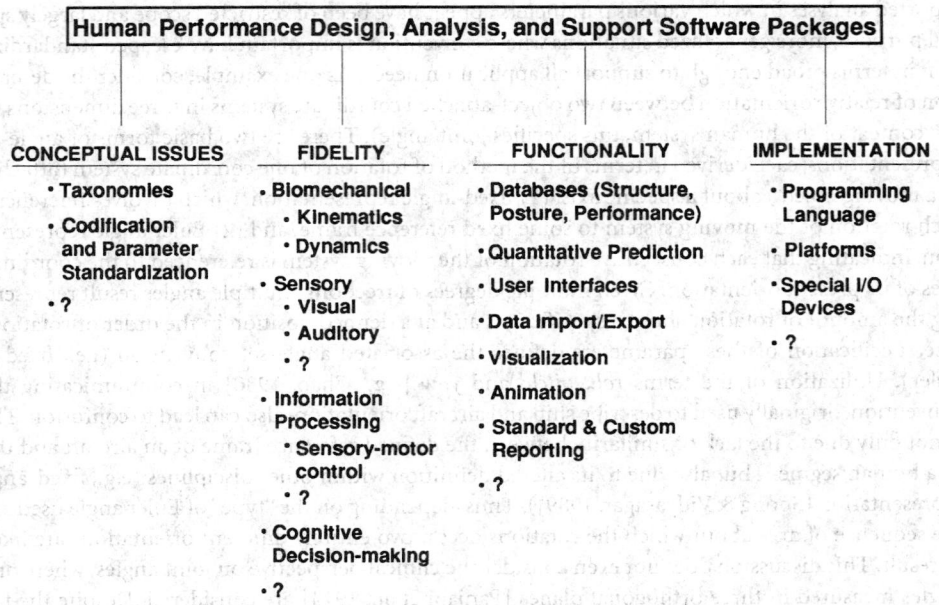

FIGURE 154.1 Related aspects of human design and performance software describe the diversity and scope of underlying issues.

parameter choices and codification (e.g., hierarchical level of representation, identification in structured input/output file formats), and compliance with or deviation from accepted standards with the varied communities that deal with human performance. They may well deserve special recognition given the impressionable developmental stage of the class of software tools addressed. Perhaps because developers are so familiar with a given perspective or body of knowledge, key conceptual issues are often overlooked or incorporated de facto from previous work (e.g., research studies) that is similar (but perhaps not identical) to the intended purpose of a given package, which is frequently broader and more general than the research efforts or projects that inspired it. Software packages impose on users the constructs on which they are based, and this may result in conflicts within an already structured environment. Conceptual foundations and approaches are not yet as cleanly defined in human performance as they are in disciplines such as electrical and mechanical engineering. This is further complicated by the wide variety of disciplines (and therefore educational backgrounds) represented by those with interest in participating in software development. Clear and complete disclosure of the conceptual foundation used by developers is thus helpful to both users (potential and actual) and developers.

The concept and scope of fidelity in the present context were delineated earlier and are further represented by the subtopics in Fig. 154.1. We have chosen to apply them here in their broadest sense. In a fairly recent National Research Council panel on human performance modeling [Baron et al., 1990], recommendations were made toward problems regarding design and implementation issues. Though not specifically addressing computer software, the extension of the discussion is natural given present technology and implementation methods. While it was concluded that an all-inclusive model (i.e., high fidelity, in the sense that biomechanical, information-processing, sensory, and perceptual aspects, etc. are represented) might be desirable, it is highly unlikely that it could be achieved or would be useful, since the inherent complexity would impede effective usage. The basic recommendation made was to pursue more limited scope submodels. The implication is that two or more computer-based versions of such submodels could be integrated to achieve a wide range of fidelity, with the combination selected to meet the needs of particular situations. However, there is neither a general framework nor a set of guidelines for developers of submodels (i.e., an *open-architecture concept*) that would facilitate integration of relatively independent software development efforts. Thus integration is left to the end user, and typically only cumbersome methods are available.

Fidelity should be considered in combination with productivity, and both must be carefully assessed against needs. For example, a package that provides the user with control over a large number of parameters (e.g., joint stiffness, balance control, etc.) that define the human system under analysis typically allows for greater intrinsic fidelity and can be valuable if the ability to specify parameters at that level of detail is an absolute user requirement. If not, this level of specificity only increases the number of prerequisites steps to achieve a given analysis and leads to a more complex program in terms of operation and function (which is perhaps most evident in the user interface). Furthermore, more accurate results are not necessarily obtained. Programs that are structured to automatically rely on default parameter values that can be inspected or changed when desired serve both types of needs. However, concern is typically raised that "lazy" users will forego the entry of values more appropriate to the situation at hand. Thus, while software developers can provide features that greatly simplify procedures and recommendations regarding their proper use, users bear the responsibility of choosing when to invoke such features. Fidelity issues are often viewed as "either-or" choices, when many times a "both or all" approach is quite feasible. This gives the user the decision-making power and responsibility for decisions that may effect quality of results. Such approaches also typically result in a greater user pool for a given package. How such flexibility is implemented, however, is critical. For example, if fidelity decisions are likely to be made once in a given installation, schemes that require decision making with each analysis can prove to be cumbersome and ineffective.

Functionality can be considered in terms of basic and special subcategories. Far too often, attention is given to special features while those which are more basic (such as import/export capabilities) are ignored. Most items listed in Fig. 154.1 under the "functionality" category are self-explanatory, although it should be noted that features such as importing and exporting are more complex in the present context than one might anticipate due in part to the lack of standards for parameters representation (see above). Developers must carefully select functionality, and potential users must carefully evaluate the impact of these choices against their specific needs. For example, the processing power required to display and animate contoured multisegment human figures in real time and in three dimensions is substantial. Programs with this ability typically require high-end platforms and also require that a large fraction of the programming effort and user interface be used for this functionality. The addition of processes such as a dynamic analysis places even a greater stress on processing power and complexity. Visualization of human figures in three dimensions along with some environmental components is essential for some applications. For many applications, such as those in which numeric results are required and conveyed with simple printed reports, such visualizations are not required or contribute little to achieving the desired end purpose (although they are almost always viewed as "attractive" by potential users). Functionality options are further developed and exemplified in the discussion of actual software packages below.

The last of these four categories describes the support structure upon which the software packages are built. Software implementation in today's ever-changing computer market requires careful thought. In addition to host platform and standard accessories, special input/output interfaces are often necessary (e.g., to allow direct access to laboratory acquired kinematic data). Support software for such special hardware is not always available on all platforms, preventing operation with analytical software in the same environment. Choices of programming language (supporting modules and libraries, platform diversity) and the operating system (Macintosh, Windows, Unix, etc.) are also critical. As exemplified below, no existing packages run on all platforms and under all operating systems, leaving users who wish to employ multiple packages with cumbersome and often costly solutions.

As computing power at the single-user level (i.e., personal computer) increases, there is little doubt that a full set of state-of-the-art features covering a broad scope of human performance and data needs *could* be integrated into a single package. At present, though, limitations are real and necessary. These are the result of specific tradeoffs that must be considered during development when determining target users. Operational costs include software acquisition, maintenance, basic platform acquisition and outfitting, and training costs. A large feature set and high performance are not always indicative of a software tool's value. Value is lost if a user's requirements are either unfulfilled or greatly exceed by the functionality and/or performance of a program. Unfortunately, general tradeoffs that are acceptable within different groups of users have not yet become evident.

154.3 Functional Overview of Representative Packages

In this section a selected set of different types of software packages intended specifically for human design and performance analysis applications is described. At least one example of each type exists and is noted for reference to illustrate the types of functionality developers are addressing in response to perceived needs. No endorsement of any example cited is implied. The packages included vary widely in function and performance and should not be considered to be directly comparable. Operational costs reflect this diversity, ranging from relatively inexpensive (e.g., approximately $100 plus the price of a moderately equipped DOS-based PC) to the level defined by high-end workstations (e.g., in excess of $2000 for software plus the cost of a Unix-based workstation). As with desktop computer applications, such as word processors and spreadsheets, the packages used to illustrate functionality are under constant development, and changing feature sets, performance, and cost are to be anticipated.

The types of packages included illustrate fundamental options with regard to general or dedicated analysis (e.g., user-defined tasks versus gait), different levels of analysis (e.g., "muscle" versus "joint" levels in biomechanical analyses), body-function-specific or general-purpose analysis (e.g., gait versus user-defined function), fidelity in terms of scope (e.g., biomechanical, sensory, neuromotor control, etc.), and target-user orientation (medical versus nonmedical design, although overlap is possible). It should be noted that while particular packages are highlighted under certain categories, underlying features and functions are common across many applications.

Human Parameter Databases

The need for data is evident in all aspects of human-related computer-aided design and the analysis of human performance. In certain situations, requirements may be for a specific individual or a representative population. In the former case, there are certain parameters that are not readily attainable (e.g., location of center of mass for a segment, inertia, etc.) and therefore must be estimated, as in the latter case, from normative values derived from studies. For a number of years, these estimates have been available in book form primarily as lookup tables. This format, however, does not take advantage of current technology and is not sufficient for use with software-based analytical tools. Some currently available packages, in addressing this need, have included limited data tables accessible from within the program. *Mannequin* (described in more detail below), for example, provides a significant database of anthropometric measures for various populations that is incorporated into the architecture of its graphic figures. Though the user specifies design parameter values by choosing the gender and ethnic origin representative of the desired population, database values for specific aspects can only be directly obtained by viewing parameters of specific segments from the complete figure. Thus the information is, in effect, proprietary to the software package and unavailable for direct access by other computer-based applications (understandably so). In contrast, Biomechanics Corporation of America, Inc., the supplier of Mannequin, also has produced a stand-alone ergonomics database called *Ergobase*. This software system provides on-screen access to 44 global civilian and military populations, including detailed data on wheelchair users, pregnant women, and the aging. Additionally, Ergobase provides a visual image display library, a glossary of anthropometric, ergonomic, and medical terms, as well as data on selected strengths and aerobic capacities.

In addition to measures such as segment lengths, parameters including reach and range of motion for selected postures are frequently provided in databases (e.g., horizontal sitting reach, etc.). Because it is prohibitive (if not impossible) to measure and report all possible situations, this issue may be more adequately addressed through the use of parametric data models. Data derived from such models would provide estimates for all possible conditions as well as having the additional advantage of requiring lesser storage and management requirements. Caution is warranted with regard to issues such as model validity, statistical sample sizes and variations, combinatory effects of merging databases or data models, and traceability of data to original sources.

Biomechanical, Muscle-Level Modeling and Analysis

SIMM is a graphics-based tool for modeling and visualizing any human or animal musculoskeletal system. This package is unique from those similar to Mannequin or Jack (described below) in that it is directed at low-level structures, i.e., individual muscles, in contrast to the function at a joint. The program allows users to model any type of musculoskeletal system using files which specify (1) the skeletal structure through polygonal surface objects, (2) the joint kinematics, and (3) the muscle architecture through specifications of a line of action for each muscle and isometric force data. SIMM contains four tools for observing and editing the model. "Model viewer" is used to visualize the model and allows the user to display or hide the individual muscles (shown as line segments) as well as joint angle manipulation and animation. Muscle forces, moment arms, and joint torques (static) can be analyzed via plots and graphs using the tool "plot maker." All the muscle parameters may be edited, including visual alteration of muscle lines of action, with "muscle editor." Finally, joint kinematics may be changed and viewed with "joint editor," which allows the user to alter the cubic splines used to control the animated joint movements. Developers claim that SIMM is aimed at biomechanics researchers, kinesiologists, workspace designers, and students who can benefit from visual feedback showing muscle locations and actions (Fig. 154.2).

MusculoGraphics, the developers of SIMM, also produce an add-on package specifically directed toward gait analysis that provides ground reaction force vectors and color-highlighted muscle activity through animation of the model. The software is designed to input data files written by movement analysis systems and can display plots of data such as muscle lengths and ground reaction forces. Still in the developmental stage (at the time of this writing) is another application, the Dynamics Pipeline, which is a general-purpose package that provides forward and inverse dynamics to calculate motions resulting from forces or torques required to generate a given motion, respectively. SIMM requires a Silicon Graphics workstation for operation.

Body-Function-Specific Tools

Gait Lab is a DOS-based software package that allows fundamental parameters of human gait to be derived, analyzed, and inspected. The program is divided into two main sections (i.e., subprograms that run under the "shell" of the main application): (1) a mathematics section that provides processes for generating text files representing various gait parameters throughout a gait cycle and (2) a graphics section that creates plots of the parameters as well as a representation of gait through an animated stick figure. The Gait Lab package is a combination of a gait parameterization software package, operation manual, and book [Vaughan et al., 1992] on the theories, analysis methods, and parameters of human gait. The book covers the gait parameters and equations associated with the software package as well as the underlying principles for their use in gait analysis. The software accepts four different, custom-formatted data files (ASCII text) based on direct measurements of a human subject. These include anthropometric, kinematic (i.e., three-dimensional positions of anatomic landmarks), force plate, and EMG measures. Sample files are included for a healthy adult male, female, and an adult male with cerebral palsy. From these data, text files are created for lower extremity body segment parameters (mass, center of gravity position, and moment of inertia), linear kinematics (joint center, heel and toe locations, segment reference frames), center of gravity

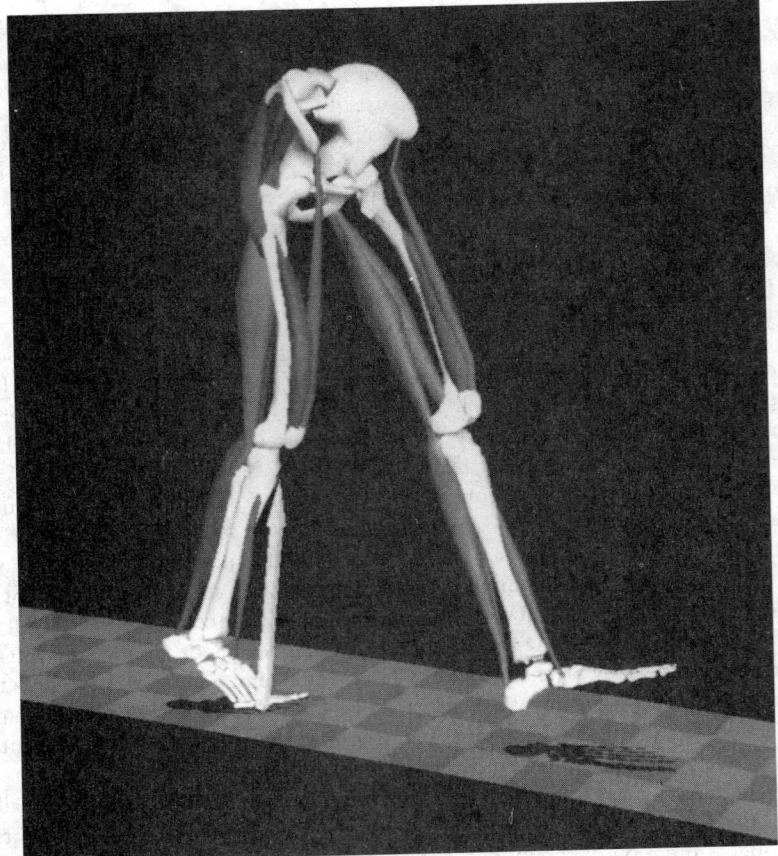

FIGURE 154.2 Muscle attachments and activation (indicated by shading) for the lower extremities during gait, created and displayed using SIMM software. (Reprinted with permission from MusculoGraphics, Inc. Portions of model developed by Lisa Schutte, Gillette Children's Hospital.)   PAGE 2344

(position, velocity, and acceleration), angular kinematics (joint angles, angular velocity and acceleration), and dynamics (joint forces and torques). The package also can display up to three simultaneous plots of these parameters in any combination. Time, percent of gait cycle, and marker position scales are also available for plotting against any of the variables.

Gait Lab provides a useful function in its ability to generate the above-mentioned parameters and is effective with its simplistic stick figure animation, allowing minimal processing power/speed requirements while providing the nuances of lower limb movement pertinent to gait analysis. The software tested (no version number was indicated, copyright 1992), while certainly not published pre-Windows, forces the user into the key-command mode (no mouse interface is provided) of using the enter, arrow, and function keys to operate menus and functions. Though not difficult to become acquainted with, it is not intuitive in layout or operation relative to today's user-interface standards. Also, with the exception of the anthropometry file, which can be created from within the software, no means is provided for editing data files. If new files are to be utilized, they must be in the required format (which must be inferred by inspection of the example files provided with the package).

Biomechanical, Joint-Level, Total Human Analysis

ADAMS is a software package designed for mechanical design and system simulation in general. It is an extensive package incorporating specific components for both modeling and kinematic/

dynamic analysis. What sets ADAMS apart from other non-performance-based simulation/dynamics packages is the availability of a module, ADAMS/Android, specifically designed to allow the user to create a human model. The human model may be edited as needed but is provided in a default configuration of a 15-joint body architecture with anthropometric parameters based on the 75th percentile male. Because the package focuses on mechanical systems in general, a great deal of control is provided to the user over the parameters of the model, including contact forces, joint friction, damping, and nonlinear stiffness, as well as control parameters. Having this capability, the human model is able to affect control over objects in its environment as well as responding biomechanically to contact. Supplemental toolsets may be (custom) developed to provide proper control over model parameters such as motion-resistance relationships, joint strength and range-of-motion limits, and delays in neuromuscular response. For a given model, kinematic or dynamic simulations may be run, and values for any parameter can be plotted on screen. Both forward and inverse dynamic analyses are available, and graphically based facilities such as the specification of trajectories via mouse input are available. Modules for animation and optimization are being developed at present but are expected to be released by the time this *Handbook* is published.

Because ADAMS' capabilities are so extensive, it has become one of the most widely used mechanical system simulation packages. Outside the realm of human performance analysis, the package is targeted at engineers and scientists who require complete observation and control of the model parameters across many hierarchical levels. While this format affords great fidelity and specificity in the analysis, a great deal of complexity and detail also must be addressed in every new simulation run. Though performance assessment is not an inherent or recognized feature in the package, custom modules may be incorporated that would allow for direct comparison of system resource utilization and stress against the demands of the task.

Visualization for Low-End Computer Platforms

Mannequin, while having inherent database functionality, is essentially a visualization tool that allows users to quickly create three-dimensional humanoid figures that may be represented in stick-figure form, as a wireframe "robot" with polygonal segments, or, as its name implies, a mannequin with contoured (shaded) segments. These figures may be postured within preset (i.e., noneditable) range-of-motion limits, as well as viewed from many different perspectives. They are created automatically by the program according to user-defined structural aspects chosen from a list of specifications for gender, population percentile, body type, age, and nationality. The package also provides a modest drawing (CAD-type) tool for creating various objects to be placed in the scene with the figure. Two additional features extend Mannequin beyond the domain of a "simple" object-rendering tool. The first is provided through animation effects, allowing the mannequin to walk via an internally generated gait sequence (a specific path may be defined through a virtual workspace), reach to a specific location, or move through any sequence of positions created on a frame-by-frame basis by the user. The second feature allows the user to specify forces acting on the mannequin's hands or feet from which static torques are calculated for both left and right wrists, elbows, shoulders, neck, back, hips, knees, and ankles.

As a visualization tool, Mannequin provides a needed capability for a modest price and requires only a personal computer to run. Figures are easily produced to the anthropometric specifications available, and posing, reaching, and walking functions, though limited, are simple to control. The package is primarily operated from mouse input with standard point, click, and drag operations that should be familiar to most users of current commercial software. A toolbox resides on the screen which enables the user to access most drawing and viewing functions, although much of the standard functionality of the package is accessed from pull-down menus. Manipulation of the figures (i.e., changing the angle of a joint) is performed using slider bars for rotation of the chosen segment about each axis of the workspace. Several three-dimensional shapes are available for rapid object prototyping as well as lathe and extrusion functions for adding depth to two-dimensional figures. Once the scene is created with humans and objects in their workspace, it is up to the user to extract any information regarding function and performance from the visual images presented by the package. These features, as well as others, are also contained within the software package Jack (described below), which provides greater functionality but is targeted toward workstation environments. In sum, Mannequin, with a good price-to-performance ratio, is an effective tool when human visualization with moderate graphics is required at the single-user platform level.

Extended Visualization for High-End Workstations

Jack is a high-end CAD-oriented design and visualization package developed within the University of Pennsylvania Center for Human Modeling and Simulation [Badler et al., 1993]. Similar in function to Mannequin (above), but with considerably more flexibility and detail, Jack is designed to allow human factors engineers to place a human in a workstation while still in the design phase. Jack extends far beyond the capabilities of Mannequin, trading simplicity for specificity, in that Jack provides users with control over a large range of variables regarding many aspects of the human figure and its virtual environment. The human model includes a 17-segment flexible torso, positionable socketed eyes, and fully articulated 16-joint hands. User-definable anthropometric parameters include segment dimensions, joint limits, moments of inertia, and strength. The figure can be positioned as desired through either mouse or keyboard interface by manipulation (rotation and translation) of a single joint or by dragging an end-effector. The total functionality of the package is far too great to list the individual aspects here, but examples include reach, hand gripping, balance (including reorientation behavior), collision detection, light and camera (view) manipulation, animation, and real-time posture tracking of a human operator through position and orientation sensors. In addition, a moderate library of CAD objects is available and editable for inclusion in the Jack environment, and many standard CAD file formats are supported (Fig. 154.3).

Similar to the functionality of ADAMS, Jack provides a great deal of control over the design and manipulation of the human figure, as would be anticipated from its 20+ years of development. Because of the large number of controllable parameters and the difficulty involved in providing an interface allowing three-dimensional manipulation of high-end graphics in a two-dimensional environment, the majority of Jack users will require training (estimated by the developers to be, on average, 2 days). Jack requires a Silicon Graphics workstation to run.

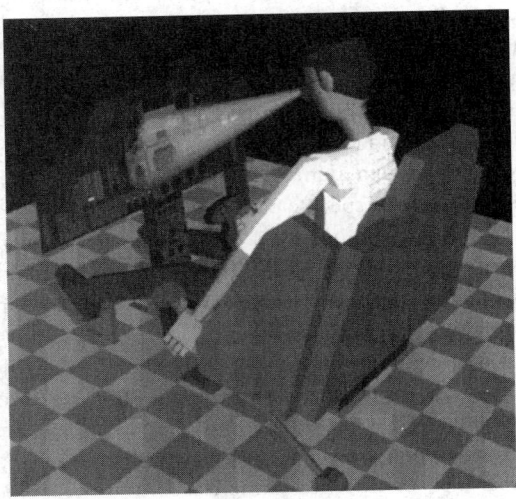

FIGURE 154.3   A human/workspace figure created and displayed using Jack software. (Reprinted with permission from the Center for Human Modeling and Simulation at the University of Pennsylvania.)

Total Human, Performance-Based, Human-Task Interface Analysis

While now under development, *HMT-CAD* represents yet a different perspective in that it is based primarily on performance modeling constructs [e.g., Kondraske, 1995] and is aimed at producing bottom-line assessments regarding human-to-task, human-to-machine, and eventually machine-to-task interfaces using logic similar to that used by systems-level designers. In a joint effort between Photon Research Associates, Inc. and The University of Texas at Arlington Human Performance Institute, performance models and decision-making strategies are combined with advanced multibody dynamic analysis.

HMT-CAD's initial development emphasized a top-down approach that set out with the goal of realizing a shell that would allow systematic incorporation of increasingly higher fidelity in a modular, stepwise fashion. The initial modules encompass biomechanical and neuromuscular aspects of performance that bases analyses on knowledge of range/extremes of motion, torque, and speed capacities. Gross total human (23 links and 41 degrees of freedom) and hand link models (16 links and 22 degrees of freedom each) are included. The Windows-based tool provides a predefined framework for specifying human structure and performance parameters (e.g., anthropometry, strength, etc.) for individuals or populations. A task library is included based on an object-oriented approach to task analysis. HMT-CAD attempts to help communicate information about many parameters via a custom graphic-button interface. For example, one analysis result screen shows a human figure surrounded by buttons connected to body joints. Button color (e.g., red or green) communicates whether an analysis found limiting factors for the specified person in the specified task associated with that joint system. Using computer mouse input, clicking on red buttons produces a new window showing a list of performance capacities and stress levels associated with systems of that joint. Maximally stressed performance resources are tagged. HMT-CAD uses the same systems level modeling constructs for human and artificial systems. A novel technique that transparently draws on as large a set of data models as needed is used to provide "the best analysis possible" with the data provided by the user. This allows users to directly specify values for all parameters, if desired, but does not require this for each analysis (Fig. 154.4).

In the present prototype, analysis scope is very limited (upper extremity, object moving tasks). Databases are being populated to allow a similar fidelity of analysis for trunk and lower extremity analyses. Development of an optimization engine based on minimizing stress across performance resources [Kondraske & Khoury, 1992] to solve problems in which redundant approaches are possible is under way. No capability is currently provided for animation of human movement, since binary assessments (e.g., red and green buttons) and numeric results (stress levels on performance capacities) are emphasized. However, an interface to emerging general-purpose animation tools is planned. Long-term development will proceed to increase fidelity in a stepwise fashion by the inclusion of performance capacities for other major systems (e.g., information processing associated with motor control) as well as additional performance capacities for major systems represented at any given time (e.g., the inclusion of neuromuscular endurance limits).

154.4 Anticipated Developments

While it is relatively easy to outline the functionality and unique aspects of the software discussed above, it is a great deal harder to describe the level of difficulty required to achieve a desired end result and to characterize how well functions are performed. On-line "help" systems, multimedia components, associated software development tools, improved parameter measurement tools, and higher-fidelity models will no doubt impact these aspects.

As mundane as it may seem, perhaps nothing is more important to the overall advancement of this class of software tools than the development of standards for parameters used, parameter conventions, and data formats. It is likely that de facto standards will emerge from individual commercial endeavors. Due to the diversity of professionals involved, it is difficult to envision the

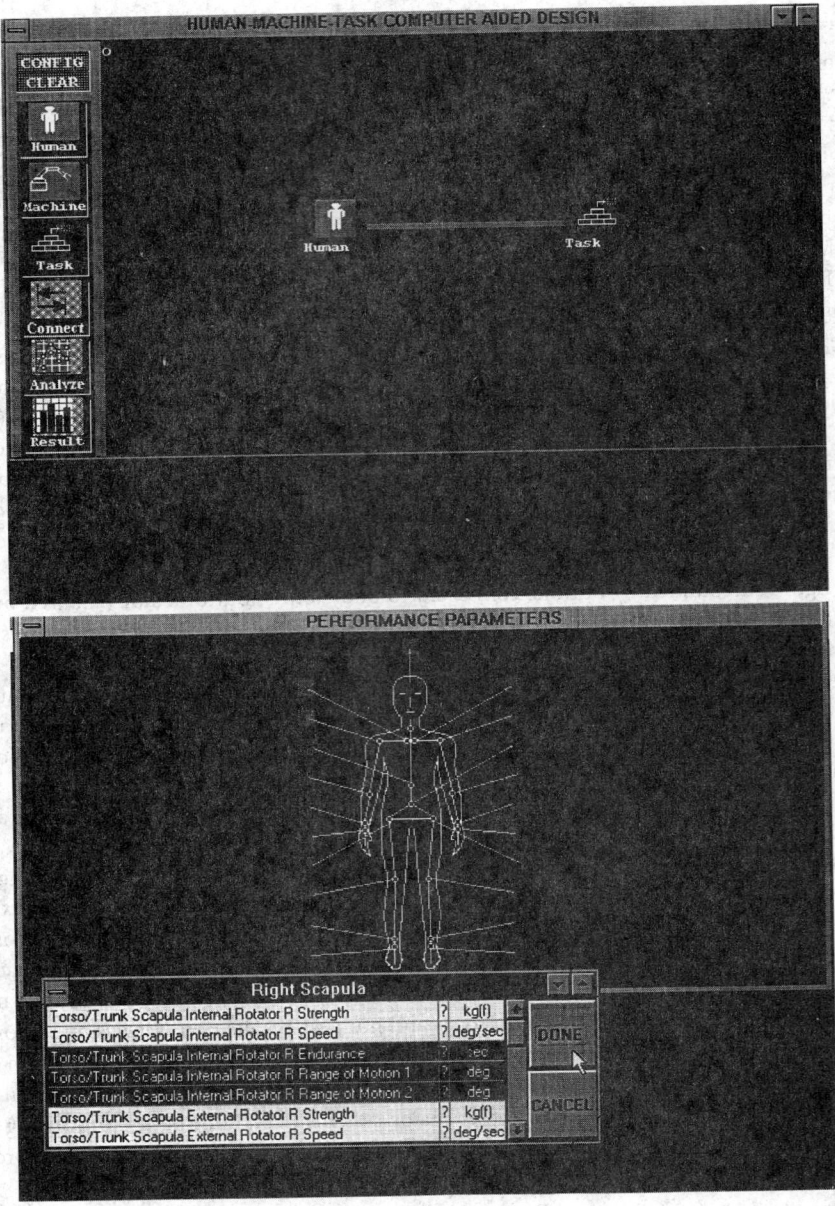

FIGURE 154.4 A desktop environment of the HMT-CAD performance assessment package including system model development and analysis result reporting.

evolution of "standards by committee." Observation of success stories in analogous efforts also supports this opinion. This, in turn, will enable progress to be made in database and data model development, which is vital to the many of the more routine functions such software will perform. Combined with modular object-oriented programming techniques, the emergence of true multitasking operating systems on desktop computers, and the support for interprocess communication (such as dynamic data exchange) will encourage developers. Many new tools, both similar to and completely different from those described here, can be anticipated.

Defining Terms

Channel capacity: The maximum rate of information flow through a specific pathway from source to receiver. In the context of the human, a sensorimotor pathway (e.g., afferent sensory nerves, processors, descending cerebrospinal nerve and α-motoneuron) is an example of a channel through which motor-control information flows from sensors to actuators (muscle).

Data model: A mathematic equation derived as a representation of the relationship between a dependent variable and one or more independent variables. Similar in function to a database, data models provide parameter values across conditions of other related parameters.

Human-task interface: The common boundary between the human and a task specified by the demands of a task on the respective resources of the human and the capacities of the human's resources involved in performing the task.

Linked multibody system: A system of three or more individual segments joined (as an open or closed chain) in some manner with the degree of freedom between any two segments defined by the characteristics of the corresponding hinge.

Open-architecture concept: A general methodology for the development of functional modules that may be readily integrated to form a higher-level system through well-defined design and interface constructs.

Parameter conventions: Aspects and/or usage of a parameter that are specifically defined with respect to general implementation.

Performance assessment: The process of determining the level or degree in which a system can perform a specific task given the demands required and the availabilities of the resources of the system which are involved in performing the task.

Performance resource: Defined as a functional unit and an associated dimension of performance (e.g., knee extensor strength) that is available to a system.

Virtual workspace: A representation of a three-dimensional physical workspace generated by computer software and displayed on a video monitor or similar device. This enables, for example, the inclusion and manipulation of computer-generated objects within the virtual workspace such that designs can be tested and modified prior to manufacturing.

References

Allard P, Stokes IAF, Blanchi JP (eds). 1994. Three-Dimensional Analysis of Human Movement. Champaign, Ill, Human Kinetics.

Badler NI. 1989. Task-oriented animation of human figures. In GR McMillan, D Beevis, E Salas (eds), Applications of Human Performance Models to System Design. New York, Plenum Press.

Badler NI, Phillips CB, Webber BL. 1993. Simulating Humans: Computer Graphics Animation and Control. New York, Oxford University Press.

Baron S, Kruser DS, Huey BM (eds). 1990. Quantitative Modeling of Human Performance in Complex, Dynamic Systems. Washington, National Academy Press.

Chao EYS. 1980. Justification of triaxial goniometer for the measurement of joint rotation. Biomechanics 13:989.

Craig JJ. 1989. Introduction to Robotics Mechanics and Control, 2d ed. Reading, Mass, Addison-Wesley.

Delp SL, Loan JP, Hoy MG, et al. 1990. An interactive graphics-based model of the lower extremity to study orthopedic surgical procedures. IEEE Trans Biomed Eng 37(8):757.

Fitts P. 1954. The information capacity of the human motor system in controlling the amplitude of movement. J Exp Psychol 47:381.

Hick W. 1952. On the rate of gain of information. Q J Exp Psychol 4:11.

Hyman R. 1953. Stimulus information as a determinant of reaction time. J Exp Psychol 45:423.

Jiang BC, Ayoub MM. 1987. Modelling of maximum acceptable load of lifting by physical factors. Ergonomics 30(3):529.

Khan C. 1991. Humanizing AutoCAD. Cadence, June.

Kondraske GV. 1988. Experimental evaluation of an elemental resource model for human performance. In Proceedings, Tenth Annual IEEE Engineering in Medicine and Biology Society Conference, New Orleans, pp 1612–1613.

Kondraske GV. 1995. A working model for human system-task interfaces. In JD Bronzino (ed), Handbook of Biomedical Engineering. Boca Raton, Fla, CRC Press.

Kondraske GV, Khoury GJ. 1992. Telerobotic system performance measurement: Motivation and methods. In JD Erickson (ed), Cooperative Intelligent Robotics in Space III (Proc. SPIE 1829), pp 161–172. New York, SPIE.

Lachman R, Lachman JL, Butterfield EC. 1979. Cognitive Psychology and Information Processing: An Introduction. Hillsdale, NJ, Erlbaum.

McConville JT, Churchill TD, Kaleps I, et al. 1980. Anthropometric Relationships of Body and Body Segment Moments of Inertia. Air Force Aerospace Medical Research Laboratory, AFAMRL-TR-80-119, Wright-Patterson Air Force Base, Ohio.

Panjabi MM, White AA III, Brand RA. 1974. A note on defining body parts configurations. J Biomech 7(4):385.

Pheasant ST. 1986. Bodyspace: Anthropometry, Ergonomics and Design. Philadelphia, Taylor and Francis.

Remington RD, Schork MA. 1985. Statistics with Applications to the Biological and Health Sciences. Englewood Cliffs, NJ, Prentice-Hall.

Spong MW, Vidyasagar M. 1989. Robot Dynamics and Control. New York, Wiley.

Vasta PJ, Kondraske GV. 1994. Performance prediction of an upper extremity reciprocal task using non-linear causal resource analysis. In Proceedings, Sixteenth Annual IEEE engineering in Medicine and Biology Society Conference, Baltimore, pp 305–306.

Vaughan CL, Davis BL, O'Connor JC. 1992. Dynamics of Human Gait. Champaign, Ill, Human Kinetics.

Winter DA. 1990. Biomechanics and Motor Control of Human Movement, 2d ed. New York, Wiley.

Further Information

For explicit information regarding the software packages included in this chapter, the developers may be contacted directly as follows:

ADAMS: Mechanical Dynamics, West Coast Consulting Group, Six Venture, Suite 100, Irvine, CA 92718, (714) 727-0430

Ergobase/Mannequin: Biomechanics Corp. of America, 1800 Walt Whitman Road, Melville, NY 11747, (516) 752-3568

Gait Lab: Human Kinetics, 1607 N. Market St., Box 5076, Champaign, IL 61825, (217) 351-5076

HMT-CAD: Human Performance Institute, The University of Texas at Arlington, P.O. Box 19180, Arlington, TX 76019, (817) 273-2335

Jack: Center for Human Modeling and Simulation, The University of Pennsylvania, 200 South 33rd St., Philadelphia, PA 19104, (215) 898-1488

SIMM: MusculoGraphics, Inc., 1840 Oak Ave., Evanston, IL 60201, (708) 866-1882

A broad perspective of issues related to those presented here may be found in M. Matilla and W. Karwowski (eds). 1992. Computer applications in ergonomics, occupational safety, and health. In *Proceedings of the International Conference on Computer-Aided Ergonomics and Safety '92*, Tampere, Finland, North-Holland Publishers, Amsterdam.

Additionally, periodic discussions of related topics may be found in the following publications: *CSERIAC Gateway,* published by the Crew System Ergonomics Information Analysis Center (for subscription information, contact AL/CFH/CSERIAC, Bldg. 248, 2255 H St., Wright-Patterson Air Force Base, Ohio, 45433); *IEEE Transactions on Biomedical Engineering* or *IEEE Engineering in Medicine and Biology Magazine* (for further information, contact IEEE Service Center, 445 Hoes Lane, P.O. Box 1331, Piscataway, NJ, 08855-1331).

Also, discussions regarding topics relating to biomechanical analysis may be found on the Internet bulletin board BIOMCH-L. Further information can be obtained by sending the command "send biomch-1 guide" to LISTSERV@HEARN.BITNET or LISTSERV@NIC.SURFNET.NL or by anonymous FTP from hearn.nic.surfnet.nl (directory BIOMCH-L).

155

Human Performance Engineering: Challenges and Prospects for the Future

George V. Kondraske
University of Texas at Arlington

Human performance engineering is a dynamic area with rapid changes in many facets and constantly emerging developments that affect application possibilities. Material presented in other chapters of this section illustrates the breadth and depth of effort required as well as the variety of applications in this field. At the same time, the field is relatively young, and as is often the case in such instances, some "old" issues remain unresolved and new issues emerge with new developments. With the other material in this section as background, this chapter focuses on selected issues of a general nature (i.e., cutting across various human subsystem types and applications) in three major areas vital to the future of the field: (1) human performance modeling, (2) measurement, and (3) data-related topics. In addition to the identification of some key issues, some speculation is presented with regard to the lines along which future work may develop. Awareness of the specific issues raised is anticipated to be helpful to practitioners who must operate within the constraints of the current state of the art. Moreover, the issues selected represent scientific and engineering challenges for the future that will require not only awareness but also the collaboration of researchers and practitioners from the varied segments of the community to resolve.

155.1 Models

It is important to distinguish various types of models encountered in human performance. They include conceptual, statistically based predictive models, predictive models based on cause and effect, and data models [e.g., Vasta and Kondraske, 1995]. Issues related to data models are described later in this chapter, while those related to the remaining types are discussed in this section.

Traditionally, a tremendous amount of activity in various segments of the human performance community has been directed toward development of statistically based predictive models (e.g.,

0-8493-8346-3/95/$0.00+$.50

regression models). This remains the most popular approach. By their very nature, each of these is very application-specific. Even within the intended application, success of these models has ranged mostly from poor to marginal, with a few reports of models that look "very good" in the populations in which they were tested. However, the criteria for "good" have been skewed by the early performance achieved with these methods, and statistically significant *r* values of 0.6 have come to be considered "good." Even if predictive performance was excellent, the long-term merit of statistically based prediction methods can be questioned on the basis that this approach is intrinsically inefficient. A unique and time-consuming modeling effort, requiring new data collection with human subjects, is required for every situation. At the same time, powerful computer-based tools are commonly available that facilitate the generation of what is estimated to be hundreds and perhaps thousands of these regression models on an annual basis. It appears that many researchers and practitioners have forgotten that one purpose of such statistical methods is to provide insight into the cause-and-effect principles at play and into generalizations that might be more broadly applied. Statistically based regression models will continue to serve useful purposes within the specific application contexts for which they are developed. However, the future of predictive modeling in human performance engineering must be based on cause-and-effect principles. The sentiment for the need to shift from statistical to more physically based models is present and growing in several of the related application disciplines, as evidenced by a sampling of quotations from the literature presented in Table 155.1.

A National Research Council panel on human performance modeling [Baron et al., 1990] conducted one of the more broad-looking investigations regarding complex human performance models; i.e., those which consider one or more major attributes (e.g., biomechanical, sensory, cognitive, structural details, etc.) of a total or near-total human. The convening of this panel itself underscored the interest in and need for human performance models. As an interesting aside, while the panel's focus was on modeling, a large fraction of the efforts cited as background represented major software packages, most of which were developed to support defense industry needs. A major application for such models is in computer simulation of humans in various circumstances, which could be used to support prediction and other analysis needs. A series of useful recommendations was included in panel's report regarding the direction that should be taken in future work. However, recommendations were quite general in nature, and no specific plans were outlined regarding how some of these objectives might actually be achieved. Nonetheless, it was clear from the choice of previous work cited and from the recommendations that development of cause-and-effect that general-purpose models should receive priority. The working model presented for this section of this text [Kondraske, 1995] is one example of a causal, integrative model that reflects an initial attempt to incorporate many of this panel's recommendations.

TABLE 155.1. Representative Quotations Illustrating the Need for a Shift Toward the Development of Causal Models

Quote	Field	Reference
"… there has been little advancement of the science of ergonomics … the degree of advancement is so low that, in my opinion, ergonomics does not yet qualify as a science … There has been no progress in the accumulation of general knowledge … because nearly all studies have not been general studies."	Human factors	Smith, 1987
"… experiments are performed year after year to answer the same questions, those questions—often fundamental ones—remain unanswered … the methodology employed today is a hodgepodge of quick fixes that evolved over the years into a paradigm that is taught and employed as sacrosanct, when in fact it is woefully inadequate and frequently incompetent …"	Human factors	Simmon, 1987
"… authors and users of these instruments lacked a conceptual model … lack of a well-developed conceptual model is unfortunately characteristic of the entire history of the field …"	Rehabilitation	Frey, 1987

Whether primarily statistical or causal in nature, frustration with what has been characterized or perceived as "limited success" achieved to date in efforts to unlock and formalize the underpinnings of complex human functions such as speech, gait, lifting, and memory have led to attacks in recent years on the basic reductionistic approach that has been pursued most aggressively. In fact, reductionism has been characterized as a "dead end" methodology—one that has been tried and has failed [Bunge, 1977; Gardner, 1985], as further evidenced by the following somewhat representative quote [Weismer & Liss, 1991]:

> This view held the scientific community spellbound until people started looking past the technological issues, and asking how well the reductionist observations were doing at explaining behavior, and the answer was, miserably. Many microscopic facts had been accumulated, and incredible technological advances had been made, but the sum of all of these reductionist observations could not make good sense of macroscopic levels of movement behavior.

Prior to total abandonment, it is perhaps wise not only to characterize the performance of reductionism but also to question why it might have failed *thus far*. For example, it may be prudent to entertain the proposition that reductionism may be "a correct approach" that has failed to date because of a problem with one or more components associated its implementation. Are we certain that this is not the case?

One potential explanation for an apparent failure of reductionism is simply the manner in which manpower has been organized (i.e., the research infrastructure) to attack problems of the magnitude of those considered, for example, by the National Research Council panel noted above. With some exceptions, the majority of funded research efforts are short term and involve very small teams. Is it possible that the amount of information "to reduce" is too much to produce results that would be characterized as "success" (i.e., does the equivalent of an undercapitalized business venture exist)? It is further observed that the value of *reduction* is often only demonstrable by the ability to *assemble*. As noted, the prime tool of assembly thus far has been statistical in nature, and relatively few causal models have been seriously entertained. With regard to human systems, it is clear that there are many such "items" to assemble and many details to consider if "assembly"—with high fidelity—is to result. Furthermore, it is clear that tools (i.e., special computer software) are needed to make such assembly efforts efficient enough to consider undertaking. Has the data management and analytical power of computers, which have only been readily available in convenient-to-use forms and with required capacities for less than a decade, been fully exploited in a "fair test" of reductionism?

Reductionism is clearly a methodology for understanding "that which is." Drawing by inference from engineering design in general, a close relationship can be observed with systems engineering synthesis methods used to define "that which will be." In artificial systems (as opposed to those which occur naturally, such as humans), reverse engineering (basically a reductionistic method) has been used quite successfully to create functionally equivalent replicas of products. The methodology employed is guided by knowledge of the synthesis process. The implementation of reductionism in human performance modeling can possibly benefit from the reverse mental exercise of "building a human," which may not be so abtract given current efforts and achievements in rehabilitation engineering. In looking toward the future, it is fair to ask, "To what extent have those who have attempted to apply reductionism, or who have dismissed it, attempted to bring to bear methods of synthesis?"

The issue of biologic variability is also frequently raised in the context of the desire to develop predictive models of human performance. It is perhaps noteworthy that variability is an issue with which one must deal in the manufacture of man-made products (i.e., particularly with regard to quality assurance in manufacturing), which are designed almost exclusively using causal principles. Taguchi methods [Bendell et al., 1988], a collection of mathematics and concepts, have been used in widespread fashion with remarkable success in modeling and controlling variability in the characteristics of a final product which is based on the combination of many components, each of which has multiple characteristics with values that also range within tolerance bands. Similarity of these circumstances suggests that Taguchi methods also may be valuable in human performance engineering. Investigations of this nature are likely to be a part of future work.

155.2 Measurements

Standardization of Variables and Conditions

Human performance literature is replete with different measures that characterize human performance. Despite the number and magnitude of efforts where human performance is of interest, a standard set of measurement variables has yet to emerge. Relatively loose, descriptive naming conventions are used to identify variables reported, leading to the perception of differences when, upon careful inspection, the variables used in two different studies or modeling efforts are the same. In other cases, the names of variables are the same, but conditions under which measures are acquired are different or not reported with enough detail to evaluate if numeric data are comparable (across the reports in question) or not.

The needs of science and engineering are considerably different. Although standardization is generally considered to be desirable in both arenas, the former stresses only that methods used be accurately reported so that they may be replicated. There has been, unfortunately, little motivation to achieve standardization in any broad sense in the human performance research world. In traditional areas of engineering, it is the marketplace that has forced the development of standards for naming of variables such as performance characteristics of various components (e.g., sensors, actuators, etc.) and for conditions under which these variables are measured. In more recent years, product databases (e.g., for electronic, mechanical, and electromechanical components) and systems-level modeling software (i.e., computer-aided design and computer-aided manufacturing), along with the desire to reduce concept-to-production cycle times, have further increased the levels of standardization in these areas.

Despite the somewhat gloomy circumstance at present, there are some signs of potential improvement. An increasing number of research groups are beginning to attack problems of larger scale, and interest is growing with regard to the ability to exchange data and models. Several small standards development efforts have surfaced recently in specific areas such as biomechanics to develop, for example, standards for kinematic representation of various body joints. The advent of an increasing number of commercially available measurement tools also has driven a trend to similarity in conventions in some specific subareas. However, the quest for standardization in measurement that is often voiced is still a distant vision. A willingness to suffer the inconvenience of "standardizing" in the short run in exchange for a greater convenience and "power" over the long run must be recognized by a critical mass of researchers, instrument manufacturers, and practitioners before a significant breakthrough can occur. The large number of different professional bodies and societies that may potentially become involved in promulgating an official set of standards will most likely contribute to slow progress in this area.

New Instruments

Instruments to acquire measures of both human structure and performance have been improving at a rapid pace, commensurate with the improvement of base technologies (e.g., sensors, signal conditioning, microprocessors, and desktop computer systems, etc.). Compared with one decade ago, a practitioner or researcher can today assemble a relatively sophisticated and broad-based measurement laboratory with commercially available devices instead of facing the burden of fabricating his or her own instruments. However, a considerable imbalance still exists across the profile of human performance with regard to commercial availability of necessary tools. This imbalance extends to the profile of tools seen in use in contexts such as rehabilitation and sports training. In particular, devices that measure sensory performance capacities are not nearly as commonplace or well developed as those which measure, for example, strength and range of motion. Likewise, there are few commercially available instruments that measure aspects of neuromotor control in any general sense other than, for example, in a selected task such as maintaining stable posture. The complexity and diversity of higher-level human cognitive processes also have hindered development of measurement instruments in this domain that possess any true degree of commonality in content across products. A wide variety of computer-based test batteries has been proliferating that are more or less implementations of the great number of tests formerly administered in paper-pencil format.

From a practitioner's perspective, prospects for the future are both good and bad. There is some evidence that suppliers of instruments that cover areas of the performance where there has been vigorous competition (e.g., dynamic strength) are experiencing market saturation and uncertainty on the part of consumers regarding what is "the best way" to acquire necessary information. This may force some groups to drop product lines, while others are expressing subtle interests in expanding measurement instrument product lines to fill empty niches. This latter behavior is good in that it will likely increase the scope of measurement tools that are commercially available. However, problems associated with standardization often confuse potential users, and this, in general, has slowed progress in the adoption of more objective measurement instruments (compared with subjective methods) in some application areas. This, in turn, has inhibited product providers from taking the risks associated with introduction of new products.

Compared with the commercial availability of tools that characterize the performance of various human subsystems, instruments that quantify task attributes are much less prevalent. However, the perception that increased emphasis on this area will increase the utility of measures that characterize the human will likely motivate a substantial increase in the number and variety of products available for task characterization. In addition, factors such as the Americans with Disabilities Act (ADA), which encourages work-site evaluations and modifications to facilitate employment of individuals with disabilities, and the increase in work-site related injuries such as carpal tunnel syndrome have led to an increased demand for such tools.

There has been a subtle but noticeable developing sense of awareness in the various communities that there is room for more than one kind of instrument to measure a given variable. Thus debates regarding "the correct approach" which were commonplace are beginning to be replaced with debates concerned with determining "the best approach for a given situation." A prime example is in the area of strength measurement. Devices range from relatively inexpensive hand-held dynamometers that provide rapid measurements and meaningful results with neurologic patients to expensive devices with electric or hydraulic servomotor systems that are more suited, for example, for use in sports medicine contexts. This trend is quite healthy and is likely to spread.

Measuring and Measurements

Reliability and *validity* have been the key words associated with characterizing the quality of measures of human structure and performance [e.g., Potvin et al., 1985]. Often, these terms are used in a manner that implies that a given test "has it" or "does not have it" (i.e., reliability or validity) when in fact both should be recognized as continuums.

There are traditional, well-known methods used in academic circles to quantify reliability. The result produced implies an interpretation of "how much" reliability a given test has, but there is no corresponding way to determine how much is needed (in the same terms that reliability of a test is measured) so that one could determine if one has "enough." Other aspects of the academic treatment of human performance measurement quality are similarly troublesome with regard to the implications for widespread, general use of measurements. For example, there is an inherent desire (and need) to generalize the results of a given reliability study for a given instrument and, at the same time, a reluctance on the part of those who conduct such studies to do so in writing. The strictly academic position is that one can *never* generalize a reliability study; i.e., it applies only to a situation which is identical to that reported (i.e., that instrument, those subjects, that examiner, that room, that time of day, etc.). Thus one may ask, "What is the value of reporting any such study?" The purely academic view may be the most correct, but strict interpretation is completely useless to a practitioner who needs to reach a conclusion regarding the applicability of a given instrument in given application. The mere fact that reliability studies are reported implies that there is an expectation of generalization to *some* degree. The question is, "How much generalization can one make?" This issue has not been adequately addressed from a general methodological standpoint. However, awareness of this issue and the need for improved methods are growing.

What is the general "quality" of measurement available today? The following is offered as a reasonably "healthy" perspective on this complex issue:

1. Technology has advanced to the point where it is now possible to measure many of the basic physical variables employing measurements such as time, force, torque, angles, linear distance, etc. very accurately, repeatably, and with high resolution without significant difficulty.

2. Most of the differences on test-retest are due to limitations on how well one can reasonably control procedures and actual variability of the parameter measured—even in the most ideal test subjects.

3. Many studies have been conducted on the reliability of a wide variety of human performance capacities. Some true generalization can be achieved by looking at this body of work as a whole and not from attempts to generalize from only single studies.

4. Across the many types of variables investigated, results of such studies are amazingly quite similar. Basically, they say that if your instrumentation is good, and if you carefully follow established, optimal test administration procedures, then it should be possible to obtain results on repeat testing that are within a range of 5% to 20% of each other. The exact location achieved in this range depends in large part on the particular variable in question (e.g., repeated measures associated with complex tasks with many degrees of freedom such as lifting or gait will differ more than repeated measures of hinge joint range of motions, for example). In addition, the magnitude of the given metric will influence such percentage characterizations, since errors are often fixed amounts and independent of the size of the quantity measured. Thus, when measuring quantities with small magnitudes, a larger variability (i.e., more like 20%) should be anticipated. One can usually determine an applicable working value in these straightforward, usable terms (e.g., 5% or 20%) that allows direct comparison with an evaluation of needs by careful review of the relevant reliability studies.

A major point of this discussion is to illustrate that traditional methods used to "measure the measurements" do not adequately communicate the information that current and potential users of measurements often need to know. While traditional methods were valuable to a degree in providing relative indicators within the context of academic group studies, methods that are more similar to those used to characterize measurement system performance in physics and other traditional engineering areas (e.g., accuracy, signal-noise-ratio concepts, etc.) are needed for practitioners who must make single measurements on individual subjects (i.e., not populations) to support clinical decision making. As the manner in which measurements are used continues to change to include more of the latter, new interest and methods for quantifying the quality of measurements can be anticipated.

155.3 Databases and Data Modeling

Much research has been conducted to define measurements of human structure and performance and to collect and characterize data as bases to increase understanding and make inferences in different contexts. A large number of problems of major medical and other societal significance require the use of such data (1) for diagnostic purposes (i.e., when assessing measures obtained from a subject under test, such as to determine the efficacy of an intervention or treatment in a medical context), (2) for modeling and simulation (e.g., analyses for return-to-work decisions of injured employees, to support job-site modifications for individuals with disabilities, to design specifications for virtual reality systems), (3) for status/capacity evaluations (e.g., disability determinations for insurance settlements, worker's compensation claims, etc.), (4) to obtain a better understanding of disease and aging processes (e.g., associated with such problems as falls in elderly populations, etc.), (5) to gain insight into the impact of environmental and occupational factors (e.g., as in epidemiologic studies, such as in lead toxicity or carpal tunnel syndrome), and (6) to support ergonomic design of consumer products and living environments for use by the public in general. Despite such a diverse range in needs for basically the same information, there has been little—if any—attempt to organize, integrate, and represent available data in a compact, accessible form that can serve the cited needs.

Figure 155.1 illustrates the scope of the general problem and infers a potential approach to integration. At the most basic level, individual measurements for a given variable must be collected and databased. In addition, databases from published studies are required to identify specific gaps that limit either analytic functionality or fidelity in the types of tasks that data must support. Data from the literature are typically available only in summary form, i.e., in terms of means and standard deviations for defined populations. Future research is required to define and validate methods for integrating data (for example) from multiple studies to form a single, more robust data model for a given performance or structure parameter. This will involve testing data models developed from databases of individual measures and databases of studies against each other. Development of data warping methods (e.g., to adapt predictions of expected performance levels to subject's of different body sizes and/or ages) is required to provide models that would be transparent operationally and would allow analyses to proceed in data-limited situations with predictable tradeoffs in fidelity. In many areas, especially with regard to practitioners such as occupational and physical therapists, performance characterization has been viewed only unidimensionally. More multidimensional perspectives are needed for an adequate representation of fidelity [e.g., Kondraske, 1995]. Another major aspect of data modeling therefore involves the development of multivariate models of performance envelopes [Kondraske, 1995] for individual human subsystems (e.g., knee flexors, visual information processors, etc.). Such models would support, for example, prediction of available torque production capacity under different specified conditions (e.g., joint angle, speed, etc.). In summary, a basic strategy is required for harvesting the vast amount of previously collected data to obtain compact, accessible representations. Means must be incorporated in this strategy to allow for integration of data from multiple sources and continuous update as new data are collected to enhance fidelity and range of applicability of composite models.

As previously noted, individuals within the human performance community typically adopt a variety of terms or identification schemes for structures and parameters employed in both the execution and communication of their work. The sheer number of parameters and variety of combinations in which they may be required to meet analysis needs may be sufficient to justify a more formal approach [e.g., Kondraske, 1993], thereby facilitating the development of common data structures. The engineering contexts in which data models can be envisioned to be used require more rigor and stability. Computer-based models and analyses beg for codification of terms and parameters (i.e., for databases, etc.). In this regard, these emerging applications bring to light the lack of precision in terminology and confusion in definitions. Moreover, the ability to integrate models and analysis modules developed independently within more narrow subsets of the field to address more complex problems requires standardized notation if for no other reason than for efficiency. Development of a standardized systematic notation is compelling; it is postulated that without such a notation, progress to the next level of sophistication cannot occur.

55.4 Summary

A relatively high degree of sophistication currently exists with regard to the science, engineering, and technology of human performance. The field is, nonetheless, relatively young and undergoing nat-

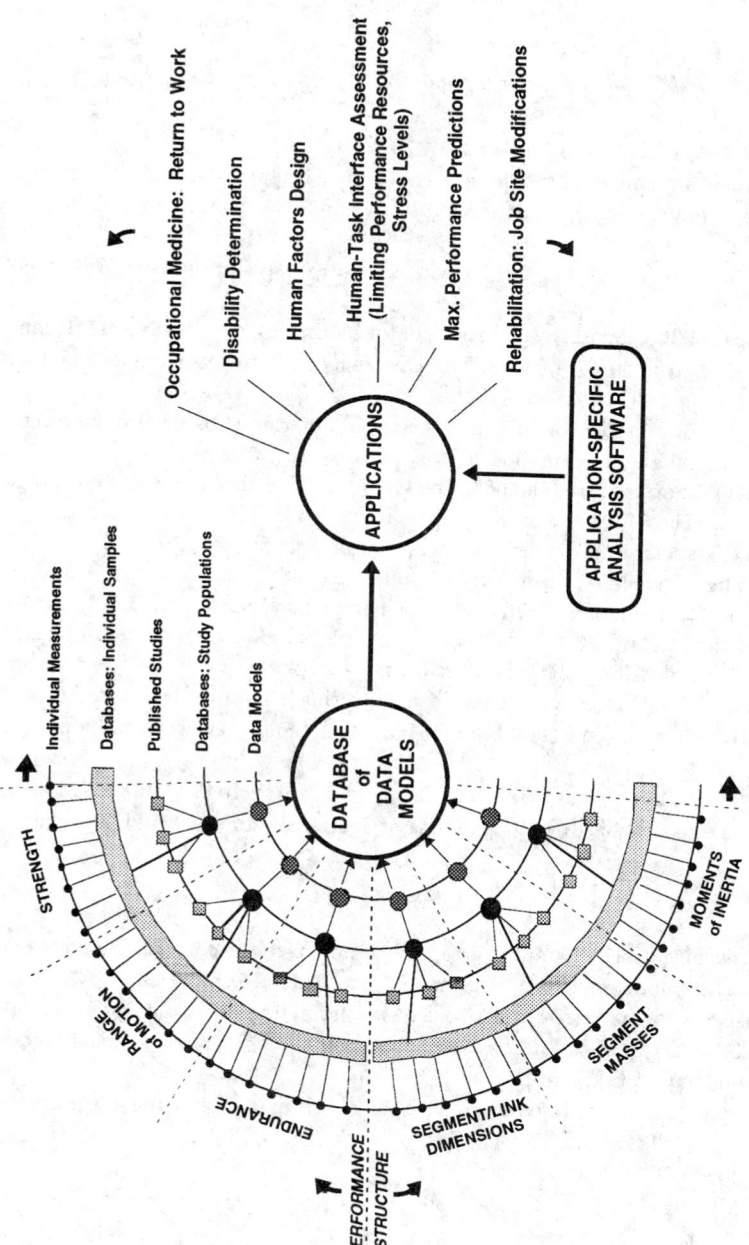

FIGURE 155.1 Summary of the complexity of the problem associated with integrating human structural and performance data to realize compact representations (i.e., parametric data models) to support analyses in multiple application areas.

ural maturation processes. Remaining needs in terms of both conceptual underpinnings and tools (which are not independent) are enormous relative to what can be envisioned. Future progress, however, is likely to be more dependent on collaborative efforts of different types. The magnitude and nature of problems that are at the forefront demand the achievement of agreement among a critical mass of researchers and practitioners. Both the challenges and prospects for the future are significant.

References

Bendell A, Disney J, Pridmore WA. 1988. Taguchi Methods: Applications in World Industry. London, IFS Publishing.

Bunge M. 1977. Levels and reduction. Am J Physiol 233:R75.

Frey WD. 1987. Functional assessment in the '80's: A conceptual enigma, a technical challenge. In AS Halpern, MJ Fuhrer (eds), Functional Assessment in Rehabilitation. Baltimore, Paul H Brookes.

Gardner H. 1985. The Mind's New Science: A History of Cognitive Revolution. New York, Basic Books.

Kondraske GV. 1993. The HPI Shorthand Notation System for Human System Parameters (technical report 92-001R V1.5). Arlington, Texas, The University of Texas at Arlington, Human Performance Institute.

Kondraske GV. 1995. A working model for human system-task interfaces. In JD Bronzino (ed), Handbook of Biomedical Engineering. Boca Raton, Fla, CRC Press.

Potvin AR, Tourtellotte WW, Potvin JH, et al. 1985. The Quantitative Examination of Neurologic Function. Boca Raton, Fla, CRC Press.

Simmon CW. 1987. Will egg-sucking ever become a science? Hum Fact Soc Bull 30(6):1.

Smith LL. 1987. Whyfore human factors. Hum Fact Soc Bull 30(2):1.

Vasta PJ, Kondraske GV. 1992. Standard Conventions for Kinematic and Structural Parameters for the "Gross Total Human" Link Model (technical report 92-003R V1.0). Arlington, Texas, The University of Texas at Arlington Human Performance Institute.

Vasta PJ, Kondraske GV. 1995. Human performance engineering computer-based design and analysis tools. In JD Bronzino (ed), Handbook of Biomedical Engineering. Boca Raton, Fla, CRC Press.

Weismer G, Liss JM. 1991. Reductionism is a dead-end in speech research. In CA Moore, KM Yorkston, DR Beukelman (eds), Dysarthria and Apraxia of Speech. Baltimore, Paul H Brookes.

Further Information

The section of this *Handbook* entitled "Human Performance Engineering" contains chapters that address human performance modeling and measurement in considerably more detail. Manufacturers of instruments used to characterize different aspects of human performance often provide technical literature and bibliographies of studies related to measurement quality, technical specifications of instruments, and application examples.

Future articles of relevance can be expected on a continuing basis in the following journals:

American Journal of Occupational Therapy
The American Occupational Therapy Association, Inc.
1383 Piccard Drive
Rockville, MD 20850-4375

Archives of Physical Medicine and Rehabilitation
Suite 1310
78 East Adams Street
Chicago, IL 60603-6103

Human Factors
The Human Factors Society, Inc.
P.O. Box 1369
Santa Monica, CA 90406

IEEE Transactions on Rehabilitation Engineering and
IEEE Transactions on Biomedical Engineering
IEEE Service Center
445 Hoes Lane
P.O. Box 1331
Piscataway, NJ 08855-1331

Journal of Biomechanics
American Society of Biomechanical Engineers
345 East 47th St.
New York, NY 10017

Journal of Occupational Rehabilitation
Subscription Department
Plenum Publishing Corporation
233 Spring St.
New York, NY 10013

Physical Therapy
American Physical Therapy Association
1111 North Fairfax St.
Alexandria, VA 22314

Rehab Management
4676 Admiralty Way
Suite 202
Marina Del Rey, CA 90292

Rehabilitation Research and Development
Scientific and Technical Publications Section
Rehabilitation Research and Development Service
103 South Gay St., 5th floor
Baltimore, MD 21202-4051

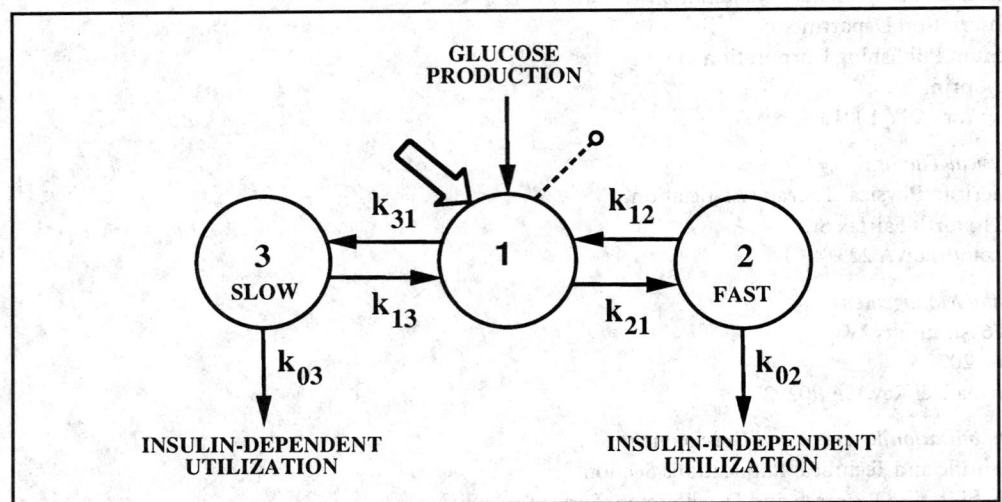

The linear compartmental model of glucose kinetics.

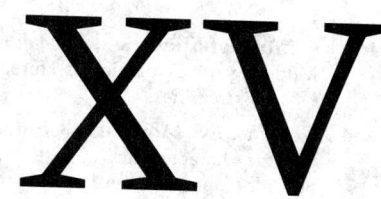

Physiologic Modeling, Simulation, and Control

Howard Jay Chizeck
Case Western Reserve University

THE USE OF THE WORDS *model* and *simulation* are common in many engineering disciplines. They convey images of mathematical equations, electrical and mechanical analogs, and computer programs designed to describe/mimic the dynamic performance of specific engineering devices and systems. These terms are of particular importance to the biomedical engineers and to those engaged in a host of biologic research projects designed to increase understanding of the underlying mechanisms responsible for, as well as the behavior of, a particular physiologic system. In essence the major attribute of the biologic model/simulation lies in its utility in suggesting to researchers/experimenters the most efficient, meaningful and creative avenues of investigation. The following section provides not only the fundamental principles of model building but also specific examples to demonstrate its utility.

The first chapter, "Modeling Strategies in Physiology," introduces the various approaches that have been used in modeling dynamic physiologic systems. The authors present examples of lumped parameter, transmission line, and integrated models using muscle and cardiovascular system dynamics, demonstrating the distinction between quantitative models capable of predicting new information and simulations based on curve fitting.

"Compartmental Models of Physiologic Systems" describes a class of dynamic models widely used for studying the kinetics of materials in physiologic systems. The production, distribution, transport and interaction of materials, such as drugs or hormones, are best studied using these types of models. A detailed mathematical description of both linear and nonlinear compartmental models are presented, highlighting specific processes, including parameter estimation, optimal experiment design and validation.

The chapter on cardiovascular models and control focuses on the use of cardiovascular (CV) modeling for use in closed-loop drug delivery systems, such as IV infusion of anesthetics and other pharmacologic agents. It provides insights into the use of computer simulation software, especially "desktop patients" to develop CV models, as well as detailed descriptions of the idealized segment of artery, vein, the heart and the combined heart and vascular system.

The chapter on respiratory models and controls emphasizes the use of models to study the continual interaction of the respiratory mechanical system and the pulmonary gas exchange process. After briefly reviewing the structure of the respiratory control system, considerable attention is placed upon specific models, including the "chemoreflex," which is useful in studying the closed-loop control of ventilation and the chemical plant; and the "respiratory control pattern generator," which incorporates control of breathing pattern upon the respiratory mechanical plant. These models include neural network and optimization approaches.

In "Neural Networks for Physiologic Control," the emphasis shifts solely to the use of neural network control systems and their use in modeling physiologic systems. Following a detailed description of the basic concepts underlying the use of neural networks, specific applications are provided. These neural networks include "supervised control," i.e., they mimic and eventually replace an existing control system, and "adaptive control" to address the problem of controlling nonlinear systems.

"Methods and Tools for Identification of Psychologic Systems" focuses on specific methods and tools that can be employed to determine the system model from experimental data, i.e., the system identification process. Considerable insights are provided regarding how to perform this processing using both parametric and nonparametric approaches.

The chapter "Clinical Care of Patients with Closed-Loop Drug Delivery Systems" provides a detailed presentation of closed-loop drug delivery (CLDD) systems. It focuses on specific approaches in control theory that have been used to study these systems. The control theory approaches described include *classical control, fuzzy control*, and *adaptive control*. After providing the theoretical background, the chapter gives specific examples of CLDD systems.

The chapter "Control of Movements" focuses on modeling the dynamics of human extremities. Following some basic definitions of rigid body mechanics, dynamic analysis of the resultant mechanical configurations, e.g., chain mechanisms, is discussed. Specific applications include *reaching and tracking control*, and *grasping control*.

The final chapter in the section, "The Fast Eye Movement Control System" is devoted to a specific physiologic system, i.e., fast eye movement or *saccade*, which enables one to move the eye quickly from one image to another. This type of eye movement, which is very common, is encountered in reading when the eyes move from the end of a line to the beginning of another. Following a description of the fast eye-movement system, saccade models are presented from the earliest to more complex and accurate models.

156
Modeling Strategies in Physiology

Joseph L. Palladino
Trinity College

Gary M. Drzewiecki
Rutgers University

Abraham Noordergraaf
University of Pennsylvania

In physics and chemistry a multitude of experimental observations can be captured in a small number of concepts, or *laws*. A law is a statement of the relation between quantities which, as far as is known, is invariable within a range of conditions. For example, Ohm's law expresses the ratio between the voltage difference across and the current through an object as a constant. In physiology, experimental observations can likewise be ordered by relating them to natural laws. In such complex systems, several laws may play their part, and the process is then referred to as development of a model, or *modeling*. Model design, therefore, must meet stringent requirements and serves to rein in undisciplined speculation. Modeling attempts to identify the mechanism(s) responsible for experimental observations and is fundamentally distinct from simulation, in which anything that reproduces the experimental data is acceptable.

A successful model provides guidance to new experiments, which may modify or generalize the model, in turn suggesting new experiments (Fig. 156.1). The quest for understanding a body of experimental observations (block 1) leads to tentative conceptual interpretation (block 2), which is transformed into quantitative statements by invoking established natural laws. The resulting mathematical model (block 3) consists of a set of equations, which are solved, generally with the aid of a computer. The equation solutions are quantitative statements about experimental observations, some of which were not part of the original body of experiments, extending knowledge about the system under study. Consequently, new experiments become specified (block 4), adding to the store of experimental data. The enlarged body of experimental observations may cause modification of the investigator's conceptual interpretation, which in turn may give reason to modify the mathematical model. This iterative process should weed out flawed experiments and misconceptions of the mathematical model. If the entire effort is successful, a comprehensive, quantitative, and verified interpretation of the relevant experimental observations will result.

The first case study of this chapter outlines the development of an arterial system model by a hybrid approach. Features of two separate, flawed classical methods are combined to interpret a wide range of previously unexplained experimental observations. In the course of interaction between model and experimentation, inclusion of greater detail may expand model complexity and size, rendering it too unwieldy as a component to a larger physiologic system. Reduction in size, distinct from simplification, may be necessary. The former is based on understanding, allowing intelligent sepa-

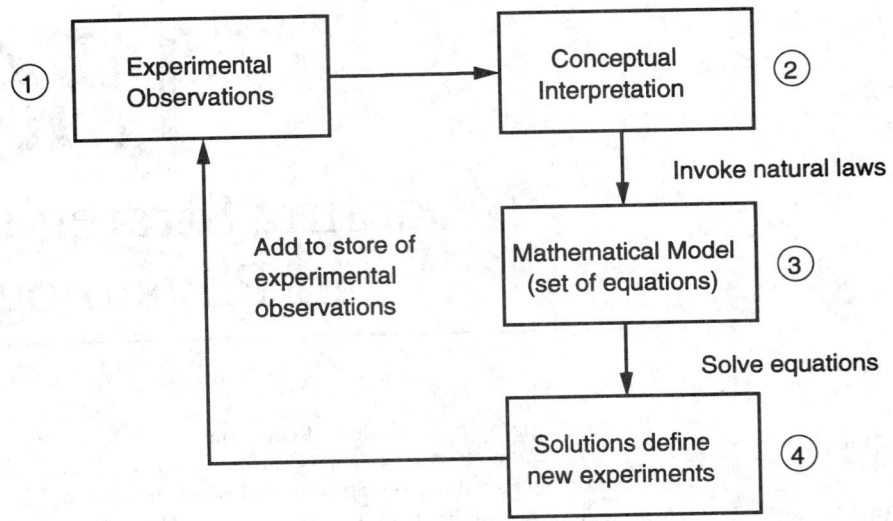

FIGURE 156.1   Iterative interrelationships between models and experiments.

ration of major and minor effects. The latter implies arbitrary action based on intuition. This case study closes by introducing systematic reduction of the arterial model.

A major challenge in the biosciences is the integration of a large body of molecular level information, with the ultimate goal of understanding organ function. Two different, novel modeling approaches to this goal are next presented. The first shows how a model based on muscle structure can predict a molecular mechanism responsible for muscle's mechanical properties (function). The second presents an approach for predicting ventricular hypertrophy (structure) based on cardiac metabolic function. Discussion is limited to the main points; however, details are available in the original research papers cited.

156.1 Hybrid Approaches and Model Reduction: Arterial Dynamics

Hales [1733] believed that the aorta and major vessels act as a "compression chamber" which transforms pulsatile inflow from the heart into steady flow into the organs. Frank [1895] called this compression chamber a *windkessel* after firefighting pumps, which produce steady flow despite oscillating pumping. An early focus was to develop a noninvasive method to measure cardiac output with the aid of a windkessel model of the systemic arterial circulation. In practice, the compliance of this windkessel is measured via the experimental pressure curve and the measured, finite, pulse wave velocity c. Since all arterial properties are lumped, c is assumed infinite. Consequently, the pulse wave velocity is assumed to be both finite and infinite in the same model. This contradiction leads to errors in stroke volume of up to a few hundred percent. A large number of efforts to improve accuracy by modifying this model has achieved little [Noordergraaf, 1978].

The interpretation of pulse wave speed has fascinated many researchers. Initially considering the aorta as a simple uniform, infinitely long transmission line, the Webers [1850, 1866] proposed the second version of a finite wave propagation theory. The transmission line approach describes pressure in a uniform, cylindrical vessel and predicts a frequency-independent wave velocity. Experimental measurements show c to be highly frequency-dependent. In spite of many attempts, the conflict between theory and experiment proved unresolvable, even if the vessel was given a finite length [Kenner & Wetterer, 1962].

Broadening the view from pulse wave velocity to include other phenomena, experimental studies show that the arterial flow pulse decreases as it moves away from the heart, as expected for a passive transmission line. The arterial pressure pulse, however, increases, seemingly violating energy conservation. Further, input impedance $Z_{in} = P_{in}/Q_{in}$ is frequency-dependent, similar to wave velocity. An arterial model capable of describing all of these features results by combining the windkessel and transmission line ideas [Noordergraaf, 1978].

The actual arterial system has bifurcations which should produce reflected pressure and flow waves. It is unfeasible to describe each branching vessel due to the very large number (10^9) of them. A compromise is to take a finite number of interconnected uniform (lumped) segments. Each of 130 segments is represented by an electrical analog equivalent, described by two partial differential equations in pressure and flow. The resulting transmission line, built of finite windkessel-like segments, was constructed as an electric analog, well before the digital computer was sufficiently advanced. This model was the first to demonstrate c and Z_{in} correctly [Westerhof et al., 1969]. The increasing pressure paradox was shown to be the result of constructive wave summation. Thus, the modification of the model to include branching proved to be the crucial step that allowed interpretation of a wide range of puzzling experimental observations.

The level of insight achieved with this large, distributed model answered the question of whether its size could be reduced, retaining the desired distributed system properties with a much-reduced number of equations. A specific example [Noordergraaf, 1969] allows study of pulse wave transmission between the carotid and renal arteries. This model reduces the number of equations from 260 to fewer than 40 by lumping large areas of the system outside the area under study. If distributed system properties such as pulse wave reflection are not of interest, the arterial system load seen by the heart can be further reduced to a simple, three-element windkessel [Westerhof et al., 1971]. This concise model, named the Westkessel after its founder, is the most widely used arterial load representation today.

156.2 Predicting Function from Structure: Muscle Contraction

Description of muscle contraction has essentially evolved into two separate approaches—lumped whole muscle models and specialized crossbridge models of the sarcomere. The former seek to interpret muscle's complex mechanical properties with a single set of model elements. Muscle force generation is believed to arise from the formation of crossbridge bonds between thick and thin myofilaments within the basic building stone of muscle, the sarcomere. These structures, in the nm–μm range, must be viewed by electron microscopy or x-ray diffraction, limiting study to fixed, dead material. Consequently, muscle contraction at the sarcomere level must be described by models that integrate metabolic and structural information.

Early whole muscle models based on a purely elastic element were refuted on thermodynamic grounds [Fick, 1891]. Expansion to a spring-dashpot viscoelastic model was subsequently rejected for thermodynamic reasons as well when Fenn [1923], reported that energy released by the muscle differs for isometric or shortening muscle. Subsequently, Hill [1939] developed the *contractile element*, embodied as an empirical hyperbolic relation between muscle force and shortening velocity. Current whole muscle models have, in general, incorporated Hill's contractile element, an empirically derived black-box force generator, in networks of traditional springs and dashpots [e.g., Montevecchi & Pietrabissa, 1987]. Since model elements are not directly correlated to muscle structure, there is no logical reason to stop at three elements—models with at least nine have been proposed [Parmley et al., 1969].

Crossbridge models focus on mechanics at the sarcomere level. Prior to their actual observation, Huxley [1957] proposed a model whereby muscle force is generated by the formation of crossbridge bonds between myofilaments. This model was subsequently shown unable to describe muscle's transient mechanical properties. Extension of Huxley's ideas to multiple-state crossbridges has been very limited in scope, e.g., the Huxley and Simmons [1973] two-state model does not include crossbridge attachment, detachment or filament sliding, but rather describes only the mechanics of a single set of overlapping actin and myosin filaments. In general, crossbridge models dictate bond attachment and detachment by probability or rate functions. This approach has shifted emphasis away from muscle mechanics toward increasingly complex rate functions [e.g., Eisenberg et al., 1980].

A large-scale, distributed muscle model based on ultrastructural kinetics, possessing direct anatomic and physiologic relevance, was developed [Palladino, 1990]. Muscle's dynamic mechanical properties arise from the dynamic model structure rather than from adaptation of a particular force-velocity curve describing the contractile element, or of a particular bond attachment or detachment function as for previous models. Crossbridge bonds are described as linear viscoelastic material, each represented by a 3-element spring-dashpot model (Fig. 156.2). During activation, the attached crossbridge head rotates, stretching the bond and generating force. A sarcomere is mechanically represented as myofilament masses interconnected by a matrix of permanently attached passive viscoelastic bonds. During activation, dynamically attached active bonds are formed as calcium ion and energy (ATP) allows.

The sarcomere model is extended to a muscle fiber by taking N sarcomeres in series with M parallel pairs of active bonds, currently 50 series sarcomeres, each with 50 parallel pairs of crossbridges. Bond formation is taken to be distributed in two dimensions due to muscle's finite electrical propagation speed and the finite diffusion rate of calcium ions from the sarcoplasmic reticulum. The large set of resulting differential equations (5300) is solved by digital computer. Since the instantaneous number of crossbridge bonds, and therefore the number of model system equations, is continuously changing, the resulting model is strongly nonlinear and time-varying, despite its construction from linear, time-invariant components. Crossbridge bonds are added in a raster pattern due to the distributed system properties. After all bonds have been added, no further conditions are imposed. Crossbridge bonds subsequently detach simply from the small internal movements of myofilaments. Consequently, the model relaxes without separate assumptions.

Transient loading provides dynamic information from muscle and critically tests muscle models. Quick release and stretch experiments subject muscle to small, rapid changes in muscle length during otherwise isometric contractions. Fig. 156.3 shows quick releases of muscle length imposed on the model fiber during isometric contractions early, at the midpoint, and late during a twitch. For both the computed and experimental curves, very small ($\leq 5\%$), rapid changes in muscle length yield profound force deactivation, consistent with x-ray diffraction studies [Huxley et al., 1983]. This deactivation functional phenomenon is present in the model solely from the original structural assumptions.

This model was subjected to a wide range of loading conditions. A single set of model parameters is sufficient to describe the main features of isometric, isotonic, and quick release and stretch experiments. The model is sensitive to mechanical disturbances, consistent with experimental evidence from muscle force curves, aequorin measurements of free calcium ion [Allen et al., 1988], and high-

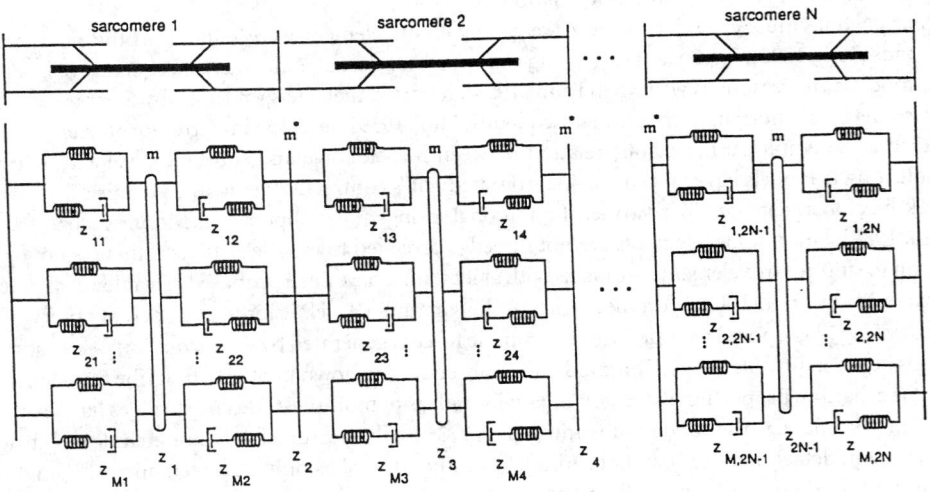

FIGURE 156.2 Schematic representation of a muscle fiber for N series sarcomeres, each with M parallel pairs of active, viscoelastic bonds.

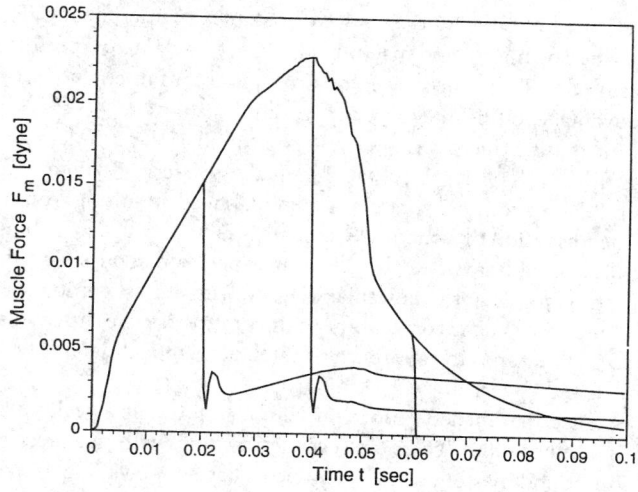

FIGURE 156.3 Quick release computed from the distributed muscle fiber model.

speed x-ray diffraction studies [Huxley et al., 1983]. The model is also consistent with sarcomere length feedback studies [Huxley & Simmons, 1973] where reduced internal motion delays relaxation.

The distributed model proposes that internal myofilament vibrations should be enhanced by ultrasound irradiation, thereby encouraging bond detachment and muscle relaxation. This prediction led to animal experiments which demonstrate the depressant effect of ultrasound on the contractile process, opening a new direction of experimental research in force deactivation via ultrasound in the heart [Dalecki, 1993].

This modeling strategy proposes a structural mechanism for the origin of muscle's complex mechanical properties and predicts new features of the contractile mechanism. Consideration of muscle's distributed properties suggests a mechanism for muscle force deactivation and for muscle relaxation. This approach serves to bridge understanding from crossbridge theories at the ultrastructural level and from muscle fiber mechanics. The main model limitation is its computational complexity. Further, muscles of different size and shape exhibit similar mechanical properties. Currently, model size is directly related to muscle fiber size. There should be some minimum model size that still retains the desired distributed system properties. This reduced configuration is especially needed for its application to describe the ventricle.

156.3 Predicting Structure from Function: Cardiac Hypertrophy

The preceding methods of modeling provide a picture of a specific physiologic system in a given state. Generally, the values of system parameters must be determined from physical and quantitative experimentation. Alternatively, it is useful to understand how these parameters arise, that is, to understand nature's design. For this purpose, it is necessary to allow the system to respond to its external demands and vary over time, denoted system *adaptation*. Because of adaptive processes, an organ system is usually in a constant state of synthesis and desynthesis. The balance of these processes results in the system's current structure or system constraints. This type of modeling obviates knowing every parameter from measurements, providing theoretical insight outside the realm of conventional experimentation.

Often, models become increasingly complex in an effort to provide the required level of structural details. Ultimately, there is a baseline level of structure where function is known, e.g., a cell or cardiac sarcomere, referred to as the *microdynamic unit*. The arrangement or structural assembly of these units that constitute the organ system is denoted the *macrodynamic unit*. The arrangement and interaction between both dynamic units yields complexity in modeling. This section demonstrates an example whereby micro- and macrodynamics are integrated, while the structure is varied to identify structural rules. These rules, even for a complex set of interactions, can often be simple, offering another advantage to this integrative approach.

The concept of integrating micro- and macro- levels of physiologic function has been presented earlier by Taylor and Weibel [1981]. They stated in qualitative terms that an organ system achieves "a state of structural design commensurate to functional needs resulting from regulated morphogenesis, whereby the formation of structural elements is regulated to satisfy but not exceed the requirements of the functional system." Recent trends in experimental physiology have focused on the lower levels of structure, particularly molecular biology, with almost complete exclusion of organismic physiology. It may now be the correct time to integrate these two different scales of functional knowledge. This section outlines the approach of integrative modeling, illustrated with the example of cardiac growth and hypertrophy.

It is generally assumed that the left ventricle attempts to normalize peak wall stress during diastole and systole [Grossman, 1980]. There are several difficulties with this theory. First, the anatomical locations of systolic and diastolic stress transducers have not been identified. Second, the value of wall stress (*set point*) cannot be determined from basic physical knowledge. Finally, the theory cannot explain ventricular size alterations due to metabolic disturbances, in contrast to mechanical disturbances. The integrative approach can resolve these difficulties by using a more general theory.

It was hypothesized that cardiac size could be determined from a single observable quantity at the sarcomere level of structure (microfunction) [Drzewiecki et al., 1992]. The cardiac sarcomere was represented in this model as the *sarcounit* (Fig. 156.4), a constant-volume structure capable of axial stress generation. Sarcounit function was defined by its active (maximal) and passive force-length curves. Activation stress was modulated via a sinusoidal time function during systole and taken as zero during passive diastole. Initial ventricular shape was approximated as a cylinder, dictating geometry by length (L), radius (r) and wall thickness (W). The sarcounits were arranged in series and in parallel, with radius determined by the number of series units, and wall thickness and length by the number of parallel units.

Macrofunction was defined by the cardiac output or mean aortic pressure and vascular load impedance (*Westkessel load*), determined by integrating the sarcounit stress and length over the cylindrical structure. Consequently, ventricular pressure and volume are obtained from sarcounit stress and length at any instant of time. Heart rate was allowed to vary as necessary to provide regulated aortic pressure. The rate of myocardial oxygen consumption MVO_2 was chosen as a measure of microfunc-

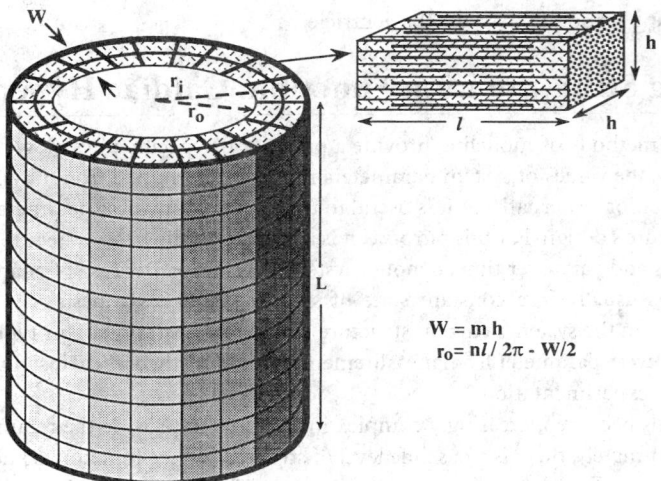

$$W = m\,h$$
$$r_0 = n l\,/\,2\pi - W/2$$

FIGURE 156.4 Cardiac sarcounit (upper right) and arrangement to form a cylindrical left ventricule. (Adapted from Drzewiecki et al., 1992.)

tion. Ventricular radius and wall thickness were then varied while analyzing MVO₂. A minimum in MVO₂ occurred at a specific cylinder (ventricle) shape (Fig. 156.5). The minimum in MVO₂ at the level of available oxygen supply was concluded to provide a unique size and shape of the left ventricle.

The results of this model were compared with known experimental patterns of cardiac hypertrophy (wall thickening). The model ventricle size was found consistent with a dog heart, for which the ventricular arterial load was chosen. Second, a pressure overload was created by requiring elevated mean pressure. This yielded the classic wall thickening and increased wall-thickness-to-radius ratio observed with pressure overload, denoted *concentric hypertrophy*. Finally, volume overload was imposed by elevating cardiac output. This change resulted in increased ventricle radius with relatively little increase in the W/r ratio, denoted *eccentric hypertrophy*. Eccentric hypertrophy was also produced by reducing the oxygen supply at the sarcounit level.

The modeling approach integrating micro- and macrodynamics was applied to the problem of cardiac growth. The theory that cardiac shape can be determined by the regulation of a single quantity at the sarcomere level, MVO₂, was illustrated by this methodology. This resulting theory and model is more general than previous wall stress–related theories as it predicts a growth response to metabolic overload, as well as to mechanical overloads. As a main benefit, this approach permits theoretical analysis that may be otherwise impossible or impractical to perform. For example, it is impossible to directly alter the ventricular wall thickness in an animal.

156.4 Summary

This chapter has focused on modeling as a tool to identify and quantify the mechanism(s) responsible for observed phenomena in physiology. The rather strict rules to which the modeling process is subject generally lead to the formulation of new, specific experiments, thereby broadening the pool of experimental data and the database for modeling. On occasion, this process leads to areas of experimentation and the development of concepts originally judged to lie outside the scope of the original problem definition. Consequently, successful modeling can deepen a researcher's insight and breadth of view.

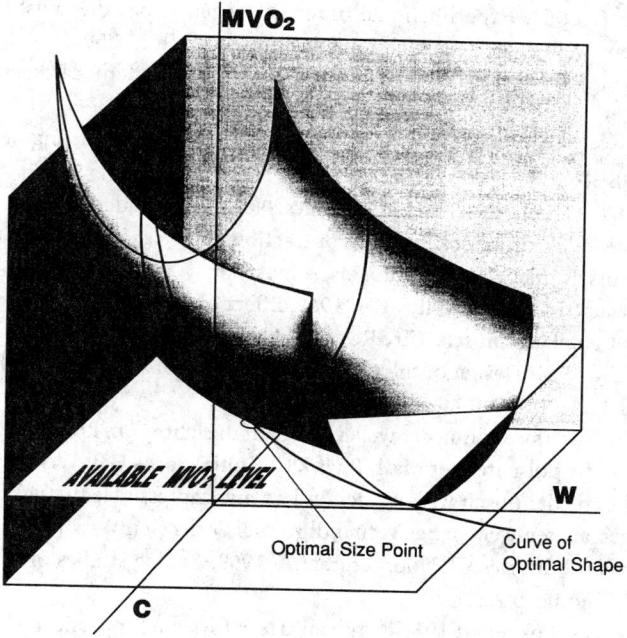

FIGURE 156.5 Sarcounit myocardial oxygen consumption MVO₂ versus the circumference (*c*) and wall thickness (*W*) of the ventricular model. (Adapted from Drzewiecki et al., 1992.)

References

Allen DG, Smith GL, and Nichols CG. 1988. Intracellular calcium concentration following length changes in mammalian cardiac muscle. In HEDJ ter Keurs and MIM Moble (eds.), Starling's Law of the Heart Revisited. Dordrecht, Kluwer Academic Publishers.

Dalecki D. 1993. Mechanisms of interaction of ultrasound and lithotripter fields with cardiac and neural tissues. Ph.D. dissertation, University of Rochester, Univ Microforms, Ann Arbor.

Drzewiecki GM, Karam E, Li J K-J, Noordergraaf A. 1992. Cardiac adaptation of sarcomere dynamics to arterial load: A model of hypertrophy. Am J Physiol 263:H1054–1063.

Eisenberg E, Hill TL, and Chen Y. 1980. Cross-bridge model of muscle contraction. Biophys J 29:195–227.

Fenn WO. 1923. Quantitative comparison between energy liberated and work performed by isolated sartorius muscle of the frog. J Physiol 58:175–203.

Fick A. 1891. Neue beitrage zur kentniss von der wärmeentwicklung im muskel. Pflügers Arch 51:541.

Frank O. 1895. Zur dynamik des herzmuskels. Z Biol (Munich) 32:370 [Eng. trans., see CB Chapman and E Wasserman, Am Heart J 58:282–317, 467–478 (1959)].

Grossman W. 1980. Cardiac hypertrophy: Useful adaptation or pathologic process? Am J Med 69:576–584.

Hales S. 1733. Statistical Essays vol. 2, London, Innys and Manby.

Hill AV. 1939. The heat of shortening and dynamic constants of muscle. Proc Roy Soc 126:136.

Huxley AF. 1957. Muscle structure and theories of contraction. Prog Biophys 7:255–318.

Huxley AF, Simmons RM. 1973. Mechanical transients and the origin of muscle force. Cold Spring Harbor Symp Quant Biol 37:669–680.

Huxley HE, Simmons RM, Faruqi AR, Kress M, Bordas J, Koch MHJ. 1983. Changes in the x-ray reflections from contracting muscle during rapid mechanical transients and their structural implications. J Mol Biol 169:469–506.

Kenner T, Wetterer E. 1962. Experimentalle untersuchungen ueber die pulsformen und eigenschwingungen zweiteiliger schalauchmodelle. Pflugers Arch 275:594.

Montevecchi FM, Pietrabissa R. 1987. A model of multicomponent cardiac fiber. J Biomech 20(4):365–370.

Noordergraaf A. 1969. Hemodynamics. In HP Schwan (ed), Biological Engineering, New York, McGraw-Hill.

Noordergraaf A. 1978. Circulatory System Dynamics. New York, Academic Press.

Palladino JL. 1990. Models of cardiac muscle contraction and relaxation. Ph.D. dissertation, University of Pennsylvania, Univ Microforms, Ann Arbor.

Parmley WW, Brutsaert DL, Sonnenblick EH. 1969. Effect of altered loading on contractile events in isolated cat papillary muscle. Circ Res 24:521.

Taylor CR, Weibel ER. 1981. Design of the mammalian respiratory system I: Problem and strategy. Resp Physiol 44:1–10.

Weber E. 1850. Ueber die anwendung der wellenlehre auf die lehre vom kreislaufe des blutes und ins besondere auf die pulsehre. Ber Math Physik Cl Königl Sächs Gen Wiss 18:353.

Weber W. 1866. Theorie der durch wasser oder andere inkompressibele flüssigkeiten in elastischen röhren fortgeplanzten wellen. Ber Verhandl Königl Sächs Gen Wiss 18:353.

Westerhof N, Bosman F, deVries CJ, Noordergraaf A. 1969. Analog studies of the human systemic arterial tree. J Biomech 2:21.

Westerhof N, Elzinga G, Sipkema P. 1971. Artificial arterial system for pumping hearts. J Appl Physiol 31:776.

157

Compartmental Models of Physiologic Systems

Claudio Cobelli
University of Padua

Maria Pia Saccomani
University of Padua

Compartmental models are a class of dynamic, i.e., differential equation, models derived from mass balance considerations which are widely used for quantitative studying of the kinetics of materials in physiologic systems. Materials can be either exogenous, such as a drug or a tracer, or endogenous, such as a substrate or a hormone, and kinetics include processes such as production, distribution, transport, utilization, and substrate-hormone control interactions.

Compartmental modeling was first formalized by Sheppard [1948] in the context of isotopic tracer distribution kinetics. Over the years it has evolved and grown as a formal body of theory [Anderson, 1983; Atkins, 1969; Brown, 1985; Carson et al., 1983; Godfrey, 1983; Jacquez, 1985; Rescigno & Segre, 1966; Sheppard, 1962].

157.1 Definitions and Concepts

Let's start with some definitions: A *compartment* is an amount of material that acts as though it is well mixed and kinetically homogeneous. A *compartmental model* consists of a finite number of compartments with specified interconnections among them. The interconnections represent a flux of material which physiologically represents transport from one location to another or a chemical transformation or both. An example of a compartmental model is illustrated in Fig. 157.1 where the compartments are represented by circles and the interconnections by arrows.

Given the introductory definitions, it is useful before explaining *well-mixed* and *kinetic homogeneity* to consider possible candidates for compartments. Consider the notion of a compartment as a physical space. Plasma is a candidate for a compartment; a substance such as plasma glucose could be a compartment. Zinc in bone could be a compartment also, as could thyroxine in the thyroid. In some experiments, different substances could be followed in plasma: plasma glucose, lactate, and alanine provide examples. Thus in the same experiment, there can be more than one plasma compartment, one for each of the substances being studied. This notion extends beyond

0-8493-8346-3/95/$0.00+$.50

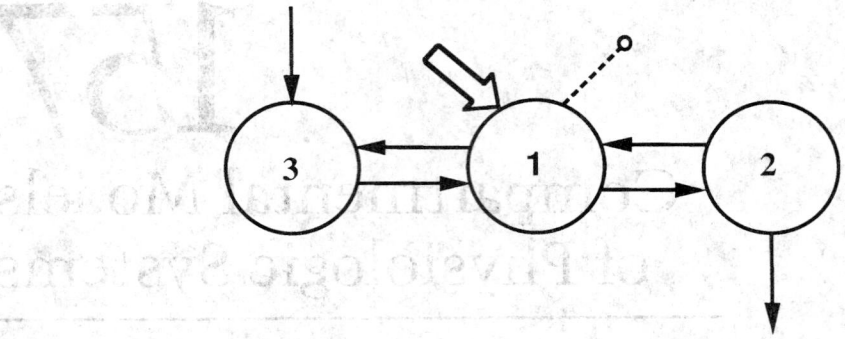

FIGURE 157.1   A three-compartment model. The substance enters de novo compartment 3 (arrow entering a compartment from "outside") and irreversibly leaves from compartment 2 (arrow leaving a compartment to the "outside"). Material exchanges occur between compartments 3 and 1 and compartments 1 and 2 and are represented by arrows. Compartment 1 is the accessible compartment: test input and measurement (output) are denoted by a large arrow and a dashed line with a bullet, respectively.

plasma. Glucose and glucose-6-phosphate could be two different compartments inside a liver cell. Thus a physical space may actually represent more than one compartment.

In addition, one must distinguish between compartments that are accessible and nonaccessible for measurement. Researchers often try to assign physical spaces to the nonaccessible compartments. This is a very difficult problem which is best addressed once one realizes that the definition of a compartment is actually a theoretical construct which may in fact lump material from several different physical spaces in a system; to equate a compartment with a physical space depends upon the system under study and assumptions about the model.

With these notions of what might constitute a compartment, it is easier to define the concepts of well-mixed and kinetic homogeneity. What *well-mixed* means is that any two samples taken from the compartment at the same time would have the same concentration of the substance being studied and therefore be equally representative. Thus the concept of well-mixed relates to uniformity of information contained in a single compartment.

Kinetic homogeneity means that every particle in a compartment has the same probability of taking the pathways leaving the compartment. Since, when a particle leaves a compartment, it does so because of metabolic events related to transport and utilization, it means that all particles in the compartment have the same probability of leaving due to one of these events.

The notion of a compartment, i.e., lumping material with similar characteristics into collections that are homogeneous and behave identically, is what allows one to reduce a complex physiologic system into a finite number of compartments and pathways. The number of compartments required depends both on the system being studied and on the richness of the experimental configuration. A compartmental model is clearly unique for each system studied, since it incorporates known and hypothesized physiology and biochemistry. It provides the investigator with insights into the system structure and is as good as the assumptions that are incorporated in the model structure.

157.2 The Compartmental Model

Theory

Let Fig. 157.2 represent the ith compartment of an n-compartment model; $q_i \geq 0$ denotes the mass of the compartment. The arrows represent fluxes into and out of the compartment: the input flux into the compartment from outside the system, e.g., de novo synthesis of material and/or exogenous test input, is represented by $u_i \geq 0$; the flux to the environment and therefore out of the system by F_{oi}; the flux from compartment i to j by F_{ji}, and the flux from compartment j to i by F_{ij}. All F_{hk} are ≥ 0. The general equations for the compartmental model are obtained by writing the mass balance equation for each compartment:

$$\dot{q}_i = \sum_{j \neq i} F_{ij} - \sum_{j \neq i} F_{ji} - F_{oi} + u_i \qquad q_i(0) = q_{io} \qquad (157.1)$$

The fluxes u_i are generally constant or functions of only time. The fluxes F_{ij}, F_{ji} and F_{oi} can be functions of $q_1, \ldots, q_n$ (sometimes also of time).

It is usually possible to write

$$F_{ji}(\boldsymbol{q}) \equiv k_{ji}(\boldsymbol{q}) q_i \qquad (157.2)$$

where $\boldsymbol{q} = [q_1, \ldots, q_n]^T$ is the vector of the compartmental masses. As a result, Eq. (157.1) can be written as

$$\dot{q}_i = \sum_{j \neq i} k_{ij}(\boldsymbol{q}) q_j - \left(\sum_{j \neq i} k_{ji}(\boldsymbol{q}) + k_{oi}(\boldsymbol{q}) \right) q_i + u_i \qquad q_i(0) = q_{io} \qquad (157.3)$$

The k_{ij}'s are called *fractional transfer coefficients*. Equation (157.3) describes the *nonlinear* compartmental model. If the k_{ij}'s are constants (or functions only of time) the compartmental model becomes *linear*.

Defining $k_{ii} = -\left(\sum_{j \neq i} k_{ji} + k_{oi} \right)$ we can now write Eq. (157.3) as

$$\dot{q}_i = \sum_j k_{ij}(\boldsymbol{q}) q_j + u_i \qquad q_i(0) = q_{io} \qquad (157.4)$$

and the model of the whole system as

$$\dot{\boldsymbol{q}} = K(\boldsymbol{q}) \boldsymbol{q} + \boldsymbol{u} \qquad q(0) = \boldsymbol{q}_o \qquad (157.5)$$

where K is the *compartmental matrix* and $\boldsymbol{u} = [u_1 \ldots u_n]^T$ is the vector of input fluxes into the compartments from outside the system.

For the linear case, i.e., K constant, the model is

$$\dot{\boldsymbol{q}} = K\boldsymbol{q} + \boldsymbol{u} \qquad q(0) = \boldsymbol{q}_o \qquad (157.6)$$

The entries of the compartmental matrix K, for both the nonlinear (157.5) and the linear (157.6) model, satisfy

$$k_{ii} \leq 0 \text{ for all } i \qquad (157.7)$$

$$k_{ij} \geq 0 \text{ for all } i \neq j \qquad (157.8)$$

$$\sum_{i=1}^{n} k_{ij} = \sum_{i \neq j} k_{ij} + k_{jj} = -k_{oj} \leq 0 \text{ for all } j \qquad (157.9)$$

K is thus a (column) diagonally dominant matrix. This is a very important property, and in fact the stability properties of compartmental models are closely related to the diagonal dominance of the compartmental matrix. For instance, for the linear model Eq. (157.6) one can show that no eigenvalues can have positive real parts and that there are no purely imaginary eigenvalues: This means that all solutions are bounded and if there are oscillations they must be damped. The qualitative theory of linear and nonlinear compartmental models has been reviewed in Jacquez and Simon [1993], where also some new stability results on nonlinear compartmental models are presented.

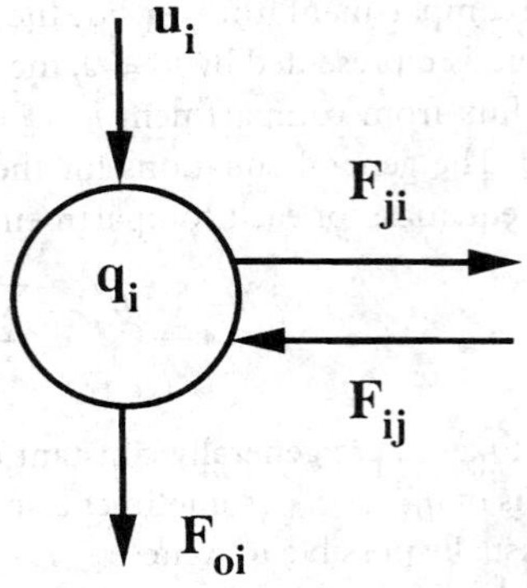

The Linear Model

The linear model, Eq. (157.6), has become very useful in applications due to an important result: The kinetics of a tracer in a constant steady-state system, linear or nonlinear, are linear with constant coefficients. An example is shown in Fig. 157.3 where the three-compartment model by Cobelli and coworkers [1984b] for studying tracer glucose kinetics in steady state at the whole-body level is depicted. Linear compartmental models in conjunction with tracer experiments have been extensively used in studying distribution of materials in living systems both at whole-body, organ, and cellular level. Example and references can be found in Berman and coworkers [1982], Carson and coworkers [1983], and Jacquez [1985].

An interesting application of linear compartmental models at the organ level is in describing the exchange of materials between blood, interstitial fluid, and cell of a tissue from multiple tracer indicator dilution data. Compartmental models provide a finite difference approximation in the space dimension of a system described by partial differential equations which may be easier resolvable from the data. These models are discussed by Jacquez [1985], and an example of a model describing glucose transport and metabolism in the human skeletal muscle can be found in Cobelli and colleagues [1989].

FIGURE 157.2   The i-th compartment of an n-compartmental model.

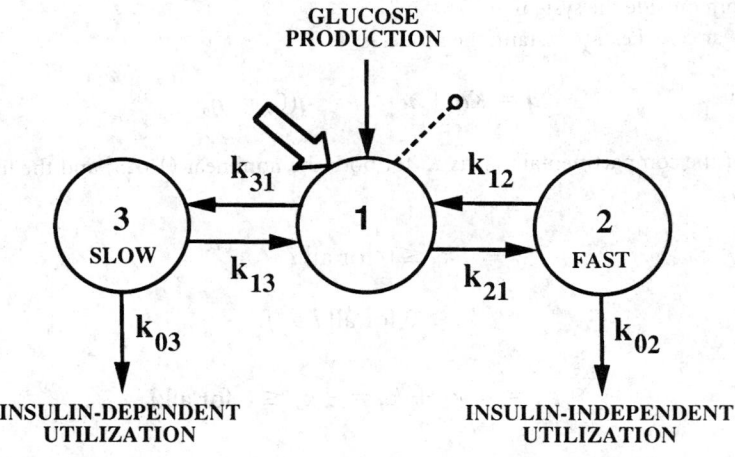

FIGURE 157.3   The linear compartmental model of glucose kinetics by Cobelli, Toffolo, and Ferrannini [1984b].

The Nonlinear Model

Also the nonlinear model, Eq. (157.5) is frequently found in applications. For such models the entries of K are functions of q, most commonly k_{ij} is a function of only a few component of q, often q_i and q_j. Examples of k_{ij} function of q_j and q_i only are the Michaelis-Menten and Langmuir nonlinearities described respectively by:

$$k_{ij}(q_j) = \frac{\alpha}{\beta + q_j} \tag{157.10}$$

$$k_{ij}(q_i) = \left(1 - \frac{q_i}{\gamma}\right) \tag{157.11}$$

where α, β, γ are constants.

Other interesting examples arise in describing substrate-hormone control systems. For instance, the model of Fig. 157.4 has been proposed [Caumo & Cobelli, 1993] to describe the control of insulin on glucose distribution and metabolism during a glucose perturbation which brings the system out of steady state. Since there is no direct interconversion, one has to have two separate compartmental models, one for glucose and one for insulin kinetics. The two models interact via a control signal which emanates from the remote insulin compartment and affects the transfer rate coefficient, k_{02}, responsible for insulin-dependent glucose utilization. In this case one has

$$k_{02}(q_3) = \delta + q_3 \tag{157.12}$$

where δ is a constant.

Additional examples and references on nonlinear compartmental models can be found in Carson and coworkers [1993], Godfrey [1993], and Jacquez [1985].

The Measurement Equation

Equations (157.5) and (157.6) define the structure of the compartmental model. There is the need to model the measurement configuration. Measurements in multicompartmental models are usually described by a linear algebraic equation

$$y = C q \tag{157.13}$$

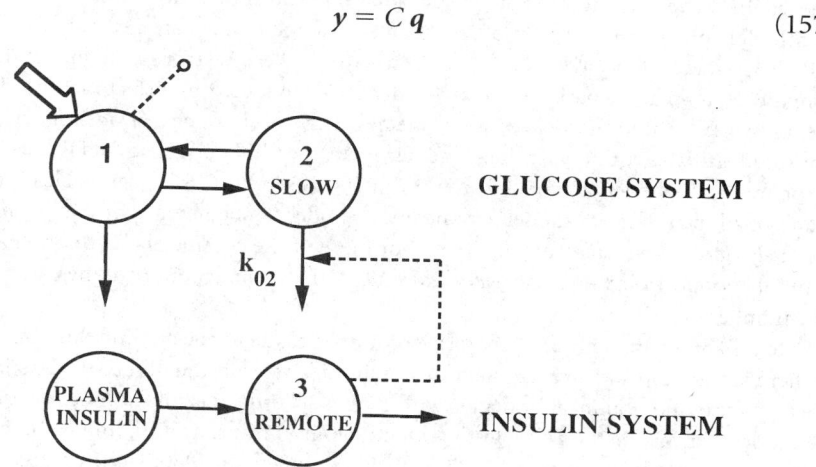

FIGURE 157.4 The nonlinear compartmental model of insulin control on glucose distribution and metabolism by Caumo and Cobelli [1993]. The dashed line denotes a control signal.

where $y = [y_1 \ldots y_m]^T$ is the vector of m model outputs and C is a constant matrix. Since model outputs are often concentrations, the entries of C are inverse of compartment volumes. Note that usually only a small number of compartments is accessible to measurement.

Real data are noisy, thus an error term e is usually added to y in Eq. (157.13) to describe the actual measurements

$$z = y + e \qquad\qquad\qquad (157.14)$$

e is usually given a probabilistic description, e.g., errors are assumed to be independent and often gaussian. Data are usually collected at discrete time instants $t_1 \ldots t_N$ so that the measurements are not continuous functions of time $z(t)$ (assuming that only one output variable is observed), as in Eq. (157.14), but are denoted $z(t_1) \ldots z(t_N)$.

Equations (157.13) and (157.14), together with Eq. (157.5) or (157.6), define the compartmental model of the system, i.e., the model structure and the input-output experimental configuration.

157.3 Identifiability

Let's assume that a compartmental model structure has been postulated to describe the physiologic system, i.e., the number of compartments and the connections among them have been specified. This is the most difficult step in compartmental model building.

The structure can reflect a number of facts: There may be some a priori knowledge about the system which can be incorporated in the structure; one can make specific assumptions about the system which are reflected in the structure; one can arrive at a structure by testing via simulation what is needed to fit the data. The result at this stage is a nonlinear, Eq. (157.5) or linear, Eq. (157.6), model which has as unknowns the parameters of the compartmental matrix K and often those of the observation matrix C in Eq. (157.13).

Before performing the experiment to collect the data to be analyzed using the model or, if the experiment is already completed, before using the model to estimate the unknown parameters from the data, the following question arises: Do the data contain enough information to estimate all the unknown parameters of the postulated model structure? This question is usually referred to as the *identifiability* problem. It is set in the ideal context of error-free model structure and noise-free measurements, and is an obvious prerequisite to determine if parameter estimation from real data is well-posed. In particular, if it turns out in such an ideal context that the postulated model structure is too complex for the particular set of ideal data, i.e., some model parameters are not identifiable from the data, there is no way in a real situation—where there is error in the model structure and noise in the data—that the parameters can be identified. To focus on the fact that the identifiability problem is worked out in the ideal context, one normally speaks of *a priori identifiability*.

A priori identifiability thus examines whether, given the ideal noise-free data y, Eq. (157.13), and the error-free compartmental model structure, Eqs. (157.5) or (157.6), it is possible to make unique estimates of all the unknown model parameters. A model can be *uniquely (globally) identifiable* or *nonuniquely (locally) identifiable*—that is, one or more of the parameters has more than one but a finite number of possible values—or *nonidentifiable*—that is, one or more of the parameters has an infinite number of solutions.

The identifiability problem is in general a large nonlinear algebraic one and thus difficult to solve, since there is the need to solve a system of nonlinear algebraic equations which is increasing in number of terms and nonlinearity degree with the model order, i.e., the number of compartments in the model. Various methods for testing identifiability of linear and nonlinear compartmental models are available [Carson et al., 1983; Cobelli & DiStefano, 1980; Godfrey, 1983; Godfrey & DiStefano, 1987; Jacquez, 1985; Walter 1982]. For linear compartmental models, various specific methods based, e.g., on transfer function, similarity transformation, and graph topology, have been developed. Explicit identifiability results on catenary and mamillary compartmental models

[Cobelli et al., 1979] and on the three-compartmental model [Norton, 1982] are also available. A parameter-bound strategy for dealing with nonidentifiable compartmental models has also been developed [DiStefano, 1983]. For nonlinear compartmental models, the problem is more difficult, and for small models the output series expansion method [Pohjanpalo, 1978] is usually employed.

However, all the proposed methods apply to models of relatively low dimension; when applied to large models, the methods involve nonlinear algebraic equations too difficult to be solved even by resorting to symbolic algebraic manipulative languages (e.g., Reduce, Maple). These difficulties have stimulated new approaches to study global identifiability based on computer algebra. In particular, for nonlinear models, approaches based on differential algebra have been investigated [D'Angió et al., 1994; Ljung & Glad, 1994], while for linear compartmental models a method based on the transfer function and Groebner basis algorithm has been proposed [Saccomani et al., 1994].

If a model is a priori uniquely or nonuniquely identifiable, then identification techniques (e.g., least squares) can be used to estimate from the noisy data z, Eq. (157.14), the numerical values of the unknown parameters. If a model is a priori nonidentifiable, then not all its parameters can be estimated using identification techniques. Various strategies can be used, e.g., derivation of bounds for nonidentifiable parameters, model reparameterization (parameter aggregation), incorporation of additional knowledge, or design of a more informative experiment. An example on the use of some of these approaches for dealing with a nonidentifiable model of glucose kinetics is given in Cobelli and Toffolo [1987].

From the above considerations it follows that a priori unique identifiability is a prerequisite for well-posedness of parameter estimation and for reconstructability of state variables in nonaccessible compartments. It is a necessary step, but, because of the ideal context where it is posed, it does not guarantee a successful estimation of model parameters from real input-output data.

157.4 Parameter Estimation

Given a uniquely identifiable parameterization of the compartmental model, one can proceed by estimating the values of the unknown parameters from the set of noisy real data. Usually the input-output experiment provides a limited set of discrete-time measurements Eq. (157.14), for estimating the unknown parameters of the nonlinear, Eq. (157.5), and linear, Eq. (157.6) compartmental model. Problems arise in parameter estimation as a result of various sources of error, e.g., measurement error—e in Eq. (157.13)—and error in model structure—K in Eq. (157.5) or Eq. (157.6). It is normally not possible to consider explicitly errors in model structure: Alternative model structures can be analyzed in order to minimize this error. The simplest situation is to consider the noisy real data as reflecting model output corrupted by an additive measurement error, like in Eq. (157.14). Parameter estimates are then obtained by nonlinear least squares or maximum likelihood together with their precision, i.e., a measure of a posteriori or numerical identifiability. Details and references on parameter estimation of physiologic system models can be found in Carson and coworkers [1983] Landaw and DiStefano [1984], and Jacquez [1985].

Weighted nonlinear least squares is mostly used, and both direct and gradient-type search methods are implemented in estimation schemes. A correct knowledge of the error structure is needed in order to have a correct summary of the statistical properties of the estimates. This is a difficult task. Measurement errors are usually independent, and often a known distribution, e.g., gaussian, is assumed. However, many properties of least squares hold approximately for wide class of distributions if weights are chosen optimally, i.e., inverse of known variances or of their relative values if variances are known up to a proportionality constant. Under these circumstances an asymptotically correct approximation of the covariance matrix of parameter estimates can be used to evaluate precision of parameter estimates. The approximation becomes exact for a sufficiently large sample size and/or decreasing variances of the measurement error. If measurement errors are gaussian, then this approximation is the Cramer-Rao lower bound (inverse of the Fisher information matrix), i.e., the optimally weighted least squares estimator is also the maximum likelihood estimator. Care must be taken in not using lower-bound variances as true parameter variances. Several factors corrupt these variances, e.g., inaccurate knowledge of error structure, limited data set. Monte Carlo studies are needed to assess robustness of Cramer-Rao lower-bound in specific practical applications.

To examine the quality of model predictions to observed data, in addition to visual inspection, various statistical tests on residuals are available to check for presence of systematic misfitting, nonrandomness of the errors, and accordance with assumed experimental noise. Model order estimation, i.e., number of compartments in the model, is also relevant here, and for linear compartmental models criteria such as F-test, and those based on the parsimony principle like the Akaike and Schwarz criteria, can be used if measurement errors are gaussian.

157.5 Optimal Experiment Design

At this point one has a compartmental model structure, a description of the measurement error, and a numerical value of the parameters together with the precision with which they can be estimated. It is now appropriate to address the optimal experiment design issue. The rationale of optimal experiment design is to act on design variables such as number of test input and outputs, form of test inputs, number of samples and sampling schedule, and measurement errors so as to maximize, according to some criterion, the precision with which the compartmental model parameters can be estimated [Carson et al., 1983; DiStefano, 1981; Landaw & DiStefano, 1984; Walter & Pronzato, 1990]. The Fisher information matrix J, which is the inverse of the lower bound of the covariance matrix, is treated as a function of the design variables and usually the determinant of J (this is called D-optimal design) is maximized in order to maximize precision of parameter estimates, and thus numerical identifiability.

The optimal design of sampling schedules, i.e., the determination of the number and location of discrete-time points where samples are collected, has received much attention as it is the variable which is less constrained by the experimental situation. Theoretical and algorithmic aspects have been studied, and software is available, for both the single- and multioutput case [Cobelli et al., 1985; D'Argenio, 1981; DiStefano, 1981; Landaw, 1982]. Optimal sampling schedules are usually obtained in an iterative manner: One starts with the model obtained from pilot experiments, and the program computes optimal sampling schedules for subsequent experimentation. An important result for single-output linear compartmental models is that D-optimal design usually consists of independent replicates at P distinct time points, where P is the number of parameters to estimate.

Optimal sampling schedule design has been shown to improve precision as compared to schedules designed by intuition or other convention [DiStefano, 1981; DiStefano et al., 1982]; to optimize the cost effectiveness of a dynamic clinical test by reducing the number of blood samples withdrawn from a patient without significantly deteriorating their precision [Cobelli & Ruggeri, 1989, 1991]; and to obtain less dispersion in population parameter estimates [D'Argenio, 1981].

The optimal input design problem has been relatively less studied, but some results are available on equidose rectangular inputs (including the impulse) for parameter estimation in compartmental models [Cobelli & Thomaseth, 1987, 1988a, 1988b].

157.6 Validation

Validation involves assessing whether the compartmental model is adequate for its purpose. This is a difficult and highly subjective task in modeling of physiologic systems, because intuition, understanding of the system, and so on play an important role. It is also difficult to formalize related issues such as model credibility, i.e., the use of the model outside its established validity range. Some efforts have been made, however, to provide some formal aids for assessing the value of models of physiologic systems [Carson et al., 1983; Cobelli et al., 1984a]. A set of validity criteria, i.e., empirical, theoretical, pragmatic, and heuristic, have been explicitly defined, and validation strategies have been outlined for two classes of models, broadly corresponding to simple and complex models. This operational classification is based on a priori identifiability and leads to clearly defined strategies as both complexity of model structure and extent of available experimental data are taken into account. For simple models quantitative criteria based on identification, e.g., a priori identifiability, precision of parameter estimates, residual errors, can be used in addition to physiologic plausibility. In contrast with simple models, complex simulation models are essentially incomplete, as there will naturally be a high degree of uncertainty with respect to both structure and parameters. Therefore validation will necessarily be based on less solid grounds. The following aids have been suggested: increasing model testability through model simplification; improved experimental design and model decomposition; adaptive fitting based on qualitative and/or quantitative feature comparison and time-course prediction; and model plausibility.

157.7 Applications and Software

Compartmental models have been widely employed for solving a broad spectrum of physiologic problems related to the distribution of materials in living systems in research, diagnosis and therapy both at whole-body, organ, and cellular level. Examples and references can be found in books [Berman et al., 1982; Carson et al., 1983; Cobelli & Bergman, 1981; Cobelli & Mariani, 1989; Cramp, 1982; Gibaldi & Perrier, 1982; Jacquez, 1984, 1985] and reviews [Berman, 1982; Carson & Jones, 1979; Cobelli, 1984, 1987; Cobelli et al., 1990; Radziuk & Hetenyi, 1982]. Purposes for which compartmental models have been developed include:

- Identification of system structure, i.e., models to examine different hypotheses regarding the nature of specific physiologic mechanisms
- Estimation of unmeasurable quantities, i.e., estimating internal parameters and variables of physiologic interest
- Simulation of the intact system behavior where ethical or technical reasons do not allow direct experimentation on the system itself
- Prediction and control of physiologic variables by administration of therapeutic agents, i.e., models to predict an optimal administration of drug in order to keep one or more physiologic variables within desirable limits
- Optimize cost effectiveness of dynamic clinical tests, i.e., models to obtain maximal information from the minimum number of blood samples withdrawn from a patient
- Diagnosis, i.e., models to augment quantitative information from laboratory tests and clinical symptoms, thus improving the reliability of diagnosis
- Teaching, i.e., models to aid in the teaching of many aspects of physiology, clinical medicine, and pharmacokinetics

The use of compartmental models in physiology and pathophysiology has been made easier by the availability of the SAAM program and its interactive version CONSAM [Foster & Boston, 1983], a software specifically designed for compartmental models which can be used both for simulation and fitting of models to data. Application of compartmental models is now even easier, since an entirely new version of SAAM called SAAM II [Saam II, 1994] has been developed. SAAM II retains the philosophy of the original version but has a user-friendly graphical user interface, is fully menu driven, and has an expanded computational functionality. The formulation of compartmental model structures and the description of experimental protocols associated with the models are therefore greatly facilitated.

References

Anderson DH. 1983. Compartmental Modeling and Tracer Kinetics. Berlin, Springer.
Atkins GL. 1969. Multicompartmental Models for Biological Systems. London, Methuen.

Berman M. 1982. Kinetic analysis and modeling: Theory and applications to lipoproteins. In M Berman, SM Grundy, BV Howard (eds), Lipoprotein Kinetics and Modeling, pp 3–36, New York, Academic Press.

Berman M, Grundy SM, Howard BV (eds). 1982. Lipoprotein Kinetics and Modeling, New York, Academic Press.

Brown RF. 1985. Biomedical System Analysis, Cambridge, Mass, Abacus Press.

Carson ER, Cobelli C, Finkelstein L. 1983. The Mathematical Modelling of Metabolic and Endocrine Systems, New York, John Wiley.

Carson ER, Jones EA. 1979. The use of kinetic analysis and mathematical modeling in the quantitation of metabolic pathways in vivo: Application to hepatic anion metabolism. N Eng J Med 300:1016.

Caumo A, Cobelli C. 1993. Hepatic glucose production during the labelled IVGTT: Estimation by deconvolution with a new minimal model. Am J Physiol 264:E829.

Cobelli C. 1984. Modeling and identification of endocrine-metabolic systems. Theoretical aspects and their importance in practice. Math Biosci 72:263.

Cobelli C. 1987. Identification of endocrine-metabolic and pharmacokinetic systems. In M Nalecz (ed), Control Aspects of Biomedical Engineering, pp 235–249, Oxford, Pergamon Press.

Cobelli C, Bergman RN (eds). 1981. Carbohydrate Metabolism, Chichester, John Wiley.

Cobelli C, Bier DM, Ferrannini E. 1990. Modelling glucose metabolism in man: Theory and practice. In J Schrezenmeir, EW Kraegen, J Beyer (eds), Computers and Quantitative Approaches to Diabetes, pp 1–10,

Cobelli C, Carson ER, Finkelstein L, et al. 1984*a*. Validation of simple and complex models in physiology and medicine. Am J Physiol 246:R259.

Cobelli C, DiStefano JJ III. 1980. Parameter and structural identifiability concepts and ambiguities: A critical review and analysis. Am J Physiol 239:R7.

Cobelli C, Lepschy A, Romanin Jacur G. 1979. Identifiability results on some constrained compartmental systems. Math Biosci 47:173.

Cobelli C, Mariani L (eds). 1989. Modelling and Control of Biomedical Systems, Oxford, Pergamon Press.

Cobelli C, Ruggeri A. 1989. Optimal design of sampling schedules for studying glucose kinetics with tracers. Am J Physiol 257:E444.

Cobelli C, Ruggeri A. 1991. A reduced sampling schedule for estimating the parameters of the glucose minimal model from a labelled IVGTT. IEEE Trans Biomed Eng 38:1023.

Cobelli C, Ruggeri A, DiStefano JJ III, et al. 1985. Optimal design of multioutput sampling schedules: Software and applications to endocrine-metabolic and pharmacokinetic models. IEEE Trans Biomed Eng 32:249.

Cobelli C, Saccomani MP, Ferrannini E, et al. 1989. A compartmental model to quantitate in vivo glucose transport in the human forearm. Am J Physiol 257:E943.

Cobelli C, Thomaseth K. 1987. The minimal model of glucose disappearance: Optimal input studies. Math Biosci 83:127.

Cobelli C, Thomaseth K. 1988*a*. On optimality of the impulse input for linear system identification. Math Biosci 89:127.

Cobelli C, Thomaseth K. 1988*b*. Optimal equidose inputs and role of measurement error for estimating the parameters of a compartmental model of glucose kinetics from continuous— and discrete—time optimal samples. Math Biosci 89:135.

Cobelli C, Toffolo G. 1987. Theoretical aspects and practical strategies for the identification of unidentifiable compartmental systems. In E Walter (ed), Identifiability of Parametric Models, pp 85–91, Oxford, Pergamon.

Cobelli C, Toffolo G, Ferrannini E. 1984*b*. A model of glucose kinetics and their control by insulin. Compartmental and noncompartmental approaches. Math Biosci 72:291.

Cramp DG, (ed). 1982. Quantitative Approaches to Metabolism, Chichester, John Wiley.

D' Angió L, Audoly S, Bellu G, et al. 1994. Structural identifiability of nonlinear systems: algorithms based on differential ideals. In M. Blanke, T. Söderström (eds), Proceedings of the 10th IFAC Symposium on System Identification, vol. 3, pp 13–18. Danish Automation Society, Copenhagen.

D' Argenio DZ. 1981. Optimal sampling times for pharmacokinetic experiments. J Pharmacokin Biopharm 9:739.

DiStefano JJ III. 1981. Optimized blood sampling protocols and sequential design of kinetic experiments. Am J Physiol 9:R259.

DiStefano JJ III. 1983. Complete parameter bounds and quasiidentifiability conditions for a class of unidentifiable linear systems. Math Biosci 65:51.

DiStefano JJ III, Jang M, Malone TK, et al. 1982. Comprehensive kinetics of triiodothyronine (T_3) production, distribution and metabolism in blood and tissue pools of the rat using optimized blood sampling protocols. Endocrinology 110:198.

Foster DM, Boston RC. 1983. The use of computers in compartmental analysis: The SAAM and CONSAM programs. In J Robertson (ed), Compartmental Distribution of Radiotracers, pp 73–142, Boca Raton, Fla, CRC Press.

Gibaldi M, Perrier D. 1982. Pharmacokinetics, 2d ed, New York, Marcel Dekker.

Godfrey K. 1983. Compartmental Models and Their Application, London, Academic Press.

Godfrey KR, DiStefano JJ III. 1987. Identifiability of model parameters. In E Walter (ed), Identifiability of Parametric Models, pp 1–20, Oxford, Pergamon Press.

Jacquez JA (ed). 1984. Berman memorial issue, Math Biosci 72(2).

Jacquez JA. 1985. Compartmental Analysis in Biology and Medicine, 2d ed, Ann Arbor, Mich, University of Michigan Press.

Jacquez JA, Simon CP. 1993. Qualitative theory of compartmental systems. Siam Rev 35:43.

Landaw EM. 1982. Optimal multicompartmental sampling designs for parameter estimation: Practical aspects of the identification problem. Math Comput Simul 24:525.

Landaw EM, DiStefano JJ III. 1984. Multiexponential, multicompartmental, and noncompartmental modeling: II. Data analysis and statistical considerations. Am J Physiol 246:R665.

Ljung L, Glad T. 1994. On global identifiability for arbitrary model parametrizations. Automatica 30:265.

Norton JP. 1982. An investigation of the sources of non-uniqueness in deterministic identifiability. Math Biosci 60:89.

Pohjanpalo H. 1978. System identifiability based on the power series expansion of the solution. Math Biosci 41:21.

Radziuk J, Hetenyi G Jr. 1982. Modeling and the use of tracers in the analysis of exogenous control of glucose homeostasis. In DG Cramp (ed), Quantitative Approaches to Metabolism, pp 73–142, Chichester, John Wiley.

Rescigno A, Segre G. 1966. Drug and Tracer Kinetics. Waltham, Mass, Blaisdell.

SAAM II User Guide 1994. SAAM Institute FL-20, University of Washington, Seattle.

Saccomani MP, Audoly S, D' Angio' L, et al. 1994. PRIDE: A program to test a priori global identifiability of linear compartmental models. In M Blanke, T Söderström (eds), Proceedings of the 10th IFAC Symposium on System Identification, vol 3, pp 25–30. Danish Automation Society, Copenhagen.

Sheppard CW. 1948. The theory of the study of transfer within a multicompartment system using isotopic tracers. J Appl Physics 19:70.

Sheppard CW. 1962. Basic Principles of the Tracer Method, New York, John Wiley.

Walter E. 1982. Identifiability of State Space Models, Berlin, Springer.

Walter E, Pronzato L. 1990. Qualitative and quantitative experiment design for phenomenological models—a survey. Automatica 26:195.

158

Cardiovascular Models and Control

William D. Timmons
University of Akron

This chapter reviews cardiovascular (CV) modeling for use in controller design, especially for closed-loop drug delivery systems (IV infusions of vasodilators, inotropes, anesthetics, neoplastic agents, and so on) and other pharmacologic applications. This first section describes the advantages and disadvantages of employing CV models for design and control and presents a brief history of CV modeling. The next section describes the basic principles and techniques for modeling the CV system, as well as the uptake, distribution, and action of cardio- and vasoactive pharmaceuticals. A short, annotated bibliography follows the references section for those interested in further reading.

158.1 Advantages and Disadvantages of Desktop Patients

More and more industries are coming to rely on computer simulations to increase productivity and decrease costs as well as to increase reliability and safety of resulting products. The defense, automotive, and aerospace industries come most quickly to mind, but the medical field is rapidly gaining ground in this area, too. Recent ARPA* initiatives for defense technology conversion are probably most responsible for the recent surge in computer-aided health care. Today, computerized simulators teach medical students everything from basic anatomy to techniques in radial keratotomy, and skilled surgeons design, evaluate, and practice new and risky procedures without ever cutting into a single patient. Thanks to the ARPA initiative, telesurgery will soon be viable, so that in the near future, surgeons may operate on patients from half a world away. From the calculation of simple-dosage regimens to the design of sophisticated blood pressure controllers, cardiovascular medicine also benefits from this technology. CV models can be used to prove initial feasibility, reduce development time, decrease costs, and increase reliability and safety of cardiovascular devices and therapeutics.

The increasing speed and decreasing costs of computers are having an enormous impact on controller design. There is a veritable explosion in the number of control designs as well as the theory to go with them. The ready availability of powerful computer workstations and sophisticated

*The Advanced Research Projects Agency of the U.S. Department of Defense, chair of the Defense Technology Conversion Council which administers the Technology Reinvestment Project.

0-8493-8346-3/95/$0.00+$.50
© 1995 by CRC Press, Inc.

engineering design packages (e.g., MATLAB, MATRIXx, CC) allow for the interactive design of high-performance, robust controllers. Engineers can tweak a controller or perturb a system, then immediately assess the effect. When combined with modern visualization techniques, these tools allow one to readily see problems and solutions that might otherwise have taken years to find and solve. Furthermore, such capabilities allow for exhaustive testing and debugging, so that the transition from the workbench to the field becomes smooth. Many companies and agencies have reported flawless transitions from the simulator to the field, most notably NASA, with its many satellites and probes that have had to work right the first time. Various companies are using simulations to improve or correct equipment and systems already in the field. A recent example is BAE Automated Systems Inc. of Dallas, Texas, which is using simulations to help debug and correct the troubled baggage system at the new Denver International Airport [Geppert, 1994].

The risk of failure or the fear of malpractice often precludes the design and evaluation of controllers in live humans, so that devices and treatments are often tested on computer and animal models first. In the past, animals have been the preferred choice, but this approach is continually being reevaluated. Whereas most researchers readily agree that animal experimentation has been and will continue to be necessary for the advancement of medical science, most would welcome methods and procedures that might reduce or even eliminate the use of animals. Furthermore, animals are rarely perfect models of human diseases and conditions. Thus, there has been and will continue to be a demand for alternative models and procedures. Tissue cultures are beginning to fill some of this need, and it is likely that computer modeling and simulation may also fill this need.

Desktop patients, if used to complement animal studies, can actually increase the reliability and applicability of certain animal tests, while also reducing the number of required experiments. In certain instances, computer modeling may be the only way to test a device prior to human use, since some human conditions are extremely difficult if not impossible to reproduce in animals. Indeed, as computers become more powerful and models become better, it may be that some day computers will be used *in place of* certain animal and human trials. Meanwhile, computer models can be used to (1) demonstrate feasibility, (2) increase confidence in controller designs by complementing animal studies, (3) help design better animal and clinical experiments, and (4) reduce the number of required animal and human experiments.

The disadvantage of using computer simulation is that available models will almost certainly need to be tailored to the application at hand. Since there is generally no predefined method for modeling or for modifying an existing model, the accuracy and reliability of the resulting model will depend heavily on the skill of the modeler, the appropriateness of the modifications, and the model's intended scope. Furthermore, modeling typically requires a good understanding of the physics of the problem, and this in turn requires supporting data and experimentation. Thus, modifications to include new pharmaceuticals may be problematic, since their mechanisms may only be poorly understood. And, even if supporting data are available, if a basic model does not yet exist, a significant time commitment may be required to develop one. Despite this up-front cost, model development may save tremendous time and costs later in the development process.

Fortunately, there are a large number of CV models to pick from, and experienced modelers can determine which, if any, is best for a given application. Once determined, the model can usually be converted easily to a form compatible with the development platform. Once converted, model integrity and suitability must be checked. Modifications can then be made, after which the model integrity must again be checked to ensure that it has not been compromised. Once a model is obtained and suitably modified, adequate thought must be given to program flow. Ideally, program flow should be designed such that the controller code is the same for real time and for simulation. This may be facilitated by treating all facets of data acquisition as part of the controlled system, instead of as part of the controller. With this approach, all software for I/O and calibration would be bundled separately from the controller software. Windows-based systems facilitate this separation even further by allowing the controller and plant software to be compiled and run as two separate programs.

Other issues that must be considered involve the practical aspects of computer simulation. Even if a well-designed and validated model exists, many factors can affect the accuracy of the simulation.

Stiffness, machine precision, program coding, integration method, step size, and even computer language can affect the results. Probably more insidious than all these factors is the operation of the model in regions outside its scope. This happens most often in large, complex programs when a variable takes on values outside its intended range. For example, a sudden increased cardiac preload may shift the end diastolic volume of the heart into a nonlinear region of the diastolic pressure-volume relationship. If the nonlinear behavior is not included in the model, misleading results might be produced. Finally, even in the best commercial code (let alone home-brewed code), bugs may affect simulation accuracy. For example, many commercial simulation packages are particularly poor at handling discrete events (such as a bolus infusion of a drug) when variable step-size algorithms are used to integrate continuous time models [Gustafsson, 1993].

158.2 History of Cardiovascular Modeling

William Harvey in the early 17th century was probably the first to clearly and convincingly demonstrate the role of the heart as a pump which caused the blood to flow in a unidirectional closed circuit through the systemic and pulmonary circulations. Prior to Harvey, the Galenic viewpoint from the 2d century AD predominated,* namely, that the blood ebbed to and fro in the veins to provide nutrition to the rest of the body, that the arteries (from the Greek *arteria,* meaning windpipe) carried air, that the lungs cooled the heart and removed sooty impurities from new blood as it entered from the intestines, and that the heart contained pores to allow spirit or gaseous exchange across the septum [Acierno, 1994].

It was Stephen Hales in his *Statical Essays* nearly a century later who considered arterial elasticity and postulated its buffering effect on the pulsatile nature of blood flow [Hales, 1733]. He likened the depulsing effect to the fire engines of his day, in which a chamber with an air-filled dome ("inverted globe") acted to cushion the bolus from the inlet water pump so that "a more nearly equal spout" flowed out the nozzle. This analogy became the basis of the first modern cardiovascular models and antedated the ARPA movement by quite a few decades! In the translation from English to German, Hales's inverted globe became a *windkessel* (air kettle); his idea later became known as the Windkessel theory when it was more formally developed and propounded by the German physiologist Otto Frank (of the Frank-Starling law of the heart) near the beginning of our century [Noordergraaf, 1978].

Frank was initially a strong proponent of the Windkessel theory, and his work spawned the interest of many subsequent investigators and led to a proliferation of modified Windkessel-type models. A critical review of these early models can be found in Aperia [1940]. The development of the analog computer shortly after World War II lead to another burst in CV modeling, based on more sophisticated segmental and transmission line theories. Grodins [1959] was probably one of the first to use these new machines to simulate cardiovascular hemodynamics. Interestingly, another early analog computer model, PHYSBE [McLeod, 1966], became a popular benchmark that is still used today to evaluate computers and simulation languages. About the mid-1970s, the advent of the inexpensive digital computer led to another revolution in CV modeling, which has continued to the present with ever-increasing detail and scope. As Rideout [1991] observed, model complexity seems to have been limited only by computer technology. If this trend continues, we can expect to see highly detailed models emerging within the next few years as parallel computers become economical.

The major criticism of the pure Windkessel theory is that it does not allow for finite wave propagation and reflection in the arteries. Whereas blood flow in the arterial vasculature is more properly formulated in terms of space and time, the Windkessel theory ignores spacial considerations and instead lumps all the vasculature into a single point, or compartment, in space. Attempts to correct this shortcoming include adding inertial and damping factors as well as collapsible components. In addition, the great arteries can be partitioned into sections to produce segmental models, or, when electrical network theory is invoked, transmission line models. Frank himself realized

---

*Galen, in turn, based many of his beliefs on those of the hippocratic era scholars—Hippocrates, Aristotle, Polybus, and Diocles (4th century BC).

that the Windkessel theory was flawed, and so he too added modifications to include traveling waves and reflections [Milnor, 1989; Noordergraaf, 1978; Rideout, 1991].

Despite its flaws, the pure Windkessel theory is still useful as a teaching tool because of its simplicity and clear, intuitive imagery. Furthermore, as mean pressure accounts for approximately 90% of the power in the arterial pressure waveform, it performs surprisingly well and displays many of the interesting phenomena seen in the vasculature. Add to this the fact that the equations are readily extended to include spacial effects (the segmental and transmission line models), and one can see why the theory has persisted into the late 20th century. Of course, one must keep in mind that any of these approaches is only an approximation; the segmental and transmission line approaches are in many ways only a mathematical convenience that allows one to fit an arbitrarily high-order model to observed data. These approaches do not necessarily lend themselves to extrapolations and predictions regarding the physiology.

Even before Frank, there was great interest in the pure mathematics of blood flow in distensible vessels. Many a famous mathematician and scientist explored wave propagation, reflection, and pressure-flow relations in blood vessels, including: Bernoulli, Euler, Young (of Young's modulus), Poiseuille, Navier and Stokes, the Weber brothers, Resal, Moens and Korteweg, Lamb, and Witzig; more recent investigators include Morgan and Kiely, and Womersley and McDonald [Fung, 1984; Milnor, 1989; Noordergraaf, 1978]. Womersley and McDonald's students continue to be influential in cardiovascular modeling today. Early studies of theoretical hemodynamics greatly influenced the field of fluid mechanics and paved the way for modern pulse-wave propagation and reflection models of the vasculature. These models are treated in the texts by Noordergraaf [1978], Fung [1985], Li [1987], and Milnor [1989].

The hydrodynamic pulse-wave CV models are not without criticisms either. For example, they are limited to short segments of the arterial or venous tree for which input and terminal impedances must be supplied. This restriction makes them currently impractical for the analysis of long-acting pharmaceutical agents and their feedback effects on the cardiovascular system. Pharmaceuticals with vaso- and cardio-active effects usually require the tracking of drug concentrations throughout the body, which, for these models, would require an exceedingly large number of components and would result in huge programs requiring large computers, with the simulations invariably being slow and cumbersome. Furthermore, numerical techniques such as the finite-element method must be used to solve many of the hydrodynamic equations, which over extended periods might incur significant round-off and integration errors. Nevertheless, this approach will certainly form the basis of future pharmacologically linked CV models as faster and more sophisticated computers and algorithms are developed.

Because of the current shortfall in computational technology, most pharmacologic simulations requiring a CV model employ simplified or reduced-order models mentioned earlier. Besides the segmental and transmission line approaches, purely black box models are also used. The reduced segmental and transmission line models are probably most appropriate for simulations of fast-acting CV pharmaceuticals, whereas compartmental models (see Chapter 157) are more appropriate for slower-acting drugs.

The distinction between segmental and transmission line models has become increasingly blurred, especially as elements of both are often combined into the same model. Transmission line models were used as early as 1905 by Frank, although Westerhof and Noordergraaf (1969) were probably most influential in promoting the transmission line approach. As a result, these models are often called Westkessel models. They employ black box, two-terminal circuits (Westkessel terminations) to reproduce the input impedances of lumped vascular trees. Segmental models, however, are generally three terminal circuits, with two terminals representing inertial flows and viscous resistances and the third representing the compliance of the segment with respect to an external reference (typically atmospheric pressure). The segmental approach is described in more detail below.

As mentioned above, reduction in model order is typically achieved by combining segmental and transmission line models. The idea here is to represent critical, nonlinear components by segments, while the less critical, more linear components are lumped together and represented by Westkessel terminations. Unfortunately, the black box Westkessel sections lose their physiologic meaning, which may present a problem in certain applications.

The highly simplified black box models are even worse in this regard. They are less concerned with the physiology than with the input-output relationships of the system and typically employ linear dynamics fit to observed patient responses. Though easy to implement, once defined, physiologically relevant perturbations may be difficult to produce. Furthermore, these models should not be used to infer properties or behaviors outside the range of the data sets. This is a potentially crippling drawback, especially when designing and evaluating CV controllers. However, if the goal is to generate clinically observed behaviors irrespective of the pathophysiology, then these models make an excellent choice.

Another potential drawback, which applies to both simplified and reduced-order models, is the loss of phenomena associated with pulse propagation and its effects on cardiac-arterial coupling and energetics. These effects are usually considered minor from a pharmacologic point of view, but their omission may lead to potentially serious design flaws when the resulting controller is used in certain patient populations. For example, isolated systolic hypertension (ISH) significantly contributes to strokes and heart disease in the elderly, and O'Rourke [1993] suggests that the therapy of choice, as well as the goal of treatment, should be different for ISH than for diastolic and mean arterial hypertension. It may be prudent, then, for control applications aimed at this population to be evaluated on more detailed models.

158.3 Cardiovascular Modeling

In this section, the concepts behind the segmental CV approach are described. Neurohumoral controls are also briefly discussed, as is the inclusion of pharmacokinetics and pharmacodynamics for drug uptake, distribution, and action.

An Idealized Segment of Artery

A short segment of artery can be modeled by an elastic, isobaric chamber attached to a rigid inlet and outlet tube (Fig. 158.1). The ability of the chamber to store fluid depends on its compliance, C, which is defined as

$$C = \frac{dV_c}{dP_c} \qquad (158.1)$$

where V_c is total segment (chamber) volume and P_c is chamber pressure. Many modelers prefer to use the reciprocal of compliance (termed stiffness, S, or elastance, E). Here, viscoelastic (stress

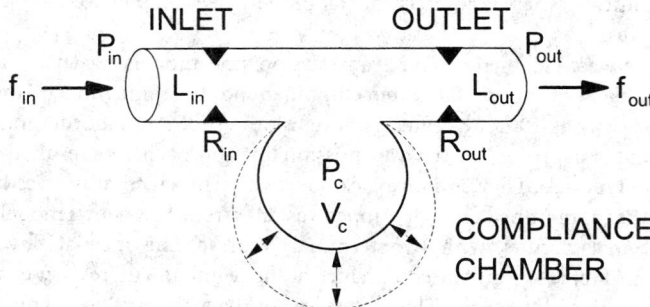

FIGURE 158.1   Idealized segment of artery approximated by an elastic, isobaric chamber attached to a rigid inlet and outlet tube. P_{in}, P_{out}, and P_c are *inlet*, *outlet*, and chamber pressures; f_{in} and f_{out} are flows; L_{in} and L_{out} are inertances; R_{in} and R_{out} are viscous resistances to flow; and V_c is total segment (chamber) *volume*. Compliance C is defined in the text.

relaxation) effects are assumed negligible, so that compliance is not an explicit function of time. Thus, compliance becomes an instantaneous variable which can be obtained from the experimentally determined, steady-state pressure-volume (P-V) relationship of the segment. Furthermore, model order can now be reduced, as pressure can be mathematically represented as an empirical function of volume, either by a piecewise linear approximation, a polynomial quotient, or some other function fit to the P-V relationship. A typical P-V curve is illustrated in Fig. 158.2, along with its piecewise linear approximation.

In arteries, pressure is usually positive with small oscillations about a nominal operating point (point A in Fig. 158.2). Hence the piecewise linear approximation can be reduced to a single line with constant slope $1/C$:

$$P_c = \frac{(V_c - V_{cu})}{C} \tag{158.2}$$

where V_{cu} is the unstressed volume (the idealized zero-pressure volume intercept). Of course, if pressure fluctuates outside this region, then additional straight-line sections should be included.

Assuming that blood is incompressible and newtonian, that the flow profile is parabolic and unchanging with axial distance along a straight rigid tube, then flow (poisenillean) is linearly proportional to the pressure gradient across the ends of the tube. Hence, flow into and out of the chamber in Fig. 158.1 may be calculated given P_{in} and P_{out} (the inlet and outlet pressures); P_c; L_{in} and L_{out} (the inertances due to fluid mass); and R_{in} and R_{out} (the resistances due to viscous drag)

$$L_{in} \frac{df_{in}}{dt} + R_{in} f_{in} = P_{in} - P_c$$

$$L_{out} \frac{df_{out}}{dt} + R_{out} f_{out} = P_c - P_{out} \tag{158.3}$$

where f_{in} and f_{out} are the flows into and out of the segment. Volume can now be calculated from the difference between the inlet and outlet flows:

$$\frac{dV_c}{dt} = f_{in} - f_{out} \tag{158.4}$$

P_c, V_c, f_{in}, and f_{out} can now be uniquely determined at any time given P_{in}, P_{out}, and the initial conditions of the segment. Determination of the parameters L and R are more problematic. They can be

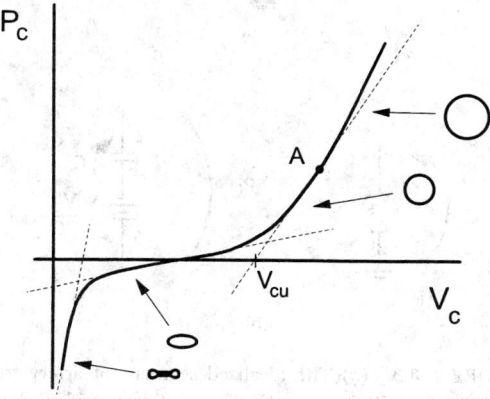

FIGURE 158.2 Static pressure-volume (P-V) relationship of a segment of artery.

derived analytically, although probably because the modeling assumptions are not completely correct, an empirical fit generally produces better segmental properties.

The simplified segmental structure can be represented as an RLC circuit as shown in Fig. 158.3a. Tsitlik and coworkers [1992] remind us that each capacitor should contain a residual charge to simulate the respective segment's unstressed volume (V_{cu}). This can be achieved most easily by inserting a battery between a standard capacitor and ground (Fig. 158.3b) [Tsitlik et al., 1992]. Or, if the unstressed volume for the segment remains constant (say, because the pharmacologic drug of interest has little effect on it), then the unstressed volume (and the battery) can be eliminated by subtracting it from the total vascular blood volume. The segment will then contain the stressed volume only (V_c-V_{cu}), so that an ordinary capacitor will suffice (again assuming operation near point A on the P-V curve).

An Idealized Segment of Vein

In most of the venous circulation, the pressure inside the vessels is greater than the external pressure, so that the pressure-flow relationship is like that in the arteries. However, in the vena cava, in certain organs such as the lungs and during certain procedures such as resuscitation or measurement of blood pressure using a cuff, venous collapse may occur [Fung, 1984]. Thus, in contrast to an artery in which only one condition normally exists, two additional conditions must be considered for a vein.

The first condition occurs when the inlet and outlet transmural pressures are *positive*. [Transmural pressure is defined as the pressure gradient across the vessel wall (P_{inside}-$P_{outside}$).] In this instance, the vein can be treated as discussed above for an artery. A second condition occurs when the inlet and outlet transmural pressures are *negative*. In this instance, the vein will collapse, and flow will stop or be greatly reduced.

The third condition occurs when the *inlet* transmural pressure is *positive* and the *outlet* transmural pressure is *negative*. In this instance, blood flows into the chamber but not out because the outlet will be collapsed. As blood flows in, the pressure inside rises until it exceeds the external pressure, forcing the outlet open and allowing blood to flow out. But, as blood flows out, the internal pressure decreases, so that the outlet transmural pressure may become negative again, collapsing the outlet, and commencing the next cycle. This cycling is called flutter, and the collapsing at the out-

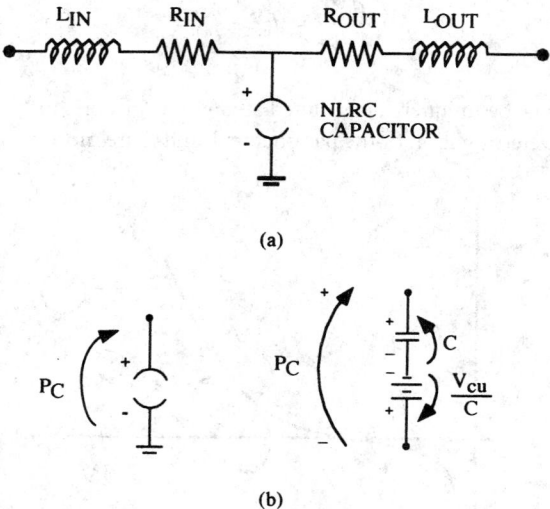

FIGURE 158.3 (*a*) The idealized segment of artery from Fig. 158.1 as an RLC circuit. (*b*) The nonlinear residual charge capacitor in (*a*). After Tsitlik et al. [1992].

let, choking. Besides flutter, a limited steady-state flow is also possible if the outlet is not completely choked off [Fung, 1984]. Limited flow is the predominant (and likely the only) effect occurring under physiologic conditions [Noordergraaf, 1978].

Purmutt and colleagues [1962] described this effect as a vascular waterfall. Water flowing over a falls depends only on conditions at the top, not on the length of the drop. In 1994 Holt used the term flow regulator for this effect in his seminal work on the collapsible penrose tube, and Conrad in 1969 called it a negative impedance conduit [Noordergraaf, 1978]. Starling in 1915 also made use of this concept when he used a collapsible tube, now known as a Starling resistor, to control peripheral resistance in his heart-lung preparations. Once flutter was found to be absent in the human physiology, Brower in 1970, Brower and Noordergraaf in 1973, and Griffiths in 1975 developed simplified equations of the pressure-flow relationship [Noordergraaf, 1978]. Snyder and Rideout [1969] also developed a model of collapsible vein. They employed a two-line approximation of the *P-V* curve—one for the uncollapsed region and one for the collapsed region. Then, based on modifications of the Navier-Stokes equations for an elliptical tube (the cross-sectional shape of a collapsing vessel), and assuming a flat flow profile, they were able to relate flow to pressure and volume in terms of nonlinear inertances, resistances, and compliances in Eqs. (158.2) and (158.3). They also included the effects of gravity and external pressures in the model.

Arterial and Venous Trees

By using the output of one segment as the input to a second, and the output of the second as the input to a third, and so on, differential equations for arbitrary lengths of vessel can be constructed (Fig. 158.4a). This method also allows bifurcations to be added. Another approach can be used to derive these same equations. First, partial differential equations are formulated to define flow along the desired length of vessel. The spacial differentials are then changed to finite differences, leaving only time derivatives [Noordergraaf, 1978].

Similar to an arterial section, the resulting lumped model of the vascular tree can be represented as an electrical circuit if desired (Fig. 158.4b), and nearby resistors and inductances can be combined to form Γ, T, or Π sections. A similar approach can be used for the venous circulation. To prevent ringing and other problems due to sudden impedance changes, it is often useful to add intermediate

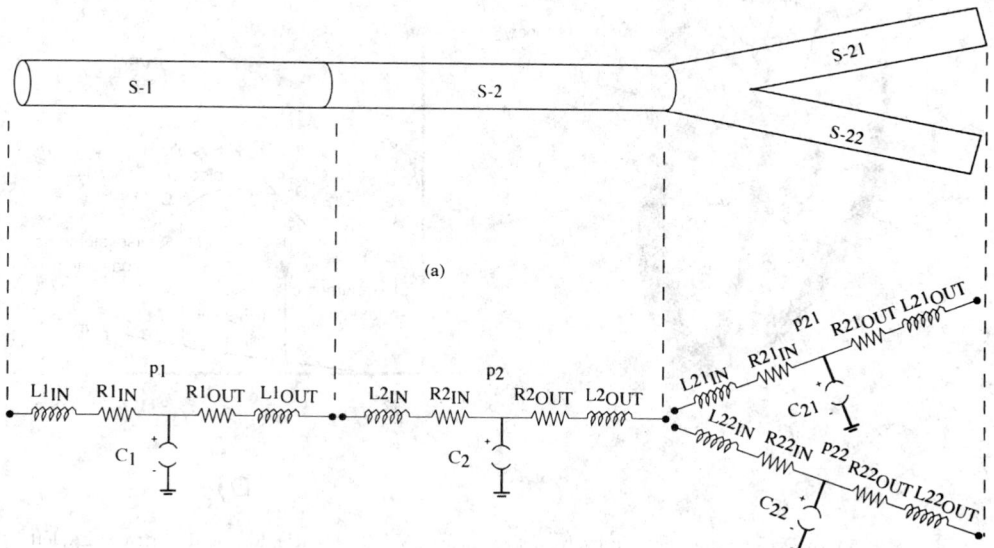

FIGURE 158.4   (*a*) A segmented, arbitrary length of vessel. (*b*) The equivalent RLC circuit.

segments to taper the impedances between the heart and the capillaries [Rideout, 1991]. That is, the impedances of the large arteries should be tapered to match the higher resistive impedances of the arterioles and capillary beds and then reduced back again from the capillary beds to the large veins.

Arterial and venous branching can be roughly grouped by vessel size (large, medium, and small arteries, arterioles, capillaries, etc.) or by organ system (heart, head, legs, liver, fat, skin, muscle, etc.). Vessel grouping is useful when the model needs to track drug concentrations at whole-body effector sites, such as nitroprusside concentration in the systemic arteriolar and venous compartments. Organ grouping is useful when the model needs to track drug concentrations in certain organs, such as insulin in the liver, glucose in the pancreas, or antineoplastic agents in diseased tissues. Note that within each organ, the flows can be broken down further by vessel size or by regional or conceptual intraorgan blood flows. Once the desired organs and vessels are described, Westkessel-type impedances can be used for the rest of the vasculature.

Models of the Heart

The heart is a muscular pump with four chambers intimately linked into one organ (Fig. 158.5*a*). Nevertheless, in modeling the heart, each chamber is usually modeled independently of the others. Each is typically set up as an elastic compartment with inertance and resistance similar to an artery or vein (see above). The differences are (1) that valves are included to constrain flow to one direction, and (2) that elastance (the inverse of compliance) is treated as a time-varying parameter.

The valves are straightforward and are often implemented as ideal diodes (for electrical circuit models) or as IF-THEN-ELSE statements (for algorithmic models) to keep all flows nonnegative. Defects in the valves can be added to simulate heart defects (e.g., leaky diodes for regurgitation). Other types of heart defects are just as easily simulated. For example, Blackstone and coworkers (1976) placed an impedance between the atrial chambers to simulate a septal opening.

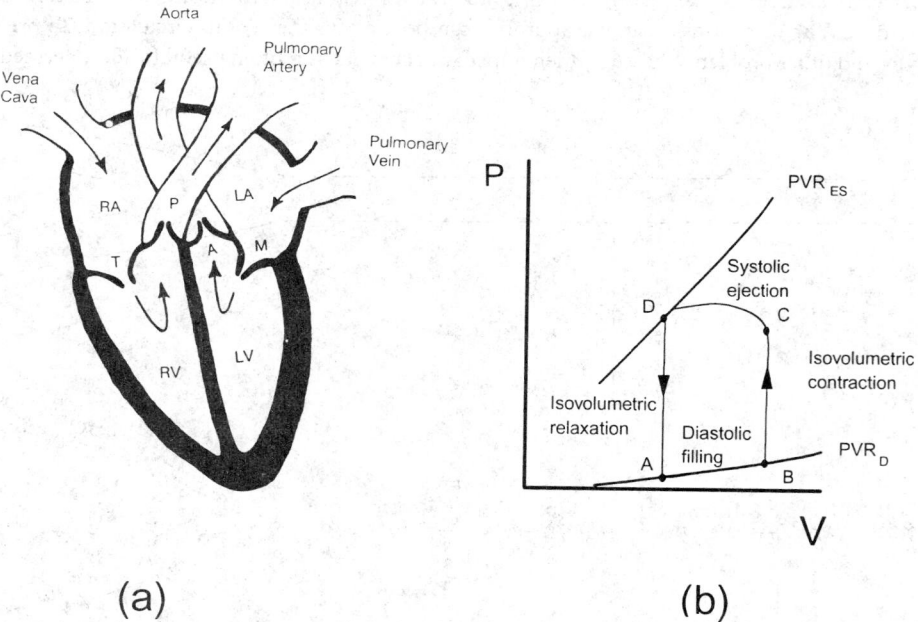

(a)   (b)

FIGURE 158.5   (*a*) The chambers and valves of the heart. LV, left ventricle; RV, right ventricle; LA, left atrium; RA, right atrium; M, mitral valve; A, aortic valve; T, tricuspid valve; P, pulmonary valve. (*b*) The left ventricular cardiac cycle in the *P-V* plane. See text.

Mathematical representation of the time-varying elastance is more complicated and is generally based on the characterization of the cardiac work cycle in the pressure-volume plane. In the *P-V* diagram in Fig. 158.5*b*, the time course of the left ventricular cardiac cycle proceeds as follows.

During diastolic filling (A to B), ventricular pressure is below atrial and aortic pressures, so the mitral valve (between the left atrium and the left ventricle) is open, and the aortic valve (between the left ventricle and the aorta) is closed. Blood therefore flows from the atrium into the ventricle, based on the pressure gradient and the inertances and resistances of the inlet. Note that the pressure gradient will decrease as the ventricle fills due to the passive compliance of the chamber and the drop in pressure in the atrium.

After diastole, the ventricle is stimulated to contract so that pressure rises above the atrial pressure, closing the mitral valve. In this state, pressure is too low for the aortic valve to open, so that both valves are closed and no blood flow occurs. Meanwhile, the ventricle continues to contract, raising ventricular pressure. This period (B to C) is termed isovolumetric contraction. Here, the muscle contraction can be thought of as decreasing the compliance of the chamber.

Once ventricular pressure exceeds the pressure in the aorta, the aortic valve opens and systolic ejection commences (C to D). Blood flows out from the ventricle into the aorta based on the pressure gradient, the inertances, and the resistances of the outlet. The muscle continues to contract until the cardiac action potentials have run their course.

As the muscle begins to relax, pressure will drop until it falls below the aortic pressure. At this time, the aortic valve closes, and again blood flow ceases. Meanwhile, the ventricle continues to relax, decreasing the ventricular pressure. This period (D to A) is termed isovolumetric relaxation. Here, muscle relaxation can be thought of as *increasing the compliance* of the chamber. Finally, ventricular pressure falls below atrial pressure, the mitral valve opens, and the cycle begins anew.

Suga and Sagawa [1972, 1974] identified and characterized several key properties of the time-varying compliance in the pressure-volume plane. In their experiments, they varied preload, afterload, stroke volume, cardiac contractility, and heart rate for both ejecting beats (heart valves patent) and isovolumic beats (heart valves sewn shut). Four observations should be noted. First, the *P-V* point at the end of systole (Fig. 158.6*a*, points D_1–D_4) nearly always lies along the static *P-V* curve for activated myocardium. Second, the end systolic *P-V* curve is unaffected by changes in preload and afterload (Fig. 158.6*a*); however, it is affected by changes in cardiac contractility (Fig. 158.6*b*). Third, t_{max}, the time to end systole (point D), is also unaffected by changes in preload and afterload; however, it is affected by changes in cardiac contractility and heart rate. And fourth, the ventricular filling phase follows the static *P-V* curve for relaxed myocardium, as expected. There are some

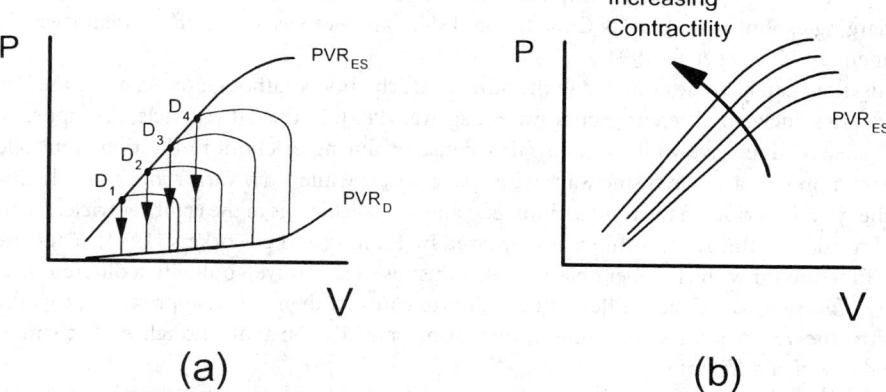

FIGURE 158.6 (*a*) Heart cycles with varying preload and afterload. (*b*) The end-systolic *P-V* curve with increasing contractility of the heart.

deviations from these observations, but over normal ranges these behaviors are fairly reliable [Maughan et al., 1984; Sunagawa & Sagawa, 1982].

Based on these observations, a continuum of static *P-V* relationships can be visualized as spanning the space between the fully relaxed and the fully contracted curves, say, as a linear combination of the two. The active curve at any time could then be construed as a function of the activity level of the myocardium, α, which itself could be a function of time and t_{max}, and which would range from zero (inactive) to one (fully active):

$$PVR(\alpha(t,t_{max})) = \alpha(t,t_{max}) \cdot PVR_{ES} + (1 - \alpha(t,t_{max})) \cdot PVR_D \qquad (158.5)$$

Here, *PVR (pressure-volume relationship)* is the active *P-V* curve, and PVR_{ES} and PVR_D are the end systolic and diastolic *P-V* curves, respectively. Using this approach, the PVR_{ES} curve would be parameterized in terms of the inotropic state of the myocardium, and t_{max} would be a function of inotropic state and heart rate.

Suga and Sagawa (1972) originally approximated the two curves, PVR_{ES} and PVR_D, with two straight lines that intersected in a common point on the volume axis (V_d, the unstressed, or dead, volume). This was a reasonable approximation, since, in their original experiments, the nonlinear portions of the *P-V* curves were not encountered. Based on this approach, the elastance *E* as a function of time becomes greatly simplified:

$$E(t) = \frac{P(t)}{V(t) - V_d} \qquad (158.6)$$

With this formulation, $\alpha(t,t_{max})$ maps to $E(t)$ by the relation

$$E(t) = \alpha(t,t_{max}) \cdot E_{max} + (1 - \alpha(t,t_{max})) \cdot E_{min} \qquad (158.7)$$

where E_{min} and E_{max} are the minimum and maximum elastances. E_{max} sets the inotropic state, and E_{min} sets the diastolic filling curve. A later modification allowed each curve to have its own dead volume [Sunagawa & Sagawa, 1982].

A common definition of $\alpha(t,t_{max})$ is a squared sine wave, time scaled and shifted to fit its first half-period into the systolic time interval, and zeroed elsewhere, e.g., see Martin and coworkers [1986]. Another common definition uses the first half-period of a sine wave, time-scaled and shifted to fit into the systolic interval. It is sometimes clipped and sometimes modified with a second harmonic to skew the waveform, e.g., see Rideout [1991]. Still others have approximated $\alpha(t,t_{max})$ as a square wave [Warner, 1959], a triangle wave [Katona et al., 1967; McLeod, 1966], a sum of charging and discharging exponentials [Sun & Chiaramida, 1992], and even as a sum of gaussian (bell-shaped) exponentials [Chung et al., 1994].

Pulsations can likewise be added to the other heart chambers, although the shape of the elastance curves are somewhat different [Sunagawa & Sagawa, 1982]. In the left ventricle, $E(t)$ appears more like a skewed sine wave while $V_d(t)$ is fairly constant during ejection; in the right ventricle, $E(t)$ appears more like a squared sine wave with a larger E_{max} while $V_d(t)$ varies continuously throughout the systolic period; in the right atrium, $E(t)$ and $V_d(t)$ behave as in the right ventricle. A common simplification of this relationship was employed by Leaning and coworkers [1983]. They used the same function for each chamber's elastance (in this case a sine wave), but with a different E_{min}, E_{max}, and t_{max} for each, as well as a different time shift to contract them when appropriate, e.g., the atria prior to the ventricles. As is common, they also made V_d constant, though each chamber was provided with a different value.

Since the activation function is typically time-scaled to fit within the heart period, the effect of a changing heart rate, say, due to neural reflexes, can be explored. However, this requires that the heart period itself be partitioned into diastolic and systolic intervals. Various partitioning schemes exist.

For the left ventricle, some fix the duration of systole [Grodins, 1959] or set it to a percentage of the heart period, with diastole taking up the rest of the period [Rideout, 1991]. A general clinical rule allocates one-third to systole and two-thirds to diastole. However, Beneken and DeWit [1967], after summarizing several publications, suggest that ventricular systole is better approximated by one-fifth the heart period plus 0.16 s. Likewise, they determined the duration of atrial systole as 9/100 the heart period plus 0.1 s. These formulae have gained considerable popularity, e.g., see Leaning and coworkers [1983] and Rideout [1991].

In many drug-delivery applications, the time constants of interest are on the order of minutes to hours. In these situations, a pulsatile heart is not needed and can be traded advantageously for a mean flow model. Mean flow models are based either on the Frank-Starling law of the heart or on the pulsatile model above. In the Frank-Starling approach, a family of flow curves is constructed based on experimental observations of the heart under various conditions of preload and afterload (Fig. 158.7) [Sagawa, 1967]. These are then used to calculate stroke volume for each beat. In the other approach, the stroke volume is derived analytically from the equations of the pulsatile heart [Rideout, 1991]. When using the Frank-Starling law, attenuation factors are used to impose the effects of inotropic state and heart rate. Examples of nonpulsatile heart models include those by Sagawa [1967], Greenway [1982], Möller and coworkers [1983], and Tham and coworkers [1990]. The Guyton-Coleman model [Guyton et al., 1972, 1980] is also nonpulsatile, though it uses a very different approach (see below).

Some models of the uptake and distribution of slow-acting drugs do not explicitly use a heart, or, for that matter, a circulation. These fall under the category of purely compartmental models. In these models, the heart and circulation are subsumed into an assumption that each compartment in the model is uniformly mixed (see Chapter 157).

Models of Combined Heart and Circulation

Whole-body CV models couple a model of the heart to models of the vasculature. The complexity of the coupling depends on the particular need and can give rise to nonpulsatile left side (*left side* meaning the systemic circulation) only, nonpulsatile left and right side (*right side* meaning the pulmonary circulation), and pulsatile left and right side models [Rideout, 1991].

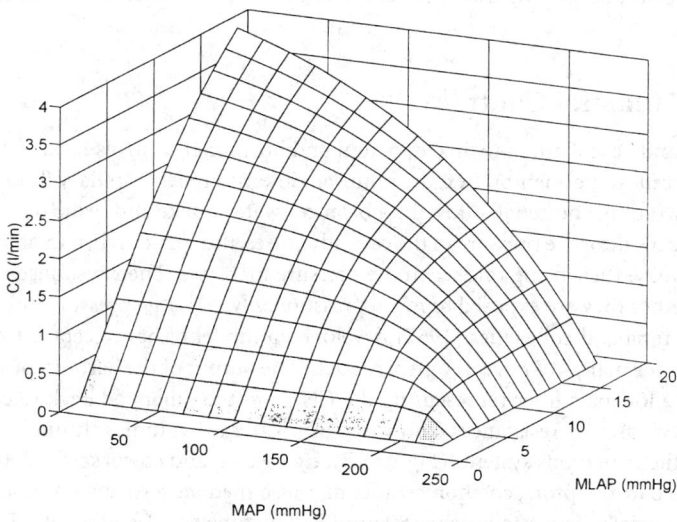

FIGURE 158.7 The Frank-Starling law of the heart: 3-D plot of Sagawa's [1967] left-ventricle equation for a 10-kg dog; CO, cardiac output; MAP, mean arterial pressure; MLAP, mean left atrial pressure.

Left-side-only models are justified when the pharmaceutical agents of interest have little effect on the pulmonary circulation. In these cases, the right side is considered a follower circuit and hence can be eliminated to provide computational savings. Even if the agents of interest do affect the pulmonary circulation, an occamistic left-side-only model may still suffice. This approach may work for two reasons: Either the model order is high enough that the right-side effects are inadvertently captured in the left-side model, or the drug effects are essentially the same on both sides. Keep in mind that these models have limited scope and hence should be used with care.

As an example of the modeling considerations for drug delivery, consider the following two drugs: propranolol, a beta blocker; and sodium nitroprusside (SNP), a vasodilator. Propranolol has a time constant on the order of 33 min, primarily affects the heart, and has only minor effects on the pulmonary circulation (although it may constrict the airways) [Ewy & Bressler, 1992; Gilman et al., 1993]. Hence, for propranolol, a nonpulsatile left-side-only model should be adequate for controller design. SNP, however, has a transport delay of 0.5 min and a time constant between 0.25 and 0.50 min. It affects the arterioles, the venous unstressed volume, and venous compliance. It also significantly decreases pulmonary wedge pressure [Ewy & Bressler, 1992; Gilman et al., 1993; Greenway, 1982]. Hence, for SNP, a nonpulsatile model is questionable, though it may be adequate. Furthermore, a two-sided model should be used, since SNP may have a significant effect on the pulmonary circulation. Greenway's [1982] two-sided nonpulsatile model seems to function adequately, although other investigators have switched to two-sided pulsatile models, e.g., see Yu et al., 1990.

Interestingly, Martin et al. (1986) may have finessed the field of nonpulsatile models by overcoming the speed limitations associated with pulsatile models. They did this by solving the pulsatile model equations semi-analytically, and were thus able to significantly reduce simulation time. Their model currently makes an attractive choice for studying and designing automated drug-delivery systems.

Despite the emphasis here on nonlinear CV-based modeling, probably the most used model for the design of blood pressure controllers is the model by Slate and Sheppard [1982]. It is based on a linear, first-order impulse response of the effects of nitroprusside on mean arterial blood pressure. The model includes a recirculation effect, as well as an occasionally observed nonlinear reflex (possibly due to the chemoreceptors). It has gained wide acceptance probably because of its simplicity. Nevertheless, it has severe limitations: It lumps the effects of the primary neural and humoral reflexes as well as the patient drug sensitivity into one gain; it does not account for the effect of changing cardiac output on drug transport; and it is not easily extended to include additional drugs or disease states.

Neural and Humoral Control

Once the heart and vasculature are linked, neural and hormonal controls need to be added. These include the baroreflex, the chemoreflex, the renin-angiotensin reflex, capillary fluid shift, autoregulation, stress relaxation, and renal–body-fluid balance (water intake and urine output).

Baroreceptors monitor the pressure in the carotid sinuses, the aortic arch, and other large systemic arteries and increase their firing rate when the pressure increases. Their response is nonlinear and depends on whether they are exposed to mean pressure only, pulsatile pressure only, or a combination of both. Katona and colleagues [1967] developed a model of baroreceptor feedback that has become the basis for many CV neural control models. The output of the baroreceptor model is often passed through a low pass filter representing the CNS and then mapped back to changes in heart rate, contractility, vascular resistances, and vascular unstressed volumes through the sympathetic and parasympathetic nervous systems (Fig. 158.8), e.g., see Yu and coworkers [1990].

In addition to baroreceptors, chemoreceptors may also mediate a strong CV response, especially when systemic arterial pressure falls below 80 mmHg [Guyton et al., 1972; see also Dampney, 1994]. This reflex, through the CNS, increases cardiac activity and peripheral resistance. Strangely, few models include this effect, although Slate and Sheppard [1982] may have inadvertently included it in their simplified black box model.

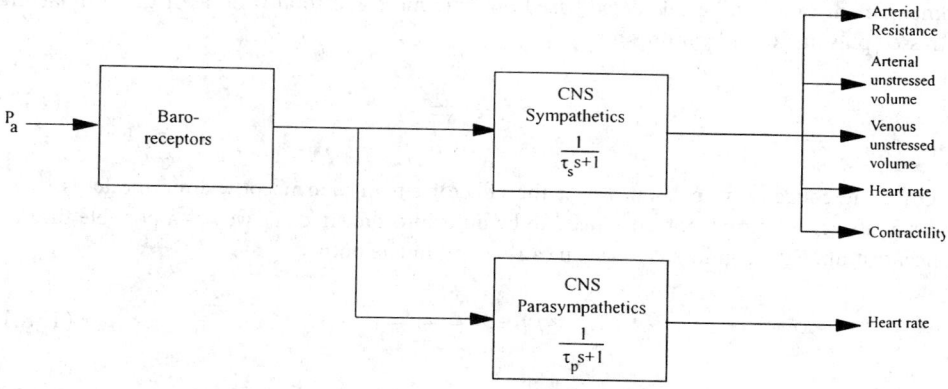

FIGURE 158.8 Baroreceptor firing rate is passed through a low-pass filter representing the CNS and then mapped back to changes in heart rate, contractility, vascular resistances, and vascular unstressed volumes.

The renin-angiotensin reflex is mediated hormonally through the kidneys. When pressure falls below normal, renin is secreted into the blood stream by the kidneys, which then causes the release of free angiotensin. Angiotensin causes marked vasoconstriction and thus increases peripheral resistance and arterial pressure. This reflex is often included in models because it plays an important role in many forms of hypertension and heart failure.

The other CV control reflexes are only sometimes included, although these and others are elucidated and modeled by Guyton and his coworkers [1972, 1980]. In his elaborate model, there are five main empirically derived physiologic function blocks with many subcomponents. The model has nearly 400 parameters and is quite remarkable in its scope. Given current computer technology, however, it is somewhat cumbersome for drug delivery applications, although it promises to have great utility in the future.

Combined CV and Pharmacologic Models

For pharmacologic control studies, CV models readily lend themselves to the calculation of drug uptake and distribution to the various parts of the body (pharmacokinetics). Once the transport model has been built, models of drug action (pharmacodynamics) then need to be linked and related back to the CV model. Other models must also be linked if necessary. For example, models of inhalational anesthetic uptake, distribution, and effect on the respiratory and CV systems require not only a CV and pharmacologic model but also a lung model. Combined models such as these are known as multiple models, a term coined by Rideout's group [Beneken & Rideout, 1968; Rideout, 1991]. Again, the time course of the agents and their effects on the heart and circulation determine whether a pulsatile or nonpulsatile model is needed, as well as the requisite level of vascular detail.

To calculate drug uptake and transport, mass balance equations can be set up for each segment and compartment in the CV model. Additional compartments, such as a tissue or an effects compartment, can also be added (see Chapter 157). For example, given a particular compartment (or segment), the mass of drug in the compartment is calculated as follows:

$$\frac{dq_i}{dt} = f_{in,i}\, c_{i-1} - f_{out,i}\, c_i \qquad (158.8)$$

where i identifies the compartment, q is the mass of drug, c is its concentration, f_{in} is the rate of blood flow into the compartment (normally equal to the flow out of the previous compartment), and f_{out} is the rate of blood flow out of the compartment. The instantaneous concentration in any compartment can then be calculated based on drug mass and total volume of the compartment (stressed plus unstressed volumes):

$$c_i = \frac{q_i}{V_i} \tag{158.9}$$

Once the concentration is known at the effector site, a pharmacodynamic model is used to describe its action. Saturation may need to be built into the effect, as well as a possible threshold concentration. Hill's sigmoidal equation can accommodate both:

$$EFF = \frac{c_e^n}{c_{50}^n + c_e^n} \tag{158.10}$$

where EFF is the normalized pharmacologic effect ($0 \le EFF \le 1$), c_e is the concentration at the effector site, c_{50} is the half-max concentration, and n parameterizes the steepness of the sigmoid. Hill's equation becomes the Michaelis-Menten equation when $n = 1$.

Once calculated, the drug effect can be used to modify parameters in the CV model, much like the neural and humoral reflexes. Resistances, compliances (including the unstressed volumes) of each segment, neural and humoral feedback gains, heart rate, and contractility are all typically modified by drugs. For example, sodium nitroprusside causes vasodilation and blood pooling; therefore it would be made to primarily increase the compliance and unstressed volume of the veins, as well as to decrease arteriolar (peripheral) resistance [Greenway, 1982; Yu et al., 1990].

158.4 Conclusions

For designing controllers to automate cardiovascular therapeutics, the nonlinear, cardiovascular-linked pharmacologic models are well worth the added effort and time needed to construct and interface them to the design platform. Not only can they help prove initial feasibility, but they can also speed up the overall design process. For example, they can be used for interactive controller design; they can be used to design improved animal and human experiments, which can potentially reduce the total number of experiments; and they can be used to simulate human conditions that are not easily produced in animals.

The reduced compartmental and combined segmental and transmission line models are probably the most practical model form at this time given current computer technology. However, as computer technology grows, we can expect to see increasingly detailed pharmacologic models that include additional cardiovascular features such as pulse wave propagation and reflection as well as multiple short- and long-term neurohumoral feedback loops.

Acknowledgments

The author is indebted to Mr. F. Casas and Mr. S. Kumar for help in collecting the references; to Mr. F. Casas and Ms. O. Huynh for help in preparing the figures; and to Dr. S. E. Rittgers for his comments on the text.

References

Acierno LJ. 1994. The History of Cardiology, Pearl River, NY, Parthenon.

Aperia A. 1940. Hemodynamical studies. Scand Arch Physiol Suppl 83:1.

Beneken JEW. 1963. Investigation on the regulatory system of the blood circulation. In A Noordergraaf, GN Jager, N Westerhof (eds), Circulatory Analog Computers, pp 16–28, Amsterdam, North-Holland.

Beneken JEW. 1972. Some computer models in cardiovascular research. In DH Bergel (ed), Cardiovascular Fluid Dynamics, vol 1, pp 173–223, New York, Academic Press.

Beneken JEW, DeWit B. 1967. A physical approach to hemodynamic aspects of the human cardiovascular system. In EB Reeve, AC Guyton (eds), Physical Bases of Circulatory Transport, pp 1–45, Philadelphia, W.B. Saunders.

Beneken JEW, Rideout VC. 1968. The use of multiple models in cardiovascular system studies: Transport and perturbation methods. IEEE Trans BME 15(4):281.

Blackstone EH, Gupta AK, Rideout VC. 1976. Cardiovascular simulation study of infants with transposition of the great arteries after surgical correction. In L Dekker (ed), Simulation of Systems, pp 599–608, Amsterdam, North-Holland.

Carson ER, Cobelli C, Finkelstein L. 1983. The Mathematical Modeling of Metabolic and Endocrine Systems, New York, John Wiley & Sons.

Chung DC, et al. 1994. A mathematical model of the canine circulation. In BW Patterson (ed), Modeling and Control in Biomedical Systems: Proceedings of the IFAC Symposium, pp 109–112, Galveston, Tex,

Dampney RAL. 1994. Functional organization of central pathways regulating the cardiovascular system. Physiol Rev 74(2):323.

Dick DE, Rideout VC. 1965. Analog simulation of left heart and arterial dynamics. Proc 18th ACEMB, p 78, Philadelphia.

Ewy GA, Bressler R. 1992. Cardiovascular Drugs and the Management of Heart Disease, 2d ed, New York, Raven Press.

Frank O. 1899. Die Grundform des arteriellen Pulses. Z Biol 37:483.

Fung YC. 1984. Biodynamics: Circulation, New York, Springer-Verlag.

Geppert L. 1994. Faults & failures. IEEE Spectrum 31(8):17.

Gilman AG, Rall TW, Nies AS, et al. 1993. Goodman and Gilman's The Pharmacological Basis of Therapeutics, 8th ed, New York, McGraw-Hill.

Greenway CV. 1982. Mechanisms and quantitative assessment of drug effects on cardiac output with a new model of the circulation. Pharm Rev 33(4):213.

Grodins FS. 1959. Integrative cardiovascular physiology: a mathematical synthesis of cardiac and blood vessel hemodynamics. Q Rev Biol 34:93.

Gustafsson K. 1993. Stepsize selection in implicit Runge-Kutta methods viewed as a control problem. Proc. 12th IFAC World Cong 5:137.

Guyton AC. 1980. Arterial Pressure and Hypertension, Philadelphia, W.B. Saunders.

Guyton AC, Coleman TG, Cowley AW, et al. 1972. Systems analysis of arterial pressure regulation and hypertension. Ann Biomed Eng 1:254.

Hales S. 1733. Statical Essays: Containing Haemastaticks, vol 2, London, Innys and Manby (Pfizer Laboratories, 1981).

Isaka S, Sebald AV. 1993. Control strategies for arterial blood pressure regulation. IEEE Trans BME. 40(4):353–363.

Katona PG. 1988. Closed loop control of physiological variables. Proc 1st IFAC Symp Modelling Control Biomed Sys, Venice.

Katona PG, Barnett GO, Jackson WD. 1967. Computer simulation of the blood pressure control of the heart period. In P. Kezdi (ed), Baroreceptors and Hypertension, pp 191–199, Oxford, Pergamon Press.

Kono A, Maughan WL, Sunagawa K, et al. 1984. The use of left ventricular end-ejection pressure and peak pressure in the estimation of the end-systolic pressure-volume relationship. Circulation 70(6):1057.

Leaning MS, Pullen HE, Carson ER, et al. 1983. Modelling a complex biological system: the human cardiovascular system—1. Methodology and model description. Trans Inst Meas Contr 5(2):71.

Li JK-J. 1987. Arterial System Dynamics, New York, New York University Press.

Linkens DA, Hacisalihzade SS. 1990. Computer control systems and pharmacological drug administration: A survey. J Med Eng Tech 14(2):41.

Martin JF, Schneider AM, Mandel JE, et al. 1986. A new cardiovascular model for real-time applications. Trans Soc Comp Sim 3(1):31.

Maughan WL, Sunagawa K, Burkhoff D, et al. 1984. Effect of arterial impedance changes on the end-systolic pressure-volume relation. Circ Res 54(5):595.

McDonald DA. 1974. Blood Flow in Arteries, 2d ed, Baltimore, Williams & Wilkins.

McLeod J. 1966. PHYSBE ... a physiological simulation benchmark experiment. Simulation 7(6):324.

Melchior FM, Srinivasan RS, Charles JB. 1992. Mathematical modeling of human cardiovascular system for simulation of orthostatic response. Am J Physiol 262 (Heart Circ Physiol 31):H1920.

Middleman S. 1972. Transport Phenomena in the Cardiovascular System, New York, John Wiley & Sons.

Milnor WR. 1989. Hemodynamics, 2d ed, Baltimore, Williams & Wilkins.

Möller D, Popović D, Thiele G. 1983. Modeling, Simulation and Parameter-Estimation of the Human Cardiovascular System, Friedr, Braunschweig, Vieweg & Sohn.

Noordergraaf A. 1978. Circulatory System Dynamics, New York, Academic Press.

O'Rourke MF. 1982. Arterial Function in Health and Disease. New York, Churchill Livingstone.

O'Rourke, MF. 1993. Hypertension and the conduit and cushioning functions of the arterial tree. In ME Safar, MF O'Rourke (eds), The Arterial System in Hypertension, pp 27–37, the Netherlands, Kluwer Academic Pub.

Purmutt S, Bromberger-Barnea B, Bane HN. 1962. Alveolar pressure, pulmonary venous pressure, and the vascular waterfall. Med Thorac 19:239.

Rideout VC. 1991. Mathematical and Computer Modeling of Physiological Systems, Englewood Cliffs, NJ, Prentice-Hall (now distributed by Medical Physics Pub., Madison, WI).

Sagawa, K. 1967. Analysis of the ventricular pumping capacity as a function of input and output pressure loads. In EB Reeve, A.C. Guyton (eds), Physical Bases of Circulatory Transport, pp 141–149, Philadelphia, W.B. Saunders.

Sagawa K. 1973. Comparative models of overall circulatory mechanics. In JHU Brown, JF Dickson III (eds), Advances in Biomedical Engineering, vol 3, pp 1–95, New York, Academic Press.

Slate JB, Sheppard LC. 1982. Automatic control of blood pressure by drug infusion. IEE Proc., Pt. A 129(9):639.

Snyder MF, Rideout VC. 1969. Computer simulation studies of the venous circulation. IEEE Trans BME 16(4):325.

Suga H, Sagawa K. 1972. Mathematical interrelationship between instantaneous ventricular pressure-volume ratio and myocardial force-velocity relation. Ann Biomed Eng 1:160.

Suga H, Sagawa K. 1974. Instantaneous pressure volume relationships and their ratio in the excised, supported canine left ventricle. Circ Res 35:117.

Sun Y, Chiaramida S. 1992. Simulation of hemodynamics and regulatory mechanisms in the cardiovascular system based on a nonlinear and time-varying model. Simulation 59(1):28.

Sunagawa K, Sagawa K. 1982. Models of ventricular contraction based on time-varying elastance. Crit Rev Biomed Eng 9:193.

Tham RQY, Sasse FJ, Rideout VC. 1990. Large-scale multiple model for the simulation of anesthesia. In DPF Moller (ed), Advanced Simulation in Biomedicine, pp 173–195, New York, Springer Verlag.

Tsitlik JE, Halperin HR, Popel AS, et al. 1992. Modeling the circulation with three-terminal electrical networks containing special nonlinear capacitors. Ann Biomed Eng 20:595.

Westenskow DR. 1986. Automating patient care with closed-loop control. MD Comput 3(2):14.

Westerhof N, Noordergraaf A. 1969. Reduced models of the systemic arteries. Proc 8th Int Conf Med Eng, Chicago.

Yu C, Roy RJ, Kaufman H. 1990. A circulatory model for combined nitroprusside-dopamine therapy in acute heart failure. Med Prog Tech 16:77.

Further Information

The text by Rideout [1991] has a particularly good tutorial on cardiovascular modeling and even includes ACSL source code. McDonald's [1974] and Noordergraaf's [1978] texts are classics, thoroughly reviewing cardiovascular physiology and the physical principles useful in modeling it. More recent texts on the cardiovascular system with a bioengineering slant include those by Milnor [1989], Li [1987], and Fung [1984]. Also, Guyton's 1980 text provides a detailed review of his model and its application for the analysis of hypertension and is well worth reading. Along this same line, Safar and O'Rourke's [1993] text, as well as O'Rourke's earlier work [1982], are also worth reading and provide many insights into hypertension and cardiovascular modeling. Melchior, Srinivasan, and Charles [1992] also present an overview of cardiovascular modeling, though with an emphasis on orthostatic response.

For historical interest, *The History of Cardiology* by Acierno [1994] provides fascinating reading, going back beyond even the early Greeks. In more recent history, a review of early CV models (early 1900s up to 1940) can be found in Aperia's monograph [1940], and a review of the post–World War II era models (late 1950s to early 1970s) that set the tone for almost all modern CV models can be found in Sagawa [1973].

For those interested in pharmacologic modeling, along with examples using the CV system, Carson, Cobelli, and Finkelstein's 1983 text is a good source. Middleman's 1972 text specifically targets transport in the CV system, but it is somewhat dated. The current understanding of the anatomic and functional organization of the neurohumoral regulation pathways can be found in Dampney [1994].

For a survey of blood pressure controllers, the reader is referred to the recent article by Isaka and Sebald [1993]. Linkens and Hacisalihzade [1990], Katona [1988], and Westenskow [1986] also survey blood pressure controllers as well as other CV control applications.

159

Respiratory Models and Control

Chi-Sang Poon
Harvard University/
Massachusetts Institute
of Technology

The respiratory system is a complex neurodynamical system. It exhibits many interesting characteristics that are akin to other physiologic control systems. However, the respiratory system is much more amenable to modeling analysis than many other systems for two reasons. First, the respiratory system is dedicated to a highly specific physiologic function, namely, the exchange of O_2 and CO_2 through the motor act of breathing. This physiologic function is readily distinguishable from extraneous disturbances arising from behavioral and other functions of the respiratory muscles. Second, the respiratory control system is structurally well organized, with well-defined afferent and efferent neural pathways, peripheral controlled processes, and a central controller. The functional and structural specificity of the respiratory system—and the diverse neurodynamic behaviors it represents—make it an ideal model system to illustrate the basic principles of physiologic control systems in general.

Like any closed-loop system, the behavior of the respiratory control system is defined by the continual interaction of the controller and the peripheral processes being controlled. The latter include the respiratory mechanical system and the pulmonary gas exchange process. These peripheral processes have been extensively studied, and their quantitative relationships have been described in detail in previous reviews. Less well understood is the behavior of the respiratory controller and the way in which it processes afferent inputs. A confounding factor is that the controller may manifest itself in many different ways, depending on the modeling and experimental approaches being taken. Traditionally, the respiratory control system has been modeled as a closed-loop *feedback/feedforward regulator* whereby homeostasis of arterial blood gas and pH is maintained. Alternatively, the respiratory controller may be viewed as a *central pattern generator* in which rhythmic respiratory activity is produced in response to phasic afferent feedback. Finally, there is increasing evidence that the respiratory controller may function as an *adaptive self-tuning regulator* which optimizes breathing pattern and ventilation according to certain performance measure.

0-8493-8346-3/95/$0.00+$.50
© 1995 by CRC Press, Inc.

Each modeling approach reveals a separate "law" of a multifaceted controller. However, these control laws must be somehow related to one another because they are governed by the same neural network that forms the respiratory controller. It is therefore instructive to examine not only how the various models work but also how they might be fit together to encompass the myriad of response behaviors of the respiratory control system.

159.1 Structure of the Respiratory Control System

The respiratory control system is a nonlinear, multioutput, delayed-feedback dynamic system which is constantly being perturbed by unknown physiologic and pathologic disturbances (Fig. 159.1). Rhythmic respiratory activity is produced by a respiratory central pattern generator (RCPG) which consists of a network of neuronal clusters in the medulla oblongata and pons areas of the brain stem. The RCPG forms the kernel of the respiratory controller. The control problem is defined by the characteristics of the controlled processes (plants) and the control objective.

Chemical Plant

Pulmonary Gas Exchange

The chemical plant is propelled by the ventilation of the lung, $\dot{V}_E$, which determines the alveolar PCO_2 and PO_2 according to the following mass-balance equations:

$$V_LCO_2 \cdot \frac{d}{dt} P_ACO_2 = \dot{V}_E\left(1 - \frac{V_D}{V_T}\right)(P_ICO_2 - P_ACO_2) + 863\, \dot{V}CO_2 \quad (159.1)$$

$$V_LO_2 \cdot \frac{d}{dt} P_AO_2 = \dot{V}_E\left(1 - \frac{V_D}{V_T}\right)(P_IO_2 - P_AO_2) - 863\, \dot{V}O_2 \quad (159.2)$$

The input-output relationships of the chemical plant are subject to several endogenous and exogenous disturbances. For example, increases in the metabolic production of CO_2 during muscular

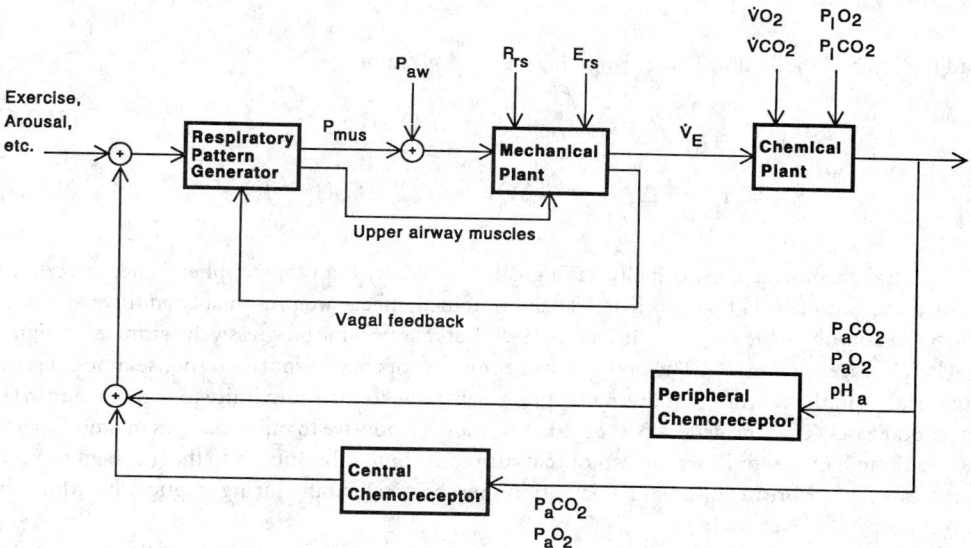

FIGURE 159.1   Block diagram of the respiratory control system.

exercise, PCO_2 in the inspired air, and respiratory dead space during rebreathing all contribute to an increase in CO_2 load to the lung. The added CO_2 is eliminated by an increase in pulmonary ventilation, but the effectiveness of the control action in restoring P_ACO_2 varies considerably with the type of disturbance. The input-output sensitivity $S_{pco2} \equiv \delta P_A CO_2 / \delta \dot{V}_E$ of the plant is highest with metabolic CO_2 load and lowest with inhaled CO_2 load, whereas the plant dynamics is slowest with dead space load.

In pulmonary disease the efficiency of the plant in removing CO_2 is further decreased because of pulmonary ventilation/perfusion maldistribution [Poon, 1987a]. Another source of disturbance is metabolic acidosis and alkalosis which alter arterial blood gas tensions and pH through acid-base buffering in blood. All these disturbances interact nonlinearly with the plant and are not directly sensed. How does the controller cope with such variety of disturbances effectively if its only means is to alter $\dot{V}_E$? Not surprisingly, the controller responds quite differently to the various forms of CO_2 disturbance and their combinations [Juratsch et al., 1982; Oren et al., 1981; Poon & Greene, 1985; Poon, 1989a, 1989b, 1992b; Sidney & Poon, 1991].

Chemosensory Feedback

The peripheral (arterial) chemoreceptors response to changes in P_aCO_2 may be modeled by linear first-order dynamics [Bellville et al., 1979]

$$\tau_p \cdot \frac{d}{dt} A_p = -A_p + G_p[P_aCO_2(t - T_p) - I_p] \qquad (159.3)$$

where τ_p, G_p, I_p, are the time constant, gain, threshold of the peripheral chemoreceptor and T_p is the lung-to-chemoreceptor transit delay of blood flow. Similarly, the central (intracranial) chemoreceptor is responsive to brain tissue PCO_2

$$A_c = G_c\{P_bCO_2 - I_c\} \qquad (159.4)$$

where the brain tissue PCO_2 is given by

$$V_bCO_2 \cdot \frac{d}{dt} P_bCO_2 = \dot{Q}_b\{P_aCO_2(t - T_c) - P_bCO_2\} + \frac{\dot{M}_bCO_2}{KCO_2} \qquad (159.5)$$

and the cerebral blood flow [Vis & Folgering, 1980] is given by

$$\dot{Q}_b(t) = \dot{Q}_0 + \Delta \dot{Q}_b(t) \qquad (159.6)$$

$$\tau_b \cdot \frac{d}{dt} \Delta \dot{Q}_b = -\Delta\dot{Q}_b + G_b \cdot P_aCO_2(t - T_c) \qquad (159.7)$$

The central chemoreceptor normally has a greater sensitivity than the peripheral chemoreceptors (which may be silenced by hyperoxia). Their combined effects are presumably additive at low to moderate stimulation levels [Heeringa et al., 1979] but may become progressively saturated at higher levels [Eldridge et al., 1981]. The peripheral chemoreceptors have a shorter response time constant and delay than the central chemoreceptor, presumably due to their proximity to the lung and arterial blood gases. They are generally thought to be more responsive to rapid changes in blood chemistry, although the central chemoreceptor may also contribute substantially to the transient respiratory response to breath-to-breath fluctuations in chemical input during eupneic breathing in wakefulness [Bruce et al., 1992].

The dynamic response of the peripheral chemoreceptors to P_aO_2 may be modeled in a similar fashion but the steady-state response is hyperbolic [Cunningham et al., 1986]. Furthermore, hypoxia and hypercapnia have a multiplicative effect on carotid chemoreceptor discharge [Fitzgerald & Lahiri, 1986], although the effect of changes in pH is presumably additive [Cunningham et al., 1986]. Prolonged hypoxia has a depressant effect on central respiratory neurons [Neubauer et al., 1990] which may offset the stimulatory effect of peripheral chemosensitivity.

Inputs from the peripheral chemoreceptors are temporally gated throughout the respiratory cycle. Stimuli are effective only if they are delivered during the second half of the inspiratory or expiratory cycle [Eldridge & Millhorn, 1986; Hildebrandt, 1977; Teppema et al., 1985]. The effect of such stimuli on medullary respiratory neurons is excitatory during the inspiratory phase and inhibitory during the expiratory phase [Lipski & Voss, 1990]. The gating effect may be modeled by a gated time function

$$A_{cpg} = gate\{A_p(t)\} \qquad (159.8)$$

where gate $\{\cdot\}$ is a windowing function which reflects the phasic activity of peripheral chemoreceptor inputs.

The intrinsic transient delay and nonlinearity in the transduction of chemical signals are undesirable from an automatic control perspective. However, the nonlinear behavior may represent neural preprocessing in the sensory nervous system. Such transformations in the feedback path may have important bearing on the controller's ability to achieve the control objective.

Mechanical Plant

Respiratory Mechanics

Pulmonary ventilation results from tidal expansion and relaxation of the lung. The equation of motion is:

$$R_{rs} \cdot \frac{dV}{dt} = -E_{rs} \cdot V + P_{aw}(t) - P_{mus}(t) \qquad (159.9)$$

Both R_{rs} and E_{rs} may be nonlinear. The mechanical load of the respiratory muscles is increased by airway constriction or lung restriction in pulmonary disease, or by the imposition of external resistance and elastance which cause a back pressure P_{aw} at the airway opening. Increases in ventilatory load may elicit a compensatory response in P_{mus} so that $\dot{V}_E$ is largely restored [Poon 1987b, 1989a, 1989b] except under severe ventilatory loading. Reverse compensatory responses are observed during ventilatory unloading [Poon et al., 1987a,b; Ward et al., 1982].

Respiratory Muscles

The mechanical plant is propelled by the respiratory muscles which serve as a mechanical pump. Normally, P_{mus} is sustained by the inspiratory muscles (principally the diaphragm and, to a lesser extent, the external intercostal and parasternal muscles). During hyperpnea or with increased expiratory load the expiratory muscles may be recruited [Marroquin, 1991], as are accessory muscles which may contribute significantly to the generation of P_{mus} in paraplegics.

Paradoxically, the respiratory muscles may also act to reduce ventilation. During quiet breathing some postinspiratory inspiratory activity may persist during the early expiratory phase, retarding lung emptying [Poon et al., 1987b]. In disease states inspiratory activity may also be recruited during the expiratory phase to prevent lung collapse [Stark et al., 1987] or overinflation [Poon & Kolandaivelu, 1994]. The upper airways abductor muscles may be activated by the controller or higher brain centers to increase R_{rs} in disease states [Stark et al., 1987] or in sleep [Phillipson & Bowes, 1986]. In awake states, respiration may be interrupted by behavioral, emotional, or defensive activities which compete for the respiratory apparatus under cortical or somatic sensory commands.

The mechanical efficiency of the respiratory muscles is limited by the force-velocity and force-length relationships which may be modeled as linear "active" resistance and elastance, respectively

[Milic-Emili & Zin, 1986]. Neuromechanical efficiency may be impaired in respiratory muscle fatigue or muscle weakness, resulting in diminished P_{mus} for any given neural drive.

Thus the respiratory pump is equipped with various types of actuators to regulate $\dot{V}_E$ in the face of many exogenous and endogenous mechanical disturbances. Such disturbances are detected by mechanoafferents originating in the lungs, thorax, and airways.

Mechanosensory Feedback

Among the various types of mechanoafferents, vagal slowly adapting pulmonary stretch receptors (SAR) input exerts the greatest influence on respiration by inhibiting inspiratory activity and facilitating expiratory activity (Hering-Breuer reflex). Vagal SAR volume feedback is crucial for the compensatory response of the RCPG to mechanical disturbances.

The SAR characteristic is linear at low lung volumes but may exhibit saturation nonlinearity at elevated volumes. Also, at any given lung volume SAR discharge increases with increasing rate of lung inflation [Pack et al., 1986]. To a first approximation vagal volume feedback may be modeled by

$$vag(t) = sat\{a_0 + a_1 V(t) + a_2 \dot{V}(t)\} \tag{159.10}$$

where $sat\{\cdot\}$ is a saturation function; a_0 denotes tonic vagal activity [Phillipson, 1974]; and a_1, a_2 are sensitivity parameters.

Control Objective

It is generally assumed that the prime function of respiration is to meet the metabolic demand by the exchange of O_2 and CO_2. The control problem is to accomplish this objective within some prescribed tolerance, subject to the physical as well as environmental constraints of the respiratory apparatus. Various models of the controller have been proposed as possible solutions to the control problem [Petersen, 1981], each representing a separate control strategy and degree of modeling abstraction. In what follows we provide a synopsis of the various modeling approaches and their physiologic significance.

159.2 Chemoreflex Models

The simplest controller model is a proportional controller [Cunningham et al., 1986; Grodins & Yamashiro, 1978]. In this approach attention is focused on the control of the chemical plant; the RCPG and the mechanical plant are lumped together to form a constant-gain controller. The control signal is taken to be $\dot{V}_E$, and the effects of the breathing pattern and vagal feedback are often neglected. Thus the controller is assumed to be a fixed relay station that regulates $\dot{V}_E$ via the chemoreflex loop. These simplifications allow quantitative closed-loop analyses of the chemoreflex system.

Feedback Control

In the chemoreflex model the respiratory control system acts like a chemostat. This is consistent with the well-known experimental observation that ventilation increases with increasing chemical stimulation. The steady-state ventilatory response to CO_2 inhalation is given by:

$$\dot{V}_E = \alpha(PaCO_2 - \beta) \tag{159.11}$$

This empirical relationship is in agreement with the chemoreflex model which assumes that ventilatory output is proportional to the sum of chemosensory feedback:

$$\dot{V}_E = G_0(A_c + A_p) \tag{159.12}$$

Equation (159.11) follows from the steady-state solutions to the model Eqs. (159.3)–(159.7) and (159.12), provided that the effect of changes in cerebral blood flow may be neglected. The effects of hypoxia and hypoxic-hypercapnic interaction may be modeled in a similar fashion by a hyperbolic relation [Cunningham et al., 1986].

A comprehensive model of the dynamical chemoreflex system is due to the classic work of Grodins and coworkers [1967]. The dynamical response to CO_2 is given by the transient solutions of the system equations, Eqs. (159.3)–(159.7) and (159.12). Under closed-loop conditions system dynamics is also influenced by the nonlinear dynamical response of the chemical plant, Eq. (159.1), as well as CO_2 uptake in body tissues. Therefore, measurement of the CO_2 response curve, Eq. (159.8), is often a slow and tedious procedure. Open-loop conditions may be achieved by dynamic forcing of end-tidal PCO_2 with servo-control of P_ICO_2 which obviates the nonlinearity and slow equilibration of the lung and other body tissue stores. This technique has been used to experimentally estimate the model parameters in normal and peripheral-chemoreceptor denervated subjects by means of system identification techniques [Bellville et al., 1979]. Another open-loop technique is the CO_2 rebreathing procedure [Read, 1967] which causes a metabolically induced ramp increase in P_aCO_2 and, hence, a similar increase in $\dot{V}_E$ by way of chemoreflex. The rebreathing technique is much simpler to use than dynamic end-tidal PCO_2 forcing and is therefore suitable for clinical applications. However, this technique may not accurately determine the steady-state CO_2 response, presumably because of the variability in cerebral blood flow induced by changing P_aCO_2. More reliable techniques using pulse-step [Poon & Olson, 1985] or step-ramp [Dahan 1990] P_ICO_2 forcings have been proposed for rapid determination of the steady-state CO_2 response with minimal experimental requirements.

Stability of the chemoreflex model may be studied by linearization of the system about some nominal state. Instability may occur if the loop gain and phase shift exceed unity and 180°, respectively. This may explain the periodic breathing phenomena found in hypoxia or high altitude where peripheral chemoreceptor gain is increased and congestive heart failure in which transit delay is prolonged [Khoo et al., 1982]. However, chemical instability alone does not account for the periodic episodes in obstructive sleep apnea which may also be influenced by fluctuations in arousal state [Khoo et al., 1991].

Feedforward Control

The chemoreflex model provides a satisfactory explanation for the chemical regulation of ventilation as well as respiratory instability. However, it fails to explain a fundamental aspect of ventilatory control experienced by everyone in everyday life: the increase in ventilation during muscular exercise. Typically, $\dot{V}_E$ increases in direct proportion to the metabolic demand ($\dot{V}CO_2$, $\dot{V}O_2$) such that the outputs of the chemical plant, Eqs. (159.1) and (159.2), are well regulated at constant levels from rest to exercise. As a result, homeostasis of arterial blood chemistry is closely maintained over a wide range of work rates. The dilemma is: If increases in metabolic rate are not accompanied by corresponding increases in chemical feedback, then what causes exercise hyperpnea?

One possible explanation of exercise hyperpnea is the so-called set-point hypothesis [Defares, 1964; Oren et al., 1981] which stipulates that P_aCO_2 and P_aO_2 are regulated at constant levels by the chemoreflex controller. However, a set point is not evident during hypercapnic and hypoxic challenges where the homeostasis of P_aCO_2 and P_aO_2 is readily abolished. Furthermore, to establish a set point the controller gain must be exceedingly high, but this is not found experimentally in the hypercapnic and hypoxic ventilatory sensitivities. Finally, from a control systems perspective a high gain controller is undesirable because it could drive the system into saturation or instability.

Another possible explanation of exercise hyperpnea is that the proportional controller may be driven by two sets of inputs: a chemical feedback component via the chemoreflex loop and a feedforward component induced by some exercise stimulus [Grodins & Yamashiro, 1978]. The "feedforward-feedback control" hypothesis offers a simple remedy of the chemoreflex model, but its validity can be verified only if the postulated "exercise stimulus" is identified. Unfortunately, although many such signals have been proposed as possible candidates [Wasserman et al., 1986], none of them has so far been unequivocally shown to represent a sufficient stimulus for exercise.

Among the variously proposed mechanisms of exercise hyperpnea, the "PCO_2 oscillation" hypothesis of Yamamoto [1962] has received widespread attention. According to this hypothesis, the controller may be responsive not only to the mean value of chemical feedback but also to its oscillatory waveform which is induced by the tidal rhythm of respiration. This hypothesis is supported by the experimental finding that alterations of the temporal relationship of the P_ACO_2 waveform could profoundly modulate the exercise hyperpnea response [Poon, 1992b].

Regardless of the origin (or even existence) of the exercise stimulus, there is evidence that exercise and chemical signals are processed by the controller in a multiplicative fashion [Poon & Greene, 1985; Poon, 1989a, 1989b]. The input-output relationship of the controller may therefore be written as

$$\dot{V}_E = G_0(A_c + A_p)A_{ex} + G_{ex}A_{ex} \tag{159.13}$$

Note that $\dot{V}_E$ vanishes when A_{ex} is reduced to zero, in agreement with the finding of Phillipson and colleagues [1981].

159.3 Models of Respiratory Central Pattern Generator

Although the chemoreflex model is useful in studying the closed-loop control of ventilation and the chemical plant, it is lacking as to the control of breathing pattern and the mechanical plant. Models of the RCPG are often studied under open-loop conditions with chemical feedbacks being held constant while vagal volume feedback is experimentally manipulated. Modeling and analysis of the RCPG in closed-loop form are difficult because the input-output relationships of the RCPG and the mechanism of pattern generation are poorly understood. Several modeling approaches have been used to characterize its behavior under specific conditions.

Phase-Switching Models

The breathing cycle consists of two distinct phases: inspiration and expiration. It is therefore natural to model each phase separately and then combine them with a model of phase switching (for review, see Younes and Remmers [1981]). Each phase is controlled by a separate "center" which generates ramplike central inspiratory and expiratory activity, respectively. The resulting lung expansion and collapse are sensed by SAR, which causes the RCPG to switch from inspiration phase to expiration phase, or vice versa, when the volume-time relationship reaches some inspiratory or expiratory off-switch threshold. The off-switch mechanisms are dependent on both the threshold values and the corresponding volume-time histories. Also, inspiratory and expiratory off-switches may be mechanistically linked, as suggested by the correlation between inspiratory and expiratory durations in consecutive breaths. Both the rate of rise of inspiratory activity and the inspiratory off-switch threshold increase with increasing chemical stimulation. Throughout the inspiratory phase, vagal volume feedback exerts graded and reversible inhibition on inspiratory activity until immediately before the inspiratory off-switch where inspiratory termination becomes irreversible [Younes et al., 1978]. Perturbations of the mechanical plant, such as increases in ventilatory load, alter respiratory rhythm by changing the volume-time profiles and off-switch thresholds (Fig. 159.2). These effects are abolished by vagotomy such that the RCPG always oscillates with a fixed rhythm. Various neuronal models of phase switching have been proposed [Cohen & Feldman, 1977], and putative phase-switching neurons in the medulla have been identified [Oku et al., 1992].

The two-phase respiratory cycle may be expanded into three phases if the expiratory phase is subdivided into an early postinspiratory inspiratory phase (stage I) and a late expiratory phase (stage

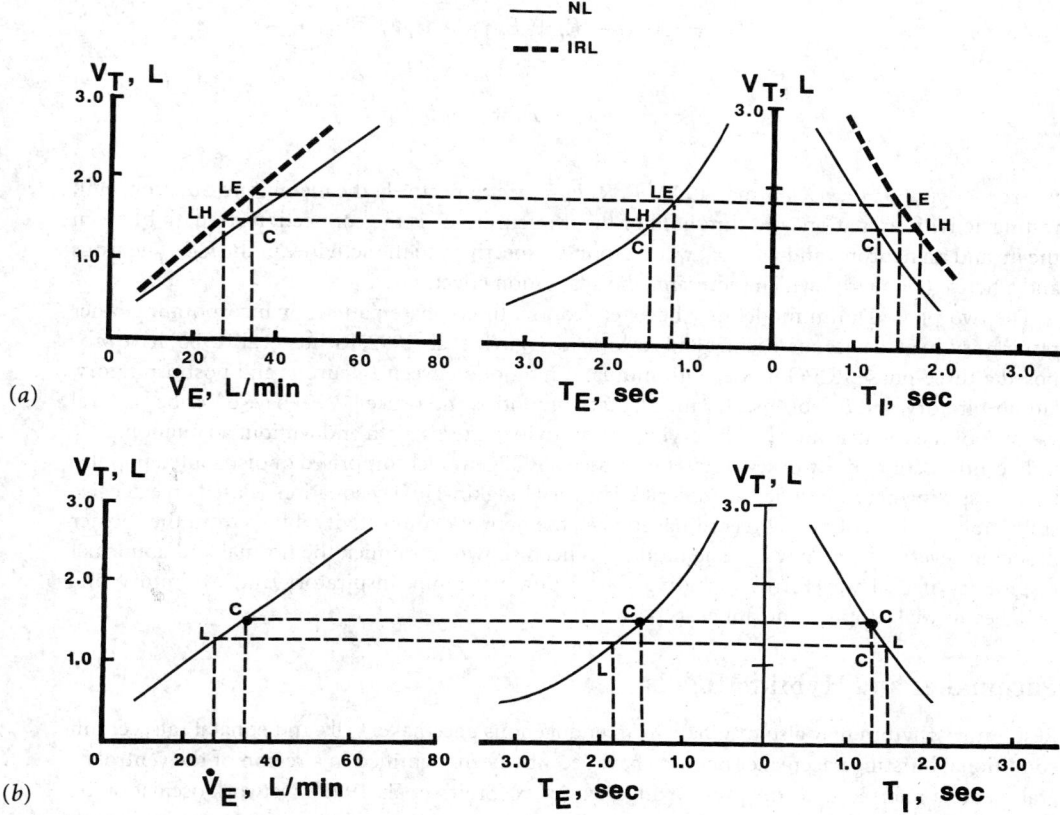

FIGURE 159.2 Stylized diagrams illustrating the Hey plots (*left*) and respiratory phase-switching curves (*right*) for subjects breathing normally (NL) or: (*a*) under an inspiratory resistive load (IRL): (*b*) under an inspiratory elastic load (IEL) at rest or during exercise. In (*a*), IRL causes the normal operating point (*C*) to move to a new point *LE* if the inspirate is free of CO_2, or to a point *LH* if CO_2 is added. In (*b*), IEL moves the operating point to the same point *L* whether CO_2 is present in the inspirate. Thus, the consequence of load compensation is highly dependent on the background CO_2 and the type of load. Relative scales only are shown on all axes. *Source:* Poon [1989a, 1989b], with permission.

II). Vagal feedback has differential effects on neural activities during the two stages of expiration [St. John & Zhou, 1990].

An important link between RCPG and chemoreflex models is the Hey plot [Hey et al., 1966] which suggests that $\dot{V}_E$ and V_T are linearly related except when V_T approaches vital capacity. The slope of the Hey plot is altered by resistive loads but not elastic loads to ventilation (Fig. 159.2).

Neural Network Models

Respiratory rhythmicity is an emergent property of the RCPG resulting from mutual inhibition of inspiratory and expiratory related neurons. A minimal model due to Duffin [1991] postulated the early-burst inspiratory (I) neurons and Bötzinger complex expiratory (E) neurons to be the mutually inhibiting pair. Adaptation of the I neurons (e.g., by calcium-activated potassium conductance) results in sustained relaxation oscillation in the network under constant chemical excitation. Both neuron groups are assumed to have monosynaptic inhibitory projections to bulbospinal inspiratory (I_R) output neurons (Fig. 159.3). The model equations are:

$$T_i \frac{dx_i}{dt} + x_i = R_i + E_i + \sum_j C_{ij} y_{ij}$$

$$T_f \frac{dx_f}{dt} + x_f = R_f + C_{fI} x_1 \tag{159.14}$$

where $y_i \equiv g(x_i - H_i)$; $g(X) \equiv \max(0, X)$; T_i, R_i, E_i, H_i are respectively the membrane time constant, resting activity, excitation, and threshold of the ith neuron; C_{ij} is the connection strength between the ith and jth neurons; and x_1, x_2, x_3, x_f correspond respectively to the activities of the I, E, I_R neurons and a fictive (F) neuron which represents the adaptation effect.

The two-phase Duffin model may be extended to a three-phase pattern by incorporating other respiratory-related neurons. Richter and coworkers [Ogilvie et al., 1992; Richter et al., 1986] have proposed a three-phase RCPG model with mutual inhibition between I neurons and postinspiratory, late-inspiratory, and E neurons, all with adaptations. Botros and Bruce [1990] have described several variants of the Richter model with varying connectivity patterns, with and without adaptation.

Recently, Balis and coworkers [1994] proposed a RCPG model comprised of distributed populations of spiking neurons which are described by the Hodgkin-Huxley equations. Based on extensive spike-train analysis of neural recordings in vivo, the network connectivity differs from the Richter model in several essential ways. The model has been shown to mimic the normal and abnormal respiratory neural waveforms including the inspiratory ramp, inspiratory and expiratory off-switches, as well as apnea and apneusis.

Pacemaker and Hybrid Models

Respiratory rhythm may also originate from endogenous pacemaker cells. In neonatal rats, certain conditional bursting pacemaker neurons have recently been identified in a region of the ventrolateral medulla referred to as the pre-Bötzinger complex [Smith et al., 1991]. Network oscillation by mutual inhibition is difficult in neonates because of immaturity of the GABAergic inhibitory system. During the postnatal developmental stage there may be progressive transformation from pacemaker to network oscillation with possibly some form of hybrid operation in the transition period [Smith, 1994]. A hybrid RCPG model composed of a neural network oscillator driven by a pacemaker cell (Fig. 159.3) has been proposed [Matsugu et al., 1994].

Nonlinear Dynamics

An empirical (black-box) approach to studying rhythmic behavior is to model the oscillation as limit cycles of a nonlinear oscillator. A classic example of limit-cycle oscillation is the Van der Pol oscillator:

$$\ddot{V} = \epsilon \left\{ 1 - \left(\frac{V}{a} \right)^2 \right\} \dot{V} - V \tag{159.15}$$

where ϵ and a are shape and amplitude parameters, respectively. This model has been shown to mimic the phase resetting and phase singularity properties of the RCPG [Eldridge et al., 1989] which are typical of any oscillator with isolated limit cycles. Similar properties are exhibited by a network oscillator model of RCPG [Ogilvie et al., 1992] which produces similar limit cycles.

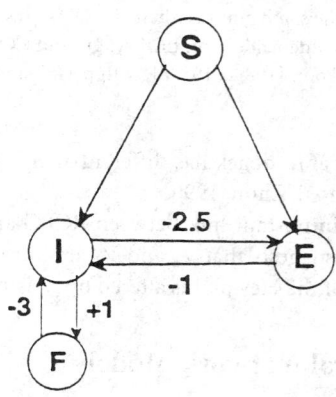

FIGURE 159.3   A minimal neural network model of RCPG. *I* and *E* denote respectively the early-burst inspiratory neurons and Bötzinger complex expiratory neurons; *F* is a fictive adaptation neuron; *S* is an excitation neuron or pacemaker cell. Not shown is the bulbospinal output neuron (I_R). Numbers denote connection strengths. *Source:* Matsugu and coworkers [1994], with permission.

Another property of nonlinear oscillators is that they may be entrained by (or phase-locked to) other oscillators that are coupled to them. The respiratory rhythm has been shown to be entrained by a variety of oscillatory inputs including locomotion, mechanical ventilation, blood gas oscillation, and musical rhythm.

A third property of nonlinear oscillators is that the limit-cycle trajectory may bifurcate and become quasiperiodic or chaotic when the system is perturbed by nonlinear feedback or other oscillatory sources. The resting respiratory rhythm is highly rhythmic in vagotomized animals but may become chaotic in normal humans [Donaldson, 1992] and vagi-intact animals [Sammon & Bruce, 1991] especially when lung volume is reduced [Sammon et al., 1993]. Both entrainment quasiperiodic and chaotic regimes have been demonstrated in a network oscillator model of the RCPG that is driven by periodic inputs [Matsugu et al., 1994].

159.4 Optimization Models

All control systems are meant to accomplish certain (implicit or explicit) control objectives. It is perhaps too simplistic to assume that the sole objective of respiration is to meet the metabolic demand; a complex physiologic system may subserve multiple objectives that are vital to animal survival. One approach to understanding respiratory control is therefore to discover the innate control objective that fits the observed behavior of the controller.

Optimization of Breathing Pattern

Any given level of ventilation may be produced by a variety of breathing patterns ranging from deep-and-slow to shallow-and-rapid breathing. How is the breathing pattern set for each ventilatory level? Rohrer [1925] was among the first to recognize that respiratory frequency at rest may be chosen by the controller to minimize the work rate of breathing, a notion that was subsequently advanced by Otis and colleagues [1950]. Mead [1960] showed that the resting frequency may be determined more closely on the basis of optimal inspiratory pressure-time integral, a measure of the energy cost of breathing. Neither the work nor energy measure, however, correctly predicts the inspiratory flow pattern [Bretschger, 1925; Ruttimann & Yamamoto, 1972]; such discrepancy has led to the suggestion that the optimization criterion may consist of a weighted sum of work and energy expenditures [Bates, 1986] or some higher-order terms [Hämäläinen and Sipilä, 1984; Yamashiro & Grodins, 1971].

Similarly, the optimization principle has also been applied to the prediction of airway caliber and dead space volume [Widdicombe & Nadel, 1963] as well as end-expiratory lung volume and respiratory duty cycle [Yamashiro et al., 1975]. In most cases, the cost functions are generally found to be relatively flat in the resting state but may become much steeper during CO_2 or exercise stimulations [Yamashiro et al., 1975]. This may explain the observed variability of breathing pattern which is generally more pronounced at rest than during hyperpnea or ventilatory loading.

Optimization of Ventilation

The classical optimization hypothesis of Rohrer [1925] and Bretschger [1925] suggests that conservation of energy may be an important factor in the genesis of breathing pattern. It thus appears that the controller is charged with two opposing objectives: to meet the metabolic demand by performing the work of breathing, and to conserve energy by minimizing the work. How does the controller reconcile such conflict? One possible solution is to establish priority. In a hierarchical model of respiratory control, metabolic needs take priority over energetic needs. At the higher hierarchy (outer/chemical feedback loop) ventilatory output is set by feedforward/feedback proportional control of the chemical plant to meet the metabolic demand, whereas at the lower hierarchy (inner/vagal feedback loop) breathing pattern is optimized by the RCPG for efficient energy utilization by the mechanical plant at a ventilation set by the higher hierarchy.

A potential drawback of such a hierarchical system is that it is nonrobust to perturbations. Changes in ventilatory load, for example, would disrupt the ventilatory command from the feed-forward signal. This is at variance with the experimental observation of a load compensation response of the controller which protects ventilation against perturbations of the mechanical plant at rest and during exercise [Poon, 1989a, 1989b; Poon et al., 1987a, 1987b]. Furthermore, if the prime objective of the controller were indeed to meet the metabolic demand (i.e., to maintain chemical homeostasis), then the hierarchical control system seems to perform quite poorly: it is well-known that arterial chemical homeostasis is readily disrupted by environmental changes.

Another form of conflict resolution is compromise. Poon [1983a, 1987] proposed that an optimal controller might counterbalance the metabolic needs versus energetic needs of the body, and the resulting compromise would determine the ventilatory response. The tug-of-war between the two conflicting control objectives may be represented by a compound optimization criterion which reflects the balance between the chemical and mechanical costs of breathing:

$$J \begin{cases} = J_c + J_m \\ = \{\alpha(P_aCO_2 - \beta)\}^2 + \ln\dot{W} \end{cases} \qquad (159.16)$$

The power (quadratic) form and logarithmic form for J_c and J_m correspond, respectively, to the classical Steven's law and Fechner-Weber law of sensory perception [Milsum, 1966]. Assuming that the work rate of breathing $\dot{W} \sim \dot{V}_E^2$, Eq. (159.16) yields an optimal ventilatory response that conforms with the normal hypercapnic ventilatory response during CO_2 inhalation and the isocapnic ventilatory response during exercise [Poon, 1983a, 1987]. Furthermore, by generalizing Eq. (159.16) to include other chemical and work rate components, it is possible to predict the normal ventilatory responses to hypoxia and acidosis [Poon, 1983a], mechanical loading [Poon, 1987b], as well as breathing pattern responses to chemical and exercise stimulation [Poon, 1983b].

The ventilatory optimization model [Poon, 1983a, 1983b, 1987b] has several interesting implications. First, it provides a unified and coherent framework for describing the control of ventilation and control of breathing pattern with a common optimization criterion. Second, it offers a parsimonious explanation of exercise hyperpnea and ventilatory load compensation responses, without the need to invoke any putative exercise stimulus and load compensation stimulus. Third, it suggests that disruption of chemical homeostasis (e.g., during CO_2 inhalation) may represent an optimal response as much as maintenance of homeostasis during exercise.

Energetics of breathing is only one of many constraints that conflict with the metabolic cause of respiration. Another is the sensation of dyspnea which may be a limiting factor at high ventilatory levels [Oku et al., 1993]. A general optimization criterion may therefore include both energetic and dyspneic penalties as follows:

$$J = \{\alpha(P_aCO_2 - \beta)\}^2 + 2\ln\dot{V}_E + k\,\dot{V}_E^2 \qquad (159.17)$$

where k is a weighting factor. At low to moderate ventilatory levels the energetic component (logarithmic term) dominates, and at high ventilatory levels the dyspneic component ($k \cdot \dot{V}_E^2$) dominates in counterbalancing the chemical component. In addition, the ventilatory apparatus may also be constrained by other factors such as behavioral and postural interference, which may further tip the balance of the optimization equation. It has been suggested that the periodic breathing pattern at extremely high altitudes may represent an optimal response for the conservation of chemical and mechanical costs of hypoxic ventilation [Ghazanshahi & Khoo, 1993].

Optimization of Neural Waveform

The neural output of the controller has been traditionally described in terms of measurable quantities such as breathing pattern and ventilation. A more accurate representation of the control signal is $P_{mus}(t)$ which drives the respiratory pump. The resulting continuous inspiratory and expiratory airflow, Eq. (159.9), then determine $\dot{V}_E$ and all other ventilatory patterns. The control problem the RCPG must solve is how to optimize $P_{mus}(t)$ in order to deliver adequate ventilation without incurring excessive energy (or other) losses. It has been shown by Poon and colleagues [1992] that many interesting characteristics of the RCPG conform to a general optimal control law that calls for dynamic optimization of $P_{mus}(t)$.

The model of Poon and coworkers [1992] assumes a compound optimization criterion, Eq. (159.16), with a mechanical penalty given by a weighted sum of the work rate of inspiration and expiration

$$\dot{W} = \dot{W}_I + \lambda \dot{W}_E \qquad (159.18)$$

where

$$\dot{W}_I = \frac{1}{T_T} \int_0^{T_I} \frac{P_{mus}(t)\dot{V}(t)}{[1 - P_{mus}(t)/P_{max}]^n \, [1 - \dot{P}_{mus}(t)/\dot{P}_{max}]^n} \, dt$$

$$\dot{W}_E = \frac{1}{T_T} \int_{T_I}^{T_T} P_{mus}(t)\dot{V}(t) \, dt \qquad (159.19)$$

The terms P_{max} and $\dot{P}_{max}$ denote the limiting capacities of the inspiratory muscles, and n is an efficiency index. The optimal $P_{mus}(t)$ output is found by minimization of J subject to the constraints set by the chemical and mechanical plants, Eqs. (159.1) and (159.9). Because $P_{mus}(t)$ is generally a continuous time function with sharp phase transitions, this amounts to solving a difficult dynamic nonlinear optimal control problem with piecewise smooth trajectories. An alternative approach adopted by Poon and coworkers [1992] is to model $P_{mus}(t)$ as a biphasic function

$$P_{mus}(t) \begin{cases} = a_0 + a_1 t + a_2 t & 0 \le t \le T_1 \\ = P_{mus}(T_1)\exp\left[-\dfrac{(t - T_1)}{\tau}\right] & T_1 \le t \le T_T \end{cases} \qquad (159.20)$$

where a_0, a_1, a_2 and τ are shape parameters; T_1 is the duration of the inspiratory phase of neural activity. The optimal P_{mus} waveform is given by the set of optimal parameters a_0^*, a_1^*, a_2^*, τ^*, T_1^*, T_T^* that minimize Eq. (159.16).

Poon and colleagues [1992] have shown that the dynamic optimization model predicts closely the $P_{mus}(t)$ trajectories under various conditions of ventilatory loading as well as respiratory muscle fatigue and weakness (Fig. 159.4). In addition, the model also accurately predicts the ventilatory and breathing pattern responses to combinations of chemical and exercise stimulation and ventilatory loading [Poon et al., 1992], all without invocation of any putative exercise stimulus or load compensation stimulus. The generality of model predictions strongly supports the hypothesis that neural processing in the RCPG is governed by an optimization law.

159.5 Self-Tuning Regulator Models

Optimization models suggest an empirical objective function that might be obeyed by the controller. They do not, however, reveal the mechanism of such neural optimization. Priban and Fincham [1965] suggested that an optimal operating point for arterial pH, PCO_2, and PO_2 might be achieved by a self-adaptive controller which seeks the optimal solution by a process of hill climbing. There is increasing evidence that the respiratory system is an adaptive control system [Poon, 1992a].

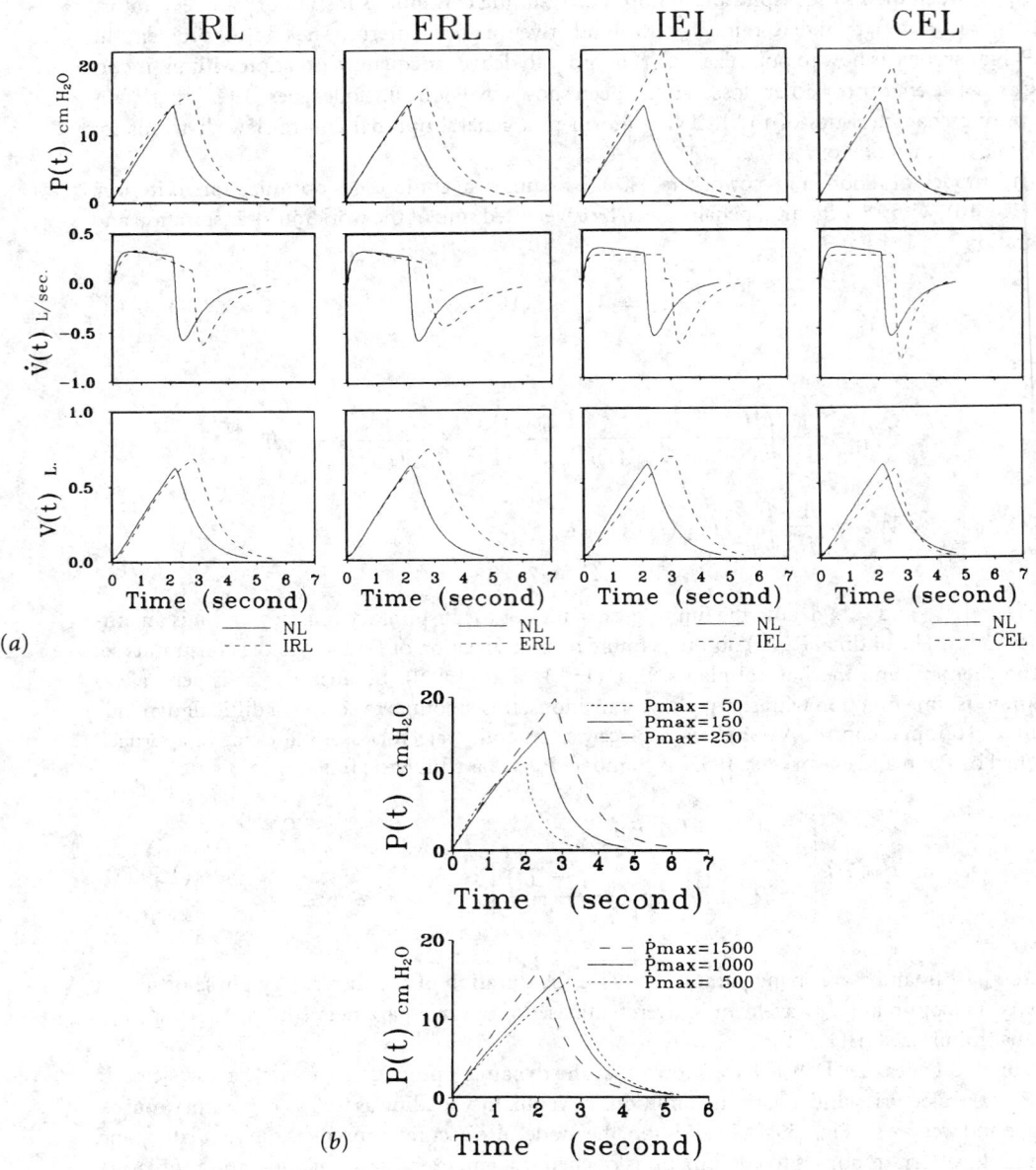

FIGURE 159.4 (*a*) Optimal waveforms for respiratory muscle driving pressure, $P(t)$; respiratory airflow, $\dot{V}$; and respired volume, V, during normal breathing (NL) or under various types of ventilatory loads: IRL and ERL, inspiratory and expiratory resistive load; IEL and CEL, inspiratory and continuous elastic load. (*b*) Optimal waveforms for $P(t)$ under increasing respiratory muscle fatigue (amplitude limited; *upper* panel) and muscle weakness (rate limited; *lower* panel). *Source:* Poon and coworkers [1992], with permission.

There are two basic requirements in any adaptive system. The first is that in order to adapt to changes, the system signals must be constantly fluctuating or persistently exciting. This should be readily satisfied by the respiratory system which is inherently oscillatory [Yamamoto, 1962] and chaotic [Donaldson, 1992; Sammon & Bruce, 1992]. Another requirement is that the system must be able to learn and then memorize the changes in the environment. Learning and memory in neuronal circuits are generally believed to result from synaptic modifications in the form of long-term or short-term potentiation which are mediated by NMDA receptors [Bliss & Collingridge, 1993]. Evidence for learning and memory in the RCPG is provided by the recent discoveries of both short-term potentiation [Fregosi, 1991; Wagner & Eldridge, 1991] and long-term potentiation [Martin & Mitchell, 1993] in vivo and the same in vitro [Fortin et al., 1992]. Also, neonatal mice which lack functional NMDA receptors have been found to suffer severe respiratory depression [Poon et al., 1994]. It has been shown that learning and memory in the brain are sufficient to achieve an optimal behavior characterized by the chemoreflex response and isocapnic exercise response [Poon, 1991].

One form of synaptic modification—correlation Hebbian learning [Sejnowski & Tesauro, 1989]—has been suggested to be compatible with the ventilatory optimization model [Poon, 1993]. According to this neuronal model, variations in the chemical feedback and mechanical feedback signals converging at a Hebbian synapse in the RCPG may induce short-term potentiation if they are negatively correlated, or short-term depression if they are positively correlated. In other words, the controller gain may be adaptively increased or decreased depending on the coupling between the cause and effect of respiration. During exercise, ventilatory neural output and chemical feedback are strongly negatively correlated (since S_{pco2} has a large negative value) so that the controller learns to increase its gain, G_0, in proportion to metabolic load. During CO_2 inhalation, $\dot{V}_E$ and P_aCO_2 are only weakly correlated (i.e., S_{pco2} is small), and the controller gain remains unchanged. Such a neural controller is analogous to a self-tuning regulator [Åstrom & Wittenmark, 1975] which regulates the output by adaptive adjustment of system parameters.

Implicit in such a self-tuning regulator model is the assumption that afferent inputs may up- or downregulate the RCPG by inducing synaptic potentiation or depression of neural transmission. Respiratory short- and long-term potentiation have been variously reported as indicated above. The possibilty of synaptic depression was recently demonstrated in the nucleus tractus solitarius of the medulla [Zhou et al., 1995].

Similarly, it is possible that some form of synaptic learning might be at work in the RCPG to modulate pattern generation, thereby resulting in an optimal $P_{mus}(t)$. However, experimental and simulation data are presently lacking for verification of this conjecture.

159.6 Conclusion

Many empirical and functional models have been proposed to describe various aspects of the respiratory control system. The classical chemostat model is useful in describing chemoreflex responses but may be too simplistic to explain the variety of system responses to exercise input and mechanical disturbances. The recent discovery of various complex behaviors of the controller such as nonlinear dynamics, optimization, and learning suggest that the RCPG may be endowed with highly sophisticated computational characteristics. Such computational capability of the RCPG may be important for the maintenance of optimal physiologic conditions under changing environments. The computational problem—which amounts to dynamic optimal control of a nonlinear plant—is a very difficult one even by the standard of modern digital computers but seems to be solved by the RCPG from instant to instant with relative ease. This remarkable ability of the respiratory neural network is interesting from both biologic and engineering standpoints. Understanding how it works may shed light on not only the wisdom of the body [Canon, 1932] but also on the design of novel intelligent control systems with improved speed, accuracy and economy.

Nomenclature

A_c, A_p: Activity of central, peripheral chemoreceptor
α, β: Slope and intercept of CO_2 response curve; L/min/mmHg, mmHg
J_c, J_m, J: Chemical, mechanical, and total costs of breathing
KCO_2: Solubility constant of CO_2 in blood; $mmHg^{-1}$
M_bCO_2: Metabolic CO_2 production in brain tissues; L/min STPD
P_ACO_2, P_AO_2: Alveolar partial pressure of CO_2, O_2; mmHg
P_aCO_2, P_aO_2: Arterial partial pressure of CO_2, O_2; mmHg

P_bCO_2: Brain tissue PCO_2; mmHg

P_ICO_2, P_IO_2: Inspired partial pressure of CO_2, O_2; mmHg

P_{aw}: Airway pressure; cmH_2O

P_{mus}: Respiratory muscle driving pressure; cmH_2O

$\dot{Q}_b$: Cerebral blood flow; L/min

RCPG: Respiratory central pattern generator

R_{rs}, E_{rs}: Total respiratory resistance, elastance; $cmH_0/L/s$, cmH_2O/L

S_{pco2}: Input-output sensitivity of chemical plant, $SP_ACO_2/S\dot{V}_E$ mm Hg/L/min

T_I, T_E, T_T: Inspiratory, expiratory, and total respiration duration; s

V: Lung volume above relaxation volume; L

V_bCO_2: Brain tissue store of CO_2; L

$\dot{V}CO_2, \dot{V}O_2$: Whole-body metabolic CO_2 production, O_2 consumption; L/min STPD

V_D/V_T: Ratio of respiratory dead space to tidal volume

V_LCO_2, V_LO_2: Lung tissue store of CO_2, O_2; L

$\dot{V}_E$: Total ventilation of the lung; L/min BTPS

$\dot{W}$: Work rate of breathing

References

Åstrom KJ, Wittenmark B. 1975. On self-tuning regulators. Automatica 9:185.

Balis UJ, Morris KF, Koleski J, et al. 1994. Simulations of a ventrolateral medullary neural network for respiratory rhythmogenesis inferred from spike train cross-correlation. Biol Cybern 70:311.

Bates JHT. 1986. The minimization of muscular energy expenditure during inspiration in linear models of the respiratory system. Biol Cybern 54:195.

Bellville JW, Whipp BJ, Kaufman RD, et al. 1979. Central and peripheral chemoreflex loop gain in normal and carotid body-resected subjects. J Appl Physiol 46:843.

Bliss TVP, Collingridge GL. 1993. A synaptic model of memory: Long-term potentiation in the hippocampus. Nature 361:31.

Botros SM, Bruce EN. 1990. Neural network implementation of the three-phase model of respiratory rhythm generation. Biol Cybern 63:143.

Bretschger HJ. 1925. Die geschwindigkeitskurve der menschlichen atemluft. Pflügers Arch für die Gesellsch Physiol 210:134.

Bruce EN, Modarreszadeh M, Kump K. 1992. Identification of closed-loop chemoreflex dynamics using pseudorandom stimuli. In Y Honda, Y Miyamoto, K Konno, et al. (eds), Control of Breathing and Its Modeling Perspective, pp 137–142, New York, Plenum Press.

Canon WB. 1932. The Wisdom of the Body, New York, Norton.

Cohen MI, Feldman JL. 1977. Models of respiratory phase-switching. Federation Proc 36:2367.

Cunningham DJC, Robbins PA, Wolff CB. 1986. Integration of respiratory responses to changes in alveolar partial pressures of CO_2 and O_2 and in arterial pH. In NS Cherniack, JG Widdicombe (eds), Handbook of Physiology, sec 3, The Respiratory System, vol 2: Control of Breathing, part 2, pp 475–528, Washington, DC, American Physiological Society.

Dahan A, Berkenbosch A, DeGoede J, et al. 1990. On a pseudo-rebreathing technique to assess the ventilatory sensitivity to carbon dioxide in man. J Physiol 423:615.

Defares JG. 1964. Principles of feedback control and their application to the respiratory control system. In WO Fenn, H Rahn (eds), Handbook of Physiology. Respiration, sec 3, vol 1, pp 649–680, Washington, DC, American Physiological Society.

Donaldson GC. 1992. The chaotic behavior of resting human respiration. Respir Physiol 88:313.

Duffin J. 1991. A model of respiratory rhythm generation. NeuroReport 2:623.

Eldridge FL, Gill-Kumar P, Millhorn DE. 1981. Input-output relationships of central neural circuits involved in respiration in cats. J Physiol 311:81.

Eldridge FL, Millhorn DE. 1986. Oscillation, gating, and memory in the respiratory control system. In NS Cherniack, JG Widdicombe (eds), Handbook of Physiology, sec 3, The Respiratory

System, vol 2, Control of Breathing, part 2, pp 93–134, Washington, DC, American Physiological Society.

Eldridge FL, Paydarfar D, Wagner P, et al. 1989. Phase resetting of respiratory rhythm: effect of changing respiratory "drive." Am J Physiol 257:R271.

Fitzgerald RS, Lahiri S. 1986. Reflex responses to chemoreceptor stimulation. In NS Cherniack, JG Widdicombe (eds), Handbook of Physiology, sec 3, The Respiratory System, vol 2, Control of Breathing, part 1, pp 313–362, Washington, DC, American Physiological Society.

Fortin G, Velluti JC, Denavit-Saubié M, et al. 1992. Responses to repetitive afferent activity of rat solitary complex neurons isolated in brainstem slices. Neurosci Lett 147:89.

Ghazanshahi SD, Khoo MCK. 1993. Optimal ventilatory patterns in periodic breathing. Ann Biomed Eng 21:517.

Grodins FS, Buell SJ, Bart AJ. 1967. Mathematical analysis and digital simulation of the respiratory control system. J Appl Physiol 22:260.

Grodins FS, Yamashiro SM. 1978. Respiratory Function of the Lung and Its Control. New York, Macmillan.

Hämäläinen RP, Sipilä A. 1984. Optimal control of inspiratory airflow in breathing. Optimal Control Applications Methods 5:177.

Heeringa J, Berkenbosch A, de Goede J, et al. 1979. Relative contribution of central and peripheral chemoreceptors to the ventilatory response to CO_2 during hyperoxia. Respir Physiol 37:365.

Hey EN, Lloyd BB, Cunningham DJC, et al. 1966. Effects of various respiratory stimuli on the depth and frequency of breathing in man. Respir Physiol 1:193.

Hildebrandt JR. 1977. Gating: A mechanism for selective receptivity in the respiratory center. Federation Proc 36:2381.

Juratsch CE, Whipp BJ, Huntsman DJ, et al. 1982. Ventilatory control during experimental maldistribution of $\dot{V}_A/\dot{Q}$ in the dog. J Appl Physiol 52(1):245.

Khoo MCK, Kronauer RE, Strohl KP, et al. 1982. Factors inducing periodic breathing in humans: A general model. J Appl Physiol 53:644.

Khoo MCK, Gottschalk A, Pack AI. 1991. Sleep induced periodic breathing and apnea: A theoretical study. J Appl Physiol 70:2014.

Lipski J, Voss MD. 1990. Gating of peripheral chemoreceptor input to medullary inspiratory neurons: Role of Bötzinger complex neurons. In H Acker, A Trzebski, RG O'Regan, et al (eds), Chemoreceptors and Chemoreceptor Reflexes, pp 323–329, New York, Plenum Press.

Marroquin E Jr. 1991. Control of Respiration under Simulated Airway Compression. Thesis, Harvard-MIT Division of Health Sciences and Technology, Harvard Medical School, Boston.

Martin PA, Mitchell GS. 1993. Long-term modulation of the exercise ventilatory response in goats. J Physiol 470:601.

Matsugu M, Duffin J, Poon C-S. 1994. Entrainment and chaos in a respiratory neural network model. In BW Patterson (ed), Modeling and Control in Biomedical Systems, pp 21–22, Madison, Wis, Omnipress.

Mead J. 1960. Control of respiratory frequency. J Appl Physiol 15:325.

Milic-Emili J, Zin WA. 1986. Relationship between neuromuscular respiratory drive and ventilatory output. In PT Macklem, J Mead (eds), Handbook of Physiology, sec 3, The Respiratory System, vol 3, Mechanics of Breathing, part 2, pp 631–646, Washington, DC, American Physiological Society.

Milsum JH. 1966. Biological Control Systems Analysis, New York, McGraw-Hill.

Neubauer JA, Melton JE, Edelman NH. 1990. Modulation of respiration during brain hypoxia. J Appl Physiol 68(2):441.

Oku Y, Saidel GM, Altose MD, et al. 1993. Perceptual contributions to optimization of breathing. Ann Biomed Eng 21:509.

Ogilvie MD, Gottschalk A, Anders K, et al. 1992. A network model of respiratory rhythmogenesis. Am J Physiol 263:R962.

Oku Y, Tanaka I, Ezure K. 1992. Possible inspiratory off-switch neurones in the ventrolateral medulla of the cat. NeuroReport 3:933.

Oren A, Wasserman K, Davis JA, et al. 1981. Regulation of CO_2 set point on ventilatory response to exercise. J Appl Physiol 51:185.

Otis AB, Fenn WO, Rahn H. 1950. The mechanics of breathing in man. J Appl Physiol 2:592.

Pack AI, Ogilvie MD, Davies RO, et al. 1986. Responses of pulmonary stretch receptors during ramp inflations of the lung. J Appl Physiol 61(1):344.

Petersen ES. 1981. A survey of applications of modeling to respiration. In JG Widdicombe (ed), International Review of Physiology. Respiratory Physiology III, vol 23, ed. pp 261–326, Baltimore, University Park Press.

Phillipson EA. 1974. Vagal control of breathing pattern independent of lung inflation in conscious dogs. J Appl Physiol 37(2):183.

Phillipson EA, Bowes G. 1986. Control of breathing during sleep. In NS Cherniack, JG Widdicombe (eds), Handbook of Physiology, sec 3, The Respiratory System, vol 2, Control of Breathing, part 2, pp 649–689, Washington, DC, American Physiological Society.

Phillipson EA, Duffin J, Cooper JD. 1981. Critical dependence of respiratory rhythmicity on metabolic CO_2 load. J Appl Physiol 50(1):45.

Poon C-S. 1983a. Optimal control of ventilation in hypoxia, hypercapnia and exercise. In BJ Whipp, DM Wiberg (eds), Modelling and Control of Breathing, pp 189–196, New York, Elsevier.

Poon C-S. 1983b. Optimality principle in respiratory control. Proc Am Control Conf. 2nd, pp 36–40.

Poon C-S. 1987a. Estimation of pulmonary $\dot{V}/\dot{Q}$ distribution by inert gas elimination: State of the art. In C Cobelli, L Mariani (eds), Modelling and Control in Biomedical Systems, pp 443–453, New York, Pergamon Press.

Poon, C.-S. 1987b. Ventilatory control in hypercapnia and exercise: Optimization hypothesis. J Appl Physiol 62(6):2447.

Poon C.-S. 1989a. Effects of inspiratory elastic load on respiratory control in hypercapnia and exercise. J Appl Physiol 66(5):2400.

Poon C.-S. 1989b. Effects of inspiratory resistive load on respiratory control in hypercapnia and exercise. J Appl Physiol 66(5):2391.

Poon C-S. 1991. Optimization behavior of brainstem respiratory neurons: A cerebral neural network model. Biol Cybern 66:9.

Poon C-S. 1992a. Introduction: Optimization hypothesis in the control of breathing. In Y Honda, Y Miyamoto, K Konno, et al (eds), Control of Breathing and Its Modeling Perspective, pp 371–384, New York, Plenum Press.

Poon C-S. 1992b. Potentiation of exercise ventilatory response by CO_2 and dead space loading. J Appl Physiol 73(2):591.

Poon C-S. 1993. Adaptive neural network that subserves optimal homeostatic control of breathing. Ann Biomed Eng 21:501.

Poon C-S, Greene JG. 1985. Control of exercise hyperpnea during hypercapnia in humans. J Appl Physiol 59(3):792.

Poon C-S, Kolandaivelu K. 1994. Phase reversal of respiratory rhythm during assisted mechanical ventilation. In Modelling and Control of Ventilation (in press).

Poon C-S, Li Y, Li SX, et al. 1994. Respiratory rhythm is altered in neonatal mice with malfunctional NMDA receptors. FASEB J 8(4):A389.

Poon C-S, Lin S-L, Knudson OB. 1992. Optimization character of inspiratory neural drive. J Appl Physiol 72(5):2005.

Poon C-S, Olson RJ. 1985. A simple quasi-steady technique for accelerated determination of CO_2 response. Federation Proc 44:832.

Poon C-S, Ward SA, Whipp BJ. 1987a. Influence of inspiratory assistance on ventilatory control during moderate exercise. J Appl Physiol 62(2):551.

Poon C-S, Younes M, Gallagher CG. 1987b. Effects of expiratory resistive load on respiratory motor output in conscious humans. J Appl Physiol 63(5):1837.

Priban IP, and Fincham WF. 1965. Self-adaptive control and the respiratory system. Nature Lond 208:339.

Read DJC. 1967. A clinical method for assessing the ventilatory response to carbon dioxide. Australasian Ann Med 16:20.

Richter DW, Ballantyne D, Remmers JE. 1986. How is the respiratory rhythm generated? A model. News Physiol Sci 1:109.

Rohrer F. 1926. Physiologie der Atembewegung. In ATJ Bethe, G von Bergmann, G Embden, et al (eds), Handbuch der normalen und pathologischen Physiologie, vol 2, pp 70–127, Berlin, Springer-Verlag.

Ruttimann U, Yamamoto WS. 1972. Respiratory airflow patterns that satisfy power and force criteria of optimality. Ann Biomed Eng 1:146.

Sammon MP, Bruce EN. 1991. Vagal afferent activity increases dynamical dimension of respiration in rats. J Appl Physiol 70(4):1748.

Sammon M, Romaniuk JR, Bruce EN. 1993. Bifurcations of the respiratory pattern associated with reduced lung volume in the rat. J Appl Physiol 75(2):887.

Sejnowski TJ, Tesauro G. 1989. The Hebb rule for synaptic plasticity: algorithms and implementations. In JH Byrne, WO Berry (eds), Neural Models of Plasticity, pp 94–103, New York, Academic Press.

Sidney DA, Poon C-S. 1995. Ventilatory responses to dead space and CO_2 breathing under inspiratory resistive load. J Appl Physiol 78(2):555.

Smith JC. 1994. A model for developmental transformations of the respiratory oscillator in mammals. FASEB J 8(4):A394.

Smith JC, Ellenberger HH, Ballanyi K, et al. 1991. Pre-Bötzinger complex: A brainstem region that may generate respiratory rhythm in mammals. Science 254:726.

St. John WM, Zhou D. 1990. Discharge of vagal pulmonary receptors differentially alters neural activities during various stages of expiration in the cat. J Physiol 424:1.

Stark AR, Cohlan BA, Waggener TB, et al. 1987. Regulation of end-expiratory lung volume during sleep in premature infants. J Appl Physiol 62:1117.

Teppema LJ, Barts PWJA, Evers JAM. 1985. The effect of the phase relationship between the arterial blood gas oscillations and central neural respiratory activity on phrenic motoneurone output in cats. Respir Physiol 61:301.

Vis A, Folgering H. 1980. The dynamic effect of Pet_{CO2} on vertebral bloodflow in cats. Respir Physiol 42:131.

Wagner PG, Eldridge FL. 1991. Development of short-term potentiation. Respir Physiol 83:129.

Ward SA, Whipp BJ, Poon C-S. 1982. Density dependent airflow and ventilatory control during exercise. Respirat Physiol 49:267.

Wasserman K, Whipp B, Casaburi R. 1986. Respiratory control during exercise. In NS Cherniack, JG Widdicombe (eds), Handbook of Physiology, sec 3, The Respiratory System, vol 2, Control of Breathing, part 2, pp 595–619, Washington, DC, American Physiological Society.

Widdicombe JG, Nadel JA. 1963. Airway volume, airway resistance and work, and force of breathing—theory. J Appl Physiol 35:522.

Yamamoto WS. 1962. Transmission of information by the arterial blood stream with particular reference to carbon dioxide. Biophy J 2:143.

Yamashiro SM, Daubenspeck JA, Lauritsen TN, et al. 1975. Total work rate of breathing optimization in CO_2 inhalation and exercise. J Appl Physiol 38(4):702.

Yamashiro SM, Grodins FS. 1971. Optimal regulation of respiratory airflow. J Appl Physiol 18:863.

Younes M, Remmers JE. 1981. Control of tidal volume and respiratory frequency. In TF Hornbein (ed), Regulation of Breathing, part 1, pp 621–671, New York, Marcel Dekker.

Younes M, Remmers JE, Baker J. 1978. Characteristics of inspiratory inhibition by phasic volume feedback in cats. J Appl Physiol 45:80.

Zhou Z, Champagnat J, Poon C-S. 1995. Synaptic short-term depression in nucleus tractus solitarius (NTS) of rat brainstem in vitro. FASEB J, in press.

160

Neural Networks for Physiologic Control

James J. Abbas
*Catholic University
of America*

This chapter is intended to provide a description of neural network control systems and of their potential for use in biomedical engineering control systems. Neural network techniques have been used by the engineering community in a variety of applications, with particular emphasis on solving pattern recognition and pattern classification problems [Carpenter, 1989; Grossberg, 1988a, 1988b; Hecht-Nielsen, 1989; Nerrand et al., 1993; Pao, 1989; Sanchez-Sinencio & Lau, 1992; Zurada, 1992]. More recently, there has been much research into the use of these techniques in control systems [Antsaklis, 1990; Miller et al., 1990b; White & Sofge, 1992]. Much of this research has been directed at utilizing neural network techniques to solve problems that have been inadequately solved by other control systems techniques. For example, neural networks have been used in adaptive control of nonlinear systems for which good models do not exist. The success of neural network techniques on this class of problems suggest that they may be particularly well suited for use in a wide variety of biomedical engineering applications. It should be emphasized that the field of neural network control is a relatively new area of research and that it is not intended to replace traditional engineering control. Rather, the focus has been on the integration of neural network techniques into control systems for use when traditional control systems alone are insufficient.

There are several textbooks available on neural networks that provide good presentations of the implementation and applications of neural network techniques [Sanchez-Sinencio & Lau, 1992; Simpson, 1990; Zurada, 1992]. Recently, a few books have been published that review the application of neural network techniques to control systems problems [Miller et al., 1990b; White & Sofge, 1992]. This chapter is intended to provide an introduction to neural network techniques and a guide to their application to biomedical control systems problems. The reader is referred to recently published textbooks and numerous journal articles for the specific information required to implement a given neural network control system.

160.1 Neural Network Basics

The term *neural networks* is used to refer to a class of computational algorithms that are loosely based upon the computational structure of the nervous system. There is a wide variety among various neural network algorithms, but the key features are that they have a set of inputs and a set

0-8493-8346-3/95/$0.00+$.50

of outputs, they utilize distributed processing, and they are adaptive. The basic idea is that computation is collectively performed by a group of distinct units, or *neurons* (sometimes referred to as processing elements), each of which receives inputs and performs its own local calculation. These units interact by providing inputs to each other via synapses, and some units interact with the environment via input-output signals. The connectivity of various units determines the structure, or *architecture,* of the network. Adjustments to the strengths of the synapses (i.e., adjustments to the synaptic weights) modify the overall input-output properties of the network and are adjusted via a learning algorithm. The design of a neural network includes the specification of the neuron, the architecture, and the learning algorithm.

Most neural networks are based on a model of a neuron that captures the most basic features of real neurons: A neuron receives inputs from other neurons via synapses, and the output from a neuron is a nonlinear function of a weighted summation of its inputs. There are many different sets of equations that capture these basic features; the following set of equations are commonly used:

$$y_j = \sum_{i=1}^{n} w_{ij} x_i \tag{160.1}$$

$$z_j = 1/(1 + e^{-my_j}) \tag{160.2}$$

where y_j is the weighted summation of inputs to neuron j, x_i is the input from neuron i, n is the number of neurons providing synaptic input to neuron j, w_{ij} is the synaptic weight from neuron i to neuron j, z_j is the output from neuron j, and m is the slope of the sigmoidal output function. Note that in this set of equations, the output of a neuron is a static nonlinear function of the weighted summation of its inputs. Some commonly used variations on this model include the use of different nonlinear output functions [Lippman, 1987], the use of recurrent inputs (i.e., past values of a neurons output would be included in the input summation) [Pineda, 1989; Williams & Zipser, 1989], and the use of dynamic neurons (i.e., Eq. (160.1) would be a differential equation rather than an algebraic one) [Carpenter, 1989; Grossberg, 1988a; Hopfield, 1982]. The use of recurrent inputs and/or dynamic neuron models may be particularly important for applications in the control of dynamic systems because these models provide the individual neurons with memory and temporal dynamics [Pineda, 1989].

Most applications use networks of neurons that are arranged in layers. The most commonly used architecture is a three-layer network which has an input layer, a hidden layer, and an output layer. A feedforward neural network architecture is one in which each neuron receives input from neurons in the previous layer. The number of neurons in each layer must be specified by the designer. There are some heuristic rules, but no solid theory, to guide the designer in specifying the number of neurons [Zurada, 1992]. Some commonly used variations on this architecture include: the use of only a single layer of neurons [Kohonen, 1989; Widrow, 1962], the use of bidirectional connections between layers [Carpenter, 1989], the use of intralayer connections [Kohonen, 1989], the use of pruning techniques which cut some of the connections for greater efficiency [Zurada, 1992], and the use of heterogeneous networks in which more than one neuron model is used to describe the various neurons in the network [Hecht-Nielson, 1989].

A general form of a neural network learning algorithm is given by

$$\Delta w_{ij} = f(\eta, z_i, z_j, e_{ij}) \tag{160.3}$$

This equation states that the change in synaptic weight is a function of the learning rate (η), the activation of the presynaptic neuron (z_i), the activation of the postsynaptic neuron (z_j), and a training signal (e_{ij}). Several different learning algorithms have been developed [Fogel, 1990; Grossberg, 1988a; Hecht-Nielsen, 1990; Hinton, 1989; Rumelhart & McClelland, 1988], most of which fit into this general form but may not use all the terms. An example is Hebbian learning [Brown et al., 1990;

Hebb, 1949] in which the change in weight is proportional to the product of the presynaptic activation and the postsynaptic activation. Often, gradient descent techniques are used to adjust the synaptic weights. The most commonly used learning algorithm, error backpropagation, uses an error gradient descent technique and passes the output error backward through the network to determine the training signal for a given neuron [Pineda, 1989; Rumelhart, 1988; Vogl, 1988]. Most of the commonly used learning algorithms are classified as supervised learning algorithms because they use a specification of the desired output of the network to determine the output error of the network. Other learning algorithms, such as reinforcement learning (discussed below) can be used when it is not possible to directly specify the desired output of the network.

In most engineering applications, the neural network is used to perform a nonlinear mapping from the space of network inputs to the space of network outputs. In addition to the internal specifications of the network discussed above, the engineer using a neural network must select the signals to be used as input to the network and the signals to be used as output from the network. Although this decision appears to be trivial, in many applications it is not. For applications in control systems, the selection of input and output signals depends on how the neural network fits into the overall structure of the system. Several different options are described below.

160.2 Neural Network Control Systems

Neural networks have often been applied in control systems where, at a block diagram level, the neural network replaces one component of the control system. Typically, the motivation for utilizing the neural network lies in the ability to perform nonlinear mappings, in the ability to handle a wide range of model structures, and/or in the ability of the network to adapt. Although there has been activity in the development of a theoretical framework for neural network control systems, most applications to date have been heuristically based to one degree or another [Farotimi et al., 1991; Miller et al., 1990b; Nguyen & Widrow, 1990; Quinn & Espenschied, 1993; Wang et al., 1992; White & Sofge, 1992]. The field of neural network control has been described as bridging the gap between mathematically based control systems engineering and heuristically based artificial intelligence [Barto, 1990].

In designing a neural network control system, one must select the overall structure of the system and decide which components will utilize neural network algorithms. Several examples of control system structures are provided below, each of which utilizes one or more neural networks as described above. This section of the chapter provides a brief overview of some neural control systems that have potential for application in biomedical control systems. For excellent, thorough reviews of recent developments in neural network control systems the reader is referred to Miller, Sutton, and Werbos [1990b] and White and Sofge [1992].

Supervised Control

In this structure (Fig. 160.1), the neural network is used to mimic, and eventually replace, an existing control system. Here, the neural network is used in a traditional feedback arrangement where it performs a mapping from the system outputs to the system inputs. The network would be trained using data collected from the actual system or a computer-simulated model with the original controller active. The training signal for the network would be the difference between the output of the original controller and the output of the network. After the net-

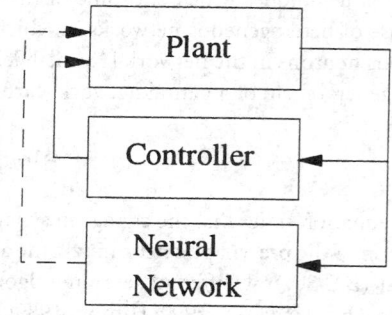

FIGURE 160.1 Supervised control system structure.

work learns to adequately mimic the original controller, the training is completed, the synaptic weights would no longer be adapted, and the original control system would be replaced by the neural network. This type of an arrangement could be useful where the neural network could perform the task less expensively or more efficiently than the original one. One situation would be when the original control system requires such heavy computation that it is impractical for real-time use on an affordable computer system. In this case, the neural network might be able to learn to perform the same (or functionally equivalent) operation more efficiently such that implementation on an affordable general purpose computer or on specialized neural network hardware would be practical. A second situation would be when the original control system is a human operator who might be either expensive or prone to error. In this case the neural network is acting as an adaptive expert system that learns to mimic the human expert [Werbos, 1990]. A third situation would be when the neural network could learn to perform the control using a different, and more easily measured, set of output variables [Barto, 1990]. This type of application would be particularly well suited for biomedical applications in which an invasive measurement could be replaced by a noninvasive one.

Direct Inverse Control

In direct inverse control (Fig. 160.2), the neural network is used to compute an inverse model of the system to be controlled [Levin et al., 1991; Nordgren & Meckl, 1993]. In classical linear control techniques, one would find a linear model of the system and then analytically compute the inverse model. Using neural networks, the network is trained to perform the inverse model calculations, i.e., to map system outputs to system inputs. This approach can be effective, but it does require a sufficient set of system input-output data for training purposes.

A variety of neural network architectures can be used in this direct inverse control system structure. A multilayer neural network architecture with error backpropagation learning could be used off-line to learn an inverse model using a set of system input-output data. If on-line learning is desired, a feedforward model of the system can be trained while a feedback controller is active [Miller et al., 1990a; Miyamoto et al., 1988]. This technique, referred to as *feedback error learning* [Miyamoto et al., 1988], uses the control signal coming from the feedback controller as the training signal for the feedforward controller update. The idea used here is that if the feedforward control is inadequate, the feedback controller would be active and it would lead to updates in the feedforward controller. To achieve the rapid learning rates that would be desirable in on-line feedback error learning, typically single-layer networks have been used, or the learning has been constrained to occur at one layer. This type of an approach is particularly useful in applications where on-line fine tuning of feedforward controller parameters is desired.

Backpropagation Through a System Model

For many control applications, system output error can be readily measured, but in order to adapt the controller parameters one needs to relate system output error to controller output (system input) error. One strategy would be to use the derivative of the system's output error with respect to its input to perform gradient descent adaptation of the controller parameters. However, there is no direct way of calculating the derivative of the system's output error with respect to its input, and therefore it must be approximated. To implement such an approximation, a pair of multilayer neural networks (Fig. 160.3) have been used: one for identification of a forward model of the plant, and

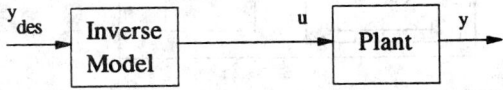

FIGURE 160.2 Direct inverse control system structure.

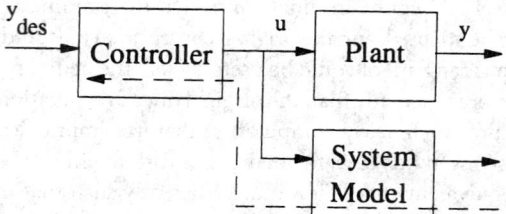

FIGURE 160.3 Backpropagating system output error through the system model.

one for implementation of the controller [Barto, 1990]. The forward model is used to provide a means of computing the derivative of the model's output with respect to its input by backpropagating the error signal (the actual plant output-tracking error) through the model of the plant to estimate the error in the control signal. The error in the control signal can then be backpropagated through the controller neural network. As described here, the backpropagation algorithm is used to minimize the output error of the system, which is a special case of maximization of utility. Although this is a very powerful technique with potential applications in a wide variety of nonlinear control problems, its primary limitation for many biomedical applications is the relatively slow training rate achieved by the back propagation algorithm.

Model Reference Adaptive Control

Neural networks have also been used in model reference adaptive control (MRAC) structures (Fig. 160.4) [Narendra & Parthasarathy, 1990; Narendra, 1992]. This approach builds upon established techniques for adaptive linear control and incorporates neural networks to address the problem of controlling nonlinear systems. The MRAC approach is directed at adapting the controlled system such that it behaves like a reference model, which is specified by the control system designer. In the structure shown in Fig. 160.4 the identification model is a model of plant dynamics, the parameters of which are identified on-line using the identification error (the difference between the actual and the estimated plant outputs) as the training signal. The controller uses the estimates of the plant parameters, reference inputs, and system outputs to determine inputs to the system. In the neural network version of the control system structure, neural networks can be used for the identification of the system model, for the controller, or for both. Multilayer neural networks using error back-propagation or a modified version of error back propagation, termed *dynamic backpropagation,* have been used for adaptive control of nonlinear systems [Narendra & Parthasarathy, 1990; Narendra, 1992].

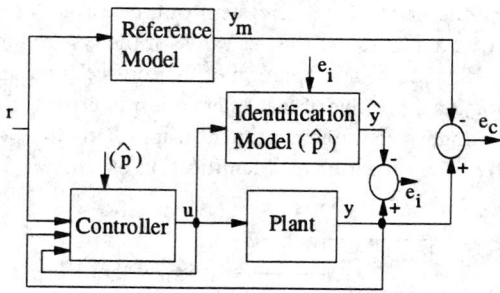

FIGURE 160.4 Indirect adaptive control system structure.

Adaptive Critics

All the approaches to control discussed thus far have utilized supervised learning techniques. The training signal used for adaptation in these techniques is an error vector that gives the magnitude of the error in the system output signal and the direction in which it should change. For many complex, multivariable control problems this type of system output error information is not readily available. The only measure available might be a scalar measure of system performance that is not directly related to the system outputs in a way that is understood by the control system designer. In such cases, a directed search of the control system parameter space could be performed in order to maximize (optimize) the scalar performance measure. Dynamic programming is a control systems engineering technique that has been used for optimal control of linear systems, but these techniques are not well suited for large-scale systems or nonlinear systems. Neural networks have been used in an approach that is similar to dynamic programming in order to optimize system performance of large-scale nonlinear systems. These techniques, termed *adaptive critic methods,* utilize a structure (Fig. 160.5) in which a critic module provides an evaluation signal to the controller module. The controller module utilizes a reinforcement learning algorithm in order to optimize performance. The details of this class of neural network controllers are beyond the scope of this chapter, but descriptions and example applications are given in Barto [1990, 1992] and Werbos [1992].

Adaptive critic algorithms may be particularly useful in several biomedical engineering control systems where the relationship between system performance and measurable system outputs are ill-defined. Although these methods that use reinforcement learning may be attractive because they are general and do not require detailed information about the system, this increased generality comes at a cost of increased training times [Barto, 1990]. Supervised learning methods, when they can be used, can be more efficient than reinforcement learning methods.

Neurophysiologically Based Approaches

All neural network systems are based upon neurophysiologic models to some degree, but in most cases this biologic basis is very superficial, as is evident in the description given above. *Computational neuroscience* is a term used to describe the development of computational models of the nervous system [Koch & Segev, 1989; Schwartz, 1990]. Such models are intended to be used by neuroscientists in their basic science efforts to understand the functioning of the nervous system. Several examples of neural network control system designs have utilized models developed in the field of computational neuroscience [Abbas & Chizeck, 1991; Beer et al., 1993; Bullock & Grossberg, 1988; Houk et al., 1990; Taga et al., 1991]. These designs have extended the notion of "mimicking the ner-

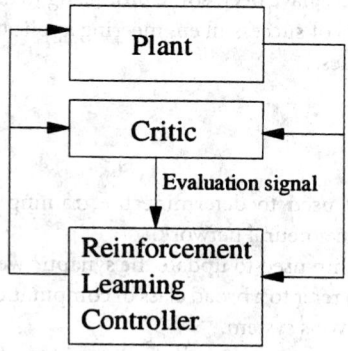

FIGURE 160.5 Adaptive critic control system structure.

vous system" beyond what is used in most neural networks. The reasoning behind this approach is based upon a view that biologic systems solve many problems that are similar to, or exactly the same as, those faced in many engineering applications and that by mimicking the biologic system we may be able to design better engineering systems. This reasoning is similar to the motivation for much of the work in the neural network field and for the recent emphasis in biomimetic techniques in other engineering disciplines.

One approach to incorporating a stronger neurophysiologic foundation has been to utilize an architecture for the overall control system that is based upon neurophysiologic models, i.e., mimicking the neurophysiologic system at a block diagram level. This type of approach has led to the development of hierarchical control systems that are based upon the hierarchical structure of the human motor control system [Kawato et al., 1987; Srinivasan et al., 1992].

A second approach to incorporating a stronger neurophysiologic foundation has been to utilize more realistic models of neurons and of their interconnections in the design of the neural network [Beer, 1990; Houk et al., 1990]. An example of this approach is the design of a coupled oscillator neural network circuit that is based upon the locomotor control system of the cockroach [Beer et al., 1992; Quinn & Espenschied, 1993]. In this neural network, some of the neurons are capable of endogenously oscillating due to intrinsic membrane currents, and the network is heterogeneous in that each neuron is not described by the same model. Most of the parameters of the models are fixed. This network has been used to robustly generate patterns for statically stable gaits at various speeds.

A biomedical control system that utilizes a neurophysiologically based approach has been developed for use in functional neuromuscular stimulation (FNS) systems [Abbas & Chizeck, 1991, 1994]. FNS is a rehabilitation engineering technique that uses computer-controlled electrical stimuli to activate paralyzed muscle. The task of a control system is to determine appropriate stimulation levels to generate a given movement or posture. The neural network control system utilizes a block diagram structure that is based on hierarchical models of the locomotor control system. It also utilizes a heterogenous network of neurons, some of which are capable of endogenous oscillation. This network has been shown to provide rapid adaptation of the control system parameters [Abbas & Chizeck, 1991] and has been shown to exhibit modulation of reflex responses [Abbas & Chizeck, 1994].

160.3 Summary

This chapter presents an overview of the relatively new field of neural network control systems. A variety of techniques are described, and some of the advantages and disadvantages of the various techniques are discussed. The techniques described here show great promise for use in biomedical engineering applications in which other control systems techniques are inadequate. Currently, neural network control systems lack the type of theoretical foundation upon which linear control systems are based, but recently there have been some promising theoretical developments. In addition, there are numerous examples of successful engineering applications of neural networks to attest to the utility of these techniques.

Defining Terms

Backpropagation: A technique used to determine the training signal used for adjusting the weights of a given neuron in a neural network.

Learning algorithm: An algorithm used to update the synaptic weights in a neural network.

Neural network: A term used to refer to a broad class of computational algorithms that are loosely based on models of the nervous system.

Reinforcement learning algorithms: Learning algorithms that utilize a system performance measure (that may or may not have a direct, known relationship to output error of the neural network) as a training signal for the neural network.

Supervised learning algorithms: Learning algorithms often used in neural networks that use the output error of the neural network as a training signal.

Synaptic weight: A scaling factor on the signal from one neuron in a network to another.

Acknowledgments

The author gratefully acknowledges the support of the National Science Foundation (NSF-BCS-9216697) and the School of Engineering at The Catholic University of America.

References

Abbas JJ, Chizeck HJ. 1991. A neural network controller for Functional Neuromuscular Stimulation Systems. Proc IEEE/EMBS Conf Orlando, Fla, 13:1456.

Abbas JJ, Chizeck HJ. 1994. Phase-dependent reflexes in a neural network control system. Proc S Biomed Eng Conf 13:494.

Antsaklis PJ. 1990. Neural networks in control systems. IEEE Control Systems Magazine, 10(3):3.

Barto AG. 1990. Connectionist learning for control: An overview. In WT Miller, RS Sutton, PJ Werbos (eds), Neural Networks for Control, pp 5–58, Cambridge, Mass, MIT Press.

Barto AG. 1992. Reinforcement learning and adaptive critic methods. In DA White, DA Sofge (eds), Handbook of Intelligent Control: Neural, Fuzzy and Adaptive Approaches, pp 469–492, New York, Van Nostrand Reinhold.

Beer RD. 1990. Intelligence as Adaptive Behavior: An Experiment in Computational Neuroethology, Boston, Academic Press.

Beer RD, Chiel HJ, Quinn RD, et al. 1992. A distributed neural network architecture for hexapod robot locomotion. Neural Computation 4:356.

Beer RD, Ritzmann RE, McKenna T. 1993. Biological Neural Networks in Invertebrate Neuroethology and Robotics, New York, Academic Press.

Brown TH, Kairiss EW, Keenan CL. 1990. Hebbian synapses: Biophysical mechanisms and algorithms. Annu Rev Neurosci 13:475.

Bullock D, Grossberg S. 1988. Neural dynamics of planned arm movements: Emergent invariants and speed-accuracy properties during trajectory formation. In S Grossberg (ed), Neural Networks and Natural Intelligence, pp 553–622, Cambridge, Mass, MIT Press.

Carpenter G. 1989. Neural network models for pattern recognition and associative memory. Neural Networks 2(4):243.

Farotimi O, Dembo A, Kailath T. 1991. A general weight matrix formulation using optimal control. IEEE Trans Neural Networks 2(3):378.

Fogel D, Sebald AV. 1990. Use of evolutionary programming in the design of neural networks for artifact detection. Proc IEEE/EMBS Conf 12:1408.

Grossberg S. 1988a. Neural Networks and Natural Intelligence, Cambridge, Mass, MIT Press.

Grossberg S. 1988b. Nonlinear neural networks: Principles, mechanisms and architectures. Neural Networks 1:17.

Hebb DO. 1949. The Organization of Behavior, a Neuropsychological Theory, NY, John Wiley.

Hecht-Nielson R. 1989. Neurocomputing, New York, Addison-Wesley.

Hinton GE. 1989. Connectionist learning procedures. Artificial Intelligence 40:185.

Hopfield JJ. 1982. Neural networks and physical systems with emergent collective computational abilities. Proc Natl Acad Sci USA 79:2554.

Houk JC, Singh SP, Fisher C, et al. 1990. An adaptive sensorimotor network inspired by the anatomy and physiology of the cerebellum. In WT Miller, RS Sutton, PJ Werbos (eds), Neural Networks for Control, pp 301–348, Mass, MIT Press, Cambridge.

Kawato M, Furukawa K, Suzuki R. 1987. A hierarchical neural-network model for control and learning of voluntary movement. Biol Cybern 57:169.

Koch C, Segev I. 1989. Methods in Neuronal Modeling: From Synapses to Networks, Cambridge, Mass, MIT Press.

Kohonen T. 1989. Self-Organization and Associative Memory, New York, Springer-Verlag.

Levin E, Gewirtzman R, Inbar GE. 1991. Neural network architecture for adaptive system modeling and control. Neural Networks 4:185.

Lippman RP. 1987. An introduction to computing with neural nets. IEEE Mag on Acoustics, Signal and Speech Proc April:4.

Miller WT, Hewes RP, Glanz FG, et al. 1990a. Real-time dynamic control of an industrial manipulator using a neural-network-based learning controller. IEEE Trans Robotics & Automation 6(1):1.

Miller WT, Sutton RS, Werbos PJ. 1990b. Neural Networks for Control, Cambridge, Mass. MIT Press.

Miyamoto H, Kawato M, Setoyama T, et al. 1988. Feedback-error-learning neural network for trajectory control of a robotic manipulator. Neural Networks 1:251.

Narendra KS. 1992. Adaptive control of dynamical systems using neural networks. In DA White, DA Sofge (eds), Handbook of Intelligent Control: Neural, Fuzzy and Adaptive Approaches, pp 141–184, New York, Van Nostrand Reinhold.

Narendra KS, Parthasarathy K. 1990. Identification and control of dynamical systems using neural networks. IEEE Trans Neural Networks 1(1):4.

Nerrand O, Roussel-Ragot P, Personnaz L, et al. 1993. Neural networks and nonlinear adaptive filtering: Unifying concepts and new algorithms. Neural Computation 5:165.

Nguyen DH, Widrow B. 1990. Neural networks for self-learning control systems. IEEE Control Systems Magazine 10(3):18.

Nordgren RE, Meckl PH. 1993. An analytical comparison of a neural network and a model-based adaptive controller. IEEE Trans Neural Networks 4(4):685.

Pao YH. 1989. Adaptive Pattern Recognition and Neural Networks, Reading, Mass, Addison-Wesley.

Pineda FJ. 1989. Recurrent backpropagation and the dynamical approach to adaptive neural computation. Neural Computation 1:161.

Quinn RD, Espenschied KS. 1993. Control of a hexapod robot using a biologically inspired neural network. In RD Beer, RE Ritzmann, T McKenna (eds), Biological Neural Networks in Invertebrate Neuroethology and Robotics, pp 365–382, New York, Academic Press.

Rumelhart DE, McClelland JL. 1988. Parallel Distributed Processing: Explorations in the Microstructure of Cognition, Cambridge, Mass, MIT Press.

Sanchez-Sinencio E, Lau C. 1992. Artificial Neural Networks: Paradigms, Applications and Hardware Implementations, New York, IEEE Press.

Schwartz EL. 1990. Computational Neuroscience, Cambridge, Mass, MIT Press.

Simpson PK. 1990. Artificial Neural Systems, New York, Pergamon Press.

Srinivasan S, Gander RE, Wood HC. 1992. A movement pattern generator model using artificial neural networks. IEEE Trans BME 39(7):716.

Taga G, Yamaguchi Y, Shimizu H. 1991. Self-organized control of bipedal locomotion by neural oscillators in unpredictable environment. Biol Cybern 65:147.

Vogl TP, Mangis JK, Rigler AK, et al. 1988. Accelerating the convergence of the back-propagation method. Biol Cybern 59:257.

Wang H, Lee TT, Graver WA. 1992. A neuromorphic controller for a three-link biped robot. IEEE Trans Sys Man Cyber 22(1):164.

Werbos PJ. 1990. Overview of designs and capabilities. In WT Miller, RS Sutton, PJ Werbos (eds), Neural Networks for Control, pp 59–66, Cambridge, Mass, MIT Press.

Werbos PJ. 1992. Approximate dynamic programming for real-time control and neural modeling. In DA White, DA Sofge (eds), Handbook of Intelligent Control: Neural, Fuzzy and Adaptive Approaches, pp 493–526, New York, Van Nostrand Reinhold.

White DA, Sofge DA. 1992. Handbook of Intelligent Control: Neural, Fuzzy, and Adaptive Approaches, New York, Van Nostrand Reinhold.

Widrow B. 1962. Generalization and information storage in networks of adaline "neurons." In MC Yovitz, TG Jacobi, G Goldstein (eds), Self-Organizing Systems. pp 435–461, Washington, DC, Spartan Books.

Williams RJ, Zipser D. 1989. A learning algorithm for continually running fully recurrent neural networks. Neural Computation 1:270.

Zurada JM. 1992. Artificial Neural Systems, New York, West.

Further Information

A good introduction to neural network basics is given in *Artificial Neural Systems* by Jacek M. Zurada. Detailed descriptions of the neural network control systems described in this chapter are provided in *Neural Network Control Systems* edited by Miller, Sutton, and Werbos and *The Handbook of Intelligent Control* edited by White & Sofge.

For journal articles on neural network theory and applications, the reader is referred to *IEEE Transactions on Neural Networks, Neural Computation* (MIT Press), and *Neural Networks* (Pergamon Press). For occasional journal articles on biomedical applications of neural networks, the reader is referred to *IEEE Transactions on Biomedical Engineering*.

161

Methods and Tools for Identification of Physiologic Systems

Vasilis Z. Marmarelis
University of
Southern California

The problem of *system identification* in physiology derives its importance from the need to acquire *quantitative models* of physiologic function (from the subcellular to the organ system level) by use of experimental observations (data). Quantitative models can be viewed as summaries of experimental observations that allow scientific inference and organize our knowledge regarding the functional properties of physiologic systems. Selection of the proper (mathematical or computational) form of the model is based on existing knowledge of the system's functional organization. System identification is the process by which the system model is determined from data. This modeling and identification problem is rather challenging in the general case of a physiologic system, where insufficient knowledge about the internal workings of the system or its usually confounding complexity prevents the development of an explicit model. The models may assume diverse forms (requiring equally diverse approaches) depending on the specific characteristics of the physiologic system (e.g., static/dynamic, linear/nonlinear) and the prevailing experimental conditions (e.g., noise contamination of data, limitations on experimental duration). This chapter will not address the general modeling issue, but rather it will concentrate on specific methods and tools that can be employed in order to accomplish the system identification task in most cases encountered in practice. Because of space limitations, the treatment of these system identification methods will be consistent with the style of a review article providing overall perspective and guidance while deferring details to cited references.

Since the complexity of the physiologic system identification problem rivals its importance, we begin by demarcating those areas where effective methods and tools currently exist. The selection among candidate models is made on the basis of the following key functional characteristics: (1) static or dynamic; (2) linear or nonlinear; (3) stationary or nonstationary; (4) deterministic or stochastic; (5) single or multiple inputs and/or outputs; (6) lumped or distributed. These classification criteria do not constitute an exhaustive list but cover most cases of current interest. Furthermore, it is critical to remember that contaminating noise (be it systemic or measurement-related) is always present in an actual study, and experimental constraints often limit experimentation time and the type of data obtainable from the system. Finally, the computational requirements for a practicable identification method must not be extraordinary, and the obtained results (models) must be amenable to physiologic interpretation, in addition to their demonstrated predictive ability.

0-8493-8346-3/95/$0.00+$.50
© 1995 by CRC Press, Inc.

A critical factor in determining our approach to the system modeling and identification task is the availability and quality of prior knowledge about the system under study with respect to the mechanisms that subserve its function. It can be said in general that, if sufficient knowledge about the internal mechanisms subserving the function of a system is available, then the development of an explicit model from first (physical or chemical) principles is possible, and the system modeling and identification task is immensely simplified by reducing to an estimation problem of the unknown parameters contained in the explicit model. Although the ease of this latter task depends on the manner in which the unknown parameters enter in the aforementioned explicit model, as well as on the quality of the available data, it is typically feasible. Furthermore, the obtained model is amenable to direct and meaningful physiologic interpretation. Unfortunately, it is rare that such prior knowledge (of adequate quality and quantity) is available in systems physiology. It is far more common that only limited prior knowledge is available, relative to the customary complexity of physiologic systems, that prevents the development of an explicit model from first principles and necessitates the search for a model that is compatible with the available input-output data.

Thus, the system identification problem is typically comprised of two tasks:

1. *Model Specification:* the selection or postulation of a model form suitable for the system at hand
2. *Model Estimation:* the estimation of the unknown parameters or functions contained within the specified model, using experimental data

All prior knowledge about the system under study is utilized in the model specification task. This includes results from specially designed preliminary experiments, which can be used to establish, for instance, whether the system is static or dynamic, linear or nonlinear, and so on. The model estimation task, however, relies on the quality of the available data (e.g., spectral characteristics, noise conditions, data length) and may set specific data-collection requirements.

This article will focus on practicable methods to perform both the model specification and model estimation tasks for systems/models that are *static or dynamic* and *linear or nonlinear*. Only the stationary case will be detailed here, although the potential use of nonstationary methods will be also discussed briefly when appropriate. In all cases, the models will take deterministic form, except for the presence of additive error terms (model residuals). Note that stochastic experimental inputs (and, consequently, outputs) may still be used in connection with deterministic models. The cases of multiple inputs and/or outputs (including multidimensional inputs/outputs, e.g., spatio-temporal) as well as lumped or distributed systems, will not be addressed in the interest of brevity. It will also be assumed that the data (single input and single output) are in the form of evenly sampled *time-series,* and the employed models are in discrete-time form (e.g., difference equations instead of differential equations, discrete summations instead of integrals).

In pursuing the model specification task, two general approaches have developed: *parametric* and *nonparametric.* In the parametric approach, algebraic or difference equation models are typically used to represent the input-output relation for static or dynamic systems, respectively. These models are accordingly linear or nonlinear, and contain a (typically small) number of unknown parameters. The latter may be constant or time-varying depending on whether the system or model is stationary or nonstationary. The precise form of these parametric models (e.g., degree/order of equation) must be determined in order to complete the model specification task. This precise form is either postulated a priori or guided by the data (in which case it is intertwined with the model parameter estimation task) as outlined in the following section.

In the nonparametric approach, the input-output relation is represented either analytically (in convolutional form through Volterra-Wiener expansions where the unknown quantities are kernel functions), computationally (i.e., by compiling all input-output mapping combinations in look-up tables) or graphically (in the form of operational surfaces/subspaces in phase-space). The graphical representation, of course, is subject to the three-dimensional limitation for the purpose of visual inspection. The model specification requirements for the Volterra-Wiener formulation consist of the order of system nonlinearity and system memory, and, for the computational or graphical approach, they consist of defining the appropriate phase-space mapping dimensions, as discussed below. Of the nonparametric approaches, the Volterra-Wiener (kernel) formulation has been used more extensively in a nonlinear context and will be the focus of this review, since nonlinearities are ubiquitous in physiology. Note that the nonparametric model estimation task places certain requirements on the experimental input (i.e., sufficient coverage of the frequency bandwidth and amplitude range of interest in each application) in order to secure adequate probing of the system functional characteristics.

An important hybrid approach has also developed in recent years that makes use of *block-structured* or *modular* models. These models are composed of parametric and/or nonparametric components properly connected to represent reliably the input-output relation. The model specification task for this class of models is more demanding and may utilize previous parametric and/or nonparametric modeling results. A promising variant of this approach, which derives from the general Volterra-Wiener formulation, employs *principal dynamic modes* as a canonical set of filters to represent a broad class of nonlinear dynamic systems. Another variant of the modular approach that has recently acquired considerable popularity but will not be covered in this review is the use of *artificial neural networks* to represent input-output nonlinear mappings in the form of *connectionist models*. These connectionist models are often fully parametrized, making this approach affine to parametric modeling, as well.

The relations among these approaches (parametric, nonparametric, and modular) are of critical practical importance and the subject of several recent studies [Marmarelis, 1994]. Considerable benefits may accrue from the combined use of these approaches in a cooperative manner that aims at securing the full gamut of distinct advantages specific to each approach.

In the following sections, an overview of these methodologies will be presented and the relative advantages and disadvantages in practical applications will be briefly outlined. The ultimate selection of a particular methodology hinges upon the specific characteristics of the application at hand and the prioritization of objectives by the individual investigator. Two general comments are in order:

1. No single methodology is globally superior to all others, i.e., excelling with regard to all criteria and under all possible circumstances. Judgment must be exercised in each individual case.
2. The general system identification problem is not solvable in all cases at present, and challenging problems remain for future research.

161.1 Parametric Approach

Consider the input and output time-series data, $x(n)$ and $y(n)$, respectively. If the system is *static and linear*, then we can employ the simplest (and most widely used) model of linear regression

$$y(n) = ax(n) + b + \epsilon(n) \tag{161.1}$$

to represent the input-output relation for every n, where $\epsilon(n)$ represents the noise or error term (or model residual) at each n. The unknown parameters (a,b) can be easily estimated through least-squares fitting, using a well-developed set of linear regression methods (e.g., ordinary least-squares or generalized least-squares depending on whether $\epsilon(n)$ is a white sequence).

This model can be extended to multiple inputs $\{x_1, x_2, \ldots, x_k\}$ and outputs $\{y_i\}$ as

$$y_i(n) = a_1 x_1(n) + a_2 x_2(n) + \ldots + a_k x_k(n) + b + \epsilon(n) \tag{161.2}$$

and well-developed multiple linear regression techniques exist that can be used for estimation of the unknown parameters $(a_1, a_2, \ldots, a_k, b)$ for each output y_i. Although these estimation methods are widely known and readily available in the literature—see, for instance, Eykhoff [1974] and Soderstrom and Stoica [1989]—they will be briefly reviewed at the end of this section.

In the event of nonstationarities, the regression coefficients (model parameters) will vary through time and can be estimated either in a piecewise stationary fashion over a sliding time window (batch processing) or in a recursive fashion using an adaptive estimation formula (recursive processing). The latter has been favored and extensively studied in recent years [Goodwin & Sin, 1984; Ljung, 1987; Ljung & Soderstrom, 1983], and it is briefly outlined at the end of this section.

If the system is *static and nonlinear,* then a nonlinear input-output relation

$$y(n) = \sum_{j=1}^{J} c_j P_j[x(n)] + \epsilon(n) \tag{161.3}$$

can be used as a parametric model, where the $\{P_j\}$ functions represent a set of selected nonlinear functions (e.g., powers, polynomials, sinusoids, sigmoids, exponentials or any other suitable set of functions over the range of x), and $\{c_j\}$ are the unknown parameters that can be easily estimated through linear regression—provided that the $\{P_j\}$ functions do not contain other unknown parameters in a nonlinear fashion. In the latter case, nonlinear regression methods must be used (e.g., the gradient steepest-descent method) that are well developed and readily available [Eykhoff, 1974; Ljung, 1987; Soderstrom & Stoica, 1989], although their use is far from problem-free or devoid of risk of misleading results (e.g., local minima or noise effects). Naturally, the choice of the $\{P_j\}$ functions is critical in this regard and may depend on the characteristics of the system or the type of available data.

These cases of static systems have been extensively studied to date but have only limited interest or applicability to actual physiologic systems, since the latter are typically dynamic—i.e., the output value at time n depends also on input and/or output values at other previous times (lags). Note that the possible dependence of the present output value on previous output values can be also expressed as a dependence on previous input values. Thus, we now turn to the all-important case of dynamic systems.

For linear (stationary) dynamic systems, the discrete-time parametric model takes the form of an *auto-regressive moving average with exogenous variable* (ARMAX) equation:

$$\begin{aligned}
y(n) = {} &\alpha_1 y(n-1) + \ldots + \alpha_k y(n-k) + \beta_0 x(n) + \beta_1 x(n-1) \\
&+ \ldots + \beta_l x(n-l) + w(n) + \gamma_1 w(n-1) \\
&+ \ldots + \gamma_m w(n-m)
\end{aligned} \tag{161.4}$$

were $w(n)$ represents a white noise sequence. This ARMAX model is a difference equation that expresses the present value of the output, $y(n)$, as a linear combination of k previous values of the output (AR part), l previous (and the present) values of the input (X part), and m previous (and the present) values of the white noise disturbance sequence (MA part) that compose the model residual (error). When $\gamma_i = 0$ for all $i = 1, \ldots, m$, the residuals form a white sequence, and the coefficients $(\alpha_1, \ldots, \alpha_k, \beta_0, \beta_1, \ldots, \beta_l)$ can be estimated through the ordinary least-squares procedure. However, if any γ_i is nonzero, then unbiased and consistent estimation requires generalized or extended least-squares procedures, similar to the one required for the multiple regression model of Eq. (161.2) when $\epsilon(n)$ is a nonwhite error sequence (reviewed at the end of the section).

Although the estimation of the ARMAX model parameters can be straightforward through multiple linear regression, the model specification task remains a challenge. The latter consists of determining the maximum lag values (k, l, m) in the difference equation (161.4) from given input-output data, $x(n)$ and $y(n)$. A number of statistical procedures have been devised for this purpose (e.g., weighted residual variance, Akaike information criterion), all of them based on the prediction error for given model order (k, l, m) compensated properly for the remaining degrees of freedom (i.e., the total number of data minus the number of parameters). It is critical that the prediction error (typically, in mean-square sense) be evaluated on a segment of input-output data distinct from the one used for the estimation of the model parameters. Application of these criteria is repeated successively for ascending values of the model order (k, l, m), and the model specification process is completed when an extremum (minimum or maximum, depending on the criterion) is achieved [Soderstrom & Stoica, 1989].

For nonlinear (stationary) systems, the ARMAX model can be extended to the NARMAX model (nonlinear ARMAX) that includes nonlinear expressions of the variables on the right side of Eq. (161.4) [Billings & Voon, 1984]. For instance, a second-degree multinomial NARMAX model of order $(k = 2, l = 1, m = 0)$ with additive white-noise residuals takes the form

$$
\begin{aligned}
y(n) = {} & \alpha_1 y(n-1) + \alpha_2 y(n-2) + \alpha_{1,1} y^2(n-1) + \alpha_{1,2} y(n-1)y(n-2) \\
& + \alpha_{2,2} y^2(n-2) + \beta_0 x(n) + \beta_1 x(n-1) + \beta_{0,0} x^2(n) \\
& + \beta_{0,1} x(n)x(n-1) + \beta_{1,1} x^2(n-1) + \gamma_{1,0} y(n-1)x(n) \\
& + \gamma_{2,0} y(n-2)x(n) + \gamma_{1,1} y(n-1)x(n-1) \\
& + \gamma_{2,1} y(n-2)x(n-1) + w(n)
\end{aligned}
\tag{161.5}
$$

Clearly, the form of a NARMAX model may become rather unwieldy, and the model specification task (i.e., the form and degree of nonlinear terms, as well as the number of input, output, and noise lags involved in the model) is very challenging. Several approaches have been proposed for this purpose [Billings & Voon, 1984, 1986; Haber & Unbenhauen, 1990; Korenberg, 1988; Zhao & Marmarelis, 1994], and they are all rather involved computationally. However, if the structure of the NARMAX model is established, then the parameter estimation task is straightforward in a manner akin to multiple linear regression—since the unknown parameters enter linearly in the NARMAX model.

It is evident that all these multiple linear regression problems defined by Eqs. (161.2)–(161.5) can be written in a vector form:

$$
y(n) = \boldsymbol{\phi}^{\mathrm{T}}(n)\boldsymbol{\theta} + \boldsymbol{\epsilon}(n)
\tag{161.6}
$$

where $\underline{\phi}(n)$ represents the vector of all regression variables in each case, and θ denotes the unknown parameter vector. For a set of data points $(n = 1, \ldots, N)$, Eq. (161.6) yields the matrix formulation

$$
y = \Phi\boldsymbol{\theta} + \boldsymbol{\epsilon}
\tag{161.7}
$$

The ordinary least-squares (OLS) estimate of θ

$$
\hat{\boldsymbol{\theta}}^{\mathrm{OLS}} = [\Phi^{\mathrm{T}}\Phi]^{-1}\Phi^{\mathrm{T}}\boldsymbol{y}
\tag{161.8}
$$

yields unbiased and consistent estimates of minimum variance, if $\epsilon(n)$ is a white sequence; otherwise, the generalized least-squares (GLS) estimator

$$
\hat{\boldsymbol{\theta}}^{\mathrm{GLS}} = [\Phi^{\mathrm{T}}\Sigma^{-1}\Phi]^{-1}\Phi^{\mathrm{T}}\Sigma^{-1}\boldsymbol{y}
\tag{161.9}
$$

ought to be used to achieve minimum estimation variance, where Σ denotes the covariance matrix of ϵ. Practical complications arise from the fact that Σ is not a priori known and, therefore, must be either postulated or estimated from the data. The latter case, which is more realistic in actual applications, leads to an iterative procedure that may not be convergent or yield satisfactory results (i.e., start with an OLS estimate of $\boldsymbol{\theta}$; obtain a first estimate of ϵ and Σ; evaluate a first GLS estimate of the $\boldsymbol{\theta}$; obtain a second estimate of ϵ and Σ; and iterate until the process converges to a final GLS estimate of $\boldsymbol{\theta}$). As an alternative to this iterative procedure, an estimate of the *moving-average model* of the residual term:

$$\epsilon(n) = w(n) + \gamma_1 w(n-1) + \ldots + \gamma_m w(n-m) \tag{161.10}$$

may be obtained from initial OLS estimation, and the covariance matrix Σ may be estimated from Eq. (161.10). Although this alternative approach avoids problems of convergence, it does not necessarily yield satisfactory results due to the dependence on the noise model estimation of Eq. (161.10). Equivalent to this latter procedure is the *residual whitening* method, which amounts to prefiltering the data with the inverse of the transfer function corresponding to Eq. (161.10) (*prewhitening filter*), prior to OLS estimation. Finally, the parameter vector may be augmented to include the coefficients $\{\gamma_i\}$ of the moving-average model of the residuals in Eq. (161.10), leading to a *pseudo-linear* regression problem [since the estimates of $w(n)$ depend on $\hat{\theta}$] that is operationally implemented as an iterative *extended least-squares* (ELS) procedure [Billings & Voon, 1984, 1986; Ljung, 1987; Ljung & Soderstrom, 1983; Soderstrom & Stoica, 1989].

In the presence of nonstationarities, the parameter vector θ may vary through time, and its estimation may be performed either in a piecewise stationary manner (with segment-to-segment updates that may be obtained either recursively or through batch processing) or by introducing a specific parametrized time-varying structure for the parameters and augmenting the unknown parameter vector to include the additional parameters of the time-varying structure (e.g., a pth degree polynomial structure of time-varying model parameters will introduce p additional parameters for each time-varying term into the vector θ, that need be estimated from the data via batch processing).

Any batch processing approach folds back to the previously discussed least-squares estimation methods. However, the recursive approach requires a new methodological framework that updates continuously the parameter estimates on the basis of new data. This adaptive or recursive approach has gained increasing popularity in recent years, although certain important practical issues (e.g., speed of algorithmic convergence, effect of correlated noise) remain causes for concern in certain cases [Goodwin & Sin, 1984; Ljung, 1987; Ljung & Soderstrom, 1983]. The basic formulae for the recursive least-squares (RLS) algorithm are

$$\hat{\theta}(n) = \hat{\theta}(n-1) + \Psi(n) [y(n) - \phi^{T}(n) \hat{\theta}(n-1)] \tag{161.11}$$

$$\Psi(n) = \gamma(n) P(n-1) \phi(n) \tag{161.12}$$

$$P(n) = P(n-1) - \gamma(n) P(n-1) \phi(n) \phi^{T}(n) P(n-1) \tag{161.13}$$

$$\gamma(n) = [\phi^{T}(n) P(n-1) \phi(n) + \alpha(n)]^{-1} \tag{161.14}$$

where the matrix $P(n)$, the vector $\Psi(n)$ and the scalar $\gamma(n)$ are updating instruments of the algorithm computed at each step n. Note that $\{\alpha(n)\}$ denotes a selected sequence of weights for the squared prediction errors in the cost function and is often taken to be unity. This recursive algorithm can be used for on-line identification of stationary or nonstationary systems. A critical issue in the nonstationary case is the speed of algorithmic convergence relative to the time-variation of the system/model parameters. Its initialization is commonly made as: $\hat{\theta}(0) = 0$ and $P(0) = c_0 I$, where c_0 is a large positive constant (to suppress the effect of initial conditions) and I is the identity matrix.

It is important to note that when output autoregressive terms exist in the model, the regression vector $\phi(n)$ is correlated with the residual $\epsilon(n)$, and, thus, none of the aforementioned least-squares estimates of the parameter vector will converge to the actual value. This undesirable correlation weakens when the predicted output values are used at each step for the autoregressive lagged terms (*closed-loop mode* or one-step predictive model) instead of the observed output values (*open-loop mode* or global predictive model). To remedy this problem, the *instrumental variable* (IV) method has been introduced that makes use of a selected IV that is uncorrelated with the residuals but strongly correlated with the regression vector $\phi(n)$ in order to evaluate the least-squares estimate [Soderstrom & Stoica, 1989]. The IV estimates can be computed in batch or recursive fashion.

In closing this section, we should note that a host of other estimation methods has been developed through the years and that these methods are operationally affine to the foregoing ones (e.g., prediction-error methods, stochastic approximation, gradient-based methods) or represent different statistical approaches to parameter estimation (e.g., maximum likelihood, bayesian approach) including the state-space formulation of the problem, that cannot be detailed here in the interest of space [for review, see Eykhoff, 1974; Goodwin & Payne, 1977; Goodwin & Sin, 1984; Ljung, 1987; Ljung & Soderstrom, 1983; Soderstrom & Stoica, 1989].

161.2 Nonparametric Approach

In the linear stationary case, the discrete-time nonparametric model takes the convolutional form:

$$y(n) = \sum_{m=0}^{M} h(m)\, x\,(n - m) + \epsilon(n) \qquad (161.15)$$

where $\epsilon(n)$ is an output-additive error/noise term and $h(m)$ is the discrete impulse response of the linear time-invariant (stationary) system with memory extent M. For finite-memory systems (i.e., when $h(m)$ becomes negligible for $m > M$ and M is finite), the estimation of $h(m)$ from input-output data can be accomplished by multiple regression, since the model of Eq. (161.15) retains the form of a parametric model with no autoregressive terms. Note that any stable ARMAX model can be put in the form of Eq. (161.15), where $M \to \infty$ and $h(m)$ is absolute-summable. The estimation of $h(m)$ can be also accomplished in the frequency domain via discrete Fourier transforms (DFTs, implemented as FFTs), observing the fact that convolution turns into multiplication in the frequency domain. Particular attention must be paid to cases where the input DFT attains very small values to avoid numerical or estimation problems during the necessary division. In actual physiologic practice, many investigators have chosen to perform experiments with specific input waveforms to facilitate this identification task, i.e., the use of an impulsive input of unit strength directly yields $h(m)$, or the use of sinusoidal inputs of various frequencies yields directly the values of the DFT of $h(m)$ at the corresponding frequencies (covering the entire frequency range of interest).

In the nonlinear stationary case, the most widely used methodology for nonparametric modeling is based on the Volterra functional expansions and Wiener's theory that employs a gaussian white noise (GWN) test input in conjunction with a modified (orthogonalized) Volterra functional expansion. Wiener's critical contribution is in suggesting that GWN is an *effective test input* for identifying nonlinear systems of a very broad class and in proposing specific mathematical procedures for the estimation of the unknown system descriptors (kernels) from input-output data, as outlined below [for more details, see Marmarelis & Marmarelis, 1987; Rugh, 1981; Schetzen, 1980].

The input-output relation of a causal nonlinear stationary system in discrete time is seen as a mapping of a vector comprised of the input past (and present) values onto the (scalar) present value of the output:

$$y(n) = F[x(n'), n - M \le n' \le n] \qquad (161.16)$$

were M is the system memory and F is a fixed multivariate function representing this mapping—note that, in continuous time, F is a functional. If the system is nonstationary, the function F varies through time. If the function F is analytic and the system is stable, then a discrete-time Volterra series expansion exists of the form:

$$y(n) = \sum_{i=0}^{\infty} \sum_{m_1=0}^{M} \cdots \sum_{m_i=0}^{M} k_i(m_1, \ldots, m_i)\, x\,(n - m_1) \ldots x(n - m_i) \quad (161.17)$$

This series converges for any stable system within the radius of convergence defined by the input ensemble. If the multivariate function F is not analytic but is continuous, then a finite-order Volterra model can be found that achieves any desirable degree of approximation (based on the Stone-Weierstrass theorem).

The multiple convolutions of the Volterra model involve kernel functions $\{k_i(m_1, \ldots, m_i)\}$ which constitute the descriptors of the system nonlinear dynamics. Consequently, the system identification task is to obtain estimates of these kernels from input-output data. These kernel functions are symmetric with respect to their arguments.

When a sinusoidal input is used, then the ith order Volterra functional (i.e., the i-tuple convolution in the Volterra model) gives rise to output harmonics of order i, $(i - 2), \ldots, (i - 2j)$ where j is the integer part $i/2$. When an impulse $A\delta(n)$ is used as input, then the ith order Volterra functional is contributing the term $A^i k_i(n, \ldots, n)$ to the output. This suggests that the Volterra kernels of a general system cannot be separated from each other and directly determined from input-output data, unless the Volterra expansion is of finite order. For a finite-order Volterra expansion, kernel estimation can be achieved through least-squares fitting procedures [Korenberg, 1988; Stark, 1968; Watanabe & Stark, 1975] or by use of specialized test inputs such as multiple impulses or step function [Schetzen, 1965; Shi & Sun, 1990; Stark, 1968] and sums of sinusoids of incommensurate frequencies [Victor et al., 1977], although the testing and analysis procedures can be rather laborious in those cases. The latter method yields estimates of the system kernels in the frequency domain at the selected input frequencies (and their harmonic/intermodulation frequencies) with increased accuracy but with limited frequency resolution.

The inability to estimate the Volterra kernels in the general case of an infinite series prompted Wiener to suggest the orthogonalization of the Volterra series when a GWN test input is used. The functional terms of the Wiener series are constructed on the basis of a Gram-Schmidt orthogonalization procedure requiring that the covariance between any two Wiener functionals be zero. The resulting Wiener series expansion takes the form:

$$
\begin{aligned}
y(n) &= \sum_{i=0}^{\infty} G_i[h_i; x(n'), n' \leq n] \\
&= \sum_{i=0}^{\infty} \sum_{j=0}^{[i/2]} \frac{(-1)^j i! P^j}{(i - 2j)! j! 2^j} \sum_{m_1} \cdots \sum_{m_i} h_i(m_1, \ldots, m_{i-2j}, l_1, l_1, \ldots, l_j, l_j) \\
&\qquad\qquad x(n - m_1) \ldots x(n - m_{i-2j})
\end{aligned} \tag{161.18}
$$

where $[i/2]$ is the integer part of $i/2$ and P is the power level of the GWN input. The set of Wiener kernels $\{h_i\}$ is, in general, different from the set of Volterra kernels $\{k_i\}$, but specific relations exist between the two sets [Marmarelis & Marmarelis, 1978].

The Wiener kernels depend on the GWN input power level P (because they correspond to an orthogonal expansion), whereas the Volterra kernels are independent of any input characteristics. This situation can be likened to the coefficients of an orthogonal expansion of an analytic function being dependent on the interval of expansion. It is therefore imperative that Wiener kernel estimates be reported in the literature with reference to the GWN input power level that they were estimated with. When a complete set of Wiener kernels is obtained, then the complete set of Volterra kernels can be evaluated. Approximations of Volterra kernels can be obtained from Wiener kernels of the same order estimated with various input power levels. Complete Wiener or Volterra models can predict the system output to *any* given input. When the Wiener or Volterra model is incomplete, the accuracy of the predicted output will be, in general, different for the two models and will depend on each specific input.

The orthogonality of the Wiener series allows decoupling of the various Wiener functionals and the estimation of the respective Wiener kernels from input-output data through cross-correlation [Lee & Schetzen, 1965]

$$h_i(m_1, \ldots, m_i) = \frac{1}{i!P^i} E[y_i(n)x(n - m_1) \ldots x(n - m_i)] \qquad (161.19)$$

where $y_i(n)$ is the ith response residual

$$y_i(n) = y(n) - \sum_{j=0}^{i-1} G_j(n) \qquad (161.20)$$

The simplicity and elegance of the cross-correlation technique led to its adoption by many investigators in modeling studies of nonlinear physiologic systems [see McCann & Marmarelis, 1975; Marmarelis, 1987, 1989, 1994; Marmarelis & Marmarelis, 1978; Stark, 1968].

Since the ensemble average of Eq. (161.19) is implemented in practice by time-averaging over a finite data-record, and since GWN is not physically realizable, many important practical issues had to be explored in actual applications of the cross-correlation technique. To name but a few: the generation of appropriate quasi-white test signals (that adequately approximate the ideal and not physically realizable GWN); the choice of input bandwidth relative to the system bandwidth; the accuracy of the obtained kernel estimates as a function of input bandwidth and record length; the effect of extraneous noise and experimental imperfections. An extensive study of some of these practical considerations can be found in Marmarelis and Marmarelis [1978] and in Marmarelis [1979].

A broad class of effective quasi-white test signals (CSRS) has been introduced that can be easily generated on the computer and may follow any zero-mean symmetric (discrete or continuous) amplitude probability density function [Marmarelis, 1977]. The use of this type of test signal allows through analysis of kernel estimation errors via cross-correlation and the optimization of the input bandwidth B (for given record length N) on the basis of a total mean-square error (TMSE) criterion for the ith-order kernel estimate given by:

$$(\text{TMSE})_i = \frac{a_i}{B^4} + \frac{b_i B^{i-1}}{N} \qquad (161.21)$$

where a_i and b_i are positive constants characteristic of the ith-order kernel [Marmarelis, 1979].

The cross-correlation technique results in considerable variance in the kernel estimates, unless very long data-records are available, because of the stochastic nature of the input. This has prompted the use of pseudo-random m-sequences [Billings & Fakhouri, 1981; Moller, 1983; Ream, 1970; Sutter, 1992]—which can reduce considerably the data-record requirements and yield improved estimation accuracy, provided that proper attention is given to certain problems in their high-order autocorrelation functions. To the same end, frequency-domain methods have been proposed for kernel estimation [Brillinger, 1970; French, 1976; Victor et al., 1977] yielding computational savings in some cases and offering a different perspective for the interpretation of results.

To reduce the requirements of long experimental data records and improve the kernel estimation accuracy, least-squares methods also can be used to solve the classical linear *inverse problem* described earlier in Eq. (161.6), where the parameter vector $\boldsymbol{\theta}$ includes all discrete kernel values of the finite Volterra model of Eq. (161.17), which is linear in these unknown parameters (i.e., kernel values). Least-squares methods also can be used in connection with orthogonal expansions of the kernels to reduce the number of unknown parameters, as outlined below. Note that solution of this inverse problem via OLS requires inversion of a large square matrix with dimensions $[(M + I + 1)!/((M + 1)!I!)]$, where M is the kernel memory and I is the (maximum) nonlinear order of the Volterra model. Since direct inversion of this matrix may require considerable computing effort and be subject to conditioning problems, it is often expedient to solve this inverse problem by use of QR decomposition that offers certain computational and numerical advantages. One such implementation is Korenberg's *exact orthogonalization method* [Korenberg, 1988], which estimates the discrete kernel values through least-squares fitting of a sequence of orthogonal vectors built from input values in accordance with the Volterra expansion (effectively forming the Q orthogonal matrix of the QR decomposition). Other numerical methods also can be used for matrix inversion, depending on the requirements of each application. Likewise, a variety of orthogonal bases can be used for kernel expansion in order to obtain a more concise representation of the kernels in each particular application. The use of the Laguerre orthogonal basis typically results in reduction of the number of unknown parameters for most physiologic system kernels (due to their built-in exponential structure), with consequent improvement in estimation accuracy [Marmarelis, 1993; Watanabe & Stark, 1975]. Thus, if $\{b_j(m)\}$ is a complete orthonormal basis defined over the system memory $[O, M]$, then the ith-order Volterra kernel can be expanded as

$$k_i(m_1, \ldots, m_i) = \sum_{j_1} \cdots \sum_{j_i} c_i(j_1, \ldots, j_i) b_{j_1}(m_1) \ldots b_{j_i}(m_i) \qquad (161.22)$$

Then the Volterra model of Eq. (161.17) takes the form:

$$y(n) = \sum_i \left\{ \sum_{j_1} \cdots \sum_{j_i} c_i(j_1, \ldots, j_i) v_{j_1}(n) \ldots v_{j_i}(n) \right\} \qquad (161.23)$$

where,

$$v_j(n) = \sum_{m=0}^{M} b_j(m) x(n - m) \qquad (161.24)$$

and the expansion coefficients $\{c_i(j_1, \ldots, j_i)\}$ of the unknown kernels can be estimated through multiple regression of $y(n)$ on the multinomial terms composed of the known functions $\{v_j(n)\}$. The kernel estimates are then reconstructed on the basis of Eq. (161.22). This kernel estimation method has been shown to be far superior to the conventional cross-correlation technique in terms of estimation accuracy and robustness to noise or experimental imperfections [Marmarelis, 1993].

Based on this observation, a general model for the Volterra class of systems can be proposed that is comprised of a set of parallel linear filters with impulse response functions $\{b_j(m)\}$ whose outputs are fed into a multi-input static nonlinearity, $y = f(v_1, v_2, \ldots)$, to produce the system output. It was Wiener who first proposed the use of Laguerre functions (albeit in continuous-time form) for the set $\{b_j(m)\}$, since they are defined over the interval $[0, \infty)$ compatible with causal systems and can be generated in analog form—a fashionable mode at the time—by a simple RC ladder network. He also suggested that the multi-input static nonlinearity be expanded in terms of orthogonal hermite functions to yield a system characterization in terms of the resulting Hermite expansion coefficients that are estimated through covariance computations. For a review of this approach, see Schetzen [1980]. This approach has been viewed as rather unwieldy and has not found many applications to date. However, the use of the Laguerre expansions of kernels (in discrete time) in conjunction with least-squares fitting has been shown to be rather promising for practical kernel estimation from short and noisy data records [Marmarelis, 1993] and consequently suitable for experimental studies of physiologic systems.

The greatest obstacle to the broader use of the Volterra-Wiener approach has been the practical limitations in estimating high-order kernels due to two reasons: (1) The amount of required computations increases geometrically with the order of estimated kernel; (2) kernel functions of more than three dimensions are difficult to inspect or interpret meaningfully. As a result, application of this approach has been limited to weakly nonlinear systems (second or third order).

A practical way of overcoming this limitation in the order of estimated kernels has been recently presented as a spin-off of studies on the relation between Volterra models and feedforward artificial neural networks [Marmarelis & Zhao, 1994]. According to this approach, a perceptronlike network with polynomial activation functions is trained with the experimental data using a modified version of the back-propagation algorithm. The parameters of the resulting network can be subsequently converted to kernel estimates of arbitrary high order (although the network itself is a nonlinear model of the system on its own right). This alternative to current kernel estimation algorithms seems to hold significant promise, since it relaxes many of the requirements of existing methods (e.g., input whiteness and low-order models) at the only apparent cost of greater computing effort.

In the event of nonstationarities, the kernels become dependent on time, and their estimation can be accomplished either in a piecewise stationary manner (when the nonstationarity is slow relative to the system dynamic bandwidth) or through truly nonstationary estimation methods. In the former case, the piecewise stationary estimates can be obtained over adjacent segments or using sliding (overlapping) windows along the time record. They can be subsequently displayed in a time-ordered sequence (revealing the time-varying pattern), under the assumption of system quasi-stationarity over the data segment or sliding window. Kernel estimation through truly nonstationary methods may be accomplished by: (1) *adaptive methods,* employing the recursive least-squares formulae previously reviewed, which track changes in least-squares kernel estimates by continuous updating based on the output prediction error at each discrete step [Goodwin & Sin, 1984]; (2) *ensemble-averaging methods,* employing direct averaging of results obtained from many repetitions of identical experiments, which are rarely used because the latter is seldom feasible or practical in a physiologic experimental setting; (3) *temporal expansion methods,* employing explicit kernel expansions over time to avoid the experimental burden of the ensemble-averaging approach and the methodological constraints of adaptive methods, which utilize a single input-output data record to obtain complete nonstationary model representations under mild constraints [Marmarelis, 1981].

We note that the Volterra-Wiener approach has been extended to the case of nonlinear systems with multiple inputs and multiple outputs [Marmarelis & McCann, 1973; Marmarelis & Naka, 1974; Westwick & Kearney, 1992] where functional terms are introduced, involving cross-kernels which measure the nonlinear interactions of the inputs as reflected on the output. This extension has led to a generalization for nonlinear systems with spatio-temporal inputs that has found applications to the visual system [Citron et al., 1981; Yasui et al., 1979]. Extension of the Volterra-Wiener approach to systems with spike (action potential) inputs encountered in neurophysiology also has been made, where the GWN test input is replaced by a Poisson process of impulses [Krausz, 1975]; this approach has found many applications including the study of the hippocampal formation in the brain [Sclabassi et al., 1988]. Likewise, the case of neural systems with spike outputs has been explored in the context of the Volterra-Wiener approach, leading to efficient modeling and identification methods [Marmarelis et al., 1986; Marmarelis & Orme, 1993].

The mathematical relations between parametric (NARMAX) and nonparametric (Volterra) models have been explored, and significant benefits are shown to accrue from combined use [Zhao & Marmarelis, 1994]. These studies follow on previous efforts to relate certain classes of nonlinear differential equations with Volterra functional expansions in continuous time [Marmarelis, 1989; Rugh, 1981]

Only brief mention will be made of the computational and graphical nonparametric methods of phase-space mappings. The computational method requires prior specification of the number of input and output lags that are needed to express the present output value as

$$y(n) = G[y(n-1), \ldots, y(n-k), x(n), x(n-1), \ldots, x(n-l)] \quad (161.25)$$

where $G[\bullet]$ is an unknown function which maps the appropriate input-output vector $\mathbf{z}(n) = [y(n-1), \ldots, y(n-k), x(n), \ldots, x(n-l)]$ onto the present value of the output $y(n)$. Then, using experimental data, we compile on the computer a list of correspondences between $z(n)$ and $y(n)$ in the form of an empirical model that can predict the output for a given z by finding the closest correspondence within the compiled list (look-up table) or using a properly defined interpolation scheme.

The graphical method is based on the notion that the mathematical model of a discrete-time finite-order (stationary) dynamic system is, in general, a multivariate function $f(\bullet)$ of the appropriate lagged values of the input-output variables

$$f[y(n), y(n-1), \ldots, y(n-k), x(n), x(n-1), \ldots, x(n-l)] = 0 \quad (161.26)$$

This function (model) is a "constraint" among these input-output lagged (and present) values at each time instant n. The number of variables that partake in this relation and the particular form of $f(\bullet)$ are characteristic of the system under study. Therefore, in a geometric sense, the system (and its model) are represented by a subspace in a multidimensional space defined by the *coordinate system* of these variables. If one can define the appropriate space by choosing the relevant variables, then a model can be easily obtained by following the vector point corresponding to the data through time—provided that the input is such that the data cover the model subspace densely. If the input is ergodic, then sufficiently long observations will allow reliable estimation of the system model.

Although this is an old and conceptually straightforward idea, it has not been widely used (except in some recent studies of chaotic dynamics of autonomous systems, where no input variable exists) because several important practical issues must be addressed in its actual implementation, e.g., the selection of the appropriate coordinate variables (embedding space) and the impracticality of representation in high-dimensional spaces. If a low-dimensional embedding space can be found for the system under study, this approach can be very powerful in yielding models of strongly nonlinear systems. Secondary practical issues are the choice of an effective test input and the accuracy of the obtained results in the presence of extraneous noise.

161.3 Modular Approach

The practical limitations in the use of Volterra-Wiener models for strongly nonlinear systems have led some investigators to explore the use of block-structured or modular models in the form of cascaded or parallel configurations of linear subsystems (L) and static nonlinearities (N). This model representation often provides greater insight into the functional organization of the system under study and facilitates the identification task by allowing separate estimation of the various component subsystems (L and N), thereby avoiding the computational burden associated with the dimensionality of high-order kernel functions. The advantages afforded by this approach can be had only when prior specification of the structure of the modular model is possible.

Simple cascade models (e.g., L-N, N-L, L-N-L) have been studied extensively, yielding estimates of the component subsystems with moderate computational effort [Billings & Fakhouri, 1982; Korenberg & Hunter, 1986; Marmarelis & Marmarelis, 1978; Shi & Sun, 1990]. Distinctive kernel relationships (e.g., between first-order and second-order kernels) exist for each type of cascade model, which can be used for validation of the chosen modular model on the basis of the kernel estimates obtained from the data—a task that is often referred to as *structural identification*. Thus, the combined use of the modular and nonparametric approaches may yield considerable benefits. This idea can be extended to more complicated modular structures entailing multiple parallel and cascaded branches [Chen et al., 1990; Korenberg, 1991]. The case of nonlinear feedback in modular models attracts considerable interest, because of its frequent and critical role in physiologic control and autoregulation. A case of weak nonlinear feedback in sensory systems has received thorough treatment [Marmarelis, 1991]. Naturally, the analysis becomes more complicated as the complexity of the modular model increases. Particular mention should be made of a rather complex model of parallel L-N-L cascades (usually called the S_m model) that covers a broad class of nonlinear systems [Billings & Fakhouri, 1981; Rugh, 1981].

A method for the development of a general model for the Volterra-Wiener class of systems, which assumes a modular form, was originally proposed by Wiener and his associates and is reviewed in Schetzen [1980]. A general modular model, comprised of parallel L-N cascades, also has been proposed by Korenberg [1991], and another, employing *principal dynamic modes* as a filterbank whose outputs feed into a multi-input static nonlinearity, has been recently proposed by Marmarelis [1994].

This latter general model evolved from the original Wiener modular model. It was first adapted to studies of neural systems that generate spikes (action potentials), whereby a threshold-trigger is placed at the output of the general modular model that obviates the use of high-order kernels and yields a parsimonious complete model [Marmarelis & Orme, 1993]. The importance of this development is found in that, ever since the Volterra-Wiener approach was applied to the study of spike-output neural systems, it had been assumed that a large number of kernels would be necessary to produce a satisfactory model prediction of the timing of output spikes, based on the rationale that the presence of a spike-generating mechanism constitutes a *hard nonlinearity*. Although this rationale is correct if we seek to reproduce the numerical binary values of the system output using a conventional Volterra-Wiener model, the inclusion of a threshold trigger in our modular model yields a compact and complete model (of possibly low order) that predicts precisely the timing of the output spikes [Marmarelis et al., 1986]. This also led to a search for the principal pathways of dynamic transformations of neural signals using eigen-decomposition of a matrix composed of the Laguerre expansion coefficients of the first- and second-order kernels [Marmarelis & Orme, 1993]. The estimation of these principal dynamic modes is accomplished via the aforementioned eigen-decomposition [Marmarelis, 1994] or through the training of a specific artificial neural network (a modified perceptron with polynomial activation functions) using a modified back-propagation algorithm [Marmarelis & Zhao, 1994]. The latter method holds great promise in providing a practical solution to the ultimate problem of nonlinear system identification, because it is not limited to low-order nonlinearities and does not place stringent requirements on the necessary input-output data, but it does retain a remarkable degree of robustness in the presence of noise.

Acknowledgment

This work was supported in part by Grant No. RR-01861 awarded to the Biomedical Simulations Resource at the University of Southern California from the National Center for Research Resources of the National Institutes of Health.

References

Billings SA, Fakhouri SY. 1981. Identification of nonlinear systems using correlation analysis and pseudorandom inputs. Int J Systems Sci 11:261.

Billings SA, Fakhouri SY. 1982. Identification of systems containing linear dynamic and static nonlinear elements. Automatica 18:15.

Billings SA, Voon WSF 1984. Least-squares parameter estimation algorithms for non-linear systems. Int J Systems Sci 15:601.

Billings SA, Voon WSF. 1986. A prediction-error and stepwise-regression estimation algorithm for non-linear systems. Int J Control 44:803.

Brillinger DR. 1970. The identification of polynomial systems by means of higher order spectra. J Sound Vib 12:301.

Chen H-W, Jacobson LD, Gaska JP. 1990. Structural classification of multi-input nonlinear systems. Biol Cybern 63:341.

Citron MC, Kroeker JP, McCann GD. 1981. Non-linear interactions in ganglion cell receptive fields. J Neurophysiol 46:1161.

Eykhoff P. 1974. System Identification: Parameter and State Estimation. New York, Wiley.

French AS. 1976. Practical nonlinear system analysis by Wiener kernel estimation in the frequency domain. Biol Cybern 24:111.

Goodwin GC, Payne RL. 1977. Dynamic System Identification: Experiment Design and Data Analysis. New York, Academic Press.

Goodwin GC, Sin KS. 1984. Adaptive Filtering, Prediction and Control. Englewood Cliffs, NJ, Prentice-Hall.

Haber R, Unbenhauen H. 1990. Structure identification of nonlinear dynamic systems—a survey of input/output approaches. Automatica 26:651.

Korenberg MJ. 1988. Identifying nonlinear difference equation and functional expansion representations: The fast orthogonal algorithm. Ann Biomed Eng 16:123.

Korenberg MJ. 1991. Parallel cascade identification and kernel estimation for nonlinear systems. Ann Biomed Eng 19:429.

Korenberg MJ, Hunter IW. 1986. The identification of nonlinear biological systems: LNL cascaded models. Biol Cybern 55:125.

Krausz HI. 1975. Identification of nonlinear systems using random impulse train inputs. Biol Cybern 19:217.

Lee YW, Schetzen M. 1965. Measurement of the Wiener kernels of a nonlinear system by cross-correlation. Int J Control 2:237.

Ljung L. 1987. System Identification: Theory for the User, Englewood Cliffs, NJ, Prentice-Hall.

Ljung L, Soderstrom T. 1983. Theory and Practice of Recursive Identification. Cambridge, Mass, MIT Press.

Marmarelis PZ, Marmarelis VZ. 1978. Analysis of Physiological Systems: The White-Noise Approach, New York, Plenum. Russian translation: Mir Press, Moscow, 1981. Chinese translation: Academy of Sciences Press, Beijing, 1990.

Marmarelis PZ, McCann GD. 1973. Development and application of white-noise modeling techniques for studies of insect visual nervous system. Kybernetik 12:74.

Marmarelis PZ, Naka K-I. 1974. Identification of multi-input biological systems. IEEE Trans Biomed Eng 21:88.

Marmarelis VZ (ed). 1987. Advanced methods of physiological system modeling: Volume I, Biomedical Simulations Resource, University of Southern California, Los Angeles.

Marmarelis VZ (ed). 1989. Advanced Methods of Physiological System Modeling: Volume II, New York, Plenum.

Marmarelis VZ (ed). 1994. Advanced Methods of Physiological System Modeling: Volume III, New York, Plenum.

Marmarelis VZ. 1977. A family of quasi-white random signals and its optimal use in biological system identification: I. Theory. Biol Cybern 27:49.

Marmarelis VZ. 1979. Error analysis and optimal estimation procedures in identification of nonlinear Volterra systems. Automatica 15:161.

Marmarelis VZ. 1981. Practicable identification of nonstationary nonlinear systems. Proc IEE, Part D 128:211.

Marmarelis VZ. 1989. Identification and modeling of a class of nonlinear systems. Math Comp Mod 12:991.

Marmarelis VZ. 1991. Wiener analysis of nonlinear feedback in sensory systems. Ann Biomed Eng 19:345.

Marmarelis VZ. 1993. Identification of nonlinear biological systems using Laguerre expansions of kernels. Ann Biomed Eng 21:573.

Marmarelis VZ. 1994. Nonlinear modeling of physiological systems using principal dynamic modes. In VZ Marmarelis (ed), Advanced Methods of Physiological System Modeling: Volume III, pp. 1–28, New York, Plenum.

Marmarelis VZ, Citron MC, Vivo CP. 1986. Minimum-order Wiener modeling of spike-output systems. Biol Cybern 54:115.

Marmarelis VZ, Orme ME. 1993. Modeling of neural systems by use of neuronal modes. IEEE Trans Biomed Eng 40:1149.

Marmarelis VZ, Zhao X. 1994. On the relation between Volterra models and feedforward artificial neural networks. In VZ Marmarelis (ed), Advanced Methods of Physiological System Modeling: Volume III, pp. 243–260, New York, Plenum.

McCann GD, Marmarelis PZ (eds). 1975. Proceedings of the First Symposium on Testing and Identification of Nonlinear Systems, Pasadena, Calif, California Institute of Technology.

Moller AR. 1983. Use of pseudorandom noise in studies of frequency selectivity: The periphery of the auditory system. Biol Cybern 47:95.

Ream N. 1970. Nonlinear identification using inverse repeat m-sequences. Proc IEEE 117:213.

Rugh WJ. 1981. Nonlinear System Theory: The Volterra/Wiener Approach. Baltimore, Johns Hopkins University Press.

Schetzen M. 1965. Measurement of the kernels of a nonlinear system of finite order. Int J Control 2:251.

Schetzen M. 1980. The Volterra and Wiener Theories of Nonlinear Systems, New York, Wiley.

Sclabassi RJ, Krieger DN, Berger TW. 1988. A systems theoretic approach to the study of CNS function. Ann Biomed Eng 16:17.

Shi J, Sun HH. 1990. Nonlinear system identification for cascade block model: An application to electrode polarization impedance. IEEE Trans Biomed Eng 37:574.

Soderstrom T, Stoica P. 1989. System Identification, London, Prentice-Hall International.

Stark L. 1968. Neurological Control Systems: Studies in Bioengineering, New York, Plenum.

Sutter E. 1992. A deterministic approach to nonlinear systems analysis. In RB Pinter, B Nabet (eds), Nonlinear Vision, pp. 171–220, Boca Raton, Fla, CRC Press.

Victor JD, Shapley RM, Knight BW. 1977. Nonlinear analysis of retinal ganglion cells in the frequency domain. Proc Natl Acad Sci 74:3068.

Watanabe A, Stark L. 1975. Kernel method for nonlinear analysis: Identification of a biological control system. Math Biosci 27:99.

Westwick DT, Kearney RE. 1992. A new algorithm for identification of multiple input Wiener systems. Biol Cybern 68:75.

Yasui S, Davis W, Naka KI. 1979. Spatio-temporal receptive field measurement of retinal neurons by random pattern stimulation and cross-correlation. IEEE Trans Biomed Eng 26:263.

Zhao X, Marmarelis VZ. 1994. Identification of parametric (NARMAX) models from estimated Volterra kernels. In VZ Marmarelis (ed), Advanced Methods of Physiological System Modeling: Volume III, pp 211–218, New York, Plenum.

162

Clinical Care of Patients with Closed-Loop Drug Delivery Systems

Eileen A. Woodruff
PA Consulting Group

A closed-loop drug delivery system applies control theory techniques to assist the clinician in providing clinical care to the patient. Drug is administered to a patient for either clinical therapy or diagnosis. The drug is administered from a drug delivery device (e.g., infusion pump), and the drug infusion rate is adjusted by the closed-loop algorithm or controller.

Typical components of a closed-loop drug delivery system are the patient, a monitor, a pump, and a control algorithm (Fig. 162.1). The patient receives drug from the pump and provides a pharmacologic response to the drug. This drug response from the patient is captured by the monitor. The monitor contains a transducer that converts the measured physical quantity into its electrical equivalent. An algorithm within the monitor calculates the numeric value of the patient's response to the drug. This response is a feedback parameter to the control algorithm. The control algorithm uses this feedback parameter value along with clinician-supplied parameters (e.g., setpoint, time or ramp to setpoint, cumulative drug dose) to determine the next infusion rate. A supervisor or safety shell may oversee the control algorithm to ensure that the closed-loop system remains stable and does not become a nonminimum phase or positive feedback system.

Closed-loop drug delivery (CLDD) systems are developed for therapeutic and diagnostic purposes. Therapeutic CLDD systems assist the clinician in administering a drug to achieve specific clinical objectives. These drugs usually have a narrow therapeutic index. Examples of clinical objectives for CLDD systems are to improve cardiovascular performance of patient, to annihilate reproduction of cancer cells through chemotherapy, to regulate glucose levels in Type-1 diabetics, and to regulate depth of anesthesia. The therapeutic CLDD system objectives are to improve patient care, improve quality of life for patients, and improve patient outcome. These objectives can be accomplished by diminishing the site and frequency of undershoots and overshoots of drug delivered and feedback parameter, and decreasing cumulative dose (especially for drugs that have toxic effects such as sodium nitroprusside with cyanide toxicity). Diagnostic CLDD systems deliver a drug to create a controlled perturbation in the patient's physical state to aid in clinical diagnosis. Examples of patient diagnoses are coronary artery disease and myocardial ischemia.

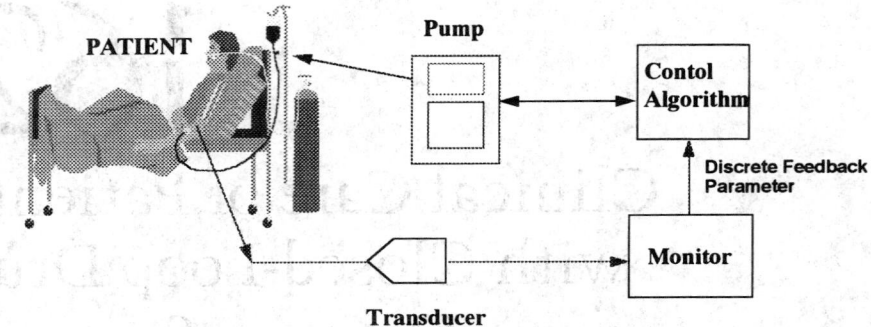

FIGURE 162.1   Illustration of closed-loop drug delivery system.

Developments of CLDD systems began in the early 1970s. All these early CLDD systems were for patient therapy. Among the pioneers that developed these therapeutic CLDD systems were Louis Sheppard, Bernard Widrow, and Michael Albisser.

Louis Sheppard used measurements of left atrial pressures to control the rate of blood replacement [Sheppard, 1980]. A short time later, Slate and Sheppard [1982] developed a mean arterial pressure using sodium nitroprusside.

Bernard Widrow [1971] with the support of Cristy Shade [1973] used adaptive control techniques to regulate mean arterial pressure while infusing vasoconstrictor drugs to canines. This research was performed at Stanford University in the early 1970s.

Michael Albisser and coworkers measured arterial blood glucose concentrations and infused intravenous insulin to control blood glucose levels in type-1 diabetics. This prototype was the first computer-controlled artificial pancreas at the Hospital for Sick Children in Toronto, Canada [Brunetti, 1991]. The first report of clinical application was at the annual meeting of the American Diabetes Association in 1973.

The effort required to develop a CLDD system depends on whether it is intended to be a commercial product. Typically, noncommercial products are developed in a university setting to be used at an affiliated medical institution. The rules and regulations for product development for noncommercial and commercial devices are distinctly different. In the former case, the institutional review board of the medical institution approves testing and uses of the product. In the latter case, the companies are governed by regulatory agencies (e.g., Food and Drug Administration) and must abide by the guidelines and code of federal regulations for manufacturing and marketing a commercial product. Examples of noncommercial and commercial products are presented later in this chapter.

The major issues surrounding development of CLDD devices are: (1) availability of less invasive biosensor technology; (2) availability of multidrug controllers, that require multiple input/multiple output control laws; and (3) acceptance by the medical community that a machine is capable of delivering dangerous drugs. Furthermore, if the CLDD system is implantable, there are two additional issues: (1) biocompatibility of material used in implantable system; and (2) drug stability.

162.1 Fundamentals of Closed-Loop Drug Delivery

A closed-loop delivery control system adjusts its output response in accordance to a control input or reference signal and the feedback signal from the monitor (Fig. 162.2). This feedback signal from the monitor is compared to the reference signal to calculate an error signal. The control algorithm adjusts its output in order to reduce the error signal to zero. Control theory provides many mathematical approaches for transforming the error signal into a control output. This theory encompasses

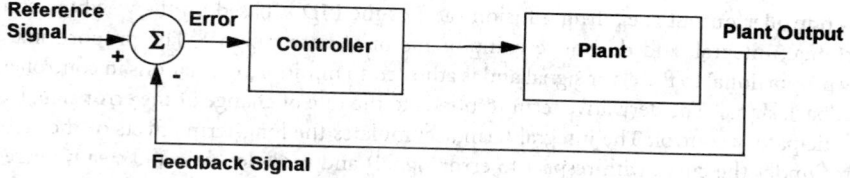

FIGURE 162.2　Block diagram of general closed-loop system.

four input-output controller structures that are: (1) single input, single output (SISO), (2) single input, multiple output (SIMO); (3) multiple input, single output (MISO); and (4) multiple input, multiple output (MIMO).

There are several classes of controllers used in control theory to adjust the controller outputs based on the controller inputs (i.e., reference signal, feedback parameter). Figure 162.3 describes these controller classes that are either classical, modern, or fuzzy. In these controller classes, the controller parameters are fixed and do not adapt to varying system dynamics caused by inter- and intrapatient variability. Adaptive control theory provides a mechanism to adapt the control parameters to changing plant dynamics.

The control laws that have been applied to medical applications are described in this chapter. These controller classes are proportional-integral-derivative (PID), adaptive, and fuzzy/rule-based. There is a significant discussion on adaptive control, since it has been most widely used in CLDD. There are other classical control laws—such as state-variable feedback and series compensators—and modern control laws for optimal control that are not discussed as they have not been used extensively in development of closed-loop drug delivery systems.

Classical Control

Classical control theory includes proportional-integral-derivative (PID), state variable feedback (SVF), and series compensation for control laws. These control laws are defined in both the continuous (*s*-plane) and discrete (*z*-plane) domains. Furthermore, these controllers are used when the plant or system dynamics are well defined under all operating conditions. The most frequently used classical controller used for closed-loop drug delivery systems is the PID controller.

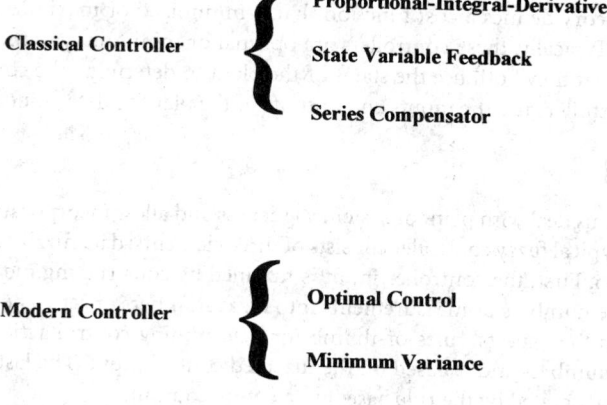

FIGURE 162.3　Classical and modern control law classes.

The controller output (i.e., drug infusion rate) of the PID is based on the weighted sum of the proportional, integral, and derivative components of the error signal. The proportional term is directly proportional to the error signal and is adjusted to minimize oscillations in controller output and feedback signal. The derivative term responds to the rate of change of the error signal and provides anticipatory control. The integral term accumulates the long-term effects of the error signal (i.e., area under the curve with respect to error signal) and provides slow and steady correction to control output.

The continuous form of the PID control law is:

$$u(t) = K_p e(t) + K_d \frac{de(t)}{dt} + K_i \int_0^t e(t) \qquad (162.1)$$

where K_p, K_d, K_i are the proportional, derivative, and integral gains of the PID control law; $e(t)$ and $u(t)$ are the error signal and the control output.

One form of a discrete PID controller is

$$u(k) = K_p \bullet e(k) + \frac{K_d}{h} \bullet [e(k) - e(k-1)]$$

$$+ \left\{ \frac{K_i \bullet h}{2} [e(k) + e(k-1)] + I_{k-1} \right\} \qquad (162.2)$$

$$I_k = \frac{K_i \bullet h}{2} [e(k) + e(k-1)]$$

where h is the sampling interval; k is the discrete time index; K_p, K_d, and K_i are the proportional, derivative, and integral controller gains; $e(k)$ is the error signal at discrete time index k and is referred to as the controller input; and $u(k)$ is the infusion rate at discrete time index k and is referred to as the controller output. In this control law the derivative was computed using 2-point central difference, and the integral applying trapezoidal integration. This is one form of a discrete PID control law; however, this controller may have different mathematical representations based on the implementations of derivative and integration components of this control law.

Modern Control

Modern control theory defines a cost function that is minimized or maximized to determine the controller output. Typically, these controllers are optimal or minimum variance. Optimal control resembles SVF in that they both use the states of the plant to determine the control output. Minimum variance controllers use the inputs and outputs of the plant to determine the control output.

Fuzzy Control

Fuzzy control systems deal with plant or system vagueness and allow incorporation of expert's rules into controller. A typical fuzzy controller consists of three elements: data fuzzification, rule base, and data defuzzification. First, the controller input is fuzzified by constructing membership functions that convert precise numbers or measurements into fuzzy numbers or sets. The rule base of a fuzzy controller contains the experts' rules-of-thumb for determining control action. This rule base is specified in fuzzy numbers and is based on the fuzzified control input. The last step is to defuzzify the control values generated by the rule base into a control output.

Adaptive Control

Adaptive control theory is the most practical technique for closed-loop drug delivery systems because the plant dynamics vary between and within patients. All the control classes may include an adaptation mechanism to modify the controller parameters as the plant dynamics change.

An adaptive control system combines a parameter estimator with a control law. In this case, the control law considers the parameter estimates to be the true parameters. This concept of using the parameter estimates as true parameters for design purposes is called *certainty equivalence adaptive control*. Adaptive controllers account for variability in system dynamics and disturbance characteristics.

A block diagram of an adaptive control system is illustrated in Fig. 162.4. There are two major classifications of adaptive control systems that are referred to as *direct* and *indirect*. In the indirect approach, the system parameters are estimated on-line, and the design calculations for the control law are based on the estimated parameters. This is called the indirect method because the control law evaluation is achieved via the system model.

In the direct method, the system model parameters are directly characterized by the controller parameters. This approach simplifies the design calculations by directly updating control law parameters.

Four frequently used adaptive controllers used in CLDD systems are gain scheduling (GS), multiple model adaptive control (MMAC), model reference adaptive system (MRAS), and self-tuning regulator (STR). Gain scheduling (Fig. 162.5) is the simplest form of adaptive control. It requires little knowledge of plant dynamics, and controller parameters can be changed very quickly. However, this technique has no feedback to compensate for an incorrect schedule and may provide sluggish control.

MMAC (Fig. 162.6) is a technique that has built-in constraints on parameter estimates because there is a bank of models that estimate plant dynamics. This technique uses an a posteriori probability function to determine the model in the model bank that is nearest to the plant dynamics. The disadvantages of this technique are a significant amount of a priori knowledge of plant dynamics, only a finite number of models are available within constraints, and for MIMO control the number of models in the model bank increases significantly.

MRAS (Fig. 162.7) requires minimal a priori knowledge of the plant dynamics. However, there is no guarantee of stability for parameter estimates of plant dynamics. An STR (Fig. 162.8) is extremely flexible and requires little a priori knowledge of plant parameters. Its disadvantage is that there is no guarantee of stability for parameter estimates of plant dynamics.

The MMAC, MRAS, and STR all require a model of plant dynamics to update the controller parameters. The model of plant dynamics is dependent on the a priori information available. For instance, MMAC needs to have adequate knowledge of the plant dynamics in order to develop the model bank. This bank of models will incorporate the knowledge of the plant dynamics and is not a black box model. In the MRAS and STR adaptive controllers, there is little a priori knowledge of the plant dynamics, so a black box model is used to estimate plant dynamics.

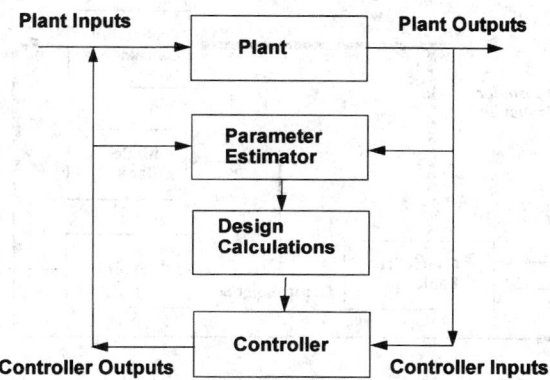

FIGURE 162.4 Block diagram of general adaptive control system.

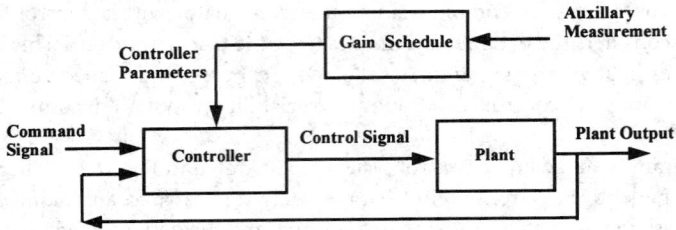

FIGURE 162.5   Block diagram of a gain-scheduling (GS) adaptive control system.

Linear black box model structures that are typically used to estimate plant dynamics are autoregressive (AR), autoregressive with inputs (ARX), autoregressive moving average (ARMA), and an autoregressive moving average with inputs (ARMAX).

The most common linear black box model used in CLDD is ARMA or ARMAX. An ARMAX model has the form:

$$y(k) = \frac{B(q^{-1})u(k)}{A(q^{-1})} + \frac{C(q^{-1})e(k)}{A(q^{-1})}$$

$$A(q^{-1}) = 1 + a_1 q^{-1} + a_2 q^{-2} + \ldots + a_n q^{-n}$$

$$B(q^{-1}) = 1 + b_1 q^{-1} + b_2 q^{-2} + \ldots + b_l q^{-1} \tag{162.3}$$

$$C(q^{-1}) = 1 + c_1 q^{-1} + c_2 q^{-2} + \ldots + c_m q^{-m}$$

In Eq. 162.3, A, B, and C are polynomials in the discrete shift operator q where a_i, b_j, and c_l are coefficients in these polynomials; $u(k)$, $y(k)$ and $e(k)$ are the model input, model output, and noise, respectively, at discrete time index k. In the ARMA structure $B(q^{-1}) = 1$; in the AR implementation $B(q^{-1})$ and $C(q^{-1}) = 1$; and in the ARX implementation $C(q^{-1}) = 1$.

Most of the adaptive controllers require an unconstrained or constrained parameter estimation technique to estimate the model and/or controller parameters. Unconstrained parameter estimation algorithms include least-squares (LS), extended least-squares (ELS), maximum likelihood (ML), and Kalman filter (KF). Constrained estimation techniques include a projection algorithm

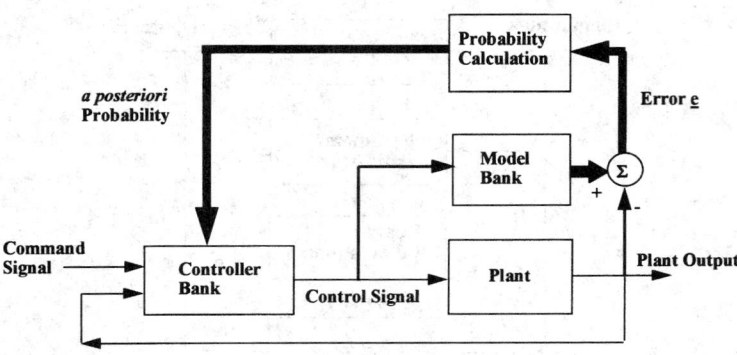

FIGURE 162.6   Block diagram of a multiple model adaptive control (MMAC) system.

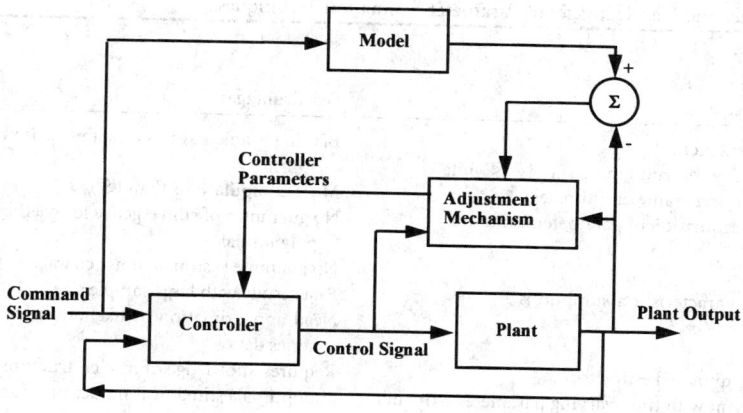

FIGURE 162.7 Block diagram of a model reference adaptive control (MRAC) system.

and constrained least-squares. Table 162.1 lists the advantages and disadvantages of the unconstrained and constrained parameter estimation techniques.

Supervisor

Control theory design does not account for the unphysiologic disturbances that occur in the clinical environment. So, a supervisor (Fig. 162.9) oversees the controller conditions and provides intelligence in the control system to avoid overaggressive or sluggish control caused by unphysiologic disturbances (e.g., arterial line flush or blood draw, change of drug concentration, low levels of anesthesia allowing pain stimuli, drug concentration in syringe or bag may change after start of delivery). Furthermore, the supervisor provides the intelligence to switch between different control laws if available, inject learning signals to identify the plant dynamics, and provide rules for controller output (e.g., maximum infusion rate) as defined by manufacturer's drug-specific labeling.

162.2 Applications and Examples of a Closed-Loop Drug Delivery System

This section provides examples of recent noncommercial and commercial CLDD systems that have been tested in the clinical environment. This section is not a comprehensive review of all closed-loop drug delivery systems or devices.

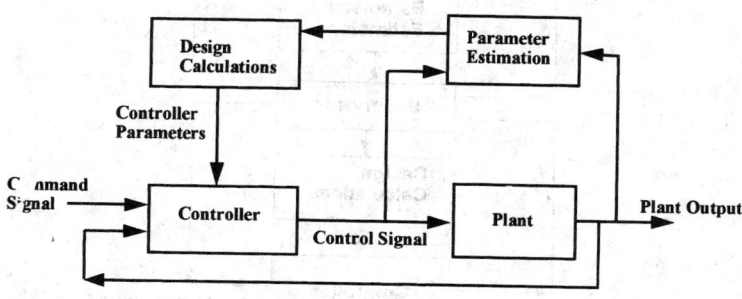

FIGURE 162.8 Block diagram of a self-tuning regulator (STR) adaptive control system.

TABLE 162.1   Advantages and Disadvantages of Parameter Estimation Techniques.

Parameter Estimation Technique	Advantages	Disadvantages
LS	Easy to implement Always find global minimum, if noise is white	Bias in parameter estimates if noise is not white
ELS	Reduce bias in parameter estimates Improved estimation of parameter estimates	More computations than LS No guarantee of convergence for coefficients in $C(q^{-1})$ polynomial No guarantee estimate noise characteristic correctly
ML	No noise-characteristic assumptions	Best results with large sample size Need approximation to likelihood function for time series data
KF	Best linear unbiased estimator Improvement with time-varying parameter estimates Excellent with short data records	Requires knowledge of model structure Suboptimal estimator if model structure is nonlinear
Constrained	May eliminate divergence of parameter estimates due to outliers or large perturbations	Significantly increases number of numerical computations Potential increase in covergence time of parameter estimate

Noncommercial CLDD Systems

Several noncommercial CLDD systems that have been used in the clinical environment were developed for patient therapy. No investigators have developed CLDD systems for diagnostic purposes. Noncommercial CLDD systems have been developed to control blood pressure and neuromuscular blockade.

Many investigators [Colvin & Kenny, 1989; Martin, 1987; Packer, 1987; Ruiz, 1993; Reid & Kenny, 1987] have developed closed-loop drug delivery systems for blood pressure. There are two reasons for this vast interest in blood pressure CLDD systems: (1) The blood pressure transducer is available; and (2) the early pioneers developed systems for blood pressure.

Packer [1987] developed a rule-based controller with an adaptive gain-tuning mechanism to regulate mean arterial pressure by titrating several drugs—sodium nitroprusside (SNP), nitroglycerin, dopamine, dobutamine, norepinephrine, and epinephrine. Adaptation was included in the control scheme to account for inter- and intrapatient variability in drug sensitivity. The model used for the

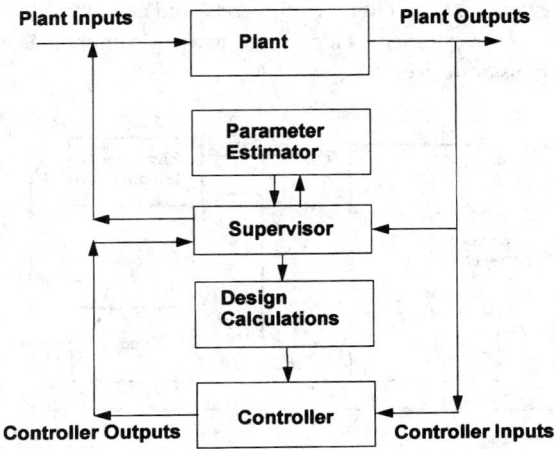

FIGURE 162.9 Block diagram of adaptive closed-loop system with supervisor.

adaptation mechanism of SNP was based on Slate's model [1980]. The control sample period is 2 min and an incremental infusion rate was computed based on the look-up table. This look-up table was defined by a manual control protocol. The feedback parameter, mean arterial pressure (MAP), was sampled every 5 s. This frequency of sampling MAP provided the opportunity to determine the quality of the blood pressure signal. McKinley [1991] reported that this closed-loop system is more effective than manual control in managing acute disturbances in the seriously ill patients. This conclusion resulted from clinical study of 74 patients in general and open heart ICUs at Royal Melbourne Hospital, Victoria, Australia.

Ruiz [1993] developed a ruled-based closed-loop controller that incorporates fuzzy logic to infuse SNP for the regulation of MAP. The fuzzy logic accounts for uncertainty as a means for including clinical expertise in this algorithm. Four distinct areas surround the MAP setpoint or target of which the most important is the target gap. The target gap is 10 mmHg wide and is above the target MAP. As long as the MAP is within the target gap there is no error. The control sample rate is 20 s, and the blood pressure sampling frequency is 200 samples per second. Infusion rate is updated in two consecutive steps. The first step uses a rule-base with fuzzy logic to determine what control approach to implement. The second step implements the control approach determined by the first step. The control law implemented in the second step has two modes—transient and optimal. The transient controller calculates a new infusion rate when the MAP is outside the target gap. The optimal control mode computes infusion rate when MAP is within the target gap. A clinical trial with this controller was conducted in 60 patients (20 with manual control) requiring SNP therapy for systemic arterial hypertension following cardiac surgery. This author reported that the closed-loop SNP controller enhanced patient care by improving blood pressure control and reducing nursing time for manual SNP titration.

Reid and Kenny [1987] developed a nonlinear PID controller to regulate systolic pressure by administering SNP. The control law was nonlinear because a set of rules defined a means for updating the controller gain. This approach was similar to the technique developed by Slate and Sheppard [1982]. They performed a clinical study of 60 patients (30 automatic and 30 manual control) to examine clinical benefits of system. The results of this study indicated that automatic titration of systolic blood pressure was controlled within a narrower range than that achieved in manual control. Colvin and Kenny [1989] extended the controller developed by Reid and Kenny [1987] to control two drugs—sodium nitroprusside and glyceryl trinitrate (nitroglycerin). This controller was tested in 24 patients who required vasodilator therapy after cardiopulmonary bypass. Fourteen of these patients were controlled with nitroglycerin. The remaining 10 patients required supplemental SNP therapy. These investigators demonstrated the use of the dual drug delivery system and suggested that glyceryl trinitrate might be sufficient to control hypertension.

Martin [1987] developed an MMAC with a Smith predictor and a series compensator coupled with PI control for control law. The model bank of the MMAC contained nine models that were developed from a modified Slate model. Nineteen patients were tested with this controller during cardiac surgery [Martin 1992]. This controller used a supervisor to provide a safe clinical environment by minimizing the effects of disturbances when calculating infusion rate. This investigator reported that the controller performed satisfactorily in the difficult clinical environment of cardiac surgery.

Olkkola and Schwilden [1991] developed an adaptive self-tuning controller for neuromuscular blockade (NMB) using vecuronium and atracurium. They defined a two-compartment open mamillary model of plant dynamics (pharmacokinetic and pharmacodynamics of drug). The initial conditions of the compartmental model were generated from mean population kinetics. The degree of NMB was based on the ratio of the first twitch in the train of four to the control value. When the measured NMB was within 2% of the desired NMB, the infusion was computed with current model parameters to keep blockade at its current level. Otherwise, the model parameters were updated, using the error between the predicted and measured NMB, prior to calculating the infusion rate. The closed-loop system was activated following a drug-loading dose or bolus with a sample period of 20 s. Two clinical trials, one using vecuronium and the other atracurium, were performed to examine controller performance. In the vecuronium clinical trial, 15 patients underwent NMB with this controller to setpoints of 70%, 80%, and 90%. In the atracurium clinical trial [Olkkola et al., 1991], 15 patients underwent NMB therapy to setpoints of 50%, 70%, and 80%. In both trials, the investigators reported that this controller provided reasonable control of muscle relaxation and provided a solution for adapting the pharmacokinetic and pharmacodynamic parameters to individuals using mean data as starting values for therapy.

Commercial Devices

Five commercial devices have been or are being developed for CLDD. Four of the five devices are therapeutic CLDD systems. Hook Lane Nyetimber, a company based in the United Kingdom, developed an oxytocin device to initiate labor. In this device, the intrauterine pressure is measured every 15 minutes during delivery of oxytocin with closed-loop controller. The infusion of oxytocin is increased gradually until labor is underway, then the infusion rate is reduced by half. Additional decreases in infusion rate occur when the controller detects increased patient sensitivity to oxytocin. Furthermore, this device can initiate labor with one-fifth the total dose of oxytocin when compared with manual intervention [Westernskow, 1986].

Life Sciences Instruments Division of Miles Labs in the United States developed a glucose control system to regulate intravenous glucose in type-1 or brittle diabetics by infusing insulin. This device was developed as a tool to investigate the carbohydrate metabolism and regulatory deficiencies in diabetes [Clemens, 1979]. The control algorithm principal was virtually unchanged from the Toronto prototype [Brunetti, 1991].

An Italy-based company, Esaote Biomedica, developed a glucose CLDD device for type-1 diabetics. This product infused insulin to regulate intravenous glucose concentrations and is referred to as BetaLike. The operating principle of this controller is similar to the Toronto prototype [Brunetti 1991].

IVAC Corporation developed a CLDD device to titrate sodium nitroprusside to regulate mean arterial pressure in postoperative cardiac patients. Bedviarski and coworkers [1990] evaluated the clinical applicability of this device to compare its efficacy with manual control in treatment of postoperative hypertension. Thirty patients (20 in automatic and 10 in manual control) were enrolled into this clinical trial. These investigators reported that this device was superior to manual titration for blood pressure control in adult patients after open heart surgery. Chitwood and coworkers [1992] evaluated the clinical impact of this device on 1089 patients (557 in automatic and 532 in manual) after cardiotomy, in a prospective trial that was conducted at nine centers. This trial included patients that underwent automatic and manual control. These investigators reported that the automated group showed a significant reduction in the number of hypertensive episodes per patient; and chest tube drainage, percentage of patients receiving transfusion, and total amount transfused were all reduced significantly by the use of this device. In addition, investigators reported that the data suggest the automatic control of nitroprusside infusion may result in improved patient outcome through more effective control of hypertension, a decreased incidence of therapy-induced hypertension, a reduction in postoperative bleeding, decreased transfusion requirements, and probable decreased incidence of reexploration caused by postoperative bleeding.

There is one diagnostic CLDD device that has been developed by Gensia, Inc. in the United States and is awaiting regulatory agency approvals to market the device internationally. The purpose of this device is to diagnose coronary artery disease by a pharmacologic stress test in patients that cannot perform an exercise stress test. In order to elevate the heart rate, which occurs in an exercise stress test, a catecholamine is titrated to heart rate. The control algorithm was defined as a rule-based gain scheduling algorithm [Valcke, 1992] where the parameters of the linear controller were changed depending on the operating region. In addition, an on-line parameter estimation scheme estimates the parameters of the pharmacodynamic model. This device appears to be very promising in diagnosing coronary artery disease in patients who are not able to use an exercise stress test to elevate the heart rate.

Defining Terms

Adaptive control: A special type of feedback control in which the states of the controller or model parameters are adjusted on line to adapt to changing plant conditions.

ARMA: A linear black box model that defines an *autoregressive moving average* structure. This model structure is used in adaptive control to estimate plant dynamics.

Feedback control: An operation in the presence disturbances that reduces the difference between the plant output and reference input or desired state.

Fuzzy control: A technique that incorporates experts' decision making into the controller. This controller has three steps: fuzzify input data, rule base, and defuzzify data to generate control output.

GS: An adaptive controller that uses gain scheduling as an adaptation mechanism.

MMAC: An adaptive control law for *multiple model adaptive control*.

Parameter estimation: A technique used to update parameters of plant dynamics or controller parameters.

PID: Proportional-integral-derivative control law that exists in classical control theory.

Plant: Any physical object or system to be controlled by feedback control.

STR: Self-tuning regulator is a specific form of an adaptive controller.

Supervisor: A hierarchical control system that oversees controller conditions and provides intelligence to controller to avoid overaggressive or sluggish control caused by nonphysiologic disturbances.

References

Astrom KJ, Wittenmark B. 1989. Adaptive Control, Reading, Mass, Addison Wesley.

Bednarski P, Siclari F, Voigt A, Demertzis S, Lau, G. 1990. Use of a computerized closed-loop sodium nitroprusside titration system for antihypertensive treatment after open heart surgery. Crit Care Med 18(10):1061.

Brunetti P, Benedetti MM, et al. 1991. Closed-loop delivery systems for insulin therapy. Int J Artif Organs 14(4):216.

Chitwood RW, Cosgrove DM, Lust RM, and the Titrator Multicenter Study Group. 1992. Multicenter trial of automated nitroprusside infusion for postoperative hypertension. Ann Thorac Surg 54:517.

Clemens AH. 1979. Feedack control dynamics for glucose controlled insulin infusion system. Med Prog Tech 6:91.

Colvin JR, Kenny GNC. 1989. Automatic control of arterial pressure after cardiac surgery. Anaesthesia 44:37.

Ljung L. 1987. System Identification: Theory for the User, Englewood Cliffs, NJ, Prentice-Hall.

Ljung L, Soderstrom T. 1983. Theory and Practice of Recursive Identification, Cambridge, Mass, MIT Press.

McKinley S, Cade JF, Siganporia R, et al. 1991. Clinical evaluation of closed-loop control of blood pressure in seriously ill patients. Crit Care Med 19(2):166.

Martin JF, Schneider AM, Quinn ML, et al. 1992a. Improved safety and efficacy in adaptive control of arterial blood pressure through use of a supervisor. IEEE Trans Biomed Eng 39:381.

Martin JF, Schneider AM, Quinn ML, et al. 1992b. Supervisory adaptive control of arterial pressure during cardiac surgery. IEEE Trans Biomed Eng 39:389.

Martin JF, Schneider AM, Smith NT. 1987. Multiple-model adaptive control of blood pressure using sodium nitroprusside. IEEE Trans Biomed Eng 34:603.

Olkkola KT, Schwilden H. 1991. Adaptive closed-loop feedback control of vecuronium-induced neuromuscular relaxation. Eur J Anaesth 8:7.

Olkkola KT, Schwilden H, Apffelstaedt C. 1991. Model-based adaptive closed-loop feedback control of atracurium-induced neuromuscular blockade. Acta Anaesthesiol Scand 35:420.

Packer JS, Mason DG, Cade JF, et al. 1987. An adaptive controller for closed-loop management of blood pressure in seriously ill patients. IEEE Trans Biomed Eng 34:612.

Reid JA, Kenney GNC. 1987. Evaluation of closed-loop control of arterial pressure after cardiopulmonary bypass. Br J Anaesth 59:247.

Ruiz R, Borches KD, Gonzalez A, et al. 1993. A new sodium-nitroprusside-infusion controller for the regulation of arterial blood pressure. Biomed Instr Tech 27:244.

Schade CM. 1973. An automatic therapeutic control system for regulating blood pressure. Proc San Diego Biomed Symp 47.

Sheppard LC. 1980. Computer control of the infusion of vasoactive drugs. Ann Biomed Eng 8:431.

Slate JB. 1980. Model-based Design of a Controller for Infusing Sodium Nitroprusside during Postsurgical Hypertension. Ph.D. dissertation. University of Wisconsin, Madison.

Slate JB, Sheppard LC. 1982. Automatic control of blood pressure by drug infusion. IEEE Proc 29:639.

Valcke CP. 1992. Closed-loop drug delivery for cardiac stress testing. IEEE/BME Proc Paris, France, 2309.

Westenskow DR. 1986. Automating patient care with closed-loop control. MD Computing 3(2):14.

Widrow B. 1971. Adaptive model control applied to real-time blood pressure regulation. Pattern Recognition Machine Learning, 310.

Further Information

The Physiological Models and Control section of the monthly journal IEEE Transactions on Biomedical Engineering reports advances in biomedical applications of closed-loop drug delivery systems. The International Journal of Bio-Medical Computing, Medical Progress through Technology, and the Medical & Biological Engineering & Computing journals describe advances in biomedical sciences and medicine. The Journal of Clinical Monitoring reports advances in new devices that have been evaluated in the preclinical and clinical environments. The journals IEEE Transactions of Automatic Control, International Journal of Control, and Automatica describe advances in control theory research and applications.

163

Control of Movements

Dejan B. Popović
*University of Miami
and University of Belgrade*

Control of movements in humans is a very complex task dealing with a *large scale, nonlinear, time-variable, dynamically nondetermined, redundant* system. Control implies: (1) an object, the plant, which may be hard, soft, biologic, or mechanical, whose behavior can be modified by the input; (2) the set of allowed inputs consisting of at least two options; (3) the set of desired outputs; and (4) an optimization criterion. If any element is missing, control is not realizable. Control has no meaning if only a single input is available.

The concept of optimization is crucial for the understanding of the control. A dynamic system may change its states in a continuous way. Without an optimization criterion, all trajectories of a system are equivalent. Let us point out that *trajectory* has a broad meaning in the control jargon. It does not refer only to motion trajectories but, in general, to the way the system coordinates vary in the course of transition from the current to the next state. An optimization criterion assigns to each transition trajectory, or a subset of trajectories, a value so that they can be arranged in the order of preference. In some cases, the trajectories of the dynamic system may be well ordered so that a single solution stands in front. Such a trajectory is given the name the *optimal solution.* Instances when optimal solutions of control tasks exist, or can be analytically determined, are relatively rare, although this term is used rather loosely in everyday life.

Once the control task has been fixed, its solution procedure, whether heuristic, computer, or analytic, must be determined. Development of optimization procedures appropriate for different classes of control problems is the main concern of control theory. What the phrase *solution of the control problem* means is easily understood from the definition of *control.* Solution procedures for the control task must be able to assign value tags, numerical or not, to the allowed set of transition trajectories of the plant so that they can be partially or well ordered. The controller then enforces the plant to follow the desired course. It goes without saying that different optimization criteria will induce different ordering relations of control inputs. This fact is crucial for the understanding of dynamic processes. Per se, all potential transition trajectories are equivalent. Only under the impact of an optimization criterion do some of the otherwise equivalent plant responses become privileged. Without control, the systems, mechanical or biologic, are free to evolve along any of the feasible courses.

When it comes to the implementation of control, then some general features of the controller, human or machine, must be considered. The requirement for the so-called real-time control is essential. Real-time control pertains to dynamic systems. Such plants evolve in time with a speed which is inherent to their nature. The term *real-time control* refers to the matching of decision dynamics and system dynamics.

0-8493-8346-3/95/$0.00+$.50
© 1995 by CRC Press, Inc.

Acting, so to say, against the real-time control is the size of the plant. As the number of controlled variables increases, the processing and decision time of the controller grows in a nonlinear way. This sets a practical limit to the size of controllable plants no matter how fast the controller reacts. Such a situation is typical of biologic systems where large in-flow of sensory information has to be transmitted and processed by the nervous multilevel structure.

The capability of the controller, human or machine, to match the plant size sets the limit to growth of control tasks. The nature and the human creativity have found nonetheless an elegant way to bypass the so-called curse of dimensionality. The answer to the size challenge is the multilevel control and the principle of hierarchy. Applying such mechanisms, the limits to growth of control tasks have been increased by many orders of magnitude with respect to the one-level approach. The term *large system* refers in the control theory to those plants which generate so much state-related information that the controller cannot process it in the straightforward manner.

Large systems come into existence either by human activity or by design, or they evolve by integration of subsystems. The reason that subsystems tend to integrate is due to a fundamental law of the large-system optimization. Namely, by more integration improved optimization for each subsystem may be realized that would otherwise not be feasible in isolation.

The properties of multilevel systems can be interpreted in terms of general control concepts previously introduced. Multilevel control implies:

1. The plant must be modeled at each control level in a more and more abstract way, i.e., by a reduced number of synthetic features.
2. Each level has its own optimization criterion which is encompassing the lower-level criteria.
3. Criterion functions of subsystems may be conflicting, in which case the optimal solution is nonexistent. Only the preferred solutions may be singled out.
4. Hierarchy implies that the higher-level controller may override the lower-level controllers and exercise directly the control over the subsystems.

Control theory of large systems must deal with problems not encountered in the design of conventional control structures. How to derive synthetic information relevant for the higher level controllers or how to synthesize the global optimization criterion out of the local ones are but a few of new problems arising in the control of large systems. Instead of the variational calculus, value judgments are instrumental in the decision processes pertaining to large systems. Heuristics, creativity, domain-oriented experience are the main approaches used by humans in running multi-level organizations. Analytical tools and computer methods appear now not as means of automatic control but as servants to the decision maker.

163.1 Modeling the Dynamics of Human Extremities

From the control engineering point of view, human extremities appear as the plant involved in the execution of functional motions. Their modeling is, thus, the prerequisite for the synthesis of control when the dynamics of functional motions is in question. However, human extremities are unlike any other plant encountered in control engineering especially in terms of joints, actuators, sensors. This fact must be kept in mind when applying the general equations of mechanics to model the dynamics of functional motions. A simple extension of analytical tools used for the modeling of mechanical plants to the modeling of biomechanical systems may easily produce results in sharp discrepancy to reality. The role of this section is to warn against inadequate modeling of the dynamics and control of functional motions.

A basic problem in motor control of human extremities is in *planning* of motions to solve a previously specified task, and, then, *controlling* the extremity as it implements the commands. In terms of mechanics, extremities are linked structures with muscles that can set the joint angle to any value in its range. Muscles can also set the desired angular velocity, acceleration, joint stiffness by their cocontraction and reciprocal inhibition. The motions of extremities are called *trajectories* and consist of a sequence of positions, velocities, and accelerations of any part of the system (e.g., hand, finger tip). It is anticipated that by using laws of mechanics one can determine necessary muscle forces to follow the given trajectory.

The discussion will be started with basic definitions of rigid body mechanics. The term *rigid body* relates to a set of material points with the distances between points being fixed. A skeletal bone is a good example of a rigid body exposed to forces within its physiologic limits. However, the body segment consisting of a bone, muscles, tendons, and ligaments can hardly be represented as a single rigid body. Inertial properties of a rigid body are its mass and the inertia tensor. The inertia tensor for a single rigid body is constant if expressed for central principal axes, and it provides information on inertial properties of the body when rotating around the center of the mass. The body segment motion is generated by the muscle contraction, with simultaneous antagonistic muscle stretch and triggering reflexes; hence, the inertial properties will change in two ways: The center of mass is shifted, and the inertia tensor varies with the position of the body part.

The second issue in the modelling of human extremities relates to the joint structure. A joint is modeled as a *kinematic pair*. The theory of mechanisms defines connection of neighboring segments as kinematic pairs having up to five degrees of freedom (DOF). Typical human joint is a rotational kinematic pair having up to three DOF forming either a pin or a ball joint. Through evolution, nature evolved many different bone segment interfaces. All these interfaces are frequently simplified in modeling and reduced to rotational joints. There are joints that fit this hypothesis, but many movements cannot be simplified to a pure pin or ball joint. Some joints are actually double joints (e.g., ankle joints have one joint for internal-external rotation and inversion-eversion and a second one for movements, flexion-extension), in sagittal plane, or the elbow joint where three bones join, forming one joint). In some cases the rotation cannot be associated with the joint but results from more complex structures such as two parallel bones in the forearm and shank (e.g., supination-pronation of the forearm is not the result of rotation at the elbow or wrist but is due to the twisting of the ulna and radius bones). Most joints are not single-axis structures (e.g., the knee joint is a spatial polycentric joint, and the displacement of the center of rotation results in the virtual change of thigh and shank segment lengths for different leg positions). There are other polycentric joints, and in all these cases inertia properties of both neighboring segments will be changed.

One needs to distinguish the *forward kinematics* from the *inverse kinematics*. The direct kinematics is concerned with the determination of the position of body parts in the absolute reference frame given joint angles, whereas the inverse kinematics computes joint angles for a given position of the body part. Of these two, the direct kinematic analysis is the simplest by far, with a straightforward solution for the unique end point of the body part corresponding to the given joint angles. However, the feasibility of an inverse kinematics solution depends on the redundancy of the structure as well as offsets and constraints. The redundancy is an important feature in biologic systems. For example, rapid movements will use some joints, but some slow postural changes produce an entirely different strategy, as explained later in the text.

The concept of *redundancy* requires a distinction between a degree of freedom and the permissible motions (e.g., rotations). The term *degree of freedom* pertains exclusively to that permissible motion which is independent from other permissible motions. A free rigid body has a maximum of six DOF, and a rigid body connected to another rigid body by a ball joint can have a maximum of three DOF; thus, any body segment has fewer than three DOF. Speaking of a structure as a whole, the total number of permissible rotations is termed system DOFs. For example, the wrist and forearm have three DOF, all three rotations, allowing the hand to assume almost any orientation in the space. The issue can be further clarified by asking the question how many DOF has the wrist, regarded as a point with respect to the shoulder joint. The shoulder joint allows for three rotations; the elbow and two forearm bones allow for two more rotations. Consequently, two of these rotations are redundant, and an infinite number of movement strategies exists which may bring the wrist in the desired position in space (within the working space). If two rotations of a wrist are added to the above five DOF of the arm, then it becomes evident that the hand can be positioned and oriented in the space by controlling seven independent variables. However, some permissible rotations are not independent such as two parallel hinges. It is difficult to determine which permissible rotations should be controlled and which will be constrained by themselves due to anatomic and physiologic limitations. Anatomic and physiologic constraints are imposed by biarticular muscles that flex one joint while extending the neighboring one, reflexive activities (e.g., contralateral extension), and so on.

The inverse kinematics includes a math problem, which is distinct from the redundancy, due to the singularity of the model. The analytic form of equations for inverse kinematics has a denominator that can be zero; thus, the equation may become undefined. Inverse kinematics relates to geometry, velocity, and acceleration.

Dynamic analysis of a chain mechanism representing the model of an extremity is performed by decomposing the linked structure into a set of single rigid bodies (links). Internal forces (muscle actions) of the linked structure become now external forces and torques when the dynamics of a single link is analyzed. In order to design a controller for muscle actions, it is essential to begin with a good *muscle model*. The muscle is a linear actuator, with a very complex behavior. Many parallel and serial elements contribute to the force generation, and they all depend on the length of the muscle, velocity of shortening, firing rate, recruitment, and type of the given muscle.

Muscle models [Zahalak, 1992] can be grouped in three classes: (1) cross-bridge models including sarcomere-microscopic, conventional cross-bridge and unconventional cross-bridge models; (2) fiber models; and (3) whole-muscle macroscopic models (viscoelastic and black box models). The distinctions between these classes are not absolute (e.g., micro-macro).

Macroscopic viscoelastic models started from the observation that the process of electrical stimulation transforms the viscoelastic material from a compliant, fluent state into the stiff, viscous state. Levin and Wyman [1927] proposed a three-element model—damped and undamped elastic element in series. Hill's work [1938] demonstrated that the heat transfer depends upon the type of contraction (isometric, slow contracting, and so on). The model includes the force generator, damping, and elastic elements. This model includes a series elastic element and a contractile element, in parallel with the damping element, and in parallel with another elastic element. Ignoring the parallel elastic element the equation is:

$$\dot{L} = C(P)\dot{P} - F(P; P_0) \qquad \textit{Hill model}$$

where L is muscle length, P the force, $C(P)$ the compliance of the elastic element, and $F(P, P_0)$ the shortening velocity of the contractile element as a function of force. The parameter P_0 is a measure of activation of the contractile tissue and is defined as the force exerted by the contractile element when it is neither shortening nor lengthening, that is $F(P_0, P_0) = 0$. The P_0 is called the isometric force. More generally, P_0 depends on the history of stimulation and time and is often called the *active state*.

$$F(P, P_0) = b\,\frac{P_0 - P}{a + P}$$

where a and b are constants characteristic of a given muscle.

This model provoked many experiments and development. The Hill model was originally formulated to describe shortening muscle at maximal stimulation over a small range of muscle lengths near the mean length of the muscle in the body, but it is further developed for other cases. Hatze used Hill's model as a microscopic model and came to very interesting results which include both the rate and size principles (recruitment). This is a very complex model (28 parameters). Winters [1990] generalized Hill's model in a simple enhancement of the original, which makes no claim to be based on the microstructure. Winters's model deals with joint moments

$$M = M_0 - B\dot{\Theta} \,,\; M_0 = AM_{0m}f(\Theta)$$

M is the muscle moment exerted about the joint, M_0 is the isometric moment (active state) with a maximum possible value M_{0m}, θ is the joint angle corresponding to the current contractile element length (which is in general not equal to the actual joint angle because of the presence of a compliant SE elements), A is a normalized activation variable ($A = 0$ for relaxed muscle, $A = 1$ for a tetanized muscle), $f(\Theta)$ is the normalized tetanic length-tension relation, and B is a variable damping coefficient. For shortening muscle

$$B = \frac{M_0(1 + \alpha)}{(\dot{\Theta} + \alpha\dot{\Theta}_0)} \qquad \dot{\Theta}_0 < \dot{\Theta} < 0$$

whereas for lengthening muscle

$$B = \frac{M_0(1 - \beta)}{(\dot{\Theta} + \gamma\dot{\Theta}_0)}, \dot{\Theta} > 0$$

where α, β, and γ are constants.

Zajac [1989] proposed an appealing new version of the Hill model designed primarily for use in studies of mechanical interactions in multiple muscle systems. Muscles are connected to a skeleton with tendons, and they have springlike behavior when stretched. A variety of different nonrigid structures are included in the musculoskeletal system (e.g., ligaments) adding different elastic and damping effects.

Dynamic analysis deals with two problems: determination of forces and torques when desired laws of motion are known (*forward dynamics*), and determination of trajectories and laws of motion when torques and forces are prescribed (*inverse dynamics*). Forward dynamics is a simple problem, and the only difficulty comes from error generated through numerical derivation on noisy input data. Using laws of mechanics (D'Alembert principle, Newton-Euler method, Lagrange equations, basic theorems of mechanics, and so on) in inverse dynamics works only for open-chain structures like an arm when reaching, or a leg during swinging, but it is not applicable for closed-chain structures such as legs during the double support phase in walking, or the arm when contacting an immobile object, or in redundant systems. Every closed, chained structure is dynamically undetermined, and the only possibility for determining forces and torques is to use the theory of elasticity. The theory of elasticity assumes that the elements of the structure are solid (not rigid), and it is inappropriate for control design because of its extreme complexity. Approximate solution of the dynamics of a closed-chain mechanism assumes how forces and torques are distributed in the structure. In the case of locomotion, it is necessary to introduce at least three equations (constraints) in order to be able to determine the dynamics of the process. In most cases the model of a system is limited to a small number of admissible rotations. The reason for simplification is twofold: the problem can be solved, and the simulation results can be interpreted.

The complexity of a body segment dynamic model depends on number and types of body segments, the joints connecting the segments, and the interaction among the segments and the environment (Fig. 163.1). How complex a model is required for dynamic analysis of externally controlled walking, standing, manipulation, and grasping? Some decisions on how complex the model should be are simple and others are not. For instance, lower limbs can be assumed rigid during standing. The decision on how many segments should be assumed and how many DOF should be assumed for each joint is controversial [Chizeck et al., 1988; Gordon, 1990; Hatze, 1980; Jaeger, 1986; Khang, 1988; Townsend & Seirig, 1973; Yamaguchi, 1990].

163.2 Control of Upper Extremities

The objective of an upper extremity assistive system must be directed toward establishing independence to the user. Most effort in upper extremity FES has been directed toward the individual with

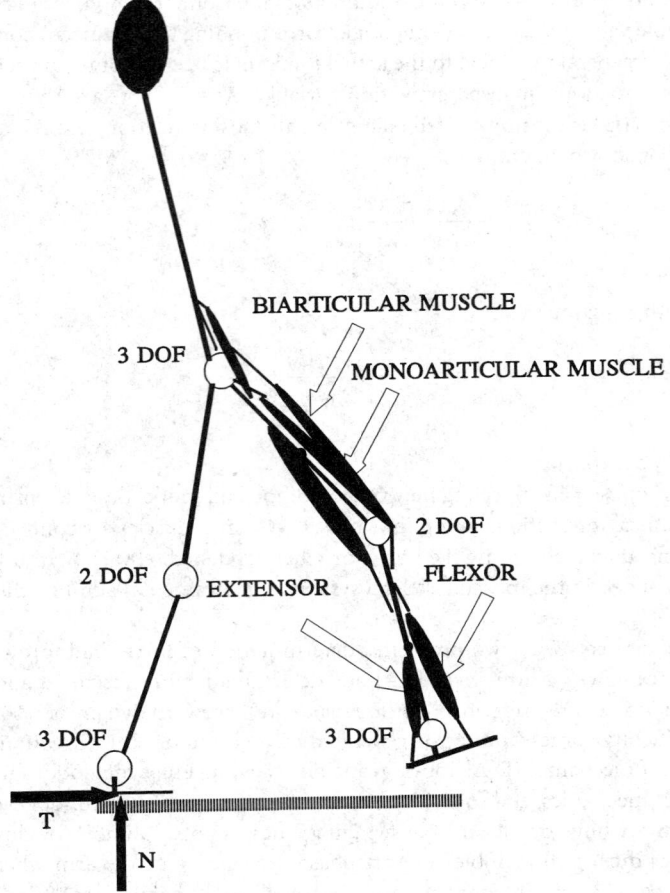

FIGURE 163.1   A sketch of the model of a human body with 13 degrees of freedom (DOF). Biarticular muscles are acting upon two neighboring joints, while monoarticular act upon a single joint. Flexor and extensor muscles regulate the stiffness of the joint, from loose to locked state, and control flexion and extension of the joint (in the case of the ankle joint they are called *plantar* and *dorsal flexion*). *T* (friction force) and *N* are projections of the ground reaction force to the direction of progression and vertical.

diminished, but preserved, shoulder and elbow functions, with lack of wrist control and grasping ability [Peckham & Keith, 1992].

Reaching and Tracking Control

What are the motor commands that generate movements to a target in space, and how is sensory information used to control and coordinate such movements? The neural system that is involved in the production of each of these movements must deal with aspects that are practical to that task, and specialized reviews are available on each of these topics [Georgopoulos, 1986; Knudsen et al., 1987; Simpson 1984; Sparks, 1988].

Arm movements to a spatial target also utilize sensory information that is initially represented in different frames of reference, and the sensory signals that specify target location need to be transformed into motor commands to arm muscles [Soechting & Flanders, 1992]. Arm movements illustrate an additional aspect of sensorimotor transformations; a distinction must be made between forces and the movements that the forces produce. In arm movements the direction of force and movement do not coincide. The transformation between kinematics and kinetics is nontrivial in the case of arm motion. Not much is known about how this transformation might be implemented by neural circuits. Mathematical formulations of the problem have been provided by several investigators [Hollerbach & Flash, 1982; Hoy & Zernicke, 1986; Zajac & Gordon, 1989]. Other investigators have quantified biomechanic factors, such as muscle stiffness [Mussa-Ivaldi et al., 1985] and the changes in the muscle lever arms with posture, which also affect the relationship between force and movement. Arm muscle activation onset [Hasan & Karst, 1989] and activation waveforms [Flanders, 1991] have been empirically related to the direction of movement.

The automatic control of the arm-reaching motion to accomplish grasping has been discussed in great detail [e.g., Desoer & Vidyasagar, 1975; Hollerbach & Bennett, 1992; Rugh, 1981]. Imperfect models, wrong initial conditions, unmodelled perturbations, and computational difficulties are serious problems in implementing analytical closed-loop control methods [Bennett, 1990; Eppinger & Seering, 1987; Jacobsen et al., 1989; Stein, 1992].

A simplified control method for reaching while grasping has been proposed [Popović & Popović, 1994]. This approach follows a so-called extended physiologic proprioception (EPP) control developed for bilateral amputees in Scotland [Simpson, 1975]. The number of control variables, by establishing a synergy between joint angles, can be reduced to a single input.

To move to a target accurately in the absence of visual guidance, the starting point of the movement, as well as the desired final point, must be sensed [Bizzi et al., 1984; Hogan, 1985]. Information about the target is provided by the visual system, whereas proprioceptors are adequate to signal initial arm posture. Because proprioceptors sense muscle length and joint angles [McCloskey, 1978], the initial frames of reference for kinesthesis are fixed to the limb segments, i.e., elbow joint angles are initially sensed in the frame of reference fixed to the upper arm [Soechting & Ross, 1984].

Grasping Control

The command interface to the assistive system must provide simple and complete control of reach and grasp functions without interference with other activities. For the existing assistive systems the command task requires both a proportional signal for grading the strength of the grasp and logic signals to change the state of the control function. The states that are controlled are on/off, lateral/palmar grasp, and active control/hold.

The first grasping system used to provide prehension and release [Long & Masciarelli, 1963] used a splint with a spring for closure and electrical stimulation of the thumb extensor for release. This attempt was unsuccessful mostly because of the state-of-the-art technology used, but also because of the muscle fatigue and erratic contractile response. Reberšek and Vodovnik [1973] suggested the use of a simple two-channel stimulation system and a position transducer (sliding potentiometer) for open-loop control of grasp with visual feedback. The shift of the potentiometer forward from its neutral position caused opening by stimulating finger flexors, and backward caused stimulation of finger extensors. One paralyzed hand was devoted to control the grasping of the other paralyzed hand. The follow-up of the initial use of the FES system was systematically continued in Japan. The Japanese research approach in functional grasping relates to subjects lacking not only hand functions but also the elbow control, and the system uses either a voice or suck/puff control and preprogrammed EMG-based stimulation patterns. This preprogrammed EMG-based stimulation is developed by detailed studies of muscle activities with intramuscular electrodes in able-bodied subjects while reaching and grasping [Handa et al., 1989; Hoshimiya & Handa, 1989].

The approach taken by Nathan [1989] uses a voice-controlled multichannel surface electrode system. As many as 12 bipolar stimulation channels and a splint are used to control elbow, wrist, and hand functions. The use of surface EMG recordings from the muscle which is stimulated [Holländer et al., 1987] has been proposed. The aim of this device is to enhance the grasping using weak muscles.

Hence, in principle it could be possible to use retained recordings from volar side of the forearm to trigger on and off the stimulation of the same muscles. In this case it is essential to eliminate the stimulation artifact, and the evoked potential caused by the stimulus, in order to eliminate positive feedback effects which will generate a tetanic contraction that cannot be turned off using the method presented.

Prochazka [1993] suggested the use of wrist position to control the stimulation of muscles to enhance the tenodesis grasping. A custom-built glove with a sensor is used to detect wrist movement, and it contains the contacts for three channels of surface stimulation electrodes. A microcomputer is built into the battery-operated stimulation unit which detects wrist movements and controls three different muscle groups. All the described techniques can be classified into open-loop control methods (Fig. 163.2).

The Case Western Reserve University (CWRU) fully implantable system has a switch to turn the system on and off and select the grasp and a joystick to proportionally control aperture of the hand for palmer and lateral grasp. These two grasps are synthesized using a preprogrammed synergy, and a cocontraction of several agonists and antagonists (Fig. 163.3). The joystick mounted on the contralateral shoulder voluntarily control the preprogrammed sequence of stimulation.

However, the lack of feedback limits somewhat the performance with devices described, hence a tremendous amount of research is dedicated to include closed-loop control. By introducing the feedback, the exercise moves to the nature and quality of sensors and applicability in real time. Two different feedback approaches exist: (1) natural sensors (e.g., myoelectric activity, peripheral nerve recordings, cortical recordings) as a source of control signals, and (2) artificial sensors. By application of pattern recognition methods or correlation techniques, functional motions can be created if adequate interface is used [Graupe & Kohn, 1988; Hoffer & Haugland, 1992; Popović & Raspopović, 1992]. The group in Aarlborg, Denmark [Sinkjaer, personal communication] recently implanted nerve cuff electrodes on the digital nerve of the index finger, following their original implantable cuff electrode on the sural nerve in a stroke subject. It is to be seen how effective these devices are in a long run, but initial results and long-term experience with animal models suggest that this is an important contribution.

Human-machine systems require the use of specific artificial sensors [Crago et al., 1986; Webster, 1988] that are not available at this time. What actually matters is not just the output of sensors but their overall properties. Human-machine systems are in great need of distributed matrix type, sensory systems with high resolution. Sensory information derived in the above way must be adequately preprocessed before it is used for control.

163.3 Control of Lower Extremities

Many control algorithms for synthesis of bipedal locomotion have been developed in the last decade. The first control algorithms applied to assistive systems for gait restoration were of the open-loop type. Open-loop control assumes a complete knowledge of the system and its behavior in different environmental conditions. Only a simplified "hand switch" control and preprogrammed automatic control mechanisms have been applied so far. Available data on gait performance of paralyzed individuals are often inadequate, which makes the application of the open-loop controllers in rehabilitation very difficult. In addition to the difficulties mentioned above, individ-

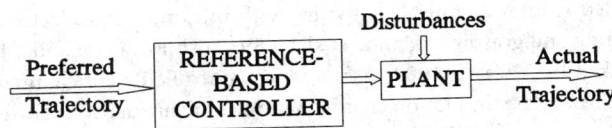

FIGURE 163.2   Open-loop (reference-based) control.

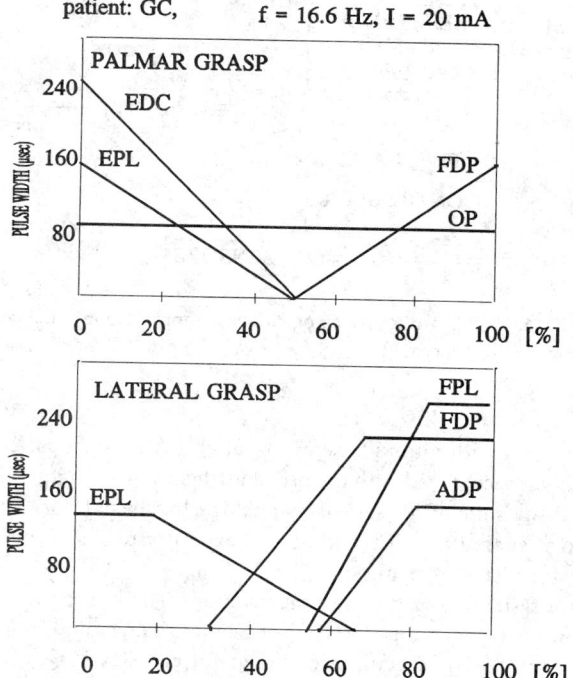

FIGURE 163.3 Preprogrammed control strategy for palmar and lateral grasp in a tetraplegic subject. EDC—extensor digitorum communis muscle, EPL—extensor pollicis longus m., FDP—flexor digitorum profundus m., OP—opponens pollicis m., FPL—flexor pollicis longus, and ADP—adductor pollicis. The subject volitionally controls the Hall effect transducer positioned at his chest from 0 (open hand) to 100 (closed hand).

ual properties such as muscle fatigue, spasticity, joint contractures, muscle denervation, etc., must be modelled quantitatively for the synthesis of an open-loop controller. Most control systems adopted the principle of memorized and triggered motor sequences. These sequences are based on recorded average EMG patterns in normal individuals [Marsolais et al., 1983; Thoma et al., 1987]. Direct, computer-controlled electrical stimulation was proposed by the Cleveland group [Chizeck et al., 1988], emphasizing muscular properties and a discrete event model with control goals for restoring locomotion functions.

Some investigators have introduced formal modelling to solve global issues such as standing stability, control strategies, feedback design [Khang & Zajac, 1989] or synthesis of rhythmic joint trajectories for gait. It is important to mention that the open-loop control relates to activation of the lower extremities, but the upper part of the body, including the hands and arms over the parallel bars, walker or crutches, actually works as a correction mechanism and provides closed-loop control. The preserved voluntary motor control above the lesion allows the use of open-loop control, because the compensatory forces and movements can be accomplished. A certain programming (feedforward) control is required for fast movements and it is essential for cyclic motions. The second approach suggested, but not used for present assistive applications, involves closed-loop control (Fig. 163.4).

Tomović [1984] proposed a nonnumeric control method, called *artificial reflex control* (ARC). ARC (Fig. 163.5) refers to a skill-based expert using rules that have an *if-then* structure [Popović et al., 1991]. The cyclic locomotor activity is presented as a sequence of discrete events. Each of these

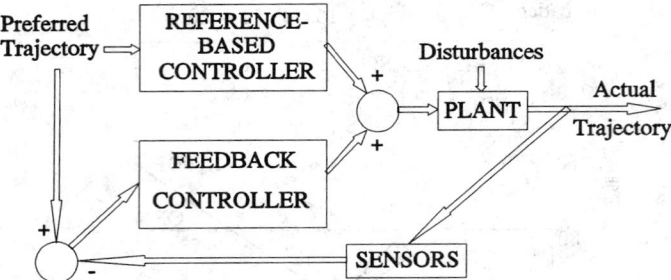

FIGURE 163.4   Closed-loop (error driven) control about the desired (reference-based) trajectory.

discrete events is associated with a unique sensory pattern. A sensory pattern occurring during particular motor activity is recognized with the use of artificial and/or natural sensors. The specific discrete event is called the *state of the system* by analogy to the state of a finite-state automata [Tomović, 1984; Tomović et al., 1987]. This skill-based expert system is of the *on-off* type and does not consider explicitly the system dynamics.

A rule-based control system has a hierarchical structure. The highest level is under volitional control of the user. Automatic adaptation to environmental changes and modes of gait is realized using artificial reflex control. The execution of the artificial reflex has to be tuned for smooth functional movements. Digital closed-loop methods using proportional (P) and proportional plus integral (PI) controllers should be used at the lowest actuator level of control [Chizeck et al., 1988].

Advantages of this hierarchical control method are: (1) adaptivity, (2) modularity, (3) ease of application and possibility of integration into a human-machine system. Rule-based control was tested in hybrid assistive systems [Andrews et al., 1989; Mulder et al., 1991; Phillips, 1990; Popović et al., 1990; Tomović et al., 1990; Veltink et al., 1990].

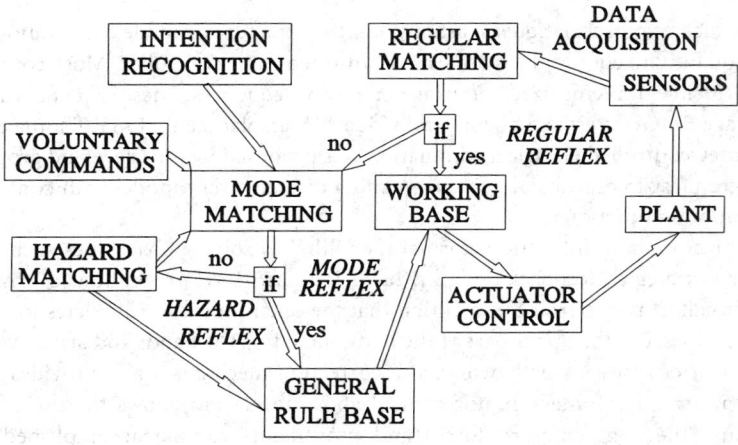

FIGURE 163.5   A scheme of the organization of the skill-based multilevel control for locomotion. Regular reflexes are sequences of system states connected with conditional *if-then* expressions within a single mode of the gait, mode reflexes relate to the change of the mode of the gait (level, slope, steps, etc.), and hazard reflexes are for situations where software or hardware cannot drive the system upon the preferred sequence of system states.

Defining Terms

Artificial reflex control: An expert system that uses production rules to control movements.

Closed-loop system: Control system which uses information about the output to correct the control parameters to minimize the error between the desired and actual trajectory.

Degree of freedom: Possible rotation or translation between two neighboring segments. A free rigid body has six degrees of freedom, a ball joint three, and a hinge joint one.

Dynamic analysis: Analytic simulation of movements of the system considering forces, torques, and kinematics. Forward dynamics uses the geometry and kinematics as input and provides forces and torques as outputs; inverse dynamics starts from forces and torques and determines kinematics and geometry of the system.

Hierarchical control: Multilevel control allowing the vertical decomposition of the system.

Kinematic analysis: Analytic simulation of movements of the system considering positions, velocities, and accelerations.

Kinematic pair: Connection of two neighboring segments.

Open-loop control: Control method that uses a prestored trajectory and the adopted model of the system to control the plant.

Production rule: A conditional expression *if-then* used in experts systems.

Rigid body: A set of material points with the distances between points being fixed.

References

Andrews BJ, Barnett RW, Phillips GF, et al. 1989. Rule-based control of a hybrid FES orthosis for assisting paraplegic locomotion. Automedica 11:175.

Bennett DJ. 1990. The Control of Human Arm Movement: Models and Mechanical Constraints, Ph.D. thesis, Massachusetts Institute of Technology, Cambridge, Mass.

Bizzi E, Accornero N, Chapple W, et al. 1984. Posture control and trajectory formation during arm movement. J Neurosci 4:2738.

Chizeck HJ, Kobetić R, Marsolais, EB, et al. 1988. Control of functional neuromuscular stimulation system for standing and locomotion in paraplegics. Proc IEEE 76:1155.

Crago PE, Chizeck HJ, Neuman MR, et al. 1986. Sensors for use with functional neuromuscular stimulation. IEEE Trans Biomed Eng BME-33:256.

Desoer CA, Vidyasagar M. 1975. In Feedback Systems: Input-Output Properties, New York, Academic Press.

Eppinger SD, Seering WP. 1987. Understanding band-width limitations in robot force control. Proc IEEE Int Conf Robotics Automation 904.

Flanders M. 1991. Temporal patterns of muscle activation for arm movements in three-dimensional space. J Neurosci 11:2680.

Georgopoulos AP. 1986. On reaching. Annu Rev Neurosci 9:147.

Gordon ME. 1990. An Analysis of the Biomechanics and Muscular Synergies of Human Standing. Ph.D. thesis, Stanford University, Stanford, Calif.

Graupe D, Kline WK. 1975. Functional separation of EMG signals via ARMA identification methods for prosthesis control purposes. IEEE Trans System Man Cybernetics SMC-5:252.

Handa Y, Ohkubo K, Hoshimiya N. 1989. A portable multi-channel functional electrical stimulation (FES) system for restoration of motor function of the paralyzed extremities. Automedica 11(1–3):221.

Hasan Z, Karst GM. 1989. Muscle activity for initiation of planar, two-joint arm movements in different directions. Exp Brain Res 76:651.

Hatze H. 1980. Neuromuscular control system modelling—a critical review of recent developments. IEEE Trans Automatic Control AC-25:375.

Hill TL. 1938. The heat of shortening and the dynamic constants of muscle. Proc R Soc London Biol 126:135.

Hoffer JA, Haugland MK. 1992. Signals from tactile sensors in glaborous skin: recording, processing and applications for restoring motor functions in paralyzed humans. In RB Stein et al (eds), Neural Prostheses: Replacing Motor Function after Disease or Disability, pp 99–125, New York, Oxford University Press.

Holländer HJ, Huber M, Vossius G. 1987. An EMG controlled multichannel stimulator. In D Popović (ed), Advances in External Control of Human Extremities IX, pp 291–295, Belgrade, Yugoslav Committee for ETAN.

Hoshimiya N, Naito A, Yajima M, et al. 1989. A multichannel FES system for the restoration of motor functions in high spinal cord injury patients: A respiration-controlled system for multijoint upper extremity. IEEE Trans Biomed Eng BME-36:754.

Hogan N. 1985. The mechanics of multijoint posture and movement control. Biol Cybern 52:325.

Hollerbach JM, Flash T. 1982. Dynamic interactions between limb segments during planar arm movement. Biol Cybern 44:67.

Hollerbach JM, Bennett DJ. 1992. Feed-forward vs. feedback control of limb movements. In RB Stein et al (eds), Neural Prostheses, Replacing Motor Function after Disease or Disability, pp 129–147, New York, Oxford University Press.

Hoy MG, Zernicke RF. 1986. The role of intersegmental dynamics during rapid limb oscillations. J Biomech 19:867.

Jacobsen SC, Smith CC, Biggers KB, et al. 1989. Behavior based design for robot effectors. In M Brady (ed), Robotics Science, pp 505–539, Cambridge, Mass, MIT Press.

Jaeger RJ. 1986. Design and simulation of closed-loop electrical stimulation orthoses for restoration of quiet standing in paraplegia. J Biomech 19:825.

Khang G. 1988. Paraplegics Standing Controlled by Functional Neuromuscular Stimulation: Computer Model, Control-System Design, and Stimulation Studies. Ph.D. thesis, Stanford University, Stanford, Calif.

Khang G, Zajac FE. 1989. Paraplegic standing controlled by functional neuromuscular stimulation: Part I. Computer model and control system design. IEEE Trans Biomed Eng BME-36:873.

Knudsen EI, duLac S, Esterly S. 1987. Computational maps in the brain. Annu Rev Neurosci 10:41.

Levin A, Wyman J. 1927. The viscous elastic properties of muscle. Proc R Soc London Biol 101:218.

Long C II, Masciarelli CV. 1963. An electrophysiologic splint for the hand. Arch Phys Med Rehabil 44:499.

Marsolais EB, Kobetić R. 1983. Functional walking in paralysed patients by means of electrical stimulation. Clin Orthop Rel Res 175:30.

McCloskey DI. 1978. Kinesthetic sensibility. Physiol Rev 58:762.

Morasso P. 1981. Spatial control of arm movements. Exp Brain Res 42:223.

Morasso P. 1983. Three dimensional arm trajectories. Biol Cybern 48:187.

Mulder AJ, Boom HBK, Hermens HJ, et al. 1990. Artificial reflex stimulation for FES induced standing with minimum quadriceps force. Med Biol Eng Comp 28:483.

Mussa-Ivaldi FA, Hogan N, Bizzi E. 1985. Neural, mechanical and geometric factors subserving arm posture in humans. J Neurosci 5:2732.

Nathan RH. 1989. An FNS-based system for generating upper limb function in the C4 quadriplegic. Med Biol Eng Comp 27:549.

Peckham PH, Keith MW. 1992. Motor prosthesis for restoration of upper extremity function. In RB Stein et al (eds), Neural Prostheses: Replacing Motor Function after Disease or Disability, pp 162–190, New York, Oxford University Press.

Phillips GF. 1990. Finite state description language: A new tool for writing stimulator controllers. In D. Popović (ed), Advances in External Control of Human Extremities X, pp 39–54, Belgrade, Nauka.

Popović D, Raspopović V. 1992. Afferent recording in digital palmar nerves. In Proceedings of the 4th Vienna International Workshop on FES, pp 105–108, Vienna.

Popović M, Popović D. 1994. A new approach to reaching control for tetraplegic subjects. J Electromyography Kinesiology 4:242–253.

Popović D, Schwirtlich L, Radosavljević S. 1990. Powered hybrid assistive system. In D Popović (ed), Advances in External Control of Human Extremities X, pp 177–187, Belgrade, Nauka.

Popović D, Tomović R, Schwirtlich L, et al. 1991. Control aspects of an active A/K prosthesis. Int J Man-Machine Stud 35:750.

Prochazka A. 1993. Life with the electric glove. Newsletter Alberta Heritage Foundation for Medical Research, 6.

Reberšek S, Vodovnik L. 1973. Proportionally controlled functional electrical stimulation of hand. Arch Phys Med Rehabil 54:378.

Rugh WJ. 1981. The Volterra/Wiener approach. In Non-linear System Theory, Baltimore, Johns Hopkins University.

Simpson, DC. 1974. The choice of control system for the multimovement prosthesis: extended physiological proprioception (e.p.p.). In P Herberts (ed), The Control of Upper-Extremity Prostheses and Orthoses, chap 15, London, C Thomas.

Simpson JI. 1984. The accessory optic system. Annu Rev Neurosci 7:13.

Soechting JF, Flanders M., 1992. Moving in three dimensional space: Frames of reference, vectors and coordinate systems. Annu Rev Neurosci 5:167.

Soechting JF, Ross B. 1984. Psychophysical determination of coordinate representation of human arm orientation. Neuroscience 13:595.

Sparks DL. 1988. Neural cartography: Sensory and motor maps in the superior colliculus. Brain Behav Evol 31:49.

Stein RB. 1992. Feedback control of normal and electrically induced movements. In RB Stein et al (eds), Neural Prostheses, Replacing Motor Function after Disease or Disability, pp 281–297, New York, Oxford University Press.

Thoma H, Frey H, Holle J, et al. 1987. Functional neurostimulation to substitute locomotion in paraplegia patients. In JD Andrade, et al (eds), Artificial Organs, pp 515–529, New York, VCH.

Tomović R. 1984. Control of assistive systems by external reflex arcs. In D Popović (ed), Advances in External Control of Human Extremities VIII, pp 7–21, Belgrade, Yugoslav Committee for ETAN.

Tomović R, Popović D, Tepavac D. 1987. Adaptive reflex control of assistive systems. In D Popović (ed), Advances in External Control of Human Extremities IX, pp 207–214, Belgrade, Yugoslav Committee for ETAN.

Tomović R, Popović D, Tepavac D. 1990. Rule-based control of sequential hybrid assistive systems. In D Popović (ed), Advances in External Control of Human Extremities X, pp 11–20, Belgrade, Nauka.

Townsend MA, Seirig AA. 1973. Effect of model complexity and gait criteria on the synthesis of bipedal locomotion. IEEE Trans Biomed Eng BME-20:443.

Veltink PH, Koopman AFM, Mulder AJ. 1990. Control of cyclical lower leg movements generated by FES. In D Popović (ed), Advances in External Control of Human Extremities X, pp 81–90, Belgrade, Nauka.

Webster JG. 1992. Artificial sensors suitable for closed-loop control of FNS. In RB Stein et al (eds), Neural Prostheses: Replacing Motor Function after Disease or Disability, pp 88–98, New York, Oxford University Press.

Winters JM. 1990. Hill-based muscle models: A systems engineering prospective. In JM Winters, SL-Y Woo (eds), Multiple Muscle Systems: Biomechanics and Movement Organization, pp 66–93, New York, Springer-Verlag.

Yamaguchi GT. 1990. Performing whole-body simulations of gait with 3-D dynamic musculoskeletal models. In: JM Winters, SL-Y Woo (eds), Multiple Muscle Systems: Biomechanics and Movement Organization, pp 663–679, New York, Springer-Verlag.

Zahalak GI. 1990. Modeling muscle mechanics (and energetics). In JM Winters, SL-Y Woo (eds), Multiple Muscle Systems: Biomechanics and Movement Organization, pp 1–23, New York, Springer-Verlag.

Zajac FE. 1989. Muscle and tendon properties: Models, scaling, and application to biomechanics and motor control. CRC Crit Rev Biomed Eng 17:359.

Zajac FE, Gordon ME. 1989. Determining muscles' force and action in multi-articular movement. In K Pandoff (ed), Exercise Sport Science Review, vol 17, pp 187–230, Baltimore, Williams and Wilkins.

Further Information

The *IEEE Transactions on Robotics and Automation,* IEEE Press, *IEE Transactions on Rehabilitation Engineering,* IEEE Press, *and IEEE Transactions on Biomedical Engineering,* IEEE Press, are all good sources for further investigation, as are the following works:

Stein RB, Peckham HP, Popović DB (eds). 1992. Neural Prostheses: Replacing Motor Function after Disease or Disability, London, Oxford University Press.

Winters JM, Woo SL-Y (eds). 1990. Multiple Muscle Systems: Biomechanics and Movement Organization, Springer-Verlag, New York.

Yugoslav Committee for Electronics and Automation. 1964–1990. Advances in External Control of Human Extremities I–X, Belgrade, Yugoslavia.

164

The Fast Eye Movement Control System

John Denis Enderle
University of Connecticut

This chapter presents a broad overview of the fast eye movement control system. A fast eye movement is usually referred to as a saccade, and involves quickly moving the eye from one image to another image. This type of eye movement is very common and is observed most easily while reading when the end of a line is reached, the eyes are moved quickly to the beginning of the next line. A qualitative description of the fast eye movement system is given first in the introduction and then followed by a brief description of saccade characteristics. Next, the earliest quantitative saccade model is presented, followed by more complex and physiologically accurate models. Finally, the saccade generator, or saccade controller, is then discussed on the basis of anatomic pathways and control theory. The purpose of this review is focused on mathematical models of the fast eye movement system and its control strategy, rather than on how visual information is processed. The literature on the fast eye movement system is vast, and thus this review is not exhaustive but rather a representative sample from the field.

The oculomotor system responds to visual, auditory, and vestibular stimuli, which results in one of five types of eye movements: fast eye movements, smooth pursuit eye movements, vestibular ocular movements, vergence eye movements, and optokinetic eye movements. Each of these movements is controlled by a different neuronal system, and all these controllers share the same final common pathway to the muscles of the eye. In addition to the five types of eye movements, these stimuli also cause head and body movements. Thus, the visual system is part of a multiple input–multiple output system.

Regardless of the input, the oculomotor system is responsible for movement of the eyes so that images are focused on the central 1/2° region of the retina, known as the *fovea*. Lining the retina are photoreceptive cells which translate images into neural impulses. These impulses are then transmitted along the optic nerve to the central nervous system via parallel pathways to the superior colliculus and the cerebral cortex. The fovea is more densely packed with photoreceptive cells than the retinal periphery; thus a higher resolution image (or higher visual acuity) is generated in the

0-8493-8346-3/95/$0.00+$.50
© 1995 by CRC Press, Inc.

fovea than the retinal periphery. The purpose of the fovea is to allow us to *clearly* see an object, and the purpose of the retinal periphery is to allow us to *detect* a new object of interest. Once a new object of interest is detected in the periphery, the saccade system redirects the eyes, as fast as possible, to the new object. This type of saccade is typically called a *goal-directed saccade*.

During a saccade, the oculomotor system operates in an open-loop mode. After the saccade, the system operates in a closed-loop mode to ensure that the eyes reach the correct destination. The reason that the saccade system operates without feedback during a fast eye movement is simple—information from the retina and muscle proprioceptors is not transmitted quickly enough during the eye movement for use in altering the control signal.

The oculomotor plant and saccade generator are the basic elements of the saccadic system. The oculomotor plant consists of three muscle pairs and the eyeball. These three muscle pairs contract and lengthen to move the eye in horizontal, vertical, and torsional directions. Each pair of muscles acts in an antagonistic fashion due to reciprocal innervation by the saccade generator. For simplicity, the models described here involve only horizontal eye movements and one pair of muscles, the lateral and medial rectus muscle.

164.1 Saccade Characteristics

Saccadic eye movements, among the fastest voluntary muscle movements the human is capable of producing, are characterized by a rapid shift of gaze from one point of fixation to another. The usual experiment for recording saccades is for subjects to sit before a horizontal target display of small light emitting diodes (LEDs), with instructions to maintain their eyes on the lit LED by moving their eyes as fast as possible to avoid errors. A saccade is made by the subject when the active LED is switched off and another LED is switched on. Saccadic eye movements are conjugate and ballistic, with a typical duration of 20–100 ms and a latency of 150–300 ms. The latent period is thought to be the time interval during which the CNS determines whether to make a saccade, and if so, calculates the distance the eyeball is to be moved, transforming retinal error into transient muscle activity.

Generally, saccades are extremely variable, with wide variations in the latent period, time to peak velocity, peak velocity, and saccade duration. Furthermore, variability is well coordinated for saccades of the same size; saccades with lower peak velocity are matched with longer saccade durations, and saccades with higher peak velocity are matched with shorter saccade durations. Thus, saccades driven to the same destination usually have different trajectories.

To appreciate differences in saccade dynamics, it is often helpful to describe them with saccade main sequence diagrams [Bahill et al., 1975]. The main sequence diagrams plot saccade peak velocity–saccade magnitude, saccade duration–saccade magnitude, and saccade latent period–saccade magnitude. Shown in Fig. 164.1 are the main sequence characteristics for a subject executing 54 saccades. Notice that the peak velocity–saccade magnitude is basically a linear function until approximately 15°, after which it levels off to a constant for larger saccades. Many researchers have fit this relationship to an exponential function. The solid lines in Fig. 164.1*a* include an exponential fit to the data for positive and negative eye movements. The lines in the first graph are fitted to the equation

$$V = \alpha_i \left(1 - e^{-\frac{x}{\beta_i}} \right) \tag{164.1}$$

where V is the maximum velocity, x the saccade size, and the constants α_i and β_i evaluated to minimize the summed error squared between the model and the data. Note that α_i is to represent the steady state of the peak velocity–saccade magnitude curve and β_i is to represent the time constant for the peak velocity–saccade magnitude curve. For this data set, α_i equals 825 and 637, and β_i equals 9.3 and 6.9, for positive and negative movements, respectively. The exponential shape of the peak velocity–saccade amplitude relationship might suggest that the system is nonlinear, if one assumes a step input to the system. A step input would provide a linear peak velocity–saccade

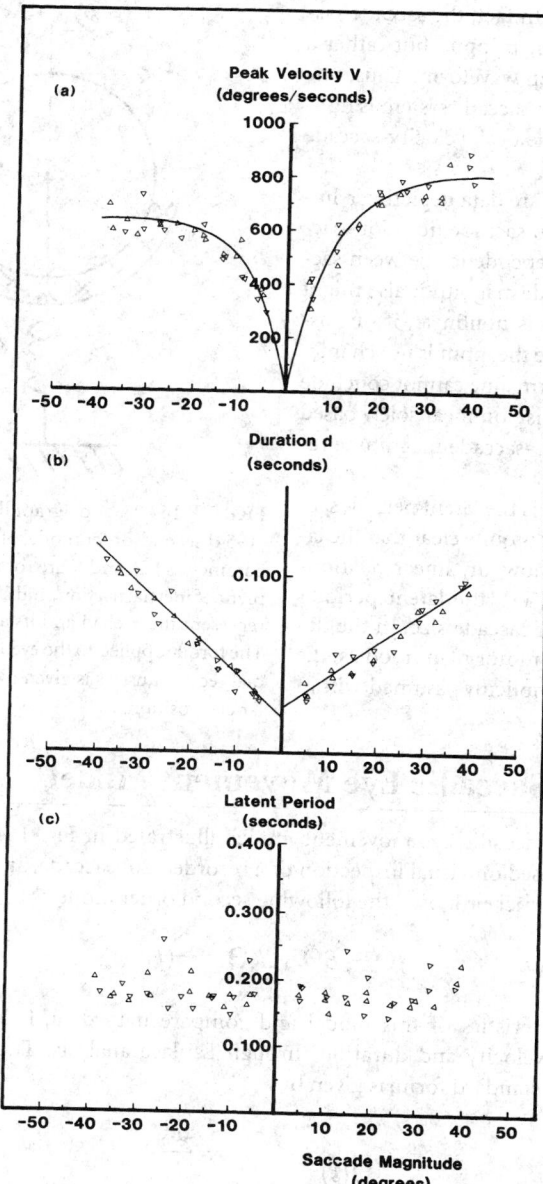

FIGURE 164.1 Main sequence diagrams. (*a*) peak velocity–saccade magnitude, (*b*) saccade duration–saccade magnitude, and (*c*) latent period–saccade magnitude for 54 saccadic eye movement by a single subject. *Source:* Enderle JD. 1988. Observations on pilot neurosensory control performance during saccadic eye movements. *Aviat Space Environ Med* 59:309. With permission.

amplitude relationship. In fact, the saccade system is not driven by a step input, but rather a more complex pulse-step waveform. Thus, one cannot conclude that the saccade system is nonlinear solely based on the peak velocity-saccade amplitude relationship.

Shown in Fig. 164.1*b* are data depicting a linear relationship between saccade duration–saccade magnitude. The dependence between saccade duration and saccade magnitude also might suggest that the system is nonlinear, if one assumes a step input. Since the input is not characterized by a step waveform, one cannot conclude that the saccade system is nonlinear solely based on the saccade duration–saccade magnitude relationship.

Shown in Fig. 164.1*c* is the latent period–saccade magnitude data. It is quite clear that the latent period does not show any linear relationship with saccade size, i.e., the latent period's value is independent of saccade size. In the development of the oculomotor plant models, the latent period will be implicitly assumed within the model.

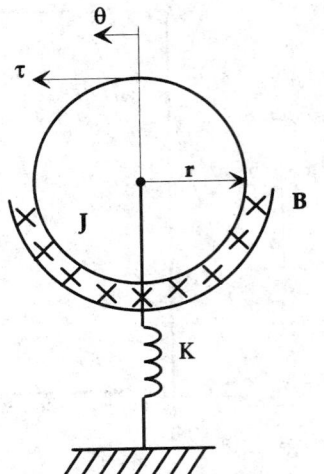

FIGURE 164.2   A diagram illustrating Westheimer's [1954] second-order model of the saccade system. The parameters J, B, and K are rotational elements for moment of inertia, friction, and stiffness, respectively, and represent the eyeball and its associated viscoelasticity. The torque applied to the eyeball by the lateral and medial rectus muscles is given by $\tau(t)$, and θ is the angular eye position.

164.2 Westheimer's Saccadic Eye Movement Model

The first quantitative saccadic eye movement model, illustrated in Fig. 164.2, was published by Westheimer [1954]. Based on visual inspection of a recorded 20° saccade, and the assumption of a step controller, Westheimer proposed the following second order model:

$$J\ddot{\Theta} + B\dot{\Theta} + K\Theta = \tau(t) \tag{164.2}$$

To analyze the characteristics of this model and compare it to data, it is convenient to solve Eq. (164.2) for peak velocity and duration through Laplace analysis. The transfer function of Eq. (164.2), written in standard form, is given by

$$H(s) = \frac{\Theta(s)}{\tau(s)} = \frac{\dfrac{\omega_n^2}{K}}{s^2 + 2\zeta\omega_n s + \omega_n^2} \tag{164.3}$$

where $\omega_n = \sqrt{\dfrac{K}{J}}$, and $\zeta = \dfrac{B}{2\sqrt{KJ}}$. Based on the saccade trajectory for a 20° saccade, Westheimer estimated $\omega_n = 120$ radians per second, and $\zeta = 0.7$. With the input $\tau(s) = \dfrac{\gamma}{s}$, $\Theta(t)$ is determined as

$$\Theta(t) = \frac{\gamma}{K}\left[1 + \frac{e^{-\zeta\omega_n t}}{\sqrt{1 - \zeta^2}} \cos(\omega_d t + \phi)\right] \tag{164.4}$$

where

$$\omega_d = \omega_n\sqrt{1 - \zeta^2} \quad \text{and} \quad \phi = \pi + \tan^{-1}\frac{-\zeta}{\sqrt{1 - \zeta^2}}$$

Duration, T_p, is found by first calculating

$$\frac{\partial \Theta}{\partial t} = \frac{\gamma e^{-\zeta \omega_n t}}{K \sqrt{1 - \zeta^2}} [-\zeta \omega_n \cos(\omega_d t + \phi) - \omega_d \sin(\omega_d t + \phi)] \qquad (164.5)$$

then determining T_p from $\left. \dfrac{\partial \Theta}{\partial t} \right|_{t=T_p} = 0$, yielding

$$T_p = \frac{\pi}{\omega_n \sqrt{1 - \zeta^2}} \qquad (164.6)$$

With Westheimer's parameter values, $T_p = 37$ ms for saccades of all sizes, which is independent of saccade magnitude and not in agreement with the experimental data that have a duration which increases as a function of saccade magnitude.

Predicted saccade peak velocity, $\dot{\Theta}(t_{mv})$, is found by first calculating

$$\frac{\partial^2 \Theta}{\partial t^2} = \frac{-\gamma e^{-\zeta \omega_n t}}{K \sqrt{1 - \zeta^2}} (-\zeta \omega_n (\zeta \omega_n \cos(\omega_d t + \phi) + \omega_d \sin(\omega_d t + \phi))$$

$$+ (-\zeta \omega_n \omega_d \sin(\omega_d t + \phi) + \omega_d^2 \cos(\omega_d t + \phi))) \qquad (164.7)$$

and then determining time at peak velocity, t_{mv}, from $\left. \dfrac{\partial^2 \Theta}{\partial t^2} \right|_{t=t_{mv}} = 0$, yielding

$$t_{mv} = \frac{1}{\omega_d} \tan^{-1} \left(\frac{\sqrt{1 - \zeta^2}}{\zeta} \right) \qquad (164.8)$$

Substituting t_{mv} into Eq. (164.5) gives the peak velocity $\dot{\Theta}(t_{mv})$. Using Westheimer's parameter values, and with the saccade magnitude given by $\Delta \Theta = \frac{\gamma}{K}$ [based on the steady-state value from Eq. (164.3)], we have from Eq. (164.5)

$$\dot{\Theta}(t_{mv}) = 55.02 \Delta \Theta \qquad (164.9)$$

that is, peak velocity is directly proportional to saccade magnitude. As illustrated in the main sequence diagram shown in Fig. 164.1a, experimental peak velocity data have an exponential form and are not a linear function as predicted by the Westheimer model.

Westheimer noted the differences between saccade duration–saccade magnitude and peak velocity–saccade magnitude in the model and the experimental data and inferred that the saccade system was not linear because the peak velocity–saccade magnitude plot was nonlinear, and the input was not an abrupt step function. Overall, this model provided a satisfactory fit to the eye position data for a saccade of 20°, but not for saccades of other magnitudes. Interestingly, Westheimer's second-order model proves to be an adequate model for saccades of all sizes, if one assumes a different input function as described in the next section. Due to its simplicity, the Westheimer model of the oculomotor plant is still popular today.

164.3 Robinson's Model of the Saccade Controller

In 1964, Robinson performed an experiment to measure the input to the eyeballs during a saccade. To record the input, one eye was held fixed using a suction contact lens, while the other eye performed a saccade from target to target. Since the same innervation signal is sent to both eyes during a saccade, Robinson inferred that the input, recorded through the transducer attached to the fixed eyeball, was the same input driving the other eyeball. He estimated that the neural commands controlling the eyeballs during a saccade are a pulse plus a step, or simply, a pulse-step input.

It is important to distinguish between the tension or force generated by a muscle, called *muscle tension,* and the force generator within the muscle, called the active-state tension generator. The active-state tension generator creates a force within the muscle that is transformed through the internal elements of the muscle into the muscle tension. Muscle tension is external and measurable, and the active-state tension is internal and unmeasurable. Moreover, Robinson [1981] reported that the active-state tensions are not identical to the neural controllers, but described by low-pass filtered pulse-step waveforms. The neural control and the active-state tension signals are illustrated in Fig. 164.3. The agonist pulse input is required to get the eye to the target as soon as possible, and the step is required to keep the eye at that location.

Robinson [1964] also described a model for fast eye movements (constructed from empirical considerations) which simulated saccades over a range of 5–40° by changing the amplitude of the

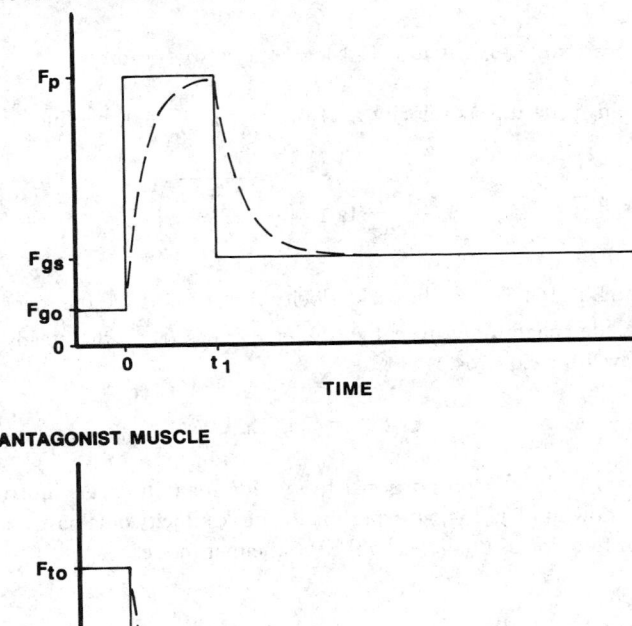

FIGURE 164.3   Agonist and antagonist neurologic control signals (solid lines) and the agonist and antagonist active-state tensions (dashed lines). Note that the time constant for activation is different from the time constant for deactivation. *Source:* Enderle JD, Wolfe JW. 1987. Time optimal control of saccadic eye movements. IEEE Trans Biomed Eng 34(1): 43. With permission.

pulse-step input. Simulation results were adequate for the position-time relationship, but the velocity-time relationship was inconsistent with physiologic evidence. To correct this deficiency of the model, physiologic studies of the oculomotor plant were carried out during the 1960s through the 1970s that allowed the development of a more homeomorphic oculomotor plant. Essential to this work was the construction of oculomotor muscle models.

164.4 A Linear Homeomorphic Saccadic Eye Movement Model

In 1980, Bahill and coworkers presented a linear fourth-order model of the oculomotor plant, based on physiologic evidence, that provides an excellent match between model predictions and eye movement data. This model eliminates the differences seen between velocity predictions of the model and the data and the acceleration predictions of the model and the data. For ease in presentation, the modification of this model by Enderle and coworkers [1984] will be used.

Figure 164.4 illustrates the mechanical components of the oculomotor plant for horizontal eye movements, the lateral and medial rectus muscle, and the eyeball. The agonist muscle is modeled as a parallel combination of an active state tension generator F_{AG}, viscosity element B_{AG}, and elastic

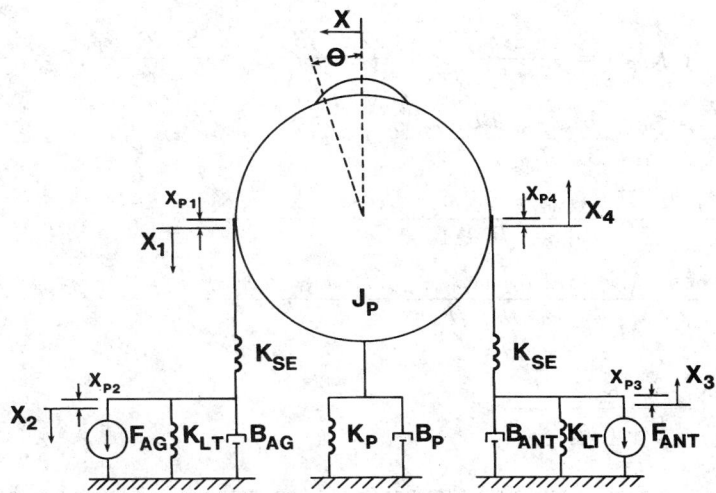

FIGURE 164.4 This diagram illustrates the mechanical components of the oculomotor plant. The muscles are shown to be extended from equilibrium, a position of rest, at the primary position (looking straight ahead), consistent with physiologic evidence. The average length of the rectus muscle at the primary position is approximately 40 mm and at the equilibrium position is approximately 37 mm. θ is the angle the eyeball is deviated from the primary position, and variable x is the length of arc traversed. When the eye is at the primary position, both θ and x are equal to zero. Variables x_1 through x_4 are the displacements from equilibrium for the stiffness elements in each muscle. Values x_{p1} through x_{p4} are the displacements from equilibrium for each of the variables x_1 through x_4 at the primary position. The total extension of the muscle from equilibrium at the primary position is x_{p1} plus x_{p2} or x_{p3} plus x_{p4}, which equals approximately 3 mm. It is assumed that the lateral and medial rectus muscles are identical, such that x_{p1} equals x_{p4} and x_{p3} and x_{p2}. The radius of the eyeball is r. *Source:* Enderle JD, Wolfe JW, Yates JT. 1984. The linear homeomorphic saccadic eye movement model—a modification. IEEE Trans Biomed Eng 31:717. With permission.

element K_{LT}, connected to a series elastic element K_{SE}. The antagonist muscle is similarly modeled as a parallel combination of an active-state tension generator F_{ANT}, viscosity element B_{ANT}, and elastic element K_{LT}, connected to a series elastic element K_{SE}. The eyeball is modeled as a sphere with moment of inertia J_P, connected to viscosity element B_P and elastic element K_P. The passive elasticity of each muscle is included in spring K_P for ease in analysis. Each of the elements defined in the oculomotor plant is ideal and linear.

Physiologic support for this model is based on the muscle model by Wilkie [1968], and estimates for the **extraocular** muscle elasticities and the passive tissues of the eyeball are based on experiments by Robinson [1981], Robinson and coworkers [1969], and Collins [1975], and studies of extraocular muscle viscosity by Bahill and coworkers [1980].

By summing the forces at junctions 2 and 3 (the equilibrium positions for x_2 and x_3) and the torques acting on the eyeball, using Laplace variable analysis about the operating point, the linear homeomorphic model, as shown in Fig. 164.4, is derived as

$$\delta(K_{SE}(K_{ST}(F_{AG} - F_{ANT}) + B_{ANT}\dot{F}_{AG} - B_{AG}\dot{F}_{ANT}))$$
$$= \ddddot{\Theta} + P_3\dddot{\Theta} + P_2\ddot{\Theta} + P_1\dot{\Theta} + P_0\Theta \tag{164.10}$$

where

$$K_{ST} = K_{SE} + K_{LT}, J = \frac{57.296 J_P}{r^2}, B = \frac{57.296 B_P}{r^2}, K = \frac{57.296 K_P}{r^2}, \delta = \frac{57.296}{r J B_{ANT} B_{AG}},$$

$$C_3 = \frac{J K_{ST}(B_{AG} + B_{ANT}) + B B_{ANT} B_{AG}}{J B_{ANT} B_{AG}}$$

$$C_2 = \frac{J K_{ST}^2 + B K_{ST}(B_{AG} + B_{ANT}) + B_{ANT} B_{AG}(K + 2 K_{SE})}{J B_{ANT} B_{AG}}$$

$$C_1 = \frac{B K_{ST}^2 + (B_{AG} + B_{ANT})(K K_{ST} + 2 K_{SE} K_{ST} - K_{SE}^2)}{J B_{ANT} B_{AG}}$$

$$C_0 = \frac{K K_{ST}^2 + 2 K_{SE} K_{ST} K_{LT}}{J B_{ANT} B_{AG}}$$

The agonist and antagonist active-state tensions are given by the following low-pass-filtered waveforms

$$\dot{F}_{AG} = \frac{N_{AG} - F_{AG}}{\tau_{AG}} \quad \text{and} \quad \dot{F}_{ANT} = \frac{N_{ANT} - F_{ANT}}{\tau_{ANT}} \tag{164.11}$$

where N_{AG} and N_{ANT} are the pulse-step waveforms shown in Fig. 164.3, and $\tau_{ag} = \tau_{ac}[u(t) - u(t - t_1)] + \tau_{de}u(t - t_1)$ and $\tau_{ant} = \tau_{de}[u(t) - u(t - t_1)] + \tau_{ac}u(t - t_1)$ are the time-varying time constants [Bahill et al., 1980].

Based on an analysis of experimental evidence, Enderle and Wolfe [1988] determined parameter estimates for the oculomotor plant as: $K_{SE} = 125$ Nm^{-1}, $K_{LT} = 32$ Nm^{-1}, $K = 66.4$ Nm^{-1}, $B = 3.1$ Nsm^{-1}, $J = 2.2 \times 10^{-3}$ Ns^{2}m^{-1}, $B_{AG} = 3.4$ Nsm^{-1}, $B_{ANT} = 1.2$ Nsm^{-1}, and $\delta = 72.536 \times 10^6$, and the steady-state active-state tensions as

$$F_{AG} = \begin{cases} 0.14 + 0.0185\Theta \; N \; for \; \Theta < 14.23° \\ 0.0283\Theta \; N \; for \; \Theta \geq 14.23° \end{cases} \tag{164.12}$$

$$F_{ANT} = \begin{cases} 0.14 - 0.00980\Theta \; N \, for \; \Theta < 14.23° \\ 0 \qquad\qquad\; N \, for \; \Theta \geq 14.23° \end{cases} \qquad (164.13)$$

Since saccades are highly variable, estimates of the dynamic active-state tensions are carried out on a saccade-by-saccade basis. One method to estimate the active-state tensions is using the system identification technique, a conjugate gradient search program carried out in the frequency domain [Enderle & Wolfe, 1988]. Figures 164.5–164.7 show the system identification technique results for an eye movement response to a 15° target movement. A close fit between the data and model prediction is seen in Fig. 164.5. Figures 164.6 and 164.7 further illustrate the accuracy of the final parameter estimates for velocity and acceleration. Estimates for agonist pulse magnitude are highly variable for saccade to saccade, even for the same size—see Fig. 9 of Enderle and Wolfe [1988]. Agonist pulse duration is closely coupled with pulse amplitude; as the pulse amplitude increases, the pulse duration decreases for saccades of the same magnitude. Reasonable values for the pulse amplitude for this model range from about 0.6N–1.4N. The larger the magnitude of the pulse, the larger the peak velocity of the eye movement.

164.5 Another Linear Homeomorphic Saccadic Eye Movement Model

The previous linear model of the oculomotor plant is derived from a nonlinear oculomotor plant model by Hsu and coworkers [1976] and based on a linearization of the force-velocity curve [Bahill et al., 1980]. Muscle viscosity traditionally has been modeled with a hyperbolic force-velocity relationship. Using the linear model of muscle reported by Enderle and coworkers [1991], it is possible to avoid the linearization and derive an updated linear homeomorphic saccadic eye movement model.

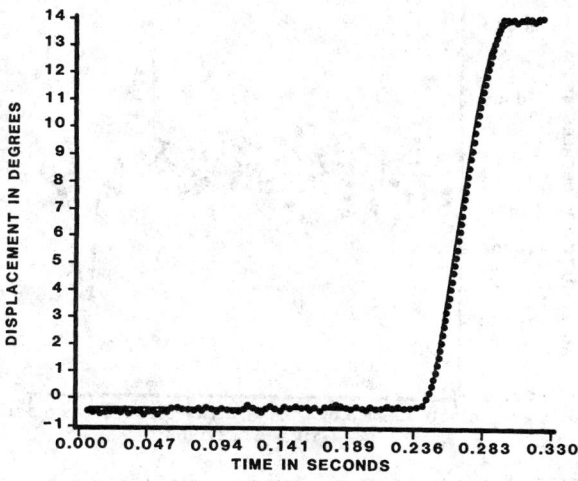

FIGURE 164.5 Saccadic eye movement in response to a 15° target movement. Solid line is the prediction of the saccadic eye movement model with the final parameter estimates computed using the system identification technique. Dots are the data. *Source:* Enderle JD, Wolfe JW. 1987. Time-optimal control of saccadic eye movements. IEEE Trans Biomed Eng 34(1):43. With permission.

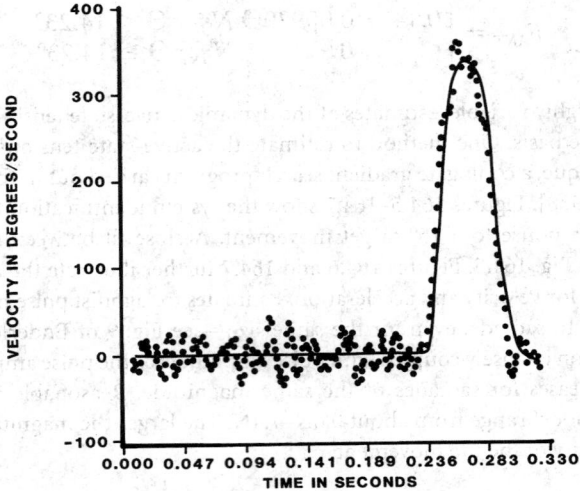

FIGURE 164.6 Velocity estimates for the saccadic eye movement illustrated in Fig. 164.5. Solid line is the saccadic eye movement model velocity prediction with the final parameter estimates computed using the system identification techniques. The dots are the two-point central difference estimates of velocity computed with a step size of 3 and a sampling interval of 1 ms. *Source:* Enderle JD, Wolfe JW. 1987. Time-optimal control of saccadic eye movements. IEEE Trans Biomed Eng 34(1):43. With permission.

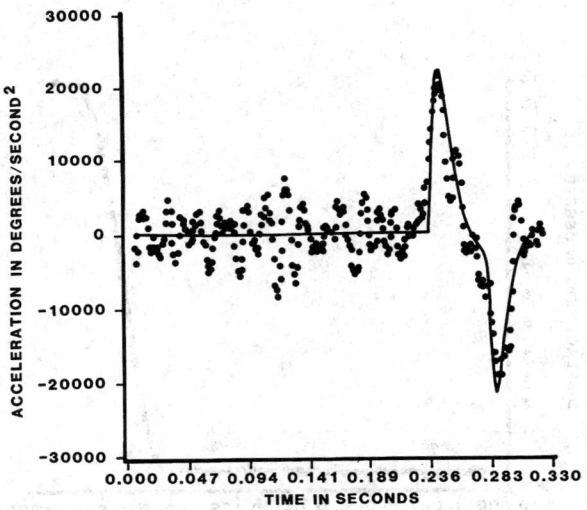

FIGURE 164.7 Acceleration estimates for the saccadic eye movement illustrated in Fig. 164.5. Solid line is the saccadic eye movement model acceleration prediction with the final parameter estimates computed using the system identification techniques. The dots are the 2-point central difference estimates of velocity computed with a step size of 4 and a sampling interval of 1 ms. *Source:* Enderle JD, Wolfe JW. 1987. Time-optimal control of saccadic eye movements. IEEE Trans Biomed Eng 34(1):43. With permission.

The linear muscle model has the static and dynamic properties of rectus eye muscle, a model without any nonlinear elements. The model has a nonlinear force-velocity relationship that matches muscle data using linear viscous elements, and the length tension characteristics are also in good agreement with muscle data within the operating range of the muscle. Some additional advantages of the linear muscle model are that a passive elasticity is not necessary if the equilibrium point $x_e = -19.3°$, rather than 15°, and muscle viscosity is a constant that does not depend on the innervation stimulus level.

Figure 164.8 illustrates the mechanical components of the updated oculomotor plant for horizontal eye movements, the lateral and medial rectus muscle, and the eyeball. The agonist muscle is modeled as a parallel combination of viscosity B_2 and series elasticity K_{SE}, connected to the parallel combination of active state tension generator F_{AG}, viscosity element B_1 and length tension elastic element K_{LT}. Since viscosity does not change with innervation level, agonist viscosity is set equal to antagonist viscosity. The antagonist muscle is similarly modeled with a suitable change in active state tension to F_{ANT}. The eyeball is modeled as a sphere with moment of inertia J_p, connected to a pair of viscoelastic elements connected in series; the update of the eyeball model is based on observations by Robinson [1981]. Each of the elements defined in the oculomotor plant is ideal and linear.

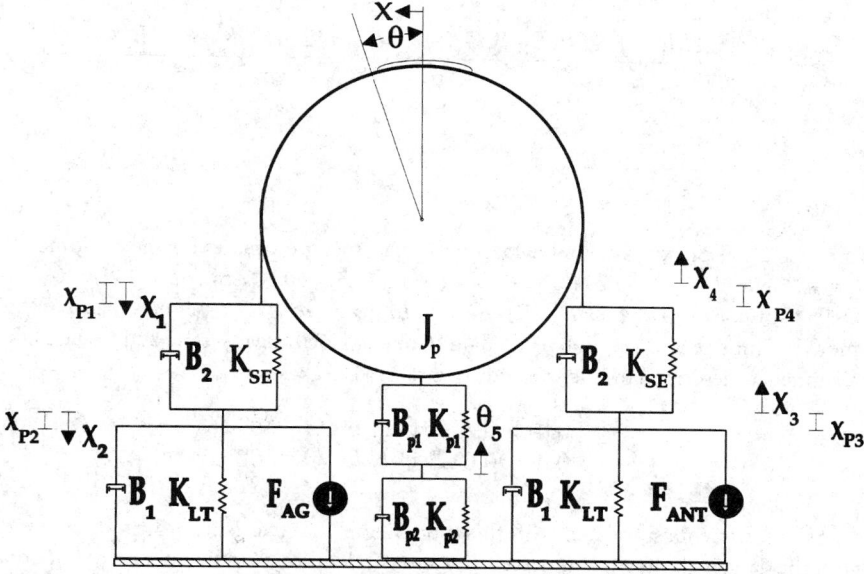

FIGURE 164.8 This diagram illustrates the mechanical components of the updated oculomotor plant. The muscles are shown to be extended from equilibrium, a position of rest, at the primary position (looking straight ahead), consistent with physiologic evidence. The average length of the rectus muscle at the primary position is approximately 40 mm and at the equilibrium position is approximately 37 mm. θ is the angle the eyeball is deviated from the primary position, and variable x is the length of arc traversed. When the eye is at the primary position, both θ and x are equal to zero. Variables x_1 through x_4 are the displacements from equilibrium for the stiffness elements in each muscle, and θ_5 is the rotational displacement for passive orbital tissues. Values x_{p1} through x_{p4} are the displacements from equilibrium for each of the variables x_1 through x_4 at the primary position. The total extension of the muscle from equilibrium at the primary position is x_{p1} plus x_{p2} or x_{p3} plus x_{p4}, which equals approximately 3 mm. It is assumed that the lateral and medial rectus muscles are identical, such that x_{p1} equals x_{p4} and x_{p3} equals x_{p2}. The radius of the eyeball is r.

The differential equation describing oculomotor plant model shown in Fig. 164.8 is derived by summing the forces acting at junctions 2 and 3 and the torques acting on the eyeball and junction 5, and using Laplace variable analysis about the operating point, and given by

$$\delta(K_{SE}K_{12}(F_{AG} - F_{ANT}) + (K_{SE}B_{34} + B_2K_{12})(\dot{F}_{AG} - \dot{F}_{ANT})$$

$$+ B_2B_{34}(\ddot{F}_{AG} - \ddot{F}_{ANT})) = \overset{....}{\Theta} + P_3\overset{...}{\Theta} + P_2\ddot{\Theta} + P_1\dot{\Theta} + P_0\Theta \qquad (164.15)$$

where

$$J = \frac{57.296J_p}{r^2}, B_3 = \frac{57.296B_{p1}}{r^2}, B_4 = \frac{57.296B_{p2}}{r^2}, K_1 = \frac{57.296K_{p1}}{r^2}, K_2 = \frac{57.296K_{p2}}{r^2},$$

$$B_{12} = B_1 + B_2, B_{34} = B_3 + B_4, K_{12} = K_1 + K_2, \delta = \frac{57.296}{rJB_{12}B_4}$$

$$C_3 = \frac{B_{12}(JK_2 + B_3B_4) + JB_4K_{ST} + 2B_1B_2B_{34}}{JB_{12}B_4}$$

$$C_2 = \frac{JK_{ST}K_2 + B_3B_4K_{ST} + B_{12}B_3K_2 + 2K_{SE}B_{34}B_1 + K_1B_{12}B_4 + 2B_2K_{LT}B_{34} + 2B_1K_{12}B_2}{JB_{12}B_4}$$

$$C_1 = \frac{K_{ST}(B_3K_2 + K_1B_4) + K_1K_2B_{12} + 2K_{LT}K_{SE}B_{34} + 2B_1K_{12}K_{SE} + 2B_2K_{LT}K_{12}}{JB_{12}B_4}$$

$$C_0 = \frac{2K_{LT}K_{SE}K_{12} + K_1K_{ST}K_2}{JB_{12}B_4}$$

Based on an analysis of experimental data, suitable parameter estimates for the oculomotor plant are: $K_{SE} = 125 \text{ Nm}^{-1}, K_{LT} = 60.7 \text{ Nm}^{-1}, B_1 = 4.6 \text{ Nsm}^{-1}, B_2 = 0.5 \text{ Nsm}^{-1}, J = 2.2 \times 10^{-3} \text{ Ns}^2\text{m}^{-1}, B_3 = 0.538 \text{ Nsm}^{-1}, B_4 = 41.54 \text{ Nsm}^{-1}, K_1 = 26.9 \text{ Nm}^{-1},$ and $K_2 = 41.54 \text{ Nm}^{-1}$. Based on the updated model of muscle and length tension data [Collins, 1975], steady-state active-state tensions are determined as described in Enderle and coworkers [1991] as

$$F = \begin{cases} 0.4 + 0.0175\Theta \text{ N for } \Theta \geq 0° \\ 0.4 - 0.0125\Theta \text{ N for } \Theta < 0° \end{cases} \qquad (164.16)$$

Saccadic eye movements simulated with this model have characteristics which are in good agreement with the data, including position, velocity and acceleration, and the main sequence diagrams.

164.6 Saccade Pathways

Clinical evidence, lesion and stimulation studies all point toward the participation of vitally important neural sites in the control of saccades, including the cerebellum, superior colliculus, thalamus, cortex, and other nuclei in the brain stem; evidence shows also that saccades are driven by two parallel neural networks. From each eye, the axons of retinal ganglion cells exit and join other neurons to form the optic nerve. The optic nerves from each eye then join at the optic chiasm, where fibers from the nasal half of each retina cross to the opposite side. Axons in the optic tract synapse in the lateral geniculate nucleus (a thalamic relay) and continue to the visual cortex. This portion of the saccade neural network is concerned with the recognition of visual stimuli. Axons in the optic tract also synapse in the superior colliculus. This second portion of the saccade neural network is concerned with the location of visual targets and is primarily responsible for goal-directed saccades.

Saccadic neural activity of the superior colliculus and cerebellum, in particular, have been identified as the saccade initiator and terminator, respectively, for a goal-directed saccade. The impact of the frontal eye field and the thalamus, while very important, have less important roles in the generation of goal-directed saccades to visual stimuli. The frontal eye fields are primarily concerned with voluntary saccades, and the thalamus appears to be involved with corrective saccades. Shown in Fig. 164.9 is a diagram illustrating important sites for the generation of a conjugate goal-directed horizontal saccade in both eyes [Enderle, 1994]. Each of the sites and connections detailed in Fig. 164.9 are fully supported by physiologic evidence. Some of these neural sites will be briefly described.

The superior colliculus (SC) contains two major functional divisions: a superficial division and an intermediate or deep division. Inputs to the superficial division are almost exclusively visual and originate from the retina and the visual cortex. The deep layers provide a convergence site of convergence for sensory signals from several modalities and a source of efferent commands for initiating saccades. The SC is the initiator of the saccade and thought to translate visual information into motor commands.

The deep layers of the superior colliculus initiate a saccade based on the distance between the current position of the eye and the desired target. The neural activity in the superior colliculus is organized into movement fields that are associated with the direction and saccade amplitude, and does not involve the initial position of the eyeball whatsoever. The movement field is shown in Fig. 164.10 for a 20° saccade. Neurons active during a particular saccade are shown as the dark circle, representing a desired 20° eye movement. Active neurons in the deep layers of the superior colliculus generate a high-frequency burst of activity beginning 18–20 ms before a saccade and ending sometime toward the end of the saccade; the exact timing for the end of the burst firing is quite random and can occur slightly before or slightly after the saccade ends. Each active bursting neuron discharges maximally, regardless of the initial position of the eye. Neurons discharging for small saccades have smaller movement fields, and those for larger saccades have larger movement fields. All the movement fields are connected to the same set of LLBN.

The cerebellum is responsible for the coordination of movement and is composed of a cortex of gray matter, internal white matter and three pairs of deep nuclei: fastigial nucleus, the interposed and globose nucleus, and dentate nucleus. The deep cerebellar nuclei and the vestibular nuclei transmit the entire output of the cerebellum. Output of the cerebellar cortex is carried through Purkinje cells. Purkinje cells send their axons to the deep cerebellar nuclei and have an inhibitory effect on these nuclei. The cerebellum is involved with both eye and head movements, and both tonic and phasic activity are reported in the cerebellum. The cerebellum is not directly responsible for the initiation or execution of a saccade but contributes to saccade precision. Sites within the cerebellum important for the control of eye movements include the oculomotor vermis, fastigial nucleus, and the flocculus. Consistent with the operation of the cerebellum for other movement activities, the cerebellum is postulated here to act both as the coordinator for a saccade and to as a precise gating mechanism.

The cerebellum is included in the saccade generator as a time-optimal gating element, using three active sites during a saccade: the vermis, fastigial nucleus, and flocculus. The vermis is concerned with the absolute starting position of a saccade in the movement field and corrects control signals for initial eye position. Using proprioceptors in the oculomotor muscles and an internal eye position reference, the vermis is aware of the current position of the eye. The vermis is also aware of the signals (dynamic motor error) used to generate the saccade via the connection with the NRTP and the superior colliculus.

With regard to the oculomotor system, the cerebellum has inputs from superior colliculus, lateral geniculate nucleus (LGN), oculomotor muscle proprioceptors, and striate cortex via NRTP. The cerebellum sends inputs to the NRTP, LLBN, EBN, VN, thalamus, and superior colliculus. The oculomotor vermis and fastigial nuclei are important in the control of saccade amplitude, and the

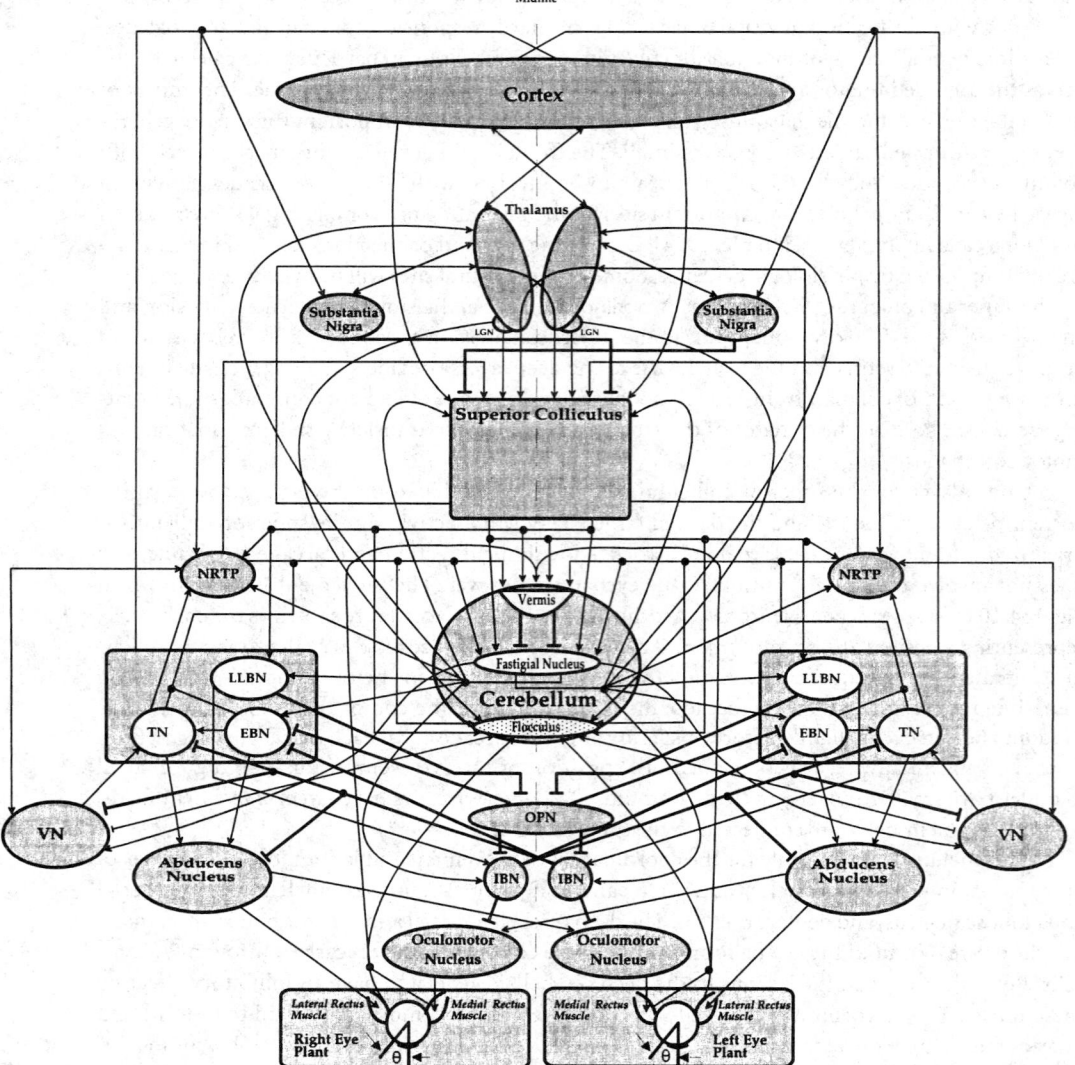

FIGURE 164.9 Shown is a diagram illustrating important sites for the generation of a conjugate horizontal saccade in both eyes. It consists of the familiar premotor excitatory burst neurons (EBN), inhibitory burst neurons (IBN), long lead burst neurons (LLBN), omnipause neurons (OPN), tonic neurons (TN), and the vestibular nucleus, abducens nucleus, oculomotor nucleus, cerebellum, substantia nigra, nucleus reticularis tegmenti pontis (NRTP), the thalamus, the deep layers of the superior colliculus (SC), and the oculomotor plant for each eye. Excitatory inputs are shown with an arrow, inhibitory inputs are shown with a ⊥. Consistent with current knowledge, the left and right structures of the neural circuit model are maintained. This circuit diagram was constructed after a careful review of the current literature. Each of the sites and connections is supported by firm physiologic evidence. Since interest is in goal-directed visual saccades, the cortex has not been partitioned into the frontal eye field and posterior eye field (striate, prestriate, and inferior parietal cortices).

flocculus, perihypoglossal nuclei of the rostral medulla, and possibly the pontine and mesencephalic reticular formation, are thought to form the integrator within the cerebellum. One important function of the flocculus may be to increase the time constant of the neural integrator for saccades starting at locations different from primary position.

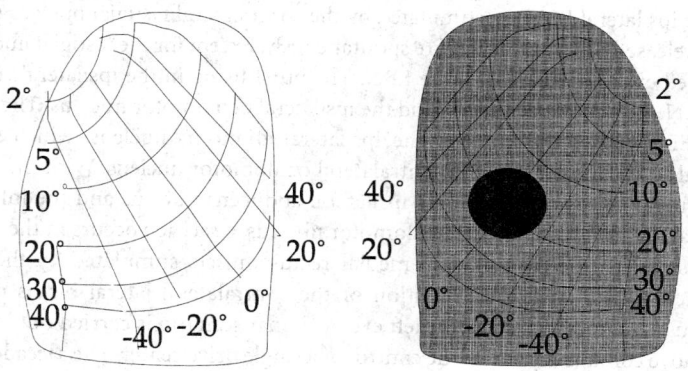

FIGURE 164.10 Movement fields of the superior colliculus.

The fastigial nucleus receives input from the superior colliculus, as well as other sites. The output of the fastigial nucleus is excitatory and projects ipsilaterally and contralaterally as shown in Fig. 164.9. During fixation, the fastigial nucleus fires tonically at low rates; 20 ms prior to a saccade, the contralateral fastigial nucleus bursts, and the ipsilateral fastigial nucleus pauses and then discharges with a burst. The pause in ipsilateral firing is due to Purkinje cell input to the fastigial nucleus. The sequential organization of Purkinje cells along beams of parallel fibers suggests that the cerebellar cortex might function as a delay, producing a set of timed pulses which could be used to program the duration of the saccade. If one considers nonprimary position saccades, different temporal and spatial schemes, via cerebellar control, are necessary to produce the same size saccade. It is postulated here that the cerebellum acts as a gating device which precisely terminates a saccade based on the initial position of the eye in the orbit.

The PPRF has neurons that burst at frequencies up to 1000 Hz during saccades and are silent during periods of fixation and neurons that fire tonically during periods of fixation. Neurons that fire at steady rates during fixation are called *tonic neurons* (TNs) and are responsible for holding the eye steady. The TN firing rate depends on the position of the eye (presumably through a local integrator type network). The TNs are thought to provide the step component to the motoneuron. There are two types of burst neurons in the PPRF called the *long-lead burst neuron* (LLBN) and a *medium-lead burst neuron* (MLBN); during periods of fixation, these neurons are silent. The LLBN burst at least 12 ms before a saccade and the MLBN burst less than 12 ms (typically 6–8 ms) before the saccade. The MLBN are connected monosynaptically with the abducens nucleus.

There are two types of neurons within the MLBN, the excitatory burst neurons (EBN) and the inhibitory burst neurons (IBN). The EBN and IBN labels describe the synaptic activity upon the motoneurons; the EBN excite and are responsible for the burst firing, and the IBN inhibit and are responsible for the pause. A mirror image of these neurons exists on both sides of the midline. The IBN inhibit the EBN on the contralateral side.

Also within the brain stem is another type of saccade neuron called the *omnipause neuron* (OPN). The OPN fires tonically at approximately 200 Hz during periods of fixation and is silent during saccades. The OPN stops firing approximately 10–12 ms before a saccade and resumes tonic firing approximately 10 ms before the end of the saccade. The OPN are known to inhibit the MLBN and are inhibited by the LLBN. The OPN activity is responsible for the precise timing between groups of neurons that causes a saccade.

Qualitatively, a saccade occurs according to the following sequence of events within the PPRF. First, the ipsilateral LLBN are stimulated by the SC, initiating the saccade. The LLBN then inhibits the tonic firing of the OPN. When the OPN cease firing, the MLBN is released from inhibition and begins firing (these neurons fire spontaneously and also stimulated by the fastigial nucleus). The ipsilateral IBN are stimulated by the ipsilateral LLBN and the contralateral fastigial nucleus of the cerebellum. The ipsilateral EBN are stimulated by the contralateral fastigial nucleus of the cerebellum and, when released from inhibition fire spontaneously. Except for the fastigial nucleus, there are no other accepted excitatory inputs to the EBN. The burst firing in the ipsilateral IBN inhibit the contralateral EBN and abducens nucleus and the ipsilateral oculomotor nucleus. The burst firing in the ipsilateral EBN causes the burst in the ipsilateral abducens nucleus, which stimulates the ipsilateral lateral rectus muscle and the contralateral oculomotor nucleus. With the stimulation of the ipsilateral lateral rectus muscle by the ipsilateral abducens nucleus and the inhibition of the ipsilateral medial rectus muscle via the oculomotor nucleus, a saccade occurs in the right eye.

Simultaneously, with the contralateral medial rectus muscle stimulated by the contralateral oculomotor nucleus, and with the inhibition of the contralateral lateral rectus muscle via the abducens nucleus, a saccade occurs in the left eye. A similar scenario is carried out in the right eye. Thus the eyes move conjugately under the control of a single drive center. The saccade is terminated with the resumption of tonic firing in the OPN via the fastigial nucleus.

164.7 Saccade Control Mechanism

Although the purpose for a saccadic eye movement is clear, that is, to quickly redirect the eyeball to the destination, the neural control mechanism is not. Until quite recently, saccade generator models involved a ballistic or preprogrammed control to the desired eye position based on retinal error alone. Today, an increasing number of investigators are putting forth the idea that visual goal-directed saccades are controlled by a local feedback loop that continuously drives the eye to the desired eye position. This hypothesis first gained acceptance in 1975 when Robinson suggested that saccades originate from neural commands that specify the desired position of the eye rather than the preprogrammed distance the eye must be moved. The value of the actual eye position is subtracted from the desired position to create an error signal that completes the local feedback loop that drives a high-gain burst element to generate the neural pulse. This neural pulse continuously drives the eye until the error signal is zero.

Subsequently, a number of other investigators have modified the local feedback mechanism proposed by Robinson [1975] to better describe the neural connections and firing patterns of brainstem neurons in the control of horizontal saccadic eye. In addition to the Robinson model, two other models describe a saccade generator [Enderle, 1994; Scudder, 1988]. All the models involve three types of premotor neurons: burst, tonic, and pause cells, as previously described, and involve a pulse-step change in firing rate at the motoneuron during a saccadic eye movement.

Although the general pattern of motoneuron activity is qualitatively accepted during a saccadic eye movement, there is little agreement on a quantitative discharge description. The saccade generator models by Robinson and Scudder are structured to provide a control signal that is proportionally weighted (or dependent) to the desired saccade size, as opposed to the saccade generator model structured to provide a control signal that is independent of saccade amplitude. Using time-optimal control theory and the system identification technique, Enderle and Wolfe [1988] investigated the control of saccades and reported that the system operates under a first-order time-optimal control. The concepts underlying this hypothesis are that each muscle's active-state tension is described by a low-pass filtered pulse-step waveform in which the magnitude of the agonist pulse is a maximum regardless of the amplitude of the saccade and that only the duration of the agonist pulse affects the size of the saccade. The antagonist muscle is completely inhibited during the period of maximum agonist stimulation. The saccade generator illustrated in Fig. 164.9 operates under these principles and provides simulations which match the data very well.

Saccadic eye movements were simulated using TUTSIM, a continuous time simulation program, for the saccade generator model presented in Fig. 164.9, and compared with experimental data. Neural sites (nucleus) are described via a *functional* block diagram description of the horizontal saccade generator model as shown in Fig. 164.11 and 164.12. Table 164.1 summarizes additional firing characteristics for the neural sites. The output of each block represents the firing pattern at each neural site observed during the saccade; time zero indicates the start of the saccade and *T* represents

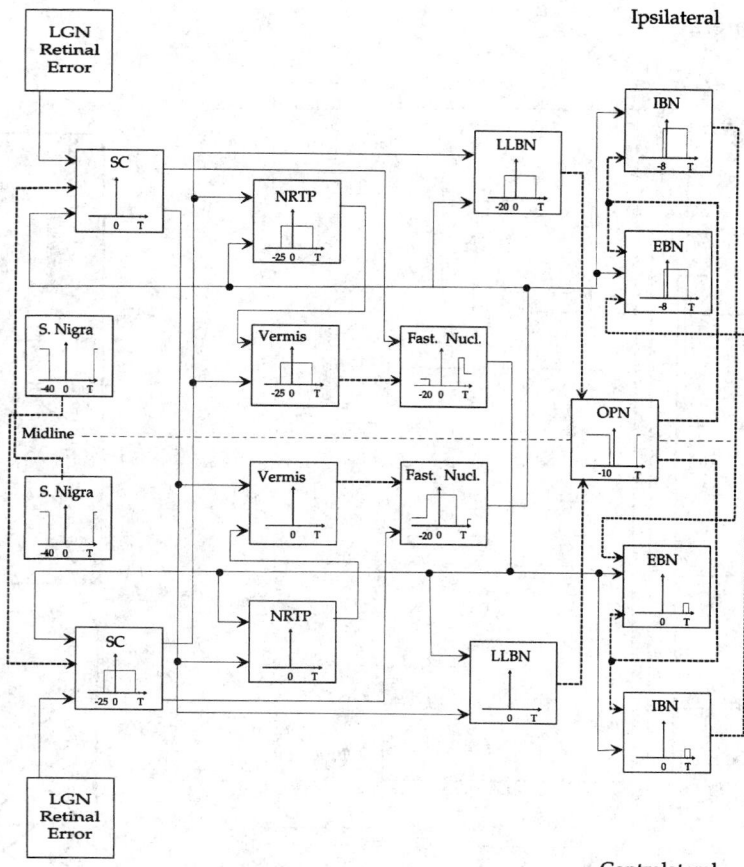

FIGURE 164.11 A functional block diagram of the saccade generator model. Solid lines are excitatory and dashed lines are inhibitory. This figure illustrates the first half of the network.

the end of the saccade. Naturally, the firing pattern observed for each block represents the firing pattern for a single neuron, as recorded in the literature, but the block represents the cumulative effect of all the neurons within that site. Consistent with a time optimal control theory, neural activity is represented within each of the blocks as pulses and/or steps to reflect their operation as timing gates. The superior colliculus fires maximally as long as the dynamic motor error is greater than zero, in agreement with the first-order time optimal controller and physiologic evidence. Notice that the LLBNs are driven by the superior colliculus as long as there is a feedback error maintained by the cerebellar vermis. In all likelihood, the maximal firing rate by the superior colliculus is stochastic, depending on a variety of physiologic factors such as the interest in tracking the target, anxiety, frustration, stress, and other factors. The actual firing patterns in the superior colliculus, the burst neurons in the PPRF (LLBN, EBN, and IBN) and abducens nucleus are simulated with filtered pulse signals, consistent with the physical limitations of neurons. For the superior colliculus and the LLBN, this involves a single pulse, for the EBN and IBN, this involves two pulses with different filters (the first pulse describes the brief rise and subsequent fall within the first 10 ms during a saccade, and the second pulse describes the steady state pulse during the saccade) to match the electrophysiologic data.

Illustrated in Fig. 164.13 is an extracellular single unit recording for the EBN, eye position data, and a simulation for a 20° saccade. Details of the experiment are given in Enderle [1994]. A 20° saccade was simulated by using EBN data as input and the oculomotor plant in Fig. 164.8. Few differences between the data and the simulation results are observed for this movement, as well as other

Ipsilateral

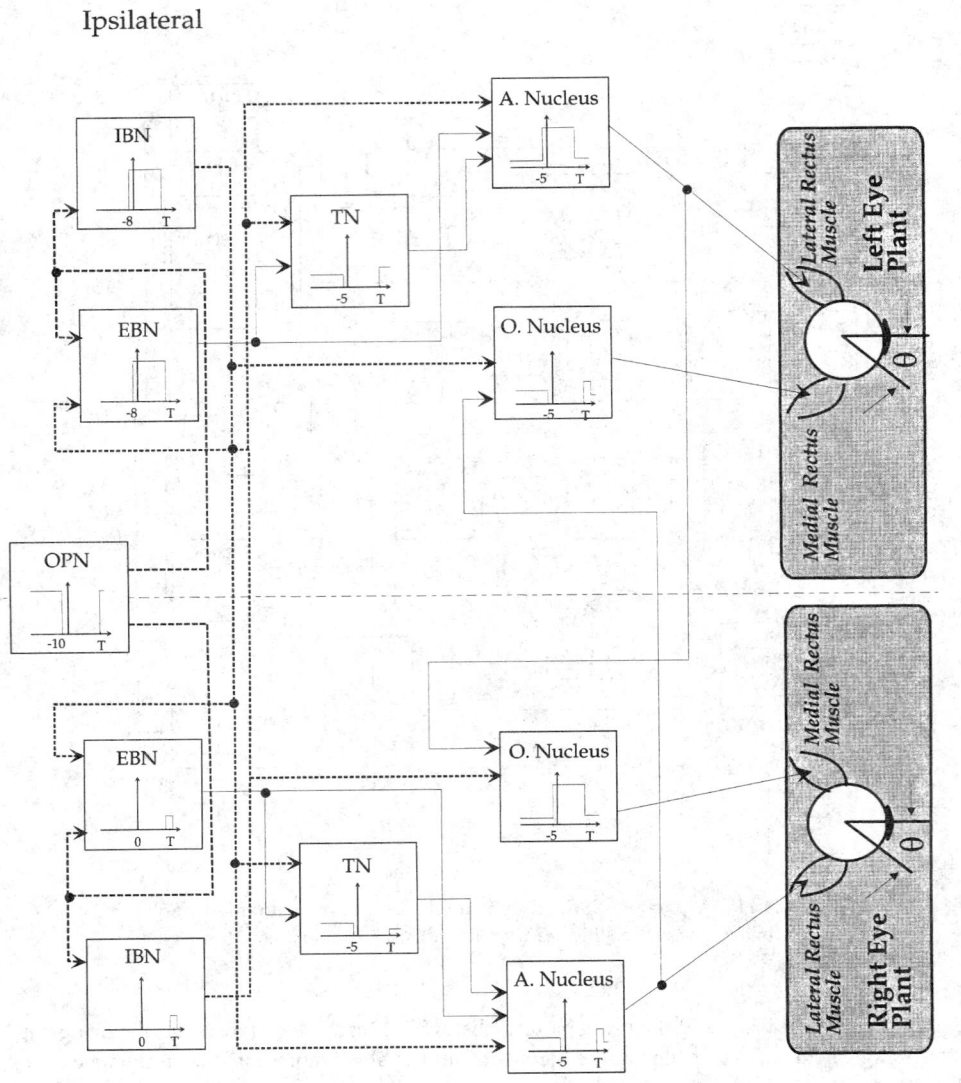

Contralateral

FIGURE 164.12   A functional block diagram of the saccade generator model. Solid lines are excitatory and dashed lines are inhibitory. This figure illustrates the second half of the network.

eye movements. The saccade generator model in Fig. 164.9 also provides an excellent description of the saccade system and matches the data very well for all naturally occurring saccades, including saccades with dynamic overshoot and glissadic behavior, without parametric changes [Enderle, 1994].

164.8 Conclusion

This chapter has focused on quantitative models and control of the fast eye movement system. Each of the oculomotor plant models described here are linear. Beginning with the most simple quanti-

TABLE 164.1　Activity of Neural Sites During a Saccade

Neural Site	Onset Before Saccade	Peak Firing Rate	End Time
Abducens nucleus	5 ms	400–800 Hz	Ends approx. 5 ms before saccade ends
Contralateral fastigial nucleus	20 ms	200 Hz	Pulse ends with pause approx. 10 ms before saccade ends, resumes tonic firing approx. 10 ms after saccade ends
Contralateral superior colliculus	20–25 ms	800–1000 Hz	Ends approx. when saccade ends
Ipsilateral cerebellar vermis	20–25 ms	600–800 Hz	Ends approx. 25 ms before saccade ends
Ipsilateral EBN	6–8 ms	600–800 Hz	Ends approx. 10 ms before saccade ends
Ipsilateral fastigial nucleus	20 ms	Pause during saccade, and a burst of 200 Hz toward the end of the saccade	Pause ends with burst approx. 10 ms before saccade ends, resumes tonic firing approx. 10 ms after saccade ends
Ipsilateral FEF	>30 ms	600–800 Hz	Ends approx. when saccade ends
Ipsilateral IBN	6–8 ms	600–800 Hz	Ends approx. 10 ms before saccade ends
Ipsilateral LLBN	20 ms	800–1000 Hz	Ends approx. when saccade ends
Ipsilateral NRTP	20–25 ms	800–1000 Hz	Ends approx. when saccade ends
Ipsilateral substantia nigra	40 ms	40–100 Hz	Resumes firing approx. 40–150 ms after saccade ends
OPN	6–8 ms	150–200 Hz (before and after)	Ends approx. when saccade ends

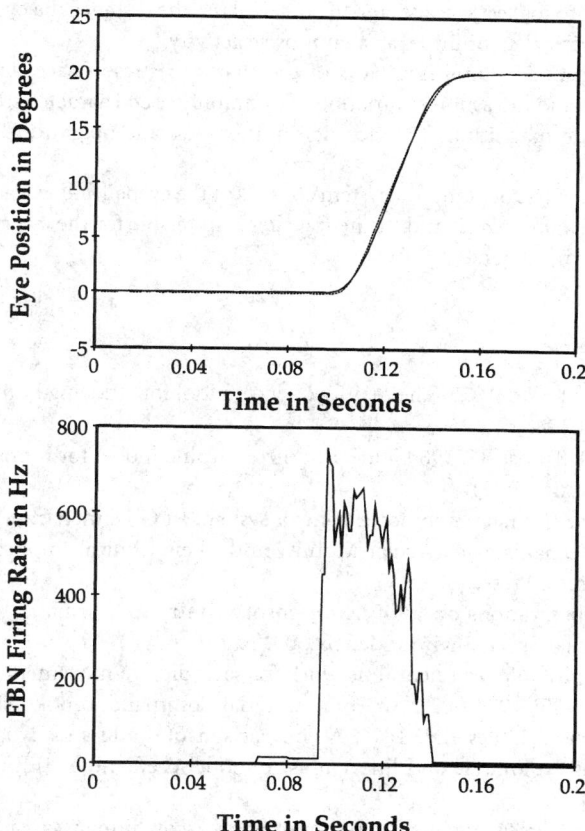

FIGURE 164.13 Simulated eye position in solid line shown in top graph, generated with EBN saccade data (shown in lower graph) and the oculomotor plant in Fig. 164.8. Actual eye movement data recorded with the EBN data during a saccadic eye movement, shown as dashed line in top graph. Data provided by Dr. David Sparks from his laboratory at the University of Alabama.

tative model of saccades by Westhiemer [1954], important characteristics of saccades were determined as a means of evaluating the quality of saccade models. Next, models of increasing complexity were presented with the end goal of constructing a homeomorphic saccade model of the oculomotor plant. These plant models were driven by improved models of muscle that ultimately provided an excellent match of the static and dynamic properties of rectus eye muscle. Finally, the control of saccades was considered from the basis of systems control theory and anatomic considerations. Many nonlinear models of the oculomotor plant exist, and readers interested in learning about them should consult Robinson [1981].

Defining Terms

Active-state tension generator: The active-state tension generator describes the element within the muscle that creates a force. This force is different from muscle tension, which is the force due to the active-state tension generator and all the other elements within the muscle.

Extraocular muscles: The six muscles attached directly to the outside of the eyeball, consisting of the medial, lateral, superior, inferior recti, and the superior and inferior oblique muscles.

Homeomorphic: As close to reality as possible.

Latent period: The latent period is thought to be the time interval during which the CNS determines whether to make a saccade, and, if so, calculates the distance the eyeball is to be moved, transforming retinal error into transient muscle activity.

Main-sequence diagrams: Summary plots of the characteristics of saccades that allow one to compare inter- and intrasubject variations. Commonly used characteristics include: (1) peak velocity–saccade magnitude, (2) saccade duration–saccade magnitude, and (3) latent period–saccade magnitude.

Oculomotor system: The oculomotor system consists of the eyeball and extraocular muscles (also called the *oculomotor plant*) and the neural sites responsible for the eye movement.

Saccade: A fast eye movement.

References

Bahill AT, Clark MR, Stark L. 1975. The main sequence, a tool for studying human eye movements. Math Biosci 24:194.

Bahill AT, Latimer JR, Troost BT. 1980. Linear homeomorphic model for human movement. IEEE Trans Biomed Eng 27:631.

Collins CC. 1975. The human oculomotor control system. In G Lennerstrand and P Bach-y-Rita (eds), Basic Mechanisms of Ocular Motility and Their Clinical Implications, pp 145–180, Oxford, Pergamon Press.

Enderle JD. 1988. Observations on pilot neurosensory control performance during saccadic eye movements. Aviat Space Environ Med 59:309.

Enderle JD. 1994. A physiological neural network for saccadic eye movement control. Armstrong Laboratory/AO-TR-1994-0023. Air Force Material Command, Brooks Air Force Base, Texas.

Enderle JD, Engelken EJ, Stiles RN. 1991. A comparison of static and dynamic characteristics between rectus eye muscle and linear muscle model predictions. IEEE Trans Biomed Eng 38:1235.

Enderle JD, Wolfe JW. 1988. Frequency response analysis of human saccadic eye movements. Comput Biol Med 18(3):195.

Enderle JD, Wolfe JW, Yates JT. 1984. The linear homeomorphic saccadic eye movement model—a modification. IEEE Trans Biomed Eng 31(11):717.

Hsu FK, Bahill AT, Stark L. 1976. Parametric sensitivity of a homeomorphic model for saccadic and vergence eye movements. Comput Methods Programs Biomed 6:108.

Robinson DA. 1964. The mechanics of human saccadic eye movement. J Physiol (London). 174:245.

Robinson DA. 1975. Oculomotor control signals. In G Lennerstrand, P Bach-y-Rita (eds), Basic Mechanisms of Ocular Motility and their Clinical Implication, pp 337–374, Oxford, Pergamon Press.

Robinson DA. 1981. Models of mechanics of eye movements. In BL Zuber (ed), Models of Oculomotor Behavior and Control, pp 21–41, Boca Raton, Fla, CRC Press.

Robinson DA, O'Meara DM, Scott AB, et al. 1969. Mechanical components of human eye movements. J Appl Physiol 26:548.

Scudder CA. 1988. A new local feedback model of the saccadic burst generator. J Neurophysiol 59(4):1454.

Westheimer G. 1954. Mechanism of saccadic eye movements. AMA Arch Ophthalmol 52:710.

Wilkie DR. 1968. Muscle: Studies in Biology, vol 11, London, Edward Arnold.

Further Information

Readers interested in additional information on the subject of fast eye movements should consult the following books. In addition, many journals publish articles on saccadic eye movements—for a sample of these journals, see the references listed within the following books as well.

Bahill AT. 1981. Bioengineering, Biomedical, Medical and Clinical Engineering, Englewood Cliffs, NJ, Prentice-Hall.

Carpenter RHS. 1988. Movements of the Eyes, 2d rev ed, London, Pion Ltd.

Wurtz RH, Goldberg ME. 1989. The Neurobiology of Saccadic Eye Movements, New York, Elsevier.

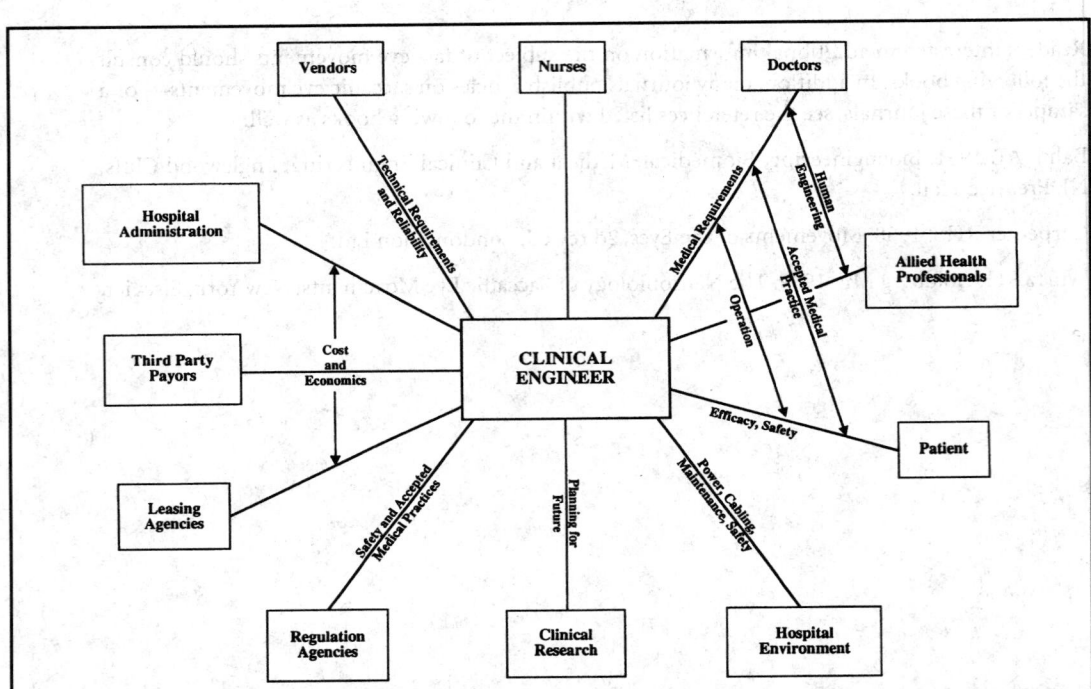

Human interactions of the clinical engineer.

XVI

Clinical Engineering

Yadin David
Texas Children's Hospital

O VER THE PAST 100 YEARS, the health care system's dependence on medical technology for the delivery of its services has grown continuously. To some extent, all professional care providers depend on technology, be it in the area of preventive medicine, diagnosis, therapeutic care, rehabilitation, administration, or health-related education and training. Medical technology enables practitioners to intervene through integrated interaction with their patients in a cost-effective, efficient, and safe manner. As a result, the field of clinical engineering has emerged as the discipline of biomedical engineering that fulfills the need to manage the deployment of medical technology and to integrate it appropriately with desired clinical practices.

The health care delivery system presents a very complex environment where facilities, equipment, materials, and a full range of human interventions are involved. It is in this clinical environment that patients of various ages and conditions, trained staff, and the wide variety of medical technology converge. This complex mix of interactions may lead to unacceptable risk when programs for monitoring, controlling, improving, and educating all entities involved are not appropriately integrated by qualified professionals.

This section on clinical engineering focuses on the methodology for administering critical engineering services that vary from facilitation of innovation and technology transfer to the performance of technology assessment and operations support and on the management tools with which today's clinical engineer needs to be familiar. With increased awareness of the value obtained by these services, new career opportunities are created for clinical engineers.

In this section the authors have attempted to provide a description of the wide range of responsibilities clinical engineering professionals encounter. After presenting the evolution of the field of clinical engineering, Chapter 165 gives specific attention to the primary function of clinical engineers. Chapter 166 describes technology management and assessment in considerable detail, using examples and case studies in a large medical center. Chapter 167 focuses on a particular technology management tool for assessing the medical equipment risk factor that can help clinical engineers effectively manage/prioritize the services to be provided to each piece of equipment under their control. Chapter 168 takes an expansive view of career opportunities for clinical engineers, while Chapter 169 focuses on one particular role, namely, that of innovator and product developer. To further assist clinical engineers in managing their equipment, Chapters 170 and 171 examine an establishment of program indicators that can lead to quality improvement. The clinical engineering program can be based in a single community hospital, in a teaching medical center, within a chain of hospitals, as part of a government agency, or as a shared service organization. Chapter 172 describes the use of coordinated services as they are offered by the West of Scotland Health Board, and Chapters 173 and 174 present a review of the standards and regulatory agencies of interest to clinical engineers. Global programs present different challenges to practitioners in developing countries because the resources and logistics are different than they are in the United States. Chapter 175 looks at specific clinical engineering issues from the perspective of developing countries.

In addition to highlighting the important roles that clinical engineers serve in many areas, the section focuses on those areas of the clinical engineering field that enhance the understanding of the "bigger picture." With such an understanding, the participation in and contribution by clinical engineers to this enlarged scope can be fully realized. The adoption of the tools described here will enable clinical engineers to fulfill their new role in the evolving health care delivery system.

All the authors in this section recognize this opportunity and are here recognized for volunteering their talent and time so that others can excel as well.

165

Clinical Engineering: Evolution of a Discipline

Joseph D. Bronzino
Trinity College/The Hartford Graduate Center

165.1 What Is a Clinical Engineer?

As discussed in the introduction to this *Handbook,* biomedical engineers apply the concepts, knowledge, and techniques of virtually all engineering disciplines to solve specific problems in the biosphere, i.e., the realm of biology and medicine. When biomedical engineers work within a hospital or clinic, they are more properly called *clinical engineers.* But what exactly is the definition of the term *clinical engineer?* In recent years, a number of organizations, e.g., the American Heart Association [1986], the American Association of Medical Instrumentation [Goodman, 1989], the American College of Clinical Engineers [Bauld, 1991], and the *Journal of Clinical Engineering* [Pacela, 1991], have attempted to provide an appropriate definition for the term *clinical engineer.* For the purposes of this handbook, a *clinical engineer* is an engineer who has graduated from an accredited academic program in engineering or who is licensed as a professional engineer or engineer-in-training and is engaged in the application of scientific and technological knowledge developed through engineering education and subsequent professional experience within the health care environment in support of clinical activities. Furthermore, the clinical environment is defined as that portion of the health care system in which patient care is delivered, and clinical activities include direct patient care, research, teaching, and public service activities intended to enhance patient care.

165.2 Evolution of Clinical Engineering

Engineers were first encouraged to enter the clinical scene during the late 1960s in response to concerns about patient safety as well as the rapid proliferation of clinical equipment, especially in academic medical centers. In the process, a new engineering discipline—clinical engineering—evolved to provide the technological support necessary to meet these new needs. During the 1970s, a major expansion of clinical engineering occurred, primarily due to the following events:

- The Veterans' Administration (VA), convinced that clinical engineers were vital to the overall operation of the VA hospital system, divided the country into biomedical engineering districts, with a chief biomedical engineer overseeing all engineering activities in the hospitals in that district.

- Throughout the United States, clinical engineering departments were established in most large medical centers and hospitals and in some smaller clinical facilities with at least 300 beds.
- Clinical engineers were hired in increasing numbers to help these facilities use existing technology and incorporate new technology.

Having entered the hospital environment, routine electrical safety inspections exposed the clinical engineer to all types of patient equipment that was not being maintained properly. It soon became obvious that electrical safety failures represented only a small part of the overall problem posed by the presence of medical equipment in the clinical environment. The equipment was neither totally understood nor properly maintained. Simple visual inspections often revealed broken knobs, frayed wires, and even evidence of liquid spills. Investigating further, it was found that many devices did not perform in accordance with manufacturers' specifications and were not maintained in accordance with manufacturers' recommendations. In short, electrical safety problems were only the tip of the iceberg. The entrance of clinical engineers into the hospital environment changed these conditions for the better. By the mid-1970s, complete performance inspections before and after use became the norm, and sensible inspection procedures were developed [Newhouse et al., 1989]. In the process, clinical engineering departments became the logical support center for all medical technologies and became responsible for all the biomedical instruments and systems used in hospitals, the training of medical personnel in equipment use and safety, and the design, selection, and use of technology to deliver safe and effective health care.

With increased involvement in many facets of hospital/clinic activities, clinical engineers now play a multifaceted role (Fig. 165.1). They must interface successfully with many "clients," including clinical staff, hospital administrators, regulatory agencies, etc., to ensure that the medical equipment within the hospital is used safely and effectively.

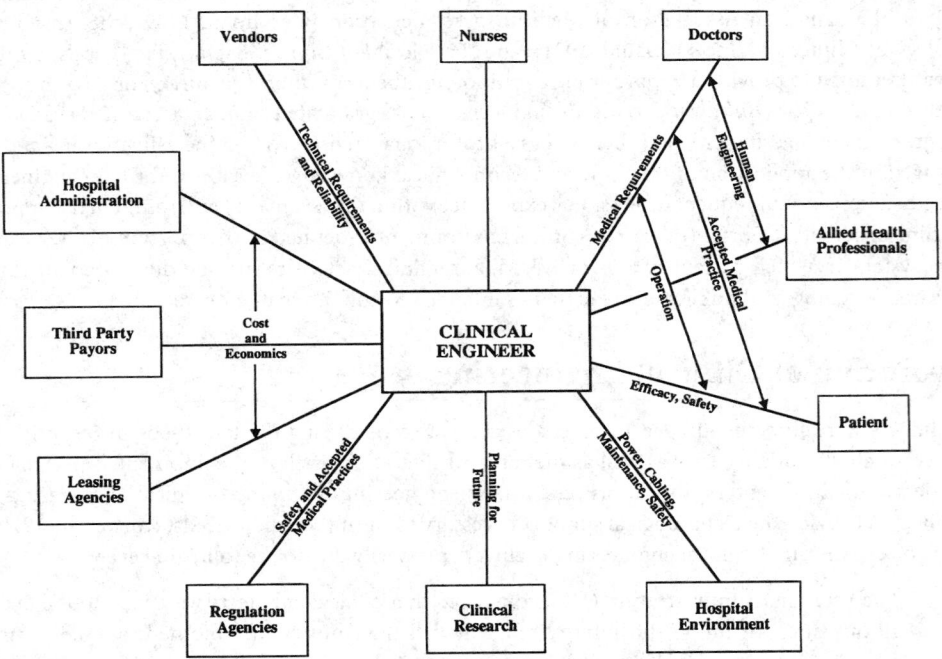

FIGURE 165.1   Diagram illustrating the range of interactions of a clinical engineer.

Today, hospitals that have established centralized clinical engineering departments to meet these responsibilities use clinical engineers to provide the hospital administration with an objective opinion of equipment function, purchase, application, overall system analysis, and preventive maintenance policies. Some hospital administrators have learned that with the in-house availability of such talent and expertise, the hospital is in a far better position to make more effective use of its technological resources [Bronzino, 1986, 1992]. By providing health professionals with needed assurance of safety, reliability, and efficiency in using new and innovative equipment, clinical engineers can readily identify poor-quality and ineffective equipment, thereby resulting in faster, more appropriate utilization of new medical equipment.

Typical pursuits of clinical engineers, therefore, include

- Supervision of a hospital clinical engineering department that includes clinical engineers and biomedical equipment technicians (BMETs)
- Prepurchase evaluation and planning for new medical technology
- Design, modification, or repair of sophisticated medical instruments or systems
- Cost-effective management of a medical equipment calibration and repair service
- Supervision of the safety and performance testing of medical equipment performed by BMETs
- Inspection of all incoming equipment (i.e., both new and returning repairs)
- Establishment of performance benchmarks for all equipment
- Medical equipment inventory control
- Coordination of outside engineering and technical services performed by vendors
- Training of medical personnel in the safe and effective use of medical devices and systems
- Clinical applications engineering, such as custom modification of medical devices for clinical research, evaluation of new noninvasive monitoring systems, etc.
- Biomedical computer support
- Input to the design of clinical facilities where medical technology is used, e.g., operating rooms (ORs), intensive care units, etc.
- Development and implementation of documentation protocols required by external accreditation and licensing agencies.

Clinical engineers thus provide extensive engineering services for the clinical staff and, in recent years, have been increasingly accepted as valuable team members by physicians, nurses, and other clinical professionals. Furthermore, the acceptance of clinical engineers in the hospital setting has led to different types of engineering-medicine interactions, which in turn have improved health care delivery.

165.3 Hospital Organization and the Role of Clinical Engineering

In the hospital, management organization has evolved into a diffuse authority structure that is commonly referred to as the *triad model*. The three primary components are the governing board (trustees), hospital administration (CEO and administrative staff), and the medical staff organization [Bronzino and Hayes, 1988]. The role of the governing board and the chief executive officer are briefly discussed below to provide some insight regarding their individual responsibilities and their interrelationship.

Governing Board (Trustees)

The Joint Commission on the Accreditation of Healthcare Organizations (JCAHO) summarizes the major duties of the governing board as "adopting by-laws in accordance with its legal accountability and its responsibility to the patient." The governing body, therefore, requires both medical and paramedical departments to monitor and evaluate the quality of patient care, which is a critical success factor in hospitals today.

To meet this goal, the governing board essentially is responsible for establishing the mission statement and defining the specific goals and objectives that the institution must satisfy. Therefore, the trustees are involved in the following functions:

- Establishing the policies of the institution
- Providing equipment and facilities to conduct patient care
- Ensuring that proper professional standards are defined and maintained (i.e., providing quality assurance)
- Coordinating professional interests with administrative, financial, and community needs
- Providing adequate financing by securing sufficient income and managing the control of expenditures
- Providing a safe environment
- Selecting qualified administrators, medical staff, and other professionals to manage the hospital

In practice, the trustees select a hospital chief administrator who develops a plan of action that is in concert with the overall goals of the institution.

Hospital Administration

The hospital administrator, the chief executive officer of the medical enterprise, has a function similar to that of the chief executive officer of any corporation. The administrator represents the governing board in carrying out the day-to-day operations to reflect the broad policy formulated by the trustees. The duties of the administrator are summarized as follows:

- Preparing a plan for accomplishing the institutional objectives, as approved by the board
- Selecting medical chiefs and department directors to set standards in their respective fields
- Submitting for board approval an annual budget reflecting both expenditures and income projections
- Maintaining all physical properties (plant and equipment) in safe operating condition
- Representing the hospital in its relationships with the community and health agencies
- Submitting to the board annual reports that describe the nature and volume of the services delivered during the past year, including appropriate financial data and any special reports that may be requested by the board

In addition to these administrative responsibilities, the chief administrator is charged with controlling cost, complying with a multitude of governmental regulations, and ensuring that the hospital conforms to professional norms, which include guidelines for the care and safety of patients.

165.4 Clinical Engineering Programs

In many hospitals, administrators have established clinical engineering departments to manage effectively all the technological resources, especially those relating to medical equipment, that are necessary for providing patient care. The primary objective of these departments is to provide a broad-based engineering program that addresses all aspects of medical instrumentation and systems support.

Figure 165.2 illustrates the organizational chart of the medical support services division of a typical major medical facility. Note that within this organizational structure, the director of clinical

MEDICAL SUPPORT SERVICES DIVISION

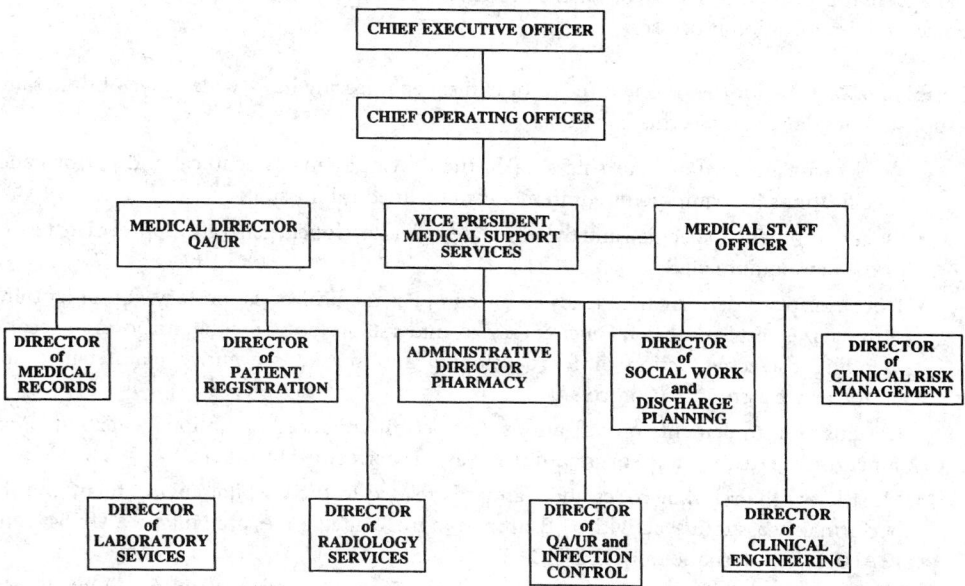

FIGURE 165.2 Organizational chart of medical support services division for a typical major medical facility. This organizational structure points out the critical interrelationship between the clinical engineering department and the other primary services provided by the medical facility.

engineering reports directly to the vice-president of medical support services. This administrative relationship is extremely important because it recognizes the important role clinical engineering departments play in delivering quality care. It should be noted, however, that in other common organizational structures, clinical engineering services may fall under the category of "facilities," "materials management," or even just "support services." Clinical engineers also can work directly with clinical departments, thereby bypassing much of the hospital hierarchy. In this situation, clinical departments can offer the clinical engineer both the chance for intense specialization and, at the same time, the opportunity to develop personal relationships with specific clinicians based on mutual concerns and interests [Wald, 1989].

Once the hospital administration appoints a qualified individual as director of clinical engineering, that person usually functions at the department-head level in the organizational structure of the institution and is provided with sufficient authority and resources to perform the duties efficiently and in accordance with professional norms. To understand the extent of these duties, consider the job title for "clinical engineering director" as defined by the World Health Organization [Issakov et al., 1990].

General Statement. The clinical engineering director, by his or her education and experience, acts as a manager and technical director of the clinical engineering department. The individual designs and directs the design of equipment modifications that may correct design deficiencies or enhance the clinical performance of medical equipment. The individual also may supervise the implementation of those design modifications. The education and experience that the director possesses enables him or her to analyze complex medical or laboratory equipment for purposes of defining corrective maintenance and developing appropriate preventing maintenance or performance assurance protocols. The clinical engineering director works with nursing and medical staff to analyze new medical equipment needs and participates in both the prepurchase planning process and the incoming acceptance testing process. This individual also participates in the equipment management process through involvement in the system development, implementation, maintenance, and modification processes.

Duties and Responsibilities.   The director of clinical engineering has a wide range of duties and responsibilities. For example, this individual

- Works with medical and nursing staff in the development of technical and performance specifications for equipment requirements in the medical mission.
- Once equipment is specified and the purchase order developed, generates appropriate testing of the new equipment.
- Does complete performance analysis on complex medical or laboratory equipment and summarizes results in brief, concise, easy-to-understand terms for the purposes of recommending corrective action or for developing appropriate preventive maintenance and performance assurance protocols.
- Designs and implements modifications that permit enhanced operational capability. May supervise the maintenance or modification as it is performed by others.
- Must know the relevant codes and standards related to the hospital environment and the performance assurance activities. (Examples in the United States are NFPA 99, UL 544, and JCAHO, and internationally, IEC-TC 62.)
- Is responsible for obtaining the engineering specifications (systems definitions) for systems that are considered unusual or one-of-a-kind and are not commercially available.
- Supervises in-service maintenance technicians as they work on codes and standards and on preventive maintenance, performance assurance, corrective maintenance, and modification of new and existing patient care and laboratory equipment.
- Supervises parts and supply purchase activities and develops program policies and procedures for same.
- Sets departmental goals, develops budgets and policy, prepares and analyzes management reports to monitor department activity, and manages and organizes the department to implement them.
- Teaches measurement, calibration, and standardization techniques that promote optimal performance.
- In equipment-related duties, works closely with maintenance and medical personnel. Communicates orally and in writing with medical, maintenance, and administrative professionals. Develops written procedures and recommendations for administrative and technical personnel.

Minimum Qualifications.   A bachelor's degree (4 years) in an electrical or electronics program or the equivalent is required (preferably with a clinical or biomedical adjunct). A master's degree is desirable. A minimum of 3 years' experience as a clinical engineer and 2 years in a progressively responsible supervisory capacity is needed. Additional qualifications are as follows:

- Must have some business knowledge and management skills that enable him or her to participate in budgeting, cost accounting, personnel management, behavioral counseling, job description development, and interviewing for hiring or firing purposes. Knowledge and experience in the use of microcomputers are desirable.
- Must be able to use conventional electronic trouble-shooting instruments such as multimeters, function generators, oscillators, and oscilloscopes. Should be able to use conventional machine shop equipment such as drill presses, grinders, belt sanders, brakes, and standard hand tools.

- Must possess or be able to acquire knowledge of the techniques, theories, and characteristics of materials, drafting, and fabrication techniques in conjunction with chemistry, anatomy, physiology, optics, mechanics, and hospital procedures.
- Clinical engineering certification or professional engineering registration is required.

Major Functions of a Clinical Engineering Department

It should be clear by the preceding job description that clinical engineers are first and foremost engineering professionals. However, as a result of the wide-ranging scope of interrelationships within the medical setting, the duties and responsibilities of clinical engineering directors are extremely diversified. Yet a common thread is provided by the very nature of the technology they manage. Directors of clinical engineering departments are usually involved in the following core functions:

Technology Management. Developing, implementing, and directing equipment management programs. Specific tasks include accepting and installing new equipment, establishing preventive maintenance and repair programs, and managing the inventory of medical instrumentation. Issues such as cost-effective use and quality assurance are integral parts of any technology management program. The director advises the administrator of the budgetary, personnel, space, and test equipment requirements necessary to support this equipment management program.

Risk Management. Evaluating and taking appropriate action on incidents attributed to equipment malfunction or misuse. For example, the clinical engineering director is responsible for summarizing the technological significance of each incident and documenting the findings of the investigation. He or she then submits a report to the appropriate hospital authority and, according to the Safe Medical Devices Act of 1990, to the device manufacturer, the Food and Drug Administration (FDA), or both.

Technology Assessment. Evaluating and selecting new equipment. The director must be proactive in the evaluation of new requests for capital equipment expenditures, providing hospital administrators and clinical staff with an in depth appraisal of the benefits/advantages of candidate equipment. Furthermore, the process of technology assessment for all equipment used in the hospital should be an ongoing activity.

Facilities Design and Project Management. Assisting in the design of new or renovated clinical facilities that house specific medical technologies. This includes operating rooms, imaging facilities, and radiology treatment centers.

Training. Establish and deliver instructional modules for clinical engineering staff as well as clinical staff on the operation of medical equipment.

In the future, it is anticipated that clinical engineering departments will provide assistance in the application and management of many other technologies that support patient care, including computer support, telecommunications, and facilities operations.

Defining Terms

JCAHO, Joint Commission on the Accreditation of Healthcare Organizations: Accrediting body responsible for checking hospital compliance with approved rules and regulations regarding the delivery of health care.

Technology assessment: Involves an evaluation of the safety, efficiency, and cost-effectiveness, as well as consideration of the social, legal, and ethical effects, of medical technology.

References

AHA. 1986. American Hospital Association Resource Center, Hospital Administration Terminology, 2d ed. Washington, American Hospital Publishing.

Bauld TJ. 1991. The definition of a clinical engineer. J Clin Eng 16:403.

Bronzino JD. 1986. Biomedical Engineering and Instrumentation: Basic Concepts and Applications. Boston, PWS Publishing.

Bronzino JD. 1992. Management of Medical Technology: A Primer for Clinical Engineers. Boston, Butterworth.

Goodman G. 1989. The profession of clinical engineering. J Clin Eng 14:27.

ICC. 1991. International Certification Commission's Definition of a Clinical Engineer, International Certification Commission Fact Sheet. Arlington, Va, ICC.

Issakov A, Mallouppas A, McKie J. 1990. Manpower development for a healthcare technical service. Report of the World Health Organization, WHO/SHS/NHP/90.4.

Newhouse VL, Bell DS, Tackel IS, et al. 1989. The future of clinical engineering in the 1990s. J Clin Eng 14:417.

Pacela A. 1990. Bioengineering Education Directory. Brea, Calif, Quest Publishing.

Wald A. 1989. Clinical engineering in clinical departments: A different point of view. Biomed Instr Technol 23:58.

Further Information

Bronzino JD. 1992. Management of Medical Technology: A Primer for Clinical Engineers. Boston, Butterworth.

Journals: Journal of Clinical Engineering, Journal of Medical Engineering and Physics, Biomedical Instrumentation and Technology.

166

Management and Assessment of Medical Technology

Yadin David
Texas Children's Hospital

Thomas M. Judd
Texas Children's Hospital

As medical technology continues to evolve, so does its impact on patient outcome, hospital operations, and financial efficiency. The ability to plan for this evolution and its subsequent implications has become a major challenge in most decisions of health care organizations and their related industries. Therefore, there is a need to adequately apply those management tools which optimize the deployment of medical technology and the facilities that house it. Successful management of technology and facilities will ensure a good match between the needs and the capabilities of staff and technology, respectively. While different types and sizes of hospitals will consider various strategies of actions, they all share the need to manage how well they utilize their limited resources. Technology is one of these resources, and while it is frequently cited as the culprit behind cost increases, the well-managed technology program contributes to a significant containment of the cost of providing quality patient care. Clinical engineer's skills and expertise are needed to facilitate the adoption of an objective methodology for implantation of a program that will match the hospital's needs and operational conditions.

Whereas both the knowledge and practice patterns of management in general are well organized in today's literature, the management of the health care delivery system and that of medical technology in the clinical environment has not yet reached that same high level. However, as we begin to understand the relationship between the methods and information that guide the decisions regarding the management of medical technology that are being deployed in this highly complex environment, the role of the qualified clinical engineer becomes more valuable. This is achieved by reformulating the technology management process, which starts with the strategic planning process, continues with the technology assessment process, leads to the equipment planning and procurement processes, and finally ends with the assets management process. Definition of terms used in this chapter are provided at the end of the chapter.

166.1 The Health Care Delivery System

Societal demands on the health care delivery system revolve around cost, technology, and expectations. To respond effectively, the delivery system must identify its goals, select and define its priorities, and then wisely allocate its limited resources. For most organizations, this means that they must acquire only appropriate technologies and manage what they have already more effectively. To improve performance and reduce costs, the delivery system must recognize and respond to the key dynamics in which it operates, must shape and mold its planning efforts around several existing health care trends and directions, and must respond proactively and positively to the pressures of its environment. These issues and the technology manager's response are outlined here: (1) technology's positive impact on care quality and effectiveness, (2) an unacceptable rise in national spending for health care services, (3) a changing mix of how Americans are insured for health care, (4) increases in health insurance premiums for which appropriate technology application is a strong limiting factor, (5) a changing mix of health care services and settings in which care is delivered, and (6) growing pressures related to technology for hospital capital spending and budgets.

Major Health Care Trends and Directions

The major trends and directions in health care include (1) changing location and design of treatment areas, (2) evolving benefits, coverages, and choices, (3) extreme pressures to manage costs, (4) treating of more acutely ill older patients and the prematurely born, (5) changing job structures and demand for skilled labor, (6) the need to maintain a strong cash flow to support construction, equipment, and information system developments, (7) increased competition on all sides, (8) requirement for information systems that effectively integrate clinical and business issues, (9) changing reimbursement policies that reduce new purchases and lead to the expectation for extended equipment life cycles, (10) internal technology planning and management programs to guide decision making, (11) technology planning teams to coordinate absorption of new and replacement technologies, as well as to suggest delivery system changes, and (12) equipment maintenance costs that are emerging as a significant expense item under great administrative scrutiny.

System Pressures

System pressures include (1) society's expectations—highest-quality care at the lowest reasonable price, where quality is a function of personnel, facilities, technology, and clinical procedures offered; (2) economic conditions—driven often by reimbursement criteria; (3) legal pressures—resulting primarily from malpractice issues and dealing with rule-intensive "government" clients; (4) regulatory—multistate delivery systems with increased management complexity, or heavily regulated medical device industries facing free-market competition, or hospitals facing the Safe Medical Devices Act reporting requirements and credentialing requirements; (5) ethics—deciding who gets care and when; and (6) technology pressures—organizations having enough capabilities to meet community needs and to compete successfully in their marketplaces.

The Technology Manager's Responsibility

Technology managers should (1) become deeply involved and committed to technology planning and management programs in their system, often involving the need for greater personal responsibilities and expanded credentials, (2) understand how the factors above impact their organization and how technology can be used to improve outcomes, reduce costs, and improve quality of life for patients, and (3) educate other health care professionals about how to demonstrate the value of individual technologies through analysis involving financial, engineering, quality of care, and management perspectives.

166.2 Strategic Technology Planning

Strategic Planning Process

Leading health care organizations have begun to combine strategic technology planning with other technology management activities in a program that effectively integrates new technologies with their existing technology base. This has resulted in high-quality care at a reasonable cost. Among those who have been its leading catalysts, ECRI (formerly the Emergency Care Research Institute) is known for articulating this program [4] and encouraging its proliferation initially among regional health care systems and now for single or multihospital systems as well [5]. Key components of the program include clinical strategic planning, technology strategic planning, technology assessment, interaction with capital budgeting, acquisition and deployment, resource (or equipment assets) management, and monitoring and evaluation. A proper technology strategic plan is derived from and supports a well-defined clinical strategic plan [15].

Clinical and Technology Strategic Plan

Usually considered long-range and continually evolving, a clinical strategic plan is updated annually. For a given year, the program begins when key hospital participants, through the strategic planning process, assess what clinical services the hospital should be offering in its referral area. They take into account health care trends, demographic and market share data, and space and facilities plans. They analyze their facility's strengths and weaknesses, goals and objectives, competition, and existing technology base. The outcome of this process is a clinical strategic plan that establishes the organization's vision for the year and referral area needs and the hospital's objectives in meeting them.

It is not possible to adequately complete a clinical strategic plan without engaging in the process of strategic technology planning. A key role for technology managers is to assist their organizations throughout the combined clinical and technology strategic planning processes by matching available technical capabilities, both existing and new, with clinical requirements. To accomplish this, technology managers must understand why their institutions' values and mission are set as they are, pursue their institutions' strategic plans through that knowledge, and plan in a way that effectively allocates limited resources. Although a technology manager may not be assigned to develop an institution's overall strategic plan, he or she must understand and believe in it in order to offer good input for hospital management. In providing this input, a technology manager should determine a plan for evaluating the present state of the hospital's technological deployment, assist in providing a review of emerging technological innovations and their possible impact on the hospital, articulate justifications and provisions for adoption of new technologies or enhancement of existing ones, visit research laboratories and exhibit areas at major medical and scientific meetings to view new technologies, and be familiar with the institution and its equipment users' abilities to assimilate new technology.

The past decade has shown a trend toward increased legislation in support of more federal regulations in health care. These and other pressures will require that additional or replacement medical technology be well anticipated and justified. As a rationale for technology adoption, the Texas Children's Hospital focuses on the issues of clinical necessity, management support, and market preference. Addressing the issue of clinical necessity, the hospital considers the technology's comparison against medical standard of care, its impact on the level of care and quality of life, its improvement on intervention's accuracy and/or safety, its impact on the rate of recovery, the needs or desires of the community, and the change in service volume or focus. On the issue of management support, the hospital estimates if the technology will create a more effective care plan and decision-making process, improve operational efficiency in the current service programs, decrease liability exposure, increase compliance with regulations, reduce workload and dependence on user skill level ameliorate departmental support, or enhance clinical proficiency. Weighing the issue of market preference, the hospital contemplate if it will improve access to care, increase customer convenience and/or satisfaction, enhance the organization's image and market share, decrease the cost of adoption and ownership, or provide a return on its investment.

Technology Strategic Planning Process

When the annual clinical strategic planning process has started and hospital leaders have begun to analyze or reaffirm what clinical services they want to offer to the community, the hospital can then conduct efficient technology strategic planning. Key elements of this planning involve (1) performing an initial audit of existing technologies, (2) conducting a technology assessment for new and emerging technologies for fit with current or desired clinical services, (3) planning for replacement and selection of new technologies, (4) setting priorities for technology acquisition, and (5) developing processes to implement equipment acquisition and monitor ongoing utilization. "Increasingly, hospitals are designating a senior manager (e.g., an administrator, the director of planning, the director of clinical engineering) to take the responsibility for technology assessment and planning. That person should have the primary responsibility for developing the strategic technology plan with the help of key physicians, department managers, and senior executives" [4].

Hospitals can form a medical technology advisory committee (MTAC), overseen by the designated senior manager and consisting of the types of members mentioned above, to conduct the strategic technology planning process and to annually recommend technology priorities to the hospital strategic planning committee and capital budget committee. It is especially important to involve physicians and nurses in this process.

In the initial technology audit, each major clinical service or product line must be analyzed to determine how well the existing technology base supports it. The audit can be conducted along service lines (radiology, cardiology, surgery) or technology function (e.g., imaging, therapeutic, diagnostic) by a team of designated physicians, department heads, and technology managers. The team should begin by developing a complete hospital-wide assets inventory, including the quantity and quality of equipment. The team should compare the existing technology base against known and evolving standards-of-care information, patient outcome data, and known equipment problems. Next, the team should collect and examine information on technology utilization to assess its appropriate use, the opportunities for improvement, and the risk level. After reviewing the technology users' education needs as they relate to the application and servicing of medical equipment, the team should credential users for competence in the application of new technologies. Also, the auditing team should keep up with published clinical protocols and practice guidelines using available health care standards directories and utilize clinical outcome data for quality-assurance and risk-management program feedback [6].

While it is not expected that every hospital has all the required expertise in-house to conduct the initial technology audit or ongoing technology assessment, the execution of this planning process is sufficiently critical for a hospital's success that outside expertise should be obtained when necessary. The audit allows for the gathering of information about the status of the existing technology base and enhances the capability of the medical technology advisory committee to assess the impact of new and emerging technologies on their major clinical services.

All the information collected from the technology audit results and technology assessments is used in developing budget strategies. Budgeting is part of strategic technology planning in that a 2- to 5-year long-range capital spending plan should be created. This is in addition to the annual capital budget preparation that takes into account 1 year at a time. The MTAC, as able and appropriate, provides key information regarding capital budget requests and makes recommendations to the capital budget committee each year. The MTAC recommends priorities for replacement as well as new and emerging technologies that over a period of several years guides the acquisition that provides the desired service developments or enhancements. Priorities are recommended on the basis of need, risk, cost (acquisition, operational and maintenance), utilization, and fit with the clinical strategic plan.

166.3 Technology Assessment

As medical technology continues to evolve, so does its impact on patient outcome, hospital operations, and financial resources. The ability to manage this evolution and its subsequent implications has become a major challenge for all health care organizations. Successful management of technology will ensure a good match between needs and capabilities and between staff and technology. To be successful, an ongoing technology assessment process must be an integral part of an ongoing technology planning and management program at the hospital, addressing the needs of the patient, the user, and the support team. This facilitates better equipment planning and utilization of the hospital's resources. The manager who is knowledgeable about his or her organization's culture, equipment users' needs, the environment within which equipment will be applied, equipment engineering, and emerging technological capabilities will be successful in proficiently implementing and managing technological changes [7].

It is in the technology assessment process that the clinical engineering/technology manager professional needs to wear two hats: that of the manager and that of the engineer. This is a unique position, requiring expertise and detailed preparation, that allows one to be a key leader and contributor to the decision-making process of the medical technology advisory committee (MTAC).

The MTAC uses an ad hoc team approach to conduct technology assessment of selected services and technologies throughout the year. The ad hoc teams may incorporate representatives of equipment users, equipment service providers, physicians, purchasing agents, reimbursement managers, representatives of administration, and other members from the institution as applicable.

Prerequisites for Technology Assessment

Medical technology is a major strategic factor in positioning and creating a positive community perception of the hospital. Exciting new biomedical devices and systems are continually being introduced. And they are introduced at a time when the pressure on hospitals to contain expenditures is mounting. Therefore, forecasting the deployment of medical technology and the capacity to continually evaluate its impact on the hospital require that the hospital be willing to provide the support for such a program. (*Note:* Many organizations are aware of the principle that an in-house "champion" is needed in order to provide for the leadership that continually and objectively plans ahead. The champion and the program being "championed" may use additional in-house or independent expertise as needed. To get focused attention on the technology assessment function and this program in larger, academically affiliated and government hospitals, the position of a chief technology officer is being created.) Traditionally, executives rely on their staff to produce objective analyses of the hospital's technological needs. Without such analyses, executives may approve purchasing decisions of sophisticated biomedical equipment only to discover later that some needs or expected features were not included with this installation, that those features are not yet approved for delivery, or that the installation has not been adequately planned.

Many hospitals perform technology assessment activities to project needs for new assets and to better manage existing assets. Because the task is complex, an interdisciplinary approach and a cooperative attitude among the assessment team leadership is required. The ability to integrate information from disciplines such as clinical, technical, financial, administrative, and facility in a timely and objective manner is critical to the success of the assessment. This chapter emphasizes how technology assessment fits within a technology planning and management program and recognizes the importance of corporate skills forecasting medical equipment changes and determining the impact of changes on the hospital's market position. Within the technology planning and management program, the focus on capital assets management of medical equipment should not lead to the exclusion of accessories, supplies, and the disposables also required.

Medical equipment has a life cycle that can be identified as (1) the innovation phase, which includes the concept, basic and applied research, and development, and (2) the adoption phase, which begins with the clinical studies, through diffusion, and then widespread use. These phases are different from each other in the scope of professional skills involved, their impact on patient care, compliance with regulatory requirements, and the extent of the required operational support. In evaluating the applicability of a device or a system for use in the hospital, it is important to note in which phase of its life cycle the equipment currently resides.

Technology Assessment Process

More and more hospitals are faced with the difficult phenomenon of a capital equipment requests list that is much larger than the capital budget allocation. The most difficult decision, then, is the one that matches clinical needs with the financial capability. In doing so, the following questions are often raised: How do we avoid costly technology mistakes? How do we wisely target capital dollars for technology? How do we avoid medical staff conflicts as they relate to technology? How do we control equipment-related risks? and How do we maximize the useful life of the equipment or systems while minimizing the cost of ownership? A hospital's clinical engineering department can assist in providing the right answers to these questions.

Technology assessment is a component of technology planning that begins with the analysis of the hospital's existing technology base. It is easy to perceive then that technology assessment, rather than an equipment comparison, is a new major function for a clinical engineering department [8]. It is important that clinical engineers be well prepared for the challenge. They must have a full understanding of the mission of their particular hospitals, a familiarity with the health care delivery system, and the cooperation of hospital administrators and the medical staff. To aid in the technology assessment process, clinical engineers need to utilize the following tools: (1) access to national database services, directories, and libraries, (2) visits to scientific and clinical exhibits, (3) a network with key industry contacts, and (4) a relationship with peers throughout the country [9].

The need for clinical engineering involvement in the technology assessment process becomes evident when recently purchased equipment or its functions are underutilized, users have ongoing problems with equipment, equipment maintenance costs become excessive, the hospital is unable to comply with standards or guidelines (i.e., JCAHO requirements) for equipment management, a high percentage of equipment is awaiting repair, or training for equipment operators is inefficient due to shortage of allied health professionals. A deeper look at the symptoms behind these problems would likely reveal a lack of a central clearinghouse to collect, index, and monitor all technology-related information for future planning purposes, the absence of procedures for identifying emerging technologies for potential acquisition, the lack of a systematic plan for conducting technology assessment, resulting in an inability to maximize the benefits from deployment of available technology, the inability to benefit from the organization's own previous experience with a particular type of technology, the random replacement of medical technologies rather than a systematic plan based on a set of well-developed criteria, and/or the lack of integration of technology acquisition into the strategic and capital planning of the hospital.

To address these issues, efforts to develop a technology microassessment process were initiated at one leading private hospital with the following objectives: (1) accumulate information on medical equipment, (2) facilitate systematic planning, (3) create an administrative structure supporting the assessment process and its methodology, (4) monitor the replacement of outdated technology, and (5) improve the capital budget process by focusing on long-term needs relative to the acquisition of medical equipment [10].

The process, in general, and the collection of up-to-date pertinent information, in particular, require the expenditure of certain resources and the active participation of designated hospital staff in networks providing technology assessment information. For example, corporate membership in organizations and societies that provide such information needs to be considered, as well as subscriptions to certain computerized database and printed sources [11].

At the example hospital, an MTAC was formed to conduct technology assessment. It was chaired by the director of clinical engineering. Other managers from equipment user departments usually serve as the MTAC's designated technical coordinators for specific task forces. Once the committee accepted a request from an individual user, it identified other users that might have an interest in that equipment or system and authorized the technical coordinator to assemble a task force consisting of users identified by the MTAC. This task force then took responsibility for the establishment of performance criteria that would be used during this particular assessment. The task force also should answer the questions of effectiveness, safety, and cost-effectiveness as they relate to the particular assessment. During any specific period, there may be multiple task forces, each focusing on a specific equipment investigation.

The task force technical coordinator cooperates with the material management department in conducting a market survey, in obtaining the specified equipment for evaluation purposes, and in scheduling vendor-provided in-service training. The coordinator also confers with clinical staff to determine if they have experience with the equipment and the maturity level of the equipment under assessment. After establishment of a task force, the MTACs technical coordinator is responsible for analyzing the clinical experiences associated with the use of this equipment, for setting evaluation objectives, and for devising appropriate technical tests in accord with recommendations from the task force. Only equipment that successfully passes the technical tests will proceed to a clinical trial. During the clinical trial, a task force–appointed clinical coordinator collects and reports a summary of experiences gained. The technical coordinator then combines the results from both the technical tests and the clinical trial into a summary report for MTAC review and approval. In this role, the clinical engineer/technical coordinator serves as a multidisciplinary professional, bridging the gap between the clinical and technical needs of the hospital. To complete the process, financial staff representatives review the protocol.

The technology assessment process at this example hospital begins with a department or individual filling out two forms: (1) a request for review (RR) form and (2) a capital asset request (CAR) form. These forms are submitted to the hospital's product standards committee, which determines if an assessment process is to be initiated, and the priority for its completion. It also determines if a previously established standard for this equipment already exists (if the hospital is already using such a technology)—if so, an assessment is not needed.

On the RR, the originator delineates the rationale for acquiring the medical device. For example, the originator must tell how the item will improve quality of patient care, who will be its primary user, and how it will improve ease of use. On the CAR, the originator describes the item, estimates its cost, and provides purchase justification. The CAR is then routed to the capital budget office for review. During this process, the optimal financing method for acquisition is determined. If funding is secured, the CAR is routed to the material management department, where, together with the RR, it will be processed. The rationale for having the RR accompany the CAR is to ensure that financial information is included as part of the assessment process. The CAR is the tool by which the purchasing department initiates a market survey and later sends product requests for bid. Any request for evaluation that is received without a CAR or any CAR involving medical equipment that is received without a request for evaluation is returned to the originator without action. Both forms are then sent to the clinical engineering department, where a designated technical coordinator will analyze the requested technology maturity level and results of clinical experience with its use, review trends, and prioritize various manufacturers' presentations for MTAC review.

Both forms must be sent to the MTAC if the item requested is not currently used by the hospital or if it does not conform to previously adopted hospital standards. The MTAC has the authority to recommend either acceptance or rejection of any request for review, based on a consensus of its members. A task force consisting of potential equipment users will determine the "must have" equipment functions, review the impact of the various equipment configurations, and plan technical and clinical evaluations.

If the request is approved by the MTAC, the requested technology or equipment will be evaluated using technical and performance standards. Upon completion of the review, a recommendation is returned to the hospital's products standard committee, which reviews the results of the technology assessment, determines whether the particular product is suitable as a hospital standard, and decides if it should be purchased. If approved, the request to purchase will be reviewed by the capital budget committee (CBC) to determine if the required expenditure meets with available financial resources and if or when it may be feasible to make the purchase. To ensure coordination of the technology assessment program, the chairman of the MTAC also serves as a permanent member of the hospital's CBC. In this way, there is a planned integration between technology assessment and budget decisions.

166.4 Equipment Assets Management

An accountable, systematic approach will ensure that cost-effective, efficacious, safe, and appropriate equipment is available to meet the demands of quality patient care. Such an approach requires that existing medical equipment resources be managed and that the resulting management strategies have measurable outputs that are monitored and evaluated. Technology managers/clinical engineers are well positioned to organize and lead this function. It is assumed that cost accounting is managed and monitored by the health care organization's financial group.

Equipment Management Process

Through traditional assets management strategies, medical equipment can be comprehensively managed by clinical engineering personnel. First, the management should consider a full range of strategies for equipment technical support. Plans may include use of a combination of equipment service providers such as manufacturers, third-party service groups, shared services, and hospital-based (in-house) engineers and biomedical equipment technicians (BMETs). All these service providers should be under the general responsibility of the technology manager to ensure optimal equipment performance through comprehensive and ongoing best-value equipment service. After obtaining a complete hospital medical equipment inventory (noting both original manufacturer and typical service provider), the management should conduct a thorough analysis of hospital accounts payable records for at least the past 2 years, compiling all service reports and preventative maintenance–related costs from all possible sources. The manager then should document in-house and external provider equipment service costs, extent of maintenance coverage for each inventory time, equipment-user operating schedule, quality of maintenance coverage for each item, appropriateness of the service provider, and reasonable maintenance costs. Next, he or she should establish an effective equipment technical support process. With an accurate inventory and best-value service providers identified, service agreements/contracts should be negotiated with external providers using prepared terms and conditions, including a log-in system. There should be an in-house clinical engineering staff ensuring ongoing external provider cost control utilizing several tools. By asking the right technical questions and establishing friendly relationships with staff, the manager will be able to handle service purchase orders (POs) by determining if equipment is worth repairing and obtaining exchange prices for parts. The staff should handle service reports to review them for accuracy and proper use of the log-in system. They also should match invoices with the service reports to verify opportunities and review service histories to look for symptoms such as need for user training, repeated problems, run-on calls billed months apart, or evidence of defective or worn-out equipment. The manager should take responsibility for emergency equipment rentals. Finally, the manager should develop, implement, and monitor all the service performance criteria.

To optimize technology management programs, clinical engineers should be willing to assume responsibilities for technology planning and management in all related areas. They should develop policies and procedures for their hospital's technology management program. With life-cycle costs determined for key high-risk or high-cost devices, they should evaluate methods to provide additional cost savings in equipment operation and maintenance. They should be involved with computer networking systems within the hospital. As computer technology applications increase, the requirements to review technology-related information in a number of hospital locations will increase. They should determine what environmental conditions and facility changes are required to accommodate new technologies or changes in standards and guidelines. Lastly, they should use documentation of equipment performance and maintenance costs along with their knowledge of current clinical practices to assist other hospital personnel in determining the best time and process for planning equipment replacement [12].

Technology Management Activities

A clinical engineering department, through outstanding performance in traditional equipment management, will win its hospital's support and will be asked to be involved in a full range of technology management activities. The department should start an equipment control program that encompasses routine performance testing, inspection, periodic and preventive maintenance, on-demand repair services, incidents investigation, and actions on recalls and hazards. The department should have multidisciplinary involvement in equipment acquisition and replacement decisions, development of new services, and planning of new construction and major renovations, including intensive participation by clinical engineering, materials management, and finance. The department also should initiate programs for training all users of patient care equipment, quality improvement (QI), as it relates to technology use, and technology-related risk management [13].

Case Study: A Focus on Medical Imaging

In the mid-1980s, a large private multihospital system contemplated the startup of a corporate clinical engineering program. The directors recognized that involvement in a diagnostic imaging equipment service would be key to the economic success of the program. They further recognized that maintenance cost reductions would have to be balanced with achieving equal or increased quality of care in the utilization of that equipment.

Program startup was in the summer of 1987 in 3 hospitals that were geographically close. Within the first year, clinical engineering operations began in 11 hospitals in 3 regions over a two-state area. By the fall of 1990, the program included 7 regions and 21 hospitals in a five-state area. The regions were organized, typically, into teams including a regional manager and 10 service providers, serving 3 to 4 hospitals, whose average size was 225 beds. Although the staffs were stationed at the hospitals, some specialists traveled between different sites in the region to provide equipment service. Service providers included individuals specializing in the areas of diagnostic imaging [x-ray and computed tomography (CT)], clinical laboratory, general biomedical instrumentation, and respiratory therapy.

At the end of the first 18 months, the program documented over $1 million in savings for the initial 11 hospitals, a 23% reduction from the previous annual service costs. Over 63% of these savings were attributable to "in-house" service of x-ray and CT scanner equipment. The mix of equipment maintained by 11 imaging service providers—from a total staff of 30—included approximately 75% of the radiology systems of any kind found in the hospitals and 5 models of CT scanners from three different manufacturers.

At the end of 3 years in 1990, program-wide savings had exceeded 30% of previous costs for participating hospitals. Within the imaging areas of the hospitals, savings approached and sometimes exceeded 50% of initial service costs. The 30 imaging service providers—out of a total staff of 62—had increased their coverage of radiology equipment to over 95%, had increased involvement with CT to include nine models from five different manufacturers, and had begun in-house work in other key imaging modalities.

Tracking the financial performance of the initial 11 hospitals over the first 3 years of the program yields the following composite example: A hospital of 225 beds was found to have equipment service costs of $540,000 prior to program startup. Sixty-three percent of these initial costs (or $340,000) was for the maintenance of the hospital's x-ray and CT scanner systems. Three years later, annual service costs for this equipment were cut in half, to approximately $170,000. That represents a 31% reduction in hospital-wide costs due to the imaging service alone.

This corporate clinical engineering operation is, in effect, a large in-house program serving many hospitals that all have common ownership. The multihospital corporation has significant purchasing power in the medical device marketplace and provides central oversight of the larger capital expenditures for its hospitals. The combination of the parent organization's leverage and the program's commitment to serve only hospitals in the corporation facilitated the development of positive relationships with medical device manufacturers. Most of the manufacturers did not see the program as competition but rather as a potentially helpful ally in the future marketing and sales of their equipment and systems. What staff provided these results? All service providers were either medical imaging industry or military trained. All were experienced at troubleshooting electronic subsystems to component level, as necessary. Typically, these individuals had prior experience on the manufacturer's models of equipment under their coverage. Most regional managers had prior industry, third party, or in-house imaging service management experience. Each service provider had the test equipment necessary for day-to-day duties. Each individual could expect at least 2 weeks of annual service training to keep appropriate skills current. Desired service training could be acquired in a timely manner from manufacturers and/or third-party organizations. Spare or replacement parts inventory was minimal because of the program's ability to get parts from manufacturers and other sources either locally or shipped in overnight.

As quality indicators for the program, the management measured user satisfaction, equipment downtime, documentation of technical staff service training, types of user equipment errors and their effect on patient outcomes, and regular attention to hospital technology problems. User satisfaction surveys indicated a high degree of confidence in the program service providers by imaging department managers. Problems relating to technical, management, communication, and financial issues did occur regularly, but the regional manager ensured that they were resolved in a timely manner. Faster response to daily imaging equipment problems, typically by on-site service providers, coupled with regular preventive maintenance (PM) according to established procedures led to reduced equipment downtime. PM and repair service histories were captured in a computer documentation system that also tracked service times, costs, and user errors and their effects. Assisting the safety committee became easier with the ability to draw a wide variety of information quickly from the program's documentation system.

Early success in imaging equipment led to the opportunity to do some additional value-added projects such as the moving and reinstallation of x-ray rooms that preserved existing assets and opened up valuable space for installation of newer equipment and upgrades of CT scanner systems. The parent organization came to realize that these technology management activities could potentially have a greater financial and quality impact on the hospitals' health care delivery than equipment management. In the example of one CT upgrade (which was completed over two weekends with no downtime), there was a positive financial impact in excess of $600,000 and improved quality of care by allowing faster off-line diagnosis of patient scans. However, opportunity for this kind of contribution would never have occurred without the strong base of a successful equipment management program staffed with qualified individuals who receive ongoing training.

166.5 Equipment Acquisition and Deployment

Process of Acquiring Technology

Typically, medical device systems will emerge from the strategic technology planning and technology assessment processes as required and budgeted needs. At acquisition time, a needs analysis should be conducted, reaffirming clinical needs and device intended applications. The "request for review" documentation from the assessment process or capital budget request and incremental financial analysis from the planning process may provide appropriate justification information, and a capital asset request (CAR) form should be completed [14]. Materials management and clinical engineering personnel should ensure that this item is a candidate for centralized and coordinated acquisition of similar equipment with other hospital departments. Typical hospital prepurchase evaluation guidelines include an analysis of needs and development of a specification list, formation of a vendor list and requesting proposals, analyzing proposals and site planning, evaluating samples, selecting finalists, making the award, delivery and installation, and acceptance testing. Formal request for proposals (RFPs) from potential equipment vendors are required for intended acquisitions whose initial or life-cycle cost exceeds a certain threshold, i.e., $100,000. Finally, the purchase takes place, wherein final equipment negotiations are conducted and purchase documents are prepared, including a purchase order.

Acquisition Process Strategies

The cost-of-ownership concept can be used when considering what factors to include in cost comparisons of competing medical devices. Cost of ownership encompasses all the direct and indirect expenses associated with medical equipment over its lifetime [15]. It expresses the cost factors of medical equipment for both the initial price of the equipment (which typically includes the equipment, its installation, and initial training cost) and over the long term. Long-term costs include ongoing training, equipment service, supplies, connectivity, upgrades, and other costs. Health care organizations are just beginning to account for a full range of cost-of-ownership factors in their technology assessment and acquisition processes, such as acquisition costs, operating costs, and maintenance costs (installation, supplies, downtime, training, spare parts, test equipment and tools, and depreciation). It is estimated that the purchase price represents only 20% of the life-cycle cost of ownership.

When conducting needs analysis, actual utilization information from the organization's existing same or similar devices can be very helpful. One leading private multihospital system has implemented the following approach to measuring and developing relevant management feedback concerning equipment utilization. It is conducting equipment utilization review for replacement planning, for ongoing accountability of equipment use, and to provide input before more equipment is purchased. This private system attempts to match product to its intended function and to measure daily (if necessary) the equipment's actual utilization. The tools they use include knowing their hospitals' entire installed base of certain kinds of equipment, i.e., imaging systems. Utilization assumptions for each hospital and its clinical procedural mix are made. Equipment functional requirements to meet the demands of the clinical procedures are also taken into account.

Life-cycle cost analysis is a tool used during technology planning, assessment, or acquisition "either to compare high-cost, alternative means for providing a service or to determine whether a single project or technology has a positive or negative economic value. The strength of life-cycle cost analysis is that it examines the cash flow impact of an alternative over its entire life, instead of focusing solely on initial capital investments" [15].

"Life-cycle cost analysis facilitates comparisons between projects or technologies with large initial cash outlays and those with level outlays and inflows over time. It is most applicable to complex, high-cost choices among alternative technologies, new services, and different means for providing a given service. Life-cycle cost analysis is particularly useful for decisions that are too complex and ambiguous for experience and subjective judgment alone. It also helps decision makers perceive and include costs that often are hidden or ignored, and that may otherwise invalidate results" [12].

"Perhaps the most powerful life-cycle cost technique is net present value (NPV) analysis, which explicitly accounts for inflation and foregone investment opportunities by expressing future cash flows in present dollars" [12].

Examples where LCC and NPV analysis prove very helpful are in deciding whether to replace/ rebuild or buy/lease medical imaging equipment. The kinds of costs captured in life-cycle cost analysis include decision-making costs, planning agency/certificate of need costs (if applicable), financing, initial capital investment costs including facility changes, life-cycle maintenance and repairs costs, personnel costs, and other (reimbursement consequences, resale, etc).

One of the best strategies to ensure that a desired technology is truly of value to the hospital is to conduct a careful analysis in preparation for its assimilation into hospital operations. The process of equipment prepurchase evaluation provides information that can be used to screen unacceptable performance by either the vendor or the equipment before it becomes a hospital problem.

Once the vendor has responded to informal requests or formal RFPs, the clinical engineering department should be responsible for evaluating the technical responses, while the materials management department should evaluate the financial responses.

In translating clinical needs into a specification list, key features or "must have" attributes of the desired device are identified. In practice, clinical engineering and materials management should develop a "must have" list and an extras list. The extras list contains features that may tip the decision in favor of one vendor, all other factors being even. These specification lists are sent to the vendor and are effective in a self-elimination process that results in a time savings for the hospital. Once the "must have" attributes have been satisfied, the remaining candidate devices are evaluated technically, and the extras are considered. This is accomplished by assigning a weighting factor (i.e., 0 to 5) to denote the relative importance of each of the desired attributes. The relative ability of each device to meet the defined requirements is then rated [15].

One strategy that strengthens the acquisition process is the conditions-of-sale document. This multifaceted document integrates equipment specifications, performance, installation require- ments, and follow-up services. The conditions-of-sale document ensures that negotiations are completed before a purchase order is delivered and each participant is in agreement about the product to be delivered. As a document of compliance, the conditions-of-sale document specifies the codes and standards having jurisdiction over that equipment. This may include provisions for future modification of the equipment, compliance with standards under development, compliance with national codes, and provision for software upgrades.

Standard purchase orders that include the conditions of sale for medical equipment are usually used to initiate the order. At the time the order is placed, clinical engineering is notified of the order. In addition to current facility conditions, the management must address installation and approval requirements, responsibilities, and timetable; payment, assignment, and cancelation; software requirements and updates; documentation; clinical and technical training; acceptance testing (hospital facility and vendor); warranty, spare parts, and service; and price protection.

All medical equipment must be inspected and tested before it is placed into service regardless of whether it is purchased, leased, rented, or borrowed by the hospital. In any hospital, clinical engi- neering should receive immediate notification if a very large device or system is delivered directly into another department (e.g., imaging or cardiology) for installation. Clinical engineering should be required to sign off on all purchase orders for devices after installation and validation of satis- factory operation. Ideally, the warranty period on new equipment should not begin until installa- tion and acceptance testing are completed. It is not uncommon for a hospital to lose several months of free parts and service by the manufacturer when new equipment is, for some reason, not installed immediately after delivery.

Clinical Team Requirements

During the technology assessment and acquisition processes, clinical decision makers analyze the following criteria concerning proposed technology acquisitions, specifically as they relate to clinical team requirements: ability of staff to assimilate the technology, medical staff satisfaction (short term and long term), impact on staffing (numbers, functions), projected utilization, ongoing related supplies required, effect on delivery of care and outcomes (convenience, safety, or standard of care), result of what is written in the clinical practice guidelines, credentialling of staff required, clinical staff initial and ongoing training required, and the effect on existing technology in the department or on other services/departments.

Defining Terms

Appropriate technology [1]:　A term used initially in developing countries, referring to selecting medical equipment that can "appropriately" satisfy the following constraints: funding shortages, insufficient numbers of trained personnel, lack of technical support, inadequate supplies of consumables/accessories, unreliable water and power utilities/supplies, and lack of operating and maintenance manuals. In the context of this chapter, appropriate technology selection must take into consideration local health needs and disease prevalence, the need for local capability of equipment maintenance, and availability of resources for ongoing operational and technical support.

Clinical engineers/biomedical engineers:　As we began describing the issues with the management of medical technology, it became obvious that some of the terms are being used interchangeably in the literature. For example, the terms *engineers, clinical engineers, biomedical equipment technicians, equipment managers,* and *health care engineers* are frequently used. For clarification, in this chapter we will refer to clinical engineers and the clinical engineering department as a representative group for all these terms.

Cost-effectiveness [1]:　A mixture of quantitative and qualitative considerations. It includes the health priorities of the country or region at the macro assessment level and the community needs at the institution micro assessment level. Product life-cycle cost analysis (which, in turn, includes initial purchase price, shipping, renovations, installation, supplies, associated disposables, cost per use, and similar quantitative measures) is a critical analysis measure. Life-cycle cost also takes into account staff training, ease of use, service, and many other cost factors. But experience and judgment about the relative importance of features and the ability to fulfill the intended purpose also contribute critical information to the cost-effectiveness equation.

Equipment acquisition and deployment:　Medical device systems and products typically emerge from the strategic technology planning process as "required and budgeted" needs. The process that follows, which ends with equipment acceptance testing and placement into general use, is known as the *equipment acquisition and deployment process.*

Health care technology:　Health care technology includes the devices, equipment, systems, software, supplies, pharmaceuticals, biotechnologies, and medical and surgical procedures used in the prevention, diagnosis, and treatment of disease in humans, for their rehabilitation, and for assistive purposes. In short, technology is broadly defined as encompassing virtually all the human interventions intended to cope with disease and disabilities, short of spiritual alternatives. This chapter focuses on medical equipment products (devices, systems, and software) rather than pharmaceuticals, biotechnologies, or procedures [1]. The concept of technology also encompasses the facilities that house both patients and products. Facilities cover a wide spectrum—from the modern hospital on one end to the mobile imaging trailer on the other.

Quality of care (QA) and quality of improvement (QI):　Quality assurance (QA) and Quality improvement (QI) are formal sets of activities to measure the quality of care provided; these usually include a process for selecting, monitoring, and applying corrective measures. The 1994 Joint Commission on the Accreditation of Healthcare Organizations (JCAHO) standards require hospital QA programs to focus on patient outcomes as a primary reference. JCAHO standards for plant, technology, and safety management (PTSM), in turn, require certain equipment management practices and QA or QI activities. Identified QI deficiencies may influence equipment planning, and QI audits may increase awareness of technology overuse or underutilization.

Risk management: Risk management is a program that helps the hospital avoid the possibility of risks, minimize liability exposure, and stay compliant with regulatory reporting requirements. JCAHO PTSM standards require minimum technology-based risk-management activities. These include clinical engineering's determination of technology-related incidents with follow-up steps to prevent recurrences and evaluation and documentation of the effectiveness of these steps.

Safety: Safety is the condition of being safe from danger, injury, or damage. It is judgment about the acceptability of risk in a specified situation (e.g., for a given medical problem) by a provider with specified training at a specified type of facility equipment.

Standards [1]:   A wide variety of formal standards and guidelines related to health care technology now exists. Some standards apply to design, development, and manufacturing practices for devices, software, and pharmaceuticals; some are related to the construction and operation of a health care facility; some are safety and performance requirements for certain classes of technologies, such as standards related to radiation or electrical safety; and others relate to performance, or even construction specifications, for specific types of technologies. Other standards and guidelines deal with administrative, medical, and surgical procedures and the training of clinical personnel. Standards and guidelines are produced and/or adopted by government agencies, international organizations, and professional and specialty organizations and societies. ECRI's *Healthcare Standards Directory* lists over 20,000 individual standards and guidelines produced by over 600 organizations and agencies from North America alone.

Strategic technology planning: Strategic technology planning encompasses both technologies new to the hospital and replacements for existing equipment that are to be acquired over several quarters. Acquisitions can be proposed for reasons related to safety, standard-of-care issues, and age or obsolescence of existing equipment. Acquisitions also can be proposed to consolidate several service areas, expand a service area to reduce cost of service, or add a new service area.

Strategic technology planning optimizes the way the hospital's capital resources contribute to its mission. It encourages choosing new technologies that are cost-effective, and it also allows the hospital to be competitive in offering state-of-the-art services. Strategic technology planning works for a single department, product line, or clinical service. It can be limited to one or several high-priority areas. It also can be used for an entire multihospital system or geographic region [4].

Technology assessment: Assessment of medical technology is any process used for examining and reporting properties of medical technology used in health care, such as safety, efficacy, feasibility, and indications for use, cost, and cost-effectiveness, as well as social, economic, and ethical consequences, whether intended or unintended [2]. A primary technology assessment is one that seeks new, previously nonexistent data through research, typically employing long-term clinical studies of the type described below. A secondary technology assessment is usually based on published data, interviews, questionnaires, and other information-gathering methods rather than original research that creates new, basic data.

In technology assessment, there are six basic objectives that the clinical engineering department should have in mind. First, there should be ongoing monitoring of developments concerning new and emerging technologies. For new technologies, there should be an assessment of the clinical efficacy, safety, and cost/benefit ratio, including their effects on established technologies. There should be an evaluation of the short- and long-term costs and benefits of alternate approaches to managing specific clinical conditions. The appropriateness of existing technologies and their clinical uses should be estimated, while outmoded technologies should be identified and eliminated from their duplicative uses. The department should rate specific technology-based interventions in terms of improved overall value (quality and outcomes) to patients, providers, and payers. Finally, the department should facilitate a continuous uniformity between needs, offerings, and capabilities [3].

The locally based (hospital or hospital group) technology assessment described in this chapter is a process of secondary assessment that attempts to judge whether a certain medical equipment/product can be assimilated into the local operational environment.

Technology diffusion [1]: The process by which a technology is spread over time in a social system. The progression of technology diffusion can be described in four stages. The *emerging* or applied research stage occurs around the time of initial clinical testing. In the *new* stage, the technology has passed the phase of clinical trials but is not yet in widespread use. During the *established* stage, the technology is considered by providers to be a standard approach to a particular condition and diffuses into general use. Finally, in the *obsolete/outmoded* stage, the technology is superseded by another and/or is demonstrated to be ineffective or harmful.

Technology life cycle: Technology has a life cycle—a process by which technology is created, tested, applied, and replaced or abandoned. Since the life cycle varies from basic research and innovation to obsolescence and abatement, it is critical to know the maturity of a technology prior to making decisions regarding its adoption. Technology forecast and assessment of pending technological changes are the investigative tools that support systematic and rational decisions about the utilization of a given institution's technological capabilities.

Technology planning and management [3]: Technology planning and management are an accountable, systematic approach to ensuring that cost-effective, efficacious, appropriate, and safe equipment is available to meet the demands of quality patient care and allow an institution to remain competitive. Elements include in-house service management, management and analysis of equipment external service providers, involvement in the equipment acquisition process, involvement of appropriate hospital personnel in facility planning and design, involvement in reducing technology-related patient and staff incidents, training equipment users, reviewing equipment replacement needs, and ongoing assessment of emerging technologies [4].

References

1. ECRI. Healthcare Technology Assessment Curriculum. Philadelphia, August 1992.
2. Banta HD, Institute of Medicine. Assessing Medical Technologies. Washington, National Academy Press, 1985.
3. Lumsdon K. Beyond technology assessment: Balancing strategy needs, strategy. Hospitals 15:25, 1992.
4. ECRI. Capital, Competition, and Constraints: Managing Healthcare in the 1990s. A Guide for Hospital Executives. Philadelphia, 1992.
5. Berkowitz DA, Solomon RP. Providers may be missing opportunities to improve patient outcomes. Costs, Outcomes Measurement and Management May-June: 7, 1991.
6. ECRI. Regional Healthcare Technology Planning and Management Program. Philadelphia, 1990.
7. Sprague GR. Managing technology assessment and acquisition. Health Exec 6:26, 1988.
8. David Y. Technology-related decision-making issues in hospitals. In IEEE Engineering in Medicine and Biology Society Proceedings of the 11th Annual International Conference, 1989.
9. Wagner M. Promoting hospitals high-tech equipment. Mod Healthcare 46, 1989.
10. David Y. Medical Technology 2001. CPA Healthcare Conference, 1992.
11. ECRI. Special Report on Technology Management, Health Technology. Philadelphia, 1989.
12. ECRI. Special Report on Devices and Dollars. Philadelphia, 1988.
13. Gullikson ML, David Y, Brady MH. An autoated risk management tool. JCAHO, Plant, Technology and Safety Management Review, PTSM Series, no 2, 1993.
14. David Y, Judd T, ECRI. Special Report on Devices and Dollars. Philadelphia, 1988. Medical Technology Management. SpaceLabs Medical, Inc., Redmond, Wash 1993.
15. Bronzino JD (ed). Management of Medical Technology: A Primer for Clinical Engineers. Stoneham, Mass, Butterworth, 1992.

167

Risk Factors, Safety, and Management of Medical Equipment

Michael L. Gullikson
Texas Children's Hospital

167.1 Risk Management: A Definition

Inherent in the definition of *risk management* is the implication that the hospital environment cannot be made risk-free. In fact, the nature of medical equipment—to invasively or noninvasively perform diagnostic, therapeutic, corrective, or monitoring intervention on behalf of the patient—implies that risk is present. Therefore, a standard of acceptable risk must be established that defines *manageable risk* in a real-time economic environment.

Unfortunately, a preexistent, quantitative standard does not exist in terms of, for instance, mean time before failure (MTBF), number of repairs or repair redos per equipment item, or cost of maintenance that provides a universal yardstick for risk management of medical equipment. Sufficient clinical management of risk must be in place that can utilize safeguards, preventive maintenance, and failure analysis information to minimize the occurrence of injury or death to patient or employee or property damage. Therefore, a process must be put in place that will permit analysis of information and modification of the preceding factors to continuously move the medical equipment program to a more stable level of manageable risk.

Risk factors that require management can be illustrated by the example of the "double-edge" sword concept of technology (see Fig. 167.1). The front edge of the sword represents the cutting edge of technology and its beneficial characteristics: increased quality, greater availability of technology, timeliness of test results and treatment, and so on. The back edge of the sword represents those liabilities which must be addressed to effectively manage risk: the hidden costs discussed in the next paragraph, our dependence on technology, incompatibility of equipment, and so on [1].

For example, the purchase and installation of a major medical equipment item may only represent 20% of the lifetime cost of the equipment [2]. If the operational budget of a nursing floor does not include the other 80% of the equipment costs, budget constraints may require cutbacks where they appear to minimally affect direct patient care. Preventive maintenance, software upgrades that address "glitches," or overhaul requirements may be seen as unaffordable luxuries. Gradual equip-

0-8493-8346-3/95/$0.00+$.50
© 1995 by CRC Press, Inc.

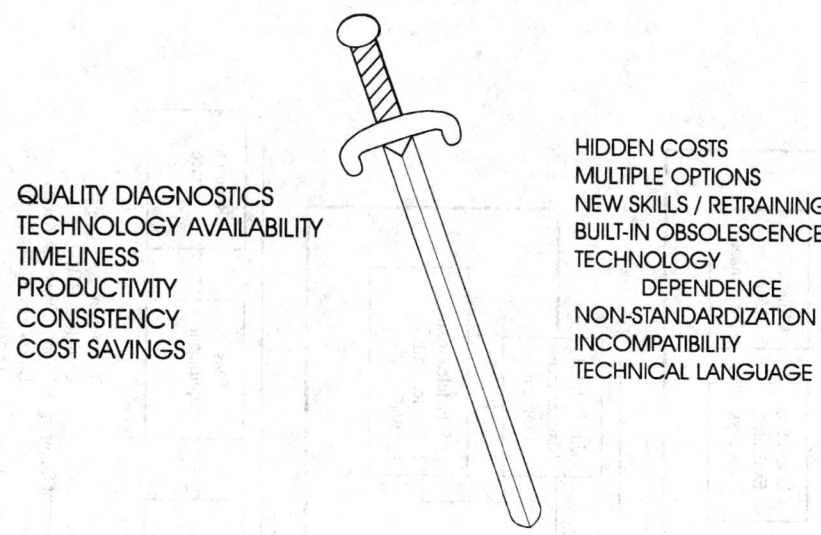

QUALITY DIAGNOSTICS
TECHNOLOGY AVAILABILITY
TIMELINESS
PRODUCTIVITY
CONSISTENCY
COST SAVINGS

HIDDEN COSTS
MULTIPLE OPTIONS
NEW SKILLS / RETRAINING
BUILT-IN OBSOLESCENCE
TECHNOLOGY
    DEPENDENCE
NON-STANDARDIZATION
INCOMPATIBILITY
TECHNICAL LANGUAGE

FIGURE 167.1   Double-edged sword concept of risk management.

ment deterioration without maintenance may bring the safety level below an acceptable level of manageable risk.

Since economic factors as well as those of safety must be considered, a balanced approach to risk management that incorporates all aspects of the medical equipment lifecycle must be considered.

The operational flowchart in Fig. 167.2 describes the concept of medical equipment life-cycle management from the clinical engineering department viewpoint. The flowchart includes planning, evaluation, and initial purchase documentation requirements. The condition of sale, for example, ensures that technical manuals, training, replacement parts, etc. are received so that all medical equipment might be fully supported in-house after the warranty period. Introduction to the preventive maintenance program, unscheduled maintenance procedures, and retirement justification must be part of the process. Institutional-wide cooperation with the life-cycle concept requires education and patience to convince health care providers of the team approach to managing medical equipment technology.

This balanced approach requires communication and comprehensive planning by a health care team responsible for evaluation of new and shared technology within the organization. A medical technology evaluation committee (see Fig. 167.3), composed of representatives from administration, medical staff, nursing, safety department, biomedical engineering, and various services, can be an effective platform for the integration of technology and health care. Risk containment is practiced as the committee reviews not only the benefits of new technology but also the technical and clinical liabilities and provides a 6-month followup study to measure the effectiveness of the selection process. The history of risk management in medical equipment management provides helpful insight into its current status and future direction.

167.2 Risk Management: Historical Perspective

Historically, risk management of medical equipment was the responsibility of the clinical engineer (Fig. 167.4). The engineer selected medical equipment based on individual clinical department consultations and established preventive maintenance (PM) programs based on manufacturers' recommendations and clinical experience. The clinical engineer reviewed the documentation and

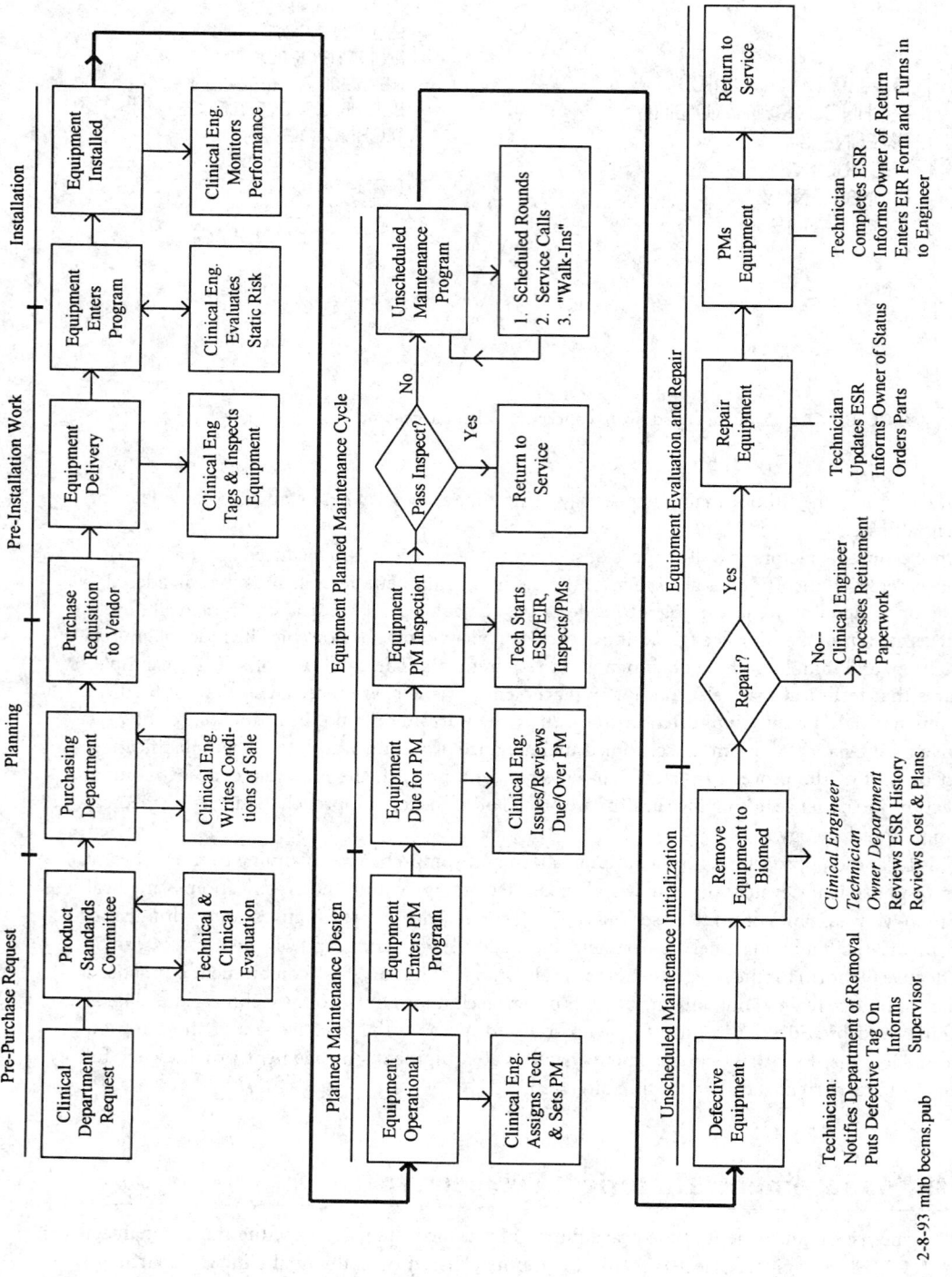

FIGURE 167.2   Biomedical engineering equipment management system (BEEMS).

"spot-checked" equipment used in the hospital. The clinical engineer met with biomedical supervisors and technicians to discuss PM completion and to resolve repair problems. The clinical engineer then attempted to analyze failure information to avoid repeat failure.

However, greater public awareness of safety issues, increasing equipment density at the bedside, more sophisticated software-driven medical equipment, and financial considerations have made it more difficult for the clinical engineer to singularly handle risk issues. In addition, the synergistic interactions of various medical systems operating in proximity to one another have added another dimension to the risk formula. It is not only necessary for health care institutions to manage risk using a team approach, but it is also becoming apparent that the clinical engineer requires more technology-intensive tools to effectively contribute to the team effort [3].

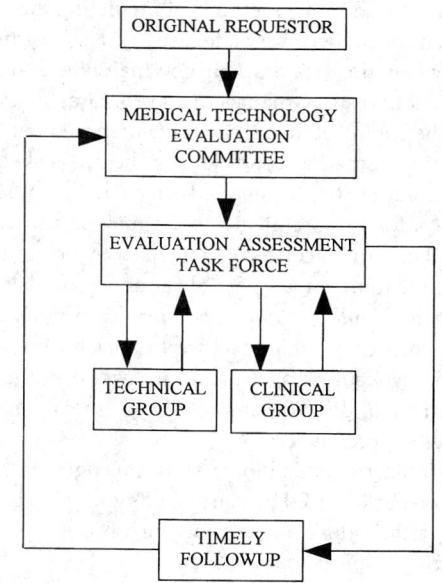

FIGURE 167.3 Medical technology evaluation committee.

167.3 Risk Management: Strategies

Reactive risk management is an outgrowth of the historical attitude in medical equipment management that risk is an anomaly that surfaces in the form of a failure. If the failure is analyzed and proper operational procedures, user in-services, and increased maintenance are supplied, the problem will disappear and personnel can return to their normal work. When the next failure occurs, the algorithm is repeated. If the same equipment fails, the algorithm is applied more intensely. This is a useful but not comprehensive component of risk management in the hospital. In

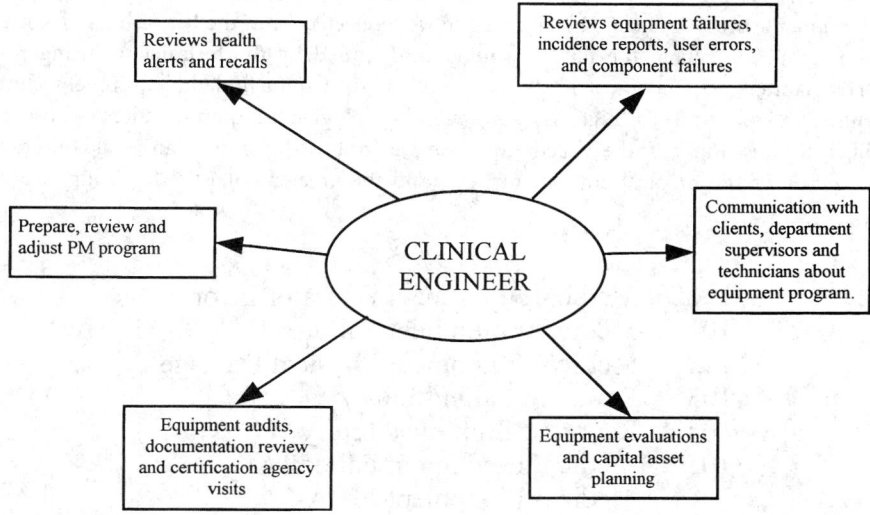

FIGURE 167.4 Operational flowchart.

fact, the traditional methods of predicting the reliability of electronic equipment from field failure data have not been very effective [4]. The health care environment, as previously mentioned, inherently contains risk that must be maintained at a manageable level. A reactive tool cannot provide direction to a risk-management program, but it can provide feedback as to its efficiency.

The engine of the reactive risk-management tool is a set of failure codes (see Fig. 167.5) that flag certain anomalous conditions in the medical equipment management program. If operator training needs are to be identified, then codes 100, 102, 104, and 108 (MBA equipment returned within 9 days for a subsequent repair) may be useful. If technician difficulties in handling equipment problems are of concern, then 108 may be of interest. The key is to develop failure codes not in an attempt to define all possible anomaly modalities but for those which *can clearly be defined and provide unambiguous direction for the correction process*. Also, the failure codes should be linked to equipment type, manufacturer/model, technician service group, hospital, and clinical department. Again, when the data are analyzed, will the result be provided to an administrator, engineer, clinical department director, or safety department? This should determine the format in which the failure codes are presented.

A report intended for the clinical engineer might be formatted as in Fig. 167.6. It would consist of two parts, sorted by equipment type and clinical department (not shown). The engineer's report shows the failure code activity for various types of equipment and the distribution of those failure codes in clinical departments.

Additionally, fast data-analysis techniques introduced by NASA permit the survey of large quantities of information in a three-dimensional display [5] (Fig. 167.7). This approach permits viewing time-variable changes from month to month and failure concentration in specific departments and equipment types.

The importance of the format for failure modality presentation is critical to its usefulness and acceptance by health care professionals. For instance, a safety director requests the clinical engineer to provide a list of equipment that, having failed, could have potentially harmed a patient or employee. The safety director is asking the clinical engineer for a clinical judgment based on clinical as well as technical factors. This is beyond the scope of responsibility and expertise of the clinical engineer. However, the request can be addressed indirectly. The safety director's request can be addressed in two steps: first, providing a list of high-risk equipment (assessed when the medical equipment is entered into the equipment inventory) and, second, a clinical judgment based on equipment failure mode, patient condition, and so on. The flowchart in Fig. 167.8 provides the safety director with useful information but does not require the clinical engineer to make an unqualified clinical judgment. If the "failed PM" failure code were selected from the list of high-risk medical equipment requiring repair, the failure would be identified by the technician during routine preventive maintenance and most likely the clinician still would find the equipment clinically efficacious. This condition is a "high risk, soft failure" or a high-risk equipment item whose failure is *least* likely to cause injury. If the "failed PM" code were not used, the clinician would question the clinical efficacy of the medical equipment item, and the greater potential for injury would be

100	Medical Equipment Operator Error
101	Medical Equipment Failure
102	Medical Equipment Physical Damage
103	Reported Patient Injury
104	Reported Employee Injury
105	Medical Equipment Failed PM
108	Medical Equipment MBA

FIGURE 167.5   Failure codes.

10514 PULMONARY INSTR TEXAS CHILDREN'S HOSP

Source	Total PM	Fail PM Items	% Fail	Reported Fail-OK	Physical Damage	Patient Injury	Employee Injury	Machine Back Again	# of Equip Fail Count	Total Equip Count	% Fail
1 NON-TAGGED EQUIPMENT	0		0.00		5				14	14	0.00
1280 THERMOMETER, ELECTRONIC	2		0.00	1					1	99	1.01
1292 RADIANT WARMER, INFANT	1		0.00						3	63	4.76
1306 INCUBATOR, NEONATAL	0	2	0.00		7				9	56	16.07
1307 INCUBATOR, TRANSPORT, NEONATAL	9	3	33.33		1			1 *	4	9	44.44
1320 PHOTOTHERAPY UNIT, NEONATAL	4		0.00						2	28	7.14
1321 INFUSION PUMP	35		0.00	15	9			3 *	34	514	6.61
1357 SUCTION,VAC POWERED,BODY FLUID	0		0.00						4	358	1.12
1384 EXAMINATION LIGHT, AC-POWERED	11		0.00						1	47	2.13
1447 CARDIAC MONITOR W/ RATE ALARM	0		0.00	1	1			1 *	1		0.00
1567 SURGICAL NERVE STIMULATOR /LOC	0		0.00						2	15	13.33
1624 OTOSCOPE	73		0.00						1	101	0.99
1675 OXYGEN GAS ANALYZER	0		0.00						3	44	6.82
1681 SPIROMETER DIAGNOSTIC	0		0.00						1	8	12.50
1703 AIRWAY PRESSURE MONITOR	1		0.00					1 *	7	9	77.78
1735 BREATHING GAS MIXER	13		0.00					1 *	4	38	10.53
1749 HYPO/HYPERTHERMIA DEVICE	1		0.00						1	3	33.33
1762 NEBULIZER	25		0.00						1	56	1.79
1787 VENTILATOR CONTINUOUS	96	7	7.29		1			1 *	11	99	11.11
1788 VENTILATOR NONCONTINUOUS	1		0.00		1				3	27	11.11
2014 HEMODIALYSIS SYSTEM ACCESSORIE	0		0.00						3	1	300.00
2051 PERITONEAL DIALYSIS SYS & ACC	4		0.00						1	5	20.00
2484 SPECTROPHOTOMETER, MASS	0		0.00						2	3	66.67
2695 POWERED SUCTION PUMP	16		0.00		1			1 *	1	32	3.13
5028 PH METER	0		0.00						1	4	25.00
5035 COMPUTER & PERIPHERALS	0		0.00						3	18	16.67
5081 OXYGEN MONITOR	0		0.00		1				15	102	14.71
5082 RESPIRATION ANALYZER	1		0.00	3	1				1	5	20.00
5097 EXAM TABLE	75		0.00						1	86	1.16
5113 PRINTER	2		0.00						1	12	8.33
5126 ADDRESSOGRAPH	2		0.00						4	1	400.00
9102 STADIOMETER	0		0.00						1	8	12.50
17211 ANESTHESIA MONITOR	23		0.00						2	23	8.70
90063 POWER SUPPLY, PORTABLE	20		0.00						1	25	4.00
Total for TEXAS CHILDREN'S HOSP	415	12		20	28			9	144	1899	

FIGURE 167.6 Engineer's failure analysis report.

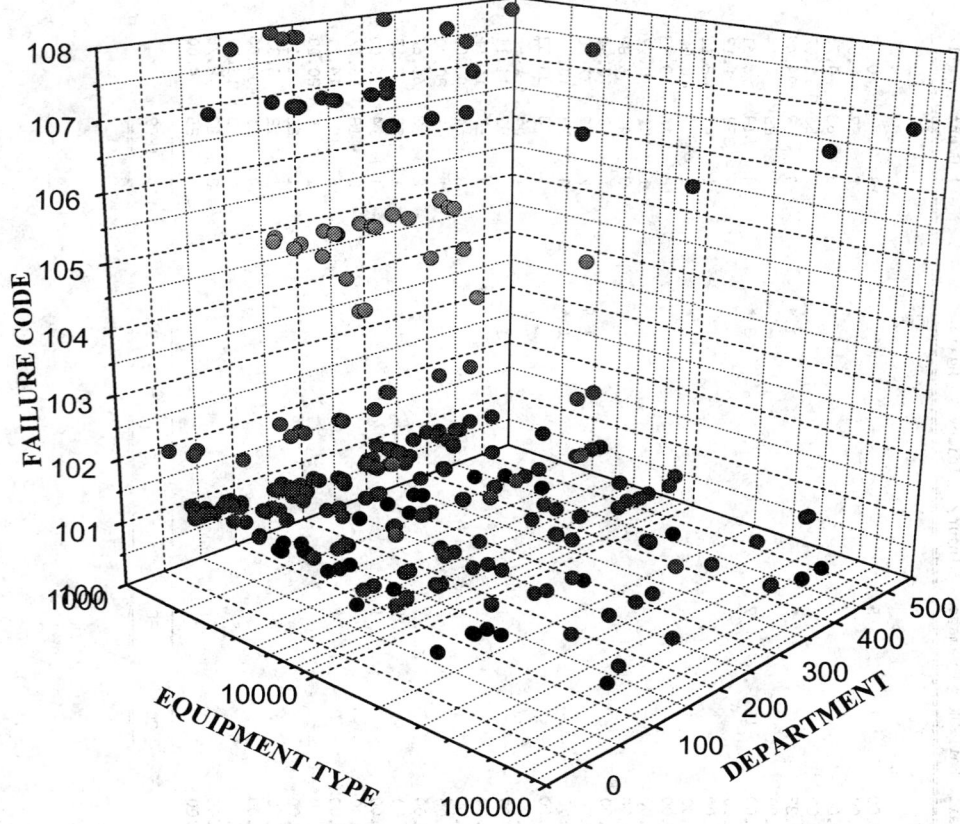

FIGURE 167.7   Failure code analysis using a 3-D display.

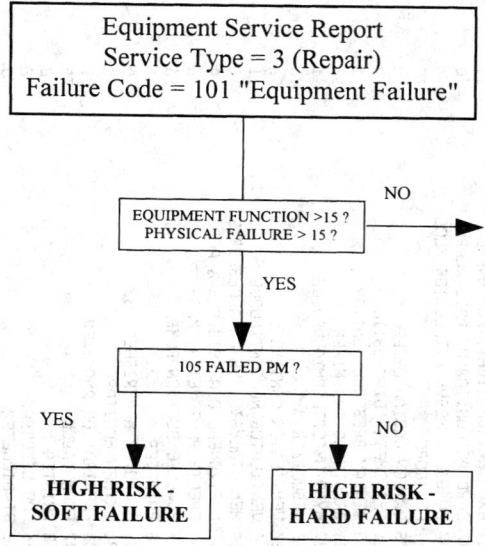

FIGURE 167.8   High-risk medical equipment failures.

identified by "high risk, hard failure." Monitoring the distribution of high-risk equipment in these two categories assists the safety director in managing risk.

Obviously, a more forward-looking tool is needed to take advantage of the failure codes and the plethora of equipment information available in a clinical engineering department. This proactive tool should use failure codes, historical information, the "expert" knowledge of the clinical engineer, and the baseline of an established "manageable risk" environment (perhaps not optimal but stable).

The overall components and process flow for a proactive risk-management tool [6] are presented in Fig. 167.9. It consists of a two-component static risk factor, a two-component dynamic risk factor, and two "shaping" or feedback loops.

The static risk factor classifies new equipment by a generic equipment type: defibrillator, electrocardiograph, pulse oximeter, etc. When equipment is introduced into the equipment database, it is assigned to two different static risk (Fig. 167.10) categories [7]. The first is the equipment function that defines the application and environment in which the equipment item will operate. The degree of interaction with the patient is also taken into account. For example, a therapeutic device would have a higher risk assignment than a monitoring or diagnostic device. The second component of the static risk factor is the physical risk category. It defines the worst-case scenario in the event of equipment malfunction. The correlation between equipment function and physical risk on many items might make the two categories appear redundant. However, there are sufficient equipment types where this is not the case. A scale of 1 to 25 is assigned to each risk category. The larger number is assigned to devices demonstrating greater risk because of their function or the consequences of device failure. The 1 to 25 scale is an arbitrary assignment, since a validated scale of risk factors for medical equipment, as previously described, is nonexistent. The risk points assigned to the equipment from these two categories are algebraically summed and designated the static risk factor. This value remains with the equipment type and the individual items within that equipment type permanently. Only if the equipment is used in a clinically variant way or relocated to a functionally different environment would this assignment be reviewed and changed.

The dynamic component (Fig. 167.11) of the risk-management tool consists of two parts. The first is a maintenance requirement category that is divided into 25 equally spaced divisions, ranked by least (1) to greatest (25) average manhours per device per year. These divisions are scaled by the maintenance hours for the equipment type requiring the greatest amount of maintenance attention. The amount of nonplanned (repair) manhours from the previous 12 months of service reports is totaled for each equipment type. Since this is maintenance work on failed equipment items, it correlates with the risk associated with that equipment type.

If the maintenance hours of an equipment type are observed to change to the point of placing it in a different maintenance category, a flag notifies the clinical engineer to review the equipment-type category. The engineer may increase the PM schedule to compensate for the higher unplanned maintenance hours. If the engineer believes the system "overreacted," a "no" decision adjusts a scaling factor by a -5%. Progressively, the algorithm is "shaped" for the equipment maintenance program in that particular institution. However, to ensure that critical changes in the average manhours per device for each equipment type is not missed during the shaping period, the system is initialized. This is accomplished by increasing the average manhours per device for each equipment type to within 5% of the next higher maintenance requirement division. Thus the system is sensitized to variations in maintenance requirements.

The baseline is now established for evaluating individual device risk. Variations in the maintenance requirement hours for any particular equipment type will, for the most part, only occur over a substantial period of time. For this reason, the maintenance requirement category is designated as a "slow" dynamic risk element.

The second dynamic element assigns weighted risk points to *individual* equipment items for each unique risk occurrence. An *occurrence* is defined as when the device

- Exceeds the American Hospital Association Useful Life Table for Medical Equipment or exceeds the historical MTBF for that manufacturer and model

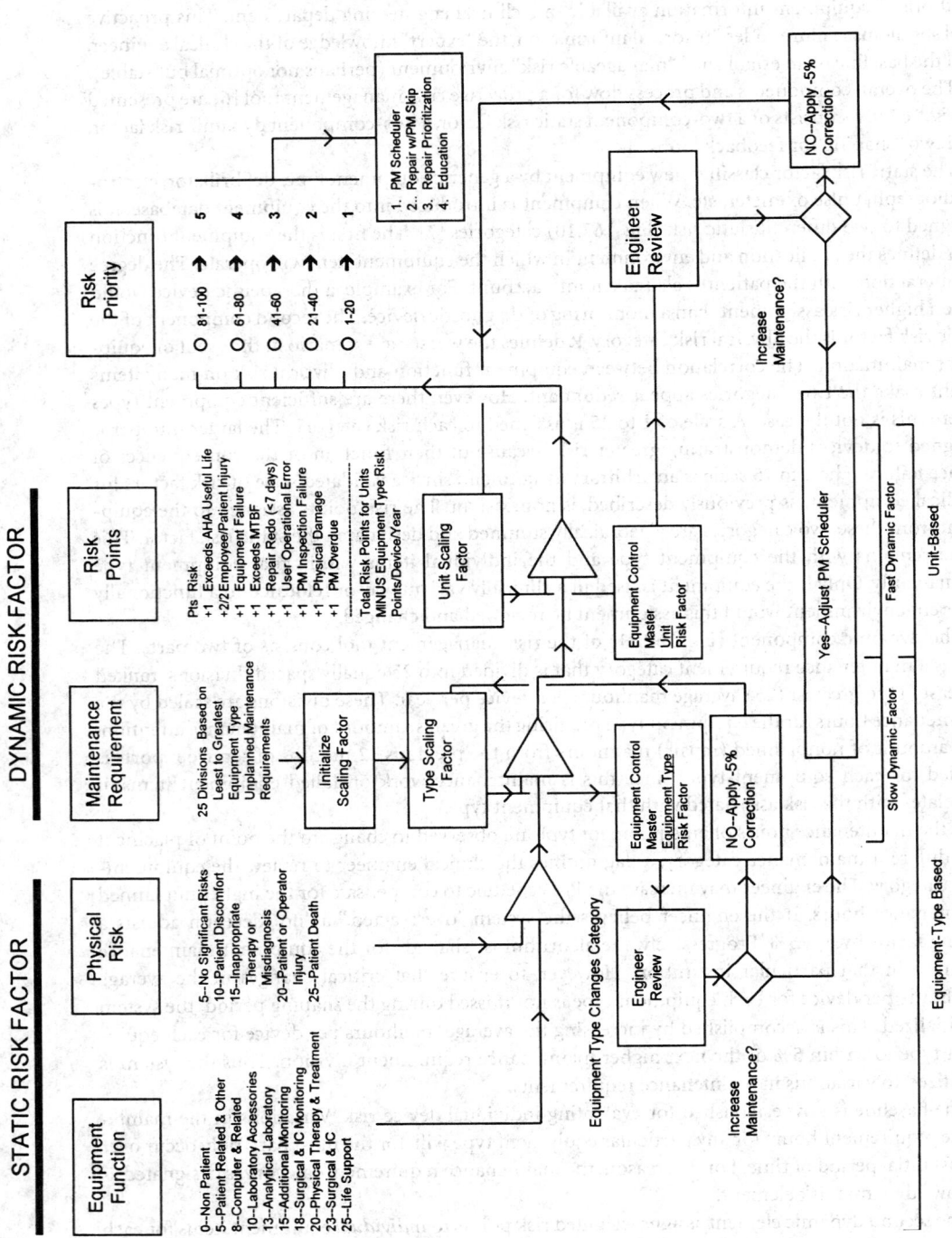

FIGURE 167.9 Biomedical engineering risk-management tool.

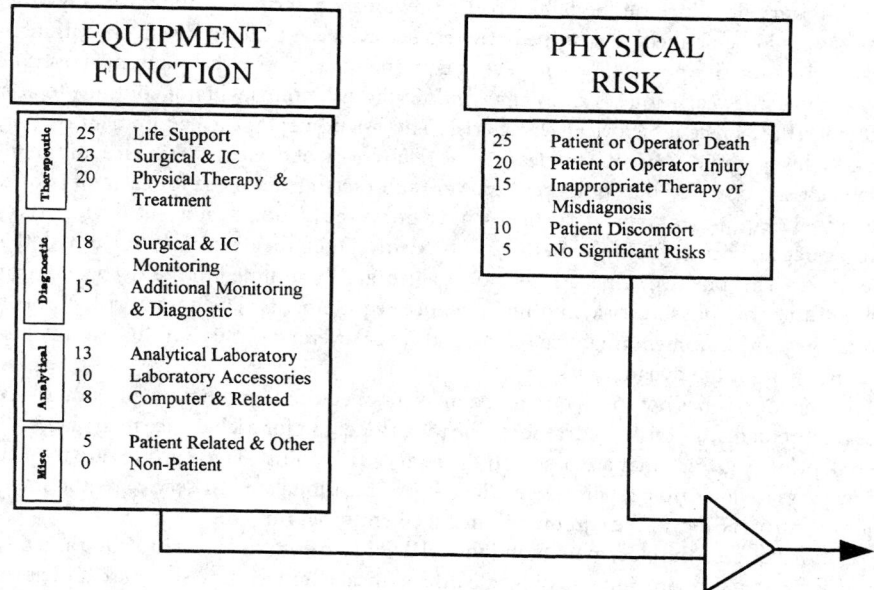

FIGURE 167.10   Static risk components.

- Injures a patient or employee
- Functionally fails or fails to pass a PM inspection
- Is returned for repair or returned for rerepair within 9 days of a previous repair occurrence
- Misses a planned maintenance inspection
- Is subjected to physical damage
- Was reported to have failed but the problem was determined to be a user operational error

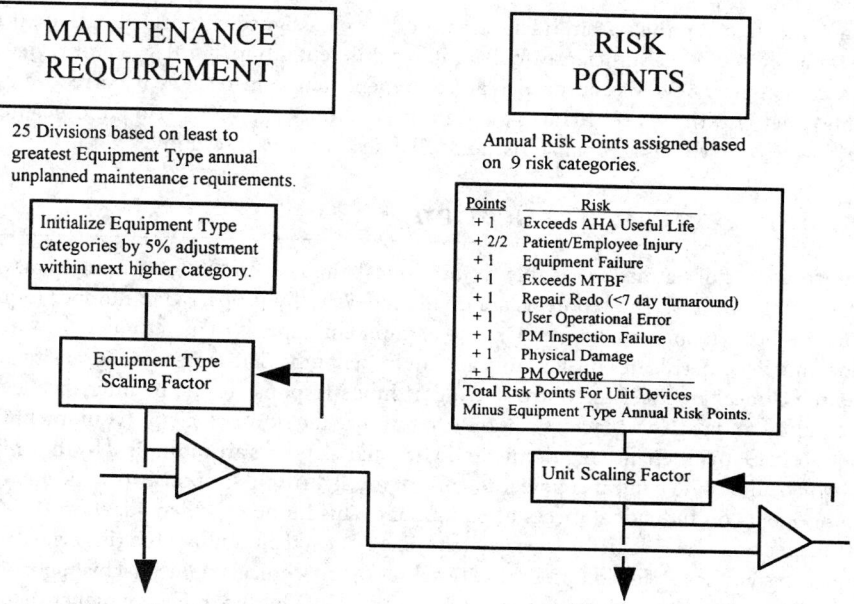

FIGURE 167.11   Dynamic risk components.

These risk occurrences include the failure codes previously described. Although many other risk occurrences could be defined, these nine occurrences have been historically effective in managing equipment risk. The risk points for each piece of equipment are algebraically summed over the previous year. Since the yearly total is a moving window, the risk points will not continue to accumulate but will reflect a recent historical average risk. The risk points for each equipment type are also calculated. This provides a baseline to measure the relative risk of devices within an equipment type. The average risk points for the equipment type are subtracted from those for each piece of equipment within the equipment type. If the device has a negative risk point value, the device's risk is less than the average device in the equipment type. If positive, then the device has higher risk than the average device. This positive or negative factor is algebraically summed to the risk values from the equipment function, physical risk, and maintenance requirements. The annual risk points for an individual piece of equipment might change quickly over several months. For this reason, this is the "fast" component of the dynamic risk factor.

The concept of risk has now been quantified in terms of equipment function, physical risk, maintenance requirements, and risk occurrences. The total risk count for each device then places it in one of five risk priority groups that are based on the sum of risk points. These groups are then applied in various ways to determine repair triage, PM triage, educational and in-service requirements and test equipment/parts, etc. in the equipment management program.

Correlation between the placement of individual devices in each risk priority group and the levels of planned maintenance previously assigned by the clinical engineer have shown that the proactive risk-management tool calculates a similar maintenance schedule as manually planned by the clinical engineer. In other words, the proactive risk-management tool algorithm places equipment items in a risk priority group commensurate with the greater or lesser maintenance as currently applied in the equipment maintenance program.

As previously mentioned, the four categories and the 1 to 25 risk levels within each category are arbitrary because a "gold standard" for risk management is nonexistent. Therefore, the clinical engineer is given input into the dynamic components making up the risk factor to "shape the system" based on the equipment's maintenance history and the clinical engineer's experience. Since the idea of a safe medical equipment program involves "judgment about the acceptability of risk in a specified situation" [8], this experience is a necessary component of the risk-assessment tool for a specific health care setting.

In the same manner, the system tracks the unit device's assigned risk priority group. If the risk points for a device change sufficiently to place it in a different group, it is flagged for review. Again, the clinical engineer reviews the particular equipment item and decides if corrective action is prudent. Otherwise, the system reduces the scaling factor by 5%. Over a period of time, the system will be "formed" to what is acceptable risk and what deserves closer scrutiny.

167.4 Risk Management: Application

The information can be made available to the clinical engineer in the form of a risk assessment report (see Fig. 167.12). The report lists individual devices by property tag number (equipment control number), manufacturer, model, and equipment type. Assigned values for equipment function and physical risk are constant for each equipment type. The maintenance sensitizing factor enables the clinical engineer to control the algorithms's response to the maintenance level of an entire equipment type. These factors combine to produce the slow risk factor (equipment function + physical risk + maintenance requirements). The unit risk points are multiplied by the unit scaling factor, which allows the clinical engineer to control the algorithm's response to static and dynamic risk components on individual pieces of equipment. This number is then added to the slow risk factor to determine the risk factor for each item. The last two columns are the risk priority that the automated system has assigned and the PM level set by the clinical engineer. This report provides the clinical engineer with information about medical equipment that reflects a higher than normal risk factor for the equipment type to which it belongs.

Manager: PHYSIOLOGICAL GROUP

Equip Control Number	Manuf	Model	Equipment Type	Equip Func	Phys Risk	Maint Requir	Avg Hours	Maint Sensitiz Factor	Slow Risk Factor	Unit Risk Points	Unit Scaling Factor	Risk Factor	Risk Priority	Equip Type Priority
17407	322	4000A	NIBP SYSTEM	18	15	1	1.66	1.78	38	6.62	1.00	41	3	2
17412	322	4000A	NIBP SYSTEM	18	15	1	1.66	1.78	38	6.62	1.00	41	3	2
17424	322	4000A	NIBP SYSTEM	18	15	1	1.66	1.78	38	6.62	1.00	41	3	2
17431	322	4000A	NIBP SYSTEM	18	15	1	1.66	1.78	38	6.62	1.00	41	3	2
15609	65	BW5	BLOOD & PLMA WARMING DEVICE	5	5	1	2.51	1.17	14	10.64	1.00	22	2	1
3538	167	7370000	HR/RESP MONITOR	18	15	1	0.10	29.47	35	8.69	1.00	43	3	2
3543	167	7370000	HR/RESP MONITOR	18	15	1	0.10	29.47	35	7.69	1.00	42	3	2
15315	167	7370000	HR/RESP MONITOR	18	15	1	0.10	29.47	35	7.69	1.00	42	3	2
17761	167	7370000	HR/RESP MONITOR	18	15	1	0.10	29.47	35	6.69	1.00	41	3	2
18382	574	N100C	PULSE OXIMETER	18	15	1	0.70	4.21	35	7.54	1.00	42	3	2
180476	574	N100C	PULSE OXIMETER	18	15	1	0.70	4.21	35	7.54	1.00	42	3	2
16685	167	7275217	2 CHAN CHART REC	18	15	1	0.42	7.02	37	6.83	1.00	41	3	2

I have reviewed this risk analysis report and have investigated these equipment items for which the risk priority factor has exceeded the average risk for that equipment type. I have taken one of two actions:

   1. investigated the equipment item and implemented changes to the maintenance program intended to reduce the risk priority value OR

   2. indicated on the printout that the dynamic risk factor program has "overreacted" and the risk factor should be reduced by 5%.

ENGINEER: _____

DATE: _____

FIGURE 167.12   Engineer's risk-assessment report.

The proactive risk management tool can be used to individually schedule medical equipment devices for PM based on risk assessment. For example, why should newer patient monitors be maintained at the same maintenance level as older units if the risk can be demonstrated to be less? The tool is used as well to prioritize the planned maintenance program. For instance, assume a PM cycle every 17 weeks is started on January 1 for a duration of 1 week. Equipment not currently available for PM can be inspected at a later time as a function of the risk priority group for that device. In other words, an equipment item with a risk priority of 2, which is moderately low, would not be overdue for 2/5 of the time between the current and the next PM start date or until the thirteenth week after the start of a PM cycle of 17 weeks. The technician can complete more critical overdue equipment first and move on to less critical equipment later.

Additionally, since PM is performed with every equipment repair, is it always necessary to perform the following planned PM? Assume for a moment that unscheduled maintenance was performed 10 weeks into the 17 weeks between the two PM periods discussed above. If the equipment has a higher risk priority of three, four, or five, the equipment is PMed as scheduled in April. However, if a lower equipment risk priority of one or two is indicated, the planned maintenance is skipped in April and resumed in July. The intent of this application is to reduce maintenance costs, preserve departmental resources, and minimize the wear and tear on equipment during testing.

Historically, equipment awaiting service has been placed in the equipment holding area and inspected on a first in, first out (FIFO) basis when a technician is available. A client's request to expedite the equipment repair was the singular reason for changing the work priority schedule. The proactive risk-management tool can prioritize the equipment awaiting repair, putting the critical equipment back into service more quickly, subject to the clinical engineer's review.

167.5 Case Studies

Several examples are presented of the proactive risk-assessment tool used to evaluate the performance of medical equipment within a program.

The ventilators in Fig. 167.13 show a decreasing unit risk factor for higher equipment tag numbers. Since devices are put into service with ascending tag numbers and these devices are known to have

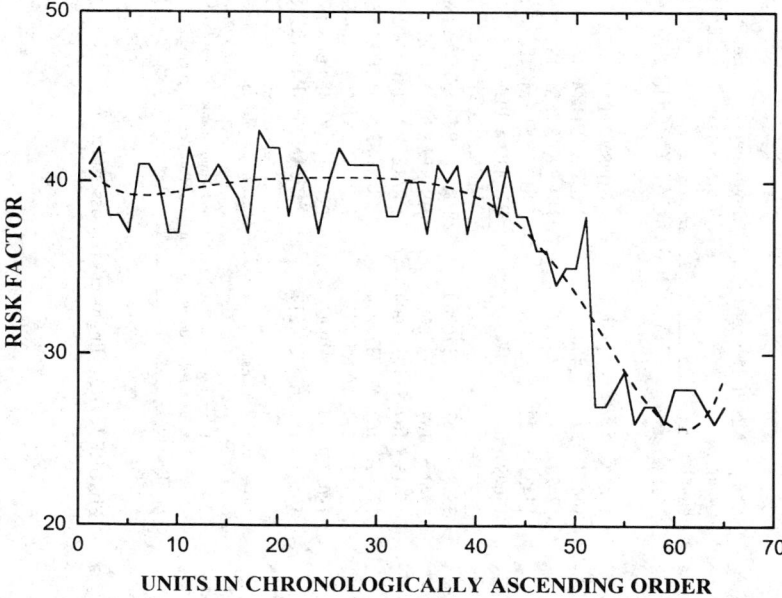

FIGURE 167.13   Ventilator with time-dependent risk characteristics.

been purchased over a period of time, the X axis represents a chronological progression. The ventilator risk factor is decreasing for newer units and could be attributable to better maintenance technique or manufacturer design improvements. This device is said to have a *time-dependent risk factor*.

A final illustration uses two generations of infusion pumps from the same manufacturer. Figure 167.14 shows the older vintage pump as *Infusion Pump 1* and the newer version as *Infusion Pump 2*. A linear regression line for the first pump establishes the average risk factor as 53 with a standard deviation of 2.02 for the 93 pumps in the analysis. The second pump, a newer version of the first, had an average risk factor of 50 with a standard deviation of 1.38 for 261 pumps. Both pumps have relatively time-independent risk factors. The proactive risk-management tool reveals that this particular brand of infusion pump in the present maintenance program is stable over time and the newer pump has reduced risk and variability of risk between individual units. Again, this could be attributable to tighter manufacturing control or improvements in the maintenance program.

167.6 Conclusions

In summary, superior risk assessment within a medical equipment management program requires better communication, teamwork, and information analysis and distribution among all health care providers. Individually, the clinical engineer cannot provide all the necessary components for managing risk in the health care environment. Using historical information to only address equipment-related problems, after an incident, is not sufficient. The use of a proactive risk-management tool is necessary.

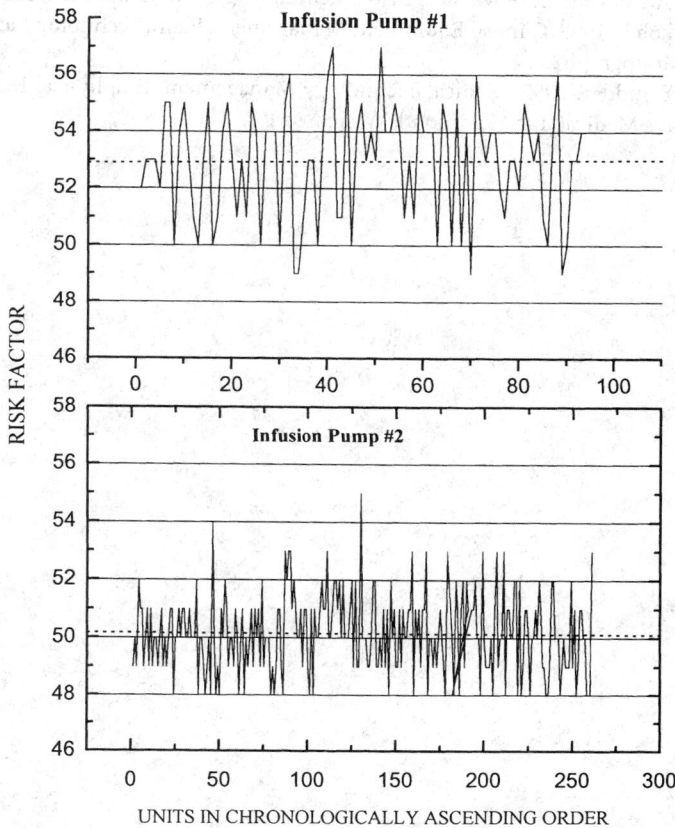

FIGURE 167.14 Time-independent risk characteristics infusion pump #1.

The clinical engineer can use this tool to deploy technical resources in a cost-effective manner. In addition to the direct economic benefits, safety is enhanced as problem equipment is identified and monitored more frequently. The integration of a proactive risk-assessment tool into the equipment management program can more accurately bring to focus technical resources in the health care environment.

References

1. Gullikson ML. 1994. Biotechnology Procurement and Maintenance II: Technology Risk Management. Third Annual International Pediatric Colloquim, Houston, Texas.
2. David Y. 1992. Medical Technology 2001. Health Care Conference, Texas Society of Certified Public Accountants, San Antonio.
3. Gullikson ML. 1993. An Automated Risk Management Tool. Plant, Technology, and Safety Management Series, Joint Commission on the Accreditation of Healthcare Facilities (JCAHO) Monograph 2.
4. Pecht ML, Nash FR. 1994. Predicting the reliability of electronic equipment. Proc IEEE 82(7):990.
5. Gullikson ML, David Y. 1993. Risk-Based Equipment Management Systems. The 9th National Conference on Medical Technology Management, American Society for Hospital Engineering of the American Hospital Association (AHA), New Orleans.
6. Gullikson ML. 1992. Biomedical Equipment Maintenance System. 27th Annual Meeting and Exposition, Hospital and Medical Industry Computerized Maintenance Systems, Association for the Advancement of Medical Instrumentation (AAMI), Anaheim, Calif.
7. Fennigkoh L. 1989. Clinical Equipment Management. Plant, Technology, and Safety Management Monograph 2.
8. David Y, Judd T. 1993. Medical Technology Management. Biophysical Measurement Series. Spacelabs Medical, Inc., Redmond, Wash.

168

Career Opportunities for Clinical Engineers

Wayne A. Morse
SpaceLabs Medical, Inc.

This chapter describes the broad spectrum of opportunities available to clinical engineering professionals, many of which exist in the medical device industry. Within that industry, college graduates in biomedical/clinical engineering can engage in such activities as product design, field service, regulatory affairs, consulting, clinical trial testing, marketing, quality assurance, technology management, or incident investigation. Other opportunities include work in the federal government (e.g., for the Food and Drug Administration, the Veteran's Administration, or any of the armed services), for nonprofit or for-profit hospitals, for shared service organizations, or as an entrepreneur.

The amount of work an engineer must do to further his or her career in clinical engineering is frequently underestimated. Before you can start a career, you need to develop short-term and long-term career goals. An important aspect of health care is knowing how the field might change in the near future. One way to do this is to read the most recent journals, trade publications, and magazines in clinical engineering. For example, salary and job responsibility data are published each year in the *Journal of Clinical Engineering*. Part of knowing your career goals is knowing what strengths you want to develop. Vertical movement, going up in job responsibilities or title, requires additional education and training. Horizontal movement, taking a position that may have new duties, requires new job duties with basically the same responsibilities. As you look to the future, remember that education increases your chances for a better job. If you have a bachelor's degree, consider a master's degree in engineering or management.

168.1 Careers in the Medical Device Industry

Most engineers work in the industrial sector of our economy. Initially recruited by industrial representatives on college campuses, the new engineer's first job typically begins in an industrial setting where he or she can learn about a company, apply skills, and gain experience. Clinical engineers, however, may be employed initially in hospitals. After gaining experience within a hospital, these professionals could then work in the medical device industry.

The medical device industry has become one of the strongest sectors of the U.S. economy. Employment in the U.S. health care technology industry grew at an annual rate of 3.4% from 1988 to 1992. During that same period, employment in private industry as a whole grew only 0.4% and employment in general manufacturing decreased 1.9% [1].

The medical device industry is very diverse, encompassing the manufacture of a wide range of products, from small medical disposables to highly sophisticated diagnostic systems. The industry has invested heavily in research and development (R&D). These R&D funds, when combined with those allocated by educational institutions and the federal government, have been substantial. For example, R&D by publicly traded medical device companies grew from 3.9% of sales in 1979 to 6.2% in 1988, nearly double the U.S. industrial average. This investment has paid off handsomely; since 1989 alone, the industry introduced nearly 5000 new products that have improved the quality of life for millions of people around the world [2].

Overall R&D expenditures by the medical device industry compare favorably with those of other industry sectors. Of the 41 industries tracked in *Business Week's* 1989 "R&D scoreboard," medical products and services ranked eighth. The only other industrial sectors that invested more in R&D were high-technology electronics industries [2] (see Table 168.1).

Several medical device manufacturers have taken a new position on the utilization of biomedical and clinical engineers. For example, a 1993 advertisement by Medtronic, Inc., stated that it had several openings for tachyrhythmia field clinical engineers throughout the United States. "Primary responsibilities include product performance studies by presenting protocols, providing technical assistance during product implants, and assisting clinical investigators in product application and troubleshooting. The field clinical engineer will also function as district technical expert to the electrophysiologist community. The position requires a B.S. in Engineering (prefer electrical or biomedical) or B.S. in Sciences (M.S. in biomedical engineering preferred), 3 to 6 years work experience in electrophysiology (assisting in ICD implants, EPS studies, mapping/ablation studies, etc.). In addition, a proven track record in teaching/education and excellent communication skills are required" [3].

This advertisement exemplifies the interest the medical device industry has in clinical engineers.

"Industry" implies research, development, and manufacture of products. Figure 168.1 illustrates the typical work flow for a medical device manufacturer.

168.2 Careers in Research

Today, basic or applied research is one of the more exciting and stimulating functions of engineering. In conducting research, the engineer is free to explore the nature of matter, explore processes to better produce and use engineering materials, and search for new applications of existing technology and applications of new medical devices. In many instances, the work of the scientist and the engineer will overlap. Although the objective of the research scientist is to *discover truths*, while the research engineer explores *applications*, on many occasions they both engage in similar activities [4].

For example, consider a clinical engineer who is working on the development of a system to dissolve kidney stones. During this activity, the clinical engineer will have to become familiar with the composition of kidney stones and investigate substances that will dissolve them. Once the substance has been identified, the clinical engineer must then develop a system to deliver the substance in minute quantities and remove excess fluid. This is *applied research*.

To engage in this activity, research engineers must be perceptive and clever. They must be able to work patiently at tasks never before accomplished and must be able to recognize and identify phenomena previously unnoticed. An inquiring mind and an innate curiosity are desirable, and in the case of the clinical engineer, a thorough training in clinical research techniques is essential. Because much of research is trial and error (laboratory experiments), engineers engaged in this activity understand that results usually occur only after long hours of painstaking and often discouraging work.

TABLE 168.1 Top 10 Research and Development–Intensive Industries, 1989 (percent of sales)

Industry	R&D
Software and services	13.2
System design	10.1
Pharmaceutical	10.1
Computer communications	9.8
Semiconductors	9.3
Computers	9.0
Disk and tape drives	6.4
Medical products and services	*6.2*
Instruments	5.8
Data processing	5.4

Source: U.S. Commerce Report.

Until the last few decades, almost all research was accomplished through the independent work of individuals. However, with the rapid expansion in the fields of chemistry, physics, and biology, it became apparent that groups or *research teams* of scientists, engineers (electrical, biomedical, and clinical), and clinicians could better accomplish their goals by pooling their efforts and knowledge. Within such teams, the group enthusiasm and team competition with other laboratories provide added incentives that serve to push the work forward. Because each person contributes from her or his own specialty, new discoveries are often facilitated.

If one asks the question "Is a career as a research engineer common for a clinical engineer?" the answer can be found in the scientific literature, which clearly shows that practicing clinical engineers are active on many research teams. For example, while working on pulse oximetry sensor technology, the clinical engineer serving on a team developed validation procedures, supervised the field trial testing, implemented product protocols, and assisted with clinical environment testing. This "team approach" saved the company time and money, but more important, product issues, serviceability, and human factors—all important if the device is to be used by clinical staff—were resolved at the beginning of the product conception, not at the end.

168.3 Careers in Development

After a basic discovery is made, the next step involves the development of the idea into a new process or device. In many organizations, the functions of research and development are so interrelated

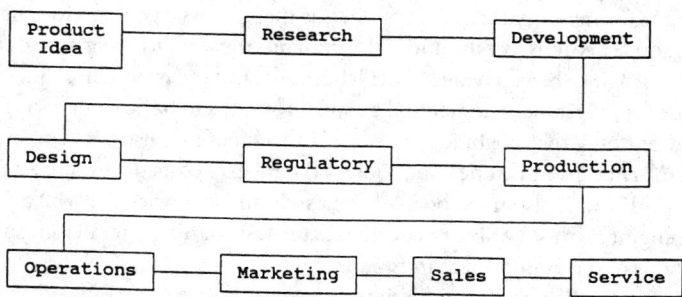

FIGURE 168.1 Typical work flow associated with product development and distribution.

that the individuals and/or department performing this work are simply part of a unified R&D program [4].

The engineering aspects of the development process are concerned with the actual construction, fabrication, assembly, layout, and testing of scale models or prototypes. While the research engineer is concerned more with making a discovery, the development engineer is interested primarily in producing a process, an assembly, or a system that will work.

Development engineers do not always deal with new discoveries from research. A major part of their work involves using well-known principles and processes or machines to perform new or unusual functions. This has major financial benefits for the individual and the company, because much of the activity in the field of development is patentable. For instance, within a very short period of time after the announcement of the discovery of the laser in 1960, a number of patents were issued on surgical devices employing the new laser technology. The lag between the discovery of new knowledge and its application has received considerable attention recently in discussions related to *technology transfer,* i.e., translation of a new idea into a new product improvement [2]. A clinician, for example, might have decided that a new type of device is necessary to determine, at all times, the location of cardiac patients having a telemetry device. First, the development engineer would determine the desired specifications. Clinical engineers, in this case serving as a development engineers, would work with the clinician to define the specifications for the particular hospital environment. The clinical engineer would investigate size, weight, and comfort level of the transmitter, acceptable battery life, and operating specifications for the central station monitor.

The next step would be to determine the availability of any device to meet the medical staff's requirements. To accomplish this task, the clinical engineer would explore the literature for information pertaining to existing designs. Such information may come from library material on processes, principles, and methods of accomplishing the task or related tasks or from literature supplied by specific manufacturers. The literature search might reveal a device that can accomplish the task with little or no modification. If this is not the case, it may be possible to use existing modules or components to accomplish the desired result. If this is not possible, the clinical development engineer might decide to formulate plans to construct a prototype for testing using results from previous research.

Development engineers are able to demonstrate the feasibility of their ideas by working them out on a trial-and-error basis so that the prototype may be modified and tested. When the system or device is in a workable state, the development engineer must then refine it and package it for use by others. The clinical engineer can then incorporate packaging ideas and human factors relevant to the clinical environment. A device that works satisfactorily in a laboratory, when manipulated by skilled technicians, may be hopelessly complex and unsuited for clinical use.

168.4 Careers in Manufacturing Design

After a development engineer has assembled and tested a device or process and it has evolved to be one that is desirable for mass-market production, it is then necessary to develop the final details to facilitate production. This activity falls under the domain of *manufacturing design engineering.*

In their role of bridging the gap between the laboratory and the production line, manufacturing engineers must be very versatile. They should be well grounded in basic engineering principles and must understand not only the capabilities of specific machines but also the temperament of those who operate them. They also must be conscious of the relative costs of producing items. Not only must the device work, but it also must be made in a style and at a price that will attract customers. The production engineer must be able to coordinate the tests of his or her design so that the device functions acceptably and is produced at minimum cost.

Engineers engaged in the production design process soon come to realize that there is usually more than one acceptable way to solve a design problem. Unlike an arithmetic problem with fixed numbers and only one correct answer, any design problem usually has many answers and many ways of obtaining a solution, and all may be acceptable. Regardless of the method used, however, the solution to a problem must take into account fabrication, costs, and sales.

Production design engineers must be creative, because every design usually embodies a departure from what has been done before. At the same time, they must be knowledgeable in fundamental engineering and be familiar with basic principles of economics, both from the standpoint of employing people and using machines. Furthermore, if they take on supervisory and management duties, principles of psychology and economics become important. For this reason, production design engineers usually will have more need for management training than will research or development engineers.

Clinical engineers often contribute greatly to the production design process and to the design engineering team. Consider the design of an ambulatory blood pressure device. Within the device, a computer controls the pump and stores each blood pressure reading every 30 minutes. The production design engineer, working with a clinical engineer, must make decisions about how to compare the new medical device with those techniques presently available to measure blood pressure. Because it is critical that clinical trials be conducted, the production design engineer (working with a clinical engineer) also will determine how many patients are required, the age groups to be used, and other aspects of a testing protocol. At this level, clinical engineers not only assist in defining the protocols, they conduct the clinical trials, collect the data, and statistically determine if the device is effective and efficient.

168.5 Regulatory Activities

The regulatory department is medical device manufacturing company's representative to the Food and Drug Administration (FDA). The role of the department is to ensure that products are designed, tested, manufactured, and distributed in a controlled manner that will deliver a consistently safe and reliable device to the public. Part of this assurance lies in the monitoring, testing, and clinical trials that may be necessary to qualify the equipment for FDA clearance to market the product.

To receive FDA approval, the product must be qualified using *clinical trials*. Clinical engineers (who understand the clinical environment) design the trials, determine the proper controls, and determine how to do the monitoring. This step is important for the company because these procedures can be costly. For example, if the clinical engineer overdesigns the clinical trial, i.e., if too many subjects are required for the study or they are followed for too long, both money and time have been wasted.

Significant problems also can occur if the FDA does not fully understand the nature of the study and gives approval to the clinical trial. Suppose, for example, the clinical engineer commits 100 patients to the study, follows them for 6 months, wraps up the study, collects the data, and submits the results to the FDA, and then the FDA responds with, "What about the long-term effect on these people?" At the onset, it is important to know what effects the FDA is interested in. What constitutes *long term, 6 months, 1 year*, or *5 years?* This needs to be clear at the very beginning of the clinical trial.

168.6 Production Careers

In the field of *production*, the engineer is more directly associated with technicians, inspectors, and assemblers. Engineers engaged in production must take the drawings or models and supervise assembly of the device.

Usually, engineers engaged in production are associated closely with the processes of estimating and controlling jobs. In this work, they employ their knowledge of structural materials, fabricating processes, and general physical principles to estimate both the time and cost to accomplish set tasks.

Usually, the term *project engineer* is given to individuals who have overall responsibility and supervision of the work from the standpoint of materials, labor, and money. The project engineer must employ whatever tools are needed for the work, set up a schedule for production, be able to answer questions that the technicians may raise concerning features of the design, and be prepared to advise design engineers concerning desirable modifications that will aid in the fabrication processes.

Preparation of a schedule for production is an important task of these engineers. In the case of a medical device, all planning for the procurement of raw materials and parts is based on the production schedule.

Qualifications for engineers engaged in production include a thorough knowledge of basic engineering principles and the ability to visualize the parts of an operation, whether it be the fabrication of a solid-state computer circuit or the building of an artificial limb. Based on an understanding of all the operations involved, these individuals must be able to arrive at a realistic schedule of time, materials, and manpower. Therefore, emphasis should be placed on courses in engineering designs, economics, business law, and psychology.

168.7 Careers in Operations

In *operations*, the medical device is actually assembled. In this process, the *manufacturing engineer* (not be confused with the production engineer) and a *quality engineer* are involved. While the manufacturing engineer develops and maintains processes used during the manufacturing cycle, the quality engineer develops and maintains inspection criteria. Both engineers must be able to resolve problems as they occur on the assembly line.

New processes, such as *just-in-time* (JIT) manufacturing techniques, are implemented by the quality and manufacturing engineers. The pragmatic version of JIT focuses on the concrete details of the production process. The manufacturing engineer uses JIT engineering techniques to facilitate changeovers and for cleaner plant layouts, quality-control training, scheduled maintenance, and simpler product designs.

Along with process control, the manufacturing and quality engineers educate the technicians and assemblers. They present new information on process techniques, and the assemblers, in turn, provide feedback on how to improve the processes. Clinical engineers involved in the education program can explain how and why the medical device is used in the clinical environment, and the assemblers explain how the medical device is assembled and tested.

Qualifications for a quality or manufacturing engineer include a thorough knowledge of basic engineering principles. He or she must have the ability to communicate effectively and enjoy working with people. This individual also must be knowledgeable in practical fundamental engineering in a wide range of subjects.

168.8 Careers in Sales

An important (and sometimes unrecognized) function of engineers is *applications* and *sales*. Because so many new medical devices have been developed within the past few years, there is considerable opportunity for engineers to demonstrate the use of new products to prospective customers.

Engineers in sales usually assume the role of a teacher. In many instances, they must present the product from an engineering standpoint. If the audience is composed primarily of engineers, the sales engineer can "talk their language" and answer their technical questions. If the audience includes nonengineers, however, then the features of the product must be presented in terms they can comprehend.

In addition to understanding the engineering features of one's own product, the sales and application engineer also must be familiar with the clinical environment. This is important from two standpoints. First, he or she should be able to show how the product will fit into the specific clinical environment. At the same time, the engineer can point out the limitations of the product. For example, a new cardiac output medical device may be available, but for a customer to use it in the cardiac care unit, a special catheter is deemed necessary. In this case, the customer would get a modification for his or her use and be trained for the proper insertion techniques for the catheter as well.

The sales and application engineer must be familiar with the clinical areas in specific hospitals because this is where equipment needs are generated. By finding an application area in which no apparatus is available to do the work, the sales engineer can report a possible need to the marketing department, suggesting that a development operation should be undertaken to produce a device or process to meet the need.

To accomplish these tasks, engineers engaged in sales and applications must have a basic knowledge of engineering principles and should, of course, have detailed knowledge of their own products. The ability to perform detailed work on abstract principles is less important than the ability to present one's ideas clearly. A genuine appreciation of people and a friendly personality are desirable personal attributes. In addition to basic technical subjects, courses in psychology, sociology, and human relations will prove valuable to the sales and applications engineer.

Usually an engineer will spend several years in a manufacturer's facility learning the details of its operation and management policies before becoming a member of the sales staff. Because sales engineers represent their company to the customer, they must present a pleasing appearance and provide a feeling of confidence in their engineering ability.

168.9 Careers in Marketing

Marketing is a vital part of every company's operations. Consequently, the marketing division is assigned a broad range of duties and responsibilities, including advertising, display, product planning, marketing research, pricing, and training.

Typically, each product line has a *marketing manager* assigned. The marketing manager, like the *sales engineer,* must have a thorough understanding of the clinical environment. In a design review with the engineering department, the marketing manager must be able to "talk engineering language" and answer clinical questions. A marketing manager must present the features of the product in terms the customer can comprehend. The marketing manager also will assist in the development of operator manuals for the equipment. Finally, the marketing manager often will train the sales representatives, who, in turn, train the clinician.

Clinical engineers have become successful marketing managers in the medical device industry. Their years of experience in the clinical environment can assist the manufacturer in understanding the complexity of the clinical environment. For example, consider the clinical engineer who assumes the role of a marketing manager for the services provided by the manufacturer. In this situation, the clinical engineer can determine the needs of the manufacturer's service organization, in light of a hospital's service capabilities. As a result, service programs can be developed that meet the needs of the hospital and create a market for the manufacturer.

The outcome of such a program can be seen at SpaceLabs Medical, with the introduction of the *Biophysical Measurement Series* books. A need was identified regarding clinical training tools for the Biomedical Department. The clinical engineer at the firm recognized the need and developed a plan to publish books dealing with cardiac output, blood pressure, electrocardiography, respiration, EEG/EMG, technology management, and advanced electrocardiography.

168.10 Careers in Service

The typical service organization is structured according to its major functions. The following paragraphs outline these functions and discuss their clinical engineering opportunities.

Field operations, often divided into regions, districts, and branches, is responsible for the actual delivery of service to hospitals. In densely populated areas, a branch office may have 10 to 20 field engineers; in more rural areas, an "office" may consist of a single field engineer working from his or her home. Field engineers are responsible for diagnosing and repairing defective equipment in the clinical environment. They generally command high salaries, commensurate with their knowledge and expertise.

Field service managers organize and supervise the field engineers, handle the administrative affairs of their offices, and manage spare parts inventories. In addition, they are responsible for customer relations.

Technical support is most often supplied on a national basis by the *technical support organization* (TSO). The personnel of the TSO are the most experienced technicians for each of the products the manufacturer services. In many cases, these product experts do not come to the TSO from the field but from engineering. In small companies the TSO may consist of two to five people, while in large companies there may be a staff of 50 or more.

The job of the increasing important *technical support specialist* is to help field service engineers solve the more difficult problems, via phone consultation or, if necessary, by visiting the site to help customers solve operational and technical problems. The technical support specialist is also responsible for technical publications that discuss engineering enhancements to the products and for reports about recurring problems that are sent to the engineering departments.

Technical training provides seminars for the field service engineers and the customers. The instructors at the seminars provide lectures and hands-on troubleshooting so that the student will be able to maintain the medical device. The instructor's experience includes either work in the hospital environment or in the field as a field service engineer.

The major goal of field service is to satisfy the customer. If one compares the field service representative's job description with that of a hospital biomedical equipment technician, similarities would exist. However, career opportunities for a clinical engineer working in a service organization are different from those in a hospital. The clinical engineer working for a service organization has more technical management potential but will be removed from day-to-day contact in the clinical environment.

Several medical device manufacturers have taken a new position on the utilization of clinical engineers. They have created independent clinical engineering departments rather than employ clinical engineers within the departments described above (see Fig. 168.1).

168.11 Management Careers

Results of recent surveys show a trend today for corporate leaders in the United States to have backgrounds in engineering and science [6]. It has been predicted that within 10 years, the majority of corporation executives will be individuals who are trained in engineering and science, as well as in business and humanities, and who can bridge the gap between these disciplines.

In previous years, it was assumed that only persons trained and educated in business administration should aspire to management positions. Now it is recognized that the education and other abilities that make a good engineer also provide the background to make a good management executive. The training for correlating facts and evaluating courses of action in making engineering decisions can be carried over to management decisions on equipment, computers, people, and money. In general, the engineer is technically strong but may be quite naive in the realm of business practicability. Therefore, it is in business operations that the engineer usually must work to develop his or her skills.

The engineer in management is more closely concerned with the long-range effects of policy decisions. Where the design engineer considers first the technical phases of a project, the engineer in management must consider how a particular decision will affect those who produce the product and how the decision will affect the people who provide the financing for the operation. It is for this reason that the management engineer is concerned less with the technical aspects of the profession and relatively more with the financial, legal, and labor aspects.

This does not mean that engineering aspects should be minimized or deleted. The growing need for engineers in management shows that the type and complexity of the machines and processes used in today's plants require a blending of technical and business training in order to carry forward effectively. This trend is particularly noted in the medical device industry, where many executive managerial positions are occupied by engineers and scientists.

The education of an engineer in management should be identical to the basic education received in other engineering fields. Management engineering requires applying engineering principles in supervisory work involving large numbers of people and large amounts of money. The individual might start out as a research engineer, a design engineer, a clinical engineer, or a sales engineer, but the ability to influence others to his or her way of thinking and a genuine liking for people and a consideration for their responses will indicate capabilities as a manager.

168.12 Careers in the Veterans Administration

The Veterans Administration (VA) is the largest employer of clinical engineers in a hospital setting. There are 172 VA hospitals throughout the continental United States. The majority of these hospitals require a clinical engineer for the biomedical department manager position. The national VA biomedical engineering program, located in Washington, D.C., provides support, leadership, policy, and staff training to all the VA hospitals.

The VA has $1.7 billion worth of medical equipment. Eighty percent of that equipment is maintained in-house, with backup assistance from either third parties or the equipment manufacturer. The VA spends almost $100 million a year on medical equipment maintenance [7].

There is an engineering training center in Little Rock, Arkansas, that provides an array of continuing education programs for biomedical technicians and engineers located throughout the United States. The center trains up to 200 technicians a year and offers one continuing course for clinical engineers on a current topic, such as nuclear medicine, radiology, maintenance management, or diagnostic ultrasound [8].

The Engineering Service Center in St. Louis, Missouri, provides service manuals, resolves difficulties with manufacturers, and provides consultation on unusual and specific device problems. The center is equipped to meet the needs of the VA hospital biomedical staff with equipment problems and service questions.

168.13 Careers in the FDA

The Food and Drug Administration's (FDA) *Bureaus of Radiological Health and Medical Devices* were consolidated in 1982. The FDA is the federal government's watchdog department that inspects, approves, recalls, and regulates the use of health care technology. The FDA is responsible for enforcing the *good manufacturing practices* (GMP) and the guidelines that govern the approval process for devices to be marketed.

A clinical engineer at the FDA has the opportunity to make a contribution to public health and safety by dealing with new and advanced technology and by applying his or her talents to making sure those products are safe and effective.

168.14 Other Careers in Government

Clinical engineers are hired by a number of government agencies and departments, including the National Institutes of Health (NIH) and the military. All government employers require the applicant to fill out a standard form 171 (the "government resumé"). Individuals interested in military employment should contact the military branch recruitment office directly. Each institute of the NIH has its own personnel office. To get more information about standard form 171 and employment with NIH, call their recruitment branch at (301) 496-2404.

168.15 Hospital Clinical Engineering Careers

Engineers were first encouraged to enter the hospital environment during the late 1960s because of a very justifiable concern about the safety and performance of hospital instrumentation. Electrical safety hazards existed, though sometimes were exaggerated, thus obscuring the true need for clinical engineering. At the onset, the duties of the clinical engineer were to monitor hospital equipment, to supervise its repair, and to supervise and control its purchase.

Today, the American College of Clinical Engineering (ACCE) defines a *clinical engineer* as one who "enhances patient care by applying engineering skills in health care technology. Clinical engineers frequently manage resources including people, space, and budgets in the cost-effective application of technology. A clinical engineer has at least a bachelor's degree in engineering or a related discipline or has proven through professional practice to have the knowledge and skills of an engineer" [7].

Clinical engineering is a relatively new profession, with a formal curriculum developed in colleges and universities during the 1980s and a professional organization started in 1990. The majority of practicing clinical engineers have a bachelor's degree in biomedical engineering.

Management training is usually obtained "on the job." Clinical engineers often attend short courses and seminars covering a variety of management topics. Management courses are offered at a variety of educational institutions or through professional societies. Optimally, management training is included at the graduated school level.

After a clinical engineer has received his or her undergraduate formal education, job opportunities are available in a variety of work environments. In the hospital environment, many clinical engineers are involved in the engineering aspect of equipment management programs. These programs include the preparation of specifications and requests for proposals, evaluation, selection, installation, operator training, applications assistance, interfacing devices, corrective and scheduled maintenance, and developing enhancements.

"Clinical engineers are further involved with incident investigations and management of equipment hazard recalls and service support for medical systems, instrumentation, and devices. In these activities, considerable attention is given to the cost-effective management of technologies and smart buildings used in health care delivery. The clinical engineer may manage physicists, safety engineers, nurses, biomedical equipment technicians, and others who provide engineering services. Equipment building systems managed by clinical engineers include patient monitoring systems, clinical laboratory equipment, systems used with respiratory therapy, anesthesiology, ultrasonic, and nuclear imaging, radiographic imaging, therapeutic radiation, clinical and administrative computer systems, communications and paging systems, lasers and other diagnostic and therapeutic equipment" [8].

168.16 Other Opportunities

Entrepreneur

When Arnold Beckman attempted to solve the problem of testing the ripeness of citrus fruit by measuring its pH, the only method available was titration. His breakthrough—a direct measurement of the electric potential arising at a special electrode immersed in the juice—has had far-reaching effects. Beckman and others have taken that one design for a pH electrode and expanded it into an entire industry for chemical instrumentation [9].

This kind of entrepreneurial startup is the most creative domain in U.S. enterprise. The individual who builds a company from scratch acquires an understanding of his or her company work that an imported chief executive cannot immediately command. The entrepreneur gains a dynamic and integrated view of his or her company and a realistic view of enterprise in general.

If the entrepreneur started in competition against established firms, he or she bears a natural skepticism toward previously existing expertise. Decisions have to be made before all the information is in, so the individual recognizes that enterprise always consists of action in uncertain circumstances. A new enterprise is an aggressive action, not a reaction. When it is launched successfully, the rest of society—government, labor, other businesses—will have to react. In a sense, entrepreneurship is the creation of surprises.

The entrepreneur must be able to accept failure, learn from it, and act boldly. "He [or she] inhibits a realm where the last become the first, where supply creates demand, where belief precedes knowledge. It is a world where expertise may be a form of ignorance and the best possibilities spring from a consensus of impossibility. It is a world where service of others, solving their problems and taking on new ones, is the prime source of leadership and wealth. It is a world where bankruptcies can serve as an index of growth, large setbacks as a portent of large gains, and stability as a precursor of failure, where other people's garbage is your wealth and sand is often a richer resource than gold. It is a world where unit losses can indeed be made up by volume, where low profit margins lead to the largest profits, and where giving is the rule of highest returns" [9].

Independent Service Organizations

As independent service organizations, a number of hospital clinical engineering programs have begun providing technical services for groups of smaller or rural hospitals. Here, the engineer has the opportunity to become an entrepreneur. Other clinical engineers have started their own independent service organizations.

Consultant

Few individuals consider the profession of *consulting engineering*. Consulting engineers are unique in that they are required to be, in the jargon of the sports world, "triple threats." They must be technically qualified in clinical engineering, they must maintain the high standards of conduct expected of professionals, and they must be capable of managing a business enterprise so that it returns a profit.

Technical competence is critical to consulting engineers. A sound reputation for quality project management is essential. It enables the company to keep the customers it has and to obtain new ones, thus ensuring a reasonably steady backlog of work.

Professionalism is important to consulting engineers because of their relationship with their customers and with the public at large. Consulting engineers have a duty to their clients to fill their needs and to represent them without conflict of interest. As professionals serving the public, they must be registered as professional engineers by the states in which they practice, and they bear a responsibility to protect the health, safety, and welfare of the general public.

Consulting engineers must be effective business managers. Because their services are furnished to clients for a fee, they need to be able to manage money and run their business soundly. Clinical engineers will not remain in private practice very long if they are unable to market their services, to contract for those services in prudent terms, to manage the production of the work contracted for, to charge and collect adequate fees, and to manage the assets that accrue from the business.

As a member of a *consulting organization,* the newly graduated clinical engineer will be provided with work assignments and the possibility of working in the clinical environment. Most education, which must continue for a lifetime, will be provided by on-the-job experience. Such continuing education is needed for study and research to solve the problems inherent in each work assignment. As the clinical engineer gains experience, his or her expertise can be sharpened, leading to recognition as an authority with opportunities for advancement into management.

Job opportunities for the clinical engineer include preaccreditation surveys, incident investigation, technology management, medical device design, bid package definition and evaluation, service contract evaluation, and expert witness.

168.17 Conclusions

This chapter has described the specific training needed in the different career opportunities in clinical engineering. All require a fundamental scientific knowledge of physical principles and mathematics. However, research and management each require different educational preparation.

For work in research, emphasis in on theoretical principles and creativity, with little emphasis on economic and personal considerations. On the other hand, in management, primary attention is given to financial and labor problems and relatively little to abstract scientific principles. Between these two extremes are careers having varying degrees of emphasis on the research-oriented or management-oriented concepts.

In all cases, the clinical engineer is a *problem solver*. Whether it be a mathematical abstraction that may have an application to a blood pressure reading or a meeting with JCAHO at a conference table, the clinical engineer confronts problems that must be reduced to their essentials and the alternatives explored to reach a problem solution. The clinical engineer then must apply knowledge and inventiveness to select a reasonable method to achieve a result, even in the face of vague and sometimes contradictory data. The engineer's ability to accomplish this is generally developed and proven by a long record of successful engineering management and productivity.

References

1. AAMI News. 1994. Health Care Technology Leads U.S. in 1988–92 Job Growth, Arlington, Virginia.
2. U.S. Department of Commerce. 1991. Growth Prospects of the U.S. Medical Device Industry in a Changing Healthcare Environment. Washington, Office of Science and Electronics.
3. Pacela AF. 1991. 1991 survey of hospital salaries and job responsibilities for clinical engineers & biomedical technicians. J Clin Eng 16(3):241.
4. Beakley GC. 1986. Engineering—A Creative Career. New York, Macmillan.
5. Goodman GR. 1991. Technology assessment, transfer and management: The implications to the professional development of clinical engineering. J Clin Eng 16(2):117.
6. Knight K. 1990. Interview: Arnold Bierenbaum. Second Source 5(5):44.
7. ACCE. 1991. Board meeting minutes, American College of Clinical Engineering, 24 February, Houston, Texas.
8. Bronzino JD. 1992. Clinical Engineering Fundamentals, p 28. St Louis, Mosby.
9. Gilder G. 1984. The Spirit of Enterprise. New York, Simon and Schuster.

169

Clinical Engineers as Innovators and Product Developers

P. Åke Öberg
Linköping University

Engineers who are active in the health care sector have great opportunities to contribute to long-term quality development, thereby developing new techniques or improving existing ones. By working daily with commercially available instruments and methods, the clinical engineer can build up a considerable knowledge bank regarding how to improve existing techniques or how to resolve completely new method problems. He or she often has a perspective on developmental requirements that is extremely valuable in order to function as an innovator. The proximity to health care gives ample opportunities for trying-out a new product in the end-user environment. Medical expertise is often extremely interested in collaborating in method development work.

Traditionally, most clinical engineering departments have not devoted very much time to product development. The reason is probably that the more routine activities in a department do not permit time-demanding development projects. The available personnel must be used to resolve the immediate daily tasks. Inventions and technical development work have a low priority. Even if extremely good competence exists in the clinical engineering departments, it is usually the case that this sector of the collective competence seldom is utilized.

The need for improved or new products for health care is the major driving force for innovations and industrial production of medical devices. New medical products are born in the light of new clinical requirements and new technical possibilities. To be able to identify the new needs and possibilities, a high degree of competence, in both the engineering and medical fields, is required.

To develop new products takes time. A 5- to 10-year period from the idea state to commercialization is not unrealistic. The interpretation of future trends and markets is very important in successful product development. Where will health care be 10 years from now? Which new techniques will emerge in the meantime? The needs we see today will not necessarily be the same 10 years ahead. To correctly assess future trends and needs is of the utmost importance in the development of new products that will be successful on the commercial market. The world market for medical and health care products is approximately $150 billion today, of which pharmaceuticals is $100 billion and the rest, $50 billion, is instrumentation and medical devices [OECD, 1992].

Today, health care and the biomedical industry use highly sophisticated technology in their products. It is reasonable to assume that technological progress will find early and advanced applications in the health care field.

It is therefore of interest to discuss which personal qualities and knowledge are important if you, as a clinical engineer, wish to devote yourself to innovation activities and product development.

169.1 From Inventor to Innovator

An *innovation* is defined as a new device (or invention) that has been marketed successfully and has reached a stage of commercial success [Fölster, 1991]. Usually we make a distinction between an inventor and an innovator. The role of an innovator is much more demanding than that of an inventor. An inventor is strongly focused on the technology and the technical development of his or her invention, the product. He or she seldom finds the commercialization of his or her invention very exciting and avoids creating the contacts necessary for further business development of the product.

An inventor must educate himself or herself to become a successful innovator and entrepreneur. The following fields are particularly important:

- *Marketing*—to be able to do simpler market assessments and to understand the essentials of marketing new products.
- *Economy*—to be able to do simpler types of project budget plans.
- *Law*—especially various forms of contracts and business negotiations.
- *Patents*—to be able to write patent applications and to understand the type of protection a patent gives.

169.2 The Innovator as a Person

Concepts such as innovations, innovator, inventor, product ideas, and creativity are commonly used when the importance of product development is discussed. Some of these concepts are regarded in daily language as synonyms, but sometimes we need a short and practically oriented discussion of these concepts.

Creativity has many hundreds of definitions in the literature. In most cases they can be summarized as "the ability to generate something new and/or useful." For others, the word *useful* can be exchanged for *interesting, attracting,* or even *selling.* In the case of technical innovations, the degree of *utility* is defined as something that can be sold on a market or can be exploited financially. Within the OECD, the concept of *innovation* has been taken to mean a technical idea that has been realized in the form of a product that has been successful on a market.

Creativity is the willingness and ability to produce something new, which is closely related to curiousness, an inherent human attribute. In addition, the inclination and the necessity to invent, to explore, are deeply satisfying and rewarding activities for the inventor, also to see solutions to problems, to create, and to develop new ideas. One reward is to see the ideas realized, a satisfaction related to that of an artist over a finished painting or sculpture. Creativity is also a necessity, a compulsion. The inventor is often obsessed by thoughts around a problem. It seems impossible not to come back to the problem repeatedly.

Creative persons may have many unique qualities that are easily identified:

- Flexibility
- Sensitivity to problems
- Originality

- Motivation to create
- Endurance
- Concentration on the task

A visionary mind is crucial, i.e., a talent to see ahead and to foresee scenarios in the future. But a visionary mind is not enough. The ability to get things done and the expertise to control project development are important talents. The innovator must always educate himself or herself in a variety of fields that all are important in the process of developing an idea into a product on a market. These fields include marketing, economics, visualization, law, and patents.

169.3 The Life Cycle of a Product

Every product has a life cycle. It is born, it matures, it reaches a maximal sales figure, and finally, it disappears from the market. The life-cycle curve of a product is a well-known concept within marketing, product development, and market research. The life cycle curve shows the sold quantity of a product as a function of time from its introduction on the market to the time when the product no longer is marketed.

The life-cycle curve is usually divided into the phases shown in Fig. 169.1 [Ohlsson, 1992]:

- *Introduction*—when the product is first introduced on a market and the first sales take place.
- *Sales growth*—when the product has been on the market for some time and the awareness of its existence spreads and increasing numbers of the product are sold.
- *Maturity*—where the consumers interested in the product already have bought and sales no longer increase.
- *Decline*—where the demand for the product decreases.

The duration of the life cycle can vary between a few months and many decades. The life-cycle curve is a useful instrument by which the future market potential for a product can be analyzed. If the sales of a particular product are studied, one can usually say in which of the phases the demand will be at that moment. Usually the introduction and development phases are more interesting than the saturation and decline phases. The future total consumption also can be calculated by means of the life-cycle curve. Today's data can be used to understand the future market potential.

169.4 Patenting and Publishing

Good patent protection is often very important for anyone who wishes to industrially exploit an invention, to dare to invest in it, or to manufacture it. The patent is a guarantee that no one else,

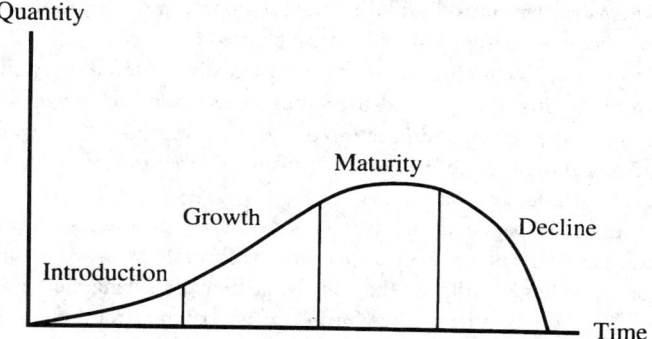

FIGURE 169.1   The life-cycle curve of a product.

without risking some form of legal punishment, can exploit the original idea for commercial profit.

In order to get a patent for an invention, it must be "new." If you make public the idea by means of the written word or a lecture, seminar, etc., then a new-product obstacle arises; i.e., the patenting possibilities are voided.

At university hospitals and other research-oriented hospitals, there are often visible differences in outlook between the academic researchers who will publish, or give lectures on, their new results and the innovators who will patent new ideas as a basis for industrial development.

Often both groups can be satisfied by first patenting and then publishing somewhat later. By this procedure, the publishing is marginally delayed, while at the same time the great commercial value of such a patent can be utilized.

169.5 Strategic Assessments for Effective Product Development

A preliminary assessment of a new product idea must always include the following considerations:

- Market analysis
- Technology assessment
- Other analyses

The results from these preliminary assessments are important cornerstones in the management of product development projects leading to a commercial success.

Market Analysis

Early market assessments will answer the two very important questions [Committee of Science and Technology, 1980]:

- Is there a need (a "market") for the product under study?
- Is the market large enough to make an investment in a development project profitable?

Irrespective of if we are developing simpler or more complicated technology, we should aim at getting a good overview of the market. An early and preliminary view of a potential market helps the innovator to plan for the long-range development of his or her invention.

Technology Assessment

Technology assessment includes analysis of problems related to product technology as well as production technology. Product technology assessment is particularly important for medical products in the clinical environment. Safety considerations are, of course, key questions. The technical design of a medical instrument must fulfill the actual standards and the national and international regulations. Already accepted design principles must be used.

An important part of the technology assessment is to involve external persons not familiar with the project for handling tests or to get end-user input. Very often such an involvement results in major improvements in the design and function of a device. Technology assessments of a shorter series of devices (5 to 10) used in the "real world" (hospitals, laboratories) will often affect the final design of the product in a decisive way.

Involvement of "external" persons in the product assessment must necessarily include some type of secrecy protection in terms of a secrecy declaration or contract in which the involved person(s) are prohibited from revealing or utilizing the knowledge they get during their evaluation work.

The assessment of production technology problems is very important before mass production starts. The choice of proper production technologies can strongly affect the market price of a product. If new production equipment must be set up, then large investments may be necessary, which will affect the economy of the whole project. Thus, by a production technology–oriented design, large savings can be made when longer series of the device are produced. This advice is particularly true for an inventor in a university or hospital environment who usually does not have extensive experience in industrial production techniques. The initiation of close and early collaboration between the inventor and the final (industrial) producer of the device is strongly recommended. Such collaboration often shortens the route to the market considerably and reduces production costs.

Economic Assessment

An innovation must, according to its definition, involve an economic success on a market. Thus it is essential that the project costs are followed up regularly and that, as early as possible, a conception of project feasibility is developed.

At an early stage this can only involve rough calculations. Such calculations should be based on the costs for product sales as well as an estimate of how large the product's market share must be for the product to be a financial success.

Concept Testing

Before technically and commercially starting to exploit a new idea, it should be investigated to ascertain if it really is completely new. Very often the same or similar ideas have been ventilated previously, and then they are often found in patent documentation. The motives for concept testing can be several:

- Is my idea a new one?
- Will I infringe on another patent on commercial exploitation?
- Can I get my idea patented?
- What has been done in this area lately?
- Where does the knowledge-bound main focus lie (company, land, orientation)?

Concept testing can be carried out partly by screening patents in areas in the proximity of the current invention. A good conception of the "state of the art" also can be gained by searching databases of different types. Libraries have large databases where correctly formulated questions in the form of search profiles can give adequate guidance on innovations in the current area of work. Published scientific literature can give interesting information on the news value of an invention but also, for example, on the diagnostic value of the investigation one can carry out with the invented method and thereby indirectly the market size, etc.

Prototype Development

Prototype design is an important part of the innovation process. To be able to test the strength of an idea from a technical and an economic point of view, to evaluate the response of a market, and to be able to calculate the production cost mean that prototype development is an important step toward mass production.

It is usually a long way from the prototype stage to mass production. Very often it is practical to proceed in several steps:

- Sketches—show the idea from a functional and technical point of view in terms of drawings or technical diagrams.
- Models—a three-dimensional presentation of the product idea in wood, metal, or plaster without any functional demands. This form is especially good for marketing purposes.
- Functional model—a three-dimensional model like the one mentioned above but, in addition, one that can demonstrate how the idea is expected to work.

- Prototype—the prototype is an exact model of the product as it will function and appear in mass production.
- 0-series—a smaller series of the product often used for demonstration or evaluations by tentative customers and experts.
- Mass-produced products—products from a production line.

169.6 Forms of Exploitation

Commercial exploitation of an invention can take place in many different ways. The two most usual are

- Licensing
- Starting new companies

Licensing entails selling the rights of the invention to an entrepreneur who is responsible for continued development and commercial introduction. Generally, the inventor has, when choosing the form of licensing, strong patent protection as a basis for negotiations with the entrepreneur. Without strong patent protection, the licensing negotiations are difficult, since it generally is the patent which, at this time, is the only tangible feature in the negotiation. In some cases it can be advantageous to *start a new company* that conducts the development work and is responsible for market launching. If the invention to be exploited concerns completely new areas where few or no established companies are active, then the startup of a new company for commercialization can be a quick route to the market. After successful product development and market launching, the company can be sold off. On starting a new company, the question of patent is generally of lesser

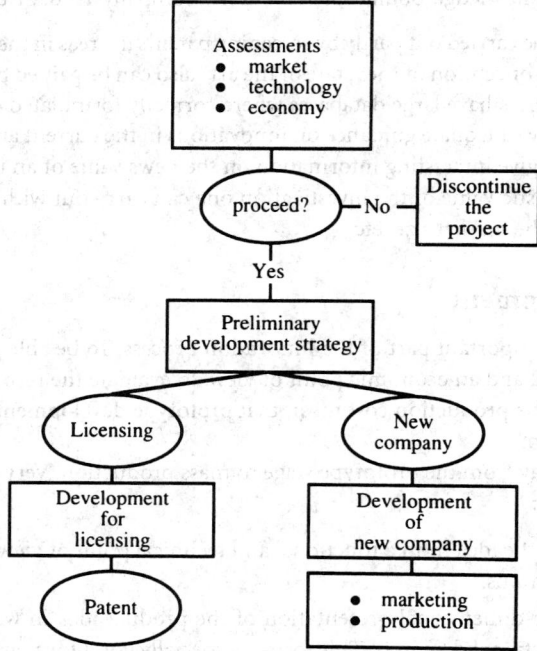

FIGURE 169.2   Strategy on choosing the form of exploitation for an invention.

TABLE 169.1 Comparison of Activities on Exploiting an Invention

	Demand	
Activity	New Company	Licensing
Patenting	Less	More
Prototype design	Same	Same
Marketing	More	Less
Manufacturing	More	Less
Financing	Same	Same
Organization	More	Less
Time span	Better	Worse
Risks	Same	Same

importance, while matters concerning marketing and manufacturing are of greater importance. When the invention has been assessed from a market, technical, and economic viewpoint, it is time to decide on the form for full-scale exploitation.

Often it is the inventor's own disposition that decides which form of exploitation is chosen. If you are more interested in the continuous development of a new technique, then you would choose licensing, i.e., transfer of the marketing and financial problems to someone else. If, however, you find it stimulating to work with the entire production process from technical development work through to sales, then you would choose to start a company. For a clinical engineer employed by a hospital, the hospital's policy also influences the choice of form of exploitation (see Fig. 169.2).

The differences between the two forms of exploitation can be described by Table 169.1.

References

Committee of Science and Technology. 1980. Small, High-Technology Firms and Innovation. Washington. US Government Printing Office.

Fölster S. 1991. The Art of Encouraging Invention. Stockholm, IUI.

OECD. 1992. Innovation Policy: Trends and Perspectives. Paris, OECD.

Ohlsson L. 1992. R&D for Swedish Industrial Renewal (DS 1992:109). Stockholm, Utbildningsdepartementet.

Further Information

The book *Inventors at Work,* by K.A. Brown, contains interviews with 16 notable American inventors (Tempus Books, 1988) and gives interesting perspectives on the invention process. The journals *Medical and Biological Engineering and Computing, Physiological Measurements, Medical Engineering and Physics,* and a few more currently publish papers on new instrument ideas. Usually national authorities give advice and recommendations on how to start new companies.

170

Clinical Engineering Program Indicators

Dennis D. Autio
Oregon Health Sciences University

Robert L. Morris
Oregon Health Sciences University

The role, organization, and structure of clinical engineering departments in the modern health care environment continue to evolve. During the past 10 years, the rate of change has increased considerably faster than mere evolution due to fundamental changes in the management and organization of health care. Rapid, significant changes in the health care sector are occurring in the United States and in nearly every country. The underlying drive is primarily economic, the recognition that resources are finite.

Indicators are essential for survival of organizations and are absolutely necessary for effective management of change. Clinical engineering departments are not exceptions to this rule. In the past, most clinical engineering departments were task-driven and their existence justified by the tasks performed. Perhaps the most significant change occurring in clinical engineering practice today is the philosophical shift to a more business-oriented, cost-justified, bottom-line-focused approach than has been generally the case in the past.

Changes in the health care delivery system will dictate that clinical engineering departments justify their performance and existence on the same basis as any business, the performance of specific functions at a high quality level and at a competitive cost. Clinical engineering management philosophy must change from a purely task-driven methodology to one that includes the economics of department performance. Indicators need to be developed to measure this performance. Indicator data will need to be collected and analyzed. The data and indicators must be objective and defensible. If it cannot be measured, it cannot be managed effectively.

Indicators are used to measure performance and function in three major areas. Indicators should be used as internal measurements and monitors of the performance provided by individuals, teams, and the department. These essentially measure what was done and how it was done. Indicators are essential during quality improvement and are used to monitor and improve a process. A third important type of program indicator is the benchmark. It is common knowledge that successful businesses will continue to use benchmarks, even though differing terminology will be used. A business cannot improve its competitive position unless it knows where it stands compared with similar organizations and businesses.

Different indicators may be necessary depending on the end purpose. Some indicators may be able to measure internal operations, quality improvement, and external benchmarks. Others will have a more restricted application.

It is important to realize that a single indicator is insufficient to provide the information on which to base significant decisions. Multiple indicators are necessary to provide cross-checks and verification. An example might be to look at the profit margin of a business. Even if the profit margin per sale is 100%, the business will not be successful if there are few sales. Looking at single indicators of gross or net profit will correct this deficiency but will not provide sufficient information to point the way to improvements in operations.

170.1 Department Philosophy

A successful clinical engineering department must define its mission, vision, and goals as related to the facility's mission. A mission statement should identify what the clinical engineering department does for the organization. A vision statement identifies the direction and future of the department and must incorporate the vision statement of the parent organization. Department goals are then identified and developed to meet the mission and vision statements for the department and organization. The goals must be specific and attainable. The identification of goals will be incomplete without at least implied indicators. Integrating the mission statement, vision statement, and goals together provides the clinical engineering department management with the direction and constraints necessary for effective planning.

Clinical engineering managers must carefully integrate mission, vision, and goal information to develop a strategic plan for the department. Since available means are always limited, the manager must carefully assess the needs of the organization and available resources, set appropriate priorities, and determine available options. The scope of specific clinical engineering services to be provided can include maintenance, equipment management, and technology management activities. Once the scope of services is defined, strategies can be developed for implementation. Appropriate program indicators must then be developed to document, monitor, and manage the services to be provided. Once effective indicators are implemented, they can be used to monitor internal operations and quality-improvement processes and complete comparisons with external organizations.

Monitoring Internal Operations

Indicators may be used to provide an objective, accurate measurement of the different services provided in the department. These can measure specific individual, team, and department performance parameters. Typical indicators might include simple tallies of the quantity or level of effort for each activity, productivity (quantity/effort), percentage of time spent performing each activity, percentage of scheduled IPMs (inspection and preventive maintenance procedures) completed within the scheduled period, mean time per job by activity, repair jobs not completed within 30 days, parts order for greater than 60 days, etc.

Process for Quality Improvement

When program indicators are used in a quality-improvement process, an additional step is required. Expectations must be quantified in terms of the indicators used. Quantified expectations result in the establishment of a threshold value for the indicator that will precipitate further analysis of the process. Indicators combined with expectations (threshold values of the indicators) identify the opportunities for program improvement. Periodic monitoring to determine if a program indicator is below (or above, depending on whether you are measuring successes or failures) the established threshold will provide a flag to detect whether the process or performance is within acceptable limits. If it is outside acceptable limits for the indicator, a problem has been identified. Further analysis may be required to better define the problem. Possible program indicators for quality improvement might include the number of repairs completed within 24 or 48 hours, the number of callbacks for repairs, the number of repair problems caused by user error, the percentage of hazard notifications reviewed and acted on within a given time frame, meeting time targets for generating specification, evaluation or acceptance of new equipment, etc.

An example might be a weekly status update of the percentage of scheduled IPMs completed. Assume that the department has implemented a process in which a group of scheduled IPMs must be completed within 8 weeks. The expectation is that 12% of the scheduled IPMs will be completed each week. The indicator is the percentage of IPMs completed. The threshold value of the indicator is 12% per week increase in the percentage of IPMs completed. To monitor this, the number of IPMs that were completed must be tallied, divided by the total number scheduled, and multiplied by 100 to determine the percentage completed. If the number of completed IPMs is less than projected, then further analysis would be required to identify the source of the problem and determine solutions to correct it. If the percentage of completed IPMs were equal to or greater than the threshold or target, then no action would be required.

External Comparisons

Much important and useful information can be obtained by carefully comparing one clinical engineering program with others. This type of comparison is highly valued by most hospital administrators. It can be helpful in determining performance relative to competitors. External indicators or benchmarks can identify specific areas of activity in need of improvement. They offer insights when consideration is being given to expanding into new areas of support. Great care must be taken when comparing services provided by clinical engineering departments located in different facilities. There are a number of factors that must be included in making such comparisons; otherwise, the results can be misleading or misinterpreted. It is important that the definition of the specific indicators used be well understood, and great care must be taken to ensure that the comparison utilizes comparable information before interpreting the comparisons. Failure to understand the details and nature of the comparison and just using the numbers directly will likely result in inappropriate actions by managers and administrators. The process of analysis and explanation of differences in benchmark values between a clinical engineering department and a competitor (often referred to as *gap analysis*) can lead to increased insight into department operations and target areas for improvements

Possible external indicators could be the labor cost per hour, the labor cost per repair, the total cost per repair, the cost per bed supported, the number of devices per bed supported, percentage of time devoted to repairs versus IPMs versus consultation, cost of support as a percentage of the acquisition value of capital inventory, etc.

70.2 Standard Database

> In God we trust . . . all others bring data!
> Florida Power and Light

Evaluation of indicators requires the collection, storage, and analysis of data from which the indicators can be derived. A standard set of data elements must be defined. Fortunately, one only has to look at commercially available equipment management systems to determine the most common data elements used. Indeed, most of the high-end software systems have more data elements than many clinical engineering departments are willing to collect. These standard data elements must be carefully defined and understood. This is especially important if the data will later be used for comparisons with other organizations. Different departments often have different definitions for the same data element. It is crucial that the data collected be accurate and complete. The members of the clinical engineering department must be trained to properly gather, document, and enter the data into the database. It makes no conceptual difference if the database is maintained on paper or using computers. Computers and their databases are ubiquitous and so much easier to use that usually more data elements are collected when computerized systems are used. The effort required for analysis is less and the level of sophistication of the analytical tools that can be used is higher with computerized systems.

The clinical engineering department must consistently gather and enter data into the database. The database becomes the practical definition of the services and work performed by the department. This standardized database allows rapid, retrospective analysis of the data to determine specific indicators identifying problems and assist in developing solutions for implementation. A minimum database should allow the gathering and storage of the following data:

Service Provided. It is important that departments catalog within the database the types of services provided to customers. The services provided should be broken down into the specific types of services provided, and these should be further subdivided into nature of complaint, action taken, and probable cause. Types of services provided typically fall into three broad categories: equipment maintenance tasks, including repairs, hazard notification reports, inspection and periodic maintenance (IPM), instrument or device modification and fabrication, operator error, modification, design, and fabrications; equipment management tasks, including installation, incoming inspections, acceptance testing, development of IPM procedures, hazard notification, incident investigation, risk management, service contract review and management, operator training, equipment inventory and maintenance, and management of the database to maintain equipment histories and provide review and analysis of the data; and technology management tasks, including consultation, technology assessment, prepurchase equipment evaluations, and specification development.

In-House Labor. This consists of three elements: the number of hours spent providing a particular service, the associated labor rate, and the identity of the individual providing the service. The labor cost is not the hourly rate the technician is paid multiplied by the number of hours spent performing the service. It should include the associated indirect costs, such as benefits, space, utilities, test equipment, and tools, along with training, administrative overhead, and many other hidden costs. A simple, straightforward approach to determine an hourly labor rate for a department is to take the total budget of the department and subtract parts' costs, service contract costs, and amounts paid to outside vendors. Divide the resulting amount by the total hours spent providing services as determined from the database. This will provide an average hourly rate for the department.

Vendor Labor. This should include hours spent and rate, travel, and zone charges and any perdiem costs associated with the vendor supplied service.

Parts. Complete information on parts used is important for any retrospective study of services provided. This information is similar for both in-house and vendor-provided service. It should include the part number, a description of the part, and its cost, including any shipping.

Timeliness. It is important to include a number of time stamps in the data. These should include the date the request for service was received, data assigned, and date completed.

Problem Identification. Both a code for rapid computer searching and classification and a free text comment identifying the nature of the problem and description of service provided are important. The number of codes should be kept to as few as possible. Detailed classification schemes usually end up with significant inaccuracies due to differing interpretations of the fine gradations in classifications.

Equipment Identification.   Developing an accurate equipment history depends on reliable means of identifying the equipment. This usually includes a department- and/or facility-assigned unique identification number as well as the manufacturer, vendor, model, and serial number. Identification numbers provided by asset management are often inadequate to allow tracking of interchangeable modules or important items with a value less than a given amount. Acquisition cost is a useful data element.

Service Requester.   The database should include elements allowing identification of the department, person, telephone number, cost center, and location of the service requester.

170.3 Measurement Indicators

Clinical engineering departments must gather objective, quantifiable data in order to assess ongoing performance, identify new quality-improvement opportunities, and monitor the effect of improvement action plans. Since resources are limited and everything cannot be measured, certain selection criteria must be implemented to identify the most significant opportunities for indicators. High-volume, high-risk, or problem-prone processes require frequent monitoring of indicators. A new indicator may be developed after analysis of ongoing measurements or feedback from other processes. Customer feedback and surveys often can provide information leading to the development of new indicators. Department management, in consultation with the quality-management department, typically determines what indicators will be monitored on an ongoing basis. The indicators and resulting analysis are fed back to individuals and work teams for review and improvement of their daily work activities. Teams may develop new indicators during their analysis and implementation of solutions to quality-improvement opportunities.

An *indicator* is an objective, quantitative measurement of an outcome or process that relates to performance quality. The event being assessed can be either desirable or undesirable. It is objective in that the same measurement can be obtained by different observers. This indicator represents quantitative, measured data that are gathered for further analysis. Indicators can assess many different aspects of quality, including accessibility, appropriateness, continuity, customer satisfaction, effectiveness, efficacy, efficiency, safety, and timeliness.

A program indicator has attributes that determine its utility as a performance measure. The reliability and variability of the indicator are distinct but related characteristics. An indicator is reliable if the same measurement can be obtained by different observers. A valid indicator is one that can identify opportunities for quality improvement. As indicators evolve, their reliability and validity should improve to the highest level possible.

An indicator can specify a part of a process to be measured or the outcome of that process. An outcome indicator assesses the results of a process. Examples include the percentage of uncompleted, scheduled IPMs, or the number of uncompleted equipment repairs not completed within 30 days. A process indicator assesses an important and discrete activity that is carried out during the process. An example would be the number of anesthesia machines in which the scheduled IPM failed or the number of equipment repairs awaiting parts that are uncompleted within 30 days.

Indicators also can be classified as sentinel event indicators and aggregate data indicators. A performance measurement of an individual event that triggers further analysis is called a *sentinel-event indicator*. These are often undesirable events that do not occur often. These are often related to safety issues and do not lend themselves easily to quality-improvement opportunities. An example may include equipment failures that result in a patient injury.

An aggregate data indicator is a performance measurement based on collecting data involving many events. These events occur frequently and can be presented as a continuous variable indicator or as rate-based indicators. A continuous variable indicator is a measurement where the value can fall anywhere along a continuous scale. Examples could be the number of IPMs scheduled during a particular month or the number of repair requests received during a week. A rate-based variable indicator is the value of a measurement that is expressed as a proportion or a ratio. Examples could be the percentage of IPMs completed each month or the percentage of repairs completed within one workday.

General indicators should be developed to provide a baseline monitoring of the department's performance. They also should provide a cross-check for other indicators. These indicators can be developed to respond to a perceived need within a department or to solve a specific problem.

170.4 Indicator Management Process

The process to develop, monitor, analyze, and manage indicators is shown in Fig. 170.1. The different steps in this process include defining the indicator, establishing the threshold, monitoring the indicator, evaluating the indicator, identifying quality-improvement opportunities, and implementing action plans.

Define Indicator. The definition of the indicator to be monitored must be carefully developed. This process includes at least five steps. The event or outcome to be measured must be described. Define any specific terms that are used. Categorize the indicator (sentinel event or rate-based, process or outcome, desirable or undesirable). The purpose for this indicator must be defined, as well as how it is used in specifying and assessing the particular process or outcome.

Establish Threshold. A threshold is a specific data point that identifies the need for the department to respond to the indicator to determine why the threshold was reached. Sentinel-event indicator thresholds are set at zero. Rate indicator thresholds are more complex to define because they may require expert consensus or definition of the department's objectives. Thresholds must be identified, including the process used to set the specific level.

Monitor Indicator. Once the indicator is defined, the data-acquisition process identifies the data sources and data elements. As these data are gathered, they must be validated for accuracy and completeness. Multiple indicators can be used for data validation and cross-checking. The use of a computerized database allows rapid access to the data. A database management tool allows quick sorting and organization of the data. Once gathered, the data must be presented in a format suitable for evaluation. Graphic presentation of data allows rapid visual analysis for thresholds, trends, and patterns.

Evaluate Indicator. The evaluation process analyzes and reports the information. This process includes comparing the information with established thresholds and analyzing for any trends or patterns. A *trend* is the general direction the indicator measurement takes over a

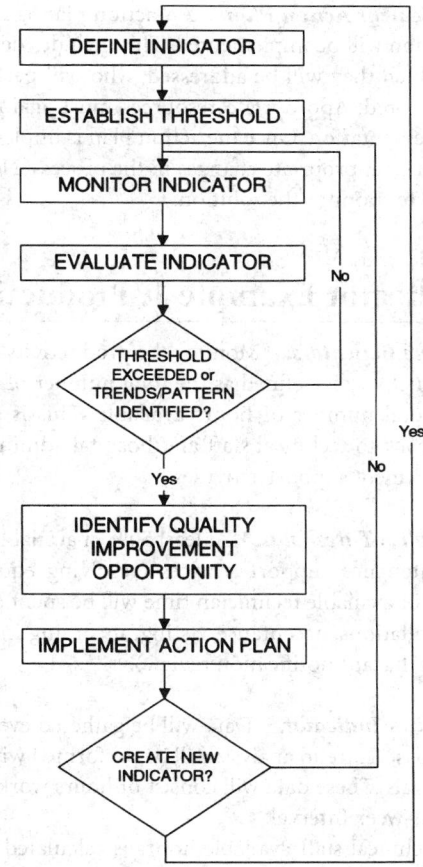

FIGURE 170.1 Indicator management process.

period of time and may be desirable or undesirable. A *pattern* is a grouping or distribution of indicator measurements. A pattern analysis is often triggered when thresholds are crossed or trends identified. Additional indicator information is often required. If an indicator threshold has not been reached, no further action may be necessary, other than continuing to monitor this indicator. The department also may decide to improve its performance level by changing the threshold.

Factors may be present leading to variation of the indicator data. These factors may include failure of the technology to perform properly, failure of the operators to use the technology properly, and failure of the organization to provide the necessary resources to implement this technology properly. Further analysis of these factors may lead to quality-improvement activities later.

Identify Quality-Improvement Opportunity. A quality-improvement opportunity may present itself if an indicator threshold is reached, a trend is identified, or a pattern is recognized. Additional information is then needed to further define the process and improvement opportunities. The first step in the process is to identify a team. This team must be given the necessary resources to complete this project, a timetable to be followed, and an opportunity to periodically update management on the status of the project. The initial phase of the project will analyze the process and establish the scope and definition of the problem. Once the problem is defined, possible solutions can be identified and analyzed for potential implementation. A specific solution to the problem is then selected. The solution may include modifying existing indictors or thresholds to more appropriate values, modifying steps to improve existing processes, or establishing new goals for the department.

Implement Action Plan. An action plan is necessary to identify how the quality-improvement solution will be implemented. This includes defining the different tasks to be performed, the order in which they will be addressed, who will perform each task, and how this improvement will be monitored. Appropriate resources must again be identified and a timetable developed prior to implementation. Once the action plan is implemented, the indicators are monitored and evaluated to verify appropriate changes in the process. New indicators and thresholds may need to be developed to monitor the solution.

170.5 Indicator Example 1: Productivity Monitors

Define Indicators. Monitor the productivity of technical personnel, teams, and the department. Productivity is defined as the total number of documented service support hours compared with the total number of hours available. This is a desirable rate-based outcome indicator. Provide feedback to technical staff and hospital administration regarding utilization of available time for department support activities.

Establish Thresholds. At least 50% of available technician time will be spent providing equipment maintenance support services (resolving equipment problems and scheduled IPMs). At least 25% of available technician time will be spent providing equipment management support services (installations, acceptance testing, incoming inspections, equipment inventory database management, hazard notification review).

Monitor Indicator. Data will be gathered every 4 weeks from the equipment work order history database. A trend analysis will be performed with data available from previously monitored 4-week intervals. These data will consist of hours worked on completed and uncompleted jobs during the past 4-week interval.

Technical staff available hours is calculated for the 4-week interval. The base time available is 160 hours (40 hours/week $\times$ 4 weeks) per individual. Add to this any overtime worked during the interval. Then subtract any holidays, sick days, and vacation days within the interval.

CJHOURS: Hours worked on completed jobs during the interval

UJHOURS: Hours worked on uncompleted jobs during the interval

AHOURS: Total hours available during the 4-week interval

$$\text{Productivity} = (\text{CJHOURS} + \text{UJHOURS})/\text{AHOURS}$$

Evaluate Indicator.   The indicator will be compared with the threshold, and the information will be provided to the individual. The individual team member data can be summed for team review. The data from multiple teams can be summed and reviewed by the department. Historical indicator information will be utilized to determine trends and patterns.

Quality-Improvement Process.   If the threshold is not met, a trend is identified, or a pattern is observed, a quality-improvement opportunity exists. A team could be formed to review the indicator, examine the process that the indicator measured, define the problem encountered, identify ways to solve the problem, and select a solution. An action plan will then be developed to implement this solution.

Implement Action Plan.   During implementation of the action plan, appropriate indicators will be used to monitored the effectiveness of the action plan.

170.6 Indicator Example 2: Patient Monitors IPM Completion Time

Define Indicator.   Compare the mean time to complete an IPM for different models of patient monitors. Different manufacturers of patient monitors have different IPM requirements. Identify the most timely process to support this equipment.

Establish Threshold.   The difference between the mean time to complete an IPM for different models of patient monitors will not be greater than 30% of the lessor time.

Monitor Indicator.   Determine the mean time to complete an IPM for each model of patient monitor. Calculate the percentage difference between the mean time for each model and the model with the least mean time.

Evaluate Indicator.   The mean time to complete IPMs was compared between the patient monitors, and the maximum difference noted was 46%. A pattern also was identified in which all IPMs for that one particular monitor averaged 15 minutes longer than those of other vendors.

Quality-Improvement Process.   A team was formed to address this problem. Analysis of individual IPM procedures revealed that manufacturer X requires the case to be removed to access internal filters. Performing an IPM for each monitor required removing and replacing 15 screws for each of the 46 monitors. The team evaluated this process and identified that 5 minutes could be saved from each IPM if an electric screwdriver was utilized.

Implement Action Plan.   Electric screwdrivers were purchased and provided for use by the technician. The completion of one IPM cycle for the 46 monitors would pay for two electric screwdrivers and provide 4 hours of productive time for additional work. Actual savings were greater because this equipment could be used in the course of daily work.

170.7 Summary

In the ever-changing world of health care, clinical engineering departments are frequently being evaluated based on their contribution to the corporate bottom line. For many departments, this will require difficult and painful changes in management philosophy. Administrators are demanding quantitative measures of performance and value. To provide the appropriate quantitative documentation required by corporate managers, a clinical engineering manager must collect available data that are reliable and accurate. Without such data, analysis is valueless. Indicators are the first step in reducing the data to meaningful information that can be easily monitored and analyzed. The indicators can then be used to determine department performance and identify opportunities for quality improvement.

Program indicators have been used for many years. What must change for clinical engineering departments is a conscious evaluation and systematic use of indicators. One traditional indicator of clinical engineering department success is whether the department's budget is approved or not. Unfortunately, approval of the budget as an indicator, while valuable, does not address the issue of predicting long-term survival, measuring program and quality improvements, or allowing frequent evaluation and changes.

There should be monitored indicators for every significant operational aspect of the department. Common areas where program indicators can be applied include monitoring internal department activities, quality-improvement processes, and benchmarking. Initially, simple indicators should be developed. The complexity and number of indicators should change as experience and needs demand.

The use of program indicators is absolutely essential if a clinical engineering department is to survive. Progress and survival are now determined by the contribution of the department to the bottom line of the parent organization. Indicators must be developed and utilized to determine the current contribution of the clinical engineering department to the organization. Effective utilization and management of program indicators will ensure future department contributions.

References

AAMI. 1993. Management Information Report MIR 1: Design of Clinical Engineering Quality Assurance and Risk Management Programs. Arlington, Va, Association for the Advancement of Medical Instrumentation.

AAMI. 1993. Management Information Report MIR 2: Guideline for Establishing and Administering Medical Instrumentation Maintenance Programs. Arlington, Va, Association for the Advancement of Medical Instrumentation.

AAMI. 1994. Management Information Report MIR 3: Computerized Maintenance Management Systems for Clinical Engineering. Arlington, Va, Association for the Advancement of Medical Instrumentation.

Bauld TJ. 1987. Productivity: Standard terminology and definitions. J Clin Eng 12(2):139.

Betts WF. 1989. Using productivity measures in clinical engineering departments. Biomed Instrum Technol 23(2):120.

Bronzino JD. 1992. Management of Medical Technology: A Primer for Clinical Engineers. Stoneham, Mass, Butterworth-Heinemann.

Coopers and Lybrand International, AFSM. 1994. Benchmarking Impacting the Bottom Line. Fort Myers, Fla, Association for Services Management International.

David Y, Judd TM. 1993. Risk management and quality improvement. In Medical Technology Management, pp 72–75. Redmond, Wash, SpaceLabs Medical.

David Y, Rohe D. 1986. Clinical engineering program productivity and measurement. J Clin Eng 11(6):435.

Downs KJ, McKinney WD. 1991. Clinical engineering workload analysis: A proposal for standardization. Biomed Instrum Technol 25(2):101.

Fennigkoh L. 1986. ASHE Technical Document No 055880: Medical Equipment Maintenance Performance Measures. Chicago, American Society for Hospital Engineers.

Furst E. 1986. Productivity and cost-effectiveness of clinical engineering. J Clin Eng 11(2):105.

Gordon GJ. 1995. Break Through Management—A New Model For Hospital Technical Services. Arlington, Va, Association for the Advancement of Medical Instrumentation.

Hertz E. 1990. Developing quality indicators for a clinical engineering department. In Plant, Technology and Safety Management Series: Measuring Quality in PTSM. Chicago, Joint Commission on Accreditation of Healthcare Organizations.

JCAHO. 1990. Primer on Indicator Development and Application, Measuring Quality in Health Care. Oakbrook, Ill, Joint Commission on Accreditation of Healthcare Organizations.

JCAHO. 1994. Framework for Improving Performance. Oakbrook, Ill, Joint Commission on Accreditation of Healthcare Organizations.

Keil OR. 1989. The challenge of building quality into clinical engineering programs. Biomed Instrum Technol 23(5):354.

Lodge DA. 1991. Productivity, efficiency, and effectiveness in the management of healthcare technology: An incentive pay proposal. J Clin Eng 16(1):29.

Mahachek AR. 1987. Management and control of clinical engineering productivity: A case study. J Clin Eng 12(2):127.

Mahachek AR. 1989. Productivity measurement: Taking the first steps. Biomed Instrum Technol 23:16.

Selsky DB, Bell DS, Benson D, et al. 1991. Biomedical equipment information management for the next generation. Biomed Instrum Technol 25(1):24.

Sherwood MK. 1991. Quality assurance in Biomedical or clinical engineering. J Clin Eng 16(6):479.

Stiefel RH. 1991. Creating a quality measurement system for clinical engineering. Biomed Instrum Technol. 25(1):17.

171

Quality Improvement and Team Building

Joseph P. McClain
Walter Reed Army Medical Center

In today's complex health care environment, quality improvement and team building must go hand and hand. This is especially true for clinical engineers and biomedical equipment technicians as the diversity of the field increases and technology moves so rapidly that no one can know all that needs to be known without the help of others; therefore, it is important that we work together to ensure quality improvement. Ken Blanchard the author of the *One Minute Manager* series has made the statement that "all of us are smarter than any one of us"—a synergy that evolves from working together. Throughout this chapter we will look closely at defining quality and the methods for continuously improving quality, such as collecting data, interpreting indicators, and team building. All this will be put together, enabling us to make decisions based on scientific deciphering of indicators.

Quality is defined as conformance to customer or user requirements. If a product or service does what it is suppose to do, it is said to have high quality. If the product or service fails its mission, it is said to be of low quality. Dr. W. Edward Demings, who is known to many as the "father of quality," defined it as surpassing customer needs and expectations throughout the life of the product or service.

Dr. Demings, a trained statistician by profession, formed his theories on quality during World War II while teaching industry how to use statistical methods to improve the quality of military production. After the war, he focused on meeting customer or consumer needs and acted as a consultant to Japanese organizations to change consumers' perceptions that "Made in Japan" meant junk. Dr. Demings predicted that people would be demanding Japanese products in just 5 years, if they used his methods. However, it only took 4, and the rest is history.

0-8493-8346-3/95/$0.00+$.50
© 1995 by CRC Press, Inc.

171.1 Deming's 14 Points

1. Create constancy of purpose toward improvement of product and service, with an aim to become competitive and to stay in business and provide jobs.
2. Adopt the new philosophy. We are in a new economic age. Western management must awaken and lead for change.
3. Cease dependence on inspection to achieve quality. Eliminate the needs for mass inspection by first building in quality.
4. Improve constantly and forever the system of production and service to improve quality and productivity and thus constantly decrease costs.
5. Institute training on the job.
6. Institute leadership: The goal is to help people, machines, and gadgets to do a better job.
7. Drive out fear so that everyone may work effectively for the organization.
8. Break down barriers between departments.
9. Eliminate slogans, exhortations, and targets for the workforce.
10. Eliminate work standards (quotas) on the factory floor.
11. Substitute leadership: Eliminate management by objective, by numbers, and numerical goals.
12. Remove barriers that rob the hourly worker of the right to pride of workmanship.
13. Institute a vigorous program of education and self-improvement.
14. Encourage everyone in the company to work toward accomplishing transformation. Transformation is everyone's job.

171.2 Zero Defects

Another well-known quality theory, called *zero defects (ZD)*, was established by Philip Crosby. It got results for a variety of reasons; however, the main ones are the following:

1. A strict and specific management standard. Management, including the supervisory staff, did not use vague phrases to explain what it wanted. It made the quality standard very clear: *Do it the right way from the start.* As Philip Crosby said, "What standard would you set on how many babies nurses are allowed to drop?"
2. Complete commitment by everyone. Interestingly, Crosby denies that ZD was a motivational program, but ZD did work because everyone got deeply into the act. Everyone was encouraged to spot problems, detect errors, and prescribe ways and means for their removal. This commitment is best illustrated by the ZD pledge: "I freely pledge myself to make a constant, conscious effort to do my job right the first time, recognizing that my individual contribution is a vital part of the overall effort."
3. Removal of actions and conditions that cause errors. Philip Crosby claimed that at ITT, where he was vice-president for quality, 90% of all error causes could be acted on and fully removed by first-line supervision. In other words, top management must do its part to improve conditions, but supervisors and employees can handle problems right in the department. Errors, malfunctions, and/or variances can best be corrected where the rubber hits the road—at the source.

171.3 TQM (Total Quality Management)

The most recent quality theory that has found fame is called *TQM (total quality management)*. It is a strategic, integrated management system for achieving customer satisfaction which involves all managers and employees and uses quantitative methods to continuously improve an organization's processes. *Total quality management* is a term coined in 1985 by the Naval Air Systems Command to describe its management approach to quality improvement. Simply put, total quality management is a management approach to long-term success through customer satisfaction. Total quality management includes the following three principles: (1) achieving customer satisfaction, (2) making continuous improvement, and (3) giving everyone responsibility. TQM includes eight practices. They are (1) focus on the customer, (2) effective and renewed communications, (3) reliance on standards and measures, (4) commitment to training, (5) top management support and direction, (6) employee involvement, (7) rewards and recognition, and (8) long-term commitment.

171.4 CQI (Continuous Quality Improvement)

Step 8 of the total quality management practices leads us to the quality concept coined by the Joint Commission on Accreditation of Healthcare Organizations and widely used by most health care agencies. It is called *CQI (continuous quality improvement).* The principles of CQI are as follows:

Unity of Purpose

- Unity is established throughout the organization with a clear and widely understood vision.
- Environment nurtures total commitment from all employees.
- Rewards go beyond benefits and salaries to the belief that *"We are family"* and *"We do excellent work."*

Looking for Faults in the Systems

- Eighty percent of an organization's failures are the fault of management-controlled systems.
- Workers can control fewer than 20% of the problems.
- Focus on rigorous improvement of every system, and cease blaming individuals for problems (the 80/20 rule of J. M. Juran and the nineteenth-century economist Vilfredo Pareto).

Customer Focus

- Start with the customer.
- The goal is to meet of exceed customer needs and give lasting value to the customer.
- Positive returns will follow as customers boast of the company's quality and service.

Obsession with Quality

- Everyone's job.
- Quality is relentlessly pursued through products and services that delight the customer.
- Efficient and effective methods of execution.

Recognizing the Structure in Work

- All work has structure.
- Structure may be hidden behind workflow inefficiency.
- Structure can be studied, measured, analyzed, and improved.

Freedom Through Control

- There is control, yet freedom exists by eliminating micromanagement.
- Employees standardize processes and communicate the benefits of standardization.
- They reduce variation in the way work is done.
- Freedom comes as changes occur resulting in time to spend on developing improved processes, discovering new markets, and other methods to increase productivity.

Continued Education and Training

- Everyone is constantly learning.
- Educational opportunities are made available to employees.
- Greater job mastery is gained and capabilities are broadened.

Philosophical Issues on Training

- Training must stay tuned to current technology.
- Funding must be made available to ensure that proper training can be attained.
- Test, measurement, and diagnostic equipment germane to your mission must be procured and technicians trained on its proper use, calibration, and service.
- Creativity must be used to obtain training when funding is scarce.
  —Include training in equipment procurement process.
  —Contract with manufacturer or education facility to bring training to your institution.
  —Use local facilities to acquire training, thus eliminating travel cost.
  —Allow your employees to attend professional organization seminars where a multitude of training is available.

Teamwork

- Old rivalries and distrust are eliminated.
- Barriers are overcome.
- Teamwork, commitment to the team concept and partnerships are the focus.
- Employee empowerment: Is critical in the CQI philosophy and means that employees have the authority to make well-reasoned, data-based decisions. In essence, they are entrusted with the legal power to change processes through a rational, scientific approach.

Continuous quality improvement is a means for tapping knowledge and creativity, applying participative problem solving, finding and eliminating problems that prevent quality, eliminating waste, instilling pride, and increasing teamwork. Further it is a means for creating an atmosphere of innovation for continued and permanent quality improvement. Continuous quality improvement as outlined by the Joint Commission on Accreditation of Healthcare Organizations is designed to improve the work processes within and across organizations.

171.5 Tools Used for Quality Improvement

The following are tools that will assist in developing quality programs, collecting data, and assessing performance indicators within the organization. These tools include several of the most frequently used and most of the **seven tools of quality.** The seven tools of quality are tools that help health care organizations understand their process in order to improve them. The tools are the cause-and-effect diagram, check sheet, control chart, flowchart, histogram, Pareto chart, and scatter diagram. Additional tools shown are the Shewhart cycle (PDCA process) and the bar chart. The clinical engineering manager must access the situation and determine which tool will work best for their situational needs.

Two of the seven tools of quality are not listed, and they are the scatter diagram and the check sheet. The scatter diagram is a graphic technique to analyze the relationship between two variations, and the check sheet is a simple data-recording device. The check sheet is custom designed by the user, which facilitates interpretation of the results. Most biomedical equipment technicians use the check sheet on a daily basis when performing preventive maintenance, calibration, or electrical safety checks.

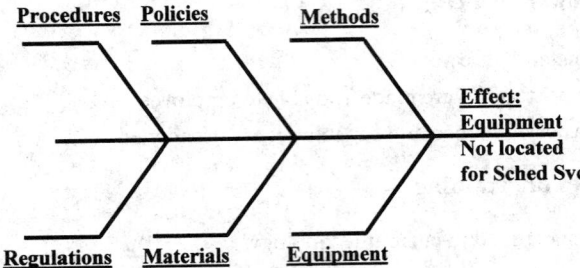

FIGURE 171.1 Cause-and-effect or Ishikawa chart.

Cause-and-Effect or Ishikawa Chart

This is a tool for analyzing process dispersion (Fig. 171.1). The process was developed by Dr. Kaoru Ishikawa and is also known as the *fishbone diagram* because the diagram resembles a fish skeleton. The diagram illustrates the main causes and subcauses leading to an effect. The cause-and-effect diagram is one of the seven tools of quality.

The following is an overview of the process:

- Used in group problem solving as a *brainstorming tool* to explore and display the possible causes of a particular problem.
- The *effect* (problem, concern, or opportunity) that is being investigated is stated on the right side, while the contributing *causes* are grouped in component categories through group brainstorming on the left side.
- This is an extremely effective tool for focusing a group brainstorming session.
- Basic components include environment, methods (measurement), people, money, information, materials, supplies, capital equipment, and intangibles.

Control Chart

A control chart is a graphic representation of a characteristic of a process showing plotted values of some statistic gathered from that characteristic and one or two control limits (Fig. 171.2). It has two basic uses: as a judgment to determine if the process is in control and as an aid in achieving and maintaining statistical control. (This chart was used by Dr. W. A. Shewhart for a continuing test of statistical significance.) A control chart is a chart with a baseline, frequently in time order, on which measurement or counts are represented by points that are connected by a straight line with an upper and lower limit. The control chart is one of the seven tools of quality.

Flowchart

A flowchart is a pictorial representation showing all the steps of a process (Fig. 171.3). Flowcharts provide excellent documentation of a program and can be a useful tool for examining how various steps in a process are related to each other. Flowcharting uses easily recognizable symbols to represent the type of processing performed. The flowchart is one of the seven tools of quality.

Histogram

A graphic summary of variation in a set of data is a histogram (Fig. 171.4). The pictorial nature of the histogram lets people see patterns that are difficult to see in a simple table of numbers. The histogram is one of the seven tools of quality.

Equipment Not Located During Scheduled Services.

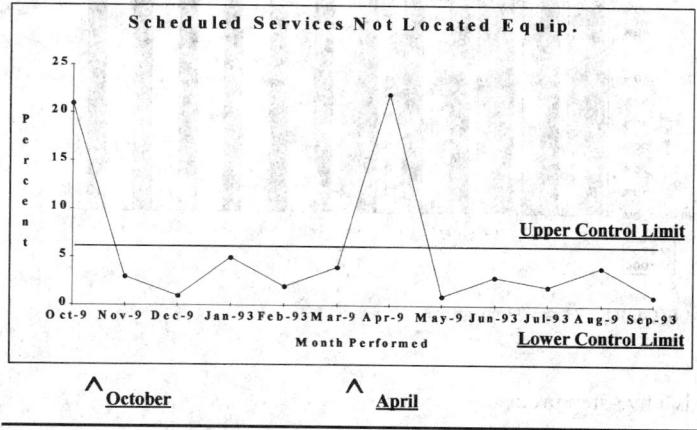

FIGURE 171.2 Control chart.

Pareto Chart

A Pareto chart is a special form of vertical bar graph that helps us to determine which problems to solve and in what order (Fig. 171.5). It is based on the Pareto principle, which was first developed by J. M. Juran in 1950. The principle, named after the nineteenth-century economist Vilfredo Pareto, suggests that most effects come from relatively few causes; i.e., 80% of the effects come from 20% of the possible causes.

Doing a Pareto chart, based on either check sheets or other forms of data collection, helps us direct our attention and efforts to the truly important problems. We will generally gain more by working on the tallest bar than tackling the smaller bars. The Pareto chart is one of the seven tools of quality.

The Plan-Do-Check-Act or Shewhart Cycle

This is a four-step process for quality improvement that is sometimes referred to as the *Deming cycle* (Fig. 171.6). One of the consistent requirements of the cycle is the long-term commitment required. The Shewhart cycle or PDCA cycle is outlined here and has had overwhelming success when used properly. It is also a very handy tool to use in understanding the quality cycle process. The results of the cycle are studied to determine what was learned, what can be predicted, and appropriate changes to be implemented.

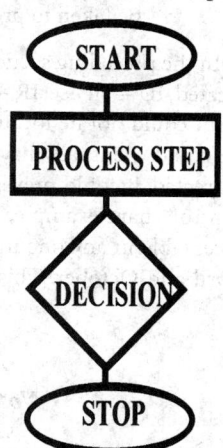

FIGURE 171.3 Flowchart.

171.6 Quality Performance Indicators (QPI)

An *indicator* is something that suggests the existence of a fact, condition, or quality—an omen (a sign of future good or evil.) It can be considered as evidence of a manifestation or symptom of an incipient failure or problem. Therefore, quality performance indicators are measurements that can be used to ensure that quality performance is continuous and will allow us to know when incipient failures are starting so that we may take corrective and preventive actions.

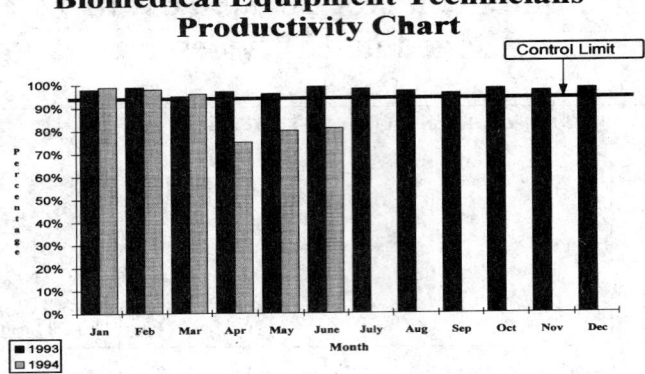

FIGURE 171.4   Histogram.

QPI analysis is a five-step process:

Step 1: Decide what performance we need to track.

Step 2: Decide the data that need to be collected to track this performance.

Step 3: Collect the data.

Step 4: Establish limits, a parameter, or control points.

Step 5: Utilize MBE (management by exceptions)—when a performance exceeds the established control limits, it is indicating a quality performance failure, and corrective action must be taken to prevent the problem.

In the preceding section, there were several examples of QPIs. In the Pareto chart, the NL = not located, IU = in use, IR = in repair. The chart indicates that during the year 1994, 35% of the equipment could not be located to perform preventive maintenance service. This indicator tells us that we could eventually have a serious safety problem that could impact on patient care, and if not corrected, it could prevent the health care facility from meeting accreditation requirements. In the control chart example, an upper control limit of 6% not located equipment is established as acceptable in any one month; however, this upper control limit is exceeded during the months of April and October. This QPI could assist the clinical and/or biomedical equipment manager in

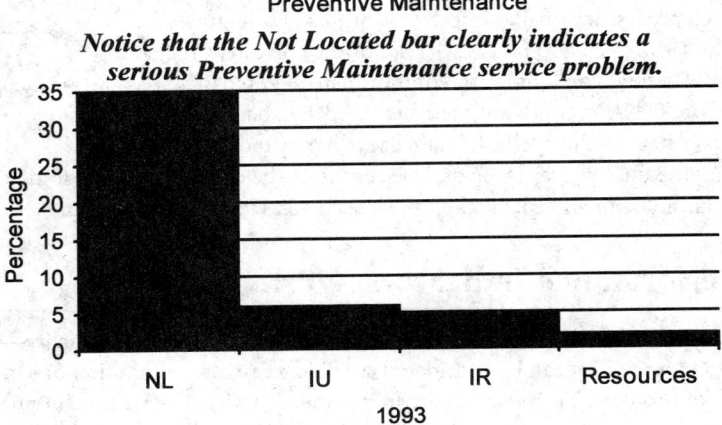

FIGURE 171.5   Pareto chart.

- Step 1 - Plan (P): Collect data upon which a plan can be constructed.
- Step 2 - Do (D): Take the necessary actions that further the developed plan.
- Step 3 - Check (C): Check the results of our actions by collecting data to make sure that we have achieved what we planned.
- Step 4 - Act (A): Act by making necessary changes to achieve Customer Satisfaction.

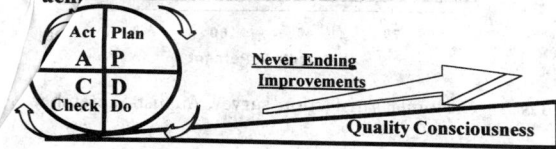

FIGURE 171.6 The Shewhart cycle.

...he problem down to a 2-month period. The histogram example established a lower narrit for productivity at 93%; however, productivity started to drop off in May, June, and corQPI tells the manager that something has happened that is jeopardizing the performance J her organization. Other performance indicators have been established graphically in Figs. nd 171.8. See if you can determine what the indicators are and what the possible cause might u may wish to use these tools to establish QPI tracking germane to your own organization.

...eams

A *team* is a formal group of persons organized by the company to work together to accomplish certain goals and objectives. Normally, when teams are used in quality improvement programs, they are designed to achieve the organization's vision. The organization's vision is a statement of the desired end state of the organization articulated and deployed by the executive leadership. Organizational visions are inspiring, clear, challenging, reasonable, and empowering. Effective visions honor the past, while they prepare for the future. The following are types of teams that are being used in health care facilities today. Some of the names may not be common, but their definitions are very similar if not commensurate.

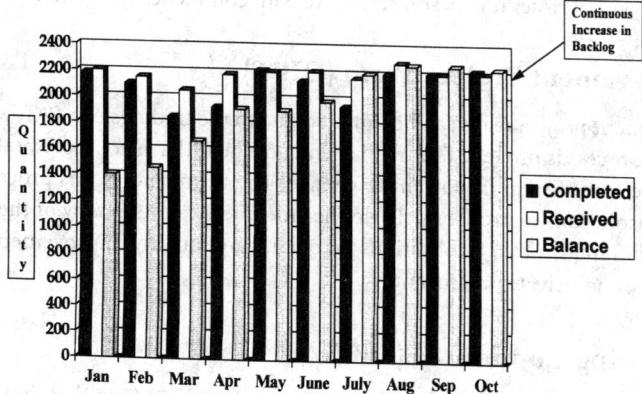

FIGURE 171.7 Sample repair service report.

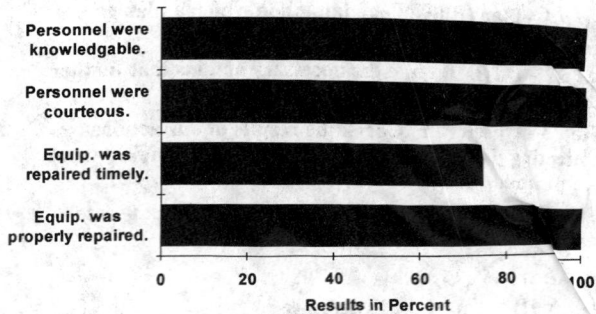

FIGURE 171.8 Customer satisfaction survey, August–September 1994.

Process Action Teams (PAT)

Process action teams are composed of those who are involved in the process being investi̥ members of a PAT are often chosen by their respective managers. The primary consideratiorhe membership is knowledge about the operations of the organization and the process being sͯ The main function of a PAT is the performance of an improvement project; hence custome. often invited to participate on the team. PATs use basic statistical and other tools to analyze a pro and identify potential areas for improvement. PATs report their findings to an executive steeri̥ committee or some other type of quality management improvement group. ("*A problem well defineɩ is half solved.*" John Dewey, American philosopher and educator; 1859–1952.)

Transition Management Team (TMT)

The transition management team (see *Harvard Business Review,* Nov–Dec 1993, pp. 109–118) is normally used for a major organizational change such as restructing or reengineering. The TMT can be initiated due to the findings of a PAT, where it has been indicated that the process is severely broken and unsalvageable. The TMT is not a new layer of bureaucracy or a job for fading executives. The TMT oversees the large-scale corporate change effort; it makes sure that all change initiatives fit together. It is made up of 8 to 12 highly talented leaders who commit *all* their time to making the transition a reality. The team members and what they are trying to accomplish must be accepted by the power structure of the organization. For the duration of the change process, they are the CEO's version of the National Guard. The CEO should be able to say, "I can sleep well tonight; the TMT is managing this." In setting up a TMT, organizations should adopt a fail-safe approach: Create a position to oversee the emotional and behavioral issues unless you can prove with confidence that you do not need one.

Quality Improvement Project Team (QIPT)

A quality improvement project team can be initiated due to the findings of a PAT, where it has been indicated that the process is broken. The main agenda of the QIPT is to improve the work process that managers have identified as important to change. The team studies this process methodically to find permanent solutions to problems. To do this, members can use many of the tools described in this chapter and in many other publications on quality and quality improvement available from schools, bookstores, and private organizations.

Executive Steering Committee (ESC)

This is an executive-level team composed of the chief executive officer (CEO) of the organization and the executive staff that reports directly to the CEO. Whereas an organization may have numerous QMBs, PATs, and QIPTs, it has only one ESC. The ESC identifies strategic goals for organizational quality-improvement efforts. It obtains information from customers to identify major product and service requirements. It is through the identification of these major requirements that quality goals for the organization are defined. Using this information, the ESC lists, prioritizes, and determines how to measure the organization's goals for quality improvement. The ESC develops the organization's improvement plan and manages the execution of that plan to ensure that improvement goals are achieved.

Quality Management Board (QMB)

This is a permanent cross-functional team made up of top and midlevel managers who are jointly responsible for a specific product, service or process. The structure of the board is intended to improve communication and cooperation by providing vertical and horizontal "links" throughout the organization.

171.8 Summary

Although quality can be simply defined as conformity to customer or user requirements, it has many dimensions. Seven of them are described here: (1) performance, (2) aesthetics, (3) reliability (how dependably it performs), (4) availability (there when you need it), (5) durability (how long it lasts), (6) extras or features (supplementary items), and (7) serviceability (how easy it is to get serviced). The word *PARADES* can help you remember this:

PARADES: Seven Dimensions of Quality

1. *Performance:* A product or service that performs its intended function well scores high on this dimension of quality.
2. *Aesthetics:* A product or service that has a favorable appearance, sound, taste, or smell is perceived to be of good quality.
3. *Reliability:* Reliability, or dependability, is such an important part of product quality that quality-control engineers are sometimes referred to as *reliability engineers.*
4. *Availability:* A product or service that is there when you need it.
5. *Durability:* Durability can be defined as the amount of use one gets from a product before it no longer functions properly and replacement seems more feasible than constant repair.
6. *Extras:* Features or characteristics about a product or service that supplement its basic functioning (i.e., remote control dialing on a television).
7. *Serviceability:* Speed, courtesy, competence, and ease of repair are all important quality factors.

Quality Has a Monetary Value!

Good quality often pays for itself, while poor quality is expensive in both measurable costs and hidden costs. The hidden costs include loss of goodwill, including loss of repeat business and bad-mouthing of the firm. High-quality goods and services often carry a higher selling price than do those of low quality. This information is evidenced by several reports in the *Wall Street Journal, Forbes Magazine, Money Magazine, Business Week Magazine,* etc. A good example is the turnaround of Japanese product sales using quality methodologies outlined in *The Deming Guide to Quality and Competitive Position,* by Howard S. and Shelley J. Gitlow. As Dr. Demings has stated *quality improvement* must be *continuous!*

Quality is never an accident; it is always the result of intelligent energy.

John Ruskins, 1819–1900
English art critic and historian
Seven Lamps of Architecture

References

Bittel LR. 1985. What Every Supervisor Should Know, 5th ed, pp 455–456. New York, Gregg Division/McGraw-Hill.

DuBrin AJ. 1994. Essentials of Management, 3d ed. Cleveland, South-Western Publishing Co.

Duck JD. 1993. Managing change—The art of balancing. Harvard Business Review, November–December 1993, pp 109–118.

Gitlow HS, Gitlow SJ. 1987. The Deming Guide to Quality and Competitive Position. Englewood Cliffs, NJ, Prentice-Hall.

Goal/QPC. 1988. The Memory Jogger. A Pocket Guide of Tools for Continuous Improvement, Massachusetts, Goal/QPC

Ishikawa K. 1991. Guide to Quality Control. New York, Quality Resources (Asian Productivity Organization, Tokyo, Japan).

Joint Commission on Accreditation of Healthcare Organizations. 1991. Using Continuous Quality Improvement Approaches to Monitor, Evaluate, and Improve Quality. Chicago, Joint Commission on Accreditation of Healthcare Organizations.

Juran JM. 1979. Quality Control Handbook, 3d ed. New York, McGraw-Hill.

Katzenbach JR, Smith DK. 1994. The Wisdom of Teams. New York, Harper Business, A Division of Harper Collins Publishers.

Mizuno S. 1988. Management for Quality Improvement. The Seven New QC Tools. Boston, Productivity Press.

Scholtes PR. 1993. The Team Handbook. How to Use Teams to Improve Quality. Madison, Wisc, Joiner Associates, Inc.

Walton M. 1986. The Deming Management Method. New York, Putnam Publishing Group.

172

Clinical Engineering: Coordinated Services

J.O. Rowan
Glasgow Royal Infirmary

In different parts of the world, the terms *clinical engineering services* and *bioengineering services* have been used to identify medical equipment management activities that have been established to ensure that medical and scientific equipment is kept functioning appropriately and safely for the benefit of patients.

Equipment management services in hospitals and other health care institutions require detailed systematic organization. Enunciations of global strategy and mission statements need to be under-pinned with a well-defined structure and action plan. A hospital is, in general, a hostile environment for technology, and if cognizance is not taken of this fact malfunctions, hazards, as well as running costs, may escalate, leading to reduction in standards of health care.

Ideally, equipment management services should be comprehensive in nature, starting with spec-ification of the equipment that is thought to be required, through procurement, acceptance testing, calibration, safety testing, planned preventive maintenance, corrective maintenance, modification, quality audit of equipment servicing, and final replacement. To be truly effective in this area, a coordinated approach is required.

172.1 Defining the Problem

The range, application, level of sophistication, quantity, and cost of individual items of medical tech-nology are extremely variable from equipment such as infusion pumps at one end of the spectrum to diagnostic tomographic imagers and therapy linear accelerators at the other. Continuous devel-opment is taking place throughout the range. As a consequence, some teams in the support organi-zation need to be generalist by nature, while others need to be more specialized.

Information is required on who uses the various services and the pattern of usage. Resources uti-lized must be related to the output and associated costing systems developed. The service should be planned on the basis of this information and cost savings identified, leading to overall improvements in the service organization.

Staffing costs inevitably form a large fraction of the overall costs involved. Therefore, all grades of staff should be used to their full potential. Training programs should be designed to ensure that this potential is fully developed.

An accurate asset register capable of being updated regularly is an essential requirement, as is a quality assurance program. Equipment should be purchased with reference to appropriate safety standards and regular testing carried out to ensure continuing compliance with these standards. It has to be recognized that the concept of quality control includes accuracy, demand management, resource utilization, speed of response, and appropriate advice to clinical users.

172.2 Managing the Problem

Equipment Procurement

A well-organized equipment management services department should be directly involved with clinical users and hospital administrators in medical equipment procurement. This can help to ensure that the equipment purchased matches the proposed application and in addition can lead to substantial budget savings and as a consequence permit additional projects to be funded.

Following prioritization of equipment bids, a generic specification should be prepared in consultation with the clinical users. This should involve both a clinical specification and a technical specification. At this time, a list of potential suppliers and additional costs can be identified.

Using this information, an invitation-to-tender document can then be prepared and sent out to suppliers by the appropriate hospital purchasing organization detailing special requirements such as technical training and provision of technical servicing manuals. The companies involved may then respond by providing quotations and completing standard specification sheets. Once the tenders for a particular project have been received, they can be sent to the equipment management services department for evaluation, and the various possibilities can be considered in consultation with the users. A letter of recommendation should then be sent to the purchasing department. Further discussions may be necessary with that department before despatch of a formal purchase order to the chosen supplier is authorized. Once the equipment has been delivered and installed, acceptance tests involving safety, calibration, and clinical performance checks can be carried out. On satisfactory completion of these tests, an equipment acceptance certificate can be signed.

Acceptance Testing

Acceptance testing and commissioning of equipment involve the initial electrical, mechanical, and, where appropriate, radiation safety tests, installation, and calibration. If required, the item can be interfaced with other equipment. Checks are then carried out to verify compliance with the technical performance specification and, in collaboration with the user, compliance with the clinical performance specification. Checks should be carried out to ensure compliance with appropriate standards, e.g., BS 5724, Electrical Safety Code for Hospital Laboratory Equipment, Ionizing Radiations Regulations, etc. The manuals supplied should be checked to ensure that they are complete, and if appropriate, arrangements should be made for the disposal of equipment being replaced.

Details for the equipment inventory should be recorded, such as

1. Equipment category
2. Manufacturer
3. Model number
4. Serial number
5. Purchase date
6. Maintenance arrangements, e.g., in-house, collaborative contract, commercial contract

An asset register number also should be allocated.

Once the equipment acceptance certificate has been signed, the equipment should be supplied to the user with appropriate manuals and details of the program for user training.

User Training

This should be carried out in situ, in the form of "live" demonstrations based on the user manual. Potential errors and faults commonly found should be highlighted together with details of the appropriate corrective action.

Maintenance Arrangements

Preventive maintenance, involving inspection and timely replacement of vulnerable components, increases equipment reliability and reduces the likelihood of major faults. It also may extend the equipment lifetime.

A number of types of maintenance arrangements can be considered, and each piece of equipment should be assessed with a view to advising users of the most cost-effective option. In some cases, the clinical engineering staff may carry out full in-house maintenance. Alternatively, a cooperative "contract" can be taken out with the manufacturer in which the clinical engineering staff carries out most preventive maintenance and first-line fault maintenance, with the manufacturer providing the necessary backup. In some instances, mainly where major items are concerned, it can be more cost-effective to take out a manufacturer's comprehensive maintenance contract. This contract should be supervised by local clinical engineering staff, who can screen calls (saving the call-out charges for "faults" due to operator error) and ensure that the appropriate work is carried out within the agreed time scale.

Equipment Assessment

This is best coordinated centrally but can be carried out to advantage in various hospital sites. It involves identifying newly available equipment, arranging demonstrations or extended loans, and obtaining capital and revenue cost information. Objective performance measurements can be made and comparisons with other equipment carried out in order to provide recommendations to users.

Equipment Inventory

An inventory of all equipment for which the equipment management teams have responsibility is an essential requirement. It can be used for the provision of reference data for the development of equipment replacement programs and for the determination of associated revenue costs. Other uses include the rapid location of equipment covered by hazard warning notices and safety action bulletins, the establishing of suppliers and product ranges for specific types of equipment, and comparison of maintenance arrangements.

Infection Control

Although each individual is responsible for his or her own personal safety and for the safety of colleagues, it is important that guidelines are drawn up to help minimize the risk of infection to staff involved in the servicing of patient-connected and hospital laboratory equipment. Ultimate responsibility for advice will, of course, rest with the locally based bacteriologist, occupational health officer, and infection-control nurse.

A "permit to work" system for all equipment is not practical, nor would it completely eliminate infection risk. Any system that is adopted must take into account the fact that staff are called on to check equipment at its point of use. However, this should be put into perspective, since the hospital environment in general presents a high risk of infection. The most effective way to control the situation is to ensure that all hospital staff adopt good working practices. Good communications should exist between staff involved with the patient and the equipment. The guidelines should identify the risk factors, outline general precautions, and list detailed precautions necessary when dealing with specific equipment.

Modifications to Equipment

If it is intended to modify equipment, the manufacturer should be consulted about the possible effects of the modifications on safety and performance. Manufacturers who provide scheduled servicing under contract might offer modifications that have been designed and developed to improve equipment performance or safety. These modifications sometimes arise out of reported defects, e.g., in a hazard warning. Equipment management services involved in in-house maintenance should have an established procedure for obtaining information concerning modifications that relate to performance and safety and for incorporating such modifications as soon as possible. Users should be notified when such modifications have been carried out.

Quality Assurance

A procedure for auditing the equipment management services both internally and externally should be established. In essence, this means that the servicing organization should be accredited with reference to a standard. The trend in the United Kingdom is to seek BSI approval with reference to BS 5750 (ISO 9000 to ISO 9006). In general, three quality-assurance manuals are produced that deal, respectively, with policy, procedures, and working instructions. The basic concept is that the level of service to be provided is defined and audits are carried out to ensure that this level of service is being delivered.

Items used for spare parts need to be traced back to the supplier not only for what is held in store but also for items that have been used in the repair of the equipment. In this context, it may be decided to use only approved suppliers.

All test equipment must be calibrated, with such calibration traceable to national standards. The frequency of calibration will be defined in the quality-assurance manual and the date of the last calibration check indicated on the test instrument.

It is essential that a call-logging system is in place whereby the process involving the service request to final handover is documented at every stage. The call-log system ensures that as much information about the equipment is available before a repair is started. Ability to identify the equipment location avoids wasting time either in the servicing laboratory or in transit to and from the requesting department.

A quality-control manager should be appointed to oversee the operation of the overall quality system.

172.3 Methodology

To provide an efficient and cost-effective equipment management service involving all the activities detailed above and covering many hospitals over a wide area, a coordinated approach is recommended. Such a service has been developed by the West of Scotland Department of Clinical Physics and Bio-Engineering and operated over many years. The major elements are now described in detail.

The department in total has a staff of 76 physics/engineering graduates and 200 medical-technical officers participating in activities such as radiotherapy physics, radiation physics (ionizing and nonionizing), nuclear medicine, radiation protection, electronic design and development, and mechanical engineering design, as well as a range of equipment management services. Equipment management is the principal activity of about 80 staff members.

Most of these staff members are based in individual hospitals, but there are, in addition, a number of core service groups providing a specific service to all hospitals. Staff members based in hospitals are under local day-to-day management and respond rapidly to local needs with respect to a wide range of equipment. However, an equipment services manager exercises general supervision and coordination of the activity.

Although the technical officers scattered through the various hospitals can tackle a very wide range of equipment, for some types of major, rare, or more specialized equipment, it is better to have a single, centrally based team that can acquire particular expertise and hold a stock of expensive spare parts. For example, one of these core service teams provides in-depth servicing of ultrasound imaging equipment, while another offers a full in-house service for medical laboratory equipment such as clinical chemistry analyzers, blood culture systems, tissue processors, and centrifuges. None of the teams accepts equipment for full in-house servicing programs unless it can be shown that in-house operational costs, with appropriate overheads included, are at a level that is competitive with those of the manufacturer and/or supplier.

All core service teams offer planned preventive maintenance programs and same-day emergency call-out. A limited amount of loan equipment is available and in certain circumstances may enable a clinical service to be maintained during the breakdown of a component part of a system such as an imager, transducer, or peripheral. Clearly, these loans can only be made for a defined period.

These core services are supported by the local hospital-based teams who are able to provide a technical filter and where appropriate carry out first-line servicing when a repair is necessary. Because of the nature of the equipment involved and the economics that can be achieved through central control of spare parts and loan modules, the establishment of core teams for these services is highly beneficial. Like the locally based teams, the core service maintenance teams provide either a full in-house service or a defined service under the terms of a collaborative contract with an equipment supplier. Cooperative contract agreements are specific to individual manufacturers, the all-round benefit being rapid response times.

In addition to these core service maintenance teams, the department's electronic and mechanical engineering development sections provide additional support for development and calibration of test equipment, electronic circuit design, and mechanical engineering development.

Obviously, in such a widespread organization, communication is vitally important. Regular meetings are held to discuss detailed issues, including safety matters, exchange information on equipment problems, establishment of standards of technical practice, and allocation of special projects, thereby avoiding duplication of effort. This coordinated approach permits efficient organization and dissemination of information. Potential hazards are identified and rectified quickly. These meetings involve a representative from each of the major hospitals, and formal minutes are taken so that appropriate follow-up action can be initiated.

Safety information such as hazard warnings and safety action bulletins are coordinated centrally through the manager of the service, who also arranges for staff training updates. Working groups are convened to examine certain issues in more detail, e.g., studying the right balance between planned preventive maintenance, routine safety checks, user training, and repair.

With the number of staff involved, manufacturers' training courses can be held at a central location, allowing significant numbers of staff to be trained at the one time and at much reduced cost. Certain maintenance contracts can be arranged centrally, thereby allowing maximum discount to be obtained.

172.4 Support Services

Equipment Inventory and Equipment Advisory Service

In order to obtain information concerning commercially available equipment with a view to preparing recommendations in terms of selection, a database containing information from over 3000 British and overseas manufacturers covering over 2000 types of products was developed.

An asset register for equipment located in hospitals and other health care establishments in Glasgow also has been developed. This uses the same product category index as the equipment advisory database and contains around 30,000 items with a total replacement value of approximately £140 million.

The equipment advisory database and the equipment inventory share the same computer. In addition to the provision of support to the equipment management services activities, the system provides information for strategic and financial management.

Maintenance Records

Because of the quantity of maintenance data that has to be collected, it makes sense to acquire and hold these data on section-based computers. Such a system is able to provide detailed costing for the maintenance service and adequate information on the service history of each item of equipment.

The financial information recorded permits

1. Measurement of the cost-effectiveness of individual groups carrying out equipment management services compared with outside agencies. This helps to ensure that only cost-effective in-house work is carried out.
2. Control over external contracts so that only work that is absolutely necessary is carried out.
3. Quotation of costs to departmental budget holders at the beginning of each contract year.
4. Provision of details of maintenance costs for specific models of equipment so that this can be accounted for in future equipment purchases.

The technical information recorded permits

1. Provision of information that allows compliance with BS 5750.
2. Assessment of the quality of the equipment management services provided in terms of factors such as response and "down" time. It is essential that a uniform system is in operation throughout the organization so that staff can be readily moved between maintenance bases, thereby ensuring that an optimal service is provided with the minimum number of staff.

172.5 Training

There are two levels of in-house medical-technical officer staff training. Program 1 for trainee medical-technical officers and program 2 for medical-technical officers at the basic level.

Program 1 is carried out over a period of 2 years and consists of six 4-month modules, *viz.*, basic electronic engineering, basic mechanical engineering, radionuclide laboratory practice, instrumentation and clinical measurement, bioengineering services, and nuclear medicine. A syllabus outlining the details of each module is given to the trainee at the beginning of each 4-month period, together with a workbook containing notes outlining background theory and detailing a number of practical exercises. The trainee is expected to keep a log book of his or her activities up-to-date. This is checked by the appropriate supervisor on a regular basis. Day release is given for college study to allow the trainee to obtain nationally recognized vocational qualifications.

Program 2 covers a period of 3 years and is made up of three 1-year placements in contrasting posts falling under the headings of bioengineering services, electronic design, and radiation physics. Day release is given to obtain higher-level, nationally recognized vocational qualifications.

Training placements, details of training given, and training assessments are recorded. At higher-grade medical-technical officer posts, further specialized training is arranged in conjunction with equipment manufacturers.

There is also in existence within the organization a training and overseas support group consisting of scientific and technical staff with substantial experience in teaching and training engineering students from abroad. Many have worked overseas on behalf of the department as development managers and advisers assisting in the design, construction, and equipping of health care facilities and in training local personnel. These instructors can call on other colleagues in the organization to provide specialized tuition and arrange appropriate training attachments.

The courses are provided in modular form so that various programs can be designed to meet the needs of individual students. Each trainee is assessed prior to commencement of the course, and an introductory training program arranged if appropriate.

A basic premise underlying all training programs is that technical training for work in hospitals should be carried out in a medical environment by an organization fully committed to a service role in health care establishments. This ensures that trainees gain practical experience in an actual working environment where true work-related technical and organization problems occur. This type of training avoids the limitations of purely theoretical instruction in such a way that the student acquires the relevant practical skills that can be put into immediate use and learns to appreciate the organizational issues that influence the successful operation of a clinical engineering service. The training is provided by staff who are practicing the techniques which they teach, with the result that the courses are being continually updated in the light of new developments.

The aim of the courses is to train the student to be able to provide a complete equipment management service. The programs consist of lectures, audiovisual presentations, discussion groups, equipment construction exercises, equipment calibration, and practical fault-finding exercises. The trainees also spend time attached to hospital service centers and centrally based equipment management teams to receive practical on-the-job training.

Missions abroad are undertaken by the staff of the overseas support group to give advice on the management, operation, maintenance, and the selection of hospital equipment and the training of hospital equipment management personnel.

172.6 Conclusions

A coordinated comprehensive equipment management service permits the establishment of hospital-based engineering teams who can deal effectively and rapidly with a wide range of local hospital equipment problems. In addition, it permits the creation of product- and model-specific teams that can be utilized to deal with complex medical and scientific equipment. Such an organization enables a forum to be established for developing practical policies in response to current issues. Real cost savings can be achieved through the development of supra-area contracts with equipment manufacturers where this is appropriate. Training programs at all levels from basic engineering skill induction to model-specific maintenance procedures can be developed economically for a range of staff.

In such an organization, a good communication system is essential involving both formal and informal exchanges, thereby ensuring that all concerned contribute effectively.

The major strengths of a coordinated approach to the provision of a comprehensive equipment management service can be summarized as follows:

1. Cost-effective use of resources in terms of utilization of manpower and space.
2. Flexible use of resources by redeploying skilled staff to provide crisis cover when faced with major equipment failure, key post vacancies, sickness, leave, etc.
3. Professional oversight of all activities, facilitating internal audit and the maintenance of high professional standards.
4. Pooling of expertise in different facets of a complex problem in order to rapidly provide a solution.
5. Maintenance of professional awareness by keeping staff informed of issues related to other areas outwith the immediate remit of their own post, leading to better troubleshooting.
6. Staff can act as facilitators with a range of external agencies, e.g., in specifying and evaluating contracts.

7. Training can be carried out effectively, resulting in the availability of a pool of up-to-date knowledge and skill and ensuring that staff potential is fully developed.

Further Information

British Standards Institution. 1987. BS 5750: Part 2: Quality Systems. London, England.

British Standards Institution. 1989. BS 5724: Part 1: Specification for safety of medical electrical equipment. London, England.

Corner GA, Shaw A. 1989. Infection control when servicing medical and laboratory equipment. J Med Eng Technol 13:177.

Health Equipment Information Bulletin No. 95. 1981. Code of practice for acceptance testing of medical equipment. HMSO.

Health Equipment Information Bulletin No. 98. 1991. Management of Medical Equipment and Devices. HMSO.

McKie J, Shaw A, Feasey CM. 1987. A medical inventory. Br J Health Care Comp 4:47.

173

A Standards Primer
for Clinical Engineers

Alvin Wald
Columbia-Presbyterian
Medical Center

The development, understanding, and use of standards are important components of clinical engineering activities. Whether involved in industry, a health care facility, governmental affairs, or commercial enterprise, one way or another the clinical engineer will encounter standards as a significant aspect of his or her professional duties. With the increasing emphasis on health care cost containment and efficiency, standards will be viewed both as a mechanism for reducing expenses and as another obstacle in providing quality patient care. In any case, standards must be addressed in their own right, in terms of technical, economic, and legal considerations.

It is important for the clinical engineer to fully understand how standards are developed, how they are used, and most important, how they affect the entire spectrum of health-related matters. Standards exist that address systems (protection of the electrical power distribution system from faults), individuals (means to reduce potential electric shock hazards), and protection of the environment (disposal of deleterious waste substances).

From a larger perspective, standards have existed since biblical times. In the Book of Genesis (Chap. 6, ver. 14), Noah is given a construction standard by God, "Make thee an ark of gopher wood; rooms shalt thou make in the ark, and shalt pitch it within and without with pitch." Standards for weights and measures have played an important role in bringing together human societies through trade and commerce. The earliest record of a standard for length comes from ancient Egypt, in Dynasty IV (circa 3000 B.C.). This length was the royal cubit, 20.620 in (52.379 cm), as used in construction of the Great Pyramid.

The importance of standards to society is exemplified in the Magna Carta, presented by the English barons to King John in 1215 on the field at Runnimede. Article 35 states:

> There shall be standard measures of wine, beer, and corn—the London quarter—throughout the whole of our kingdom, and a standard width of dyed, russet and halberject cloth—two ells within the selvedges; and there shall be standard weights also.

The principles of this article appear in the English Tower system for weight and capacity, set in 1266 by the assize of Bread and Ale Act:

> An English penny called a sterling, round and without any clipping, shall weigh thirty-two wheatcorns in the midst of the ear; and twenty ounces a pound: and eight pounds do make a gallon of wine, and eight gallons of wine do make a bushell, which is the eighth part of a quarter.

In the United States, a noteworthy use of standards occurred after the Boston fire of 1689. With the aim of the rapid rebuilding of the city, the town fathers specified that all bricks used in construction were to be 9 × 4 × 4 inches. An example of standardization to promote uniform manufacturing practices was the contract for 10,000 muskets awarded to Eli Whitney by President Thomas Jefferson in 1800. The apocraphyl story is that Eli Whitney (better known to generations of grammer school children for his invention of the cotton gin) assembled a large number of each musket part, had one of each part randomly selected, and then assembled a complete working musket. This method of production, the complete interchangeability of assembly parts, came to be known as the *armory method,* replacing hand crafting, which at that time had been the prevailing method of manufacturing throughout the world.

173.1 Definitions

A general definition of a standard is given by Rowe [1983]: "A standard is a multi-party agreement for establishing an arbitrary criterion for reference." Each word used in here corresponds to a specific characteristic that helps to define the concept of a standard. *Multi* means more than one, party, organization, group, government, agency, or individual. *Agreement* means that these parties have come to some understanding of the issues involved and of ways to resolve them. This understanding has been confirmed by via some mechanism such as unanimity, consensus, ballots, or any other means. *Establishing* defines the purpose of the agreement—to create the standard. *Arbitrary* emphasizes the understanding by the parties that there are no absolute criteria in creating the standard. Rather, the conditions and values chosen are based on the most appropriate knowledge and conditions available at the time the standard was established. *Criteria* are features and conditions that the parties to the agreement have chosen as the basis for the standard.

A different type of definition of a standard is given in the United States Office of Management and Budget circular A-119:

> . . . a prescribed set of rules, conditions, or requirements concerned with the definition of terms; classification of components; delineation of procedures; specifications of materials, performance, design, or operations; or measurement of quality and quality in describing materials, products, systems, services, or practices.

In general, a *code* is a compilation of standards relating to a particular area of concern. For example, local government health codes contain standards relating to providing health care to members of the community. A *regulation* is an organization's way of specifying that some particular standard must be adhered to. Standards, codes, and regulations may or may not have legal implications, depending on whether the promulgating organization is governmental or private.

173.2 Standards for Clinical Engineering

There is a continually growing body of standards that affects health care facilities and hence clinical engineering. The practitioner of health care technology must constantly search out, evaluate, and apply appropriate standards. The means to reconcile the conflicts of technology, the different jurisdictions involved, and the implementation of the various standards are not necessarily apparent. One technique that addresses these concerns and has proven to yield a consistent practical approach is a structured framework of the various levels of standards. This hierarchy of standards is a conceptual model that the clinical engineer can use to evaluate and to apply to the various requirements that exist in health care technology.

Standards have different purposes, depending on their particular applications. A hierarchy of standards can be used to delineate those conditions for which a particular standard applies. There are four basic categories, any one or all of which may be in simultaneous operation: (1) *local* or *proprietary standards* (perhaps more properly called *regulations*) are developed to meet the internal needs of a particular organization; (2) *common-interest standards* serve to provide uniformity of product or service throughout an industry or profession; (3) *consensus standards* are agreements among interested participants to address an area of mutual concern; and (4) *regulatory standards* are mandated by an authority having jurisdiction to define a particular aspect of concern. In addition, there are two categories of standards adherence: (1) *voluntary standards*, which carry no inherent power of enforcement but provide a reference point of mutual understanding, and (2) *mandatory standards*, which are incumbent on those to whom the standard is addressed and enforceable by the authority having jurisdiction.

The hierarchy of standards model can aid the clinical engineer in the efficient and proper use of standards. More important, it can provide standards developers, users, and the authorities having jurisdiction in these matters with a structure through which standards can be effectively developed, recognized, and used to the benefit of all.

173.3 A Hierarchy of Standards

Local or proprietary standards are developed for what might be called internal use. An organization that wishes to regulate, control, or oversee certain of its own activities issues its own standards. Thus the standard is local in the sense that it is applied in a specific venue, and it is proprietary in that it is the creation of a completely independent administration. For example, an organization will standardize on a single type of a particular monitor. This standardization can refer to a specific brand or model, or to specific functional or operational features. In a more formal sense, a local standard often may be referred to as an institutional *policy* and *procedure*. The policy portion is the why of it; the procedure portion is the how. It must be kept in mind that standards of this type that are too restrictive will limit innovation and progress, in that they cannot readily adapt to novel conditions. On the other hand, good local standards contribute to lower costs, operational efficiency, and a sense of coherence in the organization.

Sometimes, local standards may originate from requirements of a higher level of standards. For example, the Joint Commission for Accreditation of Healthcare Organizations (JCAHO) [formerly the Joint Commission for Hospital Accreditation (JCAH), a voluntary organization, but an organization that hospitals belong to for various reasons, e.g., accreditation, reimbursement, approval of training programs] does not set standards for what equipment should be used. Rather, the JCAHO requires that each hospital set its own standards on how equipment is selected and maintained. To monitor compliance with this requirement, the JCAHO inspects whether the hospital follows its own standards. In one sense, the most damaging evidence that can be adduced against an organization (or an individual) is that it (he or she) did not follow its (his or her) own standards.

Common-interest standards are based on a need recognized by interested parties that will further their own interests. Such standards are generally accepted by affected interests without being made mandatory by an authority having jurisdiction; hence they are one type of voluntary standard. These standards are often developed by trade or professional organizations to promote uniformity in a product or process. This type of standard may have no inducement to adherence except for the benefits to the individual participants. For example, if you manufacture a kitchen cabinet that is not of standard size, it will not fit into the majority of kitchens and thus it will not sell. Uniformity of screw threads is another example of how a product can be manufactured and used by diverse parties and yet be absolutely interchangeable. More recently, various information-transfer standards allow the interchange of computer-based information among different types of instruments and computers.

Consensus standards are those which have been developed and accepted in accordance with certain well-defined criteria so as to assure that all points of view have been considered. Sometimes, the adjective *consensus* is used as a modifier for a *voluntary standard*. Used in this context, *consensus* implies that all interested parties have been consulted and have come to a general agreement on the provisions of the standard. The development of a consensus standard follows an almost ritualistic procedure so that fairness and due process are maintained. There are various independent voluntary and professional organizations that sponsor and develop standards on a consensus basis (see below). Each such organization has its own particular rules and procedures to ensure that true concensus is achieved in developing a standard.

In particular, in the medical products field, standards are sometimes difficult to implement because of the independent nature of manufacturers and their high level of competition. A somewhat successful standards story is the adoption of the DIN configuration for ECG lead-cable connection by the Association for the Advancement of Medical Instrumentation (AAMI). The impetus for this standard was the accidental electrocution of several patients brought about by use of the previous industry standard lead connection (a bare metal pin, as opposed to the new recessed socket). Most (but not all) manufacturers of ECG leads and cables now adhere to this standard. Agreement on this matter is in sharp contrast to the inability of the health care manufacturing industry to implement a standard for ECG cable connectors. Even though a standard does exist (AAMI ECGC, 5/83), the physical configuration of the connector is not necessarily used by manufacturers in production, nor is it demanded by medical users in purchasing. Each manufacturer uses a different connector, leading to numerous problems in supply and incompatibility for users.

However, even though there have been some failures in standardization of product features, there also has been much progress in generating performance and test standards for medical devices. A number of independent organizations sponsor development of standards for medical devices. For example, the American Society for Testing and Materials (ASTM) has developed *Standard Specification for Minimum Performance and Safety Requirements for Components and Systems of Anesthesia Gas Machines* (F1161–88). Even though there is no statutory law that requires it, manufacturers no longer produce and thus hospitals can no longer purchase anesthesia machines without the built-in safety features specified in this standard. The Association for the Advancement of Medical Instrumentation has sponsored numerous standards that relate to performance of specific medical devices, such as defibrillators, electrosurgical instruments, and electronic sphygmomanometers. These standards are compiled in the AAMI publication *Essential Standards for Biomedical Equipment Safety and Performance*. The National Fire Protection Association (NFPA) publishes *Standard for Health Care Facilities* (NFPA 99), which covers a wide range of safety issues relating to facilities. Included are sections that deal with electricity and electrical systems, central gas and vacuum supplies, and environmental conditions. Special areas such as anesthetizing locations, laboratories, and hyperbaric facilities are addressed separately.

Mandatory standards have the force of law or other authority having jurisdiction. Mandatory standards imply that some authority has made them obligatory. Mandatory standards can be written by the authority having jurisdiction, or they can be adapted from documents prepared by others as proprietary or consensus standards. The authority having jurisdiction can be a local hospital or even a department within the hospital, a professional society, a municipal or state government, or an agency of the federal government that has regulatory powers.

In the United State, hospitals are generally regulated by a local city or county authority and/or by the state. These authorities set standards in the form of health codes or regulations, which have the force of law. Federal jurisdiction of medical devices falls under the purview of the Department of Health and Human Services, Public Health Service, Food and Drug Administration (FDA), Center for Devices and Radiological Health. Under federal law, manufacturers and distributors of medical devices are regulated under the Medical Device Amendments of 1976 (Public Law 94-295) and the

Radiation Control for Health and Safety Act of 1968 (Public Law 90-602). In addition, the Safe Medical Devices Act of 1990 (Public Law 90-629) requires that users of medical devices report adverse patient events that may be related to a medical device to the manufacturer or to the FDA in the case of a patient death. In addition, the FDA has established a voluntary program for reporting device problems that may not have caused an untoward patient event but have the potential for such an occurrence.

Section 513 of the 1976 act establishes three classifications for medical devices intended for human use:

Class I. General controls regulate devices for which controls other than performance standards or premarket approvals are sufficient to assure safety and effectiveness. Such controls include regulations that (1) prohibit adulterated or misbranded devices; (2) require domestic device manufacturers and initial distributors to register their establishments and list their devices; (3) grant FDA authority to ban certain devices; (4) provide for notification of risks and of repair, replacement, or refund; (5) restrict the sale, distribution, or use of certain devices; and (6) govern Good Manufacturing Practices, records, reports, and inspections. These minimum requirements apply also to Class II and Class III devices.

Class II. Performance Standards apply to devices for which general controls alone do not provide reasonable assurance of safety and efficacy, and for which existing information is sufficient to establish a performance standard that provides this assurance.

Class II devices must comply not only with general controls, but also with an applicable standard developed under Section 514 of the Act. Until performance standards are developed by regulation, only general controls apply.

Class III. Premarket Approval applies to devices for which general controls do not suffice or for which insufficient information is available to write a performance standard to provide reasonable assurance of safety and effectiveness. Also, devices which are used to support or sustain human life or to prevent impairment of human health, devices implanted in the body, and devices which present a potentially unreasonable risk of illness or injury. New Class III devices, those not "substantially equivalent" to a device on the market prior to enactment (May 28, 1976), must have approved Premarket Approval Applications (Section 510k).

Even though the Medical Device Amendments of 1976 call for federal standards to be written for medical devices, no such standards have been proposed by the FDA (see Class II above). Instead, the FDA has promulgated a more general type of standard, which is applicable to all types of products, i.e., a general controls provisions (see Class I above). The actual requirements can be found in the *Code of Federal Regulations*, Title 21, parts 800 to 895.

New devices can be introduced by two pathways. For devices that perform a new function or operate on a new principle, the FDA requires premarket approval (510k process). This process requires a "reasonable assurance of safety and effectiveness" before the item can enter the commercial market. For a device that duplicates the function of a device marketed in interstate commerce prior to May 28, 1976, except for certain high-risk items (see Class III above), the FDA will grant approval if the device is found to be "substantially equivalent" to the existing device. With either pathway, there can be a difference in interpretation of the law's key requirement phrases by the FDA and by the manufacturer, leading to delays in obtaining approval. Investigational and research devices that may be used clinically are not under FDA jurisdiction but rather are sanctioned by institutional review boards (IRB) via clinical trials protocols.

American National Standards

The tradition in the United States is that of voluntary standards. However, once a standard is adopted by an organization, it can be taken one step further. The American National Standards

Institute (ANSI) is a private, nongovernment, voluntary organization that acts as a coordinating body for standards development and recognition in the United States. If the development process for a standard meets the ANSI criteria of open deliberation of legitimate concerns, with all interested parties coming to a voluntary consensus, then the developers can apply (but are not required) to have their standard designated as an *American National Standard*. Such a designation does not make a standard any more legitimate, but it does offer some recognition as to the process by which. it has been developed. ANSI also acts as a clearinghouse for standards development so as to avoid duplication of effort by various groups that might be concerned with the same issues. ANSI is also involved as a U.S. coordinating body for many international standards activities.

An excellent source that lists existing standards and standards-generating organizations, both nationally and internationally, is the annually revised *Guide to Biomedical Standards* [Huang et al., 1993].

173.4 International Standards

Most sovereign nations have their own internal agency to set and enforce standards. However, in our present world of international cooperation and trade, standards are tending toward uniformity across national bounderies. This internationalization of standards is especially true since formation of the European Common Market. The aim here is to harmonize the standards of individual nations by promulgating directives for medical devices that address "essential requirements" [Freeman, 1993].

There are two major international standards-generating organizations, both based in Europe, the International Electrotechnical Commission [Commission Electrotechnique Internationale (CEI)] and the International Organization for Standardization.

The International Electrotechnical Commission (IEC), founded in 1906, oversees, on an international level, all matters relating to standards for electrical and electronic items. Membership in the IEC is held by a national committee for each nation. The U.S. National Committee (USNC) for IEC was founded in 1907 and since 1931 has been affiliated with ANSI. USNC has as its members representatives from professional societies, trade associations, testing laboratories, government entities, other organizations, and individual experts. The USNC appoints a technical advisor and a technical advisory group for each IEC committee and subcommittee to help develop a unified U.S. position. These advisory groups are drawn from groups that are involved in the development of related U.S. national standards.

Standards are developed by technical committees (TC), subcommittees (SC), and working groups (WG). IEC TC62, *Electrical Equipment in Medical Practice*, is of particular interest here. One of the basic standards of this technical committee is document 601-1, *Safety of Medical Electrical Equipment*, Part 1: *General Requirements for Safety*, 2d edition (1988) and its Amendment 1 (1991), along with document 601-1-1, *Safety Requirements for Medical Electrical Systems* (1992).

The International Organization for Standardization (ISO) oversees aspects of device standards other than those related to electrotechnology. This organization was formed in 1946 with a membership comprised of the national standards organizations of 26 countries. The purpose of the ISO is to "facilitate international exchange of goods and services and to develop mutual cooperation in intellectual, scientific, technological, and economic ability." ANSI has been the official U.S. representative to ISO since its inception. For each committee or subcommittee of the ISO in which ANSI participates, a U.S. technical advisory group (TAG) is formed. The administrator of the TAG is, typically, that same U.S. organization that is developing the parallel U.S. standard.

Technical committees (TC) of the ISO concentrate on specific areas of interest. There are technical committees, subcommittees, working groups, and study groups. One of the member national standards organizations serves as the secretariat for each of these technical bodies.

173.5 Compliance with Standards

Standards that were originally developed as voluntary standards may take on mandatory aspects. For example, consider the case cited above of the anesthesia machine standard developed by the

American Society for Testing and Materials. Manufacturers produce machines that comply with this standard for fear of not being able to sell nonstandard items and, perhaps more so, in fear of lawsuits in the event of an untoward event that implicates their product. The fact that manufacturers now only produce machines that meet this standard, in effect, makes this standard mandatory for new equipment.

Compliance with standards is often driven, at least in part, by monetary concerns, as noted above. Another example of such considerations are the Joint Commission for Accreditation of Healthcare Organizations' standards (requirements). This organization is a private body that hospitals accept as an accrediting agent. However, various health insurance organizations and physician specialty boards for resident education use accreditation by the JCAHO as a touchstone for minimum quality of activities. Thus an insurance company might not pay for care in a hospital that is not accredited, or a specialty board might not recognize resident training in such an institution.

A third means by which voluntary standards can become mandatory is by incorporation. Existing standards can be incorporated into a higher level of standards or codes. For example, various state and local governments incorporate standards developed by voluntary organizations, such as the National Fire Protection Association, into their own building and health codes. These standards then become, in effect, mandatory government regulations and have the force of (civil) law.

Finally, standards will be enforced and adhered to if they meet the needs of those who are affected by them. For example, consider a standard for safety and performance for a defibrillator. For the manufacturer, acceptance and sales are a major consideration in both the domestic and international markets. People responsible for specifying, selecting, and purchasing equipment may insist on adherence to the standard so as to guarantee safety and performance. The user, physician or other health care professional, will expect the instrument to have certain operational and performance characteristics to meet medical needs. Hospital personnel want a certain minimum degree of equipment uniformity for sureness of operation and ease of maintenance. The hospital's insurance company and risk manager want equipment that meets or exceeds recognized safety standards. Third-party payers, i.e., private insurance companies or government agencies, insist on equipment that is safe, efficacious, and cost-effective. Accreditation agencies, such as local health agencies or professional societies, often require equipment to meet certain standards. More basically, patients, workers, and society as a whole have an inherent right to fundamental safety. Finally, in our litigatious society, there is always the threat of civil action in the case of an untoward event in which a "nonstandard," albeit "safe," instrument was involved. Thus, even though no one has stated that "this standard must be followed," it is highly unlikely that any person or organization will have the temerity to manufacture, specify, or buy an instrument that does not "meet the standard."

173.6 Limitations of Standards

Standards are generated to meet the expectations of society. They are developed by organizations and individuals to meet a variety of specific needs, with the general goal of promoting safety and efficiency. However, as with all human activities, problems with the interpretation and use of standards do occur. Under such conditions, engineering judgment is often required to provide answers. Thus the clinical engineer must consider the limits of standards, a boundary that is not clear and is constantly shifting. Yet clinical engineers must always employ the highest levels of engineering principles and practices. Some of the limitations and questions of standards and their use will be discussed below.

Noncompliance with a Standard

Sooner or later, it is likely that a clinical engineer will either be directly involved with or become aware of deviation from an accepted standard. The violation may be trivial, with no noticeable effect, or there may be serious consequences. In the former case, either the whole incident may be ignored, or nothing more may be necessary than a report that is filed away, or the incident can trigger corrective actions. In the latter case, there may be major repercussions involving investigation, censure, tort issues, or legal actions. In any event, lack of knowledge of the standard is generally not a convincing defence. Anyone who is in a position to require knowledge of a standard should know about that standard. More commonly, one might know the provisions of the standard and understand the potential risks of noncompliance. Nonetheless, noncompliance with that standard, in whole or in part, may be necessary to prevent a greater risk or to increase a potential benefit to the patient. In an emergency, drastic needs require drastic measures. In any event, noncompliance with a standard may have validity if reasonable evidence is offered to support the action. For example, when no other recourse is available, it would be defensable to use an electromagnet, condemned for irrepairable excessive leakage current, to save the eye of an injured person. Even if use of this device resulted in a physical injury or equipment damage, the potential benefit is a compelling argument for transgression of the applicable standard. A general disclaimer making allowance for emergency situations is often included in policy statements relating to adherence to a standard.

Standards and the Law

Standards that are mandated by a government body are not what is called "black letter law," i.e., a law actually entered into a criminal or civil code. Standards are typically not adopted in the same manner as laws, i.e., approved by a legislative body, ratified by an elected executive, and then sanctioned by the courts. The usual course for a mandated standard is via a legislative body enacting a law that establishes or assigns to an executive agency the authority to regulate the activities addressed. This agency, under the control of the executive branch of government, then issues standards that follow the mandate of its enabling legislation. The third branch of government, the judiciary, often must interpret the intent of the legislation in comparison with its implementation. This type of law falls under civil rather than criminal enforcement.

Nonadherence to a mandated standard does not necessarily lead to imprisonment or fine or even to a reprimand. The penalty for noncompliance with a standard is not criminal or even necessarily civil prosecution. Instead, there are administrative methods of enforcement as well as more subtle and powerful methods of coercion. The state has the power (and the duty) to regulate matters of public interest. Thus the state can withhold permits for construction, occupancy, or use. Possibly more effective, the state can withhold means of finance or payment to violators of its regulations.

Incorporation

Because of advances in technology and increases in societal expectations, standards are typically revised periodically. For example, the National Fire Protection Association revises and reissues its *Standard for Health Care Facilities* (NFPA 99) every 3 years. Other organizations follow a 5-year cycle of review, revision, and reissue of standards. These voluntary standards, developed in good faith, may be adapted by governmental agencies and made mandatory, as discussed above. When a standard is incorporated into a legislative code, it is generally referenced as to a particular version and date. It is not always the case that a newer version of the standard is more restrictive. For example, ever since 1984, the National Fire Protection Association *Standard for Health Care Facilities* (NFPA 99) does not require the installation of isolated power systems (isolation transformers and line isolation monitors) in anesthetizing locations that do not use flammable anesthetic agents or in areas that are not classified as wet locations. A previous version of this standard, *Standard for the Use of Inhalation Anesthetics (Flammable and Nonflammable)* (NFPA 56A-1978) did require isolated power. However, many state hospital codes have incorporated, by name and date, the provisions of NFPA 56A. Thus isolated power is still specified in new construction of all anesthetizing locations despite the absence of this requirement in the latest version of the standard that addresses this issue.

Safety

The primary purpose of standards in clinical practice is to ensure the safety of patient, operator, and bystanders. However, it must be fully appreciated that there is no such thing as absolute safety. The more safety features and regulations attached to a device, the less useful and the more cumbersome and costly may be its actual use. In the development, interpretation, and use of a standard, there are questions that must be asked: What is possible? What is acceptable? What is reasonable? Who will benefit? What is the cost? Who will pay?

None can deny that medical devices should be made as safe as possible, but some risk will always remain. In our practical world, absolute safety is a myth. Many medical procedures involve risk to the patient. The prudent physician or medical technologist will recognize the possible dangers of the equipment and take appropriate measures to reduce the risk to a minimum. Some instruments and procedures are inherently more dangerous than others. The physician must make a judgment, based on professional knowledge and experience, if using a particular device is less of a risk than using an alternative device or doing nothing. Standards will help—but they do not guarantee complete safety.

Liability

Individuals who serve on standards development committees, as well as organizations involved in such activities, are justifiably concerned with their legal position in the event that a lawsuit is instituted as a result of a standard that they helped to bring forth. Damages claimed in such a suit may not be limited to restraint of trade but can include any injury due to an act of commission or of omission relating to the standard. Organizations that sponsor standards or that appoint representatives to standards developing groups often have insurance for such activities. Independent standards committees and individual members of any standards committees may or may not be covered by insurance for participation in such activities. Although in recent times only one organization and no individual has been found liable for damages caused by improper use of standards, even the possibility of being named in a law suit will intimidate even the most self-confident "expert." Thus it is not at all unusual for an individual who is asked to serve on a standards development committee first to inquire as to liability insurance coverage. Organizations that develop standards or appoint representatives also take pains to ensure that all their procedures are carefully followed and documented so as to demonstrate fairness and prudence.

An organization that develops standards for general use throughout the country must abide by the law. The dark side of standards is the implication that particular individuals or groups issue a standard for their own benefit, e.g., to dominate sales in a particular market. If standards are developed or interpreted in an unfair manner or give an unfair advantage to one segment, then restraint-of-trade charges can be made. Organizations that sponsor standards that are in this sense unfair are held responsible. In 1982, the U.S. Supreme Court, in the *Hydrolevel* case [Perry, 1982], ruled that the American Society of Mechanical Engineers was guilty of antitrust activities because of the way some of its members, acting as a committee to interpret one of its standards, issued an opinion that limited competition in sales so as to unfairly benefit their own employers. This case remains a singular reminder that standards development and use must be inherently fair.

Inhibition

Another charge against standards is that they inhibit innovation and limit progress [Flink, 1984]. Ideally, standards should be written so that minimum requirements for safety, performance, and efficacy are met. Improvements or innovations would still be permitted so long as the basic standard is followed. From a device user's point of view, a standard that is excessively restrictive may limit the scope of permissible professional activities. If it is necessary to abrogate a standard in order to accommodate a new idea or to extend an existing situation, then the choices are to try to have the standard changed, which may be very time consuming, or to act in violation of the standard and accept the accompanying risks.

Ex Post Facto

A question continually arises as to what to do about old equipment (procedures, policies, facilities) when a new standard is issued or an old standard is revised so that existing items become obsolete. One approach is to do nothing, the theory being that the old equipment was acquired in good faith and conformed to the then-existing standards. As long as that equipment is usable and safe, there is no need to replace it. Another approach is to upgrade the existing equipment to meet the new standard. However, such modification may be technically impractical or financially prohibitive. Finally, one can simply throw out all the existing equipment (or sell it to a second-hand dealer, or use the parts for scrap) and buy everything new. This approach would bring a smile of delight from the manufacturer and a scream of outrage from the hospital administrator. Usually what is done is a compromise, incorporating various aspects of these different approaches.

Costs

Standards cost both time and money to propose, develop, promulgate, and maintain. Perhaps the greatest hindrance to more participation in standards activities by interested individuals is the lack of funds to attend meetings where the issues are discussed. Unfortunately, and perhaps with some truth, it is often said that organizations that can afford to sponsor individuals to attend such meetings have too much of an influence in the development of that standard. On the other hand, those organizations which do have a vital interest in a standard should have an appropriate say in its development. A consensus of all interested parties tempers the undue influence of any one of them.

Standards also increase the costs of manufacturing devices and carrying out procedures. This incremental cost is, in turn, passed on to the purchaser of the goods or services. Whether or not the increased cost justifies the benefits of the standard is not always apparent. However, it can be stated that, in general, standards have made a valuable contribution to progress, in the broadest sense of that word.

173.7 Conclusions

Standards are just like any other human activity; they can be well used or a burden, depending on their conditions of use. The danger of standards is that they will take on a life of their own and rather than serve a genuine need will exist only as a justification of their own importance. This view is expressed in the provocative and iconoclastic book by Bruner and Leonard [1989] and in particular in their Chapter 9, "Codes and Standards: Who Makes the Rules?" However, the raison d'être of standards is to do good. It is incumbent on clinical engineers not only to understand how to apply standards properly but also how to introduce, modify, and retire standards as conditions change. Furthermore, the limitations of standards must be recognized in order to get the maximum benefit from their use. No standard can replace diligence, knowledge, and a genuine concern for doing the right thing.

References

American Society for Testing and Materials (ASTM), 1916 Race Street, Philadelphia, PA 19103.
Association for the Advancement of Medical Instrumentation (AAMI), 3330 Washington Boulevard, Suite 400, Arlington, VA 22201.

Bruner JMR, Leonard PF. 1989. Electricity, Safety and the Patient. Chicago, Year Book Medical Publishers.

Flink R. 1984. Standards: Resource or constraint?, IEEE Eng Med Biol Magazine 3(1):14.

Freeman M. 1993. The EC medical devices directives. IEEE Eng Med Biol Magazine 12(2):79.

Huang LG, Brush LC, Nighswonger G, Pacela AF. 1993. The Guide to Biomedical Standards. LaBrea, Calif, Quest Publishing Co.

International Organization for Standardization (ISO), Central Secretariat, Case Postale 56, CH-1211, Geneva 20, Switzerland.

International Electrotechnical Commission (IEC), Central Office, 3, rue de Varembe, CH-1211 Geneva 20, Switzerland.

Joint Commission on Accreditation of Healthcare Facilities (JCAHO), 1 Renaissance Boulevard, Oakbrook, IL 60181.

National Fire Protection Association (NFPA), Batterymarch Park, Quincy, MA 02269.

Perry TS. 1982. Antirust ruling chills standards setting. IEEE Spect 19(8):52.

Rowe WD. 1983. Design and performance standards. In CA Caceres et al (eds), Medical Devices: Measurements, Quality Assurance, and Standards, pp 29–40. Philadelphia, American Society for Testing and Materials.

174

Regulatory and Assessment Agencies

Mark E. Bruley
ECRI

Vivian H. Coates
ECRI

Effective management and development of clinical and biomedical engineering departments (hereafter called *clinical engineering departments*) in hospitals require a basic knowledge of relevant regulatory and technology assessment agencies. Regulatory agencies set standards of performance and record keeping for the departments and for the technology they are responsible for. Technology assessment agencies are information resources for what should be an ever-expanding role of the clinical engineer in the technology decision-making processes of the hospital's administration.

This chapter presents an overview of regulatory and technology assessment agencies in the United States, Canada, Europe, and Australia that are germane to clinical engineering. Due to the extremely large number of such agencies and information resources, we have chosen to focus on those of greatest relevance and/or informational value. The reader is directed to the references and sources of further information presented at the end of the chapter.

174.1 Regulatory Agencies

Within the health care field, there are over 23,000 applicable standards, clinical practice guidelines, laws, and regulations [ECRI, 1994]. Voluntary standards are promulgated by over 600 organizations; mandatory standards, by numerous state and federal agencies. Many of these organizations and agencies issue guidelines that are relevant to the vast range of health care technologies within the responsibility of clinical engineering departments. Although many of these agencies also regulate the manufacture and clinical use of health care technology, such regulations are not directly germane to the management of a clinical department and are not presented.

For the clinical engineer, many agencies promulgate regulations and standards in the areas of, for example, electrical safety, fire safety, technology management, occupational safety, radiology and nuclear medicine, clinical laboratories, infection control, anesthesia and respiratory equipment, power distribution, and medical gas systems. In the United States, medical device problem reporting is also regulated by many state agencies and by the U.S. Food and Drug Administration (FDA) via its MEDWATCH program. It is important to note that, at present, the only direct regulatory authority that the FDA has over U.S. hospitals is in the reporting of medical device–related accidents that result in serious injury or death. The prior chapter in this section by Alvin Wald discusses in

0-8493-8346-3/95/$0.00+$.50
© 1995 by ECRI. Reprinted with permission.

detail many of the specific agency citations. Presented below are the names and addresses of the primary agencies whose codes, standards, and regulations have the most direct bearing on clinical engineering and technology management.

American Hospital Association
840 North Lake Shore Drive
Chicago, IL 60611
(312) 280-6374

American National Standards Institute
11 West 42nd Street
13th Floor
New York, NY 10036
(212) 642-4900

American Society for Hospital Engineering
840 North Lake Shore Drive
Chicago, IL 60611
(312) 280 5223

American Society for Testing and Materials
1916 Race Street
Philadelphia, PA 19103
(215) 299-5400

Association for the Advancement of
    Medical Instrumentation
3330 Washington Boulevard
Suite 400
Arlington, VA 22201
(703) 525-4890

Australian Institute of Health and Welfare
GPO Box 570
Canberra, ACT 2601
Australia
(61) 06-243-5092

British Standards Institution
2 Park Street
London, W1A 2BS
United Kingdom
(44) 071-629-9000

Canadian Hospital Association
17 York Street
Suite 100
Ottawa, ON K1N 9J6
Canada
(613) 238-8005

Canadian Standards Association
178 Rexdale Boulevard
Rexdale, ON M9W 1R3
Canada
(416) 747-6776

Compressed Gas Association, Inc.
1725 Jefferson Davis Highway
Suite 1004
Arlington, VA 22202
(703) 412-0900

ECRI
5200 Butler Pike
Plymouth Meeting, PA 19462
(610) 825-6000
(610) 834-1275 fax

Environmental Health Directorate
Health Protection Branch
Health and Welfare Canada
19th Floor, Jeanne Mance Building
Tunney's Pasture
Ottawa, ON K1A 0L2
Canada
(613) 954-0291

Food and Drug Administration
MEDWATCH, FDA Medical Products
Reporting Program
5600 Fishers Lane
Rockville, MD 20857-9787
(800) 332-1088

Institute of Electrical and Electronics
    Engineers
445 Hoes Lane
P.O. Box 1331
Piscataway, NJ 08850-1331
(908) 562-3800

Int'l Electrotechnical Commission
Box 131
3 rue de Varembe, CH 1211
Geneva 20
Switzerland
(41) 022-734-0150

International Organization for Standardization
1 rue de Varembe
Case postale 56, CH 1211
Geneva 20
Switzerland
(41) 022-347-6755

Joint Commission on Accreditation
  of Healthcare Organizations
One Renaissance Boulevard
Oakbrook Terrace, IL 60181
(708) 916-5600

Medical Device Directorate
Department of Health
Room 222
14 Russell Square
London, WC1B 5EP
United Kingdom
(44) 71-636-6811

National Council on Radiation Protection
  and Measurements
7910 Woodmont Avenue, Suite 800
Bethesda, MD 20814
(310) 657-2652

National Fire Protection Association
1 Batterymarch Park
Quincy, MA 02269-9101
(617) 770-3000

Nuclear Regulatory Commission
11555 Rockville Pike
Rockville, MD 20852
(301) 492-7000

Occupational Safety and Health Administration
U.S. Department of Labor
Office of Information and Consumer Affairs
200 Constitution Avenue, NW
Room N3647
Washington, DC 20210
(202) 219-8151

ORKI
National Institute for Hospital
  and Medical Engineering
Budapest dios arok 3, H-1125
Hungary
(33) 1-156-1522

Russian Scientific and Research Institute
Russian Public Health Ministry
EKRAN, 3 Kasatkina St.
Moscow
Russia 129301
(44) 071-405-3474

Society of Nuclear Medicine, Inc.
136 Madison Avenue
8th Floor
New York, NY 10016
(212) 889-0717

Standards Association of Australia
GPO Box 105
Strathfield, NSW 2135
Australia
(61) 02-746-4600

Underwriters Laboratories, Inc.
333 Pfingsten Road
Northbrook, IL 6062
(708) 272-8800

VTT
Technical Research Center of Finland
Postbox 316
SF-33101 Tampere 10
Finland
(358) 31-163300

174.2 Technology Assessment Agencies

Technology assessment is the practical process of determining the value of a new or emerging technology in and of itself or against existing or competing technologies using efficacy, effectiveness, outcome, risk-management, strategic, financial, and competitive criteria. Technology assessment also considers ethics and law as well as health priorities and cost-effectiveness compared with competing technologies. A *technology* is defined as devices, equipment, related software, drugs, biotechnologies, procedures, and therapies and systems used to diagnose or treat patients. The processes of technology assessment are discussed in detail in Chap. 1660

Technology assessment is not the same as technology acquisition/procurement or technology planning. The latter two are processes for determining equipment vendors, soliciting bids, and systematically determining a hospital's technology-related needs based on strategic, financial, risk-management, and clinical criteria. The informational needs differ greatly between technology assessment and the acquisition/procurement or planning processes. This section focuses on the resources applicable to technology assessment.

Worldwide, there are nearly 300 organizations (private, academic, and governmental) providing technology assessment information, databases, or consulting services. Some are strictly information clearinghouses, some perform technology assessment, and some do both. For those which perform assessments, the quality of the information generated varies greatly from superficial studies to in-depth, well-referenced analytical reports.

Language limitations are a significant issue. In the ultimate analysis, the ability to undertake technology assessment requires assimilating vast amounts of information, most of which exists only in the English language. Technology assessment studies published by the International Society for Technology Assessment in Health Care (ISTAHC), by the World Health Organization, and by other umbrella organizations are generally in English. The new International Health Technology Assessment (IHTA) database being developed by ECRI in conjunction with the U.S. National Library of Medicine contains more than 20,000 citations to technology assessments and related documents.

Below are the names and addresses of some of the most prominent organizations undertaking technology assessment studies:

Agence Nationale pour le Developpement
   de l'Evaluation Medical (ANDEM)
5 bis, rue Pérignon, 75015
Paris, France

American Association of Preferred
   Provider Organizations
601 13th Street, NW
Suite 370 South
Washington, DC 20005
(202) 347-7600

American College of Obstetricians and
   Gynecologists
409 12th Street, SW
Washington, DC 20024
(202) 863-2518

American College of Radiology
1891 Preston White Drive
Reston, VA 22091
(703) 648-8900

American Hospital Association
840 N Lake Shore Drive
Chicago, IL 60611
(312) 280-6374

American Medical Association
515 North State Street
Chicago, IL 60610
(312) 464-5000

Australian Institute of Health and Welfare
GPO Box 570
Canberra, ACT 2601
Australia
(61) 06-243-5092

Battelle Medical Technology Assessment
   and Policy Research Center (MEDTAP)
901 D Street, SW
Washington, DC 20024
(202) 479-0500

British Columbia Office of Health
Technology Assessment
Centre for Health Services and Policy
   Research
S 184 Koerner Pavilion
2211 Westbrook Mall
University of British Columbia
Vancouver, BC
Canada
(604) 822-7049

Canadian Coordinating Office for Health
   Technology Assessment
110-955 Green Valley Crescent
Ottawa ON K2C 3V4
Canada
(613) 226-2553

Center for Medical Technology Assessment
Linköping University
5183 Linköping, Box 1026 (551-11)
Sweden
(46) 13-281-000

Conseil d'Evaluation des Technologies
   de la Santé de Québec
800 Tour de la Place Victoria
Bureau 4205, 42e
Boite postale 215
Montreal, PQ H4Z 1E3
Canada
(514) 873-2563

ECRI
5200 Butler Pike
Plymouth Meeting, PA 19462
(610) 825-6000

Ferno-Washington, Inc.
70 Weil Way
Wilmington, OH 45177-9371
(513) 382-1451

Frost and Sullivan, Inc.
106 Fulton Street
New York, NY 10038-2786
(212) 233-1080

Health Council of the Netherlands
Gezondheidsraad
P.O. Box 90517
2509 LM
The Hague
The Netherlands
(31) 70-347-1441

Health Services Directorate
Health Services Systems Division
Health and Welfare Canada
R 660, Jeanne Mance Building
Tunney's Pasture
Ottawa, ON K1A 1B4
Canada
(613) 941-6391

Hong Kong Institute of Engineers
9/F Island Centre
No. 1 Great George Street
Causeway Bay
Hong Kong

Institute for Clinical PET
2111 Wilson Boulevard
Suite 850
Arlington, VA 22201
(703) 516-9255

Institute of Medicine (U.S.)
2102 Constitution Avenue, NW
Washington, DC 20418

Medical Alley
1550 Utica Avenue, South
Suite 725
Minneapolis, MN 55416
(612) 542-3077

Medical Devices Directorate
Department of Health
Room 222
14 Russell Square
London, WC1B 5EP
United Kingdom
(44) 071-636-6811

Miller Freeman, Inc.
600 Harrison Street
San Francisco, CA 94107
(415) 905-2200

National Center for Nursing Research, NIH
9000 Rockville Pike
Building 38
Bethesda, MD 20892
(301) 496-4000

National Committee of Clinical Laboratory
   Standards (NCCLS)
771 E. Lancaster Avenue
Villanova, PA 19085
(215) 525-2435

New York Department of Health
Tower Building
Empire State Plaza
Albany, NY 12237
(518) 474-7354

Office Tecnica d'Avaluacio Technologica
Medical (OTATM), Ministry of Health
Catalonia
Barcelona, Spain

Physician Payment Review Commission
   (PPRC) (U.S.)
2120 L Street NW
Suite 510
Washington, DC 20037
(202) 653-7220

Saskatchewan Association of Health
   Organizations
Urban Hospital Branch
1445 Park Street
Regina, SK S4N 4C5
Canada
(306) 347-5500

Swedish Council on Technology
Assessment in Health Care
Box 16158
S-103 24 Stockholm
Sweden
(46) 08-611-1913

Swiss Institute of Public Health
Health Technology Program
Pfrundweg 14
CH-5001 Aarau
Switzerland

TNO Health Research
Center for Medical Technology
Zernikedreef 9
P.O. Box 430
2300 AK Leiden
The Netherlands
(31) 71-18-18-18

University Hospital Consortium
2001 Spring Street
Suite 700
Oakbrook, IL 60521
(708) 954-1700

University of Leeds
School of Public Health
30 Hyde Terrace
Leeds L52 9LN
United Kingdom

University of York
Center for Health Economics
Heslington, York
England

University of York
Centre for Health Services
York Y01 5DD
United Kingdom

U.S. Agency for Health Care Policy and Research
Office of Health Technology Assessment
6000 Executive Boulevard
Suite 309
Rockville, MD 208052
(301) 443-2403

U.S. Office of Technology Assessment
600 Pennsylvania Avenue
Washington, DC 20003
(202) 224-8996

U.S. Preventive Services Task Force
Office of Disease Prevention and Health
   Promotion
330 C Street SW
Room 2132
Washington, DC 20201
(202) 205-8611

Voluntary Hospitals of America, Inc.
220 East Las Colinas Boulevard
Irving, TX 75014
(214) 830-0000

References

ECRI. 1994. Healthcare Standards Official Directory. ECRI, Plymouth Meeting, Pa.
Eddy DM. 1992. A Manual for Assessing Health Practices and Designing Practice Policies: The Explicit Approach. Philadelphia, American College of Physicians.

Goodman C (ed). 1988. Medical Technology Assessment Directory. Washington, National Academy
      Press.
Marcaccio KY (ed). 1993. Gale Directory of Databases, vol 1: Online Databases. London, Gale
      Research International.
van Nimwegen Chr (ed). 1993. International List of Reports on Comparative Evaluations of Medical
      Devices. Leiden, The Netherlands, TNO Centre for Medical Technology.

Further Information

A comprehensive listing of health care standards and the issuing organizations is presented in the
Healthcare Standards Directory published by ECRI. The directory is well organized by keywords, organizations and their standards, federal and state laws, and legislation and regulations and contains
a complete index of names and addresses.

   The IHTA database is produced by ECRI. A portion of the database is also available in the U.S.
National Library of Medicine's new database called HSTAR (health services technology assessment
research).

175

Clinical Engineering Issues in Developing Countries

Hashem Odeh Al-Fadel
King Faisal Specialist Hospital and Research Center

Many of the developing countries of today were involved in developing medical devices hundreds of years ago when Europe was still in the dark ages. For example, genius medical scientists and engineers developed acupuncture instrumentation in China over 1000 years ago, while other well-defined instruments and devices were developed by the Arabs, Indians, and even much earlier by the ancient Egyptians, Romans, and Greeks.

With the rapid development that was achieved by the industrialized world, due to its wealth in resources, knowledge, research, and organization, the health care system became the most developed in the world, thereby creating an enormous demand for better, newer, and more technologically advanced equipment. And in order to meet this rapidly expanding demand, medical equipment manufacturing has flourished and, in the process, has developed various new types of medical equipment in order to meet the needs of health care institutions.

In recent times, particularly during the fourth quarter of the twentieth century, sophisticated medical equipment has become the main reason and factor in the advancement of health care technology. With this trend, diffusion of this technology began to spread throughout the world. Governments started to pay attention to health care support, and as a result, the death rates among infants, children, and adults have declined. Even though medical instrumentation has spread to developing countries, it is still far insufficient as compared with developed countries, but with this spread, many countries are not keeping up with the support requirement, as will be pointed out in this chapter.

Currently, different types of medical equipment of various levels of technology or stages of development are found in developing countries. It is often found that technology of the 1930s is mixed with that of the 1990s. With the existence of extreme shortages of resources, poor condition of equipment, and lack of proper support, much of the existing equipment in developing countries is found idle or not properly utilized.

Although clinical engineering departments exist in many countries, they may be found to be equivalent to that in the United States 20 years ago. Many hospitals do not have clinical engineering departments, and equipment support has *never* been taken into consideration. Also, the clinical engineering departments that do exist, lack support, recognition, and adequate training. This is also due to numerous other constraints and problems facing this field.

The purpose of this chapter is to provide an overview of clinical engineering issues in developing countries. Even though these issues may differ from country to country, they are predominately found in developing countries. The issues to be presented are related to medical equipment, clinical engineering, and related constraints. In addition, possible solutions will be discussed.

175.1 Medical Equipment

Developing countries spend far less of a percentage of their GNP on the health care system compared with the industrialized world due to limited resources and insufficient hard currency. It is estimated to be 0.5% to 1.5% compared with 5% to 15% [3] in the more developed countries. Medical equipment purchasing is not well regulated but is controlled mainly by the individual hospitals themselves and the local government agencies, i.e., ministries of health. Table 175.1 illustrates a survey conducted by the author and other colleagues who worked for an international health care organization in China, (1987–1989). The table shows the amount of equipment with a value of over $2700 (10,000 Yuan, 1989 rate). Even though the survey is not comprehensive, it shows, in general, the level of medical equipment availability.

The role of clinical engineers in prepurchasing evaluations in most of the developing countries is very limited. The majority of equipment purchasing decisions are decided by the director of the hospital either alone or with clinicians. As a result of improper prepurchase planning, equipment utilization and proper installation/operation are far from optimal, since they require technical knowledge and expertise. In many cases, you find a large percentage of the available equipment in hospitals not installed or not used due to lack of training, consumables, or accessories to keep them running. Other equipment is also not used primarily due to lack of proper maintenance [2]. In some cases, it is not surprising to find that a machine is not being used because the operator's manual is in a different language.

Fast developing countries with good resources (some of which can be considered developed countries) usually give more emphasis to health care, and thus some hospitals are well equipped and the equipment is purchased in a more appropriate way as compared with developing countries. For example, in Saudi Arabia, there are hospitals, such as the King Faisal Specialist Hospital, with health care support level and facilities that may even exceed those of many hospitals in the industrial world.

Most equipment in developing countries is imported from the industrial world. Table 175.2 provides the source of medical equipment imports in Chinese hospitals in 1991 as an example.

In addition to purchased medical equipment, donated equipment is very common in many of the developing countries' hospitals. Most equipment is donated randomly by the industrialized world without taking into consideration the specific needs and requirements. As a result, most of the equipment is found idle and/or not properly used. Consequently, this causes space shortages and

TABLE 175.1 Survey of Reported Available Equipment

Hospital	No. of Pieces of Equipment	No. of Beds	BME Dept.
Shanghai No. 9	120	757	
Beijing First	98	1073	
Beijing People's	74	414	
Beijing Stomatology	28	100	
Beijing Third	79	543	
Hangzhou Children's	55	460	X
Xian Dental	79	100	
Beijing Mental Hospital	5	100	
Ruijin Shanghai	89	1140	X
Second Hospital Hangzhou	72	600	X
Xinhua Shanghai	86	1036	X
TOTAL	785	6323	

TABLE 175.2 Chinese Medical Equipment Imports, 1991

	Electromedical Equipment	X-Ray Apparatus
United States	54,116 (38.4%)	26,001 (26.8%)
Japan	44,259 (31.4%)	42,081 (43.4%)
Germany	19,177 (13.6%)	20,097 (20.7%)
Hongkong	6,240 (4.4%)	1,342 (1.4%)
Netherlands	2,246 (1.6%)	2,092 (2.2%)
Other	14,848 (10.5%)	5,389 (5.6%)
WORLD	140,886 (100.0%)	97,002 (100.0%)

Note: Import market share (figures in U.S. $000).
Source: International Medical Equipment Services. 1993. A World Review [2].

other problems. The reason behind this situation includes lack of training, inappropriate power requirements, the equipment requires supplied and consumables that are hard to obtain, some pieces of equipment were donated defective from their origin, and lack of proper support and service. In order to make sure that equipment will be used effectively, it is important to take into consideration (when donating equipment) that it must be working properly, simple to operate in nature, and have a minimum or no requirement for consumables and accessories. Also, it is important that service and operation manuals accompany the equipment in simple English. Otherwise, the donated equipment will become a burden rather than a help to these countries.

It is important to note that manufacturers also should take into consideration various design factors when making equipment to be sold to developing countries. Equipment must not be sophisticated with a large number of bells and whistles that will complicate its operation because clinicians and nurses, in general, lack familiarity with advanced technology, since their education provides little opportunity for hands-on training. Another important design consideration is the ability to handle extreme environmental conditions, since in many countries, air-conditioning and heating are not available, in addition to large quantities of dust, dirt, sand, and extreme levels of temperature and humidity. And last but not the least, the lack of and difficulty in obtaining spare parts and consumable supplies also should be taken into consideration.

175.2 Clinical Engineering

Clinical engineering departments are qualified for equipment support tasks if given the opportunity, resources, and administrative support. Similar to what existed in the United States over 20 years ago, clinical engineering departments in many developing countries today exist as fix-it shops that concentrate on repairing simple equipment, and only major hospitals may include such capabilities. Programs such as preventive maintenance, incoming inspection, prepurchase evaluations, etc. are very limited or for the most part nonexistent. Even though some of them are called departments, most of them are part of other departments such as plant engineering, engineering, and purchasing departments.

As illustrated in Table 175.1, only four clinical engineering departments existed in these 11 teaching hospitals until 1989. These hospitals represent a very small number of the 62,000 hospitals and health centers in China (50,000 rural and 12,000 general/teaching hospitals) with a total of approximately 2.6 million beds [4].

Education

The technical staff members of the biomedical departments are usually graduates of local universities or vocational colleges. Many universities and colleges started teaching biomedical engineering in the late seventies and early eighties. Many curricula are based on programs that are taught in the United States and Europe. However, hands-on laboratory experience is limited as compared with that in the industrial world. It is essential that the developing world should have its own dedicated curricula based on needs that varies from those in the industrialized world, where students are prepared for industry, research, hospitals, and other areas [1]. Education needs to be focused on hands-on laboratory education with appropriate theoretical background and appropriate practical courses. Even though internships are found, they are limited and not developed; they need to be organized, structured, and practical, and such programs must be a part of the requirements in every program in biomedical engineering in order to meet the practical needs of the health care system.

Services

The major types of equipment are normally maintained by local vendors under the "supervision" of the user departments with little or no involvement from the clinical engineering staff. An independent third-party service industry is mostly nonexistent.

The clinical engineering shops are often called by various names, in which *biomedical engineering* is by far the predominant title. The number of technical staff members varies from department to department and is not dependent on any particular criterion. The number of staff members needed should not be dependent on bed size but rather on equipment number that can be maintained and the range, type, and complexity of equipment that will be maintained. The reason is based on the work hours of the week, training level, motivation, availability of staff at work, long vacations, and other factors. Repair service is usually troubleshot to the component level, which may take days or weeks to complete, and therefore, more staff members would be required as compared with hospitals in developed countries. Responsibilities per technician could range from 25 to 150 pieces of equipment with a value of over $2000 each.

Training

In general, factory service training is very limited, since it rarely is considered at the time of purchase. Some international health care organizations (based in the industrial world) started in the late seventies to provide clinical engineering training programs in a number of developing countries. Consequently, different types of training programs have been provided, including the following:

1. *Long-term/short-term consultant training programs.* Consultants usually assist in establishing clinical engineering departments in hospitals and provide assistance in setting up and providing training programs. Long-term training of 1 year or more usually is more effective than a few weeks/months training visit. The training programs also include setting up and assisting in the establishment and support of clinical engineering education in vocational colleges and universities. Even though the effectivity of such programs may vary from one country to another or one university/college to another, in general, their effectivity is far from optimal. The university training side is, however, more effective than that of hospital clinical engineering, since hospital administration usually places clinical engineering issues at the lower end of its priority list. Usually, such training programs can succeed as long as they are being supported by international organizations. Once an organization leaves after making the program reach a certain level, the chance that it will go back to square one is most likely expected, since many of the trained engineers will find better paid positions in the private sector and less emphasis will be given to clinical engineering from the administrators' side.

2. *Sending engineers to be trained in one or more hospitals in the industrial world.* As expected, this will have the least effect from many countries; either many of the staff who are sent for training will not likely go back to their home country, or if they return, they eventually will go to the private sectors or other types of work.

3. *Establishing a manufacturer/host joint venture training center in the host country to be affiliated with one of the teaching hospitals or universities.* This is another approach to training. Vendors can participate in exhibiting their products and establish workshops to provide service support. Students and engineers can then get training in these established service centers. In

return, they can assist the vendors in supporting their equipment, at least during the warranty period, and may get some incentives as well, if allowed. This program can prove to be the most beneficial if supported by hospitals and/or the ministry of health.

4. There are other types of training that are organized for developing countries either in the developed countries or locally. This includes sending factory-trained engineers and specialists to hold service training seminars to train and repair a large number of defective devices. In addition, others conduct training workshops for developing countries' technical staff, which has already been started by the American College of Clinical Engineering.

175.3 Clinical Engineering's Constraints

Some of the constraints that face the development of clinical engineering have already been pointed out briefly in the preceding sections. In this section, an overview of major issues that hinder the development of clinical engineering support to hospitals will be provided.

1. *Shortage of monetary resources and lack of budget support.* This is due to a shortage of hard currencies and limited budgets that eventually affect the establishment of an effective clinical engineering operation. As such, staff members are poorly paid, and resources for test equipment parts, etc. are not easily available because allocated budget for support is small or nonexistent. Therefore, the motivation of engineers and technicians, in most cases, is low, and equipment support will, of course, suffer. Due to this shortage and a lack of awareness by administrators about equipment-related issues, clinical engineering support is rarely considered. It is not surprising to notice in some countries that buying a replacement machine could be easier than buying the part to get one fixed instead. This, of course, is contrary to the source of the problem.

2. *Logistical difficulties in obtaining spare parts.* In addition to the difficulties of obtaining funds to get parts, ordering, approving, custom clearing, and receiving may take a very long time in various countries due to red tape, in addition to improper storage and handling of spare parts. Also, manufacturers and their representatives sometime use spare parts distribution as a threat against in-house support.

3. *Extreme temperature and humidity level.* In many countries, imported equipment specifications do not meet the temperature and humidity requirements.

4. *Lack of trained technical staff members.* Trained personnel to support modern equipment are in short supply. The most skillful personnel leave for higher-paid jobs in the private sector. Many technical graduates choose other higher-paid jobs than clinical engineering. For example, some biomedical engineers may go for computer operators or other related fields.

5. *Lack of acceptance of hands-on work by engineers.* Most engineers do not prefer hands-on work because they associate their jobs with other traditional engineering professionals, such as mechanical or civil engineers. However, there is a trend recently in accepting more hands-on jobs due to equipment complexity, the opportunities for training, and the need for initial employment. In most countries, the word *engineer* is a title similar to *doctor*.

6. In some countries, clinical engineering personnel hold more than one job to meet their living standard requirements. This multiple employment causes less productivity and less dedication.

7. Cultural problems (that may not exist in the industrial world) have some negative impact on clinical engineering development. This includes the status gap between physicians, engineers, and technicians. This often results in less cooperation in technology support. For instance, physicians in many hospitals will not allow engineers to work on "their" equipment even for repair, let alone preventive maintenance, due to the lack of trust and cooperation. It is also not surprising to find a technician performing trivial nontechnical tasks.

8. Other political constraints result from possible conflict of interests in purchasing decisions which can limit the participation of the clinical engineering staff.

The constraints pointed above are not all present in every developing country but may vary from one country to another. Therefore, different solution strategies will be required on a per-case basis.

175.4 Future Outlook

The issues in developing countries that were presented in this chapter are not impossible to solve, even though they seem very difficult. Since clinical engineering support provides savings, reliability, longer life cycle of equipment, and safety, it is not difficult to provide justification to top officials in order to raise its priority, after which proper technology support can eventually be achieved. This can be done by strategic solutions on the national and local levels. Some of the solutions for a brighter future outlook for clinical engineering involvement are as follows.

First, government institutions need to establish effective, long-standing policies for health care systems to include equipment acquisition, support, and utilization among other important factors that do not change when a top official is replaced. This could be in a form of a certifying agency to certify hospitals for accepted practice. Such groups could establish policies and procedural guidelines for various health care aspects and provide career paths, career structures, and appropriate monitory and nonmonitory incentives (such as salaries and benefits).

Second, establishing or updating clinical engineering education programs and vocational technical training to meet the required needs and to be more practical. Education must include appropriate and organized internship programs.

Third, in-house clinical engineering departments should be established and developed to perform the required functions. Hospital administration support is crucial in order to meet this objective. The role of these departments should include prepurchasing evaluation, incoming inspection, preventive maintenance, repair, and training, among other functions. Management should support and approve, when needed, test equipment, spare part kits, and training requirements as part of the purchase from the original budget. Service and operation manuals are a must with every piece of equipment purchased. Otherwise, the purchased equipment will end up idle or not utilized shortly after purchase. Clinical engineering leaders should press these issues and provide regular awareness meetings and seminars to management and users on the importance and impact of these issues.

Lastly, cooperation of various hospitals in group purchasing and in supporting the current technology is important if political difficulties between them are ironed by higher authorities. As such, cooperation between departments such as clinical engineering from different hospitals will be very beneficial. Forming societies, associations, or clubs to start regular professional gatherings for arranging presentations on new technology to study and provide solutions to existing problems will have a positive impact if support is given by top management or high-level officials. With these organizations, innovative preventive solutions can be found toward proper technology support in order to solve some of the problems mentioned earlier.

The clinical engineering support system can be viewed as the "heart" of medical equipment technology effectiveness. It is important to make this "heart" pump effectively and to solve any occlusion that could prevent it from functioning properly. The survival/establishment of clinical engineering in developing and developed countries is the best indicator for an effective and cost-saving health care technology system.

References

1. Morahold FA. 1992. Biomedical R&D: The Venezuelan experience. IEEE Eng Med Biol 11(3):26.
2. Mridha, et al. 1988. Clinical engineering challenges and problems with medical instrumentations in Bangladesh. J Clin Eng 13(4):275.
3. Schmitt JM, Al-Fadel H. 1989. Design of medical instrumentation for application in developing countries. J Clin Eng 14(4):299.
4. International Medical Equipment Services. 1993. A World Review, 1994, vol 1, no 1, pp 22–27.

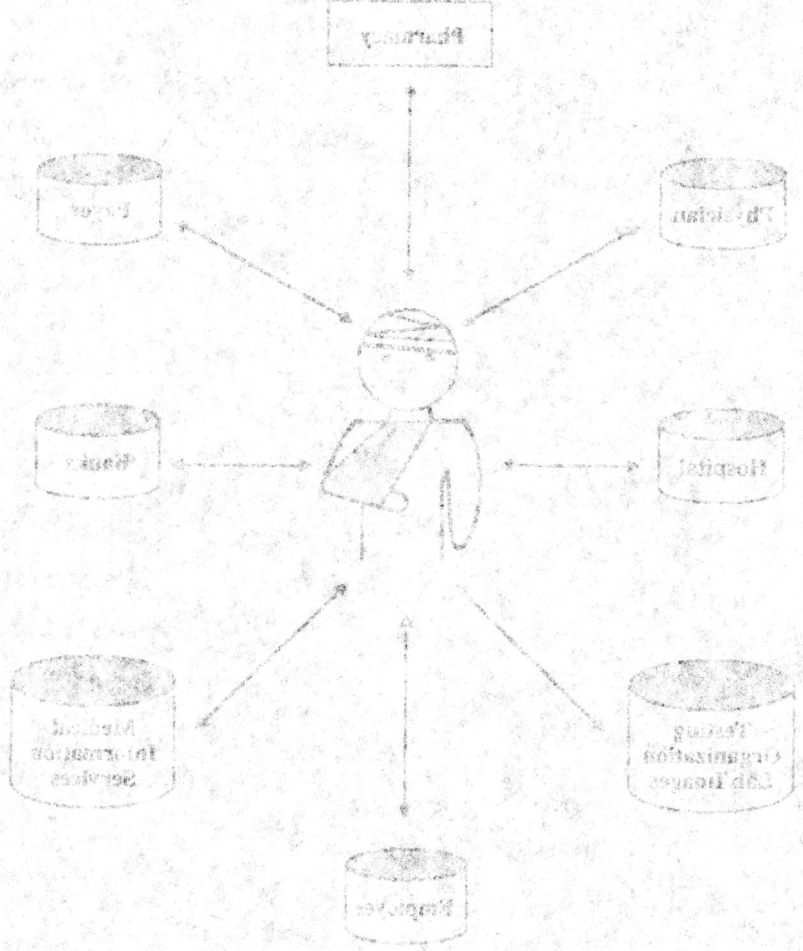

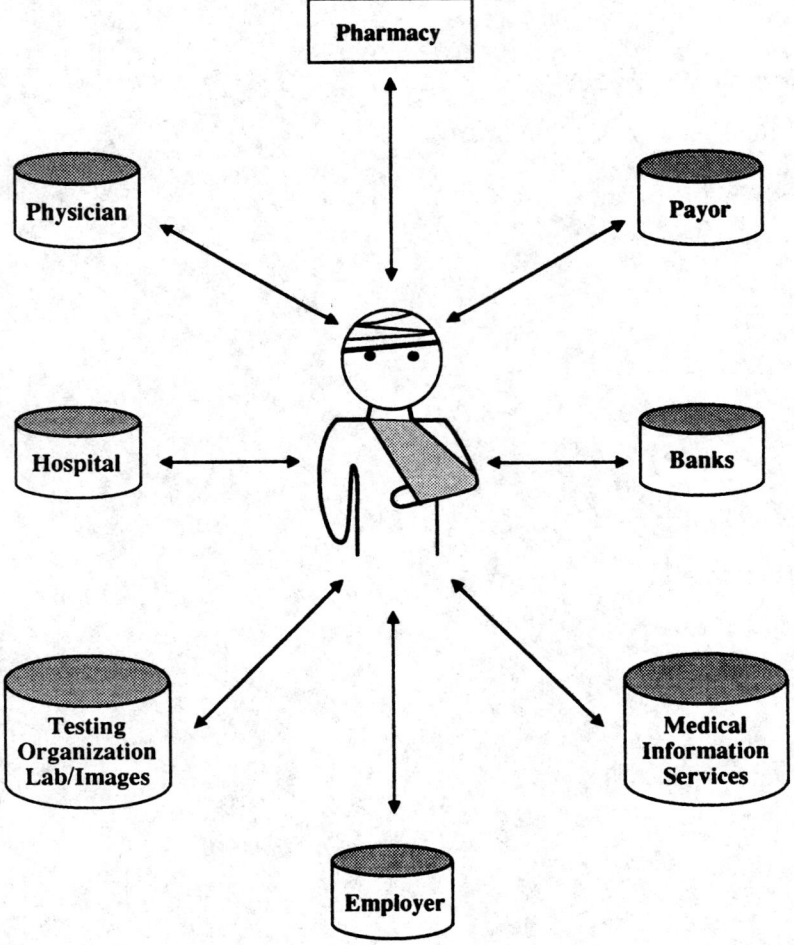

Patient-generated medical and financial data.

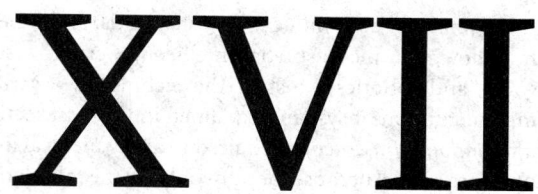

XVII

Medical Informatics

Luis G. Kun
Cedars-Sinai Medical Center

I N THE LAST 20 YEARS the field of medical informatics has grown tremendously both in its complexity and in content. As a result, two sections will be written in this *Handbook*. The first one, represented in these chapters, will be devoted to areas that form a key "core" of computer technologies. These include: hospital information systems (HIS), computer-based patient records (CBPR or

CPR), imaging, communications, standards, and other related areas. The second section includes the following topics: artificial intelligence, expert systems, knowledge-based systems, neural networks, and robotics. Most of the techniques described in the second section will require the implementation of systems explained in this first section. We could call most of these chapters the *information infrastructure* required to apply medical informatics' techniques to medical data. These topics are crucial because they not only lay the foundation required to treat a patient within the walls of an institution but they provide the roadmap required to deal with the patient's lifetime record while allowing selected groups of researchers and clinicians to analyze the information and generate outcomes research and practice guidelines information.

As an example a network of associated hospitals in the East Coast (a health care provider network) may want to utilize an expert system that was created and maintained at Stanford University. This group of hospitals, HMOs, clinics, physician's offices, and the like would need a "standard" computer-based patient record (CPR) that can be used by the clinicians from any of the physical locations. In addition in order to access the information all these institutions require telecommunications and networks that will allow for the electronic "dialogue." The different forms of the data, particularly clinical images, will require special devices for displaying purposes, and the information stored in the different HIS, Clinical Information Systems (CIS), and departmental systems needs to be integrated. This multimedia type of record would become the data input for the expert system which could be accessed remotely (or locally) from any of the enterprise's locations. On the application side, the expert system could provide these institutions with techniques that can help in areas such as diagnosis and patient treatment. However, several new trends such as: total quality management (TQM), outcomes research and practice guidelines could be followed. It should be obvious to the reader that to have the ability to compare information obtained in different parts of the world by dissimilar and heterogeneous systems, certain standards need to be followed (or created) so that when analyzing the data the information obtained will make sense.

Many information systems issues described in this introduction will be addressed in this section. The artificial intelligence chapters which follow should be synergistic with these concepts. A good understanding of the issues in this section is *required prior* to the utilization of the actual expert system. These issues are part of this section of medical informatics, other ones, however, e.g., systems integration and process reengineering, will not be addressed here in detail but will be mentioned by the different authors. I encourage the reader to follow up on the referenced material at the end of each chapter, since the citations contain very valuable information.

Several current perspectives in information technologies need to be taken in consideration when reading this section. One of them is described very accurately in the book entitled *Globalization, Technology and Competition (The Fusion of Computers and Telecommunications in the 1990s)* by Bradley, Hausman and Nolan (1993). The first chapter of this book talks about new services being demanded by end users which include the integration of computers and telecommunications. From their stages theory point of view, the authors describe that we are currently nearing the end of the micro era and at the beginning of the network era. From an economy point of view, the industrial economy (1960s and 1970s) and the transitional economy (1970s and 1980s) is moving into an information economy (1990s and beyond). Also a leadership survey done in 1994 by the Healthcare Information and Management Systems Society (HIMSS) on trends in health care computing to mainly chief information officers, directors, and the likes of health care providers showed the following results:

1. In a market driven by cost containment, the most important forces driving increased computerization in health care were: (*a*) movement to manage care (25%), (*b*) outcomes data requests (24%) and (*c*) movement to health care networks (17%).
2. The most important information systems priority for the next 2 years: (*a*) integrating across separate facilities (31%), (*b*) implementing a computer-based patient record (CPR) (19%), and (*c*) integrating departmental systems (13%) and reengineering to patient focused care (13%).

3. 56% felt that the information superhighway was essential for health care.
4. In the next 3 years the most significant health-care-related computer development affecting the average consumer would be: (*a*) more streamlined health care encounters (49%), (*b*) access to health information/services from home (20%), and (*c*) health care "smartcards" (17%).
5. Although 49% claimed to use the Internet, their health care facilities are using it for: (*a*) point-to-point E-mail (81%), (*b*) clinicians querying research databases (69%), (*c*) consumer-provider exchange (31%), and (*d*) two-way medical consultations (22%).
6. Clinicians will share computerized patient information in a nationwide system: (*a*) by the year 2000 (39%), (*b*) not happen for at least ten years (38%), and (*c*) within 1 to 3 years (14%). Many other questions and answers reflected some of the current technological barriers and users needs. Because of these trends it was essential to include in this *Handbook* technologies that today may be considered state of the art but when read about 10 years from now will appear to be transitional only. Information technologies are moving into a multimedia environment which will require special techniques for acquiring, displaying, storing, retrieving, and communicating the information. We are in the process of defining some of these mechanisms.

In some instances such as imaging, this *Handbook* contains a full section dedicated to the subject. That section contains the principles, the associated math algorithms, and the physics related to all medical imaging modalities. The intention in this section is to address issues related to imaging as a form of medical information. These concepts include issues related then to acquisition, storage/retrieval, display and communications of document and clinical images, e.g., picture archival and communications systems (PACS). From a CPR point of view, clinical and document images will become part of this *electronic chart*, therefore many of the associated issues will be discussed in this section more extensively.

The state of telecommunications has been described as a revolution; data and voice communications as well as full-motion video have come together as a new dynamic field. Much of what is happening today is a result of technology evolution and need. The connecting thread between evolutionary needs and revolutionary ideas is an integrated perspective of both sides of multiple industries. This topic will also be described in more detail in this section.

In the first chapter Allan Pryor provides us with a tutorial on hospital information systems (HIS). He describes not only the evolution of HIS and departmental systems and clinical information systems (CIS), but also their differences. Within this evolution he follows these concepts with the need for the longitudinal patient record and the integration of patient data. This chapter includes patient database strategies for the HIS, data acquisition, patient admission, transfer and discharge functions. Also discussed are patient evaluation and patient management issues. From an end-user point of view, a terrific description on the evolution of *data-driven* and *time-driven* systems is included, culminating with some critical concepts on HIS requirements for decision support and knowledge base functionality. His conclusions are a good indication of his vision.

Michael Fitzmaurice follows with "Computer-Based Patient Records" (CBPR or CPR). In the introduction, it is explained what is the CPR and why it is a necessary tool for supporting clinical decision making and how it is enhanced when it interacts with medical knowledge sources. This is followed by clinical decision support systems (CDSS): knowledge server, knowledge sources, medical logic modules (MLM), and nomenclature. This last issue in particular is one which needs to be well understood. The nomenclature used by physicians and by the CPRs differ among institutions. Applying *logic* to the wrong concepts can produce misinterpretations. The scientific evidence in this chapter includes patient care process, CDSS hurdles, CPR implementation, research data bases, telemedicine, hospital and ambulatory care systems. A table of hospital and ambulatory care computer-based patient record systems concludes this chapter.

In the next chapter Murray Loew covers "Informatics and Clinical Imaging." As explained earlier imaging is treated here from the context of patient-related information. This chapter starts with the motivation and goals, applicable areas: image acquisition, image transmission, archiving and retrieval, image display, and software. From an application point of view the following four areas are explained: diagnosis, teleconsultation, treatment planning, research, and teaching. The issues encountered in this field include compression, resolution, soft versus hard copy reading. The state-of-the-art section incorporates standards for transmission of images, compression benefits, archiving technologies, databases, and structures. Finally, the future prospects are discussed: high-performance computers and communications initiative, automatic feature extraction, diagnostic aids, content-based retrieval. A very useful table of imaging modalities provides the reader with information of network bandwidth and archive-storage requirements model for the archiving, communications, and displaying (PACS) of clinical images.

Today it is impossible to separate computers and telecommunications (communications and networks). Both are part of information systems. Soumitra Sengupta provides us in this chapter with a tutorial-like presentation which includes an introduction and history, impact of clinical data, information types, and platforms. The importance of this section is reflected both in the contents reviewed under current technologies—LANs, WANs, middleware, medical domain middleware; integrated patient data base, and medical vocabulary—as well as in the *directions and challenges* section which includes improved bandwidth, telemedicine, and security management. In the conclusions the clear vision is that *networks* will become the de facto fourth utility after electricity, water, and heat.

"Non-AI Decision Making" is covered by Ron Summers and Ewart Carson. This chapter includes an introduction which explains the techniques of procedural or declarative knowledge. The topics covered in this section include: *analytical models,* and *decision theoretic models,* including *clinical algorithms and decision trees.* The section that follows covers a number of key topics which appear while querying large clinical databases to yield evidence of either diagnostic/treatment or research value: statistical models, database search, regression analysis, statistical pattern analysis, bayesian analysis, Dempster-Shafer theory, syntactic pattern analysis, causal modelling, artificial neural networks. In the summary the authors clearly advise the reader to read this section in conjunction with the *expert systems* chapters that follow.

The standards section is closely associated with the CPR chapter of this section. Jeff Blair does a terrific job with his overview of standards related to the emerging health care information infrastructure. This chapter should give the reader not only an overview of the major existing and emerging health care information *standards* but an understanding of all current efforts, national and international, to coordinate, harmonize, and accelerate these activities. The introduction summarizes how this section is organized. It includes *identifier* standards (patient's, site of care, product, and supply labeling), *communications* (message format) standards, *content and structure* standards. This section is followed by a summary of *clinical data representations,* guidelines for *confidentiality, data security, and authentication.* After that *quality indicators* and *data sets* are described along with *international* standards. Coordinating and promotion organizations are listed at the end of this chapter including points of contact which will prove very beneficial for those who need to follow up.

Design issues in developing clinical decision support and monitoring systems by John Goethe and Joseph Bronzino provide insight for the development of *clinical decision support systems.* In their introduction and throughout this chapter the authors provide a step-by-step tutorial with practical advice and make recommendations on design of the systems to achieve end-user acceptance. After that a description of a clinical monitoring system, developed and implemented by them for a psychiatric practice, is presented in detail. In their conclusions the *human engineering* issue is discussed.

The authors of this section represent industry, academia and government. Their expertise in many instances is multiple from developing to actual implementing these technical ideas. I am very grateful for all our discussions and their contributions.

176

Hospital Information Systems: Their Function and State

T. Allan Pryor
University of Utah

The definition of a hospital information system (HIS) is unfortunately not unique. The literature of both the informatics community and the health care data processing world is filled with descriptions of many differing computer systems defined as an HIS. In this literature, the systems are sometimes characterized into varying level of HISs according to the functionality present within the system. With this confusion from the literature, it is necessary to begin this chapter with a definition of an HIS. To begin this definition, I must first describe what it is not. The HIS will incorporate information from the several departments within the hospital, but an HIS is not a departmental system. Departmental systems such as a pharmacy or a radiology system are limited in their scope. They are designed to manage only the department that they serve and rarely contain patient data captured from other departments. Their function should be to interface with the HIS and provide portions of the patient medical/administrative record that the HIS uses to manage the global needs of the hospital and patient.

A clinical information system is likewise not an HIS. Again, although the HIS needs clinical information to meets its complete functionality, it is not exclusively restricted to the clinical information supported by the clinical information system. Examples of clinical information systems are ICU systems, respiratory care systems, nursing systems. Similar to the departmental systems, these clinical systems tend to be one-dimensional with a total focus on one aspect of the clinical needs of the patient. They provide little support for the administrative requirements of the hospital.

If we look at the functional capabilities of both the clinical and departmental systems, we see many common features of the HIS. They all require a database for recording patient information. Both types of systems must be able to support data acquisition and reporting of patient data. Communication of information to other clinical or administrative departments is required. Some form of management support can be found in all the systems. Thus, again looking at the basic functions of the system one cannot differentiate the clinical/departmental systems from the HIS. It is this confusion that makes defining the HIS difficult and explains why the literature is ambiguous in this matter.

0-8493-8346-3/95/$0.00+$.50

The concept of the HIS appears to be, therefore, one of integration and breadth across the patient or hospital information needs. That is, to be called an HIS the system must meet the global needs of those it is to serve. In this context, if we look at the hospital as the customer of the HIS, then the HIS must be able to provide global and departmental information on the state of the hospital. For example, if we consider the capturing of charges within the hospital to be an HIS function, then the system must capture all patient charges no matter which department originated those charges. Likewise all clinical information about the patient must reside within the database of the HIS and make possible the reporting and management of patient data across all clinical departments and data sources. It is this totality of function that differentiates the HIS from the departmental or restricted clinical system, not the functions provided to a department or clinical support incorporated within the system.

The development of an HIS can take many architectural forms. It can be accomplished through interfacing of a central system to multiple departmental or clinical information systems. A second approach which has been developed is to have, in addition to a set of global applications, departmental or clinical system applications. Because of the limitations of all existing systems, any existing comprehensive HIS will in fact be a combination of interfaces to departmental/clinical systems and the applications/database of the HIS purchased by the hospital.

The remainder of this chapter will describe key features that must be included in today's HIS. The features discussed below are patient databases, patient data acquisition, patient admission/bed control, patient management and evaluation applications, and computer-assisted decision support. This chapter will not discuss the financial/administrative applications of an HIS, since those applications for the purposes of this chapter are seen as applications existing on a financial system that may not be an integral application of the HIS.

176.1 Patient Database Strategies for the HIS

The first HISs were considered only an extension of the financial and administrative systems in place in the hospital. With this simplistic view many early systems developed database strategies that were limited in their growth potential. Their databases mimicked closely the design of the financial systems that presented a structure that was basically a "flat file" with well-defined fields. Although those fields were adequate for capturing the financial information used by administration to track the patient's charges, they were unable to adapt easily to the requirement to capture the clinical information being requested by the health care providers. Today's HIS database should be designed to support a longitudinal patient record (the entire clinical record of the patient spanning multiple inpatient, outpatient encounters), integration of all clinical and financial data, and support of decision support functions.

The creation of a longitudinal patient record is now a requirement of the HIS. Traditionally the databases of the HISs were encounter-based. That is, they were designed to manage a single patient visit to the hospital to create a financial record of the visit and make available to the care provider data recorded during the visit. Unfortunately, with those systems the care providers were unable to view the progress of the patient across encounters, even to the point that in some HISs critical information such as patient allergies needed to be entered with each new encounter. From the clinical perspective, the management of a patient must at least be considered in the context of a single episode of care. This episode might include one or more visits to the hospital's outpatient clinics, the emergency department, and multiple inpatient stays. The care provider, to manage properly the patient, must have access to all the information recorded from those multiple encounters. The need for a longitudinal view dictates that the HIS database structure must both allow for access to the patient's data independent of an encounter and still provide for encounter-based access to adapt to the financial and billing requirements of the hospital.

The need for integration of the patient data is as important as the longitudinal requirement. Traditionally the clinical information tended to be stored in separate departmental files. With this structure, it was easy to report results from each department, but the creation of reports combining data from the different departments proved difficult if not impossible. In particular in those systems where access to the departmental data was provided only through interfaces with no central database, it was impossible to create an integrated patient evaluation report. Using those systems the care providers would view data from different screens at their terminal and extract with pencil onto paper the results from each department (clinical laboratory, radiology, pharmacy, and so on) the information they needed to properly evaluate the patient. With the integrated clinical database the care provider can view directly on a single screen the information from all departments formatted in ways that facilitate the evaluation of the patient.

Today's HIS is no longer merely a database and communication system but is an assistant in the management of the patient. That is, clinical knowledge bases are an integral part of the HIS. These knowledge bases contain rules and/or statistics with which the system can provide alerts or reminders or implement clinical protocols. The execution of the knowledge is highly dependent on the structure of the clinical database. For example, a rule might be present in the knowledge base to evaluate the use of narcotics by the patient. Depending on the structure of the database, this may require a complex set of rules looking at every possible narcotic available in the hospital's formulary or a single rule that checks the presence of the class narcotics in the patient's medical record. If the search requires multiple rules, it is probably because the medical vocabulary has been coded without any structure. With this lack of structure there needs to be a specific rule to evaluate every possible narcotic code in the hospital's formulary against the patient's computer medication record. With a more structured data model a single rule could suffice. With this model the drug codes have been assigned to include a hierarchical structure where all narcotics would fall into the same hierarchical class. Thus, a single rule specific only to the class "narcotics" is all that is needed to compare against the patient's record.

These enhanced features of the HIS database are necessary if the HIS is going to serve the needs of today's modern hospital. Beyond these inpatient needs, the database of the HIS will become part of an enterprise clinical database that will include not only the clinical information for the inpatient encounters but also the clinical information recorded in the physician's office or the patient's home during outpatient encounters. Subsets of these records will become part of state and national health care databases. In selecting, therefore, an HIS, the most critical factor is understanding the structure and functionality of its database.

176.2 Data Acquisition

The acquisition of clinical data is key to the other functions of the HIS. If the HIS is to support an integrated patient record, then its ability to acquire clinical data from a variety of sources directly affect its ability to support the patient evaluation and management functions described below. All HIS systems provide for direct terminal entry of data. Depending on the system this entry may use only the keyboard or other "point and click" devices together with the keyboard.

Interfaces to other systems will be necessary to capture a complete patient record. The physical interface to those systems is straightforward with today's technology. The difficulty comes in understanding the data that are being transmitted between systems. It is easy to communicate and understand ASCII textual information, but coded information from different systems is generally difficult for sharing between systems. This difficulty results because there are no medical standards for either medical vocabulary or the coding systems. Thus, each system may have chosen an entirely different terminology or coding system to describe similar medical concepts. In building the interface, therefore, it may be necessary to build unique translation tables to store the information from one system into the databases of the HIS. This requirement has limited the building of truly integrated patient records.

Acquisition of data from patient monitors used in the hospital can either be directly interfaced to the HIS or captured through an interface to an ICU system. Without these interfaces the acquisition of the monitoring data must be entered manually by the nursing personnel. It should be noted that whenever possible automated acquisition of data is preferable to manual entry. The automated acquisition is more accurate and reliable and less resource intensive. With those HISs which do not have interfaces to patient monitors, the frequency of data entry into the system is much less. The frequency of data acquisition affects the ability of the HIS to implement real-time medical decision logic to monitor the status of the patient. That is, in the ICU where decisions need to be made on a very timely manner, the information on which the decision is based must be entered as the critical event is taking place. If there is no automatic entry of the data, then the critical data needed for decision making may not be present, thus preventing the computer from assisting in the management of the patient.

176.3 Patient Admission, Transfer, and Discharge Functions

The admission application has three primary functions. The first is to capture for the patient's computer record pertinent demographic and financial/insurance information. A second function is to communicate that information to all systems existing on the hospital network. The third is to link the patient to previous encounters to ensure that the patient's longitudinal record is not compromised. This linkage also assists in capturing the demographic and financial data needed for the current encounter, since that information captured during a previous encounter may need not to be reentered as a part of this admission. Unfortunately in many HISs the linkage process is not as accurate as needed. Several reasons explain this inaccuracy. The first is the motivation of the admitting personnel. In some hospitals they perceive their task as a business function responsible only for ensuring that the patient will be properly billed for his or her hospital stay. Therefore, since the admission program always allows them to create a new record and enter the necessary insurance/billing information, their effort to link the patient to his previous record may not be as exhaustive as needed.

Although the admitting program may interact with many financial and insurance files, there normally exists two key patient files that allow the HIS to meet its critical clinical functions. One is a master patient index (MPI) and the second is the longitudinal clinical file. The MPI contains the unique identifier for the patient. The other fields of this file are those necessary for the admitting clerk to identify the patient. During the admitting process the admitting clerk will enter identifying information such as name, sex, birth date, social security number. This information will be used by the program to select potential patient matches in the MPI from which the admitting clerk can link to the current admission. If no matches are detected by the program, the clerk creates a new record in the MPI. It is this process that all too frequently fails. That is, the clerk either enters erroneous data and finds no match or for some reason does not select as a match one of the records displayed. Occasionally the clerk selects the wrong match causing the data from this admission to be posted to the wrong patient. In the earlier HISs where no longitudinal record existed, this problem was not critical, but in today's system, errors in matching can have serious clinical consequences. Many techniques are being implemented to eliminate this problem including probabilistic matching, auditing processes, postadmission consolidation.

The longitudinal record may contain either a complete clinical record of the patient or only those variables that are most critical in subsequent admissions. Among the data that have been determined as most critical are key demographic data, allergies, surgical procedures, discharge diagnoses, and radiology reports. Beyond these key data elements more systems are beginning to store the complete clinical record. In those systems the structure of the records of the longitudinal file contain information regarding the encounter, admitting physician, and any other information that may be necessary to view the record from an encounter view or as a complete clinical history of the patient.

176.4 Patient Evaluation

The second major focus of application development for the HIS is creation of patient evaluation applications. The purpose of these evaluation programs is to provide to the care giver information about the patient which assists in evaluating the medical status of the patient. Depending on the level of data integration in the HIS, the evaluation applications will be either quite rudimentary or highly complex. In the simplest form these applications are departmentally oriented. With this departmental orientation the care giver can access through terminals in the hospital departmental reports. Thus, laboratory reports, radiology reports, pharmacy reports, nursing records, and the like can be displayed or printed at the hospital terminals. This form of evaluation functionality is commonly called *results review*, since it only allows the results of tests from the departments to be displayed with no attempt to integrate the data from those departments into an integrated patient evaluation report.

The more clinical HISs as mentioned above include a central integrated patient database. With those systems patient reports can be much more sophisticated. A simple example of an integrated patient evaluation report is a diabetic flowsheet. In this flowsheet the caregiver can view the time and amount of insulin given, which may have been recorded by the pharmacy or nursing application, the patient's blood glucose level recorded in the clinical laboratory or again by the nursing application. In this form the caregiver has within a single report, correlated by the computer, the clinical information necessary to evaluate the patient's diabetic status rather than looking for data on reports from the laboratory system, the pharmacy system, and the nursing application. As the amount and type of data captured by the HIS increases, the system can produce ever-more-useful patient evaluation reports. There exist HISs which provide complete rounds reports that summarize on one to two screens all the patient's clinical record captured by the system. These reports not only shorten the time needed by the caregiver to locate the information, but, because of the format of the report, can present the data in a more intuitive and clinically useful form.

176.5 Patient Management

Once the caregiver has properly evaluated the state of the patient, the next task is to initiate therapy that ensures an optimal outcome for the patient. The sophistication of the management applications is again a key differentiator of HISs. At the simplest level management applications consist of order-entry applications. The order-entry application is normally executed by a paramedical personnel. That is, the physician writes the order in the patient's chart, and another person reviews from the chart the written order and enters it into the computer. For example, if the order is for a medication, then it will probably be a pharmacist who actually enters the order into the computer. For most of the other orders a nurse or ward clerk is normally assigned this task. The HIS records the order in the patient's computerized medical record and transmits the order to the appropriate department for execution. In those hospitals where the departmental systems are interfaced to the HIS, the electronic transmission of the order to the departmental system is a natural part of the order entry system. In many systems the transmission of the order is merely a printout of the order in the appropriate department.

The goal of most HISs is to have the physician responsible for management of the patient enter the orders into the computer. The problem that has troubled most of the HISs in achieving this goal has been the inefficiency of the current order-entry programs. For these programs to be successful they have to compete favorably with the traditional manner in which the physician writes the order. Unfortunately, most of the current order-entry applications are too cumbersome to be readily accepted by the physician. Generally they have been written to assist the paramedic in entering the order resulting with far too many screens or fields that need to be reviewed by the physician to complete the order. One approach that has been tried with limited success is the use of order sets. The order sets have been designed to allow the physician to easily from a single screen enter multiple orders. The use of order sets has improved the acceptability of the order-entry application to the physician, but several problems remain preventing universal acceptance by the physicians. One problem is that the order set will never be sufficiently complete to contain all orders that the physician would want to order. Therefore, there is some subset of patients orders that will have to be entered using the general ordering mechanism of the program. Depending on the frequency of those orders, the acceptability of the program changes. Maintenance issues also arise with order sets, since it may be necessary to formulate order sets for each of the active physicians. Maintaining of the physician-specific order sets soon becomes a major problem for the data processing department. It becomes more problematic if the HIS to increase the frequency of a given order being present on an order set allows the order sets to be not only physician-defined but problem-oriented as well. Here it is necessary to again increase the number of order sets or have the physicians all agree on those orders to be included in an order set for a given problem.

Another problem, which makes use of order entry by the physician difficult, is the lack of integration of the application into the intellectual tasks of the physician. That is, in most of the systems the physicians are asked to do all the intellectual work in evaluating and managing the care of the patient in the traditional manner and then, as an added task, enter the results of that intellectual effort into the computer. It is at this last step that is perceived by the physician as a clerical task at which the physician rebels. Newer systems are beginning to incorporate more efficiently the ordering task into other applications. These applications assist the physician throughout the entire intellectual effort of patient evaluation and management of the patient. An example of such integration would be the building of evaluation and order sets in the problem list management application. Here when the care provider looks at the patient problem list he or she accesses problem-specific evaluation and ordering screens built into the application, perhaps shortening the time necessary for the physician to make rounds on the patient.

Beyond simple test ordering, many newer HISs are implementing decision support packages. With these packages the system can incorporate medical knowledge usually as rule sets to assist the care provider in the management of patients. Execution of the rule sets can be performed in the foreground through direct calls from an executing application or in the background with the storing of clinical data in the patient's computerized medical record. This latter mode is called *data-driven execution* and provides an extremely powerful method of knowledge execution and alerting. That is, after execution of the rule sets, the HIS will "alert" the care provider of any outstanding information that may be important regarding the status of the patient or suggestions on the management of the patient. Several mechanisms have been implemented to direct the alerts to the care provider. In the simplest form notification is merely a process of storing the alert in the patient's medical record to be reviewed the next time the care provider accesses that patient's record. More sophisticated notification methods have included directed printouts to individuals whose job it is to monitor the alerts, electronic messages sent directly to terminals notifying the users that there are alerts which need to be viewed, and interfacing to the paging system of the hospital to direct alert pages to the appropriate personnel.

Execution of the rule sets are sometimes *time-driven*. This mode results in sets of rules being executed at a particular point in time. The typical scenario for time-driven execution is to set a time of day for selected rule set execution. At that time each day the system executes the given set of rules for a selected population in the hospital. Time drive has proven to be a particularly useful mechanism of decision support for those applications that require hospitalwide patient monitoring.

The use of decision support has ranged from simple laboratory alerts to complex patient protocols. The responsibility of the HIS is to provide the tools for creation and execution of the knowledge base. The hospitals and their designated "experts" are responsible for the actual logic that is entered into the rule sets. Many studies are appearing in the literature suggesting that the addition of knowledge base execution to the HIS is the next major advancement to be delivered with the HIS. This addition will become a tool to better manage the hospital in the world of managed care.

The inclusion of decision support functionality in the HIS requires that the HIS be designed to support a set of knowledge tools. In general a knowledge bases system will consist of a knowledge base and an inference engine. The knowledge base will contain the rules, frames, and statistics that are used by the inference applications to substantiate a decision. We have found that in the health care area the knowledge base should be sufficiently flexible to support multiple forms of knowledge.

That is, no single knowledge representation sufficiently powerful to provide a method to cover all decisions necessary in the hospital setting. For example, some diagnostic decisions may well be best suited for bayesian methods, whereas other management decisions may follow simple rules. In the context of the HIS, I prefer the term *application manager* to *inference engine*. The former is intended to imply that different applications may require different knowledge representations as well as different inferencing strategies to traverse the knowledge base. Thus, when the user selects the application, he or she is selecting a particular inference engine that may be unique to that application. The tasks, therefore, of the application manager are to provide the "look and feel" of the application, control the functional capabilities of the application, and invoke the appropriate inference engine for support of any "artificial intelligence" functionality.

176.6 Conclusion

Today's HIS is no longer the financial/administrative system that first appeared in the hospital. It has extended beyond that role to become an adjunct to the care of the patient. With this extension into clinical care the HIS has not only added new functionality to its design but has enhanced its ability to serve the traditional administrative and financial needs of the hospital as well. The creation of these global applications which go well beyond those of the departmental/clinical systems is now making the HIS the *patient-focused* system. With this global information the administrators and clinical staff together can accurately assess where there are inefficiencies in the operation of the hospital from the delivery of both the administrative and medical care. This knowledge allows changes in the operation of the hospital that will ensure that optimal care continues to be provided to the patient at the least cost to the hospital. These studies and operational changes will continue to grow as the use of an integrated database and implementation of medical knowledge bases become increasingly routine in the functionality of the HIS.

References

1. Pryor TA, Gardner RM, Clayton PD, et al. 1983. The HELP system. J Med Syst 7:213.
2. Pryor TA, Clayton PD, Haug PJ, et al. 1987. Design of a knowledge driven HIS. Proc. 11th SCAMC, 60.
3. Bakker AR. 1984. The development of an integrated and co-operative hospital information system. Med Inf 9:135.
4. Barnett GO. 1984. The application of computer-based medical record systems in ambulatory practice. N Engl J Med 310:1643.
5. Bleich HL, Beckley RF, Horowitz GL, et al. 1985. Clinical computing in a teaching hospital. N Engl J Med 312:756.
6. Whiting-O'Keefe QE, Whiting A, Henke J. 1988. The STOR clinical information system. MD Comput 5:8.
7. Hendrickson G, Anderson RK, Clayton PD, et al. 1992. The integrated academic information system at Columbia-Presbyterian Medical Center. MD Comput 9:35.
8. Safran C, Slack WV, Bleich HL. 1989. Role of computing in patient care in two hospitals. MD Comput 6:141.
9. Bleich HL, Safran C, Slack WV 1989. Departmental and laboratory computing in two hospitals. MD Comput 6:149.
10. ASTM E1238-91. 1992. Specifications for transferring clinical observations between independent computer systems. Philadelphia, American Society for Testing and Materials.
11. Tierney WM, Miller ME, Donald CJ. 1990. The effect on test ordering of informing physicians of the charges for outpatient diagnostic tests. N Engl J Med 322:1499.
12. Stead WW, Hammond WE. 1983. Functions required to allow TMR to support the information requirements of a hospital. Proc 7th SCAMC 106.

13. Safran C, Herrmann F, Rind D, et al. 1990. Computer-based support for clinical decision making. MD Comput 7:319.

14. Tate KE, Gardner RM, Pryor TA. 1989. Development of a computerized laboratory alerting system. Comp Biomed Res 22:575.

15. Orthner HF, Blum BI (eds). 1989. Implementing Health Care Information Systems, Springer-Verlag.

16. Dick RS, Steen EB (eds). 1991. The Computer-Based Patient Record, National Academy Press.

177

Computer-Based Patient Records

J. Michael Fitzmaurice
*U.S. Department of Health
and Human Services*

The objective of this chapter is to present the computer-based patient record (CPR) as a powerful tool for organizing patient care data to improve patient care and strengthen communication of patient care data among health care providers. The CPR is an even more powerful when it retrieves applicable medical knowledge to support clinical decision making. Evidence exists that the use of CPR systems (CPRS) can change both physician behavior and patient outcomes of care.

The primary role of the CPR is to support the delivery of medical care to a particular patient. Serving this purpose, ideally the CPR brings past and current information about a particular patient to the physician, promotes communication among health caregivers about that patient's care, and documents the process of care and the reasoning behind the choices that are made. Thus, the data in a CPR should be acquired as part of the normal process of health care delivery, by the providers of care and their institutions to improve data accuracy and timeliness of decision support.

The CPR can also be an instrument for building a clinical data repository that is useful for collecting information about which medical treatments are effective in the practice of medicine in the community and for improving population-based health care. Additional applications of CPR data beyond direct patient care can improve population-based care. These applications bring personal and public benefits but also raise issues that must be addressed by health care policy makers. Clinical data standards and communication networks, critical for using CPRs effectively, are treated separately in other sections in this chapter.

177.1 Computer-Based Patient Record

A CPR is a collection of data about a patient's health care in electronic form. The CPR is part of a system (a CPRS, usually maintained in a hospital or physician's office) that encompasses data entry and presentation, storage, and access to the clinical decision maker—usually a physician or nurse. The data are entered by keyboard, dictation and transcription, voice recognition and interpretation, light pen, touch screen, hand-held computerized notepad (perhaps wireless) with gesture and character recognition and grouping capabilities, and other means. Entry also may be by direct instrumentation from electronic patient monitors and bedside terminals, nursing stations, analysis by other computer systems such as laboratory autoanalyzers and magnetic resonance imagers, or another provider's CPRS.

Patient care data collected by a CPRS may be stored centrally or it may be stored in many places (distributed) for retrieval at the request of an authorized user through a database management system. The CPR may present data to the physician as text, tables, graphs, sound, images, full-motion video, and signals. The CPR may also point to the location of additional patient data that cannot be easily incorporated into the CPR.

In many current clinical settings (hospitals, physicians' offices, and ambulatory care centers), data pertaining to a patient's medical care are recorded and stored in a paper medical record. If the paper record is out of its normal location, accompanying the patient during an offsite study or procedure, it is not available to the nurse, the attending physician, or the expert consultant. In paper form, data entries are often illegible and not easily retrieved and read by multiple users. In electronic form, however, legible, clinical information can be available to all users simultaneously, improving timely access to patient care data and communication among care providers.

Individual hospital departments (laboratory or pharmacy, for example) often lose the advantages of automated data when their own computer systems print the computerized results onto *paper*. The pages are then sent to the patient's hospital floor and assembled into a paper record. The lack of standards for the electronic exchange of these data hinders the integration of departmental systems. Searching electronic files is often, but not always, easier than searching through paper. Weaknesses of paper medical record systems for supporting patient care and health care providers have been detailed [Korpman, 1990, 1991].

Many of the functions of a CPR and how it operates within a health-care information system to satisfy user demands are explained in the Institute of Medicine's report, *The Computer-Based Patient Record: An Essential Technology for Health Care* [1991].

177.2 Clinical Decision Support Systems

Another role of the CPR is to enable a clinical decision support system (CDSS)—computer software designed to aid clinical decision making—to provide the physician with medical knowledge that is pertinent to the care of the patient. Diagnostic suggestions, testing prompts, therapeutic protocols, practice guidelines, alerts of potential drug-drug and drug-food reactions, treatment suggestions, and other decision support services can be obtained through the interaction of the CPR with a CDSS.

Knowledge Server

Existing knowledge about potential diagnoses and treatments, practice guidelines, and complicating factors pertinent to the patient's diagnosis and care is needed at the time treatment decisions are made. The go-between that makes this link is a *knowledge server*, which acquires the necessary information for the decision maker from the knowledge server's information sources. The CPR can provide the knowledge server proper context, i.e., specific data and information about the patient's identification and condition [Tuttle et al., 1994].

Knowledge Sources

Knowledge sources include a range of options, from internal development and approval by a hospital's staff, for example, to sources outside the hospital, such as the practice guidelines sponsored by the Agency for Health Care Policy and Research, the Physicians Data Query program at the National Cancer Institute, other consensus panel guidelines sponsored by the National Institutes of Health, and guidelines developed by medical and other specialty societies. Additional sources of knowledge include the medical literature, which can be searched for high-quality, comprehensive review articles and for particular subjects using the "Grateful Med" program to explore the MEDLINE literature database available through the National Library of Medicine.

Medical Logic Modules

If medical knowledge needs are anticipated, acquired beforehand, and put into a medical logic module (MLM), software can provide rule-based alerts, reminders, and suggestions for the care provider at the point (time and place) of health service delivery. One format for MLMs is the Arden Syntax, which standardizes the logical statements [ASTM, 1992]. For example, an MLM might be interpreted as, "If sex = female, and age is greater than 50 years, and no Pap smear test result appears in the CPR, then recommend a Pap smear test to the patient." If MLMs are to have a positive impact on physician behavior and the patient care process, then physicians using MLMs must agree on the rules in the logical statements or conditions and the recommended actions that are based on interactions with patient care data in the CPR.

Nomenclature

Because MLMs are independent, the presence or absence of one MLM does not affect the operation of other MLMs in the system. If done carefully and well, MLMs developed in one health care organization can be incorporated in the CPRSs of other health care organizations. However, this requires much more than using accepted medical content and logical structure. If the medical concept terminology (the nomenclature used by physicians and by the CPR) differs among organizations, the knowledge server may misinterpret what is in the CPR, apply logic to the wrong concept, or select the wrong MLM. Further, the physician receiving its message may misinterpret the MLM [Pryor & Hripcsak, 1994].

For widespread use of CDSSs, a uniform medical nomenclature consistent with the scientific literature is necessary. Medical knowledge is information that has been evaluated by experts and converted into useful medical concepts and options. For CDSSs to search through a patient's CPR, identify the medical concepts, retrieve appropriate patient data and information, and provide a link to the relevant knowledge, the CDSS has to recognize the names used by the CPR for the concepts [Cimino, 1993]. Providing direction for coupling terms and codes found in patient records to medical knowledge is the goal of the Unified Medical Language System (UMLS) project of the National Library of Medicine.

177.3 Scientific Evidence

Patient Care Processes

Controlled trials have shown the effectiveness of CDSS for modifying physician behavior using preventive care reminders. In a review of the scientific literature up to February 1992, Johnston and coworkers [1994] reported that controlled trials of CDSSs have shown significant, favorable effects on care processes from (1) providing preventive care information to physicians and patients [McDonald et al., 1984; Tierney et al., 1986], (2) supporting diagnosis of high-risk patients [Chase et al., 1983], (3) determining the toxic drug dose for obtaining the desired therapeutic levels [White et al., 1987], and (4) aiding active medical care decisions [Tierney, 1988]. Johnston found clinician performance was generally improved when a CDSS was used and, in a small number of cases (3 of 10 trials), significant improvements in patient outcomes were seen.

In a randomized, controlled clinical trial, one which randomly assigned some teams of physicians to computer workstations with screens designed to promote cost-effective ordering (for example, of drugs and laboratory tests), Tierney and coworkers [1993] reported patient lengths of stay were 0.89 days shorter and charges generated by the intervention teams were $887 lower than for the control teams of physicians. These gains were not without an offset. Time and motion studies showed that intervention physician teams spent 5.5 min longer per patient during 10-h observation periods. This study is a rare controlled trial that sheds light on the resource impact of a CDSS.

In this setting, physician behavior was changed and resources used were reduced by the application of logical algorithms to computer-based patient record information. Nevertheless, a different hospital striving to attain the same results would have to factor in the cost of the equipment, installation, maintenance, and software development plus the need to provide staff training in the use of a CDSS.

Malpractice

In some emergency rooms, CDSS are used to prompt physicians to document the patient's record and to suggest the possibility of missed diagnoses—ones that could lead to serious patient harm and malpractice liability—such as myocardial infarctions. In 1990, all emergency room physicians in Massachusetts were offered lower malpractice premiums if they regularly used a particular CDSS [Institute of Medicine, 1991]. An additional benefit of a CDSS in ambulatory settings can be faster decisions and reduced time for the patient in the emergency room (for example, for triage of patients with symptoms of acute cardiac ischemia) [Sarasin et al., 1994].

Evaluation

CDSSs should be evaluated according to how well they enhance the user's performance in the user's environment [Nykanen et al., 1992]. Extending this concept, society should judge CDSSs not only on enhanced physician performance but also on whether patient outcomes are improved and systemwide health care costs are contained.

CDSS Hurdles

In a review of medical diagnostic decision support systems, Miller [1994] examines the development of CDSSs over the past 40 years and identifies several hurdles to be overcome before large-scale, generic CDSSs grow to widespread use. These hurdles include determining: (1) how to support medical knowledge base construction and maintenance over time, (2) the amount of reasoning power and detailed representation of medical knowledge required (e.g., how strong a match of medical terms is needed to join medical concepts with appropriate information), (3) how to integrate CDSSs into the clinical environment to reduce the costs of patient data capture, and (4) how to provide flexible user interfaces and environments that adjust to the abilities and desires of the user (e.g., with regard to typing expertise and pointing devices).

CPR Implementation

The real and perceived barriers to implementing a CPR include physicians' reluctance to enter data. Yet direct physician interaction with the system is important because it reduces transcription errors and allows the system to respond to the physician with preventive medicine prompts, drug contraindication alerts, and other reminders during routine patient care. During Beth Israel Hospital's transition to a CPR, data entry may not have been as large a barrier as the burden of recording clinical data on *both* paper and a CPR. Moreover, there is reason to believe that physicians have a greater concern about the confidentiality and privacy of their text notes than about other clinical data in the CPR [Rind & Safran, 1994]. Older physicians may make significantly fewer CPR system inquiries per case than younger physicians, but Clayton and coworkers [1994] reported that physician age explained only a small amount of variation (3 percent) in CPR use. In contrast, he found the average use by physicians categorized by hospital department (medical specialty) to vary by a factor of 10 between high- and low-utilization departments.

Although Massaro [1993a, 1993b] and Dambro and coworkers [1988] report on the problems faced and lessons learned during the installation period of their information technology systems, there is generally insufficient documentation in the medical literature about identifying and overcoming the barriers to successfully installing comprehensive, integrated clinical information systems in hospitals and physicians' offices.

Research Databases

CPR can have great value for developing research databases, medical knowledge, and quality assurance information that would otherwise require an inordinant amount of manual resources to obtain in their absence. An example of CPR use in research is found in a study undertaken at Latter Day Saints (LDS) Hospital. Using the HELP CPR system to gather data on 2847 surgical patients, this study found that administering antibiotics prophylactically during the 2-h window before surgery (as opposed to earlier or later within a 48-h window) minimized the chance of surgical wound infection. It also reduced the surgical infection rate for this time category to 0.59 percent, compared to the 1.5 percent overall infection rate for all the surgical patients under study [Classen et al., 1992].

The same system was used at LDS Hospital to link the clinical information system data (including a measure of nursing acuity) with the financial system's data. Using clinical data to adjust for the severity of patient illness, Evans and coworkers [1994] measured the effect of adverse drug events due to hospital drug administration on hospital length of stay and cost. The attributable difference per patient due to adverse drug events among similar patients was estimated to be an extra 1.94 patient days and $1939 in costs.

Telemedicine

A CPR may hold and exchange radiologic and pathologic images of the patient taken or scanned in digital form. The advantage is that digital images may be transferred long distances without a reduction in appearance quality. This allows patients to receive proficient medical advice even when they and their local family practitioner are far from their consulting physicians.

However, interpreting digital representations (images that are scanned, not originally digital) of radiographs, or X-ray images, although feasible, is inferior in some applications to reading conventional radiographs. Radiologists prefer customary X-ray films and view boxes to their digitized images and would require significant training and specialized experience to achieve optimal performance with digitized images. Digital images, such as magnetic resonance images (MRIs), should appear no different whether viewed at the patient's site of care or by a radiologist hundreds of miles away from the patient—if the algorithms for compressing (to reduce the costs of data transmission) and decompressing the digital data do not result in a discernable loss of quality. This feature lends itself to the development of expert systems for reading MRIs of difficult cases, for example, particularly when a patient's medical facility is isolated from academic medical centers. For the most part, only radiology and pathology applications of telemedicine have been extensively evaluated and found medically feasible. The cost-effectiveness of these applications has not been rigorously evaluated [Grigsby & Kaehny, 1993].

Telemedicine is, of course, more than teleradiology and telepathology. Much can be accomplished with telephone, facsimile machines, and teleconferencing that may not require substantial technical support or training. The financial concern is that payment for telemedicine services may increase the cost of care without improving patient outcomes. Research and project evaluation findings are needed to show where telemedicine applications improve the quality of care and are cost-effective.

In addition, when personally identifiable health care data are transported electronically across state borders for telemedicine uses, the applicability of state laws regarding confidentiality and privacy of these data is not often obvious. This raises legal questions for organizations that wish to move these data over national networks for patient management, business, or analytical reasons. A federal privacy protection law that applies generally to medical data about patients does not now exist [Waller, 1991], nor is there a federal law or licensing system to protect physicians and their patients against the consequences of telemedicine-failure malpractice.

177.4 Hospital and Ambulatory Care Systems

A review of the literature to identify CPRS studies (with a focus on ambulatory care and on the research use of their data) revealed the systems shown in Table 177.1 [Agency for Health Care Policy and Research, 1993]. Table 177.1 presents the system acronym, its meaning, its location, and a brief description. Some systems have been in use for over 25 years; they were, for the most part, developed in academic medical centers. In some cases, they are actually data registry systems. Six of these

TABLE 177.1 Hospital and Ambulatory Care Computer-Based Patient Record Systems

Private Sector Systems

ARAMIS	Arthritis, Rheumatism, and Aging Medical Information System [TOR (time-oriented record) is the collection instrument]; Stanford University Medical Center (MA); national chronic disease data bank.
ATHOS	AIDS Time-Oriented Health Outcome Study; Stanford University Medical Center (CA); national chronic disease data bank.
BICS	Brigham and Women's Hospital Integrated Computing System; Brigham and Women's Hospital (MA); hospital and ambulatory care patient record.
BIHS	Beth Israel Hospital System; Beth Israel Hospital (MA); hospital and ambulatory care patient record.
CIS	Clinical Information System; Columbia-Presbyterian Medical Center (NY); hospital and ambulatory care patient record.
COSTAR	Computer-Stored Ambulatory Record; Massachusetts General Hospital (MA); ambulatory care patient record (also commercial).
DIOGENE	University Hospital of Geneva (Switzerland); Hospital and ambulatory care patient record (non-U.S. but identified in AHCPR [1993]).
HCHP/AMRS	Harvard Community Health Plan Ambulatory Medical Record; HCHP (MA); ambulatory care patient record
HELP	Health Evaluation Through Logical Processing; LDS Hospital (UT); hospital and ambulatory care patient record (also commercial).
MARS	Medical Archival System; University of Pittsburgh (PA); hospital and ambulatory care patient record (under development).
PIMS/PIPS	Patient Information Management System/Patient Information Protocol System: Loyola University Medical Center (IL); hospital and ambulatory care patient record.
RMRS	Regenstrief Medical Records System; Indiana University Medical Center (IN); hospital and ambulatory care patient record.
RPMS	Resource and Patient Management System; Indian Health Service (AZ); hospital and ambulatory care patient record.
STOR	Summary Time-Oriented Record; University of California at San Francisco (CA); ambulatory care patient record.
THERESA	Grady Memorial Hospital (GA); hospital and ambulatory care patient record.
TMR	The Medical Record; Duke University Medical Center (NC); hospital and ambulatory care patient record.
VIPOR	Vermont Integrated Problem-Oriented Record; University of Vermont Health Center (VT); ambulatory care patient record.

Federal CPR systems

DCHP	Decentralized Hospital Computer Program; Department of Veterans Affairs; hospital patient record.
CHCS	Composite Health Care System; Department of Defense; hospital patient record (6 modules).
IHS	Indian Health Service, Department of Health and Human Services; hospital and ambulatory care patient record.

well-studied systems—COSTAR, TMR, HELP, STOR, BIHS, and RMRS—have built vast patient databases derived from the regular delivery of patient care [Tierney & McDonald, 1991]. Two of these systems, COSTAR and HELP, are also commercial systems.

There are numerous commercial computerized hospital information systems. Most of them focus primarily on administrative functions (admission, discharge, transfer, scheduling, and billing) and secondarily on order entry and results reporting. Although no one commercial HIS is operating today that integrates all the patient's clinical data from all sources and makes the data easily accessible to clinicians, nine commercial HIS vendors offering systems were identified in a study by Abt Associates, Inc. [1993, p. 2]. These systems that

are designed to be used by clinicians (especially physicians), are comprehensive in functionality and well integrated or take a unique approach to integration, and that meet moderately rigorous standards for integration of clinical, financial, and analytic information are: 3M (HELP), Bell Atlantic (StatLAN Oacis), Cerner (CareNet), Health Data Sciences (Ulticare), IDX (OCM), Meditech (HIS), Phamis (LastWord), SMS (Invision), and TDS (7000).

177.5 Extended Uses of CPR Data

Data produced by such systems have additional value beyond supporting the care of specific patients. For example, subsets of individual patient care data from CPRs can be used for research purposes, quality assurance purposes, developing and assessing patient care treatment paths (planned sequences of medical services to be implemented after the diagnoses and treatment choices have been made), assessments of treatment strategies across a range of choices, and assessments of medical technologies in use in the community after their approval by the Food and Drug Administration. When linked with data measuring patient outcomes, CPR data may be used to help model the results achieved by different treatments, providers, sites of care, and organizations of care.

If these data were uniformly defined, accurately linked, and collected into databases pertaining to particular geographical areas, they would be useful for research into the patient outcomes of alternative treatments for specific conditions treated in the general practice of medicine and for developing information to assist consumers, health care providers, health plans, payers, public health officials, and others in making choices about treatments, technologies, sites and providers of care, health plans, and community health needs. This is currently an ambitious vision considering the presently limited use of CPRs and insufficient incentives for validating and storing electronic patient record data. Many such decisions are now based on data of inferior quality, but the importance of these decisions to the health care market is driving higher the demand for uniform, accurate clinical data.

177.6 Federal Programs

Uniform, electronic clinical patient data could be useful to many federal programs that have responsibility for improving, safeguarding, and financing U.S. health. For example, the Agency for Health Care Policy and Research (AHCPR) is charged with undertaking research to "identify the most effective methods for preventing, diagnosing, treating, and managing various health conditions" in community settings and to facilitate the development of "condition-specific practice guidelines" [PL 101–239, 1989]. To examine the influence on patient outcomes of alternative treatments for specific conditions, this research needs to account for the simultaneous effects of many patient risk factors, such as diabetes and hypertension. Health insurance claims data do not have sufficient clinical detail for many research, quality assurance, and evaluation purposes. Therefore, claims data must be supplemented with data abstracted from patients' medical records. In many cases, the data must be identified and collected prospectively from patients to ensure availability and uniformity. The use of a CPR could reduce the burden of this data collection, support practice guideline development, and, by comparing medical review criteria based on condition-specific guidelines with information in the CPR, could support the evaluation of these guidelines.

Medical effectiveness research could benefit from access to uniform, accurate, nationwide data from CPRs—for example, on the last 20,000 cases of a given condition such as benign prostatic hyperplasia, low back pain, or cataracts. Because CPRs do not typically contain information on patient outcomes after discharge from a hospital (or a physician's office), CPR data would have to be supplemented with patient outcome measures.

Other federal, state, and local health agencies also could benefit from CPR-based data collections. For example, the Food and Drug Administration, which conducts postmarketing monitoring to learn the incidence of unwanted effects of drugs after they are approved, could benefit from analyzing the next 10,000 cases in which a particular pharmaceutical is prescribed, using data collected in a CPR. The Health Care Financing Administration could provide guidance and information to its professional review organizations (PROs) about local and nationwide medical practice patterns founded on analysis of national and regional CPR data about Medicare beneficiaries; the state-based, Medicare PROs could analyze these data from CPRs in their own states to provide constructive, quality-enhancing feedback to hospitals and physicians. As a further example, the Centers for Disease Control and Prevention could quickly and completely monitor the incidence and prevalence of communicable diseases with access to locally available CPR data on patient care. State and local public health departments could allocate resources quickly to address changing health needs with early recognition of a community health problem. Many of these uses require linked data networks and data repositories (that the communities trust with their health data).

177.7 Selected Issues

Whereas there are personal and public benefits to be gained from extended use of CPR data beyond direct patient care, the use of personal medical information for these uses, particularly if it contains personal identification, brings with it some requirements and issues that must be faced. Some of the issues that must be addressed by health care policy makers, as well as by private markets, are as follows.

Standards are needed for the nomenclature, coding, and structure of clinical patient care data; for the content of data sets for specific purposes; and for the electronic transmission of such data to integrate data efficiently across departmental systems within a hospital and data from the systems of other hospitals and health care providers. If benefits are to be realized from rapidly accessing and transmitting patient care data for managing patient care, consulting with experts across long distances, linking physician offices and hospitals, undertaking research, and other applications, data standards are essential [Fitzmaurice, 1994a]. The Computer-based Patient Record Institute has taken an active interest in the development of such standards, and the Healthcare Informatics Standards Planning Panel of the American National Standards Institute has coordinated the standard developing organizations that work on such standards in the United States and provided an official link to standards organizations in other countries, such as the European Standards Committee (CEN). The Board of Directors of the American Medical Informatics Association [1994] has recommended specific approaches for many patient data standards' areas—adopt the best of what exists and move quickly toward continued refinement.

Confidentiality and *privacy* of individually identifiable patient care and provider data are very likely the most important issues. For most purposes, including much research, the user does not need to know patient identities if the data have been accurately linked by a trusted party. The benefits from extended uses of these data must be balanced against the opportunities for personal harm from unwanted disclosure (which must be avoided). A federal privacy law that spells out the allowable uses of personally identifiable health care data and the conditions under which they can be used, with civil and criminal punishments for violating disclosure or redisclosure prohibitions, might appropriately address this issue. It should establish safeguards for privacy based on uniform and fair information practices [Gostin et al., 1993; Privacy Protection Commission, 1977; Secretary's Advisory Committee on Automated Personal Data Systems, 1973].

The quality of stored clinical data may be questioned in the absence of organized programs to assess the reliability, validity, and sufficiency of these data for undertaking research and for providing useful information to consumers, medical care organizers, and payers. For proper analysis, the data should be sufficient to measure and assess the relevant risk factors influencing patient outcomes.

Electronically stored records in one state may be considered to be legally the same as paper records, but not in another state. In law, regulation, and practice, many states require pen and ink recording and signatures, apparently ruling out electronic records and signatures. This inconsistency and uncertainty creates a barrier for the electronic communication and legal acceptance of patient care data, images, medical advice, and claims across state boundaries for medical and other publicly acceptable purposes [Waller, 1991].

Standard unique identifiers for patients, health care providers, institutions, and payers are needed to obtain economies and accuracy when linking patient care data at different locations and patient care data with other relevant data.

Malpractice concerns arise as telemedicine technology allows physician specialists to give medical advice across state borders electronically to other physicians, other health-care providers, and patients. Physicians are licensed by a state to practice within its own state borders. Does a physician who is active in telemedicine need to obtain a license from each state in which he or she practices medicine from outside the state? If the expert physician outside the patient's state gives bad advice, which state's legal system has jurisdiction for malpractice considerations?

System security and *integrity* become important as more and more data and information for patient treatment and other uses are exchanged through national networks. This issue relates not only to purposeful violations of privacy but also to the accuracy of medical knowledge for patient benefit. If the system fails to transmit accurately what was sent to a physician—for example, an MRI, a practice guideline, or a clinical research finding—and if a physician's judgment and recommendation is based on a flawed image or other misreported medical knowledge, who bears the legal responsibility for a resulting inappropriate patient outcome?

Benefit-cost analysis methodologies must be developed and applied to inform investment decision makers about the most productive applications of CPR systems. There is a need for a common approach to measuring the benefits and the costs to be able to compare alternative applications. Accurate research findings applied to business risk and benefit assessments can advance commercial progress for developing and implementing CPR applications.

Regional health data repositories for the benefit of employers, hospital groups, consumers, and state health and service delivery programs raise issues about the ownership of patient care data, the use of identifiable patient care data, and the governance of the data repository. A study by the Institute of Medicine [1994] examines the power of regional health data repositories for improving public health, supporting better private health decisions, recognizing medically and cost-effective health care providers and health plans, and generally providing the information necessary to improve the quality of health care delivery in all settings. Some of the data in these repositories may be based on CPR data. These data may include personally identifiable data and move outside the environment in which they were created.

177.8 National Information Infrastructure

The development of a national information infrastructure (NII) to bring widespread benefits to the users of CPRSs must address many of these issues. Early in 1993, the federal government articulated the vision of an NII [Clinton & Gore, 1993], followed by the creation of a White House information infrastructure task force (IITF) to identify the obstacles to an NII and propose federal policies to overcome them. The NII involves high-speed computers, broad national data networks, community networks, supporting software, and human interaction, linked for the good of the nation.

In late 1993, the IITF identified four areas in which it expected NII benefits: telemedicine, unified electronic claims, personal health information systems, and computer-based patient records [Information Infrastructure Task Force, 1993]. In 1994, the IITF expanded its vision of NII applications in health care and raised issues that must be addressed to bring about this vision [Fitzmaurice, 1994*b*].

A part of the NII, the Federal High Performance Computing and Communications (HPCC) program was established in 1991 to expedite the development of high-performance computers and networks. In 1994, the HPCC expanded its scope to accelerate the development and deployment of NII technologies. An HPCC national challenge in health care aims to improve health care system quality and efficiency. This national challenge envisions linking health facilities to share medical data and imagery, visualization technology, virtual reality applications, patient treatment in remote areas, medical knowledge access, and database technology for storing and obtaining patient care data while safeguarding personal privacy [Committee on Information and Communication, 1994, p. 28].

177.9 Health Care Professional Workstation

To access patient care data in a CPR as well as medical knowledge found in diverse sites around the world linked on a global network, the worldwide information superhighway, health care professionals require an intelligent workstation. This is a computer, screen, and software that assists data entry and retrieval and provider decision making in the office, the hospital, and other places where patient care is delivered. The workstation is the technological embodiment of CPRs and CDSSs that assist the delivery of care to the patient. As it develops, the workstation must adopt to the care environment and the characteristics of the professional that improve work productivity and satisfaction. Silva and Ball [1994] state, "The intelligent workstation will learn how individual professionals work, anticipate their information needs, and provide context-relevant information 'at their fingertips.'" For additional information, see the proceedings of the International Medical Informatics Association (IMIA) Conference on the health care professional workstation [IMAI, 1994].

Acknowledgments

The author is director, Office of Science and Data Development, Agency for Health Care Policy and Research, in the U.S. Department of Health and Human Services. He appreciates the helpful comments given by Robert Esterhay, M.D., and Kathleen McCormick, Ph.D., R.N.

References

Abt Associates Inc. 1993. Overcoming Barriers to Integration and Implementation of Clinical Information Management Systems: Feasibility Study, Washington, DC, AHCPR Contract Final Report 282-92-0064, NTIS Accession No. PB 94 159886.

Agency for Health Care Policy and Research. 1993. Automated Data Sources for Ambulatory Care Effectiveness Research, ML Grady, HA Schwartz (eds), Washington, DC, Agency for Health Care Policy and Research.

ASTM. 1992. E1460-92: Standard Specifications for Defining and Sharing Modular Health Knowledge Bases (Arden Syntax for Medical Logic Modules), Philadelphia, ASTM.

Board of Directors of the American Medical Informatics Association. 1994. Standards for medical identifiers, codes, and messages needed to create an efficient computer-stored medical record. J Am Med Informatics Assoc. 1:1.

Brannigan VM. 1994. Protection of patient data in multi-institutional medical computer networks: Regulatory effectiveness analysis. AMIA Proceedings. Seventeenth Annual Symposium on Computer Applications in Medical Care, pp 59–63, New York, McGraw-Hill.

Chase CR, Vacek PM, Shinozaki T, et al. 1983. Medical information management: Improving the transfer of research results to presurgical evaluation. Med Care 21:410.

Cimino JJ. 1993. Saying what you mean and meaning what you say: Coupling biomedical terminology and knowledge. Acad Med 68(4):257.

Classen DC, Evans RS, Pestotnik SL, et al. 1992. The timing of prophylactic administration of antibiotics and the risk of surgical wound infection. NEJM. 326(5):281.

Clayton PD, Pulver GE, Hill CL. 1994. Physician use of computers: Is age or value the dominant factor? AMIA Proceedings. Seventeenth Annual Symposium on Computer Applications in Medical Care, pp 301–305, New York, McGraw-Hill.

Clinton WJ, Gore A. 1993. Technology for America's Economic Growth, a New Direction to Build Economic Strength, Washington, DC. Executive Office of the President.

Committee on Information and Communication, National Science and Technology Council. 1994. High Performance Computing and Communications: Technology for the National Information Infrastructure, Washington, DC, Executive Office of the President.

Dambro MR, Weiss BD, McClure CL et al. 1988. An unsuccessful experience with computerized medical records in an academic medical center. J Med Ed 63:617.

Donaldson MS, Lohr KN (eds). 1994. Health Data in the Information Age: Use, Disclosure, and Privacy, Washington, DC, National Academy Press.

Evans RS, Pestotnik SL, Classen DC, et al. 1993. Development of an automated antibiotic consultant. MD Comput 10(1):17.

Evans RS, Classen DC, Stevens MS, et al. 1994. Using a health information system to assess the effects of adverse drug events. *AMIA Proceedings. Seventeenth Annual Symposium on Computer Applications in Medical Care,* pp 161–165, New York, McGraw-Hill.

Fitzmaurice JM. 1994a. Health care data standards are required for medically effective use of workstations. Int J Biomed Comput 34(1–4):331.

Fitzmaurice JM. 1994b. Health care and the NII. In Putting the Information Infrastructure to Work: Report of the Information Infrastructure Task Force Committee on Applications and Technology, pp 41–56, Gaithersburg, MD, National Institute of Standards and Technology.

Gostin LO, Turek-Brezina J, Powers M, et al. 1993. Privacy and security of personal information in a new health care system. JAMA 270(20):2487.

Grigsby J, Kaehny MM. 1993. Analysis of expansion of access to care through use of telemedicine and mobile health services. In Report 1: Literature review and analytic framework, Denver, Center for Health Policy Research (report to the Health Care Financing Administration under Contract No. 500-92-0046 in September 1993).

Information Infrastructure Task Force. 1993. The National Information Infrastructure: Agenda for Action. Washington, DC, Executive Office of the President.

Institute of Medicine. 1991. The Computer-Based Patient Record: An Essential Technology for Health Care, RS Dick, EB Steen (eds), Washington DC, National Academy Press.

Institute of Medicine. 1994. Health Data in the Information Age: Use, Disclosure, and Privacy, MS Donaldson, KN Lohr (eds), Washington, DC, National Academy Press.

International Medical Informatics Association. 1994. Special issue: The health care professional workstation. Int J Biomed Comput 34(1–4).

Johnston ME, Langton KB, Haynes RB, et al. 1994. Effects of computer-based clinical decision support systems on clinician performance and patient outcome. Ann Intern Med 120:135.

Korpman RA. 1990. Patient care automation: The future is now: Part 2. The current paper system—can it be made to work? Nurs Econ 8(4):263.

Korpman RA. 1991. Patient care automation; the future is now, part 8. Does reality live up to the promise? Nurs Econ 9(3):175.

Massaro TA. 1993a. Introducing physician order entry at a major academic medical center: I. Impact on organizational culture and behavior. Acad Med 68(1)25.

Massaro TA. 1993*b*. Introducing physician order entry at a major academic medical center: II. Impact on medical education. Acad Med 68(1):20.

McDonald CJ, Hui SJ, Smith DM, et al. 1984. Reminders to physicians from an introspective computer medical record. A two-year randomized trial. Ann Intern Med 100:130.

Miller RA. 1994. Medical diagnostic decision support systems—past, present, and future. J Am Med Informatics Assoc 1(1):8.

National Coordination Office for High Performance Computing and Communication. 1994. *HPCC FY 1995 Implementation Plan*, Washington, DC, Executive Office of the President.

Nykanen P, Chowdhury S, Wiegertz O. 1992. Evaluation of decision support systems in medicine. Yearbook of Medical Informatics 1992, 301.

Privacy Protection Study Commission. 1977. Personal Privacy in an Information Society, Washington, DC, US Government Printing Office.

Pryor TA, Hripcsak G. 1994. Sharing MLMs: An experiment between Columbia-Presbyterian and LDS Hospital. AMIA Proceedings. Seventeenth Annual Symposium on Computer Applications in Medical Care, pp 399–403, New York, McGraw-Hill.

Public Law 101–239, the Omnibus Budget Reconciliation Act of 1989. 42 U.S.C. 299–299c–6.

Rind DM, Safran C. 1994. Real and imagined barriers to an electronic medical record. AMIA Proceedings. Seventeenth Annual Symposium on Computer Applications in Medical Care, pp 74–78, New York, McGraw-Hill.

Sarasin FP, Reymond J, Griffith JL, et al. 1994. Impact of the acute cardiac ischemia time-insensitive predictive instrument (ACI-TIPI) on the speed of triage decision making for emergency department patients presenting with chest pain: a controlled clinical trial. J Gen Intern Med 9:187.

Secretary's Advisory Committee on Automated Personal Data Systems. 1973. Records, Computers and the Rights of Citizens, Washington, DC, U.S. Department of Health, Education & Welfare.

Silva JS, Ball MJ. 1994. The professional workstation as enabler: Conference recommendations. Int J Biomed Comput 34(1–4):3.

Tierney WM, McDonald CM. 1991. Practice databases and their uses in clinical research. Stat Med 10:541.

Tierney WM., McDonald CJ, Hui SJ, et al. 1986. Computer predictions of abnormal test results. Effects on outpatient testing. JAMA 259:1194.

Tierney WM, Miller ME, Overhage JM, et al. 1993. Physician inpatient order writing on microcomputer workstations. JAMA 269(3):379.

Tuttle MS, Sherertz DD, Fagan LM, et al. 1994. Toward an interim standard for patient-centered knowledge-access. AMIA Proceedings. Seventeenth Annual Symposium on Computer Applications in Medical Care, pp 564–568, New York, McGraw-Hill.

Waller AA. 1991. Legal aspects of computer-based patient records and record systems. In RS Dick, EB Steen (eds), The Computer-Based Patient Record: An Essential Technology for Health Care, pp 156–179, Washington, DC, National Academy Press.

White KS, Lindsay A, Pryor TA, et al. 1984. Application of a computerized medical decision-making process to the problem of digoxin intoxication. J Am Coll Cardiol 4:571.

White, RH, Hong R, Venook AP, et al. 1987. Initiation of warfarin therapy: Comparisons of physician dosing with computer-predicted dosing. J Gen Intern Med 2:141.

178

Informatics and Clinical Imaging

Murray H. Loew
George Washington University

178.1 Motivation

Since the earliest uses of medical images, it was clear that the information contained in them contributed significantly to decisions made in the diagnosis and treatment of medical problems. Images and their interpretations were integral parts of the patient's record. As the development of the computer-based patient record (CPR) proceeds, it will become evident that the record is incomplete without the presence of the images. This will be due to the diagnostic and treatment value of the images and also to the need to evaluate the quality of the decisions that were based on the image data; the effect of the inclusion of images in the informatics context will be different for the various departments.

Some of the clinical specialties that produce and use medical images, from among the multiple modalities (employing light and/or ionizing radiation), are radiology [e.g., plain films, computerized tomography, magnetic resonance (MR) imaging, ultrasound, radioisotope imaging], ophthalmology, cardiology (e.g., angiography), dermatology, dentistry, and pathology. Often, a series of images is made for a given patient (e.g., a set of axial slices in tomography, or in dentistry, a set of films that includes all the teeth); we refer to one or more images taken at one time as a *study*.

In a recent report from the Institute of Medicine [1], the primary recommendation of the review committee was that the CPR should be adopted as the standard for medical and all other records related to patient care. Images thus must be in digital form to be a legitimate part of the CPR. The report identified several desired attributes of a CPR, including its linkage with other records to provide a longitudinal patient record; its linkage to knowledge, literature, and bibliographic databases; and its inclusion of the clinician rationale for patient care decisions. It is essential, therefore, that the capability exists to retrieve and display images reliably, quickly, and accurately and that tools are available for measurement and comparison of images.

178.2 Goals

Applicable Areas

The capabilities stated above must be offered by any informatics system. Its proper concerns include all the links in the imaging chain. So it is necessary to establish goals for performance in each of a number of areas, including *image acquisition*—accuracy (i.e., resolution in space and intensity, gray-scale or color, noise and distortion) and speed; *image transmission, archiving, and retrieval*—compression ratio and type (lossy, or lossless with measure of effect on diagnosis), speed and bandwidth (effect on worst-case time to retrieve a study), reliability (e.g., effect of single or multiple disk failures), capacity (effect on retrieval time as function of age of study), compatibility of format (effect on ability to exchange data between and among imaging equipment and user workstations). Other areas for performance goals include *image display*—accuracy (pixel size and shape, screen flatness, number of gray-scale values possible per pixel), brightness, and number of images to be viewed simultaneously, and at what sizes; and *software*—user interface (effect on ease of use: navigation among images in a study; manipulation of images, individually and severally), database structure (effect on query types and response times), links with other information systems [e.g., hospital (HIS) and radiology (RIS)] (effect on accuracy of diagnosis and treatment), image processing: enhancement, registration and comparison, image fusion, feature extraction, classification (effect on diagnosis and treatment planning), and image visualization (interactive and dynamic 2-, 3-, and 4-D representations of image sequences and multiple modalities).

Applications of Interest

The goals must be defined with respect to the applications of interest, each of which has its own specific considerations.

Diagnosis

Linkage with the other parts of the medical record should be rapid and easy to establish from anywhere in the system; rapid retrieval of a patient's recent image studies from the archive is a vital component. Related cases (for use, e.g., in teaching or consultation) can be made available via a larger (national, regional) network, and image processing tools must be available for enhancement and identification of important features, for classification (e.g., tissue identification in ultrasound, characterization of plaque type in MR vessel images), and for image registration and quantitative comparison (e.g., in image fusion: combining information from several sources).

Teleconsultation

Retrieval and transmission of images from one site to another permits physicians who are geographically separated to discuss a given image that is presented to them simultaneously. This allows specialized expertise—that often would otherwise have been unavailable—to be brought to bear on difficult and unusual cases. To provide maximum benefit, the system must offer real-time audio and video, and a pointing device (e.g., mouse) with a corresponding unique screen cursor, for each user. Speed and ease of use are important characteristics of a consultation system.

Treatment Planning

Radiation therapy is an example of a treatment modality requiring the accurate display of, and interaction with, images. The goal is to use the images to define, in three dimensions, the location and orientation of beams for delivering sufficient energy to a tumor to cause it to regress, while sparing adjacent healthy tissue [8]. A 3-D rendering of the underlying image data is required, on which are superimposed the beams and the estimates of doses delivered to various regions of tissue. Clearly, the user interface, and the image-processing and visualization tools are of central importance (as is the availability of hardware with great processing capability).

Research and Teaching

The database and archiving capabilities of an informatics system are of most concern here, as it will be desired to find images having certain characteristics, perhaps not all well-defined. Thus the query-construction method and the ability of the software to examine image content are important. The latter capability is needed because it is impossible to predict all needs in advance, and the header information will of necessity be incomplete. Registration and measurement of images also will be useful for pedagogical and research purposes.

178.3 Issues

Discussed below are some of the issues that must be addressed by any informatics system intended for use with images.

Compression

Compression is desirable because it reduces the required archive capacity and permits more-rapid transmission of images between users and between the archive and users. [Table 178.1 lists typical study sizes in gigabytes (GB) and volumes for a university hospital that performs 150,000 studies per year.] Lossless compression techniques (allowing perfect recreation of the original image) typically yield maximum compression ratios of 2.5:1 to 3:1 on radiological images. And although some users report that a 10:1 lossy compression ratio (see below) may be used prior to diagnosis in the case of computed radiography [3], in most cases newly acquired images are diagnosed using only lossless compression.

Preservation of diagnostic information is the first requirement, and for the case of lossy compression there does not exist a general measure that can be applied to the (imperfect) re-created image to assess its diagnostic value. That is best evaluated by a receiver-operating-characteristic clinical study [e.g., 5], a lengthy and detailed process for which no simpler general substitute has yet been found. The issue is the choice of lossless or lossy compression, and what the compression type and ratio should be.

Resolution

Present plain-film systems for radiography (except mammography) yield resolutions on the order of 5–7 line-pairs/mm, implying an image size of about 3500 by 4500 pixels for a 14-by-17-in film, or approximately 16 million pixels. It is possible to digitize films at corresponding resolutions in space (typically 70–150 micrometers) and grayscale (12–16 bits/pixel); on a laser digitizer, the process takes 1–2 min per film. Since, however, there are not yet available displays that can present an entire image of that size, acquisition resolution often is limited to 200 micrometers, which reduces the pixel (and

TABLE 178.1 Typical Study Sizes

Imaging Modality	Edge Size (pixels), and Number of Bytes per Pixel	MB per Image	Mean Study Size, MB per Patient
Conventional radiographs	2048, 2	8	16
Computed tomography (per slice)	512, 2	0.5	22
Nuclear medicine	32–512, 2	0.002–0.5	4
Ultrasound	512, 1	0.25	7
MRI (per slice)	256, 2	0.125	13
Mammography	4096, 2	32	150
Specials (neuro and visceral)	1024, 2	2	19 (V), 120 (N)
Fluoroscopy	1024, 1–2048, 2	1–8	57

Source: Table adapted from [2].

byte) count to about one-quarter of their previous values. Alternatively, the entire image is displayed at lower resolution, and the user can move a quarter-image window through it at full resolution.

The issue is the resolution in space and gray level of the acquisition and display equipment and the effect on diagnostic performance. Additionally, resolution in time must be considered in systems that acquire sequences of images.

Soft- versus Hard-Copy Reading

Medical personnel are accustomed to reading medical images on (negative) film and on black-and-white and color prints. The transition to grayscale cathode-ray tube (CRT) monitors has been evaluated in numerous studies in radiology [6,7]. They indicate that the requirement ranges from a 19-in 2048-by-2560-pixel (sometimes called "2K") monitor to a 20-in 1024-by-1280-pixel ("1K") monitor. The actual requirement will depend on whether the display is to be used for a variety of image types, or for just one. Relatively low-resolution source images (e.g., nuclear medicine, ultrasound, MR) can be viewed effectively and individually on 1K monitors. (*Studies,* however, customarily viewed on film as sets of from 6–15 images, would require higher resolution.) Mammograms either must be viewed at reduced resolution or examined by panning through the data set and displaying sections on a 2K monitor.

Monitor luminance is another important consideration. A typical monitor may provide 206 candela/m^2 (60 foot-lamberts) when new, but this can decline to as little as 52 cd/m^2 after 6 months. The conventional light box, however, maintains 500 to 700 cd/m^2, which complicates comparison of the two methods. Adjustment of the monitor's center-luminance value and dynamic range usually makes it possible to view the darker regions of the image.

Recent developments in printer technology have made it possible to print gray-scale (not halftone) images on paper at resolutions of 300 dots per inch, thus offering an alternative to film for reading images that are routinely written from digital modalities such as CT and MR. Currently under evaluation by several radiology departments, this technology may find acceptance as a cost-effective hard-copy medium.

178.4 State of the Art

Standards for Transmission of Images

The Digital Imaging and Communications in Medicine (DICOM) 3.0 Standard [9] is a result of collaboration between the National Electrical Manufacturers' Association (the MedPACS Section of which represents many manufacturers of medical-imaging-related equipment) and the American College of Radiology. The standard describes a means of formatting and exchanging images and associated information and applies to the operation of the interface which is used to transfer data in and out of an imaging device. The standard also provides for formatting the data for transmission and for network connections with other devices; it supports the ISO OSI protocol and TCP/IP. Although DICOM does not yet have the status of an international standard, it is already a de facto standard for numerous manufacturers and is being used in several PACS installations.

Compression

Lossless compression techniques (e.g., run-length coding or Huffman coding) typically yield maximum compression ratios of 2.5:1 to 3:1 on radiologic images. Higher values can be achieved with a variety of lossy techniques (e.g., a modification of the standard [4] created by the Joint Photographic Experts Group [JPEG] yields about 10:1), but it is essential to match the technique and the ratio to the modality and intended use. Recent research in image compression has been stimulated by the medical applications, and new techniques based on wavelets [10] including the Gabor transform [11] and on fractals [12].

In addition to compression within a frame, opportunities exist in *sequences* of images for *inter-frame* compression. Predictive methods of various orders [13] are useful for pixel-to-pixel compression as the sequence progresses; other approaches use the neighborhood (typically, 3-D) to predict the value of an adjacent pixel.

Archiving Technologies

The capacity and speed requirements of archives depend on the uses to which they will be put: Storage of images for current patients, for example, would require 50–100 GB, and a transfer rate of from 0.3 (average) to 4 MB/s (peak) to ensure that radiologists can receive high-resolution images within 2 s [14]. Those requirements will increase with the expected number of simultaneous users, and decrease with the use of compression. A 7-year storage period for archived images would imply a need for long-term capacity (uncompressed) of approximately 16 TB. The required transfer rate could be considerably lower than for current patients, however, because advance scheduling would permit overnight retrieval.

Storage technologies include optical disks in changers ("jukeboxes"); magneto-optical disks; high-speed tapes (with transfer rates up to 32 MB/s) in changers having capacities to 27 TB and beyond; parallel-transfer disks; and redundant arrays of inexpensive disks (RAIDs). The capacities, access times, and transfer rates for various data-block sizes all differ across the technologies, as do the reliability [14] and ability to recover from the failure of a single unit. Trade-offs with cost usually must be made and will depend on the user's requirements.

Databases and Structures

Databases for medical images are needed to provide ready access to patients' current and previous studies. Existing film libraries are able at most to retrieve only those films that are not checked out; and misfiled films are essentially unavailable until they are discovered and filed correctly. Digital imaging and storage can ensure that images are available at all times and simultaneously to as many locations as necessary.

Speed is important, and *prefetching* is one approach to making retrievals faster. In one implementation [15], the archiving system is linked to the radiology information system so that as soon as arrival of a patient is detected, a retrieval is initiated that collects historical images, patient demographics, and other important information. Those data are then distributed to the workstation in use by the clinical people attending to that patient. That system uses an archive server, an optical-disk library, a database system, and a communication network. Clearly, historical exams can support the diagnosis of the current examination: Broken bones being examined for healing, for example, will have pictures of the original break fetched, while chest exams of lung nodules will have earlier views available to assess changes. The prefetch mechanism is software-driven, based on a look-up table composed of examination type, disease category, section radiologist, and referring physician.

Elsewhere, studies [16] of this type of approach indicate that an estimated 70% of the exams may be fetched from the archive during the night. Various strategies for limiting the extent of searches have been tried: fetch up to a certain number of exams, or fetch exams up to a certain exam age. More complex strategies can be used to reduce further the number of images retrieved.

Medical databases are heterogeneous. Linkages vary among items depending on circumstances; time specification varies with setting and purpose; images have intrinsic properties that might not have been summarized in the radiologist's report; images may be viewed as single objects over time, or as set of objects at a given time. Many standard database structures do not support the relationships present [17]. Hybrid techniques will be required. Knowledge-based image retrieval [18] is being used to predict the related images that a radiologist will require for review in a given clinical case. Distributed and object-oriented architectures offer advantages in performance and ease of expansion.

No less than other medical records, image data suffer from the variety of ways in which the same concepts are expressed in the various information sources and by the users themselves. This variety creates barriers between information and its potential users. One approach to breaking down those barriers is the Unified Medical Language System (UMLS) being developed with support from the U.S. National Library of Medicine (NLM). The two categories of UMLS components [19] are knowledge sources or databases and functional features or components. It is expected that at least three new knowledge sources will be needed for a fully-functioning UMLS: (1) a Metathesaurus representing terms and concepts present in a variety of biomedical vocabularies and classifications; (2) a semantic network identifying the useful and permissible relationships among the broad categories of semantic types (e.g., "medical device," "disease of syndrome") assigned to all Metathesaurus terms; and (3) an information sources map describing available machine-readable information sources and containing scripts that support successful automated connections to them.

The first version of the Metathesaurus, Meta-1, contains about 64,123 concepts and about 208,559 unique terms, including synonyms and slight variations. Each Meta-1 record contains three types of information: (1) basic facts about the main concept name including the vocabulary sources in which it appears, its semantic type, part of speech, lexical type (e.g., eponym, trade name, acronym), and in many cases, a definition; (2) associated terms from the Meta-1 source vocabularies including lexical variants, synonyms, related terms, and hierarchical contexts; and (3) usage information including the occurrence of the main concept name, its lexical variants, or synonyms in MEDLINE (R) or other database systems.

The UMLS would seem to be useful for image data as well as text records. It should permit linking to external databases, retrieval of patient data, and the structuring of patient records to facilitate image retrieval.

178.5 Prospects

The future of informatics in imaging will have many directions. Several of them are described briefly below. No list can be complete, because as users gain experience with these systems, new applications and new research areas will be identified.

Current efforts to create large information "superhighways" (such as those being implemented under the aegis of the United States' High Performance Computing and Communications program) are providing the infrastructure through which the searches, retrievals, and comparisons described above can be carried out. Researchers, consultants, and students will have access to extremely large databases. The utility of those databases will depend strongly on the power and convenience of the associated software.

Extraction of *features* from images is likely to become routine as large sets of images become available. A feature is a characteristic, extracted from an image or a portion of an image, that helps to describe that image. The goal is to identify features that are invariant to changes; the changes may be either intrinsic (e.g., variations in scale, in orientation, and among individuals) or extrinsic (noise, nonlinearities, scattering). Areas, shapes, textures, moments, histogram descriptors, and other measurements often are used as features, and their automatic extraction will make for repeatable, reliable characterization of images.

Once feature extraction is available, it then becomes possible to consider aids to diagnosis. Large sets of images of known classes yield probability density functions for the features. Knowledge of those densities permits several kinds of statistical decision procedures to be used and probabilities of decision error to be estimated. The procedures therefore could be used to assist the clinician by providing, for example, a list of possible diagnoses, ranked by relative likelihood. The list would be modified as nonimaging clinical data were added.

Retrieval of archived images is based at present on the availability of a unique descriptor (name, number) of a patient, possibly augmented by a date or a diagnosis. In the very near future, the range of descriptors will be great and will include anatomic, pathologic, and other information, all or any of which will be used to define and refine the search. Ultimately, however, such searches are limited by the descriptors applied to the images at the time of their archiving. Future users, however, may have needs not now apparent, leading to the need for *content-based* retrieval. The images in the database would be examined for attributes defined *at the time of the search,* possibly by use of examples as well as by explicit statements. Knowledge-based techniques are likely to play a large role in this kind of retrieval.

References

Abbreviations used in the references refer to PACS 93: Medical Imaging 1993: PACS Design and Evaluation, edited by RG Jost, Proceedings of SPIE 1899 (1993); PACS 94: Medical Imaging 1994—PACS: Design and Evaluation, edited by RG Jost, Proceedings of Society of Photo-Optical Instrumentation Engineers 2165 (1994); ACPR: Aspects of the Computer-Based Patient Record, edited by MJ Ball, MF Collen, New York, Springer (1992).

1. Dick RS, Steen EB (eds). 1991. The Computer-Based Patient Record: An Essential Technology for Health Care. Washington, National Academy Press.
2. Huda W, Honeyman JC, Frost MM, et al. 1993. Network bandwidth and archive-storage requirements model for PACS, PACS 93, pp 14–23.
3. Smith DV, Smith S, Bender GN, et al. 1994. Lessons learned and two years clinical experience in implementing the Medical Diagnostic Imaging Support (MDIS) System at Madigan Army Medical Center, PACS 94, pp 538–555.
4. Pennebaker WB, Mitchell JL. 1993. JPEG Still Image Data Compression Standard, New York, Van Nostrand Reinhold.
5. Collins CA, Lane D, Frank MS, et al. 1994. Design of a receiver operating characteristic (ROC) study of 10:1 lossy image compression. In HL Kundel (ed), Medical Imaging 1994: Image Perception, pp 149–158.
6. Horii SC. 1992. Electronic imaging workstations: ergonomic issues and the user interface. RadioGraphics 12: 773.
7. Ramaswamy MR, et al. 1994. Use of personal computer technology in supporting a radiological review workstation. PACS 94, pp 27–37.
8. Mohan R, Barest G, Brewster LJ, et al. 1988. A comprehensive three-dimensional radiation treatment planning system. Int J Radiat Oncol Biol Phys 15:481.
9. DICOM V3.0 Standard (NEMA PS 3). 1993. Washington, DC, National Electrical Manufacturers' Association.
10. Chui CK. 1992. Wavelets: A Tutorial in Theory and Applications, Boston: Academic Press.
11. Anderson MP, Loew MH, Brown DG. 1993. Gabor function based medical image compression. In HH Barrett, AF Gmitro (eds), Information Processing in Medical Imaging, Berlin, Springer-Verlag.
12. Fisher Y, Jacobs EW, Boss RD. 1992. Fractal image compression using iterated transforms. In JA Storer (ed), Image and Text Compression, Norwich, Mass, Kluwer.
13. Habibi A. 1971. Comparison of nth-order DPCM encoder with linear transformations and block quantization techniques. IEEE Trans Com COM-19 (6): 948.
14. Chen YP, Kim Y. 1993. Cost-effective data storage/archival subsystem for functional PACS. PACS 93, pp 131–142.
15. Wong AWK, Huang HK, Arenson RL. et al. 1994. Automated prefetch mechanism: Design and implementation for a radiology PACS. PACS 94, pp 102–111.
16. Wilson DL, Smith D, Rice B. 1994. Intelligent prefetch strategies for historical images in a large PACS. PACS 94 pp. 112–123.
17. Stead WW, Wiederhold G, Gardner R, et al. 1992. Database systems for computer-based patient records. ACPR, pp 83–98.
18. Liu Sheng OR, Wei C-P, Hu PJ-H, et al. 1994. Knowledge-based image retrieval: A new generation design. PACS 94, pp 137–148.
19. Lindberg DAB, Humphreys BL. 1992. The Unified Medical Language System (UMLS) and computer-based patient records. ACPR, pp. 165–175.

179
Computer Networks in Health Care

Soumitra Sengupta
Columbia University

Computer technology plays a prominent role today in health care delivery centers throughout the world. Information technology is gradually transforming the basic practice of medicine by improving the quality and quantity of information used by clinicians and administrators. The fundamental computer technology that accomplishes transparent and efficient flow of information from the creators of the information to the ultimate end users is *Computer Networking* [Tanenbaum 1988].

In a medical center, and to a lesser degree, in a health care practice center, computers are used for many purposes: in ancillary, departmental settings such as laboratory, pharmacy, radiology, pathology; in administrative contexts such as billing, patient management, transportation, payroll; in clinical and scholarly purposes such as electronic medical records, imaging, searching for medical references; and in basic research functions such as molecular modeling, genetics, robotics surgery [Rennels 1989; Duisterhout et al., 1991]. The concept of distributed computing is fast becoming a reality in medical domains, and it deals with the collection, integration and presentation of data distributed over several computers. Seamless information exchange requires the ubiquitous presence of a network, which, comprised of hardware and software components or layers, interconnects these computers. Well-defined methods and rules to communicate between computers are called *communication protocols*, and a collection of specific layers and protocols with its implementation is called a *communication standard*. Several communication standards, proprietary and open, exist today.

179.1 History

During the 1970s and the early 1980s, computing at hospitals was targeted to administrative needs. Central mainframe computers were employed for financial data processing. Even then, laboratory functions were starting to be automated due to their sheer volume and importance to the clinical community. Advent of personal computers (PCs) truly opened up automation opportunities for the ancillary departments as it became cost-effective to collect both departmental data for billing purposes and clinical data for clinical purposes. During the late 1980s, these stand-alone systems became permanent fixtures.

0-8493-8346-3/95/$0.00+$.50
© 1995 by CRC Press, Inc.

The networking technology also matured in the latter part of the 1980s. Networks' initial deployment within health care practice, however, was haphazard at best because of the large capital cost of laying cables and little understanding of the benefits at that time. Stand-alone systems started to need data from other systems: A single bill has to be sent to a patient for all services even though pharmacy and laboratory are different departments; ancillaries want to use the same demographic information that was entered in the hospital patient management system, and so on. Individual departments experimented with networking and succeeded in creating local solutions. This eventually became a problem when networks came to be appreciated as institutional resources and the local islands of information had to be rearranged for the larger institutional goals of networking efficiency and reliability.

179.2 Impact of Clinical Data

Clinical computing addresses the need for data related to patient care. These data must be delivered to the providers (physicians, nurses, technicians, therapists, social workers) in a timely fashion. The data must be accurate and be delivered in patient care settings such as bedside or nursing stations, intensive care units (ICUs), emergency rooms, operating theaters, clinics, and physicians' offices with varying degree of delivery efficiency. The needs for data in ICUs, for example, are more stringent than in a clinic. The primary data of importance in an inpatient setting are laboratory results. Other important sources of data include pharmacy, radiology, pathology, cardiology, vital signs, neurology, nursing documentation, obstetrics/gynecology, operative reports, discharge summaries, and visit notes. Whereas the paper-based patient chart has traditionally served the need for such information, it is clear that computers are far more efficient and accurate in organizing, maintaining and disseminating these records. The ability to use clinical information to support automated decision-making applications does not exist in paper-based systems. Hence, the concept of an all-electronic medical record has become popular in the past few years.

The delivery of clinical data from many different ancillary systems to diverse end-user settings requires a reliable networking infrastructure to transport the data. Clinical data may be collected from different sources and stored in a (conceptually) central clinical database. Here, a network is necessary to interconnect ancillary systems to a back-end central repository. In another scenario, a front-end workstation may query individual ancillaries and may dynamically construct an integrated view for a provider. Here, a network is necessary to connect ancillary systems to a front-end workstation. In reality, a comprehensive network that connects all computing entities within an institution enables all scenarios.

179.3 Information Types

Health care data have tremendous variety, all of which are important in patient care and have different implications for the performance required of a network. Most of the clinical data available today are in textual form as narrative reports. Radiology, pathology, and so on generate reports about specific tests; discharge summaries explain the entire episode of the patient's stay in the hospital; operative reports explain the procedure followed during operations. These reports range anywhere from a few sentences (in a specific type of pathology report) to several pages (autopsy reports).

Laboratory data tend to be in coded form, where each data item is represented as a code (alphanumeric, integers). This is very useful as providers need to look at trends in data over time (examples include temperature readings and anion count in blood). Furthermore, for computer-based clinical decision support, more data need to be in coded form so that a computer-based expert system can understand the values and act upon them to send alerts to providers, if necessary. Coded data, in general, are small in size, but in some cases such as an EKG tracing, each point may be a code, and thus the report may be of substantial size.

Hospitals also use a large amount of multimedia data. All radiologic tests are performed as visual interpretation of images and video sequences (X-ray images, CAT scans, PET scans, SPECT scans). To a lesser degree, ultrasound sonograms, pathology slides, gated blood pool studies, and neurology are other sources of these data. The size of these data is at least two orders of magnitude larger than that of coded and text data. A network that can support these kinds of data requires special consideration and design and is also more expensive.

In academic institutions, a large amount of computer-based educational information is graphical and video-based. Many stand-alone educational products are being actively used today. Looking toward the future, these data (depicting topics such as how to conduct a "physical and history" examination on a patient and how to conduct an arthroscopic surgery of the knee) will be available over the same network and on demand to all students, faculty, and practitioners.

179.4 Platforms

Individual departments have typically purchased turnkey systems (or have purchased hardware and then developed the necessary software themselves) that are *best-of-breed* variety for their applications. Once the benefits of data exchange were understood, networking has become one of the key considerations for these systems. Since there are several standards of networking, and not all are supported by all systems, heterogeneity of computing platforms has become an issue. The solutions include *application gateways,* computers that translate from one protocol to another while passing the data between them transparently. Gateways are acceptable as an exception, but too many gateways cause severe performance and reliability problems in the network. The current norm is to choose a restricted set of protocol standards that are fully supported within an institution. A strict control on resources helps in addressing the network needs of the majority.

179.5 Current Technologies

Networks are usually defined as a set of *layers,* each layer providing service to the layer above it. The networking infrastructure suitable in a campus environment today is called a *local area network* (LAN). An organization has full control over its LANs. In contrast, when communication is required over long distances (e.g., and organization which has offices all over the world), services from a long-distance carrier company are required to establish what is called a *wide area network* (WAN). The protocols at higher layers work transparently over LANs and WANs, thus providing transparency to applications. Currently, software solutions are appearing that use distributed programs in order to achieve total network transparency and data integration from the end-user viewpoint. These are popularly termed *middleware*. Finally, there are specific solutions and standards pertinent to the health care environment which address medical domain problems which may be called *medical domain middleware*. In the following, we elaborate further on each of these concepts.

Local Area Networks

The lowermost layer in networking is the *physical* medium, which can be copper cables (with different degrees of insulation, twists, and impedance), fiber cables (with different diameter and refraction indices), or even the atmosphere in the case of wireless communication based on radio-frequency transmissions. Examples of physical medium standards include 10BaseT, 10Base5, and STP. The next higher layer, the *link* layer consists of electronics or optics to drive signals on the physical layer. The most popular LAN standards in this layer today are Ethernet (or IEEE 802.3) at a rated 10Mbits/s speed (or bandwidth) and Token Ring (IEEE 802.5) at 4 or 16 Mbits/s speed. Above these layers, several proprietary protocols and layer stacks may coreside in typical medical practice center LANs. These include IBM SNA and NetBIOS, Novell SPX/IPX, DEC DECNet and LAT, and Apple AppleTalk. Among open protocols, the TCP/IP stack is the most popular standard.

The *topology* of a LAN is the layout of networking segments (e.g., Ethernet, Token Ring) and their interconnections by devices such as repeaters, bridges, and routers. Some of the factors that influence topology design are traffic estimates and patterns, redundancy, isolation and security, physical plant including building and cabling layout, and organizational structure. A practical topology is that of redundant campus backbone segments that then connect to building segments, thus forming a hierarchy of segments. A medical center LAN needs to accommodate heterogeneous sets of computers and consequently needs to support several higher-layer protocols. The choice of higher-layer protocols also influences the choice of bridges and router devices. Although initially driven by the integration of existing systems, a medical center LAN settles on a small subset of protocols for most of its mainstream communication, which is practically motivated by the support and maintenance issues.

In addition to medical domain applications, users require the usual file and print services for day-to-day applications such as spreadsheets, word processors, presentation programs, and electronic mail. As networked PCs have become popular as user workstations, Novell SPX/IPX in the IBM PC world and Apple AppleTalk in the Apple Macintosh world protocols are increasingly used to provide these services. A widely used application on the PCs today is terminal emulation by which a PC behaves as a terminal to an ancillary or central computer on the network, and thus subsequently has access to all medical applications on that application server computer. LANs, instead of the traditional point-to-point connections, have become the primary vehicle for computer communication at health care practice centers to the extent that all new computers are expected to be LAN-compatible. A special group of LAN specialists is required to support the LANs. Since LAN technology is constantly evolving toward better and faster communications, it is important to maintain up-to-date knowledge in this field.

Wide Area Networks

Health care centers employ WANs mainly for three purposes: to connect networks at physically distant buildings, offices, or clinics; to connect networks to different organizations (affiliated hospitals, insurance agencies, state or federal government regulatory bodies) or services (Internet, disaster recovery backup locations); and to provide dial-in and dial-out capabilities for employees. The difference between the first two purposes is that of control and security: access to medical information requires better control when connected to an external organization. The concept of a *firewall* as part of networking topology has become popular when connecting to the Internet in order to deter unwarranted access. A physician's office may connect to insurance networks for billing, as well as to on-line services to connect to the larger Internet. In all cases, an external telecommunications carrier's service is used to provide underlying long-distance, point-to-point communications capability.

The aggregate bandwidth in a WAN connection is typically much smaller than the LAN bandwidth because of the higher costs of WAN connections. Popular leased line connections have speeds ranging from 56 Kbits/s to 1.56 Mbits/s (T-1 circuits) to 45 Mbits/s (T-3 circuits), and fractions thereof. Other modes of such connections are accomplished by dedicated microwave or laser communications. In all cases, end devices such as modems are required to drive these connections. Additionally, multiplexers are employed to effectively use the available bandwidth. It is common to extend the LAN protocols to run over the WAN connections, so that applications run transparently regardless of location, but perhaps at a slower speed due to the restricted bandwidth.

Dial-in and dial-out access is provided over asynchronous phone lines with speeds ranging from 1200 bits/s to 28.8 Kbits/s. Integrated Services Digital Network (ISDN) solutions (at 64 Kbits/s) are becoming available and cost-effective. With implementations of the point-to-point protocol (PPP) standard, the dialing-in PC will become a full peer node on the organizational network, instead of becoming a terminal to some computer or going through a surrogate PC on the network.

Middleware

At higher layers of networking, the client-server computing paradigm is becoming an alternative to central host-based computing. By distributing the work over several nodes on the network, more efficient and flexible solutions are created. These solutions integrate data for the end-users at the front end while hiding the multiplicity of origins of the data at the back end. A reliable, distributed file system, distributed printing services, consolidated directory services, network-based security service, and transparent invocation of applications residing elsewhere are examples of middleware. In the medical center context, it is extremely important to establish standards at this level to effectively tame the heterogeneity. Specific examples of middleware include Open Software Foundation's Distributed Computing Environment (DCE), SUN's Open Network Computing (ONC), OSI X.500 directory services, MIT kerberos security service, and OMG Common Object Request Broker Architecture (CORBA).

Medical Domain Middleware

With the availability of standard networks, applications, and enabling middleware technologies, clinical computing concentrates on the collection, integration, and dissemination of clinical data. In addition, the major focus is to convert data into knowledge in order to help the provider make better clinical decisions. In order to accomplish these transformations, several medical domain middleware tools and concepts need to be constructed and understood to operate in a distributed computing environment.

Integrated Patient Database

A comprehensive clinical information system requires construction of a logically integrated repository of all clinical information for each patient. As stated previously, clinical data originate at many ancillary systems. All data may be collected at a single, physically central repository, using the network as and when data are produced at the ancillaries. In this case, a data review application needs only to query (over the network) the central repository for all data, which reduces the complexity at the front end. Alternatively, data review applications may query several ancillaries dynamically at the time a specific patient's data are being reviewed, thus creating a virtual patient repository. In either case, data integration is transparent to the end-user.

Networks permit very efficient distributions of the patient database. Since, from a clinical viewpoint one patient's data are completely independent of another patient's data, each patient's data constitutes a separate database. Therefore, it is possible to isolate a specific patient database (or a set of patient databases) on one host. One logical distribution strategy is that of dedicating a fully functional database for each nursing station within a hospital with a well-defined strategy of migrating patients from one database to another. Once again, however, the operations must be transparent to the end-user, and the explicit reference to hosts and patient information must be hidden within the database functions.

The need for clinical and hospital data exchange among heterogeneous systems has required the creation of common standards for the definition of medical events, the collection of data associated with these events, and the recognition of events that may be useful to participating systems [McDonald & Hammond, 1989]. The only practical standard today is *Health Level 7* (HL-7), commonly followed by many vendors today. Examples of events defined in HL-7 include admit, discharge, transfer, order, and order results. The use of the standard avoids the need to make unnecessary translations.

The success of these early databases has raised the interesting question: How can a patient's information be collected from many institutions (doctor's office, clinics, hospitals) to create a comprehensive record that is readily available over the network regardless of the patient's geographic location? Many efforts in electronic medical records at the national level include discussion of the pros and cons of merging of information for clinical care of the patient as well as for epidemiological research for the society at large.

Medical Vocabulary

A common medical vocabulary is fast becoming a necessity within clinical information systems. The vocabulary addresses the problem of understanding the semantics of medical concepts, answering questions about whether two concepts are the same or different, and if the latter, how so [Cimino et al., 1994]. For example, cardiomegaly and enlargement of heart are the same concepts, a fact that cannot be derived syntactically. A medical vocabulary defines medical concepts as entities and supports links between entities that collectively define that concept. In the exchange of information between systems, the vocabulary serves as the semantic standard of the meaning of the data items exchanged, much as HL-7 serves as the syntactic standard. Without the vocabulary, the end-user must know how each medical concept is described in each of the ancillaries to formulate his queries correctly. With the vocabulary, the concepts are semantically translated to either a canonical code or to the native ancillary code for that concept. The vocabulary makes the heterogeneity of terminology introduced by several ancillary systems transparent to the user.

Directions and Challenges

Medical computing will continue to take advantage of the ever-increasing expansion of the computing technology. Options not viable in the past are quickly becoming mainstream in the areas of improved networking bandwidth. In addition, the current changes in the health care business dictate more efficient forms of care delivery, which may be facilitated only by adopting information technologies. In the following sections, we discuss a few directions and challenges in this field.

Improved Bandwidth

The currently prevalent networks with 4, 10, and 16 Mbits/s bandwidth are inadequate for pervasive imaging and multimedia applications. Due to the richness of medical information, these applications are extremely important and have a tremendous impact on the required network bandwidth. Existing high-speed networks at 100 Mbits/s, primarily Fiber Distributed Data Interface (FDDI), have been used as the campus backbones but have failed to capture the marketplace due to the high cost of fiber cable deployment and adapter cards. Instead, new standards of 100 Mbits/s communication (100Base-T or Fast Ethernet, 100VG-AnyLAN) are fast becoming reality. These technologies use the same cables (UTP grade 5, STP) as for the slower networks, but at a higher cost of equipment. If fiber optic cables are used, then communication can reach Gigabits/s (1000 Mbits/s) range, although most implementations today support 155 Mbits/s. This is being accomplished by the new standard of *asynchronous transfer mode* (ATM) communication and corresponding devices called ATM switches. The long-distance carriers are standardizing on interfaces called synchronous optical network (SONET) or synchronous digital hierarchy (SDH) that support variable speeds ranging from 1.56 Mbits/s (T-1 circuits) to 155 Mbits/s (OC-3c) to 655 Mbits/s (OC-7c) over fiber optic cable. Since ATM switches can use SONET connections, ATM may be the enabling technology that allows LANs and WANs to work together seamlessly at high speeds without any performance penalties.

ATM technology is available in various forms. It can be used as a campus LAN backbone switch that connects routers, servers, and other switches. The second form is that of LAN extenders, whereby an Ethernet or Token Ring is extended to another location over high-speed ATM connections; in this form, ATM switches work as virtual LAN repeaters. ATM adapters are available for many workstations such as SUN SparcStations, IBM RS/6000, HP 9000, and DEC AlphaStations. The technology itself is flexible in that it can be supported over any type of cable (copper and fiber). The communication occurs over fixed length *cells* of 53 bytes (as opposed to variable length *packets* in X.25), which makes it possible to guarantee service to time-dependent (or isochronous) applications and allows very fast hardware-based cell switching to route the cells through the switches. ATM networking also capitalizes on today's high speed, reliable communication links by forgoing error/detection/correction at each intermediate node within the network.

The ATM standard, set by the International Telegraph and Telephone Union Telecommunications Sector (ITU-T), is promoted by an ATM Forum consisting of over 500 members. The Forum has also set standards for interfaces required to communicate between various ATM nodes, and between ATM layers and other protocols. Residing within the traditional link layer, several parallel stacks called *ATM adaptation layers* (AAL) define protocols and quality of services for voice circuit emulation (AAL 1), timing-sensitive video/audio transfer (AAL 2), connection-oriented and connectionless data transfer for bursty data (AAL 3/4), and simple and efficient adaptation layer for local, high speed LAN installations (AAL 5). Although the ATM technology has great potential, the ATM solutions must integrate with the legacy networks in an orderly fashion to achieve a smooth transition. The accelerated integration of ATM technology into the desktop, hubs, bridges, and routers indicates that ATM has a high probability of dominating the marketplace.

At many institutions today, campus backbones are composed of fiber optic cables, and some institutions even have fiber optic cables at the desktops. At a few well-known radiology centers, *picture archiving communications systems* (PACS), a technology for creating, storing, and disseminating radiologic images, have been installed using networks exclusively dedicated to PACS information exchange. The PACS systems may be considered one of the ancillary systems serving one department's needs. As faster networking technologies become universally available and as workstations become powerful enough to provide on-the-fly decompression, a true multimedia view of patient information may be constructed for the first time at the provider's desktop.

Another example of applications requiring higher bandwidth is *telemedicine.* It is a concept whereby health care may be delivered remotely over computer networks by providers who are physically far away from the patient [Halpern et al., 1992]. This technology is being actively pursued by the federal government and by several state governments through the National Information Infrastructure initiative and through statewide information highway initiatives. Several tertiary-care institutions are arranging affiliation with primary and secondary care institutions to provide expert referral services. The concept is also popular in rural settings, where more sophisticated care may be available at a limited number of locations.

One of the fundamental requirements for telemedicine is a networking bandwidth that is capable of supporting simultaneous video, audio, image and data transfer in real time. Technologies such as ATM and SONet promise to be the solutions to this problem. Today, telemedicine is restricted to asynchronous referral services for medical images, remote review of clinical information, and occasional video conferences. In prototype situations, however, complicated scenarios involving telesurgery have been shown to be possible using remote robotic hands and head-mounted displays in an augmented reality setting.

Security

Networks have made flexible data access possible. Recently data interconnections have exploded among care facilities, private physicians' offices, nursing homes, insurance agencies, health maintenance organizations, research institutions, and state and federal regulatory agencies. Internet is the precursor to the eventual information super-highway. The problem of security has become ever more important in this new world of accessible yet confidential patient information—including issues of who owns the data, how to protect the data, how to convert it securely to meet societal needs for statistical information, and so on. Smart cards, encryption, digital signatures, guaranteed authentication and authorization, and constant accounting and auditing are several techniques being considered in intense discussions addressing the security aspects of medical information networking [US Congress 1993].

Management

Managing networks and distributed applications is orders-of-magnitude harder than managing a single, monolithic system. It is, however, extremely important to invest in and learn how to manage the hundreds of networking and computing components that bring value to the networks. Although there are some good tools and standards available to monitor the lower layers of networks and devices such as bridges and routers, there is a total lack of management capabilities for middleware and nascent medical domain middleware. Monitoring of applications helps determine future demands for resources, performance guarantees, and opportunities to make a system more reliable. The primary management communication standard is simple network management protocol (SNMP), which is not yet at the advanced stage of managing higher-layer protocols and applications.

179.6 Conclusions

The use of networks at health care practice centers has provided value by increasing data availability, flexibility, and efficiency of operations. The graphical-user-interface-based applications, along with client-server paradigms of computing, have begun to appear on these networks. The next generation of multimedia applications will require higher bandwidth networks, which have already begun to appear. In addition, the national efforts to link health care industries and providers in order to improve efficiency will now be possible due to the networks that have become the fourth utility—after electricity, water, and heat—in many medical centers. Individual doctor's offices, clinics, and practice settings are connecting to computer networks that accomplish the communication functions of the larger health care business networks.

Defining Terms

Communication protocols: A set of rules and methods by which computers communicate with each other.

Ethernet, Token Ring: Examples of specific kind of communication protocols suitable for local area networks.

Fiber distributed data interface (FDDI), asynchronous transfer mode (ATM): High-speed communication protocols suitable for both local and wide area networks.

Local area network: Computer networking infrastructure suitable for a campus (or smaller) environment where the owning organization controls connection and protocols.

Medical domain middleware: Middleware addressed specifically to transparently access health care information on the network.

Middleware: Software components that help create a transparent access to resources regardless of their physical location in the network.

Network topology: A detailed map of physical and conceptual connections among networking devices.

Unshielded or shielded twisted pair (UTP, STP): Types of cables with different electrical characteristics and prices.

Wide area network: Computer networking infrastructure that connects several local area networks distributed over great geographical distances using external services.

References

Cimino JJ, Clayton PD, Hripcsak G, et al. 1994. Knowledge-based approaches to the maintenance of a large controlled medical terminology. J Am Med Informatics Assoc 1:35.

Duisterhout JS, Hasman A, Salamon R (eds). 1991. Telematics in Medicine, Amsterdam, Elsevier Science Publishers.

Halpern EJ, Newhouse JH, Amis ESJ, et al. 1992. Evaluation of teleradiology for interpretation of intravenous urograms. J Digital Imaging 5(2):101.

McDonald CT, Hammond WE. 1989. Standard formats for electronic transfer of clinical data. Ann Intern Med 110:333.

Rennels GD, Shortliffe EH. 1987. Advanced computing for medicine. Sci Am 257(4):154.

Tanenbaum AS. 1988. Computer Networks, 2d ed, Englewood Cliffs, NJ, Prentice-Hall.

US Congress, Office of Technology Assessment. 1993. Protecting Privacy in Computerized Medical Information, OTA-TCT-576. Washington, DC, US Government Printing Office.

180

Overview of Standards Related to the Emerging Health Care Information Infrastructure

Jeffrey S. Blair
IBM Health Care Solutions

As the cost of health care has become a larger percentage of the gross domestic product of many developed nations, the focus on methods to improve health care productivity and quality has increased. To address this need, the concept of a health care information infrastructure has emerged. Major elements of this concept include patient-centered care facilitated by computer-based patient record systems, continuity of care enabled by the sharing of patient information across information networks, and outcomes measurement aided by the greater availability and specificity of health care information.

The creation of this health care information infrastructure will require the integration of existing and new architectures, products and services. To make these diverse components work together, health care information standards (classifications, guides, practices, and terminology) will be required [ASTM, 1994]. This chapter will give you an overview of the major existing and emerging health care information standards, and the efforts to coordinate, harmonize, and accelerate these activities. It is organized into the major topic areas of:

- Identifier standards
- Communications (message format) standards
- Content and structure standards
- Clinical data representations (codes)

0-8493-8346-3/95/$0.00+$.50
© 1995 by CRC Press, Inc.

- Confidentiality, data security, and authentication
- Quality indicators and data sets
- International standards
- Coordinating and promotion organizations
- Summary

180.1 Identifier Standards

There is a universal need for health care identifiers to uniquely specify each patient, provider, site of care and product; however, there is not universal acceptance and/or satisfaction with these systems.

Patient Identifiers

The social security number (SSN) is widely used as a patient identifier in the United States today. However, critics point out that it is not an ideal identifier. They say that not everyone has an SSN; several individuals may use the same SSN; and the SSN is so widely used for other purposes that it presents an exposure to violations of confidentiality. These criticisms raise issues that are not unique to the SSN. A draft document has been developed by the American Society for Testing and Materials (ASTM) E31.12 Subcommittee to address these issues. It is called the "Guide for the Properties of a Universal Health Care Identifier" (UHID). It presents a set of requirements outlining the properties of a national system creating a UHID, includes critiques of the SSN, and creates a sample UHID (ASTM E31.12, 1994). Despite the advantages of a modified/new patient identifier, there is not yet a consensus as to who would bear the cost of adopting a new patient identifier system.

Provider Identifiers

The Health Care Financing Administration (HCFA) has created a widely used provider identifier known as the Universal Physician Identifier Number (UPIN) [Terrell et al., 1991]. The UPIN is assigned to physicians who handle Medicare patients, but it does not include nonphysician care givers. The National Council of Prescription Drug Programs (NCPDP) has developed the standard prescriber identification number (SPIN) to be used by pharmacists in retail settings. A proposal to develop a new national provider identifier number has been set forth by HCFA [HCFA, 1994]. If this proposal is accepted, then HCFA would develop a national provider identifier number which would cover all caregivers and sites of care, including Medicare, Medicaid, and private care. This proposal is being reviewed by various state and federal agencies. It has also been sent to the American National Standards Institute's Health Care Informatics Standards Planning Panel (ANSI HISPP) Task Force on Provider Identifiers for review.

Site-of-Care Identifiers

Two site-of-care identifier systems are widely used. One is the health industry number (HIN) issued by the Health Industry Business Communications Council (HIBCC). The HIN is an identifier for health care facilities, practitioners, and retail pharmacies. HCFA has also defined provider of service identifiers for Medicare usage.

Product and Supply Labeling Identifiers

Three identifiers are widely accepted. The labeler identification code (LIC) identifies the manufacturer or distributer and is issued by HIBCC [HIBCC, 1994]. The LIC is used both with and without bar codes for products and supplies distributed within a health care facility. The universal product code (UPC) is maintained by the Uniform Code Council and is typically used to label products that are sold in retail settings. The national drug code is maintained by the Food and Drug Administration and is required for reimbursement by Medicare, Medicaid, and insurance companies. It is sometimes included within the UPC format.

180.2 Communications (Message Format) Standards

Although the standards in this topic area are still in various stages of development, they are generally more mature than those in most of the other topic areas. They are typically developed by committees within standards organizations and have generally been accepted by users and vendors. The overviews of these standards below were derived from many sources, but considerable content came from the Computer-based Patient Record Institute's (CPRI) "Position Paper on Computer-based Patient Record Standards" [CPRI, 1994] and the Agency for Health Care Policy and Research's (AHCPR) "Current Activities of Selected Health Care Informatics Standards Organizations" [Moshman Associates, 1994].

ASC X12N

This committee is developing message format standards for transactions between payors and providers. It is rapidly being accepted by both users and vendors. It defines the message formats for the following transaction types [Moshman Associates, 1994]:

- 834—enrollment
- 270—eligibility request
- 271—eligibility response
- 837—health care claim submission
- 835—health care claim payment remittance
- 276—claims status request
- 277—claims status response
- 148—report of injury or illness

ASC X12N is also working on the following standards to be published in the near future:

- 257, 258—Interactive eligibility response and request. These transactions are an abbreviated form of the 270/271.
- 274, 275—patient record data response and request. These transactions will be used to request and send patient data (tests, procedures, surgeries, allergies, etc.) between a requesting party and the party maintaining the database.
- 278, 279—health care services (utilization review) response and request. These transactions will be used to initiate and respond to a utilization review request.

ASC X12N is recognized as an accredited standards committee (ASC) by the American National Standards Institute (ANSI).

American Society for Testing and Materials (ASTM) Message Format Standards

The following standards were developed within ASTM Committee E31. This committee has applied for recognition as an ASC by ANSI.

- ASTM E1238 standard specification for transferring clinical observations between independent systems. E1238 was developed by ASTM Subcommittee E31.11. This standard is being used by most of the largest commercial laboratory vendors in the United States to transmit laboratory results. It has also been adopted by a consortium of 25 French laboratory system vendors. Health Level Seven (HL7), which is described later in this topic area, has incorporated E1238 as a subset within its laboratory results message format [CPRI, 1994].

- ASTM E1394 standard specification for transferring information between clinical instruments. E1394 was developed by ASTM Subcommittee E31.14. This standard is being used for communication of information from laboratory instruments to computer systems. This standard has been developed by a consortium consisting of most U.S. manufacturers of clinical laboratory instruments [CPRI, 1994].
- ASTM E1460 specification for defining and sharing modular health knowledge bases (Arden Syntax). E1460 was developed by ASTM Subcommittee E31.15. The Arden Syntax provides a standard format and syntax for representing medical logic and for writing rules and guidelines that can be automatically executed by computer systems. Medical logic modules produced in one site of care system can be sent to a different system within another site of care and then customized to reflect local usage [CPRI, 1994].
- ASTM E1467 specification for transferring digital neurophysical data between independent computer systems. E1467 was developed by ASTM Subcommittee E31.17. This standard defines codes and structures needed to transmit electrophysiologic signals and results produced by electroencephalograms and electromyograms. The standard is similar in structure to ASTM E1238 and HL7; and it is being adopted by all the EEG systems manufacturers [CPRI, 1994].

Digital Imaging and Communications (DICOM)

This standard is developed by the American College of Radiology–National Electronic Manufacturers' Association (ACR-NEMA). It defines the message formats and communications standards for radiologic images. DICOM is supported by most radiology Picture Archiving and Communications Systems (PACS) vendors and has been incorporated into the Japanese Image Store and Carry (ISAC) optical disk system as well as Kodak's PhotoCD. ACR-NEMA is applying to be recognized as an accredited organization by ANSI [CPRI, 1994].

Health Level Seven (HL7)

HL7 is used for intrainstitution transmission of orders; clinical observations and clinical data, including test results; admission, transfer, and discharge records; and charge and billing information. HL7 is being used in more than 300 U.S. health care institutions including most leading university hospitals and has been adopted by Australia and New Zealand as their national standard. HL7 is recognized as an accredited organization by ANSI [Hammond, 1993; CPRI, 1994].

Institute of Electrical and Electronic Engineers, Inc. (IEEE) P1157 Medical Data Interchange Standard (MEDIX)

IEEE Engineering in Medicine and Biology Society (EMB) is developing the MEDIX standards for the exchange of data between hospital computer systems [Harrington, 1993; CPRI, 1994]. Based on the International Standards Organization (ISO) standards for all seven layers of the OSI reference model, MEDIX is working on a framework model to guide the development and evolution of a compatible set of standards. This activity is being carried forward as a joint working group under ANSI HISPP's Message Standards Developers Subcommittee (MSDS). IEEE is recognized as an accredited organization by ANSI.

IEEE P1073 Medical Information Bus (MIB)

This standard defines the linkages of medical instrumentation (e.g., critical care instruments) to point-of-care information systems [CPRI, 1994].

National Council for Prescription Drug Programs (NCPDP)

These standards developed by NCPDP are used for communication of billing and eligibility information between community pharmacies and third-party payers. They have been in use since 1985 and now serve almost 60% of the nation's community pharmacies. NCPDP has applied for recognition as an accredited organization by ANSI [CPRI, 1994].

180.3 Content and Structure Standards

Guidelines and standards for the content and structure of computer-based patient record (CPR) systems are being developed within ASTM Subcommittees E31.12 and E31.19. They have been recognized by other standards organizations (e.g., HL7); however, they have not matured to the point where they are generally accepted or implemented by users and vendors.

A major revision to E1384, now called a *standard description for content and structure of the computer-based patient record*, has been made within Subcommittee E31.19 [ASTM, 1994]. This revision includes work from HISPP on data modeling and an expanded framework that includes master tables and data views by user.

Companion standards have been developed within E31.19. They are E1633, A Standard Specification for the Coded Values Used in the Automated Primary Record of Care (ASTM, 1994), and E1239-94, A Standard Guide for Description of Reservation/Registration-A/D/T Systems for Automated Patient Care Information Systems (ASTM, 1994). A draft standard is also being developed for object-oriented models for R-A/D/T functions in CPR systems. Within the E31.12 Subcommittee, domain specific guidelines for nursing, anesthesiology, and emergency room data within the CPR are being developed [Moshman Associates, 1994; Waegemann, 1994].

180.4 Clinical Data Representations (Codes)

Clinical data representations have been widely used to document diagnoses and procedures. There are over 150 known code systems. The codes with the widest acceptance in the United States include:

- International Classification of Diseases (ICD) codes, now in the ninth edition (ICD-9), are maintained by the World Health Organization (WHO) and are accepted worldwide. In the United States, HCFA and the National Center for Health Statistics (NCHS) have supported the development of a clinical modification of the ICD codes (ICD-9-CM). WHO has been developing ICD-10; however, HCFA projects that it will not be available for use within the United States for several years. Payers require the use of ICD-9-CM codes for reimbursement purposes, but they have limited value for clinical and research purposes due to their lack of clinical specificity [Chute, 1991].

- Current Procedural Terminology (CPT) codes are maintained by the American Medical Association (AMA) and are widely used in the United States for reimbursement and utilization review purposes. The codes are derived from medical specialty nomenclatures and are updated annually [Chute, 1991].

- The Systematized Nomenclature of Medicine (SNOMED) is maintained by the College of American Pathologists and is widely accepted for describing pathologic test results. It has a multiaxial (11 fields) coding structure that gives it greater clinical specificity than the ICD and CPT codes, and it has considerable value for clinical purposes. SNOMED has been proposed as a candidate to become the standardized vocabulary for computer-based patient record systems (Rothwell et al., 1993).

- Digital Imaging and Communications (DICOM) is maintained by the American College of Radiology–National Electronic Manufacturers' Association (ACR-NEMA). It sets forth standards for indicies of radiologic diagnoses as well as for image storage and communications [Cannavo, 1993].

- Diagnostic and Statistical Manual of Mental Disorders (DSM), now in its fourth edition (DSM-IV), is maintained by the American Psychiatric Association. It sets forth a standard set of codes and descriptions for use in diagnoses, prescriptions, research, education, and administration [Chute, 1991].

- Diagnostic Related Groups (DRGs) are maintained by HCFA. They are derivatives of ICD-9-CM codes and are used to facilitate reimbursement and case-mix analysis. They lack the clinical specificity to be of value in direct patient care or clinical research [Chute, 1991].
- Unified Medical Language System (UMLS) is maintained by the National Library of Medicine (NLM). It contains a metathesaurus that links clinical terminology, semantics, and formats of the major clinical coding and reference systems. It links medical terms (e.g., ICD, CPT, SNOMED, DSM, CO-STAR, and D-XPLAIN) to the NLM's medical index subject headings (MeSH codes) and to each other [Humphreys, 1991; Cimino et al., 1993].
- The Canon Group has not developed a clinical data representation, but it is addressing two important problems: clinical data representations typically lack clinical specificity and/or are incapable of being generalized or extended beyond a specific application. "The Group proposes to focus on the design of a general schema for medical-language representation including the specification of the resources and associated procedures required to map language (including standard terminologies) into representations that make all implicit relations 'visible,' reveal 'hidden attributes,' and generally resolve . . . ambiguous references" [Evans et al., 1994].

180.5 Confidentiality, Data Security, and Authentication

The development of computer-based patient record systems and health care information networks have created the opportunity to address the need for more definitive confidentiality, data security, and authentication guidelines and standards. The following activities address this need:

- During 1994, several bills were drafted in Congress to address health care privacy and confidentiality. They included the Fair Health Information Practices Act of 1994 (H.R. 4077), the Health Care Privacy Protection Act (S. 2129), and others. Although these bills were not passed as drafted, their essential content is expected to be included as part of subsequent health care reform legislation. They address the need for uniform comprehensive federal rules governing the use and disclosure of identifiable health information about individuals. They specify the responsibilities of those who collect, use, and maintain health information about patients. They also define the rights of patients and provide a variety of mechanisms that will allow patients to enforce their rights.
- ASTM Subcommittee E31.12 on Computer-based Patient Records is developing Guidelines for Minimal Data Security Measures for the Protection of Computer-based Patient Records [Moshman Associates, 1994].
- ASTM Subcommittee E31.17 on Access, Privacy, and Confidentiality of Medical Records is working on standards to address these issues [Moshman Associates, 1994].
- ASTM Subcommittee E31.20 is developing standard specifications for authentication of health information [Moshman Associates, 1994].
- The Committee on Regional Health Data Networks convened by the Institute of Medicine (IOM) has completed a definitive study and published its findings in a book entitled *Health Data in the Information Age: Use, Disclosure, and Privacy* [Donaldson & Lohr, 1994].
- The Computer-based Patient Record Institute's (CPRI) Work Group on Confidentiality, Privacy and Legislation has completed white papers on "Access to Patient Data" and on "Authentication," and a publication entitled "Guidelines for Establishing Information Security: Policies at Organizations using Computer-based Patient Records" [CPRI, 1994].
- The Office of Technology Assessment has completed a two-year study resulting in a document entitled "Protecting Privacy in Computerized Medical Information." It includes a comprehensive review of system/data security issues, privacy information, current laws, technologies used for protection, and models.

- The U.S. Food and Drug Administration (FDA) has created a task force on Electronic/ Identification Signatures to study authentication issues as they relate to the pharmaceutical industry.

180.6 Quality Indicators and Data Sets

The Joint Commission on Accreditation of Health Care Organizations (JCAHO) has been developing and testing obstetrics, oncology, trauma, and cardiovascular clinical indicators. These indicators are intended to facilitate provider performance measurement. Several vendors are planning to include JCAHO clinical indicators in their performance measurement systems [JCAHO, 1994].

The Health Employers Data and Information Set (HEDIS) version 2.0 has been developed with the support of the National Committee for Quality Assurance (NCQA). It identifies data to support performance measurement in the areas of quality (e.g., preventive medicine, prenatal care, acute and chronic disease, and mental health), access and patient satisfaction, membership and utilization, and finance. The development of HEDIS has been supported by several large employers and managed care organizations [NCQA, 1993].

180.7 International Standards

The International Organization for Standardization (ISO) is a worldwide federation of national standards organizations. It has 90 member countries. The purpose of ISO is to promote the development of standardization and related activities in the world. ANSI was one of the founding members of ISO and is the representative for the United States [Waegemann, 1994].

ISO has established a communications model for Open Systems Interconnection (OSI). IEEE/ MEDIX and HL7 have recognized and built upon the ISO/OSI framework. Further, ANSI HISPP has a stated objective of encouraging compatibility of U.S. health care standards with ISO/OSI. The ISO activities related to information technology take place within the Joint Technical Committee (JTC) 1.

The Comite Europeen de Normalisation (CEN) is a European standards organization with 16 technical committees (TCs). Two TCs are specifically involved in health care: TC 251 (Medical Informatics) and TC 224 WG12 (Patient Data Cards) [Waegemann, 1994].

The CEN TC 251 on Medical Informatics includes work groups on: Modeling of Medical Records; Terminology, Coding, Semantics, and Knowledge Bases; Communications and Messages; Imaging and Multimedia; Medical Devices; and Security, Privacy, Quality and Safety. The CEN TC 251 has established coordination with health care standards development in the United States through ANSI/HISPP.

In addition to standards developed by ISO and CEN, there are two other standards of importance. United Nations (U.N.) EDIFACT is a generic messaging-based communications standard with health-specific subsets. It parallels X12 and HL7, which are transaction-based standards. It is widely used in Europe and in several Latin American countries. The READ Classification System (RCS) is a multiaxial medical nomenclature used in the United Kingdom. It is sponsored by the National Health Service and has been integrated into computer-based ambulatory patient record systems in the United Kingdom [CAMS, 1994].

180.8 Standards Coordination and Promotion Organizations

In the United States, two organizations have emerged to assume responsibility for the coordination and promotion of health care standards development: the ANSI Health Care Informatics Standards Planning Panel (HISPP) and the Computer-based Patient Record Institute (CPRI). The major missions of ANSI HISPP are:

1. To coordinate the work of the standards groups for health care data interchange and health care informatics (e.g., ACR/NEMA, ASTM, HL7, IEEE/MEDIX) and other relevant standards

groups (e.g., X3, X12) toward achieving the evolution of a unified set of nonredundant, non-conflicting standards.

2. To interact with and provide input to CEN TC 251 (Medical Informatics) in a coordinated fashion and explore avenues of international standards development.

The first mission of coordinating standards is performed by the Message Standards Developers Subcommittee (MSDS). The second mission is performed by the International and Regional Standards Subcommittee. HISPP also has four task groups: (1) Codes and Vocabulary, (2) Privacy, Security and Confidentiality, (3) Provider Identification Numbering Systems, and (4) Operations. Its principle membership is comprised of representatives of the major health care standards development organizations (SDOs), government agencies, vendors, and other interested parties. ANSI HISPP is by definition a planning panel, not an SDO (Hammond, 1994: ANSI HISPP, 1994).

The CPRI's mission is to promote acceptance of the vision set forth in the Institute of Medicine Study report "The Computer-based Patient Record: An Essential Technology for Health Care." CPRI is a nonprofit organization committed to initiating and coordinating activities to facilitate and promote the routine use of computer-based patient records. The CPRI takes initiatives to promote the development of CPR standards, but it is not an SDO itself. CPRI members represent the entire range of stakeholders in the health care delivery system. Its major work groups are the: (1) Codes and Structures Work Group; (2) CPR Description Work Group; (3) CPR Systems Evaluation Work Group; (4) Confidentiality, Privacy, and Legislation Work Group; and (5) Professional and Public Education Work Group [CPRI, 1994].

Two work efforts have been initiated to establish models for principle components of the emerging health care information infrastructure. The CPR Description Work Group of the CPRI is defining a consensus-based model of the computer-based patient record system. A joint working group to create a common data description has been formed by the MSDS Subcommittee of ANSI HISPP and IEEE/MEDIX. The joint working group is an open standards effort to support the development of a common data model that can be shared by developers of health care informatics standards [IEEE, 1994].

The CPRI has introduced a proposal defining a public/private effort to accelerate standards development for computer-based patient record systems [CPRI, 1994]. If funding becomes available, the project will focus on obtaining consensus for a conceptual description of a computer-based patient record system; addressing the need for universal patient identifiers; developing standard provider and sites-of-care identifiers; developing confidentiality and security standards; establishing a structure for and developing key vocabulary and code standards; completing health data interchange standards; developing implementation tools; and demonstrating adoptability of standards in actual settings. This project proposes that the CPRI and ANSI HISPP work together to lead, promote, coordinate and accelerate the work of SDOs to develop health care information standards.

The Workgroup on Electronic Data Interchange (WEDI) is a voluntary, public/private task force which was formed in 1991 as a result of the call for health care administrative simplification by the director of the Department of Health and Human Services, Dr. Louis Sullivan. They have developed an action plan to promote health care EDI which includes: promotion of EDI standards, architectures, confidentiality, identifiers, health cards, legislation, and publicity [WEDI, 1993].

180.9 Summary

This chapter has presented an overview of major existing and emerging health care information infrastructure standards and the efforts to coordinate, harmonize, and accelerate these activities. Health care informatics is a dynamic area characterized by changing business and clinical processes, functions, and technologies. The effort to create health care informatics standards is therefore also dynamic. For the most current information on standards, refer to the "For More Information" section at the back of this chapter.

References

American National Standards Institute's Health Care Informatics Standards Planning Panel, 1994. Charter statement. New York.

American Society for Testing and Materials (ASTM). 1994. Guide for the properties of a universal health care identifier. ASTM Subcommittee E31.12, Philadelphia.

American Society for Testing and Materials (ASTM). 1994. Membership information packet: ASTM Committee E31 on computerized systems, Philadelphia.

American Society for Testing and Materials (ASTM). 1994. A standard description for content and structure of the computer-based patient record, E1384-91/1994 revision. ASTM Subcommittee E31.19, Philadelphia.

American Society for Testing and Materials (ASTM). 1994. "Standard guide for description of reservation registration-admission, discharge, transfer (R-ADT) systems for automated patient care information systems, E1239-94. ASTM Subcommittee E31.19, Philadelphia.

American Society for Testing and Materials (ASTM). 1994. A standard specification for the coded values used in the automated primary record of care, E1633. ASTM Subcommittee E31.19, Philadelphia.

Cannavo MJ. 1993. The last word regarding DEFF & DICOM. Healthcare Informatics 32.

Chute CG. 1991. Tutorial 19: Clinical data representations. Washington, DC, Symposium on Computer Applications in Medical Care.

Cimino JJ, Johnson SB, Peng P, et al. 1993. From ICD9-CM to MeSH Using the UMLS: A How-to-Guide, SCAMC, Washington DC.

Computer Aided Medical Systems Limited (CAMS). 1994. CAMS News 4:1.

Computer-based Patient Record Institute (CPRI). 1994. CPRI-Mail 3:1.

Computer-based Patient Record Institute (CPRI). 1994. Position paper on computer-based patient record standards. Chicago.

Computer-based Patient Record Institute (CPRI). 1994. Proposal to accelerate standards development for computer-based patient record systems. Version 3.0, Chicago.

Donaldson MS, Lohr KN (eds). 1994. Health Data in the Information Age: Use, Disclosure, and Privacy. Washington, DC, Institute of Medicine, National Academy Press.

Evans DA, Cimino JJ, Hersh WR, et al. 1994. Toward a medical-concept representation language. J Am Med Informatics Assoc 1(3):207.

Hammond WE. 1993. Overview of health care standards and understanding what they all accomplish. HIMSS Proceedings, Chicago, American Hospital Association.

Hammond WE, McDonald C, Beeler G, et al. 1994. Computer standards: Their future within health care reform. HIMSS Proceedings, Chicago, Health Care Information and Management Systems Society.

Harrington JJ. 1993. IEEE P1157 MEDIX: A standard for open systems medical data interchange. New York, Institute of Electrical and Electronic Engineers.

Health Care Financing Administration (HCFA). 1994. Draft issue papers developed by HCFA's national provider identifier/national provider file workgroups. Baltimore.

Health Industry Business Communications Council (HIBCC). 1994. Description of present program of standards activity. Phoenix.

Humphreys B. 1991. Tutorial 20: Using and assessing the UMLS knowledge sources. Symposium on Computer Applications in Medical Care, Washington, DC.

Institute of Electrical and Electronics Engineers (IEEE). 1994. Trial-use standard for health care data interchange—Information model methods: Data model framework. IEEE Standards Department, New York.

Joint Commission on Accreditation of Healthcare Organizations (JCAHO). 1994. The Joint Commission Journal on Quality Improvement. Oakbrook Terrace, Ill.

Moshman Associates, Inc. 1994. Current activities of selected health care informatics standards organizations. Bethesda, MD. Office of Science and Data Development, Agency for Health Care Policy and Research.

National Committee for Quality Assurance. 1993. Hedis 2.0: Executive summary. Washington, DC.

Rothwell DJ, Cote RA, Cordeau JP, et al. 1993. Developing a standard data structure for medical language—The SNOMED proposal. Washington, DC, SCAMC.

Terrell SA, Dutton BL, Porter L., et al. 1991. In search of the denominator: Medicare physicians—How many are there? Baltimore, Health Care Financing Administration.

Waegemann CP. 1994. Draft—1994 resource guide: Organizations involved in standards and development work for electronic health record systems. Newton, Mass, Medical Records Institute.

Workgroup for Electronic Data Interchange (WEDI). 1993. WEDI report: October 1993. Convened by the Department of Health and Human Services, Washington DC.

Further Information

For copies of standards accredited by ANSI, you can contact the American National Standards Institute, 11 West 42d St., NY, NY 10036, (212) 642-4900. For information on ANSI Health Care Informatics Standards Planning Panel (HISPP), contact Steven Cornish, (212) 642-4900.

For copies of individual ASTM standards, you can contact the American Society for Testing and Materials, 1916 Race Street, Philadelphia, PA 19103-1187, (215) 299-5400.

For copies of the "Proposal to Accelerate Standards Development for Computer-based Patient Record Systems," contact the Computer-based Patient Record Institute (CPRI), Margaret Amatayakul, 1000 E. Woodfield Road, Suite 102, Schaumburg, IL 60173, (708) 706-6746.

For information on provider identifier standards and proposals, contact the Health Care Financing Administration (HCFA), Bureau Program Operations, 6325 Security Blvd., Baltimore, MD 21207, (410) 966-5798. For information on ICD-9-CM codes, contact HCFA, Medical Coding, 401 East Highrise Bldg., 6325 Security Blvd., Baltimore, MD 21207, (410) 966-5318.

For information on site-of-care and supplier labeling identifiers, contact the Health Industry Business Communications Council (HIBCC), 5110 N. 40th Street, Suite 250, Phoenix, AZ 85018, (602) 381-1091.

For copies of standards developed by Health Level 7, you can contact HL7, 3300 Washtenaw Avenue, Suite 227, Ann Arbor, MI 48104, (313) 665-0007.

For copies of standards developed by the Institute of Electrical and Electronic Engineers/Engineering in Medicine and Biology Society, in New York City, call (212) 705-7900. For information on IEEE/MEDIX meetings, contact Jack Harrington, Hewlett-Packard, 3000 Minuteman Rd., Andover, MA 01810, (508) 681-3517.

For more information on clinical indicators, contact the Joint Commission on Accreditation of Health Care Organizations (JCAHO), Department of Indicator Measurement, One Renaissance Blvd., Oakbrook Terrace, IL 60181, (708) 916-5600.

For information on pharmaceutical billing transactions, contact the National Council for Prescription Drug Programs (NCPDP), 2401 N. 24th Street, Suite 365, Phoenix, AZ 85016, (602) 957-9105.

For information on HEDIS, contact the National Committee for Quality Assurance (NCQA), Planning and Development, 1350 New York Avenue, Suite 700, Washington, D.C. 20005, (202) 628-5788.

For copies of ACR/NEMA DICOM standards, contact David Snavely, National Equipment Manufacturers Association (NEMA), 2101 L. Street N.W., Suite 300, Washington, D.C. 20037, (202) 457-8400.

For information on standards development in the areas of computer-based patient record concept models, confidentiality, data security, authentication, and patient cards, and for information on standards activities in Europe, contact Peter Waegemann, Medical Records Institute (MRI), 567 Walnut Street, P.O. Box 289, Newton, MA 02160. (617) 964-3923.

181

Non-AI Decision Making

Ron Summers
City University, London

Ewart R. Carson
City University, London

Non-AI decision making can be defined as those methods and tools used to increase information content in the context of some specific clinical situation without having cause to refer to knowledge embodied in a computer program. Theoretical advances in the 1950s added rigor to this domain when Meehl argued that many clinical decisions could be made by statistical rather than intuitive means [1]. Evidence of this view was provided by Savage [2] who was responsible for reintroducing bayesian decision analysis to clinical problems. Ledley and Lusted provided further support by demonstrating that medical reasoning could be made explicit and represented in decision theoretic ways [3]. Decision theory also provided the means for Nash to develop a "Logoscope," which can be considered as a mechanical diagnostic aid [4].

The information system developed using non-AI decision-making techniques may comprise procedural or declarative knowledge. Procedural knowledge maps the decision-making process into the methods by which the clinical problems are solved or clinical decisions made. Examples of techniques which form a procedural knowledge base are those which are based on algorithmic analytical models, clinical algorithms, or decision trees. Information systems based on declarative knowledge comprise what can essentially be termed a database of facts about different aspects of a clinical problem; the causal relationships between these facts form a rich network from which explicit (say) cause-effect pathways can be determined. Semantic networks and causal probabilistic networks are perhaps the best examples of information systems based on declarative knowledge. There are other types of clinical decision aid, based purely on statistical methods applied to patient data, for example, classification analyses based on logistic regression, relative frequencies of occurrence, pattern-matching algorithms, or neural networks.

The structure of this chapter mirrors to some extent the different methods and techniques of non-AI decision making referred to above. A difference is distinguished between analytical models based on quantitative or qualitative mathematical representations and decision theoretic methods typified by the use of clinical algorithms, decision trees, and set theory. The majority of these techniques add to the information base by use of procedural knowledge. Following this, the myriad of techniques which have statistical methods of decision making as their underpinning principle of analysis are investigated. This section begins with discussion of simple linear regression models and pattern recognition, but then more complex statistical techniques are introduced, for example, the use of

0-8493-8346-3/95/$0.00+$.50
© 1995 by CRC Press, Inc.

bayesian decision analysis which leads to the introduction of causal probabilistic networks. The majority of these techniques add information by use of declarative knowledge.

Particular applications are used throughout to illustrate the extent to which non-AI decision making is used in clinical practice.

181.1 Analytical Models

In the context of this chapter, the analytical models considered are qualitative and quantitative mathematical models that are used to predict future patient state based on present state and a historical representation of what has passed. Such models could be representations of system behavior that allow test signals to be used so that response of the system to various disturbances can be studied, thus making predictions of future patient state.

For example, Leaning and coworkers [5,6] produced a 19-segment quantitative mathematical model of the blood circulation to study the short-term effects of drugs on the cardiovascular system of normal, resting patients. The model represented entities such as the compliance, flow, and volume of model segments in what was considered a closed system. In total, the quantitative mathematical model comprised 61 differential equations and 159 algebraic equations. Evaluation of the model revealed that it was fit for its purpose in the sense of heuristic validity, that is it could be used as a tool for developing explanations for cardiovascular control, particularly in relation to the CNS.

Qualitative models investigate time-dependent behavior by representing patient state trajectory in the form of a set of connected nodes, the links between the nodes reflecting transitional constraints placed on the system [7]. The types of decision making supported by this type of model are both diagnostic assessment and therapy planning. In diagnostic assessment, the precursor nodes and the pathway to the node (decision) of interest define the causal mechanisms of the disease process. Similarly, for therapy planning the optimal plan can be set by investigation of the utility values associated with each link in the disease-therapy relationship. These utility values refer to a cost function, where cost can be defined as the monetary cost of providing the treatment and cost benefit to the patient in terms of efficiency, efficacy, and effectiveness of alternative treatment options.

Both quantitative [8] and qualitative [9] analytical models can be realized in other ways to form the basis of rule-based systems; however that excludes their analysis in this chapter.

181.2 Decision Theoretic Models

Clinical Algorithms

The clinical algorithm is a procedural device which mimics clinical decision making by structuring the diagnostic or therapeutic decision processes in the form of a classification tree. The root of the tree represents some initial state, and the branches yield the different options available. For the operation of the clinical algorithm the choice points are assumed to follow branching logic with the decision function being a yes/no (or similar) binary choice. Thus, the clinical algorithm comprises a set of questions which must be collectively exhaustive for the chosen domain, and the responses available to the clinician at each branch point must be mutually exclusive. These decision criteria pose rigid constraints on the type of medical problem that can be represented by this method as the lack of flexibility is appropriate only for a certain set of well-defined clinical domains. Nevertheless, there is a rich literature available; examples include the use of the clinical algorithm for acid-base disorders [10] and diagnosis of mental disorders [11].

Decision Trees

A more rigorous use of classification tree representations than the clinical algorithm can be found in decision tree analysis. Although from a structural perspective, decision trees and clinical algorithms are similar in appearance, for decision tree analysis the likelihood and cost-benefit for each choice are also calculated in order to provide a quantitative measure for each option available. This allows the use of optimization procedures to gauge the probability of success for the correct diagnosis being made or for a beneficial outcome from therapeutic action being taken. A further difference between the clinical algorithm and decision tree analysis is that the latter has more than one type of decision node (branch point): at *decision* nodes the clinician must decide on which choice (branch) is appropriate for the given clinical scenario; at *chance* nodes the responses available have no clinician control, for example, the response may be due to patient specific data; and *outcome* nodes define the chance nodes at the "leaves" of the decision tree. That is, they summarize a set of all possible clinical outcomes for the chosen domain.

The possible outcomes from each chance node must obey the rules of probability and sum to unity; the probability assigned to each branch reflects the frequency of that event occurring in a general patient population. It follows that these probabilities are dynamic, with accuracy increasing as more evidence becomes available. A utility value can be added to each of the outcome scenarios. These utility measures reflect a trade-off between competing concerns, for example, survivability and quality of life, and may be assigned heuristically.

Again, there is a rich literature describing potential applications, but practical applications have not kept pace [12].

181.3 Statistical Models

Database Search

Interrogation of large clinical databases yields statistical evidence of diagnostic value and in some representations form the basis of rule induction used to build expert systems [13]. These systems will not be discussed here. However the most direct approach for clinical decision making is to determine the relative frequency of occurrence of an entity, or more likely group of entities, in the database of past cases. This enables a prior probability measure to be estimated [14]. A drawback of this simple, direct approach to problem solving is the apparent tautology of the more evidence available leading to fewer matches in the database being found—this runs against common wisdom that more evidence leads to an increase in probability of a diagnosis being found. Further, the method does not provide a weight for each item of evidence to gauge those which are more significant for patient outcome.

Regression Analysis

Logistic regression analysis is used to model the relationship between a response variable of interest and a set of explanatory variables. This is achieved by adjusting the regression coefficients, the parameters of the model, until a 'best fit' to the data set is achieved. This type of model improves upon the use of relative frequencies, as logistic regression explicitly represents the extent to which elements of evidence are important in the value of the regression coefficients. An example of clinical use can be found in the domain of gastroenterology [15].

Statistical Pattern Analysis

The recognition of patterns in data can be formulated as a statistical problem of classifying the results of clinical findings into mutually exclusive but collectively exhaustive decision regions. In this way, not only can physiologic data be classified but also the pathology that they give rise to and the therapy options available to treat the disease. Titterington [16] describes an application in which patterns in a complex data set are recognized to enhance the care of patients with head injuries. Pattern recognition is also the cornerstone of computerized methods for cardiac rhythm analysis [17].

The methods used to distinguish patterns in data rely on discriminant analysis. In simple terms, this refers to a measure of separability between class populations.

In general, pattern recognition is a two stage process as shown in Fig. 181.1. The pattern vector, P, is an n-dimensional vector derived from the data set used. Let Ω_p be the pattern space, which is the set of all possible values P may assume, then the pattern recognition problem is formulated as finding a way of dividing Ω_p into mutually exclusive and collectively exhaustive regions. For example, in the analysis of the electrocardiogram the complete waveform may be used to perform classifications of diagnostic value. A complex decision function would probably be required in such cases. Alternatively (and if appropriate), the pattern vector can be simplified to investigation of subfeatures within a pattern. For cardiac arrhythmia analysis, only the R-R interval of the electrocardiogram is required which allows a much simpler decision function to be used. This may be a linear or nonlinear transformation process:

$$X = \tau P$$

where X is termed the feature vector and τ is the transformation process.

Just as the pattern vector P belongs to a pattern space Ω_p, so the feature vector X belongs to a feature space Ω_x. As the function of feature extraction is to reduce the dimensionality of the input vector to the classifier, some information is lost.

Classification of Ω_x can be achieved using numerous statistical methods including: discriminant functions (linear and polynomial); kernel estimation; k-nearest neighbor; cluster analysis; and bayesian analysis.

Bayesian Analysis

Ever since their reinvestigation by Savage in 1954 [2], bayesian methods of classification have provided one of the most popular approaches used to assist in clinical decision making. Bayesian classification is an example of a parametric method of estimating class conditional probability density functions. Clinical knowledge is represented as a set of prior probabilities of diseases to be matched with conditional probabilities of clinical findings in a patient population with each disease. The classification problem becomes one of a choice of decision levels which minimizes the average rate of misclassification or to minimize the maximum of the conditional average loss function (the so-called *minimax* criterion) when information about prior probabilities is not available. Formally, the optimal decision rule which minimizes the average rate of misclassification is called the *Bayes rule;* this serves as the inference mechanism that allows the probabilities of competing diagnoses to be calculated when patient specific clinical findings become available.

Advantages of bayesian classification are a large clinical database of past cases is not required, thus allowing the time taken to reach a decision to be faster than comparable database search techniques; and errors of misclassification due to the use of inappropriate clinical inferences are quantifiable. However a drawback of this approach to clinical decision making is that the disease states are considered as complete and mutually exclusive, whereas in real life neither assumption may be true.

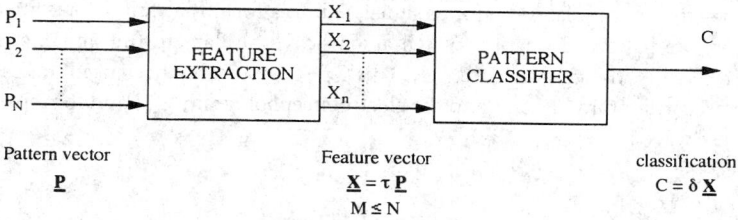

FIGURE 181.1 Statistical pattern recognition.

Nevertheless, bayesian decision functions as a basis for differential diagnosis have been used successfully, for example, in the diagnosis of acute abdominal pain [18]. Although de Dombal first described this system in 1972, it took another 20 years or so for it to be accepted via a multicenter multinational trial.

Dempster-Shafer Theory

One way to overcome the problem of mutual exclusive disease states is to use an extension to bayesian classification put forward by Dempster [19] and Shafer [20]. Here, instead of focusing on a single disorder, the method can deal with combinations of several diseases. The key concept used is that the set of all possible diseases is partitioned into *n*-tuples of possible disease state combinations. A simple example will illustrate this concept. Suppose there is a clinical scenario in which four disease states describe the whole hypothesis space. Each new item of evidence will impact on all the possible subsets of the hypothesis space and is represented by a function, the *basic probability assignment*. This measure is a belief function that must obey the law of probability and sum to unity across the subsets impacted upon. In the example, all possible subsets comprise: one which has all four disease states in it; four which have three of the four diseases as members; six which have two diseases as members; and finally, four subsets which have a single disease as a member. Thus, when new evidence becomes available in the form of a clinical finding, only certain hypotheses, represented by individual subsets, may be favored.

Syntactic Pattern Analysis

As demonstrated above, a large class of clinical problem solving using statistical methods involves classification or diagnosis of disease states, selection of optimal therapy regimes, and prediction of patient outcome. However, in some cases the purpose of modelling is to reconstruct the input signal from the data available. This cannot be done by methods discussed thus far. The syntactic approach to pattern recognition uses a hierarchical decomposition of information and draws upon an analogy to the syntax of language. Each input pattern is described in terms of more simple subpatterns which themselves are decomposed into simpler subunits, until the most elementary subpatterns, termed the *pattern primitives*, are reached. The pattern primitives should be selected so that they are easy to recognize with respect to the input signal. Rules which govern the transformation of pattern primitives back (ultimately) to the input signal are termed the *grammar*.

In this way a string grammar, *G*, which is easily representable in computer-based applications, can be defined:

$$G = \{V_T, V_N, S, P\}$$

where, V_T are the terminal variables (pattern primitives); V_N are the nonterminal variables; S is the start symbol; and P is the set of production rules which specify the transformation between each level of the hierarchy. It is an important assumption that in set theoretic terms, the union of V_T and V_N is the total vocabulary of G, and the intersection of V_T and V_N is the null (empty) set.

A syntactic pattern recognition system therefore comprises three functional subunits (Fig. 181.2): a preprocessor—this manipulates the input signal, *P*, into a form that can be presented to the pattern descriptor; the pattern descriptor which assigns a vocabulary to the signal; and the syntax analyser which classifies the signal accordingly. This type of system has been used successfully to represent the electrocardiogram [21, 22] and the electroencephalogram [23] and for representation of the carotid pulse wave [24].

Causal Modeling

A causal probabilistic network (CPN) is an acyclic multiply-connected graph which at a qualitative level comprises nodes and arcs [25]. Nodes are the domain objects and may represent, for example,

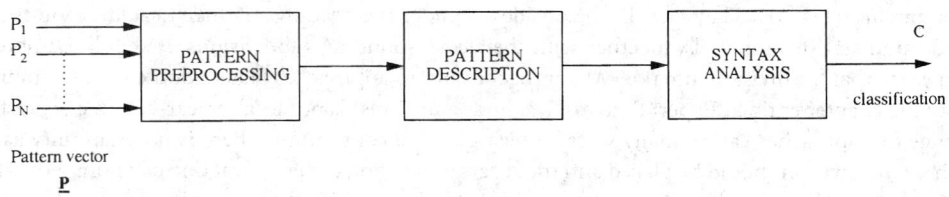

FIGURE 181.2   Syntactic pattern recognition.

clinical findings, pathophysiologic states, diseases, or therapies. Arcs are the causal relationships between successive nodes and are directed links. In this way the node and arc structure represent a model of the domain. Quantification is expressed in the model by a conditional probability table being associated with each arc, allowing the state of each node to be represented as a binary value, or more frequently as a continuous probability distribution.

In root nodes the conditional probability table reduces to a probability distribution of all its possible states.

A key concept of CPNs is that computation is reduced to a series of local calculations, using only one node and those which are linked to it in the network. Any node can be instantiated with an observed value; this evidence is then propagated through the CPN via a series of local computations.

Thus, CPNs can be used in two ways: instantiate the leaf nodes of the network with known patterns for given disorders to investigate expected causal pathways; or instantiate the root nodes or intermediate nodes in the graphical hierarchy with, for example, test results to obtain a differential diagnosis. The former method has been used to investigate respiratory pathology [26], and the latter method has been used to obtain pathologic information only electromyography [27].

Artificial Neural Networks

Artificial neural networks (ANNs) mimic their biologic counterparts, although at the present time on a much smaller scale. The fundamental unit in the biological system is the neuron. This is a specialized cell which, when activated, transmits a signal to its connected neighbors. Both activation and transmission involve chemical transmitters which cross the *synaptic gap* between neurons. Activation of the neuron takes place only when a certain threshold is reached. This biologic system is modeled in the representation of an artificial neural network. It is possible to identify three basic elements of the neuron model: a set of weighted connecting links that form the input to the neuron (analogous to neurotransmission across the synaptic gap); an adder for summing the input signals; and an activation function which limits the amplitude of the output of the neuron to the range (typically) -1 to $+1$. This activation function also has a threshold term that can be applied externally and forms one of the parameters of the neuron model. Many books are available which provide a comprehensive introduction to this class of model [e.g., 28].

ANNs can be applied to two categories of problems: prediction and classification. It is the latter which has caught the imagination of biomedical engineers for its similarity to diagnostic problem solving. For instance, the conventional management of patients with septicaemia requires a diagnostic strategy which takes up to 18–24 h before initial identification of the causal microorganism. This can be compared to a method in which an ANN is applied to a large clinical database of past cases; the quest becomes one of seeking an optimal match between present clinical findings and patterns present in the recorded data. In this application pattern matching is a nontrivial problem as each of the 5000 past cases has 51 data fields. It has been shown that the ANN method outperforms other statistical methods such as *k*-nearest neighbor in this problem [29].

181.4 Summary

This chapter has reviewed what are normally considered to be the major categories of approach available to support clinical decision making which do not rely on what is classically termed artificial intelligence (AI). They have been considered under the headings of analytical, decision theoretic, and statistical models, together with their corresponding subdivisions. It should be noted, however, that the division into non-AI approaches and AI approaches that is adopted in this volume (see the chapter entitled Expert Systems: Methods and Tools) is not totally clear-cut. In essence the range of approaches can in many ways be regarded as a continuum. There is no unanimity as to where the division should be placed and the separation adopted; here is but one of a number that is feasible. It is therefore desirable that the reader should consider these two chapters together and choose an approach which is relevant to the particular clinical context.

References

1. Meehl P. 1954. Clinical versus Statistical Prediction, Minnesota, University of Minnesota Press.
2. Savage LJ. 1954. The Foundations of Statistics, New York, Wiley.
3. Ledley RS, Ludsted LB. 1959. Reasoning foundations of medical diagnosis. Science, 130:9.
4. Nash FA. 1954. Differential diagnosis: An apparatus to assist the logical faculties. Lancet 4:874.
5. Leaning MS, Pullen HE, Carson ER, et al. (1983). Modelling a complex biological system: The human cardiovascular system: 1. Methodology and model description. Trans Inst Meas Contr 5:71.
6. Leaning MS, Pullen HE, Carson ER, et al. 1983. Modelling a complex biological system: The human cardiovascular system: 2. Model validation, reduction and development. Trans Inst Meas Contr 5:87.
7. Kuipers BJ. 1986. Qualitative simulation. Artif Intell 29:289.
8. Furukawa T, Tanaka H, Hara S. 1987. FLUIDEX: A microcomputer-based expert system for fluid therapy consultations. In: MK Chytil, R Engelbrecht (eds), Medical Expert Systems, pp 59–74, Wilmslow, Sigma Press.
9. Bratko I, Mozetic J, Lavrac N. 1988. In D Michie, I Bratko (eds), Expert Systems: Automatic Knowledge Acquisition, pp 61–83, Reading, Mass, Addison-Wesley,
10. Bleich HL. 1972. Computer-based consultations: Electrolyte and acid-base disorders. Amer J Med 53:285.
11. McKenzie DP, McGary PD, Wallace CS, et al. 1993. Constructing a minimal diagnostic decision tree. Meth Inform Med 32:161.
12. Pauker SG, Kassirer JP. 1987. Decision analysis. N Engl J Med 316:250.
13. Quinlan JR. 1979. Rules by induction from large collections of examples. In D Michie (ed), Expert Systems in the Microelectronic Age, Edinburgh, Edinburgh University Press.
14. Gammerman A, Thatcher AR. 1990. Bayesian inference in an expert system without assuming independence. In MC Golumbic (ed), Advances in Artificial Intelligence, pp 182–218, New York, Springer-Verlag.
15. Spiegelhalter DJ, Knill-Jones RP. 1984. Statistical and knowledge-based approaches to clinical decision-support systems with an application in gastroenterology. J Roy Stat Soc A 147:35.
16. Titterington DM, Murray GD, Murray LS, et al. 1981. Comparison of discriminant techniques applied to a complex set of head injured patients. J Roy Stat Soc A 144:145.
17. Morganroth J. 1984. Computer recognition of cardiac arrhythmias and statistical approaches to arrhythmia analysis. Ann NY Acad Sci 432:117.
18. De Dombal FT, Leaper DJ, Staniland JR, et al. 1972. Computer-aided diagnosis of acute abdominal pain. Br Med J 2:9.
19. Dempster A. 1967. Upper and lower probabilities induced by multi-valued mapping. Ann Math Statistics 38:325.
20. Shafer G. 1976. A Mathematical Theory of Evidence, Princeton, NJ, Princeton University Press.

21. Belforte G, De Mori R, Ferraris F. 1979. A contribution to the automatic processing of electrocardiograms using syntactic methods. IEEE Trans Biomed Eng BME-26 (3):125.

22. Birman KP. 1982. Rule-based learning for more accurate ECG analysis. IEEE Trans Pat Anal Mach Intell PAMI-4 (4):369.

23. Ferber G. 1985. Syntactic pattern recognition of intermittant EEG activity. Meth Inf Med 24 (2):79.

24. Stockman GC, Kanal LN. 1983. Problem reduction in representation for the linguistic analysis of waveforms. IEEE Trans Pat Anal Mach Intell PAMI-5 (3):287.

25. Andersen SK, Jensen FV, Olesen KG. 1987. The HUGIN core—preliminary considerations on inductive reasoning: Managing empirical information in AI systems. Riso, Denmark.

26. Summers R, Andreassen S, Carson ER, et al. 1993. A causal probabilistic model of the respiratory system. In: Proc. IEEE 15th Annual Conference of the Engineering in Medicine and Biology Society, New York, pp 534–535.

27. Jensen FV, Andersen SK, Kjaerulff U, et al. 1987. MUNIN: On the case for probabilities in medical expert systems—a practical exercise. In J Fox, M Fieschi, R Engelbrecht (eds), Proceedings First Conference European Society for AI in Medicine, pp 149–160, Heidelberg, Springer-Verlag.

28. Haykin S. 1994. Neural Networks: A Comprehensive Foundation, New York, Macmillan.

29. Worthy PJ, Dybowski R, Gransden WR, et al. 1993. Comparison of learning vector quantization and *k*-nearest neighbour for prediction of microorganisms associated with septicaemia. In: Proceedings IEEE 15th Annual Conference of the Engineering in Medicine and Biology Society, New York, pp 273–274.

182

Design Issues in Developing Clinical Decision Support and Monitoring Systems

John W. Goethe
The Institute of Living

Joseph D. Bronzino
Trinity College/The Hartford Graduate Center

As discussed in previous chapters, health care facilities presently use computers to support a wide variety of administrative, laboratory, and pharmacy activities. However, few institutions have installed computer systems that provide ongoing monitoring of care and assist in clinical decision making. Despite some promising examples of the use of artificial intelligence to enhance patient care, very few products are routinely used in clinical settings [Morelli et al., 1987; Shortliffe & Duda, 1983]. One of the important factors that has limited the acceptance of decision support tools for clinicians is the lack of medical staff input in system development. Thus, a major task for designers of computer systems that are to be incorporated into the daily clinical routine is to involve practitioners in the design process. This chapter presents a set of design recommendations, the goal of which is to ensure end-user acceptance, and describes a comprehensive clinical system that was designed using this approach and is now in routine use in a large psychiatric hospital.

182.1 Design Recommendations

The design phase of any initiative requires attention to the social and organizational context in which the new product or program will exist. Although a full discussion of the issue is beyond the scope of this chapter, it has been extensively covered in a number of texts. (See especially Peters and Tseng [1983] for a theoretical overview of the theory and illustrative case studies.) In addition to these general principles of organizational change, several specific design steps are critical to end-user acceptance.

Establish a Project Team. The composition of the project team should reflect the scope of the activities within the facility and the organizational structure (hierarchy). It should include at least one outside consultant and at least one member of the medical/professional staff who will serve as the liaison to a clinician task force representing all practitioners.

0-8493-8346-3/95/$0.00+$.50
© 1995 by CRC Press, Inc.

Establish a Clinician Task Force. In addition to the project team, which represents the entire institution, it is important to form a clinician task force of five to seven members of the medical/professional staff. In some facilities all care is provided by physicians while in other settings psychologists, social workers, nurses, and other professionals function as primary clinicians. The task force must represent *all* these professionals.

Meetings of the task force must begin well before the hardware and software decisions have been made so that there will be adequate time to incorporate suggestions from the clinical staff. The implementation schedule must allow time for resolution of the issues raised by the end-users. (*Resolution* here does not imply that *all* parties will be pleased with *all* decisions, but the design team should ensure adequate time for discussion of each issue raised by the clinical staff and for reaching closure.)

Know the Limits within Which the Project Team Must Work. Part of the design task is to determine the limitations present and the level of expectation for system use. For example, is the number of terminals and their location sufficient for all clinicians to have easy access? Does the administration expect clinicians to type rather than dictate patient summaries? If an administrator is not on the project team, interviews with the key executives should be held as soon as possible, with follow-up meetings regularly scheduled.

Identify All Institutional Initiatives and Needs. It is important for system designers to be aware of all institutional plans. For example, the facility may have recently modified its clinical documentation procedures in response to a change in reimbursement regulations or as part of a new managed care contract. Many of these changes will have an impact on the system design, and some may create opportunities for cost or time savings through automation.

Identify the Types of Patient Care Activities Typical for the Institution. Using the language/action approach of Winograd [1987] one can classify all clinical care activities within an institution. As discussed by Morelli, and coworkers [1993] all actions in a psychiatric hospital can be grouped into six categories: assessment notation, medication order, nonmedication order, notification of a critical event, request by the clinician for additional information (consultation), and request of the clinician for additional information (e.g., to justify a treatment or hospital admission). This list, while not necessary applicable to all clinical settings, is useful as a template. (See Lyytinen [1987] for a review of other approaches to understanding the component activities within an organization.) Once all possible clinical actions are categorized, list those that the system is intended to support. Such detailed assessment of the structure and nature of clinician actions allows designers to determine prior to implementation how the system will affect existing practices. For example, will clinicians be expected to use the computer to enter orders, eliminating the need for nurse transcription of handwritten orders? Will clinicians have to respond to computer notices and document why a treatment standard was not followed?

Illustrate How the New System Will Be Integrated into the Existing Environment. Computerization of one aspect of clinical care may have an unexpected impact on other areas of practice. Thus, a detailed map of the interactions involved in formulating and executing medical orders is a useful step [Morelli et al., 1993]. Even desirable changes in the clinical routine, such as reducing handwritten progress notes, must be examined since the existing nonautomated methods may have served some additional (e.g., educational) purpose not evident without careful mapping of the interaction. Both automated and manual procedures should appear logical and relevant to the staff. Screen formats and input/retrieval features, for example, must follow practices acceptable to the facility. Interactions with the computer must be viewed as nonintrusive and must not require extensive data entry by clinicians.

Clinician Interaction with the Terminal Should Be Part of Daily Clinical Activity. A computer system should not be a stand-alone tool; rather, it should be fully integrated into the clinical routine.

For example, clinicians should have direct and easy access to on-line displays of current medications and results of laboratory tests. Furthermore, clinicians should be able to query the system for additional information when laboratory or other data indicate a potential problem.

The System Should Provide Real-time Feedback to Clinicians. The timeliness of an information system is a critical factor in health care applications. Although all functions do not have to operate literally in real time, they do have to operate in a manner consistent with clinician practice. For example, the system should notify clinicians immediately of events such as drug-drug interactions, but in other situations (e.g., a reminder that a follow-up test is due) a notification within 2 days may be sufficient. Laboratory results and treatment data must reflect the orders entered as of the day the system is being queried.

Conduct Site Visits to Assess Computer Use in the Delivery of Clinical Service. Important aspects of system design may be overlooked if unique characteristics of a given site are not taken into account. For example, the system designers may plan to install a computer terminal in the area from which medications are dispensed in each nursing station. If on one unit, because of size or location, this area cannot accommodate a standard terminal, an alternative device may have to be purchased or architectural changes made.

Include Support for Key Administrative as well as Clinical Care Tasks. Administrative activities directly related to clinician practice are quality assurance, peer review, continuing medical education (including information dissemination and needs assessment), drug utilization evaluations, patient outcomes assessment, and continuous quality improvement programs. Since both administrative and clinical tasks are intended to serve a common purpose, the delivery of the best available services to the patient, they should be integrated whenever possible. A detailed listing of all such tasks, specifying the structure of each and the individuals involved, may identify important areas in which the clinical information system can be usefully applied.

Evaluate the System Prior to Implementation. Once the design is complete, an evaluation step is necessary to test the utility of the system in an actual clinical practice.

The System Must Be Adaptable to Individual Clinician and Program Needs. Since rapid changes are commonplace in health care, the system must be able to be modified and updated without extensive additional programming.

182.2 Description of a Clinical Monitoring System

The Institute of Living's Clinical Evaluation and Monitoring System (CEMS) was developed to provide comprehensive support for clinical services in a psychiatric hospital. It represents an extension of earlier work that resulted in a prototype psychopharmacology monitoring system described elsewhere [Bronzino et al., 1989]. The current system provides decision support and/or automated monitoring for each key component of care (assessment, diagnosis, and treatment) and consists of four modules: treatment standards ("pharmacotherapy guidelines"), diagnostic checklists (DCLs), information alerts, and outcome assessment. Table 182.1 shows the components of care that are supported by each of the four modules of the CEMS.

The treatment standards are accessed from the menu available to all clinical staff. This document summarizes key information about the use of selected psychiatric medications (dosages, therapeutic serum levels, indications, and side effects) and presents decision trees to guide drug selection. The manual is continuously updated and serves as both a reference and a vehicle for dissemination of new information. It is not linked electronically to the other modules, but the content is the database for the decision rules in the information alerts (described below).

TABLE 182.1 Clinical Evaluation and Monitoring System (CEMS)

CEMS Modules	Components of Care				
	Assessment				
	Pt. History/Symptoms	Labs	Outcome	Diagnosis	Treatment
Treatment standards		X		X	X
DCLs*	X		X	X	
Information alerts	X	X		X	X
Outcome assessment			X		X

*DCLs = diagnostic checklists

The diagnostic checklists (DCLs) provide an automated method for assuring documentation of the key symptoms and behavioral issues that support the assigned diagnosis and for noting at subsequent evaluation points (e.g., at discharge) the degree of change in each symptom/behavior. In contrast to diagnostic assessments in other specialties, there are few procedures or laboratory tests that definitively establish a psychiatric diagnosis. The Diagnostic and Statistical Manual (DSM) of the American Psychiatric Association [1987] and the International Classification of Diseases (ICD) published by the World Health Organization [1978] provide standard criteria on which to base diagnoses. In both DSM and ICD there is a specific algorithm that includes the type, number, and intensity of symptoms required for each diagnosis. The algorithm for all DSM diagnoses, modified to provide additional data, are used in the CEMS, and there is a separate 1-page checklist for each disorder. The clinician's admission diagnosis determines which form is presented. The form can be completed by the clinician at the terminal or a paper version can be used with subsequent input by clerical staff. The clinician indicates if each symptom/behavior is present or absent, thereby ensuring complete documentation of the findings relevant to that diagnosis. If the symptoms specified fail to meet DSM criteria for the disorder selected, a message is generated along with an explanation. The DCL is also completed at the time of discharge, at which time the system generates a new version of the form that contains only those items that the clinician indicated were present on admission. (For implementation in settings with longer periods of treatment, the DCLs could also be used for serial assessments prior to discharge.)

The information alerts are computer-generated notifications that assist in ensuring compliance with practice guidelines and medication protocols. Clinicians may respond to these notices by changing the treatment plan or diagnosis or by following up on missing or abnormal laboratory orders as directed by the alert (i.e., the clinician is then in compliance with the treatment standard). The system also allows clinicians to document the reason for deviating from the standard. This step is initiated via a function key (see Screen 1); an item is then selected from a list of reasons for "nonstandard" practice or a free-text explanation is entered (see Screen 2). The alert statement with the attached explanation is printed on the next *treatment plan review,* a medical records form summarizing treatments and patient progress that the clinician must sign. Thus, the information alerts provide ongoing monitoring and critical event notification and ensure documentation of the rationale for any nonstandard practice. (All notifications and the clinician responses are reviewed by the medical director or designee daily.) The direct feedback provided by the alerts also serves an educational and information dissemination function. New information about medications, for example, can be incorporated into one or more alerts as well as added to the treatment guidelines described above.

The system currently has 130 alerts and can be expanded to search as many as 2000 records for up to 200 critical events each day. Additional alerts can be added without additional programming, and changes in the specifications for an existing alert (e.g., dosage parameters) can be made by accessing the appropriate table from the *maintenance* screen. Alerts can include data elements on any medication prescribed, any laboratory value, any psychiatric diagnosis or a variety of histori-

```
┌─────────────────────────────────────────────────────────────────────────────┐
│  TM0197-01I. A.              ALERT REVIEW BY CLINICIAN            DIAL700B     │
│  GOETHE, JOHN DR.                                          Alert Details as of 7/12/94 │
│                                                                               │
│          Alert Nbr:   76                                                      │
│        Description:   SUBSTANCE USE DX; ON BENZODIAZEPINE                      │
│                                                                               │
│           Notified:   DR. GOETHE                                              │
│                                                                               │
│          Issued on:   07/11/94   00:50                                        │
│    Last Notified on:  07/12/94   00:41                                        │
│   Notification Nrb:   2                                                       │
│                                                                               │
│       Patient Name:   Doe, John Q.                                            │
│              MRNR:    123456                                                  │
│            Account:   123456789                                              │
│                                                                               │
│        Patient DOB:   1/1/01                                                  │
│               Sex:    M                                                       │
│                                                                               │
│                  F3: LAB      F5: RESTART    F11: SUSPEND    F13: HELP         │
│       F2: MEDS    F4: DIAG    F6: HISTORY    F10: RETURN     F14: GUIDE        │
└─────────────────────────────────────────────────────────────────────────────┘
```

SCREEN 1

```
┌─────────────────────────────────────────────────────────────────────────────┐
│  TM0197-01I. A.              ALERT REVIEW BY CLINICIAN            DIAL710A     │
│  GOETHE, JOHN DR.                                          Alert Details as of 7/12/94 │
│                                                                               │
│            Patient:   Doe, John Q.                                            │
│              MRNR:    123456                                                  │
│            Account:   123456789                                              │
│           Alert #12   MAJOR DEPRESSION NO ANTIDEPRESSANT                       │
│                                                                               │
│                       Suspension Reasons                                      │
│                01:    Medical work-up in progress to rule out organic cause of depression │
│                02:    Unable to tolerate antidepressants                       │
│                03:    Refusing antidepressants                                 │
│                04:    Washout period                                          │
│                05:    Drug-free trial                                         │
│                06:    Patient's affective episode characterized by prominent thought and/or perceptual │
│                       disturbance, and is receiving a trial of antipsychotic medication │
│                07:    Patient is receiving an antidepressant from an outside pharmacy │
│          Selection:   Type:                                                   │
│                                                                               │
│    F1: SELECT              F5: RESTART              F7: NXPG                    │
│                           F10: RETURN              F14: GUIDE                  │
└─────────────────────────────────────────────────────────────────────────────┘
```

SCREEN 2

cal/demographic items (e.g., gender, age). The limitation in the last of these four categories is the amount of information from the medical record that is currently on-line. With a completely electronic medical chart, this system could generate an alert for almost any clinical event.

182.3 Outcome Assessment

At admission, discharge, and regular intervals postdischarge nursing staff complete a functional assessment survey on all patients. These data are entered into the system using an optical scanner. Regular feedback is provided to hospital staff and used to evaluate clinical services and practice.

In a typical scenario a clinician, after logging on, would select "Show My Alerts" from the menu (Screen 3). Alerts for all of the patients assigned to that clinician are displayed as shown on Screen 4. (The medical director or other supervising clinician can select all active alerts by type, by practitioner, or by patient.) Patient name and alert message are given, but no further detail can be obtained nor can a direct response to the alert be made without selecting a specific patient and a specific alert for that patient. When the clinician goes to a specific alert, there is the option (Screen 1) to suspend the alert as described above or to query the system about the patient's diagnosis, current medication, laboratory values, or the "history" of that alert (i.e., if the alert has previously been issued, a log of all activity on that alert is given). From the current medication and laboratory screens there is an additional option that allows access to all *historical* lab values/medications. This historical feature is especially valuable for tracking patients who require frequent drug serum level determinations (e.g., with lithium carbonate) or who have medical disorders that necessitate periodic laboratory tests (e.g., chronic kidney or liver disease).

```
TM0197-01                        GUIDE                         PSEC030A
GOETHE, JOHN DR.              MEDICAL STAFF                 12 JUL 94 09:19


   01:  CHART REQUEST                11:  OUTPATIENT ACTIVITY
   02:  CLINICAL DATA REVIEW         12:  PATIENT EDUCATION MODULE

   03:  CLINICIAN PATIENT LIST       13:  SHOW MY CHART DEFICIENCIES
   04:  DAY HOSPITAL ATTENDANCE REVIEW   14:  SHOW MY PATIENTS

   05:  I.A. SHOW MY STANDING ALERTS
   06:  INPATIENT ACTIVITY

   07:  INPATIENT LOCATOR
   08:  LIST MY PATIENTS (CLINICIAN)

   09:  O.E. LAB ORDER REVIEW
   10:  O.E. PATIENT DATA R/O

   SELECTION: 0
   **END OF LIST


   F1: SELECT
```

SCREEN 3

```
┌─────────────────────────────────────────────────────────────────────────┐
│  TM0197-01I. A.              ALERT REVIEW BY CLINICIAN        DIAL700A     │
│  GOETHE, JOHN DR.                              Alert Details as of 7/12/94 │
│                                                                           │
│                                                                           │
│   Date          Count   Patient     Alert   Description                   │
│                                                                           │
│   01:07/11/94    2      Doe, John    10      NO LITHIUM LEVEL > 10 DAYS    │
│   02: 06/24/94   10     Doe, Mary     5      ANTIPSYCHOT+ANTIDEPRESSANT+ANTIPARK │
│                                                                           │
│   03: 07/12/94   1      Smith, John  12      MAJOR DEPRESSION NO ANTIDEPRESSANT │
│   04: 07/05/94   6      Jones, J.P.  13      ANTIPSYCHOTIC NO PSYCHOTIC DIAG │
│                                                                           │
│   05: 07/08/94   3      Brown, Jane  69      THYROID FUNCTION TEST ABNORMAL │
│                                                                           │
│   Selection:                                                              │
│                                                                           │
│                                                                           │
│   F1: SELECT   F3: LAB    F5: RESTART    F11: SUSPEND    F13: HELP         │
│   F2: MEDS     F4: DIAG   F6: HISTORY    F10: RETURN     F14: GUIDE        │
└─────────────────────────────────────────────────────────────────────────┘
```

SCREEN 4

182.4 Conclusion

Computers are increasingly *user* friendly, but the clinical environment may often not be computer friendly. In addition to the obvious computer engineering tasks, there is a sizable human engineering issue that must be addressed if automated tools are to be accepted and fully utilized in clinical settings. Thus, designers must take into account the social and organizational structure of the health care delivery network the system is intended to serve, involve clinician staff in its development, and adhere to a design strategy that will ensure end-user acceptance. Although the system outlined in this chapter was developed for psychiatric practice, the components of care described are common to all branches of medicine, and the design steps recommended are applicable for a wide range of clinical settings.

Acknowledgments

Many elements of the system now in place at the Institute of Living represent extensions of the earlier efforts of a number of individuals. Peter Ericson, former head of the Department of Information Services at the Institute, Bernard C. Glueck, Jr., M.D., former director of research, were among the pioneers in applying information systems to clinical care. Major contributors to one or more components described in this chapter include Pawel Zmarlicki, David Cole, David Warchol, Russell Dzialo-Evans, Bonnie Szarek, R.N.

Defining Terms

Decision trees: Decision trees or flow charts are a common way to present medical information that is intended to support the decision-making process. Many decisions are hierarchical in nature, but there may be more than one acceptable option at each nodal point on the decision tree.

Language/action model: The language/action model of human-computer communication is a term taken from the work of Winograd, who introduced the term "conversation for action" to describe how human behavior is coordinated within an organization. To quote Winograd, "We work together by making commitments so that we can successfully anticipate the actions of others and coordinate them with our own." According to this model, computer systems are part of the conversational structure of the organization and, along with the human employees, engage in a variety of well-defined interactions (communications). Winograd's approach is based on earlier work by J. L. Austin and J. R. Searle.

Map: A map of the interactions is a detailed assessment, often diagrammatically expressed, of how the work of the organization is accomplished. In a medical facility, the steps involved include the physical assessment of the patient by the clinician, various procedures performed on the patient, and the recording, storage, retrieval, and analysis of data. Such maps can be informed by but do not necessarily have to follow Winograd's language/action approach (described above) or any other formal model of analysis.

References

American Psychiatric Association. 1987. Diagnostic and Statistical Manual of Mental Disorders, 3d ed rev. Washington, DC, American Psychiatric Association.

Bronzino JD, Morelli RA, Goethe JW. 1989. Overseer: A prototype expert system for monitoring drug treatment in the psychiatric clinic. IEEE Trans Biomed Eng 36:533.

Lyytinen K. 1987. Different perspectives on information systems: Problems and solutions. ACM Computer Survey 19:5.

Morelli RA, Bronzino JD, Goethe JW. 1987. Expert systems in psychiatry: A review. Proceedings 20th Hawaii International Conference System Science, 3:84.

Morelli RA, Bronzino JD, Goethe JW. 1993. Conversations for action: A speech act model of human-computer communications in a psychiatric hospital. J Intelli Sys 3:87.

Peters JP, Tseng S. 1983. Managing Strategic Change in Hospitals, Chicago, American Hospital Association.

Shortliffe EH, Duda R. 1983. Expert systems research. Science 220:261.

Winograd T. 1987. A language/action perspective on the design of cooperative work. Report No. STAN-CS-87-1158, Stanford University.

World Health Organization. 1978. Mental Disorders: Glossary and Guide to Their Classification in Accordance with the Ninth Revision of the International Classification of Disease, Geneva, World Health Organization.

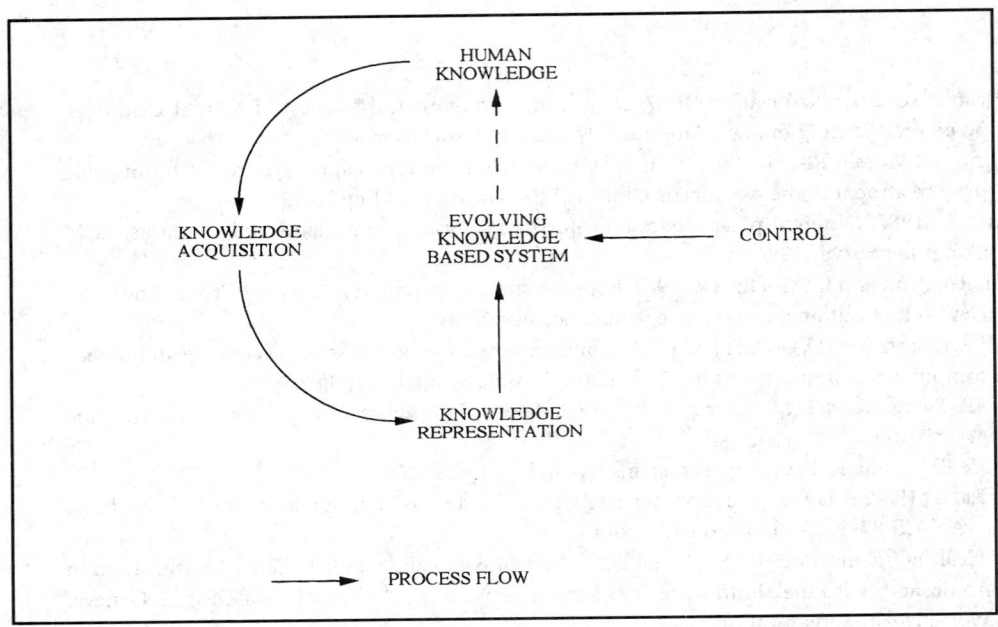

Basic steps in the development of an expert system.

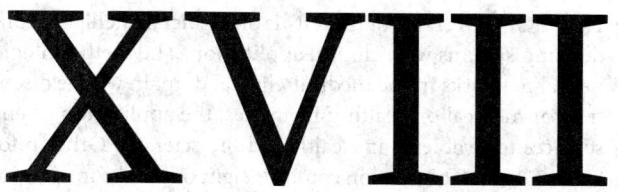

XVIII

Artificial Intelligence

Stanley M. Finkelstein
University of Minnesota

THE FOCUS OF THIS SECTION is on artificial intelligence and its use in the development of medical decision systems with clinical application. The methodologic basis for expert systems and artificial neural networks in the medical/clinical domain will be discussed. This is one aspect of the growing field of medical or health informatics, the application of engineering, computer, and information sciences to problems in health and life sciences. Other informatics applications are addressed in Section XVII. This section contains eight original contributions that cover the history, methods, and future directions in the field. It intentionally omits specific computer hardware and software details related to currently available systems because they continue to change as technology changes and are likely to be outdated even as this *Handbook* goes to press. Furthermore, chapters representing complete examples of specific clinical decision systems are not included in this section. Numerous examples can be found in the current literature, and many have been cited in the chapters of this section to illustrate particular aspects of decision system structure, knowledge acquisition and representation, the user interface, and system evaluation and testing

In Chapter 183, Dr. Kulikowski presents the history of the development of artificial intelligence (AI) methodology for medical decision making, from the early statistical and pattern-recognition methods of the 1960s to the continuing development of knowledge-based systems of the 1990s. Dr. Kulikowski has described the evolution of these AI applications in four overlapping stages. The early applications explored various approaches to handling knowledge within the specific domains of interest, utilizing either causal networks, modular rule-based reasoning, or frame/template representation of the knowledge describing the clinical domain. These varied approaches all pointed out the difficulties involved in the actual acquisition of the domain expertise needed for each application and generated research investigations into acquisition strategies ranging from literature review, case study evaluation, and detailed interviews with the experts. These efforts related to knowledge acquisition and learning were a part of the second stage of evolution, as was the development of general frameworks for building expert systems, so that each new application did not require the reinvention of the basic blocks needed for system implementation. Dr. Kulikowski characterizes the third stage as transitional, with further interest on the medical reasoning process and the computer representation of this process. Currently, in the fourth stage, there is active interest in qualitative reasoning representation, the importance of the temporal framework of the decision process, and the effort to move toward more practical systems that embody decision support for diagnostic or treatment protocols rather than the fully automated decision system. Dr. Kulikowski points out that expert clinical systems have not become the indispensible clinical tool that many had predicted in the early days of AI in medicine, describes reasons for this shortfall, and looks forward to advanced software environments and medical devices that are beginning to routinely incorporate these ideas and methods in their development.

In Chapter 184, Drs. Micheli-Tzanakou and Zahner focus on artificial neural network (ANN) methodologies and their applications in the medical and health care arena. ANNs consist of a large number of interconnected neurons or nodes that can process information in a highly parallel manner. They are specified by their processing-element characteristics, their network topology, and the training rules they use to learn how to achieve correct pattern classification from an array of multiple inputs. Drs. Micheli-Tzanakou and Zahner provide the mathematical details for the backpropagation and ALOPEX training algorithms and discuss the benefits and deficiencies of these approaches in teaching the ANN to correctly classify input patterns presented to the system. Finally, the performance of several ANN approaches in mammography and chromosome and genetic sequence classification applications are reviewed and compared.

The contribution by Nykänen and Saranummi (Chapter 185) also provides a history of AI applications in medical decision systems but focuses on both development and user acceptance problems, why they are so critical in the clinical environment, and what problem solutions could be implemented so that such systems will find greater acceptance beyond the laboratories in which they were developed. The early introduction of expert system shells provided a strong impetus for system development and indeed resulted in many published applications. The availability of inexpensive and powerful microcomputers and dedicated workstations for knowledge engineering also has contributed to the development of medical expert systems. The authors point out that data and knowledge are often less quantitative and consistent in clinical medicine than in the physical sciences and that the lack of standards for coding and representation make it difficult to exchange knowledge in the expert system context among potential system users. Appropriate, objective, and standardized evaluation and testing are often lacking as a part of the system development process, as discussed in this chapter, and this lack contributes to the acceptance question for these systems. Finally, the authors address the question of system integration within the user environment and its relationship to system acceptance and portability.

The chapter by Summers and Carson (Chapter 186) discusses specific methodologies used in expert system development and provides some general examples of rule-based and semantic network approaches to knowledge representation in medical applications. The authors use MYCIN and CASNET, two of the earliest medical expert system applications to achieve widespread recognition and serve as models for subsequent developments, to demonstrate and compare these two approaches for knowledge representation. MYCIN uses production rules to represent causal relationships between knowledge items to diagnose and treat microbial infections. CASNET uses causal or semantic networks to represent knowledge relationships in the diagnosis and treatment of glaucoma.

Dr. Garbay's contribution (Chapter 187) continues along these directions by providing a somewhat more conceptual approach to the question of knowledge domains, acquisition, and representation. Knowledge-acquisition techniques are reviewed, and several knowledge-acquisition tools designed to assist in the process are described. The ideas of shallow and deep knowledge systems are introduced from the perspective of the system's explanation facilities. Shallow knowledge systems rely primarily on reasoning based on experience and experimental results, while deep knowledge systems are based on detailed knowledge regarding the structure and function of the underlying system such as those employing physiologic models within the knowledge base. Methods for handling uncertain and imprecise reasoning are also presented.

A new and expanding application area involving intelligent patient monitoring and management in critical care environments is discussed in Chapter 188, by Dr. Dawant. Such systems involve the context-dependent acquisition, processing, analysis, and interpretation of large amounts of possibly noisy and incomplete data. These systems can be viewed within four distinct functional levels. At the signal level, the system acquires raw data from patient monitors, which include analog-to-digital conversion and some low-level signal processing. Data validity checks and artifact removal occur at the validation level. The transformation from numerical features that characterize the signals to a symbolic representation, such as normal or abnormal, is performed at the signal-to-symbol level. Finally, the inference level consists of the reasoning elements described in previous chapters to arrive at diagnoses, explanations, prediction, or initiation of control actions. Examples of both shallow and deep knowledge systems developed for patient monitoring are presented.

Systems development and widespread dissemination often have been stymied by the lack of standardization of knowledge representation, as described in all the preceding contributions. The last two chapters look at this question from the perspective of medical terminology and the status of natural language processing in biomedicine.

In discussing applications of medical knowledge bases, Dr. Kerkhof (Chapter 189) states that while technological advances in computer processors and storage media permit virtually unlimited storage and fast retrieval capability, the interpretation of natural language constitutes a major obstacle in the advancement of knowledge-based systems in medicine. In this chapter, classification and coding systems are identified, and their content is described. The richness and depth of natural language often are the focus of difficulties when attempting to develop such systems, encountering differences in such elementary concerns as definitions, spelling, usage, and precision. Dr. Kerkhof offers several approaches to handling linguistic problems associated with such systems, but all have their own inherent limitations.

In Chapter 190, Dr. Johnson describes the techniques of natural language processing as a means to bridge the gap between textual and structured data so that users can interact with the system using familiar natural language, while computer applications can effectively process the resulting data.

Applications are classified according to the levels of language competence embodied in their design. Speech-recognition and -synthesis systems deal with basic data representation, while lexical, syntactic, and discourse systems function at increasing levels of complexity from single words to entire discourses.

While the specific applications described in this section relate to biomedical concerns, the definitions and methods overview relate to the development and utilization of expert systems and artificial neural networks for a wide variety of decision systems. Detailed implementation protocols for such systems are beyond the scope of this section but can be found in the references cited at the conclusion of each chapter.

183

History and Development of Artificial Intelligence Methods for Medical Decision Making

Casimir A. Kulikowski
Rutgers University

Artificial intelligence (AI) for medical decision making and decision support is usually associated with the knowledge-intensive expert consultation systems that were introduced in the early 1970s. These differed considerably from the data-intensive statistical and pattern-recognition methods that had been applied to medical reasoning problems since the 1960s and which saw a resurgence in the 1980s as new types of computationally more powerful artificial neural networks (ANNs) were developed and more sophisticated models of bayesian and other belief networks were designed to capture the nuances of clinical reasoning. In the 1990s there is increasing recognition that a large variety of approaches will probably be needed to make computer-based medical decision systems more useful and effective, since despite three decades of research and methodological innovation, they have yet to become indispensable tools within the clinical setting. On the positive side, however, advanced software environments increasingly and routinely incorporate AI ideas and methods as they seek to facilitate the tasks of building, validating, and testing medical knowledge bases.

0-8493-8346-3/95/$0.00+$.50
© 1995 by CRC Press, Inc.

183.1 Evolution of Artificial Intelligence in Medicine—Overview

The evolution of artificial intelligence (AI) methods in medicine (AIM) can be approximately divided into four stages. At the beginning of the first stage, which can be roughly dated from 1968 to 1976, there were precursor analyses of diagnostic decision making in terms of its problem-solving characteristics [Kleinmuntz and McLean, 1968; Gorry, 1970], together with a highly influential article by Schwartz [1970] on the potential of computer-based methods to transform medical practice, enabling the physician to concentrate on patient care, while computer recall systems would handle the "encyclopedic" aspects of medicine. He proposed that automatic decision-making methods would help formalize the as-yet-informal rules of medical practice and also help disseminate rare and costly speciality expertise far beyond the narrow confines of academic medical centers to general-practice settings.

The first knowledge-intensive general frameworks for representing medical reasoning about disease processes followed, with the introduction of causal networks for describing disease processes in CASNET [Kulikowski and Weiss, 1972], modular rule-based reasoning in MYCIN [Shortliffe et al., 1974], hierarchical networks in DIALOG/INTERNIST [Pople et al., 1975], and frames or templates for disease definition in PIP [Pauker et al., 1976]. These systems, like the non-AI ones that preceded them, were designed as consultative tools to assist the nonexpert physician, nurse, or other health care practitioner by capturing some of the rules of reasoning of expert physicians in a specialty. The success of these prototypes helped shift AI research to a paradigm of knowledge-based systems, requiring knowledge engineering for their construction. This development in turn focused attention on the expert nature of the knowledge needed in such systems and gave rise to the Japanese Fifth Generation Project as well as the proliferation of expert systems, first custom-crafted to particular applications and later generalized in their knowledge representation frameworks.

In the medical domain, a second phase of evolution for AI systems can be dated from about 1977 to about 1983, when general frameworks for building expert knowledge bases, such as EMYCIN [van Melle, 1979], EXPERT [Weiss and Kulikowski, 1979], and AGE [Nii and Aiello, 1979], were developed and applied in a wide variety of medical problems from instrument control in the ICU [Fagan et al., 1979] and laboratory test interpretation [Weiss et al., 1983] to advising on the diagnosis and treatment of many different types of diseases [Lindberg, 1980; Kulikowski and Ostroff, 1980]. The problems of knowledge acquisition and learning were also first approached in a systematic way during this period [Davis, 1979; Politakis and Weiss, 1980], and the categorical nature of much of the reasoning within expert systems was recognized [Szolovits and Pauker, 1978]. A contemporary overview of the early AIM systems can be found in [Kulikowski, 1980].

From about 1981–1982, the development and dissemination of expert systems ideas and "shells" for the general representation of knowledge and decision heuristics (mainly for classification problems) became a growing cottage industry in academia while spawning large numbers of commercial companies. Many ideas from AI (such as rules and frames) gradually penetrated into software environments in this way [Waterman, 1986].

The period of 1982–1987 can be characterized as a transitional one, during which AIM researchers explored the complexities of medical reasoning and developed unique ways of representing them on the computer: critiquing as a modality of reasoning [Miller, 1983], qualitative explanatory models of clinical reasoning [Swartout, 1981; Clancey and Letsiufer, 1981], and underlying physiologic processes [Patil et al., 1981; Kuipers, 1985], and the elaboration of rule-base updating and refinement methods [Politakis and Weiss, 1984]. Contemporaneously, and in contrast to the knowledge-engineering approach, new and more computationally powerful neural networks were introduced [Rumelhard and McClelland, 1986] and later applied in medical decision making [Hudson et al., 1991].

The fourth phase of medical AI systems (from about 1987 to the present) can be characterized by continuing development of knowledge-based representations with greater structure and generic task dependencies [Chandrasekaran, 1986] based on Newell's principle that systems should be designed at the knowledge level [Newell, 1982]. There have been ongoing experiments in qualitative reasoning [Long, 1991; Widman, 1992] and modeling and control of time critical processes, as in intensive care units (ICUs) [Summers et al., 1993], and the representation of temporal reasoning [Kahn, 1991]. Most notably there has been a revival of interest in statistical approaches to decision making, linked now to more abstract models of underlying processes represented in influence diagrams [Farr and Shachter, 1992]. Work on bayesian belief nets and decision analytical methods [Speigelhalter and Lauritzen, 1990; Cooper, 1993] and continuing developments in the application of neural nets [Hudson et al., 1991; Sittig and Orr, 1992; Cho and Reggia, 1993], fuzzy pattern matching [Pedrycz et al., 1991], and a variety of learning methods [Weiss and Kulikowski, 1991] for decision making characterize the increasing complexity and diversity of an active field of research in evolution. Over the past decade there also has been a redefinition of goals by many researchers to more achievable objectives for medical decision systems. This involves much less emphasis on full-fledged automatic consultation and much more on the decision support that such systems can provide in answering queries by the user about diagnostic or treatment protocol choices. A recent review of decision support systems is found in Miller [1994].

183.2 Early Models of Medical Decision Making

The earliest efforts to formalize medical decision making involved the application of statistical decision methods (ROC curves) in radiographic interpretation. Precursor attempts at automating the logic of diagnostic reasoning by sorting symptoms and selecting diagnoses that matched a particular combination involved multiple slide-rule and early card and computer sorting techniques.

As computers became more powerful and easily programmable, they were the natural tool for representing diagnostic and treatment decision making. A watershed article by Ledley and Lusted in *Science* [1959] described the reasoning bases for medical decision making in both logical and statistical terms. The main paradigm for representing medical decisions in the 1960s was statistical, whether bayesian, hypothesis testing, or discriminant function analysis. Summary reviews of these can be found in Kulikowski [1980] and Miller [1994]. The growth of standardized laboratory test panels and multiphasic screening methods had a great effect in popularizing statistical techniques as an objective approach to the selection of decision thresholds. Bayesian methods were predominant and allowed incorporation of subjective estimates of prior probability into the calculation of diagnostic probabilities. Likelihood-ratio (hypothesis-testing) methods did not but required instead a determination of sensitivity/specificity tradeoffs with threshold selection dependent on a choice of clinically tolerable levels for them. There also were heuristic pattern-recognition methods being developed if more flexibility was required, but all these approaches at that time suffered from a common drawback. While they might perform very well for circumscribed problems with well-defined statistics or adequate samples from which to estimate the statistics, they were rarely acceptable to practicing physicians beyond their site of origin. A reason frequently given for this was the difficulty of explaining decisions based on strictly computational theories of probability in terms of the qualitative language and arguments familiar to physicians.

During the 1960s, the alternative to formal statistical methods was the coding of the sequence of expert decisions in a branching logic diagram or flowchart, often described as a *clinical decision algorithm*. This approach had the advantages of clarity and ease of explanation but was usually too rigid to capture the nuances of context without becoming very large, complex, and computationally expensive.

During this period, most mainstream AI research appeared to have little to offer medical decision making, since it was concerned primarily with the computer representation and reasoning for very general problem solving without considering explicit representations of uncertainty. Examples are means-ends analysis and search strategies and general representations of knowledge such as state spaces and memory models. Their application was usually to fairly small, well-circumscribed problems, such as block worlds or game situations. On the other hand, a very specific problem-solving paradigm was developed for the realistically complex problem of natural language understanding.

None of these approaches had immediate or obvious applicability to medical consultation problems, where the reasoning was characterized by the necessity of making choices under conditions of both risk and uncertainty, with goals often only specified imprecisely and at a very general level, such as "select an additional piece of evidence," "choose the most likely diagnoses," or "choose a treatment that covers the most likely confirmed diagnoses."

183.3 Emergence of the Knowledge-Based AI Methods for Medical Consultation

In the early 1970s, several groups involving both AI and biomedical researchers decided to explore different, more knowledge-intensive approaches to interpretive problem solving, including medical decision making. Several common themes emerged from the work of the four groups that initiated these efforts at Rutgers University, Stanford University, the University of Pittsburgh, and the MIT/Tufts collaborative group. All of them, at about the same time, recognized some of the shortcomings of existing methods and proposed a set of alternative representation and inferencing approaches that involved

- Representing uncertainty more flexibly and qualitatively than appeared possible with probabilities
- Representing more of the medical knowledge that motivated and justified a diagnostic, prognostic, or therapeutic decision
- Developing a descriptive component of medical knowledge to which some general problem-solving or inferencing strategy could be applied

Early prototypes of AI consultation systems that incorporated distinct approaches to medical decision making were CASNET [Kulikowski and Weiss, 1972], MYCIN [Shortliffe et al., 1974], DIALOG/INTERNIST-1 [Pople et al., 1975], the Present Illness Program (PIP) [Pauker et al., 1976], and the Digitalis Advisor Program [Gorry et al., 1978].

That a domain-specific model could be used as the basis for interpretive decision making was first demonstrated in the DENDRAL system [Buchanan et al., 1970]. DENDRAL interpreted mass spectra by using rules that were constrained by a model of the possible chemical structures that could have given rise to the observed spectral data. This was quite different from the domain-independent, pattern-recognition approaches previously applied to the problem.

The first AI approach to decision making in medicine itself evolved within the Rutgers Research Resource on Computers in Biomedicine, which was established in 1972. One of the goals of our research group was to find general methods of representing medical reasoning that would take advantage of the knowledge of specific diseases in ways similar to those used by medical specialists. In a collaboration with Dr. Aran Safir, an ophthalmologist at the Mt. Sinai School of Medicine (New York), we explored methods for describing and applying medical knowledge for computer-based diagnosis and management. With Sholom Weiss, who worked on his doctoral dissertation on this project, we found that a very natural way for characterizing the underlying mechanisms of disease was through cause-and-effect relations. A network of causal links among pathophysiologic conditions (or abnormal physiologic states) could then be used to describe the many pathways through which a disease might manifest itself. Each pathophysiologic state could be inferred independently from the patient's condition and asserted with some degree of confidence depending on its pattern of supportive evidence. A prototype system for testing these ideas was developed in the area of glaucoma diagnosis and management. This proved to be a good problem, because glaucoma is a major cause of loss of vision and blindness with mechanisms that are sufficiently well understood to determine the course of management yet at the same time sufficiently complex that advice on difficult cases (particularly those resistant to conventional treatment) must frequently be sought from specialist consultants.

A variety of reasoning strategies seemed to apply to different stages of the consultation. For example, while starting to gather data on a patient, the major problem for a consultant is to elucidate the patient's problem and develop diagnostic leads by asking the right questions and acquiring the relevant data. When enough data have accumulated, a different mode of reasoning is characteristically needed. The findings must be attributed to specific causes, whether single or multiple. Finally, all these explanations must be combined into a differential diagnosis. This serves to predict what will happen if the patient remains untreated (prognosis) and suggests possible ways of managing the disease (treatment or therapeutic planning). As we gained experience in extracting the knowledge from the expert practitioners, it became clear that different management strategies relied on different types of medical knowledge, and these strategies had to be sufficiently general and independent of the particular disease being modeled. Weiss built a prototype system called CASNET (for *casual associational network*) based on these ideas [Weiss, 1974; Weiss et al., 1978]. We were fortunate in being able to draw on the expertise of leading glaucoma specialists, who provided the in-depth knowledge needed to describe the disease and tested the system independently in their own laboratories. After 2 years of improving the initial prototype, the system was given a blind test by presenting it with new, previously unseen cases during a panel discussion at the major national meeting of the Academy of Ophthalmology in 1976. CASNET made no errors in its recommendations, though it was unable to answer some questions for which the knowledge was absent in the computer model [Lichter and Anderson, 1977].

During the early 1970s, another kind of biomedical AI resource was established at Stanford as the result of the DENDRAL project collaboration that had developed between AI researchers (E. Feigenbaum and B. Buchanan) and biomedical researchers (J. Lederberg and S. Cohen). This SUMEX-AIM Resource, established in 1974, provided advanced time sharing on a PDP-10 computer to a national network of investigators in AI in medicine, with appropriate systems and AI language support for what was then a very novel computational mode, serving an initial nucleus of investigators, including those at Rutgers and the University of Pittsburgh [Freiherr, 1979].

The medical component of the SUMEX-AIM research centered around the consultation system for infectious disease treatment developed by Shortliffe [Shortliffe et al., 1974; Shortliffe, 1976]. Its representation of medical knowledge was in the form of heuristic rules with a new certainty factor formalism, which decoupled the way in which positive and negative evidence was credited toward a hypothesis, thus providing more heuristic flexibility than previous probabilistic frameworks. The system's strategy was goal driven for gathering the data needed to reach the diagnostic conclusions necessary to choose the appropriate covering therapies. The modularity of MYCIN's rules turned out to be a critical design choice, since it was soon found that it was easy to modify the rules independently of the reasoning strategy and its inference engine, giving rise to a very flexible and updatable knowledge base. The certainty-factor model turned out to be less long-lived, since it was soon found to implicitly involve assumptions and constraints that did not adequately represent the complex dependencies that often exist among data and hypotheses. However, MYCIN, by providing an easy means of directly and modularly encoding the rules of medical reasoning (without an underlying disease model as in CASNET), gave rise to the most powerful representation for the first generation of knowledge-based AI systems—the rule-based paradigm [Buchanan and Shortliffe, 1984].

Another group to work intensely on AI approaches to medical decision making was that of Gorry at MIT and Pauker and Schwartz at Tufts, who led the development of the Digitalis Advisor Program [Gorry et al., 1978]. This system introduced two interesting new concepts: a patient-specific model (PSM) and a mathematical model for describing the mechanism being regulated and interpreted (digitalis uptake). The PSM grouped together all the information known about a patient during a consultation session (the findings, history, test results, etc.), as well as the hypotheses about the patient (diagnostic, prognostic, and therapeutic) produced by the computer diagnostic/therapeutic model. The mathematical model was a compartmental model of digitalis uptake, which was able to relate dosages to their expected therapeutic and toxic effects.

In a related AIM project, Pauker and Kassirer joined Gorry and Schwartz in formulating the Present Illness Program (PIP) [Pauker et al., 1976], which was designed to focus in on a medical problem based on a brief description of the patient's complaints (the present illness). Here, Minsky's frame formalism [Minsky, 1975], which had been developed to describe a template of expected objects in computer vision recognition tasks, was used as a template for grouping typical or characteristic information about a disease. Each frame contained slots that had to be filled with descriptors of the disease, with some of these slots containing rules for reasoning about the disease. In this way, diseases were related through rules, but these rules were grouped by their respective frames. An interesting observation that came from this work was that the probabilistic scoring of hypotheses, while important in diagnostic reasoning, is often overshadowed by the use of categorical or deterministic reasoning, which has to be flexible and suitably richly represented to be useful [Szolovitz and Pauker, 1978]. Subsequently, the ABEL system for modeling acid-base balance problems [Patil et al., 1981] took advantage of many of the ideas from PIP and combined them with a causal description of disease at multiple levels of abstraction and aggregation, which helped provide a more detailed description of pathophysiologic processes.

Also contemporaneously, Dr. Harry Pople at the University of Pittsburgh had been investigating biomedical applications of AI—specifically abductive reasoning with causal graphs for scientific theory formation [Pople, 1973]. In a collaboration with Dr. Jack Myers, an eminent internist, Pople began a very broad and ambitious project: to capture all of Dr. Myers' diagnostic knowledge of internal medicine into a system that could reason automatically from the facts of a case. Over the next few years, they developed a taxonomic and causal representation for characterizing diseases and their manifestations and proceeded to develop a set of alternatives for describing the various strategies of diagnostic reasoning: the preliminary assessment of findings, the attribution of causes and explanations for each of the findings, the computation of confidences and resulting ranking of diagnostic hypotheses, the development of a differential diagnosis, and the confirmation of a diagnosis once it is already strongly indicated (through specialized tests). The DIALOG system was developed to test these ideas and codify Dr. Myers' knowledge [Pople et al., 1975]. Its later version, called INTERNIST-1 [Pople, 1977; Miller, 1984], demonstrated how the very large domain-specific knowledge base of internal medicine could be assembled and validated with complex cases of disease, both from the clinic and journal CPC reports.

Research in AI in medicine (AIM) was initially presented in a series of AIM workshops, starting at Rutgers University [Ciesielski, 1978], subsequently rotating among the AIM community. Later workshops were organized in conjuction with the American Association for Artificial Intelligence (AAAI) as part of its spring symposia, while sessions on medical expert systems were to be increasingly found at most relevant scientific, engineering, medical, and informatics conferences (AAAS, IEEE, IJCAI, AAAI, SCAMC, etc.).

183.4 The Transition to Expert Systems and the Ascendancy of Rule-Based Systems—1976–1982

As mentioned earlier, the experience in developing, testing, and disseminating the prototypes of the first-generation medical consultation systems, combined with similar experiences of AI researchers outside medicine, led to a shift in AI research away from general problem solving to more domain-specific knowledge-intensive problems. Feigenbaum [1978] defined generalizations of the MYCIN system for dealing with any problem where advice-giving knowledge could be captured in the form of rules. He emphasized the separation of rule-based systems from the inference engine that reasoned with them and coined the term *knowledge engineering* to describe the art of building a knowledge-based system. This process was centered around the interviewing of domain specialists by knowledge engineers (typically computer scientists or engineers), who would attempt to understand the problem being modeled, learn about the expertise that the specialist applied in solving it, and finally formalize all this into a computer representation of the problem-solving or consultative knowledge. The early stages of the process, usually called *knowledge acquisition,* frequently became the major bottleneck in developing an expert system, particularly if the knowledge engineer had difficulties in understanding the field of expertise or came with preconceived notions about it that did not match the expert's own. Another difficulty with first-generation expert system shells was that the knowledge had to be fitted to a predetermined computer representation, which might or might not match that of the domain problem. Most shells worked well with advice-giving reasoning that involved classification-type problems that could be reduced to the selection of one or several alternatives from a large set of candidate hypotheses. In this sense, their overall problem-solving paradigm did not differ much from the statistical and pattern-recognition methods that preceded them. Their major departure was in the architectural modularity of the rule base, flexible choice of reasoning strategies, and the representation of intermediate hypotheses and reasoning constructs with which to support and assemble a final conclusion. Researchers interested in the cognitive processes of human expert diagnosticians analyzed the problem-solving behavior of experts confronted with real and simulated cases to discern their reasoning strategies [Elstein et al., 1978; Kassirer and Gorry, 1978]. These were usually found to be sufficiently complex that they did not have an effect on the design of the rapidly spreading rule-based systems of the time. Rather, they influenced the development of more sophisticated systems based on deeper medical knowledge in the following decade.

The years 1976–1978 saw the testing, critiquing, and elaboration of the prototype systems. This resulted in changes and generalizations of the initial designs, leading to the first general system-building frameworks (EXPERT [Weiss and Kulikowski, 1979], EMYCIN [van Melle, 1979], AGE [Nii and Aiello, 1979]). These came about because in the course of the research it became clear that incorporating expert knowledge about advice-giving consultation could be carried out with various kinds of reasoning: either or both hypothesis- and data-driven strategies, with corresponding backward or forward chaining of rules. Furthermore, inferences incorporated into the rules could be either interpreted (as in EMYCIN) or compiled (as in EXPERT), and knowledge could be chunked or clustered by subtasks of the problem solving with the aid of various other representational devices (context trees in EMYCIN, knowledge sources in AGE, rule clusters in EXPERT, and frames in PIP).

Building various expert systems capitalized on the increasing experience with alternative ways of representing knowledge. For example, the IRIS system at Rutgers [Trigoboff, 1976] applied a semantic network model (as was being developed in PROSPECTOR [Hart and Duda, 1977]) to rerepresent glaucoma consultation knowledge with multiple strategies of inference; the CRYSALIS system [Englemore and Terry, 1979], which explicated the structure of chemical substances from x-ray diffraction data, used the blackboard model from speech understanding; the VM system developed a real-time variant of a rule-based system for ventilation management [Fagan et al., 1979]; and the MDX system pursued a distributed conceptual model for diagnosis [Chandrasekaran et al., 1979]. The CENTAUR system [Aikins, 1979] showed that both rules and frames could be usefully combined to represent expert reasoning, and AI/RHEUM [Lindberg, 1980] demonstrated how rule-based systems with specialized medical semantics could be adapted to represent already-formalized knowledge found in rheumatologic diagnostic criteria tables. Meanwhile, many other systems were developed showing that rule-based methods could be widely and systematically applied [Reggia et al., 1980; Horn et al., 1980; Speedie et al., 1981; Buchanan and Shortliffe, 1984; Weiss and Kulikowski, 1984].

The evaluation of the first-generation systems was pursued for CASNET [Lichter and Anderson, 1977], MYCIN [Yu et al., 1979], the Digitalis Advisor [Swartout, 1981], and INTERNIST-1 [Pople, 1977]. Critical examination of knowledge structures in INTERNIST-1 led to their being rerepresented in INTERNIST-2 [Pople, 1977]. General methodologies for evaluating clinical predictions also were being developed [Shapiro, 1977]. This testing and evaluation led to the first efforts at automating knowledge acquisition and maintenance of the rule bases. For instance, the TEIRESIAS system was designed to improve the performance of MYCIN through heuristic analysis of individual cases, leading to changes in rules that were incorrectly invoked or designed [Davis, 1979].

Likewise, Politakis and Weiss [1980] developed methods for testing and improving EXPERT rule bases by providing analytical/statistical performance evaluation and rule-modification tools in an interactive environment. In 1980, a first workshop on general expert systems was held to compare the different techniques for knowledge representation and the systems that implemented them. A common problem was selected in advance without the knowledge of the different research groups and presented to them at the workshop for implementation in their system. The results of this experiment are summarized in Hayes-Roth et al. [1983]. While all the existing shells were able to represent a complex advice-giving problem (the diagnosis and tracking of a chemical spill), those with fixed inference engines proved the easiest to use for rapid prototyping. As might have been expected, the more general AI languages designed to capture expertise did permit more flexible, expressive, and detailed descriptions of the problem but at the cost of a much greater investment of time and effort in building both knowledge bases and specialized inference procedures.

The development and assessment of rule-based and frame-based systems demonstrated that while they could effectively capture large quantities of domain-specific expertise, there were still many unanswered questions about how the expertise should be best applied to specific problems while at the same time abstracting out general representations of knowledge. The complexity of human problem-solving processes revealed by cognitive analyses and simulations of clinical reasoning [Elstein et al., 1978] pointed to the difficulties of reconciling these goals.

183.5 Exploration of Alternative Representations for Medical AI and the Search for Performance—1983–1987

Two almost opposite trends in medical AI emerged from the generalization of expert systems, which continue to the present. On the one hand, driven by the goal of practical clinical applications, researchers tried to adapt existing representations and obtain high performance from them. This led to various systems with very specific goals, such as the interpretation of laboratory tests, which even reached commercial implementation and dissemination [Weiss et al., 1983]. At the opposite end of the spectrum, dissatisfaction with the oversimplified cognitive style of rule-based expert systems and the inadequate coverage and performance of large knowledge bases led to research into alternative representations of deeper medical knowledge [Chandrasekaran et al., 1979].

Explanation and Early Knowledge Level Work in AI systems

In an attempt to reuse the MYCIN knowledge base for tutorial purposes in the GUIDON system [Clancey, 1989], it was found that generating explanations from the original rule base was not only difficult but also revealed that all kinds of implementational details for consultative inferencing were mixed in with the more abstract, descriptive medical knowledge that supported the inferences. Besides adding metarules for guiding the discourse involved in tutoring, the experience in building GUIDON led Clancey to reconsider the generality of the MYCIN rule base and its representation. The NEOMYCIN system [Clancey and Letsinger, 1981] completely separated descriptive medical knowledge from details of reasoning task implementation so that it would better match the problem-solving tasks of human experts. This coincided with Newell's more general observation across AI systems: that they need to describe problem solving at the knowledge level, free of the encumberances of specific programming details [Newell, 1982]. In medicine, a similar experience had been reported in a follow-up to the digitalis project by Swartout, who designed the XPLAIN system [Swartout, 1981] as an automatic programming approach for generating a consultation model from the specification of abstract system goals. Explanations and justifications would then be automatically built into the performance system.

The role of explanatory reasoning became a major focus of attention for many medical AI groups during this period. One of the earliest and major motivations for the AI approaches to reasoning was that they were able to explain their logic in terms that were much closer to the arguments of physicians. However, by the end of the first decade, most AIM researchers found that the explanatory capabilities of their systems, while useful for tracing logical connections through their systems, left much to be desired in terms of naturalness and flexibility. Traditional statistical decision systems could produce an explanation by accounting for each manifestation's contribution to the total probability (or weight) of a diagnosis. In CASNET, an explanation could be generated by tracing the pathway of confirmed causal states that led to the final diagnosis. The confidence in the confirmation of each state could, in turn, be explained by the pattern of observed evidence that supported it. In MYCIN and other derived rule-based systems, explanations could be easily generated by tracing the rules involved in producing a decision. In the Digitalis Advisor, an explanation could be generated in terms of the causal underpinnings of the patient-specific model, while in INTERNIST-1, the diagnostic strategy could be traced in terms of the sequence of manifestations activated or covered by a particular set of hypotheses. All these approaches, while initially satisfying to the developers, upon further consideration proved to be inadequate. Tracing every detail of logic by which a system arrived at a diagnostic or therapeutic conclusion could be very useful for debugging the knowledge base during system development, but it rapidly became tedious to the expert reviewer or the practitioner using the system. What was missing was a clear summary of the underlying justification of the reasoning. A major reason for this was that the first-generation representations, in their emphasis on symbolic and qualitative descriptions of knowledge, as opposed to the earlier numerical representations, failed to separate or abstract out information at the true knowledge level from the finer-grained symbolic details of the implementation.

NEOMYCIN [Clancey and Letsinger, 1981] showed the need to reorganize the knowledge in a rule base in order to be able to produce "intelligently studied reasons" for a decision. The ABEL system demonstrated the critical importance of hierarchical causal descriptions using composition and decomposition operators to explain interactions among subprocess contributing to an overall pathophysiologic disease process [Patil, 1983]. In a restructuring of the INTERNIST-1 knowledge base, Pople [1982] showed how combinations of very elementary operators (causal, hierarchical) could be used to construct and explain alternative complexes of hypothesis with different interpretations for the same set of confirmed states. MDX stressed the importance of describing problem-solving tasks in diagnosis and using procedural knowledge to capture the knowledge of expert practitioners [Chandrasekaran et al., 1979]. This research, applied to several liver diagnostic problems and a red cell identification problem [Smith et al., 1985], among others, led Chandrasekaran [1986] to develop a theory of generic problem-solving tasks in order to advance our understanding of diagnostic and other expert reasoning processes.

A completely different form of reasoning was implemented in the ATTENDING system [Miller, 1983]. Rather than modeling consultative reasoning directly, Miller analyzed and critiqued the plans that physicians had developed for anesthesia administration, using an augmented transition network of states. This novel departure helped define a new type of critiquing system that was very useful for instructional purposes and therefore more likely to be used by physicians who either felt threatened by automated consultative systems or else found them lacking and not essential to their practice.

The Search for Performance

In trying to deal with practical clinical problems, many AIM researchers found that the first general expert systems shells did not satisfy their requirements. The shells frequently had many options that would never be used in a particular application while being difficult to adapt to problem-specific reasoning methods and domain-specific knowledge structures. Furthermore, for an expert system to be really useful, they found that design of easy-to-use human interfaces, while not scientifically rewarding at first glance, was actually quite essential. In this regard, the next major medical project of the Heuristic Programming Project at Stanford, the ONCOCIN system [Shortliffe et al., 1981], demonstrated that well-engineered interfaces mimicking on a screen the input of charts, images, and other data for cancer treatment protocols, could directly improve data acquisition and were essential in guiding the application of the protocols. Knowledge acquisition for ONCOCIN was provided by a very flexible graphics-oriented system, called OPAL [Musen et al., 1986]. An important representational issue also was settled in the ONCOCIN experiments: the need for event-driven reasoning as well as goal-driven reasoning in rule-based MYCIN-like systems, as had been earlier advocated in the EXPERT scheme.

Exploiting other, natural knowledge representations became a theme in an application of the EXPERT system for building a rheumatology knowledge base [Lindberg et al., 1983]. Here it was found that domain-specific decision rules had already been defined by the American Rheumatological Association in the form of diagnostic criteria tables. These, however, needed more detailed elaboration in terms of observational criteria for findings, as well as customization of the diagnostic criteria within a working expert system—AI/RHEUM [Kingsland et al., 1983].

The goal of producing high-performance systems led researchers during this period to experiment with technology transfer, disseminating the knowledge of experts within the medical community. The first expert system on a chip was pioneered at Rutgers with the SPE/EXPERT system for serum protein electrophoresis analysis [Weiss et al., 1983]. In this system, a knowledge base was developed by a leading specialist in the field, using the high-level EXPERT language, and then automatically translated into algorithmic form and compiled into the assembly language of the ROM that existed to process signals from the scanning densitometer of the Cliniscan instrument (TM-Helena Laboratories, Beaumont, Texas). Similar technology was used to develop an advice-giving system for primary eye care on one of the earliest hand-held computers [Kastner et al., 1984].

In a very large undertaking, the INTERNIST-1 knowledge base was recast into a form that would make it more easily accessible by flexible querying in the QMR system [Miller, 1984], rather than being restricted to the consultative mode it had been before. The intelligent retrieval facilities of QMR have made it one of the most widely disseminated results of expert system research [Miller, 1994]. In a similar trend, other earlier non-AI systems were reengineered to have more modular architectures, as with the HELP system, which provided advice as part of the medical information system at the Latter Day Saints Hospital. Its successor, the ILLIAD system, has subsequently become an integral part of quality-assurance functions in the hospital network [Lau and Warner, 1992]. Likewise, the DXplain general decision support system was made widely available to physicians through the AMA/NET in the 1980s [Barnett et al., 1987].

With the increasing dissemination of AIM systems came parallel efforts to test and evaluate their performance while exploring new ways of dealing with the difficult issues of reasoning in uncertain environments.

An empirical approach to performance evaluation was taken with the AI/RHEUM system testing and resulted in the first system for refining a rule base using the accumulated experience of expertly solved cases [Politakis and Weiss, 1984]. This system, called SEEK, employed performance heuristics to suggest potential improvements in the rules (generalizations and specializations) and which could be tested by incorporation into the model and evaluation over the entire data base of cases. In SEEK 2, this work was extended to generate automatically and test the potential improvements, selecting the most successful improvements for inclusion in an updated knowledge base [Ginsberg, 1986]. Related to these approaches is the basic problem of uncovering underlying causal relations through the analysis of time-oriented data, such as was carried out in the RX system [Blum, 1982]. During this period, causality became a major concern of researchers seeking strong theoretical underpinnings that would explain reasoning in complex diagnostic consultation models [Patil, 1986].

The Search for Formal Theories of Reasoning
Under Uncertainty in Medicine

Many different formal methods of inference were explored and applied in knowledge-based medical decision making. These included the application of multihypothesis bayesian methods [Ben-Bassat et al., 1980], of fuzzy logic as in the CADIAG family of systems [Addlassnig and Kolarz, 1982] and the SPHINX system [Fieschi et al., 1983], or of the Dempster-Shaffer theory of evidence to structured medical problems [Gordon and Shortliffe, 1985]. Reggia et al. [1983] devised set covering strategies to parsimoniously explain diagnostic hypotheses within a probabilistic framework [Peng and Reggia, 1987].

Two major interrelated problems afflicting the handling of uncertainty in clinical decision making were how to combine evidence from multiple related sources in a non-mutually-exclusive multihypothesis inference problem and how to represent the flow of uncertainty among intermediate causal and hierarchically related hypotheses. These problems had existed from the very beggining of medical AI, and their formal treatment was avoided through the use of empirical, heuristic methods in the first generation of systems. Now researchers embarked on a more principled search for solutions. The Dempster-Shaffer theory provided a good formalism for incorporating partial belief information into a complex network of hypotheses. However, in practice, it often proved computationally expensive or might produce very broad and uninformative confidence bounds on hypotheses at the end of long reasoning chains. In an attempt to provide a link between the semantics of hypotheses related at different levels of causation and abstraction, Pearl [1987] developed methods for propagating uncertainty within a structured bayesian framework of statistical decision making. The more systematic application of these techniques in medical systems and the exploration of their implications for specific medical reasoning problems, however, are still ongoing.

The revival of interest in connectionist, neural network methods for learning and decision making was strongly stimulated around this time by the introduction of backpropagation methods [Rumelhard and McClelland, 1986]. These used differentiable nonlinear threshold functions that enabled the learning of much more complex decision rules from data than had been possible with the simpler perceptron methods of the 1960s. As researchers and practitioners came to realize that the expert systems and knowledge-engineering approaches required large amounts of investment by the most costly and indispensable consultants in the specialty being modeled, efforts again began to emphasize methods that learned directly from data through ANNs, as well as even simpler decision structures, such as decision trees [Breiman et al., 1984].

183.6 The Recent Past—Structure, Formalism, and Empiricism

Deep Medical Knowledge for Representation and Problem Solving

The trends described above continued through the 1987–1994 period as researchers continued to work on representations for the deeper medical knowledge that could help explain and justify medical decisions. One approach has continued to emphasize the centrality of causal reasoning and simulation in providing knowledge-based explanations for the physiologic underpinnings of medical reasoning [Kuipers, 1985; Long, 1987, 1991; Hunter and Kirby, 1991; Widman, 1992].

More generally, Newell's knowledge-level approach [Newell, 1982] has become the inspiration for what are usually called *second-generation* expert systems, which emphasize the multilevel nature of modeling problem-solving and related interacting knowledge structures [Chandrasekaran and Johnson, 1993].

Applications of Newell's SOAR architecture [Smith and Johnson, 1993] enables a very general type of problem-solving mechanism (chunking) to roam over flexible spaces of goals, tasks, and specific knowledge structures, thereby providing a common framework for reasoning about decisions in individual cases or with groups of cases, as for learning rules or other changes to the knowledge base. In this, as in the KADS approach [Wielinga et al., 1992], there is a view of expertise as a dynamic process that cannot be captured in strictly static knowledge structures but rather evolves as part of an ongoing interactive modeling of systems, agents, problems, and environments [Clancey, 1989]. A discussion of how this problem-solving cognitive approach affects medical decision making can be found in Kleinmuntz [1991]. Meanwhile, many of the lessons have been applied to recent knowledge-based explanation and system-building activities [Bylander et al., 1993; Koton, 1993; Swartout and Moore, 1993]. The relationship between abductive reasoning and temporal reasoning is discussed in Console and Torasso et al. [1991], and an epistemologic framework for structuring medical problem solving is found in Ramoni et al. [1992]. It is interesting to note that a related cognitive approach to eliciting and structuring medical knowledge grew up independently in the former Soviet Union through the work of Gelfand and collaborators [Gelfand et al., 1987; Gelfand, 1989].

Formal Decision-Making Methods and Empirical Systems

Formal decision-making approaches to medical reasoning took off in the 1980s with the founding of the journal *Medical Decision Making,* which involved physicians as well as decision scientists in the process of understanding how formal statistical and logical methods can apply to the modeling and interpretation of medical problems. This renewed interest in the modeling of reasoning under risk and uncertainty was motivated by the twin needs of evaluating decision-support systems and of modeling more general epidemiologic effects of medical interventions, with and without computer-based systems being involved. While not directly related to knowledge-based AI approaches, this trend nevertheless interacted with developments in operations research (OR) and AI through the confluence of the influence diagram representation of abstract states for describing processes [Shachter, 1986] and belief network representations for reasoning with causal structured hypothesis networks [Pearl, 1987]. Together, they helped make bayesian belief networks a practical tool for modeling many of the dynamic aspects of clinical cognition [Cowell et al., 1991] and provided a combined statistical-structural representation for decision-making preferences in computer-based systems [Lehman and Shortliffe, 1990; Farr and Shachter, 1992; Heckerman and Shortliffe, 1992; Jimison et al., 1992; Neapolitan, 1993]. The related use of the decision theoretic approach to integrate knowledge-based and judgmental elements also has been an important development in assisting the evaluation of systems [Cooper, 1993], and knowledge-based tools for specifying large expert system models [Olesen and Andreassen, 1993] and building decision models are also becoming more prevalent [Sonneberg et al., 1994]. In addition, tools from meta-analysis have begun to be applied to assess conflicting results from related though different clinical studies [Littenberg and Moses, 1993] and merge diagnostic accuracy results [Midgette et al., 1993]. The temporal nature of medical processes and data also has led to some initial models for decision making that make temporal dependencies explicit in their representation [Kahn, 1991; VanBeek, 1991; Hazen, 1992; Cousins et al., 1993]. Practical systems in the ICU or other monitoring situations typically have to use a temporal representation in the context of on-line expert systems [Schecke et al., 1991; Mora et al., 1993; Rutledge et al., 1993; Lehmann et al., 1994].

With more sophisticated methods for learning in artificial neural networks (ANNs), the last few years have seen a concomitant increase in their application to the modeling and learning of medical decisions [Barreto and DeAzevedo, 1993; Cherkassy and Lari-Najafi, 1992; Cho and Reggia, 1993; Forsstrom et al., 1991a; Hudson et al., 1991; Sittig and Orr, 1992]. Logic-based methods also have seen some popularity in structuring and building knowledge bases in medicine, particularly in Europe and Japan [Fox et al., 1990; Krause et al., 1993; Lucas, 1993].

The evaluation of expert systems and decision support systems remains an important ongoing research and practical problem [Miller, 1986; Potoff et al., 1988; Willems et al., 1991; Bankowitz et al., 1992; Nohr, 1994], to which a variety of machine learning techniques can be applied for the performance assessment [Weiss and Kulikowski, 1991], knowledge base refinement [Widmer et al., 1993], and the retrospective analysis of results [Forsstrom et al., 1991b].

183.7 Present and Future of Medical AI

As we approach the mid-1990s, methodological developments in both the representation of knowledge and inferencing methods in medicine, however impressive in terms of their improvements over those of 20 or 30 years ago, have still not resulted in systems that are routinely used in the clinic. A recent comparative study of four of the most widely disseminated diagnostic decision support systems [Berner et al., 1994] resulted in an editorial comment to the effect that their overall rating left much to be desired—a grade of C [Kassirer, 1994]. However, it is fair to point out that the systems reviewed were diagnostic aids, which most physicians find less than indispensible given their own training. Furthermore, these systems generally did not have to perform complex modeling or numerical computations, where computer-based assistance is often indispensible. Fields such as treatment dosage review, instrumentation monitoring and control, and multimodality imaging all suggest more essential domains for the application of AI methods, whether knowledge- or data-derived [DeMelo et al., 1992; Mora et al., 1993; Gong and Kulikowski, 1992].

The present situation, then, can be characterized as one of consolidation in integrating a variety of methods and techniques for different types of medical decision tasks while at the same time involving considerable reassessment and change in terms of expectations about the imminent application of decision-making systems within health care environments. On the one hand, the forthcoming increase in networking of various knowledge sources, digital libraries, and multimedia information opens up a whole new set of opportunities for filtering knowledge to the overwhelmed practitioner, whether in medicine, law, engineering, or other professions. On the other hand, the hard issues of understanding the role of human judgment and responsibility for clinical decisions and actions when using increasingly complex computerized instrumentation and systems presents an ongoing challenge to researchers in medicine, biomedical engineering and computer science, medical informatics, and all other fields essential to the solution of these problems.

References

Adlassnig KP, Kolarz G. 1982. CADIAG-2: Computer-Assisted Medical Diagnosis Using Fuzzy Subsets. Approximate Reasoning in Decision Analysis, 219–247.

Aikins J. 1979. Prototype and production rules: An approach to knowledge representation for hypothesis information. In Proc. 6th Int. Joint Conf Artificial Intel, pp 1–3. Tokyo, Japan.

Bankowitz RA, Lave JR, McNeil MA. 1992. A method for assessing the impact of a computer-based decision support system on health care outcomes. Meth Inform Med 31:3.

Barnett GO, Cimino JJ, Hupp JA, Hoffer EP. 1987. DXplain: An evolving diagnostic decision-support system. JAMA 258:67.

Barreto JM, DeAzevedo FM. 1993. Connectionist expert systems as medical decision aid. Artif Intell Med 5(6):515.

Ben-Bassat M, Carlson RW, Puri VK, et al. 1980. Pattern-based interactive diagnosis of multiple disorders: The MEDAS system. IEEE Trans Pat Anal Mach Intel (PAMI) 2(2):148.

Berner ES, Webster GD, Shugerman AA, et al. 1994. Performance of four computer-based diagnostic systems. N Engl J Med 330(25):1792.

Blum R. 1982. Discovery confirmation and incorporation of casual relationships from a large time-oriented data base: The RX project. Comput Biomed Res 15:164.

Breiman L, Friedman J, Olshen R, Stone C. 1984. Classification and Regression Trees. Monterey, Calif, Wadsworth.

Buchanan BG, Sutherland G, Feigenbaum EA. 1970. Rediscovering some problems of artificial intelligence in the context of organic chemistry. In B Meltzer, D Michie (eds), Machine Intelligence, pp 209–254. Edinburgh, Edinburgh University Press.

Buchanan BG, Shortliffe EH. 1984. Rule-Based Expert Systems: The MYCIN Experiments in the Stanford Heuristic Programming Project. Reading, Mass, Addison-Wesley.

Bylander T, Weintraub M, Simon SR. 1993. QUAWDS: Diagnosis using different models for different subtasks. In J-M David et al (eds), Second Generation Expert Systems, pp 110–130. Berlin, Springer-Verlag.

Chandrasekaran B, Gomez F, Mittal S, Smith J. 1979. An approach to medical diagnosis based on conceptual schemes. In Proc. 6th Int Joint Conf Artif Intell, pp 134–142. Tokyo, Japan.

Chandrasekaran B. 1986. Generic tasks in knowledge-based reasoning: High-level building blocks for expert system design. IEEE Expert Intelligent Systems and Their Applications 1(3):23.

Chandrasekaran B, Johnson TR. 1993. Generic tasks and task structures: History, critique and new directions. In J-M David et al (eds), Second Generation Expert Systems, pp 232–272. Berlin, Springer-Verlag.

Cherkassky V, Lari-Najafi H. 1992. Data representation for diagnostic neural networks. IEEE Expert 7(5):43.

Cho S, Reggia JA. 1993. Multiple disorder diagnosis with adaptive competitive neural networks. Artif Intell Med 5(6):469.

Ciesielski V (ed). 1978. Proceedings of the Fourth Annual AIM Workshop, Rutgers University Technical Report.

Clancey WJ. 1979. Tutoring rules for guding a case method dialogue. Int J Man-Machine Studies 11:25.

Clancey WJ, Letsinger R. 1981. NEOMYCIN: Reconfiguring a rule-based expert system for application to teaching. In Proc 7th Int Joint Conf Artif Intel, pp 829–836.

Clancey WJ. 1989. The knowledge level reinterpreted: Modeling how systems interact. Machine Learning 4:285.

Clarke K, O'Moore R, Smeets R, et al. 1994. A methodology for evaluation of knowledge-based systems in medicine. Artif Intell Med 6(2):107.

Console L, Torasso P. 1991. On the co-operation between abductive and temporal reasoning in medical diagnosis. Artif Intell Med 3(6):291.

Cooper G. 1993. Probabilistic and decision-theoretic systems in medicine. Artif Intell Med 5(4):289.

Cousins SB, Chen W, Frisse ME. 1993. A tutorial introduction to stochastic simulation algorithms for belief networks. Artif Intell Med 5(4):315.

Cowell RG, Dawid AP, Hutchinson T, Spiegelhalter DJ. 1991. A bayesian expert system for the analysis of an adverse drug reaction. Artif Intell Med 3(5):257.

Davis R. 1979. Interactive transfer of expertise: Acquisition of new inference rules. Artif Intell 12:121.

DeMelo AS, Gramer J, Bronzino JD. 1992. SPINEX: An expert system to recommend the safe dosage of spinal anesthesia. In Proceedings of the 14th Annual Int Conf of the IEEE Eng in Med and Biol Soc, pp 902–903. Paris, France.

Duda RO, Hart PE, Nilsson NJ. 1976. Subjective bayesian methods for rule-based inference systems. In Proc Natl Comput Conf, New York.

Elstein AS, Shulman LS, Sprafka SA. 1978. Medical Problem Solving: An Analysis of Clinical Reasoning. Cambridge, Mass, Harvard University Press.

Englemore RS, Terry A. 1979. Structure and function of the Crysalis system. In Proceedings Sixth Int Joint Conf on Artif Intell, pp 250–256.

Fagan LM, Kunz JC, Feigenbaum EA, Osborn JJ. 1979. Representation of dynamic clinical knowledge: Measurement interpretation in the intensive care unit. In Proc 6th Int Joint Conf Artif Intell, pp 250–256.

Farr BR, Shachter RD. 1992. Representation of preferences in decision-support systems. Comput Biomed Res 25(4):324.

Feigenbaum EA. 1978. The art of artificial intelligence: Themes and case studies of knowledge engineering. In Proc Natl Comput Conf, p 221. New York.

Fieschi M, Joubert M, Fieschi D, et al. 1983. A production rule expert system for medical consultations. Medinfo 83:503.

Forsstrom J, Eklund P, Virtanen H, et al. 1991a. DIAGAID: A connectionist approach to determine the diagnostic value of clinical data. Artif Intell Med 3(4):193.

Forsstrom J, Nuutila P, Irjala K. 1991b. Using the ID3 algorithm to find discrepant diagnoses from laboratory databases of thyroid patients. Med Decision Making 11(3):171.

Fox J, Glowinski A, Gordon C, et al. 1990. Logic engineering for knowledge engineering: Design and implementation of the Oxford system of medicine. Artif Intell Med 2(6):323.

Freiher G. 1979. The seeds of artificial intelligence: SUMEX-AIM. In Div Res Res, pp 80–2071. NIH.

Gelfand IM, Rosenfeld BI, Shifrin A. 1987. Data Structuring in Medical Problems. Moscow, USSR Academy of Sciences.

Gelfand IM. 1989. Two archetypes in the psychology of man. Kyoto Prize Lecture.

Ginsberg A, Weiss SM, Polikakis P. 1985. Seek-2: A generalized approach to automatic knowledge base refinement. In Proc 9th Int Joint Conf Artif Intell.

Ginsberg A. 1986. A metalinguistic approach to the construction of knowledge base refinement systems. Proc AAAI 86:436.

Gong L, Kulikowski CA. 1992. Knowledge-based experimental design for planning biomedical image analysis. Medinfo 628.

Gordon J, Shortliffe EH. 1985. The Dempster-Shaffer theory of evidence in rule based expert systems. In BG Buchanan, EH Shortliffe (eds), Rule-Based Expert Systems, pp 272–292. Reading, Mass, Addison Wesley.

Gorry GA. 1970. Modeling the diagnostic process. J Med Ed 45:293.

Gorry GA, Silverman H, Pauker SG. 1978. Capturing clinical expertise: A computer program that considers clinical responses to digitalis. Am J Med 64:452.

Hart PE, Duda RE. 1977. PROSPECTOR—A computer-based consultation system for mineral exploration. SRI Tech Rep 155.

Hayes-Roth F, Waterman D, Lenat D. 1983. Building Expert Systems. Reading, Mass, Addison-Wesley.

Hazen GB. 1992. Stochastic trees: A new technique for temporal medical decision modeling. Med Decision Making 12(3):163.

Heckerman DE, Shortliffe EH. 1992. From certainty factors to belief networks. Artif Intell Med 4(1):35.

Horn W, Buchstaller W, Trappl R. 1980. Knowledge structure definition for an expert system in primary medical care. In Proceedings of the Seventh International Joint Conference on Artificial Intelligence, pp 850–852.

Hudson DL, Cohen ME, Anderson MF. 1991. Use of neural network techniques in a medical expert system. Int J Intell Syst 6:213.

Hunter J, Kirby I. 1991. Using quantitative and qualitative constraints in models of cardiac electrophysiology. Artif Intell Med 3:41.

Jimison HB, Fagan LM, Shachter RD, Shortliffe EH. 1992. Patient-specific explanation in models of chronic disease. Artif Intell Med 4(3):191.

Kahn MG. 1991. Modeling time in medical decision-support programs. Med Decision Making 11(4):249.

Kahn MG, Fagan LM, Sheiner LB. 1989. Model-based interpretation of time-varying medical data. In Proc Thirteenth Annual Symp on Computer Applications in Medical Care, pp 28–32. Washington, IEEE Computer Society Press.

Kassirer JP. 1994. A report card on computer-assisted diagnosis—The grade: C. N Engl J Med 330(25):1824.

Kassirer JP, Gorry GA. 1978. Clinical problem solving: A behavioral analysis. Ann Intern Med 89:245.

Kastner JK, Dawson CR, Weiss SM, et al. 1984. An expert consultation system for frontline health workers in primary eye care. J Med Syst 8:389.

Kim JH, Pearl J. 1987. CONVINCE: A conversational inference consolidation engine. IEEE Trans Syst Man Cybernet et al. 17:120.

Kingsland L, Sharp G, Capps R, et al. 1983. Testing of a criteria-based consultant system in rheumatology. Medinfo 514.

Kleinmuntz B, McLean RS. 1968. Diagnostic interviewing by digital computer. Behav Sci 13:75.

Kleinmuntz B. 1991. Computers as clinicians: An update. Comput Biol Med 22(4):227.

Koton PA. 1993. Combining causal models and case-based reasoning. In J-M David et al (eds), Second Generation Expert Systems, pp 69–78. Berlin, Springer-Verlag.

Krause P, Fox J, O'Neil M, Glowinski A. 1993. Can we formally specify a medical decision support system? IEEE Expert 8(3):56.

Kuipers BJ. 1985. The limits of qualitative simulation. In M Kaufmann (ed), Proc Ninth Int Joint Conf on Artif Intell, pp 128–136. Los Altos, Calif.

Kuipers BJ. 1987. Qualitative simulation as causal explanation. IEEE Trans Syst Man Cybernet 17:432.

Kulikowski CA, Weiss S. 1972. Strategies of data base utilization in sequential pattern recognition. Proc IEEE Conf Decision Control, 103.

Kulikowski CA. 1980. Artificial intelligence methods and systems for medical consultation. IEEE Trans Pat Anal Mach Intell (PAMI) 2(5):464.

Kulikowski CA, Ostroff J. 1980. Constructing an expert knowledge base for thyroid disease using generalized AI techniques. In Proc 4th Annual Symp Comp Health Care, pp 175–180.

Lau LM, Warner HR. 1992. Performance of a diagnostic system (lliad) as a tool for quality assurance. Comput Biomed Res 25(4):314.

Lehmann ED, Deutsch T, Carson ER, Sonksen PH. 1994. Combining rule-based reasoning and mathematical modelling in diabetes care. Artif Intell Med 6(2):137.

Lehmann HP, Shortliffe EH. 1990. Thomas: Building bayesian statistical expert systems to aid in clinical decision making. In Proc 14th Symp Applic Med Care, pp 58–64. New York, IEEE Press.

Lichter P, Anderson D. 1977. Discussions on Glaucoma. New York, Grune and Stratton.

Lindberg DA. 1980. Computer based rheumatology consultant. Medinfo 80:1311.

Lindberg DA, Sharp GC, Kay DR, et al. 1983. The expert consultant as teacher. Moebius 3:30.

Littenberg B, Moses LE. 1993. Estimating diagnostic accuracy from multiple conflicting reports. Med Decision Making. 13(4):313.

Long WJ. 1987. The development and use of a causal model for reasoning about heart failure. In Proc 11th Symp Comp Applic Med Care, pp 30–36.

Long WJ. 1991. Flexible reasoning about patient management using multiple methods. Artif Intell Med 3:3.

Lucas PJF. 1993. The representation of medical reasoning models in resolution-based theorem provers. Artif Intell Med 5(5):395.

Mora FA, Passariello G, Carrault G, LePichon JP. 1993. Intelligent patient monitoring and management systems: A review. IEEE Eng Med Biol 12:23.

Midgette AS, Stukel TA, Littenberg B. 1993. A meta-analytic method for summarizing diagnostic test performances. Med Decision Making. 13(3):253.

Miller PL. 1983. Attending: Critiquing a physician's management plan. IEEE Trans Pat Anal Mach Intell (PAMI) 5:449.

Miller PL. 1986. The evaluation of artificial intelligence systems in medicine. Comput Meth Prog Biomed 22:5.

Miller RA, Pople HE, Myers JD. 1982. An experimental computer based diagnostic consultant for general internal medicine. N Engl J Med 307:468.

Miller RA. 1984. Internist-I/Caduceus: Problems facing expert consultant programs. Meth Inform Med 23:9.

Miller RA. 1994. Medical diagnostic decision support systems: Past, present, and future: A threaded bibliography and commentary. J Am Med Info Assoc 1(1):8.

Minsky N. 1975. A framework for representing knowledge. In P Winston (ed), The Psychology of Computer Vision. New York, McGraw-Hill.

Musen MA, Fagen LM, Combs DM, Shortliffe EH. 1986. Facilitating knowledge entry for an oncology therapy advisor using a model of the application area. Medinfo 46.

Neapolitan RE. 1993. Computing the confidence in a medical decision obtained from an influence diagram. Artif Intell Med 5(4):341.

Newell A. 1982. The knowledge level. Artif Intell 18:87.

Nii HP, Aiello N. 1979. AGE: A knowledge-based program for building knowledge-based programs. In Proc 6th Int Joint Conf Artif Intel, pp 645–655. Tokyo, Japan.

Nohr C. 1994. The evaluation of expert diagnostic systems—How to assess outcomes and quality parameters? Artif Intell Med 6(2):123.

Olesen KG, Andreassen S. 1993. Specification of models in large expert systems based on causal probabilistic networks. Artif Intell Med 5(3):269.

Patil, RS, Szolovitz, P, Schwartz WB. 1981. Causal understanding of patient illness in medical diagnosis. In Proc Seventh Int Joint Conf Artif Intell, pp 893–899.

Patil R. 1983. Role of causal relations in formulation and evaluation of corporate hypotheses. IEEE Med Comp.

Patil R. 1986. Review of causal reasoning in medical diagnosis. In Proc 10th SCAMC, pp 11–16.

Pauker SG, Gorry GA, Kassirer JP, Schwartz WB. 1976. Towards the simulation of clinical cognition: Taking a present illness by computer. Am J Med 60:981.

Pearl J. 1987. Probabilistic Reasoning in Intelligent Systems: Networks or Plausible Inference. San Mateo, Calif, Morgan Kaufmann.

Pedrycz W, Bortolan G, Degani R. 1991. Classification of electrocardiographic signals: A fuzzy pattern matching approach. Artif Intell Med 3(4):211.

Peng Y, Reggia JA. 1987. A probabilistic causal model for diagnostic problem solving: Integrating symbolic causal inference with numeric probabilistic inference. IEEE Trans Syst Man Cybernet 17:146.

Politakis P, Weiss SM. 1980. A system for empirical experimentation with expert knowledge. In Proc 15th HICCS, pp 675–683.

Politakis P, Weiss SM. 1984. Using empirical analysis to refine expert system knowledge bases. Artif Intell 22:23.

Pople HE. 1973. On the mechanization of abductive logic. In Proc Int Joint Conf Artif Intell, pp 147–152.

Pople H, Myers J, Miller R. 1975. DIALOG: A model of diagnostic logic for internal medicine. In Proc 4th Int Joint Conf Artif Intell, pp 848–855.

Pople H. 1977. The formation of composite hypotheses in diagnostic problem solving. In Proc 5th Int Joint Conf Artif Intell, pp 1030–1037.

Pople H. 1982. Heuristic methods for imposing structure on ill-structured problems: The structuring of medical diagnoses. In P Szolovits (ed), Artificial Intelligence in Medicine. Boulder, Westview Press.

Potthoff P, Rothemund M, Schwefel D, et al. 1988. Expert Systems in Medicine. Cambridge, England, Cambridge University Press.

Ramoni M, Stefanelli M, Magnani L, Barosi G. 1992. An epistemological framework for medical knowledge-based systems. IEEE Tran Sys Man Cybernet 22(6):1361.

Reggia JA, Pula TP, Price TR, Perricone BT. 1980. Towards an intelligent textbook of neurology. In Proceedings of the Fourth Annual Symposium on Computer Applications in Medical Care, pp 190–199. Washington.

Reggia JA, Nau DS, Wang PY. 1983. Diagnostic expert systems based on a set covering model. Int J Man-Machine Studies 19:437.

Rumelhart DE, McClelland JL. 1986. Parallel Distributed Processing: Explorations in the Microstructure of Cognition. Cambridge, Mass, MIT Press.

Rutledge GW, Thomsen GE, Farr BR, et al. 1993. The design and implementation of a ventilator-management advisor. Artif Intell Med 5(1):67.

Schecke TH, Rau G, Popp HJ, et al. 1991. A knowledge-based approach to intelligent alarms in anesthesia. IEEE Eng Med Biol 10:38.

Schwartz WB. 1970. Medicine and the computer: The promise and problems of change. N Engl J Med 283:1257.

Shachter RD. 1986. DAVID: Influence diagram processing system for the macintosh. In Proc Workshop on Uncertainty in Artificial Intelligence, AAAI, Philadelphia, Pa, pp 311–318.

Shapiro AR. 1977. The evaluation of clinical predictions: A method and initial application. N Engl J Med 296:1509.

Shortliffe EH, Axline SG, Buchanan BG, Cohen SN. 1974. An artificial intelligence program to advise physicians regarding antimicrobial therapy. Comput Biomed Res 6:544.

Shortliffe EH. 1976. Computer-Based Medical Consultation: MYCIN. New York, Elsevier.

Shortliffe EH, Scott AC, Bischoff MB, et al. 1981. An expert system for oncology protocol management. In Proc 7th Int Joint Conf Artif Intell, pp 876–881.

Sittig DF, Orr JA. 1992. A parallel implementation of the backward error propagation neural network training algorithm: Experiments in event identification. Comput Biomed Res 25(6):547.

Smith JW, Svirbely J, Evans C, et al. 1985. RED: A red-cell antibody identification expert module. J Med Syst 9(3):121.

Smith JW, Johnson TR. 1993. A stratified approach to specifying, designing, and building knowledge systems. IEEE Expert 8(3):15.

Sonnenberg FA, Hagerty CG, Kulikowski CA. 1994. An architecture for knowledge based construction of decision models. Med Decision Making. 13(30):27.

Speedie SM, Palumbo FB, Knapp DA, Beardsley R. 1981. Rule-based drug prescribing review: An operational system. In Proceedings of the Fifth Annual Symposium on Computer Applications in Medical Care, pp 598–602. Washington.

Summers R, Carson ER, Cramp DG. 1993. Ventilator management. IEEE Eng Med Biol 12:50.

Swartout WR. 1981. Explaining and justifying expert consulting programs. In Proc 7th Int Joint Conf Artif Intell, pp 815–822.

Swartout WR, Moore JD. 1993. Explanation in Second Generation Expert Systems. In J-M David et al (eds), Second Generation Expert Systems, pp 543–615. Berlin, Springer-Verlag.

Szolovits P, Pauker SG. 1978. Categorical and probabilistic reasoning in medical diagnosis. Artif Intell 11:115.

Uckun S, Dawant BM, Lindstrom DP. 1993. Model-based diagnosis in intensive care monitoring: The YAQ approach. Artif Intell Med 5(1)31.

VanBeek P. 1991. Temporal query processing with indefinite information. Artif Intell Med 3(6):325.

van Melle W. 1979. A domain independent production-rule system for consultation programs. In Proc 6th Int Joint Conf Artif Intell, pp 923–925, Tokyo, Japan.

Weiss SM. 1974. A system for model-based computer-aided diagnosis and therapy. Thesis, Rutgers University.

Weiss S, Kulikowski C, Amarel S, Safir A. 1978. A model-based method for computer-aided medical decision-making. Artif Intell 11:145.

Weiss S, Kulikowski C. 1979. EXPERT: A system for developing consultation models. In Proc 6th Int Joint Conf Artif Intell, pp 942–950. Tokyo, Japan.

Weiss SM, Kulikowski CA, Galen RS. 1983. Representing expertise in a computer program: The serum protein diagnostic program. J Clin Lab Automation 3:383.

Weiss SM, Kulikowski CA. 1984. A Practical Guide to Designing Expert Systems. Totowa, Rowman and Allenheld.

Weiss SM, Kulikowski CA. 1991. Computer Systems That Learn. San Mateo, Calif, Morgan Kaufmann.

Widman LE. 1992. A model-based approach to the diagnosis of the cardiac arrhythmias. Artif Intell Med 4(1):1.

Widmer G, Horn W, Nagele B. 1993. Automatic knowledge base refinement: Learning from examples and deep knowledge in rheumatology. Artif Intell Med 5(3):225.

Wielinga BJ, Schreiber AT, Breuker JA. 1992. KADS: A modelling approach to knowledge engineering. Knowledge Acquisition 4:5.

Willems JL, Abreu-Lima C, VanBemmel AP, et al. 1991. The diagnostic performance of computer programs for the interpretation of electrocardiograms. N Engl J Med 325:1767.

Yu VL, Buchanan BG, Shortliffe EH, et al. 1979. An evaluation of the performance of a computer-based consultant. Comput Progr Biomed 9:95.

184

Artificial Neural Networks: Definitions, Methods, Applications

Daniel A. Zahner
Rutgers University

Evangelia Micheli-
Tzanakou
Rutgers University

The potential of achieving a great deal of processing power by wiring together a large number of very simple and somewhat primitive devices has captured the imagination of scientists and engineers for many years. In recent years, the possibility of implementing such systems by means of electro-optical devices and in very large scale integrations has resulted in increased research activities.

Artificial neural networks (ANNs) or simply neural networks (NNs) are made of interconnected devices called *neurons* (also called *neurodes, nodes, neural units,* or simply *units*). Loosely inspired by the makeup of the nervous system, these interconnected devices look at patterns of data and learn to classify them. NNs have been used in a wide variety of signal-processing and pattern-recognition applications and have been applied successfully in such diverse fields as speech processing [1–4], handwritten character recognition [5–7], time-series prediction [8–9], data compression [10], feature extraction [11], and pattern recognition in general [12]. Their attractiveness lies in the relative simplicity with which the networks can be designed for a specific problem along with their ability to perform nonlinear data processing.

As the neuron is the building block of a brain, a neural unit is the building block of a neural network. Although the two are far from being the same, or from performing the same functions, they still possess similarities that are remarkably important. NNs consist of a large number of interconnected units that give them the ability to process information in a highly parallel way. The brain as well is a massively parallel machine, as it has been long recognized. As each of the 10^{11} neurons of the human brain integrates incoming information from all other neurons directly or indirectly connected to it, an artificial neuron sums all inputs to it and creates an output that is carrying information to other neurons. The connection from one neuron's dendrites or cell body to another neuron's processes is called a *synapse*. The strength by which two neurons are influencing each other is called a *synaptic weight*. In an NN, all neurons are connected to all other neurons by synaptic weights that can have seemingly arbitrary values, but in reality, these weights show the effect of a stimulus on the neural network and the ability or lack of it to recognize that stimulus.

In the biologic brain, two types of processes exist: static and dynamic. *Static* brain conditions are those which do not involve any memory processing, while *dynamic* processes involve memory processing and changes through time. Similarly, NNs can be distinguished into static and dynamic: the former being such that do not involve any previous memory and only depend on current inputs and the latter having memory and being able to be described by differential equations that express changes in the dynamics of the system through time.

All NNs have certain architectures, and all consist of several layers of neuronal arrangements. The most widely used architecture is that of the perceptron first described in 1958 by Rosenblatt [13]. In the sections that follow we will build on this architecture, but not necessarily on the original assumptions of Rosenblatt.

Since there are many names in the literature that express the same thing and usually create a lot of confusion for the reader, we will define the terms to be used and use them throughout the chapter. Terminology is a big concern for those involved in the field and for organizations such as IEEE. A standards committee has been formed to address issues such as nomenclature and paradigms. In this chapter, whenever possible, we will try to conform to the terms and definitions already in existence.

Some methods for training and testing of NNs will be described in detail, although many others will be left out due to lack of space, but references will be provided for the interested reader. A small number of applications will be given as examples, since many more are discussed in another chapter of this *Handbook* and it would be redundant to repeat them here.

184.1 Definitions

Neural nets (NNs) go by many other names, such as *connectionists models, neuromorphic systems,* and *parallel distributed systems,* as well as *artificial NNs* to distinguish them from the biologic ones. They contain many densely interconnected elements called *neurons* or *nodes,* which are nothing more than computational elements nonlinear in nature. A single node acts like an integrator of its weighted inputs. Once the result is found, it is passed to other nodes via connections that are called *synapses.* Each node is characterized by a parameter that is called *threshold* or *offset* and by the kind of nonlinearity through which the sum of all the inputs is passed. Typical nonlinearities are the hardlimiter, the ramp (threshold logic element), and the widely used sigmoid.

The simplest NN is the single-layer perceptron [13,14], and it is a simple net that can decide whether an input belongs to one of two possible classes. Figure 184.1 is a schematic representation of a perceptron the output of which is passed through a nonlinearity called an *activation function.* This activation function is of different types, the most popular being a sigmoidal logistic function.

Figure 184.2 is a schematic representation of some activation functions such as the hardlimiter (or step), the threshold logic (or ramp), a linear, and a sigmoid. The neuron of Fig. 184.1 receives

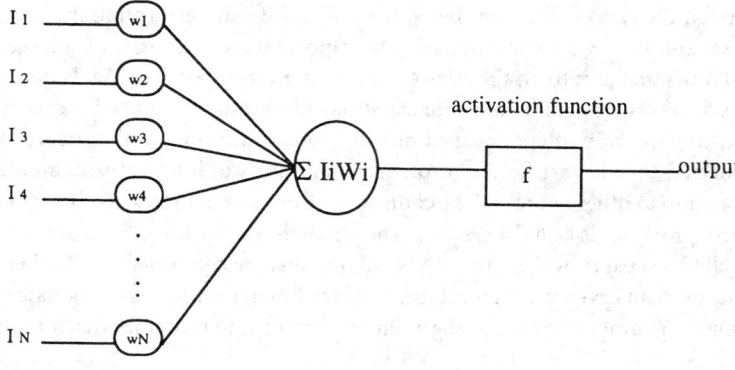

FIGURE 184.1 Artificial neuron.

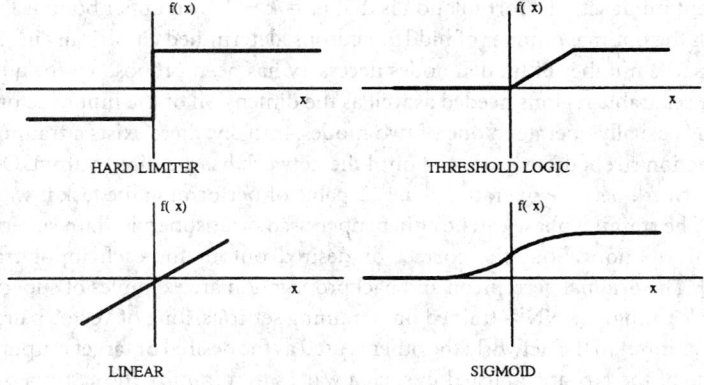

FIGURE 184.2   Typical activation functions.

many inputs I_i each weighted by a weight $W_i(i = 1, 2, \ldots, N)$. These inputs are then summed. The sum is then passed through the activation function f, and an output y is calculated only if a certain threshold is exceeded. Complex artificial neurons may include temporal dependencies and more complex mathematical operations than summation [15]. While each node has a simple function, their combined behavior becomes remarkably complex when organized in a highly parallel manner.

NNs are specified by their processing element characteristics, the network topology, and the training or learning rules they follow in order to adapt the weights W_i. Network topology falls into two broad classes: feedforward (nonrecursive) and feedback (recursive) [16]. Nonrecursive NNs offer the advantage of simplicity of implementation and analysis. For static mappings, a nonrecursive network is all one needs to specify any static condition. Adding feedback expands the network's range of behavior, since now its output depends on both the current input and network states. But one has to pay a price: longer times for teaching the NN to recognize its inputs.

Obviously, the NN of Fig. 184.1 is quite simple and inadequate in solving real problems. A multilayer perceptron (MLP) is the next choice. A number of inputs are now connected to a number of nodes at a second layer called the *hidden layer*. The outputs of the second layer may connect to a third layer and so on, until they connect to the output layer. In this representation, every input is connected to every node in the next layer, and the outputs of one hidden layer are connected to the nodes of the next hidden layer, and so on. Figure 184.3 depicts a three-layer feedforward network, the simplest MLP.

The optimal number of hidden neurons needed to perform arbitrary mapping is yet to be determined. Methods used in practice are mainly intuitive determination or are found by trial and error. Recent work has attempted to formulate bounds for the number of hidden nodes needed [17]. Mathematical derivation proves that a bound exists on the number of hidden nodes m needed to

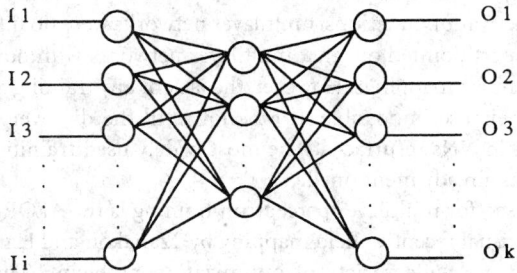

FIGURE 184.3   Three-layer feedforward network.

map a k-element input set. The formulation is that $m = k - 1$ is an upper bound. These results are consistent with the optimal number of hidden neurons, determined empirically in Kung et al. [18]. In other works, the number of hidden nodes necessary has been proposed to be a function of the number of the separable regions needed as well as the dimension of the input vector [19].

Artificial NNs usually operate in one of two modes. Initially, there exists a training phase where the interconnection strengths are adjusted until the network has a desired output. Only after training does the network become operational, i.e., capable of performing the task it was designed and trained to do. The training phase can be either supervised or unsupervised. In supervised learning, there exists information about the correct or desired output for each input training pattern presented [20]. The original perceptron and backpropagation are examples of supervised learning. In this type of learning, the NN is trained on a training set consisting of vector pairs. One of these vectors is used as input to the network; the other is used as the desired or target output. During training, the weights of the NN are adjusted in such a way as to minimize the error between the target and the computed output of the network. This process might take a large number of iterations to converge, especially because some training algorithms (such as backpropagation) might converge to local minima instead of the global one. If the training process is successful, the network is capable of performing the desired mapping.

In unsupervised learning, no a priori information exists, and training is based only on the properties of the patterns. Sometimes it is also called *self-organization* [20]. Training depends on statistical regularities that the network extracts from the training set and represents them as weight values. Applications of unsupervised learning have been limited. However, hybrid systems of unsupervised learning combined with other techniques produce useful results [21–23]. Unsupervised learning is highly dependent on the training data, and information about the proper classification is often lacking [21]. For this reason, most NN training is supervised.

184.2 Training Algorithms

After McCulloch and Pitts [24] demonstrated, in 1943, the computational power of neuron-like networks, much effort was given to developing networks that could learn. In 1949, Donald Hebb proposed the strengthening of connections between presynaptic and postsynaptic units when both were active simultaneously [25]. This idea of modifying the connection weights, as a method of learning, is present in most learning models used today. The next major advancement in neural networks was by Frank Rosenblatt [13,14]. In 1960, Widrow and Hoff proposed a model, called the *adaptive linear element* (ADALINE), which learns by modifying variable connection strengths, minimizing the square of the error in successive iterations [26]. This error-correction scheme is now known as the *least mean square (LMS) algorithm,* and it has found widespread use in digital signal processing.

There was great interest in NN computation until Minsky and Papert published a book in 1969 criticizing the perceptron. This book contained a mathematical analysis of perceptron-like networks, pointing out many of their limitations. It was shown that the single-layer perceptron was incapable of performing the XOR mapping. The single-layer perceptron was severely limited in its capabilities. For linear activation functions, multilayer networks were no different from single-layer models. Minsky and Papert pointed out that multilayer networks with nonlinear activation functions could perform complex mappings. However, the lack of any training algorithms for multiple-layer networks made their use impossible. It was not until the discovery of multilayer learning algorithms that interest in NNs resurfaced. The most widely used training algorithm is the *back-propagation algorithm,* as already mentioned.

Another algorithm used for multilayer perceptron training is the ALOPEX algorithm. ALOPEX was originally used for visual receptive field mapping by Tzanakou and Harth in 1973 [28–30] and has since been applied to a wide variety of optimization problems. These two algorithms are described in detail in the next subsections.

Backpropagation Algorithm

The backpropagation algorithm is a learning scheme where the error is backpropagated layer by layer and used to update the weights. The algorithm is a gradient-descent method that minimizes the error between the desired outputs and the actual outputs calculated by the MLP. Let

$$E_p = \frac{1}{2} \sum_{i=1}^{N} (T_i - Y_i)^2 \tag{184.1}$$

be the error associated with template p. N is the number of output neurons in the MLP, T_i is the target or desired output for neuron i, and Y_i is the output of neuron i calculated by the MLP. Let $E = \Sigma E_p$ be the total measure of error. The gradient-descent method updates an arbitrary weight w in the network by the following rule:

$$w(n + 1) = w(n) + \Delta w(n) \tag{184.2}$$

where

$$\Delta w(n) \propto - \eta \frac{\partial E}{\partial w(n)} \tag{184.3}$$

where n denotes the iteration number, and η is a scaling constant. Thus the gradient-descent method requires the calculation of the derivatives $\partial E/[\partial w(n)]$ for each weight w in the network. For an arbitrary hidden-layer neuron, its output H_j is a nonlinear function f of the weighted sum of all its inputs (net_j):

$$H_j = f(net_j) \tag{184.4}$$

where f is the activation function. The most commonly used activation function is the sigmoid function given by

$$f(x) = \frac{1}{1 + e^{-x}} \tag{184.5}$$

Using the chain rule, we can write

$$\frac{\partial E}{\partial w_{ij}} = \frac{\partial E}{\partial net_j} \frac{\partial net_j}{\partial w_{ij}} \tag{184.6}$$

and since

$$net_j = \sum_{j=1}^{n} w_{ij} I_i \tag{184.7}$$

we have

$$\frac{\partial net_j}{\partial w_{ij}} = I_i \tag{184.8}$$

and thus Eq. (184.6) becomes

$$\frac{\partial E}{\partial w_{ij}} = \frac{\partial E}{\partial net_j} I_i \tag{184.9}$$

$$\frac{\partial E}{\partial net_j} = \sum_{k=1}^{m} \frac{\partial E}{\partial net_k} \frac{\partial net_k}{\partial H_j} \frac{\partial H_j}{\partial net_j} \tag{184.10}$$

Recalling that

$$net_k = \sum_{j=1}^{n} w_{jk} H_j \tag{184.11}$$

it follows that

$$\frac{\partial net_k}{\partial H_j} = w_{jk} \tag{184.12}$$

Also,

$$\frac{\partial H_j}{\partial net_j} = f'(net_j) \tag{184.13}$$

Therefore,

$$\frac{\partial E}{\partial net_j} = f'(net_j) \sum_{k=1}^{n} \frac{\partial E}{\partial net_k} w_{jk} \tag{184.14}$$

Assuming f to be the sigmoid function of Eq. (184.5), then

$$f'(net_j) = Y_i(1 - Y_i) \tag{184.15}$$

Equation (184.14) gives the unique relation that allows the backpropagation of the error to all hidden layers. For the output layer,

$$\frac{\partial E}{\partial net_j} = \frac{\partial E}{\partial H_j} f'(net_j) \tag{184.16}$$

$$\frac{\partial E}{\partial H_j} = -(T_i - Y_i) \tag{184.17}$$

In summary, then, first, the output Y_i for all the neurons in the network is calculated. The error derivative needed for the gradient-descent update rule of Eq. (184.2) is calculated from

$$\frac{\partial E}{\partial w} = \frac{\partial E}{\partial net} \frac{\partial net}{\partial w} \tag{184.18}$$

If j is an output neuron, then

$$\frac{\partial E}{\partial net_j} = -(T_i - Y_i) Y_i (1 - Y_i) \tag{184.19}$$

If j is a hidden neuron, then the error derivative is backpropagated by using Eqs. (184.14) and (184.15). Substituting, we get

$$\frac{\partial E}{\partial net_j} = Y_i(1 - Y_i) \sum_{k=1}^{m} \frac{\partial E}{\partial net_k} w_{jk} \tag{184.20}$$

Finally, the weights are updated as in Eq. (184.2).

There are many modifications to the basic algorithm that have been proposed to speed the convergence of the system. *Convergence* is defined as a reduction in the overall error below a minimum threshold. It is the point at which the network is said to be fully trained. One method [31] used is the inclusion of a momentum term in the update equation such that

$$w(n + 1) = w(n) - \eta \frac{\partial E}{\partial w(n)} + \alpha \Delta w(n) \tag{184.21}$$

η is the learning rate and is taken to be 0.25. α is a constant momentum term that determines the effect of past weight changes on the direction of current weight movements.

Another approach used to speed the convergence of backpropagation is the introduction of random noise [32]. It has been shown that while inaccuracies resulting from digital quantization are detrimental to the algorithm's convergence, analog perturbations actually help improve convergence time.

One of these variations is the modification by Fahlman [33], called the *quickprop*, that uses second-derivative information without calculating the hessian needed in the straight backpropagation algorithm. It requires saving a copy of the previous gradient vector, as well as the previous weight change. Computation of the weight changes use only information associated with the weight being updated:

$$\Delta w = \frac{\nabla w_{ij}(n)}{\dfrac{\nabla w_{ij}(n-1) - \nabla w_{ij}(n)}{\Delta w_{ij}(n-1)}} \tag{184.22}$$

where $\nabla w_{ij}(n)$ is the gradient vector component associated with the weight w_{ij} at iteration n. This algorithm assumes that the error surface is parabolic, concave upward around the minimum, and that the slope change of the weight $\nabla w_{ij}(n)$ is independent of all other changes in weights. There are obviously problems with these assumptions, but Fahlman suggests a "maximum growth factor" μ in order to limit the rate of increase of the step size, namely, that if $\Delta w_{ij}(n) > \mu \Delta w_{ij}(n-1)$, then $\Delta w_{ij}(n) = \mu \Delta w_{ij}(n-1)$. Fahlman also used a hyperbolic arctangent function to the output error associated with each neuron in the output layer. This function is almost linear for small errors, but it blows up for large positive or large negative errors. Quickprop is an attempt to reduce the number of iterations needed by straight backpropagation, and it succeeded doing so by a factor of 5, but this factor is problem-dependent. This method also requires several trials before the parameters are set to acceptable values.

Backpropagation has achieved widespread use as a training algorithm for NNs. Its ability to train multilayer networks has lead to a resurgence of interest in the field. Backpropagation has been used successfully in applications such as adaptive control of dynamic systems and in many general NN applications. Dynamic systems require monitoring of time in ways that monitor the past. In fact, the biologic brain performs in an admirable way just because it has access to and uses values of different variables from previous instances. Backpropagation through time is another extension of the original algorithm proposed by Werbos in 1990 [34] and has been applied previously in the "truck backer-upper" by Nguyen and Widrow [35]. In this problem, a sequence of decisions must be made without an immediate indication of how effective these steps are. No indication of performance exists until the truck hits the wall. Backpropagation through time solves the problem, but it has its own inadequacies and performance difficulties. Despite its tremendous effect on NNs, the algorithm is not without its problems. Some of the problems have been discussed above. In addition, the complexity of the algorithm makes hardware implementations of it very difficult.

The ALOPEX Algorithm

The ALOPEX process is an optimization procedure that has been demonstrated successfully in a wide variety of applications. Originally developed for receptive field mapping in the visual pathway of frogs, ALOPEX's usefulness and flexible form have increased the scope of its applications to a wide range of optimization problems. Since its development by Tzanakou and Harth in 1973 [28], ALOPEX has been applied to real-time noise reduction [36], pattern recognition [37], adaptive control systems [38], and multilayer NN training, to name a few.

Optimization procedures, in general, attempt to maximize or minimize a function $F()$. The function $F()$ is called the *cost function,* and its value depends on many parameters or variables. When the number of parameters is large, finding the set $(x_1 \ x_2 \ \ldots \ x_N)$ that corresponds to the optimal (maximal or minimal) solution is exceedingly difficult. If N were small, then one could perform an exhaustive search of the entire parameter space in order to find the "best" solution. As N increases, intelligent algorithms are needed to quickly locate the solution. Only an exhaustive search can guarantee that a global optimum will be found; however, near-optimal solutions are acceptable because of the tremendous speed improvement over exhaustive search methods. ALOPEX iteratively updates all parameters simultaneously based on the cross-correlation of local changes ΔX_i and on the global response change ΔR, plus an additive noise. The cross-correlation term $\Delta X_i \Delta R$ helps the process move in a direction that improves the response. Table 184.1 shows how this can be used to find a global maximum of R.

All parameters X_i are changed simultaneously at each iteration according to

$$X_i(n) = X_i(n - 1) + \gamma \Delta X_i(n) \Delta R(n) + r_i(n) \tag{184.23}$$

The basic concept is that this cross-correlation provides a direction of movement for the next iteration. For example, take the case where $X_i\downarrow$ and $R\uparrow$. This means that the parameter X_i decreased in the previous iteration, and the response increased for that iteration. The product $\Delta X_i \Delta R$ is a negative number, and thus X_i would be decreased again in the next iteration. This makes perfect sense because a decrease in X_i produced a higher response; if you are looking for the global maximum, then X_i should be decreased again. Once X_i is decreased and R also decreases, then $\Delta X_i \Delta R$ is now positive, and X_i increases.

These movements are only tendencies, since the process includes a random component that will act to move the weights unpredictable, avoiding local extrema of the response. The stochastic element of the algorithm helps it to avoid local extrema at the expense of a slightly longer convergence or learning period.

The general ALOPEX updating equation (Eq. 184.23) is explained as follows: $X_i(n)$ are the parameters to be updated, n is the iteration number, and $R()$ is the cost function, of which the "best" solution in terms of X_i is sought. Gamma (γ) is a scaling constant, and $r_i(n)$ is a random number from a gaussian distribution whose mean and standard deviation are to find the "best" solution. As N increases, intelligent algorithms are needed to quickly locate the solution. Only an exhaustive search can guarantee that a global optimum is found; however, near-optimal solutions are acceptable because of the tremendous speed improvement over exhaustive search methods.

Backpropagation, described earlier, being a gradient-descent method, often gets stuck in local extrema of the cost function. The local stopping points often represent unsatisfactory convergence points. Techniques have been developed to avoid the problem of local extrema, with simulated annealing [39] being the most common. Simulated annealing incorporates random noise, which acts to dislodge the process from local extrema. Crucial to the convergence of the process is that the random noise be reduced as the system approaches the global optimum. If the noise is too large, the system will never converge and can be mistakenly dislodged from the global solution. ALOPEX is another process that incorporates a stochastic element to avoid local extremes in search of the global optimum of the cost function. The cost function or re-

TABLE 184.1

	ΔX		ΔR	$\Delta X \Delta R$
$X\uparrow$	+	$R\uparrow$	+	+
$X\uparrow$	+	$R\downarrow$	−	−
$X\downarrow$	−	$R\uparrow$	+	−
$X\downarrow$	−	$R\downarrow$	−	+

sponse is problem-dependent and is generally a function of a large number of parameters. ALOPEX iteratively updates all parameters simultaneously based varied, and $\Delta X_i(n)$ and $\Delta R(n)$ are found by

$$\Delta X_i(n) = X_i(n-1) - X_i(n-2) \qquad (184.24)$$

$$\Delta R(n) = R(n-1) - R(n-2) \qquad (184.25)$$

The calculation of $R()$ is problem-dependent and can be easily modified to fit many applications. This flexibility was demonstrated in the early studies of Harth and Tzanakou [29]. In mapping receptive fields, no a priori knowledge or assumptions were made about the calculation of the cost function; instead, a "response" was measured. By using action potentials as a measure of the response [28,29,40,41], receptive fields could be determined by using the ALOPEX process to iteratively modify the stimulus pattern until it produced the largest response.

It should be stated that due to its stochastic nature, efficient convergence depends on the proper control of both the additive noise and the gain factor γ. Initially, all parameters X_i are random, and the additive noise has a gaussian distribution with mean 0 and standard deviation σ initially large. The standard deviation σ decreases as the process converges to ensure a stable stopping point. Conversely, γ increases with iterations. As the process converges, ΔR becomes smaller and smaller, and an increase in γ is needed to compensate for this.

Additional constraints include a maximal change permitted for X_i for one iteration. This bounded step size prevents the algorithm from drastic changes from one iteration to the next. These drastic changes often lead to long periods of oscillation, during which the algorithm fails to converge.

Two-Dimensional Template Matching with ALOPEX

In this application, ALOPEX is used in template matching. A pattern is compared with a list of j templates, and for each template j, a response R_j is calculated. ALOPEX then iteratively modifies the initial pattern according to the global response calculation, local changes in the pattern, and an additive noise element. The updating equations are as described in the preceding subsection (Eqs. 184.23 to 184.25). An explanation of the response calculation used in template matching follows. $X_i(n)$ are the parameters to be optimized, and φ_{ij} are the stored templates; j is the number of the templates.

The response, in this case, is given by

$$R_j(n) = \sum_{i=1}^{N^2} X_i(n)\varphi_{ij} \qquad (184.26)$$

$$R(n) = CR'(n) \qquad (184.27)$$

where $$R'(n) = \text{Max}[R_j(n)] \qquad (184.28)$$

Other methods [40] of calculating $R'(n)$ include making it equal to a weighted sum of all the R_j:

$$R'(n) = \sum_{j=1}^{M} R_j(n)W_j(n) \qquad (184.29)$$

where $$W_j(n) = \frac{R_j(n)}{\sum\limits_{j=1}^{M} R_j(n)} \qquad (184.30)$$

The weighting of R_j by W_j and summing tends to slow the convergence of the algorithm, and hence Eq. (184.28) is used to select $R(n)$ from all $R_j(n)$.

Using the simple response calculation in Eq. (184.26) for a pixel-by-pixel multiplication between the pattern and template j, good results were obtained for binary (two-valued) images. The algorithm has certain constraints that dictate how it finds the maximum response. However, when multivalued templates were used, there was no longer proper convergence.

Using a response calculation based on pixel-by-pixel correlation is not suited for intermediate-valued optimization. In binary-valued optimization, the tendency to lump the maximum allowed luminance into a single pixel does not exist; therefore, the problem can go undetected. The basic problem is that in supervised learning the ideal image or solution should have maximal response, and for the example shown above, this was not the case.

To solve this problem, a new response calculation had to be implemented. Understanding the previous problem and goal of any optimal response calculation, a new function was used. The new response function given by

$$R_j(n) = \sum_{i=1}^{N^2} - (X_i - \varphi ij)^2 + \varphi ij \qquad (184.31)$$

defines a downward-facing parabola with its apex (or maximum) occurring only when $X = \varphi$. This is basically a least square error calculation that has been inverted so as to produce a maximum instead of a minimum. Also, the maximum contribution for each pixel is exactly φ; this is important because now the maximal response of $R_j(n)$ is simply equal to the total luminance. $R(n) = CR'(n)$ and $R'(n) = \text{Max}[R_j(n)]$ are the same as before. Using the new response calculation, much better convergence was achieved.

Multilayer Perceptron Network Training by ALOPEX

An MLP also can be trained for pattern recognition using ALOPEX. A response is calculated for the jth input pattern based on the observed and desired output

$$R_j(n) = \mathbf{O}_k^{des} - [\mathbf{O}_k^{obs}(n) - \mathbf{O}_k^{des}]^2 \qquad (184.32)$$

where $\mathbf{O}_k^{obs}$ and $\mathbf{O}_k^{des}$ are vectors corresponding to O_k for all k. The total response for iteration n is the sum of all the individual template responses $R_j(n)$:

$$R(n) = \sum_{j=1}^{m} R_j(n) \qquad (184.33)$$

In Eq. (184.33), m is the number of templates used as inputs. ALOPEX iteratively updates the weights using both the global response information and local weight histories, according to the following:

$$W_{ij}(n) = r_i(n) + \gamma \Delta W_{ij}(n)\Delta R(n) + W_{ij}(n - 1) \qquad (184.34)$$

$$W_{jk}(n) = r_i(n) + \gamma \Delta W_{jk}(n)\Delta R(n) + W_{ik}(n - 1) \qquad (184.35)$$

where γ is an arbitrary scaling factor, $r_i(n)$ is an additive gaussian noise, ΔW represents the local weight change, and ΔR represents the global response information. These values are calculated by

$$\Delta W_{ij}(n) = W_{ij}(n - 1) - W_{ij}(n - 2) \qquad (184.36)$$

$$\Delta W_{jk}(n) = W_{jk}(n - 1) - W_{jk}(n - 2) \qquad (184.37)$$

and

$$\Delta R(n) = R(n - 1) - R(n - 2) \qquad (184.38)$$

Besides its universality to a wide variety of optimization procedures, the nature of the ALOPEX algorithm makes it suitable for VLSI implementation. ALOPEX is a biologically influenced optimization procedure that uses a single-value global response feedback to guide weight movements toward their optimum. This single-value feedback, as opposed to the extensive error-propagation schemes of other NN training algorithms, makes ALOPEX suitable for fast VLSI implementation.

184.3 VLSI Applications of Neural Networks

Much debate exists as to whether digital or analog VLSI design is better suited for NN applications. In general, digital designs are an easier to implement and better-understood methodology. In digital designs, computational accuracy is only limited by the chosen word length. While analog VLSI circuits are less accurate, they are smaller, faster, and consume less power than digital circuits [42]. For these reasons, applications that do not require great computational accuracy are dominated by analog designs.

Learning algorithms, especially backpropagation, require high precision and accuracy in modifying the weights of the network. This has led some to believe that analog circuits are not well suited for implementing learning algorithms [43]. Analog circuits can achieve high precision, at the cost of increasing the circuit size. Analog circuits with high precision (8 bits) tend to be equally large as their digital counterpart [44]. Thus high-precision analog circuits lose their size advantage over digital circuits. Analog circuits are of greater interest in applications requiring only moderate precision.

Early studies show that analog circuits can realize learning algorithms, provided that the algorithm is tolerant to hardware imperfections such as low precision and inherent noise. In a paper by Macq et al. [45], a full analog implementation of a Kohonen map [20], one type of neural network, with on-chip learning is presented. With analog circuits having been shown capable of the computational accuracy necessary for weight modification, they should continue to be the choice of NN research.

Size, speed, and power consumption are areas where analog circuits are far superior to digital circuits, and it is these areas that constrain most NN applications. To achieve greater network performance, the size of the network must be increased. The ability to implement larger, faster networks is the major motivation for hardware implementation, and analog circuits are superior in these areas. Power consumption is also of major concern as networks become larger [46]. As the number of transistors per chip increases, power consumption becomes a major limitation. Analog circuits dissipate less power than digital circuits, thus permitting larger implementations.

One of the leaders in the field of analog VLSI neural systems is Carver Mead, who has presented a methodology for implementing biologically inspired networks in analog VLSI [47]. A silicon retina modeled after the biologic retina is constructed from simple analog circuits. These simple analog circuits function as building blocks and have been used in many other designs. Some of Mead's other work includes the design of a tracker [48], a sensorimotor integration system, capable of tracking a bright spot of light. An artificial cochlea for use in auditory localization also has been designed in analog VLSI [49].

Other methodologies of VLSI design of NNs include an analog/digital hybrid approach using pulse-stream networks. Pulse-stream encoding has been used in communication systems for many years and was first reported in the context of NNs by Murray and Smith in 1987 [50]. NN pulse-stream techniques attempt to combine the size and speed efficiency of analog circuits with the accuracy of digital circuits [51].

Recently, a digital VLSI approach to implementing the ALOPEX algorithm was undertaken by Pandya et al. [52]. Results of their study indicated that ALOPEX could be implemented using a single-instruction multiple-data (SIMD) architecture. A simulation of the design was carried out, in software, and good convergence for a 4×4 processor array was demonstrated.

In our laboratory, an analog VLSI chip has been designed to implement the ALOPEX algorithm by Zanher et al. [53]. By making full use of the algorithm's tolerance to noise, an analog design was chosen. As discussed earlier, analog designs offer larger and faster implementations than do digital designs.

184.4 Applications in Biomedical Engineering

Expert Systems and Neural Networks

Computer-based diagnosis is an increasingly used method that tries to improve the quality of health care. Systems that depend on artificial intelligence (AI), such as knowledge-based systems or expert systems, as well as hybrid systems, such as the above combined with other techniques, like NNs, are coming into play. Systems of this sort have been developed extensively in the last 10 years with the hope that medical diagnosis and therefore medical care would improve dramatically. Hatziglyger-oudis et al. [54] are developing such a system with three main components: a user interface, a database management system, and an expert system for the diagnosis of bone diseases. Each rule of the knowledge representation part is an ADALINE unit that has as inputs the conditions of the rule. Each condition is assigned a significance factor corresponding to the weight of the input to the Adaline unit, and each rule is assigned a number, called a *bias factor,* that corresponds to the weight of the bias input of the unit. The output is calculated as the weighted sum of the inputs filtered by a threshold function.

Hudson et al. [55] developed an NN for symbolic processing. The network has four layers. A separate decision function is used for layer three and a threshold for each node in the same layer. If the value of the decision function exceeds the corresponding threshold value, a certain symbol is produced. If the value of the decision function does not exceed the threshold, then a different symbol is produced. The so generated symbols of adjacent nodes are combined at layer four according to a well-structured grammar. A grammar provides the rules by which these symbols are combined [56]. The addition of a symbolic precessing layer enhances the NN in a number of ways. It is, for instance, possible to supplement a network that is purely diagnostic with a level that recommends further actions or to add additional connections or nodes in order to more closely simulate the nervous system.

With increasing network complexity, parameter variance increases, and the network prediction becomes less reliable. This difficulty can be overcome if some prior knowledge can be incorporated into the NN to bias it [57]. In medical applications in particular, rules can either be given by experts or can be extracted from existing solutions to the problem. In many cases the network is required to make reasonable predictions before it has gone through any sufficient training data, relying only on a priori knowledge. The better this knowledge is initially, the better is the performance and the shorter is the training [58,59].

Applications in Mammography

One of the leading causes of death of women in the United States is breast cancer. Mammography has been proved to be an effective diagnostic procedure for early detection of breast cancer. An important sign in its detection is the identification of microcalcifications of mammograms, expecially when they form clusters. Chan et al. [60] have developed a computer-aided diagnosis (CAD) scheme based on filtering and feature-extracting methods. In order to improve on the false-positive results, Zhang et al. [61] applied an artificial NN that is shift-invariant. They evaluated the performance of the NN by the "jack-knife" method [62] and receiver operating characteristic analysis [63,64]. A shift-invariant NN is a feedforward NN with local, spatially invariant interconnections similar to those of the neocognitron [65] but without the lateral interconnections. Backpropagation also was used for training for individual microcalcifications, and a cross-validation technique also was used in order to avoid overtraining. In this technique, the data set is divided into two sets, one used for training and the other for validating the predetermined intervals. The training of the network is terminated just before the performance of the network for the validating set decreases. The shift-invariant NN was proven to be much better in dropping the false-positive classifications by almost 55% over previously used NNs.

In another study, Zheng et al. [66] used a multistage NN for detection of mirocalcification clusters with almost 100% success and only one false-positive result per image. The multistate NN consists of more than one NN connected in series. The first stage is called the *detail network*, with inputs the pixel values of the original image, while the second network, the *feature network*, gets as inputs the output from the first stage and a set of features extracted from the original image. This approach has higher sensitivity of classification and a lower false-positive detection than the previous reports.

Another approach was used by Floyd et al. [67], where radiologists read the mammograms and come up with a list of eight findings, which were used as features for an NN. The results from biopsies were taken as the truth of diagnosis. For indeterminate cases, as classified by radiologists, the NN had a performance index of 0.86, which is quite high.

Downes [68] used similar techniques to identify stellate lesions. He used texture quantification via fractal-analysis methods instead of using the raw data. In mammograms, specific textures are usually indicative of malignancy. The method used for calculating the fractal dimension of digitized images was based on the relationship between the fractal dimension and the power spectral density.

Giger et al. [69] aligned the mammograms of left and right breasts and used a subtraction technique to find initial canditate masses. Various features were then extracted and used in conjunction with NNs in order to reduce false-positive assessments resulting from bilateral subtraction. Receiver operating characteristic (ROC) analysis was applied to evaluate the output of the NN. The methods used were evaluated using pathologically confirmed cases. This scheme yielded a sensitivity of 95% at an average of 2.5 false-positive detections per image.

Chromosome and Genetic Sequences Classification

Several clinical disorders are related to chromosome abnormalities that are difficult to identify accurately and also classify the individual chromosome. Automated systems can greatly help the human capabilities in dealing with some of the problems involved. One way to deal with this problem is the use of NNs. Several studies have already been done toward enhancing the ability of an automated computerized system to analyze chromosome identification [70]. One such study by Sweeney and Musavi [71] analyzes the metaphase of chromosome spreads employing probablistic NNs (PNNs), which have been used as alternatives to various classification problems. First introduced by Specht [72,73], PNNs are combinations of a kernel-based estimator for estimation of probability densities and the Bayes rule for classification decision. The estimation with the highest value specifies the correct class. Thus training of PNNs means to find appropriate kernel functions, usually taken to be gaussian densities, and therefore, the problem is reduced to the selection of a scalar parameter, namely, the standard deviation, of the gaussian. A way to improve the accuracy of a PNN for chromosome classification is to use the knowledge that there can be a maximum of only two chromosomes assigned to each class. This knowledge can be easily incorporated into the NN. Similar or better results were obtained to the classic backpropagation-trained NN.

A hybrid symbolic/NN machine learning algorithm was introduced by Noordewier et al. [74] for the recognition of genetic sequences. The system uses a knowledge base of hierarchically structured rules to form an artificial NN in order to improve the knowledge base. They used this system in recognizing genes in DNA sequences. The learning curve of this system was compared with that of a randomly initialized, fully connected two-layer NN. The knowledge-based NN learned much faster than the other one, but the error of the randomly initialized NN was slightly lower (5.5% versus 6.4%). Methods also have been devised to investigate what the NN has learned by an automatic translation into symbolic rules of trained NN initialized by the knowledge-based method [75].

Medial axis transform (MAT)–based features as inputs to an NN have been used in studying human chromosome classification [76]. Prenatal analysis, genetic syndrome diagnosis, and others make this research very important. Human chromosome classification based on NN requires no a priori knowledge or even assumptions on the data. MAT is a widely used method for transformations of elongated objects and requires less storage and time while preserving the topologic properties of the object. MAT also allows for a transformation from a 2D image to a 1D representation of it. The so obtained features are then fed as inputs to a two-layer feedforward NN trained by backpropagation, with almost perfect results in classifying chromosomes. An optimization on an MLP also was done [77].

References

1. Mueller P, Lazzaro J. 1986. Real time speech recognition. In J Dember (ed), Neural Networks for Computing. New York, American Institute of Physics.

2. Bourland H, Morgan N. 1990. A continuous speech recognition system embedding a Multi-Layer Perceptron into HMM. In D Touretzky (ed), Advances in Neural Information Processing Systems 2, pp 186–193. San Mateo, Calif, Morgan Kauffman.

3. Bridle JS, Cox SJ. 1991. RecNorm: Simultaneous normalization and classification applied to speech recognition. In RP Lippman et al (eds), Advances in Neural Information Processing Systems 3, pp 234–240.

4. Lee S, Lippman RP. 1990. Practical characteristics of neural networks and conventional classifiers on artificial speech problems. In DS Touretzky (ed), Advances in Neural Information Processing Systems 2, pp 168–177. San Matea, Calif, Morgan Kauffmann.

5. Fukushima K. 1983. Neocognition: A neural network model for a mechanism of visual pattern recognition. IEEE Trans Syst Man Cybernet SMC-13(5):826.

6. Dasey TJ, Micheli-Tzanakou E 1994. An unsupervised system for the classification of hand-written digits, comparison with backpropagation training. IEEE Trans Neural Networks (submitted).

7. LeCun Y, Boser B, Denker JS, et al. 1989. Backpropagation applied to handwritten ZIP code recognition. Neural Comp 1(4):541.

8. Hakim N, Kaufman JJ, Cerf G, Medows HE. 1990. A discrete time neural network model for system identification. Proc of IJCNN 90 (V3):593.

9. Hesh D, Abdallah C, Horne B. 1991. Recursive neural networks for signal processing and control. In Proceedings of the First IEEE-SP Workshop on Neural Networks for Signal Processing, Princeton, NJ, pp 523–532.

10. Cottrell GW, Munro PN, Zipser D. 1989. Image compression by backpropagation: A demonstration of extensional programming. In Advances in Cognitive Science, vol 2. Norwood, NY, Ablex.

11. Oja E, Lampinen J. 1994. Unsupervised learning for feature extraction. In JM Zurada et al (eds), Computational Intelligence Imitating Life. New York, IEEE Press.

12. Fogelman Soulie F. 1994. Integrating neural networks for real world applications. In JM Zurada et al (eds), Computational Intelligence Imitating Life. New York, IEEE Press.

13. Rosenblatt F. 1958. The perceptron: A probabilistic model for information storage and organization in the brain. Psychol Rev 65:386.

14. Rosenblatt F. 1962. Principles of Neurodynamics. New York, Spartan Books.

15. Lippman, RP. 1987. An introduction to computing with neural nets. IEEE ASSP Mag 4–22.

16. Moore K. 1992. Artificial neural networks: Weighing the different ways to systemize thinking. IEEE Potentials 23.

17. Huang S, Huang Y. 1991. Bounds on the number of hidden neurons in multilayer perceptrons. IEEE Trans Neural Networks 2(1):47.

18. Kung SY, Hwang J, Sun S. 1988. Efficient modeling for multilayer feedforward neural nets. Proc IEEE Conf Acoustics, Speech Signal Processing, New York, pp 2160–2163.

19. Mirchandani G. 1989. On hidden nodes for neural nets. IEEE Trans Circuits Syst 36(5):661.

20. Kohonen T. 1988. Self-Organization and Associative Memory. New York, Springer-Verlag.

21. Hecht-Nielsen R. 1987. Counterbackpropagation networks. In Proc of the IEEE First International Conf on Neural Networks, vol 2, pp 19–32.

22. Dasey TJ, Micheli-Tzanakou E. 1992. The unsupervised alternative to pattern recognition: I. Classification of handwritten digit. In Proc 3rd Workshop on Neural Networks, Auburn, Ala, pp 228–233.

23. Dasey TJ, and Micheli-Tzanakou E. 1992. The unsupervised alternative to pattern recognition: II. Detection of multiple sclerosis with the visual evoked potential. In Proc 3rd Workshop on Neural Networks, Auburn, Ala, pp 234–239.

24. McCulloch WC, Pitts W. 1943. A logical calculus of the ideas immanent in nervous activity. Bull Math Biophys 5:115.

25. Hebb D. 1949. The Organization of Behavior. New York, Wiley.

26. Widrow B, Lehr MA. 1990. 30 years of adaptive neural networks: Perceptron, Madaline, and backpropagation. Proc IEEE 78(9):1415.

27. Minsky M, Papert S. 1969. Perceptrons: An Introduction to Computational Geometry. Cambridge, Mass, MIT Press.

28. Tzanakou E, Harth E. 1973. Determination of visual receptive fields by stochastic methods. Biophys J 15:(42a).

29. Harth E, Tzanakou E. 1974. Alopex: A stochastic method for determining visual receptive fields. Vis Res 14:1475.

30. Tzanakou E, Michalak R, Harth E. 1979. The ALOPEX process: Visual receptive fields by response feedback. Biol Cybernet 35:161.

31. Rumelhart DE, McClelland JL (eds). 1986. Parallel Distributed Processing Cambridge, Mass, MIT Press.

32. Holstrom L, Koistinen P. 1992. Using additive noise in backpropoagation training. IEEE Trans Neural Networks 3(1):24.

33. Fahlmann SE. 1988. Faster learning variations of backpropagation: An empirical study. In D Tonretzky et al (eds), Proc of the the Connectionist Models Summer School. San Mateo, Calif, Morgan Kaufmann.

34. Werbos PJ. 1990. Backpropagation through time: What it does and how to do it. Proc IEEE 78(30):1550.

35. Nguyen D, Widrow B. 1989. The truck backer-upper: An example of self-learning in neural networks. In Proc of the Int Joint Conf Neural Networks, vol II, pp 357–361. New York, IEEE Press.

36. Ciaccio E, Tzanakou E. 1990. The ALOPEX process: Application to real-time reduction of motion artifact. Annu Int Conf IEEE EMBS 12(3):1417.

37. Dasey TJ, Micheli-Tzanakou E. 1990. A pattern recognition application of the Alopex process with hexagonal arrays. In Int Joint Conf Neural Networks, vol II, pp 119–125.

38. Venugopal K, Pandya A, Sudhakar R. 1992. ALOPEX algorithm for adaptive control of dynamical systems. Proc IJCNN 2:875.

39. Kirkpatrick S, Gelatt CD, Vecchi MP. 1983. Optimization by simulated annealing. Science 220:671.

40. Micheli-Tzanakou E. 1984. Non-linear characteristics in the frog's visual system. Biol Cybernet 51:53.

41. Micheli-Tzanakou E. 1983. Visual receptive fields and clustering. Behav Res Methods Instrum 15(6):553.

42. Mead C, Ismail (eds). 1991. Analog VLSI Implementation of Neural Systems. Boston, Kluwer Academic Publishers.

43. Ramacher and Ruckert (eds). 1991. VLSI Design of Neural Networks. Boston, Kluwer Academic Publishers.

44. Graf HP, Jackel LD. 1989. Analog electronic neural network circuits. IEEE Circuits Devices Mag 44.

45. Macq D, Verlcysen M, Jespers P, Legat J. 1993. Analog implementation of a Kohonen map with on-chip learning. IEEE Trans Neural Networks 4(3):456.

46. Andreou A, et al. 1991. VLSI neural systems. IEEE Trans Neural Networks 2(2):205.

47. Mead C. 1989. Analog VLSI and Neural Systems. Reading, Mass, Addison-Wesley.

48. Maher M, Deweerth S, Mahowald M, Mead C. 1989. Implementing neural architectures using analog VLSI circuits and systems. 36(5):643.

49. Lazzaro J, Mead C. 1989. Silicon models of auditory localization. Neural Comput 1(1):1.

50. Murray AF, Smith A. 1987. Asynchronous arithmetic for VLSI neural systems. Electron Lett 23(12):642.

51. Murray AF, Corso D, Tarassenko L. 1991. Pulse-stream VLSI neural networks mixing analog and digital techniques. IEEE Trans Neural Networks 2(2):193.

52. Pandya AS, Shandar R, Freytag L. 1990. An SIMD architecture for the Alopex neural networks. SPIE Parallel Architectures for Image Processing 1246:275.

53. Zahner AD. 1994. Design and implementation of an analog VLSI, adaptive algorithm with applications in neural networks, Master's thesis, Rutgers University.

54. Hatziglygeroudis I, Vassilakos PJ, Tsakalidis A. 1994. An intelligent medical system for diagnosis of bone diseases. In Proc of the Int Conf on Med Physics and Biomed Eng., Cyprus, vol 1, pp 148–152.

55. Hudson DL, Cohen ME, Deedwania PC. 1993. A neural network for symbolic processing. In Proc of the 15th Annual Int Conf of the IEEE/EMBS, vol 1, pp 248–249.

56. Hoperoft JE, Ullman JD. 1969. Formal Languages and Their Relation to Automata. Reading Mass, Addison-Wesley.

57. Roscheisen M, Hofmann R, Tresp V. 1992. Neural control for running mills: Incorporating domain theories to overcome data deficiency. In Advances in Neural Information Processing Systems 4.

58. Towell GG, Shavlik JW, Noordemier MO. 1990. Refinement of approximately correct domain theories by knowledge-based neural networks. In Proc of the 8th National Conf Artif Intell, pp 861–866.

59. Tresp V, Hollatz J, Ahmad S. 1994. Network structuring and training using rule-based knowledge. In Advances in Neural Information Processing Systems 5, pp 871–878.

60. Chan H-P, Doi K, Vyborny CJ, et al. 1990. Improvement in radiologists' detection of clustered microcalcifications on mammograms: The potential of computer aided diagnosis. Invest Radiol 25:1102.

61. Zhang W, Giger ML, Nishihara RM, Doi K. 1994. Application of a shift-invariant artificial neural network for detection of breast carcinoma in digital mammograms. In Proc of the World Congress on Neural Networks, vol I, pp 45–52.

62. Fukunaga K. 1990. Introduction to Statistical Pattern Recognition, 2nd ed. New York, Academic Press.

63. Metz CE. 1988. Current problems in ROC analysis. In Proc Chest Imaging Conf Madison Wisc, pp 315–336.

64. Metz CE. 1989. Some practical issues of experimental design and data analysis in radiological ROC studies. Invest Radiol 24:234.

65. Fukushima K, Miyake S, Ito T. 1983. Neocognitron: A neural network model for a mechanism of visual pattern recognition. IEEE Trans Syst Man Cybernet SMC-13:826.

66. Zheng B, Qian W, Clarke LP. 1994. Artificial neural network for pattern recognition in mammography. In Proc of the World Congress on Neural Networks, vol. I, pp 57–62.

67. Floyd CE Jr, Yun AJ, Lo JY, et al. 1994. Prediction of breast cancer malignancy for difficult cases using an artificial neural network. In Proc of the World Congress on Neural Networks, vol I, pp 127–132.

68. Downes P. 1994. Neural network recognition of multiple mammographic lesions. In Proc of the World Congress on Neural Networks, vol I, pp 133–136.

69. Giger ML, Lu P, Huo Z, Zhang W. 1994. Application of artificial neural networks to the task of merging feature data in computer-aided diagnosis schemes. In Proc of the World Congress on Neural Networks, vol I, pp 43–46.

70. Piper J, Granunn E, Rutovitz D, Ruttledge H. 1990. Automation of chromosome analysis. Sig Proc 2(3):109.

71. Sweeney WP Jr, Musavi MT. 1994. Application of neural networks for chromosome classification. In Proc of the 15th Annual Int Conf of the IEEE/EMBS, vol 1, pp 239–240.

72. Specht DF. 1988. Probabilistic neural networks for classification mapping or associative memory. In Proc of the IEEE Int Conf on Neural Networks, vol 1, pp 525–532. New York, IEEE Press.

73. Specht DF. 1990. Probabilistic neural networks. 3(1):109.

74. Noordewier MO, Towell GG, Shavlik JW. 1993. Training knowledge-based neural networks to recognize genes in DNA sequences. Adv Neural Info Proc Sys 3:530.

75. Towell GG, Graven M, Shavlik JW. 1991. Automated interpretation of knowledge-based neural networks. Tech rep Univ of Wisc Computer Sci Dept, Madison, Wisc.

76. Lerner B, Rosenberg B, Levistein M, et al. 1994. Medical axis transform based features and a neural network of human chromosome classification. In Proc of the World Congress on Neural Networks, vol 3, pp 173–178.

77. Lerner B, Guterman H, Dinstein J, Romem Y. 1994. Learning curves and optimization of a multilayer perceptron neural network for chromosome classification. In Proc of the World Congress on Neural Networks, vol 3, pp 248–253.

185

Clinical Decision
Systems

Pirkko Nykänen
VTT Information Technology

Niilo Saranummi
VTT Information Technology

Clinical decision systems are cognitive tools, computer-based systems that are planned to support and aid medical professionals in clinical decision-making tasks. These tools are planned to enhance the performance of the clinical team; they are instruments for the users, not protheses that replace or substitute missing human abilities or cognitive skills.

The value of clinical decision systems in medicine depends on their envisioned role or contribution to the patient care process. The role of a clinical decision system may be to work as a reference material or as a watch-dog to screen routines or detect deviations; they may remind the user of extreme possibilities or forecast outcomes of different alternatives. Additionally, they may produce information from data by interpretation, work as a tutoring or guidance system for the user, and represent a more experienced consultant for an unexperienced user.

185.1 Clinical Decision Making

Health care is based on a complex interdisciplinary medical science that comprises both pure natural science, technological and clinical research, and aspects of social science and humanities. These different theories and methods are modified and focused by the common goal to understand, treat, and prevent human disease. To understand medical research and knowledge, it is necessary to have this complex structure in mind. The huge system of medical knowledge, theories, and methods is focused around a common perception of human disease and clinical practice.

In medical practice, a clinician is involved in an extremely complex cognitive task where he or she applies different kinds of knowledge on several cognitive and epistemic levels. Therefore, it is necessary for a clinician to develop, on a basic natural-science level, an understanding of fundamental physiologic and pathologic processes, to develop diagnostic methods and procedures, and to investigate the effects of drugs and new treatments on real clinical cases. The clinician must have a precise representation of the clinical state of the patient and of the relevant physiologic processes going on in the patient. He or she must have a clear understanding of the purpose of his or her activity and the system of possible actions he or she is able to initiate.

Representations of these cognitive structures are based on clinical and paraclinical observations, case records, and other kinds of available empirical data (e.g., information related to hospital procedures and possibilities). All these observations constitute the empirical foundations of the representation of the patient, but they would not make much sense without a comprehensive theoretical interpretation. It is through deep theoretical processing of the data that the clinician is able to understand the state of the patient [Pedersen et al., 1993].

The role of theoretical representations has been verified experimentally by several studies. It is especially well documented in studies of differences between novices and experts. For instance, Groen and Patel [1988] have shown that when interpreting a case, experts make more inferences than novices. Inferences serve two purposes. On the one hand, they are used to distinguish between relevant and irrelevant observations. In principle, it is possible to acquire an infinite amount of information from a concrete case. Theoretical frameworks are used as a device to delimit data to a manageable and relevant set. On the other hand, inferences are made with the purpose of retaining the meaning of the data, which in many cases would be incomprehensible or even inconsistent if only interpreted on a surface level. This fact that theoretical inferences are used to filter data has been documented in many different domains, e.g., in physics, engineering, and medicine. It is true for many different kinds of cognitive tasks, especially for diagnosis and scientific work.

The central goal of medical research is to improve clinical practice. This can be achieved in many different ways. The focus may be on improving the theoretical understanding of the physiologic and pathologic processes on a high level of abstraction, on concentrating in the study of diagnostic methods, on evaluating new therapies, on developing preventive measures, etc.

A medical decision maker acquires and manages several different forms of knowledge. In some situations, he or she develops a dynamic model of the phenomena he or she is studying; in other situations causal graphs and goal structures are represented in his or her mind. These representations are only meaningful when seen on the background of deeper biomedical knowledge which has its own characteristic forms. It is part of scientific expertise to be able to develop and select exactly that kind of representation that is most relevant in a given situation. That is, an expert has available a certain amount of knowledge of these characteristic kinds, and he or she is trained in such a way that he or she is able to select or develop the most appropriate representation in a given situation. These representations constitute the basis of both scientific reasoning and selection of data-reduction methods [Pedersen et al., 1993].

185.2 Clinical Decision Systems History

The first approaches to provide computer support for medical decision making were based on bayesian statistics. Programs for diagnostic problems showed that impressive diagnostic accuracy could be achieved if the computer programs were supported by reliable data [Shortliffe, 1988]. However, the demand of independence between variables in these approaches was found to be too restrictive in medicine, and a lot of problems were related to the accessibility of reliable data. It also was noticed that to be able to tackle the information problem in medicine and health care, simultaneous perspectives from other information sciences—decision theory, linguistics, mathematical modeling, and cognitive psychology—are needed [Gremy, 1988].

Research with artificial intelligence (AI) in medicine started on 1960s based on the understanding that when computer systems are used to emulate medical decision-making steps, they need relevant medical knowledge, and this knowledge has to be represented in a context-sensitive way. Much of this knowledge must be extracted from experts in the field; the statistical data approach is not enough. The symbolic reasoning methods of AI are needed. The early work resulted in medical software called *knowledge-based systems*, like MYCIN [Shortliffe, 1976], INTERNIST [Miller et al., 1982], PIP [Pauker et al., 1976], and CASNET [Weiss et al., 1978].

The focus of this early work was in the development of methodologies and tools to support modeling of a domain, knowledge acquisition including machine learning approaches, modeling of reasoning strategies, and knowledge representations. Interests in reasoning strategies were focused on causal, temporal, heuristic, strategic, and anatomic reasoning and reasoning from multiple sources of knowledge. Issues of validation of knowledge and evaluation of prototype systems also were raised. The term *expert system* was introduced, and much of the research was focused on how to represent expert knowledge, how to acquire it, and how to use it in problem solving. Certainty factors and other heuristic scoring measures were developed to be able to manipulate probabilities and weights of evidence. Also, issues related to the users and environments of these systems were tackled: human computer interaction and interfaces to databases and database management systems, integration of natural language processing with knowledge-based systems, and integration of medical decision analysis with AI techniques [Buchanan and Shortliffe, 1984; Clancey and Shortliffe, 1984; Miller, 1988; Shortliffe et al., 1990].

In late 1980s, the big change originated from the rapid evolution both in hardware and software for AI. The expert system shells, which are tools to develop expert systems and where the inference engine is separated from the knowledge base, were introduced and got widespread use. Cheap and effective microcomputers as well as dedicated professional workstations for knowledge engineering offered powerful integrated and interactive environments of the development of expert systems. Microcomputers allow placement of the developed systems in the physician's office at an acceptable cost. The developments in computer graphics, graphic interfaces, and image processing also have supported the developments in AI applications.

The focus shifted to attempts to find general solutions to problems through modeling approaches. The final result of the development of a knowledge-based system was seen to be a model of expertise which in turn was implemented in the knowledge base. These models of expertise may incorporate assumptions about knowledge representations, knowledge base contents, problem-solving methods, and application tasks [Musen, 1989]. The knowledge-level modeling was widely recognized to be the major way to generalize and structure domain and task knowledge. The knowledge-level model describes the problem-solving process in terms of general abstract conceptualizations without reference to the implementations [Newell, 1982].

The term *expert system* is no longer widely used based on the understanding that the knowledge-based systems are seldom planned to replace human expertise and that the capabilities to develop systems that perform at the expert level are restricted. The role of these systems is to work as augmented devices; therefore, the term *clinical decision system* is closer to the function of these systems in clinical practice.

The major problems in developments have been how to go from the knowledge level to the knowledge-use level [Newell, 1982; Steels, 1990]. The possible frameworks to look at the developments at these levels are heuristic classification with the focus on the inference structures [Clancey, 1985], distinction between deep and shallow knowledge at the knowledge level [Keravnou and Washbrook, 1989; Chandrasekaran and Mittal, 1982], problem-solving method approach focusing on how the problem might be solved at the knowledge-use level [Bennet, 1985; Clancey, 1985], and finally, the generic task approach where the analysis of expertise is performed in terms of the tasks and ordering of the tasks [Chandrasekaran, 1986].

185.3 Clinical Application Areas

The first application areas were diagnosis and treatment planning. Diagnosis is often said to be the main task of the physician, and a lot of attempts have been made to model the diagnostic process. On the other hand, it has been suggested that the diagnostic process as a monolithic process does not exist. Each clinician has his or her own pathways to diagnosis, and these vary from clinician to clinician, from patient to patient, and depend on some external factors such as urgency of the situation, difficulty of the case, and the role that the physician assumes on each occasion [DeDombal, 1978]. Medical problem solving has been shown to include several features that cause difficulties in building general models. The essential features are that hypotheses are generated early and that they are considered in a decision-making situation in a limited number. The most common error in interpretation of signs and symptoms of illness is overinterpretation. The competence of the medical experts may be case-related, and the basic elements of competence are information and experience [Elstein et al., 1979]. From the process point of view, medical reasoning may be modeled by fundamental medical tasks, e.g., diagnosis, therapy planning, and monitoring. A clinical decision system requires formulation of an inference model (i.e., the reasoning process) that exploits an appropriate ontology (i.e., the medical process). An architecture, then, provides a conceptual description of these components at the knowledge and computational levels [Stefanelli, 1993].

The scope of current developments has broadened from diagnostic systems to systems addressing tasks such as treatment planning, monitoring, and follow-up of patients, diseases and treatments, especially in the domains of chronic diseases and intensive care. Applications today cover medical, managerial, administrative, and financial decisions in health care. Current clinical function areas of AI in medicine are summarized as follows [van Eimeren, 1989]: strategy and planning for total quality assurance, environmental surveillance, screening and prevention, population surveillance, disease prevention, patient diagnosis, patient treatment, patient follow-up, patient monitoring, patient rehabilitation, population and patient education, health professionals education and training, and health services management.

Most systems are still planned for highly specialized hospital environments; very rarely have problems of community care, primary care, or occupational health been touched. The scope of the development is primarily dependent on an understanding of the domain problem and the purpose and role of the system in clinical practice.

Medicine is a complex area for knowledge-based systems. The complexity arises from many sources. Medicine is not a formal science; it has an empirical basis. We have shallow or limited understanding of many of the disease processes as well as of medical decision making. The amount of knowledge that is relevant for decision-making situations is huge, even in restricted subspecialties of medicine [Miller, 1988]. The scientific foundations of clinical reasoning are apparently less developed than what was formerly believed. Medical expertise is developing through experience, and the difference between novices and experts is found on this basis [Musen, 1988; Dreyfus and Dreyfus, 1986]. Medical data and knowledge lack consistency and precision; they are soft, and there do not exist standards for coding, representation, and exchange of knowledge. The utilization of medical knowledge in clinical decision systems requires formalization of knowledge, i.e., standardized languages and terminologies [Rector et al., 1992].

185.4 Evaluation of Clinical Decision Systems Development

The evaluations of clinical decision systems performed and reported in the literature show that there does not exist a global, generally accepted methodology for evaluation. The reported results have been subjective, and evaluations have been performed without generally accepted objectives and standards.

In a study by Wyatt [1987], 14 medical decision support systems were evaluated according to a three-stage procedure where in stage 1, the main consideration, was the system's clinical role, stage 2 considered if the system had been tested with a proper sample with predefined goals for accuracy and utility, and stage 3 considered if the performance of the physician was tested when he or she was aided or not aided by the system. The result was that only three systems had the clinical role defined, seven systems had paper tests, and only one system had been subjected to a field test. Medical experts were used as the "gold standard"; in most cases, only one expert had been used. Of these 14 systems, only 2 have ever been used in practice. Another study [Lundsgaarde, 1987] comes to the same conclusion about the status of actual evaluations. Only about 10% of the medical decision support systems described over the 10 years have been tested in a laboratory environment. Also in a study of 64 medical decision support systems [Pothoff et al., 1988], the conclusion was that most of the systems were still in their developmental stage; only 8 systems were developed to a stage where they could enter routine clinical use. Some explanations for the status of the actual evaluations can be found in the following: Most systems have been developed to study and experiment with AI techniques and tools in medical domains, and the user requirements analysis as well as domain and task analyses before the development have been poor. No resources have usually been reserved for evaluation, and more important, the importance of evaluation has not been understood until quite recently. Also, evaluation methodologies are still lacking, as well as skills on how to apply them.

Most of the decision support systems are planned to work as supporting devices for clinicians, and thus they have to be integrated with the user's environment. Evaluation of the fitness of the system into the user's environment has been repeatedly neglected in actual evaluations. The only example on the effectiveness of the system in the user's environment concerns the SPHINX system [Botti et al., 1987, 1989]. The general practitioners were using the system for 6 months to get experience on how it fitted into their working environment. Though this system was used by the practitioners via the French MINITEL network, the legal issues were not considered in the studies. Data security should, however, be of particular importance for a system operating on a network [Clarke et al., 1994].

It has been suggested that evaluation of the system in the user environment should at least consider whether the system helps the user to improve the outcome of his or her work in the clinical setting, it is easy to use, and is cost-effective [Rossi-Mori et al., 1990]. In a clinical setting, it is also important to know how well the knowledge base is tuned to the local patient population and the specific disease panorama of the local area or country. The fact that medical data are soft and subject to variability and inaccuracy is well known.

185.5 Requirements and Critical Issues for Clinical Decision Systems Development

Clinical decision systems can be successful if they are planned to support human professionals in their clinical tasks. In most cases it is reasonable that the computer support does not cover the whole decision-making process but rather parts of it. For example, information enhancement is needed in many decision-making situations to be able to take the next decision step. Clinical decision support requires that reliable data and knowledge are available, preferably via the integrated information systems environment. The system must have access to all data needed. Representational issues, both semantic and syntactic, have to be solved in such a way that no misunderstandings or misinterpretations are met. We have to be conscious also of the system's brittleness, because the model implemented is always an abstraction and approximation of the reality.

The key for the successful development is the user-involvement approach. Knowledge acquisition is a bottleneck problem in the development of such systems. We need understanding on how medical expertise is achieved, how it is used in clinical situations, and how it can be captured and modeled. Modeling operations are activities where users should be involved, and the importance of the domain theory in validating these models during development has to be understood. Users need tools that enable them to analyze, structure, and visualize domain knowledge without a strong support by a knowledge engineer, i.e., tools that support modeling and reasoning strategies and system architectures for different tasks, domains, and environments [Brender et al., 1993].

The usability and utility of these systems in the health care environment are crucial; the systems must be acceptable to the users, and the needs of the users must be fulfilled. Explanation facilities are important for acceptability by users. These explanation facilities serve educational purposes, and through them, the basis of the system's output is made clear for the user. Mode of consultation also affects acceptability by users. For example, the critiquing approach seems to be an acceptable mode for users [Miller, 1982]. In this approach, the system does not give advice to the user but takes the user's proposal and discusses the pros and cons in relation to other possibilities.

A very important issue is the existence of an information processing and management infrastructure as well as computerized transactions and user culture for computer systems. Clinical decision systems need to be integrated with the health care data and information environment. The interfacing with hospital information systems and literature databases makes it possible to utilize all the existing data and information in decision making and data entry only once. The usability of integrated or embedded systems is better than that of stand-alone systems. There is evidently a need to plan and coordinate computing activities inside organizations, especially for networking and data and knowledge exchange management [Shortliffe, 1988].

A new discipline suggested for the development of clinical decision systems is the computer-supported cooperative work (CSCW) approach [Nykänen and Saranummi, 1992]. CSCW is defined as "the design of computer-based technologies with explicit concern for socially organized work practices of their intended users" [Suchmann, 1990]. CSCW tries to couple knowledge of the work situation and working practices with technological advances and to pay attention to human-computer interaction and computer-mediated communication issues [Bannon, 1986]. This approach seems promising because a medical decision maker is a member of a clinical team and this team has an organization, goals, and tasks defined in the health care process. Successful development requires analysis and definition of the tasks of team and team members, how different tasks contribute to the health care process, and finally, how these tasks can be supported with computer systems and programs.

Evaluation and validation have been recognized as necessary tasks to perform during development and before accepting the systems into use [Clarke et al., 1994]. Evaluation and validation are means to control the development and guarantee the quality of the results; thus they support development of good clinical practices. The users need guidance and support to perform evaluations, and the developer or the vendor of the system must provide the user with all the necessary material needed for evaluation [Nykänen, 1990]. Evaluation and validation lack comprehensive methodologies, standards, and guidelines still today. The impacts of these systems on patients, physicians, health care environment, organizations, quality of health care, and health care delivery should be analyzed. The cost-benefit analysis and effectiveness of these systems on health care problems need consideration. It is completely impossible today to foresee all the legal implications of the introduction of decision support systems into clinical practice. The general conclusion today has been that the use of these systems does not reduce the risk for producers or users [Kilian, 1988]. A general interpretation of the liability principle has been that decisions suggested or supported by a computer system are also ultimately the responsibility of the physician who puts them into effect.

185.6 Summary

The future of artificial intelligence in medicine is challenging, and the barriers for success are said to be logistical and related to institutional infrastructure [Shortliffe, 1988]. The use of clinical decision systems in routine is, however, expected to produce tremendous changes in today's health care systems. Some physicians and computer scientists anticipate that computers will change the role of physicians and affect the total structure, process, and outcome of medical care [Pothoff et al., 1988]. Many physicians have a fear that these systems will constrain the physician's options by eliminating the challenge of independent problem solving that has attracted many physicians to medical practice. However, an improved understanding of the role that patient-specific advice can play in helping physicians to reach good decisions, while still maintaining the ultimate authority in patient management, will increase the acceptance of these systems [Shortliffe, 1989, 1990].

References

Bannon L. 1986. Computer-mediated communication. In D Norman, SW Draper (eds), User-Centered System Design: New Perspectives on Human-Computer Interaction. Hillsdale, NJ, Lawrence Elbaum.

Bennet JS. 1985. ROGET: A knowledge-based system for acquiring the conceptual structure of a diagnostic expert system. J Automatic Reasoning 1:49.

Botti G, Michel C, Proudon D, et al. 1987 Feasibility study of the expert system SPHINX. In A Serio et al (eds), Proceedings of the Medical Informatics Europe, pp 957–966. Rome, EDI Press.

Botti G, Joubert M, Fieschi D, et al. 1989. Experimental use of the medical expert system SPHINX by general practitioners: Results and analysis. In B Barber et al (eds), Proceedings of the Sixth Conference on Medical Informatics (MEDINFO), pp 67–71. Amsterdam, North-Holland.

Brender J, Talmon J, Nykänen P, et al. 1993. KAVAS-2: Knowledge acquisition, visualisation and assessment system. In S Andreassen et al (eds), European Conference on Artificial Intelligence in Medicine, pp 417–420. Amsterdam, IOS Press.

Buchanan BG, Shortliffe EH (eds). 1984. Rule-Based Expert Systems: The MYCIN Experiments of the Stanford Heuristic Programming Project. Reading, Mass, Addison-Wesley.

Chandrasekaran B, Mittal S. 1982. Deep versus compiled knowledge approaches to diagnostic problem solving. In Proceedings of American Association of Artificial Intelligence '82, pp 349–354.

Chandrasekaran B. 1986. Generic tasks in knowledge-based reasoning: High building blocks foe expert systems. IEEE Expert, Fall 1986:23.

Clancey WJ. 1985. Heuristic classification. Artif Intell 27:289.

Clancey WJ, Shortliffe EH (eds). 1984. Readings in Medical Artificial Intelligence: The First Decade. Reading, Mass, Addison-Wesley.

Clarke K, O'Moore R, Smeets R, et al. 1994. A methodology for evaluation of knowledge based systems in medicine. Int J Artif Intell Med 6(2):107.

DeDombal FT. 1978. Medical diagnosis from a clinician's point of view. Methods Inform Med (17):28.

Dreyfus HL, Dreyfus SE. 1986. Mind Over Machine: The Power of Human Intuition and Expertise in the Era of Computer. New York, The Free Press.

Elstein AS, Shulman LS, Sprafka SA. 1979. Medical Problem Solving: An Analysis of Clinical Reasoning. Cambridge, Mass, Harvard University Press.

Gremy F. 1988. The role of informatics in medical research. In Data, Information and Knowledge in Medicine, Developments in Medical Informatics in Historical Perspective. Methods Inf Med Special Issue, pp 305–309.

Groen GJ, Patel VL. 1988. The relationship between comprehension and reasoning in medical expertise. In M Chi et al (eds), The Nature of Expertise. Hillsdale, NJ, Lawrence Erlbaum.

Keravnou E, Washbrook S. 1989. Deep and shallow models in medical expert systems. Artif Intell Med 1:11.

Kilian W. 1988. Liability for deficient medical expert systems. Workshop paper in 33rd Annual Meeting of the GDMS, EFMI Special Topic Meeting, Hannover, Germany.

Lundsgaarde HP. 1987. Evaluating medical expert systems. Soc Sci Med 24(10):805.

Miller RA, Pople HE, Myers JD. 1982. Internist-1: An experimental computer-based diagnostic consultant for general internal medicine. N Engl J Med 307:468.

Miller PL (ed). 1988. Selected Topics in Medical Artificial Intelligence. New York, Springer-Verlag.

Musen MA. 1989. Generation of model-based knowledge acquisition tools for clinical trial advice systems. Ph.D. dissertation, Stanford University.

Newell A. 1982. The knowledge level. Artif Intell 18:87.

Nykänen P (ed). 1990. Issues in evaluation of computer-based support to clinical decision making. Report of the SYDPOL-5 Working Group, Oslo, Oslo University Press, Research Report 127, Oslo.

Nykänen P, Saranummi N. 1993. Medical decision support: Where, when, how? In JP Morucci et al (eds), Proceedings of 14th Ann Int Conf IEEE Eng Med Biol Soc (EMBS), Paris, France, 29 Oct–1 Nov, 1992, pp 883–885.

Pauker SG, Gorry GA, Kassirer JP. 1976. Towards the simulation of clinical cognition: Taking a present illness by computer. Am J Med 60:981.

Pedersen SA, Jensen PF, Nykänen P. 1993. Epistemological analysis of deep medical knowledge in selected medical domain. Public Report of the KAVAS-2 (A2019) Project, Commission of the European Communities, Telematic Systems in Health Care.

Pothoff P, Rothemund M, Schwebel D, et al. 1988. Expert systems in medicine: Possible future effects. Int J Technol Assess Health Care 4:121.

Rector A, Nowlan W, Kay S. 1992. Conceptual knowledge: The core of medical information systems. In K Lun et al (eds), Seventh World Congress of Medical Informatics (MEDINFO), Geneva 1992, pp 1420–1428. Amsterdam, North-Holland.

Rossi-Mori A, Pisanelli DM, Ricci FL. 1990. Evaluation stages and design steps for knowledge based systems in medicine. Med Informatics 15(3):191.

Shortliffe EH. 1976. Computer-Based Concultations: MYCIN. New York, American Elsevier.

Shortliffe EH. 1988. Editorial: Medical knowledge and medical decision making. In Data, Information and Knowledge in Medicine, Developments in Medical Informatics in Historical Perspective. Methods Inform Med Special Issue 1988:209.

Shortliffe EH. 1989. Testing reality: The introduction of decision support technologies for physicians. Methods Inform Med 28(1):1.

Shortliffe EH, Perreault LE, Wiederhold G, Fagan L (eds). 1990. Medical Informatics: Computer Applications in Health Care. Reading, Mass, Addison-Wesley.

Steels L. 1990. Components of expertise. AI Magazine, Summer 12:28.

Stefanelli M. 1993. European research efforts in medical knowledge-based systems. Int J Artif Intell Med 5:107.

Suchman L. 1989. Notes on computer support for cooperative work. Working Paper WP-12, University of Jyväskylä, Finland.

van Eimeren W. 1989. Decision support systems. AIM-MIR Report, October 1989, Commission of the European Communities.

Weiss S, Kulikowski CA, Safir A. 1978. Glaucoma consultation by computer. Comput Biol Med (8):24.

Wyatt J. 1989. The evaluation of clinical decision support systems: A discussion of the methodology used in the ACORN project. In J Fox et al (eds), Proceedings of the Artificial Intelligence in Medicine, pp 15–24. Berlin, Springer-Verlag.

186

Expert Systems: Methods and Tools

Ron Summers
City University, London

Ewart R. Carson
City University, London

Biomedical engineering is a fertile domain for the application of computer-based techniques that have the potential to enhance patient care. These techniques come in many forms and can be classified according to the level of processing required. Low-level processing includes techniques such as signal interpretation, where, for example, a threshold value has to be reached before an appropriate action is taken. This type of system uses a shallow data model to transform data into a more useful form. However, in this chapter, the systems of interest are those which provide a further transformation, that of information into knowledge, via appropriate explanation and justification of concepts used. These so-called expert systems have various synonyms, including *intelligent systems, knowledge-based systems,* and *decision-support systems.*

Expert systems have an interesting historical development. The 1970s saw much of the work concentrated on the problem of knowledge representation. As the introduction of the ubiquitous personal computer aided dissemination of the technology on smaller hardware platforms, the work in the 1980s looked much more deeply into the issues involved in knowledge acquisition. By the 1990s, even with commercial exploitation, the number of expert systems in everyday use is disappointingly small. Research into their evaluation may be one way in which their use will eventually be accepted.

There are no methods and tools that cover every phase of expert system development (Fig. 186.1), so to aid the reader this chapter is subdivided into sections for knowledge acquisition and knowledge representation, respectively; a final catch-all section is used for those methods and tools which did not fit into either section.

186.1 Expert System Process Model

Before embarking on an investigation of the tools and methods available for expert system design and implementation, it is important to identify the distinct phases in their development (see Fig. 186.1). The problem is one in which knowledge from a human expert (or a set of experts) must be transferred to a computer program for dissemination. Domain-specific knowledge is elicited from the human expert by knowledge-acquisition methods. The output of this phase of expert

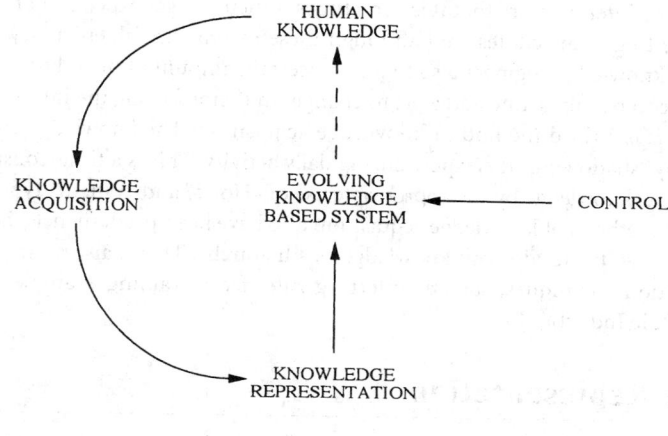

FIGURE 186.1   Knowledge engineering design.

system design is a "paper-based" system. To be of any use, this system must be represented in a form that can be implemented as a computer program. A number of methods and tools are available to perform such tasks; these are detailed below.

A different type of knowledge is required for the control strategy, i.e., decisions on when to use, or "fire," specific rules in the knowledge base. In practice, these procedures are equated with different types of search strategies, such as depth-first, breadth-first, or various implementations of optimized search strategies.

What is not captured in Fig. 186.1 are issues dealing with evaluation of the system or human-computer interactions. These are interesting topics worthy of investigation but are outside the scope of this chapter.

186.2 Knowledge Acquisition

The classic method of knowledge acquisition is the interview. Both experts and knowledge engineers are very familiar with the method because it is a part of everyday routine. However, it is not very efficient in capturing and formalizing the knowledge required for an expert system. To try and preserve the interview situation, a more formal method termed a *structured interview* is employed. In this method, the expert is given a list of variables used to describe the domain (e.g., clinical findings) and a second list that contains all possible outcomes of the system (e.g., disease states). The expert is asked to link the two lists, from which a set of production rules can be generated (see "Rule-Based Systems" below for a description of a production rule). It is crucial that all rules are formalized; although a rule of thumb suggests that 90% of the rules are captured in 10% of the development time, it is important that the remaining 10% of the knowledge base is captured. To aid this process, the second stage of the structured interview involves the expert looking at the paper-based rule set generated thus far. The knowledge engineer goes through each rule to test for conditions that affect their appropriateness. From the use of this procedure new rules may be generated.

Advantages of this method are that the experts enjoy the process, which is not too demanding of their time (experts tend to be busy), and it can be used for any type of domain. Disadvantages of the technique, as of any interview, are that it is sometimes difficult to get experts to obey instructions; experts are prone to give anecdotes, and although these may be useful, efficiency of the method deteriorates. The knowledge engineer also requires a certain amount of prior knowledge about the domain to be able to remain astute and alert to changes in theme during the interview.

Protocol analysis is a third method of knowledge acquisition. The knowledge engineer records routine activity by "shadowing" the expert during daily activity. This is a time-consuming method that generally elicits knowledge by the appropriate use of "How?" and "When?" type queries.

Graphic-based methods of knowledge acquisition also have been tried, such as the laddered grid technique, which investigates domain knowledge as a hierarchy. This is also a favored method for automatic elicitation techniques, such as inferring rules from training examples using the ID3 algorithm (see "Rule Induction").

186.3 Knowledge Representation

Knowledge representation has two main formats: rule-based systems, which take advantage of production rule technology, and semantic networks, which provide a graphic representation of the knowledge base. Below are case studies in both areas, and although dated, it can be argued that they still convey the best exemplar material of their genre. The DENDRAL system was certainly one of the first functioning expert systems, which provided a landmark for further research. MYCIN is one of the most cited expert systems in the literature and one can infer the most well known. CASNET, with its semantic net representation, provides a link with Chapter 181. Further development of this type of model provided the basis for causal probabilistic networks and other statistical network approaches to problem solving.

Rule-Based Systems

DENDRAL interpreted mass spectographic data and worked at a high intellectual level. Although the scope of the system was very narrow, it assumed expert knowledge in what was a difficult task domain [1]. At the time of its first implementation, DENDRAL was a precursor to expert systems and was responsible for the foundation of many of the techniques used in knowledge engineering. These include both knowledge elicitation and knowledge representation. The former was identified to be a "bottleneck" in the design and implementation of expert systems, because it needed prior knowledge of the expertise to be embodied. This expertise could only be elicited in discrete stages due to the time demands made on the human experts involved.

MYCIN was developed by Shortliffe and others at Stanford University [2]. The domain of interest was aiding the identification and recognizing the significance of organisms causing microbial infection and then recommending an optimal treatment protocol.

MYCIN is an example of an expert system that uses "production rules" to represent the causal relationships between individual items of factual knowledge held on the knowledge base. The form of a production rule is as follows:

IF premise assertions are true

THEN consequent assertions are true

with confidence weight *X*.

Notice that each production rule has associated with it a measure of certainty. This aids in the reasoning strategy of the system, where a value of -1 represents complete disbelief and a value of $+1$ represents complete belief in the consequent assertion(s). The assertions can be boolean combinations of clauses, each of which consists of a predicate statement triple: (attribute, object, value). For example, (Gram stain, *E. coli*, gramneg), indicates that the Gram stain of the *E. coli* organism is gram-negative.

The uniformity of representation for both domain-specific inferences and reasoning goals makes it possible for MYCIN to use a very general and simple control strategy, i.e., a goal-directed backward-chaining of the production rules. This approach can be described in the following way: The first rule to be evaluated is the one that contains the highest-level goal, which for MYCIN is "To determine if there are any organisms, or classes of organisms, that require therapy." To deduce the need for therapy requires knowledge of the infections, which is usually unknown in the first instance. Therefore, the system tries to satisfy subgoals that originate in the premise of the top goal that will allow the infections to be inferred. *Rule chaining* is the name given to the process in which the production rule hierarchy is linked together; the premise portion of each subgoal rule fires a new set of subgoals. This process is repeated until the most fundamental level of the hierarchy is reached, where the rules become assertions that can only be confirmed or denied by directly questioning the user for the appropriate information.

After MYCIN determines the significant infections, found by assessing the overall certainty factor that combines the individual degrees of confidence associated with each production rule, the organisms that account for the infections are found deterministically. Then, if appropriate, the system proceeds to recommend an antimicrobial therapy. To reach its decision, the MYCIN therapy selector uses a description of the infection(s) present, the causal organisms together with a ranking of drugs by their sensitivity, and a set of drug-preference categories. The algorithm used within the therapy selector also calculates the drug dose required and contains knowledge to modify the value if, for example, the patient is in renal failure. An advantage of this therapy selection system is that it can accept and critique a treatment protocol proposed by the user. The therapy selector has an appropriate facility to generate explanation and justification for its choice of action. "Why?" queries are dealt with by displaying the rule it is trying to imply, and if "Why?" is asked again, the query is answered by ascending the goal-tree hierarchy. "How?" queries are interpreted as the chain of rules that are fired to get to that particular conclusion, and if "How?" is repeated, the query is answered by descending the goal-tree hierarchy.

An advantage of using a production rule system is that each rule is a small "packet" of knowledge, each one being independent of all the others. This has two consequences: (1) changing or adding knowledge to the MYCIN knowledge base is relatively easy, and (2) addition of new rules is facilitated by having a modular data structure.

The MYCIN system can deal with both inexact and incomplete information. Inexact information is inherent in this domain because many test results are qualitative in nature, and relatively few statements can be made with absolute certainty. Incomplete information may arise from the time constraints involved in the identification of an organism, i.e., the time taken for an identifying laboratory test to be completed and the result of it made known to the clinician, which in some cases can be the order of 24 to 48 hours.

A disadvantage of the system is that disease states cannot always be adequately described by a rule. Also, it may not always be possible to map a series of desired actions into a set of production rules. Another disadvantage is that although new knowledge can be added by inserting a new rule, this may not interact with the existing rules in the anticipated way.

The MYCIN system is encoded in LISP, and a normal consultation takes on average 20 minutes, which includes time allowed for the optional use of the explanation facility. MYCIN has been evaluated as having a diagnostic success rate of 72%. This relatively poor performance (for an *expert* system) combined with clinician suspicion and resistance to new technology contributed to the fact that the system was not used in a clinical setting. However, as a research tool it was the subject of extensive interest in the AI fraternity, being responsible for a number of successful descendants. One of these, the PUFF system, developed to interpret pulmonary function test results, is one of the few medical expert systems in daily clinical use [3].

Network-Based Systems

CASNET is an expert system for consultation in the diagnosis and therapy of glaucoma [4]. A feature of this system is that the medical knowledge used in the patient-specific reasoning process is encompassed in a causal-associational network model of the specific disease process. Such a network, termed a *semantic net,* allows the structure of the medical knowledge covered by the system to be more coherent. A semantic network comprises nodes connected by links, where nodes correspond to either the condition or action part of the rules and the links are the inferences between the two. The model of disease is separate from the decision-making strategy, which allows the updating of both data structures to be facilitated more easily (compare with "Causal Probabilistic Modeling" in Chapter 181).

The CASNET model has a descriptive component that comprises four sets of elements as follows: observations (these consist of symptoms and laboratory test results, etc. and form the direct evidence that a disease is present), pathophysiologic states (these describe internal abnormal conditions or mechanisms that can directly cause the observed findings; the causal relations between states are of the form

$$n_i \xrightarrow{a_{ij}} n_j$$

where n_i and n_j are pathophysiologic states, and a_{ij} is the causal frequency with which state n_i, when present in a patient, leads to state n_j, disease categories (each category consists of a pattern of states and observations and is therefore conceptually at the highest level of abstraction), and treatment plans and therapies (composed of sets of related treatments or treatment plans).

Other components of the CASNET model are the decision rules, which state the degree of confidence with which an inference of a pathophysiologic state can be made from an observed pattern of findings. In rule form, this translates to

$$t_i \xrightarrow{Q_{ij}} n_j$$

where t_i is a finding (or observation) or boolean combination of findings, n_j is a pathophysiologic state as before, and Q_{ij} is a number in the range -1 to $+1$ representing the confidence with which t_i is believed to be associated with n_j. The value of Q is a certainty factor that indicates the belief that the patient is in state n_j. A threshold function is then used to determine whether or not the certainty factor confirms, denies, or leaves undetermined a particular state. Rules for associating disease categories and pathophysiologic states to treatment protocols are in the form of a classification table that consists of ordered triples,

$$(n_1, D_1, T_1), (n_2, D_2, T_2), \ldots, (n_i, D_i, T_i)$$

where n_i is the pathophysiologic state, D_i is the disease process arising from it, and T_i are the preferred treatment regimes for disease D_i.

The pathogenesis and mechanisms of a disease process are described in terms of cause-and-effect relationships between pathophysiologic states. In this way, complete or partial disease processes can be characterized by pathways through the network. When a set of cause-and-effect relationships is specified, the resulting network can be described as an acyclic graph of states. This state network is defined by a four-tuple (S, F, N, X), where S is the set of starting states (i.e., those states which have no antecedent causes), F is the set of final states, N are the number of states visited between S and F, and X are the causal relationships between the states visited (in the form of a list).

An important test for any expert system is how it copes with contradictory information. This can occur in the CASNET system, e.g., when a particular state is confirmed even though all its potential causes in the network are denied. When such a situation occurs, the CASNET system advises the user that this has happened. There are two explanations for the origin of this contradictory information: The model of the disease process may be incomplete (i.e., one or more nodes together with their respective causal relationships are missing from the knowledge base), or it may be that the threshold function associated with one of the existing causal links has been set at an inappropriate level. The modular structure of the knowledge base enables easy access to the underlying reason for the contradiction, so updating of the knowledge base can be facilitated.

An advantage of the CASNET system is that it can present alternative expertise derived from different consultants. It is this, coupled with the fact that glaucoma is a well-defined clinical problem, that results in an accuracy of diagnosis, which contributed to its relative success. The diagnostic accuracy of CASNET has been evaluated at greater than 75% for particularly difficult cases and greater than 90% for cases that constitute a broad clinical spectrum. Unfortunately, the clinical utility of the system was not assessed as high, which resulted in CASNET never being used in a routine clinical environment. However, the system was a very useful tool for research into AI in medicine and spawned further interest in other approaches to causal modeling.

186.4 Other Methods and Tools

Blackboard Architectures

The HEARSAY-II speech understanding system is a research program of Carnegie-Mellon University [5]. A feature of this system is its general problem-solving framework, termed the *blackboard architecture,* which has become the basic control model for real-time intelligent signal understanding systems [6]. The blackboard architecture contains four elements: *entries* (which is the name given to intermediate by-products of the problem-solving strategy), *knowledge sources* (these are diverse and independent subprograms that are capable of solving a specific problem efficiently; they can be thought of as a condition-action duplex, where the condition premise describes the situations to which each knowledge source can contribute, and the action component specifies the interaction of that particular knowledge source in the overall problem-solving strategy; it is the activated knowledge sources that produce the entries), the *blackboard* itself (which can be considered as a structured database; it serves two roles: first, it represents intermediate states of problem-solving activity, and second, since all communication between the individual knowledge sources is carried out via the blackboard, it can accommodate hypotheses from one particular knowledge source that may activate a number of others), and an *intelligent control mechanism* (which has sufficient knowledge embodied within it to decide if and when any particular knowledge source should be activated, thus generating entries that are recorded on the blackboard).

The blackboard control structure supports a hierarchical arrangement of knowledge sources. For instance, in the HEARSAY-II system, the top level of the hierarchy is the spoken sentence, followed by phrase, word sequence, word, syllable segment, and phoneme, respectively. The control postulate is that of "establish-and-refine," i.e., each activated knowledge source in the hierarchy tries to confirm or reject itself. If it is confirmed, then it refines itself by calling on the next immediate layer in the hierarchy to enter the same cycle. This procedure continues until (if successful) the bottom layer of the hierarchy is reached. Once the phonemes have established themselves, the spoken sentence has been modeled completely. The spoken sentence is then recognized as syntactically valid, which is one of the definitions used for speech "understanding." Further signal-processing techniques can be applied to obtain a more comprehensive understanding, such as translation into another language or paraphrasing an argument.

The blackboard architecture has been used successfully in providing interpretation of the results of blood-gas analysis [7].

Rule Induction

An expert system shell based on the rule-induction method of knowledge acquisition and representation is available and is based on the ID3 induction algorithm [8]. The original goal of the ID3 algorithm was to seek out the valuable information from large volumes of data by means of a classification rule. ID3 uses known results described in terms of a fixed set of attributes and produces a decision tree that is able to classify all possible results correctly. To optimize the decision function, the concept of "information entropy" is used.

These features are faithfully reproduced in the 1st Class Expert System shell (registered trademark of 1st Class Expert Systems, Inc.). A hypertext facility is added to provide explanation or justification as well as further information for any attribute or result obtained. Using optimization of the decision function ensures that the minimum set of questions are asked of the user to obtain the required result. As a consequence, this method is often more efficient and thorough than the human expert. The system based on the 1st Class Expert System shell is robust to missing and conflicting data. When classification is not possible, explanations can be provided by the hypertext facility. This system has been used in biomedical engineering applications such as machine malfunction, where alarms generated by the expert system are quicker and more informative than those set by the manufacturer.

186.5 Summary

The process of knowledge engineering design has been discussed in some detail. The phases of knowledge acquisition and knowledge representation have been presented, and the methods used in each phase have been discussed. The advantages of the structured interview method of knowledge acquisition over other available methods can be deduced. Knowledge representation is presented as a choice between rule-based systems and semantic networks.

MYCIN is an example of a procedural expert system, to be compared with CASNET, which is an example of a declarative expert system. The distinction between the two types hinges on the relationship between the encoded knowledge representation and the control algorithm. In systems where the knowledge representation and control algorithm are combined, then a procedural definition applies. This is exemplified by the production rule methodology, where causality is implicit in the IF . . . THEN rules. The ability to provide explanation of action, one of the prerequisites of an expert system, cannot naturally be accommodated. However, to overcome this problem, context-sensitive explanations can be used. These are a set of fixed files, each one specific to a particular production rule, which can be fired whenever the production rule they represent is used. A disadvantage of this approach is that the explanation can appear "stale" to an experienced user of the system. In systems where the knowledge representation and control algorithm are separate, then a declarative definition applies. The knowledge representation is explicitly defined, allowing a set of algorithms to act on it. This can include the test and hypothesis diagnostic cycle, an explanation-generating algorithm, and an algorithm that produces text which constitutes computer-based advice.

References

1. Lindsay RK, Buchanan BG, Feigenbaum EA, Lederberg J. 1980. Applications of Artificial Intelligence for Organic Chemistry: The DENDRAL Project. New York, McGraw-Hill.
2. Shortliffe EH. 1976. Computer-Based Medical Consultations: MYCIN. New York, Elsevier.
3. Aikins JS, Kunz JC, Shortliffe EH, Fallat RJ. 1983. PUFF: An expert system for interpretation of pulmonary function data. Comput Biomed Res 16:199.
4. Weiss S, Kulikowski CA, Amarel S, Safir A. 1978. A model-based method for computer-aided medical decision making. Artif Intell 11:145.
5. Erman LD, Hayes-Roth F, Lesser VR, Reddy DR. 1980. The Hearsay-II speech understanding system: Integrating knowledge to resolve uncertainty. Comput Surv 12:213.
6. Hayes-Roth F, Waterman DA, Lenat DB. 1983. Building Expert Systems. Reading, Mass, Addison-Wesley.
7. Chelsom JJL. 1990. The interpretation of data in intensive care medicine: An application of knowledge-based techniques. Ph.D. thesis, City University, London.
8. Quinlan JR. 1979. Rules by induction from large collections of examples. In D Michie (ed), Expert Systems in the Microelectronic Age. Edinburgh, Edinburgh University Press.

187

Knowledge Acquisition and Representation

Catherine Garbay
Laboratoire TIMC/IMAG

The scope of designing knowledge-based systems in medicine has evolved during these last few years from pure decision-making automata to open environments able to acquire, formalize, validate, and handle and disseminate elements of human expertise. The application fields have correlatedly expanded from the sole field of symbolic processing to data analysis, information management, simulation, and planning.

Therefore, the scope of knowledge acquisition and representation has been shifted from the mere transcription of expert knowledge to the modeling of pathophysiologic phenomena of increasing complexity [Stefanelli, 1993]. To reflect such evolution, the notion of model is made central in this chapter. The nature and specificity of medical expertise are addressed in the first section. Knowledge acquisition is considered afterwards, in the framework of its evolution from interviewing techniques to full designing methodologies. Knowledge representation issues are finally discussed by sucessively considering domain knowledge, control knowledge, and high-level-modeling approaches.

187.1 Medical Expertise: Domain and Control Knowledge

Expert knowledge is usually described as involving domain knowledge and control knowledge [Schreiber, 1993]. Domain knowledge is meant to represent the various elements, e.g., facts, features, relations, and concepts, that are used to represent a case, while control knowledge is meant to represent the expert know-how, i.e., the way to reason about a case.

Domain Knowledge

Domain knowledge may be seen as a kind of formal knowledge tying names, properties, and relations to the whole empirium of data, facts, observations, hypotheses, or results that are extracted from a case. Domain ontologies are used to structure and organize domain knowledge according to well-identified knowledge types or relations.

Taxonomic ontologies have been widely used in medicine because of their capacity to classify and organize diseases into hierarchical structures. As may be seen in Fig. 187.1, paroxysmal vertigo is classified as a particular kind of vertigo and may be further characterized as benign paroxysmal vertigo of childhood, benign paroxysmal positional vertigo, or paroxysmal vertigo due to vascular disorder [Schmid, 1987].

"Part of" hierarchies make it possible to describe the compositional characteristics of concepts and are particularly useful for describing anatomic properties. As may be seen in Fig. 187.2, a mammary gland lobule may be described as composed of stroma cells and acini, which in turn are composed of a basement membrane, epithelial and myoepithelial cells, and a lumen [Garbay and Pesty, 1988].

Knowledge also may be organized according to its role in the reasoning process. According to Patel et al. [1989], this process is decomposed into several levels from the empirium (the whole universe of medical problem-solving data) to the global complex level (complete understanding of the patient case). Several intermediate levels are distinguished in terms of observations, findings, facets (complex gathering of findings understood as the consequence of a pathophysiologic process), and diagnostic level, as summarized in Fig. 187.3.

Current research emphasizes the notion of causal ontologies (see Fig. 187.10), where a deep functional understanding of the process leading to a disease is sought [Jensen et al., 1987; Stefanelli, 1993].

Control Knowledge

Reasoning may be seen as the process of handling facts, observations, and hypotheses to reach a final understanding of a situation. Various mental abstraction levels are traversed in this process, which may involve different inference schemes, depending on the type of data to be processed (e.g., uncertain, geometric, or temporal) and on the type of inferencing to be applied (e.g., deductive, inductive, or nonmonotonic).

An epistemologic model of diagnostic reasoning is proposed by Lanzola and Stefanelli [1992] in terms of abstraction, abduction, deduction, and eliminative induction (Fig. 187.4). The abstraction corresponds to identification of the clinical features that diagnosis should be able to explain. The abduction corresponds to formulation of a set of hypotheses from which expected manifestations are deduced. Eliminative induction is finally used to reduce uncertainty of inferred hypotheses by matching their consequences against observed data.

The global approach to a case is nowadays often formalized in terms of tasks [Bylander and Chandrasekaran, 1987; Steels, 1990; Schreiber et al., 1993], which makes it possible to structure the overall reasoning process in terms of goals and subgoals and thus to organize knowledge and know-how according to problem-solving rationale [Newell, 1982].

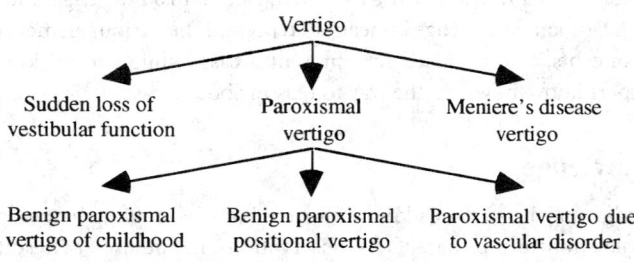

FIGURE 187.1 Vertigo taxonomy (partial view). (From Schmid [1987].)

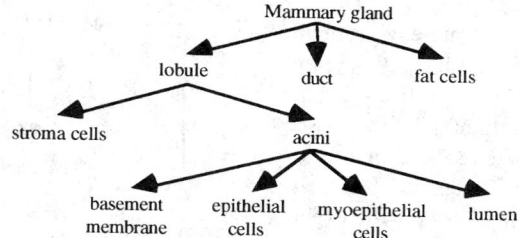

FIGURE 187.2 A part of hierarchy example (partial view). (From Garbay and Pesty [1988].)

187.2 Knowledge Acquisition

Knowledge acquisition implies the expert knowledge to be extracted, analyzed, transcribed into a computer-usable form, and then finally implemented. This complex process critically depends on the knowledge engineering tool at hand, since most representation formalisms convey a restrictive and rigid semantics, which does not refer to a clear ontology [Schreiber, 1993].

Knowledge-acquisition techniques have evolved recently from the mere interviewing techniques to the design of computerized tools and integrated environments. Current trends are to consider knowledge acquisition as an integral part of the design process.

Interviewing Techniques

Knowledge is usually acquired through direct interaction with a human expert but also may be obtained from many other sources, such as textbooks, reports, databases, or case studies [Buchanan et al., 1983]. A systematic and structured approach is necessary to ensure the completion and consistency of the interviewing process, which is usually driven by a knowledge engineer. Other techniques are often used to complement the mere interviewing approach, such as observing the expert in daily working situations, writing scenarios and reports, or filling out questionaires.

Knowledge-Acquisition Tools

Several computerized tools have been designed in the past to assist the knowledge-acquisition/transcription process. The reference work done in TEIRESIAS [Davis and Lenat, 1982] and ETS [Boose, 1985] appears to bring complementary solutions to this difficult problem. TEIRESIAS is rather meant to support the testing and refinement of a "MYCIN-like" system. It proceeds by searching for missing or inconsistent information and may suggest the generation of new inference rules. ETS, on the contrary, is meant to support direct elicitation of expert knowledge. It is based on bipolar constructs structuring the perception of the world (e.g., the grade of a tumor allows the organization of diseases according to their prognostic significance). The acquired knowledge is then represented by means of so-called repertory grids tying concepts and their properties. Distances between concepts may then be computed, as well as the discriminatory power of a given characteristic. Production rules are then generated and submitted to the expert to be modified or tested.

Knowledge-Acquisition Environments

Knowledge-acquisition environments have been designed to integrate several acquisition tech-

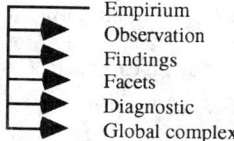

Empirium
Observation
Findings
Facets
Diagnostic
Global complex

FIGURE 187.3 Organizing knowledge according to its role in the reasoning process. (From Patel et al. [1989].)

niques. The expert is usually assisted by a cognitive engineer to use the software environment.
AQUINAS [Boose and Bradshaw, 1987] and
MORE [Kahn et al., 1985] are particularly representative of this approach. AQUINAS is based
on the cooperation between several interviewing methods and has been designed as an extension of ETS. MORE may interview the expert
according to eight different strategies and integrates several facilities such as a rule generator,
an inference engine to test the rules, and on-line assistance to the user.

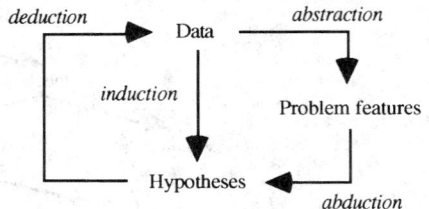

FIGURE 187.4 An epistemologic model of diagnostic reasoning. (From Lanzola and Stefanelli [1992].)

Knowledge-Acquisition Methodologies

The term *knowledge-acquisition methodologies* refers to approaches aiming at a close integration
between knowledge acquisition and system design, in which knowledge acquisition is considered as
a modeling process rather than as an extraction/transcription problem. The modeling approach
permits the investigator to work at the "right" abstraction level, often called the knowledge level
[Newell, 1982], to refer to a level at which knowledge may be expressed without referring to any
implementation constraint [Schreiber et al., 1993]. It is formulated in opposition to symbol-level
approaches, which support implementation-level modeling.

  KADS (KBS Analysis and Design Structured methodology) is among the best known methodologies [Breuker and Wielinga, 1987] and has been conceived to guide the whole process of expert
system design. It permits the progressive evolution from real world to implementation by the building of four successive models that organize the domain ontology into four knowledge levels: domain
level (description of concepts and relation between them), inference level (reasoning primitives),
task level (reasoning steps, goals and ways to reach them, structured task), and strategy level (control
and goal scheduling).

187.3 Knowledge Representation

The representation of medical knowledge is a very active research field characterized by a variety of
modeling issues and approaches. As a matter of fact, a growing range of problems must be faced,
which includes the design of deformable anatomic models, the heuristic modeling of the expert
reasoning, the causal modeling of a pathophysiologic process, as well as the task-oriented modeling
of clinical protocols. The representation of domain and control knowledge is discussed first. High-
level models (e.g., task-oriented and agent-oriented models) are then presented.

Representation of Domain Knowledge

Domain knowledge may be represented in two different ways depending on whether the emphasis
is on the structure and properties of concepts or on their mutual relations. Both representation styles
(e.g., frames and semantic networks) are usually combined. We do not cope in this section with the
numerical modeling of anatomic structures.

Frame Representations and Object-Oriented Languages

Frame-based representations have been introduced as a way to organize prototypical knowledge
about the world [Minsky, 1975]. A *frame* defines the prototypical description of concepts sharing
similar properties and behavior. It is defined as a set of slots describing the concept attributes and
their values. A variety of other slots may be introduced, including procedures, default and current
values, or type/value constraints. The frames are organized in hierarchies, tying classes and

instances. The basic inference mechanism is *instanciation*, in which the attribute values of the new instance are obtained either by inheritance, by computation (using the procedural attachments), or by default.

In a knowledge-based system to diagnose HIV pneumonias [Fiore et al., 1993], frames are used to describe the physiopathologic states of the disease for each particular pneumonia in terms of several slots describing the epidemiologic data, clinical picture, laboratory tests, and diagnosis (Fig. 187.5).

Object-oriented languages stem from classic software engineering issues involving debugging and maintenance, modularity, protection, and reusability. The basic idea is to organize the data and their processing methods around one entity: the object. It has been used by von Mulligen et al. [1991] as a general framework to integrate commercially available applications (e.g., information systems, statistical and graphic packages, as well as word-processing facilities) in the design of medical workstations. The object-oriented paradigm is nowadays increasingly considered as a way to cope simultaneously with knowledge modeling and software engineering issues, as in HELIOS [Coignard et al., 1992]. HELIOS has been conceived as a software engineering environment to facilitate the development of medical applications. It provides a core set of medical classes from which to build a new application. Several services are also provided, which include the acquisition and management of medical information, the processing of natural-language queries, as well as data-driven decision support.

Semantic Networks and Conceptual Graphs

Semantic networks [Quillian, 1968] have been proposed as a flexible formalism to represent the semantics of concepts (the nodes in the network) and their relations (the arcs) in the framework of a graphlike structure. The reasoning proceeds by unification between an unknown fact and a known concept or subgraph in the network.

The approach has been extended rapidly to represent causal relationships as well as hierarchical taxonomies and to include frames. It has been applied successfully to numerous applications in medicine, as in CASNET [Weiss et al., 1978], a consultation system for glaucoma, INTERNIST [Pople, 1977], a diagnostic consultant in internal medicine, and PIP [Pauker et al., 1976], a system devoted to renal disease. The reasoning strategy in these systems is of the event-driven type: Initial data triggers a number of hypotheses, which are then to be confirmed [Kulikowski, 1984]. The sub-

Frame Cytomegalovirus

- sort-of   intestitial pneumonia

- epidemiological data

     • other kind of pneumonia   yes

     • CD4   less than 200/mmc

- clinical picture

     • symptoms   fever, non-productive cough, dyspnea

     • signs   cyanosis tachypnea

- laboratory tests

     • PO2   lowering

     • LDH   growing

FIGURE 187.5 Using frames to represent diagnostic knowledge. (From Fiore et al. [1993].)

graph of confirmed or undetermined hypotheses constitutes a patient-specific model. Various weights and scores are usually introduced to render the reasoning strategy more flexible.

Conceptual graphs [Sowa, 1984] have been designed as an extension of the previous formalism in which an explicit representation of the links between concepts is sought. A *conceptual graph* is a directed graph comprising two kinds of nodes: concept nodes and conceptual relationships nodes. The representation is grounded on first-order logic and is currently being applied in a number of projects for the modeling and representation of medical terminology, as in GALEN [Alpay et al., 1993]. One major goal of GALEN (Generalized Architecture for Languages, Encyclopedias, and Nomenclatures in medicine) is to form a general terminology server able to conciliate a number of classifications and nomenclatures. It is based on a semantic encyclopedia of terminology connected to a multilingual information module. Conceptual graphs are used in this project to generate natural-language expressions from information coded according to the GALEN master notation.

Conceptual graphs also may be used as a formalism that supports both expressiveness and classification purposes, i.e., as a knowledge representation formalism able to integrate both terminologic and domain knowledge, as shown in Fig. 187.6 [Bernauer and Goldberg, 1993].

In the example in Fig. 187.6, the composite concept "simple oblique diaphyseal fracture of the right femur" is described as a nested set of 2-tuples each tying a relation (:loc, for example) and a composite concept (diaphysis, for example). Taxonomic as well as compositional relations are used to support classification. The equivalent nested notation for the graph in Fig. 187.6 is the following:

> (fracture
>
>   (:loc   (diaphysis   (:part (femur (:side (right))))))
>
>   (:morph   (oblique))
>
>   (:compl   (simple)))

Representation of Control Knowledge

Control knowledge may be approached from two different viewpoints, the expert and the domain viewpoints. According to the expert viewpoint, control knowledge is meant to reflect the expert way to approach a case, e.g., its consultation protocol and reasoning style. According to the domain viewpoint, on the contrary, control knowledge is meant to reflect deep pathophysiologic processes as well as their relations to the findings and disease hypotheses at hand. The expert reasoning is considered first; it is examined sucessively as the capacity to compare and retrieve learned situations (so-called case-based reasoning) and as the ability to apply well-experimented inference schemes

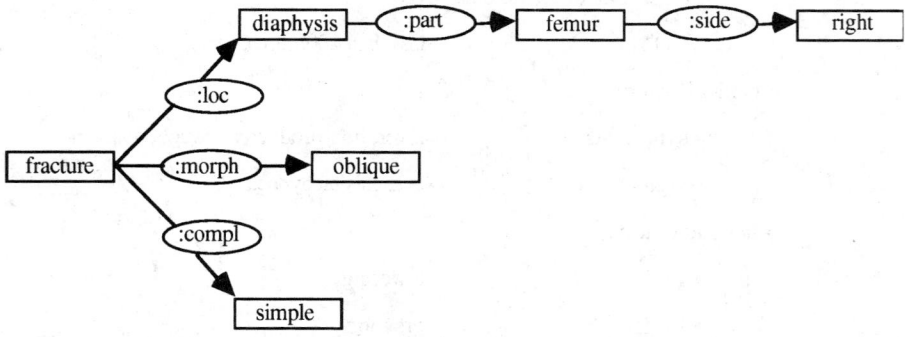

FIGURE 187.6 Conceptual graph representing the concept "simple oblique diaphyseal fracture of the right femur." (From Bernauer and Goldberg [1993].)

(usually represented by rules). One main feature of human reasoning, i.e., its capacity to handle uncertain and imprecise information, is also considered. Causal modeling of pathophysiologic processes is finally presented.

Case-Based Reasoning

Case-based reasoning is based on the hypothesis that new situations are analyzed by reference to past experience, i.e., by considering their similarity to well-experimented situations. The notion of similarity is made central in this kind of reasoning [Campbell and Wolstencroft, 1990]. The idea has received much attention recently because of the possibility to reason directly about cases without the need to acquire generic control knowledge [Goos and Schewe, 1993]. However, the choice of the similarity measure turns out to be critical with respect to the reasoning accuracy. The structuration of the case base also has to be carefully considered in order to avoid combinatorial search [Gierl et al., 1993].

Rule-Based Reasoning

The use of if-then rules (also called *production rules* or *condition-action pairs*) is a straightforward and popular way to represent the expert know-how. A rule example is given in Fig. 187.7, in which a deduction is made about the presence of bacteroids based on a composite observation.

This type of knowledge is often said to be shallow or heuristic, since it is a largely empirical and nonformalized representation mechanism. Given a set of facts, the reasoning process is then modeled as the successive activation of rules, which in turn produce new facts to be considered, until no applicable rule can be found.

The rules are handled by means of an inference engine, which may work under two inferencing modes, the data-driven or goal-driven mode. In the data-driven mode, the reasoning is modeled as a deductive process proceeding from given premises to some conclusion. In the goal-driven mode, on the contrary, the reasoning is modeled as an inductive process proceeding backwards from some hypothesized conclusion to the conditions to be verified. Both inference schemes are usually combined to implement complex hypothesis and test strategies. In addition, metarules are often used to structure the reasoning process by constraining the application of the rules. A metarule example is given in Fig. 187.8, which permits one to predict that some rules will be poorly informative, given the nonsterility of the culture site.

MYCIN, a system for diagnosing and treating infectious blood diseases, is one of the earliest and most widely known expert system in medicine [Shortliffe, 1976].

Uncertain and Imprecise Reasoning

How to model the uncertainty and imprecision that is central to the human reasoning style has raised a number of research activities during the last decades [van Ginneken and Smeulders, 1988]. The bayesian model has been for a long time the primary numerical approach to uncertain reasoning. It is based on assigning a probability distribution to each of the variables representing the problem at hand. These probabilities express the uncertainty and likelihood of occurrence of symptoms as well as diseases. Given $P(Di)$, the a priori probability of disease Di, given $P(S|Di)$, the probability that symptom S may occur in the context of disease Di, Bayes' rule (Eq. 187.1) allows one to compute $P(Di|S)$, the probability that disease Di occurs when S is observed, according to the following formula:

$$P(Di|S) = \frac{P(S|Di)P(Di)}{\sum_{j} P(S|Dj)P(Dj)}$$

(187.1)

The most important assumption underlying the use of Bayes' rule is that all disease hypotheses must be mutually exclusive and exhaustive. It means that only one disease is assumed to be present.

IF	the infection is primary-bacteremia
and	the site of the culture is one of the sterile sites
and	the suspected portal of entry of the organism is the gastrointestinal tract
THEN	there is suggestive evidence (0.7) that the identity of the organism is bacteroids.

FIGURE 187.7   A production rule example from MYCIN. (From Shortliffe [1976].)

If this condition is met, Bayes has a completely predictable performance and guarantees a conclusion with minimum overall error [van Ginneken and Smeulders, 1988].

Some intuitive methods for the combination and propagation of these numbers have been suggested and used, as in MYCIN (see the rules in Figs. 187.7 and 187.8, where coefficients are used to weight their conclusions). The empirical character of the approach has often been criticized. However, it is consistent with the heuristic style that is inherent to rule-based modeling.

The theory of possibility [Zadeh, 1978] has been used in medicine to represent the vagueness of clinical predicates, such as "young," "rather young," "infected," or "mostly infected." These vague predicates are represented by means of a fuzzy set and a possibility distribution. Fuzzy reasoning may then be implemented by means of rules handling fuzzy facts, as in the example in Fig. 187.9 [Buisson et al., 1987]. In this example, two fuzzy predicates are used, namely, "weight loss rather ≥ 2 kg" and "age rather <30." They are represented by means of two different possibility distributions, according to which the two predicates are "evaluated," given some weight and age values in the fuzzy set.

The necessity for experts to codify their knowledge is currently the major limitation of these approaches.

Causal Reasoning

One major drawback of heuristic or shallow diagnostic systems is in the weakness of their explanation abilities, since explanations are provided in terms of a succession of rules of frame instantiations, which may look a bit unnatural to the expert. In opposition to this, deep causal models are meant to provide an explicit representation of the structure and behavior of the physiopathologic process under consideration, thus supporting sound explanation abilities [Console et al., 1987].

There are at least two alternative ways to represent causal knowledge [Ramoni et al., 1992]. The first method is based on a network representation, where nodes represent states or events occurring in the patient and links represent a causal relation between them. MUNIN [Jensen et al., 1987], an expert system in electromyography, is representative of the approach. The domain knowledge is embedded in a causal probabilistic network and is further divided into three levels, representing diseases, pathophysiologic features, and findings. These levels are linked by causal relations: Diseases cause certain affections in muscles. These affections, in turn, cause expectations for certain findings. A partial view of the causal network is given in Fig. 187.10. Diseases are grouped into a single node (on the left) and characterized by their grades. The disease node is connected to several pathophysiologic nodes describing the pathophysiologic status of a muscle in terms of discrete properties (the muscle structure is rather normal, there is no myotonia, and no muscle loss). Some expectations regarding, for example, the muscle force and atrophy or the presence of spontaneous myotonic distrophy are finally obtained. Probabilities are used to characterize each state in the network (the horizontal bars in the figure) and propagated through the causal links.

An alternative way is to represent both the structure and behavior of a physiologic system [Ironi et al., 1993]. The system structure is simply given in terms of variables and relations. The system

IF	the site of the culture is one of the nonsterile sites
and	there are rules which mention in their premise a previous organism which may be the same as the current organism
THEN	it is definite (1.0) that each of them is not going to be useful.

FIGURE 187.8   A metarule example from MYCIN (From Shortliffe [1976].)

IF weight loss rather >= 2 kg and age rather < 30

THEN presumptive evidence of insulino-dependent diabetes (0.7)

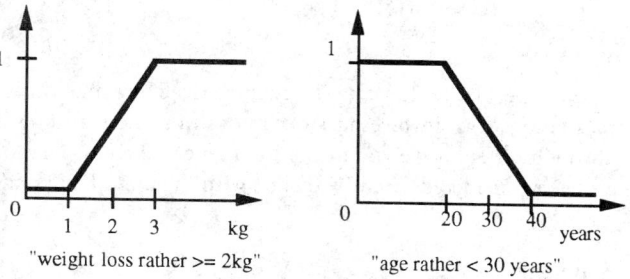

"weight loss rather >= 2kg" "age rather < 30 years"

FIGURE 187.9 Fuzzy predicates examples. (From Buisson et al. [1987].)

behavior is then modeled by a set of mathematical equations tying related variables, which represent potential perturbations of the system state. Compartmental system theory is often used in this respect because it provides a robust modeling framework based on differential calculus. It implies, however, that a precise quantitative modeling of the pathophysiologic phenomena is possible. Qualitative models, on the contrary, allow one to cope with the fuzziness and incompleteness of pathophysiologic knowledge. Among these, QSIM is the most widely applied formalism in medicine [Stefanelli, 1993]. This formalism provides a descriptive language to represent the structure of a physiologic system and a simulation algorithm to infer its qualitative behavior. The language consists in qualitative constraints that abstract the relationships in a differential equation. This approach has been applied to a variety of fields in medicine [Ironi et al., 1990]

Some tentative efforts have been made to combine the flexibility of heuristic modeling with the robustness of deep modeling, as in CHECK [Console et al., 1987]. CHECK (Combining Heuristic and Causal Knowledge) is a two-level diagnostic expert system in the field of hepatology. Heuristic knowledge (a combination of frames and production rules) is used first to produce a disease hypothesis. Causal knowledge is used in a second step to confirm and explain the diagnosis.

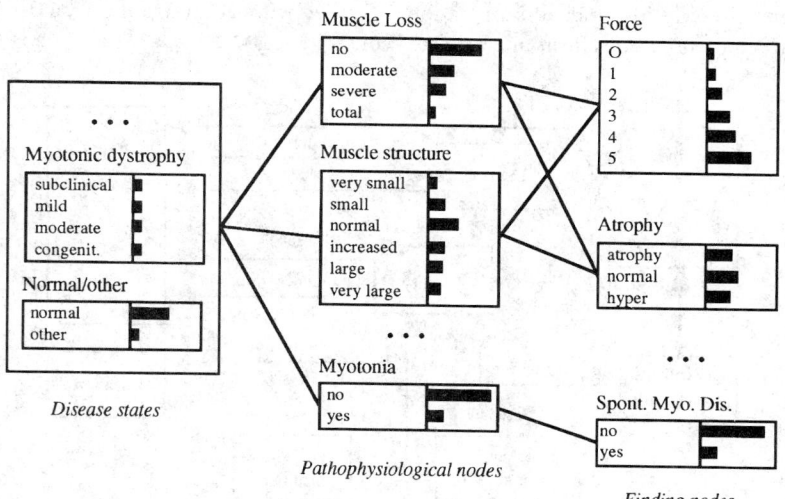

FIGURE 187.10 The domain knowledge in MUNIN (partial view). (From Jensen et al. [1987].)

It should be noted that representing pathophysiologic knowledge requires a special emphasis on the notion of time [Stefanelli, 1993], a problem early addressed by Fagan [1979]. In addition, specific knowledge-acquisition issues are raised that have been only recently addressed [Ironi et al., 1993].

High-Level Modeling

As mentioned above, the expert know-how may be characterized by a dual capacity: (1) structuring the solving of complex tasks, which involves task decomposition and planning, and (2) analyzing a complex situation through different viewpoints and inference schemes. Task-oriented and agent-based modeling have been considered recently to cope with the underlying issues of structuration and cooperation.

Task-Oriented Modeling

Task-oriented modeling has been proposed to model general problem-solving methods. The notion of generic task [Bylander and Chandrasekaran, 1987; Chandrasekaran, 1987] has been introduced in this respect as a combination of knowledge structures and inference strategies that are known to be efficient for solving certain (generic) types of problems. These generic tasks are then instanciated to cope with the specificity of given expertise domains. This notion may be used as a model to drive knowledge acquisition and system design, since knowledge and know-how specific to a task are specified at the right abstraction level [Steels, 1990].

This approach is finding a growing interest in medicine, where decision support systems are increasingly meant to cope with broad patient management issues, in opposition with their traditional conception as mere diagnostic automata [Barahona et al., 1994]. Issues of increasing complexity are raised in this respect, and there is a need for agreed and detailed care protocols for the planning of patient management [Gordon et al., 1993].

Knowledge-based systems offer a powerful medium for the dissemination of consensus guidelines in that field. A generic modeling of clinical protocol has been developed in DILEMMA [Gordon et al., 1993], a system delivering guideline-based decision support for shared care in oncology, cardiology, and primary care. A *protocol* is a formal description of a way to achieve an objective or goal, given a class of problem. It is used as a template from which to derive the specific activity to be performed for a given clinical context. Figure 187.11 depicts a data model of a prescription activity in which precise information is given about the patient, the agent responsible for the drug prescription and administration, together with administration guidelines and a description of potential side effects and expected consequences.

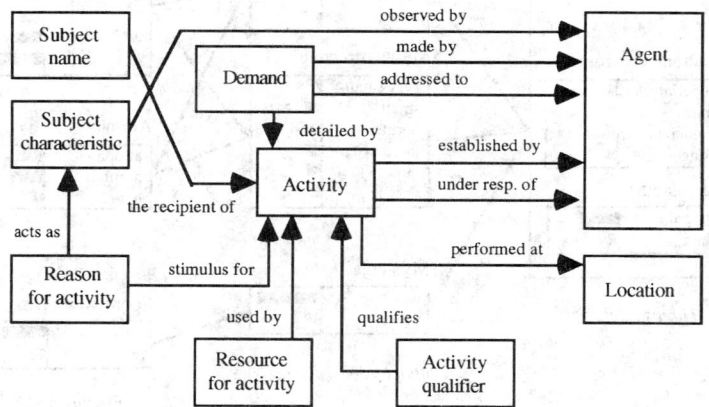

FIGURE 187.11   Model of a prescription activity in primary care (partial view). (From Gordon et al. [1993].)

Such modeling is meant to be used in the framework of a protocol decision support system able to guide the user in the accurate and correct application of protocols. The system also would offer high-quality advice on the adequacy of a given protocol or on how to apply several protocols concurrently to a single patient [Gordon et al., 1993].

Agent-Oriented Modeling

Agent-oriented modeling has developed as an extension of the object paradigm to cope with engineering and modeling issues of increasing complexity [Shoham, 1993]. The problem-solving tasks in this approach are distributed among intelligent autonomous entities that cooperate, pooling their skills and their expertise to reach a common goal [Durfee et al., 1989].

Considering the engineering viewpoint, there is a growing demand for a better integration in existing hospital information systems, which implies the capacity to handle and access knowledge sources from different modalities (e.g., texts, images, graphics, and voices) and to integrate them into a single multimedia system. Moreover, telematic capacities will increasingly be needed to allow the exchange and dissemination of data, advice, reference books, and articles, as well as the remote execution of decision support systems [Barahona et al., 1994]. In addition, multiagent systems are meant to be physically distributed, which reveals major importance with respect to criteria involving efficacity, reliability, and surety in operation but still raises unsolved issues in some areas such as privacy, legacy, and confidentiality.

Considering the modeling viewpoint, there is a growing need for the integration of multimodal knowledge representation and reasoning schemes. Such integration is needed for at least two complementary reasons, i.e., the need to analyze data from different modalities and abstraction levels and the need to dynamically adapt the knowledge representation formalism and inference scheme to the situation at hand and to the current problem-solving state. The first viewpoint is adopted in systems such as KIDS [Ovalle and Garbay, 1991], a system devoted to the interpretation of breast cytologic images, and AMNESIA [O'Hare et al., 1992], a system devoted to the diagnosis of memory-related disorder illnesses. In both systems, the knowledge and reasoning skills are distributed among several specialists that cooperate toward the solving of the problem. Each specialist in this kind of approach is devoted to handling a precise knowledge domain or task, such as, for example, validate a specimen, select a field of interest, represent the cell morphology, identify the cell type, or propose a diagnosis hypothesis [Ovalle and Garbay, 1991]. The second viewpoint has been emphasized in NEOANEMIA, a system able to recognize disorders causing anemia [Ramoni et al., 1992]. An abductive inference scheme is first of all applied to generate an initial set of hypotheses. A deductive inference scheme is then applied to compute the expected manifestations, which is based on a separate and explicit representation of taxonomic and causal ontology. Inductive resoning is finally used to prune the hypotheses set by matching the expected manifestations against the available data.

It should be noticed finally that challenging knowledge-acquisition issues are raised by this new technology [Ovalle et al., 1993].

187.4 Conclusions

The acquisition and representation of knowledge have been presented as an actively evolving research field characterized by modeling and software engineering issues of increasing complexity. Representing domain ontologies has been shown to raise a variety of issues, such as using conceptual graphs to represent the semantics of medical terms, using frames to describe domain taxonomies, or modeling pathophysiologic processes through causal networks. Modeling the expert control knowledge has been considered in terms of reasoning as well as planning abilities, which in turn leads to specific modeling issues.

In addition, the scope of designing knowledge-based systems in medicine currently evolves from the mere diagnostic task to the broader issue of patient management, which implies a better integration in existing hospital information systems. To this end, powerful multimedia workstations have to be conceived that support the remote access to knowledge sources from different modalities and the cooperative activation of distributed processing and reasoning packages. New software engineering issues are raised as a consequence that appear critical with respect to the well-known "gold standards" of usability, efficacy, and reliability.

Defining Terms

Control knowledge: The know-how by which to handle domain knowledge and to reason about a case.

Domain knowledge: Formal knowledge about the application domain theory as well as actual knowledge about the data, facts, observations, hypotheses, or results that are attached to a given case.

Generic modeling, generic task: A way to describe a concept, or a task, that is domain-dependent in the sense that it is related to a medical domain but that is generic in the sense that it may apply to several application areas in medicine.

Heuristic knowledge: Knowledge that reflects an empirical and nonformalized way to reason about a situation or solve a problem.

Knowledge level: A notion introduced by Newell to express the rationale behind the exploitation of knowledge in terms that are free from any implementation constraint.

Model, modeling approach: A formal representation of the concepts, relationships, and reasoning schemes that constitute the domain and control knowledge of the application domain at hand; a designing approach that is driven by a formal representation of the domain and control knowledge in which a close integration of the knowledge-acquisition process is performed. This approach allows one to work at a level that is free from any implementation constraints, the knowledge level.

Ontology (domain, taxonomic, causal):   The domain ontology characterizes the structure of the domain knowledge in terms of concepts and relationships. Taxonomic and causal ontologies are two major methods for organizing domain knowledge; taxonomic ontologies emphasize the hierarchical relations between concepts, while causal ontologies emphasize their deep causal relations.

Shallow (versus deep) knowledge: Shallow knowledge is often used in opposition to deep knowledge, a knowledge based on a formal theory of the domain under interest (e.g., knowledge of a pathophysiologic process). The term *shallow* refers to shortened reasoning schemes that are often gained by experience.

References

Alpay L, Baud R, Rassinoux AM, et al. 1993. Interfacing conceptual graphs and the Galen master notation for medical knowledge representation and modelling. In S Andreassen et al (eds), Artificial Intelligence in Medicine, pp 337–347. Amsterdam, IOS Press.

Barahona P, Durinck J, Florin C, et al. 1994. Knowledge processing for decision support in the health sector: A perspective for the next decade. In P Barahona, JP Christensen (eds), Knowledge and Decision in Health Telematics, pp 3–60. Amsterdam, IOS Press.

Bernauer J, Goldberg H. 1993. Compositional classification based on conceptual graphs. In S Andreassen et al (eds), Artificial Intelligence in Medicine, pp 348–359. Amsterdam, IOS Press.

Boose JH, Bradshaw JM. 1987. Expertise transfer and complex problems: Using AQUINAS as a knowledge acquisition workbench for knowledge-based system. Int J Man-Machine Studies 26:3.

Boose JH. 1985. A knowledge acquisition program for expert systems based on personnel construct psychology. Int J Man-Machine Studies 23:495.

Breuker J, Wielinga B. 1987. Use of models in interpreting verbal data. In A Kidd (ed), Knowledge Elicitation for Expert Systems: A Practical Handbook, pp 17–44. New York, Plenum Press.

Buchanan BG, Barstow, D, Bechtel R, et al. 1983. Construction of an expert system. In F Hayes-Roth et al (eds), Building Expert Systems, pp 127–167. Reading, Mass, Addison-Wesley.

Buisson JC, Farreny H, Prade H, et al. 1987. TOULMED, an inference engine which deals with imprecise and uncertain aspects of medical knowledge. In J Fox et al (eds), AIME 87: Proceedings of the European Conference on Artificial Intelligence in Medicine, Lecture Notes in Medical Informatics, pp 123–140. Berlin, Springer-Verlag.

Bylander T, Chandrasekaran B. 1987. Generic tasks for knowledge-based reasoning: The "right" level of abstraction for knowledge acquisition. Int J Man-Machine Studies 26:231.

Campbell JA, Wolstencroft J. 1990. Structure and significance of analogical reasoning. Artif Intell Med 2:103.

Chandrasekaran B. 1987. Towards a functional architecture for intelligence based on generic information processing tasks. In Proc 10th IJCAI, pp 1183–1192. New York, IEEE Computer Society Press.

Coignard J, Jean F, Degoulet P, et al. 1992. HELIOS: Object-oriented software engineering in medicine. In Health Technology and Informatics, vol 2, pp 141–149. Amsterdam, IOS Press.

Console L, Fossa M, Torasso P, et al. 1987. Man-machine interaction in CHECK. In J Fox et al (eds), AIME 87: Proceedings of the European Conference on Artificial Intelligence in Medicine, Lecture Notes in Medical Informatics, pp 205–212. Berlin, Springer-Verlag.

Davis R, Lenat D. 1982. Knowledge-Based System in Artificial Intelligence. New York, McGraw-Hill.

Durfee EH, Lesser VR, Corkill DD. 1989. Trends in cooperative distributed problem solving. IEEE Trans Know Data Eng 1:63.

Fagan LM. 1979. Representation of dynamic clinical knowledge: Measurement interpretation in the intensive care unit. In Proc of the 6th IJCAI, pp 260–262. Stanford, Calif, Stanford University, Department of Computer Science.

Fiore M, Sicurello F, Vigano M, et al. 1993. A knowledge-based system to classify and diagnose HIV-pneumonias. In S Andreassen et al (eds), Artificial Intelligence in Medicine, pp 185–190. Amsterdam, IOS Press.

Garbay C, Pesty S. 1988. Expert systems for biomedical image interpretation. In J Demongeot et al (eds), Artificial Intelligence and Cognitive Sciences, pp 323–345. Manchester, England, Manchester University Press.

Gierl L, Schmidt R, Pollwein B. 1993. ICONS: Cognitive basic functions in a case-based consultation system for health care. In S Andreassen et al (eds), Artificial Intelligence in Medicine, pp 230–236. Amsterdam, IOS Press.

van Ginneken AM, Smeulders AWM. 1988. An analysis of five strategies for reasoning in uncertainties and their suitability in pathology. In ES Gelsema, LN Kanal (eds), Pattern Recognition and Artificial Intelligence, pp 367–379. New York, Elsevier Science.

Goos K, Schewe S. 1993. Case based reasoning in clinical evaluation. In S Andreassen et al (eds), Artificial Intelligence in Medicine, pp 445–448. Amsterdam, IOS Press.

Gordon C, Herbert SI, Jackson-Smale A, Renaud-Salis JL. 1993. Care protocols and health informatics. In S Andreassen et al (eds), Artificial Intelligence in Medicine, pp 289–309. Amsterdam, IOS Press.

Hayes-Roth B. 1985. A blackboard architecture for control. Artif Intell 26(3):251.

Ironi L, Stefanelli M, Lanzola G. 1990. Qualitative models in medical diagnosis. Artif Intell Med 2:85.

Ironi L, Cattaneo A, Stefanelli M. 1993. A tool for pathophysiological knowledge acquisition. In S Andreassen et al (eds), Artificial Intelligence in Medicine, pp 13–31. Amsterdam, IOS Press.

Jensen FV, Andersen SK, Kjaerulff U, Adreassen S. 1987. MUNIN: On the case for probabilities in medical expert systems—A practical exercise. In J Fox et al (eds), AIME 87: Proceedings of the European Conference on Artificial Intelligence in Medicine, Lecture Notes in Medical Informatics, pp 149–160. Berlin, Springer-Verlag.

Kahn G, Nowlan S, McDermott J. 1985. MORE: An intelligent knowledge acquisition tool. In Proc AAAI '85, pp 581–584.

Kulikowski CA. 1984. Artificial intelligence methods and systems for medical consultation. In WJ Clancey, EH Shortliffe (eds), Readings in Medical Artificial Intelligence, pp 72–97. Reading, Mass, Addison-Wesley.

Lanzola G, Stefanelli M. 1992. A specialized framework for medical diagnosis knowledge-based systems. Comput Biomed Res 25:351.

McGraw KL, Harbison-Briggs K. 1989. Knowledge Acquisition: Principles and Guidelines. Englewood Cliffs, NJ, Prentice-Hall.

Minsky M. 1975. A framework for representing knowledge. In PH Winston (ed), The Psychology of Computer Vision, pp 211–277. New York: McGraw-Hill.

van Mulligen EM, Timmers T, van Bemmel JH, van den Heuvel F. 1991. A framework for uniform access to data, software and knowledge. In PD Clayton (ed), Fifteenth Annual Symp on Computer Applications in Medical Care, pp 496–500. New York, McGraw-Hill.

Newell A. 1982. The knowledge level. Artif Intell 18:87.

O'Hare et al. 1992. AMNESIA: Implementing a distributed KBS using RAPIDO. In Bramer MA, Milne RN (eds), Proc 12th Annual Int Conf of the British Computer Society Specialist Group on ES, pp 1–29. Cambridge, England, Cambridge University Press.

Ovalle AD, Garbay C. 1991. KIDS: A distributed expert system for biomedical image interpretation. In ACF Colchester, DJ Hawkes (eds), Information Processing in Medical Imaging, Lectures Notes in Computer Science, pp 419–433. Berlin, Springer-Verlag.

Ovalle A, Hugonnard E, Garbay C. 1993. Medical system design and knowledge acquisition using cooperating intelligent agents: A case study for breast cancer diagnosis. In S Andreassen et al (eds), Artificial Intelligence in Medicine, pp 247–258. Amsterdam, IOS Press.

Patel VL, Evans DA, Kaufman DR. 1989. A cognitive framework for doctor-patient interaction. In DA Evans, VL Patel (eds), Cognitive Science in Medicine, pp 257–312. Cambridge, Mass, MIT Press.

Pauker SG, Gorry GA, Kassirer JP, Schwartz WB. 1976. Towards the simulation of clinical cognition: Taking a present illness by computer. Am J Med 60:981.

Pople H. 1977. The formation of composite hypothesis in diagnostic problem solving: An exercise in synthetic reasoning. In Proc of the 5th IJCAI, pp 1030–1037. Pittsburgh, Carnegie-Mellon University, Department of Computer Science.

Quillian MR. 1968. Semantic memory. In M Minsky (ed), Semantic Information Processing, pp 216–270. Cambridge, Mass, MIT Press.

Ramoni M, Stefanelli M, Barosi G, Magnani L. 1992. An epistemological framework for medical knowledge-based systems. IEEE Trans Syst Man Cybernet 22:1361.

Schmid R. 1987. An expert system for the classification of dizziness and vertigo. In J Fox et al (eds), AIME 87: Proceedings of the European Conference on Artificial Intelligence in Medicine, Lecture Notes in Medical Informatics, pp 45–53. Berlin, Springer-Verlag.

Schreiber ATh, van Heijst G, Lanzola G, Stefanelli M. 1993. Knowledge organisation in medical KBS construction. In S Andreassen et al (eds), Artificial Intelligence in Medicine, pp 394–405. Amsterdam, IOS Press.

Shoham Y. 1993. Agent-oriented programming. Artif Intell 60:51.

Shortliffe EH. 1976. Computer-Based Medical Consultations: MYCIN. New York: American Elsevier.

Sowa JF. 1984. Conceptual Structures: Information Processing in Mind and Machine. Reading, Mass, Addison-Wesley.

Steels L. 1990. Components of expertise. AI Magazine, Summer 1990.

Stefanelli M. 1993. European research efforts in medical knowledge-based systems. Artif Intell Med 5:107.

Weiss SM, Kulikowski C, Safir A. 1978. Glaucoma consultation by computer. Comput Biol Med 8(1):25.

Zadeh LA. 1978. PRVF: A meaning representation language for natural "languages." Inter J of Man Machine Studies 4:395–460.

Further Information

Artificial Intelligence in Medicine is a bimonthly journal published by Elsevier Science Publishers. This international journal publishes articles concerning the theory and practice of medical artificial intelligence. Of particular interest is the special issue *ARTMED* 5(2):89–184, which was published in April 1993. Five articles are presented in this issue which present the state of the art and discuss future directions of the field.

The Addison-Wesley Series in Artificial Intelligence also represents an important source of information, among which is *Readings in Medical Artificial Intelligence*, a book edited by W. J. Clancey and E. H. Shortliffe in 1984.

Studies in Health Technology and Informatics is a series published by IOS Press, in which the proceedings of the 4th Conference on Artificial Intelligence in Medicine Europe, edited by S. Andreassen, R. Engelbrecht and J. Wyatt in 1993, gives an excellent outlook of the most recent advances of the field throughout Europe.

A good introduction to knowledge acquisition may be found in *Knowledge Acquisition: Principles and Guidelines*, by K. L. McGraw and K. Harbison-Briggs (Prentice-Hall, 1989). The book is meant to provide a practical view of the knowledge-acquisition process, its methodologies, and techniques, based on experiences building large and small expert systems in research and industrial settings.

188

Knowledge-Based Systems for Intelligent Patient Monitoring and Management in Critical Care Environments

Benoit M. Dawant
Vanderbilt University

Patient monitoring and control in critical care environments such as intensive care units (ICUs) and operating rooms (ORs) involve estimating the status of the patient, reacting to events that may be life-threatening, and taking actions to bring the patient to a desired state. It is a complex process involving physicians, nurses, and a wide variety of information ranging from clinical observations to laboratory results to on-line data provided by bedside monitoring and life-supporting equipment. New on-line monitoring devices provide the health care professionals with unsurpassed amounts of information to support his or her decision. Ironically, rather than facilitating the task of these professionals, the amount of information generated and the way this information is presented may overload their cognitive skills and lead to erroneous conclusions and inadequate actions. New solutions and systems are thus called for to manage and process the continuous stream of information and provide the health care professionals with efficient and reliable decision support tools.

Patient monitoring and management can be conceptually organized in four layers [Coiera, 1993]: (1) the *signal level,* concerned with the acquisition and low-level processing of the raw data, (2) the *validation level,* in charge of removing artifacts from the data, (3) the *signal-to-symbol transformation level,* which maps detected features to symbols such as normal, low, or high, and (4) the *inference level,* which relies on the existence of physiologic and pathophysiologic models to derive possible diagnoses, explanations of observed behaviors, predictions about future pathophysiologic states, or control actions. In addition to these four layers, systems designed to assist the health care professionals also need to be fitted with carefully designed interfaces to provide them with the information needed for rapid and accurate situation assessment.

A number of systems have been developed over the years to address some of the problems faced by clinicians in critical care environments. These range from low-level signal analysis algorithms for the detection of specific features in the monitored signals to complete architectures for signal acquisition, processing, interpretation, and advice giving. As always, specificity and generality are conflicting requirements. Systems developed for a specific application are usually successful in their limited domain of expertise. Generalization of the lessons and problem-solving strategies learned in one domain are, however, difficult to transfer to others. Generic architectures, on the other hand, aim at providing support for modeling and developing a wider range of applications. Flexibility, modularity, and ease of expansion are objectives guiding their development. Often, these architectures do, however, sacrifice specificity for flexibility and ease of expansion [Uckun, 1993]. This chapter will review some of the problems associated with each of these layers and systems that have been proposed to address these difficulties.

188.1 Intelligent Patient Monitoring and Management

Signal Acquisition and Low-Level Processing

Signals typically available in critical care environments include vital signs (ECG, EEG, arterial pressure, intracranial pressure, etc.) and information provided by therapeutic devices, infusion pumps, and drainage devices. Beside raw information, modern monitoring devices are also capable of providing derived and computed data. In heavily instrumented patients, it is not rare to see up to 20 medical devices producing up to 100 pieces of clinically relevant information. More often than not, these instruments are still stand-alone, and their interconnection requires the in-house development of dedicated software. To address this problem, the IEEE standards committee IEEE P1073 has been working since 1984 on developing a standard for handling data communication within critical care environments (Fig. 188.1). This project aims at developing standards for vendor-independent real-time interconnection of medical devices. Although this committee has been working for over 10 years, and despite long-term efforts by individual institutions [Gardner et al., 1992], a standard adhered to by major medical devices manufacturers is still lacking. This lack of interconnectivity remains a major obstacle to the development, implementation, and fielding of intelligent monitoring systems capable of using the redundancy and complementarity of the information provided by the bedside instruments.

Current bedside monitors provide information about instantaneous values for the monitored variables. To complement this information, numerous algorithms have been proposed to detect features in the signals. In particular, the detection of significant trends has received a lot of attention in the last few years. A review of trend-detection methods can be found in Avent and Charlton [1990]. Since then, methods based on median filters [Makivirta et al., 1991] and fuzzy logic [Sittig et al., 1992; Steinman and Adlassnig, 1994] also have been proposed. However, because trend detection is relatively new in critical care environments, interpreting the output of these algorithms and assessing the clinical significance of the information they provide is an ongoing task.

Data Validation

As the amount of acquired information increases, so does the risk of noise contamination, inadequate wiring, or instrument failure. In very dynamic situations, unreliable information drastically reduces the capability of the practitioner to rapidly assess the situation and to take appropriate actions. Similarly, the repeated occurrence of false alarms reduces the confidence he or she puts in the instrumentation, often leading to the complete disabling of bedside instrument alarms. To address these problems, validation of the information and so-called intelligent alarming schemes are currently being developed.

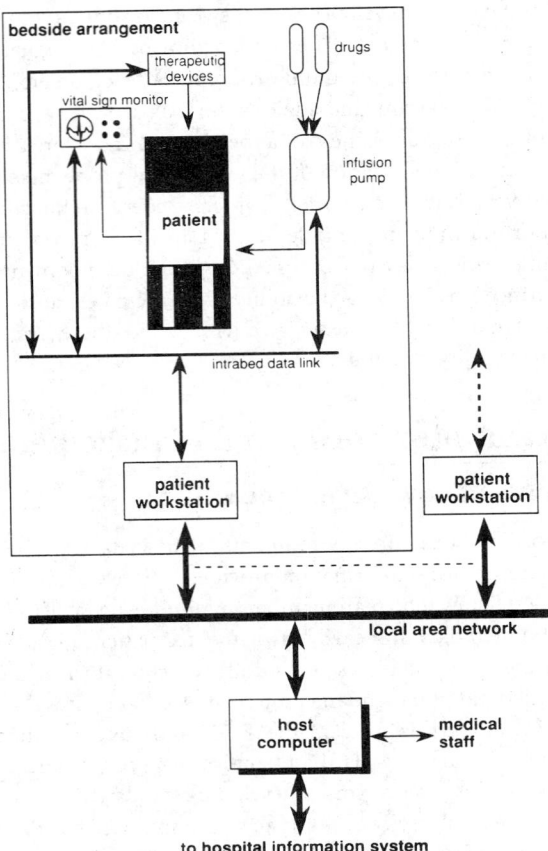

FIGURE 188.1   IEEE Standard IEEE P1073 proposition for handling data communication problems within critical care environments. (Reprinted from Mora et al. [1993].)

Methods relying on data redundancy and correlation (and thus assuming some level of interconnectivity between bedside instruments) as well as contextual information to eliminate false alarms, validate data, and diagnose malfunctions in the monitoring equipment have been proposed. Rule-based systems [Jiang, 1991; van der Aa, 1990] and neural networks [Orr, 1991] have been developed for detecting faults and malfunctions in the breathing circuit during anesthesia. Garfinkel et al. [1989] have implemented a rule-based approach for intelligent alarming for respiratory and circulation management in the operating room. Navabi et al. [1991] used a combination of heuristic rules and neural networks to integrate information from various monitors in the operating room and to reduce the number of false alarms. Arcay et al. [1993] propose a rule-based real-time system capable of modifying the frequency at which it acquires and process data, depending on patient status. Schecke et al. [1992] have developed a rule-based system combined with a fuzzy-logic scheme to handle uncertainty for patient monitoring in cardioanesthesia. Their system is also capable of providing therapy recommendations. Laursen [1994] relies on causal probabilistic networks to eliminate false alarms in the ICU. In addition to these systems specifically designed for data validation and false-alarm rejection, diagnostic and advice-giving systems (see next subsection) often include a data-validation step in their overall strategy.

The setting of appropriate and dynamic alarming thresholds is also an area of active research. These thresholds are the result of a compromise. Alarm levels should be narrow enough to alert the physician as soon as the behavior of monitored variables departs from their expected course. They should be wide enough to reduce the number of false and spurious alarms. To be most efficient, these levels should not only be adjusted for every patient to reflect demographic information, patient history, and diagnosis information, but they should also be adjusted dynamically to reflect the evolution of the patient or the intended effect of therapeutic actions.

Signal-to-Symbol Transformation and Advice Giving

The next level in the information flow involves transforming numerical values into symbolic information and the use of these symbols for diagnosis and advice giving. An exhaustive review of systems developed for patient management and advice giving is outside the scope of this chapter, but a representative sample of these systems is discussed for illustration purposes. For a more complete compilation, the reader is referred to Uckun [1993]. Although a strict taxonomy of diagnostic and advice-giving systems is difficult to create, systems with so-called shallow and deep knowledge will be distinguished. *Shallow* knowledge expresses empirically based, experiential knowledge [Mora et al., 1993] generally called *heuristics*. Reasoning in these systems is mostly associative, and the knowledge they contain is usually represented in terms of IF (antecedent) THEN (action) form. Systems developed following this formalism exhibit a high degree of competence in their limited domain of application. Their major disadvantage, however, is a rapid performance degradation for problems at the edge of their area of expertise. At the other end of the spectrum, *deep* knowledge refers to knowledge about the structure, behavior, or function of a system. Model-based reasoning involves using this knowledge to diagnose, predict, or explain the behavior of the system over time.

Shallow Knowledge Systems

These systems are typically designed to perform a very specific task and follow the same general architecture: a module responsible for transforming quantitative data into qualitative or symbolic information, a module capable of translating symbolic information into patient state, and a module designed to provide therapeutic advice based on the estimated patient state.

Among the tasks facing intensive care clinicians and following the pioneering efforts of Fagan et al. [1984] on the VM project, the problem of ventilator management is the one that has received the most attention over the years. VM was developed in the late 1970s as an extension of the rule-based MYCIN formalism to interpret on-line quantitative data in the ICU setting and to provide assistance for postoperative patients undergoing mechanical ventilation. VM addressed the important problem of adjusting the interpretation of the data in light of the patient status.

Compas [Sittig et al., 1989] was designed to provide assistance for the management of patients with adult respiratory distress syndrome (ARDS). It was built following the blackboard architecture and has three major types of knowledge sources (KS): (1) the data-processing KSs are in charge of computing derived information from the primary data (e.g., computing cardiopulmonary parameters), (2) the data-classification KSs transform numerical information into symbolic information, and (3) the protocol-instruction KSs suggest therapeutic actions. A rule-based formalism has been used to represent the necessary knowledge. The raw data level of Compas consists of information provided by clinical or blood gas laboratories, x-ray departments, and respiratory therapists. Compas is not in use any more. The knowledge it contains has, however, served as a basis for a system that is now in routine clinical use [Henderson et al., 1992].

AIRS (an Artificial Intelligent Respirator System) provides three levels of decision support to match three phases of ventilation [Summers et al., 1993]: (1) the startup phase of ventilatory support, which matches the patient state to one of 14 predetermined patient states and recommends initial ventilator settings, (2) the maintain phase provides context-dependent values for setpoint and trend alarms, and (3) the weaning phase contains knowledge represented as premise-actions rules in PROLOG to provide advice in the weaning process. The weaning module is the most knowledge-intensive component in AIRS. Its rule base is organized into four main categories: the weaning, progression, regression, and termination rules. These rules are used to move the patient from CMV (controlled mandatory ventilation) to spontaneous breathing through a series of intermediate states of synchronized intermittent mandatory ventilation (SIMV). AIRS is currently working off-line and is being evaluated retrospectively.

Vie-Vent [Miksch et al., 1993] is an advice-giving system for the monitoring and management of mechanically ventilated neonates. It consists of three modules. The data-acquisition and validation module performs simple range checking and measurements correlation, and the data-abstraction module translates numerical values into normal, low, and high ranges based on predetermined transformation rules. These rules are adapted to reflect the site of measurement and the mode of ventilation. Based on qualitative values for pH, P_{CO_2}, and P_{O_2}, the rule-based therapy-planning module proposes ventilator settings. Vie-Vent is connected to the mechanical ventilator and receives data every 10 seconds. The system is currently being clinically evaluated.

Patricia [Moreet-Bonillo et al., 1993] is a system designed to assist in monitoring and managing mechanically ventilated patients in ICUs. It consists of two main components: the deterministic and the heuristic modules. The deterministic module transforms incoming information into symbolic ranges. It uses so-called natural contexts, which include demographic information, patient history, and diagnosis information, to provide patient-dependent ranges for the symbolic variables. Based on these symbolic values, the rule-based heuristic module infers patient status and prescribes therapeutic advice. The system performs data validation both in the deterministic and the heuristic modules. It is also capable of determining prealarm situations by checking the temporal evolution of the monitored parameters. Patricia underwent a retrospective evaluation study and is still working off-line.

Other systems developed for ventilator management include ESTER [Hernandez-Sande et al., 1989], KUSIVAR [Rudowski et al., 1989] developed for the management of patients with acute ARDS, and WEANPRO [Tong, 1991] designed for assisting physicians in weaning postoperative cardiovascular patients. Expert-system methodology also has been applied to the monitoring and management of patients in the cardiac care unit (CCU) [Mora et al., 1993].

As opposed to the systems discussed before, GANESH [Dojat et al., 1992] has been designed to be used as a closed-loop controller. Its domain of application is the weaning of patients under pressure-supported ventilation (PSV). Based on the respiratory rate, tidal volume, and end-tidal partial pressure of carbon dioxide, a rule-based controller determines the patient status, determines the action to be taken, and acts on the ventilator. Preliminary clinical evaluation of the system has shown its ability to maintain patients in the region of comfort and to progressively reduce the pressure of weanable patients.

Blom [1991] also proposes the use of an expert-system approach for the closed-loop control of arterial pressure during surgery. In this approach, heuristic rules supervise a PID controller and adjust its parameters. This approach results in a robust controller capable of coping with artifacts in the signal, low signal-to-noise ratio, and patient sensitivity to sodium nitroprusside used to achieve controlled hypotension during surgery.

Deep Knowledge Systems

Despite its advantage over associative reasoning for explanation robustness, and prediction, model-based reasoning has been used in only few medical systems. In a recent review of model-based reasoning in medicine, Uckun [1992] suggests that the cause may be attributed to the relatively shallow level of knowledge we have about most disease processes and the complexity and inherent variability of human anatomy, physiology, and pathophysiology. These difficulties still challenge our ability to develop accurate models, be they quantitative, qualitative, or hybrid. Despite the difficulties involved, several model-based reasoning systems have been proposed for patient monitoring.

VentPlan [Rutledge et al., 1993] is a system designed to make recommendations for ventilator settings in the ICU. It has three main components: a belief network, a mathematical modeling module, and a plan evaluator. The belief network is used to compute probability distributions for the physiologic model parameters from qualitative and quantitative information. Using these and the value of the ventilator settings, the model predicts the distribution of future values for the dependent variables. This approach offers the capability to simulate the evolution of important variables under various ventilator settings and thus to evaluate proposed therapy plans. The plan evaluator uses predictions for Pa_{CO_2} and oxygen delivery to rank therapy plans according to a multiattribute scoring system and to propose ventilator settings.

Coiera [1989] proposes the use of QSIM [Kuipers, 1986] to diagnose acid-base balance disturbances. He has developed an approach in which the temporal behavior of several diseases (called *disease histories*) are simulated independently. The global behavior of interacting disease histories is obtained with a new technique that permits the addition of qualitative histories. The main advantage of this approach over traditional QSIM applications is that individual disease behaviors can be identified within the complete interaction behavior. The diagnose of acid-base balance disturbances was presented as a proof of principle for this approach, and the system only underwent a limited retrospective evaluation.

The patient model component of SIMON [Uckun et al., 1993; Dawant et al., 1993] is built on an extension of the qualitative process theory (QPT) [Forbus, 1984]. It has been developed for the diagnosis of neonates suffering from respiratory distress syndrome (RDS), to predict the patient's evolution, and to provide a monitoring context used to adjust alarm limits and thresholds. As opposed to QPT, this modeling approach does not produce a total envisionment (i.e., a prediction of all qualitatively distinct states the system may reach), which is of little use in an environment in which external variables (ventilator settings) do not remain constant. It also uses numerical information for prediction and ambiguity resolution, it permits the use of history information for diagnosing patient status based on the temporal evolution of clinical events, and it permits modification of the model based on discrepancies between observed and predicted values. As was the case for the previous system, the approach only underwent a limited retrospective evaluation.

KARDIO [Lavrac et al., 1985] and CARDIOLAB [Siregar et al., 1993] are examples of models developed for model-based ECG simulation, prediction, and interpretation. Based on the relation between the ECG and 30 elementary arrhythmias, KARDIO is used to generate a qualitative description of the ECG signal corresponding to various possible combinations of arrhythmias. Using this model, 2419 possible arrhythmias and 140,966 ECG descriptions were automatically generated. Observed ECGs can then be compared with the generated descriptions, and the associated arrhythmias can be retrieved from the database. Without a model permitting its automatic generation, the creation of an exhaustive database associating arrhythmias with ECG description would be a daunting, if not impossible, task. In its current state, KARDIO cannot be used on-line because it relies on the qualitative description of the ECG signal for its inference. CARDIOLAB is designed as a simulator and a tool for reasoning about cardiac processes. The heart model of CARDIOLAB relies on a qualitative-analog approach. It consists of 21 of interconnected components representing nodal and muscle tissues. Parameters driving the dynamics of each element can be determined by the user, and adjacent components interact by means of "inferrent impulses." The response of a component to an impulse is a function of both its state and the value of its prespecified parameters. Although CARDIOLAB can be used for what-if simulation, it cannot be used to provide diagnoses given an ECG recording. To do so, the authors suggest that their model could be used to generate (arrhythmia-ECG descriptions) pairs, as was KARDIO.

188.2 Toward Computer Architectures for Real-Time Intelligent Monitoring

The discussion so far has highlighted the fact that patient monitoring is a complex and multifaceted task and that many years of research have been invested to address and propose solutions to facilitate the tasks of health care professionals. Yet, despite such efforts, only some of the systems described earlier are in limited clinical use in the institution in which they were developed. None of them has been fielded and tested in other institutions. This may be imputed to the specificity of these systems and to the difficulty of modifying their structure for slightly different applications. Rather than focusing on specific tasks, other researchers are attempting to develop generic architectures that can support the development and implementation of a wider range of applications. These architectures are designed to support diverse reasoning schemes, guarantee real-time response, and permit the integration of the entire spectrum of tasks required for intelligent patient monitoring and management. The following paragraphs describe systems that have been designed for this purpose.

GUARDIAN [Hayes-Roth et al., 1992] is a blackboard system. It was developed as an application of a general architecture for intelligent agents, and it is currently applied to respiratory and cardiovascular monitoring domains. This system emerges from a long history of research on reasoning and problem solving, and much emphasis is put on the generic problem of coordinating and selecting one among possible perceptual, cognitive, or action operation while maintaining real-time constraints. It is designed to integrate heuristic, structural, or functional knowledge of (1) common respiratory problems, (2) respiratory, circulatory, metabolic, and mechanical ventilator systems, and (3) generic flow, diffusion, and metabolic systems. Its tasks range from interpreting sensed data, detecting clinical events, predicting future states and events, planning therapy actions, explaining its reasoning, and carrying closed-loop control. The systems is capable of modifying the priority of these tasks and performing the most critical ones while maintaining real-time response. The system is currently running in a simulated intensive care environment.

The Intelligent Cardiovascular Monitor (ICM) [Factor et al., 1991] is an application of the multitrellis software architecture to cardiovascular monitoring. The multitrellis software architecture supports the modeling of real-time tasks in terms of an acyclic hierarchical network of decision processes. Each decision process can be arbitrarily complex and involves its own problem-solving strategy. In the ICM application, the lowest level corresponds to the raw data, and information is abstracted along the hierarchy in a way reminiscent of the information flow in a blackboard architecture. The highest level corresponds to physiologic processes or events. Processes at the lowest level implement signal-processing algorithms for the extraction of features from the signal. Processes at higher levels contain knowledge and combination rules to interpret the output of lower-level processes. As opposed to GUARDIAN, the process trellis architecture assumes sufficient resources to execute the entire program and meet real-time constraints. The multitrellis software architecture has also been used for the development of DYNASCENE [Cohn et al., 1990]. DYNASCENE models the occurrence of hemodynamic abnormalities in terms of "scenes" and temporal relationships between scenes. Each scene corresponds to one physiologic process (e.g., increased pericardial pressure) and is related to modules designed to compute specific information from the incoming data. Neither DYNASCENE nor the ICM are fitted with patient models and are thus incapable of predicting patient behavior.

SIMON [Dawant et al., 1993] is a framework designed to support the development of real-time intelligent patient monitoring systems. It is organized around three main modules: the patient model, the data-acquisition and abstraction module, and a reconfigurable user interface. The patient model is responsible for (1) estimating the physiologic state of the patient, (2) predicting the temporal evolution of the monitored variables, and (3) providing the system with a monitoring *context*. The context includes normal and abnormal ranges for monitored variables, expected temporal evolutions of these variables, significant values and patterns to be detected in the incoming signals (events), and display configuration information (i.e., critical information to be displayed). The data-abstraction module uses the context to adjust alarm limits and thresholds and to implement strategies to detect the specified events. These may involve one or several variables and temporal relationships between events detected on each individual variable. SIMON is also capable of scheduling its activity to maintain real-time response and to dedicate its resources to the most crucial tasks. SIMON has been applied to the problem of monitoring neonates in the intensive care unit.

Following the recommendations of the INFORM project [Hunter et al., 1991], Sukuvaara et al. [1994] propose an object-oriented framework to implement systems based on the blackboard approach to problem solving. Data on the blackboard are separated into four main categories: source data (i.e., data acquired from the monitoring instruments as well as diagnostic, demographic, or laboratory data), preprocessed variables, physiologically interpreted variables, and patient status. Preprocessing knowledge sources span the two first levels and extract features from the incoming data (long- and short-term trends, instantaneous value, etc.). Transformation knowledge sources span the second and third levels in the blackboard hierarchy. They map values of preprocessed variables in a $[-1, 1]$ interval. In this scheme, -1 indicates an extremely low value and $+1$ an extremely high value. Patient state assessment knowledge sources get their input from the physiologically interpreted data and determine the patient state. The system also assumes sufficient resources to execute all its knowledge sources and meet real-time constraints.

188.3 Discussion and Conclusions

As discussed in the introduction, intelligent patient monitoring and management are complex tasks involving all aspects of information processing. They necessitate the context-dependent acquisition, processing, analysis, and interpretation of large amounts of possibly noisy and incomplete data. Systems described in this chapter all address some of the issues involved with intelligent patient monitoring and control systems. All of them fall short of addressing every aspect.

Intelligent alarm systems typically focus on a few subsystems and correlate information in a purely bottom-up fashion. Feedback from upper layers is not used to provide the alarm detection schemes with contextual information related to patient status, thus reducing their specificity. Dynamic information with the exception of simple trend information is also rarely utilized. Systems designed to transform quantitative information into symbols and to provide advice often assume the availability of reliable information, as if the problem of artifact rejection was a solved issue. Complete and robust artifact rejection schemes, however, will require a synergy between the low-level signal-processing stage and the system's component responsible for establishing the overall monitoring context.

The systems presented in this chapter illustrate the fact that, in the case of patient monitoring, the choice between specificity and generality is not an easy one. Systems that have been clinically evaluated or are being evaluated are typically developed for a very narrow, specific application for which rule-based systems are well adapted. Often too narrow in scope, however, these systems are of limited clinical utility. Research aiming at developing deeper models from which a wider range of behaviors can be inferred, on the other hand, has failed to produce convincing results. While it is clear that models capable of predicting patient behavior or response to therapeutic actions or capable of supporting what-if scenarios are desirable, none are available today except for very limited and constrained situations. Original modeling methods and approaches have been proposed, but assumptions are generally made that either drastically reduce the scope of the model or make it unrealistic for clinical purposes.

Complete architectures aim at identifying the essence of patient monitoring tasks and at providing support for the development of a class of systems. These systems should permit experimentation with a number of problem-solving strategies, the integration of diverse reasoning mechanisms, and should ultimately be capable of spanning the entire spectrum of tasks required for efficient and reliable patient monitoring. However, to move from the research laboratory to the clinical arena, these systems will have to be fitted with rich and flexible modeling tools capable of overcoming the complexity of generic architectures.

Reflecting on the fact that despite years of research and development, intelligent monitoring systems have failed to make a significant impact on the quality of patient care, Coiera [1994] suggests that current systems are not adapted to their task. He notices that a major effort has been put into developing systems assisting the physician in making diagnoses and taking therapeutic actions. He suggests, however, that the main problem facing health care professionals is not choice (i.e., diagnostic or selection of therapeutic actions) but rather establishing a clear picture of the world leading to these choices. Following this observation, he advocates the creation of a "task" layer designed to provide a good match between displayed information and the cognitive processes of physicians and nurses. More research on the way clinicians interact with intelligent monitoring devices is, however, necessary to support the design of these interfaces.

The design of intelligent monitoring systems is thus an ongoing task. The context-based acquisition, processing, analysis, and display of the information are an essential concept in these systems. Elements defining this context are, however, diverse. On the one hand, patient status and history define one interpretation and monitoring context. This context can be used to determine normal and abnormal limit values, trends, normal relations between observed variables, as well as significant events to be detected in the signals. Models could automatically establish these contexts, which, in turn, could be used to configure the monitoring system. On the other hand, the cognitive tasks (e.g., trying to assess pulmonary or cardiac function, etc.) the clinician is facing dictate the type and form of the information to be presented. This information-processing context may be more difficult to automate and will require the development of good interaction mechanisms between the system and its users. The successful development and acceptance of new generations of monitoring devices will thus be possible only through a tight cooperative effort between systems designers and users.

References

Arcay-Varela B, Hernandez-Sande C. 1993. Adaptive monitoring in the ICU: A dynamic and contextual study. J Clin Eng 18(1):67.

Avent RK, Charlton JD. 1990. A critical review of trend-detection methodologies for biomedical monitoring systems. Crit Rev Biomed Eng 17(6):621.

Blom JA. 1991. Expert control of the arterial blood pressure during surgery. Int J Clin Monit Comput 8(1):25.

Coiera EW. 1989. Reasoning with qualitative disease histories for diagnostic patient monitoring. Ph.D. dissertation, School of Engineering and Computer Science, University of New South Wales.

Coiera EW. 1993. Intelligent monitoring and control of dynamic systems. Artif Intell Med 5:1.

Coiera EW. 1994. Designing for decision support in a clinical monitoring environment. In Proceedings of the International Conference on Medical Physics and Biomedical Engineering, Nicosia, Cyprus, pp 130–142.

Cohn AI, Rosenbaum S, Factor M, Miller PL. 1990. DYNASCENE: An approach to computer-based intelligent cardiovascular monitoring using sequential scenes. Methods Inform Med 29:122.

Dawant BM, Uckun S, Manders EJ, Lindstrom DP. 1993. The SIMON project: Model-based signal acquisition, analysis, and interpretation in intelligent patient monitoring, IEEE Eng Med Biol Mag 12(4):92.

Dojat M, Brohard L, Lemaire F, Harf A. 1992. A knowledge-based system for assisted ventilation of patients in intensive care units. Int J Clin Monit Comput 9:239.

Factor M, Gelertner DH, Kolb CE, et al. 1991. Real-time data fusion in the intensive care unit. IEEE Comput 24(11):45.

Fagan LM, Shortliffe EH, Buchanan BG. 1984. Computer-based medical decision making: From MYCIN to VM. In WJ Clancey, EH Shortliffe (eds), Readings in Medical Artificial Intelligence: The First Decade, pp 241–255. Reading, Mass, Addison-Wesley.

Forbus KD. 1984. Qualitative process theory. Ph.D. dissertation, Massachusetts Institute of Technology, Cambridge.

Gardner RM, Hawley WL, East TD, et al. 1992. Real time data acquisition: Recommendations for the medical information bus (MIB). Int J Clin Monit Comput 8:251.

Garfinkel D, Matsiras P, Lecky JH, et al. 1988. PONI: An intelligent alarm system for respiratory and circulation management in the operating rooms. In Proceedings of the 12th Symposium on Computer Applications in Medical Care, pp 13–17.

Hayes-Roth B, Washington R, Ash D, et al. 1992. Guardian: A prototype intelligent agent for intensive-care monitoring. Artif Intell Med 4:165.

Henderson S, Crapo RO, Wallace CJ, et al. 1992. Performance of computerized protocols for the management of arterial oxygenation in an intensive care unit. Int J Clin Monit Comput 8:271.

Hernandez-Sande C, Moret-Bonillo V, Alonzo-Betanos A. 1989. ESTER: An expert system for management of respiratory weaning therapy. IEEE Trans Biomed Eng 36(5):559.

Hunter J, Chambrin M-C, Collinson P, et al. 1991. INFORM: Integrated support for decisions and activities in intensive care. Int J Clin Monit Comput 8:189.

Jiang A. 1991. The design and development of a knowledge-based ventilatory and respiratory monitoring system. Ph.D. dissertation, Department of Biomedical Engineering, Vanderbilt University.

Kuipers B. 1986. Qualitative simulation. Artif Intell 29:289.

Laursen P. 1994. Event detection on patient monitoring data using causal probabilistic networks. Methods Inform Med 33:111.

Lavrac N, Bratko I, Mozetic I, et al. 1985. KARDIO-E: An expert system for electrocardiographic diagnosis of cardiac arrhythmias. Expert Syst 2(1):46.

Makivirta A, Koski E, Kari A, Sukuvaara T. 1991. The median filter as a preprocessor for a patient monitor limit alarm system in intensive care. Comput Methods Progr Biomed 34:139.

Miksch S, Horn W, Popow C, Paky F. 1993. VIE-VENT: Knowledge-based monitoring and therapy planning of the artificial ventilator of newborn infants. In Andreassen S, et al (eds), Artificial Intelligence in Medicine: Proceedings of the 4th European Conference (AIME-93), pp 218–229. Amsterdam, IOS Press.

Mora A, Passariello G, Carrault G, Le Pichon J-P. 1993. Intelligent patient monitoring and management systems: A review. IEEE Eng Med Biol Mag 12(4):23.

Moret-Bonillo V, Alonso-Betanos A, Martin EG, et al. 1993. The PATRICIA project: A semantic-based methodology fore intelligent monitoring in the ICU. IEEE Eng Med Biol Mag 12(4):59.

Navabi MJ, Watt RC, Hamerof SR, Mylrea KC. 1991. Integrated monitoring can detect critical events and improve alarm accuracy. 16(4):295.

Orr JA. 1991. An anesthesia alarm system based on neural networks. Ph.D. dissertation, University of Utah.

Rudowski R, Frostell C, Gill H. 1989. A knowledge-based support system for mechanical ventilation of the lungs: The Kusivar concept and prototype. Comput Methods Progr Biomed 30:59.

Rutledge GW, Thomsen GE, Farr BR, et al. 1993. The design and implementation of a ventilator-management advisor. Artif Intell Med 5(1):67.

Schecke T, Langen M, Popp H-S, et al. 1992. Knowledge-based decision support for patient monitoring in cardioanesthesia. Int J Clin Monit Comput 9:1.

Siregar P, Coatrieux JL, Mabo P. 1993. How can deep knowledge be used in CCU monitoring. IEEE Eng Med Biol Mag 12(4):92.

Sittig DF, Pace NL, Gardner RM, et al. 1989. Implementation of a computerized patient advice system using the HELP clinical information system. Comput Biomed Res 22:474.

Sittig DF, Cheung K-H, Berman L. 1992. Fuzzy classification of hemodynamic trends and artifacts: Experiments with heart rate. Int J Clin Monit Comput 9:251.

Steinman F, Adlassnig K-P. 1994. Clinical monitoring with fuzzy automata. Fuzzy Sets Syst 61:37.

Sukuvaara T, Sydanma M, Nieminen H, et al. 1993. Object-oriented implementation of an architecture for patient monitoring. IEEE Eng Med Biol Mag 12(4):69.

Summers R, Carson ER, Cramp DG. 1993. Ventilator management: The role of knowledge-based technology. IEEE Eng Med Biol Mag 12(4):50.

Tong DA. 1991. Weaning patients from mechanical ventilation: A knowledge-based systems approach. Comput Methods Progr Biomed 35:267.

Uckun S. 1992. Model-based reasoning in biomedicine. Crit Rev Biomed Eng 19(4):261.

Uckun S, Dawant BM, Lindstrom DP. 1993. Model-based diagnosis in intensive care monitoring: The YAQ approach. Artif Intell Med 5:31.

Uckun S. 1993. Intelligent systems in patient monitoring and therapy management: A survey of research projects. Technical report KSL 93-32, Knowledge Systems Laboratory, Stanford University.

van der Aa JJ. 1990. Intelligent alarms in anesthesia: A real time expert system application. Ph.D. dissertation, Division of Medical Electrical Engineering, Eindhoven University of Technology.

Windyga P, Almeida D, Passariello G, et al. 1991. Knowledge-based approach to the management of serious arrhythmia in the CCU. Med Biol Eng Comput 29:254.

189

Medical Terminology and Diagnosis Using Knowledge Bases

Peter L. M. Kerkhof
University of Utrecht

... this man with two blue hands and abnormal blood gases and a negative chest x-ray. And high blood pressure.... [one physician] said he didn't know what the hell was going on. Would I take a look at him? Just a curbside consultation—that's all. Just an opinion. I said O.K.—be glad to. It was entirely appropriate. I was a physician of record.

From Two Blue Hands, by Berton Roueché

The basic goal of the use of computers in medicine concerns communication between human beings via an electronic medium; this medium is expected to enhance and facilitate such interaction. In the example given by Roueché, the consulting physician could be replaced by a computer system that stores and handles information that was previously obtained from a number of experts in various medical specialties. Ideally, the victim described here carries a patient data card which in an emergency case presents valuable information to the physician. The Medical Records Institute [1981] is an instrumental force in the movement toward an electronic patient record.

In technical jargon, this computer-mediated process has been clearly described by Williams [1982]: Knowledge-base (KB) systems are used for interpretation of data about a specific problem, in the light of knowledge represented in the KB, to develop a problem-specific model and then to construct plans for problem solution. The KB contains the descriptive or factual knowledge pertaining to the domain of interest. Candidate hypotheses are then derived through some pattern-matching system. Next, a reasoning "engine" (also termed *inference machine*) carries out the manipulation specified to reach a decision.

Williams [1982] continues that knowledge obviously can be represented in several ways; it can be characterized by symbols, plain words, definitions, and their interrelations. Knowledge may be expressed by spoken or written words, flowcharts, (mathematical) equations, tables, figures, and so forth, depending on the level of abstraction.

Aspects of language and text interpretation are central issues in artificial intelligence (AI). Language is regarded as a metaphor of thought. When it provides the primary abstraction of knowledge about reality, then it seems reasonable to expect that a powerful abstraction of language also should provide a powerful representation of knowledge. Various strategies have been explored. Semantic networks offer a versatile tool for representing knowledge of virtually any type that can be captured in words by employing nodes (representing things) and links (referring to meaningful relationships between things), thus expressing causal, temporal, taxonomic, and associational connections. Other approaches (such as frame systems and production systems) also have been investigated. *Conceptual graphs* [Sowa, 1984] are an emerging standard for knowledge representation (ANSI X3H4), and the method is particularly suited to the representation of natural-language semantics.

An ideal medical KB must be comprehensive (while integrating text, graphics, video, and sound), accurate and verifiable, easily accessible where doctors see patients, and the system should be adaptable to the doctors' own preferred terms or abbreviations [Wyatt, 1991]. Future developments will certainly include the use of artificial neural networks [Baxt, 1991], and examples realized thus far include myocardial infarction, diabetes mellitus, epilepsy, bone fracture healing, appendicitis, dermatology diagnosis, and EEG topography recognition.

This chapter addresses several approaches employed to represent medical definitions and knowledge. First, a survey will be presented on available coding systems, and next, an overview is given of current KB systems that primarily refer to the process of establishing a diagnosis. Finally, an anthology concerning problems related to medical terminology is presented, along with directions for solving them.

189.1 Classification and Coding Systems

With the exception of one British system, all classification or coding systems have been developed in the United States. This survey lists all projects along with some of their characteristics.

- The ICD [International Classification of Diseases, 1978] system now enters its tenth version. With approximately 8000 codes in the ninth edition, it is applied worldwide for classifying diagnoses and also permits DRG (diagnosis-related group) assignment employed for billing and reimbursement purposes.

- Another widely accepted system is called SNOMED [Systematized Nomenclature of Medicine, 1993], which offers a structured nomenclature and classification for use in human as well as in veterinary medicine. Currently, it consists of 11 modules with multiple hierarchies covering about 132,600 records, with a printed as well as a CD-ROM version available.

- CPT [Physicians' Current Procedural Terminology, 1992] provides uniform language for diagnostic as well as surgical and other interventional services. The system now presents its fourth edition, which is distributed by the American Medical Association (AMA) and has been incorporated in the Medicare program.

- MeSH [1993] is a systematic terminology hierarchy that is used to index the MEDLINE medical publications system. It forms the standard for coding keywords related to the contents of articles in the field of medicine. The system is updated yearly and is expanded in accordance with the growth of knowledge in the medical field.

- The NLM (National Library of Medicine in Bethesda, Md.) in 1986 started a project called UMLS (Unified Medical Language System) [Lindberg et al., 1993]. The project aims to address the fundamental information-access problem caused by the variety of independently constructed vocabularies and classifications used in different sources of machine-readable biomedical information. The UMLS approach will be to compensate for differences in the terminologies or coding schemes used in different systems, as well as for differences in the language employed by system users, rather than to impose a single standard vocabulary on the biomedical community. The metathesaurus contains 311,000 terms and maintains cross-references to CPT [Physicians' CPT, 1992], ICD-9-CM [ICD, 1978], SNOMED [SNOMED, 1993], and other indexes. NLM encourages broad experimentation with the fourth edition, and the tools are (with certain provisions) available on the basis of a 1-year agreement. The complete files are distributed on four CD-ROMs, while the application programs are limited to browsing tools for the metathesaurus.

- Dr. Gabrieli [1992] constructed a computer-oriented medical nomenclature based on taxonomic principles. His system covers 150,000 preferred terms and a similar number of synonyms. The partitioning method employed for medical classification readily permits replacement of English names with terms of any other language, thus creating the perspective of a worldwide standard.

- Dr. Read from the United Kingdom designed a classification for various computer applications [Chisholm, 1990]. It is designed in accordance with six key criteria: to be comprehensive, hierarchical, coded, computerized, cross-referenced, and dynamic. The system is closely connected with the British NHS (National Health Service) and is presently not commercially available outside the United Kingdom. Version 2 includes 100,000 preferred terms, 250,000 codes, and 150,000 synonyms.

189.2 An Electronic Medical Encyclopedia at Your Fingertips: Knowledge Bases and Diagnosis

In our era, most information (as stored in written documents or computer records) consists of *natural-language text.* Traditional retrieval systems use sets of keywords (index terms). It is called a *full-text retrieval system* when all (nontrivial) words of that text are indexed for future identification during search procedures. Information requests can then be formulated with the aid of *boolean operators* (namely, *and, or, not*). Synonymous terms can be specified by employing the *or* operator. The *fuzzy-set retrieval model* still uses boolean logic but refines the query process by assigning different weight factors to the individual index terms. As an attractive alternative, the *vector space processing system* evaluates the similarity where both the index terms and the stored texts are represented by weighted-term vectors [Salton, 1991]. The assumption that index terms are independent (i.e., orthogonal vector space) obviously implies a shortcoming of this retrieval method.

Within the domain of medicine, various KB systems have been developed, and current systems will be briefly characterized here. Again, all projects in this area originate in the United States, with the exception of two (namely, OSM and Medwise). One approach (namely, CONSULTANT) addresses the field of veterinary medicine. A tabulated survey of the situation in the year 1987 has been published before [Kerkhof, 1987]. An occasional system is in the public domain, whereas others sell at a single-user price anywhere between $125 and $2000 depending on configuration, discount, and other factors.

- *CMIT,* developed by the American Medical Association [Finkel, 1981], forms a reference for the selection of preferred medical terms including certain synonyms and generic terms with built-in arrangements to provide maximum convenience in usage, currency, and timely publication. Thus CMIT is both a system of reference and a "distillate of a vast amount of medical knowledge." The system is available in electronic form.

- Blois was the first physician to apply CMIT as a diagnostic tool in his *RECONSIDER* project [Blois, 1984]. The application was released in 1981 and covered 3262 disease entities, while 21,415 search terms were listed in a directory along with their frequency of occurrence (which number served as an indicator of impact for each search term).

- *DXplain* [Barnett et al., 1987] is also based on CMIT [Finkel, 1981] and was released in 1986. The project had close connections with the AMA, and information was distributed using the

AMA/NET nationwide communications network. The KB contains information on 2000 diseases and understands over 4700 terms, with 65,000 disease-term relationships.

- *QMR* patient diagnostic software [Middleton, 1991] covers some 600 disease profiles and is the personal computer version of the INTERNIST-1 prototype. The program is versatile, easy to use, and offers an attractive user interface, but unfortunately, the size of its disease KB remained remarkably constant over the last few years.

- The program *MEDITEL* [Waxman and Worley, 1990] addresses the issue of diagnosis in adults and was marketed by Elsevier Publishers. Over the last few years, not much news was reported in the literature.

- *ILIAD* version 4.0 [Bergeron, 1991] is a popular software package designed to aid students and residents in their clinical decision logic. The ILIAD project is an outgrowth of the HELP (Health Evaluation through Logical Processes) system developed at LDS Hospital in Salt Lake City. The KB includes 1300 diseases and 5600 manifestations and is built on the experience of experts in nine subspecialties of internal medicine. The KB is updated semiannually for revision and expansion. Future versions will support access to video laser discs, thereby providing an actual view of x-rays, echocardiograms, skin lesions, and other physical findings.

- The *Oxford System of Medicine (OSM)* project was initiated by the Imperial Cancer Research Fund for use in primary care and to help general practitioners during routine clinical work to support decision-making tasks such as diagnosing illnesses, planning investigations and patient treatment schedules, prescribing drugs, screening for disease, assessing the risk of a particular disease, and determining referral to a specialist [Krause et al., 1993].

- *Medwise* is a medical KB founded in 1983 and now covering some 3900 disease entities, with 29,000 different keywords [Kerkhof et al., 1993b]. It includes a separate KB with almost 500 equivalent terms that each on average refer to three related terms, e.g., extremity, leg, and limb. Equivalents are automatically generated to assist the user during the process of data entry. The matrix structure of the Medwise KB permits semantic differentiation of particular observations, e.g., lymphadenopathy as detected during palpation versus lymphadenopathy as interpreted from an x-ray picture. In the Medwise system, both refer to different elements of the matrix, and their corresponding weight factors are individually incorporated when calculating the score for disease profile matching. For obvious reasons, the language employed is English, but a complete dictionary that offers translations into Dutch is available [Kerkhof, 1993].

- The *Framemed* system [Bishop and Ewing, 1993] divides medical information into 26 domains (comparable with the matrix in Medwise [Kerkhof et al., 1993]) and arranges the items in a hierarchical sequence; formation of the hierarchies yields a logical framework for a standardized terminology that is in the public domain. The objective is to achieve a standard coded terminology to which all existing systems can relate, with obvious use as an electronic encyclopedia and for differential diagnosis. Framemed offers synonyms and claims as an advantage a simple overall structure that facilitates updating.

- *STAT!-Ref* [STAT, 1994] offers the contents of a first-choice medical library (including several standard textbooks, e.g., on primary care) as well as Medline (either primary care, cardiology, or oncology) on CD-ROM.

- *MD-Challenger* [MD-Challenger, 1994] offers a clinical reference and educational software for acute care and emergency medicine (everything from abdominal pain to zygoapophyseal joint arthritis), with nearly 4000 annotated questions and literature references. The system also includes CME (Continuing Medical Education) credits.

- *Labsearch/286* is a differential diagnosis program allowing input of up to two abnormal laboratory findings plus information on symptoms and signs. Laboratory data concentrate on body fluids (blood, urine, cerebrospinal, ascitic, synovial, and pleural fluids) entered as high or low [Labsearch, 1994]. The system includes 6500 diseases and 9800 different findings. No details are available on its diagnostic performance, although the restriction of only two laboratory data certainly will limit its potential.

- Dr. White at Cornell University (in Ithaca, N.Y.) developed a KB for veterinary medicine, called *CONSULTANT* [White and Lewkowicz, 1987]. This database for computer-assisted diagnosis and information management is available on a fee-for-service basis and is actually used in hundreds of private practices and institutions in North America.

- *Griffith and Dambro* [1993] compiled a book (approximately $49.50 with more than 1150 pages) that is intended to be updated annually. The first edition appeared in 1993 and indeed contains a realm of chartlike presented practical information on a thousand topics with reference to their ICD-9-CM code. The preface duely states that the book aptly lends itself to publication using electronic media, and the reader is advised to watch for pertinent announcements. Although the index included in the book is fairly extensive, it yet may be anticipated that the retrieval potential will be formidably enhanced once digital searching strategies become available. Close inspection of the printed version discloses a striking similarity with CMIT [Finkel, 1981]; occasionally (e.g., page 162, which presents the causalgia syndrome: ICD-9-CM 354.4), the resemblance is so perfect that it can be regarded as a straight copy of the corresponding elements as listed in CMIT. Unfortunately, decimal subdivisions within a single ICD code are not always separately described, e.g., typhus fevers. Similar to the design of Framemed [Bishop and Ewing, 1993], the information is compiled by a group of contributing authors whose names are listed in conjunction with each disease profile.

- The *Birth Defects Encyclopedia*, edited by Buijse [1992], has the significant subtitle "The Comprehensive, Systematic, Illustrative Reference Source for the Diagnosis, Delineation, Etiology, Biodynamics, Occurrence, Prevention and Treatment of Human Anomalies of Clinical Relevance." A unique feature of this printed encyclopedia is the BDFax service, which allows anyone in the world to call the center [Buyse, 1992] and request a current, daily updated version of any article in the KB. The information will then be faxed. Furthermore, BRS Information Technologies makes the full text available for on-line search and retrieval. Finally, the related BDIS (Birth Defects Information System) is a sophisticated computer-based profile matching system that reduces the research and diagnostic assistance tasks associated with complex syndromes.

189.3 Problems Related to Medical Terminology

kiotomy (ki-ot'o-me) excision of the vulva
in *Dorland's Pocket Medical Dictionary*, 21st ed., p. 342; cf. vulvectomy on p. 684

Inspection of other sources suggests that in the word *vulva* one letter *v* should be replaced by the letter *u*, followed by rearrangement of letters to obtain an anagram, namely
uvula (being a portion of the soft palate).

Medical language forms one of the greatest obstacles for the practical use of any type of KB designed for application in the field of medicine [Kerkhof, 1992]. Just imagine the confusion introduced when a visiting surgeon from an exotic country (where *cyrillarabispanic* is the native language) is requested to perform a kiotomy and consults the above-mentioned popular dictionary to look up what is supposed to be excised. Complete panic among the OR employees is the least devastating option.

Natural language often has remote roots; e.g., adrenaline and epinephrine are the same chemical substances. Similarly, (pontine) angle tumor, acoustic (nerve) neurinoma, and acoustic neurilemmoma all mean the same [Kerkhof, 1993a].

But what's in a name? Various words can be used in two senses: as noun and as adjective, e.g., antipyretic and adrenal. The Latin word *os* means both "mouth" and "bone." Also, several English words have dual meanings, e.g., apprehension, aromatic, attitude, aural, auricle, bladder, capsule, cast, cervical, chlorine, conus, crack, cream, cure, cystectomy, etc.

And next, what's in a phrase? "*. . . a neurologist found a nonfluent dysphasia, without circumlocution or paraphasias*" (Is there a single term for computer entry?) Or "*The CT scan showed accentuation of the peripheral margins of the bilateral parieto-occipital forceps major, and splenium low-absorptive abnormalities.*" (What does it mean, anyway?) [Case 45, 1988]. These examples illustrate the problem of translating medical phrases into concise "computer-storable language."

Besides problems inherent to the understanding of natural language, additional difficulties pertaining to medical terminology can be indicated:

- *American versus British spellings.* Two standard differences are evident, namely, the use of the diphtongue/digraph in British spelling (e.g., anaemia versus anemia) and preference for using *c* (e.g., in *leucocyte*) rather than *k* (as in the American word *leukocyte*). However, combination of both rules does not apply in the British equivalent of the American spelling of the word *leukemia,* where the anglicized version is spelled as *leukaemia.* Remarkably, the adjective of *humour* is *humoral* [Kerkhof, 1993]. Contrary to expectation, spelling in American and British is identical in the case of (an)aerobic.

- *Preferred terminology.* In radiology, *air* means gas within the body, regardless of its composition or site, but the term should be reserved for inspired atmospheric gas. With reference to pneumothorax, subcutaneous emphysema, or the contents of the gastrointestinal tract, the preferred term is *gas.* Sometimes the preferred terminology refers to simplicity; there is no virtue in talking about *the lower extremity* if we mean *leg* or *male siblings* if we mean *brothers.* On other occasions the preferred terminology pertains to technical vocabulary that permits high precision and resolution descriptions if the available information is extremely exact. In these circumstances, a valuable tool is blunted, if carelessness creeps in. For example, the word *clumsiness* describes defective coordination of movement, whereas the term *dysdiadokokinesis* refers to the well-defined phenomenon of a defect in the ability to perform rapid movements of both hands in unison [Murphy, 1976].

- *Different expressions and their exact meanings.* A straightforward example is tympanism, tympanites, tympanitis, and tympany, particularly in relation to tympanal, tympanic, tympanous, and tympanitic [Kerkhof, 1993a]. We present one annotated example:

  heterogenous: not originating in the body;

  heterogeneous: not of uniform composition, quality or structure;

  heterogenetic: pertaining to asexual generation

  Heterogenic, finally, has the same meaning as *heterogeneous.*

- *Meaning within a certain context.* The quality *blue* primarily refers to a particular color and strictly in terms of physics to a certain range of frequencies of electromagnetic radiation. The actual meaning in medical language may, however, reach beyond the single aspect of color if the adjective is employed in relation to a specific noun, e.g., blue asphyxia, blue baby, blue bloater, blue diaper syndrome, blue dome, blue line, blue nevus, blue pus, blue sclera, blue stone, and blue toe syndrome [Kerkhof, 1993].

- *Implicit information.* A particular statement may imply a multitude of information components; e.g., if urinalysis is found to be normal, then the preceding examination implies (at least) the absence of the quadruplet proteinuria, hematuria, glucosuria, and casts. Also *mirror-terms* may apply: *dry cough* implies "no productive cough" (which can be entered as a negative finding). Likewise, *leukopenia* in particular implies "no leukocytosis." This mutual-exclusion principle applies to all antonyms, especially all terms beginning with hypo- or hyper-.

- *Imprecise terminology* [Yu, 1983]. Some terms may carry a vague meaning, e.g., tumor, swelling, mass, and lump. To a large extent, however, the use of such terms reflects the uncertainty around an observation. In this respect, it refers to a justifiable "law of preservation of uncertainty." In other words, it would be incorrect to specify an observation in greater detail than the facts permit. This notion has consequences for the selection of equivalents.

- *Certainty versus uncertainty.* Decision analysis itself does not reduce our uncertainty about the true state of nature, but as long as we must make some choice, it does enable us to make rational decisions in the light of our uncertainty [Weinstein and Fineberg, 1980]. Yet another aspect of certainty versus uncertainty deserves mentioning, namely, where percentwise figures about prognosis or outlook are subjectively interpreted [Eraker and Politser, 1982]. Reduction of the probabilities by a factor of one-tenth completely reversed the preferences of a set of respondents. This *certainty effect* shows that outcomes perceived with certainty are overweighted relative to uncertain outcomes. Thus the formulation of information affects its interpretation by humans.

- *Limited scope of a thesaurus.* No agreement exists regarding directives for coding diseases. Major sources are organized in different ways, e.g., in ICD-9-CM [1978] one finds "Bladder, see condition (e.g., Leukoplakia)," whereas CMIT [Finkel, 1981] reads "Leukoplakia (of bladder), see bladder." Notably, "leukoplakia of the bladder" as such is not listed in MeSH [1993].

- *Knowledge engineering* implies various levels of translation. The expert formulates as precisely as possible his or her thoughts, the engineer provides feedback using the own phrases to ensure an exact match between both minds, and subsequently the resulting expression is translated to a format usable for the computer program. These three steps involve transformations of language while yet assuming that the occasional user of the program appreciates the full scope of the original thoughts of the expert.

- *Information source versus actual patient* [Kerkhof, 1987]. Current medical information sources tend to adhere to preference terminology to promote the use of uniform medical language. However, such standard vocabulary is not used by the average patient to describe the individual health problems [Hurst, 1971]. Then it is left to the clinician to transpose, e.g., "puffy face" and "moon face," if appropriate. Indeed, better health care can be realized by educating the patient about the value of structured communication with the physician [Verby and Verby, 1977].

- *Synonyms.* For some reason, *icterus* is identical to *jaundice;* it is not all that difficult, but the major problem is that you have to recall this every time you use either of them. *Leukopenia* means the same as *leukocytopenia. Thrombocytosis* and *thrombocythemia* are two words to indicate that the number of platelets in the peripheral circulation is in excess of 350,000 per microliter.

- *Subspecialty-dependent interpretation of terms.* In chest radiology, *type I bulla* means the same as *bleb* or *air cyst,* while *pneumatocele* is not regarded as a proper synonym [Glossary, 1989]. When naming a "hollow space," you may choose anything out of the following set: cavity, crypt, pouch, gap, indentation, dell, burrow, crater, concavity, excavation, gorge, pocket, cave, cavern, cistern, or lacuna. However, every expression may exhibit a nuance within a certain context. Then there is a jargon: The terms *show, engagement, lightening,* and *station,* for example, have a particular meaning within the field of obstetrics [Kerkhof, 1993]. The term *streaking* has a meaning that differs for the microbiologist and the radiologist.

- *Eponyms.* Many disease names refer to the first author (e.g., Boeck's disease for sarcoidosis) who described the particular disorder, to the first patient analyzed in detail (e.g., Mortimer's disease, again for sarcoidosis), or to the area (e.g., Lyme disease) where the illness was first detected. An epidemiologist even attempted to replace the term *Bornholm disease* just to honor a friend (Sylvest). Geographic variations also occur: The *Plummer-Vinson syndrome* (referring to sideropenic dysphagia), as it is known in the United States and Australia, is termed *Patterson-Kelly syndrome* in the United Kingdom but *Waldenström-Kjellberg syndrome* in Scandinavia [Firkin and Whitworth, 1987].

- *Multilingual approaches.* The relation between a concept and the various corresponding terms in different languages is in general not unique. This implies that a multitude of different words from different syntactical categories may represent a single concept. Particularly the European countries are confronted with additional natural-language problems. The

Commission of the European Communities supports research activities in this area through the AIM (Advanced Informatics in Medicine) project, such as EPILEX (a multilingual lexicon of epidemiologic terms containing Catalan, Dutch, English, French, German, Italian, Portuguese, and Spanish) [Du V Florey, 1993] and the development of a multilingual natural language system [Baud et al., 1994].

- *Frequency of occurrence.* The meaning of semiquantitative indicators such as *always, often,* etc. is not transparent when screening a medical text. The intuitive interpretation of some quasi-numerical determinants is summarized elsewhere [Kong et al., 1986].

- *Noise terms in patient description.* When analyzing 104 case histories, we found for Medwise [Kerkhof et al., 1993] that the input consisted on average of 75 terms; required for establishing the primary diagnosis were only 15 terms. This implies that 80% of the input data consisted of *noise terms* that do not directly contribute to the confirmation of the correct diagnosis. Rather, such an overwhelming portion of information may blur the process of hypothesis formation and in particular when the diagnostic task is solely left to the human being who is prone to confusion if the number of contributing elements is more than about 10.

- *Illogical terminology.* Sometimes terms suggest certain implications which in reality do not exist, e.g., a patient with hayfever usually does not present with fever, while acute rheumatic fever typically is a chronic disease.

189.4 Solution for Discrepancies

> Representation of knowledge is an art, not a science.
>
> D. B. Lenat [1989]

Various scientists have described techniques to help solve language-related problems in the communication area of medicine. An on-line available medical dictionary can be an important tool for research and application in natural-language processing. Recently, *Dorland's Illustrated Medical Dictionary* has been converted to an on-line interactive computer-based version [McCray et al., 1990]. To ensure exact description of definitions, a coding system has been advocated because of ease of handling, redundancy to avoid errors, specificity, indication of relationships (e.g., by using common code groups for similar terms), equating equivalent terms and linking them in different languages, and the feasibility to cross-link terms on the basis of common portions of their codes [Bishop and Dombrowski, 1990].

Attempts also have been made to automatically translate existing medical terminology systems [Cimino and Barnett, 1990]. For example, using a semantic network for mapping, the closest match between the MeSH term *portography* was *portal contrast phlebogram* in the ICD-9 procedures directory.

In our view, two independent routes are available to attack the majority of linguistic problems related to a medical KB:

1. Use uniform input data; i.e., force the user of the KB to enter only controlled terms as they already exist in the KB, that is, terms allowed by the editorial committee responsible for the KB. This route implies tedious work for the user, and the job of selecting recognizable entries has to be carried out every time the KB is consulted.

2. Apply an additional KB with equivalent expressions. Once the user enters a particular term, the KB automatically generates a list of equivalent expressions to choose from. The construction of such an auxiliary KB has to be realized only once, apart from the obvious updating process desired as the systems evolves. Furthermore, a matrix structure as applied in the Medwise KB proves to be helpful in organizing information and incorporating a substantial portion of semantic interpretation when dealing with medical knowledge. Running

104 actual cases in the Medwise system with use of the auxiliary KB yields a correct diagnosis in 93%. Disregarding the equivalent expressions, however, lowers the score to 82%. As expected, inclusion of the auxiliary KB also enhances user-friendliness of the system and accelerates the process of data entry [Kerkhof et al., 1993].

189.5 Discussion

While advances in computer technology permit virtually unlimited storage and fast retrieval capabilities, interpretation of natural language still constitutes a major obstacle for the application of medical KBs. Even common words often have highly ambiguous meanings [Murphy, 1976]; e.g., *weakness* can mean lethargy or paralysis. Therefore, the user of any KB should be aware of the fact that justifiable adoption of a particular equivalent expression may depend on the precise interpretation of the complete case report.

On the other hand, the use of uniform input data on the basis of a thesaurus would imply a substantial loss of refinement with respect to terminology. Ideally, there is a maximum degree of freedom in the selection of words and their nuances, both for the KB and for the description of the individual case study.

An auxiliary KB with synonyms [SNOMED, 1993; Gabrieli, 1992; Chisholm, 1990; Kerkhof et al., 1993; Lindberg et al., 1993] indeed may offer a considerable help during the process of matching input terms with information sources. In our analysis, this route yields a diagnostic score that is 11% higher compared with the situation where no equivalents are selected by the user [Kerkhof et al., 1993]. This result illustrates that an adequate solution to (at least a part of the) linguistic problems substantially enhances the performance of diagnostic computer programs.

It has been anticipated that in the future computers may replace the traditional role of the physician qua diagnostician [Mazoue, 1990]. Economic as well as ethical reasons were presented to support the new paradigm. However, such movement would imply another type of training for the new generation of clinicians, where more emphasis will be given to *the art to observe* the patient and subsequent translation into precise medical terminology. At the same time, all linguistic difficulties discussed here will be in even greater need for efficient solutions, because the interface formed by the human mediator is further removed in the model envisioned for the future.

189.6 Summary

A multitude of projects address the issue of how to handle an ever-increasing amount of medical information. Coding schemes have been designed and are regularly refined, while other approaches aim to collect, structure, and disclose this gigantic corpus of information that features an unconfined potential to thrive.

The lack of standardized medical language limits the optimal use of computers in medicine. Major obstacles concern imprecise terminology, the limited scope of a thesaurus, multilingual conversion problems, discrepancies between information sources and actual clinical cases, as well as the ever-expanding range of synonyms, acronyms, antonyms, and eponyms.

Incorporation of a separate knowledge base containing equivalent expressions appears indicated for the practical use of medical information systems. If no effective solutions are realized within the next decade, then we will be confronted with a medical analogue of the tower of Babel.

Defining Terms

AMA: American Medical Association, with headquarters in Chicago. This organization is actively involved in new developments concerning medical informatics. CMIT [Finkel, 1981] and CPT [Physicians' Current Procedural Terminology, 1992] as well as the cooperation with DXplain [Barnett et al., 1987] are prototypes of their activities.

ICD: International Classification of Diseases, a widely accepted system to organize all possible medical diagnoses. The tenth version is currently being translated for worldwide application.

UMLS: Unified Medical Language System, a project initiated by the NLM and distributed on CD-ROM. Cooperation with parties to implement the system within their own environment is encouraged but requires a contract [Lindberg et al., 1993].

References

Barnett GO, Cimino JJ, Hupp JA, Hoffer EP. 1987. DXplain, an evolving diagnostic decision-support system. JAMA 258:67.

Baud R, Lovis C, Alpay L, et al. 1994. Modelling for natural language understanding. SCAMC 93:289.

Baxt WG. 1991. Use of an artificial neural network for the diagnosis of myocardial infarction. Ann Intern Med 115:483.

Bergeron B. 1991. ILIAD, a diagnostic consultant and patient simulator. MD Comput 8:46.

Bishop CW, Dombrowski T. 1990. Coding, why and how. MD Comput 7:210.

Bishop CW, Ewing PD. 1993. Framemed, a prototypical medical knowledge base of unusual design. MD Comput 10:184.

Blois MS. 1984. Information and Medicine. Berkeley, Univ. California Press.

Buyse ML (ed). 1992. Birth Defects Encyclopedia. Dover, Mass, Center for Birth Defects Information Services.

Case 45. 1988. N Engl J Med 319:1268.

Chisholm J. 1990. Read clinical classification. Br Med J 300:1092.

Cimino JJ, Barnett GO. 1990. Automated translation between medical terminologies using semantic definitions. MD Comput 7:104.

Du V Florey C. 1993. EPILEX, a multilingual lexicon of epidemiological terms. Luxembourg, Office for Official Publications of the European Communities (ISBN 92-826-6211-X).

Eraker SA, Politser PE. 1982. How decisions are reached: Physician and patient. Ann Intern Med 97:262.

Finkel AJ (ed). 1981. Current Medical Information and Terminology, 5th ed. Chicago, American Medical Association.

Firkin BG, Whitworth JA. 1987. Eponyms. Park Ridge, NJ, Parthenon.

Gabrieli ER. 1992. A new American electronic medical nomenclature. Automedica 14:23.

Glossary of "Chest" Radiological Terms. 1989. Nomenclature Committee of the Fleischner Society.

Griffith HW, Dambro MR. 1993. The 5-Minute Clinical Consult. Philadelphia, Lea & Febiger.

Hurst JW. 1971. The art and science of presenting a patient's problems. Arch Intern Med 128:463.

International Classification of Diseases, Ninth Clinical Modification. 1978. Ann Arbor, Mich, Commission on Professional and Hospital Activities.

Kerkhof PLM. 1987. Dreams and realities of computer-assisted diagnosis systems in medicine (editorial). Automedica 8:123.

Kerkhof PLM. 1992. Knowledge base systems and medical terminology. Automedica 14:47.

Kerkhof PLM. 1993. Woordenboek der geneeskunde N/E & E/N. Houten, The Netherlands, Bohn Stafleu Van Loghum (ISBN 90-6016-858-5).

Kerkhof PLM, van Dieijen-Visser MP, Koenen R, et al. 1993. The Medwise diagnostic module as a consultant. Expert Syst Appl 6:433.

Kong A, Barnett GO, Mosteller F, Youtz C. 1986. How medical professionals evaluate expressions of probability. N Engl J Med 315:740.

Krause P, Fox J, O'Neil M, Glowinski A. 1993. Can we formally specify a medical decision support system? IEEE Expert 8:56.

Labsearch/286. Software available from REMIND/1 Corp, PO Box 752, Nashua, NH 03061.

Lenat DB, Guha RV. 1989. Building Large Knowledge Base Systems. Reading, Mass, Addison-Wesley.

Lindberg DA, Humphreys BL, McCray AT. 1993. The Unified Medical Language System. Methods Inform Med. 32:281.

Mazoue JG. 1990. Diagnosis without doctors. J Med Philos 15:559.

McCray AT, Srinivasan S. 1990. Automated access to a large medical dictionary: On-line assistance for research and application in natural language processing. Comp Biomed Res 23:179.

MD-Challenger, 70 Belle Meade Cove, Eads, TN 38028.

Medical Records Institute, PO Box 289, Newton, MA 02160.

MeSH, Medical Subject Headings. 1993. National Library of Medicine, Bethesda, Md.

Middleton B, et al. 1991. Probabilistic diagnosis using a reformulation of the INTERNIST-1/QMR knowledge base: II. Evaluation of diagnostic performance. Methods Inform Med 30:15.

Murphy EA. 1976. The Logic of Medicine. Baltimore, Johns Hopkins Univ Press.

Physicians' Current Procedural Terminology (CPT), 4th ed. 1992. Chicago, American Medical Association.

Roueché, B. 1982. The Medical Detectives, p 317. New York, Washington Square Press.

Salton G. 1991. Developments in automatic text retrieval. Science 253:974.

SNOMED International. 1993. Northfield, Ill, College of American Pathologists.

Sowa JF. 1984. Conceptual Graphs: Information Processing in Mind and Machine. Reading, Mass, Addison-Wesley.

STAT!-Ref. 1994. Available from Teton Data Systems, PO Box 3082, Jackson, Wyoming.

Verby J, Verby J. 1977. How to Talk to Doctors. New York, Arco.

Waxman HS, Worley WE. 1990. Computer-assisted adult medical diagnosis, subject review and evaluation of a new microcomputer-based system. Medicine 69:125.

Weinstein MC, Fineberg HV. 1980. Clinical Decision Analysis, p 61. Philadelphia, Saunders.

White ME, Lewkowicz J. 1987. The CONSULTANT database for computer-assisted diagnosis and information management in veterinary medicine. Automedica 8:135.

Williams BT. 1982. Computer Aids to Clinical Decisions, vol 2, pp 81–99. Boca Raton, Fla, CRC Press.

Wyatt J. 1991. Computer-based knowledge systems. Lancet 338:1431.

Yu VL. 1983. Conceptual obstacles in computerized medical diagnosis. J Med Philos 8:67.

Further Information

The fields of medical knowledge bases and medical terminology are rapidly developing. There is no single comprehensive source of information available, but the reader is advised to scrutinize the following journals for new information:

M.D. Computing, published by Springer Verlag (New York and Berlin), reports on research in the field of medical informatics. Of special interest to the clinician.

IEEE Expert appears four times a year and presents the latest on artificial intelligence and expert systems. Contact P.O. Box 3014, Los Alamitos, CA 90720. For those interested in technical details on intelligent systems and their applications, IEEE (P.O. Box 1331, Piscataway NJ 08855-1331) publishes a number of related journals, e.g., on knowledge engineering and on multimedia.

The National Library of Medicine (8600 Rockville Pike, Bethesda MD 20894) releases news bulletins and provides information on UMLS and contracts for cooperation.

Ongoing projects on medical nomenclature are surveyed elsewhere in this chapter, and the list of references contains several useful addresses. Obviously, annual meetings form the forum for presentation of the latest developments: SCAMC conferences are well known besides the world congress organized every 4 years. IMIA (the International Medical Informatics Association) publishes a *Yearbook of Medical Informatics*. This publication offers a gold mine of relevant information in that it contains a supreme collection of papers selected from almost a hundred outstanding journals. Contact Schattauer Publishers, Subscriptions Dept., P.O. Box 104545, W-7000 Stuttgart 10, Germany.

190

Natural-Language Processing in Biomedicine

Stephen B. Johnson
Columbia-Presbyterian
Medical Center

Natural language is the primary means of communication in all complex social interactions. In biomedical areas, knowledge and data are disseminated in written form, through articles in the scientific literature, technical and administrative reports, and hospital charts used in patient care. Much vital information is exchanged verbally in interactions among scientists, clinical consultations, lectures, and conference presentations. Increasingly, computers are being employed to facilitate this process of collecting, storing, and distributing biomedical information. Textual data are now widely available in an electronic format, through the use of transcription services and word processing. Important examples include articles published in the medical literature and reports dictated during the process of patient care (e.g., radiology reports and discharge summaries).

While the ability to access and review narrative data is highly beneficial to researchers, clinicians, and administrators, the information is not in a form amenable to further computer processing, e.g., storage in a database to enable subsequent retrievals. At present, the most significant impact of the computer in medicine is seen in processing *structured* information, information represented in a regular, predictable form. This information is often numeric in nature, e.g., measurements recorded in a scientific study, or made up of discrete data elements, e.g., elements selected from a predefined list of diseases.

The techniques of natural-language processing provide a means to bridge the gap between textual and structured data, allowing humans to interact using familiar natural language while enabling computer applications to process data effectively.

190.1 Linguistic Principles

Natural-language processing (or computational linguistics) is a branch of computer science concerned with the relationship between information as expressed in natural language (sound or text) and as represented in formalisms that facilitate computer processing. Natural-language *analysis* studies how to convert natural-language input into a structured form, while natural-language *generation* investigates how to produce natural-language output from structured representations.

Natural-language processing investigates and applies scientific principles of linguistics through development of computer systems. One of the most important principles is that natural language is built up from several layers of structure, each layer defined as a set of restrictions on the previous layer [Harris, 1991]:

Linguistic Layer	Description
Phonologic	Mapping of sounds to phonemes (letters)
Morphologic	Grouping of phonemes into morphemes (roots and inflections)
Lexical	Combining of morphemes into words
Syntactic	Combining of words into sentence structure
Semantic	Mapping of sentence structure into literal meanings
Pragmatic	Combining of sentence meanings into discourse meaning

These layers correspond roughly to the subfields of linguistics and to the areas of study in natural-language processing, which seeks to develop computer models of them. Knowledge about the rules of language structure at any or all of its levels is called language competence. Most natural-language processing applications in biomedicine do not even begin to approach the language competence of humans. For example, a transcription system may have knowledge about the sounds of a language but know nothing about the syntax of sentences. Similarly, a program that indexes scientific articles may know which terms to look for in the text but have no ability to express how these terms are related to one another. However, it is important to emphasize that such applications may perform extremely useful tasks, even with very limited competence.

Many natural-language processing applications exploit the fact that biomedical fields are *restricted semantic domains,* which means that natural-language information associated with that field is focused on a narrow range of topics. For example, an article about cell biology is limited to discussions of cells and tissues and is unlikely to mention political or literary issues. The natural language of a restricted semantic domain is called a sublanguage. Sublanguages tend to have specialized vocabularies and specialized ways of structuring sentences (e.g., the "telegraphic style" of notes written about patients in hospital charts) and ways of organizing larger units of discourse (e.g., the format of a technical report) [Grishman and Kittredge, 1986; Kittredge and Lehrberger, 1982].

These properties of sublanguages allow the use of methods of analysis and processing that would not be possible when processing the language of newspaper articles or novels. For example, a program that indexes medical articles can select index terms from a list of terminology known to be of interest to researchers; a speech-recognition system can exploit the fact that only certain words can be uttered by a user in response to a given prompt; a system that analyzes clinical reports can look for predictable semantic patterns that are characteristic of the given domain.

190.2 Applications in Biomedicine

There are four forms of natural-language exchange possible between human and the computer: The human can supply information to the computer using natural language; the human can retrieve information from the computer through natural language; the computer can supply information to the human in the form of natural-language output; and the computer can request information from the human using natural-language questions. Applications of natural-language processing may support one or several of these modes of exchange. For example, an automated questionnaire for patients may generate multiple-choice questions but be able to receive only numbered answers, while a database interface may be able to accept natural-language questions submitted by a researcher and return natural-language replies. Applications can be classified according to the levels of language competence embodied in their design: speech systems, lexical systems, syntactic and semantic systems, and discourse systems.

Speech Systems

Speech-recognition systems process voice data into phonemic representations (such as text), while speech-synthesis systems generate spoken output from such representations. Speech-processing applications may work only at this level of language competence, e.g., software that transcribes spoken input into text or software that generates speech when visual information cannot be employed, such as on the telephone. Applications in this category include systems that capture structured endoscopic reports [Johannes and Carr-Locke, 1992] and emergency room notes [Linn et al., 1992]. Applications also may employ speech technology as part of a larger system. Examples include interfaces to diagnostic systems [Landau et al., 1989; Shiffman et al., 1992] and systems for taking patient histories [Johnson et al., 1992].

Lexical Systems

Lexical systems work with language at the level of words and terms (short sequences of words). A *lexicon* is a special type of database that provides information about words and terms, which may include pronunciation, morphology (roots and affixes), and syntactic function (noun, verb, etc.). The Specialist Lexicon provides information about medical terms and general English words [National Library of Medicine, 1993]. A thesaurus groups synonymous terms into semantic classes, which are frequently organized into a hierarchical classification scheme. The Systematized of Nomenclature of Medicine (SNOMED) classifies medical terms in several hierarchies, such as topography, morphology, etiology, function, disease, occupation, and procedure [Rothwell et al., 1993]. Medical Subject Headings (MeSH) classifies terms used in the medical literature [National Library of Medicine, 1990]. The metathesaurus of the Unified Medical Language System (UMLS) combines SNOMED, MeSH, and other thesauri [Lindberg, 1993].

Semantic classes are used to index natural-language documents to facilitate their retrieval from a database. For example, MeSH is used to index the medical literature in the MEDLINE database [Bachrach, 1978]. Semantic classes are also used to define the set of data elements (controlled vocabulary) that can be processed by a computer application. Controlled vocabularies are used by diagnostic systems and clinical information systems—by the programs that collect data, store them in databases, and display them [Linarrson and Wigertz, 1989].

Syntactic and Semantic Systems

Lexical techniques can only approximate the meaning of an article or some text entered by the user of a computer application. One approach to obtaining deeper understanding is to produce a representation of the syntactic structure of a sentence (e.g., what is the subject, the verb, and the object) and then map this structure into a representation of its meaning (such as predicate calculus). A computer program that analyses the structure of sentences is called a parser and uses a lexicon and a grammar (a formal representation of the syntactic rules of a language). Representations of semantic content (or knowledge representation) vary, but most representations have the form of a frame, in which predefined slots are filled with information from natural-language sentences. The Linguistic String Project employs a wide-coverage grammar of English and maps sentences from discharge summaries into "information formats" [Sager et al., 1986]; the MEDSORT system maps sentences into a semantic net representation [Evans, 1987]; the METEXA [Schroder, 1992] system maps sentences from radiology reports into "conceptual graphs" [Sowa, 1984]; and the MediTAS system performs a syntactic analysis of cytopathology findings [Pietrzyk, 1991].

In highly restricted sublanguages, it is sometimes possible to map natural-language sentences into a knowledge representation in a direct manner using semantic patterns that approximate syntactic analysis [Friedman, 1994; Baud et al., 1992].

Discourse Systems

Information from the sentences of a discourse (e.g., an article or clinical report) combine in complex ways; for example, cross-references are made (e.g., using pronouns), and events are related temporally or causally. Understanding a discourse fully may require information about the context in which the natural-language exchange occurs or background knowledge of a technical field. Systems based on syntax and semantics usually carry out an analysis of the discourse and context information as a subsequent stage. Other systems attempt to approximate the semantic analysis of sentences using medical knowledge to guide the overall processing of a text by defining the possible sequences of topics and subtopics characteristic of the domain. Domains in which these methods have been attempted include the history and physical sections of a patient chart [Archbold and Evans, 1989], echocardiography reports [Canfield et al., 1989], discharge summaries [Gabrieli and Speth, 1987], and radiology reports [Ranum, 1988].

Natural language is also a convenient mode for the output of applications, e.g., in producing clinical reports [Kuzmak and Miller, 1983]. Some expert systems have used natural language to express their recommendations [Rennels et al., 1989], and to provide explanations of their reasoning process [Lewin, 1991].

190.3 Challenges

The technology of speech systems is still evolving. Many systems are not speaker-independent and require substantial training. Recognition of continuous speech is an extremely difficult process, and the more robust systems require speakers to pause between words. In addition, the number of words that can be discriminated successfully by most speech systems is still too small to satisfy the requirements of all biomedical applications.

The design of controlled vocabularies is an important area of research [Cimino et al., 1989]. As yet, no comprehensive vocabulary for clinical medicine exists, and the effort to create one is beyond the means of any single institution. Indexing of articles and reports is currently a labor-intensive process, and quality control is a significant problem. Index terms are a poor approximation of the meaning of a text. Similarly, systems that capture clinical information through the entry of individual findings fall short of capturing the patient history. Natural-language processing systems with greater understanding of syntax and semantics may help by providing richer information representations.

No natural-language processing system currently covers the complete range of language interaction with significant competence at all levels—from speech to discourse. In the near future, the systems with the greatest practical success will specialize in performing selected language-processing tasks in well-defined domains.

Defining Terms

Controlled vocabulary: A set of well-defined data elements intended for use in a computer application.

Grammar: A formal representation of language structure, usually syntactic structure.

Language competence: Knowledge about the rules of a language.

Lexicon: A formal compilation of the words of a language, with information about phonetics, morphology, syntax, and semantics (depending on requirements of computer applications).

Morphology: Field studying how sounds combine into morphemes and how morphemes combine to form words.

Parser: A computer program that uses a grammar and lexicon to analyze sentences of a language, producing a syntactic or semantic representation.

Phonology: Field studying the rules that govern the sounds used in languages.

Pragmatics: Field studying how sentences are combined to form larger units of discourse and how to represent meaning in the context of a situation.

Semantics: Field studying the relation between natural-language sentences and formal representations of meaning.

Structured data: Data that has a explicit, unambiguous, and regular structure, making it amenable to computer processing.

Sublanguage: The natural language of a restricted semantic domain that is focused on a specific set of tasks or purposes, e.g., interpreting x-ray images.

Syntax: Field studying how words combine to form sentences.

References

Allen J. 1981. Natural Language Understanding. Menlo Park, Calif, Benjamin/Cummings.

Archbold A, Evans D. 1989. On the topical structure of medical charts. In Proceedings of the 13th Annual SCAMC, pp 543–547. Washington, IEEE Computer Society Press.

Bachrach CA, Chaen T. 1978. Selection of MEDLINE contents, the development of its thesaurus, and the indexing process. Med Informat 3(3):237.

Baud RH, Rassinoux AM, Scherrer JR. 1992. Natural language processing and semantical representation of medical texts. Methods Inform Med 31(2):117.

Bernauer J, Gumrich K, Kutz S, et al. 1991. An interactive report generator for bone scan studies. In Proceedings of the 15th Annual SCAMC, pp 858–860. Washington, IEEE Computer Society Press.

Canfield K, Bray B, Huff S, Warner H. 1989. Database capture of natural language echocardiography reports: A Unified Medical Language System approach. In Proceedings of the 13th Annual SCAMC, pp 559–563. Washington, IEEE Computer Society Press.

Cimino JJ, Hripcsak G, Johnson SB, et al. 1989. Designing an introspective, multi-purpose controlled medical vocabulary. In Proceedings of the 13th Annual SCAMC, pp 513–518. Washington, IEEE Computer Society Press.

Covington MA. 1994. Natural Language Processing for Prolog Programmers. Englewood Cliffs, NJ, Prentice-Hall.

Evans D. 1987. Final Report on the MedSORT-II Project: Developing and Managing Medical Thesauri. CMU-LCL-87-3. Pittsburg, Laboratory for Computational Linguistics, Carnegie Mellon University.

Friedman C, Alderson PO, Austin HM, et al. 1994. A general natural language text processor for clinical radiology. JAMIA 1(2):161.

Gabrieli E, Speth D. 1987. Computer processing of discharge summaries. In Proceedings of the 11th Annual SCAMC, pp 137–140. Washington, IEEE Computer Society Press.

Grishman R, Kittredge R (eds). 1986. Analyzing Language in Restricted Domains: Sublanguage Description and Processing. Hillsdale, NJ, Erlbaum Associates.

Harris Z. 1991. A Theory of Language and Information: A Mathematic Approach. Oxford, England, Clarendon Press.

Johannes RS, Carr-Locke DL. 1992. The role of automated speech recognition in endoscopic data collection. Endoscopy 24(suppl 2):493.

Johnson K, Poon A, Shiffman S, et al. 1992. A history taking system that uses continuous speech recognition. In Proceedings of the 16th Annual SCAMC, pp 757–761. Washington, IEEE Computer Society Press.

Kittredge R, Lehrberger J (eds). 1982. Sublanguage: Studies of Language in Restricted Semantic Domains. New York, De Gruyter.

Kuzmak PM, Miller RA. 1983. Computer-aided generation of result text for clinical laboratory tests. In Proceedings of the 7th Annual SCAMC, pp 275–278. Washington, IEEE Computer Society Press.

Landau JA, Norwich KN, Evans SJ. 1989. Automatic speech recognition: Can it improve the man-machine interface in medical expert systems? Int J Biomed Comput 24(2):111.

Lewin HC. 1991. HF-Explain: A natural language generation system for explaining a medical expert system. In Proceedings of the 15th Annual SCAMC, pp 644–648. Washington, IEEE Computer Society Press.

Lindberg DAB, Humphreys BL, McCray AT. 1993. The Unified Medical Language System. In van Bemmel JH, McCray AT (eds), Yearbook of Medical Informatics, pp 41–51. Amsterdam, International Medical Informatics Association.

Linarrson R, Wigertz O. 1989. The data dictionary: A controlled vocabulary for integrating clinical databases and medical knowledge bases. Methods Inform Med 28(2):78.

Linn NA, Rubenstein RM, Bowler AE, Dixon JL. 1992. Improving the quality of emergency room documentation using the voice-activated word processor: Interim results. In Proceedings of the 16th Annual SCAMC, pp 772–776. New York, McGraw-Hill.

National Library of Medicine. 1990. Medical Subject Headings (NTIS NLM-MED-90-01. Bethesda, Md, National Library of Medicine.

National Library of Medicine. 1993. The Specialist Lexicon. Bethesda, Md, Natural language systems group, National Library of Medicine.

Pietrzyk PM. 1991. A medical text analysis system for German: Syntax analysis. Methods Inform Med 30(4):275.

Ranum D. 1988. Knowledge based understanding of radiology text. In Proceedings of the 12th Annual SCAMC, pp 141–145. Washington, IEEE Computer Society Press.

Rennels G, Shortliffe E, Stockdale F, Miller P. 1989. A computational model of reasoning from the clinical literature. AI Magazine 10(1):49.

Rothwell DJ, Palotay JL, Beckett RS, Brochu L (eds). 1993. The Systematized Nomenclature of Medicine: SNOMED International. Northfield, Ill, College of American Pathologists.

Sager N, Friedman C, Lyman M. 1987. Medical Language Processing: Computer Management of Narrative Data. Reading, Mass, Addison-Wesley.

Scherrer JR, Cote RA, Mandil SH. 1989. Computerized Natural Language Medical Processing for Knowledge Representation. Amsterdam, North Holland.

Schroder M. 1992. Knowledge-based processing of medical language: A language engineering approach. In Advances in Artificial Intelligence, 16th German Conference on AI, pp 221–234. Berlin, Springer Verlag.

Shiffman S, Lane CD, Johnson KB, Fagan LM. 1992. The integration of a continuous speech recognition system with the QMR diagnostic program. In Proceedings of the 16th Annual SCAMC, pp 767–771. Washington, IEEE Computer Society Press.

Sowa JF. 1984. Conceptual Graphs: Information Processing in Mind and Machine. Reading, Mass, Addison-Wesley.

Further Information

For general information about the field of natural language processing, see Allen [1981] and Covington [1994]. Surveys of research in sublanguage can be found in Kittredge and Lehrberger [1982] and Grishman and Kittredge [1986]. A variety of papers on medical language processing are collected in Scherrer et al. [1989].

Historical Perspectives 5
Electroencephalography

Leslie A. Geddes
Purdue University

Historical Background

Hans Berger (1929) was the first to record electroencephalograms from human subjects. However, before then, it was well known that the brain produced electrical signals. In fact, in Berger's first paper there is a short history of prior studies in animals. Interestingly, the first person to demonstrate the electrical activity of the brain did not make recordings. In 1875, Richard Caton in the United Kingdom used the Thomson (Kelvin) sensitive and rapidly responding reflecting telegraphic galvanometer to display the electrical activity of exposed rabbit and monkey brains. His report [Caton, 1875], which appeared in the *British Medical Association Journal,* occupied only 21 lines of a half-page column. In part, the report stated:

> In every brain hitherto examined, the galvanometer has indicated the existence of electric currents. The external surface of the grey matter is usually positive in relation to the surface of a section through it. Feeble currents of varying direction pass through the multiplier [galvanometer] when the electrodes are placed on two points of the external surface, or one electrode on the grey matter, and one on the surface of the skull. The electric currents of the grey matter appear to have a relation to its function. When any part of the grey matter is in a state of functional activity, its electric current usually exhibits negative variation. For example, on the areas shown by Dr. Ferrier to be related to rotation of the head and to mastication, negative variation of the current was observed to occur whenever those two acts respectively were performed. Impressions through the senses were found to influence the currents of certain areas; e.g., the currents of that part of the rabbit's brain which Dr. Ferrier has shown to be related to movements of the eyelids, were found to be markedly influenced by stimulation of the opposite retina by light.

No recordings of the movement of the spot of light on the scale of the Kelvin galvanometer have been found, perhaps because, at that time, telegraphic operators used to read the dots and dashes of the Morse code by watching the movements of the spot of light on the galvanometer scale. Nonetheless, Caton's description clearly shows that he witnessed the fluctuating potentials that we now know exist. Also important is the fact that Caton was the first to report visual-evoked potentials.

Berger, a psychiatrist in Jena, Germany, was aware of the several prior electroencephalographic animal studies and had conducted experiments using dogs. The only recording devices available to him were the string galvanometer, developed by Einthoven [1903] for electrocardiography and the capillary electrometer developed by Marey [1876]. Although there were a few mirror-type oscillographs available for recording waveforms from alternating current (50 to 60 Hz) generators and

0-8493-8346-3/95/$0.00+$.50
© 1995 by CRC Press, Inc.

transformers, the sensitivity of such devices was very low, and they could not be used for bioelectric recording without a vacuum-tube amplifier.

The voltage appearing on the scalp produced by the brain is only about one-tenth that of the ECG detected with limb leads. To enable recording brain activity with the string galvanometer, the tension in the string was reduced, which increased the sensitivity but reduced the speed of response. This was the method used by Berger when he found that the capillary electrometer was unsatisfactory.

Apart from problems of the lack of sensitivity and speed of response in the recording apparatus, Berger faced severe electrode problems. Because of the low amplitude of the cortical signals, the electrodes had to be very stable, producing no voltages that could be seen on the electrocortical recordings. In other words, the electrode noise and stability had to be in the low-microvolt range. Zinc electrodes were popular at that time, and Berger used them in his first dog studies just after the turn of this century. For human use, he used zinc-plated needles (insulated down to the tip) and inserted them through existing trephine holes or skull defects so that the tip was epidural. The electrodes were sterilized with 10% formalin solution. Berger first used the single-string Edelmann galvanometer designed for electrocardiography. Later he used a two-string unit of the type shown in Fig. HP5.1 so that he could record the ECG along with the EEG. Such units also were equipped

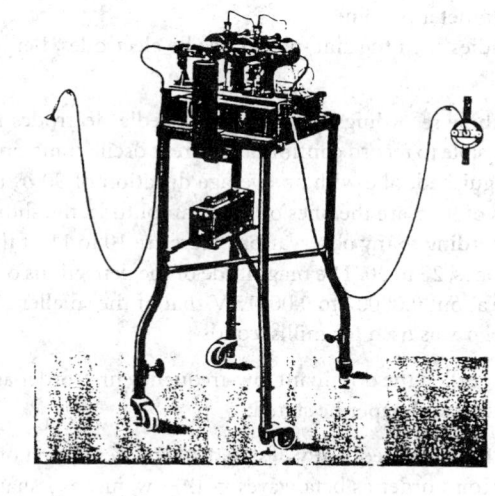

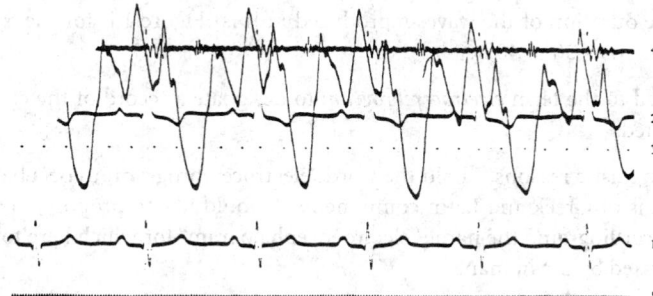

FIGURE HP5.1 (*a*) The Edelmann double-string galvanometer of the type used by Berger. On the left is a funnel for detecting the arterial or venous pulse and on the right is a device for detecting the heart sounds, all of which can be recorded along with the two channels of ECG and a time signal on 12-cm-wide photographic paper. (*b*) The phonocardiogram, venous-pulse record, and two recordings of the ECG. (From Zusatz apparate zum Elektrokardiographen, Siemens-Reiniger-Veifa Berlin ca. 1926.)

with devices to record the venous or arterial pulses and heart sounds. The photographic recording paper was 12 cm wide and 50 m in length.

The string galvanometer is a current-drawing device; therefore, a low electrode-subject resistance was necessary for adequate sensitivity. Berger stated that it was difficult to obtain a low resistance and reported a value of 1600 Ω for his needle electrodes when placed 5 to 6 cm apart with the tips in the epidural space. A high-resistance electrode pair would reduce the amplitude of the recorded activity. Later Berger used chlorided silver needle electrodes to help solve this problem.

Difficulties with the zinc-plated needle electrodes led Berger to develop very thin lead-foil electrodes, wrapped in flannel, and soaked in 20% NaCl solution. The combination of saline-soaked flannel and the use of a rubber bandage to hold the electrodes to the scalp permitted recording the EEG for hours without the saline evaporating. The resistance measured between a pair of such electrodes ranged from 500 to 7600 Ω depending on the size of the electrodes.

Berger's final improvement to his recording equipment consisted of placing a capacitor in series with the electrodes and string galvanometer to block the steady potential difference due to slight electrochemical differences in the two lead electrodes. Recall that the amplitudes being recorded were in the range of tens of microvolts, and any steady difference in electrode potential would cause a steady deflection of the baseline of the recording. With the capacitor, this steady offset potential did not deflect the galvanometer baseline.

Describing his first studies with the zinc-plated needle electrodes, Berger stated [translation by Gloor, 1969]:

> As a general result of these recordings with epidural needle electrodes I would consequently like to state that it is possible to record continuous current oscillations, among which two kinds of waves can be distinguished, one with an average duration of 90 σ, the other with one of 35 σ. The longer waves of 90 σ are the ones of larger amplitude, the shorter, 35 σ waves are of smaller amplitude. According to my observations there are 10 to 11 of the larger waves in one second, of the smaller ones, 20 to 30. The magnitude of the deflections of the larger 90 σ waves can be calculated to be about 0.00007 to 0.00015 V, that of the smaller 35 σ waves, 0.00002 to 0.00003 V. [The symbol σ was used for milliseconds.]

In his first paper, Berger called the dominant low-frequency first-order and the higher-frequency waves second order. In his second paper he stated:

> For the sake of brevity I shall subsequently designate the waves of first order as alpha waves = $\alpha - w$, the waves of second order as beta waves = $\beta - w$, just as I shall use "E. E. G." as the abbreviation for the electroencephalogram and "E. C. G." for the electrocardiogram.
>
> The average duration of the waves reproduced in [his] Figure 1 is for the $\alpha - w = 120 \sigma$ and for the $\beta - w = 30$ to 40 σ.

Berger objected to the term *electrocerebrogram* to designate a record of the electrical activity of the brain. He stated:

> Because for linguistic reasons, I hold the word "electrocerebrogram" to be a barbarism, compounded as it is of Greek and Latin components, I would like to propose, in analogy to the name "electrocardiogram," the name "electroencephalogram" for which here for the first time was demonstrated by me in man.

Berger's papers contain many EEGs from patients, but those from his son Klaus are discussed frequently. In fact, Klaus was used as a subject for electrode testing. For example, Berger wrote:

> Klaus' records were taken with every other possible type of electrodes: silver, platinum, lead electrodes, etc.; also, different arrangements of these on the skin surface of the head were used. However, time and again it was found that the best arrangement was that with electrodes placed on the forehead and occiput. Of Klaus' many records, I only want to show another small segment of a curve obtained in this manner [Fig. HP5.2]. In this instance lead band electrodes were applied

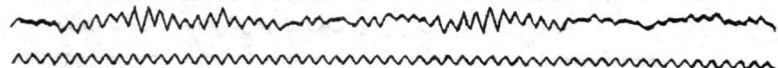

FIGURE HP5.2 Klaus at the age of 15. Double-coil galvanometer. Condenser inserted. Recording from forehead and occiput with lead band electrodes. (*Top*) The record obtained from the scalp; (*bottom*) time in 1/10 second.

to the forehead and occiput and were fixed with rubber bandages. From these lead band electrodes records were taken with galvanometer 1 of the double-coil galvanometer; galvanometer 2 was set at its maximum sensitivity and was used as a control to make sure that no outside currents were entering the galvanometer circuit to disturb the examination. At that time I was still very distrustful of the findings I obtained and time and again I applied such precautionary measures. The record of galvanometer 2 ran as completely straight line, without any oscillation.

From the lengthy discussions in Berger's papers, it is easy to see that few believed that his recordings originated in the brain. To dispel some of the uncertainty, Berger usually recorded the ECG along with the EEG. Occasionally, he recorded heart sounds and the arterial pulse. In addition to the electrical activity of the heart, various critics proposed that Berger's recorded activity was due to friction of blood in the cerebral arteries, pulsations of the brain and/or scalp, respiration, contraction of piloerector or skeletal muscle, and glandular activity. Berger dealt with all the potential artifacts, pointing out that their time course and frequency were different from those of the EEG and showed that the EEG continued with transient slowing of the heart rate. Finally, he stated (perhaps in exasperation):

> I therefore believe I have discussed all the principal arguments against the cerebral origin of the curves reported here which in all their details have time and again preoccupied me, and in doing so I have laid to rest my own numerous misgivings.

Among the first to publish an English-language verification of Berger's observations were Jasper and Carmichael [1935], then at Brown University in the United States. Silver electrodes (1 to 2 cm in diameter), covered with flannel and soaked in saline, were connected to an amplifier/mirror-oscillograph system. They were able to confirm Berger's findings and extend them, showing that with a two-channel system used to record the EEG of a girl with a convulsive disorder, the alpha wave frequency was 10 per second on the left side of the head and 6 to 8 per second on the right side, one of the early indications that the EEG was altered by brain pathology. Figure HP5.3*a* shows one of the records obtained by Jasper and Carmichael.

Jasper later came to the Montreal Neurological Institute (McGill University) and created the Eletrophysiological Laboratory, which was formally opened with a celebration meeting held on February 24–26, 1939. In attendance were the world leaders in electrophysiology.

Clinical EEG at the Montreal Neurological Institute was inaugurated using a machine built by Andrew Cipriani. The inkwriter was of unique design and featured a strong magnetic field produced by an electromagnet. In this field was a circular coil coupled to an inkwriting pen. It is interesting to observe that this principle had been used by d'Arsonval [1891] with pneumatic coupling to a tambour that caused a pen to write on a rotating drum, as shown in Fig. HP5.4*a*. Later in the 1930s, this coil design was coupled to a conical diaphragm and became the first dynamic loudspeaker. The pen motor devised by Cipriani is sketched in Fig. HP5.4*b*. A small vane, affixed to the writing stylus, dipped into an oil chamber (dashpot) to provided damping. This four-channel instrument was in routine use when the author first came in contact with Jasper in the early 1940s; it was replaced in 1946 by a six-channel model III Grass EEG.

Meanwhile, at Harvard University (Boston, Mass.), Gibbs, Davis, and Lennox [1935] were pursuing their interest in epilepsy. Recognizing the potential of the EEG for the diagnosis of epilepsy, they initiated a series of studies that would occupy the next many decades. Their recorder consisted

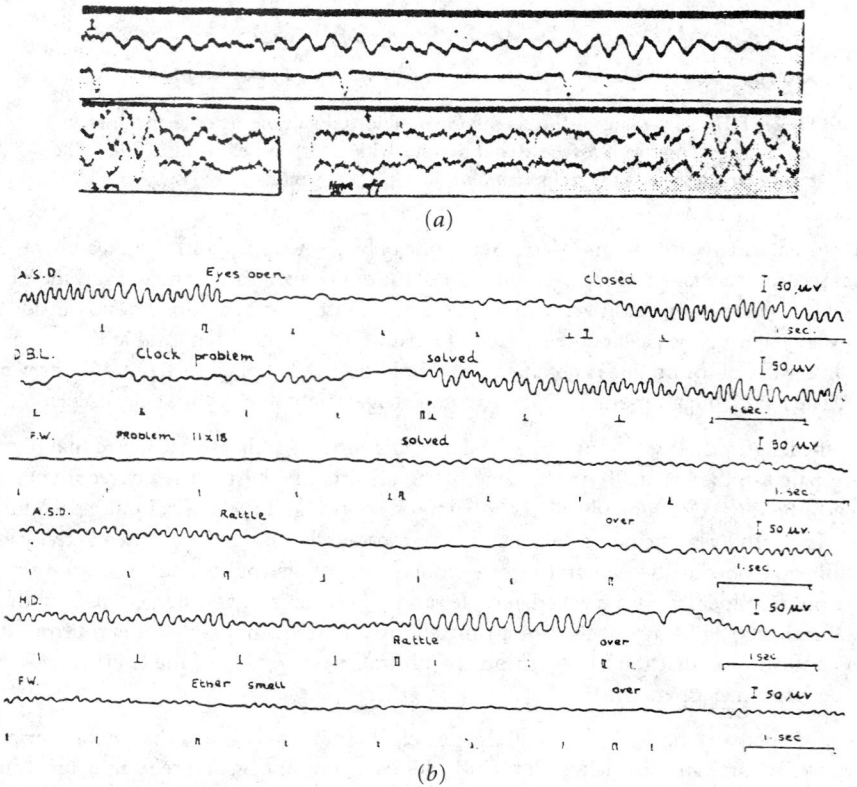

(a)

(b)

FIGURE HP5.3   The first U.S. records of the EEG to confirm Berger's report. (*a*) The records obtained by Jasper and Carmichael (1935). The first channel shows the alpha waves, and the second shows the electrical activity detected by electrodes on the leg above the knee. The second record shows alpha inhibition by illumination of the retina, and the third record shows return of the alpha waves when the light was extinguished. (*b*) The first records published by Gibbs et al. (1935) showing alterations in normal subjects by various types of sensory stimulation eyes open and closed, problem solving, noise (rattle), and smelling ether. (Both by permission.)

of an ink-writing telegraphic recorder called the Undulator. In December of 1935, they published their first paper on EEG which carried a footnote that read: "This paper is no. XVII in a series entitled *Studies in Epilepsy*." Citing the Berger papers and that by Jasper and Carmichael, Gibbs et al. stressed the importance of direct-inking pens for immediate viewing of the EEG so that the effect of environmental factors could be identified immediately. They reported:

> The method is exceedingly simple. Electrical contact is made to two points on the subject's head. Except for the study of grand mal epileptic seizures we regularly employ as electrodes two hypodermic needles inserted one into the scalp at the vertex of the skull and the other into the lobe of the left ear. Enough procaine hydrochloride is injected previously to insure the continued comfort of the subject.

Figure 3*b* is a reproduction of the first EEG obtained by Gibbs et al. Soon Gibbs produced his well-known *Atlas of Electroencephalography*, which first appeared in 1941 and became the "bible" for training electroencephalographers.

The first recording equipment used by Gibbs et al. [1935] was built by Lovett Garceau. It consisted of a four-stage, single-sided, resistance-capacity–coupled amplifier made with high-grain, screen-grid tubes driving a direct-inking telegraphic recorder called the Undulator (*U* in Fig. 5) obtained

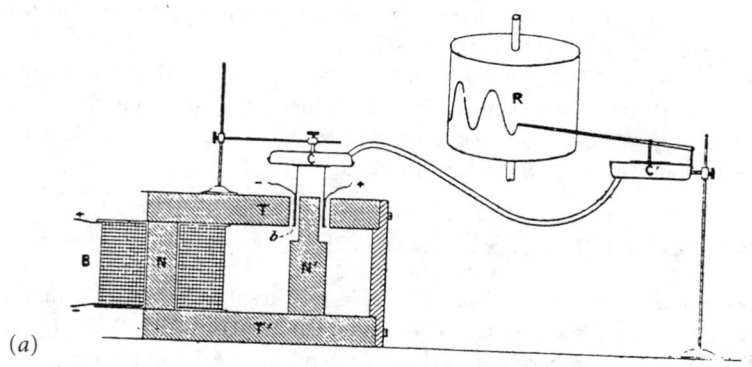

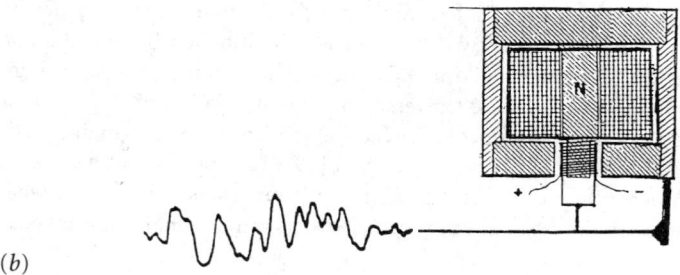

FIGURE HP5.4 Electropneumatic inkwriter described by d'Arsonval (1891) (*a*) and sketch of moving-coil inkwriter devised by Cipriani in the late 1930s for EEG at the Montreal Neurological Institute (*b*).

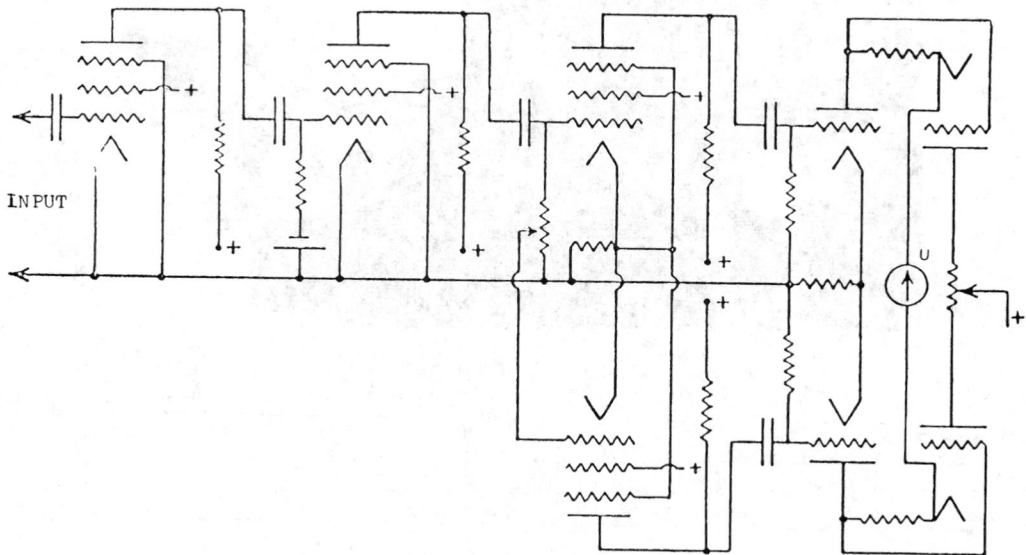

FIGURE HP5.5 The single-sided, five-stage, resistance-capacitor–coupled amplifier developed by Gareau to drive the Western Union inkwriting telegraphic recorder (Undulator) used by Gibbs et al. to record EEGs. (From Garceau et al. 1935. Arch Neurol Psychiatry. With permission.)

from the Western Union Telegraph Company; Fig. 5 shows the circuit diagram. The overall high-frequency response extended to 25 Hz [Grass, 1984].

Slightly earlier, in Germany, Toennies [1932] had developed a direct-inking recorder that he called the Neurograph. Fig. HP5.6 shows a picture of the instrument and a record of the human electro-cardiogram and the response of canine eyes to light. Note that the chart is running in the opposite direction to conventional recordings. The time marks are 1/5 second.

Commercial Production of EEG Machines

The excellent collaboration between Gibbs and Grass in 1935 resulted in replacement of the Undulator telegraphic inkwriter with a robust, d'Arsonval-type inkwriter in early 1936. Meanwhile, the Grass Instrument Company had been founded (1935) to produce electrophysiologic equipment at the well-known address, 101 Old Colony Avenue, Quincy, Mass.; the address is the same today.

In 1937, Grass adopted folding chart paper and by 1939 was providing three-, four-, and six-channel EEGs. The Model III shown in Fig. HP5.7 is the machine recognized by all and founded many EEG laboratories. It featured a knee-hole console with the pens at the right and ample viewing space for the record as it evolved. The chart speed was 30 mm/s, which ultimately became the standard.

At about the same time Grass was building EEG machines in Quincy, Mass., Franklin Offner, a research associate of Ralph Gerard at the University of Chicago, started his own company at 5320 North Kedzie Avenue, Chicago, to produce an EEG using the Crystograph, a high-speed, piezoelectric inkwriter that was described by Offner and Gerard [1936]. It consisted of two slabs of rochelle salt crystals; three corners of each were clamped, and the fourth was free to move when a voltage was applied to electrodes on the crystals. The moving corners were mechanically linked by a slender

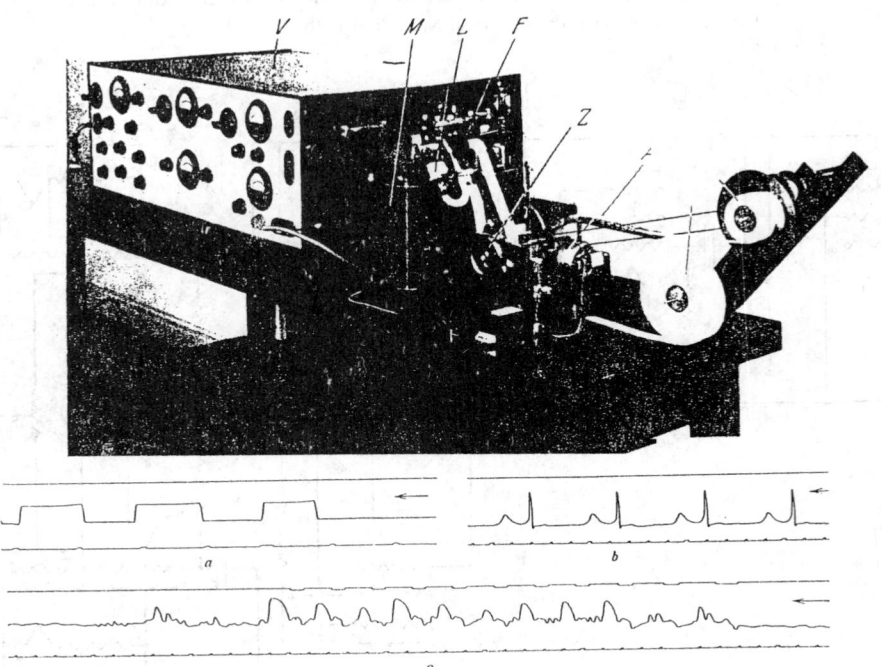

FIGURE HP5.6 Toennies Neurograph and recordings showing a 1-mV calibration, the human ECG, and electrical activity from the canine eye; time marks 1/5 s. (From Toennies [1932].)

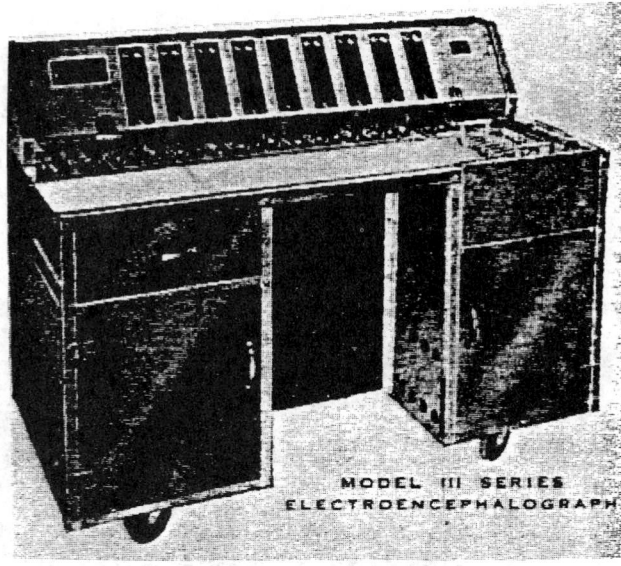

FIGURE HP5.7   The Grass Model III EEG, *circa* late 1940s. (Courtesy Brass Instrument Co., Quincy, Mass.)

brass belt that caused motion of the rod that carried the inkwriting stylus. The sinusoidal frequency response extended uniformly to 100 Hz; the chart speed was 25 mm/s, the same as for ECG. However, a gear shift provided chart speeds above and below 25 mm/s.

The Crystograph was used with the first Offner EEG machines, and it was ideally suited for high-efficiency energy transfer from vacuum-tube amplifiers because of its high impedance. The differential amplifiers were housed in two 19-in relay racks, as shown in Fig. HP5.8*a;* the Crystograph rested on an adjacent table; a six-channel Crystograph is illustrated. Damping was adjusted by a series variable resistor to achieve an excellent response to a step function. The record shown in Fig. HP5.8*a* was produced by a 3-μV (peak-peak) square wave, showing the excellent transient response and the remarkably low internal noise level of the amplifiers.

Although the Crystograph EEG produced elegant records, temperature and humidity played havoc with the rochelle salt crystals, and Offner replaced it with the Dynagraph, shown in Fig. HP5.8*b,* the recorder being a low-impedance, robust d'Arsonval-type moving-coil inkwriter.

Efficient coupling between the output amplifier stage and the moving-coil inkwriter was always a problem that was solved by Offner in his Dynagraph. A synchronous vibrator sampled the signal from the preamplifier, amplified the pulses, and recombined them after passing through a step-down transformer, thereby providing an efficient impedance match between the amplifier output stage and penwriter. Fig. HP5.8*b* is an illustration of the Offner Dynagraph that featured a sit-down console for viewing the record. The antiblocking feature of this design is shown at the bottom of Fig. HP5.8*b* by a sine wave record in which a transient, 100 times larger than the recording, was presented and the recording was restored a fraction of a second after the transient. Offner later replaced the vacuum tubes with transistors, bringing out the first transistorized EEG.

In the late 1940s, Warren Gilson, who was a pioneer in devising physiologic instruments, started production of EEGs in Madison, Wisc.; Fig. HP5.9 is a photograph of one of his later instruments (*circa* 1959).

It is noteworthy that following the Grass Model III EEG, all subsequent instruments were of the console type with the penwriter at the right end of the desktop of the console. Not easily identified in any of the foregoing figures are the two rotary switches for each channel. Each switch could connect each side of the differential amplifier input to any of the 21 electrodes of the 10–20 system.

(a)

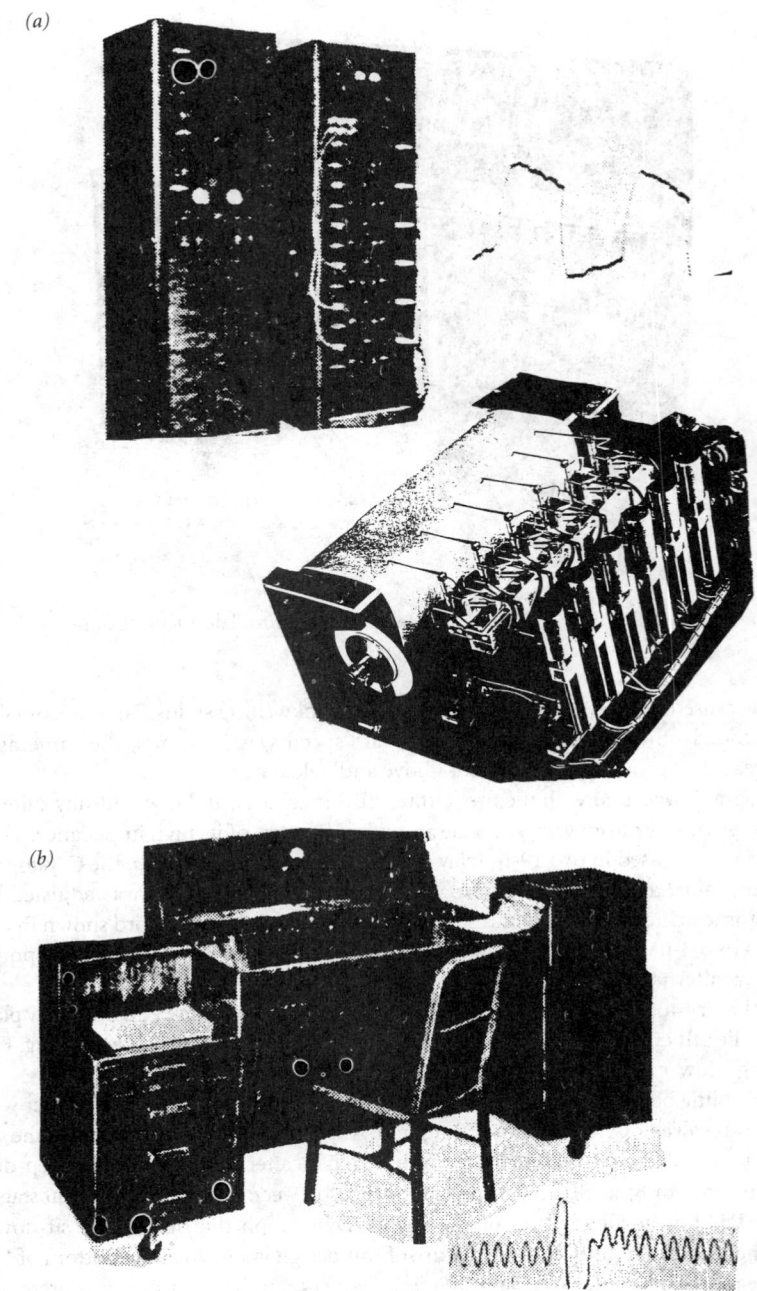

(b)

FIGURE HP5.8   The Offner EEG which used the Crystograph recorder (*a*) and the Offner Dynagraph EEG (*b*), *circa* late 1940s. (Courtesy of Franklin Offner.)

Switching also was provided to apply a step-function calibrating signal to all channels simultaneously, the step function typically being produced by depressing a pushbutton or rotating a knob. In addition, a low-current ohmmeter was provided to permit measurement of the resistance of any pair of electrodes. Some EEGs included a high-frequency filter for each channel to exclude muscle artifacts often seen when patients clenched their jaws.

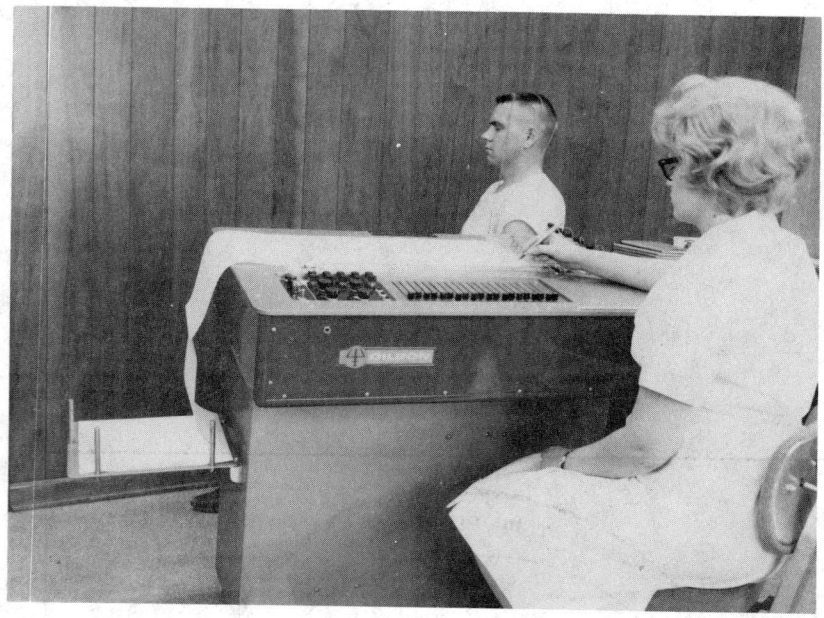

FIGURE HP5.9　　The Gilson EEG, *circa* 1950. (Courtesy of Warren Gilson.)

Electroencephalographs have changed little since their development in the post-World War II days. Transistors have replaced the vacuum tubes, but the chart speed and frequency response are the same as those established by the first manufacturers of EEG machines, although many new recording techniques have been introduced.

References

Caton R. 1875. The electric currents of the brain. Br Med J 2:278.

d'Arsonval A. 1891. Galvanograph et machines producant des courants sinusoidaux. Mem Soc Biol 3(new series):530.

Einthoven W. 1903. Ein neues Galvanometer. Ann Phys 12(suppl 4):1059.

Gibbs FA, Davis H, Lennox WG. 1935. The electroencephalogram in epilepsy as in conditions of impaired consciousness. Arch Neurol Psychiatry 34(6):1135.

Gloor P. 1969. Hans Berger on the electroencephalogram. EEG Clin Neurophysiol (suppl 28):350.

Grass AM. 1984. The Electroencephalographic Heritage. Quincy, Mass, Grass Instrument Co.

Jasper HH, Carmichael L. 1935. Special article: Electrical potentials from the intact human brain. Science 81:51.

Marey EJ. 1876. Des variations electriques des muscles du coeur en particulier etudiee au moyen de l'ectrometre d M. Lippmann. C R Acad Sci 82:975.

Offner F, Gerard RW. 1936. A high-speed crystal inkwriter. Science 84:209.

Toennies JF. 1932. Der Neurograph. Die Naturwiss 27(5):381.

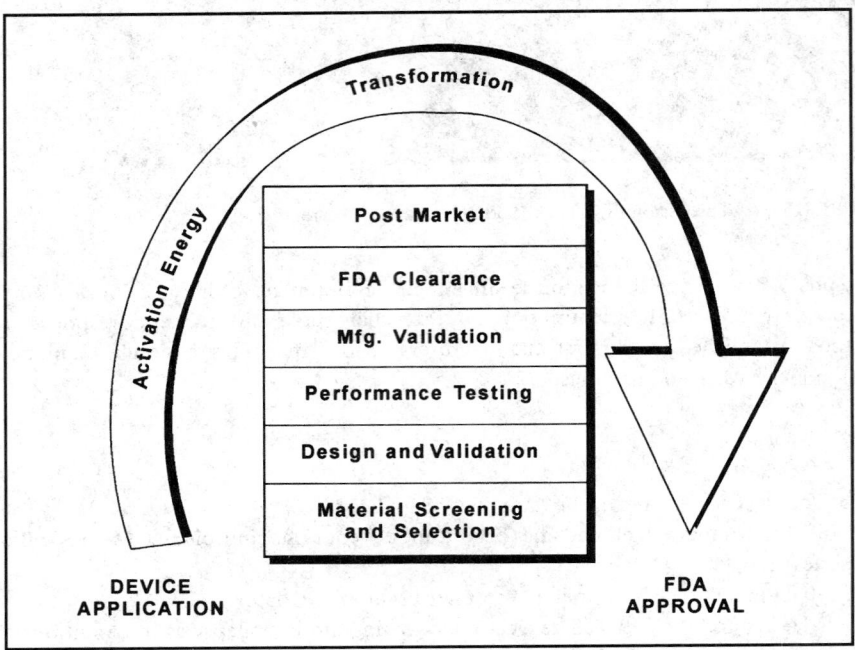

The barrier of device regulations.

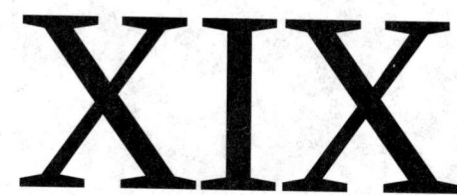

Regulations and Organizations

Joseph D. Bronzino
Trinity College/The Hartford Graduate Center

191

The Role of Professional Societies in Biomedical Engineering

Swamy Laxminarayan
New Jersey Institute
of Technology

Joseph D. Bronzino
Trinity College/The Hartford
Graduate Center

Jan E. W. Beneken
Eindhoven University
of Technology

Shiro Usai
Toyohashi University
of Technology

Richard D. Jones
Christchurch Hospital

Professionals have been defined as an aggregate of people finding identity in sharing values and skills absorbed during a common course of intensive training. Parsons [1954] stated that one determines whether or not individuals are professionals by examining whether or not they have internalized certain given professional values. Friedson [1971] redefined Parson's definition by noting that a professional is someone who has internalized professional values and is to be recruited and licenced on the basis of his or her technical competence. Furthermore, he pointed out that professionals generally accept scientific standards in their work, restrict their work activities to areas in which they are technically competent, avoid emotional involvement, cultivate objectivity in their work, and put their clients' interests before their own.

The concept of a profession that manages technology encompasses three occupational models: science, business, and profession. Of particular interest is the contrast between science and profession. Science is seen as the pursuit of knowledge, its value hinging on providing evidence and communicating with colleagues. Profession, on the other hand, is viewed as providing a service to clients who have problems they cannot handle themselves. Science and profession have in common the exercise of some knowledge, skill, or expertise. However, while scientists practice their skills and report their results to knowledgeable colleagues, professionals—such as lawyers, physicians, and engineers—serve lay clients. To protect both the professional and the client from the consequences of the layperson's lack of knowledge, the practice of the profession is regulated through such formal institutions as state licensing. Both professionals and scientists must pursuade their clients to accept their findings. Professionals endorse and follow a specific code of ethics to serve society. On the other hand, scientists move their colleagues to accept their findings through persuasion [Goodman, 1989].

Consider, for example, the medical profession. Its members are trained in caring for the sick, with the primary goal of healing them. These professionals not only have a responsibility for the creation, development, and implementation of that tradition, they also are expected to provide a service to the public, within limits, without regard to self-interest. To ensure proper service, the profession itself closely monitors licensing and certification. Thus medical professionals themselves may be regarded as a mechanism of social control. However, this does not mean that other facets of society are not involved in exercising oversight and control over physicians in their practice of medicine.

Professional Development. One can determine the status of professionalization by noting the occurrence of six crucial events: (1) the first training school, (2) the first university school, (3) the first local professional association, (4) the first national professional association, (5) the first state license law, and (6) the first formal code of ethics [Wilensky, 1964; Goodman, 1989; Bronzino, 1992].

The early appearances of the training school and the university affiliation underscore the importance of the cultivation of a knowledge base. The strategic innovative role of the universities and early teachers lies in linking knowledge to practice and creating a rationale for exclusive jurisdiction. Those practitioners pushing for prescribed training then form a professional association. The association defines the task of the profession: raising the quality of recruits, redefining their function to permit the use of less technically skilled people to perform the more routine, less involved tasks, and managing internal and external conflicts. In the process, internal conflict may arise between those committed to established procedures and newcomers committed to change and innovation. At this stage, some form of professional regulation, such as licensing or certification, surfaces because of a belief that it will ensure minimum standards for the profession, enhance status, and protect the layperson in the process.

The last area of professional development is the establishment of a formal code of ethics, which usually includes rules to exclude the unqualified and unscrupulous practitioners, rules to reduce internal competition, and rules to protect clients and emphasize the ideal service to society. A code of ethics usually comes at the end of the professionalization process.

In biomedical engineering, all six critical steps mentioned above have been clearly taken. Therefore, biomedical engineering is definitely a profession. It is important here to note the professional associations across the globe that represent the interests of professionals in the field.

191.1 Biomedical Engineering Societies in the World

Globalization of biomedical engineering (BME) activities is underscored by the fact that there are several major professional BME societies currently operational throughout the world. The various countries and continents to have provided concerted "action" groups in biomedical engineering are Europe, the Americas, Canada, and the Far East, including Japan and Australia. While all these organizations share in the common pursuit of promoting biomedical engineering, all national societies are geared to serving the needs of their "local" memberships. The activities of some of the major professional organizations are described below.

American Institute for Medical and Biological Engineering (AIMBE)

The United States has the largest biomedical engineering community in the world. Major professional organizations that address various cross sections of the field and serve over 20,000 biomedical engineers include (1) the American College of Clinical Engineering, (2) the American Institute of Chemical Engineers, (3) the American Medical Informatics Association, (4) the American Society of Agricultural Engineers, (5) the American Society for Artificial Internal Organs, (6) the American Society of Mechanical Engineers, (7) the Association for the Advancement of Medical Instrumentation, (8) the Biomedical Engineering Society, (9) the IEEE Engineering in Medicine and Biology

Society, (10) an interdisciplinary Association for the Advancement of Rehabilitation and Assistive Technologies, and (11) the Society for Biomaterials. In an effort to unify all the disparate components of the biomedical engineering community in the United States as represented by these various societies, the American Institute for Medical and Biological Engineering (AIMBE) was created in 1992. The AIMBE is the result of a 3-year effort funded by the National Science Foundation and led by a joint steering committee established by the Alliance for Engineering in Medicine and Biology and the U.S. National Committee on Biomechanics. The primary goal of AIMBE is to serve as an umbrella organization "for the purpose of unifying the bioengineering community, addressing public policy issues, identifying common themes of reflection and proposals for action, and promoting the engineering approach in society's effort to enhance health and quality of life through the judicious use of technology" [Galetti, 1994].

AIMBE serves its role through four working divisions: (1) the Council of Societies, consisting of the 11 constituent organizations mentioned above, (2) the Academic Programs Council, currently consisting of 46 institutional charter members, (3) the Industry Council, and (4) the College of Fellows. In addition to these councils, there are four commissions, Education, Public Awareness, Public Policy, and Liaisons. With its inception in 1992, AIMBE is a relatively young institution trying to establish its identity as an umbrella organization for medical and biologic engineering in the United States. As summarized by two of the founding officials of the AIMBE, Profs Nerem and Galletti:

> What we are all doing, collectively, is defining a focus for biological and medical engineering. In a society often confused by technophobic tendencies, we will try to assert what engineering can do for biology, for medicine, for health care and for industrial development. We should be neither shy, nor arrogant, nor self-centered. The public has great expectations from engineering and technology in terms of their own health and welfare. They are also concerned about side effects, unpredictable consequences and the economic costs. Many object to science for the sake of science, resent exaggerated or empty promises of benefit to society, and are shocked by the sluggish or misdirected flow from basic research to useful applications. These issues must be addressed by the engineering and medical communities. For more information, contact the Executive Office, AIMBE, 120 G Street, N.W., Suite 800, Washington, D.C. 20005. (Tel: 202-434-8737; fax: 202-434-8707)

IEEE Engineering in Medicine and Biology Society (EMBS)

The Institute of Electrical and Electronic Engineers (IEEE) is the largest international professional organization in the world and accommodates 37 different societies under its umbrella structure. Of these 37, the Engineering in Medicine and Biology Society represents the foremost international organization serving the needs of nearly 8000 biomedical engineering members around the world. The field of interest of the EMB Society is application of the concepts and methods of the physical and engineering sciences in biology and medicine. Each year, the society sponsors a major international conference while cosponsoring a number of theme-oriented regional conferences throughout the world. Plans are currently under way to organize such regional conferences in 1995 in India, Taiwan, and New Zealand. A growing number of EMBS chapters and student clubs across the major cities of the world have provided the forum for enhancing local activities through special seminars, symposia, and summer schools on biomedical engineering topics. These are supplemented by EMBS's special initiatives that provide faculty and financial subsidies to such programs through the society's distinguished lecturer programs as well as the society's International Activities Committee. Other feature achievements of the society include its premier publications in the form of two monthly journals (*Transactions on Biomedical Engineering* and *Transactions on Rehabilitation Engineering*) and a bi-monthly *EMB Magazine* (the *IEEE Engineering in Medicine and Biology Magazine*). EMBS has recently become a transnational voting member society of the International Federation for Medical and Biological Engineering. For more information, contact the Secretariat, IEEE EMBS, National Research Council of Canada, Room 393, Building M-55, Ottawa, Ontario K1A OR8, Canada. (Tel: 613-993-4005; fax: 613-954-2216; email: soc.emb@ieee.org)

Canadian Medical and Biological Engineering Society

The Canadian Medical and Biological Engineering Society (CMBES) is an association covering the fields of biomedical engineering, clinical engineering, rehabilitation engineering, and biomechanics and biomaterials applications. CMBES is affiliated with the International Federation for Medical and Biological Engineering and currently has 272 full members. The society organizes national medical and biologic engineering conferences annually in various cities across Canada. In addition, CMBES has sponsored seminars and symposia on specialized topics such as communication aids, computers, and the handicapped, as well as instructional courses on topics of interest to the membership. To promote the professional development of its members, the society has drafted guidelines on education and certification for clinical engineers and biomedical engineering technologists and technicians. CMBES is committed to bringing together all individuals in Canada who are engaged in interdisciplinary work involving engineering, the life sciences, and medicine. The society communicates to its membership through the publication of a newsletter as well as a recently launched academic series to help nonengineering hospital personnel to gain better understanding of biomedical technology. For more information, contact the Secretariat, The Canadian Medical and Biological Engineering Society, National Research Council of Canada, Room 393, Building M-55, Ottawa, Ontario K1A OR8, Canada. (Tel 613-993-1686; fax: 613-954-2216)

European Society for Engineering in Medicine (ESEM)

Most European countries are affiliated organizations of the International Federation for Medical and Biological Engineering (IFMBE). The IFMBE activities are described in another section of this chapter. In 1992, a seperate organization called the European Society for Engineering in Medicine (ESEM) was created with the objective of providing opportunities for academic centers, research institutes, industry, hospitals and other health care organizations, and various national and international societies to interact and jointly explore BME issues of European significance. These include (1) research and development, (2) education and training, (3) communication between and among industry, health care providers, and policymakers, (4) European policy on technology and health care, and (5) collaboration between eastern European countries in transition and the western European countries on health care technology, delivery, and management. To reflect this goal, the ESEM membership constitutes representation of all relevant disciplines from all European countries while maintaining active relations with the Commission of the European Community and other supranational bodies and organizations.

The major promotional strategies of the ESEM's scientific contributions include its quarterly journal *Technology and Health Care, ESEM News,* the Society's Newsletter, a biennial European Conference on Engineering and Medicine, and various topic-oriented workshops and courses. ESEM offers two classes of membership: the regular individual (active or student) membership and an associate grade. The latter is granted to those scientific and industrial organizations which satisfy the society guidelines and subject to approval by the Membership and Industrial Committees. The society is administered by an Administrative Council consisting of 13 members elected by the general membership. For more information, contact the Secretary General, European Society for Engineering in Medicine, Institut für Biomedizinische Technik, Seidenstrasse 36, D-70174 Stuttgart, Germany. (Fax: 711-121-2371)

French Groups for Medical and Biological Engineering

The French National Federation of Bioengineering (*Genie Biologique et Medical, GBM*) is a multidisciplinary body aimed at developing methods and processes and new biomedical materials in various fields covering prognosis, diagnosis, therapeutics, and rehabilitation. These goals are achieved through the creation of 10 regional centers of bioengineering, called the *poles*. The poles are directly involved at all levels, from applied research through the industrialization to the marketing of the product. Some of the actions pursued by these poles include providing financial seed support for innovative biomedical engineering projects, providing technological help, advice, and assistance, developing partnerships among universities and industries, and organizing special seminar and conferences. The information dissemination of all scientific progress is done through the *Journal of Innovation and Technology in Biology and Medicine.* For more information, contact the French National Federation of Bioengineering, Coordinateur de la Federation Francaise des Poles GBM, Pole GBM Aquitaine-Site Bordeaux-Montesquieu, Centre de Resources, 33651 Martillac Cedex, France.

International Federation for Medical and Biological Engineering (IFMBE)

Established in 1959, the International Federation for Medical and Biological Engineering (IFMBE) is an organization made up from an affiliation of national societies including membership of transnational organizations. The current national affiliates are Argentina, Australia, Austria, Belgium, Brazil, Bulgaria, Canada, China, Cuba, Cyprus, Slovakia, Denmark, Finland, France, Germany, Greece, Hungary, Israel, Italy, Japan, Mexico, Netherlands, Norway, Poland, South Africa, South Korea, Spain, Sweden, Thailand, United Kingdom, and the United States. The first transnational organization to become a member of the federation is the IEEE Engineering in Medicine and Biology Society. At the present time, the federation has an estimated 25,000 members from all of its constituent societies.

The primary goal of the IFMBE is to recognize the interests and initiatives of its affiliated member organizations and to provide an international forum for the exchange of ideas and dissemination of information. The major IFMBE activities include the publication of the federation's bimonthly journal, the *Journal of Medical and Biological Engineering and Computing,* the *MBEC News,* establishment of close liaisons with developing countries to encourage and promote BME activities, and the organization of a major world conference every 3 years in collaboration with the International Organization for Medical Physics and the International Union for Physical and Engineering Sciences in Medicine. The IFMBE also serves as a consultant to the United Nations Industrial Development Organization and has nongovernmental organization status with the World Health Organization, the United Nations, and the Economic Commission for Europe. For more information, contact the Secretary General, International Federation for Medical and Biological Engineering, AMC, University of Amsterdam, Meibergdreef 15, 1105 AZ Amsterdam, the Netherlands. (Tel: 20-566-5200, ext. 5179; fax 20-691-7233; email: ifmbe@amc.uva.nl)

International Union for Physics and Engineering Sciences in Medicine (IUPESM)

The IUPESM resulted from the IFMBE's collaboration with the International Organization of Medical Physics (IOMP), culminating into the joint organization of the triennial World Congress on Medical Physics and Biomedical Engineering. Traditionally, these two organizations held their conferences back to back from each other for a number of years. Since both organizations were involved in the research, development, and utilization of medical devices, they were combined to form IUPESM. Consequently, all members of the IFMBE's national and transnational societies are also automatically members of the IUPESM. The statutes of the IUPESM have been recently changed to allow other organizations to become members in addition to the founding members, the IOMP and the IFMBE.

International Council of Scientific Unions (ICSU)

The International Council of Scientific Unions is a nongovernmental organization created to promote international scientific activity in the various scientific branches and their applications for the benefit of humanity. ICSU has two categories of membership: scientific academies or research councils, which are national, multidisciplinary bodies, and scientific unions, which are international disciplinary organizations. Currently, there are 92 members in the first category and 23 in the second. ICSU maintains close working relations with a number of intergovernmental and non-governmental organizations, in particular with UNESCO. In the past, a number of international programs have been launched and are being run in cooperation with the UNESCO. ICSU is particularly involved in serving the interests of developing countries.

Membership in the ICSU implies recognition of the particular field of activity as a field of science. Although ICSU is heralded as a body of pure scientific unions to the exclusion of cross and multi-disciplinary organizations and those of an engineering nature, IUPESM attained its associate membership in the ICSU in the mid-1980s. The various other international scientific unions that are members of the ICSU include the International Union of Biochemistry and Molecular Biology (IUBMB), the International Union of Biological Sciences (IUBS), the International Brain Research Organization (IBRO), and the International Union of Pure and Applied Biophysics (IUPAB). The IEEE is an affiliated commission of the IUPAB and is represented through the Engineering in Medicine and Biology Society [ICSU Year Book, 1994]. For more information, contact the Secretariat, International Council of Scientific Unions, 51 Boulevard de Montmorency, 75016 Paris, France. (Tel: 1-4525-0329; fax: 1-4288-9431; email: icsu@paris7.jussieu.fr)

Biomedical Engineering Societies in Japan

The biomedical engineering activities in Japan are promoted through several major organizations: (1) the Japan Society of Medical Electronics and Biological Engineering (JSMEBE), (2) the Institute of Electronics, Information and Communication Engineering (IEICE), (3) the Institute of Electrical Engineers of Japan (IEEJ), (4) the Society of Instrument and Control Engineers (SICE), (5) the Society of Biomechanisms of Japan (SBJ), (6) the Japanese Neural Network Society (JNNS), (6) Japan Ergonomics Research Society (JERS), and (7) the Japan Society of Ultrasonics in Medicine (JSUM). The various special sister societies that are affiliated under the auspicies of these organizations mainly focus on medical electronics, biocybernetics, neurocomputing, medical and biologic engineering, color media and vision system, and biologic and physiologic engineering. The JSMEBE has the most BME concentration, with two conferences held each year in biomedic engineering and three international journals that publish original peer-reviewed papers. The IEICE, which is now 77 years old, is one of the largest international societies, constituting about 40,000 members. The aim of the society is to provide a forum for the exchange of knowledge on the science and technology of electronics, information, and communications and the development of appropriate industry in these fields.

BME Activities in Australia and New Zealand

The BME activities in Australia and New Zealand are served by one transnational organization called the Australasian College of Physical Scientists and Engineers in Medicine (ACPSEM) covering Australia and New Zealand and a national organization called the College of Biomedical Engineers of the Institute of Engineers, (CBEIE) serving the Australian member segment.

The Australasian College of Physical Scientists and Engineers in Medicine was founded in 1977 and comprises 6 branches and 339 members. The membership is made up of 76% from Australia, 17% from New Zealand, and the rest from overseas. A majority of members are employed in public hospitals, with most of these in departments of medical physics and clinical engineering. The primary objectives of the college are (1) to promote and further the development of the physical sciences and engineering in medicine and to facilitate the exchange of information and ideas among members of the college and others concerned with medicine and related subjects and (2) to promote and encourage education and training in the physical sciences and engineering in medicine. Entry to ordinary membership of the college requires applicants to have an appropriate 4-year bachelor's degree and at least 5 years of experience as a physical scientist or engineer in a hospital or other approved institution.

Bioengineering in Latin America

Latin American countries have demonstrated in the past decade significant growth in their bioengineering activities. In terms of IEEE statistics, Latin America has the fastest growing membership rate. Currently, there are over 10,000 IEEE members alone in this region, of which about 300 are members of the Engineering in Medicine and Biology Society. In an effort to stimulate this growth and promote active international interactions, the presidents of the IEEE EMBS and the IFMBE met with representatives of biomedical engineering societies from Argentina, Brazil, Chile, Columbia, and Mexico in 1991 [Robinson, 1991]. This meeting resulted in the formation of an independant Latin American Regional Council on Biomedical Engineering, known by its spanish and portugese acronym as CORAL (*Consejo Regional de Ingenieria Biomedica para Americana Latina*). Both the EMBS and the IFMBE are the founding sponsoring members of the CORAL. The main objectives of CORAL are (1) to foster, promote, and encourage the development of research, student programs, publications, professional activities, and joint efforts and (2) to act as a communication channel for national societies within the Latin American region and to improve communication between societies, laboratories, hospitals, industries, universities, and other groups in Latin America and the Caribbean. Since its inception, CORAL has already provided the centerpiece for bioengineering activities in Latin America through special concerted scientific meetings and closer society interactions both in a national and an international sense. For more information, contact the Secretary General, CORAL, Centro Investigacion y de Estudios, Avanzados Duel Ipn, Departamento Ingenieria Electrica, Seccion Bioelectronica, Av. Instituto Politecnico Nacional 2508, Esg. Av. Ticoman 07000, Mexico Apartado Postal 14-740, Mexico.

191.2 Summary

The field of biomedical engineering, which originated as a professional group on medical electronics in the late fifties, has grown from a few scattered individuals to a very well-established organization. There are approximately 50 national societies throughout the world serving an increasingly growing community of biomedical engineers. The scope of biomedical engineering today is enormously diverse. Over the years, many new disciplines such as molecular biology, genetic engineering, computer-aided drug design, nanotechnology, and so on, which were once considered alien to the field, are now new challenges a biomedical engineer faces. Professional societies play a major role in bringing together members of this diverse community in pursuit of technology applications for improving the health and quality of life of human beings. Intersocietal cooperations and collaborations, both at national and international levels, are more actively fostered today through professional organizations such as the IFMBE, AIMBE, CORAL, and the IEEE. These developments are strategic to the advancement of the professional status of biomedical engineers. Some of the self-imposed mandates the professional societies should continue to pursue include promoting public awareness, addressing public policy issues that impact research and development of biologic and medical products, establishing close liaisons with developing countries, encouraging educational programs for developing scientific and technical expertise in medical and biologic engineering, providing a management paradigm that ensures efficiency and economy of health care technology [Wald, 1993], and participating in the development of new job opportunities for biomedical engineers.

References

Fard TB. 1994. International Council of Scientific Unions Year Book, Paris, ICSU.

Friedson E. 1971. Profession of Medicine. New York, Dodd, Mead.

Galletti PM, Nerem RM. 1994. The Role of Bioengineering in Biotechnology. AIMBE Third Annual Event.

Goodman G. 1989. The profession of clinical engineering. J Clin Eng 14:27.

Parsons T. 1954. Essays in Sociological Theories. Glencoe, Ill, Free Press.

Robinson CR. 1991. Presidents column. IEEE Eng Med Bio Mag.

Wald A. 1993. Health care: Reform and technology (editors note). IEEE Eng Med Bio Mag 12:3.

192

Health Technology Assessment: The Evidentiary Base of Medical Practice

Thomas V. Holohan
Agency for Health Care Policy and Research, U.S. Public Health Service

The recent and dramatic evolution of biomedical technology has profoundly transformed the practice of medicine. While this phenomenon has created some remarkable opportunities for improving medical care, it has simultaneously posed difficulties regarding the evaluation of the proper roles of the various interventions available. Health technology assessment is a discipline that emerged in response to a need for appraising the risk/benefit ratio, the specific and the comparative clinical utility, and the effective application of medical technologies. This chapter will provide a brief description of health technology assessment activities of the Public Health Service, indicate areas of recent congressional interest in this discipline, and suggest how these activities are likely to evolve in the near future.

192.1 Development of the Assessment Program

In the federal sector, the growth of governmentally funded biomedical research and medical care programs provided a strong impetus to determine which factors need be considered to permit the selection of the most appropriate technologies in the various clinical circumstances confronting physicians and their patients. Following establishment of the Medicare program, the Health Care Financing Administration (HCFA) began requesting consultation of the Public Health Service (PHS) as to whether particular technologies were "reasonable and necessary" and thus eligible for coverage. The National Center for Health Care Technology (NCHCT) was established in 1978 as the specific entity in the PHS designated to respond to such requests. The center had only a short existence and was disbanded when the Reagan administration withheld budget authorization in 1981 [Perry, 1982]. However, the continuing need for medical and scientific consultation on the part of the Medicare program resulted in the establishment of a successor to NCHCT; this smaller unit, the Office of Health Technology Assessment (OHTA), was formed in 1981. In 1989, Public Law 101-239 established the Agency for Health Care Policy and Research (AHCPR), with OHTA as one of its

0-8493-8346-3/95/$0.00+$.50
© 1995 by CRC Press, Inc.

components. AHCPR was required by that statute to evaluate the "safety, efficacy, and effectiveness, and as appropriate, . . . the legal, social and ethical implications and appropriate uses of health care technologies." AHCPR also was expected to make recommendations as to whether specific health care technologies should be reimbursable under federally financed health programs, including any "conditions or requirements" under which reimbursements should be made. OHTA/AHCPR has defined *health technologies* broadly to include any discrete service, procedure, or diagnostic or therapeutic modality used to diagnose or treat illness, prevent or mitigate disease, promote patient well-being, or facilitate the provision of health care services.

192.2 The Assessment Process

A full description of the process employed in conducting technology assessments and formulating recommendations for coverage has been published in the *Federal Register* [1993]. It should be appreciated that this technology assessment program is distinct from the responsibilities of the Food and Drug Administration (FDA), which regulates medical devices, drugs, and biologics and has the authority to grant approval to market such regulated products under the Food, Drug and Cosmetic Act and the Medical Device Amendments. The Medicare program considers approval by the FDA a necessary but not always a sufficient condition for coverage. While some have claimed that the FDA and OHTA processes are redundant, that belief is a misapprehension of both the proper role of each organization and the purpose of the assessment process. Stated in the simplest terms, the major programmatic differences can be considered in four general domains:

1. *Legal authority:* FDA authority extends to regulated products but not medical or surgical procedures or services.
2. *Data:* For drugs and biologics, the FDA requires submission of original data unique to their requirements and does not ordinarily accept studies published in the medical literature as a basis for approval. Approval of medical devices under the premarket approval process is most often based on original studies whose protocols have been directed toward FDA requirements. However, devices also may be approved if they are considered as "substantially equivalent" to devices that were on the market prior to the 1976 Device Amendments, and in those instances clinical trial data may not be required [the so-called 510 (k) approval].
3. *Labeling:* FDA approval is limited to use as specified in the manufacturer's product label.
4. The FDA approval process is not intrinsically based on comparison with alternative technologies; i.e., approval is not contingent on demonstration of superiority or equivalence to alternative products.

The last of these is a particularly significant distinction; for example, different medical devices intended to treat the same or similar clinical conditions may be approved for marketing if they are judged to be safe and effective for their labeled indications. However, in clinical use the devices may vary in their overall and comparative usefulness, risk/benefit ratios, or utility for specific patient categories or clinical characteristics and may be associated with diverse outcomes when used in dissimilar environments. Moreover, a given disease or disorder may be treated with medical devices, drugs, surgery, or a combination of these approaches. In these circumstances, technology assessment provides a unique perspective; e.g., the OHTA review of laparoscopic cholecystectomy compared the risks and benefits of that technology with those of open cholecystectomy (laparotomy), gallstone-dissolution drugs, and the external shock wave biliary lithotripter [Holohan, 1991].

While the FDA evaluates devices employed in laparoscopy, the agency's responsibilities do not reach to the clinical utility of the particular surgical procedures in which the devices may be employed. FDA also evaluates and approves drugs intended for gallstone dissolution (e.g., urso- and chenodeoxycholic acid) but does not evaluate their safety and effectiveness in comparison with alternative surgical procedures. The shock wave lithotripter had not been approved by the FDA; it was included in OHTA's review on the basis of European use in a large number of patients. The assessment process may therefore address questions concerned with the overall clinical effectiveness of a technology, comparative effectiveness of alternative technologies, patient or institutional selection criteria, or other conditions or circumstances that may affect the safety, efficacy, or effectiveness of a health technology.

Assessment requests are usually made of OHTA by federally funded medical programs. The issues may originate in various entities, which have included programs' regional offices, Medicare carriers, professional societies, manufacturers or trade associations, Congress, and others. In 1990, OHTA reviewed Medicare data to determine both the types of technologies evaluated and the original source of the inquiries that eventuated in assessment requests during the years 1981–1990. Nearly all technologies assessed could be classed as devices, nonsurgical procedures, or surgical procedures (Medicare has only rarely requested assessments involving drug products). It was found that 72% of the requests were directed toward medical devices, 19% toward nonsurgical procedures, and 9% toward surgical operations. With regard to the most common sources of the requests for assessments of devices, 35% originated with the manufacturer and 24% with the Medicare regional offices. However, the rates were not constant during the decade: Manufacturers' inquiries initiated the process in 27% of the cases from 1981 to 1985, and this proportion increased to 67% during the years 1986–1990. Since the establishment of AHCPR in December of 1989, 28 assessments have been completed or are in progress; 15 involve devices, and 7 address surgical procedures.

After receipt of a request for an assessment, OHTA/AHCPR consults with other components of the PHS to determine if the issues in question are appropriate to the assessment process. Depending on the nature of the medical or scientific questions raised by the inquiry, the adequacy of the available evidence, or the time frame available for response, a formal technology assessment may be initiated, a briefer technology review process may be selected, or the questions may be referred back to the requesting agency for review.

If a formal assessment is deemed appropriate, notice is published in the *Federal Register* announcing the initiation of an assessment and inviting public comment and the submission of information regarding the technology. OHTA also routinely contacts nongovernmental groups and organizations to solicit data on the technology in question. For example, at the time of initiation of the assessment of pancreas-kidney transplant, letters soliciting information and inviting participation in the assessment process were sent to every U.S. transplant center that performed pancreas transplants or had expressed an interest in doing so according to the United Network for Organ Sharing. Consultation is routinely requested from other PHS agencies such as the National Institutes of Health (NIH), FDA, and others as required by the issue under consideration. A comprehensive review of the published medical and scientific literature is undertaken, and that material is considered in conjunction with the data obtained in response to the *Federal Register* notice and from the solicitation of various organizations and other PHS agencies.

The review of this information comprises the essential function of the assessment process, and consequently, the quality of the evidence is of paramount importance in preparing the assessment. The significance of this factor can hardly be overemphasized. While all data are considered, greater weight is given to well-designed studies in which the results are less likely to be affected by measurement artifact, deficiencies in study design, bias, or misinterpretation. Statistically significant results may be reported that on analyses prove to be due to imprecision, errors in measurement, patient selection criteria, etc. and therefore may not reflect an actual effect on patient outcome. Moreover, an adequate description of the methodology used in the conduct of a study is necessary to permit a conclusion as to the generalizability of the results to the patient population of interest. OHTA believes that expert opinion, in the absence of substantiating objective data, is not an adequate basis for a conclusion as to a technology's clinical effectiveness. Several examples of the critical nature of evidence quality and study methodology are discussed in the case studies section below.

When the assessment is completed in draft form, it is reviewed by all professional staff of OHTA and, after appropriate revisions, is forwarded for peer review to other agencies of the PHS. Review is always requested of the NIH and FDA; consultation with other agencies may be solicited as the subject demands. Each PHS agency independently selects reviewers on the basis of their expertise in the technology or the clinical conditions under evaluation. While in particular instances outside nongovernmental experts may be consulted, review of draft assessments is not a public process.

If the entity that requested the assessment is a federally funded health program [e.g., Medicare or the Office of Civilian Health and Medical Programs of the Uniformed Services (OCHAMPUS)], a memorandum recommending whether the technology should be reimbursable is prepared for the signature of the administrator of AHCPR. Public Laws 101–239 of 1989 and 102–410 of 1992 require that the administrator make such recommendations and in so doing must "cooperate and consult" with the commissioner of the FDA, the director of the NIH, and other appropriate PHS agency heads. Consequently, the memorandum is reviewed at a meeting of the OHTA director and staff involved in the assessment preparation and representatives of PHS agencies who have provided information or review of the assessment. PHS personnel other than those assigned to OHTA or AHCPR are not expected to endorse the coverage recommendations on behalf of their agencies. Rather, they are asked if they are aware of any objective data that contradict a statement made in the recommendation. When the coverage recommendation is finalized, it is forwarded to the requestor along with the completed assessment. While the assessment documents are ultimately published as an official agency document, the coverage recommendations are not considered public documents by Medicare or by OCHAMPUS. The Medicare and OCHAMPUS programs are bound by neither the findings of the assessment nor the coverage recommendations, since they retain sole authority to make coverage decisions. The more circumscribed technology reviews that are prepared by OHTA are not accompanied by a coverage recommendation.

192.3 New Legislative Requirements

Public Law 102–410 significantly altered the assessment process, and additional obligations were mandated for OHTA. All new assessments must now include a cost-effectiveness analysis "where cost data are available and reliable." This may significantly increase the workload imposed by each assessment. Nonetheless, interest in the cost-effectiveness of medical care is rapidly increasing, and the congressional concern and intent are reflected in the law. The first assessment OHTA will publish that incorporates cost-effectiveness analysis (CEA) is the review of simultaneous and sequential combined kidney-pancreas transplantation.

Health technology assessment is a medical research discipline and not intrinsically directed toward economic considerations. Moreover, CEA is only applicable to circumstances wherein the technology is found to be clinically effective and when alternative technologies exist. Nevertheless, addition of CEA to the assessment process may prove to be a powerful tool in comparing the costs and benefits of competing technologies. In fact, some Western industrialized nations now require preparation of a CEA by manufacturers prior to the granting of product marketing approval.

An additional responsibility of the OHTA/AHCPR imposed by the new law is the requirement that technologies be selected for assessment on the basis of a formal prioritization process. The selection criteria specified in the statute include

(A) the prevalence of the health condition for which the technology aims to prevent, diagnose, treat, and clinically manage;

(B) variations in current practice;

(C) the economic burden posed by the prevention, diagnosis, treatment, and clinical management of the health condition, including the impact on publicly-funded programs;

(D) aggregate cost of the use of [the] technology;

(E) the morbidity and mortality associated with the health condition; and

(F) the potential of an assessment to improve health outcomes or affect costs associated with the prevention, diagnosis, or treatment of the condition.

The law did not restrict the process to these criteria, and as a result of public meetings on this issue, OHTA/AHCPR agreed to include as an additional criterion the ethical, legal, and social considerations attendant to specific technologies.

This statute required AHCPR to publish, in 1994, a full description of the methodology to be employed in the prioritization; this recently appeared in the *Federal Register* [1994]. The process is based on a report of the Institute of Medicine (IOM) [Institute of Medicine, 1992] that was commissioned by AHCPR. Briefly, weights are assigned to each of the prioritization criteria, and a set of candidate technologies is selected. For each technology, the required background information for the criteria is obtained (e.g., prevalence of the health condition, economic burden, aggregate cost of the use of the technology, etc.). These quantitative or semiquantitative data are scaled, multiplied by the respective criteria weights, and an aggregate score is calculated for each technology in question. The relative rank of each technology in the prioritization listing is assigned on the basis of its overall score.

Preliminary criteria weights have been assigned based on detailed discussion and debate at a public meeting convened for that purpose, with subsequent review by AHCPR's National Advisory Council. A public notice in the *Federal Register* will solicit nominations of technologies, and a wide range of organizations will be directly contacted for submissions. The list of candidate technologies will be reduced to a manageable number with the cooperation of our National Advisory Council and the prioritization process entered. The final rank order will be published.

The agency believes that the process is appropriate and that the technologies subjected to assessment are likely to be those of the most importance to the public health. Implementation of this initiative will serve to improve the overall relevance and utility of the technology assessment program. The procedure will be "resistant to control by special interests" [Institute of Medicine, 1992] in the selection of technologies for review; adequate provision is made for broad public input; the process is open and explicit; and it affords a mechanism to most efficiently utilize the limited resources currently available for assessment.

Some reservations regarding technology assessment appear to derive from the belief that for novel technologies the available data may be limited, and thus early assessment is likely to impede the diffusion of a useful technology. This argument is based on two separate assumptions that should be explicitly addressed. First, it is not at all clear that rapid diffusion of a technology prior to an impartial and conscientious evaluation is likely to be beneficial to the public health; the case study of extracranial-intracranial bypass surgery discussed below is but a single illustration of this point. Second, early assessment may indicate specific deficits in the evidence base and thus provide direction for the most efficient application of future clinical research.

Finally, there are those who believe that a formal technology assessment program is inimical to their interests. Indeed, some have contended that the advocacy of such beliefs was responsible for the demise of the National Center for Health Technology Assessment [Perry, 1982]. However, the assessment process is not inhospitable to technology development; in fact, a valid and reliable assessment would likely prove advantageous to a technology for which objective evidence demonstrated a favorable position relative to alternative choices. Moreover, among the alternative strategies for addressing the serious problems associated with the costs and the benefits of the delivery of health care, technology assessment may prove to be the most palatable and the most defensible option.

192.4 Case Studies

These examples illustrate problems related to the quality of evidence and study methodology in published literature supporting the use of particular technologies assessed by OHTA.

Extracranial-Intracranial Bypass Surgery

Extracranial-intracranial (EC-IC) bypass is a surgical technique developed in the 1960s; it was intended to prevent stroke due to distal carotid artery disease. The risks and benefits of EC-IC bypass were not readily apparent in the literature. In the various published case series, perioperative morbidity and mortality could not be ascertained because of varying or absent definitions of the perioperative period. In reporting freedom from stroke after bypass, the duration of follow-up varied between studies and in some reports was never specified; likewise, the type of evaluation at follow-up varied from complete neurologic examination to contact by telephone. These deficiencies made estimation of postoperative stroke rates suspect. Additionally, despite the evidence that antiplatelet drugs were effective in stroke prevention, few studies described the antiplatelet drugs or dosing schedules employed, and some never addressed the issue of concomitant antiplatelet therapy. Outcomes following surgery were compared with historical controls, whose reported annual stroke rates varied from 3% to 4% to as high as 60% [Holohan, 1990]. Because of the resulting uncertainty as to the risks and benefits of bypass, the NIH sponsored a multicenter, prospective, randomized trial of the surgery. This study included over 1600 patients and demonstrated that not only was the operation not superior to medical therapy for prevention of stroke, but operated patients died sooner and in greater numbers than medically managed patients.

Although the operation had been claimed effective on the bases of published case series, the prospective studies were initiated due to concerns that the data available did not permit unambiguous conclusions as to the benefit of a costly procedure associated with significant morbidity and some mortality. The OHTA assessment of EC-IC bypass concluded that the procedure had not been demonstrated as safe and effective [Holohan, 1990].

Many of the surgeons advocating EC-IC bypass were highly respected leaders in their fields; there was no evidence to suggest that their primary concern was anything other than their patients' best interests. They had come to believe, on the basis of mostly retrospective summaries of selected cases compared with varying groups of historical controls, that the technology had an excellent risk/benefit ratio. Unfortunately, that belief was incorrect. Many similar instances have repeatedly demonstrated that excellent clinical skills and long experience are not sufficient to provide accurate conclusions if study design, methodology, and attention to the quality of evidence are deficient.

Diagnostic Tests

Many reports have presented apparently impressive data and concluded that particular diagnostic tests were clinically useful. Erroneous or unsubstantiated conclusions have resulted from methodologic flaws that included a disregard for the effect of the prevalence of the index disorder in the patients selected for study, inappropriate application of statistical techniques, inattention to (or misapplication of) the concepts of specificity, sensitivity, and positive/negative predictive value, comparison to a "gold standard" which in fact proves to be inadequate, etc. Such reports are unfortunately frequent in the published literature.

Thermography

Thermography was assessed in 1989 and, at the request of Medicare, was reevaluated in 1992. The preponderance of the published data supporting the technology was flawed. For example, one proponent published a study that employed thermography in 19 patients with back pain and an abnormal CT scan and in a smaller group of 15 "normals" (not further described); the thermograms were read as positive in all the patients and in 40% of normal individuals. Sensitivity (true positive rate) was reported as 100% and specificity (true negative rate) as 60%, and on that basis, thermography was recommended as a suitable screening procedure for use prior to CT imaging. However, since all the patients had both clinical symptoms and an abnormal CT, the prevalence of back disease was likely to have approached 100%, and any test positive in the majority of patients would have demonstrated a high (but meaningless) sensitivity. The actual issue addressed by this study was the likelihood of thermography being positive given the presence of back pain and an abnormal CT (i.e., a conditional probability). Such deficiencies in experimental design were quite common in the literature supporting thermography.

Cardiac Output

A number of published reports compared measures of cardiac output (CO) derived from a particular test, with CO obtained by thermodilution, a widely accepted technology. Both the test in question and thermodilution were sequentially applied to groups of patients with varying clinical conditions; results were reported in the form of correlation coefficients. These data were cited by proponents of the technology under review, and effectiveness was asserted on the basis of positive correlation. However, the actual range of the reported correlation coefficients was from $+0.17$ to $+1.0$, clearly representing mixed results. In addition, some calculations were derived from multiple measurements in the same patients, and the measurement variation within subjects was not compared with the variation between subjects. Moreover, in many cases the lower correlation coefficients were reported in the most hemodynamically unstable patients, in whom CO measurements are most critical (e.g., $+0.51$ in cardiomyopathy, $+0.55$ in sepsis or dysrhythmias). Finally, no published data related CO measurements using the newer technology to patient outcomes.

Notwithstanding, a high positive correlation alone is insufficient to demonstrate equivalent clinical utility. A perfect correlation would result if the ranked order of the subjects' cardiac output values on one test was identical to the order on the second test, regardless of the magnitudes of the individual values or the extent of their variations about the group means. Correlation techniques provide a description of the degree of simultaneous or concomitant variation of two variables; an index test may be highly correlated with a "standard" and still be variably inaccurate in quantifying a measure of interest. Therefore, correlation alone does not provide a reliable comparison of the usefulness of a diagnostic technology in actual clinical practice. This is particularly important in circumstances wherein a physician is likely to initiate risky or invasive interventions based on test results.

Polysomnography

A retrospective review of 144 patients clinically suspected of narcolepsy reported the use of two diagnostic tests, mean sleep latency (MSLT) and early sleep onset rapid eye movement (SOREMPS). Results of MSLT and SOREMPS were reported in comparison with what was described as an "ultimate clinical diagnosis." However, the specific criteria for these "ultimate" diagnoses were not provided, although the results of SOREMPS and MSLT were themselves component elements. Nevertheless, calculations of sensitivity and specificity were reported for MSLT and SOREMPS. In the 61 patients diagnosed as narcoleptic, 16% failed to exhibit diagnostic SOREMPS and 43% did not meet the MSLT criteria for narcolepsy. The authors maintained the usefulness of these tests for the diagnosis of narcolepsy and proposed that the then-current standards might be "too exclusionary" and that "center-specific norms" might be necessary. This report illustrates the employment of an undefined "gold standard" (which, however, included the tests under consideration) and calculation of therefore meaningless sensitivity and specificity, disregard of the concepts of positive and negative predictive value of a diagnostic test, and advocacy of institution-based norms in lieu of more standardized criteria.

Defining Terms

Positive predictive value: The proportion of subjects with positive test results who really have the abnormality ($a/a + b$)

Sensitivity: The ability of a test to identify an abnormality when it is in fact present ($a/a + c$)

Specificity: The ability of a test to identify the absence of an abnormality when it is in fact not present ($d/d + b$)

References

Federal Register, Dec. 3, 1993; 58(231):63988.

Federal Register, April 25, 1994; 59(79):19725-6.

Holohan TV. 1990. Extracranial-intracranial bypass to reduce the risk of ischemic stroke. Health Technology Assessment Reports, no. 6. Department of Health and Human Services, Public Health Service, Agency for Health Care Policy and Research.

Holohan TV. 1991. Laparoscopic cholecystectomy. Lancet 338:801.

Institute of Medicine. 1992. Setting Priorities for Health Technology Assessment: A Model Process. Washington, National Academy Press.

Perry S. 1982. The brief life of the National Center for Health Care Technology. N Engl J Med 307(17):1095.

193

Regulation of Biomaterials and Medical Devices

Edward P. Mueller
U.S. Food and Drug Administration

Arthur Ciarkowski
U.S. Food and Drug Administration

Ken McDermott
U.S. Food and Drug Administration

It is no secret, and perhaps no surprise, that many in the medical device industry regard the federal government's regulatory system for medical devices as a confusing and intrusive patchwork of rules, requirements, and procedures. In part, the complexity of the Food and Drug Administration's (FDA's) regulatory program for devices is inherent in the laws that authorize it. Some of this is due to the scores of interpreting regulations that, while necessary, are seen as mind-boggling by some. Without them, however, chaos would reign. Uneven regulation might well result. Regulatory enforcement could be spotty. The end result would be inadequate consumer protection.

To cope with the regulatory labyrinth, many in industry have created myths, while others have instituted business practices based on misinformation and misunderstanding. It's as if they have walled themselves into a darkened room. In their desperate search for a way out, they ignore the flashlights in their pockets to locate the exit and the keys to unlock the exit door.

Certainly not all the problems stem from industry misperception. As with any large organization, communication breakdowns do occur [HHS, 1970]. Getting caught up in the swirl of daily business has a tendency to draw people's attention inward. Government business grows insular, and as a result, frustration grows among those being regulated over the inability to get straight answers to questions about how to "play" the "regulatory game."

Those in charge of FDA's medical device program are keenly aware of the special need to be clear and open about the regulatory process. In an industry dominated by small business, it is crucial for the sake of even-handed regulation and a competitive marketplace for *everyone* to understand the "rules of the road." Since passage of the original medical device law in 1976, which mandated a small manufacturers' assistance program, FDA has made a concerted effort to demystify the regulatory maze. It is in this spirit that we offered to author this chapter.

We view this contribution as more than a service to industry. It is a public service. By elucidating what's required of manufacturers of finished medical devices and biomaterials, FDA's job becomes more straightforward. Doing so enables us to spend less time as counselor and more time as scientific evaluator. It also enables you to present the best scientific case and, assuming the merits of that case hold up, get innovative products to the market faster. In other words, a smoother-running device review system benefits regulators and the regulated industry, but most important, it benefits the American consumer.

In this chapter we give an overview of FDA's regulatory process for medical devices, explain the practical implications of the current regulatory system, and describe how the system specifically affects biomaterials used in the manufacture of medical devices.

193.1 Current Medical Device Regulatory Requirements

Historical Perspective

Enactment of the Federal Food, Drug and Cosmetic Act of 1938 provided the FDA, for the first time, with regulatory powers over medical devices. That historic law, however, limited regulatory action to devices available in interstate commerce and deemed to be either adulterated or misbranded. At that time, the law did not provide for premarket review of device safety and effectiveness [FDA, 1989b; Appler and McMann, 1990].

The postwar revolution in biomedical technology lead to a veritable explosion in new medical devices (e.g., pacemakers, heart valves, kidney dialysis machines, etc.). Under expanded human drug authority conferred by the 1962 amendments to the FFDCA, some devices were regulated as drugs, a move that was upheld by the courts. But with continual advancements in medical technology came findings by a presidentially appointed committee of patient injuries. These revelations led to sweeping legislation that broadly empowered the FDA to control the market entry of newly developed devices based on determinations of safety and effectiveness. The Medical Device Amendments of 1976 established a risk-based regulatory system with a corresponding range of enforcement "tools" to protect the public from unsafe and hazardous products [GPO, 1990].

In the years since passage of that landmark law, Congress has twice modified the 1976 law. The most substantive action occurred in 1990, with congressional approval of the Safe Medical Devices Act [FDA, 1991a; Congress, 1990a]. This action significantly broadened FDA's enforcement powers; e.g., it authorized the levying of civil penalties and created a series of postapproval controls for monitoring the performance of marketed devices throughout their clinical life.

System Overview

Taken as a whole, current authorities afford the FDA with control over virtually all life phases of a medical device, from conception throughout its useful life. The prime focus of FDA device regulation is directed at the premarket testing, manufacture, and postmarket experience of devices. In practical terms, this entails stratifying devices on the basis of risk and applying commensurate regulatory control, a process known as *classification.*

The device regulatory program also consists of manufacturer registration, product listing, premarket evaluation of newly emerging devices and oversight of clinical investigations that generate the data necessary to support premarket applications, postmarketing requirements such as product tracking and product performance studies, manufacturing controls (known as *good manufacturing practices*) site inspections by agency personnel to verify compliance with these requirements, and reporting of adverse device-related incidents by manufacturers and users [Mueller et al., 1991; FDA]. In the sections that follow, we embellish on each of these program elements.

A final but equally important element of the program relates to the device-user interface. In an age of computerization and automation, this may seem less critical, but with the advent of a greater array of over-the-counter diagnostic and therapeutic products, coupled with the broad-scale utility of some device in the clinical setting, education of device users, especially when unanticipated product failures occur, is essential to fully safeguard public health.

Classification of Medical Devices

The key to FDA's regulatory approach for medical devices is the classification system introduced by the Medical Device Amendments of 1976 [GPO, 1990; O'Reilly, 1979; Basile, 1990]. FDA identified all devices in commercial distribution prior to May 28, 1976 and classified them into class I, II, or III. When FDA receives an application for premarket evaluation, the agency classifies the device into class I or II if it is substantially equivalent to a predicate device or into class III if there is no predicate device. The class of the device determines the level of regulation or control by the agency.

The three levels of control based on device class include

> *Class I* devices (e.g., a tongue depressor) whose safety and effectiveness are ensured with a minimum level of regulation: "general controls." These include establishment (manufacturing site) registration, device listing, premarket notification, and good manufacturing practices (GMP).
> *Class II* devices (e.g., a stainless steel bone plate) subject to "special controls" as well as "general controls" requirements. Special controls include performance standards, postmarket surveillance, patient registries, guidance documents [including guidelines for the submission of clinical data in premarket notification submissions, known as 510 (k)'s], and other appropriate actions.
> *Class III* devices (e.g., a heart valve) for use in supporting or sustaining human life or for use which is of substantial importance in preventing impairment of human health. For these devices, special controls and general controls are considered insufficient to ensure the safety and effectiveness of the device.

General Controls

Regardless of the device classification, all device manufacturers must meet the following general controls requirements [unless exempt under 510 (g) of the FD&C Act]:

> Register each manufacturing location (establishment).
> List marketed medical devices.
> Submit a "premarket notification" [510 (k)] before marketing a device that is new to the firm or that has been significantly modified (except in cases where devices are considered premarket exempt or when a PMA is required).
> Manufacture devices in accordance with the good manufacturing practices (GMP) regulation.

These controls are explained below.

Establishment Registration
[Stigi and Kohler, 1990]

The owner or operator of an establishment must register with the FDA within 30 days after beginning any of these activities: manufacture, preparation, propagation, compounding, assembly, or processing of a device intended for human use. Activities requiring registration include repackaging, relabeling, importing of foreign devices, and specifications development.

Initial registration is made on the "initial registration form" (FDA 2891). Thereafter, firms will receive an "annual registration form" (FDA 2891a) from the FDA each year. If changes in registration status occur at other than the annual registration time, they must be submitted in a letter to the FDA within 30 days after they occur. Under SMDA [FDA, 1991a], distributors are also required to register with the FDA.

Listing Devices
[Stigi and Kohler, 1990]

Devices are listed on the "device listing form" (FDA 2892). Unlike registration, listing is not updated yearly. Only when a significant change occurs in one or more of the data elements on the form does the firm submit a new listing form containing the changes.

Premarket Notification
[510 (k)] [FDA, 1990; Holstein, 1990]

At least 90 days before it intends to market a device for the first time, a firm must submit to the FDA a "premarket notification," also called a "510 (k) submission." The 510 (k) submission must contain sufficient information to show that a device is substantially equivalent to a predicate device, which is legally marketed in the United States. A premarket notification also is required for a product that has been or is being marketed by a firm when a change or modification, including intended use of the device, may significantly affect its safety and effectiveness.

Clearance of the 510 (k) application to market the device is based on an evaluation of information about the manufacturer, a comparison of features (including specifications, characteristics, and labeling) between the new device and its predicate, and performance data, which may include *in vitro*, animal, and/or clinical data. If a "not substantially equivalent" determination is made, a premarket approval application must be submitted. In 1993 there were approximately 6000 510 (k)'s submitted to the FDA, and only 2% were determined to be not substantially equivalent.

While there is not a standard form for 510 (k) submissions, Section 807.87 of 21 CFR (*Code of Federal Regulations*) [FDA, 1993] outlines the information required in an application.

Good Manufacturing Practices
[FDA, 1993, 1978; Riordan and Cotliar, 1991]

The good manufacturing practices (GMP) regulation covers the methods, facilities, and controls used in preproduction design validation, manufacturing, packaging, storage, and installation of medical devices. The GMP regulation identifies the essential elements required of the quality assurance program. FDA monitors compliance with the GMP regulation during inspection of the firm's manufacturing facilities.

To address the variety and complexity of devices, the GMP regulation designates two device categories: "noncritical" and "critical." General requirements apply to all devices, but critical devices must meet additional GMP requirements.

Investigational Device Exemption
[FDA, 1989a; Canty, 1990]

To allow manufacturers of devices intended solely for investigational use to ship these devices for use on human subjects, the FD&C Act authorizes the FDA to exempt these firms from certain requirements. This exemption is known as an "investigational device exemption" (IDE) and applies only to investigational studies gathering safety and effectiveness data for a medical device when using human subjects. If a device is considered to present "significant risk," IDE applicants submit information to the FDA demonstrating that testing will be supervised by an institutional review board (IRB), that appropriate informed consent will be obtained, and that certain records and reports will be maintained. For a "nonsignificant risk" device, submission to the FDA is not necessary, but IRB approval and adherence to the IDE regulations are still required (see 21 CFR, parts 50, 56, and 812).

A "significant risk" investigational device is one that

> Is intended as an implant and presents a potential for serious risk to the health, safety, or welfare of a subject.
>
> Is purported or represented to be for use in supporting or sustaining human life and presents a potential for serious risk to the health, safety, or welfare of a subject.
>
> Is important in diagnosing, curing, mitigating, or treating disease (or otherwise preventing impairment of human health) and presents a potential for serious risk to the health, safety, or welfare of a subject.
>
> Otherwise presents a potential for serious risk to the health, safety, or welfare of a subject.

Certain types of devices are exempted from the IDE regulation. These include custom devices, certain in vitro diagnostic devices, devices solely for veterinary use, and devices that are substantially equivalent [as determined by FDA review of a 510 (k)] to preamendment devices used for the same intended purpose.

Premarket Approval
[FDA, 1986a, 1991b; Basile and Prease, 1990]

A premarket approval (PMA) application is an indepth review of the safety, efficacy, and clinical utility of a device. A major focus of a PMA application is the evaluation of the clinical performance of the device in its intended patient population to evaluate some hypothesis (e.g., does a porous coating improve the clinical results of a hip stem). The study endpoints are independent of whether the biomaterials used to fabricate the device are existing or new materials [Ely, 1984].

Preamendment devices are medical devices in commercial distribution before May 28, 1976. In the past, the agency has cleared class III preamendment devices under the authority of the 510 (k) provision. This activity is being phased out, and the agency is calling for submission of PMAs for these devices as required in the 1990 Safe Medical Devices Act. Based on the PMA, the FDA will either reclassify a device into class II or consider the device abandoned.

Before requiring a firm to have an approved PMA application in order to continue marketing a preamendment medical device, the FDA must wait 30 months from the effective data of a final classification regulation for the device or 90 days after publication of a final regulation requiring the submission of a PMA—whichever is later.

Postamendment devices are those first commercially distributed after May 28, 1976. Manufacturers of class III postamendment devices that are not substantially equivalent to preamendment class III devices are required to obtain PMA application approval before marketing their device.

Inspections
[Munsey and Holstein, 1990]

It is unlawful to refuse to permit an inspection, as allowed by the provisions of the law, of any factory or establishment in which medical devices are manufactured, processed, packed, or stored for introduction into interstate commerce.

The FDA is required to inspect manufacturers of class II and class III medical devices at least once every 2 years. A history of problems with a company or its products will influence the frequency of inspection visits. Such manufacturers will be placed on a high-priority inspection schedule, particularly for critical devices being used for lifesaving or life-sustaining applications.

The FDA compliance program covering the inspection of medical device manufacturers is designed to determine the extent to which manufacturers are complying with the good manufacturing practice requirements. The inspection involves a review and evaluation of records and data, labeling procedure, equipment, and facilities and an examination of operations and personnel. Under the government-wide quality assurance program, the FDA sometimes assigns agreements with other government agencies to make required inspections of medical device manufacturing establishments to eliminate redundancy. In those cases where an inspection has revealed deficiencies, the FDA transmits a letter, known as a "warning letter," to the company pointing out the problems. A response within 10 days is required from the manufacturer explaining how the deficiencies or violations will be corrected. If the response is judged to be inadequate or is tardy, the FDA can initiate legal action.

User Reporting

User facilities (including hospitals, nursing homes, and outpatient treatment and surgical facilities) are required to report medical device failures that resulted in death or serious injury to the manufacturer and, if a death occurs, to the FDA. User facilities must submit a semiannual report to the FDA that summarizes their reports of such incidents. This is an extension of the existing mandatory device reporting (MDR) regulation that required manufacturers to report death and serious injury information to the FDA [Yahiro, 1994].

Tracking

Manufacturers of certain high-risk medical devices are required to establish a method for tracking their products whose failure would jeopardize the health of the patient. For life-sustaining medical devices used outside a user facility and some kinds of permanent implants, SMDA [FDA, 1991a; Congress, 1990b] requires that the device manufacturer establish a system for identifying and locating a device at any given time.

All device manufacturers must report any removals or corrective actions taken to reduce the risk to the patient's health or remedy a violation of a medical device requirement. This requirement is intended to facilitate recall and notification provisions of the medical device law.

Postmarket Surveillance

The postmarket surveillance study provisions of the act are probably the most far-reaching and immediate for devices manufactured from new materials [Congress, 1990b]. Two types of studies are outlined in the new law: mandatory and discretionary. Manufacturers of permanent implant devices and life-sustaining and life-supporting devices that are brought to market after January 1, 1991 will be required to conduct postmarket studies of the performance characteristics of their products. In addition, the FDA has the discretion to require the manufacturer of any device to initiate such a study of the device's performance, regardless of when the device was first marketed. The Congress's intention for these studies was to expand the information available on the performance of the device over a larger population and for a longer period of time beyond that gathered during the premarket testing. The FDA will likely define the aspects of the device that are to be studied; i.e., specific populations may be targeted for study as high risk with the use of a new material, the qualifications of the principal investigator, and the characteristics of an acceptable study. The study protocol and the qualifications of the principal investigator require FDA approval prior to initiation of the study.

Master Files for Medical Devices (MAFs)

Various applications and forms submitted to the FDA often contain proprietary data or confidential information such as quality-control procedures, materials composition, test data, and manufacturing processes. Such trade secrets may be protected in a device master file (MAF). This is a document containing proprietary information—for FDA's eyes only—kept on file at the FDA in support of some future IDE, PMA, or 510 (k). Any company can refer to an MAF, without ever seeing it, if permission is obtained from the MAF owner. For example, a ceramic femoral ball manufacturer may permit a sponsor of a femoral stem prosthesis to reference the test data in its MAF for use with the stem. Proprietary information such as composition, structure, and manufacturing of the ball is kept secret in the MAF, yet both the ball and stem can be evaluated by FDA together.

There are various types of MAFs (e.g., biologic, drug, food, and veterinary) in addition to those intended for medical devices. The latter MAFs are designed to fulfill various functions related to manufacturing procedures and controls, synthesis and specifications for chemicals and materials used in producing devices, and packaging materials. There is a specified format and arrangement for the MAF to facilitate its easy use, storage, and retrieval. The contents of the master file may have to be modified to incorporate the latest test results and information or to account for changes in the manufacturing procedure or in the product.

Criteria for acceptance of an MAF include the following:

- The MAF must provide factual information useful to the evaluation of the device.
- The MAF is not intended to be used by manufacturers of medical devices to provide added protection for their proprietary processes and data but is to be used only when services or materials are to be made available to other device producers and would otherwise have to be duplicated.

FDA Guidance

The FDA has generated numerous guidance documents to help manufacturers and developers of new products with regulatory requirements. With regard to premarket approval requirements, over 50 device-specific guidance documents detailing what studies and data would be useful to evaluate safety and efficacy have been generated. Examples include prosthetic heart valves, PTCA catheters, cochlear implants, and ventricular assist devices. In addition, other documents useful to device developers, such as a survey of medical device standards, FDA's medical devices research agenda, and CDRH office's annual reports, are readily available [FDA, 1989c]. To facilitate dissemination of this information, FDA/CDRH has a Division of Small Manufacturers Assistance (DSMA) [Dunning, 1990] that has established an electronic docket for immediate access to the preceding documents. The electronic docket access number is 1-800-252-1366 and can be accessed by any terminal or PC with terminal emulation software via modem.

193.2 Myths of Biomaterials Regulation

FDA Inhibits the Development of New Materials

Many developers of devices that include new materials have falsely convinced themselves that the time and expense of obtaining FDA clearance will be astronomical and/or that clearance may never be obtained. This leads to an unwillingness to even try.

To avoid the appearance of being "new," developers often focus on new uses for old materials or key in on a surface treatment to an "acceptable" old material. In reality, however, the safety and effectiveness data FDA requires for a medical device implant are the same regardless of whether the device incorporates a new material or an old material with a new manufacturing process. Often, the primary problem with applications to FDA that include materials that were previously cleared is a lack of basic characterization and safety information.

As guidance to manufacturers is refined and FDA focuses in on the characteristics and properties of a device/material that are critical for different intended uses, the volume of testing will diminish.

Then FDA will begin to focus more on how the tests are done to make comparisons of data from different test laboratories on comparable devices. To accomplish this, it is important to establish standards for test methodologies and to have performance minimums and/or reference materials/devices [Horowitz, 1991; MacNeill and Altman, 1987] (more details about FDA use of standards appear in a later section). When this occurs, the FDA regulatory requirements and document processing will be less subjective and appear less chaotic.

Large resources have been committed to medical research in the United States, but only a small portion of this research is invested in the area of biomaterials development. Many developments have evolved from government-sponsored clinical research using materials developed for other nonmedical purposes. There are many computer-based materials identification and selection tools that should aid in the selection of materials as candidates for medical implantation.

FDA Has a List of Acceptable Materials

Numerous device applications to the FDA claim that a material is FDA approved; e.g., one application claimed that a device for permanent implantation into the thorax included a material that was previously approved for milk containers. Obviously, a material that is acceptable for use in a milk container may not be suitable for an implantable device that contacts blood and tissue.

The FDA does not keep a list of materials that are certified biocompatible, since biocompatibility is application-dependent. The clinical application of a device and its intended use are critical in whether or not a given material is biocompatible. Materials and other design features are interactive and so must be evaluated together. This evaluation involves biocompatibility, effects of critical manufacturing processes on significant device properties, the intended use of the device, and the physiologic exposure environment.

A corollary to this point is that the biologic performance properties of a specific material within a class of materials can vary substantially. In one application, a manufacturer claimed that its granular carbon for impregnation into a polymer was, in a biocompatibility sense, equivalent to the pyrolytic carbon used in heart valves. The only properties these two materials have in common is the name carbon and the color black. Their physical, mechanical, and chemical properties differed radically. In fact, for some type of granular carbons, there are concerns about potential carcinogenicity.

In this regard, the biocompatibility of a material is considered on a case-by-case basis. Some effort, however, is being taken to change this approach by using previous experience along with fundamental knowledge of material science. This effort is discussed below.

Once a Material Is Approved in One Device, It Is OK to Use in Any Other Device Application

FDA regulates *devices*, not biomaterials. Few implants are simple materials—most implants have dimensions and a geometry that affect its properties. The FDA does regulate biomaterials indirectly, and the level of scrutiny depends on the intended use of the device. If the device is a material (e.g., collagen, bone cement, hyaluronic acid) and it is sold with a performance claim, the FDA would regulate it according to the claim.

The FDA does not, however, directly regulate the components of a device as separate entities, though tests of only the material may be required. Such material tests include preclinical screens of biologic performance and/or properties related to durability that cannot easily be assessed in the completed device. Biocompatibility screening test data for a material may be used to support safety claims for that material used in another device, provided differences in the manufacturing processes do not significantly alter the composition, morphology, or other properties. However, in general, materials are always evaluated relative to the proposed application of the device. Therefore, it would not be appropriate to use the data to support an entirely different application for the same material.

The Material for a Device Can Only Come from a Single Supplier

Because of the perceived or real expense or poor planning associated with biomaterials selection in medical implant development, a large number of device manufacturers have come to depend on a single source of material for their product. This is illustrated by the acute problem with silicone materials when a major material supplier withdrew some of its materials from the medical implant market. This is exacerbated by other large materials suppliers who have taken actions in response to potential liability considerations.

The FDA, working with industry, developed a strategy that will facilitate the review of silicone materials from different suppliers. This strategy involves the implementation of an expedited review for devices made from silicone and the development of a characterization scheme for the materials that helped establish materials comparability. Similar strategies are being worked out for other materials expected to be withdrawn.

The Regulatory Threshold Has Been Raised Recently

From roughly 1990 to 1993, the operating procedures of the Office of Device Evaluation were under review. The reviews were conducted by internal committees and external groups to evaluate the integrity of the program, consistency of decision making, record keeping, and management of workload.

One of the findings was that the information provided in many applications did not meet the minimum requirements outlined in existing regulations, guidance documents, and office policies. To address this issue, management conducted training of the staff to review the existing requirements of the device evaluation program, instituted a uniform record keeping for device reviews, and developed a management action program.

These programs did not increase the information that was required for the evaluation of a new device but did require that information specified in the existing requirements be submitted for all devices. For example, the Tripartite Biomaterials Guidance [FDA, 1986b] was placed into effect on April 24, 1987, but applicants did not always comply fully with the requirements specified in this document, nor did the agency act consistently in all cases. Currently, manufacturers must demonstrate that the material is equivalent in every way that it is used in a predicate product or conduct tests that fulfill the intent of this guidance.

While the regulatory threshold for clearance of a new medical device has not been raised, the requirements for record keeping and assurance that all existing policies are satisfied fully are viewed by many as an increasing regulatory burden. For those manufacturers who did not completely test their devices prior to submitting an application, the threshold has been raised. For manufacturers who routinely conduct all testing recommended, there has been no change.

193.3 FDA Regulation Is a Process, Not a Barrier

Models of Regulation

For some, the premarket evaluation of a new medical device can seem to be an insurmountable obstacle or an unmanageable process (see Fig. 193.1). When the application process is viewed as a single event, the amount of information, testing, and paper work can be overwhelming. This approach is referred to as the *barrier model of device regulation*.

The Food, Drug and Cosmetic Act is one of the more lengthy and complex laws in existence. This law is accompanied by extensive regulations, guidelines, guidance documents, standards, and operating policies (see Fig. 193.2).

For the newcomer to device regulation, the requirements that must be met to market a device in the United States are substantial. The requirements imposed on medical devices by the FD&C Act

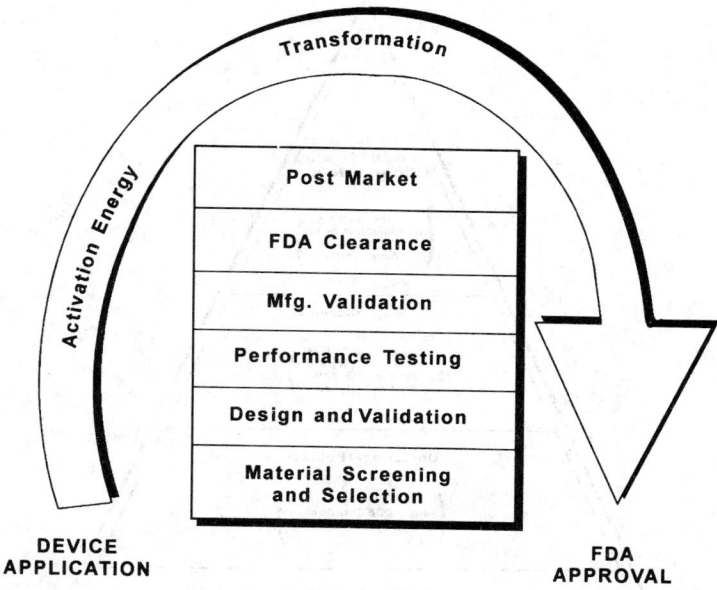

FIGURE 193.1 The barrier model of device regulation.

are no different for a large company in business for years or for a small or new company. Over 80% of U.S. medical device companies have less than 50 employees. Whether the manufacturer is large or small, the devices are used for the medical treatment of patients, and the FDA is obligated to ensure that these devices are safe and effective when used properly.

Deconvolution of the Barrier

While compliance with FDA requirements does require effort, the level of effort can be reduced if one has some knowledge of the process and a plan to manage the process. The process of gaining information and developing a plan means you are deconvolving the regulatory barrier into a manageable process (Fig. 193.3). To do this requires a strategy for acquiring information about the regulatory requirements.

The strategy for achieving this goal is basic and can be laid out in a few steps: Identify sources of information, develop connections and work with others familiar with the process, organize the information into categories that work for you, and stay abreast of events that affect you and the regulatory process.

The sources of information about the agency are numerous, including the agency itself. The FDA is part of the executive branch of government and must comply with the "sunshine laws." With the exception of proprietary information submitted by manufacturers, the agency must disclose general information in its possession and operate with open doors.

As a citizen, you have the right to request and receive information about the FDA. This right is legislated in the Freedom of Information Act (FOIA). Table 193.1 provides a number and address to request information about medical devices. Unfortunately, many requests are received daily, and information may be slow in coming. However, other avenues are available to obtain information as well (Table 193.2). Table 193.3 lists only a few of the professional groups involved in regulatory matters. In addition to these groups, many professional organizations have groups or committees involved in regulatory affairs, standards development, or practice guidelines. The agency often turns

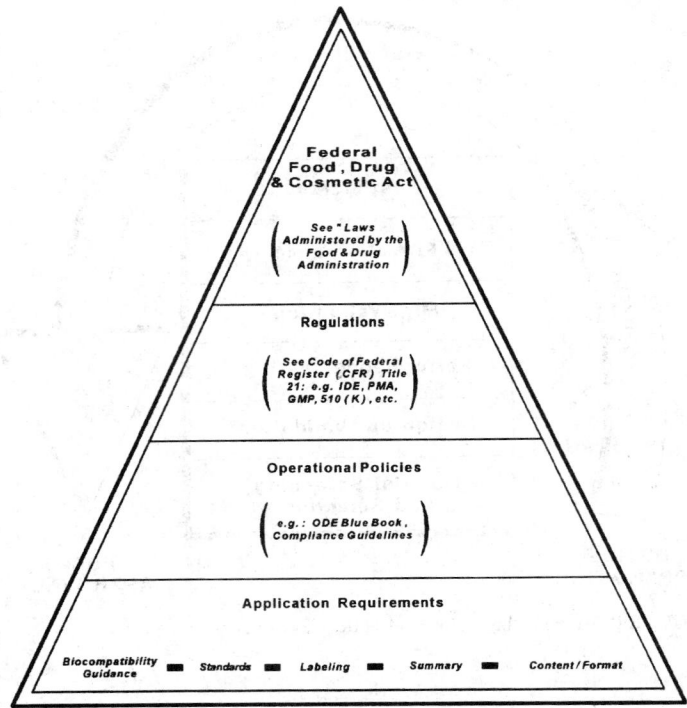

FIGURE 193.2   Hierarchy of FDA requirements.

to professional organizations for advice or assistance in solving problems or in determining options for the regulation of new medical devices. Active participation in these organizations will benefit you, others in your profession, and the regulatory agency. Table 193.4 lists several newsletters and services that track FDA activity and also provide information about the regulatory process.

Learning about the regulations is just one part of what is needed to effectively manage the regulatory process. The second part is developing a plan that will ensure that the information needed for submission to the agency is ready and available when the time comes to prepare a marketing application. The following general comments on this process should be kept in mind during the development of a new device.

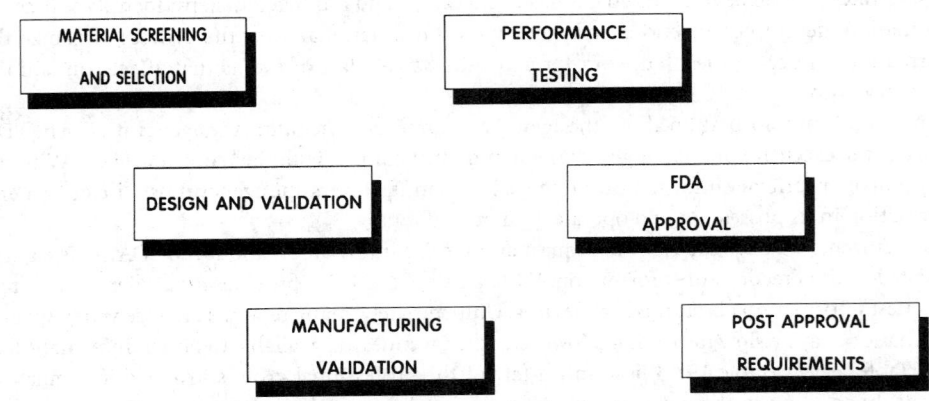

FIGURE 193.3   Steps in the regulatory process.

TABLE 193.1   Freedom of Information Requests

Freedom of Information
Food and Drug Administration (HFA-305)
5600 Fishers Lane
Rockville, MD 20857
(301) 443-6311

or

Freedom of Information
Center for Devices and Radiological Health (HFZ-82)
Food and Drug Administration
Oakgrove Building 4
2094 Gaither Rd
Rockville, MD 20857
(301) 594-4774

Materials Selection and Screening

Materials should not be selected merely because that they are used in currently marketed devices; the material problems in the old device may be duplicated in the new device. For example, small-diameter catheters used for continuous spinal anesthesia were all made out of a material with a radiopaque agent because manufacturers assumed that it must contain a radiopaque material to be approved. The catheters were not easily detected under x-rays despite the presence of the radiopaque agent because their walls were too thin. The radiopaque additive did nothing more than decrease the tensile strength of the catheters so that they fractured in patients. Thus it is important that a material should be chosen that has properties appropriate for the performance of the device.

Information also must be collected to demonstrate a material's biocompatibility. There are a couple of approaches to this phase of testing. The safest route is to perform the tests specified in the tripartite guidance. These tests are performed on the device or on a material sample that has been processed exactly the same way as the final device (including sterilization and packaging). The ISO

TABLE 193.2   Sources of Information about the
Center of Devices and Radiological Health

Division of Small Manufacturers Assistance
(800) 638-2041 or (301) 443-6597
   Automated Touch Tone Service
   (301) 443-8818 FAX

Bulletin Board Service
Access to many guidance documents
(800) 252-1346
9600 baud, 8 data bits, 1 stop bit, no parity
See attachment describing this service.

Publications
Medical Devices Bulletin (published monthly)
Contact:
   Mickie Kivel, Editor
   Center for Devices and Radiological Health (HFZ-30)
   Food & Drug Administration
   12720 Twinbrook Parkway, Building 5
   Rockville, MD 20857

TABLE 193.3   List of Societies and Organizations

Organization	Address	Phone/Fax
The Food and Drug Law Institute	1000 Vermont Avenue, NW, Washington, DC 20005	(202) 371-1420 (202) 371-0649F
Regulatory Affairs Professionals	12300 Twinbrook Parkway, Suite 630, Rockville, MD 20852	(703) 770-2920
American Association for the Advancement of Instrumentation	3330 Washington Blvd, Suite 400, Arlington, VA 22201-4598	(703) 525-4890
Health Industry Manufacturers Association	1200 G Street, NW, Suite 400, Washington, DC 20005	(202) 783-8700 (202) 783-8750F

TC-194 standards may be more appropriate in some cases, but a check with the people evaluating the device at the FDA would be prudent.

The second and more common approach to biocompatibility testing is to demonstrate that the material used is *identical* in formulation, processing, and intended use to a previous material. Though this may be the more convenient route to take, problems often occur because differences in the intended use or the technical characteristics of the device make the transfer of test results from one device to another inappropriate. The source of the material and the manufacturing process also can affect the properties of the material in the finished product.

Testing a device in its final configuration is not always possible or practical. It may be possible to rely in part on the biocompatibility tests completed by the supplier of the material. To do this requires that all the critical manufacturing processes be identified and information gathered that demonstrates how the properties of the material are altered. For example, if a plasticizer is added to polyethylene, can the process be well characterized. How much is added? Are there biocompatibility data on the additive? If not, is the additive washed out or eliminated in the final product? What data are there to demonstrate that there are no residuals in the final product? If there are residuals, are they at an abnormal level, and how do you know?

Design Validation

Design validation is a concept growing out of total quality management and is incorporated into the ISO 9000 series of standards. Over the last 9 years, the FDA has identified the lack of design controls as one of the major causes of device recalls. Recently, general design-control requirements have been added to the good manufacturing practices regulation for all class III and II devices and several class I devices.

TABLE 193.4   Newsletters

Newsletter	Address	Phone/Fax
Medical Devices and Instrumentation *The Gray Sheet*	F-D-C Reports, 5550 Friendship Blvd, Suite One, Chevy Chase, MD 20815-7278	(301) 657-9830 (301) 656-3094F
Devices and Diagnostic Letter	1117 North 19th Street, No. 20, Arlington, VA 22209-1798	(703) 247-3434 (703) 247-3421F
Medical Devices Report	PO Box 1062, Manassas, VA 22110	(703) 361-6472
Europe Drug and Devices Report	1117 North 19th Street, No. 20, Arlington, VA 22209-1798	(703) 247-3434 (703) 247-3421F
Biomedical Technology Information Services	1351 Titan Way, Brea, CA 92621-3787	(714) 738-6400
Biomedical Safety and Standards	1351 Titan Way, Brea, CA 92621-3787	(714) 738-6400
The BBI Newsletter	Biomedical Business International, 1524 Brookhollow Drive, Santa Ana, CA 92705-5426	(714) 755-5757 (714) 755-5705F
MDR Watch	1117 North 19th Street, No. 20, Arlington, VA 22209-1798	(703) 247-3434 (703) 247-3421F
Recall/Regulator Y Analysis	McVicker Associates, Inc, PO Box 6353 Silver Spring, MD 20916	(301) 460-8821

Manufacturing Validation

There are two important concepts relating to manufacturing of a device: validation of the process and identification of the critical manufacturing processes. Validation provides assurance that each step in the process achieves its desired goal. For example, if the material must go through a glass transition, is the temperature of the process adequate to achieve this transition, and how is this ensured?

Standards

A common language used by both the regulators and those regulated will make the regulatory evaluation process, particularly for biomaterial critical devices, more manageable. Another problem encountered with the regulatory process is associated with timing in the product-development cycle and with the differences of opinion over key assessment criteria. These differences can stem from the perspective of the individual involved; i.e., a developer is more critical of intended device specifications, and the regulator tends to focus more on what can go wrong. Agreement on assessment criteria early in the development cycle can save considerable time and expense [Saito, 1986].

This is being addressed to some extent with guidance documents generated by the FDA for specific products or for generic evaluations such as the tripartite biocompatibility guidance. These documents tend to be in some instances data heavy because of fear of the unknown. Another approach would be to make better use of the voluntary standards process [Marlowe and Mueller, 1991; Estrin, 1990]. Development of standards often begins years before the standard is formally published. The early draft stage of a standard focuses to a large extent on the important performance attributes of a device and how they should be measured.

These characteristics of the draft standard are much like FDA guidance documents. Perhaps FDA guidance documents could be worked on by standards-development organizations. The advantage of this is that a wider group of individuals is involved in the development of standards than in the development of guidance documents. As the guidance documents mature and minimum levels of performance are defined, they could be included in a standard, and the FDA could use the standard for regulatory evaluation.

As the economies of countries of the world become more integrated, the role of international standards is becoming much more prominent in the United States. The development and promulgation of international standards are largely concentrated in two International Organization for Standardization (ISO) Technical Committees: ISO TC-150, Implants for Surgery, and ISO TC-194, Biological Evaluation of Medical Devices.

Performance Standards for Medical Implants. Technical Committee 150 of the International Standards Organization (ISO) is responsible for developing most of the performance standards for surgical implant devices. At present, 20 foreign countries are currently participating (P) members of ISO TC-150, including the United States. The committee members meet annually to introduce, draft, and develop standards that gain international recognition and acceptance. These standards describe the materials and devices, define their property and performance requirements, and provide test methods for evaluation and characterization. The actual work is carried out in various subcommittees and working groups. These include materials, cardiovascular implants, neurosurgical implants, bone and joint replacements, osteosynthesis, terminology, certification, and retrieval and analysis of implants.

The ISO TC-150 has already published a wide variety of useful surgical device standards that include standards on specific devices such as orthopedic and cardiovascular devices, surgical instruments, and test methods and procedures. Available ISO standards can be obtained in the United States from the American National Standards Institute (ANSI) in New York.

Biocompatibility Standards. The ISO Technical Committee 194 was established to address biologic screening tests for medical devices and related materials. The initial efforts were directed at consolidating existing national methods for performing such tests as opposed to developing new techniques. Fourteen countries participate on 12 working groups to develop a series of standards in the following areas:

WG 1:   Systematic approach to biologic evaluation and terminology
WG 2:   Degradation aspects related to biologic testing
WG 3:   Animal protection aspects
WG 4:   Clinical investigations in humans
WG 5:   Cytotoxicity
WG 6:   Mutagenicity, carcinogenicity, reproductive toxicity
WG 7:   Systemic toxicity
WG 8:   Irritation, sensitization
WG 9:   Selection of tests for interactions with blood
WG 10:   Implantation
WG 11:   Ethylene oxide and other sterilization process residues
WG 12:   Sample preparation and reference materials

Presently, the FDA relies on a tripartite biocompatibility guidance for assessing medical device/material toxicity. This guidance was established at the September 1984 meeting of the Tripartite Subcommittee on Medical Devices, which was composed of officials from the health departments of the United States, Canada, and the United Kingdom. The document identified the types of biocompatibility data required to evaluate the toxicologic effects of the final product and possible leachable chemicals or degradation moieties and provided a rational framework for the application of the toxicity evaluation of medical devices. The guidance was limited to the effect of the material on the host body and did not consider the material response and distinguished the physical nature of the contact of the materials with the body from the duration of the contact. Because of the similarity between the tripartite guidance and the standard developed in WG 1 of ISO-TC-194 [ISO 10993, 1992] and the other standards generated in TC-194, harmonization of the documents is likely in the near future.

More so now than in the past, the activities in the international standards are of special interest to the medical devices community because these standards will promote understanding across national boundaries, establish requirements, facilitate foreign trade, and set acceptable levels of quality and performance for medical devices. Many countries are using international standards as a basis for developing their regulatory requirements.

193.4 Conclusions

The field of biomaterials is in transition. It is a field that is struggling to develop its own identity. The struggle to make the biomaterials field stand on its own is taking place on multiple planes. It is confronting problems in the areas of technology, regulation, product liability, and basic science funding. This chapter has attempted to address some of the regulatory issues confronting the field. Some of the problems are more based in mythical beliefs than well-founded facts. Rather than fight mythical battles, developers should direct their limited resources toward solutions to the real technological problems and objective assessments of their products.

Resolving these problems, however, is complex and needs a concerted effort by biomaterials scientists, manufacturers, medical researchers, lawyers, and government. Some of the areas where the FDA can participate is in developing consensus on the methods and criteria to assess new and existing biomaterials. The task is not easy, but each step will bring us closer to our destination.

References

Appler WD, McMann GL. 1990. Medical device regulation: The big picture. In NF Estrin (ed), The Medical Device Industry, pp 35–52. New York, Marcel Dekker.

Basile EM. 1990. In NF Estrin (ed), Overview of Current FDA Requirements for Medical Devices. New York, Marcel Dekker.

Basile EM, Prease AJ. 1990. Compiling a successful PMA application. In NF Estrin (ed), The Medical Device Industry, pp 245–264. New York, Marcel Dekker.

Canty EL. 1990. Complying with the IDE regulation. In NF Estrin (ed), The Medical Device Industry, pp 273–282. New York, Marcel Dekker.

Congress. 1990a. Conference Report No. 101-959, pp 101–959. Washington, House of Representatives.

Congress. 1990b. The Medical Device Amendments of 1976, as Further Amended by the Safe Medical Devices Act of 1990. Washington, US Government Printing Office.

Dunning HN. 1990. The FDA's role in assisting small manufacturers. In NF Estrin (ed), The Medical Device Industry, pp 95–112. New York, Marcel Dekker.

Ely JL. 1984. FDA regulations and policy regarding new materials. In J Boretos, M Eden (eds), Contemporary Biomaterials, pp 626–644. Park Ridge, NJ, Noyes Publications.

Estrin NF (ed). 1990. The Medical Device Industry. New York, Marcel Dekker.

FDA. 1978. Regulations Establishing Good Manufacturing Practices for the Manufacture, Packing, Storage, and Installation of Medical Devices (43FR 31508).

FDA. 1986a. Premarket Approval Manual (FDA 87-4214).

FDA. 1986b. Tripartite Biocompatibility Guidance for Medical Devices.

FDA. 1989a. Investigational Device Exemptions: Regulatory Requirements for Medical Devices (FDA 89-4159).

FDA. 1989b. Regulatory Requirements for Medical Devices: A Workshop Manual (FDA 89-4165).

FDA. 1989c. Research Agenda for the 1990s, FDA/CDRH—Special Publication.

FDA. 1990. Premarket Notification: 510(k)—Regulatory Requirements for Medical Devices (FDA 90-4158).

FDA. 1991a. Highlights of Safe Medical Devices Act of 1990, FDA Booklet.

FDA. 1991b. Premarket Approval (PMA) Manual Supplement (FDA 91-4245).

FDA. 1993. Code of Federal Regulations, Food and Drugs, Title 21.

FDA. In press. An Introduction to Medical Device Regulation.

GPO. 1990. Medical Device Amendments of 1976, Federal Food, Drug and Cosmetic Act as Amended and Related Laws (0-248-576QL3).

HHS. 1970. Medical Devices: A Legislative Plan.

Holstein HM. 1990. How to submit a successful 510(k). In NF Estrin (ed), The Medical Device Industry, pp 227–244. New York, Marcel Dekker.

Horowitz E. 1991. Performance standards: A role for ISR? Inst Standards Res Newsletter 2(3):1,12.

ISO (10993). 1992. Biological Testing of Medical and Dental Materials and Devices: I. Guidance and Selection of Tests. Geneva, International Standards Organization.

MacNeill C, Altman M. 1987. The government role in developing voluntary medical devices standards. ASTM Stand News 15.

Marlowe DE, Mueller EP. 1991. The FDA and ASTM. ASTM Stand News 28.

Mueller E, Kammula R, Marlowe D. 1991. Regulation of biomaterials and medical devices. MRS Bull 16(9):39.

Munsey RR, Holstein HM. 1990. FDA/GMP/MDR inspections: Obligations and rights. In NF Estrin (ed), The Medical Device Industry, pp 367–386. New York, Marcel Dekker.

O'Reilly JT. 1979. Food and Drug Administration. New York, McGraw-Hill.

Riordan JJ, Cotliar W. 1991. Complying with FDA Good Manufacturing Practice Requirements. Washington, US Government Printing Office.

Saito M. 1986. Manufacturing. In Proceedings of the 1st International Conference of Medical Device Regulatory Authorities (ICMDRA), pp 130–134.

Stigi JF, Kohler AC. 1990. In NF Estrin (ed), U.S. and Foreign Requirements: A Legal Overview. pp 855–888. New York, Marcel Dekker.

Yahiro MA. 1993. The Food and Drug Administration's MEDWatch Program: Adverse Events for Orthopedic Devices in 1993.

Index